17th edition

CECIL TEXTBOOK OF MEDICINE

Volume 2

Edited by

JAMES B. WYNGAARDEN, M.D.

Director, National Institutes of Health,
Bethesda, Maryland

LLOYD H. SMITH, Jr., M.D.

Chairman, Department of Medicine,
University of California, San Francisco, School of Medicine,
San Francisco, California

1985

W. B. SAUNDERS COMPANY Philadelphia/London/Toronto/Mexico City/Rio de Janeiro/Sydney/Tokyo

W. B. Saunders Company: West Washington Square
Philadelphia, PA 19105

1 St. Anne's Road
Eastbourne, East Sussex BN21 3UN, England

1 Goldthorne Avenue
Toronto, Ontario M8Z 5T9, Canada

Apartado 26370—Cedro 512
Mexico 4, D.F., Mexico

Rua Coronel Cabrita, 8
Sao Cristovao Caixa Postal 21176
Rio de Janeiro, Brazil

9 Waltham Street
Artarmon, N.S.W. 2064, Australia

Ichibancho, Central Bldg., 22-1 Ichibancho
Chiyoda-Ku, Tokyo 102, Japan

Listed here is the latest translated edition of this book together with the language of the translation and the publisher.

Chinese (7th Edition)—Chinese Medical Association, Shanghai, China
Italian (9th Edition)—Societa Editrice Universo, Rome, Italy
(15th Edition, in preparation)—Piccin Editore, Padova, Italy
Japanese (14th Edition)—Igaku Shoin Ltd., Tokyo, Japan
Polish (9th Edition)—Panstwowy Zaklad Wydawnictw Lekarskich, Warsaw, Poland
Portuguese (14th Edition)—DISCOS CBS Industria e Comercio Ltda., Rio de Janeiro, Brazil
Serbo-Croat (11th Edition)—Medicinska Knjiga, Belgrade, Yugoslavia
Spanish (14th Edition)—Nueva Editorial Interamericana Ltda., Mexico City
(15th Edition, in preparation)—Nueva Editorial Interamericana Ltda., Mexico City

Library of Congress Cataloging in Publication Data
Main entry under title:

Textbook of Medicine.

Simultaneously published in 1 v.
Includes bibliographies and index.
1. Internal medicine. I. Cecil, Russell L. (Russell La Fayette), 1881–1965. II. Wyngaarden, James B., 1924– . III. Smith, Lloyd H. (Lloyd Holly), 1924– . IV. Title: Cecil Textbook of Medicine.
[DNLM: 1. Medicine. WB 100 T354]
RC46.T35 1985 616 84-20225
ISBN 0-7216-9629-5 (set)
ISBN 0-7216-6927-9 (v. 1)
ISBN 0-7216-9628-7 (v. 2)

Library of Congress Cataloging in Publication Data
Main entry under title:

Textbook of Medicine.

Simultaneously published in 2 v.
Includes bibliographies and index.
1. Internal medicine. I. Cecil, Russell L. (Russell La Fayette), 1881–1965. II. Wyngaarden, James B., 1924– . III. Smith, Lloyd H. (Lloyd Holly), 1924– . IV. Title: Cecil Textbook of Medicine.
[DNLM: 1. Medicine. WB 100 T354]
RC46.T35 1985b 616 84-20226
ISBN 0-7216-9626-0

ISBN 0-7216-9626-0 Single Volume
ISBN 0-7216-9627-9 Volume 1
ISBN 0-7216-9628-7 Volume 2
ISBN 0-7216-9629-5 Set

Textbook of Medicine

Last digit is the print number: 9 8 7 6 5 4 3 2 1

CONTENTS

(Detailed Table of Contents begins on the following page)

Contents

PART XI GASTROINTESTINAL DISEASES

PART XII DISEASES OF THE LIVER, GALLBLADDER, AND BILE DUCTS

PART XIII HEMATOLOGIC DISEASES

Diseases Caused by Chlamydiae

Rickettsial Diseases

Section 3 Viral Diseases

Viral Infections of the Respiratory Tract

RNA Viral Infections Characterized by Cutaneous Lesions

Diseases Caused by Herpes-Type Viruses

Enteroviral Diseases, Raphael Dolin

Viral Disease of the Gastrointestinal Tract

Arthropod-Borne Viral Fevers

Undifferentiated Fevers

Viral Hemorrhagic Fevers

Section 4 The Mycoses, *David J. Drutz*

PART XX DISEASES CAUSED BY PROTOZOA AND METAZOA

Section 1 Protozoan Diseases

Section 2 Helminthic Diseases

The Cestodes, Martin S. Wolfe

The Trematodes

The Nematodes

Filariasis

Section 3 Arthropods and Animal Poisons

PART XXI DISEASES OF THE IMMUNE SYSTEM

PART XXII MUSCULOSKELETAL AND CONNECTIVE TISSUE DISEASES

PART XXIII NEUROLOGIC AND BEHAVIORAL DISEASES

Section 1 Clinical Study of the Patient with Neurologic Symptoms

Section 2 Disorders of Cerebral Function

Section 3 Pathophysiology and Management of Major Neurologic Symptoms

PART XXVII LABORATORY REFERENCE RANGE VALUES OF CLINICAL IMPORTANCE

CECIL
TEXTBOOK OF MEDICINE

Part XVI
NUTRITIONAL DISEASES

212. NUTRIENT REQUIREMENTS

Robert M. Russell

RECOMMENDED DIETARY ALLOWANCES

Recommended Dietary Allowances (RDAs) have been established for most essential nutrients by the Food and Nutrition Board of the National Academy of Sciences (NAS). These dietary allowances (Table 212–1) do not represent nutrient requirements for individuals; they are designed as guidelines for the daily intake of nutrients sufficient to ensure that almost all members of the population are not at risk of developing nutrient deficits. Thus, the RDAs exceed the nutrient requirements for most healthy individuals. Recommendations for energy intakes are an exception in that they represent averages ± 1 SD for particular age and sex groups.

RDAs have been determined by balance studies, measurement of the amount of a nutrient needed to result in tissue saturation, examination of the food supplies of healthy populations, examination of minimum nutrient intakes required to prevent or correct either a naturally occurring deficit or an experimentally produced deficit, epidemiologic observations, and animal studies. Precise RDAs have not been established for some nutrients (e.g., vitamin K, selenium, etc.) because of limited experimental data. However, ranges of safe intakes of these nutrients have been determined by the National Academy of Sciences and are provided in Table 212–2. Continued consumption of trace minerals above the upper limit of the recommended ranges can lead to toxic effects.

The RDAs should be met by a variety of foods for two major reasons. First, certain dietary components (e.g., carotene, fiber, and possibly others as yet undefined), which are not considered "required," may nevertheless have a beneficial effect on body functioning. For example, if an individual is limited to a diet containing only preformed vitamin A, he or she could be deprived of the alleged beneficial effects of carotene (a vitamin A precursor). Second, a monotonous diet over a prolonged period may not supply a beneficial ratio of individual nutrients (e.g., a diet of very high carbohydrate content may increase the body's need for thiamin). Many such nutrient-nutrient interactions are not fully known at present.

Body growth, body size, pregnancy, and lactation alter the RDAs. Other factors that result in an alteration of dietary needs include environmental temperature, fever, menstruation (an increased requirement for iron), malabsorptive diseases, and medications. The RDAs are not applicable to sick or traumatized patients or to individuals with metabolic disorders such as hyperthyroidism. Table 212–3 provides a guide to the possible effects of medication on nutrient requirements and the mechanisms by which these interactions occur.

Nutrient requirements and dietary recommendations for adults are defined in broad age classes in Table 212–1, namely 19 to 22 years, 23 to 50 years, and 51 years and older (76 years and older for energy). In the absence of adequate information, the present recommendations used for the elderly are the same as for the young adult population with few exceptions. However, age-related changes affect the absorption, metabolism, and excretion of many nutrients so that age-specific standards for the elderly are needed. In addition, chronic disability, illness, and the increased use of medications in the elderly introduce other variables. Despite all of these caveats, the RDAs do serve as useful guidelines for the practitioner when judging the adequacy of an individual's diet.

ENERGY

Energy needs vary with body size, growth phase, age, sex, and activity. Factors that increase energy requirements are cold exposure, pregnancy, lactation, infection, fever, hyperthyroidism, and trauma. Recommended energy allowances for all ages are presented in Table 212–4. The energy allowances for children are based on median heights of American children at different ages. The allowances for young adults are based on so-called "desirable" weights of American men and women engaged in light work (e.g., walking, shopping, playing golf, etc.). In addition to the age groups 19 to 22 and 23 to 50 years, energy recommendations for older people are divided into 57 to 75 and 75+ years. The aging process normally results in a progressive decrease in energy needs primarily as a result of a decrease in energy expenditure.

Protein and carbohydrate supply approximately four calories per gram, alcohol seven calories per gram, and fat nine calories per gram. Basal energy expenditure (BEE) may be estimated for healthy individuals using the Harris Benedict equations:

$$\text{Men: BEE} = 66 \pm (13.7 \times \text{weight in kg}) + (5 \times \text{height in cm}) - 6.8\ (\text{age in years})$$

$$\text{Women: BEE} = 65.5 + (9.6 \times \text{weight in kg}) + (1.7 \times \text{height in cm}) - 4.7\ (\text{age in years})$$

Depending on factors such as activity level or illness, energy needs may be increased many times over the basal level. For example, the energy expenditure of a 70-kg man at rest is approximately 70 kcal per hour. However, heavy labor may increase this expenditure to 600 kcal per hour. For each Celsius degree of fever, a 13 per cent increase in calories is required. In catabolic patients, 150 to 200 per cent of the BEE may be necessary to prevent further tissue breakdown. Malnutrition caused primarily by insufficient energy in the diet is known as marasmus, named from the Greek word meaning "to waste away" (Ch. 214).

PROTEIN

A constant supply of protein is needed to maintain body function and structure. On a protein-free diet, the average net loss of body protein by males is about 0.34 gram per kilogram of body weight. However, when allowance is made for incomplete utilization of dietary protein and for variability in needs, the allowance recommended for adults rises to 0.8 gram of protein per kilogram. Protein needs in part are dependent on energy intakes. Increased energy intakes result in protein conservation and decreased energy intakes result in the diversion of protein to meet energy needs. Pregnancy and lactation increase the body's protein requirement.

Dietary proteins differ in their digestibility and in their amino acid composition. Nine essential amino acids must be provided in the diet, since the human body lacks the ability to synthesize them. These proteins are lysine, leucine, isoleucine, valine, methionine, phenylalanine, tryptophan, threonine, and possibily histidine, especially for infants. The condition of malnutrition caused by inadequate protein intake is known as kwashiorkor (Ch. 214) and is seen mainly in infancy.

High-quality proteins have a high degree of bioavailability (i.e., they are easily digested and absorbed) and have a high biologic value (a measure of the efficiency of utilization of absorbed protein, which in turn is dependent on adequate amounts and proportions of essential amino acids). The highest-quality proteins are found in eggs and milk. Seeds and nuts, rice, corn, and grain proteins are of lesser quality. It is recommended that 10 to 15 per cent of caloric intake should be derived from protein. Amino acids supplied in excess of the body's requirement are not stored but are degraded to metabolic products (urea, uric acid), and the carbon skeleton is converted to carbohydrate and fat or oxidized for energy. It is important that a mixed diet be consumed so that adequate amounts of each essential amino acid are received. Some amino acids are

TABLE 212–1. FOOD AND NUTRITION BOARD, NATIONAL ACADEMY OF SCIENCES—NATIONAL RESEARCH COUNCIL RECOMMENDED DAILY DIETARY ALLOWANCES,* Revised 1980

Designed for the maintenance of good nutrition of practically all healthy people in the U.S.A.

		Weight		Height			Fat-Soluble Vitamins			Water-Soluble Vitamins							Minerals					
	Age (years)	(kg)	(lb)	(cm)	(in)	Protein (g)	Vitamin A (μg RE)†	Vitamin D (μg)‡	Vitamin E (mg α-TE)§	Vitamin C (mg)	Thiamin (mg)	Riboflavin (mg)	Niacin (mg NE)¶	Vitamin B_6 (mg)	Folacin** (μg)	Vitamin B_{12} (μg)	Calcium (mg)	Phosphorus (mg)	Magnesium (mg)	Iron (mg)	Zinc (mg)	Iodine (μg)
Infants	0.0–0.5	6	13	60	24	kg × 2.2	420	10	3	35	0.3	0.4	6	0.3	30	0.5††	360	240	50	10	3	40
	0.5–1.0	9	20	71	28	kg × 2.0	400	10	4	35	0.5	0.6	8	0.6	45	1.5	540	360	70	15	5	50
Children	1–3	13	29	90	35	23	400	10	5	45	0.7	0.8	9	0.9	100	2.0	800	800	150	15	10	70
	4–6	20	44	112	44	30	500	10	6	45	0.9	1.0	11	1.3	200	2.5	800	800	200	10	10	90
	7–10	28	62	132	52	34	700	10	7	45	1.2	1.4	16	1.6	300	3.0	800	800	250	10	10	120
Males	11–14	45	99	157	62	45	1000	10	8	50	1.4	1.6	18	1.8	400	3.0	1200	1200	350	18	15	150
	15–18	66	145	176	69	56	1000	10	10	60	1.4	1.7	18	2.0	400	3.0	1200	1200	400	18	15	150
	19–22	70	154	177	70	56	1000	7.5	10	60	1.5	1.7	19	2.2	400	3.0	800	800	350	10	15	150
	23–50	70	154	178	70	56	1000	5	10	60	1.4	1.6	18	2.2	400	3.0	800	800	350	10	15	150
	51+	70	154	178	70	56	1000	5	10	60	1.2	1.4	16	2.2	400	3.0	800	800	350	10	15	150
Females	11–14	46	101	157	62	46	800	10	8	50	1.1	1.3	15	1.8	400	3.0	1200	1200	300	18	15	150
	15–18	55	120	163	64	46	800	10	8	60	1.1	1.3	14	2.0	400	3.0	1200	1200	300	18	15	150
	19–22	55	120	163	64	44	800	7.5	8	60	1.1	1.3	14	2.0	400	3.0	800	800	300	18	15	150
	23–50	55	120	163	64	44	800	5	8	60	1.0	1.2	13	2.0	400	3.0	800	800	300	18	15	150
	51+	55	120	163	64	44	800	5	8	60	1.0	1.2	13	2.0	400	3.0	800	800	300	10	15	150
Pregnancy						+30	+200	+5	+2	+20	+0.4	+0.3	+2	+0.6	+400	+1.0	+400	+400	+150	‡‡	+5	+25
Lactation						+20	+400	+5	+3	+40	+0.5	+0.5	+5	+0.5	+100	+1.0	+400	+400	+150	‡‡	+10	+50

*The allowances are intended to provide for individual variations among most normal persons as they live in the United States under usual environmental stresses. Diets should be based on a variety of common foods in order to provide other nutrients for which human requirements have been less well defined.

†Retinol equivalents. 1 retinol equivalent = 1 μg retinol or 6 μg β-carotene.

‡As cholecalciferol. 10 μg cholecalciferol = 400 IU of vitamin D.

§α-tocopherol equivalents. 1 mg d-α-tocopherol = 1 α-TE.

¶1 NE (niacin equivalent) is equal to 1 mg of niacin or 60 mg of dietary tryptophan.

**The folacin allowances refer to dietary sources as determined by *Lactobacillus casei* assay after treatment with enzymes (conjugases) to make polyglutamyl forms of the vitamin available to the test organism.

††The recommended dietary allowance for vitamin B_{12} in infants is based on average concentration of the vitamin in human milk. The allowances after weaning are based on energy intake (as recommended by the American Academy of Pediatrics) and consideration of other factors, such as intestinal absorption.

‡‡The increased requirement during pregnancy cannot be met by the iron content of habitual American diets nor by the existing iron stores of many women; therefore the use of 30 to 60 mg of supplemental iron is recommended. Iron needs during lactation are not substantially different from those of nonpregnant women, but continued supplementation of the mother for two to three months after parturition is advisable in order to replenish stores depleted by pregnancy.

TABLE 212–2. ESTIMATED SAFE AND ADEQUATE DAILY DIETARY INTAKES OF SELECTED VITAMINS AND MINERALS*

	Age (years)	Vitamins			Trace Elements†						Electrolytes		
		Vitamin K (μg)	Biotin (μg)	Panthothenic Acid (mg)	Copper (mg)	Manganese (mg)	Fluoride (mg)	Chromium (mg)	Selenium (mg)	Molybdenum (mg)	Sodium (mg)	Potassium (mg)	Chloride (mg)
Infants	0–0.5	12	35	2	0.5–0.7	0.5–0.7	0.1–0.5	0.01–0.04	0.01–0.04	0.03–0.06	115–350	350–925	275–700
	0.5–1	10–20	50	3	0.7–1.0	0.7–1.0	0.2–1.0	0.02–0.06	0.02–0.06	0.04–0.08	250–750	425–1275	400–1200
Children	1–3	15–30	65	3	1.0–1.5	1.0–1.5	0.5–1.5	0.02–0.08	0.02–0.08	0.05–0.1	325–975	550–1650	500–1500
and	4–6	20–40	85	3–4	1.5–2.0	1.5–2.0	1.0–2.5	0.03–0.12	0.03–0.12	0.06–0.15	450–1350	775–2325	700–2100
Adolescents	7–10	30–60	120	4–5	2.0–2.5	2.0–3.0	1.5–2.5	0.05–0.2	0.05–0.2	0.10–0.3	600–1800	1000–3000	925–2775
	11+	50–100	100–200	4–7	2.0–3.0	2.5–5.0	1.5–2.5	0.05–0.2	0.05–0.2	0.15–0.5	900–2700	1525–4575	1400–4200
Adults	—	70–140	100–200	4–7	2.0–3.0	2.5–5.0	1.5–4.0	0.05–0.2	0.05–0.2	0.15–0.5	1100–3300	1875–5625	1700–5100

*Because there is less information on which to base allowances, these figures are not given in the main table of RDA and are provided here in the form of ranges of recommended intakes.

†Since the toxic levels for many trace elements may be only several times usual intakes, the upper levels for the trace elements given in this table should not be habitually exceeded.

From National Research Council: Recommended Dietary Allowances. 9th ed. Washington, DC, National Academy of Sciences, 1980.

TABLE 212–3. EXAMPLES OF DRUG-NUTRIENT INTERACTIONS

Drug	Increased Requirement	Potential Mechanism	Deficiency Symptoms
Antacids (aluminum and magnesium hydroxides)	Phosphate	Formation of insoluble salts	Malaise, paresthesias, anorexia
Anticonvulsants (phenobarbital, phenytoin)	Vitamin D	Induction of hepatic microsmal enzymes resulting in inactive vitamin D metabolites	Rickets, osteomalacia
Oral contraceptives (norethindrone/mestranol)	Folic acid	Inhibition of polyglutamic folate absorption	Megaloblastic anemia
Antituberculous drugs (isoniazid, cycloserine)	Vitamin B_6	Excretion of pyridoxal hydrazone complex	Peripheral neuropathy
Anticoagulants (coumarin, warfarin)	Vitamin K	Inhibition of vitamin K recycling	Hypoprothombinemia
Diuretics (benzothiadiazides)	Potassium	Enhancement of renal excretion	Hypokalemia

TABLE 212-4. MEAN HEIGHTS AND WEIGHTS AND RECOMMENDED ENERGY INTAKE*

Category	Age (years)	Weight (kg)	Weight (lb)	Height (cm)	Height (in)	Energy Needs (kcal)
Infants	0.0–0.5	6	13	60	24	kg × 115
	0.5–1.0	9	20	71	28	kg × 105
Children	1–3	13	29	90	35	1300 ± 400
	4–6	20	44	112	44	1700 ± 400
	7–10	28	62	132	52	2400 ± 400
Males	11–14	45	99	157	62	2700 ± 400
	15–18	66	145	176	69	2800 ± 400
	19–22	70	154	177	70	2900 ± 400
	23–50	70	154	178	70	2700 ± 400
	51–75	70	154	178	70	2400 ± 400
	76+	70	154	178	70	2050 ± 400
Females	11–14	46	101	157	62	2200 ± 400
	15–18	55	120	163	64	2100 ± 400
	19–22	55	120	163	64	2100 ± 400
	23–50	55	120	163	64	2000 ± 400
	51–75	55	120	163	64	1800 ± 400
	76+	55	120	163	64	1600 ± 400
Pregnancy						+300
Lactation						+500

*Adapted from National Research Council: Recommended Dietary Allowances. 9th ed. Washington DC, National Academy of Sciences, 1980.

complementary; for example, tyrosine may in part meet the body's requirement for phenylalanine, and cystine may in part meet the body's requirement for methionine. The ability of the body to utilize protein is impaired if one essential amino acid is missing, underscoring the need for mixed sources of dietary proteins.

In parenterally fed patients, zero nitrogen balance may be achieved with as little as 0.5 gram per kilogram per day of mixed amino acids (including all essential amino acids). However, patients with abnormal losses or increased demands (burns, trauma, wound repair) may require 1.5 to 2.5 grams per kilogram of amino acids per day.

In the clinical setting, the state of nitrogen balance can be crudely estimated by measuring the 24-hour urinary urea nitrogen level:

$$\text{Nitrogen balance} = \frac{\text{protein intake}}{6.25} - (\text{urinary urea nitrogen} + 4)$$

CARBOHYDRATE AND FAT

Because protein and fat alone can provide all the energy needs of the body, there is no fixed requirement for carbohydrate in the diet. However, carbohydrates help to make the diet palatable and comprise the main energy source for most people in the world. Further, a diet devoid of carbohydrate would be likely to result in ketosis. Fiber is an unabsorbed carbohydrate. Primarily because of epidemiologic disease patterns (e.g., for colon cancer and diverticulitis), an increase of dietary fiber to approximately 40 grams per day has been suggested.

Fat, a source of concentrated calories, serves as a carrier for fat-soluble vitamins. All body cells with the exception of the central nervous system and erythrocytes can directly utilize fatty acids as a source of energy. Deficiency of linoleic acid results in the syndrome of essential fatty acid deficiency, consisting of scaling skin and impaired growth in children. Linoleic acid deficiency has also been recognized among patients on prolonged parenteral feedings not containing fat. Three per cent of calories in the form of linoleic acid is recommended for the average daily diet.

FAT-SOLUBLE VITAMINS
(see Ch. 217 for more complete discussion)

VITAMIN A. High concentrations of preformed vitamin A are found in dairy products, fish oils, and liver. Good carotene sources include both yellow and green vegetables. The overall utilization of the provitamin, β carotene, as vitamin A is approximately one sixth that of retinol (the alcohol form of vitamin A) because of inefficient carotene absorption and hydrolysis. The vitamin A value of diets is expressed in retinol equivalents, where 1 retinol equivalent is equal to the following: 1 μg retinol, 6 μg β carotene, 12 μg of other provitamin A carotenoids, 3.33 IU of vitamin A activity from retinol, and 10 IU vitamin A activity from β carotene.

Vitamin A is essential for the integrity of epithelial tissues and for retinal function. Night blindness is one of the earliest symptoms of vitamin A deficiency, followed by follicular hyperkeratosis, xerosis, Bitot spots, corneal ulceration, and scleromalacia. Fat malabsorption increases the requirement for vitamin A and for all fat-soluble vitamins. When used regularly over prolonged periods, mineral oil may increase the dietary requirement for all fat-soluble vitamins. Acute toxicity from vitamin A may result in pseudotumor cerebri and exfoliative dermatitis. Chronic ingestion of excess vitamin A may result in a myriad of problems, the most serious of which are hepatic fibrosis and portal hypertension. The lowest reported dose of vitamin A to cause chronic intoxication is 25,000 IU over a period of 7 years.

VITAMIN D (Ch. 244). With normal exposure to ultraviolet light, the skin forms vitamin D_3 (cholecalciferol) from 7-dehydrocholesterol in amounts that are probably sufficient to meet the body's requirement. The vitamin D requirement can also be readily satisfied by diets containing vitamin D–fortified foods. Vitamin D deficiency may result in people who have little or no sunlight exposure and diets containing low amounts of animal tissue or milk that has been fortified with either vitamin D_2 (ergocalciferol) or vitamin D_3 (cholecalciferol). Vitamin D deficiency results in rickets and growth failure in children and osteomalacia in adults. Active metabolites of vitamin D are formed in the liver (25-hyroxyvitamin D) and kidney (1,25-dihydroxyvitamin D).

VITAMIN E. Vitamin E appears to play a role as an intracellular antioxidant. Although the biochemical mechanism is unclear, vitamin E also prevents cell membrane damage. Vitamin E-deficient red blood cells undergo excessive hemolysis when exposed to dilute hydrogen peroxide. Infants who are vitamin E-deficient have been reported to develop hemolytic anemia and muscle damage. Vitamin E deficiency has been described in adults undergoing prolonged parenteral nutrition, and the resulting neuropathy and retinopathy have been found to respond to the administration of vitamin E. Some of the better food sources of vitamin E include vegetable shortenings and oils, margarine, seeds, whole grains, and liver. Since other isomers of tocopherol are not necessarily as well utilized, the vitamin E content of the diet is expressed in α-tocopherol equivalents (αTE) (1α-tocopherol equivalent = 1 mg dl-α-tocopherol or 1.1 IU). Although oils in general are rich sources of vitamin E, the ingestion of a diet high in polyunsaturated fats increases the requirement for vitamin E. Vitamin E toxicity has not been described, although there is evidence that high doses of vitamin E may antagonize the vitamin K-dependent carboxylation of proteins.

VITAMIN K. The synthesis of coagulation factors prothrombin VII, IX, and X by the liver is dependent on vitamin K (Ch. 217). Vitamin K acts as a catalyst to gamma carboxylate glutamic acid residues in the precursor of prothrombin as well as other vitamin K-dependent proteins. Warfarin-type anticoagulants interfere with vitamin K recycling. Phylloquinone (vitamin K_1) is found in green leafy vegetables, and menaquinone (vitamin K_2) is found in bacteria and animals. It is uncertain whether intestinal bacterial synthesis of menaquinones alone is sufficient to meet the human requirement for this vitamin. Deficiency of vitamin K results in hemorrhage and may be seen in infants with immature gut colonization or in adults with malabsorption who are receiving antibiotics or who are on diets lacking in vitamin K. Administration of synthetic vitamin K (menadione) may cause hemolytic anemia.

WATER-SOLUBLE VITAMINS
(see Ch. 217 for more complete discussion)

THIAMIN (VITAMIN B_1). Thiamin functions in the utilization of pentose sugars in the hexose monophosphate shunt and serves as a coenzyme (thiamine pyrophosphate) in the metabolism of alpha keto acid and 2-keto sugars. Beriberi is the deficiency disease state, which involves the cardiovascular and nervous systems and is seen largely in populations subsisting on unenriched rice and wheat flour and in chronic alcoholics (as a result of poor diet, decreased absorption, and altered metabolism). Wernicke's encephalopathy and Korsakoff's psychosis among alcoholics (Ch. 17) may respond to therapeutic doses of thiamin (50 mg thiamin per day until there is stabilization). A clinical test for thiamin deficiency is the measurement of red blood cell transketolase activity.

Thiamin is easily destroyed by cooking and food processing. The best sources of thiamin include whole grains, organ meats, pork, and legumes. The dietary requirement for thiamin increases in diets high in carbohydrate and caloric content and appears to be slightly reduced in diets in which a high proportion of calories is achieved from fat.

RIBOFLAVIN (VITAMIN B_2). Dietary riboflavin sources include milk, meat and poultry, fish, and leafy green vegetables. The vitamin is very sensitive to sunlight and high cooking temperatures. Deficiency of riboflavin is accompanied by mouth lesions, angular stomatitis, cheilosis, glossitis, skin lesions (seborrhea, scrotal or vulval dermatitis), and conjunctivitis. Riboflavin functions as the active component of coenzymes (e.g., flavin mononucleotide, flavin-adenine dinucleotide) for flavo proteins involved in tissue oxidation and reduction reactions (e.g., glutathione reductase, cyclochrome c reductase, succinic dehydrogenase, amino oxidases).

NIACIN. Pellagra is caused by niacin deficiency and is manifested by dermatitis, diarrhea, and dementia, some or all of which may be present in any one patient. The deficiency state is not uncommon among peoples subsisting on corn. It is also found quite regularly among alcoholics. Niacin is needed for fat synthesis, glycolysis, and tissue respiration and is a component of nicotinamide adenine dinucleotide and nicotinamide adenine dinucleotide phosphate. Good food sources for niacin include meat, poultry, fish, whole grains, and legumes. Tryptophan is converted in the body to niacin, and the niacin requirement is inversely related to tryptophan intake. However, tryptophan cannot in practicality meet the niacin requirement since one niacin equivalent (1 mg of niacin) is equal to 60 mg of tryptophan. Ingestion of pharmacologic doses of nicotinic acid may result in dilation of blood vessels, gastrointestinal symptoms, and alterations in lipid metabolism.

PYRIDOXINE (VITAMIN B_6). Pyridoxine is one of several active forms of vitamin B_6 (pyridoxine, pyridoxamine, pyridoxal) that are involved in protein, fat, and carbohydrate metabolism. Pyridoxal phosphate and pyridoxamine act as coenzymes in decarboxylation and deamination reactions of amino acids. Convulsions have been reported among infants who are deficient in pyridoxine, and pyridoxine-responsive anemias and calcium oxalate kidney stones have been reported in adults who are deficient. Paradoxically, the neuropathy caused by isoniazid, which binds to pyridoxine, may be prevented by concurrent administration of extra pyridoxine. Neurologic damage caused by pyridoxine has been described recently among individuals ingesting large doses of this vitamin over prolonged periods. Biochemical deficiency may be diagnosed by decreased red blood cell transaminase levels.

Good food sources of vitamin B_6 include meats (particularly liver), wheat germ, potatoes, bran, and whole grain cereals. The requirement appears to be increased by high-protein diets and ingestion of oral contraceptive agents.

FOLIC ACID. Folates are a group of molecules that are metabolically interrelated and function as coenzymes for one-carbon transfers in the synthesis of DNA and the interconversions of amino acids (Ch. 135). Folate deficiency is common during pregnancy and among alcoholics and institutionalized elderly patients. Megaloblastic anemia caused by folate deficiency is also common among patients with proximal small intestinal disease (e.g., celiac sprue) or resection. Azulfidine appears to interfere with the absorption of folate from the gastrointestinal tract. Alcohol appears to directly interfere with folate metabolism. In one human study of a low-folate diet, megaloblastic anemia occurred at approximately 16 weeks.

Rich food sources of folate include liver, yeast, and green leafy vegetables. Estimates of body stores of folate range from 10 to 50 mg.

VITAMIN B_{12}. Vitamin B_{12} has essential coenzyme activity for the methylation of homocysteine to methionine and for the conversion of methyl malonyl coenzyme A to succinyl coenzyme A. Vitamin B_{12} is also essential for the regeneration of tetrahydrofolate from 5-methyl tetrahydrofolate, a link in the synthesis of DNA. The megaloblastic anemia caused by vitamin B_{12} deficiency responds to the administration of folate (Ch. 135). However, the nerve degeneration caused by vitamin B_{12} deficiency continues unabated despite folate therapy. In the absence of vitamin B_{12} enterohepatic circulation, the storage of the vitamin appears to last for two to five years. Primary dietary sources of vitamin B_{12} are animal products.

VITAMIN C. Specific biochemical reactions dependent on vitamin C activity have not been well defined. However, the vitamin appears to play a role in biological oxidation-reduction reactions, collagen formation, and iron absorption. Deficiency of vitamin C may lead to the clinical syndrome called scurvy, consisting of perifollicular hemorrhage, subperiostal hemorrhage, petechiae, ecchymosis, and bleeding gums. Smoking and oral contraceptives have been reported to decrease plasma levels of vitamin C, but the significance of these observations remains uncertain. There is no convincing evidence that large doses of vitamin C provide any benefits to humans. Hyperoxaluria has been noted occasionally as a side effect of excessive vitamin C intake.

BIOTIN. Biotin is widely distributed among many foodstuffs. Biotin is essential for the activity of many enzyme systems involved in the metabolism of fat and carbohydrate (e.g., pyruvate carboxylase, acetyl coenzyme A carboxylase). Deficiency in adults has only been produced by feeding large amounts of a biotin binder (avidin) and in patients on total parenteral nutrition. Symptoms and signs of deficiency include dermatitis, glossitis, anemia, and depression.

PANTOTHENIC ACID. Pantothenic acid is a component of acetyl coenzyme A that plays a key role in the intermediary metabolism of fats, carbohydrates, and protein. Pantothenic acid is also required for the synthesis of sterols, steroid hormones, and acetyl choline. In the absence of complicating medical conditions, dietary deficiency in man has not been recognized in populations eating a variety of foods, since pantothenic acid appears to be ubiquitous. No formal RDA has been established.

MINERALS

CALCIUM. Calcium is a major mineral constituent of the body and makes up about 2 per cent of body weight (see Ch. 243). Ninety-nine per cent of body calcium is contained in the skeleton, and the small amount of calcium that is present in intracellular and extracellular fluids plays an important role in membrane and muscle function and in blood coagulation. Milk and cheese are rich in calcium, as are shellfish and egg yolk.

Dietary constituents that decrease calcium availability include phytate, liver, oxalate, and malabsorbed fatty acids. Increased dietary protein appears to augment losses of calcium of skeletal origin in the urine. The intestine is able to increase the efficiency of calcium absorption when chronically presented with food that is low in calcium content. Vitamin D is necessary for efficient calcium absorption. There is evidence that the present RDA for calcium for adults (800 mg) is too low.

PHOSPHORUS. Dietary deficiency of phosphorus is unlikely, since nearly all foods contain phosphorus. Prolonged use of nonabsorbable antacids may result in phosphorus deficiency. Phosphorus is important for bone mineralization and for a variety of biochemical reactions in the body (e.g., energy transfer, buffering activity, oxygen transfer from hemoglobin). See Ch. 207 for more details.

MAGNESIUM. Regulation of electrical potential across nerve and muscle membranes is dependent on magnesium. The magnesium deficiency syndrome is similar to hypocalcemic tetany (see Ch. 208). In addition, many enzyme systems are magnesium-dependent. Malabsorptive diseases, alcoholism, kwashiorkor, and diabetes mellitus may all contribute to magnesium deficiency. Phytate decreases the absorption of magnesium, and diuretics promote urinary loss. Magnesium is plentiful in most foods.

IRON. Hemoglobin, myoglobin, and a number of enzymes contain iron. Gastric acidity and reducing and chelating substances such as ascorbic acid promote the absorption of iron from the gastrointestinal tract, whereas calcium and phosphate salts, tannic acid (tea), phytates, and antacids decrease iron availability. Further, heme iron has a greater bioavailability than nonheme iron. Although the normal intestine is somewhat able to adapt its efficiency in absorbing iron to low or high dietary intakes of iron, iron overload may result in hemosiderosis and hemochromatosis. Thirty per cent of body iron is in a nonfunctional storage pool that must be depleted before a reduction in hemoglobin occurs. Microcytic anemia is therefore an insensitive indicator of iron status; rather serum ferritin appears to be a more sensitive clinical indicator of body iron stores.

Trace Minerals
(see Ch. 218 for more details)

ZINC. Zinc deficiency syndrome in humans was first described in Iran and Egypt with growth stunting and hypogonadism recognized as pronounced features. Zinc is an integral part of many enzyme systems (e.g., both DNA and RNA polymerases). Functions such as taste and smell and dark adaptation may also, in part, depend on the state of zinc nutriture. Acrodermatitis enterohepatica is a childhood syndrome caused by an impaired ability of the intestine to absorb zinc. Acute zinc toxicity has been described following ingestion of lemonade mixed in galvanized containers. The syndrome includes nausea, vomiting, and diarrhea. Chronic zinc ingestion in doses of 625 mg has resulted in hypochromic anemia due to copper deficiency. Phytate and fiber are known to impair zinc absorption from the gastrointestinal tract.

COPPER. Copper is a component of numerous metalloenzymes that are critical in mitochondrial energy generation (e.g., cytochrome C oxidase), melanin synthesis, and the cross-linking of collagen. Sources of dietary copper are shellfish, organ meats, and nuts, while dietary factors that decrease the bioavailability of copper include liver, phytate, zinc, calcium, molybdenum, and sulfates. Deficiency of copper is manifested by hypochromic anemia (due to impaired iron absorption and utilization), leukopenia, and hypotonia. Inherited disorders of copper metabolism include albinism and Menkes kinky hair syndrome, wherein impaired copper absorption results in neurological degeneration, growth retardation, and brittle, sparse hair. Copper toxicity is manifested by nausea, vomiting, myalagia, and hemolysis and may occur when dietary intakes of copper exceed 10 to 12 mg per day.

IODINE, FLUORIDE, MANGANESE, SELENIUM, COBALT, CHROMIUM, MOLYBDENUM. For a discussion of iodine, fluoride metabolism, and electrolytes, see Chapters 228, 218, and 76, respectively.

In many animal species *manganese* is a component of enzymes involved in energy and protein metabolism and in mucopolysaccharide synthesis. *Chromium* (as glucose tolerance factor) may promote the action of insulin at the cell membrane level. Meat products and cheese are good dietary sources of chromium. Selenium is needed for glutathione peroxidase activity,

which protects the cell against oxidative damage. A fatal cardiomyopathy seen in Chinese children (Keshan disease) may result from *selenium* deficiency. The requirement for selenium may be higher when dietary vitamin E levels are low. A single patient with *molybdenum* deficiency has been described who, after a course of prolonged total parenteral nutrition, developed neurologic and metabolic abnormalities related to a defect in sulfur amino acid metabolism.

U.S. DIETARY GOALS
(see Ch. 13 concerning the judicious diet)

The U.S. dietary goals, prepared and published in 1977, attempt to outline a prudent diet for the relatively affluent United States public in order to avoid diseases and disabilities that appear to have a relation to diet. These goals recommend a reduction in the percent of calories ingested as fat by the U.S public from 42 per cent to 30 per cent (10 per cent saturated, 20 per cent mono- or polyunsaturated). At least 12 per cent of total calories should be ingested as protein. It further recommends that total calories ingested as carbohydrate be increased from 40 per cent to 58 per cent with an increase in complex carbohydrates (e.g., fiber) and naturally occurring sugars from 28 per cent to 48 per cent. Refined and processed sugar ingestion should be decreased to 10 per cent of the total caloric intake. As more knowledge becomes available, these guidelines may be altered in the future.

Goodhart RS, Shils ME (ed.): Modern Nutrition in Health and Disease. Philadelphia, Lea and Febiger, 1980.

National Research Council: Recommended Dietary Allowances. 9th ed. Washington DC, National Academy of Sciences, 1980.

Roe DA: Drug Induced Nutritional Deficiencies. Westport, AVI Publishing Company Inc. 1976.

Select Committee on Nutrition and Human Studies, United States Senate: Dietary Goals for the United States. US Government Printing Office, 1977.

All of the above are general references that give a broad overview of human nutrition and of recommended dietary allowances. As such they provide excellent background information as well as references concerning more specific topics.

213. NUTRITIONAL ASSESSMENT

Robert M. Russell

The recognition and treatment of malnutrition that accompanies illness plays an important role in optimizing patient care. New modes of delivering nutrients to sick patients by both the parenteral and enteral routes have reduced morbidity and mortality and have shortened the length of hospitalization for both medical and surgical patients.

Methods of nutritional assessment that have been used for some time to judge the severity of malnutrition in lesser developed countries (e.g., anthropometric measures) are now being applied to hospitalized patients in North America and Western Europe. An unexpectedly high prevalence (up to 40 per cent) of protein energy malnutrition has been identified among Western patients. Some of the reasons for the lack of recognition of malnutrition in hospitalized patients include preoccupation with the treatment of the disease process, neglect of the overall nutritional status of the patient, lack of sensitivity of casual observation in the recognition of protein energy malnutrition, absence of a single indicator for diagnosis of malnutrition, and latent onset of clinical signs of malnutrition and relative lack of specificity of these signs. A single nutrient deficiency rarely occurs in a patient; rather, a complex and confusing array of deficiencies are most often present at the same time.

The diagnosis of malnutrition should be made on the basis of dietary information, anthropometric and laboratory measurements, and clinical examination. By using all of this information, a more accurate diagnosis of the malnourished can be achieved, and an effective plan of treatment can be instituted.

DIET

It is not expected that the physician will interpret dietary records of a patient in detail. However, he or she should be aware of the key questions to ask patients, which provide clues about whether or not the patient's dietary intake requires adjustment (Table 213–1). A detailed medical and social history can alert the physician to an existing dietary problem or the likelihood of a dietary problem occurring in the future. For example, poverty, physical or mental disability, complaints of dysphagia, anorexia, nausea, abdominal pain while eating, or ill fitting dentures, and alcoholism may all be factors that prevent adequate dietary intake. Increased nutritional requirements can result from diarrhea, fever, open wounds or burns, malabsorption, diabetes, and hyperthyroidism. The physician should be able to counsel patients regarding general dietary guidelines and recognize cases for referral to a dietitian for more detailed counseling.

The elderly are a group with an increased risk of malnutrition. The reasons for this include poverty, the inability to move around easily, the accumulation of chronic disease necessitating multiple medications, social isolation, and the lack of knowledge for adequate preparation of meals (particularly among elderly men). Problems often arise when interviewing the elderly person for dietary habits if the individual is senile or has impaired short-term memory. A family member may therefore be of great assistance when obtaining dietary information. Finally, appropriate standards for judging the elderly person's diet are not currently available. The Recommended Dietary Allowances (see Table 212–1) were developed as population standards (not individual requirements) and are set to meet the needs of most healthy individuals. The standards for adults are based only on young adults. As a result, they may not be appropriate for meeting the needs of the elderly patient, who has an array of chronic diseases or aging disorders or both.

ANTHROPOMETRIC MEASUREMENTS

Sophisticated and specialized methods to assess body composition are available, e.g., underwater weighing for body density, CT scanning, neutron activation analysis, and K^{40} counting. However, none of these methods is available for widespread clinical use. Anthropometric measurements are inexpensive, quick, and convenient ways of estimating the patient's nutritional status in terms of protein and fat reserves. The most useful anthropometric measures include height, weight, triceps skinfold (actually fatfold) thickness, and midarm circumference. Accurate measurements require only three simple pieces of equipment: a beam or lever balance scale with a vertical measuring rod and a headpiece, a constant tension skinfold caliper, and a flexible measuring tape, preferably with an insertion.

TABLE 213–1. KEY QUESTIONS TO ASK AS PART OF THE NUTRITIONAL ASSESSMENT OF THE ADULT

1. Is there recent weight gain or weight loss? How much?
2. Are there alterations in appetite, sense of smell, or taste?
3. Are there problems with chewing or swallowing? Does the patient have poor dentition or poorly fitting dentures?
4. Are there symptoms of gastrointestinal disorders: diarrhea, constipation, nausea, vomiting, early satiety?
5. Does the patient live alone? If not, who prepares meals? Does he/she know how to cook?
6. What type of cooking facilities and refrigeration are in the patient's home?
7. Does the patient purchase a variety of food? If not, is it due to financial difficulties?
8. How many meals are eaten per day? How many snacks? Are one or more meals eaten outside of the home? If so, where?
9. Is the patient physically or mentally handicapped? Does this prevent the individual from shopping, cooking, or feeding herself or himself?
10. Does the patient take any dietary supplements (e.g., vitamins)?
11. How much alcohol does the patient consume?
12. Does the patient use prescription or nonprescription drugs?
13. Are there any religious or ethnic beliefs or food intolerances that prevent adequate food intake?
14. Does the patient follow a dietary restriction? Is it prescribed or self-imposed?
15. Is the patient depressed?

TABLE 213–2. REFERENCE WEIGHT/HEIGHT FIGURES DERIVED FROM ACTUARIAL (MORTALITY EXPERIENCE) DATA OF THE 1979 BUILD AND BLOOD PRESSURE STUDY*

Height		Weight			
		Male		Female	
(in)	(cm)	(lb)	(kg)	(lb)	(kg)
58	147.3	—	—	114	51.7
59	149.9	—	—	116.5	52.8
60	152.4	—	—	119	53.9
61	154.9	—	—	122	55.3
62	157.5	133	60.3	125	56.7
63	160.0	135	61.2	128	58.0
64	162.6	137.5	62.4	131	59.4
65	165.1	140	63.5	134	60.8
66	167.6	143	64.9	137	62.1
67	170.2	146	66.2	140	63.5
68	172.7	149	67.6	143	64.9
69	175.3	152	68.9	146	66.2
70	177.8	155	70.3	149	67.6
71	180.3	158.5	71.9	152	69.0
72	182.9	162	73.9	—	—
73	185.4	166	75.3	—	—
74	188.0	169.5	76.9	—	—
75	190.5	174	78.9	—	—

*Weights represent the midpoint of the middle frame for each height. These values correct the 1983 Metropolitan Tables to nude weights and heights.

WEIGHT FOR HEIGHT. Single reference weights for each inch of height have been derived from United States life insurance actuarial data on longevity and have been termed "ideal" or "optimal" by some investigators. However, these single weights should not be interpreted as "ideal," since they represent the midpoint of an acceptable range for a person of medium frame and were derived from the mortality experience of only those men and women between the ages of 20 to 59 years who could afford life insurance. These weights are neither age nor race specific and do not represent all cultural groups. Further, these reference weights cannot be applied to patients with peripheral edema or ascites. Despite the recognized flaws in using such single reference weights as standards, clinicians have found the 1983 Metropolitan Life Insurance Reference Weights for height useful for judging a patient's nutritional status reflecting caloric sufficiency. These reference weights (corrected to the nude state) are provided in Table 213–2. Using these weights for heights as a reference, 20 per cent above each weight places approximately 25 per cent of the United States population in the overweight for height or obese category, and 20 per cent below places less than 5 per cent of the population in the underweight category. Although these values were derived from a younger population, it appears that these reference values can be applied cautiously to the elderly based on data indicating that mean weights of healthy men and women from ages 70 to 90 years old closely approximate the Metropolitan weights. In children, weight and height are often used as separate measures to indicate malnutrition and are expressed as percentiles of a cross-section of American children. Weight and height tables for children can be found in most pediatric textbooks.

The amount of weight lost and the rate at which it was lost by a patient are also important for judging an individual's nutritional status. A history of weight loss of 10 per cent or greater (6 per cent in an overweight patient) over a six-month period can be indicative of malnutrition.

TRICEPS SKINFOLD THICKNESS. This measurement provides an estimate of the body's fat reserves. The measurement should be taken at a marked point on the right arm, halfway between the acromial process of the scapula and the olecranon process of the elbow. The patient's arm should be relaxed when the fatfold is grasped posteriorly between the thumb and forefinger of the examiner. The fold should be raised, allowing underlying

TABLE 213–3. RECOMMENDED ANTHROPOMETRIC MEASUREMENT STANDARDS FOR THE UNITED STATES ADULT POPULATION

	Triceps Skinfold (mm)		Mid-Arm Muscle Circumference (cm)	
	25–64 yr	*>65 yr*	*25–64 yr*	*>65 yr*
Male	12	11	27.9	26.8
Female	21	24	21.2	22.5

muscle to fall back to the bone, and the calipers applied. The measurement is useless if arm edema or paralysis is present. Age- and sex-specific standards for triceps skinfold (TSF) thickness have been published by Frisancho (1981) for all ages through 75 years (summarized in Table 213–3). A range of 40 to 190 per cent of the standard is considered an acceptable TSF measure, since large variances are found for fatfold thicknesses in the normal population. A patient whose TSF thickness is

TABLE 213–4. SUGGESTED CRITERIA TO JUDGE MALNUTRITION AND OBESITY IN THE UNITED STATES ADULT POPULATION

	Malnutrition		Obesity	
	Per Cent of Standard	*Corresponding Percentile*	*Per Cent of Standard*	*Corresponding Percentile*
WT/HT	<80	5th	>120	<5*
Triceps Skinfold	<40	5th	>190	>90th
Midarm Muscle Circumference	<80	5th	NA	NA

*Weight for height percentiles are based on the Health and Nutrition Examination Survey (HANES) of 1971–1974 comparison to Metropolitan 1983 standards. Triceps skinfold and midarm muscle circumference percentiles are derived from HANES data.

TABLE 213–5. CLINICAL SIGNS AND SYMPTOMS OF NUTRITIONAL INADEQUACY IN ADULT PATIENTS

	Clinical Sign or Symptom	Nutrient
General	Wasted, skinny	Calorie
	Loss of appetite	Protein-energy
Skin	Psoriasiform rash, eczematous scaling	Zinc
	Pallor	Folate, iron, vitamin B_{12}, copper
	Follicular hyperkeratosis	Vitamin A
	Perifollicular petechiae	Vitamin C
	Flaking dermatitis	Protein-energy, niacin, riboflavin, zinc
	Bruising	Vitamin C, vitamin K
	Pigmentation changes	Niacin, protein-energy
	Scrotal dermatosis	Riboflavin
	Thickening and dryness of skin	Linoleic acid
Head	Temporal muscle wasting	Protein-energy
Hair	Sparse and thin, dyspigmentation	Protein
	Easy to pull out	
Eyes	History of night blindness (also impaired visual recovery after glare)	Vitamin A, zinc
	Photophobia, blurring, conjunctival inflammation	Riboflavin, vitamin A
	Corneal vascularization	Riboflavin
	Xerosis, Bitot spots, keratomalacia	Vitamin A
Mouth	Glossitis	Riboflavin, niacin, folic acid, vitamin B_{12}, pyridoxine
	Bleeding gums	Vitamin C, riboflavin
	Cheilosis	Riboflavin
	Angular stomatitis	Riboflavin, iron
	Hypogeusia	Zinc
	Tongue fissuring	Niacin
	Tongue atrophy	Riboflavin, niacin, iron
	Scarlet and raw tongue	Niacin
	Nasolabial seborrhea	Pyridoxine
Neck	Goiter	Iodine
	Parotid enlargement	Protein
Thorax	Thoracic rosary	Vitamin D
Abdomen	Diarrhea	Niacin, folate, vitamin B_{12}
	Distention	Protein-energy
	Hepatomegaly	Protein-energy
Extremities	Edema	Protein, thiamin
	Softening of bone	Vitamin D, calcium, phosphorus
	Bone tenderness	Vitamin D
	Bone ache, joint pain	Vitamin C
	Muscle wasting and weakness	Protein, calorie, vitamin D, selenium, sodium chloride
	Muscle tenderness, muscle pain	Thiamin
	Hyporeflexia	Thiamin
	Ataxia	Vitamin B_{12}
Nails	Spooning	Iron
	Transverse lines	Protein
Neurologic	Tetany	Calcium, magnesium
	Paresthesias	Thiamin, vitamin B_{12}
	Loss of reflexes, wrist drop, foot drop	Thiamin
	Loss of vibratory and position sense	Vitamin B_{12}
	Dementia, disorientation	Niacin
Blood	Anemia	Vitamin E, B_{12}, folate, iron, pyridoxine
	Hemolysis	Phosphorus

less than 40 per cent of the HANES standard is considered to have depleted body fat stores, while the patient whose TSF thickness is more than 190 per cent of standard is considered obese.

MIDARM MUSCLE CIRCUMFERENCE. This derived value is used to estimate lean body or skeletal muscle mass. To calculate this value, the midarm circumference must first be measured at the same site as the triceps fatfold with the patient's right arm in a relaxed posture. The formula to calculate midarm muscle circumference (MAMC) is:

$$\text{MAMC (cm)} = \text{midarm circumference (cm)} - (0.314 \times \text{TSF (mm)})$$

Median values are summarized in Table 213–3. Twenty per cent below this standard is indicative of a depletion of lean body mass. Neither TSF nor MAMC standards have been derived for the very elderly (i.e., older than 75 years). A summary of criteria to judge malnutrition and obesity by anthropometric measurements is presented in Table 213–4.

CLINICAL ASSESSMENT

Early clinical symptoms and signs of malnutrition are rather vague and often include weakness, lethargy, irritability, and lightheadedness. Many of the symptoms and signs are nonspecific for a single nutrient deficit and may be caused by insufficiency of one of several nutrients. For example, flaking dermatitis may accompany deficiencies of protein, riboflavin, or linoleic acid. On the other hand, when certain clinical signs appear, the nutrient deficit may be very severe (e.g., scleromalacia, a leading and rapidly progressive cause of blindness due to vitamin A deficiency). Table 213–5 contains a listing of clinical presentations and the associated nutrient deficits that may cause them.

Functional and end organ testing have been advocated for diagnosis of specific nutrient deficits (e.g., dark adaptation for vitamin A, taste and smell for zinc, bone density for vitamin D, and so on). However, functional tests are not available to assess the status of most nutrients, and, as with clinical signs, the functional tests are often nonspecific. For example, impairment of dark adaptation may be caused by zinc deficiency as well as vitamin A deficiency. Taste and smell may be affected by age, smoking, and drugs as well as by zinc nutriture. Bone density is diminished in both osteoporosis and osteomalacia due to vitamin D deficiency.

As with dietary assessment, the elderly present a particular problem when evaluated for the presence or absence of clinical signs or symptoms of malnutrition. Some of the changes associated with malnutrition may also be a function of normal aging (e.g., hypogeusia, dry skin, sparse hair, atrophy of the tongue, bleeding gums from ill fitting dentures). Nevertheless, as with younger patients, clinical signs should be assessed for possible nutritional implications.

LABORATORY ASSESSMENT

Laboratory measurements are another tool that can aid the physician in making a diagnosis of malnutrition. Modern analytical instruments (e.g., high-performance liquid chromatography), techniques (e.g., radio or enzyme immunoassays), and computerization have greatly increased the capability of nutritional biochemical testing. Currently available biochemical tests for assessing nutritional status include the direct measurement of a nutrient or nutrient metabolite in blood, other body fluid (e.g., urine, saliva), or tissues (e.g., white blood cells, hair, liver) and the measurement of a biochemical function that is nutrient specific. For example, laboratory tests for pyridoxine status may include the direct measurement of pyridoxal 5′-phosphate in plasma or the enzymatic activity of erythrocyte transaminase, for which pyridoxal 5′-phosphate is a cofactor. The latter test involves the calculation of an activity coefficient whereby red blood cell transaminase activity is determined before and after the addition of pyridoxal 5′-phosphate. An activity coefficient of greater than 1 is indicative of pyridoxine deficiency.

The establishment of normal nutrient values in body fluids or tissues for each sex varies from laboratory to laboratory, and the normal range usually represents a mean ± 2 SD of a normal population. Optimally, a low biochemical nutrient value in body fluids or tissue should be coupled with a specific functional abnormality before making the diagnosis of a nutrient deficiency. However, in practice this is rarely done. One guide for interpretation of laboratory values that reflects the status of various nutrients in the blood or serum of adults is presented in Table 213–6. For some nutrients (e.g., vitamin A) children have a different normal range than adults. The reader is referred to a pediatric or nutrition text for detailed information on age-specific normal values. Normal biochemical ranges have not been established for the very old (i.e., over 75 years). The physician must rely upon values derived from younger populations to judge the nutritional biochemical parameters for this group.

TABLE 213–6. GUIDE FOR INTERPRETATION OF BIOCHEMICAL INDICES FOR SELECTED NUTRIENTS

Nutrient	Normal*	Deficient	Marginal
Albumin	3.5–5.5 g/dl	2.8–3.2	3.2–3.5
Transferrin	200–400 mg/dl	< 200	
Prealbumin	10–40 mg/dl	<10	
Ferritin	12–300 ng/ml	< 12	
Retinol	30–90 μg/dl	< 15	15–30
Carotene	40–240 μg/dl	< 40	
Vitamin E	0.5–1.8 mg/dl	< 0.5	0.5–0.7
Vitamin D (25-OH-D_3)	15–40 ng/ml		
Thiamin (erythrocyte)	0.9–1.25†	> 1.25	1.25–1.20
Riboflavin	0.9–1.39†	> 1.40	1.30–1.40
Pyridoxine	0.9–2.2†	> 2.2	
Niacin (urine 2-pyridone/N′-methyl nicotinamide—metabolite ratio)	1.0–4.0	< 1.0	
Serum Folate	6–20 ng/ml	≤ 3.0	3–6
Red Cell Folate	150–450 ng/ml	< 150	
Vitamin B_{12}	> 200 pg/ml	< 150	150–200
Vitamin C	0.3–2.0 mg/dl	< 0.2	0.2–0.3
Calcium	8.5–10.5 mg/dl	< 8.5	
Phosphorus	2.5–4.5 mg/dl	< 2.5	
Iron	50–170 μg/dl		
Zinc	70–130 μg/dl	≤ 65	65–70
Copper	70–160 μg/dl	< 70	
Magnesium	1.4–2.5 mg/dl	≤ 1.4	

*These normal values will vary with the method used and in different laboratories.
†An enzymatic assay. Values represent an activity coefficient.

Many nutrient biochemical diagnostic tests are not readily available in a hospital clinical chemistry laboratory. Nevertheless, there are several laboratory tests that are routinely performed (e.g., hemoglobin level, serum protein level) that may aid the physician in assessing the nutritional status of his or her patients. In the absence of liver disease, a low serum albumin may be used as an indicator of protein nutriture. In sick patients who are obese, silent kwashiorkor (protein malnutrition) may develop, as reflected by low serum protein values, although the patient may continue to look overnourished and anthropometric measures may be normal or exceed the normal range. Other proteins that are synthesized in the liver and that have a more rapid turnover than albumin (e.g., transferrin, prealbumin) may also be used to diagnose protein malnutrition at an earlier stage. The transferrin in serum, if not directly measured, may be estimated from the total iron binding capacity (TIBC) according to the formula: $(0.8 \times \text{TIBC}) - 43$. Protein values that are more than 20 per cent below the lower limit of the normal range are generally regarded as severely substandard. It has been suggested that elderly people have a somewhat lower normal serum albumin value and that age-specific standards for serum protein values are needed.

Muscle protein can be estimated from urinary creatinine excretion; this complements the anthropometric indicator MAMC. The amount of creatinine appearing in the urine over 24 hours is proportional to muscle mass. A crude standard for creatinine excretion can be derived by multiplying an individual's reference weight-for-height by 23 or 18 (for males and females respectively). Twenty per cent below these derived values may represent muscle protein depletion. However, several factors are known to affect creatinine excretion (e.g., kidney disease, diet, fever, strenous exercise, menstrual cycle), and the interpretation, therefore, must be carried out cautiously.

In protein energy malnutrition, the number of circulating lymphocytes diminish, and the patient demonstrates impaired delayed hypersensitivity to common skin antigens (e.g., mumps, *Candida* tuberculin). Thus, these tests also may be used in assessing the patient's nutritional status. A lymphocyte count of less than 1200 per cubic millimeter is regarded as severely substandard. The effect of advanced age on these parameters is uncertain.

Frisancho AR: New norms of upper limb fat and muscle areas for assessment of nutritional status. Am J Clin Nutr 34:2540, 1981. *This article presents American standards for athropometric measures for ages 1 to 75 years, derived from the HANES survey of 1971–1974.*

Goodhart RS, Shils ME (eds.): Modern Nutrition in Health and Disease. Philadelphia, Lea and Febiger, 1980. *This nutrition textbook provides detailed discussion of signs and symptoms of nutritional disorders.*

Jelliffe DB: The Assessment of Nutritional Status. Oxford University Press (in press). *An updated version of the World Health Organization's Manual for Nutritional Assessment of Populations.*

Paige DM (ed.): Manual of Clinical Nutrition. Pleasantville, Nutrition Publications, Inc., 1983. *This manual provides most tables and information for clinical assessment of nutritional status for pediatric and adult patients.*

Sauberlich HE, Dowdy RP, Skala JH: Laboratory Tests for the Assessment of Nutritional Status. Boca Raton, CRC Press, 1979. *This volume provides descriptions and some evaluation measures for laboratory tests used for the assessment of nutritional status.*

214. PROTEIN-CALORIE UNDERNUTRITION

Errol B. Marliss

The syndromes of protein-calorie malnutrition (PCM) were defined in the 1920's in areas where food was deficient in quantity and/or quality. The terms kwashiorkor and marasmus have retained an "exotic" ring in developed countries and rarely if ever appear in the diagnostic categories on discharge summaries, despite the fact that between 450 million and one billion humans suffer from chronic hunger and malnutrition. However, these syndromes are anything but curiosities. With a resurgence of interest in the role of nutrition in health and disease, a veritable "epidemic" has been recognized in a number of patient populations. In particular, hospitalized adult medical and surgical patients have been shown to develop signs of PCM in 25 to 50 per cent of cases within two weeks of admission. Thus PCM is not only a problem of postweaning third-world children, but is an almost ubiquitous problem that can be readily treated, but preferably prevented. This chapter emphasizes the forms most likely to be encountered in developed countries.

DEFINITION AND ETIOLOGY

Precise definitions require quantitative reference to appropriate control populations and depend upon the anthropomorphic and laboratory measures referred to in Ch. 213. "Undernutrition" is the state produced by inadequate intake of food and may have as its only manifestation retarded growth in children or loss of weight in adults. While "malnutrition" can refer to over- or undernutrition, it most commonly connotes a dietary lack of one or more nutrients, which markedly retards development in children and causes the appearance of specific, clinically recognizable deficiency states at all ages. Marasmus is the clinical syndrome resulting from prolonged limitation of intake of both protein and energy, whereas kwashiorkor results from deficiency of protein relative to energy. Caloric intake may be adequate or even excessive, and kwashiorkor may occur concurrently with marasmus. PCM is classified as primary, due to limited food supply, and secondary, due to the presence of disease(s) that prevents access to or absorption of food, causes excessive caloric loss, or increases demand for energy, or combinations of these. However, since primary PCM is often complicated, as by infection, this distinction may be difficult to make.

INCIDENCE, PREVALENCE, AND EPIDEMIOLOGY

Undernutrition is encountered with different frequencies in different age and population groups, and prevalence data vary according to diagnostic criteria. In children, decreased weight for height is taken as the diagnostic criterion but is criticized because stunting is not thereby ascertained. Similarly, mortality rates in infancy are a crude index of undernutrition because all causes are grouped together. Although in this age group diarrheal diseases are still the commonest cause of mortality world wide, they are highly correlated to poor nutritional status. Furthermore, early childhood mortality rates increase, especially with decrease below 80 per cent of normal weight for height. Thus figures of 25 per cent (in 28 developing countries) to 64 per cent (in Central America) of children with malnutrition gives indication of the enormous magnitude of this problem. In developing countries, it must be considered to be a social "disease," affecting families, communities, and geographic areas: undernourished adults show poor work performance, perhaps lower intellectual performance, suceptibility to infection, and poor reproduction performance in terms of weight gain in pregnancy, small-for-dates babies, and inadequate milk production. Thus, although fewer adults show overt clinical signs of malnutrition themselves (e.g., 8 per cent of hospital admissions in Guatemala), they are index cases of a more widespread problem. This is referred to as the "microenvironment," i.e., the family and individual level, compared to the "macroenvironment," i.e., the regional or national level. Factors in the microenvironment that lead to poor nutrition include restricted purchasing power, poor nutrition education leading to poor consumption practices, and inappropriate distribution of nutrients among family members. One distressing feature of the macroenvironment is that production on a worldwide basis is in fact adequate to feed the population, and this also applies to many individual countries with high prevalence of malnutrition. This situation is explicable by losses of food between production and utilization (30 per cent in some countries), by problems of distribution between areas of production and consumption, and by economic and political factors. Improvements especially in the "macroenvironment" had led to decreases in infant mortality over the two decades preceding the recent recession, but international economic factors have reversed this trend in recent years.

The microenvironmental factors also occur in developed countries. As improbable as it might seem, kwashiorkor has been reported in several United States centers. Some cases are due to peculiar dietary habits imposed by parents on children (e.g., unbalanced vegetarian diets), almost total elimination of protein in children considered (often incorrectly) to have sensitivity to cow's milk, and replacement of milk by low-protein nondairy creamers, as well as extreme poverty, parental alcoholism, and other social disruptions. The incidence of such cases is probably higher than reported.

Furthermore, nutritional surveys even in pediatric teaching hospitals have also revealed a striking prevalence of PCM, e.g., 37 per cent in one study. Several such surveys in hospitalized adults in the past ten years have shown both anthropomorphic and biochemical evidence for PCM; Bistrian and colleagues' data suggested 44 per cent of general medical patients and 50 per cent of surgical patients were afflicted. In patients in a medical service for two or more weeks, 79 per cent showed decreases in arm muscle circumference, 74 per cent lost weight (average 4.5 kg), 64 per cent had decreases in hematocrit, and 47 per cent had declining serum albumin (Butterworth et al). Patients at greatest risk for PCM in hospital were found to have the following: (1) gross underweight (less than 80 per cent weight for height), (2) gross overweight (because their requirements are often overlooked), (3) recent loss of more than 10 per cent body weight, (4) alcoholism, (5) "nil per os" orders for more than ten days on 5 per cent dextrose in water solutions intravenously, (6) protracted nutrient losses (gut, fistulas, dialysis), (7) increased metabolic needs, and (8) therapies with catabolic, anorexogenic, or antinutrient drugs (steroids, chemotherapy, immunosuppressants). Aged patients are likely at greatest risk because of poor premorbid nutrition, polypharmacy, and concurrent illnesses. Certain psychiatric patients in hospitals and the community are probably malnourished. Much hospital PCM is the direct result of spectacular therapeutic advances that prolong the lives of patients, while their concurrent nutrient requirements are not attended to. Other groups at risk are those who self-administer nutritionally inadequate reducing diets with the primary aim of fat mobilization. Those at all parts of the weight spectrum—the obese, those with normal weight who wish to lose weight for cosmetic reasons, and those with anorexia nervosa—may suffer PCM of variable severity and duration during such diets. The prevalence of these subsets of PCM is particularly difficult to ascertain, as are potential long-term consequences (see Ch. 215 and 216). They are likely to be common, however, given the widespread use of reducing regimens and the large numbers of individuals in these categories.

PATHOPHYSIOLOGY

METABOLIC FACTORS. Maintenance of normal body composition and energy fuel homeostasis requires regular intake of energy substrates, protein, water and electrolytes, vitamins, and other essential micronutrients. Reference values are given in Ch. 212. Specific quantitative and qualitative increments are required for growth, pregnancy, muscular exercise, severe environmental conditions, and disease. In the case of the undernourished adult, deficits in energy and protein are made up from endogenous sources, via an elegantly orchestrated set of hormonal, neural, and local tissue enzymatic responses. These appear to operate in a hierarchial fashion with highest priority on sparing protein (of which there is no known "storage" form) by use of endogenous fat stores for energy. Early in undernutrition, liver and possibly muscle glycogen are depleted but appear to be at least partly restored later—possibly constituting a short-term "emergency" energy supply. The mobilization of protein stores beyond a critical limit presumably results in death. This may well be the case in kwashiorkor, in which some fat stores remain, but in other forms of starvation, exhaustion of fat stores may be the critical step, even with some protein theoretically still available.

The best controlled data in such states are from experimental studies of total fasting. This, however, is a state rarely encountered clinically; either the individual has maintained some level of oral energy and protein intake, or some level has been provided parenterally. In total fasting increased ketogenesis provides the brain with a fuel that displaces its glucose requirement and thereby allows for sparing of the protein (which would otherwise be used for glucose synthesis). This response is not directly applicable to the starved individual, since very little carbohydrate is required to suppress ketogenesis (e.g., 50 grams per day, or a sum of protein plus carbohydrate of 100 grams per day), and the undernourished individual is not typically ketotic or even ketonuric (a highly sensitive index). Exceptions are in therapeutic hypocaloric "protein-sparing modified fasts" (see Ch. 216) with increased energy requirement and in diabetics.

Although carbohydrate alone is "protein sparing" (vis-à-vis total fasting), the fundamental law of protein homeostasis is that it requires exogenous protein. At any given protein intake, added calories either as carbohydrate or fat enhance the availability for maintenance of protein synthesis of the constituent amino acids, which would otherwise be oxidized as an energy source. Thus the protein requirement varies with concurrent energy intake, being higher in both relative (protein-energy ratio) and absolute terms when energy intake is below requirement. Furthermore, the protein quality (in terms of essential amino acid composition) is a factor. The higher the quality (animal proteins), the lower the relative requirement. Unfortunately, where malnutrition is rampant, not only quantity but quality of protein is often poor—being mainly from vegetable sources. Of protein consumed in North America, 70 per cent is from animal sources, whereas it is as low as 14 to 20 per cent in developing countries. Thus the diet most likely to be associated with malnutrition is one based on cereal grains, starchy roots, cornstarch, possibly with overdiluted milk, snack foods, and alcohol and without animal protein. Such a diet is low in animal and separated vegetable fats, with less than 10 per cent of energy from the naturally occurring vegetable fat in developing countries, but it may have a substantial fat intake in developed countries if it is based on processed foods.

In energy-balance terms such diets, even if adequate in calories, are often very low in protein of good biologic value. When total calories are restricted further, the protein inadequacy assumes even greater importance. In either case in the adult, body protein is mobilized, and in the energy-starved individual both protein and fat are depleted, the latter generally more rapidly. The body progressively adapts to this situation by decreased energy expenditure (metabolic rate) overall and per unit of lean body mass, decreased physical activity, and decreased rates of body protein turnover. If such changes result in equilibrium with intake, a fragile state of "maximal adaptation" occurs that may persist over long periods. However, once the caloric deficit is severe, basal energy expenditure may be normal or increased relative to lead body mass, which then decreases at a faster rate.

In childhood, the energy and protein deficiencies occur when requirements are high per unit of body weight. Pathophysiology of the deficits varies with age. If they occur before weaning, they are in both protein and energy, leading to retarded growth with decreased or absent fat stores. If after weaning, the replacement nutrients determine the course in one of three usual patterns: (1) Marginal protein and calories, a pattern that perpetuates undernutrition. The adapted state continues with slower than normal physical growth, but with frequent infections (e.g., measles, pertussis, parasitic infestations, diarrheal diseases) that may precipitate severe PCM. (2) Severe restriction, which results in marasmus. (3) High calorie but protein-deficient diets, which lead to the typical edematous PCM of the "sugar-baby" type. In all cases brain growth and development may well be retarded, and irreversible deficits may occur. Concurrently, head circumference may remain small, and muscle mass and muscle cell size are subnormal. Tissues with rapid cell turnover also develop impaired size and possibly impaired function. Atrophy of the gut, and deficiency of intestinal, pancreatic, and biliary secretions may compound PCM by reducing absorption of what is ingested. Those who survive to adulthood then may remain in this precariously adapted state, although with smaller body size than had the malnutrition started in adulthood.

ENDOCRINE FACTORS. The changes in endocrine and neuroendocrine function in PCM are complex and some remain controversial. Insulin is the principal hormone of anabolism, and catabolism is enhanced when its levels fall. Both postabsorptive and postchallenge (glucose, amino acids) insulin levels are lowered in PCM. These levels allow net mobilization of fatty acids from adipose tissue triglyceride and of amino acids from protein (subsequently oxidized, recycled into protein synthesis, or converted to glucose by gluconeogenesis), as well as decreased protein synthesis in many tissues. However, a stimulation of insulin secretion by carbohydrate administration during protein deficiency in PCM has been considered partly responsible for the kwashiorkor-like syndrome in malnourished hospital patients. The resulting "high" insulin levels have been postulated to restrict fat mobilization, to limit use of muscle-derived amino acids for synthesis of "visceral" proteins, and to result in more amino acid oxidation. (This hypothetical sequence could equally well be interpreted to implicate the lack of exogenous protein and ongoing caloric deficits as responsible.) Insulin responses are certainly related to the sum of carbohydrate and protein intake, but other mechanisms not as yet defined remain capable of assuring that caloric deficits are filled from endogenous fat (when present), at widely varying insulin levels. Thus, strategies of nutrient replacement should not be aimed at achieving the lowest theoretical insulin response, but must take account of the other mechanisms, as well as the impairment of insulin responsiveness, that are clearly characteristic of PCM. Insulin secretion returns to normal after recovery from PCM. Increase in glucagon levels occurs in total fasting but not necessarily in PCM, and the role of this hormone is not likely to be central.

Hypothalamic-pituitary function is also altered in a complex manner. Growth hormone levels are generally increased in PCM, although plasma somatomedins are low, especially with severe protein deficiency. The pituitary-thyroid axis may well be an important factor in the decrease in metabolic rate. Carbohydrate intake appears to play an important role in this response. When intake is decreased, although TSH and its responses to TRH are unaltered, thyroxine levels are often normal (but may be low), but its peripheral conversion to triiodothyronine is altered, in favor of the inactivating pathway to reverse triiodothyronine (Ch. 228). Interpretation of thyroid hormone values must take account of decreases in binding proteins in PCM, and of decreased synthesis of triiodothyronine receptors.

The pituitary-adrenal axis has been the focus of hypotheses to explain differences between kwashiorkor and marasmus: An increase in activity (hypercortisolemia) in marasmus was postulated to sustain flux of amino acids from muscle (increasing the wasting) to liver to support albumin synthesis, whereas the calories provided in kwashiorkor were supposed sufficient not to result in hypercortisolemia, and therefore to restrict such flux, with consequent hypoalbuminemia. While a coherent hypothesis, the data have not so far proven this to be the case. When hypercortisolemia occurs, it appears more related to impaired catabolism than to increased production, and its pathophysiologic significance is not clear.

A variety of abnormalities in pituitary-gonadal function has been reputed, including low testosterone accompanied by high FSH and LH in adult males and many reproductive disorders in females, most of which return toward or to normal after treatment.

ELECTROLYTE, MINERAL, AND MICRONUTRIENT CHANGES. The tissue loss leads to concomitant losses of body nitrogen, potassium, and phosphorus. Fluid shifts may further lead to changes of sodium and chloride and to exchange of sodium intracellularly for potassium and magnesium. In kwashiorkor, the frequent diarrhea further exacerbates losses. Extrarenal fluid and electrolyte losses are an important factor in hospital PCM, with the acid-base alterations that accompany them. The most prominent, clinically important depletions are of potassium and magnesium. Total and extracellular water and sodium are increased in kwashiorkor, related to the hypoproteinemia, and associated with increased plasma aldosterone. In severe cases, renal plasma flow, glomerular filtration rate, urine concentrating ability, and acidification are impaired. Zinc and chromium deficiencies are recognized in certain geographic regions and during prolonged parenteral nutrition, and their role in PCM is currently the subject of active study. The manifestations of vitamin deficiencies will vary with local dietary patterns or the inpatient population considered. Although clinical signs of water-soluble vitamin deficiencies may be uncommon, and serum levels normal, inadequate intake of thiamin, riboflavin, ascorbic acid, niacin, and folate may have taken place. In kwashiorkor, serum vitamin A is consistently low and may be accompanied by ocular lesions. This is often accounted for not only by poor intake of vitamin A, but also by abnormal absorption and transport. Vitamin E shows similar decreased levels and kinetic defects. Some reports have indicated elevated levels of vitamin B_{12}.

IMMUNE RESPONSES. Almost all aspects of the immune response have been shown to be impaired in PCM, with the degree of impairment related to severity. Concurrent infection, especially with loss of nutrients, exacerbates this state. Some resistance to infection is conferred during breast feeding, but this depends on the adequacy of maternal nutrition and is lost on weaning. When PCM begins at or before birth, the infant is generally immunocompromised, with decreases in IgG, IgA, IgM, and IgE, whereas in older children immunoglobulins are usually normal, or elevated when infection is present. Often a single class may be increased, e.g., IgA, perhaps reflecting the frequency of respiratory and gastrointestinal infections. Specific antibody production to many antigens is subnormal, and this causes poor responses to immunization programs, although responses to different agents vary. Not only the quantity of the antibody response, but affinities and binding capacities are reduced. In vivo and in vitro tests of cell-mediated immunity are impaired, and skin tests for delayed-type hypersensitivity give subnormal responses. The thymus is atrophic. Typically, peripheral blood lymphocyte counts are decreased, especially thymus-derived lymphocytes, with values commonly less than 1200 per cu mm. Some of the cellular immune abnormalities may be related to trace metal deficiencies, including zinc. Nonspecific defenses are abnormal, including opsonization, interferon production, bacterial killing by phagocytes (although phagocytosis itself may be normal), and neutrophil and plasma lysozyme levels. Complement components other than C_4 may be decreased. Iron deficiency may contribute to the impaired bacterial killing after phagocytosis. Frequently acute phase protein levels are elevated, including C-reactive proteins, alpha-2-macroglobulin, alpha-1-antitrypsin, and haptoglobin, related to the protein loss and infection. The critical factors that decrease resistance to infection in PCM have not been fully elucidated but are of obvious importance. Introduction of nutrients seems to reverse most if not all the abnormalities; in fact, in the hospital setting, they are largely preventable. Even in previously normal adults, immune deficits appear to develop sufficiently rapidly that preventive measures appear mandatory.

OTHER PHYSIOLOGIC CHANGES. The adrenergic limb of the sympathetic nervous system is highly responsive to both energy and protein intake, with decreased norepinephrine turnover in many tissues (as long as salt intake is maintained), possibly responsible in part for the fall in metabolic rate. Dietary amino acids have a precursor role in neurotransmitter synthesis (tyrosine for norepinephrine, tryptophan for serotonin), such that their levels and turnover decrease with protein deficiency. Electroencephalograms may show diminished voltage and excessively slow rhythmic activity. The decreases in triiodothyronine, adrenergic tone, insulin, and possibly the lack of "insulation" by subcutaneous fat are associated with decreased body temperature and decreased febrile response to infection.

Many aspects of cardiovascular function change in PCM via complex mechanisms related to serum proteins, extracellular and vascular volume, adrenergic activity, and cardiac muscle size and performance. Cardiac output declines in parallel to metabolic rate; blood pressure is reduced, although pulse rate may increase; and electrocardiograms show low voltage. Postural hypotension occurs. Renal function decreases, but usually remains adequate because of the decrease in requirements, unless an additional metabolic or infective burden is superimposed. Blood volume, the hematocrit, and erythrocyte counts decrease, producing a normochromic, normocytic anemia whose pathogenesis relates to multiple deficiencies.

Despite marked fatty changes in the liver, beginning in the periportal of the lobule and extending toward the portal vein, common tests for liver function are usually normal in the absence of hepatitis. The exocrine pancreas decreases in size and its secretions diminish, and indices of small intestinal mucosal turnover and function do likewise. These can result secondarily in malabsorption and lactose intolerance, even without bacterial overgrowth or other infections. Epidermal atrophy with varying degrees of hyperkeratosis and parakeratosis is found in the skin.

CLINICAL MANIFESTATIONS AND DIAGNOSIS (Table 214–1)

The classic syndromes of kwashiorkor and marasmus are not encountered frequently in clinical practice in developed areas. Even in developing countries in Asia, Africa, and Latin America, intermediate syndromes are in fact more common. In both settings chronic mild to moderate malnutrition is the form that predominates, and while not difficult to diagnose it is less flagrant than the "textbook" PCM usually described. In children, longstanding restriction is apparent from retardation in height and weight gain; when adapted to PCM the stunted child may even have adequate weight for height. This is not "normal but small," because immaturity in biologic development is present: deficits in lean body mass and adiposity, with relative overhydration, reduced physical activity, apathy, frequent episodes of ill-defined sickness, anorexia, diarrhea, and a higher mortality rate from common infectious diseases. Furthermore, psychomotor and mental development are retarded, although it is uncertain what contribution is from the social versus the nutritional deprivations so common in such individuals. In adults, similar body compositional changes occur, but physically the appearance is of leanness that may merge into cachexia. Since protein requirements are lower per unit of lean body mass in children, the manifestations are most often those of caloric deficits. In the aging population, especially the disadvantaged, prevalence of such changes may be very high. Symptoms are nonspecific, but the complex of weight loss (irrespective of whether prior weight was normal or elevated), decreased effort tolerance, lethargy, cold intolerance, ankle swelling, and dry flaking skin should arouse concern for nutritional status. The physical examination is similarly not diagnostic—especially if weight is still at or above normal—and is based on height, weight, midarm muscle circumference, and skinfold thickness measurements (see Ch. 213) with reference to norms and previous data from the individual. In addition, one may find easily pluckable hair, edema, and delayed wound healing. Often the clinical picture is dominated by the underlying cause in cases of secondary undernutrition. Laboratory studies in such individuals demonstrate low excretion of urea nitrogen per gram creatinine, decreased plasma levels of branched-chain amino acids, decreased hydroxyproline excretion, and small decreases in serum transferrin and albumin. With significant protein depletion the creatinine/height index is decreased. When PCM is severe it tends to follow the patterns of the two classic forms.

TABLE 214–1. INDICES OF UNDERNUTRITION*

Variable	Abnormal Status Suggested by
MINIMAL ASSESSMENT (ROUTINE CLINICAL USE)	
Anthropomorphic	
Adults	
loss of weight in 1 month	$\geq$5%
loss of weight in 6 months	$\geq$10%
Children	
body weight for height,	<80% standard
or percentile drop in weight from growth chart over 6-month period	$\geq$20 percentiles
Laboratory	
Serum albumin	$\leq$2.8 g/dl
Serum transferrin	$\leq$150 mg/dl
Lymphocyte count	$\leq$1200 cells/mm^3
COMPREHENSIVE ASSESSMENT (DETAILED FOLLOW-UP AND RESEARCH)	
Anthropomorphic	
Skinfold thickness	
Midarm muscle circumference	
Creatinine—height index	
Body composition	
underwater weighing	
multiple isotope dilution	
neutron activation analysis	
Immunologic	
Delayed cutaneous hypersensitivity	
T-cell subsets	
Immunoglobulins	
Fat Metabolism	
Cholesterol, total and fractions	
Triglycerides	
Ketone bodies	
Protein Metabolism	
Plasma individual free amino acids	
Urine total nitrogen, urea, ammonium	
Urine hydroxyproline	
Labeled amino acid turnover	
Hormones	
Insulin	
Catecholamines	
Growth hormone	
ACTH, cortisol	
TSH, thyroxine, triiodothyronine, reverse triiodothyronine	
Reproductive hormones	
Vitamins	
Vitamin A	
Vitamin E	
Folates	
Vitamin B_{12}	
Vitamin C	
Muscle Function	
Force, relaxation, fatigability	
Respiratory muscle function	
Other Circulating Proteins	
Retinol-binding protein	
Thyroxine-binding proteins	
Acute phase proteins	

*Modified from Alpers et al., 1983.

KWASHIORKOR. This form of PCM is typically found in the hospitalized adult unable to eat and/or under the stress of an acute illness or major surgery. In this setting, symptoms and signs of prior lesser degrees of malnutrition are as noted in the previous paragraph, or may be absent if the time course has been short. Hepatomegaly may be present. The child with severe kwashiorkor will have marked edema or anasarca, decreased movement of the extremities, and extreme apathy; will cry only weakly if disturbed; and will show severe anorexia and diarrhea. The "flaky-paint" lesions of the skin are pigmented, dry, hyperkeratotic, sometimes excoriated, and commonly located in the perineum, extremities, and face. They may involve the trunk. Hair becomes dry, fine, brittle, straight, and reddish or yellowish. The abdomen is distended due to flaccid muscles, ascites, and hepatomegaly. Blood pressure is decreased and the pulse may be slow. Hypothermia is common. The laboratory diagnosis is based on a sharp decline in serum albumin to less than 2.8 grams per deciliter, lymphocyte count to less than 1200 cells per cu mm, serum transferrin less than 150 mg per deciliter, and nonreactive skin tests. Those abnormalities listed above under mild malnutrition are present but are more marked. Other findings are variably present. Anemia is common, most frequently normochromic and normocytic, but varies according to other deficiencies. Liver function is not usually impaired, and enzyme levels may be below normal. The alterations in immunoglobulins, lymphocytes, neutrophils, vitamins, and other micronutrients may be as referred to earlier, and plasma glucose and lipids tend to be low. Other transport proteins, like ceruloplasmin, retinol-binding protein, and hormone-binding proteins are decreased. The hormonal changes have been described earlier. Urea nitrogen in serum and urine is low, and urine creatinine is decreased. Hypokalemia and hypomagnesemia are common, and metabolic acidosis may be present. Hypocalcemia is due to the decreased albumin. The heart is usually small and exhibits a decreased cardiac output. All of these laboratory studies are by no means necessary to establish the diagnosis or even to serve as a baseline for therapy, but when they are done for other reasons, the effect of PCM must be considered in their interpretation.

MARASMUS. The clinical picture of marasmus is dominated by growth arrest, emaciation, loss of muscle and fat, and atrophy of most organs, resulting in a "skin and bones" appearance. The sky is dry, "baggy," and decreased in turgor, although without the lesions of kwashiorkor. Hair is sparse, thin and dry, and dull in appearance. Edema is absent; appetite is adequate or increased; and while the patient is irritable, the apathy of the kwashiorkor victim is not present, although weakness may be profound. Bowel action is usually decreased, but bouts of diarrhea are not rare. Pulse, blood pressure, and temperature may be low. In contrast to kwashiorkor, fewer laboratory values are abnormal, with serum albumin greater than 2.8 grams per deciliter. Except in the severest cases, the other "visceral" proteins may be unaffected. While any of the other changes described above may be found, especially where a mixed picture of the two types is present, they may be absent. Where available, objective studies of muscle function show altered force of contraction and an increased fatigability and slowed relaxation rates in all types of malnutrition.

TREATMENT

In the case of mild to moderate PCM, the strategy is to treat the precipitating event and increase protein and energy intake calculated on the basis of actual height in children and ideal weight in adults. This will give a relatively greater intake of both than if intake is based on actual age or weight and will allow for the extra requirement for "catch-up" in children or "regrowth" in the adult. Specific supplementation of individual nutrients is indicated by the presence of signs of their deficiency.

In severe PCM, rehabilitation is pursued in two phases. The first is the resuscitation from the acute infection, water and electrolyte imbalances, or other factors that caused decompensation. The second phase is devoted to repletion of depleted protein and energy. Specific issues requiring attention in the first phase are the total body potassium depletion; the metabolic acidosis; and the risks of hypocalcemia and hypomagnesemia

while correcting acidosis and hypoalbuminemia, if calcium and magnesium replacement are insufficient. When indicated, all nutrients can be given parenterally (see Ch. 220). Introduction of nutrients into the gut of the malnourished individual can itself generate diarrhea because of the atrophy of the mucosa and the deficiency of digestive enzymes. Lipids and lactose are given sparingly for the first week, then in gradually increasing amounts. Starting at 0.8 gram of protein and 80 kcal per kilogram per day in children, the goal is to provide 4 grams of protein and 150 kcal per kilogram once tolerated and until recovery is complete. These calculations are based on actual weight. In the adult, daily initial intakes of 0.6 gram of protein and 50 kcal per kilogram are increased to 3 to 4 grams of protein and 80 to 100 kcal per kilogram. Vitamins, including folate, should be administered from the outset, including a large initial loading dose of vitamin A. When the oral or enteral route can be used but elemental formulations are preferred because of bowel disease, preparations are selected accordingly (see Ch. 219). Care must be taken in conversion from total parenteral nutrition to oral feeding, and in the introduction of normal nutrients after elemental diets.

The course of children is toward complete nutritional recovery within three to four months, with clearly measurable laboratory changes present within two to three weeks and anthropomorphic changes from three weeks onward. The changes may be slower in adults, unless the PCM was acute and of short duration. Comprehensive programs of nutrition education, psychosocial stimulation, and progressive increments in physical activity should be undertaken.

PREVENTION

In the hospitalized population, physicians should be aware of the patients who are at risk of developing PCM, as listed above. A checklist of use in assuring adequate nutrition of all patients to prevent PCM, as well as to monitor treatment of it, is presented in Table 214–2. These are easily incorporated into the nursing, dietetic, laboratory and pharmaceutical monitoring that accompanies standard medical practices. There is good evidence that both morbidity and mortality can be reduced in a cost-effective manner by such approaches. The prevention of childhood PCM, especially in developing countries, is oriented first toward prevention of severe cases, and second toward improvement of the nutrition of populations. Direct actions to achieve the first include encouragement of breast feeding and adequate supplementation of the diet of infants, together with supplements for women while pregnant and lactating and for children up to school age. Improvements of sanitary conditions and specific nutrition education are critical measures. However,

TABLE 214–2. CHECKLIST OF PROCEDURES TO PREVENT AND TREAT HOSPITAL MALNUTRITION*

1. Make an accurate record of admission height and weight and weekly follow-up weights.
2. Record specific orders regarding diet, and monitor ability to eat and amounts consumed.
3. Obtain consultation with dietician and assure follow-up collaboration on oral and tube feeding regimens.
4. Ascertain regularly whether the composition of nutrients consumed or infused is sufficient to cover basal and stress-related needs.
5. Be informed as to composition of standard nutrient preparations and supplements used in your hospital.
6. Do not wait longer than 3 to 5 days before adding protein, calories, and other nutrients to intravenous regimens. Avoid prolonged used of D5W and saline alone.
7. Use the simple anthropometric and available laboratory tests to assess and to monitor nutritional state.
8. Be cognizant that "hospital food," witholding meals for tests, and anorexia from medication can cumulatively contribute to malnutrition.
9. Consult the nutrition support service when indicated and monitor its recommended regimen.
10. Be especially vigilant with patients at high risk (see text).

*Inspired by Butterworth et al., 1980.

the solution to these problems also presupposes more effective means of distribution of available food to needy populations.

Alpers DH, Clouse RE, Stenson WF: Manual of Nutritional Therapeutics. Boston, Little, Brown and Company. 1983. *Well organized, readable, and contemporary, well-referenced how-to-do-it manual.*

Bistrian BR, Blackburn GL, Vitale J, Cochran D, Naylor J: Prevalence of malnutrition in general medical patients. JAMA 235:1567, 1976. *One of a series of studies establishing the high incidence of malnutrition in teaching hospitals.*

Butterworth CE, Jr, Weinsier RL: Malnutrition in hospital patients: Assessment and treatment. *In* Goodhart RS, Shils ME (eds.): Modern Nutrition in Health and Disease. 6th ed. Philadelphia, Lea and Febiger, 1980, p 667. *Contains more detail of the nutritional examination, strategy of therapy, and comprehensive list of effects of drugs on nutritional status.*

Chase HP, Kumar V, Caldwell RT, O'Brien D: Kwashiorkor in the United States. Pediatrics 66:972, 1980. *Occurrence and causes of the classic syndrome in the United States brought into focus.*

Crim MC, Munro HN: Protein-energy malnutrition and endocrine function. *In* DeGroot LJ (ed.): Endocrinology. New York, Grune and Stratton, 1979, p 1987. *This chapter reviews major hormones and their responses and roles in PCM and raises questions of relevance of changes found to PCM pathophysiology.*

Suskind RM (ed.): Malnutrition and the Immune Response. Kroc Foundation Series, Volume 7. New York, Raven Press, 1977. *A symposium report that covers all relevant aspects of immune response in PCM, the central issue in infection susceptibility.*

Viteri FE, Torun B: Protein-calorie malnutrition. *In* Goodhart RS, Shils ME (eds.): Modern Nutrition in Health and Disease. 6th ed. Philadelphia, Lea and Febiger, 1980, p 697. *Well-balanced review of classic syndromes of PCM.*

Waterlow JC: Childhood malnutrition—the global problem. Proc Nutr Soc 38:1, 1979. *The perspective of a renowned investigator on the world-wide impact of PCM, in a symposium on this topic.*

215. ANOREXIA NERVOSA

Gerald F. M. Russell

DEFINITION. Anorexia nervosa is a prolonged illness principally affecting young girls after puberty. It is characterized by severe weight loss which is self-induced, amenorrhea, and a specific psychopathology.

HISTORICAL NOTE. Sir William Gull described anorexia nervosa in 1868 and 1874. For a long time, confusion resulted from the concept of "Simmonds' cachexia," which embodied the mistaken view that panhypopituitarism caused loss of weight and wasting. Much needless effort was spent on the differential diagnosis of these two disorders which do not resemble each other.

ETIOLOGY. The cause of anorexia nervosa is unknown. A partial genetic contribution is favored by the finding of a significantly higher concordance of anorexia nervosa among monozygous than dizygous twins. Morbidity is also higher among sisters of patients (6.6 per cent). Anorexia nervosa used to be considered a rare illness. However, a five-fold increase in incidence was noted in Malmö, Sweden, between the 1930's and 1950's. Similar observations in Britain and the United States favor the view that culturally determined attitudes might lead to the illness. In recent years the upper social class bias for anorexia nervosa has diminished. The incidence of new cases ranges from 0.6 to 1.6 per 100,000 of the whole population, but the prevalence may be high in groups at special risk: 1 in 250 among schoolgirls aged 16 or over in England, 7 per cent of ballet students in Canada.

PSYCHOPATHOLOGY AND PATHOGENESIS. Anorexia nervosa is usually thought to be a disorder of psychogenic origin. The illness can also be viewed as a disorder of the feeding and endocrine functions normally controlled by the hypothalamus. It is important to consider simultaneously the mental and bodily disturbances in anorexia nervosa so as to comprehend their interaction as far as is possible.

The evidence for a psychogenic origin of anorexia nervosa is strong. Patients explain that they cannot eat because they feel guilty after eating, or are fearful that they will be unable to stop and hence will become unbearably fat. Disturbed family relationships or the conflicts of puberty and adolescence often play an important role. A disturbance of body image underlies the illness; for example, patients tend to overestimate the width of their own body. Food intake becomes determined by the patient's impression of the size of her own body. Because this impression is a distorted one and she imagines herself to be already too fat, she starves herself so as to acquire what she considers to be more desirable proportions.

Anorexia nervosa was originally considered to be a hypothalamic disorder on the grounds that destruction of the "feeding centers" in animals causes refusal of food. The strongest evidence for a primary hypothalamic disorder is the failure in the function of the hypothalamic–anterior pituitary–gonadal axis. Gonadotropins (FSH and LH) are not released from the anterior pituitary, the ovarian production of estrogens ceases, and ovulation fails to occur. There is a reversible hypothalamic disturbance interfering with the secretion of gonadotropin-releasing hormone and hence a diminished release of FSH and LH. As the patient regains weight, the recovery of endocrine function follows a definite sequence. First, there is a gradual increase in the levels of gonadotropins; the anterior pituitary also responds to administered LH-releasing hormones by releasing FSH and LH. Next, a return of the negative feedback effect of estrogens can be shown indirectly with clomiphene (blocking the negative feedback action), which causes a rise in basal plasma LH levels. The positive feedback effect of estrogens is last to return and can be demonstrated directly with a three-day course of ethinyl estradiol, which is followed by a peak rise in plasma LH. This final stage of recovery may be delayed, even after the patient's weight has returned to normal, but is necessary for the resumption of cyclical menstruation and ovulation. The persistence of abnormal endocrine function in anorexia nervosa is probably also dependent in part on the patient's abnormal mental state: a complete response to administered estrogens (with a positive feedback effect) is less likely to occur if there is a persistence in the psychologic disorder. These findings, together with the early onset of amenorrhea which may precede weight loss, indicate that the endocrine disorder is not wholly due to malnutrition.

A simplified diagram (Fig. 215–1) serves to emphasize the complexity of the interactions between the psychologic disorder, the endocrine disturbances, and the malnutrition in anorexia nervosa. The thickness of the lines reflects the strength of the evidence in support of each interaction. The best established pathways are those of the mental disorder causing a reduced food intake and weight loss (a), which in turn cause the endocrine disturbance and amenorrhea (b). It is also probable that weight loss and malnutrition worsen the mental disorder (c). The adverse effects of the patient's abnormal mental state on her endocrine and menstrual function support

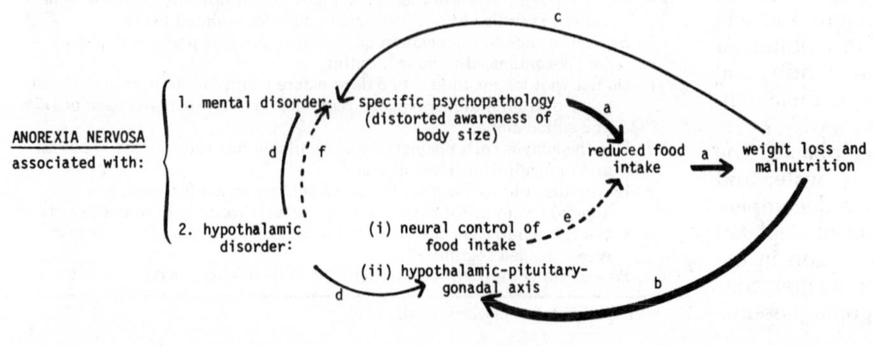

Figure 215–1. Psychologic, endocrine, and nutritional factors in anorexia nervosa. (Modified from Psychol Med 7:365, 1977.)

pathway (d). The original postulate that a disorder in the hypothalamic control of food intake might underlie the food refusal of anorexia nervosa is represented by the dotted line (e). There is no direct evidence in support of this mechanism or for the postulated link (f), representing the neural effects of a hypothalamic disorder in molding mental function so as to give rise to faulty attitudes to eating and body size. Nevertheless, it is clear that self-perpetuating disturbances play an important part in anorexia nervosa.

CLINICAL MANIFESTATIONS. The illness usually begins in a girl aged 14 to 17 years, but it can be earlier (9 to 13 years) or up to the age of the menopause. The patient's previous personality may have been normal, or there may be a preceding history of food fads or difficulty in making friendships; other signs of maladjustment are excessive tidiness or fears of meeting strangers or of taking school examinations. Loss of weight may be the first feature noticed by the parents, who draw the patient's attention to it. She is likely to explain the weight loss as the result of "dieting" for the purpose of improving her figure. Menstruation will have ceased by the time there has been a significant loss of weight, or this may happen as the first feature of the illness. There is often a change in the girl's temperament, consisting of impatience, irritability, and depression. She may become preoccupied with schoolwork or indulge in solitary exercises, thus withdrawing from her customary social life. The loss of weight can be very rapid, with a fall from 55 kg (121 pounds) to 35 kg (77 pounds) within two to three months. This is achieved mainly by avoiding carbohydrate-containing foods, but self-induced vomiting, the abuse of purgatives, and excessive exercising, in various combinations, may accelerate the loss of weight. The patient's life becomes unhappy and constricted. If she has a boyfriend, she loses interest in him and avoids any sexual contact. Relations with members of the family become strained. Parents react to their daughter's food refusal by a passive acceptance of her behavior for fear of making her condition worse. Food refusal leads to malnutrition which may persist for months or even years. The patient subsists on a diet of vegetables, fruit, and cheese, and avoids bread, potatoes, cakes, and sugar. On some days she may take only black coffee. In severe cases the patient presents a pitiable sight of emaciation, apathy, weakness, and severe depression. There is a risk of death from suicide or complications of malnutrition—especially potassium depletion or hypothermia.

In spite of progressive malnutrition, the patient may reject her parents' entreaties to see a doctor, and she minimizes the extent of her food avoidance. When she does agree to seek help, she is likely to deny that she is unwell or admit only to insomnia, constipation, sensitivity to cold, or some depression of mood.

Mental Examination. Examination of the patient's mental state may reveal a variety of disturbances. There may be depression and agitation; compulsive features may be prominent, such as elaborate feeding rituals and the counting of calories eaten daily; hysterical mechanisms may account for her assertion that she is eating well at the same time that she is hiding food or vomiting in secret. In addition, however, more specific psychologic abnormalities will be present. Their central theme is the patient's fear of becoming fat as a result of "losing control over eating." To play safe she resolves to remain thin and sets herself a sharply defined weight threshold above which she is unwilling to rise, defending her chosen weight as "right" for her. She may betray an abnormal sensitivity about the shape and size of her body, saying that fat would go to her stomach (hips, thighs, or some other part of the body). She may overestimate her weight and maintain, with all sincerity, that she eats large amounts of food. In an extreme case she may deny that she is thin, or even assert that she is fat in spite of obvious emaciation. The patient's distorted awareness of her size can be tested by getting her to estimate the width of her body. Her estimate is liable to exceed her actual measurements by as much as 50 per cent.

Physical Examination. Physical examination will reveal the signs of severe malnutrition in a young girl who has usually developed secondary sex characteristics. The malnutrition is of a calorie-deficiency type. The disappearance of subcutaneous fat leads to gaunt, hollow facial features; bony prominences stand out sharply, the limbs are reduced to sticks, the belly is flat, the breasts shrunken, and the buttocks wasted. The hands and feet remain cold and blue, even when the room temperature is warm. The central body temperature may be reduced by 1° C. The blood pressure is low (e.g., 90/60), and the heart rate is slow (50 to 60). The skin is dry, and there is an excessive growth of dry, downy hair over the nape of the neck, cheeks, forearms, and legs (lanugo hair), changes attributed to a follicular keratosis. In older patients purpuric patches resembling senile purpura may appear over the dorsum of the hands, the forearms, and the legs after minor knocks.

In patients who vomit, dehydration ensues, together with a marked fall in the level of serum potassium, but this finding and associated complications are more frequent in bulimia nervosa (see below). Serum cholesterol levels may be raised. Carotenemia may follow a high intake of carrots or spinach, and causes a yellow pigmentation of the palms and soles. Vitamin deficiencies (e.g. thiamin) occur rarely.

Endocrine Changes. Patients who are wasted show a fall in the plasma levels of LH, FSH, and estrogens. A course of clomiphene fails to raise the low plasma LH levels. Specific measures of thyroid function fall within the normal range. Plasma levels of growth hormone and cortisol are normal or elevated and can be raised further by the administration of insulin. Most of the physical abnormalities disappear when the malnutrition is corrected. An exception to this recovery is the disorder of gonadotropin activity, as described above.

Side Effects of Refeeding. Peripheral edema may occur, especially when the diet has a high content of salt, water, and carbohydrates which cause water retention. A moderate normochromic normocytic anemia may result from hemodilution, or a more severe anemia may result from hemolysis or temporary hypoplasia of the bone marrow; occasionally, moderate iron deficiency anemia may occur. Acute dilatation of the stomach is a rare but dangerous complication of too rapid refeeding.

Delayed Puberty. If the illness occurs before the menarche (e.g., 9 to 14 years), the sequence of pubertal events will probably be delayed by several years. Thus the patient has primary amenorrhea, together with a short stature and undeveloped breasts. When malnutrition is corrected and weight is adequately maintained, a full recovery often ensues with growth in height, development of breasts, and establishment of menstruation. If malnutrition is prolonged, however, there may be permanent sequelae such as a shortness in height (e.g., 152 cm) or underdeveloped breasts. Menstruation may be delayed until 21 years or later. It is therefore essential to treat these very young patients vigorously and effectively.

Anorexia Nervosa in the Male. The illness in the male closely resembles that in the female but is 10 to 20 times less common. The age of onset is usually a few years after puberty. The young boy rapidly loses weight as a result of avoiding carbohydrate-containing foods. Like the female, he expresses a fear of becoming fat and resorts to a similar abnormal behavior of food refusal, possibly with vomiting, purgation, or exercising to excess. The malnutrition in the male is more likely to be of a type combining a deficiency of calories and proteins. The endocrine disorder is analogous to that in the female. Urinary gonadotropins and blood LH levels are low; the urinary output of testosterone is reduced. Questioning will elicit loss of recently acquired sexual interest and potency. As in the female, these hormonal abnormalities can be slowly reversed by treatment resulting in weight gain.

TREATMENT. The general management of patients is empirically based but nevertheless highly rewarding: the treatments used are those which have been found to be effective in practice. The immediate aim is to treat the patient's malnutrition, which can become severe and dangerous. Even during the early stages of treatment it is desirable to try altering abnormal attitudes, for the course of the illness is much affected by the psychologic state. Thus treatment is best administered in a psychiatric unit, but it is essential that there be good nursing facilities. The long-term aim of treatment is to reduce the duration of the illness and prevent relapses.

Short-Term Treatment. SECURING THE PATIENT'S COOPERATION. The first need is to obtain as much cooperation from the patient as possible. By the time there has been severe loss of weight, admission to hospital is the only certain way of restoring her nutrition to normal. The doctor's skills must therefore be focused on persuading the patient to come into hospital. Compulsory admission, although occasionally indicated, is best avoided because the patient's continued cooperation is essential throughout the course of the illness, which may last for a few years.

NURSING TREATMENT. The refeeding of the patient is best achieved by skilled nurses. The nurse should establish a trusting relationship with the patient, but one which is not dependent on giving way to requests to avoid food and weight gain. The patient is asked to put her trust in the nurse as someone who, for the time being, takes over decisions regarding the necessary daily food intake. She is frankly told that because of her illness she will be tempted to be deceitful about eating, vomiting, or taking purgatives, so that close supervision is necessary. The nurse sits with the patient during each meal and cajoles her to finish all the food put on her plate. When the patient has regained her weight, she is complimented on her improved appearance and is encouraged to buy new clothes to fit her healthier size. In the course of treatment the nurse decides on a judicious balance of restrictions and privileges: the balance is gradually altered in favor of added privileges as rewards for continued progress.

DIET. No special diets are needed. The patient is given her own choice of food so long as she does not exclude carbohydrate-containing foods. To begin with, the food intake should be 1500 calories daily; within seven to ten days she should be persuaded to accept full meals totaling 3000 tô 5000 calories daily. Concentrated foods may be used (e.g., Complan, Metrecal, or Carnation breakfast food) by adding them to milk.

ADDITIONAL MEASURES. The nursing care described should be viewed as a form of *psychologic treatment* embodying the principles of psychotherapy and behavior therapy.

Large doses of chlorpromazine used to be advocated to reduce the patient's resistance to eating, but they can be dangerous in undernourished patients, and are not necessary. In very agitated patients the nursing task can be facilitated by administering moderate, divided doses of chlorpromazine up to a total of 300 mg daily. There is no place for tube feeding nor for leukotomy: weight gain can be achieved by conservative treatment, and the risk of suicide is increased after leukotomy.

ASSESSMENT OF PROGRESS. The patient is weighed daily before breakfast, and this provides the best check on her progress. A weight gain of up to 28 pounds (12.7 kg) in eight weeks should be possible. Figure 215–2 shows an 18-year-old patient before treatment and nine weeks later when she had gained 18.3 kg. The patient should maintain a healthy weight for about two weeks before being discharged from hospital.

Long-Term Treatment. There is less known about the efficacy of long-term treatments. After discharge from hospital, it is necessary to provide outpatient supervision. Psychotherapy should be directed to whatever emotional problems have been identified in the patient. Family therapy which involves therapeutic interviews with the whole family may be rewarding when there is evidence of disturbed relationships between its members. Even when a normal weight is maintained, amenorrhea may persist for months or years. When the patient is eager to resume normal menstruation, one or two courses of

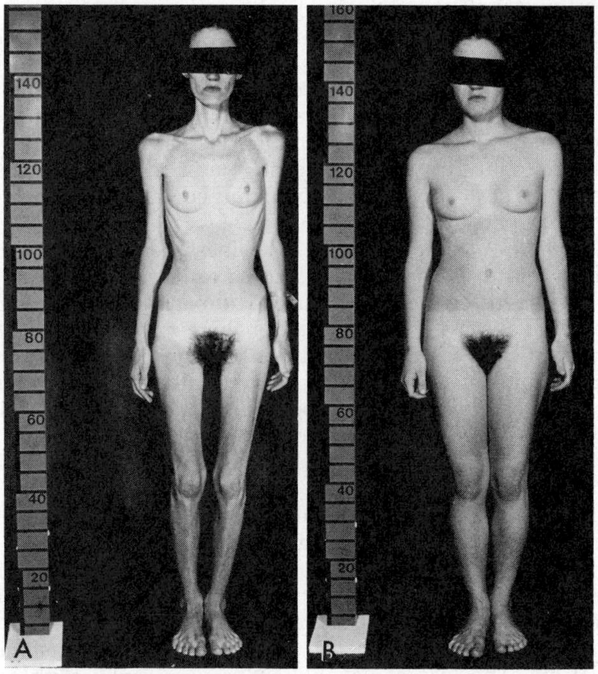

Figure 215–2. Photographs of the same patient on admission *(A)* and at the completion of treatment, nine weeks later *(B)* when she had gained 18.3 kg.

clomiphene (50 to 100 mg daily for seven days) may be effective, but only when body weight has been restored to a normal level. In the event of a serious relapse, readmission to hospital will be necessary.

PROGNOSIS. The short-term prognosis is usually excellent. Treatment should lead to a return to a normal weight; at the same time, the majority of patients show a marked improvement in their mental state. Deaths from malnutrition should not occur.

The long-term prognosis is more problematical. Relapses requiring readmissions occur in about half the patients. The illness often lasts two to three years or even longer. In a follow-up of severely ill patients who had been treated at least four years previously, 40 per cent had recovered, 27 per cent had menstrual irregularity or a moderately low body weight, 29 per cent had serious weight loss with amenorrhea, and 5 per cent had died. A proportion of the patients who fail to recover enter the chronic phase of bulimia nervosa. Poor prognostic signs are a later age of onset (early twenties as opposed to early teens) or an illness which has lasted more than five years. Even in these patients, however, good results can still be obtained from energetic treatment. In many patients the prognosis is good—their health returns to normal, and they may marry and can bear children.

BULIMIA NERVOSA

Bulimia nervosa is so called because it represents a chronic phase of anorexia nervosa, and its primary symptom consists of recurrent gorging with food. The psychopathology is the same as in typical anorexia nervosa: the patient has an exaggerated dread of becoming fat. It is this fear which leads her to get rid of the food each time she overeats. She makes herself vomit by pushing her fingers or a toothbrush down her throat. Abuse of purgatives is often combined with self-induced vomiting or may occur on its own. The resulting loss of body fluids and electrolytes leads to hypokalemia, hyponatremia, and hypochloremic alkalosis. Physical complications include erosion of dental enamel, muscular weakness, electrocardiographic abnormalities, tetany, and epileptic seizures; chronic potassium depletion may lead to urinary infections and renal failure. In contrast with typical anorexia nervosa, body weight may reach a relatively normal level, menstruation may be resumed, and fertility restored.

MENTAL EXAMINATION. The patient's morbid dread of fatness can be assessed from the weight threshold which she has set for herself, usually several kilograms below her original "healthy" weight. Signs of depression may be present.

PHYSICAL EXAMINATION. Physical examination may reveal injury to the skin over the back of the hand from rubbing against the upper incisors when inducing vomiting. Swelling of the salivary glands or signs of tetany are occasionally present. Serum potassium levels may be low (e.g., to 1.4 mEq per liter). Renal function may be impaired.

TREATMENT. Intractable self-induced vomiting and purging require admission to hospital. The nurse conveys to the patient sympathy for her preoccupation with food and controls the overeating by limiting food intake to mealtimes. This usually suffices to control vomiting; but if not, closer supervision, especially after meals, will have the desired effect. The use of purgatives must also be stopped. Potassium supplements are ineffective unless vomiting ceases, and are then unnecessary. The patient is persuaded to accept a higher body weight, which reduces the craving for food and improves the chances of maintained control over gorging and vomiting after leaving hospital. Long-term supportive psychotherapy is indicated to help the patient with interpersonal and social problems. Good results have been reported with cognitive behavioral therapy. The value of antidepressants is often limited to the relief of depressive symptoms. Prognosis for a full recovery is seldom good, and there is a risk of suicide.

Crisp AH, Palmer RL, Kalucy RS: How common is anorexia nervosa? A prevalence study. Br J Psychiat 128:549, 1976. Garner DM, Garfinkel PE: Sociocultural factors in the development of anorexia nervosa. Psychol Med 10:647, 1980. *These two references provide recent evidence supporting the relatively high prevalence of anorexia nervosa and the effects of sociocultural pressures on its incidence.*

Darby PL, Garfinkel PE, Garner DM, Coscina DV (eds.): Anorexia Nervosa: Recent Developments and Research. Neurology and Neurobiology. Vol 3. New York, Alan R. Liss, Inc., 1984. *Recent reports on psychosocial and biologic factors in anorexia nervosa and a section on treatment. There is also an article on delayed puberty.*

Garfinkel PE, Garner DM: Anorexia Nervosa: A Multidimensional Perspective. New York, Brunner/Mazel, 1982. *This is the best book for a comprehensive account of anorexia nervosa. It includes an extensive bibliography.*

Harris RT: Bulimarexia and related serious eating disorders with medical complications. Ann Intern Med 99:800, 1983. *An up-to-date review article with 44 references, better from the medical than the psychiatric point of view.*

Minuchin S, Rosman B, Baker L: Psychosomatic Families: Anorexia Nervosa in Context. Cambridge, Harvard University Press, 1978. *An account of family therapy in anorexia nervosa, including the theoretical models which have led to its introduction.*

Russell GFM: Bulimia nervosa: An ominous variant of anorexia nervosa. Psychol Med 9:429, 1979. *A detailed clinical account of a newly identified disorder closely related to anorexia nervosa.*

216. OBESITY

Edwin L. Bierman

Obesity is the most common disorder of metabolism in man and is also one of the oldest documented metabolic disturbances in recorded history. A limestone statuette dating from the Stone Age has been unearthed which appears to be the most ancient example of obesity, antedating the development of agriculture by about 10,000 years. Similar historical evidence for obesity is found in Egyptian mummies and Greek sculpture. This abnormality has persisted throughout the centuries, which have been characterized by markedly different environmental stresses and dietary habits. However, the problem of obesity has dramatically increased since the evolutionary advantage of the ability to efficiently store energy as fat has been dissipated in modern affluent societies. Thus caloric excess and sedentary habits have led to an increased prevalence of obesity and its life-shortening consequences, including cardiovascular disease, diabetes, and hypertension.

DEFINITION AND MEASUREMENT. Obesity can be defined as excess adipose tissue. However, it is still not clear whether obesity represents a "disease" or a common clinical manifestation of a group of disorders like anemia or hypertension. The definition of obesity is necessarily arbitrary, since body weight (or more accurately, quantity of body fat) is continuously distributed in populations with no clear dividing line between individuals who are obese and those who are thin. A definition of obesity could be made more easily if there were a distinct point at which a clear influence of obesity on morbidity and mortality begins. This is not the case, however, since there is a continually progressive excess mortality for increasing degrees of overweight beyond about 30 per cent. Moreover, the metabolic, physiologic, and pathophysiologic consequences appear to increase continuously with the degree of deviation above average weight.

Although it is the simplest index of obesity, body weight is not always the best reflection of the relative proportion of adipose tissue in the body or of total adipose mass that needs to be determined or estimated if exact knowledge of the degree of excess adiposity is desirable. Weight adjusted to body size gives a better indication than body weight alone. For clinical purposes, per cent ideal body weight (relative weight) based on the readily available Metropolitan Life Insurance Company tables usually gives a close approximation of the degree of adiposity (Table 216–1). Although modifications of the guide-

TABLE 216–1. GUIDELINES FOR BODY WEIGHT*

	Men (Weight in kg)			Women (Weight in kg)		
Metric Height (m)†	Average	Acceptable Weight Range		Average	Acceptable Weight Range	
1.45				46.0	42	53
1.48				46.5	42	54
1.50				47.0	43	55
1.52				48.5	44	57
1.54				49.5	44	58
1.56				50.4	45	58
1.58	55.8	51	64	51.3	46	59
1.60	57.6	52	65	52.6	48	61
1.62	58.6	53	66	54.0	49	62
1.64	59.6	54	67	55.4	50	64
1.66	60.0	55	69	56.8	51	65
1.68	61.7	56	71	56.8	52	66
1.70	63.5	58	73	60.0	53	67
1.72	65.0	59	74	61.3	55	69
1.74	66.5	60	75	62.6	56	70
1.76	68.0	62	77	64.0	58	72
1.78	69.4	64	79	65.3	59	74
1.80	71.0	65	80			
1.82	72.6	66	82			
1.84	74.2	67	84			
1.86	75.8	69	86			
1.88	77.6	71	88			
1.90	79.3	73	90			
1.92	81.0	75	93			

		Men (Weight in lbs)			Women (Weight in lbs)		
Nonmetric Height† (Ft	in)	Average	Acceptable Weight Range		Average	Acceptable Weight Range	
4	10				102	92	119
4	11				104	94	122
5	0				107	96	125
5	1				110	99	128
5	2	123	112	141	113	102	131
5	3	127	115	144	116	105	134
5	4	130	118	148	120	108	138
5	5	133	121	152	123	111	142
5	6	136	124	156	128	114	146
5	7	140	128	161	132	118	150
5	8	145	132	166	136	122	154
5	9	149	136	170	140	126	158
5	10	153	140	174	144	130	163
5	11	158	144	179	148	134	168
6	0	162	148	184	152	138	173
6	1	166	152	189			
6	2	171	156	194			
6	3	176	160	199			
6	4	181	164	204			

*Adapted from the recommendations of the Fogarty Center Conference 1973. Data from the Metropolitan Life Insurance Company tables.

†Height without shoes, weight without clothes.

lines have recently been made, the effect of age on average or ideal weight is not considered. Nevertheless, for common use, obesity can be defined as that body weight over 20 per cent above mean average body weight.

A variety of methods for assessment of total body fat, such as body density, x-ray, distribution of fat-soluble gases, total body water, and total body potassium-40, have been used for research purposes. In addition, a variety of anthropometric measurements (limb and trunk diameters and circumferences, skin-fold thicknesses) have been used to derive regression equations that correlate closely with per cent fat.

However, elaborate techniques are usually not necessary to quantify body fat for clinical purposes. The weight/height^2 index (body mass index) is one of the most useful anthropometric measurements and the simplest to obtain; it de-emphasizes the effect of stature on body weight and also correlates closely with adiposity. Obesity can be defined as a body mass index of greater than 27 (kilograms per square meter) for men and 25 for women (approximately equivalent to 120 per cent of ideal body weight). Subscapular and triceps skin-fold thickness measurements using inexpensive skin-fold calipers also provide an accurate and simple guide. On the basis of population studies, it has been suggested that triceps skin-fold thickness greater than 23 mm in men and 30 mm in women should be defined as obesity.

PREVALENCE AND EPIDEMIOLOGY. A large proportion of Western populations is obese. In the United States, using a definition of obesity based on triceps skin-fold thickness, approximately 20 per cent of middle-aged males and 40 per cent of middle-aged females are obese. In cross-sectional population surveys, the prevalence of obesity increases with age, reaching a peak by age 50 in males and somewhat later in females. The lower prevalence of obesity in older age groups may reflect the higher mortality at earlier ages associated with obesity-related diseases.

Cultural influences and socioeconomic status have a strong influence on the prevalence of obesity. Every social factor studied has been correlated with obesity, and thus there are many determinants. Socioeconomic status, based on occupation, education, and income, shows a particularly strong inverse correlation with obesity among women, i.e., the lower the socioeconomic status, the higher the prevalence of obesity.

PATHOGENESIS. ***Clinical Types.*** Although it has been clear for some time that there are two clinical types of obesity, there has been little metabolic or physiologic evidence until recently to support such a concept. In one type *(lifelong obesity)*, patients give a characteristic history. Although generally of normal birth weight, they tend to have been heavier as children, to have had a large spurt in weight gain during puberty, and (in females) to give a history of gaining weight with each successive pregnancy. These individuals usually have tried all available methods and fads promoted for caloric restriction and weight reduction to no permanent avail. After successful weight loss regardless of the program, they usually return gradually to approximately their prereduction level of overweight as though it were preset. These individuals also tend to be grossly obese (more than 175 per cent of ideal body weight) adults.

The other clinical type *(adult-onset obesity)* is much more common and represents "middle-age spread." These individuals give a history of being thin or of average weight until age 20 to 40, when weight gain associated with a more sedentary existence begins. This type of weight gain in adult life is extremely common and is seen in most affluent populations.

A possible explanation for weight gain during adult life that does not appear to be tenable is a decrease in basal energy utilization with aging. Basal oxygen consumption decreases only slightly during adult life. Body composition is changing, however, even at constant body weight. There is a larger proportion of body fat and a smaller proportion of lean body mass with age, so that basal oxygen consumption in terms of lean body mass (predominantly muscle and bone) may actually be constant with age. Although basal energy utilization may be constant, it has been suggested that obesity occurs in concert with a decline in energy utilization associated with food intake ("dietary-induced thermogenesis") and with exercise. Alternatively, adult-onset obesity simply may reflect an imbalance between caloric intake and utilization because such individuals do not reduce their caloric intake with age appropriately for their change in body composition. Ahrens has calculated that the daily caloric requirement for weight maintenance of adults decreases 43 calories per decade per square meter of surface area for males and 27 calories per decade per square meter for females.

These two broad clinical types of obesity were recognized early by Albrink, who proposed that adult-onset obesity is mainly central in location (the "middle-age spread"), whereas lifelong obesity might be peripheral as well as central. For peripheral localization of adiposity, skin-fold thickness of the forearm or the triceps is measured and compared with skin-fold thickness over the tip of the scapula. Weight gain during adult life is significantly correlated with costal, scapular, and, to a lesser extent, triceps skin-fold thickness but not with ulnar skin-fold thickness. Thus forearm fat is minimally influenced by adult-onset obesity, whereas adipose tissue of the trunk is most influenced by weight gain during adult life.

Pathophysiology. A possible pathophysiologic basis for these clinical observations was first proposed by Bjurulf, who suggested that some forms of obesity might be due to increased numbers of cells. Proof of this hypothesis was provided by the elegant experiments of Hirsch and his coworkers, who measured the cellularity of adipose tissue sampled by needle aspiration biopsy. They demonstrated that grossly obese humans (lifelong) characteristically have an increase in adipose cell number as well as adipose cell size. After weight reduction, adipose cell size shrinks, but hypercellularity remains fixed.

Adult-onset obesity (after age 20) appears to be characterized predominantly by adipose cell hypertrophy with no increase in cell number. Thus all human obesity is accompanied by cellular enlargement. Adipocyte hyperplasia becomes increasingly marked beyond body weights greater than 175 per cent of ideal. Adipose cell number appears to be determined very early in life. In studies with rats, animals subjected to overnutrition before weaning maintained larger numbers of adipose cells throughout life than did litter mates subjected to undernutrition prior to weaning. Weight changes during adult life did not influence the cell number of these animals. Studies in man also have shown that adipose cell number is determined early in life. In the nonobese, two periods of adipose cell proliferation have been identified: in the first two years and again just prior to puberty. In obese children, adipose cell number increases throughout childhood.

Experimental Obesity. Support for the concept of two types of obesity also comes from studies of experimental obesity in man by Sims and coworkers. They force-fed volunteers to produce 20 to 30 per cent increments in weights associated with central distribution of excess fat, which was predominantly due to an increase in adipose cell size without a change in adipose cell number. Prompt, spontaneous reversal of excess fat and cell size was achieved at the end of the experimental forced feeding. Thus there appears to be no change in adipose cell number during temporary overfeeding in adulthood despite changes in body weight.

Studies of experimental obesity in animals also lend some support to these concepts. Genetically transmitted obesity in rodents is characterized by adipose cell hyperplasia as well as hypertrophy, whereas experimentally induced obesity, such as that obtained by destruction of the ventromedial nucleus of the hypothalamus, is associated with hypertrophy alone. A summary of these two broad general categories of obesity is given in Table 216–2. All obesity is hypertrophic because the adipose cells are enlarged, but only certain individuals have adipose hyperplasia. Massive obesity is usually of the juvenile onset, lifelong hyperplastic type.

TABLE 216–2. TYPES OF OBESITY

	Hyperplastic	Hypertrophic
Severity	Marked	Moderate
History	Lifelong	Adult-onset
Fat distribution	Peripheral and central	Central ("middle-age spread")
Adipose cellularity	Increase in cell number and cell size	Increase in cell size only
Insulin resistance	Related to cell size	Related to cell size
Metabolic consequences	Related to cell size	Related to cell size

ETIOLOGY. Possible factors in the pathogenesis of adipose cell hypertrophy are listed in Table 216–3. No primary biochemical lesion of adipose tissue has ever been firmly documented as a cause of generalized obesity in man. Also, little is known of the etiologic basis for adipose cell hyperplasia. Genetic factors play a role, but their mechanism remains unknown. Estrogen-androgen balance also appears to influence the site and amount of adipose tissue deposition, since women and prepubertal children have a higher proportion and different distribution of subcutaneous fat than men.

Only in rare instances of hypothalamic obesity in man, in which damage to the ventromedial hypothalamic nucleus occurs as a result of tumor or trauma, can an etiology be defined and, with surgical removal of the tumor, obesity cured. This hypothalamic center appears to regulate the deposition of adipose tissue triglyceride. Formerly its role as an appetite or satiety center was emphasized, and when it was destroyed its role was related to obesity in man because inappropriate hyperphagia sometimes occurred. Recent studies, however, have shown that experimentally induced hypothalamic lesions alter insulin levels and lipogenesis independent of changes in food intake. Anomalous insulin secretion after hypothalamic injury in man has also been observed. Possibly it can be linked to the development of obesity in such individuals. In any event, the relevance to the common types of human obesity of experimental animal models whose obesity has been produced by injuring the hypothalamus is open to serious question.

Cerebral and emotional influences on eating patterns as well as cultural influences and socioeconomic status surely play a role in obesity, but, aside from overt psychiatric disturbances, the general role of altered behavioral patterns in the etiology of obesity has been difficult to define, and a specific type of personality associated with obesity has not been distinguished. No less important, habit and environment also appear to influence appetite regulation. Presumably because of decreased spontaneous activity, an obese individual will actually consume fewer calories than will his thin control counterpart.

Fatty acid mobilization from adipose tissue appears to be normal in simple obesity. There is little evidence that decreased lipolysis, or resistance to normal fat-mobilizing stimuli (hormonal, neuronal), plays an etiologic role in the usual forms of obesity (Table 216–3).

Lipoprotein lipase (the enzyme in adipose tissue responsible for assimilation of fatty acids contained in circulating triglyceride-rich lipoproteins) is increased in hypertrophic adipose cells. Increased lipoprotein lipase activity could lead to further increased deposition of dietary and endogenous fat in adipose tissue in obesity. A possible primary role for this enzyme in the etiology of obesity in some individuals is suggested by the finding that obese individuals maintain high levels of lipoprotein lipase in adipocytes after weight reduction. Also in the genetically obese rat, adipose tissue lipoprotein lipase is increased even before the animals become obese, and this increase is maintained despite food restriction. These recent findings are consistent with the idea that fat mass is regulated by as yet unknown neurohumoral factors that modulate adipose tissue lipoprotein lipase activity and provide a biochemical basis for the difficulty some obese individuals have in maintaining a weight-reduced state. Although overall basal energy utilization may be normal in obesity, subtle defects have been described in red cell sodium-potassium pump activity which correlate with the degree of obesity. The possible role of this biochemical energy-utilizing system in the etiology of obesity remains to be clarified.

TABLE 216–3. POSSIBLE FACTORS IN THE PATHOGENESIS OF OBESITY (ADIPOCYTE HYPERTROPHY)

- Excessive lipid deposition
  - Increased food intake
  - Hypothalamic lesions
  - Adipose cell hyperplasia
  - Hyperlipogenesis
  - Increased lipoprotein lipase activity
- Diminished lipid mobilization
  - Decrease in lipolytic hormones
  - Defective adipose-cell lipolysis
  - Abnormality of autonomic innervation
- Diminished lipid utilization
  - Aging
  - Defective lipid oxidation
  - Defective thermogenesis
  - Inactivity

Metabolic Abnormalities. Regardless of the cause or type of obesity, the metabolic consequences are predictable. They appear to relate directly to fat cell size, and virtually all metabolic disturbances that have been observed are inducible with weight gain and reversible with weight reduction. Thus, although numerous hormonal imbalances have been described in obesity, they are likely to be consequences of rather than causes of the obese state (Table 216–4).

The metabolic alteration with the most profound influence is the acquired resistance to the action of insulin on glucose utilization by fat and muscle cells. A predominance of abdominal adiposity in premenopausal women, similar to fat distribution in adult men, is particularly associated with insulin resistance. Insulin resistance associated with adiposity or experimental weight gain has been demonstrated both in vivo and in isolated fat cell systems. Muscle metabolism also presumably plays an important role in the insulin resistance of obesity. One of the consequences of this resistance to the action of insulin appears to be a feedback compensatory hyperinsulinism. The beta cells of the pancreatic islets are stimulated by an unknown mechanism to produce more insulin, and beta-cell hypertrophy eventually results. The signal is as yet unknown but may be neuronal or hormonal, or may involve small changes in glucose, fatty acids, or specific amino acids. In any case, the result is an increase in circulating insulin levels (both basal and in response to a variety of stimuli), which is directly related to the degree of adiposity and is reversible with weight reduction. It is not simply a matter of body weight or lean body mass that is associated with hyperinsulinemia, since very muscular individuals who are heavy do not appear to have hyperinsulinism. Circulating levels of insulin regulate their own receptors on cell surfaces. Thus obesity has been associated with fewer numbers of insulin receptors on muscle, liver, and adipose cell surfaces, thereby further contributing to insulin resistance and impaired glucose utilization by cells. However, decreased postreceptor insulin responsiveness of adipose tissue appears to be the major contributor to the insulin resistance of obesity.

TABLE 216–4. METABOLIC AND ENDOCRINE CONSEQUENCES OF OBESITY

- Decreased sensitivity to insulin (muscle, adipose tissue)
- Hyperinsulinemia
- Decreased glucose tolerance, hyperglycemia
- Hyperaminoacidemia
- Hypertriglyceridemia
- Hypercholesterolemia
- Decreased growth hormone responses
- Decreased prolactin responses
- "Resistance" to ketosis
- Increased glucocorticoid secretion

The emergence of adult-onset (non-insulin-dependent) diabetes mellitus in the population is profoundly influenced by the degree and duration of obesity. One concept is that prolonged hyperinsulinism might lead to beta-cell "exhaustion" in those individuals who are genetically susceptible. As is well known, when the pressure is off after successful weight reduction, glucose intolerance is reversed. Thus glucose intolerance in the obese adult may represent "high-output failure," in which the beta cell has failed to compensate fully for the degree of peripheral insulin resistance associated with adiposity. Abnormal regulation of growth hormone and prolactin secretion has been associated with obesity, but the significance of these findings and their relation to the glucose intolerance of obesity is not understood. These changes in insulin and growth hormone regulation in obesity can be found even in early childhood.

Another metabolic consequence of obesity is hypertriglyceridemia, which may result in part from the associated hyperinsulinism. Triglyceride levels in populations are correlated with relative body weight, with skin-fold thickness, and particularly with weight gain in adult life. In a variety of studies circulating insulin levels are consistently correlated with triglyceride levels, and insulin is one of the factors involved in endogenous triglyceride-rich lipoprotein secretion by the liver. In obese individuals, both hyperinsulinism and hypertriglyceridemia are reversible with weight reduction. The role of obesity in determining serum lipid levels is suggested by the finding that age-related curves of relative body weight, plasma triglyceride, and plasma cholesterol in comparable population groups are superimposable.

Serum cholesterol levels are less closely linked with obesity, but a significant relationship exists. This could be explained in part by the observation that the cholesterol production rate appears to be related to the degree of adiposity. This relationship may be linked to the increased propensity of obese individuals to develop gallstones. Elevated triglyceride-rich lipoprotein levels are associated with reduced levels of high density lipoprotein (HDL) cholesterol, characteristic of obesity.

The influence of obesity on glucose, lipid, and lipoprotein levels also may be related to the increased tendency of the obese to develop all the complications of atherosclerosis. Thus obesity, altered carbohydrate and fat metabolism, and atherosclerosis appear to be linked.

CLINICAL MANIFESTATIONS. The pathophysiologic consequences of obesity lead to a variety of clinical manifestations and aggravate or predispose to a number of common diseases (Table 216–5). For many of these diseases obese individuals have higher death rates than their thin counterparts affected by the same disorder.

Every major organ system appears to be involved. In the *cardiovascular system,* obesity is associated with five major risk factors for atherosclerosis, i.e., hypertension, diabetes, hypercholesterolemia, hypertriglyceridemia, and low HDL cholesterol. Therefore it is not surprising that obese individuals have more atherosclerotic manifestations and are more prone to sudden death. The effect of obesity in predisposing to atherosclerosis may be mediated by these factors rather than by more direct mechanisms related to nonspecific myocardial lesions or hemodynamic factors (increased oxygen consumption, blood volume, cardiac output, stroke volume, and cardiac work).

TABLE 216–5. DISEASES ASSOCIATED WITH OBESITY

Cardiovascular disease	Arthritis
Atherosclerotic	Osteoarthritis
Hypertensive	Gout
Cor pulmonale	Varicose veins and thromboembolism
Hypertension	Intertriginous dermatitis
Pulmonary disease	Hernias, ventral and diaphragmatic
Diabetes mellitus, adult-onset	Endometrial carcinoma
Fatty liver	Toxemia of pregnancy
Cholelithiasis and cholecystitis	Amenorrhea and oligomenorrhea

There is a close correlation between blood pressure levels and obesity in most populations. (In the markedly obese individual with large subcutaneous fat deposits in the arm, blood pressure measurements should be made with a large leg cuff which more accurately reflects arterial levels.) A large portion of the increased death rate of moderate or markedly obese individuals may be a direct or indirect consequence of hypertension (e.g., cerebrovascular accidents). Several factors have been implicated in the association between obesity and hypertension, including hemodynamic alterations resulting from increased blood volume and the need for increased perfusion of excess adipose tissue and lean body mass, and increased salt intake accompanying increased food consumption. Increased stroke volume and left ventricular hypertrophy often result. Obese individuals appear to respond to antihypertensive management as do their nonobese hypertensive counterparts with an improvement in morbidity and mortality from cerebrovascular complications.

In the *respiratory system,* alveolar hypoventilation associated with massive obesity eventually leads to carbon dioxide retention (P_{CO_2} values consistently above 48 mm Hg), daytime somnolence, chronic fatigue, dyspnea, and personality changes (the obesity-hypoventilation syndrome or pickwickian syndrome, named after a character in Dickens' *Pickwick Papers,* Fat Joe, who fell asleep at the most inopportune moments). The syndrome is initiated by the increased work of respiration necessary to move the ponderous thoracic wall and abdomen and is associated with decreased compliance of the thorax. Hypoxia, secondary polycythemia, pulmonary hypertension, and eventually cor pulmonale with cardiopulmonary failure ensue. Occasionally, sleep apnea (see Ch. 472.5) may be an associated feature. Many of these abnormalities can be partly reversed by weight loss. Although the full-blown syndrome is seen in only grossly obese adults, milder pulmonary functional abnormalities can be detected with lesser degrees of obesity, including reduction in vital capacity and expiratory reserve volume, and ventilation-perfusion disturbances resulting in mild decreases in arterial oxygenation. All these abnormalities contribute to the increased surgical risk in obesity associated with use of general anesthetics.

Obesity is the single important factor associated with the emergence of *diabetes mellitus* in populations throughout the world. In the United States more than 80 per cent of adult-onset diabetics are obese. The duration rather than the degree of obesity in individuals is more closely correlated with glucose intolerance. As indicated, certain genetically prone individuals may not be able to sustain the chronic oversecretion of insulin necessary to overcome the insulin resistance of obesity, and although absolute circulating insulin levels after carbohydrate intake may be higher than in thin individuals, they may not be high enough to compensate for the extra demand resulting from adiposity. Again, weight reduction may be dramatically successful in reducing the hyperglycemia of the adult diabetic and is the treatment of choice; however, the influence of weight gain and loss on the associated microangiopathy of diabetes is unknown.

Gastrointestinal symptoms are frequent in the obese and are usually nonspecific (bloating, dyspepsia). Diaphragmatic hernias may become symptomatic. Fatty liver is common, with associated abnormalities of liver function being detectable in as many as 85 per cent of obese patients (mild abnormalities of SGPT and LDH that become normal with weight reduction). The incidence of cholesterol-rich gallstones is strikingly related to the degree of obesity, particularly among women. Women below the age of 50 with cholelithiasis average 25 pounds heavier than women without gallstones. The mechanism presumably relates to the supersaturation of bile with cholesterol resulting from the overproduction and increased excretion of cholesterol in obesity. Weight reduction will reduce the saturation of bile with cholesterol after a new stable lower weight is achieved. However, during the period of active weight loss, bile remains supersaturated, apparently because of increased mobilization of cholesterol from large adipose tissue stores.

Thus continuous weight loss–weight gain cycles characteristic of many obese patients during their lifetime may be a potent predisposing condition for gallstone formation.

The incidence of several types of *arthritis* is increased among the obese. In populations, uric acid levels are directly related to the degree of overweight, and the prevalence of gouty arthritis is increased in obesity. Gouty arthritis may also be precipitated during treatment of obesity with carbohydrate-deficient ("ketogenic") fad diets (see Treatment) presumably related to the hyperuricemia resulting from the competition between ketone acids and uric acid for renal excretion. Osteoarthritis is also more common and severe, particularly in the spine and other joints that bear the brunt of excess weight bearing.

In addition to the arterial lesions of atherosclerosis, *varicose veins* are common, as is venous stasis and edema. This contributes to the increased postoperative morbidity caused by thrombophlebitis and pulmonary embolism in obesity.

Flabby and redundant *skin* associated with excessive subcutaneous fat produces moist folds, resulting in a propensity to fungal and yeast skin lesions (intertriginous dermatitis, particularly in the axillae, in the perineal region, and under the breasts).

Women who are obese tend to have irregular *menses* and increased morbidity associated with *pregnancy* and again after childbearing ceases. The incidence of toxemia of pregnancy and hypertension is increased. Obstetric risk is higher due to longer duration of labor, larger babies, more cesarean sections, and higher anesthetic risk. Later in life, there are more uterine fibroids and an increased risk of development of endometrial cancer directly related to the degree of obesity. The large adipose mass is associated with both increased estrogen storage and increased conversion of adrenal androgens to estrone, which may result in increased chronic hormonal stimulation of the uterus.

Surgical risk is in general greater in obesity. Mortality figures for a variety of surgical procedures may be two- to three-fold higher for the obese than for the nonobese. Contributing factors include increased anesthetic risk, technical difficulties and longer duration of procedures, and increased atelectasis, wound infection, and thrombophlebitis postoperatively.

DIFFERENTIAL DIAGNOSIS. Less than 1 per cent of obesity can be ascribed to an identifiable cause or aggravating factor (Table 216–6). There is no rationale for the use of the popular diagnostic term "exogenous" obesity, which has no pathophysiologic meaning.

Endocrine lesions as specific primary causes of adiposity are uncommon. It is clear, however, that hormones influence fat deposition. This may involve a general effect on adipocyte metabolism throughout the body (e.g., insulin, thyroid hormone) or characteristic regional effects (e.g., glucocorticoids, estrogen). Hyperinsulinism can lead to adiposity, as exemplified by patients with insulinoma. However, individuals with this tumor are rarely markedly obese.

Although much attention has been given to hypothyroidism and milder degrees of "hypometabolism" as a cause of obesity, and vast quantities of thyroid extract have been administered for treatment, there is little evidence for deficiency of thyroid hormone secretion or action as a primary cause in most cases. Most of the weight gain associated with the development of myxedema is due to the accumulation of fluid rather than to adipose mass. Furthermore, the administration of thyroid hormone to obese patients may result in a loss of lean body mass exceeding the loss of fat and in increased appetite. Circulating thyroid hormone levels, thyroidal radioiodine uptake, and Achilles reflex time are usually normal.

The fat deposition associated with hyperadrenocorticism (Cushing's syndrome) is characteristic. Helpful diagnostic clinical features, in addition to fat distribution, that distinguish the much more common obese individual with mild hypertension and glucose intolerance from obesity secondary to adrenal hypersecretion include thick rather than thin skin, pale rather than purplish striae, absence of plethora and polycythemia, preservation of muscle strength, and absence of osteoporosis. Laboratory tests are also helpful. Higher than normal urinary excretion rates of hydroxycorticoids and an increase in cortisol turnover may be present, but these changes correlate with the increase in lean body mass associated with obesity. Blood and urine cortisol levels tend to be normal in obesity and are usually suppressible, and the diurnal rhythm in adrenal steroid secretion appears to be maintained.

Gonadal deficiency certainly is not a common cause of obesity. Although in animals it has been shown that castration is often followed by obesity, this association has been much less prominent in humans. Nevertheless, it has been observed, particularly when the castration is performed after puberty. Moreover, some eunuchoid males are found to be somewhat obese and tend to lose some of the obesity after the administration of testosterone. Women with the Stein-Leventhal syndrome tend to be obese. Presumably the obesity results from the secretion by the ovary of steroids with actions similar to those of some of the adrenal steroids.

Hypothalamic syndromes are rare causes of obesity in man. Bray has collected a series of these patients and found that they were of the hypertrophic type but were characterized by unusually high insulin levels. In the case of gross lesions found in the vicinity of the hypothalamus, e.g., craniopharyngioma or lesions caused by trauma, obesity associated with hypogonadotropic hypogonadism, and in some instances with diabetes insipidus, is part of the syndrome. It is not clear to what extent impairment of the secretion of hypothalamic pituitary–releasing factors might contribute to the obesity.

Obesity rarely may be present in early childhood as part of a variety of congenital syndromes such as adiposogenital dystrophy (Fröhlich's syndrome), Prader-Willi syndrome, Laurence-Moon-Biedl syndrome, Alström's syndrome, and pseudohypoparathyroidism. The cause of the obesity in these syndromes remains unknown, although structural or functional hypothalamic defects have been postulated.

Unusual distributions of adiposity can occur. Partial lipodystrophy is a rare variation of congenital lipodystrophy (lipoatrophy), in which subcutaneous fat is totally absent from a portion of the body and hypertrophied in the remainder. In multiple lipomatosis, a familial disorder characterized by localized, discrete, subcutaneous fat deposits throughout the body, stored triglyceride in lipoma cells (indistinguishable from the more usual adipose tissue cells) appears to be unavailable for mobilization even during starvation.

TREATMENT. In general, obesity can be treated by reduction of caloric intake or increase of caloric expenditure, or both. In special circumstances, particularly as applied to lifelong obesity, surgical techniques to decrease gastrointestinal adsorption of food and to decrease fat storage capacity by resection of large amounts of tissues have been used. Weight loss can be achieved by caloric restriction, regardless of the nature of the diet. The amount of weight loss depends largely on the degree of negative energy balance that is attained. Unfortunately, oxygen consumption declines in parallel with weight loss, making it

TABLE 216–6. DIFFERENTIAL DIAGNOSIS OF OBESITY*

Endocrine syndromes	Inflammatory disease
Hypothyroidism	Increased intracranial pressure
Hyperadrenocorticism	Pseudotumor cerebri
Hypogonadism	Empty sella syndrome
Insulinoma	Adiposogenital dystrophy
Polycystic ovaries (Stein-Leventhal)	Prader-Willi syndrome
Pseudohypoparathyroidism	Laurence-Moon-Biedl syndrome
Hypothalamic syndromes	Multiple lipomatosis
Tumors	Partial lipodystrophy
Craniopharyngioma	Drugs
Others	Cyproheptadine
Trauma	Phenothiazine

*An identifiable cause such as any of those listed above is present in less than 1 per cent of cases.

more difficult to maintain a steady degree of weight loss over the long term.

Diet. Although there have been many suggestions that the macronutrient composition of the calorically restricted diet is important for successful weight reduction, there is no firm evidence that a calorie is anything more or less than a calorie, regardless of the food source from which it is derived, despite the popularity of many calorically unbalanced "fad" diets. The rate of weight loss on low calorie diets high in protein is the same as the rate on diets high in fat or high in carbohydrate. Previous observations that indicated less rapid weight loss with high-carbohydrate, low-calorie diets have been attributed to short-term treatment in which changes in salt and water balance obscure changes in weight. It is apparent that an obese individual has a marked propensity to retain sodium during weight reduction and that this tendency is transiently exaggerated by carbohydrate in the diet. Carbohydrate-depleted ("ketogenic") diets increase weight loss solely by affecting water excretion, and their long-term use associated with mild ketosis and acidosis may cause decreased bone mineralization and amenorrhea. Meal frequency may play a role in the degree of success; frequent feedings may be more likely to prompt weight loss than less frequent consumption of larger loads which may lead to abnormal eating patterns, such as the night-eating syndrome. Although obesity may be more common in individuals who eat less frequently, there is no evidence of an effect of feeding frequency on the rate of weight loss in obese subjects studied in a metabolic ward. Total starvation has been promoted as a rapid route to achieve or start weight loss. However, the additional metabolic and other consequences of prolonged total starvation, such as unexplained anemia, body potassium depletion, hyperuricemia, gout, ketosis, lactic acidosis, liver function abnormalities, arrhythmias, hypotension, and, rarely, sudden death, have limited the utility of this form of treatment. Furthermore, it has been shown that the additional weight loss achieved by total starvation or carbohydrate-deprived diets over that achieved by a 600 to 800 mixed calorie diet is achieved by a selective loss in lean body mass rather than by additional loss of fat mass. The protein-modified fast may minimize this loss, but does not influence the other side effects of starvation. Thus a minimal quantity of protein and carbohydrate in weight reduction diets appears necessary, although the body has an unusual capacity to conserve nitrogen. In principle, it is clear that the aim of a weight reduction diet should be to keep normal body composition as well as to attain normal weight or to prevent further weight gain. There is no evidence to support the superiority of any form of low-calorie diet over that of any other. Thus a practical dietary recommendation for long-term management of obesity would be 15 to 20 cal per kilogram of ideal body weight, containing 20 per cent protein, 45 per cent carbohydrate, and 35 per cent fat calories. Substitution of one or more meals each day by fixed composition liquid formulas appears to have contributed to successful initiation of weight loss in many individuals. However, unbalanced formulations, such as the high protein, "protein-sparing" formula, appear to be associated with the same untoward consequences as seen with total starvation and other carbohydrate-deprived regimens, and the use of liquid protein hydrolysates to supplement total fasting has been associated with increased mortality. When psychologic problems appear prominent, emotional support may be necessary. The success of weight reduction groups for many individuals indicates that support of the "group therapy" type may be a useful adjunct.

Exercise. The most common method for promoting caloric expenditure in obese individuals is increased exercise. Obese patients, particularly adolescent females, are consistently less active than are thin individuals. In practice, obese individuals on weight reduction diets tend spontaneously to decrease their activity further, perhaps to compensate for decreased caloric intake in an attempt to preserve their fat mass. Exercising animals appear to gain less weight than do free-eating sedentary controls as a result of both an increase in caloric expenditure and a decrease in food intake. Exercise results in a significant decrease in the percentage of body fat, with a proportional increase in lean body mass. Thus exercise does appear to influence both body composition and food intake and should be part of reducing regimens. Exercise alone, however, does not appear to be an effective means of weight reduction, since the caloric equivalent of most activities is easily nullified by small amounts of food intake.

Drugs. Appetite suppressants (usually amphetamine derivatives) are of limited utility, because their effect is transient and rarely leads to more than a 10 per cent weight reduction. Inasmuch as the treatment of obesity is lifelong, such drugs have no demonstrable role in the long-term management of obesity. However, since neural regulation of adipose mass appears likely, future development of drugs altering such mechanisms holds promise. Thyroid hormone has been widely used to increase oxygen consumption of obese patients regardless of whether they suffer from hypothyroidism or "hypometabolism." Studies of body composition have shown that the accelerated weight loss from superimposition of thyroid extract on a low-calorie diet is due to a differential loss of lean body mass rather than to loss of fat tissue. Numerous other medications have been promoted for ability to achieve weight loss in obese individuals. Evaluation of these becomes a problem, because the routine of frequent physician visits, weight measurement, emotional support, medication, and diet itself promotes weight loss, and it is difficult to ascribe success to a particular medication. Furthermore, weight loss may result predominantly from loss of fluid, as with the widely dispensed diuretics, rather than from loss of adipose mass.

Surgery. A jejunoileal bypass operation has been used as a radical form of treatment of severe and refractory obesity in an attempt to lessen morbidity and early mortality. This procedure was devised to eliminate the function of a sufficient length of jejunum and ileum to cause weight loss without producing clinical steatorrhea. The distal ileum is essentially bypassed. Unfortunately, bypass surgery has, in several instances, caused massive fatty changes in the liver, cholestasis, fibrosis, interstitial inflammation, and fatal hepatic necrosis. Other complications include high operative mortality, severe crippling diarrhea, electrolyte imbalance, arthritis, and oxalate renal stones. Because of fewer reported complications, gastric partitioning procedures have been used more recently as the preferable surgical treatment. At present, caution in use of these experimental procedures is warranted, since complications such as peripheral neuropathy are being reported. There is no rationale for adipectomy in the management of lifelong obesity, although the disorder is characterized by adipose cell hyperplasia. Experimental studies in animals lead to little optimism, because excision of large adipose deposits has been followed by compensatory hypertrophy of remaining fat cell mass.

Behavior Modification. Since there are differences in feeding behavior between lean and some obese individuals, the newer methods of behavioral control have been applied to overeating. Short-term success in small groups of patients has been reported, and this approach appears to have promise, particularly as an adjunct to other forms of therapy, but long-term success does not appear to be enhanced.

PROGNOSIS. Overall mortality rates are higher in untreated moderate or severe obesity beyond about 30 per cent overweight. Insurance company figures suggest that for 45-year-old men averaging about 30 per cent overweight, death rates are 40 per cent higher than those for all insured men. For any degree of obesity, the mortality risk is higher for males than females and is greater for obesity occurring at a younger rather than an older age. These higher mortality rates can be reversed with weight reduction.

Unfortunately, successful weight reduction over the long term is difficult to achieve. The prognosis for treatment of obesity appears to vary with the clinical type. Lifelong obesity is frustrating to treat and leads to grief on the part of both physician and patient. In view of the poor results after long-term follow-up of a variety of dietary weight reduction schemes (which may be very successful in the short term), this form of obesity may be virtually irreversible. It is a common experience in obesity clinics that less than 5 per cent of the grossly (presumably lifelong) obese patients ever attain normal weight, and few can maintain a short-term weight loss in excess of 40 pounds. The long-term prognosis after gastrointestinal surgery is as yet unknown. Reduced caloric intake in childhood may lead to short stature and delayed puberty.

On the other hand, the more common adult-onset obesity should be amenable to treatment, so that most of the metabolic and pathophysiologic consequences of enlarged adipose cell mass and its associated diseases can be reversed.

PREVENTION. As with hypertension, most obesity is "essential," because definable, preventable, and treatable causes rarely can be identified. However, focus on the most refractory form of obesity, hyperplastic or juvenile-onset, should produce additional insights leading to more effective prevention. It is premature to suggest to physicians that obesity must be prevented in childhood if there is to be an impact on obesity in the adult.

Thus it can no longer be assumed that most obesity is simply the result of overeating and that every fat person is an overfed normal one. Most slightly overweight adults are fundamentally normal, but have eaten a little too much and exercised much too little. The grossly overweight patient who has had the problem from early childhood suffers from a disorder that is not well understood and is unsuccessfully treated. Nevertheless some of the complications of obesity can be managed, and the obese individual who has experienced multiple failures in weight reduction needs sympathetic attention rather than admonition.

Alexander JK, Peterson KL: Cardiovascular effects of weight reduction. Circulation 45:310, 1972. *A study of hemodynamic variables in markedly obese patients before and after significant weight reduction, indicating that the circulatory effects of gross obesity are largely reversible with weight loss.*

Alpers DH: Surgical therapy for obesity. N Engl J Med 308:1026, 1983. *A brief review of the present status of surgical approaches with an editorial comment on the companion article concluding, on the basis of late follow-up, that jejunoileal bypass surgery is no longer justified.*

Bray GA (ed.): The Obese Patient. Philadelphia, W. B. Saunders Company, 1976. *A compendium of information about the epidemiology, pathogenesis, and metabolic and physiologic effects and treatments of obesity. A valuable source of references.*

Bray GA, Gallagher TF Jr: Manifestations of hypothalamic obesity in man. A comprehensive investigation of eight patients and a review of the literature. Medicine 54:301, 1975. *An in-depth review of one of the known causes of human obesity.*

Czech MP, Richardson DK, Smith CJ: Biochemical basis of fat cell insulin resistance in obese rodents and man. Metabolism 26:1057, 1977. *The mechanisms of impaired glucose utilization in response to insulin in fat cells isolated from obese individuals is reviewed. Emphasis is on altered metabolic activities rather than insulin receptors or the hormone effector system.*

Glass AR, Burman KD, Dahms WT, Boehm TM: Endocrine function in human obesity. Metabolism 30:89, 1981. *A comprehensive review of abnormalities of endocrine function in obesity.*

Hirsch J, Batchelor B: Adipose tissue cellularity in human obesity. Clin Endocrinol Metab 5:299, 1976. *A review of the current status of the role of adipose cell hyperplasia in obesity.*

Hubert HB, Feinleib M, McNamara PM, Castelli WP: Obesity as an independent risk factor for cardiovascular disease: A 26-year follow-up of participants in the Framingham Heart Study. Circulation 67:968, 1983. *A reexamination of the relationship of degree of obesity and the incidence of cardiovascular disease over 26 years in more than 5200 men and women indicates that obesity was a significant independent predictor, particularly among women.*

Knittle JL, Timmer K, Ginsberg-Fellner F, Brown RE, Katz DP: The growth of adipose tissue in children and adolescents. Cross-sectional and longitudinal studies of adipose cell number and size. J Clin Invest 63:239, 1979. *A detailed cross-sectional and longitudinal study of adipose cell number as a function of age in obese and nonobese children from ages 4 months to 19 years, documenting continuing hyperplasia in the obese throughout childhood.*

Lew EA, Garfinkel L: Variations in mortality by weight among 750,000 men and women. J Chron Dis 32:563, 1979. *A description of the mortality experience of 750,000 men and women in a long-term prospective study by the American Cancer Society, documenting that individuals 30 to 40 per cent heavier than average had a mortality rate 50 per cent higher than those of average weight. Mortality comparisons as a function of weight for all the common diseases are included.*

Schwartz RS, Brunzell JD: Increase of adipose tissue lipoprotein lipase activity with weight loss. J Clin Invest 67:1425, 1981. *Evidence that increased adipose tissue lipoprotein lipase activity in obesity is a metabolic abnormality not corrected by weight reduction and thus might be a primary abnormality leading to enhanced fat deposition.*

Sims EAH, Danforth E Jr, Horton ES, Bray GA, Glennon JA, Salans LB: Endocrine and metabolic effects of experimental obesity in man. Recent Prog Horm Res 29:457, 1973. *A summary of the results of a comprehensive study of the metabolic effects of experimental overfeeding in man.*

Stunkard AJ: The Pain of Obesity. Palo Alto, The Bull Publishing Company, 1976. *A review of the psychosocial aspects of obesity and the possible role of psychiatry in therapy.*

Van Itallie TB: Obesity: Adverse effects on health and longevity. Am J Clin Nutr 32:2723, 1979. *A summary of the health implications of obesity and the variety of disorders thought to be caused or aggravated by obesity.*

Van Itallie TB, Yang MU: Diet and weight loss. N Engl J Med 297:1158, 1977. *A review and a careful metabolic study of the effects of macronutrient composition of low calorie reducing diets on body composition. Carbohydrate depleted (ketogenic) diets increase weight loss solely by affecting water excretion.*

217. DISORDERS OF VITAMIN METABOLISM: DEFICIENCIES, METABOLIC ABNORMALITIES, AND EXCESSES

Richard S. Rivlin

In approaching disorders of vitamin metabolism, several considerations should be kept in mind about the properties of vitamins, their roles in biochemistry, and the shifting nature of their deficiencies that have evolved over a period of years. In general most vitamins must be acquired from dietary sources because they cannot be synthesized in the body. There are several exceptions to this rule in that certain vitamins can be synthesized in the body but in very small amounts. An example is niacin, which is formed in vivo from an essential amino acid, tryptophan. A tryptophan-poor diet cannot provide sufficient precursor to meet the metabolic needs for niacin, and niacin would have to be obtained from dietary sources in order to avoid deficiency. Other examples of vitamins synthesized by the body, or more correctly by the intestinal microflora, are vitamin K and biotin. Deficiency of these vitamins may result from long-term antibiotic therapy, which eliminates the bacterial sources. Under normal circumstances, however, endogenous supplies are not sufficient, and some must be obtained from food sources. Another example is vitamin D, which can be synthesized in the skin after exposure to light (Ch. 244).

Many vitamins, particularly the B vitamins, function as essential coenzymes required in intermediary metabolism. The dietary form of the vitamin is first converted into its active derivatives before it can serve as a coenzyme. Examples include dietary thiamin and its coenzyme derivative thiamin pyrophosphate, pyridoxine and pyridoxal phosphate, and riboflavin and flavin adenine dinucleotide. Vitamin deficiencies may arise not only because of dietary deficiencies but also because conversion of the dietary form of the vitamin to its coenzyme derivatives is diminished by drugs, diseases, or other factors. Vitamin deficiencies may also be caused by abnormalities of intestinal absorption, plasma transport, tissue storage, binding to proteins, or excretion. Assuring adequate vitamin status involves *exogenous* factors, such as dietary adequacy and food processing, preparation, and storage, as well as *endogenous* factors, that is, those that control vitamin utilization by the body.

Overt vitamin deficiencies caused by diet are seldom isolated. Although generations of students are familiar with scurvy caused by vitamin C deficiency and pellagra resulting from niacin deficiency, in common clinical practice in the United States these classical syndromes are encountered only rarely. Rather, the typical picture one encounters in hospitalized patients with protein-calorie malnutrition is that of multiple deficiencies, because a diet poor in one vitamin is usually poor in several others. Furthermore, one vitamin is often required for the metabolism of another. An example is riboflavin, which is involved in the metabolism of folic acid, pyridoxine, vitamin K, and niacin.

The clinical development of vitamin deficiencies is generally gradual; the physical examination is usually not useful in detecting deficiencies of specific vitamins early in their course. For example, by the time that perifollicular hemorrhages characteristic of scurvy have developed, vitamin C deficiency is already far advanced. Even the abnormalities detected by physical examination late in the course of the deficiency state are often not pathognomonic. Cheilosis and glossitis, typically attributed to deficiency of riboflavin, can be observed with deficiencies of a number of other B vitamins. Finding an abnormality of this kind on physical examination helps to establish the diagnosis of malnutrition but does not identify a specific nutrient as missing from the diet.

Increasing attention is now being paid to drugs and alcohol as significant causes of specific vitamin deficiencies. Drug-induced vitamin deficiencies often are poorly recognized and become evident most frequently in chronically ill long-term drug users on a marginally adequate diet. The elderly are particularly vulnerable to the deleterious effects of ethanol. This commonly used and abused substance is now established as the major cause of deficiencies of folate and thiamin among individuals 65 years of age and older, and this is probably true in younger age groups as well.

The rate at which vitamin stores are depleted following restriction of dietary intake varies widely among vitamins. The body stores of some vitamins, such as B_{12}, may not be depleted for years, whereas folic acid, thiamin, and niacin may be depleted within weeks or months. In general, the body's capacity for storage of water-soluble vitamins is limited, and when the storage capacity is exceeded, the excess is usually excreted rapidly; their tissue concentrations often cannot be increased even by massive doses given parenterally. By contrast, body stores of fat-soluble vitamins may become very great, and toxicity often develops with prolonged administration of doses greatly exceeding the recommended dietary allowances (RDA).

At present, many individuals are consuming vitamins in doses far in excess of the RDA. More than one third of individuals 65 years of age and older in the United States are estimated to be taking some kind of nutritional supplement. Toxicity frequently develops with prolonged use of megadoses of vitamins A and D. Individuals vary considerably in the rate at which they develop toxicity with prolonged use of megadoses of vitamins. Certain conditions predispose to early symptomatology. For example, individuals with a gouty diathesis may be at increased risk for renal toxicity caused by megadoses of vitamin C, and the onset of acute liver disease may precipitate vitamin A toxicity in a previously stable patient who has taken megadoses of this vitamin.

Under certain circumstances vitamins may be used appropriately as drugs. For example, ascorbic acid is widely employed to acidify the urine in cases of refractory urinary tract infections. Certain derivatives of vitamin A, in particular the 13-cis isomer of retinoic acid, have potent antikeratinizing effects that have been applied to the treatment of cystic acne. Nicotinic acid is utilized in the management of severe hyperlipoproteinemia. Thus, the therapeutic applications of vitamins extend far beyond their roles in correcting dietary deficiency.

VITAMIN B_1 (THIAMIN)

Structure and Biochemical Function

The thiamin molecule is composed of pyrimidine and thiazole moieties joined by a methylene bridge, as shown in Figure 217–1. The principal biochemical role of thiamin is that of precursor of thiamin pyrophosphate, a coenzyme required for oxidative decarboxylation of α-ketoacids to aldehydes. These reactions are widely distributed and are an important source of energy generation. In addition, thiamin pyrophosphate serves as the coenzyme for transketolase, which catalyzes the conver-

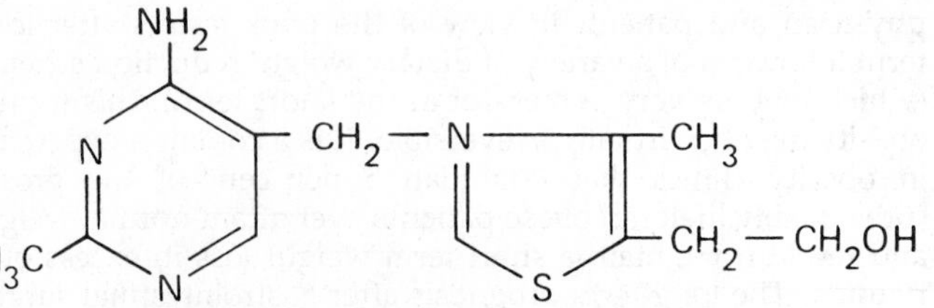

Figure 217–1. Structural formula of thiamin.

sion of the two 5-carbon sugars, xylulose-5-PO_4 and ribose-5-PO_4, to the 7-carbon sugar, sedoheptulose-7-PO_4, and the 3-carbon sugar glyceraldehyde-3-PO_4. This reaction is used as a functional index of thiamin nutritional status, as discussed later in this chapter.

In addition to serving as a coenzyme, thiamin may have a role in the neurophysiology of facilitating conduction in peripheral nerves. The initiation of nerve impulses is associated with hydrolysis of thiamin pyrophosphate or thiamin triphosphate or both.

Normal Physiology

Dietary thiamin is absorbed from the intestinal tract both by passive diffusion (high concentrations) and by active transport (low concentrations). The absorptive process is associated with phosphorylation of the thiamin molecule within the mucosal cell. In folate deficiency the absorption of thiamin is diminished. Muscle serves as the major storage organ for thiamin; most of the body stores are in the form of thiamin pyrophosphate, with lesser amounts stored as thiamin triphosphate, thiamin monophosphate, and thiamin itself. The degradation and excretion pathways of thiamin are not known with certainty, and more than 25 metabolites of the vitamin have been recovered from urine.

Requirements and Dietary Sources

The RDA for thiamin in adult males is 1.2 to 1.5 mg per day and in adult women, 1.0 to 1.1 mg per day, depending upon age, with a 50 per cent increase during pregnancy and lactation. The allowance is generally related to caloric intake as 0.5 mg per 1000 Kcals, although it is recommended that thiamin intake not go below 1.0 mg per day even with a caloric intake reduced below 2000 Kcal. The best dietary sources of thiamin are beef, pork, whole grains, enriched cereal grains, peas, beans, and nuts. Thiamin is rapidly destroyed at alkaline pH and is also heat-sensitive when not under strongly acid conditions. Some food items, particularly raw fish and seafood, are believed to contain thiaminases, which destroy the dietary supply of thiamin. A number of antithiamin factors have been identified from both plant and animal sources.

Deficiency

PATHOGENESIS. In addition to being caused by a poor diet, thiamin deficiency in the United States most commonly occurs as a result of alcoholism. Thiamin absorption is exquisitely sensitive to ingested ethanol, which significantly interferes with thiamin absorption even in healthy individuals. Repeated drinking throughout the day prevents most of the dietary thiamin from being absorbed, particularly in alcoholics, in whom some degree of malabsorption is quite common. Approximately 25 per cent of alcoholics admitted to general hospitals in the United States have evidence of thiamin deficiency either by clinical or biochemical criteria. Alcoholism is clearly the most important cause of thiamin deficiency in older age groups and probably in younger age groups as well. There is some evidence that alcohol also adversely affects the intermediary metabolism of thiamin, and chronic liver disease secondary to alcoholism may diminish the conversion of thiamin to thiamin pyrophosphate. Refeeding an alcoholic patient without thiamin may precipitate thiamin deficiency. It is likely that other factors, such as heavy coffee consumption, possibly may diminish the intestinal absorption of thiamin. Thiamin deficiency is also observed with diabetes, cancer, other chronic illnesses, and with long-term parenteral nutrition or use of intravenous fluids not containing thiamin.

CLINICAL FEATURES. Early thiamin deficiency is characterized by anorexia, irritability, and weight loss. Later, individuals experience weakness, peripheral neuropathy, headache, and tachycardia. Advanced thiamin deficiency presents with involvement of two major organ systems predominantly: the cardiovascular system (the syndrome known as "wet beriberi", i.e., beriberi heart disease) and the nervous system, both central and peripheral (known as "dry beriberi").

The following criteria are generally accepted for the diagnosis of beriberi heart disease: absence of other known etiologic factors, history of at least three months of documented dietary thiamin deficiency, associated peripheral neuritis, enlarged heart with normal sinus rhythm (usually tachycardia), peripheral edema, nonspecific ST- and T-wave changes, and rapid therapeutic response to thiamin administration. Beriberi heart disease is well recognized as a cause of high output failure, which is a consequence of the profound peripheral vasodilatation. Resting tachycardia, weakness, and weight loss often resemble the clinical features of apathetic hyperthyroidism, with which it is frequently confused.

The central nervous system manifestations of thiamin deficiency consist primarily of the Wernicke-Korsakoff syndrome (Ch. 482). The Wernicke's component is an acute disorder consisting of variable degrees of vomiting, horizontal nystagmus, ophthalmoplegia caused by weakness of the rectus muscles, fever, ataxic gait, and progressive mental impairment. Patients have died when the disease has been unrecognized and allowed to progress. The Korsakoff syndrome typically has loss of memory and confabulation as prominent features.

The peripheral nervous system abnormalities of thiamin deficiency typically consist of a symmetrical lesion that involves motor, sensory, and reflex responses. The legs are usually involved earlier and more completely than the arms. Pain and paresthesias may be particularly disabling to afflicted patients. It is possible that there is genetic variation in the susceptibility to dietary thiamin deficiency associated with differences in the binding affinity of transketolase for thiamin.

DIAGNOSIS. Thiamin status can be evaluated using bioassays, microbiologic technique, chemical analyses, and functional enzyme assays. In actual practice, the two most widely used assays are urinary thiamin excretion and the transketolase activity coefficient. Urinary thiamin can be determined accurately, but the results may be misleading if there has been recent thiamin intake in a previously deficient patient or if the patient has recently taken diuretics, which promote thiamin excretion. The results obtained under those circumstances would not yield the expected low value. Transketolase, as noted previously, requires thiamin pyrophosphate as its cofactor. In vitamin deficiency, the erythrocyte apoenzyme is not fully saturated with its cofactor, and addition of the cofactor in vitro to an erythrocyte hemolysate results in an increase in measured enzyme activity. The degree of increase in the activity coefficient (i.e., enzyme activity after incubation with the cofactor in vitro compared to that before incubation in vitro, expressed as a per cent) is an indication of the degree of unsaturation of the apoenzyme with thiamin pyrophosphate. The degree of unsaturation, in turn, is indicative of the magnitude of depletion of body stores of thiamin. An activity coefficient of 15 to 20 per cent or greater is generally regarded as reflecting significant thiamin deficiency. If these assays are unavailable, a therapeutic trial of thiamin, which provides rapid improvement (in 12 hours or less) in cardiovascular function and in ophthalmoplegia, may be regarded as supportive evidence for the diagnosis of thiamin deficiency. Cardiac output may diminish and vascular resistance increase within 30 minutes of intravenous administration of a single 100 mg dose of thiamin given to a patient with beriberi.

TREATMENT. If thiamin deficiency is suspected, rapid treatment with large doses of the vitamin is essential. Generally, 50 to 100 mg are administered intramuscularly or intravenously every day for the first few days, after which lower doses in the range of 5 to 10 mg may be given orally. Other therapeutic applications for which pharmacologic doses of thiamin are required include several rare inborn errors of metabolism: thiamin-responsive megaloblastic anemia, thiamin-responsive lactic acidosis, and thiamin-responsive branched-chain ketoaciduria, as well as subacute necrotizing encephalomyelopathy (Leigh's syndrome), a condition in which thiamin triphosphate is deficient in the brain.

Toxicity

Thiamin can be given safely by mouth in very large amounts without fear of toxicity, although the intestinal absorptive capacity is limited. When given by the intravenous route, large doses of thiamin on very rare occasions have been associated with poorly understood reactions resembling anaphylactic shock. Fortunately, these reactions occur so rarely that intravenous therapy with thiamin should not be withheld from a seriously ill thiamin-deficient patient.

Iber FL, Blass JP, Brin M, Leevy CM: Thiamin in the elderly—Relation to alcoholism and to neurological degenerative disease. Am J Clin Nutr 36:1067 (Suppl), 1982. *Discussion of effects of alcohol and drugs upon thiamin bioavailability.*

Neal RA, Sauberlich HE: Thiamin. *In* Goodhart RS, Shills ME (eds.): Modern Nutrition in Health and Disease. 6th ed. Philadelphia, Lea & Febiger, 1980. pp 191–197. *Discussion of structure, functions, requirements, and toxicity of thiamin.*

VITAMIN B_2 (RIBOFLAVIN)

Structure and Biochemical Functions

Riboflavin must be converted to its coenzyme derivatives, flavin mononucleotide (riboflavin-5'-phosphate, FMN) and flavin adenine dinucleotide (FAD), in order to be metabolically active (Fig. 217–2). These coenzymes are formed sequentially from dietary riboflavin after reacting with ATP and function as cofactors for a wide variety of enzymes in intermediary metabolism, particularly those involving oxidation-reduction reactions. FAD-dependent enzymes include α-glycerophosphate dehydrogenase, xanthine oxidase, and NADPH-cytochrome c reductase. A small fraction of tissue flavin is found in covalent linkage with protein and includes the enzymes monoamine oxidase (MAO), succinic dehydrogenase, and sarcosine dehydrogenase.

Normal Physiology

Riboflavin and FMN are absorbed from the upper gastrointestinal tract by a specific and saturable transport process. FAD, the predominant form in foods such as meat, must first be degraded to riboflavin and FMN prior to being absorbed. Covalently-bound flavins are largely unavailable as nutritional sources of riboflavin. A number of metals and drugs form complexes or chelates with dietary riboflavin and may influence the bioavailability of this vitamin. Such agents include copper, zinc, iron, saccharin, tryptophan, and ascorbic acid. After absorption, riboflavin is bound to several serum proteins and particularly to IgG during normal pregnancy. The renal tubule transports riboflavin in both directions, and in urine the predominant form detected is riboflavin rather than the coenzyme derivatives. Recently, several new metabolites of riboflavin have been identified in human urine, including 7α- and 8α-hydroxyriboflavin. The precise metabolic pathways are unknown.

Thyroid and adrenal hormones regulate the conversion of riboflavin to FMN, FAD, and covalently-bound flavins. Analogues of riboflavin interfere with certain actions of aldosterone and may possibly have potential as antihypertensive agents.

Requirements and Dietary Sources

The RDA for riboflavin in adult males is 1.4 to 1.7 mg per day and in adult females, 1.2 to 1.3 mg per day, depending upon age. Allowances are increased during pregnancy and lactation and probably should be increased with heavy exercise.

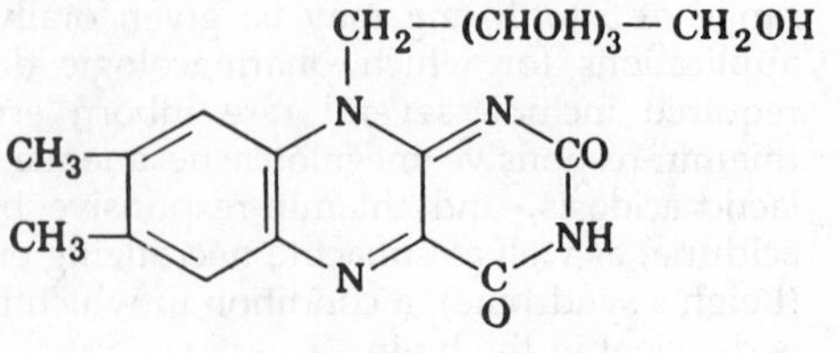

Riboflavin

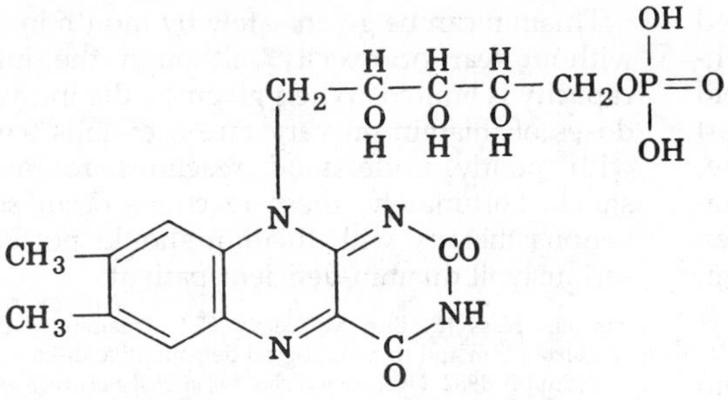

Riboflavin phosphate (flavin mononucleotide)

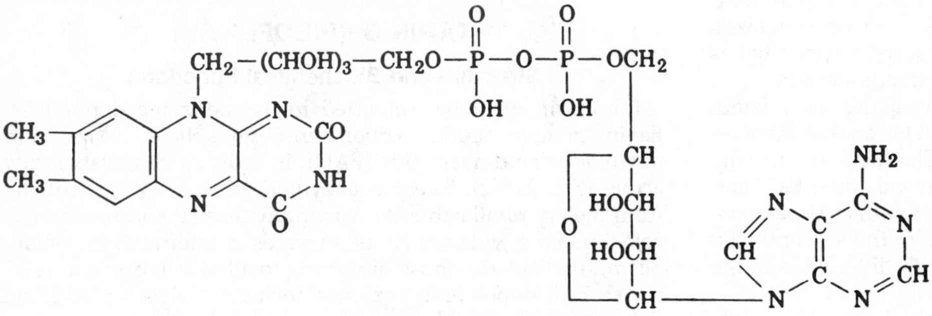

Flavin adenine dinucleotide (FAD)

Figure 217–2. Structural formulae of riboflavin (vitamin B_2) and its coenzyme derivatives.

When riboflavin is consumed in amounts greater than the RDA, increased urinary excretion occurs promptly. In the United States, milk and milk products supply close to half the daily intake of riboflavin, with meat, fish, poultry, eggs, and legumes providing another 30 per cent; the remainder comes largely from fruits, vegetables, and grain products. In developing countries, the principal sources are cereals, roots, and tubers. Riboflavin is light-, acid-, and alkali-sensitive and rapidly loses biological activity when exposed to sunlight or when treated with sodium bicarbonate, a common but unfortunate practice used to retain the color of green vegetables.

Deficiency

PATHOGENESIS. Riboflavin deficiency arises not only because of an inadequate diet, but also when hormones, drugs, or diseases impair the absorption, utilization, metabolic transformations, binding, or excretion of this vitamin. In experimental animals, hypothyroidism and the psychotropic drugs, chlorpromazine, imipramine, and amitriptyline, diminish the conversion of riboflavin to its active coenzyme derivatives, FMN and FAD. The underlying mechanism of this effect appears to be inhibition of flavokinase, the enzyme that converts riboflavin to FMN, the first of two steps in the biosynthesis of FAD. Phototherapy of newborn infants with hyperbilirubinemia may lead to some decomposition of riboflavin because of its light sensitivity. Boric acid forms a complex with riboflavin and leads to massive riboflavinuria. Ethanol may diminish both the intestinal absorption of riboflavin and its bioavailability from food sources. Deficiency of riboflavin likely results also after severe trauma, burns, surgery, chronic debilitating diseases, and severe and prolonged diarrhea. Increased riboflavin excretion may occur under conditions of negative nitrogen balance, including diabetes after withdrawal of insulin.

CLINICAL FEATURES. Early symptoms of riboflavin deficiency include soreness of the mouth, burning and itching of the eyes, and personality deterioration. Advanced riboflavin deficiency produces a constellation of findings that include cheilosis, angular stomatitis, seborrheic dermatitis, glossitis, corneal vascularization, reticulocytopenia and anemia, and retarded intellectual development. Cheilosis and angular stomatitis, once thought to be specific for riboflavin deficiency, are now known to occur frequently in other nutritional deficiencies. The clinical picture of riboflavin deficiency isolated from other deficiencies is rarely observed. Riboflavin deficiency is a major cause of congenital malformations in experimental animals, but it is unclear at present whether malformations result from human maternal riboflavin deficiency. The rate of metabolism of a number of drugs is altered in riboflavin deficiency, at least in part because the microsomal hydroxylase system requires a flavin cofactor.

DIAGNOSIS. In riboflavin deficiency, there is a reduction in urinary excretion of riboflavin as well as a reduction in the concentrations of various flavins in plasma and in erythrocytes. A functional test of riboflavin status is the activity coefficient of erythrocyte glutathione reductase, an FAD-requiring enzyme. When FAD is added in vitro to an erythrocyte hemolysate the increase in activity produced is much greater in erythrocytes from riboflavin-deficient than from riboflavin-replete individuals. As with transketolase and thiamin pyrophosphate (referred to above), this assay reflects the lesser degree of saturation of the apoenzyme with its cofactor in deficient compared with normal individuals. Results are expressed as the activity coefficient, i.e., the ratio of enzyme activity after incubation with FAD in vitro to that before incubation. Activity coefficients greater than 1.2 to 1.3 are generally considered to be indicative of a riboflavin-deficient state.

TREATMENT. Riboflavin deficiency can be treated satisfactorily with food sources high in riboflavin, such as milk, liver, meat, eggs, and certain vegetables, or with the vitamin itself. Deficient patients treated with 10 to 15 mg per day of riboflavin undergo healing of skin lesions within days to weeks of initiation of therapy. The intravenous administration of riboflavin, which may be needed in debilitated patients or in those with serious disorders of the gastrointestinal tract, is greatly restricted by its limited solubility in aqueous solution.

Toxicity

Riboflavin, FMN, and FAD are completely free of any known toxicity.

Massey V, Williams CH (eds.): Flavins and Flavoproteins. Seventh International Symposium. North Holland, NY, Elsevier, 1983. *Volume covering the latest conference proceedings of subjects related to biochemistry, chemistry, and medical aspects of riboflavin and its coenzyme derivatives.*

Merrill AH, Lambeth JD, Edmondson DE, McCormick DB: Formation and mode of action of flavoproteins. *In* Darby WJ, Broquist HP, Olson RE (eds.): Annual Review of Nutrition. Vol. 1. Palo Alto, Annual Reviews Inc., 1981, pp 281–317. *Review of the basic biochemistry of riboflavin and its derivatives and flavin enzymes.*

Rivlin RS: Riboflavin. *In* Olson RE (ed.): Present Knowledge in Nutrition. 5th ed. Washington DC, The Nutrition Foundation, 1984, pp 285–302. *Discussion of the physiology, sources, functions, and metabolic roles of riboflavin.*

NIACIN

Structure and Biochemical Function

The term niacin is used in this review to refer to two compounds, nicotinic acid and nicotinamide, and other biologically active pyridine derivatives, as shown in Figure 217–3. The term niacin is sometimes restricted to nicotinic acid only. Although niacin was formerly referred to as "vitamin B_3," this term is no longer used as an official designation. Niacin is a precursor of two coenzymes, nicotinamide adenine dinucleotide (NAD) and nicotinamide adenine dinucleotide phosphate (NADP), which function in a wide number of oxidation and reduction reactions. NAD and NADP are involved in glycolysis, pyruvate metabolism, pentose biosynthesis, and lipid, amino acid, protein, and purine metabolism. These coenzymes also have other functions, some of which are discussed in the following paragraphs. Niacin is stable both to light and to heat.

Normal Physiology

Niacin given by itself appears to be nearly completely absorbed by diffusion from the stomach and small intestine in amounts as high as 3 grams. When present in a bound form in certain foods such as corn, however, niacin has only limited bioavailability. A portion of dietary niacin occurs in a bound form (as niacinogen) in cereal grains but remains biologically available. As noted previously, niacin can be synthesized from the essential amino acid tryptophan. Under normal circumstances approximately 1.5 per cent of dietary tryptophan is converted to niacin. The efficiency of this conversion is regulated by a number of hormonal and nutritional factors and is greater under conditions of niacin deficiency. Vitamins B_2 and B_6 are required for this conversion. Niacin is present in all cells, and only small amounts can be stored in the body. Both nicotinic acid and nicotinamide, as well as certain of their metabolites, particularly N-methylnicotinamide and 2-pyridone, are excreted in urine.

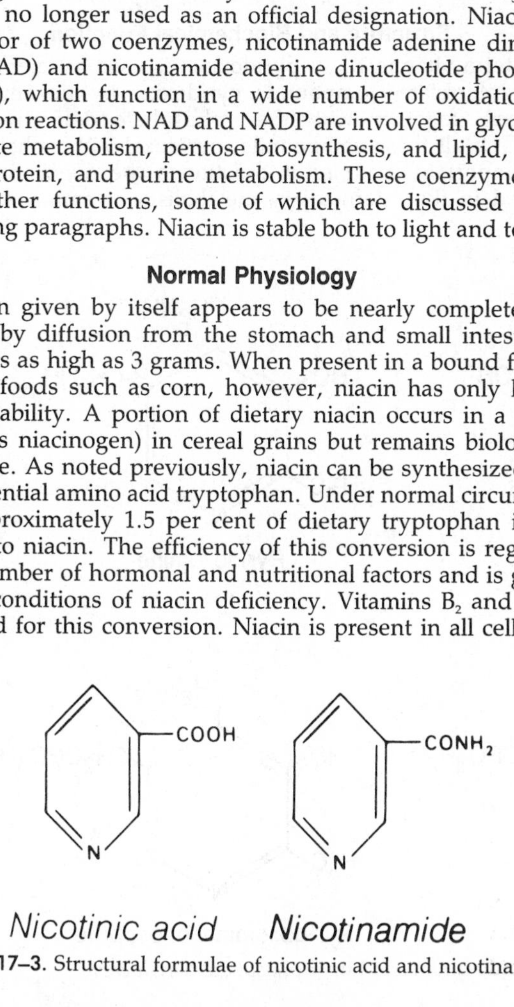

Figure 217–3. Structural formulae of nicotinic acid and nicotinamide.

Requirements and Dietary Sources

The RDA for niacin in adult males is 16 to 19 mg and in adult females, 13 to 14 mg, depending upon age, with an additional 2 mg recommended for pregnancy and 5 mg for lactation. The allowance is expressed in terms of niacin equivalents, because approximately 60 mg of dietary tryptophan are needed to form 1 mg of niacin. Proteins of animal origin such as meat, milk, and eggs have a relatively high tryptophan content and therefore are good sources of endogenously generated niacin. Vegetable proteins also supply tryptophan, but the concentration is lower than in animal proteins. Diets dependent heavily upon corn are a particular problem because not only is the tryptophan content low but also the niacin is poorly available. Niacin from wheat sources also has limited bioavailability. Pyridoxine and riboflavin deficiencies increase the dietary requirement for niacin, because these vitamins are required for the biosynthesis of niacin from tryptophan.

PATHOGENESIS. Niacin deficiency may develop because of a number of factors. First, dietary deficiency develops when corn is the major staple of the diet. Pellagra caused by consumption of corn was once very common in parts of the United States but fortunately has largely disappeared at the present time. Secondly, niacin deficiency may arise as a result of alcoholism, a condition in which diet is often poor and erratic. It is likely that in prolonged alcoholism, particularly in the presence of other nutrient deficiencies, the absorption and metabolism of niacin may be impaired. In addition, certain drugs interfere with niacin metabolism to a clinically significant degree, the best known of which is isonicotinic acid hydrazide (INH). The neurologic symptoms occurring with INH treatment can be ameliorated by administration of pyridoxine. Certain anticancer drugs, particularly 6-mercaptopurine, may produce niacin deficiency. In the rare inborn error of Hartnup's disease, pellagra may develop because of a defect in the intestinal and renal tubular transport of tryptophan and of several other amino acids (Ch. 83.3). Malnourished patients with the malignant carcinoid syndrome have been known rarely to exhibit manifestations of pellegra; under these circumstances, dietary tryptophan is diverted from niacin to serotonin (Ch. 242). Under certain conditions, excess leucine in the diet produces a deficiency by inhibiting the conversion of tryptophan to niacin.

CLINICAL FEATURES. In the early stages of niacin deficiency, clinical findings may be vague and nondiagnostic. Patients often complain of decreased appetite, loss of weight, abdominal aching and discomfort, weakness, irritability, inability to concentrate, and other nonspecific indications of illness. As the deficiency progresses, there may be epithelial changes that include glossitis, stomatitis, soreness and pain in the mouth (particularly the tongue), and eventually development of the characteristic skin lesions. These lesions, when well established, are dark, scaling, and cracking and occur over the areas of skin that are exposed to sunlight, frequently leaving a sharp line of demarcation at the unexposed skin surfaces. The lesion may resemble a necklace and is described as Casal's necklace.

In addition to the dermatitis, patients with the advanced form of niacin deficiency, that is, pellegra, have diarrhea and dementia. The diarrhea is often severe and intractable and may have a component of malabsorption that appears to be related to villous atrophy. The latter likely results from the long period of minimal food intake. Neuropsychiatric manifestations are mild at first but in advanced cases may progress to confusion, disorientation, seizures, hallucinations, and frank psychosis. Death may result in very advanced cases, usually preceded by major confusional states. Pellagra is popularly known for the four D's: dermatitis, diarrhea, dementia, and death.

Niacin deficiency secondary to drugs is generally mild and often unrecognized by clinicians. The consequences of drug-induced deficiencies of niacin and of other vitamins are much greater in the presence of a marginal or frankly deficient diet.

DIAGNOSIS. The diagnosis of advanced deficiency can often be made on clinical grounds alone if the patient exhibits the classic findings. Such patients are very unusual, however. In the early stages of the illness or in the absence of all the classic features, diagnosis may be difficult and is often missed without a high index of suspicion. Blood concentrations of NAD and NADP are reduced but may not be indicative of niacin deficiency, because reduced levels also occur in other severe, constitutional illnesses that are unrelated to niacin status. Attention has therefore turned to assay of urinary metabolites of niacin as indices of niacin nutriture. The most widely used is N-methylnicotinamide. Low urinary levels are interpreted as indicative of niacin deficiency. The excretion of another metabolite, 2-pyridone, is less widely used and requires a cumbersome assay. Some investigators have considered the ratio of these two metabolites in urine to be the most accurate index of niacin nutriture.

TREATMENT. The treatment of advanced pellagra has been accomplished satisfactorily by administering large oral doses (approximately 50 to 150 mg) of niacin as nicotinamide (the form present in most commercial vitamin formulations). The exact dose given is somewhat empirical. The therapeutic response is often dramatic, and patients may show marked improvement within several days after the start of therapy. Maintenance levels are then given together with dietary repletion. Nicotinamide is usually well tolerated under these circumstances.

Other therapeutic applications of niacin include its use as nicotinic acid in the control of elevated serum cholesterol and triglyceride levels in daily doses of 3 grams or more (Ch. 183–186). Nicotinic acid may be useful in treating patients of types II, IV, and V hyperlipoproteinemia. The mechanism of the therapeutic effect on lipid metabolism is not known, and this property is not shared by nicotinamide. With nicotinic acid treatment, HDL levels rise because of a slight decrease in synthetic rate with a large decrease in degradative rate. Because of the toxicity of nicotinic acid at high doses, treatment with this agent is generally reserved for patients with extreme lipid abnormalities. At the present time, nicotinic acid is believed to reduce the recurrence rate of nonfatal myocardial infarction but not to influence overall mortality rate.

Doses in the range of those used to treat pellagra are also needed to treat niacin deficiency in Hartnup's disease and in the carcinoid syndrome. Massive doses of niacin have not proven useful in the treatment of schizophrenia and other psychiatric disorders, despite the claims of food faddists and so-called "orthomolecular" therapists.

Toxicity

At the doses of nicotinamide used to treat niacin deficiency (described previously) there is little if any toxicity. When nicotinic acid in doses of 3 grams or more is used in the treatment of a lipid disorder, the most common side effect observed is flushing of the face due to vascular dilatation. Other common side effects of nicotinic acid may include dryness, itching and increased pigmentation of the skin, and abdominal pain. Rarely, hepatotoxicity, hyperuricemia, and worsening of peptic ulcer and glucose tolerance have been observed. The abnormalities in liver function may be severe, but both biochemical and histologic findings regress with discontinuation of nicotinic acid.

Henderson LaVM: Niacin. *In* Darby WJ, Broquist HP, Olson RE (eds.): Annual Review of Nutrition. Vol. 3. Palo Alto, Annual Reviews Inc, 1983, pp 289–307. *This review covers transport, metabolism, and physiologic and pharmacologic effects of niacin.*

Moran JR, Greene HL: The B vitamins and vitamin C in human nutrition. II. "Conditional" B vitamins and vitamin C. Am J Dis Child 133:308, 1979. *Discussion of physiology, metabolic disorders, and toxicity of niacin.*

Narasinga Rao BS, Gopalan C: Niacin. *In* Olson RE (ed.): Present Knowledge in Nutrition. 5th ed. Washington DC, The Nutrition Foundation, 1984, pp 318–331. *Review stressing metabolism, function, pathogenesis of deficiency, and therapeutic uses of niacin.*

VITAMIN B_6 (PYRIDOXINE)

Structure and Biochemical Function

The term vitamin B_6, or pyridoxine, is used to refer to three closely interrelated compounds, pyridoxine, pyridoxamine, and pyridoxal, together with their phosphate derivatives (Fig. 217–4). Of all these compounds, pyridoxal-5-phosphate is the most important, because it constitutes the major coenzyme involved in the intermediary metabolism of amino acids, in-

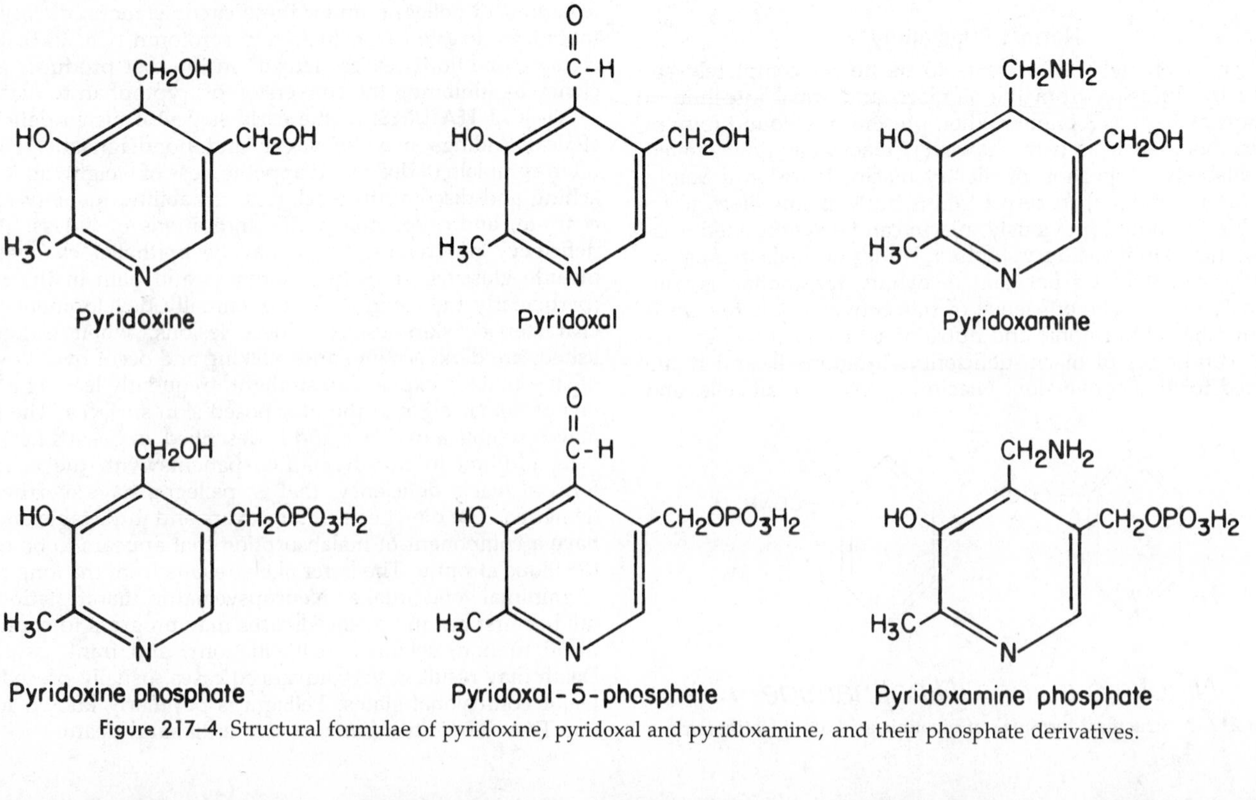

Figure 217–4. Structural formulae of pyridoxine, pyridoxal and pyridoxamine, and their phosphate derivatives.

cluding aminotransferases, decarboxylases, racemases, and synthetases. Pyridoxal phosphate is also involved in biosynthesis of heme and sphingosine. Under certain circumstances, pyridoxamine phosphate can also fulfill a coenzyme function. Pyridoxine is the major dietary source found in plants, whereas pyridoxal and pyridoxamine constitute the major forms in foods from animal sources. Pyridoxine is stable in acid solutions, but is highly light-sensitive in acid or neutral solutions. Pyridoxal and pyridoxamine are destroyed at high temperatures, particularly by autoclaving.

Normal Physiology

Dietary pyridoxine and related compounds are absorbed from the upper gastrointestinal tract probably by simple diffusion. The vitamin is widely distributed in the body; muscle constitutes an important storage organ, in which it is bound to phosphorylase, thus serving to stabilize the enzyme molecule. The various forms of pyridoxine are readily interconverted to one another by the liver under normal circumstances. Only very small amounts of dietary pyridoxine are converted to pyridoxal phosphate. In urine, pyridoxine, pyridoxal, and pyridoxamine can all be detected but at low concentrations; the major metabolite of pyridoxine, 4-pyridoxic acid, is found in urine in high concentrations.

Thyroid hormones reduce the concentrations of vitamin B_6 in various tissues, and increased sensitivity to insulin is demonstrable during B_6 deficiency.

Requirements and Dietary Sources

The RDA for vitamin B_6 is 2.2 mg per day for adult males and 2.0 mg per day for adult females, regardless of age, with a 0.5 to 0.6 mg per day increase during pregnancy and lactation. The requirement for vitamin B_6 is greater with a higher protein intake.

Vitamin B_6 is widely distributed in the food supply and can be derived from both plants and animals. Sources of vitamin B_6 are similar to those of other B vitamins and include liver, meat, wheat, nuts, beans and other vegetables, fruits, and cereals. Considerable losses occur during prolonged cooking, particularly pressure cooking. The bioavailability of vitamin B_6 from dietary sources varies widely depending upon storage, processing, and composition of food.

Deficiency

PATHOGENESIS. Dietary deficiency of pyridoxine is unusual, perhaps because of its widespread sources in the food supply. Rather, deficiency of pyridoxine is recognized increasingly as a consequence of prolonged therapy with certain medications. Foremost among these drugs is isoniazid, which complexes with pyridoxal phosphate to a clinically significant degree. Individuals with the genetic trait of inactivating isoniazid at a slow rate are particularly susceptible to B_6 deficiency from this drug. Isoniazid induces peripheral neuritis and diarrhea in adult patients; in children it produces anemia and seizures that can be prevented by coincident administration of pyridoxine. Cycloserine, another drug widely used for tuberculosis, is also a vitamin B_6 antagonist. With the widespread use of penicillamine for the treatment of rheumatoid arthritis, its B_6-antagonistic properties are of increasing clinical importance. Pyridoxine deficiency occurs frequently in alcoholism in association with other deficiencies, particularly folic acid deficiency. The increased urinary excretion of certain tryptophan metabolites, particularly xanthurenic acid, in women treated with oral contraceptives has been interpreted as indicating vitamin B_6 deficiency because B_6 is needed for conversion of tryptophan to niacin. L-DOPA, used for Parkinson's disease, may also cause B_6 deficiency over a prolonged period of time.

CLINICAL FEATURES. Deficiency of vitamin B_6 is not thought to produce a characteristic syndrome. As with deficiencies of other B vitamins, dermatitis, glossitis, cheilosis, and stomatitis may be manifestations of pyridoxine deficiency. Markedly deficient patients may have irritability, weakness, depression, dizziness, peripheral neuropathy, and seizures. As noted previously, deficiency in infants and children is typically characterized by diarrhea, anemia, and seizures. The rapidity with which drug-induced deficiency of B_6 occurs depends upon the adequacy of the patient's diet as well as the dosage and duration of drug therapy. Chronic vitamin B_6 deficiency also leads to secondary hyperoxaluria, increasing the risk of kidney stone formation (Ch. 89).

In addition to the deficiency syndromes of vitamin B_6 caused by diet or drugs or both, there is a group of disorders in which the affected patients do not display manifestations of deficiency, either clinically or biochemically, and yet require massive doses of this vitamin for adequate treatment. These disorders are known as dependency syndromes and include such diverse entities as pyridoxine-dependent convulsions, pyridoxine-responsive anemia, homocystinuria caused by cystathionine synthetase deficiency, cystathioninuria, and xanthurenic aciduria. Of these, pyridoxine-responsive anemia requires special mention because it is often confused with iron-deficient anemia; both disorders are characterized by hypochromic, microcytic red cells. In the pyridoxine-responsive anemia, however, serum iron is elevated with an increase in saturation of transferrin and an increase in iron absorption from the intestinal tract. There is evidence of iron overload, with hemosiderin deposits in bone marrow, liver, and other organs. Many patients have hepatosplenomegaly, and a hemolytic component may contribute to the anemia. It is important to differentiate this syndrome from iron-deficient anemia, because in the former inadvertent administration of iron worsens pyridoxine-responsive anemia. The blood count rises satisfactorily in response to pharmacologic doses of vitamin B_6.

DIAGNOSIS. The diagnosis of pyridoxine deficiency can be made by direct assay of vitamin B_6 in blood (normal levels generally are greater than 50 ng per milliliter) or by determining the urinary excretion of the main metabolite of pyridoxine, 4-pyridoxic acid. The excretion of less than 1.0 mg per day of this compound is generally considered suggestive of deficiency. Less frequently, the excretion of pyridoxine in urine is also determined. Functional enzyme assays, similar to those in use for diagnosing thiamin and riboflavin deficiencies, have also been developed for vitamin B_6 using aspartate aminotransferase or alanine aminotransferase in erythrocyte hemolysates. Enzyme activity is determined with and without the addition of pyridoxal phosphate in vitro. When activity coefficients (as defined previously) are greater than 1.5 for aspartate aminotransferase and 1.2 for alanine amino transferase, they are considered to be indicative of pyridoxine deficiency. These procedures have generally supplanted the tryptophan load test, in which the increased excretion of xanthurenic acid is taken as an index of B_6 nutriture.

TREATMENT. Dietary deficiency of pyridoxine can be treated satisfactorily with oral doses in the general range of 2 to 10 mg per day; doses of 10 to 20 mg per day may be needed in pregnancy. Pyridoxine deficiency occurring in association with specific drugs that inhibit pyridoxine metabolism, such as isoniazid, cycloserine, and penicillamine, requires higher doses, perhaps up to 100 mg per day, to ameliorate peripheral neuropathy. Rather than administer B_6 when symptoms develop, it is much more effective to prevent these side effects by administering vitamin B_6 when therapy with a B_6-antagonizing drug is initiated and particularly when a prolonged course of treatment is anticipated. Since iatrogenic vitamin B_6 deficiency is entirely preventable, B_6 is now routinely prescribed for patients receiving INH. Treatment with high doses of vitamin B_6 is contraindicated in patients receiving L-DOPA, however, as it may interfere with the efficacy of the drug.

Treatment of a pyridoxine-dependency syndrome requires much higher doses of B_6, and up to 1500 mg per day have been prescribed. The possible effectiveness of pyridoxine in the management of the carpal-tunnel syndrome and premenstrual tension is controversial. In some women on contraceptive steroids, vitamin B_6 has appeared to benefit depression. Pyridoxine is regarded as ineffective in treating schizophrenia, autism, and childhood hyperactivity, as well as peripheral neuropathies in which there is no known B_6 deficiency, such as in diabetes.

Toxicity

Pyridoxine has generally been considered to be safe and without toxicity. Recently, a sensory neuropathy was described in a small number of patients receiving 2 grams or more of pyridoxine per day. This potentially important finding requires confirmation and extension. At the present time, there are no indications for treatment of any disorder, even a pyridoxine-dependency syndrome, with doses of this magnitude. Thus, pyridoxine appears to be safe when prescribed in the appropriate milligram amounts needed to correct deficiency and to treat dependency states.

Henderson LM: Vitamin B_6. *In* Olson RE (ed.): Present Knowledge in Nutrition. 5th ed. Washington DC, The Nutrition Foundation, 1984, pp 303–317. *Review of B_6 stressing absorption, transport, and human requirements.*

Schaumburg H, Kaplan J, Winderbank A, et al.: Sensory neuropathy from pyridoxine abuse. A new megavitamin syndrome. N Engl J Med 309:445, 1983.

Sturman JA, Rivlin RS: Pathogenesis of brain dysfunction in deficiency of thiamine, riboflavin, pantothenic acid, or vitamin B_6. *In* Gaull GE (ed.): Biology of Brain Dysfunction. Vol. 3. New York, Plenum Press, 1975, pp 425–475. *Discussion of the pyridoxine-dependent syndromes.*

VITAMIN B_{12} (COBALAMIN)

The structure, function, pathophysiology, and therapeutic use of vitamin B_{12} are discussed in Ch. 135 in association with the megaloblastic anemias.

VITAMIN C (ASCORBIC ACID)

Structure and Biochemical Function

Ascorbic acid, a 6-carbon α-keto-lactone, resembles glucose in having several polyhydroxyl groups adjacent to one another (Fig. 217–5). Ascorbic acid can be oxidized to dehydro-L-ascorbic acid, which is also biologically active, and can be generated from the latter by reacting with reduced glutathione.

Ascorbic acid participates in oxidation-reduction reactions and in hydrogen ion transfer. This vitamin is a powerful reducing agent or anti-oxidant, particularly in lipid and vitamin metabolism, and is especially important in preventing oxidation of tetrahydrofolate. In addition, ascorbic acid enhances the intestinal absorption of nonheme iron. This vitamin is required in collagen metabolism, specifically for the synthesis of chondroitin sulfate and of hydroxyproline from proline. Defects in collagen biosynthesis are believed to be the basis for much of the symptomatology of scurvy. In the absence of vitamin C, dopamine-β-hydroxylase activity is reduced, impairing the biosynthesis of neurotransmitters. Ascorbic acid is also involved in carnitine biosynthesis, tyrosine metabolism, cholesterol metabolism, wound healing, and immune function and is a component of drug-metabolizing enzyme systems.

Prolonged storage or excessive cooking diminishes the biological activity of ascorbic acid. This highly water-soluble vitamin is also destroyed by oxidation, particularly by exposure to air in the presence of copper ion and an alkaline medium.

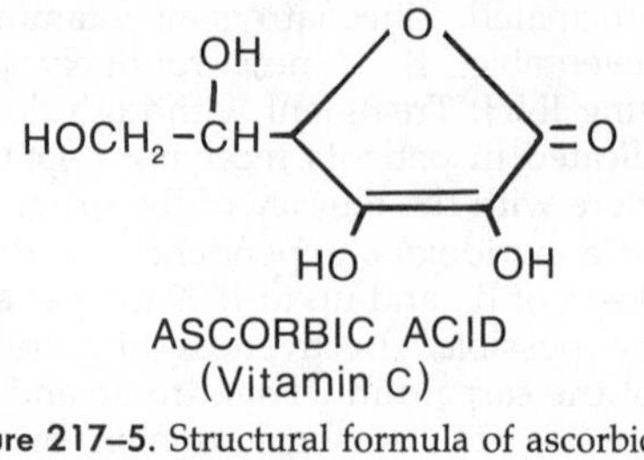

Figure 217–5. Structural formula of ascorbic acid.

Normal Physiology

Ascorbic acid is absorbed by a limited-capacity mechanism in the distal small intestine. As dietary intake of ascorbic acid increases, a progressively smaller proportion is absorbed, that is, about 95 per cent at 100 mg, 75 per cent at 1 gram, but only 20 per cent at 5 grams. Within the usual range of dietary ascorbic acid intake of 10 to 130 mg per day, the plasma level is proportional to the amount ingested. As the dietary intake increases further, however, the low renal threshold for excretion assures that excess plasma levels of ascorbic acid are promptly excreted. Another mechanism protecting against excessive accumulation of ascorbic acid is the microsomal enzyme, NADPH monodehydro-ascorbate transhydrogenase, which is induced by its substrate, ascorbic acid; in response to a large dietary load of ascorbic acid, degradative capacity is rapidly and substantially increased.

The body pool of ascorbic acid in adult males consuming about 80 mg per day is estimated to be approximately 1500 mg, and the rate of catabolism is about 3 per cent of the pool size per day. Increasing the dietary intake of ascorbic acid to more than 80 mg per day seems not to increase significantly the saturation of tissues with this vitamin. As with most B vitamins, the storage capacity for vitamin C is limited. Urinary excretion is in the form of ascorbic acid and dehydro-L-ascorbic acid, as well as several metabolites, including a sulfated derivative, ascorbate-2-sulfate, and oxalic acid.

Requirements and Dietary Sources

The RDA for ascorbic acid is 60 mg per day for all healthy adult males and females regardless of age. This allowance is generally regarded as quite generous inasmuch as 10 mg per day prevents scurvy. As noted, amounts greatly in excess of the RDA do not increase tissue stores significantly. The dietary allowance is increased by 20 mg per day during pregnancy and 40 mg per day during lactation. Human milk contains 30 to 55 mg per liter. It is especially important to maintain an adequate intake of ascorbic acid during lactation, because the vitamin concentration in milk is closely dependent upon dietary intake.

Serum ascorbic acid levels are lowered in smokers, possibly as a result of accelerated metabolism, and in users of oral contraceptive drugs, but the implications of these findings are unclear. The decreases are quantitatively small and can be corrected with a modest increase in consumption of ascorbic acid from dietary sources (about 40 mg for smokers). Patients who are exposed to cold or heat stress or who are febrile, undergoing surgery, or subjected to trauma have increased requirements for vitamin C. Patients receiving parenteral nutrition have higher requirements because of urinary losses.

The best dietary sources of ascorbic acid appear to be citrus fruits and green vegetables, especially broccoli, green peppers, tomatoes, cabbage, oranges, grapefruits, and lemons. Care must be taken during food preparation in order to avoid losses of the vitamin. Much smaller amounts are contained in milk, meats, and cereals. As noted above, ascorbic acid is heat-sensitive and is destroyed by alkali. Some decreased vitamin content is also observed with prolonged storage.

Deficiency

PATHOGENESIS. Urban poor, particularly the elderly, are at increased risk for dietary deficiency of ascorbic acid, in large measure because economic deprivation prevents them from obtaining the richest sources, namely citrus fruits, leafy vegetables, and tomatoes.

An increasingly important cause of ascorbic acid deficiency is food faddism and bizarre nutritional practices. The strict macrobiotic diet may lead to scurvy, particularly with pressure cooking of food items that have little ascorbic acid to begin with. Elderly individuals following a "tea and toast" diet are vulnerable to a number of deficiencies, particularly of ascorbic acid, as these sources are grossly inadequate. Children develop scurvy when fed unsupplemented cow's milk for the first year of life. Vitamin C deficiency progressing to scurvy is common in chronic alcoholics, probably because the diet is notably deficient in vitamin C-containing food items. Vitamin C deficiency, however, is not generally as prevalent as deficiencies of B vitamins in chronic alcoholism.

CLINICAL FEATURES. In the early stages of deficiency, symptoms and signs may be fairly nonspecific and include general malaise, lethargy, and weakness. As the disease progresses, probably one to three months after onset, patients may complain of dyspnea and pain in bones and joints, due predominantly to hemorrhages below the periosteum. Perifollicular hemorrhages, particularly about hair follicles, are indicative of advanced deficiency. Petechiae often are prominent and may appear over the arms after application of a sphygmomanometer. This finding is known as the Rumpel-Leed test. With progressive vitamin C depletion, there are ecchymoses and purpura initially at areas of trauma irritation, or pressure points. Joints, muscles, and subcutaneous tissues may become sites of hemorrhage. Swollen, bleeding gums are characteristic manifestations of advanced deficiency. Pallor and anemia may be the result of prolonged bleeding or to associated folic acid deficiency, with which scurvy commonly occurs. In children, disturbances of growth occur, and teeth, bones, blood vessels, and other collagen-rich structures develop abnormally. Preformed teeth may become loose and fall out because of alveolar bone resorption.

Wounds heal poorly, and previously healed wounds may open up again. In very advanced deficiency, edema, oliguria, and neuropathy are prominent. Should intracerebral bleeding occur, serious neurologic sequelae and even death may result.

DIAGNOSIS. The diagnosis of advanced scurvy is often made on clinical grounds alone because the skin changes may be quite characteristic. Capillary fragility is commonly abnormal. X-rays are useful in demonstrating subperiosteal elevation, disturbances of calcification of the cartilage matrix, fractures and dislocations, ground glass appearance of the cortex, alveolar bone resorption, and other findings.

Plasma ascorbic acid levels are greatly reduced in scurvy, usually to 0.1 mg per deciliter or lower. Some depression of plasma ascorbic acid levels occurs, however, in a variety of other conditions, including cigarette smoking, tuberculosis, rheumatic fever, many chronic disorders, and in some women using oral contraceptive drugs. These conditions must be considered when a low ascorbic acid level is detected.

The assay of ascorbic acid in serum or plasma can be accomplished with titrimetric, spectrophotometric, or fluorometric methods. Some laboratories prefer to make the diagnosis of scurvy by assay of platelet ascorbic acid.

TREATMENT. As little as 10 mg per day of ascorbic acid can completely prevent the clinical manifestations of scurvy. Even far-advanced cases of scurvy respond rapidly to ascorbic acid in the range of 100 to 200 mg per day. Marked improvement is to be expected within several days. Patients should also be instructed in the importance of a proper diet to prevent further recurrences.

Patients with rare inborn errors of metabolism, including tyrosinemia, osteogenesis imperfecta, and Chédiak-Higashi syndrome, have had some apparent benefit from the use of ascorbic acid in the range of 50 to 200 mg per day. Certain forms of the Ehlers-Danlos syndrome are the only disorders in which pharmacologic doses (4 grams) were reported to be effective.

Special mention must be made of two conditions in which the use of megadoses of ascorbic acid has attracted wide attention: the common cold and advanced cancer. Many studies have been performed on the possible benefits of 2 grams and higher per day of ascorbic acid on the prevention of colds and on the alleviation of symptoms once they develop. On balance, the predominance of evidence favors the view that while some individuals may receive slight benefit in terms of symptoms, probably as a result of a mild antihistamine action of ascorbic acid, no consistent, reproducible improvement occurs in the

frequency, duration, or severity of illness in the great majority of cases.

With respect to advanced cancer, there is some theoretical basis for the view that maintenance of immune function may depend upon the adequacy of vitamin C nutriture, as may wound healing and collagen formation. Nevertheless, treatment of cancer patients with megadoses of vitamin C after chemotherapy and radiation has been ineffective when evaluated in an objective manner. The use of vitamin C under no circumstances should replace established methods of treating cancer with chemotherapy, surgery, or radiation.

Vitamin C at a dose level of approximately 0.5 to 3 grams per day has been used to acidify the urine in cases of refractory urinary tract infections. Ascorbic acid is only a weak acidifying agent, and its efficacy under these circumstances is difficult to evaluate.

Ascorbic acid in amounts ordinarily contained in food may be useful in facilitating the intestinal absorption of nonheme iron. To be effective, the ascorbic acid and the iron sources must be consumed together. As little as 100 ml of orange juice, which contains 40 to 50 mg of ascorbic acid, has been reported to increase the absorption of nonheme iron more than threefold.

A potentially useful application of ascorbic acid lies in its ability to inhibit in vitro the conversion of nitrites and secondary amines to the carcinogenic nitrosoamines. Whether ascorbic acid can achieve this effect in vivo under ordinary circumstances of food consumption is important to determine.

Toxicity

At the dose range of approximately 1 gram per day and higher there is potential for toxicity. There is great variability among individuals in regard to susceptibility to the side effects of megadoses of ascorbic acid and the doses necessary to cause toxicity. In the intestinal tract, large doses (2 grams and higher) of ascorbic acid may produce pain, discomfort, and an osmotic diarrhea. Such doses of ascorbic acid give a false-negative guaiac test for blood, thereby obscuring recognition of occult bleeding. Urine tests for glucose also may be misleading when large doses of ascorbic acid are ingested, producing a false-negative Testape and false-positive Clinitest.

As oxalate is a degradative product of ascorbic acid, large amounts of this vitamin will be expected to increase the delivery of oxalate to the renal tubule, posing the potential risk of oxalate stones in susceptible individuals. The increase in oxalate excretion is small in magnitude, however, and in most cases still falls within the normal range. Uricosuria and uric acid stones are also believed to occur with increased frequency because uric acid has less solubility in an acid medium. Nevertheless, the frequency of kidney stone formation in megadose users of ascorbic acid is not known precisely at present.

There is a likelihood of exacerbating systemic acidosis in those disorders with failure of urinary acidification, such as chronic renal disease and renal tubular acidosis. Certain patients with diminished glucose-6-phosphate dehydrogenase activity may be at increased risk for hemolytic episodes with megadose ascorbic acid therapy. Scurvy has been reported in several infants of mothers who consumed large amounts of ascorbic acid during pregnancy, presumably as a result of a dependency state developing in the infant. Therefore, it is probably not advisable to treat pregnant women with large doses of vitamin C. There is some concern that ascorbic acid, which increases intestinal absorption of iron, may also increase absorption of heavy metals such as lead and mercury and accelerate the development of toxicity from these metals.

Sauberlich HE: Ascorbic acid. *In* Olson RE (ed.): Present Knowledge in Nutrition. 5th ed. Washington DC, The Nutrition Foundation, 1984, pp 260–272.

Vitler RW: Nutritional aspects of ascorbic acid: Uses and abuses. West J Med 133:485, 1980. *Useful discussion of clinical features of ascorbic acid deficiency and treatment, including risks of megadoses.*

Wooliscroft JO: Megavitamins: Fact and fancy. Disease-a-Month 29:1, 1983.
Discussion of the hazards of misuse of large doses of vitamin C and other vitamins.

VITAMIN A

Structure and Biochemical Function

The structure of vitamin A and its major derivatives is shown in Figure 217–6. Vitamin A refers to retinol, although the term is often used loosely to indicate all of these compounds. Recently, the term retinoids has been used to designate all the natural and synthetic isomers and derivatives of vitamin A. Retinol is oxidized to vitamin A aldehyde (retinal), which is critical to vision. Retinoic acid (vitamin A acid) is the major oxidative metabolite of retinol. Retinoic acid can fulfill the growth-promoting and epithelial-differentiating roles of retinol but cannot fully maintain its function in reproduction, nor can retinoic acid fulfill the functions of retinal in vision. Carotenoids are larger precursor molecules that undergo cleavage to yield retinal. The most important of the more than 30 carotenoids with pro-vitamin A activity is β-carotene (Fig. 217–6).

Of the various metabolic roles of vitamin A, the best understood is the visual process. Retinal is the prosthetic group of all the visual pigments that capture light. The human retina contains four kinds of visual pigments: rhodopsin in rods and three iodopsins in cones. In the dark-adapted retina, rhodopsin is activated by photons of light. This event initiates the visual cycle, during which retinal changes its conformation from a cis to a trans isomer, and other conformational changes occur in the protein. During dark adaptation, these processes are reversed and rhodopsin is regenerated. In view of the absolute requirement for retinal, it is not surprising that loss of highly sensitive night vision is an early symptom of vitamin A deficiency. Vitamin A probably serves additional roles in the normal functioning of the retina.

The mechanism of action of vitamin A in growth and differentiation is not known. One hypothesis is that vitamin A is similar to steroid hormones in influencing events in the genome following attachment to specific cellular binding proteins. An alternative hypothesis is that vitamin A participates in the synthesis of glycoproteins, which in turn mediate metabolic events. The striking effects of vitamin A upon differentiation, particularly of epithelial tissues, underlie the current concept that this vitamin and its derivatives may possibly have a role in the prevention of certain cancers, particularly of epithelial origin.

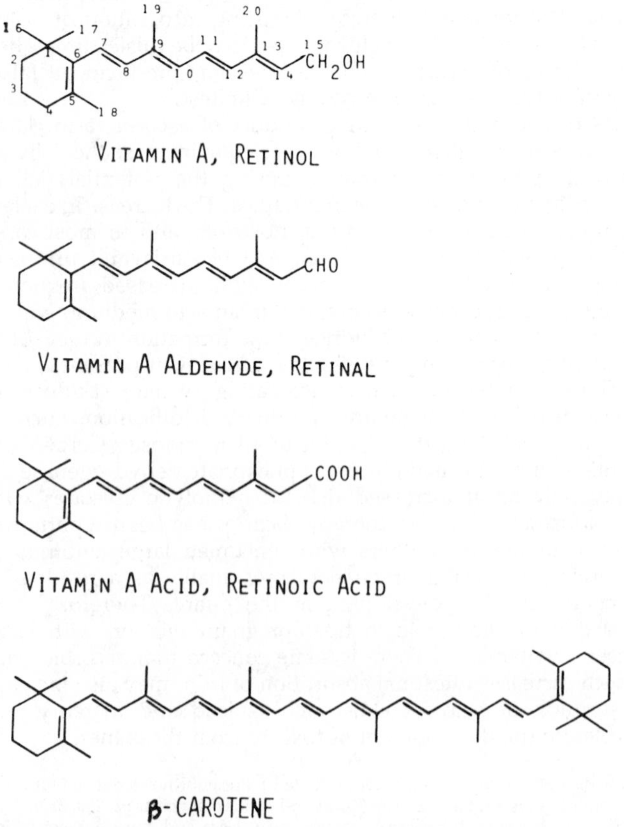

Figure 217–6. Structural formulae of retinol, retinal, retinoic acid, and β-carotene.

Retinol is fat soluble, sensitive to acid and heat, and is rapidly oxidized upon exposure to light and oxygen. β-carotene is relatively less heat-sensitive than retinol.

Normal Physiology

Foods containing retinol or carotenoids are digested by gastric pepsin and intestinal enzymes, and then both forms are absorbed by the intestinal mucosa. About 80 to 90 per cent of dietary vitamin A is absorbed. The rate of absorption of dietary β-carotene is much slower, and only 40 to 60 per cent is absorbed. Within the intestinal mucosa, β-carotene is cleaved to two molecules of retinal, which are then reduced to retinol. The retinol generated from β-carotene, as well as that absorbed directly, is esterified with palmitic acid. The retinyl esters formed are incorporated into chylomicra and transported via lymph to the general circulation, where the triglycerides in the chylomicra are degraded by lipoprotein lipase. The smaller chylomicra remnants remaining are then cleared by the liver, the major storage organ for vitamin A, which contains approximately 90 per cent of the total body reserves. Retinyl esters, mostly in the form of retinyl palmitate, are stored in the liver as a complex; hydrolysis of the retinyl esters in the liver generates retinol, which binds to a specific apo-retinol binding protein (RBP). The holo-RBP is secreted into the plasma, where it forms a 1:1 molar complex with prealbumin, a tetrameric serum protein that also binds thyroxine and triiodothyronine.

Cell surfaces recognize the RBP-retinol complex rather than retinol, and once inside the cell, retinol binds to a specific binding protein, cellular retinol binding protein (CRBP). A cellular retinoic acid binding protein (CRABP) has also been detected in a number of neonatal tissues and epithelial tumors that are sensitive to retinoic acid therapeutically.

In vitamin A deficiency, total plasma RBP levels fall to about half their normal levels and consist primarily of apo-RBP. At the same time, the liver concentration of apo-RBP is greatly increased. With vitamin A repletion, the liver apo-RBP becomes saturated, and levels of holo-RBP begin to rise in blood.

The degradative metabolism of retinol and its derivatives proceeds by a series of chain-shortening steps to yield a group of compounds of little if any intrinsic biological activity. These compounds can be detected in urine but have not been generally utilized diagnostically to characterize vitamin A nutriture.

Requirements and Dietary Sources

The RDA for vitamin A is currently 1000 μg of retinol equivalents (RE) for adult males and 800 μg for adult females. One RE is defined as 1 μg retinol or 6 μg β-carotene. The allowances are calculated in this fashion because the overall utilization of β-carotene is only about one sixth that of retinol, as a result of the relative inefficiency with which β-carotene is absorbed and converted to vitamin A.

Vitamin A allowances were formerly expressed in terms of international units (IU), and this nomenclature still appears on most commercial vitamin bottles. One retinol equivalent is equal to 3.33 IU retinol and 10 IU β-carotene. The RDA for vitamin A expressed in terms of IU is 5000 for adult males and 4000 for adult females. These figures are based upon the estimate that the U.S. diet contains approximately equal amounts of β-carotene (2500 IU = 250 RE, for males) and retinol (2500 IU = 750 RE, for males).

β-carotene is derived predominantly from plant sources, including vegetables such as carrots and sweet potatoes, leafy green vegetables, and some fruits. Palm oil is a particularly rich source of carotenes. Preformed vitamin A is derived almost exclusively from animal sources. Liver obviously is the richest source, followed by kidney, milk and milk products, and eggs. Fish liver oils have unusually high concentrations of vitamin A.

Deficiency

PATHOGENESIS. Vitamin A deficiency is a very common problem world wide, particularly in developing countries, as a consequence of famine or shortages of vitamin A-rich foods. The ocular manifestations of vitamin A deficiency are such a serious problem that they now constitute the leading cause of blindness in young children throughout the world. In such situations, a diet high in rice, wheat, maize, and tubers contain little if any β-carotene. Breast and cow's milk do not provide enough vitamin A to meet the needs of the growing child.

In the United States, vitamin A deficiency is encountered among the urban poor, the elderly, alcoholics, patients with malabsorption, and those individuals on a marginal diet. Individuals chronically using laxatives, particularly mineral oil, and certain other drugs are vulnerable to vitamin A deficiency. In alcoholism, vitamin A deficiency may develop for several reasons. Zinc deficiency, which frequently occurs in alcoholism, impairs the release of RBP from liver and probably interferes with the conversion of retinol to retinal needed in vision. Thus, alcoholism-associated zinc deficiency may intensify night blindness and other sequelae of dietary vitamin A deficiency. Also, in alcoholism the degradative enzyme, alcohol dehydrogenase, which converts retinol to retinal in the retina, may be so saturated with ethanol that retinal production is sharply diminished. Furthermore, as malabsorption develops in chronic alcoholism, dietary carotenes and vitamin A may be lost in increasing amounts in the stool.

Vitamin A deficiency may occur after long term use of mineral oil because this fat-soluble vitamin is dissolved in the oil. Other laxatives may result in vitamin A deficiency because of rapid intestinal transit and diminished intestinal absorption. Vitamin A deficiency may result also after prolonged use of drugs, such as cholestyramine, colestipol, neomycin and colchicine.

CLINICAL FEATURES. Night blindness, as noted previously, may be an early manifestation of vitamin A deficiency. It has been suggested that the frequent episodes of falling and of traffic accidents involving chronic alcoholics at night may be due to some degree to underlying night blindness. In addition, dryness or xerosis of the conjunctivae and later of the cornea may develop, leading to softening and perforation of the cornea and development of Bitot's spots (small, white patches) on the sclerae. Because of the role of vitamin A in maintaining differentiated epithelium, deficiency leads to abnormal development of epithelial tissue and keratinization, particularly in the eye, lung, sweat glands, and gastrointestinal tract. Loss of taste may also occur.

It has been suggested that decreased intake of β-carotene or vitamin A-rich foods or both may be associated with an increased prevalence of epithelial cancers, particularly lung cancers, among smokers. Also, vitamin A-deficient animals have an increased risk of chemical carcinogenesis; administration of retinoids can prevent chemically induced cancers in animals.

DIAGNOSIS. The demonstration of abnormal dark adaptation is important evidence for the diagnosis of vitamin A deficiency. Techniques are being developed that can be carried out under field conditions without expensive equipment. Retinol can be detected directly in serum by immunoassay. Normal levels are in the approximate range of 30 to 65 μg per deciliters. Serum levels may be increased by hypothyroidism, nephrotic syndrome, oral contraceptives, and other disorders of lipid metabolism. By the time serum levels of retinol begin to decrease in dietary deficiency, liver reserves are already seriously depleted.

TREATMENT. The extensive eye problems of vitamin A deficiency encountered in developing countries are best approached through a systematic plan of prevention. Such programs are increasing in scope and magnitude. Injections of vitamin A in large doses (50,000 to 100,000 IU), every four to six months are highly effective and are tolerated remarkably

well. In the United States, when dietary deficiency is advanced, it should be treated with doses similar to these but for several days only, and then maintenance doses should be administered. Water-soluble forms of vitamin A under development should provide great assistance in patient management.

Derivatives of vitamin A (referred to as retinoids), particularly 13-cis-retinoic acid (isotretinoin), have been applied recently to the treatment of cystic acne with considerable success. Investigations are continuing in other dermatologic disorders, including psoriasis, actinic keratosis, leukoplakia, and pityriasis rosea. The mechanism of action of this derivative may lie in its inhibition of keratinization, suppression of sebaceous gland secretion, or possibly to a direct anti-inflammatory effect.

The use of β-carotene or retinoids or both, especially the less toxic forms, for the possible prevention of epithelial cancers is under intense study. Smokers should be expected to benefit particularly by increasing their intake of vitamin A and/or carotenoids. The exact doses necessary to achieve preventive effects are not known, and it is possible that major benefits can be obtained simply by increasing the intake of foods rich in carotenoids or vitamin A without additional supplementation. Further research is needed to clarify these vital issues.

Toxicity

The carotenoids are generally without toxicity. Consumption of β-carotene in large amounts from foods, for example, carrots, may stain the skin a curious yellow-orange color, but this phenomenon is believed to be entirely benign. The sclerae remain white in carotenemia; thus the condition can easily be differentiated from jaundice.

Vitamin A (retinol), on the other hand, is quite toxic when taken continuously in large amounts, particularly at the level of 50,000 IU and higher, for periods of three months or more. The skin may become dry, pruritic, coarse, and scaly with fissures; hair loss may occur. It is of interest that both vitamin A excess and deficiency have adverse effects upon the skin. Sore mouth, anorexia, and vomiting may ensue. The most serious side effects of vitamin A overdosage pertain to the central nervous system: patients may develop serious headaches, drowsiness, irritability, failure to concentrate, increased intracranial pressure, and papilledema. The liver may enlarge, rarely progressing to fibrosis and cirrhosis. Generalized lymph node enlargement may become evident. There may be painful hyperostoses, and there are preliminary indications that long-term use of vitamin A in large amounts possibly may accelerate the bone loss of aging. Congenital malformations have occurred in the infants of several women consuming 50,000 IU per day during pregnancy.

In cases of vitamin A toxicity, serum vitamin A levels are increased, particularly in the form of retinyl esters. In an asymptomatic patient receiving megadoses of vitamin A, the onset of liver disease such as hepatitis may precipitate overt clinical toxicity, presumably by releasing stored retinol into the general circulation. With discontinuation of megadoses of vitamin A, the symptoms will gradually recede.

The development of synthetic retinoids with lower toxicities and greater uptake in target organs is expected to facilitate the application of these agents in the possible chemoprevention of cancer.

Goodman DS: Vitamin A and retinoids in health and disease. N Engl J Med 310:1023, 1984. *This comprehensive review highlights recent advances relating vitamin A and retinoids to clinical medicine and public health, particularly ophthalmology, nutrition, dermatology, and cancer.*

Olson JA: Vitamin A. *In* Olson RE (ed.): Present Knowledge in Nutrition. 5th ed. Washington DC, The Nutrition Foundation, 1984, pp 176–191. *Recent review of physiology, binding proteins, metabolism, and function of vitamin A.*

Olson JA, Bridges CDB, Packer L, Chytil F, Wolf G: The function of vitamin A. Fed Proc 42:2740, 1983. *Succinct review of biochemical functions of vitamin A in the retina, in differentiation, and at nuclear and extranuclear sites.*

Sporn MB, Roberts AB: The role of retinoids in differentiation and carcinogenesis. Cancer Res 43:3134, 1983. *Discussion of the recent application of vitamin A and its related compounds to the chemoprevention of certain forms of cancer.*

VITAMIN D

Vitamin D is discussed in Chapter 244 in association with calcium metabolism and metabolic bone diseases.

VITAMIN E

Vitamin E activity is derived from a series of dietary tocopherols and tocotrienols, the most potent of which is d-α-tocopherol. This vitamin serves as an antioxidant, protecting polyunsaturated fatty acids in membranes and possibly also in tissues from attack by free radicals. Vitamin E deficiency in animals increases the likelihood of membrane and cellular damage from ozone, nitrogen dioxide, and hyperbaric oxygen. Dietary selenium is a precursor of selenide, a cofactor for glutathione peroxidase, which also provides important protection against lipid peroxidation in vivo. Dietary selenium under certain circumstances may spare the requirement for vitamin E.

Intestinal absorption of tocopherols requires normal mechanisms of digestion and absorption of fat, particularly bile formation. Tocopherols are transported to the general circulation in chylomicra. Levels of tocopherols in blood correlate with those of plasma lipoproteins to which they are bound both normally and in various disease states. In contrast to vitamin A, there does not appear to be a specific carrier protein in blood for vitamin E, nor a specific organ in which it is stored. Since dietary deficiency occurs only under very unusual circumstances, cases of E deficiency have usually been identified with prolonged and severe fat malabsorption. Vitamin E deficiency has also been detected in patients receiving parenteral nutrition.

The dietary allowance for vitamin E is expressed in terms of mg α-tocopherol equivalents (α-TE), and is 10 mg per day (15 IU) for adult males and 8 mg per day (12 IU) for adult females, with increases of 2 mg per day for pregnancy and 3 mg per day for lactation. The increased requirement for vitamin E with diets high in polyunsaturated fatty acids, previously shown in experimental animals, is thought not to be clinically relevant, since the items highest in vitamin E content—soybean, corn, cottonseed, wheat germ, and safflower oils and their derivatives—are also high in polyunsaturated fatty acids.

Deficiency of vitamin E has generally not been recognized as a clearly definable syndrome. The red cell half-life may be shortened, although anemia is uncommon in the absence of other precipitating causes. Clinical and neuropathologic evidence of posterior column abnormalities have been described, with disturbances of gait, proprioception, and vibration. In premature infants, vitamin E deficiency is associated with hemolytic anemia, thrombocytosis, and edema. Diagnosis of vitamin E deficiency is usually made by measurement of plasma E levels; normal levels are generally 0.50 to 0.70 mg per deciliter and higher. In several of the hemolytic anemias, such as sickle cell anemia and G-6-PD deficiency, serum vitamin E levels tend to be low.

The therapeutic role of vitamin E remains controversial at the present time. Although vitamin E has been advocated by food faddists as an "anti-aging" vitamin, there is no evidence that it prolongs life in man. This vitamin has been claimed to enhance sexual performance, an attribute that also has not been substantiated. Some patients with intermittent claudication appear to have improved after therapy with vitamin E. Hemolytic anemia in the premature newborn is generally benefited by vitamin E therapy, and the severity but not the incidence of retrolental fibroplasia may be reduced. Large doses may prevent the neurologic complications from developing in abetalipoproteinemia and cholestatic liver disease.

There are a number of other effects of vitamin E demonstrable, in vitro, in experimental animals and in some instances in man, but their clinical relevance remains unresolved. These effects include reducing platelet aggregation, inhibiting conversion of nitrites to nitrosoamines, inhibiting prostaglandin synthesis, improving erythrocyte formation, and protecting against environmental toxicants and pollutants. Further research is needed on these important issues.

Vitamin E is certainly far less toxic than the other fat-soluble vitamins, and a daily intake in the range of 200 to 600 mg per day (20 to 60 times the RDA) is generally considered safe. Nausea, flatulence, and diarrhea have been reported at doses in excess of 600 mg. The intestinal absorption of vitamins A and K is reduced at high doses, which may be clinically significant in patients on marginal diets. Vitamin E appears to increase the vitamin K requirement, and megadoses of vitamin E administered together with the anticoagulant drug warfarin may result in overt bleeding.

Bieri JG, Corash L, Hubbard VS: Medical uses of vitamin E. N Engl J Med 308:1063, 1983. *This article reviews the rationale for treatment with vitamin E in various clinical disorders, limitations of treatment, and toxicities encountered.*

Horwitt MK: Therapeutic uses of vitamin E in medicine. Nutr Rev 38:105, 1980. *Current status of the medical uses of vitamin E.*

Lubin B, Macklin LJ (eds.): Vitamin E: Biochemical, Hematological and Clinical Aspects. New York, New York Academy of Sciences, 1982. *This volume covers the proceedings of a conference dealing with cellular biochemistry, relation to human diseases, deficiencies and therapeutic doses of vitamin E.*

VITAMIN K

Vitamin K occurs naturally in two forms, both of which are naphthoquinone derivatives, differing from one another only in their side chains. Vitamin K_1 is made by plant sources: vitamin K_2 is synthesized by normal intestinal flora. It is also contained in some foods. Vitamin K_3 (menadione) is an artificial provitamin that can be converted to menoquinone (K_2) by the liver.

The intestinal absorption of various forms of vitamin K resembles that of vitamin E in requiring bile and other normal mechanisms of fat absorption. There are differences in the absorption of vitamin K_1 and vitamin K_2: vitamin K_1 is absorbed principally in the proximal segment via a saturable energy-dependent process, whereas vitamin K_2 is absorbed by the small intestine and by the colon via a noncarrier-mediated, nonenergy-dependent process. The efficiency of absorption varies greatly and is markedly diminished by mineral oil, other fat solvents, and laxatives. In patients who have fat malabsorption that is severe and prolonged, as in sprue, regional ileitis, and other disorders, or in patients with obstruction to bile flow, vitamin K deficiency commonly develops. Deficiency also may occur after prolonged antibiotic therapy, destroying the intestinal synthesis of vitamin K.

After absorption, vitamin K is transported in plasma chylomicrons. The main excretory products of vitamin K in urine are derivatives that have undergone chain shortening and oxidation.

Vitamin K deficiency occurs frequently in newborn infants for several reasons. First, fetal stores tend to be low because very little of this vitamin is transported across the placenta. In addition, the fetal gut is sterile, and therefore the newborn lacks the supply of vitamin K that can be provided by normal intestinal flora. As the intestinal tract becomes colonized postnatally, the synthesis of vitamin K becomes appreciable.

The best sources of vitamin K are green, leafy vegetables, particularly turnip greens, broccoli, and brussels sprouts. There are moderate amounts in liver, bacon, cheese, butter, and coffee. No single recommended dietary allowance is made for vitamin K because of the important and variable contribution made by intestinal bacteria. It is recommended only that normal adults consume 70 to 140 μg per day. Dietary deficiency based upon consuming less than this amount is uncommon at the present time in the United States, because the usual diet contains ample amounts of vitamin K.

The mechanism of action of vitamin K consists of a post-translational γ-carboxylation of glutamic acid moieties in inactive precursor proteins, which confers calcium-binding properties to the proteins. The most widely known of these proteins are involved in blood coagulation. Four clotting factors are dependent upon vitamin K for this important action: prothrombin (factor II), proconvertin (factor VII), Christmas factor (factor IX), and Stuart-Prower factor (factor X). Lack of vitamin K may result in death from uncontrolled hemorrhage.

The anticoagulant drugs, warfarin and dicoumarol, inhibit the vitamin K-dependent γ-carboxylation by interfering with activation of vitamin K to its metabolically active hydroquinone form. As a result of this inhibition, the synthesis of the four clotting factors is greatly reduced.

A recent advance in the field of vitamin K research has been the identification of proteins that are involved in the mineralization of bone (osteocalcin) and possibly also in calcium resorption from the renal tubule. The vitamin K antagonists, warfarin and dicoumarol, cause a marked decrease in formation of osteocalcin, presumably by interfering with γ-carboxylation.

Vitamin K deficiency responds rapidly to the administration of vitamin K, provided that liver function is normal. A number of preparations of vitamin K are available, some of which are water soluble, for example, menadiol sodium diphosphate. These forms are more toxic than the lipid-soluble phylloquinone form. In patients with advanced liver disease, the serum prothrombin is decreased and responds poorly if at all to administration of vitamin K. Patients with low serum prothrombin caused by vitamin K deficiency can be distinguished from those with low prothrombin caused by liver disease because in vitamin K deficiency the prothrombin precursor in blood is not γ-carboxylated; normally γ-carboxylated prothrombin is found in patients with liver disease.

Olson RE: Vitamin K. *In* Goodhart RS, Shils ME (eds.): Modern Nutrition in Health and Disease. 6th ed. Philadelphia, Lea & Febiger, 1980, pp 170–180. *Thorough discussion of nutritional aspects of vitamin K, with emphasis upon biochemical mechanisms.*

Suttie JW: Current concepts of the mechanism of action of vitamin K and its antagonists. *In* Lindenbaum J (ed.): Nutrition in Hematology. Contemporary Issues in Clinical Nutrition. Vol. 5. New York, Churchill Livingstone, 1983, pp 245–270. *Discussion of the basic biochemistry of vitamin K and its relation to clotting factors.*

Suttie JW: Vitamin K Metabolism and Vitamin K-Dependent Proteins. Baltimore, University Park Press, 1980. *Comprehensive volume dealing with biochemical, nutritional, and functional aspects of vitamin K.*

218. DISTURBANCES OF TRACE MINERAL METABOLISM

Clifford Tasman-Jones

The bulk of living matter is formed by eleven elements, all of which are from the lowest part of the periodic table (H, C, N, O, Na, Mg, P, S, Cl, K, and Ca). In addition to these, there are essential minerals that are present in trace amounts. These latter include F, Si, V, Cr, Mn, Fe, Co, Ni, Cu, Zn, Se, Mo, Sn, and I.

While deficiencies of trace minerals and vitamins are uncommon in humans eating a normal diet, there is a likelihood of trace mineral deficiencies developing with the use of enteral and parenteral feeding. Deficiencies developing during parenteral nutrition have focused attention on trace mineral function in human metabolism.

Trace minerals essential for life act as essential cofactors of enzymes and as organizers of the molecular structures of the cell (e.g., mitochondria) and its cellular membrane. There is an optimal tissue concentration for trace minerals; excess can be toxic and insufficiency leads to metabolic failure.

Trace minerals are absorbed through the intestine; their bioavailability is dependent on the processing that occurs within the intestinal mucosa. In plasma, trace minerals are bound either to a specific protein or to albumin for transportation. There may be a small amount of unbound trace mineral. The excretory path varies but most are excreted into the gastrointestinal tract, many by way of bile; some are excreted in the urine and some by the sweat glands. Not all trace minerals have been shown to be clinically important. Some, such as iron and iodine, are so important in specific disorders that they are covered separately in this volume.

ZINC

METABOLISM. Although zinc represents only 0.003 per cent (1.4 to 2.3 grams) of the human body, it is an intrinsic part of at least 70 metalloenzymes and other cellular components and is essential for the synthesis of protein, DNA, and RNA.

Zinc is absorbed from the small intestine, although the exact mechanism for this remains uncertain. A low-molecular-weight zinc-binding ligand possibly secreted from the pancreas is a postulated mechanism for absorption.

In the human body, zinc has a nonuniform distribution with the highest concentrations occurring in the prostate, the skin and its appendages, the brain choroid, the liver, the pancreas, bone, and blood. In blood approximately 80 per cent of zinc is in erythrocytes, 16 per cent in plasma, 3 per cent in leukocytes, and the remaining 1 per cent in platelets. Plasma zinc is normally 12 to 20 μmol per liter, but this amount may not truly reflect tissue store. Zinc is excreted mainly in the feces, but small amounts (between 4.0 and 12.0 μmol per 24 hours) are secreted in the urine.

DEFICIENCY SYNDROMES. In man zinc deficiency has been described in a chronic form and in an acute form. In Iran and Egypt hypogonadal dwarfism in males is associated with zinc deficiency and a deficiency of dietary protein. Additionally, these children usually eat clay, which may bind zinc, making it unavailable for absorption.

Acrodermatitis enterohepatica, a rare autosomal recessive inherited disorder of zinc metabolism, represents a chronic form of pure zinc deficiency. This entity is characterized by diarrhea; an unpleasant skin rash of the extremities, face, and perineum; alopecia; mental irritability; muscle wasting; and depression. Although the nature of the disease remains in doubt, it may be caused by an absence of the ligand essential for zinc absorption. This ligand is present in human milk but not in cow's milk.

Acute zinc deficiency has been described in patients receiving parenteral nutrition. This syndrome is characterized by diarrhea; disturbance of the central nervous system with mental irritability and depression; skin lesions of the face, perineum, limbs, and skin folds; alopecia; loss of taste; and defects in the immunologic mechanisms. Treatment with zinc supplementation, usually in the form of zinc sulfate, results in a dramatic response.

Zinc deficiency may occur in inflammatory bowel disease, malabsorption, cirrhosis, and high alcohol intake, probably because of an increased excretion of zinc in the urine. In Crohn's disease, when there is severe catabolism, zincuria may be severe, depleting body stores that are needed during anabolism. Although the alcoholic has increased zinc loss, there appears to be increased absorption to compensate.

Zinc taken in excess may cause gastrointestinal upset with nausea and vomiting.

COPPER

METABOLISM. An average healthy adult has 12.6 to 18 mmol of body copper. Copper is absorbed from the stomach and proximal duodenum by complexing with amino acids. In the presence of excess intraluminal micronutrients such as zinc or cadmium, copper absorption may be reduced. Absorbed copper is bound to albumin, and after circulating through the liver, it is complexed to ceruloplasmin for distribution to body tissues. The plasma concentration of copper is 13 to 22 μmol per liter, 90 per cent of which is bound to ceruloplasmin. Plasma copper may not adequately reflect copper stores but rather reflect plasma ceruloplasmin concentrations.

The best known function of copper is its effect on erythropoiesis. It is essential for hemoglobin formation. There are many copper enzymes known. Copper is necessary for collagen formation, the functioning of the central nervous system, and skin pigmentation.

Usually copper is excreted in the bile as a form of metallocomplex. There is an additional copper loss in the urine (0.16 to 0.95 μmol per day) and saliva (0.006 to 0.008 μmol per day).

The highest concentrations of copper occur in the liver, brain, heart, spleen, kidneys, and blood. The mean daily requirement of copper is estimated to be between 5 and 15 μmol when given intravenously and between 30 and 40 μmol when given orally.

DEFICIENCY SYNDROMES. Hypocupremia occurs in a number of inherited disorders such as Wilson's disease (a disease of copper excess), Menkes' kinky hair syndrome, a syndrome of neurologic disorder with hypocupremia, and familial hypoceruloplasminemia. It may also be found with decreased copper intake, as in parenteral nutrition, or with the poor absorption or increased loss associated with protein-losing enteropathy, the nephrotic syndrome, cystic fibrosis, and other malabsorptive disorders such as coeliac disease and sprue.

Menkes' kinky hair disease is a rare X-linked genetic disorder in which there is defective connective tissue formation, gross mental retardation, imperfect keratinization of the skin, and depigmentation of the hair. Serum copper and ceruloplasmin levels are very low and return to normal when parenteral but not when oral copper is given. This therapy has no demonstrated benefit in the disease, however.

Chronic copper deficiency causes anemia, usually of a microcytic type, but sometimes it is associated with megaloblastic changes in the marrow, leukopenia, and neutropenia.

EXCESS. Hypercupremia occurs in response to inflammation and has been described in rheumatoid arthritis. The rise in copper is most probably caused by the rise in ceruloplasmin—an acute-phase reactant protein. Copper in excess may produce nausea, vomiting, myalgia, and hemolysis. *Wilson's disease*, the most important human disorder of excess copper, is described in detail in Ch. 205.

MANGANESE

METABOLISM. Manganese, a trace element essential for life, is present in an amount of approximately 12 to 20 mg in the average adult. Maximally absorbed in the duodenum by an unknown transport mechanism, magnesium is bound to transmanganin, a specific β_1 globulin transport protein. Manganese is concentrated in tissues rich in mitochondria and is widely distributed in the body with maximum concentrations in the brain, kidneys, pancreas, and liver. The blood and serum levels vary widely. Excretion of manganese is principally by the bile.

Manganese is an activator of many enzymes, but only one manganese metalloenzyme is known—pyruvate carboxylase. It appears to be intimately involved in the synthesis of DNA, RNA, and protein.

DEFICIENCY. The syndrome associated with deficiency of manganese includes the following features: impaired growth, skeletal abnormalities, abnormal reproductive function, ataxia, convulsions, and anomalies of fat metabolism. In the best described patient with manganese deficiency there were weight loss, a transient dermatitis, nausea and vomiting with changes in the color and growth of hair, and hypocholesterolemia.

EXCESS. Manganese poisoning, which usually occurs after industrial exposure, induces a syndrome that closely resembles Parkinson's disease.

CHROMIUM

METABOLISM. Chromium is an essential micronutrient required for the maintenance of normal blood glucose levels. The recommended daily intake is 50 to 200 μg, and the normal serum level is 0.5 to 9.0 μg per liter. Chromium is present in yeast, meat, and grain. Chromium complexes with nicotinamide to form the glucose tolerance factor. This factor acts as a facilitator for insulin to react at receptor sites on insulin-sensitive tissues.

DEFICIENCY. Chromium deficiency is characterized by impaired glucose tolerance, encephalopathy, and neuropathy. Because of impaired insulin activity, patients may develop hyperglycemia with hyperosmolar nonketotic coma. Chromium deficiency may give a confusional state similar to hepatic encephalopathy with ataxia and peripheral neuropathy. A suggested association between chromium deficiency and coronary artery disease awaits confirmation.

EXCESS. If too much chromium is given, symptoms of nausea, vomiting, gastrointestinal ulceration, liver damage, kidney damage, and central nervous system abnormalities with convulsions may occur.

SELENIUM

METABOLISM. Selenium has a significant biological role believed to be due to selenocysteine in the enzyme glutathionine peroxidase. This enzyme is important in protecting the lipids of the cell membrane, proteins, and nucleic acids against oxidant damage. There are significant regional differences in serum selenium concentrations in the United States, but the mean level is about 0.135 μg per milliliter. A low blood selenium concentration reflecting a low soil content has been noted in three areas: Finland, China, and New Zealand.

The daily requirement for selenium is not known. It is probably dependent on the supply of other trace minerals, including zinc, copper, magnesium, and iron and also the supply of other antioxidant substances, such as vitamin E and vitamin C. In the United States the intake is above 150 μg per day.

DEFICIENCY. *Keshan disease* is a syndrome of endemic cardiomyopathy in the People's Republic of China which is alleviated by giving oral sodium selenite. In the areas of China where Keshan disease is prevalent the dietary intake is estimated at approximately 11 μg per day. A New Zealand woman on intravenous feeding developed muscle pains and tenderness and a very low blood selenium level. The symptoms were alleviated by giving selomethionine. In Finland a reduced serum selenium concentration has been shown to correlate with cardiovascular death and acute coronary heart disease. In a prospective study the selenium level in the serum of those patients who subsequently developed malignancy was found to be significantly lower than that of controls.

EXCESS. Excess selenium is a cell toxin, and as such, selenium should be given with considerable care.

MAGNESIUM

METABOLISM. The amount of magnesium in the human body is about 1000 mmol of which about 50 per cent is contained in the skeleton and only 1 per cent is extracellular. Intracellular magnesium is the second most common cation in the human body, but the serum levels justify its inclusion in a section on trace minerals.

The recommended intake is about 15 mmol, and this comes largely from green vegetables, meat, and fish. Magnesium is absorbed in the entire small bowel but mainly from the distal part of the ileum.

Magnesium is an essential part of some 300 different enzymes and is necessary for cell membrane permeability; neuromuscular excitability; protein, nucleic acid, and fat synthesis; muscle contraction, and so on. While there is no laboratory test which unequivocally reveals magnesium deficiency, the serum magnesium level is not without value. Normal values for serum magnesium are 0.8 to 1.0 mmol per liter. Magnesium deficiency is often present without low serum magnesium levels. Urinary magnesium analysis may be of some value and is usually 3 to 5 mmol per day.

Disorders of magnesium metabolism are described in detail in Ch. 208.

VANADIUM

Analysis of vanadium is difficult. The total body vanadium is about 100 μg. Blood levels are very low and are between 0.005 and 8.4 μmol per liter.

Vanadium depresses plasma cholesterol levels, Na^+/K^+ ATPase, myosin, Ca^{++} ATPase, adenylate kinase, and phosphofructokinase, and it stimulates adenyl cyclase. Vanadium deficiency has been postulated to play a role in nutritional edema, and vanadium excess has been postulated to be a factor in manic-depressive illness. Neither of these suggestions has been confirmed.

COBALT

Cobalt in human metabolism is related to vitamin B_{12}, a topic which is covered in Ch. 135 on pernicious anemia.

NICKEL

For a long time nickel was not believed to have any biologic function. Recently, it has been shown to be a component of urease in plant cells and to be present in some bacterial hydrogenases. Its importance in normal human metabolism is not yet established.

Its importance in human medicine relates to the contact dermatitis that frequently has been associated with it.

SILICON

Silicon is found in high concentrations in tendons, aorta, and eye tissues. It is necessary for mammalian bone growth and calcification. In experimental animals, silicon appears to inhibit atheroma development. Chronic inhalation of silicon as silica (SiO_2) produces lung disease, as described in Ch. 559.

Burch RE, Sullivan JE: Symposium on trace metals. Med Clin North Am 60:653, 1976. *A general review of trace mineral metabolism in the human.*

Chan X, Yang G, Chen J, Chen X, Wen Z, Go K: Studies on the relations of selenium and Keshan Disease. Biol Trace Element Res 2:91, 1980. *An interesting study relating selenium deficiency as a major factor in a specific form of cardiomyopathy.*

Jeejeebhoy KN, Chu RC, Marliss et al.: Chromium deficiency, glucose intolerance and neuropathy reversed by chromium supplementation in a patient receiving long term total parenteral nutrition. Am J Clin Nutr 30:531, 1977. *Parenteral nutrition afforded the opportunity to identify the important role of chromium in glucose metabolism.*

Mills PR, Fell GS, Bessent TG, et al.: A study of zinc metabolism in alcoholic cirrhosis. Clin Sci 64:527, 1983. *A careful study indicating the nature of altered zinc metabolism in alcoholic liver disease.*

Salonca JT, Alfthan G, Nuttunen JK, et al: Association between cardiovascular death and myocardial infarction and serum selenium in a match-pair longitudinal study. Lancet 2:175, 1982. *Selenium deficiency appears to be one correlate with myocardial infarction in Finland.*

Tasman-Jones C: Zinc deficiency states. Adv Intern Med 26:97, 1980. *A review of zinc deficiency with particular emphasis on the acute zinc deficiency syndrome.*

Ulmer DD: Trace Elements. N Engl J Med 297:318, 1977. *A general review of the major trace minerals.*

Williams DM: Copper deficiency in humans. Semin Hematol 20:118, 1983. *Major features of normal copper metabolism and copper deficiency are summarized in a very readable form.*

219. ENTERAL NUTRITIONAL THERAPY

David H. Alpers

Enteral nutrition therapy implies modification of the usual diet and is used for two major general indications. The first is supplementation of protein and calories in a wide variety of situations with the intention of providing part or all of the daily requirements. This use is not disease-specific. The second and more traditional indication involves the use of diets for specific diseases or pathophysiologic situations. The diets used involve restricting a particular element of the diet (e.g., fat, lactose), adding a nutrient that may be required in larger amounts than are available from a well-balanced diet (e.g., calcium, potassium), or altering the consistency of the diet (e.g., high-fiber, full-liquid). These two major indications will be discussed in this chapter. Also included is a discussion about formulating a plan for calorie and protein supplementation, which will place this and the following chapter on parenteral nutrition in proper perspective.

PROTEIN AND CALORIE SUPPLEMENTATION

Initial Decisions: Completeness of Nutrient Provision and Route of Administration

The range of methods for providing protein and calorie supplements has expanded greatly beyond table foods in recent years, and likewise the range of available products for this use is very great. For many patients all that may be needed is a careful history of dietary intake, estimation of protein and caloric requirements, and adjustment of the diet to provide the needed nutrients. Whether table foods or commercial supplements are used, there are two major considerations for the physician in order to provide the most appropriate therapy for each patient: (1) Is the supplement intended as a partial fulfillment of daily needs (incomplete provision) or a total replacement of calories and protein (complete provision)? (2) Are the nutrients to be delivered by the enteral or the parenteral route? Table 219–1 summarizes these major choices. Forced enteral feeding refers to the delivery of nutrients to the small intestine via a small (7 to 8 French) polyurethane or silicone catheter (e.g., Dobbhoff, Duo-tube, Keofeed or by a surgically placed feeding tube). Parenteral supplementation by peripheral or central vein will be discussed in Ch. 220. The options listed in Table 219–1 are not mutally exclusive. For example, sometimes forced enteral feeding can be used together with peripheral vein feeding; nutritionally complete commercial supplements can be used orally in some patients to supply total macronutrient requirements; central vein feeding can be supplemented by oral intake. The choices made in formulating a support plan will depend upon a number of considerations as discussed in the following paragraph.

Formulating a Protein-Calorie Support Plan

Figure 219–1 illustrates a flow diagram useful for selecting patients in negative protein and calorie balance for intensive nutritional support. The correct choice for nutritional support (enteral vs. parenteral, oral vs. forced enteral) depends largely upon the four key questions outlined in the figure. The physician should estimate protein and caloric requirements for the individual patient. Methods for making these estimates are available in a number of handbooks. While the estimates are fairly crude, they are clinically useful, since they provide some quantitative guidelines for deciding the magnitude of supplementation needed. If the diet is meeting requirements (question 1), no further therapy is needed. If the diet is inadequate, an assessment of the patient's present nutritional status is then obtained. Caloric reserves are monitored most easily by body weight and protein reserves by serum albumin levels. Other available methods are discussed in Chapter 213. If the degree of depletion (question 2) as assessed by body weight is mild (about 5 per cent decreased) and the gastrointestinal tract is intact, oral supplements may be used. If the degree of depletion is moderate (5 to 10 per cent decreased) to severe (over 10 per cent decreased) and the anticipated duration of support is long (question 3), intensive therapy may be needed. Whether forced enteral feeding or total parenteral nutrition (TPN) via a central vein is chosen depends on the availability or adequacy of the gastrointestinal tract (question 4). The gastrointestinal tract is usually evaluated by history (the presence or absence of diarrhea or malabsorption), physical exam (normal motility or ileus), and barium radiographs. Some patients are selected for TPN because of the need for complete bowel rest. Data to support the use of this therapy have been obtained in Crohn's disease, ulcerative colitis, the postoperative adaptive period of

TABLE 219–1. STRATEGY FOR CALORIC AND PROTEIN SUPPLEMENTATION

Route of Delivery	Incomplete Provision	Complete Provision
Enteral	Oral supplementation Table foods e.g., milk, peanut butter, egg Commercial supplements Individual macronutrients (e.g., protein, fat, carbohydrate) Nutritionally complete supplement	Forced enteral feeding Nutritionally complete commercial diets Blenderized formulas
Parenteral	Peripheral (e.g., 3 per cent amino acids, 5 to 10 per cent dextrose, 10 per cent lipid emulsion)	Central (e.g., 4.25 per cent amino acid, 25 per cent dextrose, vitamins, minerals, fatty acids)

the short bowel syndrome, and severe pancreatitis (see Ch. 200). Some patients with these disorders can be treated with forced enteral feeding. Often, however, bowel rest will control symptoms more rapidly. Other considerations (social, economic) may play a role in the final choice of therapy for a given patient. The patient may be unwilling to maintain a nasal feeding tube, or hospitalization may not be possible because of cost restrictions. Finally, an occasional patient may need to be fed via gastrostomy or jejunostomy.

The following categories of patients are commonly considered for enteral nutrition therapy: (1) chronically ill patients with anorexia, (2) patients with chronic inflammatory illnesses who have increased requirements but a usual caloric intake for their size, (3) poorly or marginally nourished patients preparing for tests or intestinal surgery, and (4) patients with specific dietary needs that benefit from the special characteristics of some commercial supplements (e.g., low residue, lactose-free). Forced enteral feeding typically is used for those patients who have moderate to severe anorexia, those who cannot maintain a calorie and protein intake commensurate with their needs (e.g., burn patients), or those whose illnesses prevent them from satisfactory oral feeding (e.g., patients with neck fractures or swallowing disorders).

Choice of Supplements

Table Foods

If requirements are not great and appetite is good, table foods can be recommended as protein and calorie supplements. Each ounce of meat, fish, poultry, or cheese contains about 7 grams of protein, an egg 6 to 7 grams and one cup of milk 8 grams. One-half cup of dried beans, peas, or nuts contains 5 grams or more of protein, but these sources contain protein of a lower biologic value (sustains growth less well) and are not usually recommended for "catch up" therapy. Milk products are very useful, provided that lactose intolerance is not a problem. Meat and fish are helpful if fat is well tolerated. Otherwise, poultry without skin or tuna canned in water should be selected. Peanut butter contains 8 grams of fat and 4.2 grams of protein per tablespoon and is a good source of concentrated calories and protein. Table foods remain an excellent choice for oral supplementation, since they are tasty, esthetically and socially appealing, reasonable in cost, easily obtained, and

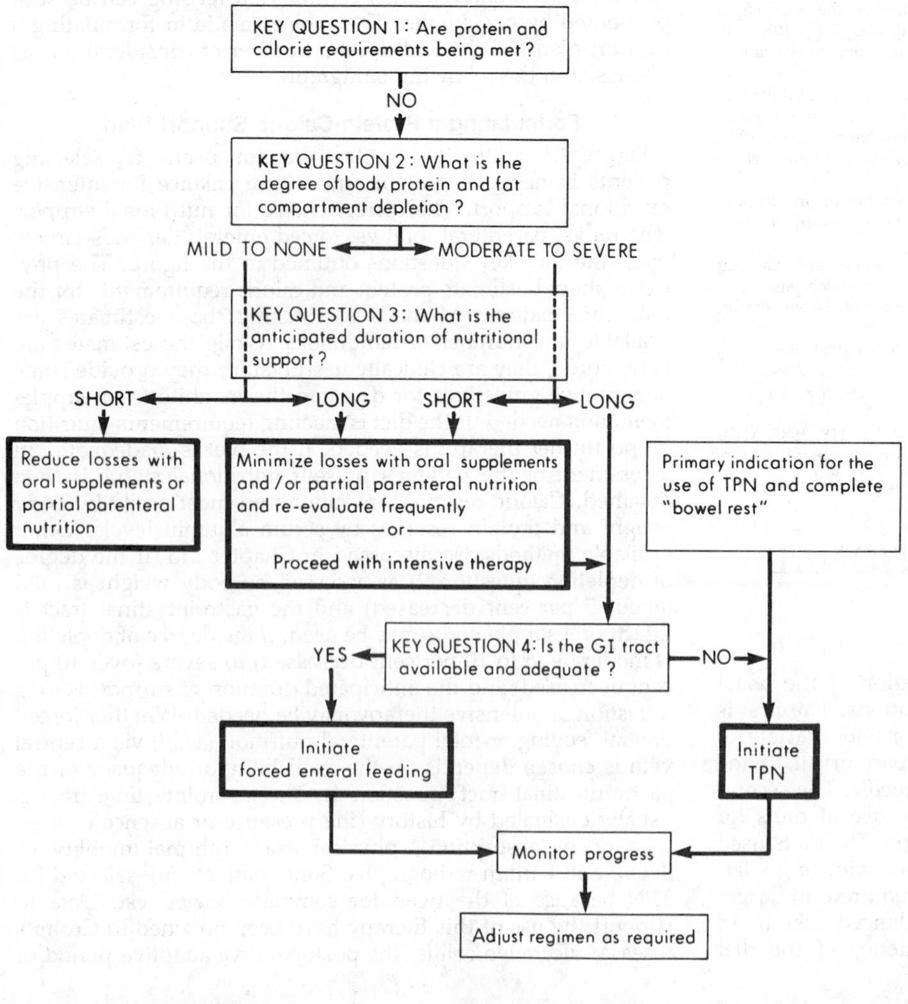

Figure 219–1. Flow diagram useful for selecting patients in negative protein and calorie balance for intensive nutritional support. TPN = total parenteral nutrition; GI = gastrointestinal.

available in a wide variety of choices. They should not be supplemented by commercial supplements unless the supplements exhibit specific properties that make them preferable.

Commercial Supplements

Commerical supplements, like table foods, display a diversity of characteristics that help the physician determine the choice for each patient (Table 219–2). These products are of high caloric density and precisely defined nutrient composition but have the disadvantages of limited esthetic and taste appeal, taste fatigue with constant use, frequent occurrence of diarrhea, and higher cost than table foods. The nutritionally incomplete supplements can be used when the deficiency is specific (protein or calorie) or the deficiency is only anticipated for a short time, as in preparation for surgery. Protein is not wisely provided without another source of calories, since about 25 to 40 nonprotein kcal per gram of protein are needed to maintain positive nitrogen balance. Otherwise, a portion of the amino acids in the protein is converted to carbohydrate to provide the energy needed for assimilation.

The nutritionally complete supplements are largely distinguished by four major characteristics: (1) the presence or absence of lactose, (2) the use of intact protein or hydrolyzed protein (or amino acids), (3) the presence of small or large amounts of fat as caloric sources, and (4) isotonic or hypertonic osmolality. Supplements that are isotonic or nearly so contain less available carbohydrate and more lipid, which is osmotically less active. This characteristic is of greatest importance when forced enteral feeding is used, but any of the hypertonic solutions may be diluted or infused at a slower rate. The other three characteristics are more important for patients with abnormal intestinal absorption. Hydrolyzed protein may be useful for patients with pancreatic insufficiency, lactose-free supplements for patients with lactose intolerance, and low-fat supplements for those with limited intestinal fat absorption. The nutritionally complete supplements just described are designed to be the sole source of daily nutrients and thus contain all needed micronutrients in adequate quantities, if deficiencies are not present and if requirements are usual. Nonprescription milk-based products also provide good sources of protein and calories in a wide variety of flavors (e.g., Metrical, Sego, and Carnation Instant Breakfast). If the patient is lactose tolerant, they may be used very successfully.

COMPLICATIONS OF ENTERAL FEEDING USING COMMERCIAL SUPPLEMENTS. The use of enteral feeding with highly concentrated supplements can be limited by side effects. The most common is diarrhea, which can be due to intolerance to one of the macronutrients (fat, lactose) or intolerance to the osmotic load. Altering the rate of delivery or the concentration of the supplement is often helpful. Complications of forced enteral feeding alone include esophagitis and tracheobronchial aspiration. Volume or sodium overload can occur, especially in the edema-prone patient.

TABLE 219–2. GENERAL CLASSIFICATION OF COMMERCIALLY AVAILABLE SUPPLEMENTS

Classification	Examples
Macronutrient specific	
Protein	Gevral, Casec
Carbohydrate	Polycose, Hy-Cal
Lipid	Lipomul-Oral, Microlipid
Protein + carbohydrate	Citrotein
Nutritionally complete	
Intact protein	
Not fat restricted	Meritene, Ensure, Precision Isotonic
Low fat (≤ 15 grams fat/1000 kcal)	Precision LR, Sustagen
Hydrolyzed protein or amino acids	Vivonex Standard, Vital
Lactose free	Most products
Isotonic	Isocal, Precision Isotonic

THERAPEUTIC DIETS FOR SPECIFIC DISORDERS OR PATHOPHYSIOLOGIC STATES

Restrictive Diets

The diets most commonly used to control symptoms are those that restrict one or another element in the diet. Diets restricted for each of the major macronutrients (fat, carbohydrate, and protein) have their individual uses (Table 219–3). As expected, these diets are helpful in altering pathophysiologic states and are not specific for any disease. Any condition causing steatorrhea can be improved symptomatically by limiting fat intake. Care must be taken with any restrictive diet to supplement any nutrients that have been secondarily limited. Thus, a fat-restricted diet must be made isocaloric by increasing carbohydrate intake. In order for this diet to be successful the patient must not have any generalized carbohydrate intolerance. Similarly, the low lactose or low available carbohydrate diet is low in calcium. Most restrictive diets do not eliminate the nutrient whose content is altered. A low-lactose diet is much easier to achieve than a truly lactose-free one and is usually sufficient to relieve symptoms. Control of symptoms is the usual goal of dietary management, and restriction of the appropriate nutrient to the point at which symptoms are altered is an acceptable goal. Thus, a low-protein diet for hepatic encephalopathy should still deliver the estimated daily protein requirement (0.5 to 0.8 gram per kilogram of body weight) to avoid protein deficiency. This concept is especially important in the management of chronic renal failure, a situation in which the protein requirement may be actually increased. When the glomerular filtration rate (GFR) falls below 25 ml per minute, the protein allowance should be not more than 1.3 grams per kilogram per day (referring to ideal body weight), and falls to 0.6 gram per kilogram per day for a GFR of 4 to 10 ml per minute. Over 50 per cent of the protein intake should be of high biologic value (with high essential amino acid content). Requirements actually increase with dialysis because of the loss of amino acids in the dialysate. The allowance rises with hemodialysis to 1 gram per kilogram per day, and to 1.2 to 1.5 grams per kilogram per day with chronic peritoneal dialysis.

Some of the diets used for therapy actually control or modify the content of macronutrients rather than restrict them. The diet for diabetes mellitus is a good example of this principle (Ch. 230). Successful management of the obese diabetic combines a weight reduction diet with regulation of the carbohydrate content. The prudent diet recommended by the American Diabetes Association still contains 40 to 50 per cent of calories as carbohydrates, but there is much less simple sugar (requiring no pancreatic digestion) and more starch than in normal diets. There is also less cholesterol and saturated fats to reduce blood lipids. These latest recommendations contain relaxed restrictions on carbohydrate intake. High starch diets are well tolerated by diabetics as long as total caloric intake is controlled. Many patients require diets that may utilize elements from diets designed specifically for weight reduction, diabetes mellitus, hyperlipidemias, and chronic renal failure.

TABLE 219–3. THERAPEUTIC DIETS CHARACTERIZED BY RESTRICTION OF DIETARY COMPONENTS

Diet	Typical Indication
Low fat (60–75 grams/day)	Steatorrhea, mild
Low fat (40–60 grams/day)	Steatorrhea, severe
Low oxalate	Enteric hyperoxaluria
Low lactose	Lactose intolerance
Low available carbohydrate	Reactive hypoglycemia
Gluten free	Celiac sprue (see Ch. 103)
Low fiber	Acute diarrhea, bowel prep
Low protein	Hepatic encephalopathy (see Ch. 127) Chronic renal failure (see Ch. 78)
Elimination	Food allergies
Controlled carbohydrate	Diabetes mellitus (see Ch. 230)
Calorie restricted	Obesity
Low sodium	Edematous states
Low fat, cholesterol, or carbohydrate according to type	Hyperlipidemia (see Ch. 183)
Low copper	Wilson's disease
Low phosphate	Chronic renal failure (see Ch. 78)

TABLE 219–4. THERAPEUTIC DIETS CHARACTERIZED BY SUPPLEMENTATION OF DIETARY COMPONENTS

Diet	Typical Indication
High fiber	Irritable bowel, prevention of recurrent diverticulitis
High calcium (milk products, $CaCO_3$, or combination)	Postmenopausal osteoporosis
High protein (high biologic value)	Chronic hemo- or peritoneal dialysis
High protein	Malabsorption
Supplemental potassium	Diuretic use

Diets That Supplement Dietary Components

Although less commonly required, diets that add a component to the normal diet are often employed. A high fiber intake has not been clearly shown to have a beneficial effect on the symptoms of the irritable bowel syndrome and on the recurrence of attacks of acute diverticulitis, although supplementation with fiber is now commonly used for these disorders. The reasons for the uncertainty are that (1) these disorders are identified mostly by clinical criteria, (2) the irritable bowel syndrome is probably a heterogeneous group of motility disorders, (3) the definition of fiber and estimation of its intake are imperfectly developed, and (4) many types of fiber supplements are used, containing different components of dietary fiber. There are limited data on the food content of the major components of dietary fiber, i.e., cellulose, hemicelluloses, pectin, mucilage and gums, and lignins. Thus, it is not always clear when an individual patient is ingesting a low-fiber diet. Most often fiber is supplemented by ingestion of commercial preparations containing psyllium seed or by the use of bran. Psyllium is rich in hemicelluloses, while bran contains more cellulose. Present practice recommends the addition of 6 to 10 grams of fiber per day (2 teaspoons of psyllium seed or one-half cup of bran) for the irritable bowel syndrome (characterized by alternating diarrhea and constipation) and for recurrent diverticulitis. Benefits of high-fiber intake (type and amount variable) have been reported for diabetes mellitus, maintenance of lower calorie intake, and lowering of serum cholesterol. At present the data do not clearly support a role for a fiber-supplemented diet in any of these disorders.

A diet low in fiber (Table 219–3) is useful in acute diarrheal illness and as a preparation for barium enema, colonoscopy, and intestinal surgery. The diet is then additionally modified in the form of a clear liquid diet (Table 219–4) for further reduction in ileal residue.

The best treatment for postmenopausal osteoporosis is still debatable, but it is generally agreed that increased calcium intake is a necessary component of the treatment plan (Ch. 249). Milk products serve this role best, as they provide protein as well as calcium. In the patient who is lactose-intolerant or who does not like milk, calcium carbonate (40 per cent calcium by weight) may be used. If achlorhydria is present, a more water-soluble form of organic calcium (e.g., glubionate or gluconate) should be used, since the carbonate salt requires an acid pH to be solubilized.

Protein supplements are needed for conditions characterized by excessive protein loss, such as protein-losing enteropathy, dialysis, and burns. These supplements can be supplied as table food or as commercial supplements. For each 10 grams of protein added, another 250 kcal from nonprotein sources must also be ingested to ensure that the amino acids will be converted into body protein.

When diuretics and low-sodium diets are used, potassium is frequently replaced as an inorganic salt, but dietary supplementation can often be used and would be more palatable. For instance, the salt substitutes often used with low-sodium diets contain about 12 mEq of potassium per gram and potassium is present in fairly high concentration in most fruits and vegetables and their juices (Table 219–5). Eight ounces of frozen orange or tomato juice contains 12 mEq of potassium, one medium orange or banana 6 to 8 mEq, and one 6 × 2 inch watermelon slice 16 mEq. Milk is also a good source of potassium, but because of its high sodium content would be an inappropriate supplement for a patient taking diuretics.

Diets That Alter the Consistency of Food

One of the most common dietary manipulations used in hospitalized patients is the *liquid diet*. The clear liquid diet provides the daily requirement for water and requires minimal digestion and intestinal motility, but it does not provide adequate amounts of protein or calories. It is also a low-fiber diet. If the patient who requires such a diet is already protein and calorie malnourished, the diet needs to be supplemented with carbohydrate, protein, or both (see Table 219–2). Even so, it is difficult to provide much more than 1000 kcal per day. For chronic use the full liquid diet is more often prescribed. If table foods from all food groups are used or the diet is enriched with commercial supplements, the diet can be nutritionally complete. Care should be given to determining the actual food ingested, however, since a full liquid diet is often used for a patient who has some difficulty in swallowing table food. Thus, the ingested food may not equal what is ordered. This precaution of course should be exercised when any diet is used for therapy, but it is particularly important when impaired food ingestion or anorexia is the cause of the prescribed diet.

The *bland diet* is often combined with a mechanical soft diet for the treatment of peptic ulcer disease. Despite this widespread use, there are no data that clearly support the value of such a diet for any clinical condition, and present practice does not favor its use (Ch. 99). Restriction of seasonings makes the food less palatable and discourages the successful use of whichever diet is being presented.

Alpers DH, Clouse RE, Stenson WF: Manual of Nutritional Therapeutics. Boston, Little, Brown and Co, 1983. *A detailed practical account of the use of diets and enteral therapy. Includes nutritional characteristics of most commercial supplements and diets.*

American Dietetic Association: Handbook of Clinical Dietetics. New Haven, Yale University Press, 1982. *A comprehensive and carefully outlined source for obtaining the details of most diets.*

Connor WE, Connor SL: The dietary treatment of hyperlipidemias. Med Clin North Am 66:485–518, 1982. *A current summary of the use of diets in five types of hyperlipidemia.*

Friedman GR: Diet in treatment of diabetes mellitus. *In* Goodhart RS, Shils MR, (eds.): Modern Nutrition in Health and Disease. Philadelphia, Lea and Febiger, 1980, pp 977–997. *A good summary of the current dietary recommendations.*

Garrow JS: Treat Obesity Seriously. London, Churchill Livingstone, 1981. *A sensible and multifaceted approach to the therapy of obesity, especially the use of diet.*

Paige DM (ed.): Lactose Digestion. Baltimore, Johns Hopkins Unitersity Press, 1981. *An up-to-date symposium covering all aspects of lactose intolerance.*

Spiller GA, Kay RP (eds.): Medical Aspects of Dietary Fiber. New York, Plenum Press, 1980. *Summarizes the evidence for the role of dietary fiber in human disease.*

TABLE 219–5. SODIUM AND POTASSIUM CONTENT OF COMMON FOODS

Food	Portion	Sodium Content (mg)	Potassium Content (mg)
Milk	cup	120	350
Meat, fish, poultry	ounce	25	100–180
Most fruits and their juices	cup	4–10	300–490
Most vegetables	½ cup	5–9	300–500

220. PARENTERAL NUTRITION

Ray E. Clouse

Parenteral nutrition includes delivery of micro- and macronutrients. Those nutrients that can rapidly become depleted in disease, such as water and major minerals (e.g., sodium, potassium), are administered routinely by vein in the hospitalized patient. In the last decade the technical feasibility of providing nutrients that become depleted more slowly, such as amino acids, calorie sources, and the essential fatty acid linoleic acid, has resulted in the ability to deliver total parenteral nutritional support not only in the hospital but also at home. The most obvious long-term usefulness of these advances has been for patients who have irreversibly inadequate small bowel absorptive capabilities either from advanced disease (such as scleroderma) or because of intestinal resection (as from mesenteric infarction). The application of short-term total parenteral nutrition (TPN), however, far exceeds the use in this small number of patients. In fact, concern has been expressed regarding the possible excessive use of this technique in patients for whom some form of enteral therapy would suffice or for whom the expected nutritional losses from acute illness would be adequately tolerated without intensive support.

Parenteral delivery of protein and calories can serve either to partially meet the daily requirement (for instance in combination with an otherwise inadequate enteral plan) or to totally meet or exceed the requirements. Thus, parenteral nutrition can be utilized in much the same way as enteral supplements or forced enteral feeding when designing an appropriate nutritional support plan (Ch. 219). The technique of delivery and the morbidity (physical, psychological, financial) of such methods are more important considerations in the choice of parenteral or enteral nutrition routes than are differences in basic concepts of energy or specific nutrient requirements.

PARENTERAL ENERGY AND PROTEIN DELIVERY

Basic Considerations

Protein and calorie requirements are closely linked. Positive nitrogen balance, reflecting net positive endogenous protein synthesis, cannot be accomplished without positive energy balance. Thus, amino acids alone, even if provided in excessive quantities, will not be adequate to promote sustained net protein synthesis. Additional caloric sources in the form of carbohydrate or fat must be provided to prevent the use of amino acids (delivered or from catabolism) as energy substrates. If nonprotein calories are provided for the average hospitalized patient in a ratio of calories to amino acid nitrogen (in grams) of $\geq$ 150:1, delivered amino acids are likely to be utilized for protein synthesis. The ratio decreases in more intense catabolic states (e.g., major burns), in which protein requirements are higher, and increases in less stressed situations. This fact is not unique to parenteral nutrition; similar energy-to-nitrogen ratios apply to enteral nutrition techniques.

Protein balance can be approximated by measuring nitrogen losses in urine and other fluids and by estimating the relatively small fecal and skin losses. Achieving positive protein (nitrogen) balance is a goal in long-term parenteral nutrition therapy for several reasons: (1) A positive nitrogen balance indirectly implies adequate energy delivery. (2) The body's proteins are all functional; there are no excess stores. Continued losses from both the visceral (metabolic proteins of the organs and circulating proteins) and somatic (largely skeletal muscle) protein compartments will eventually be detrimental to recovery from disease. (3) Many patients already have moderate to severe depletion of these protein compartments. Thus the need to begin restoration, as well as prevent further depletion, is often already present (see Ch. 219 for patient selection).

Some short-term beneficial effect is gained by providing nitrogen as amino acids without additional calories. The degree of negative nitrogen balance may be reduced, but positive balance is not achieved with this approach. Since endogenous protein catabolism is reduced, the effect is termed "protein sparing." Energy requirements are met under these circumstances from endogenous fat stores and from any additional caloric sources provided. This approach as well as the parenteral delivery of small amounts of carbohydrates in combination with amino acids can be useful in short-term management in that the degree of negative nitrogen balance will be diminished.

Practical Applications

A combination of dextrose, amino acids, and water provides the base solution for parenteral protein and calorie delivery (Table 220–1). Major and minor minerals as well as vitamins can be added to this solution. The monohydrate form of dextrose used in most commercial intravenous solutions provides 3.4 kcal per gram in contrast to 4 kcal per gram for the carbohydrate alone. When a peripheral vein is used as the access route, osmolarity limitations prevent the use of concentrated solutions that provide all the daily energy and protein requirements as dextrose and amino acids. For example, a formulation made from 800 ml of a 3 per cent amino acid solution and 200 ml of 50 per cent dextrose will provide only 340 nonprotein kcal with 24 grams of amino acids, but the osmolarity will exceed 800 mOsm per liter. Solutions with osmolarities in excess of 600 mOsm per liter often produce thrombophlebitis when continuously infused into the peripheral veins. Co-infusion of a lipid emulsion will reduce the osmolarity, since lipid emulsions are isotonic (280 to 340 mOsm per liter). Typical solutions for total parenteral nutrition have final osmolarities in excess of 2000 mOsm per liter and therefore must be infused into central veins (e.g., superior vena cava).

Lipid emulsions contain a source of calories in the form of emulsified droplets of soybean or safflower oil, which provide 9 kcal per gram, supplemented slightly by the caloric contribution of the emulsifiers (Table 220–1). Until recently, lipid emulsions were used mainly to supply the essential fatty acid linoleic acid in biweekly infusions or were co-administered with base solutions in peripheral veins to boost daily caloric delivery while reducing infusate osmolarity. Fat calories in the daily nutrition plan were not considered necessary, especially during total parenteral nutrition given by central vein where concentrated dextrose readily meets usual daily energy requirements. More recently, lipid emulsions have been utilized daily to provide 20 to 40 per cent of the total nonprotein calorie requirement, despite the knowledge that positive nitrogen and energy balance had routinely been accomplished with dextrose as the only nonprotein calorie source.

Parenteral nutrition with concentrated glucose as the calorie source results in greater CO_2 production than similar energy provided by a glucose-lipid combination. Theoretically, this could be clinically detrimental to patients with CO_2 retention or those being weaned from ventilators. Patients given calories as the lipid-dextrose combination are also less likely to develop symptomatic fatty liver than those given the same amount of calories from the carbohydrate alone. However, this can be avoided by keeping the energy provision close to the daily

TABLE 220–1. PROTEIN AND CALORIE SOURCES UTILIZED IN PARENTERAL NUTRITION

Macronutrient Category		Parenteral Form of Macronutrient	Nonprotein Caloric Value
Protein		Crystalline amino acids	
Calories	Carbohydrate	Dextrose monohydrate	3.4 kcal/g
	Fat	Lipid emulsion	10% emulsion—1.1 kcal/ml
			20% emulsion—2.0 kcal/ml

requirement. The use of lipids daily also provides a parenteral "diet" with a macronutrient composition that approximates that of the average oral diet. Resistance to the routine use of lipids is based on (1) the expense of lipid emulsions compared to dextrose; (2) the cumbersome need to piggy-back the emulsions into the parenteral nutrition line, thereby enhancing the likelihood of contamination; and (3) the risk of morbidity, albeit small, of lipid infusion. All in all, the actual superiority in the average patient of either a combination of fat and carbohydrate or carbohydrate alone as the parenteral energy source remains unresolved.

TOTAL PARENTERAL NUTRITION

Besides amino acids and calorie sources, all other recognized nutrients can be provided by a parenteral route. Total parenteral nutrition (TPN) is required for short or long periods of time by patients who either temporarily or permanently have an unusable or an inadequate small intestine. The techniques of TPN beyond the scope of this textbook are described in many monographs and handbooks. The most successful TPN programs involve the direction of a knowledgeable physician and the cooperation of informed and interested colleagues in the pharmacy, nursing, and dietetics departments.

Indications

A small number of patients require lifelong TPN because of extensive resection (e.g., from mesenteric vascular accidents, Crohn's disease, trauma) or advanced small bowel disease (e.g., scleroderma, radiation enteritis). The majority of patients with short bowel syndrome from resection, however, can eventually be managed with oral feeding after an initial adaptation period. TPN is indicated as a temporary nutritional therapy mainly for two patient groups: (1) those selected for intensive nutritional support in whom the intestinal tract is not usable for forced enteral feeding (see Ch. 219) and (2) those in whom a nothing-by-mouth regimen ("bowel rest") would be beneficial to the primary gastrointestinal disease. The majority of patients placed on TPN are those with the first indication. Figure 219–1 gives a flow diagram incorporating the various questions used in deciding which patients are indeed candidates for intensive nutritional support. In general, this group has moderate to severe protein compartment depletion at the initial evaluation and is expected to suffer significant additional losses with the current illness.

In the nothing-by-mouth regimen TPN is used for both *parenteral nutrition* and *bowel rest* in an attempt to actually assist in disease regression. Prior to the availability of TPN, regression had been observed in some patients who were not allowed to eat or who minimized input for brief periods, especially those with Crohn's disease, ulcerative colitis, enterocutaneous fistulas, and pancreatitis (Table 220–2). With TPN, regression of disease is variable but is most frequent in patients with uncomplicated Crohn's disease of the small bowel who have failed usual regimens (Table 220–2). In a prospective randomized trial, patients with acute ulcerative colitis who were managed with TPN and bowel rest in addition to usual medical measures did no better than those given oral feedings and standard intravenous fluids as the nutritional adjuvants, as judged by the number requiring colectomy or the induction of remission. However, nutritional benefits that are gained by the severely malnourished patient or nutritional deterioration that is prevented by initiating TPN in the healthier patient preoperatively will not be reflected in a small number of patients if colectomy is the only end point. In all of these diseases, the best gauge of the success of TPN is its effect on nutritional parameters (Ch. 213). TPN allows total bowel rest to be carried on for longer periods of time without the fear of nutritional deterioration, possibly improving the chances that bowel rest will be successful in aiding disease regression. An adequate TPN plan will also uniformly replete the malnourished patient in the process; any additional beneficial effects of nutritional repletion on the primary disease are difficult to assess.

TABLE 220–2. SUMMARY OF THE EFFECTS OF TOTAL PARENTERAL NUTRITION (TPN) WITH BOWEL REST IN VARIOUS DISEASES

Disease	Nutritional Maintenance or Repletion Achieved	Short-term (In-hospital) Disease Regression	Long-term Disease Regression
Ulcerative colitis*	Majority	30–50%	20–30%
Crohn's disease*	Yes	60–80%	50–60%
Subgroup with fistulas†	Yes	30–40%	10–30%
Subgroup with colitis†	Yes	60%	NA‡
Enterocutaneous fistulas (not Crohn's disease)	Yes	30–70% closure§	NA
Severe pancreatitis	Yes¶	NA	NA

*Many patients in reported series are treated with corticosteroids as well as TPN and bowel rest.
†Small patient series; subgroups not always designated.
‡Adequate data not available.
§Many patients eventually managed with surgical therapy; wide range of reported success rates.
¶Parenteral nutrition is successful and does not contribute to morbidity of pancreatitis despite theoretical concern regarding pancreatic stimulatory effects.

In patients with cancer nutritional status can be maintained or improved with an adequate TPN program, but this has not proved to be of overall benefit in enhancing tumor responsiveness to antineoplastic agents. The best candidates for intensive nutritional support are those who have tumors potentially responsive to anticancer therapy but who could not receive optimal management because of the combined detrimental effects of the planned therapy and malnutrition. Some of these patients can be managed with forced enteral nutrition rather than TPN.

Nutrients Provided During TPN (Table 220–3)

Protein requirements (as described in Ch. 212) are met with crystalline amino acids in commercially available solutions. Nonprotein calories are provided by concentrated dextrose and by lipid emulsions. Two liters of a base solution composed of equal amounts of 8.5 per cent amino acids and 50 per cent dextrose in conjunction with 500 ml of a 10 per cent lipid emulsion is a feasible daily protein-calorie prescription. This would provide approximately 80 grams of protein as amino acids, 1680 carbohydrate calories, and 550 fat calories. The resultant nonprotein calorie-to-nitrogen ratio is 170:1, with 25 per cent of the daily calories provided by fat. An alternate regimen would provide all the nonprotein calories as dextrose. The daily protein and calorie prescription should be tailored to a patient's requirements or exceed them by 20 to 40 grams of protein and 500 to 1000 kcal if restoration of depleted compartments is a goal.

Major mineral requirements vary considerably from patient to patient and during any one patient's course of TPN. In particular, potassium requirements may be initially large because of extra- to intracellular fluxes with glucose (and possibly insulin) infusion and because of reversal of the catabolic state. The ranges of major mineral requirements listed in Table 220–3 are typical for the average adult patient, but careful monitoring of serum levels is always necessary to determine the correct provision, especially in the first few weeks of TPN.

Deficiencies of trace minerals are rarely observed in patients on oral feedings because these nutrients are widely distributed among foods and the requirements are low. Deficiencies of zinc, chrominum, copper, and selenium may occur during long courses of TPN, however. Such deficiencies are now prevented

TABLE 220–3. TYPICAL DAILY NUTRIENT PROVISIONS DURING TOTAL PARENTERAL NUTRITION (TPN) FOR STABLE ADULT PATIENTS WITHOUT CARDIAC, HEPATIC, OR RENAL FAILURE

Calories	Dextrose	60–80% of requirement (see Ch. 212)
	Lipid emulsion*	20–40% of requirement
Protein	Crystalline amino acids	100% of requirement (see Ch. 212)
Minerals	Sodium	90–120 mEq
	Potassium	90–150 mEq
	Chloride	90–150 mEq
	Calcium	12–16 mEq
	Phosphorus	20–40 mmole
	Magnesium	12–16 mEq
	Iron†	
	Zinc‡	2–8 mg
	Copper	1–1.6 mg
	Chromium	10–16 μg
	Manganese	0.4–0.8 mg
	Selenium§	120 μg
	Iodine§	50–80 μg
Vitamins¶	A	3300 IU
	D	200 IU
	E	10 IU
	B_1 (thiamin)	3.0 mg
	B_2 (riboflavin)	3.6 mg
	B_3 (pantothenic acid)	15.0 mg
	B_5 (niacin)	40.0 mg
	B_6 (pyridoxine)	4.0 mg
	B_7 (biotin)	60.0 μg
	B_9 (folic acid)	400.0 μg
	B_{12} (cobalamin)**	5.0 μg
	C (ascorbic acid)	100.0 mg††
	K	5 mg/wk§§
Essential Fatty Acid¶¶	Linoleic acid	4% of total calories

*See text for a discussion of the use of lipid emulsion as a daily calorie source. May be co-administered with the base solution.

†The daily requirement (not taking phlebotomy losses into consideration) is about 1.5 mg and can be met by giving 1 ml (50 mg Fe) of iron-dextran solution intramuscularly per month. Replacement is usually dictated by indices of iron stores.

‡Requirements are increased if intestinal fluid losses are great (see Ch. 218).

§Additive usually reserved for patients on long courses of TPN.

¶Based on guidelines from the American Medical Association/Nutrition Advisory Group, 1975. These guidelines do not take into account increased requirements during metabolic stress.

**May be given by monthly intramuscular injection.

††Daily provision often increased to 50 mg or more during periods of catabolic stress.

§§Not provided by multivitamin preparation; given by separate injection.

¶¶Provided by lipid emulsions on a biweekly or triweekly basis. Linolenic acid is also present in some emulsions and may be required during long term TPN (see text).

by supplementing TPN fluid with trace minerals from the outset. Zinc, copper, chromium, and manganese are commonly provided; selenium and iodine are usually given only to patients on very long courses of TPN, such as during home TPN. See Ch. 218 for further discussion of the trace minerals.

Recommendations for vitamin supplementation are given in Table 220–3; few detrimental effects have appeared when these guidelines have been followed. More commonly, vitamin deficiency results from the inadvertent omission of folate or cobalamin, which may not be included in the multivitamin preparation used, or from omission of vitamin K, which is not included in any parenteral multivitamin formulation.

Linoleic, linolenic, and arachidonic acids cannot be synthesized by humans. However, essential fatty acid (EFA) deficiency can usually be prevented by supplying adequate quantities of linoleic acid alone. EFA deficiency is rarely observed as an isolated deficiency except during TPN. A large amount (8 to 10 per cent) of the fat in adipose tissue contains the EFAs. However, the high insulin levels observed during TPN with concentrated dextrose are believed to impair access to this store through inhibition of lipolysis. Manifestations of EFA deficiency include dry, cracked skin, coarsening of the hair, hair loss, and impaired wound healing. It is estimated that 2 to 4 per cent of the daily energy requirement should be provided by linoleic acid to prevent deficiency, and lipid emulsions (500 ml of 10 per cent emulsion triweekly) will satisfy this requirement. A report of linolenic acid deficiency in a child receiving a lipid emulsion low in this fatty acid during long-term TPN suggests that linoleic acid alone may not always be adequate to prevent essential fatty acid deficiency in humans. Use of a lipid emulsion with both linoleic and linolenic acid is currently recommended to avoid EFA deficiency during long courses of TPN.

COMPLICATIONS OF PARENTERAL NUTRITION

Both nonmetabolic and metabolic complications may occur with parenteral nutrition. Thrombophlebitis from hyperosmolar solutions is the most frequent nonmetabolic complication when a peripheral vein is used. The complications related to a central vein intravenous catheter or to its insertion include pneumothorax, hemothorax, air embolus, arterial laceration, brachial plexus injury, inappropriate tip placement, venous thrombosis, and catheter-related sepsis. Some of these complications will be detected by a chest radiograph after catheter insertion, a practice that should always be followed. Others may appear later during the course of TPN. Some degree of clinically inapparent catheter-related thrombosis may occur in as many as 50 per cent of patients. At present, only symptomatic patients (certainly < 5 per cent of those with subclavian vein catheters) are evaluated and treated for noninfected thrombosis along the catheter path. Catheter-related sepsis should also occur in no more than 5 per cent of patients treated with TPN of varying

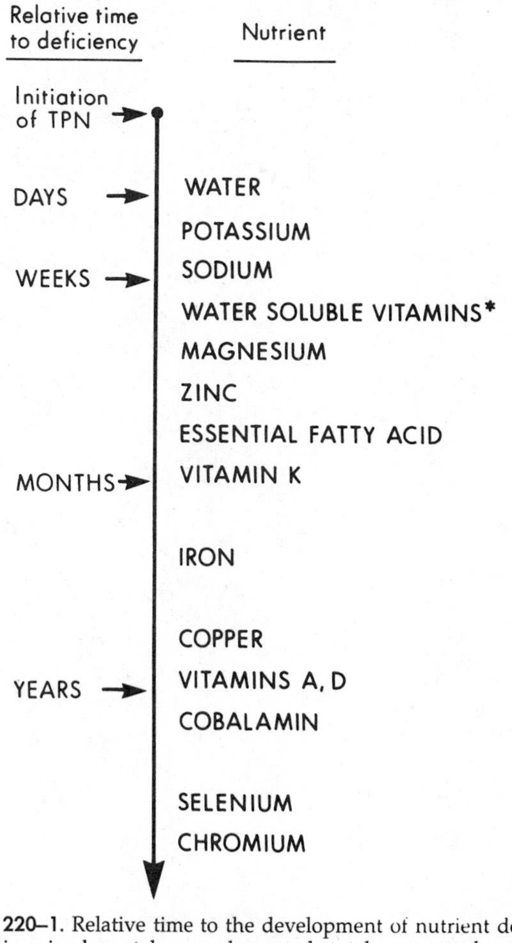

Figure 220–1. Relative time to the development of nutrient deficiencies during inadequately supplemented total parenteral nutrition (TPN). The time is proportional to body stores and inversely related to the fractional catabolic rate of the nutrient in an individual patient. Thus, the relative times given are only estimates. (*Excluding cobalamin.)

course length in a typical hospital-based program if maximal efforts are being made to prevent infection. Culturing of removed catheter tips often reveals that the source of fever was not actually an infected catheter.

Metabolic complications include the appearance of nutritional deficiencies resulting from inadequately prescribed TPN. Figure 220–1 shows the relative time to appearance of deficiencies under these circumstances. Each deficiency of course will become more quickly apparent if body stores of that nutrient were originally depleted.

Hyperglycemia is common in patients given concentrated dextrose by central vein. Regular insulin added to the base solution should be used to keep serum glucose below 200 mg per deciliter. Hypoglycemia is not likely to occur if (1) exogenous insulin is added to the base solution rather than given subcutaneously, (2) the base solution is never interrupted abruptly, and (3) termination of TPN is performed slowly over 24 hours or more with a stepwise reduction of glucose delivery rate. Incorrect provisions of major minerals can also be detected by regular laboratory monitoring, especially during the first two weeks of TPN.

Other metabolic complications include alterations in liver enzymes (usually transient and inconsequential); fatty liver; periarticular, long bone, and back pain; and gallbladder disease. The cause of the bone pain, which usually appears months into a course of TPN, remains unclear, but is likely related to altered vitamin D metabolism. Patients respond to discontinuation of TPN and to removal of vitamin D from the TPN fluid. As many as one third of patients treated with TPN for a period of two years have detectable gallstones. The prevalance is even higher (50 per cent) in the subset with ileal disease (Crohn's disease or prior resection or both). Gallbladder stasis and an increase in bile saturation with fasting are possible explanations for these higher than expected prevalences. Other metabolic complications resulting from alteration of normal physiology are likely to be recognized as more patients with potentially catastrophic small bowel resections or diseases are maintained with long courses of TPN both in the hospital and at home.

Alpers DH, Clouse RE, Stenson WF: Manual of Nutritional Therapeutics. Boston, Little, Brown and Company, 1983. *This manual outlines parenteral nutrient requirements and describes techniques of parenteral nutrition in a chapter devoted to the subject. It is also a reference source for nutrient composition of proprietary products.*

Bengoa JM, Rosenberg IH: Parenteral nutritional therapy in gastrointestinal disease. Adv Intern Med 28:363, 1983. *Provides a critical review and summary of the use of these techniques in patients with inflammatory bowel disease and other gastrointestinal disorders.*

Brennan MF: Total parenteral nutrition in the cancer patient. N Engl J Med 305:375, 1981. *The many studies examining various effects of parenteral nutrition on cancer management are reviewed. The author summarizes reasonable expectations of the use of this form of nutritional support in cancer patients. Correspondence regarding this review should also be read (N Engl J Med 305:1589, 1981).*

Grant JP: Handbook of Total Parenteral Nutrition. Philadelphia, W. B. Saunders Company, 1980. *A well-referenced monograph with a detailed review particularly of uses and complications of parenteral nutrition.*

Part XVII
ENDOCRINE AND REPRODUCTIVE DISEASES

221. PRINCIPLES OF ENDOCRINOLOGY

John D. Baxter

Multicellular organisms must communicate among their cells to maintain homeostasis, to carry out normal growth and development, and to allow for effective adaptations to stress. The endocrine system and the nervous system, both separately and through their interactions, have evolved to meet that need. In general the nervous system, of ectodermal origin, informs by the local release of neurotransmitters in the immediate vicinity of the target cell. By contrast, the endocrine glands, usually of mesodermal or entodermal origin, release hormones into the systemic circulation for a more universal distribution. However, hormones may have more restricted pathways of effective distribution; this occurs, for instance, in the portal systems of the abdomen and of the hypothalamic-hypophyseal region. Finally, both hormones and neurotransmitters can migrate to target cells through the interstitial fluid without entering the circulation (paracrine communication).

In the nervous system there is physical continuity with complex arcades of integration; the endocrine system is multifocal in form and function. Strictly speaking, it is not one "system" but a series of systems for intercellular chemical communication. There can be integration among glands in the flow of information, as illustrated by the sequential responses that follow the release of corticotropin releasing factor (CRF) by the hypothalamus. CRF triggers corticotropin (ACTH) release from the adenohypophysis (anterior pituitary gland), which stimulates cortisol release from the adrenal cortex to effect physiologic responses in the target tissues. Other endocrine glands are more freestanding. The parathyroid glands and their hormone, parathyroid hormone (PTH), function in a closed circuit to maintain extracellular calcium homeostasis independent of the nervous system, and have no known direct interactions with the pituitary gland, although they are indirectly linked to the endocrine systems of calcitonin and of vitamin D and its products.

In spite of these distinctions, the endocrine and nervous systems overlap in their functions and are closely interrelated. Thus, the ectodermal posterior pituitary gland (neurohypophysis) and adrenal medulla are arguably parts of the nervous system, although they release vasopressin and epinephrine, respectively, for systemic distribution. Further, nervous impulses can trigger hormone release and vice versa. Neurotransmitters and hormones also share common mechanisms in eliciting their actions.

Neuroendocrinology has emerged as a discipline that focuses on the interrelationships between the nervous and endocrine systems. The central role of the hypothalamus as a neuroendocrine organ has long been known, as summarized in Ch. 224. Several of its secretory products that trigger the release of hormones (e.g., ACTH, gonadotropins) from the anterior pituitary gland have been characterized and synthesized for clinical use. The peptides with opiate activity found in both the pituitary and central nervous system are discussed in Ch. 222. Even hormones previously thought to be strictly gastrointestinal (gastrin, cholecystokinin) are now known to be abundant in the central nervous system. Thus it is clear that the two major systems for communication are interrelated directly and in more subtle ways. Perhaps it is more appropriate to think instead of a single neuroendocrine integrating system with subspecialization of delivery systems into neurons, gland cells, and various mixed forms in between.

The *target cell* for hormone action must possess special mechanisms for recognizing and responding to these particular chemical signals, accepting those which are appropriate and rejecting those which are inappropriate from among the jumble of substances to which it is exposed. This specificity of recognition exists in the three-dimensional structure of unique macromolecules termed *receptors* that bind the hormone selectively and with high affinity. The target cell must also contain a mechanism to couple the hormone-receptor interaction with the subsequent steps in the cellular response to the information received.

A *hormone* therefore is a substance that is released in one tissue and travels through the circulation (usually) to the target tissue, where it elicits a particular response. There are interesting variations in this simple schema. A precursor to a hormone may be released, for example, with the final effector molecule being formed in the circulation, in the target tissue, or even in another organ. Renin substrate (angiotensinogen) is synthesized in the liver as a prohormone to be subsequently converted in the plasma to the effector substance angiotensin II by two successive modifications catalyzed by renin (kidney) and angiotensin-converting enzyme (lung and other tissues), respectively. Testosterone is converted to dihydrotestosterone, which is responsible for many androgenic actions, by 5α-reductase in the target tissue. The endogenous biosynthesis of the most active form of vitamin D_3, 1,25-dihydroxycholecalciferol, requires steps that are sequentially carried out in the skin, liver, and kidney. Also, in some cases, hormones may act in cells in which they are produced; estradiol, for instance, can affect ovarian granulosa cells.

What then are the limits of endocrinology? They are not always easy to define. Are the brain (endorphins, gastrin, releasing factors) and liver (renin substrate, 25-hydroxycholecalciferol) endocrine glands? Should the kidney be so classified based on erythropoietin, renin, prostaglandins, and 1,25-dihydroxycholecalciferol? The definitions become arbitrary and conventional. The prostaglandins are important intercellular regulators, although they are not often considered to be hormones in the strict sense, since they may serve more for local transfer of information. They are discussed together with other arachidonate metabolites in Ch. 223. By convention the major islet cell hormones have been translocated into "metabolism" and the extensive gastrointestinal hormone system has been woven into gastroenterology. Various polypeptide growth factors (nerve, epidermal, platelet derived) for specific target tissues have been identified, but are not yet generally sanctified as hormones. Further, whereas oncology is not generally considered a discipline of endocrinology, certain products of cancer genes now appear to be similar to growth factors. The thymus has emerged more into immunology than endocrinology, but thymosin might properly be considered a hormone, and, more remotely, the various lymphokines are recognized as chemical messengers as well. Since "hormone" derives from a Greek verb meaning "to set in motion" or "to spur on," what better candidate can there be than a chemotactic factor? Armed with powerful new tools for separating, purifying, and chemically defining "factors" and the cells and genes that produce them, and with exquisitely sensitive assay systems of increasing specificity, the endocrinologist has greatly enhanced means now to better understand molecule-mediated communication systems and their interrelations.

A communication system must be coupled for both emission (signal) and reception. Beyond that it should allow for an appropriate response. Classic endocrinology has been signal oriented. Attention has been devoted mostly to the release and transport of hormones and the arcades of control which govern those phenomena. This has been enormously productive in the study of normal physiology and of the pathophysiology, diagnosis, and treatment of human endocrine diseases. It seemed at one time that endocrinology, almost by definition quantifiable by measurements of hormone levels in the circulation, could be reduced to a Mendeleev-type periodic table of syndromes representing all possible combinations of "too much" or "too little" of the known hormones. As such it might be considered largely a laboratory endeavor. More recently attention has been increasingly shifted to the reception-response domain of the discipline. Pseudohypoparathyroidism was recognized as a syndrome of resistance to hormone action as early as 1942 in the classic clinical investigation carried out by Fuller Albright and his colleagues. Many examples of such resistance, both genetic and acquired, are now known, as will be described below and in specific detail in other chapters of Part XVII. The structures of hormone receptors and how they are linked to cellular responses are now becoming understood. The mechanisms that have been detected and the experimental approaches merge into molecular biology without sharp distinction. Endocrinology *within the cell* increasingly is being pursued through receptor and postreceptor mechanisms to the point of response generation. Perhaps Albright with his whimsy would have called this "endoendocrinology."

HORMONE SYNTHESIS AND RELEASE

Over 50 different hormones are produced by the body. As usually defined, these are represented by several types of molecules: (1) amino acid analogues and derivatives (thyroid hormones, catecholamines), (2) polypeptides, and (3) steroids. The arachidonic acid system (prostaglandins, leukotrienes) will not be discussed here, but is presented in Ch. 223. Endocrine glands synthesize and to some extent store their hormones for subsequent release into the circulation. This function is similar whether it is found in an anatomically separate gland (pituitary, thyroid, adrenal, parathyroids) or in specialized cells or cell clusters within other host tissues (islets of Langerhans, testis, ovary, small intestine, kidney). In some cases the endocrine function has not been found to be isolated to cells specialized for that function—e.g., the production of somatomedins or renin substrate by liver, or of erythropoietin or 1,25-dihydroxycholecalciferol by the kidney.

AMINO ACID ANALOGUES AND DERIVATIVES. Tyrosine is the unique amino acid precursor of these hormones. In the thyroid gland, tyrosine moieties within the large protein thyroglobulin are iodinated to form monoiodotyrosine (MIT) and diiodotyrosine (DIT) while still in peptide linkage. These iodotyrosines undergo oxidative condensation, which couples the respective phenolic groups through ether linkage to form the iodinated thyronines, thyroxine (T_4), and triiodothyronine (T_3). The thyroglobulin of colloid is then taken up by the cuboidal cells of the thyroid follicle in which the action of proteases and peptidases release T_3 and T_4 to be delivered into the circulation. The major secretory product, T_4, serves largely as a prohormone, since it is then further converted to the more active T_3 in the peripheral tissues by the removal of an outer ring iodine. These steps are detailed in Ch. 228 (see Fig. 228–1).

Catecholamines and dopamine, in contrast, are synthesized from free tyrosine in a series of reactions that enzymatically hydroxylate and decarboxylate the parent molecule. These reactions are summarized in Ch. 241.

POLYPEPTIDE HORMONES. Most of the polypeptide hormones are the products of particular genes and are synthesized by the steps outlined in Figure 221–1. The polypeptide gene contains sequences whose transcripts code for the hormones; these are flanked by DNA sequences important for directing the initiation and termination of transcription and in many cases the level of expression of the gene. Between the flanking sequences are "exon" sequences in the DNA whose transcripts contain the RNA sequences that are contained in the mature mRNA product of the gene. The exon sequences are usually interrupted in one or more places in the gene by intervening sequences termed "introns." When the gene is transcribed, a large precursor messenger RNA (pre-mRNA) is made. This is then processed by polyadenylation, the removal of the sequences transcribed from the introns, and splicing together of the exon sequences in the RNA to form the mature mRNA that is transported to the cytoplasm. The polypeptide hormones, like other secreted proteins, are synthesized in a larger precursor form termed a "prehormone" as the direct product translated from the mRNA. In addition to the amino acids of the hormone (or "prohormone"; see below), the prehormone contains a "signal peptide" sequence at the amino terminus that is important for transfer of the protein from the surface of the endoplasmic reticulum in the cytoplasm, where it is synthesized, into the endoplasmic reticulum. The signal peptide sequence is responsible for binding of the polyribosome complexes, containing mRNA, ribosomes, and nascent protein chains being synthesized, to the rough endoplasmic reticulum. The signal peptide sequence is subsequently removed by proteolysis, leaving either the hormone (e.g., growth hormone, prolactin) or a prohormone (e.g., proinsulin, proparathyroid hormone, proopiomelanocortin, procalcitonin). Further proteolysis of the prohormone in the endoplasmic reticulum is required to yield the hormone itself. Insulin is formed, for example, by the excision of a "C" peptide that connects the "A" and "B" chains in the nascent molecule. In the mature molecule, the latter chains are linked through disulfide bonds. ACTH is cleaved from the center of a much larger protein (proopiomelanocortin) that contains several other hormones, including β-endorphin and α- and β-melanocyte-stimulating hormone. Some hormones are further modified by glycosylation prior to their release; these include thyroid-stimulating hormone (TSH), luteinizing hormone (LH), chorionic gonadotropin (HCG), and follicle stimulating hormone (FSH). These hormones consist of two subunits, each encoded by a separate gene. The subunits bind together following their synthesis.

Variations in this scheme can sometimes result in different hormones arising from the same gene. For instance, growth hormone pre-mRNA is processed in two ways that differ in the size of one of the intervening sequences that is removed.

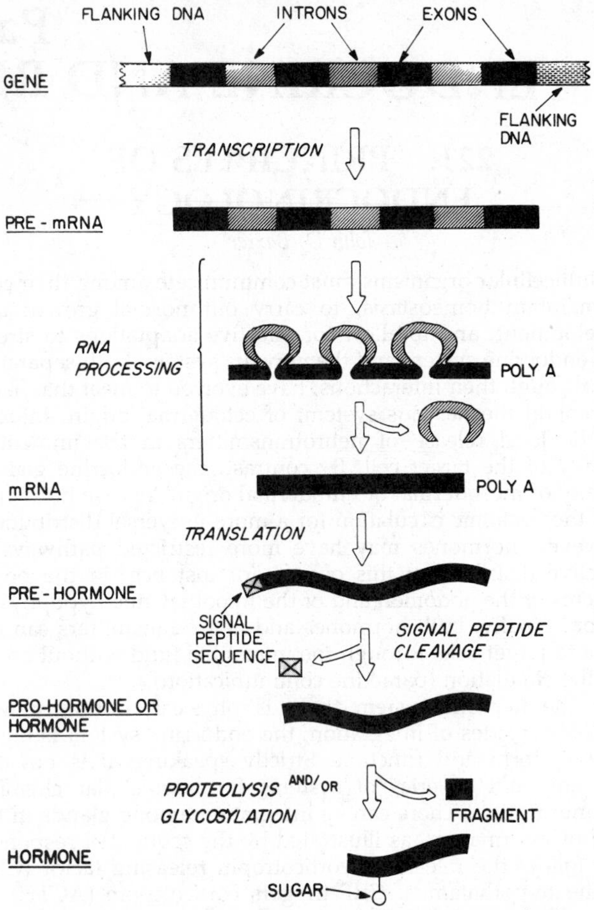

Figure 221–1. Steps in polypeptide hormone biosynthesis.

These differences result in two growth hormone mRNAs and consequent protein forms that differ somewhat in their biologic activities. The pre-mRNA that yields mRNA coding for preprocalcitonin is alternatively processed primarily in the brain to yield an mRNA that codes for a different peptide. At the post-translational level, proopiomelanocortin can be processed to yield in some cases predominantly ACTH and β-lipotropin (β-LPH) and in other cases predominantly corticotropin-like intermediate lobe peptide (CLIP) and β-endorphin.

The hormones within the cisternae of the endoplasmic reticulum are transported to the Golgi complex. This occurs either by direct transfer through the cisternae, which are in continuity with the membrane channels of the Golgi complex, or by the formation of vesicles (transition elements). Secretory vesicles (and/or secretory granules) with more condensed protein contents are formed in the Golgi complex. The hormones are then released into the extracellular fluid by exocytosis, which involves a fusion of the membrane of the granules with the plasma membrane.

STEROIDAL HORMONES. The steroid hormones are derived from cholesterol, and 7-dehydrocholesterol is the precursor to vitamin D. In a series of modification reactions, the side chain of cholesterol is cleaved to yield the 21-carbon steroid pregnenolone. The functioning steroidal hormones are then derived through a series of specific hydroxylations and other modification reactions. For example, there is placement of a 4-5 double bond in the A ring with progesterone, testosterone, cortisol, and aldosterone and aromatization of the A ring in the case of estrogens. Most of these reactions take place in the specific endocrine gland, although in some cases final modifications occur in the target tissue (testosterone→dihydrotestosterone) or in other peripheral tissues (testosterone in the female; estradiol in the male). As an example, the biosynthetic pathway for the glucocorticoids is shown in Ch. 229. Specificity in the production of steroidal hormones depends upon the presence of the appropriate enzymes. Through this mechanism almost all of the aldosterone is produced in the adrenal glomerulosa, most cortisol in the adrenal fasciculata-reticularis, and most estradiol in women in the ovary.

HORMONE STORAGE AND RELEASE. Endocrine cells store hormones to a varied extent. For example, the steroid hormones, although predominantly hydrophobic in nature, still are polar enough not to accumulate in large supply in lipid stores. By contrast, vitamin D and its metabolites accumulate in appreciable quantities in lipid stores. With many of the polypeptide hormones, the glands can store substantial quantities of the hormones. For example, a five-day supply of insulin can be stored in the pancreatic islets. Although the thyroid gland does not store thyroxine per se in appreciable quantities, the gland can have about a two-week supply of this hormone stored as a precusor in thyroglobulin. Also, nerve endings usually contain several days' supply of norepinephrine.

The stimuli to hormone production can trigger both the release of stored hormone and the synthesis of new hormone. The various mechanisms for hormone release have received relatively little attention in comparison with the extensive studies on hormone synthesis (with which it is closely linked). Some of the polypeptide hormones (insulin, glucagon, growth hormone) are released by active exocytosis of granules in which they are stored. Thyroid hormones are released by proteolysis of thyroglobulin derived from follicular stores by pinocytosis. Steroidal hormones seem only to diffuse down concentration gradients.

The pattern of release of hormones shows marked variations. The release of some hormones (ACTH, cortisol) is predominantly pulsatile in nature. The mechanisms by which this occurs are not clear; nor is it established whether these irregular bursts of secretion reflect predominantly changes in synthesis promoting release or in secretion alone. It is especially important to be aware of such episodic changes in evaluating the significance of random blood samples assayed for hormones released in this way. By contrast, the release of other hormones (PTH, prolactin) is more steady. Some hormones (e.g., insulin) display both pulsatile and steady release characteristics. Finally, a few hormones also have an overall pattern of release that is circadian (e.g., ACTH and cortisol).

REGULATION OF HORMONE PRODUCTION
(Fig. 221–2)

For the endocrine system to serve effectively its function of communicating information among cells, it must have mechanisms for regulating the release of hormones. These include not only mechanisms that affect basal and circadian release of hormones but also those that allow hormone levels to increase or decrease in response to physiologic or pathologic stimuli. The system also makes use of mechanisms that monitor whether the hormonal signal has been appropriate to attain its goals of maintenance of homeostasis, stimulation of growth and development, and response to stress.

For the most part, three types of influences govern hormone release: (1) There can be spontaneous release of hormone from the gland at a relatively constant rate (e.g., thyroxine) or in a circadian rhythm (e.g., cortisol). These patterns may be due to intrinsic activity of the gland, or to extrinsic factors that affect hormone release. (2) Hormone release can be affected by a variety of physiologic or pathologic influences that act through the same mechanisms that affect the basal release or through separate pathways. (3) "Sensor" mechanisms monitor the appropriateness of the hormonal levels or responses and provide further regulation. Three major modulators of hormone release that can act at any of the levels discussed above are other hormones, the central nervous system, and the physiologic responses produced.

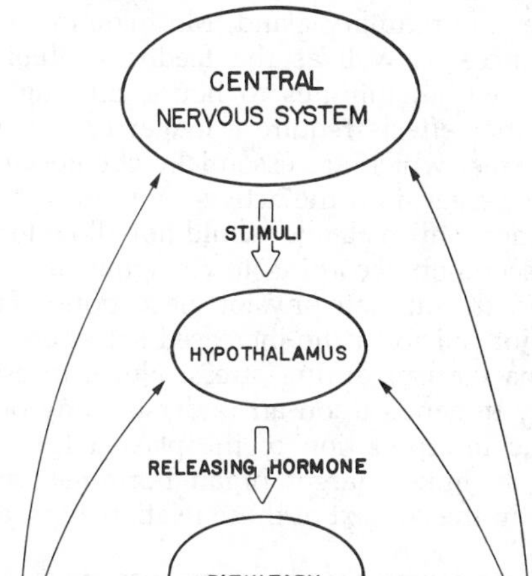

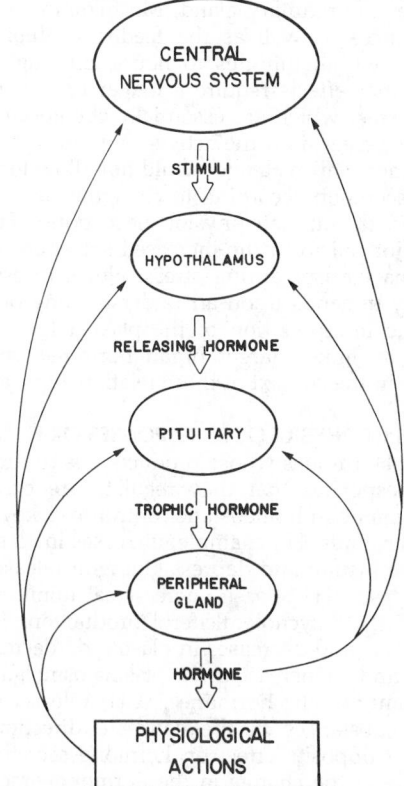

Figure 221–2. Organization of a set of endocrine glands, with interrelated regulatory elements. Shown is the flow of information from the central nervous system through the hypothalamus to the pituitary and then to the peripheral glands. Also indicated is that either the hormone product of the peripheral gland or the physiologic actions induced by the hormone can feedback-inhibit the stimuli to hormone release at any of several loci. As a rule, all of the potential regulatory influences do not operate with respect to a given set of glands, nor do all of the components shown operate for all endocrine glands.

HORMONES THAT STIMULATE THE RELEASE OF OTHER HORMONES. The primary function of several hormones is to stimulate or inhibit the release of other hormones. This is the case with the "tropic" hormones of the anterior pituitary gland (ACTH, TSH, LH) and the hypothalamic releasing factors (CRF, thyrotropin releasing hormone [TRH], gonadotropin releasing hormone [GnRH]). Some of these factors are essential for the release of the respective hormones under their control. For instance, with TSH or ACTH deficiency, thyroxine and cortisol production, respectively, drop to negligible levels and there is atrophy of the corresponding glands. By contrast, with chronic excess of these hormones there can be hyperplasia and hypertrophy of the target gland that, in addition, increases its capacity to produce hormones. Other factors are inhibitory of hormone release; their disappearance leads to an increased production of hormone by the gland. Lesions of the pituitary stalk can block the inhibitory influence of dopamine on the prolactin-producing cells of the anterior pituitary gland, resulting in an increase in the secretion of this hormone. The production of tropic hormones is usually modulated by the hormones whose production they stimulate; thus these hormones themselves measure the appropriateness of the response to the tropic hormone. For instance, feedback inhibition of ACTH release occurs in response to cortisol, inhibition of TSH release occurs in response to thyroxine, and inhibition of LH release occurs in response to testosterone. Conversely, during the menstrual cycle, the rising concentration of estradiol triggers the surge of LH and FSH release prior to ovulation (see Ch. 225). The feedback influences can be exerted either directly at the level of the pituitary or more indirectly at the level of the hypothalamus to block production of the releasing factor that stimulates the pituitary gland. Most commonly, the stimulatory influences as well as the feedback-inhibitory effects occur rapidly, within minutes to hours, although the tropic and certain other effects require a longer time. These simple servomechanisms, which are essentially chemostats, maintain the level of the free—i.e., the active—hormone at a "normal" level. These mechanisms alone would not allow for alterations in hormone secretion according to changing need, since they do not measure the ultimate physiologic response. For example, they would not call forth the increased secretion of ACTH to elevate plasma cortisol during stress. Nevertheless, much of endocrinology depends upon an understanding of these relationships. The interpretation of the plasma level of a tropic hormone or its linked target organ hormone can be made logically only in the context of these relationships, as described below.

INFLUENCES OF PHYSIOLOGIC RESPONSES OR EXTRACELLULAR SUBSTANCES. Hormones whose production is controlled by the physiologic responses that they regulate are predominantly those which maintain homeostatic control over key substances in extracellular fluids. For example, increases in plasma glucose levels increase insulin and depress glucagon release. Increases in Ca^{++} decrease PTH release, increase calcitonin release, and decrease 1,25-hydroxycholecalciferol production. Increases in extracellular Na^{+} and decreases in plasma K^{+} decrease aldosterone release, and an increase in the plasma osmolality increases vasopressin antidiuretic hormone (ADH) release. Changes in the effector substances in the converse direction have the corresponding opposite effect on hormone secretion. In each case the effect of the change in the hormone concentration is to "correct" the changes in the extracellular substance toward "normal." These mechanisms most often operate rapidly (minutes to hours), and they provide an exquisitely sensitive system for the maintenance of homeostasis. The regulation by the effector substance can occur directly on the hormone-producing cell, as with the effect of glucose on insulin or glucagon release or of K^{+} on aldosterone release, or it can occur indirectly. As an example of the latter, an increase in plasma sodium (probably through its associated Cl^{-}) depresses the release of renin by the kidney. The decreased renin level results in less angiotensin production, which in turn results in lower aldosterone production.

CENTRAL NERVOUS SYSTEM. The central nervous system (CNS) participates in the regulation of hormone release in several ways. It not only directs the spontaneous patterns of hormone secretion, but also mediates stress-stimulated secretion and other responses that interrupt the spontaneous (basal) rhythms. These influences occur through effects on the hypothalamus with consequent changes in the delivery of releasing factors to the pituitary, and they also occur through influences on the sympathetic nervous system. The influences of the CNS on the hypothalamus govern the circadian release of CRF that stimulates ACTH release, the surges in growth hormone during REM sleep, events surrounding the onset of puberty, the release of prolactin during suckling, and the release of growth hormone and ACTH with "stress." Little is known about how the spontaneous patterns are determined, although in some cases they may be due to the influences of extrinsic factors on the CNS. The circadian rhythm of ACTH release in rodents appears to be "set" predominantly by the feeding cycle. Events influenced by the CNS through the sympathetic nervous system include the release of insulin by the pancreas, of renin by the kidney, and of epinephrine by the adrenal medulla. These can be considered as part of "fight or flight" responses. Thus, the CNS is able to determine the needs of the organism for normal physiology and development, to sense when there is a need for intervention for specific purposes, and to dictate the appropriate response.

There are many aspects of the regulation of hormone synthesis and release that remain poorly understood in terms of both the mechanisms involved and why certain stimuli are effective. For instance, the release of growth hormone is influenced by the level of blood sugar or certain amino acids, but these may not be the most important physiologic determinants for its secretion. What is the function and the control of prolactin secretion in the male? What are the physiologic roles of intestinal vasoactive peptide and somatostatin?

HORMONE TRANSPORT

The polypeptide hormones circulate largely as free entities. By contrast, the steroid and thyroid hormones circulate largely bound by plasma proteins. For most of these (aldosterone is an exception), specific plasma proteins bind the hormones with high affinity such that only a small amount of the hormone (<1 to 10 per cent) is free. Thyroxine-binding globulin (TBG), thyroid hormone–binding prealbumin (TBPA), and corticosteroid-binding globulin (CBG) are examples of such specific proteins. The hormones rapidly equilibrate with their protein carriers and also rapidly dissociate from them when the free hormone concentration is lowered. The function of these proteins is unknown. They do not appear to have an obligatory role in hormone action, and genetic disorders in which the binding proteins are markedly reduced or increased are not associated with abnormal endocrine function. They do not appear to be required to "transport" the hormones, which are soluble enough at concentrations at which they are active. The plasma proteins serve to some extent as a reservoir that "buffers" the plasma against rapid fluctuations in hormone release and also tend to decrease the clearance of the circulating hormones, making them less accessible to degradative enzymes and to loss through glomerular filtration. CBG-like proteins also exist within some cell types; in the kidney, these may serve to sequester cortisol and prevent it from occupying mineralocorticoid receptors that mostly bind aldosterone (Ch. 73). In addition to the association with high-affinity plasma-binding proteins, hormones also bind with lower affinity to other proteins, particularly to albumin.

Free hormone rather than the plasma-bound hormone appears to be responsible for eliciting hormone action. Furthermore, the physiologic regulatory mechanisms that are sensitive to the concentration of hormones in plasma respond to the free rather than to the total hormone concentration.

The concentrations of the plasma binders of hormones vary both on a genetic basis and as the result of the effects of certain drugs or other factors. For instance, estrogens increase CBG and TBG. In contrast, the synthesis of these binding proteins tends to be diminished by androgens and in patients with severe liver disease, and they may be lost in the urine in the nephrotic syndrome. As noted, there are rare persons who have a genetic deficiency of a specific binding protein.

It is particularly important to be aware of plasma binding in the clinical evaluation of endocrine excess and deficiency states. Since the free hormone is biologically active and is maintained by homeostatic mechanisms, this fraction rather than the total hormone concentration reflects the state of endocrine function. Plasma assays of free hormone concentrations have been developed but are not commonly available; instead, the total plasma hormone concentration is usually measured. The total plasma concentration of a hormone will be elevated or depressed in parallel with any change in the level of its binding protein, even though the free hormone concentration will usually be maintained normal by homeostatic control mechanisms. Conversely, a patient with low binding protein levels could have a high free hormone level and endocrine hyperfunction in the face of a low total hormone concentration, and a patient with a high binding protein level could have an elevated total but a low free hormone concentration and therefore endocrine hypofunction.

METABOLISM OF HORMONES

In order for the endocrine system to be able to adapt to physiologic needs, there must be a turnover of the circulating hormones. This requires mechanisms for removal of active hormones, which may be very rapid (a few minutes for most protein hormones) or comparatively prolonged (over a week for thyroxine). As might be expected, the rapidity of removal tends to parallel the rapidity with which the specific endocrine gland is called upon to adapt its secretion to normal stimuli.

The polypeptide hormones are broken down to their component amino acids in the plasma and by tissue proteases and peptidases. To some extent this occurs intracellularly after the hormone is taken up (internalized). Inactive fragments of polypeptide hormones may circulate (e.g., fragments of PTH) and thereby constitute a problem in radioimmunoassay procedures (see Ch. 246). At present, there are no known endocrine syndromes caused by abnormalities in the metabolism of polypeptide hormones, although sometimes insulin resistance in diabetes can be due to excessive subcutaneous destruction of the injected hormone.

Thyroid hormones are metabolized largely by deiodination in peripheral tissues and to a lesser degree by the oxidative deamination and decarboxylation of the alanine side chain. Part of the metabolism of T_4 is its conversion, as a prohormone, to the more potent T_3. Some T_4 and T_3 are excreted in the bile and undergo an enterohepatic circulation. In a number of disease states (Ch. 228) the metabolism of T_4 is altered to favor initial deiodination in the inner ring to form more reverse T_3, and less T_3 is formed. This may represent part of the body's adaptation to disease by creating a state of relative hypothyroidism that reduces the metabolic demands elicited by the actions of these hormones. The metabolism of catecholamines, by O-methylation and oxidative deamination (see Ch. 241), leads to end-products (vanillylmandelic acid, metanephrine, normetanephrine) which can be readily identified in the urine and measured for diagnostic purposes.

Steroidal hormones are hydrophobic. Thus, although the free hormones are filtered by the kidney, they are mostly reabsorbed and are therefore poorly excreted. To facilitate their removal, they are metabolized to more polar forms through the reduction of double bonds, further hydroxylations, and conjugation with glucuronide or sulfate prior to excretion into the urine and to a lesser extent into the gut. As an example, the metabolic pathway for inactivation of cortisol is described in Ch. 229. An important step in this pathway, the reduction of ring A by specific hepatic enzymes, may be impaired in severe liver disease such that the half-life of cortisol and of estradiol, for instance, is significantly prolonged. Whereas plasma cortisol is maintained at a normal level, in this case by appropriate reduction in its rate of secretion by the adrenal cortex, the abnormality results in elevated estradiol levels. The obverse obtains in thyrotoxicosis: cortisol is more rapidly metabolized; however, the plasma cortisol level is maintained normal by enhanced secretion. Sometimes drugs can increase the rate of steroid metabolism.

Again, homeostatic mechanisms may operate to normalize the hormone concentration by compensatory changes in output. Such variations can be important when hormones are used in therapy either for replacement of an endocrine deficiency or for treating nonendocrine diseases with pharmacologic doses (see Ch. 229).

MECHANISMS OF HORMONE ACTION

The action of a hormone is initiated by its binding to a specific receptor protein. The polypeptide and catecholamine hormones bind to receptors that are located on the cell surface; the steroid and thyroid hormones bind to receptors within the cell. The polypeptide or catecholamine hormone-receptor interaction usually triggers changes in the production of or in the levels of intracellular mediators, which in turn are responsible for eliciting the hormone effect. The steroid and thyroid hormone-receptor interactions appear to stimulate or inhibit the transcription of particular genes. The translation products of the resulting mRNAs then mediate the hormonal effect. There are exceptions to these generalities. Certain actions of thyroid and steroid hormones may not be mediated through nuclear events, for example. Furthermore, the possibility that polypeptide hormones may act by binding to receptors inside the cell is a subject of active inquiry.

HORMONE RECEPTORS. Hormone-receptor proteins bind hormones specifically and with high affinity; this binding then triggers subsequent reactions that result in the hormone response. The binding is noncovalent in nature, is driven predominantly by hydrophobic interactions, and is facilitated by electrostatic and other ionic interactions between the hormone and the receptor. Since the hormone-receptor interaction is reversible, the laws of mass action may be applied to its study. The initial binding reaction can conform to the relationship:

$$\text{Hormone (H)} + \text{receptor (R)} \rightleftharpoons \text{[HR] complex}$$

Thus, the equilibrium dissociation constant (K_d), which is the reciprocal of the equilibrium association constant (K_a), conforms to:

$$K_d = \frac{[H]\,[R]}{[HR]} = \frac{[H]\,[R_{TOTAL} - HR]}{HR}.$$

Rearrangement of this and substituting bound (B) for HR, free (F) for H, and R_T for R_{TOTAL} yields the Scatchard equation:

$$\frac{B}{F} = \left(-\frac{1}{K_d}\right) B + \frac{R_T}{K_d}.$$

This is the equation of a straight line of which the slope is $-1/K_d$ and the intercept on the abscissa equals R_T. Thus, in a plot of B/F as a function of B, the finding of a straight line indicates that the reaction is bimolecular, and the slope and intercept of that line indicate, respectively, the affinity (K_d) and the total concentration of binding sites.

For most hormone-receptor interactions a straight line is obtained. There are exceptions, however, and these generally indicate either the presence of several independent classes of sites or of negative cooperativity. For example, with insulin and aldosterone binding, concave Scatchard plots can be generated. With insulin (especially at temperatures below physiologic), there is negative cooperativity whereby binding of the first molecule of insulin lowers the affinity of other unoccupied receptor units for binding subsequent molecules. By contrast, aldosterone binds to two molecular species, exhibiting a higher affinity binding to "mineralocorticoid" receptors that mediate sodium-retaining actions, and lower affinity binding to "glucocorticoid" receptors that mediate glucocorticoid actions.

The structure of the binding site on the receptor is such that it exhibits a high specificity for binding the major hormones that act through it. For example, glucagon receptors have a high affinity for glucagon but not insulin, and vice versa. However, there are several circumstances in which different "classes" of hormones are similar enough in structure to lead to overlapping association. This is illustrated by the weak binding of aldosterone to glucocorticoid receptors; this is probably of little consequence physiologically, since the concentration of aldosterone relative to its affinity for these receptors is too low to result in appreciable occupancy. Conversely, cortisol can bind significantly to mineralocorticoid receptors that are the primary mediators of aldosterone action. Even though cortisol has only 1 to 2 per cent of the affinity of aldosterone for these receptors, it circulates at concentrations much higher than aldosterone, and consequently cortisol probably does play some role as a salt-retaining hormone. As another example, epinephrine as a catecholamine binds to and acts through both α- and β-adrenergic receptors.

In most, if not all, cases the hormone-receptor interaction results in conformational changes in the receptor that lead to the cascade of events in the hormone response. Thus, hormone receptors are generally considered to be allosteric proteins. These properties of receptors distinguish them from other hormone-binding proteins such as the plasma hormone–binding proteins. The specific post-receptor-binding responses are described in the following sections.

The structures of the hormone receptors are beginning to be elucidated. For instance, the glucocorticoid receptor is a single polypeptide chain of about 90,000 molecular weight that contains steroid-binding, DNA-binding and "effector" domains. The insulin receptor contains four polypeptide chains linked by disulfide bonds. This receptor also is glycosylated, and these sugar moieties are critical for receptor function. This receptor can be autophosphorylated in response to insulin and phosphorylated in response to other stimuli; these phosphorylations can affect receptor-binding activity.

HORMONE AGONISTS AND ANTAGONISTS. A hormone agonist is a compound that is capable of eliciting the actions of the hormone; a hormone antagonist is a compound that can directly block agonist actions. Antagonists bind to receptors, but they do not (in contrast to agonists) trigger the subsequent steps in the hormonal response. If present in sufficient concentrations, antagonists occupy sufficient sites to block the binding of agonists by the receptors and therefore prevent agonist action. Some compounds are partial agonists in that they bind to receptors and elicit a response, but one that is not as great as that of a full agonist. If the partial agonist is present in sufficient concentration, it can block the binding and actions of an agonist, but in this case it serves as a "partial antagonist" since its partial agonist response will be observed. Hormone antagonists (e.g., the antimineralocorticoid spironolactone and the β-adrenergic blocker propranolol) can have important clinical uses.

POLYPEPTIDE AND CATECHOLAMINE HORMONES. The cell surface receptors that mediate polypeptide and catecholamine hormone action have their binding sites exposed to the outside surface of the cell. Binding of the specific hormone by the receptor alters the conformation of the receptor in a manner such that intracellular mediators are affected; these in turn are responsible for eliciting the hormonal responses. These mediators include cyclic AMP that activates serine and threonine kinases, tyrosine kinases, phospholipids, calcium ion, and possible protein mediators. Examples of hormones that appear to act through particular mechanisms are shown in Table 221–1. In numerous instances hormones utilize more than one mechanism, and as described below, these effector systems have extensive interrelations. Knowledge in this area is evolving rapidly, and the list in Table 221–1 will probably be modified. Often the tabulation reflects prevalent thinking rather than established fact.

In many cases, occupancy of only a small proportion of the receptors for polypeptide and catecholamine hormones results in a full hormonal response. In these cases, "spare receptors" are said to be present. This situation arises because the limiting factor in determining the magnitude of the hormonal response resides in some step distal to the initial hormone-receptor interaction. The spare receptors are hardly spare, however, as they are functional and allow for a greater receptor occupancy (and, as a consequence, a greater hormonal response) at lower concentrations of the hormone. This derives from the fact that the quantity of hormone-receptor complexes is proportional not only to the hormone but also to the receptor concentration.

Cyclic AMP (cAMP) and Kinase Activation. cAMP is the intracellular mediator for the actions of many hormones. These can increase or decrease cAMP levels and do so by affecting the production or, rarely, the degradation of the nucleotide. cAMP is formed from ATP by adenylate cyclase (Fig. 221–3).

At least three components are necessary for the activation or inactivation of adenylate cyclase (Fig. 221–3): the hormone receptor, a guanine nucleotide–binding regulatory protein (N protein), and a catalytic unit of the cyclase enzyme itself. There are two regulatory proteins. One stimulates and the other inhibits the activity of the enzyme in response to the hormone-receptor complex (Fig. 221–3). For activation of the cyclase the hormone binds to the membrane receptor, and the resulting receptor-hormone complex associates with N protein. This stimulates N protein to bind GTP and also activates a GTPase activity of the protein. GTP binding promotes the association

TABLE 221–1. MEDIATORS OF POLYPEPTIDE AND CATECHOLAMINE HORMONE ACTIONS

Elevate cAMP	Stimulate Phospholipid Turnover and/or Synthesis
ACTH	ACTH
β-adrenergic agonists	Angiotensin II
Calcitonin	α-adrenergic agents
HCG	HCG
CRF	EGF
FSH	FSH
GHRF	GnRH
LH	LH
PTH	Muscarinic agents
Prostaglandin E_1	PTH
TSH	TRH
Vasopressin	TSH
	Vasopressin
Lower cAMP	**Increase Intracellular Ca^{++}**
α_2-adrenergic agents	ACTH
Angiotensin II	α-adrenergic agents
Insulin	Angiotensin II
Muscarinic agents	HCG
Opiates	EGF
Oxytocin	FSH
Somatostatin	GnRH
	LH
Stimulate Tyrosine Kinase	TSH
	Vasopressin
EGF	
Insulin	
Platelet-derived growth factor	
Insulin-like growth factor 1	

ACTH, corticotropin; HCG, chorionic gonadotropin; CRF, corticotropin releasing factor; EGF, epidermal growth factor; FSH, follicle-stimulating hormone; GHRF, growth hormone releasing factor; GnRH, gonadotropin releasing hormone; LH, luteinizing hormone; PTH, parathyroid hormone; TRH, thyrotropin releasing hormone; and TSH, thyroid-stimulating hormone. The classification in this table is meant to reflect current thinking rather than established fact.

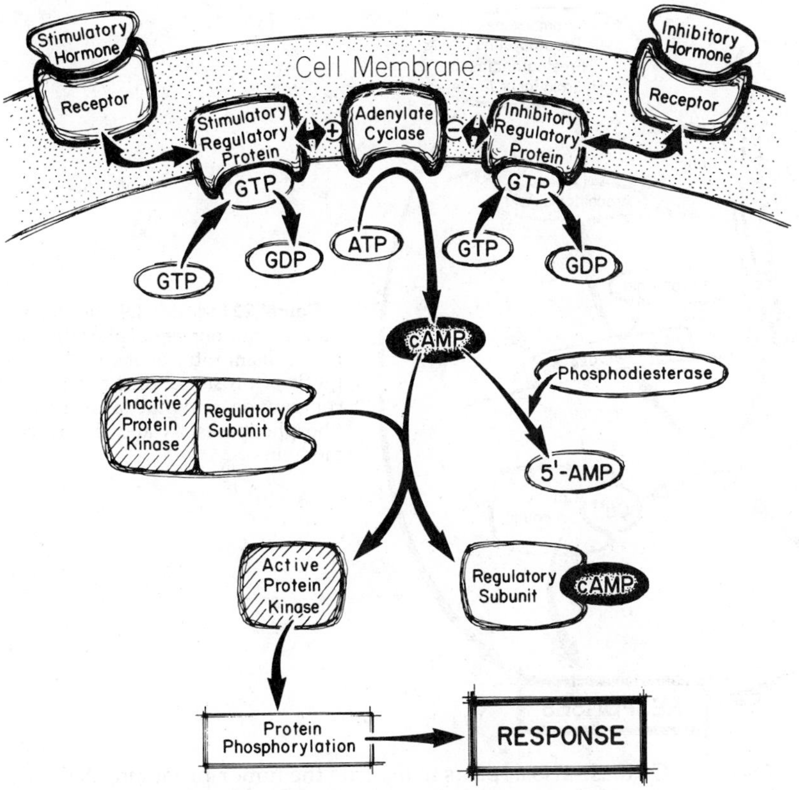

Figure 221–3. Steps in the hormonal activation or inactivation of adenylate cyclase and in the actions of cAMP.

of the N-GTP complex with the catalytic moiety of adenylate cyclase in such a way that the latter is activated to convert ATP to cAMP. The GTPase activity of N protein then converts GTP to GDP. This results in a loss of activity of the regulatory proteins, which terminates the activation. Analogous steps occur when hormones inhibit adenylate cyclase; in these cases the hormone-receptor complex binds to the inhibitory protein that in turn inhibits the activity of the cyclase.

cAMP is formed inside the cell and acts intracellularly. Some cAMP may leak into the extracellular fluid, but there is no evidence that it has any extracellular function. This extracellular cAMP can occasionally be of diagnostic usefulness; urinary cAMP measurements can provide an index of the actions of PTH on the kidney (see Ch. 246).

Most if not all of the actions of intracellular cAMP appear to be mediated through its activation of intracellular protein kinases (Fig. 221–3). These cAMP-activated protein kinases (only a small subset of the total cellular kinases) exist in an inactive basal state in association with two regulatory subunits. cAMP binds to and promotes dissociation of the regulatory subunits from the catalytic subunit, thereby activating it to stimulate the phosphorylation of specific serine and, to a lesser extent, threonine residues on proteins. Some of these phosphorylations alter the conformation and thus the enzymatic activities of proteins that in turn affect metabolic events in the cell.

cAMP is degraded by phosphodiesterases (Fig. 221–3). Since the concentration of intracellular cAMP represents a balance between its synthesis and degradation, regulation could occur at either step. Although it appears that regulation of cAMP synthesis is the predominant mechanism, there are circumstances in which phosphodiesterase is regulated; for example insulin in some cases can increase phosphodiesterase. Certain pharmacologic agents, such as the methylxanthines (caffeine, theophylline) can inhibit phosphodiesterase (although they may also have other actions) and thereby elevate cAMP levels.

Calcium as a Second Messenger. Ionized calcium also plays a role in mediating the actions of many hormones. The hormone-receptor interaction in some way affects the cellular distribution of calcium either by promoting its uptake through the cell membrane or else by stimulating its release from intracellular organelles (e.g., mitochondria or sarcoplasmic reticulum) into the cytoplasm (Fig. 221–4). In the case of cell membrane–stimulated uptake, the hormone-receptor complex may directly, or indirectly, open calcium channels, permitting the influx of ionized calcium into the cell from the extracellular space. A major stimulant for such release appears to be inositol-1,4,5-triphosphate, generated from hormone-receptor complex activation of phospholipase C, as discussed in the following section.

The actions of calcium as a hormonal second messenger are often mediated through an intracellular calcium receptor termed calmodulin (Fig. 221–4). When calmodulin binds calcium, the protein changes to a configuration in which it activates a number of enzymes, including glycogen phosphorylase kinase, Na^+/K^+ ATPase, calcium-dependent protein kinase, myosin light chain kinase, adenylate cyclase, and cAMP phosphodiesterase.

One of the best-studied actions of Ca^{++} is the activation of glycogen phosphorylase that catalyzes the breakdown of glycogen to glucose 1-phosphate. Catecholamines bind to α-adrenergic receptors in cell membranes of hepatocytes and thereby stimulate an increase in intracellular Ca^{++}. In this case, calmodulin is an integral part of the glycogen phosphorylase kinase enzyme complex, binds calcium, and is induced to activate the enzyme.

Although most hormone actions mediated by calcium appear to involve calmodulin, several other Ca^{++}-binding proteins also participate in metabolic control. For example, troponin C is a calcium-binding protein that influences the contraction of smooth muscle. In this case, acetylcholine stimulates smooth muscle contraction by increasing intracellular Ca^{++} and therefore the concentration of the troponin C-Ca^{++} complex, whereas catecholamines produce relaxation by decreasing the intracellular Ca^{++} levels.

Phospholipids. Recent work suggests that membrane phospholipids and their metabolic products appear to participate in hormone action in at least two ways: (1) as a source of arachidonic acid precursors for synthesis of prostaglandins and

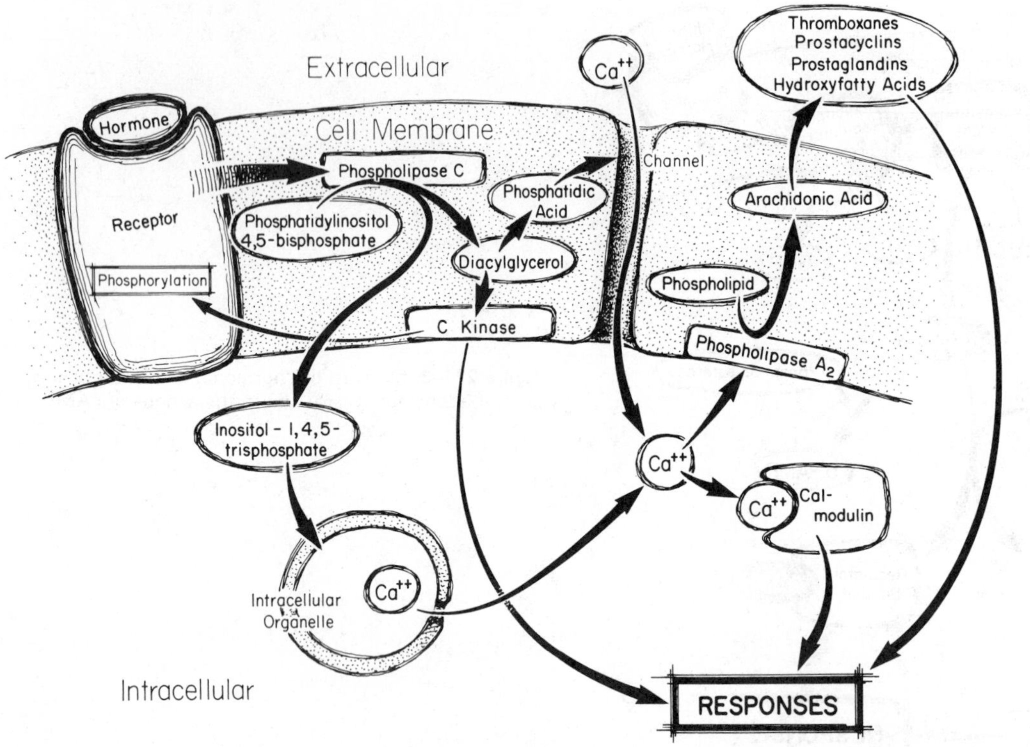

Figure 221–4. Model for the actions of hormones on phospholipid metabolism, intracellular Ca^{++}, synthesis of prostaglandins and related compounds, and the activation of phospholipases A_2 and C and calmodulin.

related compounds that secondarily have target-tissue effects and (2) by stimulating an increased turnover and/or synthesis of phosphoinositides that influence target-cell metabolism.

STIMULATION OF ARACHIDONIC ACID AND OTHER PRECURSORS OF PROSTAGLANDINS AND RELATED COMPOUNDS. Arachidonic acid—a precursor to the prostaglandins, prostacyclins, thromboxanes and hydroxy fatty acids—is released from phospholipids by phospholipase A_2 (Fig. 221–4). Several hormones (ACTH, hypothalamic releasing factors) have been shown to activate such membrane-associated phospholipases that catalyze arachidonic acid release, leading to an increase in the synthesis of the products listed above. These compounds can then elicit other actions on target cell metabolism to form important links between hormone action and prostaglandin, prostacyclin, thromboxane, and hydroxyfatty acid action (see Ch. 223). The mechanisms by which phospholipase A_2 is activated are not clear, although they may be indirect. The activation in many cases is Ca^{++} dependent, and as Figure 221–4 shows, it may be the result of hormone-induced changes in intracellular Ca^{++}. Other sites in the pathway of phospholipid metabolism may also be activated. In ovarian granulosa cells, for example, prostaglandin production is increased by LH, not by increasing arachidonic acid formation but by increasing prostaglandin synthetase activity.

STIMULATION OF PHOSPHOINOSITIDE TURNOVER (Fig. 221–4). Phosphoinositides make up a minor proportion of the membrane phospholipids. The breakdown and resynthesis and/or the synthesis of these phospholipids is enhanced by a number of hormones (Table 221–1). Phosphatidylinositol is converted to phosphatidylinositol 4-phosphate that is converted to phosphatidylinositol 4,5-bisphosphate. The latter can be converted into diacylglycerol plus inositol 1,4,5-trisphosphate catalyzed by phospholipase C (Fig. 221–4). Hormones such as vasopressin and angiotensin II may activate this reaction through influences on the enzyme or its substrates. Diacylglycerol can activate a serine and threonine kinase, termed C kinase, that differs from the cAMP-activated kinase. C kinase can phosphorylate epidermal growth factor (EGF) receptors with a consequent decrease in their affinity for EGF binding and capacity for EGF stimulation of tyrosine kinase activity (discussed below). Thus, this pathway may be involved in heterologous and homologous down-regulation of hormone responsiveness (discussed below). C kinase also appears to mediate the tumor-promoting activities of certain agents such as phorbol esters and may mediate the actions of hormones that stimulate phospholipid turnover. Inositol 1,4,5-trisphosphate appears to be capable of increasing intracellular Ca^{++} by stimulating the release of the ion from intracellular organelles, and may therefore be responsible for many of the effects of hormones that increase intracellular Ca^{++} (Fig. 221–4). Diacylglycerol can also be converted to phosphatidic acid that has been proposed to have calcium ionophore activity (Fig. 221–4). Hormones can also stimulate phosphoinositide synthesis. As is the case with effects on phospholipase A_2, these actions appear to be Ca^{++} dependent and may be secondary to other hormone effects such as those that elevate intracellular Ca^{++}. For example, actions of trophic hormones in steroidogenic tissues on phosphoinositide synthesis may participate in subsequent stimulation of steroidogenesis. Changes in phospholipid synthesis may also be stimulated by cAMP through Ca^{++}-dependent mechanisms, providing a link between adenylate cyclase activation and effects on Ca^{++}.

Activation of Tyrosine Kinase. The binding of at least four classes of hormones (Table 221–1) to their receptors results in activation of tyrosine kinase activity of the receptor. This results in phosphorylation of tyrosine moieties on the receptors and other cellular proteins. These phosphorylations may mediate subsequent events in the actions of these hormones, although the specific steps are not known. The products of certain oncogenes also have similar tyrosine kinase activity; this suggests possible similarities in the actions of growth factors and oncogene products.

Other Possible "Second Messengers." A number of other factors are currently under consideration as possible second messengers for hormones. These include cyclic GMP, changes in phospholipid methylation, other ions (K^+, Cl^-), certain other enzymes that may modify protein structure by other phosphorylations, acetylation, or methylation, for example, and peptide mediators, as for instance with insulin or prolactin action.

INTERNALIZATION OF SURFACE RECEPTORS FOR HORMONES (Fig. 221–5). Cell surface receptors and their complexes are internalized by invagination of the cell membrane into vesicles, particularly at specialized regions of the cell membrane termed coated pits. At these distinctive regions the protein clathryn accumulates on the inside portion of the membrane. Vesicles

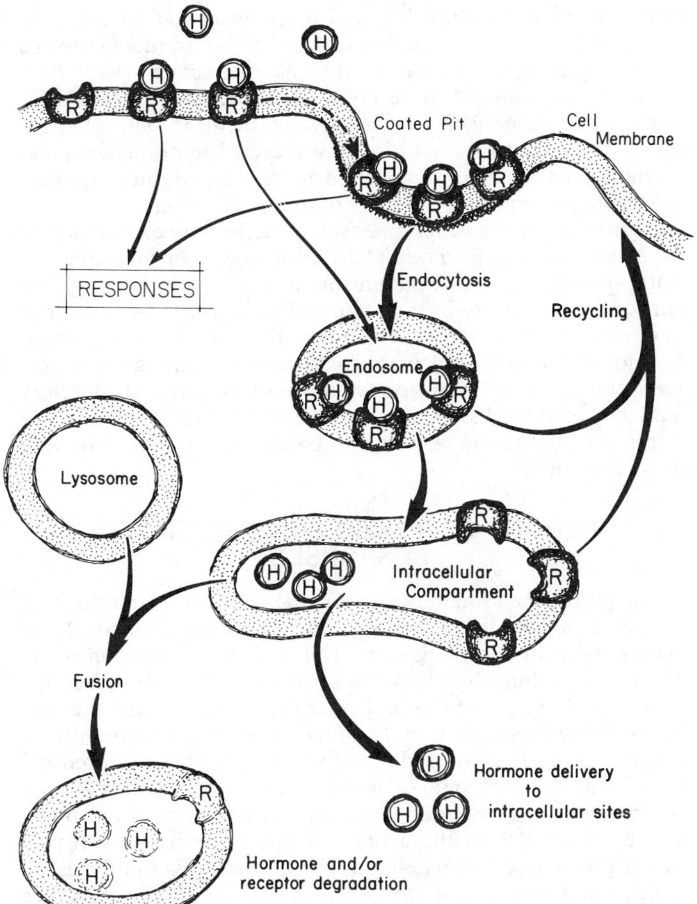

Figure 221–5. Internalization of hormone-receptor complexes and intracellular trafficking and metabolism of hormones and receptors. H = hormone; R = receptor.

from coated pits, termed endosomes, can then have a variety of fates. The endosome appears to have specialized functions such as a proton pump that can decrease the intraendosomal pH. This promotes in some cases the dissociation of the hormone from the receptor. The endosome can be returned to the cell membrane or can differentiate into other cellular compartments where the hormones and receptors can be separated. Membranes of these compartments can then pinch off and either be returned to the membrane to deliver the receptor and sometimes the hormone-receptor complex back to the cell surface or can be fused with the lysosome wherein the hormone or the receptor or both can be degraded.

The quantitative aspects of these pathways vary considerably with different hormones. For instance, most of the internalized insulin is degraded whereas most of the receptors are returned to the membrane. With EGF, most of the receptors and hormone are degraded. This provides one of the mechanisms whereby hormones can down-regulate the levels of their receptors. With iron bound to transferrin, the metal is released inside the cell and both transferrin and its receptor are returned to the membrane. With the lipoprotein receptor, cholesterol bound to lipoprotein is released inside the cell where its metabolic products feedback-inhibit cholesterol biosynthesis.

STEROID HORMONES (Fig. 221–6). Steroid hormones penetrate cells readily. The existence of transport systems has not been excluded, but if they exist, they do not appear appreciably to affect the accessibility of the hormone to the soluble intracellular receptors. In some cases (estrogens), the hormone-free receptors appear to be concentrated in the nucleus, whereas in other cases (glucocorticoids) at least some of the free receptors may be in the cytoplasm. Binding of the active steroid induces conformational changes in these receptors termed activation or transformation that stimulate their binding to the nuclear chromatin. This binding then influences the rates of transcription of specific genes. The translation products of the resulting mRNAs then mediate the response to the steroid hormone. For instance, glucocorticoids increase the synthesis of certain hepatic enzymes involved in gluconeogenesis and decrease the synthesis of proopiomelanocortin. Mineralocorticoids induce proteins that facilitate Na^+ reabsorption in the cortical collecting tubules of the kidney.

Steroid hormone–responsive genes contain specific DNA sequences on which receptor-steroid complexes act. These regulatory sequences are distinct from the promoter sequences where DNA transcription is initiated by RNA polymerase, and they can be located either fairly close to or at least up to several hundred nucleotides away from the promoter (Fig. 221–6). The regulatory sequences bind the receptor-steroid complexes (alone or in conjunction with other factors) with a much higher affinity than does random DNA. This DNA binding then results in an increased rate of initiation of transcription at the promoter of the steroid-responsive gene. The mechanisms by which the stimulation occurs are not known, but may involve a receptor-induced perturbation of chromatin structure that increases RNA polymerase accessibility to the promoter.

In some cases, steroid hormones can regulate mRNA levels through influences on mRNA stability. The mechanisms by which this occurs are not understood, but the steroids could, through transcriptional mechanisms, regulate other proteins that secondarily have effects on mRNA stability.

There is usually a close correlation between steroid binding by the receptor and the relative magnitude of the hormone

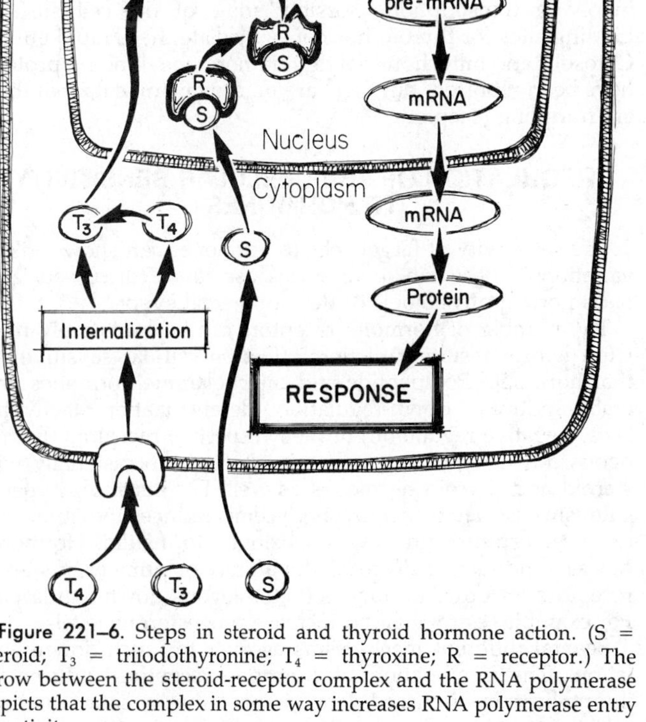

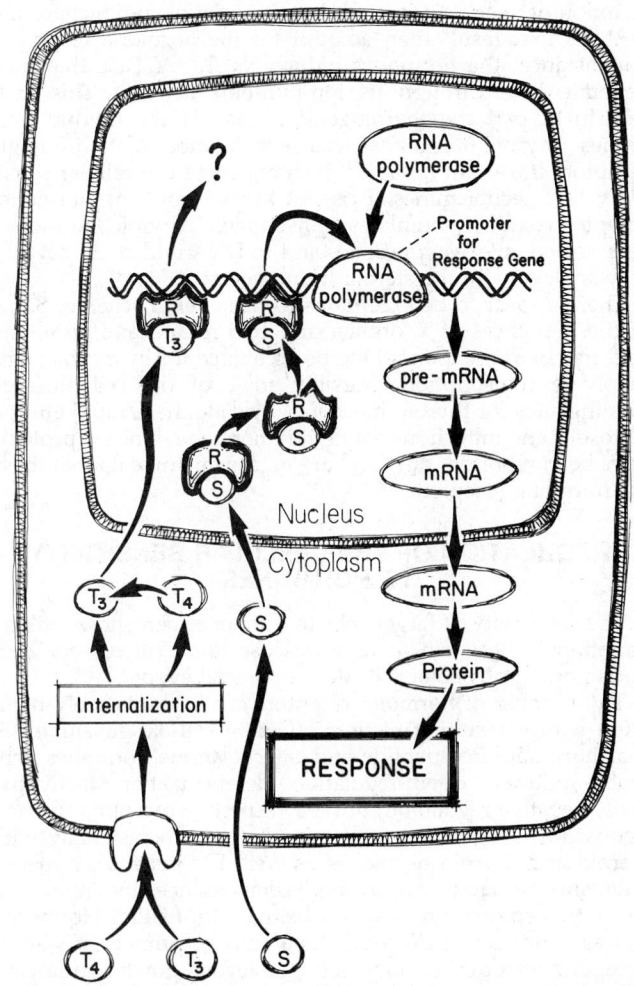

Figure 221–6. Steps in steroid and thyroid hormone action. (S = steroid; T_3 = triiodothyronine; T_4 = thyroxine; R = receptor.) The arrow between the steroid-receptor complex and the RNA polymerase depicts that the complex in some way increases RNA polymerase entry or activity.

response. This implies that the receptor rather than other elements of the response is limiting in determining the magnitude of the response.

Responses to steroid hormones are ordinarily observed several hours after administration of the hormone. This latent period represents the time required for the steroid-induced mRNAs and proteins to accumulate. Similarly, following removal of the steroid, the effect may last for a considerable period of time (hours to days). Again, this prolonged effect probably reflects the time required for degradation of the induced mRNAs and proteins. There are exceptions to these general mechanisms, but they are probably rare. Glucocorticoids inhibit ACTH release within a very few minutes, too rapidly for the effect to be due to an influence of the hormones on the transcription of DNA and its ultimate phenotypic expression. Even in this system, however, the hormone elicits other slower actions on ACTH mRNA that probably are mediated through nuclear mechanisms similar to those discussed above.

THYROID HORMONES (Fig. 221–6). Thyroid hormone receptors are found on the nuclear chromatin whether or not they are bound by the hormone. Thyroxine (T_4) and triiodothyronine (T_3) bind to sites on the cell surface and these protein-hormone complexes are internalized. This mechanism probably accounts for thyroid hormone uptake. Once inside the cell, T_4, which largely serves as a prohormone, is converted to T_3, and this newly formed T_3 plus that which had entered the cell then binds to the chromatin receptors.

The chromatin receptor–T_3 interaction stimulates the transcription of specific genes, and the translation products of the mRNAs that result then account for the hormone response. For instance, the hormones induce Na^+/K^+ ATPase that may generate heat through its ion-pumping activity. This may explain in part the thermogenic actions of the thyroid hormones. Thyroid hormones increase the number of β-adrenergic receptors in certain tissues, which enhances the cellular sensitivity to catecholamines. It is not known how the hormone-receptor complex stimulates transcription. Thyroid hormone–receptor complexes appear to bind to DNA and could act in a way analogous to the steroid hormones.

There appear to be exceptions to this overall scheme. Some of the influences of T_3 on blocking TSH release and on amino acid transport are too rapid to be accounted for by mechanisms involving transcription. Possibly some of the cell surface–binding sites for thyroid hormones mediate these rapid effects. Cytosolic and mitochondrial thyroid hormone–binding proteins have been reported, but there are no convincing data that these are hormone receptors.

REGULATION OF THE CELLULAR SENSITIVITY TO HORMONES

The sensitivity of target cells to hormones can show striking variations. These can occur in disease states (discussed later) or as normal physiologic or developmental events.

The number of hormone receptors can be extensively regulated with a resulting distinct effect on cellular sensitivity to that hormone. Polypeptide and catecholamine hormones generally induce a down-regulation (desensitization, tachyphylaxis, negative regulation) of their respective receptors (homologous down-regulation) and this can occur occasionally with steroid and thyroid hormones as well. For instance, hyperinsulinism associated with hyperglycemia reduces the number of insulin receptors and lowers sensitivity to insulin. Hormones can also increase or decrease the affinity or number of sites of receptors for other hormones (heterologous down-regulation). For example, estrogens can increase progesterone levels.

Several different mechanisms account for such down-regulation. The degradation of hormone receptors induced by internalization discussed above is operative in some cases. In other circumstances, hormones can influence receptor synthesis or degradation through different mechanisms. With catecholamine receptors, hormone binding either can induce receptors to be sequestered away from the cell membrane where they are inactive or can induce receptor phosphorylation by a cAMP-dependent mechanism that inactivates them; in both of these cases, the receptors are ultimately recycled to an active state. Homologous or heterologous hormones can induce receptor phosphorylations that can alter hormone affinity.

Regulation of the cellular sensitivity to hormones also occurs extensively owing to modulation of postreceptor mechanisms. Both synergisms and antagonisms exist. As examples, glucocorticoids are required for certain actions of the catecholamines and vice versa; certain glucocorticoid actions require thyroid hormone; glucagon, glucocorticoid hormones, and growth hormone have actions that oppose those of insulin and therefore lead to a decreased sensitivity to insulin. Magnesium deficiency diminishes the tissue response to parathyroid hormone as well as its secretion.

ACTIONS OF HORMONES: INTEGRATED RESPONSES

The endocrine system controls metabolic events in individual tissues and coordinates effects that occur simultaneously or sequentially in many tissues. The actions of hormones are diverse, affecting every tissue in some way, but with substantial selectivity in terms of the particular functions that are affected. Some tissues respond to only a few hormones, whereas others respond to many. The actions of some hormones are predominantly directed at one or a few tissues (e.g., aldosterone), whereas other hormones (cortisol, epinephrine) affect many tissues. Examples of the actions of hormones have been provided previously in this chapter, with particular emphasis on trophic hormones and on how certain hormones influence cellular sensitivity to the same or other hormones. Although any attempt to list the actions of hormones represents an oversimplification, some of the more prominent types of influences deserve emphasis.

Hormones exert major control of intermediary metabolism. Many of the responses are due to coordinated influences on several tissues and can involve several different hormones. The actions of hormones on carbohydrate metabolism are illustrative. In liver, glucagon and epinephrine promote glycogen breakdown and inhibit glycogen synthesis. These hormones and cortisol stimulate glucose production by enhancing gluconeogenesis. In fat cells, epinephrine, cortisol, and growth hormone stimulate lipolysis, providing free fatty acids (an alternative to glucose as an energy source) and glycerol, which may be converted to glucose. Epinephrine and cortisol inhibit glucose uptake by fat cells, and epinephrine stimulates glycogenolysis in muscle. Cortisol inhibits glucose uptake in lymphoid and fibroblastic tissues, and inhibits protein synthesis and stimulates protein breakdown in several tissues. The amino acids released increase the substrate available for gluconeogenesis. All of these responses tend to elevate the blood sugar and can make glucose available, for instance, during fasting. By contrast, insulin lowers the blood sugar by stimulating glycogen synthesis, by inhibiting lipolysis and stimulating lipogenesis, and by promoting protein synthesis. Thus, through its ability to recruit several different hormones and to affect multiple tissues in an integrated way, the endocrine system can be highly effective in the maintenance of homeostasis. Such an integrated system may reduce dependency on only one hormone or tissue, a feature that can facilitate compensation in disease states.

Many hormones affect growth. Prominent among these is growth hormone, which stimulates the production of yet other growth factors termed somatomedins. Epidermal growth factor, fibroblast growth factor, multiplication-stimulating activity (MSA), nonsuppressible insulin-like activity (NSILA), sex steroids, thyroid hormones, erythropoietin, and the "tropic" hormones that affect endocrine glands are also growth factors. Although in some cases the physiologic roles of these hormones are understood, in other circumstances considerable additional clarification is needed.

Hormones affect water and mineral metabolism. Thus, aldosterone regulates sodium, potassium, and hydrogen ions; vasopressin regulates water; PTH, vitamin D, and calcitonin affect calcium and phosphate ions; and prolactin affects milk production.

Hormones, especially the catecholamines, affect the cardiovascular and respiratory systems. Glucocorticoids can promote bronchodilatation in asthma. Angiotensin and vasopressin cause vasoconstriction; bradykinin produces vasodilation. Some hormonal actions on the cardiovascular system are indirect. For instance, sodium retention induced by an excess of aldosterone can cause hypertension.

Hormones are important in development and differentiation. Deficiency of thyroid hormone in childhood results in the serious and irreversible intellectual impairment of cretinism. Abnormalities in sexual maturation result from deficient androgenic effects during development. In fact, most classes of hormones have some developmental actions.

Hormones vary considerably in the rapidity with which they act. Some hormones act quickly and are more important in the minute-to-minute control of metabolism. Epinephrine, glucagon, and other "surface-active" hormones are representative of this type of hormone. Other classes of hormones regulate more long-term responses and thus tend to provide more chronic types of adaptations. Steroid and thyroid hormones generally fall into this latter category. These patterns may not be surprising based on the molecular mechanisms of action of these hormones. The surface-active hormones commonly activate enzymes by mechanisms that do not require macromolecular synthesis, whereas the slower responses to the steroid and thyroid hormones reflect the time required to change the levels of the mRNAs and proteins whose synthesis they regulate. Exceptions to these generalities occur. Thyroid and steroid hormones can have rapid actions (discussed above), and hormones that bind to surface receptors can have influences on gene transcription.

DISORDERS OF THE ENDOCRINE SYSTEM (Fig. 221–7)

Endocrinology has traditionally been signal oriented, concerning itself largely with whether hormones are secreted appropriately or inappropriately (in excess or deficit). Indeed, most recognizable disorders of the endocrine system are due to an excess or a deficiency of particular hormones, whether caused by abnormalities of endocrine glands, ectopic production of hormones, abnormal conversion of prehormones to their active forms, or iatrogenic factors. Endocrine abnormalities can also be due to changes in the responses (either enhanced or diminished) of target tissues to hormones. These disorders can occur by a variety of mechanisms.

HORMONE DEFICIENCY SYNDROMES. ***Hypofunction of Endocrine Glands.*** Endocrine glands may be injured or destroyed by neoplasia, infections, hemorrhage, autoimmune disorders, and other causes. The destruction can be acute, but commonly it is chronic with normal basal hormone production until late in the disease. The gland is usually compromised in its reserve capacity before the basal level of secretion falls and cannot respond normally in circumstances in which an increase in hormone production is needed. Such partial defects may therefore not be detected by measurement of basal hormone levels, but require other testing of the reserve function of the gland. Since many manifestations of endocrine disease require weeks or even months to develop, there can be considerable differences in the clinical presentation, depending on the rapidity of glandular destruction. In acute endocrine deficiency, chronic manifestations of the disease may not be present.

As would be expected, a deficiency of a hormone that controls the synthesis and release of another hormone may result in a syndrome which simulates a primary deficiency of that target organ. Thus, hypothalamic lesions resulting in impaired secretion of releasing hormones can be manifested by pituitary dysfunction, and the latter can result in abnormalities in the function of its various target organs (gonads, thyroid, adrenal).

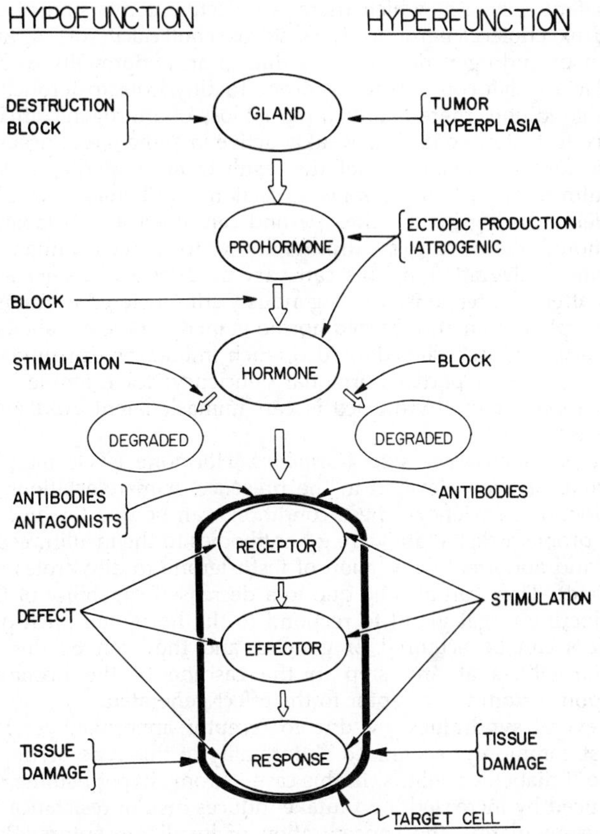

Figure 221–7. Causes of hypofunction or hyperfunction of the endocrine system.

Genetic defects can cause endocrine hypofunction, usually because of abnormalities in hormone synthesis but rarely because of the production of an abnormal hormone (as documented for insulin in a rare form of diabetes melitus). These genetic defects in hormone synthesis can be partial or complete. For example a rare form of growth hormone deficiency is due to deletion of the growth hormone gene. A partial defect may be somewhat analogous to incomplete destruction of the gland—i.e., basal hormone production may be normal, but reserve may be inadequate. In fact, sometimes genetic defects present not with the problems of hormone deficiency but with manifestations of a compensatory adaptation. For instance, partial blocks in thyroid hormone biosynthesis may result in an enlarged thyroid gland (goiter) that is due to the TSH hypersecretion that results from low levels of thyroid hormone. With the 17α-hydroxylase syndrome, there is defective cortisol production and consequent ACTH hypersecretion with an excessive production of adrenocorticosteroids that are not 17α-hydroxylated (see Ch. 229). One of these (corticosterone) substitutes for cortisol such that manifestations of cortisol deficiency are not observed. On the other hand, excessive compensatory synthesis of corticosterone and deoxycorticosterone leads to a mineralocorticoid excess syndrome with hypertension and hypokalemia.

Hormone Deficiency Secondary to Extraglandular Disorders. In principle, a number of types of extraglandular disorders could result in hormone deficiency. These could involve defective conversion of prohormones to active forms, enhanced degradation of hormones or the production of substances (antibodies, hormone antagonists) that block the actions of hormones. Impaired conversion of a prohormone to a hormone occurs in chronic renal disease and in pseudo–vitamin D resistant rickets in which there is defective conversion of 25-hydroxycholecalciferol to 1,25-hydroxycholecalciferol. A rare form of androgen deficiency is due to an abnormality in 5α-reductase that converts testosterone to dihydrotestosterone. In this condition, there is only a partial loss of androgenic effects since testosterone itself is weakly active in some target tissues. Rare forms of diabetes mellitus result from antibodies to the insulin receptor that block insulin action. Antibodies to insulin develop during insulin therapy and can affect its availability. Although there are no syndromes known to be due to enhanced hormone degradation, this can vary as discussed earlier and can affect the response to exogenously administered hormones (e.g., phenytoin and thyroid hormone increase the metabolism of certain glucocorticoids). Also, such influences can unmask or aggravate a partial hormonal deficiency; for example, the development of thyrotoxicosis can unmask latent Addison's disease.

Hyporesponsiveness to Hormones. Hormone levels may be normal or even elevated in the presence of manifestations of endocrine deficiency. These conditions can be due to some of the problems listed above (e.g., antibodies to the insulin receptor and abnormal conversion of testosterone to dihydrotestosterone). They can also be due to a decreased capability of the endocrine target gland to respond to the hormone. Such disorders can be acquired or genetic, and they can be due to abnormalities at any step in the cascade of the hormone response from the receptor to the effect generated.

Several syndromes are due to receptor abnormalities. The most commonly recognized abnormality of this type occurs in type II diabetes mellitus. In this case, chronic hyperinsulinemia induced by increased food intake induces insulin resistance by down-regulating the concentration of insulin receptors. Recognition of this problem also affects the therapy, since treatment is directed not only at correcting the hyperglycemia with insulin or other drugs but also at decreasing insulin need by dietary maneuvers. This form of diabetes also exhibits the additional and perhaps primary abnormality whereby the pancreatic islets do not release insulin normally in response to glucose, but can respond normally to other agents. In the testicular feminization syndrome there is unresponsiveness to androgens. As a consequence, a female phenotype occurs in a person with a male genotype. Most persons with this X-linked disorder have a defect in the androgen receptor.

At least one disorder is due to an abnormality in the coupling of hormone-receptor complexes to effector mechanisms. In pseudohypoparathyroidism there are symptoms and chemical derangements of hypoparathyroidism associated with elevated PTH levels and insensitivity to this hormone (see Ch. 246). In some such patients this insensitivity can be shown to be due to decreased levels of the guanyl nucleotide–binding regulatory protein that couples the PTH-receptor complex to adenylate cyclase.

Overall damage to the hormone target tissue can result in insensitivity to hormones. For instance, renal disease can lead to insensitivity to vasopressin, and liver disease can lead to insensitivity to glucagon.

There are several forms of target organ insensitivity in which the molecular mechanisms have not been elucidated. One form of dwarfism (Laron) is due to an impaired ability of growth hormone to generate somatomedin production. Vasopressin-resistant diabetes insipidus is not associated with frank renal disease. There is a syndrome of hypercortisolism with decreased sensitivity to glucocorticoids. In this case, the hypercortisolism compensates for the hyposensitivity, but the mineralocorticoid actions of the steroid also cause hypertension with hypokalemia.

Abnormal Production or Administration of Antagonists. Rarely, endogenously produced or exogenously administered substances can produce a hormone-deficient state. Antibodies to the insulin receptor can produce insulin resistance with functional insulinopenia. Cimetidine given for peptic ulcer disease can act as an androgen antagonist and produce an androgen-deficient state.

HORMONE EXCESS SYNDROMES. Hormone excess syndromes can result from hyperfunctioning endocrine glands, "ectopic" hormone production by tumors, less commonly from influences on target tissues that enhance hormone sensitivity, autoimmune disease in which antibodies cause hypersecretion of hormones or act as hormone agonists, defects in hormone biosynthesis in which precursor hormones produced in excess have deleterious consequences, and iatrogenic or therapeutic administration of hormones or substances that act like hormones.

Hyperfunction of Endocrine Glands. The most common cause of hormone excess syndromes is hyperfunction of endocrine glands secondary to tumors of the glands or to hyperplasia of several causes. Hyperfunctioning tumors of endocrine glands are usually well-differentiated adenomas (although carcinomas also occur) so that the prognosis is usually favorable with an early diagnosis. In addition to the manifestations of hormone excess, local extension of the tumor can produce symptoms. For instance, pituitary tumors can destroy the normal gland or extend into the suprasellar region to cause headaches or visual impairment.

Hyperplasia is a cause of hyperfunction of several of the endocrine glands (thyroid, adrenals, parathyroids). The most common form of thyroid hyperplasia appears to be due to an immunologic abnormality in which antibodies stimulate the gland in a manner similar to TSH. Hyperplasia of the zonae fasciculata and reticularis of the adrenal with consequent cortisol hypersecretion is usually due to ACTH hypersecretion by a pituitary tumor or an ectopic hormone-secreting tumor. The etiology in other cases of endocrine gland hyperplasia is less clear, as with hyperplasia of the adrenal zona glomerulosa with excessive aldosterone production, or of chief cell hyperplasia of parathyroid glands with PTH hypersecretion.

Ectopic Hormone Production by Tumors (see Ch. 173). Sometimes hormones are produced in excess by cells of endocrine or nonendocrine origin that are not normally the primary source of the hormone. In most cases, hormones produced ectopically by tumors are those that arise from a single gene (e.g., ACTH, growth hormone, prolactin, PTH, calcitonin, gastrin, erythropoietin), or two genes (HCG, LH, FSH). This may be due to the fact that for other hormones (e.g., steroids, thyroid hormones, catecholamines) a large number of genes not ordinarily expressed by the tumor but whose products participate in hormone biosynthesis would need to be activated to produce the hormone. Although a large number of different types of tumors can produce hormones, specific cell types are more commonly associated with certain tumors (see Ch. 173). For instance, certain cells of entodermal origin, termed *a*mine *p*recursor *u*ptake and *d*ecarboxylation (APUD) cells, are more commonly associated with ectopic hormone production. These cells are found in oat cell carcinoma of the lung, carcinoid tumors, thymomas, and others. Although a number of molecular mechanisms are now understood that could explain how genes that are ordinarily not expressed are activated in tumors, those actually causing ectopic hormone production are not understood.

Iatrogenic Causes. When hormones are used to treat nonendocrine diseases, when hormone replacement therapy is excessive, and sometimes when patients self-administer hormones (or their analogues), iatrogenic endocrine disease may occur. Patients will sometimes take excessive doses of glucocorticoids or thyroxine because these hormones produce a feeling of well-being. Rarely, administration of nonhormonal substances can cause hormone-like effects. Licorice ingestion can produce a syndrome mimicking primary aldosteronism, for example.

Tissue Hypersensitivity. Endocrine excess syndromes caused by hypersensitivity of target tissues are uncommon. Thyroid hormones increase the catecholamine receptors in certain tissues and thereby lead to excessive β-adrenergic stimulation. In this case the hyperresponsiveness is actually part of the syndrome of hyperthyroidism. Many of the manifestations of primary aldosteronism are simulated in a rare syndrome with low plasma renin and aldosterone levels in which the kidney responds as if it is excessively stimulated by aldosterone. Finally, disease of the target tissue itself can render it excessively sensitive to a hormone. For instance, cardiac arrhythmias, such as atrial fibrillation in thyrotoxicosis, probably occur most frequently in an already damaged heart.

A lingering question is whether subtle abnormalities in the sensitivity to hormones contribute to the pathogenesis of disease more than is generally perceived. With more refined methods for measuring alterations in sensitivity to hormones, it may be possible to detect more subtle abnormalities. For instance, are some forms of essential hypertension due to increased sensitivity to pressor substances or decreased sensitivity to vasodilator substances? Are some forms of osteoporosis due to abnormalities in sensitivity to estrogens or to calcium-regulating hormones? Why do glucocorticoids increase the intraocular pressure (and even precipitate glaucoma) in some persons but not in others?

Autoimmune Disease. Autoimmune disease can result in the production of antibodies that act as hormones. The most frequent situation in which this occurs is with Graves' disease, discussed in Ch. 228. Rarely, antibodies to the insulin receptor are formed that have insulin-like actions.

Hormone Biosynthetic Defects. Certain adrenal steroid biosynthetic defects (the 21α- and 11β-hydroxylase syndromes) result in overproduction of hormones proximal to the block; these syndromes are discussed in Ch. 229.

Secondary Causes of Hormone Hypersecretion. Hypersecretion of hormones may be due to excessive physiologic stimulation of glands that are basically normal. The secondary hyperaldosteronism of hepatic disease and ascites, congestive heart failure, the nephrotic syndrome, and other conditions is illustrative. The excess aldosterone can aggravate the tendency to edema in these conditions. Secondary hyperparathyroidism occurs in azotemia (see Ch. 248).

MULTIPLE ENDOCRINE SYNDROMES (see also Ch. 240). Simultaneous involvement of more than one endocrine gland can result in syndromes of hyper- or hypofunction. The most common syndrome of multiple endocrine deficiencies, sometimes termed Schmidt's syndrome, can involve the pancreatic islets, thyroid, adrenals, parathyroid glands, and gonads. The disease appears to be caused by immunologic destruction of the glands. This may result from common antigenic determinants, caused possibly by a common developmental origin of the glands.

At least three syndromes of multiple endocrine hyperfunction result from hyperplasia, adenomas, or carcinomas of endocrine tissues, termed multiple endocrine neoplasia (MEN) types 1, 2, and 3. Type 1 is associated with hyperfunction of the parathyroids, pancreatic islets, pituitary, adrenal cortex, and thyroid. In some cases more than one hormone may be produced by the tumor; islet cell tumors can produce insulin, glucagon, gastrin, vasoactive intestinal peptide (VIP), prostaglandins, ACTH, PTH, ADH, somatostatin, and serotonin. MEN type 2 is associated with pheochromocytoma (sometimes bilateral and extra-adrenal), medullary carcinoma of the thyroid, and parathyroid hyperplasia. MEN type 3 is associated with medullary thyroid carcinoma, pheochromocytoma, and other features such as neuromas. These syndromes are often familial with a dominant transmission, but the basic pathogenesis is unknown.

ABNORMALITIES OF ENDOCRINE GLANDS NOT ASSOCIATED WITH HORMONAL IMBALANCE. Tumors, nodules, cysts, infiltrative diseases, and other abnormalities may involve endocrine glands without impairing their secretory functions significantly. For instance, nodules of the thyroid gland are common but usually nonfunctioning. The major problem is that malignancy may develop in them. Sometimes particular processes have a propensity for affecting an endocrine tissue. This is the case with tuberculosis and the adrenals.

CLINICAL ASSESSMENT OF ENDOCRINE STATUS

The assessment of the endocrine status of a patient relies on findings from the history and physical examination and on laboratory testing. The latter can involve measurements of levels of hormones or their metabolites in plasma or urine either in the basal state or in response to provocative testing. Laboratory tests may also be used to measure abnormalities that result from derangements in hormonal secretion and to evaluate the patient's sensitivity to hormones.

HISTORY AND PHYSICAL EXAMINATION. Many syndromes of hormonal excess or deficiency display manifestations that are readily apparent at the time of the initial presentation, e.g., severe thyrotoxicosis or Cushing's syndrome. In other instances, the clinical presentation can be more subtle and the physician must rely on laboratory testing to establish a diagnosis. This is especially true in the early stages of most endocrine problems, in elderly persons (e.g., with thyrotoxicosis or myxedema), or when the disease presents acutely and has not been present long enough for chronic manifestations to develop. Since it is beneficial to treat these diseases early, it is important for the physician to consider endocrine diseases in patients without full-blown manifestations, despite the fact that in the early stages of many of these disorders (e.g., adrenal insufficiency, hypothyroidism, Cushing's syndrome, hyperparathyroidism) the presenting symptoms and signs are sufficiently vague to suggest more common problems. Thus, endocrine diseases should be considered in the differential diagnosis of many common problems, such as weakness, tiredness, vague gastrointestinal discomfort, hypertension, or weight loss or gain. Once the diagnosis is considered, it is usually relatively easy to establish whether or not the disorder is present. Since endocrine diseases can be caused by primary processes external to the endocrine systems, the physician should consider these in taking the history and performing the physical examination. Sometimes, the primary process (e.g., carcinoma of the lung producing ACTH, tuberculosis causing adrenal insufficiency) will dominate the clinical presentation such that hormonal abnormalities are more difficult to detect clinically.

LABORATORY TESTING. ***Hormone Levels.*** Over the past few decades, assays have been developed to measure the levels of most of the hormones in body fluids. These vary in the ease with which they can be performed and their overall reliability; some assays are generally available, whereas others are performed only in certain research institutions.

RADIOIMMUNOASSAY. The advent of radioimmunoassay, first developed for measuring plasma insulin levels, was a major breakthrough in endocrinology. Antibodies that are relatively specific for certain chemical groups or conformations on the hormone can be developed for the polypeptide hormones and also for the smaller ligands such as thyroid and steroid hormones. The success of the assay depends on the specificity of the antibody as well as its affinity for binding the hormone.

In the radioimmunoassay, the plasma or urine sample or an extract of it is incubated with the antibody to the hormone along with a tracer of radiolabeled hormone. Then the antibody-tracer complexes are quantified in a variety of ways. For instance, charcoal can be used to adsorb and thereby remove the hormone that is not bound by the antibody, and the remaining radiolabeled hormone–antibody complexes can then be assessed. The extent to which the hormones in the sample block the binding of the radiolabeled hormone by the antibody is then related to a standard curve prepared from reactions in which known quantities of the hormone are present to yield the concentration of the hormone in the sample.

In most cases, radioimmunoassay yields extremely accurate information. However, there are problems that the physician should consider in interpreting the results. The antibody may cross-react with related hormones or with precursors or metabolites of the hormone. If these compounds are present in sufficient concentration, they can give spuriously high values. For instance, some antibodies are specific for the carboxyterminal portion of PTH. This part of the molecule is present in certain circulating fragments of PTH that are biologically inactive. This is especially true in chronic renal disease, in which PTH levels by radioimmunoassay are extremely high. This problem can be obviated by the use of antibodies that are specific for other parts of the PTH molecule (see Ch. 246).

COMPETITIVE PROTEIN-BINDING AND RADIORECEPTOR ASSAYS. These assays depend on the availability of a protein that binds the hormone with high affinity and specificity. The protein can be the normal receptor for the hormone, or it can be another protein, usually a plasma hormone–binding protein (CBG, TBG, sex hormone–binding globulin [SHBG]). The assay is performed in a manner analogous to that of the radioimmunoassay.

These assays provide an indication of summed products of the affinities times the concentrations of all compounds in the sample that bind to the protein. Typically, however, only one hormone accounts for most or all of the activity that is present. Radioreceptor assays are not widely used currently, in part because it is difficult to work with receptor preparations. By contrast, several competitive protein-binding assays have come into general use. Noteworthy are the CBG-isotope and TBG assays for cortisol and thyroxine, respectively, that depend on the fact that the major chemical species in plasma that binds to CBG is cortisol and to TBG is thyroxine.

CHEMICAL ASSAYS. Many hormones can be assayed by chemical means. For example, the fluorimetric assay for cortisol depends on the fluorescence of steroids with Δ^4-3-ketone, 20-ketone, and 11β- and 21-hydroxyl groups. Ordinarily, cortisol is the only steroid present in the circulation at sufficient concentration to react significantly in this way, although in certain congenital adrenal biosynthetic defects and adrenal carcinomas, other steroids produced can contribute substantially to the assay results.

HIGH-PERFORMANCE LIQUID CHROMATOGRAPHY (HPLC). The development of more sophisticated HPLC techniques has increased their capability for routine measurements. Although these methods are not commonly used for hormone measurements, they will probably be used increasingly for the measurement of smaller molecules such as steroids, catecholamines, and small peptides.

LEVELS OF FREE HORMONE. Free hormone, rather than that which is protein bound, is usually the best index of its effective concentration in plasma. The problems with assessment of total hormone concentrations due to potential variations in the concentrations of plasma steroid and thyroid hormone–binding proteins have been emphasized earlier in this chapter.

Levels of free hormone can be assessed in several ways: (1) The free hormone can be physically separated from that which is plasma bound and measured directly, although these methods have not yet come into general use. (2) The plasma concentration of the binding protein can be measured directly. Again this approach has not been applied widely. (3) The saturation of the binding protein can be assessed. When plasma levels of binding proteins are high, the protein will be undersaturated and less of the total hormone is free, whereas the converse occurs when plasma levels are low. This approach is now used in the case of TBG. Thus, the T_3 uptake assay measures the capacity in plasma for T_3 binding, which mostly reflects the extent of saturation of TBG. By combining knowledge of the total T_4 levels with the extent of saturation of TBG, a reasonable estimate of the effective plasma hormone concentration can be obtained (see Ch. 228). (4) An index of the free hormone concentration can sometimes be obtained by measuring its urinary excretion (or that of one of its metabolites). For instance, a small fraction (less than 1 per cent) of the secreted cortisol is excreted unchanged into the urine. A measurement of the 24-hour urine free cortisol usually provides a reasonable estimate of the integrated levels of free plasma hormone. In essence this method uses the glomerular basement membrane to separate hormone that is bound from that which is free.

SECRETION AND PRODUCTION RATES. Hormone production can be assessed by more complicated assays that involve either the injection of radioactive tracers or a combined assessment of plasma levels and hormone excretion. These techniques can circumvent many of the problems in interpretation associated with sole measurements of plasma or urinary hormones. Unfortunately, these procedures are cumbersome and not generally available.

SELECTIVE SAMPLING. Sometimes more accurate indications of a hormone-excess state and the site of hormone hypersecretion can be obtained by assaying the venous effluent from a given gland or organ. For example, in renovascular hypertension, peripheral renin levels may be normal, but sampling from a catheter inserted into the renal veins may reveal renin hypersecretion from one side and hyposecretion from the other side. Pituitary venous effluent sampling from the petrosal sinuses can be useful to determine whether ACTH hypersecretion results from a pituitary adenoma or from ectopic sites.

CLINICAL INTERPRETATION. With marked hormone excess or deficiency states, plasma or urinary hormone measurements commonly provide a clear indication of the abnormality. Nevertheless, it is important to be aware of the limitations of such tests. Hormone levels increase and decrease owing to physiologic stimuli, the presence of which must be considered when evaluating the significance of a hormone determination. For instance, plasma insulin levels should be evaluated in relation to the plasma glucose concentration, and PTH levels should be considered in relation to the serum calcium levels. Basal hormone secretion may not reflect the functional capacity of the gland, as considered in more detail under Dynamic Testing, below. Hormone levels should be evaluated in relation to target cell sensitivity. For example, in maturity onset diabetes of the obese, plasma insulin levels are often elevated but may still be inappropriately low in view of the associated insulin resistance. Since the release of many hormones is not constant, random readings can be particularly misleading. Cortisol, for example, is released episodically. In Cushing's syndrome the number of these releases is increased. Although this commonly results in an elevation of the plasma cortisol throughout the day, the morning plasma levels of this steroid may be normal. Since cortisol production integrated over a 24-hour period is increased in Cushing's syndrome, the 24-hour urine free cortisol will provide a more accurate index of whether there is cortisol hypersecretion.

Although urinary measurements can sometimes be more useful than plasma assays for obtaining an integrated assessment of the production of certain hormones (especially steroids), they cannot be used in this way for other hormones (e.g., thyroid hormones) whose metabolites are not predominantly secreted into the urine. Further, urinary metabolites of steroids can sometimes be derived from several sources (e.g., 17-ketosteroids from the adrenal and gonads), and hormone excretion can be influenced by changes in renal function. There are also circumstances in which the quantities of metabolites (e.g., of aldosterone) can be primarily affected by factors that do not affect the production of the hormone.

Sometimes the significance of hormone levels can be evaluated only by the simultaneous measurement of more than one hormone. For instance, with progressive damage to the thyroid gland and impaired release of thyroid hormones, secretion of TSH increases in a compensatory fashion such that normal plasma levels of the thyroid hormones may be maintained. By simultaneously measuring thyroid hormone levels and TSH, an indication of the compensatory response can be obtained. Such a simultaneous assessment of linked hormones can also provide an indication of the site of a primary defect. Plasma estrogens are low in ovarian failure. If ovarian failure is due to disease of the ovary, plasma gonadotropins will be elevated. If ovarian failure is secondary to pituitary or hypothalamic disease, plasma gonadotropin levels will be decreased.

Dynamic Testing. Provocative testing assesses the ability of a gland to respond to stimuli as an index of its reserve capacity. This is especially useful when plasma or urinary hormone measurements are borderline. It can also yield information about the site of the endocrine defect. In some cases, a hormone is given that stimulates the release of another hormone(s). For example, the administration of gonadotropin releasing hormone (GnRH) stimulates LH and FSH release, and TRH stimulates TSH and prolactin release. In other cases hormone production is blocked to interrupt normal feedback inhibition. Metyrapone blocks cortisol production by inhibiting 11β-hydroxylation, thereby stimulating ACTH release. The elevated ACTH levels increase the release of adrenal steroids proximal to the block (e.g., 11-deoxycortisol). A normal increase in 11-deoxycortisol signifies not only a normal adrenal but also a normal hypothalamic-pituitary axis. Sometimes a physiologic stimulus to hormone release is given. Insulin-induced hypoglycemia is used to assess the ability of cells that produce ACTH and growth hormone to respond. With endocrine hyperfunction, provocative tests can assess the extent to which the normal physiologic mechanisms that control hormone release are suppressed or the degree of autonomy of the hormone-producing tumor or hyperplastic gland. In primary aldosteronism resulting from an aldosterone-producing adenoma, the plasma renin levels that are suppressed by excessive sodium retention will not rise with acute postural, salt restriction, or diuretic stimuli. In Cushing's syndrome resulting from ectopic secretion of ACTH by a tumor, the glucocorticoid dexamethasone will not ordinarily suppress the elevated ACTH levels.

Tests That Provide Indirect Information. Useful information can frequently be obtained from laboratory tests that provide an index of the actions of the hormones (or a lack of them) or else an indication of the primary process causing the endocrine disease. Thus, it is helpful to follow the blood sugar levels in diabetes, the serum calcium levels in hyperparathyroidism, and the serum potassium levels in primary aldosteronism. Such tests often provide indices of the severity of the condition even more important than the hormone level. In conditions in which immunologic processes are important, assessment of antibody levels can be particularly helpful. Other tests provide information that is more of a corroborative nature, but which nonetheless can be useful. For instance, the serum sodium is almost always greater than 139 mEq per liter in patients with an aldosterone-producing adenoma; the plasma cholesterol tends to be high in hypothyroidism and low in hyperthyroidism; the serum potassium tends to be high in Addison's disease; the alkaline phosphatase tends to be elevated in osteomalacia; and the serum phosphate levels tend to be elevated in acromegaly.

Evaluation of the Sensitivity of Target Cells to Hormones. Suspicion of hyposensitivity to a hormone is raised when manifestations of deficiency of the hormone occur in the presence of elevated hormone levels. In type II diabetes mellitus there is hyperglycemia with hyperinsulinism; in pseudohypoparathyroidism, hypocalcemia and symptoms resulting from this with elevated PTH levels; and in pseudohermaphroditism caused by the testicular feminization syndrome, decreased androgenicity with elevated plasma testosterone levels. The existence of hyposensitivity can be confirmed by administering the hormone in question and determining the presence or extent of response, although commonly it is not necessary to do this. In some cases, such as with insulin or androgen resistance, it is possible to obtain further confirmation of the hyposensitivity state by isolating cells from the patient and measuring receptors or responses, although these techniques are not generally available. Conversely, hypersensitivity to hormones is characterized by low hormone levels relative to the response. In low-renin "essential" hypertension the adrenal glomerulosa is excessively sensitive to angiotensin II. This is

reflected by normal to elevated plasma aldosterone levels in the presence of low angiotensin II levels. This sensitivity can be documented by measuring the plasma aldosterone levels following an infusion of angiotensin.

TREATMENT OF ENDOCRINE DISEASES

For endocrine deficiency syndromes, hormones are generally administered to replace the deficiency. In general the hormone that is deficient is replaced. In some cases this is not possible or expedient, and other hormones are given that help compensate for the defect. For instance, vitamin D is given instead of PTH to treat hypoparathyroidism since it can increase the extracellular Ca^{++}. In cases in which hormone resistance is present, steps are taken when possible to alleviate this, as through diet restriction in diabetes.

In hormone-excess syndromes, a variety of approaches is used. Hyperfunctioning tumors are removed when possible, and sometimes hyperplastic glands are removed. In other cases drugs are given to block hormone production (propylthiouracil in thyrotoxicosis and bromocriptine for prolactin-producing adenomas). Antagonists such as spironolactone in primary aldosteronism due to hyperplasia can sometimes be useful.

For both excess and deficiency syndromes adjunctive therapy is frequently important. Thus multiple measures are used to treat the complicatons to diabetes mellitus, and patients with Addison's disease are cautioned to avoid stress.

SUMMARY

Endocrinology in the 1980's is an open-ended discipline for the study of molecule-mediated communication and response. New systems are still being elaborated (opioids, prostaglandins, leukotrienes, vitamin D, cell growth factors); older systems are increasingly being defined in molecular terms. In addition, the clinical abnormalities that occur are being understood and the means to evaluate them are being refined to allow more rational, accurate, and beneficial approaches to diagnosis and treatment. This introductory chapter has presented a general overview of this discipline as a background for the following chapters, which will be devoted to its specific components and the disorders that occur in human endocrine diseases.

Alberts B, Bray D, Lewis J, Raff M, Roberts K, Watson JD: Molecular Biology of the Cell. New York, Garland Publishing, Inc., 1983. *Reviews in detail recent advances in cell and molecular biology, including information on gene structure and function, protein synthesis, internalization, and hormone action.*

Cohen P: The role of protein phosphorylation in neural and hormonal control of cellular activity. Nature 296:613–620, 1982. *An overview of the role of phosphorylation in hormone action.*

Felig P, Baxter JD, Broadus AE, Frohman LA (eds.): Endocrinology and Metabolism. New York, McGraw-Hill Book Company, 1981. *Provides an extensive analysis of the topics included in this chapter. The chapters by Vaitukaitis on hormone assays, by Habner on hormone biosynthesis and secretion, and by Catt and Dufau on hormone action provide much detailed information.*

Ganong WF: The brain as an endocrine organ. Acta Physiol Lat Am 32:31–44, 1982. *Provides an excellent discussion of neuroendocrine relationships.*

Greenspan FS, Forsham PH (eds.): Basic and Clinical Endocrinology. Los Altos, Lange Medical Publications, 1983. *An excellent general reference on endocrinology and metabolism.*

Hopkins CR: The importance of the endosome in intracellular traffic. Nature 304:684–685, 1983. *A concise update of the events in hormone and receptor internalization, recycling, and degradation.*

Karin M, Haslinger A, Holtgreve H, Cathala G, Slater E, Baxter JD: Activation of a heterologous promoter in response to dexamethasone and cadmium by metallothionein gene 5′-flanking DNA. Cell 36:371–379, 1984. *Discusses recent advances in understanding the mechanisms of steroid receptor function.*

Lieberman S, Greenfield NJ, Wolfson A: A heuristic proposal for understanding steroidogenetic processes. Endocr Rev 5:128–148, 1984. *A comprehensive account of the mechanisms of steroid biosynthesis.*

Verhoven GFM, Wilson JD: The syndromes of primary hormone resistance. Metabolism 28:253, 1979. *An extensive discussion of the problems of hyposensitivity to hormones and of the clinical approaches to the diagnosis of these disorders.*

Williams RH (ed.): Textbook of Endocrinology. 6th ed. Philadelphia, W. B. Saunders Company, 1981. *An excellent general reference on endocrinology and metabolism.*

222. ENDORPHINS, ENKEPHALINS, AND OTHER OPIOID PEPTIDES: THEIR SIGNIFICANCE IN PHYSIOLOGY AND MEDICINE

Roger Guillemin

INTRODUCTION. The word *endorphin,* from (end)ogenous and m(orphin)e, was originally coined to define peptides of brain origin with biologic activities similar to those of the alkaloids of opium (morphine). The word *enkephalin* (from the Greek roots for "inside the head") will be used exclusively to define two specific pentapeptides also with morphine-like activities. The word *dynorphin* (from the Greek dyna, power) refers to a family of peptides with unusually potent opiate-like activity. The necessity and significance of this nomenclature will become evident as this chapter unfolds. All these substances are also referred to as *endogenous opioid peptides.*

The hypothesis that there should be *endogenous* opioid peptides involved in the normal biochemistry and physiology of the brain evolved from the pharmacologic concept of opiate receptors in the brain. In the early 1970's, the alkaloids of opium were shown to bind specifically to so-called opiate receptors, which have the following characteristics: (1) they are protein molecules on synaptosomes from various parts of the brain; (2) binding of the opiate molecules on these receptors is stereospecific; i.e., only those stereoisomers of the opiate series that have biologic (analgesic) activity bind to the receptor; (3) the binding of the opiates is competed for by synthetic analogue antagonists such as naloxone or naltrexone; and (4) opiate receptors exist in higher concentrations in those regions of the brain where opiates are known to exert their biologic effects as analgesic agents. It seemed clear in this early conceptualization that these opiate receptors in the brain of vertebrates did not exist solely for the binding of the alkaloids of opium. It seemed more likely that they served to recognize and bind endogenous molecules, with or without structural similarities to the opiate alkaloids, which would normally be involved in the control of pain in the central nervous system. In early studies such endogenous molecules, peptidic in nature, could indeed be demonstrated in crude extracts of the brain. The original characterization of the endogenous opioid peptides did not use the receptor affinity as an assay system, but a simple pharmacologic bioassay. It had been known for years that opiate alkaloids could affect the electrically induced contraction of the smooth muscles of thin strips of guinea pig ileum (or of mouse vas deferens) kept in a simple in vitro perfusion system, and that synthetic analogues of some of these opiate alkaloids were active in this in vitro system as antagonists in roughly the same ratios as they were antagonists of the in vivo analgesic effects of opiates. In 1975, two groups, taking advantage of such simple bioassays, isolated and characterized the first endogenous opioid peptides from brain extracts and pituitary extracts. From extracts of porcine brains, Hughes, Kosterlitz, and their colleagues characterized two pentapeptides, differing by only one amino acid at the C-terminus, and which were called Met^5-enkephalin and Leu^5-enkephalin. From extracts of the neurohypophysis plus hypothalamus, Ling, Burgus, and I characterized a hexadecapeptide which was called α-endorphin, labeled α since there was evidence in the last stages of purification that several peptides with opiate-like activity were present and would eventually have to be characterized. The remarkable observation was made that the complete amino acid sequence of the pentapeptide Met^5-enkephalin was contained as the N-terminal pentapeptide of the amino acid sequence of α-endorphin. Perhaps even more remarkably, both Met^5-enkephalin and α-endorphin were found to be fragments of β-*lipotropin,* a larger 91 amino acid polypeptide which had been found in extracts of the pituitary gland by C. H. Li and collaborators in 1964. No major biologic activity had ever been found for β-lipotropin except for a minor fat-mobilizing effect in some in vitro systems, from which its name was derived. An extraordinary flurry of excitement followed these early reports. It became very rapidly obvious that a series of fragments of the 61–91 C-terminal region of β-lipotropin would show opiate-like activity in the in vitro system and also in binding assays to synaptosomes. The most potent of all of these peptides, on a molar basis, was shown to be the complete 61–91 peptide, which had been isolated from pituitary extracts and named β-*endorphin* by C. H. Li. Figure 222–1 shows the amino acid sequences of the various endorphins which have been isolated and characterized as α, β, γ, and δ, all related fragments of the C-terminal region of β-lipotropin.

BIOSYNTHESIS. *Endorphins* are located in all cells of the intermediate lobe of the pituitary gland and also in scattered cells of the adenohypophysis, as shown by immunocytochemical techniques. These same regions also contain ACTH and β-lipotropin. It is now known that the endorphins, β-lipotropin, and ACTH are synthesized as parts of a common larger glycoprotein prohormone with a molecular weight of approximately 31,000 daltons for which a complete amino acid sequence has been proposed from DNA-recombinant studies. There is now satisfactory evidence that all endorphins are actually part of this biosynthetic pathway and that they are enzymatically processed in the pituitary cells from that common precursor (Fig. 222–1).

Immunocytochemistry (Fig. 222–2*A*) and early biochemistry have shown that endorphins are also present in some neurons in a well-defined system of the brain; their biosynthesis in

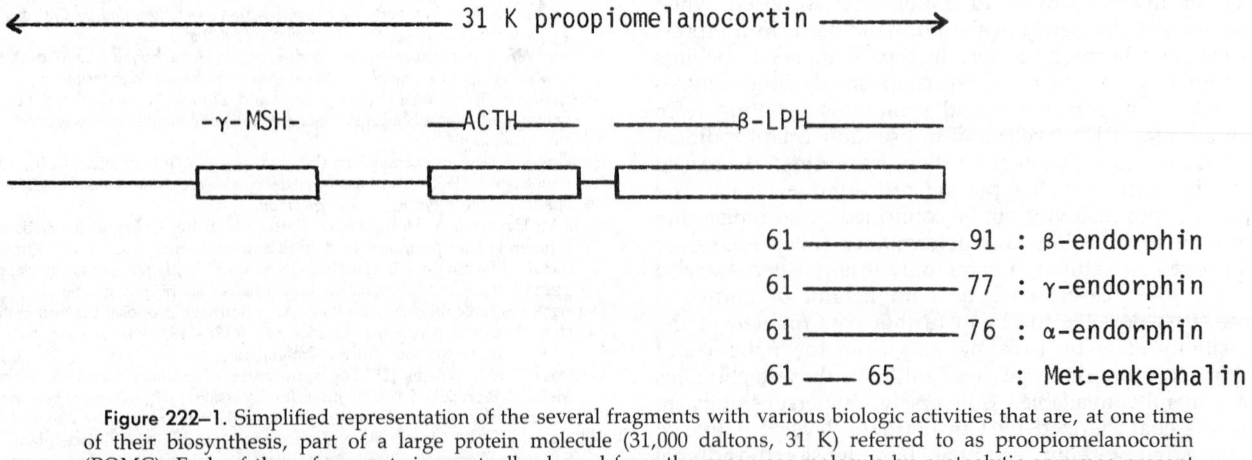

Figure 222–1. Simplified representation of the several fragments with various biologic activities that are, at one time of their biosynthesis, part of a large protein molecule (31,000 daltons, 31 K) referred to as proopiomelanocortin (POMC). Each of these fragments is eventually cleaved from the precursor molecule by proteolytic enzymes present in the pertinent pituitary cells and neurons. 61–91, etc., refer to the numbering of amino acids in the β-LPH molecule (1–91). (See Nakanishi et al. for complete details.)

these neurons is known to be identical to that in the cells of the intermediate lobe of the pituitary.

ENKEPHALINS. The biosynthetic pathway for the enkephalins is totally different. It was originally assumed that the pentapeptide enkephalins would come from the larger endorphins by enzymatic cleavage. The first evidence that enkephalins and endorphins come from different biosynthetic pathways was suggested from immunocytochemical studies showing that immunoreactive β-endorphin and enkephalins have a vastly different anatomic distribution in the brain. Further discrepancies in the biosynthetic pathways for the endorphins and the enkephalins have become evident. Immunoreactive enkephalins, not endorphins, have been observed in the gut and the adrenal medulla, in addition to the locations in the brain and spinal cord mentioned above (Fig. 222–2*B*). The adrenal medulla in particular contains several polypeptides of molecular weights ranging from 5,000 to 25,000 daltons and which, from partial amino acid sequencing, contain one or several replicates of the amino acid sequences of both Met^5-enkephalin and Leu^5-enkephalin. The enkephalin sequences in the large adrenomedullary polypeptides are usually found between pairs of basic amino acids, such as Arg-Arg or Lys-Arg, which are now recognized as the hallmark of enzymatic processing by intracellular enzymes, as in the case of proinsulin to insulin, proopiomelanocortin to ACTH, β-lipotropin, β-endorphin, etc. Moreover, several groups have now shown the presence of small peptides containing the sequence of one of the enkephalins preceded and/or followed by amino acid sequences with no relation to those of β-lipotropin. Such is the case for the recently characterized peptides *α-neoendorphin* and *dynorphin,* both of which, particularly dynorphin, appear to be endowed with extremely high opiate-like activity. They are several times more potent than β-endorphin on a molar basis, which is itself 10 to 100 times more potent than morphine on a molar basis, depending on the type of assay used. The complete nucleotide sequence of the cDNA coding for the precursor protein of each of these opioid peptides has now been established from cloning mRNA of either adrenal medulla or brain origin.

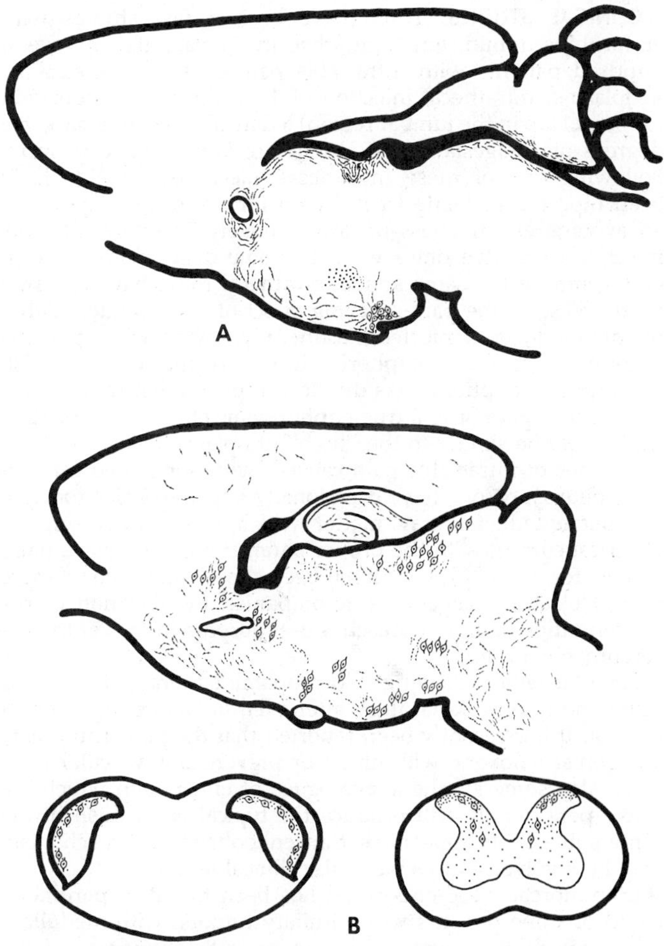

Figure 222–2. *A,* Schematic sagittal view of β-endorphin-reactive neurons and fibers in the rat brain. The neuronal perikarya in the basal hypothalamic region give rise to fibers that sweep forward along the routes indicated to enter the preoptic area and then to course within the periaqueductal region of the diencephalon and pons. *B,* Diagram of the distribution of enkephalin-containing neurons and fibers (sagittal section of the rat brain). Note also the presence of enkephalin-containing neurons in mid-brain and spinal cord.

MAPPING OF RECEPTORS FOR THE OPIOID PEPTIDES. Assays based on competition of displacement of tritiated ligands, such as tritiated morphine or normorphine, have permitted the mapping of opiate receptors in the central nervous system and other organs, while radioimmunoassays are being used to measure quantitatively the endogenous opioid peptides. Receptors for endogenous opioid peptides are mostly present in those anatomic areas of the central nervous system in which opiates have been known to exert their biologic activity as analgesic agents. These same regions correspond to those with the highest concentrations of immunoreactive endorphins or enkephalins.

Opiate receptors, as well as opioid peptides, have been found primarily in (1) the ventral hypothalamus, which is known to integrate visceral pain, a type which responds best to opiates; (2) the substantia gelatinosa of the spinal cord, also known to participate in the transmission of sensory inputs (only enkephalins, not β-endorphin, are found in the spinal cord); (3) the mid-brain nuclei corresponding to the vagus and glossopharyngeal nerves– these are known to be involved in the coughing reflex and gastric motility and secretion, events known to be affected by opiates (enkephalins and dynorphin are reported to be present in these nuclei); (4) the amygdala of the limbic system, where opiate receptors are located on nerve endings (immunocytochemistry shows the presence of β-endorphin on these nerve endings, but not in any neurons—an anatomic distribution which may be related to the participation of the limbic system in emotional behavior); and (5) the area postrema of the fourth ventricle and the periaqueductal gray matter, two regions in which electrical stimulation as well as stereotaxic placement of opiates will produce, respectively, nausea or relief from visceral pain, or both. There are also opiate receptors in the gut, and likely in the endocrine pancreas. Binding of endorphins has also been reported for some leukocytes.

In the pituitary gland the neural lobe has opiate receptors; it does not contain endorphins but appears to contain enkephalins, whereas endorphins are found in the pars intermedia and the anterior lobe, as pointed out above. The presence of opiate receptors and enkephalins in the neural lobe has been related to an enkephalinergic mechanism involved in the control of vasopressin (antidiuretic hormone) secretion.

PHYSIOLOGIC AND PATHOPHYSIOLOGIC EFFECTS OF THE OPIOID PEPTIDES. Peripheral injection of relatively high doses of enkephalins (up to 1 mg per 100 grams of body weight in laboratory animals) produces practically no observable systemic effect. This is best explained by the very short half-life of the enkephalins (a matter of seconds), owing to enzymatic degradation. A specific *enkephalinase* has been isolated and characterized. Similarly, peripheral injection of large amounts of synthetic β-endorphin does not lead to any obvious major effects in terms of analgesia. This is best explained by proposing that β-endorphin does not readily cross the blood-brain barrier, although it appears to have a rather long half-life (up to 30 minutes). Following peripheral administration of β-endorphin, there is evidence of decreased motility of the gut, with slowing of the gut transit. β-Endorphin also acutely releases growth hormone, as well as prolactin and antidiuretic hormone, probably by acting at the level of the median eminence, which is somewhat outside the blood-brain barrier. The effects on the secretion of growth hormone, prolactin, and antidiuretic hormone are not directly at the level of pituitary tissues, since β-endorphin has no such activity when added to pituitary tissues in in vitro systems.

The injection of β-endorphin directly into the cerebrospinal fluid, bypassing the blood-brain barrier (e.g., as by injection into the cisterna magna, or the lateral or third ventricle of the brain), produces far more striking biologic effects. In nanomolar quantities β-endorphin will produce, in laboratory animals, profound and complete analgesia lasting for several hours, depending on the dose administered. In rodents (rats, mice, rabbits), but not in monkeys, the same doses of β-endorphin produce an unusual state of rigid muscular immobility highly reminiscent of the clinical syndrome of catatonia. Laboratory animals also show profound hypothermia after a central administration of β-endorphin. All these effects are removed in a matter of seconds following the intravenous administration of an opiate antagonist such as naloxone. When injected intrathecally, enkephalins produce minor analgesia which is not as marked as that produced by β-endorphin and is of very short duration. The enkephalins behave more like true synaptic transmitters, which can be promptly inactivated by enzymatic mechanisms. There is no evidence of a reuptake mechanism by neurons of either enkephalins or endorphins.

SECRETION BY THE PITUITARY. β-Endorphin is secreted by the adenohypophysis simultaneously with ACTH and roughly in equimolar ratios in all acute or chronic circumstances, such as stress, which have been known to be accompanied by the classic pituitary and adrenal secretions of ACTH and glucocorticoids. This is of course best explained by the evidence presented above of the common precursor of biosynthetic origin for β-endorphin and ACTH (Fig. 222–1). Pituitary secretory granules have been shown to contain both endorphins and corticotropin, and all stimuli or secretagogues, including the hypothalamic releasing factor CRF (corticotropin-releasing factor), known to stimulate the secretion of ACTH in vivo or in vitro have been shown also to stimulate the concomitant secretion of β-endorphin. This holds true also for perturbations in the adrenal-pituitary feedback system: adrenalectomy is accompanied by chronic elevation of plasma levels of ACTH and β-endorphin, whereas acute or chronic administration of a glucocorticoid such as dexamethasone will suppress the plasma concentrations of ACTH and β-endorphin. It is of course tempting to propose, on that basis, some sort of unified theory of pituitary involvement in response to acute stress—ACTH and glucocorticoids being involved in the metabolic, somatic, stress-induced response, and the endorphins being involved with the response of the central nervous system to painful or emotionally disturbing stimuli. This would explain the age-old observation of nonresponse to, or lack of awareness of, painful stimuli at times of acute stress or emergency. If this is the case, we have to assume that pituitary endorphins, secreted during stress, somehow pass directly into the central nervous system, since intravenous injection of large amounts of synthetic β-endorphin produces no evidence of major analgesia. Pituitary endorphins could enter the third ventricle by upward flow in the hypothalamohypophyseal portal vessels. The matter is far from being settled.

In animal studies relatively small concentrations of β-endorphin injected directly into the arterial circulation of the pancreas stimulate the secretion of insulin and glucagon and concomitantly inhibit the secretion of somatostatin. These results must be mediated by opiate receptors, since they are sensitive to the administration of the antagonist naloxone.

The enkephalins are probably true neurotransmitters, particularly in the afferent systems for pain in the spinal cord. Evidence for this role is based on their size, the short duration of their biologic activity, and their location, as observed by refined immunocytochemistry. The role of the endorphins in the brain appears to be far more complex. The long duration of the effects of a single administration of β-endorphin in the central nervous system is completely different from the brief effects of classic synaptic transmitters, and is reminiscent of the role and effects of hormones.

An important question for pharmacologists, physiologists, and clinicians has been whether chronic administration of β-endorphin and/or enkephalins would lead to tolerance regarding their analgesic effects as well as to addiction, in analogy with the opiate alkaloids. The biologic half-life of the enkephalins is so short and their specific activity so limited that the question has little significance in their case. In the case of β-endorphin, which is far more potent on a molar basis than the enkephalins (approximately 100-fold), the original question must be modified by the additional requisite that it pertain to β-endorphin injected directly into the brain tissue or into cerebrospinal fluid. Studies both in laboratory animals and in a few clinical cases in which β-endorphin was injected intravenously have led to no reliable results, most likely because of the fact that β-endorphin does not readily cross the blood-brain barrier. When β-endorphin is injected repeatedly every 24 hours into the cisterna of laboratory rats for as long as ten days, there is no obvious decrease in the profound analgesic activity of the same dose of the peptide. This would imply that tolerance to the analgesic effect of endorphin, when it is injected into the cerebrospinal fluid in these relatively short studies, is absent or minimal. Reports are conflicting regarding addiction of laboratory animals to chronic doses of β-endorphin.

CLINICAL STUDIES. There have been a few studies with endorphins administered intrathecally in patients. In several hundred patients with intractable pain caused by metastatic neoplasms, intrathecal injection of 1 to 3 mg of β-endorphin (by spinal tap in the lumbar region) led in all cases to remarkable degrees of analgesia in the absence of any additive therapy. Following one of these intrathecal injections, patients have been reported as being free of pain for up to five days, with an average effectiveness of approximately 72 hours. Patients injected up to five times with the same dose of synthetic β-endorphin by the same spinal intrathecal route have reported no decrease of the pain-relieving effect of the peptide. With 3 mg of β-endorphin injected intrathecally, several of the patients reported a sense of euphoria. It is difficult to distinguish whether this euphoria was due to complete relief from severe and chronic pain or to a true euphorigenic effect of the peptide that would be similar to the "high" of opiates.

In cases of intractable pain caused by disseminated carcinomas, neurosurgeons have occasionally implanted electrodes in the periaqueductal gray matter which, upon delivering an electrical current with the proper parameters, will relieve pain, usually for up to 24 hours. It has been shown that such effective central electric analgesia is accompanied by elevation of the concentration of immunoreactive β-endorphin in the ventricular cerebrospinal fluid.

Some diabetics receiving chlorpropamide therapy develop an acute and intense facial flush after even moderate ingestion of alcohol. It has recently been reported that the powerful opiate antagonist naloxone will inhibit or prevent this vascular reaction. Also some synthetic analogues of enkephalin which are active peripherally will produce the typical facial flush in the same subjects. It appears that an enkephalinergic mechanism may be involved in this particular clinical feature.

Immunoreactive β-endorphin has been found in peripheral blood of some patients with pituitary tumors, with medullary carcinoma of the thyroid, or with oat-cell carcinomas of the lung. In all cases the immunoreactive β-endorphin was detected along with immunoreactive ACTH and usually other peptides, such as calcitonin or somatostatin. It has been proposed that the measurement of plasma immunoreactive β-endorphin could serve as a marker of the presence of neoplastic tissues.

There have been reports that peripheral administration of β-endorphin in large amounts (milligrams) has led to dramatic improvements in psychiatric patients with schizophrenia or manic-depressive psychosis. These reports, occasionally marked by sensationalism, have not been confirmed by other investigators. First of all, as noted above, β-endorphin given peripherally enters the central nervous system to a very limited degree, if at all. Furthermore, the experimental administration of the powerful opiate antagonist naloxone, which readily passes into the central nervous system, has led to conflicting reported results in schizophrenia. There have also been reports that levels of immunoreactive endorphins in the cerebrospinal fluid of schizophrenics in acute exacerbation or remission phases vary in relation to the clinical status.

None of these provocative and preliminary observations has led to any consensus. There are first of all major methodologic problems; there are also major problems in the clinical interpretations. The concept, however, that molecules such as the opioid peptides could be involved in the maintenance of normal behavior and that alterations in the normal metabolism of these opioid peptides could be accompanied by abnormalities in behavior is of such heuristic significance that it should not be discarded on the basis of preliminary conflicting evidence. One of the major requisites for such studies will, in my opinion, be a much larger number and variety of studies in man than have actually been available so far.

CONCLUSIONS. There is little doubt that endogenous opioid peptides are involved in the normal neurophysiologic processing of painful stimuli, particularly those known to be processed by the visceral system. It is possible that endorphins and/or enkephalins are involved in the normal processing of other sensory stimuli: immunoreactive enkephalins have recently been reported in some amacrine cells of the retina, and immunoreactive endorphins have been measured in extracts of peripheral nerves such as the vagus or the sciatic nerve. The role, if any, of endorphins of pituitary origin is not clear and remains to be investigated further.

Proposed roles of the brain endorphins in the central nervous system biochemistry of normal, hence also abnormal, behavior remain to be demonstrated. Interrelationships between the opioid peptides and the classic neurotransmitters (acetylcholine, dopamine, catecholamines) are just beginning to be explored. There is no dearth of working hypotheses, many of profound heuristic significance, to approach and carry out these studies.

Bloom F, Battenberg E, Rossier J, Ling N, Guillemin R: Neurons containing β-endorphin in rat brain exist separately from those containing enkephalin: Immunocytochemical studies. Proc Natl Acad Sci (USA) 75:1591, 1978. *Immunocytochemistry with the peroxidase method using antisera against β-endorphin and enkephalin, with several plates.*

Bradbury AF, Smith DG, Snell CR, Birdsall NJM, Hulme EC: C-fragment of lipotropin has a high affinity for brain opiate receptors. Nature 260:793, 1976. *Technical report on the opiate-like activity, assessed by binding to synaptosomes, of the C-terminal fragment 61–91 of the ovine pituitary β-lipotropin.*

Goldstein A: Opioid peptides (endorphins) in the pituitary and brain. Science 193:1081, 1976. *A general review by one of the earliest pharmacologists to have proposed the existence of specific opiate receptors. Covers that concept and the recent isolation of enkephalins and endorphins.*

Gubler U, Seeburg P, Hoffman BJ, Gage LP, Udenfriend S: Molecular cloning establishes proenkephalin as precursor of enkephalin-containing peptides. Nature 295:206, 1982. *The complete primary structure of the precursor protein for both Met- and Leu-enkephalins deduced from the nucleotide sequence of the corresponding cDNA of bovine adrenal origin.*

Hökfelt T, Johansson O, Ljungdahl A, Lundberg M, Schultsberg M: Peptidergic neurones. Nature 284:515, 1980. *An elegant and comprehensive review by one of the best groups of immunocytologists in the world. Includes discussions of anatomic localizations, relations between various "networks" of peptides containing neurons, and relations with the classic catecholaminergic systems. Discusses peptidergic neurons in the brain, the spinal cord, the gastrointestinal tract, and other non-central nervous system locations.*

Hughes J, Smith T, Kosterlitz H, Fothergill L, Morgan B, Morris H: Identification of two related pentapeptides from the brain with potent opiate agonist activity. Nature 258:577, 1975. *The original technical report on the isolation and characterization (amino acid sequence) of the two enkephalins, with the statement about the relationship between their amino acid sequence and that of a region of pituitary β-lipotropin.*

Kakidani H, Furutani Y, Takahashi H, Noda M, Morimoto Y, Hirose T, Asai M, Inayama S, Numa S: Cloning and sequence analysis of cDNA for porcine β-neo-endorphin/dynorphin precursor. Nature 298:245, 1982. *A technical report describing how the primary structure of a precursor protein that contains β-neo-endorphin, dynorphin, and a third leu-enkephalin sequence with a carboxyl extension was deduced from the nucleotide sequence of cloned DNA to the porcine hypothalamic mRNA encoding it.*

Leslie RDG, Pyke DA: Chlorpropamide-alcohol flushing: A dominantly inherited trait associated with diabetes. Br Med J 2:1519, 1978. *Case reports and proposal of the hypothesis.*

Lewis RV, Stern AS, Kimura S, Rossier J, Stein S, Udenfriend S: An about 50,000-dalton protein in adrenal medulla: A common precursor of [Met]- and [Leu]-enkephalin. Science 208:1459, 1980. *The first technical report on the presence in the adrenal medulla of a large protein (50,000 daltons), which, upon partial tryptic digestion, generates peptide-fragments with the (characterized) amino acid sequence of Met- and Leu-enkephalin, and also has opiate-like biologic activities.*

Li CH, Chung D: Isolation and structure of an untriakontapeptide with opiate activity from camel pituitary glands. Proc Natl Acad Sci (USA) 73:1145, 1976. *Technical report of the isolation and characterization (amino acid sequence) of a peptide from camel pituitary glands corresponding to the fragment 61–91 of β-lipotropin, with bioassay data showing its opiate-like activity.*

Ling N, Burgus R, Guillemin R: Isolation, primary structure and synthesis of α-endorphin and γ-endorphin, two peptides of hypothalamic-hypophysial origin with morphinomimetic activity. Proc Natl Acad Sci (USA) 73:3942, 1976. *The original technical report on the isolation and characterization (amino acid sequence) of the first two molecules of hypothalamic and pituitary origin, isolated on the basis of their opiate-like activity in a bioassay, and different from the enkephalins.*

Mains RE, Eipper BA, Ling N: Common precursor to corticotropins and endorphins. Proc Natl Acad Sci (USA) 74:3014, 1977. *The original technical description of the existence of multiple sizes of immunoreactive ACTH (adrenocorticotropin) and lipotropin, with the evidence that the largest molecule (31,000 daltons) is immunoreactive with both antisera to ACTH and lipotropin (more exactly β-endorphin) from a tumoral cell line of mouse pituitary origin.*

Nakanishi S, Inoue A, Kita T, Nakamura M, Chang ACY, Cohen SN, Numa S: Nucleotide sequence of cloned c-DNA for bovine corticotropin-β-lipotropin precursor. Nature 278:423, 1979. *The first report of the nucleotide sequence of cloned c-DNA for bovine corticotropin-β-lipotropin precursor, accompanied by the proposed amino acid sequence of the whole protein precursor (now called pro-opio-melano-cortin)—includes the proposal of the existence of a new form of melanotropin-γ-MSHs.*

223. PROSTAGLANDINS, THROMBOXANE A_2, AND LEUKOTRIENES

John A. Oates

Thromboxane A_2, prostacyclin, prostaglandin D_2, prostaglandin E_2, and the leukotrienes are potent compounds which participate in pathologic processes as diverse as platelet aggregation and asthma. They have in common a biosynthesis that originates with the oxygenation of arachidonic acid, but their structures and their actions differ markedly. Although there is considerable variety in the possible metabolic pathways for arachidonic acid within the body, specific cells are highly selective in the biotransformation of this fatty acid. This selectivity in arachidonic acid metabolism usually can be linked to a function of the cell.

THE CYCLOOXYGENASE PATHWAY (Fig. 223–1). The biotransformation of arachidonic acid into thromboxane A_2, prostacyclin, prostaglandin D_2, (PGD_2), PGE_2, and $PGF_{2\alpha}$ is initiated by a common enzyme, the *fatty acid cyclooxygenase* (Fig. 223–1). This enzyme catalyzes the attachment of molecular oxygen at C_{11} of arachidonic acid. There is subsequent rearrangement to a cyclic endoperoxide in which a dioxygen bridge links C_9 and C_{11}. The formation of the endoperoxide is closely coupled to the introduction of a second oxygen molecule at C_{15} to yield a 15-hydroperoxy cyclic endoperoxide (PGG_2). The subscript 2 in this and other prostaglandin nomenclature refers to the two double bonds in the structure. The cyclooxygenase enzyme is inhibited by aspirin, indomethacin, and the other nonsteroidal anti-inflammatory drugs (see Fig. 223–3). A hydroperoxidase converts the 15-hydroperoxy group of PGG_2 to a hydroxyl, yielding the 15-hydroxy-endoperoxide PGH_2 in a reaction that liberates a free radical as a byproduct. PGH_2 is the common precursor of PGD_2, PGE_2, $PGF_{2\alpha}$, thromboxane A_2, and prostacyclin (PGI_2). The enzymes which catalyze the metabolism of PGH_2 to these active products confer cellular specificity. PGH_2 is a labile intermediate which undergoes nonenzymatic breakdown in water. However, in cells which contain an appropriate

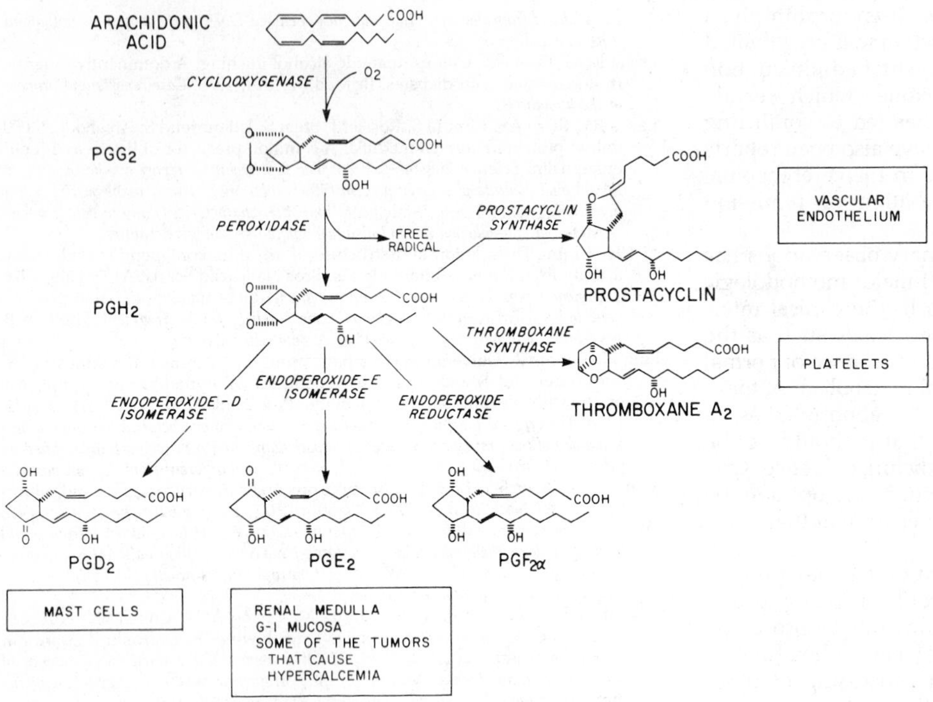

Figure 223–1. The cyclooxygenase pathway of arachidonic acid metabolism leading to the synthesis of prostaglandins.

enzyme for metabolizing PGH_2, it is rapidly converted to a specific prostaglandin, as noted below.

Thromboxane A_2. Thromboxane A_2 is the predominant product of arachidonic acid in the platelet and is formed from PGH_2 in a reaction catalyzed by thromboxane synthase (Fig. 223–1). Thromboxane A_2 is a potent aggregating agent which is released in a burst at the initiation of platelet aggregation (see Ch. 166). The inhibition of platelet aggregation by aspirin results from blockade of thromboxane A_2 biosynthesis. Thromboxane A_2 is quite labile, undergoing nonenzymatic hydrolysis to a relatively inactive product, thromboxane B_2, with a half-life of 30 seconds.

In addition to causing platelet aggregation, thromboxane A_2 contracts arterial smooth muscle, including that of the coronary and cerebral arteries.

Prostacyclin. Disruption of the vascular endothelium leads to the adherence of platelets, which release thromboxane A_2 locally to signal neighboring platelets to join in the aggregation process. Clearly some mechanism is required to restrain the further recruitment of platelets short of aggregation of the total body pool. One restraint that normal vascular endothelium imposes on the aggregation process is the release of prostacyclin, which is a potent inhibitor of aggregation. Prostacyclin is the essentially exclusive product of PGH_2 metabolism in the vascular endothelium and is produced in far smaller quantities by other cells, such as macrophages. It also is labile in aqueous solution, with a half-life of about three minutes, undergoing nonenzymatic degradation to 6-keto-$PGF_{1\alpha}$.

The inhibition of platelet aggregation by prostacyclin is accompanied by a marked rise in the concentration of cyclic AMP in the platelet. Current evidence suggests that this cyclic nucleotide mediates the inhibition of aggregation. Prostacyclin is a general inhibitor of platelet aggregation, blocking aggregation evoked by a variety of stimuli, including thrombin, ADP, and epinephrine. This is in contrast to cyclooxygenase inhibitors, such as aspirin, which inhibit the aggregation evoked by only a subset of specific stimuli. Thus, aspirin will block the aggregation evoked by collagen and will shift the dose response curve to ADP, but its effect is readily overridden by thrombin. Thrombin-induced aggregation can take place by a mechanism that is independent of thromboxane A_2.

The inhibition of aggregation by prostacyclin is illustrated by its ability to prevent almost completely the adhesion and aggregation of platelets in extracorporeal circuits such as pump oxygenators and hemodialysis units. In contrast, heparin and aspirin are relatively ineffective in preventing the trapping of platelets in extracorporeal circuits and the release of platelet aggregates from their surfaces. Prostacyclin also will prevent the formation of platelet aggregates evoked by vascular trauma or marked vascular stenosis.

In addition to inhibiting platelet aggregation, prostacyclin is a vasodilator. Its actions on platelets as well as any vasodilator role that it may have are local phenomena, for the production of prostacyclin under normal circumstances is not great enough to exert vasodilator or antiplatelet effects by acting as a circulating hormone.

Prostaglandin D_2. Prostaglandin D_2 is the principal cyclooxygenase product of arachidonic acid produced by the *mast cell* (see Fig. 438–1). Its formation from PGH_2 is catalyzed by the endoperoxide D_2 isomerase. It is released from the mast cell along with histamine when antigens bind to IgE on the mast cell surface. Like histamine, PGD_2 is a vasodilator. Its precise role in the normal immunologic responses mediated by the mast cell is unknown. Patients with systemic mastocytosis have mast cell infiltration in multiple body organs (see Ch. 438). Massive overproduction of prostaglandin D_2 participates along with histamine in the episodes of flushing, hypotension, and even shock that some patients with mastocytosis experience.

Prostaglandin E_2. The metabolism of PGH_2 to PGE_2 is catalyzed by the endoperoxide E_2 isomerase in several tissues, including the renal medulla and gastrointestinal mucosa. PGE_2 is a vasodilator. Its other actions include inhibition of gastric acid secretion and inhibition of renal tubular sodium reabsorption.

A number of solid tumors are known to produce hypercalcemia by an endocrine mechanism (see Ch. 173). In a subset of these, the hypercalcemia is evoked by an overproduction of PGE_2 by the tumor. PGE_2 evokes hypercalcemia in these patients by stimulating osteoclastic activity. The excessive production of PGE_2 can be quantified by measuring one of the urinary metabolites of this prostaglandin. Administration of aspirin or indomethacin in doses sufficient to reduce PGE_2 metabolite excretion will lower serum calcium substantially in these patients. Such a beneficial effect on serum calcium is seen only when the tumor is acting through a humoral mechanism and not after extensive metastases to bone, in which case local mechanisms for hypercalcemia supervene.

Prostaglandin $F_{2\alpha}$. $PGF_{2\alpha}$ is formed from PGH_2 via the action of endoperoxide reductase. It also is formed as a metabolite of PGD_2. $PGF_{2\alpha}$ stimulates uterine and bronchial smooth muscle and is a vasoconstrictor in some vascular beds. Neither a unique site of its formation nor a clearly defined pathophysiologic role for $PGF_{2\alpha}$ has been found. The administration of this prostaglandin is employed therapeutically to induce labor.

Additional Products. In addition to initiating the oxygenation of arachidonic acid to thromboxane A_2 and the prostaglandins, the cyclooxygenase enzyme also initiates conversion of other polyunsaturated fatty acids to corresponding oxygenated metabolites. Eicosatrienoic acid (20:3ω6) undergoes cyclooxygenation to metabolites with structures corresponding to those formed from arachidonic acid, with the exception that they have only one double bond (Δ^{13}) and are designated PGE_1, $PGE_{1\alpha}$, and so forth. Eicosapentaenoic acid (20:5ω3), a polyunsaturated fatty acid prevalent in the marine food chain, is transformed by the cyclooxygenase to corresponding metabolites with three double bonds ($\Delta^{5, 13, 17}$), e.g., PGI_3. When dietary arachidonic acid is substituted with 20:5ω3, the biosynthesis of proaggregatory thromboxanes is reduced, in part because 20:5ω3 is not efficiently converted to thromboxane A_3. This leads to reduced aggregation of platelets and prolongation of bleeding time.

FUNCTIONS OF ARACHIDONIC ACID METABOLITES. The effects of cyclooxygenase inhibitors that can be replicated by several of the drugs in this class are assumed to result from blocking the formation of one or more of the cyclooxygenase metabolites. By this approach, the functions of the metabolites of arachidonic acid, whose formation is catalyzed by cyclooxygenase, can be inferred even though the specific metabolite mediating the function is not known with certainty.

Fever. Salicylates were introduced to medicine as antipyretics, and all cyclooxygenase inhibitors will attenuate fever. The cyclooxygenase metabolite that mediates pyrexia is not known.

Inflammation. The major use of aspirin and the nonsteroidal anti-inflammatory drugs is for the treatment of noninfectious inflammatory disorders such as arthritis. The specific inflammatory mediator has not been ascertained.

The Gastric Mucosa. Certain prostaglandins, particularly PGE_2, will increase gastric mucosal blood flow and block pentagastrin-evoked acid secretion. In addition, they seem to exert a "protective" effect on the gastric mucosa through mechanisms that are unclear. When these prostaglandin-mediated effects are abolished by cyclooxygenase inhibitors, gastric erosion and ulceration may result as major adverse effects of this class of drugs. There is evidence that their deleterious effect on the gastric mucosa is enhanced if the gastric mucosa is directly exposed to large concentrations of cyclooxygenase inhibitor in addition to the lesser concentrations delivered via the circulation.

The Release of Renin. The adrenergic nervous system is a major regulator of the release of renin. An additional nonadrenergic mechanism also contributes to the control of the release of renin, as for example in renal artery stenosis. Most if not all of the nonadrenergic regulation of renin release is mediated by a cyclooxygenase metabolite of arachidonic acid. As such, the release of renin may be partially blocked by cyclooxygenase inhibitors such as indomethacin. The reduction of renin by cyclooxygenase inhibition has obvious implications in the diagnostic application of renin measurements. Furthermore, the associated decrease in aldosterone production may be deleterious for patients who are prone to hyperkalemia.

Renal Function. Inhibition of cyclooxygenase has little effect on the glomerular filtration rate in normal persons. In various disease states associated with impaired renal function, inhibition of cyclooxygenase will decrease glomerular filtration rate. Substantial diminution in glomerular filtration may be seen after the administration of cyclooxygenase inhibitors to patients with the nephropathy of systemic lupus erythematosus, Bartter's syndrome, cardiac failure, and cirrhosis. In patients with cardiac failure, the reduction in glomerular filtration rate together with inhibition of renin-mediated aldosterone production can lead to hyperkalemia.

Prostaglandin E_2, the predominant prostaglandin produced in the renal medulla, is natriuretic. In part its natriuretic action may be due to inhibition of sodium reabsorption in the distal tubule. Administration of a cyclooxygenase inhibitor will cause sodium retention for a day or two, following which sodium balance is restored despite continued treatment with the agent. This is of little consequence in normal persons, but may be of importance in those in whom sodium retention has deleterious hemodynamic effects.

Indomethacin and other cyclooxygenase inhibitors enhance the antidiuretic action of vasopressin, implicating an arachidonic acid metabolite in the elimination of water. The extent to which this is a primary action of the cyclooxygenase metabolite on water transport versus an increase in the medullary sodium content (driving force for sodium reabsorption) is not clear. Indomethacin will diminish the excessive water elimination in nephrogenic diabetes insipidus and in lithium-induced diabetes insipidus.

Patent Ductus Arteriosus. In the neonatal period, closure of a persistently patent ductus arteriosus can be achieved by inhibition of the cyclooxygenase with indomethacin. This implies that some (unknown) cyclooxygenase metabolite contributes to ductal patency. The E prostaglandins dilate the ductus, and infusion of PGE_1 has been used to maintain an open ductus in infants with pulmonary atresia and other disorders in which ductal patency is advantageous until operative intervention can be accomplished.

Asthma and Anaphylaxis Evoked by Aspirin. In some patients with bronchial asthma (about 10 per cent) aspirin will provoke attacks of bronchoconstriction. These attacks may be very severe and can be induced with small doses of aspirin, as well as with all of the nonsteroidal anti-inflammatory drugs. The bronchoconstriction therefore does not result from an allergy to aspirin, but from some consequence of cyclooxygenase inhibition. This could be the reduced formation of a prostaglandin that normally restrains the release of mediators that cause bronchoconstriction, or the shunting of arachidonic acid into other pathways such as that leading to the leukotrienes (see below).

In a subset of patients with recurrent anaphylaxis, aspirin and other cyclooxygenase inhibitors also act as triggers for the episodes of hypotension, flushing, tachycardia, and dyspnea. Some of these patients have systemic mastocytosis as an underlying disorder. Anaphylaxis provoked by cyclooxygenase inhibitors may be severe and even fatal.

THE LIPOXYGENASE PATHWAY (Fig. 223–2). In addition to the cyclooxygenase pathway described above, oxygenation of arachidonic acid also can proceed via lipoxygenation. The lipoxygenation reactions result in the insertion of an oxygen molecule at a carbon adjacent to one of the double bonds, yielding a hydroperoxy-arachidonic acid. These oxygenations are not blocked by aspirin or indomethacin. The important biologic implications of lipoxygenation emerged from studies of this pathway in leukocytes, in which a major route of arachidonic acid metabolism is 5-lipoxygenation (Fig. 223–2). The initial reaction product is 5-hydroperoxy-eicosatetraenoic acid (5-HPETE) which undergoes further transformation to either 5-hydroxy-eicosatetraenoic acid (5-HETE) or to a 5,6 epoxide which is termed leukotriene A_4 because of the conjugated triene structure that results from the formation of the 5,6 epoxide. The subscript 4 refers to the four double bonds in the structure. Leukotriene A_4 is a precursor for several other compounds with a conjugated triene structure. One of these is leukotriene B_4 (5,12-dihydroxy-eicosatetraenoic acid). Leukotriene B_4 is a potent chemotactic agent for leukocytes. Leukotriene A_4 also undergoes biotransformation to a series of compounds which constitute the mixture previously known as the "slow-reacting

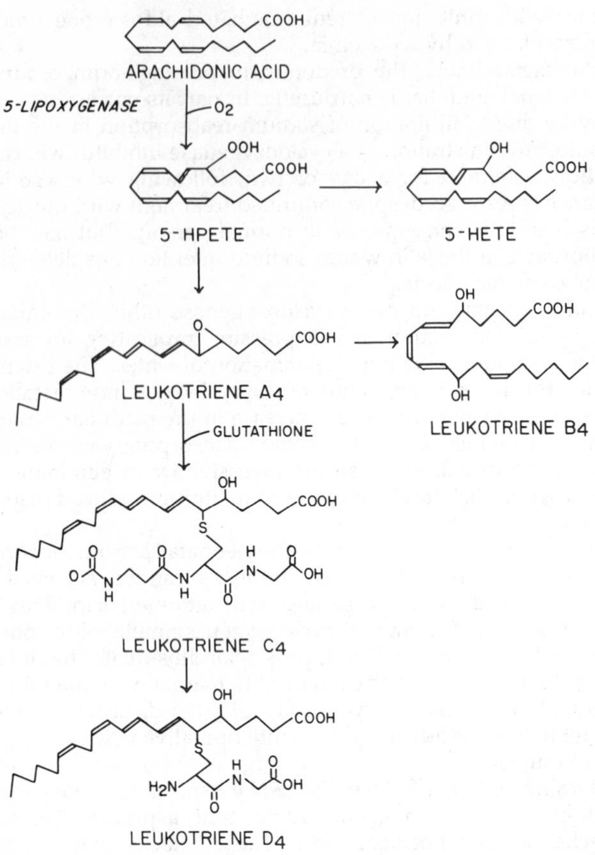

Figure 223–2. The lipoxygenase pathway of arachidonic acid metabolism leading to the formation of the leukotrienes.

substances of anaphylaxis" (SRS-A). Biosynthesis of SRS-A results from reaction of leukotriene A_4 with glutathione to form the glutathionyl adduct leukotriene C_4. Leukotriene C_4 undergoes further biotransformation by γ-glutamyl transpeptidase to yield the cysteinyl-glycine adduct, which is termed leukotriene D_4. Leukotriene D_4 is an extremely potent bronchoconstrictor, having an action approximately 1000 times the molar potency of histamine. In addition, leukotriene D_4 evokes increased vascular permeability. Leukotriene C_4 is a somewhat less potent bronchoconstrictor. Leukotriene C_4 also is a pulmonary vasoconstrictor, an action blocked by indomethacin, suggesting that this vasoconstriction may be mediated via the release of thromboxane A_2 by leukotriene C_4. There is considerable evidence that leukotrienes C_4 and D_4 contribute to antigen-evoked bronchoconstriction.

REGULATION OF BIOSYNTHESIS. None of the arachidonic acid oxygenation products described above are stored for subsequent release from cells; rather, their release is equivalent to biosynthesis. The controlling step for biosynthesis is the liberation of free arachidonic acid from lipid esters (Fig. 223–3). This has been elucidated most clearly in the platelet, where arachidonic acid is liberated from phosphatidyl inositol by an initial reaction with phospholipase C followed by diglyceride lipase to yield free arachidonic acid. In conjunction with the liberation of arachidonic acid during platelet aggregation, phosphatidyl inositol stores are depleted. It is likely that there are cells in which acyl hydrolases other than phospholipase C regulate the release of free arachidonic acid. In most instances, the liberation of arachidonic acid from phospholipids is calcium dependent.

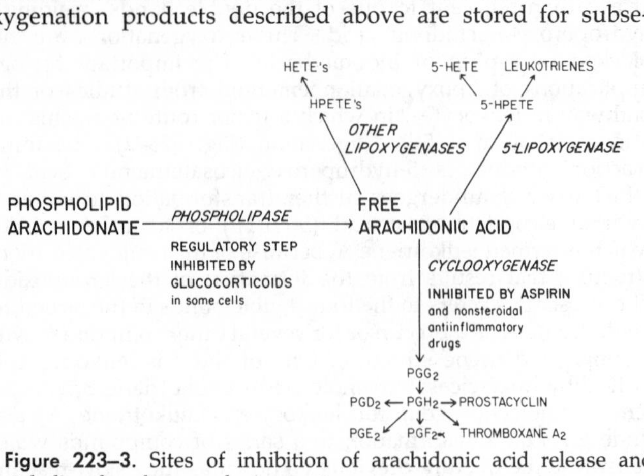

Figure 223–3. Sites of inhibition of arachidonic acid release and metabolism by pharmacologic agents.

PHARMACOLOGIC INHIBITION OF BIOSYNTHESIS. It is possible to inhibit the fatty acid cyclooxygenase clinically with a number of drugs, including aspirin, salicylic acid, indomethacin, phenylbutazone, oxyphenbutazone, ibuprofen, fenoprofen, tolmetin, piroxicam, sulfinpyrazone, and sulindac. There are important differences among these drugs, however. Whereas indomethacin and the other nonsteroidal anti-inflammatory drugs are competitive inhibitors of the cyclooxygenase in vivo and therefore inhibit for a limited duration, aspirin covalently acetylates the enzyme, producing irreversible inhibition. As the platelet is incapable of synthesizing new enzymes, the irreversible inhibition of platelet cyclooxygenase by aspirin persists throughout the life span of the circulating platelet. Because small doses of aspirin (approximately 300 mg) almost completely inhibit the platelet cyclooxygenase, a daily dose in this range is sufficient to maintain a high degree of cyclooxygenase inhibition. Other tissues, including the vascular endothelium, can synthesize new cyclooxygenase, and the effect of low dose aspirin on these nonplatelet sites is more transient. Thus it seems likely that a low dose of aspirin would be preferable if the aim is to inhibit platelet thromboxane A_2 production with a less protracted effect on prostacyclin synthesis by the endothelium, and indeed, 324 mg of aspirin daily has been shown to reduce the incidence of myocardial infarction and death in men with unstable angina. Another tissue that may be selectively affected by the irreversible inhibition of cyclooxygenase by aspirin is the mucosa of the stomach and duodenum. If aspirin is given in a pharmaceutical preparation that undergoes dissolution in the stomach, the mucosa is exposed briefly to larger concentrations of aspirin and thereby to a higher degree of irreversible inhibition of the cyclooxygenase than are tissues which receive the drug through the systemic circulation. In contrast, salicylic acid and other competitive inhibitors of cyclooxygenase exert a greater inhibition on the gastric mucosa for only the brief period in which they are present in the stomach. Sulfinpyrazone and sulindac are prodrugs that inhibit the cyclooxygenase only slightly, but undergo metabolic transformation by the intestinal flora to potent cyclooxygenase inhibitors. Effects of these prodrugs on gastric mucosa are equivalent to those at other tissue sites.

Sharing the common action of inhibiting cyclooxygenase, this class of drugs is composed of a diverse array of chemical structures, and their therapeutic actions and adverse effects are not all identical.

In some cells, the liberation of arachidonic acid from phospholipids is inhibited by glucocorticoids, but this is not the universal effect of glucocorticoids in all cell types. Release of arachidonic acid during platelet aggregation, for example, is not inhibited by glucocorticoids. In those cells in which glucocorticoids do inhibit arachidonic acid mobilization, the formation of both cyclooxygenase and lipoxygenase products is inhibited, whereas the effects of aspirin-like drugs are limited to blocking the cyclooxygenase pathway. This provides an attractive hypothesis for the broader range of anti-inflammatory effects of glucocorticoids, the proof of which is still forthcoming.

Kuehl FA Jr, Egan RW: Prostaglandins, arachidonic acid and inflammation. Science 210:978, 1980. *A review of the metabolism of arachidonic acid as it relates to inflammation, including information on the action of anti-inflammatory drugs. The references provide an excellent entrée to the original articles in this area.*

Moncada S, Vane JR: Mode of action of aspirin-like drugs. Adv Intern Med 24:1, 1979.
Moncada S, Vane JR: Prostacyclin and the cardiovascular system. Adv Prostaglandin Thromboxane Res 6:43, 1980. *Overviews of the biosynthesis and pharmacology of prostacyclin by the discoverers of this prostaglandin.*
Samuelsson B: Leukotrienes: Mediators of immediate hypersensitivity and inflammation. Science 220:568, 1983. *A review describing the structure and biosynthesis of the leukotrienes (slow-reacting substances of anaphylaxis).*

224. NEUROENDOCRINE REGULATION AND ITS DISORDERS

Lawrence A. Frohman

NEUROENDOCRINE REGULATION

The central nervous system exerts profound regulatory control over hormonal secretion and metabolic events. The integration of this control is focused in the region of the ventral hypothalamus and consists of three major systems:

1. A classic neuronal pathway traveling through the base of the brain, through the autonomic nervous system pathways of the spinal cord, and terminating in the liver, gastrointestinal tract, pancreas, adrenal medullae, and adipose tissue. The pathway, which consists of bidirectional fibers, is involved in neurometabolic regulation, and its greatest effects are on blood glucose and fatty acid regulation and on metabolic homeostasis, i.e., appetite control (satiety), temperature control (thermoregulation), and body fat stores.
2. A neurosecretory pathway from the anterior hypothalamus that traverses the floor of the ventral hypothalmus and pituitary stalk and terminates in specialized neuronal elements called pituicytes, located in the posterior pituitary. The system is involved in osmoregulation, through the production of vasopressin, and in parturition and nursing, through the secretion of oxytocin. A detailed discussion of this system is provided in Ch. 226.
3. A neuroendocrine system involving clusters of peptide- and monoamine-secreting cells in the anterior and mid-portion of the ventral hypothalamus whose products are transported along nerve fibers to terminals in the outer layer of the median eminence, from where they are released into the capillary vessels of the hypothalamic-hypophyseal portal system and transported to the pituitary to regulate the secretion of the hormones of the anterior pituitary.

Neuroendocrine Anatomy

In contrast to tissues outside the central nervous system and even within many portions of the brain, much of the functional morphology of the hypothalamus cannot be precisely defined in terms of its anatomic structure. The neurometabolic function of the hypothalamus can be divided into those components associated with the sympathetic or the parasympathetic branches of the autonomic nervous system. Medial sympathetic and lateral parasympathetic zones of the hypothalamus have been defined on the basis of extensive studies in laboratory animals and pathologic findings in patients with anatomically defined diseases of the hypothalamus who exhibit disorders of neurometabolic regulation (i.e., temperature control and nutrient homeostasis). However, the cellular elements (neuronal perikarya) involved in a particular function cannot be precisely localized to one specific nuclear region. Neurons involved in the inhibitory control of food intake (satiety) are located more medially, and those responsible for appetite stimulation are located more laterally. This distinction probably explains why destructive lesions of the hypothalamus, which frequently occur in the midline, are more likely to result in obesity than in starvation. A second reason is that fibers from the hypothalamic controlling centers cross the midline, and thus bilateral hypothalamic destruction is necessary for interruption of normal regulatory control.

Neurons of the neurohypophyseal system represent a more anatomically distinct entity with cell bodies located in the paraventricular and supraoptic hypothalamic nuclei. Within these areas there are also neurons producing a variety of other neuropeptides. The posterior pituitary hormones, oxytocin and vasopressin, are synthesized in the cell bodies as part of a precursor molecule, which also contains a specific carrier protein (neurophysin), and transported along axonal fibers through the ventral hypothalamus and pituitary stalk, during which time the hormones are cleaved from the precursor. In the pituicytes of the posterior pituitary they are packaged into storage granules to be released in response to stimulation (e.g., osmotic, barometric) of receptors on the cell bodies in the hypothalamus. The posterior pituitary is therefore functionally an integral part of the brain.

The cell bodies of the neuroendocrine system are diffusely distributed throughout the mediobasal hypothalamus in an area known as the hypophysiotropic region. Although the releasing hormone–secreting neurons receive input from other brain regions in response to changes in the external environment, they continue to function even in the absence of extrahypothalamic input, indicating that their most important homeostatic stimuli are blood borne. Thyrotropin releasing hormone (TRH)- and somatotropin release inhibiting factor (SRIF)-secreting cells that regulate pituitary function are located in the anterior hypothalamus, while those secreting growth hormone releasing factor (GRF) are concentrated in the region of the ventromedial and arcuate nuclei. Gonadotropin releasing hormone (GnRH)-secreting cells are more widely distributed with cell bodies in both the anterior hypothalamus and the arcuate nuclei. Cell bodies of corticotropin releasing factor (CRF) neurons terminating in the median eminence are located predominantly in the paraventricular nucleus.

The releasing and inhibiting hormones are stored in nerve terminals in the median eminence where their concentrations are 10 to 100 times as great as elsewhere in the hypothalamus. Since the portal blood flow to the pituitary is not compartmentalized, i.e., various cells types in the pituitary are distributed throughout the gland, releasing and inhibiting factors secreted into the portal system have access to all cell types of the anterior pituitary. Specificity of action is achieved not by anatomic segregation but by the presence of specific receptors on individual pituitary cell types.

The cells of both the neuroendocrine and neurohypophyseal systems have been called transducer cells, containing both neuronal and endocrine characteristics. They respond to classic neurotransmitter-mediated signals, yet they respond by releasing peptide hormones into a regional or systemic circulation.

PORTAL VASCULAR SYSTEM. The vascular supply of the anterior pituitary is unique in that there are no direct connections with the arterial system. All of the arterial blood flows through the hypothalamic arteries and forms a capillary plexus within the outer layer of the median eminence in juxtaposition to nerve terminals of the hypophysiotropic neurons. In contrast to most other brain regions, the blood-brain barrier in the area of the median eminence is incomplete, permitting protein and peptide hormones as well as other charged particles access to the intercapillary spaces and the nerve terminals contained therein. These terminals respond to changes in concentrations of circulating hormones and metabolic signals as well as to classic neuronal stimuli by secreting releasing and inhibiting factors into the portal system.

The portal capillaries coalesce into a series of veins that descend through the pituitary stalk and form a second capillary plexus that bathes the cells of the anterior pituitary. Venous drainage from the anterior pituitary passes through the posterior pituitary and from there into systemic veins. Some reverse blood flow occurs from the posterior pituitary to a variable length up the pituitary stalk but does not reach the median eminence, and thus its physiologic significance is uncertain.

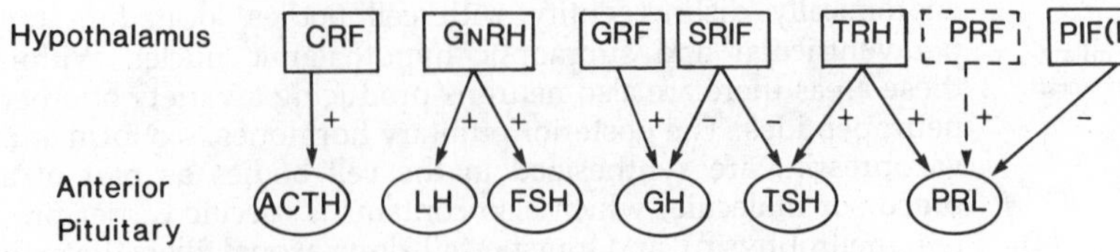

Figure 224–1. Interrelationships between hypothalamic and pituitary hormones. Solid lines denote hormones, the structures of which have been determined. Interrupted lines indicate factors, the identity of which is still unknown.

Releasing and Inhibiting Hormones

The hypothalamic hormones that control the secretion of anterior pituitary hormones and their effects on pituitary hormone secretion are shown in Figure 224–1. Several different patterns of control exist: (1) a single hypothalamic hormone stimulating release of a single pituitary hormone (CRF: ACTH), (2) a single hypothalamic hormone stimulating release of several pituitary hormones (GnRH: luteinizing hormone [LH] and follicle-stimulating hormone [FSH], TRH: thyroid-stimulating hormone [TSH] and prolactin), and (3) several hypothalamic hormones affecting a single pituitary hormone (GRF and SRIF: growth hormone [GH]).

With one exception, the predominant influence of the hypothalamic hormones on the pituitary is stimulatory. Interference with the integrity of the hypothalamic-pituitary connection results in decreased secretion of pituitary hormones. The exception is prolactin, the secretion of which is increased when hypothalamic influence is removed.

All of the hypothalamic hormones whose structures have been determined are, again with one exception, peptides with sequence length ranging from 3 to 44 amino acids. Their structures, shown in Figure 224–2, were identified over a 14-year period, beginning in 1969, and resulted in awarding of a Nobel Prize to the two pioneers in the field: Roger Guillemin and Andrew Schally. As the complexity of the structures increases, both multiple forms of the peptide (see section on somatostatin and GRF) and marked species variation in sequence occur. Whereas the structures of TRH, GnRH, and SRIF are identical in all mammalian species studied to date, and for TRH, in amphibia as well, those of GRF and CRF exhibit marked species specificity. The structures of rat GRF and CRF differ from their human and ovine counterparts by 14 and 7 amino acids respectively. The structure of human CRF has been determined from its gene sequence and is identical in structure to rat CRF. The existence of a separate PRF is still controversial, though a candidate for this title is vasoactive intestinal polypeptide (VIP). The one nonpeptide hypophysiotropic hormone is dopamine. In addition to its major role as a neurotransmitter, dopamine is the most important physiologic inhibitor of prolactin.

ROLE OF BIOGENIC AMINES AND NEUROPEPTIDES IN THE REGULATION OF HYPOTHALAMIC HORMONE SECRETION. The major neurotransmitter systems utilized for intercellular communication within the central nervous system consist of monoamines and peptides. Neurotransmitters can influence the hypothalamic hormone-secreting neurons at several sites (Fig. 224–3). These include axodendritic connections (site 1) and axoaxonic connections involving presynaptic receptors on the hormone-containing nerve terminals (site 3). Multiple neurotransmitters may also participate in the regulation of hormone secretion through intermediary neurons (site 2), and neurotransmitters may be released directly into the portal system to modify the effect of hypothalamic hormones on the pituitary (site 4). Major advances in the understanding of hypothalamic-pituitary function have occurred as a consequence of the availability of neuropharmacologic compounds that selectively alter neuro-

STRUCTURES OF HYPOPHYSIOTROPIC HORMONES

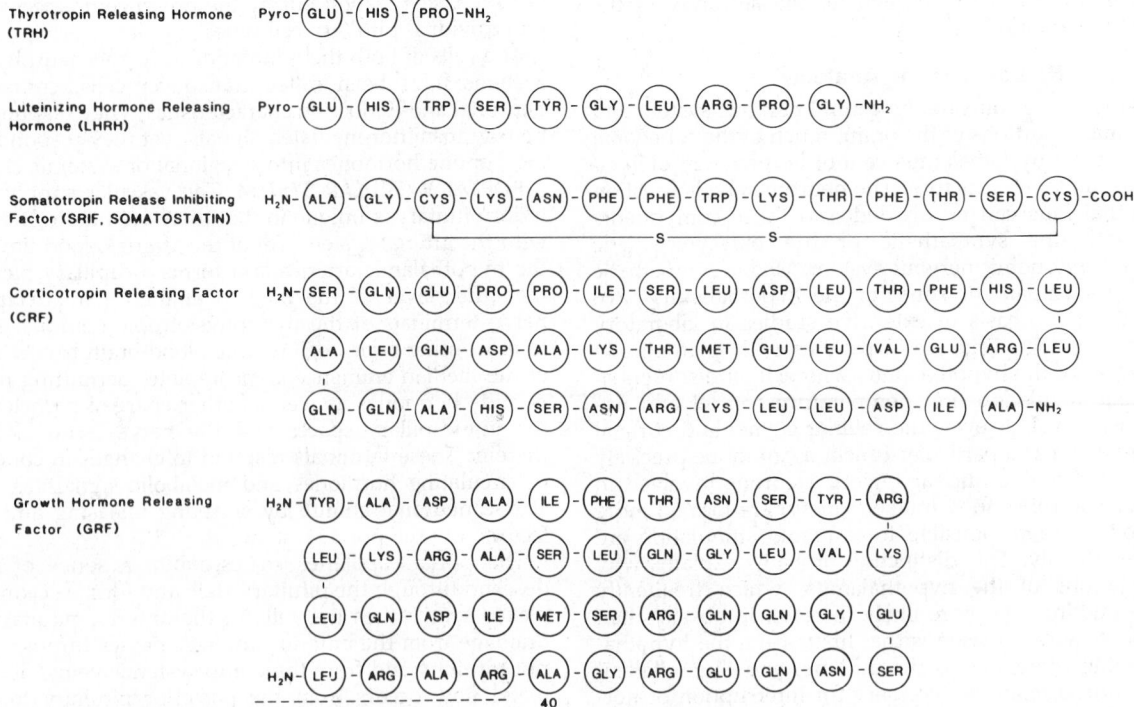

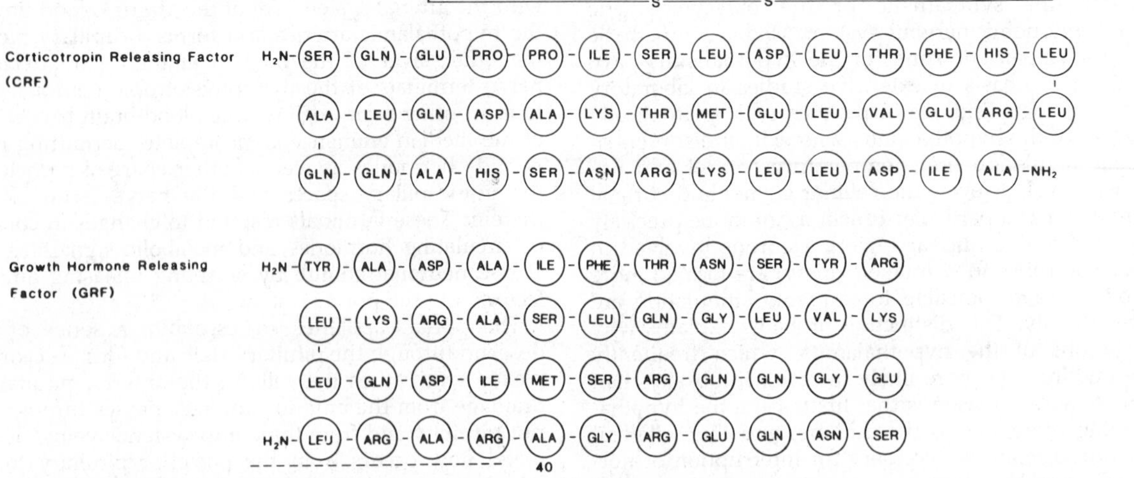

Figure 224–2. Structures of hypothalamic hormones. The sequences of TRH, GnRH, and somatostatin are believed to be similar in all mammalian species, whereas those of CRF (shown as ovine) and GRF (shown as the human sequence derived from a pancreatic tumor) exhibit considerable variability.

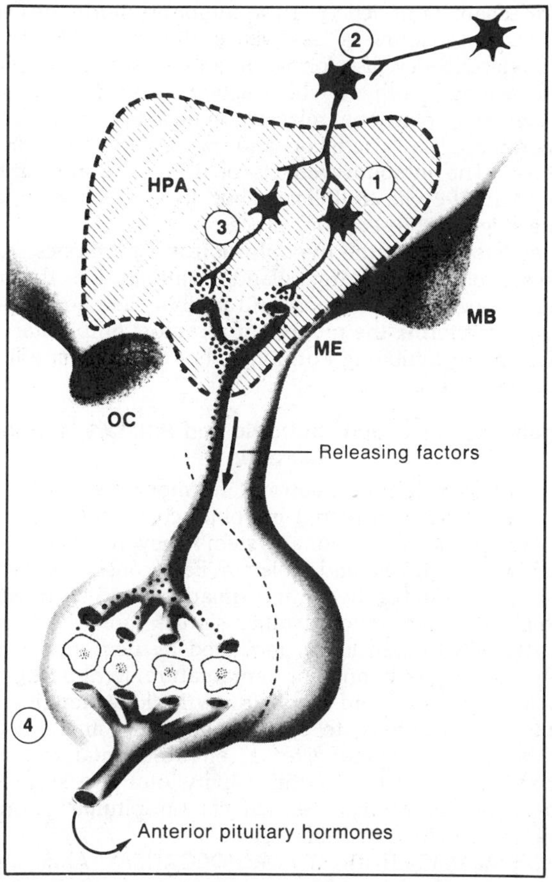

Figure 224–3. Sites of potential neurotransmitter effects on hypothalamic releasing and inhibiting hormone secretion and function. HPA = hypophysiotropic area; OC = optic chiasm; ME = median eminence; MB = mamillary body. Refer to text for description of effects at each site. (Reprinted with permission from Frohman LA: Clinical neuropharmacology of hypothalamic releasing factors. N Engl J Med 286:1391, 1972.)

transmitter function. Information resulting from techniques with only limited application to human investigation has been supplemented by the use of the neuropharmacologic probes that can be safely studied in man. A brief review of biogenic amine neurotransmitters is provided to indicate where selective neuropharmacologic agents can be used to alter neurotransmitter effects, and in turn, hypophysiotropic hormone function.

Catecholamines (Dopamine, Norepinephrine, Epinephrine). The common precursor for the catecholamines is tyrosine, which is actively transported from the blood into catecholaminergic neurons in the CNS. Tyrosine is converted to dihydroxyphenylalanine (L-dopa) by tyrosine hydroxylase, which, because of its low concentration, represents the rate-limiting step in catecholamine biosynthesis. It is therefore the enzyme most susceptible to pharmacologic blockage by tyrosine analogues such as α-methylparatyrosine. L-dopa is rapidly decarboxylated by aromatic L-amino acid decarboxylase to dopamine (5-hydroxytryptamine). This enzyme can be inhibited by L-dopa analogues such as α-methyldopa and α-methyldopahydrazine (carbidopa). In dopaminergic neurons, dopamine is stored in secretory granules and released as a neurotransmitter, while in noradrenergic and adrenergic neurons it is further hydroxylated by dopamine β-hydroxylase to form norepinephrine. Copper-chelating agents such as disulfiram are potent inhibitors of this step and impair the conversion of dopamine to norepinephrine. In noradrenergic neurons, this transmitter is packaged similarly to that of dopamine, whereas in selective neurons it is converted to epinephrine by phenylethanolamine-N-methyltransferase. See Ch. 241 also for a discussion of catecholamine metabolism.

In nerve endings, newly synthesized catecholamines are stored in secretory granules that protect them from enzymatic degradation. There are at least two distinct pools of neurotransmitters that are differentially susceptible to releasing stimuli. A long-lasting depletion of catecholamines can be produced by reserpine, which causes a slow but constant release of the monoamines and inhibits reuptake. Catecholamine release occurs in response to nerve stimulation by fusion of the secretion vesicle membrane with the cell membrane and extrusion of the amine directly into the intercellular space. Once released, catecholamines bind to postsynaptic receptors that appear to be similar in the hypophysiotropic neurons to those demonstrated in other neural sites. In addition, they bind to presynaptic receptors on the nerve terminals to effect a feedback regulation. Alterations in presynaptic and postsynaptic receptor activity are accomplished by the use of receptor agonists and antagonists. The specificity of most of the available agents, however, is not absolute. Catecholamine action terminates by reuptake of the neurotransmitter into the presynaptic neuron, removal into circulation, or by metabolic degradation. The first mechanism is the most important one. Drugs such as cocaine, tricyclic antidepressants, or nomifensine inhibit reuptake, resulting in enhancement of catecholamine effects. Metabolic degradation occurs by two enzymes: monoamine oxidase (MAO) and catechol-O-methyltransferase. Catecholamine action is therefore enhanced by MAO inhibitors such as pargyline and tranylcypromine.

Indolamines (Serotonin, Melatonin). Tryptophan, the precursor of serotonin, is actively transported from blood to brain. Since tryptophan hydroxylase activity is not saturated at physiologic concentrations, fluctuations in plasma tryptophan levels determine the rate of brain serotonin synthesis. After hydroxylation, 5-hydroxytryptophan is converted to serotonin by aromatic L-amino acid decarboxylase. Serotonin functions as a neurotransmitter and, in the pineal, also serves as a precursor of melatonin. Serotonin synthesis can be inhibited by p-chlorophenylalanine, which inhibits tryptophan hydroxylase, and by L-dopa, which competes with 5-hydroxytryptophan for decarboxylation. The storage, release, and uptake of serotonin are similar to that of norepinephrine with many of the same agents (i.e., amphetamine) releasing both compounds. Tricyclic antidepressants inhibit serotonin uptake, though in contrast to norepinephrine, imipramine and amitriptyline are more potent than their desmethyl derivatives (desmethylimipramine and nortriptyline). Alteration of serotonin receptor activity can be produced by agonists such as quipazine and LSD and by antagonists (methysergide and cyproheptadine). Termination of serotonin effects occurs by pre-synaptic reuptake and metabolic degradation involving MAO. Drugs interfering with MAO activity also enhance serotonin effects.

Acetylcholine. Acetylcholine is synthesized from acetyl-CoA and choline. The source of choline is probably phosphatidylcholine which, after crossing the blood-brain barrier, is partially degraded to choline. Choline is then converted to acetylcholine by choline acetyltransferase. There are two types of acetylcholine receptors, muscarinic and nicotinic, which have different anatomic distribution and physiologic function. Arecoline and atropine, a muscarinic agonist and antagonist, respectively, cross the blood-brain barrier and modify acetylcholine receptor activity.

Gamma-Aminobutyric Acid (GABA). In the mammalian hypothalamus GABA is an inhibitory neurotransmitter. It is formed by the decarboxylation of L-glutamate and is metabolized by transamination. Numerous agents inhibit GABA synthesis and degradation, but none is specific or useful clinically in altering neuroendocrine function.

Histamine. Histamine is synthesized within the CNS from histidine by a specific decarboxylase and the nonspecific aromatic L-amino acid decarboxylase. Alteration of histamine effects is brought about primarily by histamine receptor antagonists. There are two classes of histamine receptors: H_1 and H_2. Drugs such as diphenhydramine and cyproheptadine inhibit

TABLE 224–1. NEUROPEPTIDES WITH POTENTIAL EFFECTS ON HYPOTHALAMIC RELEASING HORMONES

Somatostatin
Thyrotropin releasing hormone
Vasoactive intestinal polypeptide
Cholecystokinin
Gastrin
Substance P
Neurotensin
Bombesin/gastrin releasing peptide
Secretin
Motilin
Insulin
Glucagon
Pancreatic polypeptide
Methionine-leucine-enkephalin
Beta-endorphin
Alpha-melanocyte–stimulating hormone
Neuropeptide PYY
Neuropeptide PHI
Calcitonin
Angiotensin
Bradykinin

H_1 receptors, while cimetidine and ranitidine inhibit H_2 receptors.

Neuropeptides. A large number of neuropeptides have been identified in the hypothalamus, and their role in the regulation of neuroendocrine function is, at present, only incompletely understood. A list of neuropeptides with potential effects on releasing and inhibiting hormones is provided in Table 224–1. Many of these peptides are widely distributed in extrahypothalamic CNS and function as neurotransmitters or neuromodulators in other pathways. Of particular significance is a group of peptides common to both the CNS and the gastrointestinal tract. Although the function of these peptides within the CNS remains to be determined, they may have a role in a number of integrative systems relating to homeostatic mechanisms. Their presence throughout evolution and as far back as unicellular organisms underscores their essential role in intercellular communication. With the exception of analogues of enkephalin capable of crossing the blood-brain barrier and of TRH, neuroendocrine effects of peptides other than hypophysiotropic hormones have not been documented in man. Limited information is available concerning biosynthesis, storage, secretion, and metabolism of hypothalamic neuropeptides. Peptidases capable of degrading neuropeptides have been demonstrated, though their specificity and physiologic importance are not yet known.

MECHANISM OF ACTION OF HYPOTHALAMIC HORMONES. Hypophysiotropic hormones affect pituitary hormone secretion by several mechanisms. Specific, high-affinity receptors are present on the anterior pituitary target cells, and cyclic AMP stimulation occurs as a consequence of releasing hormone–receptor interaction. Releasing hormone action is also calcium dependent, and a convincing role now exists for Ca^{++} as a second messenger. In addition, releasing hormones stimulate RNA and protein synthesis, and excessive stimulation can lead to cellular hyperplasia and even tumor formation.

The mechanism of action of the inhibitory hormones somatostatin and dopamine is less well understood. Somatostatin inhibits adenylate cyclase formation and enhances phosphodiesterase activity, both of which actions would impair cyclic AMP–mediated hormone release. Somatostatin also inhibits transmembrane Ca^{++} transport and may have other effects on exocytosis. The inhibitory effects of dopamine appear to be independent of cyclic AMP levels, but, like somatostatin, occur at a late stage in the secretory process.

The effects of all of the hypophysiotropic hormones studied to date are modified by target gland hormones, i.e., thyroxine, cortisol, estrogens, androgens, and inhibin. The hormones act primarily by altering the number of receptors on pituitary cells for releasing or inhibiting hormones, but also exhibit effects at postreceptor sites.

Regulation of Hypophysiotropic and Pituitary Hormone Secretion

The control of hypophysiotropic hormone secretion is best appreciated when considered in conjunction with that of the five major pituitary hormone systems they regulate: ACTH, LH and FSH, TSH, GH, and prolactin. Each consists of feedback (closed loop) systems involving primarily blood-borne signals on which are superimposed other signals mostly originating within the CNS (open loop), mediated by neurotransmitters, and representing environment (temperature, light-dark), stress (pain, fear, psychic) and intrinsic rhythmicity (ranging from ultradian or short-term to diurnal, monthly, and seasonal). Thus, both internal and external environmental factors are important determinants of the activity of these systems. A summary of neurotransmitter effects on pituitary hormone secretion is provided in Table 224–2.

HYPOTHALAMIC-PITUITARY-ADRENOCORTICAL AXIS. Nearly all of the monoamine neurotransmitters have effects on CRF release. Acetylcholine stimulates CRF release predominantly through nicotinic receptors and appears to be the primary neurotransmitter mediating stress-induced CRF release. Serotonin also stimulates CRF release, but the effect is likely mediated through a cholinergic interneuron, since it can be blocked by atropine. Norepinephrine inhibits the cholinergic effects on CRF release through an α-adrenergic receptor, and GABA exerts a similar effect. Melatonin inhibits CRF release and may be responsible for the circadian pattern of CRF release that is entrained to the light-dark cycle. Enkephalins exert inhibitory effects on the pituitary-adrenal axis. This effect is believed to occur within the hypothalamus at the level of CRF release, though an additional action on the pituitary has not been excluded.

CRF stimulates ACTH release, which in turn stimulates the secretion of glucocorticoids and mineralocorticoids from the adrenal cortex. Glucocorticoids inhibit ACTH secretion by a concentration–dependent rapid feedback (minutes) and a concentration–independent delayed feedback (hours). The rapid feedback occurs primarily at the pituitary by inhibiting the response to CRF but also by inhibiting CRF release. The delayed feedback also occurs at both pituitary and hypothalamic levels and appears to reflect inhibitory effects on CRF and ACTH synthesis. In addition, ACTH exerts a "short-loop feedback" on CRF release.

TABLE 224–2. EFFECTS OF AMINERGIC AND PEPTIDERGIC NEUROTRANSMITTERS ON ANTERIOR PITUITARY HORMONE SECRETION

	Norepinephrine	Dopamine	Serotonin	Acetylcholine	Histamine	GABA	Other
ACTH	α ↑	–	↑	↑	–	–	Enkephalins ↓
LH and FSH	(↑)	↓	–	–	–	–	–
TSH	↑	↓	↑	–	–	–	Neurotensin ↓
GH	α ↑ β ↓	↑	↑	↑	–	(↑)	Neurotensin ↓ Substance P ↓ Enkephalins ↑
Prolactin	–	↓	↑	–	↑	↑	Neurotensin ↓ Enkephalins ↑ VIP ↑

NOTE: ↑ = stimulates; ↓ = inhibits; – = no effect or insufficient data; ( ) = conflicting data exist. All effects reflect CNS rather than peripheral sites of action (with the exception of dopamine). The data are derived (whenever possible) from studies in humans.

Plasma ACTH secretion exhibits a diurnal pattern, with lowest levels occurring between 6 and 11 P.M. followed by a rise in the early morning, peaking between 6 and 8 A.M. The pattern appears independent of sleep stage. Superimposed on this regulatory system are the stimulatory effects of stress, including severe trauma, pyrogens, hypoglycemia, and anxiety. Considerable interaction exists between the feedback influence of circulating corticosteroids and neurotransmitters. Phenytoin administration, for example, decreases CNS sensitivity to steroid feedback, thereby diminishing the ACTH response to metyrapone (which reduces circulating glucocorticoid levels) but also enhances pulsatile ACTH secretion while not affecting the ACTH response to stress and vasopressin. Vasopressin, once believed to be CRF, stimulates ACTH release directly as well as through a CNS-mediated mechanism and potentiates the effects of CRF.

HYPOTHALAMIC-PITUITARY-GONADAL AXIS. The major neurotransmitter effects on GnRH identified to date involve dopamine and serotonin. Dopamine stimulates the release of GnRH, though it is not clear whether this involves the tonic or cyclic release of GnRH. Serotonin exerts an inhibitory effect on both cyclic and tonic GnRH secretion. Norepinephrine may also stimulate GnRH release.

The regulation of the hypothalamic-pituitary-gonadal axis is complex, varying with age and sex. LH and FSH are present in circulation from birth, and through the early stages of puberty FSH levels gradually increase to a greater degree than do LH levels. During this period, FSH responses to GnRH are greater than LH responses, a pattern opposite to that seen following puberty, and the hypothalamus is exceedingly sensitive to the suppressive effects of gonadal steroids. In the later prepubertal period (seven to nine years) sleep-related pulsatile LH secretion begins, and synchronization occurs between LH and FSH pulses, particularly in girls. These pulses stimulate the secretion of testosterone in boys and estradiol in girls that initiates the clinical characteristics of puberty. At the same time, evidence for lessening sensitivity of hypothalamic GnRH secretion in response to steroid feedback can be demonstrated. In women, development of positive LH and FSH feedback to gonadal steroids permits the cyclic preovulatory gonadotropin surge resulting in the establishment of cyclic ovulation by the mid teens. In adult males the LH secretory pattern is characterized by 8 to 10 spikes occurring randomly through the day, and the teenage relationship to the sleep-wake pattern disappears. Similar pulsatile secretion of LH and FSH occurs in mature women, the frequency in magnitude of the pulses varying with the phase of the menstrual cycle. When ovarian follicles disappear at menopause, secretion of the major ovarian hormones stops, and the loss of negative feedback of these hormones enhances secretion of FSH and, to a lesser extent, LH. A similar increase in LH and FSH is observed in men in the seventh and eighth decade in response to decreasing testicular function.

In men, surgical stress results in a transitory rise in the level of LH followed by a prolonged fall, accompanied by a fall in testosterone levels. No changes have been observed in women, although hypothalamic anovulation is frequently seen during periods of stress. Pheromones or other environmental factors have been implicated as the cause for the synchronization of menstrual cycles seen in women living in close association.

Steroid hormones regulate LH and FSH secretion by two major mechanisms. Gonadal steroids regulate tonic secretion by a negative feedback mechanism. Testosterone appears to be more potent than estrogen in this negative feedback effect, while progesterone has an intermediate effect. Inhibin, a peptide produced by germinal epithelium, has a selective action in inhibiting FSH release, possibly by impairing the effects of GnRH. Cyclic release of LH and FSH is stimulated by a positive feedback effect of ovarian steroids during the final phases of follicular growth prior to ovulation. The preovulatory surge of LH is preceded by an increase in circulating estrogen levels in the presence of low or decreasing progesterone levels. The positive effects occur at both the hypothalamic and pituitary levels, though the latter appear to be more important. GnRH is released in a tonic pulsatile manner by the hypothalamus every 60 to 90 minutes, and this pattern of secretion is critical for its effects on the pituitary. In an individual deficient in GnRH secretion, pulsatile administration of GnRH allows restoration of normal cyclic ovulation. In contrast, constant infusion of GnRH leads to down-regulation of pituitary GnRH receptors and a loss of gonadotropin secretion. This observation has enormous implications in terms of therapy aimed at enhancing or preventing fertility. In contrast to its effects on GnRH, dopamine inhibits tonic LH secretion. The physiologic significance of this observation is unclear, since inhibitory effects on the midcycle LH surge can also be blocked by dopamine receptor blockers.

HYPOTHALAMIC-PITUITARY-THYROID AXIS. TSH secretion by the pituitary is regulated by TRH and somatostatin. For a discussion of the control of somatostatin secretion, the reader is referred to the section on the regulation of GH secretion. TRH secretion is stimulated by norepinephrine and dopamine and is inhibited by serotonin. TRH stimulates TSH secretion, which in turn enhances the release of thyroxine and triiodothyronine by the thyroid. The feedback effects of these hormones, primarily triiodothyronine, occur principally in the pituitary where they inhibit the TSH response to TRH. A reduction in circulating thyroid hormone levels leads to a prompt rise in TSH levels. TRH is not required for this acute response, though it is necessary for the full expression of TSH hypersecretion over a long time. In addition, TRH is required for maintaining basal TSH secretion. In contrast to its effects on the pituitary, triiodothyronine exerts a stimulatory effect on TRH secretion from the hypothalamus.

Acute changes in environmental conditions requiring increased metabolic activity, such as cold exposure, lead to a TRH-mediated increase in TSH secretion. This effect is readily demonstrable in infants but not in adults, in whom other mechanisms of thermogenesis (mediated by the autonomic nervous system and resulting in shivering and free fatty acid mobilization) are more important. Agents inhibiting adrenergic neurotransmission block the TSH response to cold.

Dopaminergic agents exert an inhibitory effect on TSH release by the pituitary that is most pronounced in patients with elevated TSH levels but also seen in normals. A role of endogenous dopamine in suppressing TSH secretion has also been demonstrated.

Somatostatin inhibition of TSH secretion exerts a relatively minor physiologic role under normal circumstances, but increases in hypothalamic somatostatin release as a result of elevated GH levels can suppress TSH secretion to subnormal levels.

HYPOTHALAMIC-PITUITARY-SOMATOTROPH AXIS. GH secretion is regulated by releasing and inhibiting hormones: GRF and SRIF (somatostatin). Many physiologic stimuli affect GH secretion. Intrinsic GH rhythmicity involves a diurnal pattern with stable basal patterns superimposed on which are occasional surges of GH unrelated to any known signals, the most consistent of which occurs about one hour after the onset of sleep and is associated with sleep stages 3 and 4. With age, GH secretion changes dramatically, both qualitatively and quantitatively. Extremely high levels seen in the first few days of life decrease by two weeks of age. During the pubertal period levels indistinguishable from those of adults are seen, though the GH surges occur more frequently. By the fifth and sixth decade, GH surges, both during the day and in association with sleep, are diminished. Similarly, responses to GH releasing stimuli decrease with age. Neurotransmitter regulation of GH secretion has been extensively defined. Dopamine, norepinephrine (through the alpha receptor), epinephrine, serotonin, GABA, and acetylcholine have all been shown to stimulate GH secretion. Melatonin has both stimulatory and inhibitory effects, TRH and neurotensin exhibit inhibitory effects, and endorphins/enkephalins have stimulatory effects, all mediated within the CNS. The mechanism by which these neurotransmitters affect the secretion of GRF and SRIF is not completely understood, though dopamine, norepinephrine, acetylcholine, GABA, neurotensin, substance P, and bombesin have all been reported to stimulate SRIF release.

GH secretion is profoundly affected by nutrients. Elevations of amino acid levels, decreases in free fatty acids, and hypoglycemia all stimulate GH secretion, while hyperglycemia inhibits GH release. GH secretion is increased by exercise, anxiety, and emotional or physical stress. Many hormones affect GH responsiveness. Estrogen administration increases GH responsiveness, while excesses of corticosteroid and thyroid hormone decrease responsivity. GH secretion is also decreased in states of thyroid hormone deficiency. In pubertal and prepubertal males, androgen administration also enhances GH responses.

In addition to these "open loop" stimuli, a closed loop feedback system also exists. GH stimulates the production of somatomedins (insulin-like growth factors [IGF] I and II) by the liver, and both GH and IGF-I exhibit feedback effects. IGF-I stimulates the release of somatostatin and also inhibits basal and GRF-stimulated GH release by the pituitary. GH itself stimulates somatostatin secretion at concentrations that are reached during secretory bursts. It is not yet known whether GH and IGF-I exhibit effects on GRF secretion.

HYPOTHALAMIC-LACTOTROPH-BREAST AXIS. Prolactin secretion is predominantly controlled by inhibitory CNS influences, with dopamine being the major prolactin inhibiting factor. Two peptides, TRH and vasoactive intestinal polypeptide (VIP), appear to have physiologic prolactin releasing factor (PRF) activity, though their relative importance is not yet clear. Neurotransmitter influences on prolactin secretion are extensive. Serotonin stimulates prolactin release by effects on PRF. Melatonin and histamine have stimulatory effects within the CNS as do opioid peptides and GABA. The effect of the latter two agents appears due to their inhibitory effects on the tuberoinfundibular dopaminergic system.

Prolactin secretion is increased by tactile stimulation of the breast via receptors in the nipple and areola that reach the spinal cord by the intercostal nerves. During pregnancy, prolactin levels increase as a result of estrogen stimulation. Following parturition, the rapid decline in estrogen and progesterone levels allows the unopposed action of prolactin to stimulate lactation from the estrogen-primed breast. The suckling stimulation of prolactin secretion is in part controlled by VIP. Prolactin levels return to normal after several months even during continual lactation. Prolactin is a stress-responsive hormone, and increased secretion is observed after surgical stress, exercise, and insulin hypoglycemia. Prolactin secretion is increased in states of thyroid hormone deficiency and decreased in the presence of thyroid hormone excess.

del Pozo E, Lancranjan I: Clinical use of drugs modifying the release of anterior pituitary hormones. *In* Ganong WF, Martini L (eds.): Frontiers in Neuroendocrinology. Vol 5. New York, Raven Press, 1978, pp 207–248. *A detailed review of the neuropharmacologic agents that have been used to modify pituitary hormone secretion. Both diagnostic and therapeutic uses are covered, with particular emphasis on drugs affecting dopaminergic systems.*

Epstein A: Neuroendocrinology of thirst and salt appetite. *In* Ganong WF, Martini L (eds.): Frontiers in Neuroendocrinology. Vol 5. New York, Raven Press, 1978, pp 101–134. *An extremely well-written review of neural regulation of salt and water metabolism. The studies are primarily in laboratory animals, though the principles apply to human physiology.*

Krieger DT: Neuroendocrine physiology. *In* Felig P, Baxter JD, Broadus AE, Frohman LA (eds.): Endocrinology and Metabolism. New York, McGraw Hill Book Company, 1981, pp 125–250. *A systematic in-depth presentation of the anatomy and physiology of human neuroendocrinology. Designed for the advanced medical student and clinical trainee.*

Krieger DT: Brain peptides: What, where and why? Science 222:975, 1983. *An excellent and comprehensive review of the recent developments in neural peptide research, their implications, and an attempt to explain their presence throughout evolution. Interesting for clinicians, though not of immediate use.*

Krieger DT, Brownstein M, Martin JB (eds.): Brain Peptides. New York, John Wiley & Sons, 1983. *A comprehensive collection of monographs on the role of brain peptides as transmitters, hypophyseotropic hormones, and messengers throughout the nervous system. This will be a definitive reference volume for years. Of interest to the medical student, neurobiologist, and clinical trainee.*

Krieger DT, Hughes JC (eds.): Neuroendocrinology. Sunderland, Sinauer Associates, Inc., 1980. *A collection of reviews on hypothalamic function involving normal physiology and organic and behavioral disease states. Articles are very readable and beautifully illustrated, although they do not provide in-depth coverage of subject material.*

McCann SM: The role of brain peptides in the control of anterior pituitary hormone secretion. *In* Muller EE, MacLeod RM (eds.): Neuroendocrine Perspectives. Vol 1. Amsterdam, Elsevier Biomedical Press, 1982, pp 1–22. *An up-to-date review of releasing and inhibiting factors and of other neural peptides that regulate hormone secretion by the pituitary. Results are derived from animals but form the basis for evaluating human neuroendocrine regulation as well.*

Morley JE: The endocrinology of the opiates and opioid peptides. Metabolism 30:195, 1981. *A well-documented, current review of the role of opiates and the endorphin/enkephalin family of peptides in relation to neuroendocrine function and the regulation of neurometabolic control. Both human and animal studies are discussed.*

Rivier J, Spiess J, Thorner M, Vale W: Characterization of a growth hormone releasing factor from a human pancreatic islet tumor. Nature 300:276, 1982. Guillemin R, Brazeau P, Bohlen P, Esch F, Ling N, Wehrenberg WB: Growth hormone releasing factor from a pancreatic tumor that caused acromegaly. Science 218:585, 1982. *Two papers describing the isolation and characterization of growth hormone releasing factor from pancreatic islet adenomas. The culmination of a 20-year search, with an unexpected tissue source leading to the solution.*

DISEASES OF THE CENTRAL NERVOUS SYSTEM WITH ALTERED NEUROENDOCRINE AND NEUROMETABOLIC FUNCTION

The frequent association of altered hormone secretion with disorders of the CNS has been recognized for many decades. The hypothalamus was the initial focus of attention because of its crucial role in neuroendocrine regulation. However, it is now recognized that diseases localized to extrahypothalamic brain regions as well as nonlocalized CNS disorders can also produce disturbances in neuroendocrine function. The clinical and laboratory manifestations of these disorders are frequently indistinguishable from those of hypothalamic origin, since their mediation is usually via the hypothalamus. Similarly the distinction between hypothalamic and pituitary causes of certain pituitary hormone secretory disorders may be difficult for other reasons.

Because of the reticular organization of the anatomic structure of the hypothalamus, some functions can be localized to a precise anatomic locus, whereas others require the participation of diffuse areas. In addition, neurons within a specific hypothalamic locus may be involved in several separate regulatory functions. Consequently the extent of endocrine or metabolic disturbance is more dependent on the location than the size of the hypothalamic lesion. Furthermore, slowly growing lesions tend to be silent until they have reached considerable size, whereas rapidly enlarging lesions, depending on location, can cause dramatic clinical and laboratory manifestations even when quite small.

Acute hypothalamic damage is associated with impairment of consciousness, sustained hyperthermia, and severe disturbances of cardiovascular, gastrointestinal, or respiratory function. In contrast, persistent disease in the hypothalamus results in alterations in cognition and complex homeostatic functions. Although disorders of neuroendocrine regulation can be produced by acute lesions destroying the median eminence or the pituitary stalk, they generally tend to be seen with chronic disorders and often result in inability of the endocrine system to adapt to environmental changes rather than in alteration of basal hormone secretion. Because hypothalamic neuronal projections, in contrast to those involving sensory and motor function, are generally not lateralized, unilateral damage seldom results in significant or prolonged symptoms. Thus disturbances of hypothalamic function are most commonly seen with infiltrative or inflammatory diseases that affect the region diffusely, with tumors of the midline that expand bilaterally, or with disorders affecting the median eminence, the final common effector pathway to the pituitary.

Etiology of Hypothalamic Disease

Defined anatomic disorders of the hypothalamus vary in frequency with different age groups and are summarized in

Table 224–3. In addition, disturbances of neuroendocrine or neurometabolic function are frequently unassociated with anatomic evidence of hypothalamic disease. Many have been attributed to disorders of neurochemical function, though it is currently not known whether they represent defects in receptor binding, postreceptor mechanisms, biosynthetic defects, or other disorders.

TUMORS. Hypothalamic tumors are frequently located in the region of the third ventricle. Those tumors located in the inferior portion of the third ventricle or the anterior mediobasal hypothalamus frequently produce disturbances in neuroendocrine and neurometabolic regulation. The most frequent hypothalamic tumors are craniopharyngiomas (see next section) and their variants (ependymomas and epidermoid cysts), followed by astrocytomas and dysgerminomas. Two other tumor types, hypothalamic pinealomas and hamartomas, will be considered separately because of their association with specific neuroendocrine disorders. Since they are frequently of developmental origin, the majority of hypothalamic tumors occur in patients under 25 years of age. Endocrine disturbances generally result from destruction of those neuronal elements required for normal pituitary function. The most frequently occurring manifestations are diabetes insipidus, hypogonadism, and growth retardation. Disturbances in thyroid and adrenal function are less common. The diagnosis of a hypothalamic tumor is made by standard neuroradiologic and neuro-ophthalmologic procedures, using computed tomography, visual field measurement, and visual evoked responses. The combination of an atypical visual field defect (i.e., loss of inferior visual fields), normal sellar anatomy, and intact responses to releasing hormones in a patient with hypopituitarism points to primary hypothalamic disease. The surgical treatment of hypothalamic tumors generally precludes complete removal without destruction of normal tissue critical for maintaining homeostasis. Many of these tumors, because of their developmental origin, tend to be slow growing and may even undergo spontaneous growth arrest or regression. Cystic tumors can be aspirated or marsupialized into the cerebroventricular system. Radiotherapy is also effective in many of these tumors. The loss of endocrine function is, however, rarely reversible, and replacement hormone therapy is required.

TABLE 224–3. ETIOLOGY OF HYPOTHALAMIC DISEASE

Neonates
Intraventricular hemorrhage
Meningitis: bacterial
Tumors: glioma, hemangioma
Trauma
Hydrocephalus, hydranencephaly, kernicterus
1 Month–2 Years
Tumors: glioma, especially optic glioma, histiocytosis X, hemangiomas
Hydrocephalus, meningitis
"Familial" disorders: Laurence-Moon, Bardet-Biedl, Prader-Labhart-Willi, etc.
2–10 Years
Tumors: craniopharyngioma, glioma, dysgerminoma, hamartoma, histiocytosis X, leukemia, ganglioneuroma, ependymoma, medulloblastoma
Meningitis: bacterial, tuberculous
Encephalitis: viral and demyelinating, various viral encephalitides and exanthematous demyelinating encephalitides, disseminated encephalomyelitis
"Familial" disorders: diabetes insipidus, etc.
Damage from nasopharyngeal radiation therapy
10–25 Years
Tumors: craniopharyngioma, pituitary tumors, glioma, hamartoma, dysgerminoma, histiocytosis X, leukemia, dermoid, lipoma, neuroblastoma
Trauma
Subarachnoid hemorrhage, vascular aneurysm, arteriovenous malformation
Inflammatory diseases: meningitis, encephalitis, sarcoidosis, tuberculosis
Associated with midline brain defects: agenesis of corpus callosum
Chronic hydrocephalus or increased intracranial pressure
25–50 Years
Nutritional: Wernicke's disease
Tumors: glioma, lymphoma, meningioma, craniopharyngioma, pituitary tumors, angioma, plasmacytoma, colloid cysts, ependymoma, sarcoma, histiocytosis X
Inflammatory: sarcoidosis, tuberculosis, viral encephalitis
Subarachnoid hemorrhage, vascular aneurysms, arteriovenous malformation
Damage from pituitary radiation therapy
50 Years and older
Nutritional: Wernicke's disease
Tumors: sarcoma, gliobastoma, lymphoma, meningioma, colloid cysts, ependymoma, pituitary tumors
Vascular: infarct, subarachnoid hemorrhage, pituitary apoplexy
Infectious: encephalitis, sarcoidosis, meningitis

Adapted from Plum F, Van Uitert R: Non-endocrine diseases of the hypothalamus. *In* Reichlin S, Baldessarini RJ, Martin JB (eds.): The Hypothalamus. New York, Raven Press, 1978, p 415.

Hamartomas. One type of hypothalamic tumor, the hamartoma, has been associated with increased, rather than decreased, hypothalamic function. Hamartomas consist of masses of redundant, partially disoriented glial and neuronal cells or an abnormally lodged collection of normal nerve tissue. Hamartomas associated with precocious puberty consist of encapsulated nodules in the posterior hypothalamus containing membrane-bound secretion granules similar to those in hypothalamic neurosecretory cells. Vessels in the hamartoma have fenestrations characteristic of those in the median eminence, suggesting a secretory process similar to that in the median eminence. These vessels are presumed to connect to the pituitary portal system. The secretion granules contain GnRH, which is found in high concentrations in CSF from patients with this disorder. Hamartomatous cells are believed to secrete GnRH in a pulsatile manner, but are not under normal prepubertal inhibitory influences. The resultant hormonal effects produce pubertal changes that in girls lead to menarche and cyclic ovulatory menses as early as the second year of life.

Harmartomas are present in one third of all children with this form of precocious puberty. Specific therapy aimed at the hamartoma appears unnecessary, since its course is benign with no other neuroendocrine disturbances and no loss of nonendocrine hypothalamic structure or function. Therapy of the precocious puberty, however, is of great importance both for psychologic reasons and for prevention of premature epiphyseal fusion and stunted growth. Current therapy consists of monthly injections of a long-acting progesterone that inhibits the gonadotropin response to GnRH and effectively inhibits vaginal bleeding but is only partially effective in slowing bone growth. A GnRH analogue, currently in investigational status, acts by down-regulating the pituitary GnRH receptor, resulting in diminished gonadotropin secretion, and is capable of suppressing the accelerated bone growth. The use of GnRH analogues should become standard therapy in the future.

Hypothalamic hamartomas have also been associated with acromegaly and GH-secreting pituitary tumors. They have been shown to contain GRF, which is secreted into the portal system, resulting in GH hypersecretion and somatotroph tumor formation.

Gangliocytomas. A closely related tumor, the gangliocytoma, consists of randomly oriented large ganglion cells similar to those in the hypothalamic magnocellular (large cell) nuclei. Intrapituitary gangliocytomas are also seen in association with acromegaly and GH-secreting tumors of the pituitary and contain GRF. In contrast to hypothalamic hamartomas, the axons of the intrapituitary tumors directly contact the somatotropic cells.

Pineal Tumors. Pineal tumors constitute less than 1 per cent of all intracranial neoplasms and consist of three separate tumor types: pinealomas (pineal parenchymal tissue tumor [20 per cent]), glial tumors (25 per cent), and germinomas (also called ectopic pinealomas or teratomas [55 per cent]). The neuroendocrine effects (precocious puberty) of the first two types are most likely a consequence of destruction of the normal pineal by tumor, leading to loss of pineal secretory products (possibly melatonin, arginine vasotocin, or another factor) that normally inhibit the initiation of sexual maturation. Only a small percentage of pineal tumors cause sexual precocity and usually not until they extend beyond the pineal region. Some pineal tumors are associated with delayed puberty, which may be mediated by production of an antigonadotropic factor. Precocious puberty associated with germinomas, which are similar both histologically and functionally to ovarian and testicular germ cell tumors, is caused by the production of chorionic gonadotropin. Levels as high as those seen during the first month of pregnancy are often present. Many of the "ectopic" pinealomas occur in the midline of the ventral hypothalamus and result in loss of other endocrine functions. Surgical treatment of pinealomas is generally unsatisfactory though the tumors consisting of germinal elements are exquisitely radiosensitive. The tumors frequently contain nongerminal elements (teratomas) that are relatively radioresistant.

INFILTRATIVE AND INFLAMMATORY DISEASES

Histiocytosis X (see also Ch. 161). This granulomatous disease of the histiocytic type, with eosinophilic elements, involves the ventromedial hypothalamus and is associated with diabetes insipidus, anterior hypopituitarism due to destruction of releasing hormone–secreting neurons, or both. The three clinical subgroups of the disease are Hand-Schüller-Christian disease, the most common type characterized by polyuria, exophthalmos, and skull defects; Letterer-Siwe disease, a more rapidly progressive form; and eosinophilic granuloma, in which similar pathologic findings are present in isolated bone lesions. The disease may begin with diabetes insipidus, which is present in nearly 50 per cent of patients with Hand-Schüller-Christian disease. Less commonly, growth failure, hypogonadism, and panhypopituitarism are seen. The diagnosis is established by bone or intracranial biopsy. The CNS forms of the disease may respond to high-dose glucocorticoid therapy or chemotherapy, but the impairment in neuroendocrine function appears irreversible.

Sarcoidosis (see Ch. 67). Involvement of the CNS by sarcoidosis in uncommon. When it is present, however, the hypothalamus and pituitary are frequently involved with infiltrating granulomatous nodules. Patients may develop diabetes insipidus, galactorrhea due to hyperprolactinemia, partial or total anterior pituitary insufficiency, and neurometabolic and neurovegetative symptoms such as somnolence or hyperphagia. In general, the usual treatment with glucocorticoids does not improve the endocrine dysfunction.

TRAUMA. Basal skull fractures are frequently accompanied by shearing of the pituitary stalk, leading to panhypopituitarism and diabetes insipidus. In patients who become comatose following skull fractures, impairment in the pituitary-thyroid and pituitary-gonadal axes have been reported in the absence of stalk damage. Gonadal and thyroid hormones generally return to normal upon recovery.

RADIATION-INDUCED HYPOTHALAMIC DYSFUNCTION. Radiation therapy for intracranial neoplasms, including pituitary tumors, and for nasopharyngeal and maxillary sinus carcinomas frequently leads to hypopituitarism. The interval between therapy and appearance of hormone deficiencies ranges from one to ten years or possibly longer. Children appear more susceptible than adults, and the critical dose is believed to be about 4000 rads. In children, growth failure associated with reduced GH secretion, hypogonadotropic hypogonadism, and hypothyroidism is seen. The site of the defect appears to be variable, with some patients exhibiting hypothalamic and others pituitary damage.

FUNCTIONAL DISEASES OF THE CENTRAL NERVOUS SYSTEM WITH NEUROENDOCRINE DISTURBANCES

Disturbances in neuroendocrine function manifested by both decreased and increased pituitary hormone secretion can occur in the absence of structurally detectable disease in the pituitary or CNS. With the aid of releasing hormones to test specifically the pituitary component and other stimuli to test the hypothalamic-pituitary unit, some degree of discrimination can be made as to the source of the disordered hormone secretion. The following are recognized functional disturbances that have been attributed to hypothalamic (or possibly other CNS) disease. The specific biochemical defect responsible remains to be determined.

HYPOTHALAMIC HYPOGONADISM. This disorder is defined as an impairment in pituitary-gonadal function caused by deficient or disordered secretion of GnRH. The manifestations vary according to the age of presentation.

Prepubertal. The presence of hypothalamic hypogonadism prior to puberty results in failure of normal sexual maturation. Other pituitary hormone deficiencies, also attributed to hypothalamic dysfunction, may coexist. A major subgroup of this disorder, most frequently seen in boys, includes anosmia or hyposmia (*Kallmann's syndrome* or olfactory-genital dysplasia). This syndrome may be associated with other neurologic defects such as color blindness and nerve deafness. The disorder is frequently familial, though sporadic cases have also been reported. Midline developmental defects occasionally occur, and hypoplasia in the region of the anterior commissure, olfactory bulb, and hypothalamus has been found. In some patients there is an additional defect characterized by decreased testicular response to LH. The gonadotropin responses to a single injection of GnRH are markedly impaired or absent, indicating a lack of prior GnRH function. Repeated administration of GnRH, given to prime the gonadotrophs, eventually produces a normal or supranormal gonadotropin response and serves to differentiate this disorder from that of primary gonadotroph failure. Standard therapy consists of the use of gonadal steroids for the development and maintenance of secondary sexual characteristics and gonadotropins for promoting fertility. The administration of GnRH analogues can produce both effects, provided pulsatile administration is used, by means of an intermittent infusion pump, to simulate endogenous secretion.

Postpubertal. Postpubertal hypothalamic hypogonadism affects primarily women. It is manifested clinically by secondary amenorrhea or oligomenorrhea and occasionally by infertility associated with anovulatory cycles. The terms *functional* or *psychogenic amenorrhea* and *infertility* have also been used for this disorder. Patients may exhibit normal tonic levels of gonadotropins and estradiol, resulting in maintenance of normal secondary sexual characteristics, although pulsatile secretion of LH, seen in normal women, is absent and the cyclic ovulatory surge of gonadotropins does not occur. The gonadotropin responses to a single injection of GnRH reveal enhancement of the FSH rather than the LH response. These women respond normally to clomiphene, an estrogen receptor antagonist, suggesting the defect is related to a functional derangement in the positive estrogen feedback mechanism. The disorder is usually self-limited.

Hyperprolactinemia exerts an inhibitory effect on the positive feedback effect of estradiol on GnRH secretion that has been attributed to enhanced tuberoinfundibular dopamine secretion. The negative estrogen feedback mechanism appears intact, since elevated FSH and LH levels are maintained in postmenopausal women with hyperprolactinemia. In men, hyperprolactinemia produces hypogonadism, manifested most frequently by diminished libido and potency.

In severe cases, basal estradiol levels and serum gonadotropin responses to GnRH are reduced, implying a defect in tonic as well as cyclic GnRH secretion. Similar physiologic disturbances are seen in some patients with hyperprolactinemia irrespective of cause. Marked increases and decreases in body weight are often accompanied by amenorrhea, as occurs in professional ballet dancers and female athletes; anorexia nervosa (see details later in this section); and severe obesity.

Treatment of this disorder depends on the extent of hypogonadism and the patient's desire for fertility. Restoration of ovulatory menses may be accomplished by cycles of clomiphene administration, cyclic estrogen-progestin (oral contraceptive) therapy, gonadotropin administration, or GnRH infusions, depending on the desired goal. In hypoestrogenemic women, decreased vaginal secretions, leading to dyspareunia and decreased libido, and the long-term consequences of osteopenia and metabolic bone disease warrant replacement therapy. In men, testosterone replacement therapy is indicated if endogenous hormone levels are subnormal.

Polycystic Ovary Syndrome (See also Ch. 236). The polycystic ovary (Stein-Leventhal) syndrome is characterized by amenorrhea, obesity, hirsutism, and consistently elevated LH levels. It is occasionally associated with a history of childhood CNS injury or "encephalitis." The altered hormonal secretory pattern of polycystic ovaries appears to be secondary to the increased LH secretion. This syndrome is occasionally seen in patients with hyperprolactinemia, but the causal relationship remains to be established (see Ch. 236.)

HYPOTHALAMIC HYPOTHYROIDISM. This is an uncommon disorder manifested by hypothyroidism, a low plasma TSH level, and an exaggerated and delayed response of TSH to TRH. In patients with this disorder, peak TSH responses occur at 90 to 120 minutes, in contrast to the 15- to 30-minute peak response time seen in normal subjects. Children of one subgroup have shown elevated basal TSH levels, but in most subjects basal levels are normal. Hypothalamic hypothyroidism can occur as an isolated defect or, more commonly, is seen in association with deficiencies of gonadotropin, GH, or ACTH secretion. Treatment of this disorder is with thyroxine.

HYPOTHALAMIC-ADRENAL DYSFUNCTION. Decreased ACTH secretion on the basis of hypothalamic or other CNS disorders is relatively rare. It is seen most commonly in association with other pituitary hormone dificiencies during childhood and, by inference, has been attributed to a CNS cause. Disturbances of ACTH diurnal rhythm and suppressibility of ACTH are common in patients with a variety of intracranial diseases and reflect disturbances in neuroendocrine control mechanisms. They do not have major clinical significance, but subtle effects on behavior cannot be excluded. In particular, patients with affective disorders (unipolar depression) or experiencing bereavement exhibit a lack of normal glucocorticoid suppressibility similar to that seen in Cushing's disease.

IDIOPATHIC HYPERPROLACTINEMIA. Idiopathic hyperprolactinemia (IH) is a disorder in which prolactin levels are elevated in the absence of demonstrable pituitary or CNS disease and of any other recognized cause of increased prolactin secretion. The clinical manifestations of IH consist of galactorrhea and amenorrhea. In some patients, oligomenorrhea is present, and in a few, sporadic ovulation persists. Prolactin levels are elevated but rarely exceed 150 ng per milliliter. The disease is confined to women of the childbearing age. The diagnosis remains inferential and based on exclusion of a pituitary microadenoma.

Many patients in whom IH was previously diagnosed have subsequently been found by computed tomography to harbor microadenomas. Extensive testing using neuropharmacologic probes has failed to distinguish patients with IH from those with microadenomas, suggesting that the same pathophysiologic mechanism underlies both disorders. IH has been attributed to a CNS neurotransmitter defect related to dopamine metabolism, based on the observations that drugs impairing dopaminergic neurotransmission (i.e., neuroleptic dopamine receptor antagonists) increase prolactin secretion. The major action of these drugs in elevating prolactin levels, however, appears to be at the pituitary rather than within the CNS. IH is a rather benign condition, since only a small percentage of patients followed over a period of years will subsequently show evidence of a pituitary tumor.

Therapy depends on the level of symptoms and the degree of inconvenience they produce. Bromocriptine, (2.5 mg two or three times a day) is a dopamine receptor agonist that suppresses prolactin levels, eliminates galactorrhea, and restores cyclic menses and fertility. Nearly 80 per cent of patients will experience menses within two months of initiating therapy, and 65 per cent will become fertile. The effect of the drug is of short duration, however, and hyperprolactinemia recurs following its discontinuation. In some patients, hyperprolactinemia may remit spontaneously or following a pregnancy subsequent to bromocriptine administration. There is no evidence that long-term bromocriptine therapy per se restores prolactin secretory dynamics to normal.

HYPOTHALAMIC DISORDERS OF GROWTH HORMONE SECRETION. ***Idiopathic Growth Hormone Deficiency.*** Idiopathic GH deficiency (IGHD) occurs as either an isolated hormone deficiency or in association with other anterior pituitary hormone deficiencies and as both a familial and sporadic disorder. It is a disease of childhood, the diagnosis frequently being made because of impaired linear growth when the child is between two and three years of age. Impairment in GH secretion may be complete, with basal levels barely detectable, or partial, with subnormal responses to stimuli. The absence of radiologic abnormalities of the pituitary and the frequent coexistence of TRH- and GnRH-responsive deficiencies of TSH and gonadotropins suggest the defect is located in the hypothalamus. No histologic studies of the pituitary or hypothalamus are available because of the generally benign nature of the disease. It is assumed to be due to a deficiency of GRF secretion, most likely on the basis of a neurotransmitter or biosynthetic abnormality, rather than to a structural defect in the hypothalamus. Preliminary studies with synthetic GRF have indicated subnormal GH responsiveness. The significance of these findings, however, remains to be determined. Several subgroups of GH deficiency are now recognized, including one in which partial deletion of the GH gene results in complete absence of the hormone and another in which there is spontaneous recovery of GH secretion. Therapy of IGHD is limited to the prepubertal period and consists of human GH. Hypothyroidism, if present, must also be treated. If gonadotropin deficiency is present, therapy with gonadal steroids is postponed as long as possible to avoid accelerating bone growth and producing epiphyseal closure before acceptable linear bone growth is achieved by GH.

Psychosocial Dwarfism. A pattern indistinguishable from IGHD is seen occasionally in children reared in environments with deficient maternal care and affection. Children with this disorder, also termed the emotional deprivation syndrome, exhibit impaired GH responses to stimuli when studied. Within a short time in an improved environment, however, GH secretion returns to normal, and linear growth is restored. It is presumed that the impaired GH secretion is secondary to a behaviorly associated alteration in neurotransmitter metabolism.

Cerebral Gigantism. This childhood disease is characterized by rapid growth, accelerated bone age, and mental retardation. Ventricular enlargement is present, although no focal CNS lesions have been detected. GH secretion has been normal in the few patients described with this disorder. A variant of the syndrome is associated with lipodystrophy, hyperpigmentation, hypertrichosis, hepatosplenomegaly, increased adrenal steroid production, and hyperlipemia.

CENTRAL NERVOUS SYSTEM DISORDERS OF WATER REGULATION. Organic lesions of the CNS and drug therapy can lead to "cerebral hyponatremia" or "cerebral hypernatremia," which are entities distinct from diabetes insipidus (see Ch. 226, Posterior Pituitary).

Hyponatremia. The syndrome of inappropriate secretion of antidiuretic hormone (ADH) results from the autonomous secretion of vasopressin, resulting in hyponatremia, renal sodium loss, and inability to excrete dilute urine in the presence of normal renal, pituitary, adrenal, and thyroid function; resistance to correction by hypertonic saline; and reversibility following restriction of water (see Ch. 76). The increased renal sodium excretion occurs secondary to expanded extracellular volume, resulting in suppression of aldosterone secretion. When measured, vasopressin levels in the circulation have been increased.

This syndrome has been reported in patients with carcinoma metastatic to the brain, primary brain tumors, cerebral infarction, basal skull fracture, subarachnoid hemorrhage, meningoencephalitis, and acute intermittent porphyria, but it may also occur in the absence of any underlying structural disease. Certain hypoglycemic and antineoplastic drugs can produce the same syndrome. The former, including chlorpropamide and tolbutamide, augment ADH action on the renal tubule and also stimulate ADH release. Vincristine and cyclophosphamide have direct neurotoxic effects on neurohypophyseal tissue. Other agents such as carbamazepine (Tegretol), amitriptyline (Elavil), thioridazine (Mellaril), and clofibrate also produce the syndrome, presumably by affecting endogenous vasopressin release.

Hypernatremia. Patients with intracranial lesions with or without disturbances of consciousness may exhibit hypernatremia in the presence of normal renal function, adequate fluid intake, absence of thirst, and failure of forced fluid intake to correct the hyperosmolality. This syndrome has been attributed to impaired regulation of thirst as well as vasopressin secretion, and has been described in association with histiocytosis, craniopharyngioma, optic nerve glioma, pineal tumor, encephalitis, and ruptured intracranial aneurysm. The treatment of this disorder, above and beyond that of the specific causative lesion, is similar to that for diabetes insipidus.

DISORDERS OF NEUROMETABOLIC REGULATION

Acute Disorders. Acute disturbances of metabolic regulation occur most commonly in states of stress that activate the sympathetic nervous system. Thus, patients with hypothermia, trauma, sepsis, and burns, and in the presence of general anesthesia, may exhibit hyperglycemia and hyperglucagonemia along with impaired insulin secretion. In most instances these changes represent merely an extension of normal physiologic processes, do not result in significant clinical problems, and resolve spontaneously when the stress disappears. However, when stress is prolonged, as in severe burns, the responses can produce a severe catabolic state that can be life threatening.

Stress diabetes, seen frequently in the same clinical disorders, may have several causes. Some patients may manifest true diabetes mellitus for the first time under circumstances in which there is enhanced secretion of cortisol, glucagon, catecholamines, and GH, but in other patients the marked hyperglycemia may be unrelated to true diabetes. A syndrome indistinguishable from nonketotic hyperglycemia with or without coma is associated with severe head injury, cerebral thrombosis, encephalitis, and heat stroke. The severity of the hyperglycemia and its duration predict the probability of survival following head injury. Treatment consists of hydration and small doses of insulin. Beta adrenergic blockade has been used in some patients, but should not be considered standard therapy.

Hypoglycemia is seen only rarely with hypothalamic disease. It has been reported in association with subdural hemorrage.

Chronic Disorders. Destruction of the ventromedial hypothalamus leads to a syndrome of obesity, but damage to the ventrolateral hypothalamus results in anorexia and inanition. Because bilateral destruction is necessary, inanition is infrequently observed, since the concomitant loss of other important homeostatic mechanisms is usually incompatible with prolonged survival. An anatomically identifiable hypothalamic lesion is present in only a small percentage of patients with extensive obesity or inanition. However, the remarkable similarity of clinical and biochemical features in patients with and without definable lesions suggests that many "functional" disorders of caloric homeostasis ("essential" obesity and anorexia nervosa) are caused by biochemical disturbances in hypothalamic function that are presently undefined.

HYPOTHALAMIC OBESITY. Ventromedial hypothalamic destruction resulting from encephalitis, infiltrative diseases (leukemia or histiocytosis X), trauma, vascular accidents, and tumors has been associated with obesity. Oxygen consumption, insulin secretion, body composition, and adipose metabolism are similar in patients with hypothalamic obesity and in those with "essential" obesity. Adipose tissue mass increases primarily as the result of hypertrophy rather than hyperplasia. Marked insulin resistance is present, and diabetes may develop in some patients. GH secretion is impaired, and hypogonadism is common.

A number of familial disorders (Laurence-Moon, Bardet-Biedl, Alstrom-Hallgren, Prader-Willi) are associated with extreme obesity and evidence of other hypothalamic disturbances, including hypogonadism, temperature intolerance, and loss of diurnal rhythms; and of extrahypothalamic disturbances, such as deafness, pigmentary retinopathy, hypotonia, and mental retardation.

Therapy of hypothalamic obesity is not very successful. Once true destruction has occurred, the functional alterations are almost always irreversible. In children with hypothalamic leukemic infiltrates, successful chemotherapy can lead to cessation of hyperphagia and reduction of weight to normal. In general, therapeutic measures are aimed at treatment of the morbidly obese patient.

ANOREXIA NERVOSA. This disorder has been recognized for more than 300 years, is seen almost exclusively in young women, and consists of weight loss, amenorrhea, and behavioral disturbances. See Ch. 215 for a detailed description.

Almost every neuroendocrine system is affected by the disorder. Gonadotropin secretion "regresses" to a prepubertal stage characterized by absence of pulsatile secretion of LH and altered FSH-LH responses to GnRH. GH levels are normal or, at times, elevated, particularly in the presence of severe malnutrition, in which a paradoxic response to glucose may be observed. TSH responses to TRH are reduced, but thyroid function tends to be normal. Plasma cortisol levels are elevated, but diurnal variation is generally preserved. Patients tend to be poikilothermic, exhibiting difficulty in maintaining body temperature in response to changes in the environment. Impaired vasopressin secretion can be demonstrated, but is rarely of clinical importance.

Most of the endocrine metabolic disturbances can be attributed to the severe malnutrition, and successful therapy resulting in weight gain is usually accompanied by restoration of normal neuroendocrine responses. One exception is gonadotropin secretion, which frequently remains abnormal and results in persistence of amenorrhea in up to one third of patients. Another appears to be osmoregulation, which remains discoordinated, with vasopressin being secreted for prolonged periods.

Prognosis for the reversal of cachexia and weight loss is reasonably good. Mortality is currently less than 5 per cent, and the majority of patients return to within 10 per cent of original body weight. Only 40 per cent of patients maintain their weight over a long term; the remainder exhibit moderate to severe weight loss with time.

CENTRAL NERVOUS SYSTEM BEHAVIORAL DISORDERS AFFECTING NEUROENDOCRINE FUNCTION. Disturbances of endocrine function have been observed in patients with a variety of psychiatric illnesses. The association is presumably through disordered neurotransmitter metabolism, although it is still unclear whether the same defect underlies both the behavioral and neuroendocrine dysfunction or whether altered behavior itself secondarily affects neuroendocrine function.

Of all the conditions studied, depressive affective behavior and the manic-depressive state have been most clearly shown to exhibit endocrine changes. Cortisol secretion in depressed patients is enhanced, and they are relatively resistant to dexamethasone suppression. This abnormality reverts to normal with successful treatment. In manic-depressive patients, cortisol secretion tends to be decreased during manic states and elevated during depressive periods.

Brown GM, Garfinkel PE, Grof E, Grof P, Cleghorn JM, Brown P: A critical appraisal of neuroendocrine approaches to psychiatric disorders. *In* Muller EE, MacLeod RM (eds.): Neuroendocirne Perspectives. Vol 2. Amsterdam, Elsevier Biomedical Press, 1983, pp 329–364. *A review of the recent flurry of excitement concerning the use of neuroendocrine testing to obtain indirect evidence for neurotransmitter disorders in patients with psychiatric disease. The linkage of selective neuroendocrine defects to specific diagnostic entities may provide new insights into their pathophysiology.*

Comite F, Cutler GB, Rivier J, Vale WW, Loriaux DL, Crowley WF: Short-term treatment of idiopathic precocious puberty with a long-acting analogue of luteinizing hormone-releasing hormone. N Engl J Med 305:1546, 1981. *The use of an agonist of GnRH paradoxically decreases pituitary gonadotropin secretion when given continuously, as a result of down-regulation of the pituitary GnRH receptor. This approach to treatment is the basis for future use of GnRH analogues as contraceptive agents.*

Frohman LA: Clinical aspects of hypothalamic disease. *In* Motta M (ed.): The Endocrine Functions of the Brain. New York, Raven Press, 1980, pp 419–446. *A comprehensive review of neuroendocrine and neurometabolic disorders in man. Emphasis is on the overall integration of homeostatic systems.*

Frohman LA, Krieger DT: Endocrine disorders due to central nervous system disease. *In* Felig P, Baxter JD, Broadus AE, Frohman LA (eds.): Endocrinology and Metabolism. New York, McGraw-Hill Book Company, 1981, pp 233–252. *A systematic review of neuroendocrine pathophysiology and anatomic and functional disorders. Designed for the medical student, clinical trainee, and practicing physician.*

Gold PW, Kaye W, Robertson GL, Ebert M: Abnormalities in plasma and cerebrospinal fluid arginine vasopressin in patients with anorexia nervosa. N Engl J Med 38:1117, 1983. *A careful investigation of the disturbances in water regulation in patients with anorexia nervosa. Insight is provided into some of the previously recognized features of a mild diabetes insipidus-like state.*

Hoffman AR, Crowley WF Jr: Induction of puberty in men by long-term pulsatile administration of low-dose gonadotropin-releasing hormone. N Engl J Med 307:1237, 1982. *Description of the use of pulsatile administration of GnRH to stimulate gonadotropin secretion in subjects with hypogonadotropic hypogonadism. A classic example of the transfer of information from animal physiologic studies to treat human disease.*

Jeffcoate WJ, Laurance BM, Edwards CRW, Besser GM: Endocrine function in the Prader-Willi syndrome. Clin Endocrinol 12:81, 1980. *A human model of hypothalamic obesity with careful neuroendocrine studies that provide an important characterization of the disorder.*

Lieblich JM, Rogol AD, White BJ, Rosen SW: Syndrome of anosmia with hypogonadism (Kallmann's syndrome). Clinical and laboratory studies in 23 cases. Am J Med 73:506, 1982. *An excellent clinical study of Kallmann's syndrome with detailed endocrine studies very lucidly presented.*

Scherbaum WA, Bottazzo GF: Autoantibodies to vasopressin cells in idiopathic diabetes insipidus: Evidence for an autoimmune variant. Lancet 1:897, 1983. *Circulating antibodies to hypothalamic vasopressin-secreting cells but not to vasopressin are demonstrated in one third of patients with idiopathic diabetes insipidus, suggesting the existence of a new entity.*

225. THE ANTERIOR PITUITARY

Lawrence A. Frohman

ANATOMY

The pituitary is located in a saddle-shaped cavity, the *sella turcica,* which is an integral portion of the sphenoid bone. Its anterior boundary is the midline *tuberculum sella* and the anterior clinoid processes that project posteriorly from the sphenoid wings. The posterior limit is the *dorsum sella,* which projects laterally to form the posterior clinoid processes. The lateral boundaries of the sella are nonosseous and consist of the medial wall of the cavernous sinus, in which is contained the internal carotid artery. The *diaphragma sella,* a thickened reflection of the *dura mater,* forms the roof of the sella and is attached to the clinoid processes. Only the external layer of the dura extends into the sella as a periosteal lining, and thus the pituitary is normally extradural and not in direct communication with cerebrospinal fluid. The pituitary stalk and its blood vessels pass through a foramen in this membrane that may be incomplete or fenestrated.

The shape of the sella varies from ovoid to spheroid, resulting in considerable variation in normal pituitary dimensions. The average dimensions of the pituitary are 10 mm (anterior-posterior) by 13 mm (transverse) by 6 mm (height). Pituitary weight varies from 0.5 to 0.7 grams, being slightly greater in women. The anterior lobe constitutes about 75 per cent of the total pituitary weight and during pregnancy can increase up to two-fold in size.

The arterial blood supply of the pituitary originates from the internal carotid artery via branches from the circle of Willis and hypophyseal arteries. Whereas the posterior lobe is supplied directly by the inferior hypophyseal artery, the blood supply of the anterior lobe is derived entirely from the portal vascular system (see Ch. 224). Venous drainage from the anterior lobe enters the posterior pituitary capillary bed and then the cavernous sinus. The nerve supply of the anterior pituitary consists almost exclusively of postganglionic sympathetic fibers that accompany and terminate on arteriolar vessels. The importance of these fibers in regulating pituitary blood flow is unknown. There are also nerve fibers connecting the posterior and anterior lobes, and their function is also unknown.

EMBRYOLOGY

The glandular portion of the pituitary *(adenohypophysis)* is derived from Rathke's pouch, an ectodermal evagination of the oropharynx that fuses with an outpouching of the region of the third ventricle in the developing embryo. This portion of the diencephalon eventually differentiates into the *neurohypophysis,* or posterior lobe. That portion of Rathke's pouch not in contact with the diencephalon differentiates to form the *pars anterior,* or anterior lobe. Two lateral outgrowths from the anterior lobes fuse in the midline and extend forward along the hypophyseal stalk to form the *pars tuberalis,* which in humans is limited to a small group of cells along the anterior region of the stalk. The portion of Rathke's pouch contiguous with the neurohypophysis develops less extensively and forms the *pars intermedia,* or intermediate lobe. This structure is not well defined in humans and tends to become intermingled with the anterior lobe. This combined structure has been called the *pars distalis.*

Cells of the pars anterior differentiate into cells that secrete growth hormone (GH), prolactin, corticotropin (ACTH), thyroid-stimulating hormone (TSH), luteinizing hormone (LH), and follicle-stimulating hormone (FSH). Cells of the pars intermedia secrete ACTH, lipotropin, and endorphins. Pituitary tumors developing in various regions of the pars distalis tend to reflect the predominant cell types in each region.

The lumen of Rathke's pouch is obliterated during development, although remnants may persist at the boundary of the neurohypophysis as either a cleft or small colloid-filled cysts. The connection with the oropharynx disappears early in development, because of growth of the sphenoid bone, although a few cells in the lower portion of the pouch may persist along the tract, occasionally within the sphenoid bone, and are known as the pharyngeal pituitary. These cells contain secretory granules for GH and prolactin, can be a source of "ectopic" pituitary tumor development, and conceivably could exhibit significant endocrine function subsequent to destruction or removal of the pars distalis.

The fetal pituitary anlage is first recognizable at four to five weeks of gestation, and cellular cytologic differentiation occurs between the seventh and tenth weeks. Monoamine fluorescence in the median eminence occurs by 13 weeks and is followed shortly thereafter by development of the portal vascular system. The hypothalamic-pituitary unit appears anatomically mature by 20 weeks. Pituitary hormones are detected immunochemically as early as the seventh week, and CNS control of anterior pituitary hormone secretion occurs early in gestation. In contrast, true functional maturation, including aspects of feedback regulation, do not develop until well into postnatal life.

CELL TYPES

The anterior pituitary contains many cell types, the predominant function of which is the synthesis, storage, and release of a specific hormone(s). Immunohistochemical stains have permitted distinction of specific hormone-containing granules, leading to identification of individual cell types. Secretory granules and the structure of certain cellular organelles, vary greatly between cell types. The secretion granule size within a single cell type varies considerably, depending on the functional state of the cell. The recognized anterior pituitary cell types are as follows:

SOMATOTROPHS. Originally identified as acidophilic cells, these cells secrete GH. Tumors of the cell type predominate in patients with acromegaly. The cells are located predominantly in the lateral portions of the anterior lobe.

LACTOTROPHS. Lactotrophs are also acidophilic and secrete prolactin. They tend to be located more peripherally than somatotrophs, and their secretion granules are smaller. During pregnancy and fetal life, lactotrophs are increased in number, reflecting the effects of increased estrogen levels. Virtually all of the increase in pituitary size during pregnancy can be accounted for by lactotroph proliferation. Both lactotrophs and somatotrophs appear to be derived from a common stem cell, tumors of which may secrete both GH and prolactin.

THYROTROPHS. The basophilic staining cells that secrete TSH occur most frequently at the anterior edge of the pituitary near the midline, although they are also present in deeper portions of the gland. Their secretion granules are smaller than GH and prolactin granules and exhibit considerable heterogeneity. Under normal conditions, thyrotrophs constitute only about 6 per cent of anterior lobe cells. In primary hypothyroidism, they undergo marked hypertrophy, exhibit changes indicative of increased secretory activity, and can eventually undergo neoplastic transformation.

GONADOTROPHS. These cells are located deep in the lateral portion of the gland in association with lactotrophs and secrete both LH and FHS. Although constituting only 3 to 4 per cent of anterior pituitary cells normally, they increase in number following castration and decrease during pregnancy as a result of placental gonadotropin production.

CORTICOTROPHS. This cell type, which can exhibit chromophobic or basophilic characteristics, is found in two separate locations. One group of cells resides most commonly in the medial mucoid region of the anterior lobe. A second group migrates during development to the junctional region of the anterior and posterior lobes and also to the pars tuberalis. Anterior lobe corticotrophs exhibit sparse granulation, whereas those in the pars tuberalis–posterior lobe region contain large and electron-dense granules. The same precursor molecule is present in both cell types, although processing enzyme activity varies, resulting in different ratios of hormones derived from the precursor (ACTH, melanocyte-stimulating hormone [MSH], endorphin) in the two different regions. Increases in glucocorticoid levels produce degranulation and microtubular hyalinization of corticotrophs (Crooke's changes). Anterior lobe corticotrophs increase in number with glucocorticoid deficiency, while those in the intermediate-posterior lobe region decrease, suggesting that only the former are physiologically important ACTH-secreting cells.

OTHER CELL TYPES. As many as 15 to 20 per cent of anterior pituitary cells cannot be stained by antibodies to any of the recognized anterior pituitary hormones. Some of these may represent resting degranulated cells or undifferentiated primitive secretory cells. However, some may be responsible for the secretion of other as yet uncharacterized pituitary hormones such as ovarian growth factor or exophthalmos-producing substance. In addition, a few cells are stellate, with cellular processes extending into the perivascular spaces in a manner suggestive of primitive follicle formation. These cells generally do not contain secretory granules, and their function is unknown.

ANTERIOR PITUITARY HORMONES

The anterior pituitary secretes six well-recognized hormones for which specific and sensitive radioimmunoassays are available. They can be divided into three general categories: corticotropin and related peptides, glycoprotein hormones, and somatomammotropin hormones. The chemical characteristics of these hormones are given in Table 225–1.

CORTICOTROPIN-RELATED PEPTIDES. ACTH and its related family of peptides are synthesized as a single precursor molecule, preopiomelanocortin, with a molecular weight of approximately 29,000. Following glycosylation, the molecule is differentially cleaved into an N-terminal fragment, the biologic activity of which remains uncertain; a midportion, which contains ACTH; and a C-terminal portion, β-lipotropin (LPH). Subsequent processing, which varies in the different groups of corticotrophs and also in the brain, may also cleave ACTH into α-MSH and corticotropin-like intermediate lobe peptide. β-LPH is also differentially processed further to β-endorphin and other endorphin-related peptides (Ch. 222). Although the structures of β-MSH and met-enkephalin are contained within the β-LPH sequence, the former is not synthesized in human pituitaries, and the biosynthesis of the latter occurs through a separate precursor.

ACTH. The primary effects of ACTH are stimulation of secretion of glucocorticoid, mineralocorticoid, and androgenic steroids by the adrenal cortex. ACTH binds to specific receptors on adrenocortical cell membranes and stimulates steroidogenesis by enhancing cholesterol conversion to pregnenolone. ACTH also stimulates adrenal protein synthesis, leading to cellular growth and hyperplasia.

A number of extra-adrenal effects of ACTH have also been described, including stimulation of lipolysis in adipose tissue, insulin-releasing effects on the pancreatic B cell, stimulation of GH secretion, enhancement of glucose and amino acid transport into muscles, and prolongation of cortisol half-life in plasma. Except in patients with ACTH-secreting tumors, it is unlikely that plasma ACTH levels sufficient to produce these

TABLE 225–1. ANTERIOR PITUITARY HORMONES IN HUMANS

Class	Members	Molecular Weight	Amino Acids	Carbohydrate	Other Features
Corticotropin-lipotropin	ACTH	4,500	39		All members of class derived from a single precursor
	α-MSH	1,800	13		N-terminal 13 amino acids of ACTH. In humans, found only in fetal life
	β-Lipotropin	11,200	91		
	β-Endorphin	4,000	31		C-terminal (amino acids 61–91) portion of β-LPH
Glycoprotein	LH	29,000	α subunit: 89 β subunit: 115	1% sialic acid	All have two subunits, with the α subunit being identical or nearly identical and the β subunit conferring biologic specificity
	FSH	29,000	α subunit: 89 β subunit: 115	5% sialic acid	
	TSH	29,000	α subunit: 89 β subunit: 112	1% sialic acid	
	Chorionic gonadotropin*	46,000	α subunit: 92 β subunit: 139	12% sialic acid	
Somatomammotropin	Growth hormone	21,800	191		All single-chain proteins with two or three disulfide bridges
	Prolactin	22,500	198		
	Placental lactogen*	21,800	191		

Adapted from Frohman, LA: Diseases of the anterior pituitary. *In* Felig P, Baxter JD, Broadus AE, Frohman LA (eds.): Endocrinology and Metabolism. New York, McGraw-Hill Book Company, 1981.

*Of placental origin and included for comparison purposes.

effects are ever achieved. Although ACTH has less potent pigmenting effects than α-MSH or β-MSH, it has long been considered the major pigmenting hormone in man. Recent studies, however, have indicated control of pigmentation to be a complex process, and the importance of ACTH has come under question.

ACTH is the most difficult of the pituitary hormones to measure and exhibits the greatest variability, in part because of its episodic secretion. Plasma ACTH levels in normal adults range from undetectable to 80 pg per milliliter (the lower limit of detection in most assays is approximately 10 pg per milliliter. In addition to its episodic secretion, a diurnal rhythm can be detected with lowest levels in the evening and peak levels in the early morning. Changes in plasma ACTH levels can be shown to precede those of plasma cortisol with a short lag period. With stress, plasma ACTH levels can reach several hundred picograms per milliliter. In patients with ectopic ACTH production, immunoreactive ACTH levels may be exceedingly high and consist in part of larger molecular sized forms ("big" ACTH) believed to represent partially processed precursor molecules. ACTH is rapidly eliminated from plasma; its half-life is 3 to 9 minutes, leading to an estimated secretion rate of 25 μg per day, which represents approximately 5 per cent of pituitary hormone content.

β-LPH, Endorphins, and Related Peptides. β-LPH and β-endorphin are secreted in an equimolar ratio to ACTH in response to all types of stimulation. The presence of both molecules in the same precursor as ACTH, with enzymatic cleavage immediately prior to or concomitant with the secretory process, offers an attractive explanation for this observation. The plasma levels of β-LPH and β-endorphin, however, do not necessarily parallel those of ACTH because of a slower metabolic clearance rate. β-LPH is cleared primarily by the kidneys, and its levels rise disproportionately to those of ACTH in renal failure. Since ACTH secretion is normal in this disorder, β-LPH must exert relatively little feedback effect on its own secretion or that of ACTH. The relative ease of measuring β-LPH, in contrast to ACTH, has prompted its use as a marker for the diagnosis of ACTH-secreting tumors, much as C peptide is used in the diagnosis of insulinomas. (β-LPH and β-endorphin have not been shown to have any effects peripherally at the levels normally seen in plasma).

GLYCOPROTEIN HORMONES. The pituitary glycoprotein hormones consist of an α and β subunit, each containing a peptide core with branched carbohydrate side chains that are required for biologic activity and for stability in plasma. The α subunits of the glycoprotein hormones are identical, whereas the β subunits vary, thereby providing the biologic specificity of each hormone. There is considerable homology between β subunits of the different hormones as well as cross-species homology of both α and β subunits, which explains why bovine or ovine glycoprotein hormones are active in humans. The isolated subunits have no intrinsic biologic activity. Evidence of hormone heterogeneity, related to the degree of glycosylation, has been detected and may explain the reported variations in glycoprotein bioactivity at different times in the menstrual cycle. The individual subunits are synthesized separately, and the rate-limiting step in glycoprotein hormone secretion is controlled by β subunit production. Elevations in plasma α subunit levels can be seen after both TRH and GnRH stimulation and also in occasional pituitary tumors.

TSH. TSH effects on the thyroid cells are largely analogous to those of ACTH on the adrenal cortex. High-affinity receptors are present on cell membranes, and TSH binding leads to activation of adenylate cyclase, enhanced iodine transport and binding to protein, increased thyroglobulin and thyroid hormone synthesis, and increased thyroglobulin proteolysis with release of thyroid hormones. RNA and protein synthesis are also stimulated, leading to an increase in thyroid size and vascularity.

TSH is measured by a specific assay utilizing an antibody directed to antigenic determinants on the β subunit that exhibit little or no cross-reactivity with other glycoprotein hormones. Normal levels of plasma TSH are generally reported as under 6 μU per milliliter, with most assays being unable to detect levels less than 1 μU per milliliter. Some of the more recently developed assays appear to have greater sensitivity and specificity, resulting in an upper limit of 3 μU per milliliter and the ability to discriminate normal from low levels. In primary hypothyroidism, TSH levels may increase to greater than 100 μU per milliliter. A few patients have been described with hypothyroidism and slightly elevated TSH levels in whom administration of thyrotropin releasing hormone (TRH) results in an exaggerated TSH increase and a concomitant increase in thyroxine. Evidence for a biologically less potent TSH has been found in such individuals. TSH is cleared from circulation with a half-life of 75 to 80 minutes, and the secretion rate of the hormone is 100 to 200 mU per day. In hypothyroidism, secretion rates may be increased 10 to 15 times that in normals.

LH and FSH. Gonadal function is regulated by two pituitary hormones: (1) FSH, which stimulates ovarian follicular growth, testicular growth, and spermatogenesis, and (2) LH, which promotes ovulation and follicular luteinization, stimulates testicular interstitial cell function, and enhances production of steroids in both ovary and testis. Both gonadotropins bind to receptors in the ovary and testis. In the ovary, FSH promotes growth and maturation of the primordial follicle cell, and LH stimulates progesterone production by the corpus luteum by enhancing the conversion of cholesterol to pregnenolone. In the testis, FSH acts on the Sertoli cell, where, in conjunction with testosterone, the production of an androgen-binding protein is stimulated. The target cell of LH is the Leydig cell, leading to enhanced testosterone production. The androgen-binding protein serves to transport testosterone in high concentrations into the tubular cells to stimulate spermatogenesis. (See also discussion in Ch. 234.)

The gonadotropin assays exhibit some degree of cross-reactivity between the hormone and its subunits, though this is not a practical problem. Of importance, however, is the cross-reactivity due to the great similarity between LH and chorionic gonadotropin. Most LH assays do not discriminate between the two hormones.

Plasma levels of FSH and LH in women vary with the menstrual cycle. FSH levels rise slightly and then decline progressively during the early follicular phase of the cycle, during which time LH levels are generally stable or rise slightly. An abrupt rise in LH at midcycle, initiated by increasing estrogen secretion by the developing follicle and accompanied by an FSH rise, triggers ovulation. Both hormone levels decline during the luteal phase. Levels of FSH and LH in males are similar to those in females during the follicular phase. FSH and LH levels increase in response to age-related decreases in gonadal function in both sexes. In women this occurs at menopause, and in men a gradual increase is seen during the sixth to eighth decades. The half-life of LH in circulation is approximately 30 minutes, whereas that of FSH is twice as long, the difference being attributed to the varying sialic acid content of the hormones.

SOMATOMAMMOTROPIC HORMONES. This hormonal class consists of GH, prolactin, and a structurally similar placental hormone, chorionic somatomammotropin, or placental lactogen. Extensive interspecies homology exists for both GH and prolactin, suggesting relatively limited changes in gene duplication during evolution. Despite the similarity, subprimate growth hormones are biologically inactive in humans. GH and placental lactogen exhibit 83 per cent homology in contrast to only 16 per cent homology between GH and prolactin. Despite these differences, each hormone has both intrinsic lactogenic and growth-promoting activity. The biosynthetic precursor molecules for both GH and prolactin contain an N-terminal extension of approximately 30 amino acids that is cleaved during processing and packaging in the endoplasmic reticulum. Large, molecular weight-sized hormones ("big" GH and prolactin) have been identified in both pituitary and plasma. The big hormones appear to be dimers connected by interchain disulfide linkages. They are secreted by the pituitary, bind to the hormone target cell receptors, and exhibit reduced biologic activity as compared to the monomer. There are four or five additional GH variants, including proteolytically modified forms, electrophoretic variants, and a smaller molecule ("20K variant") lacking amino acids 32 to 46, which is encoded by a separate mRNA species derived from the authentic GH gene and formed by differential splicing of pre-mRNA to mRNA. This variant, while representing 10 to 20 per cent of pituitary GH, constitutes less than 5 per cent of secreted GH, and levels in circulation do not change in response to GH secretagogues. It is of potential clinical interest because it possesses the same growth-promoting and lactogenic activity as the normal 22K GH but lacks the hyperglycemic or diabetogenic activity.

Growth Hormone. GH exhibits an important role in production of linear growth and regulation of metabolic processes. GH administration to GH-deficient patients results in positive nitrogen balance, decreased urea production, decreased body fat stores, and enhanced carbohydrate utilization. Biphasic effects on circulating glucose, amino acid, and free fatty acid levels occur in response to GH with an initial decrease and subsequent return to normal or an increase. The acute effects of GH in isolated tissues resemble those of insulin and include increased amino acid uptake and incorporation into protein, stimulation of new RNA synthesis, and enhanced glucose utilization. GH also antagonizes the lipolytic effect of catecholamines in adipose tissue. These acute effects disappear within three to four hours, by which time a series of delayed effects appears. These include enhanced triglyceride lipolysis, increased sensitivity to catecholamine-mediated lipolysis, and inhibition of glucose uptake and utilization secondary to impaired pyruvate decarboxylation. These effects form the basis of the diabetogenic action of the hormone. GH also exhibits multiphasic effects on insulin secretion. There is an acute direct stimulatory effect on the beta cell, a subsequent inhibitory effect, and a late and persistent stimulation of insulin release that occurs secondary to the impairment of carbohydrate utilization. The last effect has the greatest pathophysiologic significance in the development of diabetes secondary to GH hypersecretion.

Many GH effects cannot be produced by exposure of tissues to the hormone and are mediated by a group of GH-dependent growth factors, most of which are synthesized in the liver. GH binds to specific receptors on hepatocyte membranes to stimulate their production. The most important of these factors is somatomedin C or insulin-like growth factor I (IGF I), a peptide of about 7500 daltons that has many similarities to insulin, including structural resemblance to proinsulin and binding to insulin receptors. Somatomedin C receptors are present in many tissues, including cartilage, where sulfate incorporation into proteoglycan and amino acid uptake incorporation are stimulated. A closely related peptide, somatomedin A (IGF II), and a platelet–derived growth factor are also GH dependent, though they are less important in both mediating the growth-stimulating effects of GH and peripheral feedback of GH secretion. GH also stimulates cardiac and renal hypertrophy and production of specific hormones such as renin and aldosterone and conversion of thyroxine to triiodothyronine.

Immunoreactive measurements of GH are considered valid indicators of GH bioactivity. Mean GH levels during adolescence and adult life are generally less than 3 ng per milliliter, although the spontaneous secretory pulses of GH can produce elevations as great as 30 to 50 ng per milliliter in young adult subjects. Levels in women during the childbearing age are generally greater than in men, particularly in response to exercise or other stimuli. GH is cleared from plasma primarily by the liver and to a lesser extent by the kidney. The half-time of GH disappearance from circulation is 20 to 25 minutes, and the overall secretion in normal adults ranges from 300 to 500 μg per square meter per day.

Prolactin. The major effect of prolactin is to stimulate the synthesis of milk constituents, including lactalbumin, lipids, and carbohydrates (Ch. 238). Prolactin receptors are present on alveolar surfaces of mammary cells and, in addition, have been identified in liver and kidney. Prolactin is not required for normal breast development in humans, and pathologic elevations of the hormone are not associated with an increase in breast size. During pregnancy, prolactin, in conjunction with estrogen, progesterone, and placental lactogen, results in further breast development and milk formation. Following parturition, the abrupt decrease in estrogen and progesterone derived from the placenta permits initiation of lactation. This effect underlies the use of estrogens to inhibit lactation in the postpartum period and explains the frequent development of galactorrhea in hyperprolactinemic women after discontinuance of oral contraceptives. Continued prolactin secretion is required to maintain lactation once it is initiated, and the return of prolactin to normal levels in the postpartum period is delayed in women who nurse for prolonged periods. The actual milk let-down reflex is mediated by the release of oxytocin in the posterior pituitary rather than by prolactin. Oxytocin stimulates contraction of myoepithelial cells surrounding the terminal acinar lobules that expel their milk into the lobular ducts. Although prolactin has numerous effects on behavior and on fluid and electrolyte metabolism in lower species, no such effects have been convincingly demonstrated in humans.

Normal prolactin levels do not exceed 15 ng per milliliter in men or 20 ng per milliliter in women. There are no significant changes during the menstrual cycle, but levels decrease at menopause. During pregnancy, prolactin levels rise continuously from early gestation to values of 150 to 200 ng per milliliter at term. Prolactin is cleared from circulation with a half-time of approximately 50 minutes. The liver and, to a lesser extent, the kidney are the major sites of prolactin removal.

TESTS OF ANTERIOR PITUITARY HORMONE FUNCTION

ACTH. Since ACTH levels in normal subjects may be undetectable at times, random measurements of the hormone are of limited value. In a patient with signs and symptoms of adrenocortical insufficiency and low plasma cortisol levels, a low or even normal ACTH level is suggestive of hypothalamic-pituitary disease. The most useful test for evaluating ACTH function is that of insulin hypoglycemia. A dose of insulin calculated to decrease the fasting blood glucose to 40 mg per deciliter is administered, and plasma cortisol levels are measured over a two-hour period. A rise greater than 10 μg per deciliter or a peak level greater than 20 μg per deciliter is indicative of a normal hypothalamic-pituitary-adrenal axis. The standard dose of insulin is 0.1 U per kilogram (intravenously), although the dose should be decreased by 50 per cent when the diagnosis of hypopituitarism is strongly suspected and increased by 50 per cent in patients with anticipated insulin resistance (i.e., obesity). No treatment is necessary for mild symptoms of hypoglycemia (catecholamine-mediated phenomena), but symptoms of central glucopenia (impaired mentation or altered states of consciousness) require immediate therapy. This test must not be performed in patients with suspected primary adrenal insufficiency.

Corticotropin releasing factor (CRF) is currently being evaluated as a diagnostic agent for assessing ACTH function and, when available for general use, is expected to provide a valuable adjunct. A normal response to CRF and an impaired response to insulin hypoglycemia, for example, would suggest hypothalamic rather than pituitary disease. Impairment of normal cortisol feedback using metyrapone, an 11β-hydroxylase inhibitor, at a dose of 750 mg orally every four hours for six doses, with measurement of plasma 11-desoxycortisol or urinary 17-hydroxycorticoids, is an alternative way to test the entire hypothalamic-pituitary-adrenal axis. This test is less useful than insulin hypoglycemia in predicting normal responsiveness of the axis to stress.

The best test of suspected excessive ACTH and cortisol secretion is by dexamethasone suppression. The rapid dexamethasone suppression test involves administration of 1 mg dexamethasone orally at 11 P.M. and measurement of plasma cortisol at 8 o'clock the following morning. A level of less than 5 μg per deciliter indicates normal suppressibility. In patients in whom normal suppression is not demonstrated, a standard low-dose dexamethasone suppression test (0.5 mg orally every six hours for 48 hours) is performed. Plasma cortisol will be suppressed to less than 5 μg per deciliter, and urinary free cortisol levels will be suppressed to within the normal range in normal subjects but not in patients with pituitary ACTH hypersecretion or primary adrenocortical hypersecretion. In patients in whom suppression fails, a high-dose dexamethasone suppression test (2 mg orally every six hours for 48 hours) is then used to distinguish between pituitary and adrenal causes.

TSH. Impairment of TSH secretion should be suspected in patients with hypothyroidism in whom plasma TSH levels are not elevated. Differentiation of pituitary from hypothalamic causes of TSH deficiency can usually, but not always, be accomplished by administering TRH, 500 μg (intravenously), and measuring plasma TSH levels. In normal persons, plasma TSH increases to at least 8 μU per milliliter after TRH administration, and peak levels usually occur at 15 to 30 minutes. In patients with hypothalamic hypothyroidism, the response may be exaggerated and is frequently prolonged, with peak values occurring at 90 to 180 minutes. Since thyroxine impairs the TSH response to TRH, it is not possible to assess TSH function in patients receiving thyroid hormone replacement therapy until at least a month after discontinuation of medication.

LH AND FSH. LH and FSH deficiency should be suspected in patients with clinical evidence of hypogonadism and subnormal testosterone or estradiol levels in whom gonadotropin levels are not elevated. Gonadotropin releasing hormone (GnRH) (100 μg, intravenously) can be administered and gonadotropin responses measured. An increase of at least three- to five-fold in LH is seen in normal subjects. A single injection, however, may not distinguish between hypothalamic and hypopituitary causes, since impaired responses may be seen in both disorders and only after repeated injections does a response occur in patients with hypothalamic hypogonadism. Clomiphene, an estrogen antagonist, will stimulate gonadotropin levels in some patients with hypothalamic hypogonadism.

GROWTH HORMONE. The most frequently employed stimulus for GH secretion is the insulin hypoglycemia test. The details of testing and the cautions required are as described under ACTH testing. Peak growth hormone levels usually occur at 60 or 90 minutes, and a peak level of 9 ng per milliliter or greater is required for a normal response. Up to 30 per cent of normal subjects may not respond to insulin hypoglycemia. L-arginine (0.5 gram per kilogram intravenously during a 30-minute period), L-dopa (0.5 gram orally), and clonidine (25 μg orally) are other effective stimuli used to test GH secretory reserve. The responses are comparable in magnitude to those after insulin. Although other stimuli have been used (glucagon plus propranolol, endotoxin, vasopressin, ACTH), none has any advantage over those described. There is currently insufficient information to know whether growth hormone releasing factor (GRF) will be useful as a diagnostic test in distinguishing pituitary from hypothalamic causes of GH deficiency.

Suppressibility of GH secretion in patients with elevated GH levels is evaluated with a standard glucose tolerance test. A decrease in GH levels to less than 2 ng per milliliter is seen in normal subjects. TRH is also used in distinguishing between types of suspected GH hypersecretion. TRH has no effect on GH levels in normal subjects, whereas in 80 to 90 per cent of patients with acromegaly a rapid increase in GH levels occurs.

PROLACTIN. Impaired prolactin secretion is rarely a clinical problem. Prolactin deficiency can be suspected in patients with levels of less than 2 ng per milliliter, and the diagnosis is confirmed by the absence of a response to TRH. Elevated

prolactin levels in nearly all patients, with the exception of occasional patients with prolactin-secreting tumors and patients with chronic renal failure, can be suppressed by dopamine infusions, L-dopa, or other dopaminergic agents. These tests have limited usefulness in determining the cause of hyperprolactinemia and are generally not used.

Ezrin C, Horvath E, Kovacs K: Anatomy and cytology of the normal and abnormal pituitary gland. *In* DeGroot LJ, Cahill GF Jr, Martini L, et al (eds.): Endocrinology. Vol. 1. New York, Grune & Stratton, 1979, pp 103–121. *A well-organized and referenced presentation of pituitary structure with emphasis on the changes in human disease.*

Frohman LA: Diseases of the anterior pituitary. *In* Felig P, Baxter JD, Broadus E, Frohman LA (eds.): Endocrinology and Metabolism. New York, McGraw-Hill Book Company, 1981, pp 151–231. *A detailed systematic description of the chemistry, physiology, and pathophysiology of the pituitary. Of particular use to the clinical trainee and practicing physician.*

Frohman LA: Growth hormone releasing factor: A neuroendocrine perspective. J Lab Clin Med 103:819, 1984. *A review of the clinical studies leading to the isolation and characterization of GRF and the initial results of its use in normal human subjects and patients with GH secretory disorders.*

Jaffe RB, Monroe SE: Hormone interaction and regulation during the menstrual cycle. *In* Ganong WF, Martini L (eds.): Frontiers in Neuroendocrinology. Vol. 6. New York, Raven Press, 1980, pp 219–248. *A comprehensive review of the hormonal interactions responsible for the cyclical reproductive cycle in women. Provides a firm basis with which to understand pathophysiologic conditions.*

Lufkin EG, Kao PC, O'Fallon WM, Mangan MA: Combined testing of anterior pituitary gland with insulin, thyrotropin-releasing hormone, and luteinizing hormone-releasing hormone. Am J Med 75:471, 1983. *A clearly presented study confirming that the combined use of the three standard agents used in testing pituitary hormone function is more efficient than individual testing protocols.*

Miller WL, Eberhardt NL: Structure and evolution of the growth hormone gene family. Endocr Rev 4:97, 1983. *This review documents in great detail the recent exciting developments in molecular biology related to GH gene expression. Although of limited practical use to the clinician, this work describes concepts important for understanding recombinant DNA technology as applied to the production of human hormones.*

Orth DN, Jackson RV, DeCherney CS, DeBold CR, Alexander AN, Island DP, Rivier J, Rivier C, Spiess J, Vale W: Effect of synthetic ovine corticotropin-releasing factor. Dose response to plasma adrenocorticotropin and cortisol. J Clin Invest 71:587, 1983. *Classic study of the use of a new releasing hormone to evaluate ACTH secretion. When available for clinical use, this peptide should permit differential assessment of hypothalamic and pituitary components of the regulation of ACTH secretion.*

Scanlon MF, Lewis M, Weightman DR, Chan V, Hall R: The neuroregulation of human thyrotropin secretion. *In* Ganong WF, Martini L (eds.): Frontiers in Neuroendocrinology. Vol. 6. New York, Raven Press, 1980, pp 333–380. *An excellent review of mechanisms by which the CNS influences the secretion of TSH. The interaction of neurotransmitters, TRH, and thyroid hormones is clearly described.*

Tolis G, Stefanis C, Mountokalakis, T, Labrie F (eds.): Prolactin and Prolactinomas. New York, Raven Press, 1983. *A series of monographs on various aspects of prolactin physiology and pathophysiology with particular emphasis on hyperprolactinemic states with and without pituitary tumors.*

HYPOPITUITARISM

DISEASE STATES ASSOCIATED WITH HYPOPITUITARISM (Table 225–2). The subject's age, rapidity of onset of the disorder, and the extent of impaired hormone secretion as well as the specific pathologic process all influence the clinical manifestations. When acute and complete the disease can be life threatening, but in a mild form it can remain undetected for many years. Hypopituitarism can occur as a result of a *primary* disorder due to absence or destruction of anterior pituitary cells or *secondary* to CNS disease. In the latter, pituitary hormone deficiency occurs because of a lack of appropriate releasing factors.

The classic example of *primary hypopituitarism* is ischemic postpartum pituitary necrosis, first associated with the clinical features of hypopituitarism by Simmonds and characterized by Sheehan. The mechanism of acute ischemic necrosis is believed to relate to vasospasm of hypophyseal vessels, possibly influenced by estrogen-induced sensitivity to the vasoconstrictive stimulus of hypoxia. This disorder occurs most frequently in the immediate postpartum period and is associated with severe hemorrhage and hypotension. Some degree of hypopituitarism occurs in up to one third of women experiencing severe hemorrhage during delivery. The disorder is recognized by absence of lactation in the postpartum period and failure of normal cyclic menstruation to resume. Because of the slowly progressive nature of this disease the presence of postpartum

TABLE 225–2. ETIOLOGY OF HYPOPITUITARISM

A. Primary
- Ischemic necrosis of the pituitary
  - Postpartum (Sheehan's syndrome)
  - Diabetes mellitus
  - Other systemic diseases (temporal arteritis, sickle-cell disease and trait, arteriosclerosis, eclampsia)
- Pituitary tumors
  - Primary intrasellar (chromophobe adenoma, craniopharyngioma)
  - Parasellar (meningioma, optic nerve glioma)
- Aneurysm of intracranial internal carotid artery
- Pituitary apoplexy (almost always related to a primary pituitary tumor)
- Cavernous sinus thrombosis
- Infectious disease (tuberculosis, syphilis, malaria, meningitis, fungal disease)
- Infiltrative disease (hemochromatosis)
- Immunologic (lymphocytic hypophysitis)
- Iatrogenic
  - Irradiation to nasopharynx
  - Irradiation to sella
  - Surgical destruction
- Primary empty sella syndrome
- Metabolic disorders (chronic renal failure)
- Idiopathic (frequently monohormonal and occasionally familial)

B. Secondary
- Destruction of pituitary stalk
  - Trauma
  - Compression by tumor or aneurysm
  - Iatrogenic (surgical)
- Hypothalamic or other central nervous system disease
  - Inflammatory (sarcoidosis)
  - Infiltrative (lipid storage diseases)
  - Trauma
  - Toxic (vincristine)
  - Hormone induced (glucocorticoids, gonadal steroids)
  - Tumors (primary, metastatic, lymphomas, leukemia)
  - Idiopathic (frequently congenital or familial, often restricted to one or two hormones, and may be reversible)
  - Nutritional (starvation, obesity)
  - Anorexia nervosa
  - Psychosocial dwarfism

Adapted from Frohman LA: Diseases of the anterior pituitary. *In* Felig P, Baxter JD, Broadus AE, Frohman LA (eds.): Endocrinology and Metabolism. New York, McGraw-Hill Book Company, 1981.

lactation does not preclude development of the disorder at a later time. Since complete hypopituitarism requires at least 90 per cent destruction of the pituitary, the diagnosis may never be made in many patients with pituitary necrosis and minimal evidence of hypopituitarism. The disease is currently much less common than previously, because of the marked improvement in obstetric care during the past half century. Ischemic pituitary necrosis can be seen with other disorders, though much less commonly.

The most common cause of hypopituitarism is a pituitary tumor (discussed in the following section). Other parasellar mass lesions, including CNS tumors and internal carotid aneurysms, can also invade the sella and destroy the pituitary. Intrapituitary hemorrhage *(pituitary apoplexy)* associated with pituitary tumors may produce varying degrees of hypopituitarism. If bleeding occurs gradually, the pituitary is compressed and symptoms of hypopituitarism predominate. If the hemorrhage is sudden, presenting symptoms include headache, visual field defects or blindness, ophthalmoplegia, and subarachnoid irritation. Furthermore, a pre-existing pituitary tumor may suddenly expand. Immediate glucocorticoid therapy is essential in such patients. Most will recover without the need for surgical intervention, but it may be necessary in some to restore visual function.

Radiation therapy for treatment of malignant tumors of the head and neck frequently causes primary or secondary hypopituitarism. Growth disturbances are the most common manifestations in children, whereas hypogonadism is more common in adults. Hypopituitarism may occur within 6 to 12 months after a dose of 3000 rads or greater, and children appear to be more susceptible than adults. The disorder may not appear until several years following irradiation. Lymphocytic hypopituitarism, a recently recognized disorder, tends to occur in the postpartum period and may present as an expanding pituitary mass lesion associated with hypopituitarism (and occasionally hyperprolactinemia). Destruction of pituitary tissue with round cell infiltration has been found histologically, but the cause is unknown. Hypopituitarism may occur without detectable underlying disease and may be limited to one or two hormones rather than involving all of them. There are reports of both autosomal and X-linked recessive varieties of the disease. Partial hypopituitarism also occurs in patients with chronic renal failure and is reversible after renal transplantation.

Secondary hypopituitarism can be caused by diverse CNS disorders, all of which disrupt the delivery of releasing factors to the pituitary. The distinction between CNS and pituitary causes can frequently, but not always, be made on the basis of responses to the hypothalamic releasing hormones. Diseases of the pituitary stalk are most frequently due to trauma. Basilar skull fractures often shear the stalk, rupturing both neural and vascular connections. Parasellar tumors and aneurysms can compress the stalk sufficiently to impair blood flow to portal vessels. Disorders of the CNS, primarily the hypothalamus, that impair releasing factor secretion are described in Ch. 224.

CLINICAL FEATURES. In the most dramatic form of hypopituitarism, panhypopituitarism occurring after surgical hypophysectomy, severe pituitary apoplexy, or withdrawal of hormone therapy, clinical features are noted within a few hours (diabetes insipidus) to a few days (adrenal insufficiency). In partial hypopituitarism the signs and symptoms develop slowly and may be vague and nonspecific. The clinical features are best considered in terms of the deficiencies of individual pituitary hormones.

Hormone-specific Features

ACTH. Manifestations of ACTH deficiency are similar to those of adrenocortical deficiency. Weakness, postural hypotension, malaise, dehydration, and cold intolerance are common, though a true addisonian crisis is infrequent because some aldosterone secretion is maintained through the renin-angiotensin mechanism, which is independent of ACTH. Nausea, vomiting, and severe hypothermia can occur, and hypoglycemia associated with prolonged fasting or alcohol ingestion may be seen as a result of impaired gluconeogenesis. In contrast to Addison's disease, in which hyperpigmentation occurs, patients with ACTH deficiency frequently exhibit depigmentation and decreased tanning after exposure to sunlight. If ACTH secretion is only partially impaired, symptoms may be experienced only during periods of stress. Adrenal androgen deficiency occurs and contributes to decreased libido and to loss of axillary and pubic hair in women. In men the deficiency is of little consequence if testicular function is preserved.

TSH. The features of primary and secondary TSH deficiency are quite similar with the exception of severity. Patients experience cold intolerance, dry skin, pallor, mental slowing, bradycardia, hoarseness and constipation. True myxedema and hypercholesterolemia are seen only infrequently. Menstrual flow may be increased or more likely decreased because of associated gonadotropin deficiency. During childhood, TSH deficiency results in growth retardation which is unresponsive to GH treatment.

LH AND FSH. In women, gonadotropin deficiency results in amenorrhea and signs of estrogen deficiency, including breast atrophy, skin dryness, decreased vaginal secretions, and, occasionally, decreased libido. In males, the testes decrease in size and become softened. Decreased androgen production results in a loss of libido and potency, decreased rate of growth of secondary sexual hair, and reduced muscular strength. If the deficiency occurs prior to puberty there is total or partial impairment of secondary sexual development. If GH secretion is unaltered, failure of sex steroid–induced epiphyseal closure of the long bones produces excessive growth of limbs, leading to a eunuchoid appearance.

GROWTH HORMONE. GH deficiency in the adult is unassociated with significant clinical symptoms. Carbohydrate tolerance is impaired in GH-deficient subjects, but this disorder is distinct from diabetes mellitus and is not associated with microangiopathy. In children, GH deficiency results in growth retardation. Fasting hypoglycemia is often seen, particularly when ACTH deficiency is also present.

PROLACTIN. Prolactin deficiency results only in the absence of postpartum lactation.

VASOPRESSIN. Deficiency of vasopressin results in diabetes insipidus, described in detail in Ch. 226. The impairment of water reabsorption by the kidneys results in polyuria and polydipsia, and, if fluid intake is not maintained, severe dehydration. Extreme thirst may be present that is preferentially relieved by ice water. Polyuria may not be present when ACTH deficiency coexists because of the requirement of cortisol for free water excretion. The appearance of polyuria during ACTH or glucocorticoid administration is highly suggestive of a combined vasopressin and ACTH deficiency.

OXYTOCIN. Oxytocin deficiency is unassociated with any clinically apparent disease in humans. In particular, in women with panhypopituitarism who become pregnant, initiation of labor is normal, as is parturition.

General Clinical Features. The skin of hypopituitary patients often exhibits decreased turgor and a waxy character. Perioral and periorbital wrinkling is common, giving the appearance of premature aging. Nutrition, in general, is quite well preserved. Moderate anemia commonly occurs that is usually normochromic and normocytic, but it may be hypochromic or macrocytic and is attributed to a combination of thyroid, testosterone, and erythropoietin deficiencies. Mental slowing and apathy are quite common, as are other psychiatric symptoms, including delusions and occasionally paranoid psychosis. Carbohydrate metabolism is generally intact in nondiabetics, but in insulin-requiring diabetics, hypopituitarism necessitates reduction in insulin dosage, frequently to less than half of the original level; there is also an increased tendency for hypoglycemic reactions. These changes may persist even with full glucocorticoid replacement therapy.

The sequence of pituitary hormone loss varies among patients with hypopituitarism. In general, deficiencies of GH and gonadotropins are the earliest to occur and, thus, the most frequently observed. ACTH and TSH deficiencies are less common and are seen at a later stage in the natural history of the disease. The pattern, however, is not predictable in individual patients, thus precluding the usefulness of evaluating pituitary function by measurement of only one or two hormones.

DIFFERENTIAL DIAGNOSIS. The major categories of diseases with which hypopituitarism can be confused include (1) disorders of multiple target glands or of the CNS and (2) diseases that share the generalized features of hypopituitarism that are unassociated with endocrine dysfunction.

While measurement of pituitary hormones is indispensable in the differential diagnosis, certain clinical features have discriminatory value. Primary adrenal insufficiency is associated with hyperkalemia, hyperpigmentation, and salt craving, all of which are absent in hypopituitarism. Some patients with primary gonadal failure exhibit a discrepancy between the loss of gonadal steroid production and the loss of spermatogenesis or ovulation. Both components of gonadal function are diminished to the same extent in hypopituitarism. Primary ovarian failure often results in characteristic symptoms (hot flashes) that are usually not seen when ovarian failure is secondary to gonadotropin deficiency.

Patients with chronic malnutrition or liver disease exhibit weakness, lethargy, cold intolerance, and decreased libido, frequently raising the possibility of hypopituitarism. The presence of cachexia is important in suggesting a nonpituitary disease. Although anorexia nervosa may often be confused with hypopituitarism, the severe weight loss, psychiatric symptoms, and preservation of axillary and pubic hair are all useful discriminating factors (Ch. 215).

DIAGNOSIS. The diagnosis of hypopituitarism should be carefully and appropriately established since therapeutic decisions imply lifelong hormonal replacement therapy. In addition, studies directed at determining the etiology of the hypopituitarism (neuroanatomic studies) are an integral part of the workup and are discussed in the section on pituitary tumors.

Functional studies of each of the anterior pituitary hormones have been described in the previous section, where the specific testing details are provided. Certain general concepts used in testing are described here.

In evaluation of ACTH secretion, it is important to consider the practical implications. Testing is performed to identify patients with suspected partial adrenal insufficiency in whom an inadequate response to stress may occur. The best stimulus for this purpose is insulin hypoglycemia, in which the response to cortisol correlates well with that to surgical stress. The same test can also be used to evaluate GH responsiveness. Recent administration of glucocorticoid therapy can complicate the workup of a patient with suspected hypopituitarism. The suppressive effects of glucocorticoids on the hypothalamic-pituitary-adrenal axis can result in a subnormal response or absence of response to any of the stimuli used. Glucocorticoids should be discontinued for at least one month, if possible, prior to definitive testing.

A similar problem occurs in evaluating TSH function in patients who have been receiving long-term thyroid hormone therapy, which can impair the TSH response to TRH for at least one month.

In patients with gonadotropin deficiency, distinguishing between hypothalamic and pituitary causes is often difficult. A single GnRH challenge is frequently of little help in making this distinction and is useful primarily when neuroanatomic evidence of pituitary disease is present and the status of the gonadotrophs is being questioned.

Documentation of GH deficiency is important primarily in children of short stature when therapy with exogenous GH is being considered. Decisions concerning GH therapy require careful assessment because of the effort and expense involved. Failure of response to at least two stimuli, usually insulin hypoglycemia and arginine, is generally required before institution of GH therapy. In addition, hypothyroidism, if present, must be corrected prior to GH testing. In adults, GH deficiency serves as a marker for acquired hypopituitarism, particularly with pituitary tumors. In children and adults with obesity, GH responses to all stimuli tested are impaired, even in the presence of seemingly normal growth.

THERAPY. Hormonal replacement therapy must be determined individually, and treatment goals specifically defined. The therapeutic use of pituitary hormones is restricted to GH for correcting growth retardation and gonadotropins for inducing fertility. Potential uses of hypothalamic hormones or their synthetic analogues are at present limited to GnRH for the treatment of hypothalamic hypogonadism, though current research in this field may shortly result in other potential uses. For the most part, target organ hormones are used because of their cost advantage, ease of administration, and prolonged action.

ACTH. ACTH deficiency is treated with glucocorticoids. Cortisone (25 mg orally), hydrocortisone (20 mg orally), or prednisone (5 mg orally) given as a divided dose provides adequate therapy for most patients under normal conditions. Supplemental mineralocorticoid therapy is unnecessary because of the partial preservation of aldosterone secretion. The use of prednisone is preferred because of its reduced cost. Occasional patients may require full glucocorticoid replacement therapy (a dose 50 per cent greater than those listed), but in most patients this dose is excessive. During stress, the dose should be increased two- to three-fold and then gradually tapered. If oral medication cannot be retained, injectable steroids (hydrocortisone hemisuccinate [Solu-Cortef] for initial emergency use, 100 mg intramuscularly or intravenously), or cortisone acetate for long-term use (50 to 100 mg intramuscularly every 12 hours) is indicated. Treatment of the acutely ill hypopituitary patient requires the same dosage of hydrocortisone (100 to 300 mg per day) as used in primary adrenal insufficiency. Preoperatively, patients should receive hydrocortisone hemisuccinate 50 mg intramuscularly every 6 hours beginning the evening prior to surgery and continuing through the immediate postoperative period, followed by gradual tapering to maintenance dosage. Treatment of patients with partial ACTH deficiency without symptoms in the nonstressed state is more controversial. With adequate education, many patients will not need maintenance replacement therapy except in times of stress. Such patients in particular should wear appropriate medical identification bracelets.

TSH. TSH deficiency is treated with L-thyroxine 0.15 to 0.2 mg per day, though a lower dose may suffice in occasional patients. Clinical assessment of the patient and serum thyroxine levels during initiation of therapy are used to establish the appropriate dose. Adrenal insufficiency must be corrected prior to instituting thyroid hormone replacement therapy, and patients with partial adrenal insufficiency may require glucocorticoid replacement only after thyroid hormone replacement is started. In the presence of severe or longstanding hypothyroidism a small dose of thyroxine (0.025 mg per day) should be used initially and increased slowly to a maintenance dose. The use of triiodothyronine, particularly as long-term therapy, is not recommended, because its shorter biologic half-life results in more rapid appearance of thyroid deficiency in the event therapy is omitted.

LH and FSH. Treatment of gonadotropin deficiency requires consideration of both gonadal steroid replacement and treatment of infertility. The subjects are considered in greater detail in Ch. 234 and 236.

WOMEN. Estrogen replacement therapy is indicated in premenopausal women to maintain secondary sex characteristics and to prevent osteoporosis and possibly coronary artery disease. This can be accomplished with ethinyl estradiol 5 to 20 μg per day or conjugated estrogens (Premarin) 0.6 to 1.25 mg per day. The lowest possible dose that produces the desired clinical effects should be used. To induce cyclic bleeding, estrogen should be given for 25 days each month, accompanied on the last five days by a progestinic agent such as medroxyprogesterone 5 to 10 mg per day. Alternatively, an oral contraceptive preparation containing no more than the equivalent of 25 μg estradiol per day can be used. The advantage of replacement therapy after the menopause is still controversial, and the potential risks and benefits should be discussed with the patient to help make an appropriate decision. Estrogen therapy usually corrects the dyspareunia attributable to local estrogen deficiency in women with hypopituitarism, but decreased libido due to the absence of adrenal androgens often persists. This can be corrected by injection of a small dose of long-acting androgen such as testosterone enanthate 50 mg every one to two months or by oral administration of fluoxymesterone 5 to 10 mg once or twice weekly.

Restoration of fertility is possible in a large percentage of women with clomiphene or GnRH therapy if the cause of the disorder is hypothalamic or with combined FSH/LH preparations if pituitary disease is present. An FSH-rich preparation from postmenopausal urine is used to initiate follicular growth and maturation; it is monitored by measurement of plasma estradiol levels. Human chorionic gonadotropin is then injected to induce ovulation. This therapy is expensive, entails the risk of superovulation and multiple pregnancy, and should be undertaken only under the direction of an experienced physician.

MEN. Testosterone replacement therapy in adult males is accomplished by intramuscular injection of a long-acting testosterone preparation (testosterone enanthate or cypionate, 200 mg every three to four weeks). The endpoints are restoration of full androgenization, including beard growth, improvement in muscular strength, libido and potency. Androgen therapy should be withheld as long as possible in the adolescent with growth retardation to avoid premature epiphyseal closure, which limits the potential for future linear growth. Testosterone therapy may be required for many months before full restoration of libido and performance. If gonadotropin deficiency has developed before puberty, full androgenization may never occur. In patients with longstanding hypogonadism, psychosocial behavorial changes affecting the patient's entire lifestyle may be disrupted by initiation of testosterone therapy, leading to major adjustment problems with both sexual and nonsexual relationships.

Infertility in men with hypopituitarism can be corrected with a combination of FSH and human chorionic gonadotropin (HCG), though therapy is required for several months, and the success rate is less than 50 per cent. Current studies indicate that, in the future, GnRH analogues may provide a convenient and less expensive form of therapy for individuals with hypothalamic hypogonadism.

Growth Hormone. GH therapy is indicated for the correction of impaired linear growth, and its use is thus confined almost exclusively to childhood and adolescent years. Early establishment of the diagnosis is critical, since the probability of successful long-term therapy is inversely related to the extent of growth retardation. Treatment requires the use of human GH, which has traditionally been extracted and purified from pituitaries obtained at autopsy. Preliminary studies with GH produced by recombinant DNA technology have indicated comparable hormone biopotency, and this source should provide an unlimited supply of GH in the near future. GH is administered intramuscularly or subcutaneously in a dosage of 0.1 to 0.2 U per kilogram three times weekly; its use is continued until the final height is achieved, coincident with long-bone epiphyseal closure. A goal of 5 feet 4 inches is generally pursued but not always achieved. Careful attention must be given to concomitant hormone deficiencies, particularly thyroid. Glucocorticoids should be used sparingly because of their interference with growth-promoting effects of GH. Some physicians have proposed that small doses of oral androgens be used simultaneously to increase growth velocity, though this has not gained widespread acceptance. Estrogens are to be avoided because of their greater effect on epiphyseal closure. Gonadal steroid therapy is usually initiated during the years of puberty to avoid psychosocial problems. However, if significant catch-up growth is required, its use should be delayed. GH therapy increases height age more rapidly than bone age, may initially be associated with a decrease in body fat, and also corrects the fasting hypoglycemia of GH-deficient children.

Asa SL, Bilbao JM, Kovacs K, Josse RG, Kreines K: Lymphocytic hypophysitis of pregnancy resulting in hypopituitarism: A distinct clinicopathological entity. Ann Intern Med 95:166, 1981. Baskin DS, Townsend JJ, Wilson CB: Lymphocytic adenohypophysitis of pregnancy simulating a pituitary adenoma: A distinct pathological entity. Report of two cases. J. Neurosurg 56:148, 1982. *Two reports of a newly recognized pregnancy-related syndrome diagnosed by histological examination of pituitary tissue. Clinical differentiation from pituitary tumors is difficult, and the pathogenesis is unclear.*

Frasier SD: Human pituitary growth hormone (hGH) therapy in growth hormone deficiency. Endocr Rev 4:155, 1983. *An up-to-date assessment of the use of human GH as therapy in children with GH deficiency. Critical evaluation of various treatment protocols, necessitated because of the limited supply of GH, has resulted in effective means of assessing the responses to the hormone.*

Gharib H, Frey HM, Laws ER Jr, Randall RV, Scheithauer BW: Coexistent primary empty sella syndrome and hyperprolactinemia. Report of 11 cases. Arch Intern Med 143:1383, 1983. *The empty sella syndrome is being recognized with greater frequency, and coexisting hyperprolactinemia does not necessarily imply the presence of a pituitary microadenoma.*

Phillips JA, Parks JS, Hjelle BL, Herd JE, Plotnick LP, Migeon CJ, Seeburg PH: Genetic analysis of familial isolated growth hormone deficiency type I. J Clin Invest 70:489, 1982. *Analysis of nuclear DNA from patients with familial isolated GH deficiency has suggested the presence of genetic mutations. Similar studies can be expected in the future that may explain the pathogenesis of many isolated hormonal deficiencies.*

Sheehan HL, Summers VK: The syndrome of hypopituitarism. Quart J Med 42:319, 1949. *The classic monograph describing the clinical-pathologic correlations of hypopituitarism. Its lucid and detailed presentation make it worthwhile reading even after three decades.*

Stackpoole PW, Interlandi JW, Nicholson WE, Rabin D: Isolated ACTH deficiency: A heterologous disorder. Critical review and report of four new cases.

Medicine 61:13, 1982. *The pathogenesis of this disorder is heterologous despite similar clinical manifestations. Detailed endocrine testing is required to differentiate the various causes.*

PITUITARY TUMORS

CLASSIFICATION. Pituitary tumors are subdivided by their histologic characteristics and also by their functional activity. Specific considerations of hormone-secreting pituitary tumors will be found in the next section. The two major histologic types of primary pituitary tumors are the adenoma and the craniopharyngioma. In addition, parasellar tumors such as optic nerve glioma, meningioma, sphenoid wing sarcoma, as well as metastatic tumors can also be present within the sella turcica.

Pituitary Adenomas. This cell type constitutes greater than 90 per cent of all pituitary tumors. The classic subdivision into chromophobic and chromophilic tumors has given way to more specific identification on the basis of immunohistochemical stains for individual hormones. Using these techniques, only 10 to 20 per cent of pituitary adenomas appear to be nonfunctioning. Pituitary tumors account for 6 to 18 per cent of all brain tumors, and small adenomas, many of which are functioning, have been detected in up to 30 per cent of unselected autopsy series. The growth pattern of pituitary adenomas appears unrelated to hormone secretion. Rapidly enlarging tumors are generally recognized because of their mass lesion effects, whereas slowly growing tumors tend to allow for expression of their hormone hypersecretory effects. The peak incidence of nonfunctioning pituitary adenomas is between 40 and 50 years, and the frequency is uninfluenced by sex. Although pituitary adenomas are almost always histologically benign, they may exhibit aggressive growth behavior with invasion of surrounding structures, making their surgical removal impossible. Adenomas are generally solid with a well-defined capsule, although they may on occasion be cystic and hemorrhagic. Calcification, if present, results from organization of a previous hemorrhage.

Craniopharyngiomas. These tumors are of congenital origin, may be partly or entirely cystic, and are always benign. The cysts may contain an oily fluid with a high cholesterol content. Calcification, generally concentric, is present in 50 per cent. The tumors grow at variable rates and may remain dormant for many years. Although half of the tumors are seen during childhood, they may appear at any time during life. The site of origin of most tumors is in the midline at the upper portion of the pituitary stalk, and approximately 15 per cent involve the upper portion of the anterior lobe and are therefore intrasellar. Variations of craniopharyngiomas include ependymomas and epidermoid cysts.

CLINICAL FEATURES. The manifestations of pituitary tumors are neuroanatomic, endocrinologic, and radiologic. Presenting symptoms of pituitary tumors have changed in frequency over the years with refinements in diagnostic procedures. Whereas in nearly 90 per cent of cases diagnosed 30 years ago, patients exhibited visual disturbances, only 25 per cent do so at present. In contrast, the most common presentation today relates to impaired gonadal function, frequently associated with prolactin-secreting pituitary tumors. A small percentage of patients (less than 5 per cent) are discovered accidentally on review of skull films obtained for other purposes as a result of bony destruction of the sella turcica.

Neuroanatomic manifestations occur secondary to tumor growth causing pressure on the overlying dura and the diaphragma sellae. This results in headaches that are variable in nature, imprecisely located, generally of dull quality, unassociated with nausea or visual symptoms, unrelated to position, and inconsistently relieved by analgesics. Disappearance of headache is frequently a sign of rupture of the dura. With continued expansion the tumor exerts pressure on the optic chiasm, leading to the classic findings of bitemporal hemianopsia. At earlier stages the field defects may be asymmetric and involve only the superior temporal fields. Eventually, blindness and optic atrophy will occur. Anterior growth of the tumor may cause symptoms limited only to one eye. Papilledema occurs in one fourth of craniopharyngiomas but rarely in pituitary adenomas. Further growth results in hypothalamic compression leading to temperature instability, hyperphagia, altered sleep patterns, and emotional disturbances. Pressure on the third ventricle results in internal hydrocephalus. Rarely, temporal or frontal lobe compression may cause behavioral changes and seizures, and midbrain compression may produce long-tract signs. Lateral extension is more common and leads to compression of the third, fourth, and sixth cranial nerves in the cavernous sinus, resulting in ophthalmoplegia and diplopia. Expansion inferiorly into the sphenoid sinus may result in cerebrospinal fluid rhinorrhea. Hemorrhage into the tumor, *pituitary apoplexy,* may result in rapid expansion of the tumor and lead to the sudden appearance of headache of varying intensity that subsides after a few days. If the tumor is intrasellar, hypopituitarism often results; if extrasellar, there may be rapid deterioration of vision. "Spontaneous" cures of hormone-secreting pituitary tumors may also occur as the result of hemorrhagic tumor necrosis.

Neuroradiologic presentations consist of a deformed or enlarged sella seen on standard skull roentgenography or a mass lesion seen on computed tomography (CT) performed for unrelated reasons. In the absence of endocrine symptoms a low-density lesion suggests an empty sella (discussed below).

Endocrine symptoms include diminished function secondary to destruction of normal pituitary tissue by tumor or interference with portal blood supply and hyperfunction due to tumor or hyperplasia. The two may be combined. In addition, diminished function may occur secondary to the effects of hormone hypersecretion (i.e., hypogonadism secondary to hyperprolactinemia). The frequency of presentation and the manifestations have been described in the previous section.

DIAGNOSTIC PROCEDURES. Diagnosis of a pituitary tumor necessitates differentiation from other parasellar disorders, determination of the tumor size and extent of sellar and extrasellar destruction, and assessment of the extent of hormone deficiencies. Endocrine evaluation should be performed prior to definitive therapy, if possible, since the extent of hypopituitarism may influence the type and extent of therapy. When this is not possible, because of rapidly deteriorating vision or progressive neurologic symptoms, the patient must be considered to have panhypopituitarism and immediate treatment with glucocorticoids must be initiated.

Neuroradiologic procedures have improved remarkably during the past decade, and the definitive study is currently the CT scan, performed with intravenous contrast media, using a third or fourth generation scanner (Fig. 225–1). The best views

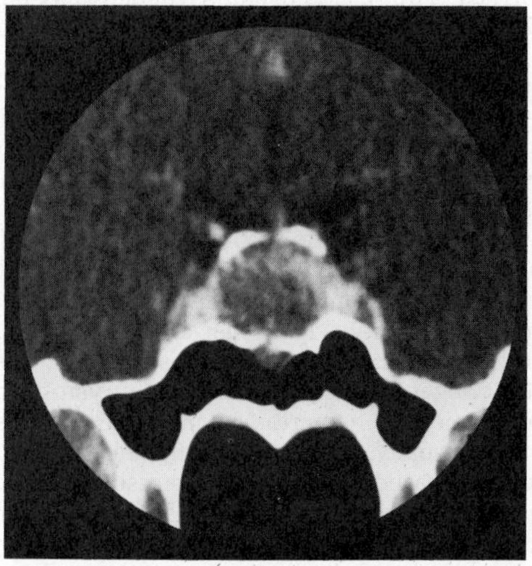

Figure 225–1. Computerized axial tomographic (CT) scan of pituitary (coronal view) demonstrating a pituitary tumor with erosion of the sellar floor and inferior extension of the tumor into the sphenoid sinus.

are obtained using coronal sections. This technique permits evaluation of the contents of the sella as well as the surrounding bony structures, which provide the only clues on routine x-ray studies. CT can also indicate the degree of extension of pituitary tumors in all directions and has precluded the need for invasive procedures such as pneumoencephalography. Digital vascular imaging is also useful as an adjunct in determining the position of the carotid arteries in relation to the tumor prior to surgical intervention and has almost entirely replaced carotid angiography.

The most important neuro-ophthalmologic study is evaluation of visual fields using Goldmann perimetry. Test objects of varying sizes and colors can provide an excellent assessment of both central and peripheral fields. The technique is reproducible and sensitive and useful in observing patients for serial changes. Bitemporal field defects are, however, not specific for pituitary tumors; they may occur with parasellar tumors, vascular abnormalities, arachnoiditis, or rarely with chiasmal prolapse into the sella associated with the empty sella syndrome. Atypical field defects may also occur, even those suggesting superior rather than inferior pressure. The visual evoked response (VER) is an even more sensitive technique for detecting early chiasmal compression by pituitary tumors. The VER measures the pattern and latency of the response from the occipital cortex produced by photic stimulation. Chiasmal pressure produces a delayed or reduced response in the crossed pathways as compared with uncrossed pathways and may provide evidence of abnormalities before they are evident on visual field examination.

DIFFERENTIAL DIAGNOSIS. Disorders that must be differentiated from pituitary tumors include the empty sella syndrome, parasellar diseases, and pituitary enlargement associated with other endocrine disorders.

The *empty sella* is partly or nearly completely filled with CSF and results from extension of the subarachnoid space into the intrasellar region. The pituitary gland is flattened along the posterior portion of the floor and the dorsum. Primary empty sella syndrome is unassociated with prior surgical or irradiation therapy and has been found in up to one quarter of autopsy series, usually unassociated with endocrine disease. The etiology is unknown, but the syndrome has been postulated to be due to incomplete formation of the diaphragma sella, permitting CSF pressure to be transmitted to the sella and gradually leading to herniation of the arachnoid and remodeling of the sella. Nearly all patients are asymptomatic, though some may have nonspecific headaches. The syndrome is seen commonly in obese women and in association with systemic hypertension, benign intracranial hypertension (pseudotumor cerebri), and CSF rhinorrhea. The sella is usually symmetrically enlarged or ballooned and may be deformed. Results of testing of endocrine function are generally normal, though patients may exhibit diminished TSH and gonadotropin secretion, hyperprolactinemia, and rarely panhypopituitarism or diabetes insipidus. The diagnosis is established by CT, which on occasion may need to be performed in conjunction with metrizamide cisternography. The empty sella may coexist with a pituitary tumor, which is usually hyperfunctional. The secondary empty sella syndrome is seen in patients following pituitary surgery or irradiation.

The signs and symptoms of parasellar disorders may mimic those of pituitary tumors. Parasellar disorders include inflammatory and granulomatous diseases (sarcoidosis, eosinophilic granuloma), degenerative disorders (aneurysms), and neoplasms (meningiomas, hamartomas, metastatic tumors). Suprasellar tumors usually present with the neurologic manifestations of increased intracranial pressure, hypothalamic symptoms, and internal hydrocephalus. Endocrine manifestations tend to follow rather than precede neurologic symptoms. CT is extremely valuable in differentiating these disorders from primary pituitary tumors.

Longstanding primary hypothyroidism or hypogonadism can result in sellar enlargement, increased TSH or gonadotropin secretion, hyperplasia of tropic hormone–producing cells, and in some patients, hormone-secreting tumors. Institution of appropriate replacement hormone therapy can reverse the hypersecretory and hyperplastic changes in their early stages.

THERAPY. Treatment of pituitary tumors is required to prevent or limit the loss of pituitary function and the consequences of extrasellar extension. The two therapeutic methods include surgery and radiation therapy.

Pituitary surgery, established as a safe and effective procedure by Cushing, is the conventional therapy for pituitary tumors. The transsphenoidal approach is currently used for all tumors except those with extensive suprasellar extension, particularly when separated from the intrasellar portion by a narrow neck. Tumors encircling optic nerves can be removed only by a transfrontal approach. Currently the operative mortality is less than 1 per cent. The transsphenoidal approach includes the use of modern fluoroscopic aids and microsurgical techniques. It provides better visualization of the sellar contents and has been instrumental in permitting selective adenomectomy to be performed. If preoperative evaluation reveals preservation of anterior pituitary function, a more conservative approach is indicated to preserve remaining pituitary hormone secretion. A small rim of adenohypophyseal tissue is often sufficient to maintain adequate pituitary function. Glucocorticoid coverage is essential for the perioperative period even for patients with intact pituitary-adrenal function and is accomplished with parenteral administration of hydrocortisone, 50 mg intramuscularly every six hours. Postoperatively the patient must be carefully observed for the development of diabetes insipidus, particularly since an obtunded patient may not perceive thirst. Transient polyuria and increased plasma osmolality commonly occur in the immediate postoperative period as a result of mild trauma to the pituitary stalk. Persistence of these findings beyond the first 48 hours usually indicates significant destruction of the stalk or posterior pituitary and permanent impairment of function. However, fluctuations in posterior pituitary function may occur for a period of several weeks, and recovery has been observed as late as several months postoperatively. Initially the patient should be treated with aqueous vasopressin (5 U subcutaneously) rather than with a long-acting preparation so the natural history of the process can be observed.

Radiation therapy can be used as an alternative to surgical excision of the pituitary tumor or as adjunct therapy. Although less popular as primary therapy, because of its delayed effects, radiation therapy using conventional high-energy sources (supravoltage) or heavy-particle (proton beam) sources is an effective method of treatment. Radiation therapy is to be avoided in patients with significant suprasellar extension or in the presence of marked visual field defects.

The recurrence rate of pituitary tumors following surgical treatment alone ranges from 25 to nearly 100 per cent in different series. Since postoperative radiographic and endocrine studies indicate that intraoperative assessment of the extent of pituitary tumor removal is often inaccurate, postoperative irradiation is indicated in all patients with pituitary adenomas unless specifically contraindicated. The dose currently employed is 4500 to 5000 rads, which can be given with minimal side effects. Some late loss of pituitary function occurs in 15 to 25 per cent of patients.

Burrow GN, Wortzman G, Rewcastle NB, Holgate RC, Kovacs K: Microadenomas of the pituitary and abnormal sellar tomograms in unselected autopsy series. N Engl J Med 304:156, 1981. *Clinically unrecognized microadenomas were found in one third of an autopsy series. Many were hormone containing but without manifestations of hypersecretion.*

Carbezudo JM, Vaquero J, Areitio E, Martinez R, De Sola RG, Bravo G: Craniopharyngiomas: A critical approach to treatment. J Neurosurg 55:371, 1981. *Increasing experience with this tumor indicates the importance of radiation therapy in addition to surgery in preventing tumor recurrence. In most patients total excision is not recommended.*

Cook DM: Pituitary tumors: Diagnosis and therapy. CA 33:215, 1983. *An excellent, well-referenced review of the recent literature that compares therapeutic effectiveness of methods as reported by others. Very readable.*

Crane TB, Yee RD, Hepler RS, Hallinan JM: Clinical manifestations and radiologic findings in craniopharyngiomas in adults. Am J Ophthalmol 94:220, 1982. *A*

comprehensive review of the clinical features in 51 patients emphasizing the predominance of visual findings.
Daniels DL, Williams AL, Thornton RS, Meyer GA, Cusick JF, Haughton VM: Differential diagnosis of intrasellar tumors by computed tomography. Radiology 141:697, 1981. Chambers EF, Turski PA, LaMasters D, Newton TH: Regions of low density in the contrast enhanced pituitary gland: Normal and pathologic processes. Radiology 144:109, 1982. *The use of CT in diagnosis of pituitary tumors is now well established. Subtleties in interpretation of the results, however, must be carefully assessed.*
Max MB, Deck MD, Rottenberg DA: Pituitary metastasis: Incidence in cancer patients and clinical differentiation from pituitary adenoma. Neurology 31:998, 1981. *A careful analysis of both autopsy and clinical series in which differentiation was facilitated by the clinical rather than the radiologic characteristics.*
Valenta LJ, Sostrin RD, Eisenberg H, Tamkin JA, Elias AN: Diagnosis of pituitary tumors by hormone assays and computerized tomography. Am J Med 72:861, 1982. *Analysis of 170 patients with endocrine abnormalities by dynamic testing and CT examination demonstrating the value of each in the diagnosis or exclusion of tumors.*
Zull DN, Falko JM: Metrizamide cisternography in the investigation of the empty sella syndrome. Arch Intern Med 141:487, 1981. *This enhancement of the standard CT has simplified the diagnosis of the empty sella and has eliminated the need for invasive radiologic techniques previously used.*

PITUITARY HYPERFUNCTION: HORMONE-SECRETING PITUITARY TUMORS

Except in the case of certain hormone-secreting tumors, pituitary hormone hypersecretion generally involves overproduction of only a single hormone. Physiologically, hormone overproduction occurs in response to altered feedback signals (i.e., hyperprolactinemia due to increased estrogen secretion in pregnancy; ACTH, TSH, and gonadotropin hypersecretion in response to diminished target organ feedback in primary hypofunction of the adrenal, thyroid, and gonads; and GH hypersecretion associated with chronic and severe caloric malnutrition). Whereas these changes begin as functional alterations, prolonged stimulation can result in hyperplastic as well as hypersecretory changes. Pathologic hyperfunction occurs in association with pituitary hyperplasia or tumor unrelated to regulatory feedback mechanisms. These disorders involve, almost exclusively, somatotrophic, lactotrophic, and corticotrophic cells.

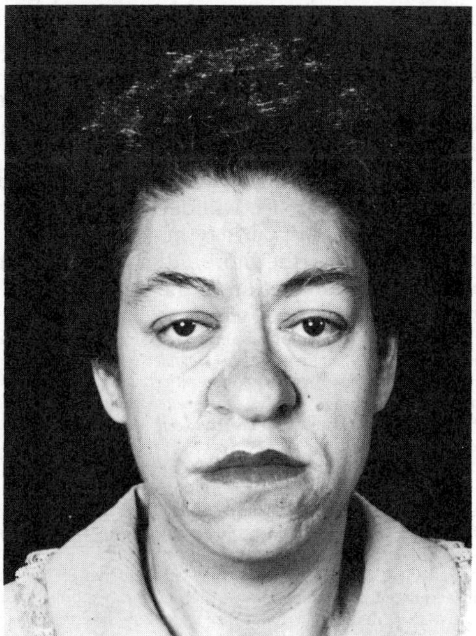

Figure 225–2. Clinical features of a 43-year-old patient with acromegaly of 15 years' duration. Coarsened features result from soft tissue overgrowth about the eyes, nose, and mouth. Lacrimal overgrowth, thickening of skin folds, and fibroma molluscum are also present. (Reprinted with permission from Frohman LA: *In* Felig P, Baxter JD, Broadus AE, Frohman LA (eds.): Endocrinology and Metabolism. New York, McGraw-Hill Book Company, 1981, p 201.)

Growth Hormone–Secreting Tumors: Acromegaly

GH hypersecretion is most commonly associated with a pituitary somatotroph tumor or rarely somatotroph hyperplasia. These tumors previously were considered eosinophilic (due to GH storage granules) or chromophobic (when little hormone was stored). Tumors with abundant hormone storage tend to be better differentiated and more slowly growing, resulting in more pronounced clinical features of GH hypersecretion, whereas the less differentiated non–hormone-storing tumors tend to grow more rapidly, leading to more pronounced effects of an expanding tumor mass.

CLINICAL FEATURES. The clinical manifestations of GH hypersecretion depend on the age at which the disorder begins. During childhood and prior to epiphyseal fusion, GH hypersecretion produces proportional skeletal growth leading to gigantism. Hypogonadism is frequently present, leading to delayed epiphyseal closure and thus a more prolonged growth period. The tallest reported patient with gigantism reached a height of nearly 9 feet. It is more common for patients to exhibit features of both gigantism and acromegaly, reflecting persistence of GH hypersecretion into adult life.

Signs and symptoms of GH hypersecretion beginning during adult life develop slowly. Soft tissue swelling and hypertrophy involving the extremities and face are the earliest findings (Fig. 225–2). These changes are usually best documented by comparing photographs taken over a one- or two-decade span. Spadelike changes develop in the fingers, and increased soft tissue volume necessitates ring enlargement and increases in glove and shoe sizes. The skin becomes thickened and leathery, and skin folds increase in prominence. A generalized increase in hair growth and pigmentation often occurs. Fibroma molluscum (pedunculated epithelial tags) and acanthosis nigricans are common. The skin becomes oily, and sebaceous cyst formation is common. Increased sweating occurs in most patients and is a sensitive biologic indicator of disease activity.

Bony changes occur more slowly and include cortical thickening, tufting of terminal phalanges, and osteophyte proliferation. Degenerated articular cartilages and ligamentous hypertrophy produce a hypertrophic arthropathy that eventually leads to deforming and crippling arthritis. Prognathism results from mandibular enlargement and causes a significant overbite of the lower incisors and increased spacing of the teeth. Bony overgrowth of the frontal, malar, and nasal bones occurs; increase in size of the paranasal sinuses together with vocal cord hypertrophy leads to deepening of the voice. Eustachian tube mucosal hypertrophy often produces obstruction and serous otitis media.

Peripheral neuropathy commonly occurs because of nerve entrapment by surrounding tissue overgrowth, most commonly affecting the median nerve and producing the carpal tunnel syndrome. Axonal demyelinization of peripheral nerves associated with perineurial and subepineurial proliferation results in palpable nerve fibers. Paresthesias, sensory losses, and proximal muscle weakness occur frequently.

Prolonged hypersecretion leads to generalized visceromegaly involving salivary glands, liver, spleen, and kidneys. Salivary gland enlargement is detectable clinically whereas that of the other organs is not, and significant hepatosplenomegaly usually implies the presence of a coexisting disease. Both secretory and reabsorptive functions of the kidney are increased in acromegaly.

Thyroid enlargement with nodule formation is common, but true hyperfunction is infrequent. Parathyroid hyperplasia and adenoma are frequently associated, explaining the hypercalciuria and nephrolithiasis often observed. Mild elevations of prolactin levels may also occur, resulting in galactorrhea, amenorrhea, and decreased libido.

The effects of GH on the cardiovascular system are controversial. Hypertension is common but generally mild and responsive to drug therapy. Cardiomegaly is routinely found, but there is no characteristic form of acromegalic heart disease. Cardiac failure, when it occurs, appears related to hypertension and not to the effects of GH hypersecretion. Yet the incidence of cardiovascular disease is increased in acromegalics, as is mortality. Weight gain is uncommon, but carbohydrate intolerance and diabetes are seen in 25 per cent of acromegalics, primarily in those with a family history of diabetes. Insulin resistance is common and the development of ketosis is occasionally noted. Diabetic microangiopathy, however, is extremely uncommon, even in longstanding disease.

LABORATORY STUDIES. The diagnosis of acromegaly is established by the finding of elevated plasma GH levels that do not respond normally to physiologic suppression and stimulation; in adults, a GH value greater than 2 ng per milliliter in males or 5 ng per milliliter in females after oral glucose administration is confirmatory. Randomly obtained samples with markedly elevated levels are also diagnostic. However, in normal children and young adults, GH levels as high as 50 ng per milliliter are sporadically exhibited, thereby necessitating dynamic studies of GH secretion in many patients. TRH stimulates GH secretion in 70 to 80 per cent of acromegalics but not in normal subjects, and this procedure is useful in following the patient after therapy as well. Plasma GH levels are paradoxically suppressed by dopaminergic agents and frequently stimulated by GnRH, but these tests are of limited clinical use. GH secretion in acromegalics differs in other ways from that in normal persons, including absence of a sleep-associated increase in GH and a tendency for wide spontaneous fluctuations in GH levels, indicating intermittent secretory activity.

Plasma somatomedin C (IGF-I) levels are also increased in acromegaly and provide good correlation with the clinical manifestations of GH hypersecretion. Determination of somatomedin C levels for assessing disease activity has been proposed, but at present its value remains as a supportive measurement.

DIFFERENTIAL DIAGNOSIS. The clinical features of acromegaly are not confused with other diseases. The question commonly raised is whether features suggestive of the disease are associated with active disease, inactive disease, or no disease. Dynamic studies of GH secretion are required to differentiate these possibilities. Gigantism during childhood occasionally occurs in the absence of GH hypersecretion (cerebral gigantism) through a yet to be determined mechanism. GH levels are elevated in patients with renal failure, cirrhosis, protein calorie malnutrition and anorexia nervosa and in the Laron dwarf (a dwarf with a defect in somatomedin generation), but in these conditions the clinical features of acromegaly are absent.

PATHOGENESIS. Acromegaly can occur as a primary disorder due to neoplastic transformation of somatotrophs within the pituitary or secondary to excessive stimulation by an ectopic GH- or GRF-secreting tumor. The vast majority of patients with acromegaly have primary pituitary disease. Selective removal of the GH-secreting adenoma is followed in most patients not only by restoration of normal GH values but by normal responses to dynamic testing. In some patients, however, GH-secreting pituitary tumors have been associated with carcinoid tumors of the bronchus and foregut, pancreatic islet tumors, and small cell carcinoma of the lung. Removal of the extrapituitary tumor has resulted in a return of GH levels to normal and regression of the pituitary tumor. GRF has been isolated from several of these tumors; in fact, its sequence was first determined from a pancreatic islet tumor rather than from the hypothalamus. Pituitary histology in patients with secondary acromegaly ranges from local or generalized somatotroph hyperplasia to actual tumor formation. In addition, neuronal tumors present in the hypothalamus (hamartomas) or in the pituitary, contiguous with the somatotroph adenoma (gangliocytoma or choristoma), may also be the source of GRF production in a few patients with acromegaly. Since excessive stimulation by GRF is capable of inducing adenomas as well as hyperplasia, it is possible that some patients now considered to have primary pituitary disease actually have a hypothalamic disorder characterized by excessive GRF production from nontumorous tissue.

Comparison of the limited numbers of reported patients with secondary acromegaly does not provide any evidence of differences in either clinical manifestations or responses to dynamic studies of GH secretion. In patients with ectopic GRF production, immunoreactive plasma GRF levels are readily detectable, in contrast to patients presumed to have primary pituitary disease in whom levels are near or beneath the limits of detectability.

THERAPY. Therapy for patients with acromegaly involves three potential methods: surgery, irradiation, and medical (pharmacologic). Considerations of the space-occupying mass and of hypopituitarism are similar to those described for nonfunctioning pituitary tumors. Prior to initiation of therapy to the pituitary itself, consideration should be given to the possibility of an extrapituitary tumor, removal of which may reverse the GH hypersecretion.

Surgical treatment of GH-secreting pituitary tumors is currently the most commonly used method. Transsphenoidal or, if necessary, transfrontal adenomectomy is indicated once the presence of the disease has been established, even though the radiologic findings are minimal. The results in published series vary, some reports indicating up to 90 per cent cure rates with small tumors. The success in returning GH levels to normal is inversely related to the size of the tumor; less favorable results occur with tumors greater than 2 cm in diameter or plasma GH levels greater than 100 ng per milliliter. The clinical features of GH, however, are frequently improved dramatically even without complete restoration of GH values to normal. In patients whose GH levels return to the normal range, tumor recurrence is infrequent (approximately 5 per cent), but with incomplete removal the recurrence rate is greater than 50 per cent if no further therapy is administered.

Radiation therapy, using methods similar to those for nonfunctioning tumors, is effective as a primary means of treatment of acromegaly. The reduction in GH hypersecretion is, however, slow, and return to normal levels may require five or even ten years, although 70 to 80 per cent of patients will exhibit normal GH levels after two years. Postoperative irradiation is indicated when GH levels remain elevated and, used in conjunction with surgery, offers the best prognosis.

Pharmacologic therapy in acromegaly is of very limited value. The only useful agent for long-term use is the dopamine agonist bromocriptine,* but it is effective in lowering GH levels to normal in only 25 per cent of patients. In approximately 5 per cent of patients the tumor size will decrease during therapy as well. Doses of up to 60 mg per day may be required, and side effects are frequent. Furthermore, therapy is effective only during continued administration of the drug.

Arosio M, Giovanelli MA, Riva E, Nava C, Ambosi B, Faglia G: Clinical uses of pre- and postsurgical evaluation of abnormal GH responses in acromegaly. J Neurosurg 59:402, 1983. *Responses to dynamic testing of GH secretion indicate that persistence of abnormal responses postoperatively even when the basal GH levels are within the normal range should be considered evidence of residual neoplastic tissue. The studies may help distinguish between reactivation of disease and true recurrence.*

Baskin DS, Boggan JE, Wilson CB: Transsphenoidal microsurgical removal of growth hormone-secreting pituitary adenomas. A review of 137 cases. J Neurosurg 56:634, 1982. *The largest published series of GH-secreting tumors to date indicating that the greatest success occurs in patients with tumors confined to the sella and with GH levels less than 40 ng per milliliter.*

Dons RF, Rieth KG, Gorden P, Roth J: Size and erosive features of the sella turcica in acromegaly as predictors of therapeutic response to supervoltage irradiation. Am J Med 74:69, 1983. *Size and basal GH levels tended to parallel one another and formed a rough predictor of the response to therapy. In all patients the decrease in GH levels occurred in proportion to the initial value.*

Frohman LA, Szabo M, Berelowitz M, Stachura ME: Partial purification and characterization of a peptide with growth hormone-releasing activity from extrapituitary tumors in patients with acromegaly. J Clin Invest 65:43, 1980. Thorner MO, Perryman RL, Cronin MJ, Rogol AD, Draznin M, Johanson A, Vale W, Kovacs K: Somatotroph hyperplasia. Successful treatment of acromegaly by removal of a pancreatic islet tumor secreting growth hormone-releasing factor. J Clin Invest 70:965, 1982. *Reports of patients with ectopic GRF secretion that led to the isolation and structural identification of GRF, the only hypothalamic releasing factor to be sequenced first from human tissue.*

*This use is not listed in the manufacturer's directive.

Melmed S, Braunstein GD, Horvath E, Ezrin C, Kovacs K: Pathophysiology of acromegaly. Endocr Rev 4:271, 1982. *Thoughtful analysis of the various characteristics of GH-secreting pituitary tumors, together with a thorough discussion of the multiple pathogenetic mechanisms resulting in acromegaly. The disease clearly has more than one cause, and the numerous possibilities are presented.*

Moses AC, Molitch ME, Sawin CT, Jackson IM, Biller BJ, Furlanetto R, Reichlin S: Bromocriptine therapy in acromegaly: Use in patients resistant to conventional therapy and effect on serum levels of somatomedin C. J Clin Endocrinol Metab 53:772, 1981. *Although this agent is not nearly as effective as in the treatment of hyperprolactinemia, most patients with acromegaly exhibit clinical improvement along with reduction of GH levels. Its use is advocated only as an adjunct in patients inadequately treated by other means.*

Schuster LD, Bantle JP, Oppenheimer JH, Seljeskog EL: Acromegaly: Reassessment of the long-term therapeutic effectiveness of transsphenoidal pituitary surgery. Ann Intern Med 95:172, 1981. *The recurrence of disease prompted a critical review of hormone measurements after surgery, leading to the conclusion that GH suppression to levels seen in normal individuals is required if the patient is to be considered cured.*

Prolactin-Secreting Tumors: Amenorrhea-Galactorrhea Syndrome

Hyperprolactinemia is the most common form of pituitary hyperfunction. It is present in as many as 25 per cent of infertile women. The incidence in men is much lower. In patients with pituitary tumors the incidence of elevated prolactin levels ranges from 60 to 80 per cent and is greater than that of any other pituitary hormone. The distinction between patients with *idiopathic hyperprolactinemia* and those with *prolactin-secreting tumors* is currently made on the basis of CT examination of the pituitary. Thus, changes in the relative frequency of the two diseases reflect primarily recent improvements in radiologic technology.

CLINICAL FEATURES. In women, hyperprolactinemia causes galactorrhea, oligomenorrhea or amenorrhea, and infertility (see Ch. 238 for a discussion of galactorrhea). Galactorrhea requires near-normal levels of ovarian steroids and is therefore not seen in all patients. It frequently occurs in association with oral contraceptive use, usually following their discontinuation. The reported incidence of galactorrhea in patients with prolactin-secreting tumors varies from 50 to 90 per cent. Oligomenorrhea or amenorrhea occurs in a similar percentage of patients and in nearly all with radiographic evidence of a pituitary tumor. The development of amenorrhea and the development of galactorrhea are not necessarily related to one another and are of no diagnostic importance. The cause of amenorrhea is related to effects of altered CNS neurotransmitters, principally dopamine, as a result of hyperprolactinemia, which interferes with a normal positive feedback effect of estradiol on GnRH secretion. The effects of anovulation include hypoestrogenemia, which results in decreased vaginal secretion, and dyspareunia, which may be responsible for diminished libido. Mild hirsutism may also occur in association with increased dehydroepiandrosterone sulfate production by the adrenals. Longstanding hyperprolactinemia has, in some women, been associated with decreased bone density, only part of which may be attributed to the hypoestrogenemia.

In men, hyperprolactinemia results in impotence and diminished libido. A defect in endogenous GnRH secretion is present, along with diminished testosterone secretion. The decreased libido is, however, not explained entirely on this basis, since it often persists despite testosterone replacement therapy. In some men oligospermia is also present.

LABORATORY STUDIES. Plasma prolactin levels in patients with prolactin-secreting tumors vary from slightly above normal (15 to 20 ng per milliliter) to values greater than 10,000 ng per milliliter. Levels less than 200 ng per milliliter are of little use in distinguishing between the various causes of the disorder, whereas levels greater than 200 ng per milliliter are invariably associated with prolactin-secreting tumors. Since prolactin is a stress-responsive hormone and levels fluctuate in normal subjects, repeated sampling in patients with moderate degrees of hyperprolactinemia is essential.

A large number of dynamic studies of prolactin secretion reveal differences between normals and pathologic hyperprolactinemics, but none is reliable in distinguishing between idiopathic hyperprolactinemia and prolactin-secreting tumors. Prolactin responses to submaximally suppressive infusions of dopamine are impaired in such patients, as compared to those with known extrapituitary disorders causing hyperprolactinemia, though the latter can usually be distinguished on clinical grounds. Patients with prolactin-secreting tumors and idiopathic hyperprolactinemia have impaired responses to dopamine receptor–blocking agents, to stimulation with TRH, to a combination of L-dopa plus the dopa decarboxylase inhibitor, carbidopa, and to cimetidine, a histamine H_2-receptor blocker.

In some patients with pituitary tumors and mild hyperprolactinemia (i.e., less than 100 ng per milliliter) the tumor does not secrete prolactin, but rather appears to interrupt hypothalamic-pituitary portal blood flow, resulting in increased prolactin secretion by normal lactotrophs.

DIFFERENTIAL DIAGNOSIS. Consideration should be given to an extrapituitary cause for hyperprolactinemia in all patients, since subtle changes on CT studies may not always indicate the presence of a pituitary tumor. This is particularly true in patients with prolactin levels less than 200 ng per milliliter. The differential diagnosis of hyperprolactinemia is given in Table 225–3. If none of the disorders listed is present and there is no history of drug ingestion, the patient with a normal radiographic examination is considered to have idiopathic hyperprolactinemia.

The many similarities between patients with idiopathic hyperprolactinemia and those with small prolactin-secreting pituitary tumors (microadenomas) have led to the belief that these entities represent different stages of the same disorder. Follow-up evaluation of idiopathic hyperprolactinemia suggests that only a small percentage of patients (under 5 per cent) progress to demonstrable pituitary tumor formation and that among cases of microadenoma, the vast majority remain stable for years with respect to both prolactin levels and tumor size.

Some patients with galactorrhea have normal or borderline elevation of prolactin levels, normal dynamic studies of prolactin secretion and ovulatory menses, and normal fertility. These patients represent the most common type of nonpuerperal galactorrhea, termed *normoprolactinemic galactorrhea,* which is attributed to enhanced sensitivity of the breast to prolactin. It can be seen as persistence of postpartum galactorrhea or following discontinuation of oral contraceptives.

PATHOGENESIS. As with GH-secreting tumors, a controversy currently exists whether prolactin-secreting tumors represent a primary pituitary disease or are secondary to altered hypotha-

TABLE 225–3. DIFFERENTIAL DIAGNOSIS OF NONPHYSIOLOGIC HYPERPROLACTINEMIA

A. Pharmacologic Agents
- Monoamine synthesis inhibitors (alpha-methyldopa)
- Monoamine depletors (reserpine)
- Dopamine receptor antagonists (phenothiazines, butyrophenones, thioxanthines)
- Estrogens (oral contraceptives)
- Narcotics (morphine, heroin)

B. Central Nervous System Disorders
- Inflammatory/infiltrative (sarcoidosis, histiocytosis)
- Traumatic (stalk section)
- Neoplastic (hypothalamic or parasellar tumors)

C. Pituitary Disorders
- Prolactin-secreting tumors
  - Macroadenomas
  - Microadenomas
- Empty sella syndrome

D. Idiopathic Hyperprolactinemia

E. Other
- Hypothyroidism
- Renal failure
- Cirrhosis
- Chest wall/breast disease or surgery
- Thoracic spinal lesions
- Nonendocrine tumors with ectopic hormone production (rare)

lamic influence. Prolactin-secreting tumors also occur in association with other tumors, in particular pancreatic islet tumors and parathyroid tumors/hyperplasia as part of the multiple endocrine neoplasia syndrome type I (Ch. 232).

A hypothalamic etiology is supported by a large number of pharmacologic studies suggesting impaired CNS dopaminergic tone. However, evidence for prolactin resistance to dopamine has also been demonstrated, though this appears to be unrelated to altered dopamine receptors. A possible role of oral contraceptives has been suggested, since idiopathic hyperprolactinemia and prolactin-secreting tumors are primarily diseases of women of childbearing age. Most studies, however, have failed to support this hypothesis.

THERAPY. The therapy for prolactin-secreting tumors has undergone considerable change in the past decade. Surgery remains the primary form of therapy for large prolactin-secreting tumors (macroadenomas). The timing of surgery in relation to pharmacotherapy is discussed below. The overall management of large tumors that either secrete prolactin or are nonfunctioning is similar, i.e., removal of the tumor mass and preservation of pituitary function. Primary therapy of small tumors (microadenomas) has also been surgical, and cure rates of 90 per cent, as judged by restoration of cyclic menses and fertility, are achieved. However, growth of microadenomas is infrequently observed, and this, plus their detection in up to one third of unselected autopsies, raises the question whether their removal is indeed necessary in all patients. In addition, long-term follow-up of presumably cured patients indicates recurrence of hyperprolactinemia in at least 25 per cent.

A frequent reason for treatment of microadenomas is infertility. The most rapid and effective means of reducing prolactin levels to normal in such patients is by use of the dopamine agonist bromocriptine, which suppresses prolactin secretion in all forms of hyperprolactinemia by an action directly on the lactotroph. Prolactin levels are decreased by more than 90 per cent and galactorrhea is improved or eliminated in most patients, even if prolactin levels remain slightly elevated. Similarly, cyclic menses and fertility may return without complete normalization of prolactin levels. The dosage required for most patients is 2.5 to 7.5 mg per day in divided doses. Some patients may require up to 15 mg per day. Side effects consist primarily of nausea and vomiting due to stimulation of the emesis center and occasionally of hypotension due to a CNS-mediated mechanism and mood changes. The side effects may be minimized by initiating therapy with a small dose and gradually increasing it, though 5 to 10 per cent of patients are unable to tolerate the drug. The incidence of congenital abnormalities in infants of women who have conceived while taking bromocriptine does not appear to be increased, and even when given throughout pregnancy the drug appears to be safe. It is, in fact, the recommended therapy for women who develop signs and symptoms of a prolactin-secreting tumor during pregnancy. Bromocriptine is effective in males with hyperprolactinemia; restoration of serum testosterone levels and of libido follows institution of therapy.

Bromocriptine also decreases the size of prolactin-secreting adenomas, most dramatically of very large tumors. In approximately two thirds of patients bromocriptine will reduce tumor size by 50 to 75 per cent. The effects are usually quite rapid, occurring within days, but in some patients tumor shrinkage may require several months. The reduction in size continues as long as the patient takes the drug, even as long as eight to ten years. Following discontinuance of bromocriptine, however, there is rapid regrowth of the tumor, and symptoms may recur within days. The drug is useful in reducing the size of very large tumors prior to surgery, in postoperative treatment of patients in whom partial tumor removal was accomplished, and in patients who are not candidates for surgery.

Bonneville JF, Poulignot D, Cattin F, Couturier M, Mollet E, Dietemann JL: Computed tomographic demonstration of the effects of bromocriptine on pituitary microadenoma size. Radiology 143:451, 1982. *Careful radiographic examinations reveal that bromocriptine shrinks microadenomas as well as macroadenomas, and in some patients the tumor can no longer be demonstrated radiographically.*

Chiodini P, Liuzzi A, Cozzi R, Verde G, Oppizzi G, Dallabonzana D, Spelta B, Silvestrini F, Borghi G, Luccarelli G, Rainer E, Horoski R: Size reduction of macroprolactinomas by bromocriptine or lisuride treatment. J Clin Endocrinol Metab 53:737, 1981. *Two thirds of macroprolactinomas are decreased in size by these dopaminergic agonists, though in none did the tumor disappear completely. The drugs are proposed as a first-stage treatment for all macroprolactinomas prior to surgery or irradiation.*

Glickman SP, Rosenfield RL, Bergenstal RM, Helke J: Multiple androgenic abnormalities, including free testosterone, in hyperprolactinemic women. J Clin Endocrinol Metab 55:251, 1982. *Adrenal androgens are increased in women with hyperprolactinemia, and an increase in free testosterone is also present, related to decreased testosterone-binding globulin. These alterations explain the increased androgenization seen in some hyperprolactinemic patients.*

Herman V, Kalk WJ, de Moor NG, Levin J: Serum prolactin after chest wall surgery: Elevated levels after mastectomy. J Clin Endocrinol Metab 52:148, 1981. *Mastectomy stimulates prolactin secretion in most subjects, with levels remaining elevated for months and explaining the frequently observed galactorrhea on the basis of neurogenic stimulation via the sucking reflex.*

Randall RV, Laws ER Jr, Abboud CE, Ebersold MJ, Kao PC, Scheithauer BW: Transsphenoidal microsurgical treatment of prolactin producing adenomas. Results in 100 patients. Mayo Clin Proc 58:108, 1983. Wilson CB, Dempsey LC: Transsphenoidal microsurgical removal of 250 pituitary adenomas. J Neurosurg 48:13, 1978. *Two large series of patients with prolactinomas treated surgically show similar results in that the cure rate is highest in microadenomas and considerably lower in large tumors and in patients with prolactin levels above 200 ng per milliliter.*

Schlechte JA, Sherman B, Martin R: Bone density in amenorrheic women with and without hyperprolactinemia. J Clin Endocrinol Metab 56:1120, 1983. *Hyperprolactinemic women have decreased bone density that is unexplained by their amenorrhea and hypoestrogenemia. The mechanism remains to be clarified.*

Serri O, Rasio E, Beauregard H, Hardy J, Somma M: Recurrence of hyperprolactinemia after selective transsphenoidal adenomectomy in women with prolactinoma. N Engl J Med 309:280, 1983. *Despite return of prolactin levels to normal following surgery, 80 per cent of patients with macroadenomas and 25 per cent of patients with microadenomas exhibit recurrent hyperprolactinemia within a few years. These results require reevaluation of the currently used methods for treating these disorders.*

Spark RF, Willia CA, O'Reilly G, Ransil BJ, Bergland R: Hyperprolactinemia in males with and without pituitary macroadenomas. Lancet 2:129, 1982. *The major clinical manifestation of hyperprolactinemia in males is impotence. Bromocriptine is effective in restoring normal testosterone levels and potency in most subjects with or without tumors.*

von Werder K, Eversmann T, Rjosk H-K, Fahlbusch R: Treatment of hyperprolactinemia. *In* Ganong WF, Martini L (eds.): Frontiers in Neuroendocrinology. Vol 7. New York, Raven Press, 1982, pp 123–160. March CM, Kletzky OA, Davajan V, Teal J, Weiss M, Apuzzo MLJ, Marrs RP, Mishell DR: Longitudinal evaluation of patients with untreated prolactin-secreting pituitary adenomas. Am J Obstet Gynecol 139:835, 1981. *These two studies report on the natural history of idiopathic hyperprolactinemia and microadenomas, followed without specific treatment. They indicate that in the vast majority (> 90 per cent) size and prolactin levels remain relatively stationary for many years, concluding that immediate surgical intervention is not required in many patients.*

Wollesen F, Anderson T, Karle A: Size reduction of extrasellar pituitary tumors during bromocriptine treatment. Ann Intern Med 96:281, 1982. *Bromocriptine treatment reduces the size of prolactin-secreting tumors, and when large doses are used, even other tumors (including nonsecreting tumors) exhibit a response, though of lesser magnitude.*

ACTH-Secreting Tumors: Cushing's Disease

Basophilic adenomas of the pituitary associated with bilateral adrenocortical hyperplasia and the features of hypercortisolism constitute a disorder first described by Cushing. The tumors, which tend to be located in the midline or near the anterior-posterior pituitary junction, are usually benign, but in contrast to other pituitary tumors, often exhibit more aggressive growth behavior, may have true malignant potential, and on rare occasions metastasize within and without the CNS. Corticotroph tumors may first become clinically apparent following bilateral adrenalectomy in patients with Cushing's disease (Nelson's syndrome). Corticotroph tumors may also be chromophobic and are found in 5 to 7 per cent of pituitaries at autopsy in patients without evidence of ACTH hypersecretion during life. Defects in the hormone secretory process may be responsible for these nonfunctioning tumors.

CLINICAL FEATURES. The clinical features of corticotroph tumors consist of those related to hypercortisolism and those caused by hypersecretion of ACTH and related peptides. The signs and symptoms of hypercortisolism are indistinguishable from those associated with adrenocortical adenomas or exogenous hormone administration and include centripetal obesity, hypertension, diabetes, amenorrhea, hirsutism, acne, osteoporosis and compression fractures, muscle atrophy, violaceous striae, capillary fragility, impaired wound healing, decreased resistance to infection, and behavorial changes. These are discussed in greater detail in Ch. 229. Increased secretion of ACTH and β-LPH produces pigmentation similar to that seen in Addison's disease. In addition to generalized pigmentation, the pressure points (knuckles, elbows, knees, belt or brassiere strap regions), areolae, genitalia, mucous membranes, and recently healed scars are particularly affected. Because ACTH production is only partially autonomous in this disease, hyperpigmentation is mild or moderate in the early stages and becomes more pronounced after adrenalectomy or in very large tumors.

LABORATORY STUDIES. Plasma cortisol levels are elevated in only about half of the patients with Cushing's disease. The 24-hour urinary free cortisol is the most reliable measurement for distinguishing patients with increased adrenocortical function. Normal values are less than 100 μg per 24 hours. Of the dynamic tests, dexamethasone suppressibility is the most reliable and widely used. In normal subjects, low-dose dexamethasone decreases urinary free cortisol to less than 20 μg per 24 hours and plasma cortisol to less than 5 μg per deciliter. Patients with corticotroph tumors exhibit impaired suppression with the low dose but at least 50 per cent suppression with the high dose. In some patients, however, larger doses may be required to demonstrate suppression. Dexamethasone does not suppress cortisol secretion fully at any dose in patients with adrenal adenomas or ectopic ACTH secretion. These conditions can be distinguished by measurement of plasma ACTH levels, which are absent in the former and exceedingly high in the latter. Patients with Cushing's disease exhibit ACTH hyperresponsiveness to CRF; those with adrenal adenomas or ectopic ACTH production do not exhibit a response. High-quality CT scanning of the pituitary will demonstrate the presence of a tumor in only 60 per cent of patients with Cushing's disease.

DIFFERENTIAL DIAGNOSIS. ACTH-secreting tumors are responsible for approximately 80 per cent of cases of endogenous hypercortisolemia. Adrenal tumors are present in about 15 per cent, and the remainder are caused by ectopic ACTH-secreting tumors. The differential diagnosis of these disorders is discussed in greater detail in Ch. 229. Ectopic ACTH production can occur in a variety of tumors, most commonly small-cell lung carcinomas, carcinoids, and pancreatic islet tumors (Ch. 173). The disease can mimic that of corticotroph tumors, though in patients with malignant diseases, weight gain is often absent and severe hypokalemia is a prominent feature. Some of these tumors have been shown to secrete CRF alone or in combination with ACTH, explaining the occasional similarity in responses to dynamic hormone testing to those in patients with corticotroph tumors. Ectopic ACTH secretion should be suspected when the clinical and biochemical features of hypercortisolism occur on a periodic or intermittent basis.

Mild elevations of plasma cortisol, loss of diurnal variation, and absence of dexamethasone suppressibility are seen in patients under stress, during periods of bereavement, and in patients with depressive illness. Biochemically it is frequently impossible to distinguish these patients from those with ACTH-secreting tumors, though the clinical features of hypercortisolism are generally absent.

PATHOGENESIS. Arguments have been made for both a hypothalamic and a pituitary cause of ACTH-secreting tumors. Hypothalamic tumors have been identified in association with Cushing's disease, suggesting tumorous overproduction of CRF. Patients with ACTH-secreting tumors generally respond to CRF, as does tumor tissue tested in vitro. Basophilic hyperplasia, rather than tumor, is occasionally found in patients with Cushing's disease. In addition, cyproheptadine, a serotonin-receptor blocker, suppresses ACTH secretion in some patients with the disorder, providing strong support for a primary CNS role. The major argument for a primary pituitary disorder is based on the successful treatment by transsphenoidal adenomectomy, which includes reestablishment not only of normal quantitative cortisol secretion but of diurnal periodicity and glucocorticoid suppressibility. It is possible that two subgroups of the disease exist that are not readily distinguishable by clinical or laboratory methods currently available.

THERAPY. Definitive treatment of ACTH-secreting pituitary tumors is indicated as soon as the diagnosis has been established. Once ectopic ACTH or CRF production has been excluded, surgical removal of the pituitary ACTH-secreting tumor is indicated. Tumors may be extremely small and difficult to identify. If the tumor cannot be located or if the patient remains hypercortisolemic following surgery, anterior hypophysectomy or bilateral total adrenalectomy is necessary, the decision being influenced by the patient's age, desire for subsequent pregnancy, and overall general health. Following pituitary adenomectomy, adrenocortical hypofunction requiring glucocorticoid replacement therapy may persist for as long as two years. A success rate of up to 85 per cent has been reported in patients with small ACTH-secreting tumors, although in those with large tumors this figure is reduced to about 30 per cent.

Radiation is also effective as primary therapy in ACTH-secreting tumors. Cure rates have been reported of 80 per cent in children and 60 per cent in adults with either conventional radiotherapy or proton beam therapy. Some long-term loss of other pituitary function has been noted after radiotherapy.

Pharmacologic therapy of Cushing's disease is directed at suppression of cortisol biosynthesis by the adrenals, using aminoglutethimide, metyrapone, or mitotane (o,p'-DDD); at neurotransmitter metabolism within the CNS; or at the pituitary directly. Detailed discussion of drugs acting on the adrenal is provided in Ch. 229. They have been used, together with radiotherapy, as an alternative to surgical treatment in selected patients. The combination of metyrapone, aminoglutethimide, and dexamethasone has been advocated for restoring cortisol secretion to normal prior to pituitary adenomectomy. This is unnecessary in most patients, but in some with severe disease it may be of use. The serotonin-receptor blocker cyproheptadine and the GABA agonist sodium valproate have been successful in a small number of patients with Cushing's disease in restoring both ACTH and cortisol secretion to normal. Responses have also been seen in patients with Nelson's disease. A few patients will also exhibit decreases in ACTH secretion during bromocriptine therapy. There is no evidence for regression of tumor size by these agents to date.

Dornhorst A, Jenkins JS, Lamberts SW, Abraham RR, Wynn V, Beckford U, Gillham B, Jones MT: The evaluation of sodium valproate in the treatment of Nelson's syndrome. J Clin Endocrinol Metab 56:985, 1983. *This GABA agonist reduced ACTH levels, produced clinical improvement, and in one patient decreased pituitary tumor size. The site of action is believed to be the hypothalamus, where it increases GABA activity, thereby inhibiting CRF release.*

Findling JW, Aron DC, Tyrrell JB, Shinsako JH, Fitzgerald PA, Norman D, Wilson CB, Forsham PH: Selective venous sampling for ACTH in Cushing's syndrome: Differentiation between Cushing's disease and the ectopic ACTH syndrome. Ann Intern Med 94:647, 1981. *The selective sampling procedure used was capable of identifying the source of elevated ACTH levels when other procedures failed to differentiate between pituitary and extrapituitary sources.*

Fitzgerald PA, Aron DC, Findling JW, Brooks RM, Wilson CB, Forsham PH, Tyrrell JB: Cushing's disease: Transient secondary adrenal insufficiency after selective removal of pituitary microadenomas: Evidence for a pituitary origin. J Clin Endocrinol Metab 54:413, 1982. *Temporary adrenal insufficiency is observed after successful removal of an ACTH-secreting tumor, providing evidence for suppression of residual pituitary corticotrophs.*

Krieger DT: Physiopathology of Cushing's disease. Endocr Rev 4:22, 1983. *A detailed review presenting the arguments pro and con for both pituitary and CNS causes of Cushing's disease. Evidence for multiple causes are supported by the author's arguments.*

Lamberts SW, de Lange SA, Stefanko SZ: Adrenocorticotropin-secreting pituitary adenomas originate from the anterior or the intermediate lobe in Cushing's disease: Differences in the regulation of hormone secretion. J Clin Endocrinol Metab 54:286, 1982. *ACTH-secreting tumors can be subdivided into two subgroups with different sites of origin, responses to dynamic testing, and probabilities of surgical cure.*

Lankford HV, Tucker HTS, Blackard WG: A cyproheptadine-reversible defect in ACTH control presenting after removal of the pituitary tumor in Cushing's disease. N Engl J Med 305:1244, 1981. *Relative resistance of cortisol feedback suppression in Cushing's disease persists after removal of the pituitary tumor and is correctable by a serotonin-receptor blocker, providing evidence for a CNS role in the pathophysiology of the disease.*

Muller OA, Stalla GK, von Werder K: Corticotropin releasing factor: A new tool for the differential diagnosis of Cushing's syndrome. J Clin Endocrinol Metab 57:227, 1983. *Patients with pituitary ACTH-secreting tumors exhibit hyper-responsiveness to CRF, while those with adrenal adenomas and ectopic ACTH-secreting tumors do not respond, providing a diagnostic test of considerable clinical importance.*

Other Hormone-Secreting Tumors

TSH and gonadotropin secretion by pituitary tumors is extremely rare. TSH-secreting tumors are detected during the workup of hyperthyroid patients with elevated rather than suppressed TSH levels. The clinical manifestations consist of hyperthyroidism and a pituitary tumor mass. Occasionally mixed pituitary cell types are present with coexisting GH or prolactin hypersecretion. TSH secretion is not completely autonomous, since suppression of thyroxine production by methimazole frequently results in an increase of TSH secretion. Treatment must be directed to removal of the tumor mass, though medical therapy to suppress the elevated thyroxine levels is required preoperatively.

FSH and FSH/LH-secreting pituitary tumors are very rare and often associated with longstanding hypogonadism. Occasionally tumors otherwise considered to be nonfunctioning may produce the isolated glycoprotein alpha subunit that is devoid of any clinical manifestations and serves primarily as a tumor marker.

Harris RI, Schatz NJ, Gennarelli T, Savino PJ, Cobbs WH, Snyder PJ: Follicle-stimulating hormone–secreting pituitary adenomas: Correlation of reduction of adenoma size with reduction of hormonal hypersecretion after transsphenoidal surgery. J Clin Endocrinol Metab 56:1288, 1983. *Convincing evidence is presented for production of FSH by pituitary tumors with concomitant reduction in serum testosterone levels presumably caused by impairment of LH secretion from normal gonadotrophs.*

Klibanski A, Ridgway EC, Zervas NT: Pure alpha subunit-secreting pituitary tumors. J Neurosurg 59:585, 1983. *Six patients with otherwise "nonfunctioning" pituitary tumors are described with elevated glycoprotein alpha subunit levels that can be used as a marker for monitoring the effects of therapy. No clinical manifestations of the secretory product have yet been recognized.*

Smallridge RC, Smith CE: Hyperthyroidism due to thyrotropin-secreting pituitary tumors. Diagnostic and therapeutic considerations. Arch Intern Med 143:503, 1983. *In a review of 33 reported cases the authors describe the characteristic laboratory findings and provide recommendations for therapy.*

226. THE POSTERIOR PITUITARY

*Thomas E. Andreoli**

ANTIDIURETIC HORMONE

The neurohypophysis of man elaborates two hormones: *arginine vasopressin* (AVP), which exhibits vasopressor and antidiuretic activity, and *oxytocin,* which is galactobolic and uterotonic. Both hormones are octapeptides of approximately 1100 daltons, with a 20-member ring structure created by disulfide bonds. The antidiuretic and vasopressor activities of AVP are each approximately 100 times as great as those of oxytocin, a difference that is related to the different tertiary conformations of the two peptides.

The posterior pituitary gland contains terminal axons whose cell bodies lie in hypothalamic cell clusters known as the *supraoptic* and *paraventricular nuclei.* Synthesis of posterior pituitary hormones occurs in these hypothalamic nuclei rather than in the posterior pituitary gland: (1) AVP can be demonstrated immunochemically in cells of both the supraoptic and the paraventricular nuclei; and (2) neurosecretory granules accumulate only on the hypothalamic side of a sectioned hypophyseal stalk.

*The author acknowledges the dialogue and constructive suggestions provided by R. Michael Culpepper, M.D., Assistant Professor of Internal Medicine, University of Texas Medical School at Houston, and Attending Physician, Hermann Hospital, for his assistance in the preparation of this chapter. T.E.A.

Vasopressin is synthesized as a prohormone in conjunction with a specific carrier protein, neurophysin II, and then is transported to the posterior pituitary gland in discrete neurosecretory granules by axonal streaming within the cytoplasm of pituicytes (see Fig. 226–1). In the posterior pituitary gland, these granules rest in terminal projections of axonal plasma membranes, which are juxtaposed to capillaries of the systemic circulation. Other pituicyte nerve fibers terminate in the median eminence and along the third ventricle, thus allowing access of vasopressin to cerebrospinal fluid.

There are two pools of AVP-containing neurosecretory granules in pituicytes: one adjacent to the cell membrane and therefore available for immediate release, and a second storage pool removed from immediate contact with the plasma membrane. Release of hormone occurs by an exocytotic process involving fusion of neurosecretory granules with pituicyte plasma membranes. In other words, AVP release is quantal. A stimulus to the hypothalamic pituicyte cell body is transmitted to the site of granule storage, where it causes cell membrane depolarization, an associated increase in calcium permeability, and rapid calcium entry into the pituicytes. This influx of calcium activates the exocytosis of AVP-containing neurosecretory granules.

RELEVANT PHYSIOLOGY. Detailed accounts of the renal and pituitary processes resulting in the formation of a dilute or concentrated urine are presented in Ch. 73 and 76. Antidiuretic hormone (ADH) exerts major physiologic effects on discrete regions of the nephron and also affects vascular smooth muscle tone. In all epithelia which respond to ADH, the hormone binds to specific receptors on the basolateral plasma membrane of the cell and, in so doing, activates the enzyme adenylate cyclase. Adenylate cyclase increases the production of 3′,5′-cyclic adenosine monophosphate (cAMP) from its substrate adenosine triphosphate (ATP). Cyclic AMP then acts as a second messenger to activate a cell-specific protein kinase, which induces the final cellular response to the hormone (see Ch. 221). ADH-stimulated adenylate cyclase is present in the collecting duct and in the medullary, but not cortical, thick ascending limb of Henle (mTALH) of mammalian kidneys.

The *cardinal* physiologic effect of ADH is to promote the formation of a hypertonic urine. The formation of a hypertonic urine depends particularly on two sets of events operating in parallel within the renal medulla. First, in the thick ascending limb of Henle, approximately 15 to 20 per cent of the filtered load of sodium chloride is absorbed. Since the mTALH is water impermeable, this process contributes simultaneously to the maintenance of a hypertonic medullary interstitium and to the formation of a dilute urine. Under normal circumstances, the osmolality of the renal medullary interstitium rises from isotonic, at the corticomedullary junction, to very hypertonic, approximately 1200 mOsm per kilogram of H_2O, at the papillary tip; and approximately 10 per cent of fluid filtered at the

SECRETION OF ADH

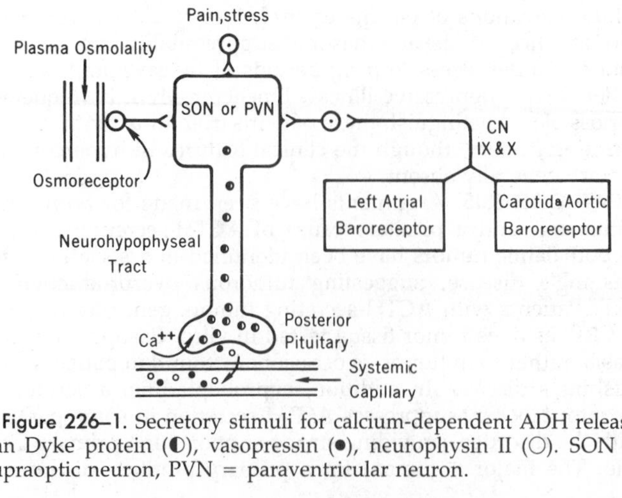

Figure 226–1. Secretory stimuli for calcium-dependent ADH release: van Dyke protein (◐), vasopressin (●), neurophysin II (○). SON = supraoptic neuron, PVN = paraventricular neuron.

glomerulus, or about 18 liters daily, reaches the early distal tubule with an osmolality of approximately 50 mOsm per kilogram of H_2O. Since the enrichment of medullary interstitial osmolality and dilution of tubular fluid both depend on sodium chloride absorption by the water-impermeable mTALH, the latter region of the nephron is commonly termed the medullary diluting segment.

When ADH is absent, the water permeability of collecting ducts is at a minimum. Thus there is reduced osmotic equilibration of fluid passing through collecting ducts with the medullary interstitium, and most of the fluid escapes unchanged as hypotonic urine. Since only 10 per cent of filtered water normally reaches the collecting duct system, the maximal degree of polyuria in a patient with complete pituitary diabetes insipidus (or complete nephrogenic diabetes insipidus) is therefore approximately 18 liters daily. During normal antidiuresis, ADH, acting through the second messenger cAMP, increases the water permeability of luminal (urinary) cell membranes of cortical and outer medullary collecting ducts. Thus in the presence of ADH, there is osmotic equilibration of hypotonic luminal fluid in collecting ducts with the hypertonic medullary interstitium and, consequently, water absorption, a reduction in urine volume, concentration of urine, and conservation of body water.

The ADH-dependent increase in the water permeability of collecting ducts is due to a hormone-dependent increase in the number of water-specific channels available for water transport through luminal membranes. These channels are rather narrow, approximately 2 Å in radius, and therefore exclude urea and NaCl. As a consequence, the luminal fluid concentrations of these two solutes increase when water is abstracted from cortical and outer medullary collecting ducts during antidiuresis. In turn, the increase in luminal urea concentration creates a favorable gradient for passive urea diffusion out of inner medullary (papillary) collecting ducts into the interstitium, thereby maintaining interstitial hypertonicity. ADH also causes a slight increase in papillary duct urea permeability, thus favoring passive movement of urea down its concentration gradient for recirculation through the medullary interstitium.

A *second ADH-mediated* event in the antidiuretic response is to increase the rate of NaCl transport in medullary, but not cortical, thick ascending limbs of Henle (mTALH). This process involves a furosemide-sensitive electroneutral cotransport of Na^+:K^+:$2Cl^-$ from luminal fluid into cells; virtually all of the potassium entering cells through this process is recycled back into luminal fluid via potassium-specific channels in luminal membranes. This potassium recycling contributes to the establishment of a lumen-positive voltage, which in turn drives the reabsorption of additional sodium through the paracellular pathway. Thus there occurs net absorption of sodium chloride by net transcellular absorption of chloride and net sodium absorption through both cellular and paracellular routes. Ultimately the energy source for this process depends on the maintenance of low concentrations of sodium and high concentrations of potassium within renal tubular cells; both of these conditions are met by the (Na^+ + K^+)-ATPase situated in basolateral membranes.

The action of ADH on increasing the rate of salt absorption in the mTALH appears to involve a hormone-dependent increase in both the functional number of Na^+:K^+:$2Cl^-$ cotransport units and potassium-specific channels in apical membranes of medullary diluting segments. Consequently, the action of ADH on the medullary diluting segment provides a means for enriching medullary interstitial osmolality.

This effect of ADH is opposed, however, by at least three other factors. First, as interstitial NaCl concentrations increase, the backleak of NaCl into the tubular lumen of the mTALH also increases, and thereby tends to reduce net NaCl absorption by the mTALH. Second, increases in interstitial osmolality down-regulate the ADH stimulation of NaCl cotransport. Finally, prostaglandins of the E series, which are produced in abundance in the renal medullary interstitium, inhibit competitively the ADH-mediated increases in the rate of intracellular cAMP formation.

Thus these latter three processes have a negative feedback on ADH enhancement of active NaCl transport in the mTALH. Consequently, the diluting power of the mTALH remains constant during either antidiuresis or water diuresis.

At levels of hormone that exceed those necessary for antidiuresis, ADH also has pressor activity (this was the first known effect of posterior pituitary extract, and provided the basis for the name vasopressin) that is the result of a direct constricting effect on vascular smooth muscle. At all but high pharmacologic doses, this pressor effect is easily overcome by compensatory vasodilatory reflexes, so that hypertension is not routinely seen during AVP replacement therapy. Lesser doses may, however, cause significant vasoconstriction of coronary arteries. Another effect of vasopressin, seen at levels that supersede those necessary for antidiuresis, is stimulation of intestinal motility. Finally, some evidence suggests that AVP released into the CSF and thalamic centers may play a role in such diverse processes as memory and regulation of corticotropin release.

OSMOTIC REGULATION OF ADH RELEASE. Verney's elegant studies demonstrated a strong antidiuretic response to perfusion of carotid vessels with hypertonic solutions of various solutes, including sodium salts and glucose; hypertonic urea solutions elicited no such response. Therefore he concluded that specific cells that acted as osmoreceptors were present within the distribution of the carotid circulation and that the plasma membranes of these cells were impermeable to sodium salts and glucose, but permeable to urea. In the presence of extracellular hyperosmolality induced by impermeable species, these osmosensing cells reached osmotic equilibrium by losing water to the hypertonic plasma. In other words, Verney deduced that osmoreceptor shrinkage, produced by raising plasma osmolality with solutes restricted to the extracellular compartment, was the stimulus for ADH release.

When the anterior wall of the third ventricle is exposed to hypertonic saline, neurons in both the anterior hypothalamus and the preoptic area have increased rates of depolarization. Concomitantly, about half of the pituicytes in hypothalamic nuclei show a characteristic depolarization pattern, and plasma antidiuretic activity increases. Therefore it is probable that the neurons in the anterior hypothalamus and preoptic areas, which depolarize in response to hypertonic saline, represent Verney's osmoreceptors.

In normal man, plasma AVP levels are undetectable below a plasma osmolality of 280 mOsm per kilogram of H_2O. Since the usual plasma osmolality in man is approximately 287 mOsm per kilogram of H_2O, secretion of AVP is tonic; the average circulating hormone levels are between 2.0 and 2.5 pg per milliliter. Vasopressin levels increase in a linear fashion with increasing plasma osmolality, such that a rise in plasma osmolality of only 1 per cent (2.9 mOsm per kilogram of H_2O) evokes a 1 pg per milliliter rise in AVP. Parallel examinations of plasma AVP and urine osmolality indicate that each unit increase in AVP allows an increase of 250 mOsm per kilogram of H_2O in urinary concentration. Since the maximal concentrating ability of the human kidney is approximately 1200 mOsm per kilogram of H_2O, maximal water conservation is therefore achieved at a plasma AVP level of 5.0 pg per milliliter.

Combining these relations yields a measure of the efficiency of the water homeostatic mechanism: for each 1 mOsm per kilogram of H_2O change in plasma osmolality there is a change in urinary concentration of 95 mOsm per kilogram of H_2O, which represents a gain of almost 100-fold. The ingestion of water sufficient to decrease plasma osmolality by only 1 mOsm per kilogram of H_2O will reduce urinary concentration by 95 mOsm per kilogram of H_2O, thus allowing the water to be excreted and osmotic balance to be restored. The opposite effect, water loss, results in stimulation of ADH release, increase in urinary concentration and conservation of body water by the same magnification phenomenon.

NONOSMOTIC REGULATION OF ADH RELEASE. Isotonic or hypotonic volume depletion of man or experimental animals results in an antidiuretic state. Evidence now exists for stretch receptors, or baroreceptors, that sense changes in vascular wall tension in both the venous (low pressure) and arterial (high pressure) circulations. Immersion and negative pressure breathing, i.e., maneuvers that augment intrathoracic blood volume, as well as balloon distention of the left atrium, all produce a water diuresis which can be overcome by administering ADH. Conversely, positive pressure breathing and upright posture, which reduce intrathoracic blood volume, or left atrial collapse, produce antidiuresis. These observations indicate that the left atrium and the pulmonary vasculature are the major loci for low pressure baroreceptors which modulate ADH release.

Hypotension, or selective clamping of major systemic arterial vessels, also produces a profound antidiuresis. These data indicate the presence of a baroreceptor system in the arterial circulation, localized to the carotid bifurcations and aortic arch, which also modulates ADH release. This type of nonosmotic ADH release is modulated by stimulatory or inhibitory signals arriving from the baroreceptors via parasympathetic pathways in the vagus and glossopharyngeal nerves. The low pressure baroreceptors are more sensitive regulators of ADH release than those in high pressure regions of the circulation. These relations are summarized in Figure 226–1.

Circulating levels of ADH rise with vascular volume depletion. However, volume-mediated, nonosmotic ADH release has a "threshold" requiring more than 7 per cent blood volume depletion, with greater degrees of blood volume contraction eliciting exponential rises in circulating ADH levels. Thus nonosmotic ADH release differs strikingly from osmotically mediated ADH release, which occurs with only a 1 to 2 per cent increase in plasma osmolality and rises linearly with further increases in plasma osmolality. With less than a 7 per cent decrease in blood volume, ADH release is governed wholly by plasma osmolality. At greater reductions in blood volume, ADH release is increasingly dominated by nonosmotic, volume-dependent stimuli. This observation explains the finding of progressive fluid dilution in patients with hypovolemia or states of decreased cardiac output.

Input from higher cortical functions also appears to influence ADH release. Pain, emotion, stress, and some psychotic states are associated with ADH stimulation or inhibition. Most common is the transient antidiuresis that occurs postoperatively.

PATHOLOGIC ALTERATION OF ADH RELEASE. A wide variety of drugs are known to affect ADH activity (Table 226–1). Nicotine, as a stimulant of ADH release, and acute alcohol ingestion, as an inhibitor of ADH release, have figured prominently in devising means to assess neurohypophyseal integrity. Stimulatory drugs such as clofibrate and chlorpropamide have been utilized to treat states of partial ADH insufficiency. Other drugs, such as lithium and demethylchlortetracycline, are prominent for their effect on the renal collecting duct, making it unresponsive to ADH, and thereby producing nephrogenic diabetes insipidus.

TABLE 226–1. DRUGS THAT ALTER ANTIDIURETIC HORMONE ACTIVITY

Drugs That Modify Release of ADH	
Enhance	*Suppress*
Vincristine	Phenytoin
Cyclophosphamide	Alcohol
Clofibrate	Narcotic antagonists
Carbamazepine	α-Adrenergic agents
Barbiturates	
Morphine and narcotic analogues	
Chlorpropamide	
Nicotine	
β-Adrenergic agents	

Drugs That Modify the ADH Effect on Collecting Ducts	
Enhance	*Suppress*
Chlorpropamide	Lithium
Biguanides	Methoxyflurane
Indomethacin	Demeclocycline

The syndrome of inappropriate antidiuretic hormone secretion (SIADH) is characterized by persistent hyponatremia, an inappropriately elevated urine osmolality, and no discernible stimulus for ADH release. A common cause for this condition is neoplastic, most notably oat cell carcinoma of lung; SIADH is due to ectopic production of ADH by the tumor, with persistent release of hormone independent of regulatory influences. Inflammatory disorders of the lung, such as pneumonia or cavitary tuberculosis, provide other sites for ectopic ADH production. The syndrome also occurs in patients with head trauma or with other diseases of the central nervous system and often terminates with recovery of neurologic function. The SIADH syndrome is discussed in detail in Ch. 76.

THIRST REGULATION. Body water content is governed not only by ADH modulation of renal water excretion but also by regulation of water intake through thirst. Both systems operate in parallel under the influence of osmotic and volume mediators. Thirst also requires an intact cerebral cortex, which transforms the urge to drink into appropriate behavior to secure water.

Hyperosmolality, and presumably shrinkage of thirst receptors, is the primary stimulus for thirst, and requires only a 2 per cent rise in plasma osmolality. The thirst "threshold" in conscious man is about 294 mOsm per kilogram, the same osmolality at which maximal urinary concentration under ADH is achieved. Hypovolemia also stimulates thirst via an angiotensin II–mediated mechanism. Indeed, hyperreninemic states such as malignant hypertension are often accompanied by pathological thirst. Phenothiazines enhance thirst and contribute to the hyponatremia seen in some patients treated with these drugs for affective disorders. Finally, prostaglandin E also stimulates thirst. The polydipsia which accompanies hypokalemia probably depends on increased production of prostaglandin E.

WATER REPLETION REACTION. It is evident from the preceding description that hyperosmolality and blood volume contraction simultaneously stimulate ADH release and thirst. The integrated activity of ADH and thirst has been termed the water repletion reaction, and may be viewed as shown in Figure 4 of Chapter 76.

Because the afferent, or positive, limbs of this system respond to 1 to 2 per cent changes in plasma osmolality, the day-to-day regulation of body water osmolality is remarkably constant, and variations in a given normal person's osmolality are negligible. The serum sodium concentration, which reflects body fluid osmolality, is therefore also constant in normal individuals. Finally, both ADH release and thirst give preference to volume maintenance at the expense of body fluid osmolality when vascular volume is reduced by more than 7 per cent. Consequently, profound volume contraction is accompanied by antidiuresis, increased thirst, and hyponatremia.

Culpepper RM, Andreoli TE: Interactions among prostaglandin E_2, antidiuretic hormone and cyclic adenosine monophosphate in modulating Cl^- absorption in single mouse medullary thick limbs of Henle. J Clin Invest 71:1588–1601, 1983. *An analysis of the interactions between prostaglandins and ADH in modulating NaCl transport in the medullary diluting segments.*

Culpepper RM, Hebert SC, Andreoli TE: Nephrogenic diabetes insipidus. *In* Stanbury JB, Wyngaarden JB, Fredrickson DS, Goldstein JL, Brown MS (eds.): The Metabolic Basis of Inherited Disease. New York, McGraw-Hill Book Company, 1982, pp 1867–1888. *A comprehensive review of the physiology of vasopressin and the renal concentrating mechanism; extensively referenced.*

Robertson GL, Shelton RL, Athar S: The osmoregulation of vasopressin. Kidney Int 10:25, 1976. *A quantitative examination of the relationships among plasma osmolality, vasopressin secretion, and urinary concentration.*

Verney EB: The antidiuretic hormone and the factors which determine its release. Proc R Soc Lond (Biol) 135:25, 1947. *A classic treatise describing a series of elegant studies which led to the notion of a central nervous system osmoreceptor for ADH secretion.*

DIABETES INSIPIDUS

Pituitary Diabetes Insipidus

DEFINITION. Pituitary diabetes insipidus is a polyuric syndrome that results from a lack of sufficient ADH to effect appropriate concentration of the urine for water conservation. The disease is identified by the persistence of an inappropriately dilute urine in the presence of strong osmotic or nonosmotic stimuli to ADH secretion, and in the absence of renal concentrating defects, and a rise in urine osmolality upon the administration of vasopressin. Pituitary diabetes insipidus may result either from destruction of the centers of ADH synthesis or from failure of the mechanisms effecting ADH release.

ETIOLOGY. Trauma to the neurohypophysis, either accidental or as a result of hypophysectomy, is the major identifiable cause of diabetes insipidus. A second major cause for pituitary diabetes insipidus is an intracranial tumor, which may be primary, as in craniopharyngioma, or metastatic, among which breast carcinoma is the most likely cause. Less frequent causes of pituitary diabetes insipidus are granulomatous lesions of the central nervous system, including tuberculosis and sarcoidosis, the histiocytoses, encephalomeningitis, or vascular lesions. There is a rare familial form of pituitary diabetes insipidus which affects either sex, occurs at any age, and is associated with extensive gliosis of neurohypophyseal nuclei. Finally, 30 to 40 per cent of all patients with pituitary diabetes insipidus have no identifiable cause for the disorder.

PATHOGENESIS. Pituitary diabetes insipidus depends on one of two different pathogenic mechanisms. Most commonly, the disorder occurs when there is atrophy or destruction of the hypothalamic centers responsible for hormone production. Neither removal of the posterior pituitary gland alone nor low section of the neurohypophyseal tract with preservation of hypothalamic nuclei is sufficient to produce a permanent polyuric state. Rather, direct trauma to the pituitary gland or low section of the neurohypophyseal tract results in a transient diabetes insipidus; for example, the polyuric state following low stalk section lasts for only one to two weeks postsurgery. Since the anterior and posterior lobes of the pituitary gland have totally separate blood supplies, infarction of the anterior pituitary gland does not disrupt posterior pituitary function.

A second group of patients has been identified, often classed under the heading "essential hypernatremia," in which osmotic stimuli fail to elicit ADH release, while nonosmotic stimuli result in antidiuresis. Although euvolemic, these patients are polyuric and excrete a hypotonic urine, and water deprivation alone fails to elicit an antidiuretic response. However, when these patients are volume contracted, a significant antidiuresis ensues. Thus in this disorder, there is selective failure of osmoreceptors to stimulate ADH release. The intact response of ADH release to nonosmotic stimulation verifies the integrity of the hypothalamic centers that produce ADH.

Nephrogenic Diabetes Insipidus

DEFINITION. The term *nephrogenic diabetes insipidus* should be applied to disorders in which renal tubular unresponsiveness to ADH, without disturbances either in solute delivery to the loop of Henle or in countercurrent multiplication or exchange processes, is responsible for polyuria and hyposthenuria. Thus nephrogenic diabetes insipidus may be due to inability of ADH to raise cellular cAMP concentrations, to inability of cAMP to increase the water permeability of luminal membranes of collecting ducts, or to a combination of these two disorders.

FAMILIAL NEPHROGENIC DIABETES INSIPIDUS. This familial disorder occurs primarily in males and exhibits a hereditary pattern of X-linked transmission with variable penetrance in females. In normal individuals or patients with pituitary diabetes insipidus, exogenous ADH can increase the rate of urinary cAMP excretion. In some patients with familial nephrogenic diabetes insipidus, comparable doses of ADH do not increase rates of urinary cAMP excretion. However, in two groups of children with nephrogenic diabetes insipidus, both basal and ADH-stimulated rates of urinary cAMP excretion exceeded those of normal children. These disparate results led to the postulate that familial nephrogenic diabetes insipidus is a heterogeneous disorder produced by either a defect in hormone receptor adenylate cyclase stimulation or a defect beyond the generation of cAMP. In patients with familial nephrogenic diabetes insipidus, however, plasma cortisol concentrations can rise in response to ADH, a finding interpreted to indicate that vasopressin stimulation of extrarenal, i.e., pituitary, cAMP formation is intact in the disease.

ACQUIRED NEPHROGENIC DIABETES INSIPIDUS. Vasopressin-resistant hyposthenuria associated with otherwise normal or nearly normal renal function may occur as a complication of drug therapy or in association with systemic diseases. Appropriately termed acquired nephrogenic diabetes insipidus, this condition is to be distinguished from the rare familial disorder described earlier.

Vasopressin-unresponsive hyposthenuria occurs in patients receiving demeclocycline; both the concentrating defect and vasopressin-unresponsiveness are reversible and disappear shortly after discontinuance of antibiotic therapy. The glomerular filtration rate in these patients is generally normal, as is the ability for maximal urinary dilution (positive free water formation), indicating that solute abstraction from the loop of Henle is probably unimpaired.

In human renal medulla, demeclocycline noncompetitively inhibits basal adenylate cyclase activity, ADH-stimulated adenylate cyclase activity, and cAMP-dependent protein kinase activity. Thus demeclocycline-induced nephrogenic diabetes insipidus may be due in part to inhibition of cAMP accumulation in collecting duct cells.

Nephrogenic diabetes insipidus may also be produced by volatile fluorocarbon anesthetics. Methoxyflurane anesthesia is complicated by a full spectrum of renal injury, ranging from vasopressin-resistant polyuria and hyposthenuria to acute tubular necrosis. Both fluoride and oxalic acid, which are metabolic products of methoxyflurane, contribute to the nephrotoxicity of the anesthetic. However, the polyuric state is related to the markedly increased serum concentration and urinary excretion of inorganic fluoride. Sodium fluoride causes vasopressin-resistant polyuria in dogs, and in rats inorganic fluoride seems to reduce collecting duct water permeability without affecting salt transport in the ascending limb.

Serum lithium concentrations of 0.5 to 1.5 mEq per liter, which are generally regarded as being in the therapeutic range for affective disorders, produce vasopressin-resistant diabetes insipidus. Nephrogenic diabetes insipidus has been observed in 12 to 30 per cent of patients receiving lithium therapy; the defect is usually reversible, and urinary concentrating ability returns toward normal when lithium is discontinued. Finally, nephrogenic diabetes insipidus characterized by persistent, vasopressin-resistant hyposthenuria and polyuria occurs rarely in certain systemic diseases, including most notably sarcoidosis and Sjögren's syndrome.

ACQUIRED POLYURIC STATES. There are also sets of disorders that may present with polyuria and relative vasopressin resistance, although not necessarily with profound hyposthenuria. Rather, these polyuric disturbances are generally characterized by inability to concentrate urine maximally in response to vasopressin, either stimulated endogenously or administered exogenously; random urine samples are ordinarily not profoundly hypotonic but are usually only slightly hypotonic or modestly hypertonic.

In general, such polyuric disorders occur most commonly in association with hypokalemic nephropathy (Ch. 76) or hypercalcemic nephropathy (Ch. 246), or as a consequence of diseases that disrupt medullary architecture and consequently impair the generation and maintenance of a hypertonic medullary interstitium. The latter disorders include those diseases that affect particularly the renal interstitium, such as sickle cell disease, pyelonephritis, analgesic nephropathy, and multiple myeloma. These diseases are considered in Ch. 81.

Finally, states characterized by osmotic, or solute, diuresis, for example, in diabetic ketoacidosis and hyperglycemic nonketotic states, may result in polyuria with isotonic urine formation and unresponsiveness to vasopressin. In these disorders, the fraction of isotonic glomerular filtrate delivered to the loop of Henle is greatly increased because of failure to absorb solute, for example, glucose, in the proximal nephron. Thus the amount of solute and water reaching the loop of Henle becomes large with regard to the diluting or concentrating ability of the loop of Henle and collecting ducts, respectively, and vasopressin-resistant polyuria and isosthenuria ensue. Consequently the polyuric state in osmotic diuresis differs from that in nephrogenic diabetes insipidus in two respects: urinary solute excretion is dramatically increased in osmotic diuresis but not in nephrogenic diabetes insipidus; and the urine osmolality is nearly isotonic in solute diuresis but rather hypotonic in nephrogenic diabetes insipidus.

PITUITARY OR NEPHROGENIC DIABETES INSIPIDUS

CLINICAL MANIFESTATIONS. The foremost clinical feature of either pituitary or nephrogenic diabetes insipidus is *polyuria,* with urine volumes ranging from 3 to 15 liters per day. Along with polyuria there is near-continuous *thirst,* often with a preference for ice cold water. The disease is almost always accompanied by *nocturia,* in contrast to persons with primary polydipsia (compulsive water drinking), in whom nocturia is usually absent. The onset of polyuria in pituitary diabetes insipidus is most often abrupt, with peak urine flow reached in one or two days. Therefore, polyuria developing over weeks or months suggests a disease other than pituitary diabetes insipidus. The polyuria of familial nephrogenic diabetes insipidus is present from birth.

The polyuria in complete diabetes insipidus, either pituitary or nephrogenic, has an upper limit of approximately 18 liters daily, or about 10 per cent of filtered water, since 90 per cent of the glomerular filtrate is normally absorbed by the nephron prior to reaching the collecting system. In partial pituitary diabetes insipidus, the daily urine volume may be considerably smaller. In contrast, persons afflicted with compulsive water drinking, often referred to as primary or psychogenic polydipsia, not infrequently ingest more than 20 liters of fluid daily. Therefore, the daily urine volume in these patients may also exceed 20 liters.

Modest degrees of volume depletion may curtail polyuria, even in complete diabetes insipidus, for two reasons. First, volume contraction will increase the fraction of glomerular filtrate absorbed by the proximal nephron, so that a smaller volume of hypotonic fluid reaches the collecting duct system. Second, even in the absence of ADH, or when collecting ducts are unresponsive to ADH, collecting ducts have a slight permeability to water; consequently, a small fraction of the water reaching the collecting duct system can be absorbed even without ADH. Since the volume of glomerular filtrate reaching the collecting duct system is reduced during volume contraction, the further absorption of relatively small volumes of water by collecting ducts during the volume-contracted state can result in dramatic reductions in polyuria.

Aside from the discomfort and inconvenience of polyuria and polydipsia, patients with pituitary or nephrogenic diabetes insipidus suffer no ill effects unless they are *deprived of access to water.* When this happens, *circulatory collapse* or *hypertonic encephalopathy* may occur. Because of the high rates of urine flow in some patients with diabetes insipidus, these complications may develop in a period of hours. For example, a patient with pituitary diabetes insipidus might excrete 5 per cent of his glomerular filtrate daily, or about 9 liters of urine. In a 70-kg man having 42 kg of body water, this loss, if not continuously replenished, would result in a 20 per cent reduction in body water in only 24 hours.

Hypertonic Encephalopathy. Both in man and in experimental animals, acute increases in extracellular fluid osmolality to levels exceeding 350 mOsm per kilogram of H_2O produced by solutes such as NaCl or glucose (in diabetes), which cross cell membranes poorly, result in central nervous system dysfunction ranging from lethargy to frank coma. Since comparable elevations of plasma osmolality produced by urea, which permeates cell membranes freely, do not produce the disorder, it is evident that hyperosmolality per se is not the basis for the disturbance. Rather, acute hypertonic encephalopathy occurs because cell membranes, being freely permeable to water, are in virtually constant osmotic equilibrium with extracellular fluid. When hypernatremia develops acutely, cellular water loss produces brain shrinkage; and the increase in brain solute content is accounted for entirely by a rise in intracellular Na^+, K^+, and Cl^- concentrations.

In children who develop acute hypernatremia and attain a serum sodium concentration above 160 mEq per liter in 24 hours, the mortality rate exceeds 40 per cent; about two thirds of the survivors have permanent neurologic sequelae. The autopsy results in these circumstances reveal widespread damage in cerebral vasculature. Vessels are markedly congested and engorged, hemorrhages are evident both in subcortical brain parenchyma and subarachnoid spaces, and venous thrombosis occurs.

When hypernatremia develops gradually, the incidence of hypertonic encephalopathy is greatly reduced, both in man and in experimental animals. This occurs because brain cells adapt to gradually developing hypernatremia by accumulating solutes intracellularly. The sum of brain Na^+, K^+, and Cl^- accounts for approximately 75 per cent of intracellular solutes; the remaining solutes, as yet unidentified, are commonly referred to as "idiogenic osmoles." Thus in chronic hypernatremia, brain accumulation of "idiogenic osmoles" minimizes the extent of water loss and consequently brain shrinkage. This in turn reduces the frequency with which encephalopathy develops.

Posthypophysectomy Course. The acute diabetes insipidus following hypophysectomy has a characteristic triphasic response. For a few hours to days following the insult, there exists a polyuric, hyposthenuric phase which depends on inhibition of ADH release. Next, there follows a period with reduced urine volume and a rise in urine osmolality. During this phase, there is persistent release of ADH from atrophying neurons, an inability to excrete a water load, and the risk of progressive hypotonicity with continued parenteral adminstration of large volumes of hypotonic fluids. The final phase, if the diabetes insipidus becomes permanent, is marked by recurrence of polyuria and hyposthenuria.

Laboratory Manifestations. Persistent hyposthenuria, with a urine specific gravity of 1.005 or less and urine osmolality less than 200 mOsm per kilogram of H_2O, is the hallmark of the diabetes insipidus syndromes. In euvolemic patients, the glomerular filtration rate (GFR) is normal. Since patients with diabetes insipidus ingest water in response to plasma hypertonicity, random plasma osmolality determinations in these patients will be, on the average, above the usual norm of 287 mOsm per kilogram of H_2O. The serum sodium concentrations are also elevated and account quantitatively for the increases in plasma osmolality. In contrast, persons with primary polydipsia have a primary aberration of the thirst mechanism and ingest water independent of physiologic stimuli. These patients often have a mild dilutional hyponatremia.

In patients whose diabetes insipidus, either pituitary or nephrogenic in origin, begins in childhood, considerable dilation of the urinary bladder, ureters, and renal pelvis may occur. This dilation has led to a reduction in GFR in some patients.

DIAGNOSIS. Based on the underlying pathophysiology, the polyuric syndromes may be grouped into the following general categories: (1) pituitary diabetes insipidus, in which there is absence or diminished production and secretion of ADH; (2)

solute diuresis, in which excessively high rates of solute delivery to the loop of Henle overwhelm quantitatively the ability of distal nephron segments to dissociate solute and water absorption; (3) nephrogenic diabetes insipidus, either familial or acquired, in which collecting duct cells are partially or completely unresponsive to ADH; (4) renal concentrating disorders, in which there is impaired generation of a hypertonic medullary interstitium by renal countercurrent multiplication and exchange processes; and (5) primary polydipsia, in which the ingestion of unusually large volumes of water results in polyuria, the appropriate physiologic response.

Disorders such as diabetes mellitus, which produces a solute diuresis, are characterized by an isotonic urine and by glycosuria. The history and laboratory data are adequate to identify disorders such as sickle cell disease or interstitial nephritis, both of which impair the ability to generate a hypertonic medullary interstitium. Routine laboratory screening readily identifies the presence of hypercalcemia or hypokalemia. Finally, congenital nephrogenic diabetes insipidus is identified by a history of having been present since birth, generally in males, and by *persistent* unresponsiveness to exogenous ADH. Acquired nephrogenic diabetes insipidus is recognized by ADH unresponsiveness combined with a history of exposure to agents, such as lithium, demeclocycline, or methoxyflurane anesthesia, which antagonize the action of ADH on collecting ducts.

The more difficult diagnostic problem is the differentiation of patients with partial or complete deficiency of ADH from those with primary polydipsia. Certain factors may point toward the most likely diagnosis. For example, a 24-hour urine volume greater than 18 liters, a random plasma osmolality determination below 285 mOsm per kilogram of H_2O, and a history of episodic polyuria all suggest compulsive water drinking as the underlying disorder. A history of head trauma or neoplasm, a history of sudden onset of unrelenting polyuria, and a random plasma osmolality determination greater than 290 mOsm per kilogram of H_2O all suggest pituitary diabetes insipidus.

The basis of all tests for pituitary diabetes insipidus rests on the ability of the kidney to excrete a hypertonic urine after an osmotic stimulus. The simplest maneuver is to produce hypertonicity of body fluids by water deprivation. The absolute level of urine concentration achieved with water deprivation is nondiagnostic, since maximal concentrating ability depends on the degree of medullary hypertonicity as well as the presence of adequate amounts of ADH. For example, Miller et al. found the maximal urine osmolality produced by water deprivation in a group of randomly selected hospitalized patients to be 764 mOsm per kilogram of H_2O as compared with 1067 mOsm per kilogram of H_2O in healthy volunteers. Presumably, the lower value for maximal urine concentrating ability in hospitalized patients reflects a reduction in medullary interstitial hypertonicity with respect to that present in normal volunteers.

However, even in patients with a reduced medullary interstitial tonicity, the maximal urine osmolality achieved with water deprivation depends on maximal degrees of endogenous ADH release in response to dehydration. Therefore, in those with intact mechanisms for ADH production and release, the administration of exogenous ADH will not produce an increase in the maximal urine osmolality achieved via water deprivation. This rationale forms the framework for a test scheme, illustrated in Figure 226–2, for distinguishing complete or partial pituitary diabetes insipidus from other polyuric syndromes.

In patients with mild polyuria, water deprivation may begin the night preceding the test; patients with severe polyuria should have water restricted during the day, to allow for close observation. The test begins with paired measurements of urine and plasma osmolality. All water intake is then withheld and hourly measurements of urine osmolality and body weight are made. When two sequential urine osmolalities vary by less than 30 mOsm per kilogram of H_2O, or when 3 to 5 per cent body weight is lost, 5 units of aqueous vasopressin is injected subcutaneously. A final urine osmolality is measured 60 minutes later.

The time required to achieve a maximal urine concentration varies from 4 to 18 hours. In normal persons, water deprivation results in a urine osmolality two to four times greater than that of plasma. More important, the subsequent administration of exogenous ADH results in a less than 5 per cent further increase in urine osmolality. Patients with primary polydipsia, who have a reduced medullary interstitial tonicity as a result of prolonged water diuresis, may concentrate the urine only slightly after water deprivation. However, they too will have stimulated endogenous ADH release maximally and will exhibit a less than 5 per cent rise in urine osmolality with supplemental ADH.

Patients with complete pituitary diabetes insipidus will not raise urine osmolality above that of plasma in response to water deprivation, but will show a greater than 50 per cent increase in urine osmolality in response to injection of ADH. Patients with partial pituitary diabetes insipidus may concentrate the urine to some degree in response to water deprivation, but they will also increase urine osmolality by at least 10 per cent after ADH injection. An interesting observation is that patients with partial pituitary diabetes insipidus often show a peak urine osmolality that decreases with further water restriction. This suggests a limited reserve of neurohypophyseal hormone

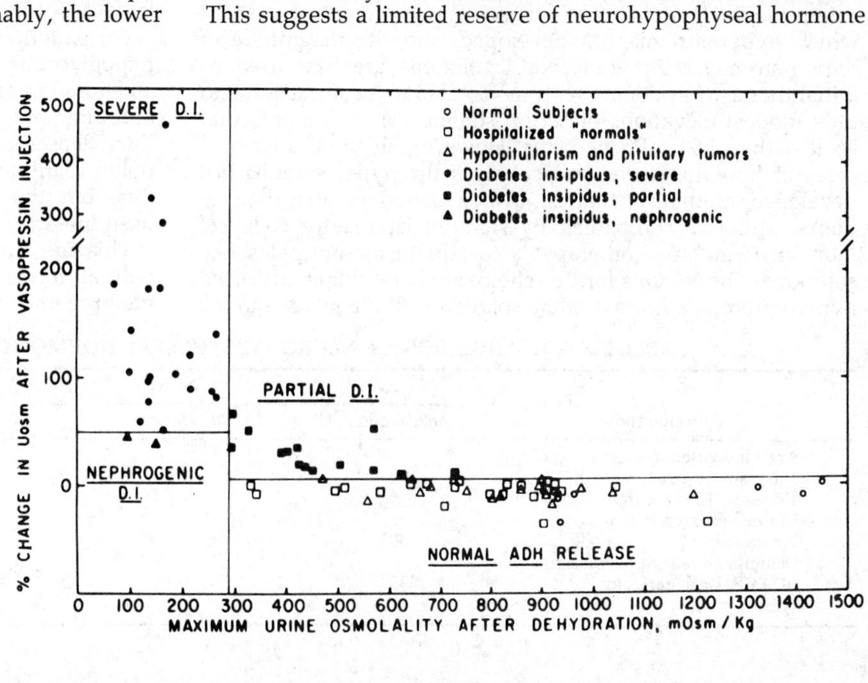

Figure 226–2. Maximal urine osmolality after dehydration versus the percentage change in urine osmolality induced by subsequent vasopressin injection. D.I. = diabetes insipidus; ADH = antidiuretic hormone. (From Miller M, et al.: Ann Intern Med 73:721, 1970. Reprinted with permission of the publisher.)

which is depleted after an initial secretory burst. Finally, patients with nephrogenic diabetes insipidus deprived of water fail to raise the urine osmolality above that of plasma even when given exogenous ADH. When a diagnosis of pituitary diabetes insipidus is made, a careful evaluation for neoplasm involving the hypothalamus or neurohypophyseal tract is mandatory.

Levels of circulating vasopressin measured by radioimmunoassay have heretofore been available only for research purposes. A commercial assay is now marketed for clinical use, but its utility is, as of now, undefined. Hypertonic saline infusions have also been utilized to test for release of antidiuretic hormone. This procedure is hazardous in patients with limited cardiac reserve, in whom volume expansion may precipitate cardiac decompensation. Moreover, the results of the test are uninterpretable if the patient develops a salt diuresis, thus fixing urine osmolality near isotonicity.

Nicotine, a nonosmotic stimulus to ADH secretion, has been used to elicit antidiuresis in those patients who have "essential hypernatremia," i.e., ADH release in response to volume contraction but not to hypertonicity. A more preferable diagnostic approach in these patients is to assess the antidiuretic response to mild volume contraction.

TREATMENT. Patients with diabetes insipidus, either pituitary or nephrogenic, may require emergency treatment of hypertonic encephalopathy or maintenance therapy for polyuria.

Hypertonic Encephalopathy. The goal in treating this medical emergency is to replenish body water, thereby restoring osmotic balance and repleting cell volume, at a rate that avoids significant complications. Since the brain adjusts to hypertonicity, at least in part, by increasing intracellular osmolar content via accumulation of "idiogenic osmoles," rapid repletion of body water with extracellular fluid dilution will cause translocation of water into cells to achieve osmotic equilibrium. The result of this water movement is cell swelling and cerebral edema. Seizures occur in up to 40 per cent of patients treated for severe hypernatremia by rapid infusions of hypotonic solutions. If water repletion is undertaken at a slower rate, brain cells lose the accumulated intracellular solutes and osmotic equilibration can occur without cell swelling. Consequently, a good rule of thumb is to adminster fluids at a rate which reduces the serum sodium concentration to normal over a 36- to 48-hour period, or to reduce the serum sodium concentration by about 1 mEq per liter every two hours.

The choice of fluid to be administered in the diabetes insipidus syndromes depends in large part on three factors: the extent to which circulatory collapse may be present; the rate at which hypernatremia has developed; and the magnitude of hypernatremia. Hypotonic NaCl solutions are best used as initial therapy in patients with modest volume contraction and only modest elevations of serum sodium concentrations, that is, less than 160 mEq per liter. However, in more advanced cases of hypernatremia, particularly if the hypernatremia has developed gradually, that is, over a period greater than 24 hours, and is accompanied by signs of circulatory collapse, more prudent initial therapy is to administer normal saline solutions. The reasons for this choice are two-fold: in advanced hypernatremia, a normal saline solution is dilute relative to the patient's body fluid osmolality and thus will dilute the latter while minimizing the risk of iatrogenic cerebral swelling; at the same time, the normal saline solution provides an effective means of volume expansion. Finally, 5 per cent glucose solutions may be used to replenish body water in acute hypernatremia without significant circulatory collapse. However, the glucose infusion rate must be less than the rate of glucose metabolism to avoid glycosuria. Otherwise, the resulting osmotic diuresis will thwart attempts to replenish body free water. The treatment of drug-induced nephrogenic diabetes insipidus consists of removal of the offending agent.

Polyuria. Patients with partial hormonal deficiency and volumes of urine output between 2 and 6 liters daily may require no treatment as long as they are assured access to water. Specific therapy for pituitary diabetes insipidus is some form of ADH replacement. A variety of hormone preparations are available which differ in the ratio of antidiuretic to vasopressor activity and the duration of biologic effect. These relations are depicted in Table 226–2.

Early preparations of dried posterior pituitary extract, termed "pituitary snuff," were given by nasal insufflation, had an effective biologic life of only a few hours, and inevitably produced chronic rhinitis, which often led to inadequate absorption of hormone. Aqueous vasopressin injections, having an activity span of only a few hours, are not practical, although nasal sprays of aqueous lysine vasopressin may provide intermittent relief of polyuria. Rhinitis, although not so severe as with dried extract, is also a frequent concomitant to this form of therapy.

The most widely used preparation has been Pitressin Tannate in oil, which is given intramuscularly. As little as 0.5 ml per day may provide adequate hormone for 24 to 48 hours. Great care must be exercised in preparing the injection by careful warming and mixing of the ampule so as to suspend the pellet of hormone in the oil. Failure to do so may result in injection of the oil vehicle alone and apparent "vasopressin resistance." Pain at injection sites and sterile abscesses are frequent complaints with this preparation. Persistent abdominal pain from the effect of ADH on intestinal motility is a not uncommon problem.

A synthetic analogue of vasopressin, dDAVP (1-deamino,8-D-arginine vasopressin), provides antidiuretic activity for 8 to 20 hours with negligible pressor effect, can be taken as a nasal spray, and is the current drug of choice. The drug is best started at night to find the lowest dose that will prevent nocturia. This dose, usually 5 to 10 μg, can be given twice daily or doubled as a single morning dose. A nasal catheter is provided, which is measured for convenient dosing in the 5 to 20 μg range. Headache may be a troublesome side effect with large doses but usually disappears with a reduction of dosage.

For patients having some residual ADH production, the oral hypoglycemic agent chlorpropamide may provide adequate amelioration of symptoms. This drug stimulates ADH secretion and augments the activity of residual ADH on the collecting duct. Doses of 250 to 500 mg daily are sufficient to reduce polyuria in most patients with partial pituitary diabetes insipidus, but the side effect of hypoglycemia limits the drug's usefulness.

Thiazide diuretics may reduce the volume of urine in patients with all forms of diabetes insipidus, that is, either pituitary or nephrogenic, by causing a state of mild salt depletion. This

TABLE 226–2. COMPARISON OF NEUROHYPOPHYSEAL HORMONES AND SYNTHETIC ANALOGUES

Preparation	Activity: Antidiuretic	:	Vasopressor	:	Oxytocic	Duration of Activity	Route of Administration
8-Arginine vasopressin							
Pitressin, Aqueous	100	:	100	:	5	2–6 hours	Intravenous
Pitressin Tannate in oil						24–48 hours	Intramuscular
8-Lysine vasopressin							
Lypressin	60	:	70	:	1	2–6 hours	Nasal insufflation
1-Deamino, 8 D-arginine vasopressin							
dDAVP, Desmopressin	290	:	0.14			6–20 hours	Nasal insufflation
Oxytocin	1	:	1	:	100		

results in a secondary increase in isotonic proximal tubular fluid absorption and a decrease in the volume of fluid delivered to the collecting duct. The effect is produced by 50 to 100 mg of hydrochlorothiazide daily, is sustained even in the absence of diuretics by salt restriction, and can be abolished by salt loading even with continued diuretic administration.

Vasopressin infusions have also been used to treat bleeding esophageal varices by reducing splanchnic blood flow. Desmopressin, a synthetic analogue of arginine vasopressin, stimulates the production of clotting factor VIII. These other actions are discussed elsewhere in this textbook.

Nephrogenic Diabetes Insipidus. The therapeutic considerations outlined above, particularly with respect to the treatment of hypertonic encephalopathy and to the value of a chronic mild salt-depleted state in minimizing polyuria, apply equally well to the care of patients with pituitary or nephrogenic diabetes insipidus. In patients with nephrogenic diabetes insipidus acquired as a consequence of drug therapy (for example, lithium or demeclocycline), the offending agent should be discontinued.

Finally, it is important to stress the need to minimize the extent of polyuria in children with congenital nephrogenic diabetes insipidus, since there is a close correlation between repeated bouts of dehydration during childhood and mental dullness in adulthood. Alternatively, in patients in whom episodes of dehydration have been minimal, both mental and physical growth retardation can be avoided.

Andreoli TE: The polyuric syndromes. *In* Andreoli TE, Hoffman JF, Fanestil DD (eds.): Physiology of Membrane Disorders. New York, Plenum Medical Book Company, 1978, pp 1063-1091. *A discussion of the physiology of the polyuric states, their differentiation one from another, and therapeutic approaches; extensively referenced.*

Arieff AI, Schmidt RW: Fluid and electrolyte disorders and the central nervous system. *In* Maxwell MH, Kleeman CR (eds.): Clinical Disorders of Fluid and Electrolyte Metabolism. New York, McGraw-Hill Book Company, 1980, pp 1409-1480. *This chapter is a superb review of the pathophysiology, manifestations, and treatment of the hyperosmolar syndrome; thoroughly referenced.*

Barlow ED, De Wardener HE: Compulsive water drinking. Quart J Med 28:235, 1959. *A thorough examination of the clinical course and pathophysiology of urinary concentration in a group of patients with primary polydipsia.*

DeRubertis FR, Michelis MF, Beck N, Field JB, David, BB: "Essential" hypernatremia due to ineffective osmotic and intact volume regulation of vasopressin secretion. J Clin Invest 50:97, 1971. *A description of patients having intact neurohypophyseal function but lacking normal regulation of ADH because of a specific defect in osmoregulation.*

Miller M, Dalakos T, Moses AM, Fellerman H, Streeten DHP: Recognition of partial defects in antidiuretic hormone secretion. Ann Intern Med 73:721, 1970. *A concise guide to testing procedures for states of ADH insufficiency and a rational scheme for interpreting the test results.*

Robertson GL: Thirst and vasopressin function in normal and disordered states of water balance. J Lab Clin Med 101:351, 1983. *A detailed account of the physiology and pathophysiology of ADH secretion and thirst in normal patients and those with polyuric disorders.*

Zerbe RL, Robertson GL: Osmoregulation of thirst and vasopressin secretion in human subjects: Effect of various solutes. Am J Physiol 244:E607, 1983. *The role of various ECF solutes on ADH release.*

THE SYNDROME OF INAPPROPRIATE ADH PRODUCTION (SIADH)

For convenience SIADH has been discussed in Ch. 76 as a major disorder producing hyponatremia.

OXYTOCIN

Oxytocin is produced in the same hypothalamic nuclei and by the same synthetic mechanism as vasopressin. AVP and oxytocin are produced in both the paraventricular and the supraoptic nuclei of the hypothalamus. However, a given neuron in these nuclei produces only one hormone. Neurophysin I is the specific carrier protein synthesized with oxytocin and has been used as a marker for oxytocin release.

PHYSIOLOGY. The primary stimuli for oxytocin secretion are nipple stimulation (suckling) and deformation of the reproductive tract (especially the vagina) in females, and muscular contraction of the reproductive organs in the male. The neural arcs serving these stimuli are not well defined, but some evidence suggests that the final synaptic transmitter is dopamine. Estrogens appear to influence secretion directly, based on observations of increased neurophysin I in blood during estrogen peaks of the menstrual cycle, or permissively, based on findings of a graded response to vaginal distention over the period of a menstrual cycle and an enhanced response with exogenous estradiol. Progesterones inhibit response to mechanical stimuli. Hypertonicity of body fluids also appears to cause oxytocin secretion, and congenitally vasopressin-deficient rats (Brattleboro strain) show little neurohypophyseal oxytocin until given vasopressin, suggesting that these animals attempt to compensate for AVP insufficiency with the weaker antidiuretic hormone, oxytocin.

BIOLOGIC ACTIVITY. In females, oxytocin initiates its primary effect by binding to specific myometrial receptors, the affinity of which increases strikingly in the presence of estrogen. Exogenously administered oxytocin elicits contractions of the fundus indistinguishable from those of labor. However, the initiation of labor is apparently oxytocin independent, with increasing secretions seen only with dilation of the birth canal. Oxytocin may play a key role in final expulsion of the fetus and placenta. The total absence of oxytocin does not prevent parturition, although prolonged labor is seen in such women. The cellular events leading to uterine contraction are unknown, but parallel an oxytocin-induced increase in ion permeability with depolarization of the myometrial cell membrane.

The milk-ejection reflex is also mediated via oxytocin. Contraction of mammary myoepithelium is stimulated, leading to a rise in intramammary pressure and expulsion of milk from alveolar channels to large sinuses, where it is accessible to the suckling infant. A true galactogenic effect of oxytocin leading to increased milk production has not been convincingly demonstrated. Absence of oxytocin abolishes the milk-ejection reflex.

In the male, oxytocin increases ejection of sperm into the semen in response to stimulation of the reproductive organs. Oxytocin retains some antidiuretic activity, about 1 per cent that of AVP, but exerts no significant antidiuretic effect at physiologic levels of secretion. Vascular smooth muscle is relaxed by oxytocin, causing a decrease in blood pressure, cutaneous flushing, and increased limb blood flow. Reflex tachycardia and sympathetic responses quickly restore hemodynamics to normal except when such reflexes are rendered inactive as in deep anesthesia.

THERAPEUTIC USE. The primary use of oxytocin (Pitocin) is to induce or to improve the quality of labor. The uterus is relatively resistant to oxytocin in early pregnancy, but infusions given with hypertonic saline injections may speed abortions of later pregnancy.

With long-term infusion of oxytocin, patients may experience sufficient antidiuretic effects to be at risk of water intoxication. Antidiuresis may be detected at oxytocin infusion rates of 15 mU per minute, and maximal urinary concentration is usually attained at rates of 45 mU per minute. Infusions for delivery and control of postpartum uterine hemorrhage may reach 20 to 40 mU per minute, and infusions for therapeutic abortions range from 20 to 100 mU per minute.

Roberts JS: Oxytocin, Vol I. Montreal, Eden Press, 1977. *This review covers the extensive work in oxytocin physiology and chemistry; very readable and fully referenced.*

227. THE PINEAL

Seymour Reichlin

The pineal gland was discovered more than 20 centuries ago, and its function has long been a matter of scientific and philosophic speculation. Arising embryologically from ependyma lining the roof of the third ventricle, the pineal consists of parenchymal cells supported by a meshwork of neuroglia.

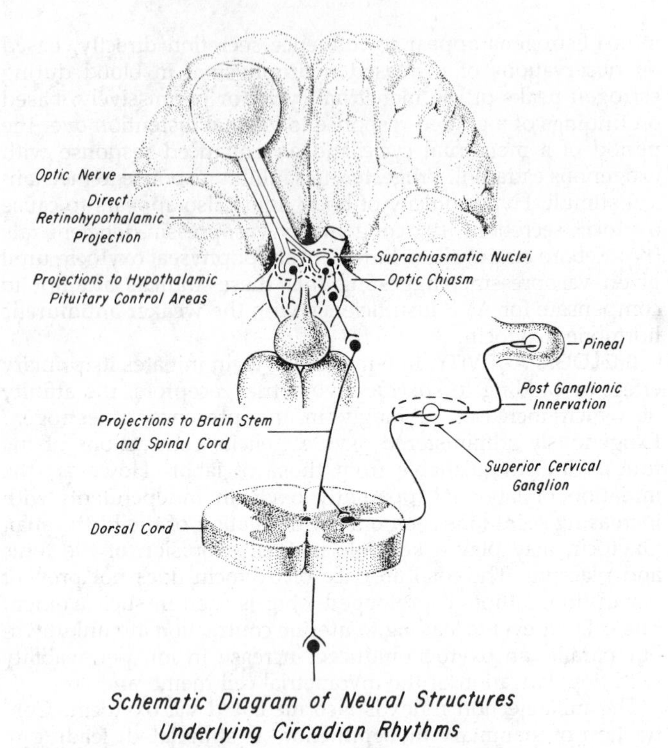

Figure 227–1. Control system for pineal regulation. Light impinging upon the retina is transduced into neural signals that reach the brain, giving both visual and nonvisual responses. This diagram outlines the nonvisual component. Those involved in endocrine regulation are mainly conducted by the direct retinohypothalamic projection to the suprachiasmatic nuclei (located in the hypothalamus). From the suprachiasmatic nuclei, nerve pathways project to the hypophysiotropic control areas of the hypothalamus and also to the spinal cord, where they influence the primary neurons of the sympathetic nerve outflow tract that terminate in the superior cervical ganglia. From the superior cervical ganglia, postganglionic sympathetic nerves (noradrenergic in function), accompanying the venous drainage of the pineal gland, enter the gland to innervate the pineal parenchymal cells. Suprachiasmatic nuclei are responsible for endogenous rhythms as well as those influenced by external lighting (see text). (Redrawn from Moore RY: *In* Yen SSC, Jaffe RB [eds.]: Reproductive Endocrinology: Physiology, Pathophysiology and Clinical Management. Philadelphia, W. B. Saunders Company, 1978, pp 3–33.)

In the adult, the gland weighs between 100 and 180 mg and is a cone-shaped organ lying in the groove formed by the superior colliculi. Although connected to the epithalamus by a peduncle, the pineal does not receive a direct nerve supply from this source. Rather, it is innervated by postganglionic nerve fibers that arise in the cervical sympathetic ganglia and travel along the great vein of Galen, the blood vessel into which pineal secretions drain. The sympathetic inflow to the pineal is in turn regulated by impulses arising in the suprachiasmatic nuclei, paired structures lying just above the optic chiasm (Fig. 227–1). This nucleus is innervated by a direct nerve pathway from the retina termed the retinohypothalamic tract. Changes in external lighting influence pineal activity (and other endocrine functions) via this pathway even when pathways mediating conscious light perception have been severed. The suprachiasmatic nucleus is also believed to serve as an internal "clock" (or biologic oscillator), regulating a number of endogenous endocrine rhythms. Circadian changes can occur even in the absence of external sensory cues, including light changes, thus indicating that there is a mechanism for determination of intrinsic rhythms. The rhythm of the endogenous oscillator can be modified by external signals such as normal light-dark cycles.

SECRETIONS OF THE PINEAL

Many different neurotransmitter substances, including norepinephrine, serotonin, histamine, melatonin, dopamine, octopamine, and gamma-aminobutyric acid, are found in the pineal. It also contains the hypothalamic peptides somatostatin and TRH. Of all these biologically active substances, only melatonin has been shown to be secreted into the blood and can be looked upon as a true hormonal secretion of the pineal. Melatonin is present in blood, cerebrospinal fluid, and urine of many species of animals, including man. Hormone levels show a marked diurnal rhythm, with night values up to ten times higher than day values. Turning lights off is a potent stimulus to melatonin release. Melatonin is believed to exert suppressive effects on a number of endocrine functions in experimental animals, the most important of which is on the release of gonadotropic hormones. When given to man in high dosage, melatonin suppresses plasma LH levels and stress-induced growth hormone secretion. Important effects of melatonin injection in man are the production of sleepiness and changes in the electroencephalogram, mainly an increase of alpha waves. Melatonin is formed by a series of enzymatic steps from tryptophan in which one of the intermediates is serotonin (Fig. 227–2). Enzymic activity of the pineal gland and its secretory function are regulated by noradrenergic nerve endings on pinealocytes. Beta-catecholamine receptors activate adenyl cyclase with the formation of cyclic AMP through the classic second messenger mechanism. The activated ATP-protein kinase is believed to promote the formation of the melatonin-synthesizing enzymes. Norepinephrine also stimulates pineal uptake of the precursor tryptophan.

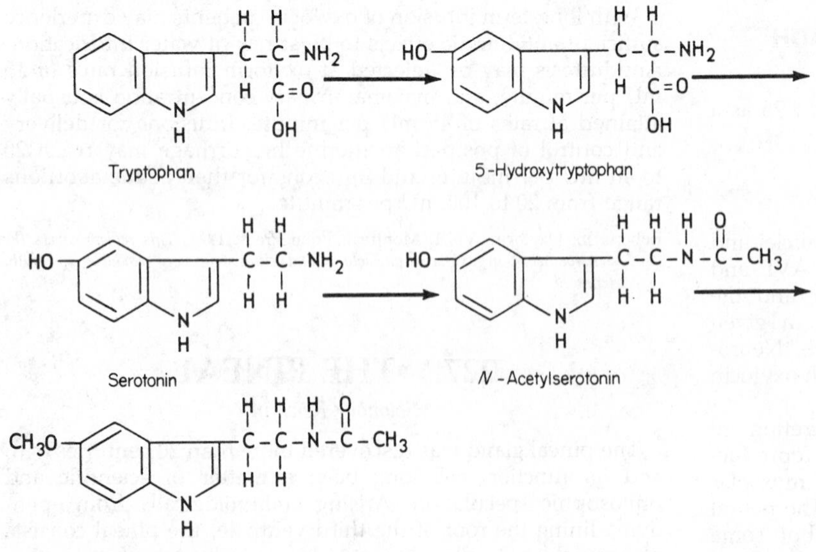

Figure 227–2. Biosynthesis of melatonin from tryptophan in the pineal gland. Step 1 is catalyzed by tryptophan hydroxylase; Step 2 by L-aromatic amino acid decarboxylase; Step 3 by N-acetylating enzyme; and Step 4 by HIOMT. (From Wurtman RJ, Axelrod J, Kelly D: The Pineal. New York, Academic Press, 1968, p 60.)

ABNORMALITIES OF THE PINEAL

The pineal gland has no known function in man but becomes of clinical significance because of the occurrence of calcification and of tumor formation. Calcific nodules termed *acervuli* form in a matrix of ground substance secreted by pinealocytes. This process begins in early childhood and becomes increasingly evident by roentgenography beginning in the second decade of life. Calcification has no known effect on pineal function.

Diseases of the pineal are rare. A few cases of hypoplasia and aplasia have been reported, and these have been associated in a relatively high proportion with genital precocity. Less than 1 per cent of intracranial neoplasms are tumors of the pineal gland, and they are seen almost exclusively in young males. The term *pinealoma* refers to a tumor of the pineal parenchymal cell, called pineoblastoma or pineocytoma according to its degree of differentiation. In one series of pineal tumor cases, only 9 of 53 fitted this category and there were 13 glial tumors, including astrocytomas and glioblastomas. The most common tumor (approximately 50 per cent) is best termed *germinoma* because it apparently arises from germ cells and not from pineal parenchymal cells. They are believed to be due to embryologic rests of germ cells. Identical tumors are found in the testis and anterior mediastinum. Approximately 10 per cent of intracranial germinomas metastasize to the spinal cord. Germinomas arising in the pineal gland may infiltrate the third ventricle and the floor of the hypothalamus, producing a characteristic triad: *diabetes insipidus, hypogonadism,* and *optic atrophy.* An identical clinical presentation can be due to germinomas arising from midline tissues at the base of the brain. X-ray of the skull rarely shows abnormality even when hypothalamic functions are grossly deranged. *Teratomas* may also arise in the pineal region, and rarely give rise to choriocarcinomas. Several cases of precocious puberty have been reported to be caused by gonadotropin-secreting choriocarcinomas of the pineal, an abnormality associated with detectable HCG in the spinal fluid.

Pineal tumors also cause sexual precocity by hypothalamic damage which destroys structures normally inhibitory to the development of puberty. Pinealomas cause precocious puberty almost exclusively in males. The most important local manifestations of pineal neoplasms are due to pressure on the quadrigeminal plate of the midbrain. An enlarging mass in the pineal region compresses the aqueduct of Sylvius and distorts the upper brainstem. Internal hydrocephalus gives rise to characteristic headache, vomiting, papilledema, and disturbed consciousness. Pressure on the superior colliculi causes paralysis of conjugate upward gaze (Parinaud's syndrome). The characteristic wide-based gait may be due to pressure on the cerebellum or brainstem.

Although a number of surgical cures have been reported, pineal tumors are rarely resectable by the time that clinical signs appear. Fortunately, the germinoma type is radiosensitive, and prolonged survival has been observed. Most workers recommend that craniotomy be carried out for diagnostic purposes, but that removal be attempted only if the lesion is favorably localized, or if it is a radioresistant lesion. Supervoltage roentgen therapy is usually given. There is little experience with chemotherapy of these tumors. In emergency situations presenting with hydrocephalus, it is usually necessary to decompress by shunting the third ventricle prior to definitive therapy.

Reichlin S: Neuroendocrinology. *In* Williams R (ed.): Textbook of Endocrinology. 6th ed. Philadelphia, W. B. Saunders. Company, 1981. *Comprehensive and systematic review of pineal function. Detailed account of clinical aspects, including diagnosis and management. Designed for medical students and fellows.*

Relkin R: The Pineal Gland. New York, Elsevier Biomedical, 1983. *A detailed basic and clinical text of greatest value because of its complete bibliography.*

Reppert SM, Klein DC (eds.): Mammalian pineal gland: Basic and clinical aspects. *In* Motta M (ed.): The Endocrine Functions of the Brain. New York, Raven Press, 1980, pp 327–371. *Detailed, authoritative review of chemistry and physiologic functions of the pineal gland.*

Schmidek HH: Pineal Tumors. New York, Masson U.S.A., 1977. *Includes excellent account of anatomy and physiology of the pineal, diseases, diagnosis, and treatment. The definitive monograph for the clinician responsible for patient care. Schmidek's views represent a comparatively conservative surgical approach.*

Wurtman RJ, Moskowitz MA: The pineal organ. N Engl J Med 296:1329, 1977. *Medical Progress review of the pineal brings the field up to date circa 1976.*

228. THE THYROID

P. Reed Larsen

Introduction

The thyroid gland secretes thyroxine, 3,5,3′,5′-tetraiodothyronine (abbreviated T_4) and small amounts of 3,5,3′-triiodothyronine (abbreviated T_3). The principal role of these substances is to regulate tissue metabolism. In infants, adequate supplies of thyroid hormone are necessary for the development of the normal central nervous system in the first one to two years of life. The absence of thyroid hormone during this period results in irreversible mental retardation, a syndrome known as *cretinism.* The hormone is also required for normal growth and bone maturation in children. Despite these important functions, the body can withstand marked reductions in thyroid hormone for long periods, although at the cost of abnormal operation of many organ systems.

EMBRYOLOGY AND ANATOMY

The thyroid develops from a combination of pharyngeal midline and bilateral primitive tissues from the fourth branchial pouch. These primitive thyroid cells migrate from the pharyngeal floor, leaving behind a residual thyroglossal duct which normally becomes obliterated. The major portion of the thyroid cell mass is derived from the median mid-pharyngeal tissue. The lateral thyroid anlagen migrate medially to fuse with median thyroid but primarily contribute the *parafollicular* or *C-cells.* The C-cells secrete thyrocalcitonin, not thyroid hormone, and do not play a role in thyroid physiology (see Ch. 228). The evolution of thyroid function occurs over the first 10 to 12 weeks of fetal life, with definite appearance of T_4 in the gland by 10 to 11 weeks. The placenta is impermeable to T_3 and T_4; the fetus depends on its own thyroid for its supply of these hormones. The adult size (15 to 20 grams) of the thyroid is reached at about age 15. The thyroid gland has the configuration of a butterfly, with the two lobes measuring about 5 × 2 cm. The lobes are composed of spherical structures called *follicles,* consisting of *colloid* surrounded by a single layer of epithelial cells enclosed by a basement membrane. Colloid consists predominantly of the protein *thyroglobulin,* which is the storage form of T_4 and T_3.

THYROID PHYSIOLOGY

The structures of the thyroid hormones and their precursors, mono-and diiodotyrosine (MIT and DIT), are shown in Figure 228–1. Iodine accounts for 65 per cent of the weight of T_4. Since this is a relatively scarce element in the earth's crust, mechanisms are present in the thyroid cell to allow it to concentrate and conserve iodine.

IODINE METABOLISM. The daily intake of iodine in man varies markedly in different areas of the world. It ranges from extremely low levels (20 μg or less per day) to as high as 600 or 700 μg per day in certain areas of the United States. The optimal iodine intake for adults is thought to be 150 to 300 μg per day. Levels appreciably below this lead to the condition known as *endemic goiter,* which is discussed later in this chapter. The high level of iodine intake in the United States is, in part, due to iodination of salt. Iodine in all forms is reduced to iodide

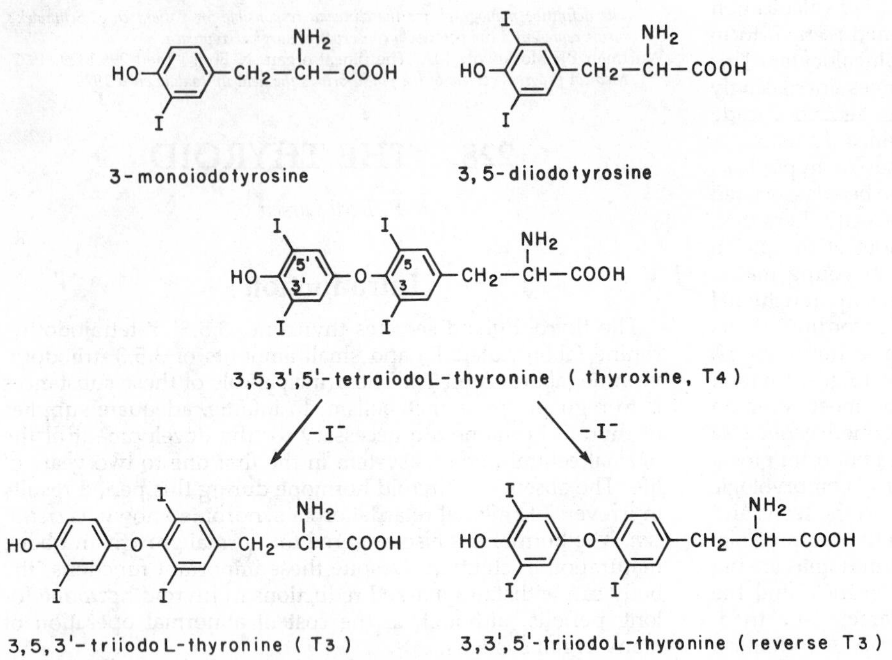

Figure 228–1. Structure of the thyroid hormones and their precursors.

(I^-) in the gastrointestinal tract and absorbed within 30 minutes of ingestion. I^- leaves the blood via two mechanisms. It is concentrated by the thyroid or excreted in the urine.

The plasma I^- concentration in man depends to a great extent on iodine intake but usually is 0.1 to 1 μg per deciliter. The thyroid clearance varies inversely with the plasma I^- and ranges from 10 to 30 ml per minute, while the urinary clearance is about 30 ml per minute. There is a wide variation in the fraction of I^- concentrated by the thyroid per 24 hours, again depending on iodine uptake. In the United States, iodine uptake by the thyroid varies from about 5 to 30 per cent.

INTRATHYROIDAL IODIDE METABOLISM. In Figure 228–2 are shown the steps involved in the synthesis of the thyroid hormones. Because the concentrations of I^- in the plasma are so low, the thyroid cell concentrates I^-, the cell:plasma ratio being about 20 to 40:1. The trapped I^- is rapidly oxidized and incorporated into protein. As a consequence, there is little I^- per se in the thyroid gland. The process of I^- oxidation and its incorporation into tyrosine is known as *organification*. The substrate for iodine is the 660,000 molecular weight glycoprotein thyroglobulin. Only about 25 per cent of the tyrosine residues of this specialized protein are available for iodination. Both mono- and diiodotyrosine are formed (MIT and DIT). In a typical molecule of fully iodinated human thyroglobulin, there are approximately 6 to 7 residues of MIT, 4 to 5 of DIT, 3 to 4 of T_4 and 0.2 to 0.3 of T_3. The T_4 and T_3 arise from the coupling of either 2 DIT residues or 1 MIT and 1 DIT residue, a reaction that requires thyroid peroxidase. This process is known as *coupling*. Both organification and coupling are inhibited by *thiourea compounds*, which are used in the treatment of patients with hyperthyroidism (see below). The thyroglobulin is iodinated at the apical border of the cell and is then exocytosed into the colloid. Under normal circumstances, T_4 and T_3 secretion occurs from this pool. The thyroid secretory process starts with phagocytosis of thyroglobulin by the apical cell membrane, leading to the formation of a *colloid droplet*. This is combined with a lysosome, and, as the colloid droplet traverses the thyroid cell, proteolysis occurs with eventual release of T_4 and T_3 at the basal cell border. Deiodination of T_4 to T_3 also occurs during this process, resulting in a ratio of T_4 to T_3 in thyroid secretion which is somewhat less than the 15:1 value found in the thyroglobulin itself. In order to conserve iodine for reuse in the thyroid cell, a *deiodinase* is present which removes the iodine from MIT and DIT, allowing it to recycle.

CIRCULATING T_4 AND T_3. Thyroid hormones in plasma exist in two forms, free and protein-bound. Although only about 0.02 per cent of total plasma T_4 and 0.3 per cent of plasma T_3 are free, it is the free hormone concentration which is maintained constant by the feedback regulatory system and which appears to parallel the rate of cellular uptake of these hormones. It is, therefore, the free hormone concentration which determines the thyroid status irrespective of the total plasma concentration. In the euthyroid person, the total hormone is determined by the quantity and affinity of certain thyroid hormone–binding proteins, which are *thyroxine-binding globulin* (TBG), *thyroxine-binding prealbumin* (TBPA), and albumin. TBG is by far the most important of these, transporting about 75 per cent of serum T_4 and T_3. It is a glycoprotein, with a

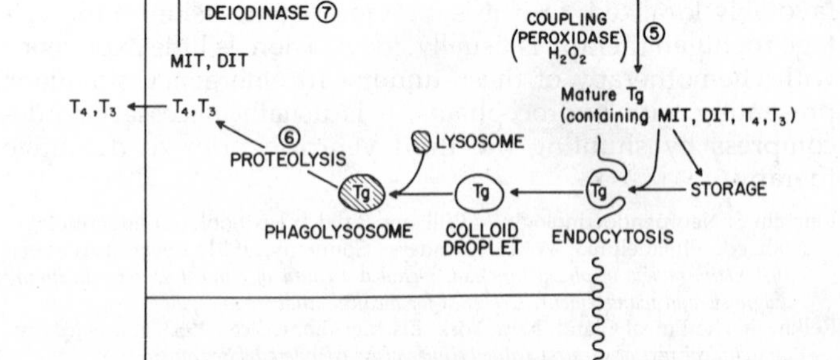

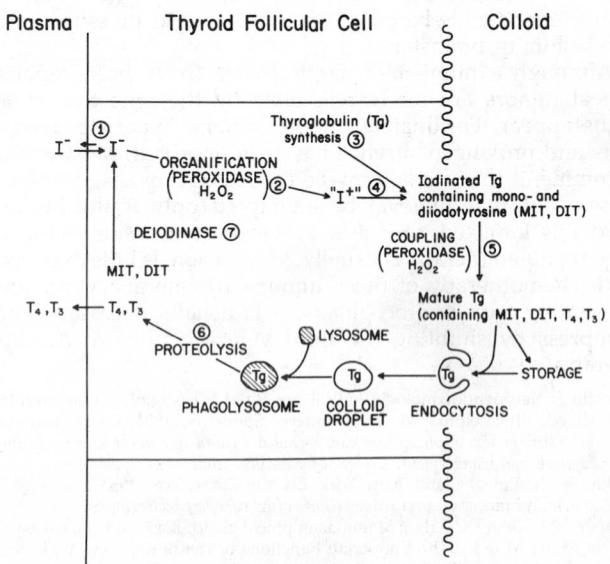

Figure 228–2. Principal steps in the synthesis and secretion of thyroid hormones. MIT = monoiodotyrosine; DIT = diiodotyrosine. The steps denoted by the numbers are those in which defects have been identified in patients with inherited abnormalities in thyroid hormone biosynthesis (see Sporadic and Endemic Goiter, below).

TABLE 228–1. CIRCUMSTANCES ASSOCIATED WITH CHANGES IN THE CIRCULATING CONCENTRATION OF THYROXINE-BINDING GLOBULIN (TBG)

Increased TBG
1. Pregnancy
2. Treatment with supraphysiologic amounts of estrogens, including oral contraceptives
3. In some patients with cirrhosis or acute hepatitis
4. As a congenital abnormality
5. In acute intermittent porphyria

Decreased TBG
1. Protein malnutrition
2. Nephrotic syndrome
3. Severe hepatic failure
4. After L-asparaginase
5. As a congenital abnormality (usually X-linked)
6. During treatment with androgenic steroids or pharmacologic doses of glucocorticoids.

molecular weight of 55,000, which is synthesized in the liver. TBG has a high affinity for both T_4 and T_3, although the affinity for T_4 is about 10- to 15-fold higher than that for T_3. There is normally sufficient TBG in serum to bind approximately 20 μg of T_4 per deciliter at a molar ratio of 1:1. The serum TBG concentrations change under many circumstances, which are listed in Table 228–1. It is important to recognize these conditions, since the resultant changes in total T_4 and T_3 may duplicate abnormalities which are found in patients with thyroid dysfunction. For example, during pregnancy, serum total T_4 and T_3 are increased but serum free T_4 and T_3 concentrations remain constant. The relationships are described in the following equation:

$$[TH] \text{ is proportional to } \frac{[TH\text{——}TBG]}{[TBG]}$$

where TH = free T_4 or T_3, [TH——TBG] = TBG-bound T_4 or T_3, and TBG = unoccupied TBG. When [TBG] increases, the bound hormone also increases until a new steady state is achieved at which [TH] is again normal. This occurs through both decreased metabolism and increased secretion of T_4 and T_3. To interpret a total serum T_4 or T_3 measurement accurately it is necessary to know the fraction of the hormone which is free; alternatively the free hormone can be measured directly or estimated (see Direct Tests of Thyroid Function later in this chapter). Certain compounds compete with T_4 and T_3 for binding to TBG. Two such drugs are salicylates and phenytoin. About a 20 to 30 per cent reduction in serum T_4 and T_3 is observed when 300 mg of phenytoin or salicylates in excess of 2.4 grams per day are given.

KINETICS OF T_4 AND T_3. Deiodination of the iodothyronines is the most significant metabolic transformation of the thyroid hormones. In the case of T_4, deiodination of the distal ring, occurring predominantly in liver and kidney, gives rise to T_3, which has approximately three to four times the metabolic potency of the parent hormone (Fig. 228–1). About 30 to 40 per cent of the 80 μg of T_4 produced per day is metabolized via this pathway (Table 228–2), giving rise to about 80 per cent of the T_3 produced daily. Loss of an iodine in the proximal ring of T_4 leads to formation of *reverse* T_3 (3,3′,5′-triiodothyronine), a compound which appears to have no metabolic effect. About 40 per cent of T_4 is metabolized via this pathway, the remainder being excreted via the biliary tract into the feces following conjugation with glucuronide. T_3 and reverse T_3 are, in turn, deiodinated in both proximal and distal rings, giving rise to the predicted mono- and diiodothyronines, none of which have physiologic effects. T_4 to T_3 conversion and reverse T_3 deiodination appear to be catalyzed by the same enzyme. If this reaction is inhibited, as it is under diverse circumstances, a reduction in serum T_3 and an increase in the serum reverse T_3 concentration occur.

TABLE 228–2. COMPARISON OF T_3 AND T_4 IN MAN

	T_3	T_4
Serum concentration		
Total (μg/dl)	0.14	8
Free (ng/dl)	0.4	1.6
Fraction of total serum hormone which is in the free form (%)	0.3	0.02
Distribution volume (liters)	35	10
Fraction intracellular (%)	64	10–20
Half-life (days)	1	7
Production rate (μg/day)	33	80
Fraction directly from thyroid (%)	20	100
Relative metabolic potency	1	0.3

The differences between T_3 and T_4 in terms of distribution volume, the intracellular fraction, and half-life can be attributed principally to the differences in the affinities of these two hormones for the plasma binding proteins (Table 228–2). The higher intracellular T_3 content explains in part its higher potency relative to T_4. Given the 3 to 4:1 ratio of metabolic potency of T_3 and T_4 and the fact that approximately one third of T_4 is converted to T_3, it appears that T_4 has little intrinsic metabolic activity in man.

REGULATION OF T_4 TO T_3 CONVERSION. The liver and kidney are the most active tissues in converting T_4 to T_3 based on in vitro studies. This enzyme, 5′-iodothyronine deiodinase, requires a sulfhydryl (SH)-containing cofactor which may be reduced glutathione. The T_3 produced by liver and kidney enters the T_3 pool. Thus, the liver and kidney are activators of T_4, producing T_3 for other tissues such as skeletal and heart muscle where this conversion occurs much more slowly. A number of factors influence the peripheral monodeiodination of T_4 to T_3 (Table 228–3). The first group includes pharmacologic agents which either are competitive inhibitors of the enzyme or interact with the SH-containing cofactor. Propylthiouracil appears to act via the latter mechanism, whereas the iodinated contrast agents used for oral cholecystography, iopanoic acid and sodium ipodate, act by the former. The latter drugs also inhibit T_4 uptake by the liver. In addition, there are significant reductions in T_4 to T_3 conversion during stress which occur because of decreased hepatic T_4 uptake, reduced SH-cofactor, and decreased enzyme content. T_4 to T_3 conversion in most tissues of the fetus is markedly reduced, probably owing to low endogenous concentrations of reduced glutathione. Many of these physiologic reductions in T_4 activation can be thought of as teleologically sound, conserving body resources in times of stress, but proof that this is so is lacking. However, reduction in the serum T_3 concentration relative to that of T_4 in all these circumstances is important when interpreting measurements of serum thyroid hormone concentrations in sick patients.

MECHANISM OF ACTION OF THYROID HORMONE. The mechanism by which thyroid hormone produces its protean effects remains obscure. In animal studies, thyroid hormone–responsive tissues contain nucleoproteins which have an extremely high affinity for thyroid hormones. These proteins, unlike those in the serum, have approximately ten-fold higher affinity for T_3 than T_4, further explaining why T_3 is the more potent hormone. Both in tissue culture and in animals, the occupancy

TABLE 228–3. PHYSIOLOGIC AND PHARMACOLOGIC INFLUENCES ON PERIPHERAL MONODEIODINATION OF T_4 TO T_3

Pharmacologic Inhibitors of T_4 to T_3 conversion
1. Propylthiouracil (not methimazole [Tapazole])
2. Iopanoic acid (Telepaque) and sodium ipodate (Oragrafin)
3. Amiodarone* (an antiarrhythmic agent)
4. Propranolol
5. Pharmacologic quantities of glucocorticoids

Physiologic situations in which T_4 to T_3 conversion is reduced
1. Fasting (particularly carbohydrate deprivation)
2. Severe acute or chronic illness of any sort or after surgery
3. In the presence of significant hepatic disease
4. In the human fetus

*Investigational drug.

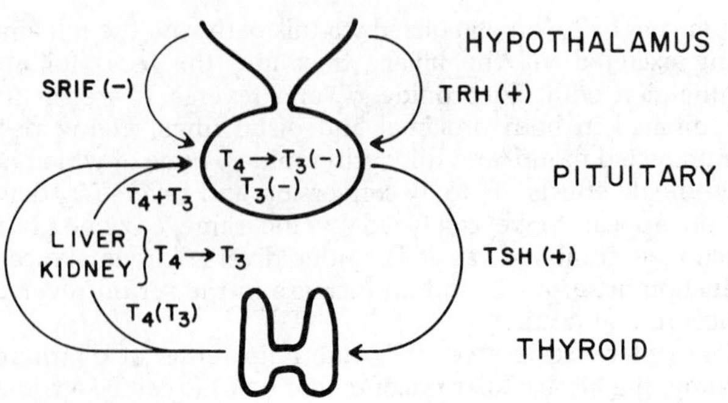

Figure 228–3. Current concepts of hypothalamic-pituitary-thyroid inter-relationships.

of these receptors by thyroid hormone can be related to changes in the rate of messenger RNA synthesis for various thyroid hormone–dependent proteins. At present, it would appear that these changes can explain virtually all the effects of thyroid hormone, although additional independent effects at the cell membrane or mitochondrion have not yet been completely excluded. The thyroid hormone nuclear receptor present in human tissues bears a close resemblance to that found in animals and appears to have the same physiologic relevance.

REGULATION OF THYROID FUNCTION. At least two tissues, anterior pituitary and cerebral cortex, are unique with respect to deiodination. In these two tissues, T_4 is monodeiodinated to T_3, but a substantial portion of the T_3 is then immediately bound to nuclear receptors without re-entering the plasma. Based on studies in the rat, at least 50 per cent of the intracellular T_3 in these two tissues originates from this source. When serum T_4 is reduced but T_3 remains constant, intracellular T_3 in these tissues will be reduced. Accordingly, the pituitary and, presumably, the cerebral cortex can recognize a decrease in serum T_4, per se, independent of changes in serum T_3.

The feedback loop for regulation of thyroid function is presented in Figure 228–3. *Thyrotropin-releasing hormone* (TRH) is secreted by hypothalamic cells and stimulates synthesis and release of thyrotropin (TSH). This hormone in turn stimulates all of the steps involved in thyroid hormone synthesis and release through activation of adenylate cyclase. T_4 and smaller amounts of T_3 are released from the gland with monodeiodination of T_4 to T_3 in liver and kidney. Both serum T_3 and T_4 (via its intrapituitary conversion to T_3) suppress the synthesis and release of TSH competing with TRH to complete the feedback loop. *Somatostatin* (SRIF) and possibly other substances such as neuropeptides and dopamine also inhibit TSH release (see Ch. 224). The role of thyroid hormones in feedback suppression at the level of the brain is poorly defined at present.

DeGroot LJ, Larsen PR, Refetoff S, Stanbury JB: The Thyroid and Its Diseases. 5th ed. New York, John Wiley & Sons, 1984. *An up-to-date revision of a classic text.*

Larsen, PR: Feedback regulation of thyrotropin secretion by hormones. N Engl J Med 306:23, 1982. *A more detailed, but clinically oriented, discussion of recent studies on the feedback regulation of TSH secretion by thyroid hormones.*

Larsen PR, Silva JE, Kaplan MM: Relationships between circulating and intracellular thyroid hormones: Physiological and clinical implications. Endocr Rev 2:87, 1981. *A recent review of the physiologic significance of intracellular T_4 to T_3 conversion and nuclear binding in various tissues.*

Oppenheimer JH: Samuels HH (eds.): Molecular basis of Thyroid Hormone Action. New York, Academic Press, 1983. *A thorough review of the evidence supporting the currently accepted mechanism for thyroid hormone action.*

Refetoff S: Thyroid hormone transport. *In* DeGroot LJ, et al. (eds.): Endocrinology, Vol I. New York, Grune & Stratton, 1979. *A comprehensive discussion of the serum thyroid hormone binding proteins.*

Werner SC, Ingbar SH: The Thyroid. 4th ed. Hagerstown, Harper & Row, 1978. *A basic text.*

Testing for Suspected Thyroid Dysfunction

The thyroid gland is unique among the endocrine organs in that symptoms may arise from two general types of problems. Hyperfunction of the thyroid (*hyperthyroidism* or *thyrotoxicosis*) or decreased secretion of thyroid hormone (*hypothyroidism* or *myxedema*) may cause the patient to seek medical help. Alternatively, physical enlargement of the thyroid *(goiter)* may cause respiratory embarassment or dysphagia or, more commonly, cosmetic abnormalities. The last-named condition may exist in the absence of any functional abnormality. Although the most severe forms are dramatic and unmistakable, milder degrees of thyroid dysfunction lead to many symptoms which are nonspecific, requiring biochemical tests for confirmation of the diagnosis.

PHYSICAL EXAMINATION OF THE THYROID

The high incidence of thyroid disease, particularly in the female (5 to 10 per cent), makes a careful examination of the thyroid gland an important part of the general physical examination. Thyroid enlargement may be the first clue to thyroid functional abnormalities in a patient with otherwise nonspecific symptoms. A cup of water is a necessity, and the patient should first be asked to swallow with the neck moderately extended while the anterior neck is inspected. Significant thyroid enlargement and thyroid nodules can often be discerned by this maneuver. The position of the trachea should then be determined, followed by palpation of the thyroid. Using the author's approach, the isthmus of the thyroid is first identified and is usually found just inferior to the cricoid cartilage. The left and right thumbs are then employed in turn to palpate the left and right lobe of the gland as the patient swallows. The normal thyroid gland is palpable in a large proportion of younger persons, although in the elderly patient it is not surprising to find the cricoid cartilage at or below the sternal notch. The pyramidal lobe, a small ridge of tissue extending vertically from the isthmus to the thyroid cartilage to the left or right of the midline, can often be palpated as well.

DIRECT TESTS OF THYROID FUNCTION

MEASUREMENT OF TOTAL SERUM THYROID HORMONE CONCENTRATIONS. Serum T_4 and T_3 are both readily quantitated by specific radioimmunoassays which require 200 μl or less of serum. Typical normal ranges for the total T_4 and T_3 concentrations are presented in Table 228–4, as well as the values in patients with alterations in TBG and in those with thyroid dysfunction.

SERUM FREE T_4 AND T_3 AND THE FREE T_4 INDEX. Since it is the concentration of free, rather than total, thyroid hormones which parallels the thyroid status, the ideal thyroid function test would be the direct determination of free thyroid hormones. The absolute serum free T_4 and T_3 can be measured either by immunoassay of a dialysate of human serum or by estimating the dialyzable (free) fraction of T_3 and T_4, multiplying this by the total hormone concentration (see Table 228–2). In patients who have abnormal total T_4 and T_3 concentrations caused by changes in serum TBG concentration but who are euthyroid, the free hormone concentrations are normal. Unfortunately, such determinations are time consuming and expensive, and an excellent indirect estimate of the free fraction of T_4 and T_3

TABLE 228–4. SERUM THYROID HORMONE CONCENTRATIONS IN NORMAL PERSONS AND PATIENTS WITH THYROID DISEASE

	Serum T_4 (μg/dl)		Serum T_3 (ng/dl)	
	Mean	*Range*	*Mean*	*Range*
Euthyroid				
Normal TBG	8	5–11	140	80–220
Increased TBG	12	8–20	190	120–320
Reduced TBG	2	<1–5	60	20–100
Infants				
Cord serum	11	8–15	48	20–80
Age six weeks	10	7–14	163	120–220
Hyperthyroidism	21	8–35	480	200–1600
Hypothyroidism	2	<1–5	50	<20–150

can be obtained from a T_3 (or T_4) *resin or charcoal uptake* test. In this test, tracer T_3 (or rarely T_4) is added to a diluted sample of unknown serum. After a brief incubation, resin or charcoal is added and the tubes centrifuged. The fraction of the tracer thyroid hormone bound to the resin or charcoal is then determined. In some tests this is expressed directly as a fraction of the total tracer added, e.g., a typical normal range is 25 to 35 per cent. In some methods anti-T_3 or T_4 antibody immobilized on a solid phase is used to bind the T_3, but the principle is identical. The result may also be normalized to those in standard samples with normal quantities of T_4 and TBG (normal range generally 0.85 to 1.15). The fraction of the tracer thyroid hormone bound to the resin or charcoal is directly proportional to the free fraction of the thyroid hormones. Since T_3 is usually bound to the same proteins as is T_4, the free fraction of T_4 can also be predicted from a test in which T_3 is used as the tracer. The similarity between the free fraction of thyroid hormones and the resin or charcoal uptake can be formalized by calculating the *free T_4 (or T_3)* index. This is the product of the normalized value for the T_3 uptake and the total serum T_4 (or T_3) concentration. The normal range for these indices in units is approximately the same as the total thyroid hormone concentrations. In the author's laboratory, the normal free T_4 index is 4.7 to 10.5. The free T_4 index is an excellent approximation of the free T_4. An alternative estimate of the free T_4 may be obtained by using one of several commercial kits. In one such method, a labeled analogue of T_4 is employed to compete with the endogenous free T_4 for binding to an antibody. The higher the concentration of free T_4, the lower is the analogue binding, and vice versa. While there are some technical advantages to these tests, they do not measure the free T_4 directly, but provide only an estimate of its concentration, as does the free T_4 index. One notable clinical situation in which both methods provide falsely high estimates of the free T_4 is in the hereditary syndrome *euthyroid dysalbuminemic hyperthyroxinemia*. In patients with this syndrome large quantities are synthesized of an albumin that binds T_4, but not T_3, with abnormally high affinity. The total T_4 value is elevated, but the free fraction of T_4 by dialysis is reduced; therefore the endogenous free T_4 concentration is normal. Neither the T_3 resin uptake nor the analogue methods reflect the reduced free T_4 fraction, since, on the one hand, T_3 does not bind to the abnormal albumin with increased avidity and, on the other, the abnormal albumin apparently competes with the antibody for the T_4 analogue. Thus, a high concentration of free T_4 is estimated and a mistaken diagnosis of hyperthyroidism is made. A T_4 uptake test would give a proper result in this syndrome. It should be noted that a "T_3 uptake test" or "T_3 resin" is *not* a measure of the serum T_3 concentration.

COMPARISON OF THE UTILITY OF T_4 AND T_3 DETERMINATIONS. The free T_4 index is the best screening test for thyroid dysfunction. It is superior to the free T_3 index by virtue of the fact that the principal thyroid secretory product is T_4. About 80 per cent of circulating T_3 derives from T_4 to T_3 conversion. Therefore, in patients who are sick or who have received any of the drugs listed in Table 228–3, the serum T_3 will invariably be reduced relative to the serum T_4, but this does not imply thyroid disease. In hypothyroidism, serum T_3 may be normal despite significant impairment of thyroid function. On the other hand, in hyperthyroidism there is a small fraction of patients in whom serum T_4 is not elevated but the concentration of serum T_3 is. This condition is called *T_3 thyrotoxicosis* (below).

SERUM REVERSE T_3 AND OTHER IODOTHYRONINES. The normal concentration of reverse T_3 is 15 to 50 ng per deciliter. It derives virtually exclusively from peripheral metabolism of T_4, and its concentration in the blood reflects a combination of that process and the rate of reverse T_3 degradation. It is not generally useful clinically, although it is an excellent barometer of the rate of T_4 to T_3 conversion. Immunoassays have been developed for both mono- and diiodinated thyronines, but these measurements do not have clinical applicability at present.

SERUM THYROID HORMONE–BINDING PROTEIN CONCENTRATIONS. The normal concentration of circulating TBG and TBPA can be measured by immunoassay or by determination of the binding capacity. The normal concentration of TBG is 1.5 mg per deciliter. This quantity of protein will bind approximately 20 μg of T_4 (1 mole T_4 per 1 mole TBG). The binding capacity of TBPA is approximately 250 μg T_4 per deciliter. These measurements are rarely necessary for clinical purposes. Virtually all of the necessary information regarding binding can be obtained from a T_3 uptake test.

RADIOACTIVE IODINE UPTAKE (RAI UPTAKE). The normal 24-hour thyroidal uptake of radioiodine ranges from 5 to 30 per cent. All the radioiodine in the thyroid at this time is in the organified form. Because of the broad normal range for this test, it is not a valid method for determining thyroid status. Its major diagnostic use is in separating patients who have hyperthyroidism caused by subacute thyroiditis from those with Graves' disease (see next section). It is contraindicated in pregnancy.

TESTS OF THYROID REGULATION

SERUM THYROTROPIN (TSH). The normal range for serum TSH by radioimmunoassay is from 1.5 to 3.5 μU per milliliter. However, for many clinical assays a normal range of up to 5 or even 10 μU per milliliter is accepted owing to the technical difficulties in attaining precise measurements. Virtually all patients with clinical symptoms attributible to primary hypothyroidism will have serum TSH concentrations >20 μU per milliliter, and many subjects with minimal symptoms or goiter alone will have results between 10 and 20 μU per milliliter. An elevation of the serum TSH concentration almost always indicates that thyroid function is impaired. It is also the critical test for separating patients with primary thyroid disease from those with hypothyroidism resulting from hypothalamic or pituitary dysfunction.

THYROTROPIN-RELEASING HORMONE (TRH) INFUSION TEST. TRH can be infused intravenously to determine the pituitary TSH reserve. This is reduced in patients with hyperthyroidism and in those with autonomous thyroid hormone production or with hypothalamic or pituitary disease. Typical normal and pathologic responses are shown in Figure 228–4. In practice, a basal serum sample is obtained, followed by intravenous infusion of 400 μg of TRH over 1 minute. A second serum sample is obtained 30 minutes after the infusion, and both are assayed for TSH. In normals, the minimal TSH increment is 2 μU per milliliter except in males over the age of 40, in the seriously ill or in patients with depression or exogenous or endogenous glucocorticoid excess in whom the normal response can be lower. The response is amplified (30-minute value >25 μU per milliliter) in patients with primary hypothyroidism. A significant increment in TSH eliminates the diagnosis of hyperthyroidism except in the extremely rare patient with the TSH-induced form of this disease.

T_3 SUPPRESSION TEST. Prior to the availability of TRH, the "T_3 suppression test" was used to determine if thyroid function was autonomous. A 24-hour RAI uptake is determined before and after the patient receives 75 to 100 μg of triiodothyronine (Cytomel) per day for one week. In normal patients, a reduction in the RAI uptake to less than 50 per cent of the original value occurs owing to suppression of endogenous TSH. In patients with hyperthyroidism or autonomous thyroid function, negligible suppression of radioactive uptake is seen. A second RAI uptake can also be determined one week after a single thyroxine dose of 3 mg. This has been reported to cause fewer symptoms and result in smaller elevations of serum T_3 in patients who have autonomous thyroid function. Neither test should be used in patients with complicating illnesses (especially of the cardiovascular system), and both have generally been superseded by the TRH test. Suppression tests can also be used in conjunction with a thyroid scan to document autonomy in thyroid nodules (see below).

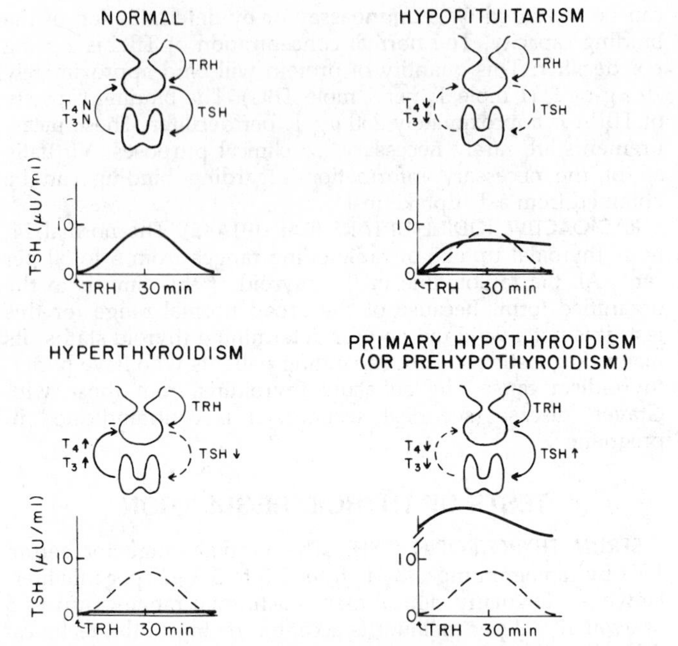

Figure 228–4. Typical responses to the infusion of TRH in patients with hyperthyroidism and primary and secondary hypothyroidism. In patients with hypopituitarism or hypothalamic disease virtually any TRH response pattern can be seen. The most pertinent diagnostic information is that serum TSH is not increased in a patient with a reduced serum free T_4 index.

METABOLIC INDICES OF THYROID STATUS

BASAL METABOLIC RATE (BMR). Since thyroid hormone is an important factor in the regulation of the rate of oxygen consumption, this test should theoretically be useful in evaluating thyroid status. However, it has given way to serum measurements, since these are more specific and usually more accurate. The normal range for the BMR is usually from −15 to +5 per cent.

DEEP TENDON REFLEX CONTRACTION AND RELAXATION TIMES. Thyroid status is reflected in the rate (not amplitude) of contraction and relaxation of skeletal muscle. These rates are more rapid in hyperthyroidism and slowed in hypothyroidism. Some clinicians have employed a kinemometer tracing to quantitate these events and have observed as high as 70 per cent diagnostic accuracy with this test. Like the BMR, it is less specific than serum hormone measurements, since hypothermia, peripheral neuropathy, gross edema, and many other conditions may slow the rate of relaxation. However, a clinically apparent delay in the relaxation phase of the deep tendon reflexes is almost invariably present in patients with significant hypothyroidism, although the more rapid relaxation in hyperthyroidism is difficult to appreciate visually.

ANATOMIC EVALUATION OF THE THYROID GLAND

THE THYROID SCAN. The capacity of the thyroid gland to trap ions such as I^- or molecules with a similar charge and configuration has provided a useful method for correlating structure and function. Of the iodine isotopes either ^{123}I or ^{131}I can be used. ^{123}I, although more expensive, is to be preferred for scanning, particularly in younger persons, since the radiation dose to the thyroid is 7.5 mrads per microcurie administered, as opposed to 800 mrads per microcurie for ^{131}I. Another isotope which gives a low radiation dose is $^{99}mTcO_4^-$ (pertechnetate), which is trapped, but not organified, by the thyroid. Because of this, a scan is performed 30 minutes after intravenous injection of this isotope. The thyroid scan is usually used to determine the functional state of a palpable thyroid nodule (see later in chapter) or in evaluating masses in the neck or upper chest to see if thyroid tissue is present.

THYROID ULTRASOUND. A determination of whether a given thyroid mass is solid or cystic can be made by ultrasonography.

NEEDLE BIOPSY OR ASPIRATION. Either a fine (21 to 26 gauge) or cutting needle (Vim-Silverman) can be used to obtain a sample of thyroid tissue for histologic examination. These techniques have received increased attention in recent years as a method for evaluation of thyroid nodules. Accurate interpretation of a fine needle aspirate requires an experienced cytologist, which has limited the experience with this simple technique to date.

OTHER TESTS SPECIFICALLY RELATED TO THYROID FUNCTION OR DISEASE

ANTITHYROID ANTIBODIES. In autoimmune thyroid disease (Hashimoto's thyroiditis or Graves' disease), antibodies which bind to various antigens of thyroid tissue are present in the serum. The most important of these is the *thyroid antimicrosomal antibody.* This antibody is found in approximately 95 per cent of patients with Hashimoto's thyroiditis and in only about 10 per cent of adults with no apparent thyroid disease. The test is generally performed by a tanned red cell hemagglutination technique, and the results are reported as the highest titer causing agglutination. Titers in excess of 1:100 are significant. About 55 per cent of patients with Graves' disease also have circulating antibodies to thyroid microsomes. *Antithyroglobulin antibodies* are also present in the serum of about 60 per cent of patients with Hashimoto's disease. Antibodies directed against the thyroid TSH receptor, present in the sera of patients with Graves' disease, can be measured either by incubation of IgG with fresh thyroid slices, quantitating the increase in cyclic AMP, or with thyroid membranes and tracer TSH in a competition technique. The result of the former method is denoted the *thyroid stimulating immunoglobulin* (TSI), and it is somewhat more specific than is the latter, called the *thyrotropin displacing activity* (TDA) (see Graves' Disease and Other Causes of Hyperthyroidism).

SERUM THYROGLOBULIN. The normal serum thyroglobulin (Tg) concentration is 2 to 20 ng per milliliter. Serum Tg may be elevated in any patient with an enlarged thyroid or following acute trauma to the thyroid whether this be a consequence of inflammation, surgery, or radiation. Thyroglobulin determinations are most useful in the follow-up of patients with metastatic thyroid carcinoma following thyroidectomy. An increase in serum Tg indicates the presence of tumor tissue, although a normal value does not eliminate this possibility.

THE EFFECTS OF NONTHYROIDAL ILLNESS ON THYROID FUNCTION TESTS

Patients with nonthyroidal illnesses can have abnormalities in serum T_4 and T_3 concentrations that may suggest underlying thyroid dysfunction. All patients will have impaired T_4 to T_3 conversion and, accordingly, have low or subnormal serum T_3 and raised serum reverse-T_3 concentrations. Most will also have slight reduction in total serum T_4 concentrations. A portion of this decrease is a result of a reduced serum TBG, especially if severe liver disease or proteinuria is present. However, about 10 per cent of patients with typical medical illnesses will have a subnormal free T_4 index. This may be due to the release of a substance that inhibits the binding of T_4 to TBG. The fracture of free T_4, as measured by equilibrium dialysis, is usually increased in such patients. Thus, the free T_4 is normal, indicating that hypothyroidism is not present. Occasionally a patient may have severe illness and an elevated level of serum T_4. Such patients should be suscepted of having underlying autonomous thyroid function and often must be treated for hyperthyroidism. This phenomenon may also occur in patients with *acute psychiatric illness* and *hyperemesis gravidarum.* Strategies for dealing with these potentially confusing situations are presented later in the chapter.

Buergi H, Wimpfheimer C, Burger A, Zaumbauer W, Rosler H, Lemarchand-Beraud T: Changes of circulating thyroxine, triiodothyronine and reverse triiodothyronine after radiographic contrast agents. J Clin Endocrinol Metab 43:1203, 1976. *The changes which occur in serum thyroid hormones and TSH following oral cholecystographic agents provide an excellent model for the effects of inhibition of T_4 to T_3 conversion on thyroid function.*

Chopra IJ, Hershman JM, Pardridge WM, Nicoloff JT: Thyroid function in nonthyroidal illnesses. Ann Intern Med 98:946–957, 1983. *A review of many of the effects of systemic illness on thyroid function.*

Docter R, Bos G, Krenning, EP, Fekkes D, Visser TJ, Hennemann G: Inherited thyroxine excess: A serum abnormality due to an increased affinity for modified albumin. Clin Endocrinol 15:363–371, 1981. *An explanation of the thyroid hormone–binding abnormalities in families with euthyroid dysalbuminemic hyperthyroxinemia.*

Kaplan MM, Larsen PR, Crantz FR, Dzau VJ, Rossing TH, Haddow JE: Prevalence of abnormal thyroid function test results in patients with acute medical illnesses. Am J Med 72:9–16, 1982. *This is a prospective study of thyroid function test abnormalities in unselected patients with acute medical illnesses.*

Schimmel M, Utiger RD: Thyroidal and peripheral production of thyroid hormones: Review of recent findings and their clinical implications. Ann Intern Med 87:760, 1977. *A discussion of the relationships between serum T_4, T_3, and reverse T_3 in the clinical setting.*

Graves' Disease and Other Causes of Hyperthyroidism

DEFINITION. The clinical syndrome of hyperthyroidism is one of the most dramatic in clinical medicine. The major symptoms associated with this syndrome are predominantly a reflection of the hypermetabolism resulting from excessive quantities of circulating thyroid hormone. The many disorders that can be associated with this syndrome are listed in Table 228–5 in their approximate order of frequency. Graves' disease accounts for over 85 per cent of such patients. Toxic nodular goiters, both multinodular *(Plummer's disease)* and uninodular, and subacute thyroiditis account for the bulk of the remainder.

GRAVES' DISEASE

In 1835, Robert Graves described a clinical syndrome including hypermetabolism, diffuse enlargement of the thyroid gland, and *exophthalmos* (forward displacement of the eyes). In continental Europe, the same condition is known as Basedow's disease after von Basedow's description in 1840. In addition to thyroid involvement and ophthalmopathy, patients may have a dermatologic condition, *pretibial myxedema.* As presently defined, patients with Graves' disease may have only one of these three major clinical manifestations, and the only common denominator is likely to be the presence of thyroid-stimulating antibodies in the serum.

ETIOLOGY AND PATHOGENESIS. The precise etiology of Graves' disease is still not known, but it seems likely that it is an autoimmune disorder. Hyperthyroidism is its principal manifestation, yet TSH is suppressed and no intrinsic regulatory abnormalities in the thyroid have been identified. Thus the thyroid stimulation seems likely to be a consequence of a circulating, non-TSH, thyroid stimulator. In 1956, Adams and Purves identified a substance in the serum of many patients with Graves' disease which caused thyroid stimulation in a mouse bioassay. Because the thyroid stimulation from this substance lasted longer than did TSH-induced stimulation, it was called *long-acting thyroid stimulator (LATS).* LATS is now known to be a 7-S gamma globulin. The LATS hypothesis was initially received with enthusiasm, but soon lost popularity as patients were found with hyperthyroidism who did not have detectable LATS. In addition, some LATS-positive patients were not hyperthyroid. Many of the latter cases may be explained by the coexistence of thyroid destruction caused by a chronic thyroiditis (Hashimoto's disease; see Thyroiditis). Recent studies have provided a more inclusive hypothesis. Serum LATS activity is decreased on exposure to thyroid tissue, suggesting that the antibody binds to a thyroid antigen. In sera from certain hyperthyroid patients who were LATS negative, a gamma globulin was found that neutralized the capacity of thyroid tissue to bind the LATS in positive sera. This antibody, called *LATS protector,* stimulated human thyroid tissue in vivo or thyroid tissue from chicks even though it did not stimulate the mouse thyroid. This observation suggested that one of the limitations in previous studies was a restriction of the bioassay to the mouse, which could well have different, albeit overlapping, antigenic sites from human thyroid tissue. In subsequent studies it has been found that LATS, LATS protector, and similar proteins present in Graves' disease patients' sera interfere with the binding of TSH to the human thyroid cell membrane, suggesting that these proteins are antibodies to the TSH receptor. These substances activate adenylate cyclase in human thyroid cell membranes, providing a plausible mechanism for thyroid stimulation in this condition. Several assays are now available to quantitate what are termed *thyroid-stimulating immunoglobulins* (TSI) or *thyrotropin-displacing activity* (TDA) (see Testing for Suspected Thyroid Function). TSI or TDA is found in 85 to 90 per cent of patients with Graves' disease. The negative sera may be explained by residual difficulties in the assay technique. The stimulus for the antibody production in these subjects remains obscure.

The etiology of Graves' exophthalmopathy is not known. Patients with exophthalmos and particularly those with dermopathy almost invariably have high titers of circulating TSI, suggesting that these two clinical manifestations represent the most severe form of this disease. Antibodies to soluble human eye muscle antigens were found in 17 of 23 patients with Graves' ophthalmopathy, but not in Graves' patients without this manifestation and rarely in those with Hashimoto's thyroiditis. This suggests a similar autoimmune etiology for ophthalmopathy and for hyperthyroidism. It has also been proposed that Tg–anti-Tg circulating immune complexes may bind to eye muscles and play a pathogenic role. Further studies will be required to resolve this question.

Emotional Factors in the Etiology of Hyperthyroidism. The emotional lability of the patient with hyperthyroidism has led many clinicians to question the role of psychologic trauma in the pathogenesis of this disease. Numerous anecdotes have been cited to suggest that emotional trauma may somehow trigger the onset of overt hyperthyroidism. If this is so, it would still appear to require participation of the immune system, since circulating TSI is such a constant feature of the clinical picture. In the author's mind, it seems more likely that an episode of physical or emotional trauma brings the patient to medical attention, at which time preexisting hyperthyroidism is recognized.

INCIDENCE. Graves' disease is common, affecting as many as 1.9 per cent of the female population and about a tenth that number of males, according to a population survey in northern England. It reaches its peak incidence in the third and fourth decades. The reason for the female predominance in this as in all thyroid diseases is not known. There is a strong familial component to Graves' disease with a family history of autoimmune thyroid disease (Graves' disease, Hashimoto's thyroiditis, or "goiter") in a significant fraction of patients. The importance of genetic inheritance in the predisposition to this syndrome has been confirmed by finding a higher relative risk of this

TABLE 228–5. DISEASES OR CLINICAL SYNDROMES ASSOCIATED WITH THYROTOXICOSIS

Graves' disease
Toxic multinodular goiter
Toxic adenoma
Iodide-induced hyperthyroidism
Subacute thyroiditis
Factitious (exogenous) thyrotoxicosis
Neonatal thyrotoxicosis (mother with Graves' disease)
TSH-secreting pituitary tumor
Nontumorigenic pituitary-induced hyperthyroidism
Choriocarcinoma (uterine or testicular origin) or hydatidiform mole
Struma ovarii
Hyperfunctioning thyroid carcinoma (usually metastatic)

TABLE 228–6. COMMON SYMPTOMS AND SIGNS OF HYPERTHYROIDISM (THYROTOXICOSIS)

Symptoms	Signs
Nervousness and/or tremor	Tachycardia or atrial fibrillation
Weight loss (usually with increased appetite)	Widened pulse pressure with increased systolic and decreased diastolic pressures
Palpitations	Hyperdynamic precordium and accentuated S1
Heat intolerance and excessive perspiration	Warm, smooth skin
Emotional lability	Tremor
Muscle weakness	Proximal muscle weakness
Hyperdefecation	Thyroid enlargement or abnormality

condition in patients with the histocompatibility antigens HLA-B8 and in Caucasians with HLA-DR3 and in Japanese and Chinese populations with HLA-B35 and HLA-Bw46, respectively.

PATHOLOGY. The thyroid of the patient with Graves' disease is diffusely enlarged and hypercellular. In patients undergoing thyroidectomy without prior treatment with antithyroid drugs or iodine, a diffusely hyperplastic epithelium is noted with little or no colloid present and often with lymphocytic infiltration, varying from minimal to extensive. In some specimens it is impossible to distinguish the microscopic picture from Hashimoto's thyroiditis (a condition sometimes called hashitoxicosis). If the patient receives iodide preoperatively, the gland contains large amounts of colloid, cells are of normal height, and the vascularity is markedly reduced. Other tissues show no specific changes except in severely hyperthyroid patients. In those situations there may be edema and focal necrosis in the liver with cellular infiltration.

In hyperthyroid patients with mild eye manifestations of Graves' disease such as lid retraction and stare, no significant orbital pathology is found, and these changes probably are due to the hyperthyroidism per se. In more severe cases, edema of the extraocular muscles occurs in association with infiltration with lymphocytes, plasma cells, and neutrophils. In addition, hydrophilic mucopolysaccharide collects in the orbital tissues. The conjuctivae may show perivascular lymphocytic infiltration and edema *(chemosis).* The end-stage of these processes is fibrosis, which most often involves the inferior eye muscles, causing restriction of upward globe movement.

CLINICAL PICTURE. The common clinical symptoms of thyrotoxicosis are listed in Table 228–6. These occur in any patient with excessive thyroid hormone secretion whether this be due to Graves' disease or some other cause. They are a consequence of the stimulatory effect of thyroid hormone on the metabolic rate and on many other tissues, especially the heart and central nervous system. The typical patient with Graves' disease is in her mid-20's with symptoms that can often be dated to six to twelve months previously. The patient is nervous, anxious, and fidgeting, and speaks rapidly. She will complain of her agitated fatigue, palpitations, and, in warmer climates, heat intolerance. There may be weight loss despite increased appetite, or the patient may merely report success in her efforts at weight control. An increased frequency of bowel movements and, rarely, diarrhea, may be noted. Emotional lability is often apparent during the interview, and a history of deteriorating domestic or occupational relationships may be obtained. A history of neck swelling (often not noted first by the patient) may be present. Amenorrhea or oligomenorrhea is not uncommon. Rarer manifestations of hyperthyroidism include pruritus and urticaria. About 5 per cent of males may experience gynecomastia, and even less commonly *hypokalemic periodic paralysis* may occur. For unknown reasons, this condition is much more common in males of Oriental extraction.

Apathetic or Masked Hyperthyroidism. The symptoms given in Table 228–6 are those generally found in the younger patient. The clinician should be aware that in some patients, particularly the elderly, the clinical symptoms and signs of hypermetabolism may not be so dramatic. Rather than appearing agitated, the elderly patient with hyperthyroidism may be depressed. Weight loss and symptoms of congestive heart failure can be the predominant manifestations of the hypermetabolic syndrome. Often this is complicated by atrial fibrillation or other supraventricular tachyarrhythmia, leading to suspicion that the heart, rather than the thyroid, is the source of the problem. Because of the subtlety of this clinical form of hyperthyroidism it is recommended that any patient with the recent onset of atrial fibrillation have tests of thyroid function. In this way a reversible cause of congestive heart failure and/or recurrent arrhythmias may be recognized and appropriate treatment instituted.

Graves' Ophthalmopathy. Eye symptoms are present in more than 50 per cent of patients with Graves' disease but, except for modest lid lag and stare, are rare in patients with other causes of hyperthyroidism. This is a useful point in establishing the diagnosis. Common complaints are protruding eyes, easy tearing, especially on exposure to wind or cold, photophobia, a gritty foreign body sensation in the eyes, and, less commonly, diplopia. (Fig. 228–5). The patient with significant *proptosis* (exophthalmos) may complain of irritation, particularly on arising, since the eyelids do not completely cover the sclera when the patient is sleeping *(lagophthalmos).* Rarely, severe chemosis, inflammation, and periorbital edema occur (malignant exophthalmos). Eye complaints are usually bilateral but may be unilateral, and Graves' disease is one of the most common causes of unilateral exophthalmos.

Pretibial Myxedema. In a few patients with Graves' disease (1 to 2 per cent) a brawny, nonpitting swelling of the pretibial area, ankles, and/or feet is present. This can appear in plaques. It has an orange-skin appearance and is usually not tender. This dermopathy, found exclusively in Graves' disease, is termed *pretibial myxedema.* The name derives from the histologic similarity of the mucopolysaccharide infiltration of the subcutaneous tissues to that found in advanced hypothyroidism (myxedema).

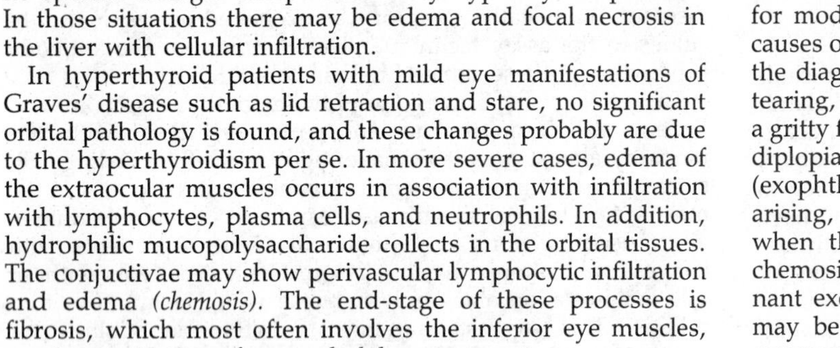

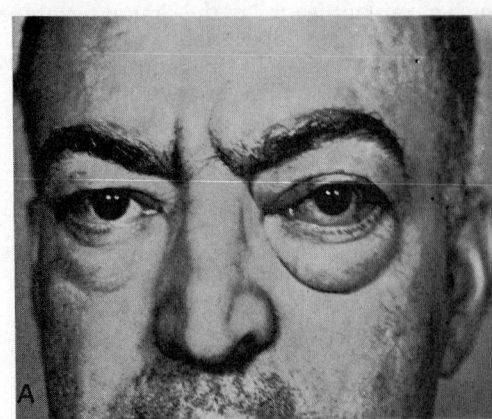

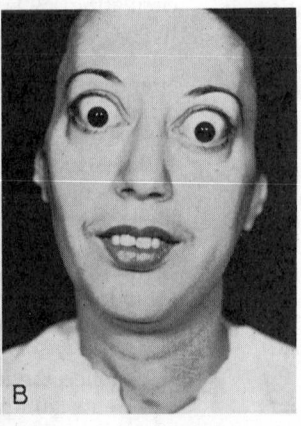

Figure 228–5. Two patients showing the typical ophthalmopathy characteristic of Graves' disease. Patient A demonstrates marked periorbital swelling, exophthalmos, chemosis, and conjunctival injection. The proptosis, limitation of extraocular movements, and other manifestations of ophthalmopathy are much more severe in Patient A than in Patient B. Patient B has marked widening of the palpebral fissures owing to lid retraction and also has significant proptosis. Patient A is euthyroid; Patient B is mildly hyperthyroid. (From Williams RH (ed.): Textbook of Endocrinology. 6th ed. Philadelphia, W. B. Saunders Company, 1981, p 189.)

Euthyroid Graves' Disease. In a small fraction of patients with Graves' disease, eye manifestations (unilateral or bilateral) with or without pretibial myxedema appear but hyperthyroidism is not present. This can arise because of destruction of the thyroid as a result of coexistent Hashimoto's disease or hyperthyroidism may be delayed in its appearance for months or years after the first eye symptoms. In many such patients, appropriate testing will often reveal subtle evidence of thyroid dysfunction.

PHYSICAL SIGNS. In younger patients, tachycardia is almost universal. The systolic blood pressure is elevated primarily because of the increased inotropic effect of thyroid hormone on the heart. The diastolic pressure is reduced owing to a decrease in peripheral vascular resistance associated with increased skin capillary blood flow. Body temperature is usually normal. The skin is smooth, warm, and moist, and the patient may radiate heat. A fine tremor of the outstretched hands and occasionally *onycholysis* of the fourth and fifth fingers or clubbing *(thyroid acropachy)* are observed. The thyroid is almost always diffusely enlarged from 1.5 to 5 to 6 times normal. One third of elderly patients will not have a detectable goiter. The gland may be soft or firm, depending on the degree of hyperthyroidism and the level of iodine intake. Auscultation of the neck may reveal a multitude of sounds. In the younger patient a *venous hum* may be heard over the external jugular vein, particularly with the patient in the sitting position. Third or fourth heart sounds are heard easily in the neck, and a carotid bruit is not uncommon. In addition, a bruit over the thyroid gland is present in some patients, a manifestation of the high blood flow to this organ. A diffuse lymphadenopathy may be present in hyperthyroidism, and splenomegaly is found in 10 per cent of patients. The liver is not enlarged except in elderly patients with congestive failure. The neurologic examination shows tremor and proximal muscle weakness. Eye signs include lid lag, a failure of the upper lid to cover the upper margin of the iris as the globe traverses from upward to downward gaze, a widened palpebral fissure so that the sclera is visible above and/or below the iris, conjunctival injection and chemosis, periorbital swelling, and proptosis. The last-named finding is determined by measuring the distance from the lateral portion of the bony orbit to the cornea, using the *exophthalmometer*. In whites this distance is 17 mm or less, with an upper limit of normal of 20 mm (22 mm for blacks). The difference between the two eye measurements should not be more than 3 mm. In addition to these moderate abnormalities, there may be impairment of globe movement. The most common restriction is in upward and/or outward gaze. This is due not to weakness of the superior eye muscles but to swelling and fibrosis of the inferior rectus and inferior oblique muscles beneath the globe. In addition, abduction and convergence may also be affected. Eye signs may be absent or mild, are usually bilateral when present, but may be asymmetric.

LABORATORY DIAGNOSIS OF HYPERTHYROIDISM. The various steps to be followed in establishing the laboratory diagnosis of hyperthyroidism are outlined in Figure 228–6. The initial screening test is to determine the free T_4 index. In virtually all patients an elevation in the free T_4 index is present. In the hospitalized patient the diagnosis may be somewhat more complicated if the patient is severely ill or has received any of the agents, listed in Table 228–3, which cause inhibition of T_4 to T_3 conversion. In these patients an impairment of T_4 clearance or inhibition of T_4 to T_3 conversion may lead to an elevation in the serum free T_4 index without hyperthyroidism. Other causes of an elevated free T_4 index, not necessarily indicating hyperthyroidism, are *euthyroid dysalbuminemic hyperthyroxinemia* (see Testing for Suspected Thyroid Dysfunction), hyperemesis gravidarium and acute psychosis. In the last two conditions, the increase in the free T_4 index is usually transient.

In such patients and in patients in whom the clinical suspicion of hyperthyroidism is present but the free T_4 index is normal or equivocal, a serum T_3 determination should be performed. The ratio of T_3 to T_4 is increased in the thyroid gland in patients with Graves' disease. As a consequence, the T_3 production rate and the fraction of T_3 coming directly from the thyroid are increased. Thus, the serum T_3 is elevated to a greater extent than is the serum T_4 (see Table 228–4). Patients in whom serum T_3 is elevated but the serum free T_4 index is

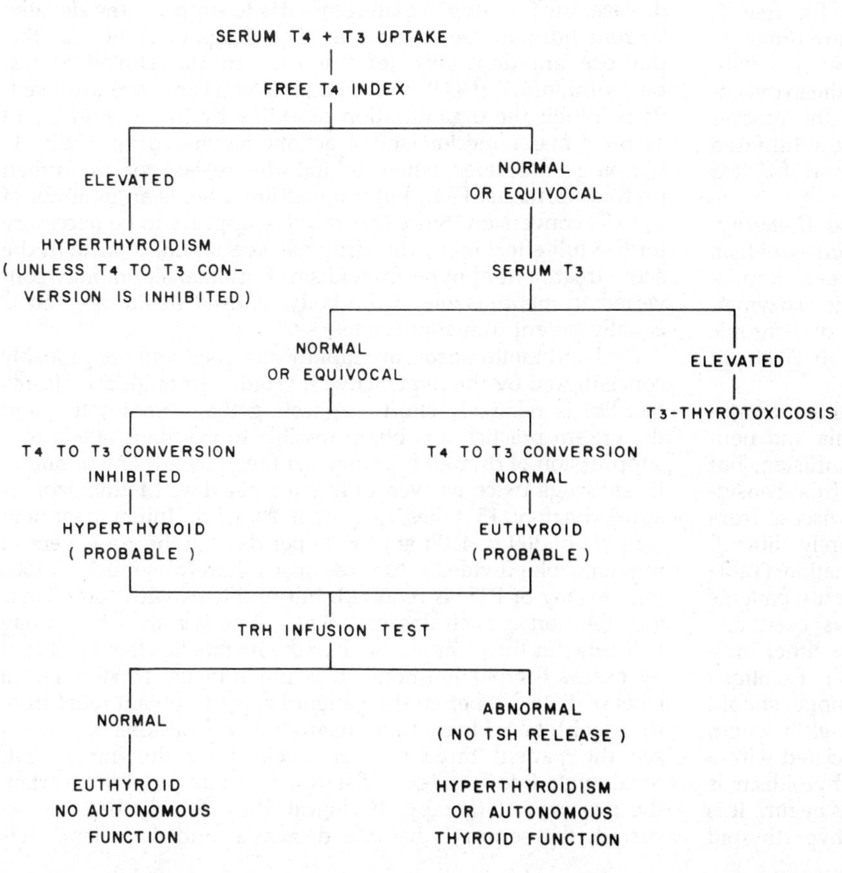

Figure 228–6. Laboratory diagnosis of hyperthyroidism.

not have T_3 *thyrotoxicosis,* which occurs in 3 to 5 per cent of patients in the United States but more commonly in areas where dietary iodine is lower. The diagnosis of hyperthyroidism cannot be eliminated until the free T_3 index (as well as the free T_4 index) has been found to be normal. Even in hyperthyroidism, a substantial fraction of T_3 derives from peripheral T_4 to T_3 conversion. Impairment of this process from any of the causes listed in Table 228–3 can lead to a reduction in serum T_3. However, in hyperthyroidism, even with severe illness, the serum T_3 is rarely depressed to less than 100 ng per deciliter.

In equivocal situations, it may be necessary to perform a TRH infusion test, (see Testing for Suspected Thyroid Dysfunction). A normal increase in TSH unequivocally eliminates all forms of hyperthyroidism except those associated with increased TSH secretion, which are extremely rare (see below). Since patients with fixed or autonomous, but not supranormal, thyroid hormone production may also have pituitary TSH depletion, an abnormal test does not indicate the presence of hypermetabolism and the need for treatment. However, particularly in patients who have only eye manifestations, the discovery of abnormalities in pituitary-thyroid regulation is consistent with the diagnosis of Graves' disease as the cause of the eye symptoms. A T_3 or T_4 suppression test (see Testing for Suspected Thyroid Dysfunction) will provide similar information.

In patients with a classic history and laboratory abnormalities, an RAI uptake and thyroid scan are not necessary to establish the diagnosis. However, if the hyperthyroidism is of brief (less than three months') duration, if the thyroid is not enlarged or palpable, or if it is tender, subacute thyroiditis must be considered, and an uptake and scan should be performed after pregnancy has been excluded. These tests are also required when nodular goiter is suspected or when factitious thyrotoxicosis is to be considered (Table 228–5).

Unilateral Ophthalmopathy. Since Graves' ophthalmopathy may be unilateral and not associated with frank hyperthyroidism, local pathology such as orbital tumor, pseudotumor of the orbit, cavernous sinus–carotid aneurysm, and sphenoid ridge meningioma must be considered. In addition to the free T_4 index, serum T_3, and TRH test, such patients require orbital x-rays, ultrasound, and CT scan. In almost all patients with Graves' ophthalmopathy, bilateral involvement of the extraocular muscles will be found even though clinically the process appears unilateral. Positive serum tests for TSI or antithyroid microsomal antibodies will provide further support for this diagnosis.

Other Chemical Abnormalities Associated with Hyperthyroidism. In 5 to 20 per cent of patients with hyperthyroidism any of the following may be found: modest hypercalcemia, increased alkaline phosphatase (bone or hepatic isozyme), increased direct bilirubin, and a mild anemia of "chronic disease." Modest neutropenia may occur (1000 to 2000 per cubic millimeter).

DIFFERENTIAL DIAGNOSIS. There are few clinical syndromes which mimic hyperthyroidism. Pheochromocytoma and neurocirculatory asthenia may cause some clinical confusion, but appropriate laboratory testing will eliminate these from consideration. Differentiation of patients with Graves' disease from those with other forms of hyperthyroidism is rarely difficult based solely on the history and physical examination (Table 228–5). The use of the RAI uptake and scan to identify patients with subacute thyroiditis or nodular disease has been discussed. Iodine-induced hyperthyroidism is due to either multinodular goiter or Graves' disease (Jod-Basedow). Factitious thyrotoxicosis, the ingestion of excess thyroid hormone, should be considered particularly in paramedical personnel in whom symptoms and laboratory manifestations are associated with a nonpalpable thyroid gland. TSH-induced hyperthyroidism is often diagnosed retrospectively after treatment has begun. It is so rare that it is not cost-effective to screen all hyperthyroid patients for this disease. Chorionic gonadotropin–induced hyperthyroidism is confirmed by the elevation in serum HCG in association with molar pregnancy or choriocarcinoma.

TREATMENT. The treatment of patients with Graves' disease must be considered in the context of its natural history. From 10 to 50 per cent of patients, depending on the series, return to normal thyroid function (remission) in association with (but probably not because of) drug treatment directed at the thyroid, not at the apparent primary defect in the immune system. If the patient destined to remit could be identified, a rational treatment approach for this disease could be developed. At present this is difficult, though some studies have suggested that patients with HLA-B8 and HLA-DR-3 antigens are less likely to have spontaneous remission than are those with other genetic backgrounds. Reduction in circulating TSI or TDA generally accompanies remission, and it may be possible to employ such assays in the future to guide definitive therapy. Currently TSI and TDA assays are available primarily as a research tool. Early studies suggested that if patients were given antithyroid drugs for 12 to 18 months, approximately 50 per cent would remain euthyroid after their discontinuation. More recently that fraction may have decreased to 10 to 20 per cent. The reason for the apparent change in the natural history of hyperthyroidism in the United States is not clear. One possible explanation is the recent increase in iodine intake. Since antithyroid drugs markedly deplete thyroidal iodine, the capacity to re-establish excessive secretion of thyroid hormone could be influenced by the iodine supply. In patients with Graves' disease who undergo a remission, hypothyroidism may occur some 20 to 30 years later. This is presumably autoimmune in origin, further emphasizing the similarities between Graves' disease and Hashimoto's thyroiditis. Lastly, patients in remission may have a relapse months to years later.

As the underlying cause for Graves' disease is not known, no specific therapy for this condition is available. There are two phases of the treatment of the hyperthyroidism of Graves' disease. The first is acute therapy with the goal of re-establishing euthyroidism. The second phase is definitive therapy, the induction of a permanent alteration in thyroid function.

Acute Treatment of Hyperthyroidism. ANTITHYROID DRUGS. In a typical patient with hyperthyroidism caused by Graves' disease, the first step in management is to suppress the elevated thyroid hormone secretion rate. The drugs of choice for this purpose are derivatives of thiourea. In the United States, propylthiouracil (PTU) and methimazole (Tapazole) are used. Both inhibit the organification of iodine by the thyroid gland as their major mechanism of action. Neither drug affects I^- trapping, nor does either inhibit the release of preformed thyroid hormone. PTU, but not methimazole, is an inhibitor of T_4 to T_3 conversion. Since this reaction appears to be necessary for the full effect of T_4, this drug has special importance in the acute treatment of hyperthyroidism. Carbimazole, rapidly converted to methimazole in the body, is used in Europe and is equally potent to methimazole.

PTU and methimazole are rapidly absorbed and are probably concentrated by the hyperactive thyroid. Although the plasma half-life is relatively short, suggesting the need for frequent dosage, in practice it is often possible to maintain satisfactory suppression of thyroid hormone synthesis by administration of these drugs twice or even only once per day. Methimazole is approximately 15 times as potent as PTU. Initial treatment consists of 300 to 450 mg of PTU per day (or the equivalent of methimazole) divided into three doses. Rarely as much as 1600 mg per day of PTU is required, but problems with compliance are common at such dosages. Since there is a five- to ten-day half-time for the disappearance of the metabolic effects induced by excess thyroid hormone, it is not unusual for the serum level of T_4 to fall before the patient begins to obtain relief from the symptoms of hyperthyroidism. It is the author's practice to see the patient three to four weeks after the initial visit, obtaining a free T_4 index and serum T_3 at that point to ascertain the progress of therapy. If clinical improvement has not occurred, the serum T_4 has not decreased and compliance has been maintained, the dose of antithyroid drug should be increased. After the first months of treatment, the dose of antithyroid drug can be reduced to a level of 100 to 300 mg per day of PTU, and the patient seen at two- to three-month intervals. In patients to be treated for six to eighteen months, therapy can be monitored by both clinical and laboratory parameters. The serum T_3:T_4 ratio will be increased because of intrathyroidal iodine deficiency and the increased thyroidal T_3:T_4 ratio in Graves' disease. Therefore both serum T_3 and the free T_4 index should be monitored. Serum TSH may increase if the serum T_4 falls below normal even if serum T_3 is normal. This is undesirable since it can lead to further thyroid enlargement and possibly an exacerbation of eye symptoms.

Thiourea derivatives have several side effects. A maculopapular rash occurs in 2 to 8 per cent of patients but does not usually require discontinuation of the drug. Both agents can rarely cause hepatocellular damage, and PTU can cause vasculitis. The most serious side effect of both agents is agranulocytosis. This occurs in 2 to 5 of 1000 patients and can be fatal if not recognized. Since this reaction may be abrupt in onset and is so rare, it is not, in the opinion of many experts, necessary to monitor the white blood count at frequent intervals. Instead, a baseline WBC and differential are obtained, and the patient is cautioned on each visit about the symptoms and significance of agranulocytosis. The patient is instructed to report immediately if infection occurs and to stop the medication. If this happens, the WBC and differential are repeated and the drug discontinued permanently if necessary. The reaction may appear at any time during therapy and does not appear to be dose related (except at extremely high doses). It is seen most commonly in the first few months of therapy. If such a reaction occurs, the drug should be withdrawn and appropriate supportive care provided. Recovery occurs in almost all patients, and an alternative treatment modality should then be used. Special precautions about the use of antithyroid drugs in pregnancy are discussed below.

The benefits of bed rest, adequate diet, and the extrication of the patient from the usual occupational or domestic pressures cannot be overemphasized. Remarkable clinical improvement is often noted within one to two days simply as a result of hospitalization. The acute treatment of severe hyperthyroidism is discussed below under Thyroid Storm.

β-ADRENERGIC BLOCKING AGENTS. The similarity of the symptoms of hyperthyroidism to those of catecholamine excess is striking. The molecular basis for this similarity is not clearly established. Although animal studies have shown thyroid hormone–induced increases in β-adrenergic receptors in cardiac tissue, the receptor number is normal in lymphocytes from patients with thyrotoxicosis. Plasma catecholamine concentrations are normal in hyperthyroidism. Nevertheless, blockade of β-adrenergic receptors by propranolol may result in symptomatic improvement prior to a decrease in serum thyroid hormones. A dose of 20 to 40 mg of propranolol every four to six hours may be used, but patients with congestive heart failure or bronchial asthma should not receive this therapy. In most patients with mild to moderate hyperthyroidism this adjunctive therapy is not necessary and may complicate the therapeutic regimen. In patients with more profound tachycardia or with thyroid storm (see below), it may have an important beneficial effect. Propranolol, although decreasing pulse rate and cardiac output in patients with hyperthyroidism, does not alter the elevated basal metabolic rate. Therefore, the tissues continue to consume oxygen at a high rate in the presence of decreased blood supply.

The Second Phase of Hyperthyroidism Treatment. If the symptoms of hyperthyroidism are not severe or after the acute treatment of symptoms with thiourea drugs, a decision must be made as to long-term therapy. There are three choices: further antithyroid drugs with hopes of a spontaneous remission, surgery, or radioiodine. None of these is ideal, and the choice for each patient must be made individually.

CHRONIC ANTITHYROID DRUG THERAPY. If chronic antithyroid drug therapy is undertaken in anticipation of a remission, it should be continued for six to eighteen months. If the quantities of drug required to maintain euthyroidism remain relatively large (e.g., 200 mg of PTU or greater) and serum T_3 and T_4 rise when the dosage is reduced, then a remission has not occurred. If the thyroid becomes smaller and the required amount of antithyroid drug lower, then a remission is probable. Some authorities recommend a TRH test at this juncture, but the author prefers to obtain a serum T_3 and T_4, to discontinue the treatment, and to repeat these tests in four weeks. The serum T_3 is especially important, since it may become elevated prior to the T_4 when a relapse occurs. If thyroid hormones remain normal, the patient should be seen at bimonthly intervals for one year, at which time the visits can be reduced in frequency.

SURGERY. Surgical removal of a portion of the thyroid gland to regulate hyperthyroidism is a time-honored and effective treatment in the hands of expert surgeons. Hyperthyroidism rarely recurs, although roughly 50 to 60 per cent of patients will eventually become hypothyroid. In most patients, hyperthyroidism is controlled by antithyroid drugs for one to two months prior to surgery. About seven to ten days before the operation, saturated solution of potassium iodide (1 gram of potassium iodide per milliliter), 2 drops three times a day, or Lugol's solution ($\simeq$ 125 mg iodide per milliliter), 10 drops three times a day, is begun to reduce the vascularity of the thyroid gland. Iodide alone can be used in patients with allergies to thiourea drugs to suppress thyroid function for periods of 10 to 28 days, as this will inhibit preformed hormone release. In addition, the elevated intracellular I^- content will block organification (Wolff-Chaikoff effect). Treatment with I^- alone should not be given beyond two to three weeks, since the hormone release rate will often increase again (escape phenomenon).

Alternatively, propranolol alone may be used to prepare the patient, or it may be combined with $I-$. One to two weeks of pretreatment with 40 mg of propranolol every six hours has been given. This approach is still experimental and should not be employed for patients who can undertake standard preoperative therapy with thiourea drugs. Aside from hypothyroidism, other potential complications of surgery include neck hemorrhage, recurrent laryngeal nerve damage, and hypoparathyroidism. In highly experienced clinics, such complications are quite rare (<1 per cent).

RADIOIODINE. Treatment of hyperthyroidism with ^{131}I has been used since the late 1940's. The principal complication of this treatment is hypothyroidism, which occurs in about 10 per cent of patients in the first year and increases about 5 per cent per year thereafter over 20 years. Depending on the dose given, about 20 per cent of patients require a second treatment. No increased risk of thyroid carcinoma or leukemia occurs after such treatment. For many years, there was a reluctance to employ ^{131}I in the treatment of women in the childbearing age group, but the ovarian dose from a typical 10 mCi treatment is approximately 2 to 4 rads, which is in the same range as that from hysterosalpingography or a barium enema. Although any unnecessary radiation is to be avoided, the calculated increase in the gamete mutation rate from exposure in this range is only a small fraction of the spontaneous mutation rate. Thus ^{131}I therapy does not appear to offer a significant risk of fetal malformation, although it is recommended that pregnancy not be undertaken for six months after this therapy to avoid transient radiation-induced changes in the gametes.

The author will generally pretreat patients who are to have ^{131}I therapy with thiourea derivatives to provide symptomatic relief and avoid the remote chance of an exacerbation of hyperthyroidism from radiation thyroiditis. These are discontinued four days prior to determining the 24-hour ^{131}I uptake. The author's practice is to administer orally an amount of ^{131}I, which when multiplied by the RAI uptake will result in thyroidal accumulation of 5 mCi ^{131}I. This will result in an average dose of 80 to 90 μCi per gram or 6000 to 7000 rads, which is associated with resolution of hyperthyroidism in about 80 per cent of patients within six months. Therapy with thiourea drugs may be restarted after one week, although it is not usually required. Patients are seen monthly thereafter with appropriate diagnostic and therapeutic measures to maintain the euthyroid state. At least six months is allowed to elapse before considering a second treatment. Since radioiodine crosses the placenta and would be concentrated by the thyroid of the fetus at 12 weeks and older, it is imperative that possibility of pregnancy be eliminated before radioiodine is administered.

The therapist administering radioiodine is committed to the planning of adequate follow-up. This consists of thoroughly informing the patient about the risks of delayed hypothyroidism (occurring in 80 to 100 per cent), providing written documentation of the treatment and its complications, and maintaining proper communication with referring physicians as to the need for indefinite follow-up. Patients are alerted to the symptoms of hypothyroidism and instructed that after the acute phase of treatment they should be seen at least every four to six months for appropriate thyroid function testing until hypothyroidism appears and treatment is initiated.

Choice of Therapy. None of the three long-term therapies for hyperthyroidism is ideal. Some thyroidologists will not use radioiodine in patients under the age of 35 or 40 because of the fear of long-term complications, whereas others employ radioiodine routinely in the treatment of hyperthyroidism in children. The author follows an intermediate position and will employ ^{131}I in patients as young as 18 years of age. In patients under the age of 18, one to two years of therapy with antithyroid drugs are given in hopes of observing a spontaneous remission. In women with this disease, the desire to raise a family will often require a decision for definitive therapy, especially if PTU requirements are high. In those patients who are over 18 at this point, ^{131}I is given, whereas for those who do not desire ^{131}I or who are under 18, surgery is recommended. Surgery is also recommended for patients with extreme thyroid enlargement or who have coexisting nonfunctioning thyroid nodules. The physician advising patients regarding this decision must consider not only these theoretical considerations and the patient's preferences but also the availability of a skilled surgeon.

Hyperthyroidism in Pregnancy. The peak incidence of Graves' disease occurs in women during the reproductive period. Therefore, it is not uncommon to find hyperthyroidism in a pregnant patient or for pregnancy to occur during therapy with antithyroid drugs. Both PTU and methimazole cross the placenta, whereas thyroid hormones do not. Excessive quantities of antithyroid drugs may cause impairment of fetal thyroid hormone synthesis. Depending on the dose, the consequence may be a compensatory hypertrophy of the thyroid gland resulting from increased TSH or frank fetal hypothyroidism with potential impairment of normal central nervous system development. I^- crosses the placenta, and the fetal thyroid is not able to adapt to high plasma I^- levels. Therefore, I^- therapy may result in iodide-induced fetal hypothyroidism. A congenital lesion, *aplasia cutis* (a 1 to 4 cm circular lesion on the scalp in which no hair follicles or accessory skin structures are present), has been found with increased frequency in infants of mothers receiving methimazole but not PTU. Uncontrolled hyperthyroidism in pregnancy is associated with an increased risk of spontaneous abortion and may lead to thyroid storm at the time of delivery.

With these facts in mind, pregnant patients with hyperthyroidism should be seen at monthly intervals, with careful clinical examination supplemented by measurements of serum T_3, T_4, and T_3 uptake. It should be recalled that the normal range for both serum T_4 and T_3 is higher during pregnancy (see Table 228–4). PTU should be given at the lowest dosage which maintains the patient at an acceptable euthyroid state. The author does not employ supplemental thyroid hormones in the treatment of the pregnant hyperthyroid patient, as has been recommended by some. If the patient's hyperthyroid symptoms cannot be controlled on less than 300 mg of PTU per day, then subtotal thyroidectomy is recommended during the second trimester. Iodides can be given for seven to ten days in preparation for surgery.

The newborn infant of the mother with Graves' disease should be examined carefully for either hypothyroidism as a consequence of excessive antithyroid drug or hyperthyroidism resulting from transplacental passage of TSI. In either situation goiter may be present, which may lead to respiratory embarrassment. Even the most meticulously managed patients will often have infants with modest reductions in serum T_4 that quickly normalize in the first week of life. Neonatal hyperthyroidism is transient but occasionally must be treated with antithyroid drugs and digitalis for tachycardia. An exacerbation of hyperthyroidism may occur following delivery and should be anticipated. The quantities of PTU in the milk of mothers receiving 200 to 300 mg PTU per day are not great enough to cause impairment of an infant's thyroid function. It seems likely that nursing mothers could take PTU at low doses, though the infant could still be at risk for nonthyroidal complications of this drug. Methimazole (and presumably carbimazole) is present in milk in significant amounts and should not be given to nursing mothers.

Lithium. Lithium has an effect on thyroid secretion quite similar to that of I^- in that it inhibits release of preformed thyroid hormone from the thyroid, probably by inhibiting thyroglobulin hydrolysis. It may also inhibit peripheral degradation of T_4. In patients with allergies to both antithyroid drugs and iodide, lithium carbonate, 0.9 to 1.5 grams per day (serum lithium concentrations of 0.5 to 1.0 mEq per liter), may be of value in the treatment of acute thyrotoxicosis. Serum lithium levels must be closely monitored, as some of the toxic effects of lithium are similar to those of hyperthyroidism.

Thyroid Storm. Some patients with hyperthyroidism develop severe manifestations which are exaggerations of many of the symptoms listed in Table 228–6. Often these occur because of superimposed stress or infection. The patient may be febrile, have abdominal pain, and become delirious, obtunded, or psychotic. This condition, called *thyroid storm*, has a mortality of 20 to 40 per cent. Such patients should be hospitalized and treated with a protocol such as is outlined in Table 228–7. I^- is

TABLE 228–7. MANAGEMENT OF PATIENTS WITH THYROID STORM

Diagnostic

1. Serum T_3 and T_4 concentrations, resin or charcoal T_3 uptake
2. Appropriate evaluation for underlying precipitating causes such as infection, acute surgical abdomen, central nervous system lesions, or psychologic trauma
3. Baseline WBC and differential, electrolytes, Ca, P
4. Plasma cortisol

Therapeutic

1. Intravenous fluids—dextrose with or without electrolytes as indicated, multivitamins
2. Propylthiouracil, 400 mg every six hours (by nasogastric tube, if necessary), to inhibit thyroid hormone synthesis and block T_4 to T_3 conversion
3. Sodium iodide, 250 mg every six hours (orally or intravenously)
4. Hydrocortisone, 50 to 100 mg every six hours intravenously
5. External cooling and acetaminophen (300 to 600 mg) every four to six hours for severe hyperpyrexia (do not use salicylates, which increase free thyroid hormones and oxygen consumption)
6. Propranolol—in patients without asthma, chronic bronchitis, or non-arrhythmia-related, congestive heart failure, 10–40 mg may be given every four to six hours orally; a slow intravenous infusion of 1 mg per minute for two to ten minutes with careful monitoring of blood pressure and ECG may be used if oral therapy is not feasible; propranolol may precipitate pulmonary edema in a few patients with hyperthyroidism; reserpine or guanethidine would not appear to have any advantages over propranolol in this situation
7. Oxygen may be helpful
8. Digitalis glycosides should be employed for therapy of congestive failure and for blockade of a rapid ventricular response to an atrial tachyrhythmia
9. Appropriate treatment of precipitating event if any

the most effective agent for inhibiting release of preformed thyroid hormone. If it is felt that the patient has a surgical abdomen, intravenous propranolol may be used intraoperatively to control tachycardia, assuming that there are no contraindications. The line between severe hyperthyroidism and thyroid storm is nebulous. In patients with severe symptoms but without fever, I^- should be added to PTU therapy to achieve a more rapid decrease in thyroid hormones. The I^- can be discontinued after one week.

Treatment of Ophthalmopathy. In most patients with ophthalmopathy no specific therapy is needed. Return of the hyperthyroid patient to euthyroidism will often result in amelioration of many of the minor symptoms, including stare and lid lag. It is important to avoid hypothyroidism, as anecdotal data suggest that this may be associated with an exacerbation of eye symptoms. The patient may note periorbital edema, especially on arising in the morning. An extra pillow or elevation of the head of the bed will relieve this. Alternatively, a diuretic can be administered at bedtime. In patients with more severe symptoms, artificial tears (1 per cent methylcellulose) are prescribed.

A small fraction of patients with Graves' disease will have more severe problems than can be relieved by these minor therapeutic measures. In patients with severe proptosis, desiccation of the sclera or even cornea may occur at night because of lagophthalmos. Taping the lids closed at night may alleviate this symptom, although lateral tarsorrhaphy is a more permanent solution. Diplopia may be treated by prisms or, if permanent, by muscle repositioning or relief of fibrous adhesions. This procedure should not be performed until the eye disease has stabilized, often a matter of two to three years. In the patient with severe inflammation and chemosis *(malignant exophthalmos)*, prednisone is required. Although 15 to 20 mg per day may be sufficient, in many patients as much as 100 mg per day is necessary with the attendant complications of treatment. Such patients should have frequent measurements of visual acuity and visual fields. Deterioration of either test is an emergency requiring steroid treatment and ophthalmologic consultation. In the case of optic compression or persistent corneal ulceration, surgical decompression may be required. Fortunately, in most patients, the severity of the eye manifestations will abate after 12 to 18 months, although in many the proptosis will never revert to normal.

Pretibial Myxedema. The lesions of pretibial myxedema are not generally incapacitating but may be cosmetically disfiguring. They may be treated with topical application of glucocorticoids, with enhancement of absorption by occlusive dressings if necessary.

PROGNOSIS. In most patients, Graves' disease is an extremely benign disorder in which the physician can play an important role in providing considerable relief to the patient. Because of the complications of treatment and the possibility of hypothyroidism even in patients with a spontaneous remission, patients with Graves' disease require lifelong observation.

TREATMENT OF OTHER CAUSES OF HYPERTHYROIDISM

The acute treatment of hyperthyroidism associated with toxic multinodular goiter or toxic adenoma does not differ from that of patients with Graves' disease. These entities are discussed in detail later in the chapter. The hyperthyroidism associated with subacute thyroiditis (particularly the lymphocytic variety) has been a subject of great interest in the past five years. This is discussed in the section Thyroiditis.

TSH-secreting pituitary tumor must be treated by surgery or x-ray. Patients with this condition are identified and separated from the group with nontumorigenic TSH–induced hyperthyroidism by finding elevation of the value of the serum α-TSH subunit as well as elevation of the value of TSH. Nontumorigenic hypersecretion of TSH is thought to be due to a reduction in feedback sensitivity to T_3 and T_4 at the pituitary level. Such patients are treated with antithyroid drugs. In patients with choriocarcinoma or hydatidiform mole, removal of the tumor will relieve these symptoms. Extremely rare is the ovarian teratoma containing thyroid tissue, *struma ovarii.* This should be treated surgically. In general, thyroid carcinoma does not function well enough to lead to hyperthyroidism. Hyperthyroidism can occur if extensive metastases are present which retain a significant degree of function, as may be seen occasionally in follicular carcinoma. This condition is readily diagnosed and is treated with ^{131}I.

Borst GC, Eil C, Burman KD: Euthyroid hyperthyroxinemia. Ann Intern Med 98:366–378, 1983. *The differential diagnosis of individuals with an elevated serum T_4.*

Cheron RG, Kaplan MM, Larsen PR, Selenkow HA, Crigler JF, Jr: Neonatal thyroid function after propylthiouracil therapy for maternal Graves' disease. N Engl J Med 304:525–528, 1981. *A prospective study of the effects of maternal antithyroid drug treatment on newborn thyroid function.*

Dallow RL: Reliability of orbital diagnostic tests: Ultrasonography, computerized tomography and radiography. Ophthalmology 85:1218, 1978. *The author describes results of these various diagnostic techniques in 342 patients with unilateral exophthalmus.*

Davis PJ, Davis FB: Hyperthyroidism in patients over the age of 60 years. Medicine 53:161, 1974. *An excellent summary of the clinical syndrome of hyperthyroidism in the elderly patient.*

Fradkin JE, Wolff J: Iodide-induced thyrotoxicosis. Medicine 62:1,1–20, 1983. *Iodide, or drugs containing this element, can cause many confusing syndromes especially in patients with underlying thyroid disease. The spectrum of these problems is reviewed in this article.*

Holm LE, Dahlquist I, Israelsson A, Lundell G: Malignant thyroid tumors after *^{131}I therapy. N Engl J Med 303:188, 1980. In a group of 3000 patients, the authors found no increased incidence of malignant thyroid tumors after ^{131}I therapy an average of 13 years earlier.*

Morley JE, Jacobson RJ, Melamed J, Hershman JM: Choriocarcinoma as a cause of thyrotoxicosis. Am J Med 60:1036, 1976. *Three typical cases of this syndrome are presented with complete thyroid evaluation.*

Weintraub BD, Gershengorn MC, Kourides IA, Fein H: Inappropriate secretion of thyroid-stimulating hormone. Ann Intern Med 95:339–351, 1981. *A review of the pathophysiology, diagnosis and treatment of TSH-induced hyperthyroidism.*

Zakarija M, McKenzie JM, Banovac K: Clinical significance of assay of thyroid-stimulating antibody in Graves' disease. Ann Intern Med 93:28–32 (part 1), 1980. *A careful study of the correlation between remission and TSI in patients with Graves' Disease.*

Hypothyroidism and Myxedema

DEFINITION. *Hypothyroidism* is the clinical syndrome which results from a deficiency of thyroid hormone. In severe hypothyroidism a hydrophilic mucopolysaccharide substance accumulates in subcutaneous tissues, causing a nonpitting edema referred to as *myxedema.* Some authorities use the terms hypothyroidism and myxedema interchangeably, whereas others reserve the latter term for the severe form of this syndrome.

ETIOLOGY. A list of causes to be considered in patients with hypothyroidism is given in Table 228–8. *Primary hypothyroidism*, that caused by thyroid gland malfunction, accounts for over 95 per cent of such cases, of which Hashimoto's thyroiditis, idiopathic myxedema (probably a variant of Hashimoto's thyroiditis), and thyroid destruction resulting from ^{131}I therapy or surgery for hyperthyroidism account for the greatest proportion. Hashimoto's and subacute thyroiditis are discussed in the next section. Hypothyroidism after therapeutic irradiation to the thyroid area for lymphoma or Hodgkin's disease is found in from 10 to 30 per cent of these patients, usually within one to two years of treatment.

Hypothyroidism can also occur with normal or near-normal thyroid tissue when there is a superimposed stress on thyroid cell function. Hypothyroidism may be caused either by severe iodine deficiency (<25 μg iodine per day) or by naturally occurring goitrogens such as have been found in Colombia or are generated by eating the cassava plant in Africa (see Sporadic and Endemic Goiter). In patients with Graves' disease, especially after RAI treatment, or in those with mild Hashimoto's thyroiditis, iodine excess may cause hypothyroidism through the Wolff-Chaikoff effect (I^- induced inhibition of organification). These glands are unable to reduce I^- uptake in the presence of an elevated plasma I^- as normally occurs. The

TABLE 228–8. CAUSES OF HYPOTHYROIDISM

- I. Primary hypothyroidism
  - A. Acquired
    - 1. Destructive lesions
      - a. Hashimoto's thyroiditis
      - b. Idiopathic myxedema (probably the end-stage of Hashimoto's thyroiditis)
      - c. ^{131}I therapy for hyperthyroidism
      - d. Subtotal thyroidectomy, especially for Graves' disease
      - e. Therapeutic external x-ray treatment to the neck for other diseases
      - f. After subacute thyroiditis (may be transient)
      - g. Cystinosis
    - 2. Impaired function of a normal or near-normal gland
      - a. Endemic goiter—iodine deficiency or naturally occurring goitrogens
      - b. Iodine excess (>6 mg per day) in patients with underlying thyroid disease
      - c. Drug-induced; lithium carbonate, para-aminosalicylic acid, thiourea drugs, sulfonamides, phenylbutazone, and others
  - B. Congenital
    - 1. Defects in enzymes required for thyroid hormone synthesis (congenital goiter)
    - 2. Thyroid agenesis
    - 3. Thyroid dysgenesis or ectopy
    - 4. Maternal iodide or antithyroid drugs
- II. Secondary hypothyroidism
  - A. Hypothalamic dysfunction
    - 1. Neoplasms
    - 2. Eosinophilic granuloma
    - 3. Therapeutic irradiation
  - B. Pituitary dysfunction
    - 1. Neoplasms
    - 2. Pituitary surgery or irradiation
    - 3. Idiopathic hypopituitarism
    - 4. Sheehan's syndrome (postpartum pituitary necrosis)
    - 5. Dopamine infusion and/or severe illness(?)
- III. Tissue resistance to thyroid hormone

drugs listed in Table 228–8 all inhibit organification of thyroidal I^-. In most cases the hypothyroidism associated with these drugs is mild.

Screening of newborns for hypothyroidism is now widely practiced, and the incidence of this condition is about 1 in 4000 births. About 65 per cent of infants with congenital hypothyroidism in North America have thyroid agenesis or hypoplasia, 25 per cent have ectopic thyroid glands, and about 10 per cent have defects in one of the steps required for thyroid hormone synthesis (see Sporadic and Endemic Goiter).

Secondary hypothyroidism occurs as a result of hypothalamic or pituitary dysfunction. Dopamine infusion and/or severe illness may suppress TSH release sufficiently to cause a modest, transient hypothyroidism. A rare cause of hypothyroidism is tissue resistance to thyroid hormones, which may be due to an abnormality in the nuclear receptor for these hormones.

INCIDENCE. Hypothyroidism is common in adults. In one recent epidemiologic survey, 1.4 per cent of adult females and about 0.1 per cent of adult males were affected. Autoimmune destruction of the thyroid gland is the most common cause of thyroid gland failure in adults. This generally affects women over the age of 40 but can occur at any age. Hypothyroidism is also a common congenital disease, occurring in about 1 of 4000 neonates in North America and Western Europe and more frequently in areas of iodine deficiency.

PATHOLOGY. The pathology of the thyroid gland in hypothyroidism depends on the etiology of the syndrome. In "idiopathic myxedema," the thyroid tissue is generally replaced by fat with few intact follicles and lymphocytic infiltration (see also Thyroiditis). When the thyroid cells remain partly functional, the elevated serum TSH leads to hyperplasia and hypertrophy. In secondary hypothyroidism, the follicular cells are low and considerable colloid is present. The gland is small in contrast to the goiter found when thyroid cell dysfunction is present and TSH secretion is elevated.

The nonthyroidal pathology of the hypothyroid state is the same regardless of its etiology. The longer the duration and the more severe the deficiency, the greater are the changes. The accumulation of mucopolysaccharide in connective tissues has already been mentioned. This material may also appear in muscle. Effusions, which often have a high protein content, occur in various serous cavities.

CLINICAL MANIFESTATIONS. The common clinical manifestations of this syndrome in the adult are summarized in Table 228–9. These symptoms and signs can be attributed to either deceleration of cellular metabolic processes or the accumulation of the hygroscopic mucopolysaccharide in the vocal cords or oropharynx, as well as the more obvious changes in the subcutaneous tissues. The symptoms are nonspecific, particularly in the early phases, and may either pass unnoticed by the patient or be attributed to advancing age. Characteristically, the patient becomes aware of their multiplicity and severity only after thyroid hormone replacement leads to a return of normal function. This is particularly true of younger patients. In the elderly, hearing impairment, somnolence, and decreased memory and ability to calculate may occur. These may lead to an apparent psychologic withdrawal and paranoia at times requiring hospitalization. The term *myxedema madness* has been used to describe this syndrome, which can be mistaken for cerebrovascular insufficiency or senile dementia. Alternatively, the patient may confabulate or respond with humorous non sequiturs to draw the interviewer's attention from his or her limited recall of recent events. This behavior has been termed *myxedema wit*. A variety of menstrual disorders may be present, although menorrhagia is said to be the most common pattern. Pregnancy may occur in patients with hypothyroidism, and the increased hormone requirements of that condition may cause a previously borderline functioning thyroid to decompensate. Despite the developmental abnormalities associated with congenital hypothyroidism, the symptoms of hypothyroidism in infants are few. Severe thyroid hormone deficiency is associated with growth retardation in the older infant and child. In the adolescent, thyroid enlargement, *adolescent goiter*, may be the only manifestation and is usually seen in the pubertal female. In some patients in whom the hypothyroidism is of rapid onset, cramps in large muscle groups may be a prominent symptom. Such symptoms usually occur after a rapid change from a hyperthyroid to a hypothyroid state, such as after surgery for Graves' disease, a second RAI treatment for hyperthyroidism, or even vigorous antithyroid drug therapy.

Many of the common signs of hypothyroidism are the opposite of those seen in the hyperthyroid patient. Bradycardia is common and is sometimes associated with hypothermia. Systolic pressure is generally reduced and diastolic pressure increased, the latter resulting from increased peripheral vascular resistance. Myxedema is manifested by a puffy, nonpitting swelling of the subcutaneous tissue, which may particularly collect in the periorbital area. Body and scalp hair is reduced; the skin may be coarse, may have a sandpaper texture, and is usually cool and sallow. The yellow complexion is due to the accumulation of carotene in the serum in patients with significant hypothyroidism. The thyroid may be enlarged, of normal size, or not palpable, depending on the cause. The heart sounds are distant, and the heart shadow is often enlarged. The latter can be a manifestation of pericardial effusion, which is common but rarely leads to tamponade. In addition to the cortical dysfunction previously mentioned, cerebellar ataxia may be

TABLE 228–9. COMMON SYMPTOMS OF HYPOTHYROIDISM

- Weakness, fatigue, lethargy
- Dry, coarse skin
- Swelling of the hands, face, and extremities
- Cold intolerance, decreased sweating
- Coarsening or huskiness of the voice
- Modest weight gain (~10 lbs) with anorexia
- Decreased memory, hearing impairment
- Arthralgia, paresthesias
- Constipation
- Muscle cramps

present. Other neurologic signs, including delayed relaxation of the deep tendon reflexes, peripheral neuropathy, and carpal tunnel syndrome, can completely resolve with treatment. There may be few signs of hypothyroidism in the newborn, hence the need for routine screening. The most common signs are hypotonia, umbilical hernia, and skin mottling, but none is present in more than one third of infants with confirmed hypothyroidism in the first three months of life.

Certain physiologic abnormalities are characteristic of hypothyroidism. Cardiac output is reduced, although not out of proportion to the decrease in O_2 consumption. Glomerular filtration is also subnormal, leading to an impairment of the capacity to excrete free water. In addition there is evidence supporting inappropriate ADH secretion in primary hypothyroidism, which may lead to hyponatremia. Gastrointestinal motility is reduced, and occasionally the patient may develop an apparent obstruction, *myxedema megacolon*. There are important abnormalities in the medulla. The sensitivity to both hypercarbia and hypoxia is reduced, and such patients may readily develop CO_2 narcosis or cardiac arrhythmias associated with hypoxia. This is one of the chief causes of death in the severe form of myxedema, *myxedema coma*. Pituitary function is impaired in severe hypothyroidism even of the primary variety. Hypoglycemic stress does not elicit normal growth hormone or cortisol responses in such patients, so that testing pituitary function must be delayed until the hypothyroid state has been corrected. Serum prolactin is elevated in moderate to severe primary hypothyroidism, and this may lead to galactorrhea in a small percentage of patients.

LABORATORY DIAGNOSIS. The diagnosis of hypothyroidism can be easily confirmed by using the scheme outlined in Figure 228–7. When the diagnosis is not made, it is usually because the nonspecificity of signs and symptoms does not immediately suggest this cause. This disease is one of the "great imitators," and a high index of suspicion should be maintained as the condition is so readily diagnosed and treated. In all patients with hypothyroidism, the free T_4 index will be reduced. It is unlikely that significant symptoms will be present in patients with an equivocal reduction in this hormone. Once a reduced free T_4 index has been found, it is imperative to determine whether the cause of the disease is primary, i.e., owing to thyroid disease, or secondary, involving the hypothalamic-pituitary axis. An elevation in serum TSH establishes the diagnosis of primary hypothyroidism. If the serum TSH concentration is normal or borderline, then the diagnosis of pituitary or hypothalamic hypothyroidism is made and further steps are taken to evaluate the possibility of a deficiency of other pituitary hormones. It is extremely important that this be done prior to the onset of therapy, since thyroid replacement will exacerbate mild ACTH insufficiency associated with hypothalamic or pituitary disease. *If unrecognized, such patients may have an addisonian crisis provoked by thyroid hormone replacement.* There are two situations recognized in which primary hypothyroidism is not associated with an elevated serum TSH. This may occur when hypothyroidism follows shortly after a period of hyperthyroidism which causes a suppression of pituitary TSH synthesis and release lasting four to five weeks. Dopamine infusion may also cause suppression of an elevated TSH into the normal range. In the patient whose symptoms are nonspecific or borderline and in whom an equivocally reduced free T_4 index is obtained, the serum TSH may be significantly elevated. An elevated TSH is the most sensitive index of impairment of thyroid gland function. Whether or not such patients are actually metabolically hypothyroid cannot be determined by using present tests. In the case of early primary thyroid disease, an exaggerated TSH response to TRH will occur (see Fig. 228–4), the TSH being greater than 25 μU per milliliter 20 minutes after TRH infusion.

There are a few clinical situations in which the free T_4 index is reduced but serum TSH is not elevated in the absence of hypothalamic or pituitary disease. This occurs in patients receiving 2 to 3 grams per day of salicylate-containing compounds, in those receiving phenytoin (300 mg per day), and in those ingesting replacement quantities (25 μg or more) of triiodothyronine (Cytomel). Occasionally, the severely ill patient without primary thyroid disease may have a reduced free T_4 index with or without dopamine infusion. Such patients presumably have transient mild hypothyroidism, although in individual cases it may be extremely difficult to determine whether permanent hypothalamic-pituitary hypothyroidism is also present. A serum cortisol determination is indicated in these patients to eliminate the possibility of ACTH deficiency before initiating therapy with both thyroxine and glucocorti-

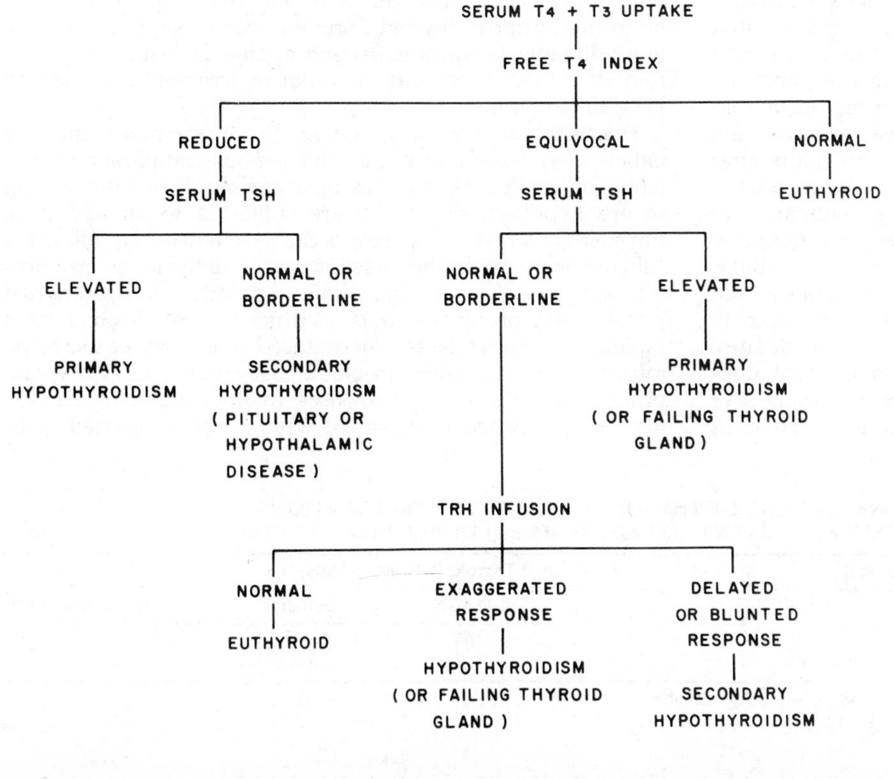

Figure 228–7. Laboratory diagnosis of hypothyroidism.

coid. A 24-hour RAI uptake test does not separate hypothyroidism from the euthyroid state, and serum T_3 concentrations may be in the normal range even in patients with significant hypothyroidism (see Table 228–4).

Other Biochemical Abnormalities and Associated Diseases in Patients with Hypothyroidism. Serum cholesterol and triglycerides, creatine phosphokinase (MM isozyme), aldolase, LDH, and SGOT may all be elevated in the patient with moderate to severe hypothyroidism. Hyponatremia with or without the inappropriate ADH syndrome is seen. There is often a modest anemia of chronic disease which may be macrocytic. Serum vitamin B_{12} should be measured in these patients because of the 3 to 6 per cent coexistence of pernicious anemia with Hashimoto's thyroiditis. Other conditions found with increased frequency in patients with autoimmune thyroid disease include idiopathic adrenocortical deficiency, diabetes mellitus, hypoparathyroidism, myasthenia gravis, and vitiligo. (Ch. 240).

DIFFERENTIAL DIAGNOSIS. There are few conditions which can masquerade as hypothyroidism in its classic form. However, patients with nephrotic syndrome or hypoalbuminemia and associated peripheral edema may be suspected of this diagnosis. Although the serum T_4 in these conditions is reduced because of hypoproteinemia, the T_3 uptake is generally quite elevated with a consequent normal free T_4 index. Patients with chronic renal disease may have symptoms entirely similar to those of hypothyroidism (including hypothermia), and laboratory tests are required to evaluate the possible coexistence of these two diseases. In patients with spontaneous primary hypothyroidism, the tests for autoantibodies to either thyroglobulin or microsomal components of the thyroid cell are generally positive. This is true even if the typical thyroid enlargement of Hashimoto's thyroiditis is not present. The other causes of hypothyroidism have already been discussed (Table 228–8), and reversible causes should be eliminated.

THERAPY. Hypothyroidism is a readily treatable disease. The preparations available for thyroid replacement are listed in Table 228–10. For many years desiccated thyroid was used quite satisfactorily, and it continues to be prescribed for about 40 per cent of the hypothyroid patients in the United States today. Although any of these substances given in the appropriate amounts are adequate to treat the major symptoms of hypothyroidism, the serum hormone results in patients receiving replacement doses of thyroxine appear to be most similar to those in normal persons. In patients receiving desiccated thyroid or the combination T_4-T_3 products, the ratio of serum T_3 to T_4 is usually higher than it is in normal subjects, since the ratio in these preparations (4:1) is higher than that in thyroid secretion. In addition, transient serum T_3 elevations above the physiologic normal range are found two to four hours after administration of desiccated thyroid and may be associated with symptoms. As noted, some tissues (e.g., pituitary and cerebral cortex) depend on serum T_4 for a significant portion of their intracellular T_3, whereas others derive most intracellular T_3 directly from the serum. Therefore, it would appear that both serum T_3 and T_4 concentrations should be normalized to fulfill the intracellular T_3 concentrations of all tissues. Because the USP standard for thyroid replacement preparations does not require specific measurement of thyroid hormones, only of organic iodine, some preparations of desiccated thyroid or thyroxine may meet these criteria without containing adequate quantities of biologically active thyroid hormone. Modifications of USP standards have been proposed to deal with this issue. The author prefers to use a brand name L-thyroxine as replacement. A dose of approximately 2.25 μg of T_4 per kilogram (1 μg of T_4 per pound), given once a day, achieves a satisfactory symptomatic and biochemical replacement in most patients. The difference between this dosage and the thyroxine production rate (≈80 to 90 μg per day) is due to the 50 to 70 per cent absorption of orally administered L-thyroxine. In patients who are in good health otherwise or whose hypothyroidism is very modest, therapy can be initiated with half-replacement doses immediately on establishing the diagnosis. This can be increased to full replacement after one month. In patients with more severe hypothyroidism, elderly patients, or those with a history of cardiovascular disease, the author prefers to begin therapy with smaller amounts (25 μg of thyroxine per day) and to increase these by 25-μg increments at four-week intervals (with due attention to symptoms) until a replacement dose is achieved. In patients with primary hypothyroidism there may rarely be an associated primary autoimmune hypoadrenalism *(Schmidt's syndrome)*. Such patients will require adequate replacement of glucocorticoid prior to institution of thyroid hormone replacement. A similar procedure must be employed in patients who have hypothalamic-pituitary disease as a cause of hypothyroidism. Biochemical evaluation of the progress of treatment of primary hypothyroidism consists of quantitation of the serum free T_4 index and TSH. The dose should be increased (symptoms permitting) until the serum TSH and free T_4 index have reached the normal range. The replacement dose of T_4 may be 20 to 40 per cent lower in elderly patients.

Hypothyroidism and Coronary Artery Disease. The patient who presents simultaneously with angina and hypothyroidism poses a serious therapeutic problem. In some patients with coronary artery disease, reintroduction of thyroid hormones results in increased myocardial oxygen demands without an adequate increase in myocardial blood flow. A trial of propranolol with small increments of thyroxine may reduce myocardial oxygen consumption without decreasing the pulse rate to unacceptably low levels. If an exacerbation of angina occurs during thyroxine therapy, T_4 to T_3 conversion may be acutely reduced in peripheral tissues with propylthiouracil (see Graves' Disease and Other Causes of Hyperthyroidism). In patients with localized coronary artery disease in whom bypass graft surgery is indicated, the frequent adverse effects of thyroxine replacement have raised the possibility that surgery should be performed prior to thyroid hormone replacement. The overall morbidity may be lower in patients operated on in the hypothyroid state than in patients in whom replacement is attempted prior to surgery.

Treatment of Myxedema Coma. In severe myxedema the patient may lapse into coma. This serious complication (mortality, 20 to 50 per cent) occurs most commonly in patients with severe hypothyroidism who are subjected to an additional physiologic stress. This may occur spontaneously, following cold exposure, or during infection, but in all too many instances it is iatrogenic. The administration of sedatives to hypothyroid patients may precipitate coma, as drugs are not metabolized as rapidly in these patients. The reduced sensitivity of the respiratory center to changes in blood gases may lead to inappropriately small ventilatory responses. In other situations, surgery may be performed in a patient who is not recognized to be

TABLE 228–10. HORMONE CONTENT OF THYROID REPLACEMENT PREPARATIONS (AMOUNTS APPROXIMATELY EQUIVALENT TO 1 GRAIN (65 mg) DESICCATED THYROID)

		Liotrix		Desiccated Thyroid (1-Grain Tablets)			
	L-Thyroxine	*Euthroid-1*	*Thyrolar-1*	*Armour*	*Proloid*	*Generics*	L-Triiodothyronine
T_4 (μg)	100	60	50	63	55	Variable*	0
T_3 (μg)	0	15	12.5	12	16	Variable*	25

*Eight generic preparations contained 9 to 59 μg T_4 and 8 to 18 μg T_3 per 1-grain tablet.
Data from Rees-Jones RW, Rolla AR, Larsen PR: JAMA 243:459, 1980.

TABLE 228–11. MANAGEMENT OF PATIENTS WITH MYXEDEMA COMA

Diagnostic
1. Serum T_4, T_3 uptake (or equivalent), TSH
2. CBC, glucose, electrolytes, blood gases, BUN, creatinine, CPK
3. Plasma cortisol before and 30 and 60 minutes after Cortrosyn, 0.25 mg, intravenous bolus
4. Careful evaluation for concomitant disease; continuous ECG and temperature monitoring

Therapeutic
1. L-Thyroxine, 2 μg per kilogram intravenously over five to ten minutes initially, and 100 μg intravenously every 24 hours thereafter
2. Cover to conserve body heat; do not rewarm externally
3. Tracheal intubation and mechanical ventilation as required
4. Intravenous fluids as determined by initial blood glucose and electrolytes and by the state of hydration; watch for water retention
5. Hydrocortisone, 100 mg by intravenous bolus, then 25 mg every six hours as a continuous intravenous drip
6. Vigorous treatment of associated and precipitating conditions such as infection

severely hypothyroid, and postoperative opiates or sedatives lead to clinical deterioration. In Table 228–11 are shown the important steps in management of patients with myxedema coma. In these emergent situations it is important to institute treatment immediately. If the serum free T_4 index is reduced, treatment is begun even if the cause of the hypothyroidism (primary versus secondary) has not been identified. Accordingly, testing for adrenal function is carried out immediately, followed by institution of glucocorticoid replacement. Because of the irregularities of either intramuscular or gastrointestinal absorption in hypothyroidism, medications should be given intravenously. Glucocorticoid replacement should not be given in pharmacologic quantities, since this will impair T_4 to T_3 conversion.

PROGNOSIS. The prognosis of hypothyroidism is excellent, provided that thyroid hormone replacement is maintained.

Withdrawal of Thyroid Hormone After Prolonged Replacement. The question sometimes arises as to whether thyroid hormone therapy is indicated in a patient already receiving it. If, based on the history, the physician is skeptical of the need for replacement, such a patient is instructed to discontinue the medication completely and return for serum free T_4 index and TSH determinations in three weeks. The patient is advised that there may be mild manifestations of low thyroid function and to notify the physician sooner if these become severe. Three weeks after cessation of treatment, a patient with normal thyroid function will have a low normal serum free T_4 index, but the serum TSH will not be elevated. If this correlates with the clinical symptomatology, the patient is instructed to return after a further three-week interval for repeat testing. The results after six weeks can be used as a reliable index of the underlying thyroid functional capacity. If the free T_4 index and TSH are normal at that time, one can exclude the diagnosis of significant hypothyroidism.

Bigos ST, Ridgway EC, Kourides IA, Maloof F: Spectrum of pituitary alterations with mild and severe thyroid impairment. J Clin Endocrinol Metab 46:317, 1978. *Mild decreases in serum T_4 with no changes in serum T_3 can be associated with significant increases in serum TSH in patients with modest impairment of thyroid function.*

Dussault JH, Walker P (eds.): Congenital Hypothyroidism. New York, Marcel Dekker, Inc., 1983. *A comprehensive discussion of the diagnosis and treatment of congenital hypothyroidism.*

Rees-Jones RW, Rolla AR, Larsen PR: Hormonal content of thyroid replacement preparations. JAMA 243:459, 1980. *Analyses of desiccated thyroid tablets show that some generic preparations have reduced quantities of T_4 and T_3 relative to those contained in brand-name products.*

Refetoff S: Syndromes of thyroid hormone resistance. Am J Physiol 243 (Endocrinol Metab 6):88–98, 1982. *A review of the various ways in which thyroid hormone-resistance may present and of the pathophysiology of these disorders.*

Sawin CT, Surks MI, London M, Ranganathan C, Larsen PR: Oral thyroxine: Variation in biologic action and tablet content. Ann Intern Med 100:641, 1984. *An example of one of the problems that may be encountered in the treatment of hypothyroid patients.*

Weinberg AD, Brennan MD, Gorman CA, Marsh HM, O'Fallon WM: Outcome of anesthesia and surgery in hypothyroid patients. Arch Intern Med 143:893–897, 1983. *Results of this experience at the Mayo Clinic suggest that patients with mild to moderate primary hypothyroidism withstand nonelective general surgery as well as do euthyroid patients.*

Thyroiditis

Thyroiditis is classified into three types: acute, subacute, and chronic. Despite the common factor of inflammation in all of these entities, there are marked differences in their clinical presentations and etiology.

ACUTE THYROIDITIS

Acute thyroiditis results from a bacterial infection of the thyroid gland with typical symptoms of such involvement, including a fever, local tenderness, and swelling. This condition is quite rare. The infection may involve the whole gland or only a portion of it. Laboratory studies generally show normal thyroid function, but there is an elevated leukocyte count with a polymorphonuclear predominance. The thyroid scan may show an area of decreased uptake corresponding to the involved portion, but the 24-hour RAI uptake is usually normal. Treatment of this condition requires proper identification of the causative agent and appropriate antimicrobial drugs. This may require a needle aspiration. If localized abscess formation occurs, it should be drained. The process usually responds rapidly to these measures.

SUBACUTE (NONSUPPURATIVE) THYROIDITIS

This condition is also referred to as *giant cell thyroiditis, granulomatous thyroiditis,* or *de Quervain's thyroiditis.* In the classic form of this disease the patient presents with an exquisitely tender thyroid, which is pathologically characterized by follicular cell destruction and by a lymphocytic and polymorphonuclear leukocyte infiltration, together with multinucleate giant cells. In recent years, a different type of subacute thyroiditis has appeared, which is often painless and associated with hyperthyroidism. It shares some pathologic features with Hashimoto's thyroiditis (see below). This condition, which will be denoted *subacute lymphocytic thyroiditis,* is discussed separately below because of its unique features. The disease described by de Quervain will be referred to as *subacute granulomatous thyroiditis.*

INCIDENCE. The incidence of subacute granulomatous thyroiditis is not known, but it is not rare. It is most common in the third to fifth decades, and females are affected about three to four times more commonly than males. It occurs with increased frequency in HLA-B35 positive individuals.

ETIOLOGY. The granulomatous form of subacute thyroiditis often follows a viral infection by several weeks. At the time of the acute illness, elevated titers of antibody to influenza virus, coxsackievirus, or adenovirus can be found. Over the next few months these fall in many patients, suggesting that an acute infection has recently occurred. In only two cases has a virus been cultured from thyroid tissue, which in both cases was mumps. Some authorities interpret the thyroiditis as being a consequence of a process set in motion by the viral illness but not representing a direct infection of the gland. The precise etiology is unknown.

PATHOLOGY. The classic pathologic picture includes the cellular infiltrate described above, along with severe destruction of the normal follicular architecture. Fibrosis appears in the latter phases. Despite the extensive destruction, complete restoration of the normal thyroid structure generally occurs.

CLINICAL MANIFESTATIONS. Subacute granulomatous thyroiditis is characterized by an often exquisitely painful two- to three-fold enlargement of the thyroid gland together with systemic symptoms, including fever, chills, and malaise. Patients often complain of neck or ear pain or dysphagia and may have had evaluation for pharyngeal infection. Symptoms of hyperthyroidism may also be present. The patient may report a prior viral illness. If symptoms of hyperthyroidism are present, they are generally of very short duration (less than two months) and are due to the release of thyroid hormones resulting from thyroid destruction. Physical examination may show fever, tachycardia, and exquisite tenderness of the slightly enlarged thyroid gland. This generally involves the whole gland but may be asymmetric.

DIAGNOSIS. The leukocyte count is mildly elevated, but there is characteristically a marked elevation of the erythrocyte sedimentation rate (ESR). This has been one of the hallmarks of this disease. The free T_4 index may be normal or increased. As would be expected from the pathology, the RAI uptake is low and the thyroid is poorly visualized on scan. The RAI uptake is the principal test for separating patients with this disease from those with hyperthyroidism resulting from Graves' disease. There may be an asymmetric involvement of the thyroid with decreased function in that area. Antimicrosomal and antithyroglobulin antibodies are absent or low in titer, although the serum thyroglobulin may be elevated, reflecting the destructive process.

TREATMENT. Since this is a self-limited disease, treatment is symptomatic. Mild analgesics such as aspirin (2 to 4 grams per day) should be given for neck discomfort. In a significant fraction of patients, this will not be sufficient, and prednisone, 20 to 40 mg per day, is required. The immediate relief associated with this therapy is almost diagnostic. The glucocorticoid should be continued for two to three weeks and then tapered over the next three weeks. There may be an exacerbation of the original symptoms during discontinuation of glucocorticoid requiring reinstitution of this therapy. Eventually this will not occur. The hyperthyroidism is usually mild but may require propranolol. Antithyroid drugs are of no use, as the serum T_4 and T_3 will decrease when the glandular supply is exhausted.

There may be transient hypothyroidism following subacute granulomatous thyroiditis, and this may be severe enough to require treatment in some patients. Therefore it is important for these patients to be followed closely during the recovery period to ascertain whether or not this complication has occurred. Replacement thyroxine can be discontinued after three to six months with appropriate biochemical monitoring to establish that thyroid function has returned to normal. In 5 to 10 per cent of patients, permanent hypothyroidism supervenes. Occasionally a patient will be seen initially in the hypothyroid phase of this illness. An elevation in serum TSH and low thyroid hormones in the absence of antimicrosomal or antithyroglobulin antibodies should alert the physician to this possibility.

SUBACUTE LYMPHOCYTIC THYROIDITIS

This disease has been referred to by a variety of descriptive terms, including *painless thyroiditis, lymphocytic thyroiditis, lymphocytic thyroiditis with spontaneously resolving hyperthyroidism, hyperthyroiditis,* and *atypical subacute thyroiditis.* This confused nomenclature reflects the principal clinical and pathologic features of the disease: hyperthyroidism which is self-limited, and lymphocytic infiltration of the thyroid.

ETIOLOGY. The etiology of the disease is unknown. There is little suggestion of a prior viral illness in these patients. The pathologic features are much closer to those of Hashimoto's disease than to those of granulomatous thyroiditis, suggesting an autoimmune etiology.

INCIDENCE. The precise incidence is not known, but one suspects that it has been increasing over the last five to ten years. This condition may account for 5 to 20 per cent of patients with hyperthyroidism. About two thirds of reported cases are in women, with patients ranging from 13 to over 80 years of age.

PATHOLOGY. Lymphocytic infiltration is the common feature in all specimens studied. Destruction of follicular architecture and fibrosis similar to that of subacute granulomatous thyroiditis is seen, but foreign body giant cells are rare. Germinal centers characteristic of Hashimoto's disease are rarely seen.

CLINICAL MANIFESTATIONS. The principal symptoms of this form of subacute thyroiditis are those of hyperthyroidism, as described in the section Graves' Disease and Other Causes of Hyperthyroidism. Nonthyroidal stigmata of Graves' disease, exophthalmos and pretibial myxedema, are not present, although a stare and widened palpebral fissure may occur as a consequence of the hyperthyroidism per se. The duration of the hyperthyroid phase is short (usually less than three months), and it is generally modest in severity. Physical signs include those typical of hyperthyroidism and a normal or slightly enlarged thyroid gland which is not tender. The gland may be firm.

The natural history of thyroid function in a patient who had a typical episode of this disease is presented in Figure 228–8.

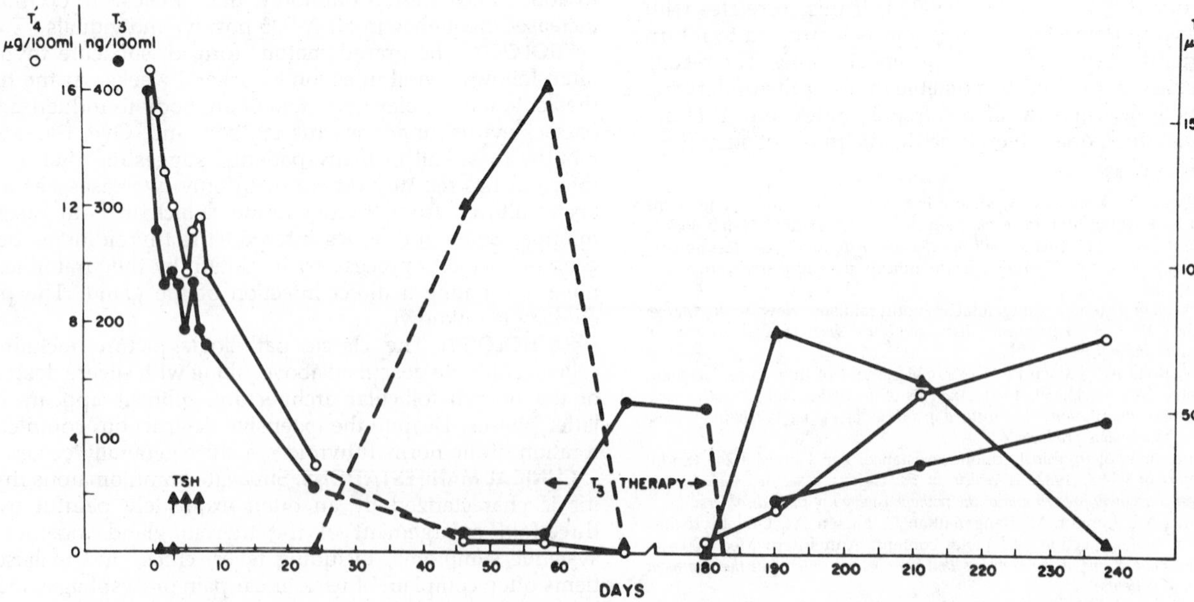

Figure 228–8. Changes in serum T_3, T_4, and TSH in a patient with subacute lymphocytic thyroiditis. The rapid decrease in serum T_3 and T_4 in the first five days is due to exhaustion of thyroidal stores as a consequence of the destructive process. Transient T_3 replacement was employed because of prolonged hypothyroidism. Normal thyroid function had returned by eight months after the initial episode. (From Larsen PR: Metabolism 23:467, 1974.)

The acute phase of hyperthyroidism resolved rapidly and spontaneously and was followed by a period of transient hypothyroidism requiring treatment. This was discontinued after three months, and, after an initial period of thyroidal resistance to TSH, normal function returned. A phase of significant hypothyroidism such as this follows the hyperthyroidism in about one third of patients. For obscure reasons, this form of thyroiditis occurs with increased frequency in the first few months postpartum.

LABORATORY DIAGNOSIS. Serum T_4 and T_3 concentrations are generally elevated, the leukocyte count normal, and the ESR normal or only slightly elevated (<50 mm at 1 hour, Westergren). This is in marked contrast to the results in the granulomatous form of the disease. The 24-hour RAI uptake is reduced and will not increase even after TSH injections. Serum thyroglobulin is elevated in the acute phase of the disease, and antimicrosomal and antithyroglobulin antibodies are usually negative or low in titer in the usual assays.

This disease must be separated from other causes of hyperthyroidism, notably Graves' disease. The best test for this is the 24-hour RAI uptake. A low uptake may occasionally also be observed in a patient with Graves' disease who has received excess iodide. This may be obvious from the history or can be eliminated by measuring the urinary iodide, which must be considerably elevated (>2 mg per 24 hours) to suppress the uptake in hyperthyroidism associated with thyroid hyperfunction. A needle biopsy will also be diagnostic. It should also be separated from Hashimoto's thyroiditis because of the difference in the natural history of these two diseases. The low antimicrosomal antibody titer will usually accomplish this, as well as the fact that hyperthyroidism is rarely seen in Hashimoto's disease. To distinguish this condition from factitious hyperthyroidism, 10 units of bovine TSH can be injected, followed in one day by a 24-hour RAI uptake. No change in the uptake is found in patients with subacute lymphocytic thyroiditis.

TREATMENT. As with subacute granulomatous thyroiditis, treatment is symptomatic. Beta-adrenergic blockade may be required for the hyperthyroid phase, but propylthiouracil is of no value except to inhibit T_4 to T_3 conversion. Glucocorticoid is not required since there is no tenderness, but more rapid resolution of the hyperthyroidism has been reported in patients given a four-week course of prednisone starting at 40 mg per day. A hypothyroid phase should be treated for three to six months, followed by withdrawal of the therapy.

PROGNOSIS. The hyperthyroid phase usually remits within a few months, and the entire history of this disease lasts less than a year. However, the potential for subsequent hypothyroidism indicates the need for annual examination of thyroid function in these patients.

CHRONIC THYROIDITIS

There are two types of chronic thyroiditis: Hashimoto's and Riedel's thyroiditis *(Riedel's struma)*.

Hashimoto's Thyroiditis

This is an apparently autoimmune disease of the thyroid gland. It appears to be closely related to Graves' disease. Synonyms for this condition are *chronic lymphocytic thyroiditis* and *lymphadenoid goiter*.

ETIOLOGY. The sera of patients with this condition contain antibodies to one or more thyroid antigens, including thyroid microsomes, thyroglobulin, or a colloid antigen which can be separated from thyroglobulin. At present it is not certain whether these antibodies are the cause or the result of this disease. The pathologic features of the condition can be reproduced in laboratory animals by immunization with thyroid tissue. However, the experimental disease is not sustained once immunizations have been discontinued, nor can the injury be induced by serum from immunized animals. Since the disease can be transferred by sensitized lymphocytes, it has been proposed that the destruction is produced by cell-mediated processes. On exposure to thyroid tissue antigens in vitro, lymphocytes of patients with Hashimoto's thyroiditis (and Graves' disease) will produce substances causing inhibition of leukocyte migration. This response is not found in patients with other forms of thyroid disease or by exposure to extracts of other tissues. Similar observations have been made in patients with idiopathic myxedema, suggesting that the atrophic thyroid found in this condition is affected by a similar process. Other evidence supporting the autoimmune hypothesis is the increased prevalence of many of the so-called autoimmune diseases in patients with Hashimoto's thyroiditis. These include Sjögren's syndrome, lupus erythematosus, idiopathic thrombocytopenic purpura, and pernicious anemia. As many as 6 per cent of patients with Hashimoto's disease have been reported to have pernicious anemia. Although rare, involvement of endocrine glands by this immunopathologic process may occur. Idiopathic Addison's disease and Hashimoto's disease may appear in the same patients. This combination is called Schmidt's syndrome (see Ch. 240). The parathyroids, the β cells of the pancreatic islets, the pituitary, and the gonads may also be involved. There are a few reports of transplacental passage of maternal thyroid antibodies leading to transient impairment of thyroid function in neonates, but such cases are the exception rather than the rule. An increased risk of the atrophic form of Hashimoto's thyroiditis is present in patients who are HLA-DR3 or HLA-B8 antigen positive.

INCIDENCE. Women are affected four to five times more frequently than men. The incidence increases with increasing age. Antimicrosomal thyroid antibodies have been found in about 10 per cent and 3 per cent of adult females and males, respectively. Ten to 20 per cent of these persons can be expected to have chemical or biochemical evidence of thyroid disease. This disease is probably the most common cause of goiter in adolescents, although the incidence is not as high as in older women.

PATHOLOGIC FINDINGS. The thyroid gland is normal or may be enlarged twofold to fivefold, depending on the degree of fibrosis. Microscopic examination reveals that varying degrees of infiltration with lymphocytes and plasma cells, fibrosis, and, in many cases, germinal centers are present. An oxyphilic change may be present in the cytoplasm of the residual thyroid follicular cells. It may be occasionally difficult to differentiate Hashimoto's disease from primary lymphoma of the thyroid gland.

CLINICAL MANIFESTATIONS. Two clinical forms of thyroid involvement are described. In the so-called atrophic form the gland is normal or reduced in size, and hypothyroidism is the prominent symptom (Table 228–9). This may well be the same syndrome as idiopathic myxedema. In other patients, variable degrees of thyroid enlargement and hypothyroidism occur, but goiter is the most common chief complaint. The gland is generally symmetrically enlarged, and often the pyramidal lobe is quite prominent, suggesting generalized hypertrophy. The thyroid is firm and may feel lobular or diffusely enlarged. Occasionally Hashimoto's disease presents as a single nodule in the thyroid gland, which represents the residual functioning thyroid tissue in a gland the remainder of which has been destroyed by this disease. The patient may have a family history of Graves' or Hashimoto's disease, pernicious anemia, or other autoimmune phenomena.

LABORATORY DIAGNOSIS. The serum free T_4 index is reduced and serum TSH elevated in many patients with this syndrome. Approximately 95 per cent of patients have positive antimicrosomal antibodies, and about 50 to 60 per cent are positive for antithyroglobulin antibodies. The PBI may be normal or elevated even in the presence of a reduced free T_4 index as a result of the presence of iodoproteins circulating in the blood. The RAI uptake may be reduced, normal, or even increased, depending on the residual thyroid cell function and the serum TSH. The thyroid scan generally reveals a heterogeneous uptake of the isotope. Occasionally a single island of functioning tissue remains. This can be differentiated from a functioning adenoma of the thyroid only by appropriate tests of thyroid function. If the diagnosis remains in doubt, a needle biopsy can be performed which will reveal the characteristic changes of lymphocytic infiltration in the majority of cases.

TREATMENT. In the early phases of Hashimoto's thyroiditis, goiter may be present, the serum TSH mildly elevated, but the free T_4 index in the lower normal range. Nevertheless, the presence of an elevated serum TSH suggests substantial decompensation of the thyroid, since in the presence of normally responsive thyroid tissue such TSH levels are quite stimulatory. Accordingly, even though the patient may have few symptoms of hypothyroidism, it is the author's practice to initiate treatment in the patient with thyroid enlargement once a secure serologic diagnosis has been established. In this way it is hoped that further thyroid enlargement and possibly surgery can be avoided. Untreated patients are also susceptible to iodide-induced myxedema and may have spontaneous fluctuation in thyroid function. Transient hypothyroidism has been noted, especially in the first few months after delivery, in women with Hashimoto's thyroiditis. More severe degrees of hypothyroidism are treated as described in the section, Hypothyroidism and Myxedema. If obstructive symptoms appear and they do not respond to TSH suppression, then surgery is required. Occasionally, the firm nature of the thyroid gland can suggest the presence of malignancy. If thyroid function is normal and there is no serologic evidence for Hashimoto's thyroiditis, then needle biopsy or surgery is required. In the younger patient, TSH suppression may cause the thyroid gland to decrease in size. On the other hand, in older subjects, particularly when fibrosis is present, little if any reduction will occur. Occasionally, Hashimoto's thyroiditis may present with hyperthyroidism ("hashitoxicosis"), which should be treated as is Graves' disease. Appropriate evaluation of the patient for the involvement of other tissues by autoimmune disease should be performed as indicated.

PROGNOSIS. The prognosis of this condition is excellent as long as thyroid hormone therapy is provided when indicated. In patients with serologic evidence of Hashimoto's thyroiditis but normal thyroid function, an annual evaluation for hypothyroidism is indicated.

Riedel's Thyroiditis

This is a rare disorder of unknown cause in which a sclerosing fibrous infiltration of the thyroid gland occurs, causing the gland to become extremely firm. As the disease progresses, local muscles in the neck and the trachea are infiltrated and hypothyroidism appears. This condition may be difficult to differentiate from carcinoma of the thyroid. It is clinically associated with both retroperitoneal fibrosis and sclerosing cholangitis. Obstruction of the trachea may occur as the fibrosis proceeds, and a surgical approach is the only satisfactory method of treatment to relieve tracheal obstruction. Glucocorticoid therapy can be beneficial to some patients.

Amino N, Mori H, Iwatani Y, Tanizawa O, Kawashima M, Tsuge I, Ibaragi K, Kumahara Y, Miyai K: High prevalence of transient post-partum thyrotoxicosis and hypothyroidism. N Engl J Med 306:14, 849–852, 1982. *A prospective survey showing a 5.5 per cent incidence of transient thyrotoxicosis or hypothyroidism post partum.*

Bartholomew LC, Cain JC, Woolner LB, et al.: Sclerosing cholangitis. Its possible association with Riedel's struma and fibrous retroperitonitis; report of two cases. N Engl J Med 269:8, 1973. *The clinical spectrum of this unusual form of thyroiditis is described.*

Nikolai TF, Brosseau J, Kettrick MA, Roberts R, Beltaos E: Lymphocytic thyroiditis with spontaneously resolving hyperthyroidism (silent thyroiditis). Arch Intern Med 140:478, 1980. *Clinical and laboratory results in 62 episodes of subacute lymphocytic thyroiditis, which these authors estimate is the cause of hyperthyroidism in 10 to 20 per cent of their patients.*

Strakosch CR, Wenzel BE, Row VV, Volpe R: Immunology of autoimmune thyroid diseases. Seminars in Medicine of the Beth Israel Hospital, Boston, N Engl J Med 307:24, 1499–1507, 1982.

Tunbridge WMG, Evered DC, Hall R, Appleton D, Brewis M, Clark F, Grimley-Evans J, Young E, Bird T, Smith PA: The spectrum of thyroid disease in a community: The Whickham survey. Clin Endocrinol 7:481, 1977. *The epidemiology of thyroid disease in an English community; this study provides a firm basis for estimates of the prevalence of Hashimoto's and Graves' disease as well as nodular goiter.*

Benign and Malignant Tumors of the Thyroid: The Solitary Thyroid Nodule

In this section are discussed those benign and malignant tumors that usually present as a solitary thyroid nodule. Multinodular goiter is discussed in the next section, Sporadic and Endemic Goiter. Virtually all tumors of the thyroid arise from glandular cells and are therefore adenomas or carcinomas. A scheme for evaluation of the patient with a solitary thyroid nodule is presented at the end of this chapter.

ETIOLOGY. The fundamental cause of thyroid tumors is unknown. However, two factors, exposure to ionizing radiation and the presence of TSH, have been found to be important for inducing thyroid tumors in animals. Similar data are available with respect to radiation exposure in man, which is responsible for an increased incidence of both benign and malignant thyroid neoplasms. A large proportion of patients presenting with thyroid carcinoma have a history of radiation delivered to the upper thorax 10 to 15 years earlier for treatment of "status thymolymphaticus," enlarged tonsils and adenoids, acne, eustachian tube dysfunction, facial hemangiomas, pertussis, and tinea capitis. In patients who receive at least 300 to 400 rads of thyroidal irradiation at less than five years of age, the incidence of thyroid carcinoma is approximately 6 per cent 10 to 20 years later. Benign thyroid tumors are about three to four times as prevalent in the same patients. For doses of external thyroid irradiation in this range, the expected incidence of carcinoma is three cases per rad per year per 1 million persons exposed. TSH stimulation per se does not appear to cause thyroid carcinoma, as this disease is not increased in areas of iodine deficiency; however, it plays a permissive role.

There are two types of familial thyroid carcinoma. The first is medullary carcinoma occurring in families with the syndrome of multiple endocrine neoplasia Type II (pheochromocytoma, parathyroid hyperplasia) or Type III (pheochromocytoma, mucosal neuroma) (Ch. 240). Papillary or follicular carcinoma may occur as part of the familial multiple hamartoma syndrome (Cowden's disease).

INCIDENCE AND PREVALENCE. Solitary thyroid nodules are common. The estimated incidence is about 1 to 3 per cent of the adult population, with a 2 to 1 preponderance of females. There is some difficulty in obtaining precise figures in this area, since a significant number of nodules which seem to be solitary by palpation are found to be dominant nodules in multinodular goiters at surgery or autopsy. Such nodules are rarely true neoplasms. The estimated incidence of thyroid nodules is 0.1 per cent per year, but since many nodules are found at autopsy that were not suspected clinically the true incidence may be higher. The incidence of thyroid carcinoma is estimated to be 36 new patients per year per 1 million persons. These two estimates would suggest that about 3 or 4 per cent of patients who develop solitary thyroid nodules have thyroid carcinoma. Many surgical series report thyroid carcinoma in from 10 to 30 per cent of resected solitary nodules, which indicates that the screening procedures employed to identify high risk patients are effective. Various autopsy series have reported an incidence of thyroid carcinoma ranging from 0.1 to 6 per cent. The higher figures are from studies in which an extremely careful search was made for microscopic carcinomas, virtually all being less than 5 mm in diameter. The clinical significance of such lesions is negligible, and this "background" of asymptomatic microscopic lesions should be kept in mind when evaluating this literature.

BENIGN NEOPLASMS

PATHOLOGY. The *follicular adenoma* is by far the most common benign thyroid tumor. It varies from microscopic to 8 to 10 cm in size and is composed of a normal-appearing thyroid epithelium arranged in a follicular structure. An intact capsule surrounds these tumors, and there is often evidence of compression of surrounding normal thyroid tissue. The follicles may range from extremely small with little colloid (*fetal adenoma* or *microfollicular adenoma*) to large distended structures (*macrofollicular adenoma*). The *embryonal* adenoma is an even more primitive-appearing structure possessing very little colloid. On occasion, the tumors may be composed of oxyphils (*oxyphil adenoma* or *Hürthle cell adenoma*). None of these differences in microscopic picture appear to bear on the functional characteristics of these nodules, nor do such nodules appear to become malignant. The hypercellular adenomas may be extremely difficult to differentiate from follicular carcinomas, especially when only a needle biopsy sample is available. Follicular adenomas have specific receptors for TSH, and these cells respond to TSH normally. However, many of these tumors do not possess the capacity for concentrating iodide or other similar substances. Since such nodules do not concentrate isotopes, they are referred to as *nonfunctioning* or *cold*.

CLINICAL MANIFESTATIONS. Thyroid adenomas fall into two categories: those that produce significant quantities of thyroid hormones, and those that do not. The latter are the more common (90 to 95 per cent). Patients with these tumors present with an asymptomatic mass in the neck. The patient may be discovered to have this tumor on routine physical examination and often is completely unaware of its existence. The tumor usually becomes palpable by the time it reaches 1 cm in diameter, but it may reach 5 to 10 cm without being noticed by the patient. Thyroid function studies in patients with nonfunctioning follicular adenomas are normal, and the thyroid scan will generally reveal an area of decreased or absent uptake of $^{123}I^-$ or $^{99m}TcO_4^-$ (a "cold" nodule). The precise diagnosis can be made only by obtaining a tissue specimen by aspiration biopsy, cutting needle biopsy (Vim-Silverman needle or its equivalent), or excision of the nodule. As these nodules may outgrow their blood supply, cystic degeneration may occur. Ultrasonography of such a lesion will reveal a cystic cavity within the nodule.

Functioning follicular adenomas may present with or without symptoms of hyperthyroidism, largely depending on their size. Lesions over 3 cm in diameter tend to cause thyrotoxicity and constitute about 50 per cent of these adenomas in patients 60 years and older. T_3 thyrotoxicosis was found in 46 per cent of such patients in one large series. More commonly, the patient is asymptomatic and a thyroid scan shows that the only area concentrating radioactivity is the nodule itself. Such patients generally have normal or high-normal serum thyroid hormone levels, and TRH infusion will not cause TSH release. Such nodules are functioning autonomously at a rate sufficient to suppress TSH synthesis in the pituitary (hence the lack of function in the remainder of the thyroid) but not at a sufficiently high level as to cause metabolic hyperthyroidism. It is the author's practice to categorize functional lesions which have suppressed TSH synthesis but not caused hyperthyroidism as *warm* nodules, whereas those associated with hyperthyroidism are called *hot* nodules. Assessment of the thyroid functional state is necessary for proper evaluation of these lesions since the thyroid scan is identical. This is especially important since Hashimoto's disease may present as a solitary focus of functioning thyroid tissue, as may congenital absence of one lobe of the thyroid. The presence of potentially functioning thyroid tissue can be demonstrated by injection of 10 units of bovine TSH, followed in 24 hours by a thyroid scan. Unlike multinodular goiters, follicular adenomas of the thyroid rarely grow large enough to cause significant physical encroachment on the trachea or esophagus.

TREATMENT. The finding of an autonomously functioning nodule virtually eliminates the diagnosis of thyroid carcinoma. Treatment at that point depends on the thyroid status. If the patient is euthyroid (a warm thyroid nodule), nothing more than an annual follow-up with appropriate thyroid function tests (including a serum T_3) need be performed. In the hyperthyroid patient, surgery or ^{131}I is available for definitive treatment, although antithyroid drugs may be necessary to control symptomatic hyperthyroidism prior to definitive therapy. The choice of treatment depends on the age of the patient and the size of the nodule. In patients under the age of 20, surgical resection should be performed, as the radiation delivered to extranodular tissue after radioiodine therapy may reach a level which is considered carcinogenic. In older patients with cosmetically disfiguring lesions or those which are compressing vital structures in the neck, surgery is also preferred. For the rest, ^{131}I is indicated. The author attempts to deliver 10 mCi of ^{131}I into the nodule. Following either surgery or radioactive iodine treatment, a period of four to six weeks is required for re-establishment of pituitary TSH secretion, following which function of the previously suppressed normal thyroid tissue should occur. The patient may need to receive thyroxine supplementation during this interim period but may not require indefinite replacement. The approach to the *nonfunctioning thyroid nodule* is described below under The Solitary Nodule.

MALIGNANT THYROID TUMORS

There are four common malignancies of thyroid tissue. About 50 per cent of thyroid carcinomas are pure papillary or mixed papillary-follicular carcinoma, 25 per cent follicular carcinoma, 15 per cent undifferentiated carcinoma, and 10 per cent medullary carcinoma. The last-named disorder is a tumor of the thyrocalcitonin-producing C cells and has no relationship to thyroid follicular epithelium.

PATHOLOGY AND NATURAL HISTORY. *Papillary carcinoma* is the most benign and the most common form of thyroid carcinoma. It is two to three times more common in women than in men and occurs with equal frequency in the third to seventh decades. Since the less well-differentiated forms of carcinoma increase with age, papillary carcinoma is the most common thyroid malignancy in younger patients. The size of these tumors varies from microscopic to several centimeters in diameter. Of the clinically apparent variety, the *occult* tumors (defined as those less than 1.5 cm in diameter) are differentiated from the *intrathyroidal* tumors, which are larger but do not extend through the thyroid surface. The tumor is classified as *extrathyroidal* if it extends through the thyroid capsule and involves surrounding tissues. Microscopically, papillary carcinoma consists of well-differentiated thyroid epithelium covering papillary fibrovascular stalks. The nuclei are frequently clear, as opposed to the denser appearance of normal nuclei. A virtually pathognomonic feature in about 40 per cent of papillary thyroid carcinomas is the so-called *psammoma body*. These calcific globules are 5 to 100 microns in diameter and are often present in the tips of the papillary projections. Their etiology is unknown, but their presence in the thyroid tumor raises the high likelihood of its carcinomatous nature. Cervical lymphatic involvement even with occult thyroid tumors is common, occurring in as many as 50 per cent. Blood-borne metastases are uncommon. The presence or absence of lymph node metastases does not seem to alter the prognosis. In a large series studied at the Mayo Clinic, the 20-year survival of patients with occult or intrathyroid papillary carcinoma was not significantly different from that of a control group. However, the 20-year survival for patients with extrathyroidal carcinoma was about 40 per cent, and this dropped to 20 per cent over the next ten years. Many thyroid cancers have areas of follicular as well as papillary structure, and blood-borne metastases may appear which have a follicular pattern even though the primary tumor is papillary. Thus, many predominantly papillary tumors have follicular elements, but the biologic behavior of these lesions seems to be a function of the predominant microscopic appearance.

Follicular carcinomas also are more common in women than in men but tend to increase in incidence with increasing age.

The tumors vary from well-differentiated, virtually normal appearing thyroid tissue to nearly solid sheets of follicular epithelium with little evidence of follicle formation. The former are differentiated from follicular adenomas only by demonstration of capsular and vascular invasion. Such a diagnosis generally cannot be made without the entire nodule for examination, and even at frozen section the carcinomatous nature of the lesion may not be recognized. Cyst formation may occur as it does in benign follicular tumors, and calcification may occur centrally. Follicular carcinomas tend to metastasize via blood vessel invasion and not, in general, via lymphatics. Metastases may not be evident at the time of initial evaluation but may appear years later despite apparent complete excision of the tumor. It is not unusual for the follicular carcinoma to concentrate radioiodine, although it does so considerably less well than does normal thyroid tissue. Thus, it is only in the absence of normal thyroid tissue and in the presence of an elevated TSH that this potential is appreciated. However, it is useful in treatment in some of these tumors (see below). Patients who have had removal of well-encapsulated, noninvasive follicular carcinomas appear to have a normal life span. On the other hand, patients with tumors which show extensive local involvement and angioinvasion at the time of initial surgery have an approximately 30 per cent ten-year survival, which is decreased to less than 20 per cent at 20 years.

The most aggressive form of thyroid carcinoma, *anaplastic carcinoma,* may appear in either small cell or giant cell varieties. The small cell carcinoma may resemble a lymphoma. The cells have a uniform appearance, often having a fibrous stroma but no amyloid. The giant-cell variety, also called a spindle-cell or carcinosarcoma, is the most highly malignant tumor of the thyroid gland. It is found almost exclusively in patients over the age of 60. The average prognosis from diagnosis to death in the giant cell tumors is less than six months, whereas patients with small cell carcinoma may have five-year survival of 20 to 25 per cent. Both tend to extend locally and often cause tracheal obstruction. Distant metastases may occur with either type.

Medullary carcinoma of the thyroid is a malignant tumor of the C cell and produces thyrocalcitonin. Its occurrence in association with multiple endocrine neoplasia syndromes has been mentioned. It may also occur spontaneously. These tumors are characterized by sheets of tumor cells separated by a hyaline-amyloid–containing stroma. The amyloid is formed by the tumor cells and deposited in the stroma. The tumors may also produce ACTH, prostaglandin, or carcinoembryonic antigen. In familial syndromes, the penetrance of this tumor is complete, so that screening of family members is indicated by use of calcium and/or pentagastrin infusions to stimulate thyrocalcitonin release from pathologic cells (see Ch. 247).

CLINICAL MANIFESTATIONS AND DIAGNOSIS OF THYROID CARCINOMA—THE SOLITARY NODULE. The approach to the patient with a solitary thyroid nodule is a matter of considerable disagreement among clinicians. For some, thyroid carcinoma is sufficiently serious to require a surgical approach to all potentially carcinomatous lesions; others feel that considerable selection should be used prior to surgery. The benign nature of the common forms of thyroid carcinoma and the relatively large number of benign nodules make a conservative approach rational. There are several clinical characteristics which dictate an open surgical approach to a nonfunctioning thyroid nodule. This includes a history of prior irradiation. Nodules in such patients carry a 20 to 25 per cent risk of carcinoma. A history of rapid growth, evidence of recurrent nerve paresis, obvious involvement of lymph nodes, or fixation of the nodule to surrounding tissues should also lead to serious consideration of immediate surgery. Statistically, the risk of a solitary cold nodule being malignant is higher in a male than in a female, since benign disease of the thyroid is much more common in females. Thyroid nodules in children are more likely to be carcinoma than those in adults.

In the absence of specific signs pointing to a diagnosis of thyroid carcinoma, there are two avenues of approach (Fig. 228–9*A* and 9*B*). If there is no obvious thyroid dysfunction (either hyperthyroidism or hypothyroidism) and an experienced cytopathologist is available, a needle aspiration can be performed (Fig. 228–9*A*). If the lesion is a simple cyst this will be curative; otherwise the cytologic report guides therapy. If carcinoma is found, then surgical exploration is indicated. If a cellular follicular aspirate is obtained that is consistent with a benign or a malignant lesion, then a ^{123}I (or ^{131}I) scan is performed. If the lesion is hypofunctional, again surgical exploration is advised. If it is warm or hot, then management is as discussed earlier under autonomous nodules. If the aspirate is benign, thyroxine replacement is given and the patient followed at six-month intervals. The need for surgery is then determined by the natural history of the individual case. Much experience with aspiration biopsy cytology has shown that false-positive results are very rare, and false-negative results, that is, a benign diagnosis in a patient with a malignant lesion, should occur in only 2 to 3 per cent of patients. This figure, however, may be higher during the early experience with this technique in a given center. In most clinics, aspiration cytology has reduced the apparent need for surgical exploration by 50 to 60 per cent. In other words, approximately 40 per cent of patients with solitary nodules will require surgical exploration because of frankly or suspiciously malignant lesions.

If a trained cytopathologist is not available, then a thyroid scan is performed followed by ultrasonography if the nodule is not hyperfunctioning (Fig. 228–9*B*). Rarely a malignant nodule will be warm by $^{99m}TcO_4^-$ but cold by iodine scan. This should be suspected and tested for when warm lesions do not suppress function in the remainder of the gland. Ultrasonography of hypofunctioning nodules is performed. A cystic lesion can be treated by aspiration and the procedure repeated twice more if the fluid reaccumulates before surgery is indicated. In the nonfunctioning solid nodule, needle aspiration cytology, cutting needle biopsy, or surgical exploration is advised. The author recommends surgical excision for patients under 20, for all males, and for those high risk patients with familial carcinoma and radiation exposure. The availability of experienced thyroid surgeons plays an important role in this approach, since serious morbidity attends inadvertent resection of the parathyroid glands or recurrent laryngeal nerve paresis. In older women and men in whom other illnesses make surgery less desirable, a diagnosis may be obtained by needle biopsy or aspiration cytology.

If these techniques are not available, the patient may be given a trial of thyroxine replacement for a period of three to six months and any change in the size of the nodule noted. Continuing enlargement in the presence of TSH suppression is an indication for surgical intervention or at least a biopsy, whereas reduction of the nodule size, although rare, is gratifying. Maintenance of the same nodule size usually justifies a continued conservative approach. If needle biopsy confirms a benign lesion, then thyroxine suppression is provided and surgery employed only if the nodule becomes physically symptomatic. Patients who have had a lobectomy should receive thyroxine replacement. The prognosis of these lesions is excellent with no evidence of malignant degeneration.

A frozen section should be performed on all solitary thyroid nodules and an attempt made to provide definitive treatment at the time of initial surgery. A reasonable approach to intrathyroidal papillary carcinoma is to perform a lobectomy with isthmectomy and explore for and remove any involved lymph nodes. An examination of the other lobe should be made for tumor, but, except in the irradiated patient, bilateral lobectomy is not required. With extrathyroidal extension of papillary carcinoma and bilateral lymph node metastases, a total thyroidectomy is performed with great care to preserve the recurrent laryngeal nerves and parathyroid glands. A follicular carcinoma is approached as are the papillary lesions, with the exception that the presence of distant lymph node metastases or extensive capsular and vascular invasion in the initial frozen section

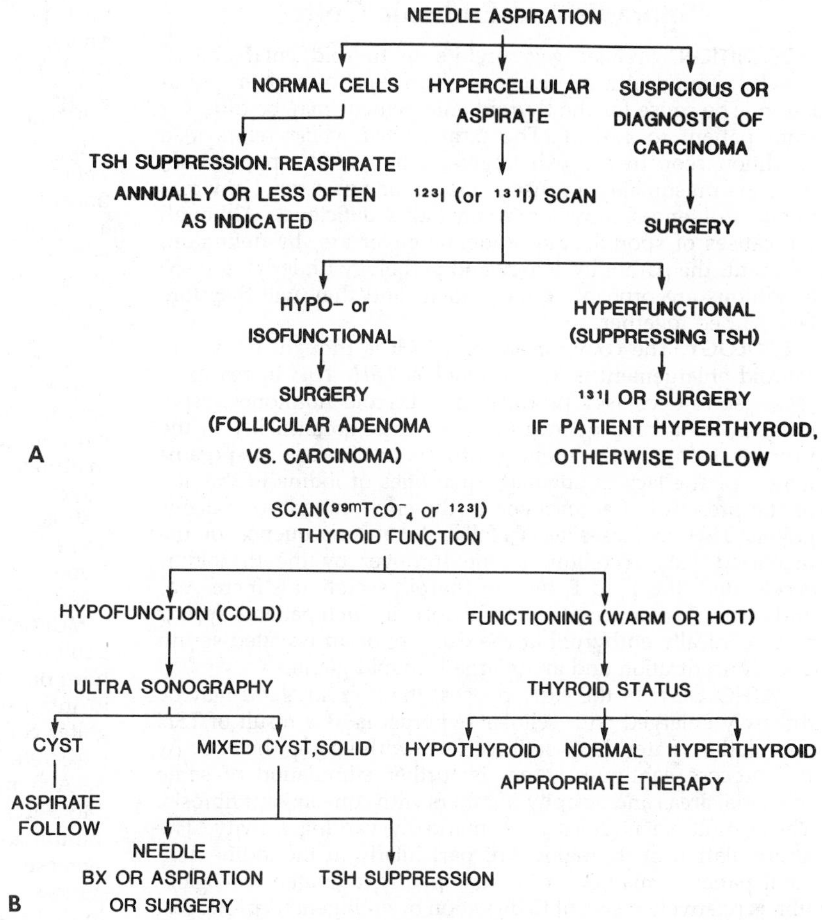

Figure 228–9. Panel *A* shows a schema for the diagnostic evaluation of a patient with a solitary thyroid nodule based on aspiration biopsy cytology. Panel *B* presents an alternative solution to the same problem starting with a thyroid scintiscan.

should lead to consideration of bilateral thyroidectomy. This is done to remove residual normal tissue to facilitate radioiodine therapy (see below). Radical neck dissection does not offer any advantage over the less-mutilating procedures described above. Medullary carcinoma of the sporadic variety may be treated as papillary carcinoma, but the familial form requires bilateral lobectomy. It is, of course, important to determine that pheochromocytoma and hyperparathyroidism are not present before undertaking surgery. Anaplastic carcinoma is rarely restricted enough to lend itself to surgical therapy with the exception of palliation to prevent tracheal compression.

RADIATION THERAPY. I^- may be concentrated to a sufficient degree as to be useful by as many as 50 to 60 per cent of well-differentiated thyroid tumors. This can be demonstrated only after the establishment of hypothyroidism with an elevation of serum TSH. In general, prophylactic therapy with radioiodine in patients with papillary carcinoma does not appear to be beneficial, although metastases may respond to this modality. In follicular carcinoma with evidence of vascular invasion or in patients with follicular metastases, particularly to the lungs, significant amelioration of symptoms and dramatic changes in the x-ray picture may be associated with this therapy. It does not appear to be as useful for patients with bone metastases. To be weighed against these beneficial effects is the increased incidence of leukemia in patients treated with large doses of ^{131}I (300 mCi and more).

The usual approach to evaluation of the feasibility of this therapeutic modality is to remove residual functioning thyroid tissue surgically or by ^{131}I administration. After this, the patient is switched to triiodothyronine (50 μg per day) for a period of approximately three weeks, following which the hormone is discontinued. Within two to three weeks, most patients will show the maximal uptake in metastatic tissue. At that time, a tracer dose of ^{131}I should be given with appropriate dosimetry of the tumor mass, bone marrow, and lungs. Following this, the maximal tolerable ^{131}I dose should be given and the patient started on TSH-suppressive therapy with thyroxine one day later. Local recurrences of papillary carcinoma can often be treated surgically by removal of involved lymph nodes. In such patients this is preferable to ^{131}I, which should be reserved for a nonresectable lesion.

Despite the poor function of thyroid tumors in terms of radioiodine trapping, carcinomatous thyroid cells have TSH receptors and respond to TSH in vitro. Accordingly, considerable effort should be made to suppress TSH to undetectable levels. A useful technique for verification that this has occurred is to perform a TRH stimulation test periodically. There should be no response. In patients who have had total thyroidectomy, serum thyroglobulin measurements may be a useful parameter of recurrence and activity of the tumor tissue.

Favus NJ, Schneider AB, Stachura ME, Arnold JE, Ryo UY, Pinsky SM, Colman M, Arnold MJ, Frohman LA: Thyroid cancer occurring as a late consequence of head and neck irradiation. N Engl J Med 294:1019, 1976. *Evaluation of roughly 1000 patients who received tonsillar or pharyngeal irradiation in childhood. The data demonstrate the increased prevalence of thyroid carcinoma in this group.*

Kaplan MM, Garnick MB, Gelber R, Li FP, Cassady JR, Sallan SE, Fine WE, Sack MJ: Risk factors for thyroid abnormalities after neck irradiation for childhood cancer. Am J Med 74:272–280, 1983. *This study shows that both benign and malignant thyroid nodules, as well as hypothyroidism, may appear 5 to 35 years after therapeutic irradiation to the neck.*

Lowhagen T, Granberg PO, Lundell G, Skinnari P, Sundblad R, Willems JS: Aspiration biopsy cytology (ABC) in nodules of the thyroid gland suspected to be malignant. Surg Clin North Am 59:3–18, 1979. *A study of the correlation between surgical and aspiration biopsy cytology diagnoses in more than 400 patients with solitary thyroid nodules.*

Mazzaferri EL, Young RL: Papillary thyroid carcinoma: A 10 year follow-up report of the impact of therapy in 576 patients. Am J Med 70:511–518, 1981. *An update of a large retrospective evaluation of the results of various treatment modalities in patients with well-differentiated thyroid carcinoma.*

Van Herle AJ, Rich P, Ljung, BME, Ashcraft MW, Solomon DH, Keeler EB: The thyroid nodule. Ann Intern Med 96:221–232, 1982. *A critical evaluation of the various approaches that can be used for patients with thyroid nodules.*

Sporadic and Endemic Goiter

DEFINITION. *Sporadic goiter* refers to thyroid enlargement, which is found in a relatively small fraction of a given population. The cause for the thyroid enlargement may be different from patient to patient. The term *endemic goiter* refers to a condition seen in a much larger fraction of the population, which is presumably a consequence of one or several environmental influences, most commonly iodine deficiency. Although the causes of sporadic and endemic goiter are, by definition, different, the pathophysiology and pathology underlying these conditions are probably quite similar, and they will therefore be grouped together.

ETIOLOGY. The common factor which is thought to lead to thyroid enlargement is *hypersecretion of TSH*. TSH increases in response to decreased production of thyroid hormones, especially T_4, as a consequence of an intrinsic abnormality in the process of thyroid hormone synthesis in the case of sporadic goiter, or the lack of adequate quantities of iodine in the diet or the presence of a goitrogen in the environment in endemic goiter. TSH increases as T_4 falls. As a consequence of the increased TSH secretion, iodine turnover by the thyroid is accelerated, the T_3 to T_4 ratio in thyroid secretion is increased, and serum T_3 may remain entirely normal. Such patients appear to be clinically euthyroid at the expense of an elevated serum TSH concentration and an enlarged thyroid gland.

PATHOLOGY. In the early phases, the thyroid gland may be diffusely enlarged with cellular hyperplasia as a result of TSH stimulation. Later, large follicles form with low epithelium. As the process continues, there is further stimulation of some thyroidal areas and atrophy of others with concomitant fibrosis. These multiple nodules have markedly varying activity. The accumulation of thyroglobulin, particularly in the iodine-deficient patients, may occur because poorly iodinated thyroglobulin is relatively resistant to digestion by endogenous proteases. To some extent, the same phenomenon may be occurring in the multinodular goiters which are sporadic and in which a specific cause has not been identified.

SPORADIC GOITER

Sporadic goiter affects about 5 per cent of the population in the United States. Females outnumber males by a 3:1 ratio. In some patients an enzymatic defect in one of the steps in thyroid hormone synthesis can be identified (see Fig. 228–2). However, in most patients no specific cause can be isolated, but it is possible that milder forms of similar enzymatic deficiencies may be present.

CONGENITAL GOITER. This condition is sometimes referred to as *sporadic cretinism.* This term refers to the syndrome of infantile myxedema characterized by growth failure, mental retardation, diffuse myxedema, and many of the signs and symptoms of hypothyroidism outlined in the section Hypothyroidism and Myxedema. Goitrous hypothyroidism can be due to a defect in any of the steps leading to the formation of thyroid hormone synthesis already discussed in the Introduction. Defects have been identified in (1) iodide transport; (2) organification of iodide due to reduction in or absence of peroxidase, to an abnormal enzyme, or to diminished peroxide generation; (3) synthesis of an abnormal thyroglobulin molecule; (4) a structural abnormality in peroxidase, impairing its function as an iodine acceptor; (5) abnormal interrelationships of iodotyrosine; (6) impaired thyroglobulin proteolysis; and, lastly, (7) a defect in iodotyrosine deiodination. The numbers given refer to the specific steps shown in Fig. 228–2. In some disorders of thyroglobulin synthesis the formation of an iodinated albumin-like protein has been described. All of these defects are rare. In North America and Europe, they constitute less than 10 per cent of the approximately 1 in 4000 infants with congenital hypothyroidism.

A detailed description of each of these various defects is beyond the scope of this general text. The most common defect is the inability to organify iodine. (defects in steps 2, 3, or 4). Such patients accumulate large amounts of I^- in the thyroid. This can be demonstrated by performance of a *perchlorate* (*ClO_4^-*) *discharge test.* If organification of I^- is defective, it is only the I^- trapping mechanism which keeps I^- in the thyroid cell. The ClO_4^- ion is concentrated by the same mechanism as is I^-, and in large quantities it will completely block the I^- trap. Therefore, if 500 mg of $NaClO_4$ is given one to two hours after tracer I^-, a marked decrease in thyroidal radioactivity will occur as the trapped I^- leaves the thyroid. In normal persons there will be no change in this parameter, since the tracer I^- has already been incorporated into protein. In some patients this condition has been found in association with eighth nerve deafness and has the eponym *Pendred's syndrome.*

Regardless of the specific defect, these patients present with goiter and hypothyroidism, the serum T_4 index is reduced, and serum TSH is elevated. Further evaluation for the type of biochemical defect requires careful laboratory investigation. The treatment of such patients is with exogenous thyroid hormone. Thyroxine treatment will cause regression of the enlarged thyroid, and mental retardation may be ameliorated or prevented if treatment is started before three months of age. Genetic counseling is desirable so that these patients will be aware of the risk of hypothyroidism in subsequent offspring.

MULTINODULAR GOITER IN THE ADULT. The hypothesis that adults with multinodular goiter have mild defects in thyroid hormone synthesis similar to the more complete forms found in infants remains to be proved. If this is the case, then the goiter could be explained by modest increases in TSH, which is secreted by the pituitary in response to the reduced serum T_4. A significant physiologic increase in TSH may be as little as 2 to 3 μU per milliliter, often below the sensitivity of the TSH immunoassay which is clinically available. The compensatory increase in the size of the thyroid gland under these circumstances results in adequate rates of thyroid hormone formation, so that the vast majority of patients with this abnormality are euthyroid.

CLINICAL MANIFESTATIONS. Patients with multinodular goiter may come to the physician because of respiratory obstruction or dysphagia. More often, the patient is asymptomatic and the enlarged multinodular thyroid is discovered on a routine physical examination. Such patients should be questioned carefully for symptoms of respiratory obstruction. The goiter often extends retrosternally; this may be demonstrated by having the patient extend the arms directly over the head. If a significant substernal goiter is present, jugular venous distention and suffusion of the face occurs *(Pemberton's sign).* Aside from physical obstruction, the most significant clinical aspect of the multinodular goiter is the tendency for hyperthyroidism to develop late in life *(Plummer's disease).* It is postulated that after decades of stimulation by TSH one or more of the nodular hyperplastic areas become autonomous. Since this condition generally appears in the elderly patient, the resulting hyperthyroidism may be of the apathetic variety (see the section Graves' Disease and Other Causes of Hyperthyroidism). In one series, administration of 50 to 100 mg of KI per day to eight patients with multinodular goiter resulted in hyperthyroidism in four patients, which required definitive treatment. The etiology of this form of iodide-induced thyrotoxicosis (probably not Jod-Basedow) is not clear, but caution is needed in administration of iodides to patients with multinodular goiter.

LABORATORY DIAGNOSIS. The physician must investigate both the anatomic and the functional nature of the thyroid pathology. Anatomic information is gained predominantly by chest and esophageal radiography and by scintiscan. ^{131}I is recommended for thyroid scanning of these patients since the γ rays emitted by $^{99m}TcO_4^-$ and $^{123}I^-$ may not be strong enough to penetrate the sternum. The scintiscan image shows patchy focal uptake of radioactivity in an enlarged thyroid gland. The significance of the nonfunctioning areas in such scintiscans is discussed below. Measurements of serum free T_4 index, T_3, TSH, and antimicrosomal and antithyroglobulin antibodies should be obtained, expecially since Hashimoto's thyroiditis may present as a multinodular goiter. A TRH test is indicated if Plummer's disease is suspected.

TREATMENT. The proper treatment depends on the clinical manifestations in the individual patient. Hyperthyroidism associated with multinodular goiter is best treated with radioactive iodine. However, because of the heterogeneity of the tissue uptake of radioiodine, a larger dose of radioiodine will be necessary (180 μCi per gram) or 10 mCi in a typical gland. The not uncommon coexistence of cardiac or pulmonary disease in this age group, together with the large size of the thyroid gland and the possibility of radiation thyroiditis, has led the author to pretreat most elderly hyperthyroid patients with antithyroid drugs prior to radiotherapy. The antithyroid drugs are discontinued approximately four to five days prior to treatment. If a high plasma I^- (low RAI uptake) does not permit the use of radioiodine, then surgical treatment must be undertaken after appropriate preparation with antithyroid drugs.

Hypothyroid patients require treatment with thyroxine as described in the section Hypothyroidism and Myxedema. Young euthyroid patients with diffuse thyroid enlargement may be started on thyroxine replacement therapy to suppress TSH, particularly if this is slightly elevated. One may block further thyroid enlargement by this treatment as well as cause regression of goiter in some. In patients over the age of 40, it is unlikely that a significant amelioration in physical symptoms will occur with TSH suppression, but this hormone may be administered on a trial basis. Great care must be exercised, particularly in the elderly, since one or more of the hyperplastic thyroid nodules may be functioning autonomously. In such circumstances, well-meaning attempts to suppress TSH can cause iatrogenic hyperthyroidism. If physical symptoms of obstruction are present or there is evidence of recurrent laryngeal nerve dysfunction, then surgical treatment is generally in order.

The Multinodular Goiter and Thyroid Carcinoma. Nodular disease of the thyroid is common and thyroid carcinoma is relatively rare. Poorly functioning areas may be present in the thyroid scintiscans of multinodular goiters, but this is not an indication for surgery for malignant disease. As heterogeneity of function is the rule, other criteria must be employed for recognition of malignancy in the multinodular goiter. Factors which raise this possibility include previous exposure to therapeutic thyroidal irradiation in childhood, a family history of thyroid carcinoma or enlargement of cervical lymph nodes, recurrent laryngeal nerve palsy, or the continuing enlargement of a single "cold" nodule in an otherwise stable gland. In situations in which doubt exists, needle biopsy may provide the requisite microscopic diagnosis to reassure the patient and the physician that conservative therapy is the appropriate course of action.

PROGNOSIS. Patients with euthyroid multinodular goiter should have thyroid function and physical findings evaluated at annual intervals. Most do not require surgery.

ENDEMIC GOITER

Iodine deficiency is the most common cause of thyroid disease in the world population, although iodination of salt has eliminated this problem in North America. Areas in which iodine intake remains low include mountainous regions such as the Andes and Himalayas. In addition, there are areas of endemic goiter in Central Africa, New Guinea, and Indonesia. Iodine prophylaxis, either in foodstuffs or in the form of iodized oil injection, has been successful in many of these countries, but iodine deficiency remains a considerable public health problem. In a few geographical locations, ingestion of a goitrogen has been implicated in the high incidence of goiter. Examples include a thiocyanate derivative from the cassava, which is eaten in large quantities in central Africa, and a goitrogenic hydrocarbon found in the water supply in parts of Colombia and in Chile.

CLINICAL MANIFESTATIONS IN ADULTS. The minimal quantity of iodine required for normal thyroid function is approximately 100 μg per day. As the level of iodine in the diet decreases below this level, there is a progressive fall in serum T_4 and a progressive rise in serum TSH. Serum T_3 concentrations remain normal or slightly elevated, a persistently elevated TSH being required for this compensation. Serum TSH concentrations may exceed 100 μU per milliliter. In the presence of lifelong stimulation of this degree, enormous hypertrophy and hyperplasia of the thyroid gland can occur. Such glands may weigh 1 to 5 kg, producing considerable physical impairment.

EFFECTS OF IODINE DEFICIENCY IN INFANTS. In areas of endemic goiter, cretinism is not uncommon. Despite the capacity of the placenta to transport I^-, in areas where iodine intake is severely reduced (25 μg per day or less) the 24-hour maternal RAI uptake is virtually 100 per cent. Infants in these areas may be born with congenital hypothyroidism as a consequence of iodine deficiency. The central nervous system may obtain a considerable portion of intracellular T_3 via conversion of T_4 to T_3 within this tissue rather than from the circulating T_3 in the serum. Although a normal serum T_3 may provide adequate levels of intracellular T_3 to tissues such as the muscles, liver, and kidney, the central nervous system, like the pituitary gland, may not be replete if T_4 is reduced and serum T_3 normal.

In areas such as the Andes or New Guinea where iodine intake may be less than 20 μg per day, a different form of *endemic cretinism* may be seen. As opposed to dwarfism and mental retardation, some children in these areas have spastic diplegia, squint, and deafness. The etiology of this syndrome is still not clarified. It may be a manifestation of the effect of iodine deficiency per se on the embryologic development of the central nervous system. Fetal or maternal hypothyroidism as a consequence of severe iodine deficiency may also contribute to this problem.

TREATMENT. The treatment of iodine deficiency is to supply this element either as a food additive or by direct injections of iodinated oil. This has often been difficult because of the inaccessibility and restricted governmental resources of those countries in which iodine deficiency is a problem. The *Jod-Basedow phenomenon* (iodine-induced hyperthyroidism) will occur in some patients receiving iodine supplementation. These presumably are individual patients with underlying Graves' (Basedow's) disease who are suddenly given adequate supplies of the substrate for thyroid hormone synthesis.

Lever EG, Medeiros-Neto GA, DeGroot LJ: Inherited disorders of thyroid metabolism. Endocr Rev 4:213–239, 1983. *A modern comprehensive review of this topic.*

Stanbury JB, Dumont JE: Familial goiter and related disorders. *In* Stanbury JB, Wyngaarden JB, Fredrickson DS, Goldstein JG, Brown MS (eds.): The Metabolic Basis of Inherited Disease. 5th ed. New York, McGraw-Hill Book Company, 1983, pp. 231–269. *A thorough review of the literature in this area with 327 references. The emphasis is on the emzymology of pathogenesis.*

Stanbury JB, Hetzel BS (eds.): Endemic goiter and endemic cretinism. New York, John Wiley & Sons, 1980. *A detailed discussion of the current state of this worldwide problem by many authorities.*

Thilly CH, Delange F, Lagasse R, Bourdoux P, Ramioul L, Berquist H, Ermans AM: Fetal hypothyroidism and maternal thyroid status in severe endemic goiter. J Clin Endocrinol Metab 47:354, 1978. *The effects of iodine deficiency on mother and newborn are described, comparing treated and untreated patients.*

Wolff J: Congenital goiter with defective iodide transport. Endocr Rev 4:240–254, 1983. *The clinical, pathophysiological and biochemical findings in patients with this form of sporadic goiter.*

229. DISORDERS OF THE ADRENAL CORTEX

J. Blake Tyrrell and John D. Baxter

Structure and Development of the Adrenal Cortex

John D. Baxter

The major function of the adrenal cortex is to provide glucocorticoid and mineralocorticoid hormones, of which cortisol and aldosterone, respectively, are the most important in man. The glucocorticoids, named for their carbohydrate-regulating properties, are essential for survival, at least in times of stress, and regulate intermediary metabolism, hemodynamic functions, and developmental processes. The mineralocorticoids regulate sodium, potassium, and hydrogen ion balance, and secondarily affect the blood pressure. Either an excess or deficiency of these steroids can have deleterious effects. Glucocorticoid excess and deficiency are termed Cushing's syndrome and Addison's disease, respectively. Aldosterone excess and deficiency are referred to as aldosteronism and hypoaldosteronism, respectively. Whereas diseases of the adrenal cortex are relatively uncommon, their clinical stigmata are part of the differential diagnosis of common problems. In addition, iatrogenic glucocorticoid excess is a common clinical problem due to the widespread usage of glucocorticoids in therapy. Secondary hyperaldosteronism is also a common problem requiring antimineralocorticoid therapy.

In addition to these two steroids the human adrenal cortex produces at least 50 other steroids. This gland is a major source of androgenic steroids in the female (Ch. 236), although in the male (Ch. 234) the importance of androgens produced by the adrenal is trivial compared to those produced by the testes. The adrenal produces only minute quantities of estrogens and progestins. Some of these steroids ordinarily produced in physiologically insignificant quantities can result in clinical abnormalities when they are produced in excess in certain pathologic states.

STRUCTURE. There are two adrenal glands, located extraperitoneally at the upper poles of each kidney lateral to the eleventh thoracic to first lumbar vertebrae. The right gland tends to be higher and more lateral than the left. The average gland weighs 4 grams and is 2 to 3 cm wide and 4 to 6 cm long. A series of small arteries arising from the abdominal aorta, renal and phrenic arteries, and occasionally from ovarian or spermatic arteries, feed the gland. Because of this, arterial infarction is unusual. The venous drainage of the gland on the left is ordinarily into the renal vein and on the right into the inferior vena cava. The gland is innervated by autonomic fibers whose roles in regulation are not understood.

The adrenal cortex comprises about 90 per cent of the gland and surrounds the centrally located medulla that produces catecholamines. The cortex has three zones. The zona glomerulosa, about 15 per cent of the cortex, is ill defined and present in foci under the capsule, contains cells with a small cytoplasmic volume and lipid content, and produces aldosterone. The remainder of the cortex, the zonae reticularis and fasciculata, can be considered as a single unit involved predominantly in cortisol and androgen production. Cells of the zona fasciculata, about 25 per cent of the cortex, appear vacuolated or clear on stained sections because of their high cholesterol content. By contrast, cells of the inner zone, the zona reticularis, are more compact with less lipid, and are responsible for basal cortisol production.

The morphology of the gland can be influenced by ACTH, angiotensin II, and potassium. Elevations of ACTH levels increase adrenal blood flow within minutes and combined weight within hours; the clear fasciculata cells lose their fat, attain the compact morphology and ultrastructural features of reticularis cells, and produce cortisol. With prolonged stimulation there is hyperplasia and hypertrophy that can double the adrenal weight. Similar increases in angiotensin II and potassium result in hypertrophy and hyperplasia of the glomerulosa cells and increased aldosterone production. With deficiency of angiotensin II there is atrophy of the zona glomerulosa and with deficiency of ACTH there is atrophy of the zonae fasciculata-reticularis; this is reversible upon restimulation. Occasionally, accessory adrenal glands may be present in a variety of locations in the abdomen or pelvis and can assume significant function in states of ACTH excess.

DEVELOPMENT. The adrenal cortex is derived from mesenchymal tissue. Cortical cells emerge to form a primitive fetal cortex around the sixth week of development. This then evolves into a fetal zone that is involved predominantly in the synthesis of androgen and estrogen precursors, and a definitive zone destined to become the adult gland. The fetal zone constitutes the major bulk of the adrenal cortex at birth; it begins to recede by the last intrauterine month and disappears around the end of the first year. The permanent cortex is formed from cells of the outer portion of the fetal gland and is not developed completely until around 3 years of age.

Synthesis, Circulation, and Metabolism of Adrenal Steroids

John D. Baxter

SYNTHESIS

The structures and steps in biosynthesis of a number of steroid hormones are shown in Figure 229–1. The letter designation for the carbon rings and the number designation of the carbon atoms are shown for pregnenolone, a key biosynthetic intermediate. α- and β- are used to designate the positions of the side groups above (β) or below (α) the plane of the molecule. The various steroids differ in the saturation of the A ring; hydroxyl and ketone groups at positions 3, 11, 17, and 21; the presence of a 3-carbon side chain at position 17; and an aldehyde group at position 18. Since the chemical nomenclature is cumbersome, trivial names for the steroids are most frequently used.

All steroids are derived from cholesterol that is either synthesized by the gland or obtained from the plasma lipoproteins. The gland is enriched in receptors that internalize low- and high-density lipoproteins. This uptake mechanism is increased when the adrenal is stimulated and provides the major cholesterol source.

Subsequent steps occur in the mitochondrion or endoplasmic reticulum. The first step is the conversion of cholesterol to pregnenolone. This step is rate limiting and is regulated by the major factors (ACTH, angiotensin II, and potassium) that stimulate steroid biosynthesis. This conversion involves several steps, catalyzed by the enzyme 20,22-desmolase (cholesterol side chain cleavage enzyme). Pregnenolone is then modified either (1) by converting its 5,6 to a 4,5 double bond with the use of 3β-hydroxysteroid dehydrogenase and Δ^5-oxysteroid isomerase, resulting in progesterone; or (2) by addition of a 17α-hydroxyl group with the use of 17α-hydroxylase, resulting in 17α-hydroxypregnenolone. The former pathway occurs in the glomerulosa, which lacks 17α-hydroxylase activity; although controversial, the latter pathway probably predominates in the fasciculata-reticularis, with subsequent conversion of 17α-hydroxypregnenolone to 17α-hydroxyprogesterone.

CORTISOL. Cortisol is synthesized by two successive hydroxylations. The first is at the 21 position, catalyzed by 21-hydroxylase, and results in 11-deoxycortisol (also called compound S). The second, at the 11 position of 11-deoxycortisol, is catalyzed by another hydroxylase and yields cortisol (also

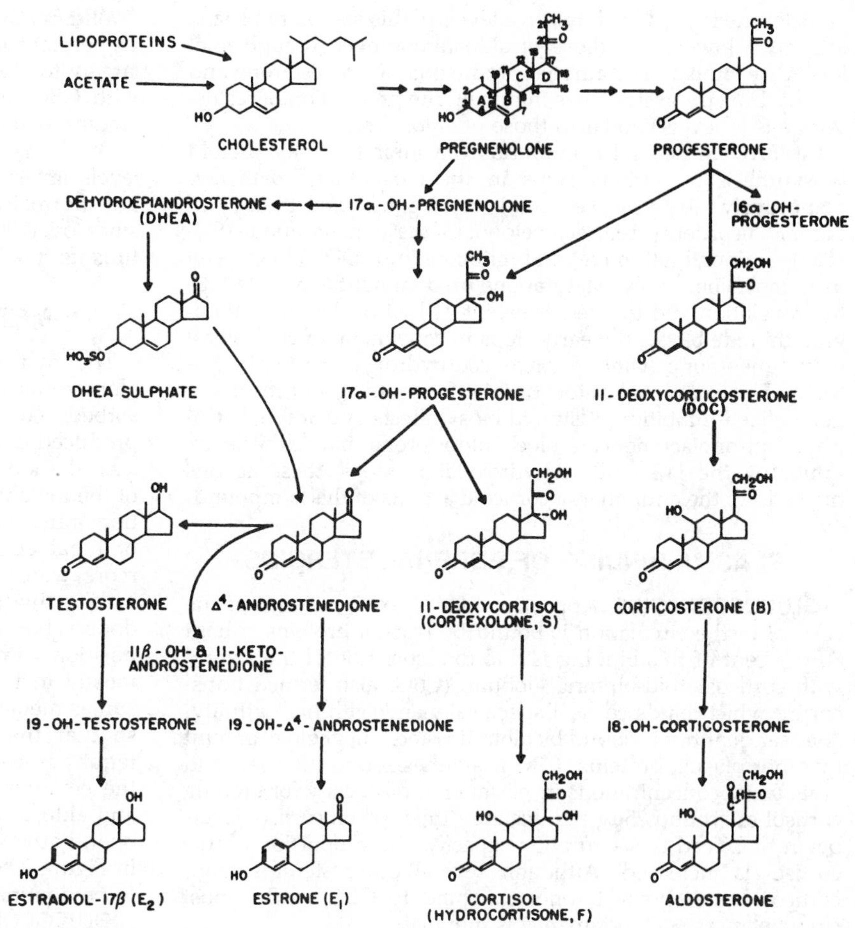

Figure 229–1. Steps in adrenal steroid biosynthesis. The numbers for the carbon atoms and the letters designating the rings of the steroid molecule are shown for pregnenolone. Arrows indicate the conversion pathways; the use of two arrows between intermediates indicates that more than one step is involved in the interconversion. (Reprinted from Baxter JD, Tyrrell JB: *In* Felig P, Baxter JD, Broadus AE, Frohman LA (eds.): Endocrinology and Metabolism. New York, McGraw-Hill Book Company, 1981, p 390.)

called hydrocortisone or compound F). These hydroxylations also require a flavoprotein dehydrogenase and cytochrome P450.

ALDOSTERONE. Aldosterone is produced by 21-hydroxylation of progesterone to form deoxycorticosterone (DOC); 11β-hydroxylation of DOC to form corticosterone; 18-hydroxylation of the latter to form 18-hydroxycorticosterone; and oxidation of the 18 CH_2OH group to an aldehyde to form aldosterone with the use of 18-hydroxycorticosteroid hydroxylase. This step is unique to the glomerulosa, explaining why aldosterone is not made by the zonae fasciculata and reticularis.

ANDROGENS. The adrenal androgens have 19 carbon atoms (C-19 steroids) and mostly serve as precursors for more potent androgens produced in peripheral tissues. These are dehydroepiandrosterone (DHEA) and its sulfate (DHEA-S), androstenedione and testosterone. DHEA is derived from 17α-hydroxypregnenolone by removal of its C-17 side chain, that leaves a keto group, with the use of C-17,20-lyase, and 17β-hydroxysteroid dehydrogenase. The sulfation of DHEA at the 3 position to DHEA-S is catalyzed by a sulfokinase. Androstenedione can be derived from either 17α-hydroxyprogesterone by removal of the C-17 side chain or from DHEA by conversion of the 5,6 to a 4,5 double bond and formation of the 3-keto group as described above. The adrenal can synthesize the C-18 steroids estradiol (from testosterone via 19-hydroxytestosterone) and estrone (from androstenedione via 19-hydroxy Δ^4-androstenedione) as outlined in Figure 229–1, but the quantities produced are minute. However, DHEA and DHEA-S synthesized by the fetal adrenal account for about 90 per cent of maternal estriol, 50 per cent of estradiol and estrone, and a substantial amount of testosterone and androstenedione production.

PRODUCTION RATES. The production rates and the blood levels under basal conditions of the major adrenal steroids are shown in Table 229–1. More cortisol is produced than any other steroid; much less aldosterone is produced. The production of DHEA plus DHEA-S is nearly as high as cortisol, although the plasma levels of DHEA are only a fraction of those of cortisol; however, plasma levels of DHEA-S are several-fold higher than those of cortisol because of the slow metabolism of DHEA-S. Corticosterone has substantial glucocorticoid activity, but is produced at much lower levels than cortisol. Similarly, DOC has substantial mineralocorticoid activity, and more DOC than

TABLE 229–1. SECRETION RATES AND PLASMA CONCENTRATIONS OF ADRENAL STEROIDS*

Steroid	24-hr Secretion (mg)	Mean Plasma Concentration (ng/ml)
Aldosterone	0.15	0.16
Androstenedione	2.4	1.5
Corticosterone	2.5	3
Cortisol	16	100
11-Deoxycorticosterone (DOC)	0.6	0.16
11-Deoxycortisol	0.4	1.7
DHEA	0.7(F), 3.0(M)	5.4
DHEA-S	7	1200
Progesterone	nil	0.2(M,F), 12(F)†
17α-Hydroxyprogesterone	nil	0.2(M), 0.6(F),2.0(F)†
Testosterone	0.2	5.6(M), 0.5(F)

*Mean values are reported for adults. Individual female (F) and male (M) values are reported only when these differ by more than two-fold. (Modified from Baxter JD, Tyrrell JB: The adrenal cortex. *In* Felig P, Baxter JD, Broadus AH, Frohman LA. (eds.): Endocrinology and Metabolism. New York, McGraw-Hill Book Company, 1981, p 394, where references to primary source material can be found.)

†Refers to the luteal phase of the menstrual cycle.

aldosterone is produced, but free levels of this steroid in plasma are much lower than those of aldosterone even though total levels are similar. The adrenal production of progesterone and 17α-hydroxyprogesterone is minimal. The production of testosterone is at levels similar to those of aldosterone.

INHIBITORS. Several compounds can inhibit adrenal steroid biosynthesis at various steps in the biosynthetic pathway, respectively. They can be useful for diagnosis and therapy of adrenal disorders (discussed below). Of these, metyrapone (SU-4885), aminoglutethimide, and mitotane (o,p′-DDD) have been used most commonly. Metyrapone predominantly inhibits 11β-hydroxylation and to a lesser extent 21-hydroxylation. Aminoglutethimide blocks the early steps in conversion of cholesterol to pregnenolone (cholesterol to 20α-hydroxycholesterol). Mitotane blocks adrenal mitochondrial functioning and results in generalized inhibition of steroid biosynthesis and adrenal atrophy. Spironolactone can block aldosterone biosynthesis by inhibiting the 11β- and 18-hydroxylation steps; these actions may add to the antimineralocorticoid actions of this compound.

PLASMA BINDING OF ADRENAL STEROIDS

GLUCOCORTICOIDS. Approximately 90 to 93 per cent of the cortisol in the circulation is bound by plasma proteins. About 80 per cent of this binding is due to association of the steroid with corticosteroid-binding globulin (CBG, also termed transcortin) which binds cortisol specifically and with high affinity. A lesser quantity is bound by albumin, and a negligible amount by other plasma proteins. CBG is synthesized in the liver, and at its usual concentrations in plasma has a capacity for binding cortisol of around 25μg per deciliter; thus, when cortisol levels begin to exceed this saturation capacity, the proportion of free cortisol is increased. Although several other steroids (e.g., corticosterone, progesterone) can bind to CBG, under most circumstances such occupancy is minimal.

CBG concentrations in plasma can vary among individuals on a genetic basis and can also be regulated by hormones and other factors. Estrogens, thyroid hormones, diabetes, and certain hematologic disorders increase CBG levels. Thus, CBG is increased in pregnancy (by almost two-fold during the third trimester), in hyperthyroidism, and by estrogens and oral contraceptives. Such effects can be maximal in three to five days and reversed by two to three weeks after cessation of therapy. CBG levels can be low congenitally and in liver disease (decreased protein production), multiple myeloma, obesity, and the nephrotic syndrome (through urinary loss).

The physiologic role of the plasma steroid–binding proteins such as CBG has not been determined. Although these have been called transport proteins, there is no obligatory need for this as cortisol is soluble at concentrations spanning its physiologic effectiveness. Similarly there appears to be no obligatory role for CBG in glucocorticoid hormone action. For instance, tissue culture cells respond to cortisol in the absence of detectable CBG. Further, the free rather than the plasma-bound steroid is physiologically active, and physiologic stimuli that regulate cortisol levels respond to the free rather than the total steroid concentration. Thus, when the CBG levels are primarily elevated or depressed, there are elevations or depressions, respectively, of the total cortisol in plasma, but the free cortisol concentration remains the same. This point is critical for evaluation of states of glucocorticoid excess or deficiency.

That CBG may have some importance is suggested by its ubiquity in mammals, even though plasma levels vary enormously, and the fact that congenital absence of CBG in man has never been found in spite of extensive screening. Recent evidence suggests that CBG or CBG-like proteins are located intracellularly, and in the kidney may sequester and therefore prevent cortisol from occupying the mineralocorticoid receptors. This would preserve the latter for the action of aldosterone as the major salt-regulating hormone. Furthermore, the protein binding of steroids in the blood may buffer rapid changes in plasma free cortisol levels that would otherwise occur as a result of episodic release of cortisol from the adrenal gland.

MINERALOCORTICOIDS. Under physiologic conditions, about 55 per cent of the total plasma aldosterone is protein bound, largely to albumin. The binding is weaker than that of cortisol with CBG, and the free rather than the plasma-bound aldosterone seems to be physiologically active.

DOC has potent mineralocorticoid activity, and its plasma levels are similar to those of aldosterone. However, DOC is not normally a physiologically important mineralocorticoid since over 95 per cent of it is bound to plasma proteins and thus its free levels are much lower than those of aldosterone.

METABOLISM OF ADRENAL STEROIDS

The hydrophobic steroids, although filtered by the renal glomerulus and excreted into the intestine, are mostly reabsorbed. For example, only about 1 per cent of the cortisol produced daily is excreted unchanged in the urine. Nevertheless, the kidneys account for over 90 per cent of the excretion of the metabolized steroids (DOC and corticosterone are exceptions); the remainder is lost in the gut. To render them capable of renal elimination, the steroids are inactivated and made more water soluble through enzymatic modifications. These involve hydroxylation of the keto groups, reduction of the double bond in the A ring, and conjugation at the 3 or 21 position with glucuronide or sulfate. These conversions occur mostly in liver, although during pregnancy the placenta assumes metabolic importance. The conversions alter the steroids so that the renal clearance of a major cortisol metabolite, tetrahydrocortisone glucuronide, is around 75 per cent that of the creatinine clearance. More than 50 metabolites of cortisol and aldosterone have been detected in humans. Although the quantitative aspects are still being refined, the pathways shown in Figure 229–2, and best studied for cortisol, appear generally to be dominant.

GLUCOCORTICOIDS. Cortisol is cleared from the plasma with a half-life of 70 to 120 minutes. About 70 per cent of infused cortisol, and presumably of that secreted, will be eliminated within 24 hours. The 11β-hydroxyl group of cortisol can be oxidized to the ketone, forming cortisone. The reaction is reversible, and in general the equilibrium is shifted to favor the 11β-hydroxyl group. However, because the adrenal produces much more cortisol than cortisone, there is substantial cortisol to cortisone conversion. These two steroids have similar subsequent metabolic fates, and roughly equivalent quantities of metabolites of these steroids are produced. Quantitatively the most important subsequent modification involves reduction of the 3-keto moiety to form dihydrocortisol and dihydrocortisone, followed by a reduction of the 4,5 double bond to form tetrahydrocortisol and tetrahydrocortisone. When the 3-hydroxyl group is formed, over 95 per cent of the products are conjugated at this position to form the glucuronide and to a lesser extent the sulfate derivatives. Conjugates of these two steroids make up around 30 per cent of the urinary cortisol metabolites. The second major site for modification involves the reduction of the 20-ketone to a hydroxyl, with subsequent reduction of the A ring, resulting in cortol (11-OH) or cortolone (11-keto). These account for approximately 25 per cent of the cortisol metabolites. Alternatively, there can be conversion of the 21-hydroxyl to a COOH; cortoic (11-hydroxyl) or cortolonic (11-keto) acid results when the A ring is reduced and the C-20-hydroxyl is formed, and they account for about 10 per cent of the cortisol metabolites. Other minor pathways involve the C-17 modifications discussed above without A-ring reduction, removal of the C-17 side chain with formation of 17-keto or 17-COOH moieties, formation of the C-21 COOH (without C-20-keto) and 6β-hydroxylation. The latter modifications constitute a major pathway in infants in whom the esterification mechanism has not been developed and for the synthetic glucocorticoids used in therapy.

MINERALOCORTICOIDS. Aldosterone is cleared with a half-

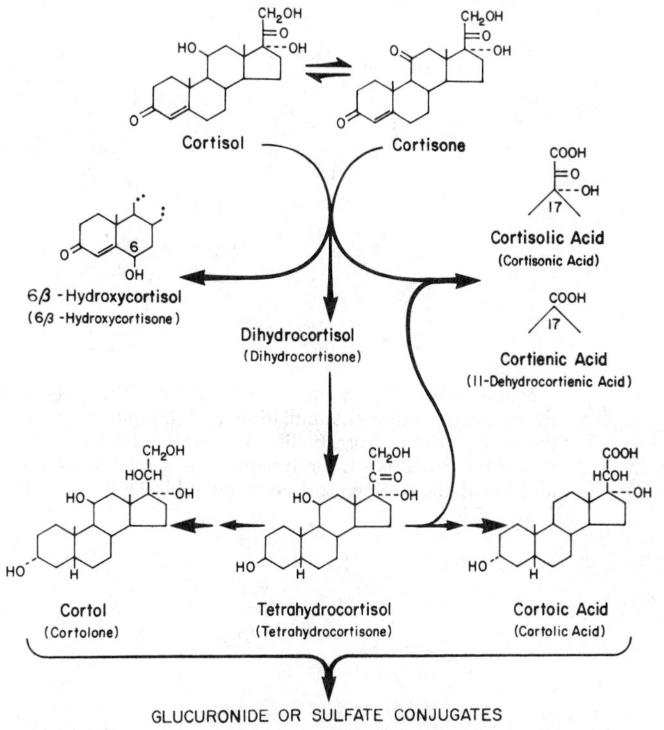

Figure 229–2. Metabolism of cortisol. See text. The interconversion of cortisol to cortisone is shown. The other steroid metabolites can be derivatives of either cortisol or cortisone. Structures shown and names are for the cortisol derivative. The names of the cortisone derivatives are shown in parentheses. In some cases, only part of the steroid molecule is shown; in these cases numbers refer to the steroid carbons for orientation. For tetrahydrocortisol, tetrahydrocortisone, and their derivatives, the 3-hydroxyl and 5-hydrogen are shown in the α and β configurations, respectively, but both α- and β-orientations occur at both positions. For a more extensive discussion and references, see Baxter JD, Tyrrell JB: *In* Felig P, Baxter JD, Broadus AE, Frohman LE (eds.): Endocrinology and Metabolism. New York, McGraw-Hill Book Company, 1981, pp 411–415.

life of around 15 minutes. Its conversion to metabolites is so effective that very little aldosterone survives passage through the liver. Less than 0.5 per cent of the aldosterone appears in the urine in the free state. The metabolism of aldosterone is similar to that of cortisol. About 35 per cent of the steroid appears as tetrahydroaldosterone glucuronide (3 position). However, two major differences are that there is much less 11β-hydroxy to 11-keto conversion, and 15 to 20 per cent of the aldosterone appears as a C-18 glucuronide that is acid labile; measurements of the urinary "aldosterone" usually reflect this metabolite.

ANDROGENS. The metabolism of androgens is discussed in Ch. 234.

VARIABLES IN RATES OF METABOLISM. The rate of steroid metabolism can be altered in certain clinical states and by various drugs. Agents that affect plasma steroid–binding proteins secondarily affect metabolism because of inhibitory influences of plasma binding on clearance. In chronic liver disease, hypothyroidism, infancy, very old age, anorexia nervosa, and protein calorie malnutrition, the rate of steroid metabolism is decreased. The converse occurs in hyperthyroidism. These states are in general not associated with abnormal free steroid levels (anorexia nervosa is an exception) because the regulatory systems tend to compensate by altering steroid production. Also, there is no major effect of renal disease (even though it does affect the clearance of some metabolites) or of most chronic diseases, obesity, and stress.

Drugs that affect steroid metabolism usually have the greatest influence on 6β-hydroxylation. Since this pathway in adults is relatively minor in terms of cortisol, these drugs do not have a major effect on endogenous cortisol. However, they can have a substantial influence on the clearance of synthetic glucocorticoids such as dexamethasone and prednisone, and this is therefore an important consideration with steroid therapy or with the use of glucocorticoids to assess the hypothalamic-pituitary-adrenal axis. These drugs include mitotane, phenytoin, rifampicin, aminoglutethimide, and barbiturates.

Regulation of Adrenal Steroid Production

John D. Baxter

Adrenal cortisol and androgen production is regulated by the hypothalamic-pituitary-adrenal axis, whereas aldosterone production is regulated predominantly by the renin-angiotensin system and by potassium (Fig. 229–3). These systems allow for basal and circadian steroid production, regulation of plasma steroid levels in normal circumstances, and increased or decreased steroid production in response to a number of specific stimuli.

REGULATION OF GLUCOCORTICOID PRODUCTION

The hypothalamus, pituitary, and adrenal comprise a neuroendocrine axis concerned with regulation of cortisol production. This axis is discussed in Ch. 224. Corticotropin releasing factor (CRF), elaborated by the hypothalamus, travels through its portal system to the anterior pituitary where it stimulates corticotropin (ACTH) release. The latter travels in the circulation to the adrenal where it stimulates cortisol production.

Three types of mechanisms are involved in regulating cortisol release: (1) circadian rhythms of secretion are established by the brain, (2) a number of types of excitatory factors can increase cortisol production, and (3) production of CRF and ACTH are regulated negatively by glucocorticoids.

ACTH AND RELATED PEPTIDES. ACTH circulates in the plasma largely as a free peptide with a half-life of around 10 minutes. It is derived from the proteolysis of proopiomelanocortin, a larger precursor pituitary protein of about 290 amino acids that also contains the sequences of several other proteins, including β-endorphin, α-, β-, and γ-melanocyte-stimulating hormones (MSH), β-lipotropin and an amino-terminal fragment (Ch. 221). Although MSH itself has the greatest pigment-stimulating activity, this activity in man is due predominantly to MSH sequences contained within ACTH (α-MSH), β-lipotropin (β-MSH) and the amino-terminal fragment (γ-MSH), as there appears to be very little MSH per se in the circulation. ACTH stimulates cortisol release by the adrenal within two to three minutes. This is due to increased cortisol synthesis primarily through stimulation of cholesterol to pregnenolone conversion, rather than through effects on secretion of stored hormone. More prolonged stimulation results in increased protein, RNA, and DNA synthesis with both hypertrophy and hyperplasia. ACTH binds to surface receptors and activates adenylate cyclase and phospholipase A_2 by a Ca^{++}-dependent mechanism. This results in increased Ca^{++} uptake, cyclic AMP generation, and phospholipid turnover. These effects increase cholesterol esterase, block cholesterol ester synthesis, increase lipoprotein uptake and stimulate cholesterol to pregnenolone conversion.

SPONTANEOUS RHYTHMS. The circadian rhythm of ACTH and cortisol results in decreasing release through the afternoon and evening. Secretion begins to increase around 3 to 4 A.M., peaks by around 8 A.M., and then begins to decline. This release occurs in pulses with intervals between them of 40 minutes to 8 hours; the changes in overall cortisol production are due to influences in the number of pulses that occur. These result in cortisol levels that vary enormously within minutes; thus, single plasma cortisol determinations may not give an adequate integrated assessment of overall cortisol production.

The spontaneous rhythm of cortisol secretion can be inter-

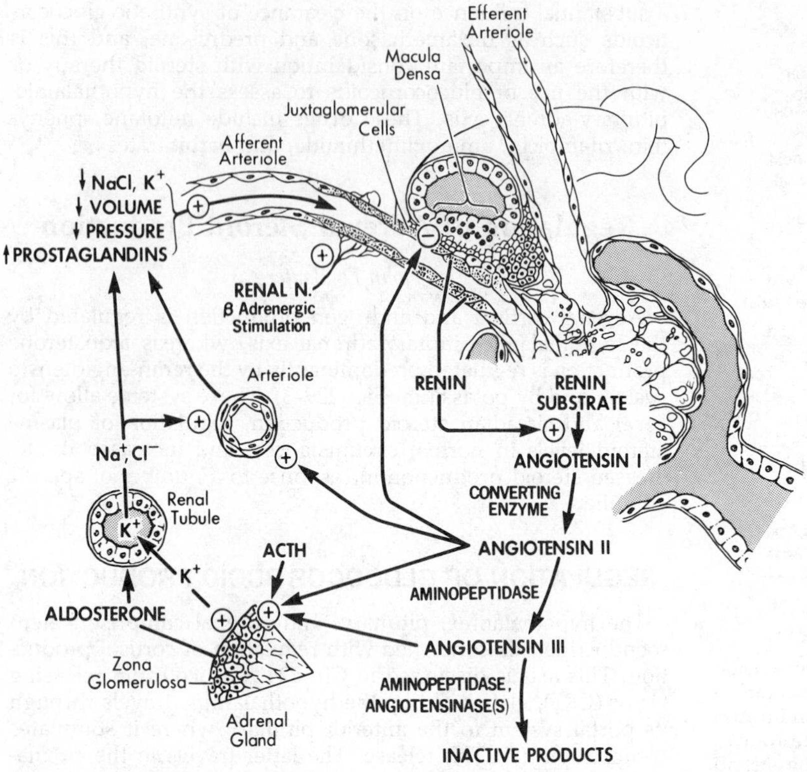

Figure 229–3. Renin-angiotensin system. The plus and minus signs indicate stimulation and inhibition, respectively. (Reprinted from Biglieri EG, Baxter JD: *In* Felig P, Baxter JD, Broadus AE, Frohman LA (eds.): Endocrinology and Metabolism. New York, McGraw-Hill Book Company, 1981, p 556.)

rupted acutely by a variety of psychologic and physical factors. These can vary from seemingly mild stresses such as the confrontation for venesection to more severe ones such as the preparation for cardiac surgery or severe anxiety. However, there are major individual variations. Major trauma or surgery, severe illness, hypoglycemia, fever, burns, and intensive exercise are illustrative of physical stresses that increase cortisol production by up to six-fold of normal. Minor illnesses such as upper respiratory infections or minor surgery can have minimal or no influence. Variations in cortisol levels can be blunted by chronic diseases such as congestive heart failure with hepatic congestion due to delayed cortisol clearance and with central nervous system disease and pituitary tumors even when they do not affect basal ACTH release. In depression, there is a circadian rhythm, but there can be increased cortisol secretion and impaired suppression by glucocorticoids. Although a number of drugs do not affect ACTH release, serotonin antagonists such as cyproheptadine inhibit both spontaneous and stimulated changes in ACTH release.

FEEDBACK INHIBITION OF ACTH RELEASE. Glucocorticoids feedback-inhibit the release of both CRF and ACTH (Ch. 221). Thus endogenous levels and stress-induced increases of cortisol and ACTH are depressed with exogenous glucocorticoid administration. ACTH levels are increased up to 10-fold to 20-fold in primary adrenal insufficiency. The feedback inhibition in response to glucocorticoids occurs within a few minutes, is progressive with continual exposure in a dose- and time-dependent fashion, affects both basal and stress-stimulated release, and is reversible. Although there are considerable individual variations, administration of a large dose of glucocorticoids for a few days does not, in general, result in suppression of pituitary function for more than a few hours; more prolonged exposure is accompanied by substantial suppression. Thus after several years of glucocorticoid therapy and then withdrawal of steroid administration, up to one year may be required for the hypothalamic-pituitary-adrenal axis to return to normal functioning. Although significant suppression occurs at both the hypothalamic and pituitary levels, the quantitative contribution of each of them has not been clarified.

REGULATION OF MINERALOCORTICOID PRODUCTION

Aldosterone production is controlled predominantly by the renin-angiotensin system and potassium, although other factors such as sodium, ACTH, and serotonin can also affect aldosterone secretion (Fig. 229–3). The renin-angiotensin system is important for adaptive blood pressure changes and is involved in the pathogenesis of some forms of hypertension.

RENIN. Renin, a glycoprotein of 340 amino acids, is produced in the juxtaglomerular cells of the afferent renal arteriole as a precursor protein (prorenin) that is cleaved to yield active renin. These cells release renin into the circulation where it has a half-life of around 15 minutes. Although renin may also be made in other tissues, the biologic role for this is uncertain, and extrarenal renin does not contribute to the plasma renin. Renin release is stimulated by lowering the blood pressure, assumption of the erect posture, salt depletion, β-adrenergic or central nervous system stimulation, and certain prostaglandins. It is inhibited by increases in blood pressure (except with malignant hypertension), salt loading, angiotensin II, vasopressin, potassium, calcium, β-adrenergic antagonists, α-methyldopa, clonidine, and by inhibitors of prostaglandin synthesis such as indomethacin.

Three types of influences mediate changes in renin release: (1) Changes in renal tubular sodium chloride concentration are detected by the macula densa, a specialized segment of the distal tubule that makes contact with the afferent arteriole just before it enters the glomerulus. This information is transmitted to the juxtaglomerular cells so that factors that reduce volume or lower the plasma sodium and chloride levels (e.g., dehydration, fluid or blood loss) increase renin release. (2) Renal baroreceptors stimulate renin release in response to decreases in renal perfusion pressure as with fluid loss or decreases in blood pressure. These receptors can function independently of innervation and salt delivery and respond more to changes in pressure than to the absolute pressure. (3) Renal sympathetic nerves that terminate in the juxtaglomerular cells and smooth muscle cells of the renal afferent arterioles secrete norepinephrine, which in turn stimulates renin release through β-adrenergic receptors. Blockage of this mechanism by agents such as propranolol probably explains how they decrease renin release. However, catecholamines can have other indirect effects on renin release through influences on renal blood flow and glomerular filtration.

Renin acts in the plasma proteolytically on renin substrate (angiotensinogen) to yield the decapeptide angiotensin I. Angiotensinogen contains over 400 amino acids and is secreted by the liver. Although its levels can be increased by estrogens and glucocorticoids, this does not appear to be an important normal mechanism of regulation. Angiotensin I is not known to have physiologically important actions; instead it serves as a substrate for production of angiotensin II.

CONVERTING ENZYME. The conversion of angiotensin I to the octapeptide angiotensin II is catalyzed by converting enzyme. Although a number of tissues have this enzyme, the lung contains much of the activity, perhaps around 50 per cent. In certain pulmonary diseases there can be decreases or increases in the plasma levels of the enzyme, although these changes do not appear to have a physiologically important effect on angiotensin II generation. Converting enzyme also catalyzes other reactions; important among these is the inactivation of bradykinin. Clinically useful inhibitors of converting enzyme are available; of these captopril has been used the most extensively. Normally, except when this enzyme is blocked pharmacologically, the rate-limiting step for angiotensin II generation is the production of angiotensin I.

ANGIOTENSIN II. Angiotensin II is the most potent vasoconstrictor known and has direct effects on arterioles. It also inhibits directly the release of renin by the juxtaglomerular cells. Finally it is a potent stimulator of aldosterone release. The hormone also has other complex effects on the kidney that affect salt balance, possibly through influences on kallikreins and prostaglandins. Plasma concentrations of angiotensin II can vary by 10-fold to 25-fold; the hormone has a half-life of only one to two minutes. There are several breakdown products of angiotensin II. One of these, angiotensin III, a polypeptide of seven amino acids, has angiotensin II activity, but its biologic importance is probably much less than that of angiotensin II.

Angiotensin II stimulates both early and late steps in aldosterone biosynthesis, resulting in increased conversion of cholesterol to pregnenolene and of corticosterone to 18-hydroxycorticosterone. Angiotensin II binds to cell surface receptors, but unlike ACTH it does not activate adenylate cyclase. It probably affects Ca^{++} influx and phospholipid turnover. Angiotensin II also has a tropic influence on the adrenal zona glomerulosa.

POTASSIUM. Increased potassium stimulates and decreased potassium inhibits aldosterone production. These effects are elicited by changes in potassium of as little as 0.1 mEq per liter in the physiologic range and are independent of sodium or angiotensin II. Prolonged hyperkalemia, like excess angiotensin II, has a tropic influence on the adrenal.

OTHER FACTORS. Other factors of lesser importance also affect aldosterone release. ACTH has a transient effect, and, rarely, aldosterone production can be blunted with chronic ACTH deficiency. Sodium deficiency decreases and sodium loading increases aldosterone release, but these influences are probably mediated through effects on renin. Dopamine agonists can inhibit and dopamine antagonists can increase plasma aldosterone. Aldosterone release is episodic and shows a tendency to a circadian rhythm that is similar to but much less prominent than that of cortisol; the mechanisms for this periodicity are not understood.

REGULATION OF ADRENAL ANDROGEN PRODUCTION

Adrenal androgen production is regulated by ACTH in a manner similar to that of cortisol. Thus plasma androgen levels tend to show the same circadian periodicity as cortisol. However, this is not the case with DHEA-S as a result of its slow turnover that tends to blunt the magnitude of increases due to episodic steroid release. Adrenal androgen release may also be affected by other factors such as during prepuberty (adrenarche); however, these are poorly understood. Finally, it should be remembered that androgens released by the testes and ovaries contribute to plasma androgen levels.

Actions of Adrenal Steroids

John D. Baxter

GLUCOCORTICOIDS

Glucocorticoids have diverse actions that in some way affect most mammalian tissues. They are also essential for survival, at least in times of stress.

INTERMEDIARY METABOLISM. Named for their carbohydrate-regulating activities, glucocorticoids have multiple influences on glucose metabolism with diverse secondary effects (Fig. 229–4). In most tissues these steroids inhibit glucose uptake. Liver, heart, brain, and erythrocytes are exceptions. In many of these tissues the steroids also block protein and nucleic acid synthesis and stimulate turnover of these macromolecules. In adipose tissue the steroids inhibit lipolysis and block lipogenesis. In liver the steroids stimulate glycogen deposition, gluconeogenesis, and the ability of other hormones to stimulate gluconeogenesis. The latter is further facilitated because of increased availability of glycerol and amino acid substrate due to the effects in peripheral tissues. The steroids also tend to stimulate the appetite, and in adrenal insufficiency there is anorexia. Finally the steroids tend to blunt the actions of insulin and decrease the affinity for insulin binding to its receptors.

The net effect of these influences is a glucocorticoid-induced tendency to hyperglycemia. This can be seen as early as 1 hour following glucocorticoid administration. However, in normal subjects the elevated levels of glucose increase insulin release that in turn tends to blunt the effects of the steroid. However,

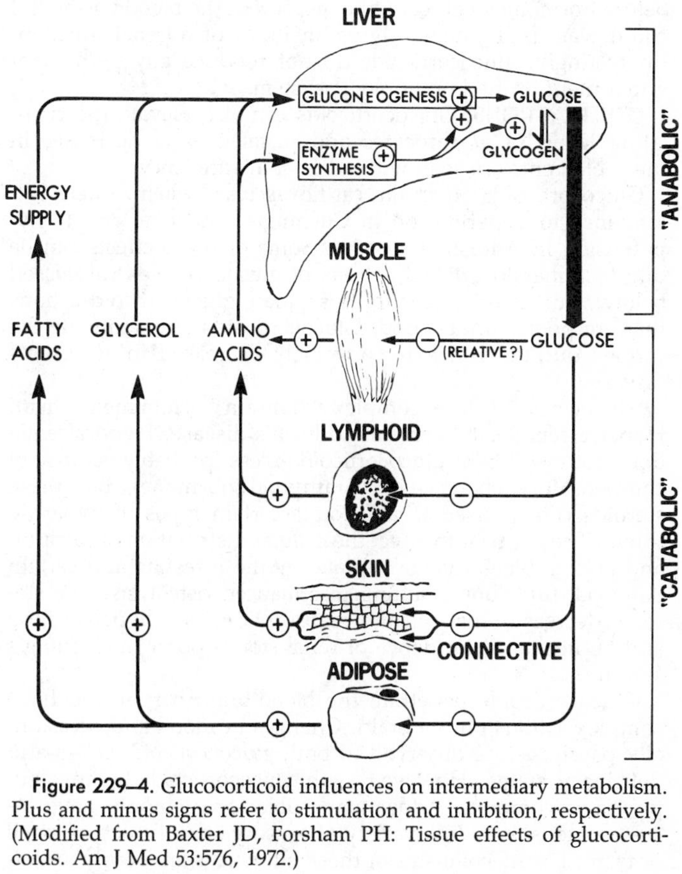

Figure 229–4. Glucocorticoid influences on intermediary metabolism. Plus and minus signs refer to stimulation and inhibition, respectively. (Modified from Baxter JD, Forsham PH: Tissue effects of glucocorticoids. Am J Med 53:576, 1972.)

in diabetes or latent diabetes, significant hyperglycemia and insulin resistance can ensue. Similarly, secondary hyperinsulinism may explain why there is a lack of fat wasting in Cushing's syndrome; lipogenesis induced by secondary increases in plasma insulin levels along with the increased food intake due to appetite stimulation may explain the truncal and sometimes generalized obesity seen in the syndrome. Conversely, in adrenal insufficiency there is a tendency to hypoglycemia; usually this is not marked, but it can be significant if there is concomitant fasting. Many of the actions of glucocorticoids on intermediary metabolism can be perceived as a protection against fasting; there is peripheral catabolism with sparing of essential tissues (heart, brain, blood cells) to make available substrate for maintenance of the blood sugar levels.

These actions of glucocorticoids on intermediary metabolism also explain many other effects of glucocorticoid excess. Thus inhibition of tissue metabolic functions may explain glucocorticoid-induced myopathy, inhibition of immunologic and inflammatory responses, and poor wound healing, thinning of the skin, striae, and osteoporosis.

INFLAMMATORY AND IMMUNOLOGIC RESPONSES. In excess, glucocorticoids suppress a number of inflammatory and immunologic responses, but it is not clear whether they normally modulate immunologic systems. In excess, glucocorticoids inhibit antigen processing, T cell function, synthesis of cellular mediators of the inflammatory response such as interleukins, plasminogen activator, lymphokines, and other active peptides, cellular migration and action at sites of inflammation, and inflammatory reactions themselves. In general they do not affect most antibody responses, although there are a few exceptions. Some populations of lymphocytes are killed by glucocorticoids; this explains the efficacy of these steroids in certain leukemias such as acute lymphoblastic leukemia of childhood. The steroids also affect mononuclear cell trafficking and tend to decrease blood monocyte, lymphocyte, and eosinophil levels and increase polymorphonuclear leukocytes; there are reciprocal changes during adrenal insufficiency. In the era before hormone levels could be measured, the blood eosinophil count was used extensively as an index of adrenal function. Interestingly, glucocorticoids do not produce any permanent impairment of the immunologic system.

OTHER ACTIONS. Glucocorticoids can also elevate the circulating levels of erythrocytes and platelets, and decreases in these elements are seen with adrenal insufficiency.

Glucocorticoids affect the cardiovascular system. There is a tendency to hypertension in Cushing's syndrome and to hypotension in Addison's disease. Some of these effects can be due to mineralocorticoid actions of glucocorticoids (discussed below), but there appear to be separate glucocorticoid actions that are poorly understood. Glucocorticoids also stimulate the cardiac output, which is conversely decreased in Addison's disease.

Glucocorticoids have complex actions on calcium metabolism. Hypercalcemia can occur in Addison's disease. Hypocalcemia does not result from glucocorticoid excess (probably because of compensatory changes in parathyroid hormone), but these steroids can be used to ameliorate certain types of hypercalcemia. They appear to affect the cellular distribution of calcium, and also to block calcium uptake by the intestine and certain bone cell functions resulting in enhanced osteolysis. The steroids decrease renal calcium reabsorption, and hypercalciuria and an increased incidence of renal stones occur in Cushing's syndrome.

Glucocorticoids penetrate the blood-brain barrier and have complex actions on the brain. Changes in mood and occasionally psychosis are observed in both glucocorticoid excess and deficiency states. However, with glucocorticoid therapy, euphoria is common. Addisonian subjects commonly have increased sensitivity to a variety of sensory stimuli such as smell or taste. The mechanisms of these influences are poorly understood. Glucocorticoids increase the intraocular pressure, probably by blocking fluid uptake by the trabecular meshwork. In susceptible individuals they can precipitate glaucoma and more rarely may result in cataract formation.

In the gastrointestinal tract glucocorticoids can inhibit DNA synthesis and tend to enhance stimuli to gastric acid secretion. They probably also enhance the tendency to form duodenal ulcers and, in high doses, the tendency to develop gastritis, although these side effects are controversial.

In excess, glucocorticoids inhibit linear growth, possibly as a result of their inhibitory influences on a number of tissues. However, glucocorticoid action appears to be required for a number of developmental processes. One particularly important process is the synthesis of surfactant in the lung. Lack of glucocorticoid induction of this factor in premature birth contributes to the respiratory distress syndrome of the newborn.

Complex interrelationships exist between glucocorticoids and other hormones. Glucocorticoids can inhibit vasopressin release; conversely, ACTH deficiency can lead to hyponatremia with water intoxication. Glucocorticoids secondarily increase insulin and parathyroid hormone (PTH) levels, and in some cases blunt the production of growth hormone, prolactin, insulin, glucagon, thyroid-stimulating hormone (TSH), and testosterone. Multiple synergisms and antagonisms between glucocorticoids and other hormones also exist at the cellular level. For example, they are synergistic with epinephrine and glucagon in stimulating hepatic gluconeogenesis. These effects are sometimes termed permissive glucocorticoid actions.

STRESS. Why glucocorticoids are essential for survival in times of stress is poorly understood. Two factors are probably operative. First, stress increases the production of a number of biologically active substances such as catecholamines, prostaglandins and other arachidonic acid metabolites, proteinases, and kinins. Glucocorticoids, by contrast, tend to blunt the production and actions of these substances, which, if left unchecked during stress, would lead to shock and vascular decompensation. Second, the stimulation of cardiovascular functions by glucocorticoids may be critical in times of stress when other compensatory systems may be less effective.

MOLECULAR MECHANISMS OF ACTION. Glucocorticoids penetrate cells and bind to intracellular receptors; the resulting hormone-receptor complexes then bind to specific sites on the DNA where they enhance the ability of RNA polymerase to stimulate transcription of glucocorticoid-responsive genes (Ch. 221). The protein products of the resulting mRNAs then mediate the glucocorticoid responses. In some circumstances the steroids probably block transcription by similar mechanisms. Also, some glucocorticoid effects occur by mechanisms that do not involve stimulation of transcription.

MINERALOCORTICOIDS

Mineralocorticoid hormones act on kidney, gut, salivary glands, and sweat glands to affect the balance of electrolytes. Direct actions on other tissues have been proposed but not clearly documented. Thus the spectrum of mineralocorticoid action is more restricted than that of glucocorticoid action.

In the kidney, the most important target organ, mineralocorticoids promote the linked reabsorption of sodium and secretion of potassium in the cortical collecting tubules of the nephron, and stimulate the secretion of hydrogen ion in the medullary collecting tubules. Thus, with mineralocorticoid excess, there is sodium retention, hypokalemia, and a tendency to alkalosis. In primary mineralocorticoid excess, hypertension develops with time. With mineralocorticoid deficiency there is sodium loss and a tendency to hyperkalemia and acidosis. The overall effects of mineralocorticoids on both sodium and potassium also depend on the level of salt intake. Increased sodium intake results in more tubular sodium for reabsorption; this enhances potassium secretion. Conversely, sodium restriction diminishes aldosterone-induced kaliuresis. In most circumstances with persistent mineralocorticoid excess, the sodium retention that occurs reaches a limit such that the body "escapes" from further sodium retention. This may be due to the secretion of other factors or hormones, or to changes in renal hemodynamics with secondary and compensating influences on sodium excretion, or to both. Exceptions are the secondary hyperaldosteronism of heart failure and of cirrhosis with ascites where sodium retention is progressive. As noted, hyperkalemia directly stimulates aldosterone secretion, which in turn enhances renal potassium excretion. This servomechanism forms an important component of the body's defense against hyperkalemia.

Mineralocorticoid actions are probably mediated through molecular mechanisms similar to those described above for cortisol, and in Ch. 221. The mineralocorticoid receptors bind aldosterone and DOC with high affinity; they also bind cortisol with 1 to 2 per cent of the affinity for aldosterone. Since plasma free cortisol concentrations are around 100-fold higher than those of aldosterone, there is probably some occupancy of mineralocorticoid receptors by cortisol, although this may be blunted by other cellular proteins that sequester cortisol. The synthetic steroid 9α-fluorocortisol binds tightly to mineralocorticoid receptors and is used for mineralocorticoid replacement therapy, since it is more stable than aldosterone after oral administration. Mineralocorticoid antagonists such as spironolactone bind to these receptors and in this way block aldosterone action.

Aldosterone stimulates the synthesis of several renal proteins that result in increases in (1) sodium permeability in the apical membrane exposed to the tubular lumen; (2) various mitochondrial enzymes that increase cellular ATP and thereby enhance the actions of the Na^+-K^+ ATPase; (3) possibly the Na^+-K^+ ATPase itself; and (4) probably other as yet unidentified factors that influence fatty acid and phospholipid metabolism. Of these the effects on the sodium channel are probably the most important. Potassium ion secretion increases secondarily to a rise in the electrochemical gradient for potassium entry into the tubular lumen, a gradient that is enhanced by the Na^+-K^+ ATPase-dependent pumping of sodium ion into the cell, thereby increasing lumen negativity.

Renal tubular transport of hydrogen ion, about which little is known, has been postulated to result from an hormonal influence on an H^+ ATPase. The mineralocorticoid-induced tendency to extracellular alkalosis is also promoted in part by hydrogen ion movement into cells in exchange for losses in potassium, leading to the dichotomy of extracellular acidosis in the presence of extracellular alkalosis. Potassium ion deficiency increases hydrogen ion excretion by decreasing Na^+-K^+ exange, which in turn increases the Na^+-H^+ exchange. As in the case of potassium, hydrogen ion loss can be blunted with sodium restriction.

The major known extrarenal targets for aldosterone are the sweat and salivary glands, ileum, and colon where the steroid promotes potassium loss and sodium retention. These actions are ordinarily minor in terms of overall salt balance. However, the aldosterone-induced changes in the salivary sodium-potassium ratio and the potential difference across the colonic epithelium have been used as diagnostic indices of mineralocorticoid activity.

Laboratory Evaluation of Adrenocortical Function

J. Blake Tyrrell

Most functions of the adrenal cortex can now be assessed by using plasma assays. Certain urinary assays remain useful, however, despite the disadvantage of 24-hour collections. Trophic hormones, e.g., ACTH, and related peptides, renin and angiotensin, can also be precisely measured and compared to adrenal secretion. The following considerations must be remembered when using these assays. (1) Current assays measure total hormone concentration, not bioactive free hormone. (2) Plasma levels of cortisol and ACTH vary greatly because of episodic secretion and many other factors (see below); thus single levels cannot always be relied upon for a definitive diagnosis. (3) In assessing adrenal function, stimulation and suppression testing provide the most definitive information.

GLUCOCORTICOID FUNCTION

ACTH AND RELATED PEPTIDES. Immunoassays for ACTH, although not always available, are extremely useful. ACTH is unstable in plasma and adheres to glass; specimens should be collected in anticoagulated plastic or silicon-coated tubes on ice, centrifuged in the cold without delay, and frozen until assayed. The normal range of plasma ACTH in the morning (8 to 9 A.M.) is 20 to 100 pg per milliliter in most current clinical assays. Values at other times of the day are lower, and consideration of this episodic secretion is important in interpretation.

Plasma ACTH levels are primarily used to differentiate pituitary, adrenal, and other causes of adrenal dysfunction. Thus, in patients with primary adrenal insufficiency (Addison's disease) elevated ACTH levels (generally greater than 250 pg per milliliter) confirm the diagnosis. Conversely, with secondary adrenal insufficiency due to hypothalamic or pituitary disease, or steroid therapy, ACTH levels will be low normal or subnormal (<50 pg per milliliter). In states of cortisol excess (Cushing's syndrome), a suppressed or undetectable ACTH level (<20 pg per milliliter) is diagnostic of an adrenal tumor hypersecreting cortisol (or of exogenous glucocorticoids). With ACTH–producing pituitary tumors (Cushing's disease), plasma ACTH levels are normal to modestly elevated (40 to 200 pg per milliliter), whereas in the ectopic ACTH syndrome they are usually elevated markedly (100 to >1000 pg per milliliter). ACTH levels in the two latter conditions may overlap, but very high (>300 pg per milliliter) values point to an ectopic tumor. Plasma ACTH levels are also elevated in congenital adrenal hyperplasia proportional to the extent of cortisol deficiency, and are markedly elevated in pituitary tumors that arise following bilateral adrenalectomy (Nelson's syndrome).

Immunoassays for other peptides derived from proopiomelanocortin are also becoming available. The available antisera usually measure both β-LPH and β-endorphin, and many reports of "beta endorphin levels" reflect in fact predominantly β-LPH that is present in the circulation in higher concentrations than β-endorphin. Reported normal morning values of immunoreactive β-LPH/β-endorphin are 20 to 200 pg per milliliter. Levels of these peptides vary similarly to those of ACTH, but because of its longer plasma half-life, β-LPH peptide levels show less episodic variability than ACTH. Also β-LPH is considerably more stable than ACTH in plasma and when frozen prior to assay. As a result, elevated β-LPH levels are seen more consistently than are elevated ACTH levels in patients with pituitary-dependent hypercortisolism. Whether measurement of β-LPH or β-endorphin will supplant measurement of ACTH levels in clinical disorders of pituitary and adrenal dysfunction remains to be determined.

PLASMA CORTISOL AND RELATED STEROIDS. Plasma cortisol is most frequently measured by radioimmunoassay; current antisera show little cross-reactivity with other natural or synthetic steroids. Competitive protein binding, fluorimetric, and high–performance liquid chromatography assays are also in use. Normal values of plasma cortisol vary with the circadian rhythm of ACTH. Mean levels at 8 A.M. are 10 to 12 μg per deciliter with a range of 3 to 20 μg per deciliter. Values at 4 to 6 P.M. are approximately 50 per cent of the morning levels, although there is great variability. Values obtained between 10 P.M. and 2 A.M. are less than 3 μg per deciliter and may be unmeasurable. (In all cases, values are 2 to 3 μg per deciliter higher than those given above when the fluorimetric assay is used.) Episodic variability and the numerous conditions increasing cortisol secretion or CBG concentrations (Table 229–2) limit the utility of single cortisol determinations; as a result, unless marked elevations are present, these values are rarely diagnostic per se.

Measurement of plasma 11-deoxycortisol (compound S) is generally available and has been used extensively in metyrapone testing of pituitary-adrenal reserve (see below).

URINARY CORTICOSTEROIDS. Measurements of urinary steroids have been traditionally used to evaluate adrenal function and provide an integrated assessment of steroid production and excretion. With the exception of urinary free cortisol, however, which is essential in the evaluation of cortisol excess, other methods are less advantageous and are being supplanted by measurements of plasma cortisol or ACTH levels.

Urine free cortisol, although less than 1 per cent of total adrenal cortisol secretion, is a useful measurement in the diagnosis of hypercortisolism. The urine is first extracted and the steroid is then measured by radioimmunoassay or competitive protein binding. Normal values range from 20 to 100 μg per 24 hours. Elevated levels are almost always present in Cushing's syndrome but not in simple obesity; this ability to separate these conditions is a major advantage. Urinary cortisol excretion is increased by any condition that increases adrenal cortisol secretion (Table 229–2) and is decreased in renal failure. Current clinical assays are insensitive at the lower range; this method is not reliable in the diagnosis of decreased cortisol production.

Urinary 17-hydroxycorticosteroids (17-OHCS) and 17-ketogenic steroids (17-KGS) measure steroid metabolites, predominantly those of cortisol and 11-deoxycortisol. These methods are currently not recommended in most situations, since the levels are altered in many disease states and the assays are subject to interference by commonly used drugs and medications.

SUPPRESSION TESTS. Suppression tests use dexamethasone, a potent synthetic glucocorticoid not measured in current cortisol assays, to inhibit ACTH and cortisol secretion. In Cushing's syndrome there is abnormal feedback by glucocorticoids, and this abnormality is diagnostic. There are two types of dexamethasone suppression tests: (1) Low-dose tests are used to document the presence of Cushing's syndrome. (2) High-dose tests are used to distinguish the various causes of Cushing's syndrome. The techniques for performing these tests and the expected responses are summarized in Table 229–3.

Low-Dose Dexamethasone Tests. The overnight 1 mg dexamethasone suppression test is an excellent screening procedure for detecting the presence of Cushing's syndrome. The test can be used on an ambulatory basis, and in this setting false-negative and false-positive responses are rare. The test is much less useful in hospitalized and chronically ill patients, of whom 25 per cent have false-positive responses. False-positive responses also occur in 15 per cent of obese patients and in a number of other conditions, including acute illness, anxiety, depression, alcoholism, estrogen therapy, and uremia. Drugs that accelerate dexamethasone metabolism, especially phenytoin and phenobarbital, also cause false-positive results. The two-day low-dose test provides the same information as the 1 mg overnight test but is more time consuming. Abnormal responses occur in about 95 per cent of patients with Cushing's syndrome. False-positive responses occur rarely in obesity or with estrogen therapy, but are seen more commonly with acute illness, depression, alcoholism, and anticonvulsant therapy.

TABLE 229–2. CONDITIONS CAUSING ELEVATED CORTISOL LEVELS

Increased CBG	Increased Secretion
Estrogen therapy	Exercise
Pregnancy	Meals
Hyperthyroidism	Physical stress
Diabetes mellitus	Anxiety
Hematologic disorders	Depression
Congenital	Starvation
	Anorexia nervosa
	Alcoholism
	Chronic renal failure

TABLE 229–3. DEXAMETHASONE SUPPRESSION TESTS

Low-dose tests

Overnight test
Dexamethasone, 1 mg p.o. at 11 P.M.; plasma cortisol at 8 to 9 A.M.
Normal response—plasma cortisol <5 μg/dl

Two-day test
Dexamethasone 0.5 mg p.o. q6h for 8 doses; plasma cortisol 6 hours after last dose and 24-hr urine free cortisol and/or 17-OHCS during second day of dexamethasone

Normal response—plasma cortisol <5 μg/dl; urine free cortisol <25 μg/24 hr; urine 17-OHCS <4 mg/24 hr or <1 mg/gram urine creatinine

High-Dose Tests

Overnight test
Dexamethasone 8 mg p.o. at 11 P.M.; plasma cortisol before and at 8 to 9 A.M. after dexamethasone

Response—Cushing's disease; suppression of cortisol to <50% of baseline; ectopic ACTH/adrenal tumors: no cortisol suppression

Two-day test
Dexamethasone 2.0 mg p.o. q6h for 8 doses; plasma cortisol before dexamethasone and after last dose; 24-hr urine free cortisol and/or 17-OHCS before dexamethasone and during second day
Response—Cushing's disease; suppression of plasma or urine steroids to <50% of baseline; ectopic ACTH/adrenal tumors: no steroid suppression

High-Dose Dexamethasone Tests. Glucocorticoids in pharmacologic doses suppress ACTH and cortisol secretion in most patients with pituitary ACTH-producing tumors, but not in patients with adrenal and ectopic tumors. Two tests are available (Table 229–3). The overnight high-dose test is simpler and more accurate than the two-day high-dose test. Approximately 90 per cent of patients with Cushing's disease have suppression of cortisol levels to less than 50 per cent of baseline levels, whereas about 95 per cent of those with adrenal tumors or the ectopic ACTH syndrome do not achieve this degree of suppression. The two-day high-dose test is more time consuming and less reliable in that 15 to 30 per cent of patients with Cushing's disease fail to achieve greater than 50 per cent suppression of urine 17-OHCS, urine free cortisol, or plasma cortisol.

STIMULATION TESTS. These procedures assess the reserve capacity of the hypothalamic-pituitary-adrenal axis and its ability to respond appropriately to stressful situations. These tests act at different sites of the axis and thus can be used to assess its different functions.

CRF Testing. Corticotropin releasing factor (CRF), currently being studied, should soon be available for the investigation of pituitary-adrenal disorders. CRF may be useful in the diagnosis of secondary adrenocortical insufficiency due to both hypothalamic-pituitary disorders and glucocorticoid therapy. However, data comparing this procedure with metyrapone stimulation or insulin-induced hypoglycemia are not yet available. CRF has already proven to be useful in the differential diagnosis of Cushing's syndrome. In states of hypercortisolism, CRF elicits responses of both ACTH and cortisol when Cushing's disease is present; in the ectopic ACTH syndrome or adrenal tumors no response is observed. Again, only limited data are thus far available, and one exception has been reported in which an ectopic tumor responded to CRF. In current protocols, CRF is generally administered intravenously in a dose of 1 μg per kilogram of body weight. ACTH and cortisol secretion peak at 30 to 60 minutes and may be sustained for several hours. Flushing and occasionally hypotension have been observed, and thus the test should be performed with the patient supine.

ACTH Testing. The administration of ACTH, which allows direct assessment of adrenal glucocorticoid reserve, is most useful in the diagnosis of adrenal insufficiency, both primary and secondary. The rapid ACTH stimulation test is best carried out with synthetic human ACTH (α1–24 ACTH), which has full biologic potency and a lesser incidence of allergic reactions than previously used ACTH preparations. The test is performed by administering 250 μg of synthetic ACTH (Cortrosyn) intravenously or intramuscularly; plasma cortisol levels are obtained prior to and at 30 or 60 minutes after ACTH administration. Normally the plasma cortisol level will be greater than 15 to 18 μg per deciliter and will have increased by at least 5 μg per deciliter. Subnormal responses to ACTH stimulation establish the diagnosis of adrenal insufficiency.

By contrast, a normal response excludes primary adrenal failure and complete secondary insufficiency, but it does not exclude partial secondary adrenal insufficiency. A normal response to ACTH in the latter case occurs when there is sufficient basal ACTH secretion to prevent adrenal atrophy but not enough pituitary reserve to respond to stress. When this infrequent situation is suspected, the issue can be resolved with the use of metyrapone or insulin hypoglycemia testing. Performance of the rapid ACTH stimulation test will delay therapy of suspected acute adrenal insufficiency by only 30 minutes, following which therapy can be administered while awaiting the results.

The rapid ACTH stimulation test gives no information regarding the cause of demonstrated adrenal dysfunction. This distinction can be made by measuring either the basal plasma ACTH level or the aldosterone response to ACTH stimulation (normally an increment in the plasma aldosterone of at least 4 ng per deciliter above baseline). The latter test is based on the fact that the zona glomerulosa responds acutely to ACTH and that this response is preserved in secondary adrenal insufficiency, but is deficient in the primary form in which the entire adrenal cortex is destroyed.

In secondary but not primary adrenal insufficiency, cortisol secretion will increase after three days of ACTH administration. Although previously useful, these tests are rarely used at present because of the availability of plasma ACTH and aldosterone measurements.

Metyrapone Testing. Metyrapone inhibits the synthesis of cortisol by blocking 11β-hydroxylation. As a result, ACTH secretion increases and drives the production of steroids proximal to the site of the block. Plasma 11-deoxycortisol is measured in response to the metyrapone test. The overnight test is most commonly used because of its rapidity and simplicity; because of the short duration of inhibition of cortisol synthesis there is little risk of precipitating acute adrenal insufficiency. In this procedure metyrapone is given at midnight with food, and plasma for 11-deoxycortisol and cortisol determinations is obtained at 8 A.M. The dose of metyrapone* is 2 grams for patients less than 70 kg; 2.5 grams for those 70 to 90 kg and 3 grams for patients weighing more than 90 kg. A plasma cortisol value <10 μg per deciliter indicates adequate 11β-hydroxylase inhibition, and in normal persons plasma 11-deoxycortisol increases to greater than 7 μg per deciliter. If assays for 11-deoxycortisol are unavailable, a three-day test can be performed in which urinary 17-OH corticosteroids, which include 11-deoxycortisol metabolites, are measured. A normal response to metyrapone requires function of both the pituitary and adrenals. A subnormal response establishes the diagnosis of adrenal insufficiency and correlates well with deficient responses to stress and hypoglycemia. The test per se does not differentiate primary and secondary causes. Since a normal response to the rapid ACTH stimulation test is usually found prior to performance of the metyrapone test, a subnormal response then indicates secondary adrenal insufficiency.

Insulin Hypoglycemia Testing (Ch. 231). Hypoglycemia elicits a central nevous system stress response that in turn stimulates CRF and ACTH secretion and, as a consequence, cortisol release. A normal cortisol response to hypoglycemia indicates a normal hypothalamic-pituitary-adrenal axis and rules out adrenal insufficiency or decreased pituitary ACTH reserve. This test is most often utilized in the evaluation of suspected hypothalamic or pituitary disorders, since growth hormone reserve can be assessed simultaneously with that of ACTH.

*This dosage is not listed in the manufacturer's directive.

OTHER PROCEDURES. Other agents such as pyrogens or vasopressin have also been used to stimulate pituitary ACTH secretion, but have achieved less acceptance. Synthetic CRF is currently being evaluated to determine if it will stimulate ACTH and cortisol release more effectively in pituitary tumors than in ectopic or adrenal tumors and can be useful to distinguish hypothalamic pituitary causes of impaired ACTH release.

MINERALOCORTICOID FUNCTION

PLASMA RENIN. Assessment of plasma renin is essential in the diagnosis of states of excess and deficient mineralocorticoid secretion; it is also helpful in the evaluation of other types of hypertension (Ch. 47). Currently used assays do not measure the plasma renin concentration directly, but instead measure the plasma renin activity (PRA) by quantifying the amount of angiotensin I generated over time in the patient's plasma. The normal values of PRA depend on the salt intake and postural status. In subjects with moderate salt intake (around 110 mEq Na^+ per day) and in the seated position, the plasma renin activity ranges from 1.5 to 5 ng of angiotensin I generated per milliliter per hour (ng A_I per milliliter per hour). In individuals in whom salt has been restricted (20 mEq Na^+ per day) for four days and who have been in the upright posture for two hours the values range from 5 to 10 ng A_I per milliliter per hour. Factors that affect renin release have been described above, since they are those that regulate mineralocorticoid production. Of those seen in clinical practice, diuretic therapy is the most commonly observed factor that increases the PRA. In patients with primary hyperaldosteronism the PRA is characteristically suppressed. With aldosterone-producing adenomas, the PRA is unresponsive or only weakly responsive to provocative stimuli, whereas in those with primary aldosteronism with bilateral hyperplasia, the PRA does respond to such stimuli.

In patients with only borderline low PRA in whom primary aldosterone excess is suspected, stimulation tests with measurement of PRA may be necessary. Patients can be subjected to salt restriction (20 mEq of sodium per day for five days) or given 40 mg of furosemide the evening and morning before sampling; blood samples are then taken after two hours in the upright posture. If the plasma renin does not increase under these conditions it is likely that primary aldosteronism is present. Caution should be exercised in performing these tests since severe and life-threatening volume depletion or hypokalemia could ensue; these risks must be weighed before the test is performed.

ALDOSTERONE MEASUREMENTS. These measurements are most often utilized in the diagnosis of primary aldosteronism and in the differentiation of its subtypes of adenoma and hyperplasia. Plasma measurements ordinarily involve extraction and chromatography of the steroid followed by radioimmunoassay. The urine measurements ordinarily quantify by radioimmunoassay the 18-glucuronide metabolite of aldosterone (about 15 per cent of the total aldosterone production). Alternatively, urinary tetrahydroaldosterone can be measured.

These measurements should be made after adequate sodium repletion (a sodium intake of at least 120 mEq per 24 hours for four days) and withdrawal of diuretics for at least two to three weeks, and in the case of plasma measurements after at least 6 hours of recumbency. Normal values for aldosterone excretion are 5 to 20 μg per 24 hours; basal plasma values in the supine patient are usually 5 to 15 ng per deciliter. Although problems with episodic steroid release are less with aldosterone than with cortisol, these may explain why measurements of plasma aldosterone levels are less reliable than are urinary assays in the diagnosis of mild aldosterone hypersecretion. Plasma aldosterone values are of greater utility in the differential diagnosis of hyperaldosteronism, as discussed under primary aldosteronism. A simple and reliable method of differentiating primary aldosteronism due to an adenoma from that due to hyperplasia is to measure the plasma aldosterone response to posture. Plasma aldosterone levels in hyperplasia, but not adenoma, are still under control of the renin-angiotensin system. Thus, the plasma aldosterone is initially measured in the supine position at 8 A.M. after four days of a sodium intake of at least 120 mEq per 24 hours and then subsequently after two to four hours in the upright posture. In patients with an adenoma there is either no increase or an actual decrease in plasma aldosterone in the upright position, whereas with hyperplasia, there is an increase in plasma aldosterone concentrations after two to four hours in the upright position.

If there is still uncertainty, additional tests can be employed. Deoxycorticosterone acetate (DOCA), 10 mg intramuscularly every 12 hours, can be given for three days to patients whose intake is 120 mEq of sodium per 24 hours and plasma or urinary aldosterone measured in relation to pretreatment values. Aldosterone is minimally or not at all suppressed in patients with an aldosterone-producing adenoma and in most patients with hyperplasia. Although some groups have given 0.3 mg of 9α-fluorocortisol orally twice for three days instead of DOCA, others have found this test to be less reliable, presumably because 9α-fluorocortisol suppresses ACTH and aldosterone production in some patients with primary aldosteronism. Saline infusion is also used; 0.5 to 2 liters of normal saline is administered over four hours and in normal persons plasma aldosterone suppresses to less than 5 ng per deciliter.

ADRENAL ANDROGENS

Plasma levels of the predominant adrenal androgens, DHEA, DHEA-S, and androstenedione, can be measured. These assays plus that of testosterone are most frequently used for the evaluation of hirsutism. Stimulation and supression tests have not been as useful as in other pituitary and adrenal disorders. Plasma free testosterone measurements usually provide a better index of total androgenicity than total levels of the hormone, since androgen excess decreases sex hormone–binding globulin and can result in a normal total level in the presence of an elevated free testosterone concentration. Measurement of androstanediol and its glucuronide, metabolic products of dihydrotestosterone, provides an index of peripheral androgen production, and may provide the best index of androgen excess.

Urinary 17-ketosteroids were traditionally measured to assess adrenal androgen production. This procedure measures mainly DHEA and DHEA-S metabolites. However, this test has limited utility since the more potent androgens such as testosterone and dihydrotestosterone contribute less than 1 per cent of the total urinary 17-ketosteroids and thus are not assessed. Furthermore, 17-ketosteroids are increased in obesity without androgen excess, and there is interference by multiple drugs and medications.

Adrenocortical Hypofunction

John D. Baxter

Adrenal insufficiency is defined by deficient production of glucocorticoids or mineralocorticoids or both. Primary adrenocortical insufficiency (Addison's disease) is due to destruction of the adrenal cortex, whereas in secondary adrenocortical insufficiency impaired cortisol production is due to deficient ACTH production. Hyporeninemia causes selective aldosterone deficiency. Selective adrenal defects due to congenital enzyme deficiencies also occur (Ch. 233).

PRIMARY ADRENOCORTICAL INSUFFICIENCY

ETIOLOGY. Primary adrenocortical insufficiency has multiple causes. In the United States over 80 per cent of the cases are due to autoimmune destruction of the adrenal. Tuberculosis is the second most frequent cause and remains a common cause of the disease in underdeveloped countries with a higher incidence of tuberculosis. Other rare causes include hemorrhage due to sepsis, anticoagulation, coagulopathies, trauma, surgery, and pregnancy; bilateral infarction, e.g., due to thrombosis or arteritis; fungal infection; invasive disorders such as lymphoma, metastatic tumors, amyloidosis, sarcoidosis, and hemochromatosis; surgery; cytotoxic agents such as mitotane; and congenital hypoplasia and hyporesponsiveness to ACTH. Nonetheless, primary adrenocortical insufficiency due to any cause is a rare disease with an estimated incidence in Western countries of around 50 per million population.

The idiopathic, presumed autoimmune form of adrenal insufficiency is 2-fold to 3-fold more common in females and is usually diagnosed in the third to fifth decades of life. Early in the disease there is lymphocytic infiltration of the gland, and there is a high association (40 to 53 per cent of patients) with disorders of other endocrine glands or with pernicious anemia or vitiligo. Antibodies to the gland are commonly present, and there is evidence for abnormal cell-mediated immunity.

The association of Addison's disease with the other disorders has been referred to as *Schmidt's syndrome,* autoimmune endocrine failure, and the polyglandular failure syndrome. Approximate associations are ovarian failure, 25 per cent of female patients (testicular failure in males is unusual); hyperthyroidism, 7 per cent (mostly female); hypothyroidism or Hashimoto's thyroiditis with goiter, 9 per cent; subclinical thyroiditis, up to 80 per cent; diabetes mellitus (type I), 12 per cent; vitiligo, 9 per cent, presumably due to immunologic destruction of melanocytes; hypoparathyroidism, 6 per cent; and, pernicious anemia, 4 per cent. Whereas these problems are common with adrenal insufficiency, patients with more common problems such as diabetes or thyroid disease only rarely develop Addison's disease. The development of autoimmune adrenocortical insufficiency shows some hereditary predisposition, and an autosomal recessive pattern of inheritance has been suggested. About 40 per cent of patients have first- or second-degree relatives with one of the associated disorders. Further, there is an increased incidence of histocompatibility antigen (HLA) types B8, Dw3 and of the haplotype HLA-A1,B8.

CLINICAL MANIFESTATIONS. The development of clinical manifestations of adrenocortical insufficiency requires loss of more than 90 per cent of the adrenal cortices. The rate of destruction varies, depending on the cause, but with the idiopathic variety this usually (but not always) requires several months. With gradual destruction, increases in ACTH secondary to the lower cortisol levels tends to stimulate the gland maximally. Thus there is a period when the gland can produce normal levels of cortisol, but when responses to stress are impaired. These patients may experience minimal symptoms unless exposed to some stressful event. In fact, in about 25 per cent of the patients symptoms first appear in a crisis or impending crisis. However, in the majority of cases destruction becomes more complete, and the patient experiences symptoms that lead to medical evaluation before a crisis occurs. The destruction of the gland results in loss of both glucocorticoid and mineralocorticoid functions and secondary increases in ACTH and in renin.

The clinical presentation depends on the rate and degree of adrenal destruction, the presence of stressful influences, and the pathology of associated or causative conditions. For these reasons it is convenient to discuss separately the chronic and acute presentations.

Chronic primary adrenocortical insufficiency may go unnoticed for some time, because of its gradual development, although retrospectively the patients frequently recall symptoms beginning months to years earlier. The major clinical features, as noted in Table 229–4, are weakness and fatigue, weight loss, anorexia, hyperpigmentation, hypotension, gastrointestinal upset (including nausea, vomiting, and less commonly diarrhea), salt craving, and postural dizziness. Weakness is generalized and not restricted to particular muscle groups. Weight loss is due both to dehydration secondary to salt loss, and to anorexia. Mild hypoglycemia is common in adults, but it is unusual for it to be severe enough to be symptomatic; however, clinically symptomatic hypoglycemia is more common in children. Fe-

TABLE 229–4. CLINICAL FEATURES OF CHRONIC PRIMARY ADRENOCORTICAL INSUFFICIENCY

	%
Weakness and fatigue	100
Weight loss	100
Anorexia	100
Hyperpigmentation	92
Hypotension	88
Gastrointestinal symptoms	56
Salt craving	19
Postural symptoms	12

From Baxter JD, Tyrrell JB: The adrenal cortex. *In* Felig P, Baxter JD, Broadus AH, Frohman LA (eds.): Endocrinology and Metabolism. New York, McGraw-Hill Book Company, 1981, p 453.

male patients can also have amenorrhea and loss of axillary hair, the latter due to decrease of adrenal androgens. Although dehydration can be significant, this is typically compensated for by increased salt intake. Hyponatremia is present in most patients, although it may be masked somewhat if there is dehydration. Mild hyperkalemia is also usually present; the presence of severe hyperkalemia should suggest concomitant renal or other disease. A normocytic, normochromic anemia is common, but can also be masked by dehydration and hemoconcentration. There tends to be neutropenia, lymphocytosis, and eosinophilia. Dehydration when present leads to increases in blood urea nitrogen and creatinine, and there may be mild acidosis. The heart tends to be small and vertical on x-ray examination; the abdominal radiograph is usually normal, but can show adrenal calcification in about 50 per cent of those cases due to tuberculosis. Calcification of the ear lobes sometimes occurs in longstanding cases.

Hyperpigmentation is an important diagnostic feature and may precede other manifestations. It is generalized, but is accentuated in sun-exposed areas, pressure points such as the elbows, knees, knuckles, and toes, and on palmar creases, nail beds, buccal mucosa, tongue, nipples, aerolae, and perivaginal or perianal mucosa, and in recent surgical scars. In blacks, pigmentation of the tongue is of diagnostic helpfulness. Hyperpigmentation is commonly misinterpreted as an excessive sun tan and the "healthy" appearance of the patient may lead to a dismissal of other symptoms.

Acute adrenocortical insufficiency is seen most commonly in a patient with either undiagnosed or diagnosed adrenocortical insufficiency who is exposed to one of the stresses discussed earlier and who therefore has an increased requirement for glucocorticoids. It can also be seen with acute adrenal destruction secondary to hemorrhage, most commonly associated with septicemia or anticoagulant therapy (adrenal apoplexy). In these cases, anorexia is often profound with nausea and vomiting that exaggerates volume depletion and dehydration. Abdominal pain is frequent and may mimic a surgical condition of the abdomen; however, these symptoms are usually vague. The blood pressure falls, and hypovolemic shock develops that is incompletely responsive to fluid replacement. Fever is common and may or may not be due to the precipitating event. Hyperpigmentation will be present or absent, depending on the duration of the disease; when present it is an important diagnostic sign. The presence of hyperkalemia, lymphocytosis, and eosinophilia should also suggest the diagnosis. Severe hypoglycemia is uncommon and is more likely to occur in children or in adults with secondary adrenal insufficiency with both ACTH and growth hormone deficiency. The diagnosis of acute adrenocortical insufficiency should be considered in any patient with unexplained shock, and the consideration of this should not be diverted by the presence of an accompanying disorder such as infection or diabetic ketoacidosis.

SECONDARY ADRENOCORTICAL INSUFFICIENCY. Secondary adrenocortical insufficiency results from inadequate ACTH production. The causes are discussed in Ch. 225. For spontaneous disease, pituitary and hypothalamic tumors are the most common cause. In these cases there is progressive loss of ACTH such that cortisol production and responses to stress are decreased, but mineralocorticoid production is almost always normal. In addition to spontaneous causes, chronic suppression of ACTH production with exogenous glucocorticoids followed by their withdrawal also causes the syndrome and is by far the most frequent cause.

The development of clinical manifestations is usually chronic but like primary adrenocortical insufficiency can be acute. The presenting features are similar to those of primary adrenocortical insufficiency with three exceptions: (1) Since hypersecretion of ACTH and related peptides is absent, there is no hyperpigmentation; in fact, patients with hypopituitarism commonly exhibit pallor of the skin. (2) The electrolyte abnormalities of hyponatremia, hyperkalemia, and mild acidosis are absent because of preservation of aldosterone secretion. Hyponatremia, if present, is due to decreased glomerular filtration rate, hypothyroidism, or increased vasopression release. (3) Other features of hypopituitarism (Ch. 225) may be present.

DIAGNOSIS. The clinical suspicion of Addison's disease should be confirmed by definitive laboratory testing. In seriously ill patients, however, therapy should not be delayed by prolonged diagnostic measures; if means for a rapid diagnosis are unavailable, therapy should be initiated if the clinical suspicion of adrenal insufficiency is significant. The diagnosis can be established or ruled out later. Diagnostic reliance on basal urine or plasma measurements is dangerous. Although an elevated plasma cortisol level (e.g., greater than 25 μg per deciliter) makes the diagnosis unlikely, normal basal cortisol levels can be present with impaired adrenal responsiveness to stress. Thus the adrenal reserve should be tested.

Figure 229–5 shows a plan of approach. If adrenocortical insufficiency is suspected, the rapid ACTH stimulation test should be performed. This test requires only 30 minutes and can be done even in most acute situations. A normal response excludes the diagnosis of primary adrenocortical insufficiency; an abnormal response establishes the presence of adrenocortical insufficiency. Only rare patients with secondary adrenocortical insufficiency will respond normally because of partial ACTH deficiency that still allows the adrenal to respond. The basal plasma ACTH level, determined prior to ACTH administration, is measured to distinguish between primary and secondary adrenocortical insufficiency. In primary adrenocortical insufficiency, the levels exceed 250 pg per milliliter and usually are greater than 400 pg per milliliter. By contrast, plasma ACTH levels in secondary adrenocortical insufficiency are inappropriately low, ranging from 0 to 50 pg per milliliter. The plasma aldosterone response to ACTH can also be used to differentiate primary from secondary adrenocortical insufficiency, but there is less extensive experience with this procedure.

Further diagnostic procedures are needed only in exceptional cases, for example, in suspected secondary adrenocortical insufficiency with a normal response to ACTH or in cases in which plasma ACTH levels are unavailable. In these cases the metyrapone or insulin hypoglycemia tests can be helpful. The latter test is usually performed in suspected hypopituitarism, since simultaneous assessment of both growth hormone and ACTH can be performed (Ch. 225). The metyrapone test is performed in patients in whom hypoglycemia is contraindicated or those with prior glucocorticoid therapy, since it provides essentially the same information and is of less potential risk to the patient. An abnormal response to metyrapone establishes the diagnosis of secondary adrenocortical insufficiency, since the primary form would have been excluded by the ACTH stimulation test. The presence of low normal or low ACTH levels further confirms this diagnosis.

In spontaneous adrenocortical insufficiency of any type, the laboratory evaluation should include a blood glucose, serum calcium and phosphorus, and thyroid function tests, including TSH and thyroid antibody determinations. If there is oligo-

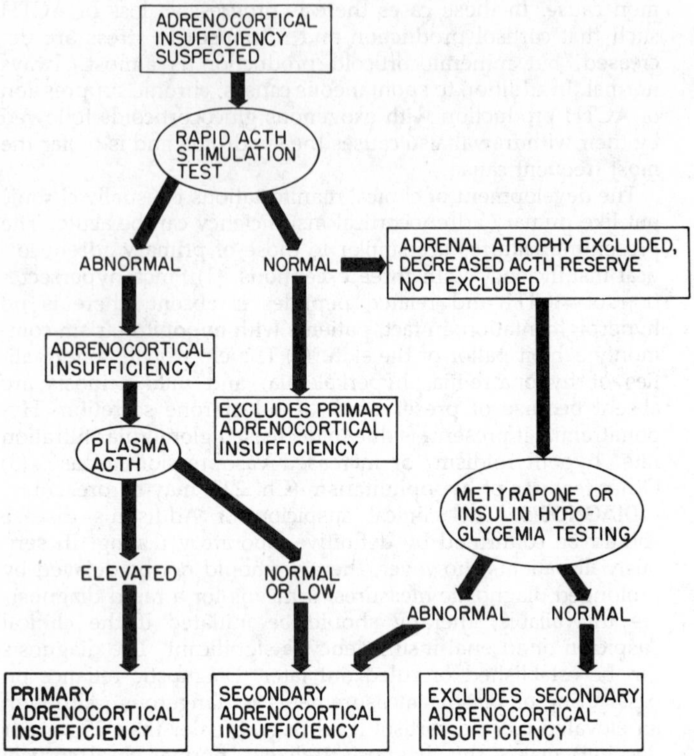

Figure 229–5. Evaluation of suspected primary or secondary adrenocortical insufficiency. Boxes enclose clinical decisions and circles enclose diagnostic tests. (Reprinted from Baxter JD, Tyrrell JB: *In* Felig P, Baxter JD, Broadus AE, Frohman LA (eds.): Endocrinology and Metabolism. New York, McGraw-Hill Book Company 1981, p 458.)

menorrhea or amenorrhea, FSH and LH levels should be determined. Finally, first- and second-degree relatives should be screened for endocrine deficiency syndromes because of the increased risk in these individuals. In secondary adrenocortical insufficiency, patients should be examined for other pituitary dysfunction, pituitary or hypothalamic tumors, and prior glucocorticoid therapy (Ch. 225). In acute adrenocortical insufficiency, the precipitating cause should be determined, since this is often infectious.

TREATMENT. *Acute Adrenocortical Insufficiency.* In an acute crisis, therapy should be instituted as soon as possible after the diagnosis is suspected (Table 229–5). A soluble glucocorticoid, such as cortisol hemisuccinate or phosphate, should be given intravenously. Volume depletion, electrolyte abnormalities, and hypoglycemia should be corrected and general supportive measures instituted. Precipitating factors should be assessed and corrected. If recovery is satisfactory, the glucocorticoid dose can then be reduced on the second day and then tapered to oral maintenance doses by the fourth to fifth days. Mineralocorticoid replacement is unnecessary when high doses of cortisol are given, but should be given if a synthetic glucocorticoid such as prednisolone or dexamethasone is used and when the cortisol dose has been tapered to near-maintenance levels.

TABLE 229–5. THERAPY OF ADRENAL INSUFFICIENCY

Acute Crisis

1. Hydrocortisone, 100 mg IV, every 6 hr for 24 hr. If stable, reduce to 50 mg every 6 hr and then taper to oral maintenance in 4 to 5 days. Maintain or increase dose to 200 to 400 mg per 24 hr if complications persist or occur.
2. Correct volume depletion, dehydration, hypotension, and hypoglycemia with intravenous saline and glucose.
3. Correct precipitating factors, especially infection.

Maintenance

1. Hydrocortisone 15 to 20 mg p.o. q A.M.; 5 to 10 mg at 4 to 6 P.M.
2. 9α-Fluorocortisol 0.05 to 0.1 mg q A.M. (primary).
3. Follow weight, blood pressure, and electrolytes.
4. Educate patient and increase cortisol dosage during stress.

Chronic Adrenocortical Insufficiency. The treatment of the primary form of this condition requires both glucocorticoid and mineralocorticoid replacement, whereas the secondary form usually requires only glucocorticoid replacement (Table 229–5). Patients must be made aware that a lifetime of replacement is necessary and of the need to increase glucocorticoid replacement in times of stress. Each patient should carry an identification bracelet or card. Cortisol at levels similar to physiologic production is given in a way that crudely approximates the circadian rhythm. Thus, for ordinary maintenance, 15 to 20 mg of cortisol are given in the early morning and 5 to 10 mg in the late afternoon. An equivalent amount of prednisolone or prednisone (about 5 mg per day) or cortisone acetate (37.5 mg per day) is also acceptable; however, the potency of dexamethasone has probably been underestimated, and this steroid is not recommended. For mineralocorticoid replacement, 9α-fluorocortisol 0.05 to 0.1 mg orally per day is recommended. Follow-up is mainly by clinical assessment of a feeling of well-being, examination of signs of glucocorticoid or mineralocorticoid excess or deficiency, and measurements of serum electrolytes. Measurements of plasma cortisol, ACTH, and renin are usually not helpful. The doses may need to be adjusted somewhat. Many of the subjective complaints of Addison's disease can be reversed within a few days; a somewhat longer time is required before strength returns to normal and hyperpigmentation subsides.

In times of stress, it is sometimes difficult to predict the need for increased glucocorticoid administration. It is best to err on the side of overreplacement rather than underreplacement. For minor illnesses such as significant upper respiratory infections, the cortisol dose should be doubled or tripled and then tapered as soon as possible. It is not usually necessary to change the 9α-fluorocortisol dose. Patients with vomiting and substantial diarrhea should seek medical attention and receive parenteral cortisol. Patients who may not have early access to medical attention should keep injectable cortisol available and be instructed in its use.

In the event of major trauma, treatment should be similar to that for adrenal crisis discussed above. In the case of elective

TABLE 229–6. STEROID COVERAGE FOR SURGERY

1. Correct electrolytes, blood pressure, and hydration if necessary.
2. Hydrocortisone phosphate or hemisuccinate, 100 mg IM, on call to operating room.
3. Hydrocortisone phosphate or hemisuccinate, 50 mg IM or IV, in recovery room and every 6 hr for the first 24 hr.
4. If progress is satisfactory, reduce dosage to 25 mg every 6 hr for 24 hr; then taper to maintenance dosage over 3 to 5 days. Resume previous 9α-fluorocortisol dose when patient is taking oral medications.
5. Maintain or increase cortisol dosage to 200 to 400 mg per 24 hr if fever, hypotension, or other complications occur.

From Baxter JD, Tyrrell JB: The adrenal cortex. *In* Felig P, Baxter JD, Broadus AH, Froham LA (eds.): Endocrinology and Metabolism. New York, McGraw-Hill Book Company, 1981, p 462.

major surgery the protocol described in Table 229–6 has been shown to be effective.

PROGNOSIS. Survival of patients in whom adrenocortical insufficiency was adequately diagnosed and treated now approximates that of the normal population. This is in sharp contrast to the period before steroids were available or when only mineralocorticoid replacement was available, at which time the survival rate was usually two years or less.

HYPOALDOSTERONISM

PATHOGENESIS. Hypoaldosteronism can occur in association with hypocortisolism or as an isolated defect. The major cause of isolated hypoaldosteronism is defective renal renin secretion (hyporeninemic hypoaldosteronism) (Ch. 76). Other rarer causes include isolated adrenal biosynthetic defects (18-hydroxylase syndrome), transient deficiency following removal of an aldosterone-producing tumor, unresponsiveness to aldosterone (pseudohypoaldosteronism) with normal or increased aldosterone production, marked potassium depletion, and heparin administration.

HYPORENINEMIC HYPOALDOSTERONISM. This is seen in patients with renal disease due to a variety of causes such as interstitial nephritis, diabetes mellitus, or multiple myeloma. It has also been observed following removal of an aldosterone-producing tumor or rarely without any apparent cause in association with hypertension. The hyporeninemia leads to decreased aldosterone production and impaired ability of the zona glomerulosa to respond to stimuli. However, the gland usually retains some capacity to secrete aldosterone through stimulation by potassium. Hypoaldosteronism results secondarily in hyperkalemia, which is disproportionate to the extent of renal disease. Chronic renal disease per se ordinarily does not lead to hyperkalemia unless the glomerular filtration rate is severely impaired (e.g., less than 15 ml per minute). In fact, hyporeninemic hypoaldosteronism is probably a common cause of hyperkalemia in patients with renal disease and creatinine clearance rates greater than 15 ml per minute. Although these patients can develop hyponatremia, in adults this is less common, probably because of the fact that the primary disease tends to favor sodium retention. These patients also tend to develop a metabolic acidosis due to the lack of H^+-secreting actions of aldosterone; this can be accentuated by a decreased glomerular filtration rate. This form of acidosis has been classified as type IV renal tubular acidosis (Ch. 83.2).

TREATMENT. The treatment of hypoaldosteronism involves therapy for the primary condition plus mineralocorticoid replacement as described above for primary adrenocortical insufficiency. However, in some patients with hypertension, treatment with 9α-fluorocortisol is not indicated and diuretics are used instead. Conversely, some patients require higher doses of mineralocorticoids, probably because the renal disease renders them more refractory to the steroid.

Cushing's Syndrome

J. Blake Tyrrell

Cushing's syndrome results from chronic glucocorticoid excess. It is seen most commonly in patients receiving long-term therapy with supraphysiologic doses of glucocorticoids. Spontaneously occurring Cushing's syndrome is a rare disorder, the precise incidence of which is unknown. It occurs as a result of either primary tumors of the adrenal gland that hypersecrete cortisol or from excess ACTH secretion that may be of pituitary or nonpituitary (ectopic ACTH syndrome) sources.

Cushing's disease, the subtype of spontaneous hypercortisolism due to excessive pituitary ACTH secretion, accounts for two thirds of reported cases. This disorder is most common in women, with a female to male ratio of at least 5:1, and usually begins clinically between the ages of 20 and 40 years.

Secretion of ACTH from ectopic tumors is found in about 15 per cent of cases with documented Cushing's syndrome. The true incidence of this disorder is probably much higher, since many patients lack the typical clinical features of cortisol excess because of the dominance of the manifestations of cancer and the rapidity of progression and thus the disorder may go undiagnosed. Because of the current predominance of oat cell carcinoma of the lung in males, the ectopic ACTH syndrome has a female to male ratio of 1:3 and an age onset most frequently between 40 and 60 years.

Primary adrenal tumors secreting cortisol account for approximately 15 per cent of cases of Cushing's syndrome. In adults there is an equal frequency of adenoma and carcinoma. In childhood prior to the age of ten years, adrenal carcinoma is the most frequent cause of Cushing's syndrome. Both adenomas and carcinomas secreting cortisol are more prevalent in women than in men. The average age at diagnosis is approximately 40 years, and 70 per cent of cases occur in adults.

PATHOLOGY. Pituitary adenomas (Ch. 225) are present in over 90 per cent of patients with Cushing's disease. These tumors are usually small; 50 per cent are 5 mm or less in diameter. They are typically basophilic and unencapsulated and contain ACTH, β-LPH, and β-endorphin. The few patients with Cushing's disease who do not have pituitary adenomas have (1) diffuse hyperplasia; (2) hyperplasia with multiple nests of adenomatous cells; (3) an adenoma or adenomatous hyperplasia of the intermediate lobe of the pituitary, or (4) no obvious pituitary disorder.

Adrenocortical hyperplasia in Cushing's disease results in modest increases in combined adrenal weight due to hyperplasia of the zonae reticularis and fasciculata. In the ectopic ACTH syndrome, adrenal enlargement and hyperplasia of the zona reticularis are usually more marked with a concomitant reduction in the number of zona fasciculata cells. Bilateral nodular hyperplasia occurs in approximately 20 per cent of cases of ACTH excess and may be due to more prolonged stimulation of the adrenal cortex by ACTH. In this case, in addition to diffuse hyperplasia of the zonae reticularis and fasciculata, there are multiple nodules that vary from microscopic to several centimeters in diameter and that contain clear cells similar to those of the zona fasciculata.

Cortisol-secreting adenomas are usually encapsulated, range from 2 to 6 cm in diameter, typically secrete cortisol alone, and are usually composed of zona fasciculata–like cells. Adrenal carcinomas that secrete cortisol are usually large at the time of diagnosis, may be palpable as abdominal masses, and may secrete a number of steroids. Histologically these tumors may appear benign or exhibit considerable pleomorphism, and the histologic appearance does not predict benign or malignant behavior. Therefore the diagnosis of adrenal carcinoma is dependent on the demonstration of either local tumor invasiveness or metastatic spread. Extension of these tumors occurs locally, and common sites of metastases are the liver and lung.

ETIOLOGY AND PATHOGENESIS. The etiology of Cushing's disease is unknown. It is possible that primary pituitary tumors arise spontaneously. In cases in which diffuse or adenomatous hyperplasia is present, it is possible that excessive secretion of CRF or some other factor stimulates the pituitary. The ectopic

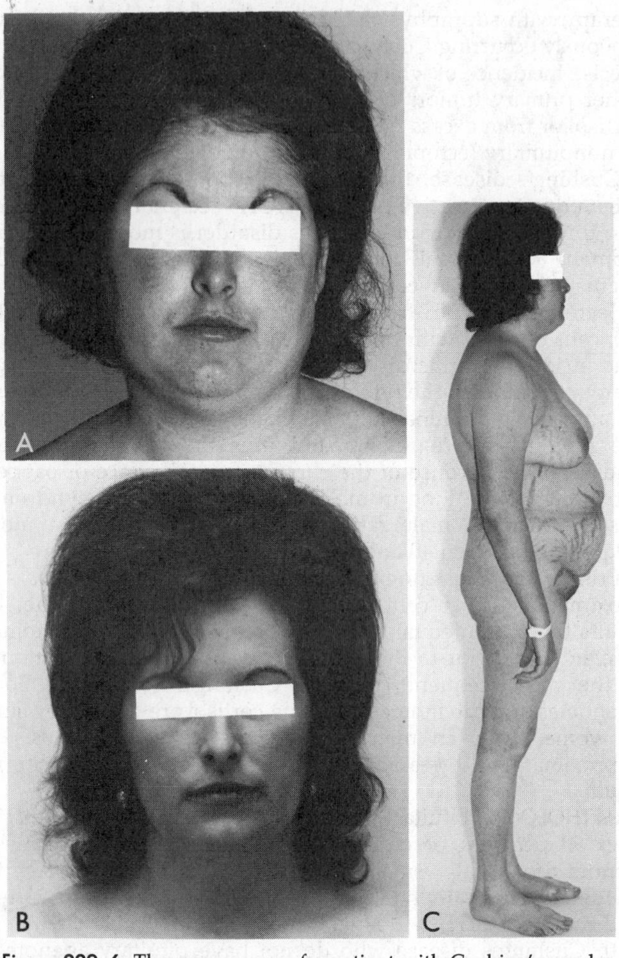

Figure 229–6. The appearance of a patient with Cushing's syndrome *(A)* before and *(B)* one year after removal of an adrenal adenoma. *(C)* Profile, before treatment.

ACTH syndrome occurs in a relatively small number of tumor types. Oat cell carcinoma of the lung, the most common, accounts for approximately 50 per cent of cases. The great production of cortisol and 11-deoxycorticosterone stimulated by the very high ACTH levels commonly results in manifestations of mineralocorticoid excess in addition to glucocorticoid excess.

Other ACTH-secreting tumors include thymomas, islet cell tumors of the pancreas, carcinoid tumors, medullary carcinomas of the thyroid, and pheochromocytomas. Many other tumors have been found to secrete ACTH, but occur very rarely. Cortisol–producing adrenal tumors arise spontaneously and are not under normal control by the hypothalamic-pituitary axis; their secretion of cortisol and the other steroids is autonomous, episodic, and random.

CLINICAL FEATURES. The classic features, most typically seen in Cushing's disease (Fig. 229–6, Table 229–7) usually develop insidiously over several years. The most common manifestation is central obesity with rounding of the face and fat accumulation around the trunk, supraclavicular areas, and dorsocervical spine. Serial photographs are sometimes helpful in recognizing these gradual changes. Whereas classically this pattern of obesity spares the extremities, generalized obesity including the extremities occurs in about 50 per cent of patients. Atrophy of the skin and underlying connective tissue is frequent. This leads to facial plethora, easy bruisability, and red to purple depressed striae. The last occur most commonly over the lower abdomen, but can also be more generalized on the trunk and upper legs. Patients also have poor healing of minor or major injuries and abrasions and an increased incidence of superficial fungal infections. Hirsutism is present in approximately 80 per cent of female patients as a result of excessive adrenal androgen secretion. Hypertension is present in the majority of patients; it is rarely accompanied by hypokalemia in Cushing's disease, although this is more common in the ectopic ACTH syndrome or adrenal carcinoma. Hypertension appears to contribute greatly to the mortality of untreated Cushing's syndrome.

TABLE 229–7. INCIDENCE OF CLINICAL FEATURES OF CUSHING'S SYNDROME

Feature	%
Obesity	94
Facial plethora	84
Hirsutism	82
Menstrual disorders	76
Hypertension	72
Muscular weakness	58
Back pain	58
Striae	52
Acne	40
Psychologic symptoms	40
Bruising	36
Congestive heart failure	22
Edema	18
Renal calculi	16
Headache	14
Polyuria/polydipsia	10
Hyperpigmentation	6

Modified from Plotz CM, et al.: Am J Med 13:597, 1952, and Ross EJ, et al: Q J Med 35:149, 1966, and reprinted from Baxter JD, Tyrrell JB: The adrenal cortex. *In* Felig P, Baxter JD, Broadus AE, Frohman LA (eds.): Endocrinology and Metabolism. New York, McGraw-Hill Book Company, 1981, p 472.

Additional common manifestations include hypogonadism in both male and female patients, psychologic disturbances (usually depression), which occur in the majority, and proximal muscle weakness. Osteopenia is present in virtually all patients and involves primarily the ribs and vertebral bodies. With more longstanding disease, frank osteoporosis is common (Ch. 249). Back pain is common, and compression fractures of the spine occur in approximately 20 per cent. Renal stones, secondary to hypercalciuria, and thirst and polyuria, which may be due to hyperglycemia or to hypercalciuria, can also occur. Routine

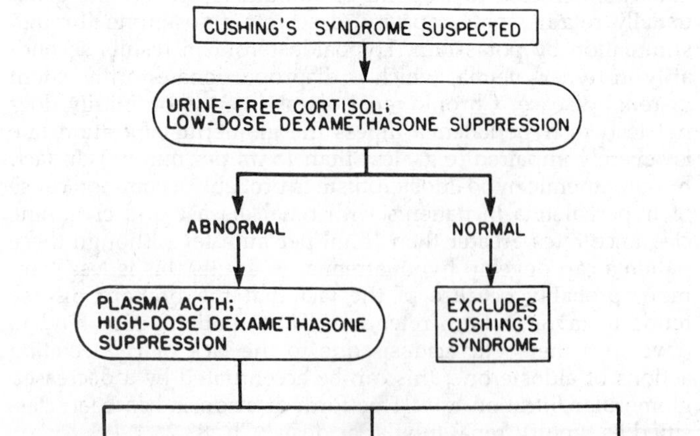

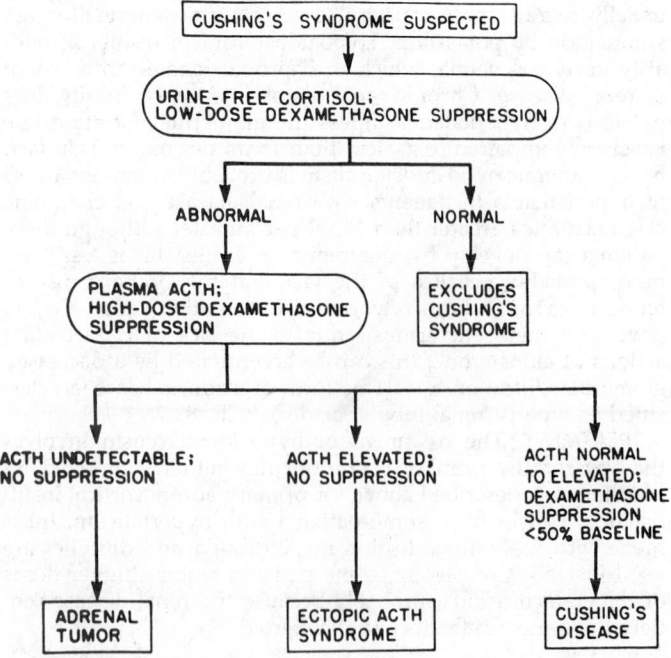

Figure 229–7. Evaluation of Cushing's syndrome. Boxes enclose clinical decisions and circles enclose diagnostic tests. See the text for details and the potential for false-positive and false-negative results. (Reprinted from Baxter JD, Tyrrell JB: *In* Felig P, Baxter JD, Broadus AE, Frohman LA (eds.): Endocrinology and Metabolism. New York, McGraw-Hill Book Company, 1981, p 475.)

laboratory tests may suggest the diagnosis but are nonspecific. These include high normal or modestly elevated values for the hematocrit, slightly elevated white cell counts, and a depressed percentage of lymphocytes and eosinophils. Electrolyte abnormalities occur only rarely in Cushing's disease, and the presence of hypokalemia should suggest the ectopic ACTH syndrome or adrenal carcinoma.

DIAGNOSIS. A suggested plan for the evaluation of suspected Cushing's syndrome is shown in Figure 229–7. If the syndrome is suspected the 24-hour urine free cortisol should be measured and the overnight 1 mg dexamethasone suppression test performed.

If results of both of these tests are normal, the diagnosis of Cushing's syndrome is excluded, with two exceptions: (1) Rare patients whose disease activity is episodic can have normal tests during periods of inactivity. In these cases, repeated evaluation during periods of disease activity will estabish the diagnosis. (2) Rare patients with Cushing's disease will have delayed clearance of dexamethasone, presumably on a genetic basis, and therefore will have a normal response to a low dose of dexamethasone. However, these patients will have elevated urine free cortisol levels.

If the 24-hour urine free cortisol level is elevated and the 1 mg overnight dexamethasone suppression test is abnormal, then spontaneous Cushing's syndrome is present provided that several abnormalities that lead to false-positive responses can be excluded. In obesity, estrogen therapy, drug therapy that increases dexamethasone metabolism (listed in Ch. 29), and chronic renal failure, results of the dexamethasone suppression test can be abnormal, although the 24-hour urine free cortisol is almost always in the normal range. In the case of obesity and estrogen therapy, the two-day low-dose dexamethasone test should be performed; the results are almost always normal in the absence of Cushing's syndrome. Response to both the 24-hour urine free cortisol and the 1 mg dexamethasone suppression tests can be abnormal in alcoholism, acute and chronic illness, depression and other states of substantial emotional stress, and anorexia nervosa. In these cases, in the absence of spontaneous Cushing's syndrome the abnormalities will subside following cessation of the condition. In any event, caution must be exercised before the diagnosis of spontaneous Cushing's syndrome is made in the presence of these conditions.

ETIOLOGIC DIAGNOSIS. Once the diagnosis of Cushing's syndrome has been established, it is essential to determine its specific cause. The two most useful procedures are the measurement of basal plasma ACTH levels and the high-dose dexamethasone suppression test. In Cushing's disease, ACTH levels are normal to modestly elevated (50 to 200 pg per milliliter) and in 90 per cent of these patients, plasma or urinary steroid levels are suppressed to less than 50 per cent of baseline values in response to the high-dose dexamethasone test. In the ectopic ACTH syndrome, plasma ACTH values are often markedly elevated and are more than 200 pg per milliliter in two thirds of patients. In about 95 per cent of these patients, hypothalamic-pituitary control of ACTH and cortisol secretion is absent, and there is no response to high-dose dexamethasone suppression. Exceptions occur in patients with relatively benign carcinoids or thymomas in whom ACTH levels may be only modestly elevated and in whom the high dose of dexamethasone may suppress ACTH release. With glucocorticoid–secreting adrenal tumors, plasma ACTH levels are suppressed to either low normal or undetectable levels, and dexamethasone suppression testing produces no reduction in cortisol levels.

Two major problems are encountered in determining the cause: (1) In approximately 10 per cent of patients with Cushing's disease the cortisol levels are not suppressed adequately in response to dexamethasone, and (2) approximately 5 per cent of patients with ectopic tumors have suppression in response to high-dose dexamethasone and thus may appear to have Cushing's disease. Testing with CRF will certainly aid in the differentiation of these two causes, since, in general,

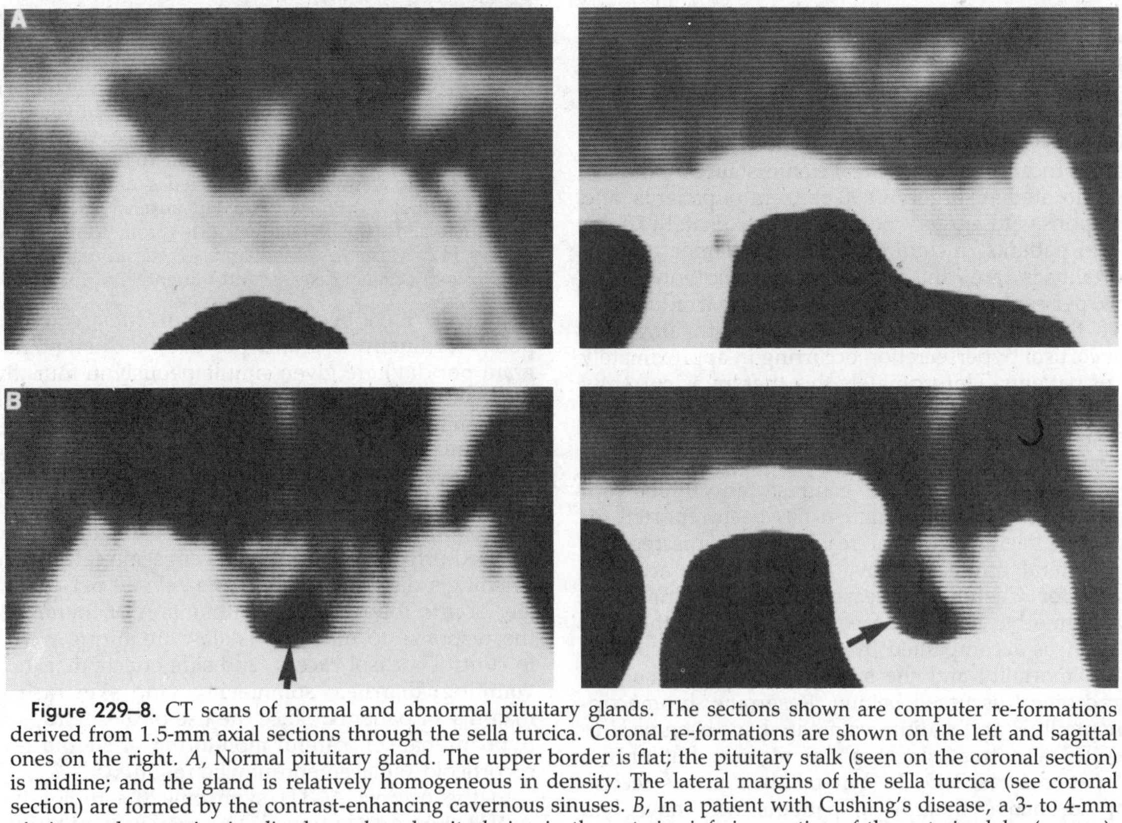

Figure 229–8. CT scans of normal and abnormal pituitary glands. The sections shown are computer re-formations derived from 1.5-mm axial sections through the sella turcica. Coronal re-formations are shown on the left and sagittal ones on the right. *A,* Normal pituitary gland. The upper border is flat; the pituitary stalk (seen on the coronal section) is midline; and the gland is relatively homogeneous in density. The lateral margins of the sella turcica (see coronal section) are formed by the contrast-enhancing cavernous sinuses. *B,* In a patient with Cushing's disease, a 3- to 4-mm pituitary adenoma is visualized as a low-density lesion in the anterior inferior portion of the anterior lobe (arrows). (Reprinted from Findling JW, Tyrrell JB: *In* Greenspan FS, Forsham PH (eds.): Basic and Clinical Endocrinology. Los Altos, Lange Medical Publications, 1983, p 59.)

responsiveness is observed in Cushing's disease but not in the ectopic ACTH syndrome. In some cases, lack of suppression with pituitary adenomas occurs with larger tumors that will be apparent when computed tomography (CT) is performed. Also, this problem is more frequent when there is nodular adrenal hyperplasia. With these cases it is necessary to use additional procedures to establish the diagnosis. These include extensive tumor screening such as the use of head and body CT, selective venous sampling of the petrosal sinuses that drain the anterior pituitary and of other suspected regions, and utilization of higher doses of dexamethasone.

Tumor Localization. In Cushing's disease high-resolution contrast-enhanced CT of the pituitary is the procedure of choice (Fig. 229–8). Because of the small size of these tumors, however, such scans allow definite tumor localization in only approximately 60 per cent of cases. Other radiologic procedures including plain sellar radiographs, polytomography, arteriography, and pneumoencephalography are of little additional utility. In the absence of a radiologically evident lesion consistent with an adenoma it is recommended that selective venous sampling for ACTH be performed prior to surgical interventions. This technique has been useful in establishing a pituitary cause of Cushing's syndrome, including in those patients with dexamethasone–nonsuppressible Cushing's disease, and in excluding a pituitary cause when an occult ectopic ACTH-secreting tumor is present. The technique requires an experienced radiologist, since sampling from the inferior petrosal sinuses is required to assess pituitary ACTH secretion adequately. A gradient of 2:1 of central to peripheral ACTH levels establishes the presence of Cushing's disease.

CT and ultrasonography of the adrenal (Fig. 229–9) should be used in patients with suspected adrenal tumors or in whom the cause is in doubt. Adrenal tumors are usually larger than 2 cm in diameter when diagnosed and thus are readily visible with those procedures. Adrenal scanning should also be performed when ACTH levels or dexamethasone studies are inconclusive. In this case they will help differentiate hyperplasia from primary adrenal tumors and may help to establish the diagnosis of nodular adrenal hyperplasia.

TREATMENT. Pituitary microsurgery with a transsphenoidal approach is the current method of choice for the initial therapy of Cushing's disease. It is critical that it be performed by a surgeon with substantial experience with the technique as it is not a common procedure. Under ideal circumstances, pituitary tumors can be located at surgery in 90 per cent of patients, and successful responses to surgery occur in approximately 80 per cent of all the patients, including those with larger tumors. Surgical mortality is rare, and significant complications occur in less than 2 per cent of patients. Heavy-particle irradiation is also effective therapy for Cushing's disease, with long-term correction of cortisol hypersecretion occurring in approximately 80 per cent of patients. Unfortunately this therapy is currently available in only one center in the United States. Conventional radiotherapy is successful in only 15 to 25 per cent of adults and should not be used as initial therapy because it precludes any further radiation therapy. In contrast, an 80 per cent response rate to conventional radiation has been reported for Cushing's disease in childhood; the reason for this discrepancy is unclear. Bilateral adrenalectomy, previously an accepted initial therapy for Cushing's disease, should be limited to patients in whom other therapies are unsuccessful. In the past, this procedure was accompanied by a high degree of surgical morbidity and mortality and the subsequent development of Nelson's syndrome (discussed below). Reserpine, bromocriptine, cyproheptadine, and sodium valproate have been used to suppress ACTH and treat Cushing's syndrome, but only a minority of patients respond. In general their use is recommended for adjunctive therapy in patients who have had unsuccessful responses to other therapy.

Drugs that inhibit adrenal cortisol secretion can also be used as adjunctive therapy or in patients in whom more definitive

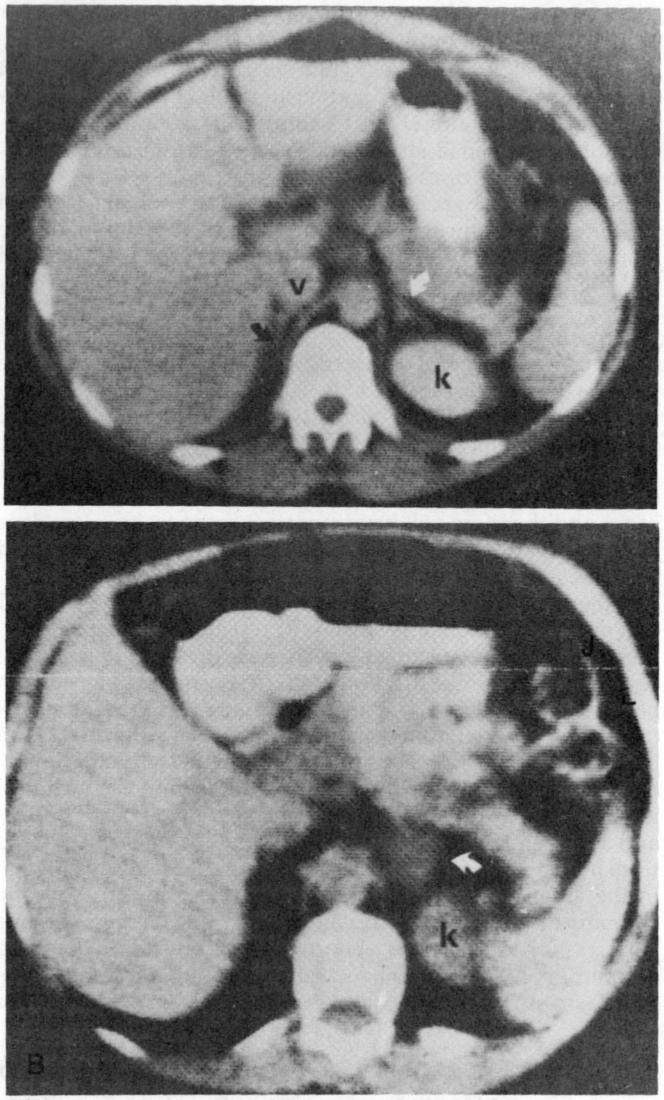

Figure 229–9. CT scans in Cushing's syndrome. *A*, Patient with ACTH-dependent Cushing's syndrome. The adrenal glands are not detectably abnormal by this procedure. The curvilinear right adrenal (black arrow) is shown posterior to the inferior vena cava (v) between the right lobe of the liver and the right crus of the diaphragm. The left adrenal (white arrow) has an inverted Y appearance anteromedial to the left kidney (k). *B*, A 3-cm left adrenal adenoma (white arrow) anteromedial to the left kidney (k). (From Korobkin M, White EA, Kressel HY, Moss AA, Montagne J-P: Computed tomographs in the diagnosis of adrenal disease. Am J Roentgenol 132:231, 1979.)

treatments have been unsuccessful. Most commonly, metyrapone* (ordinarily 2 grams per day) and aminoglutethimide (1 gram per day) are given simultaneously in four divided doses. These drugs are expensive, have frequent side effects that are predominantly gastrointestinal upsets, and result in secondary increases in ACTH levels that sometimes are sufficient to overcome the enzyme inhibition. They have not been used successfully for long-term therapy of Cushing's disease. Alternatively, mitotane, 3 to 6 grams per day in divided doses, can be used if tolerated. Although remission rates with the drug in Cushing's disease are approximately 80 per cent, relapse usually occurs following discontinuation of therapy. In addition, the response to mitotane is slow, requiring weeks to months to control cortisol excess, and side effects that include nausea, vomiting, diarrhea, somnolence, and skin rash occur in the majority of patients. Since the use of these drugs may produce hypoadrenalism, careful monitoring of steroid levels and glucocorticoid replacement may be required.

In the ectopic ACTH syndrome the tumor hypersecreting ACTH should be removed. This may be possible in the minority

*This use is not listed in the manufacturer's directive.

of patients with the more benign tumors such as thymoma, bronchial carcinoid, or pheochromocytoma. Unfortunately in the majority of patients the tumors are malignant and metastasize prior to the diagnosis of cortisol excess. In such patients, drug therapy as discussed above is used to control cortisol excess. Metyrapone and aminoglutethimide are preferred to mitotane because of their more rapid onset of action. Also hypokalemia should be corrected as required, and in some patients spironolactone therapy may be useful in blocking the mineralocorticoid effects of cortisol and 11-deoxycorticosterone. Bilateral adrenalectomy might be considered in a rare patient in whom drug therapy is inadequate and the cortisol excess rather than the tumor is life threatening.

The treatment of adrenal tumors is primarily surgical. Patients with unilateral adrenal adenoma should undergo resection of the affected adrenal. Since ACTH secretion and the contralateral adrenal are suppressed in these patients, glucocorticoid replacement therapy is required pending recovery of the normal adrenal, which frequently requires 9 to 12 months. Although surgical cure of adrenocortical carcinoma is unusual, surgical removal of the primary tumor is indicated to reduce cortisol secretion even when metastases are present. Mitotane 6 to 12 grams per day in divided doses, if tolerated, is recommended for patients with residual or nonresectable carcinoma, and approximately 75 per cent of patients achieve reduced steroid secretion. Only about one third of patients undergo reduction in tumor bulk, however, and it is not clear whether the drug prolongs survival. Metyrapone and aminoglutethimide can be used in patients who do not respond to or tolerate mitotane. The prognosis is poor with adrenal carcinoma; most patients survive less than five years following the onset of symptoms.

NELSON'S SYNDROME. Defined as the clinical progression of an ACTH–secreting pituitary adenoma following bilateral adrenalectomy for Cushing's disease, this syndrome appears to occur in at least one third of such patients. Fortunately the incidence of this disorder has dropped dramatically because of the decreased use of bilateral adrenalectomy for treatment of Cushing's disease.

The syndrome most likely results from enhanced progression of the pre-existing pituitary adenoma due to reduction of cortisol feedback inhibition of the tumor. Nelson's syndrome is seen with increasing hyperpigmentation usually within 1 to 2 years following adrenalectomy. In addition, these patients frequently exhibit local manifestations, including hypopituitarism, visual loss, headache, cavernous sinus invasion with extraocular muscle palsies, and rarely malignant changes with metastatic spread. Plasma ACTH levels are dramatically elevated and usually range from 1000 to 10,000 pg per milliliter. The majority of these tumors are greater than 1 cm in diameter and are readily localized by CT of the sella turcica.

The treatment of Nelson's syndrome is considerably less successful than that of Cushing's disease because of the large size and aggressive nature of these tumors. Although pituitary microsurgery is the preferred initial therapy, complete tumor resection is usually not possible. Heavy-particle irradiation may be utilized either as primary therapy or after surgery in patients with intrasellar tumors; however, in those with extrasellar extension, conventional postoperative radiation therapy should be undertaken. Although pharmacologic inhibition of ACTH secretion has been attempted with cyproheptadine, bromocriptine, and valproic acid, it appears that only a minority of patients respond. Nevertheless, trials of these medications are indicated if surgical and radiotherapeutic treatments are unsuccessful.

Mineralocorticoid Excess States

John D. Baxter

PRIMARY ALDOSTERONISM

Increased inappropriate production of aldosterone from the adrenal is known as primary aldosteronism, and leads to sodium retention with hypertension, suppression of plasma renin and to hypokalemia and its manifestations. It is due mainly to an adrenocortical adenoma, bilateral adrenocortical hyperplasia, or rarely to an adrenal carcinoma. The disease occurs in all age groups, with a peak incidence during the third and fourth decades. About 70 per cent of the adenomas occur in women. Although primary aldosteronism almost always results in hypertension (normotensive primary hyperaldosteronism is extremely rare), the syndrome is present in only a very small proportion (less than 2 per cent) of patients with hypertension. Nevertheless, this largely reversible form of hypertension should be considered in all hypertensive patients.

ALDOSTERONE-PRODUCING ADENOMAS. With an aldosterone-producing adenoma (Conn's syndrome), aldosterone excess leads to sodium retention and to potassium and hydrogen loss. Other steroids that are normally synthesized in the zona glomerulosa (i.e., deoxycorticosterone, corticosterone, and 18-hydroxycorticosterone) are also produced in excess, although they are probably not important in the overall pathophysiology. Sodium retention results in expansion of the extracellular fluid volume, increase in total body sodium content, and elevation of serum sodium concentration. Ultimately there is a major redistribution of fluid with an increased intracellular sodium content in tissues; this may contribute to increased vascular reactivity. Although it is clear that prolonged sodium retention is a major contributor to the associated hypertension, it has been proposed that aldosterone may have other hypertensive actions as well. The electrolyte abnormalities of hyperaldosteronism result in muscular weakness, a tendency to cardiac irritability and arrhythmia, carbohydrate intolerance, resistance to vasopressin (nephrogenic diabetes insipidus), and abnormalities in baroreceptor function. The last results in more volume-dependent hypertension. The expansion of the extracellular fluid and plasma volume is registered by the stretch receptors at the juxtaglomerular apparatus and by sodium chloride flux at the macula densa with suppression of renin release, low plasma renin levels, and unresponsiveness of renin release to the provocative stimuli that usually effect release. Thus, increased aldosterone production with a suppressed renin system defines the disorder.

Long term, the sustained hypertension leads to a bodily compensation by decreasing somewhat the plasma volume, although the hypertension continues to be aldosterone dependent. The hypertension can also lead to many of the complications of hypertension such as renal damage, stroke, and myocardial infarction.

BILATERAL ADRENAL HYPERPLASIA. Bilateral adrenal hyperplasia can be diffuse or nodular, and selectively involves the glomerulosa cells. In most series it accounts for perhaps 20 per cent of the patients in whom primary aldosteronism is diagnosed; however, its precise incidence is not known, since there is a gradient between what is termed low-renin essential hypertension without frank aldosterone excess and this syndrome. Adrenal hyperplasia is not known to precede development of an adenoma.

The pathophysiology of hyperplasia shows at least four differences from that of adenoma; (1) Even though the plasma renin is suppressed, unlike the case with an aldosterone-producing adenoma, it responds to postural and other stimuli. (2) The adrenal appears to be hypersensitive to angiotensin II, exhibiting a marked increase in aldosterone production rather than insensitivity. (3) The aldosterone hypersecretion tends to be less than with the adenoma, a feature that is useful in the differential diagnosis. By contrast the blood pressure in the two groups tends to be similar. (4) The hypertension tends not to respond to adrenalectomy, implying that common factors produce both hypertension and enhanced adrenal sensitivity to angiotensin II. Whereas the mechanism for the development of hyperplasia is unknown, it is attractive to hypothesize that there is abnormal production (or loss) of a factor that enhances adrenal and vascular sensitivity to angiotensin II.

CLINICAL PRESENTATION. Patients usually appear for treatment because of elevated blood pressure detected on routine screening or, less commonly, because of symptoms of hypokalemia. The blood pressure elevations range from mild to severe, with mean presenting pressures in the range of 200 mm Hg systolic and 120 mm Hg diastolic. Malignant hypertension is rare. A history of hypertension in pregnancy is common with female patients who develop the disorder. When present, symptoms of hypokalemia include the nonspecific complaints of tiredness, loss of stamina, weakness, nocturia, and lassitude. Symptoms of more severe depletion include alkalosis, rarely with a positive Trousseau or Chvostek sign; increased thirst and polyuria with low urine specific gravity and unresponsiveness to vasopressin; paresthesias; cardiac arrhythmias such as ventricular tachycardia; and postural hypotension with dizziness. The serum sodium is rarely less than 139 mEq per liter in the absence of diuretic therapy. In spite of fluid overload, edema is only rarely present. The heart is usually only mildly enlarged, if at all, and electrocardiographic changes are usually those of moderate left ventricular hypertrophy and potassium depletion. There tend to be fewer funduscopic changes relative to the hypertension than in other forms of hypertension.

DIAGNOSIS. The hallmarks of the disorder are hypertension with hypokalemia, suppression of the renin-angiotensin system, and increased aldosterone production. A suggested evaluation plan is shown in Figure 229–10. The initial step in diagnosis is to determine whether hypokalemia is present, since this is the hallmark of mineralocorticoid excess. All patients with hypertension should be screened, especially those with spontaneous hypokalemia, after diuretics have been withheld for at least three weeks.

The evaluation of hypokalemia requires control of the sodium balance, since sodium depletion from decreased intake or diuretics can decrease urinary potassium excretion and thus mask hypokalemia. Random serum potassium levels may be normal in up to 20 per cent of patients with primary aldosteronism, but salt loading will unmask hypokalemia in virtually all patients. If according to the dietary history the patient's usual sodium intake is 120 mEq per 24 hours or greater, measurement of normal potassium levels on three occasions obviates the need for further evaluation. If dietary intake is inadequate or unclear, the patient is instructed to consume a normal diet supplemented with 1 gram of NaCl with each meal for four days, and the serum potassium is then measured.

If the plasma potassium value is low, other causes of hypokalemia should be ruled out: diuretic therapy, gastrointestinal loss due to vomiting or diarrhea, other mineralocorticoid excess syndromes (discussed below), starvation, insulin and glucose therapy, metabolic acidosis, renal disease, and renovascular and accelerated hypertension. The tests described below should allow these to be ruled out.

Random unstimulated plasma renin activity (PRA) or plasma renin concentration (PRC) should be determined as the next step in diagnosis. In primary aldosteronism this will be suppressed even after short-term diuretic therapy, salt restriction, assumption of erect posture, or exercise, although other causes of low renin must be excluded. If PRA is normal or high, primary aldosteronism is unlikely.

If the plasma renin value is low or marginally low, 24-hour urinary aldosterone and the plasma aldosterone should be measured. Urinary measurement is superior to plasma measurement for detecting mild primary aldosteronism. Plasma measurements are elevated in most cases of primary aldosteronism, however, and are more useful in the differential diagnosis of the various forms of primary aldosteronism. It is critical to monitor the salt intake and posture, as discussed earlier, because patients with essential hypertension and a low salt intake will have increased aldosterone levels. The urinary aldosterone is increased to over 17 μg per 24 hours in most cases of primary aldosteronism regardless of the cause. With an adenoma the overnight recumbent plasma aldosterone levels will almost always exceed 20 ng per deciliter. In hyperplasia the plasma aldosterone levels are ordinarily less than 20 ng per deciliter and frequently are in the normal range. The effect of hypokalemia that decreases aldosterone secretion must also be

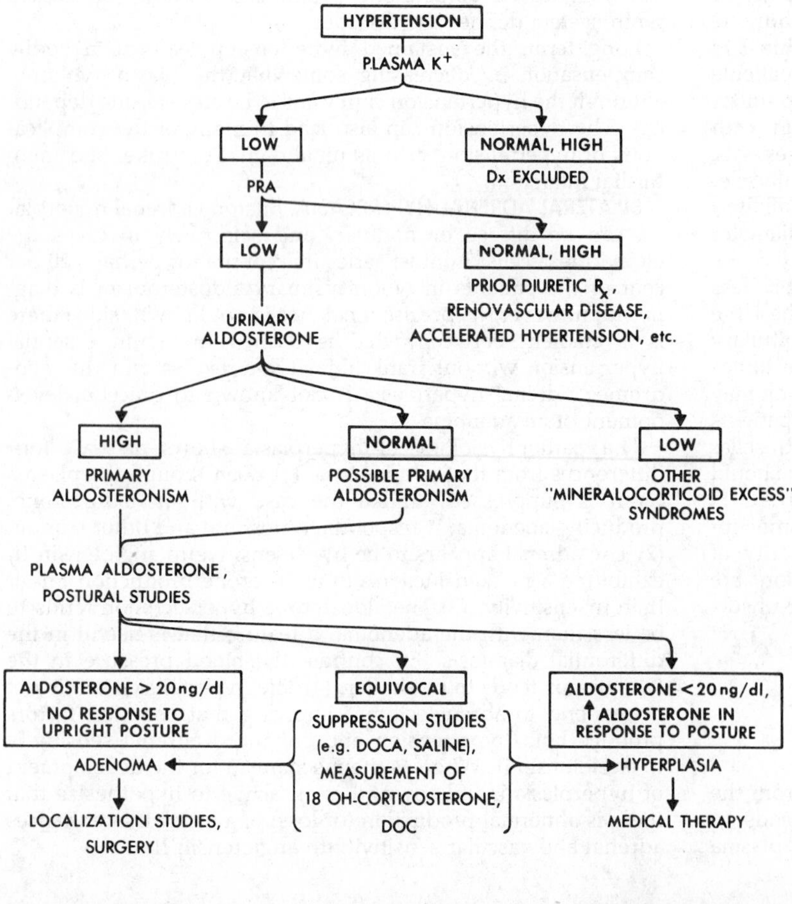

Figure 229–10. Flow diagram for the evaluation of primary aldosteronism. PRA = plasma renin activity. Dx = diagnosis. Rx = therapy. (Reprinted from Biglieri EG, Baxter JD: *In* Felig P, Baxter JD, Broadus AE, Frohman LA (eds.): Endocrinology and Metabolism. New York, McGraw-Hill Book Company, 1981, p 569.)

considered. Thus, in the presence of hypokalemia and suppressed PRA, aldosterone levels in the normal range are inappropriately high and thus abnormal.

In the presence of marginally suppressed PRC and mild elevation of plasma or urinary aldosterone, one of the stimulation tests (discussed earlier) may be necessary to diagnose primary aldosteronism. In general they are unnecessary if accurate plasma and urine aldosterone measurements can be obtained. Marginal cases are usually due to primary aldosteronism with hyperplasia, in which case antimineralocorticoid therapy is indicated. In many cases such therapy can be initiated and the case re-evaluated at a later time.

If the diagnosis of primary aldosteronism is made, it is important for therapy to distinguish between adenoma and hyperplasia. The levels of plasma aldosterone provide an initial indication; if these are substantially elevated, e.g., above 30 ng per deciliter, postural studies are unnecessary. 18-Hydroxycorticosterone measurements may even be better for discrimination, but these are not generally available. Since plasma aldosterone levels in hyperplasia but not adenoma are still under control by the renin-angiotensin system, the plasma aldosterone response to posture can be discriminatory. Patients with an adenoma will not show an increase in plasma aldosterone concentration and PRA (or at most a slight increase), whereas patients with hyperplasia will show such increases. These procedures will allow a diagnosis to be made in most instances. If uncertainty still exists, the response to DOCA, 9α-fluorocortisol, or saline can be measured and will almost always allow a distinction. More recent studies indicate that the converting-enzyme inhibitor captopril can be used alternatively. The inhibitor causes a drop in plasma aldosterone concentration in patients with hyperplasia but not adenoma.

Once an adenoma is suspected, CT of the adrenals should be performed. In most cases this will permit localization of the tumor. In the less than 20 per cent of patients in whom an adenoma is not found, selective venous sampling with measurements of aldosterone-cortisol ratios is usually helpful, can determine whether adenoma or hyperplasia is present, and can lateralize an adenoma.

TREATMENT. Unilateral adrenalectomy is indicated for aldosterone-producing adenomas. Prior to surgery the blood pressure and serum potassium should be normalized by treatment with the mineralocorticoid antagonist spironolactone (200 to 400 mg per day) or the potassium–sparing diuretic amiloride (20 to 40 mg per day). Medical therapy can be continued in the rare patient in whom surgery is contraindicated. This form of treatment also tends to reactivate the suppressed renin-angiotensin system so that the incidence of postoperative hypoaldosteronism is reduced. Also the response of the blood pressure to this therapy provides an excellent indication of the anticipated response to surgery.

Following surgery the blood pressure returns to normal in around 50 per cent of patients with reduction of hypertension in another 25 per cent. However, hypertension, but not hyperaldosteronism, returns in about 40 per cent by ten years postoperatively.

Most patients with bilateral hyperplasia will not respond to surgery; therefore medical therapy is recommended. These patients should be given spironolactone or amiloride in doses described above; this will correct the hypokalemia, but will not correct the hypertension in most cases. Additional antihypertensive medications are usually necessary. There is also a rare subgroup of patients with hyperplasia whose hyperaldosteronism is responsive to glucocorticoids; treatment of these patients with a glucocorticoid in normal replacement amounts or slightly above such amounts is recommended. Whether all patients with hyperplasia should be screened for this responsiveness is controversial.

OTHER FORMS OF HYPERTENSION ASSOCIATED WITH MINERALOCORTICOID EXCESS

There are several other mineralocorticoid-excess conditions. DOC excess can occur in the 11β- and 17α-hydroxylase syndromes (Ch. 233) and in occasional patients with Cushing's syndrome. This is particularly true when the latter is due to an ectopic ACTH-producing carcinoma. It can also be seen in certain adrenal carcinomas. In all these cases the PRC is suppressed as it is in primary aldosteronism; however, plasma aldosterone levels are usually suppressed as well in these conditions. Rarely iatrogenic causes of mineralocorticoid-excess hypertension result from excessive ingestion of licorice, carbenoxolone (for ulcer treatment), 9α-fluorocortisol for postural hypotension, or mineralocorticoid-containing nasal sprays (not available in the United States). It can be present in rare cases of relative generalized insensitivity to glucocorticoids when elevated cortisol levels have mineralocorticoid actions. There are some rare syndromes in which there are hypertension, hypokalemia, and suppressed PRC with no detectable elevations of known mineralocorticoids (e.g., Liddle's syndrome, Ch. 83.5). Some of these syndromes could represent primary hypersensitivity to mineralocorticoids. In all of these conditions there are hypertension, hypokalemia, and suppression of PRC without an associated increase of aldosterone.

SECONDARY HYPERALDOSTERONISM

Secondary hyperaldosteronism results from stimulation of the adrenal glomerulosa by extra-adrenal factors, usually the renin-angiotensin system. It can be physiologic or contribute to the pathology of disease states. A physiologic increase occurs during excessive potassium intake as part of the body's defense against hyperkalemia. Secondary hyperaldosteronism can occur during the luteal phase of the menstrual cycle and occasionally during oral contraceptive use. Aldosterone secretion increases progessively during normal pregnancy; levels are elevated by the fifteenth week of gestation and are ten times those of nonpregnant women in the third trimester. This is presumably due to an increase in renin and angiotensin, possibly due to the decrease in blood pressure that occurs in pregnancy. Interestingly, renin levels are more elevated during the first trimester, whereas plasma aldosterone levels are highest during the third trimester. This may be due to a progessive increase in sensitivity of the adrenal glomerulosa to angiotensin II. Aldosterone secretion increases when there is excessive sodium loss and when there is dietary restriction of sodium. Aldosterone increases in some patients with congestive heart failure and with significant hypoalbuminemia. Renin and aldosterone levels are commonly elevated in cirrhosis when ascites is present; this is accentuated by decreased clearance of aldosterone. The increased aldosterone further promotes sodium retention and potassium loss; this explains the rationale of using mineralocorticoid antagonists in the treatment of ascites. Elevated aldosterone levels are found in Bartter's syndrome (Ch. 83.5). Finally, secondary hyperaldosteronism and hypertension can occur with renal artery stenosis, unilateral renal ischemia, accelerated hypertension, and renin-secreting tumors.

Aron DC, Tyrrell JB, Fitzgerald PA, Findling JW, Forsham PH: Cushing's syndrome: Problems in diagnosis. Medicine 60:25, 1981. *An analysis of the problems and approaches when results do not conform to the usual norms.*

Baxter JD, Tyrrell JB: The adrenal cortex. *In* Felig P, Baxter JD, Broadus AE, Frohman LA (eds.): Endocrinology and Metabolism. New York, McGraw-Hill Book Company, 1981, pp 385–510. *An extensive review of the physiology and pathology of the adrenal cortex.*

Biglieri EG, Baxter JD: The endocrinology of hypertension. *In* Felig P, Baxter JD, Broadus AE, Frohman LA (eds.): Endocrinology and Metabolism. New York, McGraw-Hill Book Company, 1981, pp 551–598. *An analysis of the pathophysiology and approaches to diagnosis and treatment of not only primary aldosteronism but also of other types of endocrine hypertension.*

Chrousos GP, Schulte HM, Oldfield EH, Gold PW, Cutler GB Jr, Loriaux DL: The corticotropin-releasing factor stimulation test. An aid in the evaluation of patients with Cushing's syndrome. N Engl J Med 310:622, 1984. Orth ON: The old and the new in Cushing's syndrome. N Engl J Med 310:649, 1984. *These papers establish the utility of CRF in the differential diagnosis of Cushing's syndrome and are accompanied by a thoughtful editorial overview of the procedures in the differential diagnosis of cortisol excess.*

Crapo L: Cushing's syndrome: A review of diagnostic tests. Metabolism 28:955,

1979. *A detailed evaluation of the many diagnostic approaches to Cushing's syndrome. Required reading for a background in this area.*

Finkelstein M, Shaefer JM: Inborn errors of steroid biosynthesis. Physiol Rev 59:353, 1979. *This article examines the enzymology and metabolic derangements that occur in association with steroid hormone biosynthetic defects.*

Irvine WJ, Toft AD, Feek CM: Addison's disease. *In* James VHT (ed.): The Adrenal Gland. New York, Raven Press, 1979, pp 131–164. *An extensive analysis of the pathophysiology of Addison's disease and the associated disorders.*

Keeton TK, Campbell WB: The pharmacologic alteration of renin release. Pharmacol Rev 31:81, 1980. *An overview of renin release with emphasis on pharmacological factors that alter it.*

Keller-Wood ME, Dallman M: Corticosteroid inhibition of ACTH secretion. Endocr Rev 5:1, 1984. *A review of the kinetics and mechanisms whereby glucocorticoids block both CRF and ACTH release.*

Krieger DT: Physiopathology of Cushing's disease. Endocr Rev 4:22, 1983. *This analysis of Cushing's disease emphasizes its possible causes.*

Lieberman S, Greenfield NJ, Wolfson A: A heuristic proposal for understanding steroidogenic processes. Endocr Rev 5:128, 1984. *A review of the enzymology and the pathways in steroid biosynthesis.*

Munck A, Guyre P, Holbrook NJ: Physiological functions of glucocorticoids in stress and their relation to pharmacological actions. Endocr Rev 5:25, 1984. *A new proposal that explains how glucocorticoids are useful in the body's response to stress.*

Parker LN, Odell WD: Control of adrenal androgen secretion. Endocr Rev 1:392, 1980. *An excellent examination of the factors that regulate adrenal androgen production.*

230. DIABETES MELLITUS

Jerrold M. Olefsky

DEFINITION. Diabetes mellitus is a heterogeneous primary disorder of carbohydrate metabolism with multiple etiologic factors that generally involve absolute or relative insulin deficiency or insulin resistance or both. All causes of diabetes ultimately lead to hyperglycemia, which is the hallmark of this disease syndrome.

CLASSIFICATION AND DIAGNOSIS

The currently accepted classification and criteria for the diagnosis of diabetes mellitus are based on the 1979 report of the National Diabetes Data Group and are comparable to the standards set forth by the World Health Organization (Table 230–1). Diabetes can be separated into two general disease syndromes: (1) *Type I,* or *insulin-dependent diabetes mellitus* (IDDM), is present in patients with little or no endogenous insulin secretory capacity. These patients develop extreme hyperglycemia, ketosis, and the associated symptomatology unless treated with insulin, and they are therefore entirely dependent on exogenous insulin therapy for immediate survival. This form of the disease usually, but not always, develops prior to early adulthood. Older terms for this syndrome are juvenile onset, ketosis prone, or brittle diabetes. (2) *Type II,* or *noninsulin-dependent diabetes mellitus* (NIDDM), occurs in patients who retain significant endogenous insulin secretory capacity. Although treatment with insulin may be necessary for control of hyperglycemia, these patients do not develop ketosis in the absence of insulin therapy and are not dependent on exogenous insulin for immediate survival. Previous terms for this form of the disease are maturity or adult onset, nonketotic, and stable diabetes. The diagnosis of diabetes in patients with the insulin-dependent form of the disease is usually unequivocal, and the distinction between type I and type II diabetes can usually be made on clinical grounds. However, there are occasional patients with minimal, but clearly detectable, endogenous insulin secretion in whom the disease is difficult to categorize initially; when these patients are followed over longer periods, however, the necessary distinction can usually be made.

TABLE 230–1. CLASSIFICATION OF DIABETES

1. Insulin-dependent, or type I diabetes (IDDM). Formerly called juvenile-onset or ketosis-prone diabetes.
2. Noninsulin-dependent, or type II diabetes (NIDDM). Formerly called adult-onset, maturity-onset, or nonketotic diabetes.
   A. Obese (~80%)
   B. Nonobese (~20%)
3. Secondary diabetes
   A. Pancreatic disease (e.g., pancreatectomy, pancreatic insufficiency, hemochromatosis)
   B. Hormonal (excess counterinsulin hormones, e.g., Cushing's syndrome, acromegaly, pheochromocytoma)
   C. Drug-induced (e.g., thiazide diuretics, steroids, phenytoin)
   D. Associated with specific genetic syndromes (e.g., lipodystrophy, myotonic dystrophy, ataxia telangiectasia)
4. Impaired glucose tolerance (IGT). Formerly called chemical, latent, borderline, or subclinical diabetes.
5. Gestational diabetes: glucose intolerance with onset during pregnancy.

The diagnosis of NIDDM is based on a distinction between normal and abnormal levels of glycemia and therefore is less precise. Prior to the report of the National Diabetes Data Group, oral glucose tolerance tests were commonly used to establish this diagnosis. This approach is fraught with difficulties because oral glucose tolerance is affected by numerous other variables that can cause mild abnormalities of glucose metabolism independent of diabetes. Concomitant illness, stress, physical inactivity, hypocaloric or low carbohydrate intake, various drugs, and aging are among those factor that can adversely influence glucose tolerance. Therefore, when employed, glucose tolerance testing must be rigorously controlled by administering a standard oral glucose load (75 grams), insuring an appropriate antecedent diet (eucaloric with at least 200 grams carbohydrate per day), adequate physical activity, and the absence of drugs affecting carbohydrate metabolism. Even with these precautions, only a minority (15 to 25 per cent) of individuals who have normal fasting plasma glucose levels with abnormal glucose tolerance tests go on to develop overt diabetes. In recognition of the above facts, the National Diabetes Data Group recommended relatively stringent criteria for establishing the diagnosis of NIDDM: (1) fasting venous plasma glucose concentration $>$ 140 mg per deciliter on at least two separate occasions, or (2) in the absence of fasting hyperglycemia, a diagnosis of NIDDM can be made following ingestion of the standard 75-gram oral glucose tolerance test if the 2-hour venous plasma glucose and one other sample (the 30-, 60-, or 90-minute sample) exceed 200 mg per deciliter.

Impaired glucose tolerance exists if the fasting plasma glucose level is less than 140 mg per deciliter and if the 30-, 60-, or 90-minute plasma glucose concentration exceeds 200 mg per deciliter along with a 2-hour plasma glucose level between 140 and 200 mg per deciliter. Microvascular complications of diabetes rarely occur in individuals with impaired glucose tolerance, and the great majority of these cases do not deteriorate to overt diabetes in long-term follow up. Most instances of impaired glucose tolerance, therefore, are probably unrelated to the disease syndrome of NIDDM. Almost all patients who meet the criteria for NIDDM during oral glucose tolerance testing show fasting hyperglycemia (greater than 140 mg per deciliter) when they are repeatedly evaluated. Furthermore, in those few patients who meet the criteria for NIDDM in the absence of fasting hyperglycemia, most do not develop fasting hyperglycemia during prolonged follow-up, and clinical symptoms of diabetes are unusual. Thus the clinical significance of impaired glucose tolerance is unclear. As previously mentioned, only a minority (2 to 35 per cent, depending on the population examined) of these patients go on to develop overt NIDDM when followed for up to 20 years. In evaluating the meaning of impaired glucose tolerance, the real challenge is to develop markers to detect which patients with impaired glucose tolerance have a benign nonprogressive abnormality of glucose intolerance and which have a prediabetic state. Patients with impaired glucose tolerance who secrete low amounts of insulin, compared to normal individuals, have a much higher risk of developing overt diabetes (perhaps up to 40 per cent), whereas those who secrete high amounts of insulin seldom (about 5 per cent) progress to frank diabetes. In view of the above, it would seem that glucose tolerance testing is unnecessary for patient management in the absence of clinical signs and symptoms of diabetes, although this is still a highly useful procedure for epidemiologic or research purposes. An exception to this would be in a pregnant subject suspected of having gestational diabetes, since criteria for this diagnosis are less stringent and vigorous management of minimal degrees of hyperglycemia are deemed important.

Serum and plasma glucose concentrations are identical and run 10 to 15 per cent higher than whole blood determinations (the latter are infrequently performed nowadays). The glucose concentration in capillary blood is essentially identical to that in venous blood during the fasting state, but under postprandial conditions, tissues readily take up glucose and capillary blood glucose concentrations can be 10 to 30 mg per deciliter greater than concomitant venous blood glucose levels.

There is an age-related decline in glucose tolerance that has been extensively studied. Insulin secretion is not decreased in aging, whereas insulin resistance is a common finding in aged populations. This insulin resistance is due to a post-receptor binding defect in insulin action. Age-related variables such as inadequate diet, increasing adiposity with decreased lean body mass, and physical inactivity can contribute to this insulin-resistant state, but the aging process itself also plays a significant role. The glucose intolerance of aging tends to be mild and is most easily detected following an oral glucose challenge. When mild abnormalities of oral glucose tolerance tests were used to diagnose diabetes, age adjusted criteria for these tests had to be employed. However, with the current more stringent criteria noted above, this problem is largely obviated since the glucose intolerance of aging does not cause significant fasting hyperglycemia (more than 140 mg per deciliter) and only rarely would cause glucose intolerance severe enough to meet the new criteria in the absence of fasting hyperglycemia.

EPIDEMIOLOGY AND CLINICAL PRESENTATION

The prevalence of diabetes has been difficult to quantitate accurately because the criteria for the diagnosis of NIDDM have varied from survey to survey over the years; the less stringent the criteria the greater the prevalence and vice versa. It is hoped that the widely accepted, uniform, WHO and National Diabetes Data Group standards will successfully address this problem. Furthermore, the prevalence of diabetes differs widely among different populations, depending on ethnic group constituents, age, economic conditions, and probably other environmental factors. For example, the prevalence of diabetes is extremely high among Pima Indians (about 35 per cent) and certain Micronesian cultures (about 35 per cent). Indians, particularly after emigrating from their country, have a higher rate of diabetes than other ethnic groups. Thus, Indians living in South Africa, Trinidad, Singapore, Malayasia, and Fiji exhibit a higher prevalence of diabetes than the local population and than those living on the Indian subcontinent. A low prevalence of diabetes has been noted in Eskimos, Athabascan Indians (Alaska), and Chinese (although prevalence increases in Chinese populations living in Western countries). The proportion of IDDM to NIDDM also differs widely among different populations; IDDM is extremely rare in Pima Indians, Micronesians, and Eskimos, but is more common in Caucasian populations. *Overall, in the United States the prevalence of diabetes is probably between 2 and 4 per cent, with IDDM comprising 7 to 10 per cent of all cases.* The prevalence of IDDM (0.2 to 0.3 per cent) is probably more accurate than the estimates for NIDDM, because of the relative ease of ascertainment and the fact that many patients with NIDDM are asymptomatic and the disease is undiagnosed.

A few facts concerning the prevalence of major diabetes-related complications serve to underscore the enormous impact of this disease. Approximately 25 per cent of all new cases of end-stage renal failure occur in patients with diabetes. About 20,000 amputations (primarily of toes, feet, and legs) are carried out in patients with diabetes, representing approximately half of the nontraumatic amputations performed in the United States. Furthermore, diabetes is the leading cause of new cases of blindness, with approximately 5000 new cases occurring each year.

INSULIN-DEPENDENT DIABETES MELLITUS (IDDM, TYPE I). These patients have little or no endogenous insulin and usually present with relatively abrupt clinical symptoms of *polyuria*, *polydipsia*, and *polyphagia*. *Weight loss*, fatigue, and infection can often accompany the initial presentation. Because of the extreme hypoinsulinemia and hyperglucagonemia these patients readily develop *ketosis*, and the initial onset of this disease may be clinically evident as full-blown ketoacidosis. At the time of the first clinical presentations, symptoms can usually be traced back for several days to a few weeks. However, B cell destruction may have started months, or maybe even years, prior to the onset of clinical symptoms. Unfortunately, detection of this preclinical state of disease is seldom possible, so that methods to delay or prevent the full-blown clinical disease, even if such methods existed, will have limited feasibility and have not been systematically attempted. The peak age of onset of IDDM is 11 to 13 years, coinciding with early adolescence and puberty. A secondary peak is noted at age 6 to 8 years, and by the third decade of life the incidence falls to a steady, but still substantial level. It is unusual for IDDM to begin past age 40. Once IDDM is diagnosed, insulin therapy is required to achieve initial metabolic control. In many patients a "honeymoon" period follows initial treatment in which the disease remits and little or no insulin is required. This remission is due to a partial return of endogenous insulin secretion, which may last for several weeks or months and occasionally 1 to 2 years; ultimately, however, the disease recurs, and insulin therapy is required permanently.

NON-INSULIN DEPENDENT DIABETES MELLITUS (NIDDM, TYPE II). Patients with NIDDM typically present with polyuria and polydipsia of several weeks' to months' duration. Polyphagia can occur but is less common, whereas weight loss, weakness, and fatigue are frequent. Dizziness, headaches, and blurry vision are common accompanying complaints. In many patients no symptoms are apparent and the disease is diagnosed by routine blood or urine testing. In others, diabetes is advanced, and the presenting complaints are related to neuropathic, retinopathic, or vascular complications. NIDDM patients are usually but not always older than 40 at presentation and 70 to 90 per cent are overweight. Endogenous insulin secretion is relatively preserved and may even be excessive; thus, ketosis is rare, explaining why NIDDM is categorized as nonketotic or ketosis resistant.

SECONDARY DIABETIC STATES. In addition to the major categories of diabetes (IDDM and NIDDM), a large number of secondary forms of diabetes have been described. Secondary diabetes exists when some other readily identifiable primary disease entity or pathophysiologic state causes or is strongly associated with the diabetic state (Table 230–2). In general, these cases are unusual and comprise only a small proportion of the total cases of diabetes. Any disease process that limits insulin secretion or impairs insulin action can cause secondary diabetes, and numerous syndromes exist. Disorders that lead to pancreatic destruction such as chronic pancreatitis, cystic fibrosis, or hemochromatosis can reduce insulin secretion enough to cause diabetes. Conditions in which excess amounts of counterinsulin hormones are secreted, such as Cushing's disease, acromegaly, pheochromocytoma, and glucagonoma, can also produce diabetes. A number of drugs such as thiazide diuretics, glucocorticoids, and adrenergic agents can lead to, or at least exacerbate, diabetes. Many unusual genetic diseases are associated with a higher than normal incidence of diabetes through unknown mechanisms; these include muscular dystrophy, myotonic dystrophy, Friedreich's ataxia, Turner's syndrome, and others.

Finally, several rare syndromes have been recently identified, whose biochemical mechanisms are well described and which

TABLE 230–2. SOME FEATURES DISTINGUISHING BETWEEN INSULIN-DEPENDENT AND NONINSULIN-DEPENDENT DIABETES

	IDDM	NIDDM
Synonym	Type I	Type II
Age of onset	Usually <30	Usually >40
Ketosis	Common	Rare
Body weight	Nonobese	Obese (80%)
Prevalence	0.2%–0.3%	2%–4%
Genetics		
HLA association	Yes	No
Monozygotic twin studies	40%–50% concordance rate	Concordance rate near 100%
Circulating islet cell antibodies	Yes	No
Associated with other autoimmune phenomena	Occasional	No
Treatment with insulin	Always necessary	Usually not required
Complications	Frequent	Frequent
Insulin secretion	Severe deficiency	Variable: moderate deficiency to hyperinsulinemia
Insulin resistance	Occasional: with poor control or excessive insulin antibodies	Usual: due to receptor and postreceptor defects

primarily involve abnormalities of insulin-glucose physiology. Certain patients with extreme insulin resistance, acanthosis nigricans, and diabetes have been identified with circulating anti-insulin receptor antibodies. These antibodies are part of a more generalized autoimmune process, since proteinuria, leukopenia, and antinuclear and anti-DNA antibodies also exist. Other patients with the triad of acanthosis nigricans, insulin resistance, and diabetes do not have antireceptor antibodies but instead have a profound decrease in cellular insulin receptors. Typically these are young females with hirsutism and polycystic ovaries. In one such patient, several family members were also found to have decreased insulin receptors and insulin resistance, suggesting that this disorder is due to a genetically mediated decrease in insulin receptors. Patients have been reported in whom abnormal insulin products are synthesized and secreted and the specific molecular lesions identified. Familial hyperproinsulinemia involves a defect in the proinsulin molecule that prevents normal cleavage of proinsulin to insulin in the pancreatic B cell. This leads to the secretion of large amounts of proinsulin (which is biologically less active than insulin) instead of insulin. This disorder can lead to impaired glucose tolerance but has not yet been associated with overt fasting hyperglycemia. Rarely patients carry mutations in the insulin structural gene itself that lead to the secretion of insulin species with single amino acid substitutions resulting in markedly reduced biologic activity. These patients have a clinical picture of typical NIDDM. These mutant insulins are immunologically reactive and are secreted in large quantities in response to the hyperglycemic state. The clinical hallmark of this condition is the presence of hyperglycemia and marked hyperinsulinemia in a patient with normal sensitivity to exogenous insulin.

GENETICS

Diabetes has long been termed a geneticist's nightmare. The disease clearly aggregates in families and has a strong familial component. However, the precise genetic contribution to diabetes has been difficult to ascertain for at least four reasons: (1) no specific genetic marker has been identified. Glucose tolerance is the currently used method of diagnosis, but because of differences in the way tests are performed and the criteria used, it is difficult to compare one study to another; (2) There is a great deal of etiologic heterogeneity between IDDM and NIDDM and within these categories. This indicates genetic heterogeneity even though the phenotype (hyperglycemia) is comparable. It is also possible that, depending on environmental factors, there can be variable phenotypic expression of a common genotype; (3) It is likely that a "diabetogenic gene" interacts with external factors as well as with other genetic components, making the specific genetic influences underlying the final phenotypic expression of the diabetes hard to detect; (4) Actual transmission rates of diabetes from generation to generation are low.

Genetic factors are clearly important in the etiology of diabetes. This is demonstrated by classical twin studies. When twins below the age of 40 years are studied, if one twin has diabetes (mostly IDDM based on age) then the other twin develops diabetes only 50 per cent of the time. If the two pairs are concordant, the second twin usually develops diabetes within a couple of years of the first. For a purely genetic disease, concordance should be 100 per cent. This suggests that while genetic factors are important in IDDM, they are only predisposing and must interact with environmental influences if diabetes is to develop. This does not exclude the possibility that in some patients IDDM occurs entirely because of genetic or environmental factors. In twins over 40 years the concordance rate for diabetes (almost all NIDDM based on age) approaches 100 per cent. This suggests that genetic factors are more important in this form of diabetes and may be causal, or closely associated with causal mechanisms.

Despite the contribution of genetic factors, direct transmission of diabetes from parent to offspring is surprisingly low. If one parent has IDDM the risk to the offspring of developing IDDM is on the order of 2 to 5 per cent. If one child has IDDM the average risk for another sibling is 5 to 10 per cent. However, the risk is much greater if the second sibling is HLA (human leukocyte antigen) identical to the first, intermediate if HLA haploidentical, and very low if HLA nonidentical. The type of diabetes tends to run true in families, and the incidence of NIDDM in the offspring of an IDDM parent is probably not greater than normal. If one parent has NIDDM the risk is 10 to 15 per cent for offspring developing the disease. When both parents have NIDDM, the transmission risk increases but adequate data are not available to quantitate the increase in risk. If one sibling has NIDDM, the risk for another sibling is 10 to 15 per cent. These low rates of transmission make it difficult to trace models of inheritance in family studies, but the facts are clinically important in counseling and reassuring diabetic patients who wish to have children.

Strong associations have been identified between IDDM and specific HLAs coded by the major histocompatibility complex region located on the short arm of the sixth chromosome (Ch. 436). Four loci, designated A, B, C, and D, are now recognized in this region. Loci A, B, and C are defined serologically while the D locus is detected by the mixed lymphocyte (MLC) reaction. A DR locus can also be identified and typed using a serologic test. Although not proven, antigens at the D locus detected by MLC may be identical to the antigens at the DR locus identified serologically. At each of these loci numerous alleles (genes) exist, some of which confer increased risk for the development of IDDM. These high risk alleles include: HLA-DR3, HLA-Dw3, HLA-DR4, HLA-Dw4, HLA-B8, and HLA-B15 (the small w means that the antigen identified at the D locus by MLC has been provisionally accepted by the International Histocompatability Workshop; the w is deleted when identification is considered definite). The HLA-A, B, and C antigens are present on virtually all nucleated cell types, whereas the HLA-D or DR antigens or both show tissue restriction and are predominantly expressed on B lymphocytes and macrophages. It is possible that D/DR antigens are also expressed on islet cells, but this is unproven at the current time.

An HLA haplotype refers to a particular set of alleles at the four closely linked HLA loci, A, B, C, and D on one of the sixth chromosomes (each person inherits two haplotypes, one from each parent). In this system, some of the alleles are in linkage disequilibrium. This means that certain HLA antigens encoded by alleles at the different HLA loci occur together more frequently within the same haplotype than would be predicted by random statistical chance taking gene (allele) frequency into account. The antigens encoded by the HLA alleles associated with higher risk for IDDM do not directly cause or predispose to the disease. Rather, these alleles are felt to be in linkage disequilibrium with genes in the HLA region (possibly certain immune response genes) that are directly related to the etiology of IDDM. In other words, through linkage disequilibrium one "looks" at the "diabetogenic gene" via the more easily measured HLA antigens.

Current evidence indicates that the D locus is more important than the B locus because it is more closely linked to the etiologically important genes. In this event, the predictive value of the HLA-B antigen is through its linkage disequilibrium to the D locus. The relative risk for IDDM conferred by HLA-B8 or HLA-B15 is two to four times normal and is four to ten times normal for DR3/Dw3 or DR4/Dw4. Interestingly, homozygosity at any of these alleles (i.e., DR3/DR3) does not lead to greater risk than when the allele occurs on only one haplotype. However, if both sixth chromosomes bear two different diabetes-associated alleles at a particular locus (i.e., DR3/DR4) the increase in risk is more than additive. It should be kept in mind that the diabetes-associated HLA antigens are quite frequent in the nondiabetic population (although, clearly less frequent than in IDDM). For example, 30 to 35 per cent of normal persons are positive for DR3 or DR4. Thus, far more people who are positive for these antigens are normal than have IDDM (e.g., if the average risk for IDDM in a population is 0.2 per cent, and if a particular HLA haplotype confers a ten-fold increase in risk, then the risk would still be only 2 per cent for those with this haplotype). This is an important point to realize in thinking about HLA typing for screening or predictive value in a practical or clinical sense.

Despite all this information, the model of inheritance for IDDM is obscure, although it is clearly not autosomal dominant. The low penetrance of the diabetes-associated genes combined with the relative degrees of HLA associations suggests that the genetic predisposition must interact with specific environmental factors for IDDM to occur. Additionally, the disease could be multigenic, with at least two genes necessary (allelic or nonallelic) for IDDM to develop (with this model environmental factors would still be necessary).

In NIDDM no HLA associations have been identified, demonstrating the differences in etiology between the two major forms of diabetes. Although the location of the genetic component for NIDDM is not known, potentially important changes have been noted on the eleventh chromosome, which contains the insulin gene. A 1.5 to 3.4 kilobase insertion of extra DNA, about 500 base pairs upstream from the 5′ flanking end of the insulin gene, has been described as a polymorphism more frequent in patients with NIDDM compared to normal persons or patients with IDDM. If this insertion (or some more specific aspect of this polymorphism) proves to be an accurate marker for NIDDM, then this will be of great value in predicting subjects at risk and in tracing inheritance patterns. Furthermore, if this insertion influences gene regulation then it might have causal significance in terms of insulin biosynthesis. However, since NIDDM patients usually have adequate amounts of insulin within B cells, it is not readily apparent how this potential gene abnormality could influence functional dynamics of insulin secretion.

PATHOGENESIS

Before discussion of the pathogenetic aspects of diabetes it is important to review briefly some of the essential features of insulin and glucose physiology. Insulin is produced in the pancreatic B cell as the primary biosynthetic product preproinsulin containing 109 amino acid residues (MW ~ 11,500). This peptide is rapidly converted to proinsulin (86 amino acid residues, MW ~ 9000) by cleavage of the amino terminal 23 amino acid "pre" sequence. Within the B cell secretory granules, proinsulin is converted by proteolytic cleavage to insulin (51 amino acids, MW ~ 6000) and C peptide (31 amino acids, MW ~ 3000). Thus, the final B cell secretory product is 95 per cent insulin and C peptide in equimolar amounts and 5 per cent unconverted proinsulin. In familial hyperproinsulinemia, mutations in the proinsulin sequence prevent proteolytic conversion within the secretory granule, leading to release of large amounts of proinsulin having only 7 to 10 per cent of insulin's biologic activity. The regulation of insulin release is extremely complex, being influenced by glucose, amino acids, gut insulinogenic hormones, glucagon, neural influences, and other factors. However, glucose is the most important stimulus for insulin secretion.

After a brief circulating time ($t\frac{1}{2}$ 4 to 8 minutes) insulin interacts with target tissues to exert its biologic effects. At the target cell, insulin action is initiated by binding of the hormone to specific cell surface insulin receptors. Following formation of the insulin receptor complex one or more signals are propagated (second messengers) that interact with a variety of cellular effector systems such as enzymes and glucose transport proteins to produce insulin's ultimate biologic effects. Insulin exerts its major effects on carbohydrate homeostasis by stimulating peripheral glucose disposal and inhibiting hepatic glucose production. A variety of abnormalities in insulin biosynthesis, secretion, and action can lead to diabetes.

There are a number of other hormones that affect carbohydrate homeostasis termed anti-insulin or counteregulatory hormones (glucagon, growth hormone, cortisol, and catecholamines). Among these, glucagon is probably most important in terms of the pathophysiology of diabetes. Glucagon is 29 amino acids (MW ~ 3000) in length and is synthesized in the pancreatic alpha cells as proglucagon (MW ~ 9000 to 11,000). Its release is stimulated by hypoglycemia, amino acids, neural influences, and stress. Its major effect on glucose metabolism is exerted at the liver where it binds to surface receptors, stimulates cyclic AMP generation, and promotes glycogenolysis, gluconeogenesis, and ketogenesis. Its lipolytic effects are minimal in man, and glucagon has little if any effect on peripheral glucose uptake. Thus, glucagon affects glucose metabolism by influencing hepatic glucose production, and glucagon levels are absolutely or relatively increased in both IDDM and NIDDM.

NIDDM. Abnormalities of insulin and, to a lesser extent, glucagon secretion and action are central to the pathogenesis of NIDDM. Syndromes involving abnormalities of insulin biosynthesis have already been discussed. These include familial hyperproinsulinemia and mutations in the structural gene for insulin leading to secretion of a biologically defective insulin molecule. These rare syndromes lead to mild degrees of glucose intolerance or a clinical picture indistinguishable from NIDDM. Beyond these unusual syndromes, however, insulin biosynthesis is qualitatively normal in NIDDM.

Secretion of insulin is not normal in NIDDM. In some patients with impaired glucose tolerance, substantially reduced amounts of insulin are secreted in response to a glucose load. These subjects are not insulin resistant and the defect in insulin secretion appears adequately to account for their abnormal glucose metabolism. These patients have a relatively high propensity to develop overt NIDDM (up to 50 per cent) and should be followed for progression. Other patients with impaired glucose tolerance secrete normal or increased amounts of insulin, although in some cases the dynamics of secretion may be altered with a delay in release of insulin following a glucose stimulus. These patients are insulin resistant primarily because of decreased insulin receptors. This is true in both the obese and nonobese categories of this classification. In relatively few (about 5 per cent) of the hyperinsulinemic insulin-resistant patients with impaired glucose tolerance is there progression to fasting hyperglycemia.

The great majority of patients with NIDDM are both insulin deficient and insulin resistant. The decrease in insulin action exists whether they are obese or nonobese (although approximately 80 per cent are obese). Patients with NIDDM may have normal or elevated fasting insulin levels, but they almost always secrete decreased amounts of insulin following oral glucose or meals. Other functional abnormalities that have been identified include a marked decrease in early release of insulin (first phase) after intravenous administration of glucose, and much greater blunting of the insulin response to glucose compared to other insulin stimuli (amino acids, sulfonylureas, glucagon, or B agonists). These latter findings have given rise to the idea that B cell dysfunction in NIDDM may be characterized by a defect in glucose recognition by islet cells.

In addition to these abnormalities of insulin secretion, patients with NIDDM are also insulin resistant. Insulin action is a complex sequence of events beginning with binding to surface receptors; insulin resistance can be due to any abnormality at any step along the insulin action pathway. For convenience, the cellular causes of insulin resistance can be broadly divided into receptor and postreceptor defects (Fig. 230–1). A receptor defect involves a decrease in insulin binding due to a decrease in either receptor number or affinity or to both. A postreceptor defect refers to any biologically significant abnormality in the activity of effector proteins (such as insulin-sensitive enzymes or transport proteins) or an impairment in the coupling or transducing mechanisms between insulin receptor complexes and effector units. In a pure sense, a postreceptor defect is really a postbinding defect since insulin receptor function could be abnormal independent of its binding properties. In subjects with impaired glucose tolerance who are insulin resistant, receptor defects exist (decreased receptor number), but postreceptor function is normal. In NIDDM, insulin resistance exists in the great majority of patients. Although a receptor defect (decreased number) is present in most insulin-resistant NIDDM patients, this does not appear to be the major abnormality. Postreceptor defects also exist, and these appear to play the predominant role in causing the insulin-resistant state. As far as glucose homeostasis is concerned, at least one type of postreceptor defect has been biochemically defined in NIDDM; that is, these patients exhibit a decrease in the intrinsic activity of the glucose transport effector system.

Insulin deficiency and insulin resistance both contribute to the hyperglycemia of NIDDM. In addition, another abnormality also contributes to the hyperglycemia; hepatic glucose production rates are increased in NIDDM, and the magnitude of this increase is proportional to the level of fasting hyperglycemia. This hepatic abnormality is, at least partially, due to resistance to insulin's normal restraining effect on liver glucose production. Additionally, glucagon levels are often elevated, either absolutely or relatively, in NIDDM, and it is possible that excess glucagon stimulation also contributes to the increase in glucose production.

Thus, insulin deficiency, insulin resistance, and accelerated hepatic glucose production all exist in NIDDM, and all contribute to the hyperglycemia (Fig. 230–2). It is tempting to suggest a unifying pathogenetic hypothesis in which one metabolic lesion is primary and the others secondary. Unfortunately it is not possible to choose any particular sequence at this time. All three abnormalities can be generated in animal models by inducing hyperglycemia and hypoinsulinemia, and all three are at least partially reversible with weight loss, oral sulfonylureas, or insulin therapy.

IDDM. A strong genetic component is involved in the etiology of IDDM, but extragenetic factors must also contribute, at least in most patients. Several lines of evidence suggest a role for *viruses* in IDDM: (1) Autopsies of IDDM patients dying within a few months of the disease's onset have revealed an "insulitis" consisting of round cell infiltration of islet tissue. (2) A modest seasonal variation to the incidence of IDDM has been noted in some studies. (3) A clinical history of preceding viral-type illness, particularly Coxsackie B and mumps, is often reported at the onset of IDDM. (4) Increased viral titers, including coxsackievirus B4, have been reported in IDDM patients at or near the time of the disease's onset. (5) Certain diabetogenic viruses (encephalomyocarditis M, coxsackievirus B, and rheovirus) can cause diabetes when inoculated into rodents. Further, the susceptibility of different rodent strains to develop viral-induced diabetes appears to be under genetic control. (6) Diabetogenic viruses can also directly infect B cells in culture, causing cell lysis and death. (7) Finally, direct support for virus-induced diabetes has been obtained in humans. Coxsackievirus B4 was isolated from the pancreas of a boy with new-onset IDDM who died of severe ketoacidosis closely following a

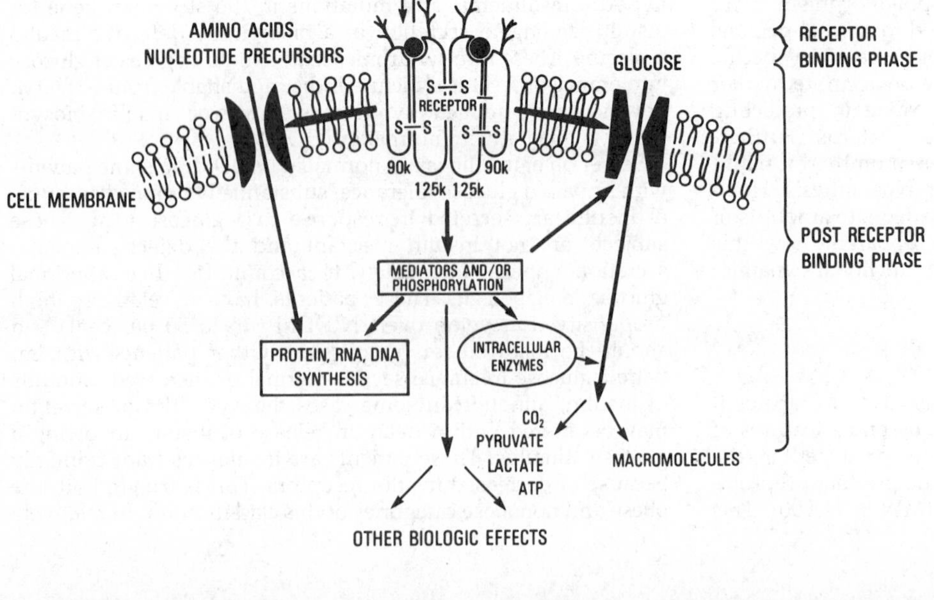

Figure 230–1. Model of insulin action and categories of insulin resistance. Abnormalities can occur at the prereceptor phase, involving biosynthesis and secretion of abnormal beta cell products; at the receptor binding phase, involving decreased insulin binding to receptors due to decreased receptor number or affinity; or at the postreceptor binding phase, involving any defect in the insulin action cascade distal to the initial binding event.

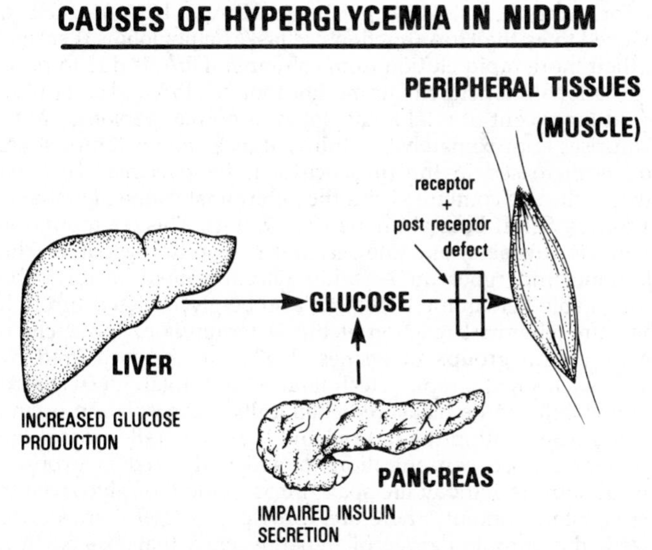

Figure 230–2. Summary of the metabolic abnormalities in NIDDM which contribute to the hyperglycemia. Increased hepatic glucose production, impaired insulin secretion, and insulin resistance due to receptor and postreceptor defects all combine to generate the hyperglycemic state.

flulike illness associated with rising serum titers of neutralizing antibody to the virus. The viral isolate was inoculated into experimental animals, producing diabetes, and viral antigens could be demonstrated in the B cells from the infected animals.

Autoimmunity may also play a role in the etiology of IDDM. Circulating antibodies to thyroid, gastric mucosa, and the adrenal are far more common in patients with IDDM than in normal persons. More importantly, up to 90 per cent of patients with new-onset IDDM have demonstrable titers of plasma islet cell antibodies. These antibodies are heterogeneous, some binding to cytoplasmic antigens common to all islet cells and others directed against the B cell surface. The latter lyse B cells in culture in the presence of complement, consistent with a pathophysiologic role in vivo. These islet cell antibodies are also observed in BB rats, an animal model that spontaneously develops an IDDM-like syndrome. In humans, titers of islet cell antibodies fall after the onset of clinical disease; by five years only 20 per cent of patients have demonstrable titers, and by 10 to 20 years the prevalence falls to 5 to 10 per cent. Patients who continue to demonstrate antibodies after several years may be examples of heterogeneity within IDDM. In these patients IDDM may represent a primary autoimmune disease, since they are largely female, show a great prevalence of other organ-specific antibodies, and have a strong family history of autoimmune disease. Patients with onset of IDDM at an older age tend to fall in this group. Genetically, they may also be different, since they have a greater prevalence of HLA-B8 and

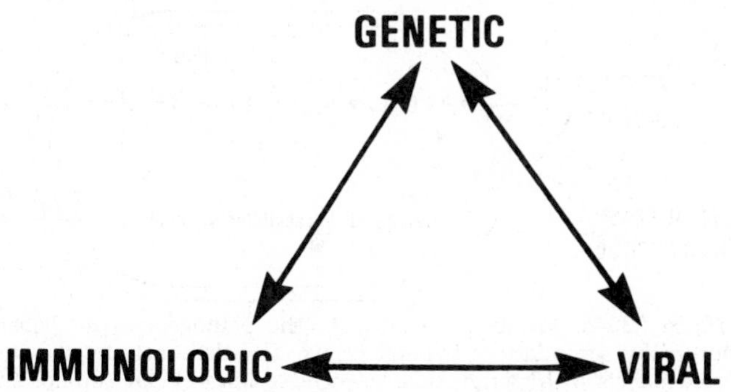

Figure 230–3. An interplay of genetic, immunologic, and viral etiologies contributes to the pathogenesis of NIDDM. The importance of each factor probably differs in subpopulations of IDDM, demonstrating the heterogeneity of this disease.

DR3. In cases of IDDM in which islet cell antibodies are cleared within one year of the disease's onset, patients are more often male, do not typically show signs of other autoimmune phenomena, experience onset of disease at a younger age, and have a higher association with HLA-B15 and HLA-DR4. Circulating antibodies may not be the only component of the immune response associated with IDDM; a cell-mediated immune response may also be involved. Increased K cells (killer lymphocytes) have been reported in IDDM along with alterations in T-lymphocyte subpopulations. Both antibody-induced and cell-mediated immune phenomena may be involved in the pathogenesis of IDDM.

Strong arguments can be made for the role of genetic susceptibility, viruses, and altered immunity in the etiology of IDDM (Fig. 230–3). However, the contribution of these factors and the sequential relationship among them cannot be stated at this time. Clearly, immune responses could provide the causal link between the HLA associations and clinical IDDM, since the HLA alleles are thought to be associated through linkage disequilibrium to immune response genes. One way to integrate these factors would be to postulate that susceptibility to IDDM is inherited through genes closely associated with the HLA loci. Given this proper genetic background, environmental agents such as certain viruses exhibiting B cell tropism and possibly chemical agents can injure and in some cases destroy B cells. Following B cell injury, an immune response (possibly antibody and cell mediated) directed against B cells occurs owing to release of B cell antigens into the circulation, alteration of B cell antigens, cross-reactivity with viral antigens, or primary modulation of the immune response. In any event, the immune response would then exacerbate or complete the initial viral or chemical B cell injury. Of course this is only one of several sequences that can be proposed, but it is consistent with most of the available data. IDDM is probably heterogeneous, and no single sequence of pathogenetic events will necessarily explain all cases. For example, IDDM patients who are HLA-B8/DR3 display other organ-specific autoantibodies and probably have a primary autoimmune disease and do not need an environmental factor to develop the disease. Based on the intertwining of genetic, viral, and immune influences, it also follows that B cell destruction in IDDM does not usually occur acutely. It is likely that this process is gradual over months to years, even though the clinical onset of metabolic decompensation is usually abrupt when destruction of B cell mass reaches a critical point or an intercurrent illness occurs. This raises the possibility of intervention therapies (immune or other) following the onset of B cell injury but prior to clinical manifestations of IDDM, since by the time IDDM appears B cell destruction may be too far advanced for effective therapy. Such an approach would require a method to detect preclinical IDDM. Such methods are currently under intense study.

C peptide is secreted in equimolar amounts compared to insulin. Since C peptide has a much longer half-life than insulin, it provides an excellent measure of insulin secretory capacity, especially in those patients with circulating anti-insulin antibodies that interfere with usual insulin radioimmunoassays. In patients with type I diabetes who have been treated with insulin for longer than five years, C peptide levels are usually undetectable. However, C peptide may be measured in many of these patients during the first years of their disease. This suggests that the loss of beta cell secretion in IDDM is not abrupt, but continues for several years after the diabetes becomes clinically apparent. For the most part, ease of diabetic management and stability of metabolic control in IDDM are correlated with the degree of the residual insulin secretion. Those patients with the highest levels of circulating C peptide are easier to treat, and those with undetectable levels are more unstable. Some of the major clinical and pathophysiologic distinctions between IDDM and NIDDM are listed in Table 230–2.

TREATMENT

In this section, details concerning the various methods of diabetic management will be discussed. However, since the severity and clinical picture of diabetes are quite variable, therapeutic methods are also varied. In particular, major differences exist in the approach to NIDDM versus IDDM, and whenever possible therapeutic distinctions for these two forms of diabetes will be made.

RELATIONSHIP BETWEEN HYPERGLYCEMIA AND COMPLICATIONS. It is important to start with more general principles and to identify overall therapeutic goals. A consideration of therapeutic goals involves one of the most important questions in the field; that is, what is the relationship between hyperglycemia and the development of diabetic complications? Simply put, are complications due to hyperglycemia or are they due to genetic factors independent of hyperglycemia? This is the central clinical question in diabetes concerning which a voluminous literature exists.

Hyperglycemia is the most obvious metabolic abnormality in diabetes. It is therefore reasonable to suspect that elevated glucose levels play a role in diabetic complications. Consistent with this is a large body of retrospective evidence showing that better control is usually associated with fewer complications. Unfortunately, in the absence of randomized, prospective studies in which significant differences in glycemic control are achieved between matched experimental and control groups over an extended period, current clinical studies can provide only nonconclusive evidence. Classical diabetic complications can occur in secondary diabetes (in which genetic aspects of diabetes are presumably missing) and in normal kidneys following transplantation into diabetic patients. Furthermore, in twin studies the degree of retinopathy is comparable in twins concordant for IDDM, whereas in discordant pairs the nondiabetic twin does not have retinopathy. Certain abnormalities seen in diabetes, such as retinal capillary leakage (as demonstrated by fluorescein angiography), slowed motor nerve conductive velocity, and microalbuminuria, can be reversed by intensive insulin therapy, but the relationship between these physiologic abnormalities and clinically significant complications has not been demonstrated. In animal experiments a number of studies have shown good correlation between the level of hyperglycemia and microvascular complications similar (but perhaps not identical) to those seen in human diabetes. In animals, these complications can also be prevented or reversed with insulin therapy.

Several biochemical mechanisms have been proposed that may link hyperglycemia to complications. Proteins can be nonenzymatically glycosylated in vivo, and the degree of this glycosylation is directly related to the degree of hyperglycemia. Chromatography of red blood cell hemolysates shows four

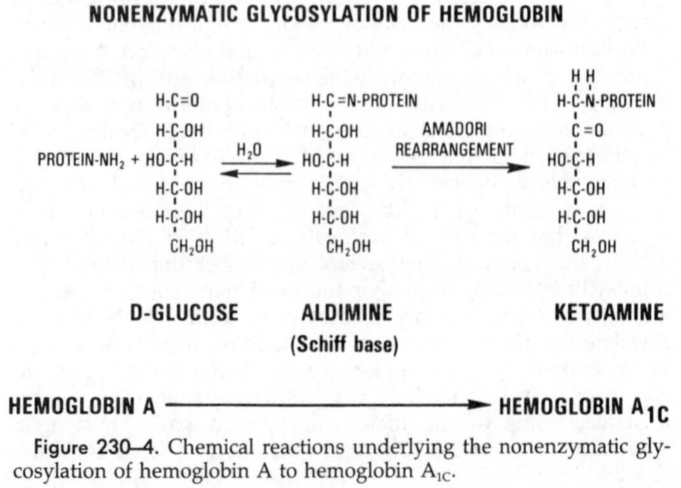

Figure 230–4. Chemical reactions underlying the nonenzymatic glycosylation of hemoglobin A to hemoglobin A_{1C}.

minor components (HbA_{1a1}, HbA_{1a2}, HbA_{1b1}, HbA_{1c}) of HbA, referred to as the HbA_1 fraction or "fast" hemoglobins (because of their more rapid elution from columns). HbA_1 is due to post-translational, nonenzymatic modification of HbA and comprises about 6 per cent of total hemoglobin in normal persons. HbA_{1c} comprises approximately two thirds of these minor components and is increased in the presence of hyperglycemia. To form HBA_{1c}, glucose combines with the N terminal valine of β chains to form a Schiff base aldimine (Fig. 230–4). This compound is relatively unstable, and the reaction is readily reversible. The aldimine undergoes an Amadori rearrangement to form the more stable ketoamine. HbA can also be glycosylated through the same chemical reaction at the N terminus of the α chain and ϵ amino groups of lysines. HbA_{1c} can be measured by various chromatographic techniques, and total glycosylated hemoglobin can be measured chemically. Glycosylation occurs continuously within the red cell and is a direct reflection of the average glucose concentration to which the cell is exposed throughout its 120-day life span. Measurement of glycosylated hemoglobin content, therefore, provides a useful means to assess the chronic degree of hyperglycemia that existed in a given patient over the preceding several weeks and is not affected by acute changes in plasma glucose level. Additionally, the nonspecific and nonenzymatic nature of hemoglobin glycosylation raises the possibility that glycosylation of other body proteins can occur, leading to structural or functional changes that may be related to chronic diabetic complications. Increased amounts of glycosylated low-density lipoprotein (LDL) molecules, for example, circulate in hyperglycemic diabetic patients and do not bind normally to LDL receptors. Since abnormal glycosylation may affect all tissues, this mechanism could be related to a variety of diabetic complications.

Additional biochemical lesions related to hyperglycemia have been proposed for nervous tissue. *Sorbitol* is a polyhydroxyl alcohol (polyol) produced from glucose by aldose reductase in nerve tissue; once formed, sorbitol can be converted to fructose (Fig. 230–5). It is theorized that this polyol pathway is particularly active in diabetes because of the hyperglycemia. This could lead to increased intracellular osmolarity (due to accumulation of sorbitol and fructose) with water influx, swelling

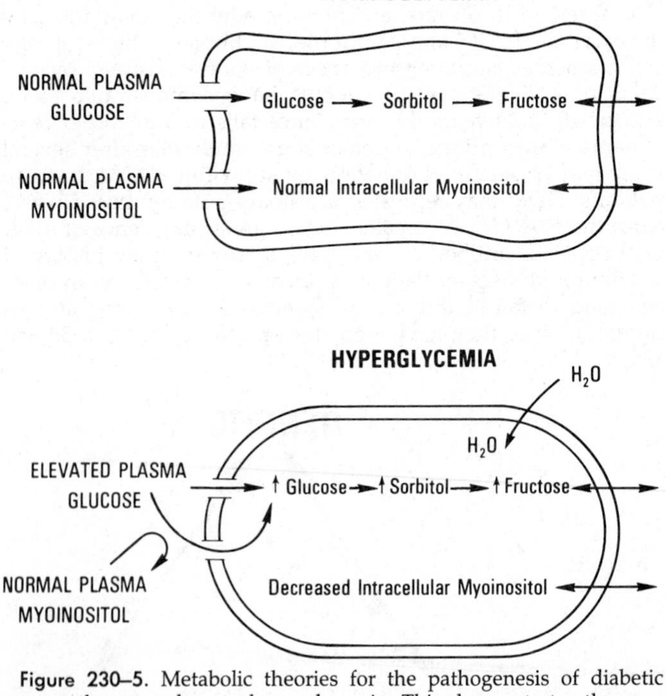

Figure 230–5. Metabolic theories for the pathogenesis of diabetic neuropathy secondary to hyperglycemia. This demonstrates the suggested effects of hyperglycemia to increase intracellular sorbitol and fructose concentrations leading to an osmotic increase in intracellular water content. In addition, it has been suggested that hyperglycemia depletes intracellular myoinositol content by competitively inhibiting the uptake of myoinositol from the extracellular space.

of Schwann cells, anoxia, and demyelination. Consistent with this, an increase in sorbitol content has been found in nerve tissue of diabetic rats, and it is reversible with insulin therapy. However, Schwann cell swelling and increased water content have not yet been demonstrated, and further testing of the polyol pathway hypothesis is necessary. Another hyperglycemia-related metabolic lesion in nervous tissue has been proposed involving *myoinositol*. Concentrations of this compound are decreased in peripheral nerves of diabetic rats, and this is associated with a decrease in nerve conduction velocity. These abnormalities can be prevented by insulin or oral myoinositol supplements. It is possible that uptake of myoinositol by nerves is inhibited by hyperglycemia, leading to depletion and pathologic sequelae. A link may exist between polyol and myoinositol metabolism in that increased activity of the polyol pathway contributes to the reduction in nerve myoinositol content.

The above discussion cites clinical and biochemical evidence supporting the relationship between hyperglycemia and complications. On the other hand, there is evidence against this relationship. For example, patients have been reported with diabetic complications at the time of onset of IDDM, when hyperglycemia should not have preexisted for a significant time. Additionally, some patients with very poor glycemic control never develop complications. Ultimately, however, the main argument against the relationship is simply that it has not been proven with certainty by well-controlled, prospective studies in man.

Taking all factors into account, it seems reasonable to me to conclude that although a definitive relationship between hyperglycemia and complications has been neither established nor disproved at present, the bulk of evidence weighs in favor of such a relationship. With this in mind it seems prudent to establish as a therapeutic goal the maintenance of plasma glucose levels as close to normal as possible in diabetic patients. The major complication of aggressive antidiabetic therapy is hypoglycemia, which, if severe enough, can unequivocally produce immediate and irreversible CNS damage. Therefore, diabetic management should be pushed until glucose levels are normal or near normal, unless recurrent, overt episodes of hypoglycemia develop. If this occurs, then compromises are necessary in the degree of glycemic control achieved. Other therapeutic goals include (1) normal growth and development in children, (2) normal pregnancy and childbirth in females, (3) reduction of diabetes-related atherosclerosis risk factors, especially in adult diabetic patients, and (4) minimal interference with normal life style in all diabetics.

DIETARY TREATMENT. Dietary treatment is an integral part of the overall therapeutic plan in all diabetic patients. In many NIDDM patients dietary therapy can be the predominant method of treatment. Dietary therapy is concerned with the total number of calories ingested, the distribution of calories throughout the day, the individual food sources that make up these calories, and maintenance of proper nutrition. Dietary therapy is much different in NIDDM and IDDM, because patients in the former are usually obese, whereas in the latter they are not, and NIDDM patients retain endogenous insulin secretion while IDDM patients do not.

Total Caloric Intake. Since most NIDDM patients are overweight, caloric restriction is advisable and can be of great benefit. The essential tenet of weight reduction is straightforward: if caloric expenditure exceeds intake, weight will be lost. There are many ways to calculate daily caloric expenditure, but on the average this amounts to 30 to 35 kcal per kilogram in normal man; 25 kcal per kilogram is attributed to the basal metabolic rate and the rest to physical activity. Daily caloric requirements are about 30 kcal per kilogram in sedentary individuals and approximately 35 kcal per kilogram in moderately active subjects. For those who engage in brisk physical exertion for prolonged intervals throughout the day caloric expenditure can exceed 35 kcal per kilogram. Another factor affecting caloric requirements (at least on a per kilogram basis) is the degree of adiposity. Adipose tissue is predominantly storage triglyceride, which is relatively inert metabolically with a decreased caloric need per unit weight. Thus, the greater the degree of adiposity, the lower the caloric requirement per kilogram. In very obese, sedentary individuals, daily caloric requirements can be as low as 25 kcal per kilogram of body weight.

A number of approaches to weight reduction exist that vary in the degree of caloric restriction and rate of weight loss, dietary constituents, as well as behaviorial and psychological support measures. These include nutritionally sound and modestly restricted diets that achieve slow gradual weight loss over several months, nutritionally balanced and very low calorie diets for rapid weight loss, and behavior modification, pharmacologic aids, and even surgical procedures (i.e., gastric plication) in the massively obese patient in whom medical therapy fails. These approaches are discussed in detail in Chapter 216.

For all these methods, inducing the initial period of weight loss is not the major problem in weight reduction, but, rather, the major problem is weight regain or recidivism. Motivated patients can usually successfully lose weight over the initial dietary period, but it is the unusual patient who successfully keeps the pounds off. The major challenge in weight reduction therapy is to develop a proper supportive environment and patient motivation to maintain weight loss after it has been achieved. In the NIDDM patient, significant caloric restriction is usually successful in lowering plasma glucose levels even before significant weight loss is achieved. Depending on the degree of obesity that was present initially and the amount of weight loss, continued beneficial effects on glycemic control can be maintained after the goal weight is achieved and a eucaloric diet is initiated. In general, the more recent the onset of NIDDM, the more responsive the patient will be to the beneficial effects of weight reduction. In patients with pronounced fasting hyperglycemia, very low calorie diets (300 to 600 kcal per day) are often useful in achieving rapid glycemic control as well as an initial rapid rate of weight loss (which can often be of important psychological and motivational benefit). Very low calorie diets usually consist of liquid formula meals and should not be utilized unless they contain adequate amounts (a minimum 30 to 40 grams per day) of high quality protein and are supplemented with vitamins and micronutrients. NIDDM patients on such diets should be supervised by a physician.

The mechanisms whereby weight reduction ameliorates hyperglycemia in NIDDM are not completely clear. Weight loss leads to a reduction in the accelerated rates of hepatic glucose production, ameliorates the degree of insulin resistance by increasing insulin receptors and reducing the magnitude of the post-receptor defect in insulin action, and possibly improves beta cell secretion. However, the precise cellular mechanisms leading to these effects are not known. Patients with IDDM are seldom obese, and an important nutritional goal is maintenance of adequate nutrition, particularly to assure normal growth and development in children and pregnant women.

Distribution of Calories. In addition to total caloric consumption, attention should also be paid to the distribution of calories throughout the day in any dietary prescription. Two principles should be kept in mind: (1) calories should be spread as evenly as possible throughout the major daily meals to avoid a large concentration of calories at any one meal and not to overwhelm the diabetic patient's impaired capacity to metabolize food; and (2) in those patients receiving exogenous insulin, caloric intake should be temporally adjusted to coincide with the time course of action of the administered insulin. The latter point highlights a major difference in dietary consideration between patients with IDDM and NIDDM. In NIDDM, endogenous insulin secretion is still present and the beta cell can respond at the appropriate times (albeit to a limited degree) to food ingestion, regardless of when it occurs throughout the day. This is even true, although to a lesser extent, in NIDDM subjects who are treated with insulin. Thus, in these patients it is sufficient to balance calories throughout the day, but the patient has a good deal of leeway to determine the timing of specific meals as long as calories are ingested at times of peak exogenous insulin action. For practical purposes, the only insulin present in patients with IDDM is that which is administered exogenously. Therefore, patients must pay close attention to the timing of meals and must be certain that there is reasonable concordance between meal ingestion and the time course of action of the insulin they have taken. To a certain extent the patient can elect a temporal pattern suitable to his lifestyle and preference and the insulin therapy regimen can then be tailored appropriately. In this way greater flexibility is allowed that improves overall patient compliance and quality of life.

Nutrient Content of Diet. A great deal of attention is currently being paid to the individual components comprising the diabetic diet. When patients consume eucaloric diets, it is important that they be properly balanced and nutritionally sound. A generally accepted protein requirement is 0.8 grams per kilogram per day for adults, but larger amounts are usually consumed in Western diets. Thus, protein usually comprises about 15 per cent of total caloric consumption. With this as a base, the proportions of fat and carbohydrate (CHO) are inversely related. Previous attempts to restrict total CHO intake are no longer deemed advisable, and most authorities now advocate liberalization of CHO intake to 50 to 55 per cent of total calories. This means that total fat intake should not exceed 30 to 35 per cent, and because diabetic patients are predisposed to macrovascular disease, saturated fat (primarily animal fat) intake should be reduced so that the polyunsaturated-saturated fat ratio is equivalent to 1:0. Ideally, cholesterol intake should not exceed 450 mg per day. The makeup of the CHO portion of the diet also requires attention. In the past it was felt that diabetics should rigorously avoid sucrose because it is rapidly absorbed and raises the blood glucose level inordinately. While this may be true when sucrose is consumed as the sole nutritive component, as in soft drinks or certain candies, it is less of a problem when modest amounts of sucrose are eaten in a mixed meal setting. Because of this, up to 5 per cent of total CHO can be consumed as sucrose, as long as it is taken in the context of a mixed meal and spaced out through the day. This allows the diabetic a wider variety of food choices, making the diet more palatable; a side benefit of this approach is that it improves patient adherence to the dietary prescription and to the other elements of the overall therapeutic plan. The remainder of the CHO predominantly consists of starches. All complex CHO cannot be lumped together as a single food group because the glycemic response to different starches differs widely, being lowest for lentils and pasta and highest for wheat and potatoes. More work needs to be done to determine the glycemic potency of a large number of foods, singly and together, in diabetic patients before the precise composition of the CHO in the diet can be recommended with certainty. At this stage it is advisable for the diabetic to consume 50 to 55 per cent of calories as CHO with a modest restriction in sucrose intake and emphasis on ingestion of those complex CHOs with low glycemic potency.

Fructose is a nutritive sweetener that may also have a place in the diabetic diet. This simple CHO is somewhat sweeter than sucrose and has similar properties when prepared in foods. Thus, fructose can be substituted for sucrose in most foods with little change in taste or texture. The advantage is that fructose is absorbed from the gastrointestinal tract more slowly than sucrose and is predominantly taken up and metabolized by the liver through non-insulin–dependent mechanisms. Within the liver, fructose is phosphorylated and eventually converted to glycogen or triglyceride through the triose phosphate intermediates. Thus, little fructose escapes hepatic uptake to enter the peripheral circulation, and only a small amount of fructose is converted to glucose for release from the liver. Ingestion of fructose leads to a minimal postprandial rise in plasma glucose or insulin levels in normal persons and in diabetics when taken alone or as part of a mixed meal. For these reasons, fructose offers some advantage in the diabetic diet, and amounts up to 75 grams per day can be safely consumed. The major exception occurs in patients with severely uncontrolled NIDDM or in poorly insulinized IDDM patients. In these conditions glycogen production is inhibited and fructose enters the gluconeogenic pathway and is ultimately released as glucose, causing hyperglycemia.

Dietary fiber can also influence CHO absorption. Glycemic excursions are reduced and insulin secretion diminished when normal persons and subjects with NIDDM consume fiber-enriched diets. This effect is mediated through delayed gastric emptying and overall slowing of the rate of CHO digestion and absorption. Since large amounts of fiber (10 to 15 grams per meal) are needed to observe these effects, major changes in dietary patterns would be necessary to achieve beneficial results. Nevertheless, when fiber is consumed as natural foods, there do not seem to be any untoward effects of increased fiber ingestion, and some studies indicate that increased fiber intake can lower serum triglyceride levels. The only potential caveat to this statement involves growing children and pregnant women, since subtle undesirable changes in micronutrient absorption due to high fiber ingestion have not been ruled out.

A minority of diabetic patients adhere to the recommended dietary regimens. To a large extent this is due to inadequate understanding on the part of the patient as well as the physician regarding dietary goals and methods. An additional factor is that dietary therapy must be individualized, taking into account each patient's life style, economic status, food preferences, and social needs. This can be a time-consuming process, and few physicians have the time or training to participate with patients in this type of detailed dietary management. For this reason it is critical to incorporate a dietitian or nutritionist trained in the principles of dietary therapy of diabetes as part of the health care team. One cannot simply give pamphlets, instructional aids, and meal plans and expect even motivated patients to adhere to the necessary regimens. Detailed instruction by a nutrition counselor is necessary to tailor the diet to each patient's special needs. Dietary therapy is a chronic treatment modality and therefore the longer view is important. Occasional deviations from recommended meal plans for special occasions are acceptable, providing the patient has a clear understanding of how this should be managed. Often, this allows for better patient compliance with the overall diet plan. Periodic meetings with a nutrition counselor are necessary to implement and maintain individualized dietary regimens.

ORAL HYPOGLYCEMIC AGENTS. Oral hypoglycemic agents are often therapeutically effective in NIDDM patients. In 1970, serious questions were raised concerning the use of these agents: results of the University Group Diabetes Program (UGDP) indicated that these drugs increased the rate of sudden death from heart disease in patients with mild NIDDM. However, because of numerous questions concerning the design and interpretation of the UGDP study, concerns about the use of oral hypoglycemic agents have greatly diminished. In patients who do not respond satisfactorily to diet and do not have severe hyperglycemia (i.e., plasma glucose levels consistently greater than 250 mg per deciliter), oral agents are an appropriate therapeutic choice. In patients with severe hyperglycemia, insulin therapy is preferable, at least initially, to gain more rapid control of clinical symptoms and to prevent hyperosmolarity. While sulfonylureas are effective in patients with NIDDM, they are ineffective in IDDM. Some have suggested that combinations of oral agents with insulin can reduce insulin requirements in IDDM; however, this has not been proven, and would be of minor clinical importance anyway.

The mechanism of action of sulfonylureas is complex. In the short term, they augment B cell insulin secretion. However, after several months of therapy, insulin levels return to pretreatment values while glucose levels remain improved. These findings led to the demonstration that sulfonylureas exert extrapancreatic effects on glucose metabolism: (1) they reduce the accelerated rates of hepatic glucose production in NIDDM; (2) they partially reverse the postreceptor defect in insulin action; and (3) they increase the number of cellular insulin receptors. These all represent significant components of the insulin resistance of NIDDM, so sulfonylureas can improve glycemia by improving insulin's effectiveness at target cells. The relative importance of each of these actions in ameliorating hyperglycemia is unclear, but it is likely that the pancreatic and extrapancreatic effects of these agents combine to produce the hypoglycemic action of these drugs.

There are several different kinds of sulfonylureas, differing primarily in potency, pharmacokinetics, and modes of metabolism as outlined in Table 230–3. *Tolbutamide* is metabolized to inert products by the liver and has a relatively short half-life, necessitating administration two or three times a day. Although it is the least potent of the available sulfonylureas on a weight basis, it has not been clearly demonstrated that any sulfonylurea produces greater hypoglycemic potency at maximal doses in diabetic patients. Therefore, for practical purposes, the differences in relative potency of the different drugs simply mean that more or less of a given agent should be used. *Tolazamide* and especially *acetohexamide* are metabolized by the liver to biologically active products that are then excreted by the kidneys. These drugs have intermediate half-lives and are usually given twice (but sometimes once) a day. Contrary to earlier data, *chlorpropamide* also undergoes considerable hepatic degradation into less active metabolites excreted in the urine. This compound can cause significant water retention and hyponatremia by potentiating ADH action on the kidney. Chlorpropamide has the longest circulating half-life and duration of action (about 60 hours) and is given only once a day. Hypoglycemia is the major complication of sulfonylureas, and this can be particularly severe with chlorpropamide because of its long duration of action. Elderly NIDDM subjects are more susceptible to hypoglycemia, especially those prone to skip meals. The route of metabolism of the different compounds may influence the choice of agent. One should be cautious about the use of chlorpropamide, acetohexamide, and, to a lesser extent, tolazamide in patients with compromised renal function because of the route of excretion. Second-generation sulfonylureas, such as *glybenclamide*, have been extensively used in Europe, but as of this writing, have not yet been released for use in the United States. These agents are metabolized by the liver and have relatively long duration of action and can be given once a day. It is claimed, but not rigorously demonstrated, that the second-generation sulfonylureas are more effective than the first-generation drugs.

The other major category of oral hypoglycemic agents consists of the biguanides, such as *phenformin*. The exact mechanism of action of these drugs is not clear, although they may interfere with hepatic gluconeogenesis. However, these drugs were strongly implicated in the development of lactic acidosis and have been prohibited from clinical use in the United States by the Food and Drug Administration. When they were used, they were often given in combination with a sulfonylurea.

In NIDDM the usual practice is to begin with a low dose of a given sulfonyluria, advancing the dose until the therapeutic response is satisfactory or a maximal dose is reached. Occasionally patients who do not respond to one drug can be switched to another with beneficial effect. Certain drug interactions occur with sulfonylureas, that is, phenylbutazone and anticoagulants compete for hepatic removal mechanisms with sulfonylureas. A disulfiram (Antabuse)-like reaction can occasionally occur following alcohol consumption by patients taking sulfonylureas. This is most frequently reported with chlorpropamide, but has not yet been noted with the second-generation agents. Potential interactions of this sort should always be kept in mind in the appropriate clinical context.

Approximately 10 to 20 per cent of NIDDM patients do not respond to oral agents, and treatment is termed primary failure. Secondary failure occurs when a patient responds initially to an oral agent, but then ceases to respond in the next year or two. This occurs in 5 to 20 per cent of patients, but these proportions obviously depend on the particular NIDDM population studied. For example, patients with new-onset diabetes respond better than those with longstanding disease. In some cases, secondary failure is due to dietary noncompliance in a patient who previously successfully adhered to a dietary regimen. However, this is often not the case, and the mechanisms of secondary failure in many patients with NIDDM remain unknown.

Debate exists as to which patients with NIDDM are appropriate candidates for oral sulfonylurea therapy. In view of the evidence implicating hyperglycemia with diabetic complications, the therapeutic goal with oral agents should be the maintenance of glucose levels as near to normal as possible. In patients with mild to moderate fasting hyperglycemia (140 to 230 mg per deciliter), dietary therapy should be tried first; if the above therapeutic goals are not achieved with this approach, then a sulfonylurea can be added. The problem arises in patients with more severe fasting hyperglycemia (more than 230 mg per deciliter) who have pronounced clinical symptoms despite dietary treatment. In these patients, some would advise an initial period of sulfonylurea therapy, and if satisfactory control is not achieved then insulin treatment should be substituted. Others would suggest an initial period of insulin therapy following which the patient is switched to sulfonylureas: if satisfactory control is achieved, the drug is continued. Alternatively, insulin can be used indefinitely in these patients. Clearly this is a gray area, and the particular approach should be individualized to each patient, taking into account the total clinical context of the patient's disease, acceptance of the various therapeutic methods, level of diabetes education, and

TABLE 230–3. CHARACTERISTICS OF SULFONYLUREAS

Generic Name	Brand Name	Dosage Range (mg)	Duration of Action (hr)	Comments
Tolbutamide	Orinase	500–3000	6–12	Metabolized by liver to inert products, given 2–3 × /day
Chlorpropamide	Diabinase	100–500	60	Metabolized by liver (~70%) to less active metabolite, and excreted intact (~30%) by kidneys; can potentiate ADH action, given 1 × /day
Acetohexamide	Dymelor	250–1500	12–24	Metabolized by liver to active metabolite given 1–2 × /day
Tolazamide	Tolinase	100–1000	10–18	Metabolized by liver to active product, given 1–2 × /day
Glyburide	Micronase	2.5–30	10–30	Metabolized by liver to inert products, given 1 × /day
Glipizide	Glucotrol	5–40	18–30	Metabolized by liver to inert products, given 1 × /day

motivation. In a patient in whom severe fasting hyperglycemia is maintained, with marked clinical symptoms and incipient hyperosmolarity, oral agents are probably not appropriate, at least initially. In these patients insulin therapy should be the primary mode of treatment and can be continued indefinitely, or a therapeutic trial of sulfonylureas can be substituted once the hyperglycemia has been brought under control by the initial period of insulin treatment. In general, response to sulfonylurea therapy is best if the onset of diabetes is recent and the patient is over 40 years of age and not thin.

INSULIN TREATMENT. Insulin is the primary mode of therapy in all patients with IDDM and in many with NIDDM (see above). The goals of therapy include: (1) normal growth and development in children, (2) normal pregnancy, delivery, and conceptus in women, (3) minimal interference with psychosocial adjustment, (4) acceptable glycemic control, with minimal hypoglycemia, and (5) prevention of complications. Little disagreement exists concerning goals 1 to 3; however, different views exist of how best to achieve goals 4 and 5. There are many different methods of insulin therapy, and the method chosen is highly dependent on one's view of goals 4 and 5. If a physician holds closely to the important relationship between control and complications, then "acceptable control" will be much more rigorously defined and a method of insulin treatment that is designed to produce the desired response will be chosen. On the other hand, those who question the link between hyperglycemia and complications are advocates of looser control and will utilize a less intensive method of insulin delivery. In general, it is quite easy to eliminate overt symptoms of hyperglycemia with any method of insulin therapy, but it is extremely difficult, and probably impossible, to achieve euglycemia on a 24-hour basis. How close one comes to this ideal depends on the method of insulin delivery chosen, which in turn depends on one's philosophy of diabetic management.

Insulin Preparations. To begin a discussion of the methods of insulin treatment, let us first consider the many different kinds of insulin available. Commerical insulin comes in concentrations of 100 units per milliliter (U-100) and 500 units per milliliter (U-500). The various insulin preparations differ in their time course of action (rapid, intermediate, and long acting), degree of purity, and source (beef, pork, beef-pork, or human synthetic insulin); these properties are outlined in Table 230–4. By adjustment of pH during preparation, the size of the zinc-insulin crystal can be modified; the larger the crystals, the slower the release after subcutaneous injection, and this accounts for the differences in time of action between semilente (rapid-acting) and ultralente (long-acting) insulin. Lente (intermediate-acting) insulin is simply a 30:70 mixture of semilente and ultralente respectively. The other method to delay the onset of action of injected insulin is to mix it with a protein (protamine) and adjust the pH. This results in NPH (intermediate) and PZI (long-acting) preparations. It should be cautioned that the values for peak onset and duration of action listed in Table 230–4 are simply estimates. There is a great deal of variability in these values from patient to patient as a result of circulating anti-insulin antibodies that alter the pharmacokinetics of insulin, variation in subcutaneous absorption, individual responses, and other factors. Additionally, absorption of insulin may be quite variable within a single patient from day to day, since absorption of subcutaneous insulin is markedly increased by vigorous exercise of the injected extremity or massage of the injection site. Differences in purity also exist. Conventional insulin preparations contain less than 10,000 parts per million (ppm) of impurities; improved single peak insulin, less than 50 ppm; and "purified" insulin, 1 to 10 ppm. The impurities mentioned are predominantly proinsulin, with smaller amounts of insulin dimers, proinsulin-like products, glucagon, pancreatic polypeptide, somatostatin, and vasoactive polypeptide. For practical purposes, commercially available insulin preparations are labeled as purified (1 to 10 ppm); if they are not specifically labeled they contain 20 to 50 ppm. The older less pure forms are no longer widely distributed. Essentially all preparations can be obtained as purified pork, beef, or beef-pork mixtures. Finally, highly purified human insulin is now available as a product of recombinant DNA biosynthesis or chemical conversion of pork to human insulin.

TABLE 230–4. PROPERTIES OF VARIOUS INSULIN PREPARATIONS

Class	Type	Peak Effect	Duration of Action (hr)
Rapid	Regular crystalline insulin (CZI)	2–4	6–8
	Semilente	2–6	10–12
Intermediate	Neutral protamine (NPH)	6–12	18–24
	Lente	6–12	18–24
Long Acting	Protamine zinc, (PZI)	14–24	36
	Ultralente	18–24	36

Methods of Treatment. The insulin regimen can be more or less intensive, depending on the number of injections per day, types of insulin used, and frequency and method of assessing control. Many NIDDM patients, and occasional IDDM patients, can achieve excellent glycemic control with a single daily (morning) injection of an intermediate-acting insulin. Occasionally, because of postbreakfast hyperglycemia, it is necessary to mix a short-acting preparation with this single dose. In most patients who realize excellent control with this regimen, endogenous insulin secretion is retained. A somewhat more intensive method to regulate glycemia involves a split-dosage regimen. This includes morning (before breakfast) and evening (before dinner) injection of mixtures of intermediate- and rapid-acting insulin. About two thirds of the total daily dose is usually given in the morning and about one third in the evening; the proportion of intermediate- to rapid-acting insulin at each injection is usually two thirds to one third. Patients receiving single-dose therapy who require more than 50 to 60 units per day should usually be tried on a split-dose regimen. In a 70-kg man, normal 24-hour insulin output has been estimated at 25 units per day. Therefore, in normal-sized diabetic subjects starting insulin therapy, it is reasonable to begin with a total daily dose of about 20 units per day with upward adjustments every several days based on the level of blood and urinary glucose. In mildly obese IDDM patients, starting doses can be 5 to 10 units per day higher. Because of insulin resistance, obese NIDDM patients requiring insulin will often need 60 to 90 units per day. With the above methods of insulin delivery, assessment of glycemic control can be carried out in several ways. Measurements of urinary glucose and ketones can be obtained before breakfast and once or twice throughout the day. Patients should be instructed to void 30 minutes before obtaining urine for glucose determination (double voiding), particularly for the morning sample, so that the urinary glucose is more representative of the corresponding blood glucose. Regardless of how carefully urinary glucose is determined, it provides only a rough approximation of blood glucose levels. Factors such as renal threshold, renal blood flow, and urine volume greatly affect the meaning of urine glucose measurements (i.e., a 4+ reaction in a concentrated urine sample is of little significance compared to a 4+ reaction in a dilute sample). For these reasons, urinary glucose is a poor way to monitor diabetic control and if at all possible should not be relied upon as the sole guide on which to base the insulin regimen. Twenty-four hour urinary glucose excretion can be periodically assessed to provide a better estimate of day-long control (less than 5 grams per day is excellent control) or glycosylated hemoglobin can be measured to assess the overall state of glycemic control during the preceding few weeks. The best current method to assess glycemic control is home-, or self-, monitoring of glucose (see below). This requires the patient to assess his own blood glucose level daily and to make appropriate adjustments in insulin dosage. This approach places a large part of the management responsibility in the hands of the patient and emphasizes the need for a continuous outpatient patient education program.

When patients with new-onset IDDM are started on insulin therapy, after an initial period of stabilization, insulin requirements frequently decrease dramatically over the ensuing few weeks. This is the so-called honeymoon phenomenon, and it is sometimes possible to maintain near-normal levels of glycemia without administering any insulin. This honeymoon phase may last for a few weeks and sometimes as long as one to two years. It is invariably followed by worsening of metabolic control with permanent recrudescence of the insulin-dependent state. Some experts have recommended that during this honeymoon period insulin administration should never be completely stopped, even if dosages have to be reduced to homeopathic levels. The reason for this is the fear that if there is a prolonged period in which insulin is not administered, once insulin therapy is reinstituted an anamnestic response with rising titers of anti-insulin antibodies might occur. However, with use of the highly purified insulin preparations now available, or with biosynthetic human insulin, this may be less of a problem.

If more intensive insulin management is required to achieve closer to normal glycemic control, then multiple daily injections of insulin or continuous subcutaneous insulin infusion (CSII) are used. At the current time these approaches are generally limited to patients with IDDM. However, if ideal control of glycemia is the therapeutic goal, there is no reason these methods could not be used in patients with NIDDM whose disease cannot be satisfactorily controlled by other means. Multiple injections involve administration of regular insulin before each meal, with the dose adjusted to the anticipated meal size. This is usually combined with either a long-acting insulin in the morning or an intermediate-acting preparation in the evening.

The most intensive method of insulin delivery is CSII. This consists of constant insulin delivery into a subcutaneous site in the abdominal wall via an open loop delivery device consisting of a small insulin pump that must be worn by the patient essentially 24 hours a day. The key to this method of therapy is the constant delivery of basal insulin. The basal insulin infusion is supplemented by a preprandial bolus of insulin given 15 minutes prior to meal ingestion. This gives the patient a fair degree of flexibility in the timing and content of meals, since the preprandial bolus is given at the patient's discretion in an amount picked to match meal size. In general, the basal insulin infusion accounts for about 50 per cent of the total daily insulin dose and usually averages 0.5 to 1 unit per hour. Typically, preprandial boluses are 5 to 10 units, depending on meal size, time of day, and proximity to time of exercise. To be successful, intensive insulin therapy regimens must be combined with home- (or self-) glucose monitoring. This requires the patient to obtain capillary blood by finger prick for glucose measurement, using a reflectance meter. There are numerous devices and algorithms for constant insulin delivery and various approaches to the frequency and method of self-glucose measurements. A detailed discussion of these issues is beyond the scope of this chapter, but suffice it to say that with properly motivated and educated patients and physicians, excellent control can be achieved in nearly all subjects. Patients generally accept this mode of therapy quite well and report an increased feeling of well-being. However, CSII should not be used indiscriminately, since pump dysfunction does occur, and hypoglycemia is a real problem, especially nocturnally. Additionally, a great deal is asked of patients when they participate in these programs in terms of dedication, education, and changes in life style.

Many other insulin treatment schedules have been proposed, all of which represent variations on the above common themes. Some of these are listed in Table 230–5. No single method is inherently superior to any other, and it is probably best for a physician to become accustomed to one or two methods and use them more or less exclusively so that he will be familiar with problems associated with insulin therapy and its individualization. All of these approaches are meant as guidelines rather than rigid algorithms, and considerable flexibility should be allowed to achieve optimal individualization.

TABLE 230–5. DIFFERENT INSULIN REGIMENS

Split dose intermediate (NPH or lente) + regular insulin		
	A.M. dose:	⅔ TDD*
		~ 70% intermediate
		~ 30% regular
	P.M. dose:	⅓ TDD
		50%–70% intermediate
		30%–50% regular
Intermediate + preprandial regular insulin		
	Breakfast:	Regular, 25%–40% TDD
	Lunch:	Regular, 25%–30% TDD
	Dinner:	Regular, 25%–30% TDD
	Night:	NPH or lente, 15%–25% TDD
Ultralente + preprandial regular insulin		
	Breakfast:	Regular, 15%–25% TDD
	Lunch:	Regular, 15%–25% TDD
	Dinner:	Regular, 15%–25% TDD
		Ultralente, 40%–60% TDD
Triple A.M. mixture: regular, lente + ultralente insulin		
Double A.M. mixture: regular + NPH (or lente) insulin		

*TDD, total daily dose

Regardless of the insulin regimen employed, an established daily dose in a given patient must not be considered to be fixed. Even long-established insulin dosages may need to be increased because of changes in growth status, subtle intercurrent illness or stress, or development of anti-insulin antibodies. Dosages may need to be decreased because of consistent increases in physical activity, dietary changes, or changes in concomitant drug therapy (e.g., stopping steroids). Additionally, absorption may vary from one anatomic site to another, and the rate of absorption of insulin can be augmented by exercise involving a particular injection site. This simply means that the physician and the patient must constantly review the treatment program and be prepared to make changes when indicated.

Complications of Insulin Therapy. Several complications are associated with insulin treatment, but the most significant of these is *hypoglycemia*. This is because even the best mode of insulin delivery is still an imperfect method to mimic the homeostatic mechanisms in normal subjects. Normal persons respond to food ingestion, exercise, and stress in such a way as to keep the blood glucose level within narrowly defined limits. One can hope to approach this, but not match it, with the methods used for delivery of exogenous insulin. For example, when normal individuals exercise, peripheral glucose uptake increases, and this is matched by a corresponding increase in hepatic glucose production. A decrease in insulin secretion allows the increase in hepatic glucose production to occur. Obviously this degree of fine tuning is difficult to achieve with exogenous insulin administration. Consequently hypoglycemia is a common complication of insulin therapy as the result of overzealous insulin administration or inappropriate timing. Most often this occurs in a situation in which tight control is attempted. Occasional mild episodes of hypoglycemia are probably acceptable if they appear in a patient in whom excellent control is generally achieved and who is fully aware of their occurrence and of methods to abort them. However, frequent and severe hypoglycemic reactions are unacceptable. These are serious and occasionally can be fatal. Furthermore, the long-term effects on the central nervous system of frequent hypoglycemic episodes have not been determined. If satisfactory control cannot be achieved without recurrence of such reactions, then compromises in the overall therapeutic plan must be made. It would seem imprudent to expose patients to known complications of hypoglycemia in the hope that superior control will prevent chronic diabetic complications in the future.

An interesting aspect of hypoglycemic episodes is the so-called *Somogyi phenomenon.* This involves rebound hyperglycemia due to excessive secretion of counterregulatory hormones following a previous episode of hypoglycemia. The classic situation involves nocturnal hypoglycemia followed by marked hyperglycemia prior to breakfast. This can induce a self-defeating cycle in which the insulin dose is progressively raised in response to the fasting hyperglycemia when a reduction in insulin dose, to prevent the nocturnal hypoglycemia, would be more appropriate.

A minority of patients beginning insulin therapy experience a variety of local allergic reactions at the injection site. Manifestations include local itching, erythematous indurated lesions, and occasional small, discrete subcutaneous nodules. These local reactions are usually self-limited and eventually disappear with continued insulin treatment. Antihistamines may be used for symptomatic relief if necessary. The frequency of these problems has decreased significantly with the use of the newer more highly purified insulins. Rare patients may develop systemic reactions, including generalized urticaria and even anaphylactic reactions. This usually occurs when insulin therapy has been stopped for a time and then reinstituted. If these symptoms cannot be controlled by antihistamines, and if insulin treatment is mandatory for the patient's well-being, then formal desensitization regimens are necessary. Other local reactions at the injection site include lipoatrophy and hypertrophy. Lipoatrophy at the injection site is a benign condition usually due to impurities in the insulin preparation. It can usually be corrected by changing to a highly purified pork insulin and injecting this into the lipoatrophic areas, which then fill in with subcutaneous fat in a normal fashion. Most likely the new highly purified human insulin preparations will also be suitable for this purpose. Insulin hypertrophy is attributed to the local lipogenic effects of the injected insulin. In advanced cases the underlying tissue can be fibrous and less vascular, making the overlying skin anesthetic. This explains why many patients prefer these areas as sites of injection. The problem can usually be corrected by carefully rotating injection sites.

FUTURE MODES OF THERAPY

Even with the most meticulous mode of insulin therapy in the most motivated patients, euglycemic control is difficult to achieve for prolonged periods. Thus the search for better, more effective, and, in some cases, curative forms of therapy continues. Transplantation of the pancreas or islet cells continues to receive extensive study. Numerous logistical, immunologic, and technical problems need to be overcome before such therapies become available for routine clinical purposes, but there are signs that some positive results might be seen in the next several years. This is the one mode of therapy that might actually be considered curative. Efforts continue to be expended in developing newer and better external or implantable insulin-delivery devices. Unquestionably the mechanical and engineering aspects of insulin-delivery devices will continue to improve dramatically over the next several years, and pumps that are smaller, safer, and more flexible will be produced. It also seems likely that reliable implantable devices are in the offing. However, unless such devices can be used to administer insulin via the portal route, the advantage of implantable pumps appears to be mostly esthetic. An additional hope for internal devices is that a closed loop system can be designed. This would require development of a reliable, fail-safe glucose sensor integrated into the appropriate algorithms for insulin delivery. If such artificial pancreases become readily available they would obviously have wide applicability. Finally, since hyperglucagonemia has been implicated in the pathogenesis of the hyperglycemia in diabetes, agents that specifically suppress glucagon secretion have been sought. Attempts to develop a glucagon-specific somatostatin derivative continue; such a compound might be a useful adjunctive therapy in the management of diabetes.

ACUTE COMPLICATIONS

A number of acute metabolic complications of diabetes exist, including diabetic ketoacidosis, hyperosmolar nonketotic coma, lactic acidosis, and hypoglycemia.

Diabetic Ketoacidosis (DKA)

DKA is due to insulin deficiency. Before consideration of the pathogenesis of this metabolic derangement, it is important to review the normal physiologic effects of insulin on carbohydrate, protein, and fat metabolism, since DKA simply represents a reversal of these normal insulin-stimulated processes.

PHYSIOLOGY OF FED AND FASTED STATE. When food is ingested, insulin functions as the major anabolic hormone facilitating the disposition of carbohydrate, protein, and fat and their synthesis into macromolecules for storage (Fig. 230–6*A*). Glucose is absorbed into the portal vein, and approximately 60 per cent of the ingested glucose-derived carbons end up in liver glycogen in the postprandial period. A significant portion of this is probably not a result of direct hepatic glucose uptake, but is due to peripheral metabolism of glucose to three-carbon fragments (lactate, pyruvate) that are then recycled to the liver where they enter the gluconeogenic pathway and are synthesized into glycogen. Glycogen then serves as the storage form of carbohydrate for later release. When glucose is metabolized via the glycolytic (anaerobic) pathway, 2 moles of ATP are generated per mole of glucose. Aerobic, or oxidative, metabolism (Krebs' cycle) is far more efficient as an energy-producing process and generates 12 moles of ATP per mole of glucose. Insulin exerts multiple anabolic effects on this process. It stimulates glucose uptake and glycogen synthesis by muscle and inhibits glycogenolysis. In liver, insulin does not directly stimulate glucose uptake, but it does actively promote glycogenesis and inhibit glycogenolysis. Although most of the ingested glucose, or glucose derived carbon, ends up in the liver in the postprandial period, the central nervous system (CNS) (primarily brain) is the predominant tissue of glucose consumption, accounting for about 70 per cent of total glucose utilization. Glucose is the primary source of energy for brain, and glucose uptake and metabolism in this tissue are independent of insulin. A major purpose of glucose homeostasis is to store glucose as liver glycogen postprandially when glucose and insulin levels are high, so that it can be released in the interprandial period for CNS consumption. Protein digestion and absorption lead to a postprandial rise in circulating amino acid levels. Insulin plays a dominant role in converting amino acids to protein by stimulating amino acid uptake in muscle and liver and by augmenting protein synthesis and inhibiting proteolysis. Fat is absorbed as chylomicrons that enter the circulation via the lymphatic system. Insulin affects fat assimilation in a number of ways. Lipoprotein lipase is an enzyme, synthesized primarily by fat and muscle tissue, that is secreted into the extracellular space and incorporated into the surface of nearby endothelial cells. In this location, lipoprotein lipase hydrolyzes fatty acids from triglyceride-rich lipoproteins (chylomicrons and very low density lipoproteins); these fatty acids are then taken up, predominantly by adipose tissue, where they are esterified into triglyceride for storage in the fat droplet of adipocytes. Insulin stimulates the synthesis and secretion of lipoprotein lipase and also strongly inhibits lipolysis of triglycerides stored in adipose tissue. Additionally, by promoting glucose uptake, insulin increases the supply of glycerol within adipocytes for esterification of fatty acids. Insulin is also lipogenic and stimulates the synthesis of fatty acids from glucose or other substrates that form pyruvate.

Many of these insulin effects are antagonized by the coun-

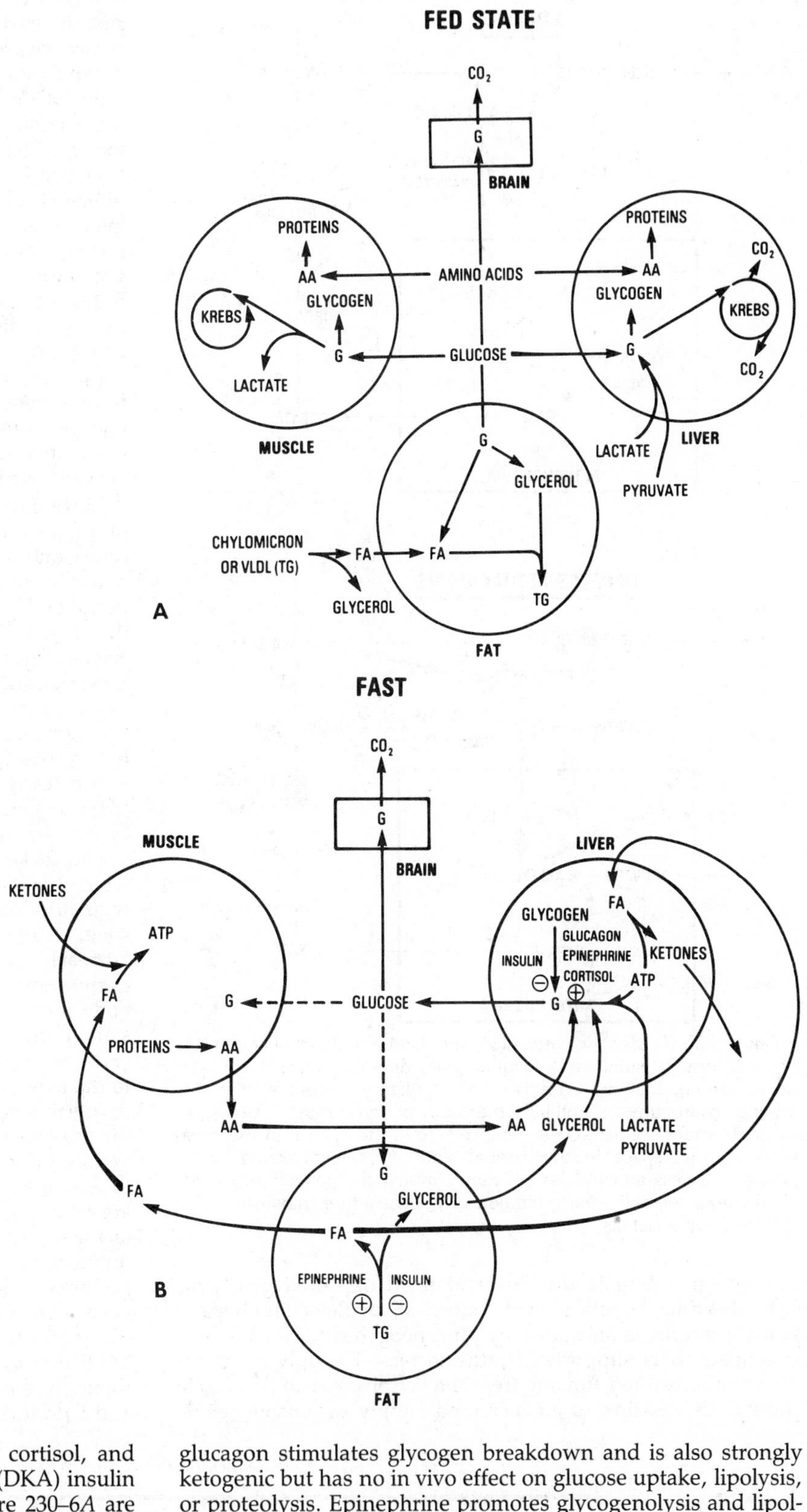

Figure 230–6. *A,* Fuel homeostasis during the immediate postprandial fed state. The key features of this diagram are the storage of glucose, amino acids, and fatty acids as the macromolecules glycogen, protein, and triglyceride in tissue depots; each of these processes is facilitated by the anabolic effects of insulin. *B,* Reversal of the anabolic effects of insulin during the insulinopenic fasting state. The major purpose of these homeostatic responses is to maintain a supply of glucose for obligate glucose uptake by the CNS while other tissues cease their consumption of glucose in favor of fatty acids from adipose tissue depots.

terregulatory hormones, glucagon, epinephrine, cortisol, and growth hormone. When mild (fasting) or severe (DKA) insulin deficiency exists, the processes outlined in Figure 230–6*A* are reversed, and characteristic metabolic derangements occur. This is illustrated in Figure 230–6*B*. A 24-hour fast causes mild insulin deficiency, and this results in a marked decrease in peripheral glucose uptake. This is accompanied by a decrease in synthesis of glycogen, protein, and triglyceride, along with increased breakdown of these storage macromolecules by accelerated glycogenolysis, proteolysis, and lipolysis. These catabolic processes increase as a result of the lack of insulin effect, but breakdown of macromolecules is also augmented by increased concentrations of counterregulatory hormones. Thus, glucagon stimulates glycogen breakdown and is also strongly ketogenic but has no in vivo effect on glucose uptake, lipolysis, or proteolysis. Epinephrine promotes glycogenolysis and lipolysis and also inhibits peripheral glucose uptake. Cortisol probably has effects that are additive or possibly synergistic with the other counterregulatory hormones and may independently stimulate proteolysis. Growth hormone probably plays a minor role in these events mediated through inhibition of glucose uptake. Taken together, insulin deficiency plus increased counterregulatory hormones lead to a marked decrease in glucose metabolism by insulin-sensitive tissues, "sparing" glucose for the obligate CNS utilization. The source of glucose in this setting is the liver. For the initial 12 to 24 hours, hepatic glucose

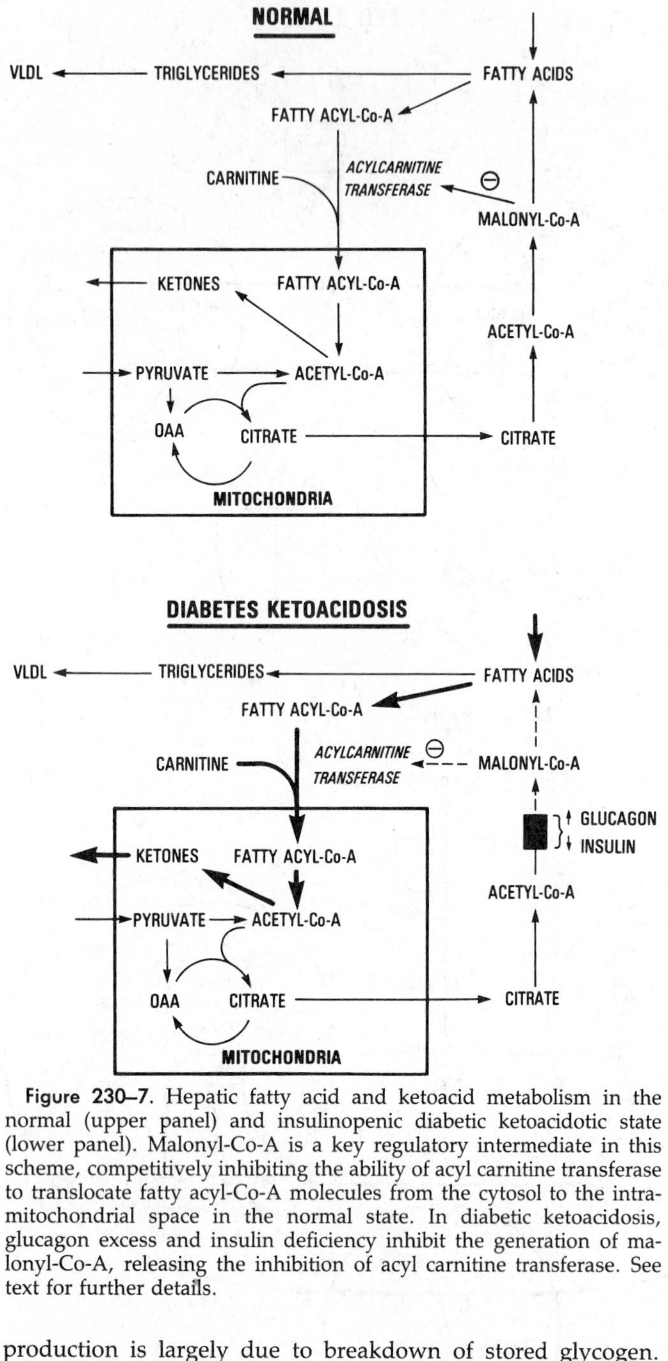

Figure 230–7. Hepatic fatty acid and ketoacid metabolism in the normal (upper panel) and insulinopenic diabetic ketoacidotic state (lower panel). Malonyl-Co-A is a key regulatory intermediate in this scheme, competitively inhibiting the ability of acyl carnitine transferase to translocate fatty acyl-Co-A molecules from the cytosol to the intramitochondrial space in the normal state. In diabetic ketoacidosis, glucagon excess and insulin deficiency inhibit the generation of malonyl-Co-A, releasing the inhibition of acyl carnitine transferase. See text for further details.

production is largely due to breakdown of stored glycogen. After this time, hepatic glycogen stores are depleted and hepatic glucose output is sustained by gluconeogenesis. Hepatic gluconeogenesis is supported by the increased supply of gluconeogenic substrates flowing from the periphery, that is, muscle proteolysis, leading to an increased supply of gluconeogenic amino acids (mainly alanine) and increased lipolysis resulting in enhanced glycerol release from adipose tissue. Some lactate and pyruvate are supplied from anaerobic metabolism of glucose in peripheral tissues (Cori cycle). Thus the liver is the central clearing house in this process by converting the breakdown products of stored fat and protein to supply glucose for the CNS in a setting (fasting) in which exogenous glucose is unavailable. In this situation the predominant energy source for non-CNS tissues is circulating free fatty acids (FFA) derived from breakdown of adipose tissue triglyceride (the CNS cannot utilize FFA as a metabolic fuel). Free fatty acids also supply the liver with the energy necessary to drive gluconeogenesis. Ketone bodies are produced in the liver from fatty acid oxidation under conditions of insulin deficiency and glucagon excess. In fasting this serves an important homeostatic purpose, since ketone bodies can be utilized by the CNS and muscle for energy, markedly reducing the need for protein breakdown to supply gluconeogenic precursors for liver glucose production. Ketone bodies provide a mechanism to convert adipose tissue energy stores into a substrate that can be metabolized in the CNS; this spares critical body proteins, allowing humans to survive relatively long-term fasts.

PATHOPHYSIOLOGY OF DKA. In DKA, all of these homeostatic processes are out of control, leading to pronounced hyperglycemia and ketonemia. The hyperglycemia is due to a combination of increased hepatic glucose production and decreased peripheral glucose uptake. The biochemical mechanisms underlying the hyperketonemia are somewhat more complex, as seen in Figure 230–7. Ketone bodies are produced in hepatocyte mitochondria by beta oxidation of fatty acids, and glucagon is the primary hormone responsible for inducing the hepatic ketogenic state. It does this by lowering malonyl coenzyme A levels, the first committed substrate in fatty acid synthesis, which leads to a marked increase in the activity of carnitine acyl transferase I. This enzyme translocates fatty acids from the cytosol to the intramitochondrial space where they are converted to ketones. Hepatic carnitine levels are also increased, which further drives this transfer step by mass action. The key regulatory point in understanding ketogenesis is that in the fed state, entry of fatty acids into the mitochondria is low, limiting fatty acid oxidation and ketogenesis in favor of fatty acid and triglyceride synthesis; thus the liver is rate limiting in ketone body formation. When insulin is low and glucagon high (as in starvation or DKA), fatty acids freely enter mitochondria to be converted to ketones, and therefore the supply of fatty acids to the liver is rate limiting for ketogenesis. Fatty acids are freely permeable across the hepatocyte plasma membrane, and thus the plasma concentration of FFA drives ketogenesis. In starvation, fatty acid levels are only moderately increased, leading to enhanced, but controlled, ketogenesis; in DKA, FFA levels are much higher, leading to uncontrolled ketogenesis. Another factor enhancing ketonemia in DKA is related to ketone body utilization. Insulin normally stimulates ketoacid uptake by peripheral tissues, and this is inhibited in DKA; additionally, very high levels of ketones may saturate the uptake mechanisms, further limiting utilization.

All of the pathophysiologic sequelae of DKA follow from hyperglycemia and hyperketonemia (Fig. 230–8). Thus, acidosis and ketonuria are directly due to the buildup of the ketoacids

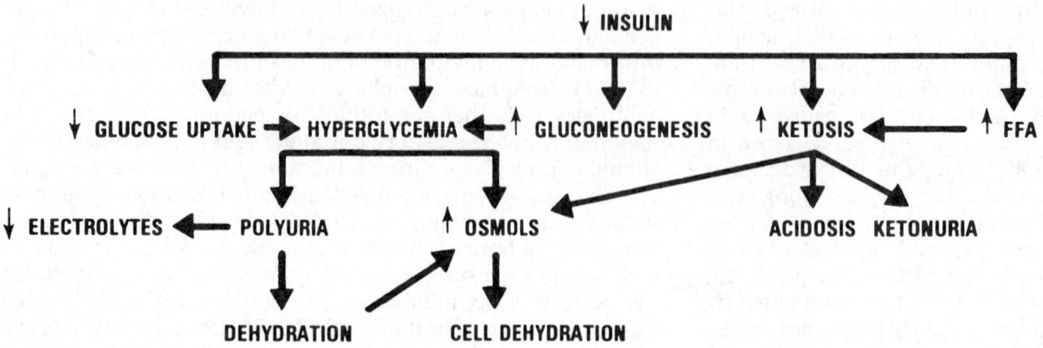

Figure 230–8. Pathophysiology of diabetic ketoacidosis. Severe insulin deficiency leads to hyperglycemia and ketonemia, and from this all of the other pathophysiologic sequelae result.

beta hydroxybutyrate and acetoacetate. The hyperglycemia and hyperketonemia produce an osmotic diuresis that causes intravascular volume depletion and dehydration and urinary electrolyte loss. The hyperosmolarity further exaggerates intracellular dehydration.

CLINICAL PICTURE. Diabetic ketoacidosis can be a life-threatening situation, and the clinical presentation is often dramatic. An antecedent history of polyuria and polydipsia for one to several days is typical, and nausea, vomiting, and anorexia are frequent accompanying symptoms. Occasionally abdominal pain is a predominant feature, sometimes mimicking an acute abdominal condition. Often this is due to gastric stasis and distention. In the obtunded patient with gastric distention, nasogastric suction should be considered to avoid vomiting with aspiration. Physical findings include tachypnea, dehydration, and disorientation, or even coma. If systemic acidosis is severe, Kussmaul respirations are present. Precipitating causes of DKA include failure of the patient to take insulin, infection, intercurrent illness, trauma, or emotional stress. When a known diabetic presents with signs and symptoms of DKA, the diagnosis is usually straightforward. However, DKA can also be the initial presenting episode of diabetes. DKA is a disease of IDDM, only rarely occurring in NIDDM, and only when precipitating causes are extreme.

Although the diagnosis of DKA can be strongly suspected on a clinical basis, confirmation is based on laboratory analyses. The diagnosis is made by demonstrating hyperglycemia and hyperketonemia in the presence of acidosis. However, the severity of these abnormalities can vary over a wide range. Occasionally the presenting episode may be severe ketonemia and acidosis and only mild hyperglycemia (200 to 400 mg per deciliter). Other patients may have severe hyperglycemia and only mild ketonemia and acidosis. Occasionally, alcoholic patients have ketonemia and hyperglycemia, and this condition, termed alcoholic ketoacidosis, must be differentiated from DKA (see next section). Direct quantitative measurements of acetoacetate and beta hydroxybutyrate are not usually readily available, and most physicians rely on reagent strips (Ketostix) or tablets (Acetest) for measurements. With this method, a nitroprusside reaction is the indicator; nitroprusside reacts mainly with acetoacetate, to a lesser extent with acetone, and not at all with beta hydroxybutyrate. Since beta hydroxybutyrate levels are much higher than acetoacetate levels in DKA, this method can sometimes be confusing. For example, when concomitant lactic acidosis exists, acetoacetate production may be inhibited in the presence of very high levels of beta hydroxybutyrate. In this setting the nitroprusside reaction may not be strongly positive. During the course of insulin therapy for DKA, beta hydroxybutyrate levels may fall out of proportion to acetoacetate levels, giving the impression that therapy is less effective than it actually is. Serum sodium levels are usually mildly decreased. This is due to the hyperglycemia- and hyperketonemia-induced hyperosmolarity, which attracts extracellular water from the intracellular space, leading to dilution of serum sodium. It should be kept in mind that the osmolar contribution of the hyperketonemia can often approach the contribution of the hyperglycemia. Serum bicarbonate levels are depressed, and the magnitude of decrease is in proportion to the degree of acidosis. BUN levels are usually modestly elevated as a result of dehydration and a component of prerenal azotemia. Serum potassium levels can be high, low, or normal, depending on the degree of dehydration and acidosis. In all cases, severe total body and intracellular potassium depletion exists. Because of cellular buffering mechanisms, which exchange intracellular potassium for extracellular hydrogen ion, extracellular potassium levels are often maintained in acidotic states. Nevertheless, greater than 95 per cent of total body potassium is intracellular, so in the presence of acidosis, extracellular potassium levels do not reflect total body potassium stores unless the potassium concentration is plotted on a nomogram related to serum pH (Fig. 230–9).

TREATMENT OF DKA. The treatment of DKA should be started as soon as it is diagnosed. The goals of therapy are to increase the rate of glucose utilization by insulin-dependent tissues, to reverse ketonemia and acidosis, and to correct the depletion of water and electrolytes. To accomplish this, treatment can be divided into four general areas: (1) insulin administration, (2) replacement of fluid and electrolytes, (3) treatment of any precipitating problems, and (4) avoidance of complications.

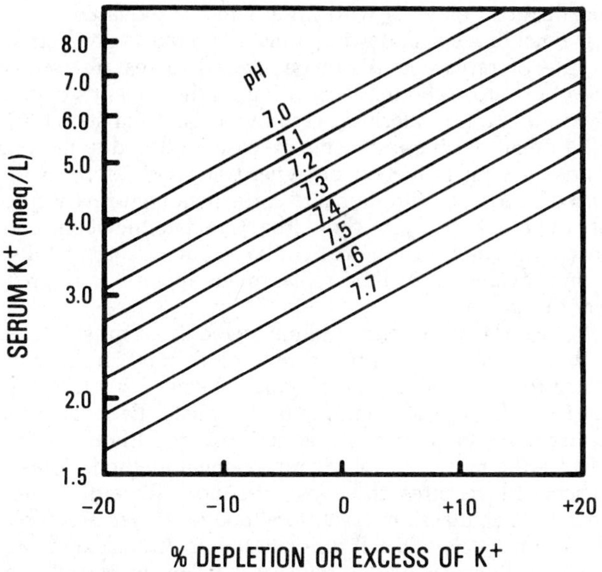

Figure 230–9. Nomogram depicting the relationship between total body potassium depletion, serum potassium, and serum pH. Per cent potassium depletion or excess is calculated by drawing a horizontal line from the ordinate intercept of the serum potassium concentration to the intersection of the diagonal line corresponding to the coexisting serum pH. From this intersection a vertical line is dropped to the abscissa and per cent potassium depletion or excess is read from the abscissal intercept. For example, at a serum potassium concentration of 4.0, at a concommitant serum pH of 7.2, an approximate 10 per cent depletion of total body potassium stores exists.

A variety of *insulin* regimens are possible, ranging from constant intravenous infusion to intermittent administration of intravenous, subcutaneous, or intramuscular boluses. The aim of all forms of insulin administration is to achieve a rapid and maximal insulin effect. In vivo insulin action is near maximal at an insulin concentration of about 200 μU per milliliter, and achieving higher levels has little further benefit. Since insulin is rapidly cleared from the circulation ($t\frac{1}{2}$ = 7 minutes), boluses must be given frequently (every 30 to 60 minutes) to maintain maximally effective insulin levels. With constant intravenous administration, serum insulin levels are maintained at a steady state throughout the infusion. In normal subjects, an infusion rate of 10 units per hour will result in an insulin level of approximately 200 μU per milliliter by 30 minutes, and if this mode of treatment is chosen a priming dose (10 to 20 units) should be given initially. Advocates of constant intravenous infusion maintain that the rate of metabolic improvement is smoother and more predictable and hypoglycemia is less common. Additionally, problems of variable or inadequate absorption from subcutaneous or intramuscular sites are avoided. One difficulty with this method occurs in the occasional patient with severe insulin resistance due to sepsis or high titers of insulin antibodies. If clear-cut metabolic improvement is not seen within the first few hours of constant insulin infusion, a bolus of insulin (20 to 30 units) should be given and the rate of insulin infusion increased.

Fluid replacement should also be started immediately. Patients with DKA are dehydrated and hypovolemic and usually have fluid deficits of 5 to 8 liters or more. Thus, rapid expansion of intravascular volume is essential, and this is achieved by an initial infusion of 1 to 2 liters of normal saline, or equivalent, over the first one to two hours. Of course, caution should be used in those patients with underlying cardiovascular or oliguric renal disease. Following initial rapid fluid administration, the rate of replacement can be slowed to restore estimated losses by 16 to 24 hours, depending on the patient's degree of dehydration and underlying cardiovascular-renal status. Much of the initial decline in plasma glucose level is due to volume expansion with reduction of hyperosmolarity, along with increased glomerular filtration and corresponding urinary glucose loss. In general, the aim should be to initiate metabolic correction rapidly, but once the patient has shown clear-cut substantial improvement, further replacement therapy can proceed more cautiously.

The electrolyte content of administered fluids must be closely monitored. Over the entire course of therapy the goal is to replace the electrolyte deficit, which averages 200 to 400 mEq each for sodium, potassium, and phosphate. Patients are usually ingesting some form of calories by 16 to 24 hours, and this provides the most physiologic replacement method. Potassium replacement requires the most attention. Regardless of the initial serum potassium level, total body reserves are depleted and serum levels will fall dramatically as acidosis and hyperglycemia are corrected. As glucose is taken up by cells under the influence of insulin, potassium is also transported intracellularly, and as acidosis is reversed the cellular buffering process exchanging intracellular potassium for extracellular hydrogen ion diminishes. To prevent hypokalemia, potassium should be included in the intravenous fluids once it is established that renal perfusion and urine flow are adequate following initial intravascular fluid expansion. To accomplish this, 40 mEq of potassium can be added to each liter of intravenous fluids as the phosphate salt. Phosphate depletion is also uniform in DKA, and some replacement is advisable, particularly if serum phosphate levels are low. This can be accomplished by administering 10 to 20 mmol per hour and can be combined with potassium replacement by giving potassium phosphate. Bicarbonate replacement should be initiated in patients with severe acidosis ($pH < 7.0$). This can be administered at the rate of 44 mEq per liter with appropriate monitoring of pH until it rises above 7.0. Three to four ampules of bicarbonate (44 mEq per ampule) will usually suffice to achieve this goal. Excessive bicarbonate replacement is contraindicated since this will exacerbate the tendency toward hypokalemia and may also result in rebound CNS acidosis. The latter occurs because carbon dioxide is more readily diffusible across the blood-brain barrier than is bicarbonate ion, causing CNS pH to fall at a time when peripheral pH is rising. This can lead to stupor and worsening of CNS status at a time when metabolic improvement is occurring.

Therapy should be monitored by frequent assessment of clinical status and laboratory measurements of urine and serum glucose and ketone levels. A fall in plasma glucose level is the earliest sign of effective therapy, and therefore plasma glucose should be frequently monitored. Once plasma glucose levels fall to approximately 250 mg per deciliter, 5 per cent glucose should be added to the intravenous fluids. Occasionally children or adolescents with DKA exhibit marked mental deterioration, including development of coma 4 to 6 hours after therapy has begun. Usually this is associated with a marked fall in hyperglycemia and serum osmolality, and cerebral edema has been noted in a few autopsy cases. Overall this is probably a rare complication of therapy. Because of the importance of plasma glucose monitoring in assessing the effectiveness of therapy, administration of glucose has no place in the initial stages of DKA treatment.

While insulin and fluid and electrolyte replacement therapy are being administered, a concomitant search for underlying precipitating factors should be undertaken. Leukocytosis often accompanies uncomplicated DKA and so should be viewed appropriately when one is searching for underlying infection. Hypothermia can be associated with DKA, and therefore fever should be a strong impetus to screen rigorously for a site of infection.

The major complications of DKA are mostly the result of treatment and include *hypokalemia, late hypoglycemia, rebound CNS acidosis*, and *CNS deterioration* (possibly due to cerebral edema). However, with proper attention to therapeutic details the former two can always be avoided, and the latter are fortunately rare. Recurrence of DKA can occur in the hospital if the vigorous phase of therapy is relaxed too soon. Maintenance of a flow chart with all therapies and laboratory tests recorded is an important means of coordination so that unexpected results do not go undetected and inappropriate therapies are not given.

Alcoholic Ketoacidosis

Alcoholic ketoacidosis can sometimes present a problem in the differential diagnosis of DKA when the patient is not a known diabetic or when a diabetic patient ingests large amounts of alcohol. This syndrome is characterized by hyperketonemia, acidosis, and dehydration. Serum glucose levels can be normal or sometimes elevated to the lower range of values seen in DKA. In the latter case a diagnostic problem can occur. The clinical picture of alcoholic ketoacidosis occurs in alcoholics following a recent, and sometimes prolonged alcoholic debauch; abstinence during the immediately preceding 12 to 24 hours is a common finding. The patient is usually anorexic, sometimes with nausea and vomiting, and some degree of starvation over the preceding one to three days is always present. The starvation, perhaps accompanied by stress-related hyperglucagonemia, creates a ketogenic state in the liver. This is accompanied by elevated FFA levels similar to those seen in starvation, which are perhaps augmented by adrenergic activation related to alcohol withdrawal, creating the metabolic environment for ketoacidosis. It is unusual for these patients to have hyperglycemia, but it can occur. When it does, the pathogenesis is unclear. In some patients, abnormalities of glucose tolerance exist after therapy, and thus the hyperglycemia may be stress related in previously glucose-intolerant patients. Alternatively, adrenergic mechanisms related to alcohol withdrawal could suppress residual endogenous insulin secretion, facilitating mild hyperglycemia. Regardless of the underlying mechanisms, the metabolic abnormalities are rapidly reversed by intravenous administration of fluids and glucose. Only occasionally is insulin needed in the early stages of treatment.

Nonketotic Hyperosmolar Syndrome

The term *nonketotic hyperosmolar coma* has frequently been applied to this syndrome, but by no means do all patients display coma or even mental obtundity. Rather, this syndrome comprises a spectrum ranging from mild degrees of hyperosmolarity with minimal CNS symptoms to severe hyperosmolarity with accompanying coma. The biochemical hallmarks are extreme hyperglycemia (mean 1000 mg per deciliter, range 600 to 2400 mg per deciliter) in the absence of overt ketoacidosis. Dehydration, hypovolemia, and disorientation are accompanying features. This syndrome usually develops over a much longer interval than DKA, with symptoms of polyuria antedating clinical presentation by several days and sometimes weeks. This syndrome usually occurs in elderly patients with NIDDM (often not previously diagnosed) who for some reason are unable to keep up with the osmotic diuresis by adequate water ingestion and this results in severe dehydration. The severe hyperglycemia is at least partly caused by decreased renal glucose excretion due either to intrinsic underlying renal disease or to decreased glomerular filtration and prerenal azotemia secondary to the marked hypovolemia and dehydration. Frequently this condition is associated with steroid, diuretic, or phenytoin therapy as a precipitating cause. Other precipitating factors include infections, cerebrovascular events, or therapeutic maneuvers such as hypertonic peritoneal dialysis or parenteral nutrition.

Serum sodium and potassium levels are usually normal while

serum bicarbonate levels are often somewhat depressed. This is usually not associated with significant ketonemia and probably reflects an underlying component of lactic acidosis due to hypovolemia. The BUN is uniformly elevated because of hypovolemia and prerenal azotemia. In these cases, though, acidosis is mild, and serum osmolality can be approximated by the formula:

$$\text{serum osmolality (mOsm per liter)} = 2 \times [\text{Na}^+ + \text{K}^+ \text{ (mEq/L)}] + \frac{\text{plasma glucose (mg/dl)}}{18} + \text{BUN (mg/dl)}/2.8.$$

However, since urea is freely diffusible across cell membranes it does not alter the effective serum osmolality, which is the clinically important factor to consider in this hyperosmolar condition. Most experts do not consider BUN levels in this calculation and prefer to estimate effective serum osmolarity as:

$$\text{Eosm} = 2 \times [\text{Na}^+ + \text{K}^+ \text{ (mEq/L)}] + \text{plasma glucose (mg/dl)}/18.$$

Values above 300 mOsm per liter are abnormal and above 320 mOsm per liter are indicative of clinically significant hyperosmolarity.

The reason ketosis is not a feature of this condition has not been satisfactorily explained. FFA levels are not as high in this syndrome as they are in DKA, and most investigators attribute the relatively lower FFA levels and decreased rates of ketogenesis to higher residual insulin levels in patients with hyperosmolar syndrome. This answer is not entirely satisfactory, however, since measured peripheral insulin levels overlap with those reported in DKA. On the other hand, peripheral insulin levels do not always reflect portal insulin concentrations, and significant differences in portal insulin levels may exist in DKA versus hyperosmolar syndrome, with the higher levels in hyperosmolar syndrome restraining hepatic ketogenesis.

In some series, the mortality has ranged up to 50 per cent. However, the relatively high mortality reflects selection criteria since mortality tends to be higher with greater severity of the hyperosmolality. The first priority of treatment should be intravascular volume expansion to restore circulatory integrity. This is accomplished by infusion of 1 to 2 liters of normal saline, or equivalent, over one to two hours, provided absolute cardiovascular contraindications do not exist. Even normal saline is hypotonic relative to serum in these patients, and therefore this therapy will initiate the correction of the hyperosmolality. As in DKA, insulin can be administered by constant intravenous infusions or bolus therapy. Since absorption of insulin administered subcutaneously or intramuscularly is variable because of dehydration and hypovolemia, and since late hypoglycemia is a more common complication of the hyperosmolar syndrome, constant intravenous administration of insulin can be very effective in this condition, leading to a predictable and fairly constant, smooth decline in plasma glucose levels. Once plasma glucose begins to decrease, and provided acceptable volume expansion and urine flow have been established, potassium phosphate salts should be added to the intravenous fluids. Subsequent to the initial volume expansion, intravenous fluids can consist of 0.5 normal saline with added potassium phosphate. Once plasma glucose levels decline to approximately 250 mg per deciliter, 5 per cent glucose should be added to the intravenous fluids. The above comments are meant more as guidelines than hard and fast rules, since, as in DKA, therapy must be individualized as far as replacement of fluids and electrolytes is concerned. This is best done by maintaining an organized flow chart with frequent measurements of plasma glucose, electrolytes, blood pressure, and urine volume. Despite even the best therapy, morbidity and mortality are high in this condition. Thrombosis and embolic events as well as infections, particularly pneumonia with accompanying adult respiratory distress syndrome, contribute significantly to adverse outcomes. In summary, rigorous but carefully monitored hydration and reestablishment of circulatory integrity are critical for successful therapy. These goals should be pursued while hyperosmolarity is corrected by administration of relatively hypotonic fluids with adequate free water along with insulin to reduce the hyperglycemia. Concomitantly a careful workup should be instituted to uncover precipitating factors with appropriate therapy when necessary.

CHRONIC OR LATE COMPLICATIONS OF DIABETES

Retinopathy

Eye disease is common in diabetes, and permanent loss of vision is one of the most striking and feared complications. Approximately 25 per cent of all newly reported cases of blindness are attributed to diabetes. When diabetics of all ages and types are considered together, the incidence of blindness from diabetic retinopathy is 0.2 per cent per year in all diabetics and 0.6 per cent per year in diabetics with retinopathy. This is 11 and 29 times greater, respectively, than the incidence of blindness from all other causes combined in the general population.

The major form of diabetic eye disease is diabetic retinopathy. Two general categories exist: nonproliferative or background retinopathy and proliferative retinopathy. Nonproliferative retinopathy can include venous abnormalities, microaneurysms, retinal hemorrhages, retinal edema, and exudates. This may progress to proliferative retinopathy, characterized by neovascularization, glial proliferation, and vitreoretinal traction. In general, diabetic retinopathy is progressive and tends to worsen with the duration of disease. However, most diabetics do not develop proliferative retinopathy. The incidence of this complication is substantially lower in NIDDM then in IDDM, even when corrected for duration of disease. However, since there are many more patients with NIDDM than IDDM, the absolute numbers of NIDDM and IDDM patients with proliferative retinopathy are roughly comparable.

NONPROLIFERATIVE RETINOPATHY. Probably the earliest retinal change is increased capillary permeability seen on fluorescein angiography. This abnormality can be readily reversed by effective glycemic control, but the relationship of this form of capillary permeability to retinopathy is unknown. Nonperfusion of retinal capillaries occurs early in diabetic retinopathy (so-called capillary dropout), and this leads to areas of retinal ischemia and infarction. Microaneurysms are small (15 to 50 μm diameter) excrescences along capillaries and are particularly prominent along the edges of areas of capillary nonperfusion. Fusiform aneurysms, or general dilatation of capillary loops, can also occur. Retinal veins are often tortuous and dilated; dilatation can be segmental, giving rise to a beaded or "sausage string" appearance. Exudates can be of two types: (1) *Hard, waxy exudates* are white to yellowish, shiny, with defined borders but without surrounding pigmentation. These exudates are due to lipid- and protein-containing fluid that has leaked from surrounding capillaries. (2) *Cotton-wool, or soft, exudates* are really areas of nonperfusion representing retinal microinfarcts and are often surrounded by microaneurysms. Clinically, an increase in cotton-wool areas indicates progressive capillary dropout and is a poor prognostic sign. Subretinal hemorrhages tend to be small and dot shaped and may resorb within a few weeks. Larger, flame-shaped hemorrhages occur in the superficial retinal layers and resorb more slowly. Preretinal hemorrhages are more serious and can impair vision if they are large or if they impinge on the macula. Following resorption, scarring and vitreous retraction or retinal detachment can occur. Edema of the retina is due to abnormal capillary permeability and ischemia. When persistent macular edema exists, vision is seriously impaired, and usual forms of therapy (photocoagulation) may not be effective. The primary pathogenetic events underlying these changes of nonproliferative background retinopathy are unclear, but loss of supporting capillary pericytes, endothelial proliferation, and hyperviscosity with red cell aggregation, together or alone, have all been proposed.

PROLIFERATIVE RETINOPATHY. The hallmark of proliferative retinopathy is new vessel formation or neovascularization. These capillary fronds or loops can grow on the surface of the retina or extend into the vitreous. Often this is accompanied by proliferation of glial elements in the region of the optic disc or along the new vessel arcades. Traction between the vitreous and the neovascular and glial elements can ultimately develop, leading to retinal detachment or large-scale hemorrhage into the vitreous. These events will lead to serious loss of vision or blindness. It has been suggested that the stimulus for neovascularization is retinal ischemia with local release of growth-promoting factors.

Photocoagulation is the therapy of choice for proliferative diabetic retinopathy. With this therapy, a light beam is focused on the retina to produce a burn or coagulum in a precisely defined area. By this means, one can selectively destroy microaneurysms, leaky vessels, neovascular elements, and areas of microinfarction or edema. Destruction of vessels prone to hemorrhage or causing traction directly prevents further deterioration. Destroying areas of retina that are poorly perfused and hypoxic may curtail the ischemic stimulus for neovascularization, preventing further proliferative changes. Regardless of the mechanism, the cooperative trial of the Diabetic Retinopathy Study Research Group clearly showed that photocoagulation decreases the incidence of retinal detachment, hemorrhage, and loss of vision. Thus, photocoagulation involves selective treatment of new vessels as well as panretinal treatment to destroy 20 to 30 per cent of the remaining retinal tissue. Whether photocoagulation therapy for preproliferative retinopathy should be undertaken is not yet clear; control studies are currently under way to resolve this question. All patients with significant diabetic retinopathy should be followed by an ophthalmologist and photocoagulation considered when new vessel formation or preretinal hemorrhage occurs. Photocoagulation early in the course of diabetic retinopathy may ultimately prove advisable. In the past, hypophysectomy was used as treatment for proliferative retinopathy. However, the therapeutic responses to this maneuver are quite variable, and significant complications exist. With the advent of photocoagulation, use of hypophysectomy has been largely abandoned. In patients with severe vitreal involvement, total vitrectomy may offer some possibility of improvement and preservation of vision.

Other Complications of Diabetes Affecting Vision

In addition to retinopathy, the eyes are affected in other ways by diabetes mellitus. Diabetics may experience temporary blurring of vision and *changes in refraction,* most likely due to osmotic changes in lens shape as a result of fluctuations in hyperglycemia. These changes can be disconcerting, but patients should be advised not to seek new refractions until a stable period of metabolic control is produced. It may take six to eight weeks before the hyperglycemia-induced changes in visual acuity subside. *Glaucoma* is also more frequent in diabetics. Rubeosis iridis is due to capillary neovascularization of the iris, which can produce closed-angle glaucoma. Usually occurring when diabetic retinopathy is advanced, this form of glaucoma is generally refractory to treatment. Open-angle glaucoma is also more frequent in diabetics, and this may relate to fibrosis or scarring of the canals of Schlemm, which drain the anterior chamber. Although *cataracts* are common in diabetes, it has not been rigorously demonstrated that the incidence of cataracts is increased in this condition. For the most part, cataracts in diabetics are indistinguishable from senile cataracts in nondiabetic patients, and the indications for surgery are the same as in nondiabetics. It is possible that the presence of diabetes accelerates the development of senile cataracts so that they occur at an earlier age than in nondiabetics. It has been postulated that hyperglycemia leads to increased sorbitol production in the lens, resulting in osmotic changes that accelerate cataract formation. While evidence in favor of this theory exists, it still remains to be proved. Opacities in the lens termed snowflake cataracts are occasionally noted in young patients whose diabetes is in poor control. This form of cataract is more specific for diabetes but can occur in other conditions and, unlike the senile cataract, can regress when glycemic control is achieved.

Nephropathy

Kidney disease is common in diabetes (See also Ch. 84 for an extensive discussion of the kidney in diabetes), and renal failure is one of the major causes of death.

PATHOLOGY. The dominant form of diabetic nephropathy is microvascular disease affecting the renal glomerulus. A number of distinct morphologic and functional abnormalities characterize diabetic glomerulopathy. Early in diabetes the kidney increases in size, and the associated glomerular hypertrophy leads to an increased glomerular filtration rate with hyperfiltration and microalbuminuria in up to 50 per cent of patients with new-onset IDDM. The hyperfiltration and increased kidney size revert to normal following effective insulin therapy and are unassociated with other glomerular lesions. Later in the disease, diffuse thickening of the glomerular basement membrane is noted along with increased mesangial volume. Patients with substantial histologic changes can exhibit normal renal function; however, impaired renal function probably does not occur in the absence of morphologic changes. Later in the disease, when decreased renal function is evident, the mesangium further expands and occupies a greater proportion of the glomerular volume while the thickness of the glomerular basement membrane is not necessarily increased. Glomerular occlusion accompanies this picture. Often characteristic nodular hyaline-like deposits, termed nodular glomerulocapillary sclerosis or Kimmelstiel-Wilson lesions, are evident in the center of peripheral glomerular capillary lobules.

CLINICAL AND FUNCTIONAL ASPECTS. The manifestations of diabetic nephropathy are quite heterogeneous. Asymptomatic, mild proteinuria can remain constant for many years. In other patients proteinuria may increase and be followed by progressive reduction in glomerular filtration and renal function. Persistent proteinuria (3 to 5 grams per day or greater) is a poor prognostic sign, usually heralding renal failure within five years. However, exceptions exist. The proteinuria may progress to include all of the classical features of the nephrotic syndrome. Once azotemia develops, progression to renal failure and uremia is inevitable within a few months to two to three years.

The diagnosis of diabetic nephropathy is usually made on clinical grounds, and renal biopsy is rarely indicated. Invasive diagnostic procedures should be aimed at detection of reversible features such as infection or obstruction. Contrast studies should not be conducted without clear indications, since rapid deterioration of renal function with acute renal failure sometimes follows intravenous pyelography or angiography in azotemic diabetic patients. When the study is performed, patients should be well hydrated before testing.

If renal failure develops in a diabetic, dialysis or transplantation must be considered. As recently as 10 to 15 years ago, uremic diabetics were thought to be extremely poor risks for dialysis with very low survival rates and high rates of complications, particularly infections and deterioration of vision. However, in recent years, results have been much better with a first-year survival of over 80 per cent and three-year survival of over 60 per cent. Additionally, far fewer cases of progressive visual impairment and blindness occur. Thus, in the absence of other negative factors, the presence of diabetes should not be considered a contraindication to dialysis, and decisions to initiate this form of therapy should generally proceed as in nondiabetic uremic patients. Chronic ambulatory peritoneal dialysis (CAPD) has been tried in some patients, but overall experience is still limited. Indications for CAPD vary widely among treatment centers, as does enthusiasm for this mode of therapy. Recent experience with renal transplantation has also been encouraging. Regardless of donor source (cadaver or related donor), survival rates after renal transplantion in diabetics approach that in nondiabetics. Interestingly, diabetic-type glomerular changes have been noted in biopsy specimens from the transplanted kidney from many of these patients.

Neuropathy

Diabetic neuropathy is perhaps the most common disabling chronic complication of diabetes. Although death seldom results from neuropathic changes alone, a great deal of morbidity and reduced quality of life can be attributed to diabetic neuropathy. The incidence and severity of neuropathy generally progress with duration of diabetes, and severe neuropathy can often exist in the absence of other chronic diabetic complications. A number of different classification schemes have been proposed, but none is entirely satisfactory, primarily because the causes of diabetic neuropathy are not known, and therefore classification must be descriptive in nature rather than based on pathogenetic mechanisms. Table 230–6 provides a simplified method of classification that may prove useful. Polyneuropathy is a diffuse symmetric disorder of peripheral nerve function. Asymmetric neuropathy implies a cluster of signs and symptoms that can be anatomically related to dysfunction of a single nerve trunk (mononeuropathy) or to more than one nerve trunk (mononeuropathy multiplex) either simultaneously or successively. It has been proposed that the symmetric or diffuse neuropathies are due to "metabolic" abnormalities of the neurons or the Schwann cells, whereas the asymmetric or focal neuropathies are due to vascular occlusion and ischemia. Diabetic neuropathy is very common in both IDDM and NIDDM, and mild to severe disease can exist in up to 50 per cent of patients. The incidence of symmetric neuropathy is comparable in IDDM and NIDDM when corrected for duration of disease, but focal neuropathies are more common in older NIDDM patients, suggesting a vascular contribution to the etiology.

SYMMETRIC DISTAL POLYNEUROPATHY. This form of diabetic neuropathy can be divided into two types: (1) relatively asymptomatic and (2) painful. The first form is diffuse, distal, usually in the lower extremities with a stocking type of distribution. It is characterized by numbness, tingling, or pins-and-needles sensation, often worse at night. Although the course may wax and wane, it is generally progressive and irreversible. Decreased sensory perception occurs and may result in neuropathic ulcers and Charcot joints. Symptoms of the painful form can range from burning or dull aching sensations to cramping or excruciating, lancinating pain. The pain is often worse at night and partially relieved by movement. Hyperesthesia can be so marked that even light touch is so painful that the patient cannot tolerate bed covers. Physical examination is similar in both types and is often rather unremarkable. The single most common finding is absence of deep tendon reflexes in the lower extremities (i.e., loss of knee and ankle jerks). Decreased perception of pain and light touch may be evident, and sometimes loss of vibratory sensation exists. The onset of pain may be abrupt or gradual and usually resolves by three months to one to two years. In some cases, institution of glycemic control coincides with resolution of pain; this may be causal. Paradoxically, insulin therapy with glycemic control can sometimes exacerbate or bring on painful neuropathic symptoms. In these cases, symptoms will subside in a few weeks if control is maintained. In some patients the decrease in pain reflects progression of the neuropathy with loss of pain sensation. A number of therapies have been tried, but these are usually unsatisfactory. Narcotic addiction may result when painful neuropathy is severe and long lasting. Combinations of B vitamins have been used, but success is unusual. Phenytoin or carbamazepine has also been used, and at least temporary or partial relief of pain and paresthesias has been reported in 25 to 50 per cent of patients. These agents should be tried at full anticonvulsant doses and discontinued if a response is not seen within two weeks. Combination therapy with amitriptyline and fluphenazine has also been advocated; there have been some reports of good results by one week. Treatment with any of these pharmacologic agents is only symptomatic and does not affect the course of the disease. Insofar as hyperglycemia causes neuropathy, maintenance of good control should be the primary emphasis. The possible role of sorbitol accumulation or myoinositol depletion in the pathogenesis of diabetic neuropathy was discussed earlier. Inhibitors of aldose reductase and oral myoinositol supplementation have been recently tried with some reports of success. Further studies will be necessary to determine the importance of these methods in the future treatment of diabetic neuropathy.

TABLE 230–6. CLASSIFICATION OF DIABETIC NEUROPATHY

1. Symmetric distal polyneuropathy
2. Asymmetric neuropathy
   A. Cranial mononeuropathy and mononeuropathy multiplex
   B. Peripheral mononeuropathy and mononeuropathy multiplex
   C. Neuromuscular syndromes
3. Autonomic neuropathy

NEUROPATHIC LESIONS AND THE DIABETIC FOOT. Loss of sensation can lead to the development of a Charcot joint as a result of repeated undetected trauma. More commonly, neuropathic ulcers develop, particularly on the plantar aspect of the foot. This can be due to weakness of the intrinsic muscles of the foot secondary to neuropathy, leading to abnormal pressure distribution. Weight bearing is then accentuated on the metatarsal heads, causing degeneration of the underlying fat pads and eventually leading to the typical open, draining neuropathic ulcer. Ulcers can also result from penetrating wounds caused by stepping on tacks or other sharp objects the patient does not feel. The best therapy is preventive. All diabetics should be trained to examine their feet daily for callous formation, blisters, or trauma. Shoes should be properly fitted; orthotic or other devices to aid in proper weight distribution are sometimes helpful. Patients should be advised never to walk barefoot. In all cases the feet should be kept clean and dry, and professional trimming of toenails and callosities is often advisable. Neuropathic foot ulcers can lead to gangrene and the requirement for amputation. Meticulous foot care substantially decreases the incidence of these ulcers and is a major form of preventive therapy that all diabetics should receive. Once open ulcers develop, healing can still occur if peripheral circulation is adequate. A high index of suspicion should be maintained for underlying osteomyelitis. Treatment is supportive with bed rest, elevation of the foot, warm (but not hot) foot soaks, debridement, and in some cases antibiotics. Protective plaster casts are sometimes advised. If these therapies fail and gangrene develops, amputation is the only recourse.

ASYMMETRIC NEUROPATHY. Diabetic mononeuropathies of the cranial nerves usually involve cranial nerve III, VI, or IV in order of frequency. This gives rise to extraocular muscle paralysis with diplopia. The most common syndrome is isolated third nerve palsy accompanied in 80 per cent of cases by sparing of the pupillary reflex. Pupillary sparing suggests that the underlying lesion is occlusion of a nutrient artery with ischemia of deep but not superficial oculomotor nerve fibers. Onset is usually abrupt and is frequently preceded by pain behind or above the eye. More than one cranial nerve is sometimes involved, and occasionally findings are bilateral. Spontaneous recovery is the rule within 3 to 12 months, but recurrences can occur. Mononeuropathies of peripheral nerves most frequently occur at sites of external pressure or entrapment (i.e., carpal tunnel). Manifestations include footdrop, wristdrop, or other symptoms related to the particular nerve involved. The clinical course is similar to that of the cranial mononeuropathies. Along with other forms of diabetic neuropathy these syndromes are usually associated with modestly increased protein content of the spinal fluid.

Another diabetic neuropathic syndrome involves *radiculopathy*. This syndrome is characterized by dysesthesias and painful hyperesthesia localized to the anatomic distribution of one or more spinal nerves. Symptoms can resemble herpes zoster, although skin lesions are seldom noted. On occasion, symptoms can be bilateral. Drug therapy similar to that used for painful symmetric polyneuropathy has been tried, but symptoms usually resolve spontaneously in weeks to months. Again, repeated episodes have been noted.

Neuromuscular syndromes related to diabetic retinopathy have been described. In the upper extremity, bilateral atrophy of the interosseous muscles as well as the thenar and hypothenar eminences of the hand can lead to profound loss of motor power with significant functional impairment. In the lower extremities, wasting and weakness of proximal leg muscles and pelvic girdle musculature have been termed diabetic amyotrophy. The clinical picture may be asymmetric, and elderly men are more commonly affected. Diabetic neuropathic cachexia is a syndrome of elderly male diabetics characterized by marked weight loss, painful peripheral polyneuropathy, and depression. The weight loss is so marked that patients appear cachectic, leading to a diagnosis of suspected underlying malignant disease. Other complications of diabetes are typically absent, and patients spontaneously recover in about one year.

AUTONOMIC NEUROPATHY. Autonomic diabetic neuropathies can be protean in their manifestations, leading to distressing clinical symptoms corresponding to the organ systems involved. Urinary bladder dysfunction is common, leading to urinary retention of large residual volumes. A definitive diagnosis can be made with a voiding cystometrogram, and therapy with cholinergic agents can sometimes be helpful. As the disease progresses, urinary tract infections become more frequent (possibly because of repeated catheterization), endangering the kidneys. In advanced cases, bladder neck resection to improve voiding may be necessary. Impotence with retrograde ejaculation is extremely common in men with longstanding diabetes. However, impotence in the diabetic male does not eliminate the need for exploration of possible psychogenic causes, which may be reversible. A variety of gastrointestinal tract syndromes can also occur. Gastroparesis diabeticorum involves delayed gastric emptying, retention, and hypotonicity. Symptoms include nausea, abdominal distention, belching, and general postprandial discomfort. Since this syndrome disrupts eating habits, control of the diabetes can be made more difficult. Treatment with metoclopramide has been useful in some but by no means all cases. Dysfunction of the small and large bowel can lead to malabsorption or diabetic diarrhea or both. Diabetic diarrhea often occurs at night, and fecal incontinence is a frequent feature. Autonomic involvement of sympathetic nervous system may lead to orthostatic hypotension and sometimes can be disabling. Attempts to expand intravascular volume with a high salt diet and sometimes mineralocorticoids are frequently effective but must be cautiously employed, since underlying cardiovascular disease is common in diabetic patients.

Cardiovascular Disease

Cardiovascular disease is the major cause of death in diabetic patients and is far more prevalent than in the nondiabetic population because of accelerated atherogenesis. Not only is cardiovascular disease more frequent, but onset is at an earlier age, and manifestations are more severe. The etiology of the accelerated atherosclerosis in diabetes is incompletely understood, but the causes are probably multifactorial. Most forms of hyperlipoproteinemia are more common in diabetic subjects, and high-density lipoprotein levels tend to be decreased in patients with uncontrolled diabetes. Furthermore, in patients with chronic hyperglycemia, circulating lipoproteins become glycosylated, adversely altering their turnover and sites of tissue deposition. This phenomenon might contribute to the increased risk of atherosclerosis in the absence of grossly elevated circulating lipid levels. Abnormalities of endothelial cell function have also been proposed that would enhance the susceptibility of arterial walls to injury. Increased platelet aggregation and hyperviscosity have also been proposed. Medical management of these risk factors is similar to that in nondiabetic subjects. Thus, specific diet and drug therapy for the various hyperlipoproteinemias should be used when indicated (Ch. 183). On occasion, lipid-lowering drugs such as nicotinic acid may accentuate glucose intolerance. Because of the high risk for atherogenesis, diabetics should be strongly encouraged to abstain from cigarette smoking. Arterial hypertension is a frequent concomitant of diabetes and should be treated promptly. Interestingly, epidemiologic studies have suggested that the existence of hypertension causes little in the way of additive risk for atherosclerosis in diabetics. The diabetic has a substantially greater risk for the development of all forms of cardiovascular disease even when hypertension and hyperlipoproteinemia are taken into account.

The pattern of coronary artery disease (CAD) has been reported to be different in diabetics and nondiabetics, exhibiting in diabetics a greater tendency toward diffuse distal lesions in addition to the usual proximal lesions. However, systematic studies have not uniformly confirmed this notion, suggesting that if this is a feature of CAD in diabetes, then only a minority of patients show diffuse distal occlusive disease. This is important, since one would expect coronary artery bypass surgery to be less successful in patients with distal disease and poor runoff. Overall the indications for myocardial revascularization are probably no different in diabetics and nondiabetics, although a greater incidence of postoperative complications is seen in diabetics. The presence of diabetes substantially eliminates the sex differences in CAD, since the incidence of CAD is roughly comparable in premenopausal diabetic women and age-matched diabetic men. Complications of myocardial infarction are more frequent in diabetics, and postinfarction survival is less. Although angina pectoris is common in diabetic patients, atypical anginal syndromes are seen more frequently than in nondiabetics. Various atypical pain patterns have been described. Painless myocardial infarction has been described in diabetes, probably due to disturbance of afferent nerve fibers. This diagnosis should be suspected in diabetic patients with the sudden onset of left ventricular failure. A syndrome of diabetic cardiomyopathy has been described and is characterized by congestive heart failure in the absence of proximal CAD. It is thought that this syndrome is due to small-vessel occlusive disease. Whether a distinct cardiomyopathy exists in diabetes in the absence of any CAD is still being debated.

Peripheral vascular disease is far more frequent in the diabetic than in the nondiabetic population, and this is particularly so for distal vascular insufficiency of the lower limbs. When combined with the neuropathic complications of diabetes, this unfortunately presents an ideal setting for the development of ischemia and gangrene, necessitating amputation. Because of the marked distal small-vessel disease, vascular bypass surgery is often unsatisfactory. Most forms of cerebrovascular disease and stroke are also seen more frequently in diabetes.

Dermatologic Lesions

Dermatologic abnormalities are common in diabetes. For example, these patients are more prone to various skin infections such as carbuncles and furuncles. These can often be extensive and difficult to treat. Vaginal candidiasis is frequent in hyperglycemic glycosuric women. Antifungal agents are effective in treating this disorder, but recurrences are common until glycosuria is effectively controlled. Necrobiosis lipoidica diabeticorum consists of round or oval, sharply defined, plaque-like lesions on the anterior surface of the lower legs. The borders of these lesions are frequently elevated, and the center may be depressed. The centers tend to be yellowish, while the borders are hyperpigmented. Although this lesion is uncommon in diabetics, when it does occur, the plaques can ulcerate upon minimal trauma. Diabetic dermopathy (shin spots) is the most frequent dermatologic lesion seen in diabetic patients, occurring in 60 per cent of males and 30 per cent of females. These lesions are common over the tibial area, but also can be observed on forearms and thighs. They begin as small reddish papules that gradually heal, leaving thin hyperpigmented atrophic areas behind. Typical xanthomatoses can occur secondary to hyperlipoproteinemia. In insulin-dependent diabetic subjects, tight waxy skin over the dorsum of the hands in conjunction with joint contractions has been observed. This may be an important clinical observation, since these patients appear to have accelerated development of other microangiopathic complications.

CONCLUSIONS

Diabetes mellitus is a chronic disease and therefore the approach to the patient and methods of management must encompass a long-term view. Patients with diabetes will be interacting with health care providers for the remainder of their lives. The patient must become well educated concerning the disease and eventually learn to individualize all the various components of therapy to his or her own personal circumstances. Ultimately many of the day-to-day therapy and management decisions rest in the hands of the patient. Since much of the treatment of diabetes involves intensive self-care, in a very real sense the patient may be his or her own most important physician. This requires education, motivation, and pycholog-ical adjustment.

Brand PW: The diabetic foot. *In* Ellenberg M, Rifkin H (eds.): Diabetes Mellitus. Theory and Practice. 3rd ed. New Hyde Park, NY, Medical Examination Publishing Co., 1983, pp 829–849. *An in-depth review of the clinical manifestations and management of diabetic foot problems.*

Bunn HF: Evaluation of glycosylated hemoglobin in diabetic patients. Diabetes 30:613, 1981. *A review of the biochemistry, clinical significance, and use of glycosylated hemoglobin in diabetes.*

Cahill GF, Jr: Starvation in man. N Engl J Med 282:668, 1970. *A classic article in which the available information on substrate and hormonal interrelationships in the fed and fasted state is synthesized into an organized homeostatic picture.*

Cudworth AG, Wolf E: The genetic susceptibility to type I (insulin-dependent) diabetes mellitus. Clin Endocrinol Metab 11:389, 1982. *A discussion of the HLA associations in type I diabetes mellitus.*

Diabetic Retinopathy Study Research Group: Preliminary report on the effects of photocoagulation. Am J Ophthalmol 81:383, 1976. *A report of the multicenter study demonstrating the utility of photocoagulation in diabetic retinopathy.*

Feig PU, McCurdy DK: The hypertonic state. N Engl J Med 297:1444, 1977. *A discussion of the pathophysiology and clinical treatment of the hyperosmolar syndrome.*

Feingold KR: Hypoglycemia: A pitfall of insulin therapy. West J Med 139:688, 1983. *An excellent clinical discussion of this important complication of the therapy of diabetes, with 56 references.*

Foster DW, McGarry JD: The metabolic derangements and treatment of diabetic ketoacidosis. N Engl J Med 309:159, 1983. *A thorough and current review of the pathogenesis and treatment of this disorder.*

Galloway JA: Insulin treatment for the early 80s: Facts and questions about old and new insulins and their usage. Diabetes Care 3:615, 1980. *A review of the biochemical and clinical features of the various insulin preparations available.*

Given BD, Mako ME, Tager H, Baldwin D, Markese J, Rubenstein AH, Olefsky J, Kobayashi M, Kolterman O, Poucher R: Circulating insulin with reduced biological activity in a patient with diabetes. N Engl J Med 302:129, 1980. *The first description of a patient producing a biologically defective insulin molecule.*

Goetz FC: Recent progress in the management of end-stage diabetic nephropathy. Clin Endocrinol Metab 11:579, 1982. *An up-to-date discussion on the relative success rates of dialysis and transplantation in end-stage diabetic nephropathy.*

Grogen CH, Lernmark A: Islet cell antibodies in diabetes. Clin Endocrinol Metab 11:409, 1982. *A literature review of islet cell antibodies in diabetes mellitus.*

Kreisberg RA: Diabetic ketoacidosis: New concepts and trends in pathogenesis and treatment. Ann Intern Med 88:681, 1978. *A discussion of pathogenetic mechanisms and a review of treatment methods in diabetic ketoacidosis.*

Lernmark A, Baekkeskov S: Islet cell antibodies—Theoretical and practical implications. Diabetologia 21:431, 1981. *A discussion of the potential role of autoantibodies directed against beta cells in the pathogenesis of diabetes.*

L'Esperance FA Jr, James SA Jr: The eye and diabetes mellitus. *In* Ellenberg M, Rifkin H (eds.): Diabetes Mellitus. Theory and Practice. 3rd ed. New Hyde Park, NY, Medical Examination Publishing Co., 1983, pp 727–757. *A general review of the ocular complications of diabetes mellitus with particular emphasis on retinopathy.*

McGarry JD, Foster DW: Regulation of hepatic fatty acid oxidation and ketone body production. Ann Rev Biochem 49:395, 1980. *Detailed review of the intermediary metabolism of ketogenesis and the pathogenesis of diabetic ketoacidosis.*

National Diabetes Data Group: Classification and diagnosis of diabetes mellitus and other categories of glucose intolerance. Diabetes 63:843, 1977. *A description of the unified classification system and methods and criteria for diagnosis of diabetes mellitus.*

Olefsky JM, Kolterman OG: Mechanisms of insulin resistance in obesity and non-insulin dependent (type II) diabetes. Am J Med 70:151, 1981. *A review of the pathogenesis and contribution of insulin resistance in NIDDM.*

Peacock I, Tattersall R: Methods of self monitoring of diabetic control. Clin Endocrinol Metab 11:485, 1982. *A review of the rationale and technique of self-monitoring of glucose in diabetes mellitus.*

Rimoin DL, Rotter JI: Genetic syndromes associated with diabetes mellitus and glucose intolerance. *In* Kobberling J, Tattersall R (eds.): Genetics of Diabetes Mellitus. New York, Academic Press, 1982, pp 149–181. *A detailed discussion of all of the genetic diseases that can be associated with diabetes mellitus.*

Rotter JI, Anderson CE, Rimoin DL: Genetics of diabetes mellitus. *In* Ellenberg M, Rifkin H (eds.): Diabetes Mellitus. Theory and Practice. 3rd ed. New Hyde Park, NY, Medical Examination Publishing Co., 1983, pp 481–503. *A review of the inheritance patterns and the genetic contributions to the etiology of type I and type II diabetes mellitus.*

Rotwein P, Chyn R, Chirgwin J, Cordell B, Goodman HM, Permutt MA: Polymorphism in the 5′-flanking region of the human insulin gene and its possible relation to type 2 diabetes. Science 213:1117, 1981. *Report of an increased frequency of a unique polymorphism of the insulin gene in NIDDM.*

Schade DS, Santiago JV, Skyler JS, Rizza RA: Intensive insulin therapy. Princeton, Excerpta Medica, 1983. *A recent monograph outlining the physiologic principles and methods of administering intensive therapy by multiple injections as well as CSII.*

Skyler JS: Complications of diabetes mellitus: Relationship to metabolic dysfunction. Diabetes Care 2:499, 1979. *A discussion of the value of glycemic control in the late complications of diabetes mellitus.*

Tattersall RB: Home blood glucose monitoring. Diabetologia 16:71, 1979. *An article dealing with measuring blood glucose instead of relying on urine values.*

Unger RH, Orci L: Glucagon and the A cell. Physiology and pathophysiology. N Engl J Med 304:1518, 1575, 1981. *A review of the physiology of glucagon secretion and action as well as its role in the pathophysiology of diabetes.*

Viberti GC, Pickup JC, Jarrett RJ, Keen H: Effect of control of blood glucose on urinary excretion of albumin and B_2 microglobulin in insulin-dependent diabetes. N Engl J Med 300:638, 1979. *A report showing the reversibility of microalbuminuria by insulin treatment in type I diabetes.*

Yoon J-W, Austin M, Onodera T, Notkins AL: Virus-induced diabetes mellitus. N Engl J Med 300:1173, 1979. *A report of a well-documented case of viral-induced diabetes.*

231. HYPOGLYCEMIC DISORDERS

F. John Service

Hypoglycemia is a pathophysiologic state and not a disease. Just as pain, fever, or vomiting requires identification of the underlying condition, hypoglycemia warrants diagnosis of the primary disorder causing the low plasma glucose level.

Hypoglycemia can be defined as a glucose concentration below the lower limit of normal. However, since hypoglycemic disorders are clinical syndromes almost invariably associated with symptoms from the low concentration of glucose, hypoglycemia is usually considered to be a glucose concentration in the range below the level at which symptoms could be expected to occur.

PHYSIOLOGY

Plasma glucose concentration is maintained within narrow bounds, in spite of intermittent food ingestion and periods of fasting, as the net balance between the rates of glucose production and utilization. Following food ingestion the increase in plasma glucose, in concert with an incretin effect from enteric factors, results in a increase in plasma insulin that accelerates glucose utilization and suppresses hepatic glucose production. As the plasma glucose concentration falls postprandially, plasma insulin decreases, which restores glucose utilization and production to the preprandial rates. There is then a transition from a state of glucose storage to one of carefully husbanded glucose production at rates designed to satisfy the obligatory needs of the body. In the postabsorptive period four to six hours after food ingestion, plasma glucose concentrations are generally 80 to 90 mg per deciliter with rates of glucose production and utilization of approximately 2 mg per kg^{-1} per min^{-1}. About half of the glucose produced is metabolized by the central nervous system. Glucose production at this time is primarily from hepatic glycogenolysis (70 to 80 per cent), with a small contribution from gluconeogenesis (20 to 25 per cent). Hepatic glycogen stores become exhausted after 24 to 36 hours of fasting.

Glycogenolysis is stimulated by epinephrine and glucagon and inhibited by insulin. Several enzymes are involved in the cleavage of glucose moieties from glycogen and the final appearance of free glucose in the circulation. Abnormalities of these enzymes may result in hypoglycemia. For example, deficient activity of glucose 6-phosphatase (von Gierke's disease) may cause severe hypoglycemia, whereas deficient activities of glycogen phosphorylase and debrancher enzyme cause milder degrees of hypoglycemia (Ch. 179). Deficiency of glycogen synthetase results in severe hypoglycemia in newborns.

Gluconeogenesis is the generation of new glucose from noncarbohydrate substrates. Defects in this process result in hypoglycemia after prolonged fasting when glycogen stores have been depleted. Lactate and pyruvate, glycerol, and amino acids account for approximately 58 per cent, 13 per cent, and 29 per cent of the glucose produced via gluconeogenesis. Defects in gluconeogenesis may arise from (1) diminished substrate availability, e.g., ketotic hypoglycemia in children; (2) altered redox state, which inhibits several important gluconeogenic enzymes, e.g., alcohol hypoglycemia; and (3) inhibition of fatty acid oxidation, which diminishes the energy source for gluconeogenesis, e.g., poisoning from the unripe ackee fruit.

Alanine and glutamine are the most important amino acids that act as glucose precursors. The carbon source of alanine is muscle-derived pyruvate, and the nitrogen source for the transamination of pyruvate to alanine is thought to be branched-chain amino acids. Impaired metabolism of leucine, a branched-chain amino acid, observed in maple syrup urine disease (see Ch. 193) is associated with reduced alanine production and sometimes with hypoglycemia.

After three days of fasting, glucose production is primarily derived from hepatic gluconeogenesis; after prolonged fasting, renal gluconeogenesis may account for approximately 50 per cent of glucose production. The effects of insulin, glucagon, catecholamines, cortisol, and growth hormone on glucose homeostasis and recovery from hypoglycemia are shown in Table 231–1. Insulin is the primary hypoglycemic hormone; the others act by a variety of mechanisms to elevate glucose concentrations. Although plasma glucagon, catecholamines, cortisol, and growth hormone increase in response to insulin-induced hypoglycemia, glucagon makes the major contribution to the acute recovery from hypoglycemia. Catecholamines can result in a modest elevation of glucose concentration in the presence of glucagon deficiency or severe hypoglycemia.

TABLE 231–1. HORMONAL CONTROL OF GLUCOSE HOMEOSTASIS

Hormone	Hepatic Glucose Production	Extrahepatic Glucose Utilization	Basal Glucose Production	Relative Importance to Recovery from Insulin-Induced Hypoglycemia
Insulin	↓	↑	↓	
Glucagon	↑	–	↑	+ + +
Catecholamines*	↑	↓	–	+
Cortisol	↑	↓	↑	–
Growth hormone†	↑	↓	–	–

NOTE: ↑ = increase; ↓ = decrease; – = no effect.

*Epinephrine is approximately ten times more potent than norepinephrine. Its action is primarily through a beta-adrenergic mechanism. In the presence of glucagon deficiency, catecholamines make a modest contribution to the recovery from hypoglycemia.

†Has an acute and transient hypoglycemic effect.

CLINICAL EVALUATION

Defects of many of the mechanisms that maintain plasma glucose in the normal range are associated with readily recognizable clinical syndromes. In some instances the symptoms and signs of the primary disorder predominate over those of hypoglycemia, or at least point to the existence of the primary disorder causing hypoglycemia. In some patients with multisystem disease, poor nutrition, or multiple-drug use, the basis for hypoglycemia may be uncertain and the patient too ill to undergo extensive evaluation. Common causes of hypoglycemia are listed in Table 231–2.

In the majority of patients with symptoms of hypoglycemia who appear healthy, screening laboratory tests should include plasma glucose, serum insulin, calcium, phosphate, uric acid, lipids, creatinine, liver function evaluation, insulin antibodies, and plasma and urine corticosteroids. Documentation of drug-induced hypoglycemia may be difficult. A detailed history must be obtained, and every medication, including nonprescription drugs, used by the patient must be examined.

When a patient is observed with symptoms of hypoglycemia, 10 to 20 ml of blood in addition to that for glucose determination should be withdrawn. The specific analyses can be determined by the clues generated from the history and physical examination. Such an opportunity may provide sufficient data to establish the cause of the hypoglycemic disorder or narrow the diagnostic possibilities. Glucose should be administered following blood withdrawal to any patient suspected of being hypoglycemic. Prompt treatment will shorten the duration of hypoglycemia, and if the patient is not hypoglycemic no harm will have been done.

In patients with asymptomatic hypoglycemia one must be alert to artifactual hypoglycemia. Whole blood glucose values may be spuriously low in polycythemia vera because of the unequal distribution of glucose between erythrocyte and plasma or excessive glycolysis by erythrocytes, or both, and in leukemia from excessive glycolysis by leukocytes. Prompt measurement of glucose in plasma in these conditions should provide accurate results.

An uncommon and challenging problem is the low plasma glucose concentration in an asymptomatic patient in whom laboratory error and spurious result have been ruled out. Such patients may have adapted to longstanding hypoglycemia or have mild symptoms that have been completely unrecognized.

A flow diagram of a clinical approach to the evaluation of a suspected hypoglycemic disorder is presented in Figure 231–1. Note that the evaluation is directed to patients who appear healthy. For those who do not appear healthy the results of the history and physical examination will determine the direction of the investigation.

Hypoglycemic disorders cause a constellation of symptoms that usually recur as discrete episodes at irregular intervals. A useful but not infallible historical aid is the timing of symptoms in relation to food intake: those occurring within six hours of food intake are the *food-stimulated hypoglycemias* and those occurring beyond six hours of food intake are the *food-deprived hypoglycemias*.

Considerable effort should be expended to obtain from the patient and family members a detailed description of symptoms and careful attention paid to their occurrence in relation to food intake. The food-stimulated hypoglycemias usually cause symptoms of catecholamine release—sweating, shakiness, anxiety, palpitations, and weakness—and rarely those of impairment of central nervous system function. The food-deprived

TABLE 231–2. COMMON CAUSES OF HYPOGLYCEMIA

Medications
Ethanol
Factitial
Insulinoma
Non–islet cell tumors
Multifactorial in sick patient
Islet dysplasia of infancy
Ketotic hypoglycemia

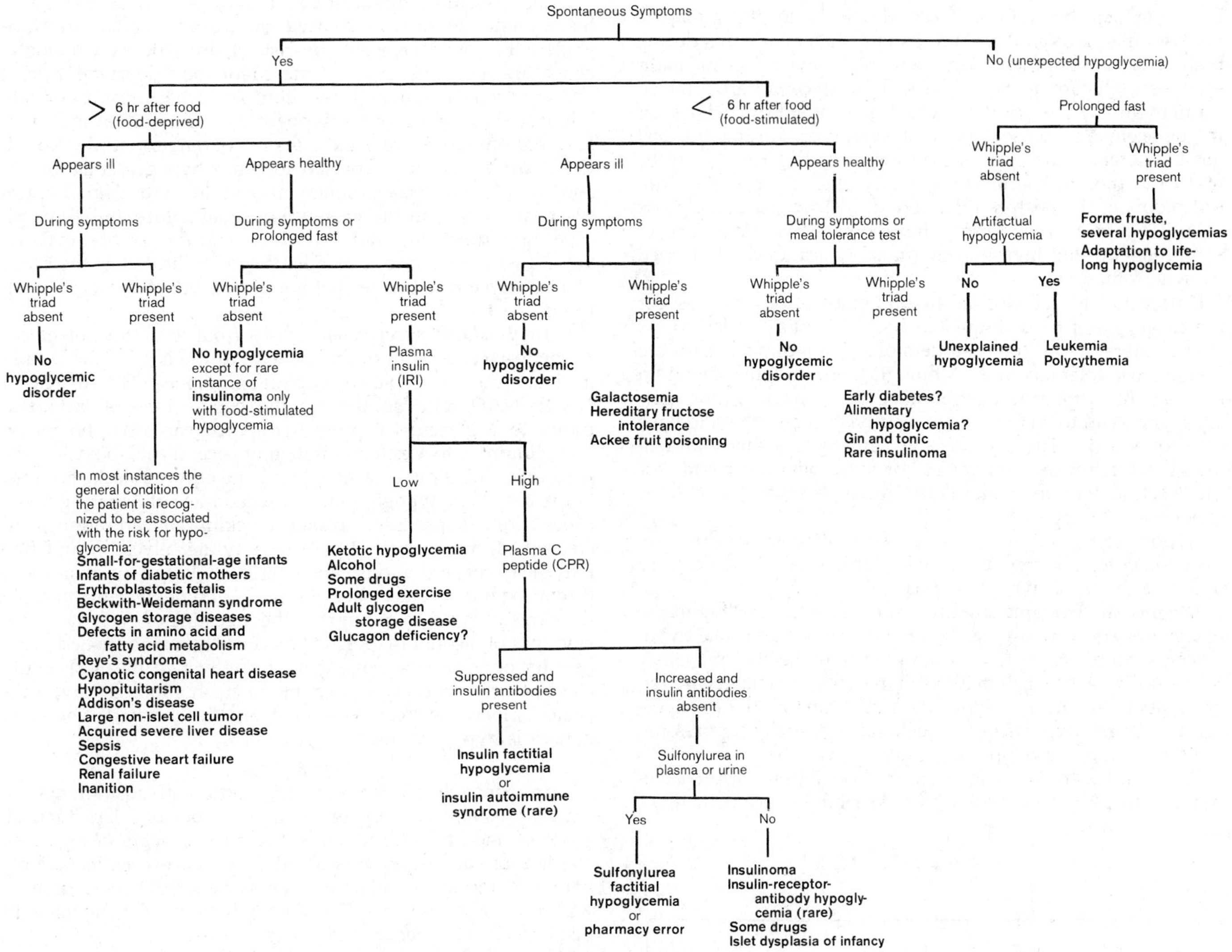

Figure 231–1. Evaluation of hypoglycemic disorders.

hypoglycemias, on the other hand, usually result in impairment of central nervous system function—reduced intellectual capacity, confusion, irritability, abnormal behavior, convulsions, and coma. Sometimes there is complicating hypothermia. Often the symptoms of catecholamine release that precede the central nervous system symptoms go unrecognized. Symptoms of hypoglycemia usually occur at plasma glucose concentrations of about 45 mg per deciliter or less (whole blood glucose of 40 mg per deciliter or less). Although some studies suggest that a rapid fall in glucose concentration results in symptoms even when plasma glucose does not decrease below 45 mg per deciliter, the weight of evidence does not support this relationship. The symptoms of hypoglycemia are nonspecific. For this reason it is necessary to demonstrate a low plasma glucose value concomitant with symptoms and subsequent relief of symptoms by correction of the hypoglycemia, i.e., *Whipple's triad.* This triad should be demonstrated before hypoglycemia can be considered to be the basis for a patient's symptoms. Although food, especially free carbohydrate, will relieve symptoms regardless of the cause of the hypoglycemia, persons without a hypoglycemic disorder may feel better after eating. It is therefore imperative to confirm that symptoms are due to hypoglycemia.

FOOD-STIMULATED HYPOGLYCEMIAS

Subsequent to the conceptualization of hyperinsulinism as a disease, after insulin became available for the treatment of diabetes, many patients with postprandial symptoms were found to have concomitant blood sugar concentrations within or even above the normal range. For such cases the term *functional hypoglycemia* was coined. Eventually reliance on a subnormal glucose concentration at the time of spontaneous symptoms came to be replaced by the oral glucose tolerance test. Reproduction of those symptoms experienced during ordinary daily activities and documentation of a plasma glucose nadir ≤50 mg per deciliter (or its equivalent) during the oral glucose tolerance test have been considered confirmation of the presence of a food-stimulated hypoglycemic disorder. Use of the oral glucose tolerance test is fraught with risk of misdiagnosis since (1) in at least 10 per cent of healthy persons the plasma glucose nadir is less than 50 mg per deciliter; (2) there is no correlation between the nadir of plasma glucose concentrations and the occurrence of symptoms of hypoglycemia in patients with symptoms suggestive of food-stimulated hypoglycemia; and (3) the results of oral glucose tolerance tests are variable upon repeated testing. Measurement of plasma cortisol responses, calculation of rates of glucose descent, and hypoglycemic indices have not improved the accuracy of the oral glucose tolerance test. Furthermore, many patients with symptoms typical of a food-stimulated hypoglycemic disorder experience symptoms after a "placebo" oral glucose tolerance test.

Recent studies have measured plasma glucose responses to mixed nutrient meals designed as more representative of the body's usual challenge to glucose homeostasis than large oral glucose loads. These results have been compared to those following standard glucose test meals (75 to 100 grams of glucose) (Fig. 231–2). Although patients had symptoms during both tests, none of the patients who had a hypoglycemic nadir after oral glucose intake evinced hypoglycemia after mixed nutrient intake. In addition, there was no EEG evidence of hypoglycemia in those who had symptoms during the test meal. Therefore the oral glucose tolerance test should not be used for the evaluation of hypoglycemia in patients with symptoms in the postprandial period. Instead, plasma glucose should be measured during the spontaneous occurrence of symptoms or after ingestion of a meal typical of that followed by symptoms.

Unfortunately, reliance on the oral glucose tolerance test for the diagnosis of food-stimulated hypoglycemia has led to extensive literature not on disorders of hypoglycemia but on the oral glucose tolerance test. Although there undoubtedly are a few patients with true postprandial hypoglycemia, most persons with symptoms following meals have been shown to have psychoneurosis. The use of low carbohydrate–high protein diets, sulfonylureas, biguanides, or anticholinergic agents for the treatment of food-stimulated hypoglycemias has limited experimental support.

Hypoglycemia following the ingestion of substances that are toxic to susceptible persons may be considered in the category of food-stimulated hypoglycemias.

The ingestion of large amounts (equivalent of three highballs) of ethanol and carbohydrate (gin and tonic) may cause hypoglycemia within three to four hours in some healthy persons.

The unripe ackee fruit may result in hypoglycemia in children or adults with chronic malnutrition by inhibiting the transport of long-chain fatty acids into mitochondria, thereby suppressing their oxidation and depressing gluconeogenesis.

Postprandial hypoglycemia occurs in children with galactosemia (Ch. 178) and hereditary fructose intolerance (Ch. 181).

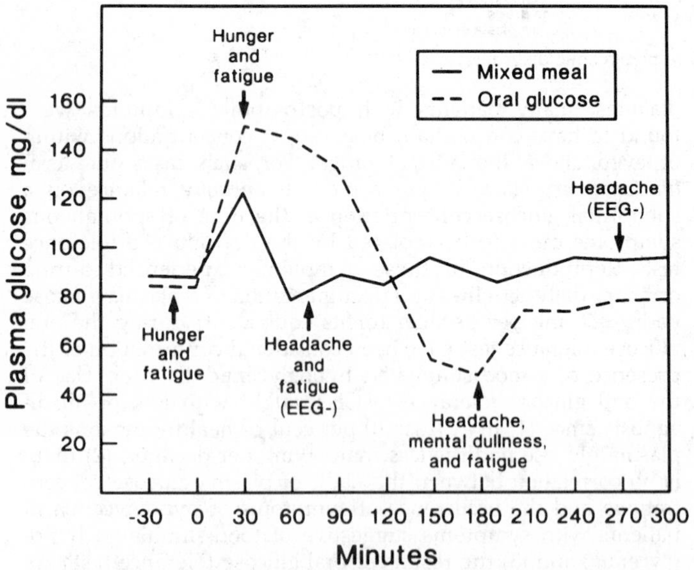

Figure 231–2. A patient with postprandial symptoms and plasma glucose responses to an oral glucose tolerance test consistent with a diagnosis of reactive hypoglycemia underwent a mixed meal study. Similar symptoms occurred in both studies; they bore no consistent relationship to the concomitant plasma glucose concentrations. Monitoring by EEG during occurrence of symptoms after the mixed meal showed no abnormalities. It was concluded that the symptoms could not be ascribed to a disorder of glucose homeostasis and that the OGTT should not be used for diagnosis of reactive hypoglycemia. (From Service FJ: *In* Hypoglycemic Disorders: Pathogenesis, Diagnosis, and Treatment. Boston, GK Hall, 1982. Reprinted with permission.)

FOOD-DEPRIVED (FASTING) HYPOGLYCEMIAS

Drug-Induced Hypoglycemias

Drugs constitute the most common cause of hypoglycemia if insulin and sulfonylureas used by diabetic persons are included. Factors increasing the risk of drug-induced hypoglycemia are extremes of age, antecedent food deprivation, and impaired renal and hepatic function. The drugs most commonly implicated as the cause for hypoglycemia in addition to insulin and sulfonylurea are salicylates, propranolol, and alcohol. Other drugs recently reported to cause hypoglycemia are disopyramide (Norpace), sulfamethoxazole, and trimethoprim (Bactrim, Septra) in the presence of renal failure and pentamidine (Lomidine)* and quinine when used for cerebral malaria. Since a wide variety of drugs has been implicated as the cause of hypoglycemia, the reader is referred to review articles on this subject.

Ethanol-induced hypoglycemia arises from inhibition of gluconeogenesis as a result of the increase in the NADH-NAD ratio in instances of depleted hepatic glycogen. The increased NADH-NAD ratio suppresses the conversions of lactate to pyruvate, α-glycerophosphate to dihydroxyacetone phosphate, and glutamate to α-ketoglutarate and several tricarboxylic cycle reactions. Infusion of ethanol into healthy subjects for four hours results in hypoglycemia, reduced rates of hepatic glucose production, suppressed plasma insulin concentrations, increased plasma lactate, β-hydroxybutyrate, glycerol, and free fatty acid concentrations, and increased lactate-pyruvate and β-hydroxybutyrate-acetoacetate ratios. Hypoglycemia usually develops within 6 to 36 hours of the ingesting of even moderate amounts of alcohol by persons chronically malnourished or by healthy persons who have missed one or two meals. Healthy children are especially susceptible to alcohol-induced hypoglycemia. Blood alcohol levels may not be elevated when the patient is hypoglycemic.

Insulinoma

Approximately 60 per cent of patients with insulinoma are female. Insulinomas are uncommon in persons less than 20 years of age and rare in those less than 5 years of age. The median age at diagnosis is about 50 years, except in patients with the multiple endocrine neoplasia (MEN) syndrome in which it is in the mid 20s. Ten per cent of patients with insulinoma are older than 70 years of age.

Of patients with insulinoma 80 per cent have single benign tumors, 11 per cent have multiple benign tumors, 6 per cent have single malignant tumors, and the remainder have multiple malignant tumors or islet hyperplasia. Ten per cent of insulinoma patients have MEN syndrome type 1 (Ch. 240), and 80 per cent of these patients have multiple insulinomas; however, only 60 per cent of patients with multiple insulinomas have the MEN syndrome.

Some tumors secrete hormones in addition to insulin: gastrin, 5-hydroxyindoles, ACTH, glucagon, and somatostatin. In rare instances, insulinomas have occurred in non–insulin-dependent diabetic persons but have never been documented in an insulin-dependent subject.

CLINICAL PICTURE. Symptoms may be present for many years prior to the diagnosis. In one series 85 per cent of patients had various combinations of diplopia, blurred vision, sweating, palpitations, or weakness; 80 per cent had confusion or abnormal behavior; 53 per cent had unconsciousness or amnesia; and 12 per cent had grand mal seizures. Twenty per cent of cases may be misdiagnosed, the belief being that the patient has a neurologic or psychiatric disorder.

Hypoglycemia usually occurs several hours after a meal, most commonly before the evening meal (Fig. 231–3). In rare instances, symptoms may occur solely in the postprandial period rather than during fasting. Symptoms may be aggravated by exercise, alcohol use, a high protein–low carbohydrate diet, treatment with sulfonylureas, and fasts. Less than 20 per cent of patients with insulinoma gain weight.

*Pentamidine (Lomidine) is an investigational drug available from the Centers for Disease Control, Atlanta, GA.

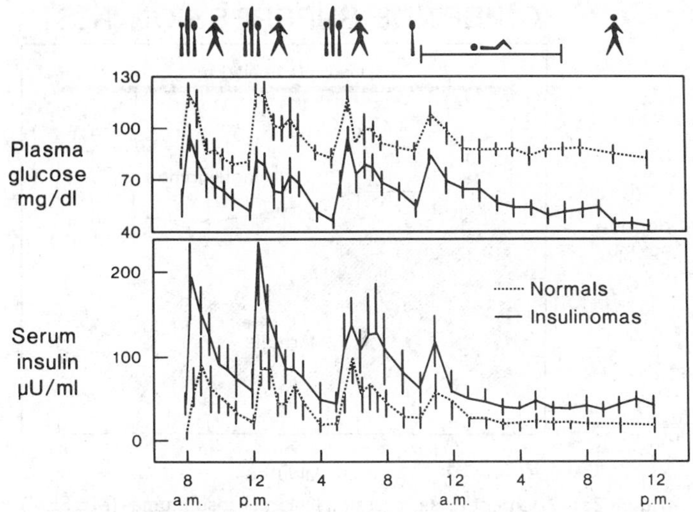

Figure 231–3. Serial measurements of plasma glucose and serum insulin in patients with insulinoma and healthy subjects under ordinary life conditions. Plasma glucose declined to hypoglycemic levels in the late postabsorptive and fasting states in those with insulinoma. Hyperinsulinemia was observed in response to meals and also in the postabsorptive and fasting states. (Fork, knife, spoon = meal; spoon = snack; standing figure = exercise; reclining figure = sleep.) (From Service FJ, Nelson RL: Insulinoma. Comp Ther 6:70, 1980. Reprinted with permission.)

DIAGNOSIS. The diagnosis of insulinoma is based on the demonstration of Whipple's triad and hyperinsulinemia or an inappropriately normal insulin level for a low glucose value. Insulin antibodies should be undetectable unless the patient has taken exogenous insulin. Useful screening tests are *daily fasting plasma glucose and insulin determinations* and the *intravenous tolbutamide test*. The latter (Fig. 231–4) has approximately a 90 per cent diagnostic accuracy. This test should be performed only in persons for whom the fasting plasma glucose is known to exceed 50 mg per deciliter on the day of the test and who have not been food deprived for several days preceding the test. Diagnostic criteria should be based on absolute values during the last hour of the test, i.e., plasma glucose <55 mg per deciliter, blood glucose <50 mg per deciliter, and serum insulin >20 μU per milliliter at the 120- to 180-minute period of the test. Diagnostic criteria will reflect local laboratory procedures and so should be generated at each institution. Diagnostic criteria based on percentage of recovery of basal plasma glucose at the end of the test are less accurate. If the plasma glucose responses to intravenous tolbutamide are normal, the insulin values give little additional information.

Prolonged supervised fasting is the single most reliable test for the diagnosis of insulinoma. During the fast the patient should be active during the day. Noncaloric beverages can be consumed. The frequency of blood sampling during the fast should be guided by the patient's history of tolerance to food withdrawal. The frequency of sampling should be increased as the plasma glucose approaches the hypoglycemic range. Whenever blood is withdrawn for glucose determination, a sample should also be drawn for determination of serum insulin and, if factitial hypoglycemia is suspected, of C peptide and sulfonylurea. During the fast the patient's intellectual status should be checked regularly by simple mathematic tasks such as serial sevens. During prolonged fasting healthy women experience lower plasma glucose concentrations than do healthy men: values as low as 42 mg per deciliter in men and 34 mg per deciliter in women may be unaccompanied by symptoms. Therefore it is essential to continue the fast to the point at which symptoms develop, or to 72 hours. Serum insulin concentrations may be in the "normal" range in about 50 per cent of determinations when the plasma glucose is in the hypoglycemic range (Fig. 231–5); 10 per cent of patients with insulinoma may have all insulin values in this normal range during hypoglycemia; however, this normal serum insulin concentration is probably excessive if it is above 6 μU per milliliter and certainly excessive if it is above 10 μU per milliliter during hypoglycemia. Various glucose-insulin ratios provide less diagnostic accuracy (Fig. 231–6).

In a large series, Whipple's triad was demonstrated within 12 hours of the last meal in 29 per cent of patients, within 24 hours in 71 per cent, within 36 hours in 79 per cent, within 48 hours in 92 per cent, within 60 hours in 97 per cent, and within 72 hours in 98 per cent. In rare instances, patients with insulinoma may not develop hypoglycemia during prolonged fasting of even up to 96 hours. At the time of hypoglycemic symptoms, plasma glucose concentrations were ≤46 mg per deciliter in 100 per cent of patients, ≤39 mg per deciliter in 75 per cent, ≤35 mg per deciliter in 50 per cent, and ≤28 mg per deciliter in 25 per cent.

The *intravenous glucagon test*, which is considered to be positive if the peak insulin response exceeds 130 μU per milliliter, has a diagnostic accuracy of 50 to 80 per cent. The *C peptide suppression test* is based on the observation that exogenous insulin-induced hypoglycemia suppresses C peptide concentration in normal persons but not in those with insulinomas (Fig. 231–7). The criteria for normal C peptide suppression will depend on the C peptide assay. The utility of other tests such as glycosylated hemoglobin, human pancreatic polypeptide, and infusions of alcohol, calcium, epinephrine and propranolol, diazoxide, and somatostatin-tolbutamide in the diagnosis of insulinoma is unproven or inadequate. Human chorionic gonadotropin or one of its subunits may be a marker for functioning

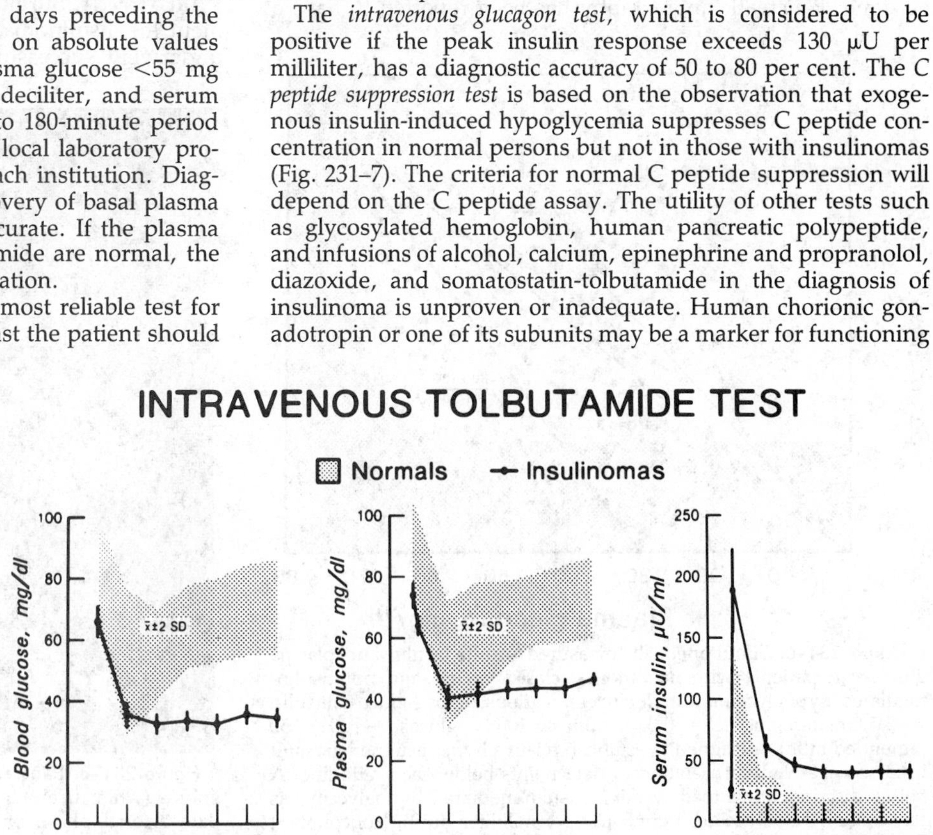

Figure 231–4. Intravenous tolbutamide test results in 34 patients with insulinoma (M ± SEM) and healthy subjects (shaded). Fourteen with insulinoma had glucose measured in whole blood; 20 had glucose measured in plasma. Criteria for diagnosis of insulinoma is a blood glucose level of 50 mg per deciliter or less, plasma glucose 55 mg per deciliter or less, and serum insulin greater than 20 μU per milliter at the 120 to 180 minute part of the test. (From Service FJ: *In* Hypoglycemic Disorders: Pathogenesis, Diagnosis, and Treatment. Boston, GK Hall, 1982. Reprinted with permission.)

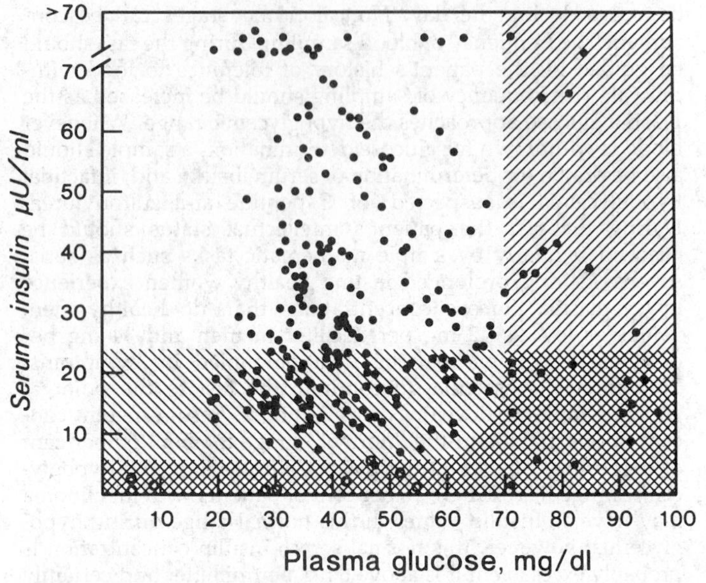

Figure 231–5. Simultaneously measured serum insulin and plasma glucose in 72 patients with insulinomas (closed circles) and six patients with noninsulin-mediated hypoglycemia (open circles). Ten per cent of those with insulinoma for whom multiple simultaneous insulin and glucose determinations were made all had insulin values in the normal range during concomitant hypoglycemia. (From Service FJ: *In* Hypoglycemic Disorders: Pathogenesis, Diagnosis, and Treatment. Boston, GK Hall, 1982. Reprinted with permission.)

malignant insulinomas. Eighty per cent of patients with insulinoma may have elevated proinsulin concentrations (>20 per cent of total immunoreactive insulin).

LOCALIZATION. Only after the diagnosis of insulinoma has been confirmed biochemically should a localization procedure be done. Pancreatic angiography has been reported to have a high rate of success if stereoscopy, magnification, and subtraction are used (Fig. 231–8). Insulinomas appear as homogeneous, intensely vascular, sharply circumscribed masses within the substance of the pancreas.

Computed tomography has had limited success in localization. Real-time high-resolution ultrasonography done both preoperatively and intraoperatively is currently demonstrating a high degree of accuracy. The indications for and value of selective venous sampling for insulin determinations done either by the percutaneous transhepatic route or directly at the time of surgery remain undetermined. Failure to localize an insulinoma by any of these techniques should not deter pancreatic exploration in a patient for whom the diagnosis has been firmly established. Surgeons experienced in insulinoma surgery are highly successful in finding the tumor even when it has not been localized preoperatively.

TREATMENT. Surgical removal is the preferred form of treatment for insulinoma. In a large series, 54 per cent of subjects underwent successful enucleation of the tumor; 38 per cent,

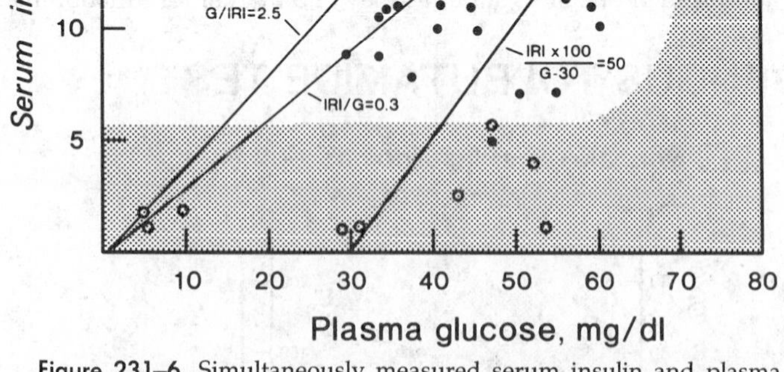

Figure 231–6. Simultaneously measured serum insulin and plasma glucose in patients with insulinoma (closed circles) and noninsulin-mediated hypoglycemia (open circles). Various ratios—glucose:insulin = 2.5, insulin:glucose = 0.3, insulin × 100 ÷ glucose − 30 = 50 (amended ratio)—designed to establish relative hyperinsulinemia result in false-negative interpretation of data points below each ratio line. A better discrimination to determine insulin-mediated hypoglycemia is any insulin value greater than 6 μU per milliliter during concomitant hypoglycemia. (From Service FJ: *In* Hypoglycemic Disorders: Pathogenesis, Diagnosis, and Treatment. Boston, GK Hall, 1982. Reprinted with permission.)

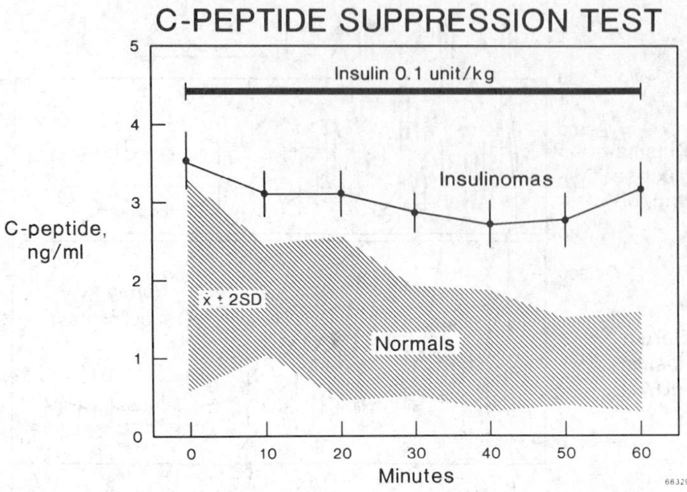

Figure 231–7. C-peptide suppression test in 17 insulinomas (M ± SEM) and controls (shaded). In response to insulin-induced hypoglycemia, insulinomas fail to suppress C-peptide. (From Service FJ, Nelson RL: Insulinoma. Comp Ther 6:70, 1980. Reprinted with permission.)

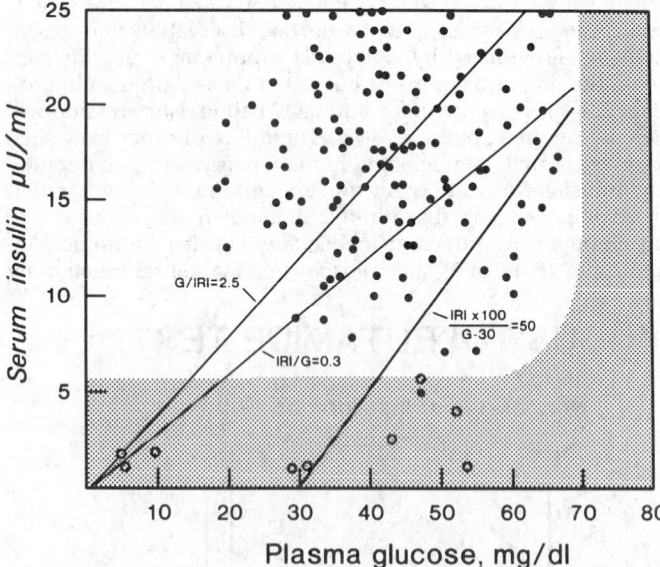

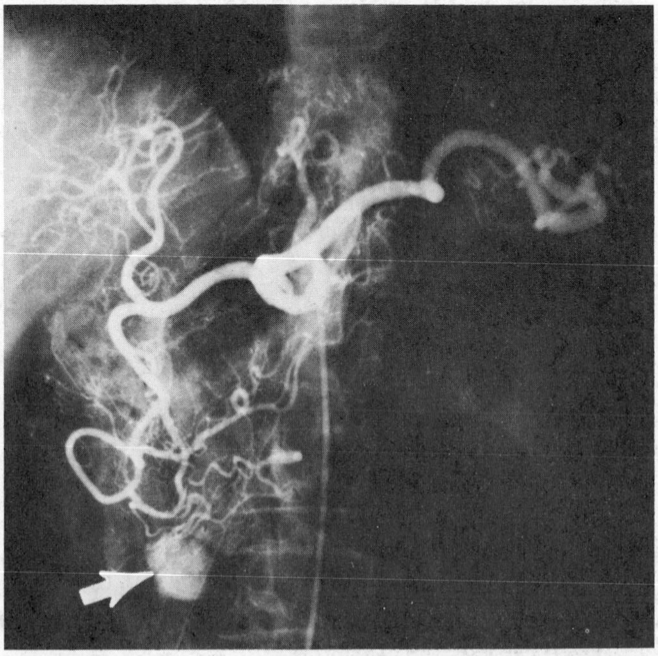

Figure 231–8. Pancreatic angiogram: intense vascular blush of insulinoma (white arrow) in the inferior portion of the head of the pancreas (late arterial phase of celiac artery injection). (From Stephens DH, Sheedy PF: Computed tomography. *In* Margulis AR, Burhenne HJ (eds.): Alimentary Tract Radiology. Vol 3. Abdominal imaging. St. Louis, CV Mosby, 1979. Reprinted with permission.)

partial pancreatectomy; and the remainder, a variety of other procedures. In the series, 84 per cent were cured, 7 per cent had diabetes, and the remainder required medical treatment to control persistent hypoglycemia from malignant insulinoma, islet hyperplasia, or a tumor missed during surgery. There was no operative mortality, and the postoperative complication rate was 10 per cent.

Intraoperative glucose monitoring should not be relied upon for surgical management, since there is a high (23 per cent) incidence of failure of plasma glucose to increase after successful insulinoma removal.

The median diameter of benign tumors has been reported to be 1.5 cm. Malignant tumors are usually large. Tumors are evenly distributed throughout the pancreas whether benign or malignant, single or multiple. Ectopically located insulinoma and islet hyperplasia are very rare. There is no correlation between the severity of symptoms and size of the insulinoma.

Treatment of persistent hypoglycemia in a patient with malignant insulinoma, in a patient in whom insulinoma cannot be found at pancreatic exploration, or in one who refuses surgery is best accomplished with diazoxide, which inhibits insulin release, although phenytoin and propranolol have been used successfully in some cases. Malignant insulinoma metastasizes primarily to local structures such as regional lymph nodes and liver; distant metastases are uncommon. The chemotherapeutic regimen of choice consists of streptozotocin and 5-fluorouracil. Survival exceeds that in adenocarcinoma of the pancreas.

Factitial and Autoimmune Hypoglycemia

Nondiabetic persons who secretly take insulin or sulfonylureas are predominantly women in the third and fourth decades of life who are employed in health-related occupations. Patients with factitial hypoglycemia have an erratic pattern in the occurrence of symptoms and may tolerate prolonged periods of fasting. With the exception of the rare instance of the insulin autoimmune syndrome, the presence of insulin antibodies is strong evidence of repeated injection of insulin. In addition, the presence of low plasma concentrations of C peptide concomitant with elevated insulin levels and hypoglycemia indicates an exogenous source of insulin. Insulin antibodies will result in spurious radioimmunoassayable plasma insulin concentrations: very high if the double-antibody assay is used and undetectable if the charcoal-coated–dextran assay is used. Results of tests for insulinoma (including the C peptide suppression test if the patient is taking a sulfonylurea) may be indistinguishable between an insulinoma patient and a patient who secretly took the hypoglycemic agent prior to the test. Concentrations of sulfonylurea should be measured in the plasma or urine if it is suspected of being the hypoglycemic agent. The clinical pattern in diabetic subjects consists of increased frequency of hypoglycemia during treatment and persistence of hypoglycemic episodes after complete cessation of use of the agent. The presence of insulin antibodies is of no help in the diagnosis in the insulin-treated patient. An inverse relation between C peptide and insulin levels during hypoglycemia is diagnostic of surreptitious insulin administration. Insulin has been used for suicide, homicide, and child abuse. Errors in filling prescriptions by substitution of a sulfonylurea for the intended medication have led to hypoglycemia.

In rare instances, patients may have hypoglycemia who apparently have never had an insulin injection but have insulin antibodies. These patients may range in age from a few days old to elderly. Hypoglycemia may be severe, occur during fasting or postprandially, and is often self-limited. Too few cases have been adequately described to ascertain whether free insulin concentrations are abnormal during episodes of hypoglycemia; free C peptide concentrations appear to be appropriately suppressed. Discrimination between autoimmune and factitial hypoglycemia rests on demonstrating differences in the characteristics of the insulin antibodies and the absence of bovine and porcine proinsulin and C peptide-specific antibodies. Neither the biochemical characteristics of this syndrome nor the mechanism of the hypoglycemia has been elucidated.

Hypoglycemia has been observed in a few persons with insulin receptor antibodies that presumably act like insulin agonists. Most of the reported patients had pre-existing insulin-resistant diabetes and evidence for autoimmune disease prior to the development of hypoglycemia. This syndrome may respond to glucocorticoid therapy but not to immunosuppressive agents or plasmapheresis.

Non–Beta Cell Tumor Hypoglycemia

A wide variety of tumors of mesenchymal or epithelial origin and some malignant hematologic diseases have been associated with hypoglycemia.

Mesenchymal tumors account for 45 to 64 per cent of the reported cases. Approximately one third of the tumors are located in the chest and two thirds are in the abdomen, usually in the retroperitoneum. They usually are large and therefore readily detectable. Hepatomas account for 22 per cent of cases.

No single pathogenetic mechanism satisfactorily explains all cases of tumor-related hypoglycemia. In some, more than one mechanism may be involved. Metastatic destruction of the adrenals or pituitary and extensive metastatic involvement of the liver can impair glucoregulatory mechanisms. Some tumors evince a high rate of glucose utilization. In others, substances such as tryptophan metabolites may impair gluconeogenesis. The conflicting data regarding the presence or absence of elevated concentrations of insulin-like growth factors in the serum of these patients may be due to methodologic differences in measuring the substances. Total or partial surgical removal of the tumor usually results in amelioration of the hypoglycemia.

Hypoglycemia in Hepatic, Renal, and Endocrine Disorders

Symptomatic hypoglycemia is uncommon in liver disease because glucose homeostasis can be maintained with as little as 20 per cent of healthy parenchymal cells, but biochemical hypoglycemia has been reported in a wide variety of acquired hepatic diseases. The hypoglycemia of congestive heart failure, sepsis, and Reye's syndrome is considered to be due to hepatic mechanisms.

Hypoglycemia is uncommon in adrenocortical insufficiency. Hypoglycemia in hypopituitarism is common in children under six years of age but less so beyond that age. Asymptomatic hypoglycemia has been observed in isolated growth hormone deficiency after prolonged fasting. Spontaneous hypoglycemia has been reported to be a frequent finding in isolated ACTH deficiency. Adults surgically deprived of epinephrine are not subject to hypoglycemia.

Hypoglycemia in nondiabetic persons with renal failure may be due to inadequate gluconeogenic substrate availability. Glucagon deficiency is a theoretic mechanism for hypoglycemia, but the existence of this disorder has not been confirmed.

Froesch ER, Zopf J, Widmer U: Hypoglycemia associated with non-islet cell tumor and insulin-like growth factors (letter). Gorden P, Kahn CR, Roth J, Megyeshi K (response to letter). N Engl J Med 306:1178–1179, 1982. *The letter and response describe the controversy regarding the concentrations of insulin-like growth factors in non–beta cell tumor hypoglycemia.*

Garber AJ, Bier DM, Cryer PE, Pagliara AS: Hypoglycemia in compensated chronic renal insufficiency. Substrate limitation of gluconeogenesis. Diabetes 23:982–986, 1974. *Data are presented indicating that hypoglycemia in chronic renal failure may be due to inadequate availability of alanine.*

Hogan MJ, Service FJ, Sharbrough F, Gerich JE: Oral glucose tolerance test compared with a mixed meal in the diagnosis of reactive hypoglycemia. A caveat on stimulation. Mayo Clin Proc 58:491–496, 1983. *The authors demonstrate the inadequacy of the oral glucose tolerance test for the diagnosis of postprandial symptoms. Patients considered to have food-stimulated hypoglycemia after oral glucose tolerance testing had no hypoglycemia after a mixed meal despite the presence of postprandial symptoms. In addition, EEG monitoring during postprandial symptoms showed no changes.*

Le-Ran A, Anderson RW: The diagnosis of postprandial hypoglycemia. Diabetes 30:996–999, 1981. *The authors report the results of oral glucose tolerance testing in a large group of healthy persons, in 10 per cent of whom the glucose nadir was ≤47 mg per deciliter. In addition, the nonspecificity of the postoral glucose symptoms is underscored by the observation of symptoms following administration of a placebo.*

Marks V: Hypoglycemia. Oxford, Blackwell Scientific Publications, Ltd., 1981. *This is an authoritative reference work on hypoglycemic disorders.*

Scarlett JA, Mako ME, Rubenstein AH, Blix PM, Goldman J, Horwitz DL, Tager H, Jaspan JB, St Jernholm MR, Olefsky JM: Factitious hypoglycemia. Diagnosis and measurement of serum C-peptide immunoreactivity and insulin-binding antibodies. N Engl J Med 297:1029, 1977. *Seven cases of surreptitious injection of insulin are described. The authors emphasize the importance of the triad of low plasma glucose and high plasma insulin levels and suppression of plasma C peptide for diagnosis of this condition. In addition, there is a useful discussion of characteristics of antibodies to insulin, proinsulin, and C peptide of human, porcine, and bovine origin for the distinction between factitial and autoimmune hypoglycemia.*

Seltzer HS: Severe drug-induced hypoglycemia: A review. Comp Ther 5:21–29, 1979. *This review is an excellent reference source regarding the drugs implicated and the conditions conducive to drug-induced hypoglycemia.*

Service FJ: Hypoglycemic Disorders: Pathogenesis, Diagnosis, and Treatment. Boston, G. K. Hall, 1983. *This book is recommended for those desiring more detailed description of hypoglycemic disorders. For those interested in hypoglycemias in the pediatric age range the chapter, Hypoglycemia in infants and children, by E. Tsalikian and M. W. Haymond, is an excellent reference source.*

Taylor SI, Greenberger G, Marcus-Samuels B, Underhill LH, Dons RF, Ryan J, Roddam RF, Rupe CE, Gorden P: Hypoglycemia associated with antibodies to the insulin receptor. N Engl J Med 307:1422–1426, 1982. *The authors report a nondiabetic patient with fasting hypoglycemia ascribed to the action of autoantibodies to the insulin receptor. Although the few other patients with this syndrome had a history of prior diabetes, evidence for coexistent autoimmune disease is a clue to the presence of antireceptor antibodies.*

232. PANCREATIC ISLET CELL TUMORS

Carl Grunfeld

THE ISLETS OF LANGERHANS

Dispersed throughout the exocrine pancreas are nests of endocrine cells, the islets of Langerhans. The islet itself is a miniature organ with a distinctive organization of individualized cells, each of which produces a single hormone (Fig. 232–1). Insulin-containing B cells form the core of the islet and make up 60 per cent of the endocrine pancreas. They are surrounded by a rim of A cells that secrete glucagon and constitute 25 per cent of the islet. In the ventral portion of the head of the pancreas, glucagon-secreting cells are rare, and the rim is predominantly made up of cells containing pancreatic polypeptide. D cells containing somatostatin or gastrin are primarily found between the A and B cells. The location and function of cells containing other hormones, such as vasoactive intestinal polypeptide, have not yet been precisely defined.

The cells of the islets are capable of communication with each other through gap junctions. These transmembrane channels permit the exchange of small signal molecules as well as some polypeptides. Complete structural integrity of the islet is probably required for normal function.

Cells of the islets may become hyperplastic in response to prolonged stimulation of hormone secretion. Thus, A cells containing glucagon are often increased in diabetes mellitus. B cells increase after prolonged excessive caloric ingestion or in the presence of insulin resistance.

ISLET CELL TUMORS

Tumors can arise from any of the hormone-producing cells of the islets of Langerhans. Patients with islet cell tumors may seek help either because of distinct syndromes due to the hypersecretion of hormones by the tumors or because of mass effects of local or metastatic tumor spread. Nearly all benign islet cell tumors and more than 80 per cent of carcinomas secrete clinically significant amounts of hormone. Some tumors, particularly those arising from more than one cell type, have been shown to produce multiple hormones. Clinical presentation usually reflects the dominance of one hormone.

The tumor is named after the hormone responsible for the syndrome or, in asymptomatic patients, the hormone found in highest concentration in the circulation or in the tumor. For example, a tumor producing insulin is known as an insulinoma, and one producing glucagon is a glucagonoma. The tumors also retain the morphologic characteristics of the cell of origin.

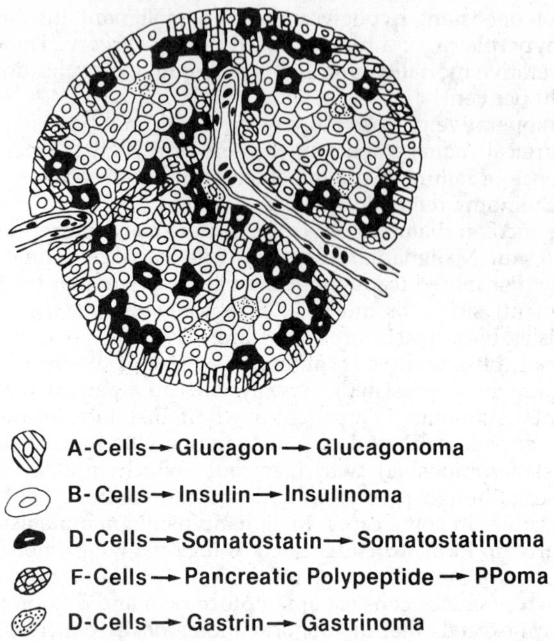

Figure 232–1. Morphology of the islets of Langerhans. This schematic representation of a typical islet demonstrates the distinctive distribution of hormone-secreting cells within the islet. Insulin-containing B cells, forming the core of the islet, are surrounded by glucagon-containing A cells. D cells are interspersed. In the posterior portion of the head of the pancreas, the proportion of cells containing pancreatic polypeptide is increased and the number of glucagon-secreting cells is strikingly decreased. Each cell type is capable of neoplastic transformation, yielding an adenoma or carcinoma that synthesizes the characteristic hormone. (Modified from Unger RH, Orci L: Glucagon and the A cell: Physiology and pathophysiology. N Engl J Med 304:1518, 1981. Reprinted with permission.)

DIAGNOSIS. Diagnosis of islet cell tumors is usually made by detecting elevated basal or fasting levels of the suspected hormone in the presence of the characteristic syndrome. Provocative tests have also been developed that use pharmacologic agents to discriminate between secretion from a tumor and from a normal pancreas. In addition, tumors usually secrete a larger proportion of prohormone or other species of high molecular weight than do normal islet cells. Once the diagnosis is made, imaging techniques such as ultrasound, computed tomography, and angiography are helpful in localizing the tumor and in detecting hepatic and lymph node metastases (see Fig. 231–8). These techniques should not be relied upon to make the diagnosis of the islet cell tumor, as there are a significant number of false-negative and false-positive results of tests. When a tumor is not readily detectable, selective venous catheterization can be used to obtain samples for radioimmunoassay, thereby identifying the area of the pancreas responsible for hypersecretion of the excess hormone. Controversy exists as to whether or not extensive preoperative tumor localization is required.

PATHOLOGY. There is no distinctive pathologic finding that can distinguish between benign and malignant islet cell tumors, although vascular invasion is suggestive of malignancy. The diagnosis of carcinoma is made when metastases are found at presentation or subsequent to resection of a solitary tumor. Elevated levels of human chorionic gonadotropin are useful in helping to establish the preoperative diagnosis of malignancy.

ASSOCIATED SYNDROMES. Pancreatic islet cell tumors may also be part of the multiple endocrine neoplasia (MEN) syndromes (see Ch. 240). It is critical to identify patients with this syndrome as they may have multiple islet cell tumors. Identification of the tumor or area of the pancreas responsible for excess secretion is essential to allow limited pancreatic resection by the surgeon. Unfortunately in patients with a MEN syndrome, tumors may continue to recur, necessitating total pancreatectomy. The presence of hypercalcemia in patients with islet cell tumors is suggestive of the MEN 1 syndrome, as 85 per cent of all patients with MEN type 1 have hyperparathyroidism at some time.

THERAPY. The primary therapy of solitary islet cell tumors is surgical resection. When a patient has islet cell carcinoma with metastasis, therapy is directed toward ameliorating the symptoms of the presenting syndrome and may include pharmacologic inhibitors of hormone secretion and action, chemotherapeutic agents, or surgical debulking. The specific agents are discussed under each tumor.

Similar syndromes resulting from hypersecretion of pancreatic hormones can occur secondary to diffuse hyperplasia of islet cells. The architecture of the pancreas may be disordered, with nests of islet cells arising from exocrine ducts. The treatment of hyperplastic syndromes is partial or near-total pancreatectomy.

The characteristic syndromes associated with islet cell tumors are outlined in Table 232–1.

Insulinoma

The most common islet cell tumor is the insulinoma, which may produce life-threatening hypoglycemia. Insulinoma is reviewed in Ch. 231.

Gastrinoma

The second most common islet cell tumor is the gastrinoma associated with Zollinger-Ellison syndrome, producing recurrent peptic ulcers due to hypersecretion of gastric acid. This syndrome is discussed in Ch. 99.

VIPoma or the Diarrheogenic Syndrome

CLINICAL PRESENTATION. VIP (vasoactive intestinal polypeptide)-oma or the diarrheogenic syndrome, associated with islet cell tumors, severe watery diarrhea, and hypokalemia, is also called pancreatic cholera, Verner-Morrison syndrome, WDHA (watery diarrhea, hypokalemia, achlorhydria) syndrome, or WDHH (watery diarrhea, hypokalemia, hypochlorhydria) syndrome. Patients have profound but intermittent secretory diarrhea, with peak diarrhea output exceeding 3 liters per day in 80 per cent. A more general discussion of secretory diarrhea is contained in Ch. 102. Unlike the diarrheal discharge of chronic laxative abuse, in this diarrhea the discharge is rich in electrolytes; fecal potassium loss can reach 300 mEq per day. Serum potassium is usually less than 3 mEq per liter and is accompanied by acidosis due to severe losses of bicarbonate.

The severe hypokalemia may lead to profound weakness, to flaccid paralysis, and to renal failure due to hypokalemic nephropathy. More than half of the patients have frank diabetes or glucose intolerance, which is probably secondary to hypokalemia, a known inhibitor of insulin secretion (see Ch. 76 for a discussion of hypokalemia). Hypercalcemia is found in half of the patients during attacks and is not usually indicative of hyperparathyroidism (and the MEN 1 syndrome), as parathyroid hormone levels are suppressed and the hypercalcemia remits with resection of the primary islet cell tumor. Despite hypercalcemia, tetany due to hypomagnesemia has been described. Dilation of the gallbladder or small intestine may be seen during radiographic examination, and flushing of the skin has been reported.

DIFFERENTIAL DIAGNOSIS. Secretory diarrhea may result from three other endocrine tumors: gastrinoma, carcinoid, and somatostatinoma. However, peak volume of diarrhea rarely exceeds 3 liters per day in these syndromes. Further, the diarrhea in Zollinger-Ellison syndrome is caused by hypersecretion of gastric acid and can be reversed by gastric suction or with cimetidine. The diarrheogenic syndrome is almost always accompanied by achlorhydria or hypochlorhydria; decreased gastric acid secretion persists when the diarrhea is in remission and the serum potassium is normal.

PATHOLOGY. Eighty per cent of the patients with the diarrheogenic syndrome are found to have islet cell tumors. Nearly half are malignant. When the diarrhea is constant, the probability of malignancy is increased. Patients without islet cell tumors often have diffuse islet cell hyperplasia. The diarrheogenic syndrome has also been reported with bronchial tumor, pheochromocytoma, and ganglioneuroblastoma.

The diarrhea probably results from excess secretion of VIP. Infusion of VIP into laboratory animals and humans results in secretory diarrhea, hypokalemia, inhibition of gastric acid secretion, and hypercalcemia. Increased plasma VIP levels have been found in patients in whom islet cell tumor, islet cell hyperplasia, bronchogenic carcinoma, ganglioneuroblastoma, or pheochromocytoma was found to be the cause of the syndrome. VIP is difficult to detect in the circulation of normal man; therefore the absence of VIP does not rule out the diagnosis. An islet cell tumor producing only pancreatic polypeptide (another presumed hormone of unknown normal function) has also been reported to be associated with this syndrome. Rare tumors have been accompanied by elevated levels of prostaglandin E_2.

THERAPY. Treatment of the diarrheogenic syndrome is primarily by surgery. Because of the profound systemic effects of this tumor, resection is considered even in the presence of metastases. When no tumor is found, subtotal pancreatectomy is usually attempted. If hyperplasia is then identified on histopathology and symptoms persist, total pancreatectomy should be considered. Metastatic tumor has been successfully treated with streptozotocin. The tumors may be transiently

TABLE 232–1. SYNDROMES ASSOCIATED WITH ISLET CELL TUMORS

Tumor	Major Findings	Minor Findings	Other Hormones in Tumor or Plasma	% Malignancy	Hyperplasia	MEN Syndrome
Insulinoma	Adrenergic: palpitations, tremor, hunger, sweating Neuroglycopenic: confusion, seizures, transient focal deficit, coma	Ischemic cardiovascular disease, permanent neurologic deficits	Gastrin, glucagon, pancreatic polypeptide, somatostatin	10	Occasional	10%
Gastrinoma	Peptic ulcers, enhanced acid secretion	Diarrhea, malabsorption, weight loss, dumping	ACTH, insulin, glucagon, VIP, 5-HIAA, MSH, somatostatin, calcitonin, pancreatic polypeptide	40–60	10%	25%
VIPoma	Watery diarrhea, hypokalemia, hypochlorhydria	Hypercalcemia, hyperglycemia, weakness, hypomagnesemia	Pancreatic polypeptide (?), prostaglandins (?)	40	20%	Rare
Glucagonoma	Rash, diabetes, weight loss, anemia	Diarrhea, abdominal pain, thromboembolic disease	Pancreatic polypeptide, 5-HIAA	60	Occasional	Occasional
Somatostatinoma	Diabetes, cholelithiasis, steatorrhea, malabsorption, weight loss	Ingestion, abdominal pain, anemia, diarrhea, ductal obstruction, hypoglycemia (?)	ACTH, gastrin, calcitonin, PGE_2, glucagon, pancreatic polypeptide, VIP, 5-HIAA, substance P	66	None reported	One case (MEN 3)

responsive to steroids, indomethacin, somatostatin, or trifluoperazine, which may be useful in preparing patients for surgery or as a palliative for metastatic disease.

Glucagonoma

CLINICAL PRESENTATION. The glucagonoma syndrome is characterized by a waxing and waning skin rash (necrolytic migratory erythema), diabetes, hypoaminoacidemia, weight loss, and anemia. The classic cutaneous lesion begins as an erythematous base, becomes indurated, and develops superficial central blistering. The blisters then erode and crust over. Healing may be accompanied by hyperpigmentation. This process takes 7 to 14 days with lesions developing in one area while others are resolving. The rash is most prominent on the perineum, along intertriginous folds, and around the mouth and nose. Glossitis, stomatitis, and cheilitis often occur in association with facial lesions. Onycholysis and brittle nails may be present.

Although cutaneous lesions were the hallmark of the first reported cases, the rash is actually present in only two thirds of patients with glucagonoma. The remaining patients usually present because of widespread metastatic disease. Rarely, patients are found during the evaluation of diabetes mellitus or are detected in the course of evaluation for the MEN 1 syndrome.

Frank diabetes occurs in 60 per cent of patients with glucagonoma, and an additional 30 per cent have glucose intolerance. Even in patients with severe hyperglycemia, diabetic ketoacidosis is rarely observed in the glucagonoma syndrome, despite the known ability of glucagon to stimulate hepatic ketogenesis. It is thought that the presence of normal or elevated levels of insulin suppresses lipolysis, limiting the free fatty acid substrates for hepatic ketone production.

Weight loss and anemia are found at the time of diagnosis in half of the patients with glucagonoma. Gastrointestinal symptoms include diarrhea, abdominal pain, and nausea and vomiting. Thromboembolic disease has also been described.

Glucagonoma is infrequently found in the MEN 1 syndrome. However, rare MEN 1 kindreds have been reported in which some members have glucagonoma and others have hyperglucagonemia without clinically detectable tumors. In addition, a familial glucagonoma syndrome has been reported in the absence of other endocrine tumors.

DIAGNOSIS. The diagnosis of glucagonoma is made by detecting elevated levels of glucagon and excluding other conditions associated with hyperglucagonemia, including diabetic ketoacidosis and hyperosmolar syndrome, chronic renal failure, cardiovascular collapse, and cirrhosis of the liver. Normal circulating levels of glucagon are 50 to 150 pg per milliliter. Most patients with glucagonoma have levels in excess of 500 pg per milliliter (occasionally as high as 10,000 pg per milliliter), while glucagon levels in the previously mentioned syndromes average 200 to 500 pg per milliliter.

Once the diagnosis of glucagonoma is confirmed, computed tomography or angiography may be helpful in localizing the tumor and detecting the presence of metastases. At the time of presentation 60 per cent of glucagonomas have metastasized, most commonly to the liver and local lymph nodes.

THERAPY. Surgery is the treatment of choice for glucagonoma confined to the pancreas. Surgery may also be indicated with metastatic disease, as debulking of the tumor mass may ameliorate the glucagonoma syndrome. Streptozotocin, with or without 5-fluorouracil and dacarbazine (DTIC), may induce significant remission. Somatostatin and its long-acting analogues consistently decrease glucagon secretion from glucagonomas. Phenoxybenzamine may also inhibit glucagon secretion from tumors.

The skin rash resolves within a few days of successful surgery and may improve during tumor remission induced by chemotherapy. The immediate cause of the cutaneous lesions is thought to be hypoaminoacidemia, found in 90 per cent of patients with glucagonoma, secondary to enhanced hepatic catabolism of amino acids. An impressive improvement of the rash occurs with hyperalimentation of amino acids, indicating that amino acid deficiency rather than hyperglucagonemia per se may be the basis of the skin lesion.

Somatostatinoma

CLINICAL PRESENTATION. Less than 20 cases of somatostatinoma have been reported; most were found incidentally during laparotomy or during the workup of obstructive jaundice, with identification made retrospectively on the basis of elevated concentrations of somatostatin in the tumor or in the patient's plasma. The tumors contain granules characteristic of D cells.

A syndrome associated with hypersomatostatinemia has been proposed that includes diabetes mellitus, cholelithiasis, steatorrhea with malabsorption, dyspepsia, and significant weight loss. Patients may also have hypochlorhydria, watery diarrhea, anemia, and flushing. The diabetes is usually mild; ketosis has not been described.

The pathophysiology of the syndrome is consistent with the known physiologic and pharmacologic effects of somatostatin. Infusion of somatostatin in man inhibits the release of multiple hormones, including insulin, glucagon, secretin, gastrin, and motilin. Hyperglycemia results from suppression of insulin secretion, but ketosis has not been noted, presumably because of the concomitant inhibition of glucagon secretion. Suppression of secretin, motilin, and gastrin, which decreases hydrochloric acid secretion, gastric emptying, and duodenal motility, tends to cause indigestion and abdominal pain. Inhibition of gallbladder contraction is thought to predispose to cholelithiasis. Malabsorption is produced by inhibition of pancreatic exocrine function.

It is difficult to make the prospective diagnosis of somatostatinoma, as all of these symptoms are nonspecific and are found more commonly in other disorders. The incidence of cholelithiasis is increased in patients with any form of diabetes. Malabsorption may occur in diabetics with chronic pancreatitis. This diagnostic difficulty is further compounded by recent reports of patients with documented somatostatinoma but with none of the components of the proposed syndrome. Three of these patients had severe hypoglycemia and were suspected of having insulinomas. Their tumors also contained small amounts of insulin, and it was proposed that secretion of small amounts of insulin from the tumors with concomitant suppression of compensatory release of glucagon from the normal pancreas resulted in hypoglycemia. Other patients presented with obstructive jaundice; no symptoms of the syndrome were elicited in retrospect.

Somatostatinomas may secrete additional hormones that modify the clinical syndrome. Striking elevations of serum calcitonin can cause watery diarrhea due to the effects of calcitonin on water and electrolyte transport in the gut. Somatostatinomas can produce ACTH, causing Cushing's syndrome. A somatostatinoma accompanied by secretion of prostaglandin E_2 was found in a patient with prominent flushing. A patient with Zollinger-Ellison syndrome was found to have an endocrine tumor of the gut secreting both gastrin and somatostatin. Hyperplasia of cells containing pancreatic polypeptide (resulting in excess secretion of this hormone) has been reported in the presence of somatostatinoma.

DIAGNOSIS. The diagnosis of somatostatinoma is made by detecting elevated basal or stimulated levels of circulating somatostatin. Tolbutamide infusion results in marked elevation of somatostatin in patients with somatostatinoma but not in controls, and has been used to detect tumors in patients with normal basal somatostatin levels.

THERAPY. Two thirds of patients with somatostatinoma have metastases at the time of presentation; this may reflect the difficulty in the clinical diagnosis of this syndrome. Streptozotocin therapy produces regression in tumor size and reduction of plasma somatostatin level.

Other Hormones Produced by Islet Cell Tumors

PANCREATIC POLYPEPTIDE. Islet cell tumors producing pancreatic polypeptide have been associated with watery diarrhea, hypokalemia, and achlorhydria. One patient had normal serum levels of VIP, but pancreatic polypeptide concentration was a thousand times normal. Pancreatic polypeptide has been detected in many endocrine tumors of the pancreas and gut, but most of these tumors usually produce higher levels of another polypeptide hormone.

ACTH. Pancreatic islet cell tumors producing ACTH account for nearly 10 per cent of cases of Cushing's syndrome due to ectopic ACTH production. Such tumors are usually found to secrete multiple hormones, including insulin, gastrin, serotonin, or somatostatin. However, it is more common to find Cushing's *disease* due to a pituitary adenoma associated with other islet cell tumors in patients with MEN type 1.

GROWTH HORMONE–RELEASING FACTOR. Acromegaly has been reported in patients with islet cell tumors secreting growth hormone–releasing factor. Although these patients often have hyperplasia of the growth hormone–secreting cells of the pituitary, it is very difficult to distinguish them from patients with classic acromegaly due to a pituitary adenoma (see Ch. 225). In either case the sella may be normal or enlarged, and growth hormone levels may show paradoxic responses to provocative testing.

SEROTONIN. Production and secretion of serotonin by islet cell tumors has been reported as a cause of the diarrheogenic syndrome. Since VIP levels were not measured, this may represent synthesis of a second hormone by a mixed adenoma. Carcinoid syndrome has also been reported in association with carcinoma of exocrine pancreatic duct cells.

Moossa AR: Tumors of the Pancreas. Baltimore, Williams & Wilkins, 1980. *Includes detailed chapters on the pathology, pathophysiology, radiology, and surgical treatment of islet cell tumors.*

Morrison AB: Islet cell tumors and the diarrheogenic syndrome. Monogr Pathol 21:185, 1980. *A complete review of all definitive and probable cases of the diarrheogenic syndrome.*

Pipeleers D, Couturier E, Gepts W, Reynders J, Sommers G: Five cases of somatostatinoma: Clinical heterogeneity and diagnostic usefulness of basal and tolbutamide-induced hypersomatostatinemia. J Clin Endocrinol Metab 56:1236, 1983. *Four of these patients with documented somatostatinoma showed none of the symptoms of the proposed somatostatinoma syndrome.*

Stacpoole PW: The glucagonoma syndrome. Clinical features, diagnosis and treatment. Endocr Rev 2:347, 1981. *A recent comprehensive review of all cases reported to date.*

233. DISORDERS OF SEXUAL DIFFERENTIATION

Julianne Imperato-McGinley

NORMAL SEXUAL DIFFERENTIATION

The fetus is bipotential for sexual differentiation. The bipotentiality includes the gonad, the internal sex structures, and the external genitalia.

Development of the Bipotential Gonad

In fetuses of both sexes an undifferentiated gonad develops during the fifth week of fetal life. A thickened area of coelomic or germinal epithelium appears on the medial aspect of the mesonephros, and proliferation of germinal epithelium cells and underlying mesenchyme produces a prominence on the medial side of the mesonephros designated the gonadal ridge. Following this, cords of cells known as primary sex cords proliferate from the epithelium into the mesenchyme. The gonad at this stage consists primarily of mesodermal cells of coelomic epithelial origin. The primordial germ cells are visible early in the third week among the endodermal cells of the wall of the yolk sac near the origin of the allantois. They are spherical and larger than mesenchymal cells, with large vesicular nuclei and abundant cytoplasm. During folding of the embryo, part of the yolk sac is incorporated into the embryo, and the primordial germ cells migrate by a combination of ameboid movement and passive transfer along the dorsal mesentery to the gonadal ridges. During migration the germ cells multiply by mitosis. By the fifth week of fetal life they begin to migrate into the underlying mesenchyme, and by the end of the sixth week the undifferentiated or bipotential gonad is formed (Fig. 233–1). The primordial germ cells develop into spermatogonia in the male and ova in the female, the sex cords become either seminiferous tubules or primary ovarian follicles, and the mesenchymal cells form either the Leydig cells or the theca and stromal cells in the female.

Gonadal Differentiation—Development of the Testes and Ovaries

Testicular or seminiferous cords evolve from primary sex cords of the indifferent gonad at approximately the seventh week of gestation in a 15- to 20-mm male embryo (Fig. 233–1). The Sertoli cells differentiate within each cord, enlarge, aggregate, and engulf the germ cells. The distal ends of the seminiferous cords then interconnect to form a network of solid cords, the rete testes, which is in direct contact with the wolffian (mesonephric) ducts. By the sixth month, the ends of the rete testes develop a lumen continuous with the mesonephric tubules, which later develop into the ductuli efferentia. The fetal Leydig cells are apparent by eight weeks of fetal life, and at three months of gestation they completely fill the interstitial spaces.

Ovarian differentiation from the indifferent gonad begins at approximately 50 days of gestation (Fig. 233–1). The primary

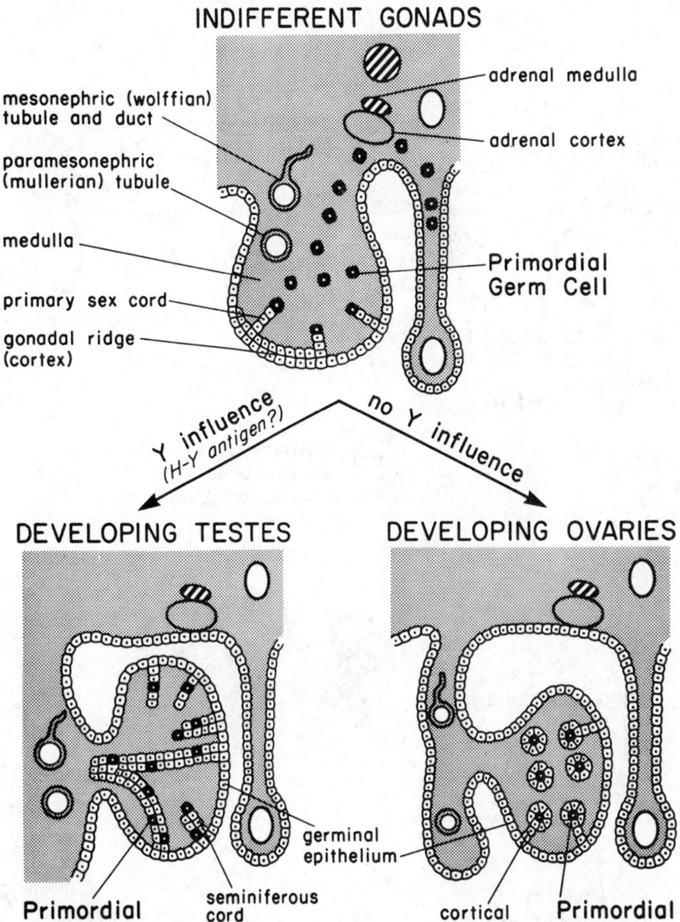

Figure 233–1. Development of the bipotential gonad from coelomic epithelium (primary sex cords) underlying mesenchymal tissue and primordial germ cells and its differentiation to either a testes or an ovary.

sex cords form irregular groups of cells called medullary cords containing primitive granulosa cells that engulf primordial oogonia. The oogonia are in the prophase of meiosis at day 50 to 55. The leptotene stage begins at day 60, the pachytene stage at approximately day 80, and by day 90 the oogonia enter the diplotene stage. As the oogonia differentiate, the primitive granulosa cells organize around them and form a single layer constituting the primordial follicle. Primary follicles are formed when the primordial follicle containing oocytes of the diplotene stage becomes separated by connective tissue. At 18 to 20 weeks of gestation, there are approximately 7 million oogonia and oocytes, whereas at birth the number decreases to approximately 2 million.

Phenotypic Differentiation

Ductal Development

In every fetus, both *wolffian (mesonephric) ducts*, which develop into epididymis, vas deferens, and seminal vesicles in the male, and *müllerian (paramesonephric) ducts*, which develop into fallopian tubes, uterus, and upper third of the vagina in the female, are present (Fig. 233–2). The wolffian ducts appear at 25 to 30 days of gestation, and the müllerian ducts at 44 to 48 days. In the male the initial event is regression of the müllerian ducts, completed at about seven and one half weeks of gestation, followed by stabilization and differentiation of the mesonephric wolffian ducts to form the epididymis, vas deferens, seminal vesicles, and ejaculatory ducts. In the female the wolffian ducts regress at approximately ten and one half weeks, and the müllerian ducts differentiate to form the fallopian tubes, uterus, and upper portion of the vagina.

Development of the External Genitalia

The external genitalia of both sexes (like the gonad) develop from common primordia, the urogenital tubercle, urogenital folds, and urogenital swellings schematically represented in Figure 233–2. In the male, external genital masculinization begins shortly after wolffian ductal differentiation. The urogenital tubercle elongates to become the glans penis, the urogenital folds fuse and become the shaft of the penis, and the urogenital

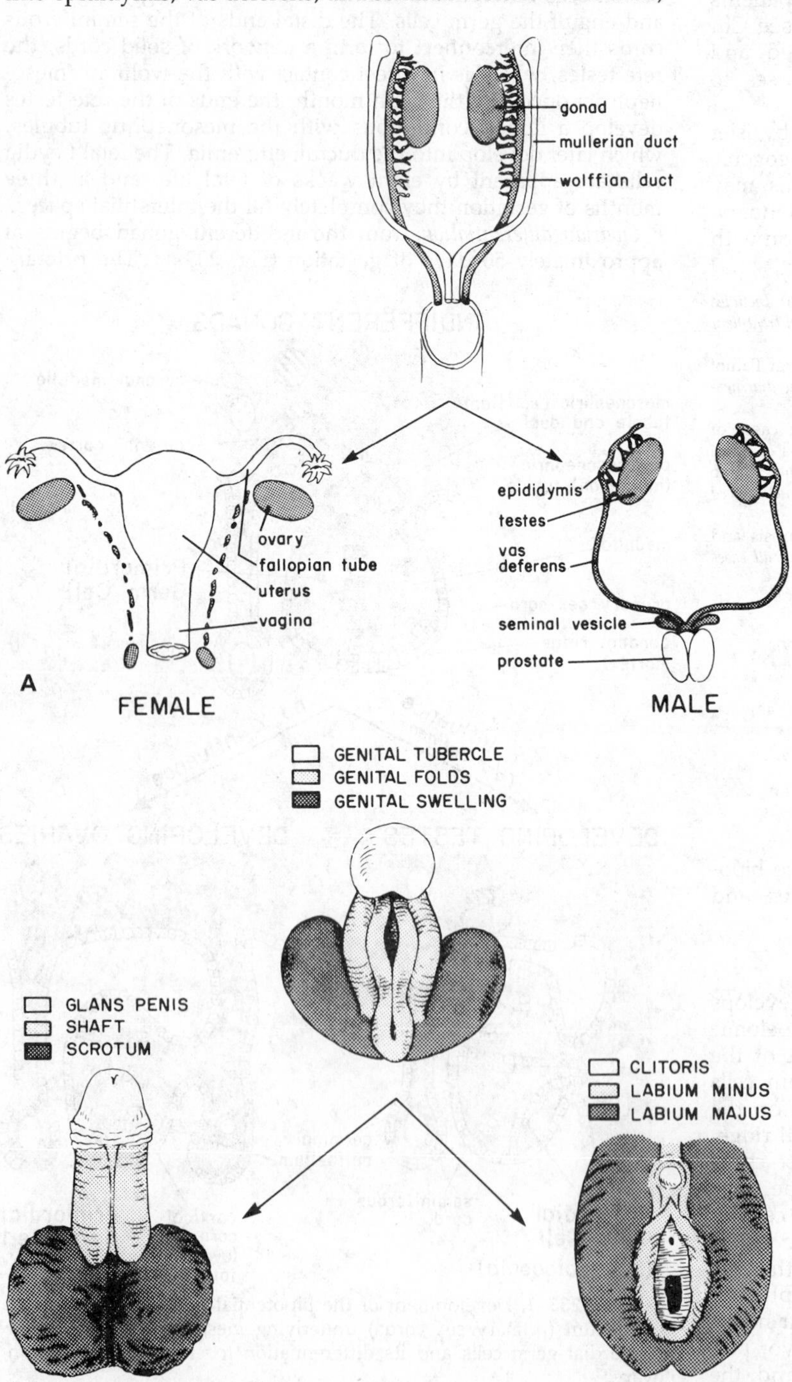

Figure 233–2. Summary of male and female sexual differentiation. *A*, Internal sexual differentiation from wolffian and müllerian ducts. *B*, Development of male and female external genitalia from common primordia.

swellings become the scrotum. The prostate arises from endodermal buds in the urethral lining at 10 weeks and grows into the mesenchyme, which forms the muscular and connective tissue components. Male external sexual differentiation is completed by 14 weeks of gestation. However, descent of the testes and growth of the penis occur between 20 weeks of gestation and term. In the female the urogenital tubercle becomes the clitoris, the urogenital swellings the labia majora, and the urogential folds the labia minora. Female differentiation occurs after the embryo has reached 10½ weeks.

Determinants of Phenotypic Differentiation

Since the fetus is bipotential, what are the determinants of the male or female phenotype?

Female Phenotypic Differentiation

Ovarian tissue containing primary follicles is found in human abortuses with a 45 XO complement. Thus, ovarian differentiation does not appear to require a 46 XX chromosomal complement. Adults, however, with a 45 XO complement no longer have ovarian follicles, and only streak gonads made of whorls of connective tissue remain. Deletion of either the long or short arm of the X chromosome will result in streak gonads. A complete 46 XX complement, therefore, although not necessary for ovarian differentiation, is essential for maintenance of normal ovarian follicular development. Deletion of the short arm of the X chromosome (XXp-) is associated with streaked gonads and the skeletal and somatic anomalies of subjects with 45 XO Turner's syndrome. In contrast, long arm deletions (XXq-) are usually associated with streak gonads and none of the stigmata of Turner's syndrome. See Ch. 236 for a complete discussion of XO and XX gonadal dysgenesis.

In the absence of gonads, either ovaries or testes, the wolffian anlagen regress and the müllerian ducts differentiate to form fallopian tubes, uterus, and upper portion of the vagina, and the external genital primordia differentiate as female (Fig. 233–2). Thus, femaleness appears to be the innate tendency of every fetus and does not require gonadal influence.

Male Phenotypic Differentiation

TESTICULAR DIFFERENTIATION. The development of the male phenotype is more complex; to initiate the process the testes must develop and function normally. Testicular influence is necessary to alter the tendency of the fetus to develop as female. In man, normal testicular differentiation is controlled by the Y chromosome. Analysis of Y chromosome structural abnormalities in man suggests that the short arm (Yp) of the chromosome near the centromere carries the gene(s) directing testicular formation. Simple absence of the (Yp) of the Y chromosome results in a female phenotype, with streak gonads.

What is the mechanism of Y chromosomal control of testicular differentiation? It has been postulated that a testicular organizing substance produced locally by cells within the gonad and under the control of the Y chromosome imposes testicular organogenesis on the gonadal primordium early in gestation, thereby preventing the undifferentiated gonad from developing as an ovary (Fig. 233–3). The inducer substance may be the H-Y histocompatibility antigen, present on the cell surface of individuals with a Y chromosome: (1) Males with two Y

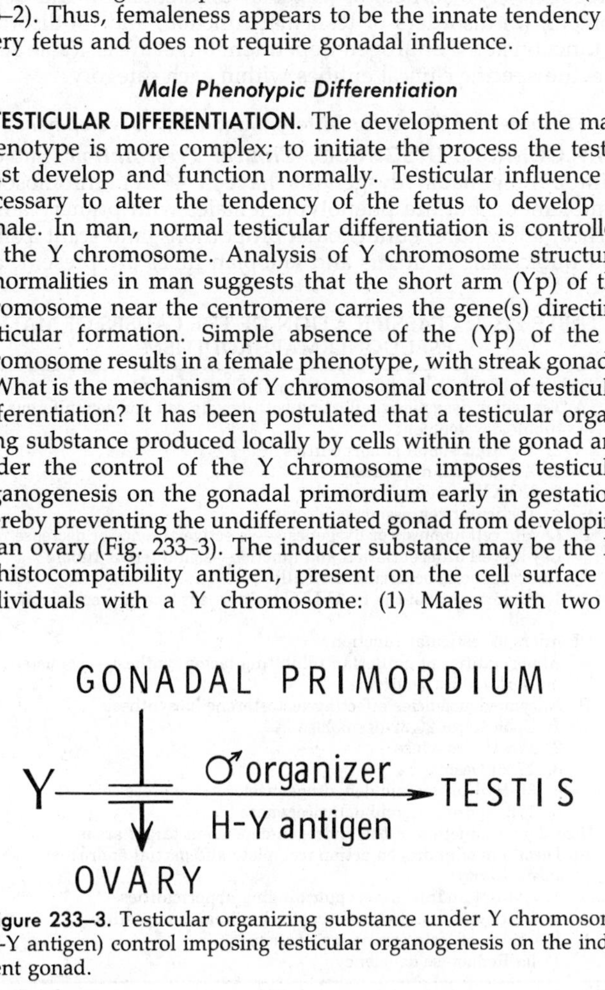

Figure 233–3. Testicular organizing substance under Y chromosome (?H-Y antigen) control imposing testicular organogenesis on the indifferent gonad.

chromosomes have more circulating H-Y antigen than normal 46 XY males. (2) In most individuals with Y chromosome deletions the H-Y gene is found on the short arm of the Y chromosome near the centromere, a region known to be testis determining. (3) In general, whenever testicular tissue is found in patients with disorders of sexual development serologic H-Y antigen is detected. Exceptions to the associations have recently been demonstrated, raising the possibility that the H-Y antigen commonly measured in neutralization reactions may not be the only form of testicular organizing factor present.

A minimum of three genes may be responsible for H-Y antigen secretion with a fourth gene controlling the gonad-specific H-Y antigen receptor. The H-Y structural gene is hypothesized to be autosomal and under the regulating influence of genes located on both X and Y chromosomes. In the presence of the Y chromosome the H-Y structural gene becomes activated. A regulator gene on the X chromosome that represses the autosomal structural gene is postulated. The action of the X-linked controlling gene must require a 46 XX complement, since a uniplex dose is insufficient for complete repression (XO subjects have been found to be H-Y antigen positive but with an intermediate titer).

DIFFERENTIATION OF MALE GENITAL STRUCTURES. Two secretions from the developing fetal testes are essential for male phenotypic differentiation, testosterone and müllerian inhibiting factor. Responsiveness to both hormones is present only during the critical period of male sexual differentiation, from the eighth to the fourteenth weeks of gestation. In the male fetus at eight weeks of gestational age the histologic appearance of differentiated Leydig cells and the onset of testosterone formation are temporally related and appear to be under the stimulation of placental chorionic gonadotropin. The initiation of testicular testosterone formation from the Leydig cells coincides with wolffian differentiation and differentiation of the male external genitalia. However, for differentiation of the external genitalia, testosterone acts as a prohormone and is converted to 5α-dihydrotestosterone by the microsomal enzyme, steroid Δ^4 5α-reductase.

Thus, testosterone and its metabolite dihydrotestosterone are essential for sexual differentiation in the male fetus, with selective roles for each hormone during embryogenesis. Testosterone acting locally mediates differentiation of the wolffian ductal system to the vas deferens, epididymis, and seminal vesicles, while the local conversion of testosterone to dihydrotestosterone mediates development of male external genitalia and prostate (Fig. 233–4). Male pseudohermaphrodites with 5α-reductase deficiency and decreased dihydrotestosterone production (see Male Pseudohermaphroditism) have defined the necessity for dihydrotestosterone in the formation of male external genitalia and prostate and have delineated specific actions for the two androgens in utero.

Both testosterone and dihydrotestosterone bind to the same high-affinity androgen receptor protein within the cells of androgen-dependent target areas. Testosterone enters the target cell by a process of passive diffusion and either binds to a cytoplasmic receptor or is converted to dihydrotestosterone, which binds to the receptor. This androgen receptor complex then binds to acceptor sites in nuclear chromatin and ultimately initiates transcription of messenger ribonucleic acid (RNA), resulting in the complex metabolic processes of androgen action (Ch. 221).

The inhibition of the müllerian anlage is not under androgen control; müllerian inhibiting factor, a high molecular weight glycoprotein, is a product of the Sertoli cells of the seminiferous tubules. Its secretion begins shortly after the initiation of seminiferous tubular differentiation and continues through the perinatal period.

In summary, normal male phenotypic development requires that the testes differentiate and function normally, so that at a critically sensitive period in utero (8 to 14 weeks) müllerian

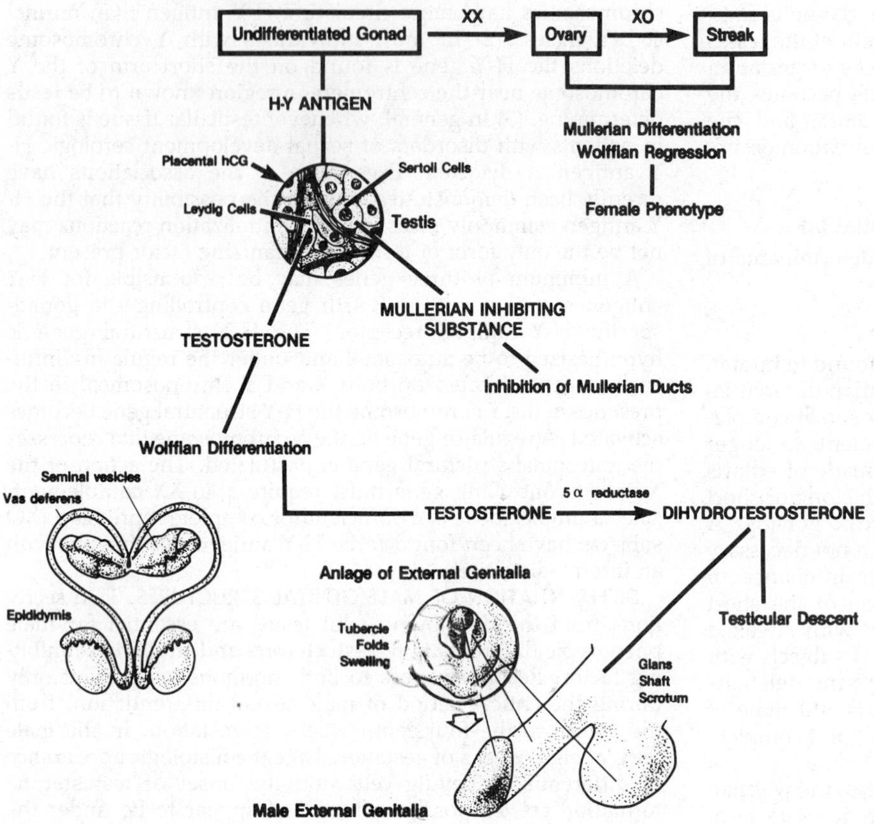

Figure 233–4. Schematic representation of the factors involved in male and female sexual differentiation.

inhibiting factor, secreted by the Sertoli cells, and testosterone, secreted by the Leydig cells, are produced in sufficient amounts. Müllerian inhibiting factor, acting locally, suppresses the müllerian anlage, and testosterone, also acting locally, causes differentiation of the wolffian anlage to epididymis, vas deferens, and seminal vesicles. Testosterone circulates and is converted by the enzyme 5α-reductase to dihydrotestosterone in the cells of the urogenital tubercle, urogenital sinus, and urogenital folds, resulting in differentiation of the male external genitalia (Fig. 233–4). Depending upon specific target tissue, either testosterone or dihydrotestosterone complexes with the cytoplasmic receptor, and this receptor-hormone complex is transferred to the nucleus to initiate androgen action.

Genetic Control of Male Sexual Differentiation

The multifactorial process of male sexual differentiation is under complex genetic control. Testicular differentiation requires the presence of gene(s) normally found on the Y chromosome. The enzymes involved in testosterone biosynthesis, as well as the the enzyme 5α-reductase converting testosterone to dihydrotestosterone, are known to be regulated by genes located on the autosomes. Genes located on the X chromosome control the cytoplasmic receptor at the androgen-dependent target areas. Inherited forms of müllerian inhibiting factor deficiency are transmitted as a recessive trait, either autosomal or X linked. Thus, normal male phenotypic development is regulated by multiple genes located on the autosomes as well as both X and Y chromosomes.

Austin CR, Edwards RG (eds.): Mechanisms of Sex Differentiation in Animals and Man. New York, Academic Press, 1981. *All aspects of sexual differentiation are covered. Chapters 4 and 5 are particularly informative.*

Wachtel S: H-Y Antigen and the Biology of Sex Determination. New York, Grune & Stratton, 1983. *The state of the art concerning H-Y antigen and sexual differentiation.*

ABNORMALITIES OF SEXUAL DIFFERENTIATION

Male Pseudohermaphroditism

The known etiologic factors in male pseudohermaphroditism or incomplete masculinization can be divided into three basic categories: (1) disorders of testicular differentiation and development; (2) disorders of testicular function; and (3) disorders of function at the androgen-dependent target areas. Table 233–1 lists the specific clinical entities within each category.

Disorders of Testicular Differentiation and Development

XY GONADAL DYSGENESIS. *Clinical Presentation.* Subjects with pure gonadal dysgenesis have a 46 XY chromosomal complement, but are phenotypic females with primary amenorrhea, tall stature, eunuchoidal proportions, and scant axillary and pubic hair. A uterus and fallopian tubes are present, and

TABLE 233–1. CLASSIFICATION OF THE CAUSES OF MALE PSEUDOHERMAPHRODITISM

I. Disorders of testicular differentiation and development
  A Testicular dysgenesis, affecting both Leydig cell and seminiferous tubule development
    1. Y chromosomal abnormalities
    2. XY gonadal dysgenesis
    3. XO/XY gonadal dysgenesis
    4. Testicular regression syndrome
  B. Leydig cell agenesis or dysgenesis—selective absence or decrease in Leydig cell differentiation and function—seminiferous tubule embryogenesis occurring normally
    1. Abnormality of the HCG-LH receptor: absence of precursor Leydig cell
II. Disorders of testicular function
  A. Abnormalities of müllerian inhibiting factor synthesis—persistent müllerian duct syndrome
  B. Enzyme deficiencies affecting testosterone biosynthesis
    1. Cholesterol 20,22-desmolase
    2. 17α-Hydroxylase
    3. 17,20-Desmolase
    4. 3β-Hydroxysteroid dehydrogenase:Δ^{5-4} isomerase
    5. 17β-Hydroxysteroid dehydrogenase
III. Disorders of function at the androgen-dependent target areas
  A. Disorders of androgen action (complete and partial androgen insensitivity)
    1. Cytosol androgen–receptor binding abnormalities
    2. Post cytosol androgen–receptor binding abnormalities
  B. Disorders of testosterone metabolism
    1. 5α-Reductase deficiency

streak gonads are found. In the incomplete forms of this condition, variable amounts of functional testicular tissue are found, and consequently at birth the subjects frequently have clitoromegaly, ambiguous genitalia, or, rarely, a penile urethra. Virilization at puberty is also variable. In pure gonadal dysgenesis, postpubertal gonadotropins are increased and in the castrate range with female levels of testosterone. However, when functioning testicular tissue is present, testosterone can be increased from slightly above the female level to a low normal male level. Additionally, if müllerian inhibiting factor is produced there may be partial or complete absence of müllerian structures (Fig. 233–5).

Pathophysiology. In pure gonadal dysgenesis the testes do not differentiate at all, and in the absence of a functional testis phenotypic development is female, with wolffian duct regression and müllerian differentiation. In the incomplete forms there is variable testicular development with varying degrees of fetal masculinization. The etiology of this condition is unknown, but it could be due to a number of theoretic causes involving testicular organizing substance (H-Y antigen). There could be a lack of, or decreased secretion of, testicular organizing substance, abnormalities in its structure, or lack or decrease in its gonadal specific receptor. Interestingly, serologic analyses of subjects with pure gonadal dysgenesis have revealed a negative H-Y antigen titer in some subjects, while others have a positive titer, suggesting genetic heterogeneity. Since H-Y antigen has been postulated to be the testicular organizing substance, the presence of streaked gonads in H-Y antigen-positive individuals has been explained by either postulating a defect in the gonadal receptor for testicular organizing H-Y antigen or by postulating the presence of a structurally inactive form of H-Y antigen.

Approximately 13 familial cases of pure gonadal dysgenesis have been described, and inheritance appears to be either X-linked recessive or autosomal dominant–sex limited. Within families there may be variable expressivity of the gene defect, with some sibs having the pure form and a female phenotype and others with ambiguous genitalia.

Management and Therapy. The streak gonads should be removed since approximately 20 to 30 per cent of subjects will develop gonadoblastomas or dysgerminomas within the streak gonads. Dysgerminomas may be malignant, and approximately 5 to 8 per cent of gonadoblastomas also contain malignant elements. In pure gonadal dysgenesis, infants are invariably reared as female and come to the attention of the physician at puberty because of lack of secondary sexual development. Estrogen and progesterone replacement therapy should be instituted after prophylactic removal of the streak gonads. In complete forms, the child should be reared in the sex that will be more functional, and appropriate surgical correction of the genitalia carried out. Intra-abdominal testicular tissue should always be removed because of the increased risk of malignancy.

MIXED GONADAL DYSGENESIS. ***Clinical Presentation.*** Classically, subjects with mixed gonadal dysgenesis have a streak gonad on one side and a testis on the contralateral side. Most demonstrate XO/XY mosaicism on chromosomal analysis. The phenotypic spectrum ranges from phenotypic females, with or without the clinical characteristics of Turner's syndrome, to subjects with ambiguous genitalia, to normal phenotypic males. The genitalia are sufficiently ambiguous in most affected subjects that approximately two thirds are raised as girls, with the stigmata of Turner's syndrome occurring in one third. Affected subjects have a uterus, and most have bilateral fallopian tubes. The vas deferens, if present, is on the side of the testis, and frequently a fallopian tube also exists adjacent to the vas deferens. Virilization generally occurs at puberty. The testes appear histologically normal before puberty. However, after puberty the seminiferous tubules demonstrate thickened walls and contain few if any germ cells. Consequently, affected subjects are infertile. If pubertal gynecomastia occurs, a gonadal tumor should be suspected.

Pathogenesis. XO/XY mosaicism in subjects with this condition can be best explained as resulting from mitotic nondisjunction or anaphase lag, resulting in loss of the Y chromosome. Perhaps the lack of testicular differentiation of the streak gonad is related to the preponderance of the XO cell line in that gonad. Despite good Leydig cell function with virilization at puberty, the testis must have been functionally dysgenetic (between the eighth to fourteenth weeks of gestation—the critically responsive period) as evidenced by absence of or incomplete virilization of the external genitalia. Theoretically a delay in testicular differentiation and function in utero could result in delayed secretion of testosterone and müllerian inhibiting factor, completely or partially missing the critically responsive period and resulting in the presence of female or ambiguous genitalia and müllerian structures.

There are subjects with an XO/XY chromosomal complement and bilaterally streaked gonads as well as XO/XY subjects with bilateral testes. Thus the classic clinical syndrome of mixed gonadal dysgenesis may be one clinical entity in a spectrum ranging from streaked gonads and a female phenotype to varied abnormalities of testicular development (symmetric or asym-

ABNORMALITIES OF TESTICULAR DIFFERENTIATION SECONDARY TO Y CHROMOSOME ABNORMALITIES

	Deletion of Y chromosome	Deletion of short arm of Y chromosome	Gene mutation(s) of short arm of Y chromosome (nonvisible damage)	Phenotype
Bilateral streaked gonads (gonadal dysgenesis)	XO	XY(p-)	XY	Female
↕	XY ↕ XO	XY(p-) ↕ XY	↕	
Asymmetric gonadal dysgenesis (MGD)	XO/XY	XY(p-)/XY	XY	Male
↕	XY ↕ XO	XY(p-) ↕ XY	↕	
Bilateral dysgenetic testes	XO/XY	XY(p-)/XY	XY	Pseudohermaphroditism
↕	XY ↕ XO	XY(p-) ↕ XY	↕	
Bilateral testes	XY	XY	XY	Normal male

Figure 233–5. Abnormalities of testicular differentiation secondary to Y chromosomal defects.

metric) and genital ambiguity, possibly depending upon the preponderance of a particular cell line, either XO or XY, within the gonad at the time of differentiation (Fig. 233–5).

Management and Therapy. Because of the increased incidence of tumor formation, an intra-abdominal testis that cannot be brought into the scrotum should be removed as well as the streak gonad. If the subject is being raised as male, a scrotal testis should be preserved. In instances in which the testes cannot be brought to the scrotum and must be removed, or the external genitalia are severely ambiguous, or both conditions exist, the sex of rearing should be female and appropriate genital surgery performed.

XY AGONADISM, TESTICULAR REGRESSION, OR VANISHING TESTES SYNDROME. *Clinical Presentation.* Typically these subjects are 46 XY phenotypic females presenting with a total absence of gonads and no müllerian or wolffian internal structures. The lack of müllerian structures, together with a total lack of gonadal remnants, separates this entity from pure XY gonadal dysgenesis. The condition appears to be secondary to regression of the differentiating testis before the onset of androgen secretion, resulting in lack of wolffian differentiation, but after the onset of secretion of müllerian inhibiting factor, resulting in inhibition of female internal structures. There is, however, a phenotypic spectrum of agonadal subjects perhaps related to testicular regression occurring at various times, during or after the critical period of male sexual differentiation. Affected subjects can therefore vary widely in phenotypes: from those with total absence of internal sex structures and female external genitalia, to subjects with ambiguous genitalia, to normal males with absent testes and a microphallus.

Pathophysiology. The etiology of the testicular regression is unknown. These subjects are unequivocally 46 XY, and chromosomal abnormalities have never been demonstrated. Familial cases of agonadism in XY subjects occur, however, suggesting that in some cases it may be an inherited condition. Variable phenotypic expression in agonadal siblings from the same kindred also occurs suggesting that this condition is a clinical, spectrum due to the time of regression of the embryonic testes.

LEYDIG CELL AGENESIS OR DYSGENESIS, GONADOTROPIN UNRESPONSIVENESS. *Clinical Characteristics.* Adult subjects with Leydig cell agenesis or dysgenesis have either normal female external genitalia or slight posterior fusion of the labia majora and have been raised as females. Two prepubertal cases have been described, one with totally female genitalia and the other with a bifid scrotum, a clitoral-like phallus, and a urogenital sinus. An epididymis and vas deferens are present in all affected subjects, indicating that little testosterone is needed at a critical period to initiate wolffian differentiation. No müllerian structures are found, confirming the fact that müllerian inhibiting factor is not secreted by the Leydig cells, but is secreted by the Sertoli cells of the seminiferous tubules. In the adults, normal appearing Sertoli cells with few spermatogonia and few or no Leydig cells are present in the testis.

Pathophysiology. In adult cases, plasma androgen levels are in the female range and do not significantly change with administration of human chorionic gonadotropin (HCG). Luteinizing hormone (LH) levels are significantly elevated, while follicle-stimulating hormone (FSH) levels are in the normal range. In the children, there is no demonstrable plasma androgen response to administration of HCG.

Theoretically the absence or decrease in Leydig cells can result from (1) an absence of or decrease in precursor cells destined to become functioning Leydig cells under HCG-LH stimulation or (2) a decrease in the HCG-LH receptor or receptor response of the precursor Leydig cells. It can also be theorized that the HCG-LH receptor mediates Leydig cell differentiation, and without these receptors, precursor Leydig cells are not formed. A complete phenotypic spectrum of subjects with this disorder can be anticipated, dependent upon the severity of the developmental defect.

Management and Therapy. Those subjects in whom the diagnosis is made in infancy or early childhood should be raised in the sex in which they will be more apt to function normally. In most instances this would be as female because of the severe genital ambiguity. Thus the testes should be removed and corrective genital surgery performed.

Those subjects in whom the diagnosis is made in adulthood who were raised as females and have a female gender identity should have the testes removed, and female sex hormone therapy should be instituted to induce and maintain breast development.

Disorders of Testicular Function

In disorders of testicular function, the testes have differentiated normally, but there is an abnormality in the secretion of either müllerian inhibiting factor or testosterone.

MÜLLERIAN INHIBITING FACTOR DEFICIENCY. *Clinical Presentation.* Males with this condition have a uterus and bilateral fallopian tubes. They have bilateral testes with normal male differentiation of wolffian structures and external genitalia and undergo normal male puberty. This entity most frequently occurs as unilateral cryptorchidism with a contralateral inguinal hernia containing müllerian structures, "uteri inguinale," and a testis. The presence of the inguinal hernia most often brings affected males to a physician's attention. Although fertility has been described, azoospermia is frequently noted. More than 70 cases of this entity have been reported, including at least 8 families with 2 affected sibs. The majority of pedigree studies suggest an X-linked or autosomal recessive inheritance. In one family study, however, inheritance was compatible with X-linked or autosomal dominant inheritance. In approximately 5 per cent of affected patients, either seminomas or other germ cell tumors occur.

Pathogenesis. This entity could be due to a number of abnormalities affecting the synthesis, structure, timing of secretion, or action of müllerian inhibiting factor. Documentation of the actual biochemical abnormality will have to await characterization of the factor or its receptor. The ultimate effect is lack of suppression of the müllerian anlage resulting in the presence of a uterus. Androgen secretion is adequate during the critical period of sexual differentiation, with normal sexual differentiation of the wolffian ducts and external genitalia.

Management and Therapy. In affected males the müllerian structures should be surgically removed if they are in the inguinal canal. Since malignant change in müllerian structures has never been reported, surgical removal is not necessary if they are located in the abdomen. The cryptorchid testes should be brought into the scrotal sac as early as possible and the patient examined frequently for the development of testicular tumors.

Imperato-McGinley J: Sexual differentiation–Normal and abnormal. Curr Top Exp Endocrinol 5:231–307, 1983. *Of particular interest in this review is the section on male pseudohermaphroditism, including an up-to-date bibliography for each clinical entity described.*

DEFICIENCIES OF TESTOSTERONE BIOSYNTHESIS. *Clinical Features.* Five enzymatic reactions convert cholesterol to testosterone; deficiencies of all have been described. These enzyme deficiencies constitute the nonvirilizing forms of the adrenogenital syndrome. The five enzymatic steps include (1) cholesterol 20,22-desmolase, (2) 3β-hydroxysteroid dehydrogenase:Δ^{5-4}isomerase, (3) 17α-hydroxylase, (4) 17,20-desmolase, and (5) 17β-hydroxysteroid dehydrogenase (Fig. 233–6). A deficiency of the enzymes cholesterol 20,22-desmolase and 3β-hydroxysteroid dehydrogenase:Δ^{5-4} isomerase also impairs production of aldosterone and cortisol. 17α-Hydroxylase deficiency impairs cortisol production, while 17,20-desmolase and 17β-hydroxysteroid dehydrogenase deficiencies affect only androgen biosynthesis. Since androgens are the precursors of estrogens, it follows that estrogen production is also low in all of the enzyme deficiencies except 17β-hydroxysteroid dehydrogenase (Table 233–2). These disorders appear to be inherited as autosomal recessive traits. Genotypic females are phenotypically normal at birth, with the exception of females with 3β-

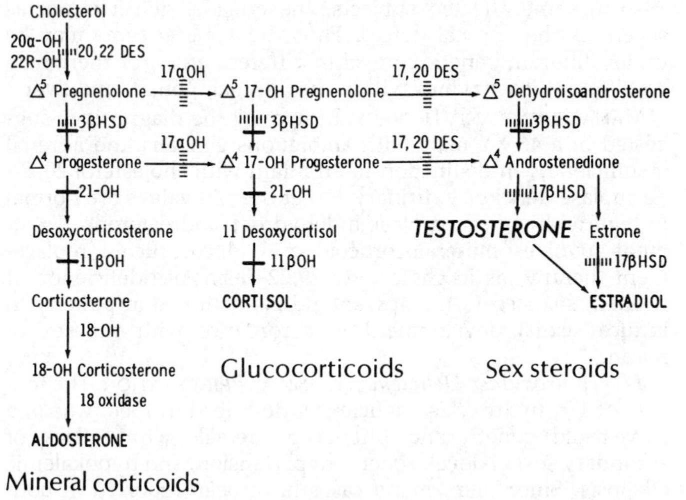

Figure 233–6. Congenital adrenal hyperplasia. *A*, Enzyme deficiencies resulting in male pseudohermaphroditism. Cholesterol 20,22-desmolase, 17α-hydroxylase, 3β-hydroxysteroid dehydrogenase:Δ^{5-4} isomerase, 17,20-desmolase, 17β-hydroxysteroid dehydrogenase. *B*, Enzyme deficiencies resulting in female pseudohermaphroditism. 21-hydroxylase, 11β-hydroxylase, 3β-hydroxysteroid dehydrogenase:Δ^{5-4} isomerase. (DES = desmolase; OH = hydroxylase; HSD = hydroxysteroid dehydrogenase.)

hydroxysteroid dehydrogenase deficiency, who may be mildly virilized.

The testes differentiate normally, and normal amounts of müllerian inhibiting factor are secreted, so that no müllerian structures are present. However, the impaired secretion of testosterone by Leydig cells at the critical period of sexual differentiation in utero (8 to 14 weeks of gestation) causes ambiguity of the external genitalia. Wolffian differentiation is usually normal. In general, the severity of the enzyme defect is reflected in the degree of external genital ambiguity at birth and the amount of virilization at puberty. Each specific enzyme deficiency, however, may show considerable variation in clinical presentation, and affected males with the same enzyme deficiency may present with totally female external genitalia or as males with mild hypospadias and cryptorchidism.

The possible causes for the abnormalities of enzymatic function include mutant genes at structural loci coding for the amino acid sequences of the enzymes changing the enzyme structure and altering its catalytic efficiency, or mutations at sites other than the structural loci. These mutations can be classified as *regulatory*, altering the rate of synthesis or degradation of the enzyme; *architectural*, affecting incorporation of enzyme molecules into active sites in the cell; or *temporal*, affecting the development of the tissue or the time of activation of regulatory systems.

Congenital Lipoid Adrenal Hyperplasia (Cholesterol 20,22-Desmolase Deficiency). In 1957, a genetic male from a consanguineous marriage was described with wolffian differentiation but with female external genitalia. The infant died in adrenal crisis at 6 days of age, and at autopsy the adrenals showed enormous accumulation of lipids in the cortical cells. Consequently the disorder was labeled congenital lipoid adrenal hyperplasia. Subsequent autopsy reports of other affected genotypic male infants have confirmed that the large, yellowish adrenals contain cells with foamy, spongy cytoplasm and stain positively for lipids.

The affected genotypic males have abdominal or inguinal testes with wolffian differentiation. There are no müllerian structures. The external genitalia are either female or severely ambiguous. As would be expected, genotypic female infants have normal female internal and external accessory sex organs.

Approximately 20 cases have been described with equal numbers of both sexes affected. Most of the affected have died in adrenal crisis in infancy, because of severe deficiencies of glucocorticoid and mineralocorticoid production. Only two children have survived to early childhood, a six-year-old male pseudohermaphrodite and an eight-year-old phenotypic female but genetic and gonadal male. Both children had severe adrenal insufficiency in infancy, and congenital adrenal hypoplasia was diagnosed. It was only with reevaluation in childhood, when they were found to have testes, that the correct diagnosis was established.

PATHOGENESIS. A deficiency in the conversion of cholesterol to pregnenolone results in decreased glucocorticoid, mineralocorticoid, and sex steroid production (Fig. 233–6). All plasma steroid values are low to unmeasurable, and little or no urinary 17-ketosteroids, 17-hydroxysteroids, or aldosterone is found (Table 233–2). In the conversion of cholesterol to pregnenolone, at least three enzymes are involved: 20α-hydroxylase, 22α-hydroxylase and 20,22-desmolase. These reactions are mitochondrial mixed-function oxidase reactions requiring a flavoprotein and non-heme iron protein that function in the transport of electrons from NADPH to cytochrome P-450 as the terminal enzyme. A cytochrome P-450 enzyme of the adrenal cortex has been shown to catalyze the formation of pregnenolone from cholesterol, 20α-hydroxycholesterol, 22R- and 22S-hydroxycholesterol, or 20,22-dihydroxycholesterol.

TABLE 233–2. XY MALE PSEUDOHERMAPHRODITISM WITH AN ENZYMATIC DEFECT IN TESTOSTERONE BIOSYNTHESIS

	Genitalia		Secretion				
Enzyme Deficiency	*Female or urogenital sinus*	*Ambiguous*	*Cortisol*	*Aldosterone*	*Androgens*	**Puberty**	**Comments**
Cholesterol 20,22-desmolase	++++	+	↓	↓	↓	↓	
3β-Hydroxysteroid dehydrogenase:Δ^{5-4} isomerase	+	++++	↓	↓	↑ DHEA	Gynecomastia despite low estrogens	Intact peripheral 3βHSD with conversion of Δ^5 to Δ^4 steroids
17α-Hydroxylase	++++	++	↓	B ↑ DOC ↑	↓	Gynecomastia despite low estrogens	Hypertension due to ↑ DOC with ↓ renin and aldosterone
17,20-Desmolase	++++	+	—	—	↓		
17β-Hydroxysteroid dehydrogenase	++++	++	—	—	↓ T ↑ Δ^4	Gynecomastia due to increased estrogen and decreased T	Peripheral conversion of androstenedione to E_1

↑ elevated; ↓ decreased; — normal; + relative frequency of occurrence; B = corticosterone; DOC = desoxycorticosterone; DHEA = dehydroepiandrosterone; T = testosterone; Δ^4 = androstenedione; 3βHSD = 3β-hydroxysteroid dehydrogenase; E_1 = estrone

In a study of adrenal tissue from a child who died with this condition, a deficiency of the enzyme 20α-hydroxylase was suggested as the cause. In another study of adrenal tissue from an affected infant, partial deficiency of cytochrome P-450, with decreased cholesterol 20,22-desmolase activity, was demonstrated. Thus there may be genetic heterogeneity in the expression of this disorder. Theoretically a deficiency of any of the three enzymes or cofactors could result in decreased conversion of cholesterol to pregnenolone.

MANAGEMENT AND THERAPY. In the newborn, signs of adrenal insufficiency with hyperkalemia and hyponatremia occur within the first two weeks, and this condition must be distinguished from 3β-hydroxysteroid dehydrogenase deficiency or congenital adrenal hypoplasia. In a phenotypic female infant, or an infant with ambiguous genitalia and adrenal insufficiency, demonstration of a 46 XY karyotype or demonstration of enlarged adrenals by a radiographic technique will help distinguish this condition from congenital adrenal hypoplasia. The finding of low urinary 17-ketosteroids and low plasma dehydroepiandrosterone levels will distinguish it from 3β-hydroxysteroid dehydrogenase deficiency. Once the diagnosis is established, glucocorticoid and mineralocorticoid therapy should be immediately instituted and is essential for survival. In genotypic males, sex hormone therapy should be instituted at puberty in accordance with the sex of rearing. In most instances, because of the severity of the genital defect, the sex of rearing would be female. Genotypic females will also require appropriate female sex hormone therapy at puberty.

3β-Hydroxysteroid Dehydrogenase:Δ^{5-4} Isomerase Deficiency. CLINICAL PRESENTATION. In 1961 the first three cases of 3β-hydroxysteroid dehydrogenase:Δ^{5-4} isomerase deficiency were described in both males and females. Affected 46 XY subjects had genital ambiguity, although mild to moderate hypospadias is more common than severe perineoscrotal hypospadias. Internal male sexual differentiation is normal, with wolffian differentiation and müllerian ductal inhibition. Curiously, genetic males who reach puberty develop gynecomastia, the etiology of which is not known. At birth affected females have normal or slightly virilized external genitalia, with clitoral hypertrophy and slight labial fusion.

Severely affected children have adrenal insufficiency and die in infancy as a result of salt-losing crisis if not adequately treated. In the milder cases sufficient cortisol and aldosterone are synthesized and consequently adrenal insufficiency is not present in infancy. A mild deficiency of the enzyme has recently been described in a genotypic female with primary amenorrhea, breast development, hirsutism, and clitoromegaly at puberty. Treatment of the adrenal defect by administration of glucocorticoids resulted in the onset of menstruation with ovulation, suggesting that the amenorrhea was secondary to the suppressive effect of excess circulating adrenal androgens on gonadotropins and that the enzymatic defect within the ovary was mild. A very subtle enzyme deficiency may be present in some women with hirsutism and menstrual irregularities.

PATHOGENESIS. In the adrenal the enzyme deficiency ultimately results in decreased cortisol production, which causes increased ACTH secretion and consequent increased production of Δ^5,3β-hydroxysteroids (Fig. 233–6). Plasma levels of pregnenolone, 17α-hydroxypregnenolone, and dehydroepiandrosterone and their sulfate conjugates are usually increased, with decreased levels of aldosterone and cortisol. The slight virilization of the external genitalia in the female is most probably due to the mild androgenic effect of the excess plasma dehydroepiandrosterone or its subsequent peripheral conversion to Δ^5-androstenediol and other androgens (Table 233–2). Surprisingly, plasma Δ^4 steroids, i.e., progesterone, 17α-hydroxyprogesterone, androstenedione, and occasionally testosterone, may be normal or even increased. These findings have been interpreted as reflecting intact hepatic and peripheral 3β-hydroxysteroid dehydrogenase:Δ^{5-4} isomerase enzyme activity. Also in some affected subjects, the gonadal defect is not as severe as the adrenal defect. Thus the same enzyme may be under different genetic control in different areas, or there may be different isoenzymes within the adrenal, gonad, and liver.

MANAGEMENT AND THERAPY. In infancy the diagnosis is suggested in a 46 XY male with ambiguous genitalia and adrenal insufficiency. In distinction to an infant with cholesterol 20,22-desmolase deficiency, urinary 17-ketosteroid values are normal to high with increased plasma dehydroepiandrosterone. Treatment involves mineralocorticoid and glucocorticoid replacement therapy, as in cholesterol 20,22-desmolase deficiency. If needed, sex steroid therapy should be instituted at puberty to induce sexual development in accordance with the sex of rearing.

17α-Hydroxylase Deficiency. CLINICAL PRESENTATION. The first case of 17α-hydroxylase deficiency, described in 1966, was in a 35-year-old genetic and phenotypic female with a lack of secondary sexual development, hypertension, and hypokalemic alkalosis. Since then, many cases have been reported in both genetic males and females. In 46 XY subjects the defect of the external genitalia is usually severe, resulting in completely female external genitalia at birth. Müllerian structures are absent, and wolffian structures are either developed or hypoplastic. Often gynecomastia develops at puberty with little or no virilization. Thus, males with this enzyme deficiency can have the same phenotype in adulthood as subjects with the complete androgen insensitivity syndrome. In 46 XX females with this condition secondary sexual development is absent at puberty and there is primary amenorrhea. Classically the affected subjects also have hypertension and hypokalemia.

PATHOGENESIS. The enzyme 17α-hydroxylase converts pregnenolone and progesterone to 17α-hydroxypregenolone and 17α-hydroxyprogesterone, respectively (Fig. 233–6). These enzymatic steps are necessary for the ultimate formation of cortisol and C19 androgens, including testosterone. Thus a deficiency results in decreased plasma cortisol, with an increase in ACTH and hypersecretion of the plasma precursor 17-deoxysteroids (pregnenolone, progesterone, desoxycorticosterone, corticosterone, 18-hydroxycorticosterone) and increased excretion of their urinary metabolites. Those steroids requiring 17α-hydroxylation are decreased, i.e., plasma 17α-hydroxypregnenolone, 17α-hydroxyprogesterone, 11-deoxycortisol, cortisol, androstenedione, dehydroepiandrosterone, testosterone, and estrogen. Consequently, urinary levels of 17-hydroxysteroids and 17-ketosteroids are low. Despite markedly impaired cortisol production, signs of glucocorticoid deficiency do not generally occur, because of the inherent glucocorticoid activity in the high levels of circulating corticosterone. Excess circulating desoxycorticosterone results in increased sodium retention with increased plasma volume, resulting in hypertension, hypokalemia, and suppression of plasma renin. The plasma aldosterone value is also low secondary to a low level of plasma renin (Table 233–2).

In affected adults, gonadotropin values are elevated, sex steroid levels are low, and in the male there is little or no testicular 17α-hydroxyprogesterone and testosterone response to HCG administration. Consanguinity has been documented in some cases, as has an occurrence of the disorder in siblings of both the same and opposite sex, supporting an autosomal recessive mode of inheritance.

MANAGEMENT AND THERAPY. Hypertension associated with hypokalemic alkalosis in an XY individual with female external genitalia or ambiguous genitalia should suggest the diagnosis. It should also be suspected in any XX female with the same symptom complex who has primary amenorrhea and lack of secondary sexual development. Glucocorticoid replacement therapy is administered to reverse the metabolic abnormality and lower the blood pressure. Appropriate sex steroid therapy concordant with the sex of rearing should be administered at puberty.

17β-Hydroxysteroid Dehydrogenase Deficiency. CLINICAL PRESENTATION. The first case of 17β-hydroxysteroid dehydrogenase deficiency was described in 1965. To date, this condition has been described only in 46 XY males. Affected subjects have either female external genitalia or mild ambiguity of the genitalia and, with few exceptions, were raised as girls. In subjects with totally female appearing external genitalia at birth, the abnormality is not noted until puberty, when virilization frequently occurs with clitoral enlargement. At puberty there are two distinct clinical presentations. Some subjects develop gynecomastia in addition to virilization, while others undergo strong virilization with a male pattern of body hair, deep voice, android build, and no gynecomastia. All subjects raised as females throughout childhood who were castrated prior to or during their teenage years have maintained a female gender identity. However 5 of 6 individuals, from four different kindreds, who were not castrated changed gender identity from female to male with virilization at puberty; also 7 of 25 affected subjects, from a large Arab kindred, with this condition changed gender role from female to male with the hormonal events of puberty.

PATHOGENESIS. 17β-Hydroxysteroid dehydrogenase is a microsomal enzyme catalyzing the conversion of androstenedione to testosterone, the final step in the synthesis of testosterone (Fig. 233–6). It also catalyzes the oxidation-reduction of estrone and estradiol, dehydroepiandrosterone, and Δ^5-androstenediol. The enzyme is not restricted to the adrenal and gonads, but is present in many tissues of the body. In affected 46 XY subjects, the enzyme deficiency results in increased circulating plasma levels of androstenedione, while plasma levels of testosterone are low to low normal (Table 233–2). Plasma luteinizing hormone is increased, while plasma follicle-stimulating hormone is normal to increased. Spermatic vein blood demonstrates an abnormally elevated ratio of androstenedione to testosterone. Approximately 90 per cent of circulating testosterone arises from the extragonadal conversion of androstenedione. Thus in the adult the defect appears to affect the testes while peripheral enzyme activity appears to be intact. However, for masculinization of the external genitalia to be minimal or absent in the fetus, peripheral conversion of androstenedione to testosterone and dihydrotestosterone in the anlage of the external genitalia must be insignificant or absent during early gestation. Thus, peripheral as well as testicular 17β-hydroxysteroid dehydrogenase activity appears deficient in utero, whereas peripheral enzyme activity appears to be intact in the adult. The elevated plasma levels of androstenedione result in increased peripheral conversion to estrone (Table 233–2). In some subjects the conversion of estrone to estradiol also appears to be as severely impaired as the conversion of androstenedione to testosterone, while in others it is impaired to a lesser degree or not at all suggesting that the 17β-hydroxysteroid dehydrogenase enzyme(s) converting estrone to estradiol and androstenedione to testosterone may be under different regulatory control. The lower the plasma testosterone-estradiol ratio, the greater the likelihood of gynecomastia developing in an affected subject at the time of puberty.

MANAGEMENT AND THERAPY. 46 XY affected subjects with female external genitalia should be raised as females and castration carried out either before or during early puberty to avoid significant virilization. Female sex hormone therapy should be instituted at puberty. In those subjects with ambiguous genitalia that can be surgically corrected, a male sex of rearing should be considered. If the diagnosis is made peripubertally or postpubertally, careful psychosexual evaluation should be performed to determine the gender identity before any therapy is instituted. If a gender change from female to male has occurred with puberty, corrective male genital surgery is needed.

17,20-Desmolase Deficiency. CLINICAL PRESENTATION. In 1972 a child with male ambiguous genitalia was described with a defect postulated to be secondary to 17,20-desmolase deficiency. A male pseudohermaphroditic cousin and maternal 46 XY "aunt" were included in the report. Since then nine cases of the enzyme deficiency in 46 XY males have been reported, all phenotypic females or subjects with severely ambiguous genitalia. Recently the first case of a genetic female with primary amenorrhea and lack of secondary sexual development has been reported.

PATHOGENESIS. Partial or complete lack of the enzyme 17,20-desmolase in the adrenal and gonads results in decreased cleavage of the two-carbon side chain from either 17α-hydroxyprogesterone or 17α-hydroxypregnenolone with a resultant decrease in androstenedione and dehydroepiandrosterone production, respectively (Fig. 233–6). This step is essential for the ultimate formation of testosterone and estrogens. Two types of 17,20-desmolase deficiency have been described, one affecting both the Δ^4 and Δ^5 pathways and one affecting the Δ^4 pathway alone, with normal plasma levels of dehydroepiandrosterone (Fig. 233–6). In prepubertal subjects with both Δ^4 and Δ^5 17,20-desmolase pathways affected, low plasma levels of dehydroepiandrosterone and androstenedione are present, which do not increase following administration of ACTH.

It is not known why the basal plasma levels of progesterone, pregnenolone, 17α-hydroxyprogesterone, and 17α-hydroxypregnenolone are elevated, particularly in prepubertal subjects with this enzyme deficiency. Since the enzyme 17,20-desmolase is not involved in cortisol biosynthesis, ACTH levels should be normal with subsequent normal amounts of the C21 precursor steroids mentioned above (Fig. 233–6).

MANAGEMENT AND THERAPY. In genotypic males the sex of rearing will depend upon the degree of ambiguity of the external genitalia. In the more severe cases, patients should be raised as females, with castration carried out in early childhood. Sex hormone therapy at puberty will invariably be necessary. In genotypic females, estrogen and progesterone supplementation will invariably be needed at the time of puberty.

Finkelstein M, and Shaeffer J: Inborn errors of steroid biosynthesis. Physiol Rev 59:353–406, 1979. *An all-encompassing review of the nonvirilizing and virilizing forms of congenital adrenal hyperplasia. A gem.*

Disorders of Function at Androgen-Dependent Target Areas

COMPLETE ANDROGEN INSENSITIVITY—TESTICULAR FEMINIZATION. ***Clinical Presentation.*** In this inherited form of male pseudohermaphroditism, genetic and gonadal males have a female phenotype and totally female psychosexual orientation. The testes differentiate normally with adequate secretion of müllerian inhibiting factor, resulting in the absence of fallopian tubes, uterus, and upper portion of the vagina. Despite normal to high-normal plasma levels of testosterone, wolffian structures are absent, and the external genitalia are totally female. Affected subjects are raised as girls, and the condition is rarely suspected prior to puberty. A prepubertal diagnosis is occasionally made when inguinal or labial masses are palpated in a phenotypic female child and are found to be testes.

Adequate breast development occurs at puberty, but pubic and axillary hair is scant to absent. Medical attention is usually sought at this time because of primary amenorrhea. A diagnosis of complete androgen insensitivity or testicular feminization should be considered in a phenotypic female with primary amenorrhea, good breast development, scantness or absence of pubic and axillary hair, a short vagina, and absence of the cervix and uterus. Rarely, patients with 17α-hydroxylase deficiency may have the same phenotypic presentation at puberty.

Pathogenesis. In patients with complete androgen insensitivity, absence of high-affinity dihydrotestosterone binding to the cytosol receptor (receptor-negative) has been demonstrated in cultured fibroblasts from genital skin. Qualitative abnormalities of the androgen receptor have also been described. Some subjects have partial cytosol receptor–binding under the usual assay conditions at 37° C, with normal binding at 26° C, demonstrating a structural alteration of the receptor at elevated temperatures that is reversible. Others show another qualitative defect demonstrated by failure of stabilization of the androgen receptor with sodium molybdate. Finally, postreceptor variants with normal cytosol receptor binding have also been demonstrated. In the latter individuals, the mutation may affect nuclear binding or the steps in the initiation of androgen action subsequent to nuclear binding, i.e., failure of RNA synthesis or an abnormality in its processing (Fig. 233–7).

It has been postulated that the X chromosomes of all mammals including man are homologous and genes X-linked in one species are X-linked in all. A defect in the receptor-negative form of complete androgen insensitivity has been found to be maternally transmitted with only males expressing the condition, suggesting inheritance as X-linked recessive or autosomal dominant–sex limited (males). Studies of genital skin fibroblasts from mothers of affected subjects demonstrate two clonal populations, one with normal dihydrotestosterone binding and one with absence of binding to the cytosol receptor, confirming X-linkage in this form of androgen insensitivity. Attempts to demonstrate linkage to known X-borne markers such as color blindness, hemophilia, XG immunoglobulin, and G6PD have been unsuccessful.

Plasma testosterone levels are normal to high with mild to moderately elevated plasma levels of luteinizing hormone (LH). A possible explanation for the elevated LH is the relative androgen insensitivity at the level of the hypothalamus resulting in partial negative feedback via conversion of testosterone to estradiol with no direct androgen inhibition. Follicle-stimulating hormone (FSH) levels are normal to elevated. Castration results in further elevation of LH and FSH levels, indicating prior partial feedback control. Urinary estrogens and plasma estradiol levels are generally in the low female range. An increased production rate has been shown for estrone and estradiol, which is mainly testicular in origin. The elevation of plasma estrogens together with the androgen unresponsiveness results in an unopposed estrogen effect that may be the cause of the breast development at puberty.

The histology of the testes cannot be distinguished from that of normal prepubertal males. Postpubertal histologic sections, however, reveal immature tubular development; they contain Sertoli cells and spermatogonia, but no evidence of spermatogenesis. Clumping of tubules with the formation of tubular adenomas is frequently found. The Leydig cells are hyperplastic with abundant smooth endoplasmic reticulum and mitochondria with tubular cristae, which correlate with the elevated plasma testosterone levels.

Management and Therapy. The frequency of testicular neoplasms in complete androgen insensitivity is approximately 2 to 5 per cent, tumors rarely occurring before the age of 25 to 30 years. For this reason the testes should be removed following puberty to allow complete breast development. Following castration, intermittent estrogen replacement therapy is necessary to maintain adequate breast turgor. In general, the vagina is adequate for normal coital function. Occasionally it is too shallow, but can frequently be enlarged with vaginal dilators, thereby bypassing the necessity for reconstructive surgery.

PARTIAL ANDROGEN INSENSITIVITY. *Clinical Presentation.* Partial forms of androgen insensitivity have been described. Affected subjects range from XY subjects with genital ambiguity and minimal to moderate pubertal virilization and gynecomastia, to those with a normal male phenotype, normal male secondary sexual development, and infertility. Within affected families the phenotype can vary, demonstrating that a single mutant gene can have variable phenotypic expression.

Pathogenesis. In general, the endocrine profile is similar to that demonstrated in subjects with complete androgen insensitivity. Plasma LH and testosterone levels are generally elevated. The total amount of 17β-estradiol produced and the quantity secreted by the testes can be greater than those found in patients with complete androgen insensitivity. However, despite increased estrogen production, the degree of feminization at puberty is not as marked as in complete androgen insensitivity, which may be a consequence of the incomplete androgen resistance with a less severe androgen and estrogen imbalance at the cellular level.

In many affected males with incomplete androgen insensitivity, the binding capacity and affinity of the androgen cytosol receptor for dihydrotestosterone is normal. Thus this condition may be a variant of complete androgen insensitivity with normal cytosol-binding activity. Other affected males, however, have a reduced number of cytosol-binding sites for dihydrotestosterone; this may represent a variant of complete androgen insensitivity with absence of androgen-binding activity. Qualitative defects in the receptor, i.e., thermolability and failure of

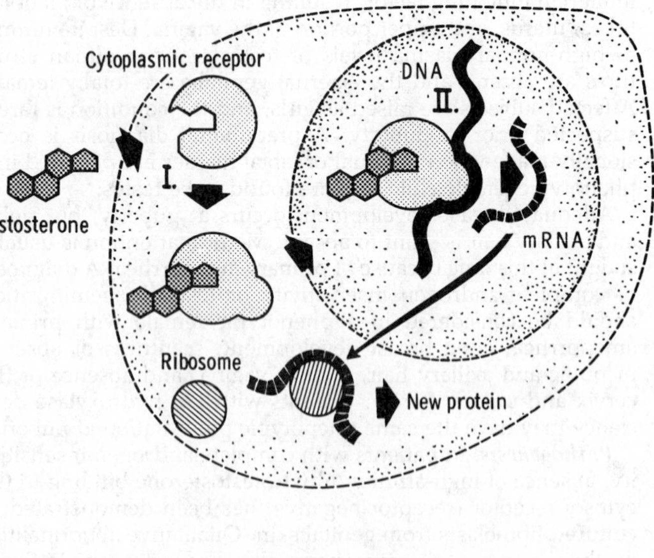

I. Abnormalities affecting binding to the cytosol receptor

A. Quantitative

1. Absent binding to cytosol receptor

B. Qualitative

1. Thermolability
2. Failure of stabilization with sodium molybdate

II. Nuclear or post nuclear receptor binding defect

Figure 233–7. Illustration of the abnormalities of androgen action resulting in androgen insensitivity.

stabilization with sodium molybdate as in complete androgen insensitivity, have also been shown.

The mildest form of incomplete androgen insensitivity may be infertility in phenotypically normal men with either azoospermia or severe oligospermia. The mean plasma levels of LH and testosterone can be either normal or elevated. The most frequent finding in cultured genital skin fibroblasts is a decrease in androgen binding capacity to the androgen cytosol receptor by over 50 per cent in comparison to that found in normal skin samples. Recently a qualitative defect affecting failure of receptor stabilization has also been identified. A major unknown in this form of androgen resistance is its frequency as a cause of infertility.

Management and Therapy. Incomplete forms of androgen insensitivity can be distinguished biochemically from male pseudohermaphroditism with defects in testosterone biosynthesis. All of these conditions can have the same phenotypic presentation prior to puberty. In the absence of a demonstrable cytosol receptor abnormality, a decrease in the anabolic response to androgen administration, i.e., decreased nitrogen retention, may help clarify the diagnosis. True hermaphrodites most commonly have an XX karyotype and can often be distinguished on that basis. Incomplete androgen insensitivity in puberty commonly results in gynecomastia and varying degrees of virilization. Following puberty, a normal to elevated plasma testosterone level with a normal androstenedione-testosterone ratio as well as normal plasma progesterone and dehydroepiandrosterone levels will distinguish subjects with this condition from subjects with 17β-hydroxysteroid dehydrogenase deficiency, 17α-hydroxylase deficiency, and 3β-hydroxysteroid dehydrogenase deficiency who can have the same appearance. Those subjects with moderate to severe defects in masculinization of the external genitalia should be raised as females and if possible castrated before puberty because of the possibility of virilization. Estrogen therapy should be added at puberty. Those with mild hypospadias can be raised as males but will require surgery for correction of both the hypospadias and the gynecomastia.

Griffin JE, Leshen M, Wilson, JD: Androgen resistance syndromes. Am J Physiol 243:E-81–87, 1982. *A comprehensive review, particularly of the biochemical abnormalities in complete and partial androgen insensitivity.*

5α-REDUCTASE DEFICIENCY. ***Clinical Presentation.*** In 1974, steroid 5α-reductase deficiency was first described as a cause of male pseudohermaphroditism in 38 subjects from a large Dominican kindred and two sibs from Dallas. This condition has subsequently been described in subjects throughout the world. Most subjects have perineal hypospadias with separate urethral and vaginal openings within a urogenital sinus. Rarely, a blind vaginal pouch opens into the urethra. The patients have an epididymis, vas deferens, and seminal vesicles. The incidence of cryptorchidism is significantly higher in childhood than adulthood, suggesting that it is not uncommon for the testes to descend during puberty in this condition.

The pubertal events include deepening of the voice, development of a muscular habitus, growth of the phallus, rugation and hyperpigmentation of the scrotum, and testicular descent. The prostate is small or absent, even in elderly subjects. Subjects have erections with ejaculation from the perineal urethra. Facial hair is decreased or absent and body hair is decreased. In only one subject has mild acne been reported, and none have temporal hairline recession.

Pathogenesis. The enzyme Δ^4,5α-reductase with NADPH as a cofactor catalyzes the reduction of the double bond at the 4–5 position of both C19 steroids, such as testosterone, and C21 steroids. It is present in high quantities in the liver and peripheral tissues, particularly the sebaceous glands, hair follicles, and skin of the external genitalia, where it actively converts testosterone to dihydrotestosterone, a more potent androgen. In subjects with 5α-reductase deficiency, the biochemical abnormality is characterized by normal to elevated levels of plasma testosterone with decreased levels of dihydrotestosterone resulting in an increased testosterone to dihydrotestosterone ratio. There is decreased production of the urinary 5α-reduced metabolites of testosterone, i.e., androsterone and androstanediol, causing elevated etiocholanolone-androsterone and etiocholanediol-androstanediol ratios. The urinary 5α-reduced metabolites of C21 and C19 steroids other than testosterone, i.e., cortisol, corticosterone, 11β-hydroxyandrostenedione, and androstenedione, are also decreased. Diminished 5α-reductase activity has been demonstrated both in skin slices and in fibroblasts cultured from genital skin. Based on consanguinity and biochemical data of parents, who demonstrate an intermediate defect in enzyme activity, an autosomal recessive inheritance has been demonstrated.

Male pseudohermaphrodites with 5α-reductase deficiency represent a unique clinical model, defining major actions for testosterone and dihydrotestosterone in male sexual differentiation and development. Since the developmental defect is limited to the external genitalia and prostate, the normal development of these structures appears to be effected through the actions of dihydrotestosterone. In contrast, wolffian differentiation develops normally and appears to be a testosterone-mediated function (Fig. 233–8). At puberty the affected males develop rugation and hyperpigmentation of the scrotum,

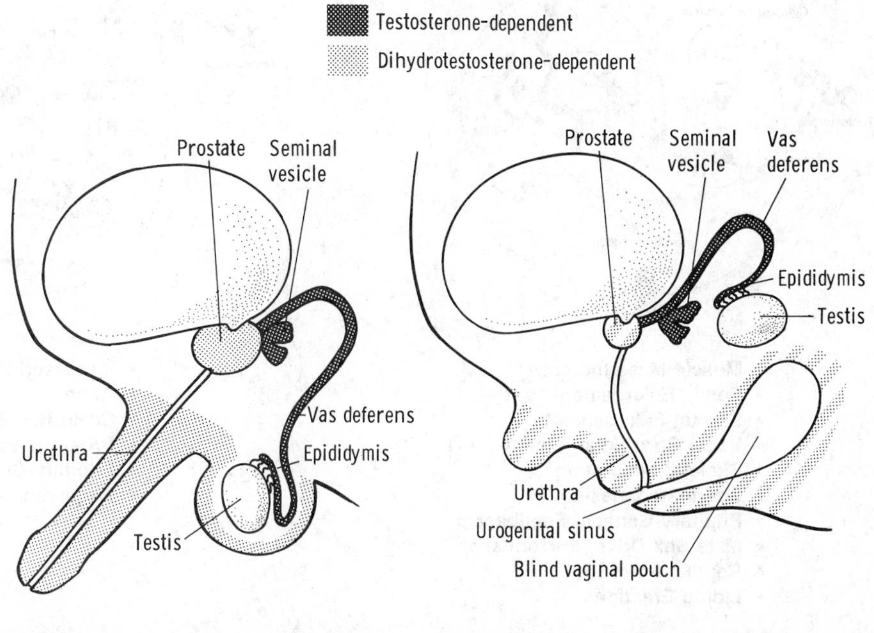

Figure 233–8. Illustration of the hypothesis for the specific actions of testosterone and dihydrotestosterone in male sexual differentiation in utero.

growth of the phallus, an increase in muscle mass, and deepening of the voice (Fig. 233–9). Their ultimate height is also similar to that of their fathers and normal male sibs. Thus the aforementioned pubertal events are mainly effected through the actions of testosterone. In contrast, prostatic development or enlargement, acne, normal male facial and body hair, and temporal recession of the hairline do not occur in affected males, and appear to be effected mainly through the actions of dihydrotestosterone.

Since both androgens share a common cytosol receptor, it is puzzling that the effects of dihydrotestosterone in dihydrotestosterone-dependent areas are not mimicked by testosterone. Two possible explanations can be submitted: (1) the cytosol receptor at certain target sites is modified so that it favors 5α-dihydrotestosterone over testosterone or (2) the 5α-dihydrotestosterone receptor complex has a higher affinity for the acceptor sites in chromatin.

In affected subjects with descended testes, testicular biopsy has demonstrated complete spermatogenesis; thus testosterone may be more important than dihydrotestosterone in the process of spermatogenesis. The question of fertility, however, remains unanswered. The cryptorchid testes of most subjects demonstrate seminiferous tubular damage with either Sertoli cells only or aberrant spermatogenesis. Plasma LH is increased despite normal to high plasma levels of testosterone, suggesting a role for dihydrotestosterone in the negative feedback control of LH. The elevated plasma LH levels correlate with the microscopic findings of Leydig cell hyperplasia. Plasma FSH levels are also elevated, which may be a consequence of the cryptorchidism with its damaging effect on spermatogenesis. Affected males have erections, with ejaculation from the perineal urethra, and thus these male sexual functions appear to be mediated through the actions of testosterone, either directly or via conversion to estradiol in the brain. Conversely, administration of pharmacologic amounts of dihydrotesterone causes a substantial decrease in plasma testosterone with subsequent loss of libido and impotence.

A documented gender change from female to male in untreated affected subjects from the Dominican kindred underscores the importance of testosterone exposure of the brain in utero, the early postnatal period, and at puberty in the determination of male gender identity. Theoretically, "masculinization" of the brain occurs under the influence of testosterone and, together with activation of testosterone-mediated puberty, a male gender identity develops, overriding the female sex of rearing. It has been proposed that gender identity becomes fixed by 18 months to 4 years of age, around the time of language development. However, from studies with these patients, it appears that the development of gender identity in man is continually evolving throughout childhood and adolescence, becoming fixed with puberty.

Imperato-McGinley J, Peterson RE, Gautier T: Male pseudohermaphroditism secondary to 5α-reductase deficiency: A review. *In* Resko J (ed.): Fetal Endocrinology. New York, Academic Press, 1981, pp 359–382. *A review of the cases reported, as well as the clinical and biochemical findings in this interesting experiment of nature.*

Imperto-McGinley J, Peterson RE, Gautier T, Sturla E: The impact of androgens on the evolution of male gender identity. *In* Kogan SJ, Hafez ESE (eds.): Clinics in Andrology: Pediatric Andrology. Vol. 7. The Hague, Matinus Nihoff, 1981, pp 99–105. *A study of gender change from female to male in a large kindred with 5α-reductase deficiency—a comprehensive theory concerning the aquisition of gender identity in males.*

XX Males and True Hermaphroditism

XX Males

Clinical Presentation. Since the first case report in 1962, reports of approximately 50 cases of XX males have been published, including members within the same family. A rare condition, the incidence in newborn males is estimated to be 1 in 20,000. Classically XX adult males have short stature, a normal-sized penis, small firm testes generally less than 2 cm, and infertility. One third have gynecomastia. The phenotypic appearance resembles that of males with Klinefelter's syndrome (XXY) with the notable exception that XX males are shorter in stature, even shorter than the average male. In general, the histologic features of the testes also resemble those of subjects with Klinefelter's syndrome. The seminiferous tubules of the testes are hyalinized and contain only Sertoli cells or occasionally a few immature spermatogonia, correlating clinically with azoospermia or oligospermia. The Leydig cells are hyperplastic. Levels of FSH and LH are elevated, with decreased plasma testosterone and increased plasma estradiol levels. More recently, XX children with bilateral testes have been reported with ambiguous genitalia, suggesting a phenotypic spectrum in this condition.

Pathogenesis. The etiologic factors for the expression of

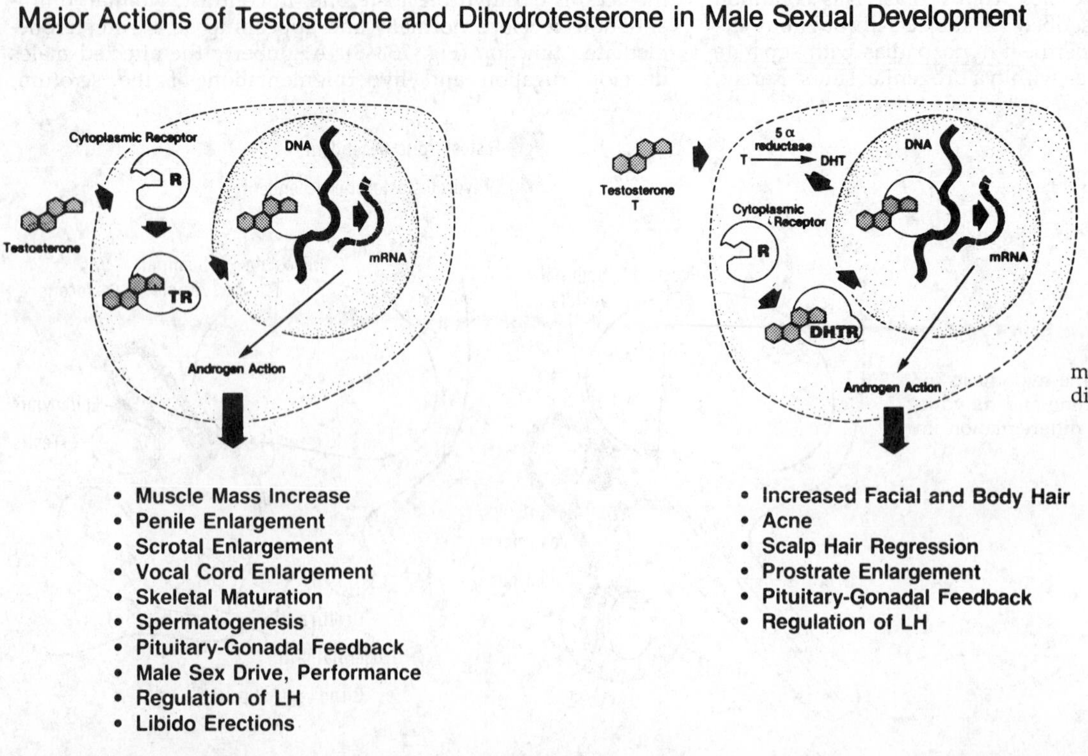

Figure 233–9. Illustration of the major actions of testosterone and dihydrotestosterone at puberty.

masculinity in XX individuals have been the subject of much speculation. Three possible mechanisms have been proposed—(1) translocation of part of the Y chromosome to the X chromosome or to an autosome, (2) undetected mosaicism XX/XY or XXY, or (3) a mutant autosomal gene determining maleness in an XX individual. Studies of H-Y antigen in subjects with this condition have revealed a positive titer. Recently, chromosome preparations from 8 of 12 46 XX males were clearly distinguishable from normal 46 XX female preparations secondary to alterations in shape, as well as an increase in the tip of the short arm of the X chromosome. DNA digests from the nuclei of cells from testes of an XX male have demonstrated Y-specific DNA fragments. Thus, the condition in a high percentage of 46 XX males appears to be a consequence of a paternal X-Y interchange affecting the testes-determining area of the Y chromosome.

True Hermaphroditism

Clinical Presentation. The morphologic expression of true hemaphroditism is the presence of both ovarian and testicular tissue, with each gonad containing its corresponding gamete. Most subjects have ambiguous genitalia, although approximately 7 per cent of true hermaphrodites have normal female external genitalia, and 12 per cent have a penile urethra; 75 per cent of affected subjects are raised as males. Although a rare form of intersex, it is relatively common among the Bantu of South Africa. The most common gonadal associations are an ovary and testis or an ovotestis and ovary, each occurring in 30 per cent of cases. Bilateral ovotestes occur in 20 per cent of the cases; an ovotestis and testis in only 10 per cent. The ovotestis frequently has ovarian and testicular tissue arranged in an end-to-end fashion. Although the ovarian portion is usually histologically normal, the testicular portion is clearly histologically abnormal, and spermatogenesis has never been observed. Gonadal tumors occur in approximately 2 per cent.

A fallopian tube is always found adjacent to an ovary. A fallopian tube is also most commonly found adjacent to an ovotestis; an epididymis is present in approximately one third of the cases. A uterus is present in approximately 90 per cent of affected subjects. In familial reports of true hermaphroditism, however, there is no uterus in the majority of those affected, and there are bilateral descended ovotestes.

With puberty, variable virilization and feminization occur. About half of affected subjects will menstruate; in those raised as males with mild or moderate hypospadias or a penile urethra, menstruation can present as cyclic hematuria. Gynecomastia will develop in 80 per cent of subjects. Pregnancy and childbirth have been reported in true hermaphrodites following removal of testicular tissue and correction of the external genitalia. A few subjects with functional testicular tissue are fertile.

Pathogenesis. A 46 XX complement is present in approximately two thirds of cases, XX/XY mosaicism in one third of cases, and 46 XY complement in one tenth of the cases. XX true hermaphrodites have been reported to be H-Y antigen positive, suggesting translocation of Y chromosomal material to either the X chromosome or an autosome, or undetected XX/XY chimerism. Although they are H-Y antigen positive, a reduced titer has been reported, suggesting random inactivation of an X chromosome that bears the translocated H-Y locus. When cells were cultured from the testicular portion of the ovotestis of an XX true hermaphrodite, they were H-Y antigen positive, whereas cells cultured from the ovarian portion were H-Y antigen negative. These observations suggest that the ovotestes arise from an H-Y+/H-Y− mosaic primordium. A reported case of true hermaphroditism in a subject whose brother and paternal uncle were XX males suggests that XX males and XX true hermaphrodites may be variants of the same condition.

Management and Therapy. The sex assignment in true hermaphroditism diagnosed in infancy and childhood is best determined by the appearance of the external genitalia, together with the gonadal tissue and internal structures. If an ovary-ovotestis and a uterus are present, the ovotestis and any male internal structures should be removed and feminizing surgery of the external genitalia performed. If bilateral ovotestes are present, and if a good line of demarcation is seen between ovarian and testicular tissue, the testicular portion should be removed, the genitalia surgically feminized, and the child raised as female. If a testis is present on one side and an ovotestis on the contralateral side, the testis should be brought into the scrotum and the child raised as male if the external genitalia can be surgically corrected. If an ovary is present on one side and a testis on the contralateral side, the sex of rearing should be decided by evaluation of the appearance of the external and internal sex structures, and appropriate surgical correction should be performed. Peripubertal or postpubertal surgical correction of the internal and external sex structures should depend exclusively upon the gender identity of the affected individual. Although testicular tumor formation is rare, if the individual is to be raised as male the testis should be brought into the scrotum, so that periodic examination can be carried out.

De La Chapelle A: The etiology of maleness in XX men. Hum Genet 58:105–116, 1981. *A review of clinical characteristics and hypotheses in the occurrence of this unique condition.*

Van Niekerk WA: True hermaphroditism—An analytic review with a report of 3 new cases. Am J Obstet Gynecol 126:890, 1976. *An extensive review of all reported cases to 1976, covering clinical presentation and etiology.*

Female Pseudohermaphroditism

Female pseudohermaphroditism can result from either fetal or maternal androgenic influences (Table 233–3). Cases of undetermined etiology have also been described.

Congenital Adrenal Hyperplasia—Virilizing Forms

Three adrenal enzyme defects, 21-hydroxylase deficiency, 11β-hydroxylase deficiency, and 3β-hydroxysteroid dehydrogenase deficiency, can result in increased androgen production in utero with virilization of the female fetus. They are the virilizing forms of congenital adrenal hyperplasia (Fig. 233–6). 21-Hydroxylase and 11β-hydroxylase deficiency can result in severe virilization of the female fetus, whereas the virilization reported with 3β-hydroxysteroid dehydrogenase deficiency is very mild. Since 3β-hydroxysteroid dehydrogenase deficiency is also a cause of male pseudohermaphroditism, it is discussed in the section Male Pseudohermaphroditism, as are the nonvirilizing forms of congenital adrenal hyperplasia. The enzyme defects causing virilization of the female fetus result in decreased cortisol production, with increased pituitary ACTH and resultant adrenal androgen overproduction. In the genotypic female, since ovaries and not testes are present, müllerian inhibiting factor is not produced, and the internal structures are female, i.e., uterus and fallopian tubes. Despite the increase in androgen production severe enough to masculinize the external genitalia, wolffian differentiation has never been described. Affected 46 XY males with either 21-hydroxylase or 11β-hydroxylase deficiency appear phenotypically normal at birth.

21-HYDROXYLASE DEFICIENCY. ***Clinical Features.*** First de-

TABLE 233–3. CLASSIFICATION OF CAUSES OF FEMALE PSEUDOHERMAPHRODITISM

I. Androgenic influences
  A. Fetal
    1. Congenital adrenogenital syndrome:
      a. 21-Hydroxylase deficiency;
      b. 11β-Hydroxylase deficiency;
      c. 3β-Hydroxysteroid dehydrogenase:Δ^{5-4} isomerase deficiency
  B. Maternal
    1. Excess maternal androgen production
    2. Maternal ingestion of virilizing substances
II. Idiopathic

scribed in 1950, 21-hydroxylase deficiency is the most common cause of ambiguous genitalia in 46 XX infants. Its incidence varies from approximately 1 in 300 births in Alaskan Eskimos to 1 in 15,000 births in Caucasians in Wisconsin. The spectrum of masculinization varies from female infants with minimal clitoromegaly and fusion of the labioscrotal folds to infants with a penile urethra and the appearance of a cryptorchid male. Classically, if affected XX children are untreated in infancy, there is rapid acceleration of growth, enlargement of the clitoris, increase in muscle mass, precocious development of pubic axillary and body hair, and advancement of bone age. Although they are tall in childhood, premature closure of the epiphyses eventually results in short stature in adulthood. At the time of expected puberty, there is absence of breast development and menstruation. Untreated males with this condition also show precocious maturation and are short in stature in adulthood. The excessive androgen production can inhibit gonadotropin secretion, so that untreated adult males, although strongly virilized, can have small soft testes and azoospermia. However, because of the adrenal androgen excess, they are capable of having erections. Frequently, however, true puberty occurs in untreated males with normal FSH and LH secretion, testicular enlargement, and spermatogenesis. ACTH-dependent testicular "tumors" have been described and can occur either unilaterally or bilaterally; most probably they are of adrenal origin.

Two forms of 21-hydroxylase deficiency have been described, a simple form and a salt-losing form. Infants with the salt-losing form usually have an adrenal crisis within the first two weeks of life. Infants with the simple form do not show signs of adrenal crisis; ambiguity of the external genitalia is the most prominent feature.

Pathogenesis. 21-Hydroxylase deficiency results in decreased synthesis of cortisol with consequent increase in ACTH and increase in plasma progesterone, 17α-hydroxyprogesterone, and C19 androgens (dehydroepiandrosterone, androstenedione, and testosterone; Fig. 233–6). In the newborn, determination of plasma 17α-hydroxyprogesterone is the test most diagnostic for this condition. The increased adrenal androgen production in the female fetus in utero results in virilization of the external genitalia. In the salt-losing form, there is a deficiency of aldosterone production. However, an additive factor in the salt loss may be due to increased production of progesterone and 17α-hydroxyprogesterone, which act as aldosterone antagonists.

The gene for 21-hydroxylase deficiency is closely linked to the HLA-B locus of chromosome 6. Obligate carrier parents and sibs predicted to be heterozygotes by HLA typing frequently demonstrate increased 17α-hydroxyprogesterone levels in response to a one-hour ACTH stimulation test. Although the tests are extremely helpful in heterozygote detection, they are not uniformly conclusive. Family members, both males and females, have also been identified who have biochemical evidence of 21-hydroxylase deficiency but are without signs of virilization, hirsutism, amenorrhea, or infertility. These individuals are designated as having a cryptic form of 21-hydroxylase deficiency. It is proposed that they are genetic compounds, the result of two recessive gene defects, a severe and a mild defect in 21-hydroxylation. Why they are clinically asymptomatic remains unanswered. A late-onset or attenuated variant of 21-hydroxylase deficiency has also recently been documented in adult women with hirsutism, or virilization and menstrual irregularities. HLA typing and ACTH testing of affected subjects' parents and sibs with this form also document linkage to the HLA-B locus of chromosome 6, as in the classic form of congenital adrenal hyperplasia.

Management and Therapy. Affected females with 21-hydroxylase deficiency have ovaries and normal internal female structures with potential for fertility. Therefore, diagnosis and treatment should be carried out early and the child appropriately treated and raised as a female. Surgical correction of the masculinized external genitalia should be performed early so that gender confusion does not occur later on in childhood and adolescence. Medical therapy involves adequate glucocorticoid replacement therapy to lower ACTH secretion and to suppress adrenal androgen excess. Overtreatment should be avoided to prevent the signs and symptoms of glucocorticoid excess, which can lead to growth retardation.

Overt salt losers must be given mineralocorticoid as well as glucocorticoid replacement therapy. Many affected subjects without overt signs of adrenal crisis have impaired mineralocorticoid production, characterized by decreased sodium content and plasma volume with resultant increase in plasma renin. The increased plasma renin has been postulated to increase release of ACTH, necessitating more glucocorticoid replacement therapy. Thus mineralocorticoid supplementation should be considered in any subject with increase of plasma renin, despite the absence of signs of adrenal insufficiency.

Assessment of adequate therapy in a child is made on the basis of maintaining normal growth velocity, without signs of excess of either androgen or exogenous glucocorticoid. Monitoring plasma 17α-hydroxyprogesterone and plasma androgens has been helpful in regulating the glucocorticoid dosage; normalization of plasma androstenedione is the most reliable predictor of optimal therapy.

11β-HYDROXYLASE DEFICIENCY. ***Clinical Features.*** In 1955 a deficiency of the enzyme 11β-hydroxylase was identified as a cause of congenital adrenal hyperplasia with hypertension. To date approximately 60 cases have been described. In females with 21-hydroxylase deficiency, the enzyme deficiency at birth results in normal female genitalia to varying degrees of masculinization of the external genitalia. Adolescence results in mild hirsutism, clitoral hypertrophy, and irregular menses to severe virilization. Males with this condition show precocious male sexual maturation but develop gynecomastia at puberty. The cause of the gynecomastia is not known, but it has been postulated to be secondary to elevated plasma desoxycorticosterone levels.

Pathogenesis. 11β-Hydroxylase deficiency results in decreased cortisol production, which causes an increase in ACTH, in C19 androgen secretion, and in desoxycorticosterone production (Fig. 233–6). Elevation of the plasma 11-desoxycortisol level is diagnostic of this enzyme deficiency and distinguishes it from 21-hydroxylase deficiency. Plasma cortisol as well as the urinary cortisol metabolites tetrahydrocortisone and tetrahydrocortisol can be normal to low. Urinary 17-ketosteroids, reflecting adrenal androgen overproduction, and urinary 17-hydroxysteroids, reflecting elevated levels of plasma 11-desoxycortisol, are increased. Excretion of pregnanetriol, a metabolite of 17α-hydroxyprogesterone, is usually normal or slightly increased. Plasma desoxycorticosterone is increased as is its urinary metabolite tetrahydrodesoxycorticosterone, while corticosterone and aldosterone are decreased. The increased production of desoxycorticosterone results in salt retention, increased plasma volume, hypertension, and decreased plasma renin. Some affected subjects are not hypertensive and have a deficiency of the enzyme that appears to be limited to the 17α-hydroxylated pathway, with normal levels of plasma desoxycorticosterone and its urinary metabolites. This has been explained by postulating the presence of either two 11β-hydroxylase enzyme systems or two different regulatory systems for 17α-hydroxylated steroids and for 17-desoxysteroids.

Management and Therapy. Glucocorticoid replacement therapy will effect biochemical normalization, decrease blood pressure, and arrest precocious development. In females, surgical correction of the external genitalia should be carried out, as in females with 21-hydroxylase deficiency.

Virilization of the Female Fetus Secondary to Excess Maternal Androgen Production or Exogenous Maternal Administration of Virilizing Hormones

Masculinization of the female infant has been demonstrated in mothers with ovarian luteomas, virilizing adrenal tumors, and untreated maternal congenital adrenal hyperplasia. Why virilization of the female fetus does not occur in all states of maternal hyperandrogenicity may be related to the onset and the degree of hyperandrogenicity and the potency of the androgens secreted. The placenta may also offer some protection for the fetus by aromatization of the maternal androgens to estrogens.

Administration of testosterone or its derivatives to pregnant women has been associated with virilization of the female fetus. These substances stimulate virilization of the external genitalia with no effect on differentiation of the wolffian ductal system. A causal relationship of the progestational agents progesterone, medroxyprogesterone, and 17α-hydroxyprogesterone has not been definitely proven. Paradoxic masculinization of the female fetus associated with maternal administration of diethylstilbestrol early in pregnancy has been reported rarely. The degree of genital masculinization is correlated with the time of initiation of treatment. The mechanism for the genital masculinization has been postulated to be secondary to inhibition of the enzyme 3β-hydroxysteroid dehydrogenase:Δ^{5-4} isomerase by diethylstilbestrol, with consequent elevation of the weak androgen dehydroepiandrosterone and possibly other Δ^5-androgenic steroids.

New M, Levine LS: Congenital adrenal hyperplasia and related conditions. *In* Stanbury JB, et al (eds.): Metabolic Basis of Inherited Disease. 5th ed. New York, McGraw Hill Book Company, 1983, Ch. 47. *Contains an excellent review of 21-hydroxylase deficiency with particular emphasis on genetics.*

234. THE TESTIS

Mortimer B. Lipsett

INTRODUCTION

Fetal Development

The primordial gonad arises in the urogenital ridge from intermediate mesoderm during the fifth week of gestation (Ch. 233). Early in its development, the bipotential primitive gonad (Fig. 234–1) is composed of two unipotential mesodermal primordia, each with a distinct physiologic as well as morphologic capacity: (1) a cortical component, consisting of the germinal epithelium; and (2) a medullary component, made up of the primary sex cords derived from the germinal epithelium, and mesonephric and blastemal elements. A third constituent, the primordial germ cell, which appears to be bipotential, arises in an extragonadal site and migrates to the gonads. Under the influence of the Y organizer, a surface protein of cells carrying the Y chromosome, the medullary component differentiates as a testis (Fig. 234–1). The cortical component can differentiate as an ovary only in the absence of Y organizer.

When the gonad destined to become a testis begins to differentiate in a male direction during the seventh to eighth week of embryonic life, the cortical component involutes. Within the medulla, seminiferous tubules form from the primary sex cords and anastomose with the rete testis and testicular ducts, and Leydig cells develop. Leydig cells proliferate predominantly during the first half of gestation, but then gradually decrease in number and involute after birth. Leydig cells acquire the capacity to synthesize testosterone, and this steroid hormone has been found in the fetal testis. At the time of pubescence morphologic differentiation of Leydig cells occurs, and testosterone production is greatly increased. Fetal development of the testis and the accessory sex structures is discussed more fully in Ch. 233.

Chemistry and Physiology of the Testicular Hormones

The testicular hormone *testosterone,* secreted from the Leydig cell, has the primary role in the development and maintenance of the male accessory sex organs, prostate, and seminal vesicles, in the elaboration of semen, and in the development of masculine secondary sexual characteristics. These properties define a class of substances, the androgens; the important androgen secreted by the testis is testosterone. The 5α-reduced derivative of testosterone, 5α-dihydrotestosterone, is the active form of the hormone at the nuclear receptor within the male accessory sex structures, and is responsible for inducing growth of these organs.

The adrenal cortex secretes little testosterone. The weak androgenic potency of adrenocortical steroids such as androstenedione and dehydroepiandrosterone can be attributed to their conversion to testosterone in small yield.

Healthy young men secrete about 7 mg of testosterone per day. Testosterone originates in the Leydig cells, although the seminiferous tubule has a weak capacity for testosterone synthesis. Clinical signs of androgen deficiency are absent and testosterone secretion is normal in certain testicular disorders in man associated with defective seminiferous tubules but with intact Leydig cells.

Pathways for the biosynthesis of testosterone by the Leydig cell resemble those in other steroid-synthesizing glands (see Fig. 233–6). Precursors such as acetate and low-density lipoprotein cholesterol are converted enzymatically to testosterone via 17-hydroxypregnenolone and 17-hydroxyprogesterone. The Leydig cell can also aromatize testosterone to estradiol. In adult men, 10 to 15 μg of estradiol is secreted daily; an additional 25 to 30 μg is produced peripherally by aromatization of testosterone and from estrone formed from adrenal androstenedione (Fig. 234–2). Blood estrogen in the male then depends on testicular secretion and rates of peripheral aromatization of adrenal and testicular precursors. Estrone, however, is predominantly a product of adrenal cortical secretions.

The liver is the main site of catabolism of testosterone and of the conjugation of its known metabolites with glucuronic or sulfuric acid; other tissues play a less important role in its metabolism. The major identifiable urinary metabolites are the 17-ketosteroids, androsterone and etiocholanolone, which are excreted principally as glucuronides and account for 20 to 40 per cent of the testosterone secreted. A small amount of testosterone (0.2 to 2 per cent) is excreted as testosterone glucuronide.

Spermatogenesis and the Sertoli Cell

SPERMATOGENESIS. About 90 per cent of the mass of the testis is due to the seminiferous tubules where spermatogenesis takes place. The seminiferous epithelium is composed of the germ cells and the nonproliferating Sertoli cells. In the human the duration of spermatogenesis is about 74 days and includes mitosis of the spermatogonia, meiosis in the subsequent generation of spermatocytes to reduce the diploid number of chromosomes to the haploid number, and finally transformation of the spermatocyte to the mature spermatozoon. These processes depend critically on normal Sertoli cell function. It has been difficult to discern clearly the effect of hormones at any specific level of spermatogenesis. The germ cell does not possess hormone receptors and thus cannot be a direct hormonal target.

SERTOLI CELL. In the human the Sertoli cell does not undergo mitosis after birth. There are inter-Sertoli cell tight junctions so that the Sertoli cells constitute a barrier between the germ cells and the external environment. Macromolecules can thus enter the Sertoli cell compartment only with difficulty. The various stages of spermatogenesis are arranged within the Sertoli cells so that the final release of the spermatogonium occurs at the apical end of the Sertoli cell into the lumen.

The Sertoli cell is a biosynthetically active tissue. It is responsible for secretion of the luminal fluid of the testis. It synthesizes a variety of proteins: androgen-binding protein, closely similar to that synthesized by the liver; plasminogen activator; ceruloplasmin; transferrin; and others of unknown function. In effect, the Sertoli cell maintains a culture medium for the germ cell, synthesizing those same proteins that have been found necessary to maintain many cells in plasma-free tissue culture.

The Sertoli cell is a target for two hormones, follicle-stimulating hormone (FSH) and androgen. FSH is apparently active

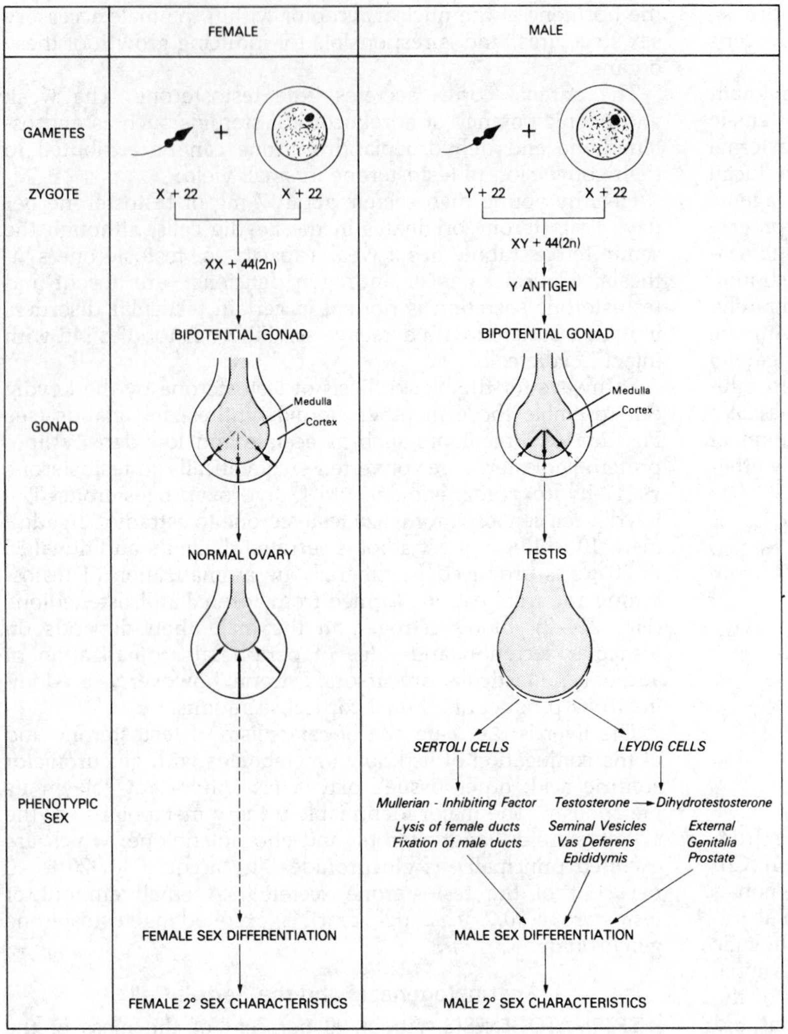

Figure 234–1. Diagrammatic scheme of human sex determination and differentiation.

only at initiation of spermatogenesis when it demonstrates the same features of other peptide hormones: surface receptors, generation of cAMP, and phosphorylation of intracellular proteins. The maintenance of Sertoli cell function and thus of spermatogenesis is dependent on high levels of androgen and the classic androgen receptor has been found in the Sertoli cell. In hypophysectomized men, spermatogenesis can be maintained by administration of human chorionic gonadotropin (HCG), intratesticular implants of androgen, or high doses of androgen, resulting in each case in a high intratesticular concentration of androgen. For optimal spermatogenesis, FSH may be needed.

There are multiple interactions between the compartments of the testis and between these compartments and the hypothalamic-pituitary unit (Fig. 234–3). The roles of the estrogen and androgen receptors in the Leydig cell during normal physiologic circumstances have not been clarified, although a high dose of estrogen can directly decrease several Leydig cell enzymes necessary for testosterone synthesis. In spite of these many new data, the relationship between luteinizing hormone (LH) and the Leydig cell remains the critical factor, and consideration of plasma levels of LH and testosterone will clarify most clinical situations.

Testosterone exerts a negative feedback on LH secretion, and it seems likely that both androgen and estrogen receptors modulate LH secretion. The hypothalamus and the pituitary have the capacity to metabolize testosterone to dihydrotestosterone and estradiol. Plasma FSH also is suppressed by testosterone, but an additional factor, inhibin, a polypeptide of about 20,000 daltons derived from the Sertoli cell, also modulates

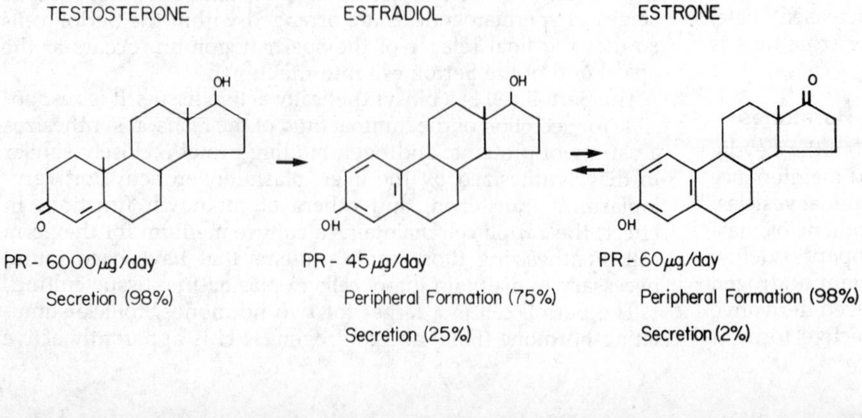

Figure 234–2. Production rates (PR) and origins of estradiol and estrone in men.

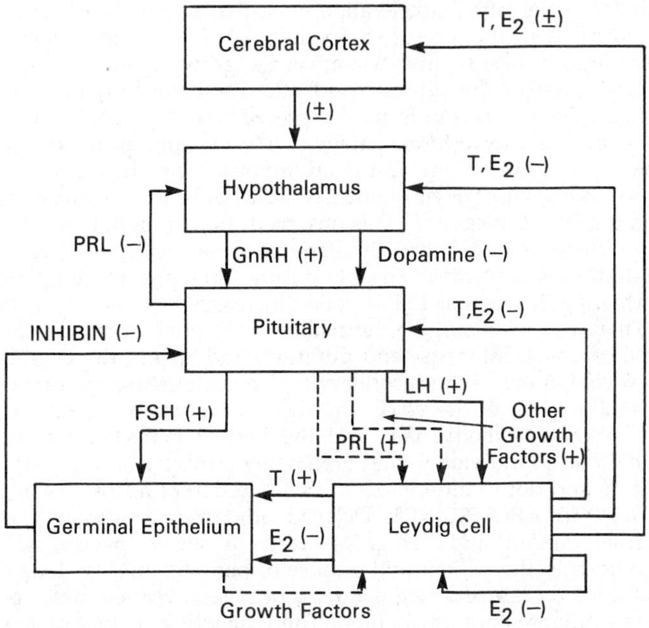

Figure 234–3. Diagram of interrelations between hypothalamus, pituitary and testis. Dotted lines indicate those actions that remain somewhat equivocal. GnRH = gonadotropin-releasing hormone; PRL = prolactin; T = testosterone; E_2 = estradiol.

FSH secretion at the pituitary level. Thus plasma FSH and LH levels are high in the absence of Leydig cell secretions, but FSH alone is increased when there is severe seminiferous tubule disease. Whether this is an important normal regulatory mechanism is not clear, but pulsatile injections of testosterone and estradiol at physiologic levels will also maintain normal plasma FSH in the castrated experimental animal. Prolactin at high levels directly inhibits the secretion of FSH and LH and may modulate Leydig cell secretions. The brain, as well, can alter hypothalamic-pituitary function.

Evaluation of Testicular Function

CLINICAL ASSESSMENT. Adequacy of androgen production can be estimated from the degree of development of the penis and scrotum, size of the prostate, general maturity and status of male secondary sex characteristics, habitus and skeletal proportions, muscular development, and sexual potency. This assessment has limitations in the mature adult, however, because regression of secondary sexual characteristics is slow even after complete loss of Leydig cell function. Furthermore, facial and body hair can be highly variable owing to genetic differences in the distribution of the pilosebaceous apparatus and differences in responsiveness of these skin appendages to hormonal stimulation. In the American Indian, the black African, and some Orientals facial and body hair is sparse or absent despite normal testicular function and plasma testosterone concentration.

URINARY 17-KETOSTEROIDS. About 80 per cent of the urinary 17-ketosteroids (17-KS) is derived from adrenocortical steroids that have little intrinsic androgenic activity. Less than 3 mg daily is derived from Leydig cell secretions. Androsterone and etiocholanolone, the principal urinary metabolites of testosterone, are also metabolites of adrenocortical 11-deoxysteroids. Thus, since urinary 17-KS are an index chiefly of adrenal cortical function, they cannot be used to assess testicular function. Testosterone, which has a hydroxyl group at carbon atom 17, is not a 17-ketosteroid.

The normal range of 17-KS excretion in men is 8 to 20 mg per day (mean, 15 mg). Before puberty only small amounts are detectable in urine. In adult men and women after the third decade, urinary 17-KS decreases gradually owing to lessening adrenal secretion of dehydroepiandrosterone. The excretion of 17-KS may be reduced in eunuchoidism, although the values obtained in such patients are often within the normal range. In panhypopituitarism the function of both the testis and the adrenal cortex is impaired, and the excretion of urinary 17-KS is greatly decreased. Low values are also frequently found in chronic debilitating disease and renal insufficiency. Measurement of urinary 17-KS has little clinical value in diseases of the testis or adrenal cortex except as a screening test for congenital adrenal hyperplasia and adrenal tumors (see Ch. 229).

PLASMA AND URINARY TESTOSTERONE. Measurement of plasma, salivary or urinary testosterone, the last as the glucuronide conjugate, provides reliable indices of Leydig cell function. The production rate of testosterone can be estimated, but the method is too cumbersome for routine use. Young adult males excrete 40 to 100 μg per day of testosterone glucuronide; women excrete less than 6 μg, and boys before puberty less than 0.5 μg. The concentration of testosterone in plasma of young adult men ranges from 0.3 to 1.2 μg per deciliter (mean 0.65 μg per deciliter), and the concentration in women varies from 0.034 to 0.06 μg per deciliter (mean, 0.054 μg per deciliter). More than 98 per cent of testosterone in plasma is bound to a specific β-globulin, sex-steroid binding globulin, and thus only 1 to 2 per cent is available for diffusion into cells. The administration of HCG to adult men induces a rise in plasma and urinary testosterone; this procedure has been used to assess the responsiveness of the Leydig cell and to distinguish between primary and secondary testicular disease.

PLASMA AND URINARY GONADOTROPINS. Gonadotropin releasing hormone (GnRH) is secreted in pulsatile fashion, and this results in marked fluctuations of plasma LH and only small changes in FSH. In normal men, there may be 8 to 15 LH secreting episodes per 24 hours, and LH levels may vary from 40 to 250 per cent of the mean level. In practice, this means that at least three measurements are necessary to estimate mean LH levels. Mean plasma FSH concentration is 12 mIU per milliliter (range, 4 to 27 mIU per milliliter). The mean LH concentration is 9 mIU per milliliter (range, 4 to 19 mIU per milliliter). Increased excretion or plasma concentrations of these hormones suggest primary testicular disease; isolated increases of FSH point to severe disease of the germinal epithelium. The lower level of sensitivity of most of the immunoassays is such that a gonadotropin concentration in the lower part of the normal range cannot be distinguished from decreased levels. Plasma LH can now be bioassayed as well, and the ratio of bioassayable LH and radioimmunologic LH will vary according to hormonal status. A case of apparently biologically inactive but fully immunoperative LH has been reported.

ASSESSMENT OF HYPOTHALAMIC-PITUITARY GONADOTROPIN RELEASE. Clomiphene citrate, an analogue of the nonsteroidal estrogen chlorotrianisene, is an estrogen antagonist and competes with estrogen at pituitary and/or hypothalamic receptors. When administered to normal men by mouth, 100 to 200 mg per day for five to seven days, it evokes a mean increase in the concentration of plasma FSH of 130 per cent and of plasma LH of 160 per cent. It also induces a rise in urinary FSH and LH and of plasma testosterone. Little or no increase in FSH or LH secretion is elicited in men with pituitary disease.

The identification and synthesis of the hypothalamic decapeptide GnRH have enabled the physician to establish pituitary responsiveness directly (see Ch. 225). It has been valuable in distinguishing between pituitary and hypothalamic disease. In general, a heightened response to GnRH indicates that there is a somewhat increased secretion of the gonadotropins and, by implication, decreased secretion of the testicular regulatory substance.

TESTICULAR BIOPSY. This procedure can be of great value in the diagnosis and prognosis of testicular disorders. It provides information concerning the gametogenic function of the testis—the status of the seminiferous tubules and the stages of spermatogenesis. Biopsy of the testis is of use in diagnosis of tubular disease, in assessing processes of sperm maturation, and in distinguishing azoospermia resulting from obstruction to the passage of sperm from azoospermia of other causes.

EXAMINATION OF SEMEN. Specimens of semen for analysis should be obtained two to three days after the last ejaculation. The volume of the specimen, the total number of sperm, and the motility and morphology of the sperm are determined. The minimal number of sperm necessary for normal fertility is unknown, but a total sperm count of 60 million may be considered normal. Less than this in general means decreased fertility. Because of the wide variations in sperm count among several specimens from the same patient, evaluation of therapy requires long control periods. Assessment of motility and morphology may require examination of many specimens to establish an accurate baseline. The quality of the sperm is only roughly quantified by these crude indices. When spermatogenesis is induced in men with hypogonadotropic hypogonadism, only a few million sperm are necessary for impregnation. The fertilizing capacity of sperm is now being assessed by penetration of the zona pellucida–free hamster ovum.

SEX CHROMATIN PATTERN. The number of X chromosomes in the sex chromosome complex can be assessed indirectly by cytologic methods because of sexual dimorphism in the nuclear structure of somatic cells. Preparations suitable for examination can be obtained from smears of buccal mucosa, skin biopsy specimens, or blood (see Ch. 35). This test is widely used in the investigation of abnormalities of sex differentiation, particularly of males with defective testes and azoospermia or severe oligospermia. When a chromatin-positive (female-type) nuclear sex chromatin pattern is detected in a phenotypic male with bilateral testes, it suggests that an associated congenital primary testicular disorder may be present.

Catt KJ, Harwood JP, Clayton RN, et al: Regulation of peptide hormone receptors and gonadal steroidogenesis. Recent Prog Horm Res 36:557, 1980. *The authors give a comprehensive review of testicular gonadotropin receptors and the events of steroid biosynthesis.*

Clermont Y: Kinetics of spermatogenesis in mammals: Seminiferous epithelium cycle and spermatogonial renewal. Physiol Rev 52:198, 1972. *This is a description of the mechanisms of spermatogenesis and provides a good framework for understanding the dynamics of the process.*

Lipsett MB: Regulation of testicular functions. Andrologia 8:43, 1976. *This article describes the interactions between steroids and gonadotropins in men.*

Lipsett MB: Physiology and pathophysiology of the Leydig cell. N Engl J Med 303:682, 1980. *The Leydig cell and its physiologic aberrations are described.*

Mainwaring WIP: The Mechanism of Androgen Action. New York, Springer-Verlag, 1977. *This monograph discusses the basic biochemistry of androgen at the cellular level.*

Parvinen M: Regulation of the seminiferous epithelium. Endocr Rev 3:404, 1982. *This is a comprehensive review of spermatogenesis in the human and the effects of hormones on the process.*

PUBERTAL DEVELOPMENT IN THE MALE

There are wide variations in the age of onset, duration, and sequence of events that characterize the biologic pattern of male puberty. In normal boys signs of puberty may appear at any age between 10 and 17 years; the average age of onset is 12 to 13 years. Once initiated, the major changes are usually completed or well advanced in three to four years; in a small percentage of normal persons, maturity is not attained until the age of 21, and rarely thereafter.

The stimulus for release of pituitary gonadotropin at puberty originates in the hypothalamus and is mediated by a neurohormonal secretion, GnRH. A certain level of physiologic maturation, presumably including the central nervous system, is necessary before this complex and incompletely understood mechanism is activated. This level of development can be best correlated with the degree of osseous and epiphyseal development (bone age) rather than with the chronologic age. Small amounts of FSH and LH are secreted by prepubertal children. The hypothalamic-pituitary-testicular negative feedback mechanism is operative and set at a low level before pubescence.

The sequence of events that marks the pubertal period starts with an acceleration in the growth of the testes and scrotum. The initial increase in testicular size, occurring between 11 and 12 years, is largely attributable to changes in the seminiferous tubules. After initial acceleration of testicular growth, there is an increase in the size of the penis, the appearance of pubic hair, which has at first a transverse growth, and gradual enlargement of the prostate and other accessory organs and glands. The increase in testis size precedes the first appearance of pubic hair by approximately two years and peak height velocity by three years, and is an important clinical feature in ascertaining onset of early puberty. With pubescence, pulsatile and increased release of LH is observed, first at night and then throughout the 24 hours. Similarly, plasma testosterone concentration is first increased only during the night, reaching its normal adult levels as LH secretion increases.

There is a wide range of normality of the pubertal process in time of onset, intensity, and duration, and also in the degree of development of the secondary sex characteristics. In normal men, the pitch of the voice, the size of the external genitalia, the amount of body hair, and the body habitus vary from individual to individual, and are largely attributable to genetic factors and not to differences in the secretion of testosterone.

DELAYED ADOLESCENCE. Delayed adolescence, although a normal variant and benign, is often a severe psychologic handicap to the patient and a cause of parental anxiety. Many of these boys are short, and a delay of several years in osseous development is not uncommon. There may be a history of late onset of puberty in other members of the family. Retardation of puberty can be due to inadequate dietary intake or to chronic illness, because these may be associated with either diminished secretion of pituitary gonadotropin or Leydig cell dysfunction.

Pubertal failure or arrest in pubertal development secondary to pituitary-hypothalamic dysfunction or gonadal disease must be excluded in cases of delayed puberty. To exclude pituitary tumor, roentgenographic examination of the skull and careful examination of the fundi and visual fields are required, as well as search for other signs of neurologic involvement in boys who are significantly delayed in their sexual development, particularly when this is accompanied by stunting of growth. It is advisable to assess other pituitary functions, especially if the delayed maturation is accompanied by short stature or a decreased rate of growth. A buccal smear for sex chromatin and determination of plasma gonadotropins may clarify the clinical situation. The response to clomiphene or to GnRH will not differentiate between delayed puberty and hypogonadotropic hypogonadism, because both groups are unresponsive to clomiphene, and GnRH causes a similar pattern of LH and FSH release in both groups.

Treatment. Treatment should be directed toward correction of the basic disturbance, e.g., measures to improve nutrition or treatment of a pituitary neoplasm. Substitution therapy with male sex hormone should be started at about 13 or 14 years of age so that the onset of the patient's maturation coincides with that of his contemporaries. The use of this regimen does not preclude subsequent induction of spermatogenesis with FSH and HCG in those individuals with hypogonadotropic hypogonadism.

Less well defined is the treatment of boys in whom no apparent etiologic factor is found. Many will mature spontaneously before 17 years of age and merely represent an extreme of the normal range. Although indiscriminate use of hormonal treatment in this group is unwise, sociopsychologic considerations may make it expedient to treat such boys. A therapeutic trial with human chorionic gonadotropin, 500 to 1000 IU three times weekly injected intramuscularly, or with a long-acting testosterone preparation 200 mg every two to three weeks for three to six months will cause virilization, and often maturation will progress after treatment is discontinued.

Marshal WA, Tanner JM: Variations in the pattern of pubertal changes in boys. Arch Dis Child 45:13, 1970. *This paper provides a detailed description of the stages in male pubertal development and variations from the normal patterns. Physicians interested in these clinical problems should read this paper.*

SEXUAL PRECOCITY

Isosexual precocity in boys is defined as the occurrence of signs of masculinization before the age of ten years. Skeletal maturation is accelerated and the epiphyses fuse at a premature age, leading to a short stature in adult life. On the other hand, mental and dental development are not precocious. Sexual precocity occurs about three times more frequently in girls than in boys. There are four main causes of isosexual precocity in boys: *cerebral, adrenocortical, testicular,* and *tumors secreting HCG.*

CEREBRAL CAUSES. *Cerebral causes of sexual precocity* are associated with premature activation of the hypothalamic-pituitary mechanism and the release of pituitary gonadotropins. This form, designated true precocious puberty or complete isosexual precocity, is manifested by maturation of the Leydig cells, enlargement of the testis, and spermatogenesis.

True precocious puberty may be caused by organic lesions of the brain either directly or indirectly involving the posterior hypothalamus, such as hypothalamic and pineal tumors, hamartoma of the tuber cinereum, craniopharyngioma, hydrocephalus, postencephalitic lesions, congenital defects, tuberous sclerosis, and neurofibromatosis. The *McCune-Albright syndrome* of sexual precocity, polyostotic fibrous dysplasia, and pigmented areas of skin is rare in boys. The mechanism whereby such lesions activate the hypothalamic-pituitary secretion of gonadotropins is unknown. Cerebral lesions, particularly tumors, accompanied by precocious puberty may affect other hypothalamic functions, causing diabetes insipidus, bulimia, obesity, somnolence, emotional lability, or disturbances in temperature regulation. The syndrome of diabetes insipidus and precocious puberty suggests *aberrant pinealoma.* Signs of puberty may precede the onset of detectable neurologic involvement, and prolonged observation with repeated careful neurologic examinations, roentgenograms of the skull, and determinations of the visual fields is necessary before it is possible to exclude cerebral neoplasm. When no organic cause is found, the condition is described as *idiopathic precocious puberty;* in some instances, it is transmitted as a sex-limited autosomal dominant trait. In the idiopathic cases, seizure disorders and abnormal electroencephalographic patterns are appreciably more frequent than in normal children.

In all varieties of precocious puberty, plasma and urinary testosterone values are increased, because either Leydig cell secretion is stimulated or testosterone is produced elsewhere. In true precocious puberty, pituitary gonadotropin is secreted in the pulsatile manner that normally occurs with pubescence. Analogues of GnRH have been shown to suppress pituitary and testicular function and are of use in true isosexual precocious puberty. Rarely secretion of HCG by extrapituitary neoplasms, such as hepatoblastoma, causes isosexual precocity.

In forms of isosexual precocity not related to intracranial causes, in contrast to the enlarged phallus the testes remain immature and true puberty does not occur. Accordingly, this type has been called *incomplete sexual precocity or precocious pseudopuberty.*

ADRENOCORTICAL CAUSES. *Adrenocortical hyperfunction* resulting from congenital virilizing adrenal hyperplasia or a virilizing adrenocortical tumor is the most common cause of precocious pseudopuberty in boys. With few exceptions the testes remain prepubertal in size despite enlargement of the penis and scrotum and development of other secondary sexual characteristics. In congenital adrenal hyperplasia ectopic nodules of hyperplastic adrenal tissue are occasionally palpable in the testis, and may be confused with Leydig cell tumor, especially in rare instances in which striking enlargement of the testis is found. The excretion of 17-KS is increased in relation to chronologic age, and plasma levels of 17-hydroxyprogesterone and its metabolite, urinary pregnanetriol, are high in congenital adrenal hyperplasia.

TESTICULAR CAUSES. *Interstitial cell tumor of the testis* is a rare cause of isosexual precocity. In almost all reported cases the tumor has been unilateral, and the contralateral testis is immature. Gynecomastia is occasionally present. The excretion of 17-KS is usually normal, although occasional high values have been reported. Plasma testosterone concentration has generally been in the low normal adult male range. Spermatogenesis has been observed in the tubules surrounding the tumor only, thereby confirming the importance of high intratesticular androgen concentrations for spermatogenesis. There are now well-documented cases of apparently autonomous Leydig cell function that had previously been attributed to hypothalamic-pituitary activation.

SECONDARY TO HCG. *Iatrogenic sexual precocity* has been produced by the administration of male sex hormone, but is seen most frequently in boys who have been treated with large doses of HCG for cryptorchidism. Ectopic production of HCG by tumors may rarely lead to precocious puberty.

HYPOGONADISM

Hypogonadism may refer to a decrease in either the endocrine or the gametogenic function of the testis or to both. Primary hypogonadism is due to testicular disease, whereas secondary hypogonadism is a result of hypothalamic-pituitary disease. The excretion or blood level of gonadotropins is normal or high in primary hypogonadism, and is decreased in secondary hypogonadism. Primary lesions of the testis involving only spermatogenesis, resulting in infertility without hypoandrogenism, occur commonly. On the other hand, whenever testosterone secretion is deficient, spermatogenesis is impaired.

ANDROGEN DEFICIENCY. The clinical signs of androgen deficiency depend upon the age of onset and upon severity and duration of the deficiency. Total loss of testicular androgenic function, usually secondary to surgical castration or congenital defects of the testes, before or during early puberty results in eunuchoidism in adulthood. Eunuchoidism causes disproportionate growth of the long bones owing to delay in epiphyseal closure. The span exceeds the height by several inches, and the distance between the symphysis pubis and the sole (lower segment) measures more than 55 per cent of the height. Tall stature is common but not invariable. (The characteristic skeletal proportions of the eunuch are not pathognomonic and may be found in otherwise normal men.) The shoulders tend to be narrow and, although the habitus may be lean or obese, excessive fat deposition often occurs about the pectoral region, hips, thighs, and lower abdomen. Muscular development is poor. Except for the appearance of sparse pubic hair, secondary sex characteristics fail to appear, and the voice remains juvenile. Gynecomastia occurs in association with Klinefelter's syndrome and with male pseudohermaphroditism. Acne and baldness do not occur. Sex drive and potency are absent or greatly reduced. The hematocrit and hemoglobin levels are characteristic of those for women and increase with administration of androgen.

The effects on somatic and sexual development of partial loss of testicular androgenic function are less striking and vary greatly in degree. Characteristic of the milder forms of eunuchoidism are the scant growth of facial hair and a female distribution of pubic hair. In men who have attained sexual maturity, castration does not result in complete regression of secondary sexual characteristics, and the signs of androgen deficiency are less conspicuous. The most common signs are reduction in prostatic size, diminished rate of growth of the beard and body hair, the appearance of fine wrinkles around the eyes, and a pasty, sallow complexion. Semen volume is reduced. Potency and libido, although usually diminished, occasionally persist. There may be vasomotor phenomena, including hot flushes.

Androgen deficiency is best treated by preparations of testosterone for intramuscular, oral, and buccal or sublingual administration. The mode of administration depends, for the most part, on the preference of the patient and the cost.

Esterification of testosterone with organic acids potentiates its activity when injected as an oily solution. Testosterone propionate in doses of 25 to 50 mg by intramuscular injection two or three times weekly is adequate for replacement therapy. However, longer-acting esters are available that can be administered less frequently. One dose of 300 mg of testosterone cyclopentylpropionate or testosterone enanthate is highly effective when injected at two- to three-week intervals.

Methyltestosterone is an effective preparation for oral and buccal or sublingual use. It is usually administered in doses of 50 mg (30 to 75 mg) orally or about 25 mg per day sublingually. It is not metabolized to 17-KS as is testosterone. Fluoxymesterone (Halotestin) in doses of 10 mg daily has also been used for substitution therapy. None of the oral androgens is as effective as the testosterone esters given by injection. No potent protein anabolic steroid lacking androgenic properties is available at present, although intensive efforts have been made to obtain one.

Undesirable effects of androgens include edema caused by retention of extracellular electrolyte (a rare effect except with use of large doses or in elderly persons with diminished cardiac reserve), polycythemia, acne, gynecomastia, and premature closure of the epiphyses. Rarely, methyltestosterone and other oral androgens cause reversible intrahepatic cholestatic jaundice. Androgen therapy may be contraindicated in patients with carcinoma of the prostate. The use of androgens by normal men to increase athletic performance remains controversial; it is certain, though, that the androgens will markedly decrease spermatogenesis.

Primary Hypogonadism (Primary Failure of the Testis)

The problem of classification of primary hypogonadism has not been entirely resolved, because the etiology of many of the disorders in this group is uncertain. Primary hypogonadism may result from genetic and developmental defects, such as seminiferous tubule dysgenesis and Laurence-Moon-Biedl syndrome, or from other causes: trauma, destruction of spermatogonia after orchitis, exposure to ionizing radiation, chemotherapy, and surgical castration. Disorders in this group may or may not be accompanied by androgen deficiency, although in some eunuchoidism is a constant or frequent feature. Disorders of spermatogenesis characterized only by oligospermia and infertility are likewise examples of primary hypogonadism. Plasma LH is increased with hypofunction of the Leydig cells as in old age or myotonic dystrophy. Plasma FSH is increased whenever tubular damage is severe enough to compromise Sertoli cell function. A high plasma FSH concentration almost always signifies irreversible infertility.

Klinefelter's Syndrome; Seminiferous Tubule Dysgenesis

This syndrome is characterized classically by small, firm testes, azoospermia, gynecomastia, and elevated urinary gonadotropins. The features become apparent during early puberty, and may include eunuchoidism. Histologically there is atrophy and hyalinization of the seminiferous tubules; Leydig cells tend to occur in large clumps and are apparently increased in number, but total Leydig cell volume is probably normal. The few remaining tubules are lined by Sertoli cells; rarely, germ cells are present. Elastic fibers in the tunica propria are absent, indicating failure of pubertal maturation. The cause of the syndrome is a developmental defect of the gonad associated with and probably resulting from a sex chromosome abnormality. Klinefelter's syndrome and its variants are now defined by the single constant finding of an increase in the number of X chromosomes in at least one cell line.

The discovery that most persons with the classic features of Klinefelter's syndrome are chromatin positive, followed by the detection of sex chromosome abnormalities, served to identify an especially well-defined disorder caused by a nonfamilial, genetically determined gonadal defect, sometimes called "seminiferous tubule dysgenesis." This disorder, which occurs sporadically, is an important cause of male infertility and a common type of sexual anomaly which occurs with a frequency in the order of 1 in 500 newborn males.

The most frequent clinical feature of Klinefelter's syndrome is the small size of the testes, the long diameter usually being less than 2 cm. The testes are firmer than normal owing to hyalinization of the tubules. Patients with this disorder are often tall, and the skeletal proportions frequently are eunuchoid as a consequence of the disproportionately long lower extremities, even though epiphyseal fusion is not delayed and skeletal maturation usually follows the normal male pattern (Fig. 234–4). Cryptorchidism and hypospadias are infrequent, and gynecomastia is present in fewer than 50 per cent of the cases. Mental retardation and psychopathic behavior are not uncommon, and there is often evidence of poor social adaptation. This disorder has been reported in association with mongolism and with leukemia. It has been suggested that chronic pulmonary disease and varicose veins are more prevalent in affected adults. The frequency of impaired glucose tolerance and of mild diabetes is increased.

In the classic form of the disease plasma FSH is increased as a result of the extensive tubular destruction. Plasma LH is usually high but may be normal in those few men with normal Leydig cell function. The plasma concentration of testosterone is often low, and may increase only slowly with the daily administration of human chorionic gonadotropin for four to five days.

The common abnormality of the sex chromosomes in Klinefelter's syndrome is a 47,XXY karyotype. Less common types of sex chromosome abnormalities in this disorder include phenotypic males with the genotypes 48,XXYY, 48,XXXY, or 49,XXXXY that have been found so far only in mentally retarded persons. Unusually tall stature has been found in the XXYY group, along with a tendency to more aggressive and delinquent behavior. The 48,XXXY sex chromosome complex is associated with two sex chromatin bodies in a proportion of diploid somatic nuclei, and the 49,XXXXY constitution with three sex chromatin bodies. In addition to mental retardation, the XXXXY men have had severe congenital malformations, including very small, usually undescended testes; hypoplastic external genitalia; minor skeletal deformities, including radioulnar synostosis; and other congenital anomalies. It seems that with increasing numbers of X chromosomes, the severity of the abnormalities increases.

Instances of sex chromosome mosaicism have also been described in which at least two populations of cells with different cell chromosome complexes were found in the same individual, e.g., XY/XXY (one cell line with an XY sex chromosome complex and another with an XXY sex chromosome complex), XY/XXXY, XX/XXY, and XXXY/XXXXY. Sex chromosome mosaics arise from a mitotic error in an early division after fertilization in a zygote that originally had either a normal or an abnormal sex chromosome constitution. The detection of a chromatin-positive sex chromatin pattern on buccal smear should not by itself be used as incontrovertible evidence of sterility. Active spermatogenesis was found in the testes of an XY/XXXXY mosaic, and additional examples of potential fertility may be found in chromatin-positive males with other forms of sex chromosome mosaicism, especially XY/XXY. In several carefully studied men with Klinefelter's syndrome, only an XX sex chromosome constitution was found. The maternal origin of the two X chromosomes suggests that a Y chromosome was present early in ontogeny and was lost or more likely translocated to an X chromosome or autosome, or that these men were mosaics and the Y-bearing cell line has escaped detection.

The typical XXY sex chromosome constitution of seminiferous tubule dysgenesis may arise from an abnormality of meiosis during gametogenesis or from a mitotic error in the fertilized zygote (see Ch. 35). The positive association of this disorder with advanced maternal age and the results of surveys of color blindness (a sex-linked recessive trait) and of the Xg blood group suggest a maternal origin with nondisjunction occurring during oogenesis. Using X-linked markers, a paternal origin of one X has been established in several informative pedigrees, nondisjunction during spermatogenesis giving rise to an XY-

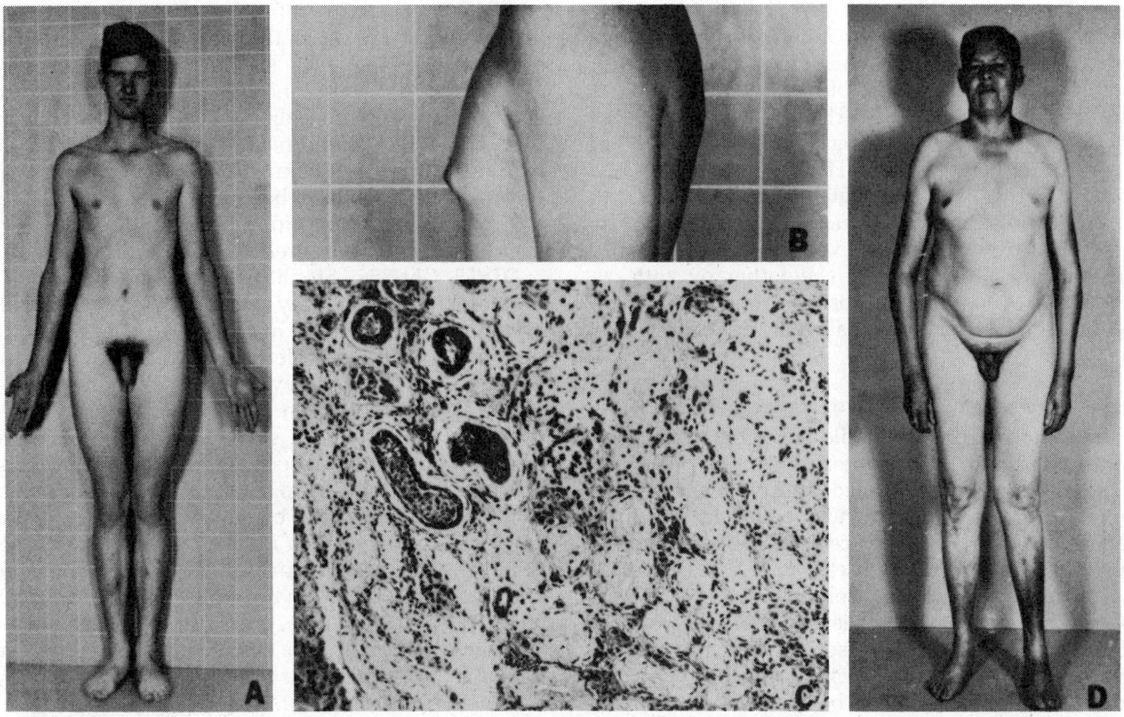

Figure 234–4. *A* and *B*, Typical 19-year-old phenotypic male with chromatin-positive seminiferous tubule dysgenesis (Klinefelter's syndrome). This patient had a positive sex chromatin pattern and an XXY karyotype. His 17-ketosteroid excretion was 11.2 mg per 24 hours, and his urinary gonadotropin excretion was more than 100 mu. These patients vary widely in their habitus and degree of virilization. This patient is well virilized, but had long extremities with eunuchoidal proportions and exhibited gynecomastia. The testes measured 1.8 × 0.9 cm and were small and firm. Testicular biopsy, *C*, revealed a severe degree of hyalinization of his seminiferous tubules and Leydig cell hyperplasia. *D*, Forty-eight-year-old man with chromatin-positive Klinefelter's syndrome who came to medical attention only because his severe leg varicosities were thought to reveal a "female trait." (From Van Wyk JJ, Grumbach MM: *In* Williams RH [ed.]: Textbook of Endocrinology. 4th ed. Philadelphia, W. B. Saunders Company, 1968.)

bearing sperm and fertilization yielding an XXY zygote. More complex sex chromosome anomalies may arise from meiotic or mitotic errors, or from a combination of both.

The gonadal defect is a consequence of the abnormal sex chromosome constitution. The single Y chromosome is a sufficiently powerful male determiner to suppress the cortical component (ovarian anlage) of the primordial gonad despite the presence of two (or even four) X chromosomes. The fetal testes that develop may have either an adequate number or a deficiency of germ cells, but bring about normal male differentiation of the genital tract. At puberty, if the function of the Leydig cells is adequate as occurs rarely, male secondary sexual characteristics develop, but the seminiferous tubules lack or are severely deficient in germ cells. Tubular hyalinization usually does not begin until the later prepubertal period. It seems likely that the characteristic appearance of the testes in adolescent and adult cases depends on the direct or indirect action of pituitary gonadotropins from the onset of puberty on an inherently defective testis, which, before this time, shows only subtle signs of an abnormal histologic structure.

TREATMENT. If there is evidence of androgen deficiency, testosterone replacement is indicated. Testosterone treatment may produce transient increase in gynecomastia and nipple tenderness. Mastectomy may be necessary in some patients, primarily for cosmetic reasons.

Chromatin-Negative Klinefelter's Syndrome

This term, a misnomer, was bestowed before the fundamental distinction was made on the basis of karyotype. The small testes and azoospermia suggest the Klinefelter phenotype. The testicular lesion resembles that of Klinefelter's syndrome, but the testis can react to injury in only a limited number of ways. The patients have none of the associated anomalies seen in Klinefelter's syndrome, but hypogonadism is sometimes present. It is probable that so-called chromatin-negative Klinefelter's syndrome is the end-stage of several different disease processes, the final result being hyalinization of the tubules with loss of spermatogonia. Some of these patients may be unrecognized mosaics with one cell line bearing an XXY karyotype and would thus be classified as having Klinefelter's syndrome. Plasma testosterone levels have varied from normal to low.

XYY Syndrome

Although the XXY syndrome is discussed under the topic of primary hypogonadism, in fact primary hypogonadism is unusual in XYY subjects. The XYY syndrome is characterized by a chromosome complement of 47 with an extra Y chromosome and a sex chromatin–negative buccal smear that contains nuclei with two small fluorescent Y chromatin masses, and is estimated to occur in 1 per 500 to 1 per 1000 male births. Newborn males and young boys with this syndrome have a normal phenotype. A number of associated characteristics have been reported in the adolescent and adult XYY male. These include tall stature (often over 6 feet), severe acne, and skeletal abnormalities, e.g., radioulnar synostosis. In studies of criminals with a history of aggressive crimes, an increased frequency of the XYY genotype has been noted. On the other hand, most adult XYY males are physically and mentally normal, and the genotype is present with greater frequency in tall men.

Although the extra Y apparently confers the potential for increased stature, Leydig cell function and plasma and urinary testosterone concentrations have been normal.

Germinal Aplasia (Sertoli-Cell-Only Syndrome)

This condition is characterized by seminiferous tubules lined with Sertoli cells, little or no tubular fibrosis, and absent germinal cells. The patients are first seen by the physician because of sterility. Leydig cell function is normal. Azoospermia is an invariable finding. The testes are somewhat reduced in size. Plasma FSH levels are increased four- to five-fold, whereas LH levels are within normal limits. There is an exaggerated response of LH to GnRH, indicating some abnormality of Leydig cell control or LH secretion. The karyotype is 46,XY. Germinal aplasia is probably a congenital disease of the Sertoli cell, and these cells are abnormal by electron microscopy. The lesion has also been described after exposure of the testes to ionizing radiation and after extensive chemotherapy with cytotoxic agents. There is no treatment for the spontaneous form, but even severe damage to the spermatogenic epithelium may be reversible.

Myotonic Muscular Dystrophy

Testicular atrophy, occurring in middle age, is found in about 80 per cent of affected men with myotonic dystrophy (see Ch. 538.1). This syndrome is characterized by myotonia, muscle wasting, frontal baldness, and lenticular opacities. Signs of androgen deficiency occur in 18 per cent of the patients and gynecomastia in 12 per cent. As the disease progresses, increasing tubular fibrosis results in high plasma FSH levels and Leydig cell failure leads to high LH levels. The testis shows tubular fibrosis, hyalinization, and disordered spermatogenesis. There are other metabolic abnormalities which, in association with the testicular findings, have been described as accelerated aging.

Anorchia

Absence of both testes in phenotypic males has been described but is exceedingly rare. Careful surgical exploration is required to establish the diagnosis. In a few cases, catheterization of the spermatic vein revealed a testosterone gradient, suggesting that a nidus of Leydig cells in the expected position of the testis remained functional. Unilateral anorchia is more common, and may result from testicular atrophy after herniorrhaphy, from attempted orchiopexy, or from a developmental disturbance, in which case there may be associated anomalies of the genitourinary tract.

Infertility

In many testicular lesions, the defect involves only spermatogenic function and results in infertility. Endocrine manifestations are absent. Either the semen lacks sperm or the number or quality of sperm is diminished. Testicular biopsy has a major role in differentiating the various disturbances in spermatogenic activity and in determining prognosis. Azoospermia is usually associated with severe tubular fibrosis, germinal aplasia, or spermatogenic arrest, and oligospermia with germinal cell desquamation, hypospermatogenesis, incomplete spermatogenic arrest, and less severe forms of tubular fibrosis. In general, only azoospermia or severe oligospermia is associated with increased plasma FSH concentrations. In most cases the cause is unknown. Azoospermia may also result from obstruction in the afferent ducts secondary to gonorrhea, tuberculosis, or a nonspecific infection. Absence or atresia of the vas deferens and a rudimentary epididymis are common bilateral lesions in boys with cystic fibrosis, but may occur spontaneously. Azoospermia in the presence of a normal FSH suggests obstructive disease and warrants biopsy and urologic consultation.

OLIGOSPERMIA. This condition is composed of many variants. There may be partial arrest of spermatogenesis at the primary or secondary spermatocyte stage or at the spermatid stage. Abnormalities of the meiotic chromosomes and reduction in chiasma formation have been noted in men with oligospermia. Sperm morphology may be abnormal. Of interest are the nonmotile sperm seen in *Kartagener's syndrome* (sinusitis, bronchiectasis, and situs inversus). The cause of immotility is the absence of the dynein arms of the microtubular elements of the sperm tail, and this defect is related to the immobility of the cilia in the bronchi. In some men with severe oligospermia the fibroblasts have only one half the normal number of androgen receptors. Thus the effect of decreased androgen action at the tubule is the putative cause of the associated infertility.

VARICOCELE. This condition is associated with decreased sperm count and infertility in 25 to 65 per cent of men, and there are varying abnormalities of sperm morphology. In general, measures of endocrine function have been normal. Results of varicocelectomy have been uneven, the incidence of restored fertility varying from 25 to 75 per cent. The role of the varicocele in producing infertility remains obscure.

OTHER CAUSES. Sterility is a common sequel of bilateral cryptorchidism and may occur in association with unilateral cryptorchidism. Sterility may follow orchitis caused by mumps, gonorrhea, brucellosis, leprosy, or occasionally other systemic infection; it may be of developmental origin, as in seminiferous tubule dysgenesis. Even relatively minor illnesses may cause profound depression in sperm count. Starvation and chronic debilitating diseases associated with inanition adversely affect spermatic function. Estrogen and androgen administration also inhibit spermatogenesis by suppression of gonadotropins with concomitant decrease in intratesticular testosterone concentration. The increasing survival and cure rates of men with lymphomas treated with multiple chemotherapeutic agents has led to assessment of testicular function after treatment. The seminiferous tubules are sensitive to alkylating agents in particular, and permanent sterility may follow therapy. Recovery of function, which occurs rarely, may be monitored by measurement of plasma FSH. If fertility is an objective after therapy, sperm banking is an option.

TREATMENT OF INFERTILITY IN THE MALE. Although important advances have been made in the evaluation of spermatogenic function, treatment of infertility caused by primary testicular disease is unsatisfactory. The results of therapy of hormonally normal men with oligospermia by the use of large doses of androgenic steroids, gonadotropins, pregnenolone, thyroid hormone, clomiphene, and vitamin preparations have been generally unsuccessful. The intermittent use of large doses of testosterone to take advantage of the "rebound effect" on spermatogenesis has not been established as efficacious, although occasional men seem to benefit. The use of testololactone, which inhibits aromatization, has been shown to increase the sperm count in some men with oligospermia. This suggests a role for intratubular estrogen in the etiology of some types of oligospermia.

Secondary Hypogonadism

Secondary hypogonadism is due to decreased secretion of gonadotropins, and may result from neoplastic, inflammatory, traumatic, vascular, or degenerative lesions involving the pituitary or hypothalamus. These lesions include such entities as pituitary adenoma, craniopharyngioma, astrocytoma, infarction, carotid aneurysm, granulomas such as tuberculosis, histiocytosis X, and hemochromatosis. In many instances, the nature of the underlying lesion is not known. A functional and reversible depression of gonadotropin secretion occurs in malnutrition, in chronic disease states associated with inanition and nutritional deficiencies, and in some patients with myxedema. High concentrations of androgen and estrogen, as in the adrenogenital syndrome, may cause secondary hypogonadism by suppression of gonadotropin secretion. Excessive estrogen, either from ingestion or an endogenous source, as from a feminizing adrenal tumor, depresses the secretion of pituitary gonadotropin. The testicular atrophy that occurs in some patients with severe liver disease is due in part to increased levels of estrogen. Decreased gonadotropin secretion may also result from the nutritional and metabolic disturbances accompanying hepatic cirrhosis. Alcohol, or its metabolite acetaldehyde, has direct toxic effects on the Leydig cell.

Decreased secretion of pituitary gonadotropins occurs either as an isolated defect, *hypogonadotropic hypogonadism,* or, more commonly, in association with a deficiency of growth hormone and other anterior pituitary hormones. On the other hand, hypoadrenocorticism or hypothyroidism secondary to pituitary failure is rarely found without concurrent involvement of gonadotropic function and secondary hypogonadism. Secondary hypogonadism is usually characterized by both inadequate androgenic function and, with rare exceptions (see below), absent or deficient spermatogenesis.

The clinical manifestations vary with age of onset, degree of the deficiency, and whether there is coexistent deficiency of other anterior pituitary hormones. Hypopituitarism occurring during childhood, commonly designated "pituitary dwarfism," results in proportionate dwarfism and complete sexual infantilism. The characteristic features of prepubertal or pubertal gonadotropic failure are eunuchoid habitus, small testes, lack of development of secondary sexual characteristics, an increased frequency of anosmia or hyposmia, low or absent gonadotropins, and low plasma testosterone concentration. The absence of gynecomastia, regarded by some as a salient feature, is of no clinical value in differentiating primary from secondary hypogonadism. It is important to detect organic disease of the pituitary region. Such evaluation should include study of the visual fields, roentgenography of the sella turcica, and, when indicated, such procedures as tomography of the sella, computed tomography, and carotid and venous angiography.

A familial form of isolated hypogonadotropic hypogonadism limited to males occurs in association with anosmia or hyposmia *(Kallmann's syndrome)* and is transmitted as either an X-linked or a sex-linked dominant trait. Aplasia of the olfactory lobes has been found in autopsied cases. Leydig cell responsiveness to HCG in some of these patients may be decreased. Both familial and sporadic forms of isolated FSH and LH deficiency are known, and these may be associated with a variety of somatic anomalies and neurologic defects. Although the initial response to GnRH has been variable, with continued administration the response becomes normal. These data suggest that hypothalamic synthesis or release of GnRH is impaired in these patients and in most patients with hypogonadotropic hypogonadism.

The testis in patients with hypogonadotropic hypogonadism remains infantile, the tubular diameter being the same as that of the fetal testis. When pituitary function is decreased in adult life, tubular collapse, fibrosis, and hyalinization occur at variable times after the onset of gonadotropic failure.

Isolated LH Deficiency. There is a group of eunuchoidal men with relatively normal-sized testes and some spermatogenic function to whom the term "fertile eunuch" has been applied. The patients are not fertile, however, because spermatogenesis is decreased, and libido and potency are absent. Leydig cells are absent or few in number, and androgen deficiency is always present. The concentration of plasma LH and the excretion of urinary LH are low or undetectable, whereas the secretion of FSH is normal. Chorionic gonadotropin stimulates Leydig cell function, ameliorates the androgen deficiency, and increases spermatogenesis. These patients have a relative deficiency of LH, which may arise from an abnormality in the hypothalamus (and the synthesis or release of GnRH) or in the pituitary gland. A kindred with two affected brothers has been reported. Rarely, a pituitary tumor or idiopathic delayed adolescence may manifest itself as isolated LH deficiency.

Treatment. A physiologic approach to the treatment of secondary hypogonadism characterized by decreased spermatogenesis requires the use of gonadotropins or GnRH. FSH preparations derived from animal sources are not consistently effective and, when injected repeatedly, stimulate antibody formation that reduces the effect of the hormones. However, gonadotropins prepared from menopausal urine have been used successfully in combination with HCG to induce spermatogenesis in patients with hypogonadotropic hypogonadism. As little as 25 IU of FSH three times a week in combination with 1000 IU of HCG three times a week has induced spermatogenesis. Impregnation often occurs with total sperm counts below 20 million. This suggests that the infertility seen in men with oligospermia whose sperm counts may be higher is due to factors other than sperm number. Spermatogenesis has been induced in hypogonadotropic hypogonadism with pulsatile injection of GnRH. Testosterone cannot be used in place of HCG, because intratesticular testosterone concentrations do not reach the levels attained when the Leydig cells are stimulated by HCG. HCG does not have a direct effect on the seminiferous tubules, although in a few instances of partial gonadotropic failure in which some FSH secretion remained, spermatogenic as well as Leydig cell function improved after its use. HCG has been effective in maintaining spermatogenesis after hypophysectomy for diabetic retinopathy, or after initiation of spermatogenesis with FSH. When only androgen substitution therapy is needed, one of the long-acting testosterone preparations is preferred.

Boyden TW, Pamenter RW: Effects of ethanol on the male hypothalamic-pituitary-gonadal axis. Endocr Rev 4:389, 1983. *A comprehensive discussion of the effects of alcohol.*

Brasel JA, Wright JC, Wilkins L, Blizzard RM: An evaluation of seventy-five patients with hypopituitarism beginning in childhood. Am J Med 38:484, 1965. *This is a comprehensive review of the clinical syndrome of hypopituitarism with many data about hypogonadism.*

Paulsen CA, Gordon DL, Carpenter RW, Gandy HM, Drucker WD: Klinefelter's syndrome and its variants: A hormonal and chromosomal study. Recent Prog Horm Res 24:321, 1968. *This is a comprehensive review of the clinical manifestations and laboratory findings of a large group of men with Klinefelter's syndrome.*

CRYPTORCHIDISM

The terms "cryptorchidism" and "undescended testes" are used synonymously to designate testes that have never descended into the scrotum. Unilateral cryptorchidism is approximately four times as common as bilaterally undescended testes. A cryptorchid testis may be situated in the abdomen, within the inguinal canal, or in an ectopic position outside the scrotum and the normal pathway of descent. The majority of undescended testes are inguinal. To avoid needless treatment, it is essential to distinguish this condition from retractile testes, which lie in the lower or upper scrotum and are withdrawn into the inguinal region and occasionally into the abdomen by slight stimulus.

The testes usually descend into the scrotum about the eighth fetal month; but occasionally descent is delayed until shortly after birth. Incomplete descent is common in premature male infants. Undescended testes are found at birth in 3 to 4 per cent of full-term male infants. During the first month of life 50 per cent of undescended testes reached the scrotum. Spontaneous descent occurs frequently during the first year of life and is less common after this age. Only 0.5 per cent of male infants have undescended testes at 12 months of age. The prevalence of unilateral and bilateral cryptorchidism in large series of adult males has been variously estimated at 0.2 to 0.4 per cent.

The etiology is not understood. Not infrequently a normal testis resides in the superficial inguinal pouch, its descent arrested by Scarpa's fascia. However, the cryptorchid testis is often dysgenetic. In rare instances, unilateral or bilateral cryptorchidism is the only overt anatomic abnormality of the external genitalia in individuals with fetal testicular dysfunction.

DIAGNOSIS. The most difficult aspect of diagnosis is distinguishing the true undescended testis from the more common retractile testis of childhood; repeated examinations may be necessary, especially in obese boys. It is important to ascertain by careful inquiry whether the testes have at any time been observed in the scrotum. In cryptorchidism the ipsilateral side of the scrotum is empty and poorly developed. The patient should be carefully examined while standing, squatting, and in a recumbent position, in a warm room and with warm hands. Bimanual examination and palpation while the patient performs a Valsalva maneuver or while the examiner applies pressure to the lower abdomen are also useful procedures. In boys with retractile testes, elicitation of the cremasteric reflex often results in a localized puckering of the scrotal skin. If the testis is palpated in the normal pathway of descent, gentle manipulation should be used in an attempt to displace it into the scrotum. Such mobile testes do not require therapy and will remain in the scrotum with the advent of puberty. Failure to palpate a testis on multiple occasions suggests that the testis is intra-abdominal, atrophic, or absent. An increase in plasma FSH and an augmented response to GnRH indicates severe Sertoli cell dysfunction.

TREATMENT. The treatment of undescended testes is a vexing and controversial subject; experienced observers differ in their approach to the problem. Major considerations are (1) the potential fertility of the undescended testis, (2) the likelihood of spontaneous descent, and (3) the propensity of the undescended testis to undergo malignant change.

During or after puberty the undescended testis shows degenerative changes that eventually proceed to atrophy. These changes have been ascribed to the deleterious effect of the higher temperature of an extrascrotal environment on the testes, especially on the germinal epithelium. The tubules gradually undergo progressive fibrosis and loss of germinal elements, although androgenic function may persist for many years. These degenerative changes may also be manifestations of a dysgenetic testis. This distinction is important, because the risk of cancer in the dysgenetic gonad is considerably greater than in the normal gonad.

Men with bilateral undescended testes are sterile. However, general agreement is lacking as to the age at which the fertility potential of the cryptorchid testis is impaired. A lag in development of the seminiferous tubules and, in some instances, a mild degree of fibrosis in undescended testes after the age of six to ten years have been observed. The significance of these changes is uncertain, but after puberty irreversible degenerative changes frequently occur.

The incidence of cancer in undescended testes is considerably greater than in scrotal testes, and more so in abdominal than in inguinal testes. The probability of cancer occurring in a cryptorchid testis is 30 to 50 times greater than in the normal testis.

The most important problem in the treatment of patients with cryptorchidism is the age at which it is advisable to attempt correction. Treatment consists of orchiopexy or of the administration of HCG followed by orchiopexy when necessary. Therapy must be started before pubescence and probably by age 6 if irreparable testicular damage is to be prevented. In the more common unilateral cryptorchidism, the scrotal testis, if normal, is adequate for fertility. Treatment is recommended for cosmetic reasons, to facilitate examination for neoplasm, and as additional insurance against infertility in the event that the scrotal testis is defective or impaired at a later age.

In bilateral cryptorchidism preservation of fertility is the major consideration, but the results of treatment are disappointing. Bilateral orchiopexy is generally followed by tubular fibrosis and atrophy. Since many undescended testes descend before puberty, it is justifiable to delay treatment until nine years of age unless the testis is ectopic or associated with a hernia.

When hormonal therapy is effective, it is probable that the testis would have descended spontaneously at puberty under the stimulus of endogenous gonadotropin. To minimize a theoretical risk of damage to the tubule, short intensive courses of 1000 units of HCG administered intramuscularly daily for three days or 1000 units three times a week for three weeks may be used. Hormonal treatment is contraindicated when the testis lies outside the normal pathway of descent.

If the undescended testis is atrophic and biopsy at the time of surgery shows irreversible changes, it is generally advisable to perform orchiectomy, provided that the contralateral testis is in the scrotum. This also applies to a testis that, despite all attempts at mobilization, cannot be brought into the scrotum.

Batata MA, Whitmore WF Jr, Chu FCH, et al: Cryptorchidism and testicular cancer. J Urol 124:382, 1980. *A review of the incidence of cancer and of the results of treatment.*

Raifer J, Walsh PC: Testicular descent: Normal and abnormal. Urol Clin N Amer 5:223, 1978. *A discussion of embryology, mechanisms and treatment.*

IMPOTENCE

Impotence is a complicated problem that may be either relative or complete and may involve any phase of the sexual act. Although it is a symptom of androgen deficiency and of genitourinary or neurologic disease, in many instances it is psychic in origin. Multiple sclerosis, tabes dorsalis, and diabetic neuropathy are commonly associated with impotence. Impotence without apparent impairment of libido has been described in patients with temporal lobe lesions. Many drugs used in the therapy of hypertension can cause impotence. When impotence is the principal complaint of a patient, it is often the result of an emotional disturbance, and in this case androgen therapy is valueless. Stress can decrease gonadotropin secretion and thereby affect androgen secretion and spermatogenesis (see Ch. 236). Increased prolactin, resulting from tumor or drugs, may produce impotence by directly suppressing LH via a "short-loop" feedback, and, consequently, testosterone secretion. Rarely primary hyperprolactinemia may cause impotence. With tests now available, specific causes of impotence can be identified more often. In one recent series, only 14 per cent of impotent men were identified as having psychogenic impotence; in an additional 7 per cent the cause was not known.

Slag MF, Morley JE, Elgon MK, et al: Impotence in medical clinic outpatients. JAMA 249:1736, 1983. *A large study of men in an outpatient clinic who were carefully studied for causes of impotence.*

"MALE CLIMACTERIC"

The male climacteric, as an analogue of the menopause, does not exist. Although during the fifth or sixth decade ovarian failure with a consequent rise in gonadotropin excretion is an anticipated physiologic accompaniment of the aging process, spontaneous testicular deficiency of sufficient degree to produce symptoms is rare. Many of the symptoms ascribed to this syndrome are common in psychoneurotic middle-aged and elderly men. The diagnosis of testicular failure should be documented by finding an increased plasma level of gonadotropin and a low level of plasma testosterone, and should be confirmed by obtaining a therapeutic response to androgen therapy but not to placebos. In healthy men there are only minor decreases in plasma testosterone concentrations with increasing age. A progressive increase in plasma LH levels after age 60 has been described, indicating mild compensated Leydig cell failure. Plasma estradiol increases with age as a result of increased conversion of testosterone to estradiol in peripheral tissues. The frequency of alterations in tubular histology increases progressively after age 30, prominent changes being thickening of the basement membrane, intratubular fibrosis, and loss of germ cells. Plasma FSH increases after age 70 in response to this seminiferous tubule damage.

ORCHITIS

Acute orchitis, a common complication of mumps, is a rare occurrence in the course of other specific infectious diseases (see Ch. 335).

Chronic orchitis is associated with painless, hard, sometimes nodular enlargement of the testis. *Syphilis*, the most common cause, may produce an interstitial orchitis in which the testis is characteristically smooth and wooden in consistency ("billiard ball" testis); involvement is frequently bilateral. Other causes include *tuberculosis*, *leprosy*, *brucellosis*, *glanders*, and certain parasitic infections such as *filariasis* and *bilharziasis*. In these diseases, Leydig cell function almost always remains intact, but severe tubular destruction may result.

TABLE 234–1. TUMORS OF TESTIS: CLASSIFICATION*

I. Primary tumors
  A. Germinal
    1. Seminoma
    2. Embryonal tumors
      a. Embryoma
      b. Choriocarcinoma
      c. Embryonal carcinoma
      d. Teratocarcinoma
      e. Adult teratoma
    3. Combinations of seminoma and embryonal tumor and of the various types of embryonal tumors
    4. Gonadal tumors in intersexes (gonadoblastomas)
  B. Nongerminal tumors
    1. Interstitial cell tumor
    2. Sertoli cell tumor
    3. Tumors of testicular stroma: fibroma, lipoma, etc.
II. Secondary tumors
  A. Lymphoma, plasmacytoma, leukemia, etc.
  B. Metastatic carcinoma

*From Melicow MM: Classification of Tumors of the Testis. J Urol 73:547, 1955.

TUMORS OF THE TESTIS

Tumors of the testis are uncommon, constituting about 0.7 per cent of all forms of cancer in the male. They occur in about 0.002 per cent of men, and frequently are malignant. The greatest incidence occurs in the third and fourth decades. Testicular tumors may arise from any of the cellular components of the testis or their embryonal precursors.

Considerable uncertainty applies to classification, especially of those neoplasms whose origin has been ascribed to the totipotent germ cell. A classification of testicular tumors is shown in Table 234–1.

Germinal Tumors

Most common are germinal tumors, and, of these, seminoma exceeds in frequency all other testicular tumors. *Seminoma,* although usually fairly uniform in cellular architecture, may contain embryonal elements such as chorionic syncytium in the primary growth or in metastatic lesions. In contrast to the embryonal tumors, which tend to invade the spermatic cord and to metastasize early, especially to lung, seminomas in general are relatively slow growing and commonly invade the iliac and periaortic lymph nodes before generalized dissemination is demonstrable. In addition, seminomas are frequently highly radiosensitive, whereas embryonal tumors are usually resistant to radiotherapy. The significantly increased incidence of germinal tumors, particularly seminoma, in undescended testes and in the dysgenetic gonads of intersexes has been discussed above.

Many patients with germinal tumors excrete increased amounts of chorionic gonadotropin. This may almost always be attributed to the presence of trophoblastic elements in the tumor. Response to therapy or evidence of recurrence may be monitored by measurement of plasma HCG levels. Other fetal protein markers such as carcinoembryonic antigens may also be secreted by these cancers.

The germ cell tumors of the testis are responsive to therapy. Removal or radiation of regional and paraortic lymph nodes has produced survival rates of 80 to 95 per cent in men with seminoma. Choriocarcinoma and embryonal cell carcinoma have responded to multiagent chemotherapeutic regimens. With the addition of cisdiamminedichloroplatinum to combinations of methotrexate, dactinomycin, and chlorambucil, response rates of 40 to 70 per cent have been achieved in men with metastatic disease. About 40 per cent of these patients are apparently in long-term remission.

Interstitial Cell Tumors

Tumors of this type are rare, occur at any age, and are usually but not invariably benign. The tumors are small and often difficult to palpate. In boys interstitial cell tumors cause sexual precocity but not true puberty, because spermatogenesis is absent in the contralateral testis. The only recognizable endocrine manifestation in the adult is gynecomastia, which has been observed in about 10 per cent of cases. Malignant interstitial cell tumors that retain their steroid-synthesizing capacities have been reported.

Fraley EE, Lange PH, Kennedy BJ: Germ-cell testicular cancer in adults. N Engl J Med 301:1370, 1979. *A review of embryology, endocrinology, and therapy of germ-cell tumors of the testis.*

Hainsworth JD, Greco FA: Testicular germ cell neoplasms. Am J Med: 75:817, 1983. *The diagnosis and treatment of these tumors is well described in this excellent review (121 references).*

235. DISEASES OF THE PROSTATE

Patrick C. Walsh

The adult prostate weighs approximately 20 grams and lies immediately below the base of the bladder surrounding the proximal portion of the urethra. This tubuloalveolar gland secretes a colorless, slightly acidic fluid that contains fibrinolysin, citric acid, acid phosphatase, spermine, potassium, calcium, and zinc. The differentiation, growth, and function of the prostate are under the regulation of testicular androgens. Testosterone, which is secreted by the testes under the control of pituitary luteinizing hormone, is the principal circulating androgen. Testosterone enters the prostatic cell by passive diffusion where it is converted to dihydrotestosterone, the principal intracellular androgen. Dihydrotestosterone then binds to a specific cytosolic receptor protein, translocates to the nucleus, and influences in a complex fashion the expression of genetic information (see Ch. 221 for details).

Unlike most other organ systems, patients with diseases of the prostate do not present with complaints referable to disorders of prostatic function. Indeed, the exact role of prostatic secretion in normal reproduction is unclear. Rather, patients present with inflammatory, congestive, or neoplastic disturbances that most often give rise to difficulties with micturition. For this reason, men are often unaware of the existence of the prostate until one of these disorders develops. Starting at puberty, the prostate increases from approximately 4 grams to 20 grams in weight by age 20. Thereafter, for the next several decades prostatitis is the most common prostatic disorder. Beyond the fifth decade, benign prostatic hyperplasia and prostatic carcinoma predominate.

PROSTATITIS

Prostatitis, which refers to any condition associated with prostatic inflammation, is the most imprecise diagnosis in all of medicine. The disease can be acute or chronic and can have either bacterial or nonbacterial causes.

ETIOLOGY AND PATHOGENESIS. Bacterial prostatitis is most commonly caused by gram-negative organisms (predominantly *Escherichia coli*) and more rarely by enterococcus. Possible routes of infection include ascending urethral infection, reflux of infected urine into the prostatic ducts that empty into the posterior urethra, invasion by rectal bacteria via direct extension or lymphogenous spread, and hematogenous infection. Whether infectious prostatitis is a sexually transmitted disease is uncertain. The etiology of nonbacterial prostatitis is unknown. Except in rare instances, the disease does not appear to be caused by fungi, obligate anaerobic bacteria, trichomonads, viral agents, T-mycoplasma, or *Chlamydia.*

CLINICAL MANIFESTATIONS, DIAGNOSIS, AND DIFFERENTIAL DIAGNOSIS. Much of the confusion concerning prostatitis is attributable to imprecise methods of diagnosis. Many male patients have multiple genitourinary complaints centered on the prostate. Often the medical history and physical findings are not helpful in the differential diagnosis. Furthermore, when done as isolated procedures, midstream urinalysis and culture offer little diagnostic assistance. The two most useful tools in forming a differential diagnosis are examination of the expressed prostatic secretions (EPS) and quantitative bacterial localization cultures. Although microscopic examination of the EPS is important, it can be misleading. The clinician should always compare the microscopic appearance of the EPS to smears of the spun sediment of the first voided 10 ml of urine (the urethral specimen) and the midstream urine (bladder specimen) to localize the site of the inflammatory response. The presence of >20 white blood cells per high power field in the EPS is abnormal. During prostatic inflammation EPS typically contain leukocytosis and abnormal numbers of lipid-laden macrophages (oval fat bodies). The most accurate and useful method of establishing the diagnosis of bacterial prostatitis is the performance of simultaneous quantitative bacterial cultures of the urethral urine, bladder urine, and EPS. Four specimens are collected: the first voided 10 ml (VB1), the midstream aliquot (VB2), the EPS, and the first voided 10 ml immediately after prostatic massage (VB3). All specimens are cultured quantitatively by surface streaking onto blood and MacConkey agar. The diagnosis of bacterial prostatitis is confirmed when the quantitative bacterial colony counts of the prostatic specimens (EPS and VB3) significantly exceed those of the urethral (VB1) and bladder (VB2) specimens by at least 1 logarithm. Based on these diagnostic maneuvers, the inflammatory diseases of the prostate have been subdivided into four categories: (1) acute bacterial prostatitis, (2) chronic bacterial prostatitis, (3) nonbacterial prostatitis, and (4) prostatodynia.

Acute bacterial prostatitis is a fulminating bacterial infection characterized by fever, chills, low back and perineal pain, and intense irritative voiding symptoms. Rectal examination usually discloses a markedly tender prostate that is swollen, firm, and warm. Prostatic discomfort and the risk of bacteremia generally make prostatic massage unwise. Because bacterial cystitis usually accompanies the disease, the pathogen can be identified by culture of a voided specimen of urine. The disease often responds dramatically to therapy with antibacterial agents.

Chronic bacterial prostatitis is one of the most common causes of relapsing urinary tract infection in men. The majority of patients complain of irritative voiding symptoms (dysuria, urgency, frequency, and nocturia) and pain in various sites (suprapubic, perineal, low back, scrotal, and penile). However, patients are usually asymptomatic until significant bacteriuria develops. Rectal palpation discloses no specific or characteristic finding. The diagnosis is based upon quantitative bacterial localization cultures. Characteristically, these patients have relapsing urinary tract infections caused by the same pathogen. Although the urine may be sterilized and symptoms may disappear during treatment with antimicrobial agents, the organism often persists unaltered in the prostatic fluid; when therapy is discontinued, reinfection of the urine and reappearance of symptoms occur.

Nonbacterial prostatitis, a disease of uncertain cause, is the most common type of prostatitis seen today. The symptoms, physical findings, and microscopic appearance of the EPS in nonbacterial prostatitis and chronic bacterial prostatitis are indistinguishable. However, the patient with nonbacterial prostatitis has no history of documented urinary tract infection, and localization cultures exclude an infectious etiology. The etiology of this disorder is unknown. Finally, some male patients complain of symptoms that mimic prostatitis, especially a painful prostate, but they have negative cultures and no history of documented urinary tract infections. Contrary to the findings in the other categories, the EPS is normal. Since these men do not actually have prostatitis, the diagnostic term *prostatodynia* has been suggested.

All patients with lower urinary tract complaints require a full evaluation. The differential diagnosis of patients with lower urinary tract irritative symptoms should include carcinoma of the bladder, urethral stricture, prostatic obstruction, pericolic abscess, neurogenic bladder, diabetes mellitus, bladder calculus, and detrusor-sphincter dyssynergia. Because the symptoms in men with nonbacterial prostatitis are identical to those of patients with flat in situ carcinoma of the bladder, urinary cytologic studies and cystoscopy should be performed in these patients to exclude the presence of a malignancy.

TREATMENT. In patients with bacterial prostatitis, the use of antibacterial agents is complicated by the fact that most of the agents that are useful against gram-negative bacteria diffuse poorly into prostatic fluid. The factors that limit diffusion include lipid solubility, pKa, protein binding, and molecular size and shape. Although trimethoprim fulfills all theoretical criteria, and experimentally high levels can be demonstrated in canine prostatic fluid, only one third of patients with chronic prostatitis are cured by treatment with trimethoprim.

In patients with acute bacterial prostatitis, hospitalization may be required. Rest in bed, sexual abstention, increased hydration, analgesics, antipyretics, stool softeners, and suprapubic bladder drainage (the latter for the rare patient who has urinary retention) have been recommended. The diffuse and intense inflammation of acute prostatitis allows many drugs to diffuse readily into the prostatic fluid. Therapy should be begun with trimethoprim-sulfamethoxazole (160 mg of trimethoprim and 800 mg of sulfamethoxazole), administered twice daily until the results of culture and sensitivity are known. Therapy with the appropriate antibiotic should then be continued for at least 30 days in an effort to prevent the evolution of chronic prostatitis. In patients with chronic bacterial prostatitis, trimethoprim-sulfamethoxazole has the best cure rate that has been documented. Among patients who receive therapy continuously for four to six weeks, the cure rate has been 32 to 71 per cent. If patients fail to respond to this treatment, therapy with erythromycin, minocycline, or oral carbenicillin indanyl sodium may be attempted. In those patients who are not cured by medical therapy, continuous suppressive treatment with low dose medication can be attempted. The most suitable choices are trimethoprim-sulfamethoxazole, 1 regular tablet daily, or nitrofurantoin, 100 mg by mouth daily. Even though the pathogen persists in the prostatic ducts, suppressive therapy usually prevents bacteriuria and controls the symptoms.

In patients with nonbacterial prostatitis, because the cause of the disease is unknown, definitive therapy is difficult. In these patients treatment is usually directed toward controlling the symptoms. A trial of clinical treatment with a tetracycline preparation or erythromycin in maximal doses is a reasonable approach to initial treatment. Most patients benefit from a frank discussion of the nature of their condition, short-term use of anticholinergic or anti-inflammatory agents, and hot sitz baths. Although prostatic massage is advocated by many, its benefits are questioned by others. The proper management of men with prostatodynia is unclear.

Feit RM, Fair WR: Prostatitis. Sex Trans Dis 5:78, 1978. *A concise article describing the diagnosis and management of the common forms of prostatitis.*

Meares EM Jr: Prostatitis syndromes: New perspectives about old woes. J Urol 123:141, 1980. *The author has provided an extensive review of the syndromes classified under the term prostatitis. The diagnosis, pathogenesis, and management of each disorder are clearly outlined. It is the most authoritative article published on this subject.*

Mears EM Jr, Barbalias GA: Prostatitis: Bacterial, nonbacterial, prostatodynia. Semin Urol 1:146, 1983. *The most up-to-date review of the subject.*

BENIGN PROSTATIC HYPERPLASIA

INCIDENCE AND PREVALENCE. Benign prostatic hyperplasia (BPH) is probably the most common neoplastic growth in men. The disease characteristically occurs in men older than age 40; few if any patients with true nodular hyperplasia have been observed before this age. In men over the age of 50, the frequency of symptomatic BPH varies from 50 to 75 per cent. The mean age of detection by race is about 65 years for whites and approximately five years earlier for blacks. The probability of a 40-year-old man's requiring an operation for BPH if he lives to 80 years of age is approximately 10 per cent.

ETIOLOGY AND PATHOGENESIS. Although the development of BPH is almost a universal phenomenon in aging men, the cause and pathogenesis of this disorder are not well understood. The two major factors necessary for the onset of BPH are the presence of the testes and aging. Consequently, much interest has been directed at identifying a hormonal etiology. There are several factors that strongly support the possibility that BPH in men is under endocrine control: (1) BPH does not occur in men who are castrated prior to puberty; (2) regression of established BPH has been reported to occur following castration; and (3) in a canine model, BPH can be produced by treatment with hormones. The prostate appears to become more sensitive to androgens as the gland enlarges and as plasma levels of testosterone decline. These observations suggest that other factors, such as estrogen induction of increased androgen receptor levels, may sensitize the prostate to adequate levels of dihydrotestosterone and accelerate growth. Medical approaches to the management of BPH must await further elucidation of these factors.

CLINICAL MANIFESTATIONS. Enlargement of the prostate causes no obvious physiologic manifestations. The disturbances that result are entirely secondary to effects on the urethra, the bladder, and the kidneys. In early cases the patient usually has minimal symptoms because the detrusor musculature is capable of compensating for the increased outlet resistance to urine flow. With increasing obstruction, however, the patient develops a constellation of symptoms called "prostatism": diminution in the caliber and force of the urinary stream, hesitancy in initiating voiding, inability to terminate micturition abruptly with postvoid dribbling, a sensation of incomplete emptying of the bladder, and occasionally urinary retention. These are *obstructive symptoms* and they must be carefully distinguished from *irritative* lower urinary tract symptoms such as dysuria, frequency, and urgency. Disastrous results can follow a prostatectomy performed on a patient whose symptoms stemmed from irritation, such as an inflammatory or infectious process, rather than from obstruction. As the amount of residual urine increases, the patient may note nocturia, diurnal frequency, a mass in the lower abdomen, and overflow urinary incontinence. In patients with slowly progressive obstruction, the patient may gradually adjust to the symptoms and present with "silent prostatism." On examination these patients may show the secondary anemia of renal insufficiency, a lower abdominal midline mass representing a distended bladder, and other findings associated with renal insufficiency (see Ch. 82).

DIAGNOSIS AND DIFFERENTIAL DIAGNOSIS. Usually there is no difficulty in establishing the diagnosis of BPH. The patient usually presents with lower urinary tract obstructive symptoms. Prior to examination the physician should observe the patient voiding to completion to document the decrease in size and force of the urinary stream. The prostate is palpated with attention to size, consistency, and shape. Hyperplasia usually produces a smooth, firm, and elastic enlargement of the prostate. However, the size of the prostate on rectal examination does not permit one to estimate the degree of bladder neck obstruction. Patients with marked enlargement of the prostate may have no urinary tract obstruction, and others with a large intravesical median lobe may have marked outflow obstructive symptoms without palpable enlargement of the gland. In addition to revealing the individual characteristics of the prostate, the rectal examination also affords the physician an opportunity to evaluate the intactness of the rectal sphincter, which indirectly reflects the state of vesical innervation.

A urinalysis and urine culture are performed to evaluate the presence of infection; a serum creatinine is obtained to evaluate renal function; and a serum acid phosphatase sample is drawn (preferably prior to prostatic examination). In patients whose disease is in an early stage and who have only mild symptoms, no further studies are necessary. However, in men with marked outlet obstructive symptoms, intravenous urography and cystourethroscopy should be performed. The intravenous urogram with a postvoiding film will document the degree of upper tract obstruction, identify the presence of bladder calculi, and estimate the degree of bladder emptying. Cystourethroscopy is valuable in confirming the presence of vesical neck obstruction, in evaluating the degree of detrusor hypertrophy (presence of trabeculation, cellules, and diverticula), and in excluding the presence of a bladder tumor.

Several other conditions produce bladder neck obstruction: carcinoma of the prostate, bladder neck contracture, urethral stricture, bladder calculus, carcinoma of the bladder, chronic prostatitis, and neurogenic bladder. The presence of irritative lower urinary tract symptoms, such as dysuria, urgency, and frequency, should alert the physician to consider conditions other than obstruction as the cause for the patient's symptoms. In the absence of a large amount of residual urine, frequency and nocturia are not caused by BPH. Bladder neck contracture, urethral stricture, bladder calculi, and bladder neoplasms are best evaluated with endoscopy.

TREATMENT AND PROGNOSIS. At present, there is no effective medical management for the treatment of BPH; surgery is the only effective form of therapy. The vast majority of men over the age of 60 have some evidence of BPH, so the mere presence of this disorder is not an indication for its treatment. The general indications for the relief of prostatic obstruction are (1) acute urinary retention, (2) hydronephrosis, (3) recurrent urinary tract infection aggravated by residual urine, (4) severe hematuria from a congestive prostate, and (5) outflow obstructive symptoms that are of sufficient concern to the patient to cause him to desire treatment. When the patient is seen early in the course of the disease, when his symptoms are mild, and before any of these relative indications are present, he is often curious about the natural history of the disease. This question is difficult to answer, because many patients who receive no treatment whatsoever will have no change in their symptoms over many years. Consequently in the group of patients that lack definitive indications for prostatectomy, it appears advisable to examine the patient periodically to observe the natural history of the disease rather than to anticipate its development by advising prophylactic prostatectomy. Simple prostatectomy can be performed in a variety of ways. However, transurethral resection of the prostate is the procedure with the least morbidity.

Walsh PC: Benign prostatic hyperplasia. *In* Harrison JH, Gittes RF, Perlmutter AD, Stamey TA, Walsh PC (eds.): Campbell's Urology. 4th ed. Philadelphia, W. B. Saunders Company, 1979, pp 949–964. *A comprehensive review of all aspects relative to the diagnosis and treatment of benign prostatic hyperplasia.*

Walsh PC, Hutchins GM, Ewing LL: The tissue content of dihydrotestosterone in human prostatic hyperplasia is not supranormal. J Clin Invest 72:1772, 1983. *Recognition that human BPH occurs in the presence of normal levels of dihydrotestosterone should focus research efforts to identify other factors that may sensitize this tissue and accelerate growth.*

Wilson JD: The pathogenesis of benign prostatic hyperplasia. Am J Med 68:745, 1980. *A concise and lucid discussion of the endocrine factors that may be responsible for the development of benign prostatic hyperplasia. Experimental studies are integrated with clinical findings to formulate a sound understanding of the pathogenesis of this common disease.*

CARCINOMA OF THE PROSTATE

INCIDENCE, PREVALENCE, EPIDEMIOLOGY. The prostate is the third leading site of cancer in males, accounting for about 17 per cent of all male cancers. The only female cancers that account for more new cancer cases per year are cancers of the breast and uterus. Approximately 5 per cent of white males and 6 per cent of nonwhite males will develop cancer of the prostate. Furthermore, it is calculated that 1.7 per cent of newborn white males and 2.3 per cent of newborn nonwhite males will eventually die of the disease. Although carcinoma of the prostate does not develop in eunuchs, there is no other evidence to suggest that a direct relationship exists between hormone levels and the development of prostatic cancer. Similarly, no relationship between the development of benign prostatic hyperplasia and prostatic cancer has been demonstrated. Furthermore, there is little relationship between prostatic cancer and industrial carcinogens, cigarette smoking, use of alcohol, disease patterns, circumcision, weight, height, blood group, or hair distribution.

PATHOLOGY. More than 95 per cent of all prostatic carcinomas are adenocarcinomas. The tumor is multifocal in 85 per cent of the cases, suggesting a multifocal rather than a single site of origin. Prostatic carcinoma can spread by local extension or by lymphatic or hematogenous dissemination. As carcinoma of the prostate progresses, the tumor extends to the urethra, the bladder neck, the seminal vesicles, and the trigone. The most common sites of lymph node metastases, in descending order of frequency, are the obturator, hypogastric, iliac, presacral, and periaortic nodes. Osseous metastases constitute the most common form of hematogenous spread. The most frequent sites of involvement are, in decreasing order, the pelvis, the lumbar spine, the femora, the thoracic spine, and the ribs. The most common sites for visceral metastases include the lung and liver. Pulmonary metastases are detected clinically or radiographically in less than 6 per cent of patients.

The prognosis of patients with prostatic cancer correlates well with the grade and stage of the tumor, although grading is somewhat difficult because most tumors exhibit a heterogeneous histologic pattern: (Table 235–1): *Stage A* disease is not palpable clinically but is found histopathologically following prostatectomy. It is subdivided into two biologically meaningful subclasses: Stage A1, focal or well differentiated carcinoma, and Stage A2, diffuse or poorly differentiated carcinoma. *Stage B* tumors are limited to the prostate and on rectal examination can be subdivided into Stage B1, a solitary nodule involving less than one lobe of the prostate, and Stage B2, cancer in which one lobe or more is involved. *Stage C* tumors extend beyond the prostatic capsule but have not metastasized. *Stage D* represents metastatic carcinoma of the prostate and includes any patient with an elevated serum acid phosphatase level. Stage D can be subdivided into Stage D1, the presence of metastatic disease in lymph nodes, and Stage D2, patients with clinical metastatic carcinoma.

CLINICAL MANIFESTATIONS AND DIAGNOSIS. Early in the clinical evolution of prostatic cancer symptoms may be entirely absent. Later, patients develop symptoms of urinary outflow obstruction or bone pain. Hematuria, lymphadenopathy, and lower extremity edema are uncommon presenting symptoms of prostatic cancer. A careful routine rectal examination is the only means of detecting prostatic cancer at an early stage. Carcinoma of the prostate characteristically has a hard consistency, felt as a region of dense induration within the substance of the prostate. With tumor penetration of the capsule, the margins of the prostate may become obscured and tumor may be palpated extending to the seminal vesicles and regions of the bladder neck. Other causes of prostatic induration include focal regions of benign hyperplasia, prostatic calculi, granulomatous prostatitis, prostatic infarction, and postoperative changes. Approximately 50 per cent of prostatic nodules are malignant.

A clinical suspicion of prostatic cancer requires histologic verification by needle biopsy. If the biopsy is positive, the patient should have a serum acid phosphatase determination, an intravenous urogram and a bone scan. Because of the lack of specificity of bone scans, skeletal radiographs should be performed of any suspicious areas. Routine lymphangiography or staging pelvic lymphadenectomy is generally unnecessary in the management of patients with prostatic cancer.

Serum acid phosphatase is elevated in most patients with bony metastases and, more rarely, with localized carcinoma. It is not sufficiently sensitive or specific for screening, so is used mainly to follow the progress of the disease. Acid phosphatase, not inhibited by l-tartrate, is characteristically elevated in the serum of patients with Gaucher's disease (Ch. 185).

TREATMENT. There is considerable debate concerning the best mode of therapy for each particular stage of carcinoma of the prostate. In selecting treatment there is often the dilemma of attempting both to maintain the quality of life and to increase the duration of survival. Men with carcinoma of the prostate are often old and suffer from other illnesses that may pose a greater threat than the cancer itself. Furthermore, although there are a variety of relatively effective therapeutic modalities from which to choose, there is little information that accurately compares their relative efficacy. Each form of treatment is associated with undesirable side effects. In selecting therapy the physician must determine the long-term threat that the tumor poses to the quality and duration of survival in each individual patient and must select a form of treatment that provides the proper balance between efficacy and morbidity.

In patients with Stage A1 prostatic cancer, observation but no further treatment is necessary. Patients with Stage A2 and B1 prostatic cancer who are less than 70 years old are ideal candidates for radical prostatectomy. In these patients, the tumor will be confined to the pathologic specimen in 84 to 95 per cent of the cases, and the long-term survival of these patients is excellent. Although the complications of radical prostatectomy are often emphasized, in the hands of the experienced surgeon the incidence of urinary incontinence should be less than 2 per cent. Previously, most patients were impotent postoperatively. However, with use of a new surgical technique this undesirable side effect can be avoided. In patients with Stage B2 prostatic cancer, 50 to 60 per cent will have involvement of the seminal vesicles. Because only 5 per cent of patients with involvement of the seminal vesicles survive 15 years free of tumor, patients with Stage B2 disease are not ideal candidates for radical surgery. For the treatment of Stage B2 and C disease, megavoltage radiation provides excellent palliation and the possibility of cure. For the treatment of Stage D disease, hormonal therapy is the preferred modality for initial treatment, but there are two major areas of controversy: (1) What are the relative merits of estrogen therapy versus therapy with bilateral orchiectomy or the combination of estrogen plus castration? (2) What is the preferred timing of endocrine treatment?

The physiologic effects of estrogen therapy and orchiectomy are similar, i.e., they produce regression of cancer of the prostate by suppressing plasma testosterone levels. Orchiectomy alone, estrogen therapy, or the combination of the two appears to be equally effective in the treatment of metastatic carcinoma of the prostate.

The second point of controversy surrounds the proper timing of endocrine therapy: Should it be instituted as soon as the diagnosis is made, or should treatment be delayed until the patient becomes symptomatic? In one study, patients with Stage A and B carcinoma of the prostate who were treated with estrogen had a higher death rate than did patients who were not receiving estrogen. The increase in death rate was caused by cardiovascular complications, suggesting that early treatment with estrogens can be harmful under some circumstances. The survival rate of patients with Stage C and D carcinoma treated with initial hormonal therapy was identical to the survival rate in those patients in whom hormonal therapy was delayed until symptoms appeared. Therefore, delaying hormonal therapy until symptoms occur has no adverse effect on the survival rate in patients with established metastatic disease. Estrogen therapy or orchiectomy should probably be delayed

TABLE 235–1. CARCINOMA OF PROSTATE

Stage (Whitmore)	Definition of Stage	Usual Treatment
A	Not palpable; found by histopathology	
A_1	Focal, well differentiated	Observation
A_2	Diffuse, poorly differentiated	Radical prostatectomy
B	Palpable, but limited to prostate	
B_1	Solitary nodule < one lobe	Radical prostatectomy
B_2	One lobe or more involved	Megavolt radiation
C	Extension beyond capsule	Megavolt radiation
D	Metastatic disease; acid phosphatase ↑	Hormonal therapy
D_1	Pelvic lymph nodes only	Rarely chemotherapy
D_2	More widespread metastases	

until symptoms appear. At that time, treatment with estrogen (diethylstilbestrol, 1 mg per day) or orchiectomy may be utilized. Reactivation of symptoms following an initial response to hormonal therapy, usually indicates a tumor no longer under hormonal control. Attempts at further endocrine therapy (adrenalectomy, hypophysectomy, or antiandrogen therapy) are usually disappointing. At present the only hope for treatment of these patients is chemotherapy. Several large scale clinical studies are currently in progress to evaluate different cytotoxic agents for the treatment of metastatic carcinoma of the prostate.

Catalona WJ, Scott WW: Carcinoma of the prostate. *In* Harrison JH, Gittes RF, Perlmutter AD, Stamey TA, Walsh PC (eds.): Campbell's Urology. 4th ed. Philadelphia, W. B. Saunders Company, 1979, pp 1085–1124. *This article provides a comprehensive review of all aspects relative to the diagnosis and treatment of carcinoma of the prostate.*

Scott WW, Menon M, Walsh PC: Hormonal therapy of prostatic cancer. Cancer 45:1929, 1980. *The hormonal therapy of prostatic cancer is approached from a physiologic standpoint. These findings are integrated with clinical studies to provide a sound basis for recommending timing and forms of treatment.*

Walsh PC, Jewett HJ: Radical surgery for prostatic cancer. Cancer 45:1906, 1980. *Radical prostatectomy for the treatment of prostatic cancer is somewhat controversial. This article provides a sound rationale for this form of treatment and identifies those patients most likely to benefit from surgical treatment.*

Walsh PC, Lepor H, Eggleston JC: Radical prostatectomy with preservation of sexual function: Anatomical and pathological considerations. Prostate 4:473, 1983. *By eliminating the fear of impotence associated with radical prostatectomy, patients and their physicians may be encouraged to diagnose prostatic cancer at an earlier stage when it is still curable.*

236. THE OVARIES

Griff T. Ross

Throughout postnatal life, normally functioning ovaries secrete sex steroid hormones and, from menarche to menopause, produce oocytes which differentiate into ova, the definitive female gametes. Since sex steroid hormones participate in the growth, differentiation, and function of a variety of extragonadal and extragenital tissues, ovarian function is not the exclusive concern of the gynecologist or the endocrinologist but of all physicians. When signs and symptoms consistent with inappropriate sex steroid hormone activity are encountered in any female patient, the physician should consider ovarian dysfunction in the differential diagnosis and proceed to determine its pathophysiologic origin.

A rational approach to the diagnosis and treatment of disorders of ovarian function depends upon knowledge of (1) the relationships of follicle growth, gametogenesis, and sex steroid hormone production; (2) regulation of these functions in health; (3) extraovarian actions of sex steroid hormones on target tissues; and (4) methods for the clinical and laboratory evaluation of these factors in health and disease. In this chapter this information will be briefly summarized and applied to the diagnosis and treatment of specific disorders of ovarian function in girls before and after puberty and in women before and after menopause.

Gross and Microscopic Anatomy

The mature ovaries are oval structures approximately 4 × 3 × 1 cm in diameter with an average combined weight of about 14 grams. Each of these structures is attached to the lateral pelvic wall by the infundibulopelvic ligament, to the posterior surface of the broad ligament by the mesovarium, and to the uterus by the ovarian ligament. Nerves, blood vessels, and lymphatics traverse the mesovarium of each ovary to enter an inner hilum, which is contiguous with a central medulla. The medulla is surrounded by an outer cortex, bounded in turn by a derivative of coelomic epithelium called the germinal epithelium (Fig. 236–1). The hilum of each ovary also contains steroid hormone–secreting cells, called hilar cells. In addition to blood vessels, the medulla of each ovary contains the cellular debris remaining after follicle maturation and regression, and the cortex contains follicle complexes in all stages of maturation.

The *follicle complex* is the indispensable structural and functional component of the human ovary; neither steroidogenesis nor gametogenesis occurs in the absence of follicles. Its cellular

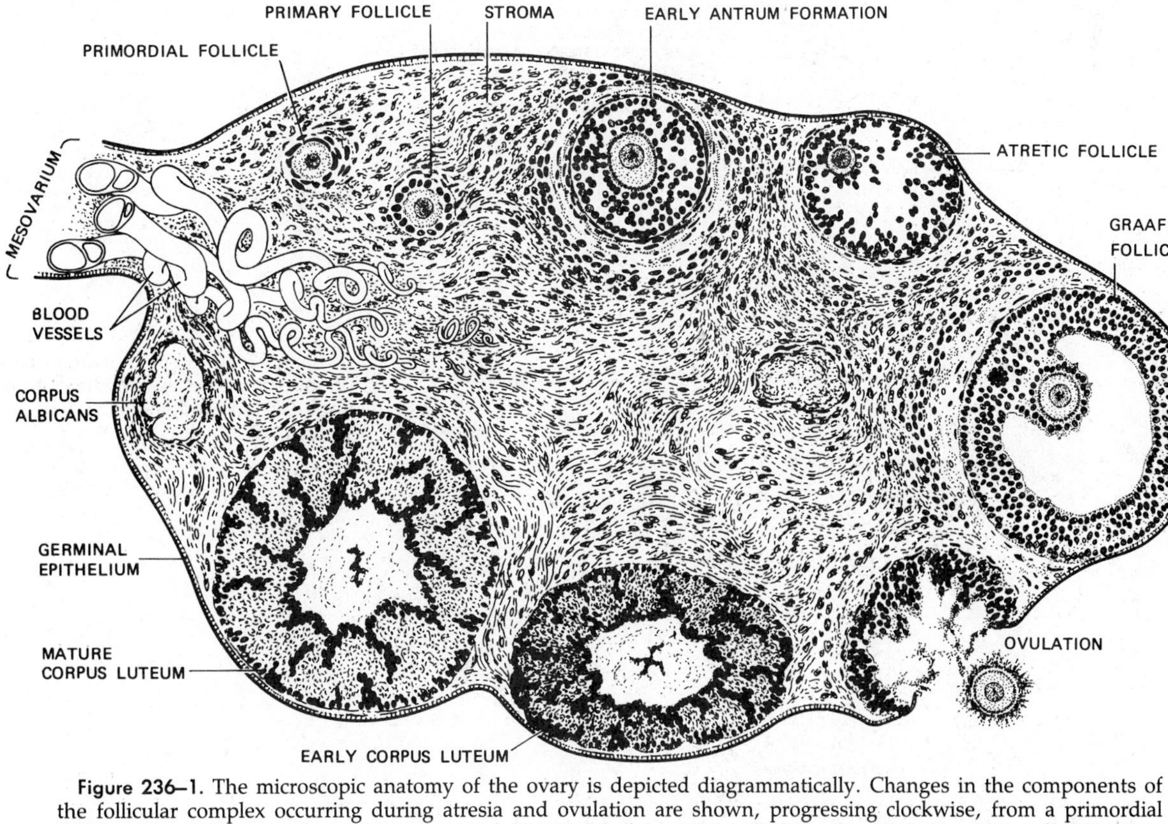

Figure 236–1. The microscopic anatomy of the ovary is depicted diagrammatically. Changes in the components of the follicular complex occurring during atresia and ovulation are shown, progressing clockwise, from a primordial follicle (upper left) to a corpus albicans (lower left). (Modified from Ross GT, Schreiber JR: *In* Yen SSC, Jaffe RB (eds.): Reproductive Endocrinology—Physiology, Pathophysiology and Clinical Management. Philadelphia, W. B. Saunders Company, 1978, pp 63–79.)

components consist of an *oocyte, granulosa cells,* and some interstitial cells called *theca cells.* Characteristic changes in the morphology of each component occur during follicle growth and differentiation. Interactions among these components give rise to the gamete (ovum) and to sex steroid hormones essential for establishing and maintaining early pregnancy should the ovum be fertilized.

The primordial follicle is bounded by a membrane, the basal lamina, which excludes blood and lymph vessels and is selectively permeable to solutes in plasma. Inside the basal lamina, less than a dozen spindle-shaped granulosa cells surround a primary oocyte, the nucleus of which is in prophase of the first meiotic division. This collection of cells is surrounded in turn by stroma, which consists of supporting connective tissue cells, contractile cells, and some steroid hormone–secreting interstitial cells, all intermingled with blood and lymph vessels (Fig. 236–1). Interstitial cells surrounding an individual follicle are called theca cells.

Morphologic Correlates of Normal Ovarian Function

From the time of their appearance in the fetal ovary until their disappearance from ovaries of postmenopausal women, selected primordial follicles begin to grow while others remain inactive. The normal progression of growth of follicles depends upon adequate stimulation by pituitary gonadotropins.

Growth and differentiation of the primordial follicle terminate in either *ovulation,* with extrusion of a secondary oocyte, or *atresia,* with retention and degeneration of the oocyte in situ. Pari passu, with either ovulation or atresia, developing follicles produce sex steroid hormones: estrogens, androgens, and progestogens. The steps in biosynthesis of sex steroid hormones are summarized diagrammatically in Figure 236–2. Two alternative pathways exist for synthesizing progestogens, androgens, and estrogens: the so-called Δ^5 pathway, in which 17α-hydroxypregnenolone and dehydroisoandrosterone are intermediates, and the Δ^4 pathway, in which pregnenolone is converted to progesterone and 17α-hydroxyprogesterone and androstenedione are the alternative intermediates. The "preferred" pathway in the human ovary is unknown.

Prior to the menarche, all developing follicles undergo atresia. After the menarche, while atresia continues, one follicle begins to grow more rapidly than its peers and moves to the surface of the cortex in preparation for ovulation. Steroid hormones secreted by this "dominant" follicle act on the hypothalamus and pituitary to stimulate a "surge" in luteinizing hormone (LH) secretion that anticipates its rupture (ovulation) by 35 to 40 hours (see Ch. 225).

This LH surge is indispensable for ovulation, but the mechanism by which it induces ovulation remains obscure. Hypotheses include an LH-induced increase in intrafollicular pressure, stimulation of contractile elements in the stroma, or proteolytic digestion of the basal lamina. Of these, the last is currently favored.

After the follicle has ruptured and the oocyte has been extruded, blood vessels and fibroblasts from the surrounding theca penetrate the basal lamina and permeate the residual granulosa cells, which rapidly differentiate into luteal cells with steroid hormone–secreting organelles. Fibroblasts, luteal cells, related thecal cells, and blood vessels together form the definitive *corpus luteum* (Fig. 236–1), which secretes increasing amounts of estrogens and progestogens for a period of about eight days. Then, unless fertilization occurs, steroid hormone production declines progressively over the last six to eight days of the cycle and menstruation begins. The corpus luteum is replaced by an avascular scar called a *corpus albicans.* If pregnancy occurs, (human) chorionic gonadotropin (hCG) produced by the conceptus stimulates continued production of estrogens

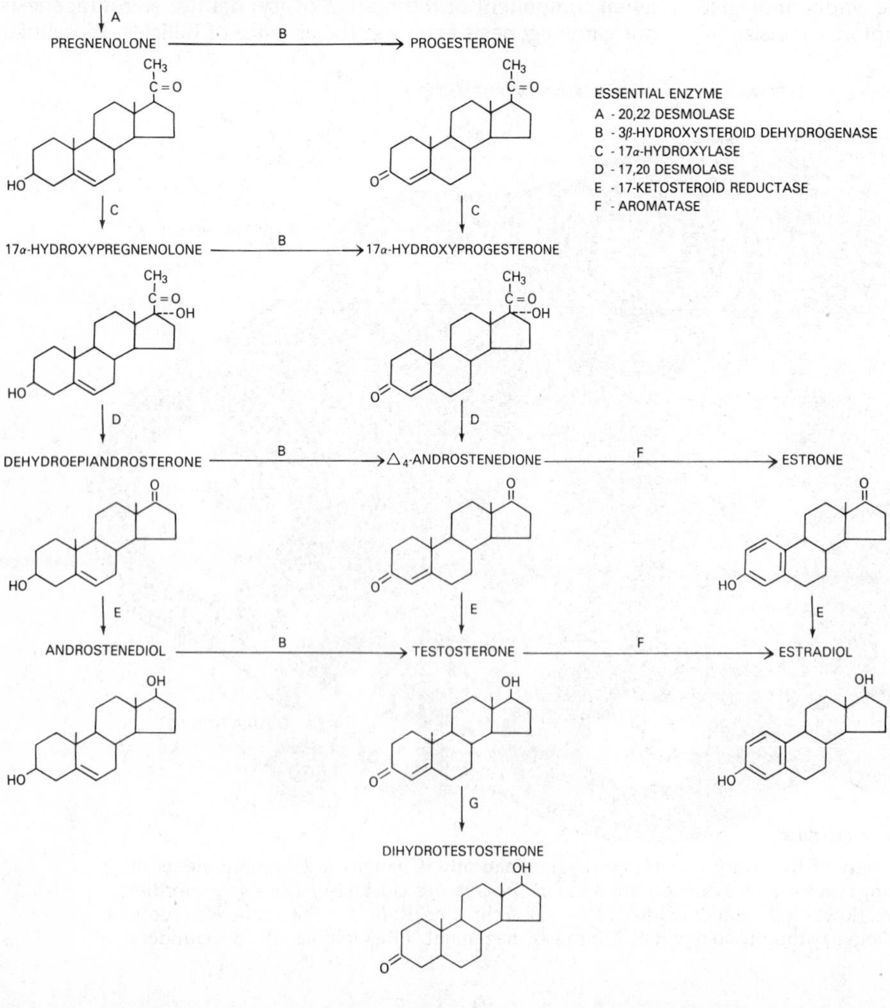

Figure 236–2. Steps in ovarian biosynthesis of steroid hormones. (Modified from data of Ross GT: *In* Rudolph AM (ed.): Pediatrics 16:1726, 1977.)

and progestogens by the corpus luteum. This persists throughout pregnancy. In addition to progesterone, hCG stimulates the corpus luteum of pregnancy to secrete relaxin, a peptide, the function of which remains obscure.

Since no oocytes are produced and no primordial follicles are formed after six months postnatally, successive cycles of atresia and ovulation deplete the supply of primordial follicles. As the number of follicles declines, the intermenstrual interval becomes irregular, anovulatory cycles occur, menses finally cease, and the *menopause* is established despite the presence of a few primordial follicles and increased pituitary gonadotropin secretion. Why these remaining follicles fail to grow or secrete steroid hormones remains unknown.

As a result of both depletion of follicles and failure of the remaining ones to mature, the ovaries shrink and ovarian weight markedly declines after the menopause. Four or five years after the last menstrual period, the last follicles disappear and only stroma persists. Ovarian estrogen synthesis ceases, but variable quantities of estrogen (mostly estrone) continue to be produced by aromatization of androgens, principally androstenedione, produced by both ovaries and adrenals, chiefly the latter. The quantity of estrone produced through this pathway is greater in obese than nonobese postmenopausal women and greater in postmenopausal than premenopausal obese women.

Hormonal Correlates of Normal Ovarian Function

The normal progression of these morphologic and functional changes requires gonadotropin secretion:

1. Once initiated, normal progression of follicle growth, steroid hormone production, ovulation, and atresia are gonadotropin dependent.

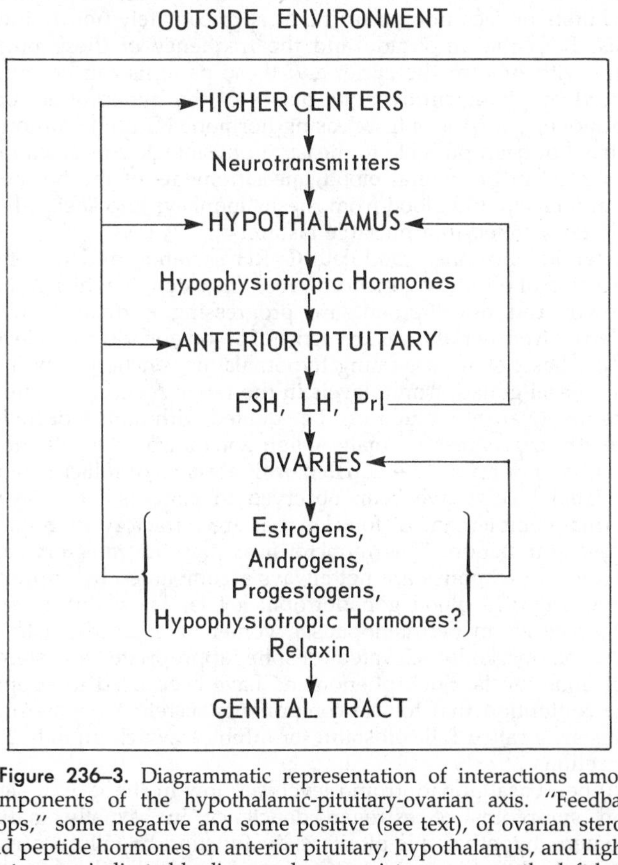

Figure 236–3. Diagrammatic representation of interactions among components of the hypothalamic-pituitary-ovarian axis. "Feedback loops," some negative and some positive (see text), of ovarian steroid and peptide hormones on anterior pituitary, hypothalamus, and higher centers are indicated by lines and appropriate arrows on the left-hand side of the figure. "Short loop feedback" of pituitary peptide hormones on hypothalamic sites, and of ovarian hormones acting locally to regulate follicular growth and development within the ovary, are indicated by lines and appropriate arrows on the right-hand side. Substances designated in lower case letters are the mediators of effects on various loci indicated in capital letters. Relevant details concerning these complex interactions will be found in the text of this chapter and in Ch. 225.

2. Sex steroid hormones produced in response to gonadotropins act locally to modulate these gonadotropin-dependent phenomena.

3. After the menarche, ovarian sex steroid hormones produced by the dominant preovulatory follicle and its successor, the corpus luteum, act systemically to coordinate functions of the hypothalamic-pituitary unit, the ovary, and the endometrium essential for maintaining ovulatory menstrual cycles and initiating pregnancy. These interactions are summarized diagrammatically in Figure 236–3.

4. The structural and functional status of follicular development (and thus of the ovaries) can be inferred from the status of sex steroid hormone production at any age throughout life. Moreover, since measures of sex steroid hormone secretion reflect the developmental status of the follicle chosen to ovulate during each cycle after the menarche, evaluation of sex steroid hormone production provides an appraisal of both steroidogenesis and gametogenesis in ovaries of women in any age group.

Sex Steroid Hormones and Clinical Evaluation of Ovarian Function

MEASUREMENTS OF SEX STEROID HORMONES. There are three major sex hormones produced by the mature human ovary: 17β-estradiol, progesterone, and testosterone. The pathways for the synthesis of these compounds and the relationship of estrogens and progesterone to follicle-stimulating hormone (FSH) and LH in the normal menstrual cycle have been shown in Figure 236–2. Table 236–1 shows the normal plasma concentrations of estrogens and progesterone during the menstrual cycle, together with their production rates.

For evaluating sex steroid hormone production, sensitive methods are available for measuring their concentrations in practical volumes of blood or aliquots of 24-hour urine specimens. These "chemical" or immunologic assays are expensive and not always easily accessible. Moreover, in a given patient, results may not be as reliable as evaluating the biologic activity of sex steroids in suitable target tissues of the hormones.

RESPONSES IN SEX STEROID HORMONE–DEPENDENT TISSUES. The sex steroid hormone target tissues include breasts, pubic and axillary hair, bone, vaginal epithelium, endocervical glands, endometrium, hypothalamus, and pituitary gland, and such metabolic processes as linear growth, basal body temperature regulation, and hepatic synthesis of some serum proteins. Responses of the target tissues to sex steroid hormones will often enable the physician to accurately assess ovarian function.

Target tissues dependent upon sex steroid hormones are responsive throughout life, but changing quantities of sex hormones produced at different times in life, coupled with limited accessibility of some of these tissues, render some end-organ responses more useful than others in the evaluation of ovarian function.

The Vaginal Epithelium. Estrogens and progestogens regulate rates of proliferation and differentiation of the stratified squamous epithelial cells which form the mucosa of the vagina. These cells exfoliate into the vagina and can be studied in smears of suitably stained vaginal secretions. The proportions of morphologically distinctive cells are altered by the prevailing sex steroid hormone milieu. Superficial cells predominate when estrogenization is adequate or excessive, whereas basal and parabasal cells predominate when estrogenization is low. Under the influence of progestogens, numbers of both superficial and basal cells decline and numbers of polymorphonuclear cells increase. This examination provides a rapid and inexpensive screen for the adequacy of estrogenic activity in the absence of vaginal infection.

The Endocervical Glands. Estrogens and progestogens regulate the amount and composition of endocervical mucus, an aqueous solution of proteins and electrolytes. Estrogens increase the quantity, the viscosity, and the elasticity or "spinnbarkeit" of the cervical mucus, as well as the tendency of

TABLE 236–1. PLASMA CONCENTRATIONS, METABOLIC CLEARANCE RATES (MCR) AND PRODUCTION RATES, AND OVARIAN SECRETION RATES OF SEX STEROID HORMONES AS A FUNCTION OF TIME IN CYCLE

Steroid	Time in Cycle	Plasma Concentration (ng/dl)	Plasma MCR (Liters/Day)	Plasma Production Rate (μg/Day)	Ovarian Secretion Rate (μg/Day)
Estradiol	Early	6	1350	81	70
	Mid-cycle	33–70		445–945	400–800
	Luteal	20		270	250
Estrone	Early	5	2210	110	80
	Mid-cycle	15–30		331–662	250–500
	Luteal	11		243	160
Estriol	Early	0.7	2100	14	18
	Luteal	1.0		23	
Progesterone	Follicular	3–10	2510	750–2500	1500
	Luteal	6–20		15,000–50,0000	24,000

electrolytes to crystallize in a "ferning" pattern (after water evaporates from smears of mucus on a glass slide). In contrast, progesterone not only inhibits endocervical mucus secretion but also reduces its viscosity, its elasticity, and its tendency to "fern." Simultaneous evaluation of endocervical mucus and vaginal epithelium enhances the value of each test.

The Endometrium. The cavity of the uterus is lined by mucosa, which consists of a superficial avascular layer of columnar epithelial cells overlying spindle-shaped stromal cells, penetrated by crypts of the surface epithelial cells and richly vascularized. Estrogens stimulate proliferation of both epithelial and stromal cells so that the mucosa thickens. In contrast, progestogens inhibit mitosis in estrogen-primed epithelial and stromal cells, stimulate secretory activity and glycogen storage in epithelial cells, increase vascularity of the stromal layer, and initiate "decidual" changes in stromal cells.

As the corpus luteum secretes less estrogen and progestogen, necrosis of stromal blood vessels is followed by multifocal necrosis and exfoliation of the epithelium which denudes the mucosa of all epithelial cells (except those lining glandular crypts). This initiates menstrual bleeding. It has been proposed that the reduction in steroids mobilizes lysosomal enzymes, which hydrolyze phospholipids. This would stimulate synthesis of prostaglandin $F_2\alpha$ which in turn is thought to stimulate endometrial necrosis and bleeding. After menses, mucosal continuity is restored by estrogen-stimulated proliferation of epithelial cells in the crypts.

Endometrial response to estrogens is sufficiently reliable to enable a pathologist to recognize the early, mid, or late proliferative (or preovulatory) phase of normal cycles. Morphologic changes in response to progesterone are sufficiently reproducible to enable a skilled observer to date the specimens in relation to an idealized 28-day cycle in which ovulation is assumed to have occurred on the fourteenth day. When the time of specimen collection is related to the onset of next menses, a discrepancy of more than two days in the actual and expected dates has been equated with inadequate corpus luteum function. For making these assessments of sex steroid hormone activity in sexually mature women, suitable specimens of endometrium can be obtained during an office visit, with minimal discomfort to the patient.

After the menarche, the appropriateness of ovarian estrogen secretion and endometrial response to the hormone can be inferred from a *progestogen withdrawal test,* performed by giving a single intramuscular injection of 100 mg of progesterone in oil, or alternatively by giving 10 mg of medroxyprogesterone acetate by mouth each day for five days. Vaginal bleeding within one week after the injection or after completing the five-day course of medroxyprogesterone has been equated with ovarian estrogen production equivalent to a mean serum estradiol level of 60 ng per deciliter, whereas failure to bleed indicates much lower serum estradiol levels of the order of 15 ng per deciliter.

The Hypothalamic Thermoregulatory Center. Estrogens reduce and progestogens increase basal body temperatures so that a progressive "thermogenic shift" of more than 0.3° C occurring after a nadir in serial basal body temperatures is a presumptive sign of ovulation, corpus luteum formation, and progesterone secretion. Although useful, this sign is not an entirely reliable test of the adequacy of corpus luteum function, since elevation of basal body temperature requires less progesterone than does adequate secretory transformation of the endometrium. Furthermore, taking body temperatures daily for five minutes before arising and recording these for 18 to 35 days is tedious, and patients often fail to comply fully.

The Hypothalamic-Pituitary Unit. The hormone concentrations in blood during a normal menstrual cycle in relation to the preovulatory LH surge or "peak" during spontaneous ovulatory cycles have been related to "feedback" effects (inhibitory or stimulatory) on pituitary cells by simultaneous changes in blood estrogen and progestogen concentrations. The smooth curves shown for FSH and LH are actually generated by pulses or bursts of secretion occurring at approximately hourly intervals. Both the amplitude and the frequency of these pulses vary with time in the cycle, and these patterns can be reproduced by giving intravenous pulses of the hypophyseotropic hormone, gonadotropin releasing hormone (GnRH). Although it has not been possible to measure physiologic concentrations of GnRH in peripheral blood, measurements of the hormone in pituitary portal blood from rhesus monkeys and sheep show it to be secreted in a pulsatile fashion.

Steroid hormones modulate GnRH secretion and therefore secretion of pituitary gonadotropins. The extent to which follicle growth and development are progressing normally can be inferred from serial measurements of blood gonadotropin levels in the basal state, assuming hypothalamic function to be normal. Basal gonadotropin levels in the range seen in castrate or postmenopausal women can be equated with failure of follicle growth to progress normally. High gonadotropin levels, however, cannot always be equated with absence of follicles, since elevated levels have been observed in patients who have a normal complement of follicles that are refractory to gonadotropic stimulation. This refractoriness may be transitory, and changes in response are not always accompanied by appropriate changes in blood gonadotropin levels. Thus, during ovulatory cycles in perimenopausal women, gonadotropin levels may be markedly elevated despite appropriate sex steroid hormone levels. Such phenomena have been used to support the contention that follicle components secrete a nonsteroidal substance called folliculostatin (or inhibin), which inhibits FSH secretion.

When basal gonadotropin levels are low in the face of signs and symptoms of estrogen deficiency in sexually mature women, hypothalamic-pituitary dysfunction or failure can be inferred. Pulsatile variations in gonadotropin levels may alter the validity of a single sample for evaluating basal secretion of the hormones. A sample taken from pooled specimens collected consecutively over the course of two to three hours will minimize this source of variation.

Bones, Breasts, and Pubic Hair. Vaginal epithelium, endocervical glands, and endometrium will respond to estrogen prior to puberty, but sampling these is not practical. Instead, response in such target tissues as bone, breasts, and pubic hair is more easily appraised. Estrogens stimulate ductular and stromal proliferation, and progestogens stimulate alveolobular development in breasts.

Estrogens stimulate growth of pubic hair, but the mechanism of hormone action is obscure.

Although the exact mechanism of action is unknown, estrogens are required for the normal formation, mineralization, and maturation of bones. Standards have been established for determining radiographically whether "bone age" is advancing appropriately in relation to chronologic age from infancy to adulthood. These standards are based on radiographs of left-sided extremities (hands, wrists, elbows, shoulders, hips, and knees) in normal children of different ages. Estrogen deficiencies retard and excesses advance bone age in relation to chronologic age, but the changes are slow to appear.

During childhood, deficiencies of estradiol are manifest by delayed or inadequate maturation and excesses by premature maturation in these steroid hormone–sensitive target tissues. During the postpubertal years, regression of breast development and osteopenia are signs of deficient, and breast engorgement and tenderness are signs of excess sex steroid hormone secretion.

Benirschke K: The endometrium. *In* Yen SSC, Jaffe RB (eds.): Reproductive Endocrinology. Philadelphia, W. B. Saunders Company, 1978, pp 241–260. *A pathologist provides a well illustrated discourse on endometrial morphology in health and disease.*

Espey LL: Ovarian contractility and its relationship to ovulation: A review. Biol Reprod 19:540, 1978. *Contains references to processes that may be involved in mechanics of ovulation.*

Knobil E: Neuroendocrine control of the menstrual cycle. Recent Prog Horm Res 36:53, 1980. *A literate treatment of results of a decade of intensive studies of hormonal events pacing the primate menstrual cycle; required reading for serious students of reproductive biology.*

Rebar RW: Practical evaluation of hormonal status. *In* Yen SSC, Jaffe RB (eds.): Reproductive Endocrinology. Philadelphia, W. B. Saunders Company, 1978, pp 469–518. *A clinician describes a systematic approach to assessing ovarian function and clinical diagnosis. Bibliography is exhaustive.*

Ross GT, Lipsett MB (eds.): Reproductive endocrinology. Clin Endocrinol Metab 7:467, 1978. *A collection of reviews on the "state of the art" of information about human ovarian function throughout life.*

Ross GT, Schreiber JR: The ovary. *In* Yen SSC, Jaffe RB (eds.): Reproductive Endocrinology. Philadelphia, W. B. Saunders Company, 1978, pp 63–79. *A treatise on ovarian morphology, physiology, and function, written by physicians for physicians.*

SEX STEROID HORMONES AND OVARIAN FUNCTION DURING INFANCY AND EARLY CHILDHOOD

Normal

Ovaries of infant and prepubertal girls respond in the same fashion as ovaries of postmenarchal women to the same gonadotropic stimulus. Ovarian follicles of prepubertal girls are smaller and secrete less steroid hormones prior to undergoing atresia because pituitary gonadotropin secretion is insufficient. The low blood estrogen levels characteristic of prepubertal girls do not elicit pituitary gonadotropin secretion comparable to that which occurs in adults following oophorectomy or primary ovarian failure. Indeed, failure of gonadotropins to rise in response to such blood estrogen levels in adults would be consistent with hypothalamic-pituitary dysfunction or failure. Ovulatory cycles are induced during chronic pulsatile administration of GnRH to prepubertal female rhesus monkeys and cease when GnRH is discontinued. In postpubertal girls, rising blood estrogens elicit an inhibition of FSH and a stimulation of LH secretion. In contrast, both FSH and LH secretion are inhibited following administration of extremely small doses of estradiol to prepubertal girls. The hypothalamic-pituitary unit during childhood is extremely sensitive to the inhibitory effects of estrogens. As puberty progresses, this sensitivity to inhibitory effects declines and gives way to a positive feedback effect of estrogens on LH secretion. Differences in hypothalamic-pituitary function therefore appear to account for differences in ovarian function before and after puberty.

Two additional observations provide circumstantial evidence for changes in steroid hormone regulation of hypothalamic-pituitary function after puberty in girls. First, pulsatile changes in blood LH levels, reflecting pulsatile secretion of LH and consistent with pulsatile secretion of GnRH, have been observed in specimens collected from pubescent girls during sleeping but not waking hours, and no such changes have been noted in clearly prepubertal girls. Second, ovulatory menstrual cycles have been induced during chronic pulsatile GnRH therapy in girls with hypogonadotropic hypogonadism, delayed puberty, and primary amenorrhea resulting from hypothalamic failure.

Abnormal

WITH NORMAL SEX STEROID HORMONE PRODUCTION. Ovarian diseases associated with normal sex steroid hormone production are uncommonly recognized during infancy and childhood. Instead, these become apparent at the expected age of puberty and will be discussed later.

WITH DECREASED SEX STEROID HORMONE PRODUCTION. Since ovarian steroid hormone production is normally low during infancy and prepubertal childhood, signs and symptoms associated with, but not resulting from, inadequate ovarian function are more useful clues for the presence of ovarian disease. These include failure to grow (the most common basis for seeking medical advice), musculoskeletal deformities, café-au-lait spots, pigmented nevi, a variety of congenital malformations, and cranial nerve deficits.

Although sex steroid hormone deficiencies produce few signs or symptoms during infancy and childhood, identification of the disorder at this time permits the physician to plan therapeutic strategies to deal with such problems as pubertal delay, primary amenorrhea, virilization at puberty, and the propensity of dysgenetic gonads to undergo malignant degeneration. All ovarian diseases associated with sex steroid hormone deficiency in infancy and childhood will be associated with sex steroid hormone deficiency later in life. Details related to specific syndromes are discussed in the next section under Delayed Puberty and Primary Amenorrhea.

WITH INCREASED SEX STEROID HORMONE PRODUCTION: PRECOCIOUS PUBERTY AND PSEUDOPUBERTY. The signs and symptoms of ovarian diseases associated with sex steroid hormone deficiency are unimpressive in infants and prepubertal girls. In contrast, the signs and symptoms of sex steroid hormone excess are dramatic, since all of the target tissues respond to stimulation in infants and children. Thus, accelerated linear growth and advanced bone age, breast growth and maturation, appearance of pubic and axillary hair, maturation of the external genitalia, and even cyclic vaginal bleeding may occur during the first year of life. The last-named event represents the syndrome of *isosexual precocious puberty,* in which premature maturation of the hypothalamic-pituitary axis results in ovulatory menstrual cycles indistinguishable from those that occur physiologically after puberty.

Similar signs may occur when the sex steroid hormone excess derives from ovarian or adrenal tumors or from normal ovaries responding to gonadotropins secreted by nonovarian tumors (so-called ectopic gonadotropin secretion). This is referred to as *isosexual precocious pseudopuberty.* In some instances pubertal changes may proceed along heterosexual, virilizing lines. The premature maturation of secondary sexual characteristics in these patients is referred to as *heterosexual precocious pseudopuberty.*

Target tissue responses to androgen excess in virilizing syndromes of heterosexual precocious pseudopuberty may be dramatic. Oily skin, severe acne, pubic and axillary hair growth, excessive facial and body hair, temporal hair recession, clitoral enlargement, and even episodic vaginal bleeding may occur in these girls. These syndromes rarely result from ovarian diseases but more commonly from adrenal cortical hyperplasia secondary to genetically determined deficiencies in enzymes required for the biosynthesis of cortisol (see Ch. 229). Ordinarily these are diagnosed during the neonatal period, but mild allelic variants associated with milder deficits occasionally escape detection until later.

Isosexual precocious puberty is rarely associated with life-threatening disease. Iso- and heterosexual precocious pseudopuberty may be associated with either life-threatening or reversible benign diseases. Thus, making the distinction promptly has important implications for treatment. Distinguishing the syndromes, however, may be difficult for at least two reasons.

First, the sequence of maturational events in the syndromes of both precocious puberty and precocious pseudopuberty is similar to that occurring during spontaneous puberty. In these syndromes, as in spontaneous puberty, breast and pubic hair development are the first changes to appear. Premature development of breasts (premature thelarche) or pubic hair (premature pubarche or adrenarche) may occur as isolated self-limited events with no further progression of pubertal maturation. Distinguishing among these alternatives early in the clinical course of any of them is often difficult.

Second, periodic vaginal bleeding may occur in isosexual precocious puberty and in both iso- and heterosexual precocious pseudopuberty. In these instances, only clear-cut presumptive indicators of ovulation which develop late in the clinical course will distinguish between these two syndromes.

CLINICAL EVALUATION OF PATIENTS WITH PRECOCIOUS PUBERTY AND PSEUDOPUBERTY. Fortunately, in some instances the history and physical examination will provide information useful for distinguishing isosexual precocious puberty from isosexual and heterosexual precocious pseudopuberty.

The History. The first element to explore carefully in eliciting the history is the temporal sequence in which signs and symptoms of sex steroid hormone excess appeared. Breast budding usually appears before or very shortly after pubic hair growth begins during normal pubescence. If pubic hair growth is not followed shortly by breast budding, the sequence suggests a diagnosis of premature adrenarche. Conversely, breast hypertrophy persisting for months without appearance of pubic hair suggests premature thelarche.

Careful questioning of the mother and other women with whom an infant or child has intimate contact may reveal a source of either inadvertent oral ingestion (oral contraceptive pills, for example) or percutaneous absorption (cosmetics or powders containing steroids) of estrogens or androgens. A diagnosis of *factitious pseudopuberty* on this basis eliminates the need for more complicated and expensive diagnostic tests.

A history of seizures or seizure equivalents provides presumptive evidence for an intracerebral tumor that may be associated with precocious puberty if the tumor stimulates pituitary gonadotropin secretion.

The Physical Examination. The physician should look very carefully for evidences of virilization. When present, virilizing signs exclude the diagnosis of isosexual precocious puberty. In their absence, however, a diagnosis of pseudopuberty cannot be excluded, since virilizing signs take a finite period of time to develop. Moreover, isosexual changes may result from estrogens produced by peripheral aromatization of androgens secreted by adrenal or ovarian tumors.

Physical examination of organ systems that are not estrogen targets may provide valuable clues for distinguishing among the etiologic variants of precocious puberty and pseudopuberty. The constellation of cutaneous café-au-lait spots, facial asymmetry, polyostotic fibrous dysplasia, and other skeletal abnormalities such as sclerotic changes in the base of the skull and cranial nerve deficits suggests a diagnosis of the *McCune-Albright syndrome* in a girl with signs of precocious puberty (see Ch. 251). Other neurologic deficits may be associated with central nervous system tumors such as phakomas, hamartomas, and neoplasms of the floor of the third ventricle which initiate isosexual precocious puberty. As noted, neurologic deficits are more likely to be associated with precocious puberty.

Signs and symptoms of thyroid hormone deficiency have been observed in girls with precocious puberty associated with thyroid-stimulating hormone (TSH)-deficient hypothyroidism. Thyroid hormone replacement therapy halts progression of the pubertal changes in these girls, and they will subsequently undergo puberty at the usual time.

Careful abdominal and rectal examination is helpful in distinguishing true precocious puberty from pseudopuberty, since most adrenal and ovarian tumors associated with iso- or heterosexual precocious pseudopuberty are palpable. Benign adrenal adenomas secreting androgens or estrogens may not be large enough to be palpated, but functioning adrenal carcinomas are almost always palpable. Ovarian cysts may also secrete sufficient estrogen to initiate isosexual pseudopuberty. Ovarian cysts may occur prior to development of ovulatory cycles in true isosexual precocity. Hence, the presence of these cysts does not exclude a diagnosis of true isosexual precocious puberty, and laparotomy is indicated to assure that the lesion is not an ovarian tumor.

When vaginal bleeding is the only sign or symptom of precocity, vaginal inspection is essential to rule out bleeding secondary to local irritation from infection or foreign bodies and to eliminate bleeding vaginal or cervical neoplasms. This examination should be done prior to embarking on more complex diagnostic studies, since vaginal bleeding as the first sign of precocious puberty is exceedingly uncommon.

TABLE 236–2. SIGNS USEFUL IN DIAGNOSING SYNDROMES OF PRECOCIOUS PUBERTY AND PSEUDOPUBERTY*

	Breast Enlargement	Pubic Hair	Vaginal Bleeding	Virilizing Signs	Advanced Bone Age	Neurologic Deficits	Abdominopelvic Masses
Premature thelarche	+	−	−	−	−	−	−
Premature adrenarche	−	+	−	−	±	−	−
Precocious puberty							
Idiopathic	+	+	+	−	+	−	Rarely
Due to CNS tumor	+	+	+	−	+	+	−
McCune-Albright syndrome†	+	+	+	−	+	+	−
Primary hypothyroidism‡	+	Rarely	+	−	−	−	Rarely
Isosexual precocious pseudopuberty							
Ovarian tumors	+	+	+	−	+	−	+
Adrenal tumors§	+	+	+	−	+	−	+
Ovarian cysts	+	+	+	−	+	−	+
Factitious¶	+	+	+	−	+	−	−
Heterosexual precocious pseudopuberty							
Ovarian tumors	+	+	+	+	+	−	Rarely
Adrenal tumors§	+	+	+	+	+	−	+
Congenital adrenal hyperplasia	+	+	+	+	+	−	−

*Modified from data of Ross GT, Vande Wiele RL: *In* Williams, RH (ed.): Textbook of Endocrinology. 5th ed. Philadelphia, W. B. Saunders Company, 1974, pp 368–422.

†Facial asymmetry and other musculoskeletal abnormalities are diagnostic.

‡Retarded bone age is diagnostic.

§Mass in upper abdomen is suggestive.

¶History of exposure is essential.

A summary of physical findings and tests useful for distinguishing entities associated with precocious puberty and precocious pseudopuberty is summarized in Table 236–2. Table 236–3 provides a scheme for further evaluating patients with and without physical signs of virilization.

Diagnostic Tests. In addition to the history and physical examination, useful maneuvers include ultrasonic scanning of adrenals and ovaries and computed tomographic (CT) scans of adrenals for confirming impressions obtained by palpation. CT scans of the head are indicated when a history of seizures is elicited or neurologic deficits are discovered in a patient with signs of precocious puberty or pseudopuberty.

Radiographic determination of bone age should be made. Plain skull films are useful in screening for pituitary and parapituitary tumors.

On occasion, measurement of steroid and peptide hormone concentrations in blood will provide diagnostically useful information. High blood levels of 17-OH-progesterone or 11-deoxycortisol which decline following oral administration of suppressive doses of dexamethasone (see Ch. 229 and 237) are useful for distinguishing adrenal cortical hyperplasia from adrenal cortical adenomas and carcinomas or from ovarian tumors secreting androgens. High levels of serum testosterone suggest an ovarian source of excess androgen, whereas high levels of dehydroisoandrosterone (DHA) or its sulfate ester (DHAS), the principal precursors of urinary 17-ketosteroids, are more consistent with adrenal sources of excess androgen.

Blood immunoreactive LH levels in excess of those encountered in any physiologic state in women and girls are diagnostic of ovarian dysgerminomas and teratomas which secrete hCG that is antigenically and biologically similar to LH and stimulates ovarian steroid hormone secretion and pseudopubertal changes in prepubertal girls. Blood FSH:LH ratios compatible with those in sexually mature women are helpful for diagnosing precocious puberty. If obtaining blood specimens is impractical, determining gonadotropin concentrations in timed urine collections serves the same purpose.

TABLE 236–3. SCHEMA FOR DIAGNOSTIC EVALUATION OF PATIENTS WITH PRECOCIOUS PUBERTY AND PSEUDOPUBERTY

I. Virilizing signs present
  A. With palpable abdominal or pelvic masses
    1. If location suggests adrenal tumor:
      a. Do CT scan to rule out bilateral tumors
      b. Look for metastases in chest, liver
    2. If location suggests ovarian tumor
      a. Confirm mass with ultrasonic scanning
      b. Examine under anesthesia and explore surgically
  B. Without palpable abdominal or pelvic masses: measure serum androgens and androgen precursors: DHA, DHAS, T
    1. If all elevated, do Decadron suppression test
      a. If suppressible, suspect congenital adrenal hyperplasia due to 11- or 21-hydroxylase deficiency; measure 17-OHP, 11-DOC to distinguish
      b. If not suppressible, suspect adrenal carcinoma or rare ovarian tumor; use scans appropriately, measure hormones in venous effluent to lateralize before surgery
    2. If testosterone is disproportionately elevated, suspect ovarian tumor, and use ultrasonic scan to lateralize before surgery
II. Virilizing signs absent
  A. With palpable abdominal or pelvic masses
    1. If location suggests adrenal tumor, proceed as in I.A.1
    2. If location suggests ovarian tumor, proceed as in I.A.2
  B. Without palpable abdominal or pelvic masses
    1. If vaginal bleeding has occurred, inspect vagina for infection, foreign body, tumor
    2. If vaginal bleeding has not occurred, do complete neuroophthalmologic exam
      a. If abnormal, involve neurosurgeon in choice of further studies for intracerebral tumors likely to produce precocious puberty
      b. If normal, determine bone age by x-ray
        (1) If retarded, diagnostic of precocious puberty due to primary hypothyroidism
        (2) If normal or advanced, measure serum DHA, DHAS
          (a) If values consistent with age, consider premature thelarche, early precocious puberty, factitious pseudopuberty, forme fruste of McCune-Albright syndrome
          (b) If values increased for age, consider premature adrenarche, early precocious puberty, pseudopuberty due to occult ovarian or adrenal tumor

TABLE 236–4. CRITERIA FOR DISTINGUISHING TANNER STAGES 1 THROUGH 5 IN BREASTS AND PUBIC HAIR MATURATION*

For Breasts	Stage	For Pubic Hair
No palpable glandular tissue; areola not pigmented; except for nipple, breast does not project from anterior chest wall	1	None
Glandular tissue is palpable at least coextensively with the diameter of the areola; nipple and breast project as a single mound from anterior chest wall	2	Occasional wispy strands, usually along the labia
Increased glandular tissue to palpation; breasts enlarged; areola increasing in diameter and becoming more darkly pigmented, but contours of breast and areola remain in a single plane	3	More, darker, coarser hair extending superiorly over the pubis
Further enlargement; increased areolar pigmentation; areola and nipple form a secondary mound above level of the breast	4	Dark, coarse, curly hair, covering the mons pubis in the adult pattern, but not extending to medial aspects of thighs
Areola and nipple no longer project but have receded to make a smooth contour in profile view	5	Mature; extends to thighs but otherwise remains in female pattern

*Modified from data of Ross GT, Vande Wiele, RL: *In* Williams, RH (ed.): Textbook of Endocrinology. 5th ed. Philadelphia, W. B. Saunders Company, 1974, pp 368–422.

SEX STEROID HORMONES AND OVARIAN FUNCTION DURING LATE CHILDHOOD

Normal

NORMAL PUBERTY. To determine if the extent of pubertal development is normal for a girl's chronologic peer group, it is necessary to know the mean age and range of ages associated with the onset of breast and pubic hair development and the rates of progression in maturation, as well as the mean age and age ranges of the normal pubertal growth spurt and of normal menarche. To give the assessment an objective, quantitative dimension, degrees of breast and pubic hair development have been assigned numbers ranging from 1 (least mature) to 5 (adults). Criteria for these states are listed in Table 236–4.

The pubertal growth spurt, manifested by acceleration in the rate of linear growth, is an important landmark. It usually begins after breast development has been initiated and is often completed by the time maturation has progressed to Stage 3.

Menarche marks the completion of pubertal change. It appears at a mean age of 12.6 years, with a standard deviation of 1.2 years. The age range of menarche is 9 to 16 years in the United States population. Thus, *the occurrence of menarche before the age of 9 or failure to occur after the age of 16 merits evaluation.* Since the beginning of breast maturation anticipates the menarche by one to two years, failure to initiate changes in sexual characteristics by age 12 merits study.

DELAYED PUBERTY. In some girls who will undergo puberty spontaneously, delays in both the age at onset and rates of progression of pubertal changes exceed three standard deviations from the means for normal girls. These delays may create psychologic problems, generate parental anxiety, and pose problems in diagnosis and management. Unfortunately, the diagnosis is confirmed only by spontaneous onset and completion of puberty, and a decision to temporize can be justified only after excluding other diagnosable entities.

As an alternative to temporizing, sex steroid hormones can be used to induce pubertal changes in secondary sexual characteristics when the psychologic burden of delay is intolerable. Although no apparent permanent damage to fertility results from giving sex steroid hormones, the extent of linear growth may be compromised if treatment is too aggressive.

Abnormal

DYSFUNCTIONAL UTERINE BLEEDING. Prolonged and severe vaginal bleeding associated with endometrial hyperplasia and anovulation may occur after the menarche. In these girls no response in plasma LH is seen following 1 mg injections of estradiol benzoate, a manipulation which elicits an increase in blood LH levels in normal postpubertal girls. Progestogens will sometimes induce a "medical curettage" and stop bleeding. If this fails, a gynecologist should be consulted.

PRIMARY AMENORRHEA. During later childhood, when pubescence normally begins, the majority of ovarian diseases present with signs and symptoms suggestive of decreased ovarian sex steroid hormone production. In addition to short stature, these include retarded development of secondary sexual characteristics (delayed puberty) or primary amenorrhea or both. The relationships between sex steroid hormone production and primary amenorrhea are shown in Table 236–5.

WITH NORMAL SEX STEROID HORMONE PRODUCTION. When pubertal changes have begun at an appropriate age and secondary sexual characteristics have matured fully and in proper sequence but menses have not appeared, primary attention should be directed to the genital tract. Müllerian dysgenesis and amenorrhea traumatica are major considerations.

Müllerian Dysgenesis. Müllerian ducts normally give rise to fallopian tubes, the uterus, the cervix, and the upper vagina in genetic females (Fig. 233–2). For unknown reasons, one or more of the derivatives may not develop, and the failure may go unrecognized until the age of puberty. The anomalies vary in severity from an imperforate hymen to complete aplasia of all müllerian duct derivatives with vaginal atresia. Although aplasia usually involves all of the derivatives, single component defects have been described. Thus, vaginal aplasia associated with absence of the uterus and cervix is the most common defect, with an estimated frequency of 1 per 4000 female infants. In about 10 per cent of cases, vaginal aplasia is associated with a functionally normal uterus and cervix. Congenital absence of the cervix associated with a functionally normal uterus and patent vagina is extremely rare, less than 20 cases having been reported.

Normal ovarian sex steroid hormone secretion induces cyclic endometrial growth and shedding after menarche. In girls with a normal uterus but cervical aplasia, vaginal aplasia, or an imperforate hymen, the menstrual effluent is retained, producing endometriosis and cyclic abdominal pain without external evidence of menses. Examination under anesthesia is essential for determining the extent of the defect and should be done by a surgeon experienced in creating vaginas for these patients. When the defect consists of an imperforate hymen only, restoration of normal function is accomplished by incising the hymenal membrane. Attempts at plastic reconstruction of a functional vagina and a patent outflow tract have met with variable success, and successful pregnancy has been reported only rarely.

Amenorrhea Traumatica. In addition to müllerian dysgenesis, endometrial synechiae associated with endometrial resistance to estrogenic and progestational steroid hormone stimulation and withdrawal may result in primary amenorrhea. Endometritis, usually tuberculous, is the predisposing etiology.

WITH DECREASED SEX STEROID HORMONE PRODUCTION FETALLY AND POSTNATALLY. ***Errors in Genital Differentiation.*** Errors in gender assignment to genetic males during the neonatal period account for about 50 per cent of cases of primary amenorrhea. These errors are usually based on gross abnormalities in genital differentiation.

Virilization of gonaductal and genital anlagen in genetic males is dependent upon two secretory products of fetal testes: (1) testosterone, which stimulates development of wolffian duct derivatives and virilization of derivatives of the urogenital sinus and genital tubercle (following its conversion to dihydrotestosterone in the target tissues); and (2) müllerian regression factor, which results in degeneration of müllerian ducts. Abnormalities are discussed in Ch. 233.

Errors in Gonadal Development. GONADAL DYSGENESIS. The term "gonadal dysgenesis" is used to designate the most common error in fetal gonadal differentiation, occurring with an estimated frequency of 1 per 5000 to 7000 newborns or 1 per 2700 newborn phenotypic females. The gonads are streaks composed of fibrous stroma and devoid of gametogenic components. In most instances sex chromosomal aberrations are found in karyotypes prepared from cultures of somatic cells and presumably predispose to reduction in the number of germ cells available at the time of follicle formation during fetal life. The limited number of follicles formed is depleted by atresia prior to puberty in most instances. Occasionally, a few will persist postnatally, mature, and produce sufficient estrogen to initiate pubertal changes. Rarely, these will be sufficient for completing puberty, and there are case reports of ovulation followed by pregnancy and delivery of normal infants at term.

Streak gonads also occur in persons in whom there are no detectable morphologic abnormalities of the sex chromosomes, suggesting that other factors may result in depletion of germ cells and reduction in number of follicles formed. Thus, there are two familial varieties of gonadal dysgenesis caused by gene mutations, both of which occur sporadically as well. A paucity of follicles has been seen in ovaries of fetuses and infants with trisomy 13 or 18 syndromes (see Ch. 35). A paucity of primordial follicles and failure of maturation of these have been described in ovaries of girls with ataxia telangiectasia (see Ch. 492). Whether chromosomal breakage and immunoglobulin deficiencies, both characteristic manifestations of the latter

TABLE 236–5. SEX STEROID HORMONE PRODUCTION AND PRIMARY AMENORRHEA

I. With normal sex steroid hormone production
  A. Müllerian dysgenesis
  B. Amenorrhea traumatica
II. With decreased sex steroid hormone production
  A. Disorders of fetal development and differentiation
    1. Of the genitalia
      a. Male pseudohermaphroditism due to deficient testosterone synthesis
        (1) 20,22-Desmolase
        (2) 3β-Hydroxysteroid dehydrogenase
        (3) 17α-Hydroxylase
        (4) 17,20-Desmolase
        (5) 17-Ketosteroid reductase
      b. Male pseudohermaphroditism due to 5α-reductase deficiency
      c. Male pseudohermaphroditism due to androgen resistance
        (1) Complete testicular feminization
        (2) Incomplete testicular feminization
        (3) Familial incomplete male pseudohermaphroditism
      d. Female pseudohermaphroditism with fetal and postnatal androgen excess
    2. Of the gonads
      a. Gonadal dysgenesis with stigmata of Turner's syndrome
      b. Mixed gonadal dysgenesis
      c. Pure gonadal dysgenesis
      d. True hermaphroditism
  B. Congenital and acquired disorders
    1. Follicular insensitivity to gonadotropins
      a. 17-hydroxylase deficiency
      b. "Resistant ovaries"
    2. Hypothalamic pituitary diseases
      a. Familial hypogonadotropic hypogonadism
      b. Pituitary and parapituitary tumors
      c. Idiopathic panhypopituitarism
      d. Anorexia nervosa
    3. Miscellaneous systemic diseases
III. With increased sex steroid hormone production
  A. Androgen secreting ovarian and adrenal tumors
  B. Male pseudohermaphroditism due to 5α-reductase deficiency
  C. Polycystic ovarian disease

syndrome, predispose to a reduction in oocytes and follicles remains to be determined.

The syndrome of sexual infantilism, short stature, musculoskeletal abnormalities, and streak gonads, referred to as *Turner's syndrome,* is associated with abnormalities of sex chromosome number or morphology. Among these patients, one of virtually every variety of chromosomal breakage, with or without reunion, has been described (see Ch. 35). However, the most common karyotype is 45,X, in which the second sex chromosome is totally deleted. Short stature and other somatic stigmata associated with chromatin-negative nuclear sex without "F" bodies (see Ch. 35) in a patient with female external genitalia and failure to achieve puberty are diagnostic of the 45,X syndrome. Many of the somatic stigmata of Turner's syndrome occur in Noonan's syndrome, in arthrogryposis, in the Klippel-Feil syndrome (see Ch. 523), and in a variety of other syndromes in which sex chromosomes are normal. Girls with these latter disorders have chromatin-positive nuclear sex (Barr bodies) and 46,XX karyotypes.

MIXED GONADAL DYSGENESIS. The term "mixed gonadal dysgenesis" has been used to designate asymmetrical gonadal development with a germ cell tumor or a testis on one side and an undifferentiated streak, a rudimentary gonad, or no gonad on the other side. Gonaductal differentiation is usually concordant with gonadal differentiation, but the extent of genital virilization is variable. In patients with germ cell tumors, 90 per cent of whom are reared as females, virilization is mild, and some breast development occurs at puberty. In contrast, among patients with a testis and a streak, only 70 per cent are raised as females, virilization at puberty is marked, and no breast development occurs. Short stature and other stigmata associated with a 45,X karyotype in Turner's syndrome are less commonly observed among patients with tumors than among patients with testes.

Nuclear sex is usually chromatin negative. "F" bodies should be sought, but failure to demonstrate an "F" body is not a definitive test for the Y chromosomes, since Y chromosomes that do not fluoresce have been identified among patients with 45,X/46,XY sex chromosomal mosaicism and mixed gonadal dysgenesis. Thus, to rule out the presence of cell lines containing "Y" chromosomes in patients with anomalous external genitalia and chromatin-negative nuclear sex but no "F" bodies, the karyotype should be determined.

No endocrine tests are diagnostic of either tumor or testis. Visualization, biopsy, and removal of all gonadal tissue seem indicated to remove sources of androgen in girls with X/XY karyotypes in whom virilization occurs at puberty and to eliminate the neoplastic potential of dysgenetic gonads. Suitable sex steroid hormone replacement therapy should be undertaken at the appropriate time.

PURE GONADAL DYSGENESIS. The term "pure gonadal dysgenesis" has been used to distinguish sexually immature taller girls (>150 cm) with bilateral streak gonads and minimal extragenital extragonadal somatic stigmata from sexually immature shorter girls (<150 cm) with streak gonads associated with the musculoskeletal defects usually regarded as manifestations of Turner's syndrome. This distinction is clinically useful in view of the high incidence of gonadal tumors in patients with pure gonadal dysgenesis and an XY karyotype.

Pure gonadal dysgenesis is a genetic disorder occurring in siblings, whereas Turner's syndrome is rarely observed in siblings. Heredofamilial gonadal dysgenesis can be associated with either an XY or XX karyotype, and the disorder is sometimes referred to as familial XX or XY gonadal dysgenesis. The two karyotypes are transmitted differently, and there are some other distinguishing clinical features. The 45,XY syndrome, transmitted as an X-linked recessive trait (see Ch. 35), is associated with gonadal tumors in about 25 per cent of cases and clitoral hypertrophy in 10 to 15 per cent of cases. These changes are found in less than 5 per cent of patients with the XX syndrome. The high incidence of tumors of germ cell origin among persons with an XY genotype mandates gonadectomy in these patients.

Sex chromosomal aneuploidy is less common among patients with pure gonadal dysgenesis. Mosaic karyotypes such as 45,X/46,XX have been described in sporadic cases of pure gonadal dysgenesis.

TRUE HERMAPHRODITISM. Gonadal differentiation may proceed differently on the two sides, giving rise to a unilateral testis or ovary or ovotestis, with an ovary or a testis or an ovotestis on the other side. When both sperm and oocytes are found in these gonads, true hermaphroditism is diagnosed. Hermaphroditism is further discussed in Ch. 233.

Disorders Due to Follicular Insensitivity to Gonadotropins. 17-HYDROXYLASE DEFICIENCY (see also Ch. 229). Failure of follicle growth to progress normally results in primary amenorrhea in women congenitally unable to synthesize estrogen because of deficiency of 17-hydroxylase. In these women steroid hormone synthesis does not progress beyond progesterone (Fig. 236–2), and estrogen deficiency gives rise to sexual infantilism and primary amenorrhea associated with increased serum and urinary gonadotropins. Furthermore, excessive synthesis of an adrenal cortical salt-retaining steroid hormone, desoxycorticosterone, predisposes to hypertension with hypokalemic alkalosis. Ovarian biopsies show numerous large cysts and numerous primordial follicles with complete failure of orderly follicular maturation despite high serum gonadotropin levels. The association of sexual infantilism and primary amenorrhea with hypertension suggests the diagnosis. When present, high serum levels of progesterone and desoxycorticosterone (DOC) are diagnostic. The hypertension may respond to glucocorticoid replacement therapy.

RESISTANT OVARIES. Some sexually immature normotensive girls with high serum and urinary gonadotropins have ovaries that contain primordial follicles that neither mature nor secrete estrogens despite stimulation with massive doses of exogenous gonadotropins. Since ovulation may follow administration of estrogens, the defect possibly lies in the inability to initiate estrogen synthesis prior to antrum formation.

Disorders Due to Hypothalamic-Pituitary Dysfunction or Failure. The pituitary must secrete sufficient quantities of gonadotropins to stimulate ovarian follicular maturation and sex steroid hormone secretion. If it does not, secondary sexual characteristics do not mature and no menses occur. Failure may result from inadequate hypothalamic stimulation or from primary pituitary diseases (such as neoplasms or granulomas) that adversely affect pituitary function. All varieties of sexual immaturity resulting from inadequate pituitary gonadotropin secretion are referred to as syndromes of *hypogonadotropic hypogonadism.* It is important to distinguish among them in order that treatment be directed toward the specific underlying disease (see Ch. 225).

FAMILIAL HYPOGONADOTROPIC HYPOGONADISM (see also Ch. 234). Kallmann's syndrome is a familial disorder characterized by anosmia or hyposmia secondary to dysplasia of the rhinencephalon, sexual immaturity, and variable expression of midline defects. The trait is transmitted as an X-linked recessive or male-limited autosomal dominant trait, although genetic heterogeneity may occur. Ovaries of these women contain numerous primordial follicles, but follicular maturation is severely retarded even when compared to that in ovaries of neonates. Successful pregnancies after induction of ovulation with gonadotropins support the contention that the hypogonadism results from inadequate gonadotropin secretion. Successful induction of ovulation after chronic pulsatile administration of gonadotropin-releasing hormone to persons with this syndrome suggests that the disease is of hypothalamic rather than pituitary origin.

ANOREXIA NERVOSA. Primary amenorrhea resulting from hypothalamic dysfunction occurs as a complication of anorexia nervosa. Anorexia nervosa is discussed extensively in Ch. 215.

SECONDARY TO PITUITARY AND PARAPITUITARY TUMORS. Disorders of hypothalamic control of pituitary hormone secretion, including gonadotropins, are associated with third ventricle tumors and parapituitary tumors. Destruction of anterior pituitary tissue by primary pituitary neoplasms or by metastatic infiltration of other neoplasms may result in hypogonadism and primary amenorrhea associated with signs and symptoms of deficiencies of other pituitary hormones (see Ch. 225 and 511). Neurologic and neuroradiologic examinations are essential for proper evaluation. Surgical ablation is indicated when feasible.

SECONDARY TO SYSTEMIC DISEASE. The hypothalamic-pituitary unit may fail to function appropriately in a number of debilitating, stressful, systemic diseases that interfere with somatic growth and development. Chronic renal failure is perhaps the most common of these. It would be rare indeed for such a disease process to be discovered during the course of an evaluation for primary amenorrhea.

WITH INCREASED SEX STEROID HORMONE PRODUCTION. The quantities of testosterone and of dihydrotestosterone produced normally in female fetuses are inadequate to effect virilization of the primordia of the urogenital sinus and external genitalia. Excessive androgen arising endogenously from the adrenals or exogenously from hormonal therapy of pregnant women will produce virilization of the external genitalia and result in female pseudohermaphroditism. The extent of anomalous genital differentiation varies from an enlarged clitoris to ambiguity sufficient to make gender assignment by inspection hazardous.

Excessive maternal ovarian androgen production during gestation sometimes results in virilization of the urogenital sinus and genital tubercle derivatives in genetic females with normal ovaries.

Excessive fetal adrenal androgen secretion is usually associated with defective cortisol synthesis, and failure to suppress pituitary adrenocorticotropin secretion results in congenital adrenal hyperplasia and excessive adrenal androgen secretion (see Ch. 229). In female fetuses with deficiencies of either the 11β-hydroxylase or 21-hydroxylase enzyme system, excessive adrenocortical androgen secretion not only results in virilization of the external genitalia, and occasionally the urogenital sinus as well, during fetal life but also stimulates development of heterosexual precocious pseudopuberty and suppresses pituitary gonadotropin secretion postnatally.

Ordinarily, signs and symptoms of adrenal cortical insufficiency in these girls during the neonatal period lead to recognition and appropriate treatment at that time. Allelic variants associated with milder enzyme deficits may not be recognized until signs and symptoms of heterosexual precocious pseudopuberty, primary amenorrhea, or severe acne and hirsutism lead to recognition of the pathophysiologic basis of the disorder. Chromatin-positive nuclear sex eliminates the diagnosis of male pseudohermaphroditism. Other diagnostic tests are discussed in Ch. 229 and 237.

Male Pseudohermaphroditism Due to 5α-Reductase Deficiency. Male pseudohermaphrodites with 5α-reductase deficiency are usually raised as girls. However, at puberty breasts fail to develop, pubic hair and beard develop, no menses occur, virilization of the external genitalia takes place, and these persons assume male gender roles. By standards for girls at puberty, testosterone production is increased (see Ch. 233).

Polycystic Ovarian Disease. A syndrome of primary amenorrhea with hirsutism, other virilizing signs, insulin-resistant diabetes, acanthosis nigricans, and obesity has been shown to be associated with enlarged polycystic ovaries secreting excessive androgen. The diabetes seems to result from circulating antibodies directed toward plasma membrane receptors for insulin, suggesting an autoimmune component in the etiology of the disorder. The disease must be distinguished from androgen-secreting ovarian and adrenal tumors which are associated with primary amenorrhea and sometimes with diabetes.

Jaffe RB: Disorders of sexual development. *In* Yen SSC, Jaffe RB (eds.): Reproductive Endocrinology. Philadelphia, W. B. Saunders Company, 1978, pp 271–296. *A concise but comprehensive summary of the literature relevant to errors in fetal genital differentiation and neonatal gender assignment.*

Kulin HE: The maturation of ovulatory potential in man. Horm Res 12:46, 1980. *Applications of timed urine collections to the study of disorders of puberty are discussed in detail.*

Marshall WA, Tanner JM: Variations in pattern of pubertal changes in girls. Arch Dis Child 44:291, 1969. *A classic paper, required reading for all serious students.*

Rosenfield RL: The ovary and female sexual maturation. *In* Kaplan SA (ed.): Clinical Pediatric and Adolescent Endocrinology. Philadelphia, W. B. Saunders Company, 1982, pp 217–268. *A scholarly treatment of prepubertal, peripubertal, and early postpubertal ovarian function in health and disease.*

Styne DM, Grumbach MM: Puberty in the male and female: Its physiology and disorders. *In* Yen SSC, Jaffe RB (eds.): Reproductive Endocrinology. Philadelphia, W. B. Saunders Company, 1978, pp 189–240. *A well-organized discussion with excellent bibliography relevant to normal or abnormal sex steroid hormone production before and after puberty in boys and girls.*

SEX STEROID HORMONES AND OVARIAN FUNCTION AFTER THE MENARCHE

Normal

Regular ovulatory menstrual cycles and fertility provide the best evidence that ovarian function is normal after the menarche; and since ovulatory menstrual cycles require normal hypothalamic, pituitary, and uterine interactions as well, one can infer that all components of the system are functioning normally. Conversely, menstrual disorders and infertility are the most common signs that ovarian function is abnormal in women after the menarche. In women with cyclic menses and infertility and in women with secondary amenorrhea, abnormal ovarian function may result in normal, decreased, or increased sex steroid hormone production. Table 236–6 provides a systematic framework for evaluating ovarian function in these women. In this table, as before, causes are stratified on the basis of sex steroid hormone production. Although measurements of plasma sex steroid hormone concentrations are not always necessary, the range of normal values which takes cyclic changes into account is summarized in Table 236–1.

Abnormal

INFERTILITY (WITH CYCLIC VAGINAL BLEEDING). ***With Normal Sex Steroid Hormone Production.*** Prior to undertaking diagnostic evaluation of women with infertility, ejaculates obtained from their husbands should be examined for abnormalities of sperm number, morphology, and motility. When sex steroid hormone production is normal and menses are regular, infertility is not due to any known ovarian disease. Since determining the cause of infertility in these women involves invasive procedures, a gynecologist with experience in evaluating such patients should be consulted. This referral is particularly appropriate now that in vitro fertilization and embryo transfer are regarded as acceptable methods for treating infertility due to tubal factors in women who ovulate. Moreover, recently in women in whom oocytes are not produced, pregnancies have been established by transferring embryos recovered from donor women artificially inseminated with sperm provided by the husband of the infertile woman.

With Decreased Sex Steroid Hormone Production. Infertility may result from anovulation or luteal insufficiency, both of which occur in women with cyclic bleeding.

LUTEAL INSUFFICIENCY. Corpus luteum function inadequate for establishing and maintaining early pregnancy has been shown to be the cause of infertility or repeated early abortions in some women with regular menstrual cycles. Mean luteal phase blood progesterone concentrations in these women are reduced when compared with those in fertile women who carry pregnancies to term. When rigid criteria based on endometrial morphology have been used for diagnosis, replacement therapy with progesterone has resulted in term pregnancies with delivery of normal infants, suggesting that inadequate luteal phase progesterone is the basis for the problem in some of them.

Inadequate (short) luteal phases occur frequently in women

who continue to ovulate and menstruate despite elevated blood prolactin levels, so that pituitary adenomas should be considered among the diagnostic possibilities in women with luteal insufficiency.

ANOVULATION. Anovulation can be associated with cyclic vaginal bleeding. Monophasic basal body temperature charts, serum progesterone consistent with follicular phase levels, and endometrial biopsies showing proliferative endometrium after the onset of bleeding are diagnostic. Anovulation may also be associated with excessive vaginal bleeding secondary to persistent proliferative endometrium resulting from estrogenic stimulation uninterrupted by progesterone. The syndrome is referred to as anovulatory *dysfunctional uterine bleeding,* and as in prepubertal girls with this disorder, giving estradiol benzoate fails to elicit an appropriate increase in LH secretion in these women. Endometrium should be sampled; if bleeding does not stop after giving progesterone, curettage may be necessary.

With Increased Sex Steroid Hormone Production. Although rare, persistent cyclic vaginal bleeding, ovulation, and fertility are consistent with ovarian and adrenal sources of excess androgen sufficient to cause virilization in a woman. More commonly, however, this constellation is associated with secondary amenorrhea (see below).

SECONDARY AMENORRHEA. Abnormalities at any level of the hypothalamic-pituitary-ovarian-uterine axis can interrupt ovulatory menstrual cycles. When menses fail to recur for six to twelve months in nonpregnant or parturient women who are not breast-feeding, a diagnosis of secondary amenorrhea is established. Secondary amenorrhea is not a disease entity but a sign that function has been compromised in one or more components of the hypothalamic-pituitary-ovarian-uterine axis. In all cases, sufficient diagnostic tests should be done to exclude pregnancy or life-threatening disease from the list of possible causes. Subsequent evaluation should be directed toward longitudinal monitoring to assure that the problem is not secondary to a serious disease, or to restore fertility if the patient wishes to become pregnant.

As in women with cyclic vaginal bleeding and infertility, sex steroid hormone production may be classified as normal, decreased, or increased (see Table 236–6). In these women, an objective test of estrogen production, based on endometrial response to progesterone administration and withdrawal, and, when indicated, determinations of blood FSH, LH, and prolactin can be used to assist in identifying the possible etiologic factors.

With Normal Sex Steroid Hormone Production. Amenorrhea in the face of cyclic changes in ovarian steroid hormone levels and activities consistent with those occurring during ovulatory cycles, or failure to bleed after receiving estrogens and progestogens, indicates failure of endometrial response to steroid hormone stimulation and withdrawal, obstruction of the outflow tract, or total absence of endometrium. When outflow tract obstruction and hysterectomy have been eliminated, endometrial refractoriness must be the cause. Cervical stenosis and intrauterine synechiae resulting from postpartum, postabortal, or tuberculous endometritis or following myomectomy or cesarean section must be considered. Surgical correction of these lesions is followed by resumption of menses in most cases.

With Decreased Sex Steroid Hormone Production. In women with secondary amenorrhea, decreased sex steroid hormone production results from either primary or secondary ovarian failure. In primary ovarian failure, decreased steroid hormone production results from physiologic or pathologic depletion of follicles, from transitory failure of follicles to respond to gonadotropic stimulation in young women, or from combinations of the two phenomena during the perimenopausal period. Low estrogen activity and high blood gonadotropins are characteristically seen.

In secondary ovarian failure, reduced ovarian sex steroid hormone production results from inadequate gonadotropic stimulation of follicles. Reduced blood FSH and LH levels and sometimes increased blood prolactin levels are indicative of dysfunction or failure of the hypothalamic-pituitary unit. Measurements of blood FSH and LH, high in primary failure but normal to low in secondary ovarian failure, distinguish the two categories.

When secondary ovarian failure is diagnosed, the cause of the hypothalamic-pituitary dysfunction must be determined. The process may be intrinsic to the hypothalamus or the pituitary or extrinsic to these organs, and other diagnostic measures are required to differentiate the two types (see Ch. 225).

"Postpill" amenorrhea persisting for more than a year after a woman discontinues oral contraceptives requires an evaluation to exclude other causes of secondary amenorrhea. These include pregnancy, premature ovarian failure, polycystic ovarian disease, and pituitary tumors. Ovulatory cycles will be resumed spontaneously in most women in whom these other causes have been excluded. Moreover, in women in whom amenorrhea persists without other demonstrable causes, normal pregnancies have followed ovulation induction, and postpartum, spontaneous, ovulatory menstrual cycles have resumed.

With Increased Sex Steroid Hormone Production. Ovarian tumors autonomously secreting estrogens or androgens or both may cause amenorrhea during the reproductive years. Ovarian secretion of androstenedione provides substrate for estrogen production by peripheral aromatization. The quantities of androgen derived from the androstenedione may be insufficient to produce signs of virilization but sufficient to stimulate estrogen production. The pathophysiologic basis of the amen-

TABLE 236–6. SEX STEROID HORMONE PRODUCTION AND OVARIAN DYSFUNCTION AFTER THE MENARCHE

I. Sex steroid hormone production and infertility
  A. With normal sex steroid hormone production
  B. With decreased sex steroid hormone production
    1. Luteal insufficiency
    2. Anovulation
  C. With increased sex steroid hormone production
II. Sex steroid hormone production and secondary amenorrhea
  A. With normal sex steroid hormone production
    1. Amenorrhea traumatica
      a. Postinfectious
      b. Postoperative
    2. Hysterectomy
  B. With decreased sex steroid hormone production
    1. Primary ovarian failure (gonadotropins elevated)
      a. Due to depletion of follicles
        (1) In gonadal dysgenesis
        (2) In autoimmune diseases
        (3) After chemotherapy
        (4) After irradiation
        (5) After surgery
        (6) After toxic exposure (smoking)
      b. Due to follicle resistance to gonadotropins
    2. Secondary ovarian failure (gonadotropins normal or low)
      a. Hypothalamic-pituitary dysfunction or failure with hyperprolactinemia
      b. Hypothalamic-pituitary dysfunction or failure with euprolactinemia
        (1) Due to primary hypothalamic or pituitary disorders
          (a) Tumors
          (b) Postoperative
          (c) Postirradiative
          (d) Posttraumatic
          (e) Postinfectious
          (f) Postinfarctional
          (g) The "empty sella"
        (2) Due to secondary hypothalamic or pituitary disorders
          (a) Psychogenic amenorrhea
          (b) Anorexia nervosa and excessive weight reduction
          (c) "Postpill" amenorrhea
          (d) Nonovarian endocrinopathies; thyroid diseases, adrenal diseases, diabetes
          (e) Systemic diseases
  C. With increased sex steroid hormone production
    1. Ovarian tumors secreting androgens or estrogens
    2. Adrenal tumors secreting androgens
    3. Increased peripheral aromatization of androgens
    4. Polycystic ovarian disease

orrhea is similar to that seen when ovarian estrogen or androgen production is excessive, and results from the integrated effect of sustained peripheral estrogen production on the hypothalamic-pituitary unit and the steroid hormone–dependent target organs.

Polycystic Ovaries (Stein-Leventhal Syndrome). Grossly, the ovaries are sometimes enlarged with a glistening surface and a cortex thickened by excessive collagen deposition. Microscopically, these ovaries contain numerous follicular cysts with thecal hyperplasia and hypertrophy (sometimes called hyperthecosis). "Lutein cells" are sometimes seen in the stroma. The microscopic appearance of these follicles is consistent with that of follicles undergoing atresia in response to excessive stimulation by interstitial cell–stimulating hormone (LH or hCG).

High concentrations of androstenedione have been found in venous effluent from these ovaries, and antral fluid from the follicular cysts contains more androgens and less estrogens and progestogens than antral fluid from follicles destined for ovulation.

The constellation of thecal hypertrophy, stromal lutein cells, and elevated antral fluid androgen levels are consistent with the observation that peripheral blood LH levels are higher and FSH levels lower than those seen in samples collected during the follicular phase of ovulatory cycles in normal women.

Despite levels of androgens in ovarian venous and peripheral blood that are frequently sufficient to produce hirsutism, or rarely, virilization, there is considerable evidence of estrogenic activity in target tissues from these women. The endometrium is hyperplastic and sometimes undergoes neoplastic changes (atypical for young women); pituitary FSH secretion is decreased and LH secretion is increased, both consistent with normal hypothalamic-pituitary response to estrogenic stimulation. Production of estrogens results from peripheral aromatization of androstenedione so that daily estrone production rates are increased two- to four-fold over those seen in the follicular phase of women with ovulatory menstrual cycles.

The following pathogenetic sequence is consistent with the clinical observations: (1) Estrone acts on the hypothalamic-pituitary unit to suppress FSH secretion and stimulate LH secretion. (2) Inhibition of FSH secretion reduces FSH-dependent aromatase induction so that less estradiol is produced. (3) Increased LH secretion stimulates thecal and stromal hyperplasia, hypertrophy, and androstenedione secretion. (4) Increased ovarian androstenedione production stimulates atresia, inhibits follicle growth and estradiol production in the ovaries, and produces signs of androgen excess in the extraovarian tissues. (5) Increased peripheral aromatization of androstenedione leads to increased estrone production. (6) Estrone acts upon target tissues to produce chronic anovulation and "continuous estrus," with signs of androgen excess.

How the cycle of events originates remains speculative. Among others, increased adrenal androstenedione production prior to the menarche, leading to increased estrone production in the periphery, remains a viable possibility.

Ovarian enlargement and continuously increased androstenedione and estrone production also occur in women with ovarian tumors, adrenal tumors, Cushing's syndrome, and virilizing congenital adrenal hyperplasia. Discussion of how the distinction can be made will be deferred until diagnosis and treatment of hirsutism are discussed (see Ch. 237). The clinical features of polycystic ovarian disease with hirsutism are similar to those for idiopathic hirsutism. In both syndromes, ovarian function may be deranged. To minimize repetition in relation to diagnosis and treatment of these disorders, the reader is referred to Ch. 237.

Evaluating the Patient with Secondary Amenorrhea. The History. In eliciting the medical history of a woman with secondary amenorrhea, the physician should make a candid appraisal of coital habits, including contraceptive methods used and, if parous, a detailed review of events during prepartum, intrapartum, and postpartum periods of all pregnancies. These data are essential for correctly interpreting results of assays for chorionic gonadotropin in blood or urine, and in deciding about the need for further tests to distinguish pregnancy from gestational trophoblastic neoplasms, or tumors of ovaries or other tissues which secrete chorionic gonadotropins and threaten the woman's life.

Intra- or postpartum hemorrhages requiring blood transfusions, coupled with failure to lactate or to resume menses, are consistent with presumptive diagnosis of Sheehan's syndrome (postpartum pituitary necrosis), whereas persistent galactorrhea and amenorrhea after weaning are suggestive of a pituitary tumor secreting prolactin. Galactorrhea and amenorrhea unrelated to parturition have similar implications. Postpartum endometritis or vigorous dilatation and curettage predisposes to intrauterine synechiae and amenorrhea traumatica (Asherman's syndrome).

Probing dietary habits may provide presumptive evidence for hypothalamic dysfunction secondary to precipitous weight reduction or the syndrome of anorexia nervosa (see Ch. 215). Drugs, including psychotropic agents, antihypertensives, and oral contraceptives, predispose to amenorrhea with or without galactorrhea in some women, and careful questioning about medications is relevant. Secondary amenorrhea is more common among women who participate in marathon running and other strenuous forms of exercise than among their sedentary peers. Along with inquiry about nonovarian endocrinopathies, evidence should be sought for hypothalamic-pituitary dysfunction or failure from postoperative, postirradiative, post-traumatic, postinfectious, and postinfarctive insults. Signs and symptoms of estrogen deficiency, including vasomotor instability, reduction of vaginal secretions, vaginitis, and dyspareunia, suggest a diagnosis of primary ovarian failure resulting from premature or physiologic menopause.

The Physical Examination. Some diagnostically useful signs which should be kept in mind during physical examination include (1) general nutritional status; (2) amount, type, and distribution of hair; (3) cutaneous manifestations of thyroid, ovarian, and adrenal cortical disease, including oiliness, acne, excessive dryness, cutis marmorata, melanotic pigmentation, telangiectasia, bruising, and striae; (4) volume of breasts and presence of galactorrhea; (5) neurologic deficits, including visual field defects and other evidence for pituitary, parapituitary, or other intracerebral tumors; (6) abdominal masses suggestive of adrenal tumors; and (7) quality of vaginal mucosa, cervical mucus, size of uterus, and ovarian and parametrial masses.

Diagnostic Tests. No diagnostic tests should be performed until pregnancy has been eliminated as a cause of secondary amenorrhea. Sensitive methods for measuring chorionic gonadotropin in blood or urine are indispensable.

Prevailing levels of estrogen significantly influence endometrial responses to exogenous progestogens so that presence or absence of withdrawal bleeding following progestogens provides a useful screening test of ovarian sex steroid hormone production and thus of ovarian function in women with secondary amenorrhea. Moreover, when coupled with measurements of blood FSH, LH, and prolactin concentrations, the test provides a rational basis for categorizing the etiologic varieties of secondary amenorrhea.

To minimize the effects of exogenous sex steroid hormones on basal gonadotropin concentrations, specimens of blood (see above) should be collected on the first visit and retained until results of the progestogen withdrawal test are known. If bleeding occurs, five conclusions are valid: (1) the hypothalamic-pituitary unit responds to changes in the sex steroid hormone milieu, (2) the pituitary secretes FSH and LH, (3) ovarian follicles respond to the gonadotropins, (4) the endometrium responds to both stimulation and withdrawal of estrogens and progesterone, and (5) the outflow tract is patent. Measurements of sex steroid hormone or gonadotropin levels are not useful in women who bleed following progesterone. However, since about 15 per cent of patients with prolactin-secreting tumors will bleed following progesterone, measuring prolactin is indicated.

If bleeding does not occur, 50 μg of ethinyl estradiol or equivalent amounts of other estrogens should be administered for 21 days and the progesterone withdrawal test repeated. Failure to bleed can be equated with a refractory endometrium, and measuring blood hormone concentrations is not necessary. Instead, the patient should be referred to a gynecologist for further evaluation and treatment.

In every patient in whom bleeding fails to occur following progesterone alone but does occur after giving estrogen and progestogen, blood FSH, LH, and prolactin concentrations should be measured. High levels of FSH and LH are consistent with primary ovarian disease, whereas low or normal levels suggest secondary ovarian failure resulting from hypothalamic-pituitary dysfunction or failure.

Increased levels of prolactin are suggestive of hypothalamic-pituitary dysfunction associated with prolactin-secreting pituitary adenomas, and the higher the prolactin levels, the greater the likelihood that a tumor is present. Plain skull films should be obtained in all cases and complemented with computed tomography as indicated. Skull x-rays should be examined for signs of an "empty sella" resulting from a congenitally abnormal diaphragma sella which permits the subarachnoid space to extend into the sella turcica, forming a cavity around which pituitary tissue is molded (see Ch. 225). The empty sella may also be associated with euprolactinemic amenorrhea (see below).

When blood prolactin is normal in a patient with signs of decreased sex steroid hormone production and low blood FSH and LH concentrations, primary hypothalamic or pituitary disorders that result in tissue destruction must be distinguished from secondary hypothalamic-pituitary disorders, nonovarian endocrinopathies, and systemic diseases. To choose tests which will assist in distinguishing hypothalamic and pituitary tumors from an empty sella and other causes of hypothalamic-pituitary dysfunction or failure, consultation should be obtained with colleagues in neurology, neurosurgery, and radiology (see Ch. 225).

Davajan V, Israel R: Infertility: Causes, evaluation, and treatment. *In* DeGroot LJ, et al. (eds.): Endocrinology, Vol 3. New York, Grune & Stratton, 1979, pp 1459–1472. *A lucid, logical approach to evaluating infertile couples.*

DiZerega GS, Ross GT: Luteal phase dysfunction. Clin Obstet Gynaecol 8:733, 1981. *A clinically oriented review of an important cause of infertility.*

Ross GT, Hillier SG: Luteal maturation and luteal phase defect. Clin Obstet Gynaecol 5:391, 1978. *A review of hormonal control of corpus luteum function in mammals, including humans.*

Ross GT, Vande Wiele RL: The ovaries. *In* Williams RH (ed.): Textbook of Endocrinology. 5th ed. Philadelphia, W. B. Saunders Company, 1974, pp 368–422. *An extensive discussion of the physiology and pathophysiology of ovarian function to facilitate clinical diagnosis and treatment of disorders in these throughout life.*

Toaff R, Balla S: Traumatic hypomenorrhea-amenorrhea (Asherman's syndrome). Fertil Steril 30:379, 1978. *An informative discussion of these phenomena for clinicians.*

Yen SSC: Chronic anovulation. *In* Yen SSC, Jaffe RB (eds.): Reproductive Endocrinology. Philadelphia, W. B. Saunders Company, 1978, pp 297–323. *An interpretation of the pathophysiologic bases for anovulation, amenorrhea, and dysfunctional uterine bleeding in the light of disorders of "feedback" mechanisms which the author's research has illuminated.*

SEX STEROID HORMONES AND OVARIAN FUNCTION AFTER THE MENOPAUSE

Normal

When the primordial follicles remaining in the ovary cease to mature in response to gonadotropins, ovarian estrogen secretion declines markedly. However, some estrogen continues to be produced by extraovarian conversion (aromatization) of androstenedione to estrone, and estrone becomes the major circulating estrogen after the menopause. The adrenals contribute more androstenedione than do the ovaries in postmenopausal women.

As a result of decreased estrogen production, estrogenic effects are reduced at the target tissues. Thus, the vaginal epithelium thins, cervical mucus declines, vaginal secretions decrease, endometrium atrophies, the breasts atrophy, hypothalamic thermoregulatory function alters, pituitary gonadotropin secretion rises, and osteoporotic changes in bone accelerate. These changes, however, become sufficiently severe to warrant estrogen replacement therapy in no more than 25 per cent of postmenopausal women. Except for the thermoregulatory dysfunction which results in "hot flushes," the changes are insidious and may never reach symptomatic levels.

Abnormal

WITH NORMAL OR DECREASED SEX STEROID HORMONE PRODUCTION. Since decreased ovarian estrogen secretion is normal after the menopause, it is difficult to know where to draw the line between "normal" and "decreased" ovarian steroid hormone production in postmenopausal women.

Intolerable symptoms of "decreased" ovarian steroid hormone production include hot flushes and vaginitis. Subjective sensations of hot flushes are associated with average maximal increments of about 2.5° C in peripheral skin temperatures. These may recur at hourly intervals, persist for about half an hour, are usually preceded by pulsatile increments in blood LH concentrations, and usually subside spontaneously after a year or two. Vaginitis and dyspareunia, related to thinning and reduction in glycogen content of vaginal epithelium, are unlikely to subside spontaneously.

WITH INCREASED SEX STEROID HORMONE PRODUCTION. Syndromes associated with increased steroid hormone production are easily recognized in postmenopausal women. If the steroid is estrogen, breast engorgement and tenderness, increased vaginal secretions, and vaginal bleeding are common signs and symptoms. On the other hand, if increased androgen production occurs, virilizing signs such as male pattern balding, oily skin, acne, increased libido, clitoral enlargement, changes in the larynx and voice, and hirsutism may occur singly or in combination. These excess steroids are almost invariably produced by adrenal cortical or ovarian tumors, and most of these are palpable. Endometrial carcinomas give rise to vaginal bleeding, and these occur more commonly in women with increased estrogen production, whether secreted by ovarian tumors or resulting from excessive aromatization of androstenedione secreted by normal or neoplastic adrenal tissue. Obesity, age, and liver disease all enhance aromatization in postmenopausal women.

Korenman SG, Sherman BM, Korenman JC: Reproductive hormone function: The perimenopausal period and beyond. Clin Endocrinol Metab 7:625, 1978. *A clinician who has studied hormonal events during and following the menopause examines the clinical relevance of these studies.*

MacDonald PC, Edman CD, Hemsell DL, Porter JC, Siiteri PK: Effect of obesity on conversion of plasma androstenedione to estrone in postmenopausal women with and without endometrial cancer. Am J Obstet Gynecol 130:448, 1978. *Contains references to the pioneering observations by MacDonald and Siiteri et al. on the phenomenon of extraglandular aromatization as a source of estrogens after the menopause.*

OVARIAN TUMORS

Ovarian tumors may give rise to signs and symptoms of ovarian dysfunction in any age group. They will be discussed as a group to minimize repetition.

Ovarian tumors include the following major types: (1) common "epithelial" tumors derived from coelomic epithelial cells; (2) sex cord stromal tumors consisting of theca cells, granulosa cells, stromal cells, Sertoli cells, Leydig cells, or their progenitors; (3) lipid cell tumors composed of cells similar but not identical to Leydig cells, lutein cells, and adrenal cortical cells; (4) germ cell tumors, which include dysgerminomas; and (5) gonadoblastomas composed of cells resembling germ cells, granulosa cells, and Sertoli cells. Each of these major classes includes a number of different histologic variants, too numerous to mention here. Cells of the common epithelial tumors, the most frequently occurring ovarian tumors, rarely secrete hormones, but some cells in each of the other varieties may produce hormones in quantities sufficient to stimulate target tissue responses suggestive of excess ovarian steroid hormone secretion.

Although only 5 per cent of ovarian tumors secrete sufficient hormone to produce overt signs and symptoms of response in the appropriate target tissues, a larger proportion of them secrete small amounts of hormones, which may include estrogens, androgens, progesterone (rarely), chorionic gonadotropin (which stimulates steroid hormone production by the nontumorous portion of the ovaries), thyroxine, serotonin, or, more rarely, other peptide hormones (see Ch. 172). In addition to hormone secretion by tumor cells per se, both primary and metastatic ovarian tumors appear to stimulate surrounding normal ovarian stroma to "luteinize" and secrete sex steroid hormones, particularly androgens.

Some tumors are associated with clinical manifestations of decreased hormone production. The prolonged periods of amenorrhea caused by steroid hormone suppression of gonadotropins may alternate with periods of excessive vaginal bleeding secondary to endometrial hyperplasia.

Ovarian tumors occur in all age groups, but most of them are less common in younger persons, especially infants and children. Steroid hormone–secreting ovarian tumors produce overt manifestations of pseudopuberty in a small proportion of girls with the syndrome. Amenorrhea and erratic bleeding may occur in association with tumors during the reproductive years. In postmenopausal women increased estrogens, either secreted by the tumor or produced by aromatization of androgens secreted by the tumor, stimulate endometrial proliferation and are often accompanied by bleeding and occasionally by changes suggestive of endometrial neoplasia.

Some clinical features of ovarian tumors producing hormones are summarized in Table 236–7. Fortunately most of them are palpable, and scanning with ultrasound makes it possible to identify some too small to palpate. Whenever a pelvic mass is discovered during evaluation of ovarian dysfunction in any girl or woman, it is the physician's responsibility to determine the nature of the mass and treat it appropriately.

In addition to frank neoplasms, there are some "tumor-like" conditions characterized by ovarian enlargement and sex steroid hormone secretion similar to that seen with bona fide tumors (from which they must be differentiated). These include the following: (1) pregnancy luteomas (nodular theca–lutein hyperplasia) that result in virilization of the mother (and occasionally her female fetus as well) and regress spontaneously post partum; (2) ovarian stromal hyperplasia and hyperthecosis, sometimes associated with virilizing syndromes; (3) multiple luteinized follicle cysts or corpora lutea which result from excessive gonadotropic stimulation by hCG, secreted by gestational trophoblastic neoplasms, or by mixtures of menopausal gonadotropins and hCG used in ovulation induction; (4) inclusion cysts, containing surface epithelium (germinal epithelium); (5) simple cysts without lining cells; and (6) paraovarian cysts.

Ovarian enlargement resulting from multiple follicle cysts, excessive ovarian androgen secretion, and ovarian enlargement are seen in patients with polycystic ovaries or the Stein-Leventhal syndrome. Since coincidental ovarian tumors occur in patients with the Stein-Leventhal syndrome, diagnostic evaluation should include visualization of the ovaries.

Sometimes ovarian enlargement, caused by endometrial cysts, occurs in women with endometriomas. Around the menarche and around the menopause, cysts may increase and decrease in size in relation to the menstrual cycle; they require close surveillance and repeated examination to exclude the possibility of neoplasms.

Babaknia A, Calfopoulos P, Jones HW Jr: The Stein-Leventhal syndrome and coincidental ovarian tumors. Obstet Gynecol 47:233, 1976. *Coincidental neoplasma were found in 28 of 181 patients with surgically proven Stein-Leventhal syndrome.*

Scully RE: Ovarian tumors with endocrine manifestations. *In* DeGroot LJ, et al. (ed.): Endocrinology, Vol 3. New York, Grune & Stratton, 1979, pp 1473–1488. *An excellent discussion of the clinical manifestations of ovarian tumors for any physician who undertakes the medical care of women.*

TREATMENT OF OVARIAN DYSFUNCTION

Sex steroid hormone replacement therapy is virtually the only treatment of primary ovarian failure; other alternatives are available for restoration of ovarian function in persons with secondary ovarian failure. None of the available regimens is without hazard. The physician and the patient should have a candid discussion of the risks, benefits, and alternatives prior to electing the modality to be used.

Complications of Sex Steroid Hormone Therapy

WITH ORAL CONTRACEPTIVES IN PREMENOPAUSAL WOMEN. Oral contraceptive preparations containing a combination of estrogens and progestogens produce a hormonal milieu similar to that found during the luteal phase of an ovulatory menstrual cycle, or during early pregnancy. The term "pseudopregnancy" is used sometimes to describe the condition, since the metabolic effects of this hormonal mixture of estrogens and progestogens mimic those seen during pregnancy. For example, blood levels

TABLE 236–7. CLINICAL FEATURES OF HORMONE-PRODUCING OVARIAN TUMORS*

		Incidence					
		Age in Years					
Tumor	Hormones Produced†	Peak	Range	Malignancy	Bilaterality	Size Range in cm (per cent) Palpable)	Miscellaneous
Androblastoma (arrhenoblastomas)	*Androgens*, estrogens	20–40	4–69	20%	Rare	< 5– > 25 (85)	Most common virilizing ovarian neoplasm
Dysgerminoma	Androgens, *chorionic gonadotropin*	10–30	6–76	100%	15%	3–50 (60)	May be "mixed" with other tumors originating from germ cells
Gonadoblastoma	*Androgens*, estrogens	10–30	6–38	50%	40%	< 1– > 30 (?)	Usually occur in genetic males with female external genitalia
Granulosa-theca cell	*Estrogens*, androgens, progestogens	30–70	< 1–92	5–20%	10–15%	< 1– > 30 (80–90)	Most common functioning ovarian neoplasm
Hilar cell	*Androgens*, estrogens	45–75	4–86	Rare	Rare	1–9 (50)	Hypertension in 50%, diabetes in 50%
Lipoid cell (adrenal-like)	*Androgens*, estrogens	20–50	6–78	20%	Rare	0.5–30	Diabetes associated with lesion in 50%
Teratomas, benign	Serotonin, thyroxine	10–40	< 1–78	Rare	10%	2–45 (90)	Carcinoid syndrome only in patients with large carcinoid tumors
Teratomas, malignant	Chorionic gonadotropin	6–15	6–42	100%	Rare	> 5 (100)	Not all secrete chorionic gonadotropin

*Modified from data of Rose GT, Vande Wiele, RL: *In* Williams RH (ed.): Textbook of Endocrinology, 5th ed. Philadelphia, W. B. Saunders Company, 1974, pp 368–422.

†When more than one hormone is secreted, the major one is *italicized*.

of carrier proteins such as cortisol-binding globulin, thyroid hormone–binding proteins, transferrin, and ceruloplasmin are elevated as they are in pregnancy. This results in increased "total" blood levels of the ligands but seems to have little pathophysiologic significance.

The contraceptive steroid preparations may reproduce the syndrome of *idiopathic recurrent jaundice,* related to disorders in bile conjugation and excretion, and therefore are contraindicated in patients with a history of recurrent jaundice of pregnancy. There is a two-fold increase in the incidence of *gallstones* associated with alterations in the composition of bile, particularly increased cholesterol content of bile (see Ch. 129).

Benign hepatic adenomas and *focal nodular hyperplasia of the liver* have an increased incidence in women taking oral contraceptive preparations. The tumors are rare but are prone to rupture with exsanguinating hemorrhage.

There is no convincing evidence that oral contraceptives increase the incidence of breast cancers. In contrast, an association of increased incidence in *endometrial cancers* with estrogens (endogenous and exogenous) seems to be established for women receiving estrogens after menopause (see below). Close surveillance is therefore indicated. Oral contraceptives may stimulate rapid growth of uterine leiomyomas, requiring surgical intervention. If these agents are given to a woman who has these tumors, the uterine size should be assessed frequently.

The most serious complication of using oral contraceptives is an increased incidence of *thromboembolic phenomena,* originally thought to be due exclusively to the estrogen component but now known to involve the progestogens as well. The incidences of *cerebrovascular thrombosis* and *hemorrhage* are increased ninefold and twofold, respectively, among women using oral contraceptives. Spontaneous incidence of these cerebrovascular accidents is extremely low in a control population of the same age. Other cerebrovascular effects include induction or *intensification of migraine* headaches among women with this diathesis. *Thrombophlebitis, pulmonary embolism,* and also *hepatic vein thrombosis* have been reported to be increased in frequency. Alternative methods of contraception should be prescribed for women with a history of thromboembolic disorders.

Hypertension associated with the use of oral contraceptives may now be the most frequent form of endocrine hypertension and seems to be related to activation of the renin-angiotensin system. The incidence of induced hypertension rises with duration of use to levels of 5 per cent of users after five years. Hypertension usually regresses after discontinuation of the drugs in women who were normotensive prior to taking the agents. The blood pressure should therefore be followed closely. Conversely, in any woman found to be hypertensive, an inquiry must be made about the use of such hormonal preparations.

The incidence of *abnormal glucose tolerance tests* rises with duration of use. In women with diabetes severe enough to require insulin, dosage must be adjusted upward after taking the agents. Fasting blood glucose concentrations and urine tests for glucose should be done at least annually in women receiving oral contraceptives, particularly women at increased risk for developing diabetes.

Estrogens *increase serum triglyceride levels,* and the pathologic consequences of this action appear to be amplified by smoking, obesity, hypertension, and diabetes. These effects are particularly evident among older women. Serum lipids should be measured prior to instituting this form of therapy, which is contraindicated in those having pre-existing hyperlipidemia.

There is no evidence that using oral contraceptives affects subsequent fertility adversely; 85 per cent of nulliparous and 93 per cent of parous women in one large series conceived during the two years immediately after discontinuation of oral contraceptive use. "Postpill" amenorrhea has been discussed earlier.

A potpourri of other side effects includes salt and water retention, increased nitrogen retention and weight gain, nausea, vomiting, bloating, depression, and sleep disturbances. These all contribute to the unwillingness of some women to use oral contraceptives and compel consideration of alternative methods.

Although the incidence of certain complications is increased, the absolute risk is still low and may be tolerable if the benefit is likely to be significant. An agreement on the need for close surveillance, adhered to scrupulously by physician and patient alike, will reduce the likelihood of serious morbidity if complications occur.

WITH ESTROGENS IN POSTMENOPAUSAL WOMEN. The therapeutic use of estrogens in postmenopausal women can be summarized as follows: (1) The minimal effective dose of estrogens should be given for as short a time as required for symptomatic relief of hot flushes if the severity of symptoms and the patient's assessment of the need for symptomatic relief are sufficient. (2) Estrogens can be used successfully in relieving vaginitis and dyspareunia, but establishing relative merits of topical and systemic administration requires further study. (3) If given around the time of the menopause, estrogens may retard bone loss, but it has not been shown that this will prevent subsequent development of fractures related to osteoporosis (see Ch. 249). (4) There is no convincing evidence for usefulness of estrogens in treating primary psychologic problems in this age group.

With regard to risks, the following summary represents a reasonable current consensus: (1) There are no persuasive data that customary doses of estrogens alter the incidence of thromboembolic phenomena, stroke, or heart disease in women undergoing a natural menopause. (2) Estrogens stimulate cystic hyperplasia of the endometrium, a premalignant condition. (3) The spontaneous incidence rate of endometrial cancer (1 per 1000 women not receiving estrogens) is increased several-fold after using conjugated estrogens (estrone sulfate) in doses of 0.625 to 1.25 mg per day for two to four years. These cancers tend to be low grade and in early stages when detected, and are associated with a high cure rate. Progestogens given for several days during treatment cycles decrease the incidence of cystic hyperplasia, but this regimen has not been shown to reduce the incidence of endometrial cancer. The endometrium should be sampled prior to beginning treatment and whenever bleeding supervenes. The effectiveness of endometrial sampling in the absence of bleeding is questionable. (4) In postmenopausal as in premenopausal women, estrogens increase cholesterol content of the bile and double the incidence of gallstones. (5) There is no convincing evidence that giving estrogens increases the incidence of carcinoma of the breast in postmenopausal women.

In postmenopausal women, then, it appears that the risk of giving estrogens is tolerable, particularly if therapy is deemed necessary by doctor and patient alike. The recommendations and assessments cited above were arrived at by a national Consensus Development Conference in 1979.

Consensus: Estrogen Use and Postmenopausal Women. National Institutes of Health Consensus Development Conference Summary, Vol 2, No 8, September 13–14, 1979. *A consensus on the state of the art as relates to risks and benefits.*

Mishell DR Jr: Contraception. *In* DeGroot LJ, et al. (eds.): Endocrinology, Vol 3. New York, Grune & Stratton, 1979, pp 1435–1450. *An authoritative discussion of the risks and benefits of contraceptive modalities.*

Schenker JG, Weinstein D: Ovarian hyperstimulation syndrome: A current survey. Fertil Steril 30:255, 1978. *A comprehensive review, sufficient in itself for the needs of many clinicians, but with references for those interested in pursuing the subject further.*

Weinstein M: Estrogen use in postmenopausal women: Costs, risks, and benefits. N Engl J Med 303:308, 1980. *A critical evaluation of risks and benefits of the use of estrogens in postmenopausal women.*

Regimens of Treatment

Once the physician has determined whether steroid hormone production is normal, decreased, or increased, and has ascertained the locus of the problem, treatment is generally directed toward restoring manifestations of ovarian function to normal for the peer group. Accordingly, therapy will be considered in relation to the age group of a patient.

PRIOR TO THE MENARCHE. ***With Normal Sex Steroid Hormone Production.*** In those instances in which attention is drawn to müllerian dysgenesis by signs or symptoms unrelated to ovarian function (e.g., in girls with Klippel-Feil syndrome), a route of egress of menstrual fluids is established, but reconstruction of a vagina is usually delayed until the patient contemplates marriage.

With Decreased Sex Steroid Hormone Production. When delayed pubertal changes are due to primary ovarian failure, sex steroid hormone replacement therapy must be used judiciously to assure a girl some parity with her peers in development of secondary sexual characteristics such as breasts and pubic hair. The girl and her parents should be prepared to cope with problems of irregular vaginal bleeding which complicate initiation of replacement therapy with estrogens. Ethinyl estradiol (30 to 50 μg per day), or a biologically equivalent dose of some other oral estrogen, is given continuously for periods of 90 days, coupled with a progestogen such as medroxyprogesterone acetate for the last seven days of this period. This is followed by a week to ten days of no treatment, during which vaginal bleeding should occur. The use of GnRH to induce pituitary gonadotropin secretion is under study and promises to be effective when delayed pubertal changes are due to ovarian failure secondary to hypothalamic-pituitary dysfunction or failure. As noted, it is sometimes wise to temporize rather than use sex steroid hormones for initiating pubertal changes in girls with idiopathic delayed puberty.

With Increased Sex Steroid Hormone Production. When the source of sex steroid hormone excess is an ovarian or adrenal tumor, surgical removal of the tumor must be attempted. When congenital adrenal hyperplasia is the cause, suppression of ACTH secretion with exogenous glucocorticoids will slow advancing pubertal changes (see Ch. 229).

Regimens available for inhibiting progression of isosexual precocious puberty, preventing premature closure of epiphyses and thus preventing short stature, are unsatisfactory. Although menses can be suppressed effectively with progestogens in children with precocious puberty, other stigmata such as advancing bone age with premature closure of epiphyses and short stature progress. Moreover, this therapy is often complicated by signs and symptoms of glucocorticoid excess. Giving long-acting analogues of GnRH inhibits the effects of endogenous pulses of this hypophysiotropic hormone with the result that signs of precocious puberty, including advancing bone age, regress. To date, there are no untoward results of this treatment. Furthermore, pubertal changes are resumed when the drug is discontinued.

AFTER THE MENARCHE. ***With Normal or Decreased Sex Steroid Hormone Production.*** If sex steroid hormone production is normal, then therapy must be directed toward whatever problem gives rise to the patient's concerns. As long as ovarian sex steroid hormone production and ovulatory menstrual cycles persist, a woman engaging in sexual intercourse is at risk for pregnancy, desired or undesired, and prevention of pregnancy may be the reason for consulting a physician.

The oral contraceptives that suppress ovulation by suppressing gonadotropin secretion provide the most effective protection against unwanted or unplanned pregnancies. However, side effects such as nausea (sometimes with vomiting), weight gain, fluid retention, hypertension, hyperglycemia and glycosuria, gallstones, hepatic adenomas, and thrombophlebitis complicate use of these substances. Moreover, ethical constraints limit their usefulness in some women, and inability to follow the prescribed regimen limits their effectiveness in others.

In some of these latter women, intramuscular injections of large doses of long-acting progestogens are effective, but, again, side effects such as "breakthrough" vaginal bleeding have limited their acceptability. In others, intrauterine devices, which permit ovulation and menstruation to continue but prevent implantation, provide a satisfactory alternative. However, pregnancies occurring with the device in situ and increased infections complicate use of intrauterine devices.

If sex steroid hormone is decreased as a consequence of primary ovarian failure, sex steroid hormone replacement may be indicated. On the other hand, if the cause of decreased sex steroid production is secondary ovarian failure, a series of options exist, and choices depend upon the patient's concerns. The first option is to do nothing if reassurance is all the patient requires. However, if cyclic vaginal bleeding is important to the woman's self-image and there are no contraindications, cyclic administration of sex steroid hormones, preferably a combination of estrogens and progestogens, will result in cyclic bleeding. Finally, if a woman wishes to become pregnant, her husband is fertile, and her ovaries contain responsive follicles, a number of other choices are available.

Infertility and early abortions secondary to euprolactinemic luteal insufficiency have been reversed successfully with vaginal suppositories of progesterone. In women with hyperprolactinemic luteal insufficiency or anovulation, suppression of prolactin secretion with ergolines, such as bromocriptine, has been used effectively to induce ovulation followed by pregnancy with delivery of normal infants at term (see Ch. 238). If there is a prolactin-secreting pituitary tumor, surgical removal of the tumor results in resumption of ovulatory menstrual cycles in 60 to 90 per cent of young women, depending on its nature and size.

In euprolactinemic women with decreased sex steroid hormone production and low to normal gonadotropins who bleed following progesterone withdrawal, stimulating pituitary gonadotropin secretion will result in ovulation followed by normal pregnancies. The use of clomiphene citrate, an estrogen antagonist which blocks the feedback inhibition of gonadal steroids on the hypothalamus, has induced ovulations followed by pregnancies. In recent clinical investigations, pulsatile injections of GnRH around the clock for 20 days or more have also induced ovulation in such patients. Pregnancy rates appear to be lower than those associated with spontaneous ovulations.

If attempts at inducing ovulation by stimulating pituitary gonadotropin secretion fail, follicle growth can be stimulated by daily injections of menopausal gonadotropins containing FSH and LH in ratios around 1:1 until serum estradiol levels, determined daily, rise to levels consistent with those seen in late follicular phase of spontaneous cycles (400 to 600 pg per milliliter). Then follicle rupture and corpus luteum function are stimulated by one or more injections of hCG, a surrogate for LH. Morbidity may result from multiple ovulations with multiple fetuses or from a syndrome of massive ovarian enlargement, ascites, hydrothorax, hemorrhage resulting from intravascular coagulation and fibrinolysis, and hypovolemia and shock following administration of hCG, particularly in women who conceive. Monitoring estrogen levels in blood or urine daily during ovulation induction and withholding hCG when these become excessive reduce the incidence to acceptable levels but do not eliminate these complications.

With Increased Sex Steroid Hormone Production. Methods for distinguishing ovarian from adrenal tumors secreting excess androgens are discussed in relation to treatment of hirsutism (see Ch. 237). In these women, signs and symptoms of excess steroid hormone production will disappear slowly following complete removal of the tumor. When excess steroid hormone secretion is gonadotropin dependent, oral contraceptives containing mixtures of estrogens and progestogens will suppress pituitary gonadotropin secretion, reduce steroid hormone production, and ameliorate signs and symptoms. The usefulness of potent, long-acting GnRH antagonists for this purpose is under study.

When excess steroid hormone production is ACTH dependent, glucocorticoids given orally will suppress pituitary ACTH secretion. However, chronic suppression renders the pituitary–

adrenal cortical axis incapable of responding to stress with increased glucocorticoid production so that the patient is vulnerable to the hazards of acute adrenal cortical insufficiency (see Ch. 237). Treatment of women with polycystic ovarian disease is sufficiently complex to merit separate consideration. If restoration of fertility is the primary goal, clomiphene or exogenous gonadotropins may be used to induce ovulation. In some instances in which clomiphene has not been effective, surgical resection of a significant amount of ovarian tissue has resulted in resumption of spontaneous ovulatory menstrual cycles and restoration of fertility. Since these salutary results of surgery do not always persist for the remainder of the patient's reproductive life, surgical intervention is not the treatment of choice when alternative therapies are effective.

When the objectives of treatment relate to control of hirsutism, the principles outlined in Ch. 237 are applicable to patients with polycystic ovarian disease.

AFTER THE MENOPAUSE. ***With Normal or Decreased Sex Steroid Hormone Production.*** Except for occasional neoplasms not affecting sex steroid hormone production, there are no ovarian disorders associated with normal sex steroid hormone production in postmenopausal women.

Few well-designed prospective studies have been done to establish either the safety or the efficacy of giving sex steroid hormones to all postmenopausal women in order to prevent signs and symptoms of reduced sex steroid hormone production in some of them. As noted, the existence of a "syndrome" to which all women are equally susceptible is questionable.

Complications of osteoporosis occurring after the menopause are major medical problems of aging in women. Although the hormonal milieu is contributory, the pathophysiologic basis of osteoporosis after the menopause is multifactorial (see Ch. 249). Other factors contributing to the risk include smoking, low body weight, decreased dietary calcium, inadequate vitamin D intake, and inadequate exercise, and these should be corrected in any event.

In the face of the multiplicity of factors contributing to osteoporosis after the menopause, it is not surprising that it would be difficult to establish either prophylactic or therapeutic benefit from giving estrogens. However, the consensus is that daily low doses (0.625 to 1.25 mg of conjugated estrogen) or equivalent doses of others should be used. Alternatives to oral routes of administration are under study.

In contrast to osteoporosis, the efficacy of estrogens for relief of intolerable hot flashes, dyspareunia, and vaginal infections is easily demonstrated. The dose of estrogens should be the minimal amount required for relief, and the need for continuing treatment indefinitely once the symptoms have been ameliorated is questionable. Attempts should be made to progressively reduce and finally stop treatment altogether.

With Increased Sex Steroid Hormone Production. Treatment of disorders resulting in excess steroid hormone secretion after the menopause is identical to that recommended for use prior to the menopause.

Consensus: Estrogen Use and Postmenopausal Women. National Institutes of Health Consensus Development Conference Summary, Vol 2, No 8, Sept. 13–14, 1979. *A consensus on the state of the art as it relates to risks and benefits.*

Mishell DR, Jr: Contraception. *In* DeGroot LJ, et al. (eds.): Endocrinology, Vol 3. New York, Grune & Stratton, 1979, pp 1435–1450. *An authoritative discussion of the risks and benefits of contraceptive methods.*

Research on the menopause. Technical report series 670. World Health Organization, Geneva, 1981. *A summary of the world literature on the menopause.*

Schenker JG, Weinstein D: Ovarian hyperstimulation syndrome: A current survey. Fertil Steril 30:255, 1978. *A comprehensive review, sufficient in itself for the needs of many clinicians, but with references for those interested in pursuing the subject further.*

Weinstein M: Estrogen use in postmenopausal women. Costs, risks, and benefits. N Engl J Med 303:308, 1980. *A critical evaluation of risks and benefits of the use of estrogens in postmenopausal women.*

ACKNOWLEDGMENT

The skillful assistance given by Mrs. Ollie S. Monger in preparing the original and by Mary Gilliland and A.M. Ross in preparing the revised manuscript is gratefully acknowledged.

237. HIRSUTISM

D. Lynn Loriaux

DEFINITIONS. ***Normal Hair Growth.*** Except for the palms of the hands and the soles of the feet, the bodies of men and women are covered with hair follicles. The hairs growing from these follicles are of two types, *vellous* and *terminal*. Vellous hair is the soft, downy hair that is characteristic of the faces of children. Terminal hair (the hairs of the scalp and eyebrows being examples) is usually more deeply pigmented, of greater diameter, and stiffer. Androgens induce follicles to change the nature of the hair produced from vellous to terminal (or vice versa, as in male pattern baldness) in certain areas of the body, including the mons pubis, axillae, chest, and face (mustache and beard). There is a spectrum of androgen-dependent hair follicle response, the mons pubis being the most sensitive and the beard hairs usually being the least sensitive. In other areas, notably the arms and legs, increased androgen stimulation is not obligatory for the change from vellous to terminal hair. These follicles are considered to be partially androgen dependent.

Hirsutism. In women, excessive growth of body hair is called hirsutism. This is not a disease per se, but it may be a sign of disease. Certain patterns of hair growth can be said to be clearly abnormal in women, e.g., terminal hair on the upper abdomen or shoulders and upper back. Only 3 per cent of women have terminal hair over the sternum. Thus, terminal hair in these locations suggests an underlying disorder. More often, however, women complaining of hirsutism come to the physician not with hair in these abnormal locations, but with the subjective impression that either the rate of hair growth or the distribution of hair, or both seems to be changing. This can be an early indication of serious illness. In the majority of patients, however, no underlying disease can be found.

ETIOLOGY. Etiologically, hirsutism can be divided into two categories: androgen-independent hirsutism and androgen-dependent hirsutism. Ordinarily, the distinction between the two varieties can be made on clinical grounds.

In *androgen-independent hirsutism* the hair is usually vellous and evenly distributed over both androgen-independent areas, such as the forehead, and androgen-dependent areas, such as the chin and upper lip (Fig. 237–1). The more common causes of androgen-independent hirsutism are listed in Table 237–1.

In *androgen-dependent hirsutism*, the hair is of the terminal type and the distribution is restricted to androgen-responsive areas such as the chin, upper lip, and chest. Androgen-dependent hirsutism, caused by androgen excess, may be found in association with other signs of androgen effects, as noted below. The causes of androgen-dependent hirsutism are listed in Table 237–2. Since androgens in women are secreted only by the adrenal glands and by the ovaries, one or the other of these two glands must be the source of the excess androgen, except in cases of factitious hirsutism caused by exogenous androgen administration.

PATHOGENESIS OF ANDROGEN-DEPENDENT HIRSUTISM. Androgen-dependent hirsutism is the result of an elevated plasma protein unbound testosterone concentration. The pathophysiologic mechanism underlying the increased plasma testosterone concentrations found in the adrenal causes of hirsutism, such as adrenal cancer and virilizing adrenal adenomas, and the ovarian causes of hirsutism, including ovarian neoplasms, polycystic ovarian disease, and idiopathic hirsutism, is the excessive secretion of testosterone and/or its immediate precursor, androstenedione. Androstenedione contributes to plasma testosterone by being converted to testosterone in the liver and other peripheral tissues.

The syndromes of congenital adrenal hyperplasia (CAH) also cause hirsutism through increased androgen secretion, but the mechanism is more complex (see Ch. 229). The more common of these virilizing syndromes, 21-hydroxylase deficiency, results

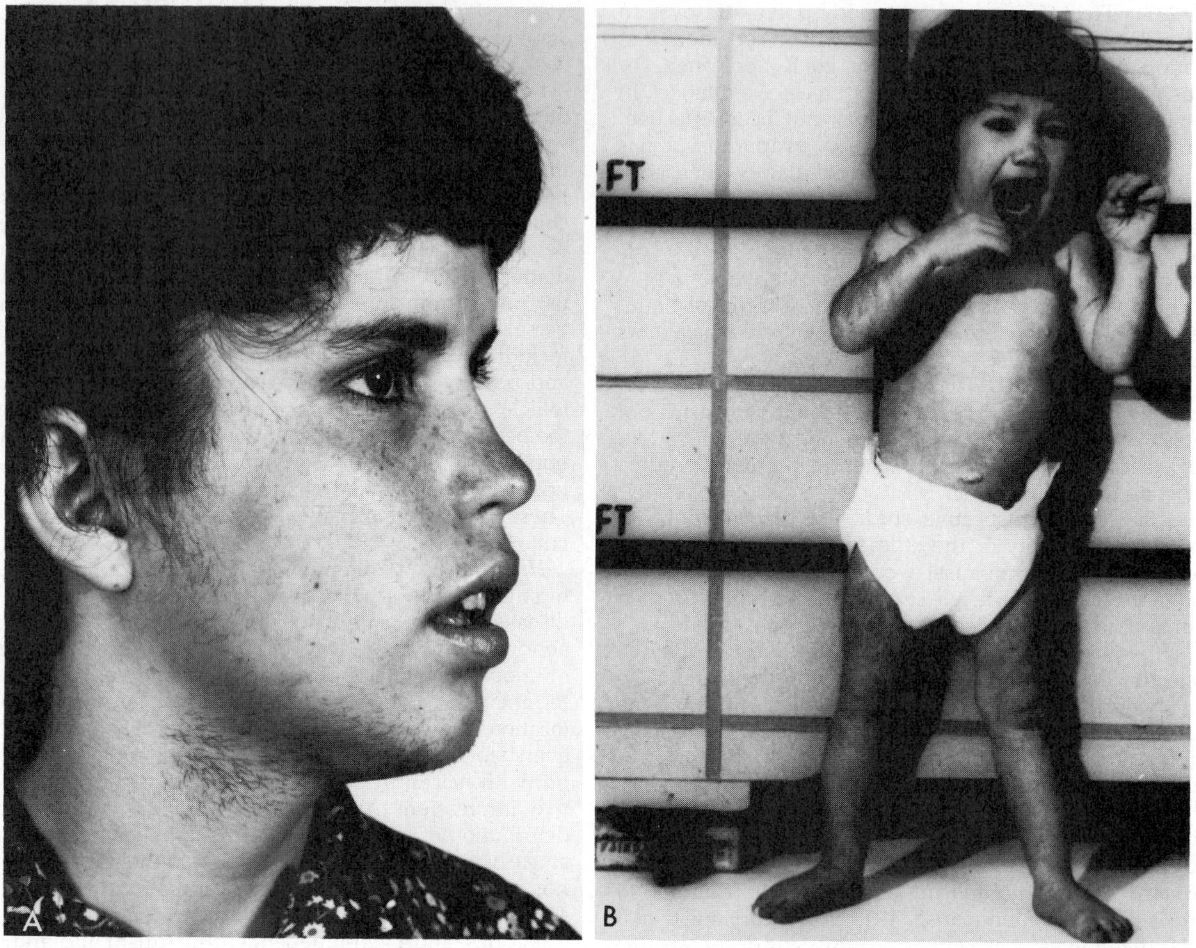

Figure 237–1. Examples of androgen-dependent and androgen-independent hirsutism. *A,* Androgen-dependent hirsutism in a woman with the polycystic ovarian syndrome. The terminal hairs are confined to the beard and mustache areas. *B,* A child with androgen-independent hirsutism induced by diazoxide. Note the even distribution of the hair over arms, legs, abdomen, chest, and face.

in the impaired ability of the adrenal gland to synthesize cortisol. Impaired cortisol production causes increased ACTH stimulation of the adrenal gland with resultant overproduction of 17-hydroxyprogesterone, the substrate for 21-hydroxylase activity, and its metabolic product androstenedione (see Fig. 233–6). Androstenedione is partially converted to testosterone, the hormone responsible for hirsutism and virilization. A second and less common form of CAH, 11-hydroxylase deficiency, is also associated with excessive testosterone production. This presumably results from the conversion of 11-deoxycortisol, the cortisol biosynthetic intermediate just before the 11-hydroxylase block, to androstenedione and thence to testosterone (see Fig. 233–6).

CLINICAL MANIFESTATIONS. The consequences of elevated plasma testosterone concentrations include hirsutism, acne, temporal balding, increased muscle strength, altered libido, and, in virilized patients, clitoral enlargement and deepening of the voice. There is usually also defeminization with amenorrhea, decrease in the size of the breasts, and change from the female body habitus. The various disorders leading to androgen excess vary primarily in the time of onset of the symptoms and the degree to which they progress.

TABLE 237–1. CAUSES OF ANDROGEN-INDEPENDENT HIRSUTISM

1. Medications:
Phenytoin
Diazoxide
Glucocorticoids
Minoxidil
2. Metabolic disorders:
Starvation (anorexia nervosa)
Porphyria cutanea tarda
Hypertrichosis lanuginosa
3. Genetic disorders
Cornelia de Lange syndrome
Seckel's dwarfism
Congenital hypertrichosis

TABLE 237–2. CAUSES OF ANDROGEN-DEPENDENT HIRSUTISM

1. Ovarian causes:
Neoplastic
Sertoli-Leydig cell tumors (arrhenoblastoma)
Granulosa-stromal cell tumors
Gynandroblastoma
Lipoid cell tumor
Gonadoblastoma
Non-neoplastic
Polycystic ovarian disease
Hyperthecosis
Idiopathic hirsutism
2. Adrenal abnormalities:
Neoplastic
Adrenocortical carcinoma
Virilizing adrenal adenoma
Non-neoplastic
Congenital adrenal hyperplasia
21-Hydroxylase deficiency
11-Hydroxylase deficiency
Cushing's disease
3. Medications:
Androgens (such as Danazol, Halotestin)
"19-Nor" progestins

Idiopathic hirsutism and polycystic ovarian disease tend to present a similar clinical picture, and in fact there may be a continuous spectrum between them. Patients with these disorders rarely become virilized and as such do not have clitoral enlargement or masculinization of the larynx. The hirsutism is usually first noticed in the peripubertal period and tends to stabilize after one to two years of progressive worsening. Menses are often irregular in polycystic ovarian disease and may cease altogether with time. On physical examination hirsutism and the frequent occurrence of enlarged ovaries are usually the only abnormal findings.

Hirsutism that has its onset before or after the pubertal period is suggestive of more serious disease. Adrenal carcinoma can appear at any time in life. These tumors are generally inefficient in producing steroid hormone and hence are large at the time of presentation. Forty per cent are palpable, 90 per cent are detectable by intravenous pyelography, and perhaps all are detectable with computed tomography. The rare virilizing adrenal adenomas, on the other hand, are quite efficient in the synthesis of steroid hormones and are usually only a few centimeters in diameter at the time that symptoms first appear.

Congenital adrenal hyperplasia usually becomes clinically apparent at birth or during childhood. It is characterized, in girls, by rapid growth, by heterosexual precocious puberty, and by hypertension in those having the 11-hydroxylase–deficient variety. Rarely, congenital adrenal hyperplasia may first become clinically apparent at the time of puberty or thereafter. When this occurs, the major clinical manifestations are hirsutism, acne, and menstrual irregularity.

Ovarian neoplasms with manifestations of excessive androgen secretion usually occur in adults (Table 237–2). Most will lead to overt virilization with time, and the majority are palpable on pelvic examination.

DIAGNOSIS. Important historical points include age at onset of hirsutism, rate of progression of hirsutism, the body areas involved, the menstrual history, libidinal changes, changes in appetite and weight, and the family history regarding hirsutism. Important physical findings include the nature of the hair (vellous versus terminal), the hair distribution, and the presence or absence of the signs of virilization noted above. Additionally, a careful examination for abdominal and pelvic masses must be made.

The laboratory evaluation of the hirsute woman relies on the measurement of plasma testosterone and plasma 17-hydroxyprogesterone, and on the imaging of the adrenal glands with computed tomography and the ovaries with ultrasonography.

In normal women, the upper limit of plasma testosterone concentrations is about 80 ng per deciliter. Values in excess of 200 ng per deciliter are rarely associated with idiopathic hirsutism or polycystic ovarian disease but are frequently associated with adrenal and ovarian tumors. Hence, values in this range make the diagnosis of an adrenal or ovarian neoplasm much more likely. Additionally, testosterone values in this range will ultimately lead to virilization, making definitive diagnosis and treatment imperative. Plasma testosterone values of less than 200 ng per deciliter are more likely to be associated with a benign process, but periodic re-evaluation (i.e., at three- to six-month intervals) is necessary to ensure that those patients with a progressive disorder will be identified as early as possible.

The measurement of plasma 17-hydroxyprogesterone is the single best test for the diagnosis of congenital adrenal hyperplasia resulting from 21-hydroxylase deficiency. Plasma 17-hydroxyprogesterone values are less than 200 ng per deciliter in normal women. Most patients with 21-hydroxylase deficiency have values at least five times this level. The most reliable diagnostic test for this disorder is determination of the plasma level of 17-hydroxyprogesterone 30 minutes after an intravenous injection of 250 μg synthetic ACTH. In normal subjects the value rarely exceeds 400 ng per deciliter. Patients with 21-hydroxylase deficiency achieve levels of 3000 ng per deciliter or greater. Since 17-hydroxyprogesterone can also be secreted by certain ovarian and adrenal neoplasms, it is essential that plasma 17-hydroxyprogesterone levels be shown to normalize after three days of adrenal suppressive therapy, using 0.5 mg of dexamethasone four times daily to document the adrenal origin of the abnormality.

The diagnosis of 11-hydroxylase deficiency depends, similarly, upon the measurement of plasma 11-deoxycortisol. Because this steroid is also secreted by adrenal neoplasms, distinguishing the 11-hydroxylase type of congenital adrenal hyperplasia from adrenal neoplasms again requires the demonstration that adrenal suppression with dexamethasone lowers the plasma 11-deoxycortisol into the normal range.

Adrenal neoplasms should be sought with computed tomography or ultrasonography, but pelvic ultrasonography is sufficient for diagnosing most virilizing ovarian tumors and does not expose the ovaries to ionizing radiation. If an adrenal or ovarian mass is found and congenital adrenal hyperplasia has been excluded, surgical exploration should be undertaken for definitive diagnosis and initial treatment.

TREATMENT. The treatments of Cushing's disease, adrenal neoplasms, and congenital adrenal hyperplasia are discussed in Ch. 229. Patients with congenital adrenal hyperplasia should be treated with 12 to 15 mg of hydrocortisone per square meter per day, or its equivalent, given preferably at bedtime, to suppress ACTH secretion and thus adrenal androgen production.

The treatment of idiopathic hirsutism and polycystic ovarian disease is less well defined. Many treatment regimens have been proposed. These include hypothalamic-pituitary-ovarian suppression with oral contraceptives, adrenal suppression with exogenous glucocorticoids, electrolysis, wax and chemical depilatories, and simple shaving. Antiandrogens such as cyproterone acetate have been employed in European countries.

Since the extent of hirsutism in women with idiopathic hirsutism and polycystic ovarian disease is usually stable and rarely progresses to virilization, the problem is primarily a cosmetic one with its attendant psychologic ramifications. Although the psychologic discomfort associated with these disorders may be great, it is difficult to justify potentially dangerous hormonal therapies for the treatment of these patients. Thus, the potential complications of treatment with oral contraceptives, glucocorticoids, and antiandrogens should be carefully considered before treatment with these agents is initiated.

The disadvantages of electrolysis include expense, potential scarring, and the need to continue the treatment on a regular basis for an indefinite period. Using wax or chemical depilatories can be painful and untidy. Shaving, on the other hand is safe, effective, and inexpensive. Although shaving is alleged to exacerbate hirsutism, this is not borne out by clinical study. Many women will reject shaving on the basis that it is unfeminine. They will often relent, however, when it is pointed out that they have no such misgivings about shaving their legs and underarms. On balance then, shaving is the cheapest, safest, and most effective form of treatment for idiopathic hirsutism and should be employed whenever possible.

PROGNOSIS. Since hirsutism is a symptom of many different disorders, prognosis for remission is linked to the efficacy of treatment for these maladies. It should be emphasized again that most patients complaining of hirsutism have no serious underlying disorder. Complete extirpation of an androgen-producing neoplasm can be expected to result in the resolution of hirsutism. However, the recovery period may be as long as two years, and patients should be warned not to expect a dramatic decrease in hair growth immediately following therapeutic intervention.

Hirsutism tends to progress to a given level and to stabilize without treatment in idiopathic hirsutism and polycystic ovarian disease. Patients are often aware that the process does not seem to be progressing, but the assurance that it probably will not progress is often helpful in allaying anxiety.

Blankstein J, Faiman C, Reyes FI, et al.: Adult onset familial adrenal 21-hydroxylase deficiency. Am J Med 68:441, 1980. *The best documented cases of this rare cause of hirsutism.*

Chrousos GP, Loriaux DL, Mann DL, Cutler GB: Late-onset 21-hydroxylase deficiency mimicking idiopathic hirsutism or polycystic ovarian disease. Ann Intern Med 96:143, 1982. *Clinical and laboratory description of a rare genetic disorder associated with hirsutism with review of the literature and 80 references.*

Ferriman D, Gallway M: Clinical assessment of body hair in women. J Clin Endocrinol Metab 21:1440, 1961. *Delineates normal and abnormal hair growth patterns in women.*

Kirschner MA, Zucker IR, Jespersen D: Idiopathic hirsutism, an ovarian abnormality. N Engl J Med 294:637, 1976. *The best pathogenetic study of idiopathic hirsutism.*

Korobkin M, White EA, Kressel HY, et al.: Computed tomography in the diagnosis of adrenal disease. Am J Roentgenol 132:231, 1979, *An up-to-date discussion of the power of this technique for diagnosing adrenal mass lesions.*

Lipsett MB: Benign masculinizing adrenal adenomas. N Engl J Med 289:802, 1973. *A concise discussion of this rare disorder.*

238. NONMALIGNANT DISEASES OF THE BREAST

George Tolis

Diseases of the breast are important in medical practice. In this chapter some of the developmental aspects and the function (lactation) of the breast will be reviewed briefly as a background for more extensive discussions of two clinically important disorders, gynecomastia and galactorrhea. Carcinoma of the breast, by far the most important disease of that organ, will be discussed in Ch. 239.

DEVELOPMENTAL ASPECTS OF THE MAMMARY GLAND. The human breast has a tubuloalveolar structure and consists of 15 to 25 lobes radiating from the nipple. Each lobe is subdivided into lobules from which emerge lactiferous ducts. The mammary line is well developed in the five-week embryo, but it is not until the fifth gestational month that both the nipple and the secondary buds develop. Until puberty the human mammary gland does not develop unless a pathologic condition occurs (e.g., feminizing adrenal carcinoma). With the onset of puberty, the areola enlarges and becomes pigmented and a significant growth of the tubular duct of the female breast ensues. Estrogens primarily stimulate the development of the mammary duct; progesterone seems to play a major role in alveolar growth. The role of other factors (such as growth hormone, insulin, somatomedins, epidermal growth factor, glucocorticoids, and thyroxine) in the normal growth of the mammary gland is incompletely understood.

INITIATION AND MAINTENANCE OF LACTATION. The hormonal factor absolutely required for lactation is prolactin. In the absence of adequate circulating prolactin, lactation does not occur or ceases if previously established. Furthermore the experimental administration of a specific antiserum to prolactin inhibits galactopoiesis. For prolactin activity to be fully expressed, optimal concentrations of other hormones (such as estrogens, thyroxine, and insulin) are also required. The effects of prolactin upon the female breast are modulated by various factors such as age, hormones, and medications. The adminstration of estrogens in the postpartum period will suppress lactation in many women by a mechanism independent of serum prolactin levels. Since serum prolactin concentrations do not decrease, it appears that in this situation estrogens block the action of prolactin. In contrast, the suppression of lactation by bromocriptine, a dopamine analogue, is due to the inhibition of prolactin release from the pituitary gland. In the breast-feeding mother basal serum prolactin levels fall gradually, yet the amount of milk secreted increases. Although no association exists between the resting serum prolactin levels and the amount of milk produced, there may be a correlation between the amount of lactation and the degree of prolactin increment induced by vigorous suckling.

GALACTORRHEA

Nonpuerperal lactation or galactorrhea is an abnormal physical sign which occurs in both men and women. The amount of milk secreted forms the basis of the grading system used in quantitating the disorder. Grades I and II: Milk can be expressed manually but the patient may not necessarily be aware of it otherwise. Grades III and IV: Copious milk secretion occurs in an intermittent or continuous manner. The degree of galactorrhea so defined does not correlate with the pathologic significance of the underlying disorder (i.e., pituitary tumors may be associated with Grade II galactorrhea; the use of psychotropic drugs may lead to Grade IV galactorrhea). Galactorrhea usually is of benign significance. It becomes an important clinical sign especially when it is associated with disturbances of menstruation or impairment of fertility.

ETIOLOGY AND PATHOGENESIS. The classification of galactorrhea is more meaningful if it takes into account the serum prolactin (PRL) levels (Table 238–1). *Normoprolactinemic galactorrhea* is usually benign as far as hypothalamic-pituitary pathology is concerned. In acromegaly secondary to a growth hormone–secreting tumor, excess milk production may be due to the intrinsic lactogenic activity of growth hormone or to a circulating PRL of different molecular form than that measured by the standard radioimmunoassay. Even when serum PRL is in the normal range, the level may be inappropriately increased for a particular individual, since further lowering of the PRL with bromocriptine may be effective treatment. It has also been speculated that prior to the development of galactorrhea there may have been an increase in PRL which led to an increase in the number of lactogenic receptors and therefore to enhanced sensitivity.

Hyperprolactinemic galactorrhea should prompt a thorough investigation. Increased serum levels of PRL can result either from a decrease in its metabolic clearance (e.g., in liver failure or hypothyroidism) or from an increase in PRL production. The latter can result from conditions decreasing the inhibitory

TABLE 238–1. CAUSES OF NONPUERPERAL GALACTORRHEA

- I. Central origin
  - A. Organic
    - 1. Suprahypophyseal lesions
      - a. Hypothalamic disorders—infiltrative processes (histiocytosis, metastatic diseases); masses (craniopharyngioma, meningioma); infarction; embolism
      - b. Pituitary stalk lesions—section; impingement by tumors (all types with suprasellar extension); vascular insult
    - 2. Hypophyseal tumors
      - a. Prolactin secreting* (solitary; part of multiple endocrine adenomatosis syndrome mixed with GH, TSH, ACTH)
  - B. Functional
    - 1. Drug related
      - a. Psychotropic (butyrophenones, phenothiazines)*
      - b. Antihypertensive (reserpine, alpha-methyldopa)
      - c. Cannabinoids (morphine, heroin)
      - d. Contraceptives
      - e. Antigastroplegics (metoclopramide)*
    - 2. Unclassified (idiopathic, stress, empty sella syndrome)
- II. Peripheral origin
  - A. Due to pituitary prolactin
    - 1. Due to primary failure of target endocrine gland
      - a. Hypothyroidism
      - b. Addison's disease
    - 2. Due to excess estrogen formation from target endocrine glands
      - a. Feminizing adrenal carcinoma
      - b. Polycystic ovarian syndrome
    - 3. Due to decreased metabolic clearance of PRL
      - a. Renal failure
      - b. Liver failure
      - c. Hypothyroidism
    - 4. Due to local breast conditions
      - a. Mechanical stimulation or suckling
      - b. Thoracic and/or breast trauma, burn
      - c. Inflammation, i.e., mastitis, herpes zoster
  - B. Due to ectopic prolactin production
    - 1. Renal neoplasia
    - 2. Bronchogenic neoplasia

*Most common causes of highest serum PRL levels.

hypothalamic (dopaminergic) control of the pituitary or from the presence of a prolactin-secreting pituitary tumor. A decrease in the hypothalamic suppression of the secretion of PRL by the pituitary can be due either to lesions in the hypothalamus (e.g., gliomas, craniopharyngioma, histiocytosis, infarction) or to disruption of the hypothalamic-pituitary neurovascular connections (e.g., pituitary stalk section, tumoral impingement on the stalk such as by suprasellar extension of pituitary tumor). Functional causes of decreased dopaminergic control are mainly due to the intake of drugs which may (1) inhibit dopamine synthesis (e.g., alpha-methyl paratyrosine); (2) deplete the pool of catecholamine (e.g., reserpine); (3) dilute the catecholamine content in the presynaptic neurons (e.g., the false neurotransmitter methyldopa); or (4) occupy the postsynaptic receptor sites (e.g., haloperidol). Other drugs which stimulate the pituitary lactotrope are exogenous opiates and contraceptive steroids, especially those with high estrogen content. In susceptible animals, administration of a large dose of estrogen may induce pituitary prolactin-secreting tumors and result in hyperprolactinemia.

Galactorrhea and hyperprolactinemia may occur in primary myxedema or in Addison's disease. The mechanism whereby hypothyroidism leads to hyperprolactinemia is unknown, but it is believed to be mediated via excessive thyrotropin-releasing hormone (TRH) secretion. Whether excess corticotropin releasing factor (CRF) accounts for the hyperprolactinemic galactorrhea of Addison's disease or Cushing's syndrome is unknown. Other conditions leading to excess PRL secretion include the polycystic ovary syndrome and adrenal carcinoma, presumably because of the excess estrogen production found in these syndromes.

Excess production of PRL has been reported in patients with bronchogenic or renal neoplasms. Ectopic sources of PRL should be considered in the differential diagnosis.

CLINICAL PRESENTATION AND DIFFERENTIAL DIAGNOSIS. The clinical presentation of galactorrhea is highly variable, with milk production anywhere on the scale of I to IV (see above). There may be no other symptoms, or the patient may present the signs or symptoms of any of the disorders listed in Table 238–1. It is particularly important to determine carefully any drugs the patient may be taking.

In humans, the incidence of prolactin-secreting tumors (prolactinomas) is far higher in women then in men. A more general discussion of pituitary tumors has been presented in Ch. 225. Galactorrhea associated with amenorrhea is the most common presentation of a prolactinoma in women. Galactorrhea alone is found in less than one third of patients with prolactinoma. Prolactinomas in men produce galactorrhea much more rarely and, partly because of this, tend to present later as larger, space-occupying tumors.

One should measure serum PRL in every patient with galactorrhea. If the level is elevated and there is no evidence of psychotropic drug intake or primary hypothyroidism, one should exclude the presence of a pituitary tumor. If the tumor is non-prolactin-secreting and impinges upon the stalk, then the administration of TRH (500 μg intravenously) will provoke an increase of at least two-fold in serum PRL in the majority of patients (see Ch. 224 for normal response of PRL to TRH). If the tumor is composed of prolactin-secreting cells, then the diagnosis can be established with a combination of radiologic techniques and hormonal assays. If serum PRL levels exceed 500 ng per milliliter, a macroadenoma of the pituitary will generally be demonstrable by a plain skull film of the sella turcica by both the anteroposterior and lateral views. If the levels are between 100 and 500 ng per milliliter, the plain skull film may be normal but complex motion tomography will demonstrate a microadenoma in 85 per cent of the patients. In as many as 20 per cent of such patients TRH may elicit a doubling of serum PRL levels. If the levels of PRL are less than 100 ng per milliliter, no sella pathology may be detected even when high resolution computed tomography is utilized. In these cases a larger proportion of patients may respond to TRH. If PRL is not released by TRH in patients with hyperprolactinemia, the diagnosis of an autonomously secreting adenoma is strongly suspected. In our series surgical exploration successfully identified a tumor in 14 out of 16 patients who had equivocal radiologic examination of the sella but who did not respond to TRH with an increase in serum PRL.

TREATMENT. The treatment of the patient with galactorrhea depends on the primary disease. Discontinuation of medications or treatment of conditions such as hypothyroidism should lessen milk secretion. In persistent hyperprolactinemia without radiologic evidence for prolactinoma, bromocriptine will often be sufficient therapy (see below for treatment schedule). In such patients annual evaluation by sella radiology may be necessary if, upon discontinuation of the medication, hyperprolactinemia again supervenes. If a microadenoma is strongly suspected, the same strategy can be followed even for the woman who desires pregnancy. Small (10 mm or less) noninvasive microadenomas do not seem to grow rapidly during the gestational period. If there are signs of tumor growth despite bromocriptine treatment, transsphenoidal tumor resection is the preferred treatment. If during bromocriptine treatment there is no radiographic evidence of growth of the tumor, if the serum PRL is maintained within normal limits, and if the clinical abnormality is corrected, the patient can be kept on this regimen indefinitely. Reasons for discontinuation of medical therapy are (1) patient noncompliance, (2) cost of the medication, (3) development of side effects, and (4) failure of the medication to control the clinical and hormonal disorder (e.g., continuation of galactorrhea-amenorrhea and nonsuppression of serum PRL). In these instances, which are not uncommon, transsphenoidal resection of the pituitary adenoma could be undertaken in specialized centers. Pituitary tumor irradiation is the alternative to surgery. For those patients with galactorrhea and large adenomas, with or without parasellar and suprasellar extension, a combination of surgery, radiotherapy, and bromocriptine offers the best results. There have been reports of rapid decrease in tumor size with the use of bromocriptine alone, but there have been other reports to the contrary. Bromocriptine should not be the sole treatment of prolactin-secreting macroadenomas.

The management of patients with idiopathic normoprolactinemic galactorrhea is very difficult. Reports of the efficacy of pyridoxine and cyproheptadine in the treatment of these patients are not convincing and may represent only a placebo effect. Bromocriptine has been used to treat normoprolactinemic galactorrhea, but the number of "responders" not unexpectedly is smaller than in hyperprolactinemic patients. A trial of bromocriptine in normoprolactinemic galactorrhea may be warranted, based on the reasoning that (1) the levels of PRL, although within the normal range, may be inappropriately high for a given patient, and (2) there may be a discrepancy between the biologically active versus the immunologically detectable PRL molecule.

Bromocriptine should be administered carefully in the treatment of galactorrhea. Our custom is to begin with 1.25 mg (occasionally even with half that dose) every night for one week, and then to increase it by 1.25 mg every week until a dose of 2.5 mg twice daily is reached. A total daily dose of 10 mg is rarely exceeded, although the dose can be increased to 20 mg per day. Bromocriptine is taken with a meal, and the patient is asked to avoid abrupt postural change in order to prevent orthostatic hypotensive episodes. Nausea and behavioral changes (of the manic type) are other side effects. Currently there is no evidence for teratogenicity or other defects in the offspring of mothers who conceived while receiving bromocriptine. The drug passes the placental barrier, however, and exposed children have been followed for less than ten years. It is probably prudent, therefore, for women to discontinue the medication on the days of planned insemination and during pregnancy.

GYNECOMASTIA

Gynecomastia is defined as a palpable, firm mass, measuring at least 2 cm in diameter in the subareolar region. It represents excessive development of the male breast with a feminine appearance, and is the most common disorder of the male breast; about 85 per cent of male breast masses are due to gynecomastia. Pathologically it may be florid with proliferation of glandular or fibrous elements, characterized by increase of stromal tissue. The florid type may regress or progress to the fibrous type; the fibrous type is typically irreversible.

Gynecomastia usually begins at puberty when it may be unilateral or bilateral. When gynecomastia is unilateral it is more commonly on the left side for reasons unknown. Approximately 40 per cent of pubescent boys may develop some transient gynecomastia, with the highest incidence being between 14 and 15.5 years of age. Autopsy studies of elderly men have revealed true gynecomastia in as many as 40 per cent of subjects. The development of gynecomastia from late puberty to male senescence may signal a serious underlying disorder, such as adrenal or testicular tumor, and in such cases early diagnosis and treatment may be lifesaving.

ETIOLOGY AND PATHOPHYSIOLOGY. A classification of gynecomastia is contained in Table 238–2. The pathophysiology of gynecomastia has been partly clarified. For the majority of patients it seems to be associated with a disturbance in the balance of estrogenic-androgenic effects on the mammary epithelium. The pathogenesis of gynecomastia may be complex. For example, both increased estrogen production and aromatization of secreted androgens to estrogens may occur in adrenal

TABLE 238–2. CLASSIFICATION OF THE CAUSES OF GYNECOMASTIA

All true gynecomastia is caused by an estrogenic effect on the male breast. This may result from excessive estrogen or from deficient androgen.

I. Physiologic—newborn, puberty, senescence
II. Pathologic
  A. Increased estrogen secretion
    1. Hermaphroditism
    2. Klinefelter's syndrome
    3. Congenital adrenal hyperplasia
    4. Neoplastic
      a. Adrenal carcinoma
      b. Testicular tumor (Sertoli cell, Leydig cell, choriocarcinoma)
      c. Paraneoplasms secreting human chorionic gonadotropin (lung, liver, kidney, stomach, lymphopoietic system)
  B. Increased conversion of androgens to estrogens
    1. Adrenal carcinoma
    2. Liver disorders (failure secondary to infectious or nutritional causes, carcinoma)
    3. Nutritional (refeeding after starvation)
    4. Thyrotoxicosis
  C. Decreased androgen secretion
    1. Primary testicular failure (anorchia, Klinefelter's syndrome, enzymatic defects in testosterone synthesis)
    2. Secondary testicular failure (castration; infectious orchitis; mumps and other viruses, lepromatous, tuberculous; neurologic disorders: paraplegia, muscular dystrophy; renal failure; panhypopituitarism; prolactin-secreting tumors)
  D. Decreased androgen activity due to receptor protein abnormalities
    1. Complete testicular feminization
    2. Incomplete testicular feminization
    3. Reifenstein's syndrome
III. Pharmacologic—a combination of mechanisms
  A. Cannabinoid—methadone and marijuana
  B. Psychotropics—phenothiazine, butyrophenone, reserpine
  C. Antihypertensives—reserpine, alpha-methyldopa, spironolactone
  D. Cardiac—digitalis
  E. Gastrointestinal—cimetidine, metoclopramide, domperidone
  F. Antituberculous—isoniazid
  G. Hormonal
    1. Sex steroids—estrogens, androgens
    2. Gonadotropins—human chorionic gonadotropin
    3. Antiandrogens
  H. Cytotoxic—cyclophosphamide, mustine, vincristine, mitotane
  I. Miscellaneous—penicillamine
IV. Idiopathic

tumors and congenital adrenal hyperplasia. In nonadrenal neoplasms associated with human chorionic gonadotropin (HCG) production, the excess estrogen levels are due to increased secretion of estrogens by the testes. Finally, the estrogen level may be only relatively increased in comparison to the testosterone level, as in Klinefelter's syndrome or in testicular failure, with an increased estrogen-androgen ratio. An increased extraglandular formation of estrogens from androgens is believed to play a significant role in the gynecomastia seen in patients with chronic liver disease, starvation, and thyrotoxicosis. In these conditions, as a result of decreased hepatic extraction, there is increased androgen available for peripheral conversion to estrogens. The latter mechanism seems to be operative in some patients with idiopathic gynecomastia but its significance in that syndrome has not been fully elucidated.

Peptide hormones may contribute to the genesis of gynecomastia directly or indirectly. Human placental lactogen (HPL) is secreted by some testicular tumors, but its role in the proliferation of mammary epithelium is not clear. Some patients with hyperprolactinemia associated with prolactin-secreting pituitary tumor have gynecomastia. This is probably secondary to a decrease in androgen secretion (suppression of gonadotropins), possibly to a decrease in the peripheral conversion of testosterone to its active metabolite dihydrotestosterone.

In the syndrome of complete testicular feminization, androgen production by the testes is normal but pituitary luteinizing hormone (LH) output is enhanced (because the absence of cytoplasmic androgen receptors in the pituitary impairs feedback control) and leads to testicular estrogen production. The increased estrogen, coupled with a defect in the action of androgen owing to the lack of the receptor in the mammary gland, leads to excessive estrogenic expression and gynecomastia. A similar mechanism has been invoked in incomplete

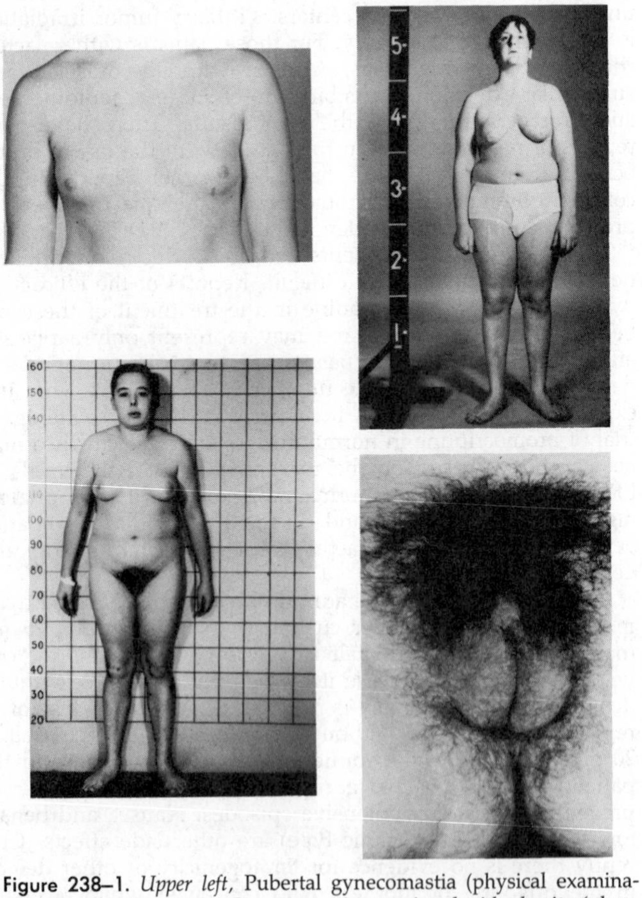

Figure 238–1. *Upper left,* Pubertal gynecomastia (physical examination: normal). *Upper right,* Gynecomastia associated with obesity (physical examination: normal except for increased adiposity). *Lower left and right,* Phenotypic appearance of body habitus and external genitalia in a genetically male patient with the syndrome of incomplete testicular feminization (physical examination: female escutcheon, hypospadias, bifid scrotum, normal-sized testes). (Courtesy of Dr. H. Guyda.)

testicular feminization and in Reifenstein's syndrome. Perhaps variations in hormone receptor levels may account for other cases of gynecomastia associated with normal circulating levels of estrogens and androgens.

Gynecomastia occurs in patients receiving various drugs, in particular estrogens (orally, parenterally, or as ointments). Other drugs, however, can also lead to gynecomastia by altering the effective estrogenic-androgenic ratio of activity in the breast. Some lead to decreased testosterone synthesis (e.g., chemotherapeutic agents, high doses of spironolactone) or interfere with testosterone action (e.g., cyproterone, low doses of spironolactone). They may cause increased estrogen production (e.g., HCG) or may themselves have an estrogen-like effect (digitalis, tetrahydrocannabinol).

DIAGNOSIS AND DIFFERENTIAL DIAGNOSIS. It is obviously important to be sure that true gynecomastia is present. The most common error is to confuse the "false gynecomastia" of obesity with true gynecomastia. The obese breast lacks glandular elements on palpation. Palpation will also differentiate gynecomastia from such disorders as carcinoma or neurofibroma. It should be evident that even the presence of true gynecomastia with onset at the time of puberty does not call for a major medical investigation in view of its high incidence (see above) and benign prognosis.

The differential diagnosis of gynecomastia may be accomplished on the basis of history and physical examination. In most instances laboratory studies will be important as well. For example, examination of the head and neck may reveal the presence of signs of compression of the anterior visual pathways consistent with suprasellar extension of a pituitary tumor, or diplopia, lid lag, or goiter consistent with Graves' disease. Examination of the breasts may reveal the presence of galactorrhea, in which case measurement of serum prolactin (PRL) is mandatory. The skin and abdomen may reveal signs of liver failure and examination of the testes may establish microrchidia, in which case a chromosomal disorder should be suspected (e.g., Klinefelter's syndrome). Alternatively, asymmetrical enlargement of a testis raises suspicion of a malignant process.

Laboratory studies will be selected in part based on the clinical circumstances revealed by the history, physical examination, and the age of the patient. A study of liver function is usually indicated. Useful hormone assays include the determination of serum estrogens (estrone and estradiol), androgens (androstenedione and testosterone), and luteinizing hormone (LH), and of urinary 17-ketosteroids. Excess serum estrogens are found in patients with Leydig cell tumors and adrenal carcinoma; in such patients serum LH and testosterone levels are low. Elevated serum LH is found in primary testicular failure (in which case testosterone levels are low) and in HCG-secreting tumors (due to cross-reaction of HCG in the assay for LH if a specific HCG assay is not done). If HCG is elevated, serum testosterone may be normal but serum estrogens tend to be elevated. Abnormally high LH occurs in the syndrome of peripheral androgen resistance and is accompanied by normal or elevated testosterone levels. Finally, excessive excretion of 17-ketosteroids almost invariably reflects disease of the adrenal cortex. Inability to demonstrate abnormal values in any of the aforementioned measurements does not exclude a metabolic cause of gynecomastia. More elaborate methods are required to facilitate in vivo study of the binding or the biologic action of sex steroids in order to elucidate further the cases of idiopathic gynecomastia.

Radiologic studies can be of significant help in selected cases. Four radiographic patterns have been identified: (1) the presence of ductlike structures (54 per cent incidence in one series); (2) marked proliferation of the ducts occupying almost the entire breast; (3) homogeneous density occupying either or both subareolar breast areas; and (4) nonhomogeneous density in subareolar or most breast regions. The last appearance was found more often in adults, whereas homogeneity was more prevalent in pubertal gynecomastia. Xeromammography in a patient with a breast mass raises strong suspicions for cancer when the mass is solid, spiculated, and located eccentrically in relation to the nipple; benign gynecomastia, by contrast, is symmetrical in relation to the nipple.

TREATMENT. Regression of gynecomastia can occur in the majority of patients. It is spontaneous in the pubertal cases (up to 90 per cent regress within one to three years). In the rest of the patients, removal of the offending agent or appropriate drug treatment will result in significant improvement when utilized not too late in the course of the abnormality. Thus, impressive improvement occurs with the removal of a sex steroid–producing tumor or treatment of thyrotoxicosis, whereas poor results are obtained in longstanding cases of Klinefelter's or fibrous gynecomastia. In cases of androgen deficiency, androgen administration certainly leads to improvement; however, the active biotransformation of aromatizable androgens to estrogens sustains gynecomastic changes. Attempts to use nonaromatizable androgens or dihydrotestosterone may have promise. As well, independent or combined administration of antiestrogens could theoretically protect the breast tissue from the estrogenic side effects; well-documented series are not as yet reported. If gynecomastia is long lasting, the ensuing fibrotic changes are irreversible, so that even the removal of the causative agent (e.g., drug withdrawal) may not lead to a return of the breasts to normal size. Cosmetic mastectomy may be the preferred mode of "treatment," depending upon the wishes of the patient.

Galactorrhea

Friesen HG, Tolis G: The use of bromocriptine in the galactorrhea-amenorrhea syndromes. Clin Endocrinol 6S:91, 1977. *An important document in the North American literature. It is based on the Canadian Cooperative Study and should be a standard reference.*

Kleinberg DL, Noel GH, Frantz AG: Galactorrhea: A study of 235 cases, including 48 with pituitary tumors. N Engl J Med 296:589, 1977. *This study confirms and extends previous observations. It is among the most comprehensive reports on etiologic entities associated with galactorrhea.*

Koppelman MCS, Jaffe MJ, Rieth KG, Caruso RC, Loriaux DL: Hyperprolactinemia, amenorrhea and galactorrhea. Ann Intern Med 100:115, 1984. *The authors report on their experiences with 25 patients with this syndrome and emphasize its benign clinical course. Because of this they advocate conservative treatment.*

Tolis G: Galactorrhea. *In* Krieger DT, Bordin WC (eds.): Current Therapy in Endocrinology 1983–1984. Toronto and St. Louis, B.C. Decker and C.V. Mosby Companies, 1983, pp 427–428. *Report based on author's data and literature review of normoprolactinemic and hyperprolactinemic galactorrhea.*

Tolis G, Franks S: Prolactin pathophysiology. *In* Clinical Neuroendocrinology: A Pathophysiological Approach. New York, Raven Press, 1979, pp 291-318. *This paper is based primarily on numerous studies reported by the authors during the last decade. It contains an extensive review of work that has been amply confirmed.*

Tucker A: Control of lactation. Semin Perinatol 3:199, 1979. *A scholarly analysis of the current concepts of lactogenesis.*

Yen SSC: Lactogenesis and lactation. *In* Yen SSC, Jaffe RB (eds.): Reproductive Endocrinology. Philadelphia, W. B. Saunders Company, 1978, pp 165-167. *Lucid description of current knowledge with regard to control of lactation in humans. The whole chapter on prolactin must be read even by the advanced reader.*

Gynecomastia

Chandrakant CK, Parekh NJ: The male breast. Radiol Clin North Am 21:137, 1983. *A thorough review and presentation of the authors' own series of radiologic issues in the evaluation of gynecomastia.*

Large DM, Anderson DC: Twenty-four hour profiles of circulating androgens and estrogens in male puberty with and without gynecomastia. Clin Endocrinol 11:505, 1979. *A significant contribution. It documents the long-held view that there is an estrogen-androgen imbalance associated with pubertal gynecomastia.*

Large DM, Jones JM, Shalet SM, Scarffe JH, Gibbs AC: Gynaecomastia complicating the treatment of myeloma. Br J Cancer 48:69, 1983. *A detailed hormonal study of patients with gynecomastia receiving cytotoxic agents.*

Wilson JD, Aiman J, MacDonald P: The pathogenesis of gynecomastia. Adv Intern Med 25:1, 1980. *This review is based on the authors' longstanding experience in the steroid field and presents a "state of the art" contribution with regard to the pathophysiology of gynecomastia.*

239. CARCINOMA OF THE BREAST

George P. Canellos

Carcinoma of the breast is the most common malignant tumor of women, accounting for approximately 35,000 annual deaths. It is estimated that 1 of every 13 women in the United States will develop breast cancer at some time in her life—approximately a 7 per cent chance. Greater public awareness and increased application of self-examination and mammographic screening are now identifying about 105,000 new cases annually in the United States.

ETIOLOGY. Hormonal and genetic factors predispose to the development of this tumor. A maternal history of breast cancer increases the risk three-fold; the tumor tends to occur at an earlier age in descendants of patients who have had breast cancer. Ovarian function and estrogenic hormones have been implicated as causative factors. Elevated blood levels of estradiol plus estrone and prolactin have been found in the daughters of breast cancer patients. In some experimental animals the estrogens estradiol and estrone are carcinogenic. A generally increased risk for breast cancer has been associated with nulliparity, late first pregnancy, and premenstrual symptoms of breast swelling. A decreased risk has been associated with castration before the age of 40. Multiparity, especially beginning before 20 years of age, and prolonged lactation with long-term nursing exert a protective effect probably related to suppression of ovulation.

The incidence of breast cancer rises progressively from age 30 to 90, although the greater number of cases occur between 45 and 59. Mortality from the disease is much higher in Western and/or developed countries. It is rare in Japan, and when it occurs the course tends to be more benign than that seen in the United States. There is no clear explanation for the different incidence between Japanese and American women, although the Western high fat diet and obesity are thought to affect storage and metabolism of estrogens. Certain defined ethnic groups, such as the Parsis of India, have a higher than expected incidence of breast cancer.

The same etiologic factors which contribute to the development of breast cancer may participate in the genesis of benign breast disorders such as fibroadenoma and fibrocystic disease, since patients with breast cancer tend to have had a higher frequency of benign breast disease. The hazards of radiation exposure have been debated in light of the use of mammography. A direct linear relationship seems to exist between the amount of radiation exposure and the risk of breast cancer and amounts to less than 1 per cent increased risk per rad. These estimates were derived from studies of atomic bomb survivors, women treated with radiation for acute postpartum mastitis, and those who received repeated fluoroscopic examinations of the chest.

PATHOLOGY. Carcinoma of the breast is a neoplasm of the ductal epithelium in over 90 per cent of cases. The presence of fibrosis confers its scirrhous character. Neoplastic degeneration can occur in the lobules (lobular carcinoma), usually as low grade tumor or carcinoma in situ, and can often be bilateral. This form of breast carcinoma and noninfiltrating (intraductal) carcinoma constitute 5 to 10 per cent of all breast cancer and rarely ever disseminate. Another relatively benign variant of ductal epithelium is medullary carcinoma, which occurs in about 20 to 25 per cent of cases. This tumor has a significantly higher ten-year survival (84 per cent). There is an equal frequency of nodal metastases but a better prognosis when nodes are positive when compared to other infiltrating ductal cancers.

Paget's disease of the breast (nipple) is a crusted, eczematoid lesion caused by subareolar intraductal carcinoma which begins in the minute ducts of the nipple and grows up toward the skin. Large, clear vacuolated tumor cells (Paget's cells) occur in the deeper layers of the epidermis.

Inflammatory carcinoma represents a particularly malignant variant. It is characterized by erythema, pain, and fullness of the breast owing to dermal lymphatic invasion of anaplastic tumor cells. The median survival of such patients is usually less than 18 months.

The biologic behavior of human breast cancer is highly variable, as reflected in measured mean tumor volume doubling times of 105 to 212 days with a wide range of 15 to 1869 days.

CLINICAL MANIFESTATIONS. ***Primary Disease.*** The majority of patients present with a painless breast mass which was self-detected. Unfavorable prognostic signs include skin involvement, inflammatory signs, fixation to the chest wall, tumor size in excess of 5 cm, palpable axillary nodes, and nipple involvement. The prognosis for development of subsequent metastases can be determined from the extent of axillary node involvement. Patients with negative nodes have a 20 to 30 per cent chance of relapse over ten years. The frequency of relapse rises 66 per cent when one to three nodes are involved and to 85 per cent when more than three nodes are involved. A number of histologic findings have been reported to increase the likelihood of axillary metastases. These include poor differentiation, blood vessel invasion, and lack of lymphoid infiltration of the tumor.

The present clinical staging system incorporates the features described above:

Stage I—tumor <2 cm without skin involvement and with no clinically suspicious axillary nodes.

Stage II—tumor <2 cm with clinically suspicious nodes; any tumor 2 to 5 cm with or without clinically suspicious nodes.

Stage III—any tumor >5 cm; skin involvement or chest wall attachment; any sized tumor with clinically fixed axillary nodes; edema of arm; infraclavicular nodes.

Stage IV—metastatic disease.

The accuracy of clinical diagnosis for isolated breast masses is about 70 per cent. The use of low dose mammography has an accuracy of about 90 per cent. The currently recommended guidelines for screening mammography restrict its use to women 50 years old or older. Women aged 40 to 49 years should have the technique used for annual screening only if they have a prior history of breast cancer or if their mother or sister(s) has breast cancer. In the 35 to 39 age group, women should have annual mammography only if there is prior history of breast cancer, since these patients have a 10 per cent chance of developing cancer in the contralateral breast.

Metastatic Disease. There is a risk of metastatic disease at any time up to at least 20 years postmastectomy, although the majority of metastases are clinically evident by five to seven years. The most common sites of metastases in patients who have positive axillary nodes include the locoregional area, the bones, and the viscera. Routine bone scans at the time of surgery have not been useful in identifying metastatic disease, since only about 6 per cent are abnormal in Stage I or Stage II patients. The incidence of positive scans rises to 25 per cent in Stage III patients. The use of brain scans as a survey technique for metastases is equally inefficient, since about 98 per cent are normal even in the presence of recurrent disease. Biochemical markers have rarely been useful in the detection of clinically undetectable metastatic disease. The serial measurement of alkaline phosphatase, carcinoembryonic antigen, and gamma glutamyl transpeptidase has been proposed as useful in the early detection of metastatic disease, since abnormalities in at least one of these three tests may precede clinical detection by three months. Preoperative measurement of carcinoembryonic antigen (CEA) is not of diagnostic value in early breast cancer, since the incidence of minimal elevation (30 per cent) is approximately the same as for normal women. Persistent postoperative elevation, however, has correlated with the likelihood of relapse. Sixty-eight per cent of patients with metastatic disease have an elevated CEA, with the highest frequency in those with hepatic metastases (93 per cent).

ESTROGEN RECEPTOR PROTEIN (ERP) (Table 239–1). It is possible to measure cytoplasmic proteins which function as receptors to bind and transfer estrogens to the nuclei of cells. These can be measured as femtomoles of ^{3}(H) estradiol bound per milligram of cytosol protein. Approximately 60 per cent of

TABLE 239–1. SOME FEATURES OF THE ESTROGEN RECEPTOR PROTEIN (ERP)

Occurs in breast cancer (male and female), but also in some other tumors, e.g., melanoma
Cytoplasmic protein with 4S, 8S peaks (8S peak correlates with response), expressed as femtomoles of ^3H estradiol bound per milligram of protein
Fifty to 60 per cent of tumors will have levels >3 femtomoles per milligram of protein; 50 to 60 per cent ERP-positive tumors respond to endocrine ablation, hormone therapy, or antiestrogen
Breast tumors are positive in 30 per cent of premenopausal patients and 70 per cent of postmenopausal patients
ERP status of metastatic lesion usually reflects value of primary tumor—unchanged by chemotherapy
ERP-negative tumors tend to have higher kinetic (labeling) indices and to recur sooner than ERP-positive tumors

primary breast tumors have measurable ERP, usually >10 femtomoles per milligram. The presence and the quantity of ERP tend to vary with the menstrual status. Approximately 30 per cent of breast carcinomas in premenopausal women and >60 per cent of such tumors in postmenopausal women contain measurable ERP. The concordance for the presence or absence of ERP between primary and metastatic tumor is high (80 per cent), as it is between multiple metastatic sites. The level is unaffected by chemotherapeutic agents. There is a positive correlation between the presence of the ERP and response to hormonal manipulation: approximately 50 to 60 per cent ERP-positive patients experience objective tumor regression; less than 5 per cent of ERP-negative patients benefit from hormonal treatment. ERP-positive tumors tend to be more differentiated, have lower mitotic activity, and are associated with a longer time interval between primary treatment and metastases in those who subsequently relapse.

The ERP is heterogeneously distributed in the cells of a breast tumor. ERP-positive tumors which recur following endocrine treatment tend to have low or absent ERP. The subsequent response to chemotherapy does not appear to be affected by ERP status or response to previous hormonal treatment. In addition to receptors for estrogen, the cytosol of breast tumors contains receptor proteins for progesterone (PRP) in about 50 per cent of cases. The presence of both ERP and PRP is associated with the highest response rate to hormonal treatment. Tumors lacking both receptors (30 per cent of all cases) rarely respond.

TREATMENT (Table 239–2). ***Primary Therapy.*** There has been a gradual departure from the classic Halsted radical mastectomy to more conservative surgery for primary breast tumors. The modified radical mastectomy with preservation of the pectoralis major muscle and removal of axillary nodes has been the standard approach to Stage I and II tumors. An increasing body of evidence suggests that simple mastectomy alone may suffice in patients with small primary tumors and clinically uninvolved axillary nodes. The routine use of postoperative radiation therapy following either modified radical mastectomy or simple (total) mastectomy does not improve survival but does decrease local recurrence. Exploration (or sampling) of ipsilateral axillary nodes for evidence of microscopic involvement remains an important procedure to identify patients at higher risk of developing distant metastases. An alternative to mastectomy has been the use of primary radiation therapy following excision of the tumor ("lumpectomy"). External beam radiation and iridium needle implants are capable of delivering 8000 to 10,000 rads to the tumor. The local control rate for small primary tumors appears comparable to mastectomy.

Stage III tumors have a high potential for local recurrence and distant metastases with a five-year survival between 20 and 30 per cent. Such tumors are treated primarily by radiation therapy preceded or followed by some form of systemic therapy. In some instances mastectomy can be performed after radiation, but extensive skin infiltration, ulceration, attachment to chest wall, or inflammatory changes require radiation and/or chemotherapy as the initial form of therapy.

In some instances reconstructive surgery with insertion of a prosthesis can be accomplished following radical surgery.

Hormonal Treatment. In all instances a measurement of ERP should be made on all primary tumors, since subsequent metastases would be expected to have a similar ERP constitution. Lacking an ERP measurement, certain clinical features predict response to hormonal treatment: (1) a disease-free interval in excess of two years; (2) a small tumor; (3) metastatic disease confined to bone, skin, lung, and nodes; and (4) the patient's being more than five years postmenopausal.

The likelihood of response to hormonal treatment can be predicted from the height of the ERP value as well as the presence of progesterone receptors. The preferred initial approach to hormonal treatment of premenopausal patients is oophorectomy. Without knowledge of the ERP status, about 33 per cent of patients will respond for a mean duration of 12 to 16 months and are likely to survive almost two years longer than nonresponders. In the past, response to oophorectomy could be used to predict subsequent benefit from further endocrine ablation such as adrenalectomy or hypophysectomy. Although criteria for response are variable, response to adrenalectomy is likely in 40 to 60 per cent of those who have responded to oophorectomy and in <30 per cent of nonresponders. Metastases to the central nervous system and liver rarely respond to either oophorectomy or adrenalectomy.

Transsphenoidal hypophysectomy is about as effective as adrenalectomy in patients who have responded to previous hormonal treatment. The mean duration of response to either mode of therapy is about 18 months, although responses up to five years have been noted in a minority of patients. Measurement of pituitary hormones suggests that transfrontal hypophysectomy is superior to the transsphenoidal approach. Antitumor response may be seen without complete ablation of pituitary endocrine function as measured by radioimmunoassay of serum levels of pituitary hormones in basal or stimulated states. Endocrine ablation in postmenopausal patients has been gradually replaced by antiestrogen therapy with tamoxifen or "medical adrenalectomy" with aminoglutethimide.

Medical Adrenalectomy. Aminoglutethimide will inhibit adrenal estrogen synthesis in castrated or postmenopausal women by inhibiting adrenal conversion of cholesterol to pregnenolone. This results in a marked but not complete inhibition of the synthesis of progesterone, testosterone, androstenedione, and other Δ^4 class steroids. An additional action of the drug is inhibition of the conversion, in peripheral extra-adrenal tissues, of androstenedione to estrone (aromatization), which is a precursor to estradiol. The extra-adrenal sources normally account for almost all of the estrogen produced in postmenopausal women. The adrenal production of cortisol is also suppressed, resulting in a compensatory rise of ACTH, which can overcome the blockade by aminoglutethimide. Effective suppression of estrogen production by aminoglutethimide must therefore in-

TABLE 239–2. THERAPEUTIC APPROACH TO BREAST CANCER

Stage I—Optimal local treatment	
ERP +	No further therapy (in pre- and postmenopausal); hormone therapy is investigational
ERP −	Adjuvant chemotherapy (optional in premenopausal)
Stage II—Optimal local treatment	
ERP +	Premenopausal: adjuvant chemotherapy; addition of hormonal therapy is investigational
ERP +	Postmenopausal: adjuvant chemotherapy and/or hormone therapy is recommended but remains investigational
ERP −	Adjuvant chemotherapy recommended for premenopausal and most postmenopausal patients
Stage III—Locally advanced	
	Optimal local treatment with radiation and surgery if possible. This may be preceded and followed by chemotherapy.
Stage IV	
ERP +	Skin, soft tissue, bone, lymph nodes, pleura: hormonal therapy
ERP +	Liver, lymphangitic spread to lung, multiple metastatic sites (three): chemotherapy plus hormonal therapy
ERP −	Chemotherapy

clude the addition of glucocorticoid, preferably hydrocortisone rather than dexamethasone. Metabolism of the latter steroid can be accelerated by aminoglutethimide. Clinical trials of aminoglutethimide, employing 250 mg four times a day with 40 mg of hydrocortisone daily, have demonstrated a 30 to 40 per cent objective response rate of breast carcinoma in postmenopausal women. The response rate is somewhat higher in women with ERP-positive tumors. Comparative trials show a response rate equivalent to that obtained by surgical adrenalectomy or hypophysectomy. Toxic side effects, which occur in about 20 per cent of cases, include dizziness, somnolence, rash, or a combination, which generally improve over a few days but may not wane for one or two weeks.

Additive Hormone Therapy. Estrogens, androgens, and progestational agents have been used to treat advanced breast cancer in postmenopausal women. Prior to the introduction of antiestrogens the most commonly used hormonal agents were the estrogens, and among these the usual preparation was diethylstilbestrol, 5 mg three times a day.

Response is usually slow, occurring over several weeks and lasting about 12 to 14 months. A positive response is more likely to occcur in women ten years beyond the menopause. The general response rate is about 30 per cent, but this rises to about 50 per cent in ERP-positive patients. Carcinoma in the skin, lymph nodes, and breast is more likely to respond than osseous metastases. Anorexia, nausea, and vomiting may occur at the initiation of therapy, but these symptoms can be relieved by changing to other estrogenic preparations. The chronic toxicity of estrogens includes fluid retention, softening of skin, and breast engorgement. The most troublesome side effect, usually seen at the beginning of treatment, is increased bone pain and/or hypercalcemia, which can be controlled by hydration, diuresis, and/or mithramycin. If the hormone is continued, the flare reaction can actually herald an antitumor response. Patients whose disease progresses while they are receiving estrogens may respond to the sudden cessation of treatment. This rebound regression can occur in up to 30 per cent of treated patients and usually predicts response to other forms of endocrine therapy.

Androgenic hormones are usually less effective than estrogens in postmenopausal patients with soft tissue metastases. They are equal to or superior to estrogens in the treatment of osseous metastases. The usual preparations are testosterone propionate, 100 mg intramuscularly three times a week, or fluoxymesterone, 10 mg by mouth twice a day. The side effects are mainly virilization, erythrocytosis, and increased libido. The mechanism of the therapeutic action of estrogens and androgens in breast carcinoma is unknown, although suppression of pituitary function as well as a direct toxic effect on the cancer cell has been proposed.

Progestational agents in high dosage have also been used successfully, especially in patients who have previously responded to estrogens or androgens. Progestational hormones are less toxic than sex steroids, but they have not been as extensively studied as primary hormonal treatment. The tumor response rate varies from 5 to 25 per cent, but response rarely occurs in patients refractory to other hormones. The use of sex steroid hormones as first line endocrine treatment must be weighed against the fact that safe and effective antiestrogen therapy, with tamoxifen, can achieve comparable responses. Corticosteroids offer the potential of transient antitumor benefit by virtue of their suppression of pituitary ACTH and secondary decrease of adrenocortical function. The toxicity of long-term corticosteroids reduces the usefulness of this form of hormonal therapy.

Antiestrogen Therapy. A number of antiestrogen compounds, such as nafoxidine, clomiphene, and tamoxifen, have the ability to interfere with the effect of estrogen on certain target tissues. The most commonly used and safest antiestrogenic drug is tamoxifen, which competes with estradiol for the high affinity cytoplasmic receptor, binds to it, and makes it refractory to subsequent estrogenic stimuli. In a dosage of 20 to 40 mg per day the drug is capable of inducing remissions of metastatic breast carcinoma, with a duration of response equal to or exceeding that seen with androgens, estrogens, and hypophysectomy. Eventual refractoriness to tamoxifen or other hormonal therapy does not preclude a subsequent hormonal response if that patient is crossed-over to the alternative therapy.

Antitumor response in premenopausal women with advanced cancer has been noted with tamoxifen, although it has not replaced oophorectomy as primary treatment of the ERP-positive patient. The drug is primarily indicated for ERP-positive postmenopausal women. As with other forms of hormonal treatment, responses are most frequent for lesions of soft tissue, lymph nodes, and bone. A tumor which is positive for ERP and which has responded to prior endocrine therapy can be predicted to have a 60 to 80 per cent response rate to tamoxifen, lasting 12 to 18 months on the average. The side effects of tamoxifen are minimal. There is transient nausea or vomiting in about 10 per cent of cases. If a "flare" consisting of increased bone pain and hypercalcemia occurs, it is usually short lived and, as with estrogen treatment, usually heralds an antitumor response.

The primary hormonal therapy for premenopausal women with ERP-positive metastatic disease is oophorectomy followed by antiestrogen therapy or endocrine ablation. Postmenopausal patients with ERP-positive tumors are usually treated with antiestrogens, followed by medical or surgical adrenalectomy for previous hormonal responders. The combination of medical adrenalectomy and antiestrogen therapy is still investigational.

Cytotoxic Chemotherapy. A variety of cytotoxic agents of differing biochemical mechanism of action have demonstrated antitumor activity in advanced breast cancer.

The most commonly used agents include cyclophosphamide, L-phenylalanine mustard (L-PAM), methotrexate, 5-fluorouracil, and doxorubicin (Adriamycin). Each drug used as a single agent can induce a partial regression in about 20 to 30 per cent of cases, but complete responses are rarely seen. When active agents are used in combination chemotherapy programs, the results are superior to the single agents in overall responses, as well as in the achievement of complete remissions. Combination chemotherapy is particularly effective in patients with extensive metastatic disease in the liver and lymphangitic pulmonary metastases, two sites which rarely respond to hormonal therapy. All metastatic sites are capable of responding to combination chemotherapy regimens, including osseous lesions. Neither the previous response to endocrine therapy nor the ERP status influences the response to cytotoxic chemotherapy, and, conversely, prior administration of chemotherapy does not negate a subsequent hormonal response. About 20 per cent of patients achieve a complete remission with combination chemotherapy, which is rarely seen with hormonal therapy or single agent cytotoxic drugs. The more commonly used combination chemotherapy regimens include cyclophosphamide or L-PAM, methotrexate, and 5-fluorouracil (CMF or PMF). An alternative regimen substitutes doxorubicin for methotrexate (CAF). Among the variety of programs available, no one of them has clearly emerged as superior. Cytotoxic chemotherapy in advanced disease can induce remissions lasting in excess of 12 months but rarely exceeding 24 months. It is rare also that all drug therapy can be discontinued in patients with complete remission.

As with hormonal therapy, bone films in patients treated with drugs can often show an increase in osteoblastic reaction as part of the healing process, and this may be falsely interpreted as disease progression. The simultaneous addition of cytotoxic chemotherapy to hormonal therapy, either endocrine ablation or tamoxifen, has shown no clear improvement in survival over the sequential use of these methods. Marked osteolytic destruction of the femur or humerus may necessitate insertion of a prosthesis to prevent pathologic fracture.

Radiation therapy has an important palliative role in metastatic cancer. Metastatic lesions to the brain or meninges can often be effectively treated with complete disappearance of radiographic abnormalities. Intrathecal chemotherapy may also be required when meningeal infiltration is the predominant abnormality. Pain resulting from metastatic bone lesions can be relieved, as well as impending spinal cord compression by tumor.

Adjuvant Therapy. Patients can be identified as being at high risk for developing metastatic disease according to the presence of microscopic involvement of axillary lymph nodes by tumor. Two categories of risk include those with one to three positive nodes (moderate risk) and those with more than three nodes (high risk). Chemotherapy given as an adjuvant to primary treatment is intended to eradicate or significantly retard the growth of microscopic metastases. The current information suggests a definite role for adjuvant combination chemotherapy of premenopausal women in the moderate and high risk groups. Disease-free survival has been significantly prolonged in premenopausal women by the use of combination chemotherapy. The latter is superior to single-agent treatment. More recent trials have shown similar advantages of adjuvant chemotherapy for postmenopausal patients. The addition of hormonal agents to cytotoxic drugs will enhance the disease-free survival of patients with ERP-positive tumors, but overall survival may not be superior to the sequential use of these methods. Some postmenopausal patients in similar risk categories may also benefit, but further controlled trials are required to establish the definite value of adjuvant chemotherapy in postmenopausal patients.

MALE BREAST CANCER. Carcinoma of the male breast is rare, accounting for 0.9 per cent of all breast cancer. The epidemiology, clinical presentation, and primary therapy are very similar to those of female breast cancer. The etiology is unknown, although abnormalities of estrogen metabolism have been reported. Carcinoma of the breast occurs in higher frequency in patients with Klinefelter's syndrome. The management of metastatic disease includes castration as the primary approach, which will yield a response rate in excess of that seen following oophorectomy in premenopausal women (40 to 60 per cent). Similarly, adrenalectomy and hypophysectomy can effectively palliate metastatic disease. ERP has been noted in male breast cancer, but the results of additive hormonal therapy are considerably less than in female breast cancer.

Casebeer K, et al.: Recommendations of the consensus development panel on breast cancer screening. Cancer Res 38:476, 1978. *The proceedings of the NCI-sponsored meeting on the medications for mammography screening.*

Crichlow RW: Breast cancer in man. Semin Oncol 1:145, 1974. *A concise review of the literature on this rare form of breast cancer.*

Henderson IC, Canellos GP: Cancer of the breast. The past decade. N Engl J Med 302:17, 78, 1980. *Comprehensive review of the literature concerning primary and metastatic disease treatment.*

Legha SS, Davis HL, Muggia FM: Hormonal therapy of breast cancer: New approaches and concepts. Ann Intern Med 88:69, 1978. *A review of the approaches to hormonal treatment.*

Legha SS, et al.: Complete remissions in metastatic breast cancer treated with combination drug therapy. Ann Intern Med 91:847, 1979. *The natural history of a series of patients who achieved complete remission with combination chemotherapy.*

McCarthy KS Jr, Silva JS, Cox EB, Leight GS Jr, Wells SA Jr, McCarthy KS Sr: Relationship of age and menopausal status to estrogen receptor content in primary carcinoma of the breast. Ann Surg 197:2, 1983. *Up-to-date study of ERP and age.*

Rosen PP, Saigo PE, Braun DW, Weathers E, Kinne DW: Prognosis in stage II ($T_1N_1M_0$) breast cancer. Ann Surg 194:5, 1981. *The Memorial Hospital experience with this common stage.*

Rossi A, Bonadonna G, Valagussa P, Veronesi U: Multimodal treatment in operable breast cancer: Five-year results of the CMF programme. Br Med J 282, 1981. *The most recent review of the Milan data.*

Senn HJ: Current status and indications for adjuvant therapy in breast cancer. Cancer Chemother Pharmacol 8:139, 1982. *A comprehensive and critical statement on adjuvant therapy.*

Wolmark N, Fisher B: Surgery in the primary treatment of breast cancer. Breast Cancer Res Treat 1:339, 1982. *The NSABP experience with primary treatment.*

Wynder EL, MacCormack FA, Stellman SD: The epidemiology of breast cancer in 785 United States caucasian women. Cancer 41:2341, 1978. *A review of demographic and hormone-related risk factors with a good review of the literature.*

240. POLYGLANDULAR DISORDERS

John N. Loeb

A number of different syndromes are characterized by autonomous hyperfunction or hypofunction of more than one endocrine gland. Although the majority of these syndromes are clearly of genetic origin, the fundamental mechanisms leading to hyperfunction or hypofunction thus far remain unknown in any instance. The syndromes to be considered in this chapter are those in which dysfunction appears to be autonomous within the affected endocrine glands themselves; multiple glandular abnormalities resulting from primary abnormalities in the hypothalamic-pituitary axis or to various locally infiltrative processes are discussed elsewhere.

SYNDROMES CHARACTERIZED BY MULTIPLE ENDOCRINE GLAND HYPERFUNCTION OR NEOPLASIA

The major syndromes characterized by multiple endocrine hyperfunction are those of multiple endocrine adenomatosis (MEA) or multiple endocrine neoplasia (MEN). A number of these syndromes are clearly inherited as autosomal dominant traits and are clinically distinct. The term MEN is now generally preferred because it is more inclusive, comprising both hyperplastic and carcinomatous as well as adenomatous abnormalities. Table 240–1 compares the clinical features of some of these syndromes.

MULTIPLE ENDOCRINE NEOPLASIA, TYPE 1 (WERMER'S SYNDROME). In 1954 Wermer reported the familial occurrence of *multiple tumors of the anterior pituitary, parathyroid glands, and pancreatic islet cells* in association with a high incidence of peptic ulcer. This complex of abnormalities is now most commonly referred to as multiple endocrine neoplasia, type 1 (MEN 1). The syndrome may also include tumor or hyperfunction of the adrenal and thyroid glands, but the relation of these latter endocrinopathies to the underlying genetic abnormality is less well defined. Although it has been proposed that the fundamental defect in MEN 1 is an abnormal differentiation of neural crest tissue, current evidence in support of this hypothesis is by no means conclusive (see also below, under MEN 2).

More than half of patients with MEN 1 have adenomas of two or more different endocrine glands, and involvement of three or more different glands is seen in up to 20 per cent of affected individuals. The approximate frequencies of glandular involvement in patients exhibiting any manifestation of endocrine hyperfunction are, in descending order, parathyroids (90 to 95 per cent), pancreatic islet cells (30 to 35 per cent), and anterior pituitary (15 to 20 per cent). Less commonly there may be hyperfunction (adenomas) of the adrenal cortex and thyroid gland; carcinoid tumors have been reported occasionally. Initial manifestations are most commonly detected in middle age, and many years may elapse between the manifestation of the first endocrine abnormality and ensuing ones. The clinical course is highly variable, depending in part upon which glands are affected and whether the neoplasm results in hypersecretion or instead in compression of surrounding normal glandular tissue with concomitant loss of function. By far the greatest majority of patients (over 90 per cent) have problems related to hypercalcemia, peptic ulcer, hypoglycemia, or pituitary dysfunction. In patients with pituitary neoplasms symptoms are most commonly attributable to pituitary enlargement, with headache or visual-field abnormalities, or to hypopituitarism. Acromegaly, the galactorrhea-amenorrhea syndrome with hyperprolactinemia, and, considerably more rarely, Cushing's syndrome, may also be seen.

Parathyroid gland involvement is by far the most common manifestation of MEN 1 but may be clinically "silent" for many years. Patients may have a history of kidney stones or progressive renal failure as the first manifestation of hyperparathyroidism, or, much more commonly, hypercalcemia may be detected incidentally upon routine screening. All four parathyroid glands are frequently abnormal, and pathologic study may reveal either hyperplasia or multiple adenomas. Parathyroid carcinoma is rare.

Islet cell tumors of the pancreas can be either adenomas (generally multiple) or carcinomas; they may be preceded by diffuse hyperplasia of islet tissue and most typically secrete excess gastrin. Hypersecretion of gastrin may give rise to the *Zollinger-Ellison syndrome* (see Ch. 99) characterized by marked hypersecretion of hydrochloric acid, peptic ulceration (sometimes involving esophageal, distal duodenal, or jejunal sites), and, often, diarrhea. Abdominal pain, bleeding, and perforation are more common than in ordinary instances of peptic ulcer, and radiographic signs consistent with hypersecretion of gastric acid (e.g., hypertrophied gastric rugae) are frequently seen. Many patients in whom the Zollinger-Ellison syndrome initially appears in isolation represent a subset of individuals with MEN 1; approximately half of such patients ultimately develop manifestations of additional endocrine neoplasms.

TABLE 240–1. COMPARISON OF THE CLINICAL FEATURES OF THE MAJOR SYNDROMES CHARACTERIZED BY MULTIPLE ENDOCRINE GLAND HYPERFUNCTION

Endocrine Abnormality	MEN 1*	MEN 2 ("2A")*	MEN 3 ("2B")*
Hyperparathyroidism [Hyperplasia or multiple adenomas]	90–95%, with high incidence of hypercalcemia and nephrolithiasis	25–30%, but only 10% with frank hypercalcemia or nephrolithiasis	Rare
Pancreatic islet cell hyperfunction [Hyperplasia, adenomas, or carcinoma, with hypersecretion (*e.g.*, of gastrin or insulin)]	30–35%	—†	—
Pituitary adenomas ["Nonfunctioning" or with hypersecretion of prolactin (common) or growth hormone (rare)]	15–20%	—	—
Multiple cutaneous lipomas	20%	—	—
Thyroid adenomas, adrenal cortical adenomas, carcinoid tumors	Rare	—	—
Thyroid C-cell hyperplasia with hypersecretion of calcitonin ± medullary carcinoma	—	"100%"‡	"100%"‡
Pheochromocytoma	—	Probably > 20%	Probably > 20%
Multiple mucosal neuromas; marfanoid habitus	—	—	Characteristic
Inheritance	Autosomal dominant	Autosomal dominant	Autosomal dominant, but frequently "sporadic"

*Percentages indicate approximate frequencies among affected individuals manifesting hyperfunction of at least one endocrine gland.
†— = *not* part of the syndrome.
‡Generally taken to be an essential component of the syndrome.

Hypersecretion of insulin by islet cell neoplasms may produce hypoglycemia as an initial manifestation, whereas the elaboration of other substances may, considerably more rarely, result in a variety of other syndromes. Vasoactive intestinal peptide and prostaglandins have been proposed as agents possibly responsible for the intractable watery diarrhea that can be seen even in the absence of hypersecretion of gastrin and the Zollinger-Ellison syndrome, and hypersecretion of glucagon with hyperglycemia, weight loss, and a characteristic skin rash ("necrotizing migratory erythema") has been reported. Islet cell tumors may also secrete pancreatic polypeptide or, rarely, ACTH or serotonin.

Symptoms caused by *pituitary adenomas* in MEN 1 are most commonly due to local encroachment of tumor on other structures, with headache or visual-field abnormalities, or to deficiency of one or more of the tropic hormones. Many of these tumors secrete prolactin and may give rise to the galactorrhea-amenorrhea syndrome. More rarely there is hypersecretion of growth hormone with resulting acromegaly. Hypersecretion of ACTH in MEN 1 is almost always attributable to an ectopic (pancreatic) site.

Adrenocortical hyperfunction may be due to ectopic production of ACTH or to independently functioning adrenal adenomas or carcinomas. Functioning adenomas most commonly elaborate hydrocortisone, giving rise to signs of glucocorticoid excess, but predominant secretion of aldosterone has been reported in rare instances. Hyperfunction of the *thyroid* gland has been reported least frequently of all, and, in part owing to the high incidence of thyroid abnormalities in the population at large, it is possible that sporadic instances of thyroid hyperfunction in MEN 1 represent incidental occurrences unrelated to the underlying genetic abnormality. Adenomas, thyroiditis, and rarely papillary and follicular cell carcinomas have all been reported in association with MEN 1; medullary carcinomas are *not* a part of this syndrome (cf. MEN 2, below). *Other tumors* that can form a part of the clinical picture of MEN 1 include schwannomas, multiple cutaneous lipomas, thymomas, and both bronchial and small intestinal carcinoids.

Management of the various manifestations of MEN 1 is, for the most part, similar to management of the identical manifestations when they occur in sporadic form and hence is considered elsewhere in this textbook. As indicated above, parathyroid involvement, when it occurs, frequently involves more than one gland, and histopathology far more commonly reveals diffuse hyperplasia than a single adenoma. In such instances a number of surgeons now advocate total parathyroidectomy with reimplantation of a glandular fragment in a location conveniently accessible to subsequent exploration if necessary (e.g., the muscle of the forearm). Management of severe peptic ulceration in MEN 1 requires either long-term cimetidine therapy or near-total gastrectomy—rather than an attempt to eliminate the source of excess gastrin—since hypersecretion of gastrin by islet-cell tissue in this syndrome is almost always attributable to either multiple tumors or diffuse hyperplasia.

Because of the sporadic nature of the sequential manifestations of this syndrome, it is important to follow affected individuals with particular attention to the development of new abnormalities. Once the diagnosis has been established in a given patient and baseline films of the sella turcica and prolactin levels have proved to be normal, the major requisite is a careful interval history and a periodic (e.g., yearly) determination of the serum calcium and phosphorus. Because of the high incidence of affected first-degree relatives, such family members should be carefully evaluated for evidence of the syndrome.

MULTIPLE ENDOCRINE NEOPLASIA, TYPE 2 (SIPPLE'S SYNDROME). A second and entirely distinct syndrome, multiple endocrine neoplasia, type 2 (MEN 2 or MEN 2A), is characterized by *medullary carcinoma of the thyroid, pheochromocytoma, and parathyroid hyperplasia.* First partially described by Sipple in 1961, this syndrome, like MEN 1, is inherited as an autosomal dominant trait. The pheochromocytomas are frequently multiple, involving both adrenal glands as well as extra-adrenal sites, and the medullary carcinoma of the thyroid generally appears to be multifocal in origin. A particularly convenient and virtually constant feature of the medullary thyroid carcinomas is the hypersecretion of calcitonin, which serves as a useful marker for the presence of this neoplasm. Elevated levels of calcitonin, either under basal conditions or in response to the provocative stimuli of calcium and pentagastrin infusions, are an indication of parafollicular C-cell hyperplasia in the thyroid gland and may herald the presence of the genetic abnormality well before pathologic changes appear that are unequivocally malignant. As in the instance of the pancreatic adenomas in MEN 1, the medullary carcinomas of the thyroid in MEN 2 may secrete a variety of hormones that are not secreted by the corresponding normal tissues: ACTH, prolactin, histaminase, vasoactive intestinal peptide, serotonin, and a number of prostaglandins. Only rarely does medullary carcinoma of the thyroid present as a palpable mass. Pheochromocytoma is observed in only about one half of affected individuals, and hyperparathyroidism in about one quarter. Only about 10 per cent of individuals with MEN 2 exhibit hypercalcemia or nephrolithiasis (cf. the much higher incidence of overt hyperparathyroidism in MEN 1). Glial tumors and meningiomas may also be seen in MEN 2, but occur far less frequently.

It has been suggested that MEN 2 represents a form of neuroectodermal dysplasia in which so-called APUD cells (cells capable of *a*mine *p*recursor *u*ptake and *d*ecarboxylation and possessing rather characteristic histologic staining properties)—following their normal embryonic migration to the foregut and subsequent localization in a variety of endocrine tissues—later become neoplastic and secrete excessive amounts of hormone in response to a specific genetic defect. Although the evidence for a common APUD cell origin is somewhat better for MEN 2 than it is for MEN 1, it is still by no means wholly convincing. In particular, the high incidence of parathyroid involvement is difficult to reconcile with this theory, since the bulk of present evidence suggests an epithelial rather than a neural crest origin for this tissue.

The pheochromocytomas of MEN 2 are generally benign and are treated surgically. Because they are frequently bilateral, an anterior surgical approach is often recommended; CT scan, multiple-site venous sampling for catecholamines, and angiography can all be helpful in planning surgery. Medullary carcinoma of the thyroid, on the other hand, runs a typically malignant course, and, because of its multifocal nature, requires total thyroidectomy. Elevated levels of calcitonin per se constitute a sufficient indication for total thyroidectomy, even when the tumor is otherwise clinically silent. The tumor is frequently slowly growing, and limited node dissection is thus justified; completeness of tumor removal and the possibility of subsequent recurrence are both conveniently monitored by serum calcitonin levels. The isolated finding of medullary carcinoma of the thyroid should prompt a particularly careful inquiry into the family history since it is likely that at least 10 per cent of such tumors are familial.

MULTIPLE ENDOCRINE NEOPLASIA, TYPE 3 (MUCOSAL NEUROMA SYNDROME). This syndrome (MEN 3 or MEN 2B) resembles MEN 2 but differs in four important respects: (1) The medullary carcinoma of the thyroid and the pheochromocytomas may be accompanied by striking and often disfiguring neuromas of the lips, buccal mucosa, and tongue, as well as by ganglioneuromas of the gastrointestinal tract, thickened corneal nerves visible upon slit-lamp examination, and cafe-áu-lait spots, neuromas, or neurofibromas of the skin; (2) the body habitus may somewhat resemble that seen in patients with Marfan's syndrome; (3) parathyroid hyperplasia sufficient to result in frank hyperalcemia is rare; and (4) mean survival time in MEN 3 is considerably shorter than that in MEN 2 (30 versus 60 years). In contrast to MEN 1 and MEN 2, MEN 3 is frequently sporadic, a history of affected family members being obtainable in not more than half of the cases.

McCUNE-ALBRIGHT SYNDROME. In 1937, McCune and Albright and their associates both described a syndrome characterized by a triad of *polyostotic fibrous dysplasia, cafe-áu-lait pigmentation of the skin* (typically over the forehead, nuchal or sacral areas, or buttocks), and *precocious puberty of the female.* The precocious puberty, although predominantly seen in the female, may occur in males as well. This syndrome may be accompanied by a variety of other endocrine abnormalities, including pituitary hyperfunction (with Cushing's syndrome, acromegaly, or gigantism), bilateral pheochromocytomas, hyperthyroidism, and hypercorticism resulting from adrenal adenoma. Frank malignant disease has not been described. Although the sexual precocity appears to be hypothalamic in origin, patients with adrenal adenomas and hyperthyroidism have been found to have low plasma levels of ACTH and TSH, respectively. The cause of the bone lesions is unknown. The disease appears to be sporadic.

SYNDROMES CHARACTERIZED BY MULTIPLE ENDOCRINE GLAND HYPOFUNCTION

Syndromes characterized by hypofunction of multiple endocrine organs will be discussed under the separate headings of Schmidt's syndrome and the syndrome of polyglandular deficiency associated with mucocutaneous candidiasis. As noted below, however, evidence that the two syndromes actually represent different entities is incomplete. Table 240–2 compares the clinical features of these syndromes.

MULTIPLE ENDOCRINE DEFICIENCY SYNDROME (SCHMIDT'S SYNDROME). In 1926, Schmidt described two patients with biglandular failure characterized by *idiopathic Addison's disease and lymphocytic thyroiditis.* This syndrome has subsequently been expanded to include "primary" failure of other endocrine glands, including the gonads, parathyroids, and endocrine pancreas, as well as a number of nonendocrine abnormalities of presumed autoimmune origin (see below). Virtually any

TABLE 240–2. COMPARISON OF THE CLINICAL FEATURES OF THE MAJOR SYNDROMES CHARACTERIZED BY MULTIPLE ENDOCRINE GLAND HYPOFUNCTION

	Multiple Endocrine Deficiency Syndrome (Schmidt's Syndrome)	Polyglandular Deficiency with Mucocutaneous Candidiasis
Hypoadrenalism	Common	Common
Hypothyroidism	Common	Less common
Hypoparathyroidism	Less common	Common
Gonadal failure	Less common	Less common
Diabetes mellitus	Less common	Rare
Pituitary insufficiency	Rare	Rare
Autoantibodies to endocrine tissues and gastric parietal cells	Often present	Often present
Sex distribution	Strong female predominance	Female preponderance about 4 : 1
Inheritance	Usually "sporadic"; relatively high frequency of certain HLA alleles	Generally inherited as autosomal recessive; no apparent HLA association
Time of onset	Usually becomes evident during adult life	Typically becomes evident during childhood preceded by chronic mucocutaneous moniliasis
Other associated "autoimmune" diseases and characteristics	Pernicious anemia; celiac disease; alopecia; vitiligo; antibody-mediated IgA deficiency; myasthenia gravis; isolated red-cell aplasia	Pernicious anemia; celiac disease; alopecia; vitiligo; IgA deficiency; hypergammaglobulinemia; chronic active hepatitis; proliferative glomerulonephritis

combination of the foregoing endocrine deficiencies may appear in a single individual. The order of appearance is extremely variable; a lag of as much as 17 years has been observed in the manifestation of sequential deficiencies. Hypothyroidism and hypoadrenalism are particularly common; diabetes mellitus, hypoparathyroidism, and gonadal failure are somewhat less so. The frequencies of the different glandular failures probably vary greatly with ascertainment; if one considers juvenile-onset diabetes mellitus as part of the syndrome, the association of this with autoimmune thyroid disease may be the most commonly encountered combination.

Characteristic of this syndrome is the presence of autoantibodies to endocrine tissue and at times to gastric parietal cells as well. Such antibodies are often detectable before the appearance of clinical glandular insufficiency and are a hallmark of syndromes of "idiopathic" endocrine failure. Their presence has been implicated in the pathogenesis of the glandular destruction itself rather than merely as reflecting an immune response to tissue antigens released during antecedent glandular degeneration. Thus, for example, approximately two thirds of patients with idiopathic Addison's disease are reported to have autoantibodies to adrenal tissue, whereas such antibodies are generally absent in patients whose adrenal insufficiency is secondary to tuberculous destruction. About twice as many females are affected with idiopathic adrenal insufficiency as males. Although most cases of multiple deficiency syndromes are sporadic, their occasional appearance in kindreds, as well as the relatively high gene frequency of the HLA-B8 and HLA-Dw3 alleles in affected persons, provides strong evidence for a genetic component contributing to the pathogenesis of polyglandular failure. Other "autoimmune" diseases that may accompany the aforementioned endocrine deficiencies include pernicious anemia, celiac disease, myasthenia gravis, alopecia, vitiligo, isolated red-cell aplasia, and antibody-mediated IgA deficiency. Because it occurs in the same families and has the same HLA associations, Graves' disease is considered by many to be another facet of the syndrome.

Although the constellation of adrenal, thyroid, and gonadal failure in a single patient can easily be confused with primary pituitary insufficiency, measurement of the appropriate tropic hormones now permits a ready differentiation of the two syndromes. Occasionally the simultaneous presence of hyperpigmentation in such an individual suggests a diagnosis of primary adrenal failure on "clinical" grounds alone. Because of the sporadic appearance and variable sequence of subsequent endocrine deficiencies, patients with a proven idiopathic endocrine deficiency should be periodically screened for evidence of additional endocrine involvement.

POLYGLANDULAR DEFICIENCY ASSOCIATED WITH MUCOCUTANEOUS CANDIDIASIS. A clinical picture somewhat different from that of Schmidt's syndrome is presented by patients with the so-called candidiasis-endocrinopathy syndrome. Characteristically this syndrome is dominated by the presence of extensive mucocutaneous candidiasis that appears in early childhood and is followed by the development of idiopathic adrenal insufficiency or hypoparathyroidism or both. Most typically, but not invariably, the appearance of these endocrinopathies postdates the acquisition of chronic monilial infection (mean age of onset, 13 versus 3 years, respectively). As in Schmidt's syndrome, antibodies against endocrine tissues are frequently demonstrable, and pernicious anemia with antibodies against gastric parietal cells may also be present. Diabetes mellitus, in contrast, is relatively rare. Also contrasting with Schmidt's syndrome, which most typically becomes evident in adult life, is the fact that there is no apparent association with the presence of specific HLA alleles, and the apparent inheritance of the syndrome as an autosomal recessive trait. Chronic active hepatitis and proliferative glomerulonephritis have also been reported. The mucocutaneous candidiasis is associated with hypergammaglobulinemia, IgA deficiency, and anergy to *Candida albicans*, and typically is relatively resistant to therapy. No evidence for disseminated candidiasis has been found in autopsied individuals, nor has *Candida* yet been cultured from an affected endocrine gland.

Albright F, Butler AM, Hampton AO, Smith P: Syndrome characterized by osteitis fibrosa disseminata, areas of pigmentation and endocrine dysfunction, with precocious puberty in females. N Engl J Med 216:727, 1937. *One of the two classic descriptions of the McCune-Albright syndrome. Excellent figures.*

Eisenbarth GS, Wilson PW, Ward F, Buckley C, Lebovitz H: The polyglandular failure syndrome: Disease inheritance, HLA type, and immune function. Ann Intern Med 91:528, 1979. *Excellent review summarizing evidence for association of the syndrome of familial polyglandular failure with the HLA-B8 allele.*

Irvine WJ, Barnes EW: Adrenocortical insufficiency. Clin Endocrinol Metab 1:549, 1972. *Exhaustive review contrasting the characteristics of idiopathic and other types of primary adrenal insufficiency. Contains a wealth of material on the association between idiopathic Addison's disease and other examples of idiopathic end-organ failure.*

Marx SJ, Spiegel AM, Levine MA, Rizzoli RE, Lasker RD, Santora AC, Downs RW Jr, Aurbach GD: Familial hypocalciuric hypercalcemia: The relation to primary parathyroid hyperplasia. N Engl J Med 307:416, 1982. *Excellent review of hereditary causes of primary parathyroid hyperplasia, including explicit discussion of the different MEN syndromes.*

Prosser PR, Karam JH, Townsend JJ, Forsham PH: Prolactin-secreting pituitary adenomas in multiple endocrine adenomatosis, type I. Ann Intern Med 91:41, 1979. *Evidence for a high incidence of prolactin-secreting pituitary tumors in MEN I.*

Schimke RN: Syndromes with multiple endocrine gland involvement. Prog Med Genet (ns) 3:143, 1979. *Concise review providing a rationale for the current classification of polyglandular disorders. Useful bibliography.*

Schimke RN: Genetic aspects of multiple endocrine neoplasia. Annu Rev Med 35:25, 1984. *A useful recent review.*

Trence DL, Morley JE, Handwerger BS: Polyglandular autoimmune syndromes. Am J Med 77:107, 1984. *An up-to-date recent review of these interesting disorders supplemented by 110 references.*

241. THE ADRENAL MEDULLA AND THE SYMPATHETIC NERVOUS SYSTEM

Philip E. Cryer

The sympathochromaffin system consists of two components: (1) the sympathetic nervous system and (2) the chromaffin tissues, including the adrenal medulla. The primary endocrine, neurotransmitter and perhaps paracrine products of the sympathochromaffin system are the catecholamines—epinephrine (Adrenaline), norepinephrine (noradrenaline), and dopamine. Cells of the sympathochromaffin system also contain, and in some instances are known to synthesize and release, a variety of peptides of potential biologic importance, including enkephalins. Their pathophysiologic roles, if any, are unknown.

Catecholamine excess commonly results in hypertension along with typical symptoms. It has long been suspected, but is still not proven, that increased sympathetic nervous system activity is the cause of primary (essential) hypertension. Catecholamine overproduction from chromaffin cell tumors—pheochromocytomas—is an uncommon, but curable, cause of hypertension. Deficient sympathetic neuronal norepinephrine release results in postural (orthostatic) hypotension, a sharp decrease in blood pressure when a person stands. Under certain conditions, deficient adrenomedullary epinephrine secretion results in hypoglycemia. These three prominent examples of sympathochromaffin pathophysiology are discussed in the paragraphs that follow. Possible roles of the sympathochromaffin system in the pathophysiology of a variety of human disorders—such as cardiac, hepatic, and renal failure, diabetes, asthma, thyroid disease, myocardial infarction, and cardiac arrhythmias, among others—are emerging but will not be discussed here.

PHYSIOLOGY OF THE SYMPATHOCHROMAFFIN SYSTEM

CATECHOLAMINE BIOSYNTHESIS. The term *catecholamines* is often used to refer to epinephrine and norepinephrine, although dopamine is also a catecholamine, i.e., has the dihydroxyphenyl ("catechol") ring structure and an amine side chain (Fig. 241–1). The catecholamines are synthesized from the amino acid tyrosine, which is derived from the diet or formed by hydroxylation of the essential amino acid phenylalanine. Tyrosine hydroxylase, the enzyme that converts tyrosine to dihydroxyphenylalanine (dopa), is the rate-limiting enzyme in catecholamine biosynthesis. In the presence of a nonspecific decarboxylase, dopa is converted to dopamine, which is the final product in some systems (e.g., interneurons in the sympathetic ganglia). After transport into cytoplasmic vesicles (storage granules), dopamine can be converted to norepinephrine in the presence of dopamine β-hydroxylase. Norepinephrine is the final product in sympathetic postganglionic neurons. Other tissues, such as the adrenal medulla, have cells that also contain phenylethanolamine-N-methyltransferase, the enzyme that converts norepinephrine to epinephrine, which is the final product of those cells.

Catecholamines are stored in cytoplasmic granules and released from the cell by exocytosis in response to neural stimulation. The major determinants of tyrosine hydroxylase activity and synthesis, and thus of catecholamine biosynthesis, are product inhibition and the frequency of transsynaptic neural stimulation of catecholamine-releasing cells. Product inhibition decreases the activity of tyrosine hydroxylase; repetitive stimulation increases synthesis of the enzyme.

CATECHOLAMINE DEGRADATION AND ELIMINATION. Catecholamines are degraded by two principal enzyme systems, catechol-O-methyltransferase (COMT) and monoamine oxidase (MAO) (Fig. 241–1). COMT converts norepinephrine and epinephrine to their respective O-methyl derivatives, the metanephrines (normetanephrine and metanephrine). MAO converts norepinephrine and epinephrine to dihydroxymandelic acid. These intermediates, the metanephrines and dihydroxymandelic acid, can then serve as substrates for MAO and COMT respectively, resulting in their conversion to the major end product of extra-CNS catecholamine metabolism, vanillylmandelic acid (VMA). Dopamine metabolism (not shown in Figure 241–1) by MAO and COMT leads to the formation of

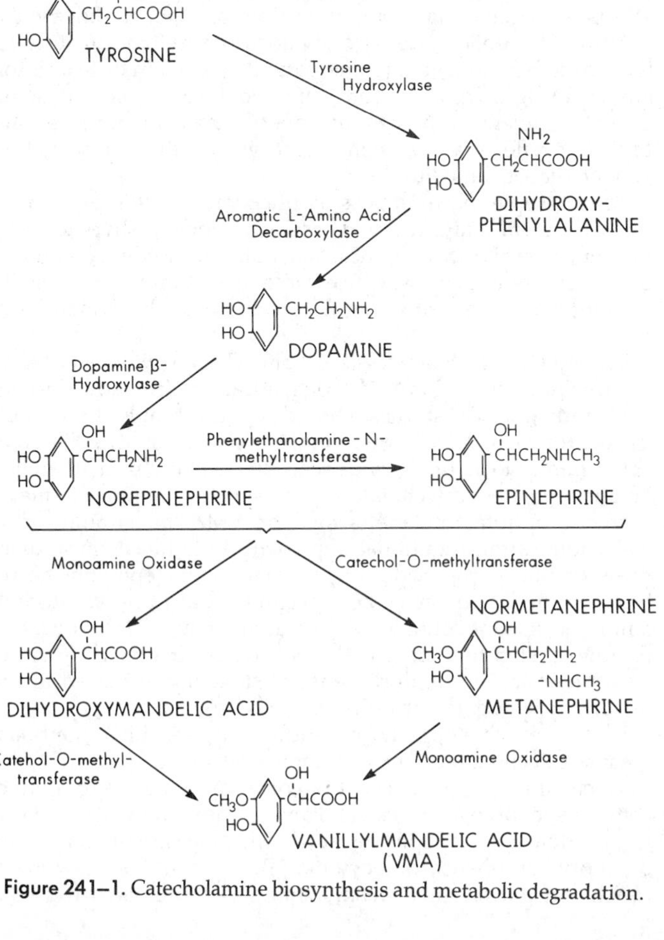

Figure 241–1. Catecholamine biosynthesis and metabolic degradation.

homovanillic acid (HVA), which is identical to VMA except that it lacks a hydroxyl group on the β carbon of the side chain.

In general, catecholamine degradation within the sympathochromaffin cells is via MAO, whereas that of released catecholamines is via COMT. Released catecholamines are also conjugated, largely to sulfate in humans, and this may be another important route of inactivation. The relative importance of conjugation in relation to cellular uptake and degradation by MAO and COMT remains to be established. Nonetheless, 60 to 80 per cent of plasma epinephrine and norepinephrine and roughly half of the catecholamines excreted in the urine are conjugated.

Catecholamines are cleared rapidly from the circulation. Plasma half-times are 1 to 2 minutes. Clearance is largely extrarenal; less than 5 per cent appears in the urine unaltered.

BIOLOGIC ROLES OF THE CATECHOLAMINES. Epinephrine, norepinephrine, and dopamine are neurotransmitters in the CNS. Outside of the CNS, epinephrine is a hormone of the adrenal medulla, and norepinephrine is primarily the neurotransmitter of sympathetic postganglionic neurons. Dopamine is probably also a neurotransmitter, although its physiologic role has not been defined clearly.

Neurally regulated secretion of epinephrine from extra-adrenal chromaffin tissue (not sympathetic neurons) occurs, but in the absence of the adrenal medulla even stimulated plasma epinephrine levels in adults are not high enough to produce measurable biologic effects. Biologic actions of extra-adrenal epinephrine, if any, must be paracrine/neurotransmitter, not hormonal, in nature, at least in adults. Thus, epinephrine functions primarily as a hormone of the adrenal medulla and its plasma concentration is a valid index of its secretion.

Norepinephrine is released from axon terminals of sympathetic postganglionic neurons in direct relation to adrenergic receptors on innervated target cells. Most released norepinephrine is dissipated locally by reuptake into an axon terminal ($uptake_1$), where it is either stored in vesicles or metabolized, or by uptake into other cells adjacent to the synaptic cleft ($uptake_2$), where it is metabolized. Only a small fraction escapes into the circulation. The plasma norepinephrine concentration is a reasonable index of sympathetic neural activity under common physiologic conditions, at least in the basal state and during upright activity in humans. However, under some conditions, such as hypoglycemia, substantial amounts of norepinephrine (along with large amounts of epinephrine), are released from chromaffin tissues, specifically the adrenal medulla. Under such conditions the plasma norepinephrine concentration is clearly not an index of sympathetic neural activity. During vigorous physical activity and in a variety of pathologic states such as surgery, acute myocardial infarction, and diabetic ketoacidosis, circulating norepinephrine is probably derived from both the sympathetic nerves and the adrenal medulla, and its concentrations can be high enough to produce measurable effects. Under these conditions norepinephrine may function as a hormone as well as a neurotransmitter.

This physiology is relevant to the clinical use of plasma catecholamine measurements. Norepinephrine release from sympathetic neurons in amounts sufficient to produce biologically active norepinephrine concentrations in the synaptic cleft can be associated with very small, even undetectable, increments in its plasma concentration. On the other hand, if norepinephrine is released directly into the circulation (as from a pheochromocytoma) substantial increments in its plasma concentration are required to produce biologically active synaptic cleft concentrations.

BIOLOGIC ACTIONS OF THE CATECHOLAMINES. Catecholamines produce a variety of hemodynamic and metabolic effects. These are the result of catecholamine occupancy of adrenergic receptors (adrenoceptors) on the surface of target cells and a consequent series of intra-membrane and intracellular biochemical events. Adrenergic receptors are divided into α- and β-adrenergic receptors, which are subdivided into α_1- and α_2-adrenergic receptors and β_1- and β_2-adrenergic receptors on the basis of measurements of the responses to various agonists and antagonists and the binding of a variety of ligands (generally antagonists) and competition for binding of these ligands by agonists and antagonists in vitro. In general, β-adrenergic receptors are linked through a stimulatory guanine nucleotide regulatory protein to adenylate cyclase, and α_2- (but not α_1-) adrenergic receptors are linked through an inhibitory protein to adenylate cyclase. A discussion of adrenergic receptors is beyond the scope of this chapter although selected examples are given.

Catecholamines increase the rate and force of myocardial contraction (β_1) and produce vasoconstriction (α) in most vascular beds, although vasodilatation (β_2) occurs in some vascular beds, e.g., those of skeletal muscle. Norepinephrine produces increased vascular resistance and blood pressure (systolic and diastolic); the increased blood pressure reflexively limits the increase in heart rate. Probably because it has a higher affinity than norepinephrine for β_2-adrenergic receptors, epinephrine normally produces a somewhat different pattern: increased systolic, but not diastolic, blood pressure and increased heart rate.

Catecholamines increase the plasma glucose concentration through complex actions. These involve both stimulation of hepatic glucose production and limitation of glucose utilization and are mediated by both direct and indirect mechanisms. Foremost among the indirect mechanisms is limitation of insulin secretion (α). The direct actions are largely β mediated. Catecholamines also stimulate lipolysis, ketogenesis, glycolysis, and mobilization of amino acids such as alanine. They also increase thermogenesis.

Symptoms that occur when the sympathochromaffin system is activated include palpitations, anxiety, headache, and diaphoresis. All but the last are attributable to released catecholamines; diaphoresis has been attributed to a sympathetic cholinergic mechanism.

PHEOCHROMOCYTOMA

Pheochromocytomas are catecholamine-releasing tumors that typically produce hypertension. They are an uncommon cause of hypertension; fewer than 1 in 200 hypertensive patients harbors a pheochromocytoma. Yet it is important to detect a pheochromocytoma for several reasons: (1) Hypertension due to a pheochromocytoma is usually curable by surgical removal of the tumor. (2) Patients with a pheochromocytoma are at risk for a lethal hypertensive paroxysm. (3) Some pheochromocytomas (probably less than 5 per cent) are malignant; early detection and removal would be expected to reduce the frequency of metastatic disease. Parenthetically, malignancy is established convincingly only by proven metastases; histologic criteria in the primary tumor are not reliable. (4) The presence of pheochromocytomas can be a clue to the presence of associated endocrine and nonendocrine familial disorders (Ch. 240). Pheochromocytomas are components of the multiple endocrine neoplasia type 2 (MEN 2) and type 3 (MEN 3) syndromes. These familial disorders are inherited as autosomal dominant traits. MEN 2 includes medullary carcinoma of the thyroid, primary hyperparathyroidism, and pheochromocytoma. MEN 3 includes medullary carcinoma of the thyroid, multiple mucosal neuromas, and pheochromocytoma. Pheochromocytomas are not a component of the MEN 1 syndrome (pituitary and pancreatic adenomas and hyperparathyroidism). Familial pheochromocytomas also occur as an isolated disorder, in neurofibromatosis, and in the von Hippel-Lindau syndrome.

PATHOLOGY. Pheochromocytomas arise from chromaffin cells. Chromaffin cells are widespread and associated with sympathetic ganglia during fetal life. Postnatally most chromaffin cells degenerate; the major residual clusters of chromaffin cells comprise the adrenal medulla. Thus, it is not surprising that approximately 90 per cent of pheochromocytomas arise from the adrenal medulla. Extra-adrenal pheochromocytomas (paragangliomas) have been found in sites ranging from the carotid body to the pelvic floor. However, the majority are associated with sympathetic ganglia in the abdomen and most of the others with ganglia in the posterior mediastinum. Multiple pheochromocytomas, including bilateral adrenomedullary tumors, occur in up to 10 per cent of apparently sporadic cases. Bilateral adrenomedullary pheochromocytomas, with or without extra-adrenal tumors, are the rule in familial pheochromocytoma. Bilateral adrenomedullary hyperplasia, thought to be a precursor to pheochromocytoma, has been found in members of affected families.

The vast majority of pheochromocytomas release norepinephrine, and most also release some epinephrine. Rarely, a pheochromocytoma releases epinephrine predominantly or even exclusively.

CLINICAL MANIFESTATIONS. The clinical manifestations of pheochromocytomas are commonly due to the effects of released catecholamines and only rarely to the mass effect of the tumor. Common symptoms are *headache, palpitations,* and *diaphoresis.* Less common symptoms include abdominal or chest pain, gastrointestinal symptoms, weakness, or visual symptoms. Symptoms are typically paroxysmal and associated with increments in blood pressure. Hypertension is sometimes truly intermittent. In many cases, hypertension is sustained, but exhibits marked fluctuations with peak values occurring during symptomatic episodes. In general, these paroxysmal clinical expressions can be explained by episodic catecholamine release. Plasma catecholamine levels are higher during symptomatic, hypertensive episodes than during asymptomatic, less hypertensive, or even normotensive intervals. The event(s) that precipitates episodic catecholamine release is usually not identifiable. However, the relationship between plasma catecholamine concentrations and blood pressure is not tight. This may reflect contrasting effects of norepinephrine and epinephrine but raises the possibility that hypertension in a patient with a pheochromocytoma may not be exclusively the result of direct effects of circulating norepinephrine on the cardiovascular system. Metabolic features of pheochromocytoma include an increased metabolic rate (some patients complain of heat intolerance, weight loss, or both) and an insulin-resistant state. Glucose intolerance occurs, but overt diabetes is unusual and probably reflects a coexistent defect in insulin secretion, i.e., genetic diabetes mellitus.

The rare epinephrine-releasing pheochromocytomas can produce different paroxysms. These may include hypotension, prominent tachycardia, noncardiac pulmonary edema, and cardiac arrhythmias. It is conceivable that tumor products in addition to epinephrine might contribute to these manifestations.

DIAGNOSIS. The diagnosis of pheochromocytoma is based upon clinical suspicion and biochemical confirmation. In general, radiographic studies should be used only to localize pheochromocytomas known to be present on the basis of clinical and biochemical evidence. Fluorometric measurements of unconjugated catecholamines or spectrophotometric measurement of total metanephrines or VMA in 24-hour urine collections is the traditional approach to the biochemical diagnosis of pheochromocytoma. If predominant epinephrine release is suspected on clinical grounds, the urinary catecholamines can be fractionated. The frequency of false-negative findings is slightly higher with VMA determinations. Nonetheless, the excretion of all three is substantially increased in the majority of patients with pheochromocytomas.

With the development of sufficiently sensitive methods, plasma catecholamine measurements have been effectively introduced into the diagnosis of pheochromocytoma. From direct comparison of plasma catecholamine measurements and 24-hour urinary metanephrine and VMA measurements in the diagnosis of pheochromocytoma, Bravo and his co-workers concluded that plasma catecholamine measurements were superior because there was less overlap in the data between affected and unaffected hypertensive patients (Fig. 241–2). However, the two approaches yield somewhat different information. Urinary measurements provide an index of catecholamine release integrated over time. Thus they might reflect intermittent plasma catecholamine elevations that could be missed by plasma measurements that provide information relevant only to a time frame of a few minutes. Conceptually similar is the measurement of catecholamines in platelets.

Most patients with a pheochromocytoma have markedly elevated plasma catecholamine values. Three points warrant emphasis, however. First, occasional patients with pheochromocytomas and typical histories of paroxysms have normal plasma catecholamine concentrations during an asymptomatic, normotensive interval. Second, some patients, commonly those investigated because of family history of pheochromocytoma, have no symptoms or signs and have normal plasma catecholamine concentrations, but are found to have pheochromocytomas. These are not innocent tumors; lethal hypertensive paroxysms have occurred in such patients. Third, patients thought to have predominant epinephrine-secreting pheochromocytomas on clinical grounds can also have substantial overproduction of norepinephrine.

Strict attention to the details of sample collection, handling and storage, the sources of possible biologic variation, and the effects of drugs is critical if diagnostic error is to be avoided in the biochemical assessment of patients with suspected pheochromocytomas. Patients should be studied in the drug-free state if at all possible. Elevated plasma catecholamine concentrations are to be expected during physical or mental stress and in any acute illness. Elevations, at times marked, have been well documented in patients with acute myocardial infarction, shock, burns, diabetic ketoacidosis, and cerebrovascular accidents, as well as during and immediately after surgery. Stable plasma catecholamine elevations also occur in patients with chronic disorders—for example, hypothyroidism, congestive heart failure, chronic obstructive pulmonary disease, anemia, duodenal ulcer, and depression. Lastly, elevated plasma catecholamine concentrations have been found in some, but certainly not all, patients thought to have essential hypertension.

It is my practice to obtain samples for determination of plasma norepinephrine and epinephrine in the basal state, with the patient supine, when pheochromocytoma is suspected. Substantial elevations over reference values provide strong support for the diagnosis of pheochromocytoma and are commonly found in affected patients. Samples are also obtained during symptomatic paroxysms. However, the interpretation of such values is more judgmental since reference values cannot be defined precisely. Patients without pheochromocytoma might be expected to have somewhat elevated plasma norepinephrine and epinephrine levels during such symptomatic episodes. Thus the biochemical diagnosis of pheochromocytoma is more convincingly supported if plasma catecholamine levels are elevated in the basal state and rise further during symptomatic episodes.

It is useful to record the blood pressure and whether or not symptoms are present when plasma samples for catecholamine measurements are drawn from a patient suspected of having a pheochromocytoma. Clearly, normal plasma (or urinary) catecholamine values obtained when the patient is normotensive and free of symptoms do not exclude the presence of a pheochromocytoma. Theoretically, 24-hour urinary catecholamine or metabolite measurements might detect intermittent catecholamine release missed by plasma sampling, so these measurements as well as plasma norepinephrine and epinephrine measurements should be obtained unless the diagnosis is obvious.

Substantial plasma norepinephrine elevations are required to produce hypertension in normal humans (e.g., venous plasma norepinephrine elevations to approximately 1000 pg per milliliter are required to raise the diastolic pressure, and elevations to approximately 2000 pg per milliliter are required to produce diastolic hypertension). Plasma epinephrine elevations within the physiologic range do not raise the diastolic blood pressure. It is reasonable, therefore, to consider normal or even moderately elevated plasma catecholamine levels obtained when the patient is hypertensive to be strong evidence against the diagnosis of pheochromocytoma.

Most patients ultimately found to have pheochromocytomas have distinctly elevated plasma and urinary catecholamine levels. The considerations raised in the preceding paragraphs also apply to patients in whom the diagnosis is less clear cut and to the always difficult problem of the degree of certainty of a negative conclusion. Obviously one can never be absolutely certain during life that a given patient does not have a pheochromocytoma. As in many other areas of medicine, clinical judgment must be based upon probability.

Recently, oral clonidine (0.3 mg) has been found to suppress plasma catecholamine levels in hypertensive patients without pheochromocytoma but not in patients with pheochromocytoma. Thus the clonidine suppression test has been suggested to distinguish patients with primary hypertension with elevated basal plasma norepinephrine levels from those with hyperten-

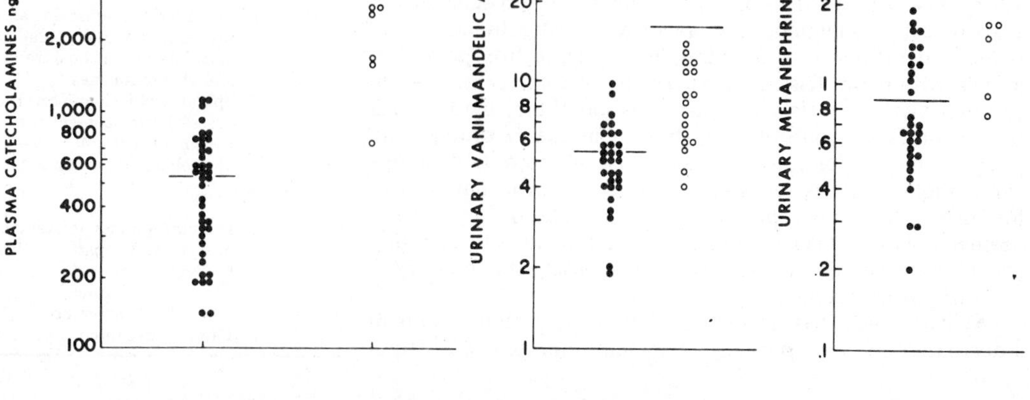

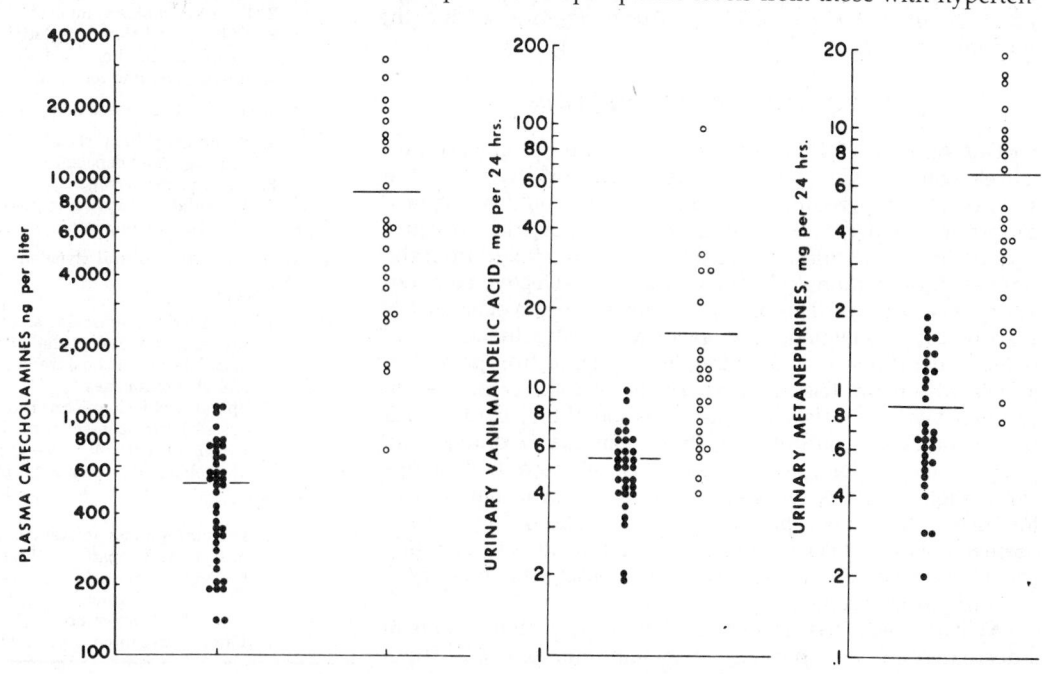

Figure 241–2. Plasma total catecholamine concentrations and urinary vanillylmandelic acid and metanephrine excretions in patients with pheochromocytomas (open symbols) and in hypertensive controls (closed symbols). Note the semi-logarithmic scales. (From Bravo EL, Tarazi RC, Gifford RW, Stewart BH: Circulating and urinary catecholamines in pheochromocytoma. N Engl J Med 301:682, 1979, with permission.)

sion due to a pheochromocytoma. Definition of the utility of this test awaits further experience. False negatives have already been reported. Further, hypotension can follow administration of 0.3 mg clonidine.

LOCALIZATION. Given biochemical confirmation of pheochromocytoma, anatomic localization is desirable. Normal adrenal glands can usually be imaged with modern computed tomography (CT) and the majority of adrenomedullary pheochromocytomas can be seen with this technique. CT is the recommended initial localizing procedure. It is conceivable that ultrasonography of the adrenals might be positive despite negative CT scans in an unusually thin patient. External scanning after the injection of radioactive agents that localize in pheochromocytomas has the conceptual advantage of measuring function rather than anatomy and the practical advantage of permitting scanning of the entire trunk of the body and might, therefore, be expected to localize extra-adrenal pheochromocytomas better than CT scans. The initial experience with [^{131}I]-m-iodobenzylguanidine (MIBG) scans has been encouraging in this regard.

TREATMENT. Treatment is surgical removal of the pheochromocytoma. Patients are usually prepared for surgery by administration of an α-adrenergic antagonist, such as phenoxybenzamine or prazosin, in doses sufficient to produce normal blood pressure and to prevent paroxysms. These drugs can also be used to treat chronic catecholamine excess in patients with metastatic tumor, although they do not influence the growth of a malignant pheochromocytoma. A β-adrenergic antagonist, such as propranolol, can be added to the preoperative regimen if arrhythmias are, or become, a problem.

Most patients are cured by surgery. The differential diagnosis of persistent hypertension includes a missed pheochromocytoma, a surgical complication resulting in renal ischemia, and underlying primary hypertension.

OTHER NEURAL CREST TUMORS. Pheochromocytomas are tumors of differentiated neural crest cells, the chromaffin cells. Tumors of more primitive cells also occur. These include neuroblastoma, a rather common malignant tumor of infancy and early childhood, usually arising in the adrenal medulla, and ganglioneuroma, a generally benign tumor often arising in sympathetic ganglia. These tumors commonly synthesize catecholamines, but usually do not release catecholamines in sufficient quantities to produce clinical manifestations. Presumably the catecholamines are largely inactivated within the tumor. Nonetheless, measurements of catecholamine metabolites such as HVA and VMA are useful, particularly in assessing the response to therapy.

AUTONOMIC HYPOFUNCTION

NORMAL PHYSIOLOGY. Assumption of the upright position causes a sharp reduction in venous return to the heart. In the absence of compensatory mechanisms this would result in a corresponding decrease in cardiac output, in arterial pressure, and in blood flow to the brain. Syncope would result from the simple act of standing. Obviously there are effective compensatory mechanisms. The primary compensatory mechanism is a baroreceptor-initiated, CNS-mediated, sympathetic neural reflex that results in a norepinephrine release from axon terminals within the tissues. This results in a sharp increase in systemic vascular resistance (and limitation of the fall in venous return and cardiac output) and, thus, maintenance of the blood pressure in the standing position. Postural activation of this sympathetic reflex is reflected in a rapid, approximately twofold rise in plasma norepinephrine concentrations. Thus, measurement of the plasma norepinephrine response to standing provides a relatively simple means of assessing the integrity of this sympathetic reflex.

PATHOPHYSIOLOGY. Defective postural adaptation results in a decrement in blood pressure upon standing, termed postural (orthostatic) hypotension. Conceptually, postural hypotension can be caused by one or more of three general mechanisms: (1) absolute or relative intravascular volume contraction; (2) resistance to the cardiovascular actions of norepinephrine; and (3) an afferent, central or efferent defect in the sympathetic neural reflex arc. Patients with postural hypotension due to intravascular volume contraction or resistance to the action of norepinephrine exhibit an exaggerated plasma norepinephrine response to standing. They have *hyper*adrenergic postural hypotension. In contrast, patients with postural hypotension due to a defect in the sympathetic reflex arc have a blunted plasma norepinephrine response to standing. They have *hypo*adrenergic postural hypotension.

HYPERADRENERGIC POSTURAL HYPOTENSION. The causes of hyperadrenergic postural hypotension are listed in Table 241–1. These should be considered in all patients with postural hypotension, including those with overt autonomic disease, because they are commonly treatable. A given patient can have multiple hypotensive mechanisms; correction of one can result in clinical improvement. For example, in a patient with relatively mild autonomic hypofunction, otherwise trivial sodium depletion may result in symptomatic postural hypotension that can be treated by sodium repletion.

HYPOADRENERGIC POSTURAL HYPOTENSION. Hypoadrenergic postural hypotension can result from afferent, central or efferent lesions in the sympathetic neural arc. Diseases recognized to cause secondary hypoadrenergic postural hypotension produce lesions in the brain, spinal cord, or peripheral nerves (Table 241–1). Diabetes is a common cause. In the absence of such diseases, autonomic hypofunction is considered to be idiopathic or primary. Undoubtedly a heterogenous group of disorders of unknown etiology, primary autonomic dysfunction can be divided into two clinical and pathophysiologic syndromes. *Primary autonomic dysfunction type 1,* most commonly referred to as idiopathic orthostatic hypotension, is characterized by autonomic hypofunction in the absence of central nervous system disease. In addition to a blunted plasma norepinephrine response to standing, common to both the type 1 and type 2 disorders, as a group patients with the type 1 disorder have low basal plasma norepinephrine concentrations. They are thought to have lesions of the peripheral autonomic nerves.

TABLE 241–1. DIFFERENTIAL DIAGNOSIS OF POSTURAL HYPOTENSION

I. Hyperadrenergic postural hypotension
   - A. Intravascular volume contraction
     1. Hemorrhage
     2. Severe chronic anemia
     3. Sodium (and water) depletion—aldosterone deficiency, diuretics, gastrointestinal or renal diseases
     4. Relative volume contraction—pregnancy
   - B. Resistance to released norepinephrine
     1. Sodium depletion (see above)
     2. Glucocorticoid deficiency
     3. Bartter's syndrome
     4. Vasodilator drugs—nitroglycerin; hydralazine and minoxidil; prazosin, bromocriptine, and other α-adrenergic antagonists

II. Hypoadrenergic Postural Hypotension
   - A. Secondary
     1. Brain lesions—vascular accidents involving the brainstem, toxic/nutritional encephalopathies, demyelinating and degenerative disorders, neoplasms, trauma, infections, tricyclic antidepressants, and phenothiazines
     2. Spinal cord lesions—cervical transection, mass lesions (tumor, abscess), syringomyelia, combined systems disease, tabes dorsalis
     3. Peripheral nerve lesions—diabetic adrenergic neuropathy, alcoholism, amyloidosis, porphyria, vincristine
   - B. Primary
     1. Primary autonomic dysfunction
        - a. Type 1: Idiopathic orthostatic hypotension
        - b. Type 2: Idiopathic orthostatic hypotension with somatic neurologic deficit (Shy-Drager syndrome, multiple system atrophy)
     2. Familial dysautonomia (Riley-Day syndrome)

Primary autonomic dysfunction type 2 is perhaps best known as the Shy-Drager syndrome; it has also been referred to as multiple system atrophy or idiopathic orthostatic hypotension with somatic neurologic deficit. In addition to autonomic hypofunction, patients with the type 2 disorder have degenerative central nervous system disease most commonly manifested as parkinsonism. Such patients have normal basal plasma norepinephrine concentrations and their autonomic lesions are thought to be in the central nervous system.

Impairment of both sympathetic and parasympathetic neural functions is the rule in primary autonomic dysfunction. Thus a variety of symptoms, such as diminished sweating and heat intolerance, difficulty in focusing, gastrointestinal symptoms, urinary and fecal incontinence and impotence, in addition to postural symptoms, occur commonly.

Treatment involves correction of the underlying cause of postural hypotension (Table 241–1) when possible. Symptomatic treatment approaches include sodium loading (NaCl) tablets plus fludrocortisone, (0.1 to 0.3 mg daily), which can produce hypokalemia and might precipitate cardiac failure in a patient with heart disease. Although not approved by the FDA at this writing, the agonist midodrine (which constricts veins as well as arterioles) appears to be an effective drug.

EPINEPHRINE DEFICIENCY

Glucagon normally plays a primary role in promoting glucose recovery from *hypoglycemia*. Epinephrine is not critical when glucagon secretion is intact but compensates largely, and becomes critical, when glucagon secretion is deficient. Glucose recovery from hypoglycemia fails to occur only in the absence of both glucagon and epinephrine.

In patients with insulin-dependent diabetes mellitus (IDDM), glucagon secretory responses to hypoglycemia are commonly blunted or absent. This defect occurs relatively early in the course of the disease and is selective for the response to plasma glucose decrements. Its mechanism is unknown. To the extent that they have deficient glucagon secretory responses, patients with IDDM are dependent upon epinephrine to promote recovery from hypoglycemia. If deficient epinephrine secretory responses also develop, as they sometimes do late in the course of the disease (or if the hyperglycemic actions of epinephrine are blocked as with propranolol administration), patients can become defenseless against hypoglycemia. Studies have shown that patients judged to have inadequate glucose counterregulation on the basis of an insulin infusion test and subsequently found to have recurrent, severe hypoglycemia during intensive treatment of their diabetes, have combined deficiencies of glucagon and epinephrine secretion in response to glucose decrements. In contrast, patients judged to have adequate glucose counterregulation, and subsequently found to have few severe hypoglycemic episodes during intensive treatment, have comparably deficient glucagon secretion but normal epinephrine secretion. Thus, inadequate glucose counterregulation due to combined deficiencies of glucagon and epinephrine secretion results in a 25-fold increase in the risk of severe hypoglycemia during intensive therapy of IDDM.

Bravo EL, Tarazi RC, Fouad FM, Vidt DG, Gifford RW Jr: Clonidine suppression test: A useful aid in the diagnosis of pheochromocytoma. N Engl J Med 305:623, 1981. *A suppression test for the diagnosis of pheochromocytoma.*

Cryer PE: Physiology and pathophysiology of the human sympathoadrenal neuroendocrine system. N Engl J Med 303:436, 1980. *A review from the perspective of plasma norepinephrine and epinephrine measurements.*

Cryer PE: Diseases of the adrenal medullae and sympathetic nervous system. *In* Felig P, Baxter JD, Broadus AE, Frohman LE (eds.): Endocrinology and Metabolism. New York, McGraw-Hill Book Company, 1981, pp 511–550. *A more detailed discussion of sympathochromaffin physiology and pathophysiology.*

Cryer PE, Gerich JE: The relevance of glucose counterregulatory systems to patients with diabetes: Critical roles of glucagon and epinephrine. Diabetes Care 6:95, 1983. *Review of hypoglycemic glucose counterregulation in normal and diabetic persons.*

Manger WM, Gifford RW Jr: Hypertension secondary to pheochromocytoma. Bull NY Acad Med 58:139, 1982. *An extensive clinical experience.*

Schirger A, Sheps SG, Thomas JE, Fealey RD: Midodrine. A new agent in the management of idiopathic orthostatic hypotension and Shy-Drager syndrome. Mayo Clin Proc 56:429, 1981. *A promising drug for the treatment of hypoadrenergic postural hypotension.*

Thomas JE, Schirger A, Fealey RD, Sheps SG: Orthostatic hypotension. Mayo Clin Proc 56:17, 1981. *An extensive clinical experience.*

White NH, Skor D, Cryer PE, Bier DM, Levandoski L, Santiago JV: Identification of type 1 diabetic patients at increased risk for hypoglycemia during intensive therapy. N Engl J Med 308:485, 1983. *Demonstration that combined glucagon and epinephrine deficiencies result in a 25-fold increased risk of severe hypoglycemia during intensive treatment of insulin-dependent diabetes mellitus.*

Zweiffler AJ, Julius S: Increased platelet catecholamine content in pheochromocytoma. N Engl J Med 306:890, 1982. *An alternative to plasma catecholamine measurements in the diagnosis of pheochromocytoma, although seldom necessary.*

242. THE CARCINOID SYNDROME

Philip E. Cryer

Carcinoid tumors arise from enterochromaffin (Kulchitsky) cells that are located predominantly in the gastrointestinal mucosa. Enterochromaffin cells have the potential to produce a variety of biologically active amines and peptides, including serotonin, bradykinin, and histamine, as well as prostaglandins. Carcinoid tumors are relatively common. Those that release sufficient quantities of mediators into the systemic circulation to produce the clinical carcinoid syndrome—flushing often with diarrhea and sometimes with wheezing or cardiac failure—are rare. Carcinoid tumors are most commonly found in the appendix or rectum, but these rarely produce the carcinoid syndrome. The tumors that produce the syndrome typically arise in the ileum, although the carcinoid syndrome can also result from tumors of the stomach, bile duct, duodenum, pancreas, lung, or even the ovary. Despite the release of a variety of mediators, the biochemical common denominator of the carcinoid syndrome is the overproduction of serotonin and the excretion of its major metabolite, 5-hydroxyindoleacetic acid (5-HIAA).

A variety of ectopic humoral syndromes have been associated with histologic carcinoid tumors. These include Cushing's syndrome (ACTH) and dilutional hyponatremia (vasopressin) with bronchial carcinoids, gynecomastia (chorionic gonadotropin) with gastric carcinoids, and hypoglycemia (insulin) with pancreatic carcinoids. Typically, such patients do not have the carcinoid syndrome.

BIOSYNTHESIS AND DEGRADATION OF SEROTONIN. Serotonin is synthesized from dietary tryptophan (Fig. 242–1). In the

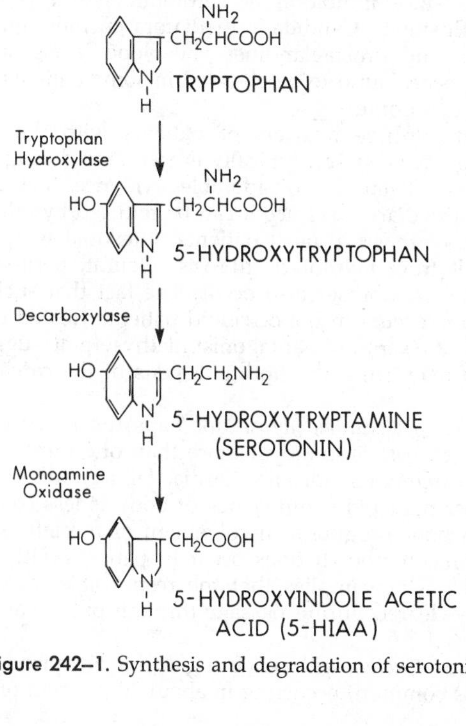

Figure 242–1. Synthesis and degradation of serotonin.

presence of tryptophan hydroxylase, tryptophan is converted to 5-hydroxytryptophan, which, in the presence of aromatic L-amino acid decarboxylase, is converted to 5-hydroxytryptamine (serotonin). Through a series of reactions, including that involving the enzyme monamine oxidase, 5-hydroxytryptamine is converted to 5-hydroxyindoleacetic acid.

Approximately 90 per cent of serotonin in the body is normally found in the gut. Serotonin synthesis accounts for only 1 per cent of the metabolism of tryptophan in normal individuals. This may be as high as 60 per cent in patients with the carcinoid syndrome. Indeed, a pellagra-like skin rash has been attributed to diversion of tryptophan from nicotinic acid synthesis in such patients. Normal individuals excrete less than 10 mg of 5-HIAA per 24 hours. Patients with the carcinoid syndrome commonly excrete 50 to 100 mg per 24 hours.

CLINICAL MANIFESTATIONS. Clinical carcinoid syndrome is usually associated with an ileal carcinoid tumor that has metastasized to the liver. Although carcinoids in sites, such as the lung or ovary, that do not drain into the portal circulation can rarely produce the carcinoid syndrome without evident hepatic metastases, carcinoid syndrome due to an ileal carcinoid is almost invariably associated with overt hepatic metastases. Presumably the liver clears mediators released from the tumor, and this clearance is impaired by metastatic tumor, resulting in the clinical syndrome.

More than 90 per cent of patients with the carcinoid syndrome have episodes of *cutaneous flushing*. The flush usually begins in the face and may spread to the trunk or even the extremities. It is red initially and then becomes purple; it commonly lasts only a few minutes, but may continue for hours. *Telangiectasias* of the face can result from frequent flushing. The heart rate increases and the blood pressure tends to decrease during a flush. This is in contrast to patients with pheochromocytomas who typically have episodes of pallor with hypertension. Bronchial carcinoids may be associated with more intense and long-lasting flushing episodes. In patients with gastric carcinoids, flushing tends to be patchy initially and may be anywhere on the body. Headache commonly follows the flush.

Flushing can be precipitated by alcohol, food, stress, or palpation of the liver, or it may follow the administration of catecholamines, pentagastrin, or reserpine. A single mediator that causes the carcinoid flush has not been identified. It is not serotonin, since inhibition of serotonin synthesis does not prevent flushing. Candidate mediators include bradykinin, histamine, and prostaglandins. The blood levels of each of these has been found to be elevated in some patients with the carcinoid syndrome.

More than three quarters of patients with the carcinoid syndrome have *diarrhea*, typically exacerbated during episodes of flushing. There is considerable evidence that serotonin mediates the diarrhea, since it can be reduced by inhibition of serotonin synthesis in most patients. Intestinal symptoms can also result from mesenteric fibrosis. Pleural, peritoneal, and retroperitoneal fibroses also occur. The fact that such fibrosis occasionally occurs in noncarcinoid patients treated for a long term with the serotonin antagonist methysergide suggests that serotonin may cause the fibrotic lesions of the carcinoid syndrome.

Right-sided endocardial fibrosis, perhaps the result of chronic serotonin excess, is found in more than one third of patients with the carcinoid syndrome. Cardiac failure, due to pulmonic stenosis or tricuspid insufficiency or both, is less common but implies a poor prognosis. Involvement of the left side of the heart is uncommon. It does occur in patients with bronchial carcinoids, which implies that the responsible mediator(s) is ordinarily cleared during passage through pulmonary capillaries.

Bronchoconstriction with wheezing during an episode of flushing is less common, occurring in about 20 per cent of patients. Like flushing, but unlike diarrhea, bronchoconstriction is not prevented by inhibition of serotonin synthesis.

Somatostatin has been reported to decrease flushing, diarrhea, and bronchoconstriction in patients with the carcinoid syndrome. The mechanism(s) of this effect is not known.

DIAGNOSIS. Diagnosis is based upon clinical suspicion—usually a history of flushing and diarrhea—associated with markedly increased urinary 5-hydroxyindoleacetic acid excretion. Metastatic hepatomegaly is common. Since carcinoid tumors produce the carcinoid syndrome rarely, the histologic diagnosis of a carcinoid tumor does not establish the presence of the carcinoid syndrome. Platelet serotonin levels are elevated in most patients with the carcinoid syndrome. Gastric carcinoids appear to have low decarboxylase activity since 5-hydroxytryptophan, rather than serotonin, is the major product of indole metabolism in some such patients.

Provocative tests, such as the precipitation of episodes with intravenous administration of epinephrine, are seldom necessary and potentially dangerous, since severe hypotension and bronchoconstriction can occur.

False-positive urinary 5-HIAA determinations are common and should be suspected particularly when the values are minimally elevated, e.g., 10 to 20 mg per 24 hours. Increased 5-HIAA excretion can follow the ingestion of chocolate, bananas, tomatoes, pineapples, walnuts, and avocados and the use of drugs, including mephenesin, methocarbamol, reserpine, acetaminophen, and glyceryl guaiacolate (the last in some cough syrups). Increased values have also been reported in Whipple's disease and nontropical sprue.

Computed tomography, radionuclide scans, ultrasonography, and conventional barium contrast x-ray studies can be used to define tumor anatomy. Despite widespread metastases, the primary tumor can be small and difficult to demonstrate.

TREATMENT. In the presence of documented metastases, resection of a primary ileal carcinoid tumor is not indicated. It may become necessary because of intestinal obstruction or because of intussusception. Rarely, surgical removal of an isolated tumor (e.g., a bronchial or ovarian carcinoid) is curative. Devascularization of metastatic tumor by percutaneous arterial embolization has been reported to produce symptomatic relief in some patients.

Survival of less than five years after the onset of the carcinoid syndrome is the rule, but survival for more than 20 years is well documented. Thus, high-risk attempts at curative therapy are generally not indicated. Carcinoid tumors are not radiosensitive. Low-risk chemotherapy has not been very effective.

Symptomatic therapy includes nutritional support plus the provision of nicotinamide to prevent pellagra. Diarrhea has been treated with serotonin antagonists such as methysergide or cyproheptadine as well as with opiates. The drug parachlorophenylalanine, a tryptophan hydroxylase inhibitor, reduces diarrhea. However, allergic reactions and CNS side effects have occurred, and the drug remains experimental. No drug is consistently effective in preventing flushing; H_1 and H_2 histamine antagonists, including cimetidine, are often tried. Phenothiazines and the α-adrenergic antagonist phenoxybenzamine have also been used, as have glucocorticoids. Recently, treatment with leukocyte interferon was reported to decrease flushing and diarrhea in six of nine patients with the carcinoid syndrome. Symptomatic improvement, reduction of 5-HIAA excretion, and reduction in tumor size was reported in a patient treated with tamoxifen.

Frolich JC, Margolius HS: Prostaglandins, the kallikrein-kinin system, Bartter's syndrome and the carcinoid syndrome. *In* Felig P, Baxter JD, Broadus AE, Frohman LE, (eds.): Endocrinology and Metabolism. New York, McGraw-Hill Book Company, 1981, pp 1247–1274. *A more detailed discussion of the carcinoid syndrome.*

Melia WM, Nunnerly HB, Johnson PJ, Williams R: Use of arterial devascularization and cytotoxic drugs in 30 patients with the carcinoid syndrome. Br J Cancer 46:331, 1982. *Promising symptomatic responses to tumor devascularization but not to cytotoxic drugs.*

Oberg K, Funa K, Alm G: Effects of leukocyte interferon on clinical symptoms and hormone levels in patients with mid-gut carcinoid tumors and carcinoid syndrome. N Engl J Med 309:129, 1983. *Unanticipated clinical and biochemical responses with demonstrable reductions in tumor size.*

Part XVIII
DISEASES OF BONE AND BONE MINERAL METABOLISM

243. MINERAL AND BONE HOMEOSTASIS

Claude D. Arnaud

THE INTEGRATED CALCIOTROPIC HORMONE SYSTEM

A highly integrated and complex endocrine system maintains calcium, phosphate, and magnesium homeostasis in all vertebrates. It involves an interplay between two polypeptide hormones, parathyroid hormone (PTH) and calcitonin, and a sterol hormone, 1,25-dihydroxycholecalciferol [$1,25(OH)_2D$]. Biosynthesis and secretion of the polypeptide hormones are regulated by a negative feedback mechanism that involves calcium ion activity in the extracellular fluids (Fig. 243–1). Biosynthesis of $1,25(OH)_2D$ from the major circulating metabolite of vitamin D, 25-hydroxycholecalciferol (25OHD), takes place in the kidney and is regulated by PTH and calcitonin as well as by the extracellular fluid concentrations of calcium and phosphate. Other hormones, such as insulin, growth hormone, somatomedin, cortisol, thyroxine, epinephrine, estrogen, testosterone, and inorganic phosphate, together with some compounds not yet identified and certain physical factors, undoubtedly play roles in the modification and regulation of organ responses to PTH, calcitonin, and $1,25(OH)_2D$.

Parathyroid hormone, calcitonin, and $1,25(OH)_2D$ regulate the flow of minerals into and out of the extracellular fluid compartment through their actions on intestine, kidney, and bone (Fig. 243–1, Table 243–1). The target cells of these organs function as a barrier between the extracellular fluid compartment and the intestinal lumen, the renal tubular lumen, and the bone fluid compartment (Fig. 243–2). These target cells are highly specialized for solute transport against a concentration gradient and thus are often described as being polarized.

PARATHYROID HORMONE. Under normal circumstances, PTH prevents serum calcium from falling below physiologic concentrations by stimulating calcium movement from the bone fluid compartment and the intestinal and renal tubular lumina into the blood. Whereas its effects on bone and kidney are direct, PTH acts indirectly on the intestine, through the mediation of vitamin D. The hormone stimulates the conversion of 25OHD to $1,25(OH)_2D$ via a 1α-hydroxylase in the mitochondria of the renal tubule (this stimulation works directly and indirectly through a decrease in serum phosphate levels). The $1,25(OH)_2D$ thus formed stimulates intestinal absorption of calcium via a vitamin D–dependent calcium pump.

Parathyroid hormone also prevents serum phosphate levels from rising above normal physiologic concentrations by increasing renal tubular excretion of phosphate. This regulatory action is important because phosphate, like calcium, is also released into the blood by PTH-induced bone resorption. This function can be particularly appreciated in patients with end-stage renal failure and associated severe hyperparathyroidism. These patients develop hyperphosphatemia because large quantities of phosphate are released from bone and the kidney can no longer excrete it.

CALCITONIN. Calcitonin prevents abnormal increases in both serum calcium and serum phosphate. It decreases the translocation of calcium from the renal tubule and bone fluid compartment into the blood and thus can be considered as a counterregulator of PTH in this regard. The effects of calcitonin on the intestinal absorption of calcium and vitamin D metabolism are uncertain.

VITAMIN D. Vitamin D, as $1,25(OH)_2D$, acts primarily to maintain the cellular calcium transport system in the intestine, which causes the active extrusion of calcium against a concentration gradient from the interior of the cell (ionized calcium concentration = 10^{-7} to 10^{-6} M), across the antiluminal membrane, and into the extracellular fluid (ionized calcium concentration = 10^{-3} M) (Fig. 243–3). Thus, PTH and $1,25(OH)_2D$ are interdependent. The renal production of $1,25(OH)_2D$ depends upon the prevailing concentration of PTH in the blood, and the ability of PTH to increase plasma calcium depends upon a calcium transport system maintained by $1,25(OH)_2D$.

CONTROL MECHANISMS. Figure 243–1 shows the relationships among the different components involved in maintaining a normal level of plasma calcium. Each of the three overlapping feedback loops involves one of the target organs of the calciotropic hormones and the four controlling elements—i.e., plasma calcium, PTH, calcitonin, and $1,25(OH)_2D$. The left limbs of the loops depict physiologic events that increase plasma calcium, and the right limbs events that decrease plasma calcium. Under physiologic conditions, there are small fluctuations in plasma calcium. Decreases in plasma calcium increase

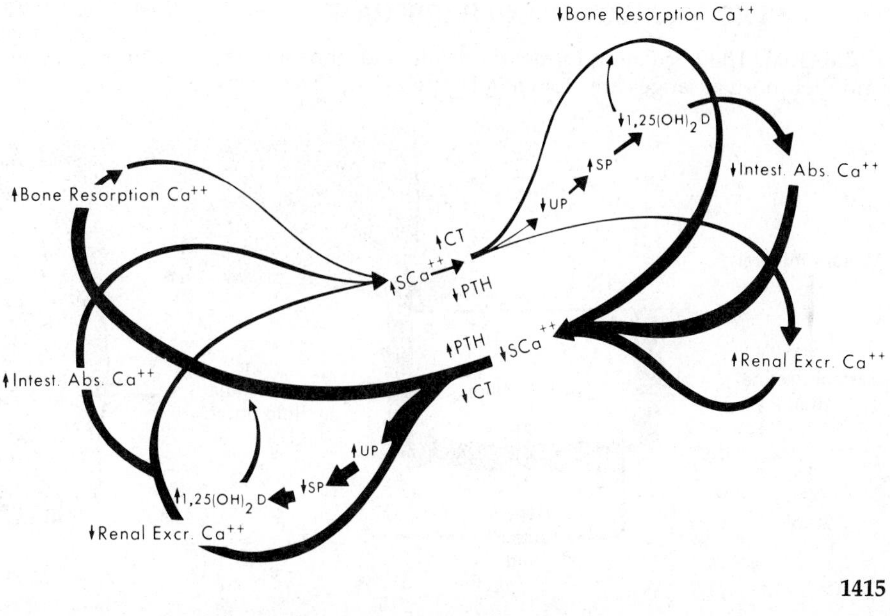

Figure 243–1. Schema of calcium homeostasis, consisting of three overlapping control loops that interlock and relate to one another through the level of blood concentrations of ionic calcium, parathyroid hormone, and calcitonin. Each loop involves a calciotropic hormone target organ (bone, intestine, kidney). The limbs on the left depict physiologic events that increase the blood concentration of calcium, and the limbs on the right, events that decrease this concentration. See text for detailed descriptions. (From Arnaud CD: Calcium homeostasis: Regulatory elements and their integrity. Fed Proc 37:2558, 1978.)

TABLE 243–1. ACTIONS OF MAJOR CALCIUM-REGULATING HORMONES

	Bone	Kidney	Intestine
PTH	Increases resorption of calcium and phosphate.	Increases resorption of calcium; conversion of 25OHD to $1,25(OH)_2D$. Decreases resorption of phosphate; resorption of bicarbonate.	No direct effects.
Calcitonin	Decreases resorption of calcium and phosphate.	Decreases resorption of calcium and phosphate. Questionable effect on vitamin D metabolism.	No direct effects.
Vitamin D	Maintains Ca^{2+} transport system.	Decreases resorption of calcium.	Increases absorption of calcium and phosphate.

Adapted from Arnaud CD, Kolb FO: The calciotropic hormones and metabolic bone disease. *In* Greenspan FS, Forsham PH (eds.): Basic and Clinical Endocrinology. Los Altos, Lange Medical Publications, 1983, p 188.

PTH secretion and decrease calcitonin secretion. These changes in hormone secretion lead to increased bone resporption, decreased renal excretion of calcium, and increased intestinal calcium absorption (via PTH stimulation of $1,25(OH)_2D$ production; left side of Fig. 243–1). As a consequence of these events, plasma calcium rises slightly above physiologic levels, inhibiting PTH secretion and stimulating calcitonin secretion. These changes in plasma hormone concentrations decrease bone resorption, increase renal excretion of calcium, and decrease intestinal absorption of calcium (right side of Fig. 243–1), causing plasma calcium to fall below the physiologic level. This sequence of events probably occurs within milliseconds, so that plasma calcium is maintained at physiologic levels with minimal oscillation. The "butterfly" scheme in Figure 243–1 not only shows the relationships among elements that control mineral homeostasis under physiologic conditions but also suggests how potential pathogenetic mechanisms and adaptive responses elicited by disease or treatment would operate in this system.

PLASMA CALCIUM AND PHOSPHATE

CALCIUM. The circulating forms of calcium and phosphorus and their normal ranges are shown in Figure 243–4. Calcium is distributed in three major fractions: ionized, protein-bound, and complexed. The ionized form (Ca^{2+}), the only biologically active species, constitutes 46 to 50 per cent of total calcium. The protein-bound fraction, roughly equivalent to the ionized fraction in amount, is biologically inert. However, the calcium bound to albumin (80 per cent) and globulin (20 per cent) is important because it provides a readily available reservoir of this important cation. Since the binding of calcium to these proteins obeys the mass-law equation, calcium can dissociate from its binding sites to provide a first-line defense against hypocalcemia. Moreover, hyperproteinemia (e.g., hyperglobulinemia in myelomatosis) can increase and hypoproteinemia (e.g., hypoalbuminemia in cirrhosis of the liver or nephrosis) can decrease total plasma calcium without changing the concentration of ionized calcium. Formulas have been developed to estimate the percentage of calcium bound to the plasma proteins based on the differential binding affinities of albumin and globulin; for example,

$$\text{Per cent protein-bound Ca} = 8 \times \text{albumin (grams per deciliter)} + 2 \times \text{globulin (grams per deciliter)} + 3.$$

Such formulas permit the calculation of diffusible calcium (see below) by subtracting protein-bound from total calcium. Such estimates can be notoriously inaccurate, however, especially in patients with low plasma protein concentrations. The only accurate means of determining the plasma concentration of ionized calcium in hypo- or hyperproteinemic states is to measure it directly by an ion-selective electrode procedure. The fraction of plasma calcium that is complexed to organic (e.g., citrate) and inorganic (e.g., phosphate or sulfate) acids is small (approximately 8 per cent), and, like the ionized fraction, it is ultrafilterable (diffusible). Complexed calcium probably has little importance as a reservoir for ionized calcium, but in states of hyperphosphatemia, such as chronic renal failure, excessive complexing of calcium with phosphate may contribute to the decrease in plasma ionized calcium observed in this condition.

The normal range for serum calcium (Fig. 243–4) is small (1.2 mg per deciliter) compared to the total concentration of serum calcium (8.9 to 10.1 mg per deciliter), and the same is true for the ionized fraction. Thus, values for total calcium below 8.9 mg per deciliter, assuming that plasma protein concentrations are normal, reflect clinically significant hypocalcemia, and values above 10.1 mg per deciliter reflect hypercalcemia. In recent years, serum calcium has been measured with reasonable accuracy in most clinical laboratories. However, stored plasma samples may yield artifactual decreases in circulating calcium concentrations, and contaminated serum samples may yield artifactual increases. The latter problem is most frequently caused by inadvertent contamination of the blood-drawing tubes with calcium when they are manufactured or contamination of laboratory equipment by airborne calcium carbonate dust from laboratory chalk boards. Thus, it is important to use *fresh serum* for calcium measurements and eliminate sources of calcium contamination in order to obtain reliable measurements of calcium.

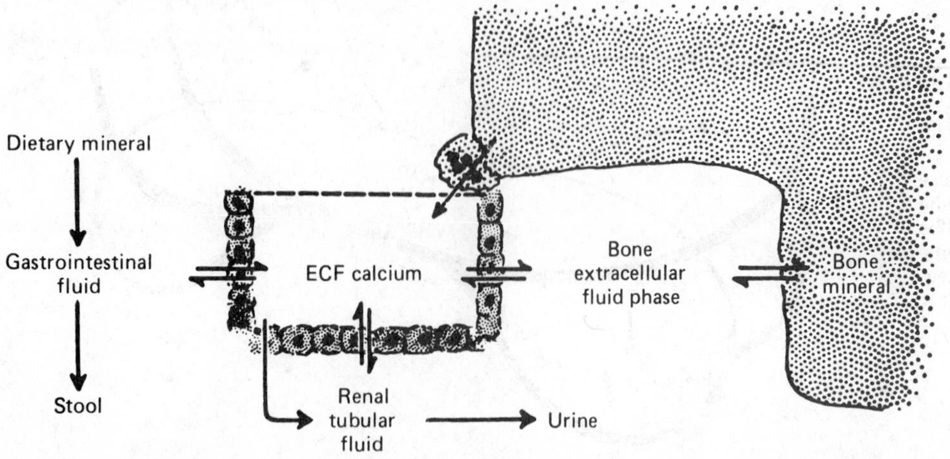

Figure 243–2. Cellular barrier separating the extracellular fluid compartment from the intestinal lumen, the renal tubular lumen, and the bone fluid compartment. PTH, calcitonin, and $1,25(OH)_2D$ act on these cells (directly or indirectly) to regulate the flow of calcium into and out of the extracellular fluid. (From Rasmussen H, et al.: Effect of ions upon bone cell function. Fed Proc 29:1191, 1970.)

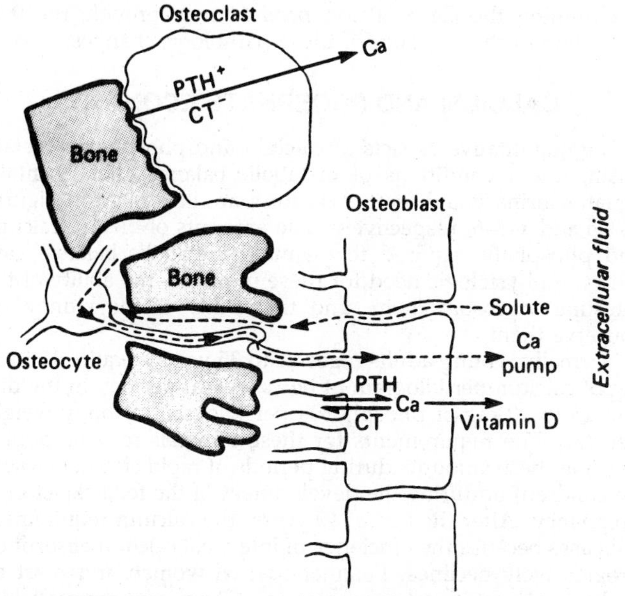

Figure 243–3. Relationships between calciotropic hormones, bone cells, and calcium transport. Bone crystal is represented by the shaded areas. The osteoclast, with an active "ruffled border," is shown resorbing bone—a process stimulated by PTH^+ and inhibited by calcitonin (CT^-). The osteoblasts are actively extruding calcium (Ca) from the bone fluid (between cells and crystals) under the influence of hormones. Processes connecting deep osteocytes are shown participating in calcium transport (dotted arrows). (From Arnaud CD, Kolb FO: The calciotropic hormones and metabolic bone disease. *In* Greenspan FS, Forsham PH (eds.): Basic and Clinical Endocrinology. Los Altos, Lange Medical Publications, 1983, p 189.)

The plasma calcium concentration varies little in spite of large changes in dietary calcium because of the adaptive alterations in the endocrine system regulating this mineral. Minor diurnal changes (decreases in the afternoon) have been recorded. In addition, plasma calcium decreases with age in men but not in women, probably due to a decrease in the serum albumin concentration in men. Total (but not ionized) serum calcium also decreases during pregnancy, and this change may also be due to the well-documented decrease in the serum albumin concentration in this condition.

Hypocalcemia produces a myriad of symptoms, and when severe can result in tetany and possibly convulsions (see Ch. 510). *Hypercalcemia* can produce functional changes in most organ systems, and these changes may lead to a confusing variety of symptoms and objective findings (see Ch. 246).

PHOSPHORUS. Only 15 per cent of plasma phosphate is bound to proteins in the blood (Fig. 243–4). The rest is ultrafilterable and consists mainly of free HPO_4^{2-} and $NaHPO_4^-$ (85 per cent), with free $H_2PO_4^-$ making up the remainder (15 per cent). By convention, plasma phosphate is expressed in terms of the amount of elemental phosphorus involved.

In comparison to calcium, phosphate has a wider range of normal plasma values (2.5 to 4.5 mg per deciliter) (Fig. 243–4). Moreover, increases or decreases in dietary phosphate are promptly reflected in changes in the same direction in serum phosphorus and urinary phosphorus excretion. There are also marked diurnal variations in serum phosphorus and urinary phosphorus excretion, even during a fast, which are caused in part by diurnal changes in plasma cortisol. Serum phosphorus concentrations in young children are almost double those in adults, and they increase slightly with age in women.

Serum phosphorus can be measured accurately and precisely in most laboratories. However, spuriously high values may be obtained if (1) serum extracts or dialysates are exposed to acid longer than is prescribed (resulting in hydrolysis of organic compounds containing phosphorus) or (2) hemolyzed serum is used (red blood cells contain phosphorus).

Hyperphosphatemia. Acute, severe hyperphosphatemia, as might be induced by intravenous phosphate infusion, can cause hypocalcemia sufficiently severe to result in tetany and even death. The less severe hyperphosphatemia induced by phosphate ingestion rarely causes symptoms; however, if the patient has an associated disorder in which there is a tendency toward hypocalcemia (e.g., mild hypoparathyroidism or chronic renal failure), frank hypocalcemia may develop.

Hypophosphatemia (see also Ch. 207). Acute respiratory alkalosis, the administration of a large quantity of carbohydrate, and insulin administration all cause a rapid decrease in serum phosphorus. Severe hypophosphatemia may occur during the treatment of diabetic ketoacidosis or forced nutrition of undernourished patients and can cause both skeletal myopathy and cardiomyopathy. These conditions may lead to rhabdomyolysis, as evidenced by increases in serum creatine phosphokinase (Ch. 76). The levels of 2,3-diphosphoglyceric acid and

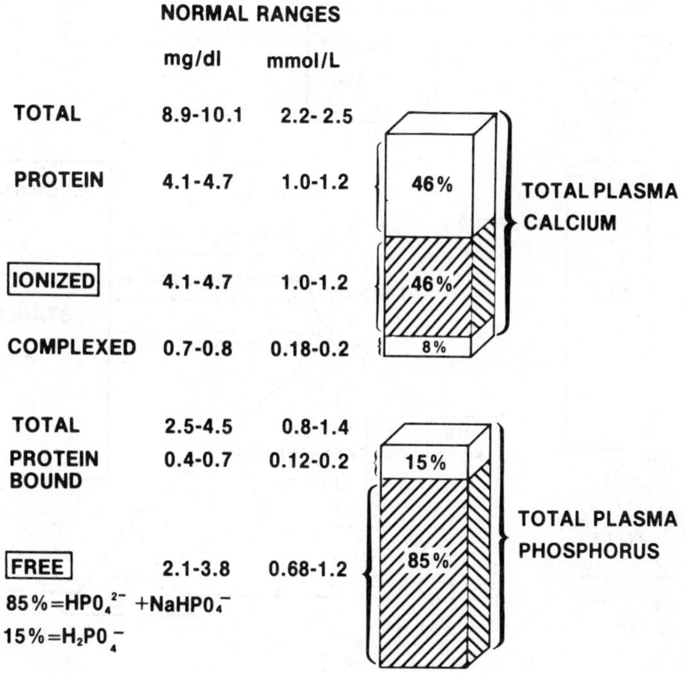

Figure 243–4. Distribution and normal ranges of calcium and phosphorus in the plasma.

adenosine triphosphate (ATP) in erythrocytes may also decrease; the decrease in 2,3-diphosphoglyceric acid in turn may decrease oxygen delivery to tissues, and the decrease in ATP may cause hemolytic anemia. Chronic, moderate hypophosphatemia frequently results in osteomalacia or rickets, as in the genetic disorder X-linked hypophosphatemia (Ch. 207). Generally, restoration of serum phosphate concentrations to normal corrects abnormal organ function in hypophosphatemic conditions, except in X-linked hypophosphatemic rickets, which requires regimens specially tailored for individual patients.

INTERRELATION OF PLASMA CALCIUM AND PHOSPHATE

The physiologic importance of the relationship between the circulating concentrations of ionized calcium and diffusible (free) phosphate is poorly understood, especially with regard to the formation and dissolution of amorphous calcium phosphate ($Ca_3(PO_4)_2$) and hydroxyapatite ($Ca_{10}(PO_4)_6(OH)_2$) in bone. However, available evidence indicates that the ion product of normal plasma concentrations of calcium and phosphate (the Ca × P ion product) is considerably higher than that necessary to form these two compounds. Thus, in comparison to bone, plasma is saturated with calcium and phosphate, and this can be considered an important driving force in bone mineralization. The positive effect of vitamin D on bone mineralization is probably indirect and resides in its ability to maintain the Ca × P ion product in the normal range by increasing calcium and phosphate absorption by the gut and their resorption by bone (Fig. 243–1).

The biologic significance of the Ca × P ion product has been questioned in recent years, but it is important to recognize that products below 20 mg per deciliter (0.7 mmol per liter) usually reflect a mineralization defect in bone, and products above 70 mg per deciliter (2.2 mmol per liter) a propensity toward soft tissue calcification. There are exceptions to these numerical guidelines that will become apparent in future chapters, but, short of directly measuring changes in bone formation in bone biopsy specimens or changes in calcium content in soft tissues, determining the Ca × P ion product may provide the best indication of the presence of these pathologic changes.

CALCIUM AND PHOSPHATE ECONOMY

The quantitative aspects of calcium and phosphorus metabolism, under conditions of metabolic balance (dietary intake equal to urinary and fecal excretion), are illustrated in Figures 243–5 and 243–6, respectively. The amounts of dietary calcium and phosphate required to maintain metabolic balance vary with the physiologic need for these minerals, the ability of the intestine to absorb them, and the ability of the kidneys to conserve them.

Normally, young adults (ages 21 to 35 years) require 12 to 15 mg of calcium per kilogram of body weight per day in the diet and 15 to 20 mg of phosphorus per kilogram of body weight per day. The requirements for these minerals may be double or triple these amounts during periods of rapid skeletal growth (in children) or during the development of the fetal skeleton in pregnancy. After the age of 40 years, the calcium requirement increases because the efficiency of intestinal calcium absorption progressively declines. Postmenopausal women and most elderly men must ingest approximately 50 per cent more calcium than young adults to avoid negative balance.

Dietary deprivation of calcium or phosphorus induces adaptive changes in the production and secretion of the calciotropic hormones that minimize the development of negative balance. In the case of calcium, only 30 to 50 per cent of ingested calcium is normally absorbed (Fig. 243–5). With decreased intake, serum calcium decreases slightly, and the sequence of events depicted in the left limbs of the feedback loops in Figure 243–1 is activated. In severe, chronic dietary deficiency of calcium in normal subjects, PTH stimulates an increase in plasma $1,25(OH)_2D$ levels, which can increase fractional calcium absorption up to 75 per cent; hence, the total body calcium is minimally perturbed. However, this adaptive response requires a chronic increase in plasma concentrations of PTH. The destructive effects of such hyperparathyroidism on bone (see Ch. 246) may be of little consequence to the young adult, in whom the net loss of total body calcium is minimal, but they may be devastating to individuals with high calcium requirements (e.g., young children and pregnant women) or to patients who cannot

CALCIUM POOLS AT BALANCE

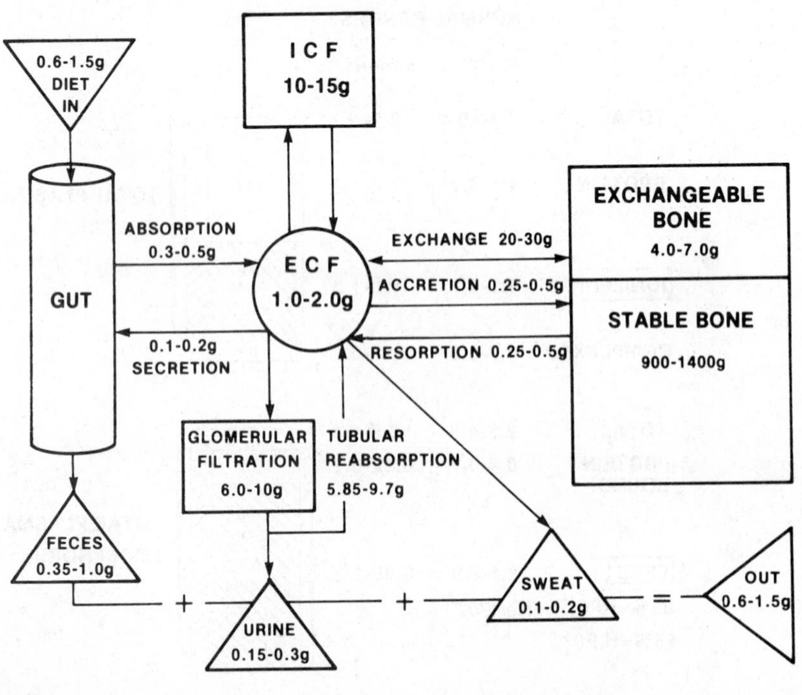

Figure 243–5. Normal distribution of calcium in the body. ICF denotes intracellular fluid, and ECF extracellular fluid.

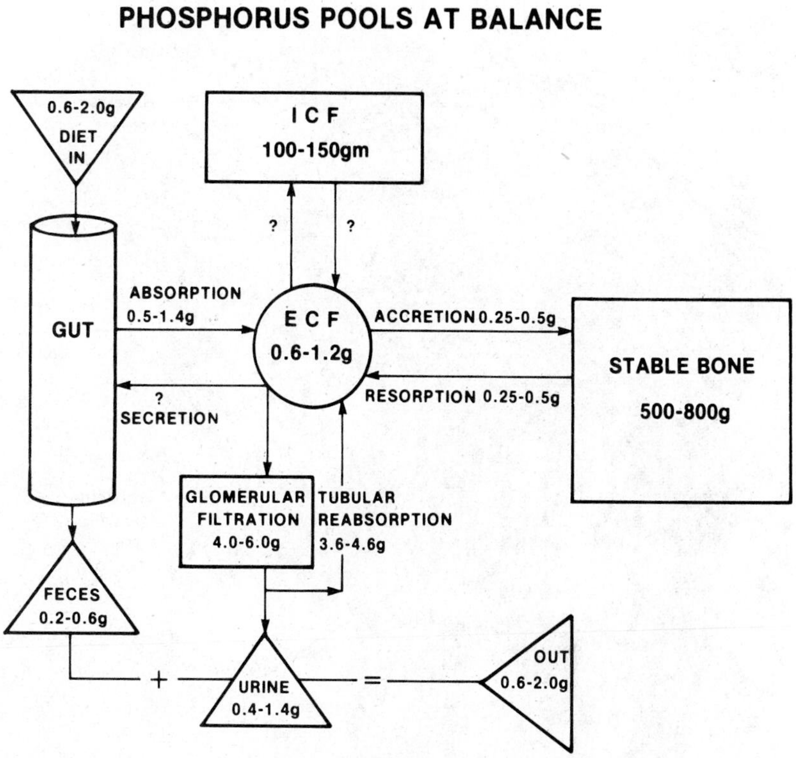

Figure 243–6. Normal distribution of phosphorus in the body. ICF denotes intracellular fluid, and ECF extracellular fluid.

adapt adequately to calcium deprivation by increasing intestinal absorption of calcium (e.g., the elderly).

Whereas the intestine plays the major role in the body's adaptation to a dietary deficiency of calcium, the kidney, with its ability to rapidly reduce urinary phosphate excretion, plays the major role in maintaining phosphate balance during a dietary deficiency of this mineral. Normally, 70 to 80 per cent of dietary phosphorus is absorbed, and therefore any increase in its fractional absorption during deprivation would have little influence in preventing the development of negative balance. However, 80 per cent or more of absorbed phosphorus is normally excreted in the urine; thus, decreasing excretion by 50 per cent, for example, would have an effect comparable to that of almost tripling dietary intake.

The mechanism(s) involved in the decrease in urinary excretion of phosphorus in response to dietary deprivation is not entirely understood. Hypophosphatemia in this condition is associated with increased production of $1,25(OH)_2D$, increased intestinal absorption of calcium, mild hypercalcemia, and decreased PTH secretion (Fig. 243–1, left middle limb). Any one or a combination of these changes could account for part or all of the decrease in urinary excretion of phosphorus. However, it is also possible that other, as yet undescribed, factors may also play a role.

BONE

Function of Bone

Bone has four major functions: (1) Bones provide rigid support to extremities and to the body cavities that contain vital organs. When bone is weak or defective, erect posture may be impossible and vital organ function may be compromised. (An example is the cardiopulmonary dysfunction that occurs in patients with severe kyphosis due to vertebral collapse.) (2) Bones are crucial to locomotion in that they provide efficient levers and sites of attachment for muscles. With bony deformities, these levers become defective, and severe abnormalities of gait develop. (3) Bone provides a hospitable environment for the dispersed hematopoietic system. (4) Bone provides a large reservoir of ions, such as calcium, phosphorus, magnesium, and sodium, that are crucial for life and can be mobilized when the external environment fails to provide them.

Structure of Bone

Two thirds of the weight of bone is mineral; the remainder is water and collagen. Minor organic components, such as proteoglycans, lipids, noncollagenous proteins, and acidic proteins that contain γ-carboxyglutamic acid, are probably important, but their functions are poorly understood.

There are two types of bone mineral. The major form consists of hydroxyapatite in crystals of varying maturity. The remainder is amorphous calcium phosphate, which lacks a coherent x-ray diffraction pattern, has a lower calcium-to-phosphate ratio than pure hydroxyapatite, occurs in regions of active bone formation, and is present in larger quantities in young bone.

As a living tissue, bone is unique in that it is not only rigid and resists forces that would ordinarily break brittle materials but is also light enough to be moved by coordinated muscle contractions. These characteristics are a function of the strategic location of two major types of bone (Fig. 243–7). Cortical bone, composed of densely packed, mineralized collagen laid down in layers, provides rigidity and is the major component of tubular bones. Trabecular (cancellous) bone is spongy in appearance, provides strength and elasticity, and constitutes the major portion of the axial skeleton. Defective or scanty cortical bone leads to fractures of the long bones, whereas defective or scanty trabecular bone leads to vertebral fractures. Fractures of long bones may also occur because normal reinforcement by trabecular bone is lacking.

Microscopically, there are two types of bone structure: woven and lamellar. Both may be found in either cortical or trabecular bone. Woven bone is a normal constituent of embryonic bone but in adult bone usually reflects the presence of disease. Lamellar bone is stronger than woven bone and is formed more slowly. It progressively replaces woven bone as the skeleton develops from birth. Whereas woven bone has nonparallel collagen fibers, many osteocytes per unit area of matrix, and mineral that is poorly incorporated into collagen fibrils, lamellar bone has a parallel arrangement of collagen fibers, few osteocytes per unit area of matrix, and mineral that is well incorporated into collagen fibrils. Cortical lamellar bone is present in

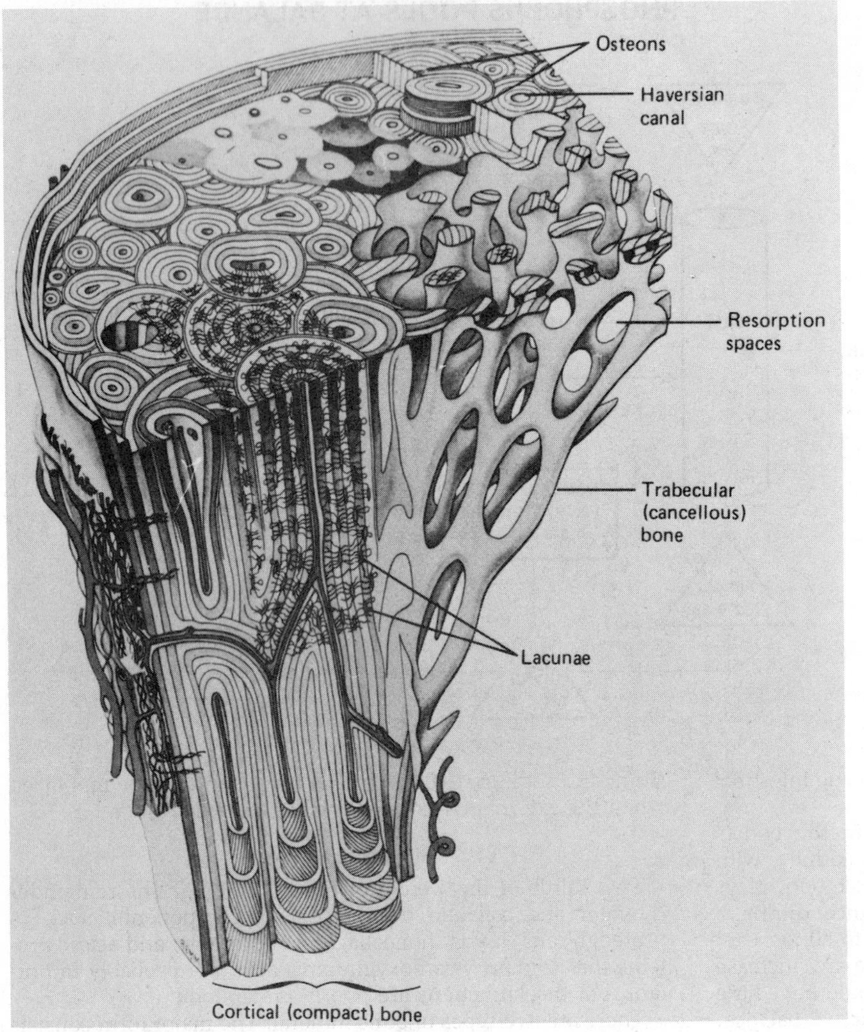

Figure 243–7. Diagram of some of the main features of the microstructure of mature bone seen in both transverse (top) and longitudinal sections. Areas of cortical (compact) and trabecular (cancellous) bone are included. The central area in the transverse section simulates a microradiograph, with the differences in density reflecting variations in mineralization. Note the general construction of the osteons, the distribution of the osteocyte lacunae, the haversian systems, resorption spaces, and the different views of the structural basis of bone lamellation. (Adapted from Warwick R, Williams PL [eds.]: Gray's Anatomy. 35th ed. Edinburgh, Churchill Livingstone, 1973, p 217.)

concentric layers surrounding the vascular channels that compose the haversian systems of cortical bone (osteons) (Fig. 243–7). In contrast, the lamellar bone of trabeculae is present in layers and is laid down in long sheaves and sheets (Fig. 243–8).

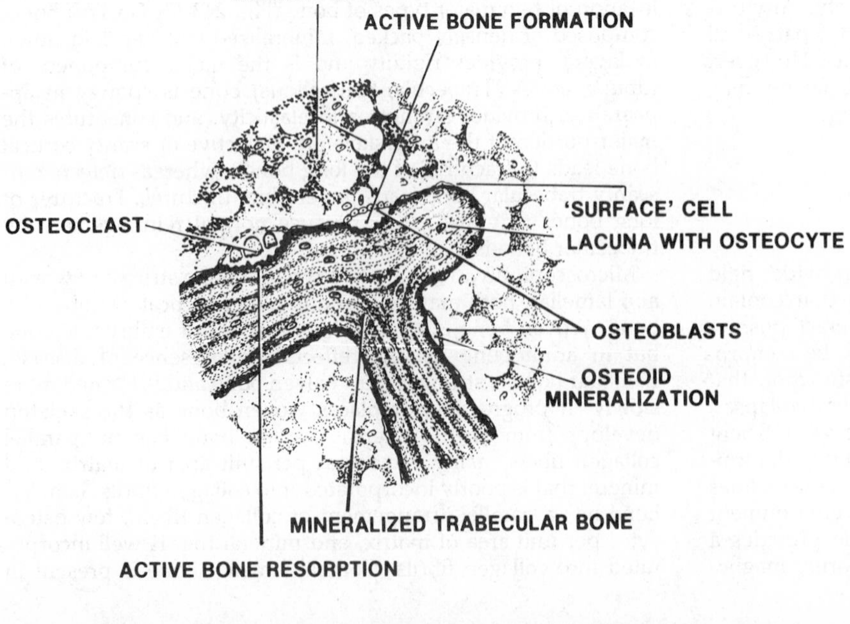

Figure 243–8. Schema of typical microscopic appearance of a section of undemineralized trabecular bone showing active bone resorption and formation.

Formation and Resorption of Bone

Bone is formed and resorbed continuously throughout life. These important processes depend upon three major types of bone cells, each with different functions.

OSTEOBLASTS. Osteoblasts are thought to be derived from a population of dividing cells, present on bone surfaces, that arise from mesenchymal cells in the connective tissue in bone. These specialized cells form new bone on bone surfaces previously resorbed by osteoclasts and have alkaline phosphatase activity. The exact role of alkaline phosphatase in osteoblast function remains uncertain. Osteoblasts are actively involved in the synthesis of the components of bone matrix (primarily collagen) and probably facilitate the movement of mineral ions between extracellular fluid and the bone surface (Fig. 243–3). The evidence supporting such ion transport by osteoblasts is sparse, but there is widespread agreement that osteoblast-mediated transport of calcium and phosphate is involved in the mineralization of collagen, which in turn is crucial for the formation of bone. In the process of bone formation, osteoblasts gradually become encased in the bone matrix they have produced.

OSTEOCYTES. Once trapped in the mineralized matrix, the functional and morphologic characteristics of osteoblasts change, and they are then called osteocytes. Protein synthesis decreases markedly, and the cells develop multiple processes that reach out through lacunae (Figs. 243–3, 243–7, and 243–8) in bone tissue to "communicate" with processes of other osteocytes within a unit of bone (osteon) and with the processes of surface osteoblasts (Fig. 243–3). The physiologic importance of osteocytes is controversial, but it is believed that they permit mineral movement in and out of regions of bone that are removed from surfaces.

OSTEOCLASTS. Osteoclasts are multinucleated giant cells that are responsible for the resorption of bone (Figs. 243–3 and 243–8). They are probably derived from circulating mononucleated macrophages, which differentiate into the mature osteoclasts by fusion in the bone environment. These cells contain all of the enzymatic components that, when secreted into their environs, solubilize matrix and release calcium and phosphate. Once released, mineral is transported through the osteoclasts into the extracellular fluid and ultimately into blood. Opinion has varied over the years concerning the relative importance to extracellular homeostasis of osteoclastic resorption of bone and the translocation of mineral from the surface of bone into the extracellular space by surface osteoblasts. It is likely that the major role of osteoclastic bone resorption is in bone remodeling (see below).

Dynamics of Bone

The term "modeling," as applied to bone, denotes processes involved in the formation of the macroscopic skeleton. Thus, modeling ceases at maturity (age 18 to 20). The term "remodeling" denotes those processes, occurring at bone surfaces before and after adult development, that are required to maintain the structural integrity of bone.

Abnormalities of remodeling are responsible for metabolic bone diseases. These abnormalities involve alterations in the balance between bone formation and resorption, which lead to diminished structural integrity of bone and ultimately compromise its functions. Normally, in spite of continuous bone remodeling, there is no net gain or loss of skeletal mass after longitudinal growth has ceased (Figs. 243–5 and 243–6). This has led to the view that bone resorption and formation are closely coupled and that this coupling is the result of the coordinated activity of "packets" of interacting osteoblasts and osteoclasts. These packets have been termed "basic multicellular units." The activity of such a unit is characterized by osteoclastic resorption of a defined quantity of bone (on the surface in trabecular bone and by actual excavation in cortical bone), followed by repair of the defect by osteoblasts. During the repair process, collagen (osteoid) is laid down and subsequently mineralized.

Using timed, sequential labeling of bone with orally administered tetracycline (which binds to recently mineralized collagen) and histomorphometric analysis of transiliac bone biopsies from normal adult humans, it has been possible to time the activities of a basic multicellular unit. Estimates indicate that osteoclastic resorption proceeds for about one month in a normal 30-year-old adult, and osteoblastic repair for about three months. The term "sigma" is used to denote the total duration of activity of a typical basic multicellular unit. The concept of sigma has added a new dimension to the understanding of the pathogenesis of metabolic bone disease. Thus, an imbalance between bone formation and resorption could be due not only to alterations in the relative numbers and activities of osteoblasts and osteoclasts but also to abnormalities in the relative duration of the activities of these two cell types.

General Evaluation of Patients with Metabolic Bone Disease

The early detection and treatment of metabolic bone disease is important because it may be difficult or impossible to restore skeletal mass after bone has been lost. This is particularly true of the bone loss that occurs in postmenopausal women and the elderly. It is insidious but causes symptoms only when skeletal mass has decreased to the point that fractures occur with minimal trauma. Establishing bone loss can be difficult because available techniques cannot always detect a decrease in skeletal mass in individual patients. It is necessary, therefore, to have a high index of suspicion for the presence of metabolic bone disease in patients at risk for its development, so that treatment can be instituted early. Since specific metabolic bone diseases are discussed in other chapters, this section will provide only a broad overview of the evaluation of patients with these disorders.

Any one or a combination of the risk factors listed in Table 243–2, especially if accompanied by symptoms such as back pain and muscular weakness or a history of bone fracture with minimal trauma, should raise the question of whether a patient has metabolic bone disease. The extent and type of investigation done should be determined by the specific metabolic bone disease suspected. More than one pathologic process may be involved in producing skeletal disease in an individual patient. Thus, once metabolic bone disease is discovered, the clinician should evaluate the patient for the presence of all of the diseases and risk factors that could alter skeletal metabolism and aggravate the bone disease.

In postmenopausal or elderly patients who have sustained a

TABLE 243–2. MAJOR RISK FACTORS FOR THE DEVELOPMENT OF METABOLIC BONE DISEASE

A. Physiologic Factors
   1. Non-black race
   2. Postmenopausal
   3. Aging
B. Dietary, Environmental, and Physical Factors
   1. Decreased calcium intake
   2. Decreased phosphate intake
   3. Decreased vitamin D intake
   4. Sunlight deprivation
   5. Immobilization
C. Drugs
   1. Corticosteroids
   2. Thyroid hormone
   3. Anticonvulsants
   4. Alcohol
   5. Antacids containing aluminum
   6. Heparin
   7. Cancer chemotherapy
D. Diseases
   1. Endocrinologic
      a. Hyperparathyroidism
      b. Hyperthyroidism
      c. Hyperadrenocorticism
      d. Sex hormone deficiency
   2. Gastrointestinal
      a. Intestinal malabsorption
      b. Malabsorption due to gastric or intestinal resection
      c. Chronic obstructive biliary disease
   3. Renal
      a. Functional impairment of any cause
      b. All tubular disorders resulting in calcium or phosphate loss
      c. ? Nephrosis

recent fracture with minimal trauma, the cause of the osseous demineralization underlying the fracture should be investigated. Although a generalized decrease in skeletal mass due to the osteoporosis associated with menopause or aging is the most likely cause, the first diagnostic consideration should be osseous malignancy, and such patients should be investigated for multiple myeloma (using immunoelectrophoresis of serum and urine protein, Ch. 163) and metastatic malignancy (using radionuclide bone scans). The clinician should also assess vitamin D nutritional status and parathyroid function (serum measurements of calcium, phosphorus, magnesium, alkaline phosphatase, 25OHD, and immunoreactive PTH). Hypercalcemia, if found, should be investigated as described in Chapter 246. Hypocalcemia, especially if it is accompanied by hypophosphatemia, suggests the presence of vitamin D deficiency and osteomalacia. Such a diagnosis is confirmed if serum concentrations of 25OHD are low and serum concentrations of immunoreactive PTH and alkaline phosphatase are increased. These findings should prompt an investigation of possible causes of vitamin D deficiency, such as intestinal malabsorption (e.g., a 72-hour stool fat measurement).

If the noted serum measurements are normal and no evidence for malignancy can be found, the next major objective is to establish the extent and location of bone demineralization so that the effects of treatment can be assessed over time. The only clinical measurement of value is patient height. Decreased height usually reflects the progression of spinal crush fractures and is probably the best indication of disease activity. Although lateral x-rays of the spine, done serially, show only gross decreases in bone mineral, they are the only means of directly assessing new vertebral crush fractures. They should be performed initially and repeated routinely every two years or if there is significant recurrence of back pain. Roentgenograms of the proximal femur yield information about the integrity of the femoral neck and trochanter, which are major sites of osteoporotic fractures that can result in permanent incapacitation and even death (10 to 20 per cent) in the elderly. Disappearance of the superior trabecular pattern that traverses the greater trochanter (arrow in Grade 3 sketch, Fig. 243–9) signals that osteoporosis is sufficiently severe to place the patient at increased risk for hip fracture. It is probably wise to obtain x-rays of these areas at the initial evaluation of postmenopausal or elderly patients for two reasons. First, if grade 2 or 3 trabecular patterns are present, patients should be cautioned to eliminate hazards that may cause falls in their home environments. Second, they provide a basis for comparison with similar x-rays obtained during long-term follow-up and treatment.

There are several clinically applicable techniques for measuring bone mass. The first involves careful x-rays of the hands and measurement of the endosteal and periosteal diameters of the second to fourth metacarpal bones with a precision caliper. The combined cortical thickness of bones is then determined by subtracting the internal from the external diameter. The precision of this measurement is about ± 2 per cent, and values obtained are reasonable reflections of appendicular skeletal mass. The second technique, single photon absorptiometry, measures the attenuation by bone (usually the radius) of a gamma ray beam generated by a ^{125}I or ^{247}Am source. The precision of this measurement is also about ± 2 per cent, and values obtained reflect predominantly appendicular skeletal mass.

Two recently developed techniques can directly measure the mineral content in almost any bone in the body, although both have been used mainly to assess the axial skeleton. The first technique, dual photon absorptiometry, measures the combined mineral content of several vertebrae in both cortical and trabecular bone, as well as that present in overlying structures (e.g., in calcified abdominal aorta). It uses equipment that can be modified from equipment available in most nuclear medicine units. The second technique, which uses computer-assisted tomography, is much more selective than the first, measuring the mineral content of only vertebral trabecular bone. Both techniques are amazingly precise. Although these techniques are currently available only at larger centers, recent advances should make them generally available soon.

The clinical usefulness of techniques that measure bone mineral content is unclear. Unfortunately, they cannot definitely exclude the presence of osteoporosis because there is a large overlap in measurements between patients with proved osteoporotic fractures and age-matched subjects without fractures. However, it may be possible to use single measurements to estimate the fracture risk in individual patients, once data concerning the incidence of fracture are available from long-term, prospective follow-up of such patients.

Presently, histomorphometric analysis of transiliac bone biopsies has achieved almost the status of a fine art. The procedure is most useful in establishing a diagnosis of osteomalacia (Ch. 245) and in determining if, in a given patient, diminished bone density is associated with significant changes in the duration of bone formation or resorption.

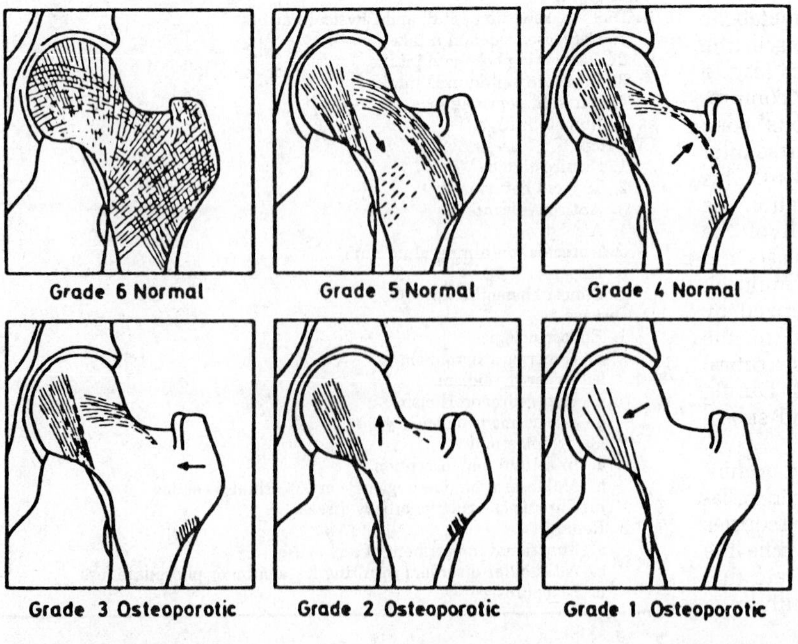

Figure 243–9. The effects of increasingly severe osteoporosis on the pattern of trabecular bone in the upper end of the femur. Arrows show progressive radiologic disappearance of trabecular groups. (Adapted from Singh M, et al.: Femoral trabecular-pattern index for evaluation of spinal osteoporosis. Ann Intern Med 77:64, 1972.)

Arnaud CD: Calcium homeostasis: Regulatory elements and their integration. Fed Proc 37:2557,1978. *Original description of "butterfly" diagram of calcium homeostasis and its usefulness in understanding pathogenic schemes and predicting effects of treatment.*

Aurbach GD, Marx S, Spiegel AM: Parathyroid hormone, calcitonin and the calciferols. *In* Williams RH (ed.): Textbook of Endocrinology. Philadelphia, W. B. Saunders Company, 1981, pp 922–1031. *Focuses on the calciotropic hormones and diseases associated with their abnormal production, secretion, and metabolism.*

Avioli L, Raisz L: Bone metabolism and disease. *In* Bondy PK, Rosenberg LE (eds.): Metabolic Control and Disease. Philadelphia, W. B. Saunders Company, 1980, pp 1709–1786. *Provides an excellent, in-depth description of bone metabolism and disease.*

DeGroot LJ (ed.): Endocrinology. Vol 2. New York, Grune & Stratton, 1979, pp 551–692. *Comprehensive review of the basic science of the mineral-regulating hormones, arranged in 13 chapters written by internationally renowned experts. Topics include parathyroid hormone, calcitonin, and vitamin D chemistry, biosynthesis, secretion, metabolism, and action.*

244. VITAMIN D

Daniel D. Bikle

Vitamin D is a steroid hormone with two molecular forms: vitamin D_3 (cholecalciferol) and vitamin D_2 (ergocalciferol). Vitamin D_3 is produced in the skin of animals, including humans. Vitamin D_2 is derived from the plant sterol ergosterol. It differs from vitamin D_3 in that the side chain has a double bond at C22–23 and a methyl group attached to C24. Vitamin D_2 is the usual form of vitamin D available for pharmaceutical use, although both vitamin D_2 and D_3 are used as food supplements. Despite subtle differences in physiology and biochemistry, vitamin D_2 and D_3 have equivalent potency and mechanisms of action in humans. Therefore, in the ensuing discussion, lack of a subscript after the D indicates that both forms of vitamin D are implied.

To achieve biologic potency, vitamin D must be metabolized further. Two of these metabolites, 25-hydroxyvitamin D (25OHD) and 1,25-dihydroxyvitamin D (1,25(OH)$_2$D), are produced by successive hydroxylations; the hepatic enzyme vitamin D 25-hydroxylase acts at the C25 position to form 25OHD, and the renal enzyme 25OHD 1-hydroxylase acts at the C1 position to form 1,25(OH)$_2$D. Both 25OHD (calcifediol) and 1,25(OH)$_2$D (calcitriol) are available in drug form to treat disorders of calcium homeostasis. A third metabolite, 24,25-dihydroxyvitamin D (24,25(OH)$_2$D), also shows promise as a therapeutic agent but as yet is available only for investigational purposes. 24,25(OH)$_2$D, like 1,25(OH)$_2$D, is produced from 25OHD principally in the kidney.

VITAMIN D ENDOCRINE SYSTEM

The vitamin D endocrine system can be divided into three levels (Fig. 244–1): bioavailability of vitamin D from skin and gut, metabolism of vitamin D to its active forms principally by the liver and kidney, and the action of these metabolites on target tissues.

BIOAVAILABILITY. Vitamin D_3 production in the skin is a multistep process. Irradiation of 7-dehydrocholesterol by ultraviolet (UV) light converts it to previtamin D_3, which then undergoes thermal isomerization to vitamin D_3. No clear regulation of vitamin D_3 production, other than the amount of UV irradiation that reaches the 7-dehydrocholesterol in the epidermis, has been observed.

Vitamin D is also available from the diet, as it is commonly used as a food supplement in dairy products. Vitamin D is absorbed principally in the jejunum by a process (chylomicron formation) that is facilitated by bile salts, fatty acids, and monoglycerides. Most of the vitamin D absorbed passes through the lymphatic system before entering the bloodstream. The hydroxylated metabolites of vitamin D (i.e., 25OHD and 1,25(OH)$_2$D) depend less on chylomicron formation for their absorption.

Vitamin D and its metabolites are transported in blood bound mainly to an alpha globulin (molecular weight, 58,000) called vitamin D binding protein (DBP). This protein has a higher affinity for 25OHD and 24,25(OH)$_2$D than for vitamin D and 1,25(OH)$_2$D. Since the amount of DBP in blood (5×10^{-6}M) far exceeds that of vitamin D and its metabolites (see accompanying table), 1 per cent or less of the total amount of these metabolites is actually free to diffuse into cells. It is unclear whether DBP serves principally as a circulating reservoir for the vitamin D metabolites in blood or whether it facilitates the transport of these metabolites into target tissues. Changes in DBP levels

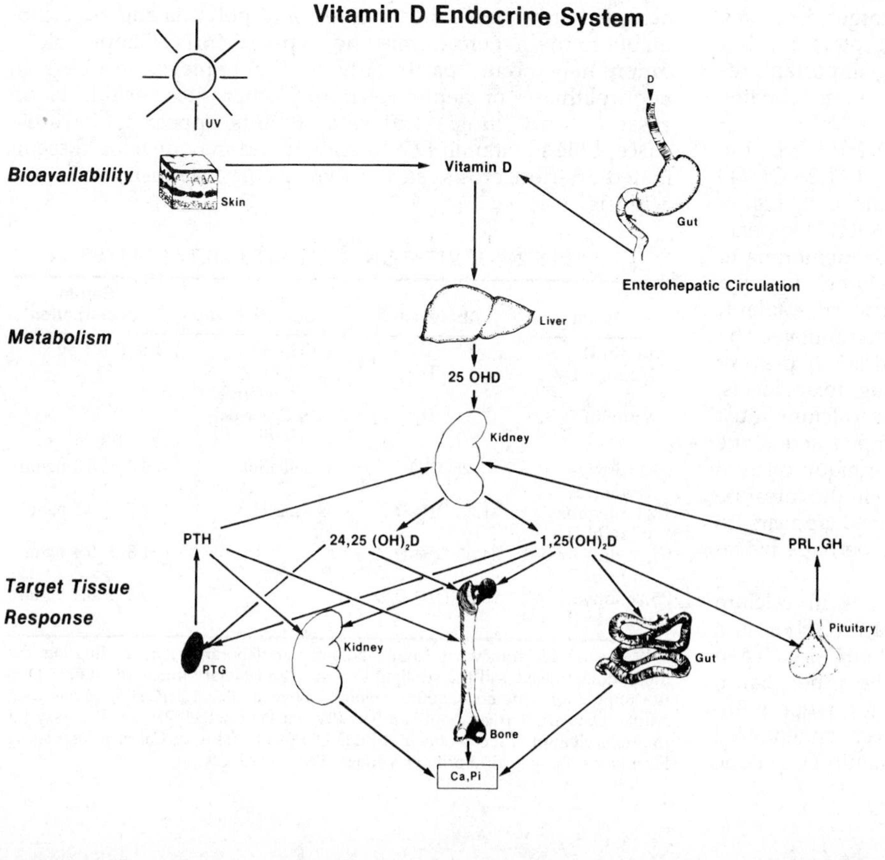

Figure 244–1. The vitamin D endocrine system. Vitamin D is made available to the body by photogenesis in the skin and absorption from the intestine. Vitamin D is then hydroxylated in the liver to 25OHD, then in the kidney to 1,25(OH)$_2$D and 24,25(OH)$_2$D. The active vitamin D metabolites act on different tissues to produce a variety of responses. The three target tissues principally responsible for calcium (Ca) and phosphate (Pi) homeostasis are kidney, bone, and intestine. Endocrine tissues such as the parathyroid gland (PTG) and anterior pituitary are also target tissues. Their hormones, parathyroid hormone (PTH), prolactin (PRL), and growth hormone (GH), help regulate vitamin D metabolism in the kidney; in addition, PTH has a direct effect on bone and kidney regulation of calcium and phosphate homeostasis. (Reproduced with permission from Bikle DD: The vitamin D endocrine system. *In* Stollerman GH, et al. (eds.): Advances in Internal Medicine, Volume 27. Copyright © 1982 by Year Book Medical Publishers, Inc., Chicago.)

(pregnancy and estrogen increase DBP, and liver disease and proteinuria decrease DBP) affect total concentrations of vitamin D metabolites without necessarily affecting the free concentrations. The relative importance of free and total concentrations of the vitamin D metabolites has not been established.

METABOLISM. ***Liver.*** The first step in the bioactivation of vitamin D occurs in the liver, where vitamin D 25-hydroxylase converts vitamin D to 25OHD. This cytochrome P450 mixed function oxidase is found in both microsomes and mitochondria. Since 25OHD production is governed principally by the supply of substrate (i.e., vitamin D), circulating 25OHD levels are a good indicator of vitamin D bioavailability. Hepatic production of 25OHD appears to be well preserved in all but the most severe cases of liver disease unless the vitamin D stores are depleted. However, compounds such as phenytoin and phenobarbital, which induce drug-metabolizing enzymes in the liver, alter the hepatic metabolism of vitamin D in such a manner as to lead to clinical bone disease.

Kidney. The 25OHD produced by the liver is further metabolized to $1,25(OH)_2D$ and $24,25(OH)_2D$, principally in the kidney, by 25OHD 1-hydroxylase and 24-hydroxylase, respectively. Little if any $1,25(OH)_2D$ is produced outside the kidney (except by the placenta) under normal circumstances, although other tissues, such as bone, cartilage, skin, and intestine, may produce $25(OH)_2D$ under some circumstances. Lymphomatous or sarcoid tissue may also contain 1-hydroxylase activity. Both 1-hydroxylase and 24-hydroxylase are cytochrome P450 mixed function oxidases located exclusively in the mitochondria of the proximal renal tubule. Their activities are closely regulated by a variety of ions and hormones, the most important of which are calcium, phosphate, $1,25(OH)_2D$ itself, and parathyroid hormone (PTH). Low serum calcium and phosphate levels and elevated PTH levels stimulate $1,25(OH)_2D$ production. High $1,25(OH)_2D$ levels inhibit $1,25(OH)_2D$ production but increase $24,25(OH)_2D$ production.

TARGET TISSUE RESPONSE. Although bone, gut, and kidney are the primary target tissues for vitamin D, many other tissues, including the pituitary, parathyroid glands, pancreas, brain, and skin, contain a specific receptor for $1,25(OH)_2D$ and respond to it by a change in function. Muscle contains no receptors for $1,25(OH)_2D$ but appears to be a target tissue for 25OHD. Whether all tissues that contain receptors for the vitamin D metabolites have a physiologically important response to normal circulating concentrations of the metabolites has not been established.

Intestine. Of the various tissues affected by $1,25(OH)_2D$, the intestine has been the most extensively studied. $1,25(OH)_2D$ regulates calcium transport across the intestine in a highly integrated sequence of events. First of all, $1,25(OH)_2D$ appears to increase the permeability of the brush border membrane to calcium, permitting calcium to enter from the lumen into the intestinal epithelial cell down a steep electrochemical gradient. The calcium that enters the cell must be accumulated by subcellular organelles, such as the mitochondria, to prevent cytosolic calcium concentrations from reaching toxic levels; $1,25(OH)_2D$ stimulates this accumulation. The calcium must then be transported through the cell and pumped across the basolateral membrane into the bloodstream. A unique calcium binding protein (CaBP), induced by $1,25(OH)_2D$ in the intestine as well as in a number of other target tissues, appears to modulate intracellular calcium concentrations, perhaps by facilitating the removal of calcium from the cell.

Bone. The role of the vitamin D metabolites in calcium movement in and out of bone is less clear. $1,25(OH)_2D$ is a potent stimulator of bone resorption and inhibitor of collagen production (bone formation) in vitro. On the other hand, $24,25(OH)_2D$ may stimulate bone and cartilage formation without stimulating bone resorption. These results have engendered a controversy as to whether all the effects of vitamin D on bone are mediated by $1,25(OH)_2D$ or whether other metabolites, $24,25(OH)_2D$ in particular, have a unique biologic role.

Although the vitamin D metabolites may play a role, independent of PTH, in regulating renal calcium and phosphate excretion, this role has not been well defined.

MEASUREMENT IN SERUM

Most assays for the vitamin D metabolites use naturally occurring binding proteins. Radioimmunoassays employing poly- or monoclonal antibodies and a bioassay evaluating bone resorption from cultured bone in vitro have also been developed. The principal difficulty in measuring vitamin D metabolites is that chromatographic separation of the metabolites from each other and from other interfering substances is required. Nevertheless, most laboratories generally agree on the measurements of 25OHD and $1,25(OH)_2D$ (Table 244–1). Measurement of vitamin D itself remains difficult because of its poor solubility in aqueous solutions and modest affinity to the binding proteins used in the assays.

HYPOVITAMINOSIS D

Vitamin D deficiency results from insufficient vitamin D in the diet, insufficient production of vitamin D in the skin, inadequate absorption of vitamin D from the diet, or abnormal conversion of vitamin D to its bioactive metabolites. Vitamin D deficiency appears clinically as rickets in children and osteomalacia in adults. This subject is discussed in detail in the chapter on Osteomalacia (Ch. 245).

HYPERVITAMINOSIS D

Hypervitaminosis D may occur in three general settings: (1) excessive consumption, usually for therapeutic purposes, of vitamin D, vitamin D analogues (such as dihydrotachysterol), or vitamin D metabolites; (2) the abnormal conversion of vitamin D to its biologically active metabolites, as occurs in sarcoidosis and possibly other granulomatous diseases; or (3) a change in the sensitivity of the target tissue to vitamin D, as can occur with the remission of a variety of gastrointestinal diseases associated with calcium malabsorption. The initial signs and symptoms of vitamin D intoxication include weakness, lethargy, headaches, nausea, and polyuria and are attributable to the hypercalcemia and hypercalciuria. Ectopic calcification may occur, particularly in the kidneys, resulting in nephrolithiasis or nephrocalcinosis; other sites include blood vessels, heart, lungs, and skin. Infants appear to be quite susceptible to vitamin D intoxication and may develop disseminated arteriosclerosis, supravalvular aortic stenosis, and renal acidosis.

TABLE 244–1. VITAMIN D AND ITS METABOLITES

Name	Abbreviation	Generic Name	Serum Concentration*
Vitamin D	D	Calciferol	1.6 ± 0.4 ng/ml
Vitamin D_3	D_3	a) Cholecalciferol	
Vitamin D_2	D_2	b) Ergocalciferol	
25 hydroxyvitamin D	25OHD	Calcifediol	26.5 ± 5.3 ng/ml
1,25 dihydroxyvitamin D	$1,25(OH)_2D$	Calcitriol	34.1 ± 9.8 pg/ml
24,25 dihydroxyvitamin D	$24,25(OH)_2D$		1.3 ± 0.4 ng/ml
25,26 dihydroxyvitamin D	$25,26(OH)_2D$		0.5 ± 0.1 ng/ml

*Values differ somewhat from laboratory to laboratory, depending on the methodology used and the sunlight exposure and dietary intake of vitamin D in the population studied. Children tend to have higher $1,25(OH)_2D$ levels than adults. Data are derived from Lambert PW, Fu IY, Kaetzel DM, et al.: Assay for multiple vitamin D metabolites. *In* Bikle DD (ed.): Assay of Calcium Regulating Hormones. New York, Springer-Verlag, 1983, pp 99–124.

The dose of vitamin D required to produce toxicity varies among patients, reflecting differences in absorption, storage, and subsequent metabolism of the vitamin as well as in target tissue response to the active metabolites. For example, an elderly patient with senile osteoporosis and a low turnover rate for bone also tends to have a reduced ability to absorb calcium in the intestine and a reduced ability to produce $1,25(OH)_2D$ in the kidney. Such a patient can usually ingest 50,000 to 100,000 IU of vitamin D per day without developing hypercalcemia or hypercalciuria. In contrast, a patient of similar age with a similar degree of osteoporosis but in whom the osteoporosis develops as a result of primary hyperparathyroidism would almost certainly be harmed by this amount of vitamin D. In the latter patient the ability of vitamin D to stimulate bone resorption and intestinal calcium absorption is enhanced in part because of the greater rates of $1,25(OH)_2D$ production and bone turnover observed in primary hyperparathyroidism. Patients with sarcoidosis appear to develop vitamin D intoxication because $1,25(OH)_2D$ production in the abnormal tissue apparently is not subject to the normal feedback mechanisms that regulate renal production of $1,25(OH)_2D$. Analogues of vitamin D, such as dihydrotachysterol, or the renal metabolite of vitamin D, $1,25(OH)_2D$, which bypass the normal rate-limiting step of vitamin D bioactivation (the renal 1α-hydroxylase), are more likely than vitamin D or 25OHD to result in hypercalcemia if used in excess.

Hypervitaminosis D is treated by stopping the administration of vitamin D or its analogues or metabolites. If the hypercalcemia is severe, the patient should be placed on a low calcium diet and given glucocorticoids (e.g., 60 mg of prednisone every day) and generous amounts of fluids. Acute hypercalcemia, when symptomatic, can be treated with saline and furosemide diuresis, as described under the general management of hypercalcemia. Hypercalcemia lasts only for a few days when caused by $1,25(OH)_2D$ excess, but it may persist for weeks or months when caused by vitamin D excess. The hypercalcemia of sarcoidosis tends to respond within days to glucocorticoid therapy.

Barbour GL, Coburn JW, Slatopolsky E, Norman AW, Horst RL: Hypercalcemia in an anephric patient with sarcoidosis: Evidence for extrarenal generation of 1,25-dihydroxyvitamin D. N Engl J Med 305:440, 1981. *An instructive case of an anephric patient with sarcoidosis in whom hypercalcemia and elevated $1,25(OH)_2D$ levels developed in parallel and then decreased in parallel following prednisone therapy.*

Bikle DD: The vitamin D endocrine system. Adv Intern Med 27:45, 1982. *A review of the physiology and pathophysiology of the vitamin D endocrine system.*

Bikle DD (ed.): Assay of Calcium Regulating Hormones. New York, Springer-Verlag, 1983.

Bikle DD, Morrissey RL, Zolock DT, Rasmussen H: The intestinal response to vitamin D. Rev Physiol Biochem Pharmacol 89:63, 1981. *A comprehensive discussion of intestinal calcium and phosphate transport and the role of $1,25(OH)_2D$ in this process.*

Fraser DR: Regulation of the metabolism of vitamin D. Physiol Rev 60:551, 1980. *A thorough, well-balanced review of vitamin D metabolism in the liver and kidney.*

Haddad JG Jr: Transport of vitamin D metabolites. Clin Orthop 142:249, 1979. *A good review of the vitamin D binding protein in blood.*

Lee DBN, Zawada ET, Kleeman CR: The pathophysiology and clinical aspects of hypercalcemic disorders. West J Med 129:278, 1978. *This article discusses all the major hypercalcemic disorders, including the diagnosis and treatment of hypervitaminosis D.*

Mason RS, Frankel T, Chan Y-L, Lissner D, Posen S: Vitamin D conversion by sarcoid lymph node homogenate. Ann Intern Med 100:59, 1984. *Provides direct evidence that sarcoid tissue in a lymph node may be capable of metabolizing 25OHD to $1,25(OH)_2D$ and $25,26(OH)_2D$.*

245. OSTEOMALACIA AND RICKETS

Daniel D. Bikle

DEFINITIONS

Osteomalacia and rickets are caused by the abnormal mineralization of bone. Osteomalacia refers to the defect that occurs in bone in which the epiphyseal plates have closed (i.e., in adults), whereas rickets refers to the defect that occurs in growing bone (i.e., in children). Abnormal mineralization in growing bone affects the transformation of cartilage into bone at the zone of provisional calcification. As a result, an enormous profusion of disorganized, nonmineralized, degenerating cartilage appears in this region, leading to widening of the epiphyseal plate (observed radiologically as a widened radiolucent zone) with flaring or cupping and irregularity of the epiphyseal-metaphyseal junctions. This latter problem gives rise to the clinically obvious beaded swellings along the costochondral junctions (rachitic rosary) and the swelling at the ends of the long bones. Growth is retarded by the failure to make new bone. Once bone growth has ceased (i.e., after closure of the epiphyseal plates), the clinical evidence for defective mineralization becomes more subtle, and special diagnostic procedures may be required for its detection.

PATHOGENESIS

The best known cause of abnormal bone mineralization is vitamin D deficiency. Vitamin D, through its biologically active metabolites, insures that the calcium and phosphate concentrations in the extracellular milieu are adequate for mineralization to occur. Vitamin D also may permit osteoblasts to produce a bone matrix that can be mineralized, and then allows them to mineralize that matrix in a normal fashion. Phosphate deficiency is another condition that can cause defective mineralization. It may act independently or in conjunction with other predisposing abnormalities since most hypophosphatemic disorders associated with osteomalacia or rickets also affect the vitamin D endocrine system. Dietary calcium deficiency has been implicated recently as a cause of rickets and may contribute to the osteomalacia and osteoporosis found in elderly patients. Osteomalacia or rickets may develop despite adequate levels of calcium, phosphate, and vitamin D if the bone matrix cannot undergo normal mineralization. For example, the deficiency in alkaline phosphatase in patients with hypophosphatasia can cause a defect in mineralization. This enzyme cleaves pyrophosphate, an inhibitor of bone mineralization, and a deficiency results in reduced removal of this inhibitor. Finally, drugs such as etidronate and heavy metals such as aluminum can interfere with mineralization and lead to osteomalacia or rickets.

Table 245–1 lists diseases associated with osteomalacia and rickets according to the presumed mechanism responsible for the mineralization defect. Diseases that appear under multiple headings affect bone mineralization via multiple mechanisms. It is important to understand the mechanism by which a particular disease interferes with bone mineralization in order to choose appropriate diagnostic procedures and therapy.

Disorders in the Vitamin D Endocrine System

The exact mechanism or mechanisms by which vitamin D maintains normal bone development is unknown, but disorders in the vitamin D endocrine system are the leading cause of rickets and osteomalacia through decreased bioavailability of vitamin D, abnormal metabolism of vitamin D, and abnormal response of target tissues to the biologically active vitamin D metabolites.

Decreased Bioavailability

REDUCED SUNLIGHT EXPOSURE. The human skin can generate adequate amounts of vitamin D if exposed to sufficient ultraviolet irradiation. However, in countries with limited sunlight or where the population dresses in a fashion that reduces sunlight exposure, circulating levels of vitamin D metabolites are often low. These low levels may help explain why the incidence of osteomalacia is higher in Great Britain, the Scandinavian countries, the Middle East, and India than in the United States.

NUTRITIONAL VITAMIN D DEFICIENCY. The fortification of dairy products with vitamin D has made nutritional vitamin D-

TABLE 245–1. THE OSTEOMALACIC SYNDROMES*

A. Disorders in the vitamin D endocrine system
  1. Decreased bioavailability
    - Insufficient sunlight exposure
    - Nutritional vitamin D deficiency
    - Nephrotic syndrome (urinary loss)
    - Malabsorption (fecal loss)
      - Billroth type II gastrectomy
      - Sprue
      - Regional enteritis
      - Jejunoileal bypass
      - Pancreatic insufficiency
      - Cholestatic disorders
      - Cholestyramine
  2. Abnormal metabolism
    - Liver disease
    - Chronic renal failure
    - Vitamin D dependent rickets type I
    - Tumoral hypophosphatemic osteomalacia
    - X-linked hypophosphatemia
    - Hypoparathyroidism (?)
    - Chronic acidosis (?)
    - Anticonvulsants
  3. Abnormal target tissue response
    - Vitamin D dependent rickets type II
    - Gastrointestinal disorders

B. Disorders of phosphate homeostasis
  1. Decreased intestinal absorption
    - Malnutrition
    - Malabsorption
    - Antacids containing aluminum hydroxide
  2. Increased renal loss
    - X-linked hypophosphatemic rickets
    - Tumoral hypophosphatemic osteomalacia
    - De Toni-Debré-Fanconi (phosphaturia, aminoaciduria, glycosuria, bicarbonaturia)
    - Cystinosis
    - Oculocerebralrenal syndrome (Lowe's syndrome)
    - Paraproteinemias
    - Wilson's disease
    - Glycogen storage diseases
    - Galactosemia
    - Tyrosinemia
    - Cadmium poisoning
    - Neurofibromatosis

C. Calcium deficiency
  1. Dietary insufficiency
  2. Excessive renal loss (?)
  3. Malabsorption of calcium (?)

D. Primary disorders of bone matrix
  1. Hypophosphatasia
  2. Fibrogenesis imperfecta ossium
  3. Axial osteomalacia

E. Inhibitors of mineralization
  1. Aluminum
    - Chronic renal failure
    - Total parenteral nutrition
  2. Etidronate
  3. Phenytoin (?)
  4. Fluoride (?)

*This table categorizes diseases that produce osteomalacia according to the presumed mechanism(s) by which bone mineralization is inhibited. A question mark indicates that the association of the disease to osteomalacia or the mechanism by which it produces osteomalacia is not established.

deficient rickets uncommon in the United States, although it is still prevalent in other parts of the world. Even in the United States vitamin D deficiency may occur in children of vegetarian mothers who avoid milk products (and presumably have reduced vitamin D stores) and in children who are not weaned to vitamin D-supplemented milk by age 2. The contribution of nutritional vitamin D deficiency to osteomalacia in elderly people is unknown. Osteomalacia has been observed in 25 to 30 per cent of bone biopsies from elderly patients who have suffered hip fractures in Scandinavia and Great Britain. Most likely, both reduced vitamin D intake and reduced sunlight exposure contribute to the development of osteomalacia in the elderly.

NEPHROTIC SYNDROME. Even when vitamin D intake is adequate, vitamin D and its metabolites can be lost in the urine. The vitamin D metabolites in serum are tightly bound to an alpha globulin called vitamin D binding protein (DBP), which has a molecular weight of 58,000. Patients with the nephrotic syndrome may lose substantial amounts of DBP into their urine and consequently have very low circulating levels of the vitamin D metabolites. The incidence of osteomalacia in patients with the nephrotic syndrome is unknown; osteomalacia has only recently been recognized as a complication of this renal disease.

MALABSORPTION. Fecal loss of vitamin D and its metabolites occurs in patients with malabsorption for several reasons. Ingested vitamin D is absorbed primarily in chylomicrons; disorders that involve the biliary tract, pancreas, or mid to distal portions of the small intestine reduce the efficiency of this process. Endogenous vitamin D and its metabolites undergo enterohepatic circulation; disorders of the distal small bowel disrupt this circulation. In cholestatic disorders, urinary excretion of vitamin D metabolites is increased and intestinal absorption is decreased. Drugs, such as cholestyramine, that are used in the treatment of cholestatic disorders may compound the problem by binding to the vitamin D metabolites and enhancing their fecal excretion. The resulting bone disease is often a combination of osteomalacia and osteoporosis. The extent of osteomalacia in patients with cholestatic and gastrointestinal disorders varies from country to country. It appears to be higher in Great Britain and Northern Europe than in the United States. Fully 25 to 50 per cent of British and European patients who have undergone Billroth type II gastrectomy or jejunoileal bypass or who have cholestatic liver disease or inflammatory bowel disease have osteomalacia when evaluated by bone biopsy. Pancreatic insufficiency appears to be associated with a lower incidence of osteomalacia than these other forms of gastrointestinal disease.

Abnormal Metabolism

LIVER DISEASE. The hepatic production of 25-hydroxyvitamin D (25OHD) is not tightly controlled. Neither cholestatic nor parenchymal liver disease has much effect on 25OHD production. The low levels of circulating 25OHD found in patients with liver disease can usually be attributed to reduced hepatic synthesis of DBP, poor nutrition, or malabsorption rather than to failure by the liver to metabolize vitamin D. Regardless of the mechanism, patients with chronic liver disease are predisposed to developing osteomalacia.

CHRONIC RENAL FAILURE (also see Ch. 78). Metabolism of 25OHD to 1,25-dihydroxyvitamin D ($1,25(OH)_2D$) and 24,25-dihydroxyvitamin D ($24,25(OH)_2D$) in the kidney is tightly regulated. Renal disease results in reduced circulating levels of both these metabolites. With the reduction in $1,25(OH)_2D$ levels, intestinal calcium absorption falls and bone resorption appears to become less sensitive to parathyroid hormone (PTH)—a result that leads to hypocalcemia. Phosphate excretion by the diseased kidney is decreased, resulting in hyperphosphatemia and aggravation of the hypocalcemia. As a consequence, hyperparathyroidism develops, possibly facilitated by the fact that the levels of the vitamin D metabolites are too low to inhibit parathyroid hormone (PTH) secretion. The net effect of deficient $1,25(OH)_2D$ and $24,25(OH)_2D$ and excessive PTH on bone is complex. Patients may have osteitis fibrosa (reflecting excessive PTH), osteomalacia (in part reflecting vitamin D deficiency), or a combination of the two. One particularly debilitating form of renal osteodystrophy is found in a small percentage of patients in whom only osteomalacia occurs. These patients have normal or only modestly elevated levels of PTH and alkaline phosphatase; hypercalcemia, especially after small doses of $1,25(OH)_2D$, and refractoriness to $1,25(OH)_2D$ therapy are often found. Such patients appear to have increased aluminum content in their bones, particularly in the zone where mineralization is occurring (calcification front).

VITAMIN D-DEPENDENT RICKETS TYPE I. Vitamin D-dependent rickets type I, or pseudo-vitamin D deficiency, is a rare, autosomal recessive disease in which there is a low level of $1,25(OH)_2D$ resulting from a selective deficiency in the renal production of $1,25(OH)_2D$. Although affected patients do not respond to doses of vitamin D that are adequate to treat vitamin D deficiency (i.e., 400 to 4000 IU per day), they do respond to moderate doses (4000 to 40,000 IU per day) of vitamin D or physiologic doses (0.5 to 1.0 μg per day) of $1,25(OH)_2D$.

TUMOR-INDUCED HYPOPHOSPHATEMIC OSTEOMALACIA. Certain unusual tumors (usually mesenchymal) produce osteomalacia associated with low serum levels of phosphorus and $1,25(OH)_2D$ and increased phosphaturia. The cause of this syndrome is unknown, but it is presumed that a humoral product of the tumor suppresses both $1,25(OH)_2D$ production and phosphate reabsorption in the kidney. Removal of the tumor reverses the abnormalities.

X-LINKED HYPOPHOSPHATEMIA. X-linked hypophosphatemia (vitamin D-resistant rickets, or VDRR) is characterized by renal phosphate wasting, hypophosphatemia, and a subtle decrease in $1,25(OH)_2D$ production. Although most cases are diagnosed in childhood and have an X-linked dominant form of inheritance, sporadic adult cases and autosomal transmission occur. Most patients have $1,25(OH)_2D$ levels that are inappropriately low for the degree of hypophosphatemia, which ordinarily increases $1,25(OH)_2D$ production. Treatment with oral phosphate and vitamin D suppresses $1,25(OH)_2D$ to even lower levels. The primary abnormality in these patients is thought to be a defect in renal tubular phosphate transport, resulting in renal phosphate wasting. This defect may secondarily alter vitamin D metabolism. X-linked hypophosphatemia is a fairly common form of metabolic bone disease that should be suspected in all individuals who have low levels of serum phosphate and evidence of bone disease.

HYPOPARATHYROIDISM. Parathyroid hormone is a major stimulator of $1,25(OH)_2D$ production. One would expect osteomalacia to develop when the hormone is absent, because of the reduction in $1,25(OH)_2D$ production. However, osteomalacia appears to be a rare complication of hypoparathyroidism.

CHRONIC METABOLIC ACIDOSIS. Acute metabolic acidosis results in reduced $1,25(OH)_2D$ production. Although chronic metabolic acidosis is associated wih osteomalacia, especially when accompanied by renal loss of phosphate and bicarbonate (as in proximal renal tubular acidosis), it is unclear whether chronic metabolic acidosis has a direct effect on the renal metabolism of vitamin D. Distal renal tubular acidosis and chronic respiratory acidosis are not associated with osteomalacia.

ANTICONVULSANTS. Phenytoin and phenobarbital induce drug-metabolizing enzymes in the liver that alter the hepatic metabolism of vitamin D. This effect may account for the lower circulating levels of 25OHD found in patients treated with anticonvulsants. Surprisingly, these drugs do not lead to a reduction in $1,25(OH)_2D$ levels. Institutionalized children and adults treated with anticonvulsants have a high incidence of rickets or osteomalacia. Outpatient studies of adults treated with anticonvulsants suggest a lower but still substantial incidence of osteomalacia by biochemical criteria, although large studies that incorporate bone biopsy evaluations have not been performed. Clinically debilitating osteomalacia is unusual in outpatient populations treated with anticonvulsants.

Abnormal Target Tissue Response

VITAMIN D-DEPENDENT RICKETS TYPE II. Vitamin D-dependent rickets type II is a rare condition that occurs in childhood and is not responsive to even huge doses of vitamin D. Unlike patients with vitamin D-dependent rickets type I (see Abnormal Metabolism, above), children with type II disease have high circulating levels of $1,25(OH)_2D$. Their problem appears to be a deficiency of normal intracellular receptors for $1,25(OH)_2D$.

GASTROINTESTINAL DISORDERS. Less exotic examples of abnormal target tissue response include a variety of gastrointestinal diseases, such as sprue, short bowel, and regional enteritis, in which calcium and phosphate malabsorption occur not only because of vitamin D deficiency but also because of decreased absorptive surface, steatorrhea, and rapid transit time.

Disorders of Phosphate Homeostasis (also see Ch. 207)

Chronic hypophosphatemia may lead to rickets or osteomalacia independently of other predisposing abnormalities. However, the principal diseases in which hypophosphatemia is associated with osteomalacia or rickets also include other abnormalities that can interfere with bone mineralization. Chronic phosphate depletion is caused by decreased intestinal absorption or increased renal clearance. Acute hypophosphatemia can result from movement of phosphate into cells (e.g., after infusion of insulin and glucose), but this condition is transient and does not result in bone disease (see Ch. 207).

Decreased Intestinal Absorption

MALNUTRITION. Seventy to 90 per cent of dietary phosphate is absorbed, primarily in the jejunum. This process is not tightly regulated, although vitamin D, at least in animal models, stimulates phosphate absorption. Meat and dairy products are the principal dietary sources of phosphate, and vegetarian diets that exclude them can result in phosphate deficiency. The incidence of osteomalacia in vegetarians who avoid all meat and dairy products is unknown. However, since these dietary practices also lead to decreased vitamin D intake, such individuals may be predisposed to bone disease.

MALABSORPTION. Intrinsic small bowel disease and surgical rearrangement of the small bowel interfere with phosphate absorption and, if coupled with diarrhea or steatorrhea, can result in phosphate depletion. The hypophosphatemia may contribute to the osteomalacia seen in such patients, especially when vitamin D levels are reduced (see Decreased Bioavailability of Vitamin D, above).

ALUMINUM HYDROXIDE ANTACIDS. A number of widely used antacids (for example, Mylanta, Maalox, Basaljel, and Amphojel) contain aluminum hydroxide, which binds phosphate and prevents its absorption. Patients who ingest large amounts of these antacids may become depleted in phosphate. This mechanism may contribute to the severity of the osteomalacia observed in patients with chronic renal failure, and in patients who have undergone partial gastrectomy but who continue to ingest large quantities of antacids (see Ch. 248).

Increased Renal Loss

Eighty-five to 90 per cent of the phosphate filtered by the glomerulus is reabsorbed, primarily in the proximal tubule. This process is regulated by PTH, which reduces renal tubular phosphate reabsorption, and probably also by vitamin D, which appears to increase renal tubular phosphate reabsorption. Many diseases that affect renal handling of phosphate are associated with osteomalacia. X-linked hypophosphatemia and tumoral hypophosphatemic osteomalacia have been described above. The De Toni-Debré-Fanconi syndromes are also associated with osteomalacia (Ch. 83.5). They include a heterogeneous group of unusual disorders that are characterized by phosphaturia, aminoaciduria, glycosuria, and bicarbonaturia, and frequently by mild acidosis and hypercalciuria. In general, the osteomalacia or rickets associated with these proximal tubular disorders responds only to large doses of vitamin D. The associated bone disease is most likely the result of a combination of systemic acidosis, hypophosphatemia, and abnormal vitamin D metabolism.

Calcium Deficiency

Calcium deficiency may contribute to the mineralization defect that complicates gastrointestinal disease and proximal tubular disorders, but it is less well established as a cause of osteomalacia than is vitamin D or phosphate deficiency. However, in one carefully performed study of children who ingested a low-calcium diet, there was clinical, biochemical, and histologic evidence of osteomalacia. The serum phosphate and 25OHD levels were normal but the serum calcium levels were low. Since intestinal absorption of calcium decreases with age, the daily requirement for calcium increases from approximately 800 mg in young adults to 1400 mg in the elderly. Calcium deficiency can result not only from inadequate dietary intake but also from excessive fecal and urinary losses.

Primary Disorders of the Bone Matrix

Intrinsic disorders of bone in which matrix is produced but not mineralized are rare. Three diseases appear to fit this category, but none are well understood.

Hypophosphatasia

Hypophosphatasia is a familial disease that is transmitted in an autosomal recessive pattern. Children with this disease usually present with a severe form of rickets, whereas adults may present merely with a predisposition to fractures. The biochemical hallmarks are low serum (and tissue) levels of alkaline phosphatase and increased urinary levels of phosphoethanolamine. The reason why these patients develop osteomalacia or rickets is unclear, but the following mechanism has been suggested. Skeletal alkaline phosphatase cleaves pyrophosphate, an inhibitor of bone mineralization; patients deficient in alkaline phosphatase may be unable to hydrolyze this inhibitor and so develop a mineralization defect.

Fibrogenesis Imperfecta Ossium

Fibrogenesis imperfecta ossium is a rare, painful disorder that affects middle-aged males in what appears to be a sporadic fashion. Serum alkaline phosphatase is increased. The bones have a dense, amorphous, mottled appearance radiologically and a disorganized arrangement of collagen with decreased birefringence, histologically. Presumably, the disorganized collagen matrix retards normal bone mineralization.

Axial Osteomalacia

Unlike fibrogenesis imperfecta ossium, axial osteomalacia is not painful, involves only the axial skeleton, shows no disorganization of collagen on bone biopsy, and is not associated with increased serum alkaline phosphatase. The reason for the mineralization disorder in this rare disease is uncertain.

Inhibitors of Mineralization

Several drugs are known to cause osteomalacia or rickets by inhibiting mineralization, but in no case is the mechanism fully understood.

Aluminum

Patients on hemodialysis are exposed to aluminum in the dialysate if tap water is used and through the antacid preparations used to control serum phosphate. Most develop bone disease. Bone biopsies show a correlation between the extent of osteomalacia in these patients and the amount of aluminum deposited in bone. It is likely that the aluminum blocks normal mineralization. Severely affected patients respond to a reduction in their exposure to or body stores of the metal.

Many patients who are treated by total parenteral nutrition for extended periods of time develop bone disease characterized by osteomalacia. In some cases the aluminum content of the casein hydrolysate used to provide amino acids is high. Replacement of casein hydrolysate with purified amino acids may correct or prevent this complication.

Etidronate

Etidronate, the only diphosphonate available for clinical use in the United States, produces osteomalacia at doses greater than 5 to 10 mg per kilogram of body weight. Therefore, the dose must be limited. Etidronate affects osteoblast function and inhibits calcium phosphate crystallization. It is unclear why this drug and not other diphosphonates results in osteomalacia.

Phenytoin

As discussed previously (see Anticonvulsants), phenytoin therapy may cause osteomalacia by inducing enzymes that alter the hepatic metabolism of vitamin D. In addition, phenytoin directly and adversely affects bone mineral metabolism in animals. This effect may also contribute to bone disease.

Fluoride

Fluoride stimulates bone formation, but if it is administered in high doses without adequate calcium supplementation, the bone is poorly mineralized. The mechanism or mechanisms by which fluoride alters osteoblast function and bone mineralization is unknown.

DIAGNOSIS

In children the presentation of rickets is generally obvious from a combination of clinical and radiologic evidence. The diagnostic challenge is to determine the etiology. The most common causes—malabsorption, liver disease, chronic renal failure, X-linked hypophosphatemic rickets, and vitamin D deficiency—are readily distinguished on the basis of history, clinical findings, and routine analyses of blood and urine. In adults the clinical, radiologic, and biochemical evidence for osteomalacia is often subtle. In situations in which osteomalacia should be suspected (malnutrition, liver disease, malabsorption, renal failure, and unexplained osteopenia), the clinician must decide whether to biopsy the bone for histomorphometric examination. When bone biopsy is performed, the information obtained is valuable both for planning and for following therapy. However, this definitive procedure is not yet widely available. When bone biopsy is not used, diagnosis is less certain, but the radiologic and biochemical tests discussed in the paragraphs that follow are still useful in selecting patients for a therapeutic trial of vitamin D, calcium, or phosphate, or all three.

Clinical Features

The clinical presentation of rickets depends on the age of the patient and, to some extent, the etiology of the syndrome (Fig. 245–1). The affected infant or young child may be apathetic, listless, weak, hypotonic, and growing poorly. A soft somewhat misshapen head with widened sutures and frontal bossing may be observed. Eruption of teeth may be delayed, and teeth that do appear may be pitted and poorly mineralized. The enlargement and cupping of the costochondral junctions produce the "rachitic rosary" on the thorax. The tug of the diaphragm against the softened lower ribs may produce an indentation at the point of insertion of the diaphragm—Harrison's groove. Muscle hypotonia can result in a pronounced pot belly and a waddling gait. The limbs may become bowed, and joints may swell because of flaring at the ends of the long bones (including phalanges and metacarpals). Pathologic fractures may occur in patients with florid rickets.

Adult patients with osteomalacia may complain of poorly localized bone pain that is characterized as a constant, dull ache. Muscle weakness, usually of the proximal muscles, may be present, and severely affected patients may be unable to walk. A fracture, often of the hip, may be the initial presentation. In general, however, it is difficult to diagnose osteomalacia on clinical grounds alone.

Radiologic Features

The radiologic features of rickets, like the clinical manifestations, can be quite striking, especially in the young child. In growing bone, the radiolucent epiphyses are wide and flared, with irregular epiphyseal-metaphyseal junctions. Long bones

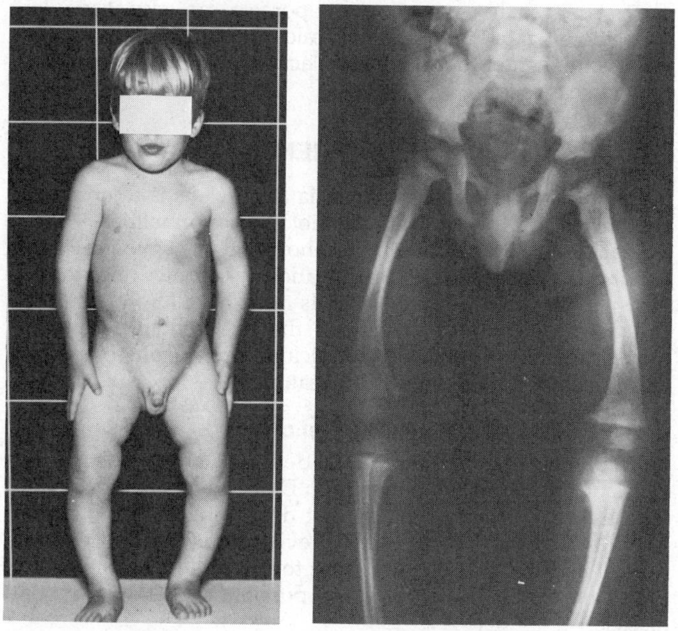

A B

Figure 245–1. The clinical (*A*) and radiologic (*B*) appearance of a young boy with X-linked hypophosphatemic rickets. The most striking abnormalities are the bowing of the legs, apparent in both femora and tibiae, with flaring of the ends of these bones at the knee. (Photographs courtesy of Dr. Sara B. Arnaud.)

may be bowed. The cortices of the long bones are often indistinct. Occasionally, evidence of secondary hyperparathyroidism—subperiosteal resorption in the phalanges and metacarpals and erosion of the distal ends of the clavicles—is observed. Pseudofractures (also known as Looser's zones or Milkman's fractures) are an uncommon but nearly pathognomonic feature of rickets and osteomalacia (Fig. 245–2). These radiolucent lines are most often found along the concave side of the femoral neck, the pubic rami, the ribs, the clavicles, and the lateral aspect of the scapulae. Pseudofractures may result from unhealed microfractures at points of stress or at the entry point of blood vessels into bone. They may progress to complete fractures that go unrecognized and thereby lead to substantial deformity and disability. Bone density is not a reliable indicator of osteomalacia, since bone density can be decreased in patients with vitamin D deficiency or increased in patients with chronic renal failure. In adults with normal renal function, radiologic evidence of a mineralization defect is often subtle and not readily distinguishable from osteoporosis.

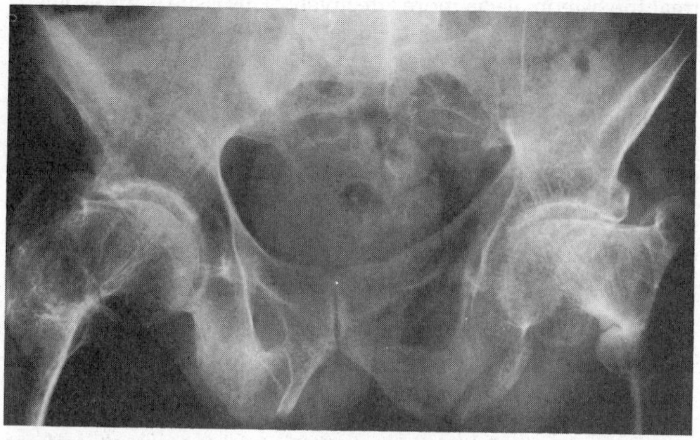

Figure 245–2. Roentgenogram of the pelvis of an elderly female with severe osteomalacia. This film reveals marked bowing (varus deformity) of both femoral necks, with pseudofractures of the medial aspect of the femoral necks and the superior aspect of the left pubic ramus. (Photograph courtesy of Dr. Harry K. Genant.)

Biochemical Features

The multiple etiologies of rickets and osteomalacia do not produce a single pattern of biochemical abnormalities. Furthermore, osteomalacia may be found on bone biopsy with no abnormality in serum or urinary levels of minerals and electrolytes. However, certain general patterns can be recognized.

Vitamin D Deficiency

Vitamin D deficiency, whether it is caused by nutritional deficiency, malabsorption, or abnormal metabolism, results in decreased intestinal absorption of calcium and phosphate. In conjunction with the resulting secondary hyperparathyroidism, vitamin D deficiency leads to increase in bone resorption, urinary phosphate excretion, and urinary calcium reabsorption. The net result tends to be a low normal serum calcium level, low serum phosphate level (unless chronic renal failure prevents phosphaturia), elevated serum alkaline phosphatase level, increased PTH level, decreased urinary calcium level, and increased urinary phosphate level. Finding a low 25OHD level in combination with these other biochemical alterations confirms the diagnosis of vitamin D deficiency. Caution is necessary in interpreting such biochemical data, however. Other factors, such as age and diet, must also be considered. For example, serum phosphate values are normally lower in adults than in children, and alkaline phosphatase levels are lower and are less reliable indicators of vitamin D deficiency in adults than in children. Dietary history is important, since urinary phosphate excretion and, to a lesser degree, urinary calcium excretion reflect dietary phosphate and calcium content. Since phosphate excretion depends on the filtered load (the product of the glomerular filtration rate [GFR] and serum phosphate), urinary phosphate levels may be normal if either the GFR or serum phosphate levels are reduced, despite the presence of hyperparathyroidism. Expressions of renal phosphate clearance that account for these variables (e.g., renal threshold for phosphate, or TmP/GFR) are a better indicator of renal phosphate handling than is total phosphate excretion.

Chronic Renal Failure (Ch. 78)

Most patients with chronic renal failure and renal osteodystrophy have osteitis fibrosa alone or in combination with osteomalacia. If not well controlled, these patients will have a low serum level of calcium and high serum levels of phosphate, alkaline phosphatase, and PTH. A few patients develop severe secondary hyperparathyroidism in which the PTH level increases dramatically, with restoration of the serum calcium to normal or even elevated levels (sometimes called tertiary hyperparathyroidism). Another small subset of patients with renal osteodystrophy present with normal or low serum levels of PTH and alkaline phosphatase. Their serum calcium levels are often elevated after treatment with small doses of 1,25$(OH)_2$D. These patients have pure osteomalacia on bone biopsy and are thought to suffer from aluminum intoxication (see Ch. 248). Regardless of the type of bone disease, most patients with chronic renal disease have low 1,25$(OH)_2$D and 24,25$(OH)_2$D levels and, unless treated with vitamin D, tend to have low 25OHD levels as well.

Vitamin D–Dependent Rickets Types I and II

In these rare diseases, serum and urinary levels of calcium and phosphate resemble those in vitamin D–deficient rickets. However, serum 25OHD levels are normal or high. In type I patients, serum 1,25$(OH)_2$D levels are low in comparison to serum 25OHD levels, whereas in type II patients, serum 1,25$(OH)_2$D levels may be extraordinarily high.

Anticonvulsants

Patients on long-term anticonvulsant therapy tend to have the biochemical findings of mild vitamin D deficiency, including a low serum 25OHD level. Since these patients have normal serum $1,25(OH)_2D$ levels, some investigators have suggested that anticonvulsants may directly inhibit calcium transport in intestine and bone.

Hypophosphatemic Disorders

A low serum phosphate level and high renal clearance of phosphate are characteristic of diseases such as X-linked hypophosphatemic rickets, tumoral hypophosphatemic osteomalacia, and the variety of proximal renal tubular disorders that are associated with osteomalacia. Serum calcium is generally normal. In both X-linked hypophosphatemic rickets and tumoral hypophosphatemic osteomalacia, serum $1,25(OH)_2D$ is inappropriately low for the serum phosphate, although it is often in the low normal range. The proximal tubular diseases that present with the full De Toni-Debré-Fanconi syndrome also result in increased urinary levels of bicarbonate, amino acids, and glucose, as well as metabolic acidosis. Levels of the vitamin D metabolites have not been reported in large series of such patients.

Calcium Deficiency

In one study children suspected of having rickets on the basis of calcium-deficient diets had normal serum levels of 25OHD and phosphate, elevated serum levels of alkaline phosphatase, and low serum and urinary levels of calcium. Additional studies of calcium deficiency are necessary to confirm these observations.

Mineralization Disorders

Disorders attributed to an intrinsic defect in mineralization of the bone matrix do not produce the biochemical abnormalities observed in vitamin D deficiency. For example, patients who have developed osteomalacia as a result of long-term hemodialysis or total parenteral nutrition frequently are found to have hypercalcemia and hyperphosphatemia with low or normal levels of PTH. It is possible that the skeleton in these patients is unable to adequately buffer calcium and phosphate from the intestine, total parenteral nutrition solutions, or dialysate, resulting in marked oscillations of serum calcium and phosphate.

Histologic Features

Because of the difficulty in diagnosing osteomalacia in adults by clinical and radiologic means, transcortical bone biopsy is becoming increasingly popular. The rib and iliac crest are the sites generally biopsied. To assess osteoid content and appositional rate, the bone biopsy specimen is processed without decalcification. This requires special equipment.

In osteomalacia, bone is mineralized poorly and slowly, resulting in wide osteoid seams ($\sim 12\mu$) and a large fraction of bone covered by unmineralized osteoid. States of high bone turnover (increased bone formation and resorption), such as hyperparathyroidism, can also cause wide osteoid seams and increased osteoid surface, producing a superficial resemblance to osteomalacia. Therefore, the rate of bone turnover should be determined by labeling bone with tetracycline which provides a fluorescent marker of the calcification front. When two doses of tetracycline are given at different times, the distance between the two labels divided by the time interval between the two doses equals the appositional rate of bone formation. Normal appositional rate is approximately 0.74 μ per day. Mineralization lag time, the time required for newly formed osteoid to be mineralized, can be calculated by dividing osteoid seam width by the appositional rate. It is normally about 20 to 25 days. Because tetracycline labels the calcification front, the fraction of the osteoid surface undergoing active mineralization (normally about 60 per cent) can also be determined. Depressed appositional rate, increased mineralization lag time, and reduced calcification front clearly distinguish osteomalacia from high turnover states such as hyperparathyroidism. Low turnover states such as senile osteoporosis can also have low appositional rates and reduced calcification fronts, but these are distinguished from osteomalacia by normal or reduced osteoid seam width.

TREATMENT

The goal in treating osteomalacia and rickets is to normalize the clinical, biochemical, and radiologic abnormalities without producing hypercalcemia, hyperphosphatemia, hypercalciuria, nephrolithiasis, or ectopic calcification (especially nephrocalcinosis). To realize this goal, patients must be followed carefully, and as the bone lesions heal or the underlying disease improves, the dose of vitamin D, calcium, or phosphate needs to be adjusted to avoid such complications.

Vitamin D Deficiency

Simple nutritional vitamin D deficiency responds to oral doses of 2000 to 4000 IU of vitamin D per day, taken for several months, followed by replacement doses of 200 to 400 IU per day. Radiologic and biochemical evidence of healing requires several months. If the patient fails to respond to treatment, the physician should consider other possible causes of the bone disease.

Intestinal Malabsorption and Liver Disease

Patients with intestinal malabsorption or liver disease may respond to large doses of oral vitamin D (25,000 to 100,000 IU per day), or they may require parenteral administration of the vitamin. Since patients with steatorrhea absorb 25OHD (calcifediol) better than they do vitamin D, 50 to 100 μg of calcifediol per day or every other day should be tried if large doses of vitamin D fail to raise circulating levels of 25OHD into the high normal range. Vitamin D therapy should be supplemented with 1 to 3 grams of calcium per day. Only the osteomalacic component of the bone disease associated with these conditions responds to vitamin D; the osteoporotic component does not. Consequently, patients must be carefully selected for vitamin D treatment and carefully followed. Histomorphometric evaluation of bone biopsies is particular useful in this regard.

Chronic Renal Failure

Most patients with renal osteodystrophy respond to $1,25(OH)_2D$ (calcitriol, 0.5 to 1.0 μg per day) or dihydrotachysterol (DHT, 0.25 to 0.5 mg per day), calcium supplementation (1 to 3 grams per day), and phosphate restriction (dietary restriction supplemented with phosphate binders such as aluminum hydroxide). The goal is to achieve and maintain normal serum levels of calcium, phosphate, PTH, and alkaline phosphatase. This regimen treats osteitis fibrosa more effectively than the osteomalacia. Some authorities recommend the use of calcifediol rather than calcitriol or DHT since calcifediol may treat the osteomalacia more effectively. This issue is unresolved. Patients with only osteomalacia usually fail to respond to $1,25(OH)_2D$ alone, but they have responded to $1,25(OH)_2D$ in combination with $24,25(OH)_2D$, a metabolite not yet available for clinical use. The osteomalacia in renal osteodystrophy also appears to respond to the removal of aluminum with deferoxamine, a drug approved for the treatment of iron overload. Neither $24,25(OH)_2D$ nor deferoxamine has been approved by the United States Food and Drug Administration for the treatment of renal osteodystrophy, and both must currently be considered investigational drugs for this purpose.

Hypophosphatemia

The bone disease in patients with X-linked hypophosphatemia responds to the combination of phosphate (1 to 3 grams per day) and either large doses (25,000 to 100,000 IU) of vitamin D or more physiologic doses (0.25 to 1.0 μg per day) of $1,25(OH)_2D$. Neither phosphate nor vitamin D alone is as effective. Unfortunately, oral phosphate preparations also act as laxatives, and tolerance of full doses is therefore sometimes difficult to achieve. Less information is available regarding the efficacy of vitamin D and phosphate in other hypophosphatemic syndromes. When hypophosphatemia is associated with metabolic acidosis, as it often is in the De Toni-Debré-Fanconi syndrome, correction of the acidosis with bicarbonate may improve the associated metabolic bone disease.

Calcium Deficiency

Calcium supplements (1 to 3 grams per day) are useful in the treatment of calcium deficiency resulting from deficient diets, intestinal malabsorption, and aging. The amount of calcium should be adjusted to achieve adequate intestinal absorption, as monitored by urinary calcium excretion and serum levels of calcium and PTH.

Inhibitors of Mineralization

Restricting the use of aluminum-containing antacids in patients with chronic renal failure or peptic ulcer, removing aluminum and other impurities from the water used in hemodialysis, and substituting purified amino acids for the aluminum-containing casein hydrolysate in total parenteral nutrition solutions should reduce the incidence of aluminum intoxication. Chelation and removal of aluminum from the body with deferoxamine shows promise as a remedy of the future.

Patients on long-term anticonvulsant therapy may benefit from the prophylactic use of 2000 to 4000 IU of vitamin D per day and 500 and 1000 mg of calcium per day, especially if their serum 25OHD levels are low.

Etidronate, which is used in the treatment of Paget's disease, should be limited to a dose of 5 mg per kilogram and restricted to therapeutic periods of six months with at least six months between treatment periods.

Fluoride, which is currently under investigation for the treatment of osteoporosis, must be accompanied by 1 to 2 grams of calcium per day.

Bikle DD: Calcium absorption and vitamin D metabolism. Clin Gastroenterol 12:379, 1983. *An up-to-date review of the effect of vitamin D on the intestine and the gastrointestinal diseases that lead to osteomalacia.*

Contrib Nephrol 18, 1980. *This entire issue is devoted to renal oseodystrophy and the role of the vitamin D metabolites in its treatment.*

Frame B, Parfitt AM: Osteomalacia: Current concepts. Ann Intern Med 89:966, 1978. *An excellent review of osteomalacia, with a complete list of the diseases that produce it and a full description of the mineralization defect.*

Fukumoto Y, Tarui S, Tsukiyama K, et al: Tumor-induced vitamin D-resistant hypophosphatemic osteomalacia associated with proximal renal tubular dysfunction and 1,25-dihydroxyvitamin D deficiency. J Clin Endocrinol Metab 49:873, 1979. *A good description of a case of tumoral hypophosphatemic osteomalacia.*

Glorieux FH, Marie PJ, Pettifor JM, Delvin EE: Bone response to phosphate salts, ergocalciferol, and calcitriol in hypophosphatemic vitamin D-resistant rickets. N Engl J Med 303:1023, 1980. *This article describes modern therapy for this disorder.*

Goldstein DA, Haldimann B, Sherman D, Norman AW, Massry SG: Vitamin D metabolites and calcium metabolism in patients with nephrotic syndrome and normal renal function. J Clin Endocrinol Metab 52:116, 1981. *This article describes the pathogenesis of osteomalacia in the nephrotic syndrome.*

Hahn TJ, Halstead LR: Anticonvulsant drug-induced osteomalacia: Alterations in mineral metabolism and response to vitamin D_3 administration. Calcif Tissue Int 27:13, 1979. *This review describes the mechanisms by which anticonvulsants produce osteomalacia.*

Klein GL, Targoff CM, Ament ME, et al.: Bone disease associated with total parenteral nutrition. Lancet 2:1041, 1980. *This article describes the development of osteomalacia in patients on long-term total parenteral nutrition.*

Long RG, Sherlock S: Vitamin D in chronic liver disease. Prog Liver Dis 6:539, 1979. *This review of hepatic osteodystrophy emphasizes the abnormalities of the vitamin D endocrine system observed in and the recommended treatment for patients with liver disease.*

Mankin HJ: Rickets, osteomalacia, and renal osteodystrophy. Parts I and II. J Bone Joint Surg Am 56A:101, 352, 1974. A thorough review with an excellent accounting of the history of the subject, an excellent description of the clinical presentation of rickets, and a complete list of the etiologies of bone mineralization disorders.

Marie PJ, Pettifor JM, Ross FP, Glorieux FH: Histological osteomalacia due to dietary calcium deficiency in children. N Engl J Med 307:584, 1982. *This study indicates that calcium deficiency alone may be sufficient to cause osteomalacia.*

Parfitt AM, Gallagher JC, Heaney RP, Johnston CC, Neer R, Whedon GD: Vitamin D and bone health in the elderly. Am J Clin Nutr 36:1014, 1982. *A review of the importance of adequate vitamin D intake in adults, discussing among other issues the high incidence of osteomalacia found in patients with hip fractures.*

Rasmussen H, Bordier P: Vitamin D and bone. Metab Bone Dis Relat Res 1:7, 1978. *A mechanistic discussion of the effect of vitamin D and its metabolites on bone, emphasizing the concept that different vitamin D metabolites have different biologic effects.*

Scriver CR, Reade TM, DeLuca HF, Hamstra AJ: Serum 1,25-dihydroxyvitamin D levels in normal subjects and in patients with hereditary rickets or bone disease. N Engl J Med 299:976, 1978. *This report contains a good description of vitamin D-resistant rickets (X-linked) and vitamin D-dependent rickets type I.*

246. THE PARATHYROID GLANDS, HYPERCALCEMIA, AND HYPOCALCEMIA

Claude D. Arnaud

PARATHYROID HORMONE

STRUCTURE AND SYNTHESIS. *Parathyroid hormone (PTH),* an 84 amino acid, linear polypeptide with a molecular weight of 9500, is the principal regulator of the concentration of ionic calcium in extracellular fluid. The biosynthesis and intracellular processing of the hormone are complex (Fig. 246–1). The original hormonal gene product of the parathyroid cell is a 115 amino acid precursor termed pre-proparathyroid hormone. Like other exportable proteins, it is synthesized on ribosomes bound to the membrane of the endoplasmic reticulum and discharged vectorially into its cisternal space. When the growing polypeptide chain attains a length of 20 to 30 amino acids, the first two amino-terminal methionine residues of the "pre" sequence are removed by a putative methionyl amino peptidase. With further growth of the chain, the hydrophobic 23 amino acid "pre" sequence acts to bind the polyribosome-precursor complex to the reticular membrane. This process provides the precursor access to the cisternal space of the endoplasmic reticulum and, presumably, to the enzyme ("clipase") that removes the pre-sequence, leaving the 90 amino acid proparathyroid hormone structure. Proparathyroid hormone is converted to parathyroid hormone in the Golgi apparatus by proteolytic removal ("tryptic clipase") of the remaining 6 amino acids at the amino terminus. Here, the 84 amino acid polypeptide is readied for secretion either in a secretory granule or in its free form. There is no evidence that either of the parathyroid hormone precursor molecules or the "pre" or "pro" peptide sequence normally finds its way into the circulation.

In contrast to the rapid regulation of secretion, hormone biosynthesis is only slowly influenced by changes in concentrations of extracellular ionic calcium. Intracellular stores of parathyroid hormone may be regulated by a degradative pathway that is stimulated by high and inhibited by low extracellular calcium. This degradative pathway is of considerable current interest. Not only may it provide an important mechanism for regulating parathyroid hormone economy, as noted later, but the fragments of the hormone produced during its intracellular degradation may also provide a major source for the multiple immunoreactive forms of the hormone known to circulate in the blood (see below).

The amino acid sequences of bovine, porcine, and human parathyroid hormone have been determined (Fig. 246–2). The differences among them prevent complete immunologic cross-reactivity. This probably accounts for the difficulties that have been encountered in developing radioimmunoassays for the measurement of human parathyroid hormone, using antisera directed against bovine or porcine peptides, which previously were more readily available than the human peptide. All of the structural information required for full biologic activity of native, 84 amino acid parathyroid hormone lies within the 34 amino acids at the amino terminus. The active fragments of the bovine and human hormones, multiple fragments of the mid and carboxyl regions of the bovine and human hormones, and recently the full sequence of human parathyroid hormone have been synthesized and are commercially available for investigational use. Limited studies of the mid- and carboxyl-region fragments have shown them to be biologically inert.

CONTROL OF SECRETION. Parathyroid hormone is rapidly

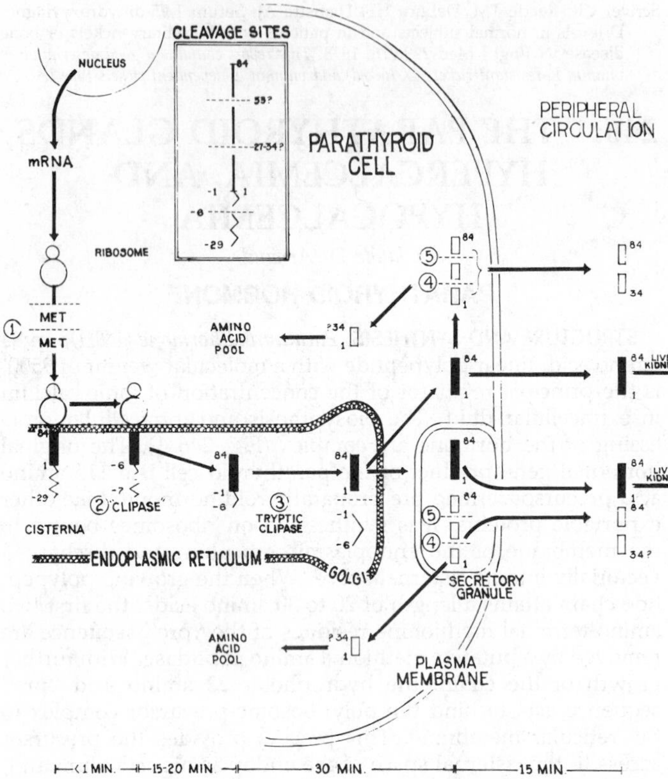

Figure 246–1. Proposed intracellular pathway for the biosynthesis of parathyroid hormone. Pre-proparathyroid hormone (Pre-ProPTH), the initial product of synthesis on the ribosomes, is converted into proparathyroid hormone (ProPTH) by removal of (1) the NH_2-terminal methionyl residues and (2) the NH_2-terminal sequence (-29 through -7) of 23 amino acids during synthesis and within seconds afterwards, respectively. The conversion of Pre-ProPTH probably occurs during transport of the polypeptide into the cisterna of the rough endoplasmic reticulum. By 20 minutes after synthesis, ProPTH reaches the Golgi region and is converted into PTH by (3) removal of the NH_2-terminal hexapeptide. PTH is either stored in a secretory granule or released into the cell cytoplasm, where it remains until it is released into the circulation in response to a fall in the blood concentration of calcium. Intact PTH [PTH(1-84)] undergoes at least two cleavages while in the secretory granule (and possibly in the cytoplasm) (4,5). These cleavages generate amino-, mid-, and carboxyl-region fragments. The mid- and carboxyl-region fragments are secreted into the circulation along with PTH(1-84), whereas the amino-region fragments are further degraded by the cell. The PTH(1-84) released into the circulation undergoes metabolic degradation in the liver and kidney (6), and this adds to the pool of circulating fragments. The time needed for these events is given below the schema. (Adapted from Habener JF, et al.: Biosynthesis of parathyroid hormone. Rec Prog Hormone Res 33:287, 1977.)

released from the parathyroid glands in response to a fall in plasma ionic calcium. It acts on kidney, intestine (indirectly, see below), and bone to restore the concentration of this cation to just above a normal set point, which, in turn, inhibits the secretion of the hormone. This negative feedback cycle is depicted in the "butterfly" diagram shown in Figure 243–1, in which the cycle is dissected into three loops, each involving one of the major target organs of parathyroid hormone. The concentration of extracellular ionic calcium is the major regulator of parathyroid hormone secretion. A more general discussion of calcium metabolism and its homeostasis is provided in Ch. 243. Other factors influence secretion only indirectly. For

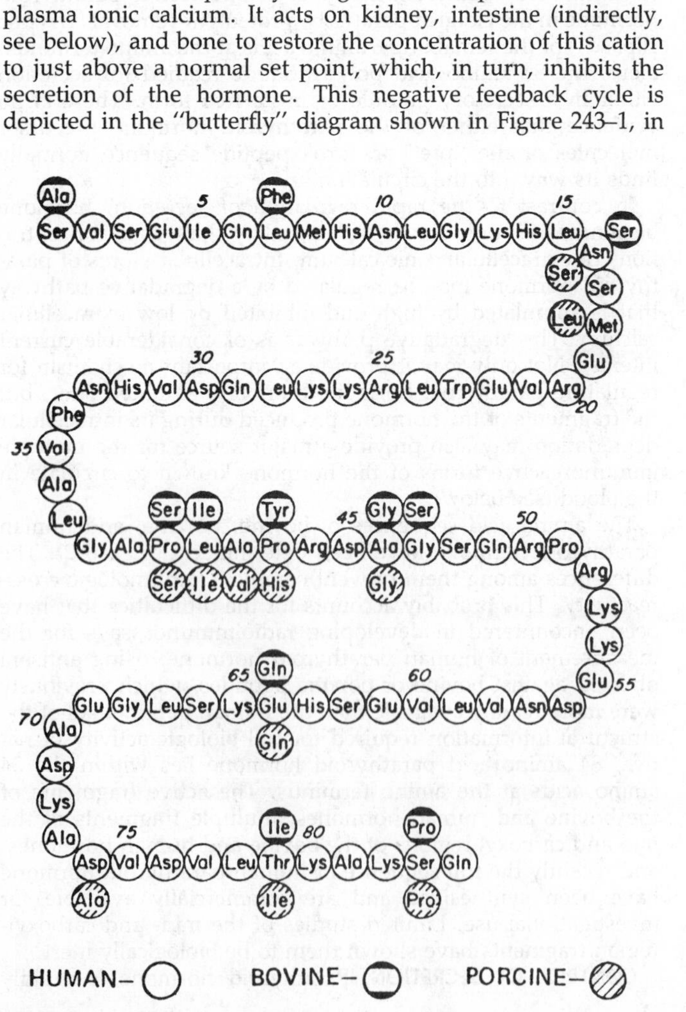

Figure 246–2. Parathyroid hormone. The figure shows the structure of human PTH and indicates at which positions the amino acid residues differ for bovine and porcine PTH. (Reprinted with permission from Keutmann HT, et al.: Complete amino acid sequence of human parathyroid hormone. Biochemistry 17:5728, 1978. Copyright 1978 American Chemical Society.)

example, plasma phosphate alters the degree to which calcium is complexed, and blood pH, the degree to which it binds to albumin. The effects of extracellular magnesium concentrations on secretion are qualitatively similar to those of ionic calcium but are physiologically less important. Paradoxically, severe, prolonged hypomagnesemia markedly inhibits secretion of parathyroid hormone and may be associated with hypocalcemia (see below). Known, direct parathyroid hormone secretagogues of questionable physiologic importance include β-adrenergic agonists, prostaglandins, and histamine. These agents, as well as decreased ionic calcium, stimulate the production of cyclic 3′5′-adenosine monophosphate (cyclic AMP) in parathyroid cells in vitro, and it is presumed that this compound mediates their actions on hormone secretion.

THE CIRCULATING HORMONE. Circulating parathyroid hormone is heterogeneous. It consists of the intact 84 amino acid polypeptide and multiple fragments of the hormone. These fragments are derived from the mid and carboxyl regions of the hormone molecule and therefore are likely to be biologically inactive. There is no evidence that biologically active fragments are secreted by the parathyroid gland or that they are present in the circulation. It is not possible at present to determine precisely the relative quantities of intact parathyroid hormone and of its fragments in serum, but grossly there are more circulating fragments than intact hormone. This difference is due primarily to the fact that the fragments survive longer in the circulation. The fragments are derived both from the degradative metabolism of intact parathyroid hormone (Fig. 246–1) and from glandular secretion, but the quantitative importance of these sources is uncertain.

Biologically active parathyroid hormone normally circulates in the blood at extremely low concentrations (<50 pg per milliliter). It is likely that there are individual, constitutionally derived "set point" values for the plasma ionic calcium above which glandular secretion rates are decreased and below which they are increased. However, steady state levels of parathyroid hormone are probably determined primarily by the degree to which the parathyroid glands must adapt to individual, chronic, environmentally induced changes in the level of plasma ionic calcium (e.g., dietary calcium and phosphate). There is an inverse relationship between fasting levels of serum calcium and serum immunoreactive parathyroid hormone (iPTH) in normal subjects (Fig. 246–3). Serum iPTH also increases with age (Fig. 246–4).

ACTION OF PARATHYROID HORMONE. The major function of PTH is to defend against hypocalcemia. It carries out this function by promoting virtually all of the actions that could be teleologically postulated: (1) release of calcium from bone, (2) conservation of calcium by the kidney, (3) enhanced absorption of calcium from the gut (indirectly via vitamin D), and (4) reduction in plasma phosphate. These physiologic effects of parathyroid hormone will be described after a brief summary of what is known concerning its mechanism of action.

MECHANISM OF ACTION OF PTH. Parathyroid hormone binds to specific plasma membrane receptors of target cells. These occupied receptors interact with a membrane-bound protein that is regulated by guanyl nucleotides; this protein in turn activates membrane-bound adenylate cyclase to convert ATP to cyclic AMP (Fig. 246–5). Cyclic AMP, by virtue of its ability to initiate a cascade of enzyme-activating intracellular phosphorylations, is considered to be one of possibly several intracellular "second messengers" responsible for mediating the final expression of the action of the hormone. The details of these enzyme activations and the manner in which they relate to discrete effects of the hormone are unknown. Other potential second messengers of parathyroid hormone (e.g., calcium itself) that might act in concert with or modulate the actions of cyclic AMP are under investigation. A more general description of the mechanisms by which polypeptide hormones act on target cells is contained in Ch. 221.

Information concerning the structural requirements for the action of parathyroid hormone at the site of its receptor is rapidly becoming available. The region of the molecule essential for receptor binding is the amino acid sequence 25-30, and for receptor activation, the 1-7 sequence. Recently, two analogues of bovine PTH that are truncated at the amino terminus have been developed. One of these, [8]Nle,[18]Nle,[34]Tyr bovine PTH(3-

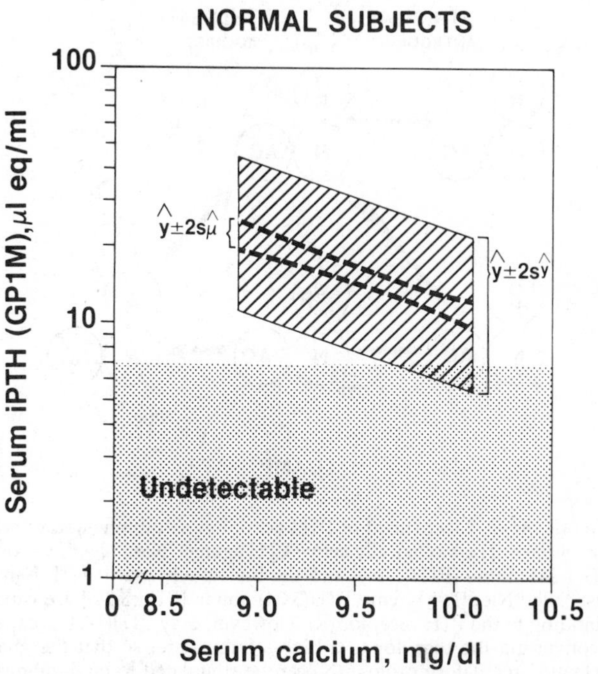

Figure 246–3. Serum immunoreactive parathyroid hormone (iPTH) (log scale) as a function of serum total calcium in 150 normal subjects (r = −0.424; p <0.001). (From Purnell D, et al.: Treatment of primary hyperparathyroidism. Am J Med 56:801, 1974.)

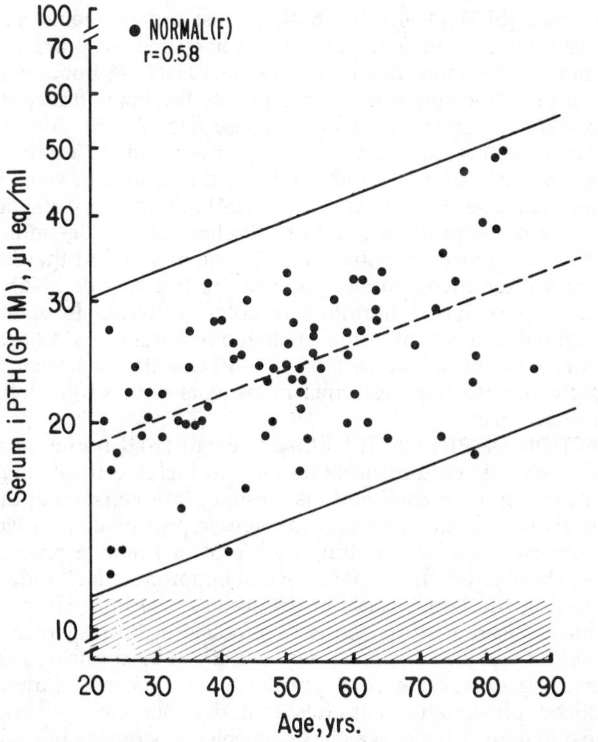

Figure 246–4. Serum immunoreactive parathyroid hormone (iPTH) as a function of age in 78 normal Caucasian women. Cross-hatched area at bottom represents limit of assay detectability. Mean increase in serum iPTH between age 20 and 90 is 80 per cent and is significant (p <0.001). (From Gallagher JC, et al.: The effect of age on serum immunoreactive parathyroid hormone in normal and osteoporotic women. J Lab Clin Med 95:376, 1980.)

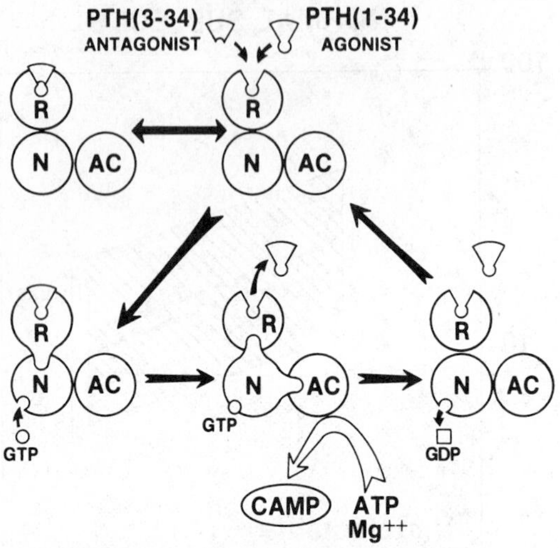

Figure 246–5. Mechanism of PTH action on membrane-bound adenylate cyclase. The biologically active PTH agonist ^{8}Nle,^{18}Nle,^{34}Tyr bovine PTH(1-34) amide [PTH(1-34)] and the biologically inactive PTH antagonist ^{8}Nle,^{18}Nle,^{34}Tyr bovine PTH(3-34) amide [PTH(3-34)] are capable of binding to the PTH receptor (R). However, only PTH(1-34) is capable of converting the receptor to a high-affinity state, so that the guanyl nucleotide regulatory protein (N) can be stimulated to bind guanosine triphosphate (GTP). The binding of GTP to N converts R to a low-affinity state, inducing dissociation of PTH(1-34) *and* the formation of an N-adenylate cyclase (AC) complex, leading to the activation of this enzyme and the increased production of intracellular cAMP. In contrast, the binding of PTH antagonist to R does not change the affinity of R; consequently, R cannot interact with N or induce activation of AC. (From Arnaud CD, Kolb FO: The calciotropic hormones and metabolic bone disease. *In* Greenspan FS, Forsham PH (eds.): Basic and Clinical Endocrinology. Los Altos, Lange Medical Publications, 1983, p 193.)

34) amide [bPTH(3-34)], has both agonist and antagonist properties in vitro. It binds to parathyroid hormone receptors in the kidney to the same degree as bovine PTH(1-34) but is much less potent in converting the receptor to the high-affinity state necessary to activate adenylate cyclase (Fig. 246–5). Although bPTH(3-34) acts as an antagonist in vitro, it fails to antagonize concomitantly administered parathyroid hormone in vivo. The other analogue, ^{34}Tyr bovine PTH(7-34) amide, has antagonist but no agonist properties in vitro. Preliminary studies indicate that it antagonizes parathyroid hormone in vivo but that large doses are required, possibly due to the fact that its ability to bind to parathyroid hormone receptors is weak. In spite of this, the development of this analogue represents an important advance in the effort to design a PTH antagonist that can rapidly reverse hypercalcemia in patients with severe hyperparathyroidism.

ACTION OF PTH ON THE KIDNEY. Parathyroid hormone acts most immediately on the kidney (1) to increase renal tubular reabsorption of calcium and magnesium, thus conserving these two divalent cations, and (2) to increase phosphate and bicarbonate excretion by inhibiting their proximal tubular reabsorption. These latter effects have several important, albeit indirect, effects on the homeostasis of extracellular calcium. Hormone-induced bicarbonaturia tends to produce acidosis, which decreases the ability of circulating albumin to bind calcium, thus increasing ionic calcium by physiochemical means. Hormone-induced phosphaturia assures that the increased release of phosphate from bone, which occurs obligately during hormone-induced calcium mobilization from bone, does not produce hyperphosphatemia. Increased serum phosphate would tend to complex calcium and thereby counteract the physiologic effect of parathyroid hormone to increase plasma ionic calcium.

The most important indirect effect of the phosphaturic action of the hormone is illustrated in the intestinal feedback loop in Figure 243–1. Parathyroid hormone, either directly or by its hypophosphatemic action, stimulates renal tubular 25OH 1α-hydroxylase to convert the major circulating metabolite of vitamin D, 25-hydroxycholecalciferol (25OHD), to its major, biologically active metabolite, 1α,25-dihydroxycholecalciferol [$1,25(OH)_2D$]. This latter metabolite acts directly on the intestinal mucosal cell to increase calcium absorption and on bone to increase resorption (see arrow between the intestinal and bone loops in Fig. 243–1). The metabolism of vitamin D is discussed in detail in Ch. 244.

In the process of stimulating adenylate cyclase in renal tubular cells, parathyroid hormone increases the urinary excretion of cyclic AMP. Presumably, cyclic AMP is simply released into the tubular fluid following its intracellular synthesis, since it has no known extracellular function. Urinary cyclic AMP is increased by the administration of other hormones active in the kidney, including epinephrine and glucagon, but its renal production and excretion are almost entirely due to parathyroid hormone. It can therefore be used as an indirect measure of the action of parathyroid hormone on the kidney, as noted below.

ACTION OF PTH ON BONE. Parathyroid hormone increases the net release of calcium and phosphate from bone into extracellular fluid. In this defense of calcium homeostasis the hormone influences the differentiation and activities of bone cells. These cellular events appear to depend upon a permissive effect of biologically active vitamin D metabolites (e.g., $1,25(OH)_2D$), but the precise mechanism involved in this important relationship between parathyroid hormone and vitamin D is poorly understood. The physiology and pathophysiology of mineral metabolism demonstrate a wide range of interactions between parathyroid hormone (tropic) and vitamin D (permissive), as will be noted here and in the chapters on metabolic bone diseases.

ASSAY IN BIOLOGIC FLUIDS. The major tool for measuring parathyroid hormone in biologic fluids is radioimmunoassay. Values for serum iPTH vary from laboratory to laboratory, however, because of the differences in the source (bovine or human) and purity of the parathyroid hormone preparations used as standards and in the specificity of the antisera. Therefore, interpretation of serum iPTH values requires knowledge of the normal range for each assay system. Until recently, most radioimmunoassays of human PTH have used ^{125}I-labeled bovine PTH as the radioligand and cross-reacting antisera directed against porcine or bovine PTH. Use of synthetic human PTH or its fragments, which have recently become commercially available, may help to minimize some of the inconsistencies in the future. However, variations in the specificities of antisera used in different assays will continue to result in different iPTH values for the same serum sample. Such differences reflect true differences in the concentrations of the various forms of circulating parathyroid hormone.

At present, all available antisera that have a sufficiently high affinity for parathyroid hormone to be useful in radioimmunoassays are multivalent and contain antibodies directed at multiple regions of the PTH molecule. Antisera directed against the mid or carboxyl region of the PTH molecule recognize inactive mid- or carboxyl-region fragments and intact, biologically active PTH, and antisera directed against the amino region recognize amino-region fragments and intact PTH. Because the quantities of mid- and carboxyl-region fragments in the circulation are greater than those of amino-region fragments or intact PTH, values for serum iPTH are higher in mid- and carboxyl-region assays than in amino-region assays.

Mid- and carboxyl-region assays have provided surprisingly good diagnostic tools in the evaluation of patients suspected of having parathyroid disease, even though the resulting values for serum iPTH primarily reflect circulating, biologically inactive hormone (i.e., mid- and carboxyl-region fragments) (see below). This is fortunate because the concentrations of intact PTH in the circulation are so low that, with rare exception, they are beyond the sensitivity limits of all the amino-region assays yet developed.

Ideally, radioimmunoassays for parathyroid hormone should do the following: (1) be able to measure serum iPTH in over 95 per cent of normal subjects, (2) demonstrate an inverse relationship between serum iPTH and total serum calcium over the normal range of serum calcium (Fig. 246–3), (3) show consistently low or undetectable serum iPTH values in all patients with hypoparathyroidism as well as in all patients with hypercalcemia of nonparathyroid origin, other than cancer, and (4) demonstrate iPTH values greater than the upper limits of normal in 90 per cent of patients with surgically proved primary hyperparathyroidism.

Until recently, bioassays for parathyroid hormone lacked sufficient sensitivity for the study of circulating parathyroid hormone. This obstacle has now been overcome by two novel approaches. One is a cytochemical bioassay that is based on the PTH-specific stimulation of glucose-6-phosphate dehydrogenase in guinea pig renal slices. This assay is extremely sensitive, measuring femtogram amounts of parathyroid hormone. Its disadvantage is its technical complexity. The other assay, which is more convenient, uses a nonhydrolyzable analogue of guanosine triphosphate, 5'guanyl-imidodiphosphate [Gpp(NH)p], to greatly augment the sensitivity of adenylate cyclase to parathyroid hormone in canine kidneys in vitro. In the presence of Gpp(NH)p, as little as 10 pg per milliliter of intact PTH elicits significant stimulation. However, even with this sensitivity, the measurement of parathyroid hormone in normal serum requires the immunoextraction of 3 ml of serum. This assay is accurate, precise, and simple and can be performed rapidly.

DeGroot LJ (ed.): Endocrinology. Vol 2. New York, Grune & Stratton, 1979, pp 587–636, 713–716. *Comprehensive review of PTH chemistry and physiology.*

Goltzman D, Henderson B, Loveridge N: Cytochemical bioassay of parathyroid hormone: Characteristics of the assay and analysis of circulating hormonal forms. J Clin Invest 65:1309,1980. *Describes the clinical application of the cytochemical bioassay of serum PTH for the evaluation of patients with parathyroid dysfunction.*

Nissenson RA, Abbott SR, Teitelbaum AP, Clark OH, Arnaud CD: Endogenous biologically active human parathyroid hormone: Measurement by a guanyl nucleotide-amplified renal adenylate cyclase assay. J Clin Endocrinol Metab 52:840,1981. *Describes the guanyl nucleotide-amplified adenylate cyclase bioassay of serum PTH.*

Nissenson RA, Teitelbaum AP, Abbott SR, Pliam N, Silve C, Zitzner L, Nyiredy K, Arnaud CD: Parathyroid hormone receptors in kidney and bone: Relation to adenylate cyclase activation. *In* Cohn DV, Talmage RV, Mathews JL (eds.): Hormonal Control of Calcium Metabolism. Amsterdam, Excerpta Medica, 1981, pp 44–54. *Review of the current knowledge about the interaction between PTH receptors and adenylate cyclase.*

PRIMARY HYPERPARATHYROIDISM

DEFINITION. Primary hyperparathyroidism describes a disorder or group of disorders resulting from excessive, relatively uncontrolled secretion of parathyroid hormone by a single or multiple parathyroid glands. The actions of parathyroid hormone on bone and kidney usually result in hypercalcemia, the biochemical hallmark of the disorder, but this fails to inhibit PTH secretion normally. Most patients are now detected by routine measurement of the serum calcium while relatively asymptomatic and without other readily demonstrable manifestations of the disease. When present, symptoms can be remarkably varied and vague and are related to hypercalcemia, hypercalciuria (nephrolithiasis), or osteitis fibrosa cystica (bone pain).

ETIOLOGY. The etiology of primary hyperparathyroidism is unknown. In several families the disease has been inherited as an autosomal dominant trait. Patients studied for the detection of thyroid carcinoma following previous neck x-irradiation have incidentally shown a greater than expected number of cases of primary hyperparathyroidism. It is difficult to interpret such studies, however, because information about the general incidence and natural history of primary hyperparathyroidism is incomplete.

Calcium infusions in the hyperparathyroid patients with mild hypercalcemia incompletely suppress serum immunoreactive parathyroid hormone levels. This strongly suggests that increased hormone secretion in these patients is due, at least in part, to a set point error in the level of ionic calcium at which abnormal tissue is suppressed. This defect can be demonstrated in vitro. Higher concentrations of calcium are required in the medium to decrease parathyroid hormone secretion from parathyroid cells isolated from abnormal glands than are required for cells isolated from normal glands.

INCIDENCE. Routine, automated measurement of serum calcium has vastly increased the detection of primary hyperparathyroidism. The incidence of primary hyperparathyroidism increases in both men and women after age 50, but it is two to four times more common in women. The disease is rare in children. In a careful epidemiologic study of cases detected in Rochester, Minnesota, over a ten-year period, the age-adjusted incidence rate was estimated to be 42 per 100,000. Studies of selected populations (mostly older than 40 years of age) have revealed prevalence rates of primary hyperparathyroidism as high as 1 in 1000 to 1 in 200 of those surveyed.

PATHOLOGY. Histologically, abnormal parathyroid glands from patients with primary hyperparathyroidism have been characterized as being hyperplastic, adenomatous, or malignant. Unfortunately, it is often difficult, if not impossible, to distinguish between an adenoma and chief cell hyperplasia in a given gland, and, occasionally, abnormal parathyroid tissue that is benign has many of the histologic features of malignant tissue. Thus, it has generally been necessary to revert to the gross pathology observed at surgery to classify parathyroid lesions. The surgeon determines the number of abnormal glands present on the basis of their size and gross appearance, and the pathologist determines whether the biopsy specimens are parathyroid tissue. Single gland involvement ("adenoma") is observed in about 80 per cent of patients and multiple gland involvement ("hyperplasia") in about 20 per cent. Less than 2 per cent of hyperfunctioning glands are carcinomatous as judged by a combination of gross appearance, histology, and the ultimate biologic behavior of the abnormal tissue. Multiple glands are almost always involved in familial primary hyperparathyroidism and the hyperparathyroidism associated with multiple endocrine neoplasia (MEN) syndromes. Abnormal parathyroid glands usually weigh between 0.2 and 2.0 grams (25 to 75 mg is normal) and have a characteristic yellow-red color and "bulging" appearance in situ. Occasionally, very large glands (e.g., >10 grams) are observed. The severity of the clinical manifestations, especially the degree of hypercalcemia, is generally proportional to the quantity of hyperfunctioning tissue present and the level of serum immunoreactive PTH (iPTH). The predominant cell type in most abnormal glands is the chief cell, although so-called "water-clear cells" and oxyphilic cells may be admixed, and very occasionally either of these cells may predominate. The secretory capabilities of the "water-clear" and oxyphilic cells are unknown.

Virtually all patients with primary hyperparathyroidism have histomorphometric evidence of excess parathyroid hormone action in bone biopsies from the iliac crest, although most of these patients do not have radiographic evidence of bone disease. An increase in the amount of bone surface undergoing resorption, increased numbers of osteoclasts, osteocytic osteolysis, and, in moderate to severe cases, marrow fibrosis are characteristic of this lesion, which is termed osteitis fibrosa cystica. Only far advanced disease is associated with classic bone cysts and fractures. It is not uncommon to observe extensive evidence of a mineralization defect characterized by large quantities of unmineralized osteoid and disorganized (woven versus lamellar) bone.

Between 20 and 30 per cent of patients have nephrolithiasis, not infrequently complicated by pyelonephritis. Gross nephrocalcinosis or calcification of the renal papillae is unusual, but careful microscopic examinations of kidneys with special calcium stains occasionally reveal peritubular and tubular calcifications at autopsy. The incidence of such soft tissue calcification in patients with mild to moderate disease is unknown; however, it may be relatively frequent because chondrocalcinosis and calcific tendinitis can be demonstrated on x-ray in approximately 7.5 to 18 per cent of cases. Calcification of other organs such as stomach, lung, and heart has been observed in patients with hyperparathyroid crisis (serum calcium >15.0 mg per deciliter).

Myopathy is relatively common in primary hyperparathyroidism, and muscle biopsy may show neuropathic atrophy of both Type I and Type II muscle fibers. These histologic changes parallel clinical, neurologic, and electromyographic dysfunction.

PATHOPHYSIOLOGY. The excessive release of parathyroid hormone from hyperfunctioning parathyroid tissue causes exaggerated physiologic responses of target organs (see Fig. 243–1) and inappropriately raises the concentration of ionized calcium in extracellular fluid. In contrast to other hypercalcemic states, in primary hyperparathyroidism the first lines of defense against hypercalcemia (increased renal and intestinal loss of calcium) are not fully operative, since the kidney and intestine are target organs for PTH and are themselves contributing to the pathogenesis of the hypercalcemia. Early in the course of the disease, when serum calcium values are <11.5 mg per deciliter (normal range, 8.9 to 10.1 mg per deciliter), urinary calcium is often relatively low for the degree of hypercalcemia and may be normal. When serum calcium values exceed 12.0 mg per deciliter, the increased filtered load of calcium overwhelms renal tubular reabsorption and hypercalciuria develops. This assists in limiting the further rise of plasma calcium but at the cost of producing kidney stone diathesis secondary to continued hypercalciuria, along with other changes in urine composition (e.g., increased pH resulting from bicarbonaturia).

Factors other than urinary loss may tend to limit the degree of hypercalcemia in primary hyperparathyroidism. First, calcium may be "lost" from the extracellular fluid by being deposited in soft tissues. This metastatic calcification may cause symptoms (e.g., joint pain owing to calcific tendinitis and chondrocalcinosis) or compromise function (e.g., nephrocalcinosis leading to renal failure). Secondly, the permissive effect of vitamin D is necessary for the action of parathyroid hormone; in its absence patients with even severe hyperparathyroidism become either eucalcemic or nearly so. In fact, stores of vitamin D may become depleted in a patient who previously was marginally replete because of the increased renal conversion of 25OHD to $1,25(OH)_2D$, which is caused by excessive parathyroid hormone. As a result, such patients may have severe osteomalacia in addition to osteitis fibrosa cystica. Finally, hypercalcemia per se may increase the degradation of biologically active forms of parathyroid hormone peripherally (i.e., in the liver and possibly the kidney) and in the parathyroid tissue itself. In this way plasma calcium not only may regulate parathyroid hormone secretion but also may be an important factor in determining the relative quantities of circulating, biologically active parathyroid hormone and inactive hormone fragments. Increased secretion of calcitonin might be expected to play an important role in correcting the hypercalcemia of primary hyperparathyroidism (see Fig. 243–1), but this seems not to occur in the majority of patients. In fact, the secretory reserve of calcitonin often appears to be depleted.

Parathyroid hormone decreases renal tubular reabsorption of phosphate, and in excess tends to cause hyperphosphaturia and hypophosphatemia. Normally, these effects both support mineral homeostasis (by stimulating $1,25(OH)_2D$ production) and protect it (by clearing from the blood phosphate that is removed from bone during resorption of calcium). In patients with primary hyperparathyroidism, however, hypophosphatemia tends to worsen hypercalcemia by causing increased production of the hypercalcemic compound $1,25(OH)_2D$ and decreased complexing of blood ionic calcium by phosphate.

Patients with primary hyperparathyroidism generally have mild to moderate hyperchloremic acidosis, primarily because excess hormone decreases urinary hydrogen ion excretion and increases urinary bicarbonate excretion. These effects also tend to aggravate existing hypercalcemia by decreasing the ability of blood albumin to bind ionic calcium, and by increasing the dissolution of bone mineral.

Urinary cyclic AMP is increased in as many as 80 per cent of patients with primary hyperparathyroidism. Presumably, increased hormonal occupancy of renal receptors stimulates adenylate cyclase to produce an increase in this intracellular second messenger. Interestingly, the phosphaturic and cyclic AMP responses to exogenously administered parathyroid hormone are blunted in patients with primary hyperparathyroidism, suggesting refractoriness or "desensitization" of one or more of the cellular components responsible for these effects. This desensitization, as well as the increased excretion of nephrogenous cyclic AMP, has been used as a diagnostic test for the presence of hyperparathyroidism.

Patients with radiologic evidence of osteitis fibrosa cystica (a bone lesion caused by excess PTH), almost always have increased serum concentrations of the bone isoenzyme of alkaline phosphatase. This enzyme is produced by osteoblasts and probably constitutes one of several enzymes involved in osseous mineralization. These patients also excrete in their urine greater than normal quantities of small peptides that contain hydroxyproline. This amino acid is unique to collagen, which is the major structural protein in bone. Combined increases in serum alkaline phosphatase and urinary excretion of hydroxyproline reflect grossly increased bone turnover, which can be documented further by studies of the dynamics of intravenously administered, isotopically labeled calcium (^{47}Ca, ^{45}Ca).

SYMPTOMS. Most patients with primary hyperparathyroidism are relatively asymptomatic when the diagnosis is made, or else they have nonspecific symptoms, especially those of weakness and easy fatigability. When symptoms do occur, they can generally be attributed to either hypercalcemia with associated hypercalciuria or to osteitis fibrosa cystica.

Hypercalcemia. The symptoms attributable to hypercalcemia involve a number of systems: (1) Central nervous system—impaired mentation, loss of memory for recent events, emotional lability, depression, anosmia, somnolence, and even coma. (2) Neuromuscular—weakness (especially of the proximal musculature), arthralgias, severe pruritus (which may be due to metastatic calcification in the skin), and the restless leg syndrome (no comfortable position for legs when attempting to sleep). The joint pains may be due to associated gout, intra-articular deposition of calcium pyrophosphate crystals (pseudogout), calcific tendinitis, or chondrocalcinosis. (3) Gastrointestinal—anorexia, nausea, vomiting, dyspepsia, constipation, and possibly an increased incidence of peptic ulcer and acute pancreatitis. (4) Renal—polyuria, nocturia, and susceptibility to calcium oxalate or calcium phosphate stones, which sometimes leads to renal failure from calcium nephropathy, with associated symptoms of uremia. (5) Cardiovascular—increased frequency of hypertension. In general, all of these abnormalities are related to the degree of increase in ionized calcium in extracellular fluid, but the correlation is a crude one. One patient may be severely incapacitated at a level of serum calcium that produces only moderate symptoms in another.

Osteitis Fibrosa Cystica. Bony abnormalities can be demonstrated by special techniques in biopsy specimens from the iliac crest in most patients with primary hyperparathyroidism. However, symptomatic bone disease is now rare in this disorder. Patients may infrequently complain of diffuse or localized (e.g., to the back) bone pain. Very rarely patients may have a pathologic fracture through a bone cyst. The radiographic changes in osteitis fibrosa cystica are described later.

PHYSICAL SIGNS. Most patients with primary hyperparathyroidism have no abnormal physical signs of the disorder. When present, such signs are usually confined to the neuromuscular system or to organ systems in which soft tissue calcification can be noted. Neurologic abnormalities are nonspecific and include impaired mentation, hyperactive deep tendon reflexes, sensory loss for pain and vibration, proximal muscle weakness (particularly the thighs), abnormal tongue movements (resembling fasciculations), glossal atrophy, and ataxic gait.

Soft tissue calcification can result in arthritis (chondrocalcinosis or calcific tendinitis), conjunctivitis (conjunctival calcium phosphate crystals), and "band keratopathy," which is characterized by deposition of opaque calcium phosphate in vertical lines parallel to and within the ocular limbus, usually laterally (3 o'clock) in the cornea. These ocular signs, which can be best seen with slit lamp examination, are rare in hyperparathyroidism unless the serum phosphate is elevated, as occurs after the onset of renal failure.

Primary hyperparathyroidism is a prominent component of the rare multiple endocrine neoplasia syndromes (MEN I or IIa), which are described in Ch. 240. The clinician should look for evidence of these abnormalities—e.g., acromegaly, hypopituitarism, pheochromocytoma, and medullary carcinoma of the thyroid—during the physical examination.

Enlarged parathyroid glands are only rarely demonstrable on physical examination. In fact, even in the presence of primary hyperparathyroidism, a nodule felt in the neck is almost certainly one of the thyroid rather than the parathyroid.

Rarely, patients may exhibit bone tenderness on examination, and even more rarely bone deformities, fractures through an osteoclastic cyst, or the presence of an epulis (brown tumor of the jaw).

RADIOGRAPHIC MANIFESTATIONS. The most specific and frequent radiographic sign of osteitis fibrosa cystica is that of subperiosteal bone resorption. This sign is best demonstrated in magnified, fine grain, industrial radiographs of the fingers (particularly the index finger) (Fig. 246–6*A*). Particular attention should be paid to the radial surface of the phalanx, where the cortex is almost completely resorbed, leaving only a lacey edge. Other radiographic manifestations of the disease range from generalized osteopenia to bone cysts ("brown tumors") and erosion of distal phalangeal tufts or the distal ends of the clavicles. Figure 246–6*B* provides an example of severe osteitis fibrosa cystica involving the skull.

Soft tissue calcifications (e.g., calcific tendinitis, chondrocalcinosis, nephrocalcinosis, and pulmonary calcifications) may be detected on routine films incidentally. The latter two are demonstrated best with bone scanning techniques, using radioactively labeled diphosphate compounds.

Nephrocalcinosis is rarely seen radiographically, but lithiasis is common. Since the stones are usually radiopaque (i.e., calcium oxalate and calcium phosphate stones), nephrotomograms are helpful in identifying, localizing, and measuring them. This procedure is important in determining the "activity" of the stone disease (see Ch. 89). An increase in stone diameter with time can be taken as objective evidence of "active" stone disease and is probably an additional indication for treatment of hyperparathyroidism (see below). Primary hyperparathyroidism may also be associated, although less commonly, with uric acid stones (not radiopaque). Thus, x-ray examination of the urinary tract with contrast material is also important.

DIFFERENTIAL DIAGNOSIS. In general, the major problem in the differential diagnosis of primary hyperparathyroidism is distinguishing this disease from other conditions associated with hypercalcemia. Hypercalcemia associated with thiazide

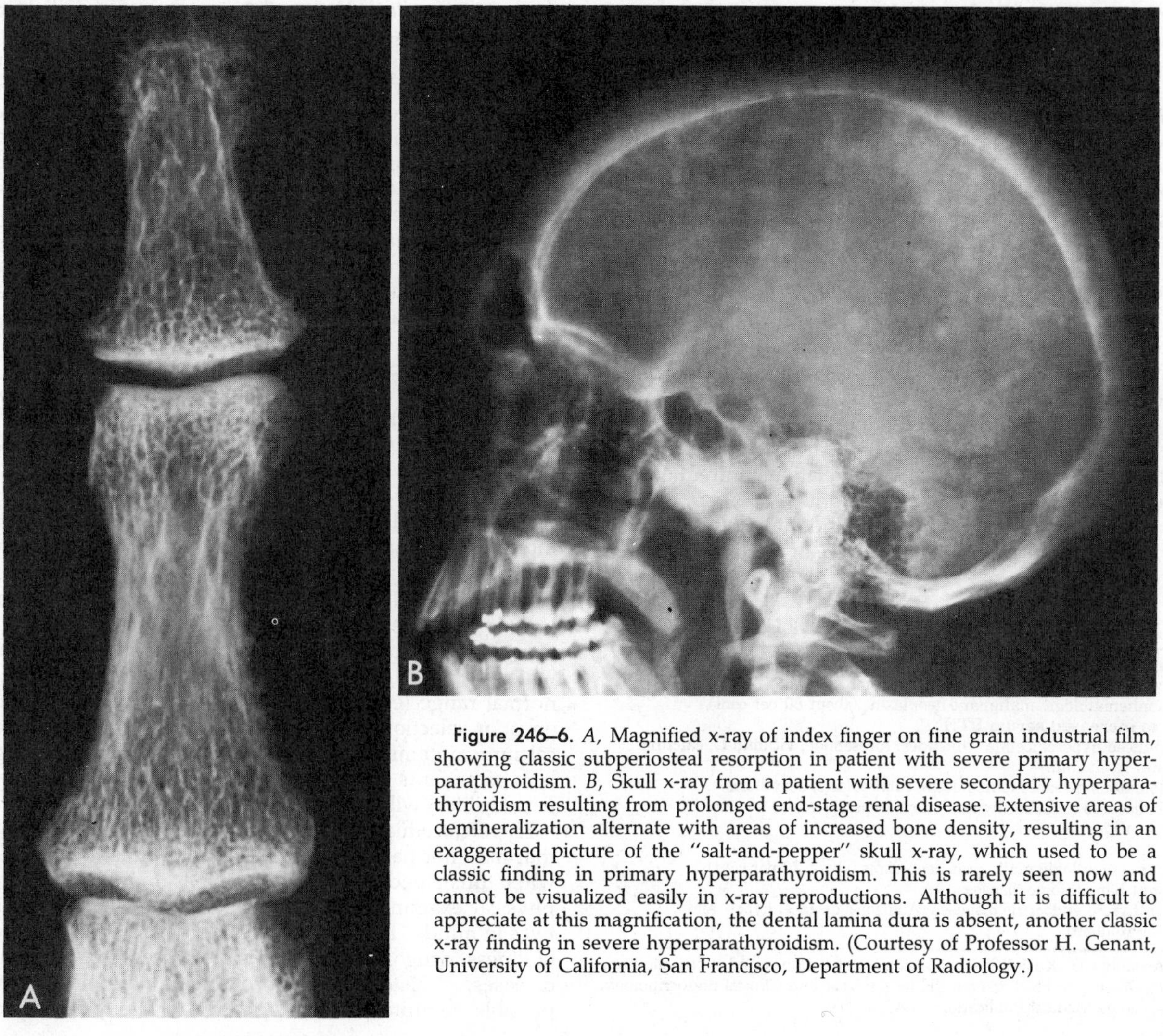

Figure 246–6. *A*, Magnified x-ray of index finger on fine grain industrial film, showing classic subperiosteal resorption in patient with severe primary hyperparathyroidism. *B*, Skull x-ray from a patient with severe secondary hyperparathyroidism resulting from prolonged end-stage renal disease. Extensive areas of demineralization alternate with areas of increased bone density, resulting in an exaggerated picture of the "salt-and-pepper" skull x-ray, which used to be a classic finding in primary hyperparathyroidism. This is rarely seen now and cannot be visualized easily in x-ray reproductions. Although it is difficult to appreciate at this magnification, the dental lamina dura is absent, another classic x-ray finding in severe hyperparathyroidism. (Courtesy of Professor H. Genant, University of California, San Francisco, Department of Radiology.)

diuretic therapy and with nonhematologic malignancy are the most frequently encountered among these. Other important causes of hypercalcemia are (1) hematologic malignancies involving bone (myeloma, lymphoma, and leukemia); (2) granulomatous diseases (sarcoidosis, tuberculosis, and berylliosis); (3) endocrine disorders, including thyrotoxicosis and acute adrenal insufficiency; (4) familial hypocalciuric hypercalcemia (a genetic disorder formerly called benign familial hypercalcemia); (5) excessive ingestion of calcium, vitamin D, or vitamin A; (6) extensive skeletal immobilization (e.g., spica body cast) in normal young people and prolonged bed rest in patients with osteolytic metabolic bone disease; and (7) idiopathic hypercalcemia of infancy.

Pathophysiologically, hypercalcemic disorders can be segregated into those caused by excess parathyroid hormone and those caused by factors other than parathyroid hormone (Table 246–1). Only patients with primary hyperparathyroidism and certain patients with malignant diseases have both hypercalcemia and elevated levels of circulating parathyroid hormone. In all other patients with hypercalcemia the secretion of parathyroid hormone is suppressed.

The underlying causes of the hypercalcemia in conditions without increased secretion of parathyroid hormone are varied and for the most part uncertain. They are discussed below under "Nonparathyroid Causes of Hypercalcemia." The most important among these, in terms of the differential diagnosis of primary hyperparathyroidism, are the hypercalcemia of malignancy and familial hypocalciuric hypercalcemia.

Hypercalcemia of Malignancy. It is unlikely that metastases to bone produce chronic hypercalcemia simply by physical displacement of bone. Rather, malignant tumors probably produce osteolytic humoral factors that act either systemically or locally in the immediate vicinity of a metastasis. These factors include parathyroid hormone–like substances, prostaglandins, osteoclast-activating factor (OAF), and probably other factors yet to be discovered. Any one or a combination of these factors might be secreted systemically by a tumor or released locally by its bony metastases in sufficient quantities to stimulate osteolysis and produce hypercalcemia. Osteoclast-activating factor is largely responsible for the production of hypercalcemia in patients with hematologic malignancies, especially multiple myeloma. Ectopic secretion of prostaglandins of the E_2 series may be associated with hypercalcemia, as documented by the presence of prostaglandin metabolites in urine, and more specifically by the response of the hypercalcemia to treatment with inhibitors of prostaglandin synthesis, such as indomethacin (see Ch. 223). Extensive experience now shows, however, that the primary involvement of prostaglandins in the production of hypercalcemia of malignancy is relatively infrequent, so that other humoral factors must be sought.

More than 35 years ago, Fuller Albright postulated that parathyroid hormone was the major cause of the hypercalcemia of malignancy. In the absence of renal failure, a large proportion of patients with this disease have the same degree of hypophosphatemia as do patients with moderate to severe primary hyperparathyroidism. In my experience, as many as 70 to 80 per cent of hypercalcemic patients with nonhematologic malignancies exhibit normal (80 per cent) to increased (20 per cent) values for serum immunoreactive parathyroid hormone (iPTH). The presence of immunoreactive parathyroid hormone in the serum of a hypercalcemic patient is considered to be abnormal. Other laboratories using different assays have reported lower frequencies for measurable levels of iPTH in the hypercalcemia of malignancy. Serum values for iPTH tend to be much higher in patients with primary hyperparathyroidism than in patients with malignancy with equal degrees of hypercalcemia. These results suggest (1) that the iPTH measured in the sera of patients with malignancy-associated hypercalcemia is an incidental finding and not pathogenetically related to the hypercalcemia, or (2) that the iPTH is quantitatively misrepresented by assays used to detect it and that, in fact, sufficient quantities of a biologically active parathyroid hormone–like compound with low PTH immunoreactivity circulates in the plasma of these patients to explain the hypercalcemia. I favor the latter alternative, based on studies concerning the heterogeneity of circulating PTH in patients with ectopic hyperparathyroidism and on the fact that such patients usually excrete increased nephrogenous cyclic AMP in amounts comparable to that found in patients with primary hyperparathyroidism. Patients with the ectopic syndrome have not only greater hypercalciuria but also much lower values for serum $1,25(OH)_2D$ than do patients with primary hyperparathyroidism. This suggests that the range of biologic actions of the parathyroid hormone–like substance in patients with ectopic disease may be different from that of native parathyroid hormone.

Benign Familial Hypercalcemia. Benign familial hypercalcemia (or familial hypocalciuric hypercalcemia) is probably the second most important consideration in the differential diagnosis of primary hyperparathyroidism. This recently described condition is rare and is inherited as an autosomal dominant trait. It is characterized by asymptomatic hypercalcemia, hypocalciuria, a tendency toward mild hypermagnesemia, and normal to low levels of serum iPTH. Histologically, the parathyroid glands either are normal or show equivocal "hyperplasia," and subtotal parathyroidectomy has consistently failed to restore eucalcemia. The response of nephrogenous cyclic AMP to exogenous and endogenous parathyroid hormone is greater in patients with familial hypocalciuric hypercalcemia than in normal subjects or in patients with primary hyperparathyroidism. The hypercalcemia in this familial syndrome may be due, at least in part, to renal hypersensitivity to the hypocalciuric effects of parathyroid hormone. In this sense then, familial hypocalciuric hypercalcemia could be considered to be a form of hyperparathyroidism. However, the notable absence of the characteristic sequelae of primary hyperparathyroidism (e.g., renal stones and osteitis fibrosa cystica) in these patients clearly indicates that tissue hypersensitivity to parathyroid hormone is probably not generalized.

DIAGNOSTIC INVESTIGATIONS. *General.* The presence of hypercalcemia is established when at least three measurements of total serum calcium are increased above the normal range, which is 8.9 to 10.1 mg per deciliter. If laboratories use a wider normal range (e.g., 9.0 to 11.0 mg per deciliter), based either on poor selection of normal control subjects or problems with calcium contamination in the laboratory (Ch. 243), large numbers of patients with mild hypercalcemia (i.e., 10.2 to 11.0 mg per deciliter) will go undetected.

Hypercalcemia generally reflects serious underlying disease that may not have been suspected on initial evaluation. Thus, when unsuspected hypercalcemia is found, the history and physical examination should be repeated with specific objectives in mind. These include detailed evaluation of the duration of illness, drug intake, the possible presence of other endocrine diseases, a history of nephrolithiasis with documentation if possible, symptoms of malignancy, a family history of endo-

TABLE 246–1. DIFFERENTIAL DIAGNOSIS OF HYPERCALCEMIA

Due to increased serum PTH
Primary and "tertiary" hyperparathyroidism
Some nonhematologic malignant neoplasms (about 80 per cent)
Not due to increased serum PTH
Drug-induced hypercalcemia (thiazides, furosemide, vitamin D, calcium, vitamin A, lithium)
Granulomatous diseases (sarcoidosis, tuberculosis, berylliosis)
Genetic diseases (familial hypocalciuric hypercalcemia)
Immobilization
"Idiopathic"
Some nonhematologic malignant neoplasms (about 20 per cent)
Malignant hematologic diseases
Nonparathyroid endocrine diseases (Addison's disease, hyper- and hypothyroidism)

From Arnaud CD, Kolb FO: The calciotropic hormones and metabolic bone disease. *In* Greenspan FS, Forsham PH (eds.): Basic and Clinical Endocrinology. Los Altos, Lange Medical Publications, 1983, p 208.

crine and mineral disorders, and the possible presence of palpable lymph nodes or masses, unusual skin pigmentation or lesions, and an enlarged thyroid, liver, or spleen.

Illness of long duration associated with kidney stones but no weight loss favors primary hyperparathyroidism; illness of short duration associated with weight loss without nephrolithiasis favors a nonparathyroid cause for hypercalcemia, particularly malignancy. A history of thiazide intake might explain an increase in serum calcium to 11.0 mg per deciliter, but higher values usually indicate that the effects of this drug have augmented the hypercalcemia of another condition (e.g., mild hyperparathyroidism). Patients who are taking thiazides and are hypercalcemic should be re-evaluated one month after discontinuing the drug. Vitamin D in doses exceeding 50,000 units per day can cause hypercalcemia in adults, and its ingestion may not have been elicited in the initial history. Hypercalcemic patients may be abnormally sensitive to vitamin D. Thus, intake of less than 50,000 units per day may aggravate existing hypercalcemia in sarcoidosis or primary hyperparathyroidism. What may appear initially to be a severe form of the primary disorder may prove to be relatively mild when vitamin D intake is curtailed. Excess calcium ingested in the form of antacids containing calcium carbonate (>5 grams per day) can cause severe hypercalcemia in susceptible individuals, especially when coupled with additional intake of alkali (bicarbonate) as in the "milk-alkali syndrome." This condition is rare in the absence of other abnormalities. Many patients actually have underlying primary hyperparathyroidism and are taking calcium carbonate and alkali for associated gastric hyperacidity.

The family history may hold the key to both the correct diagnosis and the correct treatment of a hypercalcemic patient. Systematic inquiry regarding a history of neck exploration and the presence of hypercalcemia, nephrolithiasis, metabolic bone disease, intractable peptic ulcer disease, and endocrine tumors in family members is essential. There is no specific family history in the syndrome of familial hypocalciuric hypercalcemia, although a history of unsuccessful parathyroid surgery in more than one hypercalcemic relative is characteristic of this condition. The diagnosis can be made definitive only by documenting hypercalcemia in the immediate relatives of the patient. If a multiple endocrine neoplasia syndrome or familial hyperparathyroidism is present, the patient will almost certainly have enlargement ("hyperplasia") of all four glands, and subtotal parathyroidectomy (removal of three and one half glands), as opposed to single gland removal, would be indicated.

Radioimmunoassay of Parathyroid Hormone. The availability of sensitive and specific radioimmunoassays of parathyroid hormone in serum has revolutionized the approach to the diagnosis of primary hyperparathyroidism during the past few years. Previously, patients were first extensively evaluated for nonparathyroid disorders that could cause hypercalcemia, and the diagnosis of hyperparathyroidism was one of exclusion. Now measurements of serum iPTH and calcium allow the assignment of patients either to a group that is very likely to have a surgically resectable parathyroid lesion(s) or to groups that require further diagnostic evaluation for the cause of hypercalcemia (Fig. 246–7).

The author's experience in the diagnosis of primary hyperparathyroidism, using a radioimmunoassay of serum parathy-

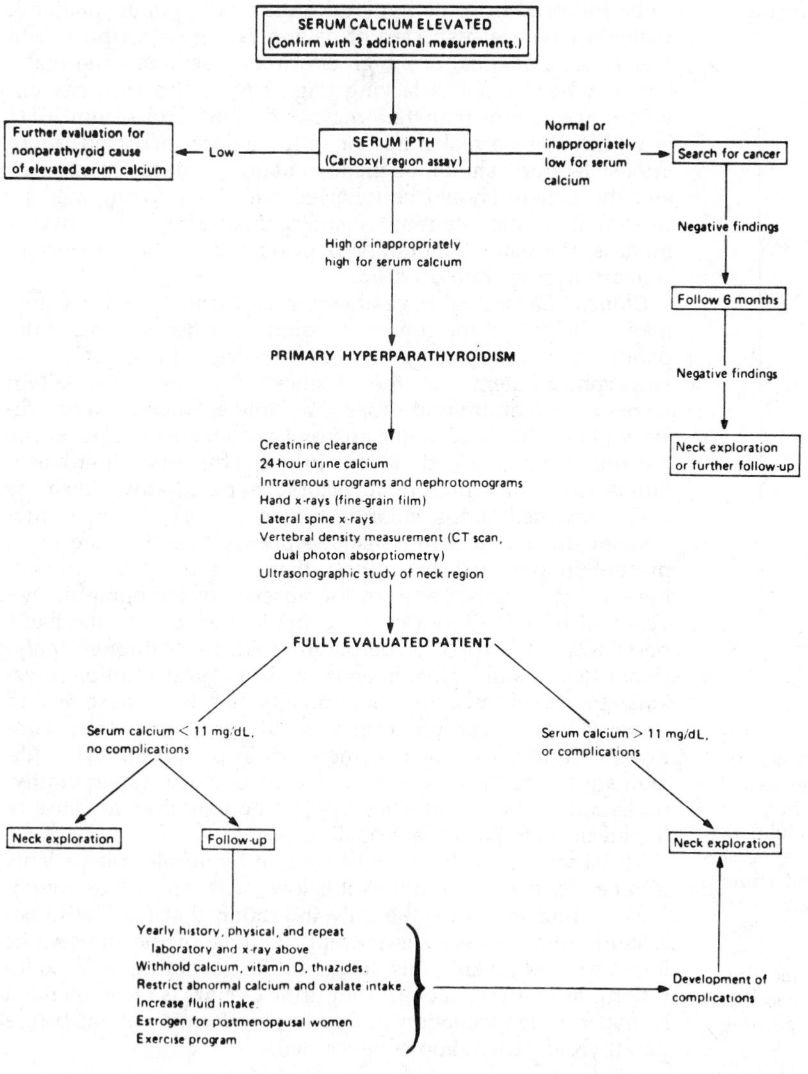

Figure 246–7. Use of PTH radioimmunoassay in the diagnosis and management of patients with hypercalcemia. (From Arnaud CD, Kolb FO: The calciotropic hormones and metabolic bone disease. *In* Greenspan FS, Forsham PH (eds.): Basic and Clinical Endocrinology. Los Altos, Lange Medical Publications, 1983, p 211.)

roid hormone that is specific for the mid region of the molecule, is illustrated in Figure 246–8. Ninety per cent of patients with surgically proved disease had values of serum iPTH that exceeded the upper limit of normal, and 10 per cent had values that were in the upper range of normal but inappropriately high for the total calcium concentration. Not shown are serum iPTH values in patients with nonparathyroid hypercalcemia (e.g., sarcoidosis and vitamin D intoxication). These are low or undetectable except in ectopic hyperparathyroidism caused by nonparathyroid cancer (see below). Thus, it is possible, by measuring calcium and iPTH in a single morning fasting serum sample, to categorize correctly 80 to 90 per cent of the hypercalcemic patients who have a potentially resectable hyperfunctioning parathyroid gland(s) and to categorize a similar percentage of the patients who have nonparathyroid hypercalcemia and who therefore require further study to discover the underlying cause of this derangement (see below). The advantages of using the serum iPTH as the principal laboratory probe to "triage" the hypercalcemic patient are clear. In the majority of patients with primary hyperparathyroidism, a correct diagnosis can be made in an outpatient setting, eliminating the costs and inconveniences of hospitalization and the multiple indirect tests required for a similar, less definitive diagnosis by exclusion.

Values of serum iPTH, measured with an assay specific for the mid or carboxyl region, are much lower for a given serum calcium in malignancy-associated hypercalcemia than in primary hyperparathyroidism (Fig. 246–9). This interesting phenomenon is probably due to the fact that patients with the hypercalcemia of malignancy have relatively low serum quantities of carboxyl- and mid-region fragments in comparison to

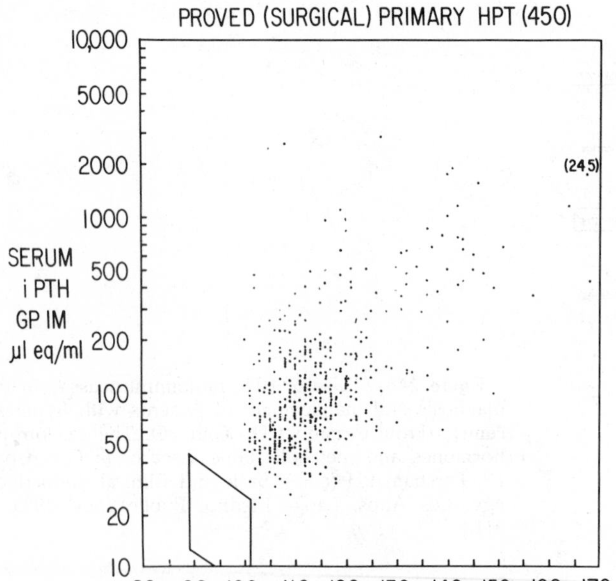

Figure 246–8. Serum iPTH values as a function of serum calcium concentration in 450 patients with surgically proved primary hyperparathyroidism. The area enclosed by the solid lines represents the normal range ± 2 SD for serum iPTH and serum calcium. Note that there is a 10 per cent overlap of serum iPTH with the normal range. Greater than 95 per cent of normal sera and all hyperparathyroid sera have measurable iPTH. Formal discriminative analysis of serum iPTH and serum calcium separates 100 per cent of hyperparathyroid patients from normal subjects. (From Arnaud CD, et al.: Human parathyroid hormone: Biologic and immunologic activities of its synthetic (1-34) tetratriacontapeptide and the utility of a carboxyl-terminal-specific radioimmunoassay in assessment of hyperparathyroid syndromes. Excerpta Medica International Congress Series No. 346, Calcium-Regulating Hormones, 1975, p 19.)

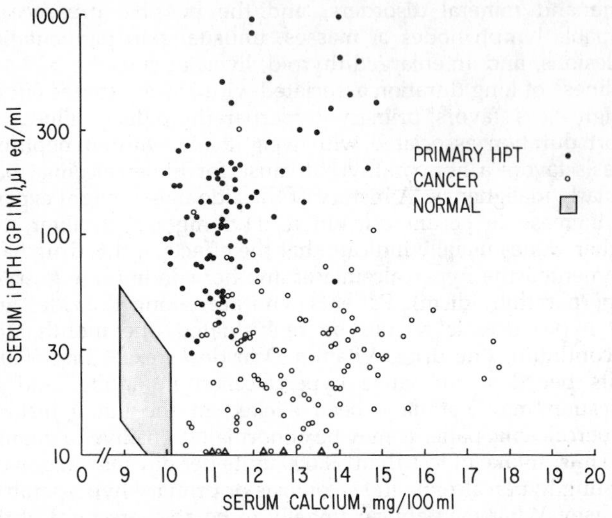

Figure 246–9. Relationship between serum iPTH and serum calcium in primary hyperparathyroid patients (●) and hypercalcemic patients with cancer(○). Note that for a given serum calcium value, serum iPTH is lower in patients with cancer. Of 105 patients with cancer, 5 had undetectable serum iPTH (Δ). Area enclosed with solid lines indicates normal range ± 2 SD for serum iPTH and serum calcium. (From Benson RC, Jr, et al.: Radioimmunoassay of parathyroid hormone in hypercalcemic patients with malignant disease. Am J Med 56:823, 1974.)

patients with primary hyperparathyroidism, but essentially equivalent quantities of intact parathyroid hormone. Irrespective of the pathophysiology involved, the relationships shown in Figure 246–9 help greatly in determining the course of action to be followed in some hypercalcemic and hypophosphatemic patients who are suspected of having cancer (e.g., those with weight loss, anemia, or a high erythrocyte sedimentation rate) but in whom proof is lacking (Fig. 246–7). If serum calcium values are greater than 12.5 mg per deciliter and serum iPTH is within the normal range or only slightly increased, more intensive efforts should be made to identify a neoplastic lesion, and the patient should be followed with temporizing medical treatment. If the situation is not clarified after six to twelve months, the patient should be re-evaluated for the presence of primary hyperparathyroidism.

Clinical Chemistry. Several serum and urine measurements may be helpful in the course of assigning patients to either the parathyroid or the nonparathyroid categories of hypercalcemia. Hyperphosphatemia in the absence of severe renal failure favors a nonparathyroid cause. Hypophosphatemia, when dietary phosphate is adequate and oral phosphate binding agents are not being ingested, favors primary hyperparathyroidism but is frequently present in ectopic hyperparathyroidism as well. Increased serum chloride favors primary hyperparathyroidism. Increased serum alkaline phosphatase is more often present in patients with cancer than in those with primary hyperparathyroidism and, in the absence of radiographic evidence of osteitis fibrosa cystica, should alert one to the likely possibility of ectopic hyperparathyroidism. Although polyclonal hypergammaglobulinemia might suggest multiple myeloma or sarcoidosis, this abnormality has been observed in primary hyperparathyroidism with disappearance after parathyroidectomy. Anemia and increases in the erythrocyte sedimentation rate have been recorded in primary hyperparathyroidism, but these findings suggest a nonparathyroid cause of hypercalcemia, particularly malignancy.

Measurement of the urine calcium in hypercalcemic patients is generally not useful unless it is low (<100 mg per 24 hours). This finding may give the only indication that familial hypocalciuric hypercalcemia is present. Because of the therapeutic importance of making this diagnosis (i.e., avoiding neck exploration), measurement of 24-hour urine calcium is recommended in the routine evaluation of any hypercalcemic patient before parathyroid exploration is performed.

Nephrogenous Cyclic AMP. Approximately 40 to 50 per cent of the cyclic AMP excreted in the urine is derived from the renal tubular cell. Its production and cellular release into the urine are almost entirely under the control of parathyroid hormone (see above). This component of urinary cyclic AMP can be accurately estimated and is termed nephrogenous cyclic AMP. It is increased above normal in 80 per cent of patients with primary hyperparathyroidism and in a large proportion of patients with the syndrome of ectopic hyperparathyroidism. Thus, it is not helpful in distinguishing between these two common disorders. Because low levels of nephrogenous cyclic AMP are present in patients with nonparathyroid hypercalcemia (excluding ectopic hyperparathyroidism), the test is useful in those patients whose serum iPTH is equivocally increased. In such patients, a low level of nephrogenous cyclic AMP would suggest that the serum iPTH value was artifactual and would argue against primary hyperparathyroidism, whereas a normal or increased level would confirm the validity of the serum iPTH value and favor this condition.

Other Diagnostic Tests. The glucocorticoid suppression test may be used in the rare event that the results of all the diagnostic tests already discussed are equivocal. It is based on the empirical observation that the hypercalcemia of conditions such as vitamin D intoxication, sarcoidosis, lymphoproliferative syndromes, and myeloma generally responds to the administration of 300 mg of cortisone or 60 mg of prednisone given daily in divided doses for ten days, whereas the same treatment only rarely results in a decrease in serum calcium in primary or ectopic hyperparathyroidism. The mechanisms involved in steroid-induced suppression of hypercalcemia are poorly understood, and variables other than steroids (e.g., hydration) may influence the level of serum calcium during the ten days of the test. A positive test (i.e., a significant decrease in serum calcium) should argue against neck exploration and for intensive investigation for another cause of hypercalcemia. A negative test would be consistent with primary or ectopic hyperparathyroidism.

Other diagnostic tests used less frequently include measurement of phosphate clearance (which is increased in primary hyperparathyroidism) and measurement of nephrogenous cyclic AMP after PTH administration (which is decreased in primary hyperparathyroidism, most likely because of a desensitization mechanism).

Finally, radiographs of the hands on fine grain industrial film should be obtained whenever hypercalcemia presents a diagnostic problem. Although the finding of definitive subperiosteal bone resorption is relatively unusual (approximately 8 to 10 per cent of patients with primary hyperparathyroidism), it is diagnostic of hyperparathyroidism and is probably the most reliable and readily available evidence supporting the need for neck exploration in patients with severe, life-threatening hypercalcemia.

PREOPERATIVE LOCALIZATION OF ABNORMAL PARATHYROID TISSUE. The abnormal parathyroid tissue causing primary hyperparathyroidism will be discovered and excised in greater than 90 per cent of initial neck explorations performed by an experienced parathyroid surgeon. Thus, there is no need for preoperative localization prior to first surgery except under unusual circumstances. In general, localization procedures are reserved for those patients in whom the first neck exploration was unsuccessful or for those who suffer recurrent disease. Noninvasive procedures include esophagography, ultrasonography, computed tomography, and isotopic scanning with thallium. Invasive procedures include arteriography, differential venous catheterization with measurement of iPTH in the serum samples obtained, and needle aspiration of a tumor with ultrasonic guidance.

Esophagography may occasionally identify a relatively large parathyroid gland, deep in the tracheoesophageal groove, which was inadvertently missed on first exploration because of its aberrant shape. Generally, however, the procedure is unrewarding. It is now possible to identify parathyroid lesions that are less than 1 cm in diameter by ultrasound examination of the neck or by thallium scanning. Further technological development in these areas is expected, and, because of the simplicity of the procedures, evaluation prior to initial neck exploration may become routinely advisable. Ultrasonography has not proved useful in identifying mediastinal parathyroid lesions, but computed tomography has. These noninvasive procedures may also have diagnostic value in the patient with severe hypercalcemia who has not undergone previous neck exploration. When a mass lesion(s) is identified in a location(s) consistent with normal or aberrant parathyroid tissue, the patient probably has primary hyperparathyroidism, and neck exploration should be performed early, before values for serum iPTH are available (usually requires several days) if the patient's condition is sufficiently serious.

Of the invasive procedures, thyroid arteriography is the most useful to the surgeon when a lesion is identified. As with the noninvasive procedures, the results are specific only in the sense that the location of an identified lesion is consistent with that of a normal or aberrant parathyroid gland. This procedure is not without risk, since neurologic complications such as transient occipital blindness and hemiplegia have been recorded.

Differential catheterization of the thyroidal and mediastinal veins for the purpose of obtaining serum for iPTH analysis can be performed after the veins have been identified during arteriography. The procedure is simple if a lesion has been identified by arteriography, since all that is required of iPTH analysis of the blood draining the lesion is confirmation that it is parathyroid in origin. If arteriography has not identified a lesion, all of the small veins should be entered and sampled. It is frequently difficult to obtain proper blood samples from small veins because the lumen may be obstructed by the catheter tip and because the sample may be diluted with blood from larger veins. It is important that a bioassay for PTH or a radioimmunoassay of PTH that recognizes only intact PTH (assays specific for the amino region or intact PTH) be used for measurements of iPTH in sera obtained during differential venous catheterization. Step-up differences in iPTH concentrations between peripheral sera and sera from veins draining parathyroid lesions are greater using such assays because of the relatively low concentrations of intact PTH in the peripheral circulation. By contrast, mid- and carboxyl-region specific assays measure the high concentrations of mid- and carboxyl-region fragments in the peripheral circulation and provide smaller step-up increases.

TREATMENT. The medical treatment of hypercalcemia is described in detail below ("Nonparathyroid Causes of Hypercalcemia"). The discussion here will be confined to the definitive treatment of hyperparathyroidism per se. The surgical removal of abnormal parathyroid tissue should be considered in all patients in whom the diagnosis of primary hyperparathyroidism has been established. Although patients with only biochemical abnormalities do not always develop clinically significant sequelae, they often do. Furthermore, the majority of these patients have histologic evidence of hyperparathyroidism in bone biopsies. This should be kept in mind before a long-term medical follow-up program is embarked upon, especially in older women who may have already suffered considerable bone loss as a result of age-related factors. Age per se should not be a contraindication to neck exploration. In fact, it is better to perform elective parathyroidectomy in an older person than to face hypercalcemia later as a complication of another age-related, serious illness (e.g., myocardial infarction).

If surgery is withheld and one embarks on following a patient who has hyperparathyroidism with only biochemical abnormalities, there remains a group of compelling indications for neck exploration: (1) radiographic evidence of metabolic bone disease, (2) demonstration of decreasing renal function, (3) active nephrolithiasis, (4) serum calcium concentrations greater than 11.0 mg per deciliter, and (5) the development of one or more "complications" of hyperparathyroidism, such as serious psychiatric disease, peptic ulcer that is resistant to treatment, pancreatitis, or severe hypertension. In any patient proposed for long-term follow-up, certain follow-up studies should be done systematically (Fig. 246–7). At a minimum, these should include a yearly history and physical examination, determinations of serum calcium and creatinine clearance, x-rays of the hand on fine grain industrial film to detect subperiosteal bone resorption, and a plain film of the abdomen to detect renal calcifications. If inactive nephrolithiasis has been detected on initial examination, nephrotomograms should be done to determine if new stones have developed or old stones have increased in size. By definition, either of these would be interpreted as the recrudescence of active stone disease, which would in turn be an indication for surgery.

The most critical consideration in the surgical treatment of patients with primary hyperparathyroidism is the selection of the surgeon. He should not only have extensive experience in parathyroid surgery but also be able to recognize an abnormal, enlarged parathyroid gland—a difficult skill to attain. The surgeon usually attempts to identify all four parathyroid glands (using biopsy if absolutely necessary), with the plan of removing a single enlarged parathyroid gland or three and one half parathyroid glands if multiple glands are involved. Less commonly, one side of the neck is explored first and any single enlarged parathyroid gland is removed. If the second parathyroid gland on the same side is normal, the other side of the neck is not explored. If the second parathyroid gland is abnormal, it is removed and the other side of the neck is explored and all the parathyroid tissue removed except for one half of a gland. The second approach has the advantage of leaving the unoperated side without scar tissue and easier to explore at a future time for recurrent hyperparathyroidism, but has the disadvantage of not firmly establishing whether multiple glands are enlarged.

Autotransplantation of parathyroid tissue to the muscles of the forearm may be of considerable value in special circumstances, such as when the last known parathyroid gland is removed because of recurrent primary hyperparathyroidism. Such patients are likely to be rendered hypoparathyroid without successful transplantation. The functioning of such transplants can be easily assessed by determining if there is a step-up in the concentration of parathyroid hormone in venous blood from the ipsilateral forearm in comparison with the other forearm.

Approximately 20 per cent of abnormal parathyroid glands are in the mediastinum, but the great majority of these (approximately 95 per cent) are high enough that they can be readily identified and removed during routine neck exploration. In the remaining cases abnormal parathyroid tissue is located elsewhere in the mediastinum and can be approached for excision only by splitting the sternum. Before the advent of localization procedures (see above), the success rate in removing abnormal parathyroid tissue from the mediastinum was only 50 per cent. The decision to carry out mediastinal exploration depends to a large extent on the accuracy and completeness of the information obtained during initial neck exploration. If the exploration was inadequate or the records are incomplete, neck surgery probably should be repeated.

Postoperatively, serum calcium concentrations decrease to within the normal range or below within 24 to 48 hours. It is possible to determine if all of the abnormal parathyroid tissue has been removed by measuring urinary cyclic AMP (which should be decreased) within two hours of parathyroidectomy. Patients who have significant bony demineralization may develop significant hypocalcemia postoperatively, presumably owing to the avidity of demineralized bone for extracellular fluid calcium. This "hungry bone syndrome" can be distinguished from hypoparathyroidism by the absence of hyperphosphatemia and the presence of increased concentrations of serum iPTH. Treatment of this syndrome, which may be difficult, requires very large quantities of intravenous calcium given continuously by infusion and administration of calcium carbonate by mouth in doses of 1 to 5 grams per day, depending upon the serum calcium response. Administration of vitamin D (usually 50,000 to 100,000 units daily) is of equivocal value but should be given. The biologically active metabolite of vitamin D $1,25(OH)_2D$ may prove to be an effective therapeutic agent in the future.

Most patients who develop hypocalcemia and mild hyperphosphatemia have temporary hypoparathyroidism, as evidenced by low normal values for serum iPTH. A small percentage of these patients will develop permanent hypoparathyroidism requiring treatment (see below).

Worsening of renal function (either temporary or permanent), metabolic acidosis, hypomagnesemia, pancreatitis, and gout or pseudogout are other complications that may occur in the postoperative period. Deterioration in renal function should be anticipated in patients who have abnormal renal function preoperatively, and prophylactic mannitol infusions should be given early in the postoperative period to initiate an osmotic diuresis. Likewise, a flaring of gout or pseudogout should be anticipated in patients with intra-articular calcification or a history of prior arthritic attacks.

PROGNOSIS. The natural history of primary hyperparathyroidism is not known. This is because the majority of patients, once the diagnosis is established, are subjected to neck exploration and removal of the abnormal parathyroid glands and are cured.

A large proportion of patients have "biochemical" hyperparathyroidism—i.e., only a slightly increased serum calcium (10.1 to 11.0 mg per deciliter) and no clinical manifestations of the disease. In a large prospective study (150 patients), relatively few (10 to 30 per cent) progressed to a more severe form of the disease within five years. In this study, no clinical or biochemical abnormality was found to be predictive of such a progression.

It is presumed that patients with mild to moderately severe manifestations of primary hyperparathyroidism represent progression from a previously "biochemical" form of the disease. A relatively small portion of this group of patients also attains some degree of disease stability; some patients have been observed for as long as 10 to 15 years without apparent progression. Except for a very small number who progress to severe disease, the remaining patients in this group probably progress slowly in the signs and symptoms of the disease and suffer a gradual deterioration of renal function. Patients with severe primary hyperparathyroidism (serum calcium >15 mg per deciliter) will almost certainly die of their disease unless it is detected and appropriately treated.

Surgical resection of benign parathyroid lesions is generally curative in primary hyperparathyroidism. Recurrences are rare in patients who have single gland disease, but relatively common when multiple glands are involved. The calcium nephropathy of hyperparathyroidism may be irreversible; whether improvement in hypertension occurs after successful treatment of hyperparathyroidism has not been estabished. Active nephrolithiasis generally becomes inactive unless factors other than primary hyperparathyroidism are present to perpetuate this problem. There have been anecdotal reports that severe psychiatric symptoms may disappear after the removal of abnormal parathyroid glands. All but the more severe forms of osteitis fibrosa cystica demonstrate improvement within months of parathyroidectomy and essentially complete resolution within a year. At present it is not known if the surgical treatment of hyperparathyroidism in patients who also have postmenopausal or senile osteoporosis results in improvement of the osteopenic disease. However, this will be important to determine because as many as 8 to 10 per cent of patients with age-related osteopenia have increased circulating levels of immunoreactive parathyroid hormone and may suffer from some form of curable hyperparathyroidism.

Arnaud CD, Clark OH: Primary hyperparathyroidism. *In* Krieger DT, Bardin CW: Current Therapy in Endocrinology 1983–1984. Philadelphia and St. Louis, B. C. Decker, Inc., and C. V. Mosby Company, 1983, pp 277–282. *Review of the medical and surgical treatment of primary hyperparathyroidism.*

Benson RC Jr, Riggs BL, Pickard BM, Arnaud CD: Radioimmunoassay of parathyroid hormone in hypercalcemic patients with malignant disease. Am J Med 56:821,1974. *Prospective study of serum calcium and serum PTH in 108 unselected patients with the hypercalcemia of cancer and 87 patients with primary hyperparathyroidism. Cancer patients had a lower serum PTH for a given degree of hypercalcemia than did patients with primary hyperparathyroidism.*

Christensson T, Hellström K, Wengle B, Alveryd A, Wikland B: Prevalence of hypercalcemia in health screening in Stockholm. Acta Med Scand 200:131, 1976. *In this study at least 3 per cent of 15,903 residents of Stockholm (predominantly middle-aged) had "asymptomatic hypercalcemia" and, most probably, primary hyperparathyroidism.*

DeGroot LJ (ed.): Endocrinology. Vol 2. New York, Grune & Stratton, 1979, pp 693–737. *Extensive and inclusive review of primary hyperparathyroidism by internationally renowned experts. The subjects discussed include clinical features, differential diagnosis, parathyroid hormone radioimmunoassay, localizing techniques, medical management, and surgical management.*

Foley TP Jr, Harrison HC, Arnaud CD, Harrison HE: Familial benign hypercalcemia. J Pediatr 81:1060, 1972. *First description of the syndrome of familial benign hypercalcemia, or familial hypocalciuric hypercalcemia.*

Heath H III, Hodgson SF, Kennedy MA: Primary hyperparathyroidism: Incidence, morbidity and potential economic impact in a community. N Engl J Med 302:189, 1980. *Only available systematic, epidemiologic study of the incidence of primary hyperparathyroidism in a well-characterized general population.*

Reading CC, Carboneau JW, James EM, Karsell PR, Purnell DC, Grant CS, van Heerden JA: High-resolution parathyroid sonography. Am J Roentgenol 139:539,1982. *An evaluation of high-resolution ultrasonography in the localization of pathologic parathyroid tissue.*

Stark DD, Moss AW, Gooding GAW, Clark OH: Parathyroid scanning by computed tomography. Radiology 148:297,1983. *An evaluation of computed tomography in the localization of pathologic parathyroid tissue.*

HYPOPARATHYROIDISM

DEFINITION. Hypoparathyroidism, or deficient secretion of parathyroid hormone, is characterized clinically by symptoms of neuromuscular hyperactivity and biochemically by hypocalcemia, hyperphosphatemia, and diminished to absent levels of circulating immunoreactive parathyroid hormone.

ETIOLOGY. There are three types of hypoparathyroidism: surgically induced, idiopathic, and functional. *Surgically induced hypoparathyroidism,* the most common of these, may occur after any surgical procedure in which the anterior neck is explored, including thyroidectomy, removal of abnormal parathyroid glands, and excision of various malignant lesions in the neck. Parathyroid glands need not actually be removed for hypoparathyroidism to ensue. In such cases it is presumed that the blood supply to the parathyroid glands has been compromised.

Idiopathic hypoparathyroidism occurs spontaneously and can be categorized according to whether it appears early or late in life. Aside from congenital absence of the glands, as in DiGeorge's syndrome (see Ch. 429), the syndromes occurring at an early age are genetic and are transmitted most frequently as an autosomal recessive trait. This type of hypoparathyroidism is called multiple endocrine deficiency–autoimmune–candidiasis (MEDAC) syndrome or juvenile familial endocrinopathy–hypoparathyroidism–Addison's disease–moniliasis (HAM) syndrome. Hypoparathyroidism, Addison's disease, and mucocutaneous candidiasis characterize the disorder. Circulating antibodies specific for parathyroid and adrenal tissues are frequently present, but they correlate poorly with clinical manifestations. Sporadic cases of MEDAC syndrome have been reported, as well as cases that have an autosomal recessive mode of inheritance. The majority of these are generally seen at a later age, and some have hypoparathyroidism only. This syndrome is described in Ch. 240. The late onset form of idiopathic hypoparathyroidism occurs sporadically and circulating glandular antibodies are absent. The cause of parathyroid gland destruction in these cases is unknown.

Functional hypoparathyroidism occurs in patients with severe and prolonged hypomagnesemia of whatever cause (see Ch. 208). Since magnesium is required for release of parathyroid hormone from the glands, serum iPTH is characteristically low or undetectable in this syndrome. Infusion of magnesium increases serum iPTH rapidly (within minutes), and restoration of magnesium to normal levels ultimately restores eucalcemia. Magnesium is probably also required for the peripheral action of parathyroid hormone; the hypocalcemia in patients with functional hypoparathyroidism may be due, in part, to the failure of PTH to act normally on its target tissues.

Neonatal hypoparathyroidism occurs in infants of mothers who have primary hyperparathyroidism. It is presumed that in utero exposure to maternal hypercalcemia results in prolonged suppression of fetal parathyroid glands and failure of the parathyroid glands to respond to hypocalcemic stimuli after birth.

PATHOLOGY. Patients with MEDAC syndrome may have lymphocytic infiltration and fibrosis of glands. In the few patients with late onset idiopathic hypoparathyroidism who have been examined, fatty infiltration, fibrosis, and atrophy have been found. Longstanding cases of hypoparathyroidism have characteristic soft tissue calcifications in the lens and basal ganglia of the brain. All types of bone cells are diminished, and both formation and resorption surfaces in bone are decreased.

PATHOPHYSIOLOGY AND CLINICAL CHEMISTRY. The pathophysiology and biochemical consequences of parathyroid gland removal can be appreciated by referring to the "butterfly" diagram (Fig. 243–1). In hypoparathyroidism the right limbs of the three feedback loops predominate. There is (1) decreased bone resorption; (2) decreased renal phosphate excretion, increased serum phosphate, decreased $1,25(OH)_2D$, and decreased intestinal absorption of calcium; and (3) increased excretion of calcium for the prevailing serum concentration of calcium. Patients have hypocalcemia and generally hyperphosphatemia, provided that dietary phosphate has been normal. Urinary calcium is usually low unless eucalcemia has been restored with treatment. In that case, urinary calcium is generally inappropriately high for the level of serum calcium and occasionally reaches hypercalciuric levels. Nephrogenous cyclic AMP is decreased but increases briskly with the administration of parathyroid hormone.

Hypocalcemia and mild alkalosis (resulting from decreased bicarbonate excretion), if sufficiently severe, cause increased neuromuscular excitability with consequent tetany and, rarely, convulsions.

CLINICAL MANIFESTATIONS. The clinical manifestations of hypoparathyroidism depend upon the severity of the disease (degree of hypocalcemia) and its chronicity. The rate of decrease in the serum calcium appears to be a major determinant in the development of the neuromuscular complications (see below) of hypocalcemia. Thus, these symptoms are more likely to occur within one to two days after parathyroidectomy, when serum calcium decreases acutely, and at serum calcium values that may be considerably higher (e.g., 8.0 mg per deciliter) than might be found in patients who have had more severe hypocalcemia (e.g., 6.0 mg per deciliter) for a longer time. It is therefore important to observe patients carefully for the development of the clinical signs heralding tetany, immediately and for several days after neck surgery, in the region of the parathyroid glands, rather than relying entirely on the absolute concentration of the serum calcium.

Hypocalcemia causes a decreased threshold of excitation, repetitive responses to a single stimulus, reduced accommodation, and, at the extreme, continuous activity of nervous tissues. Such neural activity occurs spontaneously in both sensory and motor fibers in hypocalcemic states and gives rise to neuromuscular symptoms and signs. Symptoms include numbness and tingling around the mouth, in the tips of the fingers, and sometimes in the feet. An attack of tetany usually begins with this prodrome and is followed by muscle spasms in the extremities and face. The hands, forearms, and, less commonly, feet become contorted in a characteristic way (Fig. 246–10). First, the thumb is strongly adducted, followed by flexion of the metacarpophalangeal joints, extension of the

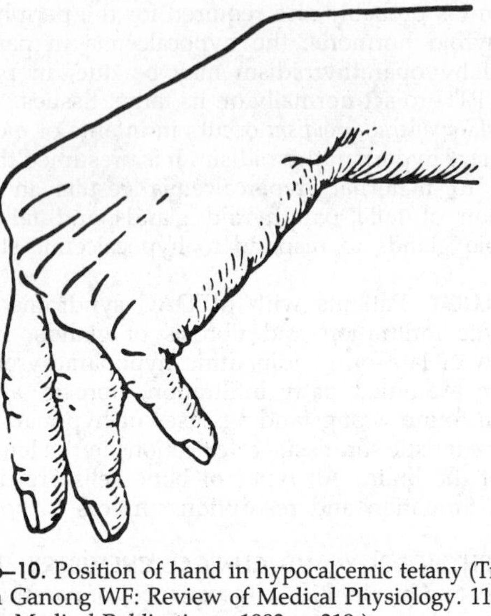

Figure 246–10. Position of hand in hypocalcemic tetany (Trousseau's sign). (From Ganong WF: Review of Medical Physiology. 11th ed. Los Altos, Lange Medical Publications, 1983, p 319.)

interphalangeal joints (with fingers together), and flexion of the wrist and elbow joints. This somewhat grotesque spastic condition may be quite painful but is more alarming than dangerous. Because of its alarming quality, patients may hyperventilate and secrete more epinephrine. Hyperventilation causes hypocapnia and alkalosis and worsens hypocalcemia by increasing the binding of ionic calcium to plasma proteins. Increased epinephrine secretion produces further anxiety, tachycardia, sweating, and peripheral and circumoral pallor. Prolonged hyperventilation in normal subjects can lower serum ionic calcium and produce tetany, but great care should be exercised in attributing such findings to hyperventilation alone.

Patients with hypoparathyroidism may have convulsions, especially during childhood. A more generalized form of tetany may be followed by prolonged tonic spasms, or the patient may have a typical epileptiform seizure (grand mal, jacksonian, focal, or petit mal), with characteristic associated electroencephalographic (EEG) findings. Because restoration of eucalcemia results in a decrease in the number of seizures without improvement in the EEG findings associated with seizures, it is thought that hypocalcemia lowers the excitation threshold of pre-existing epilepsy in such patients. The characteristic EEG changes associated with hypocalcemia per se do disappear after restoration of eucalcemia. Laryngeal spasm and stridor may occur during tetany and may precipitate seizures because of hypoxia. The relatively unusual finding of papilledema and increased intracranial pressure resulting from hypocalcemia in association with convulsions may suggest the diagnosis of brain tumor.

Latent tetany can be detected by several relatively specific physical signs. *Chvostek's sign* is elicited by tapping the facial nerve just anterior to the ear lobe, just below the zygomatic arch, or between the zygomatic arch and the corner of the mouth. The response ranges from twitching of the lip at the corner of the mouth to twitching of all of the facial muscles on the stimulated side. Simple twitching at the corner of the mouth occurs in 25 per cent of normal subjects, but more extensive muscle contraction (ala nasi and orbital muscles) is a reliable sign of latent tetany.

Trousseau's sign is demonstrated with a sphygmomanometer cuff inflated about the arm to above the systolic blood pressure for at least two minutes. A positive response consists of the development of typical ipsilateral carpal spasm (Fig. 246–10), with relaxation only occurring five to ten seconds after the cuff is deflated. Apparent spasm disappearing instantly should be regarded with suspicion. Trousseau's sign is the most reliable physical finding of latent tetany, and serial tests for this sign should be done and the results recorded in the immediate postoperative period after anterior neck surgery.

Beyond the neurologic manifestations described above, there are a number of other possible manifestations of hypocalcemia: (1) basal ganglia calcification and occasional extrapyramidal neurologic syndromes; (2) papilledema and increased intracranial pressure; (3) psychiatric disorders; (4) skin, hair, and fingernail abnormalities; (5) susceptibility to *Candida* infections; (6) inhibition of normal dental development; (7) lenticular cataracts; (8) intestinal malabsorption; (9) prolongation of the Q-T_c and S-T intervals of the electrocardiogram, in rare cases 2:1 heart block, and even more rarely heart failure requiring digitalis and diuretics; and (10) increased serum concentrations of creatine phosphokinase and lactic dehydrogenase.

Extrapyramidal neurologic syndromes, including classic parkinsonism, may occur in patients with chronic hypoparathyroidism. Such manifestations are presumably caused by the basal ganglia calcification observed in the majority of such patients. Many untreated patients without extrapyramidal syndromes are unduly sensitive to the dystonic side effects of phenothiazine drugs, suggesting that calcification of the ganglia may have more general pathologic importance than was once believed. Treatment of hypocalcemia usually improves the neurologic disorder, and decreases in basal ganglia calcification have been documented radiologically.

Psychiatric disorders occur but are unusual in defined populations of hypoparathyroid patients. Mental retardation occurs in about 20 per cent of children with the disease, but this condition improves with restoration of eucalcemia in some. Tooth development is impaired in many children with the disease; hypoplasia of enamel, increased susceptibility to caries, delayed eruption, gaps between the teeth, and dysplastic dentin have been observed.

Lenticular cataracts are the most common sequelae of hypoparathyroidism. Visual impairment is observed only after five to ten years of cataract development. Fully mature cataracts in hypoparathyroidism are confluent and produce total opacity of the lens. Such cataracts are different from senile cataracts, which are frequently confined to one segment of the lens. Successful treatment of hypocalcemia generally halts the progress of cataracts, and, rarely, opacities may diminish in size.

The skin of patients with longstanding hypoparathyroidism may be dry and scaling, the nails ridged longitudinally, and the hair coarse, dry, friable, and falling. An occasional patient will suffer exfoliative dermatitis or atopic eczema, and existing psoriasis may be made worse. All of these lesions tend to improve and disappear with restoration of eucalcemia. *Candida* infections can complicate skin, nail, and hair abnormalities. They also improve with treatment of hypocalcemia but may require specific antifungal therapy as well.

Intestinal malabsorption with steatorrhea occurs in rare cases of longstanding untreated hypoparathyroidism. The disorder is presumed to be due to decreased serum calcium because it is reversed by successful treatment of hypocalcemia but not by a gluten-free diet. The problem is particularly difficult to manage because the treatment of hypoparathyroidism largely depends upon the ability to increase calcium transport across a normal gastrointestinal tract with drugs. Conversely, malabsorption may cause functional hypoparathyroidism by producing magnesium deficiency.

Hypocalcemia causes prolongation of the Q-T_c interval in the electrocardiogram, but clinical cardiac abnormalities are rare in hypoparathyroidism. Congestive heart failure, requiring digitalis and diuretics, has been reported, but this condition usually reverses following successful treatment of hypocalcemia.

DIAGNOSIS. The detection of hypoparathyroidism depends upon maintaining a high index of suspicion in certain clinical situations. Serum calcium should be measured yearly in patients who have had anterior neck surgery or who are suspected of having the MEDAC syndrome. Cutaneous candidiasis, cataracts, incidental discovery of basal ganglia calcification, convulsions, numbness and tingling of the fingers, facial muscle spasm (spontaneous or self-induced), delayed dentition, and developmental retardation should all prompt serum calcium measurement.

In the absence of renal failure, the diagnosis of hypoparathyroidism is virtually certain if hypocalcemia and hyperphosphatemia are found. However, some patients may be actually relatively depleted in phosphate because of dietary restriction or the ingestion of aluminum hydroxide gels. In addition, in patients who have undergone parathyroidectomy for primary hyperparathyroidism, bone uptake of minerals may be so great as to produce hypophosphatemia (the "hungry bone syndrome"). The measurement of serum iPTH is crucial for diagnosis. Increased values in a range appropriate to the degree of hypocalcemia would essentially exclude the presence of hypoparathyroidism and suggest the possibility of end-organ resistance to parathyroid hormone (i.e., pseudohypoparathyroidism [see below], vitamin D deficiency, and vitamin D dependency) or secondary hypoparathyroidism resulting from such disorders as dietary deficiency of calcium, intestinal malabsorption of calcium, or excessive intake of drugs containing absorbable phosphate.

Undetectable serum iPTH confirms the diagnosis of hypoparathyroidism, provided that the assay used is sufficiently sensitive to measure serum iPTH in the large majority of normal subjects. Serum iPTH may be barely detectable in some patients with hypoparathyroidism if the assay employed is very sensitive, but such low values may be due to nonspecific effects of serum per se in radioimmunoassays that do not adequately control for this factor.

Patients with functional hypoparathyroidism resulting from hypomagnesemia also have low to undetectable levels of serum iPTH. Detection of this condition depends upon the measurement of serum magnesium and its diagnosis upon the demonstration that successful treatment with magnesium salts restores eucalcemia and increases serum iPTH (see Ch. 208).

TREATMENT. Theoretically, the most appropriate therapy for hypoparathyroidism would be the physiologic replacement of parathyroid hormone. This approach is impractical at present because the hormone must be administered parenterally and because synthetic human parathyroid hormone is too expensive. Such treatment might become practical in the future for some patients who are poorly controlled on conventional regimens.

Because of the absence of parathyroid hormone and the consequent hyperphosphatemia, the renal enzyme that converts 25OHD to $1,25(OH)_2D$, 1α-hydroxylase, is relatively inactive in patients with hypoparathyroidism. Conversion of circulating 25OHD to $1,25(OH)_2D$ is poor, and serum levels of this most active vitamin D metabolite are low or undetectable. In fact, hypoparathyroid patients are resistant to pharmacologic quantities of vitamin D for this reason.

The lowering of serum phosphate levels, using diets low in phosphate (i.e., restricting dairy products and meat) and oral aluminum hydroxide gels to bind intestinal phosphate, might be expected to increase the conversion of 25OHD to $1,25(OH)_2D$, but such treatment has received little attention. Rather, treatment with pharmacologic doses of vitamin D_2 or its more potent analogue, dihydrotachysterol, in combination with oral calcium, has been the mainstay regimen for many years. Unfortunately, unpredictable hypercalcemic episodes sometimes occur with this therapeutic regimen unless serum calcium is monitored at least once per month. A single episode of vitamin D intoxication can irreversibly impair renal function and can last from weeks to months because the body stores vitamin D and its metabolite 25OHD. The treatment of the vitamin D intoxication is similar to that described for severe hypercalcemia (see below), but with the additional use of corticosteroids (60 mg of prednisone or 300 mg of cortisone in four divided doses per day), which appear to antagonize vitamin D action.

Tetany caused by hypoparathyroidism requires emergency treatment with intravenous calcium to prevent laryngeal stridor and convulsions, the occurrence of which cannot be predicted.

A 10 per cent solution of calcium gluconate (10 to 20 ml) should be given slowly (not more than 10 ml per minute) intravenously until symptoms are relieved or until serum calcium rises above 7 mg per deciliter. Hypercalcemia should be avoided; maintaining calcium levels between 7.5 and 9.0 mg per deciliter is adequate. Caution should be exercised in patients taking digitalis because calcium potentiates the action of this drug on the heart. Electrocardiographic monitoring during intravenous administration of calcium is prudent. It may be necessary to maintain serum calcium at levels that prevent tetany for several days before treatment with vitamin D or its metabolites or analogues (see below) becomes effective. This is accomplished by combining oral with intravenous calcium administration. Oral calcium is begun as soon as possible, starting with 200 mg of elemental calcium (as the gluconate or chloride salt) every two hours, increasing to 500 mg with each dose. If serum calcium falls below 7.5 mg per deciliter after six hours of the combined intravenous and oral regimen, continuous calcium infusion should be started. Five hundred ml of 5 per cent glucose and water containing 10 ml of 10 per cent calcium gluconate (1 gram) is given over six hours initially, with the quantity of calcium increased in increments of 5 ml (0.5 grams) every six hours until satisfactory control is achieved. In patients with hyperparathyroidism and bone disease who have undergone successful excision of a hyperfunctioning parathyroid gland(s), hypocalcemia may be profound and extremely resistant to treatment. As much as 10 grams of elemental calcium administered intravenously by infusion over 24 hours may be required to increase serum calcium above 7.5 mg per deciliter. Such patients are notoriously resistant to vitamin D.

Most patients with severe hypoparathyroidism require some form of long-term treatment with vitamin D. An effective regimen is as follows: dihydrotachysterol, 4 mg per day for two days, then 2 mg per day for two days, then 1 mg per day until dose adjustment is required, as judged by serum calcium values. Ideally, serum calcium should be maintained between 8.5 and 9.0 mg per deciliter, leaving a margin for the calcium to fluctuate upward to levels that are still not dangerous. The major advantage of dihydrotachysterol is its relatively rapid onset of action and short half-life. With regard to the latter, hypercalcemia caused by inadvertent overdosage is relieved within one to three weeks after the drug is discontinued; in comparison, the hypercalcemic effects of overdoses of vitamin D persist for 6 to 18 weeks. Dihydrotachysterol offers another advantage in that parathyroid function can be tested fairly soon after withdrawal of the drug. Hypocalcemia occurring within two weeks of withdrawal proves the persistence of hypoparathyroidism. The disadvantage of dihydrotachysterol is its cost.

The only natural vitamin D preparation currently available for general clinical use is ergocalciferol, or vitamin D_2, which is derived from plant sources (vitamin D_3 is the naturally produced compound in humans). In initiating vitamin D_2 therapy, the development of hypercalcemia can best be avoided by giving small doses initially (0.2 mg [8,000 units] to 0.5 mg [20,000 units]), with gradual increases only after steady state levels of serum calcium are achieved at each dose level. Most patients can be managed successfully with 1.0 mg (40,000 units) to 3.0 mg (120,000 units) of vitamin D_2 daily. The occasional patient who requires more than 3.0 mg per day is a candidate for the shorter acting analogues or metabolites of vitamin D.

Relatively little information is now available concerning the long-term management of hypoparathyroidism with the vitamin D_3 metabolites 25-OH-D_3 (calcifediol) or $1,25(OH)_2D_3$ (calcitriol). Both appear to be biologically effective and superior to vitamin D_2 with respect to the rapidity of onset and termination of action. Neither seems to have major advantages over dihydrotachysterol, except in patients who are particularly difficult to manage. The initiation and termination of action appears to be faster for $1,25(OH)_2D_3$ than for dihydrotachysterol. Both metabolites are even more expensive than dihydrotachysterol.

Since vitamin D acts primarily to increase intestinal calcium absorption, dietary calcium must be adequate: an approximate total (dietary and supplemented) intake of 1.0 gram daily in patients under 40 and 2 grams in patients over 40. Supplements can be provided by administering calcium as the gluconate, chloride, or carbonate salt. There are disadvantages to each. Calcium gluconate tablets contain relatively small quantities of calcium (9 per cent by weight), so that a large number of tablets must be given. Calcium chloride tablets contain larger quantities of calcium (27 per cent) but tend to produce gastric irritation. Calcium carbonate tablets also contain large quantities of calcium (40 per cent) but tend to produce alkalosis, which may aggravate hypocalcemia.

Patients with milder hypoparathyroidism may require only calcium supplementation (1 to 5 grams daily) and moderate degrees of phosphate restriction (including aluminum hydroxide gels) to maintain serum calcium in a therapeutic range. This treatment should be tried whenever a successful outcome is thought to be possible in order to avoid vitamin D intoxication entirely.

Long-term restoration of serum calcium to normal or nearly normal levels usually results in improvement in most manifestations of surgical and idiopathic hypoparathyroidism, including the skin disorders and associated candidiasis. Unfortunately, the latter appears to persist in the MEDAC syndrome, and resolution usually can be achieved only with iodoquinol or with systemic amphotericin (alone or combined with transfer factor) therapy.

Hypercalciuria can complicate successful restoration of a normal plasma calcium owing to the absence of the influence of parathyroid hormone to maintain normal renal tubular reabsorption of calcium. Accurate measurement of 24-hour urine calcium is therefore mandatory as serum calcium approaches the normal range during calcium and vitamin D treatment in order to avert possible renal stone formation. Thiazide diuretics, which cause increased renal tubular reabsorption of calcium, may be useful in such patients and may have the added advantage of partially restoring eucalcemia as a result of this action.

Anast CS, Mohs JM, Kaplan SL, Burns TW: Evidence for parathyroid failure in magnesium deficiency. Science 177:606, 1972. *First definitive demonstration of functional hypoparathyroidism in a magnesium-deficient patient with a selective intestinal defect in the absorption of magnesium.*

Attie JM, Kafif RA: Preservation of parathyroid glands during total thyroidectomy. Improved techniques utilizing microsurgery. Am J Surg 130:399, 1975. *Describes techniques in thyroid surgery that should help prevent destruction of the parathyroid glands and consequent hypoparathyroidism.*

Avioli LV: The therapeutic approach to hypoparathyroidism. Am J Med 57:34, 1974. *An important review of the problems encountered in the treatment of hypoparathyroidism.*

Harrison HE, Lifshitz F, Blizzard RM: Comparison between crystalline dihydrotachysterol and calciferol in patients requiring pharmacologic vitamin D therapy. N Engl J Med 276:894, 1967. *A classic review of the relative merits of vitamin D and dihydrotachysterol in the treatment of vitamin D resistant states, including hypoparathyroidism.*

Hunt G, Morgan DB: The early effects of dihydrotachysterol on calcium and phosphorus metabolism in patients with hypoparathyroidism. Clin Sci 38:713, 1970. *A careful evaluation of the effects of dihydrotachysterol in patients with hypoparathyroidism.*

Neer RM, Holick MF, DeLuca HF, Potts JT Jr: Effects of 1α-hydroxyvitamin D_3 and $1,25(OH)_2D_3$ on calcium and phosphorus metabolism in hypoparathyroidism. Metabolism 24:1403, 1975. *These authors investigated the acute effects of 1αOHD₃ and 1,25(OH)₂D₃ in five patients with surgical hypoparathyroidism and found that these compounds are rapid acting. Since urinary hydroxyproline levels did not increase, they concluded that these compounds act on the intestine rather than on bone to increase serum calcium.*

Nusynowitz ML, Frame B, Kolb FO: The spectrum of the hypoparathyroid states: A classification based on physiologic principles. Medicine 55:105, 1976. *Broad and in-depth evaluation of all forms of hypoparathyroidism.*

Parfitt AM: The incidence of hypoparathyroid tetany after thyroid operations. Relationship to age, extent of resection and surgical experience. Med J Aust 1:1103, 1971. *Detailed compilation of the factors involved in the production of hypoparathyroidism resulting from thyroidectomy.*

Parfitt AM: The spectrum of hypoparathyroidism. J Clin Endocrinol Metab 34:152, 1972. *This detailed analysis of serum calcium values in hypoparathyroid patients formed the basis for the author's classification of the severity of the disease.*

Parfitt AM: Adult hypoparathyroidism. Treatment with calcifediol. Arch Intern Med 138:874, 1978. *A systematic study of the therapeutic efficacy of 25OHD in hypoparathyroid patients for a total of 19 patient-years.*

Parfitt AM: Surgical, idiopathic, and other varieties of parathyroid hormone–deficient hypoparathyroidism. *In* DeGroot LJ (ed.): Endocrinology. Vol 2. New York, Grune & Stratton, 1979, pp 755–768. *Comprehensive review of parathyroid hormone–deficient hypoparathyroidism.*

PSEUDOHYPOPARATHYROIDISM AND PSEUDOPSEUDOHYPOPARATHYROIDISM

DEFINITIONS. *Pseudohypoparathyroidism* describes a rare clinical state of hypoparathyroidism that results from target tissue resistance to parathyroid hormone, associated with a secondary, hypocalcemia–induced increase in parathyroid gland function. Patients with pseudohypoparathyroidism classically have a variety of congenital defects in growth and skeletal development, including short stature and foreshortened metacarpal and metatarsal bones (Fig. 246–11). Patients with *pseudopseudohypoparathyroidism* have analogous developmental defects without clinical hypoparathyroidism. Some patients with pseudohypoparathyroidism have target tissue resistance to the hormone but no developmental abnormalities, and others with developmental abnormalities have spontaneous remission of clinical hypoparathyroidism. Very rarely, patients have developmental abnormalities and clinical hypoparathyroidism with typical osteitis fibrosa cystica, a syndrome described by the barbarism "pseudohyperhypoparathyroidism."

ETIOLOGY AND GENETICS. It is difficult to conceive that all these combinations of manifestations could be ascribed to a single underlying biochemical defect. Although abnormal target tissue responses to parathyroid hormone may be the underlying theme, it is likely that an array of separate, rate-limiting steps, from receptor binding of parathyroid hormone to final expression of the cellular actions of the hormone (see Fig. 246–5) could be involved.

In some patients with pseudohypoparathyroidism, the guanyl nucleotide–sensitive regulatory protein (N protein), which couples parathyroid hormone–occupied receptors to adenylate cyclase, is decreased by 50 per cent in the red blood cells (see Fig. 246–5). In such patients this defect appears to produce resistance to several other hormones that apparently exert their actions by stimulating the increased production of cellular cyclic AMP (e.g., vasopressin and glucagon). Other possible mechanisms, as yet largely untested, include the secretion of a biologically inert form of parathyroid hormone, an intrinsic abnormality of parathyroid hormone receptors, autoantibodies to the parathyroid hormone receptor, a defect in adenylate cyclase, a disturbance in the process by which parathyroid hormone alters the distribution of ions across membranes, abnormalities of cellular protein kinases or other hormone-dependent enzymes, or gross cellular abnormalities that permit all of the actions of the hormone except the actual transfer of minerals from the cell to the blood.

Patients with pseudohypoparathyroidism generally fail to respond normally to the administration of large doses of parathyroid hormone with an increase in urinary phosphate excretion and nephrogenous cyclic AMP. A few have normal cyclic AMP responses but diminished phosphate responses, whereas others may have the reverse. The implication is that cyclic AMP may not be involved in the biologic actions of PTH. However, these results can be explained by several alternative explanations, including the possibility that urinary excretion of cyclic AMP does not accurately reflect all of the cyclic AMP–related cellular events critical to parathyroid hormone action and that only small changes in intracellular cyclic AMP are required for parathyroid hormone action.

Levels of $1,25(OH)_2D$ have been reported to be low in pseudohypoparathyroidism, and, because of this, defective conversion of 25OHD to $1,25(OH)_2D$ has been suggested as the mechanism involved in the abnormal mineral homeostasis in these patients. Support for this argument is derived from the success achieved in restoring serum calcium and urinary phosphate excretion to normal levels with $1,25(OH)_2D$ administration in patients with pseudohypoparathyroidism. Again, alter-

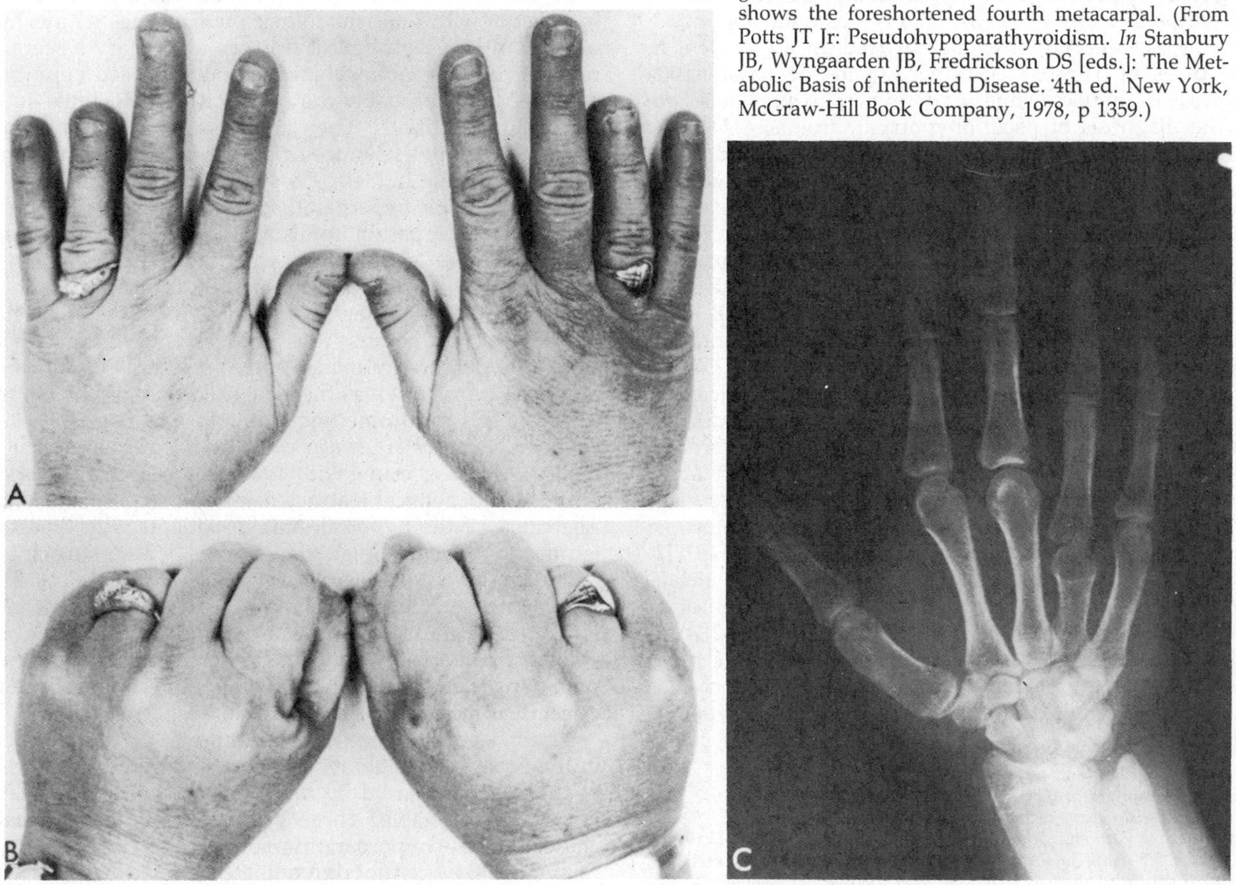

Figure 246–11. Hands of patient with pseudohypoparathyroidism. *A,* Note the shortened fourth finger. *B,* Note the "absent" fourth knuckle. *C,* Film shows the foreshortened fourth metacarpal. (From Potts JT Jr: Pseudohypoparathyroidism. *In* Stanbury JB, Wyngaarden JB, Fredrickson DS [eds.]: The Metabolic Basis of Inherited Disease. 4th ed. New York, McGraw-Hill Book Company, 1978, p 1359.)

native explanations for these observations are not only possible but likely. Increased renal tubular cyclic AMP may be involved in the stimulation of 1-α hydroxylation of 25OHD. If this is true, normal tissue responsiveness to parathyroid hormone may be necessary for the production of 1,25$(OH)_2$D. This would account for the low levels of serum 1,25$(OH)_2$D found in pseudohypoparathyroidism. Likewise, 1,25$(OH)_2$D might be expected to improve the responsiveness of bone to parathyroid hormone in patients with deficient production of 1,25$(OH)_2$D simply because the hypercalcemic action of parathyroid hormone depends upon the presence of biologically active metabolites of vitamin D. Finally, the phosphaturia induced in pseudohypoparathyroidism by 1,25$(OH)_2$D administration could be due to the restoration of eucalcemia; it is well known that phosphaturia occurs when the serum calcium is restored to normal in patients with surgical hypoparathyroidism.

Although pseudohypoparathyroidism is inherited, the mode of its transmission is unclear. A sex-linked dominant mechanism is possible, since there is a female-to-male ratio of 2:1 for the disease. It is difficult to explain how the developmental defects of pseudohypoparathyroidism can be inherited without abnormalities occurring in the adenylate cyclase system. Furthermore, four cases of male-to-male transmission of the developmental defects have been recorded.

PATHOPHYSIOLOGY AND CLINICAL CHEMISTRY. The biochemical findings in patients with pseudohypoparathyroidism are identical to those observed in patients with surgical or idiopathic hypoparathyroidism, except that serum iPTH is increased appropriately for the degree of hypocalcemia. The pathophysiology of the disease can be visualized best by referring to Figure 246–1. Parathyroid hormone action is blocked in all three of the left limbs of the feedback loops. The result in the right limbs is (1) decreased bone resorption caused by decreased bone cell responsiveness to parathyroid hormone; (2) increased serum phosphate caused by decreased renal tubular responsiveness to the phosphaturic action of PTH, which in turn decreases production of 1,25$(OH)_2$D and intestinal calcium absorption; and (3) increased renal excretion of calcium for the degree of hypocalcemia, which is caused again by decreased renal tubular responsiveness to the hypocalciuric effects of parathyroid hormone. The consequent hypocalcemia stimulates parathyroid hormone secretion.

PATHOLOGY. In patients who are hypocalcemic, the parathyroid glands are hyperplastic. Aside from the unique developmental abnormalities noted under Clinical Manifestations, below, the findings are the same as in surgical hypoparathyroidism.

CLINICAL MANIFESTATIONS. Most of the symptoms and signs of pseudohypoparathyroidism are the same as those of surgical and idiopathic hypoparathyroidism, and are due almost entirely to hypocalcemia. However, there are certain unique developmental features. Many patients are mentally retarded, have short stocky builds, are obese, have rounded faces, and display one or more short metacarpal or metatarsal bones. A classic sign of the brachymetacarpia, usually most marked in the fourth and fifth metacarpals, is the formation of a dimple over the head of the involved metacarpals when the patient makes a fist (Fig. 246–11). The fingers may be foreshortened. The calvarium is thickened in one third of patients, and there may be delayed dentition, defective enamel, and absence of teeth. There also may be exostoses, coxa vara, coxa valga, and bowing of the radius, tibia, and fibula.

DIAGNOSIS. The diagnosis of pseudohypoparathyroidism or pseudopseudohypoparathyroidism is likely when the described developmental abnormalities are discovered. When normal serum calcium and phosphorus are found in such a patient, the diagnosis of pseudopseudohypoparathyroidism is almost certain, although many of the same developmental abnormalities seen in pseudopseudohypoparathyroidism are present in unusual cases of Turner's, Gardner's, and the basal nevus syndromes. If hypocalcemia and hyperphosphatemia are found, the diagnosis of pseudohypoparathyroidism is highly likely. Increased serum iPTH and markedly diminished phosphaturic and nephrogenous cyclic AMP responses to parathyroid hormone distinguish pseudohypoparathyroidism from surgical, idiopathic, and functional hypoparathyroidism in patients with equivocal signs of the developmental abnormalities. If serum phosphorus is normal or low in such patients, secondary hyperparathyroidism resulting from vitamin D deficiency, dietary calcium deficiency, or intestinal malabsorption of calcium must be excluded. Measurement of serum 25OHD should help determine the presence of vitamin D deficiency, and dietary history or analysis, the presence of dietary calcium deficiency. The third underlying cause, intestinal malabsorption of calcium, may present difficulties because hypocalcemia per se may produce malabsorption (see above), and, unless magnesium deficiency is present, patients with intrinsic intestinal malabsorption usually have increased levels of serum iPTH. Therapeutic tests may be needed. When treatment of malabsorption with a gluten-free diet restores eucalcemia, the diagnosis is probably gluten-sensitive enteropathy (see Ch. 103). If correction of hypocalcemia with a regimen used in the treatment of hypoparathyroidism cures the malabsorption syndrome, the underlying diagnosis is probably pseudohypoparathyroidism.

Albright F, Burnett CH, Smith PH, Parson W: Pseudohypoparathyroidism—an example of "Seabright-Bantam syndrome." Endocrinology 30:922, 1942. *First description of pseudohypoparathyroidism.*

Chase LR, Melson GL, Aurbach GD: Pseudohypoparathyroidism: Defective excretion of 3′5′-AMP in response to parathyroid hormone. J Clin Invest 48:1832, 1969. *First demonstration of renal blockade of parathyroid hormone–stimulated cyclic AMP excretion in pseudohypoparathyroidism.*

Drezner MK, Burch WM: Altered activity of the nucleotide regulatory site in the parathyroid hormone-sensitive adenylate cyclase from the renal cortex of a patient with pseudohypoparathyroidism. J Clin Invest 62:1222, 1978. *Demonstration that the addition of GTP to renal cortical membranes from a patient with pseudohypoparathyroidism restores their sensitivity to parathyroid hormone stimultion of adenylate cyclase in vitro. These results suggest that the molecular defect in some patients with this disease may be an abnormality of the regulatory protein that couples parathyroid hormone to adenylate cyclase.*

Farfel Z, Brickman AS, Kaslow HR, Brothers VM, Bourne HR: Defect of receptor-cyclase coupling protein in pseudohypoparathyroidism. N Engl J Med 303:237, 1980. Levine MA, Downs RW Jr, Singer M, Marx SJ, Aurbach GD, Speigel AM: Deficient activity of guanine nucleotide regulatory protein in erythrocytes from patients with pseudohypoparathyroidism. Biochem Biophys Res Commun 94:1319, 1980. *The work described in these two papers was done simultaneously and independently by two different groups. The results are essentially the same: the activity of the guanyl nucleotide regulatory protein in the red blood cell membranes of some patients with pseudohypoparathyroidism was significantly reduced. Taken with the results of the study by Drezner and Burch (see above), they support the hypothesis that deficient activity of this protein is the molecular basis for hormone resistance in some patients with this inherited disorder.*

Potts JT Jr.: Pseudohypoparathyroidism. *In* DeGroot LJ (ed.): Endocrinology. Vol 2. New York, Grune & Stratton, 1979, pp 769–776. *Comprehensive review of pseudohypoparathyroidism.*

HYPERCALCEMIA AND ITS TREATMENT

Many diseases and conditions of nonparathyroid origin are associated with hypercalcemia (Table 246–1). Malignancy-associated hypercalcemia and familial hypocalciuric hypercalcemia are discussed extensively in relation to the differential diagnosis of primary hyperparathyroidism (see above), because these disorders frequently resemble primary hyperparathyroidism in their clinical presentation and biochemical characteristics. This section will describe the spectrum of disorders that can produce hypercalcemia by mechanisms unrelated to parathyroid hormone (these are listed in Table 246–1 under the category of hypercalcemia "not due to increased serum PTH"). This section will also discuss the medical treatment of hypercalcemia, whether of parathyroid or nonparathyroid origin.

Nonparathyroid Causes of Hypercalcemia

Malignancy

As discussed above, the underlying cause of hypercalcemia in patients with nonhematologic malignancies who exhibit the other common biochemical features of primary hyperparathyroidism (i.e., hypophosphatemia and increased nephrogenous cyclic AMP) is probably the secretion of a PTH-like substance by malignant tissue. The cancers that are most commonly associated with this syndrome are bronchogenic carcinoma and carcinoma of the kidney. Thus, although not strictly accurate, the term "ectopic hyperparathyroidism" has been used (as well as pseudohyperparathyroidism) to segregate these patients from those with malignancy-associated hypercalcemia who do not have hypophosphatemia and increased nephrogenous cyclic AMP. This segregation appears to be justified on therapeutic grounds because the hypercalcemia in patients with ectopic hyperparathyroidism rarely responds to corticosteroid administration, whereas the hypercalcemia in patients who do not have this syndrome frequently does respond.

Carcinoma of the breast accounts for approximately half of the malignancies associated with hypercalcemia. It is not associated with the biochemical features of ectopic hyperparathyroidism. The cause of the hypercalcemia in patients with breast cancer is uncertain. Many other solid tumors secrete substances that stimulate the cellular elements in bone to increase bone resorption. However, cultured breast cancer cells can increase the release of calcium from devitalized bone in vitro in a manner similar to osteoclasts. Thus, the direct interaction of tumor cells with bone (i.e., metastasis) may be required to produce hypercalcemia in patients with breast cancer.

Serum levels of phosphate are normal or slightly increased in hypercalcemic patients with breast cancer, and serum levels of iPTH (as measured by mid- or carboxyl-region assays) are low or undetectable. These biochemical findings usually exclude primary hyperparathyroidism as a cause of hypercalcemia, but they cannot differentiate between ectopic hyperparathyroidism and breast cancer associated with hypercalcemia. The measurement of nephrogenous cyclic AMP may be helpful in this regard. It is almost always increased in patients with the syndrome of ectopic hyperparathyroidism and normal or decreased in patients with breast cancer. The hypercalcemia of patients with breast cancer usually responds to corticosteroids.

The finding of increased serum levels of iPTH and hypophosphatemia in hypercalcemic patients with a history of successfully treated breast cancer or with active disease almost certainly reflects associated primary hyperparathyroidism. Successful treatment of the latter (see above) may completely resolve the hypercalcemia. Frankly increased levels of serum iPTH in hypercalcemic patients with nonhematologic malignancies other than breast cancer should be interpreted similarly. As described in Figure 246–9, serum iPTH (as measured by mid- or carboxyl-region assays) is either normal or slightly increased in most patients with the syndrome of ectopic hyperparathyroidism. Thus, values of serum iPTH that are greater than two times the upper limit of normal in such patients indicate the coexistence of malignancy and primary hyperparathyroidism.

Multiple myeloma is the most common of the hematologic malignancies causing hypercalcemia. Approximately 20 to 30 per cent of patients with this disease have increased calcium levels. As in breast cancer, serum phosphate is normal or slightly increased, and corticosteroid administration frequently resolves the hypercalcemia. Patients with multiple myeloma often present with vertebral compression fractures and can be mistakenly diagnosed as having idiopathic osteoporosis. Roentgenograms of the spine may not distinguish between these two diseases. Interestingly, radionuclide bone scans often do not identify the bony lesions of multiple myeloma; a "positive scan" is more consistent with metastatic malignancy. A definitive diagnosis of multiple myeloma can usually be made if immunoelectrophoresis of serum or urine protein shows immunoglobulin abnormalities or if bone marrow biopsies show increased plasma cells.

The underlying cause of the hypercalcemia in patients with multiple myeloma is probably increased osteoclastic osteolysis induced by the local elaboration by myeloma cells of a small, as yet uncharacterized, peptide, osteoclast-activating factor (OAF) (Fig. 163–2). However, in some patients with this disease, the hypercalcemia may not be due to osteolysis but to extensive binding of calcium by the high circulating concentrations of myeloma proteins, which results in an increase in the protein-bound, biologically inert fraction of the plasma calcium (Ch. 243).

Hypercalcemia is unusual in other hematologic or lymphoproliferative malignancies, but it can occur in acute lymphocytic leukemia and more rarely in Hodgkin's disease, lymphosarcoma, and reticulum cell sarcoma. Although it has not been proved, the cause of hypercalcemia in these conditions is thought to be osteolysis induced by osteoclast-activating factor (or a similar substance) that is elaborated by tumor deposits (accumulations of malignant cells) in bone. Such lesions are common in patients with acute leukemia (50 to 90 per cent), but the incidence of hypercalcemia is quite low (5 per cent), suggesting that leukemic cells only rarely develop the capacity to produce significant quantities of osteolytic substances. High serum levels of 1,25-dihydroxyvitamin D have been reported in three patients with non-Hodgkin's lymphoma and hypercalcemia; it was speculated that the increased 1,25 dihydroxyvitamin D was synthesized in the neoplastic tissue.

Drugs

Thiazide diuretics regularly cause small increases in the plasma levels of total and ionized calcium in normal subjects by increasing serum protein concentrations (hemoconcentration due to volume depletion) and increasing renal tubular reabsorption of calcium. The widespread use of these agents for hypertension and as diuretics has complicated the diagnosis of hypercalcemia. Two simple rules are valuable in the evaluation of such patients. First, thiazide diuretics rarely increase serum calcium levels above 11.0 mg per deciliter, and therefore patients with higher values probably have a hypercalcemic disorder that is not related to thiazide administration. Secondly, serum calcium should be restored to the normal range (8.9 to 10.1 mg per deciliter) in normal patients within three weeks of discontinuing thiazides. There is no evidence that the mild hypercalcemia caused by thiazide diuretics causes adverse effects.

Furosemide, a diuretic commonly used in the treatment of severe hypercalcemia (see below), has been reported to cause mild hypercalcemia when administered chronically. There is no explanation for this apparent paradox.

Vitamin D was once used in large doses (>50,000 units per day) to treat rheumatologic conditions; not surprisingly, vitamin D intoxication (see Ch. 244) and consequent hypercalcemia were common complications of that type of therapy. It is relatively rare now but should be considered in the differential diagnosis of hypercalcemia, particularly in those patients treated with large doses of vitamin D or its metabolites (e.g., for hypoparathyroidism and renal osteodystrophy) and in individuals who are prone to self-medication with large doses of vitamins and minerals. The hypercalcemia associated with vitamin D intoxication usually is accompanied by slight to moderate increases in serum phosphate unless there is some independent reason for phosphate depletion. As with other nonparathyroid disorders, this biochemical feature helps distinguish vitamin D intoxication from primary hyperparathyroidism, but the diagnosis can be confirmed by demonstrating decreased or undetectable serum levels of iPTH and serum levels of 25OHD that are greater than 300 ng per milliliter. Corticosteroids characteristically reverse the hypercalcemia of vitamin D intoxication, as they do the hypercalcemia of breast cancer and hematologic malignancies.

Vitamin A, when ingested in doses of 50,000 to 100,000 units daily (10 to 20 times the minimum daily requirement), may result in hypercalcemia and diffuse bone pain. It is presumed that increased bone resorption underlies these abnormalities, even though skeletal x-rays are generally normal. In some cases these films may show multiple calcifications of the periosteum along the shafts of the phalanges and metacarpals. The diagnosis is confirmed by demonstrating that serum vitamin A levels are two to three times higher than normal. Symptoms, skeletal lesions, and hypercalcemia resolve rapidly after discontinuation of the vitamin.

Lithium, used in doses typical for manic-depressive illness, can cause mild hypercalcemia, which resolves after the drug is discontinued. The mechanism by which lithium induces hypercalcemia is unclear, although increased serum iPTH levels have been demonstrated recently in patients taking this drug. Further investigation is needed to determine whether increased secretion of PTH plays an important role in the hypercalcemia associated with lithium treatment.

Milk-Alkali Syndrome (Burnett's Syndrome). Ingestion of antacids that contain large amounts of calcium (i.e., >5 grams per day) can produce hypercalcemia in susceptible individuals and should be suspected, particularly in neurotic or psychiatrically ill patients who may be medicating themselves surreptitiously. If excessive calcium intake and the resulting hypercalcemia continue for a long time, the kidney may be damaged and renal failure may occur. This course of events was more frequent many years ago when the treatment of peptic ulcer included the use of large quantities of calcium in the form of milk or calcium carbonate and soluble alkali.

Granulomatous Diseases

Hypercalcemia occurs in 10 to 20 per cent of patients with *sarcoidosis* but is rare in other granulomatous diseases. When hypercalcemia is present, serum levels of phosphate and alkaline phosphatase are generally increased and hypercalciuria is common. Other manifestations of the sarcoidosis, such as hilar lymphadenopathy, enlarged liver or spleen, peripheral lymphadenopathy, skin lesions, and hyperglobulinemia, are usually present. An increased serum level of angiotensin-converting enzyme in a hypercalcemic patient is highly suggestive of sarcoidosis (see Ch. 67), and the demonstration of noncaseating granulomatous lesions in a biopsied lymph node (e.g., the scalene) is confirmatory.

The presence of low serum levels of phosphate and increased serum levels of PTH in a hypercalcemic patient with sarcoidosis indicates primary hyperparathyroidism. Diagnosis may be difficult in such patients when sarcoidosis involves the kidneys and compromises renal function.

Patients with sarcoidosis are very sensitive to the hypercalcemic effects of vitamin D. They have an increased ability to convert vitamin D to its biologically active form, $1,25(OH)_2D$. The site of this increased conversion may be the abnormal granulomatous tissue that these patients harbor. This tissue appears capable of hydroxylating 25OHD to form a compound that has chromatographic properties similar to those of $1,25(OH)_2D$. Although proof is lacking at present, it is presumed that the mechanism underlying the hypercalcemia in other granulomatous diseases is similar to that responsible for the hypercalcemia in sarcoidosis. Treatment with corticosteroids lowers serum calcium levels in hypercalcemic patients with sarcoidosis in the same way as in vitamin D intoxication.

Nonparathyroid Endocrine Diseases

Hyperthyroidism frequently (in 20 per cent of patients) causes mild hypercalcemia, which resolves soon after treatment for the hyperthyroidism is instituted. The hypercalcemia is accompanied by normal or slightly increased concentrations of serum phosphate, decreased concentrations of serum iPTH, and increased excretion of hydroxyproline. As might be expected, bone biopsies from patients with hyperthyroidism are hypercellular and show increases in both formation and resorption surfaces of bone. It is presumed that the hypercalcemia in these patients is due to the uncoupling of bone formation and resorption so that resorption predominates. Serum levels of calcium above 11.5 mg per deciliter are rare in patients with hyperthyroidism; when they occur, they suggest the presence of another hypercalcemic disorder.

Acute adrenal insufficiency may be associated with hypercalcemia. Although the mechanism is poorly understood, increases in serum protein concentrations associated with severe hemoconcentration may be involved. Glucocorticoid replacement restores serum calcium concentrations to normal.

Familial Hypocalciuric Hypercalcemia
(See above, p. 1438.)

Immobilization

Immobilization of patients in body casts or by quadraplegia frequently causes hypercalcemia as a result of increased dissolution of bone. Hypercalcemia is generally mild in adults but can be severe in children (e.g., >15.0 mg per deciliter). This difference in severity is probably due to the higher turnover rate of bone in children. The mechanism responsible for enhanced dissolution of bone in immobilized patients is unclear, but available evidence from histomorphometric examination of bone biopsies from these patients suggests that bone formation surfaces are decreased and bone resorption surfaces are increased. The hypercalcemia associated with immobilization usually resolves rapidly when patients can bear weight with their lower extremities (as little as one or more hours per day). Treatment of hypercalcemia in adults is rarely needed because it is mild. However, the severe hypercalcemia seen in immobilized children requires prompt treatment using the measures detailed below (i.e., increased fluids, sodium chloride, phosphate, and possibly calcitonin).

Idiopathic Hypercalcemia of Infancy

Idiopathic hypercalcemia of infancy is rare. It is associated with several congenital cardiovascular and facial defects. Hypersensitivity to vitamin D is suspected as the cause of the hypercalcemia because corticosteroids can lower the serum calcium concentrations in these patients. Moreover, there may be increased conversion of vitamin D to $1,25(OH)_2D$ in affected infants.

Neonatal primary hyperparathyroidism, also a rare disease, is easily confused with idiopathic hypercalcemia of infancy. The treatments for these two diseases are different and depend completely upon the correct diagnosis. Measurement of serum iPTH is key in this latter regard; levels are increased in primary hyperparathyroidism and decreased or undetectable in idiopathic hypercalcemia.

Renal Failure and Renal Transplantation

Hypercalcemia may occur during the development of severe secondary hyperparathyroidism caused by chronic renal failure or after renal transplantation. The pathogenesis and treatment of the hypercalcemia associated with these conditions is described in Ch. 248. Hypercalcemia is a frequent complication of acute renal failure, but its cause is poorly understood. It is usually managed successfully by hemodialysis with dialysis baths that contain low concentrations of calcium.

Medical Treatment of Hypercalcemia

Acute Severe Hypercalcemia

The medical treatment of acute severe hypercalcemia (>13.0 mg per deciliter) should be started immediately, because the condition is life-threatening. Serum levels of calcium, magnesium, sodium, and potassium must be monitored every two to four hours. If possible, patients should remain ambulatory, since immobilization may increase serum calcium in some patients. In patients with heart disease who are in danger of developing heart failure due to volume overload from fluid administration, central venous pressure should be monitored so that appropriate measures can be taken if the pressure increases.

The diagnostic approach to determining the underlying cause of hypercalcemia outlined here should be instituted early so that the cause of hypercalcemia can be specifically identified and treated.

In addition to these measures, dietary calcium should be restricted, and all drugs that might cause hypercalcemia (e.g., thiazides or vitamin D) discontinued. If the patient is taking digitalis, it may be wise to reduce the dose because the hypercalcemic patient may be more sensitive to the toxic effects of this drug. Ideally, the patient should be admitted to an intensive care unit for electrocardiographic monitoring while antihypercalcemic measures are instituted. Beta-adrenergic blockade is useful in protecting the heart against the adverse effects of severe hypercalcemia, especially serious arrhythmias.

The mainstay of therapy is a regimen of hydration, initially with normal saline, plus forced diuresis using furosemide or ethacrynic acid. The objective is to increase the urinary excretion of calcium rapidly, thus decreasing the exchangeable calcium pool and the serum calcium concentration. Saline is given to increase sodium excretion because sodium clearance parallels calcium clearance during water or osmotic diuresis. Furosemide and ethacrynic acid inhibit the tubular reabsorption of calcium and aid in maintaining diuresis. Approximately 4 to 6 liters of isotonic saline (sometimes as much as 12 liters are needed) should be given intravenously each day, along with 20 to 100 mg of furosemide or 10 to 40 mg of ethacrynic acid every 1 to 2 hours (intravenously or orally). Such a regimen usually increases urinary calcium excretion to 500 to 1000 mg per day and lowers serum calcium by 2 to 6 mg per deciliter after 24 to 48 hours. Potassium and magnesium depletion are complications of therapy, and appropriate replacement should be instituted early.

After serum calcium has decreased to a reasonably safe level (<13 mg per deciliter), a chronic regimen may be instituted. At the minimum, this should consist of a daily oral regimen of 40 to 160 mg of furosemide or 50 to 200 mg of ethacrynic acid, 400 to 600 mEq of sodium chloride (in tablet form), and 3 liters of fluid. Serum calcium, magnesium, and potassium should be monitored daily at first, and then weekly when serum calcium has stabilized. Magnesium and potassium should be replaced as necessary. Patient compliance with this regimen can be monitored by measuring 24 hour urinary excretion of sodium (which should exceed 300 mEq per day) and 24 hour urinary volume (minimum required is 2500 ml per day).

Chronic Treatment of Moderately Severe Hypercalcemia

Whereas the acute treatment of severe hypercalcemia (>13.0 mg per deciliter) is nonspecific and relatively straightforward, requiring primarily hydration and saline diuresis (see below), the chronic treatment of moderately severe hypercalcemia (<13.0 mg per deciliter) requires knowledge of the underlying disease and involves trial and error in formulating an effective drug regimen. The problem is less difficult in diseases of nonparathyroid origin because treatment of the underlying disease (e.g., hyperthyroidism), discontinuation of drugs (e.g., thiazide diuretics), or treatment with corticosteroids (e.g., 300 mg of cortisone or 60 mg of prednisone given daily in divided doses for sarcoidosis, multiple myeloma, or vitamin D intoxication) usually results in satisfactory resolution of hypercalcemia. However, the medical treatment of hypercalcemia in those diseases associated with excess circulating levels of PTH or PTH-like substances is considerably more difficult. The drugs that are available may not be completely effective and may have serious side effects.

All patients with moderately severe hypercalcemia should maintain a high fluid intake (3 to 5 liters per day) and, unless contraindicated because of associated diseases, a sodium chloride intake of at least 300 to 400 mEq per day. These measures increase the renal excretion of calcium while maintaining the concentration of urinary calcium below that conducive to renal stone formation. Periodic measurements of serum electrolytes should be made because this regimen can cause magnesium and potassium depletion. These ions should be replaced if their serum concentrations decrease. Except in patients with breast cancer, in whom the administration of estrogens or androgens may induce hypercalcemia for unknown reasons, hypercalcemic postmenopausal women with either primary hyperparathyroidism or the syndrome of ectopic hyperparathyroidism should be given cyclic estrogen-progestin therapy (as described in Ch. 249). Estrogens suppress bone resorption and have been used successfully in the long-term management of mild hypercalcemia in women with primary hyperparathyroidism.

If hypercalcemia is not controlled (10.0 to 11.0 mg per deciliter) using these simple measures, other agents may be tried. Oral phosphate, either as neutral or potassium phosphate, may be given in doses as high as 2 to 4 grams of elemental phosphorus per day. Initial doses should be relatively low (1 to 2 grams per day in divided doses every 6 hours) because gastrointestinal side effects (e.g., nausea and diarrhea) may occur; these should disappear, however, with time. During treatment with phosphate, serum levels of calcium, phosphate, and creatinine should be monitored to determine whether the serum calcium level has decreased and whether hyperphosphatemia or impaired renal function has developed. Increases in serum phosphorus above 5 mg per deciliter should be avoided because extraskeletal calcifications (e.g., in the kidney) may be induced. Phosphate should be discontinued if the serum creatinine level increases significantly.

If phosphate therapy fails, the only effective approach to the treatment of hypercalcemia is to use mithramycin. This cytotoxic antibiotic has been used to treat testicular tumors but also ameliorates hypercalcemia by dramatically inhibiting bone resorption, presumably by killing osteoclasts. However, the drug is associated with renal and hepatic toxicity, thrombocytopenia, nausea, vomiting, stomatitis, and facial swelling. Therefore, it is usually reserved for hypercalcemic patients with malignancy. The intravenous administration of 15 to 25 μg of mithramycin per kilogram of body weight generally restores serum calcium to nearly normal levels within a few days. The duration of this effect varies, but it can last as long as a month. When hypercalcemia recurs, mithramycin can be administered again, provided that thrombocytopenia has not occurred and renal and hepatic function have not been impaired. Lower doses (10 to 15 μg per kilogram of body weight) can be tried, with the expectation that there will be fewer side effects. In general, the toxic effects of mithramycin can be reversed by discontinuing the drug.

The treatment of hypercalcemia with calcitonin, although rational, has been disappointing, and there is no convincing evidence that it is effective in the chronic management of hypercalcemia in these patients.

Indomethacin, given orally in doses of 25 mg every 6 hours, may be tried, but it is rarely effective. The rationale for its use is that the hypercalcemia may be due to increased bone resorption caused by excess prostaglandin released by the cancer.

Bilezikian JP: Hypercalcemia. *In* Krieger DT, Bardin CW: Current Therapy in Endocrinology 1983–1984. Philadelphia and St. Louis, B. C. Decker, Inc., and C. V. Mosby Company, 1983, pp 272–277. *Brief but incisive review of the treatment of hypercalcemia.*

Rodman JS, Sherwood LM: Disorders of mineral metabolism in malignancy. *In* Avioli LV, Krane SM (eds.): Metabolic Bone Disease. Vol 2. New York, Academic Press, 1978, pp 577–631. *A systematic assessment of the diagnosis, etiology, and management of patients with malignancy-associated hypercalcemia.*

Suki WN, Yium JJ, Von Minden M, Saller-Herbert C, Eknoyan G, Martinez-Maldonado M: Acute treatment of hypercalcemia with furosemide. N Engl J Med 283:836,1970. *Classic paper outlining the acute treatment of hypercalcemia.*

Symposium on the etiology and medical management of hypercalcemia. Metab Bone Dis 2:143,1980. *A series of review articles describing recent advances in understanding the causes and medical treatment of hypercalcemia.*

247. THE ULTIMOBRANCHIAL CELLS AND CALCITONIN

Claude D. Arnaud

INTRODUCTION. The ultimobranchial cells develop from neural crest tissue in the ultimobranchial cleft during embryonic life. They form a discrete organ in submammalian vertebrates called the ultimobranchial gland. In the mammal, the anlage of the cells merges with the embryonic thyroid gland, ultimately becoming dispersed in the central region of each lobe (of the thyroid gland), adjacent to the follicular cells.

Calcitonin, a 32 amino acid, 3700 molecular weight polypeptide with a 1-7 disulfide bridge, is biosynthesized and secreted by the ultimobranchial (parafollicular or "C") cells. It is synthesized as a large molecular weight precursor.

Calcitonin is rapidly released by the "C" cells in response to small increases in plasma ionic calcium. It acts on kidney and bone to restore the level of this cation to just below a normal set point, which in turn inhibits the secretion of the hormone. Calcitonin is a physiologic antagonist to parathyroid hormone, and these agents presumably act in concert to maintain the normal concentration of ionic calcium in the extracellular fluid. These relationships are illustrated in Figure 243–1.

The actual importance of calcitonin in the calcium homeostasis of adult humans is not established. An excess or deficiency of parathyroid hormone or vitamin D produces dramatic clinical disorders. In contrast, an excess (medullary carcinoma of the thyroid) or deficiency (post-thyroidectomy) of calcitonin produces few discernible and no serious abnormalities in mineral metabolism. The basal plasma levels of calcitonin and its responsiveness to induced hypercalcemia or pentagastrin injection are lower in women than in men and decrease with age. In adult humans, calcitonin may function primarily to restrain the bone resorptive effects of parathyroid hormone. If so, the long-term combination of a progressive decrease in calcitonin secretion and reserve and an increase in parathyroid hormone secretion may contribute to the osteoporosis of aging.

Calcitonin exists in multiple molecular forms in ultimobranchial tissue and plasma. In contrast to parathyroid hormone, however, the major circulating species are not hormone fragments but immunoreactive forms with molecular weights larger than 32 amino acid calcitonin. It is likely that some of these forms represent polymers of calcitonin with disulfide molecular links. The different antisera used in radioimmunoassays recognize these forms differently, and therefore the normal range for plasma calcitonin must be established for each assay. The concentrations of calcitonin are extremely low (<100 pg per milliliter). Induced hypercalcemia and pentagastrin injection cause an increase in plasma calcitonin in approximately 40 to 50 per cent of normal women and 70 to 80 per cent of normal men. However, it is unlikely that gastrin is a physiologic calcitonin secretagogue. Other calcitonin secretagogues of unproved physiologic significance include glucagon, β-adrenergic agonists, and alcohol.

When bone turnover rates are high, calcitonin administration produces rapid and profound hypocalcemia and hypophosphatemia. This is largely due to the fact that the hormone decreases bone resorption. Calcitonin also increases urinary excretion of calcium and phosphate, but its action on the kidney is transient and variable. Calcitonin stimulates adenylate cyclase in bone and kidney, but whether cyclic AMP is the major intracellular mediator of calcitonin action has not been established. It is also unclear whether calcitonin influences intestinal calcium absorption.

HYPOCALCITONINEMIA

No clinical condition has been reported to date in which hypocalcitoninemia plays a definitive role, except possibly the osteoporosis of aging (see above).

MEDULLARY CARCINOMA

DEFINITION. Medullary carcinoma, a malignancy of the parafollicular cells of the thyroid gland, is the only recognized disorder in which calcitonin is inappropriately secreted in excess. It occurs sporadically but also may be inherited as an autosomal dominant trait as part of the multiple endocrine neoplasia (MEN) syndromes, Types II and III. These syndromes include medullary carcinoma of the thyroid gland and pheochromocytoma. Patients with MEN II have a normal appearance but a high incidence of hyperparathyroidism, most frequently resulting from enlargement of multiple parathyroid glands. Patients with MEN III have a striking appearance owing to ganglioneuromas of the labia and mucosae, a marfanoid habitus, and other somatic abnormalities. Hyperparathyroidism is unusual.

INCIDENCE. Medullary carcinoma constitutes between 3.5 and 10 per cent of all thyroid malignancies. The incidence in males and females is almost equal, there being a male-to-female ratio of 1.3:1 in sporadic cases and 1:1 in familial cases. In general, familial cases present at a younger age than do sporadic cases.

PATHOLOGY. Medullary carcinoma manifests as a solid, often hard mass confined to but not encapsulated in the substance of the thyroid gland. In sporadic cases, it is often unilateral, but in familial cases it is frequently bilateral. It is composed of sheets of cells with granular cytoplasms, and usually contains irregular masses of amyloid and fibrous tissue. Most patients who present with a thyroid mass have metastases to cervical lymph nodes. Some lesions spread to the upper mediastinum. Spread beyond the mediastinum, usually delayed until late in the natural history of the disease, is most commonly to lungs, liver, bones, and the adrenal glands.

PATHOPHYSIOLOGY. Medullary carcinomas secrete large quantities of calcitonin and respond to provocative stimuli such as increased serum calcium or intravenous pentagastrin. Although calcitonin produces hypocalcemia and hypophosphatemia in experimental animals, these biochemical findings are unusual in patients with medullary carcinoma in spite of extremely high levels of immunoreactive calcitonin. This paradox is probably due to a combination of factors, including homologous desensitization of tissues that normally respond to calcitonin.

Medullary carcinoma may secrete many other bioactive substances in addition to calcitonin, each with the potential of causing clinical symptoms. These substances include biogenic amines, ACTH and corticotropin-releasing hormone, prostaglandins, nerve growth factor, and possibly a prolactin-releasing hormone. Diarrhea is present in 20 per cent of patients. It relents after surgical excision of the tumor and is therefore thought to be humorally mediated. Cushing's syndrome is present in about 5 per cent of cases and is secondary to secretion of excessive ACTH.

CLINICAL MANIFESTATIONS AND DETECTION. The majority of patients with sporadic medullary carcinoma present with an asymptomatic thyroid mass. Patients with MEN III may complain of the neuromas they harbor and their marfanoid habitus. Hypercalcemia may be detected on routine blood screening in patients with MEN II and primary hyperparathyroidism. Most important, hypertension in patients with MEN II and III may lead to the diagnosis of pheochromocytoma, which is more life threatening than is medullary carcinoma.

Paraneoplastic syndromes, such as Cushing's syndrome or intractable diarrhea, should alert the physician to the possible existence of medullary carcinoma. Certainly, a history of more than one family member with thyroid cancer should raise suspicion in a patient with bizarre symptoms.

Other neural manifestations in MEN III include medullated nerves on slit lamp examination of the eye and ganglioneuromas of the gastrointestinal tract. The latter can cause gastrointestinal obstruction as well as megacolon.

Medullary cancers occasionally calcify. The discovery of a calcified thyroidal mass does not indicate that it is benign; rather, it is probably an indication for the measurement of serum immunoreactive calcitonin (see below).

DIAGNOSIS. The cornerstone for the investigation of patients suspected of having medullary carcinoma is the radioimmunoassay of calcitonin in plasma. Although not specific for this tumor, increased levels of immunoreactive calcitonin in patients with a thyroid mass, pheochromocytoma, or a family history of medullary carcinoma virtually assure the diagnosis. Serum immunoreactive calcitonin may be increased in many other conditions, however, including other malignancies that secrete calcitonin ectopically (especially small cell carcinoma of the lung), chronic renal failure, gastrointestinal disorders such as tumors of the pancreas and pernicious anemia, subacute Hashimoto's thyroiditis, and pregnancy. These conditions should be considered in the interpretation of a high value.

The diagnostic power of the calcitonin radioimmunoassay is greatly enhanced when combined with provocative tests. For example, as many as 30 per cent of members of a family with MEN II who actually harbor small medullary carcinomas will have normal unstimulated plasma levels of immunoreactive calcitonin. They can only be detected by intravenous administration of 0.5 μg of pentagastrin* per kilogram of body weight over five to ten seconds, or 150 mg of calcium chloride over ten minutes. Plasma levels of immunoreactive calcitonin increase abnormally in the majority of these patients, thus establishing the diagnosis; surgery can then be performed before metastatic spread occurs. The calcitonin radioimmunoassay should be able to measure normal plasma levels of immunoreactive calcitonin (males, <100 pg per milliliter; females, <70 pg per milliliter). Without such sensitivity it is unlikely that the assay will be able to detect relatively small increases above the stimulated normal range, thus making the test impossible to interpret.

To rule out familial medullary carcinoma, immunoreactive calcitonin should be measured during a provocative test in all primary relatives of all patients with medullary carcinoma, regardless of family history. In a few affected patients with minimal parafollicular cell disease, false-negative results will be obtained with any of the tests outlined. Provocative testing should therefore be performed yearly in primary relatives with previous negative tests, since approximately 50 per cent of the members of a given family with MEN II should eventually develop medullary cancer. Its timely detection will permit definitive surgical treatment.

TREATMENT. After exclusion or treatment of pheochromocytoma, total thyroidectomy is mandatory. This is especially true in patients with MEN II because medullary carcinoma is almost always bilateral and polycentric. Lymph nodes in the midline compartment should be removed and those in both internal jugular chains sampled. If jugular lymph nodes are involved, a modified neck dissection should be performed. Postoperatively, all patients should be studied with a provocative test(s) to determine if residual tumor is present and should be given thyroid hormone replacement. The overall prevalence of residual medullary cancer after such surgery is about 35 per cent. The majority of these patients are older and have had regional metastases at surgery. Long-term follow-up with provocative tests every year is advised for all patients. Although it is usually difficult to determine the location of metastases responsible for a positive result in a provocative test, local recurrences are likely and can be dealt with surgically. There is no known effective chemotherapeutic, isotopic, or radiologic treatment for medullary carcinoma.

PROGNOSIS. Patients with sporadic medullary carcinoma have the least favorable prognosis. Metastases are usually present, and only 46 per cent of these patients survive for ten years. Patients with MEN II appear to fare better, with few having been recorded as dying from their disease. Conversely, in the Mayo Clinic series of patients with MEN III, 67 per cent have had residual disease after surgery, and 18 per cent have died of medullary cancer. The reasons for the apparent difference in the prognosis of MEN II and MEN III are unknown.

---

*This use is not listed in the manufacturer's directive.

THERAPEUTIC USE OF CALCITONIN

Calcitonin is used to treat Paget's disease of bone and hypercalcemia of all causes (see Ch. 250). The preparation most frequently employed is synthetic salmon calcitonin because this species is about 30 times more potent in lowering serum calcium than are mammalian calcitonins (porcine, human). The rationale for its use in both Paget's disease and hypercalcemia is its inhibitory effect on bone resorption. In unusual cases, high titers of circulating antibodies are formed against salmon calcitonin. These antibodies may block the action of the hormone and its beneficial effects. In such cases, synthetic human calcitonin may be successfully substituted, but this species of the hormone is not readily available commercially at present.

Austin L, Heath H III: Calcitonin: Physiology and pathophysiology. N Engl J Med 304:269, 1981. *Lively review of recent advances in calcitonin research in health and disease.*

Gagel RF, Melvin KEW, Tashjian AH Jr, Miller HH, Feldman ZT, Wolfe HJ, DeLellis RA, Cervi-Skinner S, Reichlin S: Natural history of the familial medullary thyroid carcinoma–pheochromocytoma syndrome and the identification of preneoplastic stages by screening studies: A five-year report. Trans Assoc Am Physicians 88:177, 1975. *The first description of the diagnostic power of the calcitonin radioimmunoassay in the diagnosis of familial medullary carcinoma.*

Sizemore GW, Carney JA, Heath H III: Epidemiology of medullary carcinoma of the thyroid gland: A five year experience (1971–1976). Surg Clin North Am 57:633, 1977. *Describes this group's extensive experience with both the familial and sporadic forms of medullary carcinoma of the thyroid gland.*

Williams ED: Medullary carcinoma of the thyroid. *In* DeGroot LJ (ed.): Endocrinology. Vol 2. New York, Grune & Stratton, 1979, pp 777–792. *Comprehensive review of medullary cancer of the thyroid gland.*

248. RENAL OSTEODYSTROPHY

Eduardo Slatopolsky

Renal osteodystrophy is a generic term that describes the complex lesions of bone that are present in the majority of patients with advanced renal failure. The main components of renal osteodystrophy are osteitis fibrosa and osteomalacia. A lesser role is played by osteosclerosis and osteoporosis. Osteitis fibrosa, a consequence of increased parathyroid hormone activity, is characterized by an increase in the number of osteoclasts, an increase in bone resorption, and marrow fibrosis. Osteomalacia, a condition secondary in part to alterations in vitamin D metabolism, is characterized by a decreased mineralization rate of osteoid tissue shown histologically by an abnormal calcification front in bone. Osteosclerosis is caused by localized areas of mineralized woven bone, which appears as increased bone density on radiographic studies. Osteoporosis is defined as a decrease in the mass of normally mineralized bone and represents only an infrequent and minor component of renal osteodystrophy.

OSTEITIS FIBROSA (also see Chapter 246)

Secondary hyperparathyroidism is a universal complication of chronic renal disease. Chief cell hyperplasia of the parathyroid glands and high levels of immunoreactive parathyroid hormone (i-PTH) are among the earliest findings affecting mineral metabolism in patients with chronic renal failure. The factors that contribute to the development of secondary hyperparathyroidism in renal insufficiency include (1) phosphate retention, (2) altered vitamin D metabolism, (3) skeletal resistance to the calcemic action of PTH, (4) impaired degradation of parathyroid hormone, and (5) altered feedback regulation between ionized calcium and the secretion of PTH.

PHOSPHATE RETENTION. Considerable evidence supports an important role of phosphate retention in producing secondary hyperparathyroidism. Long-term feeding of a diet high in phosphate to animals with normal renal function can produce secondary hyperparathyroidism. Conversely, restriction of dietary phosphate can prevent the development of secondary hyperparathyroidism in chronic renal failure. The effect of phosphate retention is mediated via lowering ionized calcium concentration. This effect probably is caused by a combination of factors, such as complexing ionized calcium, decreasing the production of 1,25-dihydroxycholecalciferol ($1,25(OH)_2D_3$), the active metabolite of vitamin D, and decreasing bone calcium mobilization from the skeleton. In patients with far advanced renal failure (glomerular filtration rate [GFR] less than 20 ml per minute), correction of hyperphosphatemia alone does not completely reverse secondary hyperparathyroidism, since many other factors also contribute to the increased PTH levels in blood.

ALTERATIONS IN VITAMIN D METABOLISM (see Ch. 244). Renal osteodystrophy may arise in part because of defective renal production of the active form of vitamin D in advanced renal failure. The liver hydroxylates vitamin D_3 to 25-hydroxycholecalciferol ($25(OH)D_3$), the predominant form of vitamin D_3 present in plasma. $25(OH)D_3$ is further hydroxylated to $1,25(OH)_2D_3$ by the enzyme 25-hydroxycholecalciferol-1α-hydroxylase, which is localized in the mitochondrial fraction of the proximal tubular cells (Fig. 244–1). Parathyroid hormone and low-phosphate diets play a key role in the stimulation of 1α-hydroxylase. On the other hand, lack of parathyroid hormone or hyperphosphatemia decreases the activity of 1α-hydroxylase. The evidence that alterated vitamin D metabolism contributes to abnormal calcium metabolism in advanced renal failure is considerable. Metabolic balance studies and radioisotopic techniques have shown reduced intestinal absorption of calcium in patients with far advanced renal insufficiency. Low levels of $1,25(OH)_2D_3$ in serum and calcium malabsorption are usually present in patients with a GFR of less than 40 per minute.

SKELETAL RESISTANCE TO THE ACTION OF PARATHYROID HORMONE. Skeletal resistance to the calcemic action of PTH may also play a role in the development of hypocalcemia seen in patients with renal insufficiency. Higher circulating levels of PTH may be needed for the maintenance of a normal plasma calcium in patients with renal failure.

IMPAIRED DEGRADATION OF PTH SECONDARY TO REDUCED RENAL FUNCTION. The liver and the kidney play key roles in the metabolism of parathyroid hormone. The uptake of i-PTH by the liver is selective for the intact hormone. The liver does not remove either amino terminal or carboxy terminal PTH fragments from the circulation. The kidney, on the other hand, removes both intact PTH and amino and carboxy terminal fragments from the circulation. Thus, in patients with chronic renal insufficiency, the high levels of circulating i-PTH result in part from increased PTH secretion, caused by chief cell hyperplasia, and in part from a decreased catabolism secondary to a decreased number of nephrons and decreased hepatic metabolism of intact PTH.

ALTERED FEEDBACK REGULATION BETWEEN IONIZED CALCIUM AND THE SECRETION OF PARATHYROID HORMONE. The control of the secretion of PTH by ionized calcium levels in plasma may be blunted in patients with chronic renal insufficiency. Hyperplastic parathyroid glands display less sensitivity to calcium than do normal tissues. This suggests that the mechanism for increased PTH levels may be caused by a shift in the set-point for calcium as well as the increased tissue mass. The set-point is defined as the amount of calcium necessary to suppress the secretion of parathyroid hormone by 50 per cent. Thus, a normal concentration of plasma calcium may not be sufficient to suppress hyperplastic glands, and plasma calcium may have to be increased to or even above the upper limits of normal to control the release of PTH in patients with secondary hyperparathyroidism.

OSTEOMALACIA (see Ch. 245)

Osteomalacia is defined as an increase in the osteoid seam width accompanied by a decrease in the mineralization front. The presence of excess osteoid per se does not necessarily indicate osteomalacia. An increase in osteoid tissue may be secondary to abnormalities in mineralization (osteomalacia) or caused by an increased rate of bone collagen synthesis, which is normally mineralized. The use of double tetracycline labelling of the calcification front in vivo can differentiate between these two possibilities. Therefore, the use of this technique and quantitative bone histology are critical for the diagnosis of osteomalacia. The mechanisms whereby altered vitamin D metabolism leads to impaired mineralization of bone are poorly understood. Whether vitamin D or $1,25(OH)_2D_3$ can directly stimulate bone mineralization or whether they lead to mineralization by increasing the levels of calcium and phosphate in the extracellular fluid surrounding bone remains a matter of controversy. Although the plasma levels of $1,25(OH)_2D_3$ are reduced in patients with far-advanced renal insufficiency, overt osteomalacia is found in only a small fraction of patients with end-stage uremia and may be absent even in anephric patients. Thus other factors, such as the plasma level of phosphorus, could also participate in the pathogenesis of osteomalacia in uremic patients. Hypophosphatemia per se can produce severe osteomalacia even in patients with normal renal function. Additional factors include alterations in collagen synthesis and maturation, defective bone crystal maturation, increased bone magnesium, elevated levels of pyrophosphate, and diminished calcium carbonate. The combination of these factors may play a role in the maturation of the bone and potentially contribute to the development of osteomalacia. Acidosis also contributes to the skeletal disease. In chronic renal insufficiency the skeleton plays an important role in buffering the hydrogen entering the body. Administration of bicarbonate and correction of the acidosis in azotemic patients can reduce fecal calcium excretion.

There is another type of osteomalacia that usually does not respond to any metabolite of vitamin D. Patients with this type of osteomalacia have pathologic fractures and complain of severe bone pain, and characteristically they have low levels of parathyroid hormone. When biopsies have been performed in these patients and the tissue stained appropriately, deposition of aluminum in the interface between the osteoid tissue and the calcification front has been found. Aluminum has a toxic effect on the osteoblast. The source of the aluminum may be a high aluminum content in the water or the ingestion of phosphate-binders containing aluminum or both. Finally, the lack of parathyroid hormone in patients who have had total parathyroidectomy leads to low bone turnover and rarely may precipitate the development of osteomalacia.

CLINICAL MANIFESTATIONS

Most of the symptoms related to renal osteodystrophy appear only when renal failure is advanced. On the other hand, certain biochemical alterations may appear early in the course of renal insufficiency. Knowledge of the presence of these alterations may help the physician to introduce treatment early in the course of renal failure and aid in the prevention of severe complications in bone and mineral metabolism.

Bone pain can develop and progress slowly to a point at which the patient becomes bedridden. Moreover, this can occur whether the skeletal pathology is osteitis fibrosa or osteomalacia. The bone pain is generally vague and commonly located in the lower back, hips, knees, and legs. Low-back pain may arise from the collapse of the vertebral body, and sharp chest pain may indicate spontaneous rib fracture. Physical findings are frequently lacking.

Muscular weakness when present is usually proximal, appears slowly, and progresses with time. Plasma levels of the muscle enzymes, creatinine phosphokinase and transaminase, are usually normal, and the electron micrographic changes are nonspecific. The pathogenesis of such muscular weakness is uncertain. In patients with myopathy, electron micrography has revealed localized disorganization of the myofibrils and dispersion of the Z-band material, which reverts to normal following treatment with $25(OH)D_3$.

Pruritus due to calcium deposition in skin is a common symptom in uremic patients, particularly with severe secondary hyperparathyroidism. Peripheral ischemic necrosis and vascular calcification also have been reported in these patients. The lesions may involve the tips of the toes and fingers, and the skin becomes violaceous. Ulcerations and scar formation may occur with clear demarcation of the lesions from the surrounding skin.

Calcific periarthritis, which is associated with acute pain and swelling around one or more joints, may be caused by deposition of hydroxy apatite crystals and is accompanied by marked hyperphosphatemia. *Skeletal deformities* are common in azotemic children who are growing. Bowing of the tibia and femur and deformities from slipped epiphyses are not uncommon. Children with renal rickets sometimes exhibit typical radiographic findings of viamin D deficiency. In adults with renal failure, particularly those with osteomalacia, marked skeletal deformities with lumbar scoliosis, thoracic kyphosis, and deformity of the thoracic cage may be observed. *Growth retardation* is usually seen in young children before and during maintenance hemodialysis.

BIOCHEMICAL FEATURES

One of the early changes in patients with renal insufficiency (GFR 60 to 80 ml per minute) is the presence of elevated levels of circulating i-PTH. As the disease progresses (GFR less than 40 ml per minute), hypocalcemia and low levels of $1,25(OH)_2D_3$ are present in these patients. In patients with advanced renal insufficiency the serum calcium may remain close to normal and values below 7.5 mg per deciliter are infrequent. Usually hypocalcemia is more marked in those patients who have severe osteomalacia and in those with profound metabolic acidosis. Occasionally, hypercalcemia may be observed in uremic patients, particularly those undergoing long-term dialysis. This can arise from severe hyperparathyroidism, from the ingestion of large amounts of calcium and vitamin D, from unrelated diseases such as sarcoidosis or malignancies, or from a "pure" mineralizing defect. This has been described in patients who have osteomalacia secondary to aluminum retention.

Hyperphosphatemia is usually common in patients with a GFR of less than 25 ml per minute. The degree of hyperphosphatemia depends on the amount of phosphate ingested in the diet, the fraction absorbed in the intestine, and the amount excreted in the urine. Obviously, if the patient ingests phosphate binders, the serum phosphate level may remain normal despite advanced renal insufficiency. Patients with severe hyperparathyroidism and advanced renal insufficiency usually have higher concentrations of serum phosphate in plasma.

Hypermagnesemia occurs in patients when renal insufficiency is very advanced, usually with a GFR of less than 15 ml per minute. The increase in serum magnesium levels is usually associated with an increased content of magnesium in bone, a factor that may affect crystal formation.

Total serum alkaline phosphatase levels are commonly higher in uremic patients with osteitis fibrosa than in those with osteomalacia. Coexistent liver disease should be excluded as a cause of elevated alkaline phosphatase levels.

RADIOGRAPHIC FEATURES

The main radiographic feature of secondary hyperparathyroidism is *osteitis fibrosa,* manifested as an increase in bone resorption, more commonly seen on the subperiosteal surfaces of bone (Fig. 246–6). Erosions that occur in conjunction with formation of new bone may appear as cysts or osteoclastomas (brown tumors). The presence of subperiosteal erosion correlates with serum i-PTH and histomorphometric features of osteitis fibrosa on bone biopsy. Subperiosteal resorption of the phalanges may be the most sensitive radiographic sign of secondary hyperparathyroidism. The tuft of the terminal phalanx or the second or third digit commonly shows resorption. With severe tuft erosion there may be a collapse of the soft tissue and a change in the contour of the tuft so that the finger appears to show clubbing. Bone erosions may also occur at the upper end of the tibia, the neck of the femur or the humerus, and the lower surface of the medial end of the clavicle. In the skull, resorption leads to the mottled and granular appearance commonly associated with altering areas of osteosclerosis.

Osteosclerosis is thought to be another feature of osteitis fibrosa arising from an increase in the thickness and number of trabecula in spongy bone. Osteosclerosis can lead to a typical "rugger jersey" appearance of the spine.

The x-ray features of *osteomalacia* are far less distinctive than those of secondary hyperparathyroidism. The Looser zone or pseudofracture are the only pathognomonic findings of osteomalacia in the adult (Fig. 245–2). A typical x-ray feature of rickets, that is, widening of the epiphyseal growth plate, cannot develop after epiphyseal closure and, hence, is limited to children. With mechanical stress and severe prolonged vitamin deficiency, a Looser zone may extend across the full width of the bone and produce a true fracture with displacement of fragments. Uremic patients with osteomalacia commonly have secondary hyperparathyroidism with concomitant x-ray features of the latter. Thus, a diagnosis of osteomalacia rests on histologic examinations, and one can only be certain of this diagnosis from bone therapy.

EXTRASKELETAL CALCIFICATIONS. The factors that predispose to the appearance of soft tissue calcification include an increase in the calcium phosphate product in plasma, the degree of secondary hyperparathyroidism, the magnitude of alkalosis, and the degree of local tissue injury. Three major varieties include (1) calcification of the medium sized arteries, (2) articular or tumoral calcifications, and (3) visceral calcifications affecting the heart, lung, and kidney.

TREATMENT

The objectives of the treatment of patients with renal osteodystrophy are (1) to return the blood levels of calcium and phosphorus to normal, (2) to suppress secondary hyperparathyroidism, (3) to reverse the histologic abnormalities in the skeleton, and (4) to prevent and reverse extraskeletal deposits of calcium and phosphate. It is very important to begin measures for the control of the abnormal mineral metabolism of renal disease early in the course, when the GFR is 30 to 40 ml per minute. Guidelines for the management of renal osteodystrophy are summarized in Table 248–1.

TABLE 248–1. GUIDELINES FOR MANAGEMENT OF RENAL OSTEODYSTROPHY

A. *Control of serum phosphate* (P) (3.5–5.0 mg/dl)

Restrict phosphorus intake in diet to 600 to 800 mg per day
Phosphate-binding antacids: aluminum carbonate or hydroxide; individualize dosage: Basalgel, Dialume, Alucap, Amphogel, 1 to 4 capsules with each meal
Hypophosphatemia should be avoided
Predialysis phosphorus: 4.5–5.5 mg/dl

B. *Adequate calcium intake*

Oral calcium supplements, providing 1 to 2 gm per day when serum P is controlled: Os-Cal, Titralac
Dialysate Ca, 6.5 to 7.0 mg per dl (3.25 to 3.5 mEq per liter)

C. *Use of vitamin D sterols*

Vitamin D_2 or D_3: 50,000 to 250,000 IU (1.25 to 6.25 mg)
Dihydrotachysterol: 0.25 to 2.0 mg per day
25-hydroxyvitamin D_3 (calcifediol): 20 to 100 μg per day (Calderol)
1,25-dihydroxyvitamin D_3 (calcitriol): 0.5 to 1.0 μg per day (Rocaltrol)

D. *Parathyroidectomy:*

Severe secondary hyperparathyroidism (bone erosions and increased i-PTH) plus any of the following:
- Persistent hypercalcemia (serum Ca > 11.5 to 12.0 mg per dl)
- Progressive or symptomatic extraskeletal calcification
- Persistently elevated serum calcium × phosphorus product
- Pruritus not responsive to medical treatment
- Calciphylaxis (ischemic ulcers and necrosis)
- Symptomatic hypercalcemia after renal transplantation

CONTROL OF PHOSPHORUS. To control phosphorus, dietary phosphate intake should be reduced to 700 to 800 mg per day by restricting the ingestion of dairy products and by decreasing the amount of protein in the diet. In addition to dietary control of phosphorus, patients with advanced renal failure very likely need phosphate-binders to reduce the intestinal absorption of phosphate. Phosphate-binders should be ingested with the meal in order to increase their efficiency in binding phosphate. One of the obstacles to the use of aluminum-containing gels is the potential development of aluminum accumulation. Therefore, they should be used with caution and if the patient develops symptoms and signs suggesting aluminum-induced osteomalacia, aluminum-containing gels should be discontinued. If the phosphorus level is not controlled, the patient will develop severe secondary hyperparathyroidism and extraskeletal calcification. The addition of calcium carbonate in a dose of 1 to 2 grams with each meal helps to bind phosphate and to reduce the amount of aluminum binders necessary for the treatment of hyperphosphatemia. Calcium carbonate also provides dietary calcium and thereby helps to correct the negative calcium balance characteristic of far advanced renal insufficiency. The goal when using phosphate binders is to reduce the serum phosphorus to near normal. If the patient is not yet receiving dialysis treatment, the serum phosphorus should be maintained between 3.5 and 4.5 mg per deciliter.

CONTROL OF CALCIUM. The plasma calcium level should be maintained at the upper limits of normal. If a patient has severe hyperphosphatemia, the administration of large amounts of calcium can aggravate the deposition of calcium phosphate salts and metastatic calcification; thus the hyperphosphatemia should be corrected before calcium administration. Supplemental calcium administration should be discontinued if the serum calcium increases above 11.5 mg per deciliter. The concentration of calcium in dialysate can clearly affect serum calcium levels in patients treated with maintenance hemodialysis. The ideal calcium concentration in the dialysate is between 6.5 and 7.0 mg per deciliter. Despite dietary control of phosphate, the use of phosphate binders, the adequate intake of calcium in the diet, and appropriate levels of calcium in the dialysate, a significant number of uremic patients still develop skeletal disease. Thus, vitamin D and its metabolites are important and effective agents in the treatment of renal osteodystrophy.

VITAMIN D. $1,25(OH)_2D_3$, the most active metabolite of vitamin D, has a short half-life, approximately 10 to 15 hours. This is the drug of choice in the treatment of hypocalcemia and secondary hyperparathyroidism. The usual dose is 0.5 to 1 microgram per day. If the main histologic lesion is osteomalacia, excellent results have been obtained with the use of $25(OH)D_3$ (20 to 100 μg per day), in addition to $1,25(OH)_2D_3$. The most common and important side effect of vitamin D and its metabolites is hypercalcemia; less frequently hyperphospatemia develops.

PARATHYROIDECTOMY. The treatment modalities outlined in the previous paragraphs can improve the homeostasis of calcium and phosphorus, reverse the symptoms of bone disease, and suppress PTH secretion. However, such measures may not be entirely successful, and parathyroidectomy may be required in some cases. Indications for parathyroid surgery include severe secondary hyperparathyroidism (bone erosions and high levels of i-PTH) plus any of the following: (1) persistent hypercalcemia, particularly when symptomatic; (2) intractible pruritus that does not respond to dialysis or other medical treatment; (3) progressive extra-skeletal calcification in conjunction with a high calcium-phosphorus product that is consistently about 75 to 80 mg per deciliter despite appropriate phosphate restriction; and (4) the appearance of calciphylaxis with ischemic lesions of the soft tissues. Because of lack of compliance, many patients are unable to control their serum phosphorus levels. In these cases, neither calcium supplements nor vitamin D or its metabolites can be recommended safely.

Moreover, this type of patient usually develops severe secondary hyperparathyroidism and surgical parathyroidectomy may be the treatment of choice.

Post-operative hypocalcemia may pose a problem if the remaining parathyroid tissue is inadequate. The chances for developing hypocalcemia are enhanced if severe osteitis fibrosa is present preoperatively. Pre-operative treatment of such patients with $1,25(OH)_2D_3$ in the dose of 1 to 2 μg per day may obviate such problems. Serum levels of phosphorus and magnesium sometimes decrease after parathyroid surgery, and aluminum-containing phosphate binders should be withheld if the serum phosphorus falls below 3.0 mg per deciliter. Rapid remineralization of the skeleton occurs during this period, and once the "hungry bones" have been mineralized, serum calcium rises. A fall in elevated plasma alkaline phosphatase level towards normal may be a clue that rapid skeletal remineralization is nearly complete and indicates that calcium supplements and vitamin D dosage may be reduced or discontinued. In the past, the removal of three and a half parathyroid glands was the procedure of choice; more recently, surgeons have gained experience with total parathyroidectomy followed by autotransplantation of parathyroid tissue into the patient's forearm. The tissue that is transplanted to the forearm is more accessible for subsequent surgical removal if necessary. Total parathyroidectomy without autotransplantation has little place in the management of renal bone disease, and this may predispose to the development of isolated mineralization defects or osteomalacia in uremic patients. Cryopreservation of removed parathyroid tissue is a useful precaution so that hypoparathyroidism may be treated by reimplantation of parathyroid tissue.

ALUMINUM-INDUCED OSTEOMALACIA. If the patient has aluminum-induced osteomalacia, phosphate binders containing aluminum should be discontinued at once. Phosphate should be controlled by using a more restrictive phosphate diet, and the serum phosphorus level may be allowed to increase to 6 mg per deciliter. Although still experimental and not approved for general use, deferoxamine, a drug known to chelate iron, also has an effect on aluminum. Preliminary reports have shown that use of this substance produced a significant improvement in patients with aluminum-induced osteomalacia.

Coburn JW, Slatopolsky E: Vitamin D, parathyroid hormone and renal osteodystrophy. *In* Brenner BM, Rector FC (eds.): The Kidney. 2nd ed. Philadelphia, W. B. Saunders Company, 1981, pp 2213–2305.

Massry SG: Divalent ion metabolism and renal osteodystrophy. *In* Massry SG, Glassock RJ (eds.): Textbook of Nephrology. Baltimore, Williams and Wilkins, 1983, pp 7.104–7.148. *These two references offer comprehensive, up-to-date reviews of the pathogenesis, diagnosis, prevention, and treatment of renal osteodystrophy. They also review the alterations in calcium and phosphate metabolism found in renal disease. Both contain extensive reference lists.*

249. OSTEOPOROSIS

B. Lawrence Riggs

GENERAL CONSIDERATIONS

DEFINITION. Osteoporosis is defined as an absolute decrease in the amount of bone to a level below that required for mechanical support or, as Fuller Albright succinctly put it many years ago, "There is too little bone." The bone that is present is normal chemically and histologically.

PATHOPHYSIOLOGY. For bone to be lost, there must be an absolute or relative increase in bone resorption over bone formation. Bone remodeling occurs at discrete foci in the skeleton, termed "bone remodeling units." A team of osteoclasts appears, constructs a resorption tunnel in cortical bone or a resorption groove on the surface of trabecular bone and then, several weeks later, is replaced by osteoblasts, which fill in the resorption space to form a new bone structural unit. The time required for completion of this sequence normally is about three months but may be longer in osteoporotic patients. Osteoporosis could be caused by an increase in the activity or duration of action of osteoclasts (leading to the excavation of a larger resorption space), by a decrease in the activity or duration of action of osteoblasts (leading to an incompletely refilled resorption space), or by a combination of both. All three mechanisms have been observed in the various types of osteoporosis. Thus, osteoporosis may be associated with low, normal, or high bone turnover.

EPIDEMIOLOGY. Osteoporosis is an enormous public health problem. About one million fractures in the United States each year are attributable to osteoporosis. Among women over age 65, 25 per cent will have one or more vertebral fractures caused by osteoporosis. By extreme old age, one woman in three and one man in six will have had a hip fracture. These fractures are associated with a mortality of 15 per cent, result in long-term domicilliary care in 50 per cent of the cases, and cost over $1 billion each year for only the short-term medical and surgical care. Indeed, falls are the leading cause of accidental death in the elderly, primarily because of hip fractures.

RISK FACTORS FOR OSTEOPOROSIS. Risk factors for bone loss are cumulative and, in any given patient, may be multiple. These can be categorized into five groups and are described in the following paragraphs.

(1) The phenomenon of age-related bone loss is perhaps most important. Beginning in early middle age, all individuals lose bone with aging. Over a lifetime, women lose about 45 per cent of the bone from their vertebrae and about 55 per cent from their proximal femur; men lose about half of this amount. The major cause of age-related bone loss appears to be insufficient bone formation in individual bone remodeling units.

(2) Insufficient accumulation of skeletal mass in young adulthood predisposes to fractures later in life as age-related bone loss ensues. Differences in bone density at skeletal maturity explain in part racial and sexual differences in the incidence of osteoporosis. White women have the lightest skeleton and black men have the heaviest; white men and black women have skeletons of intermediate density. This rank order corresponds to the rank order for occurrence of fractures. Women of short stature and of northern European extraction tend toward a more gracile skeleton and also have an increased incidence of osteoporosis later in life. Moreover, if the rate of bone loss with age is constant, those white women with the lowest bone density values at skeletal maturity are at the greatest risk for fracture in later life. The amount of bone in young adulthood has been shown to have significant genetic determinants, and osteoporotic patients often have affected relatives.

(3) Bioavailability of calcium is a third important factor. In contrast to the requirements for other mineral nutrients, the basal requirement for calcium is relatively high because of obligatory fecal and urinary losses—about 150 to 250 mg per day. When the amount of absorbed dietary calcium is insufficient to offset these losses, calcium must be withdrawn from bone, which contains 99 per cent of total body stores. Both menopause and aging increase the requirement for dietary calcium mainly by decreasing the efficiency of intestinal calcium absorption. Estimates based on metabolic balance suggest that premenopausal women require 1,000 mg of calcium per day to maintain calcium balance and postmenopausal women require 1,400 mg per day. Yet the dietary calcium intake of American women from middle life onward is only about 550 mg per day.

(4) The menopause and other abnormalities in endocrine function contribute to osteoporosis. Longitudinal studies of appendicular, mainly cortical, bone after oophorectomy have shown accelerated loss (total, about 8 per cent more than predicted) for about seven years. The extent of axial, mainly trabecular, bone loss due to estrogen deficiency is controversial but probably is somewhat more than appendicular bone loss. The negative calcium balance induced by menopause is associated with increased bone turnover—bone resorption increases more than does bone formation. It has been suggested that estrogen deficiency might increase the responsiveness of bone to circulating endogenous parathyroid hormone. Because

women have lower serum levels of immunoreactive calcitonin than men and because the menopause may further decrease calcitonin secretion, calcitonin deficiency may contribute to bone loss. Both intestinal calcium absorption and serum levels of 1,25-dihydroxyvitamin D are decreased in osteoporosis.

(5) Various risk factors for bone loss in the environment have been identified. These include high protein intake, high alcohol consumption, smoking, and decreased physical activity. Obesity is protective, possibly because of increased loading stress to the spine and, in postmenopausal women, because of increased conversion (in fat tissue) of adrenal androgens to estrogens.

SPECIFIC OSTEOPOROSIS SYNDROMES

Osteoporosis can be associated secondarily with a large number of disorders (Table 249–1). In 60 per cent of cases in men and 80 per cent in women, the disease occurs in middle-aged and older persons without any secondary abnormality. This common, primary form of the disease has been termed "involutional osteoporosis."

JUVENILE OSTEOPOROSIS. A rare syndrome of osteoporosis occurs in prepubertal children, usually between ages 8 and 14 years. The radiographic features of the syndrome are indistinguishable from those of involutional osteoporosis. Histologically, bone formation is normal or decreased but bone resorption is strikingly increased. Onset is acute, and multiple vertebral fractures occur over a period of two to four years. Then there is spontaneous remission and resumption of normal bone growth. Thus, treatment consists of protection of the spine until the remission occurs. There is no evidence that drug therapy is beneficial. Sex steroids are contraindicated because they may result in early closure of the epiphyseal growth plates. The syndrome is distinguished from osteogenesis imperfecta by lack of blue sclera and other characteristic stigmata, by the lack of a history of fractures of long bones, and by the absence of family history for bone disease. Cushing's syndrome should be excluded by adrenal function tests. Although the etiology is unknown, the temporal relationship to puberty suggests that hormonal factors may be important.

IDIOPATHIC OSTEOPOROSIS IN YOUNG ADULTS. This term is used to describe the relatively uncommon occurrence of osteoporosis in younger men or premenopausal women in whom no etiologic factor can be found. Undoubtedly, it is etiologically heterogeneous. In some patients, it runs a clinical course similar to that of involutional osteoporosis; in others, it is rapidly progressive and may lead to severe disability or even death (from respiratory failure) several years after onset. Except when the characteristic clinical features are present, it may be difficult to exclude a variant form of osteogenesis imperfecta tarda. Bone biopsy may help because patients with osteogenesis imperfecta invariably have very low bone turnover whereas patients with idiopathic osteoporosis often have high bone turnover.

TABLE 249–1. CLASSIFICATION OF CAUSES OF OSTEOPOROSIS

Primary osteoporosis	Bone marrow disorders
Juvenile	Multiple myeloma and related disorders
Idiopathic (young adults)	Systemic mastocytosis
Involutional osteoporosis	Disseminated carcinoma
Endocrine diseases	Connective tissue diseases
Hypogonadism	Osteogenesis imperfecta
Ovarian agenesis	Homocystinuria
Hyperadrenocorticism	Ehlers-Danlos syndrome
Hyperthyroidism	Marfan's syndrome
Hyperparathyroidism	
Diabetes mellitus (?)	
Gastrointestinal diseases	Miscellaneous causes
Subtotal gastrectomy	Immobilization
Malabsorption syndromes	Chronic obstructive pulmonary disease
Chronic obstructive jaundice	Chronic alcoholism
Primary biliary cirrhosis	Chronic heparin administration
Severe malnutrition	Rheumatoid arthritis (?)
Alactasia	

TABLE 249–2. INVOLUTIONAL OSTEOPOROSIS

	Type I	Type II
Age	51–65 yrs*	> 75 yrs*
Sex ratio (F:M)	6:1	2:1
Bone loss: Type	Mainly trabecular	Trabecular and cortical
Rate	Accelerated	Not accelerated
Fracture type	Mainly vertebral	Both vertebral and hip
Parathyroid function	Decreased	Increased
Calcium absorption	Decreased	Decreased
Metabolism of 25(OH)D to $1,25(OH)_2D$	Secondary decrease	Primary decrease
Major etiologic factors	Menopause	Decreased bone formation Secondary hyperparathyroidism

*Both types occur in the decade from 66 to 75 years.

INVOLUTIONAL OSTEOPOROSIS. It is becoming increasingly clear that the common variety of osteoporosis occurring in men and women with increasing frequency after middle life may consist of two distinct syndromes. Type I osteoporosis ("postmenopausal" osteoporosis) occurs in a relatively small subset of postmenopausal women who are 51 to 65 years of age. Less frequently, a similar syndrome occurs in men of comparable age. Type II osteoporosis ("senile" osteoporosis) occurs in a large proportion of women or men who are more than 75 years of age. Osteoporosis occurring in the decade from 66 to 75 years may represent a combination of both types. These two syndromes can be shown to differ with respect to epidemiology, patterns of trabecular and cortical bone loss, parathyroid function, and cause (Table 249–2).

Type I osteoporosis is the classic form of the disease described in 1940 by Fuller Albright and his associates and characteristically occurs in women within 15 years of menopause. Less commonly, men are affected with a form of osteoporosis that is otherwise indistinguishable from that occurring in postmenopausal women. Vertebral fracture is its main clinical manifestation but Colles' fracture of the distal radius occurs frequently. Both of these fracture sites contain large amounts of trabecular bone. Recent measurements of bone density have clearly established that patients with type I osteoporosis have accelerated loss of trabecular bone but their rate of loss of cortical bone is similar to or only slightly less than that for age-matched normal subjects. The accelerated bone loss leads to decreased parathyroid hormone secretion which, in turn, leads to decreased production of 1,25-dihydroxyvitamin D [$1,25(OH)_2D_3$]. The decreased circulating levels of serum $1,25(OH)_2D_3$ results in impaired calcium absorption, which may further increase bone loss. The predilection for women and the temporal proximity to menopause implicate estrogen deficiency as an etiologic agent. Yet only a relatively small subset of postmenopausal women have this form of osteoporosis, but all are deficient in estrogen. In postmenopausal women, most investigators have found no differences between those with and those without osteoporosis. Thus, some factor or factors in addition to menopause must determine individual susceptibility.

Type II osteoporosis occurs in persons 75 years of age or older and is manifested mainly by hip fracture and vertebral fracture, but fractures of the proximal humerus, proximal tibia, and pelvis may also occur. In patients with type II osteoporosis, individual bone densitometric values for the proximal femur, vertebrae, and bones of the appendicular skeleton are in the lower part of the age- and sex-adjusted normal range. Thus, type II osteoporosis is characterized by proportionate loss of both cortical and trabecular bone and a rate of loss similar to that in the general population. There may be two major causes for type II osteoporosis—impaired bone formation and secondary hyperparathyroidism. First, from the fourth decade of life onward, less bone is formed than is resorbed at individual remodeling foci, and this imbalance increases with aging. Second, the age-related increase in parathyroid function occurs concomitantly with and probably results from the age-related decrease in calcium absorption. Although serum levels of 25(OH)D are generally normal, serum levels of $1,25(OH)_2D$ decrease in the elderly and may be even lower in patients with hip fracture. These decreases may be caused by impaired metabolism of 25(OH)D to $1,25(OH)_2D$, an abnormality that has been documented in aging rats. The recent observation that overall bone turnover among women may increase with aging (as assessed by measurement of serum bone gla-protein and other biochemical markers) suggests that secondary hyperparathyroidism may increase the number of individual bone remodeling units and thus increases bone turnover at the tissue level. Because bone formation remains decreased at the level of individual remodeling units, increased bone turnover would result in increased bone loss.

ENDOCRINE DISEASES. Osteoporosis may be associated with a number of syndromes of endocrine dysfunction. *Hypogonadism* in either sex leads to an increased incidence of osteoporosis. Hypogonadism is probably the main cause of osteoporosis associated with ovarian agenesis *(Turner's syndrome)* although a genetic abnormality of bone maturation probably also is present. Endogenous or exogenous *hyperadrenocorticism* is associated with both decreased bone formation and increased bone resorption that lead to rapid bone loss. The decrease in bone formation results from inhibition of collagen biosynthesis. The increase in bone resorption may be indirectly mediated, possibly by an increased sensitivity of bone to parathyroid hormone. Patients with glucocorticoid excess also have impaired calcium absorption, and this can be reversed by administering vitamin D or its active metabolite. An effect of corticosteroids on vitamin D metabolism, however, has not been conclusively established.

Although *hyperthyroidism* consistently increases bone turnover, in most patients formation and resorption remain coupled. Symptomatic osteoporosis associated with hyperthyroidism therefore is relatively unusual and, when present, generally occurs in postmenopausal women. Although osteitis fibrosa is the characteristic skeletal abnormality associated with *hyperparathyroidism,* about 5 per cent of patients, mostly postmenopausal women, present with osteopenia and vertebral compression fractures. It has been suggested that patients with either juvenile- or adult-onset *diabetes mellitus* have an increased risk for osteoporosis, but others have challenged this view. Osteoporosis associated with *acromegaly* is believed to be rare and, when present, is the result of concomitant hypogonadism. In fact, because of the anabolic effect of growth hormone excess on the skeleton, most patients with acromegaly have an increase in both trabecular and cortical bone mass.

GASTROINTESTINAL DISEASES. These conditions can cause either osteoporosis or osteomalacia, and they generally produce a mixture of both. About 5 per cent of patients with *subtotal gastrectomy,* particularly in those with the Billroth II type, subsequently develop bone disease. *Malabsorption syndromes* impair absorption of calcium and vitamin D; usually this results in osteomalacia but, if mild, the predominant lesion may be osteoporosis. Chronic obstructive jaundice may be associated with bone disease because the enterohepatic circulation of active vitamin D metabolites is impaired. This mechanism may play a role in the osteomalacia associated with *primary biliary cirrhosis.* In the United States, however, osteoporosis associated with a profound depression in bone formation is the typical finding. Its etiology is unknown. *Severe malnutrition* involving both protein and calcium deficiency—as has been observed in prisoners of war and in patients with anorexia nervosa—may cause osteoporosis. Finally, *alactasia* has been reported in up to 30 per cent of osteoporotic subjects. This disorder may be a risk factor for osteoporosis because it produces intolerance to milk and, thus, is associated with a low calcium intake.

BONE MARROW DISORDERS. *Multiple myeloma* is associated with diffuse osteoporosis in about 10 per cent of patients and in a lesser proportion of other myeloproliferative disorders. It is mediated by an increased local production of osteoclast activating factor (a lymphokine with potent bone-resorbing properties) by bone marrow cells. Diffuse osteoporosis also may occur when *disseminated carcinoma* involves the bone marrow.

CONNECTIVE TISSUE DISEASES. An unusually severe form of osteoporosis may occur in *osteogenesis imperfecta.* This disease is usually inherited as an autosomal dominant trait and is associated with blue sclera, deafness, thin skin, and impaired biosynthesis of type I collagen. Although onset usually is in childhood, some patients present with premature spinal osteoporosis in the absence of a history of limb bone fracture. The *Marfan* and *Ehlers-Danlos syndromes* also may be associated with spinal osteopenia but less frequently include vertebral fractures. Osteoporosis commonly occurs in patients with *homocystinuria,* an autosomal recessive disorder caused by deficient cystathionine synthase activity. The resultant increase in homocysteine and other metabolites in the circulation interferes with cross-linking of collagen.

MISCELLANEOUS CAUSES. Total *immobilization,* such as occurs in traumatic quadriplegia, results in a loss of up to 1 per cent of bone per month, especially in the trabecular bone of the axial skeleton. After loss of 40 to 50 per cent of bone from the spinal column, a new steady state is reached and bone mass is maintained. Bone loss is associated with both depressed bone formation and enhanced bone resorption. Significant bone loss also occurs during total bed rest among nonparalyzed individuals. If immobilization is transient, replacement of bone mass occurs on remobilization, provided that there has been only thinning of bone trabeculae rather than loss of trabeculae and other structural elements.

Not infrequently, osteoporosis is associated with *chronic obstructive pulmonary disease.* Whether this is related to the consumption of tobacco, which is believed to be a bone toxin, or to the pulmonary disease itself is unknown. Young alcoholics also have been shown to have thinner bones than other subjects of similar age. Long-term therapy with *heparin* has been reported to cause severe loss of bone and spontaneous fractures. Heparin decreases the stability of lysosomes, and release of collagenase and other lysosomal enzymes may be responsible for the bone loss. Finally, although it has been suggested that osteoporosis may be a complication of rheumatoid arthritis, most of the bone loss in these patients can probably be accounted for by corticosteroid use and by immobilization.

CLINICAL CONSIDERATIONS

CLINICAL PRESENTATION. Osteoporosis is manifested by *back pain, loss of height* and *spinal deformity,* especially kyphosis, and *fractures of the hips, wrist,* and, less frequently, other bones. The most characteristic symptom of osteoporosis is back pain caused by vertebral compression. Typically, a woman within 20 years after menopause develops acute lumbar or thoracic back pain after some ordinary activity such as raising a window or lifting a sack of groceries. The pain may be mild or severe, and it may be localized or exhibit flank radiation. It remits in days or weeks but then recurs. After several episodes of acute intermittent pain, the patient may develop a chronic mechanical backache resulting from spinal deformity. Untreated or unsuccessfully treated patients may develop *severe kyphosis* and a loss of 4 to 8 inches of height. In severe cases, the rib cage comes to rest on the pelvic brim. The frequency of occurrence of vertebral fractures and the number of fractures that eventually occur vary widely between patients, but the average is one per year. In general, elderly women progress more slowly and commonly develop substantial dorsal kyphosis and cervical lordosis—the so-called dowager's hump—in the absence of significant pain. Half of the hip fractures in elderly men and women are spontaneous and half are associated with falls.

RADIOLOGIC FINDINGS. Roentgenograms of the spinal column show accentuation of the vertebral end-plates, prominence of the weight-bearing, vertical trabeculae (due to disappearance of the horizontal trabeculae), and loss of contrast in radiodensity between the interior of the vertebral body and adjacent soft tissue (Fig. 249–1). Vertebral deformity may take the form of collapse (reduction of anterior and posterior height), anterior wedging (reduction in anterior height, usually occurring in the thoracic spinal column), or "ballooning" (biconcave compression of the end-plates by pressure of the intervertebral discs, usually occurring in the lumbar spinal column). Also, localized herniation of the nucleus pulposus into the vertebral body (Schmorl's nodes) may occur. Osteoporosis due to glucocorticoid excess should be considered when there is associated osteoporosis of the skull, fractures of the ribs and pelvic rami, and prominent partially mineralized callus at the sites of fracture. In the absence of pseudofractures, osteomalacia may be difficult to distinguish from osteoporosis, but it often has a "ground glass" appearance rather than the characteristic "clear glass" appearance of osteoporosis. Posterior wedging of a vertebra suggests a destructive lesion rather than osteoporosis.

DIAGNOSTIC EVALUATION. All newly discovered patients with osteoporosis should have a general medical evaluation to exclude secondary diseases that may cause osteoporosis and to assess severity. Systemic symptoms or abnormal physical findings suggest the presence of an underlying disease. Serum calcium and phosphorus levels are normal in primary osteoporosis. Serum alkaline phosphatase level also is normal except for transient elevations during healing of vertebral fractures. Sustained elevation of alkaline phosphatase level, in the absence of liver disease, suggests osteomalacia or a destructive skeletal process.

Multiple myeloma may be present in the absence of symptoms and with a normal hematogram and erythrocyte sedimentation rate. Although most cases can be diagnosed by serum and urine protein electrophoresis, bone marrow examination occasionally is required (see Ch. 163). Sometimes this is necessary to diagnose some cases of disseminated carcinoma. Transiliac bone biopsy may be needed to exclude osteomalacia or to stage the abnormality in bone remodeling.

Severity of osteoporosis can be assessed most easily by determining the amount of height loss and the number of vertebral fractures, but it can be assessed more precisely by measuring vertebral density directly with either dual photon absorptiometry or quantitative computed tomography. Although currently confined to only a few research centers, these procedures should soon be widely available.

TREATMENT

GENERAL THERAPEUTIC MEASURES. Acute back pain responds to analgesics, heat, and gentle massage to alleviate muscle spasm. Sometimes a brief period of bed rest is required. Chronic back pain often is caused by spinal deformity and thus is

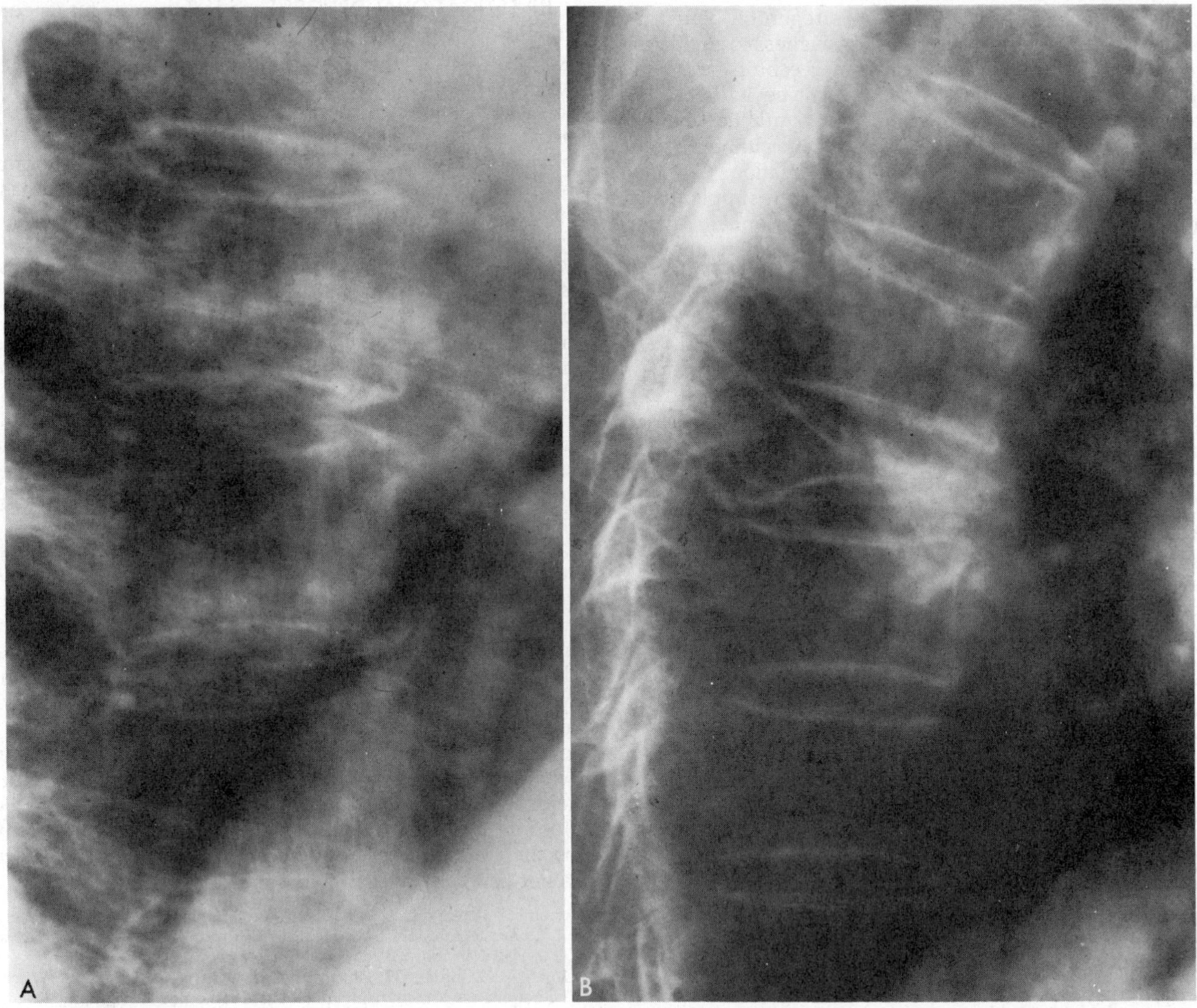

Figure 249–1. *A*, Moderate osteopenia of the thoracic spine is shown radiographically by accentuation of the cortical outlines of the vertebral body, prominence of the vertebral trabeculae, and relative lucency of the vertebral body. *B*, Advanced osteoporosis of the thoracic spine is shown radiographically by relative lucency of the vertebral bodies, accentuation of the cortical outlines, wedge deformities, and a compression fracture. (Photographs courtesy of Dr. Harry K. Genant.)

difficult to relieve completely. Instruction in posture and gait training and institution of regular back extension exercises to strengthen the flabby paravertebral muscles usually are beneficial. Occasionally, an orthopedic back brace is required. All patients with osteoporosis should have a diet adequate in calcium, proteins, and vitamins, should be reasonably active physically, and should take precautions to prevent falls.

DRUG THERAPY. Calcium, vitamin D, estrogen, anabolic steroids, and calcitonin inhibit bone resorption. When a new steady state is attained after three to six months of treatment, there is a coupled reduction in bone formation that approximates the reduction in bone resorption. Thus, the best result that can be obtained with this class of therapeutic agents is maintenance of the existing skeletal mass or slowing of its rate of loss.

Calcium, which is prescribed to offset the impaired calcium absorption that is often present in osteoporosis and to decrease parathyroid hormone secretion, is safe, well-tolerated, and inexpensive. *Vitamin D* and its active metabolites have a similar function but must be used judiciously, because the dose that increases calcium absorption is not much smaller than the dose that increases bone resorption.

Estrogen is more effective than calcium but has significant side effects. These commonly include induction of menstruation, mastodynia, and fluid retention; less common but more serious side effects are venous thrombosis, endometrial carcinoma, and cholelithiasis. The effect of estrogen on bone may be mediated by decreasing skeletal responsiveness to circulating parathyroid hormone. Because estrogen receptors have not been demonstrated in bone, its action may be indirect. The mechanism of action of androgens and synthetic anabolic agents probably is similar to that of estrogen, although some data suggest a weak stimulation of bone formation. *Calcitonin* is an effective antiresorption agent, but calcium supplementation must be given concurrently to prevent secondary hyperparathyroidism. Disadvantages include the requirement for parenteral administration, a relatively high cost, and the development of neutralizing antibodies in some patients.

Therapy for patients with involutional osteoporosis should be individualized. For patients with mild disease, particularly in those older than 75 years, only calcium supplementation (1.0 to 1.5 grams per day) need be employed. For more extensive disease, especially in women within 15 years of menopause, low-dose estrogen therapy (such as cyclic doses of 0.625 mg daily of conjugated estrogen or 0.025 mg daily of ethynyl estradiol) may be used. Because the risk of endometrial hyperplasia (and, therefore, carcinoma) is reduced or eliminated by concomitant progestin therapy, 5 mg daily of medroxyprogesterone acetate is given during the last ten days of the cycle. Even a hysterectomized woman should receive cyclic therapy. If fractures continue on this regimen, the dosage of both the estrogen and progestin should be doubled. Elderly women may prefer synthetic anabolic steroids to estrogens.

Vitamin D and its active metabolites probably should be reserved for patients with a documented or suspected impairment in calcium absorption. This can be inferred from a relatively low urinary calcium excretion rate (<75 mg per day), especially if this does not increase significantly with calcium supplementation. Calcitonin is most likely to be effective in patients with osteoporosis associated with a high bone turnover. In the absence of a bone biopsy, this can be inferred from values in the upper portion of the normal range for serum phosphorus and urinary calcium. The recommended dose is 100 units daily accompanied by at least 1.0 gram of supplementary calcium daily.

The same therapeutic approach with modifications can be used for other types of osteoporosis. Idiopathic osteoporosis occurring in young adult women often is relatively refractory to therapy. Because the women are premenopausal, there is no reason to prescribe sex steroids. Some of these patients have impaired calcium absorption, which is correctable with vitamin D therapy. The mainstay of treatment, therefore, is calcium supplementation with or without pharmacologic doses of vitamin D. Calcitonin can be added to reduce the increased level of bone resorption that may be present.

Men with osteoporosis usually do not have a deficiency of sex steroids and thus have no need for hormonal treatment. But 10 to 20 per cent have partial or complete hypogonadism from various causes. Patients with documented low plasma testosterone levels should receive replacement therapy with, for example, testosterone enanthate (Delatestryl) in a dose of 200 to 400 mg intramuscularly every four weeks. Calcium supplementation with or without pharmacologic doses of vitamin D should also be given.

The most common cause of secondary osteoporosis is chronic use of pharmacologic dosages of glucocorticoids. The single most effective measure is reduction of dosage or, if possible, complete discontinuation of the glucocorticoids. Administering the glucocorticoids once daily or on alternate days may maintain a more favorable balance between anti-inflammatory and immunosuppressive effects and the osteopenic effect. All patients should be given calcium supplements, and postmenopausal women should be given estrogens. Although glucocorticoids inhibit calcium absorption, the use of pharmacologic dosages of vitamin D or its metabolites in this circumstance is controversial and may abet the calciuric effects of glucocorticoids. There is increasing evidence that glucocorticoids do not induce major alterations in vitamin D metabolism.

INVESTIGATIONAL DRUGS. The ideal therapy for osteoporosis should result in an increase in bone formation over bone resorption and consequently an increase in bone mass. Three investigational regimens have been described that may have this effect: low-dose therapy with the synthetic 1-34 fragment of parathyroid hormone, combined oral therapy with phosphate and calcitonin, and combined therapy with fluoride and calcium. Only the last has been studied in detail and has given reproducible results.

Sodium fluoride is a potent stimulator of osteoblasts, and recent studies on bone cells *in vitro* have shown that this effect is direct. Sodium fluoride can induce a substantial increase in trabecular bone of the axial skeleton. But concurrent administration of supplementary calcium is required to prevent or minimize the incomplete mineralization that may occur when fluoride is given alone. Bone biopsy studies suggest that fluoride therapy may bypass the normal remodeling sequence and induce osteoblast formation *de novo* on previously quiescent surfaces. Although fluoridic bone may be structurally less sound than an equivalent amount of normal bone, the substantial increase in bone mass increases net bone strength.

Patients treated with fluoride at the Mayo Clinic had fewer new fractures. Unfortunately, a significant subset (25 to 40 per cent) responded to sodium fluoride therapy incompletely or not at all, possibly because they had an intrinsic abnormality in osteoblast function. At least one third of treated patients develop gastric or rheumatic side effects: the former consist of nausea or epigastric burning distress caused by gastric irritation and the latter consist of periarticular pain, particularly in the knees, ankles, and feet. Both types of symptoms disappear when treatment is discontinued and usually do not recur after reinstitution of sodium fluoride at a lower dosage. Sodium fluoride has not been approved for treatment of osteoporosis by the United States Food and Drug Administration, and so it is not generally available in a high-dose form.

Avioli LV: Osteoporosis. *In* Peck WA (ed.): Bone and Mineral Research. Annual 1. Amsterdam, Excerpta Medica, 1983, pp 280–318. *Comprehensive survey of new developments with detailed literature review.*

Genant HK, Gordan GS, Hoffman PG Jr: Osteoporosis: part I. Advanced radiographic assessment using quantitative computed tomography—Medical Staff Conference, University of California, San Francisco. West J Med 139:75, 1983. *Description of this new method for assessing density of the spine.*

Parfitt AM: Quantum concept of bone remodeling and turnover: Implications for the pathogenesis of osteoporosis. Calcif Tissue Int 28:1, 1979. *A lucid review of the role of abnormalities of bone remodeling in pathogenesis of osteoporosis.*

Parfitt AM: Morphologic basis of bone mineral measurements: Transient and steady state effects of treatment in osteoporosis. Min Electrolyte Metab 4:273, 1980. *The theoretical basis for differences in early and late effects of therapeutic agents on bone remodeling and bone density in osteoporosis.*

Riggs BL, Seeman E, Hodgson SF, et al.: Effect of the fluoride/calcium regimen on vertebral fracture occurrence in postmenopausal osteoporosis. N Engl J Med 306:446, 1982. *Effect of calcium, estrogen, and sodium fluoride, alone and in combination, on fracture occurrence.*

Riggs BL, Melton LJ III: Evidence for two distinct syndromes of involutional osteoporosis. Am J Med 75:899, 1983. *Summary of evidence that supports this concept.*

Riggs, BL, Wahner HW, Seeman E, et al.: Changes in bone mineral density of the proximal femur and spine with aging. J Clin Invest 70:716, 1982. *Bone density measurements in normal and osteoporotic subjects using dual photon absorptiometry.*

Steinbach HL: The roentgen appearance of osteoporosis. Radiol Clin North Am 2:191, 1964. *Classic article on the radiologic appearance of osteoporosis.*

250. PAGET'S DISEASE OF BONE (OSTEITIS DEFORMANS)

Frederick R. Singer

INCIDENCE AND EPIDEMIOLOGY

Paget's disease is a common bone disorder second in incidence to osteoporosis. In areas of prevalence it affects approximately 3 per cent of the population over age 40. The disease is commonly diagnosed in the United Kingdom and in the countries to which its inhabitants have migrated, including the United States, Canada, South Africa, Australia, and New Zealand. The disease also is common in France, Germany, and Italy. Patients are rarely found in China, Japan, India, or Scandinavia. There is no major predilection for either sex.

There is evidence of an autosomal dominant transmission that is linked to histocompatibility leukocyte antigens. As high as 50 per cent of patients have been reported to have at least one relative with the disease.

PATHOLOGY

Paget's disease may affect one or many bones but in the majority of patients most of the skeleton is uninvolved. The earliest phase is characterized by a localized osteolytic process in which proliferation of multinucleated osteoclasts is the dominant lesion. The osteoclasts of Paget's disease are occasionally quite large and may exhibit more than 100 nuclei in a cross-section of one cell. Adjacent to the advancing osteolytic front, the pathology is characterized by a mixed osteolytic and osteoblastic process of great intensity. Numerous plump osteoblasts line bony trabeculae that have previously been partially resorbed by osteoclasts. The marrow spaces may be devoid of hematopoietic cells and instead are filled with fibroblasts, connective tissue, and blood vessels. The resultant architecture of the bone takes on a "mosaic" pattern in which the cement lines are arranged in a haphazard pattern instead of the normal symmetry of parallel collagen fibers in both cortical and trabecular bone. Occasionally this abnormal mosaic pattern is present with little or no cellular activity. Osteolytic, mixed osteolytic and osteoblastic, and "burned out" Paget's disease may be present in a single bone. Paget's disease can usually be readily distinguished from primary hyperparathyroidism, osteomyelitis, and osteomalacia by light microscopy, but electron microscopy studies have provided evidence of a characteristic lesion. The nuclei, and at times the cytoplasm, of the osteoclasts frequently contain abnormal inclusions that resemble the nucleocapsids of viruses of the Paramyxoviridae family. Further evidence of a viral presence in these cells has been obtained by the use of immunohistologic staining. Antisera to respiratory syncytial virus and measles virus have produced positive results in the osteoclasts of Paget's disease but in no other disorder.

ETIOLOGY

Sir James Paget, in his original description of the disease, proposed that the entity was inflammatory in nature. The recent ultrastructural and immunohistologic studies support the concept of a "slow" virus infection, although definitive proof is still to be obtained. Other hypotheses for which there are insignificant supporting data include an abnormality of hormone secretion, a neoplastic state, a vascular anomaly, an autoimmune state, and an inborn error of connective tissue biosynthesis.

CLINICAL FEATURES

In many patients Paget's disease is not appreciated until an abnormal radiograph or laboratory test is encountered either in the course of a routine evaluation or during assessment of an unrelated complaint. The most common complaints of symptomatic patients are *skeletal deformity* and *musculoskeletal pain.* The bones most likely to be abnormal on physical examination are the cranium, the clavicles, and the long bones, particularly of the lower extremities. The complications associated with skull lesions include hearing loss, vertigo, tinnitus and, less commonly, headaches. Severe enlargement of the base of the skull may lead to basilar impression and compression of the spinal cord, the brain stem, the cerebellum, and the basilar and vertebral arteries. Slurred speech, impaired swallowing, diplopia, and urinary incontinence may result. Deformity of the facial bones (leontiasis ossea) is much less common in patients with Paget's disease than in patients with fibrous dysplasia, a disease which usually is diagnosed several decades earlier in life. The spine may be involved at any level, but lumbar and thoracic vertebrae are most commonly affected. One or more vertebrae, consecutive or not, can manifest the disease. Back pain may be severe and of complex origin since degenerative arthritis is common in this age group, and impingement of skeletal tissue on nerve roots or the spinal cord can occur. The sudden onset of intolerable pain suggests that a compression fracture has occurred. Disease affecting the pelvis and proximal femur produces a common severe pain syndrome, weight-bearing pain from degenerative arthritis of the hip. Ambulation may also be impaired when significant lateral or anterior bowing of the femur or tibia develops. These bones are also prone to pathologic fracture. Evidence of disease activity in long bones is manifested by increased skin temperature over the affected bone. This results from the increased cutaneous blood flow associated with the hypervascular bone beneath.

Defects in Bruch's membrane of the retina, termed angioid streaks, may be observed in about 10 per cent of patients and seldom are associated with impaired vision. Cardiac enlargement and frank congestive heart failure may be a manifestation of prior increased cardiac output, which is thought to be a consequence of increased vascularity of affected bones. This usually occurs in patients with more than 30 per cent of the skeleton affected by Paget's disease or when the skull is severely involved. Bone tumors such as osteosarcoma and giant cell tumor may develop in lesions of Paget's disease (Ch. 252). A rapid worsening of bone pain or the relatively sudden development of a mass or both are the common modes of presentation.

RADIOLOGY. The radiologic features of Paget's disease are so characteristic that it is seldom necessary to obtain a bone biopsy for diagnosis. The earliest manifestation is a localized osteolytic lesion most readily detected in the skull and at either end of a long bone. In the skull, the circumscribed radiolucent area has been termed osteoporosis circumscripta (Fig. 250–1). The osteolytic lesion in an extremity bone usually progresses with a sharply defined V-shape at an average rate of progression of 1 cm per year. Linear cortical radiolucencies may develop in the femur or tibia on the convex surface of a curved bone and may be precursors of fractures. An uncommon variant of the osteolytic lesion may occur at the distal end of the tibia in which a cystic-like expansion of the bone is seen. Osteolytic disease of the vertebral bodies is often associated with sclerotic margins

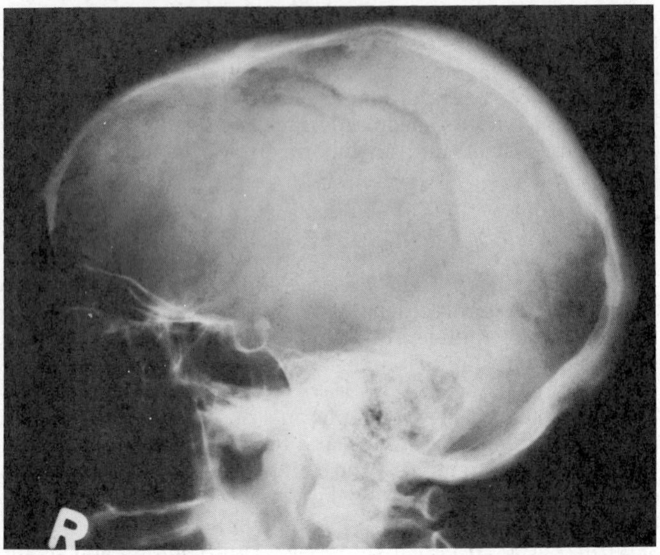

Figure 250–1. Osteoporosis circumscripta of the skull involving the frontal, parietal, and temporal bones.

giving a "picture frame" appearance. These vertebrae are prone to compression fractures.

The radiographic manifestations of osteoblastic activity generally appear years or even decades after the onset of osteolysis. In the skull a "honeycomb" appearance of patchy new bone may fill in the underlying osteoporosis circumscripta, and subsequently the classic "cotton-wool" lesions of exuberant chaotic bone formation appear with a strikingly thickened calvarium (Fig. 250–2). In the long bones, the osteolytic lesions evolve into thickened bone with irregular trabeculation. In the pelvis, thickening of the iliopectineal line, the "brim sign," is nearly pathognomonic of Paget's disease. It is also found in patients with osteopetrosis but rarely in patients with osteoblastic metastases. Enlargement of the ischial and pubic bones is also typical of Paget's disease. Sclerosis of the pagetic vertebral body may be difficult to distinguish from malignant bone involvement, but if the vertebral body is clearly larger than adjacent vertebral bodies, Paget's disease is likely. Computerized tomography of the spine is a useful means of evaluating the detailed anatomy of the spine and is particularly helpful in defining arthritic and neurologic complications in the patient with back pain.

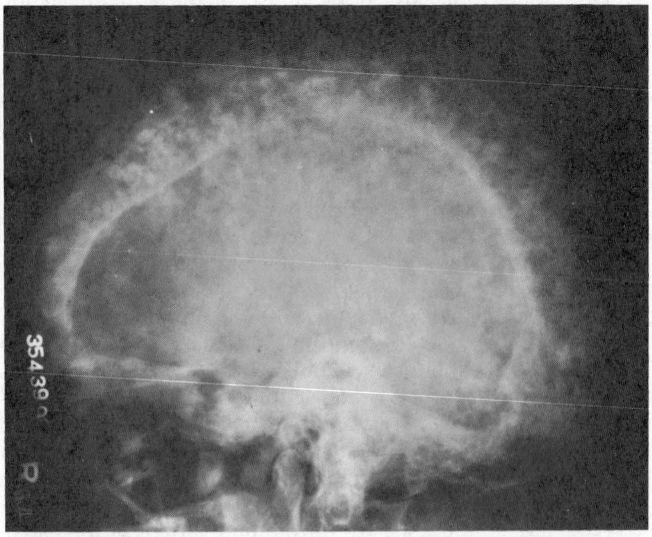

Figure 250–2. Advanced involvement of the skull with marked thickening of the entire cranial vault, areas of osteolysis, and patchy new bone formation resulting in a "cotton-wool" appearance.

The bone scan is the most sensitive means to detect active lesions of Paget's disease, although it is not a specific diagnostic test. The earliest lesions may not be discernible roentgenographically at the same time an area of increased uptake of the radiolabeled scanning agent is obvious.

BIOCHEMICAL FEATURES

The extent and activity of Paget's disease has been found to correlate reasonably well with serum alkaline phosphatase activity (an index of osteoblastic activity) and urinary hydroxyproline excretion (an index of bone matrix resorption). Patients with very limited active disease have normal biochemical parameters, whereas increases of 50-fold greater than normal sometimes occur in patients with polyostotic disease of greatest extent. The serum calcium concentration is normal except in patients who are immobilized or in whom malignancy or primary hyperparathyroidism develops. Hypercalciuria precedes hypercalcemia in these patients. Hyperuricemia, with or without clinical gout, is sometimes found and may reflect increased turnover of purines.

MEDICAL AND SURGICAL THERAPY

CALCITONIN. Most patients with Paget's disease do not require any therapy or may only require analgesic agents such as aspirin or indomethacin. Effective and safe therapy of Paget's disease only became possible in 1975 with the availability of salmon calcitonin. Subcutaneous injections of 50 to 100 MRC units daily or on alternate days produce an average decrease of 50 per cent in biochemical parameters and improve many of the manifestations of the disease. Relief of bone pain, healing of osteolytic lesions, reduction of increased cardiac output and elevated skin temperature, stabilization of auditory acuity, and reversal of various neurologic deficits have all been convincingly documented during chronic therapy. Treatment may be necessary for years in patients with active osteolytic lesions. Side effects include nausea, facial flushing, and polyuria, but they seldom require interruption of therapy. Salmon calcitonin elicits an antibody response in more than 50 per cent of patients, since its amino acid sequence differs considerably from human calcitonin. Approximately 25 per cent of patients acquire high enough antibody titers to become resistant to hormone action. These patients respond to human calcitonin (still experimental in the United States) or to other forms of therapy.

DIPHOSPHONATES. An alternate form of therapy is disodium etidronate, whose main advantage is its oral mode of administration. At a dose of 5 mg per kilogram of body weight daily for an initial treatment period of six months this drug produces benefits similar to calcitonin. However, healing of osteolytic lesions has seldom been documented. Long-term use of higher doses should be avoided because of impairment of bone mineralization and resulting susceptibility to fracture.

CYTOTOXIC AGENTS. Mithramycin is a cytotoxic antibiotic which has not been approved for therapy of Paget's disease by the FDA but has been used in selected patients because of its great potency. Dosage has not been standardized but intravenous infusions of 10 to 15 μg per kilogram daily for 10 days or once weekly have been reported to suppress many of the manifestations of the disease. The platelet, renal, and hepatic toxicity of this agent warrants great caution in its use. It should be reserved for patients with marked symptomatology who fail with other agents.

The effectiveness of medical therapy can usually be assessed by measurement of serum alkaline phosphatase activity alone at intervals of two to four months. The appropriate duration of therapy varies in respect to the type of lesions encountered in the patient and the specific drug administred.

Surgery is an important adjunct to medical therapy in selected patients. Occipital craniectomy may be necessary in patients with basilar impression, and decompression of neurologic structures affected by vertebral lesions is another procedure of critical importance. More commonly orthopedic procedures are required to enable more normal ambulation in patients with pelvic and lower extremity disease. Degenerative arthritis of the hip is a common complication that can produce severe pain and limit ambulation. Results of total hip replacement are excellent. Deformity of the tibia may also limit ambulation because of knee and ankle pain. Tibial osteotomy leading to restoration of a more normal knee-ankle alignment can also markedly alleviate joint pain and restore a near normal gait. If possible 1 to 3 months of medical therapy should be administered prior to surgery in order to reduce the amount of intra- and postoperative bleeding and to prevent immobilization hypercalcemia postoperatively.

Altman RD, Singer FR: Proceedings of the Kroc foundation conference on Paget's disease of bone. Arthritis Rheum 23:1073, 1980. *A comprehensive coverage of etiologic, metabolic, and therapeutic aspects of the disease.*

Barry H: Paget's Disease of Bone. Baltimore, Williams & Wilkins Company, 1969. *A general review of Paget's disease written by an orthopedic surgeon and emphasizing surgical and neoplastic aspects of the disease.*

Mills BG, Singer FR, Weiner LP, Suffin SC, Stabile E, Holst P: Evidence for both respiratory syncytial virus and measles virus antigens in the osteoclasts of patients with Paget's disease of bone. Clin Orth Rel Res 183:303, 1984. *A study documenting antigens of two paramyxoviridae viruses in osteoclasts of Paget's disease.*

Nagant De Deuxchaisnes C, Krane SM: Paget's disease of bone; clinical and metabolic observations. Medicine 43:233, 1964. *Excellent review of clinical and metabolic features of Paget's disease.*

Singer FR: Paget's Disease of Bone. New York, Plenum Press, 1977. *A monograph written for the practitioner that emphasizes clinical manifestations of the disease and the approach to therapy.*

251. OSTEONECROSIS, OSTEOSCLEROSIS, AND OTHER DISORDERS OF BONE

Gordon J. Strewler

OSTEONECROSIS

Osteonecrosis is synonymous with aseptic or avascular necrosis of bone; these terms describe infarction of bone, presumably resulting from ischemia. Such infarcts may be asymptomatic or associated with self-limited pain if they occur in the shaft, as in sickle cell disease or hyperbaric injury (caisson disease). Syndromes with greater morbidity occur with infarcts of subarticular bone, especially in the femoral head.

ETIOLOGY. The most common cause of osteonecrosis is fracture or dislocation of the femoral neck. Other bones susceptible to post-traumatic osteonecrosis are the proximal pole of the carpal scaphoid and the body of the talus. Nontraumatic vascular compromise, usually of the femoral head, is the likely cause of osteonecrosis in sickle cell disease (sludging of sickled erythrocytes), caisson disease (gas bubble emboli), Gaucher's disease (obstruction by histiocytes), hemophilia, and polycythemia vera. Other important etiologies are glucocorticoid therapy, cytotoxic chemotherapy, radiation injury, and renal transplantation. The prevalence of osteonecrosis after renal transplantation ranges from 3 to 41 per cent in various reports. In addition to corticosteroid therapy, precedent renal osteodystrophy and persistent secondary hyperparathyroidism may be etiologic factors. Osteonecrosis is associated with alcoholism, chronic pancreatitis, hyperuricemia, and diabetes mellitus, but diabetics seem to be relatively protected against its development after renal transplantation. The epiphyseal regions of growing bone in children are susceptible to osteonecrosis; here the relative roles of constitutional factors and trauma are poorly defined. Over 50 eponymic syndromes, collectively called osteochondroses, are associated with osteonecrosis at various epiphyseal sites. The commonest, once again, is the femoral head (Perthes' disease).

PATHOGENESIS. While in some disorders (e.g., sickle cell disease), osteonecrosis can readily be ascribed to vascular obstruction, in others, such as glucocorticoid excess, its cause is unknown. There is little support for such proposed mechanisms of steroid-induced osteonecrosis as increased intramedullary pressure with obstruction of venous outflow, fat embol-

ization, or osteopenia with nonhealing microfractures. Also poorly understood are the mechanisms by which infarction of bone leads to its eventual collapse. Dead bone does not lose mechanical stability; bone resorption occurring as part of the reparative process may weaken the infarcted area, predisposing the infarcted bone to fractures and fragmentation.

CLINICAL MANIFESTATIONS. Besides the femoral head, common sites of nontraumatic osteonecrosis include the femoral condyles, distal tibia, humeral head, and talus. The presenting symptom is pain, often of acute onset. Radiologic diagnosis may be delayed for weeks or months because dead and living bone are radiologically indistinguishable. It is mostly slow reparative processes that are visualized radiographically. Patchy lucencies reflect resorption, whereas linear subchondral lucencies reflect collapse of bone; patchy sclerosis indicates growth of new bone over the scaffolding of dead trabeculae. These reparative processes may lead to healing if fragmentation or collapse of weakened bone does not supervene. Initial therapy consists of avoidance of weight bearing, but surgery, such as transpositional osteotomy, arthrotomy with removal of fragments, or arthroplasty, may be required.

Davidson JK (ed.): Aseptic Necrosis of Bone. New York, American Elsevier, 1976. *Review of the radiology and pathology of osteonecrosis, with chapters on traumatic, dysbaric, and hemoglobinopathy-related syndromes.*

Glimcher MJ, Kenzora JE: The biology of osteonecrosis of the human femoral head and its clinical implications. III. Discussion of the etiology and genesis of the pathological sequelae; comments on treatment. Clin Orthop 140:273, 1979. *A thoughtful review of the pathogenesis of osteonecrosis and its clinical implications.*

DISORDERS OF INCREASED BONE DENSITY

Radiographic evidence of increased bone density usually reflects increased bone mass per unit volume, rather than increased mineral per unit of bone mass. This increase can result from accelerated synthesis and mineralization of the bone matrix or from decreased bone resorption. The pathogenesis of such disorders is rarely known, and their histologic characteristics are often indistinguishable; hence, they are classified in the accompanying table on the basis of their radiographic appearance. In the table the term osteosclerosis refers

TABLE 251–1. CAUSES OF OSTEOSCLEROSIS*

A. Osteosclerosis found predominantly in spongy trabecular bone
Neoplastic causes (prostatic carcinoma, breast carcinoma, gastrointestinal adenocarcinoma, carcinoid tumors, transitional cell carcinoma, myeloma, lymphoma, leukemia)
Hematologic causes (sickle cell disorders, systemic mastocytosis, myelofibrosis, polycythemia vera)
Metabolic causes (renal osteodystrophy, Paget's disease, primary hyperparathyroidism, fluorosis, vitamin D-resistant rickets)
B. Osteosclerosis involving cortical and trabecular bone
Osteopetrosis
Malignant (congenita)
Benign (tarda)
Pyknodysostosis
Sclerosteosis
C. Osteosclerosis found predominantly in compact cortical bone
Hypertrophic osteoarthropathy
Pachydermoperiostosis
Vitamin A intoxication
Progressive diaphyseal dysplasia (Camurati-Engelmann disease)
Hereditary hyperphosphatasia
Endosteal hyperostosis
Van Buchem's disease (hyperostosis corticalis generalisata)
Autosomal dominant (Worth's disease)
D. Focal osteosclerosis
Osteopoikilosis
Osteopathia striata
Melorheostosis

*Adapted from Genant HK: Review of the osteoscleroses. *In* Margulis AR, Gooding CA (eds.): Diagnostic Radiology. San Francisco, University of California, 1981, pp 109–122.

to increased bone density; as indicated, sclerosis can involve predominantly cortical or trabecular (cancellous) bone or both. Sclerosis of the cortex can produce increased width as the result of new bone formation, and this is sometimes referred to as hyperostosis. Bone shape can also be altered by disorders of modeling, the process by which bones assume their adult shape during development.

Trabecular Osteosclerosis

This form of osteosclerosis is the most frequently encountered. Its causes can be categorized as neoplastic, hematologic, or metabolic.

Neoplastic. Prostatic and breast carcinoma, as well as other neoplasms with osteoblastic metastases, can present on occasion as diffuse osteosclerosis; however, localized blastic or lytic areas are generally also present and permit radiologic diagnosis of malignancy. Generalized osteosclerosis is a rare presentation of myeloma and other hematologic malignancies.

Hematologic. In 40 per cent of cases of agnogenic myeloid metaplasia with myelofibrosis, diffuse skeletal sclerosis is seen. Osteosclerosis is also preceded by myelofibrosis when it occurs in mastocytosis and polycythemia vera. Sickle cell disease is manifested in bone by sclerosis, medullary bone infarcts, and subchondral osteonecrosis.

Metabolic. Renal osteodystrophy characteristically gives rise to sclerosis of the vertebral end-plates—the "rugger-jersey" spine—and to trabecular sclerosis in the metaphyses of long bones and the skull (Ch. 248). Cortical erosions of secondary hyperparathyroidism are also typically present. Diffuse osteosclerosis is an unusual presentation of Paget's disease and is rare in primary hyperparathyroidism. Fluorosis occurs endemically in areas of India and Africa where the fluoride content of water is high, following industrial exposure in aluminum and fertilizer plants, and, increasingly, in individuals treated for osteoporosis (see Ch. 249). Uniform sclerosis of bone is accompanied by exostoses and roughened cortical calcifications at muscle and ligamentous insertions, which suggest the diagnosis. Periarticular pain and limitation of motion are common. Histologically, thick trabeculae are covered by wide osteoid seams, which indicate the presence of osteomalacia.

Cortical and Trabecular Osteosclerosis

Osteopetrosis

Osteopetrosis (Albers-Schönberg disease or marble bone disease), a rare disorder of greatly increased bone density, occurs in several distinct forms. The malignant, autosomal recessive form (osteopetrosis congenita) results in replacement of the marrow space with bone, which causes anemia, infection, and early death. The benign, autosomal dominant form (osteopetrosis tarda) may be asymptomatic and rarely limits survival. A mild form with autosomal recessive rather than dominant inheritance is characterized by renal tubular acidosis and absence of the isozyme carbonic anhydrase II in erythrocytes. In obligate heterozygotes for this disorder, carbonic anhydrase II activity is half of normal. This is undoubtedly an important clue to the nature of osteoclast dysfunction in these individuals.

PATHOLOGY. Osteosclerosis results from defective osteoclast function with a failure of normal bone resorption. The medullary cavity is occupied by thickened bone trabeculae with central zones of entrapped calcified cartilage, which indicate a failure to resorb the primary spongiosa. Osteoclasts are abundant. In some cases defective osteoclast function is suggested by the absence of a ruffled border, the redundantly invaginated membrane structure normally adjacent to bone in actively resorbing osteoclasts.

MALIGNANT OSTEOPETROSIS. The malignant, autosomal recessive form of osteopetrosis presents in infancy with failure to thrive and delayed development. Proptosis, blindness, and frequently deafness and hydrocephalus ensue before age two,

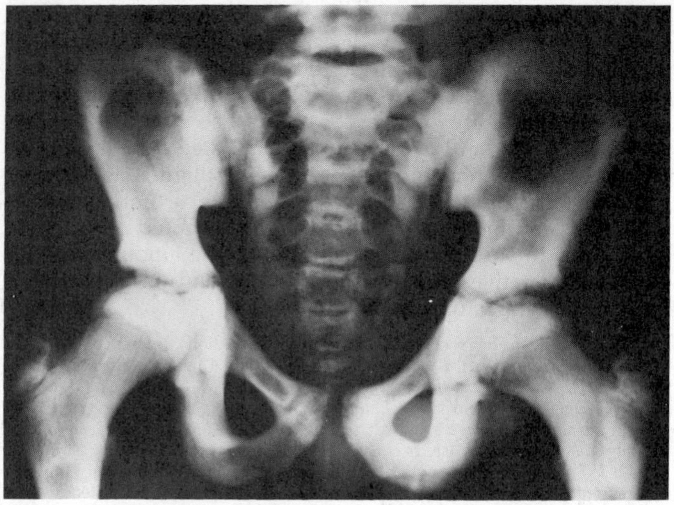

Figure 251–1. Roentgenogram of the pelvis of a teenager with the benign, autosomal recessive form of osteopetrosis.

as bone encroaches upon the cranial foramina. Despite its solid appearance, osteopetrotic bone is fragile, and fractures are frequent. Osteomyelitis is common. Obliteration of the marrow space causes extramedullary hematopoiesis, with hepatosplenomegaly and hypersplenism. Leukoerythroblastic anemia and thrombocytopenia are accompanied by elevated acid and alkaline phosphatase levels and, on occasion, hypocalcemia. Radiologically, the bone is everywhere sclerotic, often with metaphyseal bands of increased density. The long bones are poorly modeled and clublike; ragged metaphyseal-epiphyseal junctions may suggest rickets. Untreated, malignant osteopetrosis results in death from infection, bleeding, or anemia.

BENIGN OSTEOPETROSIS. This autosomal dominant variant is asymptomatic in about half of cases and is usually detected in family studies or as an incidental radiologic finding. The remainder of patients present with fractures of brittle osteopetrotic bone (about 40 per cent) or with osteomyelitis, usually of the mandible. Radiographically, the picture resembles that in the malignant form, but bones are well-modeled (Fig. 251–1). The only laboratory abnormality is an increased acid phosphatase level in some patients.

TREATMENT. Several animal models of osteopetrosis are available. The observation that the disease in mice and rats could be cured by transplantation of marrow or spleen cells has led to the successful use of bone marrow transplantation from HLA-identical sibs for treatment of malignant, autosomal recessive osteopetrosis. Establishment of a chimeric state is accompanied by remarkable regression of osteosclerosis and the reversal of anemia and incomplete nerve deficits. Defective function of killer T cells, which may predispose to infectious complications, may also be reversed by marrow transplantation. A conceptual by-product of these experiments has been the demonstration that the osteoclast originates from hematopoietic elements, thus ending a long debate about its ancestry.

Pyknodysostosis

This disease has only recently been distinguished from osteopetrosis. Inherited as an autosomal recessive trait, it is characterized by short stature and generalized osteosclerosis and is distinguished from osteopetrosis by several additional features: an obtuse mandibular angle with receding chin, multiple wormian bones with persistently open cranial fontanelles, and hypoplasia of terminal phalanges and clavicles. Fractures are common. Toulouse-Lautrec is thought to have suffered from pyknodysostosis.

Cortical Osteosclerosis

Hypertrophic Osteoarthropathy

This term describes subperiosteal formation of new bone in the long bones, secondary to some other condition. It usually occurs in conjunction with digital clubbing and arthritis (see

Ch. 461). The etiologies include pulmonary, hepatic, and intestinal disease. Bronchogenic carcinoma (except small cell carcinoma) is the commonest cause of hypertrophic osteoarthropathy and of clubbing; other causes of hypertrophic pulmonary osteoarthropathy are pleural tumors, lung abscesses, and empyema. Hypertrophic osteoarthropathy occurs in as many as 30 per cent of patients with chronic liver disease, often without clubbing. It is occasionally seen in ulcerative colitis and regional enteritis. Hypertrophic osteoarthropathy is unusual in cyanotic congenital heart disease, although clubbing is typically observed.

Hypertrophic osteoarthropathy is usually confined to the distal tibia and fibula and the distal radius and ulna. When advanced, it may involve other bones. However, it rarely involves the distal phalanges, even in the presence of clubbing. Bone pain, tenderness, and soft tissue swelling may be present, but the condition is sometimes asymptomatic. The periosteum is thickened, and subperiosteal formation of new bone is radiographically evident. Initially present as a separate stripe, new bone may eventually fuse with the cortex. The differential diagnosis includes pachydermoperiostosis, hypervitaminosis A, syphilis, and polyarteritis nodosa. The pathogenesis is unknown. However, blood flow to affected extremities is increased, and the condition sometimes responds to vagotomy; these findings suggest that central reflex changes may be operative.

Pachydermoperiostosis

Pachydermoperiostosis is an autosomal dominant condition in which periosteal formation of new bone occurs from puberty in the same distribution as in secondary hypertrophic osteoarthropathy. Also classically present are marked clubbing and thickened, oily skin. Facial features are coarse, and the thickened forehead and scalp are often marked by transverse folds (cutis verticis gyrata). The appearance may superficially resemble acromegaly. Pachydermoperiostosis is differentiated from secondary hypertrophic osteoarthropathy by the family history and lack of an antecedent cause.

Vitamin A Intoxication (Ch. 217)

Previously witnessed mostly in abusers of vitamins, this disorder is being seen more often, sometimes with hypercalcemia, in those treated with 13-cis-retinoic acid for cystic acne, ichthyosis, or malignancy. The characteristic periosteal new bone is often seen as a fusiform excrescence on the midshaft.

Progressive Diaphyseal Dysplasia

This rare disorder, also known as Camurati-Engelmann disease, is inherited as an autosomal trait. Classically, it is manifest in childhood by a thin body habitus, muscle wasting and weakness with a waddling gait, and bone pain. Serum biochemistry is usually normal, but the alkaline phosphatase level may be increased; the erythrocyte sedimentation rate is also elevated. X-rays show characteristic hyperostosis of the diaphyseal cortices with symmetrical fusiform enlargement of the long bones. The skull is sometimes involved. These changes progress with time, at a pace that slows in adulthood. Bone pain and muscle weakness sometimes respond to corticosteroids, but the bony changes do not. Like other autosomal dominant traits, progressive diaphyseal dysplasia exhibits considerable phenotypic variation; asymptomatic individuals and a mild adult variant (Ribbing disease) are common.

Hereditary Hyperphosphatasia

Hereditary hyperphosphatasia has also been called congenital hyperphosphatasia, osteoectasia with hyperphosphatasia, and juvenile Paget's disease; the last, however, is a poor term since Paget's disease is probably not heritable. Children affected by this rare, crippling, autosomal recessive condition present before age two with an enlarging skull, bowing of the extremities, bone pain, and fractures. Alkaline and acid phosphatase levels and the urinary hydroxyproline level are greatly increased. The calvaria is thickened, with focal densities that resemble cotton-wool balls. Elsewhere, bones are thickened symmetrically and may be demineralized, sometimes with loss of the normal cortex. Several patients have responded dramatically to calcitonin.

Endosteal Hyperostosis

This disease occurs in autosomal recessive (van Buchem's disease, hyperostosis corticalis generalisata) and dominant forms. The distinguishing feature is asymptomatic enlargement of the mandible from childhood, with sclerosis of the skull and thickening of the diaphyseal cortices of long bones.

Focal Osteosclerosis

Osteopoikilosis is an asymptomatic, autosomal dominant trait. Pea-sized sclerotic spots, prominent in the metaphyseal area, are accompanied in some kindreds by unique cutaneous lesions (dermatofibrosis lenticularis disseminata). These are yellowish papules or plaques with increased elastin. The combination is known as the Buschke-Ollendorff syndrome. *Osteopathia striata,* another autosomal dominant disorder of the sclerosing type, is usually asymptomatic and is characterized by symmetrical, parallel arrays of fine streaks in the long bones and pelvis. *Melorheostosis* is a progressive, painful disorder in which discrete hyperostotic areas appear to flow down the long bones like dripping wax. No hereditary predisposition is evident.

Beighton P, Cremin BJ: Sclerosing Bone Dysplasias. New York, Springer-Verlag, 1980. *A radiographic atlas with useful comments on nosology and a good bibliography.*

Coccia PF, Krivit W, Cervenka J, Clawson C, Kersey JH, Kim TH, Nesbit ME, Ramsay NCK, Warkentin PI, Teitelbaum SL, Kahn AJ, Brown DM: Successful bone-marrow transplantation for infantile malignant osteopetrosis. N Engl J Med 302:701, 1980. *The first successful treatment of this disorder.*

Murray RO, Jacobson HG: The Radiology of Skeletal Disorders: Exercises in Diagnosis. 2nd ed. Vol. 4. Edinburgh, Churchill Livingstone, 1977. *The question-answer format and a charming prose style make this an eminently readable book.*

Schneerson JM: Digital clubbing and hypertrophic osteoarthropathy: The underlying mechanisms. Br J Dis Chest 75:113, 1981. *A review of clubbing and hypertrophic osteoarthropathy, with 180 references.*

Sly WS, Hewett-Emmett D, Whyte MP, Yu Y-SL, Tashian RE: Carbonic anhydrase II deficiency identified as the primary defect in the autosomal recessive syndrome of osteopetrosis with renal tubular acidosis and cerebral calcification. Proc Natl Acad Sci USA 80:2752, 1983. *Elucidation of the probable pathogenesis of one variant of osteopetrosis.*

OTHER DISORDERS OF BONE

Fibrous Dysplasia

Fibrous dysplasia occurs in both monostotic and polyostotic forms. The latter is often associated with cutaneous café au lait spots and precocious pseudopuberty in females, and this triad is called Albright's syndrome (also the McCune-Albright syndrome).

The etiology of fibrous dysplasia is unknown. It is not heritable. Individual lesions are composed of dense fibrous tissue in medullary bone, interspersed with thin bone trabeculae (often covered by wide osteoid seams) and sometimes islands of cartilage. Radiographically, the lesions have a multilocular appearance beneath a thinned cortex (Fig. 251–2). Within, they have the appearance of ground glass, owing to their fine trabeculation. Although monostotic and polyostotic forms are histologically indistinguishable, monostotic lesions are not associated with an endocrinopathy. They commonly involve the proximal femur, tibia, or ribs, may occur at any age, and can cause bone pain, fractures, or deformity. Malignant transformation occurs in about 1 per cent of lesions.

Polyostotic fibrous dysplasia usually presents between the ages of 3 and 10. It may involve over 50 per cent of the skeleton and frequently produces "shepherd's-crook" deformity of the femur and discrepancies in leg length; skull involvement may cause gross facial disfigurement (leontiasis ossea). Fractures are common. Serum biochemistry is frequently normal except for elevation of the alkaline phosphatase level. The café au lait spots sometimes seen in polyostotic fibrous dysplasia have

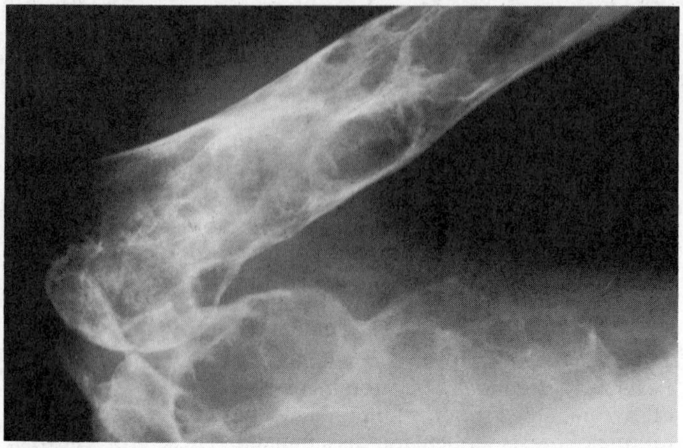

Figure 251–2. Roentgenogram of the humerus and scapula of a patient with extensive polyostotic fibrous dysplasia. Both bones are extensively involved with typical lesions.

jagged borders that Albright likened to the coast of Maine, to distinguish them from those in neurofibromatosis, which have smooth borders like the coast of California.

About half of girls with polyostotic fibrous dysplasia undergo precocious pseudopuberty, which may precede detection of the bony abnormality. Precocious pseudopuberty has also been reported in a few boys with this syndrome. Sexual maturation in both sexes is associated with low gonadotropin levels, and fertility does not occur (hence, it is termed *pseudo*puberty). Histologically, the ovaries display multiple follicle cysts. Several other endocrinopathies have been described in Albright's syndrome; these include hyperthyroidism (in about 20 per cent), gigantism with acromegaly, and Cushing's syndrome. Levels of thyroid-stimulating hormone (TSH) are suppressed in hyperthyroidism associated with Albright's syndrome, and adrenocorticotropic hormone (ACTH) is likewise suppressed when adrenal hyperfunction occurs in Albright's syndrome. In all these glands, which thus function autonomously, receptors for the respective tropic hormones—luteinizing hormone (LH), follicle-stimulating hormone (FSH), TSH, and ACTH—are coupled to adenylate cyclase. However, the nature of the regulatory defect remains to be defined and may be unrelated to the receptor-adenylate cyclase system.

In addition to these disorders of endocrine hyperfunction, hypophosphatemic osteomalacia has been described in association with Albright's syndrome.

Hereditary Multiple Exostoses

This relatively common disorder (also called diaphyseal aclasis) is inherited as an autosomal dominant trait with high penetrance. Irregular bony excrescences protrude from the expanded metaphyses of the long bones. These osteocartilaginous exostoses arise from the growth plate and grow as the bone does. They may subsequently become isolated from the epiphysis or remain in continuity, but they reproduce normal structure, with an outer cortex and an inner spongiosa continuous with that of the bone of origin. Growth ceases in adulthood. Disability results principally from limb-length discrepancies: linear bone growth decreases as the bone grows transversely. Less common are syndromes of nerve, spinal cord, and vascular compression. The exostoses undergo sarcomatous degeneration in 3 to 10 per cent of affected individuals, and this must be suspected when a lesion enlarges rapidly, especially during adulthood.

Enchondromatosis (Dyschondroplasia, Ollier's Disease)

A sporadic condition, enchondromatosis becomes symptomatic in childhood as multiple, growing, cartilaginous masses within the trabecular bone, which produce swelling and interfere with linear bone growth. As with cartilaginous exostoses, these arise from the growth plate, growth ceases at puberty, and replacement of cartilage by mature bone may follow. Enchondromas appear radiologically as radiolucent defects in the metaphyseal area of the tubular and flat bones, often with central calcific stippling. The affected area may be expanded, with thinning of the cortex. Enchondromatosis must be distinguished from hereditary exostoses and from fibrous dysplasia. Malignant degeneration is uncommon. When enchondromatosis is associated with multiple hemangiomas (Maffucci's syndrome), the enchondromas or hemangiomas undergo malignant transformation in 15 per cent of cases.

Achondroplasia

Chondrodystrophies are disorders of cartilaginous growth that typically eventuate in disproportionate short stature. The commonest of them is achondroplasia. Affected individuals are easily recognizable: the limbs are short; the trunk is of relatively normal length; and the head is large, with a bulging forehead and scooped-out nose. Achondroplasia is inherited as an autosomal dominant trait. About 80 per cent of cases represent new mutations; the mutation rate increases with paternal age. To account for short bones and a shortened cranial base but a normal cranial vault, the mutation must affect endochondral ossification, as in the limbs and chondrocranium, but not membranous ossification, as in the vault. Surprisingly, the growth plate is not grossly disorganized histologically and chondrocytes are normal ultrastructurally—the pathogenesis of achondroplasia remains an enigma. Radiographically, the cranial base and foramen magnum are small, lumbar lordosis is greatly exaggerated, and the lumbar spinal canal narrows from the upper to lower lumbar spine, as indicated by a decreasing interpeduncular distance. The long bones appear massive, owing to their disproportionately normal width. Complications can include hydrocephalus, presumably related to the small size of the foramen magnum, and spinal cord and root compression, a potential consequence of even minimal impingement by a disk or osteophyte upon the small spinal canal. Reproductive potential is limited by social factors as well as cephalopelvic disproportion. Despite its problems, achondroplasia is compatible with good health and a normal lifespan.

Grabias SL, Campbell CJ: Fibrous dysplasia. Orthop Clin North Am 8:771, 1977. *A review of clinical, radiologic, and orthopedic aspects of monostotic and polyostotic forms of fibrous dysplasia.*

McKusick VA: Heritable Disorders of Connective Tissue. 4th ed. St. Louis, CV Mosby, 1972. *This scholarly, profusely illustrated book remains an excellent source for the inherited diseases of bone.*

Rimoin DL: The chondrodystrophies. Adv Hum Genet 5:1, 1975. *Achondroplasia and a host of less common causes of disproportionate short stature are discussed.*

252. BONE TUMORS

Henry J. Mankin

PRIMARY TUMORS OF BONE

Primary bone tumors are uncommon but they are important since they are most frequent in the young (the second to the fourth decades) and they tend to be extraordinarily malignant. Beyond their random occurrence, bone tumors have been associated with (1) genetic disorders of preosseous cartilage (hereditary multiple osteocartilaginous exostoses and enchondromatosis), (2) radiation injury, (3) Paget's disease, (4) bone infarcts, and (5) chronic osteomyelitis.

CLASSIFICATION AND STAGING

Any connective tissue element that exists in the osseous or preosseous skeleton can be the cell of origin of a neoplastic process; both benign and malignant tumors may be classified according to cell type as osseous, cartilaginous, fibrous, and "other" (including vascular, neural, marrow, lipid, and tumors of unspecified origin). Furthermore, within each broad category, several radiologically, histologically, and biologically distinct types of tumors exist, providing a sometimes puzzling array of diagnoses from which to choose for a patient who presents with an obvious radiographic lesion.

Prior to treatment, all primary bone tumors must be "staged" in order to assess the local extent of the lesion (T), the grade of the tumor (G), and the presence or absence of distant metastases (M). The determination of T is best done by physical examination, radiographs, and special imaging studies, including angiography, computerized and planar tomography, and ^{99m}Tc bone scanning. The grade of the tumor can only be determined by study of biopsy material using both standard and specialized techniques. Since most bone tumors metastasize to the lungs and occasionally other bones, full lung tomograms or computerized tomography of the chest and a bone scan are required to establish "M."

BENIGN BONE TUMORS

Most benign tumors of bone present as a mass or deformity detectable on physical examination, as an incidental finding on a radiograph, or occasionally as a result of a pathologic fracture through a weakened area of the bone. With few exceptions, benign lesions are small and painless. For some, the radiographic features are so characteristic as to be easily recognizable. Benign bone tumors show well-defined cortical margins, absence of a soft tissue mass, and sclerotic bony margination separating the lesion from the normal tissues. Some lesions may require biopsy for definition, and some, particularly those that threaten the integrity of the skeleton, require treatment, which for most of these lesions is "intralesional" (such as simple excision or curettage and packing of the defect with auto- or allograft bone), resulting in a "cure" in a high percentage of the cases.

MALIGNANT PRIMARY TUMORS OF BONE

Multiple myeloma, the most common primary malignancy of bone, is discussed in Ch. 163. Other primary malignant tumors of bone are rare. The majority of these are osteosarcoma and (depending on the age group studied) chondrosarcoma; round cell tumors (Ewing's sarcoma and primary lymphoma of bone), giant cell tumors, and malignant fibrous tumors follow in order of diminishing frequency.

OSTEOSARCOMA. The peak age of incidence for osteosarcoma is in the second decade with a second lesser peak occurring in later years (in association with Paget's disease). The tumor has a predilection for the distal femur or proximal tibia of the rapidly growing child and occurs more frequently in males. Osteosarcoma in later life usually occurs as a complication of Paget's disease, irradiation injury of bone, or a bone infarct.

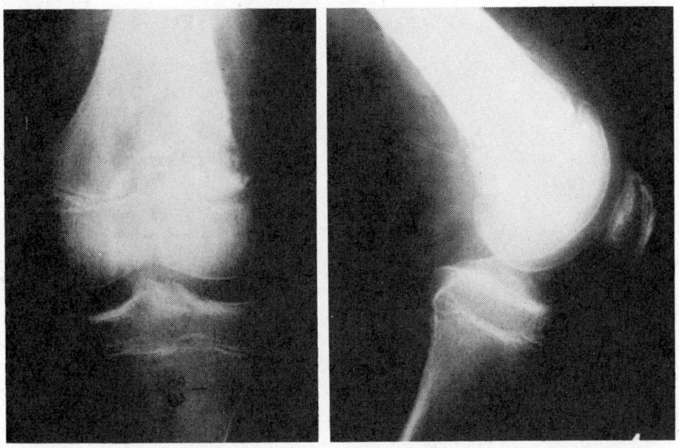

Figure 252–1. Anteroposterior lateral radiographs of the distal femur of a 10-year-old girl, showing the classic picture of an osteosarcoma. Note the destruction and blastic productive changes both within the bone and in the adjacent soft tissue mass, which is seen best extending posteriorly on the lateral film.

Pain, limitation of movement, and swelling are the principal complaints, and even at earliest observation, the radiographic findings show obvious destruction and a soft tissue mass outside the bone (Fig. 252–1). Productive changes within and without the bone suggest the presence of the osteosarcoma. Typically, the serum alkaline phosphatase level is markedly elevated. Fully one fourth of patients have metastases to the lungs at the time of the initial examination or shortly after. If left untreated, the course is fulminant with a rapid progression of the tumor, widespread metastases, and death in less than a year.

Treatment consists of wide excision of the primary tumor, which in many cases will require amputation of the extremity, but in selected instances includes a local resection and limb reconstruction with auto- or allograft or metallic implants. Chemotherapeutic agents such as doxorubicin, high dose methotrexate with citrovorum rescue or cis-platinum or both may improve the prognosis of patients with pulmonary micrometastases, with reported survival figures ranging from 50 to 80 per cent, at three years. Resection of pulmonary nodules in conjunction with aggressive chemotherapy appears to be successful in effecting cure in over 20 per cent of the patients so treated.

ROUND CELL SARCOMA. *Ewing's sarcoma* is a highly malignant tumor of unknown cytogenesis, which primarily affects teenage children and produces a very destructive, lytic tumor often of the pelvis, shaft of the femur, or other long bones. Symptoms and signs include not only local pain, swelling, and a palpable mass, but at times systemic findings such as fever, malaise, chills, and a rapid sedimentation rate. The prognosis for this tumor is particularly poor without treatment, but the lesions, like the lymphomas of bone, are remarkably radiosensitive. The combination of local radiation and chemotherapy provide a long survival rate exceeding 60 per cent. *Non-Hodgkin's lymphoma* and less frequently *Hodgkin's lymphoma* may make their appearance as a bony focus difficult to distinguish radiographically and sometimes histologically from Ewing's sarcoma. Staging of these individuals is essential to be certain that the bony tumor is solitary rather than an osseous focus of diffuse disease. The treatment is similar to that of lymphoma of other sites, depending principally on the radiosensitivity of the primary site and the response of the tumor to chemotherapeutic drugs.

CHONDROSARCOMA. The chondrosarcomas are extraordinarily variable in clinical presentation, degree of malignancy, and biological behavior. Central chondrosarcomas, most prevalent in middle age, occur most frequently in the pelvis and proximal portions of the appendicular skeleton. Both radiation and chemotherapy are relatively ineffective, particularly for large tumors. With accurate staging, however, surgery may produce a cure in up to 85 per cent of patients, depending on the stage of the disease.

METASTATIC TUMORS OF BONE

Certain of the malignant neoplasms and tumors of the hematopoietic system have a propensity for metastasis to the skeleton. At times, the presenting complaint for a patient with a primary breast, lung, prostatic, renal, or thyroid carcinoma may be pain in the spine, ribs, or long bones or a pathologic fracture through a metastatic focus. In males, the most frequent source of metastastic carcinoma is carcinoma of the prostate, followed closely by carcinoma of the lung and gastrointestinal tract; in women, carcinoma of the breast is by far the most frequent cause of metastatic bone disease. The frequency of metastatic carcinoma far exceeds that of primary tumors of bone, especially in later life, so that staging of any individual with a bone tumor should include a careful clinical, imaging, and laboratory evaluation of the more frequent sites of origin.

Conversely, patients who are under treatment for primary tumors of the organs just cited should have frequent bone scans, which are far more sensitive than radiographs in revealing the presence of distant metastases.

Radiographic findings in metastatic bone disease vary with the type of primary tumor and the bony site involved, but almost always the tumorous deposits are in the axial and proximal appendicular skeleton, are centrally placed within the bone, and are quite destructive in appearance. About 90 per cent of prostatic, 50 per cent of breast, and 25 per cent of lung carcinomatous metastases evoke a sclerotic response in the affected bone producing a mottled increase in osseous density on the radiograph. The treatment of skeletal metastases from a primary carcinoma depends on the patient's general condition, the radiosensitivity of the lesion, the site and extent of involvement, and the proximity of the tumor to vital structures such as the spinal cord. Regression and long-term remission can be achieved in some patients with carcinoma of the prostate and breast simply with the use of hormones and radiation (see Ch. 235 and 239). When the integrity of the skeletal system is threatened or a pathologic fracture of a long bone has occured, prophylactic or therapeutic open reduction and internal fixation is clearly indicated and frequently provides the patient with considerable relief of pain and restoration of function.

Enneking WF: Musculoskeletal Tumor Society. New York, Churchill Livingston, 1983. *A comprehensive text detailing the principles and technical aspects of surgical management of bone tumors.*

Huvos AG: Bone Tumors, Diagnosis, Treatment and Progress. Philadelphia, W.B. Saunders Company, 1979. *A detailed text describing the classification system, radiologic characteristics, and pathologic patterns for a variety of benign and malignant bone tumors.*

Mankin HJ: Current concept in cancer: Advances in diagnosis and treatment of bone tumors. N Engl J Med 300:543, 1979. *A review article on recent trends in diagnosis and management of bone tumors.*

Part XIX
INFECTIOUS DISEASES
Section One INTRODUCTION

253. INTRODUCTION TO MICROBIAL DISEASES

Charles C. J. Carpenter

Those diseases for which specific cures are possible and for which immunoprophylaxis is available are caused primarily by infectious agents. Throughout the developing world, acute infections, predominantly acute diarrheal illnesses and acute respiratory disease, are by far the leading causes of mortality. In more circumscribed areas of Asia, Africa, and South America, protozoal diseases (especially malaria) and helminthic infections (notably schistosomiasis and onchocerciasis) continue to affect millions of individuals and to cause hundreds of thousands of deaths annually. In the developed world, microbial disease processes remain the most common curable causes of both morbidity and mortality. Pneumococcal pneumonia, although curable by timely antimicrobial therapy, and in large part preventable by immunization of susceptible population groups, remains among the ten leading causes of death in North America. New problems associated with infectious diseases continue to make their appearance in patients immunocompromised by treatment with cytotoxic or immunosuppressive drugs, or both. Such patients are susceptible to life-threatening infections caused by a wide range of opportunistic, normally commensal, microorganisms. The great variety of unusual infections occurring in immunosuppressed patients presents a continuing diagnostic and therapeutic challenge.

Rapid progress has continued in the development and application of vaccines effective against major life-threatening viral illnesses, and the utilization of recombinant deoxyribonucleic acid (DNA) technology and hybridoma-derived antibodies give promise of yielding effective means of preventing additional bacterial, protozoal, and helminthic infections. The eradication of smallpox has been a reality for several years, and more widespread immunization against poliomyelitis has led to further decline in the incidence of this frightening disease. An effective vaccine against hepatitis B became commercially available in 1982 in quantities adequate to immunize the populations at greatest risk in North America. The preparation of the hepatitis B vaccine is unique in that it consists of an antigen derived from the serum of humans with hepatitis B antigenemia, and the lengthy purification process has made the vaccine so expensive as to limit its use to high-risk populations. Concomitant with this development, however, has been the recognition that non-A, non-B hepatitis (presumably caused by two or more viruses, for which there are no specific diagnostic tests) is now the leading cause of post-transfusion hepatitis. The availability of the remarkably effective human diploid cell rabies vaccine has greatly decreased the cost and discomfort of immunization against this uniformly fatal illness; the development of this vaccine has fortuitously occurred concomitantly with an increase in endemic sylvatic rabies in many parts of the United States. Recent in vitro studies give promise, at long last, that the development of an effective antimalarial vaccine, using recombinant DNA technology, is near fruition.

However, despite heartening progress in the prevention and treatment of a number of major microbial illnesses, new infectious diseases continue to appear, and additional previously recognized disease syndromes have been shown to be caused by microbial agents. During the past four years, two additional previously recognized illnesses, Lyme disease and adult T cell leukemia, have been shown to result from infectious processes. Furthermore, the acquired immune deficiency syndrome (AIDS) was first recognized in 1979, and its incidence has increased exponentially since that time. This illness has recently extended beyond the initially recognized susceptible population of male homosexuals, intravenous-drug users, and hemophiliacs. Recently, both children and female sexual partners of male patients with AIDS, as well as occasional transfusion recipients, have, albeit in small numbers, developed this disease. Epidemiologic data suggest that AIDS, which results in virtually complete destruction of cellular immune mechanisms, may result from an infectious agent that resembles hepatitis B in its mode of transmission. Recently, both viral isolation and serologic studies have strongly supported an etiologic role for a retrovirus in AIDS. Human T cell lymphotropic virus type III (HTLV-III) and lymphadenopathy-associated virus (LAV) have been implicated by American and French investigators, respectively, as etiologic agents. Published data do not permit a definite conclusion as to whether or not HTLV-III and LAV are identical, or closely related, retroviruses. Susceptibility to infection and the development of clinical illness following exposure to the putative etiologic virus may, however, be influenced by subclinical immunodeficiency in the groups at greatest risk. For example, male homosexuals are repeatedly exposed to a variety of agents (e.g., cytomegalovirus) that may cause transient impairment of the cellular immune response.

Once the clinical syndrome of AIDS develops, the management of this group of patients poses unique challenges from the standpoint of infectious diseases, since the patients invariably develop multiple serious infections, often with microorganisms that are resistant to available therapeutic agents (e.g., cryptosporidia, *Mycobacterium avium–intracellularis,* disseminated cytomegalovirus). Patients with fully developed AIDS have generally succumbed to the illness within two years after the diagnosis has been established. Although one or more opportunistic infections (e.g., *Pneumocystis carinii*) may respond to appropriate antimicrobial therapy, no therapeutic approach has been effective yet in correcting the defect in cellular immunity. Several trials with potentially helpful agents, including immune interferon and interleukin II, are underway. AIDS represents the most devastating of the health problems that plague the homosexual community, and the ultimate extent of this disease cannot be estimated. The frequent development of an unusually aggressive form of Kaposi's sarcoma in patients with AIDS may provide an important clue as to the relationship between altered immune function and neoplasia.

Microbial diseases have provided original models for critical studies of immune processes; recently, another newly recognized illness, Lyme disease, has been shown to be of infectious etiology and has provided a unique look at the immune interaction between host and parasite. Lyme disease is now known to be caused by a borrelia-like spirochete, which is transmitted by the tick *Ixodes dammini.* Many of the features of Lyme disease mimic those of Reiter's syndrome, another post-infectious, immunologically mediated rheumatologic illness; clinical similarities between certain cases of Lyme disease and rheumatoid arthritis have provided added impetus to the search for an infectious, and therefore potentially eradicable, etiologic agent in rheumatoid arthritis.

Because of the clear-cut etiologic role between certain retroviruses and neoplasia in experimental animals, a search for viral etiologic agents in human cancer has been under way for several decades. The first clear-cut link between a specific virus and human neoplasia has recently been established, with the demonstration of a strong epidemiologic relationship between a unique retrovirus, human T cell leukemia virus, and adult T cell leukemia in three distinct geographic locations (Southern Japan, the Caribbean, and the Southeastern United States). This demonstration provides great impetus to search for chemotherapeutic agents effective against retroviruses. It also encourages a more intensive search for viral etiologic agents in other human neoplastic processes.

In the face of rapid and sometimes bewildering changes,

both in the nature of the infectious diseases with which the clinician is confronted and the therapeutic armamentarium at his disposal, two basic principles continue to guide the physician's approach to patient management. When faced with a sick patient, a physician's primary responsibility is to determine whether or not the illness does indeed represent an acute infectious process—a decision made more complex by such factors as frequent lack of fever in elderly patients with pneumonia, lack of leukocytosis in many patients on cytotoxic drug therapy, and so forth. There is probably no situation in clinical medicine in which the thoughtful attention to all relevant details of the patient's medical history and a meticulous physical examination remain more important to the welfare of the patient. Once a physician has made the decision that a patient has an infectious process, his next responsibility must be to determine whether or not the patient has a potentially fulminant, life-threatening illness, which could cause death within the next few hours in the absence of prompt and appropriate therapy. Such illnesses obviously include such life-threatening diseases as acute bacterial meningitis, falciparum malaria, and gram-negative bacteremia but may also include such generally nonlethal illnesses as acute bacterial pneumonia. Because of the difficulty in determining which infectious processes are potentially death-dealing, it is incumbent on the physician, when faced with a patient with an acute infectious process, to establish a tentative diagnosis as rapidly as possible (e.g., with the use of Gram stained preparation in the case of acute bacterial pneumonia or purulent meningitis) and to initiate specific therapy for the presumed pathogen as rapidly as possible. In no other major group of illnesses is the rapid initiation of appropriate therapy so important as in acute infectious diseases.

Despite the prophylactic and therapeutic advances that have resulted from the rapid evolution of cellular and molecular biology, the microbial world continues to present the thoughtful physician with some of the most perplexing, and potentially rewarding, problems in the practice of medicine.

254. THE FEBRILE PATIENT

Sheldon M. Wolff

Fever is one of the most common symptoms that physicians encounter. In the vast majority of patients the fever is secondary to an infectious process, often viral in origin. In such patients, the febrile state is self-limited and relatively little is needed in terms of diagnostic workup or therapy. However, when the fever persists for more than a few days or is excessively high, a more thorough evaluation is indicated. Certain aspects of the febrile patient are worth emphasizing. For example, fever is *never* the sole manifestation of an illness. Constitutional symptoms such as headache, myalgias, or malaise almost always accompany fever. In addition, except in rare instances, the type or pattern of fever is of no diagnostic value. When a quotidian fever pattern occurs in the proper setting, then malaria should be considered. Furthermore, a Pel-Ebstein pattern should suggest Hodgkin's disease, but is not diagnostic. In fact, viral diseases can cause hectic fevers accompanied by chills and be indistinguishable from the response of patients with bacteremia or fungemia. Thus, when approaching a patient with fever, careful history taking, thorough physical examination, and close observation are all indicated.

Some patients with febrile illnesses will have persistent symptoms (and fever) for more than two weeks despite a thorough evaluation by history, physical examination, and laboratory tests, including appropriate cultures of blood, sputum, urine, and, if indicated, stools. Such patients can be considered to have a fever of unknown origin (FUO), and they require extensive evaluation.

When attempting to determine the cause of a prolonged fever, the wide spectrum of diseases that cause fever must be considered. Factors such as age, social and economic factors, geography, and recent exposure are all important determinants of the causes of prolonged fevers. In the overwhelming majority of FUO patients, an underlying cause is discovered or the patient recovers spontaneously.

CAUSES OF FEVER OF UNKNOWN ORIGIN. ***Infections.*** Approximately one third of all FUO patients will have an infectious etiology to explain their illness. Any infectious agent can be the cause of an FUO, although it is rare for a virus to be the cause of such a condition. Although most will be obvious, self-limited, or responsive to therapy, other infectious diseases may still present as an FUO. In particular, certain sites such as bone, sinuses, heart valves, subphrenic area, biliary tract and the urinary tract may be infected and not provide localizing signs.

Neoplasias. Some tumors are likely to be associated with fever and may present as an FUO. At least 20 per cent of FUO patients will have an underlying tumor as a cause of the FUO. The percentage of such patients is increasing. Examples of such neoplasms include Hodgkin's and other lymphomas, hypernephroma, preleukemia, and atrial myxoma. However, tumors of almost any origin may present as an FUO, and this may occur in the absence of metastases. In addition, the fever may precede the clinical appearance of the underlying disease by weeks or months.

Hypersensitivity Diseases. Although most collagen vascular diseases can present as an FUO, systemic lupus erythematosus, Still's disease (in children and adults), and certain of the systemic necrotizing vasculitides such as temporal arteritis are more likely than others. Certain drug reactions may present as an FUO. Scleroderma is one of the collagen vascular diseases that rarely or never presents as an FUO.

Granulomatous Diseases. There are three major granulomatous diseases of unknown etiology that may present as fevers of unknown origin. The most common of these is sarcoidosis. Most, but not all, sarcoid patients who present with an FUO have extrapulmonary disease often involving the liver. In regional enteritis, fever can sometimes be much more prominent than any gastrointestinal signs or symptoms. Many of the well-known causes of granulomatous hepatitis, such as tuberculosis, sarcoidosis, or systemic fungal infections, can present as an FUO. In addition, there is a separate group of patients with granulomatous hepatitis of unknown cause and FUO. Thus, any FUO patient whose symptoms persist despite thorough noninvasive workup should have a liver biospy.

Inherited Diseases. There are at least four inherited diseases that present as an FUO. The most common of these is familial Mediterranean fever (FMF). Although FMF is most common in Armenians, Sephardic Jews, and Arabs, it can occur in almost any ethnic group. It is in the latter situation that the diagnosis is most often missed and the patient is considered to have an FUO. Patients with an inherited hyperlipidemia (Type 1) may have fever as a presenting complaint. In patients with Fabry's disease, an X-linked inherited error of glycosphingolipid metabolism characterized by telangiectases and lancinating pain, fever may be a prominent sign. Cyclic neutropenia often presents as an FUO, and a small percentage of patients with this disease seem to have a familial form.

Factitious Diseases. A small number of patients who present with an FUO turn out to have a factitious or self-induced illness. In general, these patients are young female adults who are in the health-related professions. Such patients can be roughly separated into two groups. The first consists of patients who feign illness by manipulating thermometers and often have a bona fide febrile illness prior to the onset of their so-called FUO. The second group is predominantly in the third or fourth decade of life, and these patients have more profound psychiatric problems. They will often induce disease and in fact can do themselves considerable harm.

EVALUATION OF THE PATIENT WITH AN FUO. The approach to the patient with an FUO requires an awareness of the myriad etiologies and a willingness to demonstrate a thoroughness in the workup that few other situations in medicine demand. Careful attention to the history is required. Has there been any exposure to infectious agents? Any unusual travel? These and many other questions must be asked. If the answers are positive, then follow-up laboratory procedures will be required. A thorough and complete physical examination is mandatory. Furthermore, repeated attention must be paid to any changes, such as the appearance of septic phenomena in the skin, fundi, nailbeds, or other areas.

Approximately 10 per cent of FUO patients will defy extensive evaluation and continue to have fevers without a diagnosis forthcoming. Such patients require close observation and follow-up, and workups may have to be repeated. A patient with an ongoing active debilitating illness requires earlier re-evaluation than the patient with a chronic, slowly progressive course. The longer a patient has an FUO, the less likely he is to have an infectious or neoplastic cause for the fever.

The laboratory evaluation of the patient with an FUO should be logical and complete. Knowledge of the causes of fever directs the physician toward appropriate laboratory tests. Certain examinations are mandatory such as skin tests, liver function tests, and complete blood counts. However, tests should not be performed just for the sake of completeness if they have little or no chance of providing useful information. Appropriate cultures must be made, but again reason should prevail regarding the number and sites.

Radiographic studies must include the chest, sinuses (if headache or pain is present), the entire gastrointestinal and biliary tracts, and the urinary tract. Radionuclide scanning should be employed after the appropriate x-rays have been obtained. Finally, CT scans and ultrasonography should be obtained when indicated.

If all of these noninvasive procedures have been performed and a diagnosis still has not been made, then invasive procedures must be employed. Bone marrow and liver biopsies should be done. When indicated, other biopsies will prove of value. For example, biopsy of a skin lesion, biopsy of an enlarged node, or temporal artery biopsy may prove useful in selected patients. The availability of needle biopsy techniques and the use of scanning methods and, when indicated, peritoneoscopy make exploratory laparotomy no longer indicated in the evaluation of FUO patients.

Aduan RP, Fauci AS, Dale DC, Herzberg JH, Wolff SM: Factitious fever and self-induced infections. Ann Intern Med 90:230, 1979. *A comprehensive review of a large group of patients with factitious and self-induced diseases.*

Dinarello CA, Wolff SM: Approach to the patient with fever of unknown origin. *In* Mandell G, Bennett JE, Douglas RG (eds.): Principles and Practices of Infectious Diseases, Vol 1. New York, John Wiley & Sons, 1979, pp 421-428. *A detailed discussion of the evaluation and diagnostic procedures to be followed in patients with fevers of unknown origin.*

Dinarello CA, Wolff SM: Fever of unknown origin. *In* Mandell G, Bennett JE, Douglas RG (eds.): Principles and Practices of Infectious Diseases, Vol 1. New York, John Wiley & Sons, 1979, pp 407–421. *A categorization of the types of diseases that can present in patients with fevers of unknown origin.*

Larson EB, Featherstone HJ, Petersdorf RG: Fever of undetermined origin: Diagnosis and follow-up of 105 cases, 1970–1980. Medicine 61:269, 1982. *A comparison by Dr. Petersdorf's group of their recent experience and the data they published in 1961.*

Petersdorf RG, Beeson PB: Fever of unexplained origin. Medicine 40:1, 1961. *The classic paper on fever of unknown origin.*

Wolff SM, Fauci AS, Dale DC: Unusual etiologies of fever and their evaluation. Ann Rev Med 26:277, 1975. *A summary of a 15-year study of a large group of patients with chronic or recurring fevers.*

255. PATHOGENESIS OF FEVER

Charles A. Dinarello

DEFINITION. Fever is an elevation of temperature above the normal amplitude of daily variation. Infections are most commonly associated with fever, but several noninfectious diseases may also have fever as their primary clinical presentation. Although the vast majority of patients with elevated body temperature are experiencing fever, there are a few instances in which elevated temperature is not fever but rather hyperthermia. These include heat stroke syndromes, certain metabolic diseases, and the effects of pharmacologic agents that interfere with thermoregulation.

Fever is best understood at the hypothalamic level, and the home thermostat can be used as an analogy for hypothalamic control of body temperature. The thermoregulatory center located in the anterior hypothalamus regulates internal temperature at about 37° C (98.6° F) primarily by its ability to balance heat production and peripheral heat loss. During fever, the thermostat setting in the hypothalamic center shifts upward, e.g., from 37 to 39° C. This results in signals to increase heat production and decrease peripheral heat loss. Heat production from shivering muscles and heat conservation from peripheral vasoconstriction continue until the temperature of the blood supplying the hypothalamus matches the higher thermostat setting. In contradistinction to fever, the setting of the thermoregulatory center during hyperthermia remains unchanged at normothermic levels, while, in an uncontrolled fashion, body temperature increases and overrides the ability to lose heat. Exogenous heat exposure and endogenous heat production are two mechanisms by which hyperthermia can result in dangerously high internal temperatures. In comparison to fever, hyperthermia is a much rarer cause for elevated body temperature, but it is nevertheless important to make the distinction. Hyperthermia can be rapidly fatal, and its treatment differs from that of fever.

PATHOGENESIS. Several substances in addition to infectious agents have been recognized to cause fever. The most widespread and potent of these is the lipopolysaccharide of gram-negative bacteria, also called *endotoxin.* Endotoxin will produce fever in humans when as little as 2 ng per kilogram is injected intravenously. Other substances that produce fever include toxins from gram-positive bacteria, drugs in sensitized individuals, and incompatible blood products. It has become a custom to refer to endotoxin and other substances that produce fever as *exogenous pyrogens.* Exogenous pyrogens share no common physicochemical structure, are derived from varied sources of microbial and nonmicrobial origin, and, in general, do not directly affect the hypothalamus but rather produce fever through the action of a mediator molecule, *endogenous pyrogen.*

ENDOGENOUS PYROGEN. Endogenous pyrogen, a small molecular weight protein, was first described by Beeson in 1948. Subsequent animal and human studies established the importance of endogenous pyrogen in mediating fever and as being responsible for the upward resetting of the hypothalamic thermostat. This substance is produced in response to infections, toxic substances, or immunologic reactions. It is not species specific, and endogenous pyrogen produced from human cells causes fever in animals. Endogenous pyrogen is a product of phagocytic leukocytes but, unlike other substances released by phagocytes, it is not preformed. Following stimulation by exogenous pyrogens, phagocytes synthesize endogenous pyrogen de novo and release the substance into the circulation. Monocytes, fixed mononuclear phagocytes such as Kupffer cells of the liver, alveolar macrophages, and splenic sinusoidal cells are capable of releasing the pyrogen, but lymphocytes and neutrophils are not. In patients with severe bone marrow depression and no circulating phagocytic cells, the tissue macrophages are a potential source of endogenous pyrogen and may account for the fever observed in these individuals. Studies also suggest that certain tumors produce endogenous pyrogen in vitro. These include human lymphoma cell lines, circulating monocytic leukemia cells, and renal carcinomas. Pyrogen production by certain tumor cells may be one mechanism by which fever is produced in patients with these tumors.

Human subjects injected with endogenous pyrogen made by their blood leukocytes respond with chills and fever. The pyrogen has been demonstrated in sterile pleural, peritoneal, and joint effusions and is readily produced in vitro when human phagocytes are stimulated. The induction of endogenous pyrogen from human phagocytic cells in vitro by a variety of exogenous pyrogens is one of the methods used to study the pathogenesis of fever in humans. Most substances that produce fever when injected into humans induce the release of endogenous pyrogen in vitro.

Animal studies have shown that the preoptic area of the anterior hypothalamus is the primary site of action for the induction of fever by endogenous pyrogen. Thermosensitive cells in the preoptic anterior hypothalamus increase their rate of discharge when endogenous pyrogen is injected. In addition, there is a concomitant rise in the concentration of monoamines and prostaglandins in the third and fourth cerebral ventricles and in the vicinity of the thermoregulatory center. Synthesis of prostaglandins, particularly of the E series, is an important result of the action of endogenous pyrogen on the hypothalamus. Like endogenous pyrogen, prostaglandin E_2 produces fever when injected into the anterior hypothalamus. See Figure 255–1.

ACTION OF ANTIPYRETICS. Aspirin and other antipyretics have no effect on the synthesis and release of endogenous pyrogen from phagocytic leukocytes. Therefore, their role in reducing fever is not directly related to their peripheral anti-inflammatory properties. The potency of an antipyretic in reducing fever is proportionately related to its ability to inhibit the synthesis of brain prostaglandins, and thus the primary mechanism of antipyretics is the prevention of prostaglandin synthesis in the hypothalamus. The ability of endogenous pyrogen to raise the hypothalamic thermostat setting is due to its ability to increase the concentration of hypothalamic prostaglandin, and hence antipyretics lower fever by preventing pyrogen-induced prostaglandin synthesis. This is corroborated by the clinical observation that antipyretics do not lower normal body temperature but only the elevated temperature of fever. Corticosteroids prevent fever by reducing the amount of endogenous pyrogen released from phagocytes. Therefore, the ability of corticosteroids to reduce fever is related to their peripheral anti-inflammatory properties.

DIAGNOSIS. Individuals maintain body temperature at about 37° C despite wide variations in environmental temperatures. For some individuals, normal body temperature can be below or above 37° C without constituting a pathologic process. During a 24-hour period, body temperature varies from a low point in the early morning to the highest levels at 4 to 6 P.M. The amplitude of this daily variation, also called circadian temperature rhythm, is about 0.6° C (1° F), and individuals retain their circadian rhythm throughout life despite intervening bouts of prolonged illness. An elevation above the normal amplitude of daily temperature for an individual is considered fever. During fever, the morning low and evening high temperature pattern can still be observed. In the occasional situation in which elevated temperature is really hyperthermia, this rhythm is absent. A diagnosis of hyperthermia is often made because of a preceding history of heat exposure or use of certain drugs that interfere with normal thermoregulation. In some patients the hypothalamic set-point is elevated owing to local trauma, hemorrhage, tumor invasion, or intrinsic hypothalamic malfunction. The term "hypothalamic fever" is sometimes used to describe elevated temperature caused by abnormal hypothalamic function. However, the majority of patients with hypothalamic damage have hypothermia or do not thermoregulate properly to mild environmental termperature changes. In those patients in whom hypothalamic fever is suspected, diagnosis depends on demonstrating other abnormal hypothalamic functions, such as production of hypothalamic-releasing factors, abnormal response to cold, and absence of circadian rhythm.

MANIFESTATIONS OF FEVER. The subjective symptoms of fever include sensations of feeling cold or warm, headache, myalgias, arthralgias, and general malaise. The objective signs besides elevated temperature include increased respiratory rate, widened pulse pressure, and rapid heart rate. There are exceptions, however. Patients with typhoid fever and certain hypothalamic tumors have lower pulse rates than expected during fever. Laboratory findings are altered in fever. The most notable of these is elevated erythrocyte sedimentation rate resulting from increased haptoglobin, fibrinogen, ceruloplasmin, and C-reactive protein levels. These are often called "acute phase reactants" and account for the elevation in globulins seen on serum protein electrophoresis. In some patients the neutrophil count is elevated and young marrow forms appear in the peripheral blood, but these leukocyte changes may reflect the disease causing the infection rather than the fever itself. Serum iron and zinc levels are decreased during fever, and the low iron may play a role in the anemia that frequently accompanies chronic fever.

Metabolic rate is increased during fever (13 to 15 per cent per degree above 37° C), thus requiring more calories and increased oxygen. The metabolic consequences of fever can be detrimental. For example, muscle breakdown occurs in which the amino acids are inefficiently consumed for energy. Muscle protein breakdown appears to be triggered by endogenous pyrogen-induced PGE_2 production. Also, fever is accompanied by an increase in urinary calcium, which reflects progressive

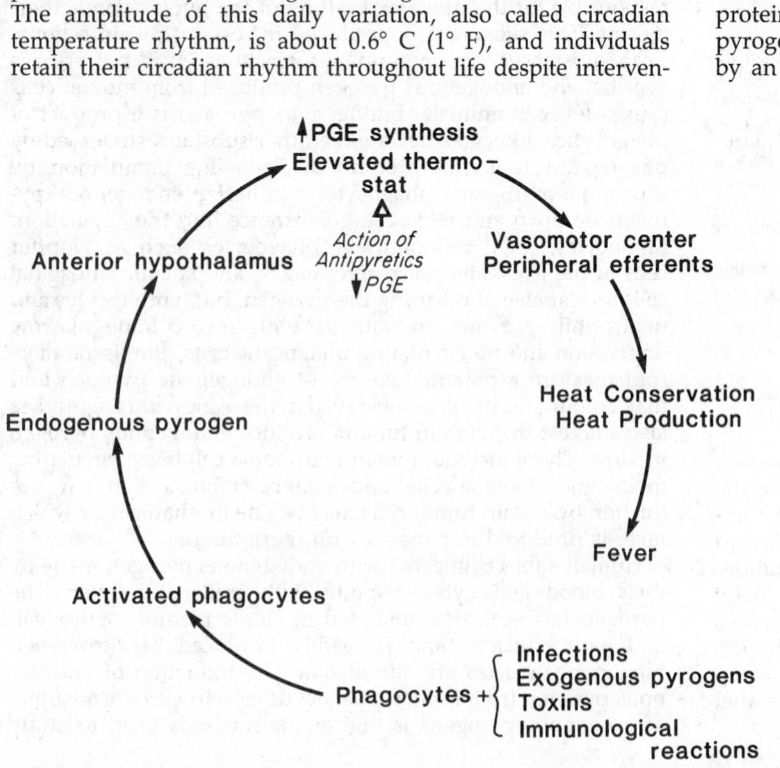

Figure 255–1. Mechanisms for the production of fever.

breakdown of bone. Aminoaciduria and proteinuria reflect the generalized breakdown of tissue during fever.

Fever caused by infectious, toxic, or immunologic diseases rarely exceeds 41.1° C (106° F), and there is clinical as well as animal evidence that the hypothalamic set-point for pyrogen response has a thermal ceiling. Extremely high fever (hyperpyrexia), however, can occur in any patient with significant disease, but it is most frequently observed in patients with central nervous system hemorrhage. In general, there are only a few clinical conditions in which moderately elevated temperature is detrimental. These are in patients with central nervous system disease, decreased cardiovascular function, and prior history of febrile seizure, and in pregnant women. The increased oxygen demand, cardiac output, and pulse rate associated with fever are particularly dangerous to patients with a compromised myocardium. Fever may also be teratogenic for the developing fetus.

TREATMENT. Most individuals with fever caused by infectious diseases, such as upper respiratory tract infections or flu syndromes, experience unpleasant symptoms and treat their fever with antipyretics. There is no evidence that moderately elevated temperature is harmful to patients who are not in one of the risk groups noted above. It is often desirable to withhold antipyretic therapy so that fever can be used as an index of improvement or worsening of a disease. On the other hand, there are no data on humans to suggest that fever is beneficial, although in some animal models survival from certain bacteremias is increased in febrile as compared with normothermic animals. Presently, there is renewed interest in the use of hyperthermia in treating disease, particularly disseminated cancers. In these situations, there may be beneficial aspects of elevated temperature for certain host defense mechanisms as well as the injurious effects of high temperature on some neoplastic cells. In most clinical settings, the use of oral antipyretics suffices to reduce fever. In febrile adults, a single oral dose (600 to 900 mg) of acetaminophen or aspirin reduces body temperature to normal levels in three to six hours. Peak plasma levels of the drugs vary and the times of peak drug concentration also vary considerably between one and five hours following oral administration.

Acetaminophen and aspirin in comparable oral doses have approximately equal ability to lower body temperature. The need to repeat the dose of antipyretics may be related to continued synthesis and release of endogenous pyrogen and the short duration of action of antipyretics. In adults, the total daily dose of acetaminophen should not exceed 3 grams under ordinary circumstances and should be lower in patients with impaired hepatic function. The dose limits in children are adjusted on the basis of body surface or weight.

Acetaminophen should be used as an antipyretic in patients who are allergic to salicylates or who have gastrointestinal intolerance to aspirin. In addition, acetaminophen is preferable to aspirin in patients with hemophilia, von Willebrand's disease, or other diseases of blood coagulation or who are being treated with oral anticoagulants. Aspirin is contraindicated in patients with peptic ulcer or asthma. However, with the exceptions cited above, there is no advantage to using acetaminophen rather than aspirin for the reduction of fever.

Several physical methods can also be used to reduce body temperature. The most common is water or alcohol sponging. The use of air-conditioned rooms, fans, and cooling blankets will also reduce core temperature by facilitating air and surface heat conduction from the skin. If physical methods are used to reduce core temperature at a time when the hypothalamic set-point remains elevated, shivering and vasoconstriction will occur as the hypothalamic drive to raise core temperature competes with the peripheral removal of heat. Thus, the ideal circumstance for reducing body temperature during fever combines the use of an antipyretic that lowers the hypothalamic set-point with physical methods that promote heat dissipation. In some circumstances, overzealous methods to reduce fever can lead to hypothermia. This is often the case when phenobarbital, chlorpromazine, or large doses of corticosteroids are administered in conjunction with antipyretics and sponging.

Any patient with fever of 41.1° C (106° F) (hyperpyrexia) requires urgent medical care. For some patients with pre-existing cardiovascular, pulmonary, or central nervous system diseases, or in children who have had a febrile seizure, the temperature at which the individual is at risk may be considerably lower. Efforts to reduce hyperpyrexia should be instituted with rapidity before physiologic changes secondary to prolonged high temperature produce significant morbidity. These may include acidosis, hypovolemia, cardiac arrhythmias, respiratory and contraction alkalosis, and electrolyte abnormalities. It is helpful to use physical methods to reduce body temperature during hyperpyrexia, but core temperature should be carefully monitored.

Dinarello CA: Interleukin-1. Rev Inf Dis 6:54, 1984. *A comprehensive review of the interrelationship between fever and the acute phase response.*

Dinarello CA, Wolff SM: Molecular basis of fever in humans. Am J Med 72:799, 1982. *A detailed review of the pathogenesis of fever with discussion of the production and action of human endogenous pyrogen.*

Atkins E: Fever: Its history, cause and function. Yale J Biol Med 55:283, 1982. *A concise review of the history and function of fever.*

Milton AS (ed.): Pyretics and Antipyretics. Berlin, Springer Verlag, 1982. *A monograph (600 pages) with over 25 recognized contributors updating the mechanisms of fever production and antipyresis.*

256. SHOCK SYNDROMES RELATED TO SEPSIS

John N. Sheagren

Sepsis is defined as the presence of various pus-forming and other pathogenic organisms or their toxins in the blood or tissues. The presumptive diagnosis of sepsis is often made on the basic of historical, physical, and laboratory data even in the absence of proof. The most serious complications are produced when infection spreads from the original focus to the bloodstream. Bacteremia can produce two very different types of complications: microbiologic and inflammatory. The microbiologic complications result from the local and systemic proliferation and seeding of the causative organism, which cause direct tissue or organ damage. The inflammatory complications are produced locally and can result in tissue or organ destruction independent of toxic factors produced by the causative organism. Bacteremia triggers intravascular activation of the same inflammatory systems that are protective within tissues. These combine with stress-generated endocrine responses to produce a sequence of metabolic events. The end stage of these events is the systemic vascular collapse traditionally termed *septic shock*.

Morbidity and mortality associated with septic shock are quite high: approximately two thirds of such patients die. Therefore, prevention of septic shock should be the primary goal. It is possible to recognize clinically the changes that occur in patients in the early stages of the septic shock syndrome. Intervention at early stages of the syndrome can reduce morbidity and mortality.

INCIDENCE AND EPIDEMIOLOGY. Infections most commonly occur in the hospital setting. Many infected patients become bacteremic. It is estimated that of 100 randomly chosen patients who appear to be infected (septic) in a hospital setting, approximately 90 per cent will actually be infected. Of those in whom infection is ultimately documented, about 20 per cent will develop some evidence of hemodynamic instability and appear, at least temporarily, "shocky." About half of that group of shocky patients (or about 10 per cent of all septic-appearing patients) will go on to frank septic shock and/or manifest serious end organ malfunction related to the septic episode such as adult respiratory distress syndrome (ARDS), renal failure, or disseminated intravascular coagulation (DIC). Since about 5 per cent of all hospital patients either are admitted with or develop an infection during hospitalization, the number of patients at risk of developing septic shock is large. The clinician must be familiar with the manifestations and differential diagnosis of the septic-appearing patient and have in mind rapid comprehensive diagnostic and therapeutic plans of action.

Shock Related to Gram-Negative as Opposed to Gram-Positive Organisms. Many authors state that septic shock more commonly follows gram-negative than gram-positive septic episodes, and many textbooks still refer to generic septic shock as gram-negative sepsis or endotoxic shock because endotoxin is found only in gram-negative bacterial cell walls. Recent studies suggest that in a theoretical group of 100 patients who are bacteremic with gram-negative microbes, the incidence of metabolic complications and shock is high (about 25 per cent). However, about 10 per cent of patients with gram-positive bacteremia, especially those infected with *Staphylococcus aureus*, develop shock. The incidence of suppurative complications (metastatic seeding to bones, joints, viscera, and so on), on the other hand, is much higher with gram-positive microorganisms. Gram-positive bacteria have the capability of adhering to endothelial cells to a much greater degree than do gram-negative organisms, so that seeding to heart valves and other organs is much more common.

PATHOGENESIS. Sepsis can cause shock in many ways, either related to the primary focus of infection or to the systemic effects of bacteremia. These mechanisms of shock are listed in Table 256–1.

The classic *septic shock syndrome* results primarily from the sequence of events triggered by bacteremia during which cell wall bacterial substances (endotoxin in gram-negative organisms and the peptidoglycan/teichoic acid complex in gram-positive organisms) activate the complement, coagulation, kinin, and ACTH/endorphin systems. This activation results in a series of metabolic events that ultimately progress to a state of shock (see Table 256–1, inflammatory-system–mediated shock). This type of shock traditionally has been erroneously referred to as gram-negative or endotoxic shock. Clinically, severe sepsis produces hemodynamic changes in two phases. Septic patients initially have hemodynamic changes primarily reflecting vasodilation. The patient is hyperdynamic with increased cardiac output and decreased systemic vascular resistance. As this hyperdynamic state develops, the peripheral processes of complement-mediated leukoagglutination and capillary damage cause a severe capillary leak syndrome. Intravascular volume begins to decrease, resulting in the "unloaded patient" in full-blown septic shock. This second phase of septic shock occurs when blood pressure falls dramatically as intravascular volume decreases, and as cardiac output, previously elevated, declines. Several factors contribute to the decline in cardiac output: peripheral resistance in late septic shock begins to increase, and several cardiodepressants are demonstrable, namely vasopressin and encephalin (one of the products of the endorphin system activation). Individual organs may be damaged independently of the hypotensive events; for example, direct pulmonary damage by the activated leukocytes may result in ARDS, or the patient may develop renal malfunction whether or not frank hypotension has occurred. Presumably these end organ manifestations are related to localized direct inflammatory damage caused by the events previously described. It is in this stage that disseminated intravascular coagulation associated with severe hypoperfusion may occur with extremely high morbidity and mortality.

TABLE 256–1. MECHANISMS OF SHOCK CAUSED BY SEPSIS

1. Shock related to a localized primary focus of infection
   Hypovolemic shock: severe local infection may
   —cause sufficient local fluid accumulation to produce systemic hypovolemia.
   —produce severe diarrhea with gastrointestinal fluid loss.
   —erode into a local vessel with mycotic aneurysm formation and rupture.
   Cardiogenic shock: extension of a pericardiac infection (usually pneumonia) into the pericardium may cause purulent pericarditis and tamponade.
   Toxigenic shock (the toxic shock syndrome): a toxin is produced locally, causing
   —endothelial cell damage with capillary leakage.
   —cardiodepression.
2. Shock related to bacteremic infections
   Cardiogenic shock: seeding of the organism through the bloodstream may cause
   —valvular malfunction (endocarditis).
   —myocarditis secondary to multiple metastatic myocardial abscesses.
   —purulent pericarditis (metastatic).
   Inflammatory-system–mediated shock: bacterial cell wall substances activate the complement, coagulation, kinin, and ACTH/endorphin systems and thus cause
   —vasodilation (roles of endorphins, kinins, and complement).
   —capillary leakage (primarily due to the intracapillary adherence and aggregation of activated polymorphonuclear leukocytes).
   —disseminated intravascular coagulation.
   —cardiodepression (encephalins, vasopressin, possibly other substances).

Figure 256–1 outlines the sequence of early events initiated from the localized focus of infection. From these events are derived the various complications of bacteremia, which include metastatic abscess formation and the metabolic complications described earlier. Antibiotics limit metastatic abscess formation (the microbiologic complications of bacteremia). However, a number of other metabolic events, when activated and independent of bacterial proliferation, still produce substantial morbidity and mortality. Therefore, anti-inflammatory therapy is recommended.

The ACTH/Endorphin System. During systemic stress, increased ACTH release occurs. For each molecule of ACTH produced, a molecule of one of the endorphins or encephalins is also produced. The endorphins are very powerful opiate-like substances that have a variety of other metabolic effects. The endorphins provide pain relief during severe stress, and high levels of circulating endorphins may have the same side effects as opiates, resulting in hypotension, changes in vascular permeability, and alterations in mentation.

Coagulation/Kinin System Activation. Bacterial endotoxins and other cell wall materials directly activate the coagulation system both by initiating platelet aggregation and by activating Hageman factor. These coagulation events are triggered simultaneously by intravascular bacterial cell wall products. Subsequently, kinin system activation (see Ch. 442) results in the production of bradykinin, a powerful vasodilator.

Complement System Activation. The complement system is also directly activated by high molecular weight bacterial and fungal polysaccharides primarily by means of the alternative pathway. A sequence of intravascular events ensues, resulting in microvascular instability as well as massive chaotic activation of circulating polymorphonuclear leukocytes (PMNs). The activated PMN has enhanced bactericidal capabilities but also an

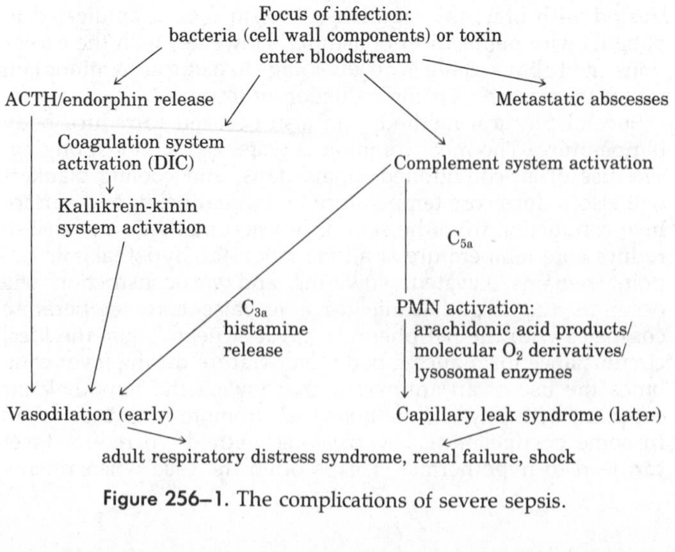

Figure 256–1. The complications of severe sepsis.

enhanced capability of damaging host tissues. The activated PMN possesses increased amounts of lysosomal enzymes and produces a variety of toxic metabolites of molecular oxygen, all of which are both bactericidal and cytocidal. Furthermore, the activated PMN produces both inflammatory prostaglandins and several products of the lipoxygenase system, many of which enhance inflammation by also producing vasodilation, capillary leakage, chemotaxis, and PMN activation. The activated PMNs adhere to each other (the *leukopenic phase* of sepsis during which PMN aggregates form in capillaries) and to endothelial cells to cause severe endothelial cell damage and capillary leakage.

CLINICAL MANIFESTATIONS. ***The Septic Patient.*** The clinical situation in which a patient is considered septic (highly likely to be infected) is common. Patients in this setting usually have fever. High fever and the presence of a chill strongly indicate that bacterial sepsis is occurring. Starting with the clinical recognition of fever, the managing physician must be constantly on the alert for signs that the patient's condition is deteriorating in a manner suggestive of septic shock. Thus, clinically it is useful to try to identify subgroups of patients who are not only likely to be infected but have additional systemic signs of toxicity that suggest that they may be toxemic or bacteremic and in danger of developing full-bown shock. When a clinical diagnosis of septic shock can be made, the mortality rate is exceedingly high. It is important to develop the concept of the "preshock phase of septic shock" predicated on identifying a subgroup of infected patients more likely than others to develop shock. Treatment before shock develops may prevent some of the morbidity and mortality associated with sepsis.

Table 256–2 lists several systemic signs and a variety of physical findings likely to be predictive of the development of septic shock. Extremes of body temperature are often associated with shock. Specifically, fever in excess of 40.6° C and hypothermia associated with sepsis should be alerting signs that hypotension may soon follow. Also, in the febrile patient with a distinct change in mentation the mortality rate is higher. In association with such a finding, primary central nervous system infection may be present, and lumbar puncture is often indicated. Febrile patients who have hemodynamic instability (who are orthostatic with a blood pressure decrease of 30 mm Hg or greater) should be considered on the verge of developing septic shock.

While it is not possible to distinguish between simple dehydration and early septic shock solely on the basis of orthostatic blood pressure changes, hemodynamic monitoring will show an increase in peripheral vascular resistance in the former case and a reduction in the latter. Also, fluid challenge alone will rapidly stabilize the condition of the purely hypovolemic patient. Sepsis is associated in the early stages with a state of "warm shock" in which there is a decrease in orthostatic blood pressure but good perfusion in the extremities (they are warm and pink rather than cool and cyanotic). Since the lung is such an important organ in systemic septic shock, tachypnea with hypoxemia or the development of a metabolic acidosis or both may be predictive of impending ARDS. The development of peripheral edema, often with a suddenly decreased serum albumin concentration, just as in toxigenic shock (see section on the Toxic Shock Syndrome in Ch. 270), is often caused by an unrecognized bacteremic event.

Laboratory Data Suggesting Bacteremia or Toxemia. Several laboratory tests are often helpful in the evaluation of a potentially septic patient (Table 256–2). The blood may show hypoxemia and a metabolic acidosis. Serum lactate elevation is highly predictive of deterioration leading to septic shock. Decreasing urine output, often associated with rising blood urea nitrogen and creatinine, may be seen early in sepsis as renal failure occurs. Serum albumin measurements may show decreases in excess of that calculated by catabolism alone. Often such patients show signs of progressive peripheral edema. In early sepsis, the total white count may be low, with most of the decrease in the PMN count, owing to complement-induced leukoaggregation. As white cells aggregate, platelets become caught up in the process. Thrombocytopenia is predictive of high risk of septic shock and ARDS.

TABLE 256–2. PHYSICAL SIGNS AND LABORATORY DATA LIKELY TO BE PREDICTIVE OF THE DEVELOPMENT OF SEPTIC SHOCK

1. Extremes of body temperature (fever >40.6° C or hypothermia)
2. Altered mental status
3. Orthostatic blood pressure decrease (>30 mm Hg)
4. Decreasing urine output
5. Unexplained edema, usually associated with a falling serum albumin concentration
6. Tachypnea with hypoxemia and/or the development of a metabolic acidosis
7. Elevated serum lactate concentration
8. Development of leukopenia (predominantly neutropenia)
9. Development of thrombocytopenia with or without petechial skin rash

In the future, assistance in clinical decision making will be provided by rapid laboratory measurements of the activation of many of the systems shown in Figure 256–1. For example, the rapid identification of a falling total complement level and elevated levels of C5a, prostaglandins, or endorphins might predict subgroups of septic patients at risk of developing shock.

DIAGNOSIS. The presumptive diagnosis of sepsis must be made when the setting and attendant clinical signs are suggestive. In general, patients with fever should be considered septic until proved otherwise. Therapy should always be initiated for high-risk febrile patients in advance of microbiologic confirmation of sepsis.

Evaluation of the Septic Patient. The setting in which the episode is occurring should be evaluated promptly. Crucial to appropriate initial decision making are the background history, which may help to define the type of host defense defect present, and prior cultural data, which might be predictive of the infecting organism. The physical examination should be directed at quickly but thoroughly searching for the septic source as well as signs of end organ failure that might indicate progression to shock such as altered mental status, progressive edema, hypotension, and so on (Table 256–2). All potentially infected foci should be appropriately sampled, and the material obtained should be Gram-stained and cultured.

Differential Diagnosis of Severe Sepsis. Having done a thorough preliminary evaluation, one can reassess the clinical situation on subsequent days and stop antibiotic therapy if the episode later seems not to be infectious. Many nonseptic events can cause high fever with or without vascular instability. For example, a variety of hypersensitivity reactions (often caused by drugs) may mimic sepsis. Vasculitic diseases may present with high fever, unstable blood pressure, and altered mentation. Pulmonary emboli occur frequently in the hospital setting, and especially if the patient develops fever the embolic event initially may be confused with sepsis. Myocardial infarction may result in hemodynamic instability, and in the subset of patients who develop higher than average fever, may lead to initial confusion with sepsis.

There are infectious syndromes against which antimicrobials are of no use in which bacterial sepsis may be suspected. For example, viral syndromes such as those caused by influenza viruses, enteroviruses, adenoviruses, cytomegalovirus, and hepatitis viruses may all have very high fever and be quite difficult to diagnosis. Malaria, common in other parts of the world, can be extremely hard to identify when it is afflicting patients in the United States. It is sometimes difficult initially to differentiate malaria from severe sepsis unless the parasite is detected on the peripheral blood smear.

TREATMENT. ***Antibacterial Therapy.*** Extremely broad coverage is required in patients with the syndrome of severe sepsis. It is best to initiate therapy with a combination of antibiotics when the infecting organism is unknown. An aminoglycoside should always be used, and gentamicin remains the aminoglycoside of choice unless other considerations (such as abnormal renal function and known microbial resistance) dictate the use of tobramycin or amikacin. In the granulocytopenic patient, the aminoglycoside should be combined with high doses of carbenicillin, ticarcillin, or mezlocillin. In the patient likely to have an anaerobic focus of infection in which *Bacteriodes fragilis* is likely to be present, such as an intra-abdominal or gynecologic infection, or decubitus and lower extremity vascular and neuropathic ulcers, clindamycin is combined with gentamicin. For all other patients, gentamicin plus cefazolin, the best first-generation cephalosporin, is the combination of choice. When cultures define the causative microbe(s) or other data point to a specific organism, therapy can be tailored to the most appropriate, most specific, least toxic, and least expensive single antibiotic.

Antishock Therapy. The most important component of the therapy of shock associated with sepsis is volume replacement. Sufficient quantities of an appropriate solute (or, where indicated, albumin or whole blood) should be administered to the septic patient in an attempt to provide adequate volume support. Hemodynamic monitoring of the patient's clinically deteriorating septic condition is mandatory and is preferably carried out in the intensive care unit (see Ch. 71 on Critical Care Medicine). For example, while fluid administration should be vigorous from the beginning, adequate volume support means administering just enough fluid to bring the patient's pulmonary capillary wedge pressure to the high normal range. As outlined in Figure 256–2, an attempt can be made to counter the adverse inflammatory sequelae of bacteremia with appropriate anti-inflammatory drug therapy. Used most commonly in severely septic patients are massive doses of methylprednisolone sodium succinate, a dose of 30 mg per kilogram being appropriate. One should not use longer acting glucocorticoids such as dexamethasone that extend the period of immunosuppression. This controversial topic has recently been extensively reviewed (see Sande and Root, chapter on "Glucocorticoid Therapy in the Management of Severe Sepsis").

The use of other anti-inflammatory drugs such as the antiprostaglandins is under active investigation. These agents may selectively suppress inflammatory damage caused by the activated PMN without interfering with the antibacterial capabilities of these important host defense cells.

Some clinicians are beginning to use naloxone in severe sepsis on the basis of the documented contribution of the

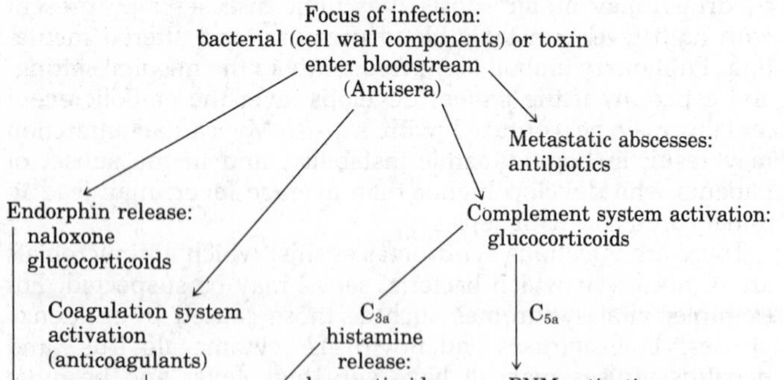

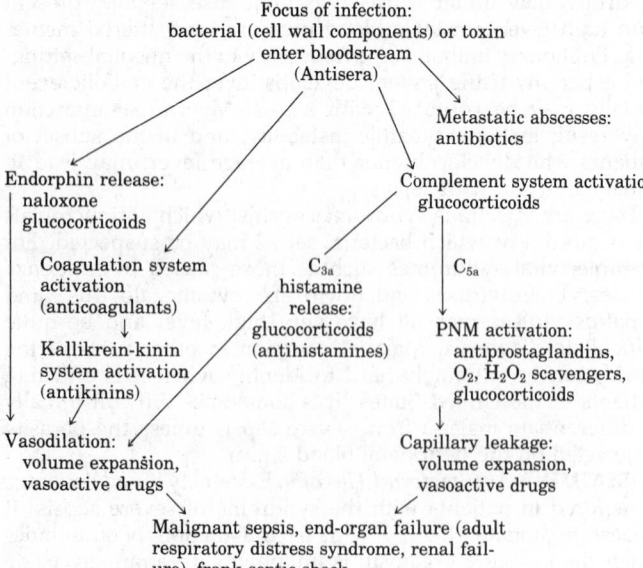

Figure 256–2. Therapy for the complications of severe sepsis.

endorphin system to hemodynamic instability in experimental models of septic shock. However, in primate models naloxone, like alpha agonists (aramine and levophed) appears to increase blood pressure without leading to improved tissue perfusion. Therefore, naloxone as routine therapy for patients with severe sepsis is premature. Further investigation of the use of naloxone in severe sepsis and septic shock is indicated.

In DIC, one should not use anticoagulant therapy when the cause is thought to be sepsis. Many other modalities of therapy are being evaluated in septic shock.

The Role of Surgery and Hyperbaric Oxygen. Surgical debridement and drainage of septic foci is especially important. All severe localized infections, especially with gas formation, should be widely debrided and drained. Hyperbaric oxygen has been used in patients with the gangrene syndromes and clostridial myonecrosis. Whether or not it stabilizes patients' conditions or influences the ultimate outcome is unknown.

Antiendotoxin Antiserum. Recently, it has been demonstrated that an antiserum against endotoxin enhances survival in patients bacteremic with gram-negative organisms. In a recent prospective randomized study, an antiserum directed against the "core" (common) lipopolysaccharide moiety of an *Escherichia coli* mutant significantly reduced mortality in severely septic patients (Ziegler, 1982). Thus, ultimately the infusion of a monoclonal antiendotoxin antiserum may be beneficial in patients showing signs of the early stages of septic shock.

PROGNOSIS. Most febrile patients lacking other signs of severe sepsis (as described in Table 256–2) will usually do well even when bacteremic. Such patients usually respond quickly to volume administration, antibacterial therapy, and drainage of the primary focus of infection. However, the presence of shock dramatically increases morbidity and mortality. Even when the inciting infection is localized, the presence of shock (with the exception of the toxic shock syndrome) is associated with a 50 per cent mortality. As noted earlier, full-blown, bacteremia-associated septic shock has greater than 70 per cent mortality. A favorable outcome in a patient in frank shock depends on the skill of management in the intensive care unit. Early diagnosis and therapy of severely septic patients will decrease the morbidity and mortality.

PREVENTION. Prevention of infection, especially in the hospital, is the key to reducing morbidity and mortality associated with septic shock. Strict adherence to the hospital infection control program with avoidance of Foley catheters and meticulous attention to the placement and maintenance of intravascular lines dramatically reduces the incidence of bacteremic infections. The concept of the preshock approach to the therapy of septic shock is useful; in all such patients fluids should be administered and broad antibiotic coverage started early. In addition, in some overtly bacteremic patients anti-inflammatory therapy will probably reduce morbidity and mortality. Controlled studies of anti-inflammatory therapy in severe sepsis are under way and better guidelines soon should be forthcoming.

Abraham E, Shoemaker WC, Bland RD, Cobo JC: Sequential cardiorespiratory patterns in septic shock. Crit Care Med 11:799, 1983. *Describes the hemodynamic patterns occurring in patients as they develop septic shock.*

Hoffman SL, Punjabi NH, Kumala S, et al.: Reduction in mortality in chloramphenicol-treated severe typhoid fever by high-dose dexamethasone. N Engl J Med 310:82, 1984. *A prospective controlled study showing significant reduction in mortality in patients in the "preshock" stage of typhoid fever who were given 6 mg per kilogram of dexamethasone along with antibiotic and volume support.*

Jacob HS, Craddock PR, Hammerschmidt DE, Moldow CF: Complement-induced granulocyte aggregation: An unsuspected mechanism of disease. N Engl J Med 302:789, 1980. *Describes how complement-induced granulocyte aggregation leads to capillary and organ damge.*

Sande M, Root RR: Septic Shock: Newer Concepts in Pathophysiology and Treatment. New York, Churchill Livingstone, Inc. (in press). *Complete up-to-date review of all aspects of septic shock including papers on the roles of endorphins, complement, prostaglandins, the PMN, and glucocorticoid therapy.*

Sheagren JN: Septic shock and corticosteroids. N Engl J Med 305:456, 1981. *A brief review of the rationale and potential problems of corticosteroid administration to patients in septic shock.*

Sprung CL, Civetta J, Rackow EC, et al.: The Pulmonary Artery Catheter—Methodology and Clinical Applications. Baltimore, University Park Press, 1983. *A complete review of the use of the Swan-Ganz catheter.*

Weissman G, Smolen JE, Dorchak HM: Release of inflammatory mediators from stimulated neutrophils. N Engl J Med 303:27, 1980. *An excellent description of the events leading to and occurring in the activated PMN.*

Zeigler EJ, McCutchan JA, Fierer J, et al.: Treatment of gram-negative bacteremia and shock with human antiserum to a mutant *Escherichia coli*. N Engl J Med 307:1225, 1982. *Describes therapy of bacteremic patients with human antiserum to endotoxin core resulting in a significant reduction in mortality.*

257. THE COMPROMISED HOST

John I. Gallin

COMPONENTS OF THE HOST DEFENSES. The host defenses comprise complex and interrelated systems, which are outlined in Table 257–1. Familiarity with these systems provides a basis for the diagnosis and management of patients with compromised defenses.

Physical Barriers. Intact skin and mucous membranes prevent microbial invasion. The skin is a complex organ, consisting of several cell types which, in addition to providing a physical barrier, produce numerous antimicrobial agents such as lactic acid, ammonia, urea, and free fatty acids. These protect the host from superficial challenges. The mucous membrane secretions, which trap inhaled microorganisms, contain soluble factors such as immunoglobulin A, lactoferrin, lysozyme, and α_1-antitrypsin, which have antibacterial activity. Proper function of the nasal and respiratory passage cilia facilitates microbial clearance. In addition, host defenses require normal anatomy of the respiratory, genitourinary, and gastrointestinal systems.

Inflammatory Response. The circulating phagocytes (neutrophils, monocytes, eosinophils, and basophils) are the central components of the inflammatory response. The phagocytes are manufactured and undergo maturation in the bone marrow, and upon appropriate stimulation are delivered to the bloodstream where they circulate and are distributed to local tissue sites. Recruitment of phagocytic leukocytes from the bloodstream involves a complex process called diapedesis or emigration. The initial step of this process is not completely understood but seems to require phagocyte aggregation and adherence to the endothelium. The phagocytic cells pass between the endothelial cells as they migrate to tissue sites. The availability of the potential space between endothelial cells through which phagocytes migrate is modulated by local tissue products of the complement cascade (the anaphylatoxins, or small molecular weight cleavage products of the third and fifth complement components, C3a and C5a) and the potent vasodilator bradykinin produced by activation of the fibrinolytic and kinin generating systems. The complement cascade and the fibrinolytic and kinin generating systems are activated by microbial products, such as endotoxin, and a variety of substances secreted by leukocytes, platelets, and fibroblasts. Locomotion of phagocytes requires cell adherence to their substratum, deformability, machinery for random locomotion, and the ability to sense a gradient of a chemical signal (chemotactic factor) and convert random locomotion (kinesis) to directed locomotion (chemotaxis). The locomotory apparatus includes an intact actin and myosin system for movement and an intact microtubule system to stabilize the cell during locomotion and organize the intracellular granules, which are secreted extracellularly during locomotion and appear to be important modulators of the inflammatory process.

TABLE 257–1. THE HOST DEFENSES

Physical barriers
Skin
Mucocus membranes
Inflammatory response
Circulating phagocytes
Humoral mediators
Reticuloendothelial system
Fixed phagocytes
Immune response
T cells (cell-mediated immunity, delayed hypersensitivity)
B cells (antibody responses)
Other mediators (i.e., lymphotoxin)

The chemotactic factors are humoral mediators and include products from activation of the complement system (C5a) and the arachidonic acid cascade (leukotriene B_4). Other chemoattractants result from activation of the kinin generating system, products from neutrophils, macrophages, lymphocytes (lymphokines), and fibroblasts (collagen and other peptides), some bacterial products, as well as oxidation products of certain fatty acids. Some chemotactic factors are highly preferential for particular cell types (i.e., histamine and other mast cell products are preferential for eosinophils, whereas an alveolar macrophage product is preferential for neutrophils). After recruitment, microorganisms that have been opsonized by complement products and immunoglobulins to facilitate adherence to the phagocyte membrane are then ingested, killed, and digested. These events require complex biochemical and biophysical events with specific mechanisms for elimination of different classes of microorganisms (see Ch. 148).

Reticuloendothelial System. The reticuloendothelial system is the major system for the clearance of circulating microorganisms from the bloodstream. The main components of the system are the tissue, or "fixed," phagocytes, consisting of splenic macrophages, alveolar macrophages, Kupffer cells, lymph node macrophages, and microglial cells in the brain. Many or perhaps all of these macrophages are derived from circulating monocytes that migrate from the bloodstream into the extravascular space where they differentiate into the tissue macrophages.

The Immune Response. The T and B lymphocytes are the main components of the immune response. T lymphocytes are the functional cells of cell-mediated immunity or delayed hypersensitivity. Mature B cells, or plasma cells, produce antibodies and are the cells of humoral immunity. The functions of T and B lymphocytes are closely related. For example, helper T cells facilitate B cell function, whereas suppressor T cells are important regulators of B cell function. The thymus gland controls the maturation of the T lymphocytes; factors controlling B cell maturation in humans are not known.

Upon appropriate signal, lymphocytes are released from the bone marrow into the circulation, where they are distributed throughout the body. The mechanism of mobilizing lymphocytes to tissue sites from the circulation is poorly understood but may involve chemotaxis. At tissue sites lymphocytes perform their specific tasks. The T lymphocytes are believed to be critical in eliminating such pathogens as *Mycobacterium tuberculosis*, *Histoplasma capsulatum*, *Candida albicans*, and certain viruses. The B cells respond to antigens (which may first have to be processed by macrophages) by synthesis of the immunoglobulins (antibodies), which have important roles in complement activation, virus neutralization, and opsonization. (For a detailed review of the various components of the immune response, see Ch. 427.)

ETIOLOGY. Infection is a major cause of morbidity and mortality in patients undergoing treatment for neoplasia or collagen vascular diseases, or therapy to prevent organ rejection following organ transplantation. In each of these clinical settings there may be an inherent defect of host defenses. However, the most common cause for the recurrent infections in each of these settings is the use of drugs which suppress the cellular and/or humoral components of the inflammatory and immune responses. Thus drugs which cause neutropenia, such as Cytoxan or myelosuppressive agents; drugs which suppress phagocytic cell function, such as corticosteroids or aspirin; drugs which suppress the T or B cell systems, such as Cytoxan (presumably inhibits T suppressor cells) or methotrexate (presumably inhibits antigen-specific lymphocyte transformation); and drugs used to prevent graft versus host disease, such as cyclosporin A (presumably inhibits antigenic triggering of immunocompetent cells), all have the potential to compromise the host defenses and predispose the patient to infection. These drug-related effects are probably the most common cause for the compromised host seen in the hospital.

A host may also be compromised as a consequence of environmental factors, such as protein-calorie malnutrition, thermal injury, alcoholism, and irradiation. Host defense defects can also result from a number of inherited and congenital disorders, as well as from acquired defects associated with numerous diseases. The particular type of infection will depend on the nature of the fundamental defect.

PATHOGENESIS AND PATHOLOGY. Pathologic models in support of predicted abnormalities of host defenses are well described for certain components of the defense system. Other examples are emerging as we understand what parameters are important to assess. Examples related to infection from penetration of the skin are obvious and include penetrating trauma and severe burns.

Mucous membrane secretions are abnormally viscid in cystic fibrosis, and mucous plug formation with obstruction and subsequent pneumonia can result. Mucociliary movement is abnormal in Kartagener's syndrome (situs inversus, chronic sinusitis, and bronchiectasis), and this is related to absence of a particuar cilial subunit (dynein arms). Mucus secretion and cilial integrity may also be damaged by decreases in temperature and humidity, exposure to inhalants such as cigarette smoke and atmospheric pollutants, supplemental oxygen, endotracheal tubes, and thermal injury. Infection by certain respiratory viruses (i.e., influenza) and *Mycoplasma pneumoniae* can damage the mucociliary system, resulting in increased susceptibility to bronchitis and pneumonia. Recurrent bacterial pneumonias result from anatomic derangement of bronchi by obstruction from neoplasm, foreign objects, mucous plugs, or local collapse secondary to bronchiectasis and from chronic aspiration.

Gastrointestinal "blind loops" following certain surgical procedures result in overgrowth with coliform bacteria which consume vitamin B_{12} or folic acid and thereby contribute to neutropenic states. Genitourinary tract infections with gram-negative bacteria are associated with congenital and acquired abnormalities such as congenital ureteral abnormalities, urethral stricture, urethral changes following pregnancy, and urethral obstruction from stones, prostatic hypertrophy, and prostatic carcinoma.

Other anatomic defects increasing susceptibility to infection include damaged heart valves following endocarditis or rheumatic fever. Aortic aneurysms can be infected with salmonellae (particularly *Salmonella choleraesuis*), staphylococci, and streptococci. Peripheral vascular disease of diabetes mellitus is associated with infection of the distal phalanges of the toes. Foreign objects, including prosthetic devices, sutures, gauze, and intravenous or Foley catheters, interfere with normal anatomic integrity and are subject to microbial colonization and subsequent microbial dissemination.

Patients who have had splenectomy are at increased risk for *Streptococcus pneumoniae* infection, especially infants and young children. The precise basis for this is not known, but decreased clearance of bacteria by the reticuloendothelial system is thought to be important. Children with sickle cell hemoglobinopathies, as well as patients with hemoglobinopathies from a variety of causes, are susceptible to *Salmonella*, *Streptococcus pneumoniae*, and *Bartonella* infection. The host defect in the hemoglobinopathies may relate to splenic dysfunction, but abnormal alternative complement pathway function and impaired phagocytosis and killing of the indicated organisms by leukocytes have been described. Splenic dysfunction is also seen in splenomegaly from a variety of causes, including passive congestion, certain collagen-vascular diseases (systemic lupus erythematosus and Felty's syndrome), and lymphomas. These examples of splenic dysfunction are associated with neutropenia from neutrophil trapping and destruction in the spleen.

A number of other conditions predispose to compromised defenses. During viral influenza there is increased susceptibility to pneumococcal and staphylococcal pneumonia. The mechanism for this is poorly understood, but impaired mucociliary function, neutropenia, and adverse effects of the virus on phagocytic cell function have been implicated. Neoplasms, malnutrition, diabetes mellitus, and effects of a variety of pharmacologic agents, especially corticosteroids and myelosuppressive agents, compromise host defenses by affecting the production, distribution, and function of leukocytes. Prolonged use of antimicrobial drugs predisposes toward colonization with microorganisms resistant to the antibiotics, particularly *Staphylococcus aureus*, resistant gram-negative bacilli such as *Pseudomonas*, *Serratia*, and the gram-negative coccobacilli *Acinetobacter* species, as well as fungi *(Candida)*, and the compromised host is more likely to become infected with these organisms.

Leukopenias. Perhaps the best evidence for a role of leukocytes in host defenses is the severe infections associated with leukopenias. Leukopenia exists when the peripheral white blood count is below 4000 per cubic millimeter. Although all leukocytes can be depressed, most frequently neutrophils are the cell type affected. In general, when the granulocyte count is below 500 to 1000 cells per cubic millimeter, patients are at increased risk of infection, and when there are fewer than 200 cells per cubic millimeter, the inflammatory response is essentially absent and severe infection is the rule. Both the degree of granulocyte depression and its duration are important variables relating to the severity and rate of infection. Lymphopenia exists when the number of lymphocytes is below 1400 per cubic millimeter in children and 1000 per cubic millimeter in adults. The complete absence of leukocytes is not compatible with life in a normal environment. The particular type of infection associated with leukopenia depends upon which leukocyte population is depressed. Absence of thymus-dependent lymphocytes or T cells, as in thymus aplasia (DiGeorge's syndrome) or thymus hypoplasia (Nezelof's syndrome), is associated with severe defects of cell-mediated immunity (see Ch. 429). Absent B lymphocytes (Bruton's X-linked agammaglobulinemia) is associated with a severe abnormality of humoral mediated immunity (see Ch. 429). Combined T and B cell lymphopenia (see Ch. 429) has a particularly poor prognosis.

The causes of leukopenias are multiple and are related to depressed marrow production (idiopathic, drug-induced, leukemias, tumor invasion of the bone marrow, and nutritional deficiencies), peripheral destruction (immune mechanisms, splenic trapping), or peripheral pooling with overwhelming bacterial infection. Leukopenia is seen following infection with bacteria (typhoid, paratyphoid fever, tuberculosis, brucellosis), viruses (influenza, measles, infectious mononucleosis, rubella), rickettsiae, and protozoa (malaria, kala-azar). (For a complete review of the leukopenias, see Ch. 150.)

Leukocyte Dysfunction. The leukocyte dysfunction syndromes also demonstrate the primary importance of leukocytes in host defenses. Patients with T cell dysfunction include those with acquired immune deficiency syndrome, mucocutaneous candidiasis, and nucleoside phosphorylase deficiency. Combined T and B cell dysfunction is seen in adenosine deaminase deficiency and the Wiskott-Aldrich syndrome (see Ch. 429). Neutrophil dysfunctions attributable to abnormal adherence, chemotaxis, degranulation, and bactericidal activity are reviewed in Ch. 149. Defects of the humoral components of the inflammatory response include abnormalities of mediators. These include deficiencies of certain complement components (C3 and C5) with abnormal anaphylatoxin, opsonin, and chemotactic factor production. Inhibitors acting on the chemotactic factors have been described in patients with Hodgkin's disease, sarcoidosis, alcoholism, and cirrhosis. Patients deficient in the late complement components (C6 and C7) have increased susceptibility to *Neisseria* infections.

CLINICAL MANIFESTATIONS. The clinical history can be very important when evaluating a patient suspected of having a host defense defect. The type, frequency, duration, and location of infections, the intensity of the inflammatory reaction, and associated illnesses or clinical problems, such as allergies or atopic dermatitis, as well as the family history, are important and are summarized in Table 257–2.

Leukopenias. The clinical manifestations of leukopenia without infection are minimal, or those of the underlying disease. With acute drug-induced leukopenia, chills, fever, and prostration may be the initial manifestations and may be attributed to invasion by bacteria. However, these symptoms may occur within an hour of administering a drug which results in a hapten-antibody type reaction, such as with aminopyrine, and may relate to release of endogenous pyrogens from immune lysis of leukocytes. The initial symptoms may transiently disappear, to be followed by recurrent fever, chills, headaches, and frequently ulceration of the oropharynx and sometimes the rectum and vagina. These ulcerations are called aphthous ulcers and may be the initial clinical manifestation of neutropenia. The ulcers often have a gray membrane, but frank pus is absent. Patients receiving cytotoxic drug therapy get similar ulcers, independent of neutropenia, which may be difficult to distinguish from aphthous ulcers. Following or concomitant with this stage there are usually symptoms of local bacterial invasion. Frequently bacterial invasion is overwhelming without impressive clinical manifestations because of lack of an inflammatory reaction. Minimal skin lesions characterized by local erythema and tenderness or minimal roentgenographic findings often are the only indications of overwhelming infection with gram-negative bacilli. Careful and frequent inspection of the patient is thus required. With agranulocytosis, regional lymph nodes become enlarged. In the absence of aggressive therapy or spontaneous remission, death from overwhelming infection (usually gram-negative bacilli) ensues. If remission of the agranulocytosis occurs, immature granulocytes appear in the circulation before mature cells.

Patients with severe leukopenia also have an increased incidence of *Pneumocystis carinii* and cytomegalovirus infection as well as infection with the systemic mycoses, including candidiasis, invasive aspergillosis, and mucormycosis. Systemic candidiasis, defined as tissue invasion with or without colonization of superficial surfaces, is the most common mycosis in the neutropenic patient. Prolonged drug therapy for a bacterial infection predisposes to candidiasis and especially *C. albicans* because of normally occurring local colonization. The presence of thrush in the mouth, vagina, or skin indicates candidiasis in these patients, and indwelling catheters may serve as portals of entry. In systemic candidiasis symptoms are usually confined to the distal esophagus or the bladder, with rare local symptoms in the lung, liver, spleen, or kidney. Symptomatic lesions in the distal esophagus in compromised hosts are usually indicative of candidiasis and are characterized by dysphagia, odynophagia, pyrosis, retrosternal pain, and gastrointestinal bleeding. On x-ray irregular scalloping of the esophageal lining is manifest. Aspergillosis (penetration of hyphae into tissues) is an infection seen in neutropenic patients who are also on corticosteroid therapy; mucormycosis is also seen in this setting, especially in patients with diabetes mellitus. Aspergillosis almost invariably involves the lung, causing symptoms suggesting pneumonia or pulmonary emboli. Pulmonary mucormycosis is almost indistinguishable from aspergillosis.

Disorders of the Inflammatory Response. Patients with defective phagocyte chemotaxis present with minimal physical findings or findings characteristic of their underlying disease. The signs and symptoms of the infection are delayed because too few phagocytes arrive too late. Patients with defective leukocyte chemotaxis frequently have severe periodontal disease and dermatologic abnormalities, and these patients have frequent sinopulmonary infections with recurrent otitis media, bronchitis, and pneumonia. *Staphylococcus aureus* is the most frequent infectious agent, but *Streptococcus pneumoniae* and *Hemophilus influenzae* are also common.

A syndrome in which defective neutrophil and monocyte chemotaxis has been an associated host defense defect is found in patients with eczematous and pustular dermatitis, markedly elevated IgE (especially against *Staphylococcus aureus* and *Candida albicans*), low grade eosinophilia, "cold" staphylococcal skin infections, and recurrent bronchitis and pneumonias with subsequent bronchiectasis (Job's syndrome and its variants). About 50 per cent of patients with this disease have mucocutaneous candidiasis. The chemotactic defect in these patients, however, is variable, and it is not clear whether this is the primary host defense defect. Many of the patients appear to have a T cell defect, although how the T cell abnormality relates to the neutrophil and monocyte chemotactic defect is presently not known. It is possible that the primary problem is related to the lymphocyte and not the phagocyte. These patients frequently have subcutaneous and lymph node abscesses requiring surgical drainage, and their facies have a characteristic broad nasal bridge. Many patients are teenagers at the time of evaluation for host defense defects, and few patients over 30 years of age have been noted. Usually these patients have had recurrent pneumonias since early childhood, and many have thoracotomy scars from lobectomy for the severe bronchiectasis, bronchopleural fistulas, and cyst formation. The syndrome appears to be familial in some cases. Similar clinical spectrums with high IgE and a chemotactic defect are seen in patients with incontinentia pigmenti and an unusual type of ichthyosis.

Defective neutrophil and monocyte chemotaxis, delayed degranulation of neutrophils, and abnormal microbial killing are also noted in patients with the Chédiak-Higashi syndrome, a rare disease with autosomal recessive inheritance characterized by partial oculocutaneous albinism, nystagmus, neutropenia, recurrent cutaneous infections (particularly with *Staphylococcus aureus*), and giant lysosomes in all cells containing lysosomes. Patients with either congenital or acquired (from thermal injury) deficiency of specific granules also have defective neutrophil chemotaxis. All of these patients usually have multiple subcutaneous scars from their recurrent infections.

An impressive list of diseases with chemotactic defects and recurrent infections has emerged in recent years and includes the following: diabetes mellitus, leukemias, malignancies (melanoma and breast carcinoma), rheumatoid arthritis, Felty's syndrome, systemic lupus erythematosus in some patients, thermal injury, bone marrow transplantation (associated with graft versus host disease and administration of antithymocyte globulin), congenital ichthyosis with *Trichophyton rubrum* infection, hypogammaglobulinemia, α-mannosidase deficiency, chronic renal failure (especially if the patient is on chronic hemodialysis), severe protein-calorie malnutrition, severe bacterial infections, and viral influenza. The mechanism for the chemotactic defect has not been delineated in most of these diseases, and it is not clear whether the chemotactic defect is a cause or effect of the recurrent infections. However, a few well documented case reports of patients with severe pyogenic infections and defective leukocyte locomotion attributable to actin dysfunction or abnormal microtubule assembly clearly illustrate the importance of leukocyte chemotaxis in the host defense system.

Other phagocyte disorders include deficient phagocytosis which can be related to abnormal opsonization as in sickle cell disease or to possible dysfunction of the fifth complement component, Leiner's syndrome, and congenital deficiency of certain complement components (C3 and C5) or immunoglobulins. Clinical manifestations of these deficiencies are recurrent otitis media, bronchitis, pneumonia, and sepsis with encapsulated bacteria. These deficiencies, as well as those with abnormal killing of bacteria, as in chronic granulomatous disease in which there is defective superoxide and hydrogen peroxide generation, are reviewed in Ch. 149.

Immune Dysfunctions. Patients with T cell abnormalities have

TABLE 257–2. INFECTIONS IN PATIENTS WITH HOST DEFENSE DEFECTS

Host Defect	Clinical Examples	Clinical Manifestation of Infections	Infectious Agents
Inflammatory response			
Neutropenia	Aplastic anemia Agranulocytosis Leukemias	Pneumonia; ulcers of skin, oral cavity, rectum, and vagina; fever; depressed inflammatory response	Gram-negative bacilli (especially *E. coli, Pseudomonas* sp., *Klebsiella, Staph. aureus)* fungi *(Candida, Aspergillus), Pneumocystis carinii*
Chemotaxis	Chédiak-Higashi syndrome Specific granule deficiency Deficiency of 110,000 dalton glycoprotein	Subcutaneous abscesses	*Staph. aureus, Strep. pyogenes*
	Job's syndrome and variants (variable chemotactic defect)	"Cold" abscesses, bronchitis, otitis, pneumonia, bronchiectasis	*Staph. aureus, C. albicans, H. influenzae*
	Newborns	Bacteremia	Gram-negative bacilli
	Protein-calorie malnutrition; others (see text)	Bacteremia	Gram-negative bacilli
Phagocytosis			
Cellular defect	Systemic lupus erythematosus, megaloblastic anemia, chronic myelocytic leukemia	Otitis, bacteremia, pneumonias, meningitis	Encapsulated bacteria
Opsonin deficiency			
C3 deficiency	Inherited or acquired (i.e., systemic lupus erythematosus)	Otitis, bacteremia, pneumonia, meningitis	*Pseudomonas, Proteus, Staph. aureus, Strep. pneumoniae*
C5 dysfunction (possible)	Leiner's syndrome of newborn infants	Generalized seborrheic dermatitis, severe diarrhea, local and systemic infections	Gram-negative bacilli
Alternative complement pathway	Sickle cell disease	Pneumonia, osteomyelitis	Salmonella, *Strep. pneumoniae*
Bactericidal activity	Chronic granulomatous disease	Recurrent infection of lymph nodes, skin, lung, liver, bone, and other tissues	Catalase (+) microorganisms *(Staphylococcus, Klebsiella, E. coli, Serratin marcescens, Pseudomonas, Proteus, Salmonella, Candida, Aspergillus, Nocardia)*
Immune response			
T cells			
Deficiency	Thymic aplasia (DiGeorge's syndrome) and thymic hypoplasia (Nezelof's syndrome)	Otitis, pneumonia	Tuberculosis, *Listeria,* BCGosis, leprosy, *Candida,* cryptococci, aspergillosis, *Pneumocystis,* toxoplasmosis, *Strongyloides,* herpes simplex, herpes zoster, cytomegalovirus, measles
	Acquired immune deficiency syndrome	Pneumonia, oral thrush, esophagitis, meningitis, disseminated infection	*Pneumocystis, Candida, Cryptococcus,* herpes simplex, cytomegalovirus, Epstein-Barr virus, *Mycobacterium tuberculosis, Toxoplasma gondii, Cryptosporidiosus*

Dysfunction	Mucocutaneous candidiasis	Candida of mucous membranes or oral cavity, esophagus, vagina, nailbeds	*Candida albicans*
	Purine nucleoside phosphorylase deficiency	Chronic pneumonias, diarrhea, candidiasis	Fungal and viral infections
B cells	Bruton's X-linked agammaglobulinemia	Bacteremia, pneumonias, sinusitis	Fulminant hepatitis, poliomyelitis, measles, chickenpox
	Dysgammaglobulinemias, agammaglobulinemia, multiple myeloma, chronic lymphocytic leukemias		
	IgA deficiency and nodular lymphoid hyperplasia of the intestine	Diarrhea, malabsorption	*Giardia lamblia*
Mixed T and B cells	Common variable hypogammaglobulinemia (may be due to excess T suppressor cells inhibiting B cells)	Sinusitis, bronchitis, pneumonia, bacteremia	High and low grade bacterial pathogens, *Pneumocystis,* cytomegalovirus
	Ataxia telangiectasia (decreased IgA and IgE)	Sinusitis, bronchitis, pneumonia	*Strep. pneumoniae, H. influenzae,* rubella, *Giardia lamblia*
	Wiskott-Aldrich syndrome (defective antibody response to polysaccharides, decreased IgE, IgM, abnormal monocyte chemotaxis)	Otitis, pneumonia	Infections seen in T and B cell dysfunction
	Severe combined immunodeficiency, adenosine deaminase deficiency	Severe infection involving multiple sites	Infections seen in T and B cell dysfunction
Mixed defects	Hodgkin's disease and lymphoma (lymphocytopenia, delayed hypersensitivity, abnormal monocyte chemotaxis)	Pneumonia, bacteremia, hepatitis	Tuberculosis, histoplasmosis, *Salmonella, Listeria, Brucella abortis, Pneumocystis,* cytomegalovirus, herpes zoster, herpes simplex, *Cryptococcus, Candida, Aspergillosis*
	Diabetes mellitus (abnormal chemotaxis, phagocytosis, compromised neurovascular supply)	Cellulitis, urinary tract infections	*Staphylococcus aureus,* gram-negative bacilli, *Candida,* mucormycosis
	Uremia (chemotactic defect, depressed, delayed hypersensitivity, lymphopenia)	Bacteremia, pneumonia, urinary tract infection	*Staph. aureus, E. coli, Klebsiella, Pseudomonas*
	Burns (chemotactic defect, necrosis)	Cellulitis, bacteremia, pneumonia	*Staphylococcus, Strep. pyogenes, Pseudomonas* sp., *Candida,* herpes simplex
	Cystic fibrosis (mucociliary dysfunction)	Bronchitis, pneumonia	*Staph. aureus, Pseudomonas*
	Splenectomy	Pneumonia and osteomyelitis	*Streptococcus pneumoniae, Salmonella*
Iatrogenic	Foreign body (intravenous catheters, prosthetic devices)	Bacteremia, local abscesses	*Staph. aureus,* gram-negative bacilli, *Candida*
	Antibiotics	Bacteremia	*Staph. aureus,* gram-negative bacilli *(Serratia, Pseudomonas, Mima-Herellea), Candida*
	Corticosteroid therapy (depressed delayed hypersensitivity, neutrophil margination and adherence)	Bacteremia, pneumonia	*Candida, Pneumocystis, Staph. aureus,* gram-negative bacilli, others

recurrent infections from intracellular bacteria such as *M. tuberculosis*, leprosy, BCGosis, *Listeria*, and *Legionella*. These patients also become infected with other fungi (cryptococcosis, *Candida* and aspergillosis), protozoa (*Pneumocystis carinii*, toxoplasmosis, and *Strongyloides*), and viruses (herpes simplex, varicella/zoster virus, cytomegalovirus, and measles). The clinical presentation of these patients is discussed in Ch. 429.

In other patients the number of T cells is normal, but there is abnormal effector cell response to antigenic stimulation. Delayed skin responses to *Candida* and other naturally occurring antigens is absent, and lymphocytes from many of the patients do not respond to in vitro stimulation with antigens, especially *Candida*, by producing lymphokines or by replication. A well defined group of patients with T cell dysfunction have mucocutaneous candidiasis with *Candida albicans* infection restricted to the skin, nails, and mucous membranes. Another small group of patients deficient in purine nucleoside phosphorylase have T cell dysfunction with recurrent viral and fungal infections.

A dramatic form of an acquired defect of cell mediated immunity is the acquired immune deficiency syndrome (AIDS) (Ch. 430). AIDS is characterized by a remarkably selective deficiency of the number and function of the T helper cells. As a consequence, these patients are susceptible to infection with *Pneumocystis carinii*, *Candida albicans* (oral thrush and esophagitis), *Cryptococcus neoformans* meningitis or disseminated disease, cytomegalovirus, herpes simplex virus, toxoplasmosis, and mycobacterial infections, especially disseminated *Mycobacterium avium-intracellulare*. The latter infection is common in AIDS patients but rare in other immunosuppressed patients.

The prototype disease for B cell deficiency is Bruton's X-linked agammaglobulinemia with absent fully developed B cells and grossly deficient synthesis and secretion of antibody. These patients are subject to infection with encapsulated virulent pathogens such as *Streptococcus pneumoniae*, *Hemophilus influenzae*, and *Pseudomonas aeruginosa*. Untreated, these infections spread rapidly, and patients have sinorespiratory infections with recurrent pneumonias and otitis media, as well as osteomyelitis, dermatitis, and meningitis. The patients usually respond to appropriate antimicrobial drugs, probably because of normal phagocyte and T cell function. Infections caused by intracellular microorganisms such as *M. tuberculosis*, *Histoplasma*, and fungi are relatively infrequent.

Diseases with combined deficiencies of T and B cells are associated with severe infections. Such patients usually succumb early in life to many different forms of infection, including *Pneumocystis carinii*, cytomegalovirus, other viruses, and bacterial pathogens of high and low grade virulence.

DIAGNOSIS. Initial evaluation of patients with recurrent infections requires a thorough history. For example, a history of contact dermatitis (poison ivy) helps eliminate T cell dysfunction, whereas a history of mucocutaneous candidiasis suggests a T cell abnormality. Aphthous ulcers may be early signs of severe neutropenia. Staphylococcal skin infections and recurrent pneumonias suggest a chemotactic defect, and a history of recurrent infections with catalase positive microorganisms suggests chronic granulomatous disease.

Tests useful in the laboratory evaluation of compromised hosts are summarized in Table 257–3. Initial laboratory screening studies can be very informative. A white blood count and differential count will serve as a screen for the leukopenias. In occasional patients in whom the clinical course suggests cyclic neutropenia, daily white blood cell counts for several months are necessary. The morphology of the white cell can be particularly helpful. For example, multilobed nuclei are seen in polymorphonuclear leukocytes in vitamin B_{12} or folate deficiency, and when considering the Chédiak-Higashi syndrome the characteristic giant lysosomes can be seen. An excellent screening test used to diagnose chronic granulomatous disease is the ability of granulocytes to reduce nitroblue tetrazolium dye. This test, which is available in most medical centers, reflects leukocyte oxidative metabolism and is markedly abnormal in chronic granulomatous disease and a few related disorders of phagocyte function (see Ch. 149). Other tests capable of detecting chronic granulomatous disease include the chemiluminescence assay as well as a new spectrofluorometric assay employing lipophilic fluorescent probes of membrane potential. The latter assay is simple and fast. An abnormality of the latter assay may reflect a fundamental defect of ion transport in leukocytes obtained from patients with chronic granulomatous disease.

TABLE 257–3. DIAGNOSTIC TESTS USED IN THE EVALUATION OF HOST DEFENSE DEFECTS

Host Defense	Test
Bone marrow production	Peripheral white blood count*
	Marrow aspirate*
	Bone marrow reserve test†
Inflammatory response	Rebuck skin window*†
	Leukocyte function
	Adherence*†
	Chemotactic response*†
	Phagocytosis‡
	Degranulation‡
	Bactericidal activity*†
	Oxidative metabolism
	Nitroblue tetrazolium dye reduction (NBT test)*†
	Hexosemonophosphate shunt activity‡
	Leukocyte glucose-6-phosphate dehydrogenase and myeloperoxidase‡
	Cytochrome b‡
	Chemotactic and opsonic activity of serum*†
	Complement levels (CH50,* C3*, C4†)
Immune response	
T cell system (cellular immunity)	Delayed hypersensitivity skin tests to common antigens*
	Sensitization to dinitrochlorobenzene‡
	Chest x-ray to assess thymus gland*
	Quantitation of T cells†
	T cell rosettes
	Specific membrane markers
	Lymphocyte transformation studies†
	Nonspecific mitogens (pokeweed, concanavalin A)
	Specific antigens (PPD, mumps, streptokinase-streptodornase, *Candida albicans*)
	Lymphokine and monokine production‡
	Chemotactic lymphokines
	Interleukins
	Macrophage migration-inhibitory factor
B cell system (humoral immunity)	Quantitative immunoglobulins*
	Immunoglobulin subclasses‡
	Kinetics of antibody synthesis following primary and secondary immunization‡
	Antibodies to common viruses†
	Specific antibody response after immunization* (typhoid H and O agglutinins)

*Screening tests.
†Generally available at major medical centers.
‡Available only in specialized laboratories.

Qualitative immunoglobulin tests assess B cell function, and in the presence of borderline hypogammaglobulinemia the capacity of patients to produce specific antibodies after immunization is important. Most hospital laboratories can measure typhoid H and O agglutinins before and after immunization with standard vaccines, and antibodies to common viruses are also usually available. In addition, antibody titers to some antigens used for childhood immunization (e.g., tetanus, diphtheria) can often be obtained through referral laboratories. T cell function can be screened by delayed hypersensitivity skin testing to common antigens (PPD, *Candida*, mumps, streptokinase, and streptodornase). A chest x-ray will help in evaluation of the thymus gland and may reveal evidence for recurrent pneumonias or bronchiectasis. Total hemolytic complement (CH50), C3, and C4 levels are available in many laboratories, although studies of individual complement components can be obtained only in a few research centers.

More specific studies are often necessary to define host defense defects. Marrow reserves can be evaluated by a bone marrow aspirate and with an etiocholanolone administration test. The inflammatory response can be estimated in vivo with a Rebuck skin window, which assesses the ability of leukocytes to accumulate at a superficial abrasion. More precise characterization of the cellular and humoral components of the inflammatory response require studies in vitro. Leukocyte adherence is measured by the ability of cells to stick to nylon wool. Locomotion can be qualitatively evaluated by looking at cells moving on glass slides and by measuring cell migration into different kinds of filter paper. Chemotactic factors are assessed by their ability to attract normal leukocytes. These studies of the inflammatory response are generally available in medical centers, as are studies for the quantitation of leukocyte phagocytosis and killing of bacteria. Studies of leukocyte hexose monophosphate shunt activity, leukocyte actin and myosin, or microtubule function are presently restricted to a few clinical research laboratories.

In-depth studies of the immune system include quantitation of T and B cells (and their subpopulations), using specific membrane markers. B cell function can be evaluated by the kinetics of antibody synthesis following primary and secondary immunization. Measurement of immunoglobulin G subclasses is also available. T cell function can be further characterized in vivo by monitoring the delayed hypersensitivity response after contact sensitization with dinitrochlorobenzene. T cell functional correlates of delayed hypersensitivity can be assessed in vitro by measuring proliferative responses (tritium incorporation) to nonspecific stimuli such as mitogens (phytohemagglutinin, pokeweed mitogen, and concanavalin A) or specific stimuli such as antigens (PPD, mumps, streptokinase-streptodornase, or *Candida albicans*). Quantitation of the release of lymphokines and monokines (i.e., migration inhibitory factor, interleukins, or chemotactic lymphokines) is generally available in medical centers. Other specific tests of T cell function are available only in highly specialized laboratories.

Particularly puzzling patients with no demonstrable defect of host defenses should raise one's suspicion of the possibility of a psychologic disorder with self-inflicted lesions. Psychologic problems can be very serious, with patients or parents of children inoculating foreign material subcutaneously or performing other manipulations that can manifest as severe abscesses or unexplained fevers; many of these patients are medical or paramedical professionals. Continual culture of fecal flora from wounds and localization of infections to conveniently reached areas (such as the left side of the body in right-handed individuals) should lead one to suspect psychologic problems.

MANAGEMENT. ***General Considerations.*** Management of the compromised host is based in part on the specific problems. Risk from environmental factors such as crowded living conditions, contaminated hospital respirators, or intravenous lines must be rigidly controlled. Intravenous lines should be used only when necessary; metal (scalp vein) devices should be used whenever possible, as microbial colonization with these is less than with plastic catheters. Similarly, all catheters, especially Foley catheters, should be used as little as possible, and they should be changed regularly. Antimicrobial agents should be carefully selected and used with as much microbial specificity as possible.

Certain procedures are associated with bacteremia or local spread of infection, and compromised hosts undergoing these procedures may be at increased risk. In particular, dental manipulation, bronchoscopy, certain gastrointestinal studies (gastroscopy, jejunal biopsy, liver biopsy, sigmoidoscopy, barium enema, retrograde cholangiograms), urinary tract manipulations (catheterization, cystoscopy, retrograde pyelogram), angiograms (cardiac catheterization), orthopedic surgery, and, on rare occasions, bone marrow aspiration have all been associated with bacteremia.

Prophylactic Antibiotics. In severely compromised hosts, administration of appropriate antimicrobials (depending on the expected bacteremia) prior to and for several hours after the procedure may prevent development of disseminated foci of infection. Oxacillin (2 grams intravenously for adults or 200 mg per kilogram intravenously for children) plus gentamicin (1.5 mg per kilogram intramuscularly or intravenously for adults or 3 to 5 mg per kilogram intramuscularly or intravenously for children) 30 to 60 minutes before and 8 and 16 hours after procedure is one regimen useful for dental or surgical patients. There is increasing evidence that oral nonabsorbable "prophylactic" antibiotics such as gentamicin, vancomycin, and neomycin may be appropriate for decreasing sepsis and pulmonary and anal-rectal infections in patients receiving induction chemotherapy for tumors. This is particularly true if the white blood cell count is less than 1000 cells per cubic millimeter for more than two weeks. However, such oral antibiotics are associated with malabsorption as well as poor patient compliance because of bad taste, often made worse by the nausea and vomiting from induction chemotherapy. Therefore, unless good patient compliance is anticipated, oral nonabsorbable antibiotics should not be used.

Considerable controversy exists regarding the necessity for isolating patients with compromised defenses. Obviously judgment is required as to which patients require isolation. Patients with severely compromised defenses (such as patients with agranulocytosis plus corticosteroid therapy) may benefit by isolation from hospital personnel, as may those with draining staphylococcal wounds or herpes zoster. However, isolation is disruptive to hospital routine and should not be continued any longer than required. Hospital personnel with minor infections, such as active oral herpetic lesions, should avoid contact with severely compromised patients such as neonates or adult patients in laminar flow facilities. Since malnourished patients have major problems with inflammatory and immune responses, adequate diet and correction of a malnourished state is often critical to the care of a compromised host.

Leukopenias. The compromised host with leukopenia, and in particular granulocytopenia, poses a particularly difficult management problem. Usually the faster the granulocytopenia evolves, the more severe the consequences. This is especially true if immunosuppressive drugs such as corticosteroids are being used concurrently. If there is any possibility of an environmental or drug-induced leukopenia, the etiologic agent should be eliminated. When infections occur, inflammatory manifestations are markedly diminished or absent, and careful and frequent examination of the patient for subtle findings of infection is required. Surveillance cultures of the oral cavity, stool, and open wounds, as well as culture of withdrawn catheter tips, can be very helpful in the selection of initial antimicrobials when these patients become infected.

A particularly difficult management problem is the granulocytopenic patient with fever. In most series, about one third of these patients will have positive cultures, one third will have sepsis, and one third will have no evidence of infection. In general, combination antibiotics such as an aminoglycoside (i.e., tobramycin), a broad-spectrum antipseudomonal penicillin (i.e., ticarcillin), and gentamicin are recommended as initial therapy. The duration of therapy is governed by the clinical response and culture results. If there is a good clinical response with a rise in granulocyte count, antibiotics can be discontinued when the patient has been afebrile for 48 hours. If a pathogen is isolated, appropriate antibiotics are selected and serum antibiotic levels are monitored; signs of local infection must be searched for repetitively. If the patient becomes afebrile but remains neutropenic, combination antibiotics are continued, although increased problems with fungal infection may result. In the setting of persistent neutropenia and positive blood cultures, white blood cell transfusions may be appropriate. If there is no clinical response and no pathogen is isolated, it is appropriate to add a cephalosporin antibiotic. If still no response is seen over an additional 48 hours, strong consideration of disseminated fungal infection should be entertained, and initiation of empiric therapy with amphotericin B is appropriate; white blood cell transfusions may then be considered.

Neutropenic patients with documented mycotic infections

require special attention. Heavy colonization with *Candida* (thrush of the mouth, esophagus, or vagina) should be treated with a topical antifungal agent such as nystatin (Mycostatin, Miconazole, or Ketoconazole). Patients with *Candida* urinary tract colonization, as judged by pseudohyphae in the urine, who have no fever or other evidence of infection and in whom a Foley catheter is required, may benefit from bladder irrigation for several days with amphotericin B (50 μg per milliliter). If a bladder catheter is not in place, oral 5-fluorocytosine should be considered, especially if the clinical situation is not urgent and renal function is normal. With severe candidiasis, intravenous amphotericin B should be used. Patients with compromised defenses who demonstrate transient candidemia that is thought to be related to contaminated intravenous lines may benefit from a short course of intravenous amphotericin B to try to prevent the establishment of disseminated foci. Fungemia in patients with malignancies and compromised defenses, especially lymphoreticular or hematopoietic malignancies, is frequently associated with disseminated fungal infection, and in these patients early use of amphotericin, sometimes prior to microbiologic confirmation, should be considered. Ketoconazole is particularly useful in the management of chronic *Candida* infection of the nails and oral cavity in patients with Job's syndrome.

Use of agents such as lithium and androgens to stimulate the bone marrow has been of use in some patients. Bone marrow transplantation to reconstitute patients with agranulocytosis and other immunodeficiencies is attractive but still under investigation and at present is restricted to only a few medical centers. Use of leukocyte transfusions to transiently correct leukopenias may prove to be beneficial. Initial studies using leukocyte transfusions are encouraging, but methods for collection and storage of leukocytes and techniques for the prevention of antileukocyte antibody formation in recipients remain particular problems.

Disorders of the Inflammatory Response. Management of patients with neutrophil dysfunction syndromes requires aggressive therapy of particular infections with careful selection of antimicrobial drugs. Aggressive use of antimicrobials and early surgical drainage of abscesses in some patients (i.e., with chronic granulomatous disease) is appropriate. Long-term chemoprophylaxis has not been established as beneficial, although it may help in selected situations; chemoprophylaxis prior to procedures commonly associated with bacteremia is appropriate. Trimethoprim-sulfamethoxazole may be useful as a prophylactic agent in selected patients with chronic granulomatous disease because it significantly prolongs infection-free intervals. Patients allergic to sulfamethoxazole appear to benefit from prophylactic trimethoprim-dicloxacillin. There is increasing evidence that leukocyte transfusions are important adjunct therapy for life-threatening infections in chronic granulomatous disease. Leukocytes used for transfusion in chronic granulomatous disease should not be irradiated since graft versus host disease is no problem in these patients and irradiation damages phagocyte function. Although bone marrow transplantation may have a role in the future, currently the severe complication of bone marrow transplantation excludes its use in patients with phagocyte defects.

Manipulation of leukocyte function with pharmacologic agents may be an important future approach to management of patients with leukocyte dysfunction. Ascorbic acid has improved granulocyte function in a few patients with the Chédiak-Higashi syndrome. Levamisole,* which previously was thought to be of use in patients with hyper IgE-recurrent infection (Job's) syndrome, has been shown to be nonefficacious and is no longer indicated. Vitamin E, which is thought to protect phagocytes from auto-oxidative damage, is under investigation for treating certain patients with phagocyte defects.

*Investigational drug.

Aside from the infectious complications of the inherited phagocyte defect syndromes, a number of other problems often appear with specific syndromes. Abnormal, chronically inflamed gingivae and a predisposition to periodontal disease are common findings in all the inherited syndromes of phagocyte dysfunction. Special attention to routine oral hygiene procedures seems to be the most reasonable approach to this chronic problem. Twice-daily tooth brushing with 3 per cent H_2O_2 and baking soda brings about dramatic improvement in the dental health of some patients.

Patients with chronic granulomatous disease can develop granulomatous inflammation, which is not obviously infectious, at any anatomic site. With time and repeated episodes, the physical size of such granulomatous masses can cause disease by mass effect; esophageal, gastric antrum, and duodenal obstruction due to such granulomatous masses have all been described. Although such obstructions usually resolve with empiric antibiotic therapy, surgical resection of involved areas has been used to clear obstruction that did not respond to antimicrobials.

Several skin conditions are commonly seen in patients with defective phagocyte function. Patients with chronic granulomatous disease often have seborrheic dermatitis involving the scalp, axillary, and pubic hair. This dermatitis tends to wax and wane in severity, and often becomes secondarily infected with common skin flora, especially *Staphylococcus aureus*. Dramatic improvement is usually seen during periods of intravenous antibiotic therapy for other infections. For chronic management of this dermatitis, daily local scrubs with hexachlorophene or iodine-containing soaps and application of hydrocortisone cream locally can be helpful. Of course, with continued use of these soaps, possible side effects from absorption of hexachlorophene or iodine must be monitored. Patients with chronic granulomatous disease also have chronic inflammation of the nares that can be severe, painful, and cause denuding of skin around the tip of the nose. When this nasal inflammation is mild, it needs no specific therapy other than good local hygiene. However, if it becomes severe, it should be treated with 7- to 10-day courses of antibiotics. Penicillinase-resistant penicillin, given orally, usually proves effective, with courses of therapy repeated as inflammation flares.

Disorders of the Immune Response. Patients with IgG immunoglobulin deficiency with recurrent bacterial infections usually benefit from replacement therapy with human gamma globulin. Maintenance of plasma IgG around 200 mg per milliliter is reported to decrease severe infections, although sinusitis, bronchitis, and otitis may persist. Intramuscular injection of IgG (100 mg per kilogram) at monthly intervals is usually adequate. Immunoglobulin also may be administered by slow subcutaneous infusion, although replacement immunoglobulin preparations that can be administered intravenously recently have become available. Globulin injection is beneficial only in patients deficient in immunoglobulin G. An alternative therapy is infusion of fresh plasma, 10 to 20 ml per kilogram, at intervals of three to four weeks. The advantage is that, in addition to replacing IgG, it replaces IgM and IgA, although the IgA never enters the secretory pools. The disadvantage is the risk of transmitting hepatitis and the volumes required. Despite gamma globulin, repeated infections and progression of pulmonary fibrosis and bronchiectasis may persist.

Attempts at immune reconstitution have also included bone marrow transplantation, infusion of histocompatible lymphocytes, and administration of alpha interferon, gamma interferon, and interleukin. Despite transient signs of improvement of several deficiencies, no impressive long-lasting cures have consistently been seen with these approaches.

Treatment of patients with T cell deficiencies is largely a research procedure. Attempts to reconstitute cell-mediated immune responses with BCG, killed *C. parvum*, cimetidine, muramyl dipeptide, lithium compounds, and interferon have had mixed success. Some patients have responded to fetal thymus graft with increased numbers of T cells and improved T cell function, especially those with the fungal infections, candidiasis, or coccidioidomycosis. Other patients have responded to immune reconstitution with transfer factor therapy. However, efficacy with transfer factor only seems to be long-lasting when it is used in combination with antifungal therapy and when the transfer factor is obtained from donors sensitive to the fungus. At present, therapeutic use of transfer factor should be considered investigational and its use restricted to investigators actively evaluating its therapeutic potential.

Dale D, Guetry D, Wewerka JR, Bull JM, Chusid MJ: Chronic neutropenia. Medicine 58:128, 1979. *A nice survey of chronic neutropenias, particularly with regard to diagnosis and natural history. Good for medical students and house officers.*

Donabedian H, Gallin JI: The hyperimmunoglobulin E-recurrent infection (Job's) syndrome. A review of the NIH experience and the literature. Medicine 62:195, 1983. *A comprehensive review of the pathogenesis and management of this complex disease.*

Easmon CSF, Gaya H: Second International Symposium on Infections in the Immunocompromised Host. London, Academic Press, 1983. *A comprehensive overview of host defenses, ranging from pathophysiology of parasitic and viral infection to therapeutic use of antiviral agents and immunopotentiators. Excellent book for fellows and established clinicians in infectious diseases with selected fine chapters for students.*

Gallin JI: Abnormal phagocyte chemotaxis: Pathophysiology, clinical manifestations and patient management. Rev Infect Dis 3:1196, 1981. *A comprehensive review of the presentation and management of these unusual patients.*

Gallin JI, Buescher ES, Seligmann BE, Gaither T, Nath J, Katz P: Recent advances in chronic granulomatous disease. Ann Intern Med 99:657, 1983. *Detailed updated review and discussion of the recent advances in the pathogenesis and management of chronic granulomatous disease.*

Gallin JI, Fauci AS: Advances in Host Defense Mechanisms. Vol. 1. Phagocytic Cells. Vol. 2. Lymphoid Cells. Vol. 3. Chronic Granulomatous Disease. New York, Raven Press, 1982–1983. *A new series designed to integrate highly sophisticated science with applicability to clinically relevant host defense mechanisms. Geared for broad readership, including students, fellows, and specialists in infectious diseases.*

Good RA (ed.): Proceedings of a workshop on intravenous immune globulin: Its use and potential. J Clin Immunol 2 (Suppl) 4S–48S, 1982. *A clearly written collection of papers analyzing the use of intravenous immune globulin. Good for fellows and specialists who need a review of this emerging therapy.*

Grieco MH (ed.): Infections in the Abnormal Host. New York, Yorke Medical Books, 1980. *A collection of chapters by leading investigators. Very complete approach. Ideal for fellows and residents.*

Lichtenstein LM, Fauci AS: Current Therapy in Allergy and Immunology, 1983–1984. New York, B.C. Decker, Inc., 1983. *Contains clearly written chapters on the management of the immunocompromised host. A practical guide for those managing these difficult patients.*

Klebanoff SJ, Clark RA: The Neutrophil: Function and Clinical Disorders. Amsterdam, North Holland Publishing Company, 1978. *An "encyclopedia" of neutrophil function and disorders. Excellent references through 1977. Ideal for fellows; selected chapters are superb for students.*

258. PREVENTION AND TREATMENT OF HOSPITAL-ACQUIRED INFECTIONS

*Richard P. Wenzel**

HISTORY. The father of infection control is Ignaz Semmelweis (1818–1865), whose observations in Vienna—prior to formulation of the germ theory—laid the foundations for hospital epidemiology. At the Allgemeines Krankenhaus, Semmelweis compiled mortality data on two obstetrics wards: on one ward (I), in which all women were attended by obstetricians and medical students, the mortality was over 8 per cent; on the other ward (II), in which all women were attended by midwives, the mortality was 2 per cent. In retrospect the cause of death with puerperal sepsis was the Group A β-hemolytic streptococcus, *S. pyogenes*. Semmelweis made two very important observations: (1) there was a lower mortality on ward I when medical students were on vacation, and (2) the odor of the autopsy room was noted on ward I whenever students were present. Furthermore, a colleague and pathologist, Professor Kolletschka, accidentally cut his own finger while performing a postmortem examination on one of the women who died of puerperal sepsis. Professor Kolletschka developed a syndrome very similar to that of the obstetric patients and died. Semmelweis reasoned that some element was carried on the hands of students and physicians from the autopsy room (where they performed postmortem examinations) to the obstetrics ward (where they examined patients). Eventually Semmelweis introduced the practice of handwashing with an antiseptic (chloride of lime) between the autopsy room and the delivery room and before the examination of each patient. Thereafter, the mortality in ward I fell to less than 2 per cent.

INTRODUCTION. Each year approximately 40 million people are hospitalized in the United States. Between 5 and 10 per cent, or 2 to 4 million patients, will develop an infection that was not present or incubating upon admission. Such infections are referred to as hospital acquired or nosocomial.† Nosocomial infections are directly responsible for an estimated 75,000 to 150,000 deaths, and lead to excess hospitalization (Table 258–1) with an economic burden of approximately 5 billion dollars per year. Several features distinguish nosocomial infections from community-acquired infections: the former are often (50 to 70 per cent) caused by aerobic gram-negative rods; they frequently occur in patients with altered host immune defenses; and they require therapy with more toxic antibiotics. Staphylococcal disease accounts for 10 to 20 per cent of hospital-acquired infections, and in some hospitals an increasing proportion of these are resistant to methicillin and other penicillinase-resistant antibiotics. The distribution of infections by anatomic site in acute care hospitals (Table 258–1) indicates that infections of the urinary tract account for 35 to 40 per cent of all nosocomial infections; postoperative wounds, 20 per cent; bloodstream, 5 to 10 per cent; lung, 15 per cent; and others, 15 to 20 per cent. Although the data on infections acquired in nursing homes are limited, estimates are that they may total 7 million or more each year.

No matter how effective an infection control program may be, it is impossible to eliminate all infections, in part because many arise endogenously in patients whose immune defense mechanisms are impaired, such as patients with leukemia and those who have received organ transplants. In addition, many patients have indwelling catheters, which provide organisms access to the body. Interspersed among such endemic infections, epidemics occur. An epidemic implies an unusual and significant increase in the incidence of a particular disease. It is estimated that 4 per cent of infected patients acquire their infections as part of a major epidemic; another 4 to 6 per cent are thought to acquire their infection as part of a cluster of epidemiologically linked infections. Both epidemic and endemic infections may result from a transient breakdown in proper technique or another common source event. Recognition of endemic infection may allow for correction of the problem before epidemic rates occur. The major point is that infection control efforts should focus on preventable infections.

Infection or colonization results when a sufficient number of organisms with ability to attach to skin or mucosal surfaces reaches a susceptible host. Colonization implies a peaceful coexistence between organism and host, whereas infection results from an altered balance of power in favor of the organism. Three major routes are recognized by which organisms are transmitted to hospitalized patients: direct contact, the air (via droplet nuclei less than 5 μ in diameter), and common source vehicles such as contaminated nebulizers. The most

TABLE 258–1. IMPACT OF HOSPITAL-ACQUIRED INFECTIONS IN ACUTE CARE INSTITUTIONS

Anatomic Site	Number of Infections per 100 Admissions	Proportion of All Hospital-Acquired Infections	Estimated Direct Mortality	Mean Number of Excess Hospital Days per Infection
Urinary tract	2.5	35–40%	<1%	2
Postoperative wound	1.5	20%	<1%	7
Pulmonary	1	15%	?*	?
Bloodstream	0.5–1	5–10%	25%	30
Others	1	15–20%	Varies with site	Varies with site

*Gross mortality was 35 per cent in an uncontrolled study at a university hospital.

*The author gratefully acknowledges the assistance of Bruce F. Farber, M.D., Division of Infectious Diseases, University of Pittsburgh Hospital, Pittsburgh, Pennsylvania.

†Nosocomial is derived from the Greek word for hospital.

likely mode of transmission of infection in the hospital is direct contact via the hands of medical personnel. Furthermore, the rate of transmission by all mechanisms is highest in patients in close proximity to the reservoir. Simple handwashing is effective in preventing direct contact transmission and remains the most important infection control measure. Additionally, infections can be minimized by elimination of the reservoir. If the reservoir is an inanimate object (e.g., a pressure monitor transducer head), infection control is readily accomplished. Unfortunately the reservoirs for most nosocomial infections are patients themselves. Thus, isolation techniques (see below) are utilized to contain certain organisms that cannot be readily eliminated.

HIGH RISK LOCATIONS. Certain areas of any hospital are likely to be the locale of high rates of endemic infections as well as of outbreaks or epidemics. The high risk areas include the critical care areas, burn units, and dialysis units. Critical care areas are usually the birthplace and area of highest prevalence of antibiotic resistance in the hospital, including methicillin-resistant *S. aureus* and aminoglycoside-resistant gram-negative rods. Recently the importance of *S. epidermidis* bloodstream infections in patients in intensive care units has been stressed.

Critical Care Areas. Medical, surgical, and neonatal critical care areas provide a concentration of patients at high risk for developing nosocomial infections. This is a reflection of patients' underlying diseases, the frequent use of invasive monitoring, and alteration of normal flora by antibiotics. Often patients are in close proximity to each other, promoting transmission by busy medical personnel who fail to wash their hands between contacts. Cross-infection has been reported to be particularly common among thermally injured patients. Furthermore, the widespread use of topical antibiotics may select for colonization and infection with multiply resistant organisms. The major pathogens include *Pseudomonas aeruginosa, Providencia stuartii,* other gram-negative rods, and, in some burn units, methicillin-resistant *S. aureus*.

Proper design of critical care units with regard to separation of patients by partitions and placement of sinks at the entranceway to individual patient cubicles, as well as optimal nursing-to-patient ratios, may minimize the risks of cross-infection. Other suggested infection control measures include (1) the notification of the infection control team by the unit of all new procedures or products and (2) use of a clinical flow sheet listing all catheters, dates of insertion, and rationale for continued use.

Dialysis Units. Both bacterial and viral infections occur with increased frequency in patients with chronic renal failure. Bacterial infections often affect fistulas and arteriovenous access shunts. With infected fistulas, up to one third of patients may have no objective signs of infection, and may complain only of intense pain. With *S. aureus* infections of fistulas or shunts, up to 20 per cent may develop secondary endocarditis. Evidence of viral infection (including both non-A non-B and type B viral hepatitis) is found in virtually all units. Often the virus is introduced by one of the blood products used. Once introduced, transmission to other patients and staff can occur by accidental needle stick exposure, contaminated dialysis equipment, and possibly other contact. Renal patients are more likely to become chronic carriers of hepatitis B surface antigen (HB_sAg) than are patients in the community who become infected with hepatitis B. Staff members working in these units are also at increased risk of infection. Recent data from the Centers for Disease Control indicate that in 1982 only 0.4 per cent of dialysis personnel and 0.5 per cent of patients acquired hepatitis B. The annual incidence of non-A non-B hepatitis in patients was 1.6 per cent. Thus, there would appear to be a dramatic reduction in hepatitis B relative to the late 1970's and a 3 to 1 ratio of non-A non-B to type B infection in dialysis patients. The infections may result in chronic liver disease, including a susceptibility to delta infection in chronic carriers of HB_sAg, and may expose offspring of pregnant workers to the risk of neonatal hepatitis. With the recent introduction of an effective vaccine for hepatitis B, susceptible hospital personnel who are exposed to blood products are advised to receive it. The vaccine is given in three 1 ml doses administered intramuscularly at times zero, one month, and six months. In addition, the risk to the staff can be minimized and epidemics identified early or prevented with proper control practices: (1) Strict handwashing procedures should be observed. (2) Serologic surveillance of patients and dialysis staff for hepatitis at three- to six-month intervals is recommended unless anti-HB_S antibody is present. (3) Protective clothing should be worn in the area. (4) Eating, drinking, smoking, and mouth pipetting should be prohibited in the unit. (5) Contaminated materials should be autoclaved or incinerated. (6) Contaminated surfaces should be washed with 0.5 to 1.0 per cent sodium hypochlorite prior to routine cleanup. (7) Needles used to draw blood should be discarded in boxes, and not recapped. (8) Pregnant staff members might consider transferring to another area of the hospital in order to avoid acquiring viral hepatitis and transmitting the infection to the baby.

SURVEILLANCE. Surveillance refers to the routine and orderly collection of information regarding the occurrence of a disease. In the hospital it is primarily used to define endemic rates and to identify high and low risk areas. Data from surveillance identify clusters and epidemics when certain threshold rates are exceeded. Thus, surveillance is the basis for alteration of existing procedures and practices. The impact of various methods of surveillance in reducing infections is currently under study. A minimal data base is necessary in order to establish priorities for a proper infection control program and to satisfy the requirements of the Joint Commission for Accreditation of Hospitals (JCAH). In general, surveillance is performed by infection control practitioners, most of whom are nurses. In addition, the practitioners gathering data often reinforce isolation procedures and identify new problems by their visibility on the wards and by communication with staff nurses and physicians. The starting point for data collection varies; review of nursing care plans, antibiotic use, bacteriology reports, and fever curves have all been used to identify patients at high risk. Once high risk patients are identified, trained practitioners can then review their charts, seeking any evidence for infection. Practitioners who wish to compare infection rates among similar categories of hospitals should use identical definitions for infection (Table 258–2). Infection rates for a defined period are later compiled by identifying the number of infections (numerator) and the total number of patients at risk (denominator). By convention, the number of patients admitted or discharged is often substituted for the number of patients at risk. Infection rates by site, service, organism, and procedure are tallied. In hospitals with sophisticated surveillance, infection rates by underlying diagnosis are also reported. In addition, a summary of antibiotic sensitivity patterns for hospital pathogens may help clinicians select proper initial antimicrobial therapy of nosocomial infections.

Analysis of data collected by surveillance requires knowledge of basic epidemiologic measurements. These include the following: (1) Incidence—the number of new cases of a disease in a population at risk over a specified unit of time. An example is the number of new cases of wound infection per 100 patients

TABLE 258–2. DEFINITIONS OF NOSOCOMIAL INFECTION* USED IN SURVEILLANCE

Anatomic Site	Criteria
Urine	≥100,000 colonies of bacteria per milliliter of urine
Postoperative wound	Pus at the incision site
Blood	Positive culture (exclude contaminant)
Pulmonary	New infiltrate on chest film associated with purulent sputum (exclude atelectasis and pulmonary embolus with infarction)
Burns	$\geq 10^6$ organisms per gram of biopsy tissue

*Infections which are not incubating or present upon admission.

at risk per month. (2) Prevalence—the number of persons with a disease (newly acquired or not) at a given time. An example is the number of patients on January 1 with an obvious wound infection per 100 patients on the ward. (3) Attack rate—the number of new cases of a disease in a particular population exposed to a particular risk. No defined unit of time is implied, although the period of risk is assumed to be limited. An example is the number of patients with a wound infection per 100 undergoing appendectomies.

Surveillance data should be summarized in a report for distribution throughout the hospital. This enables the various services to review their performance routinely and to become aware of potential problems. If a change in the infection rate appears to be significant, it is necessary to use statistical testing to be sure.

URINARY TRACT INFECTIONS. The upper and lower urinary tracts are the source of 35 to 40 per cent of all nosocomial infections. About 80 per cent of infections occur in patients who have undergone some form of instrumentation, usually catheterization.

A simple in-and-out catheterization is frequently used to obtain urine samples from patients who cannot give a clean voided sample. Although this procedure carries a relatively low risk of significant bacteriuria in healthy ambulatory men and women (2 to 3 per cent), the risk is 6 per cent in hospitalized women, 9 per cent in postpartum women, and 23 per cent in postpartum women who have had complicated labors. Although the risk may be justified in postoperative patients with transient retention, routine catheterization should be discouraged in healthy obstetric patients at the time of delivery.

Indwelling Foley catheters are used in 10 to 20 per cent of hospitalized patients. They are the major predisposing agents of nosocomially induced urinary tract infection. The risk associated with these catheters is dependent upon the length of time they remain in place: bacteriuria occurs at a rate of 5 per cent per day that the indwelling catheter is left in place. Evidence of upper tract involvement by antibody coating tests and the presence of circulating endotoxins are not infrequent in patients with catheter-related infection. In addition, urinary infections serve as the most common predisposing source for secondary gram-negative rod bacteremia. Secondary bacteremia occurs in 3 per cent of bacteriuric patients. However, recent data suggest that the rate of secondary bacteremia with *Serratia marcescens* bacteriuria is very high (16/100) and that all bacteriuric patients with the organism should be given appropriate therapy regardless of symptoms.

The principal organisms involved in nosocomial urinary tract infections are as follows: *E. coli* (33 per cent), enterococci (15 per cent), *Proteus* (15 per cent), *Klebsiella* (10 per cent), and *Pseudomonas* (10 per cent). Unlike community-acquired urinary tract infections, these organisms are usually resistant to sulfonamides and ampicillin. Newer β-lactam antibiotics and aminoglycosides are effective in most cases, but outbreaks of multiply resistant organisms have occurred.

Hematogenous spread of bacteria to the urinary tract is uncommon. In most catheter-related infections, organisms gain entrance to the system and ascend into the bladder. There are several areas where contamination is likely to occur: the junction of the catheter and urethral meatus, the internal aspect of the collection vessel tubing with retrograde flow to the bladder, and the urethra at the time of catheterization resulting from inadequate preparation or improper technique. Bacteria can migrate from the perineum along the outside of the catheter into the bladder. This is probably the major route of infection occurring within the first week of catheterization. In one well-described outbreak, the risk of acquiring a Foley catheter–related urinary tract infection was significantly greater in patients who had a catheterized roommate with a similar infection. Cross-infections seemed to occur by the hands of medical personnel, with contamination of the collection system and subsequent migration around the catheter into the bladder.

All patients requiring indwelling catheters should have closed drainage systems in an effort to maintain the sterility of the system and help prevent cross-infections among patients. Proper care of the closed system is important in minimizing the risk of infection. Basic practices include the following: (1) Aseptic insertion by trained personnel. In one study patients catheterized by specially instructed physicians had significantly less bacteriuria at 48 hours than did those catheterized by licensed practical nurses. Catheter care teams have not been shown to be cost effective or efficacious. (2) Drainage bags should be hung and kept upright below the level of the patient's bladder to prevent retrograde flow. They should never be allowed to rest on the floor or to be inverted. (3) Drainage bags should be emptied frequently to avoid distention and contamination. All vessels used to measure urine output should be disinfected between patients to avoid cross-infection. (4) The system should not be irrigated unless absolutely necessary. Small specimens of urine can be aspirated from the proximal lumen of the catheter with a sterile syringe after proper disinfection. (5) Routine changing of the catheters is probably unnecessary unless they become obstructed or encrusted.

Perineal care and use of antimicrobial lubricants either around the catheter or impregnated within the catheter are not of proven efficacy. Similarly, the use of disinfectants in the drainage bag has not reduced infections in patients catheterized one week or less. Furthermore, the practice of culturing the tip of catheters at the time of removal has been shown not to be a valuable monitor of infection.

Several authors have suggested the use of prophylactic irrigation of closed drainage systems with acetic acid or polymyxin-neomycin solutions. Their use should probably be reserved for those who require irrigation to relieve obstruction by clots. The efficacy of prophylactic antibiotics appears to be limited to the first four days of catheterization. Although this may be of value in selected patients such as those undergoing prostate surgery, prolonged or widespread use should be discouraged, since it will most likely select for resistant organisms. In addition, the efficacy of prophylactic antibiotics has not been critically evaluated in closed drainage systems.

NOSOCOMIAL PNEUMONIAS. Approximately 1 per cent of hospitalized patients will develop a nosocomial pneumonia. Hospital-acquired pneumonias tend to be more common in university than community hospitals owing to differences in patient populations. Although crude mortality for nosocomial pneumonias in university patients has been reported to be 35 per cent, prospective studies of the direct morbidity and mortality of hospital-acquired pneumonias (apart from the influence of underlying diseases) are lacking. *Pseudomonas* pneumonia appears to carry a particularly high mortality (70 per cent), as do pneumonias in the compromised hosts and those which are superinfections. A recent survey by the Centers for Disease Control's National Nosocomial Infectious Study suggested that 7 per cent of nosocomial pneumonias led to secondary bacteremias.

The most common cause of nosocomial pneumonias is the gram-negative bacilli, accounting for over 50 per cent of all cases. No study has employed transtracheal aspirates or lung aspirates to confirm the etiology of nosocomial pneumonias in a large series of patients. *Klebsiella, S. aureus, Pseudomonas aeruginosa,* and *E. coli* are frequently isolated from sputum. These organisms colonize the upper airways of up to 50 per cent of critically ill hospitalized patients, usually within four to five days of admission. Once colonized, a patient is at higher risk for the development of pneumonia; in one study of intensive care unit patients, pneumonia occurred in 23 per cent of colonized, in contrast to 3 per cent of noncolonized, patients. Factors influencing colonization are multiple and poorly understood. Organisms appear to come from exogenous sources (especially *Pseudomonas*) via respiratory care equipment or the hands of medical personnel; organisms (especially Enterobacteriaceae) may also come from the patient's own gastrointestinal tract. One measure to reduce pharyngeal colonization rates is proper handwashing to prevent cross-contamination.

Aspiration of gastric contents with subsequent pneumonitis is common in the patient with cerebrovascular disease, seizures, drug overdose, cardiopulmonary arrests, and any condition which alters the patient's respiratory clearing mechanisms. Similarly, postoperative patients are at higher risk of developing pneumonia. Chemical pneumonitis from aspiration of gastric contents generally develops immediately and may be associated with respiratory failure. The pneumonia may result in death or resolve over a five-day period. Chemical pneumonitis does not require antimicrobial therapy, and studies have demonstrated the lack of efficacy of steroid therapy. Bacterial pneumonia, however, may develop as a complication of aspiration. Bacterial infection is characterized by deterioration after a transient period of recovery.

Frequently, postoperative and seriously ill patients have endotracheal or nasotracheal tubes or tracheostomies. Although these protect the patient from aspiration, they also bypass normal defense mechanisms and predispose to tracheal injury from suctioning. Uncommonly, secretions and gastric contents may be aspirated around the tube. There are occasionally serious problems associated with respiratory therapy. Outbreaks of pharyngeal colonization and pneumonia have been associated with the use of contaminated anesthesia equipment, ventilators, and IPPB machines with medication nebulizers. Usually, the gases from oxygen and air compressors, and internal parts of the machines, do not become contaminated or promote bacterial growth. The changeable tubing and masks can become contaminated if not disinfected or sterilized between patients. The greatest source of contamination is large volume Venturi nebulizers. Nebulizers produce liquid in aerosol (droplet) form by either ultrasonic or centrifugal means. These droplets can emit aerosols containing large numbers of gram-negative rods that may be delivered to terminal bronchi, resulting in pneumonia. Contamination of the large volume cascade humidifier may occur during cleaning or replenishing water. Organisms capable of growing under these conditions include *P. aeruginosa, P. cepacia, Serratia marcescens, Acinetobacter calcoaceticus,* and *Flavobacterium meningosepticum.* Pneumonia caused by any of these suggests the possibility of exogenous contamination. The risk of contamination appears to be minimal with small volume medication nebulizers as long as the medications used are sterile. Humidifiers usually do not serve as a potential risk to patients, because bacteria are not transported by molecules of water in vapor form.

The immune compromised host with pulmonary infiltrates represents a particularly difficult diagnostic and therapeutic problem. These are generally patients whose diseases are being treated with steroids or cytotoxic agents or both. Although the most common cause for their pneumonias are aerobic gram-negative rods, up to 25 per cent may become infected with fungi, herpesviruses, *Legionella pneumophila, Legionella (tatlockia) micdadei, Nocardia,* acid-fast bacilli, and combinations of these. Optimal therapy generally requires a tissue diagnosis, often an open lung biopsy of diffuse infiltrates, or needle aspirate of solitary nodules. Hospitals with clusters of patients with *Legionella pneumophila* have usually identified water as the significant vehicle, and control of contamination has been followed by a reduction in number of cases.

A great deal of attention has been focused on the infection control practices necessary to minimize the risk of pneumonias from respiratory care equipment. Although the data are incomplete, important points include the following: (1) Large volume reservoir nebulizers should be replaced by humidifiers if possible. Water used for humidification should be sterile. (2) All medication used for respiratory therapy should be sterile and preferably administered as a single unit dose. (3) Equipment such as tubing that comes into direct contact with patients should be changed between patients and every 24 to 48 hours when in continuous use.

BLOODSTREAM INFECTIONS. Hospital-acquired bloodstream infections may be primary (without an apparent source) or secondary to infection at a distal site. The distinction is important for both epidemiologic and clinical reasons. Secondary bloodstream infections complicate 3 per cent of urinary tract infections, 5 to 7 per cent of postoperative wound and pulmonary infections, and 7 per cent of cutaneous infections. *E. coli, S. aureus, K. pneumoniae, S. marcescens,* and *P. aeruginosa* are the usual pathogens. Identification of the source allows one to treat both the underlying condition and the complicating bacteremia. For example, bacteremia developing in patients with a urinary tract infection should suggest the possibility of obstruction, which may require surgery as well as antibiotics.

When true primary bacteremias occur, even in the compromised host, one must always consider the possibility of an infusion- or instrument-related infection. Twenty-five per cent of all patients hospitalized receive intravenous infusions, and the use of hyperalimentation and arterial and Swan-Ganz catheters has increased greatly in recent years.

Infections related to intravenous fluids or intravascular devices may occur from either intrinsic or extrinsic contamination of the system (see Fig. 258–1). Contamination of the infusion or administration set at the site of manufacture (intrinsic) may be extremely difficult to detect. In the early 1970's, at least 400 cases of *Enterobacter* sepsis occurred secondary to contaminated dextrose infusions. Because only a small proportion (0.7 to 0.9 per cent) of all manufactured bottles were contaminated and because these were shipped to many different hospitals, the association of contaminated fluids and septicemia was difficult to detect. Certain clues, however, should serve as a flag for such a possibility: (1) sepsis occurring in an otherwise low risk patient receiving an intravenous solution, or (2) a cluster of primary bloodstream infections with an unusual pathogen. Only certain organisms are capable of growing well in intravenous solutions (pH as low as 4.5). *Klebsiella, Enterobacter,* and *Serratia* can readily grow in 5 per cent dextrose in water, exceeding 10^5 colonies per milliliter within 24 hours at room temperature. Thus, careful examination of intravenous infusion bags or bottles may be useful, but even when the infusion contains 10^6 organisms per milliliter, cloudiness may be difficult to detect with the unaided eye. *Pseudomonas cepacia, Citrobacter freundii,* and *Flavobacterium* species are also likely to contaminate intravenous infusions. In contrast, *Proteus* species, *Pseudomonas aeruginosa, S. aureus, E. coli, Acinetobacter* species, and *Candida* species are all unable to survive in significant numbers under these conditions.

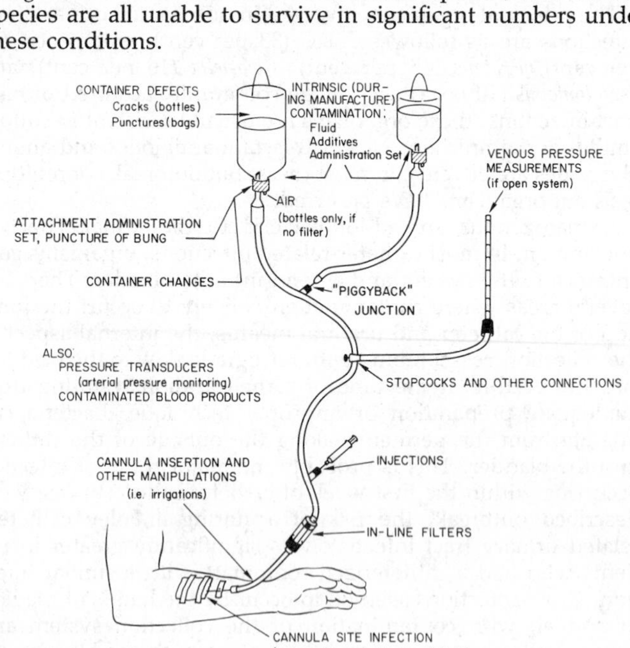

Figure 258–1. Causes of bloodstream infections. (From D. G. Maki, with permission.)

Extrinsic contamination, usually at the catheter site, is the most likely source of infusion-related infections. Steel needles carry a lower risk than plastic catheters. The incidence of a catheter-related infection rises with the length of time the catheter is left in place. Inflammation at the catheter site (a "cord," redness, swelling, pain), when present, strongly suggests catheter-associated sepsis. Catheters introduced via surgical cutdowns, femoral catheters, and devices left in place for more than 48 hours are particularly at risk. In contrast to contamination of the infusion, cannula-related sepsis is likely to be caused by gram-positive organisms, predominantly by *S. aureus* (50 per cent), *S. epidermidis*, and enterococci, although some are caused by gram-negative rods. Preliminary data suggest that intra-arterial catheters should not remain in place longer than four days. A semiquantitative technique of culturing the catheter tip when it is removed has been described by Maki et al. to aid in the diagnosis of catheter-related sepsis. The technique requires that the indwelling catheter be removed after a thorough antiseptic preparation of the insertion site. The distal section of the catheter is then cut off with a sterile scissors, beginning several millimeters inside the former skin surface–catheter interface, and placed into a sterile screw-capped container. The tip is then rolled four times back and forth on an agar plate in the microbiology laboratory. Colony counts of greater than 15 suggest the presence of a concordant catheter-related sepsis.

An unusual complication of catheters is suppurative thrombophlebitis, a purulent infection involving the entire vein, often occurring in the burn patient. Although local evidence of infection may be absent, the patients have unremitting sepsis. Therapy requires surgical excision of the vein, beginning proximal to the involved section, as well as antimicrobial therapy.

In recent years, the use of Hickman-Broviac intravenous catheters has become popular, both for infusing fluids and for withdrawing blood from selected patients. The catheters are tunneled under the skin of the chest wall midway between the nipple and sternum and enter the subclavian vein superiorly. The tip of the catheter is placed in the right atrium; the origin of the catheter on the outside of the chest wall has a Luer lock and contains heparinized saline solution when not in use. Several studies have shown an association between the use of these catheters and subsequent bloodstream infection. Although the attack rate is as high as 20 to 40 per cent of patients, the incidence of bloodstream infection is low, approximately 3 per 1000 days of use. The most frequent isolates are *S. epidermidis* (20 per cent), *S. aureus* (20 per cent), *Candida* sp. (15 per cent), and gram-negative rods. Although it is not always necessary to remove the catheter in the face of sepsis, generally it is wise to do so if the etiologic agent is *Corynebacterium*, *Nocardia*, or a fungus.

Parenteral hyperalimentation presents some unique problems regarding infection control. The hypertonic solutions require the use of central venous catheters which are left in place for prolonged periods of time. Although the high concentrations of glucose do not support bacterial growth, *Candida* species grow well in this milieu. *Candida* and other bacteria can colonize the occlusive dressings used to cover the catheter insertion site. Preparation of the solution under strict sterile technique is required. In addition, supervision of therapy by hyperalimentation teams, including surgeon, nurse, and pharmacist, seems to reduce the attack rate of fungemia from 10 to 20 per cent to 1 to 2 per cent.

The use of topical antibacterial ointments around intravenous catheter sites does not reduce the risk of infection. Their use may increase the risk of colonization by *Candida* around hyperalimentation lines. Similarly, bacterial filters have not yet been demonstrated to be efficacious in reducing fungemia. Recently the use of transparent plastic dressings for intravenous catheters has been popularized. Their efficacy in reducing catheter-related sepsis has not been established.

Recommended measures to reduce the incidence of catheter-related sepsis include strict aseptic technique in inserting a cannula after preparation of the skin, the use of steel needles for intravenous infusions whenever possible, changing arterial lines at least every four days, and changing intravenous catheter and administration sets at least every 48 hours. The use of flow sheets to keep track of the multiple monitoring devices used in intensive care areas should be encouraged.

Despite the use of control measures, bloodstream infections related to infusion therapy will occur. The following is offered as a general guide in the approach to the hospitalized patient with sepsis:

1. Determine the most likely source of infection (is it primary or secondary?). If secondary, where is the other infection site: urinary tract, lung, wound, or elsewhere?

2. What intravenous and intra-arterial devices are in place? How long have they been there? Is there any evidence of local inflammation? If the bacteremia is primary or caused by an unusual pathogen, or occurs while the patient is receiving appropriate antimicrobial therapy, the following measures should be undertaken: (a) Discontinue the intravenous device immediately. (b) After iodine prep of the latex injection port at the distal end of the intravenous tubing (allow iodine to remain at least two minutes and then remove with 70 per cent isopropyl alcohol), aspirate 10 ml of the intravenous contents. Place 5 ml into each of two blood culture bottles (one set), and send to the bacteriology laboratory. (c) Remove the indwelling catheter aseptically, and send it to the laboratory for semiquantitative culture. (d) Record the lot number of all intravenous products the patient was receiving.

3. Draw blood cultures and obtain appropriate cultures at distal sites.

4. Initiate intravenous antimicrobial therapy. Until sensitivities are available, initial antibiotic selection should be based on the surveillance data for the hospital ward(s) in which the patient has resided. This suggestion is prompted by the fact that the probability of specific aminoglycoside-resistant gram-negative rods and the probability of methicillin-resistant *S. aureus* may be different in intensive care unit areas and in the general wards.

5. Treat the underlying sources of infection. In the setting of breakthrough bacteremia (occurring while the patient is on appropriate therapy), special attention should be given to the possibility of an undrained abscess, a vascular focus of infection, or inadequate levels of antibiotic. Polymicrobial sepsis suggests the presence of a gastrointestinal, hepatobiliary, or genitourinary source, often with obstruction.

POSTOPERATIVE WOUND INFECTIONS. The rate of infection at the incision site following surgery depends on the skill of the surgeon and the degree of contamination at the time of operation. Contamination of a postoperative wound with subsequent infection can occur from either an endogenous or an exogenous source. The risk of endogenous contamination is dependent upon the type of operation being performed. Surgical fields involving the colon or other nonsterile structures are more likely to get infected than those involving clean areas such as with hip replacement. Another likely source of endogenous contamination is an active site of infection at a peripheral location. For example, an untreated urinary tract infection or infected ulcer is associated with a two to three times increased rate of postoperative wound infection and should be treated prior to elective surgery.

In contrast to endogenous contamination, exogenous contamination usually occurs from a break in technique at the time of surgery. A wide variety of sources have been described, including operating room personnel and surgical materials. In addition, certain practices appear to be associated with a higher infection rate, e.g., failure of the patient to use an antiseptic soap during the preoperative shower, and shaving of the operative site.

Prophylactic antibiotics given just prior to surgery have been shown to reduce the incidence of infection following certain procedures. Effective chemoprophylaxis requires that the antimicrobial cover only the most likely pathogens, be initiated just prior to surgery, and be given for brief periods of time (no more than 48 hours after surgery). There must be high tissue and blood levels of drug at the time of surgery. When wound infections do occur, they are generally caused by *S. aureus* or gram-negative rods. Patients with *S. aureus* infections should be placed on "contact" or "drainage/secretion" precautions to minimize the risk of cross-contamination. Treatment usually requires drainage followed by antibiotic therapy for approximately seven days.

If pus is found after surgery and no organisms are recovered from routine cultures, then a possibility exists that infection is caused by anaerobic bacteria, rapid-growing atypical mycobacteria, or a saprophytic fungus. The latter two situations are distinctly unusual and should be considered only if there are clinical or laboratory features suggesting nonvegetative bacterial infection.

Wound infections occurring unusually early (within 24 to 48 hours of surgery) should suggest the possibility of infection with β-hemolytic Group A streptococci (*S. pyogenes*), *Clostridium* species (gas gangrene) or organs causing necrotizing fasciitis. These are especially serious and life-threatening infections requiring immediate evaluation and therapy. Their management is discussed elsewhere in this text.

OTHER INFECTION SITES. A wide variety of infections occur in hospitalized patients in addition to those previously discussed. Nosocomial meningitis usually occurs following neurosurgical shunting procedures and is usually caused by *S. aureus*, *S. epidermidis*, or gram-negative rods, rarely by *Candida* as a late infection. In the compromised host, nosocomial meningitis may occur without prior surgery. *Listeria*, *Cryptococcus*, and gram-negative rods are the likely pathogens. Group B streptococci are a common cause of meningitis in the neonate, and there have been recent reports of *Citrobacter* bloodstream infection and meningitis in a few neonatal units.

Infections following the insertion of artificial joints are particularly difficult to treat. Those occurring in the hospitalized patient usually are "early onset" infections. *S. epidermidis*, *S. aureus*, and gram-negative rods are involved. In a large study of infections following total knee arthroplasty at the Mayo Clinic, the significance of anaerobes was stressed. Unless the infection is of a superficial wound, salvage of the prosthesis is infrequent. Infections with a late onset (beyond eight weeks) account for at least 50 per cent of infections involving prosthetic joints.

In the last ten years, the percentage of infants delivered by cesarean section has risen. Currently, up to 25 per cent of all deliveries are performed in this manner. In contrast to the incidence of endometritis following vaginal deliveries (1 per cent or less), that following cesarean section ranges from 20 to 30 per cent. The specific contribution to the increased infection risk by the cesarean section, underlying disease, or use of fetal monitoring is unclear.

INFECTION CONTROL COMMITTEE. In order to be accredited by the Joint Commission for Accreditation of Hospitals (JCAH), all hospitals in the United States are required to have an infection control committee that meets at least six times a year. The committee formulates and reviews hospital policies with regard to infection control practices. Usually, its members are diverse, representing the medicine, surgery, microbiology laboratory, nursing, and pharmacy departments. One member of the committee serves as the hospital epidemiologist, usually someone with training in infectious diseases or clinical microbiology who has a strong interest in infection control.

An important task of the committee is to adopt and enforce proper isolation practices to prevent the transmission of communicable diseases within the hospital. Most hospitals utilize a limited number of types of isolation based upon the route of transmission of the disease. The Centers for Disease Control (CDC) released a new set of isolation guidelines in 1983 (Table 258–3). Of note is that their earlier recommendation for "protective" isolation was deleted because efficacy has not been demonstrated. Hospitals may want to utilize the CDC guidelines verbatim or modify them for local use. An isolation manual listing the precautions and the type of isolation a specific disease requires should be distributed to each ward. Infection control practitioners then review on-ward practices to assure compliance and to prevent unnecessary isolation, which is costly and inefficient. "Isolation" is used to imply that a private room is necessary, and "precaution" is used when a private room is optional or not indicated.

INANIMATE OBJECTS. The inanimate environment of a hospital may serve as a potential reservoir for microorganisms. Water in flower vases may contain up to 10^9 organisms per milliliter (usually *Pseudomonas*), and stethoscopes are capable of being colonized. The risks associated with toilets and laundry chutes appear minimal. In one cancer hospital, fireproofing

TABLE 258–3. NEW ISOLATION PROCEDURES RECOMMENDED BY THE CENTERS FOR DISEASE CONTROL IN 1983

Isolation Category	Private Room Necessary	Masks	Gowns	Gloves	Hand-washing	Examples of Diseases for Which It Is Recommended
Strict	+	+	+	+	+	Pharyngeal diphtheria; varicella; zoster (localized in immunocompromised patient or disseminated)
Contact	+	For those in close contact	If soiling likely	If contact with infective material	+	Staphylococcal furunculosis in newborns; Herpes simplex disseminated, severe primary, or neonatal; methicillin-resistant *S. aureus*
Respiratory	+	For those in close contact	—	—	+	Measles; meningococcal pneumonia, meningitis, or meningococcemia; *H. influenzae*, pneumonia, or meningitis
Tuberculosis (AFB)	+	If patient is coughing	Only to prevent gross contamination	—	+	Tuberculosis
Enteric precautions	Only if patient's hygiene is poor	—	If soiling likely	If contact with infective material	+	Viral hepatitis A; *Salmonella*, *Shigella*, or *C. difficile* enterocolitis
Drainage/secretion precautions	—	—	If soiling likely	If contact with infective material	+	Minor or limited skin infections including those caused by *S. aureus*
Blood/body fluid precautions	Only if patient's hygiene is poor	—	If soiling with blood or body fluids likely	If contact with blood or body fluid	+	AIDS; Creutzfeldt-Jakob disease; viral hepatitis B

materials were shown to be a reservoir for *Aspergillus*, which caused deep tissue infections in patients, some of whom are only briefly immunosuppressed. In all outbreaks of nosocomial *Aspergillus* pulmonary infections, the mode of transmission was airborne.

Based on the limited amount of information available, several recommendations can be made: (1) Flower vases probably do not belong in burn units or intensive care areas. (2) Patients on isolation should be issued a single stethoscope to be used by all physicians entering the room. In addition, alcohol swabs will kill most bacteria on the stethoscope to be used on high risk patients (those with severe dermatitis or burns). (3) Prior to construction or installation of waste disposal chutes, fireproofing material, or other environment changes, an infection control specialist should be consulted. (4) In general, routine culturing of the inanimate environment should be discouraged. Only in working up an outbreak might this be essential.

STERILIZATION AND DISINFECTION. In order to reduce the number of organisms that come in contact with patients, sterilization, disinfection, and antiseptics are employed. Sterilization refers to the killing of all forms of microbiologic life, including spores. The term disinfection implies that there is a marked reduction of the number of microorganisms but that spores are not killed. Antiseptics are degerming agents which can be used on the skin.

Sterilization. Two types of sterilization are generally employed in hospitals: autoclaving and gas. The former, use of moist heat under pressure, is the more effective and less expensive method. Boiling at normal atmospheric pressure is not sufficient to sterilize (kill spores). Gaseous sterilization, using ethylene oxide, is an acceptable alternative for use on items that cannot withstand heat. The gas is effective at lower temperatures and can penetrate plastics and other materials. However, ethylene oxide is an explosive and a skin irritant, and is potentially mutagenic and carcinogenic. The Occupational Safety and Health Administration has proposed to reduce the current permissible exposure limit for ethylene oxide from 50 parts per million to 1 part per million as an eight-hour time-weighted average. Regardless of the method of sterilization used, biologic sterility testing with spore strips must be used to document adequacy of the sterilization process. *Bacillus stearothermophilus* spores are very heat resistant and are used to monitor sterilization processes using moist heat. *Bacillus subtilis* spores are used to monitor the efficacy of gas sterilization processes.

Disinfection. Several different classes of chemical disinfectants exist. Commonly used agents include chlorine, iodine, phenols, hexachlorophenes, alcohols, and second generation quaternary ammonium compounds. They vary in their ability to kill microorganisms, and the type of agent utilized depends upon the likely pathogens and the properties of the object to be disinfected. Two epidemics of idiopathic neonatal hyperbilirubinemia have been linked to excessive use of a phenolic disinfectant plus detergent. Thus, alternatives are recommended for use in the newborn area. Particular care must be taken with hepatitis B virus and the Jakob-Creutzfeldt agent. Both are resistant to killing by most disinfectants, but they are thought to be susceptible to high concentrations of hypochlorite. For the Jakob-Creutzfeldt agent, the preferred method is autoclave sterilization for unusually long times (one hour at 121° C). It has recently been suggested that if autoclave sterilization is not possible, a one-hour exposure to 1 N sodium hydroxide inactivates Jakob-Creutzfeldt agent. Furthermore, it is less corrosive than hypochlorite for all materials except aluminum.

Recently there have been reports of bloodstream infections and pseudoinfections and peritonitis traced to contaminated povidone iodine and polyximer iodine antiseptic compounds. The organisms were *Ps. cepacia* and *Ps. aeruginosa*, respectively, species that are naturally resistant to many antibiotics, have minimal growth requirements, and are ubiquitous. Their ability to survive in an iodine-containing product has stimulated research into the chemistry of these agents and an increased awareness of infectious complications with antiseptics.

With the recent isolation of *Legionella pneumophila* from cooling towers, the question of decontamination arises. The Centers for Disease Control recommend that cooling towers undergo periodic maintenance to ensure low levels of slime bacteria and algae in accordance with the American Society of Heating, Refrigeration and Air Conditioning Engineers and the Environmental Protection Agency. Field trials are being planned to evaluate the efficacy of various water additives to eliminate *L. pneumophila*.

With respect to the acquired immune deficiency syndrome (AIDS), the Centers for Disease Control (CDC) have recommended that the same precautions be used when caring for patients with viral hepatitis B, in whom blood and body fluids likely to have become contaminated with blood are considered infective. The same guidelines also hold for reusable instruments. Specifically, the CDC stated that lensed instruments should be sterilized after use on AIDS patients. A similar statement regarding endoscopes was made by the American Hospital Association's Advisory Committee on Infections Within Hospitals.

HANDWASHING. Proper and frequent handwashing is the most important control measure available in preventing the transmission of infectious diseases in hospitalized patients. The role of antiseptics is secondary in importance to standard handwashing with plain soap and water before and after routine patient contact.

The normal flora of the skin consists of a transient and permanent group of organisms. Transiently present organisms are more often the gram-negative rods and at times *S. aureus*. Permanent flora include the micrococci *S. epidermidis* and *Propionibacterium acnes*. Recent data suggest that certain gram-negative rods appear to be persistent after standard handwashing efforts and thus may be part of the permanent flora. *S. aureus* can also become part of the permanent flora of the anterior nares and thereby repeatedly colonize the hands. Soap and water appear to be generally effective in removing the transient flora. Various antiseptics, including isopropyl and ethyl alcohol, are more effective in reducing, but not eliminating, the permanent flora. Hexachlorophene is highly effective against *S. aureus*, but has little or no activity against gram-negative rods and fungi. In addition, absorption of hexachlorophene through the skin has been shown to cause vacuolization of brain tissue in some infants and experimental laboratory animals, and therefore its routine use for washing babies in the newborn and premature units is discouraged. Aqueous benzalkonium chloride (Aqueous Zephiran) is relatively ineffective and will sustain the growth of gram-negative rods. Its use as an antiseptic should be discouraged. Iodine remains an excellent antiseptic with a wide range of action, but causes local irritation. Chlorhexidine is also an effective antiseptic, but may cause dermatitis with excessive use.

EMPLOYEE HEALTH. The employee health division should be concerned with protecting both patients and employees from the transmission of infectious diseases. Problems most frequently arise regarding the transmission of tuberculosis, viral hepatitis, herpesvirus infections, and meningococcal infections.

Tuberculosis. The risk of tuberculosis is related to exposure to unsuspected cases among patients. After patients have been placed upon respiratory isolation, the risk becomes minimal. Unfortunately, routine chest x-rays are not specific or sensitive enough to screen for suspected cases. The addition of a tuberculin skin test for all patients who have respiratory symptoms or radiographic abnormalities may lead to earlier diagnosis and may prevent early transmission.

All employees should receive a tuberculin skin test (intermediate strength or 5 tuberculin units PPD-S) prior to beginning work. These are repeated yearly or three months after exposure to an initially unsuspected case. Employees who convert their PPD skin test result from negative to positive (10 mm induration or greater) should be considered for therapy with isoniazid (INH), 300 mg per day for one year.

Viral Hepatitis. Transmission of hepatitis A to employees or other patients is very unusual. Unlike hepatitis B and non-A non-B viral hepatitis, hepatitis A is transmitted almost exclusively by the oral-fecal route. In addition, peak viral excretion maximally occurs prior to the development of symptoms. Enteric precautions are probably effective in protecting medical personnel from acquiring hepatitis A from hospitalized patients with the disease.

Hepatitis B is transmitted by parenteral or mucous membrane exposure to infected blood or body fluids. Because of their frequent exposure to blood from accidental needle sticks and blood spills, medical personnel are at increased risk. The prevalence of both HB_sAg and anti-HB_s has been shown to be higher in medical personnel than in control populations: approximately 15 per cent of physicians are positive for anti-HB_s, and 1 per cent carry HB_sAg. Dentists and oral surgeons appear to be at even higher risk.

The infection control committee in conjunction with the employee health division should set up a standardized procedure with regard to the prevention of hepatitis. Despite the institution of proper isolation of infected patients, needle stick accidents will occur. Data on the best way to manage these exposures are incomplete. Currently it seems reasonable to draw blood from both the donor (source) and the recipient in order to clarify the risk of transmitting hepatitis B to a susceptible hospital employee. If the donor shows evidence of infection with hepatitis B and the recipient is susceptible, then both high titered anti-hepatitis B immunoglobulin (HBIG) and the first dose of vaccine should be offered to the hospital worker. At one month and six months, the second and third doses of vaccine should be given. A second dose of high titered globulin is *not* necessary. If there is concern about the transmission of either hepatitis A or non-A non-B hepatitis, standard immune serum globulin could be given, although its efficacy in preventing non-A non-B disease is uncertain. This virus has replaced hepatitis B as the most common cause of post-transfusion–related hepatitis, and non-A non-B is responsible for at least 80 per cent of post-transfusion hepatitis. Its exact role in needle stick associated disease, however, is unknown.

Herpes Infections. Nonimmune personnel having direct contact with the oral secretions of patients are at risk for developing herpes skin infections. Usually a nurse involved in suctioning a tracheostomy comes in contact with virus-contaminated secretions at the site of a locally traumatized or minimally lacerated finger. This exposure is followed by the development of a localized, painful, herpes simplex infection referred to as "whitlow." These infections are often misdiagnosed as bacterial infections and may get secondarily infected if incised and drained. The use of gloves will probably prevent the transmission of herpes, although personnel with vesicles should avoid contact with immunosuppressed patients.

Meningococcal Disease. Few events produce more panic among hospital employees than exposure to a patient suspected of having meningococcal disease. Nevertheless, cases among exposed medical personnel are very rare. Secondary attack rates are significantly higher in household contacts. Close contact with the index case appears to be required. Guidelines recommended by the Centers for Disease Control include the following: (1) Suspected cases of meningococcal disease should be placed on respiratory isolation immediately. (2) A contact list of those who have had *close* (possible secretion) contact with the case should be compiled. The Public Health Department should be notified immediately to supervise the identification of contact exposures made in the community prior to admission. (3) Personnel who have known close contact should be given antimicrobial prophylaxis as soon as possible, and should not await cultural confirmation of the diagnosis or susceptibility testing. Recommended prophylaxis for adults is rifampin, 600 mg orally twice daily for two days. If rifampin is not tolerated, minocycline, 100 to 200 mg orally every 12 hours, can be given for three days. Sulfonamides may be used only if the organism has been shown to be sensitive. Penicillin is not effective for prophylaxis for elimination of the carrier state. (4) Routine nasopharyngeal cultures of employees are not useful. (5) Indiscriminate use of prophylactic therapy should be discouraged (in those who have had fleeting or casual contact). (6) In the setting of an epidemic, the use of vaccines as an adjuvant to antimicrobial prophylaxis should be considered if the offending organism is in the serogroup A or C.

American Hospital Association: A hospitalized approach to AIDS. Recommendations of the Advisory Committee on Infections Within Hospitals. Infect Control 5:242, 1984.

Bennett J, Brachman S: Hospital Infections. Boston, Little, Brown & Company, 1979. Wenzel, R: Handbook of Hospital Acquired Infections. Boca Raton, Fla., CRC Press, 1981. *Two comprehensive texts devoted solely to the problem of hospital-acquired infections.*

Centers for Disease Control: Acquired immune deficiency syndrome (AIDS): Precautions for clinical and laboratory staffs. Morbid Mortal Wkly Rep 31:577, 1982.

Cundy K, Ball W: Infection Control in Health Care Facilities. Microbiologic Surveillance. Baltimore, University Park Press, 1976. *A review of the limited amount of data available regarding potential risks of inanimate objects in promoting infection.*

Garner JS, Simmons BP: CDC guidelines for isolation precautions in hospitals. Infect Control 4 (Special Suppl):245, 1983.

Kunin CM: Detection, Prevention and Management of Urinary Tract Infections. Philadelphia, Lea & Febiger, 1979. *A readable reference that provides both basic and advanced knowledge regarding all aspects of urinary tract infections.*

Maki DG, Weise EC, Sarafin HW: A semiquantitative culture method for identifying intravenous catheter related infection. N Engl J Med 296:1305, 1977. *Description of the microbiologic technique to help determine the likelihood of catheter-induced sepsis.*

Proceedings of the Second International Conference on Nosocomial Infections, Centers for Disease Control, Atlanta, August 5–8, 1980. Am J Med 70:379, 631, 899, 1981. Proceedings of the International Symposium and Workshop on Nosocomial Infection, Jerusalem, Israel, April 27 to May 2, 1980. Rev Infect Dis 3:635, 1981. Proceedings of the First International Symposium on Hospital Acquired Infections, Vienna, Austria, April 24–28, 1983. Infect Control 4:363, 440, 1983; 5:18, 1984. *Three recent conferences updating information on hospital-acquired infections.*

Russell AD, Hugo WB, Ayliffe GAJ: Principles and Practice of Disinfection, Preservation and Sterilization. Boston, Blackwell Scientific Publications, 1982. *Provides detailed discussion of the chemical agents and modes of action, as well as tests of sterility. Two chapters are devoted specifically to issues in the hospital.*

Simmons RL, Howard RJ: Surgical Infectious Diseases. New York, Appleton-Century-Crofts, 1982. *Comprehensive review of infections in surgical patients.*

259. ADVICE TO TRAVELERS

Jeffrey A. Gelfand

Travelers frequently make precise arrangements for connecting flights, hotels, theater tickets, and tours, but give little or no advance consideration to their health while traveling. This can result in disrupted plans, physical misery, serious illness, and considerable expense. Vaccination requirements for entering different countries vary and depend on where the traveler has stopped en route. There are several publications that address these issues. The Centers for Disease Control (CDC) publishes an annually updated guide, *Health Information for International Travel.* It contains a compendium of the vaccination requirements for entry into other countries, epidemiologic information, current CDC recommendations for vaccinations, chemoprophylaxis, and other helpful information. It can be obtained by writing the Superintendent of Documents, United States Government Printing Office, Washington, D.C. 20402. The publication number is the year followed by 8280 (i.e., 84–8280). Finally, local health departments and "Traveler's Clinics" (now available in a number of teaching hospitals) can provide up-to-the-minute information about changing epidemiologic and vaccination requirements.

Travel to such areas as Europe, Australia, and New Zealand poses no greater health hazard than travel in the United States and Canada. The risks of travel to other areas vary greatly from country to country and depend on the traveler's local living conditions and length of stay. In general, brief visits to large cities, with accommodations in good tourist hotels and meals in reputable restaurants, carry little risk of exotic infection. Travel to rural areas may greatly increase such risks.

GENERAL MEASURES. Gastronomic curiosity and gourmet tastes should be restrained by prudence. Meat and fish should be well cooked. Smoking, salting, and drying are not sufficient to kill tapeworm cysts. Peelable raw fruits and vegetables with unbroken skin are safe if peeled by the diner; the skin should be discarded. Lettuce is especially to be avoided because it is virtually impossible to cleanse it of protozoal cysts. In general, dairy foods, including local cheeses, should be avoided. Milk can be safely consumed after boiling. Untreated water should be avoided, as should ice. Alcohol does not confer "sterility" to local water, and many pathogens can tolerate alcohol better than can the traveler. Very hot tap water is safer but not risk-free. Bottled water is not necessarily safe, although carbonated bottled water and beverages usually are. Tea and coffee made with boiled water are safe. Beer and wine present few hazards (save for the next morning).

While recent evidence suggests that following such rules will not help the traveler evade the ever-present threat of uncomplicated traveler's diarrhea, these measures are likely to reduce the probability of developing more serious food-bourne bacterial and parasitic diseases. Swimming in fresh water in tropical areas where schistosomiasis is found should be avoided; salt water and chlorinated pools are safe. Measures to prevent insect bites (clothing, netting, repellents) should be considered where appropriate. Patients should be cautioned against taking over-the-counter medications proferred by pharmacists and physicians abroad. These medications, as well as prescription drugs, may contain agents of dubious efficacy and significant toxicity. For example, chloramphenicol may be present in cold remedies. Finally, lists of English-speaking physicians can be supplied by United States and other consulates general. Practical advice on securing such information after hours can be found in *Traveling Health—A Complete Guide to Medical Services in 23 Countries,* a traveler's guide to foreign health services.

IMMUNIZATIONS. The two immunizations occasionally required for entry into other countries are for yellow fever and cholera. In general, these vaccinations are not required for travel from the United States to Canada, Mexico, Europe, or Caribbean countries, nor for re-entry to the United States. All travelers should receive a tetanus–diphtheria toxoid booster if the tetanus immunization status is uncertain or if ten or more years have passed since the last vaccination. Poliomyelitis is a real threat in developing nations, and all travelers to such areas should receive a booster dose of trivalent oral polio vaccine (TOPV). Persons not previously immunized should receive the primary series of TOPV. Those with depressed immune function should receive inactivated polio vaccine.

Cholera. The risk of cholera to most tourists is low, and cholera vaccines are of limited effectiveness in protecting against clinical cholera. Vaccination is not recommended unless the traveler will be visiting an area experiencing an outbreak or will be living in an endemic area with poor sanitation. Travel to other countries from such areas may require vaccination as a condition of entry.

Hepatitis A. Immune serum globulin is effective in reducing the risk of hepatitis A. A dose of 5 ml is recommended for adults traveling to the developing world for periods of over three months and is repeated every four to six months. For those staying in endemic areas for a briefer period, a dose of 2 ml can be used.

Measles. For those born after 1956 without prior physician-documented history of the disease or immunization, vaccination is advised.

Plague. Plague vaccine is recommended only for those traveling to enzootic rural areas of Asia, South America, and Africa.

Rabies. Prudence would dictate that anyone anticipating exposure to animals in an enzootic or epizootic area ought to receive pre-exposure prophylaxis. Simple residence for several months in such an area is sufficient for some to advocate vaccination. A new human diploid cell vaccine is now available in the United States.

Smallpox. Smallpox vaccine should not be given for international travel.

Typhoid. Typhoid vaccination is only partially effective, and the protective effect may be overcome by large inocula. It is recommended for travelers to endemic areas experiencing an outbreak. Highly susceptible travelers (patients with achlorhydria, immunosuppression, or sickle cell disease) should be immunized.

Typhus. This vaccine should be considered only for those traveling to the highland areas of Africa, the Andes, and the Himalayas.

Yellow Fever. Yellow fever vaccination is recommended for travel to endemic areas of South America and Africa. Vaccination is also required for travel to and between such areas. It can only be given at designated yellow fever vaccination centers (travelers should check with the local board of health).

MALARIA CHEMOPROPHYLAXIS. Falciparum malaria can kill within 48 hours. Travelers to areas where malaria is endemic should receive chloroquine prophylaxis. A weekly dose of 500 mg (300 mg base) of chloroquine phosphate should be taken by adults (50 kg body weight) beginning two weeks before arrival in an endemic area and continuing while there and for six weeks after leaving. Travelers returning from prolonged, heavy exposure in areas where *P. vivax* and *P. ovale* are endemic can be given a course of primaquine phosphate during the last two weeks of postexposure chloroquine prophylaxis to prevent relapse from extraerythrocytic infection, although such therapy is not recommended for the average traveler. Glucose-6-phosphate dehydrogenase deficiency should be ruled out prior to primaquine therapy.

Travelers to areas with chloroquine-resistant falciparum malaria are advised to take a weekly dose of a fixed ratio tablet containing sulfadoxine (500 mg) and pyrimethamine (25 mg), marketed under the name Fansidar (Hoffman-LaRoche) and recently licensed for sale in the United States. This should be taken in addition to the weekly dose of chloroquine, the preferred prophylaxis for *P. vivax.* Even for countries listed as having chloroquine-resistant *P. falciparum,* the occurrence of these strains may be limited to certain areas only. More detailed references should be consulted for information about Fansidar-resistant *P. falciparum,* prophylaxis in pregnancy, and other selected topics.

TRAVELER'S DIARRHEA. Diarrhea, sufficiently severe to disrupt plans, strikes one quarter to one half of travelers to certain areas. Enterotoxigenic *E. coli* (ETEC) are associated with from 40 to 70 per cent of cases of diarrhea in travelers, depending on location and culture techniques. Other agents, notably shigellae, salmonellae, campylobacter, vibrios, *Entamoeba histolytica, Giardia,* reovirus, and Norwalk virus, may be causes. In the tropics, traveler's diarrhea usually begins in the first week and lasts on the average about three and a half days. In addition to the general measures previously recommended—which may not prevent simple traveler's diarrhea—prophylactic measures have been investigated. One agent widely used abroad, iodochlorhydroxyquin (Entero-Vioform), has been associated with severe neurotoxicity and is of dubious efficacy. Both doxycycline and trimethoprim/sulfamethoxazole (TMP/SMX) have been used and are effective prophylaxis for traveler's diarrhea. However, allergic reactions, photosensitivity reactions, and the demonstrated emergence of resistance to these drugs by ETEC lead most authorities to advise against such prophylaxis for routine travel. Bismuth subsalicylate (Pepto-Bismol), 60 ml taken four times a day during the trip, is effective and safe prophylaxis for those not already taking salicylates in high doses but is impractical for most.

Many authorities advise travelers to wait until diarrhea begins and then to institute therapy. Pepto-Bismol, 30 to 60 ml taken every half hour for eight doses, reduces the number of loose stools by about 50 per cent and increases the rate of recovery within 24 hours. A recent double-blind, controlled study demonstrated that either TMP/SMX (160 mg TMP; 800 mg SMX) or TMP alone (200 mg), taken twice daily for five days, substantially reduced the severity of traveler's diarrhea. The opiate drugs may actually intensify dysentery with shigellae and therefore should be used sparingly and only for mild disease. A reasonable approach, therefore, would be to treat mild disease with Pepto-Bismol and with judicious use of opiates to reduce periods of great inconvenience. More serious illness could be treated with either TMP/SMX or TMP alone, with the understanding that drug reactions could be a hazard with antimicrobial therapy. Finally, replacement of fluid losses is critical for therapy of severe disease. Several commercial preparations of World Health Organization rehydration salts are now commercially available.

ADVICE ON RETURNING HOME. The most important single bit of advice is to remind the traveler to include the history of travel when seeking medical attention. The clinical onset of certain diseases may be months or even years after the traveler returns home, and the traveler should be reminded of this possibility.

Centers for Disease Control: Health information for international travel, 1983. Morbid Mortal Weekly Rep 28 (Suppl), 1983. Available from the Superintendent of Documents, United States Government Printing Office, Washington, D.C. 20402, HEW Publication No. (CDC) 83–8280. *This is a thorough and very helpful guide to the medical aspects of international travel, from vaccination requirements to the importation of pets.*

DuPont HL, Galindo E, Evans DG, Cabada FJ, Sullivan P, Evans DJ: Prevention of traveler's diarrhea with trimethoprim-sulfamethoxazole and with trimethoprim alone. Gastroenterology 84:75, 1983. *A placebo-controlled, double-blind trial of TMP/SMX or TMP alone in United States students studying in Mexico. Prophylaxis was very effective.*

DuPont HL, Hornick RB: Adverse effect of Lomotil therapy in shigellosis. JAMA 226:1525, 1973. *Although the frequency of stools was diminished by this commonly used antidiarrheal agent, fever and toxemia were increased in patients with this infection by an invasive pathogen.*

DuPont HL, Reves RR, Galindo E, Sullivan PS, Wood LV, Mendiola JG: Treatment of travelers' diarrhea with trimethoprim/sulfamethoxazole and with trimethoprim alone. N Engl J Med 307:841, 1982. *This critical paper is the basis for recommending therapy with these drugs.*

DuPont HL, Sullivan P, Pickering LK, Haynes C, Ackerman PB: Symptomatic treatment of diarrhea with bismuth subsalicylate among students attending a Mexican university. Gastroenterology 73:715, 1977. *Treatment of traveler's diarrhea with Pepto-Bismol reduced loose movements and speeded recovery.*

Gorbach SL: Traveler's diarrhea. N Engl J Med 307:881, 1982. *A clear, practical, concise, and thoughtful view of the subject by an authority.*

Hillman SM, Hillman RS: Traveling Healthy—A Complete Guide to Medical Services in 23 Countries. New York, Penguin Books, 1980. *This paperback guide is a highly useful compendium. Included are practical advice, first aid, sensible suggestions for patients with pacemakers and numerous other disorders, glossaries of emergency medical terms in languages from Danish to Serbo-Croatian, and a pharmacopeia listing commonly used drugs and their equivalents abroad. An outstandingly valuable little book for travelers.*

Immunization and chemoprophylaxis for travelers. Med Lett 25:37, 1983. *Reviews current immunization requirements and recommendations and also contains a complete list of all countries with malaria risk, the nature of those risks, and malaria chemoprophylaxis recommendations.*

Portnoy BJ, DuPont HL, Pruitt D, Abdo JA, Rodriguez JT: Antidiarrheal agents in the treatment of acute diarrhea in children. JAMA 236:844, 1976. *An evaluation of two of the most commonly used agents for treating diarrhea. Neither was effective in a controlled study.*

Steffen R, Van der Linde F, Gyr K, Schär M: Epidemiology of diarrhea in travelers. JAMA 249:1176, 1983. *A retrospective analysis of 16,568 European travelers' experiences. The data suggest that dirty fingers reach the best of hotels and restaurants and that four stars do not protect a guest from diarrhea.*

Wyler DJ: Malaria-resurgence, resistance, and research. N Engl J Med 308:875;934, 1983. *A comprehensive review. Includes such problems as Fansidar-resistant P. falciparum and other topics beyond the scope of this chapter.*

Section Two BACTERIAL DISEASES

Pneumonia

260. INTRODUCTION TO PNEUMONIA

Herbert Y. Reynolds

Pneumonia is a general term denoting a group of clinical diseases that result from microbial infection of lung parenchyma. It is a commonly encountered disease and, in one form or another, continues to be a leading cause of death in the United States. Histologically, pneumonitis represents an inflammatory reaction in the interstitium of alveoli and an accumulation of exudate in alveolar lumina. Consolidation and a degree of impaired gas-exchange may occur in affected lung tissue. With successful inactivation of the infecting agent, resolution occurs and normal lung structure is usually restored. Exceptions to the complete healing phase occur in certain necrotizing pneumonias, those caused by staphylococcal or gram-negative bacteria, after which lung scars or fibrosis may develop. Bronchopneumonia denotes multiple patchy and diffuse areas of involvement and often implies that a less severe form of disease exists because signs and radiographic evidence of consolidation are absent.

Mycoplasmal, pneumococcal, certain other primary bacterial pneumonias, and the necrotizing (frequently nosocomial) pneumonias are considered in Ch. 261 to 266. Because staphylococcal pneumonia is so closely related to influenza, it is discussed under influenza (see Ch. 78), as well as under staphylococcal disease (see Ch. 270). The pneumonias caused by viruses, rickettsiae, certain fungal species, i.e., *Histoplasma*, coccidioidomycosis, *Aspergillus*, *Legionella* and other taxonomically less well defined species, such as *Pneumocystis carinii*, are considered in the individual chapters dealing with those infections.

PATHOGENESIS. Microorganisms reach lung tissue in several ways: (1) by direct inhalation of infectious particles from ambient air or by aspiration of secretions from the mouth and nasopharynx, (2) by deposition in lung vasculature following hematogenous spread from another site, and (3) by exogenous penetration of lung tissue. The last-named route includes trauma as well as iatrogenic inoculation of lung tissue with bacteria during chest surgery or from other kinds of diagnostic or therapeutic procedures, e.g., bronchoscopy. The inhalation-aspiration route is by far the most significant. Also important are the size and configuration of inhaled particles and droplets, which determine the site or level of deposition in the respiratory tract. For example, approximately 90 per cent of particles between 5 and 10 μ in diameter impact at some point along the trachea or in major bronchi, whereas those between 0.5 and 3 μ in size may escape filtration and be deposited in terminal air spaces. Particles <0.5 μ in diameter remain suspended in air and may leave the body via expired air. Because many bacteria are in this small size range, they frequently plumb the airways to the alveoli.

Of importance in developing pneumonia are the forces that can keep microorganisms in the lung. The mucosal surfaces of the nose and mouth and the gingival border possess numerous microorganisms that are considered to be normal flora; yet surprisingly few species of aerobic gram-negative bacilli routinely colonize these areas, especially the potentially pathologic gram-negative rod bacteria. With almost any alteration in health status of the host, there is a substantial increase in the recovery of Enterobacteriaceae and *Pseudomonas* bacteria in cultures or swabs taken from the naso-oropharynx. Poor nutrition, debilitation, and hospitalization itself seem to enhance colonization. An assay in vitro that allows these bacteria to react with buccal cells or nasal and tracheal ciliated epithelial cells from such patients will show increased attachment of bacteria. Common to both viruses and mycoplasmas is their injury of the ciliary epithelium lining the trachea and conducting airways. After viral infections in particular, bacteria may not be cleared normally from the lower airways owing to damage in the ciliary clearing action of the respiratory epithelium. Subsequent stasis of mucus and secretions allows for bacterial multiplication, or breaks in the cellular junctions of the lining surface may permit submucosal penetration of bacteria. Viruses shed from infected respiratory epithelium in proximal airways can be aspirated into alveoli and ingested by macrophages, thereby infecting these cells and impairing their phagocytic and bactericidal capacity. This is a well-recognized sequence predisposing to bacterial superinfection, frequently with staphylococci, with pneumonia as a common aftermath. Finally, special features of invading microorganisms can be important in establishing the beachhead of infection—a large inoculum, unusual virulence, or secretion of exo- or endotoxins and other enzymes that directly affect the function of host cells or structurally damage lung tissue. Some common bacteria (*Hemophilus spp.*, pneumococci, and *Neisseria spp.*) that colonize the airways of those with chronic bronchitis can produce an IgA protease that cleaves secretory IgA_1 and that may favor attachment to the mucosa.

LUNG HOST DEFENSES. Many microbial agents can infect the lungs and cause pneumonia, but bacteria do so most frequently. Although a common disease, bacterial pneumonia is a relatively rare occurrence in normal people, considering the burden of microorganisms in the ambient air and our frequent exposure to infectious respiratory droplets and secretions from the sneezing and coughing of fellow humans. This attests to the effectiveness of the lung host defense system. This defense system consists of a complex interrelationship between anatomic barriers and cleansing mechanisms present in the nasopharynx and upper airways and with local cellular and humoral factors operant in the terminal air-exchange units (alveoli). This might be described as the "natural defense system" of the respiratory tract. With respect to infectious agents, normal lungs are generally kept sterile beyond the first bronchial divisions.

In the upper respiratory tract and large airways, a combination of mechanisms excludes particulate material: (1) anatomic barriers such as the epiglottis and tight apical cellular junctions between epithelial lining cells, (2) frequent branching of the pulmonary tree (to effect aerodynamic filtration of inspired air), (3) mucociliary clearance of particulates that impact on the mucosa, and (4) the cough response. When infectious agents, bacteria in particular, elude the physical or mechanical defenses described above and are deposited in the alveoli, another group of host factors takes over. This switch occurs because lung structure changes at the level of respiratory bronchioles, and in the terminal units (alveolar ducts and alveoli) ciliated epithelium and mucus-secreting cells (goblet cells and mucous glands) are no longer present. Therefore, mucociliary clearance does not occur in the terminal units; nor does coughing effectively clear material from the alveoli. Thus microbial clearance and removal of other antigenic material from alveoli are dependent entirely on cellular and humoral factors.

If a bacterium of critical size reaches an alveolus (in the absence of edema fluid of either circulatory or inflammatory origin), the microbe may encounter at least three substances that conceivably might inactivate it, exclusive of its eventual inactivation by phagocytosis. First, surfactant, secreted by Type II pneumocytes, may have some antibacterial activity against staphylococci and rough colony strains of some gram-negative rod bacteria. Second, immunoglobulins, principally of the IgG class and, in lesser concentration, monomeric and secretory forms of IgA, may have specific opsonic antibody activity for the bacterium. Third, complement components, especially properdin factor B, might interact with the bacterium and trigger the alternative complement pathway. One or all of these substances can prepare the bacterium for ingestion by an alveolar macrophage, or the activated complement sequence can lyse it directly. Although alveolar macrophages avidly phagocytose some inert particles, they ingest viable bacteria with considerably less enthusiasm. Coating or opsonizing the organisms will enhance phagocytosis approximately ten-fold. Immunoglobulin G appears to be the principal substance capable of increasing alveolar macrophage phagocytosis, although complement (C3b) can function to enhance or amplify the process. Some particulates that activate the alternate complement pathway can interact with fragments of fibronectin found in the alveoli lining fluid, which in turn bind to a specific receptor on alveolar macrophages. Thus, nonimmune opsonins may aid phagocytosis. Once phagocytosis has occurred, the alveolar macrophage can inactivate susceptible organisms. Intracellular killing proceeds but often at a slower rate than that measured in PMNs and along less well studied metabolic pathways. Whereas PMNs may kill ingested bacteria with one or a combination of four antimicrobial systems (H_2O_2, superoxide anion [O_2^-], myeloperoxidase, or halide anion), the process is less certain in alveolar macrophages.

Following ingestion of bacteria, the fate of alveolar macrophages is not certain. They are long-lived tissue cells that can survive months to years and presumably are capable of handling repeated bacterial and other microbial challenges. Because they are mobile cells, they can migrate to other alveoli through the pores of Kohn or move to more proximal areas of the respiratory tract and get aboard the mucociliary escalator for elimination from the lungs. In addition, macrophages gain entry into lung lymphatics and can be carried to regional lymph nodes, which can be sites for initiating humoral and cellular immune responses for the lung. Undoubtedly, macrophages are instrumental in degrading antigenic material and presenting it to appropriate lymphocytes in these nodes. This exit also gives potential access to systemic lymphoid tissue.

Alveolar macrophages are the most numerous resident phagocytes present in the alveoli. They are the bona fide first line of cellular defense on the airside of the lower respiratory tract. A few PMNs, about one per 100 alveoli, are present, but primarily they are reserve phagocytic cells close by in the intravascular compartment. A plentiful supply of PMNs resides in the blood of lung capillaries as part of the body's pool of marginated PMNs. Even though PMNs are in close proximity to alveolar spaces, they are nonetheless separated by several planes of tissue-capillary endothelium, interstitial space, and alveolar epithelium. Depending upon the species of bacteria that is inhaled into the lungs, alveolar macrophages and/or PMNs are selected to respond to the inoculum. Experimentally in mice, a small dose of aerosolized *Staphylococcus aureus* is contained solely by macrophages, whereas *Klebsiella* and *Pseudomonas* evoke a PMN exudate in alveoli. Or, if a sufficiently large bacterial inoculum or particularly virulent microorganisms reach the lower respiratory tract, the lung parenchyma mounts an extensive inflammatory response, which is a potent mechanism to augment host defense. The development of the inflammatory response and hence pneumonia is a deliberate and controlled reaction in the lungs. The ingredients of initiation, amplification, and, finally, suppression are present. When the lung parenchyma mounts an extensive inflammatory response it may be perceived as clinical illness, and a chest roentgenogram usually reveals an infiltrate.

Granulocyte movement into the alveoli is an orderly reaction initiated from the alveolar side. This is termed directed migration or chemotaxis. At least two mechanisms for chemotactic activity exist that can set in motion the inflammatory response in the alveoli and amplify the PMN response. *The first* is best illustrated with the example of gram-negative rod bacteria known to contain lipopolysaccharide substances termed endotoxins. Some complement components, particularly factor B, are present in small amounts in bronchoalveolar fluids. Bacterial endotoxin can directly activate the alternative complement pathway, leading to the formation of fragments such as C5a that are known to be potent stimulators of PMN chemotaxis. In addition, the inflammatory response may include activation of the kinin system. This could result in generation of kallikrein, which has chemotactic activity, and bradykinin, which is capable of increasing vascular permeability and could account for the accumulation of fluid and other humoral substances in alveoli that accompany pneumonia. *The second mechanism* may emanate from the alveolar macrophage itself. Following phagocytosis of opsonized bacteria, chemotactic factors are synthesized and secreted that will selectively attract PMNs. These small molecular weight, noncomplement factors include some leukotriene substances (LTB_4) derived from arachadonic acid along its lipoxygenase pathway.

Once PMNs and other components of edema fluid have filled alveolar spaces, an exudative inflammatory reaction exists in lung parenchyma and pathologically pneumonitis is present. Ultimately lung tissues become consolidated. Proteolytic enzymes (PMN-derived elastase) are released but largely neutralized by several inhibitor proteins, $alpha_1$ proteinase and bronchial mucosal inhibitor, which minimize autodestruction of lung tissue. Pending successful containment of the infection, resolution and healing phases eventually occur. At present, however, little is known about the processes that turn off or limit the acute inflammatory reaction of pneumonia and initiate recovery. Serum-derived chemotactic factor inactivator can inhibit immune-complex deposition in animal lung tissue and modify the ensuing inflammatory response. The identification of such inhibitors and the potential for manipulating them is a part of lung immunophysiology that is still in its infancy.

CLINICAL PRESENTATION. For the physician to discover that a pneumonia, i.e., an intrapulmonary process of some sort, is present in an adult patient is not a difficult feat, but two more things are necessary—to assemble evidence that the disease is indeed microbial in origin and not an infarct or neoplasm and to identify the specific microbe that is involved. Every aspect of management—the choice of treatment, the complications to be watched for, and the hour-by-hour prognosis—depends on the nature of this information. To obtain it accurately *and in proper time* requires the physician to be wholly familiar with the various ways in which each one of the microbial pneumonias expresses itself. Some forms of pneumonia encountered relatively rarely arise as complications of familiar microbial diseases such as measles or tuberculosis or streptococcal disease. Occasionally, well-known viruses such as influenza or chickenpox cause pneumonia, or the physician may be asked to see a patient with psittacosis. In the compromised host, necrotizing pneumonias caused by *Pseudomonas* and other gram-negative bacilli are commonplace. Most of the time, in an adult patient the physician is dealing with *mycoplasmal pneumonia* or with *one of three bacterial pneumonias,* pneumococcal, staphylococcal, or some other form of necrotizing pneumonia in an obviously altered host. This narrowing of the probabilities does not really lighten the seriousness of making the correct choice, for the most effective treatment for pneumococcal pneumonia is without much value in *Klebsiella* pneumonia. A choice of therapy based on a diagnosis of mycoplasmal pneumonia when the patient actually has staphylococcal pneumonia could result in a fatality. Recently recognized bacteria (*Legionella spp.*), unexpected combinations of microbes in immunocompromised hosts (viral and lethal *Pneumocystis carinii* in homosexuals and illicit-drug users) or antibiotic-resistant strains are part of a changing spectrum of pneumonia that can be encountered in community-acquired disease or as complications in hospitalized patients. Unusual microbial etiologies are to be expected.

As indicated above, in most persons with pneumonia, the physician's opportunity for error comes not from overlooking altogether that respiratory disease is present, but from minimizing its importance ("a little bronchitis") or from lightheartedly mislabeling a quite serious *nonmicrobial* condition, such as pulmonary infarction, as "a viral pneumonia." Therefore, to establish that a pneumonic process is present and to amass evidence that it is most probably microbial in origin, two things are of importance: obtaining a relevant clinical history and using some readily available and simple laboratory techniques. Young adults often have the classic symptoms that can be readily pinpointed to the lower respiratory tract, whereas infants and the elderly may have so few respiratory symptoms as to cause concern that infection may be arising from another organ system. Elderly or severely ill patients may have an unimpressive amount of cough, scant sputum production, little evidence of respiratory symptoms, and a deceptive absence of fever. Only after excluding infection systematically in other organ systems does the respiratory tract receive greater consideration. The onset of fever and agitation or altered mentation frequently ushers in an acquired or nosocomial lung infection in a hospitalized or immunocompromised patient (see Ch. 264). Obviously, a high index of suspicion is needed, plus confirming evidence from the physical examination and other laboratory aids.

A conscientious medical history and physical examination are essential. The oral account from an ambulatory patient may be straightforward and describe a prodromal upper respiratory infection, sudden and precise onset of chills followed by fever, painful cough, fatigue and apprehension, and failure of antipyretic medication to provide relief. With a chronically ill hospitalized patient, the search for a source of a temperature spike always includes a chest radiograph, which may happen to show a new infiltrate; an extensive history is less necessary. Answers to a few specific queries are always needed; e.g., has there been prior illness, hemoptysis, use of antibiotics, chills, or pleuritic chest pain? Once the nature of respiratory illness has been determined, other problems invariably come to mind, which should be weighed appropriately. Does the patient have any obvious risk factors or underlying illnesses that make him or her susceptible to a specific bacterial infection? Are there any special epidemiologic considerations, and—of special importance—are any other members of the immediate family ill? Is this a recurrent pneumonia? What other peculiar problems of the patient may complicate medical management, such as drug allergies, compromised renal or hepatic function, poor superficial arm veins that prevent easy intravenous access, and so on? Will the patient require hospitalization or outpatient management? Some of the considerations are not relevant for every case. The point for emphasis, however, is the use of a mental checklist to organize and cover most facets of the patient's presentation. This leads to initiation of an orderly plan for the management of the particular respiratory infection.

Auscultation and percussion of the chest may reveal typical signs of lung consolidation that affirm the existence and location of infection. If the pneumonic process has been viewed on chest radiograph prior to examination of the patient, as may occur in a busy emergency room or in an intensive care unit where routine chest films are obtained, the physician may not always follow through with a detailed physical examination. This is a mistake because valuable contributory information may be missed. Appearance of the skin and mucous membranes can help assess fluid status, indicate jaundice or cyanosis, which can accompany serious pneumonia, reveal needle tracks in illicit drug users, and disclose lesions suggesting peripheral emboli. Assessment of oral hygiene, condition of the teeth and gingiva, and adequacy of the gag reflex could all point to a likely aspiration syndrome and anaerobic infection. Fingernail beds roughly reflect oxygenation, or the presence of clubbing may give a clue to underlying lung disease. Acute endocarditis can complicate pneumonia; hence auscultation of the heart and a search for signs of emboli are important. Just watching the patient breathe or observing his position in bed as he attempts to splint his chest or to minimize pleuritic pain can help one gauge the discomfort the patient is experiencing. Upper abdominal tenderness may reflect diaphragmatic irritation resulting from inflamed pleural surfaces, but the association can be confusing in the patient. High fever can cause changes in mental status, but meningitis can occasionally complicate pneumonias as well, especially those caused by gram-negative bacilli; thus a neurologic examination should also be part of the evaluation.

DIAGNOSIS AND MANAGEMENT. The physician in possession of the patient's history, the results of the physical examination, and the chest radiograph knows a lot about the setting of the illness, the likely cause, and the probable extent of involvement. A good sputum specimen, well Gram stained, may suggest a causative agent, and an elevated white blood cell count with a left shift of the differential reinforces the impression of acute disease. With this data base a good diagnosis is possible, but the final decision on the causative agent may have to await culture results. Thus, an element of uncertainty is present and antibiotic therapy is somewhat empiric. At this point in formulating a plan of action, three principles of patient management bear repeating and deserve emphasis: (1) obtain all the necessary specimens for appropriate bacteriologic cultures before antimicrobial therapy is begun so that there is a reasonable chance for laboratory recovery of the organism; (2) ensure that the drug therapy is as specific as one's certainty of the etiologic agent allows, yet sufficiently broad—temporarily at least—to cover the common yet unsuspected microorganisms as well; and (3) tailor or change the antimicrobial coverage in several days when the results of the cultures are available. A few days of a broad-spectrum antimicrobial coverage will usually not cause superinfections or selection of the drug-resistant bacteria so long as the physician discontinues unnecessary drugs and appropriately narrows the antimicrobial spectrum as soon as possible.

Since appropriate examination and culture of respiratory secretions are so necessary for the rational treatment of pneumonia, the physician should be vigorous in his attempt to get adequate specimens. If the patient is not producing sputum, an attempt to induce secretions by nebulization of ultrasonic water particles is reasonable. Such particles (which may vary in size between 0.8 and 10 μ in diameter) serve as an irritant and stimulate most subjects to cough. Attempts to obtain lung secretions by passing a small rubber catheter through the nose or mouth rarely get beyond the vocal cords of an alert patient and accomplish little more than further distressing an already sick patient in order to obtain a sample of oropharyngeal fluids.

In addition to sputum cultures, the desirability of having blood and pleural fluid (if evidence of pleural effusion is present) specimens for culture must be weighed. Several blood cultures are recommended because the causative bacterium can be obtained in a reasonable percentage of patients, especially with lobar pneumococcal pneumonia, in which the recovery rate may be 10 to 25 per cent. A parapneumonic effusion is a common occurrence, and one may be evident on initial presentation or develop in the course of the illness, despite appropriate antibiotic treatment. Indications for use of a diagnostic thoracentesis vary. On *initial* evaluation if the patient has clinical evidence of pleural space fluid, substantiated by decubitus chest radiographs or ultrasonography, a thoracentesis is indicated to determine whether the fluid is exudative or whether empyema exists. Empyema is usually associated with pneumonitis or lung abscess in adjacent lung tissue, and the fluid is exudative and like pus; microorganisms may be seen on stained smear and usually grow from cultures, especially anaerobic ones. Aside from culturing the pleural material, cellular analysis (total cell count and differential count) and certain chemical tests (pH, LDH, glucose, total protein, and on occasion lactic acid, amylase, lipids, and cytology) will identify pleural fluid to be a transudate or exudate (see Ch. 58). If an empyema exists or analysis of an exudate meets certain criteria (e.g., pH <7.2, or purulent material with high white cell count), repeated thoracenteses to drain the fluid or use of an indwelling chest tube to promote continuous drainage is usually deemed necessary to hasten healing and to prevent or minimize future pleural adhesions. *Later* in the disease course, if a parapneumonic effusion develops, thoracentesis is indicated if (1) fever persists for 72 hours after beginning treatment with appropriate antibiotics; (2) a large effusion develops that is contributing to discomfort and difficult breathing or is perceived to be increasing in size; and (3) there is evidence that once freely movable fluid has become loculated. In contrast, if a small effusion develops but the patient continues to improve and remains afebrile, it is acceptable to watch the condition, because the fluid will likely diminish and be absorbed. Needle pleural biopsy should be included with a thoracentesis procedure if the etiology of the lung infection is not definite or prior cellular analysis of pleural fluid suggests that an unsuspected primary pleural process is present. Histology and culture of pleural tissue are often invaluable in the diagnosis of carcinomatosis or mycobacterial infection.

In the patient who has a new lung infiltrate, fever, and the clinical setting of pneumonia but who is unable to provide an adequate expectorated sputum sample, the question of how vigorous to be in obtaining respiratory secretions is always difficult to resolve. The situation arises most often in the debilitated, chronically ill patient or the immunosuppressed host, and many factors such as patient tolerance, hematologic parameters, and probability of opportunistic infection dictate the decision on how invasive to be. Each of the procedures noted below carries with it some risk of producing a potentially serious complication in a patient who may be already quite sick. The use of any of these procedures should be carefully limited to those necessary situations in which the additional knowledge to be obtained could be of significant benefit to the patient. The confidence and skill with which certain procedures are performed reflect the experience of the physician involved, so that preference of one technique over another may reflect community availability of an appropriate operator.

Percutaneous transtracheal aspiration is a direct approach that eliminates much of the contaminating oral microbial flora. Aspiration is performed through a plastic angiocatheter (No. 14 or 16 needle size) and needle inserted through the cricothyroid membrane into the airway lumen, and material is aspirated after a small injection of saline solution which makes the patient cough. Transtracheal specimens can become contaminated with mouth flora and yield confusing results if shortcomings in the procedure are not recognized. However, bacteriologic data obtained are more reliable than those gotten from routine sputum samples. Both anaerobic and aerobic cultures should be planted when a tracheal aspirate is obtained. Although this procedure is generally safe, occasionally some hazard accompanies it, such as air leak, leading to subcutaneous or mediastinal emphysema, or tracheal bleeding. A review of over 1200 such aspirations found the mean incidence of complications from subcutaneous emphysema and hemorrhage (not just blood-tinged sputum) to be less than 0.5 per cent (range reported, 0 to 1.6 per cent).

The availability of *fiberoptic bronchoscopy* with bronchial lavage and brushing provides another approach to lower respiratory secretions. The risk of bronchoscopy is small even in patients with extensive pneumonia; correction of thrombocytopenia, if present, with platelet transfusions and the administration of supplemental oxygen during the procedure are indicated. Often a direct view of the affected lung anatomy, particularly if a loss of volume in the lung lobe accompanies the infection, may provide evidence of an endobronchial obstruction. Removal of secretions or a mucous plug could make the procedure therapeutic as well as diagnostic.

Usually, the lavage fluid or brush culture will contain the offending pathogen; however, microbial cultures from the bronchoscopy specimens also contain contaminating flora from the nasopharynx. Interpretation of culture results is often confusing, and identifying the predominant organism may be difficult. To date, no one has perfected a completely reliable way of collecting bronchoscopy lavage specimens that avoids this contamination, although a variety of new telescoping, protected catheters are available. Transbronchial biopsy can be added to the procedure to provide lung tissue for culture and histology. Biopsies of pieces 2 to 3 mm in size are usually obtained. Upon reviewing the diagnostic accuracy of about 230 fiberoptic bronchoscopy procedures, which included bronchial brushing and transbronchial biopsy specimens and were performed in immunocompromised hosts with lung infection, the yield of a specific etiologic diagnosis was about 50 per cent. Brushing gave the correct diagnosis in about 27 per cent and biopsy in about 40 per cent; the combination was about 50 per cent. Complications arising from bronchoscopy include hemorrhage in about 7 per cent and pneumothorax in 5 to 7 per cent. Occasionally, a chest tube is needed to treat the pneumothorax. In about 15 to 25 per cent of patients having bronchoscopy, a postbronchoscopy fever (38.3 to 38.9° C) will develop four to eight hours after the procedure. This usually lasts less than 24 hours. Fever does not seem to reflect a complicating pneumonia, although bacteria are introduced from the nose and throat into the lung with the procedure. The episode can usually be managed with antipyretic therapy alone and without an antibiotic.

Direct examination and culture of affected lung tissue is often indicated. Physicians who care for adult patients with pneumonia generally do not think in terms of needle aspiration of lung tissue. Pediatricians, on the other hand, confronted with undiagnosed pneumonias in infants, feel more comfortable with the procedure and use it frequently. Precise indications for a needle aspirate lung biopsy in an adult cannot be formulated unequivocally; however, a localized, peripheral infiltrate which is "well situated" may lend itself to a needle approach with relatively small risk of complication. Spreading microorganisms along the needle track or soiling the pleural surface is always a consideration, but in actual practice it seems to occur rarely. A small pneumothorax may complicate a needle aspiration in about 25 per cent of cases, but the frequency of this occurrence depends somewhat on the type and size of the needle used. Self-limited hemoptysis occurs in about 5 per cent of patients. Often the factor of most significance is the skill and experience of the physician doing the procedure; this usually dictates the frequency and success with which needle aspiration is used within a particular hospital or medical community. The need to do a *small open thoracotomy* to obtain lung tissue is often easier to agree upon. This approach gives the best piece of tissue and is tolerated surprisingly well by even the sickest patient. Generally thoracic surgeons are extremely skillful in managing this situation. Open lung biopsy is often necessary in the immunocompromised patient with an advancing, undiagnosed pulmonary infiltrate and pneumonia. However, two failings often are observed with the procedure. Medical personnel wait too long to get the biopsy, thus delaying appropriate antimicrobial therapy, or they do not coordinate the handling of the tissue with the microbiologist and pathologist to ensure optimal analysis. A brief presurgical consultation with all the principals is most helpful. The pathologist can often suggest the best area of lung to biopsy, and having the microbiology laboratory prepared can ensure that the most appropriate cultures are quickly planted.

Invariably the initial therapy must be chosen on the basis of the skillful interpretation of essentially *clinical* phenomena and must be heavily weighted toward protecting the patient against the most dangerous of the conceivable diagnoses in that particular set of circumstances. Antimicrobial therapy—plus appropriate support with fluids, antipyretic drugs, oxygen, suction or postural drainage, and the other modalities employed to treat serious lung infection—remains the cornerstone of medical management. Intelligent use of antimicrobial drugs is not easy, and frequent reappraisal of their choice and patient response must be practiced. Once the patient's therapy is underway, the physician can not relax but must remain alert for complications that can develop. A resurgence of fever after an initial period of defervescence is a frequent clue. One of a number of problems could be the cause. Poor coughing and an accumulation of secretions or a mucous plug can obstruct an airway, leading to partial collapse of a lung lobe or segment. Vigorous postural drainage and endotracheal suctions may remove secretions and help re-expand the lung portion and should be tried if possible for 24 hours before resorting to bronchoscopy. The development of loculated pleural fluid has been addressed already and usually requires thoracentesis and possible chest tube drainage. Secondary bacterial infection following a viral pneumonia or superinfection occurring after broad-spectrum antimicrobial therapy may cause fever and worsening of the patient's condition; thus reculturing sputum and blood is necessary. Drug allergy causing mild blood eosinophilia and lingering fever is a frequent and often unsuspected complication that requires discontinuation or substitution in the antibiotic regimen. Finally, complete resolution of the pneumonic process or closure of a lung abscess must be observed, for failure of this part of the healing phase may require additional attention. Sputum cytologies and bronchoscopy might be indicated to rule out a partially obstructing airway lesion or endobronchial tumor.

Bordelon JY, Legrand P, Gewin WC, Sanders CV: The telescoping plugged catheter in suspected anerobic infections. Am Rev Respir Dis 128:465, 1982. *Equipment not yet perfected.*

Czop JK, McGowan SE, Center DM: Opsonin-independent phagocytosis by human alveolar macrophages: Augmentation by human plasma fibronectin. Am Rev Respir Dis 125:607, 1982. *Existence of nonimmune opsonins adds another mechanism for increasing phagocytosis, a process that is becoming increasingly complex to understand.*

Fick RB, Reynolds HY: Changing spectrum of pneumonia: News media creation or clinical reality? Am J Med 74:1, 1983. *An overview of a troublesome situation. Antibiotic therapy also is discussed.*

Kilian M, Mestecky J, Kulhavy R, Tomana M, Butter WT: IgA_1 proteases from *Hemophilus influenzae, Streptococcus pneumoniae, Neisseria meningitides* and *Streptococcus sanguis:* Comparative immunochemical studies. J Immunol 124:2596, 1980. *A fascinating adaptative feature of bacteria to thwart host defenses.*

Marini JJ, Pierson DJ, Hudson LD: Acute lobar atelectasis. A prospective comparison of fiberoptic bronchoscopy and respiratory therapy. Am Rev Respir Dis 119: 971, 1979. *A pertinent clinical trial demonstrating that vigorous respiratory therapy is important.*

Matthay RA, Mortiz ED: Invasive procedures for diagnosing pulmonary infection—a critical review. Clin Chest Med 2:3, 1981. *Summarizes the literature on the diagnostic yield of bronchoscopic, transtracheal, and lung biopsy techniques to obtain lung diagnoses and bacteriologic cultures.*

Niederman MS, Rafferty TD, Sasaki CT, Merrill WW, Matthay RA, Reynolds HY: Comparison of bacterial adherence to ciliated and squamous epithelial cells obtained from human respiratory tract. Am Rev Respir Dis 127:85, 1983. *The kinetics of Pseudomonas aeruginosa binding to cells are explored. Provides good background references.*

Palmer DL, Davidson M, Lusk R: Needle aspiration of the lung in complex pneumonias. Chest 78:16, 1980. *A procedure whose time is arriving.*

Rehm SR, Gross GN, Pierce AK: Early bacterial clearance from murine lungs. Species dependent phagocyte response. J Clin Invest 66:194, 1980. *An interesting research model showing that various bacteria may be cleared in the lungs by different types of phagocytes—alveolar macrophages or polymorphonuclear granulocytes.*

Reynolds HY: Lung host defenses—status report. Chest 75:239(Suppl.), 1979. *An appraisal stressing control of the lung inflammatory response and assessing ways that immune responses are initiated in the airways.*

Reynolds HY: Lung inflammation: Role of endogenous chemotactic factors in attracting polymorphonuclear granulocytes. Am Rev Respir Dis 127:16(Suppl.), 1983. *Summarizes macrophage- and complement-derived chemotactic substances.*

261. PNEUMOCOCCAL PNEUMONIA

David T. Durack

DEFINITION. Pneumococcal pneumonia is a common bacterial infection of the lungs caused by *Streptococcus pneumoniae.* This illness is usually characterized by sudden onset, high fever, shaking chills, pleuritic chest pain, and a racking cough which raises thick, blood-stained sputum.

HISTORICAL NOTE. The pneumococcus was described simultaneously by Pasteur in France and by Sternberg in the United States in 1881. Pasteur isolated the organism from frothy saliva on the lips of a child who had died with rabies, whereas Sternberg found it in the throats of healthy people. Thus, both original isolations correctly indicated that this species could be a constituent of the normal flora of the upper airways. Weichselbaum showed that the organism caused pneumonia. The crucial discovery by Avery, MacLeod, and McCarty that DNA was the genetic material which transformed a rough, avirulent strain of pneumococcus into the smooth, virulent form led directly to the development of the science of molecular biology as we know it today. MacLeod and his colleagues demonstrated in the 1940's that a vaccine derived from pneumococcal polysaccharide provided some immunity to pneumonia. Austrian's work led to recognition of the continuing need for a vaccine in the antibiotic era, and to reintroduction of a useful vaccine in the 1970's.

MICROBIOLOGY. Pneumococci are gram-positive streptococci, each organism measuring about 0.8 μ in diameter. They associate in pairs much more often than in chains. They are not quite spherical, so that on a Gram-stained slide these diplococci look like two short, fat bullets pointing away from each other, with bases touching.

Pneumococci are facultative anaerobes. They flourish in nutrient media containing 5 to 10 per cent blood or serum, and their growth is encouraged by carbon dioxide. On blood agar plates they form circular colonies 0.5 to 1.5 mm in diameter. These are dome shaped at first, but often become umbilicated as time passes owing to autolysis of the cocci in the older, central part of the colony. Autolysis is a characteristic attribute of pneumococci; for example, a broth culture full of living pneumococci sometimes spontaneously becomes sterile, containing nothing but bacterial debris, within a day. This self-destruction is caused by the pneumococcal enzyme L-alanine muramyl amidase. Pneumococci also elaborate a hyaluronidase, but unlike other common pathogens such as staphylococci, clostridia, and pseudomonas they produce no known toxins. Colonies of pneumococci growing on blood agar are surrounded by a zone of green (alpha) hemolysis caused by a hemolysin, which under anaerobic conditions causes clear (beta) hemolysis. Pneumococci undergo rapid autolysis when exposed to bile or sodium deoxycholate, and are highly sensitive to optochin. These characteristics are exploited in the laboratory to distinguish pneumococci from other alpha-hemolytic streptococci.

Possession of a capsule is an important attribute of pneumococci. These capsules consist of a high molecular weight polysaccharide polymer that forms a glutinous coat around each bacterium. Variations in the composition of these capsular carbohydrates allow serologic differentiation of at least 83 antigenically distinct types of pneumococci. The capsule is also a crucial virulence factor. It confers resistance to ingestion by phagocytes; this can be partially or completely overcome if type-specific antibody and complement are available to opsonize the pneumococci. Encapsulated, virulent strains form smooth, glistening, mucoid colonies, whereas noncapsulated, nonvirulent strains form rough, dry, granular colonies. The Type 3 pneumococcus is a particularly virulent strain that is noted for producing an abundance of capsular polysaccharide; its colonies are therefore unusually large and mucoid. Incubation of pneumococci with specific antiserum to the capsule causes it to swell and become visible under the microscope. This is the quellung reaction, which can be used for rapid confirmation of presence of pneumococci in clinical specimens as well as for typing.

Pneumococci are ordinarily highly sensitive to a broad range of antibiotics, including the penicillins, cephalosporins, chloramphenicol, erythromycin, tetracyclines, clindamycin, and vancomycin. They are relatively resistant to aminoglycosides. For penicillin, the minimal inhibitory concentration (MIC) is usually 0.01 μg per milliliter or less, but intermediate (MIC 0.2 to 1.0 μg per milliliter) or high-level resistance (MIC 1.0 μg per milliliter or more) can occur. Penicillin resistance in pneumococci, in contrast to gonococci, is mediated by chromosomal mutations, not by plasmids. High-level resistance was extremely rare until 1977, when many resistant strains appeared among pneumococci isolated from children in Durban and Johannesburg, South Africa. Subsequently, a large number of strains that were resistant to many other antibiotics as well as to penicillin were isolated from patients and carriers in these cities. Currently intermediate resistance can be expected in 2 to 5 per cent of clinical isolates in the United States, and high-level resistance in 0.5 to 1 per cent. Therefore, sensitivity tests should be performed on isolates from blood or cerebrospinal fluid when practicable. The necessity for *routine* sensitivity testing of isolates from sputum is debatable. Because the prevalence of resistance seems to be increasing gradually, clinicians should be alert to the possibility of antibiotic treatment failures in future.

EPIDEMIOLOGY. Pneumococci are commonly present in the upper respiratory tract as part of the normal microbial flora. Various studies have found that 10 to 60 per cent of healthy people carry one or more types of pneumococci at any one time. These are most often the higher-numbered, less pathogenic types, with the exception that Type 3 is carried quite commonly by normal people. Lower-numbered, more pathogenic types are found less frequently in the oropharynx, but presumably must have been acquired transiently by patients who develop pneumococcal pneumonia.

Pneumococci cause about 50 per cent of *all* bacterial pneumonias and 90 per cent of all cases of *lobar* pneumonia. In children, Types 6, 14, 18, 19, and 23 predominate. In adults, Types, 1, 3, 4, 6, 7, 8, 12, 14, 18, 19, and 23 cause about four fifths of pneumococcal infections. Typing is not merely of academic interest, because polyvalent vaccines must include antigens from the predominant types.

The ratio of males to females among patients with pneumococcal pneumonia is about 3:2. Most cases occur during winter and early spring, when viral respiratory infections are prevalent. Pneumococcal pneumonia is generally a sporadic rather than epidemic disease; it should not be regarded as contagious. Rarely, epidemics of pneumonia have occurred in closed communities when the carriage rate of a pathogenic pneumococcus has become unusually high and a viral respiratory infection passes through the group. This observation demonstrates that pneumococci carried in the nasopharyngeal flora of normal persons can cause infection under suitable circumstances. When bacterial pneumonia complicates influenza, the pneumococcus is the most common etiologic agent, followed in frequency by staphylococci. Therefore, epidemiologists are able to monitor the advent and progress of influenza epidemics by watching the monthly death rate from pneumonia.

PATHOGENESIS. Microorganisms enter the lower airways every day in everyone. The likelihood that pneumonia will result is directly proportional to the *inoculum size* and *virulence* of the organisms, and inversely related to the adequacy of pulmonary *host defenses.* These include the epiglottal and cough reflexes, the carpet of mucus lining the large airways (which is kept moving away from the alveoli at a rate of 1 to 3 cm per hour by the cilia of the respiratory epithelium), lymphatic drainage of alveoli, alveolar macrophages, opsonins, antibodies, and neutrophil leukocytes. Partial or complete obstruction of a bronchus interferes with local defenses and strongly predisposes to infection.

Pneumonia occurs when one or more of these defenses is impaired and pneumococci are aspirated (Table 261–1). The central importance of aspiration in pathogenesis is supported by experiments in laboratory animals. Other experiments have shown that fluid-containing alveoli are far more susceptible to infection than are dry alveoli, hence the increased risk of pneumonia in patients with heart failure. Like any aspiration pneumonia, pneumococcal pneumonia shows a predilection for dependent portions of the lung: the lower lobes and the

TABLE 261–1. CONDITIONS THAT PREDISPOSE TO PNEUMOCOCCAL PNEUMONIA AND OTHER LOWER RESPIRATORY TRACT INFECTIONS BY INTERFERING WITH THE NORMAL DEFENSE MECHANISMS

Impairment of Defenses	Causes
Depressed epiglottal and cough reflexes	Unconsciousness, seizures, alcohol, anesthesia, CNS depressants, neuromuscular diseases
Decreased activity of cilia	Smoking, inhaled pollutants and toxic gases, upper respiratory infections, pertussis, chronic bronchitis, intubation, Kartagener's syndrome
Increased secretions	Common cold, other viral respiratory infections, anesthesia, bronchiectasis
Decreased lymphatic flow	Congestive heart failure, tumor
Atelectasis	Tumor or foreign body in bronchi, anesthesia, trauma
Fluid in the alveoli	Congestive heart failure, aspiration, hypoproteinemia, trauma
Abnormality of phagocytes	Neutropenia, sickle cell disease, influenza, asplenia
Abnormality of humoral immunity	Hypogammaglobulinemia, congenital or acquired, e.g., multiple myeloma; starvation, sickle cell disease, hypocomplementemia

posterior segments of the upper lobes. However, the right middle lobe is involved more often than in other forms of aspiration pneumonia.

The mouse provides a useful model for study of the pathogenicity of pneumococci. Most encapsulated strains are "mouse virulent," i.e., injection of only one to ten pneumococci into the peritoneal cavity of a mouse will result in its death from overwhelming pneumococcal bacteremia. If the capsule is removed by treatment with a polysaccharidase before inoculation, more than 1 million of the same pneumococci are needed to kill a mouse. Similarly, a rough (unencapsulated) mutant is far less virulent than its smooth parent. These observations indicate the crucial importance of the capsule as a virulence factor.

Opsonizing antibodies to the capsule are vitally important in host defense against pneumococci. This is evident from the clinical observation that patients with immunoglobulin deficiency are at increased risk for pneumococcal infections. For example, pneumococcal pneumonia occasionally provides the presenting evidence of multiple myeloma. During the first few days of an infection, only nonspecific antibodies possessing relatively weak opsonizing capacity are present in serum. If the patient survives, monospecific anticapsular antibody usually appears after five to ten days, promoting efficient phagocytosis and thus assisting in recovery. Because the issue of death or recovery is often decided before this, great efforts have been made to provide a patient with specific antibodies early enough to influence the course of illness. In the preantibiotic era, passive immunity was provided by administration of specific horse or rabbit antisera, resulting in significant improvement in outcome. Today, a degree of active humoral immunity can be provided by administering polyvalent pneumococcal vaccine to selected high-risk patients.

PATHOLOGY. Once a sufficient inoculum of sufficiently virulent pneumococci has reached the alveoli, pneumonia develops and evolves in a stereotyped fashion. First, fluid pours out from capillaries to fill the alveoli, spreading concentrically outward via the pores of Kohn and the smallest airways to fill adjacent alveoli and acini. This infected tide carries pneumococci into contiguous areas until its flow is stopped by an anatomic barrier, usually the visceral pleura investing a segment or lobe of the lung. Edema fluid containing pneumococci also enters the bronchi, by way of which it can bypass segmental anatomic divisions to involve nearby segments or other lobes. The normal smooth, slippery surface of the pleura overlying an affected segment or lobe becomes roughened as dilated vessels leak plasma and inflammatory cells, forming a patch of fibrinous pleurisy. The movements of breathing then give rise to pleuritic chest pain and a friction rub at the site. Often there is an associated exudative effusion.

Next, the interaction of pneumococci with serum opsonins and complement in the alveolar exudate generates chemotactic factors, which stimulate an outpouring of neutrophils into the alveoli. These phagocytes, together with many red cells that spill out from damaged capillaries, pack the alveoli to cause *consolidation*. Although neutrophils do not phagocytose bacteria efficiently when suspended in fluid, they can ingest pneumococci that are trapped against cell surfaces such as the alveolar wall (surface phagocytosis) or immobilized in consolidated exudate. Thus a finely balanced contest develops between the spreading pneumococcal infection and pursuing phagocytes brought to the site by the host's inflammatory reaction. Even without treatment, polymorphonuclear phagocytes will eventually contain the acute infection in a majority of patients. Therefore, antibiotic treatment should be regarded as only one of many antibacterial mechanisms working together to overcome pneumococcal infection. Antibiotics need not *kill* pneumococci to be effective; bacteriostatic agents work as well as bactericidal drugs because in this infection treatment need only tip the balance slightly in favor of the host, whose phagocytes will then effect cure. Unfavorable factors for the host include a high inoculum, a virulent infecting strain, a wide area of involved lung, lack of specific opsonizing antibody, and anatomic abnormalities such as bronchial obstruction, especially when the patient is elderly and debilitated by other diseases.

Finally, macrophages migrate into the consolidated alveoli and ingest the debris left behind as the acute infection resolves. This, together with expectoration of alveolar contents by coughing, results in ultimate resolution of the exudate. Because the alveolar wall is not destroyed when consolidation occurs, recovery is complete in most cases, with restoration of normal pulmonary anatomy.

In a fully developed case of pneumonia, all of the three main stages of the inflammatory reaction described above may be present at once. At the periphery is a spreading zone of serous edema fluid containing bacteria but few cells. Within is a zone of early consolidation, marked by hemorrhage and migration of neutrophils into alveoli, causing the pathologic appearance graphically described as "red hepatization." In the oldest part of the lesion is found a zone of advanced consolidation in which leukocytes predominate; this is termed "gray hepatization." Here the process of resolution begins.

Pneumococcal pneumonia can develop in a patchy, multifocal, and peribronchial rather than segmental or lobar distribution. This form of the disease may be termed *bronchopneumonia*. It is more common in elderly, immobile, or debilitated patients, especially those with cardiac failure, and is often a preterminal complication contributing to, or causing, death.

Spread of Infection. Pneumococci can infect contiguous pleural or pericardial spaces by direct spread from the lung. The organisms may travel via lymphatics, spread across anatomic barriers breached by inflammation, or pass through new communications such as bronchopleural fistulas. The thoracic duct, fed by lymphatic drainage from infected lung, can carry pneumococci to the bloodstream, causing *bacteremia*. Hematogenous seeding of distant susceptible sites can lead to pneumococcal meningitis, endocarditis, pericarditis, arthritis, or ophthalmitis. All these metastatic infections have become uncommon in the antibiotic era.

CLINICAL FINDINGS. The bedside examiner finds a patient suffering from a serious febrile illness, intermittently sweating, breathing fast, distressed by frequent bouts of coughing, and preoccupied with pleuritic pain. The patient may be too ill to cooperate fully with history or examination until these symptoms improve.

Many patients have had an upper respiratory infection for several days before the onset of pneumonia. This may be as mild as a common cold or as severe as influenza. Then they experience an abrupt chill, followed quickly by fever, cough, and chest pain, often with rapid progression over 12 to 24 hours. Patients may vomit once or twice early in the course. The *chill* is often severe, being accompanied by a teeth-chattering, bed-rattling rigor lasting from 10 to 30 minutes. Chills may continue intermittently, but frequently only a single episode of true rigor occurs; repeated rigors over several days are unusual unless a complication has developed. The *fever* is usually high and continuous, ranging between 39.5 and 41° C. This contributes to the patient's striking malaise, weakness, myalgia, and prostration. Temperature should be measured rectally, because the patient is usually breathing rapidly through his mouth. Anxiety, restlessness, and delirium are common.

Cough occurs in more than 90 per cent of patients; it may be dry at first, but soon the patient begins to raise sputum. This is blood tinged or bloody in about three fourths of cases. The blood is usually well mixed through the sputum rather than streaked on the surface, because bleeding occurs directly into the exudate in the alveoli. This gives the sputum a characteristic "rusty" or "prune-juice" appearance. The pneumococcal capsular polysaccharide itself may be present in the sputum in such abundance as to lend it a sticky, tenacious mucoid character, especially in Type 3 infections. In some cases the sputum is simply mucopurulent.

Chest pain is common and frequently severe. It is stabbing in nature, localized over the involved lobe, and sharply exacerbated by deep breathing or coughing. The patient often carefully adjusts his position in bed in order to "splint" the ribs, reducing chest wall movement over the area of pleurisy. Diaphragmatic pleurisy may cause upper abdominal pain or pain referred to the shoulder.

On examination, the patient's brow is usually beaded with sweat and his skin is hot. The "fever blisters" of reactivated herpes simplex virus infection are commonly present around the lips. Rapid pulse and wide pulse pressure accompany the fever. Respiratory distress is evident, with tachypnea, dyspnea, and use of the accessory muscles. Breathing may be so restricted by pleuritic pain that each shallow breath is followed by an audible, grunting expiration. Mild central cyanosis may be present owing to alveolar hypoventilation as a consequence of shallow breathing, and to shunting of venous blood through consolidated lung. Shock may supervene.

On inspection, chest wall movements may be diminished on the affected side owing to the combined effect of consolidation of the underlying lung and splinting of voluntary muscles. Palpation confirms decreased respiratory movement and will occasionally reveal a palpable pleural rib. The trachea is usually central but occasionally deviates toward the affected side if there is associated atelectasis or away from it if there is a large pleural effusion. Vocal fremitus is increased owing to conduction of vibrations from patent bronchi through solid lung.

Percussion reveals dullness over the affected lung, unless the area of consolidation is too small or too deep to be detectable. Even light percussion may cause local pain at the site of underlying pleurisy.

Auscultation over consolidated lung reveals bronchial breath sounds, increased vocal resonance, whispered pectoriloquy, egophony ("*e to a* change"), and crackling rales. A localized pleural friction rub is often present.

Other findings that may be present include *jaundice,* which occurs in a few severe cases and indicates a worse prognosis, and *abdominal distention,* which can be due to gastrectasia (acute gastric dilatation) or generalized ileus. *Neck stiffness* could be due to concomitant meningitis, and the neurologic examination should be complete enough to exclude this complication and to detect any focal neurologic signs. Signs of shock or heart failure can be present in severe cases. *Systolic murmurs* in the aortic area are common, most often signifying no more than a high cardiac output. Murmurs caused by aortic or mitral regurgitation should raise the possibility of pneumococcal endocarditis.

Many patients with pneumococcal pneumonia have milder symptoms and less striking physical signs. Not all need admission to hospital.

LABORATORY FINDINGS. The leukocyte count is usually elevated to 15,000 to 30,000 cells per cubic millimeter, with an increased percentage of mature and immature neutrophils. These often show toxic granulation. Painstaking examination of a Gram-stained smear of the buffy coat (if time is available) will show intraleukocytic pneumococci in a few cases, especially in patients who are asplenic. Leukopenia occurs in some severe cases, and is associated with a worse prognosis. The infection is usually too short lived to cause anemia; if present, anemia probably reflects a pre-existing condition. Moderate free-water depletion caused by fever and sweating is reflected by raised serum sodium concentration in most patients. Hypovolemia may occur owing to the combined effects of vomiting, vasodilatation, and ileus. The erythrocyte sedimentation rate may be elevated, but is of little value in diagnosis.

Examination of *Gram-stained sputum* is an important step in evaluation of a patient with pneumonia. Smears containing many epithelial cells associated with normal flora should be discarded, because they are heavily contaminated with saliva and can only be misleading. Presence of many polymorphonuclear leukocytes indicates that the specimen is sputum. A smear showing predominant gram-positive bullet-shaped diplococci associated with pus cells together with a positive *sputum culture* for pneumococci provides good evidence (but not proof) of pneumococcal infection in a patient with pneumonia. Interpretation of the sputum Gram stain should be tempered by the knowledge that false positives are common (because pneumococci are part of the normal flora), and that the Gram stain may not correlate with the results of sputum culture. Sputum from many patients with pneumococcal pneumonia shows only mixed flora. In practice, the sputum Gram stain is sometimes more useful by helping to rule out staphylococcal or gram-negative pneumonia than by helping to rule in pneumococcal disease.

In seriously ill patients with pneumonia, further measures to identify the causative organism may be considered necessary. Transtracheal aspiration provides a more reliable specimen for Gram stain and culture than sputum, but about one third of transtracheal specimens will yield one or more contaminating organisms from the upper airways. Direct needle aspiration of the lung will not yield contaminants, but a false-negative result is obtained in about one third of cases. Bronchoscopy is of limited value in diagnosis of acute pneumonia, except when endobronchial obstruction must be excluded. Fortunately, these techniques are not necessary for diagnosis and management of most cases of pneumococcal pneumonia.

Two *blood cultures* should be taken prior to treatment from all patients with pneumonia who are ill enough to be hospitalized. Fifteen to 25 per cent of patients with pneumococcal pneumonia have positive blood cultures. Unlike a positive sputum culture, a positive blood culture proves the diagnosis, and also indicates that the patient has a higher risk of complications and death than patients with negative blood cultures.

Counterimmunoelectrophoresis (CIE) and co-agglutination are modern techniques that can identify pneumococcal polysaccharide in clinical specimens such as cerebrospinal fluid, urine, and blood within one to three hours by utilizing specific antigen-antibody reactions. Since the lungs in pneumococcal pneumonia can contain as much as 1 to 2 grams of polysaccharide, it is not surprising that this substance can be found in patients' blood and urine. CIE will be positive on blood from half or more of patients with bacteremia. High levels indicate severe disease and a worse prognosis. Although more valuable in evaluation of meningitis than of pneumonia, CIE occasionally confirms a diagnosis missed by blood and sputum cultures and provides another means to type the pneumococcus. Polysaccharide can sometimes be detected in the urine of a patient with pneumococcal infection for days or even weeks after eradication of living pneumococci.

ROENTGENOGRAPHY. The chest x-ray usually shows a homogeneous opacity in one or more segments or lobes of the lung (Fig. 261–1). An air bronchogram is almost always present, and volume loss is slight or nonexistent. Patients with bronchopneumonia have diffuse, patchy infiltrates on x-ray rather than consolidation. In a patient with emphysema, pneumonia causes poorly defined opacities that are honeycombed with small holes, presumably emphysematous spaces that escape consolidation (Fig. 261–2). Rarely, pneumococcal pneumonia may produce a spherical opacity on the chest film.

Resolution after treatment may be rapid, progressing to completion in two weeks or less, but in some cases the radiologic appearance of consolidation persists for several weeks despite successful treatment. This may cause unjustified alarm and despondency on the part of the physician; therefore, frequent follow-up x-rays should be avoided in patients who are clinically cured. On the other hand, follow-up x-rays are mandatory for patients who do not recover promptly. They may reveal various causes of treatment failure, including tumor, lung abscess, empyema, or bronchopleural fistula.

DIFFERENTIAL DIAGNOSIS. Many other infections can simulate pneumococcal pneumonia. *Klebsiella pneumoniae* causes a form of lobar pneumonia that may be radiologically indistinguishable. Some cases show a bulging interlobar fissure on x-ray, but this sign is not specific. *Klebsiella* pneumonia shows some predilection for the upper lobes, and frequently causes necrosis

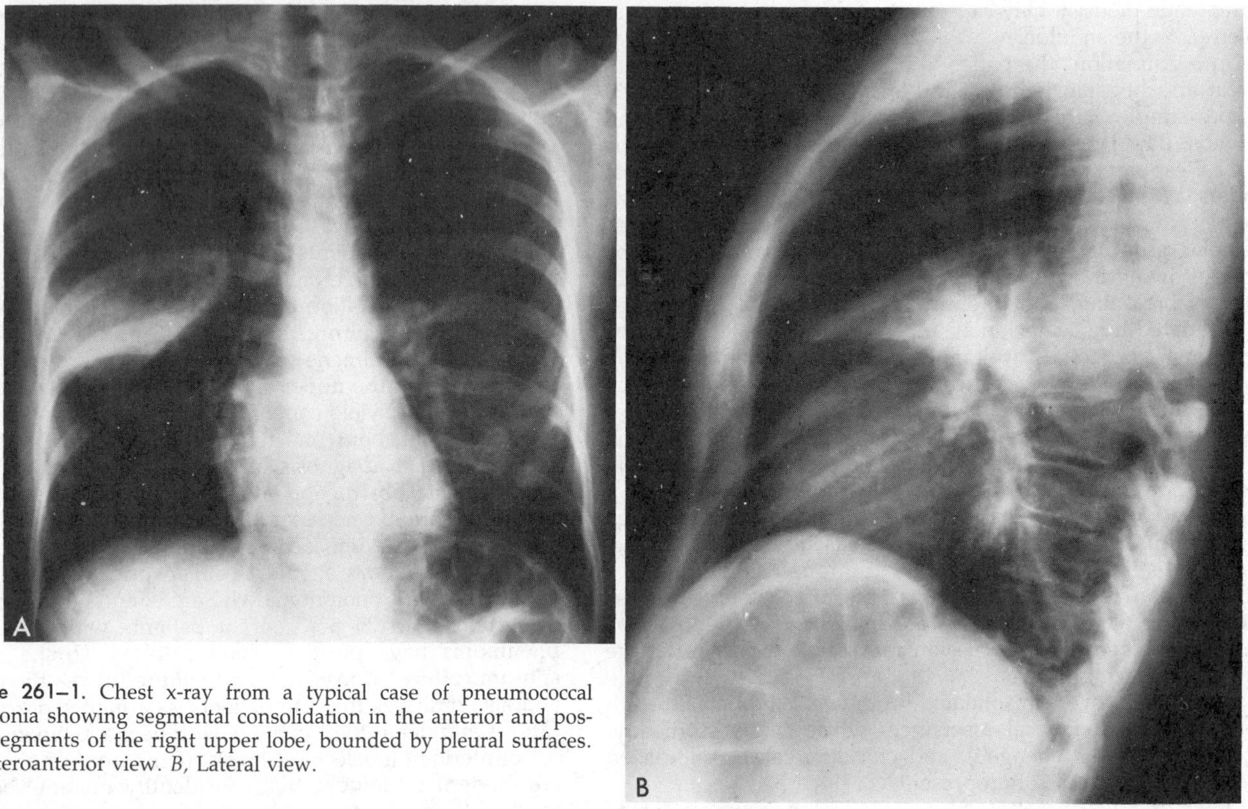

Figure 261–1. Chest x-ray from a typical case of pneumococcal pneumonia showing segmental consolidation in the anterior and posterior segments of the right upper lobe, bounded by pleural surfaces. *A*, Posteroanterior view. *B*, Lateral view.

of pulmonary parenchyma so that patients produce sputum likened to red currant jelly. Staphylococcal pneumonia occurs as a complication of influenza or as part of disseminated staphylococcal infections; it often causes multiple patchy infiltrates that may progress to form pneumatoceles or abscesses. *Hemophilus influenzae* type b pneumonia may be clinically indistinguishable from pneumococcal infection, but is much more common in children under five years of age than in adults. *Streptococcus pyogenes* and *Neisseria meningitidis* (usually group Y) are other rare causes of pneumonia that can be distinguished with certainty only by the results of culture.

Mycoplasma and chlamydial pneumonias are usually less acute in onset and less likely to cause lobar consolidation. Patients with tuberculous pneumonia show less acute prostration and are less likely to have neutrophil leukocytosis. Legionnaires' disease usually does not evolve as rapidly as pneumococcal pneumonia and is more likely to be associated with gastrointestinal upset.

The differential diagnosis between pulmonary infarction and pneumonia is frequently difficult, but must be made in order to treat these conditions correctly. Misdirected treatment of pulmonary embolus as pneumonia (or vice versa) can have serious consequences. Careful consideration of the differential features (Table 261–2) may be sufficient to clarify the diagnosis, but in some cases only pulmonary angiography can resolve the issue.

Infections below the diaphragm such as subphrenic or hepatic abscesses can cause fever, cough, low chest pain, referred pain to the shoulder, atelectasis, and pleural effusion, thus closely simulating lower lobe pneumonia. Gonococcal perihepatitis can mimic right lower lobe pneumonia.

TREATMENT. *Supportive measures* are important for the comfort and safety of patients with pneumococcal pneumonia. They should be put at bed rest, without undue disturbances except for regular checks of respiratory rate, blood pressure, and urine output until there is clearly no danger that shock will develop.

Adequate *analgesia* is needed, both to relieve distress and to allow deeper breathing and coughing to help raise secretions. Codeine tablets may suffice, but will not be adequate for some patients with severe pleurisy or those not absorbing oral drugs because of ileus. These patients should receive parenteral meperidine, 50 to 100 mg every three to six hours until relief is provided, unless there is *real* danger of harming the patient by depressing the respiratory center. In many patients with pneumonia, the benefits of parenteral narcotic treatment for

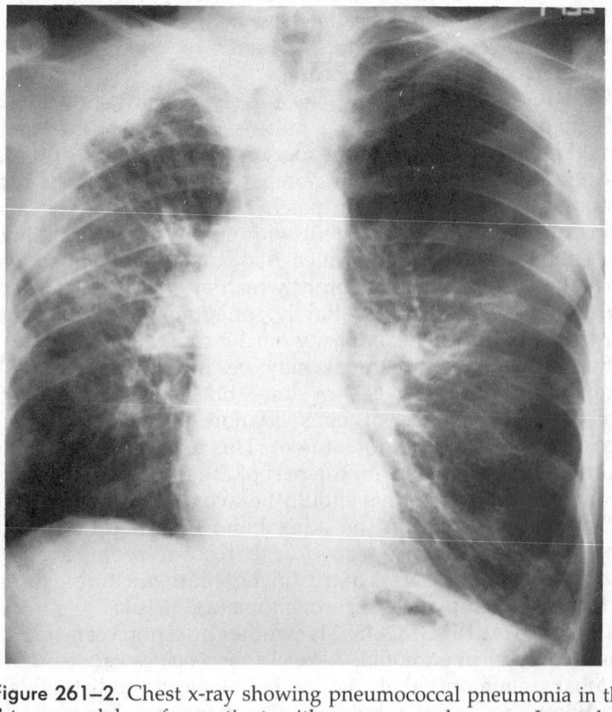

Figure 261–2. Chest x-ray showing pneumococcal pneumonia in the right upper lobe of a patient with severe emphysema. Instead of homogeneous consolidation there is diffuse, patchy ("Swiss-cheese") opacification.

TABLE 261–2. COMPARATIVE FEATURES OF PNEUMOCOCCAL PNEUMONIA AND PULMONARY INFARCTION (IN PRACTICE, EXCEPTIONS TO THESE GUIDELINES ARE COMMON, MAKING THIS A DIFFICULT DIFFERENTIAL DIAGNOSIS)

	Pneumococcal Pneumonia	Pulmonary Infarction
Predisposing factors	Alcoholism, measles, debility	Recent trauma or operation; immobility
Previous upper respiratory infection	Yes	No
Fever, sweating	Yes, usually >39.5°C	Yes, usually <39.5°C
Rigors	Yes	No
Cough	Severe, in paroxysms	Slight or none
Purulent sputum	Yes	No
Hemoptysis	Yes; rusty color, well mixed with sputum	Yes; bright red blood
Pleuritic chest pain, pleural rub	Yes	Yes
Dyspnea, cyanosis	Yes	Yes
Sputum Grain stain	Gram-positive diplococci or mixed flora; leukocytes present	Mixed flora from saliva; few leukocytes
Leukocytosis	Yes; often >15,000/mm^3	Yes; often <15,000/mm^3
Shift to the left, toxic granulations	Yes	No
Bilirubin	May be elevated	May be elevated
Arterial oxygen	Moderate reduction	Moderate reduction
Chest roentgenogram	Lobar or segmental opacity	Pleural-based, segmental, wedge-shaped opacity
Radionuclide scan	Matched ventilation and perfusion defect	Matched ventilation and perfusion defect
Pulmonary angiogram	Normal	Obstruction of pulmonary arteries

pleuritic pain far outweigh any risks, so they should not be allowed to suffer because of excessive reluctance to use a respiratory depressant. Aspirin should be avoided because it interferes with evaluation of progress by means of the temperature chart. Moreover, haphazard use of antipyretics can actually increase the patient's discomfort by subjecting him to intermittent swings in temperature with associated heavy sweats. If antipyretic therapy seems truly necessary, it should be given on a round-the-clock dosage schedule.

Because pneumococcal pneumonia is common in alcoholics, delirium tremens often develops during treatment, requiring additional nursing care, sedation, and fluid replacement. Its manifestations must be distinguished from those of unsuspected meningitis.

Oxygen should be administered to moderately or severely ill patients until improvement begins, preferably by a mask with humidification to avoid desiccation of the mucosae of the upper airways. Intubation and mechanical ventilation may be necessary if respiratory failure develops.

Intravenous fluids should not be given automatically, because some patients with mild disease have no disturbance of fluid balance. Significant fluid and electrolyte depletion should be treated, with the aim of keeping up a good urine flow with specific gravity less than 1.020, and maintaining the serum sodium below 145 mEq per liter. Because the degree of free water depletion caused by fever is usually greater than the degree of salt depletion, half-normal saline or quarter-normal saline plus 5 per cent dextrose will usually provide correct replacement therapy.

If the patient has significant distention and discomfort from ileus or gastrectasia, oral treatment should be avoided and nasogastric suction should be instituted until peristalsis returns. Otherwise, patients may be given clear liquids until improvement begins, after which a light diet can be given when the patient requests it. Because the illness is usually brief, tube feeding or hyperalimentation should not be necessary.

Even though many patients would recover completely without treatment, *antibiotics* reduce mortality, shorten the duration of illness, and prevent development of complications, especially bacteremia and metastatic infections. Therefore all patients should be treated as soon as a clinical diagnosis of pneumococcal pneumonia is made, without waiting for results of cultures.

Penicillin is the drug of choice. The selection of one of several well-tried regimens employing one of the various forms of penicillin (Table 261–3) should be based upon the severity of the illness and the convenience of the patient. Neither oral nor intramuscular therapy should be used for patients in shock. For most patients the course of penicillin need not be prolonged beyond five to seven days.

For patients allergic to the penicillins, a cephalosporin can usually be substituted, because the cross-reaction rate is very low. Care should be taken, however, to administer the first dose in a setting in which an immediate allergic reaction can be treated adequately. For added safety a simple scratch test through a drop of the cephalosporin solution placed on the skin, to look for wheal and flare reaction, may be performed. Patients who cannot tolerate either penicillins or cephalosporins may be treated with erythromycin. This antibiotic is also active against *Mycoplasma pneumoniae.* Therefore, it is particularly useful for patients with mild symptoms who could have either mycoplasmal or pneumococcal pneumonia, and who could be treated as outpatients.

Response to treatment is usually rapid, gratifying both patient and physician. Temperature often falls to normal by crisis within 24 hours, but persistence of fever with resolution by lysis over several days is *not* uncommon and need not be interpreted as treatment failure. Fever recurring or persisting after three days may be due to a focus of extrapulmonary pneumococcal infection that is more resistant to treatment, such as empyema, pericarditis, or arthritis. Other causes of fever during treatment include polymicrobial infection, drug fever, or another underlying disease that was overlooked or misdiagnosed. Failure of the pneumonia to resolve may be due to obstruction of a bronchus by tumor or foreign body, or to infection with more than one organism.

COMPLICATIONS. At least 10 to 20 per cent of patients with pneumococcal pneumonia develop a concomitant *pleural effusion.* The true incidence is considerably higher, but the effusions pass unnoticed because patients are not routinely x-rayed in the lateral decubitus position. Small effusions usually resolve spontaneously after successful treatment, and pleural aspiration is not mandatory. Pleural fluid should be obtained, cultured, and tested for pH, cell count, protein, and lactic dehydrogenase concentration in severely ill patients, in those with large effusions, in those who do not recover smoothly, and whenever empyema is suspected.

Most parapneumonic effusions resolve after treatment, but a few progress to *empyema.* This complication is more likely to

TABLE 261–3. STANDARD ANTIBIOTIC REGIMENS FOR TREATMENT OF PNEUMOCOCCAL PNEUMONIA

For patients with mild symptoms, treated outside hospital	Penicillin V, 500 mg PO four times daily for seven days *or* Erythromycin, 250 mg PO four times daily for seven days*
For inpatients with uncomplicated pneumonia	Crystalline penicillin G, 1.0 million units (600 mg) IV every six hours for five to seven days *or* Procaine penicillin G, 300,000–600,000 units IM every twelve hours for five to seven days
If the patient is allergic to penicillin	Cefazolin, 0.5 gram IM or IV every eight hours for five to seven days
If the patient is allergic to penicillin and cephalosporin	Erythromycin, 250 mg IV every eight hours for five to seven days
For inpatients with pneumonia plus meningitis, pericarditis, arthritis, or endocarditis	Crystalline penicillin G, 3.0–4.0 million units IV every four hours for ten days (meningitis) or two to four weeks (pericarditis, endocarditis)

*If etiology is uncertain, erythromycin is a good first choice because it also treats mycoplasma pneumonia.

develop in untreated cases, or in patients whose treatment was delayed or inadequate. Empyema occurs in less than 5 per cent of adequately treated patients. The clinical distinction between simple effusion and empyema is important, because most empyemas require drainage. Small or moderate effusions noted early in the course of treatment often do not require drainage, even though the fluid has the biochemical characteristics of an exudate and occasionally is infected with pneumococci. Later, if the fluid turns to thick pus composed of fibrin, serum, organisms, and disintegrating leukocytes releasing enzymes and nucleic acids, spontaneous resolution is unlikely to occur. By this time the effusion has evolved into a true empyema; loculations that cannot be drained by simple needle aspiration have usually formed, and secondary bacterial infection with anaerobes or other denizens of the oropharynx may have occurred. Drainage via a chest tube should be instituted. Because a thick, infected exudate often cannot move freely with changes in position, radiographic diagnosis of empyemas can be difficult. Loculated empyemas can be misinterpreted on x-ray as unresolved pneumonia, or tumor. Ultrasonography and needle aspiration can help to make the diagnosis.

The possibility that pneumococcal *meningitis* is present in a patient with pneumonia must be carefully considered (even though this complication is uncommon), because meningitis requires a much higher dosage of penicillin than pneumonia for cure (Table 261–3). If there is any doubt about this issue, a spinal tap should be performed. A small subgroup of patients, usually alcoholics, develop the triad of pneumonia, meningitis, and endocarditis (Austrian's syndrome). These patients are always bacteremic, and their prognosis is very grave; about 80 per cent will die despite treatment. First- or second-generation cephalosporins or erythromycin must not be used in a patient with pneumococcal meningitis; if a patient with this complication is allergic to penicillin, chloramphenicol, 1.0 gram intravenously every six hours, should be added to the treatment regimen. Alternatively, a third-generation cephalosporin that provides good concentrations in cerebrospinal fluid (such as cefotaxime 2.0 gram intravenously every four hours) could be used.

Pneumococcal pericarditis, peritonitis, endocarditis, and arthritis all may occur in association with pneumonia. These conditions are discussed in Ch. 53, 269, and 446, respectively.

PROGNOSIS. The overall case fatality rate for untreated pneumococcal pneumonia is about 25 per cent. This varies widely among subgroups: in young people without pre-existing diseases and without bacteremia, mortality would be only 1 in 20 even without treatment, whereas in bacteremic, elderly patients with chronic heart or lung disease, mortality would be about ten times higher.

Recognized adverse prognostic factors include pneumonia occurring in old age or in infancy; chronic heart, lung, or liver disease; malnutrition; debilitation; bacteremia; positive CIE for polysaccharide in blood; shock, meningitis, endocarditis, or pericarditis; alcoholism or delirium tremens; advanced pregnancy; involvement of more than one lobe; infection with virulent serotypes, e.g., Type 3; leukopenia; jaundice; and delayed treatment.

In the pre-penicillin era, both serotherapy and sulfonamide treatment improved the prognosis significantly. Penicillin further improved these figures, so that overall mortality is now about 5 per cent. However, for those patients with several major adverse prognostic factors, mortality remains higher than 20 to 30 per cent, even with penicillin treatment and modern intensive care.

PREVENTION. Even though the sputum of a patient with pneumococcal pneumonia contains the etiologic organism, there is negligible risk that medical staff and other patients who come in contact with him will "catch pneumonia." Isolation during treatment is therefore not necessary.

Antibiotic treatment given empirically for viral upper respiratory infections undoubtedly prevents or aborts some cases of pneumococcal pneumonia. However, because upper respiratory infections are hundreds of times more common than pneumonia, the cost and risks of treating all of them with antibiotics outweigh the benefit of preventing an occasional case of pneumonia. In young children with absent or hypofunctioning spleens, long-term, low-dose penicillin prophylaxis may be appropriate, but in this setting the primary aim is to prevent fulminant pneumococcal *bacteremia* rather than pneumonia.

The presently available polyvalent pneumococcal vaccine (Pneumovax 23) contains purified polysaccharide antigens derived from the 23 types most commonly recovered from infected patients. These 23 types cause about 90 per cent of pneumococcal infections, and the vaccine is estimated to be about 80 per cent effective. This means that theoretically the vaccine could prevent about two thirds of pneumococcal pneumonias, and possibly some other pneumococcal infections. Not all vaccinated persons will produce protective levels of antibody, and infections caused by types contained in the vaccine have occurred after vaccination. It does not seem to be effective in prevention of pneumococcal otitis. Children less than two years of age should not receive this vaccine, because their antibody response is inadequate. This is unfortunate because among asplenic patients, very young children are at the greatest risk for severe pneumococcal infection.

Present recommendations call for vaccination of high-risk patients over two years old, including those with sickle cell disease; patients with splenic hypofunction or asplenia; the elderly; and patients with chronic cardiac or respiratory disease. Apart from children with asplenia, this is essentially the same population that should receive influenza vaccine.

Because the vaccine consists of purified polysaccharide, there is no risk of inadvertently causing infection if an immunosuppressed patient is vaccinated. Even though such patients' antibody responses are unpredictable, it is reasonable to vaccinate them in the hope that partial protection will result. Side effects are limited to local tenderness. Immunity appears to be long lasting; patients should not be revaccinated in less than five years, lest a more severe local reaction occur.

Austrian R: Random gleanings from a life with the pneumococcus. J Infect Dis 131:474, 484, 1975. *A potpourri of interesting observations on pneumococci, by a true authority.*

Austrian R, Douglas RM, Schiffman G, Coetzee AM, Koornhof HJ, Hayden-Smith, Reid RDW: Prevention of pneumococcal pneumonia by vaccination. Trans Assoc Am Physicians 89:184, 1976. *This paper summarizes the rationale for vaccination against pneumococcal infection and gives the results of initial clinical studies proving efficacy of the currently available vaccine.*

Coonrod JD, Kunz LJ, Ferraro MJ (eds.): Direct Detection of Microorganisms in Clinical Samples. New York, Academic Press, 1983. *The title of this comprehensive volume is self-explanatory. It provides numerous references to detection of pneumococci in body fluids, including notes on counterimmunoelectrophoresis (CIE) and coagglutination.*

Fraser RG, Paré JAP: Diagnosis of Diseases of the Chest. 2nd ed. Philadelphia, W.B. Saunders Company, 1978, pp 689–695. *A standard, authoritative text that sets down the salient radiographic features of pneumococcal pneumonia.*

Heffron R: Pneumonia, with Special Reference to Pneumococcus Lobar Pneumonia. New York, Commonwealth Fund, 1939. *This is a classic description of large numbers of patients studied in the preantibiotic era. Valuable today for its superb detail on clinical findings and the natural history of pneumonia.*

Hook EW, Horton CA, Schaberg DR: Failure of intensive care unit support to influence mortality from pneumococcal bacteremia. JAMA 249:1055, 1983. *This clinical brief shows that even the most intensive modern medical care cannot save 30 to 76 per cent of patients with pneumococcal bacteremia and thus emphasizes the need for vaccines.*

Istre GR, Humphreys JT, Albrecht KD, et al.: Chloramphenicol and penicillin resistance in pneumococci isolated from blood and cerebrospinal fluid: A prevalence study in metropolitan Denver. J Clin Microbiol 17:472, 1983. *A short recent paper with current information on the prevalence of antibiotic resistance among clinical isolates of pneumococci in the United States.*

Jacobs MR, Koornhof HJ, Robins-Browne RM, et al.: Emergence of multiply resistant pneumococci. N Engl J Med 299:735, 1978. *An important report describing the emergence of a large number of strains of antibiotic-resistant pneumococci in South Africa. Emphasizes the potential for worldwide spread of resistant strains, and supports the need for an effective vaccine.*

Jay SJ, Johanson WG Jr, Pierce AK: The radiographic resolution of *Streptococcus pneumoniae* pneumonia. N Engl J Med 293:798, 1975. *This study demonstrates that radiographic changes may persist for several weeks after successful treatment of bacteremic pneumococcal pneumonia. The authors recommend follow-up x-ray not earlier than six weeks after onset for patients who are doing well.*

Lerner AM, Jankauskas K: The classic bacterial pneumonias. Disease-a-Month, February 1975, pp 1–46. *A general description of pneumococcal pneumonia, with additional comments on other bacterial pneumonias.*
Robbins JB, Austrian R, Lee C-J, et al.: Considerations for formulating the second-generation pneumococcal capsular polysaccharide vaccine with emphasis on the cross-reactive types within groups. J Infect Dis 148:1136, 1983. *An extensive review of pneumococcal serotypes, related specifically to human infection and vaccines.*

262. MYCOPLASMAL INFECTIONS

Stephen G. Baum

INTRODUCTION

The most significant human infections caused by mycoplasmas are diseases of the respiratory tract, including pharyngitis, tracheobronchitis, and pneumonia. Recently one species of mycoplasmas, *Mycoplasma hominis*, and a closely related organism, *Ureaplasma*, have been etiologically implicated in some diseases of the human urogenital tract.

The high incidence of mycoplasmal infection is not generally appreciated. Factors responsible for this include lack of familiarity with mycoplasmal syndromes; the absence of specific, rapid tests for diagnosis in the early phases of these diseases; and the relative difficulty of growing the organisms in the diagnostic laboratory.

Accurate etiologic diagnosis of mycoplasmal diseases, however, is of considerable clinical importance. Mycoplasmal infections do not respond to the antimicrobial therapies usually used for respiratory or genital infections but treatment with erythromycins or tetracyclines leads to amelioration of symptoms, decrease in the likelihood of spread, and eventually, true microbiologic cure.

HISTORY. In the late 1930's, a group of pneumonias was delineated that did not resemble typical bacterial lobar pneumonia. Because the cause of the pneumonias was unknown, and because the radiographic appearance and low mortality distinguished these cases from pneumococcal and other bacterial respiratory infections, these were called *primary atypical pneumonias*. A decade later, when sulfa drugs were in use and penicillin was hailed as a cure for all bacterial infections, it was recognized that this group of pneumonias was also atypical in its lack of response to penicillin and sulfa drugs.

In the intervening years, recognition of many new viral, bacterial, rickettsial, and chlamydial organisms has revealed the cause of some of these atypical pneumonias. In the 1950's, the organism responsible for many cases of so-called atypical pneumonia was isolated by Eaton and was shown to be similar to one causing pleuropneumonia in cattle; hence the names Eaton agent and pleuropneumonia-like organisms (PPLO). In 1962, Chanock and co-workers showed that this agent belongs to the family of mycoplasmatacea (then newly described), and so it was reclassified as *Mycoplasma pneumoniae*.

Mycoplasmas are ubiquitous in the animal kingdom. There are about ten species that colonize the respiratory or genital tract of humans. In addition, a related organism, *Ureaplasma urealyticum*, is frequently cultured from the human genital tract. Because of the ubiquity of these agents and the fact that related members of the order Mycoplasmatales infect various animals, the etiologies of a large variety of contagious, neoplastic, and inflammatory syndromes have been ascribed to infection by these organisms. However, only one species of *Mycoplasma*, *M. pneumoniae*, has been unquestionably proved to cause disease in humans.

DESCRIPTION OF THE ORGANISM AND RELATIONSHIP TO PATHOGENESIS. The mycoplasmas, members of the class Mollicutes, represent the smallest free-living forms, i.e., they do not require host cells for replication. For many years the question of whether these organisms were viruses or bacteria was debated. However, it appears that they are neither, and there is no significant deoxyribonucleic acid similarity between mycoplasmas and any known bacterium or virus.

The average diameter of mycoplasmas (125 to 150 nm) is in the size range of large viruses. They have no cell wall but are bounded by a limiting membrane containing lipid. Absence of a cell wall renders them susceptible to lysis by hypotonic solutions but insensitive to cell-wall active antibiotics such as the penicillins. Mycoplasmas and *Ureaplasma* can be grown on agar supplemented with serum proteins and sterols. Most *Mycoplasma* species form 200- to 300-μm colonies, which look much like a fried egg. They have a peripheral halo and a thicker central portion lying just below the surface of the agar. *M. pneumoniae* colonies, however, lack the halo and resemble a mulberry. *Ureaplasma* was previously called "T-strain" *Mycoplasma* because it formed tiny colonies on agar. When *M. pneumoniae* is grown on agar containing mammalian erythrocytes, it rapidly produces a clear zone of hemolysis similar to β-hemolysis of some bacteria. *M. pneumoniae* also differs from many other mycoplasmas in that it grows more slowly, ferments glucose to produce acid, adsorbs red cells to growing colonies, and reduces the dye tetrazolium under aerobic conditions. All of these characteristics have been exploited to establish a rapid microbiologic diagnosis.

When mycoplasmas contaminate tissue culture systems, as they often do, they are found intracellularly. This fact has led to speculation as to the mechanisms of persistence of these organisms in vivo. However, electron microscopic studies using tracheal organ culture systems have demonstrated most of the infecting organisms extracellularly at the base of the cilia of epithelial cells.

Two properties of *M. pneumoniae* seem to correlate extremely well with its pathogenicity in humans. *M. pneumoniae* has a selective affinity for respiratory epithelial cells and produces hydrogen peroxide. The H_2O_2 is thought to be responsible for much of the initial cell disruption in the respiratory tract. H_2O_2 also causes damage to erythrocyte membranes. In the laboratory, this damage results in hemolysis, and, in the patient, may alter erythrocyte antigens, thereby stimulating cold agglutinins. These agglutinins appear in the serum of over 50 per cent of patients who develop mycoplasmal pneumonia and are capable of clumping red blood cells in vitro at 4° C. They are different from cold precipitins or cryoglobulins occurring in other diseases. Cold agglutinins are IgM antibodies directed at the I antigen on the surface of normal erythrocytes. There is increasing evidence that cold agglutinins are antibodies to a glycolipid in the membrane of *M. pneumoniae*, which happens to cross-react with a similar erythrocyte antigen. Cold agglutinins occur rarely in other diseases, including influenza and adenoviral pneumonia.

RESPIRATORY DISEASES CAUSED BY *M. pneumoniae*

DEFINITION. Respiratory infection by *M. pneumoniae* may be asymptomatic or may lead to inflammation of the upper airways (pharyngitis or tracheitis) or lower respiratory tract (bronchitis or pneumonia). In the vast majority of cases, disease is self-limited, but proper antibiotic therapy can shorten the duration of symptoms.

EPIDEMIOLOGY. The monitoring of large populations over prolonged periods has disclosed that each year about one out of every thousand people in the United States will experience mycoplasmal pneumonia. The incidence of all other mycoplasmal upper and lower respiratory infections is probably ten times that of mycoplasmal pneumonia. Studies of selected "closed" populations such as exist in military recruit camps, boarding schools, and colleges have shown that from one quarter to three quarters of all pneumonias occurring in these groups are caused by *M. pneumoniae*.

Mycoplasmal respiratory infection is most common in children and young adults, with a peak incidence in the age range of 5 to 20 years; however, infants and elderly patients are also infected. Distribution is worldwide. Although documented epidemics have occurred primarily in the fall months, this disease does not have the marked seasonal predominance that is found with influenza.

Infection is spread from person to person by respiratory secretions expelled during bouts of coughing. The organism is present in these secretions for several days prior to the onset of symptoms and peaks in titer in the sputum during the first week of clinical illness. Of significance to the spread of this disease is the fact that *M. pneumoniae* organisms persist in the sputum, albeit in reduced numbers, for weeks after the cessation of appropriate antimicrobial therapy.

In open populations under nonepidemic conditions, the infection seems to be spread most easily between playmates and within the household. The index case is usually a child. The majority of households having an index case will experience secondary infections, and the majority of susceptible family members will become infected, with resultant symptomatic disease or asymptomatic seroconversion.

In comparison with viral respiratory disease, the incubation period for mycoplasmal infection is relatively long, averaging two to three weeks. Therefore, unless two or more people from a household are simultaneously infected from an index case, it is unusual for several family members to be ill at the same time, and the disease may take several months to run its course through a household.

CLINICAL PRESENTATIONS. Mycoplasmal infection of the upper airways is impossible to distinguish clinically from infection by other agents. On the other hand, mycoplasmal pneumonia has several characteristics that may help the physician to diagnose this disease (see Fig. 262–1). The onset of mycoplasmal pneumonia is usually insidious in contrast to the abrupt onset of adenoviral or influenzal pneumonia. Mild fever is usually the first sign of infection. The hallmark of the disease is severe, disabling, paroxysmal cough, which usually becomes prominent two or three days after the onset of fever and often requires narcotic medication for suppression. Although usually nonproductive, the cough may yield small amounts of whitish sputum. Occasionally the sputum may contain flecks of blood, but grossly purulent sputum and marked hemoptysis are rare. Production of purulent or bloody sputum is actually more prevalent in tracheobronchitis than in pneumonia.

Headache occurs commonly in conjunction with the cough. During the first week of illness, many patients complain of burning soreness in the chest, though true pleuritic pain is uncommon. Fever rarely exceeds 39.5° C (102 to 103° F), and mild myalgias and malaise occur early in the disease. A history of shaking chills, severe myalgias, or gastrointestinal complaints is unusual.

On physical examination, the pharynx may be slightly injected or inflamed. Much diagnostic emphasis has been placed on the presence of bullous myringitis in patients with mycoplasmal respiratory disease. This finding was noted in less than 25 per cent of volunteers experimentally infected with *M. pneumoniae*, and is very rare in naturally occurring mycoplasmal infection. Bacteria are much more commonly cultured than *M. pneumoniae* from patients with bullous myringitis, and the relationship between *M. pneumoniae* infection and bullous myringitis or otitis remains tenuous.

Examination of the chest usually fails to show signs of dense consolidation or fluid accumulation. Auscultation reveals fine rales either unilaterally or bilaterally, which are often not very impressive. Findings from the remainder of the physical examination are usually normal.

In this regard, the radiographic appearance of the lungs frequently presents a surprise. There is marked patchy infiltration of the lungs consistent with extensive interstitial pneumonia; bilateral involvement is evident in about one quarter of the patients. Infiltration is most prominent at the base of the lungs, although mycoplasmal pneumonia can be seen in any pulmonary segment. There may be slight blunting of the costovertebral angle on the affected side(s) in 10 to 20 per cent of patients, but large pleural effusions are rare. If thoracentesis is performed, it yields a serous or serosanguinous transudative fluid.

COMPLICATIONS. Spread of infection within the lung and pleural effusions are the most common pulmonary complications. Involvement of a number of extrapulmonary sites has been attributed to infection with *M. pneumoniae*, usually occurring as complications of pulmonary disease. Occasionally, they have been seen without pneumonia, and mycoplasmal causation has been substantiated on the basis of culture of the organism from involved organs, four-fold or greater rises in mycoplasma-specific antibodies, or demonstration (described later) of less specific cold hemagglutinins.

Three extrapulmonary complications are relatively common (occurring in 2 to 10 per cent of patients). These deserve comment because, when present, they help to confirm the diagnosis of mycoplasmal pneumonia.

Erythema Multiforme Major (Stevens-Johnson Syndrome). Some patients with mycoplasmal pneumonia develop blistering lesions involving the mouth, eyes, and skin. Usually, although the lesions look quite severe, they heal with minimal scarring. However, when the cornea is involved, blindness may ensue, and local and systemic steroid therapy is often recommended in these instances. This dermatologic syndrome has many causes, including adverse reaction to drugs. When, however, it occurs in conjunction with interstitial pneumonia in a child or young adult, its presence helps confirm the clinical diagnosis of mycoplasmal pneumonia.

The pathogenesis of this syndrome is unknown. There is one report of isolation of *M. pneumoniae* from skin lesions, but most authorities consider Stevens-Johnson syndrome an allergic reaction. A great variety of other skin rashes in mycoplasmal pneumonia has been described, but these are not diagnostically helpful.

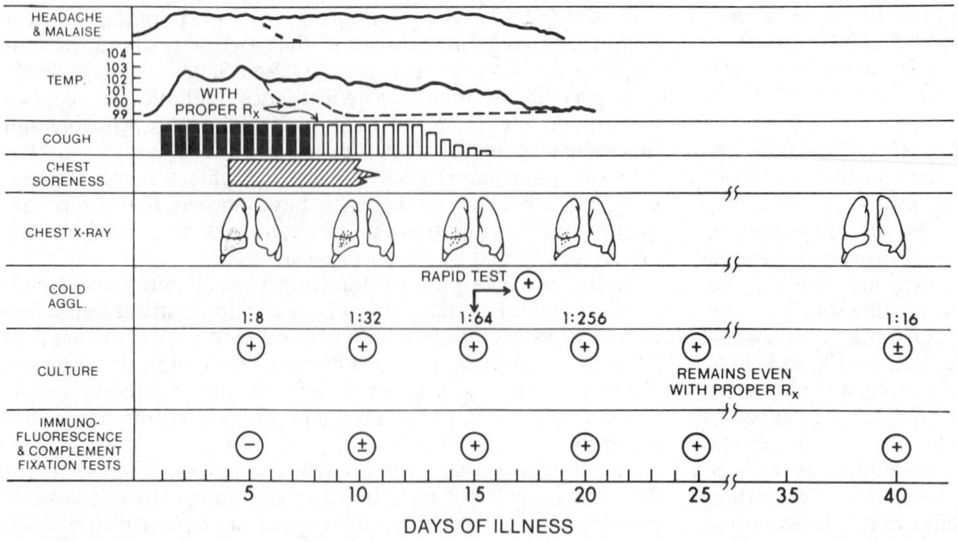

Figure 262–1. Major clinical manifestations of mycoplasmal pneumonia.

Raynaud's Phenomenon. A second syndrome, manifesting itself in the skin of fewer than 5 per cent of mycoplasmal pneumonia patients, is Raynaud's phenomenon. This consists of a painful blanching of the distal parts of fingers and toes that occurs upon exposure to a cold environment. Blanching may occur whether or not the patient has a history of Raynaud's phenomenon unrelated to mycoplasmal infection. There is no experimental evidence on the pathogenesis of this complication in *M. pneumoniae* infection. However, it is tempting to hypothesize that high titers of cold hemagglutinins could play a role by creating minute thrombi in the microcirculation of the distal extremities when exposed to cold. Patients with sickle cell disease may have particularly severe symptoms when they contract mycoplasmal pneumonia. In the presence of extremely high titers of cold agglutinins (1:20,000), gangrene of the distal parts of fingers and toes in these patients has been reported.

Hemolysis. Patients with cold agglutinin titers of greater than 1:500 may experience rapid and severe hemolysis with decreases of 50 per cent in hematocrit. This complication occurs in less than 5 per cent of patients in the second or third week of illness.

LESS COMMON COMPLICATIONS. Among the organ systems reported to be rarely involved in mycoplasmal infection are the cardiovascular, skeletal, and central nervous systems. In a very few cases involving each of these systems, the organism has been cultured directly from the affected organ. However, since mycoplasmal respiratory infection is very common (one per 100 people per year), it is quite possible that in those cases in which *Mycoplasma* was not cultured from the site, the extrapulmonary syndrome was due to a second agent and that two diseases, such as viral aseptic meningitis and mycoplasmal upper respiratory infection, occurred concurrently.

NEUROLOGIC COMPLICATIONS. Aseptic meningitis, meningoencephalitis, cranial nerve neuritis, peripheral neuritis, Guillain-Barré syndrome, transverse myelitis, and psychosis all have been reported as complications of *M. pneumoniae* infection. Most often, etiologic diagnosis is made on the basis of exclusion of other agents and antibody response to *M. pneumoniae*. Spinal fluid cell counts and glucose and protein levels are extremely variable in these cases, ranging from normal to patterns consistent with aseptic meningitis. In some cases, elevated cerebrospinal fluid proteins were found to contain antibodies to *M. pneumoniae*, but these often paralleled serum antibody levels, and it was unclear whether or not cerebrospinal fluid antibody represented diffusion from the serum. There are only two or three reports of isolation of *M. pneumoniae* from cerebrospinal fluid or neural tissue, and the prevailing hypothesis is that mycoplasmal central nervous system disease occurs on the basis of allergic reaction.

Patients with neurologic complications seem to have greater mortality than is commonly associated with mycoplasmal disease. This could signify either a group of patients at markedly increased risk of death from mycoplasmal infection or alternatively, support the hypothesis that these patients had a second (concurrent) undiagnosed disease with greater inherent mortality.

CARDIOVASCULAR COMPLICATIONS. Pericarditis and myocarditis are the most commonly reported cardiovascular complications of mycoplasmal infection. In general, the major criteria of heart disease have been congestive failure and abnormal electrocardiographic results. Large pericardial effusions have not occurred. There have been a few deaths during the acute phase of the disease, but recovery without sequellae is the rule. In most cases documentation of *M. pneumoniae* infection has been made by noting seroconversion. In one retrospective study based on seroconversion, 8 per cent of patients with *M. pneumoniae* infection had evidence of pericarditis or myocarditis. The average age of these patients was 46 years, considerably older than the mean for patients with *M. pneumoniae* infection.

MUSCULOSKELETAL COMPLICATIONS. Arthralgias are common in association with mycoplasmal pneumonia, but frank arthritis is rare. When it does occur, arthritis may continue long after the other manifestations of mycoplasmal infection are gone. Large joints seem to be preferentially affected, and the arthritis may be migratory. *Mycoplasma* has not been cultured from joint fluid of immunocompetent patients.

M. pneumoniae and other mycoplasmas have been implicated as the causative agents of a number of other connective tissue diseases, including rheumatoid arthritis, juvenile rheumatoid arthritis, and Reiter's syndrome. Nonhuman mycoplasmas have been shown to cause arthritis in the animals they infect, and *M. pneumoniae* has been cultured on sevaral occasions from the joints of immunocompromised patients. To date, however, there is no evidence that human mycoplasmas cause joint disease, except perhaps as an acute manifestation of pneumonia.

CLINICAL COURSE. Mycoplasmal respiratory disease is almost invariably self-limited and very rarely results in death. In the absence of treatment, upper respiratory infection usually lasts one to three weeks, and pneumonia may persist from four to six weeks. Recovery is gradual, with clinical improvement preceding roentgenographic clearing. Development of any of the severe cardiovascular, dermatologic, hematologic, or neurologic complications described earlier may prolong resolution. Proper treatment, which is often not begun until other antibiotics have failed, would appear to shorten the duration of symptoms by about half. Results might be even better than this if treatment were begun earlier. Relapse occurs in 5 to 10 per cent of patients. In most cases these patients receive courses of therapy less than two weeks in duration.

Two groups of patients commonly appear to develop severe disease. The first group consists of infants who, until recently, were thought not to be particularly susceptible to *M. pneumoniae* infection. Many infants develop severe respiratory distress requiring intubation and supported respiration. Fortunately, despite severe illness the prognosis for these children is excellent. The second group contains patients with sickle cell disease. In addition to digital gangrene, these patients are prone to develop large multilobar pneumonias and pleural effusions. The possibility of mycoplasmal infection should be considered in a patient with sickle cell crisis and interstitial pneumonia.

PATHOLOGY. Since death is rare in patients with mycoplasmal pneumonia, descriptions of pathologic changes in this disease rest on a very small number of specimens. The tracheobronchial tree and lungs are generally hyperemic. There is evidence of interstitial pneumonia with engorged lungs consistent with the findings on x-ray. Cellular infiltrate, usually minimal, consists mostly of mononuclear elements. Tracheal organ culture systems have been used to demonstrate that infection with *M. pneumoniae* causes a marked decrease of ciliary action, followed by complete loss of cilia and sloughing of epithelial cells.

IMMUNITY. There is a variety of antibody responses to infection with *M. pneumoniae*. It is unclear what role these immune responses play in the pathogenesis of, and recovery from, infection. Secretory IgA antibody is thought to be the most protective immunoglobulin in this disease. Individual immunity may be relatively short-lived, and there are well-documented instances of recurrent disease within two to ten years following primary infection.

DIAGNOSIS. A clinical diagnosis of mycoplasmal pneumonia should be seriously entertained whenever interstitial pneumonia occurs in a young adult. Examination of the Gram-stained sputum is helpful in that it reveals inflammation but no bacterial organisms. The peripheral leukocyte count may be normal or slightly elevated. There is minimal shift toward immature forms, and mild lymphopenia may exist. The diagnosis is substantiated by finding a cold agglutinin titer greater than 1:32 in the serum.

Hospital bacteriology or serology laboratories titrate cold agglutinins in patients' serum using Rh-positive, type O erythrocytes to avoid reactions due to major blood-group isoantibodies present in the patient's serum. However, a simple, rapid bedside procedure for finding cold agglutinins can be performed using only the patient's blood. One milliliter of freshly drawn blood is placed in a tube containing anticoagulant. The tube used for prothrombin determinations is suitable. The tube is chilled on ice for two or three minutes and then gently rotated in a horizontal position. Development of small clumps of erythrocytes, similar to those seen when typing blood, which disappear on warming the tube between the hands, indicates the presence of cold agglutinins. The agglutination-dissociation cycle can be repeated many times with the same blood sample. This differentiates the reaction from direct hemagglutination by viruses—a process that generally cannot be recycled. A positive test result correlates with a cold agglutinin titer of 1:64 or greater. When the cold agglutinin titer is extremely high, an easily dissociable clot may form in the tube. Blood from a patient with an unrelated disease should be used as a control. Cold agglutinins are usually found during the second and third weeks of illness and may peak one month or more after the onset of symptoms.

Diagnosis of mycoplasmal pneumonia should be further supported by finding rising titers of specific antibodies to the *Mycoplasma* organism. These can be measured by complement fixation, inhibition of hemadsorption, or immunofluorescence techniques. In addition, patients with mycoplasmal pneumonia may develop a false-positive test result for syphilis.

Definitive diagnosis of mycoplasmal pneumonia rests, however, on coupling an antibody rise with culturing *M. pneumoniae* from sputum. Although growth on agar may take two to three weeks, rendering results useless for initiating drug therapy, a more rapid (three to four days) presumptive diagnosis can be based on the use of a diphasic medium available in some diagnostic laboratories.

DIFFERENTIAL DIAGNOSIS. The most common respiratory infections mimicking mycoplasmal pneumonia are influenza and adenoviral and legionnaires' disease. These tend to be more fulminant in onset and are associated with more severe systemic symptoms and greater respiratory insufficiency. Patients with legionnaires' disease are likely to be older males with histories of smoking. Often one cannot definitively distinguish between these diseases, and a therapeutic trial with erythromycin (which will also treat *Legionella pneumophila*) may be warranted. Psittacosis and ornithosis (chlamydial diseases) and Q fever (a rickettsial disease) should also be considered in the diagnosis. In such cases, exposure to birds on the one hand and to cattle on the other may prove diagnostically helpful.

THERAPY. Treatment with appropriate antibiotics can terminate symptoms abruptly and usually must be begun on the basis of clinical diagnosis. Penicillins, cephalosporins, and aminoglycosides, such as streptomycin, kanamycin, and gentamicin, have little or no effect against these organisms.

M. pneumoniae is sensitive in vitro and in vivo to erythromycin and to the tetracyclines. These agents appear to be equally effective in diminishing the symptoms of the disease. Because there are fewer adverse effects, especially in children under age ten years, erythromycin is preferred. The dosage for either drug is 250 to 500 mg four times daily for two weeks. Although erythromycin and the tetracyclines are effective in ending symptoms, *M. pneumoniae* can be isolated from the sputum of patients for several weeks after the onset of therapy. The mechanism of persistence is unknown but does not depend on the emergence of drug-resistant organisms.

PREVENTION. The frequency of mycoplasmal infection makes the development of a vaccine an attractive objective. Inactivated vaccines, while producing rises in serum antibody levels, give little protection. This observation has aroused the suspicion that IgA antibodies in nasopharyngeal secretions may have more significance than serum antibodies in preventing the disease.

The possible roles of IgA antibodies and delayed hypersensitivity in combating disease have prompted the trial of intranasally administered vaccines using temperature-sensitive (ts) mutants of *M. pneumoniae*. The rationale was that these mutants would induce a localized nasopharyngeal immune response but would not replicate in the warmer lower respiratory tree and cause disease. The results of initial trials of these vaccines have been variable.

GENITAL INFECTION BY MYCOPLASMA AND UREAPLASMA

INTRODUCTION. One strain of human mycoplasmas, *M. hominis*, and a closely related organism, *Ureaplasma urealyticum*, frequently colonize the male and female genital tracts. During the past decade, there has been increasing interest in discovering the role these organisms might play in causing disease of the genitourinary system.

EPIDEMIOLOGY. *M. hominis* and ureaplasmas can be included in the group of venereally transmitted infectious agents. Infants are colonized during birth, but carriage of the organism is lost during the first year of life. After this, the prevalence of colonization increases with age and sexual experience as it does for other sexually transmitted organisms. At all ages, females seem to be more readily colonized than males, and colonization is found most frequently in patients from lower socioeconomic groups.

CLINICAL PRESENTATIONS. *M. hominis, U. urealyticum*, or both organisms have been implicated in nongonococcal urethritis and inflammatory disease of the prostate, vagina, cervix, upper urinary tract, and female pelvic organs. In addition, colonization by one or both of these organisms has been associated with male and female infertility, habitual abortion, and recurrent production of premature and underweight infants.

INFECTION OF THE LOWER URINARY TRACT. Chlamydia are responsible for a large percentage of cases of nongonococcal urethritis (NGU). *U. urealyticum* is probably the cause of many of the remaining cases of NGU. Evidence for this stems from the many patients with NGU from whom ureaplasmas are cultured and from these patients' poor clinical response to treatment with sulfa drugs, to which chlamydia are susceptible and to which *Ureaplasma* is not. *M. hominis* probably does not cause urethritis. This organism has been cultured from men with prostatitis, but its causative role is unclear.

INFECTION OF THE UPPER URINARY TRACT. *M. hominis* has been isolated from the kidneys and ureters of patients with clinical pyelonephritis. Antibody to the organism was detected in serum and urine from some of these patients, providing moderately strong evidence that *M. hominis* causes some cases of pyelonephritis. *U. urealyticum* infection has not been detected in patients with pyelonephritis, but the agent may infrequently play a role in urinary calculus formation. This relationship might be expected from the organism's ability to metabolize urea to ammonia, producing alkaline urine in which calcium is poorly soluble, a trait it shares with some *Proteus* bacteria that are also associated with urinary stone formation.

INFECTION OF THE FEMALE GENITAL TRACT. *M. hominis* probably causes a small proportion of the cases of vaginitis and cervicitis. Infection of the uterus and fallopian tubes with this organism has also been documented. *Ureaplasma* rarely, if ever, causes infection in the female pelvis.

MYCOPLASMAS AND REPRODUCTIVE ABNORMALITIES. *U. urealyticum* has been cultured from the sperm of males with fertility disorders. Treatment to eradicate *Ureaplasma* has resulted in increased motility and number of sperm as well as improved morphology. No evidence has been collected as to improvement in fertility after therapy.

Ureaplasma has also been isolated from internal organs of the products of conception of patients with repeated spontaneous abortions. In addition, in some studies *U. urealyticum* was more often isolated from the genital tracts of women with this syndrome than from control populations. Finally, treatment with tetracycline prior to conception in women with histories of habitual abortion has been reported to increase fetal salvage rate. Unfortunately, few if any of these studies took into account the presence of chlamydia, which might have been responsible for the reproductive disorders.

LOW BIRTH WEIGHT. Prior to the realization that tetracycline is contraindicated in pregnancy, it was shown that tetracycline treatment of mothers who habitually gave birth to underweight fetuses would increase birth weight. In addition, vaginal colonization by ureaplasmas was correlated with decreased birth weight. However, these studies did not take into account the presence or absence of chlamydia.

PUERPERAL INFECTION. *M. hominis* infection and septicemia have been associated with some cases of postpartum fever. This organism has been found in the blood of up to 10 per cent of women with fever after delivery, and antibody response indicating true infection has been noted in many cases.

THERAPY. Mycoplasmas and *Ureaplasma* are all susceptible to the tetracyclines. *U. urealyticum* is sensitive to erythromycin, but *M. hominis* is not. Spectinomycin, an antimicrobial agent used in cases of penicillin-resistant gonococcal disease, appears to be effective against both *M. hominis* and *U. urealyticum*. Since both *U. urealyticum* and *C. trachomatis* are sensitive to tetracycline, it is recommended that patients with NGU be treated with a tetracycline at a dose of 1 to 2 grams daily for one to two weeks. The patient should abstain from sexual intercourse during this period, and sexual partners should be evaluated for therapy.

In addition, tetracycline therapy prior to conception and erythromycin therapy during pregnancy should be considered for couples with recurrent infertility or gestational problems who are shown to harbor *U. urealyticum* in the genitourinary tract.

Episodes of postabortal and puerperal fever are usually self-limited and do not require antimicrobial therapy directed at mycoplasmas. Should such therapy be deemed necessary, tetracycline is the drug of choice.

Couch RB: Mycoplasma disease. *In* Mandell G, Douglas RG, Bennet JE (eds.): Principles and Practice of Infectious Diseases. 2nd ed. New York, John Wiley & Sons, 1984. *An up-to-date chapter dealing with both clinical and microbiologic aspects.*

Roberts DB: The etiology of bullous myringitis and the role of mycoplasmas in ear disease: A review. Pediatrics 65:761, 1980. *A definitive review of several studies indicating no significant relationship between this organism and ear disease.*

Taylor-Robinson D, McCormack WM: The genital mycoplasmas. N Engl J Med 302:1003, 1980; 302:1063, 1980. *A comprehensive two-part article on epidemiology, microbiology, clinical presentation, and therapy.*

263. PNEUMONIA DUE TO KLEBSIELLA

(Friedländer's Pneumonia)

Herbert Y. Reynolds

Within the family of Enterobacteriaceae, three related bacteria—*Klebsiella, Enterobacter,* and *Serratia*—constitute a tribe designated as Klebsielleae. The genus *Klebsiella* consists of four species: *K. pneumoniae,* which accounts for about 95 per cent of the clinical isolates; *K. ozaenae,* which occurs infrequently and is associated with a form of chronic atrophic rhinitis (ozena) and purulent infection of the mucous membrane; *K. rhinoscleromatis,* which is the cause of scleroma, a granulomatous process rarely encountered in the United States, which can involve the respiratory mucosa of the nose, paranasal sinuses, middle ear, and oropharynx; and a close variant of *K. pneumoniae, K. oxytoca.* All of the species are nonmotile lactose fermenters with cellular capsules. On solid culture media, klebsiellae produce large, mucoid colonies reflecting polysaccharide capsular material. Capsular antigens, termed K antigens rather than somatic O antigens, provide one serologic basis for distinguishing *Klebsiella* strains. Bacteriocin production by *Klebsiella* strains is another typing method that seems useful.

Klebsiella pneumoniae may be present in the oropharynx of normal persons, although the prevalence is low (1 to 6 per cent). There is no tendency for contacts to acquire the organism from a carrier, and it is difficult to implant organisms in the pharynx of healthy volunteers. As with a number of other pathogenic bacteria, the prevalence of *Klebsiella* in pharyngeal cultures increases (up to 20 per cent) in hospitalized subjects. The organism is an important cause of nosocomial infection in infants in nurseries and intensive care units. Pulmonary infections most likely arise from inhalation or aspiration of organisms from the oropharynx during circumstances in which the major pulmonary antibacterial defense mechanisms are compromised. For example, classic primary *Klebsiella* pneumonia usually occurs in patients with underlying conditions such as alcoholism, chronic obstructive airways disease (emphysema-bronchitis), or diabetes mellitus. Operationally, infections may be considered as primary if *Klebsiella* organisms are isolated from specimens obtained when the patient first seeks medical aid. The designation "secondary" is then applied to those infections that either represent superinfection of an underlying infection or are opportunistic in origin. The present chapter is concerned with the primary pneumonia. The management of the so-called "secondary" *Klebsiella* bronchopulmonary infections is essentially the same as for any nosocomial pneumonia (see Ch. 264). There are no clinical features that readily distinguish nosocomial *Klebsiella* lung infection from that caused by other aerobic gram-negative bacilli.

In patients with primary pneumonia, males predominate heavily (80 to 90 per cent) and most infections occur in middle-aged and older patients. A common coexisting disease is alcoholism (66 per cent). Both chronic bronchopulmonary disease and, to a lesser extent, diabetes mellitus appear to predispose to *Klebsiella* pneumonia.

PATHOLOGY. The outstanding characteristic of *Klebsiella* pneumonia is its destructiveness; it is a necrotizing pneumonia, leading in many instances to cavitation. In fatal cases lobar involvement most often occurs, but infection may be lobular or may be a combination of both; an upper lobe is most frequently involved. The pleural surface is covered by a fibrinous exudate, and adhesions form early. Empyema is appreciably more frequent than in pneumococcal pneumonia and probably occurs in about one fifth of cases. Microscopically, in the acute stage the alveolar walls are congested. Usually the alveoli are filled with an exudate composed of a mixture of predominantly polymorphonuclear cells. There is abscess formation in association with necrosis of the alveolar walls. Other findings at autopsy may include extrapulmonary sites of dissemination, e.g., pericarditis or meningitis. Evidence of alcoholic hepatitis and alcoholic cirrhosis is common.

CLINICAL MANIFESTATIONS. The onset is usually sudden, associated with cough productive of sputum (90 per cent), pleuritic chest pain (80 per cent), and true rigors (60 per cent). Early prostration is a usual feature. Occasionally the acute onset is preceded by a nondescript upper respiratory infection and cough. Rarely, epigastric pain and vomiting are the initial symptoms. A gray-green, blood-tinged sputum is usual, but it can be a nonputrid, homogeneous, thick mixture of blood and mucus, brick red in color, resembling currant jelly. On examination, the patient appears acutely ill, febrile, dyspneic, and often cyanotic. Tachycardia is present in proportion to the fever. Chest examination usually reveals signs of pulmonary consolidation. There may be loss of lung volume as manifested by decreased size and expansion of the involved hemithorax and diaphragmatic elevation. Auscultation may reveal suppressed breath sounds with few rales, despite evidence of considerable consolidation. Involvement of more than one lobe is frequent (in two thirds of patients), with a predilection for upper lobes.

LABORATORY AND ROENTGENOGRAPHIC FINDINGS. Peripheral leukocyte counts vary from marked leukopenia to leukocytosis, but leukopenia (and neutropenia) is a poor prognostic sign. In one quarter of patients the total leukocyte count may be in the normal range. On sputum culture, other gram-negative bacilli may be isolated in addition to *Klebsiella*. A mixed sputum flora containing other gram-negative bacilli such as *Pseudomonas spp.* is especially common in secondary infections. A pulmonary source is often incriminated in patients with *Klebsiella* bacteremia. This is an unusual association, because in other types of gram-negative bacillary bacteremia the urinary tract usually represents the major primary source, followed by the gastrointestinal tract.

The roentgenographic features are variable and include massive lobar consolidation, lobular involvement, lung abscess formation with either multiple small thin-walled or large abscess cavities, and residual parenchymal fibrosis. Bulging of a fissure, sharp advancing borders of the infiltrates, and abscess formation occur with greater frequency than in other types of pneumonia. The pneumonic infiltrate is relatively dense, but shadows of similar density can be seen with other types of bacterial pneumonia. Bronchopneumonic distribution is less characteristic but can occur, and even bilateral perihilar infiltrates are reported.

COMPLICATIONS. Rapid destruction of pulmonary tissue with suppuration or residual fibrosis occurs in as many as half of the surviving patients. Necrosis may occur within 24 to 48 hours, and abscess formation may be recognized within four days. Less common pulmonary complications include pleural effusion and pneumothorax. Rarely, massive pulmonary gangrene complicates lobar *Klebsiella* pneumonia; surgical removal of the lung tissue may be required to ensure patient survival. In the past, activation of quiescent pulmonary tuberculosis has been reported. It is believed that some of these cases actually represent a slough of localized tuberculous disease by the necrotizing *Klebsiella* pneumonia.

The course of illness is not marked by frequent extrapulmonary manifestations, but they can occur and include pericarditis, meningitis, gastroenteritis, erythematous skin rashes, and nonsuppurative polyarthritis.

PROGNOSIS AND TREATMENT. In the preantimicrobial era, the case mortality of *Klebsiella* pneumonia ranged from 51 to 97 per cent. The use of antimicrobials has markedly decreased mortality, but in some series the mortality remains nearly 50 per cent. In these series there has been a predominance of severely ill, alcoholic patients, although good results have been reported even in this group. Analysis of the mode of death frequently reveals that inadequate removal of tenacious pulmonary secretions was a significant factor. The correlation of bloodstream invasion and fatality is frequently close.

The majority of strains of *Klebsiella* are susceptible in vitro to chloramphenicol, the cephalosporins, and the aminoglycosides. Some of the "second and third generation" cephalosporins (cefoxitin and cefotaxime) and new penicillin antibiotics (piperacillin and mezlocillin) have good activity against *Klebsiella* also; however, clinical experience is still limited for some of these antibiotics in serious infections. The antimicrobial regimen of choice varies according to the gravity of the acute clinical situation and the extent of the underlying problem. Because necrosis of lung tissue can occur so rapidly, it is essential that maximally effective antimicrobial therapy be started immediately. In patients with life-threatening infection, which is at least potentially always the case, a two-drug regimen of intravenous cephalothin and an aminoglycoside (gentamicin) is recommended. After several days of such therapy, if the infection is well under control, the cephalothin may be discontinued. Meticulous measures directed at supportive care—maintenance of clear airways, adequate but not excessive ventilation and oxygenation, adequate fluid and electrolyte replacement, and often control of delirium tremens—are essential.

An emerging problem is the developing resistance of *Klebsiella* to multiple antibiotics, including gentamicin. In such a situation another aminoglycoside should be chosen, and, if possible, drug susceptibility studies should be done. Streptomycin, amikacin, and tobramycin are the principal drugs from among which a choice must be made.

CHRONIC CAVITARY KLEBSIELLA DISEASE

Occasionally chronic cavitary disease of the lung will result from infection with *Klebsiella.* In some cases this chronic disease is a known sequel to a primary pneumonia. In other cases, there is no convincing history of such an acute process and the disease appears to have persisted in subacute or chronic form for many months. Because of the rarity of this form of *Klebsiella* disease, its natural history has not been well characterized. It should be treated initially with the drug-pairing regimen of cephalothin and gentamicin, which can be appropriately modified as improvement occurs. The general treatment should be that for any other lung abscess, including surgical excision in rare cases (see Ch. 63).

Bauernfeind A, Petermuller C, Schneider R: Bacteriocins as tools in analysis of nosocomial *Klebsiella* pneumoniae infections. J Clin Microbiol 14:15, 1981. *Perhaps a simpler method of typing and good for epidemiologic studies.*

Bloomfield AL: The fate of bacteria introduced into the upper air passages. V. The Friedländer bacilli. Bull Johns Hopkins Hosp 31:203, 1920. *A historical account but still pertinent.*

Knight L, Fraser RG, Robson HG: Massive pulmonary gangrene: A severe complication of *Klebsiella* pneumonia. Can Med Assoc J 112:196, 1975. *A rare complication that requires surgical resection.*

Lerner AM: The gram-negative bacillary pneumonias. Disease-a-Month, November 1980, pp 1–56. *Excellent review.*

O'Callaghan RJ, Rousset KM, Harkness NK, Murray ML, Lewis AC, Williams WL: Analysis of increasing antibiotic resistance of *Klebsiella pneumoniae* relative to changes in chemotherapy. J Infect Dis 138:293, 1978. *An all too common problem with many bacteria.*

264. PNEUMONIA CAUSED BY OTHER AEROBIC GRAM-NEGATIVE BACILLI (Pseudomonas, Escherichia coli, and Serratia)

Herbert Y. Reynolds

Bacterial species that belong to the families Enterobacteriaceae and Pseudomonadaceae are considered together because of (1) similarities in the pulmonary infection they produce and (2) common circumstances in which they cause disease. Only a few of the bacteria that are frequently encountered as respiratory pathogens will be discussed individually. Others may be important in special instances, but statistically are less of a problem. Specialized texts on microbial diseases and the periodical literature can supply more detailed information about rare or unusual infections.

The family Enterobacteriaceae is composed of numerous interrelated bacilli, all of which are gram-negative, are nonsporulating, grow on ordinary media, and rapidly ferment glucose. The following genera are included in the family: *Shigella, Escherichia, Salmonella, Arizona, Citrobacter, Edwardsiella, Klebsiella, Enterobacter, Serratia, Proteus, Providencia,* and *Erwinia.* The nonfermenting aerobic gram-negative bacilli are recognized with almost equal frequency. Organisms in this category include *Pseudomonas aeruginosa, P. maltophilia, P. pseudomallei, P. cepacia, P. stutzeri, Acinetobacter lwoffi* (previously *Mima polymorpha*), *Acinetobacter anitratus* (previously *Herellea vaginicola* and *Achromobacter anitratus*), *Alcaligenes spp., Achromobacter spp., Flavobacterium spp., Moraxella spp.,* and *Aeromonas hydrophila.* Infections caused by *Pseudomonas pseudomallei* (melioidosis) are presented in Ch. 290.

Pulmonary infections associated with the small aerobic gram-negative bacilli belonging to the genera *Bordetella, Brucella, Hemophilus,* and *Yersinia,* as well as nonsporulating anaerobic gram-negative bacilli, e.g., *Bacteroides* and *Fusobacterium,* are discussed in the individual chapters dealing with each of these infections. Pneumonia caused by *Klebsiella* is the subject of Ch. 263.

Aerobic gram-negative bacilli are frequently the cause of respiratory infection in two groups of patients: those who develop a superinfection or acquire an infection in the hospital (nosocomial), and those who are immunocompromised. These topics are discussed in detail in Ch. 257 and 258.

NOSOCOMIAL PNEUMONIA—PREDISPOSING FACTORS

Many common aerobic gram-negative bacteria normally inhabit the human gastrointestinal tract, and a significant number of healthy, normal people have oropharyngeal colonization with a small number of these bacteria. Certain species such as *Pseudomonas aeruginosa* can be isolated from various skin sites (hands and axillae) in some instances. Since these bacteria are part of the normal microbial flora, they rarely cause primary infection. However, they are a menace for superinfection or secondary hospital-acquired infections. The magnitude of this infectious disease problem is large in terms of patient morbidity and mortality and financial burden to the health care system. Hospital-acquired infections develop in approximately 5 to 7 per cent of all hospitalized patients, with infections of the urinary tract and surgical wounds still causing most of them. However, lower respiratory tract infections account for 15 to 20 per cent of these infections in medical and surgical patients. Perhaps more disturbing than the frequency of respiratory infections is the poor success generally cited for treatment and control. Serious underlying disease is usually present, and, despite antimicrobial therapy, the case mortality from nosocomial pneumonia may approach 50 per cent, depending somewhat on the specific causative bacterium and the clinical setting of the patient. Because *Klebsiella pneumoniae, Pseudomonas aeruginosa, Serratia spp.*, and, less frequently, other gram-negative rods are the cause of severe, nosocomial respiratory infections in hospitalized and/or immunocompromised patients, some general comments about the enviromental setting and alterations in lung host defenses will be offered before focusing on individual disease entities.

Conditions which lead to nosocomial pneumonia are usually obvious. Susceptible patients invariably have one or a combination of the following: (1) chronic debilitating illness, often requiring prolonged hospitalization; (2) prior therapy with antimicrobial drugs having a broad spectrum; (3) a breach of the airway by tracheostomy or endotracheal tube; and (4) impaired host immunity (cellular and/or humoral) owing to a primary disease or as a consequence of immunosuppressive therapy.

The hospital environment itself is a prime source of opportunistic microorganisms and a good repository for some hardy drug-resistant strains. However, the term "nosocomial," strictly defined as an infection originating in a hospital or as one that is not clinically evident or incubating at the time of hospital admission, may not include all the circumstances inducing it. Other descriptions, such as iatrogenic or autogenic infection and superinfection, are often more appropriate.

Chronic illness and hospitalization per se are associated with some striking changes in patterns of bacterial colonization of the respiratory tract which seem significant. Generally the oropharynx of a normal person is not a very suitable environment for growth of aerobic gram-negative bacteria. Yet colonization develops rapidly in patients admitted to a medical intensive care unit, for example, and occurs in about half of them within a few days of admission. Patients with diabetes mellitus or alcoholism also have an increased carriage of gram-negative bacilli in their oropharynx. Such colonization of the respiratory tract apparently plays a major role in the pathogenesis of nosocomial respiratory infections through aspiration of oropharyngeal secretions which inoculate the airways. Thus, a change in nutritional milieu of the oronasopharynx induced by chronic disease, prior antibiotics, gingival disease, metabolic disease, and many other causes promotes sticking and adherence of certain bacteria to buccal mucosal cells, which may lead to colonization. Moreover, altered mentation, which depresses control of swallowing mechanisms or coughing, compounds the aspiration problem. When pharyngeal and sputum cultures become positive for Enterobacteriaceae or Pseudomonadaceae and other pathogenic bacteria, it is likely that the respiratory tract is also colonized with these microorganisms. Such a finding should alert one to impending respiratory infection. New techniques to assess adherence of bacteria to the patient's buccal mucosa cells or respiratory ciliated cells cultured in vitro may prove important in selecting patients who are susceptible to bacterial colonization. Such susceptible persons might profit from enhanced surveillance or prophylactic use of a topical antimicrobial drug in the oropharynx to prevent colonization with potential pathogens. The future will decide the usefulness of this approach.

The importance of prior antimicrobial therapy as a determinant of oropharyngeal colonization with gram-negative bacilli is not as obvious as might be expected. Some studies which recorded development of colonization in hospitalized patients have failed to find strong evidence that prior or concomitant antimicrobial use was a requisite factor, although such therapy usually increases the occurrence of colonization. On the contrary, in principle, broad-spectrum antimicrobial therapy that reduces a proportion of the normal bacterial flora of the gastrointestinal tract and naso-oropharyngeal area should improve the opportunity for more drug-resistant strains to emerge. Perhaps of greater significance is the emergence of fungal strains in the wake of a bacterial void so that colonization with these opportunistic organisms presages respiratory infection.

An interruption in the continuity of the airway with an endotracheal tube, for example, is often associated with bacterial colonization of the tracheobronchial tree and with recurrent respiratory infections. Important mechanical barriers that guard entry into the lungs are bypassed and microorganisms have direct access. Some aspiration of upper airway secretions often continues despite the inflated cuff around the tube, and the situation can be compounded if ventilatory equipment is attached that may itself contain a source of bacteria and, in fact, forcefully aerosolize them into the airway. In the time since it was demonstrated that contaminated inhalation respiratory equipment could be the source of nosocomial pneumonia, significant improvement has occurred in the general care and handling of this equipment, with the pleasing result that this form of iatrogenic infection is less frequent.

The immunocompromised patient presents a complex array of disordered host defenses, and the lungs are but one organ system at risk for infection. Predisposition to pneumonia with gram-negative bacilli occurs because a number of cellular components in the respiratory tract are vulnerable to the direct effects of various antineoplastic chemotherapy drugs and anti-inflammatory agents, or they may have been depleted because renewal from the bone marrow, for example, is inadequate. (See Lung Host Defenses in Ch. 257.)

Granulocytopenia is the most common abnormality in patients who have ineffective granulocytopoiesis or are receiving cytotoxic chemotherapy. With an inadequate systemic supply of circulating phagocytic cells, a lack of reserve or marginated granulocytes develops in capillary storage areas, such as the lung capillary vasculature. As a result the lower respiratory tract lacks secondary phagocytes that can be attracted to alveolar areas to attack bacteria, and the inflammatory response is diminished.

Although alveolar macrophages do not appear to be as easily depleted as the short-lived polymorphonuclear granulocytes in the immunosuppressed subject, subtle metabolic effects from cytotoxic drugs probably do impair their phagocytic and bactericidal capacity, thereby accounting for the greater susceptibility of the host to respiratory infections. Available evidence indicates that bone marrow–derived circulating monocytes are the precursors of tissue macrophages in the lungs. After the monocyte enters the pulmonary lymphoreticular system, it undergoes further development into a mature phagocytic macrophage which has a life span of months or years. Alveolar macrophages obtained by lung lavage from leukemia patients who have been leukopenic (monocytopenic) for several months are functionally and morphologically normal, despite intensive chemotherapy. Moreover, some human pulmonary macrophages are capable of a slow rate of replication, which suggests that the number of lung macrophages can be maintained in part by local cell proliferation when the usual influx of cells from peripheral blood and from bone marrow is absent.

Lymphoid tissue is extensive along the airways, and its alteration could directly affect the lung's handling of antigenic substances contained in respired air. Certain populations of lymphocytes are sensitive to radiotherapy (T cells) and may be eliminated when various forms of irradiation therapy are given. Cytotoxic drugs such as cyclophosphamide have various effects on both major subpopulations of lymphocytes (B and T cells). Cytotoxic agents, therefore, have the potential for blunting cell-mediated immune responses as well as for impeding the development of immunoglobulin-producing lymphocytes and plasma cells that secrete local secretory antibodies onto respiratory mucosal surfaces. Deficiencies in circulating humoral antibodies also occur in persons who are heavily immunosuppressed.

The consequence of injury to other cell types in the lung, such as surfactant-secreting Type II alveolar epithelial cells, various mucus-producing cells, and ciliated epithelial cells, is largely conjectural, because the deleterious effects of immunosuppressive agents on these cell types have not been established. Yet it seems plausible that drastic regimens of immunosuppressive therapy may impair the function of these cells. The cumulative effects of diminished surfactant production promoting lung atelectasis, altered mucus secretion, and reduced ciliary clearance all could contribute to stasis and accumulation of lung secretions which promote local bacterial growth and subsequent pneumonia.

PNEUMONIA CAUSED BY PSEUDOMONAS

Pseudomonas, which is a distinct genus of bacteria and is not included in the family Enterobacteriaceae, is widespread in the environment and is generally part of the usual bacterial flora of hospitals and intensive care units. *Pseudomonas* organisms are frequently carried on the skin (axillary and anogenital areas) of normal people and transiently may be part of the intestinal flora in a significant number (up to 20 per cent). Almost any alteration in normal health status, such as hospitalization or antimicrobial or immunosuppressive therapy, is associated with increased carriage of *Pseudomonas* organisms.

For this discussion, *Pseudomonas* respiratory infection refers to infection caused by *Pseudomonas aeruginosa,* which is the most important pathogen of the genus. The reader should remember, however, that other *Pseudomonas* species can cause serious infections (*P. pseudomallei* [melioidosis] and P. *mallei* [glanders]). Moreover, other less frequently encountered species are being implicated in human infection. *P. cepacia* has the distinction of being at least one in this group of clinical pathogens that is generally not susceptible to gentamicin, hence making drug susceptibility testing necessary for proper drug selection. Increasingly, this species is becoming a problem for those with cystic fibrosis.

PREDISPOSING FACTORS. *Pseudomonas* rarely produces infection in a normal person but is a frequent cause of sepsis and pneumonia in the abnormal host. It continues, along with *Klebsiella,* to be among the organisms most frequently isolated from patients with nosocomial pneumonia. In the past, chronic lung or heart disease apparently increased susceptibility to *Pseudomonas* pneumonia; now leukopenia (granulocytopenia) and other evidence of immunosuppressive disease or treatment is more common. *Pseudomonas* infection is likely to be an acquired or secondary pneumonia following any one of the predisposing causes already outlined. As a form of primary pneumonia, it is essentially limited to patients who are receiving inhalation therapy that incorporates reservoir nebulization. Following *Pseudomonas* bacteremia, pulmonary complications are well described, consisting of nodular areas of lung infarction with massive bacterial infiltration of arterial and venous walls. Such bacteremia produces a form of necrotizing pneumonia. This presentation may occur in illicit intravenous-drug users who develop *Pseudomonas* tricuspid endocarditis. People with cystic fibrosis (CF) have a special problem with *Pseudomonas.* This organism may not initiate lung infection and tissue destruction in CF, for staphylococci are usually the culprit, but *Pseudomonas* eventually becomes the long-term nemesis. Sputum and lungs of CF subjects are persistently colonized with the organism, which causes frequent episodes of bronchitis and pneumonia. Infection-free intervals become shorter, and multiple courses of parenteral antibiotic therapy are required to control *Pseudomonas* in the lungs. A mucoid, slime-producing strain of *P. aeruginosa* has a peculiar affinity for the CF lung.

PATHOGENESIS AND PATHOLOGY. The ubiquitous *Pseudomonas* organisms seem benign and harmless when they encounter a normal person. For the altered or compromised host, they are invasive and virulent. The bacterium is well equipped with an arsenal of extracellular toxins (exotoxin A), proteolytic enzymes (elastase and collagenase), hemolytic factors (phospholipases), leukocidin, pigments (pyocyanin and fluorescein), and cell wall endotoxin, which variously affect host tissues and inflammatory cells. Also, *Pseudomonas* has a capsular slime coat which may provide added protection. An adequate supply of granulocytes seems to be an important determinant in host resistance to infection. Once pseudomonads become enmeshed in lung tissue, they are difficult to eradicate completely, and colonization or chronic infection may persist.

On microscopic section, the intra-alveolar inflammatory exudate is a mixture of polymorphonuclear leukocytic and mononuclear cells, or the cellular infiltrates may consist predominantly of mononuclear cells admixed with fragmented pyknotic nuclei of necrotic neutrophils. At a later stage, alveolar spaces are filled with a deeply basophilic granular material containing large macrophage-like cells and dense colonies of gram-negative bacilli. In an abscess there is often focal hemorrhage. The dominant microscopic lesion is that of alveolar septal necrosis. In association with these necrotizing lesions, necrosis of arterial walls and secondary thrombosis of vessels have been encountered when the *Pseudomonas* pneumonia is of bacteremic origin or associated with nebulizing therapy equipment. In primary *Pseudomonas* pneumonia, as reported by Tillotson and Lerner (1968), vascular involvement is not a feature. *Pseudomonas cepacia* is also associated with a necrotizing granulomatous pneumonia.

CLINICAL FEATURES. In patients with *Pseudomonas* pneumonia, apprehension, toxicity, confusion, and progressive cyanosis are characteristic; hemoptysis is unusual. Relative bradycardia may occur. Alteration in diurnal temperature patterns, with the peak temperature in early morning, was noted by Tillotson and Lerner. The physical signs over the thorax are those found with any pneumonic process. The development of empyema is common and may occur in 30 to 50 per cent of patients. In CF patients with chronic and recurrent episodes of *Pseudomonas* pneumonia, cough and sputum and chest signs are evident, but they may have only low grade fever and little elevation in white blood cell count. Infection is confined to the respiratory tract, and septicemia or peripheral sites of infection virtually never occur. Roentgenograms reveal bilateral pneumonic infiltrates, usually in the lower lobe, that are often nodular and may undergo necrosis, with abscesses that may be small but are often greater than 1 cm in diameter. A pattern of interstitial infiltration may be seen. With resolution of pneumonia, areas of lung with poor expansion and residual "scarring" may be noted on follow-up chest films.

LABORATORY FINDINGS. The usual laboratory tests such as leukocyte counts are of little help, their results being either normal or moderately increased but most often reflecting the bone marrow status of an underlying disease. Cultures of sputum are of only moderate help, because *Pseudomonas* organisms are frequently present as commensals in patients who are receiving antimicrobial therapy or in those who are critically ill. Distinguishing tissue infection from colonization may be facilitated by a serum antibody response to *Pseudomonas* exotoxin A. Infection and invasive disease may elicit an antibody titer of 1:1000 in patients who are not immunosuppressed. If the situation necessitates establishing with certainty the organism involved, specimens could be collected by transtracheal aspiration or by other methods already suggested. With empyema, thoracentesis with staining and culture of the fluid will help confirm the diagnosis and facilitate the selection of optimal therapy.

PROGNOSIS AND TREATMENT. Prognosis varies with the underlying condition of the patient. Patients with CF often have chronic *Pseudomonas* infection punctuated by acute episodes of pneumonia. Although the infections can be suppressed and controlled for a variable period of time, up to many years, eventually recurrent *Pseudomonas* infections cause considerable morbidity and the demise of the patient. Case mortality rates in the range of 80 per cent are not uncommon in the immunocompromised patient with nosocomial *Pseudomonas* pneumonia, especially if bacteremia develops. However, in recent years, the mortality seems distinctly less and appears to be about 50 per cent. Several important advances have occurred. First, better antimicrobial drugs are available. The use of an aminoglycoside (gentamicin, tobramycin, or netilmicin) and carbenicillin (or ticarcillin) in combination for *Pseudomonas aeruginosa* infections has had a dramatic impact. Tobramycin seems to be the drug of choice for nonresistance strains, and amikacin is best reserved for use when resistance to another aminoglycoside develops. Several new penicillins are available as alternatives to carbenicillin and tricarcillin, if *Pseudomonas* drug resistance is a problem. These are piperacillin, mezlocillin, and azlocillin. They are active against many gram-negative bacilli but are ineffective against beta-lactamase-producing bacteria. Because *Pseudomonas* resistance can develop if one of the penicillin antibiotics is used alone, they are given in combination with an aminoglycoside. One advantage of these new penicillins is their lower sodium content. Several newer "third generation" cephalosporins have activity against *Pseudomonas* strains (cefoperazone, ceftazidin*, and cefulodin*) and may offer additional options for antibiotic selection. However, clinical use of these drugs for serious *Pseudomonas* infections is still rather limited. Undoubtedly, it will be necessary to search for additional antimicrobials in the future to keep ahead of the adaptable *Pseudomonas* strains. Second, medical personnel are much more aware of their role in the transmission of this ubiquitous microorganism, and appropriate changes in patient care techniques have been made. Third, meticulous cleanliness of respiratory ventilation equipment and use of disposable endotracheal or tracheostomy suctioning devices are routine.

Other forms of supportive care are also essential. Because *Pseudomonas* organisms are difficult to clear from infected lung tissue, patients will frequently relapse after drug therapy is discontinued, despite what is considered an adequate course of therapy. Re-treatment is usually necessary and should be done in conjunction with drug susceptibility testing. With successful treatment, *Pseudomonas* may still reappear in the sputum, making it necessary to distinguish between relapse and persistent colonization of the respiratory tract. Changing lung infiltrates and clinical signs help separate the two. Passive antibody administration of anti-*Pseudomonas* gamma globulin or prophylactic immunization of high-risk patients with *Pseudomonas* lipopolysaccharide antigens may become practical in the future. Granulocyte transfusion therapy in appropriate patients is a reasonable possibility.

PNEUMONIA DUE TO OTHER AEROBIC GRAM-NEGATIVE BACILLI (E. coli, Serratia Marcescens, and Proteus spp.)

Many bacterial species other than *Klebsiella pneumoniae* that belong to the families Enterobacteriaceae and Achromobacteraceae may produce pulmonary infection. In addition, in many

*Investigational drugs in U.S.A.

hospitals other gram-negative organisms such as *Serratia marcescens* are being encountered, especially in hospital-associated secondary pneumonia.

Primary *E. coli* pneumonia tends to be present as a scattered pneumonic process in the lower lobes. Empyema formation is less common than with *Klebsiella* or *Pseudomonas*. *E. coli* bacteremia from a urinary or gastrointestinal source results in lung infection more commonly than does bacteremia from other gram-negative bacilli.

Proteus species also produce a clinical picture similar to that of *Klebsiella* (see Ch. 263), with fever, chills, dyspnea, pleuritic chest pain, and cough productive of purulent sputum. Signs of consolidation are usual. Roentgenograms reveal dense infiltrates in the posterior segment of an upper lobe or superior segment of the right lower lobe. Progression to lung abscess or empyema is common.

Serratia infections, which are always secondary, have been associated with "pseudohemoptysis" resulting from a red pigment produced by some strains of *Serratia marcescens*. Other features may include abscess formation, empyema, or both.

Clinical experience with the other bacterial genera such as *Flavobacterium* and *Acinetobacter* is limited, but suggests that their clinical manifestations are similar to those of secondary *Klebsiella* infections.

The antimicrobial regimen of choice may be selected according to the physician's knowledge of the epidemiologic pattern of drug resistance to be anticipated in a given community, but should be confirmed, when possible, by tests on an individual patient's organism.

Doggett RG (ed.): *Pseudomonas aeruginosa*—Clinical Manifestations of Infection and Current Therapy. New York, Academic Press, 1979. *A fine book with experienced authors covering all important features of* Pseudomonas *disease.*

Fick RB, Reynolds HY: *Pseudomonas* respiratory infection in cystic fibrosis: A possible defect in opsonic IgG antibody. Bull Eur Physiopathol Resp 19:151, 1983. *More details about mechanisms of infection in these patients.*

Gilardi GL: Infrequently encountered *Pseudomonas* species causing infection in humans. Ann Intern Med 77:211, 1972. *Emphasizes that other* Pseudomonas *organisms can be pathogenic.*

Higushi JH, Johanson WG: Colonization and bronchopulmonary infection. Clin Chest Med January 1982, p 133. *By authors who have spearheaded this clinical association.*

Jonas M, Cunha BA: Bacteremic *Escherichia coli* pneumonia. Arch Intern Med 142:2157, 1982. *Still a virulent infection and perhaps overlooked among the other gram-negative pneumonias.*

LaForce FM: Hospital-acquired gram negative rod pneumonias: An overview. Am J Med 70:664, 1981. *A good update.*

Pierce AK, Sanford JP: Aerobic gram-negative bacillary pneumonias: State of the art. Am Rev Respir Dis 110:647, 1974. *Still a good review.*

Pollack M, Longfield RN, Karney WW: Clinical significance of serum antibody responses to exotoxin A and type-specific lipopolysaccharides in patients with *Pseudomonas aeruginosa* infections. Am J Med 74:980, 1983. *A new laboratory parameter that seems helpful.*

Reynolds HY, Fick RB Jr.: *Pseudomonas aeruginosa* pulmonary infections (emphasizing nosocomial pneumonia and respiratory infections in cystic fibrosis). In Sabath LD (ed.): *Pseudomonas aeruginosa*—the Organism, Diseases It Causes and Their Treatment. Bern, Hans Humber, 1980, pp 71–88. *This reference complements the present chapter. Of more importance is the book itself, which is another excellent volume on most facets of the bacterium.*

Reynolds HY, Levine AS, Wood RE, Zierdt CH, Dale DC, Pennington JE: *Pseudomonas aeruginosa* infections: Persisting problems and current research to find new therapies. Ann Intern Med 82:819, 1975. *Most helpful on the immunocompromised patient. Reviews approaches to immunotherapy.*

Tillotson JR, Lerner AM: Characteristics of pneumonias caused by *Escherichia coli*. N Engl J Med 277:115, 1967. *Best description of this infection.*

Tillotson JR, Lerner AM: Characteristics of nonbacteremia *Pseudomonas* pneumonia. Ann Intern Med 68:295, 1968. *The classic clinical description.*

265. ASPIRATION PNEUMONIA

Herbert Y. Reynolds

Pneumonitis is an important host response of the respiratory tract to a variety of substances, liquid and particulate, that can be inhaled into the airways. The nature of the inciting material dictates the degree of inflammation and the extent of its effect on the lungs. These materials can be divided for convenience into (1) inert, nontoxic substances; (2) acid gastric contents; (3) fluid admixed with food particles, which can cause mechanical obstruction to airways; and (4) oropharyngeal secretions laden with bacteria. A variety of liquids, if breathed into the lungs, cause acute pulmonary edema, including fresh and sea water (near-drowning), acid gastric juice, and halogenated aromatic hydrocarbons. Also, innumerable chemical agents inhaled as fumes or vapors cause irritation, edema, bronchorrhea, and varying degrees of alveolitis or bronchitis (see Ch. 560). Aspiration of solid foreign bodies, which usually occurs in children or in those suffering maxillofacial trauma, may be suspected if acute coughing or wheezing develops. Often the only residual clue is radiographic evidence of a persisting infiltrate or a localized area of lung collapse or of overinflation, suggesting endobronchial obstruction. Thus, there are many causes and kinds of inocula that produce a pulmonary inhalation syndrome of dyspnea, cough, airway irritation, alveolitis, pulmonary edema, and, frequently, infection. Lung infection and abscess are such frequent concomitants that their control is an important part of therapy and management (see Ch. 281).

PATHOGENESIS. With normal swallowing the tongue rises against the hard palate to propel a bolus into the pharynx, and aspiration is prevented by closure of the soft palate, glottis, and epiglottis. However, aspiration of small amounts of pharyngeal fluid is a normal occurrence, especially during deep sleep. Yet the saliva and nasal drainage, admixed with normal bacterial flora of the nose and mouth, which trickle into the trachea and bronchi incite no reaction or symptoms; presumably normal mucociliary clearance removes the secretions and microorganisms. In the absence of gastric regurgitation, which might add acid to the oral secretions, the pH of oropharyngeal fluid is neutral, and this fact may minimize irritation.

The normal microbial flora of the oral cavity is complex, and each anatomic site—mucous membranes, tooth surfaces, and gingival crevices—has elements of an individual flora. Anaerobic bacteria predominate over aerobic ones in a ten-fold ratio and the microbiota is diverse. Anaerobes isolated from the gingiva include *Bacteroides oralis, B. melaninogenicus, Fusobacterium,* and other spirochetal forms. *Streptococcus mutans* and *S. sanguis* are found on tooth surfaces and in dental plaque, whereas the tongue and buccal surfaces contain many forms of aerobic gram-positive and gram-negative bacteria such as *Streptococcus viridans, Neisseria catarrhalis,* enterococci, *S. pneumoniae, Staphylococcus aureus,* and *Hemophilus spp.* Furthermore, *Candida spp.* and certain known pathogens, such as *S. pyogenes* and *N. meningitidis,* presumably as part of a carrier state, can be recovered in asymptomatic people. Enterobacteriaceae are rare, but their carriage increases tremendously with hospitalization and serious illness. Why aspiration syndromes are particularly associated with indigenous, saprophytic, noninvasive anaerobic strains of bacteria is not completely understood. Concomitant lung tissue necrosis, presence of poorly vascularized lung or malignant tissue, plentiful facultative bacterial growth in existing bronchiectatic airways, or poor dental hygiene with an unusually large number of anaerobic bacteria in the gum tissue, coupled with malnutrition, immunosuppressive therapy, diabetes, or alcoholism, all may variously combine to make the host more susceptible to local lung growth of these organisms. Mixed infections with a variety of anaerobic and aerobic bacteria are common.

The aspiration of gastric acid secretions with low pH (<2.5) is usually thought to be an important cause of aspiration injury. Originally this entity defined the aspiration syndrome. Mendelson noted that obstetric patients who aspirated liquid gastric contents (40 of the 66 patients were so classified) developed an asthma-like syndrome which also included cyanosis, rales, rhonchi, and occasionally pulmonary edema. This developed acutely but resolved quickly (in 36 hours) with an uncomplicated recovery in 75 per cent and no mortality. This clinical sequence is less severe than the fulminant, life-threatening disease that acid aspiration produces in animal models and in nonobstetric patients, which is characterized by widespread, rapid damage from a chemical burn of the airways and alveoli. Acute pulmonary edema, hemorrhage, and degeneration of the alveolar epithelial surface occur, accompanied by necrosis of Type I pneumocytes; a few hours later, the pulmonary transudate has been replaced by an infiltration of polymorphonuclear granulocytes and deposition of fibrin in alveoli. Alveolar epithelial permeability for albumin and larger-sized molecules (>170,000 MW) is increased, so that many plasma components cross the blood-air barrier. Affected lung tissue evolves through an edematous, hemorrhagic, consolidated phase in which hyaline membranes are present if the patient or animal survives. Resolution features regeneration of bronchial epithelium, fibroblast proliferation, and resorbing inflammation. The clinical parallel of these changes is the adult respiratory distress syndrome, in which treatment is directed toward improving oxygenation in noncompliant, atelectatic lungs with poor ventilation and perfusion match-up.

What has been described is a catastrophic disease of extreme seriousness, yet the presentation usually encountered is far less severe. The animal model results from instillation of 1 to 5 ml per kilogram of dilute acid into the experimental lung. In most clinical situations, less toxic fluids or secretions are aspirated and usually in smaller quantities.

Blood may accumulate in the lung if aspiration follows hematemesis or hemoptysis; chest trauma with lung contusion is also a common source of blood in the airways. Blood may cause acute local airway obstruction and may result in areas of atelectasis and lung infiltration. The residual blood itself is eventually well handled in the lungs. Although it may cause consolidation, it incites only a moderate inflammatory response and no necrosis of lung tissue. Alveolar macrophages ingest red blood cells and degrade them within a few days; hemosiderin-laden macrophages eventually can be found in sputum. However, repeated bleeding in an area of the lung can result in chronic inflammatory changes and interstitial fibrosis.

Of more pertinence to injury mechanisms that result from aspiration are the effects of nonacid (pH >2.5) liquid containing small, nonobstructing particles of food. This combination may be the most prevalent in hospitalized patients who are being fed through nasogastric tubes, or who have endotracheal tubes or tracheostomies. Similar circumstances may pertain to patients with neurologic disabilities, esophageal motor dysfunction, or a tracheoesophageal fistula. Repeated aspirations of small quantities of regurgitated liquid and foodstuff plus inhalation of oronasopharyngeal secretions during sleep may result in frequent and chronic insults to the airways. Although periodic bouts of fever and pneumonitis occur and chest radiographs often show infiltrates or residual scarring, it is often surprising how well this type of repeated aspiration is tolerated. Neutral, nonacid, clear, inert liquids incite little inflammatory response in the lungs; however, formula feeding, dairy products, and creamy liquids or soups cause more reaction. The size of the particles, their chemical composition, and the ease with which they disintegrate or undergo phagocytosis and biodegradation determine the degree of local inflammatory response. Hemorrhagic pneumonia and a parenchymal granulomatous response can occur from these kinds of insult. Concomitant bacterial infection does not seem to be a uniform complication, but excluding it can be difficult. A chemical alveolitis can produce the same physical and roentgenographic signs as bacterial pneumonitis. Infectious complications and lung abscess are more frequent in inebriated patients and those with depressed consciousness.

CLINICAL PRESENTATION. Aspiration syndromes constitute a spectrum ranging from tracheal obstruction from a bolus of meat to bronchial obstruction from a peanut or tooth, to inhalation of vomitus or blood during an emergency intubation procedure, to aspiration of fluids leaking around an endotracheal tube with development of a localized lung infiltrate. The overt and acute situations present no problem in diagnosis, but do require prompt action to remove an obstruction or suction out the airways, to control dyspnea and cough, and to correct hypoxia. Following apparent aspiration of acid gastric contents containing partially digested food particles, a brief latent period (up to one or two hours) may occur before clinical signs of respiratory distress develop. Often the patient has a disturbance of consciousness resulting from a sedative drug or general anesthesia. Tachypnea, fever (up to 39° C), diffuse rales, and hypoxemia develop in 70 to 90 per cent of patients, whereas cough, wheezing, cyanosis, and apnea occur in about one third. In the setting of aspirated gastric contents, lung infection develops in about 25 per cent of patients and becomes evident in three to five days. Apnea and shock are ominous signs that are likely to be associated with a fatal outcome. The adult respiratory distress syndrome frequently develops.

Inapparent or subtle forms of aspiration are often difficult to detect and troublesome to manage because of uncertainty about the diagnosis or because the condition cannot be easily remedied. The process may be recurrent and chronic. Persons who have lost consciousness from drug overdoses, inebriation, generalized seizures, or neurovascular injury are often assumed to have aspirated stomach or oropharyngeal fluid, although actual evidence of foreign material in the throat or trachea may be lacking. If pneumonia develops and an infiltrate is visible on radiograph, aspiration is a reasonable assumption, provided that a specific primary infection can be excluded. Following cardiopulmonary resuscitation or emergency intubation, patients may inhale fluid or blood, and subsequent pneumonitis is reasonably ascribed to aspiration. Once a patient is intubated or has a tracheostomy in place, the danger of aspiration is not over. A bit of red-colored gelatin appearing in the endotracheal suctioning catheter is a vivid indication that the patient is aspirating around an endotracheal tube. If a few drops of Evans blue dye are placed on the tongue of an intubated patient and dye is obtained by suctioning through the endotracheal tube, aspiration is proved. Such leakage of dye into the trachea will occur in about 20 per cent of patients who are intubated with a high volume, low pressure cuffed tube. Such a balloon cuff marks a technologic improvement over the low volume, high pressure cuffed tubes in standard use until a few years ago. With the stiffer, smaller balloon tube, the incidence of pericuff aspiration of blue dye was about 56 per cent. The incidence of aspiration in patients with tracheostomies has been reduced from about 80 per cent to 15 per cent by use of large volume, low pressure cuffs.

Other factors that contribute to potential aspiration in the hospitalized patient are presence of a nasogastric tube, supine position in bed, cloudy mental status, and inadequacy of cough reflex. Nasogastric tubes have been associated with aspiration. Imprecise gastric placement and poor mechanical suction or drainage may allow fluid to accumulate; the nasogastric tube passes through both upper and lower esophageal sphincters, making them incompetent and thus providing an easy route for liquid to travel. A greater risk may be posed by a small bore "pediatric" tube inserted through the nose and esophagus for intragastric feeding with liquid formula and hypertonic fluids. With this small tube it is impossible to evacuate the stomach of residual liquid prior to the next feeding. If gastric emptying is delayed and feeding is overly zealous, gastric overflow and regurgitation may occur. Careful regulation of the amount of feeding can obviate this complication. Other factors listed can be controlled by conscientious nursing care, which protects the patient until normal reflexes to cough and to swallow return.

Problems of chronic aspiration usually have a well-defined cause related to failure of mechanical closure of the airway during swallowing or to esophageal dysphagia. Neurologic sequelae affecting striated muscles of the pharynx (bulbar palsy), laryngectomy for cancer, and a variety of esophageal diseases are common causes. Overflow regurgitation of accumulated food and fluid occur with hypopharyngeal (Zenker's) diverticulum and functional esophageal obstruction (achalasia), so that aspiration pneumonia is a common complication. The esophagus is often affected in progressive systemic sclerosis, and difficult swallowing enhances the risk of aspiration. Occasionally, tumor, chest trauma, or irradiation therapy may create a complicating tracheoesophageal fistula through which swallowed fluid and small pieces of food are directly inhaled into the airways; persistent pneumonia and lung abscess usually develop.

LABORATORY AND RADIOGRAPHIC FINDINGS. Normal oropharyngeal fluids, including saliva and tracheobronchial secretions, have a neutral pH and a low glucose content (<5 mg per deciliter). With overt aspiration of acid stomach fluid, it may be possible transiently to record a low pH in fluid recovered from the airways, but the fluid is quickly buffered by plasma components and may be neutral. Recovery of food particles in suctioned airway fluid is prima facie evidence of aspiration. Because the glucose content is normally low in airway fluid, aspiration of oral feeding formulas can significantly elevate the glucose level (>25 to 90 mg per deciliter) in tracheobronchial secretions. As with most pneumonias, the peripheral white blood cell count is usually elevated.

Sputum analysis is essential, but microbial cultures can be confusing. The patient may complain of a foul taste to the sputum; it may smell putrid and contain some blood as well. A sputum Gram stain may not show a predominant organism but rather may contain a mixture of gram-positive and gram-negative flora and inflammatory cells. Failure to isolate an aerobic bacterial pathogen on culture should make one consider anaerobic organisms. Pending the patient's initial response to empiric antibiotic therapy, suitable culture specimens obtained by transtracheal aspirate or direct needle puncture must be considered. Expectorated sputum is of no value for anaerobic cultures because of contamination by normal mouth flora. If pleural fluid is present, a thoracentesis is indicated. If an abscess is present and bronchoscopy has been performed, anaerobic cultures should be made from the irrigation fluid, but the results can be confusing owing to contamination with mouth flora.

The bacteriology from 70 prospective cases of suspected aspiration in 38 community-acquired and 32 hospital-acquired infections (cultures obtained from blood, pleural fluid, or transtracheal aspiration) has provided some important information: Mixed bacteriologic infections (anaerobic and aerobic) were found in 26 per cent of the former compared with almost 60 per cent of the latter. Aerobic infections only were highest in the hospitalized patients (19 per cent versus 8 per cent). The high incidence of aerobic organisms probably reflects the frequency of aerobic gram-negative bacilli in the oropharynx of many chronically ill, hospitalized patients. Infection with anaerobes alone occurred in 66 per cent of the community-acquired aspirations but in only 22 per cent of hospital cases. The most frequent anaerobic isolates were *Bacteroides melaninogenicus*, peptostreptococcus, *Fusobacterium nucleatum*, peptococcus, and *B. fragilis;* of aerobic bacteria the most frequent were *Streptococcus pneumoniae*, *Staphylococcus aureus*, *Klebsiella spp.*, *Pseudomonas aeruginosa*, and *E. coli.*

On the chest radiograph, certain locations of a lung infiltrate have special importance in confirming or alerting the physician to the diagnosis of aspiration pneumonitis. In a recumbent, supine position, posterior segments of the upper lobes or the superior segments of the lower lobes may be dependent; in the upright position, basal segments of the lower lobes are susceptible. With acid aspiration, multiple lobes can be involved and the entire lung fields can show evidence of infiltration and alveolar filling if widespread pulmonary edema and the adult respiratory distress syndrome ensue.

If aspiration is complicated by an anaerobic lung infection, the initial localized pneumonitis may be subpleural and may spread to adjacent segments of lung or into the pleural space. As liquefaction and necrosis occur, the center of the pneumonia becomes a thin wall abscess, resulting in a cavity; if bronchial drainage develops, there will be an air-fluid level. Radiographically, one to two weeks is required for this sequence to occur. The picture of the abscess is not specific, and similar findings can occur with fungal and tuberculous infections, with aerobic bacterial infections, and occasionally from cavitating carcinoma. In these instances, the abscess tends to have a thicker, irregular, or shaggy wall.

THERAPY AND MANAGEMENT. Because pulmonary aspiration of gastric contents poses a hazard in emergency surgical patients and obstetric patients, attempts have been made to decrease gastric acidity with an H_2-receptor histamine antagonist, such as cimetidine or ranitidine. Such prophylactic therapy will increase pH signficantly and reduce gastric fluid volume in many (80 per cent) but not all patients, so its effects must be monitored.

Massive aspiration of blood or vomitus, especially with acid liquid, is an emergency. Debris must be cleared from the throat and airways, a patent airway established with an endotracheal tube, and adequate oxygenation provided. The situation may not stabilize, and intravenous fluid therapy for shock, plus assisted mechanical ventilation with use of end-expiratory pressure and high inspired concentrations of oxygen, may be needed. The use of corticosteroid therapy in this acute situation to minimize the chemical inflammatory reaction in lung parenchyma remains controversial. With experimental acid instillation into the lung, corticosteroid action lessens the impact of injury, provided that the drug is given prior to the injury. Delayed treatment is less helpful. In the clinical situation the drug can only be given after the initiating insult. However, administration of a high dose of intravenous corticosteroid as part of the immediate therapy will not likely cause complications and might contribute positively. Such therapy should not be continued for more than 24 hours after the insult was perceived to have occurred. Use of antibiotic therapy is likewise confusing. Bacterial pneumonia may follow acid aspiration in 25 to 45 per cent of cases, typically during the first week when the patient may be recovering from chemical pneumonitis. With the initial aspirating insult, oral bacteria undoubtedly inoculate the airways, so it might seem logical to eliminate them straightaway with early antibiotic therapy. Unfortunately, prophylactic antibiotic therapy does not seem to prevent pneumonia or favorably influence mortality. Thus, the prudent course may be to withhold antibiotic therapy but *carefully* observe the patient for evidence that bacterial infection has supervened. A new fever spike, progressive chest infiltrates, purulent sputum, or cultures showing pathogenic bacteria would dictate the addition of antibiotics. Similarly, with aspiration of inert, nontoxic fluids, bacterial infection may not invariably follow, so withholding antibiotics is recommended unless a clear indication for their use develops. This approach may suffice as well for patients who regurgitate liquid food feedings or who are noted to aspirate around cuffed endotracheal tubes. Nursing care directed toward evacuating residual gastric contents before refeeding, maintaining an upright position during eating, encouraging progressive ambulation, and improving pulmonary status to hasten extubation is the preferred course.

Aspiration of oropharyngeal secretions in patients with depressed levels of consciousness in whom dental and gingival hygiene are poor may lead to a necrotizing pneumonia, lung abscess, or empyema. Infection with a variety of anaerobic bacteria is a certainty; if the patient has been hospitalized or is chronically ill, concomitant infection with aerobic bacteria is likely. Antibiotic therapy is directed initially at the anaerobes, for which intermittent, high dose parenteral penicillin G is usually sufficient. An alternative choice is clindamycin, particularly if penicillin allergy is of concern. If aerobic bacterial coverage is deemed reasonable, inclusion of an aminoglycoside and an antistaphylococcal antibiotic is indicated. In this situation a combination such as gentamicin and clindamycin or the equivalent is good. In addition, vigorous maneuvers to promote pulmonary drainage of secretions (chest wall clapping and postural drainage) are advocated. Drainage of pleural fluid is often necessary.

Usually, a pulmonary abscess will eventually close with appropriate therapy, although some weeks may be required for this to happen. Antibiotic therapy is indicated until healing occurs, and a course of three to four weeks, or possibly several months, is often needed, rather than the customary ten to fourteen days of treatment suggested for routine pneumonias. Closure of the abscess cavity should be followed radiographically; if resolution does not occur, additional diagnostic evaluation is indicated, including sputum for cytology and fiberoptic bronchoscopy. Pulmonary carcinoma can be present in such an abscess area.

With chronic aspiration syndromes often not much can be offered, and in some instances radical procedures must be contemplated. For those with esophageal disorders care with eating and mechanical dilation of obstruction to promote better emptying and flow-through of ingested food may suffice. Occasionally to remedy defects in laryngeal closure, an arytenoid-epiglottic flap is reconstructed; oversewing the larynx necessitates a tracheostomy, prevents speech, and is a drastic solution. Such patients may have persistent areas of lung infiltration on chest radiograph which change or wax and wane in appearance. Continuous low grade fever may occur. The response is a low grade reactive pneumonitis which is not attended by many systemic symptoms or overwhelming infection. Antibiotic therapy is not indicated continuously and should be reserved for well-defined episodes.

Andrews AD, Brock JG, Downing JW: Protection against pulmonary acid aspiration with ranitidine. A new histamine H_2 antagonist. Anaesthesia 37:22, 1982. *Other similar articles, including those on the use of cimetidine, should be reviewed for timing of doses and expected results.*

Bartlett JG: The triple threat of aspiration pneumonia. Chest 68:560, 1975. *A nice review with helpful classification of aspiration syndromes.*

Bartlett JG: Aspiration pneumonia. Clin Notes Respir Dis 18:3, 1980. *Update of the preceding entry with pertinent references.*

Bynum LJ, Pierce AK: Pulmonary aspiration of gastric contents. Am Rev Respir Dis 111:1129, 1976. *Good clinical review focusing only on the problem of aspirating gastric contents.*

Huxley EJ, Viroslav J, Gray WR, Pierce AK: Pharyngeal aspiration in normal adults and patients with depressed consciousness. Am J Med 65:564, 1978. *Evidence seems conclusive that normal people can aspirate during sleep.*

Lorber B, Swenson RM: Bacteriology of aspiration pneumonia. A prospective study of community and hospitalized cases. Ann Intern Med 81:329, 1974. *Complements the Bartlett references and adds details about the etiology of infection in this disease.*

Mendelson CL: The aspiration of stomach contents into the lungs during obstetric anesthesia. Am J Obstet Gynecol 52:191, 1946. *The classic description, yet this disease in pregnant patients differs in severity from that in other patients who aspirate stomach acid secretions.*

Spray SB, Zuidema GD, Cameron JL: Aspiration pneumonia—incidence of aspiration with endotracheal tubes. Am J Surg 131:701, 1976. *A common problem that has been alleviated somewhat with the new endotracheal design of a high volume, low pressure cuff.*

Winterbauer R, Durning R Jr., Baron E, McFadden M: Aspirated nasogastric feeding solution detected by glucose strips. Ann Intern Med 95:67, 1981. *Interesting approach to diagnosis.*

Wynne JW, Modell JH: Respiratory aspiration of stomach contents. Ann Intern Med 87:466, 1977. *A thorough review with detailed discussion of therapy.*

266. LEGIONELLOSIS

David W. Fraser

DEFINITION. Legionellosis refers to acute bacterial infections of humans caused by *Legionella pneumophila, L. micdadei, L. bozemanii, L. dumoffii, L. gormanii, L. longbeachae, L. jordanis, L. oakridgensis, L. wadsworthii, L. feeleii*, or *L. morrisii*. As several additional species have been identified but not yet named, the list can be expected to lengthen. Infections caused by *Legionella spp.* have occurred in two distinct forms: legionnaires' disease, which is characterized by pneumonia, involvement of other organ systems, and (at least for *L. pneumophila*) a two- to ten-day incubation period; and Pontiac fever, which is characterized by fever without pneumonia or involvement of other organ systems and an incubation period of 5 to 66 hours.

ETIOLOGY. Members of the genus *Legionella* are aerobic, weakly staining, gram-negative bacilli that will not grow on most commonly used bacteriologic media but will grow on media containing supplementary L-cysteine, ferric salts, and activated charcoal. Growth is best at 35° C, but colonies may take up to 12 days to appear on primary culture, especially if the inocula are small. They do not form spores but contain vacuoles that stain with Sudan black B. Many strains are flagellated. In tissue, *L. micdadei* is partially acid fast if the Kinyoun modification is used. In all species, 60 per cent or more of cellular fatty acids have branched chains. They are catalase-positive but do not ferment sugars. *Legionella* species can be distinguished most readily by direct immunofluorescence but phenotypic differences are seen in regard to the presence and color of colonial autofluorescence in ultraviolet light, the pattern of fatty acids in gas liquid chromatography, browning of yeast extract agar medium supplemented with L-tyrosine, ability to hydrolyze hippurate, and gelatinase and oxidase activity. Nine serogroups of *L. pneumophila* and two of *L. longbeachae* have been identified that can be distinguished by direct immunofluorescence or slide agglutination. In addition, antigens are shared among the six serogroups of *L. pneumophila*, the species of Legionellae, and other genera of gram-negative bacilli. Legionellae are found in a wide variety of watery environments. *L. pneumophila* can survive more than one year in tap water. The means by which these fastidious bacteria survive so well in water has not been established, but the presence of algae, amebae, and other bacteria may be important. Apparent variations in the virulence of strains of *L. pneumophila* have been related to the presence or absence of plasmids and particular surface antigens.

EPIDEMIOLOGY. Although only recently recognized to cause human disease, three species of *Legionella* were first isolated decades ago (*L. micdadei*, 1943; *L. pneumophila*, 1947; *L. bozemanii*, 1959). Legionellae cause outbreaks of both pneumonic and nonpneumonic disease, as well as sporadic cases of pneumonia. The incidence of sporadic *L. pneumophila* pneumonia caused by serogroups 1 or 2 has been estimated from a prospective serologic study to be 12 cases per 100,000 population per year. The incidence of pneumonia caused by the other Legionellae is unknown but is probably much lower. Five per cent of recognized pneumonia cases caused by *L. pneumophila* and most so far recognized as being caused by *L. micdadei* are nosocomial. Cases of *Legionella* pneumonia have been documented in six continents. Cases occur throughout the year but primarily in the summer. Epidemiologic factors associated with increased risk of *L. pneumophila* pneumonia include male sex, middle or old age, cigarette smoking, excessive consumption of alcohol, travel, work in construction, residence near excavation or construction, and underlying medical conditions or therapy commonly associated with immunosuppression. Immunosuppression is also common in those with *L. micdadei* pneumonia.

The only proven mode of spread of *Legionella* is the airborne route. Outbreaks have been traced to airborne spread of bacteria released in aerosols by air-conditioning cooling towers, evaporative condensers, and industrial grinding machinery and inhaled by people downwind. *L. pneumophila* infections have been traced to contamination of the hot water in potable water systems, but whether spread in these cases is by aerosolization, drinking, or mucous membrane contact is unknown. Person-to-person spread has not been documented.

Clusters of *Legionella* infections have occurred in one or two epidemiologic patterns. Outbreaks of legionnaires' disease (named for the group most affected in the 1976 Philadelphia outbreak) are characterized by attack rates of 0.1 to 5.0 per cent for people presumed to be exposed. All documented point-source outbreaks have been caused by *L. pneumophila*, and the usual incubation period has been two to ten days (mean = 5.5 days). More than 30 outbreaks have been recognized. Pontiac fever outbreaks (named for the city in which an outbreak occurred in 1968) are characterized by attack rates of 95 to 100 per cent for people intensively exposed and by incubation periods of 5 to 66 hours (mean = 36 hours). Five such outbreaks have been documented, caused by *L. pneumophila* in four and *L. feeleii* in one. No differences in the source or mode of spread of the organism appear to explain the epidemiologic (or clinical—see later discussion) differences between legionnaires' disease and Pontiac fever.

PATHOGENESIS. Legionnaires' disease appears to occur two to ten days after inhalation of *L. pneumophila*. About half of those infected develop clinical illness. The only consistent pathologic condition found is in the lung and includes areas of acute fibrinopurulent pneumonia bounded by lobular septa. The infiltrate comprises polymorphonuclear leukocytes and macrophages, many of which are necrotic, mixed with proliferating Type II pneumocytes and fibrin. Large numbers of bacteria can be demonstrated by Dieterle silver stain or direct immunofluorescence in areas of pneumonia and commonly clustered in macrophages. Bacteria can also be seen in areas of pleuritis. The lung architecture is usually intact, although focal septal necrosis is sometimes seen, and frank lung abscess may occur in immunosuppressed people. Respiratory bronchioles are affected, but larger bronchioles and bronchi (and their cilia) are spared, perhaps explaining in part the usual paucity of sputum and rarity of person-to-person spread. Healing is commonly complete, but in some patients residual fibrosis can be detected by diminished capacity to diffuse carbon monoxide.

The degree to which involvement of organs other than the lungs is due to direct invasion by *L. pneumophila* or to remote effects of the organism in lung tissue is uncertain. Rarely, *L. pneumophila* has been visualized in mediastinal lymph nodes, blood vessels, liver, spleen, bone marrow, and kidneys and has been recovered from blood. *L. pneumophila* has some of the properties of endotoxins and produces a soluble hemolysin and lymphocytotoxin, but the role of these or other toxins in the pathogenesis of disease is unclear.

L. pneumophila organisms are ingested by monocytes, including human alveolar macrophages. In unactivated macrophages, the bacteria multiply freely—apparently helped by their ability to inhibit phagosome-lysozyme fusion. In macrophages that are activated, as by incubation with lymphocytes stimulated by concanavilin A, *L. pneumophila* multiply more slowly and may indeed be killed. The intracellular location of *Legionella* may help explain the poor agreement between antibiotic sensitivities observed in vitro and in vivo. Although complement-mediated killing of *L. pneumophila*, apparently by the classic pathway, is accelerated by specific antibody in vitro, a protective effect of antibody has not been shown in humans. The possibility that opsonic activity of serogroup-specific antibody is more protective of bacterium than host has been suggested.

Little is known about the pathophysiology of the Pontiac fever syndrome of *L. pneumophila* or *L. feeleii* infection or of the cases of pneumonia caused by Legionellae other than *L. pneumophila*. Pathologically, the latter cases resemble *L. pneumophila* pneumonia. No differences have been found in *L. pneumophila* strains that cause legionnaires' disease and Pontiac fever.

CLINICAL MANIFESTATIONS. *Legionella* infections occur in at least two distinct syndromes: legionnaires' disease and Pontiac fever. Pontiac fever is an acute influenza-like illness characterized by fever, headache, and myalgia. Cough, sore throat, diarrhea, confusion, and chest pain occur but are not usually prominent. Pneumonia does not occur, although one patient had a pleural friction rub during convalescence. The illness is debilitating for two to seven days, but all patients recover completely.

Legionnaires' disease varies in severity from a mild grippe to a severe multisystem disease affecting lungs, liver, kidney, gastrointestinal tract, and central nervous system. Typically, patients have the subacute onset of malaise, weakness, anorexia, dry cough, and fever, without accompanying upper respiratory symptoms. Illness progresses over the next day or two, commonly with repeated rigors, pleuritic chest pain, headache, watery diarrhea, generalized abdominal pain, and confusion. Sputum may be expectorated but is often scant and nonpurulent and may be streaked with blood. Patients appear acutely ill, usually with temperatures of 38.9 to 40.4° C. The degree of tachypnea reflects the severity of the pneumonia, but the pulse rate is often slower than would be expected from the temperature. Pulmonary rales are common early, and signs of consolidation may appear later. Nonfocal neurologic disturbances (confusion, clumsiness, ataxia, slurred speech, and apparent hallucinations) occur and often are of a severity disproportionate to the degree of fever or metabolic derangements.

Laboratory testing shows normal or moderately elevated leukocyte counts with an excess of juvenile neutrophils. Erythrocyte sedimentation rate is greatly elevated. Modest elevations of serum concentrations of transaminases are common. Microscopic hematuria is seen in one third of patients and is often accompanied by cylindruria and proteinuria. Azotemia is found at some time during the illness in about 15 per cent of patients and occasionally necessitates dialysis. Chest radiographs may show patchy infiltrates early in the disease, which later progress to dense consolidation, often in a lobar or segmental pattern and commonly bilaterally. Cavitation is sometimes seen in the immunocompromised host. Pleural effusions are seen in up to one third of patients but are small except in occasional immunosuppressed patients. Gram staining of transtracheally aspirated material usually shows moderate numbers of neutrophils, but large numbers of bacilli are rarely seen. The protein and cellular composition of pleural fluid suggests an exudate in half and a transudate in the other half of the cases in which it is examined. Cerebrospinal fluid is usually normal, although small numbers of lymphocytes have been seen. Without specific therapy fever, pneumonia, and accompanying hypoxemia may progress for five to seven days and be complicated by the syndrome of inappropriate secretion of antidiuretic hormone. Death occurs in 15 to 20 per cent of patients and is usually the result of progressive pneumonia; however, in a few cases a syndrome resembling septic shock precedes death. With specific therapy temperature generally begins to decrease within 24 hours and may be normal within two days, although radiographically the pneumonia may continue to progress for two to five days. Radiographic resolution of *L. pneumophila* pneumonia may take many weeks, longer than for pneumococcal or *Mycoplasma* pneumonia. Residual scarring can be seen histologically and radiographically. In rare cases patients with severe neurologic involvement show mild residual aphasia and impaired memory. Amnesia for the acute illness is common.

Rare cases of *Legionella* infection localized outside the lungs have involved perirectal abscess, focal myocarditis, hemodialysis fistula infection, or pyelonephritis. Coinfection with other bacteria may occur in such sites.

DIAGNOSIS. *Legionella* pneumonia must be distinguished from pneumonia caused by other bacteria or infections caused by *Mycoplasma pneumoniae, Chlamydia psittaci, Coxiella burnetii,* influenza virus, or several other respiratory viruses. Clinical clues that are of differential value for *L. pneumophila* pneumonia include very high fever with repeated rigors, lack of preceding upper respiratory symptoms, diarrhea, unexplained impairment of mental function, hematuria, abnormal liver function, negative routine bacteriologic cultures, and failure to respond to therapy with penicillins, cephalosporins, or aminoglycosides. Epidemiologic clues (see above) may also be helpful in suggesting the diagnosis. With *Legionella* pneumonia, staining well-collected lower respiratory secretions by the Gram method reveals neutrophils accompanied by no bacteria or by weakly staining gram-negative bacilli.

Specific diagnosis is made by isolation of *Legionella* from lung tissue, respiratory secretions, pleural fluid, or blood; detection of specific antigens in lung tissue, respiratory secretions, extrapulmonary tissue, or urine; or demonstration of a significant rise in serum antibody titer during convalescence. Charcoal yeast extract (CYE) agar or buffered CYE agar supports growth of all species, but isolation of *L. pneumophila* from sputum is aided by the incorporation of cefamandole (or vancomycin), polymyxin B, and anisomycin in the agar to inhibit other organisms. A biphasic medium with CYE agar as the solid phase has been successful for culture of *L. pneumophila* from blood. Direct immunofluorescence using species- and serogroup-specific conjugated antisera is useful in detecting *Legionella* in tissue and secretions. For *L. pneumophila,* about two thirds of infected patients have organisms detectable in lower respiratory tract secretions, and they remain detectable for an average of four days after specific therapy is started. *L. pneumophila* serogroup 1 antigen can be detected in the urine of most infected patients by latex agglutination, enzyme-linked immunoassay, or radioimmunoassay and may persist for many weeks. The procedure used for serologic detection of infection is usually indirect immunofluorescence, but this procedure is not well standardized for strains other than *L. pneumophila* serogroup 1. About 80 per cent of patients with *L. pneumophila* pneumonia have a four-fold or greater rise in antibody titer to 1:128 or greater within two to six weeks after onset of symptoms. Rises in titer are not always serogroup specific and may involve IgM, IgG, or IgA. Because rises in titers to *L. pneumophila* have been found in patients with culture-confirmed plague, tularemia, or *Bacteroides fragilis* bacteremia and in patients with simultaneous rises in antibody titers to *M. pneumoniae* or *Leptospira interrogans,* it is likely that serologic diagnosis is not always specific.

THERAPY. Patients with severe *Legionella* pneumonia require supportive respiratory therapy, including supplemental oxygen and mechanical ventilation with or without positive end-expiratory pressure. Careful management of fluid and electrolytes may be necessary in cases of renal insufficiency and inappropriate secretion of antidiuretic hormone. Dialysis may be needed as a temporary measure in frank renal failure. Vasoactive amines, such as dopamine, may be helpful in managing septic shock.

Experimental studies have provided conflicting information as to antimicrobials that may be effective as specific therapy. However, assay systems suggest that erythromycin and rifampin are effective against all *Legionella* species. Retrospective studies of epidemic cases suggest that therapy of *L. pneumophila* pneumonia with erythromycin is associated with a decrease in case-fatality ratio from 24 to 5 per cent.

Recommended initial therapy for pneumonia suspected to be caused by any of the *Legionella* species is erythromycin, 2 grams per day (50 mg per kilogram per day for children) given in four divided doses orally, or in seriously ill patients, intravenously. The dose for adults can be doubled if clinical response is not prompt. Patients with confirmed disease who do not respond to high-dose erythromycin given intravenously may be given rifampin, 600 mg daily, in addition. Because of concern about development of resistance to the drug, rifampin should not be given alone. Therapy should continue for 14 days, although pulmonary cavitation may require therapy to be prolonged. The possibility of relapse after specific therapy is stopped should be remembered. In cases of relapse, erythromycin therapy should be resumed promptly. The potential value of sulfamethoxazole-trimethoprim, tetracyclines, and cefoxitin in treating *Legionella* pneumonia deserves further study.

Initial treatment of adults with pneumonias of uncertain cause but suspected to be of bacterial origin can usefully include erythromcyin—with or without an aminoglycoside—because of the relative safety of erythromycin and its broad spectrum of activity against the most common bacterial agents of pneumonia in this group. Doses are as recommended for *Legionella* pneumonia.

No specific therapy is needed for Pontiac fever.

PREVENTION. Outbreaks caused by organisms from contaminated cooling towers, evaporative condensers, or industrial grinding coolants can be stopped by turning off this equipment or perhaps by treating it with chemicals effective against *L. pneumophila,* such as calcium hypochlorite, quaternary ammonium compounds, and dibromonitrilopropionamide. Whether these chemicals would be helpful in preventive maintenance of these units is unknown. Outbreaks traced to potable water have been controlled by raising the temperature of the hot water to ≥55° C or by hyperchlorination (to ≥2 mg free residual chlorine per liter). Secretion precautions in hospitalized cases may be helpful in decreasing the theoretical possibility of person-to-person spread. In the laboratory caution should be exercised to prevent generation of aerosols of live organisms or to contain them in a biologic safety cabinet.

Edelstein PH, Meyer RD, Finegold SM: Laboratory diagnosis of legionnaires' disease. Am Rev Respir Dis 121:317, 1980. *Detailed paper from the clinical laboratory most experienced in diagnosis of legionnaires' disease; covers culturing, direct immunofluorescence staining, and serology. Complete set of references.*

Fraser DW, Tsai TR (sic), Orenstein W, Parkin WE, Beecham HJ, Sharrar RG, Harris J, Mallison GF, Martin SM, McDade JE, Shepard CC, Brachman PS, Field Investigation Team: Legionnaires' disease. Description of an epidemic of pneumonia. N Engl J Med 297:1189, 1977. *The 1976 Philadelphia outbreak.*

Horowitz MA, Silverstein SC: Intracellular multiplication of Legionnaires' disease bacteria (*Legionella pneumophila*) in human monocytes is reversibly inhibited by erythromycin and rifampin. J Clin Invest 71:15, 1983. *One of a series of papers that emphasize the role of cell-mediated immunity in legionellosis.*

Kirby BD, Snyder KM, Meyer RD, Finegold SM: Legionnaires' disease: Report of

65 nosocomially-acquired cases and review of the literature. Medicine 59:188, 1980. *The largest series of cases seen by one group of clinicians.*

Muder RR, Yu VL, Zuravleff JJ: Pneumonia due to the Pittsburgh pneumonia agent: New clinical perspective with a review of the literature. Medicine 62:120, 1983. *Clinical summary of* L. micdadei *pneumonia.*

Sathapatayavonas B, Kohler RB, Wheat LJ, White A, Winn WC Jr: Rapid diagnosis of legionnaires' disease by latex agglutination. Am Rev Respir Dis 127:559, 1983. *Utility of urinary antigen detection in diagnosis of legionellosis.*

Thornsberry C, Feeley JC, Jakubowski W, Balows A (eds.): Proceedings of Second International Symposium on *Legionella*. Washington, D.C.: American Society of Microbiology (in press). *State of the art as of June 1983. Concise reviews and helpful original papers on bacteriology, epidemiology, ecology, pathogenesis, and diagnosis.*

Wilkinson HW, Reingold AL, Brake BJ, McGibboney DL, Gorman GW, Broome CV: Reactivity of serum from patients with suspected legionellosis against 20 antigens of *Legionellaceae* and *Legionella*-like organisms by direct immunofluorescence assay. J Infect Dis 147:23, 1983. *Useful caution about interpretation of serologic tests in suspected legionellosis.*

Winn WC, Myerowitz R: The pathology of *Legionella* pneumonias: A review of 74 cases and the literature. Hum Pathol 12:401, 1981. *Documents the similarity of pneumonias caused by the various Legionellae.*

Streptococcal Diseases

267. STREPTOCOCCAL DISEASES

Richard M. Krause

Streptococci are ubiquitous, gram-positive globular bacteria that grow in chains. They were first described by Billroth in 1874 in purulent exudates from erysipelas lesions and infected wounds. Subsequently they were shown to cause different forms of streptococcal disease, including streptococcal sore throat, scarlet fever, streptococcal skin infections (impetigo or pyoderma), suppurative infections including abscesses and pneumonia, food poisoning, septicemia, bacterial endocarditis, and urinary tract infections. A single streptococcal species may be responsible for a variety of diseases, and many different kinds of streptococci may be cultured from humans and animals.

The first classification of these organisms was based on their capacity to lyse red blood cells. When streptococci are cultured on blood agar plates, three types of hemolytic reactions are observed. Streptococcal colonies surrounded by a clear zone of hemolysis are termed beta, colonies surrounded by green partial hemolysis are termed alpha, and the nonhemolytic colonies are termed gamma.

Primarily through the efforts of Lancefield, the beta-hemolytic streptococci were further differentiated into a number of immunologic categories, designated groups A to H and K to T, on the basis of specific polysaccharide antigens. Most streptococci causing pharyngitis and impetigo belong to group A. Rheumatic fever occurs only after group A pharyngitis. Streptococci belonging to certain other Lancefield groups are now recognized as important causes of infection. Alpha-hemolytic and gamma streptococci can cause sepsis with systemic illness.

Group A streptococcal pharyngitis has been intensely studied over the years because it may give rise to the delayed, nonsuppurative sequelae acute rheumatic fever (ARF) and acute glomerulonephritis (AGN). While ARF is less common in the United States today than 30 years ago, it still persists as a common cause of heart disease in much of the developing world.

CLASSIFICATION OF STREPTOCOCCI OF CLINICAL IMPORTANCE

The classification of streptococci on the basis of hemolysis patterns on blood agar plates and antigenic composition was a major advance. Nevertheless, it is frequently necessary to employ a combination of features, including growth characteristics and biochemical reactions, to fully characterize these organisms because they are such a heterogeneous group. A classification of streptococci with a clinical orientation for the most important streptococcal infections is presented in Table 267–1. While group A streptococci remain important human pathogens, beta-hemolytic non-group A, alpha hemolytic, and nonhemolytic streptococci are of increasing importance as the cause of suppurative infections in all regions of the body.

GROUP A INFECTIONS. Group A streptococci are the most common cause of streptococcal pharyngitis. They are recognized by the characteristic group A carbohydrate cell wall antigen, which is identified by serologic reactions to specific rabbit antiserum. In this way they can be distinguished from other beta-hemolytic streptococci that are also frequently isolated from the human pharynx, vagina, or skin.

GROUP B INFECTIONS. Group B streptococci are identified serologically by their characteristic cell wall polysaccharide. Group B streptococci were first recognized as a cause of bovine mastitis, but since the 1960's they have emerged as a major cause of neonatal sepsis with or without meningitis. Carriage of group B streptococci in the female genital tract is a major source of these infections.

GROUP D INFECTIONS. Group D streptococci consist of two major categories: enterococci (such as *S. faecalis*) and nonenterococci (such as *S. bovis*). Strains isolated from clinical cultures are usually nonhemolytic or alpha hemolytic, but beta-hemolytic strains are seen.

Enterococci are present in the normal intestinal flora and are a significant cause of community-acquired and hospital-acquired sepsis, as demonstrated by the cultivation of these organisms from the blood. Enterococci are a frequent cause of urinary tract infections, particularly in patients with structural abnormalities of the urinary tract. They are also a frequent cause of endocarditis. Enterococci are frequently resistant to many antibiotics, which complicates treatment. For the treatment of enterococcal endocarditis, combined therapy should be employed, including intravenously administered penicillin in high doses plus an aminoglycoside antibiotic. In combination, these drugs have a synergistic killing effect on enterococci.

In contrast to enterococci, nonenterococcal group D streptococci isolated from patients with endocarditis are extremely sensitive to penicillin. Because of these differences in antibiotic sensitivity, it may be necessary to perform additional biochemical tests to differentiate enterococci from nonenterococcal group D organisms. One simple procedure that may be useful is to attempt growth in a broth containing 6.5 per cent sodium chloride. Enterococci will usually grow under these conditions, whereas other streptococci will not.

OTHER STREPTOCOCCAL INFECTIONS. Not infrequently, the beta-hemolytic streptococci cultured from the throat or other

TABLE 267–1. CLINICAL CLASSES OF STREPTOCOCCAL INFECTIONS

Lancefield Groups	Hemolysis on Blood Agar	Representative Species	Major Clinical Syndromes	Colonization (Carriage)
A	Beta	*S. pyogenes*	Pharyngitis (scarlet fever), pyoderma, wound infection, sepsis, rheumatic fever, acute glomerulonephritis	Pharynx
B	Beta	*S. agalactiae*	Perinatal sepsis, newborn meningitis, subacute bacterial endocarditis, urinary tract infection, adult sepsis	Adult urogenital tract, gastrointestinal tract, throat, rectum, pharynx
C and G	Beta	—	Mild pharyngitis	Pharynx
D	Variable (usually nonhemolytic)	Enterococci *(S. faecalis)*	Subacute bacterial endocarditis, urinary tract infection	Bowel
		Nonenterococci *(S. bovis)*	Subacute bacterial endocarditis	
Nongroupable: viridans streptococci	Alpha (green)	*S. salivarius, S. sanguis, S. mutans*	Subacute bacterial endocarditis, caries	Oropharynx, saliva
Anaerobic (microaerophilic streptococci)	Gamma (nonhemolytic) or variable	*Peptostreptococcus*	Abscesses, gangrene, necrotizing fascitis, peritonsillar abscess	Mouth, intestine, vagina

sites are identified as group C or G organisms. Most commonly when they infect the pharynx, these organisms produce no symptoms or illness. But on occasion a low grade pharyngitis occurs, which may be exudative. A rise in the convalescent antistreptolysin O titer indicates that these groups actually can cause an infection of the pharynx and other sites and are not just passively carried. An unexpected event was the occurrence of ten cases of group C streptococcal sepsis, including meningitis, in New Mexico in the summer of 1983. In addition to group C and G, case reports indicate that under diverse circumstances streptococci belonging to most of the other groups can cause sporadic infections, including meningitis, infected heart valves, visceral abscesses, and soft tissue infections following surgical procedures. Furthermore, these less common organisms are now known to cause opportunistic infections in individuals whose resistance has been compromised by other diseases or treatments.

The predominant aerobic flora of the oral pharynx normally consists of a large variety of streptococci. These are classified as *viridans,* alpha hemolytic, or green streptococci. It is probable that they play some useful role by maintaining a favorable ecologic balance. However, they can produce disease in abnormal circumstances. They are a common cause of subacute bacterial endocarditis and enter the bloodstream most often from diseased teeth and gums.

Special interest has now centered on a species of these organisms identified as *S. mutans.* These bacteria colonize the oral cavity and have been implicated in the development of dental caries. They produce a mucoid substance that becomes part of the plaque adhering to the tooth enamel. The bacteria remain embedded in the plaque and excrete metabolic products that are a factor in the production of caries. Currently there is evidence that dental caries can be prevented by decreasing sugar in the diet to diminish the growth of these bacteria as well as by practicing proper oral hygiene to remove the plaque containing the *S. mutans* organisms. Work is also in progress on a possible vaccine.

Anaerobic streptococci are also a prominent part of the normal flora in the mouth, intestine, and vagina. It is suspected that they maintain an ecologic balance on the surface of these tissues, but the mechanism is unknown. The presence of this normal flora appears to be important, however, because when the ecologic balance is disturbed by the use of antibiotics, pathogens such as *Candida albicans* may cause infections of these sites.

Anaerobic streptococci may cause abscesses in many different regions of the body, including retropharyngeal spaces, paranasal sinuses, dental structures, and the brain. Visceral infections include lung abscesses and empyema fluids, abscesses of the liver and other intra-abdominal viscera, and perirectal and pelvic abscesses. Anaerobic streptococci are especially prone to thrive in dead or devitalized muscle, skin, or subcutaneous tissue. A rapidly progressing necrotizing fasciitis or *progressive synergistic gangrene* is usually produced by these anaerobic streptococci along with *Staphylococcus aureus.* While these anaerobic organisms are usually sensitive to penicillin, debridement and drainage of abscesses is an important aspect of treatment.

GROUP A STREPTOCOCCAL INFECTIONS

BACKGROUND AND PATHOGENESIS. Although streptococci were identified as the cause of scarlet fever and tonsillitis in 1895, determination of the origin and epidemiology of streptococcal infections stems from the serologic classification of the organisms into groups by Lancefield and into types by Lancefield and Griffith. With these developments it was possible to identify group A streptococci as the most common cause of streptococcal pharyngitis. The ability to measure serologic responses was another important advance. Most widely used has been the antistreptolysin O (ASO) test developed by Todd in 1932. This was a major achievement because a rise in an ASO titer or a markedly elevated titer was indicative of a prior streptococcal infection. These immunologic and bacteriologic developments led to the firm conclusion that ARF and AGN were nonsuppurative sequelae to group A streptococcal infections and that infections by *none* of the other streptococcal groups resulted in such sequelae. The rare exception to this rule is that on occasion group C streptococcal infections appear to cause AGN. ARF is only observed after group A pharyngitis, whereas AGN is seen after pharyngitis and other streptococcal infections such as pyoderma.

Epidemics of streptococcal disease in the armed forces have been known since the Civil War. The epidemics in World War I, World War II, and the Korean War were studied in detail, and much of the current knowledge concerning the epidemiology of group A streptococcal disease rests on this research. A major advance was the prevention of rheumatic fever by penicillin treatment of streptococcal pharyngitis and the use of penicillin prophylaxis to prevent recurrences of ARF in patients who had had prior ARF. Epidemics have not been confined to the armed forces, however. Epidemics of streptococcal sore throat and scarlet fever were once commonly observed among school children, and this resulted in extensive programs for the early detection and treatment of pharyngitis for the prevention of rheumatic fever. While epidemics of streptococcal pharyngitis are now less common, sporadic outbreaks in school or other closed populations still occur as minor epidemics. As a result occasional cases of ARF and AGN are still seen in civilian populations.

In the United States, England, and much of Europe, the incidence of streptococcal disease has declined dramatically in the last two decades. There is a belief in some quarters that this decrease is due in part to those properties of the group A streptococci that account for their ability to spread widely in a community and to produce acute disease. While such changes in streptococcal characteristics may have occurred, it is also possible that extensive use of antibiotics has decreased the reservoir of virulent streptococci and therefore their spread. It should be remembered that the untreated patient is the source of secondary spread to susceptible individuals.

Group A streptococci are subdivided into M types on the basis of an antigen known as *M protein*. More than 70 antigenically distinct M types have been identified. This substance plays a very important role in the pathogenesis of group A streptococcal infections. The M protein is a surface component of the streptococcus and is correlated with its ability to resist phagocytosis. Streptococci that have large amounts of M protein are highly resistant to phagocytosis, whereas those with no or small amounts of M protein are susceptible to phagocytosis. Following an infection with streptococci of a particular M type, homologous type-specific immunity develops, so that the individual is resistant to infection by organisms of the same M type. Because this type-specific antibody can persist for many years, reinfection with the same M type is rare. Penicillin or other antibiotic therapy can suppress the type-specific immune response, however; for this reason reinfection with the same M type has been seen in recent years. Because immunity is M-type–specific and because there are numerous M types of streptococci, repeated streptococcal infections caused by different M types are common, particularly in childhood and early adult life.

Because of the importance of M-type–specific immunity in resistance to group A streptococcal infections, intensive research has centered on the immunochemistry of the M protein and the immune response to it. The complete chemical structure of several different M proteins is now known, and with the use of recombinant deoxyribonucleic acid technology, pure type 6 M protein has been produced by *Escherichia coli*. It should now be possible to examine at the molecular level the chemical basis for the antiphagocytic properties of M protein and to explore the molecular interactions that occur when specific antibody promotes phagocytosis of group A streptococci. While these recent developments on the chemistry of M protein again have raised the possibility of a multivalent streptococcal vaccine for use in regions where streptococcal disease still flourishes, a number of theoretical and practical impediments have to be overcome before the development of such a vaccine.

The T antigen is another streptococcal surface protein that has assisted in the classification of streptococci isolated from clinical material. As with M proteins, there are multiple serotypes of T antigens. While T antigens (unlike M proteins) play no part in virulence, they have become very useful antigenic markers, particularly in the recognition of less virulent strains that have lost their M protein. The T antigen classification also has been useful in identifying strains isolated from patients with pyoderma for which an M protein has not yet been identified.

In addition to the M and T proteins, two other major elements of the streptococcal cell wall are the group-specific C carbohydrate and the backbone matrix, a peptidoglycan similar to that in many other gram-positive bacteria. When injected into animals, the backbone matrix produces many of the same biologic reactions as do the endotoxins of gram-negative bacteria. Derivatives of it are known to function as an adjuvant.

Because group A streptococcal infections have been such an important health problem in the past, the organisms and their products have been intensely studied in an effort to determine the cause of ARF and AGN, but the precise nature of the pathogenesis of these complications is unknown. (See Ch. 268 and 80.) Group A streptococci grown in vivo and in vitro produce a great variety of antigenic extracellular products such as the two hemolysins streptolysin O and streptolysin S, streptokinase, hyaluronidase, nicotinamide adenine dinucleotidase (NADase), several deoxyribonucleases (DNAses), and proteinases. The antibody responses to several of these substances are useful in diagnosis. Hemolysis surrounding colonies on the surface of blood agar plates is due primarily to the action of streptolysin S. It is not antigenic. Streptolysin O is reversibly inhibited by oxygen. Because anaerobic conditions prevail beneath the surface of the blood agar, hemolysis in this region is due to streptolysin O. Streptolysin O is produced by almost all group A strains as well as by many group C and G organisms. Since streptolysin O is a good antigen, titration of ASO antibodies in human sera is the most widely used serologic procedure in clinical practice to detect a prior group A streptococcal infection. In recent years, a test to measure anti-DNAse B antibodies has been used in the evaluation of streptococcal pyoderma.

It is assumed that extracellular products play a role in the pathogenesis of streptococcal infections, but the exact relationship is conjectural. Nevertheless, it is probable that the breakdown of fibrin and nucleic acids by streptokinase and the DNAses, respectively, produces the characteristic thin pus of streptococcal infections. It is also possible that hyaluronidase contributes to the rapid spread of the organisms through the tissues, as is seen in streptococcal cellulitis. None of these substances has been implicated in the pathogenesis of ARF or AGN. The erythrogenic toxins cause the typical erythema of scarlet fever. There are three serologically distinct toxins, each neutralized by its respective antibody. For this reason scarlet fever may occur more than once. All strains of streptococci do not produce an erythrogenic toxin. These toxins are induced by lysogeny of group A streptococci with a temperate bacteriophage.

Group A streptococci most commonly infect the tonsils, nasopharynx, and skin. A number of features of streptococcal skin infections set them apart from streptococcal tonsillitis. For this reason, the clinical features of skin infections will be considered separately.

EPIDEMIOLOGY. Streptococcal pharyngitis and tonsillitis are the most common group A streptococcal infections. Their most frequent occurrence is in children between 5 and 15 years of age, but both younger and older persons are still highly susceptible to infection. This is particularly true when special environmental circumstances enhance transmission. For example, mobilization of troops during wartime results in an increased incidence of streptococcal infections in individuals 18 to 25 years of age. The high attack rate in children and military recruits is related to the mode of transmission of group A streptococcal infections. Transmission occurs as a result of close contact between susceptible individuals and either infected persons or healthy individuals who carry contagious streptococci in the pharynx. Organisms are transmitted from one person to another on saliva droplets produced by sneezing or coughing. For this reason, transmission of this disease requires close association with an individual who harbors infectious streptococci in the pharynx. The streptococci that contaminate the fomites and dust in the environment are not the cause of pharyngeal infection even though the organisms are viable and can be cultivated on blood agar from these environmental sources.

Untreated patients are the primary source of the spread of streptococcal disease, especially during the period of acute pharyngitis and for the first several weeks of convalescence. Studies of kindergarten and school-age children indicate that an untreated child is often the source of the disease in the classroom as well as in the home. It is therefore important to identify and treat patients as soon as possible to prevent secondary spread of the disease.

Patients not treated with antibiotics may carry group A streptococci in the nasopharynx for several weeks or months. Furthermore, many individuals will acquire the organism and carry it for similar periods of time without any signs or symptoms of acute pharyngitis. Epidemiologic studies have revealed that untreated patients and asymptomatic carriers are highly infectious during the first one to three weeks after acquisition of pharyngeal group A streptococci. Throat cultures from such individuals frequently reveal large numbers of group A streptococcal colonies; these people have been labeled "dangerous" carriers. Long-term carriage for many weeks or months is seen frequently, but usually the throat culture yields only a small number of group A streptococcal colonies. Furthermore, the streptococci isolated after three weeks frequently have a diminished amount of M protein. The small number of streptococci in the throat and the loss of M protein are probably responsible for the lack of transmission of streptococci from individuals during convalescence and from those who remain persistent carriers for weeks or months.

Nasal or throat carriage (or both) of virulent streptococci is also a source of infection of open wounds and skin abrasions as well as of puerperal sepsis. Secondary infection of the lungs may occur, particularly after a respiratory infection such as influenza. Indeed, streptococcal pneumonia may be seen with greater frequency during an influenza epidemic.

A confusing aspect of streptococcal pharyngitis is that a significant number of individuals have "silent" infections that are detected by positive throat cultures *and* a rise in the ASO titer. In early studies it was learned that at least 25 to 30 per cent of all patients who developed ARF had had a preceding silent throat infection. Such silent infections complicate the control of spread of streptococcal disease in a family or community. Epidemiologic studies have shown that patients with subclinical or silent infection are capable of disseminating the streptococci to other individuals who then may develop overt disease.

Currently there is debate concerning reasons for the declining frequency of severe acute pharyngitis with exudate. Certainly the number of such patients with severe disease is much smaller than it was 30 years ago, while the mild form appears more common. It is unknown whether this change in the clinical picture is due to a decline in the virulence of the streptococci, to host factors, or to the widespread use of antibiotics to treat patients who had been infected with the more virulent forms of streptococci, thus eliminating these organisms from the reservoir of potential pathogens.

A number of epidemiologic factors influence the spread of streptococcal disease. Clearly, socioeconomic factors that promote crowding will result in close contact between individuals and therefore in the spread of streptococci. Climate, season, and geography also can enhance the spread of streptococci because of their influence in bringing people into close contact. It has already been mentioned that military recruits are susceptible because they are clustered in large camps under crowded conditions. Similarly, streptococcal disease is common in civilian populations where poverty and poor housing promote crowded living conditions and therefore the spread from one individual to another. It is probable that these factors continue to influence the widespread occurrence of streptococcal disease in developing countries. For this reason ARF and rheumatic heart disease are common in these regions.

Scarlet fever is now uncommon in the United States. The reasons for this are not clear because the decline began before the widespread use of antibiotics. Streptococcal strains that produce scarlet fever are the same as those that produce group A infections except that they are lysogenized by a bacteriophage that induces the production of erythrogenic toxin.

Whereas streptococcal pharyngitis is most common in the winter months when close contact between individuals is greatest, streptococcal pyoderma occurs in the late summer and early fall. Presumably this is due to exposure of uncovered skin during the warmer months to minor trauma and insect bites, which favor skin infections. Although streptococcal pharyngitis and streptococcal pyoderma occur worldwide, geography clearly influences the occurrence of these two diseases. Pharyngitis is more common in temperate and cold climates, and pyoderma is more frequent in hot or tropical climates.

The attack rate of ARF after streptococcal infections may vary widely. During the major epidemics of World War II and the Korean War, the attack rate was 3 per cent or more in military recruits with untreated group A streptococcal infections. Since that time, studies of children and other civilian populations, particularly those experiencing the sporadic infections that occur today, have suggested that the attack rate may be as low as 0.3 per cent or less. Two features were associated with the large military epidemics of pharyngitis in which the ARF attack rates were high: (1) the magnitude of the immune response associated with infection and (2) the long duration of convalescent carriage of strains after untreated infection. For example, patients who had very high ASO responses were more likely to have attacks of ARF than those who had low or moderate responses. The mild acute streptococcal pharyngitis seen in recent years is followed by a small increase in the ASO titer and a brief period of pharyngeal carriage. This changing pattern in the severity of pharyngitis, in combination with antibiotic therapy, may be responsible for the decreased incidence of ARF. Whatever the reasons for the decrease, this event has implications concerning methods of medical management, including the use of penicillin prophylaxis, which is a matter that will be discussed later.

The epidemiology and the bacteriology of the streptococcal infections that precede ARF differ in important respects from those of the streptococcal infections that precede AGN. In the early years of streptococcal bacteriology, ARF was seen as a complication of epidemic pharyngitis due to nearly all of the different types of group A streptococci. For example, certain M types such as 1, 3, 5, 6, 14, 18, 19, and 24 have all produced epidemics of pharyngitis in the United States that have resulted in ARF. In contrast, AGN was not a constant complication of these epidemics. The occurrence of AGN has been associated with epidemics of pharyngitis due to a limited number of M types, such as type 12. Such differences in the bacteriology of ARF and AGN have raised speculation concerning "rheumatogenic" and "nephritogenic" strains of streptococci. However, such designations become blurred on the basis of epidemiologic information. Sporadic outbreaks of AGN due to types 1, 3, and 6 have been seen, all of which have been associated with ARF. There is no doubt that certain outbreaks of type 12 pharyngitis have resulted in an unusually high incidence of AGN, but type 12 strains in the general population have not consistently resulted in outbreaks of AGN. Therefore, no single M type can be arbitrarily designated nephritogenic. Clearly the *antecedent* streptococcal infection that results in AGN must be due to an organism that has acquired some special characteristic other than a particular M protein. Despite intensive study, there is no certainty as to the nature of this special characteristic. Efforts are under way to identify streptococcal antigens in the immune complexes of patients with AGN that are associated with "nephritogenic" streptococci. It is tempting to speculate that strains acquire the "nephritogenic" property by some form of gene transfer from those streptococci that already possess the capacity to produce AGN.

As attention was focused on the epidemiology of streptococcal infections and AGN, additional M serotypes that had not been associated with pharyngitis were identified, primarily from skin infections. Nearly 20 new M serotypes have been identified from skin cultures as the cause of impetigo. AGN has been associated with skin infections due to several of these types, such as M type 49.

STREPTOCOCCAL SORE THROAT. The usual incubation period

of streptococcal pharyngitis is between two and four days. Typically in both children and adults there is a rather abrupt onset of sore throat. A particular characteristic is pain on swallowing. Hoarseness is rare. Other symptoms include headache, malaise, feverishness, and anorexia. Chilliness is common, but not rigor. Nausea, vomiting, and abdominal pain are common in children. The patient appears mildly to moderately ill, but signs and symptoms depend upon the severity of the illness. Temperature frequently exceeds 38.5° C. In the moderately severe case, examination of the throat reveals diffuse erythema, edema, and lymphoid hyperplasia of the posterior pharynx. The uvula may be edematous. The tonsils are enlarged and reddened, with either a punctate or a confluent yellow-gray exudate. There may be discrete areas of exudate about 1 to 2 mm in diameter on the posterior pharynx. The anterior cervical nodes are usually enlarged. The white blood cell count is usually greater than 12,000 per cu mm. When properly taken, the throat culture usually reveals large numbers of group A beta-hemolytic streptococci. Not uncommonly, group A streptococci are the predominant organisms observed on the culture plate. The course of streptococcal pharyngitis is usually self-limited and the fever abates within a week. The constitutional symptoms and sore throat disappear during this time.

A pharyngitis of the severity just described is typical of the infections seen in earlier years in civilian populations and during military epidemics, but such infections occur less commonly today. Most patients do not have all of the signs and symptoms just described. For example, in mild pharyngitis, there may be no exudate and the throat culture may reveal modest numbers of group A streptococci.

If antimicrobial therapy has not been used, group A streptococci persist in the pharynx for weeks or months following acute pharyngitis. A small number of patients who are treated with penicillin will carry the streptococci for several weeks. If the course of antibiotics has been adequate, these patients need not be retreated. They are unlikely to be a source of spread to other individuals.

The diagnosis of streptococcal pharyngitis in infants and small children presents a special challenge. The disease lacks a well-defined onset. Often there is rhinorrhea as a dominant manifestation. Fever is low grade. Usually the physical signs in the throat are not helpful in the differential diagnosis. A throat culture is positive when properly taken. Despite the mildness of the pharyngitis in infants, suppurative complications such as otitis media can occur.

SCARLET FEVER. Scarlet fever occurs in those patients with streptococcal pharyngitis in whom the infected organism produces an erythrogenic toxin and who are not immune to the toxin because of prior exposure. The enanthem of scarlet fever includes a tongue that may be bright red with large papillae (raspberry tongue) or coated with the red papillae protruding (strawberry tongue). These manifestations of the disease are rarely seen in adults. The rash appears shortly after the onset of the sore throat, usually within two days, and involves the neck, upper chest, and back and then spreads to the remainder of the trunk and the extremities. The palms and the soles are spared. The rash consists of a diffuse erythema that blanches on pressure, with numerous 1-mm punctate elevations that give a sandpaper texture to the skin. There is a generalized facial flush with a pale area often seen around the mouth, the *circumoral pallor*. The distribution of the rash is variable. The trunk and inner aspects of the arms and thighs are most often affected, but in milder cases the rash is seen only in the axilla or groin. Linear striations of confluent petechiae are known as *Pastia's lines*. A tourniquet applied to the arm for five minutes results in large numbers of petechiae distal to the obstruction in nearly all cases (the *Rumpel-Leede sign*). The erythema usually disappears by the sixth to ninth day after the onset of infection. Desquamation of the skin is a characteristic of scarlet fever. It begins with a fine scaling of the face and body and is usually completed during the second week. There then occurs an extensive and characteristic desquamation of the palms and soles. Eosinophilia has been observed, particularly during the period of desquamation.

SUPPURATIVE COMPLICATIONS. The most frequent suppurative complications of streptococcal pharyngitis are perinasal sinusitis, otitis media, and mastoiditis. Suppurative cervical adenitis may occur, as well as impetigo. Bacteremia was seen more commonly in earlier times prior to the use of antibiotics; this resulted in metastatic lesions in joints, bones, and other sites. Group A streptococcal meningitis is now uncommon.

An unusual and infrequent complication of streptococcal tonsillitis is *peritonsillar abscess*, or *quinsy*. While it is probable that the streptococcal infection leads to the formation of the abscess, the abscesses themselves do not contain group A streptococci but a variety of oropharyngeal flora, including anaerobic bacteria. This complication should be suspected if there is an abrupt increase in (1) soreness in the throat, (2) swelling in the neck, and (3) fever during or shortly after streptococcal pharyngitis. Inspection of the throat will reveal the displacement of the tonsil on the affected side toward the midline. A fluctuant mass may be felt in the affected area with a gloved finger; it should be treated promptly because complications arise when the infection extends further into the neck and surrounding tissues.

NONSUPPURATIVE COMPLICATIONS. The nonsuppurative complications of streptococcal disease are ARF and AGN. These are discussed in Ch. 268 and 80.

DIAGNOSIS. Group A streptococcal pharyngitis must be differentiated from pharyngitis due to other bacterial and viral agents. Gonococcal tonsillopharyngitis should be suspected if there is a history of homosexuality or fellatio. *Vincent's angina* usually has an insidious onset without the constitutional symptoms characteristic of a streptococcal sore throat. Signs of this infection, including an exudate, are commonly unilateral, whereas streptococcal pharyngitis is not. *Diphtheria* is now rare, although it should be recognized by the presence of the characteristic diphtheritic membrane as well as the other signs and symptoms of the disease.

The major confusion in the differential diagnosis will stem from viral respiratory infections, which not only occur more frequently than do streptococcal infections but which also may cause pharyngeal and tonsillar exudate. While many upper respiratory infections have a "common cold–like" quality, the symptoms may overlap considerably with those of streptococcal disease. It should be remembered that adenoviruses can cause an exudative pharyngitis that clinically is indistinguishable from that due to group A streptococci. A severe exudative pharyngitis with fever and toxicity is seen in infectious mononucleosis. The generalized symptoms and signs associated with infectious mononucleosis, however, should assist in the differential diagnosis. Pharyngitis due to group A coxsackieviruses (herpangina) or to herpes simplex will result in formation of vesicles. When these rupture they may leave shallow ulcers that can often be differentiated by inspection from streptococcal disease. Because it is frequently not possible to distinguish streptococcal from nonstreptococcal sore throat on clinical grounds, precise diagnosis requires a throat culture.

Before any antimicrobial therapy is administered, swabs should be passed through the mouth under direct vision and a good light and rubbed over the tonsils and posterior pharynx. The swab should be streaked directly, with a minimum of delay, on a sheep blood agar plate of low dextrose content. After incubation overnight, the number of hemolytic streptococci present should be recorded in a roughly quantitative manner. These organisms will be very numerous in nearly all cases if they are the cause of the infection. The presence of a few colonies does not provide convincing evidence that they are responsible for the illness, because 5 to 10 per cent of the general population may be nasopharyngeal carriers of these organisms. Serologic grouping and typing of the isolated organisms are usually not necessary for routine clinical diagnosis. Because the growth of group A streptococci is inhibited in vitro by paper discs containing less than 0.02 unit of bacitracin, some laboratories routinely determine the bacitracin susceptibility of hemolytic streptococci. Hemolytic bacteria resistant to such low concentrations of bacitracin are unlikely to be group A streptococci. On the other hand, approximately 5 per cent of non-group A hemolytic streptococci are also susceptible to this low concentration.

If the pharyngitis persists with adequate penicillin therapy, it is unlikely to be due to group A streptococci. It should be remembered, however, that viral pharyngitis is often of brief duration, and if such patients are treated with penicillin, it may appear that there has been a therapeutic response when in fact the disease has abated spontaneously.

The ASO test is not useful in the diagnosis of streptococcal pharyngitis. An elevation in titer is evidence of a recent infection and is employed in the diagnosis of patients with rheumatic fever and rheumatic heart disease.

TREATMENT. There are three reasons for treating streptococcal pharyngitis: (1) the prevention of suppurative complications, (2) the prevention of the nonsuppurative complications ARF and AGN, and (3) the prevention of spread of the disease through family contacts or to persons in small social units such as school rooms and army barracks. Prevention of ARF depends upon the eradication of the organism from the pharynx, and this requires treatment for at least ten days. Because signs and symptoms frequently subside in a few days, there is a tendency to shorten the time antibiotics are given. Brief periods of antibiotic therapy do not eliminate the streptococci from the pharynx. Patients treated briefly have a greater risk of developing ARF than do those who are adequately treated for at least ten days.

Penicillin is the drug of choice. Group A streptococci are highly susceptible to the action of penicillin. Despite its use for the last 40 years, no penicillin-resistant strains have developed. A single intramuscular injection of 1.2 million units of benzathine penicillin G provides a sufficiently prolonged level of penicillin in the blood to eradicate the organism. For children weighing less than 60 pounds, the dose is 600,000 units. If oral therapy is used, 250,000 units of penicillin G or 250 mg of penicillin V, three or four times daily, is the treatment of choice. If penicillin allergy is suspected or known to exist, erythromycin is the drug of choice, 20 mg per pound per day (not to exceed 1 gram per day) for a period of ten days. Erythromycin resistance is not yet a serious problem in the United States. Many group A streptococci have developed resistance to tetracycline, and it is no longer recommended for treatment of group A infections. Sulfonamides, when used to treat streptococcal pharyngitis, are ineffective in preventing rheumatic fever. They do not suppress the immune response, do not terminate pharyngeal carriage of streptococci, and thus do not reduce the attack rate of subsequent rheumatic fever. They may be used, however, as continuous prophylaxis to prevent new infections.

Treatment of streptococcal sore throat should be started as soon as a definite diagnosis of streptococcal infection is made. It has been shown, however, that a short delay (even for several days) in initiating antimicrobial therapy while awaiting throat culture results does not significantly interfere with rheumatic fever prevention. One exception to this statement involves the patient with a history of rheumatic fever. In such a patient, the prevention of rheumatic recurrence is not always possible unless treatment is instituted at the first clinical sign of streptococcal infection. For such a patient, any delay of therapy entails the risk of reactivation of the disease.

If severe suppurative streptococcal infections such as mastoiditis, pneumonia, wound infections, or other forms of sepsis are present, patients should receive 600,000 units of procaine penicillin G twice a day intramuscularly for several days until the illness is under control. Then a shift can be made to benzathine penicillin or oral penicillin. It may be necessary to prolong therapy for several weeks whenever pus or necrosis is present, particularly when adequate debridement is not possible, and mixed infection with anaerobes should be excluded.

STREPTOCOCCAL PNEUMONIA

Streptococcal pneumonia is now uncommon. It can be seen, however, as a complication of influenza, measles, pertussis, or varicella. It is characterized by abrupt onset of fever, chills, myalgia, dyspnea, cough, pleuritic chest pain, and hemoptysis. Patients are severely ill. Radiologically, there is usually bronchopneumonia. Lobar consolidation is less common. One characteristic feature of streptococcal pneumonia is the early and rapid accumulation of a large volume of thin empyema fluid. The pneumonic infection can extend to the mediastinum and pericardium. Bacteremia occurs in 10 to 15 per cent of the cases. Bacteriologic diagnosis depends on recovering group A streptococci from the sputum, empyema fluid, and blood. Because the patient is very ill, treatment should be started promptly. Therapy consists of 4 to 6 million units of parenteral procaine penicillin G given daily; this total daily dose is given in two to four intramuscular injections. There must also be adequate drainage of the empyema fluid. This may require insertion of a chest tube.

STREPTOCOCCAL SKIN INFECTIONS

PYODERMA. Group A streptococci can produce localized purulent skin infections known as pyoderma. While some of the lesions represent secondary infections of wounds or burns, most commonly the infection is primary and is usually referred to as *streptococcal impetigo* or *impetigo contagiosa*. Intensive studies over the past 20 years have revealed a number of important bacteriologic and epidemiologic differences between streptococcal impetigo and streptococcal pharyngitis (Table 267–2). Impetigo occurs in the summer and fall, whereas pharyngitis is seen in the winter and spring. Children between the ages of

TABLE 267–2. COMPARISON OF THE FEATURES OF STREPTOCOCCAL PHARYNGITIS AND PYODERMA*

Features	Pharyngitis	Pyoderma
Clinical Illness	Acute	Indolent
Laboratory		
Leukocytosis	Usually present	Often absent
Antistreptolysin O response	Common	Uncommon
Epidemiology		
Seasonal occurrence	Winter and spring	Late summer and early fall
Geographic distribution	More common in temperate or cold climates	Common in hot or tropical climates
Age	School-age children	Children of preschool age
Transmission	Direct spread from human reservoirs	Unknown; insects may be mechanical vectors
Carrier state	Common in pharynx of many populations	Unusual on skin
Preceding trauma	Not present	May predispose to infection
Complications		
Acute nephritis	Occurs; partially preventable (50%)	Occurs; preventability unknown
Acute rheumatic fever	Occurs; preventable	Does not occur
Treatment		
Local	Not important	Removal of crusts and scrubbing with hexachlorophene soap
Systemic	Single intramuscular injection of benzathine penicillin or oral penicillin for 10 days	May not be necessary; extensive lesions may require intramuscular benzathine penicillin

*Modified from Wannamaker LW: N Engl J Med 282:23, 78, 1970.

two and five years are more commonly infected. They are usually from underprivileged families residing in the southern United States or the tropics. Nevertheless, outbreaks can be seen among children of similar circumstances in other areas of the United States, such as those in American Indian reservations.

Epidemiologic studies have not clarified the mode of spread of streptococcal pyoderma, but it is reasonable to assume that personal contact with infected patients and perhaps insect vectors may be important. Despite the uncertainty about the mode of spread, a number of important epidemiologic and clinical facts have emerged from recent studies. In general, the streptococci that cause pyoderma are the higher numbered M types, whereas pharyngitis is usually due to M types 1 through 40. Children who develop streptococcal impetigo and who carry the higher types on the skin may then develop pharyngeal carriage of these skin strains, which are unlikely to cause pharyngitis. Such pharyngeal carriage must be taken into consideration in the diagnosis of respiratory disease in these children, because carriage of these strains alone is not indicative of streptococcal pharyngitis.

Differences have been seen also in the immune response, depending on the site of the streptococcal infection. While the ASO response is usually brisk following streptococcal pharyngitis, it is weak or absent in patients with impetigo. It has been suggested that inactivation of streptolysin O by the lipids present in the skin accounts for this feeble antibody response. Brisk antibody responses do occur, however, to DNAse B in patients with impetigo. M type-specific protective antibodies are almost always produced after streptococcal pharyngitis, but the response to the M type-specific antigens is variable in the case of impetigo. It is not surprising, therefore, that lesions due to the same serotype may persist for months if untreated.

The lesions of streptococcal impetigo occur over the exposed areas of the body. They are more common on the lower extremities, undoubtedly because abrasions of the skin are more common in these areas. The lesions begin as papules but rapidly evolve into vesicles surrounded by erythema. They may be localized but are often multiple. As the papules enlarge, they break down over five or six days to form a thick crust. The lesions heal slowly, leaving a depigmented area. While there may be some regional lymphadenitis, systemic symptoms are not usually present.

While streptococcal impetigo can be suspected from the history as well as the examination, definite diagnosis requires bacteriologic culture. The crust must be removed to obtain specimens from the base of the lesion after washing the infected area of the skin with sterile water. Soap or other detergents can kill or reduce the number of group A streptococci. Culturing the surface of the lesion itself will usually give a negative result. Culture results may show both group A streptococci and *Staphylococcus aureus*, but it is generally believed that the streptococcus is the primary pathogen. In many instances mild impetigo responds to local treatment. The crusts should be removed and the skin washed with soap and water. Topical antibiotics and other antiseptics have little or no value in treatment or prevention. When the lesions are more extensive, parenteral use of benzathine penicillin is indicated. The lesions respond well to penicillin therapy. The antibiotic regimen is the same as used for the treatment of pharyngitis. Even though the *S. aureus* present may produce penicillinase, this does not interfere with penicillin treatment. Prevention of impetigo is achieved with good personal hygiene and liberal use of soap and water.

The importance of streptococcal impetigo beyond the inconvenience and some disfiguration of the skin relates to its association with AGN. Not all strains of group A streptococci that cause impetigo and other forms of pyoderma result in AGN; nevertheless, certain M types such as 49, 55, and 57 have been associated with sporadic cases as well as large epidemics of pyoderma-associated AGN. These have occurred in many different geographic regions. Although there is evidence to suggest that treatment of streptococcal pharyngitis will prevent AGN 50 per cent of the time, there is no conclusive evidence that treatment of an individual case of pyoderma will prevent subsequent occurrence of AGN. Nevertheless, treatment of the individual is important, particularly in a setting in which AGN is occurring or has occurred in the past, because this eradicates the streptococcus from the environment. The individual is therefore not a risk to siblings and other school children.

A more severe ulcerated form of pyoderma is known as *ecthyma*. During the Vietnam conflict, this was seen in combat troops serving in the jungle. The ulcers, located on the ankle or dorsum of the foot, are circular, have a punched-out appearance and are 0.5 to 3 cm in diameter. They contain purulent material and may be covered with a yellow-gray crust. They are surrounded by a zone of erythema, and in more severe cases there may be cellulitis and lymphadenitis.

ERYSIPELAS. Erysipelas (St. Anthony's fire) is an acute infection of the skin and subcutaneous tissues caused by group A streptococci. The disease is more common in infants, young children, and elderly people. It is most commonly seen on the face and has a "butterfly" distribution when the bridge of the nose and the cheeks are involved. Eyelids are edematous and often swollen shut. The source of the infection is the patient's nasopharynx. Erysipelas may also develop from streptococcal infections elsewhere on the body, including surgical incisions and wounds. In some cases the disease has been seen in association with dermatophytosis.

As with streptococcal pharyngitis, the onset is usually abrupt, and similar systemic symptoms are frequently present. The lesion initially begins with an area of mild discomfort at the site of infection. Erythema follows and enlarges rapidly, reaching a maximum in three to six days. The lesion, pink to deep red in color, has an advancing irregular margin. It is warm to the touch. Vesicles and bullae may appear, which then rupture and become crusted. As the margin advances, the central area begins to clear and the skin returns to a normal appearance, usually with some residual pigmentation.

While recovery is usually seen in a week or ten days, this varies with the severity of the infection. High fever and bacteremia were often present before antibiotics were available, and mortality was not uncommon, particularly in patients who had bacteremia. Death is rare when the disease is adequately treated with penicillin or another appropriate antibiotic. Early diagnosis and treatment are important in infants and in elderly, debilitated, or immunosuppressed individuals. Death can occur in these cases if treatment is not prompt. Not uncommonly the disease will recur in the same site, particularly if there are areas of lymphatic obstruction.

Large numbers of group A streptococci can usually be cultured from the nasopharynx of patients with early erysipelas. Efforts to culture the streptococci from the edema fluid of the lesion are not always successful. Diagnosis is primarily made on the basis of clinical findings.

PREVENTION AND PROPHYLAXIS OF GROUP A STREPTOCOCCAL DISEASES AND THEIR NONSUPPURATIVE SEQUELAE

Views on the antibiotic treatment of streptococcal pharyngitis to prevent ARF and AGN are undergoing re-evaluation because of the decrease in the severity of streptococcal pharyngitis in recent years and the dramatic decline in the occurrence of ARF. Do the low attack rates of ARF (1 to 2 per 100,000 people per year for the age group 5 to 17 years) justify intensive efforts to detect streptococcal infections by bacteriologic cultures? Do they justify a prolonged course of antibiotic therapy for all patients in whom streptococcal infection is suspected, however mild it may be? Views are currently changing on these matters, and there is now discussion of some relaxation of the vigorous efforts used in the past to diagnose and treat streptococcal pharyngitis.

From this debate several principles are emerging. While direct proof is lacking, it is probable that the decline in the incidence of both ARF and streptococcal pharyngitis is due at least in part to the widespread use of penicillin to treat this infection during the past 25 years. It is difficult to believe that this decline in disease has occurred as a result of genetic changes in the streptococci. This would have required the simultaneous occurrence of similar genetic events in a large number of different streptococci during this interval, which seems unlikely. Certainly the decline in both diseases has been too precipitous to have been the result of changes in the genetic background of the population that would have enhanced natural immunity. These considerations suggest that the treatment of pharyngitis with penicillin has been a major factor in reducing the incidence of this infection; it follows that penicillin treatment has also influenced the decline in ARF. It seems likely that continuation of treatment in the future will maintain this low incidence. It is known that virulent group A streptococci lurk in the shadows and are the cause of occasional outbreaks of streptococcal pharyngitis. It is certainly conceivable that such outbreaks would become more common if penicillin treatment were no longer used. Therefore, arguments to discontinue the use of penicillin to treat streptococcal pharyngitis, even though the disease is less virulent today than in previous times, are reminiscent of the arguments to discontinue the use of pertussis or poliomyelitis vaccines now that these diseases are rare. We know that failure to vaccinate will result in the re-emergence of these diseases.

Until there is more evidence concerning the benign nature of the streptococcal diseases that are occurring today, it will be prudent to maintain vigilance concerning streptococcal infections. Nevertheless, a consensus is emerging that the milder forms of pharyngitis need not be treated until the diagnosis is confirmed by throat culture. Furthermore, many specialists question the value of a throat culture in all cases of upper respiratory disease. These authors would reserve the throat culture for laboratory confirmation of streptococcal disease that is suspected on clinical grounds. Current recommendations call for a second throat culture at the end of ten days of treatment to be certain that the streptococcus has been eliminated. This is probably no longer necessary in the routine case. Furthermore, throat cultures of family members in contact with the usual case of streptococcal pharyngitis seem unnecessary.

Despite the decrease in the severity of streptococcal diseases and the decrease in incidence of ARF and AGN, small outbreaks of streptococcal infection still occur that result in sporadic cases of ARF and AGN. Certainly the occurrence of an index case of either ARF or AGN should alert the physician to the possibility that an outbreak of streptococcal disease is occurring in a family or school.

It is apparent from this dicussion concerning the infrequency of ARF and the milder nature of streptococcal disease that there is probably much less risk today of the recurrence of rheumatic fever in patients with prior history of the disease following an untreated streptococcal infection. Continuous antibiotic prophylaxis has been employed in the past to prevent recurrences of rheumatic fever in such patients, and while discussions are under way concerning modification of the recommendations, the three regimens listed below are still recommended at this time.

1. Benzathine penicillin G in a single injection of 1.2 million units will provide protection for about 30 days. The disadvantages and discomfort of this regimen have to be weighed against the individual patient's susceptibility to rheumatic recurrences. Those with rheumatic heart disease, those who have had a recent attack of rheumatic fever, and those exposed to an environment in which the incidence of streptococcal infection is frequent deserve the most effective protection. For such patients, benzathine penicillin by monthly injection is recommended.

2. Sulfonamide given daily by mouth in the form of 1.0 gram of sulfadiazine or one of the other sulfapyrimidines provides satisfactory prophylaxis, but failures will occur. Toxic reactions may be observed during the first 60 days of continuous treatment. These have been rare, however, with the small doses of sulfadiazine that have been employed extensively.

3. Penicillin in oral doses of 200,000 units (125 mg) of penicillin G twice daily has been employed widely for prevention of streptococcal infections. This regimen has not been any more effective, however, than the daily dose of 1.0 gram of sulfadiazine. Indeed, 200,000 units of penicillin twice daily has not proved as yet to be clearly superior to the single dose. It is possible that the oral dose of penicillin may have to be increased to nearly therapeutic proportions to be more effective than sulfonamides, and this would increase further its expense and impracticability.

GROUP B STREPTOCOCCAL INFECTIONS

In the past, group B streptococci were primarily of interest to veterinarians because they were the cause of bovine mastitis. However, in recent years human strains of group B streptococci that appear to be distinct from the bovine strains have received considerable attention because they frequently produce neonatal sepsis. Group B streptococci are subdivided by means of surface polysaccharides into five serotypes: Ia, Ib, Ic, II, and III. Recent evidence suggests that group B streptococci normally colonize the intestine, and it is speculated that there is then secondary spread from the rectum to the vagina. This raises the possibility of sexual transmission of these organisms. Vaginal carriage is asymptomatic in postpubertal women. The incidence of carriage and of neonatal infection varies widely depending on socioeconomic status and geographic residence.

Infections due to group B streptococci are associated with perinatal events. Maternal infections include chorioamnionitis, septic abortion, and puerperal sepsis. Group B streptococci are now recognized as one of the most frequent causes of neonatal sepsis and meningitis. Extensive clinical and epidemiologic studies have delineated two forms of the disease. "Early onset disease" primarily involves infection of the lungs. The disease usually occurs within the first ten days of life, but cases after this period have been reported. The organisms are usually acquired from the maternal genital tract. This may be secondary to aspiration of infected amniotic fluid. Septicemia may be present. Early onset disease occurs as frequently as in 5 of every 1000 live births, although this varies depending upon the regions of the country and the specific hospital reporting. Early onset disease tends to occur in infants of certain high-risk pregnancies, such as those involving prematurity, prolonged rupture of membranes, and maternal infection. The other form of group B streptococcal neonatal infection has been referred to as "late onset disease." Affected infants develop meningitis and bacteremia. The infant is usually over ten days old, but cases have occurred at four or five days of age. Infection is due to nosocomial transmission. The disease has a much lower mortality rate than early onset disease. Type III organisms predominate as the cause of early and late onset disease.

Because all the evidence suggests that early onset disease in the newborn infant is acquired by vertical transmission from the mother who has vaginal colonization by group B streptococci, intravenous administration of ampicillin sodium has been used to treat such women during labor in an effort to prevent transmission. While several reports clearly indicate that transmission of group B streptococci carriage to the newborn infant has been prevented, the number of deliveries has not been sufficiently large to determine whether early onset disease has also been prevented. All newborns who acquire group B carriage in the ear, nose, umbilicus, and rectum do not develop early onset disease. Nevertheless, prevention of vertical transmission of carriage is a promising development, particularly if current studies also show the prevention of early onset disease.

Another strategy to prevent early onset disease has been penicillin treatment of all newborn infants immediately after birth. Several controlled studies involving the treatment of thousands of infants have shown a decrease in the number of cases of early onset disease due to group B streptococci, but there is also an indication that disease due to penicillin-resistant pathogens increased during this neonatal period of observation. Additional studies now in progress may clarify this matter. At this time, routine use of penicillin at birth to prevent group B streptococcal infections cannot be recommended.

While group B streptococci frequently may be cultured from the throat, they rarely if ever cause pharyngitis. Group B streptococcal infection can, however, cause urinary tract infections in both sexes. Infected men are likely to be elderly. Group B streptococci may produce suppurative gangrenous lesions in adults with insulin-dependent diabetes mellitus who have peripheral vascular insufficiency. Any large series of infectious diseases will reveal group B streptococci as a cause of endocarditis, pneumonia, empyema, meningitis, peritonitis, and terminal bacteremia in patients with malignancy.

All group B streptococci are susceptible to penicillin. It is the drug of choice for these infections. Thus far, most strains are susceptible to erythromycin. Tetracycline should not be used because the organisms have developed resistance to this antibiotic.

Baker CJ: Group B streptococcal infections. Adv Intern Med 25:475, 1980. *A brief but comprehensive review of the clinical features, epidemiology, and clinical microbiology of this most important cause of sepsis and meningitis in the newborn. Approximately 100 references are annotated.*

Holm SE, Christensen P: Basic Concepts of Streptococci and Streptococcal Diseases. Surrey, England, Readbooks Ltd., 1982. *Over 100 short papers on many aspects of the bacteriology, epidemiology, and pathogenesis of streptococcal diseases. An excellent source of recent articles in journals.*

McCarty M: Streptococci. *In* Davis BD, Dulbecco R, Eisen HN, Ginsberg HS (eds.): Microbiology. New York, Harper & Row, 1980, pp 607–622. *A good brief review of all aspects of streptococcal bacteriology and streptococcal disease.*

Read SE, Zabriskie JB (eds.): Streptococcal Diseases and the Immune Response. New York, Academic Press, 1980. *An exhaustive symposium of immunology in general and streptococcal diseases in particular by leading American and British investigators.*

Rheumatic Fever Committee, American Heart Association: Prevention of rheumatic fever. Circulation 55:s1, 1977. *Standard recommendations for the prevention of rheumatic fever, which should be basic knowledge for all physicians.*

Shulman ST (ed.): Management of Pharyngitis in an Era of Declining Rheumatic Fever. Columbus, Ohio, Ross Laboratories, 1984. *A collection of papers that thoroughly reviews the changing patterns of streptococcal diseases and the implications of these changes for treatment and management.*

Wannamaker LW: Infections of the throat and skin. N Engl J Med 282:23, 78, 1970. *A critical review of the clinical microbiology and epidemiology of "skin strains" of group A streptococci.*

Wannamaker LW: Immunology of streptococci. *In* Nahmias AJ, O'Reilly RJ (eds.): Immunology of Human Infection. Part I: Bacteria, Mycoplasmae, Chlamydiae, and Fungi. New York, Plenum Medical Book Company, 1981, pp 47–92. *An excellent review of the humoral and cellular immune responses to many different streptococcal products and antigens. Includes 400 references.*

Wood HF, Feinstein AR, Taranta A, Epstein JA, Simpson R: Rheumatic fever in children and adolescents. III. Comparative effectiveness of three prophylaxis regimens in preventing streptococcal infections and rheumatic recurrences. Ann Intern Med 60 (S5):31, 1964. *A classic controlled long-term study of the prevention of rheumatic recurrences and the relative effectiveness of the three regimens commonly in use for secondary prophylaxis.*

Yow MD, Mason EO, Leeds LJ, Thompson PK, Clark DJ, Gardner SE: Ampicillin prevents intrapartum transmission of group B streptococcus. JAMA 241:1245, 1979. *One of the first papers to demonstrate that women who are colonized with group B streptococci and are treated with intravenous ampicillin sodium during labor do not vertically transmit group B streptococci to their newborn infant.*

268. RHEUMATIC FEVER

Alan L. Bisno

DEFINITION. Rheumatic fever is a delayed, nonsuppurative sequel of upper respiratory infection with group A streptococci. The disease is characterized by inflammatory lesions involving primarily the joints, heart, and subcutaneous tissues; its pathogenesis remains obscure. The clinical manifestations include polyarthritis, carditis, subcutaneous nodules, erythema marginatum, and chorea in varying combinations. In its classic form, the disorder is acute, febrile, and largely self-limited. However, damage to heart valves may be chronic and progressive, causing cardiac disability or death many years after the initial episode. Persons who have had rheumatic fever are inordinately susceptible to recurrent episodes following group A streptococcal upper respiratory infections. Both initial and recurrent attacks of acute rheumatic fever are largely preventable by treatment or prophylaxis of the antecedent streptococcal infection.

ETIOLOGY. The development of acute rheumatic fever (ARF) requires antecedent infection with a specific organism, the group A *Streptococcus,* at a specific body site, the upper respiratory tract. Cutaneous streptococcal infection, a frequent precursor of poststreptococcal acute glomerulonephritis, has never been shown to cause rheumatic fever. The explanation for this phenomenon remains obscure. It may indicate a requirement for a site with a rich endowment of lymphoid tissue, such as the pharynx, for initiation of the disease process. It may relate to the blunted immunologic response to certain streptococcal antigens observed following skin infection. Still another possible explanation is that so-called "pyoderma" strains of group A streptococci lack rheumatogenic potential.

Strains representing a number of the more than 70 M protein serotypes of group A streptococci are capable of eliciting ARF. Whether *all* clinically virulent strains of *S. pyogenes* are equally "rheumatogenic" remains a matter of controversy. There is evidence to suggest, however, that group A streptococci may vary in their rheumatogenic potential. Analysis of epidemics of ARF caused by a variety of serotypes shows a striking absence of certain highly prevalent types (e.g., type 12) and an overrepresentation of others, particularly type 5. Reports from the preantibiotic era document epidemics of streptococcal tonsillitis, even among rheumatic subjects, in which ARF failed to appear. Prospective studies from Trinidad, where poststreptococcal acute glomerulonephritis and ARF occur simultaneously in the same indigent population, indicate that the streptococcal strains responsible for each sequel are serotypically distinct.

PATHOGENESIS. The mechanism by which group A streptococci elicit the connective tissue inflammatory response which constitutes ARF remains unknown. Various theories have been advanced: (1) direct tissue invasion by streptococci themselves or by variants of the organism with incomplete cell walls; (2) toxic effects of streptococcal products, particularly streptolysins S or O, both of which are capable of initiating tissue injury; (3) a serum sickness–like reaction mediated by antigen-antibody complexes, perhaps localized to sites of tissue injury; and (4) "autoimmune" phenomena induced by the similarity of certain streptococcal and human tissue antigens.

Efforts to discriminate among these potential pathogenetic mechanisms have been hampered by the lack of an animal model of rheumatic fever. Many authorities currently favor the theory that ARF is an "autoimmune" disorder, in which tissue damage is mediated by the host's own immunologic responses to the antecedent streptococcal infection. This theory is made more credible by the relatively long latent period between the onset of pharyngitis and ARF and by the demonstration of numerous examples of antigenic similarity between somatic constituents of the group A *Streptococcus* and human tissues. The most intensively studied of these antigenic cross-reactions has been that between streptococci and human heart. Many patients with ARF or rheumatic heart disease demonstrate in their sera antibodies that cross-react with heart tissue in a variety of test systems. These "heart reactive antibodies" (HRA) are also present, although in lower titer, in sera of some patients with uncomplicated streptococcal infection. HRA are also present in the sera of patients with postcardiotomy and postmyocardial infarction syndromes and in endomyocardial fibrosis, and it is possible that they represent a secondary response to myocardial antigenic determinants exposed or modified by tissue damage.

Two pieces of evidence suggest, however, that the presence of HRA in ARF patients is not secondary but rather is based upon cross-reactions between streptococcal and host antigens. Rabbits immunized with group A streptococcal cell walls develop antibodies that bind to sarcolemma and subsarcolemmal sarcoplasm in cardiac myofibers and skeletal muscle, as well as to smooth muscle of vessel walls and of endocardium. HRA in rheumatic patients but not in those with nonstreptococcal-related illness may be absorbed by streptococcal constituents. Antigens of the group A *Streptococcus* that share antigenic determinants with heart tissue have been localized both to the cell wall (including the M protein molecule) and to the cell membrane.

Another intriguing cross-reaction is that described between the group A carbohydrate in cell walls of *S. pyogenes* and a glycoprotein in human and bovine heart valves. The cross-reactive substance appears to be N-acetyl glucosamine, the terminal residue in rhamnose side chains of group A carbohydrate. This cross-reaction is of special interest because serum levels of antibodies to group A carbohydrate remain elevated for years in patients with rheumatic valvulitis (but not in rheumatic patients without valvulitis) and decline remarkably if valve resection is performed.

Patients with ARF have, on the average, higher titers of serum antibodies to virtually all streptococcal extracellular and somatic antigens than do patients with uncomplicated streptococcal infections. Perhaps for this reason, much of the immunologic investigation of rheumatic fever has focused upon humoral antibodies (e.g., HRA, anticarbohydrate antibodies, and anti–brain-cell antibodies) that cross-react with human and streptococcal antigens. Data relating to cellular immunity are more limited. ARF patients exhibit an exaggerated cellular reactivity to streptococcal constituents, particularly streptococcal cell membrane antigens, as demonstrated by inhibition in vitro of migration of peripheral blood lymphocytes.

Chronic remittent nodular lesions have been produced in dermal connective tissue following injection into experimental animals of a streptococcal mucopeptide-polysaccharide cell wall complex. Taken together, these and other reported antigenic cross-reactions and toxic phenomena could theoretically account for most of the manifestations of ARF. As yet, however, there is no direct evidence that any of them is of pathogenetic significance.

Several observations suggest that development of rheumatic fever may be modulated, at least in part, by the specific genetic constitution of the host. These include (1) the tendency of rheumatic fever to affect more than one member of a given family; (2) the fact that only a small percentage of all individuals experiencing an immunologically significant streptococcal infection develop ARF; (3) the tendency of rheumatic individuals to experience recurrent attacks; and (4) the propensity of rheumatic subjects to exhibit exaggerated immunologic responses to streptococcal antigens. Analyses of the relative frequencies of histocompatibility antigens in rheumatic subjects and controls have been inconclusive. A preliminary report, however, suggests that a particular B cell alloantigen is present in three quarters of rheumatic subjects but in less than 20 per cent of controls.

EPIDEMIOLOGY. The epidemiology of ARF mirrors that of streptococcal pharyngitis. The peak age incidence is 5 to 15 years, but both primary and recurrent cases are frequently seen in adults. ARF is rare in children less than 4 years of age, a fact that has led some observers to speculate that repetitive streptococcal infections are necessary to "prime" the host for the disease. There is no clear-cut sex predilection, although females are more likely to develop certain manifestations such as Sydenham's chorea and mitral stenosis.

Rheumatic fever occurs in all parts of the world; there is no known racial predisposition. In temperate climates, ARF peaks in the cooler months of the year, in the winter and early spring or shortly after schools open in the fall. The major environmental factor favoring occurrence appears to be crowding, as in military barracks or similar closed institutions and in large households. Crowding favors interpersonal spread of group A streptococci and perhaps enhances streptococcal virulence by frequent human passage. At present, ARF is primarily a disease of lower socioeconomic classes, particularly those massed in the densely populated core areas of major urban metropolitan centers. The disease remains rampant in developing areas such as the Middle East, the Indian subcontinent, and many nations of Africa and South America. It has been estimated that rheumatic heart disease causes 25 to 40 per cent of all cardiovascular disease in the third world.

The precise incidence of ARF in the United States is difficult to ascertain. In many localities the disease is not reportable. Cases manifested by carditis alone may not come to medical attention during the acute phase, and instances of polyarthritis or cardiac disease of other etiologies are frequently confused with ARF. All observers agree, however, that the incidence of ARF and the prevalence of rheumatic heart disease have declined dramatically both in America and in Western Europe over the past four to five decades. Studies of the incidence of ARF (hospitalized and nonhospitalized cases) among children aged 5 to 19 years in Baltimore and Nashville during the 1960's indicated rates in the range of approximately 24 to 34 per 100,000 population. The rate for blacks was about twice that for whites, a fact thought to be related to socioeconomic rather than to genetic factors. During roughly the same time period, the ARF attack rate among school-aged children in the most congested of Manhattan's Spanish-American neighborhoods was estimated to be 78 per 100,000. At present, however, rates of less than 2 per 100,000 school children have been reported from several centers. In the affluent suburbs of many United States cities, ARF is becoming extremely rare.

The frequency with which ARF develops following untreated group A streptococcal upper respiratory infection differs with the epidemiologic circumstances. In the years following World War II, careful prospective studies were conducted among personnel in military recruit camps suffering from exudative tonsillitis or pharyngitis caused by M typable group A streptococci. Under such circumstances, in which cases of streptococcal pharyngitis tend to be clinically severe and to appear in discrete epidemics, approximately 3 per cent of untreated patients developed ARF. Studies of endemically occurring streptococcal infection among open populations of children are complicated by the difficulties of differentiating cases of mild, nonexudative streptococcal pharyngitis from viral pharyngitis occurring in streptococcal carriers; nevertheless, the ARF attack rate in such circumstances is clearly lower than in the military experience, with an overall attack rate of less than 1 per cent.

Certain features of the antecedent streptococcal infection are associated with an increased risk of ARF. Among these are the magnitude of the ASO titer rise and the persistence of the infecting organism in the pharynx. Prospective civilian studies indicate that ARF is more likely to occur following clinically severe exudative pharyngitis than following mild, nonexudative illness. On the other hand, one third or more of cases of ARF occur after streptococcal infections which are asymptomatic or so mild as to have been forgotten by the patient.

Patients with a history of ARF are at greatly increased risk of recurrent disease following an immunologically significant streptococcal infection. In long-term prospective studies of rheumatic subjects carried out at Irvington House, a rheumatic fever sanatorium outside New York City, one of every five documented streptococcal infections gave rise to a recurrence of ARF. The risk of recurrence is greater in patients with preexisting rheumatic heart disease and in those experiencing symptomatic throat infections; the risk declines with advancing age and with increasing interval since the most recent rheumatic attack. Nevertheless, rheumatic patients remain at increased risk well into adult life, perhaps indefinitely.

PATHOLOGY. ARF is characterized by exudative and proliferative inflammatory lesions in the connective tissues, especially those of heart, joints, and subcutaneous tissues. The early lesions consist of edema of the ground substance, fragmentation of collagen fibers, cellular infiltration, and fibrinoid degeneration. In the heart, diffuse degeneration and even necrosis of muscle cells may be observed. At a slightly later stage, focal perivascular inflammatory lesions develop. These so-called *Aschoff nodules* (Fig. 268–1), considered pathognomonic of rheumatic fever, consist of a central area of fibrinoid surrounded by lymphocytes, plasma cells, and large basophilic cells, some of them multinucleate. Many of these cells have elongated nuclei with a distinctive chromatin pattern, sometimes called "caterpillar" or "owl-eye" nuclei, depending on their orientation in microscopic cross-section. Cells containing these nuclei are called "Anitschkow myocytes," despite the fact that most authorities believe them to be of mesenchymal origin.

Cardiac findings may include pericarditis, myocarditis, and endocarditis. Foci of coronary arteritis may also be observed. A thickened and roughened area ("MacCallum's patch") is frequently present in the left atrium above the posterior leaflet of the mitral valve. Valvular lesions appear early as small verrucae along the line of closure. Later, as healing occurs, the valves may become thickened and deformed, the chordae shortened, and the commissures fused. These changes result in valvular stenosis or insufficiency. The mitral valve is most commonly involved, followed by the aortic, the tricuspid, and, rarely, the pulmonic.

Pathologically, the *arthritis* of ARF is characterized by a fibrinous exudate and sterile effusion without erosion of the joint surfaces or pannus formation. *Subcutaneous nodules* have many histologic features in common with the Aschoff nodules. They consist of central zones of fibrinoid necrosis surrounded by histiocytes, fibroblasts, occasional lymphocytes, and rare polymorphonuclear cells. Inflammation of the smaller arteries and arterioles may occur throughout the body. Despite pathologic evidence of diffuse vasculitis, aneurysms and thrombosis are not typical features of ARF.

CLINICAL MANIFESTATIONS. Rheumatic fever may involve a number of different organ systems, most notably the heart, joints, skin, and central nervous system. The clinical picture of the disease may thus be quite variable, depending upon which systems are attacked, whether they are involved singly or in combination, the order in which they are affected, and the severity of the involvement. Five clinical features of the disease are so characteristic of it that they are recognized as "major manifestations" according to the revised Jones criteria (see below) for diagnosis of ARF: carditis, polyarthritis, chorea,

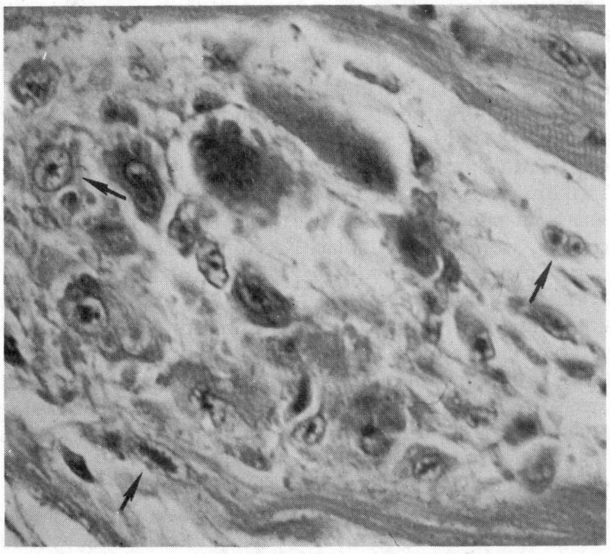

Figure 268–1. Myocardial Aschoff nodule demonstrates areas of fibrinoid degeneration and numerous large cells with polymorphous nuclei; several of the nuclei have "owl eye" or "caterpillar" configurations (arrows). (× 630.) (Courtesy of Robert Peace, M.D.)

subcutaneous nodules, and erythema marginatum. Certain other findings, frequently present but nonspecific, have been designated "minor manifestations." These include arthralgia, fever, history of previous rheumatic fever or evidence of preexisting rheumatic heart disease, and certain laboratory findings (see below).

In cases in which it can be determined, the *latent period* between the antecedent streptococcal infection and the onset of symptoms of ARF ranges between one and five weeks. The average latent period is 19 days for both primary and recurrent attacks. When acute polyarthritis is the presenting complaint, the onset is often rather abrupt and may be marked by high fever and toxicity. If isolated carditis is the initial manifestation, the onset may be insidious or even subclinical. Between these two extremes, a wide variety of gradations exists in the initial presentation of ARF. In most attacks, fever and joint involvement are the earliest clinical manifestations, although they may occasionally be preceded by abdominal pain localized to the periumbilical or infraumbilical areas. At times the location and severity of the pain, as well as fleeting signs of peritoneal inflammation, may lead to a misdiagnosis of acute appendicitis. Carditis, if it is to appear, usually does so within the first three weeks of the illness. In contrast, chorea tends to occur later in the course of the disease, sometimes after all other manifestations have subsided. Fortunately, chorea and polyarthritis almost never occur simultaneously. Epistaxis may be a feature of ARF, occurring both at the onset and throughout the acute phase of the illness; it may be quite severe.

Overall, arthritis occurs in approximately 75 per cent of first attacks of ARF, carditis in 40 to 50 per cent, chorea in 15 per cent, and subcutaneous nodules and erythema marginatum in fewer than 10 per cent. The incidence of individual manifestations, however, varies with age. Carditis is more frequent in the youngest age groups and is relatively rare in first attacks occurring in adults. Chorea occurs primarily in persons between age five years and puberty. It is seen more frequently in females and virtually never occurs in adult males. Thus, most attacks of ARF occurring in adults are manifested primarily by arthritis.

Arthritis. Joint involvement ranges from arthralgia alone to acute, disabling arthritis characterized by swelling, warmth, erythema, severe limitation of motion, and exquisite tenderness to pressure. The larger joints of the extremities are usually involved—most frequently the knees and ankles, but also the wrists and elbows. The hips and small joints of the hands and feet are affected occasionally. Involvement of shoulders and lumbosacral, cervical, sternoclavicular, and temporomandibular joints occurs in a relatively small percentage of cases. The synovial fluid contains thousands of white blood cells with a marked preponderance of polymorphonuclear leukocytes; bacterial cultures are sterile.

Characteristically, the articular involvement in ARF assumes a pattern of *migratory polyarthritis*. This does not mean that inflammation in one joint disappears before the next is attacked. Rather, a number of joints are affected in succession and the periods of involvement overlap. Inflammation in one joint may subside while another is becoming symptomatic, so that the process seems to migrate from joint to joint. In untreated cases, as many as 16 joints may be affected, and about half the patients develop arthritis in more than six joints. When effective anti-inflammatory therapy is administered early in the course of the disease, the involvement not infrequently remains monoarticular or pauciarticular.

In most instances, inflammation in any one joint begins to subside spontaneously within a week and the total duration of involvement is no more than two or three weeks. The entire bout of polyarthritis rarely lasts more than four weeks and resolves completely, leaving no residual joint damage. Some authors have described the rare occurrence of *Jaccoud's arthritis*, so-called chronic post–rheumatic fever arthropathy of the metacarpophalangeal joints, following repetitive bouts of rheumatic polyarthritis. This entity is not a true arthritis but a form of periarticular fibrosis; its relationship to rheumatic fever remains unresolved.

Carditis. Rheumatic fever may involve the endocardium, myocardium, and pericardium, and thus the disease is capable of inducing a true *pancarditis.* Carditis is the most important manifestation of ARF because it is the only one capable of causing significant permanent organ damage or death. Although the clinical picture may at times be fulminant, it is more frequently mild or even asymptomatic and may escape notice in the absence of more obvious associated findings such as arthritis or chorea. The diagnosis of carditis requires the presence of one of the following four manifestations: (1) organic cardiac murmurs not previously present, (2) cardiomegaly, (3) pericarditis, or (4) congestive heart failure. In practice, the characteristic murmurs of ARF are almost always present in cases of rheumatic carditis, unless the ability to hear them is obscured (e.g., loud pericardial friction rub, large pericardial effusion, low cardiac output, severe tachycardia). The diagnosis of carditis should be made with caution in the absence of one of the following three murmurs: apical systolic, apical mid-diastolic, and basal diastolic. Such murmurs, if they are destined to develop, do so usually within the first week and almost always within the first three weeks of illness. (An exception to this rule may occur in the patient with "pure" chorea; see later discussion.) The *apical systolic murmur* of relative or actual mitral regurgitation encompasses most of systole. It is blowing, relatively high pitched, and heard best at the apex; it radiates to the axilla and at times to the base of the heart or the back. It must be distinguished carefully by quality, location, and radiation from a variety of functional precordial systolic murmurs heard in normal individuals, especially in children. The *apical mid-diastolic* (Carey-Coombs) murmur is a low-pitched sound replacing or immediately following the third heart sound and ending distinctly before the first heart sound. It may be heard in a variety of conditions associated with increased flow across the mitral valve and is thus not pathognomonic of ARF. It may be differentiated from the diastolic rumble of mitral stenosis by the absence of an opening snap, presystolic accentuation, or accentuated first sound at the mitral area. The high-pitched, decrescendo *basal diastolic murmur* of aortic regurgitation is best heard along the upper left sternal border or over the aortic area. It may be brief and faint, best heard after expiration with the patient leaning forward.

Other prominent auscultatory findings in patients with active rheumatic carditis include tachycardia, which persists during sleep; protodiastolic, presystolic, or summation gallops; an indistinct or "mushy" quality to the first heart sound (resulting in some cases from first degree heart block); pericardial friction rub; or muffling of heart tones caused by pericardial effusion. In the early stages of congestive heart failure, rapid distention of the hepatic capsule may lead to right upper quadrant aching and tenderness over the liver. All the usual clinical findings of pericarditis or congestive failure may be observed.

A number of different rhythm disturbances may occur during the course of ARF. By far the most common is first degree atrioventricular block. Second and third degree heart block, nodal rhythm, and premature contractions may also be observed; atrial fibrillation, on the other hand, is usually a feature of chronic rather than acute rheumatic involvement. Conduction disturbances do not in themselves indicate acute carditis, and their presence or absence is unrelated to the subsequent development of rheumatic heart disease.

In cases of ARF with severe carditis, areas of patchy pneumonitis are sometimes seen. Many observers feel that these pulmonary infiltrates represent a specific *rheumatic pneumonia.* The case is difficult to prove, however, because of the confusion induced by such confounding clinical entities as pulmonary edema, pulmonary embolization, superimposed bacterial pneumonia, and the acute respiratory distress syndrome in these severely ill and toxic patients.

Sydenham's Chorea (Chorea Minor, "St. Vitus' Dance"). This neurologic syndrome occurs after a latent period which is variable but on the average longer than that associated with the other manifestations of ARF. It frequently occurs in "pure" form, either unaccompanied by other major manifestations or, after a latent period of several months, at a time when all other evidences of acute rheumatic activity have subsided. Chorea is characterized by rapid, purposeless, involuntary movements, most noticeable in the extremities and face. The arms and legs flail about in erratic, jerky, incoordinated movements which may sometimes be unilateral (hemichorea). Facial tics, grimaces, grins, and contortions are evident. The speech is usually slurred or jerky. The tongue, when protruded, retracts involuntarily, while asynchronous contractions of lingual muscles produce a "bag of worms" appearance. The involuntary motions disappear during sleep and may be partially suppressed by rest, sedation, or volition.

Patients with chorea display generalized muscle weakness and an inability to maintain a tetanic muscle contraction. Thus, when the patient is asked to squeeze the examiner's fingers, a squeezing and relaxing motion occurs which has been described as "milkmaid's grip." The knee jerk may have a pendular quality. There is no cranial nerve or pyramidal involvement, and sensory modalities are unaffected. The electroencephalogram may display abnormal slow wave activity.

Emotional lability is characteristic of Sydenham's chorea and often may precede other neurologic manifestations, leaving teachers and parents puzzled over apparently inexplicable personality changes.

Subcutaneous Nodules. These are firm, painless subcutaneous lesions which vary in size from a few millimeters to approximately 2 cm. The skin overlying them is freely movable and is not inflamed. The lesions tend to occur in crops over bony surfaces or prominences and over tendons. Sites of predilection include the extensor surfaces of elbows, knees, and wrists; the occiput; and spinous processes of the thoracic and lumbar vertebrae. Nodules are virtually never seen as the sole major manifestation of ARF; they almost always appear in association with carditis, and the cardiac involvement in such cases tends to be clinically severe. Nodules ordinarily do not appear until at least three weeks after the onset of an attack, usually lasting one to two weeks. They may appear in repeated crops in patients with protracted carditis. Similar nodules may be seen in systemic lupus erythematosus and in rheumatoid arthritis. Subcutaneous nodules in the latter disease are larger and more persistent than those in rheumatic fever.

Erythema Marginatum. The rash begins as an erythematous macule or papule, which then extends outward, while the skin in the center returns to normal. Adjacent lesions coalesce, forming circinate or serpiginous patterns (see Color plate 9). The lesions are neither pruritic nor indurated, and they blanch on pressure. They vary greatly in size, and appear mostly upon the trunk and proximal extremities, sparing the face. Erythema marginatum may be raised or flat; the latter was termed *erythema annulare* in the older literature. The lesions are evanescent, migrating from place to place, at times changing before the observer's eyes, and leaving no residual scarring. The erythema may be brought out by the application of heat. Individual lesions may come and go in minutes to hours, but the process may go on intermittently for weeks to months uninfluenced by anti-inflammatory therapy; its persistence is not necessarily an adverse prognostic sign. In the great majority of cases, erythema marginatum is accompanied by carditis; it also tends to be associated with subcutaneous nodules.

LABORATORY FINDINGS. No specific laboratory test is diagnostic of ARF. Usually there is a leukocytosis with an increase in the proportion of polymorphonuclear leukocytes. A mild to moderate normocytic normochromic anemia is the rule. In some patients the serum glutamic oxaloacetic transaminase level is elevated. Evidences of acute inflammation are prominent, including readily detectable quantities of C-reactive protein in the blood and elevation of the erythrocyte sedimentation rate. An exception is "pure" chorea, which may appear long after indices of inflammation have returned to normal. The urine may contain protein, white cells, and red cells. Biopsy studies have revealed a variety of renal abnormalities, but the classic proliferative glomerular abnormalities which characterize post-streptococcal acute glomerulonephritis occur quite rarely, if at all, in ARF. Electrocardiographic and radiographic studies may reveal evidence of rhythm disturbances, pericarditis, pericardial effusion, or congestive heart failure.

The major laboratory contribution to the workup of ARF is the documentation of recent group A streptococcal infection. Throat culture should always be performed but is positive in only a minority of cases. This is perhaps due to the time lapse of several weeks between the onset of the pharyngeal infection and the throat culture. The serum titer of antistreptolysin O (ASO) is elevated in 80 per cent or more of ARF patients. If two streptococcal antibody tests, e.g., ASO plus either anti-DNAse B or antihyaluronidase, are performed, an elevated titer of at least one will be found in 90 per cent of ARF patients. A battery of three tests will establish the presence of recent, immunologically significant streptococcal infection in more than 95 per cent of individuals experiencing an acute rheumatic attack. The definition of an "elevated" titer varies, depending upon the test employed, age of the patient, and geographic locale. In practice ASO titers greater than 200 to 250 Todd units per milliliter are generally considered elevated. At times, serial sampling may detect a rising titer of streptococcal antibodies in patients seen early in the course of a rheumatic attack.

A simple slide agglutination test (Streptozyme) is positive in high titer in over 90 per cent of ARF patients. However, the test must be performed by a technician skilled in interpreting hemagglutination reactions, and values of 1:100 to 1:200 should be considered equivocal. Care should be taken to test simultaneously controls of known titer.

COURSE AND PROGNOSIS. The average duration of an untreated attack of ARF is approximately three months. The duration tends to be longer, up to six months, in patients with severe carditis. Less than 5 per cent of patients have continuing rheumatic activity for longer than six months. In a few of these the disease is limited to chorea and is otherwise benign. Other patients exhibit evidence of persistent inflammatory activity, including arthritis, carditis, and subcutaneous nodules. "Chronic rheumatic fever" occurs more frequently in patients who have had one or more previous attacks; cardiac involvement in chronic rheumatic fever tends to be frequent and severe.

Death from intractable myocarditis during the acute phase of ARF is now very rare. Once the acute attack has subsided, the only long-term sequel is that of rheumatic heart disease, manifested primarily by insufficiency and/or stenosis of the mitral and aortic valves. The prognosis from a cardiac standpoint is very much dependent upon the clinical findings at the time the patient is first seen. In one large study, for example, 347 patients were examined during an acute rheumatic attack and again ten years later. Among patients who had been free of carditis during their acute attack, only 6 per cent had residual heart disease on follow-up. Patients with no pre-existing heart disease and with mild carditis during their acute attack (i.e., apical systolic murmur without pericarditis or heart failure) had a relatively good prognosis in that only approximately 30 per cent had heart murmurs ten years later. About 40 per cent of subjects with apical or basal diastolic murmurs and 70 per cent of subjects with failure and/or pericarditis during their acute attacks had residual rheumatic heart disease. The prognosis was worse in patients with pre-existing heart disease and in those who had experienced recurrent attacks of ARF in the ten-year interval.

The data cited above indicate that patients who do not develop carditis during an acute attack and are protected from ARF recurrences are most unlikely to suffer from rheumatic heart disease. The patient with "pure" chorea represents an exception to this rule. A significant proportion of such patients who have no evidence of carditis when first examined may develop rheumatic valvular disease on prolonged follow-up. Although the explanation for this phenomenon is unknown, it is conceivable that, in view of the long latent period associated with chorea, signs of carditis might have been present earlier but subsided by the time the neurologic abnormality became evident.

DIAGNOSIS. Although ARF is readily recognized in the individual who presents with multiple major manifestations or in epidemic circumstances, at other times the disease may be extraordinarily difficult to diagnose with confidence. This is because of the variability of its clinical presentation, the frequency with which only a single major manifestation is detected, and the fact that there is no definitive diagnostic laboratory test. Nevertheless, precise diagnosis is especially important in this disease because of the necessity to advise the patient regarding prolonged antimicrobial prophylaxis (see below).

The diagnostic criteria of T. Duckett Jones, as subsequently modified by a committee of the American Heart Association, attempt to minimize over- and underdiagnosis (Table 268–1). Two major manifestations, or one major and two minor manifestations, indicate a high probability of ARF, *provided that there is supporting evidence of recent streptococcal infection.* Although a positive throat culture for group A streptococci technically satisfies this requirement, it is important to realize that streptococcal carriage rates of 15 per cent are not uncommon among school-aged children during the fall and winter. Elevated titers of antibodies to streptococcal extracellular products, although not diagnostic of ARF, do indicate a recent, *immunologically significant* streptococcal infection. Conversely, if a battery of streptococcal antibody tests fails to reveal any evidence of recent infection, the diagnosis of ARF must be considered unlikely. This statement does *not* necessarily hold true in patients whose only rheumatic manifestation is Sydenham's chorea. Because of the long latent period associated with chorea, previously elevated antibody titers may have declined to normal.

The modified Jones criteria are of course only guidelines. They are most difficult to apply confidently when polyarthritis is the single major manifestation present. Under such circumstances, serious consideration must be given to various other entities, including rheumatoid arthritis, Still's disease, viral arthritides (e.g., rubella, hepatitis B), the early prepurpuric phase of Henoch-Schönlein purpura, and septic arthritis. The last-named entity has come to the fore with the resurgence of

TABLE 268–1. JONES CRITERIA (REVISED) FOR GUIDANCE IN THE DIAGNOSIS OF RHEUMATIC FEVER*

Major Manifestations	Minor Manifestations
Carditis	*Clinical*
Polyarthritis	Previous rheumatic fever or rheumatic heart disease
Chorea	Arthralgia
Erythema marginatum	Fever
Subcutaneous nodules	*Laboratory*
	Acute phase reactions
	Erythrocyte sedimentation rate, C-reactive protein, leukocytosis
	Prolonged P-R interval
	Plus

Supporting evidence of preceding streptococcal infection (increased ASO or other streptococcal antibodies; positive throat culture for group A *Streptococcus;* recent scarlet fever).

The presence of two major criteria, or of one major and two minor criteria, indicates a high probability of the presence of rheumatic fever if supported by evidence of a preceding streptococcal infection. The absence of such evidence should make the diagnosis doubtful, except in situations in which rheumatic fever is first discovered after a long latent period from the antecedent infection (e.g., Sydenham's chorea or low-grade carditis).

*From Circulation 32:64, 1965, with permission.

gonococcal arthritis as a relatively common cause of febrile polyarthralgia and polyarthritis in adolescent females in certain population groups.

Serum sickness is frequently a serious consideration, particularly if the patient has received penicillin or other antibiotics for a preceding respiratory infection. Systemic lupus erythematosus, sickle cell hemoglobinopathies, and infective endocarditis may involve the joints and the heart. Other differential diagnostic considerations include congenital heart lesions, viral and idiopathic forms of myocarditis and pericarditis, and functional heart murmurs. Nonfamilial forms of chorea have been described in systemic lupus erythematosus, and rarely in association with the use of birth control pills. It remains uncertain how often episodes of chorea occurring during pregnancy ("chorea gravidarum") represent attacks of rheumatic fever. Other disorders that may at times be confused with ARF are gout, sarcoidosis, Hodgkin's disease, and acute leukemia.

Following an episode of acute streptococcal pharyngitis, a small proportion of patients may experience persistent symptoms of malaise, arthralgia, low grade fever, and lymphadenopathy plus laboratory evidences of mild inflammation. It is difficult to classify such cases, but the affected individuals do not meet the criteria for diagnosis of ARF and, moreover, do not appear to be at risk for the delayed cardiac sequelae of ARF.

TREATMENT. Antibiotics neither modify the course of a rheumatic attack nor influence the subsequent development of carditis. Nevertheless, it is conventional to give a course of antibiotics designed to eradicate any group A streptococci remaining in the tonsils and pharynx, at least in part to prevent spread of the organism to close contacts. The recommended regimens are as follows: intramuscular benzathine penicillin G, 600,000 units for children less than 60 pounds and 1,200,000 units for heavier individuals; or penicillin V orally, 125 to 250 mg four times daily for ten days. Penicillin-allergic individuals may receive erythromycin. The specific dosage varies somewhat with the preparation selected but is in the range of 20 to 40 mg per kilogram of body weight per day divided in two to four equal doses. The maximum dose is one gram per day. Following completion of this therapy, continuous antistreptococcal prophylaxis should commence (see below).

Treatment with anti-inflammatory agents is effective in suppressing many of the signs and symptoms of ARF. These agents do not "cure" the disease, nor do they prevent the subsequent evolution of rheumatic heart disease. They should be avoided in very mild or equivocal cases, because, by suppressing the clinical manifestations, they may obscure the diagnosis. The two drugs most widely used are aspirin and corticosteroids. The former is used in patients with acute polyarthritis, provided that carditis is either absent or mild and there is no evidence of congestive heart failure. Aspirin is very effective in decreasing fever, toxicity, and joint inflammation. It should be given in a dosage of 90 to 100 mg per kilogram per day. This is administered in equally divided doses, every four hours for the first 24 to 36 hours; thereafter it may be given in four doses during waking hours. A salicylate level of 25 mg per deciliter is usually satisfactory. The incidence of nausea and vomiting may be minimized by starting somewhat below the optimal dosage level and gradually increasing over a few days. The patient should be observed for evidence of significant gastrointestinal bleeding and for signs and symptoms of salicylism. After two weeks, the dosage is reduced to 60 to 70 mg per kilogram per day for an additional six weeks. These dosage schedules represent general guidelines only. The precise aspirin dose must be determined by the patient's clinical response, blood salicylate levels, and tolerance of the drug.

Corticosteroids are generally reserved for patients who have severe carditis manifested by congestive heart failure, who are unable to tolerate large doses of salicylates, or whose signs and symptoms are inadequately suppressed by aspirin. As with aspirin, the dosage must be individualized. Prednisone, 40 to 60 mg per day in divided doses, may be used initially; after two to three weeks it should be withdrawn slowly over an additional three-week period. In cases of fulminating carditis with profound heart failure, intravenous corticosteroids may be employed. Aspirin should be administered for a month after discontinuation of prednisone. As is the case for other patients receiving corticosteroids, the physician should be alert to problems such as gastrointestinal bleeding, sodium and water retention, potassium depletion, and impairment of glucose tolerance. Suppression of the pituitary-adrenal axis or of the host immune system is a potential problem but not ordinarily a major one during this relatively short course of treatment. The role of nonsteroidal anti-inflammatory agents in management of ARF remains to be defined.

Following cessation of anti-inflammatory therapy, clinical or laboratory evidence of ARF may reappear. Such therapeutic "rebounds" occur more frequently after corticosteroid therapy than after treatment with aspirin. They may be minimized by prolonging salicylate therapy for 9 to 12 weeks and, when corticosteroids have been required, by continuing aspirin use for a month after corticosteroids have been discontinued.

Congestive heart failure is managed by the usual measures of bed rest, sodium restriction, diuretics, and, if necessary, oxygen and digitalis. The potential risk of digitalis-induced arrhythmias in the patient with active myocarditis must be borne in mind.

All patients should be kept at bed rest for the first three weeks of illness, during which time carditis will usually manifest itself if it is destined to appear. Bathroom privileges and an occasional period in a chair may be allowed unless arthritis or chorea make this infeasible or unless incipient or frank heart failure supervenes. Subsequently the level of physical activity should be guided by the patient's clinical status, primarily by the presence and activity of rheumatic carditis. Patients with congestive heart failure should be kept at bed rest as long as failure is present. Patients with Sydenham's chorea require a quiet environment, and sedatives such as phenobarbital may be helpful.

Once the acute attack has subsided completely, the patient's subsequent level of physical activity is dependent upon his cardiac status. Patients without residual heart disease may resume full and unrestricted activity. It is important that the patient not be subjected to unwarranted invalidism, either because of his own inaccurate perceptions of the nature of the rheumatic process or because of those of his parents, teachers, or employers.

PREVENTION. "Primary prevention" of ARF consists of accurate diagnosis and appropriate treatment of streptococcal sore throat (Ch. 267). Although straightforward in theory, primary prevention is often frustratingly difficult to achieve. In many of the densely populated, indigent communities in which the risk of ARF is greatest, children with self-limited illnesses such as sore throats may never come to medical attention, and throat culture services are usually unavailable to aid in diagnosis. Moreover, in one third or more of cases, ARF may arise after a clinically inapparent streptococcal infection.

Perhaps the most effective strategy for avoiding the mortality and chronic cardiac disability associated with ARF is that of "secondary prevention." This strategy focuses upon the group of persons who have already suffered a rheumatic attack and who are inordinately susceptible to a recurrence following an immunologically significant streptococcal upper respiratory infection. Recurrent attacks tend to be mimetic in nature so that patients who have suffered carditis with their previous attack are likely to have repetitive cardiac involvement and progressive cardiac damage. Because even patients who experienced only arthritis or chorea may develop carditis with recurrent attacks of ARF, *all* patients who have experienced a documented attack of ARF should receive continuous antimicrobial prophylaxis to prevent either symptomatic or asymptomatic streptococcal infections. The specific regimens to be used are indicated in Ch. 267. By far the most effective of these is monthly benzathine penicillin G. Rheumatic recurrences are very unusual in patients faithfully adhering to this regimen.

The total duration of rheumatic prophylaxis remains unresolved. Some authorities recommend lifelong prophylaxis. On the other hand, the risk of rheumatic recurrence is known to diminish with increasing age and increasing interval since the most recent rheumatic attack. Patients who escape carditis during their initial attack are less likely to experience rheumatic recurrences and less likely to develop carditis if a recurrence does ensue. These facts, coupled with the relative rarity of ARF itself in most parts of the United States at present, suggest that prophylaxis need not be perpetual for all rheumatic subjects. Continuous prophylaxis should be maintained indefinitely for all those with clinically significant rheumatic heart disease. Other rheumatic subjects should be protected until reaching adulthood, for at least five years after their most recent attack, and if they are in an epidemiologic circumstance which places them at high risk of streptococcal acquisition (e.g., parents of small children, school teachers, military recruits, pediatricians). The decision to remove a rheumatic subject from continuous prophylaxis should be an individualized one, based upon the physician's assessment of the risk and likely consequences of recurrence, and taken with the patient's informed consent. Patients taken off prophylaxis must be instructed to return immediately for medical follow-up whenever symptoms of pharyngitis occur.

Patients with rheumatic valvular heart disease must receive prophylaxis designed to avoid bacterial endocarditis whenever they undergo dental or surgical procedures likely to evoke bacteremia. This is not necessary in the rheumatic subject who is free of residual heart disease. The regimens for prevention of endocarditis (see Ch. 269) are entirely different from those prescribed for prevention of ARF, and the fact that a patient is receiving rheumatic fever prophylaxis in no way exempts him from endocarditis prophylaxis. This is a frequent point of confusion not only among patients but among physicians and dentists as well.

Bisno AL: The concept of rheumatogenic and non-rheumatogenic group A streptococci. *In* Read SE, Zabriskie JB (eds.): Streptococcal Diseases and the Immune Response. New York, Academic Press, 1980, pp 789–803. *Summarizes data supporting the hypothesis that group A streptococci vary in rheumutogenic potential.*

Bisno AL, Pearce IA, Wall HP, Moody MD, Stollerman GH: Contrasting epidemiology of acute rheumatic fever and acute glomerulonephritis: Nature of the antecedent streptococcal infection. N Engl J Med 283:561, 1970. *The epidemiology and bacteriology of endemically occurring streptococcal infections and their nonsuppurative sequels in an indigent, urban southern United States population.*

Committee on Rheumatic Fever and Bacterial Endocarditis, American Heart Association: Prevention of rheumatic fever. Circulation 55:1A, 1977. *Official recommendations of the American Heart Association for primary and secondary prevention of rheumatic fever. Includes specific antibiotic regimens.*

Feinstein AR, Spagnuola M: The clinical pattern of acute rheumatic fever: A reappraisal. Medicine 41:279, 1962. *An extremely careful and comprehensive analysis of the clinical patterns observed in 374 episodes of ARF admitted to the Irvington House rheumatic fever sanatorium.*

Land MA, Bisno AL: Acute rheumatic fever: A vanishing disease in suburbia. JAMA 249:895, 1983. *Up-to-date data on the occurrence of ARF in a middle-sized United States community. Discussion of recent trends in rheumatic fever incidence in the United States.*

Markowitz M, Gordis L: Rheumatic Fever. 2nd ed. Philadelphia, W. B. Saunders Company, 1972. *An excellent general textbook with authoritative coverage of areas of public health interest: epidemiology, primary prevention, and community health services.*

Sanyal SK, Thapar MK, Ahmed SH, et al.: The initial attack of acute rheumatic fever during childhood in north India: A prospective study of the clinical profile. Circulation 49:7, 1974. *The frequency of occurrence of the major clinical manifestations of ARF is carefully documented in patients admitted to a general hospital in north India, and the findings are compared with those from large series in the United States.*

Stollerman GH: Rheumatic Fever and Streptococcal Infection. New York, Grune & Stratton, 1975. *A comprehensive, extremely readable summary of all aspects of rheumatic fever. The bibliography is excellent.*

United Kingdom and United States Joint Report: The natural history of rheumatic fever and rheumatic heart disease: Ten year report of a cooperative clinical trial of ACTH, cortisone and aspirin. Circulation 32:457, 1965. *This definitive international study of the natural history of rheumatic fever relates the risk of developing rheumatic heart disease to the cardiac status during the acute attack. Long-term prognosis was not improved by the use of corticosteroids or ACTH.*

Wood HF, Feinstein AR, Taranta A, et al.: Rheumatic fever in children and adolescents. III. Comparative effectiveness of three prophylaxis regimens in preventing streptococcal infections and rheumatic recurrences. Ann Intern Med 60(Suppl 5):31, 1964. *This beautifully designed and executed Irvington House study provides definitive data on the efficacy of secondary prophylaxis.*

Endocarditis

269. INFECTIVE ENDOCARDITIS

David T. Durack

When microbes colonize the endocardium, they cause the disease termed *infective endocarditis*. The organism is usually a common bacterium, the site affected is usually one of the heart valves, and the characteristic lesion is a vegetation. For general use, the term infective endocarditis is more appropriate than *bacterial endocarditis*, because this disease also can be caused by fungi and chlamydia. Serviceable terms in general use include *subacute* and *acute bacterial endocarditis* (SBE and ABE), *native valve endocarditis* (NVE), *prosthetic valve endocarditis* (PVE), and *nonbacterial thrombotic endocarditis* (NBTE).

HISTORY. Throughout the last hundred years, infective endocarditis has fascinated students of internal medicine. Although the disease is not particularly common, it has traditionally been given prominence in textbooks and in teaching. Many notable scholars have studied and written on endocarditis, including Virchow, Osler, Thayer, Libman, Friedberg, and Beeson. Contrary to popular belief, the first systemic dose of penicillin was administered at Columbia University in 1940 to a patient with endocarditis, not in Oxford in 1941. The first demonstration that infective endocarditis (previously always fatal) could be cured in a large number of cases by administering penicillin came from Loewe and his colleagues in New York in 1944.

MICROBIOLOGY. Most of the species of bacteria that have been isolated from humans have been reported to cause endocarditis. However, a few common species account for the great majority of infections. Gram-positive streptococci and staphylococci dominate the list: together these organisms cause more than 80 per cent of infections on native valves. Table 269–1 shows representative figures for the reported frequency of the main etiologic microbes on native valves, on prosthetic valves, and in drug addicts. Individual and local experience may differ widely.

The Gram-Positive Cocci. The various alpha-hemolytic (viridans) streptococci together cause more cases of endocarditis than any other bacteria. These relatively avirulent streptococci are found in large numbers in the oropharyngeal and gastrointestinal flora. The species that cause SBE most often (in order of frequency) are *Streptococcus sanguis, S. mutans, S. intermedius,* and *S. mitis*. Next in frequency among the streptococci causing endocarditis are the Group D streptococci, *S. bovis* and *S. faecalis*. *S. bovis* bacteremia and endocarditis are strongly associated with the presence of lower gastrointestinal lesions, including polyps and colonic cancer. Therefore, recovery of this species from blood cultures should be followed up by investigation for colonic lesions, whether or not the patient has symptoms. *S. faecalis* (enterococcus) causes endocarditis in association with infections of the genital and urinary tract in women of childbearing age and of the urinary tract in elderly men with prostatic disease.

S. pneumoniae occasionally causes acute endocarditis. The triad of coexisting pneumococcal pneumonia, meningitis, and endocarditis is known as *Austrian's syndrome*. It is found in debilitated alcoholics and carries a very poor prognosis.

A few cases of endocarditis are caused by nutritionally dependent streptococci that require media supplemented with

TABLE 269–1. APPROXIMATE FREQUENCY OF VARIOUS ORGANISMS CAUSING INFECTIVE ENDOCARDITIS ON NATIVE VALVES, IN DRUG ABUSERS, AND ON PROSTHETIC VALVES*

	NVE (%)	Intravenous Drug Abusers (%)	Early PVE (%)	Late PVE (%)
Streptococci	65	15	10	35
Viridans, alpha-hemolytic	35	5	<5	25
S. bovis (group D)	15	<5	<5	<5
S. fecalis (group D)	10	8	<5	<5
Other streptococci	<5	<5	<5	<5
Staphylococci	25	50	50	30
Coagulase-positive	23	50	20	10
Coagulase-negative	<5	<5	30	20
Gram-negative aerobic bacilli	<5	15	20	15
Fungi	<5	5	10	5
Miscellaneous bacteria	<5	5	5	5
Diphtheroids, propionibacteria	<1	<5	5	<5
Other anaerobes	<1	<1	<1	<1
Rickettsia	<1	<1	<1	<1
Chlamydia	<1	<1	<1	<1
Polymicrobial infection	<1	5	5	5
Culture-negative endocarditis	5–10	5	<5	<5

*These are representative figures collated from the literature; wide local variations in frequency are to be expected.

Adapted from Durack DT: Infective and non-infective endocarditis. *In* Hurst JW (ed.): The Heart. Chap. 54. New York, McGraw-Hill Book Company, 1982, pp 1250–1277.

L-cysteine or pyridoxine for growth. These fastidious organisms can be difficult to isolate from blood cultures, and the infections they cause are more difficult to cure than infections caused by other streptococci.

Staphylococcus aureus is the leading cause of acute bacterial endocarditis, the predominant species in narcotic addicts with endocarditis, and an important cause of PVE (Table 269–1). *Staphylococcus epidermidis* rarely causes NVE. In contrast, it is a leading cause of PVE.

Other Etiologic Organisms. Gram-negative and fungal infections are described later. Endocarditis caused by *Hemophilus* species is usually associated with *H. aphrophilus, H. paraphrophilus,* or *H. parainfluenzae,* rarely with *H. influenzae. Neisseria gonorrhoeae* endocarditis, an acute disease that often involves the right side of the heart, has become rare since the introduction of penicillin. Endocarditis caused by anaerobic bacteria is also rare, accounting for less than 1 per cent of cases.

PATHOGENESIS AND PATHOLOGY. Figure 269–1 illustrates the sequence of events in pathogenesis of SBE, which usually develops on abnormal heart valves. Previously, the underlying cardiac condition was most often chronic rheumatic valvular heart disease. Today, the leading pre-existing condition for SBE in the United States is congenital heart disease in its various forms, including mitral valve prolapse. Next in frequency is rheumatic disease, but the number of such cases will decline further in the United States and other developed countries as the prevalence of chronic rheumatic heart disease in the general population continues to fall. Other important predisposing conditions are cardiac surgery (especially if a prosthetic valve has been implanted) and previous episodes of infective endocarditis. ABE can attack previously normal as well as damaged

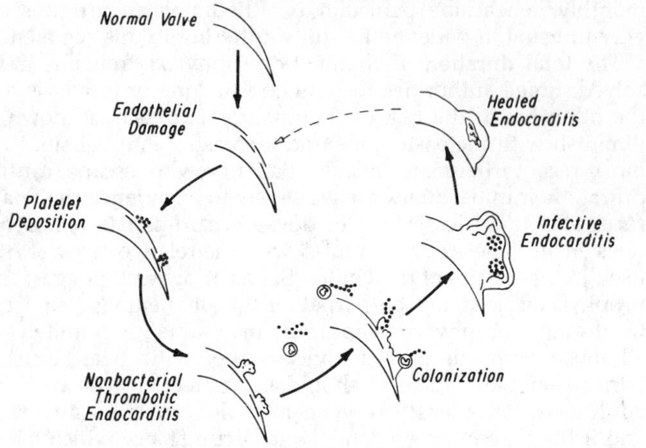

Figure 269–1. A diagram to illustrate the main events in pathogenesis of subacute bacterial endocarditis. Adapted from Durack DT: Infective and non-infective endocarditis. *In* Hurst JW (ed.): The Heart. Chap. 54. New York, McGraw-Hill Book Company, 1982.

valves. Estimates of the frequency of the main underlying heart conditions for patients of various ages with acute or subacute endocarditis are shown in Table 269–2. Table 269–3 lists estimates of the relative risks for endocarditis posed by various cardiac lesions.

The pathogenetic sequence leading to SBE begins with endothelial damage. When subendothelial connective tissue containing collagen fibers is denuded of endothelium, platelets aggregate at the site. These aggregates have been found occasionally on normal valves, but they occur more frequently on the surfaces of valves damaged by congenital or rheumatic disease or by a previous episode of infective endocarditis. These microscopic platelet thrombi may form and resolve harmlessly, but sometimes they are stabilized by deposition of fibrin and grow to form nodular sterile vegetations that are referred to as NBTE. Microscopic examination shows bundles of degenerating platelets held together by strands of fibrin, with few other cells present. This process can be induced in experimental animals by passing a catheter into the heart; NBTE forms at sites where the catheter damages the endothelium. Intracardiac pressure-monitoring catheters produce NBTE in humans in the same way. For unknown reasons, patients with cachexia caused by advanced malignancy or other wasting diseases are prone to form NBTE, which in this setting is usually termed *marantic endocarditis.* The sterile vegetations found in a few patients with systemic lupus erythematosus (Libman-Sacks endocarditis) are another form of NBTE.

The vegetations of NBTE are irregular friable white or tan masses of variable size that are usually found along the lines where valves touch upon closing. They may be so small as to be easily missed on inspection but are frequently rather large. Because there is no inflammatory reaction at the site of attachment, the vegetations of NBTE can often be picked off easily with forceps at necropsy to leave a normal-looking valve surface. These easily dislodged vegetations embolize frequently, often blocking peripheral arteries and causing infarction in myocardium, spleen, kidney, brain, gut, or extremities.

When NBTE is colonized by circulating bacteria, infective endocarditis results. Two important factors that determine

TABLE 269–2. APPROXIMATE FREQUENCY OF THE MAJOR CATEGORIES OF PRE-EXISTING CARDIAC LESIONS IN PATIENTS WITH INFECTIVE ENDOCARDITIS

	Children under 2 Years Old (%)	Children 2 to 15 Years Old (%)	Adults 15 to 50 Years Old (%)	Adults > 50 Years Old (%)	Adults, Intravenous Drug Abusers
No known heart disease	50–70	10–15	10–20	10	50–60
Congenital heart disease	30–50	70–80	20–30	10–20	10
Rheumatic heart disease	Rare	10–20	30–40	20–30	10
Degenerative heart disease	0	0	Rare	10–20	Rare
Previous cardiac surgery	5	10–15	10–20	10–20	10–20
Previous endocarditis	Rare	5	5	5–10	10–20

Adapted from Durack DT: Infective and non-infective endocarditis. *In* Hurst JW (ed.): The Heart. Chap. 54. New York, McGraw-Hill Book Company, 1982, pp 1250–1277.

TABLE 269–3. ESTIMATED RELATIVE RISK FOR INFECTIVE ENDOCARDITIS POSED BY VARIOUS CARDIAC LESIONS

Relatively High Risk	Intermediate Risk	Very Low or Negligible Risk
Prosthetic heart valves	Mitral valve prolapse	Atrial septal defects
Aortic valve disease	Pure mitral stenosis	Arteriosclerotic plaques
Mitral insufficiency	Tricuspid valve disease	Coronary artery disease
Patent ductus arteriosus	Pulmonary valve disease	Syphilitic aortitis
Ventricular septal defect	Previous infective endocarditis	Cardiac pacemakers
Coarctation of the aorta	Asymmetric septal hypertrophy	Surgically corrected cardiac lesions (without prosthetic implants, more than 6 months after operation)
Marfan's syndrome	Calcific aortic sclerosis	
	Hyperalimentation or pressure-monitoring lines that reach the right atrium	
	Nonvalvular intracardiac prosthetic implants	

Adapted from Durack DT: Infective and non-infective endocarditis. *In* Hurst JW (ed.): The Heart. Chap. 54. New York, McGraw-Hill Book Company, 1982, pp 1250–1277.

which organisms will be most likely to cause endocarditis are the frequency with which they are found in the blood and their ability to adhere to fibrin and platelet thrombi. Viridans streptococci enter the blood from the oral cavity frequently (probably daily) and adhere well. They are the leading cause of SBE (Table 269–1). In contrast, *Escherichia coli* adheres poorly and rarely causes endocarditis even though it very frequently causes bacteremia.

Once lodged upon the surface of NBTE, bacteria multiply rapidly and attain high numbers within the vegetation, after which many enter the stationary or resting phase. The presence of bacteria is a powerful stimulus for further localized thrombosis, which causes vegetations to enlarge by accretion of new layers of fibrin. Because these layers protect bacteria from phagocytes, the vegetation provides a sanctuary in which even avirulent bacteria can flourish.

Approximate figures for the frequency with which vegetations are found at various locations in the heart are given in Table 269–4. The frequency with which a cardiac valve is involved by endocarditis is related to the mean blood pressure acting upon it. Accordingly, the aortic and mitral valves are infected far more often than the tricuspid and pulmonary valves. This rule holds for SBE but not for acute endocarditis in intravenous drug abusers, in whom tricuspid valve infection is common (Table 269–4).

Endocarditis usually develops at sites where blood flows from a high-pressure source (e.g., the left ventricle) through an orifice (e.g., a ventricular septal defect) into a low-pressure sink (e.g., the right ventricle). Examples of cardiovascular conditions subject to infection that fit these criteria include mitral regurgitation, aortic stenosis, ventricular septal defect, patent ductus arteriosus, and coarctation of the aorta. Vegetations are usually located on the "downstream" side of these anatomic abnormalities, where pressure effects and turbulence favor deposition of bacteria from the swift stream of blood.

TABLE 269–4. FREQUENCY WITH WHICH ANATOMIC SITES ARE INVOLVED IN SUBACUTE ENDOCARDITIS, ACUTE ENDOCARDITIS, AND ENDOCARDITIS IN DRUG ADDICTS

	SBE (%)	ABE (%)	Endocarditis in Intravenous Drug Abusers (%)
Left-sided valves	85	65	40
Aortic	15–26	18–25	25–30
Mitral	38–45	30–35	15–20
Aortic and Mitral	23–30	15–20	13–20
Right-sided valves	5	20	50
Tricuspid	1–5	15	45–55
Pulmonary	1	Rare	2
Tricuspid and pulmonary	Rare	Rare	3
Left- and right-sided sites	Rare	5–10	5–10
Other sites (patent ductus, VSD, coarctation, jet lesions	10	5	5

Adapted from Durack DT: Infective and non-infective endocarditis. *In* Hurst JW (ed.): The Heart. Chap. 54. New York, McGraw-Hill Book Company, 1982, pp 1250–1277.

Vegetations also may develop at sites where a turbulent regurgitant jet of blood strikes the wall of a cardiac chamber, causing endothelial roughening and reactive endocardial fibrosis. These are called *jet lesions*.

The vegetations of infective endocarditis are variable in appearance. Some are small wartlike nodules, while others have the cauliflower-like polypoid appearance that gave rise to the descriptive term *vegetation*. Some are less than 1 sq mm in size, while others are so large as to block the valve orifice and cause functional stenosis. They may be white, red, tan, or gray. Vegetations in patients with ABE or fungal endocarditis are often larger than those of SBE. Microscopic examination shows colonies of bacteria or masses of fungal hyphae embedded in fibrin and platelets. Infected vegetations usually contain surprisingly few leukocytes. Inflammatory cells may accumulate at the base of the vegetation, where it attaches to the valve. This distorts the valve, superimposing new damage on any pre-existing pathology. If this reaction is severe, the valve may perforate, or an abscess may develop in adjacent tissues. Abscess formation is common in ABE and PVE but not in SBE.

Antibodies to many of the commensal organisms that cause SBE are present in low titer before infection occurs, increase in number during the course of SBE, and decrease after successful treatment. These antibodies do not arrest the progress of SBE and do not provide immunity to future endocardial infection.

The healing process begins even in untreated endocarditis but only reaches completion if antibiotic treatment kills the bacteria. Host cells move in to organize the vegetation; macrophages ingest bacterial and cellular debris; and fibroblasts lay down new collagen. The vegetations gradually shrink over a period of weeks or months and become endothelialized. Recognizable but nonviable bacteria can sometimes be found in sections of valves resected at operation or necropsy, months after infection has been eradicated. The healed valve is often scarred, thickened by fibrosis, and calcified. It may be perforated, and the supporting structures may be damaged. Residual hemodynamic dysfunction, mild or severe, is therefore likely. This condition may worsen over time, although bacteria have been eradicated by treatment long before. The scarred valve remains susceptible to reinfection for life.

CLINICAL FEATURES. All the clinical and laboratory manifestations of infective endocarditis reflect the effects of a systemic intravascular infection and the patient's physiologic and immunologic reaction to it.

History. The onset of subacute endocarditis is usually insidious, with nonspecific complaints, general malaise, anorexia, weakness, and fatigue. This nonspecific syndrome is often described as a "flu-like illness." Low grade intermittent fevers with chills and night sweats are usual. Headaches, myalgias, arthralgias, and back pain are common. A history of heart murmur, congenital heart disease, rheumatic fever, or cardiac surgery may help identify the underlying lesion. The patient may conceal intravenous drug abuse, which should be kept in mind during both interview and examination as a possible mode of infection.

Symptoms of heart failure must be carefully sought because their presence is of great prognostic significance. Embolization and infarction can cause sudden onset of neurologic symptoms such as hemiparesis or abdominal pain due to splenic, renal, or gut infarction. Embolization of a coronary artery can cause silent or symptomatic myocardial infarction. Perforation of a valve or rupture of chordae tendineae can cause sudden onset of severe heart failure.

Physical Examination. Patients with subacute endocarditis may have nonspecific symptoms of subacute systemic infection including pallor, asthenia, and sweating. A variety of interesting peripheral signs may be found on further examination, including petechiae, splinter hemorrhages, Roth's spots, Osler's nodes, Janeway's lesions, and clubbing of the fingers. Some of the characteristics of these signs are summarized in Table 269–5.

Examination of the spleen often shows moderate enlargement but no notable tenderness unless there is a splenic abscess or recent embolic infarction.

On examination of the cardiovascular system, the peripheral pulse is usually rapid because of fever, heart failure, or both. A "collapsing" pulse may be present, indicating aortic incompetence associated with pre-existing aortic valve disease or new aortic insufficiency associated with endocarditis. Individual peripheral arteries may be occluded by emboli, or they may be the site of a mycotic aneurysm.

One or more cardiac murmurs is present in virtually all patients with endocarditis. Murmurs may be caused by pre-existing heart disease, by endocarditis itself, or by both. Up to 15 per cent of patients do not have a heart murmur when first examined, but nearly all develop a murmur before the disease has run its course. New murmurs and changing murmurs are more likely to occur in acute endocarditis than in subacute disease. Development of a new murmur of aortic insufficiency during a febrile illness of unknown origin strongly suggests the diagnosis of endocarditis.

COMPLICATIONS. Heart failure is by far the most important complication of infective endocarditis because it exerts more influence on prognosis and treatment than any other complication. In one representative series, some degree of heart failure was present in 75 per cent of patients with aortic valve disease and endocarditis, in 50 per cent with mitral valve involvement, and in 19 per cent with tricuspid disease.

Arterial embolization is diagnosed in about one third of patients with subacute endocarditis and in up to two thirds of patients with acute endocarditis. Many small or large arterial emboli go undetected. Any artery may be affected. In order of frequency, arteries supplying the brain, lung, myocardium, spleen, and extremities are involved.

Neurologic manifestations of endocarditis are common and clinically important. These include toxic confusional states, stroke, meningoencephalitis, cranial or peripheral nerve lesions, and psychiatric symptoms. About 10 per cent of patients with endocarditis have complaints involving the central nervous system, while 30 to 50 per cent have nervous system involvement at some point during the course of the disease. Cerebral infarction is usually caused by embolism, while cerebral hemorrhage, which is less common than infarction, may be associated with emboli or rupture of a mycotic aneurysm. Heparin therapy increases the risk that an intracranial hemorrhage will occur during the course of infective endocarditis.

Cerebritis secondary to impaction of infected emboli or hematogenous spread of bacteria is quite common, especially in acute bacterial endocarditis caused by *S. aureus*. Cerebritis may progress to form a frank cerebral abscess, which is found in 1 to 5 per cent of cases of acute endocarditis. However, brain abscesses rarely complicate subacute endocarditis.

In up to 15 per cent of patients, examination of the cerebrospinal fluid may show reactive changes consisting of the presence of polymorphonuclear leukocytes and moderately elevated protein concentration. Such reactions are particularly common in acute staphylococcal endocarditis. In most cases cerebrospinal glucose concentrations do not decrease, cultures are negative, and true bacterial meningitis does not develop, except in a few patients with acute pneumococcal or staphylococcal endocarditis.

Mycotic aneurysm is an unusual but important complication that is diagnosed in 3 to 5 per cent of patients. The true incidence is probably higher, but a number pass undetected, especially small aneurysms in the brain. Mycotic aneurysms are caused by an inflammatory reaction in the arterial wall associated with septic microemboli to vasa vasorum or impaction of an infected embolus in the arterial lumen. The site most often involved is the proximal aorta, including the sinuses of Valsalva, followed by arteries to the viscera, extremities, and brain. Living organisms are seldom found in the wall of these aneurysms, even when the underlying endocardial infection is still active. Presumably, the damage that weakens the arterial wall was done by an earlier inflammatory reaction to infected emboli. If an aneurysm enlarges to a certain critical size (prob-

TABLE 269–5. CHARACTERISTICS OF PERIPHERAL SIGNS OF INFECTIVE ENDOCARDITIS

	Petechiae	Splinter Hemorrhages	Roth's Spots	Osler's Nodes	Janeway's Lesions	Clubbing
Appearance	Tiny red hemorrhagic spots	"Splinters" under nails; red when fresh, then brown or black	Small bright red patches with white centers	Pea-sized red or purplish nodules	Red macules	Curvature of the nails in two planes, with swelling of the terminal phalanges
Distribution	Anywhere, especially above clavicles, in mouth and in conjunctivae	Distal third of nails	Retinae	Fingers and toes; occasionally hands and feet	Palms and soles; occasionally on flanks, forearms, ankles, feet, ears	Fingers and/or toes
Incidence	Common, in both SBE and ABE	Common, in both SBE and ABE	Infrequent; usually in SBE	Infrequent; usually in SBE	Infrequent; usually in ABE	Rare; in SBE only
Pathology	Increased capillary permeability; microemboli	Blood in avascular squamous epithelium under nail; due to microemboli or increased capillary fragility	Inflammation and hemorrhage	Intracutaneous local vasculitis; bacteria rarely found; occasional abscess formation; probably embolic in origin	Origin uncertain; possibly embolic or allergic in origin	Soft tissue proliferation, occasionally periosteal new bone formation
Pain	None	None	None	Mild to moderately severe	None	Usually none; sometimes painful
Duration	Days	Weeks	Days	Days	Several hours to days	Weeks to months
Diagnostic significance	Nonspecific; also found in septicemia, after cardiac surgery, and in many other disorders	Nonspecific; found in up to 10% of normal people, and up to 40% of patients with mitral stenosis	Strongly suggestive of endocarditis but not diagnostic	Almost pathognomonic for endocarditis	Unusual in bacteremia without endocarditis	Nonspecific; found in many cardiopulmonary disorders; can be congenital

Adapted from Durack DT: Infective and non-infective endocarditis. *In* Hurst JW (ed.): The Heart. Chap. 54. New York, McGraw-Hill Book Company, 1982, pp 1250–1277.

ably about 1 cm in diameter), it is likely to continue to enlarge and eventually rupture as a result of the physical force of the arterial pressure, despite eradication of the infecting organisms by antimicrobial therapy.

Most patients with subacute endocarditis have some abnormalities in the urinary sediment. In some cases this is due to glomerulonephritis, a relatively common complication that is usually not severe enough to cause significant renal failure. Glomerulonephritis is caused by deposition of immune complexes on the glomerular basement membrane. Other inflammatory manifestations of subacute infective endocarditis that may be mediated by immune complexes include arthritis, tenosynovitis, and possibly pericarditis, Osler's nodes, and Roth's spots. In a few patients with long-term SBE, glomerulonephritis is severe enough to make dialysis necessary. Renal function usually recovers steadily within a few weeks after the start of effective treatment.

SPECIAL FORMS OF INFECTIVE ENDOCARDITIS

ACUTE BACTERIAL ENDOCARDITIS. Several important features distinguish acute from subacute bacterial endocarditis. The diagnosis is usually made within seven days from onset of symptoms. The clinical course is usually measured in days rather than in weeks or months. The associated systemic illness is more severe, and early mortality is higher.

Acute endocardial infection is usually caused by primary pathogens capable of producing invasive infection at other sites. *S. aureus* is the most common cause of acute endocarditis. This species alone accounts for 50 to 70 per cent of cases. The patient is more likely to suffer rapid destruction of the valve, including perforation, so the likelihood that valve replacement will be required is greater. Patients with acute bacterial endocarditis are also more likely to have one or more focal infections outside the heart—in brain, bone, lungs, or other sites. Such foci could be either primary (that is, the portal of entry for endocarditis) or secondary hematogenous infections. In contrast, the organisms that cause subacute bacterial endocarditis rarely cause localized hematogenous infection elsewhere in the body.

Abscesses in the fibrous cardiac skeleton or myocardium are much more likely to form in acute than in subacute endocarditis. If such abscesses are adjacent to the fibers of the conduction system, they may cause conduction defects. Abscesses may be responsible for antibiotic treatment failure.

Because acute bacterial endocarditis is caused by invasive organisms and progresses rapidly, treatment should not be delayed until blood culture results are available. It is important to clear the bloodstream of circulating organisms as soon as possible, both to reduce the risk of death from septicemia and to lessen the chances that metastatic infection will develop elsewhere. When acute endocarditis is strongly suspected, empiric antibiotic therapy should be started immediately after three blood culture samples have been drawn.

ENDOCARDITIS IN DRUG ADDICTS. Endocarditis is the most important of the many infective complications experienced by intravenous drug abusers. Salient features that distinguish endocarditis in this subgroup from the disease in general include: a younger age of onset, a higher proportion of acute cases, a correspondingly higher proportion of cases involving normal cardiac valves, and a high frequency of tricuspid valve infection. The etiologic organisms can gain entry into the bloodstream in various ways: directly, by injection of contaminated materials; or indirectly, from the patient's skin flora, from cellulitis caused by subcutaneous injection of drugs, or from suppurative thrombophlebitis or drug-related infections in other sites such as the lungs. *S. aureus* is the leading etiologic organism. Addicts also have an increased incidence of endocardial infection with gram-negative bacilli, especially *Pseudomonas* species, and fungi.

Drug addicts with acute endocarditis usually experience a brief severe illness, with heavily positive blood cultures. Because the etiologic organisms are often primary pathogens, hematogenous infection elsewhere in the body is common. A common finding on admission is multiple patches of pneumonitis visible on chest x-ray. These are caused by multiple small septic pulmonary emboli arising from vegetations on the tricuspid or occasionally the pulmonary valve. Although acute disease is typical, subacute endocarditis in addicts is not rare, especially in those who have had previous episodes of endocarditis.

The prognosis for young drug addicts with right-sided *S. aureus* infection is good, with mortality rates of less than 5 per cent. Factors that worsen the prognosis include left-sided involvement, particularly aortic, and infection with gram-negative bacilli or fungi. Recurrent episodes of endocarditis are common in addicts who continue to use drugs after their first episode of endocarditis, especially if a prosthetic valve has been inserted.

PROSTHETIC VALVE INFECTION. Prosthetic valve endocarditis should be regarded as a special category, because it differs in many ways from other forms of endocarditis. By definition, early PVE occurs within 60 days of valve placement and late PVE more than 60 days postoperatively. Early PVE occurs at a rate of about 1 per cent, although this figure varies between hospitals. Late PVE is estimated to occur at an overall rate of about 1 per cent per year. The rate for an aortic valve prosthesis is four to five times higher than for a mitral prosthesis.

The progress of PVE may be either acute or subacute, but this cannot be predicted reliably from the infecting organism. For example, even *S. epidermidis*, a nonpathogen that causes indolent chronic disease on native valves, can cause an acute syndrome in early PVE.

The spectrum of organisms causing PVE is quite distinct. *S. epidermidis*, which rarely infects native valves, is a leading cause of both early and late prosthetic valve infection. Gram-negative bacilli and fungi infect prosthetic valves notably more often than they do native valves, especially in early onset cases. The later the onset of PVE after operation, the more nearly the spectrum of etiologic organisms resembles that of native valve endocarditis.

In addition to forming vegetations, infection may spread around the circumference of the sewing ring of the prosthesis, often causing partial dehiscence and paravalvular leaks. Abscess formation in fibrous tissue or myocardium adjacent to the sewing ring is common. Despite these adverse factors, when a prosthetic valve is replaced for infection, early reinfection with the same organism is uncommon.

In general, PVE is harder to cure than most other forms of endocarditis (Table 269–6). This is due partly to the increased frequency of antibiotic-resistant organisms in PVE, and partly to the fact that a foreign body is present at the site of infection. Not surprisingly, the risk of relapse after antibiotic therapy is much higher for PVE than for native valve infection. Valve replacement is often necessary to achieve cure. Antibiotic treatment usually must be continued for a minimum of four to six weeks, sometimes for many months. In some cases in which repeated valve replacement is contraindicated, cure cannot be achieved but suppressive antibiotic therapy is continued indefinitely.

GRAM-NEGATIVE BACTERIAL ENDOCARDITIS. This term usually refers to infection with enteric or environmental gram-negative aerobic bacilli such as *Klebsiella, Pseudomonas, Serratia, Enterobacter*, and *E. coli*. (*Hemophilus* species usually cause subacute endocarditis and are not considered in this group.) Gram-negative endocarditis is a rare disease except in two settings: early prosthetic valve infection and intravenous drug addiction. In these two groups, gram-negative bacilli can account for up to 15 to 20 per cent of cases.

Gram-negative endocarditis often but not always progresses acutely. Patients may develop septic shock. The mortality rate is higher than for gram-positive infections, approaching that of fungal endocarditis. Antibiotic treatment alone is often unsuc-

TABLE 269–6. ESTIMATED BACTERIOLOGIC CURE RATES FOR ETIOLOGIC ORGANISMS TREATED WITH ANTIMICROBIAL THERAPY ALONE OR ANTIMICROBIALS PLUS SURGERY*

Native Valve Endocarditis	Antimicrobial Therapy Alone		Antimicrobial Therapy Plus Surgery	
Viridans streptococci, group A streptococci, *S. bovis*, pneumococci, gonococci	98		98	
S. fecalis	90		>90	
S. aureus (in young drug addicts)	90		>90	
S. aureus (in elderly patients with chronic underlying diseases)	50		70	
Gram-negative aerobic bacilli†	40		65	
Fungi	<5		50	
Prosthetic Valve Endocarditis	**Early PVE**	**Late PVE**	**Early PVE**	**Late PVE**
Viridans streptococci, group A streptococci, *S. bovis*, pneumococci, gonococci	‡	80	‡	90
S. fecalis	‡	60	‡	75
S. aureus	25	40	50	60
S. epidermidis	20	40	60	70
Gram-negative aerobic bacilli†	<10	20	40	50
Fungi	<1	<1	30	40

*Morbidity and mortality will be significantly greater than these figures for bacteriologic cure indicate.

†Excluding *Hemophilus* species.

‡Insufficient data to estimate rate.

Adapted from Durack DT: Infective and non-infective endocarditis. *In* Hurst JW (ed.): The Heart. Chap. 54. New York, McGraw-Hill Book Company, 1982, pp 1250–1277.

cessful, so valve replacement is frequently necessary. Treatment with combinations of two or more antibiotics for six weeks or more is often necessary. Relapse after antibiotic treatment is much more common than for gram-positive infection.

FUNGAL ENDOCARDITIS. Like gram-negative endocarditis, fungal infection of the endocardium is rare except in two groups of patients: those with prosthetic valves and intravenous drug addicts. Although a wide variety of fungal species have been recovered from patients with endocarditis over the years, only two predominate, *Candida* and *Aspergillus spp. C. albicans* endocarditis occurs in patients with central intravascular lines, especially hyperalimentation lines that are allowed to reach the level of the tricuspid valve. Therefore, these infections often involve the right side. *C. parapsilosis* and *C. tropicalis* are more likely to occur in drug addicts and can infect valves on both sides of the heart. Fungal vegetations tend to be bulky and often cause infarctions as a result of embolization of peripheral arteries. Because blood cultures are commonly negative in fungal endocarditis (see earlier discussion), surgical removal of a large embolus from an artery to one of the limbs may be diagnostic as well as therapeutic. Histologic section examination may show hyphae of the infecting fungus.

Few drugs are available for treatment of fungal endocarditis. Amphotericin B is generally used, but the chances of achieving cure with drug therapy alone is extremely low. Cure rates can be greatly increased by surgical removal of vegetations and valve replacement, but mortality remains relatively high compared with that for other forms of endocarditis (Table 269–6).

ENDOCARDITIS IN INFANTS AND CHILDREN. Infective endocarditis is an unusual occurrence in infants. When it does occur, it is most often only one component of systemic bacterial infection caused by an invasive organism such as *S. aureus*. The endocardial infection is likely to follow an acute course and is not uncommonly discovered as an unexpected finding at necropsy in an infant who has died with bacterial infection. Often a normal cardiac valve is involved, as in other forms of acute endocarditis. The remainder of cases are associated with congenital cardiac defects. Because the diagnosis is often delayed or missed, endocarditis in infants has a higher mortality than in other age groups.

In children more than one year old, infective endocarditis is not rare. Most affected children have subacute disease involving congenital cardiac defects. The spectrum of etiologic organisms and the approach to diagnosis and treatment are similar to those in adult infective endocarditis. However, the age and physical size of children must be carefully considered when choosing the best time for cardiac surgery, especially when prostheses must be implanted.

ENDOCARDITIS IN OBSTETRIC AND GYNECOLOGIC PRACTICE. Pregnancy itself poses little increased risk for infective endocarditis, but a few cases develop during delivery or in the puerperium. If the mother has pre-existing valvular disease, bacteremias associated with perinatal infective complications such as amnionitis, endometritis, parametritis, septic thrombophlebitis, or urinary tract infection can seed the endocardium. Septic abortion or pelvic infection related to intrauterine contraceptive devices can also lead to endocarditis in susceptible patients. The leading etiologic organisms in this setting are *S. faecalis, S. agalactiae* (Group B), *S. aureus*, and occasionally *Bacteroides* or gram-negative enteric bacilli.

NOSOCOMIAL ENDOCARDITIS. Intensive medical care can predispose to endocarditis in many ways. Endothelial damage can be caused by intracardiac surgery, pressure-monitoring catheters, ventriculoatrial shunts, and hyperalimentation lines if they reach into the right atrium. Portals of entry for microorganisms are provided by wounds, burns, biopsy sites, intravenous and arterial catheters and pacemakers, hemodialysis access sites, urinary catheters, and intratracheal airways. Nosocomial bacteremias are common in seriously ill patients. Therefore, it is not surprising that hospital-acquired infective endocarditis has become increasingly common in the past two decades as intensive care units have proliferated. Perhaps the highest risk is found in severely burned patients, who may sustain repeated episodes of bacteremia while pressure-monitoring catheters are kept in the right side of the heart for long periods. In contrast, diagnostic right heart catheterization for brief periods in patients in a coronary care unit, who seldom develop bacteremia, presents a very low risk for infective endocarditis.

The microbes likely to cause nosocomial endocarditis are staphylococci, *Candida* species, and gram-negative bacilli. The prognosis is worse than for most other forms of infective endocarditis. This is because the patients have serious pre-existing diseases that may obscure the symptoms and signs, thus delaying diagnosis. Also, nosocomially acquired organisms are more likely than streptococci to be resistant to antibiotics.

CULTURE-NEGATIVE ENDOCARDITIS. This term refers to the situation in which the endocardium is infected, but blood cultures remain persistently negative. Possible causes include antibiotic therapy or infection by slow-growing or fastidious microorganisms that are missed because of suboptimal blood culture technique. Culture-negative endocarditis is an uncommon disease. Therefore, when blood cultures from a patient not receiving antibiotics remain persistently negative, that patient probably does not have endocarditis. Fungal endocarditis is an exception. Blood cultures are positive in only about half of patients with *Candida* endocarditis and in less than one fifth of those with *Aspergillus* infection. When culture-negative disease does occur, it is much more likely to follow a subacute than an acute course.

If the clinical findings strongly support the diagnosis of culture-negative endocarditis, a therapeutic trial of antibiotic therapy may be given. This usually consists of a penicillin plus an aminoglycoside for subacute infection, a combination which would cover viridans streptococci, enterococci, *Hemophilus* species, and diphtheroids. If the disease is acute, treatment for *Staphylococcus aureus* must be included. To be of diagnostic value, a proper therapeutic trial must be continued for at least two weeks unless new information changes the situation.

INFECTIVE ENDARTERITIS. An infection located within an artery can mimic infective endocarditis. Possible sites of vegetations include patent ductus arteriosus, coarctation of the aorta, arteriovenous fistulas, and prosthetic vascular grafts. In the past, about one quarter of all patients with an uncorrected patent ductus arteriosus eventually developed bacterial endarteritis. Because many of the underlying lesions are surgically correctable, infective endarteritis is now uncommon in developed countries, with the exception of infections in arteriovenous shunts constructed for the purpose of hemodialysis. When bacterial endarteritis occurs in an aneurysm, the etiologic organisms are usually found within a multilayered thrombus in the lumen of the aneurysm rather than in vegetations.

RECURRENT ENDOCARDITIS. The term *recurrent endocarditis* includes both *relapses* and *reinfections.* Recurent endocarditis has been reported in from 2 to 30 per cent of cases. This wide variation is partly explained by variable duration of follow-up. Intravenous drug abusers are at higher risk than any other group for recurrent endocarditis. A few patients with more than three separate episodes of infective endocarditis have been reported.

The likelihood of relapse after treatment of different forms of infective endocarditis can be predicted from published experience (Table 269–6). Because occasional relapses occur even after optimal treatment, careful follow-up for several months after treatment is mandatory. Most relapses occur within a few days or weeks of ending treatment, but occasional late relapses occur as a result of a few organisms surviving in a metabolically inactive state deep within vegetations.

Reinfection means a new episode of endocarditis has developed after cure of a previous episode. Usually a different species or strain of etiologic organism is involved, but if the second organism is a common viridans streptococcus that appears identical to the first, one cannot be certain whether an episode of recurrent endocarditis represents reinfection or relapse.

DIFFERENTIAL DIAGNOSIS. The differential diagnosis of endocarditis is very wide because its manifestations are numerous and often nonspecific. SBE must be considered in the evaluation of every patient with fever of unknown origin. It can be confused with rheumatic fever, osteomyelitis, tuberculosis, meningitis, intra-abdominal infections, salmonellosis, brucellosis, glomerulonephritis, myocardial infarction, stroke, endocardial thrombi, atrial myxoma, connective tissue diseases, vasculitis, occult malignancy (especially lymphomas), congestive heart failure, pericarditis, and even psychoneurosis. ABE shares many manifestations with septicemias caused by *S. aureus, Neisseria,* pneumococci, and gram-negative bacilli in patients who do not have endocarditis. It may mimic pneumonia, meningitis, brain abscess, stroke, malaria, acute pericarditis, vasculitis, and disseminated intravascular coagulation.

INVESTIGATIONS. ***Routine Tests.*** Results of urinalysis are abnormal in about 50 per cent of cases, showing microscopic hematuria or slight proteinuria or both. Gross hematuria suggests that renal infarction may have occurred. Red cell casts and heavy proteinuria indicate that immune complex glomerulonephritis may be present.

The automated blood count shows only nonspecific abnormalities. Anemia is usual in SBE and fairly common in ABE. Anemia is most often of the hypoproliferative type, with a normochromic normocytic smear. ABE may cause acute hemolysis. A prosthetic valve may cause chronic low grade hemolysis in the absence of infection.

A moderate leukocytosis with some immature forms apparent on smear is often found in SBE, but in many cases the leukocyte count is normal. Patients with ABE usually show a striking neutrophilia with band forms, vacuoles, Döhle bodies, and toxic granulation. In a few cases, careful examination of a Gram-stained smear of the buffy coat will reveal organisms within neutrophils.

The erythrocyte sedimentation rate is almost always elevated, except in a few acute cases of very brief duration.

Blood Culture. This is the single most important investigation in diagnosis of endocarditis. Blood cultures should be drawn from all patients with fever and heart murmur unless their illness is clearly due to another diagnosed disease or the fever resolves quickly without recurrence. Blood cultures should also be taken if a patient with a heart lesion susceptible to endocarditis has other symptoms or signs consistent with infection.

The bacteremia of infective endocarditis is usually continuous, with between 1 and 100 organisms per milliliter of blood in subacute cases. Therefore, it is seldom necessary to draw a large number of blood cultures. The causative organism can be recovered from culture samples taken on the first day of admission in over 90 per cent of patients with culture-positive endocarditis. No more than three separate venous blood cultures should be drawn on the first day. If these show no growth by the second day, two or three further culture samples may be drawn. If the patient has received prior antibiotic therapy, further blood samples may be taken over the following week in a search for recrudescence of bacteremia after antibiotic effect has passed. Otherwise, repeated blood cultures are likely to be uninformative and wasteful.

Ten to 20 ml of blood should be drawn for each culture after careful skin preparation. Skin preparation is especially important because common skin flora (*S. epidermidis* and diphtheroids) can cause endocarditis, and their isolation from blood cultures can cause diagnostic confusion. Pour plates can help to distinguish contaminants from true positive cultures. The culture medium should be adequately supplemented to allow growth of fastidious, nutritionally variant bacteria. When endocarditis is suspected, cultures should be incubated for three weeks and stains made at intervals even if no growth is apparent on inspection.

Subacute endocarditis stimulates the humoral immune system to produce both nonspecific and specific antibodies. A positive test for rheumatoid factor is found in 40 to 50 per cent of subacute cases but rarely in ABE. It can provide a useful diagnostic clue in culture-negative cases. A polyclonal increase in gamma globulins is characteristic. Occasional false-positive serologic test results for syphilis occur.

Hemolytic complement levels may be moderately elevated, normal, or low. The lowest levels are found in patients with immune complex glomerulonephritis. Circulating immune complexes are present in more than 80 per cent of patients with either ABE or SBE but are not diagnostically important in practice. All these immunologic findings revert to normal after eradication of the organisms.

Electrocardiography. Electrocardiography may reveal evidence of otherwise silent myocardial infarction due to embolization of a vegetation to a coronary artery. When a disturbance of conduction develops during the course of endocarditis, extension of infection into the myocardium may have occurred. This could be focal myocarditis or an abscess located close to the conduction system.

Echocardiography. Echocardiography may detect valvular vegetations or help in evaluation of underlying heart disease and cardiac function. This tool can be very helpful, but its sensitivity and specificity for diagnosis of endocarditis are limited. Negative echocardiographic study results do not rule out endocarditis. Very small vegetations cannot be detected, and all the leaflets of the valves cannot be visualized in every patient. Occasionally false-positive readings for vegetations occur, particularly in patients with myxomatous degeneration of a valve.

The larger vegetations typical of acute infection in narcotic addicts and of fungal endocarditis are easier to demonstrate than the smaller lesions found in some patients with SBE. Vegetations on prosthetic valves are difficult to visualize. Sequential echocardiographic studies of vegetations during and after treatment are unreliable as a criterion for success or failure of antibiotic therapy.

Radiography. The chest x-ray is most useful in endocarditis to provide evidence of congestive heart failure. Multiple small patchy infiltrates in the lungs of an intravenous drug abuser with fever strongly suggest the diagnosis of septic emboli arising from right-sided infective endocarditis. Valvular calcification may identify a valve affected by chronic rheumatic or congenital disease. A mycotic aneurysm could cause widening of the aorta.

Abnormal motion of a prosthetic valve can be detected by fluoroscopy, indicating presence of a vegetation or partial dehiscence of the valve from the aortic root. This information can indicate that valve replacement is needed during management of PVE.

Computerized axial tomography can be very useful to define the cause of focal neurologic lesions in patients with endocarditis. Such lesions could be caused by various complications, including cerebritis, infarction, hemorrhage from a mycotic aneurysm, or brain abscess. Angiography is occasionally necessary to demonstrate mycotic aneurysms in the brain or elsewhere.

Cardiac catheterization and cineangiography are not necessary for most patients who respond well to antimicrobial therapy without developing cardiac failure. When treatment seems to be failing and/or operation is considered, cardiac catheterization can provide vital information. In one study of 35 patients who underwent cardiac catheterization during active endocarditis, the precatheterization assessment was significantly modified for 23, the diagnosis of site of valve involvement was altered for 14, and six valve ring abscesses were revealed. Surgery was postponed or cancelled for six patients when catheterization indicated only mild hemodynamic abnormalities. There were no serious complications. This study suggests that catheterization is so useful for selected patients with endocarditis that it should not be avoided for fear of dislodging emboli.

TREATMENT. ***General Measures.*** The patient should be informed of the diagnosis and treatment plan and comforted. Heart failure, if present, should be managed with bed rest, salt restriction, and drug treatment as necessary. High temperatures and headaches can be treated symptomatically.

Antibiotic Therapy. For optimal antibiotic therapy, certain microbiologic information on the infecting organism is necessary. For most bacteria, both the minimal inhibitory concentration (MIC) and minimal bactericidal concentration (MBC) of the antibiotics likely to be used should be determined. This will form the basis for choice of definitive therapy.

The serum bactericidal titer (SBT or Schlichter test) is frequently used and sometimes useful in the management of endocarditis. The infecting organism is exposed in vitro to the patient's serum, which is drawn while antibiotic therapy is being administered, to determine the maximum dilutions of serum that will inhibit and kill the organism. Clinical experience indicates that the SBT should be 1:8 or higher at intervals during each day of treatment. The SBT provides assurance that the antibiotic(s) present in the patient's serum is actually capable of killing the infecting organism. For gram-positive organisms the serum usually can kill the organism without difficulty, and SBTs are often very high (1:128 to 1:1024). In such cases, SBTs need not be measured repeatedly. The SBT is most likely to be clinically helpful when the physician is treating an unusual organism, using unusual antibiotics, using an unusual regimen (such as oral treatment), or encountering treatment failure. If treatment with unusual combinations of antibiotics is needed, further laboratory tests should be performed to find out whether they are synergistic, indifferent, or antagonistic in combination.

Bactericidal antibiotics should be used for treatment of endocarditis whenever possible. Some patients have been cured with bacteriostatic drugs, but results of treatment with these agents are usually poor, presumably because host defense mechanisms are inadequate in the vegetation. With respect to treatment, the vegetations of infective endocarditis provide a contrast to bacterial pneumonia, in which phagocytes are plentiful and bacteriostatic antibiotics are usually effective. Curative antibiotic therapy for endocarditis must eradicate organisms completely, without the help of phagocytes to eliminate microbes that are relatively resistant to antibiotics because they are in the resting phase.

Clinical experience with treatment of the common forms of bacterial endocarditis caused by gram-positive cocci is so extensive that specific therapeutic regimens can be recommended with confidence. Standard regimens for streptococcal and staphylococcal endocarditis are listed in Table 269–7. Regimens for treatment of endocarditis caused by less common organisms are not listed. For these, treatment must be chosen on the basis of more limited published experience, together with the results of tests performed upon the infecting organism in the microbiology laboratory. One of the beta-lactam antibiotics should be included in the regimen whenever possible.

Empiric Therapy. When the causative organism is unknown, the choice of empiric therapy depends upon whether the patient has acute or subacute disease. For ABE, broad-spectrum therapy that will cover *S. aureus* as well as many species of streptococci and gram-negative bacilli is required. For SBE, a regimen that will treat most streptococci including *S. faecalis* is appropriate. To meet these requirements, the following regimens are suggested (see opposite page):

TABLE 269–7. TREATMENT REGIMENS FOR INFECTIVE ENDOCARDITIS CAUSED BY GRAM-POSITIVE COCCI

Organism	Antibiotic Regimen	Duration, weeks	Comments
Alpha-hemolytic (viridans) streptococci, *S. bovis*	1. Penicillin G 2 million units every 6 hours IV plus streptomycin 10 mg per kilogram every 12 hours IM, *or*	2	For patients <65 years old without renal failure, eighth-nerve defects, or serious complications
	2. Penicillin G 2 million units every 6 hours IV *plus* streptomycin 10 mg per kilogram every 12 hours IM (for first 2 weeks only), *or*	4	For patients with complicated disease, e.g., CNS involvement, shock, moderately penicillin-resistant organism, failed previous treatment
	3. Penicillin G 4 million units every 6 hours IV, *or*	4	For patients >65 years old, with renal failure or eighth-nerve defect
	4. Cefazolin 2 grams every 8 hours IV, *or*	4	For patients allergic to penicillin
	5. Vancomycin 15 mg per kilogram every 12 hours IV	4	For patients allergic to penicillin
Group A streptococci, *S. pneumoniae*	1. Penicillin G 2 million units every 6 hours IV, *or*	2–4	These organisms are usually highly sensitive to pencillin; 2 weeks will be adequate for most cases
	2. Cefazolin 2 grams every 8 hours IV	2–4	
S. fecalis, other penicillin-resistant streptococci	1. Ampicillin 2 grams every 4 hours IV *plus* gentamicin 1.0 mg per kilogram every 8 hours IV, *or*	4–6	Four weeks will be adequate for most cases
	2. Vancomycin 15 mg per kilogram every 12 hours IV *plus* streptomycin 15 mg per kilogram every 12 hours IM	4–6	Four weeks will be adequate for most cases
S. aureus	1. Nafcillin 2 grams every 4 hours IV, *or*	4 or longer	Standard regimen
	2. Nafcillin as above *plus* gentamicin 1.5 mg per kilogram every 8 hours IV for the first 3–5 days, *or*	4 or longer	For patients with severe disseminated staphylococcal disease, gentamicin synergy may be advantageous during early stages of treatment
	3. Cephalothin 2 grams every 4 hours IV, *or*	4 or longer	For patients allergic to penicillin
	4. Vancomycin 15 mg per kilogram every 12 hours IV	4 or longer	For patients allergic to penicillin and cephalosporin; for resistant organisms

1. For ABE, a combination of nafcillin, 2 grams intravenously every four hours plus ampicillin, 2 grams intravenously every four hours plus gentamicin, 1.5 mg per kilogram intravenously every eight hours.

2. For SBE, a combination of ampicillin, 2 grams intravenously every four hours plus gentamicin, 1.5 mg per kilogram intravenously every eight hours.

These regimens should be adjusted if and when the causative organism is identified.

Duration of Therapy. Because infective endocarditis carries significant mortality even when well managed, it is important that treatment be continued long enough to ensure that relapse will not occur. On the other hand, patients with the most easily treated forms of endocarditis should not be subjected to unnecessarily long and expensive treatment in hospital. Extensive experience with treatment of the streptococci provides sufficient grounds for firm recommendations on duration of therapy for these organisms (Table 269–7).

In contrast, the natural history of *S. aureus* endocarditis is highly variable. Some patients recover swiftly without complications, but others remain febrile for several weeks, often with manifestations of disseminated staphylococcal disease such as osteomyelitis. While four weeks of therapy will be adequate for most cases, this must not be regarded as a rigid rule because some patients require treatment for six to eight weeks or longer to achieve cure. In general, the less extensive the published experience with a particular infective agent, the more one should lean toward prolonging treatment in order to provide a reasonable margin of safety. Guidelines on duration of treatment for other organisms are not listed in Table 269–7 because the duration required varies greatly according to individual circumstances.

Anticoagulants. Although the infected vegetation is essentially a thrombotic lesion, there is no evidence that anticoagulants provide a useful therapeutic effect in endocarditis. In fact, simultaneous treatment with antibiotics plus heparin carries a higher risk of serious or fatal intracerebral hemorrhage from mycotic aneurysm or infarction than treatment with penicillin alone. However, coumadin can be given to most patients with endocarditis without excessive risk.

It is therefore best to avoid use of heparin entirely in endocarditis and to discontinue or avoid anticoagulation therapy if possible. However, coumadin may be given if there is a clear-cut indication, taking care not to allow the prothrombin time to rise above 1.5 times normal values. An antibiotic treatment regimen that does not require intramuscular injections should be used if the patient is receiving anticoagulants.

Surgical Treatment. Modern operative treatment constitutes the greatest advance in management of endocarditis since the advent of antibiotics. Because surgery may be needed for any patient during the course of endocarditis, they should be managed close to a thoracic surgical unit. Consultation should be obtained early, so that immediate operation can be performed if necessary.

Aortic or mitral valvular incompetence with consequent acute left ventricular failure can occur without warning, even in the most favorable forms of endocarditis. These patients need valve replacement in order to reverse cardiac failure resulting from new or worsening valvular dysfunction. Replacement of an infected prosthesis is often necessary for cure because prosthetic valve infection is more difficult to eradicate with antibiotics than is native valve infection. Repeated major emboli constitute a relative indication for valve replacement. Occasionally, a patient remains septic despite antibiotic therapy. Operation may then be required for infection control rather than for the hemodynamic consequences of infection. Operation to close a patent ductus arteriosus or septal defect, to excise a coarctation of the aorta, or to relieve asymmetric septal hypertrophy may be required as part of treatment of endocarditis engrafted upon these lesions.

Good surgical management for endocarditis depends on correct timing for valve replacement. If operation is undertaken too soon, unnecessary operative mortality and early and late morbidity of valve replacement may result. Some patients will respond quickly to medical therapy, so that operation can be postponed indefinitely. If time is available for treatment of septicemia, renal failure, pneumonia, myocarditis, conduction defects, or other complications before valve replacement, ventricular function will improve and operative risk will be correspondingly lower. Given a few days, antibiotic therapy should eradicate or at least greatly reduce the population of organisms on the valve, thus increasing the chance that an artificial valve can be inserted without itself becoming infected. However, if surgery is delayed too long patients may die suddenly, or their hemodynamic status may deteriorate so that operation is no longer feasible. This is a tragic error, because some of these patients could have been saved by earlier operation.

Frequent re-examination of the patient, together with echocardiography and/or cardiac catheterization to extend the clinical findings, is indicated in every case in which operation may be needed. The natural history of the type of endocarditis being treated should be taken into account. Penicillin-sensitive streptococcal endocarditis can almost always be bacteriologically cured (Table 269–6), and the prognosis is good if cardiac failure does not occur. Thus, operation should usually be considered only for patients with cardiac failure who do not respond to medical treatment. Similarly, narcotic addicts with acute staphylococcal endocarditis have a relatively good prognosis, so operation should be reserved for those who develop serious heart failure. At the other end of the spectrum, the likelihood that fungal prosthetic valve endocarditis can be eradicated with antifungal drugs alone is negligible, even in the absence of heart failure (Table 269–6). Such patients usually should undergo valve replacement early, without waiting to test the remote possibility that antifungal treatment could eradicate the infection. Aortic valve involvement, staphylococcal infection in patients other than drug addicts, gram-negative infection, prosthetic valve infection, and extension of infection into the myocardium should be regarded as other relative indications favoring early valve replacement.

PROGNOSIS. Infective endocarditis is unusual among infectious diseases in that it is always fatal if untreated. Most of the rare cases of apparent recovery reported in the preantibiotic era probably did not have infective endocarditis, which can be diagnosed with absolute certainty only at operation or necropsy. The median interval between onset of symptoms and death in patients with untreated subacute endocarditis was about six months, with wide individual variation. Almost all patients with acute infective endocarditis died in less than four weeks.

Favorable prognostic factors include infection with penicillin-sensitive streptococci, a youthful patient, absence of serious pre-existing diseases, and early diagnosis and treatment. The rate of recovery for many young drug addicts with *S. aureus* infection of the tricuspid valve is excellent—greater than 95 per cent.

Heart failure is by far the most important adverse prognostic factor. Other adverse factors include aortic valve involvement, renal failure, culture-negative disease, gram-negative or fungal infection, prosthetic valve infection, and presence of an abscess in the valve ring or myocardium.

Today, bacteriologic cure can be achieved in most patients with bacterial endocarditis (Table 269–6). This is not true for infection with resistant gram-negative bacilli and fungi, but fortunately these are uncommon. Despite the ability to eradicate most organisms, both early and long-term mortality and morbidity of infective endocarditis remain significant because of damage already done before treatment. Follow-up of patients cured of infective endocarditis shows a five-year survival of only 60 to 70 per cent.

PREVENTION. Because endocarditis is a serious disease, antibiotics are usually given to susceptible patients during medical and dental procedures known to cause bacteremia, in an

TABLE 269–8. AUTHOR'S RECOMMENDATIONS FOR PROPHYLAXIS OF ENDOCARDITIS*

Types of Regimen	Indications	Drug and Dosage
Standard	For dental procedures and oral or upper respiratory tract surgery	Penicillin V 2 grams orally 1 hour before, then 1 gram 6 hours later†
Special	Parenteral regimen for high-risk patients; also for gastrointestinal or genitourinary tract procedures	Ampicillin 1 to 2 grams IM or IV *plus* gentamicin 1.5 mg per kilogram IM or IV, 0.5 hours before†
	Parenteral regimen for penicillin-allergic patients	Vancomycin 1 gram IV *slowly* over 1 hour, starting 1 hour before; *add* gentamicin 1.5 mg per kilogram IM or IV if gastrointestinal or genitourinary tract is involved†
	Oral regimen for penicillin-allergic patients (oral and respiratory tract procedures)	Erythromycin 1 gram orally 1 hour before, then 0.5 gram 6 hours later†
	Oral regimen for minor gastrointestinal or genitourinary tract procedures	Amoxicillin 3 grams orally 1 hour before, then 1.5 grams 6 hours later†
	Parenteral regimen for cardiac surgery including prosthetic valve placement	Cefazolin 2 grams IV on induction of anesthesia, repeated 8 and 16 hours later,‡ *or* Vancomycin 1 gram IV *slowly* over 1 hour, starting on induction of anesthesia, then 0.5 gram IV 8 and 16 hours later‡

*These are empiric suggestions. No regimen has been proven effective, and prevention failures may occur with any regimen. These recommendations are not intended to cover all clinical situations; practitioners should use their own judgment on safety and cost-benefit issues in each individual case. Several additional doses may be given if the period of risk for bacteremia is prolonged, but prophylaxis should not be extended for days.

†Pediatric dosages: ampicillin 50 mg per kilogram; erythromycin 20 mg per kilogram for first dose, then 10 mg per kilogram; gentamicin 2 mg per kilogram; vancomycin 20 mg per kilogram; penicillin V, cefazolin, and amoxicillin for children weighing more than 60 pounds, use same dose as for adults; for children weighing less than 60 pounds, use half the adult dose.

‡Gentamicin 1.5 mg per kilogram IV may be given with each dose only if postoperative gram-negative infections have occurred with significant frequency.

Adapted from Durack DT: Nine controversies in the management of endocarditis. *In* Petersdorf RG, et al. (eds.): Update V. Harrison's Principles of Internal Medicine. New York, McGraw-Hill Book Company, 1984, pp 35–46.

attempt to prevent this infection. Unfortunately, there is no proof that this practice is effective. Meaningful cost-benefit ratios cannot be calculated, and any recommendations are therefore necessarily empiric.

One approach is to consider two factors in each situation: (1) the relative risk for endocarditis posed by the patient's heart condition and (2) the relative risk for endocarditis posed by the procedure. If both risks are judged to be significant, prophylactic antibiotics should be given. If one or both of these risk factors is judged to be negligible, prophylaxis should be omitted. The first of these two questions can be approached by using a ranking like that shown in Table 269–3. The second can be approached by knowing something of the frequency of bacteremia after the procedure in question and the number of cases of endocarditis attributed to it. For example, if a patient with aortic stenosis were to have dental extraction or urologic surgery, attempted prevention with antibiotics would be appropriate. If the same patient were to undergo gastroscopy, antibiotics would not be indicated because that procedure poses very little risk for endocarditis.

Prophylaxis for endocarditis is probably not required to cover most gastrointestinal diagnostic procedures such as endoscopy or radiocontrast studies, nor for normal delivery, therapeutic abortion, dilation and curettage, insertion or removal of intrauterine contraceptive devices in the absence of local infection, cardiac catheterization, insertion of pacemakers, endotracheal intubation, or bronchoscopy. However, some physicians choose to cover even these low-risk procedures in patients with prosthetic valves because they are at higher risk for endocarditis.

The indication for prophylactic antibiotics in patients with mitral valve prolapse remains controversial. MVP increases an individual's risk for endocarditis by five to eight times and underlies a significant proportion of cases of subacute bacterial endocarditis. However, mitral valve prolapse is very common in the general population, while endocarditis is relatively uncommon, so prolapse should be regarded as a low-risk lesion for endocarditis. Many authorities currently recommend prophylaxis for patients with prolapse, especially those with mitral regurgitation, but an estimate of benefits in relation to costs has indicated that prophylaxis for prolapse is probably not cost-effective. In the author's opinion, it is reasonable to give prophylaxis to MVP patients undergoing procedures that cause significant bacteremia because the costs and risks of oral penicillin therapy for an individual are very low, and a serious disease may occasionally be prevented. However, use of antibiotics in this setting should be considered optional rather than mandatory. Parenteral prophylaxis for MVP patients probably should be avoided to reduce the risk of anaphylaxis.

Specific recommendations for prophylaxis of endocarditis are listed in Table 269–8.

AHA Committee Report: Treatment of infective endocarditis due to viridans streptococci. Circulation 63:730A, 1981. *A brief, authoritative statement on treatment options for endocarditis caused by streptococci.*

Bisno AL: Treatment of Infective Endocarditis. New York, Grune & Stratton, 1982. *This book deals with many aspects of endocarditis besides treatment. It provides a good source for references.*

Durack DT: Infective and non-infective endocarditis. *In* Hurst JW (ed.): The Heart. Chap. 54. New York, McGraw Hill Book Company, 1982, pp 1250–1277. *A general review of infective and noninfective endocarditis in a leading cardiology textbook (181 references).*

Durack DT: Prophylaxis of endocarditis. *In* Mandell GL, Douglas RG, Bennett JE (eds.): Principles and Practice of Infectious Diseases. New York, John Wiley & Sons (in press), 1984. *This chapter analyzes the problems of endocarditis prophylaxis in detail and reviews current recommendations (52 references).*

Karchmer AW, Dismukes WE, Buckley MJ, Austen WG: Late prosthetic valve endocarditis: Clinical features influencing therapy. Am J Med 64:199, 1978. *This paper reports on patients with late prosthetic valve endocarditis, comparing survival according to etiologic organisms and medical as opposed to surgical treatment. Various features that carry a poor prognosis are identified, and relative indications for surgery are discussed.*

Rahimtoola SH: Infective Endocarditis. New York, Grune & Stratton, 1978. *A heavily referenced book, with good material on pathogenesis, pathology, and endocarditis in addicts and fungal endocarditis.*

Reisberg BE: Infective endocarditis in the narcotic. Prog Cardiovasc Dis 22:193, 1979. *A useful review of infective endocarditis in narcotic addicts. The importance of tricuspid valve infection and the effect of different infecting organisms and the sites involved on prognosis are analyzed.*

Weinstein L: Infective endocarditis. *In* Braunwald E (ed.): Heart Disease. A Textbook of Cardiovascular Medicine. Philadelphia, W. B. Saunders Company, 1984, pp 1136–1182. *A long, detailed chapter in a major cardiology textbook (382 references).*

Staphylococcal Infections

270. STAPHYLOCOCCAL INFECTIONS

John N. Sheagren

Staphylococci are ubiquitous in nature. All humans are colonized by "nonpathogenic" staphylococci. In addition the "pathogenic" coagulase-producing *Staphylococcus aureus* is present transiently in a high percentage of people and is chronically carried by about 15 per cent of the normal population. As would be expected, staphylococci, whether causative of infection or as contaminants, are frequently isolated from cultures.

S. aureus itself is one of the most important bacterial pathogens of man. It can be aggressively invasive, spreading rapidly through soft tissues, directly invading bones and other support structures and ultimately, under conducive circumstances, seeding the bloodstream to produce a fulminant picture of septic shock and disseminated intravascular coagulation. Conversely, *S. aureus* can lie dormant deep within tissues for years without causing disease. The balance between host and parasite that results in infection with a given strain of staphylococci is not known and continues to be the subject of active research.

Staphylococci are the most important hospital-associated gram-positive organisms and rank only behind *Escherichia coli* in overall incidence of infections in the hospital setting. In the community, staphylococci, particularly *S. aureus*, are the leading cause of acute, serious, and progressive skin, soft tissue, and posttraumatic infections. A thorough understanding of the pathogenetic mechanisms and clinical manifestations of staphylococcal infections is crucial to the care of septic patients in every medical environment.

BACTERIOLOGY. Staphylococci are members of the family micrococcaceae of which there are two genera of major clinical importance, the micrococci and the staphylococci. These two genera are both catalase positive, but only staphylococci can anaerobically ferment glucose to produce acid. The staphylococci in turn have three clinically important species: *S. aureus*, *S. epidermidis*, and *S. saprophyticus*. *S. aureus* alone has the capacity to produce coagulase, which is detected by timed incubation of a sample of a broth culture with citrated rabbit plasma. This test results in the production of a clot and permits the relatively rapid separation of *S. aureus* from the coagulase-negative species (*S. epidermidis* and *S. saprophyticus*). Almost all laboratories label all coagulase-negative organisms as "*S. epidermidis*," which results in the failure to differentiate at least one clinically important subspecies, *S. saprophyticus*. *S. saprophyticus* is coagulase negative but ferments mannitol and can also be identified by resistance to novobiocin. *S. saprophyticus* is a frequent cause of urinary tract infections, almost always in young women; these organisms are sensitive to all generally prescribed urinary tract antibiotics.

As regards *S. aureus*, the word *aureus* comes from the Latin word meaning gold and refers to the fact that most *S. aureus* colonies develop a bright golden-yellow color on blood agar media. However, *S. aureus* speciation is now assigned to all strains producing coagulase, whether or not they are golden in color. In addition to the production of coagulase by *S. aureus*, almost all strains ferment mannitol and contain deoxyribonuclease (DNAase). Staphylococci grow well both anaerobically and aerobically: thus, both aerobic and anaerobic bottles in a blood culture set from a truly bacteremic patient are usually positive.

The name staphylococcus comes from the fact that these organisms grow in clusters in liquid or semisolid media or within tissues when causing infection. However, in material obtained from abscesses, the organisms can sometimes be confusing in morphology, being quite variable in size, shape, and tendency toward clustering. Occasionally the organisms may grow in pairs or even chains, and confusion with streptococci is possible. Nonetheless, to the trained eye the size and general characteristics of the organism usually permit an accurate diagnosis of a pure staphylococcal lesion when the stained smear is carefully examined.

No reproducible serologic typing schemes are available to classify staphylococci. However, bacteriophage typing has been extremely useful in identifying strain characteristics of *S. aureus* and in providing epidemiologic data. Recently, bacteriophage typing has begun to be applied to *S. epidermidis*, and over 50 per cent of recovered strains can now be typed by this system. Bacteriophages are viruses that attach to the mucopeptide-teichoic acid complex of the cell wall. Over 100 different phages are now available for use in typing *S. aureus*, and five major groups of organisms having generally similar characteristics have been designated (phage groups I through V). For example, some phage groups of staphylococci are more likely to produce certain toxins than are others. Coagulase-negative *S. epidermidis* has also been divided into subgroups, known as biotypes, based on biochemical testing.

EPIDEMIOLOGY. Staphylococci may colonize almost all animal species and, as noted earlier, *S. epidermidis* is universally present on the human skin. The carrier state of *S. aureus* is clinically important. Humans carry *S. aureus* predominantly in the nasopharynx, although some individuals can be heavily colonized in the axillae, groin, and perirectal region. The heavily colonized individual may become a source of recurrent infections both to himself and to surrounding contacts. Most humans probably carry a few *S. aureus* organisms among the normal flora of every body site but at such a low level that routine cultures rarely reveal the organism. As stated earlier, about 15 per cent of normal, non-hospital-associated persons more or less chronically carry a heavy growth of *S. aureus* in their noses.

The definition of the carrier state is a simple one: from swab culture of the anterior nares of a carrier, multiple colonies of *S. aureus* are visually identified on a blood agar culture plate. Clearly this definition is imprecise, because the more intensely one focuses attention on the organism the higher will be the percentage of normal individuals found to carry it. Nonetheless, colony counts of the nasopharyngeal flora consistently indicate a small group of persons who harbor relatively large numbers of the organism.

The factors that result in high growth rates and numbers of *S. aureus* in the nares of certain individuals and not in others are unknown. There is no evidence that the immune response to the organism (for example, secretory immunoglobulins or other inhibitory substances) plays a major role in the acquisition and loss of the organism from the nose and throat, as is the case for the meningococcus. Data indicate that the teichoic acid moiety in the cell wall of *S. aureus* mediates the adherence of the organism to nasal mucosal cells, a phenomenon of major import in mucous membrane colonization. Also, it is highly probable that the carrier state is influenced by the ability of other members of the normal bacterial flora of the nose, throat, and skin to suppress growth of a given strain of staphylococcus. Most probably, other staphylococci or micrococci (or both) will turn out to be instrumental in controlling the growth of a newly introduced staphylococcal strain. In fact, clinical use of this concept has already been attempted via the process termed *bacterial interference*. Bacterial interference is the concept that a nonpathogenic strain of staphylococcus, once established, seems to reduce the likelihood of acquisition of another, more pathogenic strain (see later section).

There is an interesting association between the nasal carriage of *S. aureus* and any condition associated with small breaks in the skin and mucous membranes. It has been known for a long time that patients with a variety of dermatoses, especially atopic dermatitis, are very likely to be heavily colonized with *S. aureus.* In fact, patients with eczematous skin diseases may be heavily colonized in the lesions but have few organisms on the intervening normal skin. Possibly related to these observations is the fact that patients who regularly use needles have an increased rate of carriage of *S. aureus.* Drug addicts, diabetics injecting insulin, patients on hemodialysis, and even patients receiving brief courses of allergy shots all have an increased rate of nasal carriage of *S. aureus.* This phenomenon is clinically important, because the organism carried in the nose and throat is often identical to that in the bloodstream of drug-abusing patients with endocarditis. Similarly, studies done years ago demonstrated that patients who entered hospitals for surgical procedures and who were carriers of *S. aureus* had increased rates of wound infections with the carried organism. Thus, the sequence of events leading to infection with *S. aureus* seems to be the following: persons who for whatever reason begin to carry the organism in the nose are at risk of seeding the organism to other bodily sites and to breaks in the skin (for example, wounds or points of insertion of intravascular catheters). From such colonized peripheral sites, the organism may invade and cause destructive and rapidly progressive local and systemic septic complications.

Carriage of staphylococci within the gastrointestinal tract has not been extensively studied. However, normally a few staphylococci can usually be isolated. *S. epidermidis* is not uncommonly isolated from the stool but probably represents contamination from the perianal skin. Staphylococci, especially *S. aureus,* may grow to very high titers in the gastrointestinal tract in the presence of antibiotic therapy and cause gastrointestinal symptoms; the presumption is that antibiotics suppress the more sensitive normal floral components that are responsible for inhibiting the growth of *S. aureus.* This rationale is similar to that for the emergence of *C. difficile* in the syndrome of antibiotic-associated colitis (see Ch. 278).

Newborn infants rapidly experience an increasing rate of colonization following birth. It is not uncommon within nurseries to note infant colonization rates of 25 to 30 per cent. Most infants remain asymptomatic; on occasion, however, outbreaks of disease within nurseries may occur, sometimes traceable to a common carrier. Adult patients become increasingly colonized with *S. aureus* the longer they remain in the hospital. Once a hospitalized individual becomes a carrier (expecially individuals with open, actively infected lesions), the nasally carried organisms may spread to other anatomic sites, to clothing and other items within the room, and to individuals with whom the patient has contact. The most effective technique for stopping transmission of staphylococci from person to person, especially in a hospital setting, is to wash one's hands meticulously immediately before and immediately after examining each patient. This process is particularly important when examining a patient with a gross, obviously staphylococcal lesion or with a chronic exudative dermatosis. Such patients should always be managed by appropriate isolation procedures while they are hospitalized.

PATHOGENESIS. Whether or not an infection develops with any microorganism depends on the balance between the aggressiveness of the organism and the level of defense provided by the host. Thus, organisms that are highly virulent may regularly infect normal hosts and, conversely, nonpathogenic (saprophytic) organisms usually only cause infection in the face of a significant impairment of host defense. The following paragraphs will first describe those microbial characteristics that lead to the presence or absence of virulence and then the primary mechanisms by which the host attempts containment.

Microbial Virulence. The factor that makes certain strains of staphylococci virulent and others nonpathogenic is unknown. A variety of extracellular enzymes is produced by *S. aureus,* many probably participating in the pathogenic capabilities of the organism. For example, in the case of streptococci, hyaluronidase probably assists the organism in its rapid spread through tissues. A variety of other enzymes may also degrade other tissue elements, may lyse inflammation-associated coagulation (coagulase), and may be directly toxic to either white cells (leukocidins) or platelets. A variety of studies in experimental models has shown a high correlation between coagulase production and organism virulence.

Numerous toxins are produced by *S. aureus.* Some have endotoxic capabilities when injected into tissues (for example, the alpha and beta toxins). *S. aureus* frequently produces an enterotoxin, and at present six enterotoxins (A through F) have been described. Enterotoxin F is identical to pyrogenic exotoxin C, the toxin involved in the toxic shock syndrome. Another well described toxin is the exfoliative toxin responsible for the staphylococcal scalded skin syndrome.

The capsular and cell wall components of *S. aureus* clearly participate in the pathogenesis of certain clinical syndromes produced by the organism. Many *S. aureus* strains have a polysaccharide capsule covering the complex rigid cell wall matrix that consists of peptidoglycan and teichoic acid (ribitol in *S. aureus* and predominantly glycerol in *S. epidermidis*). In most strains of *S. aureus* a unique substance, *protein A,* is also part of the cell wall. Protein A is an immunologically active substance having high affinity for the FC fragment of immunoglobulins, particularly subgroups of IgG. Thus, protein A binds to and aggregates IgG molecules and, interestingly, fixes complement in the process. Protein A has emerged as an extremely useful immunochemical substance for extraction or quantitation (or both) of IgG molecules from biologic specimens. Whether protein A plays some role in any of the clinical syndromes produced by *S. aureus* is unknown. However, it is intriguing to speculate that protein A interacting nonspecifically with plasma immunoglobulins and fixing complement in the process might contribute both to the pathogenesis of septic shock and to the rapid onset of glomerular damage often present in patients with staphylococcal bacteremia or endocarditis.

The presence of a capsule varies greatly from strain to strain and may explain some of the biologic differences between organisms as they invade tissues or the bloodstream. The capsule inhibits phagocytosis by interfering with the interaction between the underlying teichoic acid–peptidoglycan complex and complement, which is activated primarily via the alternative pathway. Thus, encapsulated strains are protected in tissues from the complement-mediated attack by polymorphonuclear leukocytes (PMNs). Along with the enzymes described above, the capsule undoubtedly increases the ability of *S. aureus* to protect itself as it spreads through tissues and therefore is an important virulence factor for tissue infections. Paradoxically, while unencapsulated organisms are more likely to be contained in tissues, should the bloodstream be reached (for example in a narcotics addict directly injecting carried organisms into the blood stream), the syndrome of septic shock and disseminated intravascular coagulation (DIC) may result. The syndrome of septic shock follows massive intravascular complement, coagulation system, and kinin system activation (see Ch. 256). In such a situation, unencapsulated strains of *S. aureus* produce septic shock exactly like gram-negative bacteria wherein the cell wall lipopolysaccharide (endotoxin) activates the responsible inflammatory systems.

Host Defense Aspects. The primary mechanism by which the host defends against staphylococci, expecially *S. aureus,* is via the nonspecific defense system. The specific, antibody and T cell-mediated, host defenses appear to participate very little, if at all, in defense against *S. aureus.* Thus, while antibodies are of theoretical value against encapsulated strains of *S. aureus,* no data exist to show that antibody (commonly present in the sera of most individuals against a variety of cell wall antigens and toxins of *S. aureus*) is of any clinical value. Previous attempts to develop vaccines against the organism have not yielded documented clinical benefits.

The nonspecific host defense system consists of the barrier

systems (skin and mucous membranes) plus the complement-mediated polymorphonuclear (PMN) leukocyte assault on invading organisms. Patients with defects in intracellular killing of bacteria by the PMN (for example, as in the chronic granulomatous disease of childhood or the Chediak-Higashi syndrome) are particularly prone to develop serious infections with *S. aureus*.

Certain pathologic states with highly elevated levels of IgE predispose the patient to recurrent, chronic infections with *S. aureus*. Job's syndrome is a condition wherein an elevated IgE level associated with eczematous skin changes somehow predisposes the patient to recurrent soft tissue infections. No one knows how or why staphylococcal infections are enhanced by highly elevated levels of IgE. The theory is that mast cell activation in the neighborhood of a focus of *S. aureus* infection somehow impairs normal PMN-mediated defense mechanisms. Some recent studies have shown that antihistamines may at least partially correct the defect demonstrated in these patients.

The presence of a foreign body has a dramatic effect on the development of staphylococcal infections. For example, infections with *S. epidermidis* strains are particularly common in patients harboring foreign bodies such as prosthetic heart valves, cerebrospinal fluid shunts, and artificial joints. As for *S. aureus*, the inoculum required experimentally to produce a skin infection in a healthy individual is very large (10^6 to 10^7 organisms); however, the presence of even a small foreign body such as a suture reduces the dose required to produce an infection to less than 100 organisms. Thus, foreign bodies must provide a nidus of chronic inflammation in which leukocyte accumulation is impaired. An area ripe for productive clinical investigation is how a foreign body impairs host defenses.

CLINICAL MANIFESTATIONS

This section will review two broad categories of types of human disease produced by staphylococci: first discussed will be diseases related to the production of toxins by staphylococci (exclusively *S. aureus*) and then diseases related to direct organism invasion.

TOXIN-PRODUCED DISEASES. As noted above, *S. aureus* produces a variety of toxins. Clinically, the most important toxins are the enterotoxins and exfoliative toxin. The distinction between the different types of toxins is becoming less clear: for example, the toxin involved in the toxic shock syndrome (pyrogenic exotoxin C) has recently been shown to be identical to enterotoxin F; furthermore, that toxin clearly has exfoliative properties.

Staphylococcal Gastroenteritis. While gastrointestinal disease may be caused by massive, physical overgrowth of *S. aureus* within the gastrointestinal tract, most cases of gastroenteritis follow the ingestion of foods containing a preformed toxin. The toxin itself is not produced within the gastrointestinal tract. A number of extracellular toxins are produced in large amounts when the culture media contains high amounts of carbohydrate (as in sugary and starchy foods contaminated by *S. aureus*) and when such a mixture is incubated at appropriate conditions of temperature and acidity. Toxin ingestion results in increased intestinal peristalsis, profuse nausea, vomiting, diarrhea, and in some cases fever. The organism and its preformed toxin can usually be identified in point source outbreaks from the epidemiologically implicated foodstuff. Toxin-mediated staphylococcal gastroenteritis is usually self-limited, lasting anywhere from 12 to 24 hours; however, supportive therapy (fluid and electrolyte maintenance) may on occasion be required. Antibiotics are not useful.

The Toxic Shock Syndrome (TSS). TSS is almost certainly caused by the production of a toxin at the site of a localized, often relatively asymptomatic or unnoticed infection with any strain of *S. aureus* capable of toxin production. The most common site of infection is the vagina, almost invariably in association with tampon usage. The few (less than 10 per cent) TSS cases that have not been associated with infection of the female genital tract have usually been associated with infected foreign bodies (such as sutures) in surgical wounds. As noted earlier, both enterotoxin F and pyrogenic exotoxin C were described by independent investigators as putative toxins responsible for the syndrome. Recent studies have confirmed the two substances to be identical. Toxin production by strains of *S. aureus* isolated from cases of TSS have been shown to be related to lysogeny, the presence of a temperate bacteriophage. Presumably, the clinical manifestations of the syndrome are produced when the toxin is absorbed either through mucous membranes or from a subcutaneous tissue site of colonization or infection. The toxin probably produces its systemic effects by directly damaging peripheral tissues.

The clinical syndrome that results is dramatic. The patient, almost always unaware of the focus of toxin production, experiences the abrupt onset of high fever, myalgias, and profuse nausea, vomiting and watery diarrhea. Within the first several days, a sunburn-like rash appears, and the conjunctivae become injected. On biopsy of the skin lesions, the epidermis exhibits cleavage in the basilar layers, differentiating it from the staphylococcal scalded skin syndrome (discussed later) and from viral and drug eruptions. The patient often becomes progressively more ill and is frequently in frank shock when presenting for care. A diffuse capillary leak syndrome rapidly develops, and the serum albumin concentration often plummets to less than 2 grams per 100 ml. Hypotension and frank shock are common and are often associated with the adult respiratory distress syndrome (ARDS), acute renal failure, and abnormalities in literally every organ system evaluated. For example, almost all patients exhibit an altered state of mentation, hepatocellular malfunction, elevated levels of muscle enzymes, thrombocytopenia, and a low serum calcium concentration (far out of proportion to the hypoalbuminemia). Highly elevated levels of calcitonin are present for which no explanation presently exists.

Therapy is both supportive and specific. Identification of the site of infection, drainage thereof (most frequently consisting of removal of contaminated tampons), and antibiotic therapy with beta-lactamase-resistant antistaphylococcal agents are all indicated. Antibiotics do not change the course of the initial illness but seem to prevent relapse, at least in tampon-associated cases. It is important to realize that patients with TSS are rarely bacteremic, and therefore this type of shock syndrome is different from bacteremic, inflammatory system-mediated shock (see Ch. 256), wherein complement, coagulation, and kinin system activation seem to be primary events.

The prognosis in TSS is favorable despite the fact that most patients are critically ill for a period of time in the hospital. However, between 5 and 10 per cent of patients studied so far succumb to the illness. Since recurrences, generally milder, are relatively common following tampon-associated TSS (up to 10 per cent over the subsequent three menstrual cycles), women who have recovered from TSS should avoid tampon use for at least six months following the illness.

The Staphylococcal Scalded Skin Syndrome (SSSS). SSSS is another toxin-mediated disease produced by certain strains of *S. aureus*, usually of phage group II. These organisms produce an exfoliative toxin that when injected experimentally into infant mice produces dramatic skin desquamation and mimics in every way the clinical syndrome seen in human infants. This disease is also produced by a toxin originating in a distant focus of infection: a toxin-producing organism produces and releases the exfoliative toxin that after absorption and systemic dissemination causes cleavage of the middle layers of the epidermis, bulla formation, and ultimately slippage of the superficial layer of the epithelium on gentle pressure (a positive *Nikolsky's sign*). The skin is often tender and very erythematous, producing a sunburn-like rash during the initial phase. Infants are most commonly involved, and outbreaks of this syndrome have occurred in nurseries after introduction of a toxin-producing strain. Often mild or asymptomatic omphalitis is the source.

In older children, the portal of infection can be any minor skin abrasion, furuncle, or some other infected local site. The conjunctival sac may be the source as a result of mild conjunctivitis, and this source often goes undetected. The syndrome has occasionally been reported to involve adults. The rash proceeds rapidly to desquamation, but healing is rapid and is related to how promptly the peripheral site has been treated. Mortality of SSSS is very low.

Differentiation of SSSS from viral exanthems and drug allergies is very important. The most important disease with which SSSS can be confused is *toxic epidermal necrolysis (TEN)*, an often fatal variant of erythema multiforme usually caused by a drug allergy (see Ch. 557). The two illnesses can be differentiated on skin biopsy, and therapy is very different for each: local care and antibiotics suffice to cure SSSS, whereas high dose systemic glucocorticoids are indicated in TEN, with mortality still remaining high.

DISEASES RELATED TO DIRECT INVASION AND SYSTEMIC SPREAD OF STAPHYLOCOCCI. In the following subsections, the classic clinical manifestations of invasive staphylococcal infection, bacteremia, and endocarditis are described. Under each section will be addressed not only the classic clinical manifestations but diagnostic, therapeutic, and prognostic aspects of each illness.

Dermal Infections. Most minor skin infections in man are caused either by *S. aureus* or group A beta-hemolytic streptococci. There is no way clinically to differentiate between diseases produced by the penicillin-sensitive streptococci and *S. aureus;* obviously, this is an important point, for all skin infections in which antibiotic therapy seems indicated therefore require the use of a beta-lactamase-resistant antibiotic (see Ch. 27). Direct invasion through minor breaks in skin and mucous membranes is the hallmark of disease produced by *S. aureus*. A wide variety of dermal and soft tissue infections may result, including cellulitis, local abscess formation (furuncles and carbuncles), lymphangiitis, and lymphadenitis. Direct extension then can occur to deep support structures such as bones and joints and result in primary osteomyelitis and septic arthritis. Even dermal staphylococcal infections that appear minor are important to recognize because they may become a source of bacteremia. When a patient with a localized *S. aureus* skin infection manifests fever and chills, bacteremia must be assumed to be present, and prompt diagnostic and therapeutic intervention should be initiated.

Diagnosis of dermal infections is usually relatively easy. The aspirate of a large, well developed abscess (furuncle or carbuncle) almost always reveals typical creamy pus, and on Gram stain the clustered organisms are mixed with inflammatory debris. One should not neglect performing Gram stains of materials from every dermal infection because occasionally gram-negative organisms may cause a clinical picture similar to that of gram-positive infections, especially in immunocompromised hosts, and obviously the initial therapeutic approach will be very different.

Therapy must always be initiated with a beta-lactamase-resistant antibiotic if antimicrobial therapy is indicated at all. In fact, the backbone of therapy of dermal staphylococcal infections continues to be debridement and drainage. Only large lesions associated with signs of surrounding cutaneous spread or systemic clinical symptoms need be treated with antibiotics. It is usually wise, however, before incising a large staphylococcal abscess (even when localized) to treat the patient with an oral dose of a penicillinase-resistant antibiotic (250 mg of dicloxicillin). Such a dose should be administered 30 minutes to one hour before incision and drainage is carried out.

The prognosis for most localized infections is excellent, but infections due to *S. aureus* often recur. Population surveys have found that each year most persons develop one to several isolated local lesions, most probably caused by *S. aureus*. However, not infrequently, an individual may suffer from recurrent crops of extremely debilitating local skin lesions. In this situation the patient is usually found to be carrying the causative organism in the anterior nares, the axilla or groin and/or perirectal region. Most such individuals are nasal carriers, and an attempt to eradicate nasal carriage is worth making (see later section on Treatment of Chronic Carriers).

Bone and Joint Infections. Through a variety of mechanisms, *S. aureus* commonly involves bone (osteomyelitis, see Ch. 274) and joints (see Ch. 446 on Septic Arthritis). Direct inoculation by *S. aureus* can occur in trauma or penetrating wounds. Bone and joint infections can also result from bacteremia. In children and young adults it is assumed that bacteremia originates from a minor dermal source (such as folliculitis) or somehow directly enters the bloodstream from heavily colonized mucous membranes. Seeding of *S. aureus* from the blood tends to occur to areas previously traumatized or harboring foreign bodies. In young children, the organism tends to seed into the diaphyseal plates of the long bone, areas of greatest vascularity. The affected area (usually on the ankle, knee, or shin) becomes acutely warm and swollen and may appear at first to be a primary cellulitis. Fever and shaking chills are common. Blood cultures are usually positive. In adults, the syndrome of hematogenous osteomyelitis is usually less acute, often involving the lumbar vertebrae. The individual will begin to develop low grade fever, night sweats, and back pain that gradually becomes localized to an area of point tenderness. In such cases, *S. aureus* may grow from the blood, but more commonly the organism is isolated from an aspirate of the bone or intervertebral space obtained by an orthopedic surgical consultant.

Staphylococcal septic arthritis usually involves a joint afflicted by pre-existing chronic arthritis (such as rheumatoid arthritis or osteoarthritis). Again, an episode of bacteremia causes seeding to a previously inflamed joint. The only indication in some patients is the development of increasing symptoms in one joint, usually accompanied by fever. Joint aspiration reveals a purulent effusion; Gram stains may be negative, but the organism is usually culturable. *S. epidermidis* increasingly is being described as a cause of chronic osteomyelitis, especially in debilitated patients such as those on hemodialysis or with underlying neoplastic diseases.

The diagnosis of staphylococcal bone and joint infections depends on recovering the organism from an aspirate of the involved site; every effort should be made, with the assistance of orthopedic surgeons, to aspirate or biopsy the involved area *before* antibiotics are started. Newer techniques permit core biopsies to be obtained from deep tissues and may in future permit more frequent definitive bacteriologic diagnosis of low grade, chronic bone and joint infections. The diagnosis becomes especially difficult if patients have been treated with antibiotics before appropriate culture material has been obtained. In such cases a rising or significantly elevated teichoic acid antibody titer may assist in diagnosing deep infections due to *S. aureus* (see later section on The Teichoic Acid Antibody Assay).

Treatment of osteomyelitis in adults must be prolonged. While it is becoming customary to treat children with a brief course of parenteral antibiotics, adults on oral antibiotics tend to relapse if a prolonged parenteral course of antibiotics is not administered. Four weeks of parenteral therapy is the minimun acceptable course, and most clinicians prefer to treat for six weeks. An oral antistaphylococcal agent (for example, dicloxacillin 2 grams daily) should be continued for several weeks following discharge. Gradual reduction of the dose of oral antibiotic over a three- to six-month period may leave the patient symptom-free for an extended period of time. Some clinicians treat isolated septic arthritis for only two weeks. However, it is extremely difficult to differentiate septic arthritis *without* bone involvement from that with osteomyelitis. Therefore, a four-week course of therapy with appropriate parenteral antibiotics is recommended. Staphylococcal osteomyelitis tends to relapse even after years of quiescence, and one can never be sure of complete eradication of the disease. Once a relapse has occurred, chronic recurrence will be the rule. In such situations carefully planned surgical debridement and drainage under the cover of a prolonged parenteral and oral course of antibiotics may result in extended quiescence or even apparent cure.

Staphylococcal Pneumonia and Empyema. Although most cases of *S. aureus* pneumonia follow acute viral infections of the lower respiratory tract (especially influenza), the disease occasionally occurs de novo in elderly and debilitated individuals. *S. aureus* pneumonia is most often acquired in the hospital. Primary staphylococcal pneumonia is most common in children and usually evolves radiologically from patchy pulmonary infiltrates into harder nodules and then pneumatoceles. Rapid development of pleural effusions and empyema often accompanied by pneumothorax may occur. Staphylococcal bronchitis and recurrent pneumonias are also seen in children and young adults with cystic fibrosis, and a young adult suffering from recurrent bronchitis from which *S. aureus* and/or *Pseudomonas aeruginosa* (usually with mucoid colonial morphology) are isolated should have a sweat test evaluation.

Adult patients with influenza have an increased incidence of *S. aureus* pneumonia. The patient is usually recovering from typical symptoms of influenza when the rapid onset of fever, chills, and chest pain supervenes. Gram stain of the sputum in such cases reveals large clumps of gram-positive cocci. Therapy must be intense with appropriate antibiotics. Nonetheless, such patients often do poorly and frequently develop secondary infections with gram-negative organisms, chronic respiratory failure, and progressive debility. Mortality rates remain high. Even in young people, morbidity is substantial, related to serious, rapidly progressive pulmonary disease often with empyema as well as the sequelae of the accompanying bacteremia.

In particular, pleural effusions accompanying *S. aureus* pneumonia require early drainage to prevent empyema formation. If thorough drainage cannot be accomplished by needle aspiration, a chest tube must be inserted. Every effort should be made to avoid the debilitating, prolonged sequelae that result from an extensive, multiloculated *S. aureus* infection of the pleural space.

Staphylococcal Meningitis, Cerebritis, and Brain Abscess. Meningitis due to *S. aureus* most commonly develops as a complication of a central nervous system diagnostic or neurosurgical procedure. Occasionally, however, meningitis may develop during an episode of bacteremia from a peripheral site. Many patients with staphylococcal bacteremia, with or without endocarditis, develop transient but sometimes focal central nervous system symptoms. On lumbar puncture, such patients commonly have a PMN pleocytosis with elevated protein but a normal to low normal glucose concentration and a *negative* Gram stain. These individuals probably have begun to develop multiple perimeningeal foci or areas of cerebritis (or both) and not yet frank meningitis. Almost certainly, if left untreated such patients would develop frank brain abscesses or fulminant staphylococcal meningitis. On occasion, such a patient may also exhibit purpura, disseminated intravascular coagulation, and shock in which the differentiation from *meningococcal meningitis* (see Ch. 272) is difficult. Treatment of such patients is particularly difficult, for the initial inclination is to use penicillin, an inappropriate antibiotic choice. Thus, for any patient whose Gram stain of the spinal fluid does not reveal identifiable organisms (such as meningococci or penumococci), a beta-lactamase resistant antibiotic must be included in the initial antibiotic coverage.

Brain abscesses in general are usually caused by anaerobes, but not infrequently *S. aureus* is found to accompany them. Therefore, antistaphylococcal drugs should be included with antianaerobic antibiotics in the initial coverage of such individuals. For example, nafcillin plus chloramphenicol is a combination frequently used for the patient who has a brain abscess with the source and causative organisms not yet defined. Surgical drainage is required only if the abscess is large and encapsulated.

Therapy of staphylococcal meningitis and cerebritis is usually that of the underlying syndrome (for example, endocarditis). However, even in the rare patient with an uncomplicated case of pure meningitis, therapy should be prolonged, at least four weeks parenterally, in contrast to the customary 10 to 14 days of therapy for patients with uncomplicated meningitis caused by *S. pneumoniae* or *N. meningitides.*

Staphylococcus epidermidis may cause meningeal signs and symptoms, almost always in a patient with a central nervous system shunt in place. In such instances, the infection has originated in the shunt, and the organism has proliferated and seeded back into the spinal fluid. In many such cases, the individual known to have a shunt in place simply has fever with few if any central nervous system signs. Only an aspirate of the shunt itself will reveal the organism. Therapy may result in quiescence of symptoms, but removal of the infected shunt is almost always required before cure can be accomplished.

Staphylococcal Urinary Tract Infections. Here the species spectrum changes, and coagulase-negative staphylococci become the more common infecting organisms. *S. epidermidis* may occasionally cause urinary tract infections, especially in elderly hospitalized men with obstructive urinary tract pathology or indwelling Foley catheters.

Staphylococcus saprophyticus accounts for between 5 and 10 per cent of urinary tract infections in otherwise healthy young women. Presumably the organism colonizes the genitalia and for reasons not yet ascertained may ascend the urethra to involve the bladder and cause symptomatic cystitis. *S. saprophyticus* is easily treated, being sensitive to essentially all commonly used antibiotics, including penicillin, ampicillin, sulfonamides, and cephalosporins.

S. aureus may involve the urinary tract by either of two mechanisms: first, the organism may seed to the renal cortex during an episode of staphylococcal bacteremia; second, usually in patients with lower urinary tract pathology or indwelling Foley catheters, the organism may ascend to cause a primary lower urinary tract infection. Approximately 10 per cent of patients with staphylococcal bacteremia eventually excrete the organism in the urine; other studies have found that about 25 per cent of patients with a defined urinary tract infection caused by *S. aureus* had had a preceding bacteremic episode. Thus, small cortical abscesses must occur frequently during bacteremia and ultimately rupture in some patients into the tubules and the urine. Most such patients respond promptly to therapy for the underlying disease, and renal carbuncles are now rare.

Conversely, some patients with a primary staphylococcal urinary tract infection may develop secondary bacteremia, that occurrence being reported in about 5 per cent of such patients. In some patients, the renal infection may seed to the perinephric and retroperitoneal structures, with resultant chronic infection and fibrosis. Frank perinephric abscess is a complication associated with high morbidity and mortality. This condition occurs most frequently in patients with chronic underlying renal diseases who are also often diabetic. Aggressive drainage along with prolonged antibiotic therapy is required for cure.

Staphylococcal Endocarditis. This condition follows staphylococcal bacteremia during which a nidus of infection becomes established on one or more heart valves. Endocarditis consists of two clinical syndromes (see Ch. 269): the first is "subacute" bacterial endocarditis, and the second is "acute" bacterial endocarditis.

SUBACUTE BACTERIAL ENDOCARDITIS. The patient presents with a history of days to weeks of low grade fever with or without chills, myalgias, night sweats, and weight loss. The word subacute refers to the clinical manifestations: the clinical course is one of a chronic, febrile illness. The patient almost always has a history of pre-existing organic valvular heart disease, and the species of staphylococcus involved is usually *S. epidermidis.* *S. epidermidis* accounts for approximately 5 per cent of all cases of subacute endocarditis, the vast majority being caused by streptococcal species. *S. epidermidis* is the most common cause, however, of endocarditis occurring in association with prosthetic heart valves (see Ch. 269). The organism, being a contaminant from the patient's or surgeon's skin flora, is inoculated at the time of the surgical valve replacement. Most such infections occur within the initial two months after surgery. In such instances, the outlook for therapy with antibiotics alone is poor, and reoperation with removal of the infected valve or valve ring is often required. More than half of such patients die.

ACUTE BACTERIAL ENDOCARDITIS. The word acute refers to the clinical presentation of the patient who experiences the rapid onset of fever, chills, and myalgias, often with back pain or some gastrointestinal symptoms. The fever is often quite high (103 to 105° F), and the individual at first has the feeling of developing a very bad case of the flu. In the majority of cases, the individual has not had a history of pre-existing valvular heart disease, although it is assumed that many of these individuals have had asymptomatic organic valvular lesions (such as a fenestrated or bicuspid aortic valve, mitral valve prolapse, and so forth). Frequently, therapy for such individuals, who previously had been well, is delayed because the patient and the physician do not realize the gravity of the situation.

S. aureus is almost always the cause of the syndrome of acute endocarditis. At the time of presentation, the patient may not have an obvious heart murmur or show evidence of embolic phenomenon. Thus, the differentiation between primary staphylococcal bacteremia, which may remain uncomplicated, and acute staphylococcal bacterial endocarditis is clinically difficult. The physician must closely follow every patient whose blood samples grow *S. aureus* and must examine carefully each day for the presence of a new murmur, the signs of embolic phenomena, or the observable development of vegetation(s) by echocardiography. Valve destruction, especially of the aortic valve, may progress quite rapidly (see Ch. 269 on Acute Aortic Insufficiency), and surgery may be necessary even within the first few days of presentation of a patient with an acutely insufficient aortic valve. The physician should not hesitate to operate on such a patient, because the possibility of infection of the prosthetic valve is high; over half of such patients will survive the surgical procedure and do well.

The diagnosis of staphylococcal endocarditis depends on the finding of the causative organism in the blood of a patient with one of the clinical syndromes described earlier. It is almost unheard of for a patient to have culture-negative endocarditis caused by staphylococci without having had *intensive* antibiotic therapy during the few days immediately prior to obtaining blood cultures. However, such may be the case in the postsurgical patient for whom prophylactic antibiotics may have been administered or in the drug addict who may surreptitiously have taken antibiotics.

The syndrome of *S. aureus* endocarditis in the drug addict is somewhat different from the acute bacterial endocarditis syndrome already described. In the drug abuser, the vegetation is almost always on one of the right sided heart valves, usually the tricuspid valve. Therefore, pleuritic chest pain and pulmonary infiltrates are common occurrences due to embolization. In drug-abusing patients who have surreptitiously taken antibiotics, the syndrome may be of a much lower grade and may mimic that of subacute bacterial endocarditis. In fact, it is so hard at the time of presentation to make the diagnosis of endocarditis in the drug addict that any person with a history (recent or distant) of parenteral drug abuse who presents with a fever should be considered to have bacterial endocarditis (usually with *S. aureus*) until proven otherwise.

The treatment of bacterial endocarditis must be prolonged (see Ch. 269). Four weeks of parenteral therapy is the minimum for staphylococcal endocarditis, although some authors have reported that two weeks may suffice for the drug addict, usually a young, otherwise healthy individual with right-sided endocarditis. All staphylococcal infections should be treated with a "cidal" antibiotic, and serum bactericidal levels must be monitored to guide effective therapy. For infections caused by beta-lactam antibiotic-resistant staphylococci, whether *aureus* or *epidermidis* species, a cephalosporin is not adequate therapy (see later discussion of treatment) although data may indicate sensitivity to the cephalosporins in vitro. As noted earlier, patients with prosthetic valve endocarditis often require surgery to eradicate the infection. Even those patients with prosthetic valve infections who respond to antibiotics alone probably should be treated with a prolonged course of oral therapy following the six-week course of parenteral therapy in the hospital. In patients with prosthetic valve endocarditis, usually due to *S. epidermidis*, treatment for six weeks parenterally in the hospital followed by an appropriate oral antistaphylococcal drug for a period of several months is recommended.

The prognosis for patients with staphylococcal endocarditis is guarded. Patients with prosthetic valve endocarditis have about a 50 per cent mortality rate, depending on the organism involved, how long after surgery the endocarditis develops, whether or not additional surgery is required for therapy, and the status of underlying left ventricular function. Patients with acute bacterial endocarditis caused by *S. aureus* will do well if they are young and otherwise healthy and especially if the vegetations are on the right-sided valves. The older the patient with left-sided valvular involvement, the higher the mortality (approaching 60 to 80 per cent). Pre-existing symptomatic heart disease is a particularly ominous prognostic sign. The patients who have the subacute syndrome due to *S. epidermidis* not on prosthetic valves, in which the organism is susceptible to the usual antibiotics, usually do quite well: survival rates are comparable with those of patients with streptococcal endocarditis (in the range of 80 to 90 per cent).

Staphylococcal Bacteremia. Sustained bacteremia due to *S. epidermidis* is uncommon. Although blood cultures frequently yield the organism, 80 to 90 per cent of the time it is a contaminant. The occasional case of true, sustained *S. epidermidis* bacteremia is usually caused by infection of an intravascular line or a prosthetic valve. The commonest species causing true bacteremia, especially in the hospital, is *S. aureus*.

There are two varieties of *S. aureus* bacteremia: primary and secondary. Primary bacteremia exists when a patient presenting with fever and chills grows *S. aureus* out of multiple blood cultures but does *not* have an identifiable seeding focus of infection. In this situation, the patient may have unrecognized endocarditis and should be treated accordingly. Secondary bacteremia is that associated with an obvious, peripheral focus of infection, for example, an intravascular line. Many such patients have a benign clinical course after line removal and a brief course of antibiotic treatment. The problem is to select from the overall group of such patients those that have not developed metastatic septic complications. Patients without metastatic sequelae require only a short (14-day) course of therapy. The typical patient who develops *S. aureus* bacteremia has usually been hospitalized for some other medical problem and has had a neglected peripheral or central venous or arterial access line in place. The patient suddenly develops fever and chills with or without signs of local infection at the site of the line. Other common sources are hemodialysis access shunts, postsurgical or traumatic wounds, and decubitus ulcers. The diagnosis of staphylococcal bacteremia is made when *S. aureus* grows from several blood cultures obtained before an empiric course of antibiotics is begun. Some patients already will have an obvious metastatic complication of the bacteremic episode when first examined.

The complications of an episode of *S. aureus* bacteremia are of two varieties: the first type is nonsuppurative, involving patients who develop the septic shock syndrome, including, in some, disseminated intravascular coagulation; the second type is suppurative, involving the metastatic spread of the organism via the bloodstream to heart valves or other organs. The development of endocarditis in this setting turns out to be distinctly uncommon; most suppurative spread occurs to bones, joints, and kidneys, occasionally to other deep viscera, and rarely to the meninges. Following the episode of bacteremia, the patient is placed first on broad, empiric and later on specific antistaphylococcal antibiotic therapy. Throughout this period, the patient must be examined carefully each day for metastatic suppurative sites. Laboratory evaluation may also be helpful, yielding pyuria and the organism from the urine, abnormalities of liver function, and other data. Vegetations may become demonstrable by echocardiography. Radionuclide scans may reveal infectious foci within bones, joints, or soft tissues.

Those patients who develop a clinically evident metastatic focus are treated as dictated by the type of complication that has evolved. Approximately 20 per cent of previously healthy persons who acquire *S. aureus* bacteremia develop some type of complication. In the absence of clinical findings after two weeks of observation, some experts now recommend discontinuation of antibiotics. At this point the results of a teichoic acid antibody (TA-AB) analysis reassure the clinician that no metastatic seeding had occurred. While most positive TA-AB titers will be from patients who already have developed obvious metastatic sequelae, a small subgroup of clinically well patients will also develop a positive TA-AB test. These persons probably have had subclinical suppuration and could be at risk of relapse in the days and weeks to follow. In this subgroup of patients continued parenteral therapy may be advisable with noninvasive search, despite the absence of clinical signs, for deep collections using such tests as echocardiograms, sonography, and bone, gallium, and computed tomography scans. Administration of an oral antistaphylococcal drug (dicloxacillin) should be continued for several weeks if there is any doubt about the possibility of residual metastatic abscesses.

If the following criteria are present, patients qualify for a short course (14 days) of antibiotic therapy following an episode of *S. aureus* bacteremia:

1. Host defenses are normal.
2. The patient should have no seedable sites (pre-existing valvular heart lesions, implanted prostheses, chronic arthritis).
3. The primary focus of infection should be obvious and easily managed.
4. There should be a prompt, complete response to the initial course of antimicrobial therapy.
5. The *S. aureus* recovered should be fully sensitive to the antibiotics initially chosen.
6. No clinical evidence of a metastatic, suppurative complication should be found.
7. No rise in the titer of teichoic acid antibodies should occur over a 14-day period of observation.

Septic Shock Syndromes Due to Staphylococci. Staphylococci can produce shock by five mechanisms:

1. The local infection can generate a massive inflammatory reaction resulting in sufficient "third spacing" (i.e., fluid accumulation into the area of infection) to lead to hypovolemic shock.
2. Enterotoxin producing *S. aureus* occasionally causes diarrhea severe enough to cause hypovolemia and shock.
3. Cardiogenic shock can be produced by staphylococci by causing either valve malfunction (usually aortic), multiple myocardial abscesses, or purulent pericarditis.
4. Endotoxic-like shock can be produced via intravascular complement activation (see Ch. 256 on Shock Syndromes Related to Sepsis).
5. Toxigenic shock—the toxic shock syndrome—can produce shock probably by direct capillary endothelial and end-organ damage.

Massive local infection due to staphylococci is uncommon, and such infections usually involve several organisms, usually anaerobes coinfecting with *S. aureus. S. epidermidis* may be a part of the flora in these infections but is probably not pathogenic. Specifically, patients with one of the gangrene syndromes (for example, necrotizing fasciitis or synergistic gangrene) may develop shock not caused by bacteremia but by fluid accumulation in the infected area. Such individuals require massive fluid and albumin .replacement, extensive local debridement, and broad antibiotic coverage.

Diarrhea, nausea, and vomiting may be so severe in some patients with staphylococcal food poisoning that shock may develop from hypovolemia secondary to gastrointestinal fluid loss. Hospitalization with fluid replacement may be required and will usually suffice because the disease is self-limiting.

Cardiogenic shock is self-explanatory (see Ch. 43).

During acute sepsis *S. aureus* may produce shock that in every way mimics that produced by endotoxin during gram-negative organism septicemia (See Ch. 256). Briefly, the primary event in endotoxic shock is the following: on entering the bloodstream, endotoxin activates a sequence of endocrine and inflammatory events leading first to vasodilation and subsequently to a primarily complement and PMN-mediated capillary leak syndrome resulting in full-blown septic shock. The coagulation and kinin systems also become activated, and such patients may suffer frank DIC. The presence or absence of a capsule seems to be a major factor determining whether or not a particular strain of *S. aureus* in the bloodstream will cause an endotoxic shock-like syndrome. Encapsulated organisms are virulent in tissues and are *more* likely to reach the bloodstream in the course of a peripheral infection. However, once there they are *less* likely to produce the septic shock syndrome. Unencapsulated strains activate complement readily in tissues and therefore are *more* likely to be contained and are least likely to reach the bloodstream and to cause bacteremia. Yet, these are the organisms that can cause shock when directly inoculated into the bloodstream, as by a parenteral drug user or when having colonized an intravascular line.

For a discussion of the toxigenic shock caused by *S. aureus*, refer to the earlier section on the toxic shock syndrome.

Miscellaneous Staphylococcal Infections. This section focuses on several relatively unusual infections that require special diagnostic and therapeutic considerations.

STAPHYLOCOCCAL PYOMYOSITIS. This malady is primarily a tropical disease, rare enough to be reportable in the United States. The patient develops pain, warmth, and swelling over a muscle region usually of the lower extremities and buttocks. The overlying skin may appear quite normal or may look like a mild cellulitis; however, when drainage is attempted, the surgeon discovers that the infection extends into muscle, often with extensive destruction. In the tropics, the disease afflicts malnourished individuals.

S. AUREUS EPIDURAL ABSCESS. This infection is often related to the presence of vertebral osteomyelitis wherein periosseus inflammation extends into the epidural space. The inflammation causes localized tenderness over the spine at point of infection followed by weakness and progressive neurologic signs of paraplegia. Effective therapy depends on early diagnosis and *prompt* surgical intervention and drainage.

DIAGNOSIS. The diagnosis of staphylococcal infections continues to be made clinically. Knowledgeable interpretation of the Gram stain of an adequately obtained specimen will usually suggest the presence of staphylococci. Culture of such a specimen almost always will yield the responsible staphylococcus, and absolute confirmation is provided by the presence of positive blood cultures. Some judgment is required in deciding whether *S. epidermidis* in blood cultures is a contaminant or a true infection. The presence of the organism *in more than two* consecutive blood cultures and associated with proper clinical circumstances (the presence of an indwelling intravascular catheter or a prosthetic device) strongly suggests true bacteremia. The vast majority (80 to 85 per cent) of *S. epidermidis* isolated from blood culture bottles are single organisms, usually in only one of the two bottles in a set, and are contaminants. While *S. aureus* may on occasion contaminate blood cultures, the clinician must determine the significance of the isolation of *S. aureus* from the blood under any condition. In most cases multiple blood cultures will be positive, and there is no question about the diagnosis of the true bacteremic state. If there is any doubt as to the origin of *S. aureus* either in blood, urine, or other fluid specimens, appropriate therapy should be continued.

The Teichoic Acid Antibody (TA-AB) Assay. This assay measures the presence (and titer) or absence of antibodies to staphylococcal cell wall teichoic acids. It is of no use in diagnosing infections with *S. epidermidis* because it only identifies antibodies to the ribotol teichoic acid moiety in the wall of *S. aureus*. Approximately 90 per cent of patients with *S. aureus* endocarditis develop a significant titer of teichoic acid antibodies. The test is fairly sensitive but only modestly specific for other types of serious, deep-seated *S. aureus* infections. The major role of the TA-AB assay is not primarily to diagnose *S. aureus* infections, most of which are diagnosed on clinical grounds, but to assist the clinician in deciding how long to treat bacteremic patients. Patients with *S. aureus* bacteremia who develop disseminated or metastatic abscesses will usually develop an increase in the titer of TA-AB acid antibodies as opposed to those with benign, self-limited bacteremias. The predictive value of a negative assay in someone who has experienced an episode of *S. aureus* bacteremia is high; therefore, the test is useful in *ruling out* metastatic infections in such patients. Other situations in which the teichoic acid antibody may be of some use in clinical decision making are the following:

1. For patients with endocarditis and negative blood cultures, usually because of prior antibiotic therapy (in a drug addict). A rise in TA-AB titers to a positive level confirms the diagnosis.
2. For deep tissue infections thought likely to be due to *S. aureus* but inaccessible to culturing (osteomyelitis or visceral abscesses). Again, a rising TA-AB titer is confirmatory, but a negative test does *not* rule out the involvement of *S. aureus*.
3. To determine the response to therapy of patients with endocarditis. Patients responding to therapy will have a prompt (two- to four-weeks) decrease in the titer of antibodies. A titer that remains elevated suggests an undrained focus of residual infection.
4. To detect relapse. Relapse is associated with a rapidly rising antibody titer; thus, sequential titers may help the clinician analyze febrile episodes occurring late in the course of treatment of an episode of endocarditis.

TREATMENT. Effective therapy of staphylococcal infections depends on early, effective debridement and drainage of the primary focus of infection along with the selection of antibiotics to which the organisms are susceptible. At present, 90 per cent of all organisms, whether nosocomial or community-acquired, are resistant to penicillin. Therefore, no patient suspected of having an infection with *S. aureus* should be started on a penicillinase-susceptible penicillin. Most staphylococci are still susceptible to nafcillin and oxacillin; methicillin is an antiquated drug, more toxic than either of the aforementioned parenteral alternatives. Usual doses of nafcillin and oxacillin are in the range of from 6 to 12 grams daily, and patients with endocarditis should receive between 9 and 12 grams daily. In the penicillin-allergic individual, the cephalosporins can be used in the absence of a history of an anaphylactic type of penicillin hypersensitivity; however, the most effective alternative continues to be vancomycin. Vancomycin is used in a dose of 2 to 4 grams per day parenterally and should be equal to the penicillins and cephalosporins in terms of therapeutic outcome.

Beta-Lactam Antibiotic–Resistant Staphylococci (BLARS). These organisms are usually referred to as "methicillin-resistant staphylococci." However, methicillin is simply the disc used to determine resistance of these organisms and many such organisms remain sensitive by disk and other in vitro methods to the cephalosporins. However, the clinical responses to the cephalosporins of cephalosporin-sensitive but methicillin-resistant organisms have not been good. Thus, when any species of staphylococcus has been identified as being methicillin-resistant (or, therefore, nafcillin- or oxacillin-resistant) it should be considered resistant to all beta-lactam antibiotics regardless of contrary in vitro data. The drug of choice in the treatment of BLARS is vancomycin. Alternative drugs include rifampin and trimethoprim/sulfamethoxazole (TMS). Some BLARS remain sensitive to the aminoglycosides, and aminoglycosides may provide a synergistic effect with whatever other antibiotic is used. These recommendations hold true both for *S. aureus* and *S. epidermidis*.

Treatment of Chronic Carriers. Certain individuals may suffer recurrent staphylococcal infections of the skin (furunculosis), and eradication of the nasal carrier state may be required to terminate the series of infections. Nasal carriage termination may be difficult by local means. Traditionally, individuals so afflicted have been advised to observe meticulous personal hygienic measures such as frequent bathing or showering, using pHisoHex or other bactericidal soap preparations, and the application of an antibacterial ointment such as bacitracin to the anterior nares. While such a treatment program will clear a portion of chronic carriers, many will relapse and develop recurrent crops of boils. The drug most helpful in this situation is rifampin, known to be excreted in bactericidal concentrations in external secretions. Rifampin should always be used with another oral antistaphylococcal drug that, even though present in low concentrations, will delay the emergence of rifampin resistance. Thus, a seven- to ten-day course of rifampin* (300 mg twice daily) plus, for example, dicloxacillin (125 mg four times a day) or in the penicillin-allergic patient cephalexin or TMS is very effective in eliminating nasal carriage of *S. aureus* and the associated dermal infections. A percentage of individuals will reacquire the organism and the course of therapy may have to be repeated; the physician should be sure to ascertain that the carried organism is still sensitive to rifampin. In the future, recolonization of such individuals with nonpathogenic staphylococci may play an important adjunctive role in preventing recrudescence of carriage by an aggressive organism.

Bacterial Interference. Bacterial interference is the process of recolonizing an individual with an organism in order to displace a more pathogenic microbe. Initially, investigators found that patients heavily colonized with an aggressive strain of *S. aureus* that was associated with recurrent infections (boils, omphalitis, or conjunctivitis) could be helped by being recolonized with a nonpathogenic strain (designated strain 502A) of the organism. Multiple reports in 1960's and 1970's attested to the efficacy of bacterial interference. However, from time to time, there were reports of a serious infection caused by the 502A strain of *S. aureus*. The use of bacterial interference to treat recurrent infections due to a carried strain of *S. aureus* therefore has declined. The potential usefulness of this process should be kept in mind as one considers therapeutic approaches to patients with recurrent furunculosis recalcitrant to repeated courses of therapy. It is probable that other species of truly nonpathogenic staphylococci or micrococci will also be found to interfere with *S. aureus* colonization and that clinical application of this technique will be common in the future.

PREVENTION. Prevention of nosocomial staphylococcal infections depends on breaking the chain of transmission between a carrier and a susceptible noncarrier. Transmission from person to person is interrupted by thorough handwashing before and after examination of each patient. Certain other hospital infection control recommendations and procedures apply in particular to staphylococcal infections. For example, hospitals are required to have specific recommendations about the placement and maintenance of intravascular catheters; such instructions should be followed *meticulously*. Staphylococci are among the leading causes of infection of indwelling intravascular catheters, and proper catheter maintenance substantially reduces the incidence of nosocomial infections with these organisms.

While in theory vaccines containing capsular polysaccharides

*This use of rifampin is not listed in the manufacturer's directive.

might enhance host defenses against the encapsulated strains of staphylococci, vaccines developed in the past were not shown to be of major clinical benefit. It is probable that some acquired immunity does develop against staphylococci, since the incidence of *S. aureus* infections decreases with increasing age. However, firm evidence is lacking that enhancement of humoral or cellular immunity against staphylococci significantly assists the host in its struggle with the organism.

Kaplan MH, Tenenbaum MJ: *Staphylococcus aureus*: Cellular biology and clinical application. Am J Med 72:248–57, 1982. *Reviews the clinically relevant molecular biologic aspects of S. aureus.*

Musher DM, McKenzie SO: Infections due to *Staphylococcus aureus.* Medicine 56:383–409, 1977. *A nice review of most clinical aspects of S. aureus infections.*

Sheagren JN: Endocarditis complicating drug abuse. *In* Remington JN, Swartz MN (eds.): Current Clinical Topics in Infectious Diseases. New York, McGraw-Hill Book Company, 1981, pp 211–33. *Describes the syndrome of endocarditis in the drug-abuser and highlights the role of S. aureus therein.*

Sheagren JN: Guidelines for the use of the teichoic acid antibody assay. Arch Int Med 144:250–252, 1984. *A brief summary of indications for the use of the teichoic acid antibody assay.*

Sheagren JN: *Staphylococcus aureus*—the persistent pathogen. N. Engl J Med (in press). *A complete, up-to-date review of all newer aspects of infections with S. aureus.*

Bacterial Meningitis

Morton N. Swartz

271. BACTERIAL MENINGITIS

Meningitis is an inflammation of the arachnoid, the pia mater, and the intervening cerebrospinal fluid. The inflammatory process extends throughout the subarachnoid space about the brain and spinal cord and regularly involves the ventricles. Pyogenic meningitis, considered in this chapter, is usually an acute infection due to bacteria which evoke a polymorphonuclear response in the cerebrospinal fluid (CSF). One of its major forms, that caused by meningococci, is considered in Ch. 272; less acute forms of bacterial meningitis, characterized by a mononuclear cell response in the CSF, are discussed in Ch. 298 and 497.

ETIOLOGY AND INCIDENCE. Approximately 17,500 cases of bacterial meningitis are estimated to occur annually in the United States. If all cases are included irregardless of the age of patients, data from the Centers for Disease Control in 1978 indicated that *Hemophilus influenzae* type b is the most frequent bacterial cause (46 per cent), followed by *Neisseria meningitidis* (27 per cent) and *Streptococcus pneumoniae* (11 per cent). About 70 per cent of all cases occur in children under 5 years of age.The relative frequencies with which the different bacterial species cause meningitis are age related. In the newborn, gram-negative bacilli (most frequently *E. coli,* but also other enteric bacilli and *Pseudomonas*) and group B streptococci are the principal causes. In the past 15 years the group B (type III principally) *Streptococcus* has increased in importance in neonatal meningitis; in some hospitals it is the single most frequent etiology, surpassing *E. coli.* Beyond the first month of life and extending through childhood, *H. influenzae* and *N. meningitidis* are the most frequent causes of bacterial meningitis. In adults *S. pneumoniae* and *N. meningitidis* are responsible for most cases. Meningococcal meningitis is the only type that occurs in outbreaks; its relative frequency among the meningitides will depend on whether statistics have been gathered during an epidemic period. In about 10 per cent of patients with pyogenic meningitis the bacterial cause cannot be defined. Simultaneous mixed meningitis is rare, occurring in the setting of neurosurgical procedures, penetrating head injury, or intraventricular rupture of a cerebral abscess; the isolation of anaerobes should strongly suggest the last of these.

TABLE 271–1. BACTERIAL CAUSES OF MENINGITIS

	Neonates (≤ 1 month) (%)	Children (1 month–15 years) (%)	Adults (> 15 years) (%)
S. pneumoniae	0–5	10–20	30–50
N. meningitidis	0–1	25–40	10–35
H. influenzae	0–3	40–60	1–3
Streptococci	20–40 *	2–4	5
Staphylococci	5	1–2	5–15
Listeria	2–10	1–2	5
Gram-negative bacilli	50–60 †	1–2	1–10

*Almost all isolates from neonatal meningitis are group B streptococci.
†Of all cases of neonatal meningitis, *E. coli* accounts for about 40 per cent and *Klebsiella-Enterobacter* for about 8 per cent.

Important changes have occurred in the frequencies of several types of bacterial meningitis over the past 10 to 20 years. Gram-negative bacillary meningitis has almost doubled in frequency, probably reflecting more frequent and extensive neurosurgical procedures as well as other nosocomial factors. *Listeria monocytogenes* has increased eight- to tenfold as a cause of bacterial meningitis in urban general hospitals, reflecting the enlarging immunosuppressed population at particular risk.

CLINICAL SETTINGS. The clinical setting in which meningitis develops may provide a clue to the specific bacterial cause. Meningococcal disease, including meningitis, may occur sporadically and in cyclic outbreaks; military recruits are particularly susceptible, but large urban outbreaks also occur, as in Brazil in 1971 (see Ch. 272).

Certain predisposing factors are frequently associated with the development of *pneumococcal meningitis. Acute otitis media (± mastoiditis)* occurs in about 30 per cent of patients. *Pneumonia* is present in about 25 per cent of patients with pneumococcal meningitis, a much higher frequency than in meningitis caused by *H. influenzae* or *N. meningitidis. Acute pneumococcal sinusitis* is occasionally the initial focus from which infection spreads to the meninges. A significant head injury (recent or remote) has occurred in about 10 per cent of patients with pneumococcal meningitis. CSF rhinorrhea (usually caused by a defect or fracture in the cribriform plate) is present in about 5 per cent of patients with pneumococcal meningitis. Meningitis occurring in young children with sickle cell anemia is most likely to be due to *S. pneumoniae.* A variety of defects in host defenses (primary or acquired immunoglobulin deficiencies, the asplenic state) may predispose to pneumococcal disease, particularly meningitis. Alcoholism is an underlying problem in 10 to 25 per cent of adults with pneumococcal meningitis in urban hospitals.

S. aureus meningitis is seen most commonly as a complication of a neurosurgical procedure, following penetrating skull trauma, or secondary to staphylococcal bacteremia and endocarditis. Meningitis caused by *gram-negative bacilli* takes one of three forms: neonatal meningitis, meningitis following trauma or surgery involving the central nervous system, or spontaneous meningitis in adults (e.g., bacteremic *Klebsiella* meningitis in a patient with diabetes mellitus). The most common causes of gram-negative bacillary meningitis in the adult are *E. coli* (about 30 per cent) and *Klebsiella-Enterobacter* (about 40 per cent). The most frequent causes of bacterial meningitis in patients with neoplastic disease are gram-negative bacilli (particularly *Pseudomonas aeruginosa* and *E. coli), Listeria monocytogenes, S. pneumoniae,* and *S. aureus*. Meningitis caused by *group A streptococci* is uncommon, but occasionally occurs following acute otitis media, mastoiditis, or sinusitis. *Clostridium perfringens* is a rare cause of meningitis usually secondary to a penetrating injury.

The age-related incidence (children under five years) of *H. influenzae* type b meningitis is so striking that the occurrence of this disease in an adult should raise the question of the presence of an underlying anatomic or immunologic defect, circumventing the usual barrier interposed by serum bactericidal mechanisms.

Neonatal Meningitis. The incidence of meningitis is higher in the first month of life than in any other single month. The principal cause, *E. coli* strains containing the K1 capsular antigen, is usually acquired by the neonates from their mothers who carry the organism in their stool. In the newborn the group B *Streptococcus* can produce either an "early onset" (occurring within eight days of delivery and characterized by a fulminant illness with septicemia, severe respiratory distress, and sometimes meningitis) or a "late onset" (occurring ten days to two months after delivery and presenting a more insidious, slowly progressive illness which usually includes meningitis) infection. Type III strains predominate in the latter, but in the "early onset" form the serotypes are variable. Group B streptococci are acquired by the neonate either in passage through the birth canal or through nosocomial spread in the nursery.

The clinical signs in neonatal meningitis suggest sepsis but not necessarily central nervous system involvement: fever (in only 60 per cent), jaundice, diarrhea, lethargy, poor feeding or vomiting, respiratory distress (including apnea), seizures, irritability, bulging fontanel (in only 30 per cent), and nuchal rigidity (15 per cent). Frequently, only by examination of the CSF can the presence of meningitis be ruled in or out.

PATHOLOGY. The purulent exudate is distributed widely in the subarachnoid space, most abundant in the basal cisterns and about the cerebellum initially, but also extending into the sulci over the cerebrum. The exudate in pneumococcal meningitis tends to be more evident over the convexities of the brain than in the basilar region. There is no direct invasion of cerebral tissue by the infecting organism or the inflammatory exudate, but the subjacent brain becomes congested and edematous. The effectiveness of the pial barrier accounts for the fact that cerebral abscess does not complicate bacterial meningitis. Indeed, when these two processes coexist, the sequence usually has been that of an initial abscess subsequently leaking its contents into the ventricular system, producing meningitis. Structures adjacent to the meninges may show a variety of pathologic changes secondary to bacterial meningitis. *Cortical thrombophlebitis* results from venous stasis and adjacent meningeal inflammation. Infarction of cerebral tissue may follow. *Involvement of small pial arteries* with peripheral aneurysm formation and vascular occlusion occurs occasionally in bacterial meningitis. In fulminating cases (particularly meningococcal meningitis), *cerebral edema* may be marked even though the CSF pleocytosis is only moderate. Rarely such patients develop temporal lobe and cerebellar herniation, resulting in compression of the midbrain and medulla. *Damage to cranial nerves* occurs in areas where dense exudate accumulates; the third and sixth cranial nerves are also vulnerable to damage by increased intracranial pressure. *Ventriculitis* probably occurs in most cases of bacterial meningitis; rarely this progresses to the accumulation of pus, *ventricular empyema*. *Hydrocephalus* can develop during meningitis from obstruction to CSF flow within the ventricular system (obstructive hydrocephalus) or extraventricularly (communicating hydrocephalus). *Subdural effusions* are sterile transudates which develop over the cerebral cortex in about 15 per cent of infants with bacterial meningitis. Rarely such effusions become infected, producing a subdural empyema. In the past the diagnosis has been made almost exclusively in infants, in whom abnormal transillumination or increasing head size can be detected. Now, sterile or infected (showing peripheral contrast enhancement) subdural collections can be demonstrated readily by CT scan as low density areas about the cerebrum.

PATHOGENESIS. Bacteria may reach the meninges by several routes: (1) systemic bacteremia, (2) direct ingress from the upper respiratory tract or skin through an anatomic defect (e.g., skull fracture, eroding sequestrum, meningocele), (3) passage intracranially via venules in the nasopharynx, or (4) spread from a contiguous focus of infection (infection of the paranasal sinuses, leakage of a brain abscess). Bacteremic spread to the meninges is probably the most frequent path of infection. However, not all bacteremic organisms have the same likelihood of causing meningitis. Most bacterial species causing meningitis (*H. influenzae b, N. meningitidis, S. pneumoniae, E. coli* K1, group B III *Streptococcus*) have definable capsules which are antiphagocytic. Whether the capsular polysaccharide, in addition, confers some special meningeal tropism, possibly through surface receptors, is not known. The primary focus initiating the bacteremia is usually in the upper respiratory tract or lung (pneumonia) but may be in the heart (endocarditis) or the gastrointestinal or urinary tracts. Once established in any part of the meninges, infection quickly extends throughout the subarachnoid space. In addition, evidence from animal models of bacterial meningitis suggests that a secondary bacteremia may follow meningeal infection and itself contribute to continuing further inoculation of the cerebrospinal fluid.

CLINICAL MANIFESTATIONS. ***History.*** An acute onset of fever, generalized headache, vomiting, and stiff neck are common to many types of meningitis. Although some patients develop bacterial meningitis in the absence of respiratory symptoms, the majority of patients with pyogenic meningitis of the three common causes have had an antecedent or accompanying upper respiratory tract infection, acute otitis (or mastoiditis), or pneumonia. Myalgias (particularly in meningococcal disease), backache, and generalized weakness are common symptoms. The illness usually progresses rapidly with development of confusion, obtundation, and loss of consciousness. Occasionally the onset may be less acute, with meningeal signs present for several days to a week prior to hospitalization.

General Physical Findings. Evidences of meningeal irritation (drowsiness and decreased mentation, stiff neck, positive Kernig's and Brudzinski's signs) are usually present. In certain patients the findings of meningitis may be easily overlooked; infants, obtunded patients, or elderly patients with congestive failure or pneumonia may develop meningitis without prominent meningeal signs. Their lethargy should be investigated carefully and meningeal signs should be sought; if any doubt exists, examination of the CSF is indicated.

The presence of a petechial, purpuric, or ecchymotic rash in a patient with meningeal findings almost always indicates meningococcal infection and requires prompt treatment because of the rapidity with which this infection can progress (see Ch. 272). Rarely, extensive petechial and purpuric lesions occur in meningitis caused by *S. pneumoniae* or *H. influenzae*. Very rarely skin lesions almost indistinguishable from those of meningococcal bacteremia occur in patients with acute *S. aureus* endocarditis who also have meningeal signs and a CSF pleocytosis (secondary either to staphylococcal meningitis or to embolic cerebral infarction). Usually one or two of the lesions in such a patient are those of purulent purpura; aspiration of material reveals staphylococci on Gram stain. In the summer months viral aseptic meningitis (particularly caused by echovirus 9) may produce meningeal signs, macular and petechial skin lesions, and a CSF pleocytosis of several hundred to 1000 cells, with neutrophils predominating initially.

Neurologic Findings and Complications. *Cranial nerve abnormalities,* involving principally the third, fourth, sixth, or seventh nerves, occur in 10 to 20 per cent of patients with bacterial meningitis. These usually disappear shortly after recovery. Hearing loss occurs in 20 to 25 per cent of children with bacterial meningitis. In about half of those it is a conductive loss, frequently associated with otitis media, and transient. In the other half a persistent sensorineural hearing loss (unilateral or bilateral) occurs; the most likely sites of involvement appear to be the inner ear (infection possibly spreading from the subarachnoid space along the cochlear aqueduct) and the acoustic nerve. In children permanent hearing impairment is more common following meningitis due to *S. pneumoniae* than to *H. influenzae* or *N. meningitidis.*

Seizures (focal or generalized) occur during the acute phase of bacterial meningitis in 20 to 30 per cent of patients and may be due to readily reversible causes (high fever in infants; penicillin neurotoxicity when large doses are administered intravenously in the presence of renal failure) or to focal cerebral injury. Seizures can occur during the first few days, or can appear with associated focal neurologic deficits caused by cortical vein phlebitis seven to ten days after the onset of the meningitis.

Brain swelling and increased CSF pressure are associated with seizures, third nerve dysfunction, abnormal reflexes, coma, hypertension, and bradycardia. Papilledema is rare in bacterial meningitis even with high CSF pressures. Its presence should indicate the possibility of some other associated or independent suppurative intracranial process (subdural empyema, brain abscess). Marked central hyperpnea sometimes occurs in patients with severe bacterial meningitis; CSF acidosis (principally caused by increased lactic acid levels) provides much of the respiratory stimulus.

Focal cerebral signs (hemiparesis, dysphasia, visual field defects) occur in about 15 per cent of patients with bacterial meningitis. They may develop during early meningitis secondary to occlusive vascular processes or some days later. It is important to distinguish lateralizing findings resulting from postictal changes (Todd's paralysis), which usually persist for no more than several hours.

Prompt treatment of bacterial meningitis usually results in rapid recovery of neurologic function. Persistent or late onset of obtundation and coma without focal findings suggests the development of brain swelling, subdural effusions (in the infant), hydrocephalus, loculated ventriculitis, cortical thrombophlebitis, or sagittal sinus thrombosis. The last three are commonly associated with fever and a continuing CSF pleocytosis.

Residual neurologic damage remains in 10 to 20 per cent of patients who recover from bacterial meningitis. In infants surviving neonatal meningitis, significant sequelae are much more frequent (30 to 50 per cent).

LABORATORY DIAGNOSIS. ***Cerebrospinal Fluid Examination.*** Initial CSF pressure is usually moderately elevated (200 to 300 mm H_2O). Striking elevations (over 400 mm) occur in occasional patients with acute brain swelling complicating meningitis in the absence of an associated mass lesion.

GRAM-STAINED SMEAR. By the time of hospitalization, most patients with pyogenic meningitis have large numbers (at least 10^5 per milliliter) of bacteria in the cerebrospinal fluid. Careful examination of the Gram-stained smear of the spun sediment of CSF reveals the etiologic agent in 70 to 80 per cent of cases. In most instances when gram-positive diplococci (or short chaining cocci) are observed on stained CSF smear they are pneumococci. In certain clinical settings it is important to distinguish this organism from the relatively pencillin-resistant enterococcus, which would require the addition of an aminoglycoside to penicillin in treatment. If sufficient organisms are present in the CSF, prompt identification of a pneumococcus can be made by the quellung reaction, employing pooled pneumococcal antisera. Culture of the cerebrospinal fluid reveals the etiologic agent in 80 to 90 per cent of patients with bacterial meningitis.

SPECIAL IMMUNOLOGIC AND SEROLOGIC PROCEDURES. In patients in whom the etiologic agent is not identified on Gram-stained smear of the CSF, rapid diagnosis may often be made by detection of specific bacterial antigens by latex agglutination (LA) or countercurrent immunoelectrophoresis (CIE). These techniques have been employed most extensively in the rapid diagnosis of meningitis caused by *H. influenzae* type b, but have also been used in the diagnosis of meningococcal (groups A,B,C, and Y) and pneumococcal meningitis. Antigen detection by LA is more sensitive and provides results more rapidly than CIE. Since *E. coli* K1 and *N. meningitidis* serogroup B share a common antigenic determinant, immunologic cross-reactivity may cause a false-positive reaction with the group B meningococcal reagent. Since the bacterial cause can be found on Gram-stained smear in most cases of bacterial meningitis, the role of latex agglutination appears to be as an adjunct in rapid diagnosis when no organisms are observed or in providing a specific rather than a morphologic (Gram stain) diagnosis.

The limulus gelation assay for endotoxin is positive in the CSF of patients with meningitis caused by gram-negative bacteria but not in the case of meningitis caused by gram-positive organisms.

CELL COUNT. The cell count in untreated meningitis usually ranges between 100 and 10,000 per cubic millimeter, with polymorphonuclear leukocytes predominating initially (80 per cent or more) and lymphocytes appearing subsequently. Extremely high cell counts (>50,000 per cubic millimeter) may occur rarely in primary bacterial meningitis, but should also raise the possibility of intraventricular rupture of a cerebral abscess. Cell counts as low as 10 to 20 may be observed early in bacterial meningitis (particularly that caused by *N. meningitidis* and *H. influenzae*). Occasionally, in granulocytopenic patients or in the elderly with overwhelming pneumococcal meningitis, the CSF may contain very few leukocytes and yet may appear grossly turbid because of the presence of myriads of organisms. Meningitis caused by several bacterial species *(M. tuberculosis, T. pallidum)* characteristically produces a lymphocytic pleocytosis. *Listeria monocytogenes* meningitis in infants may produce a primarily lymphocytic response in the CSF; in the adult there is usually a polymorphonuclear response, but rarely lymphocytes predominate.

GLUCOSE. The CSF glucose is reduced to values of 40 mg per deciliter or below (or less than 50 to 60 per cent of the simultaneous blood level) in over 50 per cent of patients with bacterial meningitis; this finding can be very valuable in distinguishing bacterial meningitis from most viral meningitides or parameningeal infections. A normal CSF glucose does not exclude the diagnosis of bacterial meningitis. The simultaneous blood glucose level should be determined, because patients with diabetes mellitus (or who are receiving intravenous glucose infusions) will have an elevated level of glucose in the CSF, and its significance can be appreciated only on comparison with the simultaneous blood level. However, it may take 90 to 120 minutes for equilibration to occur after major shifts in the level of glucose in the circulation. The hypoglycorrhachia characteristic of pyogenic meningitis appears to be due to interference with normal carrier-facilitated diffusion of glucose.

PROTEIN. The level of protein in the CSF is usually elevated above 100 mg per deciliter, and the higher values are more commonly observed in pneumococcal meningitis. Extreme elevations, up to 1000 mg per deciliter or more, indicate impending or actual subarachnoid block secondary to the meningitis.

OTHER ABNORMALITIES IN THE CSF. Elevated levels of lactic acid occur in pyogenic meningitis. Lactic dehydrogenase levels (particularly isozymes 4 and 5 derived from granulocytes) are commonly elevated in patients with bacterial meningitis. Although the levels of lactic dehydrogenase are higher in patients with bacterial meningitis than in those with viral infections of the central nervous system, these alterations are not of help in determining the specific etiologic agent involved.

Other Laboratory Tests. BLOOD and RESPIRATORY TRACT CULTURES. Bacteremia is demonstrable in about 80 per cent of patients with *H. influenzae* meningitis, 50 per cent of those with pneumococcal meningitis, and 30 to 40 per cent of those with meningococcal meningitis. Cultures of the upper respiratory tract have not proved helpful in establishing an etiologic diagnosis. Determination of serum creatinine and electrolytes is important in view of the gravity of the illness, the occurrence of specific abnormalities secondary to the meningitis (syndrome of inappropriate secretion of antidiuretic hormone), and problems in therapy in the presence of renal dysfunction (seizures and hyperkalemia with high-dose penicillin therapy). In patients with extensive petechial and purpuric skin lesions, evaluation for coagulopathy is indicated.

RADIOLOGIC STUDIES. In view of the frequency with which pyogenic meningitis is associated with primary foci of infection in the chest, nasal sinuses, or mastoid, roentgenograms of these areas should be taken at the appropriate time after institution of antimicrobial therapy. Computerized tomography (CT) scans are not indicated in most patients with bacterial meningitis. If a mass lesion (cerebral abscess, subdural empyema) is suspected by history, clinical setting, or physical findings (papilledema), then radionuclide or CT scans should be performed. *Bacterial meningitis is a medical emergency requiring immediate diagnosis and rapid institution of antimicrobial therapy.* Delay in performing a diagnostic lumbar puncture in order to obtain a CT scan should be avoided except on the basis of findings indicative of a parameningeal collection or other intracranial mass lesion. Changes may be observed on CT scan during meningitis itself: enlargement of the subarachnoid spaces, including the interhemispheric area; generalized contrast enhancement of the leptomeninges and the ependyma; or areas of diminished density in a patchy pattern owing to associated cerebritis and necrosis. In the patient with meningitis whose clinical status deteriorates or fails to improve, the CT scan may be helpful in demonstrating suspected complications: sterile subdural collections or empyema; ventricular enlargement secondary to communicating obstructive hydrocephalus; prominent persisting basilar meningitis; extensive areas of cerebral infarction resulting from occlusion of major cerebral arteries or veins; or marked ventricular wall enhancement, suggesting ventriculitis or ventricular empyema.

DIAGNOSIS. The diagnosis of bacterial meningitis is not difficult in a febrile patient with meningeal symptoms and signs developing in the setting of a predisposing illness. The diagnosis may be less obvious in the elderly, obtunded patient with pneumonia or the confused alcoholic patient in impending delirium tremens. Examination of the CSF should be carried out promptly under these circumstances or whenever there is any question of meningitis.

Headache, fever, vomiting, stiff neck, and CSF pleocytosis are features of meningeal inflammation and are common to many types of meningitis (e.g., bacterial, fungal, viral) and also to some parameningeal processes. The CSF findings are most helpful in distinguishing among these processes (see Ch. 496). In the patient with meningitis whose CSF does not reveal the etiologic agent on examination of Gram-stained smear, particularly when the CSF glucose is normal and the polymorphonuclear pleocytosis is atypical, certain treatable processes which can mimic bacterial meningitis should be considered in differential diagnosis: (1) *Parameningeal infections.* The presence of infections (chronic ear or nasal accessory sinus infections, lung abscess) predisposing to brain abscess, epidural (cerebral or spinal) abscess, subdural empyema, or pyogenic venous sinus phlebitis should be sought. Neurologic findings may appear in the course of primary bacterial meningitis, but their presence should alert the physician to the need for close scrutiny for the presence of a space-occupying infectious process in the central nervous system. Neurologic symptoms or findings antedating the onset of meningeal symptoms should suggest the possibility of a parameningeal infection. The isolation of an anaerobic organism should suggest the possibility of intraventricular leakage of a cerebral abscess. (2) *Bacterial endocarditis.* Bacterial meningitis may occur during bacterial endocarditis caused by pyogenic organisms such as *S. aureus* and enterococci. In subacute bacterial endocarditis sterile embolic infarctions of the brain may occur and produce meningeal signs and a CSF pleocytosis containing several hundred cells, including polymorphonuclear leukocytes. A history of dental manipulation, fever, and anorexia antedating the meningitis should be sought; careful examination for heart murmurs and peripheral stigmata of endocarditis is indicated. (3) *"Chemical" meningitis.* The clinical and CSF findings (polymorphonuclear pleocytosis and even reduced glucose level) of bacterial meningitis may be produced by chemically induced inflammation. Acute meningitis following a diagnostic lumbar puncture or spinal anesthesia may be due to bacterial (usually *Pseudomonas* species or coliform organisms) or chemical contamination of equipment or anesthetic agent. Endogenous chemical meningitis resulting from leakage into the subarachnoid space of material from an epidermoid tumor or a craniopharyngioma can produce a polymorphonuclear pleocytosis and hypoglycorrhachia. Birefringent material may be seen on polarizing microscopy of the CSF sediment.

NON-NEUROLOGIC COMPLICATIONS. ***Shock.*** When shock occurs in pyogenic meningitis it is usually a manifestation of an accompanying intense bacteremia, as in fulminant meningococcemia, rather than of the meningitis itself. Management is guided by the principles of septic shock therapy with appropriate modifications for myocardial failure (see Ch. 272).

Coagulation Disorders. Coagulopathies are frequently associated with the intense bacteremias (usually meningococcal, occasionally pneumococcal) and hypotension which can accompany meningitis. The changes may be mild such as thrombocytopenia (with or without prolongation of prothrombin and partial thromboplastin times) or more marked with clinical evidences of disseminated intravascular coagulation (see Ch. 272).

Septic Complications. ENDOCARDITIS. Previously, 5 to 10 per cent of patients with pneumococcal meningitis, particularly those with bacteremia and pneumonia as well, developed acute endocarditis, most commonly on the aortic valve. The incidence is currently much lower, as a result of earlier treatment of the initiating infection. In such patients, febrile relapse and a new murmur may appear shortly after completion of antimicrobial therapy for meningitis.

PYOGENIC ARTHRITIS. Septic arthritis may result from the bacteremia associated with meningitis caused by *S. pneumoniae, N. meningitidis,* or *H. influenzae.*

Prolonged Fever. With appropriate antimicrobial treatment of meningitis of the three most common bacterial causes, patients become afebrile within two to five days. Sometimes fever persists beyond this or recurs after an afebrile period. In the patient with persisting headache, obtundation, and cerebral findings, inadequate drug therapy or neurologic sequelae (cortical venous thrombophlebitis, ventriculitis, subdural collections) are important considerations. Re-evaluation of the CSF, particularly Gram-stained smear and culture, is essential under these circumstances. Drug fever may be responsible in the patient who continues to show clinical improvement in all other respects. Metastatic infection (septic arthritis, purulent pericarditis, thoracic empyema, endocarditis) may be the cause of continuing or recurrent fever.

A syndrome consisting of fever, arthritis, and pericarditis three to six days after initiation of effective antimicrobial therapy of meningococcal meningitis occurs in about 10 per cent of patients (see Ch. 272).

RECURRENT MENINGITIS. Repeated episodes of bacterial meningitis generally indicate a host defect, either in local anatomy or in antibacterial and immunologic defenses (e.g., recurrent *N. meningitidis* infections in patients with congenital or acquired deficiencies of complement, particularly late-acting components). *S. pneumoniae* is by far the most frequent cause of recurrent meningitis. Eleven per cent of patients with pneumococcal meningitis have had more than one episode, whereas 0.5 per cent of patients with meningitis caused by other organisms have had recurrent attacks. A history of head trauma is much more frequent in patients with recurrent meningitis. Organisms may directly enter the subarachnoid space, through a defect in the cribriform plate (the most common site), in association with the empty sella syndrome, via a basilar skull fracture, through an erosive sequestrum of the mastoid, through congenital dermal defects along the craniospinal axis (usually evident before adult life), or as a consequence of penetrating cranial trauma or neurosurgical procedures. The anatomic defect may produce a frank CSF leak (rhinorrhea or, less commonly, otorrhea) or may entrap a vascular cuff of meninges which might subsequently serve as a direct route for organisms to reach the meninges. CSF rhinorrhea may be intermittent, and meningitis may occur months or years after head injury.

Any patient with bacterial meningitis, particularly if meningitis is recurrent, should be evaluated carefully for any congenital or post-traumatic defects. The presence of CSF rhinorrhea should be sought at admission and subsequently (rhinorrhea may clear during active meningitis only to recur when inflammation has resolved). Clinical clues suggesting the presence of a CSF fistula through the cribriform plate, pericranial air sinuses, or temporal bone include (1) salty taste in the throat, (2) positionally dependent rhinorrhea (rhinorrhea only in the lateral recumbent or prone position suggests an otic or sphenoid origin), (3) anosmia (cribriform plate leak), (4) hearing loss or full feeling in the ear, often with a finding of fluid or bubbles behind the tympanic membrane (leakage into the middle ear). Demonstration of glucose in nasal secretions with glucose oxidase "sticks" (Dextrostix) suggests the presence of CSF. Quantitative determination of glucose and chloride content of nasal secretions can definitively establish the presence of CSF rhinorrhea.

Recurrent pneumococcal meningitis may occur without apparent predisposing circumstances, and cryptic CSF leaks should be sought actively in such patients by polytomography of the frontal and mastoid regions and by radioisotope techniques. (Radioiodine-labeled albumin is introduced intrathecally, and pledgets of cotton placed in the nares are subsequently examined for the radionuclide. Radioisotopic cisternography has been used successfully recently.) Intrathecal introduction of fluorescein as a visual tracer (under ultraviolet light) can be employed similarly in detecting active leaks. Surgical closure of CSF fistulas should be carried out to prevent further episodes of meningitis. Newer extracranial approaches via the ethmoid sinuses for repair of cribriform plate or sphenoid sinus dural defects are successful and avoid the higher morbidity associated with craniotomy.

In most patients with CSF otorrhea and rhinorrhea following an acute head injury, the leak ceases in one or two weeks. *Persistent rhinorrhea for more than four to six weeks is an indication for surgical repair.* Prolonged administration of penicillin will not prevent pneumococcal meningitis and may encourage infection with more drug-resistant species.

Rarely, recurrent meningitis of nonbacterial etiology may mimic bacterial meningitis. *Mollaret's meningitis* consists of repeated febrile episodes of mild meningeal symptomatology, usually without neurologic abnormalities. Initially, large "endothelial" cells may be seen in the CSF along with polymorphonuclear leukocytes, which subsequently are replaced by lymphocytes. *Behçet's syndrome,* characterized by relapsing oral and genital ulcers and ocular lesions (hypopyon), may exhibit a variety of neurologic abnormalities, including recurrent meningitis.

PROGNOSIS. The introduction of antimicrobial agents has converted bacterial meningitis from a disease that was almost always fatal to one in which the majority of patients survive without significant neurologic residua. The mortality rate for bacterial meningitis varies with the etiologic agent and the clinical circumstances. With current antimicrobial therapy the mortality rate for *H. influenzae* meningitis is below 5 per cent and that for meningococcal meningitis is about 10 per cent. The highest mortality is with pneumococcal meningitis, in which the rate is about 25 per cent. Poor prognostic factors include advanced age, presence of other foci of infection, underlying diseases (leukemia, alcoholism), coma, and delay in instituting appropriate therapy.

TREATMENT. ***Antimicrobial Agents.*** *Antimicrobial therapy should be begun promptly in this life-threatening emergency.* Treatment should be aimed at the most likely causes based on available clinical clues (age of the patient, presence of a purpuric rash, a recent neurosurgical procedure, CSF rhinorrhea). If the infecting organism is observed on examination of the Gram-stained smear of the CSF sediment, specific therapy is initiated. If the etiologic agent is not seen on smear (or not detected by CIE), treatment for bacterial meningitis of unknown etiology should be carried out (see below).

With the exception of chloramphenicol, the commonly employed antimicrobial agents do not readily penetrate the normal blood-brain barrier; but the passage of penicillin and other antimicrobials is enhanced in the presence of meningeal inflammation. Antimicrobial drugs should be administered intravenously throughout the treatment period; reduction in dosage as the patient improves should be avoided, because normalization of the blood-brain barrier during recovery reduces the CSF levels of drug that are achievable. Bactericidal drugs (penicillin, ampicillin) are preferred whenever possible in the treatment of meningitis caused by susceptible bacteria. Several antimicrobial drugs (first or second generation cephalosporins, clindamycin) which do not provide effective levels in the cerebrospinal fluid should not be used.

Meningitis of Specific Bacterial Cause. The treatment of choice for pneumococcal meningitis in the adult is penicillin (24 million units daily in divided doses every two hours) or ampicillin (12 grams daily in divided doses every two to three hours). In the patient with a major penicillin allergy, chloramphenicol (4 to 6 grams intravenously daily in the adult) is a reasonable alternative. Penicillin (ampicillin) is the most extensively studied and effective agent in the treatment of pneumococcal meningitis, but limited studies of chloramphenicol indicate that it can produce comparable therapeutic results. However, several points of caution should be made: (1) resistance to chloramphenicol has been reported from Spain in 45 per cent of pneumococcal strains, (2) the response to chloramphenicol of granulocytopenic patients may be suboptimal. Recently, isolates of *S. pneumoniae* that are relatively resistant (minimum inhibitory concentration (MIC) of 0.1 to 1.0 μg per milliliter) or highly resistant (South African strains with MIC of 4 to 8 μg per milliliter) to penicillin have been identified. In the United States, relative pneumococcal resistance to penicillin occurs in approximately 2 per cent of clinical isolates (in a few geographic areas the figures are as high as 8 or 16 per cent). In addition to cases of meningitis due to highly penicillin-resistant *S. pneumoniae* that occurred during the outbreak in South Africa in the late 1970's, seven cases of meningitis due to moderately penicillin-resistant strains (including two that were multiply-resistant) have been described in the United States and abroad. Thus, antimicrobial susceptibilities should be determined for all pneumococcal isolates from cerebrospinal fluid and blood. Chloramphenicol is a reasonable alternative to penicillin G in treatment of pneumococcal meningitis due to strains that are penicillin-resistant, provided they are not multiply-resistant. The multiply and highly penicillin-resistant strains in South Africa were susceptible only to vancomycin among the commonly employed antimicrobials. Of the currently available third-generation cephalosporins, cefotaxime has the greatest in vitro activity (MIC of 0.06 to 0.5 μg per milliliter) against moderately penicillin-resistant *S. pneumoniae,* but its effectiveness in meningitis due to such strains requires clinical evaluation.

The treatment of meningococcal meningitis is the same as for pneumococcal meningitis (see Ch. 272).

At present 25 per cent of isolates of *H. influenzae* b in the United States are ampicillin resistant. This has dictated a change in initial management of *H. influenzae* meningitis. Chloramphenicol (100 mg per kilogram intravenously daily for a child; 4 grams intravenously daily for an adult), either alone or in combination with ampicillin (300 to 400 mg per kilogram intravenously per day for a child; 12 grams intravenously per day for an adult), is the preferred treatment until drug susceptibilities are determined. If the organism proves susceptible to ampicillin, then this drug can be used alone in treatment. In the rare instance of *H. influenzae* meningitis due to a strain resistant to both ampicillin and chloramphenicol or occurring in a patient who cannot tolerate chloramphenicol, cefotaxime (180 mg per kilogram intravenously daily in divided doses every 4 to 6 hours for children) or moxalactam (100 mg per kilogram intravenously as a loading dose followed by 50 mg per kilogram every 6 hours for children) are alternatives.

Adult meningitis caused by methicillin-sensitive *S. aureus* should be treated with a penicillinase-resistant penicillin (nafcillin 10 to 12 grams intravenously per day). In the penicillin-allergic patient, vancomycin (2.0 grams intravenously in divided doses every 6 hours) is the alternative of choice. Since penetration of vancomycin into the CSF is limited, adjunctive intrathecal therapy (5,000 to 10,000 units of bacitracin slowly in 10 ml of CSF in the adult; or 5 to 20 mg of vancomycin in 10 ml of 5 per cent dextrose–0.85 per cent NaCl slowly in the adult)* has been used when CSF cultures have remained positive after 48 hours of intravenous therapy alone. For adult meningitis due to methicillin-resistant *S. aureus*, intravenous vancomycin (with adjunctive intrathecal bacitracin or vancomycin) is the treatment of choice. In refractory cases the addition of another drug for systemic therapy (rifampin or gentamicin) may be warranted.

Treatment of enterococcal meningitis in the adult involves the use of intravenous penicillin (24 million units daily) or ampicillin (12 grams daily), supplemented with parenterally administered gentamicin (3 to 5 mg per kilogram daily in divided doses every eight hours). In the patient who fails to respond promptly to parenteral therapy, adjunctive intrathecal therapy with gentamicin* (3 to 5 mg) should be considered.

The third generation cephalosporins (cefotaxime 12 grams daily intravenously in divided doses every 4 hours in adults; moxalactam 12 grams daily intravenously in divided doses every 6 hours in adults) are now being used extensively in the treatment of meningitis known to be due to susceptible gram-negative bacilli (*E. coli, Klebsiella, Proteus,* etc.). They should not be used in the treatment of meningitis due to less susceptible species such as *Pseudomonas aeruginosa* and *Acinetobacter*. Initial treatment (on the basis only of findings on Gram-stained smear of CSF) of adults with gram-negative bacillary meningitis involves either the combination of cefotaxime (or moxalactam) with an aminoglycoside (e.g., gentamicin 5 mg per kilogram daily intravenously in divided doses every 8 hours) or, alternatively, the combination of chloramphenicol (4 grams intravenously daily) with an aminoglycoside. Adjunctive intrathecal therapy with gentamicin* (3 to 5 mg administered at intervals of 24 hours for the first few days) may be indicated as well. Following identification of the specific pathogen and determination of its drug susceptibilities, alterations in antimicrobial therapy may be indicated. If the organism is *Pseudomonas aeruginosa,* parenteral and intrathecal gentamicin (or tobramycin) would be employed in combination with carbenicillin (30 to 40 grams intravenously daily).

Bacterial Meningitis of Unknown Etiology. Initial treatment of meningitis when the etiologic agent cannot be identified on Gram-stained smear of cerebrospinal fluid is based on available clinical clues. *In the neonate,* a wide range of gram-positive (group B streptococci, *Listeria*) and gram-negative organisms *(E. coli, Klebsiella, H. influenzae)* may be the cause, indicating the intravenous use of combined therapy with drugs such as ampicillin with gentamicin (or amikacin), or ampicillin with moxalactam, until results of cultures become available. *In children,* therapy is directed at the three most frequent pathogens: *H. influenzae, S. pneumoniae,* and *N. meningitidis.* The appearance of ampicillin resistance among strains of *H. influenzae* has necessitated the shift from single drug therapy (ampicillin) to a two-drug approach (ampicillin-chloramphenicol) in the treatment of meningitis of unknown cause in this age group, pending results of culture. *In adults,* therapy with ampicillin or penicillin is directed at the most common community-acquired pathogens (*S. pneumoniae* and *N. meningitidis*). However, because *H. influenzae* type b infections appear to be increasing in adults, and because of the increased incidence of gram-negative bacillary and staphylococcal meningitis in certain clinical settings, broader initial therapy may be indicated if clinical features suggest unusual organisms.

Duration of Therapy. The frequency of cerebrospinal fluid examinations depends on the clinical course, but a repeat examination should be done in 24 to 48 hours if there has not been satisfactory improvement. Routine "end-of-treatment" CSF examination is unnecessary in most patients with the common types of community-acquired bacterial meningitis. Meningococci are rapidly eliminated from the circulation and CSF with appropriate antimicrobial therapy, which should be continued for at least five to seven days after the patient becomes afebrile. If the patient has responded well, a follow-up lumbar puncture is not necesssary. *H. influenzae* meningitis should be treated for a minimum of ten days (at least for seven days after the patient becomes afebrile); re-examination of the CSF at that time usually shows cell counts of less than 60 (over 90 per cent mononuclear). Follow-up CSF examination may be omitted in those patients who have responded with very rapid and complete clinical resolution of the meningitis. Since pneumococcal meningitis produces a more intense inflammatory response, antimicrobial treatment should be continued for 10 to 14 days and follow-up examination of the CSF should be done and show resolution before discontinuing treatment. More prolonged therapy is indicated with concomitant parameningeal infection or mastoiditis. Treatment of gram-negative bacillary meningitis with parenteral antimicrobials is prolonged, usually for a minimum of three weeks (particularly in patients with a recent neurosurgical procedure) in order to prevent relapse. Repeated examinations of the CSF (particularly for cell count, Gram-stained smear, and culture) are necessary both during and at the conclusion of treatment to determine whether bacteriologic cure has been achieved.

Other Aspects of Treatment. Occasional patients with acute bacterial meningitis develop marked brain swelling (CSF pressure exceeding 400 mm H_2O), which may lead to temporal lobe or cerebellar herniation following lumbar puncture. To reduce this increased pressure, an intravenous infusion of 20 per cent mannitol solution (1.5 to 2.0 grams per kilogram) is administered over 20 to 60 minutes. Continued control of increased intracranial pressure, if needed thereafter, may be effected with mannitol, dexamethasone (10 mg intravenously, followed by 4 mg every six hours), or both. Brain swelling is about the only indication for the use of corticosteroids in the treatment of pyogenic meningitis; they should be employed only when the appropriate antimicrobial drugs are administered. Fluid restriction (1200 to 1500 ml daily in adults) is advisable during the first 24 to 48 hours to minimize brain swelling.

Patients with acute bacterial meningitis should receive constant nursing attention to ensure prompt recognition of seizures and to prevent aspiration. If seizures occur, they should be treated acutely with diazepam (Valium) administered slowly intravenously in a dose of 5 to 10 mg in the adult. Maintenance anticonvulsant therapy can be continued thereafter with intravenous phenytoin (Dilantin) until the medication can be administered orally. Sedation should be avoided because of the danger of respiratory depression and aspiration.

Surgical treatment of an accompanying pyogenic focus such as mastoiditis should be carried out when complete recovery from the meningitis has occurred, but under continuing antibiotic administration. Rarely, the mastoid infection (e.g., Bezold abscess) is so hyperacute that early drainage may be required after 48 hours or so of antibiotic therapy when the acute meningeal process will have subsided somewhat.

*Intrathecal use is not mentioned in the manufacturer's package insert approved by the U.S. Food and Drug Administration. Therefore its use in these circumstances must be considered investigational.

Berk SL, McCabe WR: Meningitis caused by gram-negative bacilli. Ann Intern Med 93:253, 1980. *Good descriptions of gram-negative bacillary meningitis occurring spontaneously and after neurosurgery.*

Carpenter RR, Petersdorf RG: The clinical spectrum of bacterial meningitis. Am J Med 33:262, 1962. *Clear description of clinical settings and findings in the common meningitides.*

Cherubin CE, Corrado ML, Nair SR, Gombert ME, Landesman S, Humbert G: Treatment of gram-negative bacillary meningitis: Role of the new cephalosporin antibiotics. Rev Infect Dis 4:S453, 1982. *Summary of results of cefotaxime treatment of 137 patients with various types of bacterial meningitis.*

Durack DT, Spanos A: End-of-treatment spinal tap in bacterial meningitis. Is it worthwhile? JAMA 248:75, 1982. *Places in perspective the role of end-of-treatment CSF examination.*

Geiseler PJ, Nelson KE, Levin S, Reddi KT, Moses VK: Community-acquired purulent meningitis: A review of 1316 cases during the antibiotic era, 1954–1976. Rev Infect Dis 2:725, 1980. *Extensive experience at one of the last contagious disease hospitals in the United States is recounted. Effects of prior antibiotic therapy on culture results are particularly well studied.*

Hand WL, Sanford JP: Posttraumatic bacterial meningitis. Ann Intern Med 72:869, 1970. *Provides a helpful approach to the problem of post-traumatic CSF rhinorrhea and meningitis.*

Hyslop NE Jr, Montgomery WW: Diagnosis and management of meningitis associated with cerebrospinal leaks. *In* Remington JS, Swartz MN (eds.): Current Clinical Topics in Infectious Diseases, Vol 3. New York, McGraw-Hill Book Company, 1982, pp 254–285. *Most complete review of the bacteriology, anatomy, diagnostic approach, and surgical repair of CSF leaks associated with meningitis.*

Mangi RJ, Holstein LL, Andriole VT: Treatment of gram-negative bacillary meningitis with intrathecal gentamicin. Yale J Biol Med 50:31, 1977. *Helpful guidance for management of this difficult-to-treat form of bacterial meningitis.*

New PFJ, Davis KR: The role of CT scanning in diagnosis of infections of the central nervous system. *In* Remington JS, Swartz MN (eds.): Current Clinical Topics in Infectious Diseases, Vol 1. New York, McGraw-Hill Book Company, 1980, pp 1–33. *Comprehensive review of the changes on CT scan in a wide variety of CNS infections. Large number of illustrative scans with good descriptions.*

Overturf GD: Treatment of the child with bacterial meningitis. *In* Remington JS, Swartz MN (eds.): Current Clinical Topics in Infectious Diseases, Vol 3. New York, McGraw-Hill Book Company, 1982, pp 218–253. *Excellent review of management of childhood meningitis.*

Rahal JJ Jr: Moxalactam therapy for gram-negative bacillary meningitis. Rev Infect Dis 4:S606, 1982. *Experience with moxalactam treatment of 20 patients with gram-negative bacillary meningitis.*

Swartz MN: Intracranial infections. *In* Rosenberg RN (ed.): The Science and Practice of Clinical Medicine, Vol 5. New York, Grune and Stratton, 1980, pp 1–40. *Comprehensive clinical review of purulent meningitis, aseptic meningitis, encephalitis, and parameningeal infections.*

Swartz MN, Dodge PR: Bacterial meningitis—a review of selected aspects. N Engl J Med 272:725, 779, 842, 898, 954, 1003, 1965. *Detailed account of experience at the Massachusetts General Hospital. Particularly good on clinical aspects, neurologic complications, and differential diagnosis.*

272. MENINGOCOCCAL DISEASE

DEFINITION. Meningococcal infections are due to *Neisseria meningitidis*. The best known syndromes are *meningococcal meningitis* ("epidemic cerebrospinal meningitis") and *fulminant meningococcemia*. Infections also occur in the upper and lower respiratory tracts, joints, pericardium, eyes, and genitourinary tract.

ETIOLOGY. *N. meningitidis* is a gram-negative coccus which appears on smears of infected fluids as biscuit-shaped diplococci, located either extracellularly or within polymorphonuclear leukocytes. Colonies are best isolated on blood, "chocolate," or enriched Mueller-Hinton agar in an atmosphere of 3 to 10 per cent CO_2. Modified Thayer-Martin selective medium is useful in detection of meningococcal carriers or in initial isolation of *N. meningitidis* from areas with an extensive indigenous flora. The organism is susceptible to drying or chilling, and specimens should be inoculated and incubated promptly.

Since other *Neisseria* species and related organisms *(Branhamella catarrhalis)*, as well as morphologically similar gram-negative coccobacilli (e.g., *Moraxella*), may be isolated from clinical specimens, biochemical and immunologic methods are needed for identification. *Neisseria* species are oxidase positive. Whereas *N. gonorrhoeae* metabolizes only glucose (but not maltose or lactose), *N. meningitidis* metabolizes both glucose and maltose (but not lactose). *N. lactamica*, a species sometimes present in throat cultures, may be mistaken for the meningococcus, since it too metabolizes both glucose and maltose; however, it also utilizes lactose. Occasional maltose-negative strains of *N. meningitidis* have been noted; fluorescent antibody or coagglutination tests or electrophoretic analysis of hexokinase isoenzymes may be helpful in distinguishing such strains from *N. gonorrhoeae*, particularly when isolated from atypical locations.

Nine serogroups of *N. meningitidis*—A, B, C, D, X, Y, Z, Z′ (also known as 29E), W135—have been defined. They differ in the structures of their capsular polysaccharides and can be identified by agglutination reactions with specific antisera. Most meningococcal disease is due to strains belonging to groups A, B, C, and Y. Twenty to 50 per cent of isolates from carriers are nongroupable (unencapsulated). Subcapsular protein antigens located in the outer bacterial membrane have been used to identify at least 15 serotypes among the various serogroups, providing a classification useful in epidemiologic studies. Serotype 2 strains are responsible for most cases of meningococcal disease due to group B (50 per cent) and group C (80 per cent) organisms (and also are associated with groups Y and W135), but they are rarely isolated from carriers not in direct contact with clinical cases. In contrast, other serotypes are commonly isolated, but primarily from carriers. Group A meningococcal strains show no variation in their outer membrane proteins and are unrelated serologically to the serotypes of other groups.

Strains of *N. meningitidis* produce extracellular proteases which cleave the IgA1 heavy chain in the hinge region. Although the role of this protease in infection is unknown, its elaboration also by the other principal causes of bacterial meningitis *(H. influenzae, S. pneumoniae)* and the importance of IgA in mucosal immunity at the pharyngeal portal for these organisms suggests a possible role in pathogenicity.

Fresh isolates of *N. meningitidis* from the pharynx of carriers and from patients with meningococcal disease contain pili, which appear to have an important role in attachment to human nasopharyngeal cells. The colonial morphology of fresh isolates of *N. meningitidis* from patients with invasive infection (transparent colonies) differs from that of isolates from asymptomatic carriers (opaque colonies). Meningococci from transparent colonies are more resistant to killing by normal serum than are meningococci from opaque colonies, suggesting that this property may be a marker for virulence.

Meningococci contain endotoxins, and these lipopolysaccharides may play a role in the purpura and other clinical features of meningococcemia.

INCIDENCE. *N. meningitidis* is second only to *H. influenzae* as a cause of bacterial meningitis reported in this country. It is estimated that 3000 to 6000 cases of meningococcal meningitis occur annually.

EPIDEMIOLOGY. The natural reservoir of *N. meningitidis* is the human nasopharynx, and transmission occurs principally through airborne droplets or close contact. Infection may occur as the asymptomatic carrier state (the most common form) or as sporadic cases, limited outbreaks, or widespread epidemics.

Carrier State. Nasopharyngeal carrier rates may fluctuate widely. In a nonepidemic period it is 3 to 10 per cent in a civilian population. The rate varies with age: 0.5 to 1.0 per cent in children 3 to 48 months of age and about 5 per cent in those 14 to 17 years of age. In the nonepidemic setting carriage usually lasts weeks to months. The carrier rate in close family contacts of a case of meningococcal disease is increased and may reach 40 per cent. In crowded populations (e.g., military training camps) the carrier rate ranges between 20 and 60 per cent and may reach 90 per cent during epidemics. Although it has often been stated that meningococcal outbreaks occur when the rate of nasopharyngeal carriage exceeds 20 per cent in a military camp, there is in reality no clear relation between the overall carriage rate in a community and the occurrence of meningococcal disease. The strain(serotype)-specific acquisition rate appears to be a more reliable indicator of an outbreak than the group-specific carriage rate.

Spread of disease appears to be mediated by carriers rather than by direct case-to-case transmission. An adult family member generally is the one who brings *N. meningitidis* into a household, where it spreads to others and often colonizes younger children and infants last. As yet unknown host and environmental factors are of decisive importance in determining whether the organism will be confined to the nasopharynx or whether dissemination will take place.

Meningococcal Disease. The annual attack rate for meningococcal disease in the United States in recent years has ranged between 0.7 and 1.3 year per 100,000 population. The highest incidence is in the first year of life (14.4 per 100,000), declining in the one- to four-year age group (4.6 per 100,000), and ultimately reaching the level of 0.3 per 100,000 in adults. During epidemics of meningococcal disease, overall annual attack rates of 5 to 24 cases per 100,000 are observed (as high as 370 per 100,000 in Sao Paulo, Brazil, in 1974). The peak incidence is in the winter and early spring.

During a nonepidemic period the risk of meningococcal illness for household contacts of an initial case is about 3 per 1000 (500- to 1000-fold higher than the overall endemic rate for meningococcal disease) and stems from the higher carriage rate in this setting. The secondary attack rate appears to be age related, with most cases occurring in younger children.

Major meningococcal epidemics, caused primarily by group A strains, tend to recur at 20- to 30-year intervals. More circumscribed outbreaks have taken place in interepidemic periods, as in Detroit in 1929, when about 750 cases occurred over an eight-month period. Aside from several minor urban outbreaks, particularly among alcoholics, in the Pacific Northwest and a small outbreak in Canada, group A strains have only rarely been implicated in meningococcal disease in North America during the past decade. However, serious epidemics caused by group A meningococci have occurred in Finland in 1973, in Brazil in 1974, and in northern Nigeria in 1977. The outbreak in Nigeria is but one of many that have occurred about once every ten years in the "meningitis belt" in sub-Saharan Africa. In the 1948–49 epidemic, about 93,000 cases were reported, with over 14,000 deaths. Although group A meningococci had been susceptible to sulfonamides in the past, resistant strains first appeared in the epidemics in Africa in the late 1960's and subsequently in Brazil and Finland.

Although group A meningococci have been involved in the most extensive epidemics of meningococcal disease, groups B and C have been responsible for more limited outbreaks and for numerous sporadic cases both in this country and abroad. In the United States in 1963 and 1964, outbreaks caused by group B meningococci (noteworthy for their frequent resistance to sulfonamides) occurred in military camps. By 1967 serogroup B was responsible for the majority of infections occurring in military and civilian populations. By the early 1970's serogroup C strains were those most frequently isolated, only to be supplanted by group B in the mid 1970's. In the period 1975–1980 the serogroups found among disease-related strains were as follows: B (56 per cent), C (19 per cent), Y (11 per cent), W135 (10 per cent), A (3 per cent), and ungroupable (1 per cent). Serogroup W135 has recently appeared as an important cause of meningococcal disease in this country (21 per cent in 1980), displacing group C as the second most frequent cause.

Just as serogrouping of meningococcal strains has been invaluable in the study of major epidemics and in the development and use of polysaccharide vaccines, serotyping can be helpful in evaluating changes in ambient strains. Between epidemics sporadic cases are caused by heterogeneous strains belonging to many serogroups and a variety of serotypes. In military recruit populations, the serogroup carried is not a valid indicator of epidemic potential. At intervals of about ten years a single serotype (e.g., serotype 2, present in most disease-related strains of groups B and C and in some strains of groups Y and W135 during this past decade) becomes pre-eminent, producing a higher endemic rate of disease, sometimes accompanied by scattered small outbreaks.

Nosocomial transmission of infection occasionally occurs. Meningococcal meningitis has developed in several physicians who gave mouth-to-mouth resuscitation to infected patients. Group Y meningococci particularly have been implicated in meningococcal pneumonia, and such patients, if not isolated, may be responsible for nosocomial spread of infection.

Immunity. The age-specific incidence of meningococcal disease is inversely proportional to the prevalence of antimeningococcal bactericidal antibodies (against serogroups A, B, C). At birth, over 50 per cent of infants have bactericidal antibody. From 6 to 24 months of age, the prevalence of antibodies is lowest, and thereafter it increases to early adulthood, when over 70 per cent of individuals have bactericidal activity. The protective role of bactericidal antibodies against *N. meningitidis* was demonstrated during an outbreak of group C meningitis among army recruits in 1968. Eleven per cent of recruits lacked serum antibody against the outbreak-associated strain, and one quarter of these susceptibles acquired this strain during their training period. Of the susceptibles exposed, 38 per cent developed systemic meningococcal disease; in contrast, only 1 per cent of the entire trainee group developed disease.

IgA antibody to meningococcal polysaccharide may have a paradoxic effect. When a large part of an individual's antibodies to a meningococcal serogroup is of this class, serum bactericidal activity of IgM and IgG is blocked, enhancing susceptibility to meningococcal disease. This odd phenomenon is observed for a short time following the induction of IgA by asymptomatic carriage of *N. meningitidis* or an immunologically related organism.

Following meningococcal meningitis serum bactericidal antibody develops, and the patient is immune to clinical reinfection with the same serogroup. However, this is not the usual means of acquiring immunity. Nasopharyngeal carriage of *N. meningitidis* is an effective immunizing process, producing rises in bactericidal antibody within five to twelve days of acquisition of the organism. About 90 per cent of carriers of group B, C, or Y meningococci develop increased serum bactericidal titers, primarily to the colonizing strain but also to heterologous strains. Similarly, nasopharyngeal carriage of nongroupable meningococci, strains rarely causing human disease, can induce antibodies against various groupable pathogenic isolates.

The group-specific capsular polysaccharides of group A and group C meningococci are good immunogens and have been used in successful vaccines. The capsular polysaccharide of group B meningococci is a polymer of α2-8–linked sialic acid and is a very poor immunogen. Human brain glycoproteins contain polysialosyl chains that cross-react immunologically with the group B capsular polysaccharide (but not with group A polysaccharide), perhaps accounting for the failure to develop an effective group B vaccine.

In young children, colonization with *N. lactamica* may induce cross-reactive antibodies to *N. meningitidis* and thus contribute to natural immunity. *N. lactamica* is relatively avirulent and has only rarely been involved in systemic infections. During the first eight years of life the age-related prevalence of meningococcal carriage is between 0.5 and 2 per cent, whereas that of *N. lactamica* is considerably higher (4 to 20 per cent).

In addition to antibody, complement is an important component of serum bactericidal activity. Isolated congenital deficiency of one of the late complement components (C5, C6, C7, or C8) is rare and has been associated with recurrent or chronic (chronic meningococcemia) infections with *N. meningitidis* or *N. gonorrhoeae*. Repeated episodes of meningococcal meningitis have occurred in patients with late complement component deficiencies in the absence of enhanced susceptibility to organisms other than *N. meningitidis*. Measurement of total hemolytic complement is helpful for screening purposes in a patient with recurrent systemic *Neisseria* infections. The course of infection, whether meningitis or meningococcemia, is not unusual, and the response to antimicrobial treatment is satisfactory. Complement deficiency, either congenital (late-acting components) or due to a complement-depleting (C1, C3, C4) underlying disease, also may be an important risk factor for the occurrence of first episodes of nonepidemic meningococcal disease: among 20 patients presenting with invasive infection 30 per cent had decreased complement function.

PATHOGENESIS AND PATHOLOGY. The factors that determine whether initial exposure to *N. meningitidis* will result in benign nasopharyngeal carriage or serious invasive infection are unclear. About one third of patients with invasive infection have had antecedent symptoms referable to the upper respiratory tract. Whether these prodromal symptoms are produced by *N. meningitidis* or a predisposing viral respiratory infection is difficult to determine, particularly since many cases of meningococcal disease occur in the winter when viral respiratory infections are frequent. A simultaneous outbreak of systemic meningococcal disease and influenza A2 infection has occurred in a closed institutional setting. The predisposing role of influenza for meningococcal lower respiratory infections may be clearer (e.g., the occurrence of numerous cases of meningococcal pneumonia complicating influenza during the 1918–19 pandemic).

The incubation period from the initiation of nasopharyngeal infection to bloodstream dissemination is difficult to determine but is probably under ten days. The incubation period may be quite short, judging by the fact that the interval between primary and secondary cases in the same household is often only one to four days. Also, among prospectively studied military recruits cultured within seven days preceding hospitalization for meningococcal disease, only about 20 per cent were carriers of the implicated strain. Once the organism has entered the circulation, the predominant (over 90 per cent) clinical expression is as meningitis or meningococcemia.

The pathologic findings in acute meningococcemia involve the microvasculature and are observed when shock and disseminated intravascular coagulation have occurred. The skin lesions show evidence of fibrin thrombi and vasculitis in small blood vessels. *N. meningitidis* can be seen in endothelial cells and in neutrophils surrounding damaged vessels. The prominent purpura has been attributed to the enhanced capacity to elicit the dermal Shwartzman reaction of its endotoxin compared to endotoxin from enteric gram-negative bacilli. Hemorrhagic adrenal infarction is often observed in patients with fulminant meningococcemia (Waterhouse-Friderichsen syndrome). Shock in this disease is a consequence of bacteremia and not of adrenal failure, since (1) fulminant meningococcemia can occur without adrenal hemorrhage, (2) serum cortisol levels are normal or elevated, and (3) patients who have recovered have not developed Addison's disease. It has been suggested that the shock, purpura, and widespread microvascular thrombi are consequences of an endotoxin-initiated generalized Shwartzman-like reaction or endotoxin-activated disseminated intravascular coagulation. Depressed levels of complement components are found in some patients with acute meningococcemia and may reflect complement activation by circulating endotoxin. Interstitial myocarditis is observed in about 70 per cent of cases of fatal meningococcal disease.

CLINICAL MANIFESTATIONS. Overt illness develops when the initial, often minimally symptomatic nasopharyngeal infection has progressed to bloodstream invasion. The subsequent clinical picture may be mild, or sudden in onset and fulminant, and may reflect principally the bacteremia or features referable to metastatic localization of infection. The most common clinical syndromes are acute meningococcemia, acute purulent meningitis, and a combination of the two (meningococcemia-meningitis).

Meningitis. Most cases occur in children between three months of age and adolescence. Isolated meningitis is less common than meningococcemia-meningitis. The clinical picture may be dominated by manifestations of either meningococcemia or meningitis. In the latter instance the findings are similar to those of meningitis caused by any of the common pyogens (see Ch. 271). Predisposing acute otitis media or pneumonia is unusual in contrast to *H. influenzae* or pneumococcal meningitis. The onset of meningeal symptomatology (1) may be rapid (less than 24 hours) without premonitory symptomatology, (2) may follow an upper respiratory infection of one or two weeks' duration, or (3) may evolve gradually over several days of upper respiratory or nonlocalizing symptoms. In the last-named instance CSF examination during this period may reveal minimal or no increase in cell count and no organisms on Gram-stained smear, but *N. meningitidis* may be isolated, indicating early meningeal involvement. A "clear" CSF in this setting should *not* preclude careful culture. The rapid onset of delirium is seen occasionally in bacterial meningitis (more frequently meningococcal), but it also may occur with a temporal lobe abscess or encephalitis. The neurologic features and complications of meningococcal meningitis are generally the same as for other bacterial meningitides.

The course of meningococcal meningitis may differ from that of other pyogenic meningitides in the occasional occurrence during convalescence of a nonseptic arthritis-pericarditis syndrome.

Meningococcemia. About 20 per cent of patients with meningococcal disease have meningococcemia without meningitis. The clinical expression of meningococcemia varies from an acute process (mild systemic illness or rapidly lethal course) to a chronic, indolent, relapsing disease that may go on for months.

MILD ACUTE MENINGOCOCCEMIA. This is the most common form of meningococcemia, characterized by the rapid development of malaise, fever, chills, myalgias, and arthralgias, often following a minor upper respiratory infection. In a few patients diarrhea has been an early symptom. The subsequent course may follow one of several paths: (1) Symptoms may abate in two or three days, and the diagnosis is made in retrospect when *N. meningitidis* is isolated from a blood culture. (2) Initial symptomatology is followed over 24 to 48 hours by recurrent chills and the appearance of erythematous macular lesions, particularly on the extremities, often accompanied by petechiae. In more severe infections, purpura and ecchymotic areas with gunmetal gray necrotic centers appear. Tachycardia and tachypnea are prominent. Mild hypotension may be present, and shock is a feature if fulminant meningococcemia ensues. In some patients headache may appear and confusion and stiff neck develop; the syndrome then becomes one of combined *meningococcemia-meningitis*. A meningoencephalopathic picture has been described in up to 15 per cent of patients. This probably represents a heterogeneous group (some with meningitis and others with fulminant meningococcemia and central nervous system changes secondary to shock), in whom confusion, delirium, or coma is striking. (3) Occasionally, initial malaise, fever, and arthralgias (accompanied by a few macular and petechial skin lesions) may persist for about a week, during which one or more joint effusions may develop. Blood cultures reveal *N. meningitidis,* and all manifestations promptly subside on treatment with penicillin.

FULMINANT MENINGOCOCCEMIA. This is the most dramatic form of infection, with an abrupt onset and extraordinarily rapid progression (occasionally less than 10 hours from onset to fatal termination). It occurs in about 10 per cent of patients with meningococcal disease. Violent chills, high fever, dizziness, headache, and profound weakness develop over a few hours. Petechiae appear initially on the extremities; they rapidly increase in number and coalesce as new ones appear in the conjunctivae and buccal mucosa. Hypotension with peripheral vasoconstriction quickly appears. Purpura soon develops (Fig. 272–1). At this point the patient may still be febrile or may have become hypothermic. As shock supervenes, restlessness, mental obtundation, and coma may follow in rapid succession. Disseminated intravascular coagulation (DIC) is commonly present, with enlarging hemorrhagic areas in the skin and sometimes mucosal and gastrointestinal bleeding. Cardiac (my-

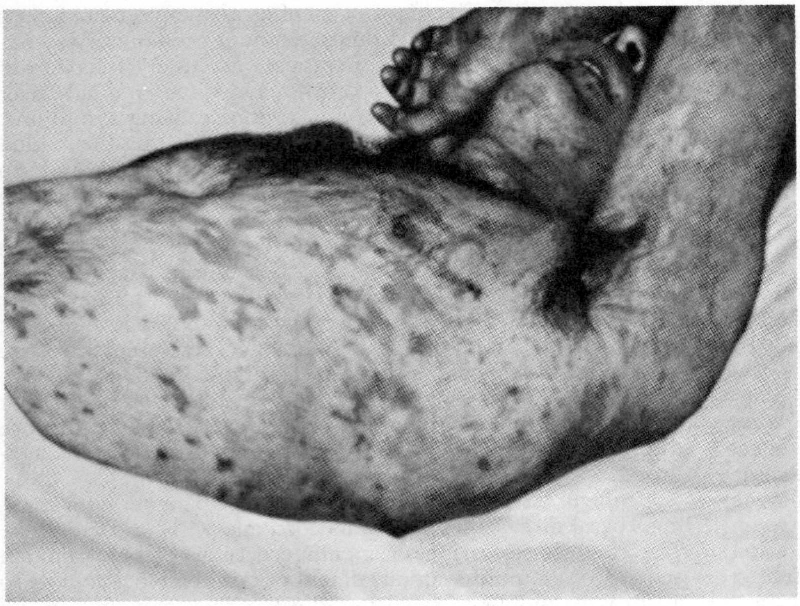

Figure 272–1. Skin lesions in fulminating meningococcemia. (Courtesy of Dr. Worth B. Daniels.)

ocarditis) and respiratory ("shock lung") failure may be terminal events. *The relentless course, once shock develops, makes mandatory early diagnosis and immediate institution of antibiotic treatment even while parts of the initial examination are being performed.*

CHRONIC MENINGOCOCCEMIA. This uncommon form of meningococcemia is characterized by intermittent febrile episodes lasting one to six days, or, rarely, by sustained fevers for several weeks. It begins with chills, migratory arthralgias (or occasionally mild arthritis), and headache, but minimal toxicity. A transient polymorphous (erythematous macules and papules, rare petechiae, and purpuric nodules) nonpruritic rash appears with each febrile episode. The total number of skin lesions is small, and Gram stain and culture only rarely reveal the etiologic agent. Biopsy reveals a leukocytoclastic angiitis, which may be mistaken for a collagen disease or allergic vasculitis. Splenomegaly is observed in 20 per cent of patients. Blood cultures are not positive during apyrexial periods and may not yield the organism until the second or third febrile episode.

Untreated, about 20 per cent of patients ultimately develop meningitis. Rarer complications include endocarditis and epididymitis.

Where the organism resides between episodes is unclear. Throat cultures frequently have not revealed meningococci. The occurrence of chronic meningococcemia in several patients with congenital late complement component deficiencies suggests a possible factor in pathogenesis.

Upper Respiratory Tract Infection. How frequently nasopharyngeal infection is symptomatic is unclear. Nasopharyngeal symptoms preceding some systemic meningococcal infections may be due to this organism or to ambient viral respiratory infections.

Pneumonia. Meningococcal pneumonia is much more often of bronchogenic than of hematogenous origin. Other than during the 1918 influenza pandemic, it has been reported only rarely until this past decade. Primary meningococcal pneumonia is most often due to group Y; in recent years among recruits pneumonia caused by group Y has become the most common form of meningococcal disease. Primary meningococcal pneumonia may be segmental, lobar, or bronchopneumonic in pattern. It sometimes follows antecedent influenza or adenoviral infection. Clinical features are similar to those of community-acquired pneumonias. The onset may be gradual or abrupt. Lower lobes are usually involved. Bacteremia occurs in about 15 per cent of cases. In some patients purulent sputum is produced, containing numerous gram-negative diplococci; in others sputum is scanty, and diagnosis is made on a transtracheal aspirate or by blood culture. Response to treatment with penicillin is prompt.

Meningococcal pneumonia occasionally develops in the course of clinical meningococcemia or meningitis, but the clinical picture is dominated by the extrapulmonary aspects.

To be distinguished from meningococcal pneumonia are occasional exacerbations of chronic bronchopulmonary infection in which the sputum may show numerous gram-negative, biscuit-shaped diplococci (usually noninvasive *Neisseria* species or *Branhamella catarrhalis*). Beta-lactamase–producing strains of *Branhamella catarrhalis* have been isolated with increasing frequency in such pulmonary infections, and they may not respond to treatment with penicillin or ampicillin.

Arthritis. Arthritis complicates 2 to 16 per cent of acute meningococcal illness and may take several forms: (1) *Isolated, acute suppurative meningococcal arthritis,* a rare type occurring in the absence of meningitis or clinical meningococcemia. The joint fluid has the characteristics of septic arthritis. (2) *Early onset (first two to three days) arthritis* during meningococcal meningitis or meningococcemia, the most common form. It is a polyarthritis with acutely inflamed joints; effusions are small or absent. It responds promptly to penicillin. (3) *Late onset (fourth to tenth day, when meningitis is subsiding) arthritis.* This is commonly a subacute mono- or oligoarthritis accompanied by joint effusions. It is associated with recrudescence of fever, pleuropericarditis, and, occasionally, new papulobullous skin lesions. Synovial and pericardial fluids are characteristically serosanguineous (but sometimes purulent) and sterile. Immunopathologic study of synovial lesions implicates immune complex formation in their genesis. Treatment involves joint aspiration and the use of anti-inflammatory agents.

Pericarditis. Pericarditis complicates 2 to 20 per cent of meningococcal disease. It may take several forms: (1) *Early onset pericarditis,* appearing in the first several days of clinical meningococcemia or meningitis, may be purulent and may be due to invasion by *N. meningitidis.* (2) *Late onset pericarditis,* developing four to ten days after onset of meningitis, may cause large sterile, serosanguineous effusions. The favorable response to anti-inflammatory agents and adrenal corticosteroids supports the proposed role of hypersensitivity in pathogenesis. (3) *Isolated purulent pericarditis,* occurring in the absence of meningitis or clinical meningococcemia, is the least common form of meningococcal pericarditis and usually presents with a purulent effusion and tamponade requiring surgical intervention.

Other Meningococcal Infections. Ocular involvement (panophthalmitis, conjunctivitis) occurs in less than 1 per cent of patients with meningococcal disease. Primary conjunctivitis, an acute purulent process, is even less common. Since dissemination develops in 10 per cent of children with primary meningococcal conjunctivitis, systemic therapy with penicillin should be employed along with topical antimicrobials.

Genital tract and anal infections with *N. meningitidis* occasionally occur, the latter in homosexual males. In the female symptomatic or asymptomatic infections of the cervix and vagina may be associated with salpingitis or subsequent clinical meningococcemia. Urethral infection is less common than anal infection but is usually symptomatic. Treatment, as for gonococcal infection, is warranted to eliminate symptomatic disease and to prevent the rare instance of disseminated infection.

COURSE AND COMPLICATIONS. Acute meningococcemia may run a varied course, from that of mild disease to that of fulminant illness with death in a day or less. Certain features (particularly if present simultaneously) indicate a poor prognosis: (1) petechiae for less than 12 hours prior to hospitalization (rapid development of crops of new petechiae and purpura from one hour to the next is ominous); (2) shock; (3) fever above 40° C; (4) absence of meningitis; (5) leukopenia; (6) thrombocytopenia or evidence of DIC; and (7) extremes of age.

Extensive purpura, acral cyanosis, hemorrhagic bullae, and peripheral gangrene are features of fulminant meningococcemia, usually occurring in the presence of shock and DIC. DIC may be evident on hospitalization or may develop precipitously in some patients who are stable initially. In acute DIC platelets, fibrinogen and factors II, V, VIII, and XIII are reduced. Abnormalities in three screening tests (prothrombin time prolongation, platelet count reduction, hypofibrinogenemia) aid in detection of DIC, which occurs to some extent in about one quarter of patients with meningococcemia. The partial thromboplastin time may also be prolonged. Confirmation is provided by demonstration of circulating fibrin degradation products in concentrations greater than 40 μg per milliliter. These coagulation defects can result in upper gastrointestinal bleeding, hematuria, and bleeding from the respiratory tract. Despite all therapeutic interventions, some patients show progressive deterioration with marked tachycardia, hyperventilation, refractory shock, metabolic acidosis, deepening coma, and "shock lung." Myocardial involvement may be manifest as either transient electrocardiographic changes or left ventricular failure.

In those who recover, resolution of the hemorrhagic or gangrenous lesions is slow and may require skin grafting. Areas of the hands and feet may remain edematous, cold, and cyanotic and may show demarcation after some weeks.

DIAGNOSIS. ***Laboratory Findings.*** Bacteriologic diagnosis is established by the finding of organisms on stained smears from an infected area (in an appropriate clinical setting), by isolation of *N. meningitidis* from blood or infected body fluids, or by demonstration by latex agglutination or counterimmunoelectrophoresis of group A, B, C, or Y polysaccharide antigen in blood or CSF. Blood cultures reveal *N. meningitidis* in about one third of patients with meningococcal meningitis and in 50 to 75 per cent with clinical meningococcemia or meningococcemia-meningitis. In rare patients with fulminant meningococcemia, diplococci can be seen on Gram-stained smears of blood or buffy coat. Demonstration of organisms on scrapings from skin lesions in acute meningococcemia has been variable: 70 per cent in one study, but much lower in more recent experience.

Since *N. gonorrhoeae* can be isolated from the pharynx and *N. meningitidis* can occasionally be found in the anogenital area, since both species may invade the bloodstream, and since gonococci and *N. lactamica* have on rare occasions been implicated in meningitis, accurate bacteriologic identification is important. However, 0.5 to 5 per cent of meningococci are maltose negative and may thus resemble gonococci and cause confusion.

Meningococcal polysaccharide antigen is demonstrated in the CSF of about 70 per cent of patients with meningococcal meningitis. Antigen is detected in the blood of 10 to 25 per cent of patients with meningococcemia, and its presence is associated with a poorer prognosis and higher incidence of late onset arthritis.

The CSF findings in meningococcal meningitis are those of pyogenic meningitis.

Differential Diagnosis. The differential diagnosis of meningococcal meningitis in the absence of clinical meningococcemia is that of acute meningitis with a purulent CSF formula. With the meningococcemia-meningitis syndrome it should be remembered that very rare instances of meningitis caused by *H. influenzae* and *S. pneumoniae* may be accompanied by petechial skin lesions. Occasional patients with enteroviral meningitis may have a brisk CSF pleocytosis (up to several thousand cells, with as many as 50 to 80 per cent neutrophils and a maculopetechial rash). Rarely, acute bacterial endocarditis caused by *Staphylococcus aureus* can produce a clinical picture almost indistinguishable from that of meningococcemia-meningitis, with a polymorphonuclear CSF pleocytosis and petechial and purpuric skin lesions. In *S. aureus* endocarditis there are a few skin lesions of purulent purpura which show the etiologic agent on Gram-stained smear. Occasionally measles or other viral exanthems may resemble early meningococcemia. Rocky Mountain spotted fever may mimic meningococcemia, but the absence of meningitis in the former, epidemiologic considerations, and demonstration of the etiologic agent aid in distinguishing between these processes.

Chronic meningococcemia, because of its protean manifestations, may be mistaken for Henoch-Schönlein purpura, acute vasculitis, gonococcemia, rheumatic fever, and subacute bacterial endocarditis.

TREATMENT. ***Antibiotic Management.*** As soon as the diagnosis is made, the patient should be put on respiratory isolation to minimize nosocomial spread of infection. Whereas practically all meningococci isolated prior to 1963 were susceptible to sulfadiazine (formerly the treatment of choice), since that time isolates resistant to sulfonamides have become common. Sulfonamide resistance in this country peaked in 1970, when 67 per cent of strains were resistant, and has since decreased (1980) to 12 per cent (8 per cent of group B, 30 per cent of group C, 4 per cent of group W135; all group Y strains susceptible). Should resistance to sulfonamides decline to less than 10 per cent, sulfonamides may again become appropriate drugs for prophylaxis.

Antimicrobial therapy should be initiated *immediately* in patients with suspected meningococcal meningitis or clinical meningococcemia because of the rapidity with which the illness may progress. Clinical isolates have been uniformly susceptible to penicillin and ampicillin (one penicillin-resistant genitourinary tract isolate, a strain with an R-factor mediated β-lactamase, has recently been described). Intravenous penicillin G is the drug of choice (24 million units daily in the adult in divided doses every two hours) for meningococcal meningitis. Alternatively, intravenous ampicillin can be employed in the adult (12 grams daily in divided doses every two to three hours). In patients allergic to penicillin, intravenous chloramphenicol (4 to 6 grams daily in the adult) is the recommended alternative, with appropriate monitoring of the hematopoietic system. The duration of treatment of meningococcal meningitis and the management of complications are considered in Ch. 271.

Intravenous penicillin G is the treatment of acute clinical meningococcemia without meningitis. Although 8 to 10 million units daily is usually adequate to sterilize the blood and most areas of metastatic infection, it may not provide therapeutic CSF levels in the patient with incipient meningitis. For this reason, initial therapy with "meningitis" doses is often employed. Treatment is continued until the patient has been afebrile for five days. Penicillin (5 to 8 million units daily intravenously in the adult) is effective treatment for chronic meningococcemia.

Other Aspects of Treatment. Treatment of severe meningococcemia requires supportive measures to deal with shock and other complications (DIC, congestive failure, metabolic acidosis, "shock lung"). These include cardiovascular monitoring in an intensive care setting, initial volume expansion, use of vasoactive agents, attention to fluid balances, maintenance of adequate oxygenation, and possible use of digitalis. A central venous pressure (CVP) catheter is placed (a flow-directed pulmonary catheter for evaluation of left atrial and ventricular filling pressures may be necessary if cardiac decompensation develops). Volume expansion (dextrose-saline infused rapidly) is necessary initially to assure that intravascular volume is optimal. If there is no sudden or progressive rise in CVP, then volume expansion (utilizing both crystalloid and colloid) is continued until shock is corrected or fluid overload (increased CVP, rales) develops. Urine output should be monitored and maintained at 40 to 50 ml per hour.

If rapid improvement does not follow volume expansion or if the CVP exceeds appropriate limits, a catecholamine should be added to enhance cardiac output and raise arterial pressure to the range of 90 to 100 mm Hg. Dopamine has been widely used because of its ability to increase renal blood flow (at dosage below 6 μg per kilogram per minute) while increasing cardiac contractility. It is administered by continuous intravenous (initial rate of 2 to 5 μg per kilogram per minute) infusion at a rate sufficient to maintain an adequate arterial pressure and urine volume.

Evidence as to whether adrenal corticosteroids have a beneficial effect in bacteremic shock is still conflicting. One or two pharmacologic doses (3 mg per kilogram of dexamethasone or 30 mg per kilogram of methylprednisolone intravenously) have been used in patients not responding to the aforementioned initial measures. Smaller maintenance doses do not appear beneficial, and continued administration predisposes to superinfection.

Adequate oxygenation is essential in a patient with shock, particularly if meningitis is also a feature (in which hypoxia can aggravate cerebral edema). Oxygen administration, and intubation with ventilatory assistance if needed, should be an integral part of therapy aiming at restoring the arterial Po_2 to appropriate levels (80 to 120 mm Hg). Acidosis should be corrected by intravenous administration of sodium bicarbonate (45 mEq) as needed. Digitalis is not of value in meningococcemic shock, but may have a possible role if fluid overload complicates volume expansion or secondary myocarditis. Generally, diuretics such as furosemide have been of more value in this acute situation.

The initial enthusiasm for heparin treatment of DIC in meningococcemia and septic shock has waned, since evidence of efficacy in reducing mortality has been conflicting despite improvement in coagulation factors. Heparin treatment on the basis of laboratory abnormalities alone is inadvisable. Reversal of hypotension is often associated with improvement in laboratory evidences of DIC and a halt in further clinical progression of the coagulopathy. Only if bleeding into deep tissues or from mucosal surfaces develops or thrombotic manifestations occur in the presence of DIC might heparinization be considered. After initiation of heparin therapy coagulation factor deficiencies can be repaired by administration of fresh frozen plasma. Once heparin is started, prothrombin time and partial thromboplastin time determinations are no longer helpful in following laboratory evidences of DIC; levels of fibrin degradation products, fibrinogen, and platelets are of greatest assistance.

PREVENTION. ***Chemoprophylaxis.*** Close contacts (e.g., same household or daycare center, medical personnel exposed by intimate contact such as mouth-to-mouth resuscitation) of a patient with meningococcal disease are at increased risk of developing systemic disease, and should receive chemoprophylaxis. Since secondary (or coprimary) cases usually occur within four days of the initial case, prophylactic treatment should begin as soon as the initial case is identified. Rifampin has been shown to be 80 to 90 per cent effective in eliminating meningococci from the nasopharynx of asymptomatic carriers, and minocycline has been almost as effective. Because of reports of vestibular side effects with minocycline, rifampin is the recommended drug for chemoprophylaxis. It is administered for two days: to adults at a dosage of 600 mg orally twice daily; to children (five to twelve years of age) at a dosage of 10 mg per kilogram twice daily; and to children three to twelve months of age, at a dosage of 5 mg per kilogram twice daily. Since even the high doses of penicillin used to treat meningococcal meningitis or meningococcemia may not eradicate nasopharyngeal carriage, rifampin should be administered also to the index patient prior to discharge from hospital. Rifampin-resistant strains appear readily and would be selected if use of the drug for prophylaxis were widespread.

Meningococcal Vaccine. Monovalent (group A or C), bivalent (groups A and C), and polyvalent (groups A, C, Y, and W135) meningococcal polysaccharide vaccines are commercially available. The vaccines are effective in adults, but they demonstrate less immunogenicity in children below two years of age. Vaccines containing group C polysaccharide have been administered routinely to all recruits in the armed forces, essentially eliminating serogroup C disease in this population. Group A vaccine has been used successfully to control epidemics in Africa, Brazil, and Finland.

The principal indication for use of meningococcal vaccines is the presence of outbreaks of meningococcal disease caused by *N. meningitidis* belonging to serogroup A or C (or more recently, Y and W135).

The routine immunization of individuals against meningococcal disease is not recommended because of the low risk of disease in the absence of outbreaks. However, vaccination should be considered for travelers to countries in which there is epidemic meningococcal disease. Since about 50 per cent of secondary cases among close contacts occur more than five days following the primary case, consideration should be given to the use of immunization as an adjunct to chemoprophylaxis to extend protection if the latter has been unsuccessful.

PROGNOSIS. The mortality from meningococcal meningitis before any treatment was available was about 75 per cent, and residual neurologic damage in the survivors was extensive. The advent of the sulfonamides brought a dramatic reduction in mortality to 5 to 15 per cent. Despite the emergence of sulfonamide-resistant *N. meningitidis,* mortality has been kept at the same low level through the use of high doses of penicillin G or ampicillin. The case-fatality ratio for patients with meningococcemia without accompanying meningitis is higher (25 per cent) than for meningococcal meningitis and reflects the fulminant course in some patients. The case-fatality ratio is highest in children under two years of age and in adults over 50.

Benoit FL: Chronic meningococcemia. Case report and review of the literature. Am J Med 35:103, 1963. *The best review of the clinical features of this fascinating entity.*

Band JD, Chamberland ME, Platt T, Weaver RE, Thornsberry C, Fraser DW: Trends in meningococcal disease in the United States, 1975–1980. J Infect Dis 148:754, 1983. *Most current review of incidence of meningococcal disease in the United States, with emphasis on the role of various serogroups and the prevalence of sulfonamide resistance.*

DeVoe IW: The meningococcus and mechanisms of pathogenicity. Microbiol Rev 46:162, 1982. *Comprehensive review of the biologic properties of* N. meningitidis *and of the epidemiologic and immunologic aspects of meningococcal disease.*

Feldman HA: Meningococcal infections. Adv Intern Med 18:117, 1972. *The best overview of the major aspects of meningococcal disease, including epidemiology, clinical aspects, treatment, and prevention. Authoritative; very well referenced.*

Greenfield S, Sheehe PR, Feldman HA: Meningococcal carriage in a population of "normal" families. J Infect Dis 123:67, 1971. *A most thorough description of the epidemiology of meningococcal carriage in a civilian urban population during a nonepidemic period.*

Goldschneider I, Gotschlich EC, Artenstein MS: Human immunity to the meningococcus. I. The role of humoral antibodies. J Exper Med 129:1307, 1969. *A most important paper, relating susceptibility to meningococcal infection to the lack of serum bactericidal activity against* N. meningitidis. *A lucid presentation of the basic facts necessary to understand the epidemiology of meningococcal disease.*

Goldschneider I, Gotschlich EC, Artenstein MS: Human immunity to the meningococcus. II. Development of natural immunity. J Exper Med 129:1327, 1969. *A second landmark paper by these authors on immunity to meningococcal infection. The role of the carrier state as an immunizing process is clearly demonstrated.*

Koppes GM, Ellenbogen C, Gebhart RJ: Group Y meningococcal disease in United States Air Force recruits. Am J Med 62:661, 1977. *A very good description of the spectrum of disease produced by group Y meningococci. The importance of pneumonia in a recruit population is emphasized.*

Peltola H: Meningococcal disease: Still with us. Rev Infect Dis 5:71, 1983. *Authoritative evaluation of the current status of meningococcal disease around the world.*

Peltola H, Makela PH, Kayhty H, et al.: Clinical efficacy of meningococcus group A capsular polysaccharide vaccine in children three months to five years of age. N Engl J Med 297:686, 1977. *A noteworthy study of a successful large-scale immunization program during a meningococcal epidemic.*

273. INFECTIONS CAUSED BY HEMOPHILUS SPECIES

DEFINITION. *Hemophilus* infections involve primarily the upper respiratory tract and the bronchopulmonary system. Invasive infections (bacteremia, meningitis, pericarditis, septic arthritis, cellulitis) may sometimes ensue; they occur predominantly in young children and are almost always due to one species, *Hemophilus influenzae* type b. Endocarditis is occasionally caused by *Hemophilus* species other than *H. influenzae* b. One *Hemophilus* species (*H. ducreyi*) is the cause of chancroid (see Ch. 305), and another (*H. vaginalis*—more recently designated *Gardnerella vaginalis*) is implicated in "nonspecific vaginitis." With the exception of these last two species, the normal habitat of the *Hemophilus* species is the upper respiratory tract.

GENERAL MICROBIOLOGIC FEATURES. The various *Hemophilus* species (Table 273–1) are similar in morphology (small, pleomorphic, gram-negative bacilli) and growth requirements (facultatively aerobic, media supplemented with blood). *H. influenzae* requires for aerobic growth both the X factor (hematin) and the V factor (NAD, NADP, or nicotinamide nucleoside) present in erythrocytes. Since some strains of *H. influenzae* grow best in 5 to 10 per cent carbon dioxide and other *Hemophilus* species have a CO_2 dependence, clinical specimens should be incubated in a CO_2 incubator. Media for isolation of *Hemophilus* species include chocolate agar, agar containing horse (but not sheep) blood, or enrichment agar (Levinthal).

H. hemolyticus rarely is isolated from sites outside the upper respiratory tract and is of dubious pathogenicity.

INFECTIONS DUE TO HEMOPHILUS INFLUENZAE. ***Etiology.*** *H. influenzae* strains are either encapsulated (typable) or unencapsulated (nontypable). The former consist of six distinguishable types, designated a to f. Nearly all strains causing invasive infection belong to type b, and the capsular polysaccharide contains both ribose and ribitol phosphate (PRP). However, encapsulated strains make up only a small percentage of clinical isolates of *H. influenzae*. Nontypable strains are more likely to be implicated in localized infections and rarely are associated with bacteremia. Encapsulated strains can be identified by a variety of methods employing antisera to their capsular antigens (immunofluorescence; production of immunoprecipitin halos ringing colonies on agar plates containing antiserum; demonstration by counterimmunoelectrophoresis of capsular antigen in culture supernatants). The outer membrane of *H. influenzae* strains contains a lipopolysaccharide with the properties of endotoxin. A classification of *H. influenzae* b into subtypes based on differences in outer membrane proteins has been developed and may be of potential use in epidemiologic studies.

Smears of clinical specimens usually show pleomorphic gram-negative coccobacilli. Occasionally, in underdecolorized gram-stained smears of spinal fluid, bipolar concentration of stain may incorrectly suggest gram-positive diplococci.

TABLE 273–1. DIFFERENTIAL PROPERTIES OF *HEMOPHILUS* SPECIES

Species	Growth Factor Requirement: X	V	CO_2 Dependence	Hemolysis
H. influenzae	+	+	−	−
H. parainfluenzae	−	+	−	−
H. aphrophilus	−, +	−	+	−
H. paraphrophilus	−	+	+	−
H. hemolyticus	+	+	−	+
H. ducreyi	+	−	−	−

Incidence and Prevalence. Nontypable *H. influenzae* are commonly carried in the nasopharynx of asymptomatic individuals. Rates of carriage for encapsulated strains (usually type b) are much lower (less than 5 per cent of children and less than 1 per cent of adults). Nasopharyngeal carriage of *H. influenzae* b may develop in some persons in the presence of circulating antibody to PRP, and successful antibiotic treatment of *H. influenzae* meningitis may not eliminate it from the upper respiratory tract. The carrier state may persist for weeks to months.

H. influenzae b is the principal (estimated 8000 to 11,000 cases annually) cause of reported cases of bacterial meningitis in the United States. The frequency of invasive infections is inversely related to age; only a small percentage of cases occur in older children or adults. In the past decade many clinicians have had the impression that systemic disease caused by *H. influenzae* b has become more frequent in adults. Systemic infection with *H. influenzae* probably should be considered in the adult in the proper setting more frequently than was formerly the case.

Epidemiology. Infections in the first two months of life are rare, probably because of transplacental transfer of maternal antibody. Most cases of meningitis, septic arthritis, and cellulitis occur in children under two years of age. The mean age of children with epiglottitis is three to five years. Host factors appearing to contribute to increased susceptibility include immune globulin deficiencies, sickle cell disease, CSF fistulas, splenectomized states, and chronic pulmonary infections. Alcoholism appears to be a risk factor in adults.

Unlike *Neisseria meningitidis*, *H. influenzae* b does not cause epidemics in the community, but it is responsible for an increased incidence of secondary cases among susceptibles in families or in day-care centers exposed to an index case. The risk of serious *H. influenzae* illness among exposed household contacts of a child with *H. influenzae* meningitis is age dependent, with an incidence of 3.8 per cent among children under two years of age, 1.5 per cent among children two to three years of age, and 0.1 per cent among children four to five years of age. The rate of infection in household contacts without regard to age represents a 600-fold increase in risk over that in the population at large.

Pathogenesis and Immunity. Most nasopharyngeal infections with *H. influenzae* are unrecognized and occur by age five years. Type b strains may occasionally invade locally, producing epiglottitis, pneumonia, or buccal cellulitis, or may be disseminated via the bloodstream, producing meningitis. Pathogenicity of type b strains is due principally to the antiphagocytic activity of its PRP capsule. Nonencapsulated strains rarely produce bacteremic infection but can produce disease involving the upper (otitis media, sinusitis) and lower (pneumonia, exacerbations of chronic bronchitis) respiratory tracts.

Since the study of Fothergill and Wright, the conventional dogma has been that susceptibility to *H. influenzae* meningitis is inversely related to the presence of serum bactericidal activity (equated with anti-PRP antibody), which in turn correlates with age. In Finland, preliminary studies of anti-PRP antibodies by radioimmunoassay indicate an inverse correlation between age-related antibody levels and incidence of bacteremic *H. influenzae* disease; 90 per cent of children (3 to 12 months of age) had antibody levels less than 150 ng per milliliter, whereas all adults had higher levels. Antibodies to outer membrane proteins also play a role in immunity, but they appear to be protective primarily against strains of the same subtype.

The antibody response to *H. influenzae* b meningitis is age related (infants responding poorly and older children and adults developing high titers) and related to PRP load and clearance rate. Antigenemia may persist for as long as several weeks in younger children; an antibody response may be delayed until antigenemia has cleared. Anti-PRP antibody responses are observed within about three months in about 80 per cent of children with meningitis.

Anti-PRP antibodies can be generated by intestinal colonization or infection with bacteria (e.g., *E. coli* 075:K100:H5) exhibiting cross-reacting surface antigens. It has been suggested that the age-related acquisition of anti-PRP antibodies is too rapid and extensive to be accounted for by the low incidence of *H. influenzae* b carriage or disease, and that cross-reacting *E. coli* strains in the intestine may serve as the primary immunogen.

Clinical Manifestations. In one survey of children with serious *H. influenzae* infections, meningitis was the most common manifestation (about 50 per cent), followed by pneumonia (15 per cent), bacteremia without definable portal (10 per cent), cellulitis (10 per cent), epiglottitis (10 per cent), and pericarditis (4 per cent). Among adults with *H. influenzae* bacteremia, pneumonia is the commonest cause. About half the isolates are nontypable, and most of the typable strains belong to type b. Other sources of *H. influenzae* bacteremia in adults include obstetric infections (nontypable strains), meningitis, occult bacteremias, cellulitis, acute sinusitis, and epiglottitis. Metastatic *H. influenzae* infections in the adult include septic arthritis and purulent pericarditis.

MENINGITIS. (See Ch. 271). *H. influenzae* type b is the preeminent cause of bacterial meningitis in childhood, most cases occurring between ages four months and two years. The clinical features are not distinctive except as they relate to pyogenic meningitis occurring at that age. The manifestations may be nonspecific (fever, irritability, listlessness, poor feeding, vomiting) initially, especially in the younger child, and there may be only minimal nuchal rigidity. If the fontanel is still open, it may not be tense, particularly if the infant is dehydrated. Subdural effusions occur more frequently (20 to 30 per cent) with *H. influenzae* meningitis, but this is related to age and ease of detection by transillumination.

EPIGLOTTITIS. This pediatric otolaryngologic emergency begins abruptly with a severe sore throat, fever, and dysphagia; progression is swift, usually requiring hospitalization (and intubation) within 12 hours of onset. In the adult the onset of epiglottitis may be more prolonged and respiratory difficulty less pronounced initially despite severe pharyngitis and dysphagia; occasionally, the clinical picture may be mistaken for that of asthma. Airway obstruction in the child develops early with a sensation of choking, inspiratory (but not expiratory) distress, drooling, and anxiety. Speech is muffled, but the barking cough observed in croup is uncommon. The patient sits leaning forward with arms, back, and neck hyperextended to provide maximal airway. Pneumonia occurs in 15 to 25 per cent of patients, but simultaneous meningitis is uncommon. *Intraoral examination of the child (particularly in the supine position) may precipitate a cardiorespiratory arrest and should be performed only with the means of establishing an airway immediately at hand.* The pharynx is reddened; the epiglottis is bright red and markedly swollen. Lateral radiographs of the neck can demonstrate swelling of the epiglottis, but are of less value in acute cases (the procedure may delay establishment of an adequate airway) than in subacute ones.

Viral croup may resemble epiglottitis but occurs in younger children (3 to 36 months), has a more gradual onset, and frequently is preceded by an upper respiratory infection; the airway obstruction is subglottic.

PNEUMONIA. Most cases occur in children, are due to type b, and are accompanied by bacteremia. Lobar consolidation occurs more commonly than bronchopneumonia, and pleural effusions (or empyema) are present in 75 per cent of cases. Lung abscess is rare. Meningitis occurs in about 15 per cent of patients.

In the adult *H. influenzae* pneumonia occurs more frequently in the setting of chronic lung disease, alcoholism, immunologic deficiency, or preceding viral respiratory tract infection, but it may develop in previously healthy individuals. The majority of sputum isolates are nontypable, as are most blood isolates from the approximately 20 per cent of patients in whom bacteremia occurs. The radiologic pattern is more often that of bronchopneumonia. Small sterile parapneumonic effusions are common. The diagnosis can be suspected on the basis of findings on Gram-stained smears of sputum, but confirmation is provided by isolation of the organism from blood, pleural fluid, or lower respiratory tract.

BRONCHITIS. *H. influenzae* (nontypable) has been associated with purulent sputum and clinical exacerbations (dyspnea, wheezing, low grade fever) of chronic bronchitis. A direct etiologic role is difficult to establish because of the frequent (20 to 80 per cent) carriage of these organisms in the upper respiratory tract of normal adults.

CELLULITIS. *H. influenzae* b causes cellulitis in children below two years of age, but recently has also been observed to cause cellulitis on rare occasions in older adults. The cheek, periorbital area, head, and neck are the most common sites. An associated ipsilateral otitis media or upper respiratory infection is a frequent precursor. It begins with fever, local pain, and increasing toxicity. The lesion develops within a few hours and progresses rapidly; it is poorly demarcated, tender, and edematous. Although usually described as having a distinctive bluish purple color, the lesion is commonly erythematous like other types of cellulitis or may occasionally resemble angioedema. Bacteremia occurs in 80 per cent of cases and can result in metastatic infection. Diagnosis is made on the basis of the appearance and location of the lesion, the patient's age, Gram-stained smears and culture of an aspirate, and blood cultures.

BACTEREMIA WITHOUT OBVIOUS PORTAL. *H. influenzae* b is responsible for about 20 per cent of cryptogenic bacteremias occurring in febrile children with mild nonspecific illnesses managed on an ambulatory basis. Such patients are at considerable risk for subsequent serious localized infection (meningitis, pneumonia, epiglottitis). Unsuspected *H. influenzae* bacteremia also occurs in patients with neoplastic disease undergoing chemotherapy. Fulminant *H. influenzae* bacteremia with fatal shock and disseminated intravascular coagulation can develop in splenectomized patients.

SKELETAL INFECTIONS. Septic arthritis accounts for 1 to 8 per cent of cases of invasive *H. influenzae* b infection in children. It is the cause of pyogenic arthritis in about half the cases in children under two years of age. Weight-bearing joints are most often involved. Most commonly pyarthrosis is secondary to bacteremic spread from an upper respiratory tract infection or otitis media, but joint involvement may result from direct spread of adjacent osteomyelitis in the first year of life.

H. influenzae is a rare cause of osteomyelitis in children, usually occurring in the first year of life.

PERICARDITIS. *H. influenzae* b is the cause of 10 to 15 per cent of cases of purulent pericarditis in children. It is a rare cause of pericarditis in adults. Pericarditis may result from either bacteremic seeding of the pericardium or contiguous spread from infected lung or pleura. Over half of the cases in children have an associated pneumonia. High fever, tachycardia, tachypnea, and the hemodynamic manifestations of cardiac tamponade are commonly present. Treatment involves pericardiocentesis for diagnosis followed by surgical drainage (closed catheter drainage or anterior pericardectomy), along with antimicrobial therapy. With treatment 85 to 95 per cent of patients recover.

OTITIS MEDIA AND SINUSITIS. *H. influenzae* is second in frequency to *Streptococcus pneumoniae* as the cause of acute otitis media in children. In most instances the *H. influenzae* strains are not typable, but type b strains can be isolated in 10 per cent of cases. Serous middle ear fluid in children with chronic low grade otitis media with effusion may be colonized by *H. influenzae,* which may contribute to its persistence. *H. influenzae* also appears to be a significant cause of otitis media in older children and adults. The manifestations of acute otitis media caused by *H. influenzae* are indistinguishable from those caused by other pyogens: otalgia, fever, hyperemia of the tympanic membrane, and middle ear fluid. Tinnitus, vertigo, and nystagmus may develop.

Acute sinusitis is more common in adults than in children. In about 25 per cent of cases *H. influenzae* (nontypable) is the cause. Acute sinusitis is often preceded by a viral upper respiratory infection. Facial pain, frontal headache, purulent nasal discharge or nasal obstruction, anosmia, and nasal speech are common features. Sinus tenderness and opacity on transillumination are helpful findings.

CONJUNCTIVITIS. Most strains of *Hemophilus* isolated from conjunctivae are unencapsulated and formerly were designated as *H. aegyptius* (Koch-Weeks bacillus) on the basis of their hemagglutinating property. Currently these strains are considered as biotypes of *H. influenzae*. *H. influenzae* mucopurulent conjunctivitis occurs principally in children, particularly in the summer. The findings of acute catarrhal conjunctivitis are present, but petechial hemorrhages on the tarsal and epibulbar conjunctivae are suggestive of *H. influenzae* or a pneumococcal cause. Transient marginal corneal infiltrates are more common with this type of infection than with those resulting from pneumococci. Diagnosis is made on the basis of Gram-stained smears of conjunctival scrapings and culture of the outer eye.

H. influenzae conjunctivitis is often self-limited, clearing in 7 to 14 days. Treatment consists of moist soaks to keep the eyelids clean and topical antimicrobials (e.g., 10 to 30 per cent sulfacetamide eyedrops).

OTHER INFECTIONS. *H. influenzae* is a very rare cause of endocarditis and brain abscess. *H. influenzae* may occasionally be the cause of nonexudative pharyngitis (with prominent pain and dysphagia), but its presence in the pharynx often merely represents colonization. Rare cases of genital tract infections (salpingitis, endometritis, puerperal sepsis) and urinary infections have occurred.

Diagnosis. Certain serious infections (purulent meningitis, epiglottitis, facial and orbital cellulitis) in young children should suggest the possibility of *H. influenzae* b as the cause. In meningitis the presence of gram-negative pleomorphic coccobacillary forms in smears of CSF is highly suggestive of *H. influenzae,* but other organisms *(Pasteurella multocida, Acinetobacter)* which only rarely cause meningitis may have a similar appearance. Rapid and sensitive methods of antigen (PRP) detection such as counterimmunoelectrophoresis (CIE), latex particle agglutination, and enzyme-linked immunosorbent assay (ELISA) have detected *H. influenzae* b antigen in initial CSF specimens of 70 to 90 per cent of cases of *H. influenzae* meningitis; they are particularly helpful in early diagnosis and in the diagnosis of patients whose cultures may be negative because of prior antibiotic therapy. Antigenemia can be demonstrated in 60 to 100 per cent of patients with *H. influenzae* b meningitis but much less frequently in children with epiglottitis and cellulitis. False-positive reactions may occur owing to cross-reactive antigens in other bacteria such as *E. coli,* but these are infrequent.

Bacteremia is commonly demonstrable in patients with invasive infections (at least 80 per cent of children with meningitis, epiglottitis, or cellulitis) caused by *H. influenzae* b. *H. influenzae* is generally isolated on cultures of the epiglottis, joint fluid, and empyema fluid when it is the cause of infection in those areas.

Treatment. Currently, about 24 per cent of strains of *H. influenzae* b isolated in this country from systemic infections are ampicillin resistant (β-lactamase producing), with some variation (13 to 36 per cent) between geographic areas. About 15 per cent of strains (usually nontypable) associated with childhood otitis media are ampicillin resistant, as are 2 to 8 per cent of strains (mostly nontypable) isolated from adults with invasive infections or chronic bronchitis. Because of this prevalence of ampicillin resistance, systemic illnesses caused by *H. influenzae* (or when this organism is suspected) should be treated with chloramphenicol alone or in combination with ampicillin (see Ch. 271) until it is determined whether the organism produces β-lactamase; if it does not, then only the ampicillin need be continued. Rare strains of *H. influenzae* resistant to chloramphenicol have been isolated from children with meningitis. Very rare cases of meningitis caused by *H. influenzae* b resistant to both ampicillin and chloramphenicol have occurred. As yet there is no reason to change the initial therapy (chloramphenicol alone or with ampicillin) for invasive disease caused by this organism. For systemic infection associated with such a doubly resistant strain, or when the presence of such an organism is suspected on the basis of clinical response to conventional therapy, treatment should involve a third generation cephalosporin such as moxalactam or cefotaxime (see Ch. 271). Antimicrobial susceptibilities of *H. influenzae* isolates from systemic diseases should be determined if possible, particularly if the response to chloramphenicol is unsatisfactory. Chloramphenicol is bactericidal against *H. influenzae* at concentrations readily achieved in humans. Although antagonism has been demonstrated in vitro and in vivo between penicillin and chloramphenicol against *S. pneumoniae,* there appears to be no antagonism between these two drugs against *H. influenzae.*

Ampicillin (50 to 100 mg per kilogram per day in four divided doses) or amoxicillin (50 mg per kilogram per day in four divided doses), because each is active against *S. pneumoniae* and most strains of *H. influenzae,* is still the drug of choice for initial treatment of otitis media in children. Alternatives include trimethoprim (TMP)–sulfamethoxazole (SMX) (40 mg TMP–200 mg SMX twice daily per 20 pounds), the combination of penicillin (or erythromycin) with a sulfonamide, or cefaclor. Treatment should be continued for 10 to 14 days. Initial treatment of *H. influenzae* pneumonia in the adult should be with ampicillin, since these infections are infrequently caused by ampicillin-resistant strains, and there is sufficient time to shift therapy (chloramphenicol, cefamandole) if the response is unsatisfactory. Based on the bacteriology (*S. pneumoniae* and *H. influenzae* are frequently identified) of acute sinusitis, ampicillin is a reasonable initial antibiotic choice. (In the patient with rapidly progressive frontal sinusitis, *S. aureus* must be considered as a cause as well, and a penicillinase-resistant penicillin should be included in the initial therapeutic program.)

Prevention. An experimental vaccine consisting of purified capsular PRP has been tested on over 50,000 children in Finland and has been found to be well tolerated, immunogenic, and capable of preventing invasive *H. influenzae* b disease above the age of 18 months. Unfortunately, for children below 18 months of age, when the incidence of *H. influenzae* meningitis is greatest, it was a poor immunogen and was not protective. This vaccine is not yet approved for use in the United States. In view of what appears to be an age-specific defect in the response of infants to thymus-independent polysaccharide antigens, promising preliminary attempts have been made to overcome this limitation by linking the PRP antigen to a protein (tetanus toxoid), thus involving T cell participation and establishing immunologic memory.

The rate of secondary cases among young children who are close contacts of a patient with invasive *H. influenzae* b infection indicates the need for an effective prophylactic antibiotic program. Since rifampin has efficacy in eliminating nasopharyngeal carriage of *H. influenzae* b, the following management of household contacts has been recommended: (1) if another child less than four years of age resides in the household of an index case, all household members (including adults) should receive rifampin (20 mg per kilogram orally once daily for four days, with a maximal daily dose of 600 mg); (2) rifampin in the same dosage should also be administered to the index patient prior to discharge from the hospital, since nasopharyngeal carriage may reappear after discontinuation of ampicillin or chloramphenicol therapy for systemic infection; (3) rifampin prophylaxis is probably not indicated if over two weeks have elapsed since illness began in the index patient or if the youngest child in the household is four years of age or older.

INFECTIONS CAUSED BY OTHER HEMOPHILUS SPECIES. ***Hemophilus Parainfluenzae.*** This *Hemophilus* species is part of the normal flora of the nasopharynx and is found in dental plaque. It is very uncommonly responsible for human disease. It has been a rare cause of meningitis, epiglottitis, otitis media, puerperal bacteremia, brain abscess, and pneumonia in adults. Ampicillin is the drug of choice, except when ampicillin resistance is present (6 per cent of isolates), in which case chloramphenicol should be used. The most common association of *H. parainfluenzae* with disease has been with infective endocarditis. It may take as long as 14 to 18 days to grow out of blood cultures. The only distinctive clinical feature (also observed with *H. aphrophilus* endocarditis) appears to be the frequent occurrence of embolic occlusion of large arteries. For endocarditis in the adult, treatment with ampicillin (12 grams daily intravenously) alone or in combination with gentamicin (4 mg per kilogram per day in divided doses every eight hours intravenously) for four to six weeks has been employed successfully.

Hemophilus Aphrophilus. This organism is part of the normal gingival flora and is a rare cause of disease, generally acting as an "opportunist." The infections it produces, often following oropharyngeal foci of infection or trauma, include abscesses (particularly brain abscess), bacteremia, and endocarditis. Most strains are susceptible to penicillin, ampicillin, cephalothin, chloramphenicol, and gentamicin. Successful treatment of endocarditis has involved the use of ampicillin or penicillin, alone or in combination with streptomycin for four to six weeks.

H. Ducreyi. See Ch. 305.

Hemophilus Vaginalis. *Hemophilus vaginalis* is now designated as a new species, *Gardnerella vaginalis*. *G. vaginalis* is found in the vaginal flora of 40 per cent of normal women but in large numbers in the vaginal fluid of over 95 per cent of patients with nonspecific vaginitis. It appears that this organism, acting in concert with certain anaerobes, causes this type of vaginal infection. Oral metronidazole, which is active against both anaerobes and *G. vaginalis*, suppresses both organisms and produces clinical improvement. Such improvement does not occur on treatment with oral ampicillin or doxycycline. Findings suggesting the diagnosis of nonspecific vaginitis include the presence of "clue" cells (vaginal epithelial cells with numerous adherent small gram-negative bacilli) in a vaginal discharge with pH 5.0 (exhibiting a "fishy" amine-like odor upon addition of potassium hydroxide). Treatment with metronidazole is effective, but its possible toxicity must be considered in view of the mildness of the disease and the possibility of reinfection.

G. vaginalis has also been a cause of puerperal fever with bacteremia, septic abortion, and neonatal bacteremia.

Hemophilus influenzae

Cherry JD: Acute epiglottitis, laryngitis, and croup. In Remington JS, Swartz MN (eds.): Current Clinical Topics in Infectious Disease, 2. New York, McGraw-Hill Book Company, 1981, pp 1–30. *Provides a particularly vivid clinical picture of acute* H. influenzae *epiglottitis. Valuable points on differential diagnosis and treatment are emphasized. A very well organized and thoroughly referenced presentation.*

Dajani AS, Asmar BI, Thirumoorthi MC: Systemic *Haemophilus influenzae* disease. J Pediatr 94:355, 1979. *This is a thorough review of an extensive pediatric experience with systemic* H. influenzae *b infections. It provides helpful data on the relative frequencies of the various clinical syndromes and an extensive bibliography.*

Feigen RD, Stechenberg BW, Chang MJ, Dunkle LM, Wong ML, Pelkes H, Dodge PR, Davis H: Prospective evaluation of treatment of *Hemophilus influenzae* meningitis. J Pediatr 88:542, 1976. *This report on 50 well-studied children with* H. influenzae *meningitis provides helpful information concerning the value of counterimmunoelectrophoresis in rapid diagnosis, the spectrum of neurologic complications, and the response to antibiotic treatment.*

Fothergill LD, Wright J: Influenzal meningitis: Relation of age incidence to bactericidal power of blood against causal organism. J Immunol 24:273, 1933. *This is the original and "classic" study demonstrating an inverse relationship between the presence of serum bactericidal antibody and the incidence of* H. influenzae *meningitis at various ages.*

Granoff DM, Ward JI: Current status of prophylaxis for *Haemophilus influenzae* infections. *In* Remington JS, Swartz MN (eds.): Current Clinical Topics in Infectious Disease, 5th ed. New York, McGraw-Hill Book Company, 1984. *Provides excellent background regarding secondary spread of* H. influenzae *infections and concrete recommendations for chemoprophylaxis of close family and day-care center contacts.*

Hirschmann JV, Everett ED: *Haemophilus influenzae* infections in adults: Report of nine cases and a review of the literature. Medicine 58:80, 1979. *This is a thorough review of the various clinical syndromes produced by* H. influenzae *in the adult. Extensively referenced.*

O'Reilly RJ, Anderson P, Ingram DL, Peter G, Smith DH: Circulating polyribosephosphate in *Hemophilus influenzae* type b meningitis. J Clin Invest 56:1012, 1975. *This is an important study showing that certain patients with impaired capacity to clear capsular polysaccharide from the blood following* H. influenzae *meningitis fail to develop the expected antibody response to PRP. Stimulating discussion.*

Peltola H, Käyhty H, Sivonen A, Mäkelä PH: *Haemophilus influenzae* type b capsular polysaccharide vaccine in children: A double-blind field study of 100,000 vaccinees three months to five years of age in Finland. Pediatrics 60:730, 1977. *This article describes a very well conducted, large scale trial of the type b capsular polysaccharide vaccine, which protected against bacteremic* H. influenzae *b disease in children older than 18 months of age but not in younger children. The data are extensive and well presented.*

Robbins JB, Schneerson R, Argaman M, Handzel ZT: *Haemophilus influenzae* type b: Disease and immunity in humans. Ann Intern Med 78:259, 1973. *This is a broad informative review of immunity to* H. influenzae *in the population and of the possible role of enteric bacteria (with cross-reacting antigens) in "natural" immunity to* H. influenzae *b.*

Spagnuolo PJ, Ellner JJ, Lerner PI, McHenry MC, Flatauer F, Rosenberg P, Rosenthal MS: *Haemophilus influenzae* meningitis: The spectrum of disease in adults. Medicine 61:74, 1982. *These 15 cases represent the largest series of cases of* H. influenzae *meningitis reported in the past 20 years. Particular emphasis is on predisposing factors in this unusual form of meningitis in adults.*

Syriopoulou V, Scheifele D, Smith AL, Perry PM, Howie V: Increasing incidence of ampicillin resistance in *Hemophilus influenzae*. J Pediatr 92:889, 1978. *Brief and to the point; ampicillin-resistance is increasing in both type b and non-b isolates of* H. influenzae *in various parts of the United States. Evidence presented is unequivocal.*

Wallace RJ Jr, Musher DM, Septimus EJ, McGowan JE, Quinones FJ, Wiss K, Vance PH, Trier PA: *Haemophilus influenzae* infections in adults: Characterization of strains by serotypes, biotypes, and β-lactamase production. J Infect Dis 144:101, 1981. *This is a detailed review of 103 cases of* H. influenzae *bacteremia or meningitis. Noteworthy is the frequency of nontypable strains among blood isolates in adults and the infrequency of ampicillin resistance in the same group.*

Hemophilus parainfluenzae and Hemophilus aphrophilus

Bieger RC, Brewer NS, Washington JA II: *Haemophilus aphrophilus:* A microbiologic and clinical review and report of 42 cases. Medicine 57:345, 1978. *A comprehensive review of the bacteriologic features, ecologic niche, and clinical impact of this uncommon cause of human disease.*

Chunn CJ, Jones SR, McCutchan JA, Young EJ, Gilbert DN: *Haemophilus parainfluenzae* infective endocarditis. Medicine 56:99, 1977. *This report from five medical centers represents the largest series described to date of* Hemophilus parainfluenzae *endocarditis. Helpful points on bacteriologic identification, distinctive clinical aspects (e.g., frequent emboli to major arteries), and antibiotic recommendations are presented.*

Oill PA, Chow AW, Guze LB: Adult bacteremic *Haemophilus parainfluenzae* infections: Seven reports of cases and a review of the literature. Arch Intern Med 139:985, 1979. *The type of infection (exclusive of endocarditis) caused by* H. parainfluenzae *and the antibiotic susceptibilities of this organism are summarized concisely.*

Gardnerella vaginalis (Hemophilus vaginalis)

Spiegel CA, Amsel R, Eschenbach D, Schoenknecht F, Holmes KK: Anaerobic bacteria in nonspecific vaginitis. N Engl J Med 303:601, 1980. *Strong circumstantial evidence implicating both anaerobic bacteria and* Gardnerella vaginalis (Hemophilus vaginalis) *in the production of "nonspecific vaginitis" is presented. Good references for those uninformed about this entity.*

Osteomyelitis

274. OSTEOMYELITIS

Francis A. Waldvogel

DEFINITIONS. Osteomyelitis is an infection of bacterial, sometimes of fungal, and exceptionally of viral origin that invades and destroys bone. Osteomyelitis is a well known, albeit rare, consequence of bacteremia (hematogenous osteomyelitis). In other situations, such as open fractures, wounds, and orthopedic procedures, the microorganism gains access to bone from a contaminated or infected contiguous structure (osteomyelitis secondary to contiguous infection). Finally, peripheral bones can also be invaded by contiguity in case of severe vascular insufficiency (osteomyelitis secondary to vascular insufficiency). In the latter case, other metabolic and neurologic factors play an important contributory role.

ETIOLOGY. Most cases of osteomyelitis are of bacterial origin, and *S. aureus* is still the most common etiologic agent, being responsible for more than 50 per cent of cases. Other etiologic agents include (1) gram-negative enteric organisms, which are often responsible for hematogenous vertebral osteomyelitis in the elderly; (2) certain *Salmonella* species, which cause osteomyelitis in patients with sickle cell disease; (3) *Pseudomonas aeruginosa,* often responsible for vertebral osteomyelitis in heroin addicts; (4) anaerobic organisms, which are sometimes isolated in pure or mixed cultures from infected bone in the vicinity of an anaerobic reservoir (maxilla, sinuses, sacrum); and (5) *Mycobacterium tuberculosis,* still a major cause of osteomyelitis of the spine in developing countries. In addition, various fungi can occasionally cause osteomyelitis after bacteremic spread, mostly in patients with intravenous access devices. Finally, rare cases of viral osteomyelitides have been described after chickenpox and smallpox.

INCIDENCE, PREVALENCE, AND EPIDEMIOLOGY. Hematogenous osteomyelitis has a biphasic incidence, occurring mainly in children, in whom it shows a predilection for the metaphysis of long bones, and in adults beyond the age of 50 years, in whom it most often involves the spine. Blunt trauma is considered by many to be a favoring factor in children. In adults, any factor favoring bacteremia (urinary tract infection, prostatitis, various skin infections, prolonged intravenous therapy, or repeated injections) can occasionally lead to hematogenous osteomyelitis of the spine. The prevalence of osteomyelitis secondary to a contiguous infection is difficult to determine and reflects the frequency of major trauma and of orthopedic procedures in a given population. It can be as high as 15 per cent in patients with multiple comminuted fractures or less than 1 per cent after total hip replacement performed under strictly aseptic conditions.

PATHOGENESIS AND PATHOLOGY. The various pathogenic mechanisms leading to bone destruction are as yet largely unknown. Since microorganisms per se are unable to destroy bone tissue, one has to postulate that the inflammatory reaction, the metabolic alterations, and the vascular changes triggered by the bacterial invasion play a preponderant role in the development of an osteomyelitic focus, i.e., in bone destruction and regeneration. From a strictly pathologic point of view, the following major changes can be identified: (1) bone necrosis, with death of the cellular constituents and disappearance of bone mass. Sometimes devitalized bone persists as a dead fragment called a sequestrum; (2) a heavy inflammatory reaction, in which granulocytes predominate initially but are replaced over time by a mononuclear infiltrate; (3) new bone apposition, originating from periosteal activation; this periosteal reaction is indeed often the first sign of osteomyelitis identified on x-rays. In some cases, this bone apposition can be exuberant and lead to bridging of two adjacent bone structures, as in vertebral osteomyelitis. In other cases, bone apposition is very modest, and x-ray examination may show only an intraosseous, punched-out radiolucent lesion, as in subacute hematogenous osteomyelitis (Brodie's abscess).

CLINICAL MANIFESTATIONS. Hematogenous osteomyelitis involving long bones starts as an acute episode with chills and fever. The young patient usually complains of an excruciating pain in the affected bone, most often the tibia or femur and more rarely the humerus or radius. Clinical examination shows normal skin over the affected limb, but the bone metaphysis is exceedingly painful on palpation. The adjacent joint is usually unaffected by the disease.

The clinical presentation is usually more progressive in hematogenous vertebral osteomyelitis: following an episode of fever, the middle-aged or elderly patient complains within the next few days or weeks of an ill-defined pain in the spine, most often in the lower dorsal or lumbar segments. On physical examination, the patient is moderately or sometimes highly febrile. There is paravertebral tenderness and spasm on palpation of the affected segment, but the overlying skin is normal. A careful neurologic examination should be carried out to exclude the possibility of a paraspinal abscess, a dreaded complication of vertebral osteomyelitis leading to paraplegia (see Ch. 496).

Osteomyelitis secondary to a contiguous focus of infection after open trauma or secondary to orthopedic reconstructive surgery is a real diagnostic challenge, since pain, low grade fever, local signs of inflammation, and x-ray findings are compatible with both postoperative changes and infection. Persistent fever and increasing signs of inflammation one week after trauma or surgery, persistent inflammation of the surgical incision with oozing of serosanguineous material, and increasing pain on weight-bearing are all helpful clinical signs in favor of infection.

DIFFERENTIAL DIAGNOSIS AND DIAGNOSIS. Whenever osteomyelitis is suspected, blood cultures should be immediately obtained. In hematogenous disease, they will yield the offending organism in 50 per cent of cases. In suspected osteomyelitis of the spine, direct aspiration or bone biopsy is often necessary for a full microbiologic diagnosis if blood cultures remain negative. In osteomyelitis secondary to a contiguous focus, careful probing of the wound with aspiration of the material under aseptic conditions for Gram stain and culture will often yield the necessary microbiologic information. Other laboratory tests are noncontributory: erythrocyte sedimentation rate is usually increased; the white blood cell count is normal or high; and blood chemical values, including alkaline phosphatases, are normal.

Radiologic changes are delayed, appearing several weeks after the onset of the disease. In hematogenous osteomyelitis

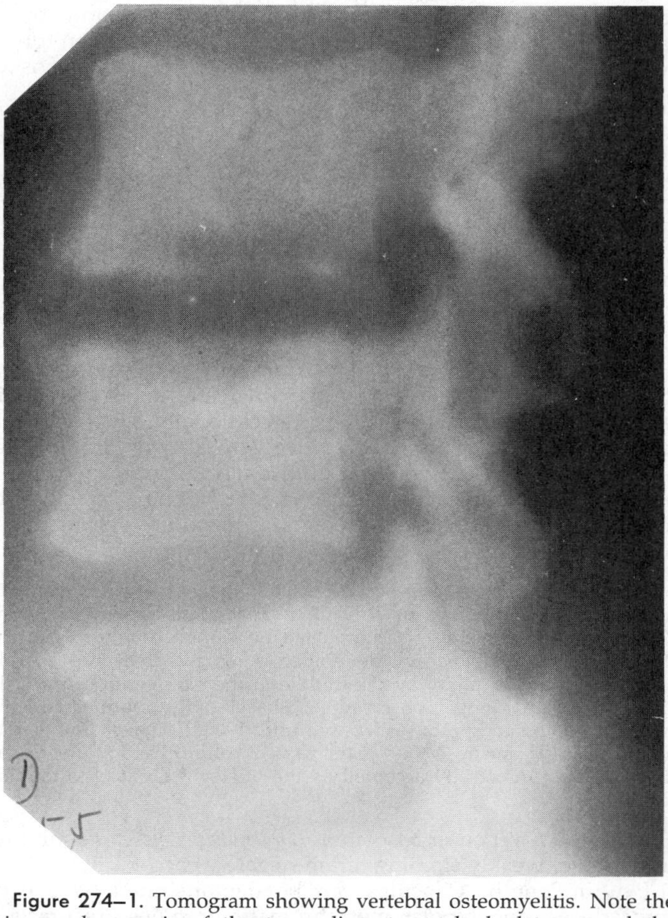

Figure 274–1. Tomogram showing vertebral osteomyelitis. Note the piecemeal necrosis of the two adjacent vertebral plateaus and the anterior bone apposition.

of long bones, periosteal elevation and subsequent bone destruction are the first changes to be observed. In vertebral osteomyelitis, progressive piecemeal destruction of two adjacent vertebral plateaus, narrowing of the intervertebral space, and progressive anterior periosteal bridging are the hallmarks of the disease, bone sclerosis being a late event (see Fig. 274–1). In tuberculous osteomyelitis of the spine, the changes just mentioned are delayed and occur over several months, periosteal reaction usually being absent.

In most cases of hematogenous osteomyelitis, ^{99m}Tc-polyphosphate uptake, although nonspecific, can be of great diagnostic help by identifying the suspected areas of infection for appropriate tomograms at a stage when conventional x-ray results are still normal. In osteomyelitis secondary to a contiguous focus of infection, radiologic techniques and bone scanning are less helpful, since they cannot distinguish between normal bone reaction and infection. Direct aspiration or biopsy for microscopical examination and culture is therefore the procedure of choice to establish the diagnosis.

Acute hematogenous osteomyelitis of long bones has to be differentiated clinically from septic arthritis, bursitis, and cellulitis. These more superficial infections are accompanied by local skin changes, and x-ray results remain normal. Osteomyelitis of the spine is a diagnostic challenge and has to be differentiated from bone tumors such as myeloma and metastases, which usually do not involve two adjacent vertebral plateaus. In case of doubt, bone biopsy may be indicated.

TREATMENT. Medical treatment of osteomyelitis includes the parenteral administration of an appropriate antibiotic, such as cloxacillin 8 grams per day* for *S. aureus* infections. As a general rule, those parenteral antibiotics used for septicemias are also effective in osteomyelitis due to the same organism if the drug is given for six weeks. Thus, osteomyelitis of the spine, which is often caused by gram-negative organisms, can be cured by ampicillin, a first or second generation cephalosporin, or an aminoglycoside (depending on sensitivity testing) given for six weeks. Bed rest is usually recommended until all signs of inflammation have abated, pain has subsided, and x-rays show signs of improvement. This is particularly true for osteomyelitis of the spine. Surgery is rarely indicated in hematogenous infection, except for drainage of intramedullary abscesses, removal of sequestra, and decompression if neurologic signs supervene in vertebral osteomyelitis. In osteomyelitis secondary to a contiguous focus of infection, careful evaluation of the situation by a skilled orthopedic surgeon is mandatory. In case of infected fractures or prostheses, stable union is a prerequisite for bacteriologic cure. Union should be achieved first despite sepsis, and infection is controlled subsequently by antibiotic therapy after removal of the foreign material. In case of nonunion of a fracture or loosening of the prosthesis, the foreign material should be removed, and if possible replaced by an external fixation device. Infected prostheses should also be removed and the infected focus cleaned out, with reinsertion of new material in a one-step or two-step procedure.

*May exceed manufacturer's recommended dosage.

PREVENTION. At present, there is no preventive treatment available for hematogenous osteomyelitis, since the occurrence of the disease after bacteremia is unpredictable. Infection rates after insertion of hip prostheses have been shown to be markedly decreased by short-term coverage (two to three days) with parenteral antistaphylococcal antibiotics. Such coverage should also be considered in high-risk operations, such as reduction of comminuted fractures, open fractures, and insertion of joint prostheses.

Kido D, Bryan D, Halpern M: Hematogenous osteomyelitis in drug addicts. Ther Nucl Med 118:356, 1973. *A concise study of 32 cases, most of them due to* Pseudomonas *species. Discusses their clinical and radiologic manifestations.*

Norden C: Experimental osteomyelitis II: Therapeutic trials and measurement of antibiotic levels in bone. J Infect Dis 124:565, 1971. *An interesting animal model allowing the study of the various pathogenic factors of osteomyelitis and the efficacy of various antibiotic regimens.*

Waldvogel FA, Medoff G, Swartz MN: Osteomyelitis: A review of clinical features, therapeutic considerations and unusual aspects I. II. III. N Engl J Med 282:198, 260, 316, 1970. *A retrospective review of 247 cases of osteomyelitis, their clinical and radiologic presentations, and their treatment.*

Waldvogel FA, Vasey H: Osteomyelitis: The past decade. N Engl J Med 303:360, 1980. *A review update of newer approaches in diagnosis and treatment of osteomyelitis, with emphasis on a combined surgical and medical approach.*

Wedge JH, Oryschak AF, Robertson DE, Kirkaldy-Willis WH: Atypical manifestations of spinal infections. Clin Orthop Rel Res 123:155, 1977. *Unusual presentations of vertebral osteomyelitis that underline its diagnostic challenge.*

Whooping Cough

275. WHOOPING COUGH (Pertussis)

Samuel L. Katz

DEFINITION. Whooping cough is an acute respiratory illness that classically affects infants and young children. The etiologic agent is usually *Bordetella pertussis;* occasionally *B. parapertussis* and rarely *B. bronchiseptica* produce a similar syndrome. The descriptive name derives from a distressing, prolonged inspiratory effort that follows paroxysmal coughing. Whooping cough is still responsible for a significant number of deaths in infants in areas where pertussis immunization is not practiced.

HISTORY. The disease was first recorded in the middle of the sixteenth century by Moulton and by DeBaillou. Sydenham applied the name "pertussis" to any illness accompanied by violent coughing, but the term became restricted to the epidemic disease that was a well-recognized clinical entity by the middle of the eighteenth century. In 1900 Bordet and Gengou observed coccobacilli in the sputum of a child with whooping cough, but it was not until 1906 that they were able to culture the organism. Many years passed before the Bordet-Gengou bacillus was universally accepted as the etiologic agent of whooping cough.

ETIOLOGY. When first isolated, *Bordetella pertussis* is a minute, nonmotile, weakly staining, gram-negative coccobacillus, 0.5 to 1.0 μ in length. Capsules can be demonstrated by special procedures, and bipolar metachromatic granules are present. The complex medium containing blood originally employed by Bordet and Gengou is still often used for cultivation. *Primary isolates, phase I organisms, will not grow on conventional laboratory media,* but will do so after prolonged passage. At the same time colonial morphology changes, marked pleomorphism of individual cells is evident, and there is an alteration in antigenic composition. This occurs in a series of phases, and the change from phase I to phase IV has been likened to the smooth to rough transition of other bacteria. Only phase I organisms are virulent, and *only phase I organisms* provide effective immunizing material.

The addition of blood to Bordet-Gengou medium is required for the growth of phase I organisms, but the blood acts to neutralize inhibitory substances, probably fatty acids, rather than to provide nutrients. Charcoal, starch, or ion exchange resins can be substituted for blood.

A single protein toxin purified from the organism's envelope is antigenic and responsible for the induction of histamine sensitization (HSF), activation of pancreatic islet cells (IAP), and lymphocytosis (LPF). Other toxins of *B. pertussis* include a heat-labile toxin and a heat-stable toxin (lipopolysaccharide). There are an extracytoplasmic adenylate cyclase, two hemagglutinins (the filamentous protein from fimbria, FHA, and the HSF-LPF-IAP hemagglutinin) as well as O and K surface and capsular antigens. The roles of these constituents in disease production and in the development of protective immunity are under investigation. The fimbrial hemagglutinin is apparently responsible for attachment of *B. pertussis* to ciliated respiratory epithelial cells. The systemic disease manifestations are likely caused by circulating HSF-IAP-LPF exotoxin secreted by bacterial cells.

Approximately 5 to 10 per cent of clinical whooping cough may be caused by *B. parapertussis*. The animal pathogen *B. bronchiseptica* is responsible for a very minor percentage of cases. These organisms can be differentiated from *B. pertussis* by growth requirements, enzyme production, and presence of species-specific antigens. It has been suggested that adenoviruses, alone or in concert with *B. pertussis*, may play an etiologic role in some cases of whooping cough.

EPIDEMIOLOGY. In communities of susceptibles the family attack rate is 80 to 90 per cent, which is extremely high for a bacterial disease, approaching that seen in varicella or measles. Transmission is by droplet infection. Carriers of *B. pertussis* are found infrequently, but persons previously immunized have been shown during outbreaks of disease to excrete the organism in the absence of clinical illness.

The mortality rate from whooping cough has fallen since the turn of this century owing to improved supportive therapy. The incidence of whooping cough, however, did not change until after the 1940's, when immunization of young children became standard practice. In the 1940's, approximately 200,000 cases of pertussis were reported annually in the United States; in 1983, 2258 cases were reported. At the same time, the fatality rate has dropped from 20 per 1000 patients to 3. The majority of deaths, over 70 per cent, occur in children under one year of age, with the preponderance in infants under the age of six months.

Neither immunization against pertussis nor natural disease provides lifelong protection. In the case of artificial immunization, an attack rate greater than 50 per cent has been reported when the interval after immunization exceeds 12 years. Thus in the face of routine immunization, it is possible that pertussis will become primarily a disease of older children and adults.

PATHOLOGY. Interpretation of pathologic material obtained at autopsy is difficult because of the common presence of complicating respiratory infections. Lesions caused by *B. pertussis* are found principally in the bronchi and bronchioles, but changes are also seen in the nasopharynx, larynx, and trachea. Masses of bacteria are intertwined with the cilia of the columnar epithelium together with mucopurulent exudate. Adherence of organisms to ciliated respiratory epithelial cells is the crucial element in pathogenesis of disease. There is also necrosis of the midzonal and basilar epithelium with infiltration of polymorphonuclear leukocytes and macrophages. Peribronchial accumulation of lymphocytes and granulocytes produces the picture of interstitial pneumonitis. Secondary atelectasis and localized emphysema are common.

CLINICAL MANIFESTATIONS. After an incubation period of 7 to 16 days, symptoms appear. It is customary to divide the clinical course into three stages, each of two weeks' duration, but variation is frequent.

Catarrhal Stage. Whooping cough begins with symptoms indistinguishable from those of a mild viral upper respiratory infection or common cold. Sneezing is frequent, the conjunctivae are injected, and a nocturnal cough appears. The temperature may be slightly elevated at this time. Infectivity is greatest at this stage.

Paroxysmal Stage. Seven to 14 days after onset, the cough becomes more frequent, diurnal, and then paroxysmal. In a typical paroxysm there is a series of 15 to 20 short coughs of increasing intensity, and then with a deep inspiration the air is drawn into the lungs, making the "whoop." A tenacious mucus plug is usually expelled, and vomiting frequently follows. Paroxysms may occur as often as every half hour, and are accompanied by signs of increased venous pressure. The conjunctivae are deeply engorged; there is periorbital edema; and petechial hemorrhages, particularly about the forehead, as well as epistaxis are common. During the attack the infant may be cyanotic until the crowing whoop occurs. In between paroxysms the child usually feels well though justifiably apprehensive.

Physical examination of the chest is usually unremarkable, although scattered rhonchi may be heard. The chest roentgenogram sometimes reveals hilar and mediastinal nodal enlargement. The presence of fever immediately suggests the development of a secondary infectious process.

Convalescent Stage. Gradually the paroxysms become less frequent and less intense; vomiting ceases, and slow recovery ensues. Often for many months even a mild, unrelated respiratory infection will induce a return of paroxysmal cough and whoop.

In very young infants the paroxysms and the whoop are often absent; instead, choking spells and apneic episodes may be the major manifestations. Second attacks of whooping cough as well as disease occurring in previously immunized individuals often present simply as an upper respiratory illness or bronchitis.

Complications. Complications may be related to the primary disease or to secondary events. Alterations in acid-base balance occur as a result of metabolic alkalosis when vomiting is severe. Recurrent vomiting can also lead to malnutrition. Anoxemic manifestations are seen when ventilation is markedly impaired. Central nervous system changes can result from cerebral anoxia or hemorrhages consequent to the elevated venous pressure. Rarely, cortical degeneration occurs, but the exact pathogenesis of the encephalopathy is unknown. A serous meningitis with lymphocytosis of the cerebrospinal fluid has been described. Localized areas of emphysema and atelectasis generally return to normal after the disease has run its course, and pneumothorax and interstitial emphysema are infrequently seen.

The major cause of death in whooping cough is complicating pneumonia or bronchopneumonia caused by other bacteria or viruses. In addition, secondary bacterial otitis media occurs frequently.

DIAGNOSIS. There is little difficulty in making the clinical diagnosis of whooping cough in a patient who, after a variable period of coryzal symptoms, develops paroxysmal coughing with a terminal inspiratory whoop. Toward the end of the catarrhal stage, or early in the spasmodic phase, leukocytosis often occurs. In contrast to the leukocytosis found in most bacterial diseases, the predominating cell type is the mature small lymphocyte. Characteristically the leukocyte count ranges from 15,000 to 30,000 per cubic millimeter, and 80 per cent of the cells are small lymphocytes. However, the leukocyte count either may be normal or may reach a level greater than 100,000 per cubic millimeter. Polymorphonuclear leukocytosis suggests a secondary bacterial complication.

Difficulty in recognizing whooping cough occurs in the catarrhal stage, in abortive or mild cases, and in young infants. Epidemiologic awareness may suggest the possibility, but microbiologic identification of the organisms is required. Physicians whose residency training was in the 1970's and 1980's may never have encountered a case of whooping cough. During the early stages *B. pertussis* can be isolated from approximately 90 per cent of patients. By the third or fourth week the organism can be recovered in only 50 per cent of cases, and in the convalescent stage it is unusual to obtain a positive culture.

Adequate specimens and appropriate media are essential if bacteriologic diagnosis is to be efficient. *Specimens are best obtained by pernasal swab rather than by the cough plate method.* A sterile cotton swab wrapped about a flexible copper wire is passed through the nares, and mucus is obtained from the posterior pharynx. The swab must not be allowed to dry out because *B. pertussis* is readily killed by desiccation. As quickly as possible the specimen is plated onto fresh Bordet-Gengou medium, to which penicillin has been added to prevent overgrowth of adventitious organisms. Incubation is at 35° C, and although the trained observer can recognize the small, bisected pearl colonies of *B. pertussis* within 48 hours, at least 72 hours of growth is usually required. Presumptive identification can be made by agglutination tests with appropriate antisera. It is virtually impossible to distinguish between *Bordetella* species on primary isolation except by serologic means.

A fluorescent antibody staining procedure that can be applied directly to clinical specimens as well as to organisms grown in culture has been utilized by many state diagnostic laboratories and the Centers for Disease Control. It greatly accelerates the identification of organisms after isolation, but is unreliable in its direct application to nasopharyngeal swabs or other clinical material.

Serologic procedures are of little help in the diagnosis of whooping cough because a rise in titer of most antibodies does not occur until at least the third week of illness. Tests are not well standardized, and few laboratories perform them.

It is difficult to distinguish abortive or mild cases of pertussis from tracheobronchitis caused by other agents except by bacteriologic means.

TREATMENT. Mild cases of pertussis require only supportive treatment. Specific therapy of severe whooping cough has been disappointing despite the in vitro susceptibility of *B. pertussis* to various antimicrobial agents and the protective effect of passively administered antibody in experimental disease.

Antimicrobials. A number of antimicrobial drugs have significant activity against *B. pertussis* in vitro. Agents that readily eradicate the organisms may shorten the course of the illness if given in the catarrhal or early paroxysmal stages. In the established paroxysmal stage the organisms can also be readily eliminated by antimicrobials, but the course of the illness is unaltered. Even in the paroxysmal stage the use of drugs may be justified in order to render the patient noninfectious.

Erythromycin, oxytetracycline, and several other drugs are effective in eliminating organisms. Erythromycin is the drug of choice. The daily dose is 50 mg per kilogram of body weight given in four divided doses. The organism is eliminated after a few days of therapy, but because bacteriologic relapse may occur, treatment should be continued for 14 to 21 days.

Immunotherapy. Hyperimmune human gamma globulin has previously been used in therapy of unimmunized patients, particularly small infants, with no efficacy demonstrated in controlled trials.

Supportive Therapy. Particularly in the young infant, supportive measures combined with careful nursing care are of paramount importance. Specific attention must be devoted to the maintenance of proper water and electrolyte balance, adequate nutrition, and sufficient oxygenation. Constant alertness for the presence of secondary infectious complications such as pneumonia is required.

PREVENTION. Unfortunately, the diagnosis is usually not made until the end of the catarrhal stage, and by then spread of the disease has already occurred. Exposed susceptibles should receive erythromycin prophylaxis, and contacts under four years of age who have been previously immunized should receive a booster dose of vaccine in addition to erythromycin. Booster doses of vaccine have been used to protect adults, such as hospital staff, but side effects tend to be frequent, and erythromycin chemoprophylaxis may be preferable.

Active Immunization. The fall in incidence of whooping cough in the very young is directly related to widespread immunization with suitable, killed suspensions of *B. pertussis*. The highest risk of serious morbidity and mortality is in the young infant. Women of childbearing age generally do not have significant levels of protective antibody in their sera, and these antibodies may be of a type (IgM) that does not cross the placenta. Consequently, newborns are not protected by maternal antibodies. Therefore active immunization is begun as early as is commensurate with the production of a satisfactory immune response. At present, it is recommended that the infant receive three injections of pertussis vaccine at eight-week intervals commencing at age two months. Each injection provides four NIH* units. The NIH unitage is based upon the ability of a vaccine to protect mice against a standard intracerebral infection. The pertussis suspension is incorporated into a triple vaccine with alum-precipitated diphtheria and tetanus toxoids (DTP). Booster injections are given one and five years after completion of the initial course. Administration of pertussis vaccine to those over six years of age is not generally recommended because of an apparent increased incidence of untoward reactions and the diminished risk of the illness itself in the older child. However, low doses have been administered to adults without incident. There is no protection against parapertussis.

As previously noted, immunization does not confer lifelong protection. Approximately 80 per cent of those vaccinated within four years of exposure will be protected, whereas 80 to 90 per cent of a matched unimmunized group with similar exposure will contact pertussis. The prophylactic efficacy of pertussis vaccine was clearly demonstrated when epidemics occurred in the United Kingdom in 1977–1979 and 1982 following a three- to five-year period during which vaccine acceptance had declined to very low levels. More than 170,000 cases of whooping cough were reported, including 42 deaths, principally among children under five years of age. Similar outbreaks have followed diminished vaccine utilization in Japan and Sweden.

Local reactions as well as fever, hyperirritability, or seizures may occur after injection of pertussis vaccine. The exact incidence of the more severe complication of encephalopathy is uncertain. A current British study suggests a risk of 1 in 300,000 immunizations for previously normal infants, with residual neurologic damage in 30 per cent of those affected. The occurrence of neurotoxicity appears to be decreasing as more refined immunizing suspensions are used, and certain components of *B. pertussis* may prove to be effective without engendering serious side effects. Despite the small, but real, incidence of neurologic complications of pertussis immunization, the risk is far less than the hazards of whooping cough in the young child. Nevertheless, in infants with a personal history of convulsions or other neurologic disorders, pertussis immunization should be deferred until the condition has stabilized and is under medical control. A Japanese vaccine containing only the two *B. pertussis* hemagglutinins, extracted, purified, and formalin-treated, is far less reactogenic than the whole bacterial cell vaccine that has been used for more than 40 years. If tests of its immunogenicity and prophylactic efficacy are convincing in field use, it may replace the killed whole cell vaccine.

Keller MA, Aftandelians R, Connor JD: Etiology of pertussis syndrome. Pediatrics 66:50, 1980. *A clarification of the interrelationships of* B. pertussis *and adenoviruses in whooping cough.*

Manclark CR, Hill JC: International Symposium on Pertussis. Washington, D.C., US Dept HEW NIH, 1979. *This 387-page volume contains informative papers on research dealing with the organism, its components, infection, disease control, and vaccine development.*

Mertsola J, Ruuskanen O, Eerola E, Viljanen MK: Intrafamilial spread of pertussis. J Pediatr 103:359, 1983. *Longitudinal household epidemiology of pertussis as influenced by prior vaccination.*

Miller DL, Alderslade R, Ross EM: Whooping cough and whooping cough vaccine: The risks and benefits debate. Epidem Rev 4:1, 1982. *Particularly cogent at this time when public confidence in pertussis vaccine has been eroded by media presentations.*

Olson LC: Pertussis. Medicine 54:427, 1975. *A time-tested review including all the "classics" among its more than 400 references.*

Sato Y, Kimura M, Fukumi H: Development of a pertussis component vaccine in Japan. Lancet 1:122, 1984. *The great hope for an improved less reactive vaccine in the 1980's.*

*National Institutes of Health.

276. DIPHTHERIA

Richard V. McCloskey

Diphtheria is an acute infectious disease caused by a bacillus, *Corynebacterium diphtheriae*. The infection usually localizes in the pharynx, larynx, nostrils, and occasionally the skin and gives rise to both local and systemic signs. The latter are related to the production of a potent, soluble exotoxin elaborated by the microorganisms multiplying at the site of infection.

HISTORY. *Corynebacterium diphtheriae* was observed in diphtheritic membrane by Klebs in 1883. Loeffler in 1884 cultivated *C. diphtheriae* and described its characteristics. The Greek name of the type species—from *Korynee,* club; *bakterion,* staff; and *diphtheria,* leather hide—describes the club-shaped bacillus that causes a leathery membrane in the pharynx. In 1888 Roux and Yersin discovered that bacillus-free filtrates from diphtheria bacillus cultures would kill guinea pigs and thus demonstrated the potent exotoxin fundamental to the pathogenesis of diphtheria. The test that first enabled physicians to distinguish between susceptible and resistant patients was described by Schick in 1913. In the same year, von Behring successfully immunized children with a toxin-antitoxin mixture. From 1923 to 1928, Glenny and Ramon treated toxin to develop toxoid. Immunization with toxoid remains the primary method for suppression of diphtheria. Between 1960 and 1970, Collier, Gill, and Pappenheimer and their colleagues described the means by which toxin disrupts protein synthesis.

ETIOLOGY. *C. diphtheriae* is a pleomorphic, unencapsulated, nonmotile gram-positive bacillus. Smears prepared with differential stains (Albert's stain) may reveal metachromatic granules. The organisms may be arranged in palisades, L or V forms, or in groups resembling "Chinese characters" when examined in stained preparations. Growth is aerobic, and potassium tellurite or coagulated serum (Loeffler's medium) promotes growth. Colonies of *Corynebacterium* species (as well as streptococci and staphylococci) growing on tellurite-containing media develop a grayish black color. *C. diphtheriae* characteristically produces both a brown-gray halo and a garlic odor when growing on Tinsdale's agar. *C. diphtheriae* cohabitates the mucous membranes of humans together with other morphologically similar saprophytic diphtheroids from which it must be distinguished, usually by differential fermentation of glycogen, starch, glucose, maltose, and sucrose. The characteristics of the three stable types of diphtheria bacillus are as follows: *gravis,* a short uniformly staining rod forming low circular coherent colonies on tellurite agar, which becomes a "daisyhead" when well developed; this type may cause slight hemolysis; *intermedius,* long pleomorphic clubbed rods forming small discrete delicate colonies on tellurite agar; *mitis,* long pleomorphic rods with prominent metachromatic granules forming "poached egg" colonies on tellurite agar.

EPIDEMIOLOGY. Intimate contact with other infected persons is required for the spread of diphtheria. Transmission is usually by way of infected droplets or nasopharyngeal secretions. Infective skin exudate is also involved in person-to-person spread. Carriers are persons harboring a toxinogenic strain of *C. diphtheriae* in the nasopharynx or on the skin. An asymptomatic carrier can only be detected by culture of the nasopharynx or skin. Attention is often directed toward carriers when close associates, siblings, or marital partners develop diphtheria. A carrier state may exist for several days before the onset of symptoms. A convalescent carrier state occurs after symptoms subside. The duration of a convalescent carrier state is greatly shortened by appropriate antibiotic treatment. Carriers constitute the reservoir from which the disease spreads to susceptible patients.

Recent surveys of diphtheria carriers show that 88 per cent have completed or partially completed a course of diphtheria immunization. In the past decade, diphtheria in the United States has been a disease of urban rather than rural populations. Diphtheria affects mainly poor persons living in crowded conditions with poor access to health care facilities. Morbidity and mortality are highest in children less than 14 years of age. In the United States, attack rates are highest among blacks and Mexican Americans between 5 and 14 years of age.

In tropical and subtropical areas, the disease is more often manifest as a skin disease than as a respiratory tract infection. Skin infections are important in maintaining endemism of *C. diphtheriae* infections in tropical and subtropical areas. Skin infections, because of greater contagiousness, result in higher environmental carrier levels of *C. diphtheriae* than does respiratory tract diphtheria. As the incidence of skin infections increases, so does the reservoir, acquisition, and transmission of *C. diphtheriae.* Such mechanisms have been thought to be important in spreading respiratory tract diphtheria in tropical and, more recently, in temperate climates.

Epidemiologists use several techniques to classify toxin-producing *C. diphtheriae* and to disrupt its method of spread. The three types—mitis, intermedius, and gravis—are identified by colonial morphologic characteristics and a number of biochemical properties. The classification does not necessarily imply that disease caused by an intermedius strain is invariably less severe than that produced by a gravis strain. Mitis strains, however, have produced less severe disease than that caused by the other two biotypes. Gravis types have produced epidemics in populations of unimmunized persons previously experiencing disease due to mitis or intermedius strains. Well-immunized populations more often experience disease caused by mitis types. Each type can cause epidemic diphtheria.

C. diphtheriae strains can be classified by patterns of bacteriophage lysis into at least 35 types. Each bacteriophage type is stable and specific. A lysotype may persist in the throats of healthy carriers for years. In a given geographic area a single lysotype may be obtained from both patients and asymptomatic carriers. Some bacteriophage types are confined to or more frequently found in certain countries, which suggests that the lysotyping scheme may reflect the adaptability of *C. diphtheriae* to selected populations. The ease with which a strain of *C. diphtheriae* can be induced to liberate the identifying bacteriophage into the surrounding medium may be directly correlated with high toxin production and high capacity to spread among a population.

Recent urban epidemics of diphtheria in the United States have been difficult to control, even though hundreds of thousands of persons completed diphtheria immunization through intensive efforts by medical personnel. Immunization with diphtheria toxoid of susceptible persons must be combined with a program that identifies carriers of diphtheria and terminates the carrier state by antibiotic treatment. Quarantine is not effective in an open urban society.

PATHOGENESIS. Myocarditis and neuritis are caused by the toxin elaborated by *C. diphtheriae* and absorbed by the infected patient. A great deal is known about the molecular mechanisms by which this toxin causes disease. The toxin is an acidic globular protein with a molecular weight of 62,000 to 63,000. It is characterized by extreme potency, a cellular site of activity, and a latent period before inhibition of cellular protein synthesis is manifest. Strains of *C. diphtheriae* infected by a lysogenic bacteriophage produce the toxin when iron is present in a critical concentration range in the medium. A fragment of toxin bypasses normal cellular digestive mechanisms and enters the cytoplasm. After crossing the cell membrane, toxin inactivates a factor *(elongation factor)* that is one of several soluble proteins needed for the translocation step of protein synthesis. The toxin catalyzes the reaction nicotine adeninedinucleotide + elongation factor = adenosine diphosphoribose–elongation factor complex + nicotinamide + hydrogen. When the elongation factor is linked with adenosine diphosphoribose, it is inactive. Translocation of peptidyl transfer ribonucleic acid (tRNA) from acceptor to donor sites on the ribosome is disrupted, and protein synthesis stops. The whole toxin is actually a proenzyme. The reaction with adenosine diphosphoribose (ribosylation reaction) is caused by a proteolytic fragment of the whole toxin (fragment A). Nontoxinogen *C. diphtheriae* elaborate a physicochemically similar but immunochemically dissimilar and biologically innocuous protein. Therefore, identification of toxin production in vitro by *C. diphtheriae* (toxinogenicity) is of paramount importance. This is usually accomplished by demonstrating immunoprecipitation lines produced by a strain of *C. diphtheriae* growing on agar on which is placed a filter paper strip containing a diluted, highly purified diphtheria antitoxin *(Elek's test)*. Other biologically active extracellular products of *C. diphtheriae* play some role in the production of diphtheria, since nontoxinogenic *C. diphtheriae* may cause clinical diphtheria although of a milder variety than that produced by toxinogenic organisms.

CLINICAL MANIFESTATIONS. Diphtheria may be a symptomless state or a rapidly fatal hypertoxic disease that devastates the heart and lungs. The primary determinants of diphtheria are the patient's immunity to diphtheria toxin, the virulence and toxinogenicity of the infecting strain of *C. diphtheriae*, and the anatomic location of the infection. Additional characteristics that may influence the symptoms elicited are age, coexisting systemic disease, and pre-existing local nasopharyngeal disease. The incubation period is usually two to six days. Most patients, excluding those with the mildest of nasal or skin infections, seek medical attention after several days of systemic illness. The speed of onset is variable. Younger patients may be desperately ill in the face of deceptively modest malaise and fatigue. The temperature gradually rises, seldom exceeding 102° F except in those most severely ill. Children are less likely than adults to complain of sore throat, which is not usually the initial complaint at any age. Other signs and symptoms depend on the extent of the local diphtheritic lesion. Further discussion may be divided on this basis.

Anterior Nasal Diphtheria. Patients with anterior nasal diphtheria may be minimally inconvenienced while producing a thick mucopurulent nasal discharge, which may irritate the external nares and upper lips. A creamy yellowish membrane, with or without crusting, may be seen in the nose. Severe intoxication from nasal diphtheria is not common.

Tonsillar (Faucial) Diphtheria. In tonsillar diphtheria the membrane begins as a thin mucilaginous structure involving one or both tonsils. It is not confined to tonsillar crypts. By the time medical advice is sought, usually there is a characteristic grayish-green color to some area of the membrane. The membrane, which is several millimeters thick, may be difficult to dislodge with a swab and when torn off often leaves a bleeding surface on the tonsil. Sometimes the membrane crosses anatomic borders and may extend beyond the anterior pillar of the tonsils, which are often enlarged. The four most common complaints during an outbreak in Texas were sore throat (85 per cent), pain on swallowing (23 per cent), nausea and vomiting (25 per cent), and headache (18 per cent). The most common sign was fever (85 per cent). Moderately tender lymph nodes, 1 to 2 cm in diameter, can usually be palpated in the anterior triangle of the neck.

Pharyngeal Diphtheria. Outside the palatine tonsil the membrane spreads to the uvula, the soft palate, and the pharyngeal wall. The marked swelling of the tonsils at this point often obscures large areas of membrane on the posterior aspect of the tonsil. The nasal mucosa may be involved and may bleed profusely. The greenish character of the membrane is more prominent. There may be necrotic black patches in those areas where the membrane first appeared. The so-called *diphtheritic fetor* is of little diagnostic value, occurring also during the course of infectious mononucleosis and Vincent's infection. A hot tender edema (bull neck) involving the anterior part of the neck may obscure the angle of the jaw, the border of the sternocleidomastoid muscle, the clavicle, and the enlarged lymph nodes, which become more prominent as the edema subsides. The child with pharyngeal diphtheria is pathetically weak, limp, unresisting, pale, and exhausted. Bleeding from the upper airway is a grave prognostic sign.

Laryngeal and Bronchial Diphtheria. The membrane may extend downward or may involve the larynx exclusively. The voice will become hoarse, inspiratory and expiratory stridor may appear, dyspnea and cyanosis occur, and accessory muscles of respiration are used. Casts of the major bronchi can be formed by the membrane. If not removed by bronchoscopy, this membrane may cause death by hypoxia.

Myocarditis. In diphtheritic myocarditis most of the electrocardiographic abnormalities appear during the first week of illness. There is a correlation between delayed conduction velocity of the median, ulnar, and common peroneal nerves and myocardial conduction system disturbances. Moreover, the delayed peripheral nerve conduction velocity precedes clinical evidence of myocarditis and myocardial conduction system abnormalities. The determination of peripheral nerve conduction delay may be used to predict the appearance of myocarditis and cardiac arrhythmias. ST-T wave changes that are destined to improve usually do so within ten days of appearance of the abnormalities.

The severity of the illness and the toxemia are roughly related to the incidence of electrocardiographic (ECG) abnormalities and acute circulatory failure. Acute circulatory failure is practically never seen with nasal diphtheria but may occur in 9 per cent with pharyngeal-laryngeal infection, largely as a consequence of the amount of toxin produced by the more extensive deeper respiratory infections. Acute circulatory failure appears as the sudden onset of pallor, hypotension, collapsed peripheral pulses, and profuse perspiration. Diphtheria with ST-T wave changes is associated with a significantly higher mortality (28 per cent) than diphtheria without ECG changes (6 to 10 per cent). Serial determinations of serum glutamic oxalacetic transaminase concentration will identify most patients with myocarditis.

Early identification of diphtheritic myocarditis is important in reducing morbidity and mortality. Patients with ECG abnormalities during diphtheria should undergo continuous monitoring in specialized cardiac units with supportive ancillary facilities. Treatment is aimed at the more serious arrhythmias and conduction disturbances. Atrioventricular (AV) block and left bundle branch block (LBBB) are ominous signs, associated with mortality of 60 to 100 per cent. Electric pacing with temporary transvenous pacing electrodes or myocardial demand pacemakers can resolve AV block and LBBB produced by diphtheritic myocarditis. Treatment regimens usually include salt restriction, careful fluid balance, and short-acting digitalis preparations if congestive heart failure is marked. Antiarrhythmic agents such as procainamide, lidocaine, and isoproterenol are used when indicated to suppress or control specific arrhythmias. High dose steroid therapy is often used in anticipation of reducing edema and fibrosis of the myocardium or conducting system, although there is no firm evidence that steroids actually accomplish these objectives.

Since patients who develop myocarditis are severely intoxicated, the physician should anticipate other toxic manifestations. Intensive nursing care may be needed to support respiration and to prevent permanent complications of peripheral neuritis. Thrombocytopenia due to platelet destruction may complicate the myocarditis, and platelet transfusions may be necessary.

DIAGNOSIS. The diagnosis of diphtheria must rest on clinical grounds alone, since treatment cannot await bacteriologic confirmation. Diphtheria must be considered whenever a membrane is present in the throat, especially if the uvula is involved. Infectious mononucleosis membrane is confined to the tonsils and remains creamy-white without necrotic patches for a longer time than diphtheritic membrane. Streptococcal pharyngitis is associated with fiery redness of the throat and white exudate. Severe throat pain and faucial distortion are not seen in uncomplicated diphtheria. The foul necrotic exudate complicating leukemia may be impossible to distinguish from diphtheria by examination alone. Vincent's angina may involve the gums and is identified by Gram stain of the exudate. Simultaneous infection with streptococci (32 per cent in a recent outbreak) does not alter the physical findings suggestive of diphtheria. The laboratory findings in diphtheria are nonspecific and include moderate leukocytosis and transient albuminuria.

TREATMENT AND PREVENTION. A patient with tonsillar or nasopharyngeal diphtheria requires isolation in the hospital with bed rest for 10 to 14 days. The early use of adequate amounts of diphtheria antitoxin (DAT) remains the most important specific mode of treatment. Every patient with diphtheria merits DAT therapy, even though a week or so may have passed since the onset of illness. Since DAT is horse serum, intradermal and conjunctival tests (or both) should be performed before administration. If either is positive, desensitization is time-consuming and hazardous but is justifiable because DAT is the only specific treatment available. The required dose of DAT may be simplified as follows: if membrane does not extend beyond the tonsil and there is no thrombocytopenia, the patient may be treated by intramuscular administration of 20,000 units. Patients with more extensive membrane require 80,000 to 100,000 units, preferably by the intravenous route. The minimum amount of DAT necessary to prevent complications is not known. Antibiotics are used to eliminate the organism from the upper respiratory tract and to terminate the carrier state. Penicillin and erythromycin are both effective. If the patient is unable to swallow, initial treatment with parenteral administration of penicillin produces less vomiting and pain at the site of administration than does parenteral erythromycin therapy. Tetracycline, rifampin, clindamycin, and ampicillin are effective in vitro against *C. diphtheriae*, but cephalexin, oxacillin, and lincomycin are not. Both benzathine penicillin and erythromycin therapy can be used to terminate the carrier state. Bed rest is strictly enforced. Airway obstruction requires tracheostomy. Bronchoscopy may be performed to remove membranes from larger bronchi. Expert nursing care is necessary to prevent pneumonia caused by gram-negative bacilli acquired in the hospital. Therapy is always expensive and not always successful.

The complications of diphtheria can be prevented by active immunization beginning in childhood, with booster immunization every ten years thereafter. Active immunization and early treatment of carriers are both necessary for control of the disease. Immunization should be begun with diphtheria-tetanus-pertussis vaccine (DTP) in infants at six weeks of age. Three 0.5-ml injections of DTP are given at monthly intervals, with a booster dose of 0.5 ml at one year. Children who have received this primary series should receive a booster dose before entry into school. For older children, primary immunization may be accomplished by two doses of pediatric diphtheria-tetanus (DT), 0.5 ml each, six weeks apart with a booster six months to one year later. Persons over 12 years of age should be primarily immunized with the same schedule, but adult-type diphtheria-tetanus vaccine (dT) should be used. Schick test are unnecessary before adult immunizations. Those heavily exposed (physicians, nurses, hospital workers) to diphtheria should receive a 0.5-ml booster dose of dT every five years. All others should receive 0.5 ml of dT at ten-year intervals. Patients exposed to a suspected case should receive a 0.5-ml dT booster dose if they have been immunized previously but have not had a booster immunization within ten years.

Barksdale L: Immunology of diphtheria. *In* Nahmias AJ, O'Reilly RJ (eds.): Immunology of Human Infection. New York, Plenum Publishing Corp. 1981, pp 171–199. *Recent and comprehensive review.*

Diphtheria, Tetanus, and Pertussis. Guidelines for vaccine prophylaxis and other preventive measures. Immunization Practices Advisory Committee. Centers for Disease Control. Ann Intern Med *95*:723–728, 1981.

Dobie RA, Tobey DN: Clinical features of diptheria in the respiratory tract. JAMA 242:2197, 1979. *A description of the signs and symptoms of diphtheritic rhinitis, pharyngitis, and laryngotracheitis.*

Koopman JS, Campbell J: The role of cutaneous diphtheria infections in a diphtheria epidemic. J Infect Dis 131:239, 1975. *An analysis of how skin infections may spread* C. diphtheriae *infections.*

McCloskey RV, Eller JJ, Green M, Smilack J: The 1970 epidemic of diphtheria in San Antonio. Ann Intern Med 75:495, 1971. *A description of clinical and epidemiologic features of an epidemic of diphtheria in a community in the United States.*

Clostridial Diseases

277. CLOSTRIDIAL MYONECROSIS AND OTHER CLOSTRIDIAL DISEASES

John G. Bartlett

Clostridia are gram-positive, spore-forming anaerobic bacteria that are widely distributed in soil and in the normal intestinal microflora of animals. Sporulation permits survival in adverse conditions so that these organisms can be isolated with ease from almost any environmental source. Concentrations vary considerably, but any fertile loam is expected to contain at least 10^3 clostridia per gram. Clostridia have been found in the intestinal tract of almost all animals examined. Most humans harbor 10^9 to 10^{10} clostridia per gram of stool; these organisms are less commonly found in the normal flora of the skin, oral cavity, and female genital tract. *C. perfringens*, the most frequent clinical isolate, is found in virtually all soil samples and, along with *C. ramosum*, is the most frequent clostridial species found in the intestinal flora of humans. Nevertheless, there are over 60 recognized species, and about 30 species have been found in human infections. Many clinical laboratories do not perform the extensive biochemical testing necessary to speciate clostridial isolates, and even when this is done, many organisms do not fit current taxonomic schema.

Clostridia cause diverse disease processes including bacteremia, localized infections at various anatomic sites, and the histotoxic clostridial syndromes. The latter refers to well-characterized syndromes caused by toxins elaborated under appropriate cultural conditions by various clostridial species (Table 277–1). The most commonly encountered histotoxic species is *C. perfringens*, which is divided into five types designated A to E on the basis of the production of the four major lethal toxins designated alpha, beta, epsilon, and iota. All *C. perfringens*, and many other species of clostridia (Table 277–1), produce alpha toxin, a phospholipase that splits lecithin to phosphoryl choline and a diglyceride. Intravenous administration of alpha toxin in experimental animals causes massive hemolysis, platelet destruction, and widespread capillary damage. Other clostridial toxins cause diseases of the intestine (enteric toxins) or

TABLE 277–1. HISTOTOXIC CLOSTRIDIAL SYNDROMES

Disease	Agent	Toxin
Enteric diseases		
Food poisoning	*C. perfringens*, type A	Enterotoxin
Antibiotic-induced diarrhea or colitis	*C. difficile*	Toxins A and B
Enteritis necroticans	*C. perfringens*, type C	Beta toxin
Neurologic syndromes		
Botulism	*C. botulinum*	Botulinal toxins A, B, E, and F
Tetanus	*C. tetanus*	Tetanospasmin
Myonecrosis (gas gangrene)	*C. perfringens, C. novyi, C. septicum, C. histolyticum, C. bifermentans, C. fallax*	Multiple toxins, especially alpha toxin

of the nervous system (neurotoxins). The toxins of *C. botulinum* and *C. tetanus* are lethal to mice in doses of 1 ng. By extrapolation, the lethal dose in the bloodstream of humans is approximately 10^{-9} mg per kilogram body weight, making these toxins the most potent poisons known. The toxins of *C. difficile* and the alpha toxin of *C. perfringens* are about 100 to 1,000 times less potent in mouse lethality testing.

Smith LDS: The Pathogenic Anaerobic Bacteria. 2nd ed. Springfield, Charles C Thomas, 1975, pp 109–324. *The author, a noted authority in the field, provides a scholarly review of clostridia, including a description of the species, their natural habitat, their toxins, and their role in disease.*

CLOSTRIDIAL MYONECROSIS

DEFINITION. Clostridial myonecrosis, or gas gangrene, is a life-threatening infection involving muscle caused by toxins produced by clostridia, usually *C. perfringens*.

ETIOLOGY. Clostridial myonecrosis usually follows wounding from trauma or surgery, contamination with histotoxic clostridia, and toxin elaboration. It is estimated that 30 to 80 per cent of serious traumatic open wounds are contaminated by clostridia, although gas gangrene remains a relatively rare infection. This experience emphasizes the decisive role of local conditions that promote toxin production primarily by decreasing the oxidation-reduction potential. Contributing factors to tissue hypoxia include vascular insufficiency, the presence of foreign bodies, tissue necrosis, and concurrent infection involving other microbes.

The most frequent pathogen, *C. perfringens*, is found in approximately 80 per cent of cases with positive cultures. Other clostridial species implicated include *C. novyi*, *C. septicum*, *C. histolyticum*, *C. bifermentans*, and *C. fallax*. In many instances, there are several clostridial species isolated from the infected site. Species causing gas gangrene produce over 20 exotoxins, including seven that are lethal to experimental animals. Perhaps the most important toxin is *alpha toxin*, a lecithinase that destroys cell membranes, alters capillary permeability, destroys platelets, and causes severe hemolysis. In appropriate environmental conditions, the histotoxic clostridia replicate and elaborate toxins that diffuse out to adjacent soft tissue and thus promote local spread as well as extensive systemic effects.

CLINICAL MANIFESTATIONS. Gas gangrene is a devastating infection characterized by prominent findings at the site of injury and profound systemic toxicity. Most cases occur in association with wounding from trauma or surgery. The usual clinical settings are: (1) traumatic injury or penetrating wound; (2) surgery, especially intestinal or biliary tract operations; (3) uterine gas gangrene, which most frequently follows septic abortions; (4) soft tissue lesions associated with vascular insufficiency; (5) intestinal gas gangrene, which is most commonly found in compromised hosts, especially patients with leukemia or colonic carcinoma; and (6) "spontaneous gas gangrene," a rare form of the disease in which there is no readily identifiable predisposing condition. The experience during peacetime among civilians in the United States is that approximately 50 per cent of cases follow severe traumatic injury and 40 per cent follow surgery. The most frequent traumatic injuries are car accidents, crush injuries, industrial accidents, and gunshot wounds. The most frequent antecedent surgical procedures are elective colon resection, nonelective colonic surgery, and biliary tract surgery. About two thirds of cases involve extremities, and one third involve the abdominal wall.

The usual incubation period from the time of wounding to the onset of symptoms is one to four days with a range of eight hours to several weeks. The first symptom is usually sudden and severe pain at the site of injury. Observations at this time typically show tense edema and tenderness. Gas may be noted in the soft tissues by palpation, x-ray, computerized tomography, or ultrasound studies. The skin is initially pale and then progresses to a magenta or bronze discoloration, and there is often cutaneous necrosis with hemorrhagic bullae. As the lesion evolves, there may be a thin, serosanguinous discharge with characteristic sweet odor. The systemic findings that accompany the evolving changes at the wound are profound. These include diaphoresis, low grade fever, and tachycardia that is disproportionate to the temperature elevation. Common complications include hemolytic anemia, hypotension, and renal failure. The patient is typically anxious throughout the disease but remains alert despite profound systemic toxicity.

DIAGNOSIS. The diagnosis of clostridial myonecrosis is based on a constellation of clinical findings, observations at the site of injury, and supporting microbiologic data. X-rays or computerized tomography studies often show gas bubbles distributed in and around muscle, and Gram stains of discharge typically show large, gram-positive bacilli with blunt ends and a paucity of polymorphonuclear leukocytes. Approximately 15 per cent of patients have clostridial bacteremia. Nevertheless, the findings on Gram stain and the detection of gas in the soft tissue cannot be considered specific. Moreover, most patients with clostridial bacteremia do not have myonecrosis. The definitive diagnostic procedure is surgical incision to expose muscle that may appear pale and edematous, beefy-red or, in the most advanced stages, black and friable. The muscle is nonviable, it fails to contract with stimulation, and the cut surface does not bleed.

The differential diagnosis includes a number of soft tissue infections that may also involve clostridia, are associated with tissue necrosis, are characterized by a fulminant course, or are associated with gas formation. Important findings in the differential diagnosis are summarized in Table 277–2.

TREATMENT. The most important facet of treatment is extensive surgical debridement with wide excision of involved muscle, amputation when an extremity is involved, or hysterectomy with uterine gas gangrene. The preferred antibiotic is aqueous penicillin G in doses of 10 to 20 million units daily for adults. Chloramphenicol in doses of 1 gram intravenously every six hours is the preferred regimen for patients with penicillin hypersensitivity. Cephalosporins and clindamycin are less active against clostridia and cannot be considered suitable substitutes for penicillin. The therapeutic value of hyperbaric oxygen is controversial. Advocates claim that this will clearly demarcate the necrotic tissue to simplify surgery and improve survival rates. Nevertheless, controlled studies to document efficacy are not available, and there may be major problems in transferring critically ill patients to centers with this type of facility. Surgery should not be delayed. Supportive measures include fluid and electrolyte replacement, control of acidosis, transfusions for severe anemia, and appropriate measures for renal failure.

PROGNOSIS. Clostridial myonecrosis is a devastating infection that often requires mutilating surgery and prolonged hospital courses. The overall mortality rate in 116 reports summarizing over 1200 cases is 25 per cent.

PREVENTION. The inoculum of *C. perfringens* required to produce gas gangrene is reduced by 10^6 organisms in experimental animals if the organism is delivered into devitalized muscle containing dirt instead of normal tissue. As noted earlier, contamination of wounds by clostridia from either soil sources or from the endogenous fecal flora is common with both traumatic injuries and surgical incisions. The incidence of clostridial myonecrosis following battlefield injury was 10 per cent in World War I, 1 per cent in World War II, and 0.01 per cent (22 cases in 139,000 battle injuries) in the Vietnam War. These figures reflect improvements in the management of battlefield injuries with major emphasis on prompt and thorough debridement. There should also be care in preserving the vascular supply, particularly with the use of tourniquets and casts. Judicious decisions regarding closure of traumatic wounds and the prophylactic use of antibiotics are also important. There is no effective means of active immunization.

TABLE 277–2. DEEP AND SERIOUS SOFT TISSUE INFECTIONS

	Gas-Forming Cellulitis	Synergistic Necrotizing Cellulitis	Gas Gangrene	"Streptococcal" Myonecrosis	Necrotizing Fasciitis	Infected Vascular Gangrene	Streptococcal Gangrene
Predisposing conditions	Traumatic	Diabetes, prior local lesion, perirectal lesion	Traumatic or surgical wound	Trauma, surgery	Diabetes, trauma, surgery, perineal infection	Arterial insufficiency	Traumatic or surgical wound
Incubation period	>3 days	3–14 days	1–4 days	3–4 days	1–4 days	>5 days	6 hours–2 days
Etiologic organism(s)	Clostridia, others	Mixed aerobic-anaerobic flora	Clostridia, esp. *C. perfringens*	Anaerobic streptococci	Mixed aerobic-anaerobic flora	Mixed aerobic-anaerobic flora	*S. pyogenes*
Systemic toxicity	Minimal	Moderate to severe	Severe	Minimal until late in course	Moderate to severe	Minimal	Severe
Course	Gradual	Acute	Acute	Subacute	Acute or subacute	Subacute	Acute
Wound findings							
Local pain	Minimal	Moderate to severe	Severe	Late only	Minimal to moderate	Variable	Severe
Skin appearance	Swollen, minimal discoloration	Erythematous or gangrene	Tense and blanched, yellow-bronze, necrosis with hemorrhagic bullae	Erythema or yellow bronze	Blanched, erythema, necrosis with hemorrhagic bullae	Erythema or necrosis	Erythema, necrosis
Gas	Abundant	Variable	Usually present	Variable	Variable	Variable	No
Muscle involvement	No	Variable	Myonecrosis	Myonecrosis	No	Myonecrosis limited to area of vascular insufficiency	No
Discharge	Thin, dark, sweetish or foul odor	Dark pus or "dishwater," putrid	Serosanguinous, sweet or foul odor	Seropurulent	Seropurulent or "dishwater," putrid	Minimal	None or serosanguinous, no odor
Gram stain	PMNs and gram-positive bacilli	PMNs, mixed flora	Sparse PMNs; gram-positive bacilli	PMNs, gram-positive cocci	PMNs, mixed flora	PMNs, mixed flora	PMNs, gram-positive cocci in chains
Surgical therapy	Debridement	Wide filleting incisions	Extensive excision, amputation	Excision of necrotic muscle	Wide filleting incisions	Amputation	Debridement of necrotic tissue

Baxter CR: Surgical management of soft tissue infections. Surg Clin North Am 52:1483, 1972. *Soft tissue infections are reviewed using three categories: infections requiring incision and drainage, infections requiring excision of tissue, and infections not requiring extensive surgery.*

Dellinger EP: Severe necrotizing soft tissue infections. JAMA 246:1717–1721, 1981. *The author reviews management principles for severe soft tissue infections and emphasizes the differential diagnosis based on clinical presentation, Gram stain, and operative inspection.*

Heimbach RD: Gas gangrene: Review and update. HBO Review 1:41, 1980. *The author reviews gas gangrene and presents an endorsement for hyperbaric oxygen treatment that may be overly enthusiastic.*

MacLennan JD: The histotoxic clostridial infections of man. Bacteriol Rev 26:117, 1962. *This is a classic monograph that summarizes the clinical, pathologic, microbiologic, and epidemiologic features of serious soft tissue infections.*

Weinstein L, Barza M: Gas gangrene. New Engl J Med 289:1129, 1972. *A review of clinical features and management recommendations for gas gangrene.*

OTHER CLOSTRIDIAL DISEASES

SEPTICEMIA. Clostridia account for up to 3 per cent of all positive blood cultures in most clinical microbiologic laboratories. The most frequent species is *C. perfringens*, which accounts for 50 to 60 per cent. On rare occasions these patients have associated findings compatible with gas gangrene. More frequently they have associated infections involving a mixed aerobic-anaerobic flora that may include clostridia at the infected site, but most often they have other conditions in which neither the source nor the significance of the clostridia is apparent. Perhaps the most important point to emphasize is that the vast majority of patients with positive blood cultures for clostridia do not have devastating soft tissue infections that require emergent surgical intervention. Special notation must be made for bacteremia with *C. septicum*. Many of these patients have a hematologic malignancy, neutropenia, or colonic carcinoma. The usual portal of entry in these cases is the distal ileum or cecum, most patients are acutely ill, and aggressive antibiotic therapy with penicillin is indicated.

MISCELLANEOUS INFECTIONS. Clostridia are frequently isolated from infections involving the host's normal flora. This situation especially applies to cases in which the infecting flora originates in the colon, such as in intra-abdominal sepsis, wound infections after intestinal surgery, and wounds or decubitus ulcers located on the lower trunk or lower extremities. These organisms are also found in 5 to 10 per cent of anaerobic pulmonary infections and with similar frequency in nonvenereal infections of the female genital tract. Such infections usually involve a mixture of aerobic and anaerobic bacteria so that the role of clostridia is uncertain. The major concern is often gas gangrene and, as already emphasized, this diagnosis is best established by supporting clinical findings. Other considerations in the differential diagnosis include soft tissue infections associated with gas formation, such as gas-forming cellulitis, necrotizing fasciitis, infected vascular gangrene, and synergistic necrotizing cellulitis. All of these may involve clostridia as well as other microbes, but they are quite different in terms of prognosis, clinical findings, and type of surgery required (Table 277–2). Penicillin G is regarded as the preferred antibiotic for clostridial infections, and chloramphenicol is appropriate for patients who have a contraindication to penicillin; clindamycin and cephalosporins are regarded as somewhat inferior.

CLOSTRIDIA ENTEROTOXEMIAS. Clostridia cause three different types of enteric disease, each of which is ascribed to a unique toxin (Table 277–1). *C. difficile*, the major cause of antibiotic-associated colitis, is discussed in Ch. 278.

C. perfringens is commonly responsible for foodborne outbreaks of a self-limited enteric disease. The cause is an enterotoxin produced by some type A strains during sporulation. The pathophysiologic mechanism is: (1) ingestion of at least 10^8 viable vegetative cells; (2) enterotoxigenic potential of the ingested strain; (3) sporulation with toxin production in the alkaline medium of the small bowel; (4) diarrhea and cramps due to fluid secretion, morphologic damage to the intestinal mucosa, and altered motility in the small bowel. The usual vehicle is meat or food made with meat, such as stews, meat pies, gravies, or casseroles. The attack rate among exposed persons is usually 30 to 60 per cent and the incubation period ranges from 7 to 15 hours. Common symptoms are diarrhea (90 per cent), abdominal cramps (80 per cent), nausea (25 per cent), fever (25 per cent), and vomiting (10 per cent). The diagnosis is suspected in any outbreak of gastrointestinal disease associated with typical symptoms and incubation period among persons sharing a common and likely food source. Confirmation requires the recovery of *C. perfringens* in concentrations of at least 10^5 per gram of epidemiologically implicated food and recovery of at least 10^6 spores per gram of stool obtained within 48 hours after onset of symptoms from victims. Nearly all patients have spontaneous resolution of symptoms within 6 to 24 hours and do not require any specific form of therapy.

Enteritis necroticans is a serious gastrointestinal disease caused by the beta toxin of *C. perfringens*, type C. This disease, once called "darmbrand," occurred in epidemic form in malnourished individuals from Norway and Germany at the end of World War II. More recently, the same condition, known locally as "pigbel," has been found to be endemic in the highlands of New Guinea. Most victims are children who have participated in pig feasts that are believed to provide the source of the organism as well as a complex set of circumstances believed necessary for pathogenesis. The toxin is susceptible to proteolytic enzymes including trypsin. However, toxin inactivation in the small bowel fails because of enzyme deficiency ascribed to protein malnutrition, excessive consumption of sweet potatoes, which contain trypsin inhibitors, or colonization with *Ascaris lumbricoides*, which secrete trypsin inhibitors. The predilection for children presumably reflects antigenic naiveté. Pathologically, enteritis necroticans is a segmental disease of the small bowel that is characterized by mucosal infarction, edema, hemorrhage, and infiltration with polymorphonuclear cells. In advanced stages the bowel is thinned, friable, and subject to perforation. Medical therapy consists of intestinal decompression, penicillin or chloramphenicol, and intravenous fluid support. About half of the patients require resectional surgery, and the overall mortality rate is 15 to 40 per cent. Prevention in the endemic area is achieved with a beta-toxoid vaccine that is currently recommended for children in the endemic area.

Alpern RJ, Dowell VR Jr.: Nonhistotoxic clostridial bacteremia. Am J Clin Pathol 33:717–722, 1971. *A review of 86 patients with clostridia bacteremia, of whom none had gas gangrene, most had self-limited disease, and 84 had no identifiable portal of entry.*

Gorbach SL, Thadepalli H: Isolation of *Clostridia* in human infections: Evaluation of 114 cases. J Infect Dis 131:S81–S85, 1975. *The authors review their experience with 152 strains of clostridia recovered from 144 patients at Cook County Hospital. Sixty-five patients had soft tissue infections, or intra-abdominal sepsis, and 84 per cent of these had polymicrobial infections. Clostridia bacteremia in 49 patients usually occurred with no apparent relation to the clinical setting.*

Lawrence G, Walker PD: Pathogenesis of enteritis necroticans in Papua New Guinea. Lancet 1:125–126, 1976. *The authors, noted authorities in the field, provide a postulate for the pathophysiology of pigbel.*

Lawrence G, Shann F, Freestone DS, Walker PD: Prevention of necrotising enteritis in Papua New Guinea by active immunization. Lancet 1:227–230, 1979. *The authors provide data from a controlled trial showing success of vaccination with beta toxin toxoid.*

Koransky JR, Stargel MD, Dowell VR Jr.: Clostridium septicum bacteremia. Am J Med 66:63–66, 1979. *A review of 59 patients with* C. septicum *bacteremia that showed 71 per cent had malignancy, most presented with a fulminant clinical course, and most died unless appropriate antibiotics were given soon after admission.*

Ramsay AM: The significance of *Clostridium welchii* in the cervical swab and blood stream in postpartum and postabortum sepsis. J Obstet Gynecol Br Commonwealth 56:247–258, 1949. *The author refers to* C. perfringens (welchii) *as a "harmless saprophyte" in a discussion of 28 women with bacteremia, since most had minimal clinical disturbance despite the fact that the majority were studied before antibiotics were available.*

Shaudera WX, Tacket CO, Blake PA: Food poisoning due to *Clostridium perfringens* in the US. J Infect Dis 147:167–170, 1983. *The authors review the Centers for Disease Control's experience with* C. perfringens *food poisoning.*

278. PSEUDOMEMBRANOUS COLITIS

John G. Bartlett

DESCRIPTION. Pseudomembranous enterocolitis is a severe gastrointestinal disease characterized by exudative plaques on the intestinal mucosa. The most commonly involved site is the colon, in which case the preferred appellation is pseudomembranous colitis rather than "enterocolitis."

ETIOLOGY. Pseudomembranous enterocolitis is usually found in association with other conditions, although occasional cases occur in healthy persons with no identifiable risk factors. This condition was initially described in the preantibiotic era when it most frequently followed intestinal surgery. Additional recognized risk factors include intestinal obstruction, uremia, the hemolytic-uremic syndrome, Hirschsprung's disease, inflammatory bowel disease, shigellosis, intestinal ischemia, and neonatal necrotizing enterocolitis. During the past three decades, the disease has been recognized most frequently as a complication of antimicrobial use.

Studies of "antibiotic-associated pseudomembranous colitis" are divided into two periods with quite different observations. Reports from the 1950's and 1960's indicated that the small intestine usually was involved ("enterocolitis"), mortality rates were high, and the most frequently implicated drugs were chloramphenicol, tetracycline, and oral neomycin. *Staphylococcus aureus* was the suspected pathogen in most cases reported at that time. More recent studies of antibiotic-associated pseudomembranous colitis show that the lesions are generally confined to the colon, different antimicrobials are usually implicated (see later discussion), and the prognosis is considerably better than previously reported. The more recent work also indicates that *Clostridium difficile* is the responsible pathogen in the majority of cases.

INCIDENCE. Most patients with pseudomembranous colitis have recent antibiotic exposure, and the other risk factors noted appear to account for less than 10 per cent of all cases. The incidence of antibiotic-associated pseudomembranous colitis depends on the frequency with which endoscopy is performed to establish the diagnosis, antimicrobial use patterns, and epidemiologic patterns. Nearly all antimicrobials with an antibacterial spectrum of activity have been implicated. The most frequent are ampicillin, clindamycin, and cephalosporins. Less frequent are penicillins other than ampicillin, erythromycin, and sulfamethoxazole-trimethoprim. Drugs rarely implicated include tetracyclines, chloramphenicol, sulfonamides, and parenterally administered aminoglycosides. *C. difficile*–induced diarrhea or colitis may occur sporadically or in clusters within institutions. Epidemiologic studies indicate that *C. difficile* may be found in the colonic flora of about 3 per cent of healthy adults, is widely distributed in the environment, and is especially common in areas subject to fecal contamination from patients who have *C. difficile*–induced diarrheal complications. This last observation provides an explanation for focal outbreaks of the disease and emphasizes the importance of appropriate precautionary measures to limit spread.

MECHANISM. *C. difficile*–induced colitis is a toxin-mediated enteric disease in which there is no microbial invasion of the intestinal mucosa.

CLINICAL MANIFESTATIONS. Virtually all patients are at risk for antibiotic-associated pseudomembranous colitis, although there appears to be an increased risk with increasing age. The most common symptom is diarrhea consisting of watery or semiliquid stools without visible blood. Stool examination may show fecal leukocytes, but this is inconsistent and nonspecific. Many patients also have fever, which is usually moderate but may reach 40° C. Other common findings are abdominal cramps, lower quadrant tenderness, leukocytosis, and hypoalbuminemia. Systemic symptoms and abdominal findings are not invariably present, and some patients simply have annoying diarrhea. Complications in severe cases include dehydration, hypoalbuminemia with anasarca, electrolyte disturbances, toxic megacolon, and colonic perforation. Symptoms may begin at any time during the course of antimicrobial treatment or up to six weeks after antimicrobials have been discontinued. The differential diagnosis includes acute and chronic diarrhea caused by enteric pathogens other than *C. difficile*, intra-abdominal sepsis, and idiopathic inflammatory bowel disease.

DIAGNOSIS. The preferred method to establish the anatomic diagnosis is endoscopy. Gross inspection of the colon typically reveals punctate, raised, yellowish-white plaques with "skip areas" of a normal mucosa or a mucosa showing erythema or edema. The plaques are usually 2 to 10 mm wide but may enlarge and coalesce over extensive segments of the colon in the late stages. Pseudomembranes are often located throughout the colon, but up to 20 per cent of patients have segmental involvement of the right side of the colon, necessitating colonoscopy rather than sigmoidoscopy. Recognition of typical lesions on gross inspection often requires an experienced endoscopist using care to wipe away mucus to detect adherent plaques. Some cases are recognized only with histologic studies of biopsy specimens. Microscopic examination shows epithelial necrosis, goblet cells distended with mucus, and infiltration of the lamina propria with polymorphonuclear cells and eosinophilic exudate. The pseudomembrane is attached to the surface epithelium and is composed of fibrin, mucin, and polymorphonuclear cells.

The preferred diagnostic test to implicate *C. difficile* is a tissue culture assay of stool to demonstrate a cytopathic toxin that is neutralized by antitoxin to *C. difficile* or *C. sordellii.* Antitoxin neutralization with antisera to *C. sordellii* reflects antigenic cross-reactivity. Toxin titers may also be performed using serial dilutions of stool specimens, although there is little correlation between the toxin titer and the severity of the disease. Nearly all patients who have this toxin in the stool will also have *C. difficile* recovered using appropriate culture techniques. However, most clinical laboratories do not have the necessary expertise to recover and identify *C. difficile,* and occasional asymptomatic patients harbor the organism without the toxin. The best clinical correlation has been with the toxin assay.

Anatomic changes in the colonic mucosa noted in patients with the diarrheal complications of antibiotic use include an entirely normal colonic mucosa, erythema or edema, and colitis with friability, ulceration, or hemorrhage. Pseudomembranous colitis is regarded as the most severe and characteristic form of this complication. The toxin of *C. difficile* has been implicated in the entire spectrum of anatomic changes, but the frequency of this toxin correlates to a large extent with the severity of the disease process. Tissue culture assays for *C. difficile* toxin are positive in over 90 per cent of patients with pseudomembranous colitis and in approximately 20 per cent of those with antibiotic-associated diarrhea and an entirely normal colonic mucosa. Thus, the tissue culture assay described reflects a mechanism and does not establish the anatomic diagnosis. There is no identifiable pathogen in most patients with antibiotic-associated diarrhea or colitis in whom the assay for *C. difficile* toxin is negative, except for occasional cases that may involve *S. aureus.*

TREATMENT. The most important therapeutic decision is discontinuation of the implicated antimicrobial agent. This approach often results in resolution of symptoms with no necessity for further diagnostic tests or therapy. Patients with severe or persistent symptoms should undergo endoscopy to define anatomic changes and stool examination to detect *C. difficile* cytotoxin. Patients with severe fluid, albumin, or electrolyte depletion often require intravenous replacement and may require hyperalimentation. The role of corticosteroids and attempts to manipulate the flora, as with oral lactobacilli or fecal enemas, is uncertain. Antiperistaltic drugs are contraindicated.

Specific therapy is available for diarrhea caused by *C. difficile,* using cholestyramine to bind the toxin or vancomycin to inhibit the pathogen. The preferred agent for seriously ill patients is orally administered vancomycin, 125 to 500 mg four times daily for 7 to 14 days. Vancomycin is active against virtually all strains of *C. difficile,* the levels in the colon with oral administration are extremely high, and systemic toxicity is nil owing to poor absorption with oral administration even in the presence of an inflamed bowel. The major problems with vancomycin are high cost, noxious taste, and relapses in about 20 per cent of patients when vancomycin is discontinued. Relapses are characterized by the recurrence of typical symptoms, positive tissue culture assays for *C. difficile* cytotoxin, and stool cultures that yield vancomycin-sensitive strains of *C. difficile.* The mechanism of relapse is presumed to be reacquisition of the organism from an environmental source or failure to eradicate the pathogen from the gastrointestinal tract because of persistence of spores.

An alternative form of treatment is cholestyramine, one 4-gram packet three times daily for five days. The mechanism of activity is binding of the toxin by the anion exchange resin. This drug is not so predictably effective for initial treatment as vancomycin and should be reserved for less seriously ill patients or those who have suffered a relapse with vancomycin therapy. Alternative antibiotics include bacitracin or metronidazole, both in doses of 500 mg orally four times daily.

PROGNOSIS. Most patients with pseudomembranous colitis eventually recover even without specific forms of therapy. However, symptoms may be prolonged and debilitating, with persistent diarrhea for several weeks or months. Reports that focus on more seriously ill patients indicate mortality rates of 10 to 30 per cent. With early institution of vancomycin therapy there is a prompt symptomatic response, and virtually all patients recover. Following recovery, there are no recurrences except with the previously noted relapses following oral vancomycin therapy or re-exposure to another antimicrobial that has been associated with this complication.

PREVENTION. The most important preventive measure is judicious use of antimicrobial agents. Patients with *C. difficile*–induced diarrhea or colitis should be isolated and placed on enteric precautions to limit spread to susceptible hosts within institutions.

Bartlett JG: Antibiotic-associated pseudomembranous colitis. Rev Infect Dis 1:123, 1979. *Summary of evidence implicating* C. difficile *and experience with assays for the toxin of this microbe.*

Bartlett JG, Gorbach SL: Pseudomembranous colitis. Adv Intern Med 22:455, 1977. *Review of the topic with extensive reference list for publications prior to evidence implicating* C. difficile.

Bartlett JG, Tedesco FJ, Shull S, Lowe B: Relapse following oral vancomycin therapy of antibiotic-associated pseudomembranous colitis. Gastroenterology 78:431, 1980. *Review of experience with vancomycin therapy for 90 patients.*

Price AB, Davis DR: Pseudomembranous colitis. J Clin Pathol 30:1, 1977. *A review of histopathologic changes.*

Fekety R, Kim K-H, Brown D, Batts DH, Cudmore M, Silva J Jr.: Epidemiology of antibiotic-associated colitis. Am J Med 70:906, 1981. *A survey of the epidemiology of* C. difficile.

279. BOTULISM

John G. Bartlett

DEFINITION. Botulism is a severe neuroparalytic disease caused by toxins of *Clostridium botulinum.* There are four recognized disease categories: (1) foodborne botulism, (2) infant botulism, (3) wound botulism, and (4) unclassified cases.

ETIOLOGY. *C. botulinum* is a gram-positive, spore-forming obligate anaerobe that is widely distributed in nature and frequently found in soil, marine environments, and agricultural products. Adults regularly ingest *C. botulinum* spores from fresh agricultural products without deleterious consequences, and this organism is not recognized as a component of the normal fecal flora. Each strain produces one of seven antigenically distinct toxins of approximately 150,000 daltons, designated A through G. Human disease is caused by types A, B, E, and rarely F. These toxins are hematogenously disseminated to peripheral cholinergic synapses where they bind irreversibly and block acetylcholine release. The result is hypotonia with a descending symmetric flaccid paralysis. Botulinal toxin is the most potent poison of man; it has an estimated lethal dose in the bloodstream of 10^{-9} mg per kilogram.

FOOD POISONING. Foodborne botulism results from the ingestion of preformed toxin in inadequately prepared food. There are an average of 15 "outbreaks" annually in the United States, most of which involve a single case. The most frequently implicated vehicle in the United States is home-canned foods, which usually have a putrefactive odor. Meat and meat products are more commonly responsible in Europe, and preserved fish is most frequent in Japan, Scandinavia, and Russia. Type

A and B organisms predominate in the United States. Type E organisms are usually, but not exclusively, associated with an aquatic source in northern latitudes, where they are found in coastal waters, lakes, and intestines of fish that inhabit these areas.

CLINICAL MANIFESTATIONS. The incubation period is usually 18 to 36 hours but may be as short as two hours or as long as eight days. Persons with the shortest incubation period usually have the most severe disease. The bulbar musculature is affected first, with resultant diplopia, difficulty in focusing to a near point, dry mouth, and dysphagia. Common gastrointestinal symptoms include nausea, vomiting, and abdominal pain. Neurologic examination shows lateral rectus muscle weakness (cranial nerve VI), ptosis, dilated pupils with sluggish reaction, decreased gag reflex, or medial rectus paresis. This is followed by descending involvement of the motor neurons to peripheral muscles, including the muscles of respiration. Some patients have only mild illness, whereas others have severe paralysis that may continue, requiring intensive supportive care for weeks. Mentation remains clear, there is no fever, and neurologic dysfunction is bilateral but not necessarily symmetric. The principle causes of death are respiratory or bulbar paralysis and infectious complications during the period of supportive care.

DIAGNOSIS. The usual laboratory test in suspected cases is analysis of serum, stool, and food suspected of harboring botulinum toxin. This is done in a mouse assay in which specimens are injected intraperitoneally to demonstrate a lethal toxin that is neutralized by type-specific antitoxin. Possibly contaminated foods and patient stool may also be cultured for *C. botulinum.* Among patients with clinical evidence of botulism, the toxin is detected in sera from one third, the toxin is found in the stool from one third, and the organism is recovered in stool from 60 per cent of patients.

Botulism should be suspected in patients with acute flaccid paralysis, especially when there is bilateral sixth cranial nerve dysfunction, associated gastrointestinal symptoms, prior ingestion of possibly contaminated food, and typical symptoms in other persons who shared this food. The differential diagnosis includes myasthenia gravis, Guillain-Barré syndrome, tick paralysis, cerebrovascular accident involving branches of the basilar artery, trichinosis, the Eaton-Lambert syndrome, hypocalcemia, hypermagnesemia, organophosphate poisoning, atropine poisoning, paralytic poisoning caused by shellfish or puffer fish, and psychiatric syndromes. Electromyography is useful in differentiating botulism from other neurologic syndromes. This shows a diminished amplitude of muscle action potentials with a single supramaximal stimulus and facilitation of action potentials using paired or repetitive stimuli. These findings do not appear until the patient develops peripheral muscle weakness and are most likely to be positive in an affected limb.

TREATMENT. Ventilatory support is most important. Elimination of the toxin from the gastrointestinal tract may be facilitated using gastric lavage, cathartics, and enemas early in the course. Antitoxin is usually given irrespective of the duration of illness, since the toxin may persist in the blood for extended periods. Treatment is initiated using two vials of the trivalent antitoxin, each containing 7500 IU type A, 5500 IU type B, and 8,500 IU type E antitoxin; this is given intravenously and repeated at two to four hours. The antitoxin is horse serum and is associated with a 20 per cent incidence of hypersensitivity reactions, the most serious being anaphylaxis in 3 to 5 per cent. Efficacy of the antitoxin is most clearly established with type E botulism. Other therapeutic considerations include guanidine hydrochloride (15 to 50 mg per kilogram daily) to enhance acetylcholine release, but efficacy has not been established. Antimicrobial agents are advocated only for infectious complications.

PROGNOSIS. The case fatality rate for foodborne botulism was formerly 60 to 70 per cent. Improved methods of management, especially support of respiratory function, have reduced the fatality rate to less than 10 per cent in recent years. Patients who survive generally have complete recovery.

PREVENTION. Foodborne botulism is caused by germination of spores in food with toxin produced by vegetative forms, although the toxin may also be produced in vivo by simultaneous ingestion of spores. The disease may be prevented by destruction of spores in the original food source, inhibition of germination, or destruction of preformed toxin. Specific measures are as follows:

1. Destruction of spores with heat or irradiation. Spores of types A and B may survive boiling for several hours, especially at high altitudes (such as in Colorado) where the boiling point may be substantially lower. These spores may be destroyed if kept at 120° C for 30 minutes using pressure cookers. Spores of type E are most heat-labile and are killed with heating at 80° C for 30 minutes.

2. Germination may be inhibited by a reduction in pH, refrigeration, freezing, drying, or addition of salt, sugar, or other inhibitory substances such as sodium nitrite.

3. Inactivation of preformed toxin is accomplished by terminal heating for 20 minutes at 80° C or for 10 minutes at 90° C.

INFANT BOTULISM. Infant botulism results from production of *C. botulinum* toxin in vivo following colonization of the gastrointestinal tract in children ages one to nine months. This is the most common form of botulism in the United States, where 30 to 80 cases are documented annually. Spores of *C. botulinum* (but not the toxin) have been found in about 10 per cent of honey supplies, which presumably account for one third of cases. The disease spectrum varies considerably, ranging from "failure to thrive" or mild changes in bowel habits to the sudden infant death syndrome or "crib death." The most commonly recognized form of the disease is the "floppy baby syndrome." Initial symptoms are lethargy, diminished suck, weakness, feeble cry, and diminished spontaneous activity with loss of head control. This is followed by extensive flaccid paralysis. The diagnosis is established with the recovery of *C. botulinum* or its toxin in stool. The toxin has rarely been detected in the serum. Fecal carriage of the organism and the toxin may persist for weeks to months following clinical improvement and hospital discharge. The major therapeutic need is supportive care with special attention to nutrition and maintenance of respiratory function. The role of antitoxin, guanidine, and antibiotics in this form of botulism has not been established, and generally their use is not advised. The mortality rate for hospitalized patients given supportive care is only 2 per cent.

WOUND BOTULISM. This is a rare form of botulism in which a traumatic wound is infected by *C. botulinum* with toxin production in vivo. Clinical features are identical to those of foodborne botulism except that the incubation period is 4 to 14 days and there is a paucity of gastrointestinal symptoms. The diagnosis is established by recovering *C. botulinum* from the wound or by detection of the toxin in serum.

UNCLASSIFIED BOTULISM. This category includes persons over the age of 12 months who have typical symptoms and signs of botulism with no identifiable vehicle. It is possible that some cases result from production of toxin in vivo by organisms colonizing the intestine in a fashion comparable to the mechanism described for infant botulism.

SPECIAL NOTE. Physicians who suspect foodborne botulism should alert their state health department and the Communicable Diseases Center (telephone 404–329–3311 on weekdays; 404–329–3644 on nights, holidays, and weekends).

Dowell VR Jr., McCroskey LM, Hathaway CL, Lombard GL, Hughes JM, Merson MH: Coproexamination for botulinal toxin and *Clostridium botulinum.* JAMA 238:1829, 1977. *Reviews methods to establish the diagnosis in foodborne botulism.*

Merson MH, Hughes JM, Dowell VR, Taylor A, Barker WH, Gangarosa EJ: Current trends in botulism in the United States. JAMA 229:1305, 1974. *Summary of the CDC experience with foodborne botulism.*

Arnon SS: Infant botulism. Ann Rev Med 31:541, 1980. *A review of infant botulism.*

280. TETANUS

John H. Kerr

Tetanus, often called "lockjaw," is a disease of the nervous system characterized by intense activity of motor neurons resulting in severe muscle spasms. It is caused by an exotoxin of *Clostridium tetani.*

ETIOLOGY. *Clostridium tetani* is an actively mobile gram-positive bacillus which, in its spore-bearing form, has a characteristic "drumstick" appearance. It is a strict anaerobe, and spores will germinate only if the oxidation-reduction potential in the environment is +0.01 volt or less at pH 7. At 37° C, *Clostridium* grows well in a cooked meat medium and on blood agar plates, where slight hemolysis is often observed. Vegetative bacilli are readily killed by antiseptics and by heat, but the spores are highly resistant to antiseptics and variably resistant to heat. To kill all spores, boiling for at least four hours or autoclaving for 12 minutes at 121° C is required.

Clostridium tetani produces two exotoxins, tetanospasmin and tetanolysin. Tetanospasmin, a protein of molecular weight 150,000, is one of the most potent neurotoxins that have been isolated. Tetanolysin can cause hemolysis on blood agar plates, but does not seem to play any significant part in the pathogenesis of the disease.

EPIDEMIOLOGY. *Clostridium tetani* is commonly found in soil and in the feces of domestic animals and humans. Spores can be recovered from dust and clothing and, in suitably dry surroundings, may survive in a viable form for many years.

Tetanus is most common in warm climates and in highly cultivated rural areas. It remains a major public health problem in economically underdeveloped countries, where it causes several hundred thousand, mostly neonatal, deaths each year. Unhygienic practices such as dressing the umbilical stump with dung and neonatal circumcision in primitive conditions tend to maintain the high incidence of neonatal tetanus, which has a fatality rate exceeding 60 per cent except in a few outstanding centers. In more temperate and economically developed areas such as Europe and North America, the disease has become extremely rare because of better hygiene, improved wound care, and high immunization rates. In these countries, neonatal tetanus is almost unknown, and tetanus has increasingly become a disease of the elderly, probably because of impaired local responses to infection and of poorly maintained immunity.

PATHOGENESIS. For tetanus to occur, *Clostridium tetani* must be introduced into and multiply within the body. Spores may be carried in through large or small wounds but will germinate only if anaerobic conditions develop. This is most likely in wounds which contain necrotic tissue or foreign bodies, or in those which are heavily contaminated with soil or manure. If these conditions persist for more than a few hours, the clostridia multiply and may produce toxins. Tetanospasmin is released by autolysis of clostridial cells and diffuses into the local tissues, from where it may be spread throughout the body in the bloodstream. Most is taken up by the peripheral endings of motor neurons, although some enters sensory and autonomic nerve fibers. The toxin then travels along nerve fibers toward the central nervous system and, after a period of time related directly to the length of the nerve and inversely to the electrical activity in the axon, reaches and is concentrated within the cell body. At this stage, the electrical and functional characteristics of the cells are unaffected by the toxin within them. The symptoms of tetanus appear only after the toxin has passed across the synaptic cleft into the presynaptic terminals of spinal inhibitory interneurons where it combines with a ganglioside and interferes with the release of the inhibitory transmitter substance. Disinhibition of both alpha and gamma motor neurons occurs, leading to the increase in muscle tone, loss of coordination, and spontaneous simultaneous contractions of both agonist and antagonist muscles that constitute tetanic spasms.

An analogous process whereby tetanospasmin migrates centripetally along the sympathetic chain to produce disinhibition in the lateral horns of the spinal cord has been demonstrated in animals and probably explains the autonomic disturbances that complicate many of the severe cases in humans. In man, pathologic lesions caused directly by tetanospasmin have not been demonstrated unequivocally, and the toxin appears to kill by disrupting neurologic coordination. Even after the most severe form of the disease, recovery, if it takes place, is complete.

CLINICAL FEATURES AND CRITERIA OF SEVERITY IN TETANUS. The criteria of severity may be established in two ways: from the history, and from the symptoms and signs.

From the History. The severity of an attack of tetanus is related to the incubation period (the period from injury to the first sign of tetanus) and the onset period (the period from the first sign to the first generalized spasm). If the former is less than nine days and the latter less than 48 hours, the attack of tetanus may be expected to be severe. The length of the onset period is, in general, the more reliable guide.

From the Symptoms and Signs. In the mild case, tetanus usually presents with rigidity of muscles, which may be generalized or affect only one limb (local tetanus). Stiffness of the jaw muscles causes trismus, and stiffness of the facial muscles may cause a change of expression. Stiffness of the muscles of the neck and back may cause discomfort or even pain on attempted flexion of the spine.

In the moderate case, the patient has more severe generalized rigidity. Trismus is pronounced, the mouth can hardly be opened, and rigidity of the muscles of the face may cause the sneering "risus sardonicus." Opisthotonos may be pronounced, but more typically the stiffness of the antagonist muscles makes the patient lie "at attention" in bed, and the muscles of the back and abdomen are hard to the touch. Muscle spasms may appear as mild exacerbations of this generalized rigidity and may arise spontaneously or more commonly as a result of stimuli. The diagnostic characteristic of the moderate case, however, is the presence of dysphagia due to involvement of the pharyngeal muscles.

The patient with severe tetanus is distinguished from the patient with moderate tetanus by the presence of reflex spasms that may be of appalling intensity. If the spasms are untreated, opisthotonos becomes extreme and the intense muscle spasm may fracture vertebrae. Spasm of the laryngeal muscles, the diaphragm, and the intercostals prevents ventilation, and cyanosis occurs. Reflex spasms that cause cyanosis and cannot be controlled except by powerful relaxants such as curare are the characteristic features of the severe case of tetanus.

Autonomic Disturbances. Disturbances of the autonomic nervous system occur frequently in severely affected tetanus patients and may prove fatal, particularly when the disease occurs in drug addicts. Younger patients often develop a fluctuating hypertension and increasing tachycardia after a few days of treatment, and cardiovascular responses to stimuli such as the aspiration of secretions from the respiratory tract become exaggerated so that systolic blood pressures of over 300 mm Hg are not uncommon. Patients sweat profusely and may become extremely vasoconstricted peripherally with a sharp line of demarcation between warm and cold skin. Hyperpyrexia occurs in the absence of significant secondary infection and probably reflects the inability of the vasoconstricted patient to lose heat. High metabolic rates have been measured in spite of muscular paralysis, and the cardiac output is often disproportionately high in relation to tissue oxygen utilization, suggesting increased neurogenic drive to the heart. Raised plasma and urine catecholamine levels occur in association with these disturbances, and it seems likely that the sympathetic nervous system is grossly overactive and incoordinate. Prolonged overactivity has been followed by supraventricular tachycardia and multifocal ventricular ectopic beats, unresponsive hypotension, sudden bradycardia, and cardiac arrest.

Perhaps fortunately, patients with severe tetanus often remember little of their illness, but may recall weird and sometimes frightening dreams. Electroencephalography usually shows a sleep pattern with activation during stimulation such as tracheal aspiration.

DIAGNOSIS. The diagnosis of the established case of tetanus is all too easy, and strychnine poisoning is the only condition which is truly similar to established tetanus. Trismus may occur from dental infections, and the author has seen one case of hysterical tetanus. Overdose with or sensitivity to the phenothiazine group of drugs can be confused with tetanus, but the movements in these conditions usually include grimacing and jaw movements in which the jaw is opened widely.

TREATMENT. Treatment in tetanus is essentially symptomatic, but all patients with the disease should receive antimicrobial drugs, active and passive immunization, and should undergo wound excision. To allow the earliest possible detection of possibly lethal manifestations of the disease, such as severe muscular or laryngeal spasms, the treatment of tetanus should be conducted in a well-lighted intensive care unit rather than in isolation in a darkened side room.

Antibiotics. Treatment with penicillin (1 million units every six hours intramuscularly) or erythromycin (500 mg every six hours intravenously) should be commenced to ensure that all clostridia are killed.

Antitoxin. Human tetanus immunoglobulin (1000 units intravenously and 2000 units intramuscularly) should be administered as early as possible to produce a high blood level. Only toxin circulating in the bloodstream and that in the tissues near the wound will be accessible to this antitoxin, since that in transit up nerve fibers and that which has entered spinal interneurons and produced symptoms cannot be neutralized by blood-borne antitoxin. In animals, intrathecal antitoxin has been shown to combine with tetanospasmin in the synaptic clefts between motor neuron and interneuron and thus prevent the development of tetanic spasms. The administration of antitoxin by this route is currently being investigated, particularly in parts of the world where tetanus is common and medical facilities are scarce. The results to date do not match those that can be expected in a fully equipped intensive care unit.

Surgical Intervention. If a focus of infection or wound is found, surgical debridement should be carried out shortly after the administration of the intravenous antitoxin so that any toxin released into the circulation at surgery will be neutralized. In about 20 per cent of tetanus cases, no source of infection is ever identified.

Active Immunization. Because an attack of tetanus does not confer immunity to tetanus, active immunization with adsorbed toxoid should be started and a full course of three injections given during the recovery period.

Symptomatic Measures. MUSCULAR HYPERTONICITY. The trismus and increased muscle tone of the mild case of tetanus can usually be controlled adequately with small doses of diazepam (10 mg every three to four hours orally or parenterally). Barbiturates and chlorpromazine have also been widely and effectively employed against these symptoms.

DYSPHAGIA AND AIRWAY MANAGEMENT. Trismus is a common early symptom in tetanus and is frequently accompanied by incoordination of the swallowing and laryngeal protective reflexes. Correct management of the airway is of vital importance, because laryngeal spasm may occur spontaneously or may be induced by attempts to swallow saliva or to pass a nasogastric tube. In addition, dysphagia may allow inhalation of infected material and saliva from the mouth so that atelectasis and pneumonia can follow; the latter remains a common cause of death in tetanus.

To minimize pulmonary complications, protection of the airway by intubation with a cuffed tube is advocated as soon as dysphagia is suspected. The symptom may be demonstrated as a tendency to cough and clear the throat after swallowing a mouthful of water, and, in more advanced form, as an inability to swallow saliva so that the patient drools or spits it out. Orotracheal intubation should be performed under general anesthesia and after muscle paralysis, allowing an elective tracheostomy with a cuffed tube. Meticulous pulmonary care should be instituted and maintained until normal pharyngolaryngeal function returns.

MUSCLE SPASMS. Muscle spasms in tetanus can be either localized or generalized and of varying severity. Sustained contraction of the muscles is exhausting, painful, and, if the respiratory muscles become involved, dangerous. When large doses of diazepam or chlorpromazine are employed in attempts to control severe spasms, oversedation may lead to hypoventilation between spasms. In this situation, and when muscle spasms themselves interfere with ventilation, therapeutic paralysis should be induced with curariform drugs and the resultant ventilatory failure treated with intermittent positive pressure ventilation (IPPV). Curare or pancuronium is given intramuscularly or intravenously and with sufficient frequency to allow IPPV to proceed freely and to keep the patient comfortable. This method of treatment has proved most satisfactory when used early in the disease rather than after prolonged attempts to manage the patient with sedative agents. Smythe et al. (1974) have reported remarkable success in neonates with similar techniques.

Once curarization and IPPV have commenced, anxiety in the conscious but paretic patient should be minimized by frequent reassurance from the nursing staff and by mild hypnosis from diazepam or a barbiturate. Some of the most severely affected patients, however, become unresponsive and appear comatose for periods of one to three weeks during the critical phase of their illness, and in this situation sedative agents and muscle relaxants should be administered only if clearly indicated. Such patients usually regain consciousness during the recovery phase and appear normal apart from amnesia. After one to four weeks of treatment, curare requirements decrease and diazepam may be reinstituted to reduce muscle stiffness during weaning from IPPV.

Nutrition. Patients with mild tetanus may be fed orally, but once dysphagia develops a nasogastric tube should be inserted while the patient is anesthetized for tracheostomy. The considerable caloric (2500 calories per day) and fluid requirements of the tetanus patient can be satisfied effectively over the two- to four-week period of dysphagia by nasogastric feeding. Paralytic ileus occurs fairly frequently in severe tetanus, but usually responds to intermittent gastric drainage followed by the instillation of antacids and gut stimulants (e.g., metoclopramide).

Fluid Balance. The maintenance of a balanced fluid status in the severely ill tetanus patient is complicated by the considerable insensible fluid losses produced by profuse sweating and by unswallowed saliva. If reliance is placed entirely upon measured fluid input and output, fluid losses may be seriously underestimated and dehydration may result.

Underhydration in an immobilized patient increases the possibility of deep venous thrombosis and of pulmonary embolism, and the latter remains a common cause of death in tetanus. Although anticoagulation, started 24 hours after tracheostomy and continued until remobilization, has been practiced without significant complication in several centers, protection against pulmonary embolism has not been complete, and avoidance of dehydration is equally important.

Insensible fluid losses are best monitored by weighing the patient each day, and dehydration is avoided by measuring the specific gravity (or osmolality) of the urine regularly. Enough fluid should be given parenterally or by nasogastric tube to produce a daily urine flow of 1.5 to 2 liters and to maintain the urine specific gravity below 1.015. Particular care must be taken to react promptly to the severe hypovolemia which may develop rapidly when overactivity of the sympathetic nervous system causes excessive sweating in association with gastrointestinal stasis.

Cardiovascular Disturbances. In some tetanus patients who show severe muscular symptoms, cardiovascular changes in the form of tachycardia, hypertension, and increased responses to therapeutic maneuvers, such as tracheal aspiration, may appear after two to five days of treatment by curarization and artificial ventilation. These changes have been controlled successfully with adrenergic blocking agents. To reduce the tachycardia resulting from the intense sympathetic stimulation of the heart, a beta-adrenergic blocking agent such as propranolol (10 mg every three to six hours via nasogastric tube) should be administered until the heart rate averages less than 100; if hypertension persists, an antihypertensive (e.g., labetalol,* 50 to 100 mg every two to six hours) should be added.

*Investigational drug in the United States.

Although other combinations of antiadrenergic agents might be more effective, short-acting drugs are preferred, because, particularly in drug addicts and in elderly patients, the pattern of autonomic disturbance may change very rapidly. In these groups of patients, episodes of profound hypotension and bradycardia may suddenly occur and, on occasion, lead to cardiac arrest. Provided that resuscitation is prompt, the cardiovascular status may be restored rapidly and repeatedly by measures such as tracheal aspiration and mildly painful stimuli

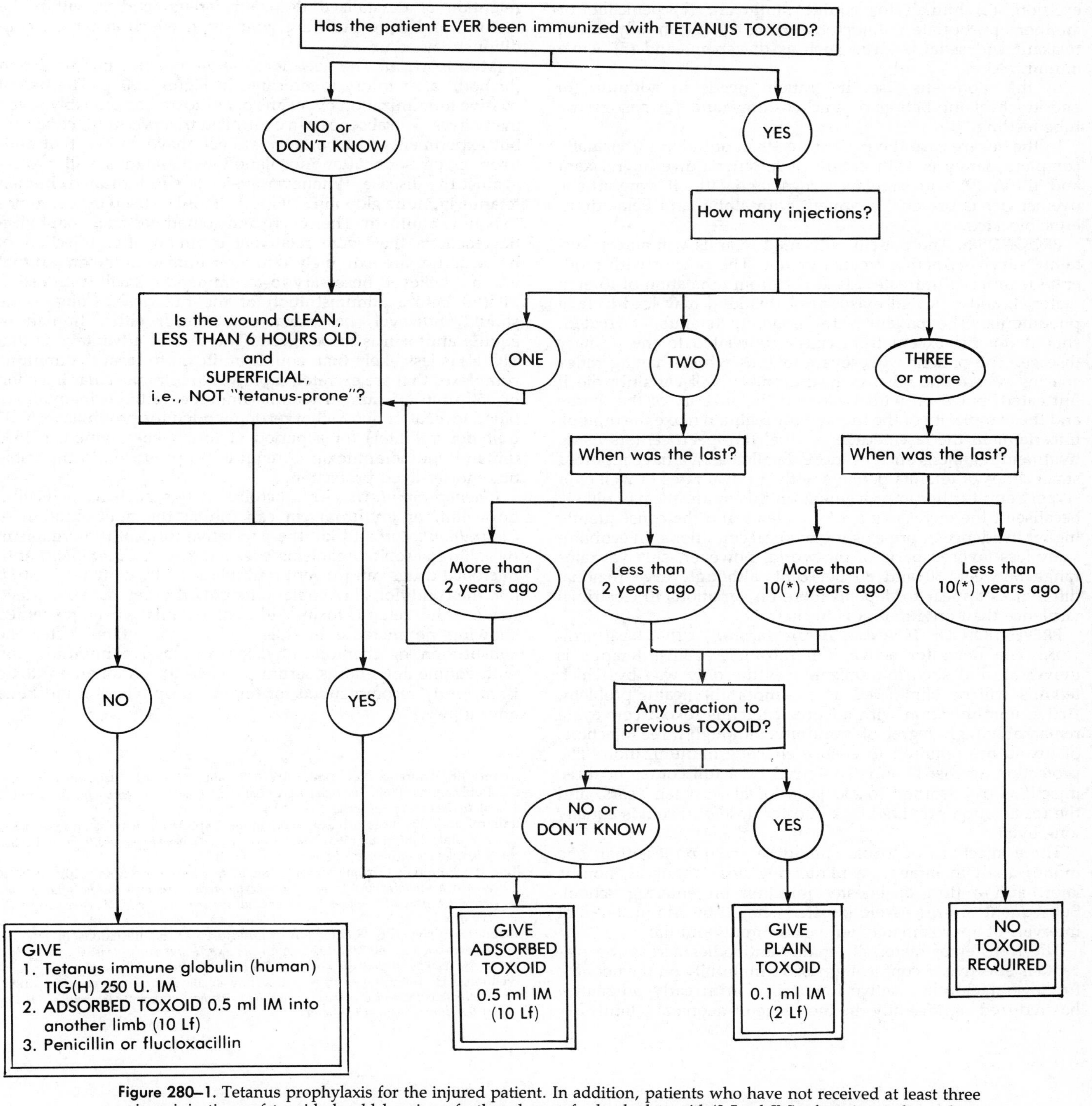

Figure 280–1. Tetanus prophylaxis for the injured patient. In addition, patients who have not received at least three previous injections of toxoid should be given further doses of adsorbed toxoid (0.5 ml IM) after six weeks and six months. The volumetric doses assume a toxoid concentration of 20 Lf per ml. (*) Five years if wound is "tetanus prone" or if patient is aged over 60 years.

which result in the release of endogenous catecholamines. These sudden and readily reversible episodes, during which the circulation appears unstimulated and dilated, must be contrasted with the unresponsive preterminal hypotension accompanied by tachycardia, vasoconstriction, and hyperpyrexia which has followed prolonged and unrelieved sympathetic overactivity. In view of the varying patterns of cardiovascular disturbance, continuous direct monitoring of heart rate and of arterial and central venous blood pressures has proved of much benefit in guiding therapy.

In summary, in a mild case the patient needs (1) wound excision, (2) human (or equine) antitoxin, (3) penicillin or another appropriate antimicrobial drug, (4) a centrally acting relaxant and sedative drug such as diazepam, and (5) active immunization.

In the moderate case the patient needs in addition (6) endotracheal intubation or tracheostomy and (7) nasogastric tube feeding.

In the severe case the patient needs in addition (8) virtually complete paralysis with curare or another powerful relaxant and IPPV, (9) anticoagulant drugs, and (10), if sympathetic overactivity is present, treatment with alpha- and beta-adrenergic blockers.

PROGNOSIS. The patient with mild tetanus will almost certainly survive whether treated or not. The patient with moderate tetanus, if untreated, is at risk from inhalation of foreign material, and repeated episodes of this kind may lead to fatal pneumonia. The patient with moderate tetanus, if treated, should not die except from causes unrelated to the primary disease. The patient with severe tetanus who is having reflex spasms severe enough to cause cyanosis will certainly die if untreated, but even with treatment the severity of the illness and the complexity of the therapeutic regimen make the outlook uncertain. In the last decade, several European centers using treatment regimens such as those detailed above have reported small series of tetanus patients with survival rates of well over 90 per cent; further improvement on this figure seems unlikely because of the increasing age of patients and the consequently higher incidence of pre-existing medical conditions. In economically less favored parts of the world, however, survival rates range between 30 and 80 per cent, although large regional differences appear to depend more on variations in clostridial virulence than on differences in therapy.

PREVENTION OF TETANUS. ***Before Injury.*** ACTIVE IMMUNIZATION. The need for active immunization against tetanus is universal, and such immunization is the only way by which tetanus will be eliminated as an important health problem. Active immunization with adsorbed tetanus toxoid conveys a remarkably high degree of immunity, although three injections of toxoid are required to ensure effective immunization. The protection against tetanus conferred by a full course of three injections of adsorbed toxoid lasts for at least ten years, and the reactivation provided by a booster dose of toxoid is equally long lived.

Three injections of toxoid should be given no less than one month apart in infancy, a reinforcing dose about 12 months later, and a fifth or booster injection on entering school. Subsequent routine toxoid boosters should be administered at intervals of approximately ten years throughout life.

The transfer of maternal tetanus antibodies across the placenta is effective in conferring passive immunity on the neonate for several months. Active immunization in early pregnancy has reduced significantly the incidence of neonatal tetanus.

After Injury. PREVENTION OF CONTAMINATION. Simple measures that prevent wound contamination can contribute significantly to the prevention of tetanus, as is shown by the effect of attention to treatment of the umbilical stump on the incidence of neonatal tetanus. The aim of surgery in prophylaxis is to remove all dead tissue and foreign bodies from a wound. This not only removes spore-bearing material but also denies the spores the anaerobic conditions necessary for their growth. Tetanus often occurs in patients in whom no wound is found, so that a precise definition of a "tetanus-prone" wound is difficult, although it is generally agreed that certain features increase the likelihood of tetanus. These features include an interval of more than six hours between injury and treatment, heavy contamination of the wound with soil or manure, the retention of devitalized tissue or foreign bodies within the wound, and deep puncture wounds in which anaerobic conditions may occur.

IMMUNIZATION. The need for passive or active immunization (or both) after injury is indicated in Figure 280–1. The use of passive immunization by means of antitoxin has probably saved many lives. The absence of a controlled trial precludes certainty, but experiments in laboratory animals have shown that antitoxin given soon after inoculation with tetanus will protect against the disease. Whenever available and indicated, human tetanus immune globulin (TIG(H)) should be used in preference to equine antitoxin. The severe and sometimes fatal anaphylactic reactions that were relatively common after injection of horse serum are extremely rare after human antitoxin, so that it is not believed necessary to recommend a small test dose of TIG(H) before administration of the full dose. Epinephrine should, however, be available whenever either human or equine antitoxin is to be given. The second advantage is that TIG(H) is less likely than equine antitoxin to form the immune complexes that are excreted rapidly. An intramuscular injection of 250 units of human tetanus immune globulin maintains a blood level at or above that recommended for prophylaxis (0.01 unit per milliliter) for a period of four weeks, whereas 1500 units of equine antitoxin is required to produce a comparable but shorter-lived protection.

Chemoprophylaxis. Antimicrobial drugs such as penicillin, floxacillin, or erythromycin can inhibit the multiplication of *Clostridium tetani* and kill the vegetative form of the organism. By killing aerobic organisms coexisting with *Clostridium,* antimicrobial drugs can prevent multiplication by denying *Clostridium* the conditions favorable to its growth; they have no effect, however, on tetanus toxin. Although data have been presented showing no increase in the incidence of tetanus after the substitution of chemoprophylaxis for passive immunization with equine antitetanus serum, the less toxic human antitoxin is currently recommended for tetanus prophylaxis if indicated after injury.

Adams EB, Laurence DR, Smith JWG: Tetanus. Oxford, Blackwell Scientific Publications, 1969. *The standard clinical text on the disease with a full bibliography up to the time of publication.*

Immunization Practices Advisory Committee: Diphtheria, tetanus and pertussis. NY State J Med 82:1563, 1982. *Current recommendations about immunization schedules and available materials.*

Kerr JH: Editorial: Current topics in tetanus. Intens Care Med 5:105, 1979. *A review which attempts to pull together the recent pathophysiologic findings and current therapeutic experience; includes all the important clinical references for the last decade.*

Tseuda K, Oliver PB, Richter RW: Cardiovascular manifestations of tetanus. Anesthesiology 40:588, 1974. *American experience with intensive care of very severe tetanus. Includes information about management in drug addiction.*

Wellhöner H: Tetanus neurotoxin. Rev Physiol Biochem Pharmacol 93:1, 1982. *Well-referenced review of the experimental work that has improved our understanding of the clinical changes in tetanus.*

281. DISEASES CAUSED BY NON-SPORE-FORMING ANAEROBIC BACTERIA

Sherwood L. Gorbach

DEFINITIONS. Anaerobic bacteria are the major constituents of the microflora that colonizes the gastrointestinal tract, upper respiratory tract, skin, and vagina. Under normal circumstances these organisms exist in a *commensal* (literal meaning "dining at the same table") relationship with their host. Anaerobic bacteria require reduced oxygen tension for growth; the more fastidious strains cannot survive exposure to atmospheric oxygen for more than five minutes. As a general rule, anaerobes associated with infectious processes are relatively aerotolerant. Teleologically, aerotolerance provides anaerobic bacteria with a survival advantage in mammalian tissues, since the extremely oxygen-sensitive forms perish almost immediately upon escape from their natural ecologic niche, while aerotolerant forms can establish a septic focus.

Regardless of the organ site, anaerobic infections have three characteristics in common. First, such infections are truly endogenous, since the pathogens originate from the normal flora of the host. Second, certain pathogenic conditions predispose to anaerobic infections by initiating spread of the normal flora beyond the confines of mucosal barriers. These inciting events also produce a low *oxidation-reduction potential* (Eh) in the tissues, thereby favoring the growth of anaerobic organisms. Compromised vascular supply, trauma, tissue destruction, and antecedent infections caused by aerobic bacteria or viruses that result in necrosis are among the situations that precede anaerobic infection. Third, the infecting flora is highly complex. Abdominal infections, for example, harbor an average of five different bacterial species, usually three anaerobes and two aerobic or facultative strains.

ANAEROBIC GRAM-NEGATIVE BACILLI. ***Bacteroides.*** *B. fragilis* is the preeminent anaerobic pathogen in humans. This distinction is based on its virulence, its ubiquity in various organ sites, and its resistance to many conventional antimicrobial drugs. The organism frequently produces abscesses and causes tissue destruction. The *B. fragilis* group has been divided into five distinct species, based on biochemical differences and DNA homology: *B. fragilis, B. distasonis, B. vulgatus, B. ovatus*, and *B. thetaiotaomicron*. Although these organisms are recognized pathogens, they all lack one of the prime virulence factors of other gram-negative organisms, endotoxin. While *Bacteroides* strains do possess a surface *lipopolysaccharide (LPS)*, this substance differs in chemical composition from LPS of other gram-negative organisms. In addition, the *B. fragilis* LPS lacks the biologic activities of classic endotoxin, such as production of septic shock and vascular collapse in experimental animals. On the other hand, *B. fragilis* contains on its outer cell membrane a specific, large molecular weight capsule composed of polysaccharide. In a purified form the capsular material is highly antigenic, and it can produce abscesses when it is injected into experimental animals.

B. fragilis causes infections in the abdominal cavity that are associated with contamination by the intestinal flora. These organisms also are found in female pelvic infections and in mixed infections of skin and soft tissue such as decubitus ulcer, diabetic foot ulcer, and gangrene of the perineum.

The *Bacteroides melaninogenicus-asaccharolyticus* group is found in the normal flora and in association with various infections. The group has seven distinct species. The major distinguishing feature of *B. melaninogenicus* is the production of a brown-black pigment, formed in the colony after five to seven days of growth on blood agar. Many strains require blood and vitamin K or its analogues for growth. Young colonies of *B. melaninogenicus* show an intense red fluorescence under ultraviolet light even before the black pigment appears. This fluorescence can also be demonstrated in wounds infected by these organisms. Infections caused by *B. melaninogenicus* are most commonly found in the respiratory tract, head and neck region, and female pelvic area.

Fusobacterium. Several species comprise the genus, of which the major ones found in clinical specimens are *F. nucleatum* and *F. necrophorum*. In Gram-stained preparations, these organisms take up the strain poorly and appear as slender spear-shaped bacilli with parallel sides and tapered ends. The LPS of *F. nucleatum* causes septic shock and vascular collapse when injected intravenously into rabbits, in contrast to the material found in *B. fragilis*, which is biologically inactive in this model. *Fusobacterium spp.* are regular constituents of the normal flora of the oral cavity, gastrointestinal tract, and female genital tract. Among the infectious processes, these organisms are major causes of pleuropulmonary infections and various abscesses of the head and neck region. They are also responsible for bacteremia. The most common sites of origin are the female genital tract, orofacial region, and lower respiratory tract.

ANAEROBIC GRAM-POSITIVE COCCI. This diverse group of organisms ranks second in importance to *Bacteroides* in frequency of isolation from infected sites. The two genera are *Peptostreptococcus* and *Peptococcus*. (There are also gram-negative cocci known as *Veillonella*, which are only rarely involved as pathogens.) Peptostreptococci form long chains of cocci in culture. They produce gas and a foul odor in the test tube and in infected sites as well. Peptococci occur as irregular clumps of gram-positive cocci that resemble *Staphylococcus aureus* in morphologic appearance. These organisms are catalase positive and produce no odor.

Anaerobic gram-positive cocci are important components of the normal flora of humans. Within the oral cavity peptostreptococci represent a significant percentage of the anaerobic isolates in saliva and dental plaque. They are also among the leading components of the fecal flora and the vaginal flora. As pathogenic organisms these anaerobic cocci are found in virtually all sites where anaerobes have been identified. Approximately 50 per cent of such isolates in a clinical bacteriology laboratory are from surgical wounds, mostly associated with abdominal operations and hysterectomies. The gram-positive cocci are also found in skin and soft tissue infections and in blood cultures. About one third of anaerobic pleuropulmonary infections are associated with these gram-positive cocci. In the female genital tract they are probably the most important cause of salpingitis and are frequently isolated in cases of pelvic abscess.

GRAM-POSITIVE NON-SPORE-FORMING BACILLI. The two leading isolates are *Propionibacterium acnes* and various species of *Eubacterium*. *P. acnes* is the most frequent anaerobe found on normal skin. Many laboratories incorrectly identify it as a diphtheroid. This organism is commonly recovered from blood cultures, most often as a contaminant. It is also isolated from wound infections as part of a mixed flora. Although these organisms have little intrinsic pathogenicity, they are important causes of infection in patients with artificial heart valves, vascular grafts, orthopedic prostheses, or ventricular shunts. *Eubacterium* is isolated from wound infections, particularly in association with *Bacteroides*. As far as can be determined, *Eubacterium* plays no pathogenic role in the infective process. The basis for this statement is that eubacteria are virtually never isolated in pure culture from an abscess; they are rarely associated with bacteremia; and they have not been isolated, as a rule, after patients have failed to respond to antibiotic treatment.

PATHOGENESIS OF ANAEROBIC INFECTIONS. ***Unitarian Compared with Synergistic Infections.*** Our theoretical models of infections are based on concepts of microbial monoetiology. Pasteur established that certain microorganisms are responsible for a specific disease state. His theory was formalized by Robert

Koch in his famous postulates. Finally, Erhlich created the concept of a single drug, the "magic bullet," designed for a specific infection. Thus, the principal states: one microbe, one disease, one drug. This concept applies to classic infections such as typhoid fever, diphtheria, and cholera. However, the classic design does not fit most infections associated with anaerobic bacteria, since these processes harbor multiple strains of organisms with varying oxygen sensitivities and undefined pathogenic potentials. Anaerobic infections follow the model of bacterial synergy, in which several bacteria behave in a cooperative fashion to produce infection. In experimental model systems of mixed infection, various microbial components contribute virulence factors or growth substances that permit other more pathogenic forms to invade the tissues. A diphtheroid, for example, adds vitamin K to a septic process, which enables *B. melaninogenicus* to cause tissue necrosis. The growth of *B. melaninogenicus* is dependent on vitamin K supplied, in this instance, by a nonpathogenic partner. Most clinical anaerobic infections are mixed, containing several species of bacteria. Since it is not clear which are the primary pathogens and which are the symbionts and commensals, it is often necessary to treat all of the potential pathogens.

Virulence Factors. The microenvironment of an anaerobic abscess has features that insure its own survival. An abscess has an Eh of -250 mv, with an extremely low concentration of oxygen. Anaerobiosis is a hostile condition for host-defense mechanisms. Within this oxygen-free zone, neutrophils are unable to kill bacteria by their oxidative metabolic pathway. Low oxygen tension also inhibits the activity of aminoglycoside antibiotics, since they require an oxidative transport system to cross the bacterial cell envelope. The abscess itself contains a large concentration of microorganisms, approximately 10^8 to 10^9 per milliliter. A high inoculum and a relatively low growth rate are adverse conditions for the activity of beta-lactam antibiotics. Thus, host defenses and antibiotic interventions are hindered in an anaerobic abscess.

Individual anaerobic microorganisms possess virulence factors that promote their survival in the host's tissues. *B. fragilis* elaborates a polysaccharide capsule that provides protection against phagocytosis by neutrophils. These organisms also elaborate extracellular enzymes, such as lipases, proteases, nucleases, and heparinases, that contribute to the formation of abscess and necrosis. Membrane-associated enzymes are found in many virulent anaerobes, including beta-lactamases and superoxide dismutase (SOD). The beta-lactamases destroy antibiotics such as penicillin and cephalosporin. SOD, an enzyme present in virtually all pathogenic anaerobes studied thus far, seems to protect the organism in its initial exposure to oxygenated tissues.

Immunologic factors are affected by anaerobic bacteria. Several species of anaerobes are more resistant to phagocytosis than coliforms and other facultative organisms. Anaerobic bacteria can also interfere with phagocytosis of aerobes when both organisms are present in a mixed infection. For example, *B. fragilis* inhibits phagocytosis and killing of *Proteus mirabilis* in vitro, but the coliforms have no effect on phagocytosis of the anaerobes. *B. fragilis* appears to influence the alternate pathway of serum complement. Cell-mediated immunity also plays a role in anaerobic infections, at least in abscess formation by *B. fragilis*.

Role of Facultative Organisms. Facultative or aerobic organisms are frequent partners in anaerobic infections. In some settings these organisms seem to initiate the infective process, perhaps by promoting early tissue necrosis or by consuming oxygen in the tissues. In abdominal infections coliforms and *Bacteroides* are often isolated together.

An animal model of intra-abdominal infection has delineated the role of these pathogens in the septic process. Following intestinal perforation, the initial phase consists of peritonitis, bacteremia, and septic shock. This phase is caused, at least in the animal model, by coliforms such as *E. coli* and *Proteus*. The later occurrence of abscess formation, however, is associated with anaerobes, particularly *Bacteroides*. Antimicrobial drugs active only against coliforms suppress the initial septicemic and shock phase but have no effect on abscess formation. Similarly, antianaerobic drugs do not protect against coliform bacteremia, but they do suppress formation of abscess. The clinical picture is complex, with overlapping of the septic shock stage and the abscess stage. However, the therapeutic implications are clear: both components of abdominal sepsis should receive appropriate antimicrobial attention.

ANAEROBIC BACTERIA IN VARIOUS INFECTIONS. Aerobic and facultative microorganisms have been traditionally considered the major pathogens in infectious diseases. Recent improvements in laboratory techniques have facilitated the identification of anaerobic bacteria, and it has become clear that these oxygen-sensitive organisms share responsibility for a significant number of infections seen in clinical practice. Certain types of infection, such as those appearing in the abdomen, chest, female genital tract, and head and neck, characteristically are caused by anaerobes. Other infections such as lobar pneumonia, acute pharyngitis, and pyogenic meningitis are rarely associated with anaerobic bacteria.

Intra-abdominal Infections. Infections within the peritoneal cavity usually are related to contamination by the intestinal flora. The microflora of the upper intestine, from the stomach to the upper ileum, consists of sparse numbers of facultative gram-positive organisms derived from the oropharynx. Relatively few coliforms and obligate anaerobes are encountered. The lower bowel, on the other hand, harbors a luxuriant flora in which anaerobes outnumber facultative organisms such as coliforms by a factor of 1000 to 1. Hence, injuries to the upper intestinal tract, such as perforated ulcer or trauma, result in a small inoculum of microorganisms and a low risk of infection. But colonic perforations release a large inoculum of bacteria, causing a high rate of infection.

Peritonitis and intra-abdominal abscess are associated with anaerobic bacteria in 95 per cent of cases. The most frequent finding is a mixture of aerobes and anaerobes. (Infection by a single facultative organism such as *E. coli* is uncommon and usually is seen in *primary peritonitis* associated with cirrhosis of the liver.) In a large series of intra-abdominal infections, an average of five different organisms were isolated from each patient, including three types of anaerobes and two aerobes. Of the anaerobes, *Bacteroides*, *Clostridium*, anaerobic cocci, and *Fusobacterium* are the major pathogens. The specific site of infection does not determine the flora, since the same pathogens are found in peritonitis, appendicitis, subphrenic abscess, and diverticular abscess.

Anaerobic Pleuropulmonary Infections. Anaerobic infections of the lower respiratory tract produce four clinical conditions: *aspiration pneumonia, lung abscess, necrotizing pneumonia,* and *empyema*. The pathogenesis of these conditions is aspiration of oropharyngeal contents, a situation associated with compromised state of consciousness, obstruction of the esophagus, and neurologic deficits. The oral flora is permitted admission to normally sterile regions of the lower respiratory tract. Approximately 90 per cent of patients with aspiration pneumonia have anaerobes as the major infecting flora. The situation applies to patients who have aspirated outside the hospital or shortly after admission, since they harbor normal oral flora. When the aspiration event occurs after hospitalization or after treatment with antibiotics, at which time the oral flora becomes colonized by gram-negative facultative organisms, the aspirated flora assumes a different character. Coliforms and *Pseudomonas* account for most cases of hospital-acquired aspiration pneumonia. Lung abscess is associated with anaerobic bacteria in over 90 per cent of cases. The aerobes that occasionally cause a solitary lung abscess include *Klebsiella* and *S. aureus*. Necrotizing pneumonia is actually an earlier stage of lung abscess in which a specific segment or lobe of the lung is extensively damaged with multiple small abscesses. In the more advanced stage these abscesses coalesce to form a single large cavity, leaving in its wake a large area of destroyed lung. Necrotizing pneumonia is a more aggressive condition than lung abscess, with higher mortality. Anaerobes are responsible for the vast majority of cases. Empyema is an infection usually associated with underlying pneumonitis or lung abscess. Nearly 75 per cent of the cases of empyema are associated with anaerobes, most frequently in patients with chronic infection. The remaining cases are caused by the classic aerobic pathogens such as staphylococci, group A streptococci, and pneumococci; these organisms produce an acute onset and a more virulent course. Formerly, most cases of empyema were caused by these aerobic gram-positive organisms, but the situation has been reversed with the advent of antimicrobial agents.

Anaerobic pleuropulmonary infections involve multiple bacterial species including *B. melaninogenicus, F. nucleatum,* and anaerobic gram-positive cocci. *B. fragilis* is found in 15 per cent of cases. The fact that these organisms are found in the same relative concentrations in the various clinical cases suggests that the inoculum of oral contents is similar in each setting. Corroboration for this hypothesis is provided by animal studies in which a spectrum of pulmonary infection is produced by the same inoculum of mixed bacteria derived from gingival scrapings.

Obstetric and Gynecologic Infections. The source of infections of the female upper genital tract is the vaginal flora, which has aerobic and anaerobic bacteria as normal constituents. The clinical conditions in which anaerobes are frequently encountered include tubo-ovarian abscess, pelvic abscess, septic abortion, endomyometritis, and postoperative wound infection (following hysterectomy). Polymicrobic bacteremia is a frequent occurrence in patients with severe pelvic infections. One important difference between pelvic abscesses derived from the female genital tract and those in the abdomen is that pure anaerobic infections—those without coliforms or other facultative forms—occur with a higher frequency in the pelvic location. The major anaerobic pathogens are *Bacteroides* (*B. fragilis,* as well as *B. bivius* and *B. disiens*), gram-positive cocci (especially *Peptostreptococcus*), *Fusobacterium,* and *Clostridium.* Pelvic inflammatory disease, also known as salpingitis, is a milder condition that is caused by an array of organisms, including gonococci, *Chlamydia,* and anaerobes, particularly *Peptostreptococcus.*

Head and Neck Infections. Since the anaerobic bacteria in the normal flora of the upper airways have limited invasive properties, they require an antecedent event that permits their movement into deeper structures. Dental manipulation, trauma, prior bacterial or viral infections, and operative interventions can provide the initiating circumstance. Necrotizing infections of the gingiva are usually associated with *B. melaninogenicus,* as well as other anaerobes. This organism is also present in endodontal infections. Spirochetes have been found at the advancing border of inflammation in histologic sections of acute ulcerative gingivitis, noma, and lung abscess. Since these organisms cannot be grown in subculture, their role in pathogenesis cannot be assessed. In patients with *sinusitis,* anaerobes are recovered from 50 per cent of patients with chronic processes. However, acute or subacute sinusitis, lasting three months or less, is rarely associated with anaerobes. *Otitis media* may be either acute or chronic. As in sinusitis, anaerobes may be present in the chronic forms but are rarely present in the more acute cases. *Space infections,* occurring in the potential spaces formed by fascial planes of the head and neck, are usually associated with three types of organisms: either *S. aureus, Streptococcus pyogenes,* or anaerobic bacteria. The first two organisms occur in space infections related to overlying skin processes such as boils or impetigo. Anaerobes are associated with space infections that arise from diseases of the mucous membrane, dental manipulations, or in those cases that occur spontaneously. *Ludwig's angina* is an example of a space infection associated with anaerobes.

Of the central nervous system infections, *brain abscess* is the one most frequently associated with anaerobic bacteria. These organisms are isolated from 85 per cent of suppurative brain abscesses unrelated to trauma or operative procedures. Gram-positive cocci, followed in frequency by *Fusobacterium* and *Bacteroides,* are the most common strains, often in association with facultative streptococci and coliforms. *Subdural empyema* may also be caused by anaerobes, particularly when it occurs in association with a parameningeal focus in an ear or nasal sinus. Classic pyogenic meningitis, however, is rarely caused by anaerobes.

Skin, Bone, and Soft Tissue Infections. The predisposing factors in anaerobic skin and soft tissue infections are trauma, ischemia, and surgery. The organisms often derive from the fecal or oral flora, particularly in wounds associated with intestinal surgery, decubitus ulcer, and human bites. The clinical presentations are *crepitant cellulitis, synergistic gangrene* or *cellulitis,* and *necrotizing fasciitis.* Anaerobes are also regularly encountered in *diabetic foot ulcers;* 75 per cent of such lesions are associated with *Bacteroides,* anaerobic cocci, and *Clostridium,* usually in mixed culture. Anaerobic *osteomyelitis* is associated with trauma or prior surgery, although some cases arise from hematogenous spread.

CLUES TO PRESUMPTIVE DIAGNOSIS OF ANAEROBIC INFECTION. Clinicians should be able to suspect the diagnosis of an anaerobic infection before the bacteriologic results are available. Such decisions are based on certain features that should suggest the presence of anaerobes in an infectious process. (1) Any infection that is contiguous or in proximity to a mucosal surface normally harboring an anaerobic flora—the gastrointestinal tract, female genital tract, and oropharynx—could potentially include anaerobes as part of the infecting flora. (2) A foul-smelling discharge is pathognomonic evidence of anaerobic infection, since the odor is caused by metabolism of these organisms. The absence of odor, however, is not helpful, because 50 per cent of anaerobic infections lack the characteristic odor. (3) The presence of severe tissue necrosis, abscess formation, fasciitis, or gangrene raises the possibility of the presence of anaerobes. (4) Gas in the tissue is highly suggestive, although not absolutely diagnostic, of anaerobic organisms. (5) A mixed infection, indicated by a Gram stain of exudate showing a polymorphic array of organisms, strongly suggests anaerobic involvement. Certain anaerobes have a characteristic appearance under the microscope, especially *Clostridium, Fusobacterium, Actinomyces,* and certain strains of *Bacteroides.* (6) The failure to recover organisms by conventional aerobic culture in the presence of clinical infection suggests that more fastidious bacteria, such as anaerobes, are present. (7) Failure to respond to antibiotics that have poor anaerobic activity, such as aminoglycosides and certain penicillins and cephalosporins, provides another clue that anaerobes may be part of the infecting flora.

TREATMENT STRATEGIES FOR ANAEROBIC INFECTIONS. Successful therapy for anaerobic infections involves rational antibiotic selection in conjunction with judicious surgical resection and drainage. The operative approach may be ultimately decisive, but it should be emphasized that surgical intervention alone may be inadequate. Anaerobic infection can continue to simmer with intermittent sepsis and insidious extension of the process unless appropriate antimicrobial agents are employed. Selection of initial antibiotic therapy should be based on knowledge of the pathogens likely to be present in a specific clinical setting. Because many anaerobic infections tend to be mixed with coliforms and other facultative organisms, it is advisable to use antimicrobial drugs active against both components. With regard to the anaerobic components, important differences are seen in infections above and below the diaphragm. Anaerobic infections above the diaphragm, including those in the central nervous system, head and neck region, and pleuropulmonary area, tend to involve organisms sensitive to penicillin. This observation is not invariably true, since certain organisms, especially *B. melaninogenicus,* can elaborate beta-lactamases, which inactivate penicillins and cephalosporins. Anaerobic infections below the diaphragm, such as those in the abdominal cavity and female genital tract, commonly involve *B. fragilis* as a major pathogen. Since this organism is commonly resistant to several antimicrobial agents, infections in these sites require special consideration for choice of antimicrobial drugs.

TREATMENT. The range of choice among antimicrobial drugs is somewhat limited with regard to anaerobic bacteria in general and even more so with *B. fragilis.* A United States survey of antibiotic susceptibility among strains of *B. fragilis* from nine medical centers was conducted during 1981. Among the 750 isolates, cefoxitin was the most active beta-lactam antibiotic with resistance rates running from 3 to 17 per cent in various centers. Piperacillin and moxalactam were the next most active beta-lactam antibiotics. Since high blood levels can be achieved with these drugs, they can be used to treat clinical infections caused by this organism. Piperacillin showed the best activity, second only to cefoxitin. Disappointing results were seen with penicillin, carbenicillin, ticarcillin, cephalothin, cefamandole, and certain third generation cephalosporins such as cefotaxime and cefoperazone. The drugs in this grouping are not considered good choices for infections associated with *B. fragilis.* Clostridia, fusobacteria, and gram-positive cocci are usually sensitive to several drugs, including penicillins, cephalosporins, clindamycin, and metronidazole.

The explanation for variations in activity of the beta-lactam drugs against anaerobes is the presence in certain strains of constitutive beta-lactamases. This enzyme is found in most strains of *B. fragilis* isolated from clinical sources. It is also found in 20 to 40 per cent of strains of *B. melaninogenicus* and in occasional strains of *Fusobacterium.* The increased activity of cefoxitin and moxalactam against *B. fragilis* is based on their apparent resistance to hydrolysis by beta-lactamase elaborated by anaerobic organisms.

Metronidazole, a bacteriocidal drug, has excellent activity against *Bacteroides, Fusobacterium, Clostridium,* and most strains of anaerobic cocci. Resistance to metronidazole among *Bacteroides* is extremely rare. Since the drug has a spectrum limited almost exclusively to anaerobes, another agent such as an aminoglycoside should be included for facultative organisms. In clinical trials metronidazole has produced excellent results in intra-abdominal infections, female pelvic infections, brain abscess, and anaerobic osteomyelitis. Many failures, however, have been noted in anaerobic pleuropulmonary infections. Such failures are probably related to the relatively poor activity against microaerophilic organisms that may accompany this infectious process.

Clindamycin is highly active against most anaerobic isolates with resistance rates among *Bacteroides* running at about 5 per cent. Some resistant isolates of *Clostridium* and *Fusobacterium* have been encountered, but they have been relatively uncommon in clinical practice. The drug is also active against streptococci, both aerobic and anaerobic, and most strains of *S. aureus.* It has very little activity against coliforms and other facultative gram-negative organisms, so a second drug is used in mixed anaerobic infections. Clindamycin has produced excellent results in intra-abdominal infections, female pelvic infections, and skin and soft tissue infections. Some authorities consider it the drug of choice for anaerobic pleuropulmonary infections, preferring it to penicillin because of apparent failures associated with penicillin treatment; however, this issue remains controversial. Erythromycin is less active than clindamycin, although resistance patterns commonly overlap. The problem with erythromycin is the difficulty in administering it parenterally. By the oral route only low serum levels of erythromycin are obtained, often below the amount needed to inhibit many anaerobic bacteria.

Tetracyclines were once touted as drugs of choice for anaerobic infections, but recently their performance against *Bacteroides* and many gram-negative cocci has considerably altered this view. Widespread tetracycline resistance has been noted in recent surveys. As a result, this class of compounds is not recommended for treatment of anaerobic infections. Chloramphenicol shows excellent activity in vitro against *Bacteroides* and most other anaerobic pathogens. It also has activity against coliforms, staphylococci, and streptococci. While some clinical trials have shown good results with chloramphenicol, others have encountered therapeutic failures. In addition, animal models of anaerobic infection have shown poor results with chloramphenicol treatment. Anaerobic organisms can inactivate chloramphenicol by at least two mechanisms, acetylation and nitroreduction. It is possible that one or both of these mechanisms is responsible for the occasional clinical failures with this drug.

Aminoglycoside antibiotics are uniformly inactive against nearly all anaerobic bacteria. These drugs are included in antimicrobial regimens for therapy of mixed infections, although their role is clearly to suppress the facultative gram-negative components.

PROGNOSIS. Prognosis of anaerobic infections is related to the site of infection, the type of pathogen, the underlying condition of the patient, and the choice of antimicrobial therapy. In general, anaerobic pleuropulmonary infections have a good outcome, especially when adequate drainage can be achieved. Penicillin G has been successful in treating these infections in the past, curing up to 95 per cent of patients with aspiration pneumonia or lung abscess, for example. Recently, some failures have been noted with penicillin, and in such instances clindamycin has been used to advantage. Metronidazole treatment has been associated with failures in lung abscess. In certain series poor outcomes are noted in 25 to 50 per cent of treated patients.

Severe intra-abdominal infections have a failure rate of 10 to 20 per cent even with optimal surgery and antimicrobial therapy. Higher failure rates in controlled clinical trials have been associated with treatment regimens using antimicrobial agents with poor activity against *B. fragilis* such as cephalothin, doxycycline, cefamandole, and cefoperazone. Infections of the female genital tract generally have a good prognosis since most patients tend to be rather healthy prior to the onset of the septic process. Good results have been reported with cefoxitin, clindamycin, and metronidazole, usually in association with another antibiotic. In one clinical trial penicillin combined with gentamicin produced a poor result in endomyometritis when compared with the alternative regimen of clindamycin and gentamicin.

In general, clinical trials with new antimicrobial agents have corroborated the findings in animal models and susceptibility testing in vitro. Because of the vast array of anaerobic organisms and their varying patterns of susceptibility, it is best to base empiric therapy on known sensitivity patterns and performance of the specific drugs in controlled clinical trials.

Bartlett JG, Finegold SM: Anaerobic infections of the lung and pleural space. Am Rev Respir Dis 110:56, 1974. *A comprehensive review of anaerobic pleuropulmonary infections, based on the authors' extensive personal experience.*

Bartlett JG, Louie TJ, Gorbach SL, Onderdonk AB: Therapeutic efficacy of 29 antimicrobial regimens in experimental intra-abdominal sepsis. Rev Infect Dis 3:535, 1981. *An experimental model of intra-abdominal infections that explains the pathophysiologic events and the rationale for antimicrobial treatments.*

Finegold SM: Anaerobic Bacteria in Human Disease. New York, Academic Press, 1977. *A compendium of information on various anaerobic bacteria and their disease manifestations.*

Gorbach SL, Bartlett JG: Medical progress: Anaerobic infections. N Engl J Med 290:1177, 1974. *The clinical and microbiologic features of anaerobic infections in many organ sites.*

Kasper DL, Weintraub A, Lindberg AA, Lonngren J: Capsular polysaccharides and lipopolysaccharides from two *Bacteroides fragilis* reference strains: Chemical and immunochemical characterization. J Bacteriol 153:991, 1983. *The chemical structure of the capsular polysaccharide, an important virulence factor of the preeminent pathogen,* Bacteroides fragilis. *This is not an article for the casual reader.*

Sweet RL: Anaerobic infections in the female genital tract. Am J Obstet Gynecol 122:891, 1975. *Good bacteriology and careful collection techniques provide the basis for this important study.*

Tally FP, Cuchural G, Jacobus NV, Gorbach SL, Aldridge KE, Cleary TJ, Finegold SM, Hill GB, Iannini PB, McCloskey RV, O'Keefe JP, Pierson CL: Susceptibility of the *Bacteroides fragilis* group in the United States in 1981. Antimicrob Agents Chemother 23:536, 1983. *A nationwide survey of antimicrobial sensitivities in this important pathogen.*

282. TYPHOID FEVER

Sherwood L. Gorbach

Typhoid ("cloudy") fever is a febrile illness of prolonged duration marked by hectic fever, delirium, enlargement of the spleen, abdominal pain, and a variety of systemic manifestations. Although caused primarily by *Salmonella typhi*, typhoidal disease occasionally is produced by other types of salmonellae. The portal of entry is the gastrointestinal tract, but typhoid fever is not truly an intestinal disease, having more systemic symptoms than those related to the bowel. There is a mortality of 1 to 5 per cent in drug-treated patients; the causes of death are intestinal perforation, hemorrhage, and severe toxemia.

EPIDEMIOLOGY. Improvements in environmental sanitation have reduced the incidence of typhoid fever in the industrialized nations. Approximately 500 cases occur each year in the United States, chiefly in young people. Most cases are sporadic, but are invariably related to a human carrier. The organism is essentially confined to humans, either in a disease state or as a carrier. Large-scale epidemics of typhoid occur on a regular basis, usually traced to contaminated food, which may be imported from an endemic area, or to contaminated water supplies. Another source of infection is the clinical bacteriology laboratory. Laboratory workers account for 2 to 5 per cent of typhoid cases each year.

Typhoid bacillus is a classic food- and waterborne pathogen. The major routes of passage are by the five F's: flies, fingers, food, feces, and fomites. *S. typhi* is extremely hardy and can survive for extended periods in polluted waters, contaminated foods, and soiled bedclothes.

Since *S. typhi* cohabits exclusively with man, the occurrence of a single case means the presence of a carrier. An investigation by public health authorities should be instituted to determine the source and the presence of other cases. Chronic carriers, as they are discovered, are registered with the health authorities. However, registered carriers represent only a minority of the potential reservoir and do not take account of the "imported" cases of typhoid, which include nearly half of the acute infections in the United States.

PATHOGENESIS AND PATHOLOGY. The pathologic events of typhoid fever are initiated in the intestinal tract following oral ingestion of typhoid bacilli. The organism penetrates the small bowel mucosa, sparing the stomach, and makes its way rapidly to the lymphatics, the mesenteric nodes, and, within minutes, to the bloodstream. There is a paucity of local inflammatory findings, which explains the lack of intestinal symptoms at this stage. This sequence of events is in marked contrast to that of other forms of salmonellosis and to shigellosis in which the intestinal findings are prominent at the onset.

The organism must survive passage through the stomach, warding off the destructive action of gastric acid. Food and beverages, the classic vehicles of typhoid fever, also serve as an excellent buffer to acid. The number of bacilli ingested is a critical determinant of infection. An inoculum of 10^9 bacilli produces disease in 95 per cent of apparently healthy people, whereas 10^3 organisms rarely cause symptoms. The higher the inoculum size, the shorter the incubation period.

Following the initial bacteremia, the organism is sequestered in macrophages and monocytic cells of the reticuloendothelial system. It undergoes multiplication, and re-emerges several days later in recurrent waves of bacteremia, an event which initiates the symptomatic phase of infection. Now in great numbers, the organism is spread throughout the host, infecting many organ sites. The intestinal tract may be seeded by direct bacteremic spread, as, for example, to Peyer's patches in the terminal ileum. Alternatively, the gallbladder contains a large number of bacilli, and contaminated bile is another method of infecting the gut.

Hyperplasia of the reticuloendothelial system, including lymph nodes, liver, and spleen, is characteristic of typhoid fever. The liver contains discrete, micronodular areas of necrosis, surrounded by macrophages and lymphocytes. Inflammation of the gallbladder is common, and may lead to acute cholecystitis. Patients with pre-existing gallbladder disease have a penchant for becoming carriers, because the bacillus becomes intimately associated with the chronic infection and may be incorporated within the gallstones themselves. Lymphoid follicles in the gut, such as Peyer's patches, become hyperplastic, with infiltration of macrophages, lymphocytes, and red blood cells. Subsequently, a follicle may ulcerate and penetrate through the submucosa to the intestinal lumen, discharging in its wake large numbers of typhoid bacilli. As the bowel wall is progressively involved, it becomes paper-thin, and is susceptible to transmural perforation into the peritoneal cavity. This occurs most commonly in the distal ileum, 25 cm from the ileocecal sphincter. Erosion into blood vessels produces severe intestinal hemorrhage.

An analogy has been drawn between the biologic effects of endotoxin and typhoid fever. Both cause chills, fever, headache, nausea, and vomiting, as well as the laboratory findings of leukopenia and thrombocytopenia. With endotoxin, however, increasing doses produce a state of tolerance in which further administration has no effect. By contrast, typhoid fever is a relentless and sustained state of illness. Administration of viable typhoid organisms to volunteers rendered tolerant to endotoxin still produces symptoms. Thus typhoid fever cannot be explained merely as a reaction to endotoxin, although this material may play some role in the disease state.

CLINICAL MANIFESTATIONS. Typhoid fever lasts about four weeks, evolving in a manner consistent with the pathophysiologic events. Classically, the illness is described as a series of one-week stages. Although in general the illness follows such a pattern, individual cases may deviate significantly, and the illness may persist (with accompanying bacteremia) with only slight improvement for four weeks or more. The *incubation period* is generally 7 to 14 days, with wide variations on either extreme. During the *first week*, the triad of fever, headache, and abdominal pain is commonly encountered. The onset usually is insidious with a stepladder rise of fever which later becomes persistent. It is accompanied by a dull headache. The pulse is often slower than would be expected for the degree of temperature elevation. Abdominal pain is localized to the right lower quadrant in most instances, although it can be diffuse. In approximately 50 per cent of patients, there is no change in bowel habits; in fact, constipation is more common than diarrhea in children. Near the end of the first week, enlargement of the spleen is noticeable. An evanescent and classic rash, "rose spots," becomes manifest at this time. It is observed in approximately 70 per cent of whites, but considerably less frequently in dark-skinned persons. Rose spots are deeply red, 2- to 4-mm macules, often present in clusters, blanching on pressure; they occur most often on the upper anterior abdominal wall and lower thorax. During the *second week*, the fever becomes more continuous. The patient looks sick and withdrawn, although he may be fully responsive. In some, marked deterioration in the mental condition, lassitude, delirium, and even coma may develop. Cough is commonly present and epistaxis is not infrequent. During the *third week*, the patient's illness continues in the "typhoidal state." There may be disoriented mentation and, in some cases, extreme toxemia. In this period there may be intestinal involvement, manifested clinically by greenish "pea-soup" diarrhea and the dire complications of intestinal perforation and hemorrhage. The *fourth week* usually but not invariably brings slackening of the fever and improvement in clinical status. The patient becomes more interested in the surroundings. There is significant weight loss, anemia, and profound fatigue. Typhoid fever is among the longest and most debilitating of microbial diseases.

Typhoid fever is a less severe illness in previously healthy persons who seek medical attention for the earliest symptoms of fever, lassitude, and headache. Prompt diagnosis and appropriate therapy interrupt the classic four-week scenario, producing an aborted illness consisting of little more than a few days of fever and malaise. Such patients should receive 14 days of antimicrobial therapy, but early discharge from the hospital can be considered, with the completion of drug treatment accomplished on an outpatient basis.

COMPLICATIONS. Since the typhoid bacillus is widely disseminated through recurrent waves of bacteremia, many organ sites are involved. Pneumonia occurs in 10 per cent of patients, although cough, without radiographic findings, is encountered in approximately two thirds. Rarely there is a small pleural effusion. During the severe toxemic phase, patients may aspirate gastric contents and develop a suppurative pneumonia. Severe headache, delirium, and even coma are often noted, but suppurative disease of the brain and meninges is quite uncommon, being seen in less than 1 per cent of patients. Typhoid pyelonephritis associated with renal pain, hematuria, and pyuria is occasionally encountered. The gallbladder and liver are often involved with inflammatory changes. Acute cholecystitis can occur during the initial period of typhoid fever. Jaundice, on the basis of diffuse hepatic inflammation, has been observed in some patients. The microorganism may spread to bone, especially ribs and spine, and to the large joints. Nerve deafness, conjunctivitis, keratitis, and optic neuritis have all been seen on rare occasions.

Although the litany of organ site involvement is long, the pre-eminent complications are intestinal hemorrhage and perforation. These events are most apt to occur in the third week and during convalescence and are not closely related to the severity of the disease. However, they tend to occur in the same patient, with the bleeding serving as a warning of a possible perforation to come. Bleeding may be sudden and severe, or a slow ooze. Prior to chemotherapy, the incidence of hemorrhage was 7 to 20 per cent in various series; it is somewhat less frequent since specific treatment has been available. The ileum is the main site of bowel perforation. The onset may be sudden with signs of acute abdominal distress. Or there may be a leak of intraluminal contents to form an abscess in the lower quadrant or pelvis, producing a more chronic, insidious course. Approximately 3 per cent of patients with typhoid fever will experience intestinal perforation.

RELAPSE. After defervescence has occurred and the patient has apparently "ridden through the storm," there remains a potential for recurrence. The relapse generally occurs eight to ten days after cessation of drug therapy and consists of a reenactment of the major manifestations such as fever, chills, skin rash, and bacteremia. Early chemotherapy of the initial infection may increase the potential for relapse because it prevents the development of natural immunity, an important feature in eventually controlling the organism within the host.

CARRIERS. After six weeks, approximately 50 per cent of typhoid victims are still shedding the organism in their feces. This figure progressively declines so that after three months only 5 to 10 per cent are excreters. A chronic carrier is defined as a person with stool cultures positive for *S. typhi* at least one year following an episode of typhoid or, in some cases, positive stool cultures without a documented history of disease. The possibility of spontaneously aborting the carrier state is very unlikely after this time. Chronic carriers are more common in older age groups, in women (a 3:1 ratio of women to men), and in people with gallbladder disease. The organism usually is harbored in the gallbladder, often forming part of gallstones, and persists in a noninflammatory symbiotic relationship with the host, causing neither local inflammation nor systemic symptoms. Occasionally, the gallbladder is free of the organism, and it is apparently carried in the large bowel. In the usual case, the bile contains enormous numbers of bacilli, up to 10^9 per milliliter, and they are discharged in the feces in varying concentrations. The organisms are viable and fully infective, so the carrier may be a source of new infection.

LABORATORY FINDINGS AND DIAGNOSIS. Many laboratory features of typhoid fever are consistent with prolonged sepsis. A normochromic, normocytic anemia persists throughout the infection; it may be made worse by intestinal blood loss or a reaction of the bone marrow to agents such as chloramphenicol. Thrombocytopenia occurs during the initial hectic period of the disease. Leukopenia is characteristic of the first week of illness, with the major depression in polymorphonuclear leukocytes.

The definitive diagnosis of typhoid fever is established by isolating the organism. During the first week, blood cultures are positive in 90 per cent of patients. If the clinical illness persists essentially unimproved, the bacteremia likewise persists, and the blood culture may be positive for several weeks or more. The blood culture thus is the primary diagnostic test. Stool cultures usually become positive in the second and third weeks when the organisms are shed from the lymphoid follicles of the intestinal wall. During the third week, urine culture yields typhoid bacilli in approximately 30 per cent of patients. Rose spots harbor the organism, and they can be sampled by small skin snips of the lesion that are cultured in nutrient broth. These are positive in two thirds of patients. A most useful source is the bone marrow, which is positive for *S. typhi* in 90 per cent of patients, even when they have received some antimicrobial therapy.

The titer of agglutinins (Widal test) against somatic (O) and flagellar (H) antigens rises during the third week of illness. An O titer of 1:80 or more in nonimmunized individuals is suggestive of typhoid fever. Higher initial titers or a four-fold rise provides stronger evidence. The H antigen is more nonspecific, and is likely to be elevated from prior immunization or infection by other enteric bacteria. There are many false-positive and occasional false-negative Widal reactions so that a diagnosis based on titer rises alone is tenuous.

DIFFERENTIAL DIAGNOSIS. In endemic regions the most perplexing diagnosis is between typhoid fever and malaria, because both diseases can cause fever, chills, splenomegaly, and neutropenia. Travelers to such areas may acquire either disease so that they present with the same diagnostic dilemma. Blood smears usually are positive in malaria, and typhoid is identified by isolating the organism in culture or, as an early clue, a positive Widal reaction. In certain parts of the world, Lassa fever or dengue is a diagnostic alternative. Other salmonellae can mimic typhoid fever. Among bacterial infections which may be confused with typhoid, tuberculosis, shigellosis, leptospirosis, and bacteremias associated with cholecystitis and pyelonephritis should be given consideration. Viral agents such as infectious mononucleosis and infectious hepatitis can present similar symptoms. Patients having delirium or coma with normal cerebrospinal fluid may be thought to have viral encephalitis rather than typhoid fever. Rickettsial diseases may be considered, but the absence of a characteristic rash would militate against this diagnosis.

TREATMENT. Drug resistance, mediated by plasmids, can occur among typhoid bacilli. Most strains are susceptible to chloramphenicol and ampicillin, although notable epidemics with strains resistant to either of these drugs have been reported in recent years. Hence, a great effort should be made in each case to isolate the organism and to perform drug susceptibility tests. Chloramphenicol remains the standard therapy because of its proved efficacy and its high activity against most clinical isolates of typhoid bacilli. The response to therapy is remarkably constant, as defervescence regularly occurs three to five days after initiating treatment. The clinical condition improves within one to two days, with decreased toxemia and slowly declining fever. In adults, chloramphenicol should be given in a total daily dose of 2 to 4 grams, administered in four equally divided doses. Occasionally in very sick patients it may be necessary to give the drug by the intravenous route, and the total daily dose of 2 to 4 grams should be used. Oral medication can then be given after improvement in the clinical status. Chloramphenicol is well absorbed from the intestinal tract, but is rather poorly absorbed from intramuscular sites. Thus the intramuscular route is to be avoided. The duration of treatment is two weeks; prolongation of this treatment does not reduce the incidence of complications or carriers. Intestinal perforation and hemorrhage can occur during what is apparently successful treatment. Relapse may follow an otherwise uneventful course and should be treated with the same drug.

Ampicillin has been recommended as alternative therapy, but it has been somewhat disappointing in comparison with chloramphenicol. The dose is 6 grams per day, intravenously, in four to six divided doses. Amoxicillin, a closely related drug, provides better absorption and increased efficacy. Several studies have shown that amoxicillin, in doses of 4 grams per day in four divided doses, has good activity, but is somewhat less effective than chloramphenicol. Sulfamethoxazole-trimethoprim has also been used effectively in the therapy of typhoid fever in a dose of 800 mg (sulfamethoxazole) and 160 mg (trimethoprim) twice daily for 14 days.

Corticosteroids are administered for severe toxemia and fever, and may produce a dramatic response in the patient with profound sepsis. The treatment should be given in high doses, 60 mg per day of prednisone divided in four doses, and rapidly tapered over the next three days. The wide experience with steroid treatment has failed to show any adverse effects, although the potentiality for masking intestinal perforation is still present. Thus steroids are best reserved for patients with severe toxicity.

Intestinal perforation is managed by standard surgical practices. All patients should be treated with nasogastric suction. Indications for operation are progressive peritoneal signs or localization of an abscess. Simple closure of the perforation is the treatment of choice. However, the ileum may be riddled with multiple perforations, and resection or exteriorization of the intestinal loop may be required.

Good nursing care plays a major role in the recovery from typhoid fever. The pyrexia can be managed with tepid baths and sponging. Salicylates and antipyretics should be used judiciously as they cause severe sweating and may lower the blood pressure.

A chronic carrier, who has been discharging *S. typhi* for longer than one year, can be treated with antimicrobials in an attempt to eliminate the infection. One regimen that works in approximately two thirds of patients is 6 grams of ampicillin per day in four divided doses for six weeks. Alternative drugs are amoxicillin and sulfamethoxazole-trimethoprim. Reappearance of the carrier state following such treatment is generally associated with gallbladder disease. In persons with gallstones or chronic cholecystitis, cholecystectomy eliminates the carrier state in 85 per cent. This procedure, however, is recommended only for those whose profession is not compatible with the typhoid carrier state, i.e., food handlers and health care providers.

PROGNOSIS. Prior to antimicrobial therapy, the case mortality of typhoid fever was around 10 to 15 per cent. The introduction of chloramphenicol has reduced this to 1 per cent, and most patients now succumb to either perforation or hemorrhage. However, in areas of the world with poor nutrition and limited medical facilities, the mortality rate may be higher. Factors that influence a lethal outcome are severity of the disease at time of admission (coma is a poor prognostic sign); age, with the very young and the very old being at greatest risk; and first infection, because a second attack, although uncommon, is less severe than the primary episode.

PROPHYLAXIS. For control of intrahospital spread, enteric precautions should be initiated; fecal, urine, and blood specimens should be disposed of by double-bag techniques and always handled with gloves. Additional precautions are unwarranted.

The currently available typhoid vaccine affords only 70 per cent protection and is associated with a high incidence of side effects, mostly at the site of injection. It is only recommended for high-risk situations and should not be given for short-term travel. Since the major forces of immunity act at the intestinal mucosal surface, an oral vaccine would offer theoretical advantages. A double mutant typhoid strain, Ty21a, lacking UDP-galactose-4-epimerase, has been developed by Professor Rene Germanier. This avirulent oral vaccine has undergone extensive field trials in Egypt and Chile. Not only has the vaccine been proven safe, it has shown a remarkable efficacy, 96 per cent, in preventing natural disease in an endemic area. A commercial product should be available sometime in the future.

Hoffman SL, Punjabi NH, Kumala S, Moechtar A, Pulungsih SP, Rivai AR, Rockhill RC, Woodward TE, Loedin AA: Reduction of mortality in chloramphenicol-treated typhoid fever by high dose dexamethasone. N Engl J Med 310:82, 1984. *In typhoid patients with delerium, obtundation, stupor, coma, or shock, dexamethasone therapy was highly efficacious.*

Hoffman TA, Ruiz CJ, Counts GW, Sachs JM, Nitskiu JL: Waterborne typhoid fever in Dade County, Florida: Clinical and therapeutic evaluation in 105 bacteremic patients. Am J Med 59:481, 1975. *Good account of an epidemic. The illness was generally mild. Chloramphenicol seemed to be superior to ampicillin for therapy.*

Hornick RB, Greisman SE, Woodward TE, DuPont HL, Dawkins AT, Snyder MJ: Typhoid fever: Pathogenesis and immunologic control. N Engl J Med 283:686, 739, 1970. *A good account of pathophysiology, including a discussion of the role of endotoxin. Human volunteer studies are reviewed.*

Johnson WD Jr, Hook EW, Lindsey E, Kaye D: Treatment of chronic typhoid carriers with ampicillin. Antimicrob Agents Chemother 3:439, 1973. *Using large doses of ampicillin orally, these authors cured ten chronic typhoid carriers.*

Kim J-P, Oh S-K, Jarret F: Management of ileal perforation due to typhoid fever. Ann Surg 181:88, 1975. *A life-threatening complication can be managed successfully by judicious surgical intervention.*

Pillay N, Adams EB, North-Coombes D: Comparative trial of amoxycillin and chloramphenicol in treatment of typhoid fever in adults. Lancet 2:333, 1975. *In a randomized clinical trial with 124 typhoid patients, chloramphenicol and amoxicillin performed equally well.*

Snyder MJ, Gonzalez O, Palomino C, Music SI, Hornick RB, Perroni J, Woodward WE, Gonzales C, Dupont HL, Woodward TE: Comparative efficacy of chloramphenicol, ampicillin, and co-trimoxazole in the treatment of typhoid fever. Lancet 2:1155, 1976. *Chloramphenicol was the superior agent for reduction of fever. Intravenous administration appears to be better than oral.*

Wahdan MH, Serie C, Cerisier Y, Sallam S, Germanier R: A controlled field trial of live *Salmonella typhi* strain Ty21a oral vaccine against typhoid: Three-year results. J Infect Dis 145:292, 1982. *An important vaccine, not only for excellent activity against an ancient enemy, typhoid fever, but also because this is the first oral bacterial vaccine.*

Wicks CB, Holmes GS, Davidson L: Endemic typhoid fever. Quart J Med 159:341, 1971. *Excellent compilation of clinical and laboratory findings in 265 patients with typhoid fever in Rhodesia.*

283. SALMONELLA INFECTIONS OTHER THAN TYPHOID FEVER

Richard B. Hornick

DEFINITION. Salmonellae comprise a large group of gram-negative bacilli that can cause a broad spectrum of disease in man and animals. The most common disorder in humans is gastroenteritis or salmonellosis, usually a mild, self-limited diarrheal illness. Systemic spread from the gut is unusual. Other patients may develop septicemia, a stubborn infection for the host to eradicate, even with antimicrobial therapy. Localized infections may present in the form of osteomyelitis, mycotic aneurysms, or abscesses. The unique human pathogen *S. typhi* produces enteric fever, an illness also caused by several other select *Salmonella* species. A prolonged carrier state which mimics that seen following infection with *S. typhi*, may result from *Salmonella* infections.

Many animals suffer fatal diarrheal disease caused by species of salmonellae that infect only animals. Some animals have an asymptomatic infection caused by strains that infect both humans and animals. Meat and eggs and other animal-derived food products serve as the most important source of infections in humans.

ETIOLOGY. Salmonellae are motile, gram-negative bacilli that do not ferment lactose or sucrose but metabolize glucose, maltose, and mannitol. They grow readily on many media.

Enrichment and transport media are useful for obtaining an increased yield from stool cultures, especially those collected as part of an epidemiologic survey.

Salmonellae contain a thick and complex lipopolysaccharide cell wall. This cell wall is the O antigen, made up of several specific O antigen types. The specificity of each of the O antigens is determined by the arrangement of the repeating sequence of sugars that constitute the outer layer of the cell wall. Strains lacking the outer layer are characterized as "rough" because of the wrinkled surface of the colonies. Such strains appear to be nonpathogenic. Antibodies directed at the R core protect against infections caused by many gram-negative bacilli. The inner or basal layer is the lipid moiety, a bridging structure between the outer two layers and the foundation of the cell wall. This whole substance is the endotoxin, the ubiquitous lipopolysaccharide material of all gram-negative bacilli that causes fever plus other severe host reactions during active disease.

There are at least 60 specific O-antigen complexes. Group-specific antibodies can be used to classify salmonellae into many serotypes. The H antigens are the flagellae of the organisms. Serotyping, using O and H antisera plus biochemical tests, has established the presence of at least 1700 species. A simplified characterization has been suggested based on host preferences and adaptations: (1) *Salmonella* serotypes highly adapted to man. These include *S. typhi, S. paratyphi A, S. schottmülleri* (paratyphi B), *S. hirschfeldii* (paratyphi C), and *S. sendai.* There is no animal reservoir for these strains, animal infection is rare, and accidental and human-to-human transmission is critical in the epidemiology of the disease they produce. (2) *Salmonella* serotypes highly adapted to specific nonhuman hosts. Most strains cause only illness in animals. *S. dublin* from cattle and *S. choleraesuis* from swine are two exceptions that often cause human disease. (3) *Salmonella* serotypes unadapted to specific hosts. This is a large group (>1400 strains), ubiquitous in nature, that usually causes gastroenteritis, rarely invades the bloodstream, and is responsible for about 85 per cent of all *Salmonella* infections in the United States. It is the strains within this last group that will be mainly discussed in this chapter. The most common serotypes involved in human disease are *S. typhimurium* (accounts for about 25 to 30 per cent of all cases), *S. enteritidis, S. heidelberg, S. newport, S. infantis, S. agona, S. montevideo, S. saint-paul,* and *S. javiana. Salmonella* infections are reportable diseases, and the ranking listed comes from the annual compilation published by the Centers for Disease Control.

EPIDEMIOLOGY. Humans ingest salmonellae primarily in contaminated food, less frequently in water, and in rare instances from exotic sources. Salmonellae can infect many species of animals. Those of greatest potential as a human health hazard are meat-producing animals and poultry. Eggs and egg products have been a consistent source of salmonellae. The organisms can be incorporated into the egg before the shell is completely calcified in the chicken, or the egg becomes contaminated during its expulsion from the chicken. Cracked or dirty eggs should raise a suspicion regarding contamination with salmonellae. An egg containing salmonellae requires at least three minutes of boiling to ensure complete bacterial killing. Poultry may become infected, have no significant disease, and yet be fecal shedders. During the processing of poultry, the carcasses may become surface contaminated from water baths or conveyer belts that were colonized by previously processed birds. Consumers handling such poultry products are at risk of infection. The organisms persist on the fingers for several hours and can be transferred to foods that can serve as culture media for further multiplication. The meat of animals usually does not contain abscesses, nor are the salmonellae isolated from mesenteric lymph nodes of meat-producing animals. Thus, most salmonellae are found on the surface of the meats and represent skin colonization from the contaminated surfaces of the processing plant. Raw milk is a persistent source of *S. dublin* for consumers. Up to 10 per cent of healthy cattle may carry this species.

Pet turtles have been an important source of salmonella infections in this country. Chickens and cattle can deposit ample salmonellae into the soil upon which the turtles feed. The legs of the common housefly can carry salmonellae, which they apparently acquire while feeding on feces. Transmission to human food is a possible but not a likely event. Carmine red dye, derived from female scale insects and larvae, has caused hospital epidemics of salmonellosis. The tainted dye was given to patients to determine intestinal transit time. Such dye has been used to color food, cosmetics, and drugs. Recently, an outbreak of salmonellosis occurred among teenagers and young adults using marijuana contaminated with *S. muenchen,* an organism isolated from poultry, swine, and cattle.

Human-to-human spread via contaminated food or water is the second most common means of transmitting salmonellae. Transient or convalescent carriers have frequently been the source of large foodborne outbreaks of gastroenteritis. Improper hand washing, inadequate refrigeration of prepared foods prior to serving, and insufficient cooking of poultry products have been common epidemiologic features of outbreaks occurring after large public feasts.

Most cases of salmonellosis occurring in healthy adults are of little medical significance. However, outbreaks in nursing homes or nurseries cause severe morbidity and unnecessary mortality. Epidemics may arise owing to contaminated hospital food; cross-infections have been documented in pediatric wards resulting from contaminated fingers or clothes of attending personnel or via aerosols from sick infants. A rare source of infection by *S. kottbus* has been infected breast milk. This unusual strain was being excreted by the donor of the milk. Faulty refrigeration allowed for multiplication of this species in the milk.

The most common form of illness produced is salmonellosis, a diarrheal disease. Children have the greatest incidence (median age, ten years), and the highest rate is in infants. In the United States, this disease occurs most frequently in the summer and early fall.

The epidemiologic characteristics of other strains causing systemic infection are also varied. *S. choleraesuis,* which is associated with swine and pork products, is an unusual isolate in the United States but is the predominant cause of localized or enteric fever syndromes. Children with this strain may develop a moderately severe form of enteric fever. Infected adults are more likely to present with bacteremia or localized infectious conditions such as abscesses in deep muscle groups, osteomyelitis, or mycotic aneurysms. This difference may be due to partial immunity developed in the adults and resulting from previous subclinical infections.

Enteric fever may be produced by *S. paratyphi A and B.* These are unusual infections in this country but are common in late-developing countries where typhoid fever is also prevalent. Patients with enteric fever induced by *S. paratyphi B* frequently respond less promptly to antibiotic treatment than do patients with typhoid fever.

PATHOLOGY. *Salmonella*-induced gastroenteritis causes death rarely. Infants and the aged are at the greatest risk. Death usually occurs as a result of the secondary effects of dehydration caused by the diarrhea. Intestinal mucosa is red and swollen and often shows petechial hemorrhages. Salmonellae induce a polymorphonuclear leukocyte infiltration in the lamina propria region. The organisms reach that area by penetrating through the epithelial cell layer. Those patients suffering from bacteremia or localized disease have collections of neutrophils in the areas of bacterial localizations. In contrast, *S. typhi* induces mononuclear cell responses in the liver or in the lamina propria and at sites of intestinal perforation. These differences in cellular responses may be due to small concentrations of endotoxin present at the sites of *S. typhi* multiplication.

PATHOGENESIS. Ingested salmonellae must penetrate through the epithelial cell layer in order to produce disease.

Stomach acid is an effective barrier to large inocula reaching the small and large intestine, where disease is initiated. Persons who are taking antacids, or who have achlorhydria because of drugs, marijuana use, surgery, or age, are at increased risk of acquiring salmonellae or other enteric pathogens. Passage through the stomach appears to be facilitated by ingestion of the bacilli in a small volume of fluid (50 ml or less). This small volume is not retained in the stomach. Nonspecific defense mechanisms in the small and large bowel such as rapid transit time, inactivation by enzymes or lysozymes, and nosocomial bacteria may decrease the number of bacteria able to penetrate through the epithelial cells.

Once the bacteria reach the lamina propria area, further penetration into the lymphatics or capillaries is impeded by the involved inflammatory response. Presumably the polymorphonuclear leukocytes effectively phagocytize and eliminate these salmonellae. Rarely does bacteremia occur in patients manifesting a diarrheal disease. Bacteremia is a more frequent event in children than in adults and may be due to a relatively incompetent immune system in the lamina propria.

The watery stools elicited by the ingestion of salmonellae probably originate in the upper small intestine, a section which has a great secretory capacity. An enterotoxin stimulates the secretion of electrolytes and fluid into the lumen. This process is similar to that associated with diarrhea induced by enterotoxigenic *E. coli.* No penetration occurs; the toxin is released on the surface of the cells and activates adenylate cyclase; secretion of chloride and sodium ions results. The inflammatory process associated with penetration in the ileum may cause diarrheal disease characterized by stools of smaller volume. These presumably result from the lesser capacity of the ileum to secrete fluid and perhaps from failure to absorb all the fluid presented to the inflamed ileum. The secretion in the ileum may be stimulated by the enterotoxins, by prostaglandins released from the inflammatory exudate, or by both. This latter mediator also activates the adenylate cyclase energy system. A smear of a small specimen of stool stained with methylene blue will reveal large numbers of neutrophils. These are indicative of involvement of the large bowel in the inflammatory process initiated by salmonellae.

The number of organisms necessary to induce gastroenteritis in man is largely unknown. Limited studies in volunteers have suggested that large doses of *S. typhimurium,* e.g., 10 million to 1 billion cells, are required to cause disease. Whether such large doses are involved in naturally occurring outbreaks is unknown. The incubation period falls within a relatively narrow range—12 to 24 hours. An inverse relationship between the size of the inoculum and the length of the incubation period probably exists, but evidence for this is lacking. The other members of the *Salmonella* genus that cause enteric fever or localized disease are ingested in the same fashion and presumably penetrate within a similar time frame, but symptoms and signs of disease do not appear for many days. During the incubation period, systemic spread is occurring and multiplication of the pathogens in the reticuloendothelial system and other organs proceeds until the spreading infection exceeds the defense mechanisms and disease is apparent. The short incubation period of salmonellosis suggests that this infection is superficial in the gut and causes disease through quick-acting substances such as enterotoxins. The self-limiting nature is consistent with rapid clearing mechanisms, e.g., short life span of the epithelial cells and efficient cellular clearing systems in the lamina propria.

Certain patients with chronic diseases are prone to *Salmonella* infections. There is a predilection for patients with sickle cell disease to develop septicemia or localized *Salmonella* infection. Osteomyelitis caused by one of the *Salmonella* strains is especially common. These patients are deficient in opsonizing capabilities, have reduced numbers of phagocytes in the spleen and elsewhere, and sustain bone and gut infarcts. Taken together, these changes can permit an easy access of salmonellae through the gut, an ability to survive in the circulation and to establish an infection in the bone. Patients with acute hemolytic processes caused by bartonellosis and malaria have an increased incidence of salmonellosis. Diseases that impair cellular immune mechanisms, e.g., leukemias and lymphomas, are associated with a high incidence of salmonellal septicemic infections. *S. typhimurium* has been one of the most frequently isolated strains from such patients. Patients with chronic *Schistosoma haematobium* infections of the genitourinary tract are prone to have chronic bacteriuria and bacteremia caused by *S. typhi* and *S. paratyphi* strains. Such patients may be chronic carriers, but also the associated obstruction of a ureter or calcification in the bladder contributes to the persistent *Salmonella* infection. Treatment of the schistosomiasis as well as the bacterial infection can be curative.

The pathogenesis of the chronic asymptomatic carrier state caused by salmonellae other than *S. typhi* is not clearly understood. A few persons will have chronic low grade infection in a diseased gallbladder identical to the typhoid carrier state. The paratyphi strains are involved in this manner. However, for those strains causing salmonellosis, carriage may persist for many months without evidence of biliary tract dysfunction. Some of those patients have received unnecessary antibiotic therapy for their diarrhea, and this can prolong the carrier state. In mice, the antibiotic eliminates part of the nosocomial flora that normally inhibits the colonization and multiplication of salmonellae. The mechanism involves the acid environment associated with the production of short chain fatty acids by the normal flora. This explanation, if applicable to the human situation, suggests that chronic carriage occurs primarily in the intestinal tract. Rarely will these patients shed salmonellae beyond eight months.

CLINICAL MANIFESTATIONS. ***Gastroenteritis.*** Gastroenteritis begins abruptly with nausea and crampy abdominal pain followed by the onset of diarrhea. The stools are watery, initially in large volume, and occasionally will contain mucus and a trace of blood. A smaller number of patients will have paste-like or semisolid stools that are associated with cramps in the lower quadrants. These stools are likely to contain mucus and blood, and white cells are seen on a methylene blue–stained specimen. Vomiting is not frequent and, if present, does not persist throughout the period of the diarrhea. Fever of 38.5 to 39° C is seen in 50 to 70 per cent of patients. Chills are noted in about 30 per cent of patients. Physical findings are few and relate to the inflammatory process in the gastrointestinal tract. Palpation tenderness resulting from contraction of loops of bowel is present but in variable locations of the abdominal cavity. Duration of symptoms in otherwise healthy adults is about two to five days. The disease persists for a longer period in patients debilitated by extremes of age, malignancy, or antibiotic or steroid therapy.

The symptoms and signs of enteric fever have been described for typhoid fever. An identical presentation is associated with disease produced by paratyphi strains.

Bacteremia. Patients with this form of salmonellal disease have a history of fever, chills, sweats, malaise, anorexia, and weight loss for several days to a week or more. Stool cultures may not reveal salmonellae, but blood cultures will be positive. A search for the source of bacteremia is mandatory but often unrewarding. Osteomyelitis, mycotic aneurysm or infection of a pre-existing aneurysm (abdominal aorta or femoral artery are common sites), pericarditis (minimal amount of exudate present), abscesses, arthritis, meningitis, pneumonia, and hepatitis are all representative of localized infections with bacteremia. Patients with solid tumors may have abscesses in these lesions that serve as a source of *Salmonella* bacteremia. Pheochromocytoma, ovarian cyst, renal cell carcinoma, uterine myomas and metastatic tumors to bone or skin are common examples of such tumors.

The isolation of *S. choleraesuis* from the blood of an adult is usually indicative of an abscess.

DIAGNOSIS. The diagnosis of any form of *Salmonella* infection is confirmed by isolation of the organism from blood or stool or both. Other isolations can be made from liver, abscesses, or localized infections when systemic disease is present. Fresh diarrheal stool specimens should be cultured. Serologic information is not helpful for salmonellosis but is useful for the systemic infections, especially enteric fever. About 65 to 70 per cent of patients with enteric fever will have a four-fold or greater increase in O and/or H antibody titers over a two- to three-week span.

Patients with gastroenteritis will have a normal white blood cell count. Hemoconcentration may occur with significant fluid loss. A smear of the diarrheal stool stained with methylene blue will often reveal numerous leukocytes, indicating colitis. Similar findings are noted with other bacteria that invade epithelial cells, e.g., *Shigella*, *Campylobacter*, *Yersinia*.

The differential diagnosis of *Salmonella* gastroenteritis includes a broad spectrum of enteric pathogens: enterotoxigenic *E. coli* (heat-stable and heat-labile toxins), *Campylobacter fetus subspecies jejuni*, *Vibrio parahaemolyticus*, *Shigella* species, *Yersinia enterocolitica*, and other bacteria associated with food-induced diarrhea. The diarrheal syndromes produced by these organisms can mimic that caused by salmonellae. Causation can be speculated on the basis of historical facts (seafood—*Vibrio parahaemolyticus;* refried rice—*B. cereus*), but confirmation requires cultural proof. Viral agents such as the parvoviruses and rotovirus can also cause the same illness; however, the highest attack rate is in infants and children. Isolation techniques for these viruses are not readily available. Unfortunately, most patients with infectious diarrhea have almost recovered from their illness when culture results are available. In certain patients, e.g., those with persistent diarrhea or those debilitated by other illness, specific cultural information is necessary to prescribe appropriate therapy. More rapid culture techniques are needed.

TREATMENT. Fluid replacement is the uniform approach to treatment of any patient with a diarrheal illness. It is especially critical in the management of patients who cannot readily tolerate a reduction in plasma volume. In most adults with salmonellosis, self-treatment with tolerated liquids is usually satisfactory. Fruit juices, broths, tea, and water are useful. Milk should be used with caution. In children an acquired lactase deficiency during the diarrhea is common, and milk can therefore prolong the diarrheal state because of the osmotic effect of undigested lactose. Intravenous fluids are necessary only for severely dehydrated patients unable to take oral replacement fluid because of nausea and vomiting.

Antibiotic treatment is not required to treat salmonellosis. Selected patients may benefit. Infants and elderly nursing-home patients who are known to be at greatest risk of mortality from this infection should be treated. A short course (three to five days) of ampicillin (4 to 6 grams per day) or amoxicillin (2 to 4 grams per day) may be used in adults. Sensitivity of the isolate to various antibiotics should be ascertained, since ampicillin-resistant strains are becoming increasingly common. Trimethoprim-sulfamethoxazole or chloramphenicol is an effective alternative. Antibiotic treatment will prolong the excretion of salmonellae in the stools and may not shorten the clinical course of the patient's illness. Adults usually recover without antibiotic therapy in two to five days.

The uncomfortable abdominal cramps may be relieved with atropine or drugs with a similar smooth muscle relaxing effect. However, such drugs have an antiperistaltic effect which can prolong the diarrhea. Thus, these drugs should be used intermittently for relief of pain only.

The treatment of the systemic forms of *Salmonella* infection requires appropriate antibiotic therapy. The approach is similar to that for typhoid fever. Three drugs have been generally effective: chloramphenicol, trimethoprim-sulfamethoxazole, and ampicillin or amoxicillin. Drainage of abscesses is mandatory. Resection of infected aneurysms is indicated, but the surgical results have been poor. Antibiotic coverage is required before, during, and after surgery.

PROGNOSIS. Gastroenteritis is a mild self-limiting infection, and recovery is complete in several days. Complications are mainly related to consequences of dehydration, e.g., azotemia, stroke, or myocardial infarction, occurring in those patients with significant arteriosclerosis or tenuous fluid balance. Mortality occurs in infants and the elderly. In some epidemics in nurseries or nursing homes, the rate has been 3 to 5 per cent. Immunity to reinfection is incomplete and repeated episodes of salmonellosis will occur following re-exposure.

The prognosis for patients with bacteremic forms of salmonellae may be poor, since many of these patients have underlying diseases. The mortality with *S. choleraesuis* infections has been reported to be as high as 20 per cent. Infants with meningitis have a mortality of 40 per cent, and residual neurologic defects are common.

PREVENTION. There is no vaccine to prevent gastroenteritis or the systemic forms of *Salmonella* infection. Typhoid fever prevention is possible with a new oral attenuated vaccine strain. Careful attention to handwashing, refrigeration of prepared foods, and proper cooking of poultry and their products can help reduce the opportunities to acquire salmonellosis.

Aserhoff B, Bennett JV: Effect of antibiotic therapy in acute salmonellosis on the fecal excretion of salmonellae. N Engl J Med 281:636, 1969. *This paper presents evidence that suggested antibiotic treatment prolongs the fecal secretion of salmonellae in patients with salmonellosis.*

Black PH, King LJ, Swartz MN: Salmonellosis: A review of some unusual aspects. N Engl J Med 262:811, 1960. *A classic paper that highlights many of the epidemiologic and clinical curiosities of* Salmonella*-induced disease.*

Giannella RA, Broitman SA, Zamcheck N: Influence of gastric acidity on bacterial and parasitic enteric infections: A perspective. Ann Intern Med 78:271, 1973. *A good review of the topic dealing with the gastric acid barrier.*

Huang CT, Lo CB: Human infection with *Salmonella choleraesuis* in Hong Kong. J Hyg 65:149, 1967. *The authors present a complete summary of the clinical manifestations of infection with this important* Salmonella *strain.*

Riley LW, DiFerdinando GT Jr, DeMelfi TM, Cohen ML: Evaluation of isolated cases of salmonellosis by plasmid profile analysis: Introduction and transmission of a bacterial clone by precooked roast beef. J Infect Dis 148:12, 1983. *A new epidemiologic tool for identifying* Salmonella *isolated from patients in scattered locations as coming from a common source.*

Other Bacterial Infections

284. EXTRAINTESTINAL INFECTIONS CAUSED BY ENTERIC BACTERIA

Charles C. J. Carpenter

Microorganisms indigenous to the gastrointestinal tract, the enteric bacteria, have become increasingly important causes of human disease over the past three decades. Bacterial infections caused by these organisms share an origin in the gut and similar epidemiologic and pathogenic characteristics and require a common approach to diagnosis, treatment, and prevention.

The enteric bacteria are the principle organisms found in infections of the abdominal viscera, peritoneum, and urinary tract, as well as frequent secondary invaders of the respiratory tract, burns, or other sites of disruption of cutaneous and mucous membrane barriers. Currently, the enteric bacteria constitute the most frequent cause of life-threatening septicemia. The majority of serious infections caused by enteric organisms may be regarded as the result of medical progress, because they have developed directly from increased use of broad-spectrum antimicrobial agents, more aggressive surgery, larger numbers of patients receiving immunosuppressive therapy, and greater use of invasive management techniques (tracheal intubation and intravenous cannulas). Antimicrobial therapy has a strong selective effect on the gastrointestinal flora and is the most important reason for the increasing role of normal colonic flora in systemic infection.

The normal human intestinal flora is extraordinarily complex and consists of over 100 bacterial species. Only a small proportion of these species is commonly involved in extraintestinal infections. The human colon contains 10^{10} to 10^{11} organisms per gram of content, and roughly 60 per cent of the bulk of the normal stool is contributed by bacteria. Ninety to 98 per cent of the normal colonic flora are obligate anaerobes. Most common among these are the gram-negative bacilli, *Bacteroides* and *Fusobacterium*, followed by gram-positive bacilli, including *Bifidobacterium, Eubacterium,* and *Corynebacterium* species, and a wide variety of anaerobic streptococci. Less common anaerobes in the colonic flora include the gram-positive spore-forming rods of the *Clostridium* species and the gram-negative cocci *Veillonella*. The aerobic gram-negative rods, most of which belong to the family Enterobacteriaceae, account for only 2 to 10 per cent of the normal colonic flora but cause the majority of life-threatening extraintestinal infections. Of these the most common are *Escherichia coli*, followed by the *Klebsiella-Enterobacter* group, *Proteus, Providencia, Edwardsiella,* and *Serratia. Salmonella, Shigella, Yersinia, Campylobacter,* and pathogenic *Vibrio* species occur only under pathologic conditions and are not constituents of the normal intestinal flora. *Pseudomonas* is an entirely unrelated species, usually found in small numbers in the colon under normal circumstances; *Pseudomonas* may, however, become far more prominent in the gut flora after antimicrobial therapy, especially in immunocompromised hosts. The same considerations apply to yeasts, especially *Candida*, which reside in small numbers in the normal large intestine but are increasingly prominent after antimicrobial therapy.

Although the upper gastrointestinal tract, from duodenum through ileum, under normal circumstances is also colonized with lesser numbers of bacteria (predominantly lactobacilli and gram-negative anaerobes), bacteria derived from the normal upper gastrointestinal tract seldom cause serious extraintestinal bacterial infections.

SPECIFIC LOCAL INFECTIONS CAUSED BY ENTERIC BACTERIA

The mixed intestinal flora participate in infections that originate from lesions of the bowel, including appendicitis, cholangitis, diverticulitis, and perforation (from diverticulitis, ileitis, colitis, or carcinoma). These lesions may lead to localized subdiaphragmatic, hepatic, and pelvic abscesses, which are frequent causes of occult fever in patients recovering from abdominal surgery or trauma; the same intestinal flora may also result in generalized peritonitis. Current data indicate that both aerobic and anaerobic bacteria play major roles in infection of the abdominal cavity. The relative importance of aerobic bacteria has been exaggerated in the past because such microorganisms as *E. coli* grow luxuriantly in both aerobic and anaerobic media and usually predominate in routine cultures. There is now compelling evidence that the anaerobic bacteria, especially *Bacteroides* species, play major roles in infection of the abdominal cavity and are largely responsible for the fecal odor of pus often obtained from such infected sites. Previous dicta have emphasized the need to suspect anaerobic bacteria when foul-smelling pus is present and when organisms can be visualized microscopically but fail to grow under routine conditions. Current data, however, indicate that anaerobes should be presumed to be present in any infection of the abdominal cavity caused by intestinal microorganisms, with the obvious implication that therapy effective against anaerobes (metronidazole or clindamycin) should be employed.

MENINGITIS AND BRAIN ABSCESS. During the first four weeks of life, purulent meningitis is frequently caused by enteric bacteria. Such cases may occur sporadically in nurseries and may be associated with septicemia and infection of any other tissue of the body. Infants with meningoceles are particularly susceptible to enteric bacterial meningitis. Meningitis caused by enteric bacteria occurs rarely in adults. Generally it develops as a complication of gram-negative bacteremia or of a neurosurgical procedure or when host immune response is impaired. Nontraumatic brain abscesses are usually caused by infection by multiple bacteria, including anaerobic bacteria similar to those found in the intestinal tract. The primary sites of infection, however, are usually chronically infected mastoid and paranasal sinuses or lung and less commonly abdominal and pelvic sites.

PERITONITIS AND BACTEREMIA ASSOCIATED WITH HEPATIC CIRRHOSIS. Occasionally individuals with cirrhosis of the liver and ascites develop *spontaneous peritonitis* without evidence of localized sepsis elsewhere. Similarly, patients with cirrhosis with or without ascites occasionally develop bacteremia that is generally caused by one of the enteric organisms, most frequently *E. coli*. The illnesses may be self-limited but should always be treated with antimicrobials active against the most likely pathogens. A definitive explanation for such spontaneous infections is lacking; possibilities include shunting of bacteria away from the liver and impairment of host humoral and cellular defense mechanisms.

PERIRECTAL ABSCESS. Perirectal abscess, in which multiple enteric bacteria are generally involved, is most often a localized infection that responds well to appropriate surgical drainage. However, perirectal abscess is a life-threatening complication in patients with marked granulocytopenia, especially leukemic patients receiving cytotoxic chemotherapy. Rectal examination should be performed gently in such patients, since bacteremia is a frequent complication, presumably because of inadequate localization of infection in the absence of adequate circulating granulocytes.

ABSCESSES AT SITES OF SUBCUTANEOUS INJECTIONS. Enteric bacilli occasionally cause abscesses in subcutaneous tissue at sites of hypodermic injections. This complication commonly affects insulin-dependent diabetic individuals. The abscesses are characterized by gas formation, which may lead to more serious clostridial infection. However, the subcutaneous infections caused by aerobic enteric bacilli usually respond well to appropriate antimicrobial therapy. Rarely *nonclostridial crepitant cellulitis*, a synergistic infection caused by intestinal aerobic and anaerobic bacteria, progresses rapidly, requiring urgent and extensive debridement as well as antimicrobial therapy.

SUPERFICIAL INFECTION. Enteric bacteria, especially *Proteus*, and environmental gram-negative bacilli, predominantly *Pseudomonas*, are commonly recovered from the surfaces of burns, varicose ulcers, decubitus ulcers, tracheostomy sites, and other unprotected surface areas. These organisms are of doubtful pathogenic significance, and satisfactory healing of surface wounds may proceed regardless of their presence. They may, however, occasionally cause fulminant gram-negative bacteremia, especially in patients with severe burns. The sinus exudate from chronic osteomyelitis or chronic otitis media often contains *Proteus* as the dominant organism, but again its pathogenic significance is doubtful.

SUPERINFECTION AND PNEUMONIA. Enteric bacteria frequently predominate in the oropharynx and bronchial secretions of patients who are elderly, chronically ill, or immunosuppressed, as well as in individuals who have been treated with antimicrobial agents. Generally, the presence of enteric bacteria in such patients simply represents superficial colonization with resistant bacterial strains after suppression of the primary flora. If tissue invasion is suspected on clinical grounds, transtracheal aspiration followed by Gram stain and culture of aspirated secretions is a useful method to distinguish between colonization of the oropharynx and true infection of the lower respiratory tract. The demonstration of elastin fibers in bronchial secretion is a reliable means of distinguishing necrotizing infections from simple colonization. Pneumonia caused by enteric bacteria is always a potentially life-threatening infection and is especially serious in patients who have difficulty clearing their secetions or require ventilator therapy. A single agent is generally responsible for the pneumonia, and successful therapy depends upon the isolation of and specific therapy for the microorganism.

URINARY TRACT INFECTIONS. Enteric bacteria are the organisms most frequently associated with urinary tract infections. *E. coli* is by far the most common microorganism in uncomplicated infections of the urinary tract. When other organisms, especially the enteric *Klebsiella-Enterobacter* group or environmental *Pseudomonas*, are involved in the absence of an indwelling urinary catheter, they usually point to structural or neurologic problems of the voiding system or to repeated instrumentation.

PROSTATIC INFECTIONS. Enteric bacilli predominate as etiologic agents in the chronic prostatitis that often accompanies prostatic hypertrophy in older men. The pathogenesis of prostatitis in such individuals is poorly understood and presents a particularly difficult therapeutic problem, since many of the agents most effective against the aerobic enteric bacilli (aminoglycosides) do not reach adequate concentrations in the prostate.

METASTATIC INFECTIONS. Despite the frequency with which enteric bacteria invade the blood and the fact that gram-negative enteric bacilli now account for the vast majority of recognized bacteremias, metastatic intravascular infection and localization of enteric bacilli on normal human heart valves remain rare. Less than 3 per cent of cases of endocarditis are caused by enteric bacilli in the absence of intravenous drug abuse. However, occasional cases of suppurative lesions such as arthritis, osteomyelitis, and panophthalmitis do occur after enteric bacteremia. Vertebral osteomyelitis occurs with increased frequency in men with prostatic disease; presumably the method of spread is by way of septic emboli through the vertebral venous plexus to the spine.

UNIQUE FEATURES OF PSEUDOMONAS INFECTIONS. *Pseudomonas*, although often responsible for infections similar to those caused by enteric gram-negative bacteria, are not truly enteric bacteria. Under certain circumstances, especially in patients on broad-spectrum antimicrobial therapy, patients with severe leukopenia with or without acute leukemia, or intravenous drug users, severe sepsis may be produced by *Pseudomonas*. In addition to the endotoxin that is in the cell wall of most gram-negative bacteria, *Pseudomonas aeruginosa* produces several enzymes, including collagenase, proteases, elastase, and an exotoxin (PA toxin) whose mode of action is similar to that of diphtheria toxin. *Pseudomonas* commonly occurs in tap water, may be resistant to antiseptics used in sterilizing instruments, and therefore frequently is introduced by cystoscopy or ventilator-associated aerosols. *Pseudomonas* is notoriously resistant to standard antimicrobial therapy and often emerges as a dominant microorganism on mucosal surfaces after eradication of the normal microbial flora by drugs. It may then become responsible for the phenomenon of superinfection, as in the bronchopulmonary infections that often complicate prophylactic antimicrobial therapy of chronic lung disease or in the urinary tract infections associated with chronic indwelling catheters.

Tissue invasion by *Pseudomonas*, most frequently recognized in patients with leukopenia or relapsing leukemia, is often characterized by a necrotizing vasculitis with bacterial invasion of the walls of arteries and veins. This may lead to the distinctive necrotic skin lesion (ecthyma gangrenosum) that may develop on any part of the body. This lesion may begin as a vesicle that later becomes necrotic; the typical lesion of ecthyma gangrenosum is a round indurated ulcer with a black center that varies from a few millimeters to 10 or more centimeters in diameter. Although not specific for *Pseudomonas* infection, the presence of ecthyma gangrenosum should make the physician suspect this microorganism.

GRAM-NEGATIVE BACTEREMIA

Bacteremia caused by gram-negative bacilli has been a problem of major importance only since the advent of antimicrobial therapy. Urinary tract infections are the source of about half of all cases of bloodstream invasion by enteric bacilli. Other causes include infections developing at the site of intravenous catheters, postoperative complications of gastrointestinal tract surgery, postpartum or postabortal sepsis, and infections of wounds, ulcers, burns, and internal prosthetic devices. Sometimes there is a clear-cut precipitating factor such as an invasive diagnostic procedure (endoscopy) or manipulation of an infected wound.

These bacteremias have clinical characteristics that closely resemble the known biologic effects of gram-negative bacterial endotoxins. The onset of symptoms often occurs with a shaking chill followed by a sharp rise in temperature. The onset is accompanied by leukopenia, but leukocytosis usually ensues within 12 hours. An important concomitant reaction may be a decrease in blood pressure with inadequate tissue perfusion. At least two factors, peripheral vasodilatation and decreased myocardial contractile force, may contribute to the circulatory dysfunction. In patients with inadequate tissue perfusion the cardiac output may be elevated or normal, associated with peripheral arterial dilatation, or it may be very low, associated with poor myocardial contractility. An initial manifestation is often hyperventilation with a consequent respiratory alkalosis, but with persistence of poor tissue perfusion metabolic acidosis ensues. The inadequate tissue perfusion may be manifested only by a modest alteration in the patient's intellectual status. Occasionally patients, especially the elderly, develop bacteremic shock without detectable elevation of temperature. For these reasons, bacteremia must always be considered in the evaluation of unexplained hypotension. Some patients with gram-negative bacteremia develop disseminated intravascular coagulation. This phenomenon is not unique to enteric bacteremia, since it also may occur with fungal, viral, rickettsial, and gram-positive bacterial infections. Although the mortality rate is high in patients with circulatory impairment associated with gram-negative bacteremia, the outcome is clearly related to a number of factors, including age, underlying disease, and antecedent cardiopulmonary status. However, with prompt diagnosis, appropriate antimicrobial therapy, hemodynamic monitoring, and correction of circulatory abnormalities, the majority of patients without major underlying disease should survive.

Generalized sepsis with enteric bacteria is one of several causes of the *adult respiratory distress syndrome (ARDS)*. This syndrome is produced by widespread damage to capillary endothelium of the lung rather than direct pulmonary infection and requires adequate oxygenation, generally including positive end-expiratory pressure.

ENDOTOXIN. Endotoxins from a wide variety of unrelated bacterial species behave similarly, regardless of the pathogenicity of the microorganisms from which they are derived. In the intact microorganism, endotoxins exist as complexes of lipid, polysaccharide, and protein. The biologic activity appears to be a property of a lipid portion. The cell wall of gram-negative bacilli may be roughly divided into three areas. The outermost region contains the chains of specific sugars that characterize the O-specific antigens that determine individual serotypes within a bacterial species. This outer region is linked to a core polysaccharide that is similar in structure among related groups of bacteria. The core polysaccharide is in turn linked through trisaccharides to the major lipid component, termed *lipid A*. The major biologic properties of endotoxin may be accounted for by the complex lipid substance. Lipid A is immunogenic, producing antibodies that cross-react among the gram-negative bacilli. Antibody prepared against lipid A protects against challenge by heterologous gram-negative bacteria in certain animal models. Better protection, however, is obtained by immunization with specific O antigens that induce opsonizing antibodies. Current data suggest that the mortality rate of patients with gram-negative bacteremia is lower in individuals with initially high titers of antibody to the lipid A component. Recent controlled studies have demonstrated that adjunctive treatment of gram-negative infections with antiserum against core lipopolysaccharide significantly increases the survival of patients with bacteremic shock.

When injected intravenously into the experimental animal, the endotoxins cause fever, leukopenia, circulatory collapse, and capillary hemorrhages. Tolerance develops after repeated injections of endotoxin. The clinical features of enteric gram-negative bacteremia may resemble the reaction of laboratory animals or humans to intravenous injection of purified endotoxic preparations. The exact role of endotoxins in the manifestation of gram-negative bacteremia remains uncertain, because chills, fever, leukocytosis, and leukopenia may also result from infection by microorganisms containing little or no biologically active endotoxin in the cell wall (*Candida, Bacteroides spp.*).

Endotoxin is believed to be pyrogenic by virtue of its ability to induce macrophages to release endogenous pyrogen. This protein is carried by the circulation to hypothalamic temperature-regulating nuclei, producing alteration in thermoregulation. In the experimental animal, frequent repeated doses of endotoxin appear to exhaust the capability of macrophages to release endogenous pyrogen. More prolonged exposure of the experimental animal to endotoxin appears to produce antibodies that block endotoxin action.

ANTIBODIES. Antibodies reacting with most Enterobacteriaceae are demonstrable in the sera of normal humans, probably because of continual absorption of small quantities of antigen by the gastrointestinal tract. Gram-negative bacteria contain a wide variety of antigenic determinants. These antigens vary in pathogenetic significance in different species. Certain enteric bacilli contain *K* or *capsular polysaccharides*. The capsular polysaccharides constitute the Vi antigens of *S. typhi*, are prominent in *Klebsiella*, and appear to contribute to the virulence of *E. coli* associated with neonatal meningitis; capsular antigens may also be related to the invasiveness of *E. coli* in pyelonephritis. Capsular polysaccharides interfere with phagocytosis and are probably responsible for the increased virulence of encapsulated bacterial strains. Antibodies to the O or somatic antigens have been most extensively studied in *E. coli*. These antibodies may provide cross-protection against a variety of other enteric microorganisms. Most enteric bacilli are susceptible to immune lysis by the combined effects of antibody and complement, both in vivo and in vitro. Presumably immune lysis is of major importance in preventing the enteric bacilli from invading the bloodstream of normal humans.

MANAGEMENT OF EXTRAINTESTINAL ENTERIC BACTERIAL INFECTIONS

GENERAL PRINCIPLES. Intestinal gram-negative enteric infections are largely iatrogenic; therefore, many of these infections are preventable, especially those arising from indwelling intravenous catheters, instrumentation of the urinary tract, and contaminated suction and ventilation equipment. Elimination of such sources of contamination is the physician's compelling responsibility. The major clinical considerations are (1) early recognition of infection and bacteremia, (2) early recognition and prompt drainage of abscesses, (3) recognition that anaerobic bacteria, not readily cultured, are almost invariably involved in certain infected sites, and (4) differentiation of true infections from superficial contamination that often requires no treatment.

GRAM-NEGATIVE BACTEREMIA. Either the clinical presumption or the documented presence of gram-negative organisms in the blood should alert the physician to initiate a meticulous search for the site of infection, including intravenous or urinary catheters and renal, pelvic, or perirectal abscesses. The successful eradication of infection can seldom be achieved without removal of infected foreign objects and drainage of abscesses. Because of the rapid downhill course of many patients with gram-negative bacteremia, treatment must be begun on the basis of the presumptive diagnosis prior to isolation of the specific causative microorganism.

In settings in which bacteremia is apt to be most rapidly fatal (severe leukopenia, acute leukemia, immunosuppressed patients), the bacteremia often occurs in hospitals where multiple drug-resistant organisms such as *Serratia, Klebsiella,* and *Pseudomonas* play prominent roles. In the febrile immunosuppressed patient, after cultures have been obtained from the blood and other suspected sites of infection, therapy should be begun with an aminoglycoside and either carbenicillin or ticarcillin. The choice of a specific aminoglycoside depends on the frequency, in a given hospital, with which endemic strains are resistant to gentamicin or tobramycin. Once the specific organism has been isolated, therapy should be altered to include the most appropriate and least toxic agents.

Modification of drug therapy is dependent on the site of infection. Gram-negative meningitis in adults often requires a third generation cephalosporin, moxalactam, or intraventricular injection of aminoglycosides via reservoir. When *Klebsiella* is strongly suspected in a pulmonary infection, a cephalosporin should generally be added to an aminoglycoside.

When anaerobes are presumed to be present in abdominal, pelvic, or anogenital infections, an agent such as metronidazole, cefoxitin, clindamycin, chloramphenicol, or moxalactam should be included, the choice being based largely on susceptibility of the patient to the toxic effects peculiar to the chosen antimicrobial agent (for example, chloramphenicol should not be used in a leukopenic individual).

Acute, nonbacteremic urinary infections are likely to respond to oral agents such as sulfamethoxazole-trimethoprim, ampicillin, or tetracycline. The selection of specific drugs should be based on in vitro sensitivity testing. Oral carbenicillin should be reserved for treatment of *Pseudomonas* urinary tract infections outside the hospital because of the danger of selecting resistant organisms in the hospital environment. In patients with indwelling urinary catheters, antimicrobial therapy is ineffective in eradicating chronic urinary infections and should be reserved for acute episodes of sepsis.

Management of bacteremic shock is complex and requires monitoring by a properly placed Swan-Ganz catheter and therapy as outlined in Ch. 43. With optimal corrective measures designed to improve tissue perfusion, survival becomes dependent on removal of any infected foreign material, drainage of abscess cavities, appropriate antimicrobial therapy, and underlying host defenses.

Kreger BE, Craven DE, McCabe WR: Gram-negative bacteremia. IV. Re-evaluation of clinical features and treatment in 612 patients. Am J Med 68:344, 1980. *A large, up-to-date, authoritative analysis of the clinical manifestations of bacteremia caused by enteric bacteria.*

McCabe WR, Treadwell TL, DeMaria A: Pathophysiology of bacteremia. Am J Med 75(1B):7, 1983. *A thoughtful and authoritative discussion of the pathogenesis, clinical manifestations, and pathophysiology of bacteremia.*

Mangi RJ, Quintiliani R, Andriole VT: Gram-negative bacillary meningitis. Am J Med 59:829, 1975. *A comprehensive review of the experience at Yale New Haven Medical Center with gram-negative bacillary meningitis over a five-year period. It demonstrates the contribution of these organisms to the overall experience with bacterial meningitis (4.2 per cent of the cases) and the frequent association with neurosurgery (69 per cent) and neonatal cases (42 per cent). It documents the importance of the nosocomial origin of these cases.*

Young LS, Martin WJ, Meyer RD, Weinstein RJ, Anderson ET: Gram-negative rod bacteremia: Microbiologic, immunologic and therapeutic considerations. Ann Intern Med 86:456, 1977. *An excellent symposium on the laboratory, epidemiologic, and biologic features of gram-negative rod bacteremia. It has an extensive (134-item) bibliography.*

Zeigler EJ, McCutchan JA, Frerer J, Glauser MP, Sadoff JC, Douglas H, Braude AI: Treatment of gram-negative bacteremia and shock with human antiserum to a mutant *Escherichia coli*. New Engl J Med 306:1225, 1982. *This careful clinical study clearly demonstrates that therapy with human antiserum against core lipopolysaccharide of gram-negative enteric bacilli greatly reduces mortality in gram-negative bacteremia.*

285. SHIGELLOSIS

Charles C. J. Carpenter

DEFINITION. Shigellosis is a specific acute bacterial infection of the human intestinal tract caused by bacteria of the genus *Shigella*, with predominant involvement of the distal colon, sigmoid, and rectum. It most commonly is manifested as a clinically nonspecific diarrhea. In the more severe cases, the initial mild diarrhea is accompanied by fever and followed by true dysentery, with cramping abdominal pain, tenesmus, and frequent stools in which mucus, leukocytes, and erythrocytes are abundant.

ETIOLOGY. Shigellae (dysentery bacilli) are nonmotile gram-negative bacilli belonging to the family Enterobacteriaceae. Four species of shigellae are recognized on the basis of antigenic and biochemical properties: *S. dysenteriae* (Group A), *S. flexneri* (Group B), *S. boydii* (Group C), and *S. sonnei* (Group D). Among these species there are over 40 types, each of which is designated by the species name followed by a specific Arabic number. With the exception of *S. flexneri* 6, they do not ferment lactose. The most common species in the United States until 1965 was *S. flexneri*; this species has largely been replaced by *S. sonnei*. *S. sonnei* is now also the most commonly isolated shigella in Western Europe and Japan. *S. boydii* is so rarely encountered in the United States that its isolation suggests exposure during foreign travel. *S. dysenteriae* is now unusual in the more developed countries.

EPIDEMIOLOGY. ***Incidence and Prevalence.*** Despite generally high standards of hygiene, there were over 14,000 cases of shigellosis reported in the United States in 1980. *S. sonnei* has been the predominant etiologic species in North America, Western Europe, and Japan for the past two decades, and the great majority of patients have been children. The true incidence is undoubtedly several times higher than the number of reported cases.

In much of Eastern Europe and in the developing areas of the world, *S. flexneri* has continued to be the predominant causative agent. *S. dysenteriae* 1 (Shiga bacillus) has nearly disappeared as a major endemic cause of dysentery but re-emerged as a major epidemic problem in Central America from 1969 to 1972. Microepidemics caused by the Shiga bacillus recur sporadically throughout the developing world.

Spread of Infection. Shigellosis is found throughout the world. Seasonal patterns vary in different regions; shigellosis characteristically peaks in the late summer and early autumn in North America. Humans and the higher primates are the only known reservoirs of *Shigella* infection. During clinical illness and for a variable period (up to six weeks) following recovery, fecal excretion of shigellae continues. Although the organisms are quite sensitive to desiccation, they may survive for several months in foods and water. Transmission most often occurs by close person-to-person contact. Children in the one- to four-year age group are at highest risk of developing shigellosis; young males are affected more often than young females. In young adults the incidence is higher in women than in men, which probably reflects closer contact of women with ill children. Intrafamilial spread is especially likely to occur when the initial case has occurred in a preschool child. Attack rates in affected families range from 10 to 80 per cent.

Custodial institutions, especially those caring for the retarded, are frequent settings for large epidemics because of difficulty in maintaining adequate hygiene in these settings. Up to 30 per cent of individuals admitted to certain custodial institutions experience an episode of shigellosis within a year of arrival. Nursery schools and day care centers have especially high attack rates whenever shigellae are introduced.

Since shigellae are transmitted by the fecal-oral route, crowded living conditions, poor water supply, and inadequate sewage facilities all correlate significantly with increased risk of infection. Within the United States, shigellosis is excessively high in urban ghettos and Indian reservations. The male homosexual population is also at great risk for shigellosis, which is one of the more common causes of the "gay bowel syndrome."

The recent pandemic spread of *S. dysenteriae* 1 (Shiga bacillus) in Central America and Mexico subsided without major extension to either North or South America. As has been true of pandemics in the past, the reasons for the development of the 1969 to 1972 Central American Shiga bacillus pandemic remain obscure.

PATHOGENESIS AND PATHOPHYSIOLOGY. Since the microorganisms are relatively resistant to acid, shigellae have less difficulty than other enteric pathogens in passing the gastric barrier. In volunteer studies, as few as 200 ingested bacilli regularly initiate disease in 25 per cent of healthy adults. This contrasts strikingly with the much larger numbers of typhoid or cholera bacilli required to produce disease in normal individuals. During the incubation period, usually 36 to 72 hours, the organisms traverse the small bowel and proliferate in the distal jejunum, ileum, and colon. In the colon shigellae reach concentrations of 10^6 to 10^{10} organisms per gram of stool. Unlike the case with certain other enteric pathogens (*V. cholerae* and enterotoxigenic *E. coli*), epithelial cell penetration is essential to the pathogenesis of shigellosis. Multiplication of bacteria occurs within epithelial cells of the colon, predominantly in the villi; this is followed by an acute inflammatory response in the subjacent lamina propria. Destruction of the villous tips, distortion of the mucosal architecture, and formation of superficial microabscesses ensue. In the more severe cases, long segments of colon may be affected with a diffuse inflammatory process that remains confined to the lamina propria. The altered mucosa is friable and is covered with an exudate of polymorphonuclear leukocytes. Stool therefore contains large numbers of erythrocytes and leukocytes. Since the inflammation is superficial, bacteremia is rare, and colonic perforation seldom occurs.

S. dysenteriae and certain strains of *S. flexneri* and *S. sonnei* produce an enterotoxin that causes secretion of isotonic fluid by the small bowel. The role of this enterotoxin in clinical shigellosis is not certain; the enterotoxin may be responsible for the watery diarrhea that often precedes full-blown bacillary dysentery. It is possible that the enterotoxin is entirely responsible for the clinical manifestations in mild cases characterized by only short-term watery nonbloody diarrhea.

CLINICAL MANIFESTATIONS. Shigellosis is often a biphasic disease, beginning with cramping abdominal pain and watery diarrhea, sometimes accompanied by fever (up to 40° C) and generalized myalgias. Fluid and electrolyte losses are greatest during the initial phase of the illness. Such losses are rarely voluminous enough to be life-threatening except in very young children and the elderly. This first phase usually lasts for one to three days; in more severely ill patients, it is followed by a second phase that in the absence of treatment may last for weeks. The second phase is that of true dysentery; the character of the stool changes, with a decrease in the volume and the appearance of bright red blood and mucus in the feces. During this phase, tenesmus may become a complicating feature, and anorexia and weight loss are common. Fever is not prominent during the second phase of the illness.

Many patients infected with shigellae are entirely asymptomatic, and a large number simply have mild cramping abdominal pain and watery diarrhea that clinically cannot be differentiated from illnesses caused by several other microorganisms. Only the more severe cases, with classic bacillary dysentery, can readily be diagnosed clinically as shigellosis. Of the *Shigella* strains now encountered in the United States, *S. dysenteriae* is the most virulent and by far the least common. *S. flexneri* is intermediate in both virulence and frequency, and *S. sonnei*, which accounts for 80 per cent of cases in the United States, presents the mildest clinical picture.

The onset of shigellosis is often more fulminant in children, who may present with unexplained high fever with or without convulsions. Neurologic symptoms and signs, including delirium, headache, nuchal rigidity, and lethargy, rarely occur in adults but are common in young children. Roughly 25 per cent of children hospitalized for shigellosis experience convulsions. The cause of the convulsions is unknown. A small proportion of children infected by *S. dysenteriae* 1 develop a severe, often fatal hemolytic-uremic syndrome; this syndrome is associated with endotoxemia and circulating immune complexes.

DIAGNOSIS. Shigellosis should be considered in any patient with acute onset of fever and diarrhea. Diagnosis is more likely in the high-risk groups just described. Examination of the stool is quite useful in the diagnosis. Blood and pus are grossly apparent in severe bacillary dysentery; even in milder forms of the disease, microscopic examination of the stool often reveals numerous leukocytes and erythrocytes. The fecal leukocyte examination should be performed with a portion of liquid stool, preferably containing mucus. A drop of stool is placed on a microscopic slide and mixed thoroughly with two drops of methylene blue. A coverslip is placed over the mixture for microscopic examination. The presence of abundant polymorphonuclear leukocytes helps in distinguishing shigellosis from diarrheal syndromes caused by enterotoxigenic *E. coli* and *Vibrio cholerae* (in which fecal leukocytes are characteristically absent). The fecal leukocyte examination is not helpful in distinguishing shigellosis from diarrheal illnesses caused by other invasive enteric pathogens (nontyphoidal *Salmonella, Campylobacter, Yersinia, Entamoeba*). The peripheral white cell count is of little diagnostic value, since it may range from less than 3000 to more than 30,000. Sigmoidoscopic examination reveals diffuse erythema and a friable mucosa, with shallow ulcers 3 to 7 mm in diameter.

Definitive diagnosis depends upon isolating shigellae by selective media. A rectal swab, a swab of a colonic ulcer obtained by sigmoidoscopic examination, or a freshly passed stool specimen should be inoculated immediately on culture plates or into carrying media. Since isolation rates of shigellae from freshly passed stools of patients with shigellosis may be as low as 67 per cent, culturing for three successive days is recommended. Stool cultures are generally positive within 24 hours after onset of symptoms and may remain positive for several weeks in the absence of antimicrobial therapy. Blood cultures are so rarely positive as to be of no diagnostic value.

Appropriate culture media include blood, desoxycholate, and salmonella-shigella (S-S) agars. Selected colonies suggestive of shigellae should be placed on triple sugar–iron agar and lysine-iron agar. Colonies showing an alkaline slant and acid butt, without gas or hydrogen sulfide in either agar, should be definitively diagnosed by agglutination with polyvalent *Shigella* antisera. S-S agar is inhibitory for the most virulent of the *Shigella* species, *S. dysenteriae* 1.

Definitive bacteriologic diagnosis becomes of critical importance in distinguishing the more severe and prolonged cases of shigellosis from ulcerative colitis, with which it may be confused both clinically and on sigmoidoscopic examination. Occasionally patients with shigellosis have been subjected to colectomy because of a mistaken diagnosis of ulcerative colitis; a positive culture should clearly prevent such a misadventure.

TREATMENT. The three steps in the treatment of shigellosis include correction of fluid and electrolyte balance, antimicrobial therapy, and symptomatic relief. Although voluminous production of diarrhea is unusual in shigellosis, fluid loss may be lethal in the very young and the very old. Fluid losses in shigellosis are qualitatively similar to those in other infectious diarrheal diseases, and the patient should be treated with appropriate intravenous or oral electrolyte repletion fluids (see Ch. 286) in quantities adequate to correct clinical signs of saline depletion. The requirement for fluids is generally small, but fluid repletion will be lifesaving in exceptional cases.

The effectiveness of antimicrobial agents in treating shigellosis has been well established. Although infections with *S. sonnei, S. flexneri,* and *S. boydii* are generally self-limited except in the very young and very old, appropriate antimicrobial therapy may decrease the duration of symptoms by 50 per cent and decrease the duration of excretion of shigellae (an important epidemiologic factor) by a far greater percentage. Infection by *S. dysenteriae* 1 may result in a 10 to 30 per cent mortality rate in the absence of antimicrobial therapy, and appropriate antimicrobials are mandatory with this pathogen. Ampicillin is currently the drug of choice for sensitive strains of shigellosis in the United States. It should be administered orally in four divided doses for a total of 2 grams a day to adults and 100 mg per kilogram per day to children for a five-day period. Because of the increasing frequency of plasmid-mediated antimicrobial resistance to *Shigella* infections, drug susceptibility testing is important. For adults with ampicillin-resistant isolates, tetracycline in a single oral dose of 2.5 grams is usually effective. Sulfamethoxazole-trimethoprim administered in standard doses twice daily for five days is now the treatment of choice for *Shigella* strains of unknown antibiotic sensitivity in both adults and children.* Certain drugs that appear effective in vitro, including amoxicillin and nonabsorbable antimicrobials such as neomycin or kanamycin, are not effective in vivo. Sulfonamide resistance is so widespread as to nullify the value of these agents.

Agents that decrease intestinal motility should not be used. Such preparations as diphenoxylate and paregoric may exacerbate symptoms, presumably by retarding intestinal clearance of the microorganisms. There is no convincing evidence that pectin- or bismuth-containing preparations are helpful.

PROGNOSIS. The mortality rate in untreated shigellosis is dependent upon the infectious strain and ranges from 30 per cent in certain outbreaks caused by *S. dysenteriae* 1 to less than 1 per cent in most *S. sonnei* infections. Even with infection caused by *S. dysenteriae* 1, mortality rates should approach zero if appropriate fluid replacement and antimicrobial therapy are initiated early. A small number of patients, especially those with histocompatibility antigen B27, develop *Reiter's syndrome* weeks or months after recovery from shigellosis.

PREVENTION. Individuals excreting shigellae should be excluded from all phases of food handling until negative cultures have been obtained from three successive stool specimens collected after completion of antimicrobial therapy. In institutional outbreaks, strict and early isolation of infected individuals is mandatory. Targeted antimicrobial chemoprophylaxis has been disappointing. The most important control measure is scrupulous handwashing by all individuals involved in handling of food. Reporting of shigellosis cases to health authorities should be mandatory.

For the traveler to countries with major *Shigella* problems, no chemoprophylactic agent is an adequate substitute for good personal hygiene and the avoidance of contaminated food and water. Although an oral attenuated vaccine has provided significant protection in volunteer studies, no effective vaccine is now commercially available.

Dupont HL, Hornick RB: Adverse effect of Lomotil therapy in shigellosis. JAMA 226:1525, 1973. *A concise discussion of clearly defined untoward effects of diphenoxylate with atropine in shigellosis.*

DuPont HL, Hornick RB, Dawkins AT, Snyder MJ, Formal SB: The response of man to virulent *Shigella flexneri* 2a. J Infect Dis 119:296, 1969. *A precise description of the clinical course and antibody response in shigellosis induced by oral administration of* Shigella flexneri, *in varying doses, to informed young adult volunteers.*

Haltalin KC, Kusmiesz, HT, Hinton LV, Nelson JD: Treatment of acute diarrhea in outpatients. Am J Dis Child 124:554, 1972. *An unequivocal demonstration of the value of appropriate antimicrobial therapy in the management of shigellosis.*

Koster F, Levin J, Walker L, Tung KSK, Gilman RH, Rahaman MM, Majid MA, Islam S, Williams RC: Hemolytic-uremic syndrome after shigellosis. Relation to endotoxemia and circulating immune complexes. N Engl J Med 298:927, 1978. *New light on the pathogenesis of this frequently lethal complication of shigellosis in children.*

Pickering LK, DuPont HL, Olarte J: Single-dose tetracycline therapy for shigellosis in adults. JAMA 239:853, 1978. *This concise, provocative study clearly demonstrates the effectiveness of single-dose tetracycline in adults infected with antibiotic-sensitive* Shigella *and strongly suggests that this therapy is also effective in adults infected by* Shigella *that demonstrate resistance to tetracycline in vitro.*

*Not recommended for children under age two months.

Stoll BJ, Glass RI, Hug MI, Khan MU, Banu H, Holt J: Epidemiologic and clinical features of patients infected with *Shigella* who attended a diarrheal hospital in Bangladesh. J Infect Dis 146:177, 1982. *Emphasizes the broad range of clinical manifestation of this disease and the continuing importance of* Shigella *as a major enteric pathogen in developed countries.*

286. CHOLERA (Asiatic Cholera)

Nathaniel F. Pierce

DEFINITION. Cholera is an acute, sometimes fulminant, diarrheal disease during which *Vibrio cholerae*, serogroup 1, are abundant in liquid stool. It occurs only in humans and varies in severity from a mild diarrheal illness to a dramatically severe disease that causes death from hypovolemic shock in a few hours owing to the passage of voluminous, watery, electrolyte-rich stools. Cholera usually occurs in epidemic form; it has caused seven pandemics in the past two centuries.

ETIOLOGY. *Vibrio cholerae* are short, slightly curved, motile gram-negative rods that grow aerobically at 37° C. There are more than 60 O serogroups of *Vibrio cholerae*, but only serogroup 1 causes epidemic cholera. Some of the others sporadically cause acute diarrhea, which is occasionally severe. *Vibrio cholerae*, serogroup 1, occurs as two serotypes, *Ogawa* and *Inaba*, which reflect differences in the somatic antigen; there are also two biotypes: the *classic* and the *eltor*. The eltor biotype is recognized by its resistance to polymyxin B and by characteristic patterns of susceptibility to vibriophage. Distinction between the two biotypes has epidemiologic importance; the eltor biotype causes a higher proportion of mild or asymptomatic infections and survives better outside the human host.

EPIDEMIOLOGY. ***The Seventh Pandemic.*** The traditional "home" of cholera is the delta region of the Ganges and Brahmaputra rivers, where thousands of cases occur during annual epidemics. During pandemics the disease has spread in Asia, Africa, Europe, and North America. The current pandemic is due to the eltor biotype; it involves Southeast Asia, the Indian subcontinent, the Middle East, Africa, and the Gulf Coast of the United States. The world total of reported cases reached its peak in 1971, and cholera now appears to be endemic in many of these recently involved areas. Cholera has also been imported to Japan, Israel, Spain, Italy, and Portugal, where it has caused isolated outbreaks. Individual cases have also occurred among travelers returning from affected areas. In the United States, cholera has occurred sporadically along the Gulf Coast since 1973. All cases were caused by the same unusual strain of *Vibrio cholerae*, which suggests that Gulf Coast waters may have been contaminated since 1973.

Mode of Spread. Cholera is largely waterborne, usually by means of fecal contamination of drinking water. However, food exposed to contaminated water may also be the vehicle for infection. Examples of the latter include fresh vegetables washed in contaminated water and shellfish harvested from contaminated water. Evidence that *Vibrio cholerae* adhere to shellfish suggests that these may prove an especially important means of spread.

Secondary cases of cholera in affected households are common because of direct contamination of water or food with infected excreta. Persons with self-limited, mild, or asymptomatic infections outnumber those with serious illness and are probably the major means by which cholera is spread from affected to nearby nonaffected communities. Prolonged gallbladder carriage also occurs in about 3 per cent of older adults convalescent from cholera; however, their role in transmission of cholera is uncertain.

Susceptibility to Cholera. The age distribution of cholera cases reflects the level of naturally acquired immunity in the population. In endemic areas, adults ingest the organism many times and develop substantial immunity; in such areas, cholera is largely a disease of children. In Bangladesh, for example, attack rates among children under five years old are ten times those of adults. In contrast, attack rates in newly affected areas, where there is no naturally acquired immunity, are nearly equal among adults and children.

Vibrio cholerae are quickly killed by pH levels below 5.5. Thus, normal gastric acidity is an important barrier to infection. Impairment of gastric acidity by mucosal atrophy, the use of antacids, or subtotal gastrectomy increases susceptibility to cholera.

PATHOGENESIS. The incubation period for cholera is usually one to two days but may vary from 12 hours to six days. Cholera occurs when *Vibrio cholerae* are ingested, survive passage through the stomach, colonize and multiply in the small bowel, and release the cholera enterotoxin. Colonization is promoted by adherence of the vibrios to the small bowel mucosa. The enterotoxin is a protein (molecular weight 84,000) composed of A and B subunits. The B subunit binds irreversibly to its receptor, GM_1 ganglioside, on the brush border of small bowel epithelial cells. This assists entry of the A subunit into epithelial cells, which causes activation of adenylate cyclase, an increase in intracellular content of 3′,5′-cyclic adenosine monophosphate, and the secretion of electrolytes into the bowel lumen. Cholera enterotoxin does not cause morphologic damage to the bowel mucosa, does not alter its permeability to serum proteins, and does not affect the active absorption of monosaccharides (e.g., glucose) or amino acids. The secreted electrolyte solution passes through the gut and emerges as watery stool, which rapidly becomes free of fecal material. Flecks of mucus give the stool its characteristic "rice-water" appearance. The stool is isotonic with plasma but has concentrations of bicarbonate and potassium greater than plasma (see Table 286–1). All of the signs, symptoms, and metabolic disorders of cholera are related to the rapid loss of this electrolyte-rich liquid stool. This loss causes hypvolemia, base-deficit acidosis, and potassium depletion.

CLINICAL MANIFESTATIONS. Cholera begins with the abrupt onset of watery diarrhea. Many cases are mild, cause little morbidity, and cannot be distinguished clinically from other types of gastroenteritis. In severe cases, however, stool loss is dramatic, sometimes exceeding 1 liter per hour. Collapse resulting from hypovolemic shock occurs when unreplaced fluid losses equal about 10 per cent of body weight. This may happen within 6 hours but usually requires 18 to 24 hours. Greater fluid losses are rapidly lethal. Vomiting, painful cramps of the gastrocnemius muscles, and severe thirst are other prominent features of severe cholera.

The outstanding physical findings in severe untreated cholera are the results of marked isotonic fluid deficit. These include collapse, poor skin turgor, weak or absent peripheral pulses, hypotension, tachycardia, and cyanosis. Eyes are sunken, the voice is faint and high-pitched, heart sounds are faint, and bowel sounds are hypoactive. Adults are usually normally oriented but apathetic. Features that occur only in children under seven years are fever and occasionally coma or convulsions.

Initial laboratory findings reflect the loss of isotonic bicarbonate-rich stool (see Table 286–1). These include increased plasma protein concentration, increased plasma-specific gravity, low arterial pH, and low plasma bicarbonate concentration.

TABLE 286–1. TYPICAL CHEMICAL VALUES IN STOOL AND PLASMA FROM PATIENTS WITH SEVERE CHOLERA

		Plasma	
	Stool	Untreated	Treated†
Sodium*	138 (105)	141	142
Chloride*	102 (90)	107	106
Potassium*	18 (25)	4.5	3.6
Bicarbonate*	45 (30)	9	21
Arterial pH	—	7.21	7.43
Plasma specific gravity	—	1.040	1.026

*Milliequivalents per liter. Stool values in parentheses are for children less than 10 years old.

†Four hours after water and electrolyte replacement.

Plasma sodium concentration is normal. Small children occasionally have severe hypoglycemia.

DIAGNOSIS. Cholera should be suspected in any acute case of watery, shock-producing diarrhea, especially in an adult. Travel to or residence in a cholera-affected area makes the diagnosis more likely. A diagnosis of cholera should also be considered in exposed persons with acute attacks of mild, painless, nonbloody diarrhea.

After treatment has begun, a direct stool examination should be performed. A fecal smear stained with methylene blue usually reveals neither erythrocytes nor leukocytes, which is a feature also characteristic of infections with enterotoxigenic *Escherichia coli* and rotavirus. Dark-field microscopy of dilute feces reveals numerous bacilli with the rapid, darting movement characteristic of vibrios. Immobilization of these organisms by addition of group-specific antisera confirms that they are *Vibrio cholerae,* serogroup 1.

Stool should also be obtained for diagnostic culture. The simplest method involves direct plating of feces on thiosulfate-citrate-bile salt-sucrose (TCBS) agar, a medium highly selective for vibrios. Opaque flat yellow colonies form on TCBS agar within 18 hours at 37° C. Confirmation of serogroup and serotype is made by direct bacterial agglutination in specific antisera. The eltor biotype is identified by its resistance to polymyxin B.

The diagnosis can be confirmed by showing significant rises during convalescence in the serum titers of *Vibrio cholerae* agglutinating antibody or of complement-dependent vibriocidal antibodies. Serodiagnostic techniques are used mostly for epidemiologic studies.

TREATMENT. The mainstay of cholera therapy is prompt, complete replacement of lost water and electrolytes. In severe cases, this should be done immediately, before diagnostic studies. Fluid replacement therapy for cholera is fully effective for cholera-like diseases sometimes caused by other bacterial or viral agents.

Water and electrolytes can be replaced intravenously or in many cases orally. The choice depends upon the patient's condition and the treatment materials available. Intravenous rehydration is required for severely hypovolemic patients and is acceptable for those less seriously ill. Oral replacement of water and electrolytes can be used throughout the course of mild cases and in severe cases after hypovolemia has been corrected by rapid intravenous replacement. Oral therapy is especially useful in rural or underdeveloped areas where intravenous fluids are in short supply.

Lactated Ringer's solution is satisfactory for intravenous rehydration. Initial treatment should aim to restore an effective blood volume as rapidly as possible. Fluid should be given through a large bore needle at 50 to 100 ml per minute until a strong radial pulse is restored. The remainder of the initial deficit is then replaced within two hours. For example, a 50-kg patient with severe dehydration has a fluid deficit of about 5 liters (10 per cent of body weight); 1 to 2 liters is replaced within 20 minutes, and the remainder (3 to 4 liters) by the end of two hours. The response to rapid rehydration is usually dramatic, patients becoming alert, comfortable, and fully cooperative within an hour. After initial rehydration, if administration of intravenous fluids is continued, the infusion should be given at a rate equal to the rate of ongoing measured stool loss until diarrhea subsides. If stool loss cannot be measured, the rate should be sufficient to maintain a strong pulse and normal skin turgor. In severe cases, stool losses may average 10 to 25 ml per kilogram per hour for the first 24 hours. Overhydration can be detected by frequent examination of the neck veins and auscultation of the lungs.

Oral therapy is effective because enteric glucose absorption and glucose-facilitated sodium absorption are intact in patients with cholera. A suitable glucose-electrolyte solution is made by adding the following (in grams per liter) to drinking water: sodium chloride, 3.5; sodium bicarbonate, 2.5; potassium chloride, 1.5; and glucose, 20. If glucose is unavailable, sucrose (40 grams per liter) is nearly as effective. Oral rehydration requires 50 to 100 ml per kilogram, depending upon the degree of dehydration. Replacement of ongoing stool losses requires 5 to 15 ml per kilogram per hour. Thirst is a valuable guide to oral fluid requirements; however, patients may need encouragement to drink the large amounts required for rehydration (up to 1000 ml per hour for adults). Vomiting may occur but does not affect the success of oral therapy unless it is severe.

The treatment of small children with cholera resembles that of adults. The same solutions may be used for oral or intravenous replacement. If lactated Ringer's solution is given, oral supplementation with glucose and potassium is needed to prevent symptomatic hypoglycemia and hypokalemia. The rate of intravenous rehydration should be slower to minimize the risk of coma or seizures caused by cerebral edema. After rapid restoration of a strong radial pulse, by infusing up to 30 ml per kilogram in 30 minutes, the remainder of the initial deficit is replaced in about six hours. Thereafter, ongoing stool losses are replaced as they occur.

Adjunctive therapy with oral antibiotics markedly reduces the duration and volume of stool loss and shortens the period of vibrio excretion. Oral tetracycline (50 mg per kilogram per day in six-hourly doses for two days, maximum daily dose 2 grams) is usually most effective. Recently, *Vibrio cholerae* resistant to tetracycline have been encountered. Furazolidone or chloramphenicol are alternative choices in such instances. A normal diet should be given as soon as appetite returns. Drinking water should be freely available and frequently offered to small children.

The complications of cholera depend largely upon the adequacy of treatment. Uncorrected hypovolemia is the major cause of death. Transient oliguria occurs in many patients, but renal failure with acute tubular necrosis occurs only when hypovolemia is poorly corrected. Inadequate potassium replacement causes cardiac arrhythmias in adults and serious paralytic ileus in children. Water and electrolyte replacement without correction of acidosis can cause pulmonary edema. Uncorrected hypoglycemia can contribute to coma or seizures in children. Severe cholera during the third trimester of pregnancy carries a high risk of fetal death.

PROGNOSIS. Mortality from serious cholera, if untreated, reaches 50 per cent. With adequate replacement therapy, however, mortality approaches zero. Despite adequate therapy, a mortality of about 1 per cent persists among small children, owing largely to complicating coma and seizures.

PREVENTION. Immunization with killed cholera vaccine (containing 10 billion bacteria per milliliter) enhances protection for about six months for adults in endemic areas but is less effective for children or persons from nonendemic areas. Cholera vaccine does not alter fecal shedding of *Vibrio cholerae* and thus does not reduce disease transmission. Tetracycline taken prophylactically by household contacts of proven cases prevents secondary cases. Safe sewage disposal and pure water supplies are the only certain means of preventing cholera.

Barua D, Burrows W: Cholera. Philadelphia, W. B. Saunders Company, 1974. *A broad review of bacteriologic, epidemiologic, immunologic, and clinical aspects of cholera written by a variety of experts.*

Blake PA, Allegra DT, Snyder JD, Barrett TJ, McFarland L, Caraway CT, Feeley JC, Craig JP, Lee JV, Puhr ND, Feldman RA: Cholera—possible endemic focus in the United States. N Engl J Med 302:305, 1980. *This article describes the recent cholera outbreak in Louisiana. It is a valuable example of how an outbreak can occur in a developed nation.*

Carpenter CCJ, Mitra PP, Sack RB: Clinical studies in Asiatic cholera. Parts I–VI. Bull Johns Hopkins Hosp 118:165, 1966. *This is an excellent series of reports concerning the pathophysiology of cholera, rational fluid replacement, and the value of antibiotic therapy.*

Hirschhorn N: The treatment of acute diarrhea in children. An historical and physiologic perspective. Am J Clin Nutr 33:637, 1980. *A thorough review of the special concerns that surround treatment of acute diarrhea, including cholera, in children. The review serves to "bridge" the traditional pediatric literature and the recent literature on cholera and related diarrheal diseases.*

Moss J, Vaughan M: Activation of adenylate cyclase by choleragen. Ann Rev Biochem 48:581, 1979. *A complete review of the cellular basis of action of cholera toxin.*

Pierce NF, Hirschhorn N: Oral fluid—a simple weapon against dehydration in diarrhea. How it works and how to use it. WHO Chron 31:87, 1977. *This is a how-to-do-it article on the use of oral glucose-electrolyte solutions for replacement therapy of acute watery diarrhea. The article was designed especially to aid workers in developing nations where medical care facilities are limited.*

Wallace CK, Anderson PN, Brown TC, Khanra SR, Lewis GW, Pierce NF, Sanyal SN, Segre GV, Waldman RH: Optimal antibiotic therapy in cholera. Bull WHO 39:236, 1966. *This article describes studies on the efficacy of several antibiotics as adjuncts in cholera therapy.*

287. YERSINIA INFECTIONS

Thomas Butler

Plague

DEFINITION. Plague is a bacterial infection of animals and humans caused by *Yersinia pestis*. The most common clinical form is *acute regional lymphadenitis*, called *bubonic plague*. Less common forms include *septicemic*, *pneumonic*, and *meningeal plague*. Mortality is high in untreated cases, but antibiotic treatment administered early in the course of the disease markedly reduces fatalities. Plague has a widespread distribution in the world with significant foci in the Americas, Africa, and Asia. The natural reservoirs of *Y. pestis* are predominantly urban and sylvatic rodents, and it is transmitted among animals and occasionally to humans by bites of infected fleas.

HISTORY. *Y. pestis* has caused devastating pandemics with high mortality rates throughout history. The fourth great pandemic in the world is presently under way. The first three are believed to have occurred in the following times: the first originated in Egypt in 542 A.D. and spread to Turkey and Europe. The second pandemic started in the 14th century in Asia Minor and Africa; after spreading to Europe the black death killed about a fourth of the continent's people. The third occurred in Europe during the 15th to 18th centuries. The present fourth pandemic began around 1860 in the Chinese province of Yunnan. It spread to the southern coast of China, reaching Hong Kong in 1894. Subsequently plague was carried by ship to India, other countries of Asia, Brazil, and California. An estimated 10 million deaths were caused by this disease in India during this century. The plague bacillus was discovered by Alexandre Yersin in 1894 in Hong Kong. It was called *Pasteurella pestis* until 1970.

ETIOLOGY. The causative agent, *Y. pestis*, belongs to the family of bacteria Enterobacteriaceae. It is an aerobic gram-negative bacillus that is readily cultured in broth or agar media with an optimal growth rate at 28° C. The plague bacillus possesses a large number of antigens and toxins that have important roles in virulence and pathogenicity. In the capsular envelope there is a protein called Fraction 1 antigen, which confers antiphagocytic activity and can activate complement proteins of the host. Fraction 1 is produced well at 37° C but not at 28° C and below, indicating that this virulence factor develops while bacteria are in their mammalian hosts but is absent while bacteria are in fleas. Another antiphagocytic antigen of *Y. pestis* is the VW antigen. In the cell walls of *Y. pestis* there is a potent lipopolysaccharide endotoxin, which like endotoxins of other gram-negative bacteria produces fever, leukopenia followed by leukocytosis, disseminated intravascular coagulation, complement activation, and many kinds of tissue damage. In experimental systems, plague endotoxin causes local and generalized Shwartzman reactions, is mitogenic for B lymphocytes, and stimulates gelation of limulus lysate. Additionally, *Y. pestis* elaborates exotoxins that may play pathogenic roles. One of these is a protein called the *murine toxin*, which is cardiotoxic in animals and produces beta-adrenergic blockade, but the role of this exotoxin in human disease is unclear.

Another important protein secreted by *Y. pestis* is a coagulase, which causes blood that is ingested by the flea to clot in the proventriculus, thus blocking the transit into the stomach of the flea. These "blocked" fleas are efficient vectors for plague infection because they regurgitate *Y. pestis* into the bite wound when they attempt to feed. The coagulase of *Y. pestis* is active at 28° C and at lower temperatures but is inactive at higher temperatures such as 35° C. This explains the cessation of plague transmission during the very hot seasons in tropical countries.

DISTRIBUTION AND EPIDEMIOLOGY. Plague is currently endemic in several countries of Africa, the Americas, and Asia. The widespread distribution of plague in the world during the last decade indicates that the infection is firmly entrenched in the world's rodent populations. Vietnam reported more cases than other countries during the 1970's, with a high of 4056 cases in 1970. After Vietnam, which reported a total of 13,786 cases during the decade, other countries with high incidences of human plague were Burma with 2795 cases, Brazil with 1464 cases, Kenya with 393 cases, Peru with 316 cases, Sudan with 226 cases, Bolivia with 219 cases, the United States with 105 cases, and Zaire with 95 cases. In the United States, plague occurs naturally in sylvatic rodents, such as ground squirrels and rock squirrels, and is geographically limited almost entirely to the Southwestern states of New Mexico, Arizona, Colorado, Nevada, and California.

Plague is primarily a zoonotic infection. It is transmitted among the natural animal reservoirs by flea bites or by ingestion of contaminated animal tissues. Throughout the world the domestic and urban rats, *Rattus rattus* and *R. norvegicus*, are the most important reservoirs of the plague bacillus. In sylvatic foci of plague, however, as occur in the United States, the important reservoirs are the ground squirrel, rock squirrel, and prairie dog. Humans are an accidental host in the natural cycle of plague and appear to play no role in the maintenance of plague in nature. Only rarely, during epidemics of pneumonic plague, is the infection passed directly from person to person. Also rarely does the infection develop in humans by the direct handling of contaminated animal tissues.

The occurrence of human plague is always linked to the transmission of plague among the natural animal reservoirs. The incidence of plague in humans for any particular locality is therefore a function of both the frequency of infection in local rodent populations and the intimacy with which the people live with the infected rodents and their fleas. Although humans develop acquired immunity after plague infection, the role of immunity in determining host susceptibility to infection of individuals in a population appears to be small.

Two other epidemiologic features of plague infection are its focal range and seasonality. Foci of active plague infection are typically limited to single villages and even to single city blocks, with the adjacent villages and blocks being entirely plague free. This striking local concentration of plague has been related to the parochial behavior of rats, which stay near one food supply for extended periods. Only during the transport of rodents by man, as on ships or trains, are infected rodents and thus epidemics of plague likely to spread to distant geographic areas.

Plague occurs predominantly in warm tropical climates. Epizootics tend to occur during humid warm seasons and are sharply curtailed during very hot seasons when average daily temperatures exceed 30° C and during very dry seasons. These seasonal fluctuations have been related to flea behavior and physiology. Humid conditions permit fleas to wait longer periods between blood meals so they can survive off the bodies of their rodent hosts during the search for new hosts. Furthermore, during the best seasons for plague transmission, fleas proliferate on their hosts, and when the flea index (ratio of fleas to rodents) exceeds 1, the conditions are usually optimal for a plague epidemic.

PATHOGENESIS AND CLINICAL FEATURES. Although plague infection of man can assume many varied clinical forms, the most common is bubonic plague, which presents a distinctive clinical picture. During an incubation period of two to eight days following a bite by an infected flea, bacteria proliferate in the regional lymph nodes. Patients are typically affected by the sudden onset of fever, chills, weakness, and headache. Usually at the same time, or after a few hours or the next day, patients notice the *bubo,* which is signaled by intense pain in one anatomic region of lymph nodes, usually the groin, axilla, or neck. A swelling evolves that is so tender that the patient typically avoids any motion that would provoke tenderness of the affected nodes.

The buboes of patients with plague are oval swellings varying from about 1 to 10 cm in length and elevating the overlying skin, which may appear stretched or erythematous. They may appear either as a smooth uniform egg-shaped mass or an irregular cluster of several nodes with intervening and surrounding edema. Palpation will typically elicit extreme tenderness. There is warmth of the overlying skin and an underlying, firm nonfluctuant mass. Usually around the lymph nodes there is considerable edema, which can be gelatinous or pitting in nature. Occasionally edema extends into the skin region drained by the affected lymph nodes. Although infections other than plague can produce acute lymphadenitis, plague is unique for the suddenness of onset of the fever and the bubo, the rapid development of intense inflammation in the bubo, and the fulminant clinical course that can produce death as quickly as two to four days after the onset of symptoms. The bubo of plague is also distinctive for the usual absence of a detectable skin lesion and likewise for the absence of an ascending lymphangitis nearby.

In uncomplicated *bubonic plague,* the patients are typically prostrate and lethargic and often exhibit restlessness or agitation. Occasionally they are delirious with high fever, and seizures are common in children. Temperature is usually in the range of 38.5 to 40.0° C, and the pulse rate is increased to 110 to 140 beats per minute. Blood pressure is characteristically low, in the range of 100/60 mm Hg, due to extreme vasodilation. Pressure determinations may be unobtainable if shock ensues. The liver and spleen are often palpable and tender.

The pathology of bubonic plague is unmistakable and characterized by hemorrhage and necrosis. The capsules of the lymph nodes are obliterated by the destructive inflammatory process that involves the periglandular tissues as much as the lymph nodes themselves. The normal architecture that separates cortex from medulla is destroyed. The lymphoid cells of the medulla are necrotic. There are large phagocytic cells, polymorphonuclear leukocytes, red cells, and a granular material that is a pure culture of plague bacilli. Blood vessels are thrombosed.

The majority of patients with bubonic plague do not have skin lesions. About a fourth of patients in Vietnam, however, did show varied skin findings. The most common were pustules, vesicles, eschars, or papules near the bubo or in the anatomic region of skin that is lymphatically drained by the affected lymph nodes. These presumably represent sites of flea bite inoculations. When these lesions are opened, they usually contain white cells and plague bacilli. These skin lesions rarely progress to extensive cellulitis or abscesses. Ulceration may lead, however, to a larger plague carbuncle.

Another kind of skin lesion in plague is purpura, which is a result of the systemic disease. The purpura may become necrotic, resulting in gangrene of distal extremities that is the probable basis of the term black death. These purpuric lesions result from vasculitis and occlusion by fibrin thrombi, resulting in hemorrhage and necrosis.

A distinctive feature of plague, in addition to the bubo, is the propensity for massive growth of bacteria in the blood. In the early acute stages of bubonic plague, all patients probably have intermittent bacteremia. Single blood cultures obtained at the time of hospital admission from Vietnamese patients were positive in 27 per cent of cases. A hallmark of moribund patients with plague is high-density bacteremia, so that a blood smear revealing characteristic bacilli has been used as a prognostic indicator in this disease. Occasionally in the pathogenesis of plague infection bacteria are inoculated and proliferate in the body without producing a bubo. Patients may actually die with bacteremia but without detectable lymphadenitis. This syndrome has been termed septicemic plague to denote plague without a bubo. Some authors have called bubonic plague with high-density bacteremia *bubonic-septicemic.*

One of the feared complications of bubonic plague is secondary pneumonia. The infection reaches the lungs by hematogenous spread of bacteria from the bubo. In addition to the high mortality, plague pneumonia is highly contagious by airborne transmission. It is characterized by fever and lymphadenopathy with cough, chest pain, and often hemoptysis. Radiographically there is patchy bronchopneumonia or confluent consolidation. The sputum is usually purulent and contains plague bacilli.

Primary inhalation pneumonia is rare now but is a potential threat to the individual exposed to a patient with plague who has a cough. The disease can be so rapidly fatal that persons reportedly have been exposed, become ill, and died on the same day. Plague pneumonia is invariably fatal when antibiotic therapy is delayed more than 20 hours after the onset of illness.

Plague meningitis is a rarer complication and typically occurs more than a week after inadequately treated bubonic plague. It results from hematogenous spread from a bubo and carries a high mortality rate when compared with uncomplicated bubonic plague. There appears to be a strong association between buboes located in the axilla and the development of meningitis. Less commonly, plague meningitis appears as a primary infection without antecedent lymphadenitis. Plague meningitis is characterized by fever, headache, meningismus, and pleocytosis with a predominance of polymorphonuclear leukocytes. Bacteria are frequently demonstrable with a Gram stain of spinal fluid sediment, and endotoxin has been demonstrated in spinal fluid by the limulus gelation assay.

Plague can produce *pharyngitis* that may resemble acute tonsillitis. The anterior cervical lymph nodes are usually inflamed, and *Y. pestis* may be recovered from a throat culture or aspiration of a cervical bubo. This is a rare clinical form of plague that is presumed to follow the inhalation or ingestion of plague bacilli. In some societies, plague pharyngitis occurs predominantly in women and has been related to their practice of searching the hair for lice or fleas and killing them by crushing between the teeth.

LABORATORY FEATURES. The white blood cell count is typically elevated in the range of 10,000 to 20,000 cells per cubic millimeter, with a predominance of immature and mature neutrophils. Patients who are most severely ill tend to have higher counts. Occasionally some patients, especially children, may develop myelocytic leukemoid reactions with white cell counts as high as 100,000 per cubic millimeter. The white blood cells in the peripheral blood typically show cytoplasmic vacuolations, toxic granulations, and Dohle bodies that are characteristic of acute bacterial infections. Blood platelet counts may be normal or low in the early stages of bubonic plague. Although a generalized bleeding tendency from profound thrombocytopenia is rare, disseminated intravascular coagulation (DIC) is common. Fibrinogen-fibrin degradation products in the serum that are indicative of DIC were detected in elevated titers in most patients tested in Vietnam.

DIAGNOSIS. Plague should be suspected in febrile patients who have been exposed to rodents or other mammals in the known endemic areas of the world. A bacteriologic diagnosis is readily made in most patients by smear and culture of a bubo aspirate. The aspirate is obtained by inserting a 20-gauge needle on a 10-ml syringe containing 1 ml of sterile saline solution into the bubo and aspirating several times until the saline solution has become blood-tinged. Because the bubo does not contain liquid pus, it may be necessary to inject some of the saline solution and to immediately reaspirate it. Drops of the aspirate should be placed on microscope slides and air-dried for both Gram and Wayson's stains. The Gram stain will reveal polymorphonuclear leukocytes and gram-negative coccobacilli and bacilli ranging from 1 to 2 μm in length. With Wayson's stain *Y. pestis* appear as light blue bacilli with dark blue polar bodies, and the remainder of the slide has a contrasting pink counterstain. Smears of blood, sputum, or spinal fluid can be handled similarly.

The aspirate, blood, and other appropriate fluids should be inoculated onto blood and MacConkey's agar plates and into infusion broth. The organism is identified in triple sugar–iron agar by an alkaline slant and acid butt without gas or H_2S, by negative urease and indole reactions, by failure to utilize citrate, and by nonmotility. For definitive identification, cultures can be mailed in double containers to the Centers for Disease Control, Plague Branch, P.O. Box 2087, Fort Collins, Colorado 80422 (telephone no.: 303-482-0213). At this same laboratory, a serologic test, the passive hemagglutination test utilizing Fraction 1 of *Y. pestis*, can be performed on acute- and convalescent-phase serum. For patients with negative cultures, a four-fold or greater increase in titer or a single titer of greater than or equal to 1:16 is presumptive evidence for plague infection.

The differential diagnosis of bubonic plague includes tularemia, streptococcal and staphylococcal lymphadenitis, secondary syphilis, and lymphogranuloma venereum. For pneumonia, the physician also should consider common forms of bacterial and viral pneumonia. For meningitis and septicemia, the common bacterial causes need to be assessed by age groups.

TREATMENT AND PROGNOSIS. Untreated plague has an estimated mortality of greater than 50 per cent and can evolve into a fulminant illness complicated by septic shock. Therefore the early institution of effective antibiotic therapy is mandatory. In 1948, streptomycin was identified as the drug of choice for the treatment of plague by reducing mortality to less than 5 per cent. No other drug has been demonstrated to be more efficacious or less toxic. Streptomycin should be administered intramuscularly in two divided doses daily, totaling 30 mg per kilogram of body weight per day for ten days. Most patients improve rapidly and become afebrile in about three days. The ten-day course is recommended to prevent relapses because viable bacteria have been isolated from buboes of patients with plague during convalescence. The risk of vestibular damage and hearing loss caused by streptomycin is minimal during a ten-day course. This antibiotic should be used cautiously, however, during pregnancy, in older patients who would have trouble adapting to vestibular damage, and in patients with previous hearing difficulty. In such patients, the course of streptomycin can be shortened to three days after the patient becomes afebrile. Renal injury as a result of streptomycin therapy is rare with this regimen; however, renal function should be monitored. If the serum creatinine concentration rises significantly, the dose of streptomycin should be reduced. In mild renal failure the recommended dose is about 20 mg per kilogram per day and in advanced renal failure 8 mg per kilogram every three days. Most preparations of streptomycin available in the United States are in an oil base and can be administered only intramuscularly.

For patients allergic to streptomycin or for whom an oral drug is strongly preferred, tetracycline is a satisfactory alternative. It is administered orally in a dose of 2 to 4 grams per day in four divided doses for ten days. Tetracycline is contraindicated in children under seven years of age and in pregnant women in order to avoid staining of developing teeth. It is also contraindicated in patients with renal failure.

For patients with meningitis who will require a drug that penetrates well into the cerebrospinal fluid and for patients with profound hypotension in whom an intramuscular injection may not be well absorbed, chloramphenicol should be administered intravenously with a loading dose of 25 mg per kilogram of body weight followed by 60 mg per kilogram per day in four divided doses. After clinical improvement oral chloramphenicol administration should be continued to complete a total course of ten days; the dosage may be reduced to 30 mg per kilogram per day to reduce the magnitude of bone marrow suppression, which is reversible after completion of therapy.

Antibiotic resistance in human isolates of *Y. pestis* has never been reported, nor has resistance emerged during antibiotic therapy. The three antibiotics streptomycin, tetracycline, and chloramphenicol given alone are clinically very effective and relapses are exceedingly rare. Therefore, there is no rationale for using multiple antibiotics to treat plague.

Because patients are febrile and often have nausea or vomiting, hypotension, and dehydration, intravenous 0.9 per cent saline solution should be given to most patients for the first few days of the illness or until improvement occurs. Patients in shock will require additional quantities of fluid with hemodynamic monitoring and the judicious use of epinephrine or dopamine. There is no evidence that corticosteroids are beneficial in plague. Although disseminated intravascular coagulation is commonly present and purpura occasionally develops in severely ill patients, therapy with heparin has no proven benefit in plague infections.

The buboes usually recede without need of local therapy. Occasionally, however, they may enlarge or become fluctuant during the first week of treatment and require incision and drainage. The aspirated fluid should be cultured for evidence of superinfection, but this material is usually sterile.

PREVENTION. All patients with suspected plague should be reported to a health department and to the World Health Organization. Patients with uncomplicated infections who are promptly treated present no health hazards to other persons. Those with cough or other signs of pneumonia must be placed in strict respiratory isolation for at least 48 hours after the start of antibiotic therapy or until the sputum culture is negative. The bubo aspirate and blood must be handled with gloves. Standard bacteriologic techniques that safeguard against skin contact with and aerosolization of infected fluids and cultures should be adequate to protect laboratory personnel.

A formalin-killed vaccine, plague vaccine U.S.P. (Cutter Laboratories, Berkeley, California 94710) is available for travelers to epidemic or hyperendemic areas, for individuals who must live and work in close contact with wild rodents, and for laboratory workers who must handle live *Y. pestis* cultures. A primary series of two injections is recommended with a one- to three-month interval between them. Booster injections are given every six months for as long as exposure continues. In addition, persons living in endemic areas should protect themselves against rodents and fleas. Measures include living in rat-proof houses, wearing shoes and garments to cover the legs, and application of insecticide dusts to houses.

The control of plague by health departments requires knowledge of the epidemiology of infected animals, vectors, and the contact of humans with these animals in any particular area. In the United States the Plague Branch of the Centers for Disease Control in Fort Collins, Colorado, has a field team of entomologists, mammalogists, and epidemiologists to investigate cases of plague. A specific approach to each case should be chosen and usually consists of insecticide use around homes, trapping of animals, and education of people to avoid contact with certain animals. Urban plague has been successfully controlled in many cities around the world by quarantine, rat control, and insecticide use.

Brubaker RR: The genus *Yersinia:* Biochemistry and genetics of virulence. Curr Top Microbiol Immunol 57:111, 1972. *A review of features of the plague bacillus that render it virulent.*

Butler T: A clinical study of bubonic plague. Observations of the 1970 Vietnam epidemic with emphasis on coagulation studies, skin histology, and electrocardiograms. Am J Med 53:268, 1972. *This paper describes clinical features of serious cases in Vietnam.*

Butler T: Plague and other *Yersinia* infections. New York, Plenum Publishing Corp., 1983. *This recent monograph gives full clinical description and contemporary literature citations.*

Pollitzer R: Plague. Mongraph Series. Geneva, World Health Organization, 1954. *This is a classic monograph covering older literature.*

Reed WP, Palmer DL, Williams RC, Kisch AL: Bubonic plague in the Southwestern United States: A review of recent experience. Medicine 49:465, 1970. *This is a good review of cases in the United States.*

Other Yersinia Infections

DEFINITION. The non-plague yersinioses are caused by *Yersinia enterocolitica* and *Y. pseudotuberculosis.* These gram-negative rod bacteria produce fever, diarrhea, and abdominal pain that can mimic acute appendicitis. The common pathologic lesions in yersiniosis are acute enteritis and mesenteric lymphadenitis. Extraintestinal disease may result from septicemia or appear as arthritis and erythema nodosum.

ETIOLOGY. The *Yersiniae* are members of the bacterial order Enterobacteriaceae. Accordingly, they are gram-negative rods that are oxidase negative and grow on agars containing bile salts. They do not ferment lactose and grow faster at 25° C than at 37° C. Of the 34 different O serotypes of *Y. enterocolitica* that have been identified, the ones most commonly associated with human disease are types 3 and 9 in Canada and Europe and type 8 in the United States. Like other gram-negative bacteria, the *Yersiniae* contain a lipopolysaccharide endotoxin in the cell wall that may be responsible, in part, for the fever and inflammation. *Y. enterocolitica* elaborates an enterotoxin that is plasmid mediated, resembles the heat-stable enterotoxin of *Escherichia coli,* and may cause the diarrhea associated with this infection.

EPIDEMIOLOGY. The yersinioses are distributed worldwide. Large numbers of confirmed cases have been reported in Europe, Canada, the United States, and Japan. This infection has also been reported from Africa and Asia, but little information is available on the incidence of infection in tropical areas. In the United States, infection with *Y. enterocolitica* appears to be rare when compared with infection with *Salmonella* and *Shigella* species, but in other countries such as Finland and Sweden the incidence of infection is higher. Both adults and children are susceptible to infection. Males acquire the infection more commonly than females. The natural reservoirs of *Y. enterocolitica* are farm animals, especially pigs and goats, and other domestic animals, including dogs and cats. The natural reservoirs of *Y. pseudotuberculosis* include birds and other diverse domestic and farm animals. These animals harbor the bacteria in their intestines and excrete them in feces. Humans become infected by ingesting food or water contaminated by animal feces or directly by the ingestion of certain fomites. Person-to-person transmission seems to be rare. In the United States, well-defined outbreaks of *Y. enterocolitica* infection have occurred in a North Carolina family with a sick dog, in a New York school at which chocolate milk was the source of infection, in members of a Brownie scout troop in Pennsylvania who ate infected bean sprouts, and in persons who drank milk from a dairy in Tennessee. There are no clear seasonal patterns of infection.

PATHOGENESIS OF CLINICAL SYNDROMES. An inoculum with as many as 10^9 organisms may be required to produce infection. During the incubation period, estimated at four to ten days, bacteria proliferate in the small bowel; invade the mucosa, especially that of the ileum; and elicit an acute inflammatory response. Ulcerations may occur and polymorphonuclear leukocytes appear in the stool. Some bacteria migrate via the lymphatics to the mesenteric lymph nodes, where inflammation occurs. The initial symptoms incude fever and either diarrhea or abdominal pain. In these instances, the corresponding pathologic finding is terminal ileitis or mesenteric lymphadenitis or both. The colon is less frequently affected, but aphthoid ulcers and hemorrhagic colitis have been described in yersiniosis. The tissues are affected by acute inflammation, thrombosis of blood vessels, hemorrhage, and necrosis. The diarrhea results from the mucosal invasion by bacteria or the action of an enterotoxin. Diarrhea varies from semisolid or watery to grossly bloody. In some patients the abdominal pain is severe and located in the right lower quadrant and may be mistaken for appendicitis; the appendix is usually normal. A few days later, some patients may develop extraintestinal complications of arthralgias, arthritis, and erythema nodosum. Since the synovial and cutaneous tissues in these syndromes are sterile, an immunologic reaction has been postulated to explain their pathogenesis. Arthritis is more likely to occur in individuals of haplotype HLA-B27, and erythema nodosum occurs more commonly in women. Septicemia is a rare complication that occurs in the setting of prior liver disease, malignancies, or immunosuppressive therapy. Rarer clinical forms of yersiniosis include pneumonia, pharyngitis, and meningitis. Antibodies appear in the blood against the O and other antigens of *Y. enterocolitica,* and nearly all infections are self-limited. However, fatalities have occurred from extensive ulceration and necrosis of the intestine and septicemia.

DIAGNOSIS. The diagnosis requires the isolation of *Yersiniae* from stool, blood, or surgical specimens. The number of bacteria in stool may be small, and a cold-enrichment technique may be required. A rectal swab or piece of stool is placed into 0.067 M phosphate-buffered saline solution at a pH of 7.6 and incubated at 4° C for four weeks. Most other stool bacteria die, whereas *Y. enterocolitica* will grow. At weekly intervals, subcultures should be made on MacConkey agar. Identification is made by finding non-lactose-fermenting colonies that on triple sugar–iron agar give an acid-acid reaction (*Y. enterocolitica*) or alkaline-acid reaction (*Y. pseudotuberculosis*) without gas or hydrogen sulfide, are positive for urease, and are motile at 25° C but nonmotile at 37° C. *Y. enterocolitica* gives a positive reaction for ornithine decarboxylase, whereas *Y. pseudotuberculosis* does not. A diagnosis can be made from serologic test results by showing a rise in agglutinin titer in paired serum specimens. The existence of cross-reacting antigens in the genera *Brucella, Vibrio,* and *Salmonella* indicates that false-positive serologic results sometimes occur.

TREATMENT AND PROGNOSIS. Yersiniosis is usually self-limited and so rarely diagnosed that it is impossible to assess the possible benefits of antibiotic treatment. Most isolates of *Y. enterocolitica* are susceptible to streptomycin, gentamicin, tetracycline, chloramphenicol, and sulfamethoxazole-trimethoprim and resistant to the penicillins and cephalosporin antibiotics. *Y. pseudotuberculosis* isolates usually have been susceptible to penicillin. It is important to suspect the diagnosis in patients with severe abdominal pain to avoid unnecessary surgery for appendicitis. The recognition that early fever accompanies yersiniosis may be helpful, as is epidemiologic information pertaining to outbreaks in the community.

PREVENTION AND CONTROL. The presumed origin of *Y. enterocolitica* infection in farm and domestic animals suggests that transmission may be similar to that of *Salmonella.* Meat and dairy products and other farm produce should periodically be examined for *Y. enterocolitica* content. During outbreaks, public health authorities should identify sources of infection in food (especially milk), water, or persons.

Bottone EJ: *Yersinia enterocolitica:* A panoramic view of a charismatic organism. CRC Crit Rev Microbiol 5:211, 1977. *A useful review of microbiologic aspects of these infections.*

Carter PB, Lafleur L, Toma S: *Yersinia enterocolitica:* Biology, epidemiology, and pathology. Contrib Microbiol Immunol 5, 1979. *This volume contains research papers given at a symposium and is excellent for the serious student of these diseases.*

Kohl S: *Yersinia enterocolitica* infections. Pediatr Clin North Am 26:433, 1979. *This clinical discussion emphasizes disease syndromes in children.*

Vantrappen G, Agg HO, Geboes K, Ponette E: *Yersinia enteritis.* Med Clin North Am 66:639, 1982. *This article contains a good clinical description of gastroenterologic features of the disease.*

288. TULAREMIA

Richard B. Hornick

DEFINITION. Tularemia is a rare infectious disease in the United States caused by a small gram-negative pleomorphic rod, *Francisella tularensis.* This organism is acquired from an animal reservoir, frequently cottontail rabbits, by direct contact with diseased animal tissues, the bite of an infected tick or deer fly, ingestion of contaminated food or water, and inhalation of aerosolized bacteria. Clinical manifestations usually include a cutaneous ulcer with enlargement of regional lymph nodes. Rarely, a pneumonitis will result from inhalation of *F. tularensis* or secondary spread from the skin ulcer and lymph nodes. Confirmation of the diagnosis by cultural technique is not advocated because of the high contagion risk to personnel handling this organism. The therapeutic response to effective antibiotic therapy is rapid.

HISTORICAL FEATURES. The typhoidal form of tularemia was first described in Japan in 1818. The disease was thought to be due to ingestion of "poisonous hare meat." In 1890 in Norway, the tularemia bacillus was isolated from ill lemmings. A clear description of the organism occurred in 1906 when McCoy uncovered a "plague-like" disease among ground squirrels in Tulare County, California. Francis coined the name tularemia to honor the American geographic site of identification and also to stress that the disease was frequently bacteremic in animals. In Japan, tularemia may be referred to as Ohara's disease, or Yato-byo (wild hare disease).

ETIOLOGY, SPECIFIC LABORATORY DIAGNOSIS, AND EPIDEMIOLOGY. *F. tularensis* is a small gram-negative pleomorphic rod-shaped bacterium. Organisms are not seen in smears of infected tissue unless special staining techniques are used. Fluorescent antibody conjugate staining and modified Dieterle staining are the best methods for demonstrating them. All tularemia strains are serologically identical, but there are biochemical and virulence differences for mammals that have allowed differentiation of two strains. These are called Jellison A and B; the former, found only in North America, is lethal for domestic rabbits *(Oryctolagus)* and causes severe disease in man. The unique biochemical capabilities of this strain—e.g., it ferments glycerol and contains citrulline ureidase—do not explain its increased virulence. Strain B lacks these biochemical features, is not lethal for cottontails, causes milder disease in man, usually is isolated from rodents or from water, and is distributed over Europe, Asia, and North America. Reasons for the differences in virulence are unknown.

Culture Methods. The direct isolation of *F. tularensis* from blood (rarely), pus from ulcers or buboes, sputum, or pharyngeal or gastric aspirations in a patient with pneumonitis can be achieved by two methods. This is a class 4 organism requiring an effective hood or an adequate isolation laboratory to prevent human disease or epizootics. The two methods for isolation are intraperitoneal inoculation of guinea pigs and direct plating of a specimen onto glucose cysteine blood agar, cystine heart agar, or eugon agar. As few as one to five viable organisms will cause death of guinea pigs in five to ten days. Appropriate facilities are needed to prevent spread of the disease to other animals. The media employed to isolate the organism usually contain drugs to suppress other flora and allow the tularemia colonies to be visible. Useful additions are 0.1 mg of cycloheximide and 20 units of penicillin per milliliter of media. The colonies are small on these media; they appear in 48 to 72 hours of incubation at 37° C.

Serologic Diagnosis. The measurement of serum agglutinating antibodies is a useful and safer method of diagnosing tularemia. Titers begin to rise in about seven to ten days and peak in three to four weeks. Paired serum specimens obtained two weeks apart and demonstrating a four-fold or greater rise are diagnostic of tularemia. However, a single specimen with a titer of 1:160 or greater in a patient thought to have tularemia on clinical grounds is diagnostic. Antibiotic therapy does not appear to dampen the antibody response. Titers remain elevated for six to eight months and then decline in the subsequent one to one and a half years to low or undetectable levels. There is a cross-reaction with brucella antigen during the early phase of the antibody response. The brucella titer falls off faster than and is never so high as the tularemia titer.

Skin Testing. A skin test antigen has proved to be reliable for diagnostic and epidemiologic purposes. A positive test result, similar in appearance to a tuberculin test response, is present during the first week of illness, frequently before the agglutinins are detectable, and remains positive for years. There is no known cross-reacting skin test antigen. The antigen is derived from *F. tularensis* by ether extraction; however, it is not commonly available. It can be obtained from the Centers for Disease Control, Atlanta. In 10 per cent of patients, the skin test antigen may boost pre-existing agglutinating antibody titers. Skin test reactivity can be shown to be associated with sensitized lymphocytes.

Epidemiology. Tularemia is a sporadic disease; man acquires it when he is bitten by an infected tick or deer fly or when he handles an infected animal. In the process of field dressing a rabbit or skinning a muskrat, the hands may become contaminated with infected blood, subcutaneous abscesses, or liver and spleen that contain millions of organisms. The act of eviscerating the animal can create an aerosol that can be inhaled. The ingestion of contaminated water or food is the least likely method of acquiring tularemia. Many carnivores such as dogs, cats, bull snakes, and others may feed on diseased rabbits. This results in contamination of the teeth and saliva. These animals are relatively resistant to tularemia. Contact with the teeth of a pet dog or cat has resulted in ulceroglandular tularemia. Studies in volunteers have quantitated the susceptibility of man to infection and disease and the virulence of *F. tularensis* for man. As few as 50 type A organisms injected subcutaneously will cause ulceroglandular disease. Pneumonic tularemia can be induced by a similar inoculum size if the aerosolized and inhaled particles are small (less than 5 microns). Type B organisms require an inoculum about 1000 times larger to induce ulceroglandular or respiratory disease in man.

The incidence of tularemia is low, fewer than 200 cases a year having been reported in each of the past ten years. The peak incidence was in 1939, when almost 2300 cases were reported. Laws passed at that time prohibited the sale of wild rabbits, especially cottontails, and this legislation plus increased public awareness of the danger of handling sick or dying wild animals has contributed to the decline. Most cases occur in the Midwest, but the disease is not restricted to any one geographic location in the United States. Cottontail rabbits in urban and suburban areas throughout the country provide the reservoir from which tularemia can occur. Epizootics among these or other animals can cause epidemics in man. Tularemia has been reported only north of the thirtieth parallel. The cottontail rabbit is not found in Europe; various rodents such as voles, muskrats, and hares carry *F. tularensis* (Jellison B type) in that part of the world. Diseased jack rabbits, found west of the Mississippi River, may be an important source of contamination of ticks and deer flies.

In the summer months, most cases of tularemia are caused by tick or deer fly bites. Ulceroglandular disease begins with an ulcer at the site of the bite, e.g., groin, axilla, or scalp. In the fall, during hunting season, sporadic cases, usually ulceroglandular, occur among hunters and trappers. In the Scandinavian countries, epidemics have occurred in the winter months when farmers handling stored hay contaminated by diseased voles inhaled *F. tularensis* and developed pneumonic tularemia.

MECHANISMS OF INFECTION AND PATHOLOGY. The most common form of tularemia results from the penetration of *F. tularensis* into the skin. This penetration may be through hair follicles or minute areas of trauma. The development of the subsequent disease takes two to six days, depending upon the number of bacteria and their virulence. The organisms multiply in the dermis and induce a marked inflammatory process consisting primarily of mononuclear cells with a perivascular distribution. This process produces an erythematous tender papule. The inflamed area continues to swell until the induced ischemia causes the skin to ulcerate. The base of the ulcer becomes black and depressed. The edges are sharply demarcated. At the time of penetration some organisms may be phagocytized and transported in the lymph to regional nodes. There is no clinically apparent lymphangitis. The nodes enlarge and become painful when caseation occurs. Histologic sections reveal geographic necrosis and disruption of the capsule. Fluctuation of the node is a late and rare event. It may then rupture.

The necrotic, purulent, painful lymph node is termed a bubo. Healing of a bubo takes months even with appropriate antibiotic treatment. Aspiration of an unruptured node may lead to an indolent draining sinus tract. *F. tularensis* may remain in the necrotic tissue and purulent drainage for many weeks. The ulcer heals slowly and usually leaves a depigmented, rounded area in the skin.

Oculoglandular tularemia may occur when the conjunctival sac is infected from an ulcer or contaminated finger. Small yellowish granulomatous lesions develop on the palpebral conjunctivae, accompanied by enlargement of the preauricular lymph nodes. In untreated patients the cornea may perforate.

Inhaled small particle aerosols (<5 microns in diameter) containing *F. tularensis* (usually type A) are ultimately deposited in the terminal bronchioles and alveoli, although infection of the trachea and large bronchi also occurs. A peribronchial inflammation develops with infiltration by neutrophils and mononuclear cells. This produces necrosis of alveolar walls and results in localized pneumonitis. In man, small areas of pneumonitis represent the most common findings on chest roentgenograms. Often these are ill defined and difficult to interpret. Lobar consolidation or lung abscesses represent extensive spread and necrosis. These are infrequent in man. Mediastinal and peritracheal lymph nodes enlarge and may be apparent on chest x-ray films. They may be partially responsible, along with the bronchitis, for the substernal burning that is common in patients with tularemic pneumonia. The incubation period for this form of tularemia varies inversely with the size and virulence of the inhaled inoculum. Following an inoculum of 10 to 50 organisms, disease appears in about four to seven days in volunteers.

Typhoidal tularemia follows systemic spread of *F. tularensis* from the oropharynx and probably the gastrointestinal tract when a huge inoculum is swallowed. Enlargement of cervical lymph nodes, and presumably nodes in the mesentery, occurs. This latter process causes abdominal pain and is associated with an ileus. This is the most unusual form of tularemia in this country.

CLINICAL MANIFESTATIONS. Disease initiated by a tick bite is manifested by an ulcer at the site or adjacent to it. The tick defecates after feeding, and the infected feces may be scratched into the epidermis. Usually the lesion will be in the inguinal, axillary, or scalp skin. If contact with tularemia organisms results from the handling of an infected animal, an ulcerative lesion evolves in the skin of the hands, frequently around a fingernail. This lesion may be so trivial that it is ignored by the patient. The ulcer is depressed into the dermis, has sharply demarcated edges, and gradually develops a black base. In the initial stage of development the lesion produces a thick, yellowish exudate. Regional lymph nodes enlarge and are tender to palpation. Fever and chills are common. The temperature curve is usually remittent or continuous in character. Without antibiotic therapy, most patients remain febrile for several weeks, the ulcer heals slowly over weeks to months, and the enlarged lymph nodes persist for months. Untreated patients may occasionally develop a secondary necrotizing pneumonia as a consequence of bacteremia. These patients may be acutely ill.

Primary tularemia pneumonia presents with the sudden development of substernal burning and a nonproductive paroxysmal cough associated with fever and chills. Headache, myalgia, photophobia, malaise, and prostration are common findings. The temperature elevates quickly to 39.4 to 40° C and remains at that level (continuous fever curve) until antibiotic treatment is given. Sixty to 70 per cent of patients will survive without specific therapy, and in these a slow defervescence occurs over several months. X-ray of the lungs may reveal ill-defined, scattered oval areas of infiltration, with enlarged peritracheal lymph nodes. Pleural effusions, lobar consolidation, and lung abscess are other manifestations of this form of tularemia. Cervical lymph nodes are palpable and tender.

DIAGNOSIS AND DIFFERENTIAL DIAGNOSIS. The diagnosis of ulceroglandular tularemia is made by the clinical manifestations and serologic studies. Paired serum specimens collected over a two- to three-week period are required to demonstrate a four-fold rise in titer. A baseline agglutinin titer of 1:160 in a patient with a history of an indolent ulcer for two or more weeks is diagnostic of tularemia. Culture of an ulcer and blood should be performed only if the hospital laboratory has appropriate protective isolation hoods. Patients with sporotrichosis or *Mycobacterium marinum* infections may have ulcers suggestive of tularemia but are usually afebrile. Enlarged lymph nodes extending centripetally as a beaded chain are a characteristic finding in sporotrichosis. Lesions of the fingers infected with staphylococci or beta streptococci usually produce more pus and may be associated with lymphangitis. *B. anthracis* can produce an ulcer (anthrax) with black-based, sharply demarcated edges similar to that initiated by *F. tularensis*. A careful history and serologic data will help in the differential diagnosis. In patients in whom any form of tularemia is suspected, the use of the skin test antigen will be helpful. The test result is usually positive prior to the development of agglutinating antibodies.

Tularemia pneumonia must be differentiated from the more common bacterial, viral, and mycoplasmal pneumonias. The history and the presence of ulceroglandular disease are helpful. Skin testing and serologic studies are diagnostic. The chest x-ray may yield suggestive findings consisting of ill-defined, small, oval, multiple infiltrates but is not diagnostic.

Patients infected with *F. tularensis* usually have a normal leukocyte count with an elevation of the sedimentation rate and a positive C-reactive protein (CRP) determination. The white count is elevated when a bubo or a lung abscess is present.

COMPLICATIONS. Pericarditis and meningitis are rare events that usually occur in patients who have been misdiagnosed and have received inappropriate treatment. Pericarditis results from direct extension of the infection from the purulent, necrotic mediastinal lymph nodes or the involved lung. Constrictive pericarditis has been reported. Meningitis develops rarely, represents a seeding of the meninges during bacteremia, and is characterized by a lymphocytic pleocytosis in the cerebrospinal fluid.

TREATMENT. Patients with all forms of tularemia respond to the following antibiotics: streptomycin, gentamicin, tetracycline, and chloramphenicol. The aminoglycoside antibiotics are recommended, since they produce a prompt cure of patients with the most severe form of tularemia. Patients with pneumonitis are afebrile within 24 to 48 hours and do not relapse. Ulcers and tender lymph nodes heal over a period of seven to ten days. Gentamicin, 5 mg per kilogram per day in divided doses, is given for ten days. Streptomycin was the principal drug for treating tularemia before gentamicin; 1 gram is given every 12 hours for ten days. Treatment with tetracycline or chloramphenicol may produce an equally rapid response, but relapses occur in 15 to 20 per cent of the patients. These drugs are not recommended unless gentamicin or streptomycin is contraindicated. Doses of 3 to 4 grams of tetracycline or 3 grams of chloramphenicol daily for ten days can be employed. Naturally acquired resistance to any of these antibiotics has not been found.

Patients with ulceroglandular tularemia respond well to these antibiotics. Fluctuant lymph nodes should not be aspirated until the patient has finished the course of the antibiotic treatment. Isolation of patients with any form of tularemia is not required; there is no evidence of person-to-person spread.

PROGNOSIS. The mortality rate for untreated ulceroglandular disease is about 5 per cent. Patients infected with type B strains and untreated probably have a mortality rate less than 1 per cent. Many of these patients probably go undiagnosed, as the disease is mild and self-limiting. Treatment with antibiotics prevents death and promotes healing in a week to ten days.

The mortality rate for pneumonic tularemia in the preantibiotic period was 30 to 60 per cent. Treatment with streptomycin or tetracycline has lowered this figure to less than 1 per cent. Healing occurs without residual lung damage or deficits in pulmonary function.

PREVENTION. Patients who recover from tularemia have a high degree of resistance to reinfection. If *F. tularensis* is reintroduced into the skin, a positive skin test reaction ensues without ulceration. Resistance to pulmonary disease may be associated with sensitized lymphocytes and alveolar macrophages.

A live attenuated strain of *F. tularensis* has been prepared as a vaccine. This can be administered by the acupuncture route, and it produces excellent immunity. The vaccine can be obtained from the Commander, U.S. Army Medical Research Institute of Infectious Diseases, Frederick, Maryland 21701. Its use is limited to persons considered at high risk such as selected laboratory workers, forest rangers, game wardens, and perhaps others known to be exposed during an outbreak. The vaccine exerts its effect through the stimulation of cellular immune mechanisms. Circulating agglutinins are not associated with resistance to disease.

Buchanan TM, Brooks GF, Brachman PS: The tularemia skin test; 325 skin tests in 210 persons: Serologic correlation and review of the literature. Ann Intern Med 74:336, 1971. *This study is an extension of the study reported by Young et al. (see below). It clearly presents proof of the efficacy of the skin test as a diagnostic test for tularemia. In addition it shows the amount of antigen stimulation needed to cause a conversion to a positive reactor.*

Francis E: The occurrence of tularemia in nature as a disease of man. Public Health Rep 36:1731, 1921. *A classic paper demonstrating the transmission experiments documenting the role of the deer fly and lice in spreading tularemia from infected animals to uninfected rabbits, also showing that nasal washings of rabbits could be a source of virulent organisms. The author cites the chronicity of tularemia in man untreated with antibiotics and reports one of the first fatal cases of ulceroglandular disease in man.*

Saslaw S, Carlisle HN: Studies with tularemia vaccine in volunteers. IV. Brucella agglutinins in vaccinated and unvaccinated volunteers challenged with *Pasteurella tularensis*. Am J Med Sci 242:70, 1961. *This was the fourth paper in the series dealing with volunteers infected with tularemia. Earlier studies documented the minimal infective dose for man, and this study differentiated serologic responses to tularemia and brucella antigens.*

Tärnvik A, Sandström G, Löfgren S: Time of lymphocyte response after onset of tularemia and after tularemia vaccination. J Clin Microbiol 10:854, 1979. *Presents evidence on the development of cellular immunity in patients with tularemia or who have received the attenuated vaccine.*

Teutsch SM, Marone WJ, Brink EW, Potter ME, Eliot G, Hoxsie R, Craven RB, Kaufman AF: Pneumonic tularemia on Martha's Vineyard. N Engl J Med 301:826, 1979. *This study illustrates the suddenness with which tularemia may appear in a geographic area. Furthermore it indicates a unique mechanism by which man can acquire pneumonic tularemia.*

Young LS, Bicknell DS, Archer BG, Clinton JM, Leavens LJ, Feeley JC, Brachman PS: Tularemia epidemic: Vermont, 1968. Forty-seven cases linked to contact with muskrats. N Engl J Med 280:1253, 1969. *This represents one of the largest outbreaks occurring in the United States in the past 20 years. It is one of the best described epidemiologic studies of infection caused by the Jellison type B organism.*

289. ANTHRAX

Philip S. Brachman

DEFINITION. Anthrax is a zoonotic disease transmitted to humans through contact with animals or animal products. Its primary forms are cutaneous, inhalational, and gastrointestinal. Occasionally, meningitis and septicemia occur, almost always secondary to one of the primary forms. In the United States, the most common form of the disease is the cutaneous lesion; inhalation anthrax occurs rarely; gastrointestinal anthrax has never been reported in the United States. Synonyms for anthrax include charbon, malignant pustule, Siberian ulcer, malignant edema, splenic fever, milzbrand, woolsorter's disease, and ragpicker's disease.

ETIOLOGY. *Bacillus anthracis* is a gram-positive, nonmotile, spore-forming bacillus (1 to 1.3 mμ × 3 to 10 mμ) that on ordinary laboratory media at 35 to 37° C produces round, grayish white, ground-glass–appearing, convex, tenacious colonies 2 to 5 mm in diameter with comma-shaped projections. Microscopic examination of artificial media growth shows long parallel chains of organisms, referred to as "boxcars." Material from a fresh lesion reveals shorter chains with individual organisms having slightly rounded ends. Fluorescent antibody staining and a specific gamma bacteriophage can be used to identify *B. anthracis*. Parenteral inoculation of mice, guinea pigs, or rabbits with agar-grown cells or washed liquid growth will result in death in 24 to 72 hours.

B. anthracis spores may persist for years in the industrial or agricultural environment.

INCIDENCE AND PREVALENCE. In 1975–1976 the worldwide incidence of anthrax was 1651 cases, undoubtedly an underestimate. Reports to the World Health Organization (WHO) concerning anthrax in countries throughout the world are inaccurate and sporadic. Cutaneous anthrax is reported to be endemic in Haiti, South Africa, and several Asiatic countries. Occasionally, inhalation anthrax is reported from some industrialized countries, primarily in Europe, and is directly related to processing hair or wool. Gastrointestinal anthrax is occasionally reported from some African and Asiatic countries and from Russia.

In the United States, the average annual occurrence in 1916–1925 was 127 cases, and in 1974–1983, 1.3 cases. Ninety-five per cent of the cases in the United States are cutaneous; the other five per cent are inhalational. Twenty of the 231 cases reported from 1955 through 1983 were fatal, for a case-fatality rate (CFR) of 8.7 per cent. Two hundred and twenty cases with 11 deaths were cutaneous (CFR, 5 per cent); 11 cases with 9 deaths were inhalational (CFR, 82 per cent). Anthrax meningitis occurs in less than 5 per cent of the cases.

EPIDEMIOLOGY. Cases are classified as either industrial (80 per cent) or agricultural (20 per cent). Industrial anthrax results from contact with animal products, usually from Asia or Africa, including goat hair, wool, hides and skin, and animal bones. Transmission is by direct contact with contaminated animal products, or by indirect contact with a contaminated environment or with airborne particles created during the processing of animal products. In some cases classified as industrial, the source of infection was clothing, yarn, insulation material, saddle pads, or fertilizer. Occasional laboratory-acquired infections are reported.

Agricultural anthrax results from contact with infected animals (cattle, horses, sheep, goats, or swine) or their discharges. Animal vaccine inadvertently injected into the injector's hand has also caused disease.

In the United States, the majority of cases are sporadic, although there are occasional epidemics. The largest epidemic occurred during ten weeks in 1957, when nine of 600 employees in a processing plant acquired anthrax; four cutaneous and five inhalation (four fatalities) cases were associated with one batch of contaminated goat hair imported from Asia.

Human-to-human transmission has not been reported.

PATHOGENESIS. Cutaneous anthrax results from the introduction of *B. anthracis* through a wound or by means of an infected animal fiber penetrating the skin. Organisms in the subcutaneous tissue germinate, multiply, and produce toxin with tissue necrosis. Organisms and toxin may be distributed by the vascular or lymphatic system, resulting in involvement of regional lymph nodes, septicemia, and toxemia.

Inhalation anthrax results from the inhalation of airborne droplet nuclei less than 5 μ in size, with subsequent deposition on the terminal alveoli, where they are phagocytized by macrophages, carried through the alveolar membranes, and deposited in the regional lymph nodes; there they germinate, multiply, and produce toxin. The resulting reaction causes necrosis of the mediastinal tissue, leading to hemorrhagic, edematous mediastinitis, a unique pathologic finding. There may be a direct toxic effect on the pulmonary capillary endothelium, causing pulmonary capillary thrombosis and respiratory failure. Primary anthrax pneumonia is not seen, although there may be secondary pneumonic involvement.

Gastrointestinal anthrax results from ingestion of contaminated meat and deposition of spores in the submucosa of the intestinal tract (commonly ileum or cecum), where they germinate, multiply, and produce toxin, with resultant edema, hemorrhage, and necrosis. A mucosal lesion may develop with hemorrhage; there may be regional lymph node involvement. Occasionally organisms are introduced through the oral mucosa (oropharyngeal anthrax) and deposited in the regional lymph nodes, where they germinate, multiply, and produce toxin.

Anthrax meningitis results from hematogenous spread of bacteria from a primary focus.

Bacillus anthracis produces a toxin consisting of three components: edema factor, lethal factor, and protective antigen. In human disease antibiotic therapy may sterilize the tissue (usually within 24 hours of initiation), but the persistence of the toxin results in continued development of clinical disease until it is metabolized.

Clinical disease probably imparts permanent immunity; purported second cases have not been confirmed.

CLINICAL MANIFESTATIONS. Cutaneous anthrax usually occurs on the upper extremities or face. There may be mild fever, malaise, and headache. After an incubation period of three to ten days (usually five to seven days), a small pruritic, painless papule (approximately 1.0 cm) develops at the site of inoculation. Several days later a small vesicle or ring of vesicles is noted; this may be surrounded by erythema and slight nonpitting edema. The lesion may enlarge to approximately 4 cm. Within several days a dark hemorrhagic area develops beneath the center of the vesicular tissue. Disruption of the tissue releases a clear or slightly serous liquid teeming with organisms. Beneath this tissue will be a well-demarcated depressed ulcer crater in the center of which a black eschar is developing. The eschar dries and separates from the tissue within one to three weeks, leaving a scar. There may be lymphangitis and regional lymphadenopathy. The lesion is not painful except when secondarily infected. Rarely the lesion is large and irregularly shaped. Significant edema may develop, particularly with lesions near the eye. Malignant edema refers to an especially serious form with spreading edema, induration, formation of bullae, high fever, and severe toxemia. Rarely, multiple simultaneous lesions have been reported, probably resulting from simultaneous coprimary infections.

Antibiotic therapy will not alter the progression of the lesion, although it may influence the development of secondary infection and of septicemia.

Inhalation anthrax has an incubation period of one to five days (commonly three to four days). This form of the disease is biphasic, with an initial phase similar to a mild upper respiratory tract infection, with mild fever, malaise, fatigue, myalgia, nonproductive cough, and occasionally a sensation of precordial oppression. The only physical finding may be rhonchi on auscultation of the chest. Within several days there may be clinical improvement, but then the second or acute phase develops with severe respiratory distress as manifested by dyspnea, cyanosis, respiratory stridor, and profuse diaphoresis. Subcutaneous edema of the chest and neck may develop. The vital signs are elevated; moist, crepitant rales may be heard; minimal pleural effusion may be evident; shock may develop. On chest x-ray, the typical finding is that of an enlarged mediastinum and possible pleural effusion. The patient usually dies within 24 hours.

Gastrointestinal anthrax has an incubation period of two to five days. In the abdominal form of the disease, the initial symptoms are nausea, vomiting, anorexia, and fever. With progression of the disease, significant abdominal pain, hematemesis, and bloody diarrhea may develop. In some instances the findings simulate an acute surgical abdomen. Ascites may be present. Further progression leads to toxemia, cyanosis, shock, and death. In the oropharyngeal form, patients develop fever, anorexia, cervical or submandibular lymphadenopathy, and edema. A primary anthrax lesion of the pharynx has also been reported.

Anthrax meningitis resembles typical hemorrhagic meningitis.

DIAGNOSIS. In cutaneous anthrax, the typical lesion is a painless, pruritic papule which progresses into a vesicle, beneath which a depressed black eschar develops. Microscopic and bacteriologic examination of fluid from a vesicle or exudate from beneath the eschar should reveal organisms. The differential diagnosis includes staphylococcal skin infections, tularemia, plague, contagious pustular dermatitis (ecthyma contagiosum or orf), and milker's nodule.

The classic physical finding of inhalation anthrax is widening of the mediastinum. The initial phase of inhalation anthrax is indistinguishable from a mild upper respiratory tract infection, and the acute phase of severe respiratory distress will resemble other diseases that cause respiratory insufficiency. Sputum cultures are not generally positive for *B. anthracis.*

Gastrointestinal anthrax has no characteristic signs and symptoms, but organisms may be demonstrable in feces or vomitus. The clinical course may resemble shigellosis or *Yersinia* gastroenteritis. Severe involvement may lead to surgery of the abdomen. Involvement of the upper gastrointestinal tract is not distinctive of infection with *B. anthracis.*

Anthrax meningitis resembles hemorrhagic meningitis or possibly a cerebrovascular accident, but there should be evidence of a primary site of infection. The organism should be demonstrable in the cerebrospinal fluid. In any of these forms of the disease, appropriate serum specimens may demonstrate a four-fold rise in indirect hemagglutination titer.

TREATMENT. The drug of choice in anthrax is penicillin; *B. anthracis* organisms resistant to penicillin have not been identified from clinical specimens. In mild cutaneous anthrax, oral potassium penicillin, 2 grams per day for five to seven days, is recommended. With extensive lesions or with significant systemic illness, intramuscular procaine penicillin, 4 to 6 million units per day for five to seven days, should be given. Tetracycline or erythromycin may also be used in oral doses of 2 grams per day for five to seven days. In malignant edema, additional therapy with intravenous hydrocortisone, 100 to 200 mg per day, has been reported to be effective.

The lesion in cutaneous anthrax should be covered with a clean dressing. Hospitalized patients should be on secretion precautions. No ointments have been shown to be effective; excision of the lesion has been reported to increase the severity of symptoms.

Therapy of inhalation anthrax is based primarily on empirical knowledge and extrapolation from animal experiments. Penicillin G should be administered intravenously in doses of 18 to 24 million units per day. Streptomycin, 1 to 2 grams per day intravenously, may also be used. Supportive therapy such as volume expanders and vasopressor agents should be used as necessary. There may be a need to ensure an adequate airway if edema results in compression of the trachea.

For gastrointestinal anthrax, the therapeutic regimen for inhalation anthrax should be initiated. Tetracycline, 1 gram per day intravenously, has also been reported to be effective.

Anthrax meningitis should be treated in the same way as inhalation anthrax.

PROGNOSIS. The case-fatality ratio for cutaneous anthrax is 20 per cent without treatment and less than 5 per cent with appropriate treatment. Inhalation anthrax is almost always fatal. Gastrointestinal anthrax has a case fatality rate of 25 to 75 per cent.

PREVENTION. Formaldehyde has been successfully used to decontaminate raw hair and wool; gamma irradiation, steam under pressure, and ethylene oxide sterilization have been used with less effectiveness. Currently, prevention is directed toward protecting the employee by use of an effective, cell-free vaccine, education, good personal hygiene, and use of protective clothing, including respirators if aerosols are created. Gastrointestinal anthrax can be prevented by education concerning the ingestion of potentially contaminated meat. Prophylactic antibiotics or hyperimmune serum have not been shown to be effective.

Agricultural cases can be prevented by practicing good animal husbandry, including annual immunization of animals.

Albrink WS, Brooks SM, Biron RE, Kopel M: Human inhalation anthrax, a report of three fatal cases. Am J Pathol 36:457, 1960. *A good review of the pathology of inhalation anthrax from personal observations.*

Brachman PS: Anthrax. *In* Evans A, Feldman H (eds.): Bacterial Infections of Humans: Epidemiology and Control. New York, Ms. Hilary Evans Publishing Company, 1982, pp 63–74. *Comprehensive summary of all aspects of anthrax, with emphasis on the epidemiology.*

Brachman PS: Inhalation anthrax, New York Academy of Science, Conference on Airborne Contagion, November 8, 1979. Ann NY Acad Sci 353:83, 1980. *An up-to-date review of all aspects of inhalation anthrax.*

Brachman PS, Plotkin SA, Bumford FH, Atchison MM: An epidemic of inhalation anthrax. II. Epidemiologic investigations. Am J Hyg 72:6, 1960. *A report on the epidemiologic investigation of an epidemic of inhalation anthrax in the United States.*

Feeley JC, Brachman PS: *Bacillus anthracis*. *In* Lenette EH, Spaulding EH, Traunt JP (eds.): Manual of Clinical Microbiology. 2nd ed. Washington, D.C., American Society for Microbiology, 1974, pp 143-147. *A thorough review of the laboratory identification of anthrax.*

Plotkin SA, Brachman PS, Utell M, Bumford FH, Atchison MM: An epidemic of inhalation anthrax. The first in the twentieth century. I. Clinical features. Am J Med 29:992, 1960. *Summarizes the clinical features of an epidemic of inhalation anthrax in the United States.*

Sirisanthana T, Navachareon N, Tharavichitkul P, Sirisanthana V, Brown AE: Outbreak of oral-oropharyngeal anthrax: An unusual manifestation of human infection with *Bacillus anthracis*. Am J Trop Med 33:144, 1984.

290. DISEASES CAUSED BY PSEUDOMONADS

Michael Barza

Melioidosis and glanders are due to closely related bacteria of the genus *Pseudomonas*. Like other pseudomonads, these are strictly aerobic, nonfermentative, gram-negative bacilli. Both species show distinctive bipolar staining with various dyes.

MELIOIDOSIS

DEFINITION. Melioidosis, caused by *P. pseudomallei*, is a rare disease which is acquired in equatorial areas. It may produce fulminant septicemia with widespread suppurative lesions or a chronic, tuberculosis-like illness with lung cavitation. Infection occurs through contact with contaminated soil or water.

ETIOLOGY. In 1912, Whitmore and Krishnaswami, while performing autopsies on derelicts in Rangoon who had died of a glanders-like illness, recovered a unique bacillus. Because of the resemblance to glanders, this bacterium came to be called *P. pseudomallei* and the disease, melioidosis.

EPIDEMIOLOGY. *P. pseudomallei* is found in a narrow belt ranging 20 degrees on either side of the equator. Most cases have been acquired in Southeast Asia, but some have been reported from the Philippines, Guam, Australia, and, rarely, Central or South America. Over 300 cases of melioidosis with 36 deaths were recorded among United States troops stationed in Vietnam.

The organism is widespread in soil and stagnant water, particularly in paddy fields. Epizootic disease occurs among sheep, goats, swine, and horses, but, in contrast to glanders, these animals do not seem to be a reservoir of human disease. Most human infections are believed to arise by contamination of skin abrasions by soil or water. This may explain the marked predilection for males. Ingestion and inhalation are occasional routes of entry. Rarely, laboratory workers have been infected in the course of working with this organism. Only one instance of human-to-human transmission has been reported.

Inapparent infection in the form of seroreactivity is common in endemic areas. Significant titers have been found in as many as 20 per cent of Vietnamese and in 1 to 2 per cent of United States soldiers who spent at least six months in Vietnam. Even higher rates were reported in soldiers wounded in Vietnam. This is of importance because of the remarkable ability of melioidosis, like tuberculosis, to become clinically manifest for the first time many years after exposure. A population of veterans in the United States is now at risk of this disease.

PATHOGENESIS AND PATHOLOGY. In acute septicemic melioidosis, organisms are disseminated widely throughout the body, particularly the lungs, liver, spleen, and lymph nodes. Lung lesions are usually due to hematogenous spread, but sometimes result from inhalation. Multiple small abscesses are formed, containing necrotic material, neutrophils, and abundant bacteria. With time, the lesions coalesce and may cavitate. A rim of hemorrhage may be evident in pulmonary abscesses.

In chronic melioidosis, the lungs and lymph nodes are most commonly affected. The lesions show a combination of central necrosis containing polymorphonuclear leukocytes, and peripheral granulomas. Giant cells may be seen. Organisms are sparse in these lesions.

CLINICAL MANIFESTATIONS. The incubation period is usually a few days, but may be as long as 20 years or more. In late-onset cases, the illness often seems to be triggered by intercurrent trauma or other disease such as diabetes mellitus, alcoholism, or cancer or by malnutrition. The most common manifestation of infection with *P. pseudomallei* is simply a positive serologic test result. Clinical disease ranges from an acute septicemic form to a subacute or chronic localized form. At both extremes, the lung is commonly involved.

Acute septicemic melioidosis causes fever, chills, tachypnea, and muscle pain, as well as signs and symptoms attributable to local abscess formation. Macroscopic abscesses are common in the liver, spleen, and lymph nodes. They are especially prominent in the lungs, chiefly in the upper lobes. Radiographic changes range from bronchopneumonia through lobar consolidation to nodular lesions which coalesce and may cavitate. There may be pleuritic chest pain and a pleural rub. Rales and rhonchi are often heard. Pustular skin lesions are sometimes seen. Routine laboratory tests show anemia and a variable polymorphonuclear leukocytosis.

Subacute or chronic melioidosis may occur in the wake of the acute infection or may arise indolently. The typical presentation is cavitary disease of the upper lobes of the lungs, resembling tuberculosis. The liver, skin, bones, and soft tissues may be affected, and sinus tracts may be formed. The general picture is of a chronic, wasting, usually febrile illness with occasional periods of remission.

Variations upon these themes may be encountered. A nodular abscess with regional lymphadenitis may occur at the site of the original infection, usually the skin. Focal and diffuse encephalitis, as well as pleural mass and effusion, have been described.

DIAGNOSIS. Melioidosis should be suspected in those who have resided in an endemic area and who manifest either an acute, febrile illness with widespread suppurative lesions, especially in the lungs and skin, or who exhibit progressive cavitary lung disease without a clear cause. Gram stain of infected material may show the organisms poorly, but Wright's, Giemsa, and other techniques usually demonstrate the bacteria and reveal the bipolar accentuation.

The laboratory should be alerted to the suspected diagnosis. The organisms usually grow well in ordinary media, although they may be sparse in chronic infections and may be overgrown by normal flora. Selective media may increase the yield. After several days of incubation, the colonies usually assume a typical "wrinkled" appearance on agar media. *P. pseudomallei* can be differentiated from other pseudomonads by a variety of biologic features. Fluorescent-antibody staining, one of the most definitive tests, cross-reacts with *P. mallei*, but the two organisms can be distinguished by the lack of motility of the latter.

Serologic studies may be helpful. The complement fixation test is suggestive at titers above 1:8 and the hemagglutination test at titers above 1:80. A four-fold rise in titer is essentially diagnostic. Serologic tests are occasionally negative in patients with active disease. Elevated titers may persist despite successful treatment of melioidosis.

TREATMENT. There is no general agreement upon an optimal regimen for the treatment of melioidosis. The choice of drugs must, to some extent, be based upon sensitivity tests. Most active in vitro are the tetracyclines, chloramphenicol, novobiocin, kanamycin, sulfonamides, and trimethoprim-sulfamethoxazole. For *acute septicemic illness,* high doses of tetracycline (80 mg per kilogram per day) *and* chloramphenicol (80 mg per kilogram per day) are recommended, together with one of the following: trimethoprim-sulfamethoxazole (9 and 45 mg per kilogram per day), sulfisoxazole (140 mg per kilogram per day), or kanamycin (30 mg per kilogram per day). Drug toxicity has been a problem at these high doses, so they should be reduced when this is feasible.

For *chronic melioidosis,* tetracycline, chloramphenicol, sulfisoxazole, or trimethoprim-sulfamethoxazole should be given in about half the dosage recommended for acute disease. One drug to which the organism is sensitive usually suffices. Because the bacteria are very difficult to eradicate, treatment for acute or chronic disease generally should be given for at least 3 months and as long as 6 to 12 months. Abscesses should be drained according to usual principles; however, surgical intervention without adequate antibiotic coverage can be dangerous. The indications for operation on patients with active lung disease are not settled.

PROGNOSIS. The mortality rate of untreated septicemic melioidosis exceeds 90 per cent, but with treatment this is reduced to about 50 per cent. Subacute or chronic infection carries a lower mortality which, with treatment, may be diminished to 10 per cent or less.

PREVENTION. No vaccine is available. It seems reasonable to recommend thorough cleansing of abrasions sustained in endemic areas. Despite the rarity of person-to-person transmission, patients with active infection, especially pulmonary infection, should probably be isolated.

Everett ED, Nelson RA: Pulmonary melioidosis. Observations in thirty-nine cases. Am Rev Respir Dis 112:331, 1975. *A thorough account of the clinical presentation of a large group of United States soldiers, most of whom had subacute or chronic pulmonary infection. Therapeutic recommendations, including the role of surgery, are discussed at length.*

Howe C, Sampath A, Spotnitz M: The pseudomallei group: A review. J Infect Dis 124:598, 1971. *An excellent review of the bacteriology and epidemiology of the disease, and of what little is known about the pathogenetic factors involved.*

John JF Jr: Trimethoprim-sulfamethoxazole therapy of pulmonary melioidosis. Am Rev Respir Dis 114:1021, 1976. *Presentation of a case and brief review of the limited information available regarding therapy of cavitary lung disease.*

Piggott JA, Hochholzer L: Human melioidosis. A histopathologic study of acute and chronic melioidosis. Arch Pathol 90:101, 1970. *A clear description of the pathologic features of this disease, based on autopsy study of ten patients with acute and six with chronic melioidosis.*

Whitmore A, Krishnaswami CS: An account of the discovery of a hitherto undescribed infective disease occurring among the population of Rangoon. Indian Med Gazette 47:262, 1912. *A fascinating account of the discovery of melioidosis among the beggars and drug addicts of Rangoon. The authors humbly describe how their simple experiments led to the gradual realization that they had stumbled onto a new disease.*

GLANDERS

DEFINITION. Glanders is primarily an infection of horses, mules, or donkeys. It is very rarely transmitted to humans but can produce an acute septicemic illness or a more chronic one involving principally the skin and lungs.

ETIOLOGY. The causative organism, *Pseudomonas mallei,* derives its species name from the Latin *malleus* (Greek *melis*), connoting "severe disease." It is a strictly aerobic, nonfermentative, gram-negative rod which closely resembles *Pseudomonas pseudomallei,* the agent of melioidosis, but is nonmotile.

EPIDEMIOLOGY. Glanders occurs almost exclusively in people handling horses, mules, or donkeys. In horses, there may be pulmonary involvement or subcutaneous nodules, especially about the head and neck ("farcy"). It is occasionally transmitted to domestic animals. In the rare instances of human infection, transmission appears to be via broken skin or possibly aerosol inhalation. Glanders has been eradicated from the United States, but cases still occur in Asia and South America. Laboratory personnel working with the organism may become infected. In contrast to melioidosis, glanders can be transmitted from person to person fairly readily.

PATHOLOGY AND PATHOGENESIS. The lesions of glanders range from acute cellulitis with necrosis and abscess formation to a chronic necrotizing process with granuloma formation.

CLINICAL MANIFESTATIONS. Within a few days of cutaneous inoculation, subcutaneous nodules appear with regional lymphadenitis. When the portal of entry is the upper respiratory tract, draining mucosal ulcers occur. Lower respiratory infection following inhalation may have a longer incubation period, 10 to 14 days, and results in a necrotizing lobar or bronchopneumonia, nodular infiltrates, or lung abscess; accompanying features include chills, myalgias, headache, and pleuritic chest pain. Systemic spread may complicate infection in any of these sites, producing a rapidly fatal illness with a generalized pustular rash.

Aside from fever and local suppuration, physical findings may include generalized adenopathy and splenomegaly. The white blood cell count may be mildly elevated. Occasionally there is severe leukopenia.

In some patients, a chronic form of disease occurs with subcutaneous or intramuscular abscesses. There may be lymphadenitis and ulceration of the nasal mucosa. Involvement of the liver, spleen, lung, eye, and central nervous system has been reported.

DIAGNOSIS. Glanders should be considered when persons handling potentially infected animals or laboratory material develop nodular, suppurative infections of the skin and upper respiratory tract or an acute, septicemic illness. Bacteria are sparse even in abscesses and may not be well seen with Gram stain. Giemsa, Wright's, or methylene blue stain, however, may reveal organisms with typical bipolar staining ("safety pin" appearance). *P. mallei* grows slowly on various standard laboratory media. The bacteria can be identified presumptively by their biochemical characteristics and lack of motility, as well as by fluorescent-antibody staining. Serologic tests (agglutination, complement fixation) may be useful.

TREATMENT. The mortality of untreated glanders is high. Experience with therapy is limited. Sulfadiazine appears to be effective. It should be administered in a dosage of 100 mg per kilogram per day for three weeks or more. By analogy with melioidosis, other drugs such as tetracycline, chloramphenicol, or an aminoglycoside might be administered concomitantly.

Infected animals should be destroyed, and infected humans should be isolated to prevent spread of the disease.

Howe C, Miller WR: Human glanders: Report of six cases. Ann Intern Med 26:93, 1947. *A review of cases which occurred among workers in a single laboratory. The diagnoses were made serologically, and all patients survived.*

291. LISTERIOSIS

Michael Barza

DEFINITION. Infection caused by *Listeria monocytogenes,* a distinctive gram-positive bacillus, occurs worldwide. The organism has a propensity to afflict people with underlying diseases but also affects previously healthy individuals. Meningitis, bacteremia, and focal infections, as well as devastating neonatal sepsis, can occur.

ETIOLOGY. In 1926, Murray, Webb, and Swann isolated a new bacterium from sick rabbits and guinea pigs. Because it produced a monocytosis in these animals, they suggested the species name *monocytogenes.* The first human isolation, in 1929, was from a patient with an illness resembling infectious mononucleosis.

EPIDEMIOLOGY. *L. monocytogenes* is widespread in soil, water, and sewage, and can survive in moist environments for months. A large variety of healthy mammals, fowl, and fish are sporadically colonized. Listeriosis is a well-recognized cause of abortion, septicemia, and encephalitis in various animal species.

Despite these observations, most infections in humans are of uncertain origin. Patients are usually urban dwellers with no evident contact with animals, unpasteurized milk, or contaminated food or water. This has led to the suspicion that asymptomatic human carriers may be important sources of infection. Indeed, colonization of the nose, throat, or genitalia of healthy individuals occasionally occurs. Moreover, the organism can be recovered from the feces of at least 1 per cent of well people and a higher proportion of household contacts of infected persons.

The frequency of listeriosis appears to be increasing. This may be due in part to heightened awareness, but probably also reflects the increasing population of patients with immunosuppressive disorders who now constitute the majority of patients with *Listeria* infection. Males are more often affected than females. In Europe two thirds of cases occur in neonates, whereas in the United States most occur in later life. The reasons for these differences in sex and geographic distribution are not known.

L. monocytogenes can be grouped into 11 serotypes, of which type 1 (usually 1b) and type 4 are the most common in the United States. Clusters of cases caused by a single serotype have occasionally been described in the community and in the hospital, suggesting that person-to-person and/or common-source spread may occur. Nursery outbreaks are well recognized.

PATHOLOGY AND PATHOGENESIS. *L. monocytogenes* shares with mycobacteria, fungi, *Salmonella* and *Brucella* the property of surviving within phagocytes, especially macrophages. Resistance to infection appears to depend mainly on the acquisition of cell-mediated immunity. Humoral immunity plays a lesser role. Accordingly, patients who have diseases which depress cellular immunity or who are taking immunosuppressive drugs are especially susceptible.

The portal of entry is not known but may be the intestine. In animals, *Listeria* multiply within epithelial cells of the gut. Presumably, bacteremia may ensue with seeding of various sites. The usual histologic response in humans is a polymorphonuclear leukocytosis with microabscess formation. However, there may occasionally be a monocytic reaction. In perinatal infection, miliary necrotizing granulomas are found in the liver, spleen, lungs, and central nervous system.

L. monocytogenes shows striking tropism for the fetus and placenta of most animals and for the central nervous system of monkeys and humans. Meningitis results in a dense, purulent reaction especially over the base of the brain. The infection sometimes extends more deeply to produce "cerebritis" or bacterial encephalitis. Brain abscess may supervene.

CLINICAL MANIFESTATIONS. After the neonatal period, listeriosis most commonly affects elderly patients, especially males. The major presentations are meningitis (55 per cent), bacteremia (25 per cent), endocarditis (7 per cent), and nonmeningitic infection of the central nervous system (6 per cent). More than one half of patients have an underlying disorder such as malignancy, cirrhosis, alcoholism, diabetes, or vasculitis, or are receiving immunosuppressive drugs such as corticosteroids. Gastrointestinal symptoms sometimes occur at the onset of the systemic illness, suggesting that the intestinal tract may be the portal of entry.

L. monocytogenes is a leading cause of bacterial *meningitis* among people with cancer, especially lymphoma and leukemia, and among recipients of renal transplants. About 30 per cent of patients have no preceding disease; however, *Listeria* accounts for fewer than 1 per cent of cases of meningitis in the population at large. The onset of illness is usually fairly sudden with headache and fever. Nuchal rigidity is present in 85 per cent of patients. Although the signs and symptoms generally resemble those of other pyogenic meningitides, coarse tremors or cerebellar ataxia may be striking. The cerebrospinal fluid in most patients (70 per cent) shows a polymorphonuclear leukocytosis and increased protein concentration; in fewer than half is the glucose decreased below 40 mg per deciliter. Occasionally, the course of *Listeria* meningitis is indolent and the spinal fluid contains a predominance of lymphocytes, leading to suspicion of tuberculous or cryptococcal infection.

Focal cerebritis or *brain abscess* may complicate the course of *Listeria* meningitis, especially in renal transplant recipients. In some patients, these focal lesions may appear without other evidence of meningitis. They usually affect the cerebral hemispheres or brainstem, causing hemiplegia or cranial nerve palsies. Aphasia, nystagmus, and dysconjugate gaze may occur as well. In the absence of meningitis, there is no nuchal rigidity and the spinal fluid abnormalities are relatively mild. Radionuclide scan and possibly computed tomographic (CT) scan may be helpful in delineating the lesions.

Bacteremia caused by *L. monocytogenes* usually affects patients under 50 years of age. About 90 per cent of patients have an underlying illness or are pregnant. There are no specific features to distinguish this from other forms of bacteremia. Fever, chills, and tachycardia are usual; hypotension and confusion may occur. Peripheral leukocytosis is the rule, but monocytosis has been reported. The major complications are meningitis and endocarditis.

Endocarditis caused by *L. monocytogenes* is rare. In contrast to other forms of listeriosis in adults, most patients have not had an immunosuppressive illness, but pre-existing valvular disease was noted in over half the cases. In several instances, infection occurred on a prosthetic valve.

Other *localized infections* include pneumonia, hepatitis, pericarditis, infected aortic aneurysm, osteomyelitis, conjunctivitis, intraocular infection, and primary skin infection. All of these are rare.

L. monocytogenes has occasionally been recovered from lymph nodes, blood, or spinal fluid of patients with a syndrome resembling infectious mononucleosis. However, this presentation is rare and is unrelated to EB-virus disease.

Perinatal infection, the most distinctive syndrome of listeriosis, may take one of two forms. In the first, the infant becomes infected in utero. The woman may be asymptomatic, or may sustain a mild influenza-like illness with fever, myalgias, diarrhea, sore throat, or urinary symptoms. Shortly thereafter, premature birth or stillbirth may occur. If the infant is born alive, signs of septicemia develop within hours. Fetal distress, pneumonia, diarrhea, seizures, and rash are common manifestations. Microabscesses, sometimes with a granulomatous component, are found in various organs. This disease, also known as "granulomatosis infantiseptica," has a very high mortality rate.

The second form of neonatal disease occurs after the first five to seven days of life. Meningitis is the usual presentation, but progressive hydrocephalus may occur. Infection is believed to be acquired during passage through the birth canal. Overall, about 10 to 20 per cent of neonatal meningitis is due to *L. monocytogenes.*

The role of listeriosis in spontaneous abortion is controversial. In one study, the organism was cultured from the cervix of 25 of 34 women who had had repeated abortions, but in none of 87 control patients. In another study, antibiotic treatment of three couples in which the wives had suffered repeated abortions resulted in successful pregnancies. However, a large body of data suggests that this sequence of events is unusual and that *Listeria* is not implicated in most instances of spontaneous abortion.

DIAGNOSIS. Beyond the neonatal period, there is little that is specific about the syndrome of listeriosis. Clearly, this organism must be suspected when meningitis occurs in a setting of diminished host defenses. However, the diagnosis rests upon bacteriologic grounds, and the key to diagnosis is awareness. Laboratories frequently misinterpret *L. monocytogenes* as diphtheroids, which are discarded as "contaminants." Gram stain of infected material may reveal the typical, pleomorphic, palisading, gram-positive bacilli. However, organisms are not seen in Gram stain of the spinal fluid in 60 to 75 per cent of patients with *Listeria* meningitis. Moreover, the organisms sometimes resemble streptococci, or in other instances, stain irregularly so that they are mistaken for *Hemophilus influenzae*. If the clinical setting is suggestive, the physician should alert the laboratory to the possibility of listeriosis. Cultures can then be examined for β-hemolysis, catalase positivity, and tumbling motility of organisms at room temperature, which distinguish *L. monocytogenes* from other agents.

Listeria is generally not difficult to grow from infected material unless the patient has received antibiotics. Selective media may be helpful with samples such as sputum and vaginal secretions that contain other bacteria. In addition to blood cultures, spinal fluid should be obtained if there is any suggestion of meningitis, for nuchal rigidity may be absent. In the newborn, material from the eye, ear, nose, throat, amniotic fluid, and meconium should be examined in addition to blood cultures.

TREATMENT. Ampicillin or penicillin G is the mainstay of therapy for listeriosis. The organisms are generally susceptible to these antibiotics as well as to trimethoprim-sulfamethoxazole, chloramphenicol, clindamycin, erythromycin, gentamicin, vancomycin, and tetracyclines, but individual strains may depart from the usual pattern. Cephalosporins should be avoided because of their limited meningeal penetration and generally poor activity against the organisms. In one retrospective study, ampicillin appeared somewhat better than penicillin G. There is some evidence that chloramphenicol, especially as a single agent, is less effective than ampicillin or penicillin G.

For initial therapy in adults, pending the results of sensitivity tests, ampicillin is recommended in a dosage of 200 mg per kilogram per day in six divided doses; alternatively, penicillin G, 300,000 units per kilogram per day in six or eight divided doses, may be used. Higher dosages may occasionally be required. There is synergy between these drugs and gentamicin or streptomycin in vitro. Thus, concomitant administration of an aminoglycoside, intrathecally for meningitis, might be considered in seriously ill patients or those who relapse. Therapy may have to be given for several weeks to prevent relapse. On the basis of activity in vitro, trimethoprim-sulfamethoxazole could be a useful alternative in the penicillin-allergic patient.

PROGNOSIS. The overall mortality of untreated listeriosis exceeds 70 per cent for meningitis or bacteremia. The outcome with treatment is influenced by coexisting diseases. In adults with meningitis, the mortality rate was 13 per cent in those without other disorders, 28 per cent in immunosuppressed patients without malignancy, and 60 per cent in those with malignancy. A low glucose concentration and high protein concentration in the cerebrospinal fluid appear to herald an unfavorable outcome of meningitis. Brain abscess or cerebritis carries a mortality rate of about 50 per cent, and residual defects are common.

Among patients treated appropriately for bacteremia with ampicillin or penicillin G, 90 per cent survive. Fatalities occur primarily among those with immunosuppressive illnesses in whom there is undiagnosed central nervous system infection. About one third of patients with endocarditis die, primarily of myocardial infarction, congestive heart failure, or subarachnoid hemorrhage.

Antibiotics have reduced the mortality rate of perinatal infection to about 50 per cent from almost 100 per cent. Patients being treated for bacteremia should be carefully watched for signs of meningitis, especially if they are being given antibiotics which penetrate the meninges poorly. Well demarcated brain abscesses require surgical drainage.

PREVENTION. There is no vaccine available to prevent listeriosis. On occasion, clusters of cases have occurred in hospitalized patients, suggesting possible cross-infection. Although such events are rare, it seems prudent to use isolation precautions for patients with listeriosis, especially if there are transplant recipients or patients with immunosuppressive disorders nearby.

It may be worthwhile to culture the cervix of women who have repeated abortions or whose infants die early in life and the blood of women who are febrile during pregnancy for the possibility of treatable *Listeria* infection.

Bottone EJ, Sierra MF: Listeria monocytogenes: Another look at the "Cinderella among pathogenic bacteria." Mt Sinai J Med 44:42, 1977. *A comprehensive review with emphasis on the bacteriologic properties and pathogenetic mechanisms of the organism.*

Green HT, Macaulay MB: Hospital outbreak of *Listeria monocytogenes* septicemia: A problem of cross-infection? Lancet 2:1039, 1978. *Just what the title says. Addresses the problem of whom, if anyone, to isolate in these circumstances.*

Lavetter A, Leedom JM, Mathies AW, Ivler D, Wehrle PF: Meningitis due to *Listeria monocytogenes*. N Engl J Med 285:598, 1971. *A retrospective comparison of the outcome of disease in 25 patients treated mainly with ampicillin or penicillin G. Although concomitant antibiotics may have skewed the results somewhat, the data suggest some advantage for ampicillin.*

Nieman RE, Lorber B: Listeriosis in adults: A changing pattern. Report of eight cases and review of the literature, 1968–1978. Rev Infect Dis 2:207, 1980. *A thorough review of the clinical aspects of listeriosis in the postnatal period, with a detailed analysis of risk factors and prognostic features.*

Perinatal listeriosis. Lancet 1:911, 1980. *A concise account of the current status of the diagnosis, treatment, and prevention of this highly fatal disease.*

Stamm AM, Dismukes WE, Simmons BP, Cobbs CG, Elliott A, Budrich P, Harmon J: Listeriosis in renal transplant recipients: Report of an outbreak and review of 102 cases. Rev Infect Dis 4:665, 1982. *An excellent review of this continuing problem. Has 110 references.*

Tuazon CU, Shamsuddin D, Miller H: Antibiotic susceptibility and synergy of clinical isolates of *Listeria monocytogenes*. Antimicrob Agents Chemother 21:525, 1982. *Stresses the lack of bactericidal activity of the penicillins (the drugs of choice) and of chloramphenicol and the excellent activity of trimethoprim-sulfamethoxazole in vitro.*

292. ERYSIPELOID

Michael Barza

DEFINITION. *Erysipelothrix rhusiopathiae* is an important cause of disease in animals. In humans, it produces a characteristic violaceous erythema of the fingers and hands known as erysipeloid (of Rosenbach). Disseminated infection and endocarditis rarely occur.

ETIOLOGY. *E. rhusiopathiae* is a slender, pleomorphic, non-spore-forming gram-positive rod which grows well on ordinary laboratory media. Its lack of motility or catalase production and its ability to form hydrogen sulfide on TSI slants help distinguish it from *Listeria monocytogenes* and *Corynebacteria* (diphtheroids).

EPIDEMIOLOGY. Erysipeloid is an occupational disease of persons exposed to infected animals or animal products. *E. rhusiopathiae* is found in various *animals,* including sheep, lamb, cattle, horses, dogs, and mice; *fish* and *shellfish;* and *fowl,* including turkeys, chickens, and ducks. It is carried by as many as 50 per cent of healthy swine and is an economically significant cause of disease in those animals and in turkeys. Swine develop septicemia, chronic arthritis with or without endocarditis, and a rhomboid urticarial skin reaction ("diamond skin"). *E. rhusiopathiae* appears to colonize the slime of fish. It survives in decaying organic matter. Although resistant to salting, pickling, and smoking, the bacteria are killed by heating at 55° C for 15 minutes.

Humans are quite resistant to infection by ingestion, but are readily infected through superficial abrasions in contact with contaminated material. Thus, the disease is most common in abattoir workers, butchers, fish-handlers, and the like. However, there is often no definite recollection of trauma.

CLINICAL MANIFESTATIONS. Within a few days of inoculation, rarely longer than a week, there is the onset of a purplish erythema, usually on the finger or hand. Pain or itching, tingling, and throbbing usually accompany and may antedate the skin lesions. The rash slowly spreads to involve other fingers, but rarely the fingertips or above the wrist. It is sharply demarcated, and there is central clearing. Vesicles and even bullae are sometimes seen. Lymphangitis or regional lymphadenitis occur in about 20 per cent of patients and constitutional symptoms such as fever in about 10 per cent. The joints in the affected extremity may be stiff and somewhat swollen. Untreated, the lesions usually resolve spontaneously over a period of weeks, but persistent sterile arthritis has been reported in up to 10 per cent of patients. In very rare instances, a generalized skin eruption occurs.

Occasionally, *E. rhusiopathiae* causes septicemia. This almost always signifies endocarditis. About half of these patients have no antecedent history of valvular disease; some have evidence of recent erysipeloid. The endocarditis may be very destructive, with a high mortality rate.

DIAGNOSIS. The characteristic skin lesion and history of animal contact point to the diagnosis. The violaceous hue, burning or painful sensation, and absence of suppuration or constitutional symptoms distinguish this from ordinary pyogenic infections. The organisms can rarely be grown from aspirates of infected material but can often (7 of 20 cases in one series) be cultured from full-thickness skin biopsy of the advancing edge. The septicemic disease is diagnosed by blood culture.

TREATMENT. The organisms are sensitive to penicillins, cephalosporins, erythromycin, clindamycin, tetracyclines, and chloramphenicol, but not to vancomycin or aminoglycosides. Uncomplicated cutaneous lesions generally respond well to oral penicillin G, although parenteral therapy is occasionally necessary. Surgical incision offers no benefit and may lead to secondary infection. A suggested regimen for endocarditis is intravenous penicillin G, 12 to 20 million units daily for four to six weeks. Valve excision may be required. With early and aggressive therapy, the survival rate is about 85 per cent.

There is no vaccine available to prevent the disease. Highly exposed persons should be advised to wear gloves and wash their hands frequently at work.

Grieco MH, Sheldon C: *Erysipelothrix rhusiopathiae.* Ann NY Acad Sci 174:523, 1970. *A concise and detailed review of the bacteriology, epidemiology, and clinical features of this disease. Many references.*

Klauder JV: Erysipeloid as an occupational disease. JAMA 111:1345, 1938. *An account of the epidemiology of the infection in 100 patients, together with a vivid, illustrated, clinical description.*

Klauder JV: *Erysipelothrix rhusiopathiae* infection in animals and in human beings. Ann NY Acad Sci 48:535, 1946. *A comparison of the disease in animals and humans, and detailed review of some unusual presentations in humans.*

Kramer MR, Gombert ME, Corrado ML, Ergin MA, Burnett V, Ganguly J: *Erysipelothrix rhusiopathiae* endocarditis. South Med J 75:892, 1982. *The first reported case in a drug addict. Points out the improved survival with current treatment, including valve replacement.*

Price JEL, Bennett WEJ: The erysipeloid of Rosenbach. Br Med J 2:1060, 1951. *A good clinical and epidemiologic description, with emphasis on the difficulties of bacteriologic diagnosis.*

293. ACTINOMYCOSIS

David J. Drutz

DEFINITION. Actinomycosis is a chronic suppurative and granulomatous bacterial infection characterized by contiguous spread, abscess formation, and sinuses that discharge grains ("sulfur granules"). There are four clinical forms: cervicofacial ("lumpy jaw"), thoracic, abdominal, and disseminated.

ETIOLOGY. Etiologic agents include *Actinomyces israelii, A. naeslundii, A. viscosus, A. odontolyticus, A. meyeri,* and *Arachnia propionica. Actinomyces bovis* produces lumpy jaw in cattle, but is virtually never a human pathogen. These filamentous bacteria are anaerobic or facultative, capnophilic, gram-positive, and non-acid-fast. Filaments may break up into coccobacilli. All are normal oral flora; none is recoverable from the environment. Sulfur granules may be found in normal tonsillar crypts in the absence of an inflammatory reaction.

Actinomycosis is characterized by "associate" bacteria (e.g., *Actinobacillus actinomycetemcomitans* or various streptococci in cervicofacial actinomycosis; *E. coli* and diverse enteric organisms in abdominal actinomycosis). Given the disruption of mucous membranes necessary for initiation of actinomycosis, their presence is not surprising. These aerobes may play a synergistic role by helping maintain the low oxygen tension necessary for growth of the actinomycetes.

EPIDEMIOLOGY. Actinomycosis occurs worldwide, and is unrelated to climate, occupation, race, or age. It may be more common in men than in women. Accurate data on incidence and prevalence are not available, but the disease is not rare. Actinomycosis occurs in many animal species, but is not transmissible to man.

PATHOGENESIS AND PATHOLOGY. The etiologic agents are poorly invasive, generally requiring a break in the mucous membrane and the presence of devitalized tissue suitable to their anaerobic growth requirements. Unlike *Nocardia* species, they are not usually opportunistic in a setting of depressed cell-mediated immunity.

In animal studies mycelia and grains are more difficult to eliminate than coccobacilli. When the suppurative response fails to eradicate the bacteria, a granulomatous reaction ensues, accompanied by intense fibrosis. Contiguous spread of infection characteristically ignores tissue boundaries, and ultimately produces draining sinus tracts and invasion of surrounding tissues.

The histopathologic picture is characterized by a mixed suppurative, granulomatous, and fibrotic process in which grains are a major distinguishing feature. When stained with hematoxylin-eosin, grains are centrally basophilic with eosinophilic rays (*Actinomyces* = "ray fungus"), terminating in pear-shaped "clubs." The clubs consist of an immune complex–derived sheath enclosing a single central filament that represents the organism itself. The grains stain well with methenamine silver, but Gram stain is needed to identify the actinomycetes.

CLINICAL MANIFESTATIONS. Cervicofacial actinomycosis accounts for 60 per cent of infections and generally occurs in a setting of tooth decay, gingival disease, dental extraction, or serious injury sufficient to disrupt mucosal integrity. Manifestations include pain (some are painless); woody-hard swelling, often in the parotid or mandibular region (attributable to fibrosis); discoloration; trismus; and multiple sinuses that discharge odorless pus containing yellow-white granules. Fever and leukocytosis may occur. The disease spreads by direct extension, and may involve tongue, salivary glands, pharynx, and larynx. Periostitis is followed by osteomyelitis. Cervical spine or cranial bone disease may lead to subdural empyema and central nervous system invasion. Cervicofacial actinomycosis may be confused with tuberculosis, nocardiosis, mycotic infections, osteomyelitis caused by other microorganisms, or neoplasm.

Thoracic actinomycosis accounts for 15 per cent of cases and may result from the aspiration of pharyngeal contents, dental plaque, or tonsillar grains; from organisms carried to the lung by a foreign body; by direct extension from cervicofacial or abdominal (especially hepatic) infection; or by hematogenous spread. There is often a history of underlying lung disease. Thoracic actinomycosis resembles other chronic inflammatory processes and malignancies. The tendency for the infection to cross pulmonary fissures and to form draining chest wall sinuses suggests the correct diagnosis. The pericardium and mediastinum may be invaded. Sulfur granules are rarely present in the sputum.

Abdominal actinomycosis accounts for about 20 per cent of cases and usually arises weeks to months following a perforation of the gastrointestinal tract. Most cases present in the right iliac fossa, reflecting a frequent association with appendicitis. Abdominal actinomycosis may spread by contiguity to other intra-abdominal structures (especially the liver), the lung, pelvis, spine, or abdominal wall. The eventual development of draining fistulas offers an important clue, and the diagnosis should be considered even in cases of perirectal abscess or fistula in ano. Abdominal actinomycosis may be confused with Crohn's disease, ulcerative colitis, tuberculosis, or malignancy. Colonization of the uterine cervix with *A. israelii* and other actinomycetes has become common with the use of intrauterine contraceptive devices (IUD's). Cases of pelvic actinomycosis have originated in this fashion.

Disseminated actinomycosis may result from the hematogenous spread of bacteria from any of the sites mentioned above, but most frequently follows thoracic disease. Hematogenous dissemination is rare. Tissues most commonly involved include the skin and subcutaneous tissues, bone, brain, liver, and kidneys.

DIAGNOSIS. The diagnosis of actinomycosis should be made by direct isolation of the infecting organism from clinical specimens, or from washed, crushed sulfur granules. Bacteriologic confirmation is achieved in less than 50 per cent of cases because of failure to obtain anaerobic cultures, or overgrowth by the "associate" bacteria. Examination of Gram-stained tissue for filamentous, branching, non-acid-fast, gram-positive organisms often provides the clue to diagnosis. The organisms can also be seen in Gram stains of crushed granules, but must be differentiated from those seen in the grains of botryomycosis, eumycetomas, or actinomycetomas (see Ch. 375). The diagnosis of pelvic actinomycosis is usually first suspected when organisms are seen on cytologic preparations from the cervix.

Transtracheal aspiration has been complicated by formation of actinomycotic neck abscess at the site of needle introduction.

There are no reliable serologic tests for actinomycosis and no skin tests. Fluorescent antibody staining techniques have been used to identify actinomycetes in tissue sections, to identify their presence in mixed cultures, and to verify their final identity after isolation. However, these tests are not generally available.

TREATMENT. Actinomycosis has a strong tendency to recur, at least partially because of inaccessibility of the disease process to antibiotic penetration. Therefore, prolonged treatment courses may be necessary. There is no generally agreed upon formula for antibiotic dose or duration, and treatment should be tailored to disease severity. Cervicofacial actinomycosis may be easier to cure than the other forms. Penicillin is the drug of choice. In severe cases, 10 to 20 million units are given intravenously daily for four to six weeks, followed by 2 to 5 million units of oral phenoxymethyl penicillin (or its equivalent) for a total of 12 to 18 months of treatment. Alternative antibiotics (given in full dosage) include tetracycline, erythromycin, lincomycin, or clindamycin. *A. israelii* is exquisitely sensitive to rifampin, but no data are available on therapy with this drug. Although *Actinobacillus actinomycetemcomitans* is not particularly susceptible to penicillin or ampicillin, patients with actinomycosis improve on these regimens. Therefore, it is not necessary to tailor therapy to the drug susceptibilities of "associate" bacteria. Adjunctive therapeutic measures for actinomycosis include surgery.

PROGNOSIS. The advent of antibiotics has greatly improved the prognosis for all forms of actinomycosis, and neither deformity nor death is common.

Berardi RS: Abdominal actinomycosis. Surg Gynecol Obstet 149:257, 1979. *A thorough and up-to-date review of all aspects of actinomycosis, with particular emphasis on the abdominal form.*

Bhagavan BS, Gupta PK: Genital actinomycosis and intrauterine contraceptive devices. Cytopathologic diagnosis and clinical significance. Hum Pathol 9:567, 1978. *An estimated 6 million women in the United States use intrauterine devices for contraception. This article discusses the role that actinomycosis may play in pelvic inflammatory disease.*

Flynn MW, Felson B: The roentgen manifestations of thoracic actinomycosis. Am J Roentgenol Radium Ther Nucl Med 110:707, 1970. *An outstanding guide to the roentgenographic diagnosis of pulmonary actinomycosis.*

Richtsmeier WJ, Johns ME: Actinomycosis of the head and neck. CRC Crit Rev Clin Lab Sci 11:175, 1979. *An excellent review, with an emphasis on infection of the head and neck.*

294. NOCARDIOSIS

David J. Drutz

DEFINITION. Nocardiosis is a subacute or chronic suppurative bacterial infection characterized by pneumonia and hematogenous dissemination, especially to the central nervous system. In immunosuppressed patients, the disease pursues a more acute, aggressive course.

ETIOLOGY. The etiologic agent is *Nocardia asteroides,* a gram-positive, aerobic actinomycete that is partially, and weakly, acid fast. Filamentous branching cells occur during logarithmic phase growth, but later fragment to small coccobacillary forms. There appear to be three subtypes of *N. asteroides,* occasionally manifesting divergent antimicrobial sensitivity patterns. There are also numerous other *Nocardia* species, and some aspects of classification are unsettled. All nocardiae contain mycolic acid and are similar to mycobacteria in this regard. All are commonly found in soil and on straw, grasses, and rotting vegetation. Nocardiae are resistant to rifampin, a useful point in taxonomy. *N. caviae, N. farcinica,* and *N. brasiliensis* can produce pulmonary and disseminated infection in man, but only rarely. *N. brasiliensis* is, however, a common cause of actinomycetoma (see Ch. 375).

INCIDENCE AND PREVALENCE. Nocardiosis occurs worldwide, in all ages, races, and climates. It is two to three times as common in men as in women, but there is no occupation-related susceptibility. Five hundred to 1000 clinical cases occur yearly in the United States, but because of underreporting the true incidence and prevalence of nocardiosis are unknown.

EPIDEMIOLOGY. Nocardiosis is presumed to result from inhalation of airborne bacteria. At least one common-source outbreak in immunocompromised patients has been reported. *N. asteroides* has been recovered from the sputum and other body sites in patients without apparent clinical disease.

Nocardiosis can occur in apparently normal persons or in those with chronic obstructive pulmonary disease, but is encountered more commonly in immunosuppressed patients. Associated clinical conditions include systemic lupus erythematosus, sarcoidosis, silicosis, alveolar proteinosis, chronic granulomatous disease, dysglobulinemias, solid or hematologic malignancies, and corticosteroid therapy. The recovery of *N. asteroides* from any immunocompromised person must be considered evidence of infection, not colonization, and must be appropriately treated.

Nocardiosis can occur as a primary cutaneous infection, usually following a local injury. Dissemination may occur.

PATHOGENESIS AND PATHOLOGY. In congenitally athymic nude mice, *N. asteroides* produces a fatal disseminated infection, but in their syngeneic thymus-bearing littermates, the disease is limited in extent and animals survive. *N. asteroides* growing in log phase prevents the phagolysosomal fusion necessary for alveolar macrophages to kill the ingested bacteria. These observations suggest that macrophages, T lymphocytes, and cell-mediated immunity play a crucial role in host defense against nocardiosis. The roles that serum factors and polymorphonuclear leukoyctes fulfill are poorly defined.

In humans, nocardiosis is characterized by suppuration and abscess formation. The intense fibrosis, extension by contiguous spread, sinus formation, grains, and granulomatous response that characterize actinomycosis and nocardial actinomycetoma are absent. Nocardiosis disseminates hematogenously, with a tendency to involve the central nervous system, kidneys, and skin. However, no organ is exempt. The histologic picture is dominated by suppuration, mimicking pyogenic bacterial infection. *N. asteroides* is usually overlooked in hematoxylin-eosin–stained tissue, but is seen with tissue Gram stain or Gomori methenamine silver (if staining time is extended). Acid-fast stains (appropriately modified to prevent overdecolorization) will demonstrate the organism, but its tendency to fragment into coccobacillary forms may cause it to be confused with *Mycobacterium tuberculosis* or atypical mycobacteria.

CLINICAL MANIFESTATIONS. Nocardiosis presents as a pneumonic process in about 75 per cent of cases; in others, the pulmonary involvement may be transient or inapparent. Fever and cough are common. The radiographic picture is characterized by segmental or lobar infiltrates, often with rapidly developing thick-walled cavities. Masses, nodules, empyema, bulging fissures, and even chest wall extension reminiscent of actinomycosis may be encountered. Other radiographic presentations include chronic solitary lung abscess or indolent progressive fibrosis. Hilar involvement and calcification are uncommon. The radiographic picture has no pathognomonic features, and is often complicated by pre-existing lung disease.

In 25 to 40 per cent of patients there is dissemination to the central nervous system. Occasionally, there is meningitis, but more frequently there are one or more space-occupying lesions, with headache and focal neurologic findings. Other common sites of dissemination include the skin and subcutaneous tissues, pleura and chest wall, kidney, eyes, liver, and lymph nodes. Fifty-five per cent of patients have no identifiable foci of secondary infection. However, dissemination is more common in the immunosuppressed, and must be aggressively sought. A negative chest film does not exclude disseminated nocardiosis.

DIAGNOSIS. In a patient with a generally intact immune system and a chronic disease course, nocardiosis may be confused with tuberculosis, mycoses, a variety of bacterial infections, or a malignancy. Repeated sputum cultures or more invasive diagnostic procedures may be required to reach the diagnosis. In the immunosuppressed patient, the disease may be confused or may coexist with any of the disorders named above, or with pneumocystosis *(P. carinii)*, Legionnaires' disease, cytomegalovirus infection, bleomycin lung, and others. In such patients, an aggressive diagnostic evaluation is indicated. Diagnostic flexibility is limited by the unavailability of reliable skin or serologic tests. Specimens of sputum, pleural fluid, tracheostomy secretions, transtracheal aspirates, bronchial washings and brushings, and transbronchial biopsy specimens should be stained and cultured. With failure of these methods, percutaneous lung aspiration or open lung biopsy should be carried out. Skin abscesses should be aspirated and smears examined for organisms. In addition, skin lesions should be biopsied, with portions submitted for histology and for culture. Computed tomographic (CT) scans of the brain should be obtained as otherwise silent cerebral abscesses or foci of cerebritis have been identified in this manner.

Nocardia asteroides will grow on most standard media. However, unless the organism is suspected, its recognition poses a practical problem because culture plates tend to be overgrown by microbial contaminants (especially in sputum) and are often discarded after 48 hours, whereas *N. asteroides* may require three to seven days for growth. As a result, the organism is more likely to be identified on media used for mycobacteria or fungi, which are observed for longer periods of time. Although chances for recovery of *N. asteroides* from the blood, urine, bone marrow, and spinal fluid are slim, cultures should nevertheless be obtained in difficult diagnostic situations.

TREATMENT. Most *N. asteroides* strains are sensitive to sulfonamides in vitro, and sulfonamides are the treatment of choice. Therapy should be initiated with 6 to 10 grams of sulfadiazine or sulfisoxazole daily. These regimens produce peak serum levels of 12 to 15 mg per deciliter. Subsequent dosage can be modified according to measured serum concentrations and clinical response. The duration of therapy is poorly standardized, but should be prolonged since relapse is common. In patients with intact host defenses, treatment should be continued for at least six weeks following clinical recovery. In the immunosuppressed, therapy should be given for at least one year. In patients with cerebral involvement, the progress of treatment should be monitored with serial CT scans. Surgery is usually required for brain abscesses and may also be necessary for subcutaneous abscesses or empyema.

Not all patients respond to sulfonamide therapy, especially those who are profoundly immunosuppressed. In these patients it may be necessary to reduce dosage of immunosuppressive drugs. It has also been common to employ supplemental drugs (cycloserine, ampicillin, tetracycline, erythromycin, streptomycin, and other aminoglycosides), but proof of efficacy of combined drug regimens is lacking. This statement also applies to co-trimoxazole, a fixed combination of one part trimethoprim to five parts sulfamethoxazole. Nevertheless, trimethoprim-sulfamethoxazole has come to be widely used, especially in immunocompromised patients or those with central nervous system involvement.

In patients unable to tolerate or not responding to sulfonamides, therapeutic alternatives include amikacin, minocycline, and chloramphenicol.

PROGNOSIS. Nocardiosis is not restricted to the immunosuppressed. However, those who are immunosuppressed have the most acute process, the greatest propensity to hematogenous dissemination, and the poorest prognosis. Prior to the sulfonamide era, only 25 per cent of patients recovered; in patients treated with a sulfonamide, the recovery rate is 54 per cent. However, Palmer et al. have recorded 75 per cent survival, even in immunosuppressed patients, when the diagnosis was established promptly and sulfonamide therapy begun. Thus, the chances for cure are directly related to the aggressiveness of management. Patients with cerebral involvement generally have a poorer prognosis.

Curry WA: Human nocardiosis. A clinical review with selected case reports. Arch Intern Med 140:818, 1980. *A current review, with valuable information concerning chemotherapy.*

Palmer DL, Harvey RL, Wheeler JK: Diagnostic and therapeutic considerations in *Nocardia asteroides* infection. Medicine 53:391, 1974. *A comprehensive literature review of 243 cases of nocardiosis (including 13 patients in their own experience) occurring between 1961 and 1972. Still the best single review on the subject.*

Simpson GL, Stinson EB, Egger MJ, Remington JS: Nocardial infections in the immunocompromised host: A detailed study in a defined population. Rev Infect Dis 3:492, 1981. *Twenty-one of 160 patients undergoing cardiac transplantation at Stanford developed nocardiosis. Percutaneous lung aspiration was of particular value in reaching the diagnosis; sputum survey cultures were rarely positive. Patients responded surprisingly well to sulfisoxazole, despite the fact that immunosuppressive therapy was not altered.*

Smego RA Jr, Moeller MB, Gallis HA: Trimethoprim-sulfamethoxazole therapy for Nocardia infections. Arch Intern Med 143:711, 1983. *This article provides an extensive literature review and argues that trimethoprim-sulfamethoxazole is likely to be superior to sulfonamides alone for patients with all forms of nocardiosis. The authors acknowledge that no direct comparative data exist but offer pharmacokinetic evidence and discussion of synergy in vitro to support the use of the combination.*

Stevens DA, Pier AC, Beaman BL, Morozumi PA, Lovett IS, Houang ET: Laboratory evaluation of an outbreak of nocardiosis in immunocompromised hosts. Am J Med 71:928, 1981. *Description of an apparent common-source outbreak of nocardiosis in a renal unit and/or possible person-to-person spread of infection.*

295. BRUCELLOSIS

*John E. Bennett**

DEFINITION. Brucellosis is an infectious disease characterized by fever, sweats, weakness, malaise, and weight loss. Infection is transmitted to man from animals or animal products containing bacteria of the genus *Brucella*.

ETIOLOGY. *Brucella suis, Brucella abortus, Brucella melitensis,* and *Brucella canis* may all cause human brucellosis. Brucellae are small, nonmotile, non-spore-forming, gram-negative rods. The four species are differentiated by biochemical and serologic reactions. Hogs are generally infected with *Br. suis,* cattle with *Br. abortus,* sheep and goats with *Br. melitensis*, and dogs with *Br. canis.* However, infections of swine with *Br. abortus* or of cattle with *Br. suis* may occur, and *Brucella* infection of caribou, deer, horses, moose, cats, and chickens has been reported. Animal-to-animal transmission is usually venereal or via ingestion of infected tissue or milk. Human infection most commonly results from ingestion of infected animal tissue or milk products, or through skin wounds directly bathed in freshly killed infected animal tissues, as in abattoir workers. Human infection via inoculation of the conjunctival sac has also been documented, and there is epidemiologic evidence to suggest rare infection via inhalation of aerosols containing *Brucella* organisms.

EPIDEMIOLOGY. Brucellosis is common in many countries of the world, with 500,000 cases per year being reported to the World Health Organization. Within the United States the number of cases reported to the Centers for Disease Control each year has gradually declined, with only 154 cases being reported in 1982. The actual number of cases in the United States is probably larger, but there is no doubt that the rigorous efforts to control brucellosis in this country have been effective.

Brucellosis most frequently occurs in persons with high rates

*This chapter is a revision of the chapter written by Thomas M. Buchanan, which appears in the 16th edition.

of exposure to *Brucella*-infected tissues, milk, or milk products. This includes slaughterhouse workers, livestock producers, veterinarians, and persons who ingest unpasteurized milk or milk products. During the ten-year period 1969–1978, 1171 (57 per cent) of the 2063 reported cases were in slaughterhouse employees.

Brucellae may remain viable in unpasteurized milk or cheese for approximately 10 or 90 days, respectively. Among the 3316 cases of brucellosis reported to the Centers for Disease Control in the 14-year period 1965–1978, ingestion of unpasteurized dairy products accounted for 8 per cent. The source of the dairy product was Mexico in 47 per cent, other foreign countries in 19 per cent, and the United States in 34 per cent. *Br. melitensis* in Mexican goat's milk cheese has been responsible for several outbreaks, including 29 cases from Texas in 1983. Isolation of *Brucella* from infected meat markedly decreases over a few days with refrigeration, and particularly with the curing and smoking processes used for ham and bacon. In the abattoir setting, persons with a combination of both high accidental cut rates and considerable exposure to the blood and lymph of freshly killed animals are most likely to develop *Brucella* infections. *Brucella* infections are often controlled by the patient's immune response, and asymptomatic infections are up to ten times more common than symptomatic disease and the clinical syndrome of brucellosis. Approximately 90 per cent of patients are immune to developing subsequent clinical brucellosis following recovery from their first infection. Therefore in populations with high exposures to potentially infected tissues (e.g., abattoir workers), most cases are seen in younger persons who have been exposed for shorter periods and are less likely to have developed immunity. Brucellosis affects men more commonly than women.

PATHOGENESIS AND PATHOLOGY. *Brucella* organisms penetrate the epithelial cells of the human skin (i.e., hands), oropharynx, conjunctivae, or lung. In the submucosa they interact with polymorphonuclear leukocytes (PMN) and/or tissue macrophages. Many are phagocytized, and, if the inoculum is sufficient, some spread via the lymphatics to regional lymph nodes. The most common sites of lymphadenitis in brucellosis are in the axillary, cervical, and supraclavicular locations, perhaps reflecting the high frequency of the hand-wound or oropharyngeal routes of infections. If the inoculum is sufficient to overcome host immune attempts at localization of *Brucella* organisms within the lymph nodes, bacteremia follows. The usual incubation period between infection and bacteremia with associated symptoms is 10 to 11 days with a heavy inoculum, and two to three weeks with a smaller inoculum. Incubation periods as short as seven days or as long as three months have been reported. Bacteremia is usually accompanied by phagocytosis of nearly all free *Brucella* organisms within a few hours by circulating PMN. These phagocytized brucellae are further localized most commonly to the spleen, liver, and bone marrow. Brucellae are located inside phagocytic vacuoles within PMN, and transient intracellular survival and even multiplication of *Brucella* organisms within phagocytes have been reported. In most instances, the inoculum is not large, the human host defenses prevail, granuloma formation does not occur, and the patient recovers. Similarly, even with a large inoculum, prompt treatment (within three to four weeks of onset of symptoms) of sufficient duration (four to eight weeks) results in rapid healing of the small granulomas and complete recovery. However, if the inoculum is large and the patient is not treated, small granulomas may fuse to form large granulomas that may eventually suppurate and serve as a source for recurrent bacteremia. Granulomas in the liver are common with infections caused by *Br. abortus* and *Br. suis,* but uncommon with hepatic involvement caused by *Br. melitensis.* Persistent bacteremia may lead to multiple system involvement, including most commonly infections and abscesses of the skeletal system (spine and joints), genitourinary tract (kidneys, bladder, epididymis, testes, urethra), optic nerve, lung, liver (abnormal liver function tests, jaundice), and cardiovascular system (endocarditis, myocarditis, pericarditis). *Br. suis* and *Br. melitensis* are more virulent than *Br. abortus,* and *Br. canis* usually causes a mild and easily treatable disease.

CLINICAL MANIFESTATIONS. Over 90 per cent of patients experience chilly sensations, sweats, and fever, accompanied by weakness and general malaise. The fever ranges from 38.3 to 40° C, and approximately 70 per cent of patients experience body aches. Over half of patients with brucellosis complain of anorexia and experience weight loss, averaging 15 to 20 pounds. Nearly 45 per cent of patients complain of headaches. Cough and/or arthralgias are present in approximately 20 to 25 per cent of patients. Diarrhea, constipation, visual disturbance, eye pain, dizziness, tinnitus, or genitourinary disturbance may occur, although less frequently. The most common signs of brucellosis in addition to fever are lymphadenopathy (up to 40 per cent), splenomegaly (up to 40 per cent), hepatomegaly (up to 8 per cent), and tenderness over the spine (up to 6 per cent), with the prevalence of each sign reflecting the chronicity of infection in the patient population studied. The average number of work days lost for an abattoir worker with brucellosis varies from 30 to 50 days. One third to one half of patients experience a sudden onset of symptoms; in the remainder the onset is gradual, over several days to weeks.

Observed complications in patients with untreated and long-standing brucellosis have included pleurisy, pleural effusion, lung abscess, millet-seed pulmonary calcification, empyema, pneumonia, chronic pulmonary granuloma, spondylitis, suppurative arthritis, osteomyelitis, hydrarthrosis, epididymitis, orchitis, cystitis, pyelitis, nephritis, optic neuritis, keratitis, uveitis, retinopathy, meningitis, encephalitis, neuritis, hemolytic anemia, thrombocytopenia or pancytopenia associated with hypersplenism, cholecystitis, pericholecystic or subdiaphragmatic abscesses, chronic cutaneous ulcers, endocarditis, myocarditis, thrombophlebitis, pulmonary embolization, and cardiac rupture. Patients suspected of central nervous system involvement with *Brucella* organisms should have cerebrospinal fluid (CSF) examined. *Brucella* meningoencephalitis or brain abscesses frequently produce increased CSF pressure and increased CSF protein levels. The CSF usually has increased gamma globulin levels and frequently contains *Brucella*-agglutinating antibodies. Many diseases more common than brucellosis have signs and symptoms that partially or almost totally mimic brucellosis. It is therefore important to exclude other more common illnesses and to obtain objective evidence of *Brucella* infection before making a diagnosis of brucellosis. Diseases that may resemble brucellosis include influenza; infectious mononucleosis; toxoplasmosis; viral hepatitis; acute pyelonephritis; ankylosing spondylitis; thyrotoxicosis; disseminated gonococcal infection; rheumatic fever; systemic lupus erythematosus; malaria; tuberculosis; sarcoidosis; leptospirosis; typhoid fever; Hodgkin's disease; lymphoblastic and lymphocytic leukemia; myeloblastic and myelocytic leukemia; metastatic carcinoma of the lung, colon, prostate, pancreas, stomach, or liver; and thiamin deficiency. If the patient has had recent exposure to animal tissue or products potentially infected with *Brucella* organisms, the clinical suspicion of brucellosis should be increased.

Objective findings useful for evaluation of possible brucellosis in a patient include physical signs, cultures, serologic data, and x-rays. The absence of at least intermittent fever of 38.3° C or higher makes a diagnosis of brucellosis extremely unlikely (less than 5 per cent of patients). Weight loss is present in approximately half of the patients; lymphadenopathy and splenomegaly are other common signs.

The definitive evidence of *Brucella* infection is the isolation of *Brucella* organisms from the patient. *However, culturing* Brucella *organisms may be dangerous to laboratory personnel. All cultures should be clearly marked "possible brucellosis." A laboratory should not undertake isolation and identification of* Brucella *unless Biosafety Level 3 facilities are available.* Early in the course of illness, particularly in association with fever and chills, the patient is likely to have *Brucella* bacteremia. Approximately 50 to 75 per cent of these patients who have not received antimicrobial drugs will yield *Brucella* organisms from their blood when one or two samples are cultured in standard blood culture bottles (containing trypticase soy broth) for one to three weeks in the presence of 5 to 10 per cent CO_2. Later in the course of the illness, bacteremia is less frequent and organisms are more likely to be isolated from infected lymph nodes, or from granulomas involving the spleen, liver, or skeletal system (most frequently, spine). During the past ten years only 15 to 20 per cent of brucellosis cases in the United States have been confirmed by culture. Most cases were diagnosed serologically.

The most reliable and standardized *serologic screening test* for brucellosis is the standard tube *Brucella* agglutination test, which measures antibodies directed predominantly at *Brucella* lipopolysaccharide antigens. A four-fold or greater rise in titer for sera drawn one to four weeks apart is indicative of recent exposure to *Brucella* or *Brucella*-like antigens. Separate sera should be tested on the same day, in the same laboratory, and under identical conditions to examine for seroconversion. Significant seroconversion is defined as four-fold or greater rise in titer from an initial titer of at least 40 or higher to an eventual titer of 160 or higher. The titer is the reciprocal of the maximal serum dilution that produces 50 per cent or more agglutination of the *Brucella* organisms under the test conditions. Most patients develop rising agglutination titers to *Brucella* antigens within one to two weeks of illness, and approximately 80 per cent of persons have an eight-fold or higher rise in their agglutinins during the acute illness. Within three weeks of illness, approximately 97 per cent of patients with brucellosis will have serologic evidence of their infection if a single serum sample is tested. With repeat testing, less than 0.7 per cent of all patients will remain seronegative (titer <160). Serum from patients infected with *Br. canis* usually fails to agglutinate the standard antigen but will react with antigen prepared from *Br. canis* or *Br. ovis*. Another cause of false negative agglutination test results is failure of the laboratory to test dilutions up to at least 1:320. The prozone phenomenon may cause lower dilutions to be negative. The maximal *Brucella* agglutination titers in sera from persons with asymptomatic *Brucella* infections may reach as high as titers in patients with clinical brucellosis. The *Brucella* skin test, cholera vaccination, or infection with *Vibrio cholerae, Pasteurella tularensis*, or *Yersinia enterocolitica* may cause seroconversion to elevated *Brucella* agglutination titers and not represent *Brucella* infection. Provided that these "cross-reactive" causes of seroconversion are ruled out, a four-fold rise in titer of *Brucella* agglutinating antibodies is indicative of current *Brucella* infection.

Significance of Elevated Antibody Titer. During the first one to two weeks of illness, the primary agglutinating antibody response to *Brucella* is of the IgM immunoglobulin class. Thereafter, IgG antibodies are formed in addition to IgM antibodies. Both IgG and IgM agglutinating antibodies are detected in the standard *Brucella* agglutination test. However, with early diagnosis and prompt treatment of sufficient duration, IgG agglutinating antibodies rarely persist beyond 6 to 12 months following onset of the disease. However, if the diagnosis is delayed for many months to years and no treatment is received, some patients (fewer than 15 per cent) will develop continuing *Brucella* infection with potentially serious complications. These patients will maintain elevated IgG *Brucella* agglutinins until diagnosed and treated. This information is useful to the clinician, because the *Brucella* agglutination performed in the presence of 0.05 M 2-mercaptoethanol (2-ME) recognizes only IgG agglutinating antibodies to Brucella. Thus in the absence of a rising agglutination titer, a single elevated 2-ME *Brucella* agglutination test titer is the most objective evidence that the patient has a current or recent infection. A titer of 160 or higher in the 2-ME test suggests either a current or recent asymptomatic infection or, if the patient is symptomatic, active infection with disease and the need for treatment. Titers of 40 to 80 in the 2-ME *Brucella* agglutination test are rarely associated with significant recent infections. In a patient with symptoms of three or more weeks' duration, a 2-ME *Brucella* agglutination titer of 20 or lower essentially eliminates the possibility that the patient's symptoms are due to brucellosis. A significant proportion of patients maintain elevated IgM agglutinating antibodies and consequently have elevated standard *Brucella* agglutination titers for many years, even after presumed complete cure of their brucellosis. In fact, standard *Brucella* agglutination titers of ≥ 160 are very common in completely asymptomatic abattoir workers. For this reason, the 2-ME *Brucella* agglutination test that measures only IgG agglutinating antibodies is the most useful indicator of whether the patient was cured (negative test). Of 92 patients with brucellosis followed recently by Buchanan and Faber for ≥ 18 months, 44 (48 per cent) retained positive standard *Brucella* agglutination test titers (≥ 160) after 18 months despite adequate treatment in nearly all cases. In contrast, only eight of these same patients retained positive titers (≥ 160) in the 2-ME *Brucella* agglutination test 12 months after treatment was initiated. None of the 84 patients with negative 2-ME titers after 12 months had significant signs or symptoms of brucellosis, and none developed chronic brucellosis. In contrast, four of the eight patients with persistent positive 2-ME titers still had signs and symptoms of brucellosis and required further treatment. Thus, the 2-ME *Brucella* agglutination test is the most useful objective indicator of whether a patient has responded to chemotherapy.

The Brucella skin test is not recommended for diagnostic purposes, because it may remain positive for many years following symptomatic or asymptomatic *Brucella* infection and it may interfere with interpretation of serologic tests by causing a rise in titer of the standard tube agglutination test.

TREATMENT. The drug of choice for brucellosis is tetracycline, given to adults as 500 mg orally four times a day and continued for four or preferably six weeks. The addition of streptomycin 1 gram intramuscularly each day for the first two weeks decreases the relapse rate and improves response in severely ill patients. Substitution of gentamicin or other aminoglycosides for streptomycin has been reported, as has usage of doxycycline instead of tetracycline. The merits of such exchanges are as yet unclear. The combination trimethoprim-sulfamethoxazole has been reasonably effective in a number of cases, particularly when the adult dose was two 80-400 mg tablets three or four times each day. Rifampin, 600 mg daily, has been a useful addition to other regimens and should be considered for cases refractory to tetracycline plus streptomycin or for patients with meningoencephalitis. Although penicillins and cephalosporins have not proven efficacious in brucellosis, moxalactam plus rifampin was reported to have cured a patient with chronic *Brucella* meningitis. With any effective treatment of brucellosis, fever may increase markedly for the first 24 hours, sometimes accompanied by delerium or shock. In severe brucellosis, concomitant administration of adrenal corticosteroids has been used for the first days of therapy to blunt this reaction. All antimicrobial regimens should be continued for four or preferably six weeks.

Relapses occur in less than 5 per cent of cases when the patient receives treatment early in the course of illness and for six weeks' duration. Relapse is more frequent when treatment is delayed or of insufficient duration. Most relapses occur within three months, and nearly all develop within ten months of completing initial therapy. Nearly all relapses rapidly respond to a repeat course of therapy.

PROGNOSIS. Brucellosis diagnosed within one month of onset of illness and treated with appropriate antimicrobial therapy for a sufficient period is a completely curable illness. Even before antimicrobial therapy was available, 85 per cent of patients recovered within three months. With chemotherapy, chronic brucellosis (illness lasting more than one year) or severe complications have become extremely rare. When either of these situations is found, it is almost invariably associated with a prolonged delay before diagnosis and/or failure to take prescribed medications. Acute brucellosis produces substantial malaise, weakness, fever, and weight loss and is frequently associated with an inability to work for one to two months, even with antimicrobial therapy. Without therapy, complications such as *Brucella* abscesses of the liver, spleen, vertebral column, heart valve, skin, meninges, lung, or bone marrow may occur, but with therapy, these complications are rare (less than 1 per cent). They almost invariably occur only in patients with continuous or intermittent fever of 38.3° C or higher and positive standard and 2-ME *Brucella* agglutination test results (titer greater than 160). When complications of brucellosis are demonstrated, they usually respond to a combination of surgical removal of the localized lesion and antimicrobial therapy. Hypersensitivity to *Brucella* antigens may occur, but in recent years it has been very unusual even among abattoir workers who are maximally exposed to potentially infected animal tissue. Therefore patients should be allowed to return to their former work, even if it means re-exposure to *Brucella* antigens, as development of hypersensitivity is unlikely. Also, immunity to reinfection follows the first *Brucella* infection in most (92 per cent) cases, and thus patients returning to work following treatment are less likely to acquire brucellosis than are previously uninfected employees. If these previously infected employees replace seronegative workers in areas of maximal exposure to freshly slaughtered animal tissues, fewer cases of brucellosis may result.

PREVENTION. Effective prevention of brucellosis in cattle results from a live attenuated *Brucella* vaccine. No vaccine is presently available for humans in the United States. The risk of acquiring brucellosis may be reduced by decreasing one's exposure to freshly killed animal tissue from potentially infected animals and by drinking only pasteurized milk and milk products. Slaughterhouse workers, meat inspectors, and veterinarians who occupationally examine large numbers of cattle and hogs may reduce their risk of infection by wearing protective gloves and goggles or eyeglasses and by avoiding hand or arm cuts that might provide a route of entry for *Brucella* organisms. Complete elimination of brucellosis in humans will first require elimination of *Brucella* infection in animals.

Buchanan TM, Faber LC: 2-Mercaptoethanol *Brucella* agglutination test: Usefulness for predicting recovery from brucellosis. J Clin Microbiol 11:691, 1980. *The most complete analysis of the standard and 2-ME* Brucella *agglutination tests, utilizing 15 to 29 sera from each of 92 patients with brucellosis who were followed closely for ≥18 months after initiation of treatment.*

Buchanan TM, et al.: Brucellosis in the United States, 1960–1972: An abattoir-associated disease. I. Clinical features and therapy. II. Diagnostic aspects. III. Epidemiology and evidence for acquired immunity. Medicine 53:403, 415, 427, 1974. *A detailed analysis of all aspects of brucellosis in 160 patients in a large Iowa abattoir.*

Cervantes F, Carbonell J, Bruguera M, Force L, Webb S: Liver disease in brucellosis. A clinical and pathological study of 40 cases. Postgrad Med J 58:346, 1982. *Biopsies and clinical features of 40 cases, mostly proved by serology, are analyzed.*

Gotuzzo E, Alarcon GS, Bocanegra TS, Carrillo C, Guerra JC, Rolands I, Espinoza LR: Articular involvement in human brucellosis: A retrospective analysis of 304 cases. Semin Arthritis Rheum 12:245, 1982. *An instructive analysis of sacroiliitis, arthritis, and spondylitis in 304 Peruvian cases, largely caused by* Br. melitensis.

Larbrisseau A, Maravi E, Aguilera F, Martinez-Lage JM: The neurological complications of brucellosis. Can J Neurol Sci 5:369, 1978. *A recent review of the neurologic complications of brucellosis, including meningoencephalitis, extradural* Brucella *granuloma, and neuritis.*

Marx A, Sandulache R, Pop A, Cerbu A: Biochemical basis of the serological cross-reactions between *Brucella abortus* and *Yersinia enterocolitica* serotype 0:9. Ann Microbiol 126B:435, 1975. *A biochemical study indicating cross-antigenicity in the lipopolysaccharide molecules of* Brucella abortus *and* Yersinia enterocolitica *serotype 0:9.*

Spink WW: The Nature of Brucellosis. Minneapolis, University of Minnesota Press, 1956. *A classic reference book detailing many aspects of brucellosis, and including an appendix of case histories of 139 bacteriologically proven cases.*

Young EJ: Human brucellosis. Rev Infect Dis 5:821, 1983. *Nine instructive cases of brucellosis are presented and the relevant literature reviewed.*

296. BARTONELLOSIS

Theodore C. Eickhoff

SYNONYMS. Synonyms for bartonellosis include Carrión's disease, Oroya fever, and verruga peruana.

DEFINITION. Bartonellosis is an insect-borne bacterial disease found only in South America, and characterized by two distinct stages. The first, Oroya fever, is an acute febrile hemolytic anemia with an appreciable mortality; the second, verruga peruana, is a benign cutaneous eruption of hemangiomatous papules and nodules.

ETIOLOGY. The disease is caused by *Bartonella bacilliformis,* a small gram-negative pleomorphic bacillus that may be cultivated readily in enriched bacteriologic media. The disease is transmitted to man by the bite of sandflies of the genus *Phlebotomus;* characteristic symptoms of Oroya fever follow an incubation period of two to six weeks.

EPIDEMIOLOGY. Although a number of epidemics have been reported, Oroya fever is more commonly seen as sporadic cases among populations of Peru, Colombia, and Ecuador, where occurrence of the disease is restricted to those who live or visit altitudes of 1500 to 9000 feet on both slopes of the Andes. This coincides in general with the ecologic zones supporting populations of the *Phlebotomus* vector.

The disease is transmitted by *Phlebotomus verrucarum,* a night-biting sandfly, and possibly by other unidentified species of sandfly. The principal reservoir of the disease appears to be man; no additional animal reservoirs have been implicated. Reports of cultivation of the agent from apparently healthy persons suggest that as much as 10 per cent of infection may be subclinical.

PATHOLOGY. In Oroya fever, the causative organism may be found in peripheral blood smears stained with Giemsa or Wright's stain, as well as in the reticuloendothelial cells. In the blood the parasite is found both free in the plasma and adherent to erythrocytes. Parasitization of the erythrocytes causes increased mechanical fragility and also increased sequestration of the cells in the spleen and liver. Because as many as 90 per cent of erythrocytes may be parasitized, a severe hemolytic anemia develops rapidly during the febrile period, erythrocyte counts decreasing within only a few days to levels of 1 to 2 million cells per cubic millimeter. Coombs' tests and tests for red cell agglutinins and hemolysins give negative results, and the mechanism of hemolysis remains poorly understood.

CLINICAL MANIFESTATIONS. The presenting symptoms of patients with Oroya fever are intermittent high fever, painful muscles and joints, tender enlarged lymph nodes, and the systemic symptoms and prostration of a severe anemia. The patient's skin color may reflect the presence of both jaundice caused by hemolysis and marked pallor caused by profound anemia. Peripheral blood films show macrocytosis, hypochromasia, poikilocytosis, Howell-Jolly bodies, and nucleated erythrocytes. Muscle and joint pain and headache may be severe. After three to six weeks, survivors begin a slow convalescence marked by disappearance of *bartonellae* from the blood and gradual normalization of temperature and red cell mass.

After a variable length of time, survivors may develop the second (verruga peruana) stage of the disease, characterized by cutaneous nodules that develop over one to two months. The "verrugas" are nodular hemangiomatous lesions, 0.5 to 2 cm in diameter, that most frequently involve exposed skin but occasionally may appear on mucous membranes or in viscera. The verrugas may persist for several months to several years in untreated persons, but mortality is infrequent. Occasional patients may experience only the fever and anemia without the skin manifestations or only the cutaneous lesions without the initial fever. Although these two aspects of the infection were once thought to be different diseases, there is ample evidence that both syndromes are manifestations of infection with the same organism. The skin lesions are believed to be an expression of developing immunity in the patient.

DIAGNOSIS. In the acute stage of Oroya fever both blood smears and blood culture usually reveal the presence of the agent. As the patient progresses toward the verruga stage of infection, the organism becomes more difficult to demonstrate in blood, but can be cultured from the cutaneous lesions.

TREATMENT AND PROGNOSIS. Mortality in the Oroya fever phase of the disease may approach 50 per cent, particularly when the infection is complicated by concurrent attacks of malaria, amebiasis, tuberculosis, or salmonellosis. The disease responds well to treatment with penicillin, tetracyclines, streptomycin, or chloramphenicol. Because of the high frequency of intercurrent *Salmonella* infections, chloramphenicol is widely used for seven or more days in a dose of 2.0 to 3.0 grams daily. Patients become afebrile in 24 to 48 hours, and, if they receive transfusions, recover strength rapidly. The mortality of the verruga stage of infection is less than 5 per cent, and the lesions respond variably to chemotherapy.

PREVENTION. Prevention requires control of the sandfly vector. Spraying of interior and exterior dwellings with residual insecticide has been helpful. Personal protection may be augmented by insect repellents and bed nets.

Archer GL, Coleman PH, Cole RM, Duma RJ, Johnston CL Jr: Human infection from an unidentified erythrocyte-associated bacterium. N Engl J Med 301:897, 1979. *Although bartonellae are the only well-characterized hemotropic bacteria known, this case report suggests the possibility that there may be others. See also the accompanying editorial by Ristic M, Kreier JP: Hemotropic bacteria, pp 937–939.*
Dooley JR: Haemotropic bacteria in man. Lancet 2:1237, 1980. Kreier JP, Ristic M: The biology of hemotrophic bacteria. Ann Rev Microbiol 35:325, 1981. *These two reviews are an excellent introduction to the broad topic of hemotrophic bacteria.*
Schultz MG: Daniel Carrión's experiment. N Engl J Med 278:1323, 1968. *A fascinating account of the young Peruvian medical student, Daniel Carrión, who demonstrated by his death that verruga peruana and Oroya fever were caused by the same etiologic agent.*

Presumptive Bacterial Disease

297. CAT SCRATCH DISEASE

Andrew M. Margileth

DEFINITION. Cat scratch disease (CSD) is usually a benign, self-limited disease characterized by tender regional chronic (≥ three weeks) lymphadenopathy and frequently preceded by a primary skin lesion following cat contact or scratches. Persistence of the adenopathy for several months in a generally healthy patient with gradual spontaneous resolution of the enlarged bubo is its natural course.

ETIOLOGY. Recently studies at the Armed Forces Institute of Pathology have implicated a small gram-negative bacillus as the causative agent of CSD. In 34 of 39 lymph nodes from patients with clinical and histopathologic criteria of CSD, pleomorphic rod-shaped bacilli were observed within the walls of capillaries, in or near areas of follicular hyperplasia, and within microabscesses. They were clearly seen with the Warthin-Starry silver impregnation stain and with immunoperoxidase stains using convalescent patient sera. Similar-appearing organisms were seen with light microscopy in the biopsied tissue of a primary inoculation cat scratch lesion on the finger of a patient with typical CSD.

EPIDEMIOLOGY. Since the initial description by Debré (1950), about 2000 patients with cat scratch disease have been reported in over 750 articles. An estimated 2000 unreported cases occur annually in the United States, primarily in children, but the true incidence is unknown. The disease is worldwide, occurring in all races with a predominance in males (61 per cent). In temperate zones, most cases have occurred during fall and winter. Seasonal variation is minimal in warmer climates. Several epidemics in the same house or geographic locality have been recorded.

TRANSMISSION AND COMMUNICABILITY. The mode of transmission is presumably by direct contact, since the bubo usually follows a scratch, bite, or lick from a young cat. Cat contact occurs in 90 per cent of patients. The disease has also developed after a dog bite or scratch and rarely after a scratch from a thorn, wood splinter, or fish bone. Person-to-person transmission has not been reported. Regional lymphadenopathy was produced experimentally in humans, monkeys, baboons, and Hartley guinea pigs after an intradermal injection of material aspirated from suppurative lymph nodes of human patients. Attempts to isolate an infectious agent from cat saliva or claws have been unsuccessful. The healthy cat—often a kitten—apparently acts as a mechanical vector for the infective agent, for skin tests with CS antigen on the implicated cats have been nonreactive. The writer's studies in family outbreaks have shown that the family cat usually transmits the causative agent no longer than two to three weeks.

PATHOGENESIS AND PATHOLOGY. No serologic test is available to measure antibodies to the causative agent. Fortunately, the cat scratch skin test is reliable and has a high degree of specificity; the reaction is a delayed hypersensitivity type. A positive reaction is usually detected at the time the clinical diagnosis is suspected; however, conversion may be delayed up to four weeks thereafter. Cutaneous reactivity lasts up to ten years. Second attacks have not been reported.

Biopsied lymph nodes may show distinct yet nonspecific stages, depending upon the interval between onset and biopsy. The early lesions reveal a reticulum cell hyperplasia followed by necrotizing granulomas, occasionally with giant cells, then multiple microabscesses, and, weeks to months later, frank abscess formation. Consequently, a presumptive histopathologic diagnosis of tularemia, brucellosis, tuberculosis, or sarcoidosis may be considered. Rarely a biopsy made before suppuration has appeared has shown histologic changes, including reticulum cell hyperplasia and granulomas, suggestive of Hodgkin's disease.

CLINICAL MANIFESTATIONS. The patient usually is not ill in spite of impressive lymphadenopathy; however, malaise, fever, sore throat, headache, and anorexia may be present. Three to ten days elapse from the time of the scratch or contact until a primary skin papule or pustule forms. It may exhibit one or more erythematous papules. Unilateral conjunctival granuloma or conjunctivitis occurred in 7 per cent of the author's 364 patients. An inoculation site (a scratch or a primary lesion, or both) may be detected in 54 to 96 per cent of patients, depending on the thoroughness of the examination and the duration of the bubo. Most primary lesions persist for one to three weeks, rarely for seven weeks. The primary lesion heals without scar formation. Regional lymphadenopathy usually develops about two weeks after the scratch (range, 3 to 50 days). Lymphangitis has not been observed. Tender nodes, present in 80 per cent of patients for the first one or two weeks, are commonly found in the head, neck, or axilla. Epitrochlear, inguinal, femoral, or popliteal areas are involved less frequently. Multiple site involvement occurred in 38 per cent of the author's cases. Node size varies from 1 to 8 cm. Enlargement persists for two to four months, rarely for 6 to 24 months. Suppuration occurs in about one tenth of patients seen in office practice and in about one quarter of those admitted to hospitals.

No clinical signs other than lymphadenopathy occurred in approximately half of the author's 707 patients observed throughout a 25-year period. In about one third of reported cases, patients had fever (38.3 to 41.2° C) lasting for 5 to 9 (1 to 30) days; 25 per cent of our 364 patients had malaise or an influenza-like syndrome lasting about 4 (1 to 21) days. Splenomegaly occurred in 16 per cent of the last 364 patients. Exanthems—maculopapular, petechial, or erythema nodosum or multiforme types—occurred in 4 per cent of the author's patients. The rash usually lasted 4 to 9 days. See Tables 297–1 and 297–2.

Unusual clinical manifestations include the oculoglandular syndrome of Parinaud (6 per cent, 42 of 707 of the author's cases), appearing as an ocular granuloma or conjunctivitis with parotid area swelling caused by preauricular lymphadenopathy;

TABLE 297–1. CLINICAL FEATURES IN 364 PATIENTS WITH CAT SCRATCH ADENOPATHY AND A POSITIVE SKIN TEST (April 1975 to January 1983)

Category	Percentage of Patients
Animal contact	
Cat	89
Dog	9
None	2
Animal scratch	
Cat	71
Dog	2
None	27
Primary lesion	
Skin papule or pustule	45
Eye granuloma	7
Mucous membrane	2
Symptoms and signs	
None except adenopathy	52
Fever (38.3–42.1° C)	33
Malaise/fatigue	25
Splenomegaly	16
Sore throat	12
Headache	11
Anorexia/emesis/weight loss	10
Exanthem	4.4
Parotid swelling	3

encephalitis (45); thrombocytopenic purpura (8); osteomyelitis (5); and primary atypical pneumonia (4).

Children with central nervous system involvement may develop encephalopathy, meningitis, radiculitis, polyneuritis, or myelitis with paraplegia. Onset of neurologic symptoms is sudden, usually with fever, and occurs within one to six weeks of the onset of adenopathy. Major symptoms and signs in 41 cases of neurologic involvement were as follows: coma or convulsions in two thirds, neurologic abnormalities, noted above, in one fourth, and lethargy and/or confusion in one sixth. In 12 of 22 patients with neurologic involvement, cerebrospinal fluid pleocytosis, elevated protein, or both were detected. Electroencephalograms were abnormal in most patients. Severe manifestations have lasted for one to two weeks, with gradual recovery to normal status in one to six months in most patients.

DIAGNOSIS. Regional lymphadenopathy developing two weeks after cat contact, and especially if a primary inoculation papule or pustule followed a scratch, suggests cat scratch disease. Three of the four following manifestations would confirm the diagnosis in a typical case, whereas all four would be necessary in an atypical case: (1) a history of animal (usually cat) contact with presence of a scratch or a primary dermal or eye lesion; (2) aspiration of sterile pus from the node (a presumptive diagnostic test) or laboratory results excluding other etiologic possibilities; (3) a positive skin test result to cat scratch antigen (5 per cent false positives occur; use of only one antigen may give a false negative result in 10 to 20 per cent of patients); (4) node biopsy revealing histopathology consistent with CSD, especially if pleomorphic rod-shaped bacilli can be demonstrated with the Warthin-Starry silver stain.

If a negative skin test result is found to one or two different cat scratch antigens applied simultaneously and again four weeks later, and if results of other studies are negative, a biopsy must be considered to rule out a benign tumor or lymphoma. The presence of tenderness favors cat scratch or a pyogenic or mycobacterial adenopathy rather than a neoplasm. Ultrasonography has been very useful in deciding whether or not to aspirate nontender or nonfluctuant cervical masses. It may also aid needle placement for cyst or abscess aspiration.

Skin Tests. A skin test using cat scratch antigen is positive in 90 per cent of patients who are clinically suspected of CSD. A negative result often occurs if the duration of illness is less than three or four weeks, and about 5 per cent of patients with typical cat scratch disease will have negative test results with one or two different antigens. The positive reaction consists of a wheal or papule with 5 mm or more of induration, with or without erythema, occurring 48 to 72 hours after intradermal inoculation of 0.1 ml of antigen. Induration may persist for five to six days or longer. A positive test result may be obtained for years (10 to 28) after the initial episode.

False-positive reactions have been reported in veterinarians (12 to 29 per cent), healthy persons (4 to 5 per cent), and family contacts; the overall incidence is 5 per cent. Thus the limit of confidence for a positive reaction is about 95 per cent. If the reaction is negative at four-week intervals, the disease can be excluded with reasonable certainty, especially if two different antigens are used. Repeated skin testing with CS antigen in the same patients has not produced positive reactions. Skin tests with PPD-T and atypical PPD mycobacterium antigens have been rarely positive in patients with cat scratch disease.

Since CS antigen is not available commercially, all aspirated pus from affected nodes should be saved to prepare test antigen (Margileth, 1968, 1971). CS antigen for medical diagnosis is usually available from the author upon written request.

Laboratory Data. Laboratory tests are not diagnostic. Eosinophilia has been reported. At the onset the number of polymorphonuclear cells may be increased with a mild leukocytosis. A sedimentation rate, usually elevated during the first few

TABLE 297–2. CAT SCRATCH LYMPHADENOPATHY IN 364 PATIENTS—CLINICAL CHARACTERISTICS OF INVOLVED NODES AND DURATION OF ADENOPATHY (April 1975 to January 1983)

Adenopathy (N = 364)	Per Cent	Size (cm) (N = 364)	Per cent
Single node	41	1.0 to < 3.0	43
Multiple nodes	21	3.0 to < 5.0	38
Multiple sites	38	≥ 5.0	19
Tender nodes	79		
Suppuration	13		
Location (N = 470)	**Per Cent**	**Duration (N = 364)**	**Per Cent**
Head: total (N = 93*)	20	Prior to diagnosis**	
Submandibular	13	2 to < 4 weeks	51
Preauricular	19	1 to < 2 months	28
Neck: total (N = 193)	41	2 to < 4 months	14
Posterior	17	4 to < 6 months	3
Anterior	21	6 to < 12 months	3
Supraclavicular	3	Regression (months, < 1.0 cm)	
Extremities: total (N = 184)	39	1 to < 2	23
Axillary	22	2 to < 6	56
Epitrochlear	5	6 to < 12	14
Inguinal	7	12 to < 24	6
Femoral	5	≥ 24	1

*Occipital = 5 (1%).
**Duration ≥ 12 months = 4 (1%).

weeks of adenopathy, suggests an inflammatory lymphadenitis.

DIFFERENTIAL DIAGNOSIS. Cat scratch disease should be considered in all patients with persistent lymphadenopathy (over three weeks), because it is the most common cause of chronic regional lymphadenitis in children or adolescents. The presence of an inoculation (dermal or ocular) lesion strongly suggests CSD. Other less common causes are sporotrichosis, primary syphilis, lymphogranuloma venereum, typical or atypical tuberculosis, other bacterial adenitis, tularemia, brucellosis, histoplasmosis, coccidioidomycosis, sarcoidosis, toxoplasmosis, infectious mononucleosis, and benign or malignant tumors. In atypical forms of cat scratch disease, one may observe benign recurrent parotid lymphosialadenopathy, Parinaud's oculoglandular disease, encephalitis, pneumonia, thrombocytopenic purpura, erythema nodosum, and osteomyelitis, as well as fluctuant lymphadenopathy simulating cystic hygroma or a thyroglossal duct cyst. If CS skin test reactions are negative, as well as appropriate cultures and serologic and PPD-T and PPD Battery skin tests, a node biopsy will usually determine the cause.

TREATMENT. The best therapy is reassurance that the adenopathy is benign and in most cases will subside spontaneously within two or three months. Management consists of appropriate follow-up examination, analgesics for pain, and aspiration if suppuration ocurs. Lack of response to antimicrobials is the rule; if cat scratch disease is suspected, antimicrobial drugs are not recommended. In the child whose node suppurates, needle aspiration on an ambulatory basis is preferred to incision and drainage. After washing with Betadine cleanser, a needle (18 or 20 gauge) is inserted through normal unanesthetized skin at the base of the mass in order to avoid a chronic sinus tract in the event that a tuberculous lesion is present. Aspiration provides material for skin test antigen, relieves painful adenopathy, and usually allows the patient to become symptom free within 24 to 48 hours. If fluid recurs, reaspiration may be necessary. Application of moist soaks to the primary lesion may facilitate drainage and shorten the duration of lymphadenopathy. The efficacy of steroid therapy in CSD is questionable, and it is not recommended. Excisional biopsy of the node may be necessary in selected patients because of persistent pain or for diagnostic purposes. Spontaneous drainage occurred in 6 per cent of our last 364 patients.

PROGNOSIS. The prognosis is excellent; lymphadenopathy usually regresses spontaneously in two to three months. One attack appears to confer lifelong immunity. Complications and sequelae are almost nonexistent. Rare patients have been reported to have had chronic adenopathy for two years.

PREVENTION. Because of the number of household pets (50 million cats in the United States), cat scratch disease will be difficult to prevent. Disposal of the suspect cat is not recommended, because the cat involved is invariably well. Four to 9 per cent of family members scratched by the same cat may develop cat scratch disease. The patient with the disease does not require isolation or quarantine. Active or passive protection is not available.

Carithers HA: Cat scratch disease associated with an osteolytic lesion. Am J Dis Child 137:968, 1983, *A case report of a child with lytic bone involvement accompanying cat scratch disease and a review of three previously reported cases.*

Carithers HA: Oculoglandular disease of Parinaud. A manifestation of cat scratch disease. Am J Dis Child 132:1195, 1978. *The diagnostic criteria compiled from 14 patients with oculoglandular cat scratch disease are presented.*

Knight PJ, Mulne AF, Vassy LE: When is lymph node biopsy indicated in children with enlarged nodes? Pediatrics 69:391, 1982. *Based on examination of 239 children who underwent peripheral lymph node biopsy, the differential diagnosis and indications for biopsy are reviewed.*

Luddy RE, Sutherland JC, Levy BE, Schwartz AD: Cat-scratch disease simulating malignant lymphoma. Cancer 50:584, 1982. *A case report of a child with oculoglandular CSD with discussion of histopathology of infectious lymphadenopathy that clinically and histologically may simulate a malignant neoplasm.*

Margileth AM, Wear DJ, Hadfield TL, et al. Cat scratch disease: Bacteria in skin at the primary inoculation site. JAMA (in press), 1984. *Five patients with CSD had biopsy or aspiration of adenopathy and biopsy of the primary inoculation skin lesion. In three patients gram-negative pleomorphic bacilli were demonstrated in the skin lesion by the Warthin-Starry silver stain, and identical bacteria were also seen in the regional lymph nodes of two of these patients.*

Wear DJ, Margileth AM, Hadfield TL, Fischer GW, Schlagel CJ, King FM: Cat scratch disease: A bacterial infection. Science 221:1403, 1983. *In a series of 39 lymph nodes studied from patients with CSD, pleomorphic rod-shaped bacilli were observed in 34 by means of special stains.*

Diseases Due to Mycobacteria

298. TUBERCULOSIS

Emanuel Wolinsky

DEFINITION. Tuberculosis is a chronic infectious disease caused by mycobacteria of the "tuberculosis complex," mainly *Mycobacterium tuberculosis*.

HISTORY. During the Industrial Revolution of the 18th and 19th centuries the disease was known as the *white plague*. It was the leading cause of death in young people all over the world. Today, despite great progress in its treatment and control, it is still an important medical problem in many developing countries. A report from the World Health Organization in 1982 indicated that there were still 7 to 10 million new cases and about 3 million deaths each year from tuberculosis. In the United States the tuberculosis mortality has decreased from a rate of 202 per 100,000 in 1900 to less than 1 in 1982. The new case rate has also declined from about 60 per 100,000 in 1950 to 11 in 1982, but the rate has tended to level off during the past few years, resulting in a decline of approximately 5 per cent per year.

The rate of infection as determined by skin test surveys remains high in many developing countries. In the United States the rate has become increasingly difficult to estimate because of the abandonment of large-scale testing in cities. Information obtained in 1977 from selected urban areas of the country indicated that the rate of infection varied from less than 3 per cent in young children to 14 to 40 per cent in adults over the age of 65. Tuberculosis is becoming more and more a disease of middle-aged and older nonwhite men in residual urban pockets of disease associated with poverty and overcrowding.

The great physicians and scientists who were associated with landmark discoveries in tuberulosis include Laennec, who early in the nineteenth century disclosed the physical signs and morbid anatomy and who suggested the concept of one disease with involvement of many organ systems; Villemin, who in 1868 showed that the infection was caused by a transmissible agent; Koch, who demonstrated the tubercle bacillus in 1882; Roentgen, whose discovery of x-rays in 1895 was the begining of diagnostic radiology and allowed recognition of cavity formation; and Waksman, whose discovery of streptomycin in 1944 provided the first agent that could be used successfully in the chemotherapy of the disease.

ETIOLOGY. The microorganism that causes tuberculosis belongs to the genus *Mycobacterium*, which is classified in the family Mycobacteriaceae of the order Actinomycetales. Other families in this order are the Actinomycetaceae, with genera *Actinomyces* and *Nocardia*, and the Streptomycetaceae, which includes the genus *Streptomyces*. Taxonomists do not agree on the further classification of the genus *Mycobacterium*, but a useful concept is that of the tuberculosis complex to include *M. tuberculosis*, *M. bovis*, and probably *M. africanum*. Some taxonomists would subdivide *M. bovis* into European, Afro-Asian, and African variants. A few suggest that there should be just one species, *M. tuberculosis*, with subclassifications of bovine type, African type, and so forth.

M. tuberculosis is an obligate intracellular parasite that shares with other mycobacteria a characteristic staining quality. The popular abbreviation *AFB* for *acid-fast bacilli* is based on this quality. Acid-fastness is the result of retention of carbol fuchsin (or certain fluorochrome dyes) after washing with acid, alcohol, or both. It is not unique to mycobacteria, since *Nocardia* and certain *Corynebacterium* strains may also be acid fast. Mycobacterial cell walls are rich in lipids, existing mainly as complexes with peptides and polysaccharides. Certain stains can form a stable complex with one of these lipid compounds, mycolic acid, provided the latter is contained within an intact cell wall structure.

In addition to the members of the tuberculosis complex, the genus *Mycobacterium* may be divided into about 30 species. Again, there is disagreement among the taxonomists on the definition of many of these species (see Ch. 299).

PATHOLOGY AND PATHOGENESIS. Tuberculosis is derived from the word tubercle, meaning a small lump or nodule. Histopathologically, the tubercle is a more or less discrete focus of granulomatous inflammation consisting of lymphocytes, epithelioid cells, macrophages, and giant cells. The granulomas seen in tuberculosis are characterized by a form of tissue necrosis known as *caseation,* so called because the caseum has the consistency of soft cheese. Prior to the time of necrosis the lesion may heal completely by resolution, but once necrosis and caseation have occurred it heals by fibrosis, encapsulation, calcification, and scar formation. Breakdown of the lesion occurs when the caseum softens and liquefies and is expelled through the bronchial system. This process results in the formation of a cavity in the lung. Spread of disease may occur by local extension, by an intrabronchial route, or through the lymphohematogenous pathway. Early in the primary infection the organisms are transported to the draining lymph nodes and may be widely disseminated throughout the body. In the apical posterior areas of the upper lobes the seeded organisms may remain dormant in inactive lesions for many years only to reactivate during a period of lowered host immunity. The processes of healing and breakdown may occur sequentially and repeatedly so that various stages of the inflammatory reaction are seen in different areas.

The primary lesion in a nonsensitized individual consists of an area of nonspecific pneumonitis in a middle or lower lung zone at the site of deposition of the inhaled droplet nuclei. The initial inflammatory response is the same as that seen in any bacterial pneumonia and consists mainly of fibrin, edema, and polymorphonuclear leukocytes. The extent of this primary exudative response varies with the number and virulence of the bacilli inhaled, the native resistance of the host, and the effectiveness of the immune response. The change to a granulomatous type of reaction occurs coincidentally with the development of delayed hypersensitivity after two or three weeks. The mechanisms of cellular immunity may allow the host to wall off the lesion and to halt the lymphohematogenous spread. It is the softening and liquefaction of the caseous focus that leads to further trouble and the provision of a favorable environment for the rapid multiplication of the mycobacteria. In the encapsulated lesion that does not soften, the bacilli slowly lose their viability.

Stages in the natural history of untreated pulmonary tuberculosis may be described as follows:

1. During the primary phase and throughout the development of the lesions there are usually no symptoms. Even in the so-called manifest primary stage, symptoms may be mild or absent despite parenchymal lesions and enlarged hilar or mediastinal lymph nodes. Pleurisy with effusion may occur. Life-threatening complications at this stage are meningitis and miliary disease.

2. The primary disease usually heals, leaving evidence of its presence in the form of a calcified pulmonary scar along with calcifications in the draining lymph nodes, which together are known as a *Ghon complex.*

3. The third stage is one of latency, during which the bacilli remain dormant but still viable within inactive lesions. This situation may exist for the remainder of the patient's life.

4. Reactivation may occur in a relatively small proportion of infected individuals. This is the mechanism by which tuberculosis in the adult usually develops, either in the lung or in an extrapulmonary site.

5. Exogenous reinfection occasionally may be documented by the demonstration of bacilli with a different phage type or drug sensitivity pattern from those of the primary infection.

EPIDEMIOLOGY. Infection is usually transmitted from person to person by the inhalation of infective droplet nuclei that result from the aerosolization of respiratory secretions. The source of the infected material usually is an adult with cavitary pulmonary tuberculosis. The most important determinants of infectivity are the concentration of organisms in the sputum and the closeness and duration of contact with the index case. Other factors of importance are the cough frequency and the personal habits of the index case, the efficiency with which aerosols are produced by such activities as singing, loud talking, and laughing, and the air circulation and ventilation in the area of contact. A situation favorable to acquisition of infection would be an overcrowded and poorly ventilated house in which there were several young children and an adult with highly positive sputum.

Ingestion is no longer a common pathway for infection, although in the days of unpasteurized milk and widespread tuberculosis in cattle this was a common route of infection for *M. bovis,* especially for the production of tuberculosis of the tonsils and subsequent involvement of the submandibular lymph nodes. Another route of infection that still may be observed, however, is primary inoculation through the skin. Laboratory workers may inoculate themselves with actively growing cultures via needle puncture or broken glass, and pathologists may sustain a penetrating injury while doing a postmortem examination.

Many localized outbreaks or mini-epidemics have been reported in the past and continue to be observed today (Lincoln, 1967; Stead, 1979). The pattern of airborne transmission in a closed environment is well described in these accounts of infections aboard ships, in day care centers, nursing homes, prisons, industrial school dormitories, and school buses, and among members of a choir.

Tuberculosis Control. Tuberculosis is perpetuated by the repeated cycle of new infections that result from the inhalation of infected droplet nuclei coughed into the air by adults with cavitary pulmonary disease. This cycle may be attacked at several points. Case finding efforts are needed to recognize individuals with active disease so that they may be placed under treatment to terminate the infectivity. Large-scale roentgenographic surveys have been abandoned in favor of contact investigation, recognition of symptomatic cases at entry points to the medical care system, and surveillance of high-risk groups such as hospital personnel, prisoners, and nursing home patients.

Protection from the complications of primary disease may be afforded by vaccination with bacille Calmette-Guérin (BCG). This was a strain of *M. bovis* attenuated by many passages on artificial media. There are now many different strains, each unique, maintained in laboratories across the world. Vaccination has been utilized mainly in areas of the world that have a high rate of tuberculosis infection. Although vaccination may protect the individual, it does not reduce the overall rate of infection in the community, since it does not prevent the transmission of infection. Its effectiveness depends on an enhancement of the immune response, which enables the host to eliminate most of the bacilli before tissue destruction and dissemination occur. The efficacy of BCG is controversial. It has not been used extensively in the United States because it interferes with the subsequent use of the tuberculin test in recognizing tuberculosis infection and because the major source of morbidity is people already infected. Nevertheless, a case could be made for BCG in certain special circumstances such as to protect the infant whose mother has active disease and to prevent infection in close contacts of an index case with drug-resistant bacilli.

Chemoprophylaxis may be used to prevent infection in close contacts with negative skin tests, to prevent disease in those already infected, and to prevent subsequent recurrences in individuals with inactive pulmonary disease. The recommended drug for prophylaxis is isoniazid, once daily, in dosage of 300 mg for adults and 10 mg per kilogram (not to exceed 300 mg) for children. When taken for one year, such treatment results in a reduction of at least 70 per cent in the appearance of primary disease in household contacts. Protection is about 90 per cent in those who actually take the drug as prescribed. The effectiveness of shorter courses of therapy has not been adequately investigated. Six months of chemoprophylaxis, while not completely ineffective, protects less well than 12 months. The two principal drawbacks to this method of control are isoniazid hepatitis and the lack of compliance of about 30 per cent of patients to take the prescribed medication.

It has been estimated that the risk of developing active disease in recent tuberculin converters of any age is about 3.3 per cent in the first year after infection. From 5 to 15 per cent may progress to active disease within five years. The risk is greater in infants. Chemoprophylaxis is recommended for close contacts of patients with recently diagnosed active disease; for persons with recent infection documented by skin test conversion within the past two years; for individuals with positive skin test results, radiographic findings consistent with inactive tuberculous disease, and neither positive bacteriologic findings nor a history of adequate chemotherapy; and for individuals with positive skin test results who have additional risk factors (such as malignancy or severe diabetes) or who are undergoing prolonged immunosuppressive or corticosteroid therapy. Although chemoprophylaxis is utilized in this country as one of the important methods of tuberculosis control, it has not been accepted in many other parts of the world. Isoniazid will not prevent disease resulting from infection with isoniazid-resistant bacilli. Rifampin has been suggested as a substitute, although no good studies of its efficacy have been published.

IMMUNOLOGY. Tuberculosis is the classic example of disease caused by an intracellular parasite. Protection is afforded by the mechanisms of cell-mediated immunity rather than by those associated with antibodies. Immunity may be natural or acquired, but in either case it is the macrophage that assumes the major burden of protection. Polymorphonuclear leukocytes have the ability to phagocytize but not to destroy mycobacteria. Although the results of some experiments are contradictory, most researchers have been able to demonstrate that macrophages from an immunized animal kill the bacilli more efficiently and at a more rapid rate than do control cells. Macrophages may be activated by immunologically specific mechanisms as well as by nonspecific stimulation. Specific stimulation occurs when sensitized T lymphocytes contact mycobacterial antigens that have been properly processed by macrophages. The lymphocytes then release a number of active chemical substances known as *lymphokines*, one variety of which activates macrophages.

Native immunity certainly has played a role in the global aspects of tuberculosis. Good examples exist in the animal kingdom; the rat and the cat are quite resistant to infection with *M. tuberculosis*, in contrast to the guinea pig and the monkey, which are highly susceptible. Lurie was able to breed two races of rabbits, one susceptible and one resistant to infection. Although it is difficult to separate the factors of social and economic conditions from those of race, the Eskimo peoples and blacks are considered by some researchers to be more susceptible. The forces of natural selection probably contributed to the decline of tuberculosis prior to the introduction of chemotherapy, although improved socioeconomic conditions played an important role. Acquired immunity may occur as a result of natural infection or by vaccination. Recovery from tuberculosis confers protection against reinfection with a new inoculum, even though the original bacilli may remain latent for many years and be capable of producing recrudescent disease. Whether acquired by natural infection or vaccination, the protection is only relative and may be overwhelmed by a sufficiently large infecting dose.

The relationship between delayed hypersensitivity and immunity is still controversial. The two functions appear at about the same time after infection and are intimately related thereafter. Nevertheless, it has been shown in experimental animals that immunity may remain despite abolition of a positive skin test result by densensitization and that immunity may be induced by ribosome preparations that do not induce a positive skin test result.

The balance between the reactions of delayed hypersensitivity and those of the humoral antibody response is very important in determining the clinical presentation and prognosis in leprosy. A similar but less dramatic situation exists in tuberculosis. A more favorable prognosis may be expected for patients who have strong reactivity in their cell-mediated immune functions than for those who are hypoergic and have abundant antibody production. Patients with nonreactive tuberculosis tend to have disseminated disease with almost unopposed multiplication of the organisms in reticuloendothelial cells and a lack of granulomatous response. The question of whether the anergic state is the cause or the result of severe tuberculosis is moot. Recovery of the compromised cell-mediated immune functions, including delayed hypersensitivity, usually accompanies clinical improvement. A patient's location in the immune spectrum usually is dynamic and changeable rather than fixed.

The Tuberculin Skin Test. The biologically active material in the liquid medium after growth of *M. tuberculosis* was named *tuberculin* by Robert Koch. This crude material was later called *Old Tuberculin (OT)*. A purified protein derivative of tuberculin *(PPD)* was made by Siebert in 1924 by precipitation with saturated ammonium sulfate. The World Health Organization adopted a large batch, designated *PPD-S*, as the international standard tuberculin. Five tuberculin units *(TU)* was defined as the biologic activity contained in a specified weight of PPD-S. Solutions with much greater stability were achieved by the addition of a wetting agent. All preparations of PPD commercially available in this country must be bioequivalent to 5 TU of PPD-S as demonstrated by comparative testing in humans.

The intracutaneous, or Mantoux, test is performed by injecting 5 TU contained in 0.1 ml of solution intracutaneously with needle and syringe. This is known as the intermediate strength test. It corresponds to 0.1 μg of the standard preparation. A more dilute solution containing 1 TU is available to test those who may be expected to have a very strong reaction, especially children. This preparation is known as first strength PPD and is essentially a five-fold dilution of the 5 TU material. Second strength PPD contains what is calculated to be 250 TU.

In the sensitized individual a reaction of redness, swelling, and induration will begin at about 6 hours, reach a maximum intensity at 36 to 60 hours, and then fade over the next several days. A positive result usually is defined as 10 mm or more of induration at 48 hours. This arbitrary definition is based on results of large-scale testing that showed that a reaction of 10 mm best separated those with from those without tuberculosis. The reading of the test is a subjective evaluation, with wide observer variation. It is only by averaging multiple readings made blindly by at least two expert readers that an accuracy within less than 3 mm may be approached.

It is unwise to have an arbitrary definition of a positive test result in the diagnostic evaluation of a sick patient. Many factors may diminish the response in a nonspecific manner. They include virus infections or live virus vaccination; immunosuppression by disease, drugs, or steroids; malnutrition; overwhelming infection of any kind; and old age. It is best to measure the induration as accurately as possible and, in addition, to describe the intensity of both the erythema and the induration. Erythema that persists for 48 hours is usually indicative of a positive test result. In case of doubt, it is often useful to repeat the test using 250 TU. If there is no reaction to the second strength material, the odds against the diagnosis of nondisseminated tuberculosis are approximately 50 to 1. It is helpful to determine the reaction to other antigens utilizing the so-called *anergy panel*. The most useful are mumps, *Candida*, trichophyton, tetanus toxoid, and a streptococcal antigen such as streptokinase. Failure to react to the panel indicates a generalized state of cutaneous anergy, which may be expected to include tuberculin. Several multiple puncture devices are available for performing a tuberculin test. Some are more reliable than others, but they should all be regarded as screening tests, and any doubtful or positive reactions should be tested with the Mantoux technique.

Intradermal administration of tuberculin in the recommended dosage does not induce an immunologic response even after repeated injections. However, a second injection from 2 weeks to 12 months after an original negative reaction may produce a booster response from recall of waning delayed hypersensitivity. To avoid the assumption that the positive reaction represents a new infection, it has been suggested that negative reactors be retested up to a week later in surveillance programs such as those for hospital personnel. Infection with any mycobacterium and probably with organisms of related genera, such as *Nocardia* and *Corynebacterium,* may give cross-reactions with the tuberculin test materials available today. Tuberculin reactivity is a quantitative function that may vary in intensity from time to time in a given person.

Factors Modifying the Course of Tuberculosis. Before chemotherapy, tuberculosis patients were considered to be at risk for recrudescent disease for the rest of their lives. Mitchell was able to follow over 2000 patients for 15 to 25 years after their moderately or far advanced disease had become inactive. He found a relapse rate of 28 per cent. Even with modern drug therapy relapse occasionally may occur, depending mainly on whether or not the patient was cooperative in taking medication. A study of 20,000 cases reported to the Centers for Disease Control in 1980 revealed that 7 to 8 per cent represented recurrent disease.

Many conditions are known to increase the risk for the recurrence of tuberculosis. Among these are emotional stress, malnutrition, drug addiction, alcoholism, immunosuppression by diseases that interfere with cell-mediated immunity, and the use of drugs such as corticosteroids. Gastric resection is a risk factor, presumably in relation to malnutrition. A risk over ten times that of suitable controls has been documented for patients with chronic renal failure on maintenance dialysis or for those with renal transplants. Influenza, pneumonia, and cancer of the lung may cause local reactivation of dormant lesions. Another local factor is the presence of pneumoconiosis, especially silicosis and coal worker's pneumoconiosis.

CLINICAL DESCRIPTION. ***Pulmonary Tuberculosis.*** Tuberculosis may involve any organ system, but the lung is the usual site of the primary lesion and the principal organ involved. In roughly one half of patients with extrapulmonary disease, however, the original pulmonary lesions may not be discernible clinically or radiographically.

PRIMARY TUBERCULOSIS. Primary tuberculosis refers to disease in a person not previously infected with a virulent mycobacterium of the tuberculosis complex. This definition excludes persons who have had BCG vaccination or infection with other mycobacteria. Primary tuberculosis formerly was seen almost exclusively in children and was known as the childhood type. At present it is not uncommon in adults of all ages. Most primary infections are subclinical and not detectable by ordinary radiographic procedures. They may be recognized, however, by a documented tuberculin skin test conversion. When accompanied by symptoms or radiographic evidence, or both, the disease is called manifest or overt primary tuberculosis. Complications of the primary infection include pleurisy with effusion, miliary disease, meningitis, bone and joint disease, and progressive primary infection. In progressive primary disease the lesions enlarge, caseate, liquefy, and cavitate. Primary disease in adults is especially prone to progression and cavity formation.

The morbidity and mortality associated with primary infection is related to age. Although usually benign in older children and adults, it is life-threatening when it occurs in infants. In a New York City study before the development of chemotherapy, tuberculosis in children less than six months of age had a mortality rate of 50 per cent. Congenital tuberculosis, often fatal, may be acquired from a mother with active disease by the hematogenous route or by the aspiration or ingestion of contaminated amniotic fluid. One of the unique findings in primary tuberculosis of young children is the development of consolidated and collapsed segmental lesions resulting from a combination of bronchial compression from enlarged hilar lymph nodes and extrusion of their caseous contents into the bronchial lumen. This situation usually is clinically benign despite the alarmingly unhealthy appearance of the chest roentgenogram. The spectrum of primary tuberculosis in adults was documented by Stead et al. in 1968. In almost half of 37 adults the disease progressed without interruption into chronic pulmonary tuberculosis.

REACTIVATION TUBERCULOSIS. This term refers to the pattern of disease in adults. It usually results from the reactivation of dormant foci in the posterior portions of the upper lobes, which had been seeded by the bloodstream during the early primary infection. Occasionally adult disease is the result of a new inoculum of tubercle bacilli in a person already sensitized by a previous infection. This condition is known as *exogenous reinfection.* Adult disease is characterized by chronicity, caseation, sloughing of liquefied caseous material, cavity formation, and the simultaneous occurrence of healing and progression in different areas of the lung. Lymph node involvement is usually minimal or absent, at least in those nodes that directly drain the pulmonary foci. Phage typing of strains recovered from different areas of the body and correlation between antimicrobial susceptibility patterns and the history of drug intake have been used to document both recrudescence of an old infection and exogenous reinfection.

The onset of disease may be *insidious, catarrhal, hemoptoic, or acute.* With insidious onset there is gradual development of fatigue, anorexia, weight loss, and other vague complaints. Later, a low grade intermittent fever may develop that is commonly associated with excessive sweating at night. The temperature elevation tends to occur in the late afternoon. The catarrhal onset is characterized by an increasingly productive cough and occasional blood streaking of the sputum. Fever and night sweats may also be noted. In the hemoptoic variety, the presenting symptom is hemoptysis either with or without some of the other symptoms already mentioned. Occasionally, the onset is acute and influenza-like with high fever, chills, myalgia, and productive cough. Pleuritic pain may be the presenting complaint, often without pleural fluid but sometimes ushering in the appearance of an effusion. Many cases of adult-type pulmonary tuberculosis in the past were discovered by routine chest films in asymptomatic persons. Some individuals might recall minor symptoms, such as slight pleurisy, night sweats, or tiredness, but others would deny all warning signs despite the presence of advanced disease. Before the advent of chemotherapy, it was not unusual for the patient to have hoarseness or perirectal abscess—both conditions being secondary to the long-term presence of highly positive sputum.

DIAGNOSIS. A careful history and physical examination often suggest the diagnosis of pulmonary tuberculosis before any laboratory test is ordered. The most characteristic physical findings of adult-type disease are rales heard posteriorly near the apex of one or both lungs. The chest radiographs will then confirm the presence of disease in the posterior portion of the upper lobes. Visualization of one or more cavities strengthens the diagnosis. In primary tuberculosis the initial pneumonic area may be anywhere in the lung, especially in the middle or lower lobes, with enlargement of the draining lymph nodes in the mediastinum. These characteristic patterns are not always seen, however. In a recent report from a large teaching hospital it was found that the diagnosis of tuberculosis was not suggested by the radiologist in 26 per cent of 100 consecutive cases. A wide variety of unusual patterns may be encountered, from mass lesions resembling malignancy to widespread interstitial disease of a nonspecific nature. Diabetics are more likely than nondiabetics to have lower lobe disease, which may also be noted as a bronchogenic spread from apical cavities.

Confirmation of the diagnosis should be sought by bacteriologic examination of the sputum. It may be necessary to obtain specimens by the inhalation of nebulized distilled water or saline solution or by gastric lavage. In addition to properly stained smears and cultures for acid-fast bacilli, it is useful to search for elastic fibers by unstained potassium hydroxide wet mounts. The presence of these fibers indicates destruction of lung tissue and should be accompanied by smears positive for AFB. Occasionally, it may be necessary to resort to bronchoscopy and even to lung biopsy to establish the diagnosis.

The tuberculin skin test is very useful in diagnosis, despite the fact that 5 to 20 per cent of those with newly diagnosed cases may have a negative response to the initial test. Transient depression of cell-mediated immune reactions may be either specific for tuberculin or a generalized anergy to all skin test antigens. For immediate diagnostic purposes in such cases, it is useful to apply a second strength PPD containing 250 TU, which will give a false negative reaction in no more than 1 to 2 per cent of patients without disseminated disease or severe debility.

Other laboratory tests are not particularly helpful. The blood count occasionally shows a leukemoid reaction, but more often there is a mild leukocytosis with a relative monocytosis. Many different serologic tests have been proposed, but none has proven useful enough at this time to be included as a diagnostic test.

DIFFERENTIAL DIAGNOSIS. Many subacute and chronic pulmonary conditions, both infectious and noninfectious, may be confused with tuberculosis. Some pulmonary mycoses, especially histoplasmosis, may present with a similar clinical and radiologic picture. Pyogenic lung abscess as well as pneumonia with a delayed resolution may be confused with tuberculosis. A pyogenic lung abscess is likely to have more fluid within it, hence a higher air-fluid level, and more dense consolidation around it. When repeated examinations of the sputum are negative for AFB, one should increase efforts at establishing another diagnosis. Tuberculomas may be confused with similar lesions arising from several different fungal infections and with pulmonary neoplasms. Sarcoidosis and tuberculosis may have similar manifestations. One third of cases of fever of unknown origin are due to infection, and extrapulmonary tuberculosis is still prominent among these cases.

TREATMENT. ***Historical Perspective.*** For many decades the physician relied upon nonspecific measures to treat tuberculosis. These measures included fresh air, good food, bed rest, and graded exercise, among others. The idea of the cottage sanatorium was started in this country in 1884 to accommodate these feeble attempts at treatment. Measures designated to collapse cavities and to put diseased portions of the lungs "at rest" included artificial pneumothorax, pneumoperitoneum, phrenic nerve crush, and various forms of thoracoplasty. Resectional surgery became popular after the introduction of effective drug therapy.

The era of chemotherapy began in 1945 with Waksman's discovery of streptomycin. In 1949 it was shown that treatment with the combination of streptomycin and para-aminosalicylic acid (PAS) delayed the emergence of streptomycin-resistant tubercle bacilli. With the introduction of isoniazid in 1952 it became possible to treat the disease with two drugs given by mouth. A course of 18 to 24 months was recommended by studies of relapse rates and the bacteriology of lesions removed at lung resection as related to duration of treatment. Ethambutol, marketed in 1961, replaced PAS because of its relative lack of annoying side effects. These drugs rendered all previous modes of therapy obsolete, and most sanatoriums in this country were closed by 1960. A study done in India in 1960 demonstrated that home treatment was not risky for the patient or his family. It was documented in 1973 that supervised intermittent treatment twice a week was just as beneficial as daily treatment, especially for the ambulatory continuation phase after a period of daily drug therapy. Such intermittent treatment is especially suited for uncooperative patients. The introduction of rifampin in 1966 provided not only another very powerful antituberculosis agent, but also the opportunity to shorten the duration of therapy by at least half. Published reports on short-course chemotherapy began to appear in 1972. It soon became obvious that the lessons learned from combination drug therapy prior to the use of rifampin did not apply to regimens containing isoniazid and rifampin. With proper combinations and rhythm of administration it is now possible to achieve excellent results with six months of treatment, provided that all doses are consumed as prescribed.

The Antituberculosis Drugs. *Isoniazid (INH)* is the most important drug in original treatment regimens. It is easily synthesized, highly stable, inexpensive, and well tolerated. The drug is well absorbed when given by mouth and may be administered parenterally. It is widely distributed throughout the body, including the central nervous system, and it reaches bacilli within cells. The drug exerts a bactericidal effect on actively multiplying bacilli. Adverse reactions may occur in approximately 5 per cent of cases with a daily dose of 5 mg per kilogram per day, usually given as 300 mg once daily for adults. A common toxicity is peripheral neuropathy, based on interference with the metabolism of pyridoxine. It is directly related to the dose and blood level and is more likely to be seen in genetically constituted slow acetylators and in malnourished individuals. Neuropathy can be prevented by the administration of 25 mg of pyridoxine daily and is not likely to occur when ordinary doses of INH are used in nonalcoholic, nondiabetic, well nourished, and relatively young patients. The most important adverse reaction is hepatitis of the hepatocellular variety. Although approximately 10 per cent of healthy individuals may have asymptomatic elevations of aminotransferases within the first two months of treatment, the enzyme levels usually return to normal despite the continued administration of the drug. The risk of hepatitis is related to age, being less than 1 per cent in those under 35 and increasing with age to 2.3 per cent at age 60. Hepatitis usually occurs within the first few months of treatment but occasionally appears in later stages. Heavy alcohol intake is associated with a greater risk of hepatitis. Several fatalities from INH hepatitis have been reported, mainly in patients whose reaction occurred late and in those who continued to take the drug despite progressive symptoms.

Some rare untoward effects include encephalopathy, loss of memory, optic atrophy, convulsions, hemolytic anemia, and purpura. The usual hypersensitivity reactions such as drug fever and skin rash occasionally may be seen. Isoniazid is one of several drugs that can produce a lupus-like syndrome. Although INH is excreted promptly and mainly by the kidneys, the half-life is prolonged only slightly in patients with renal failure.

Rifampin (RMP) is comparable to INH in its bactericidal effect on metabolically active bacilli. It is an antibiotic of the rifamycin family and is much more expensive than INH. Well absorbed when taken orally in a fasting state, the drug is widely distributed and penetrates well into cells and into the central nervous system. It differs from most of the antituberculosis drugs in that it has good activity against a variety of gram-positive and gram-negative bacteria. Its activity depends upon inhibition of DNA-dependent RNA polymerase activity. Rifampin is well tolerated by most patients in a dosage of 10 mg per kilogram per day, usually given to adults as 600 mg once daily by mouth. A parenteral preparation is not yet generally available, although it may be obtained from the manufacturer in emergency situations. Hepatitis is the most important adverse effect, occurring in about 1 per cent of patients. There are conflicting reports on the risk of hepatitis when INH and RMP are given together. Most studies now indicate no excessive risk. An exception occurs in the treatment of children, for whom a dosage of greater than 10 mg per kilogram per day of INH given with RMP is associated with a high risk of hepatitis.

Allergic reactions occasionally occur, especially in those individuals who take the drug irregularly or in those who are given intermittent treatment twice weekly in a dosage greater than 600 mg. These reactions include chills and fever and more rarely acute renal failure, thrombocytopenia, and massive hemolysis. Rifampin may induce enzymes in the liver that increase metabolic degradation of several other drugs, such as oral contraceptive agents and anticoagulants. The drug is excreted mainly by the liver and biliary tract and therefore must be given with caution to patients with liver failure.

Ethambutol (EMB) is a synthetic chemical compound of the ethylenediamine series discovered in 1961. It is well absorbed when given by mouth and is excreted mainly in the urine. Thus, the drug should be given with great care to patients with poor renal function, for whom dosage must be reduced and blood levels followed carefully. Aside from its principal toxicity, optic neuritis, there are very few adverse effects. Optic nerve toxicity is directly related to dosage and blood levels. At the recommended dosage of 15 mg per kilogram per day, optic neuritis is very rare, but some physicians administer 25 mg per kilogram per day for the first two or three months, at which dosage approximately 3 per cent of patients may have impaired visual acuity. When the higher dose is used, periodic examinations for visual acuity are indicated. The toxicity usually is reversible if administration of the drug is discontinued promptly.

Pyrazinamide (PZA) is a synthetic compound discovered in 1952 but originally rejected for general use in the United States because of excessive hepatotoxicity when given in a dosage of 40 mg per kilogram per day. It has now become an important drug because of its excellent tissue sterilizing ability when used in combination with other bactericidal drugs. Toleration is acceptable at a lower dose than that originally used. It is well absorbed from the gastrointestinal tract, widely distributed throughout the body water, and penetrates well into the central nervous system. The drug is active against only one species of *Mycobacterium, M. tuberculosis,* and then only at the low pH of 5.0 to 5.5. It is especially useful to kill tubercle bacilli within macrophages, into whose acidic environment it penetrates well. It is excreted mainly by way of the kidneys. Allergic reactions are rare, but joint pains and occasionally gout may occur as the result of a hyperuricemic effect. Hepatitis may occur in about 1 per cent of patients receiving the recommended daily dose of 20 to 30 mg per kilogram, usually 1.5 grams for small and 2.0 grams for large adults, given by mouth once daily.

Streptomycin (SM) is an aminoglycoside antibiotic that has been chemically defined and synthesized. It is not absorbed when given by mouth. The principal method of elimination is through the kidneys, so that dosage adjustment is necessary when renal function is reduced. It is distributed largely in the extracellular fluid and does not enter appreciably into the central nervous system or into macrophages. The dosage is 10 to 15 mg per kilogram per day, given intramuscularly, usually as 0.75 to 1.0 gram once daily in adults with normal renal function. As with other aminoglycosides, damage to the renal tubules is common, as manifested by cylindruria, but renal function is not compromised unless blood levels of the drug are excessive. The major toxicity is exerted against the eighth nerve, of which the vestibular division is more likely to be affected, although deafness may also be produced. The seriousness of these reactions makes periodic testing of renal and eighth nerve function advisable, especially in the elderly. Measurements of blood levels should be obtained whenever renal function is in question. Allergic reactions are fairly common, as are paresthesias of the lips and extremities immediately after injection. The drug is bactericidal against tubercle bacilli. The maximum effect is exerted at a pH of 7.7.

Kanamycin and *capreomycin* are used as substitutes for SM when the organisms are resistant to that drug or on the rare occasions when the patient cannot tolerate SM. Dosages, methods of administration, and adverse reactions are similar to those of SM. More care is needed with kanamycin since it is slightly more ototoxic and nephrotoxic than SM, especially on the cochlear division of the eighth nerve.

Ethionamide and *cycloserine* are not used for initial therapy but are reserved for retreatment cases and for special situations of drug intolerance and bacillary resistance. Both drugs are given by mouth in dosages of 10 to 15 mg per kilogram per day. The administration of ethionamide is accompanied by rather severe gastrointestinal upset and occasionally by hepatitis, and allergic reactions are common. Allergic reactions with cycloserine are rare, but aberrations of mental function and seizures are quite common.

Drug Regimens. Until the landmark short-course chemotherapy studies of the British Medical Research Council and its cooperative investigators, the conventional drug regimens for initial treatment consisted mainly of INH and EMB for one and one half to two years, supplemented by RMP or SM for the first month or two in patients with far advanced disease. An intermittent regimen consisting of supervised twice-weekly drug administration can be used after the initial two or three months of daily treatment. Dosages in mg per kilogram recommended for intermittent treatment are as follows: INH 15, SM 25 to 30, EMB 50, and RMP 10 to 15 (usually no more than 600 mg total). With a fully compliant patient and drug-sensitive bacilli, the success rate is well over 95 per cent with long-term treatment. The main problems are related to the long-term administration of a drug regimen and include insuring compliance with recommended treatment and the cost of supervision and follow-up to the local health department.

SHORT-COURSE TREATMENT. The first report of successful short-course treatment was published in 1968 and involved experience in East Africa. From the results of many other trials conducted since then, it appears that the minimum requirements include therapy with INH and RMP for at least nine months. The addition of a third drug—EMB, SM, or PZA—for the first one to three months of intensive treatment guards against the eventuality of infection with INH- or RMP-resistant bacilli. To shorten the course to six months, a third drug is necessary. That drug should be PZA for the initial two months. Treatment may then be continued with daily INH plus RMP for the remaining four months. When the patient is in a high-risk group for infection with INH-resistant or RMP-resistant organisms, use of a four-drug regimen has been suggested for the first two months (INH/RMP/PZA/SM), followed by administration of two or three drugs, depending on drug susceptibility, for four months. A modification of the six-month treatment involving only 62 doses, fully supervised, is as follows: INH/RMP/PZA/SM daily for two weeks, then twice weekly for six weeks, then INH/RMP twice weekly for 18 weeks. These intensive regimens should be considered for patients who are likely to resist treatment, such as prisoners and urban homeless alcoholics. Preliminary reports have documented the effectiveness of these regimens.

Short-course treatment has the obvious advantages of smaller amounts of drugs used and less time needed at the ambulatory health facility for supervision of treatment. Another benefit of the INH/RMP combination is more rapid sputum conversion (by approximately two to three weeks) when compared with regimens without INH/RMP, although the conversion curves usually even out by the fourth month. In addition, if relapse occurs following short-course treatment, it is usually caused by drug-susceptible organisms.

The main disadvantage of intensive three- and four-drug regimens, drug toxicity, has proved to be less troublesome than was predicted. The number of patients removed from the study because of drug intolerance has been acceptable.

Results of Treatment. The success of treatment may be judged by clinical assessment, decreased bacillary count of the sputum, and clearing of the lungs as shown on radiographs. The temperature usually returns to normal within a week or two, but in some patients who are highly febrile defervescence may not occur for many weeks. The speed of radiographic improvement depends upon the nature and extent of pulmonary disease and the age of the patient. Chronic, cavitary, and fibrotic lesions do not clear rapidly. The sputum should be examined at frequent intervals during the first few months of treatment, since a decreasing number of acid-fast bacilli is the surest indication of successful treatment. With the best of regimens, it will take four to six weeks to convert sputum cultures to negative in 50 per cent of cases; to convert 75 per cent of cases usually requires about ten weeks. The rate of conversion depends on the same factors that determine the rate of radiographic clearing. Failure of the sputum to convert to negative or a rise in the bacillary count after an initial decrease represents a treatment failure. Such failures are usually the result of poor compliance on the part of the patient but occasionally are related to bacillary drug resistance or an inappropriate drug regimen. The aim of chemotherapy is an initial success rate of 100 per cent without relapses. When relapse occurs, it is usually within a year of the completion of therapy. Rarely, relapses may occur with decreasing frequency up to five to ten years after completion of therapy. This is so infrequent after adequate drug therapy that it is no longer necessary for the local health department to carry out periodic follow-up examinations.

Corticosteroids. Corticosteroids may be a useful adjunct to chemotherapy for selected patients. They usually produce a dramatic reversal of overwhelming sepsis. Absorption of the fluid may be hastened in tuberculous pleurisy and pericarditis, although there is no evidence that late complications in the pleural and pericardial spaces are prevented. In tuberculous meningitis it was often the custom to give steroids routinely, but there is no good evidence that this is necessary. Steroids should be given for as short a time as possible, preferably for no longer than three or four weeks. A more controversial issue is whether or not to use INH prophylaxis to cover the administration of steroids in the patient with a history of tuberculosis or with a positive tuberculin skin test result. This situation is most likely to occur in patients receiving steroids to prevent rejection of transplanted organs, to help control lymphoma or leukemia, or to control severe asthma. One year of INH preventive therapy is recommended when steroids will be used on a long-term basis.

Reversal of Infectiousness. Some experts believe that it takes only about two weeks of effective chemotherapy to render patients noninfectious to others, even when large numbers of viable acid-fast bacilli are still present in the sputum. The evidence for this is inconclusive, and it is more reasonable to consider a patient with smear-positive sputum to represent a gradually diminishing risk until the smears are negative.

Drug Resistance. The phenomenon of clinical bacillary resistance was recognized soon after SM was tried as single drug therapy. The emergence of drug-resistant strains was at least delayed, if not prevented, by the use of two or more drugs in combination. Resistant populations emerge by a selective process in which resistant cells are favored that have arisen by spontaneous random mutation at the rate of about 1×10^{-8} to 1×10^{-10} per bacterium per generation.

Modern drug regimens are designed to prevent the emergence of drug resistance unless the patient is noncompliant or if infection occurs with strains already resistant to one or more drugs—a situation known as *primary drug resistance.* The rate of primary drug resistance in a community will influence the choice of drug regimens for initial treatment. Accurate figures for this country were provided by a recent study from the Centers for Disease Control, which showed that the overall rate was 7 per cent and varied in different locations from 3 to 15 per cent, depending mainly on the relative numbers of Asian and Hispanic individuals in the population. Age was another important factor; the highest rate was seen in young children. The highest single drug rate was for INH, with SM second. The study also showed that the rate diminished slightly between 1965 and 1982. The importance of the overall drug resistance problem, both primary and acquired, was highlighted by another study from the Centers for Disease Control. Forty-one per cent of unsuccessfully treated patients harbored strains resistant to at least one drug. The known contacts of an index case excreting INH-resistant tubercle bacilli should receive careful follow-up, and appropriate treatment should be given if active disease develops. Alternatively, RMP either alone or with another drug such as EMB or PZA may be used, although it has not yet been proved that RMP is effective in prophylaxis.

Retreatment. Proper therapy for initial treatment failures and disease that relapses after apparently successful treatment requires special expertise. Accurate drug susceptibility testing is a prerequisite for devising the best drug regimen, but while awaiting test results the following guidelines may be followed: A single new drug should not be added to a regimen that has failed, since this may lead to rapid emergence of resistance to the new drug. Instead, a regimen should be chosen that contains at least two drugs that the patient has never received previously. In selecting the proper drugs, all available information should be gathered from the patient, the patient's family and former physicians, and health departments. Calls should be made to whatever laboratories have been involved in testing of organisms obtained from the patient to get firsthand bacteriologic data including drug sensitivity test results. The chosen regimen should be adjusted according to any newly available information. It may be necessary to use combinations of four or more drugs, some of which have high rates of adverse reactions. After two or three relapses, especially when the infecting strain is resistant to INH, RMP, and SM, the chances of success are slim. The best way to control the problem of retreatment of patients with multiply resistant strains is to prevent this unfortunate turn of events by proper supervision of the initial course of drug therapy.

Patients with Impaired Renal and Hepatic Function. Isoniazid is excreted mainly in the urine, and it has been reported that the drug will accumulate in patients with markedly impaired renal function. However, the drug is dialyzable, and others have reported that the half-life is prolonged only slightly in patients with renal failure. It is probably not necessary to reduce the dosage, but pyridoxine supplementation should be given and patients should be monitored for hepatitis and peripheral neuropathy. It may also be advisable to assay INH serum concentrations from time to time. Rifampin is metabolized in the liver and excreted mainly in the bile. When hepatic function is impaired, the drug may accumulate to toxic levels. Thus blood levels should be monitored. Both EMB and SM are cleared by dialysis and are excreted mainly through the urine. The dosage of SM must be reduced in proportion to the renal function; serum levels should be checked frequently, and the patient should be monitored for signs of eighth nerve toxicity. In a similar fashion, the dosage of EMB must be reduced, serum levels checked, and the visual acuity monitored. Since about 20 per cent of EMB is metabolized in the liver, it would be wise to check serum levels when there is hepatic failure. There is insufficient information upon which to base recommendations for use of PZA, ethionamide, and cycloserine in patients with impaired renal or hepatic function. Since PZA and cycloserine are excreted mainly by the kidneys, the dosage should be reduced and blood levels monitored when these drugs are used in patients with poor kidney function. It is not known how ethionamide is metabolized; only a very small amount may be found unchanged in the urine. Drug levels should be monitored to avoid accumulation.

Treatment of Pregnant Women. Ethionamide and SM should be avoided, the first because of teratogenic potential, and the second because eighth nerve damage has been reported in the fetus. Cycloserine and PZA should also be avoided because of a lack of information on possible adverse effects. Rifampin crosses the placental barrier readily and inhibits RNA polymerase. It should be used with caution and only with a very strong indication, perhaps only for the first few weeks of treatment. The combination of INH and EMB is the most suitable drug therapy for pregnant women.

Treatment of Children. There are conflicting recommendations for drug regimens and dosages of individual drugs for treatment of children with tuberculosis. The most suitable combination is INH 10 mg per kilogram daily (maximum of 300 mg daily) and RMP 15 mg per kilogram daily (maximum of 600 mg daily). A third drug should be added if there is risk of infection with drug-resistant organisms. The third drug, given for the first two or three months of therapy, may be SM, EMB, or PAS. All three drugs have drawbacks: SM has a high rate of adverse effects and must be given by injection; PAS is difficult to administer to children because of stomach irritation, and the drug is no longer available in the liquid form; young children cannot be monitored for the major toxicity of EMB, optic neuritis. Ethambutol is probably the best choice of therapy. It has been used successfully in other countries in a dosage of 15 mg per kilogram daily. The duration of treatment should be one year, although preliminary reports indicate that nine months may be sufficient.

Surgical and Collapse Procedures. The need for collapse procedures such as pneumothorax, penumoperitoneum, and phrenic nerve crush and for excisional surgery with or without thoracoplasty has been virtually eliminated by the success of chemotherapy. The surgeon may still be called upon to correct late complications of previous attempts at treatment such as bronchopleural fistula or persistent empyema.

EXTRAPULMONARY DISEASE. ***Thoracic Cavity and Chest Wall.*** Tuberculosis of the pleura is almost always associated with disease of the lung, arising by contiguous spread or rupture of a subpleural tubercle. It usually begins as a localized fibrinous inflammation, which produces pleuritic chest pain. Pleurisy with effusion is often associated with primary infection. When this occurs in young adults who are untreated, approximately 75 per cent may be expected to develop overt pulmonary tuberculosis within five years. The onset may be either abrupt or insidious, with cough and fever accompanying the chest pain. Pain and friction rub often disappear as pleural fluid accumulates. Most primary tuberculous pleural effusions will resorb spontaneously, sometimes within a week or two, but the diagnosis can be made on the basis of a positive tuberculin skin test result, the exudative characteristics of the fluid, and the preponderance of lymphocytes. Tubercle bacilli are usually very scarce in the fluid so that stained smears may be negative and cultures only weakly positive. Imprints and cultures made from pleural tissue removed by closed needle biopsy are more likely than the fluid to be positive. Histologic examination also may be helpful. Pleural effusions in young adults who have positive tuberculin skin test results are best treated as tuberculosis unless some other cause can be identified. The fluid should be aspirated for diagnosis and perhaps once or twice more if it accumulates rapidly. Chest tube drainage should be avoided. Corticosteroids should not be used routinely but may be given in selected cases to hasten symptomatic improvement and absorption of the fluid. Pleural effusion may also occur in disseminated tuberculosis with multiple organ and serous membrane involvement. Tuberculous empyema may be secondary to involvement of the vertebral column or result from a bronchopleural fistula.

Endobronchial tuberculosis commonly accompanies pulmonary disease but now rarely results in identifiable symptoms and signs. In primary tuberculosis of children it is the pressure of enlarged lymph nodes together with ulceration and rupture through the bronchial wall that produce endobronchial disease. Endobronchial disease in adults usually starts as inflammatory lesions from repeated implantations of tubercle bacilli originating in lung parenchyma. These lesions may progress to ulceration and narrowing of the bronchi and eventually to cicatricial stenosis. Secondary changes include atelectasis and obstructive pneumonitis, tension cavity from involvement of the distal small bronchi or bronchioles, and accumulation of fluid within cavities. The symptoms of endobronchial disease are spasmodic coughing and a localized wheeze. Bronchial ulceration or erosion of a caseating lymph node may cause positive sputum in the absence of recognizable pulmonary disease. Bronchoscopy usually serves to identify the lesions.

Although tuberculosis of the endocardium and myocardium has been described, the most common involvement of the heart is *pericarditis.* Rupture into the pericardium of nearby caseous lymph nodes is the common route of infection, although lymphohematogenous dissemination may occur. The serofibrinous pericardial effusion usually is associated with substernal pain, fever, pericardial friction rub, and left-sided pleural effusion. Cardiac tamponade occasionally develops in the acute stage. A search for tuberculosis elsewhere and a tuberculin skin test should be performed. A thorough examination of the pericardial fluid obtained by needle aspiration or surgical drainage also may be helpful. Obtaining a pericardial biopsy sample in the operating room may be justified in obscure cases because of the importance of early drug treatment. The differential diagnosis includes benign or viral pericarditis, pyogenic infection, other granulomatous inflammations, and malignant effusion. The diagnosis is made more difficult by the facts that the skin test reaction is negative in a sizable minority; the fluid rarely contains enough organisms to be positive by smear and often not even by culture; the characteristics of the fluid are nonspecific; and about half of the individuals have no other obvious sites of tuberculosis. The administration of corticosteroids may be beneficial, but antituberculosis drugs should be used in addition even when tuberculosis is only suspected.

The most important sequela is constrictive pericarditis, which usually occurs two to four years after the acute disease. At this stage the heart is small and relatively immobile and there is a paradoxical pulse and obstruction of venous return to the heart, with congestion of the liver, peripheral edema, and later ascites. Calcification of the pericardium may be seen on x-ray films. Treatment consists of removal of the pericardium, although it is preferable to perform the operation at an earlier stage.

The chest wall may be the site of one or more subcutaneous abscesses as a result of hematogenous dissemination or sometimes as the peripheral manifestation of an empyema necessitatis as it burrows through the chest wall. Chest wall abscesses may also result from drainage of underlying caseous lymph nodes along the intercostal lymphatics.

Extrathoracic. LYMPHATIC. Tuberculous lymphadenitis is the most common manifestation of extrathoracic disease throughout the world, and the most frequently involved nodes are cervical. The disease in this location was known as *scrofula,* or the *King's Evil.* The latter name was used because the condition was supposedly amenable to cure by the royal touch. Although it was once thought that infection with *M. bovis* was responsible for most cases of scrofula, a recent study from England emphasized that *M. tuberculosis* accounted for more cases than did the bovine organism, although the latter is relatively more common in lymphatic tuberculosis than in other forms of the disease. Infection of the tonsils through the ingestion of contaminated milk was the usual route of infection for the tonsillar node high in the neck, near the angle of the jaw. At present, scrofula in young children is mainly due to infection with mycobacteria other than *M. tuberculosis* and *M. bovis* (see Ch. 299). Supraclavicular node involvement usually arises by lymphatic spread from mediastinal disease. Nodes elsewhere in the neck, as well as those in the axilla and inguinal area, the other common sites of involvement, may be the result of drainage from a primary site or from hematogenous spread.

The infected nodes are usually detectable by sight and palpation. Although the nodes usually are not painful, they may be tender during the phase of rapid enlargement early in the infection. Later they become matted together and eventually soften, slough, and drain. Draining sinuses may persist for many months, sometimes for years, with intermittent healing and breakdown. The diagnosis may be made by bacteriologic study of the pus from draining sinuses or by biopsy together with bacteriologic studies. The presence of calcific densities in the neck and axilla as seen in the chest radiograph may provide evidence of healed tuberculous adenitis.

Lymphatic tuberculosis tends to heal but often not completely, so that relapse is common even many years after the primary infection. Treatment with antituberculosis drugs is usually successful, although the tendency to late relapse may still be seen, especially with two-drug regimens that do not include RMP. Excision of large caseous nodes in accessible sites sometimes is advisable.

GENITOURINARY. The second most common site of infection is the genitourinary tract. Disease is usually centered in the kidney, which becomes seeded either during the primary infection or later. These foci may remain dormant for many years. When reactivation occurs, one or more renal abscesses are produced, followed by spread to the remainder of the urinary tract. Extensive scarring of the ureters eventually occurs. This scarring produces obstructive hydronephrosis, which together with renal caseation may destroy the kidney completely. Specific symptoms may be lacking until the hydronephrotic kidney becomes secondarily infected or until the development of tuberculous cystitis manifested by frequency and dysuria. Long before the onset of symptoms, the examination of the urine may show hematuria, pyuria, and albuminuria, along with cultures negative for pyogens. The diagnosis is made by radiographic examination of the urinary tract, cystoscopy, and demonstration of tubercle bacilli by cultures of first morning voided urines. It was found that approximately 10 per cent of a general tuberculosis patient population had positive urine cultures, and in 7 per cent of these patients the urinary tract disease was completely unanticipated. Renal tuberculosis responds well to drug treatment. According to recent recommendations, conventional long-term regimens may be replaced by six- to nine-month courses of INH, RMP, and a third drug (either EMB or PZA). The role of surgery remains controversial. Some urologists would remove destroyed kidneys and repair strictures of the ureter, while others claim that surgery is almost never indicated.

Genital tuberculosis in the male may involve the prostate, seminal vesicles, and epididymis. The acute inflammation is later replaced by induration and hard nodules, sometimes followed by obstruction, calcification, and chronic draining sinuses of the scrotum. The diagnosis is made by finding tubercle bacilli in the urine, sinus drainage, or biopsied tissues. In the female, tuberculous salpingitis is the common manifestation, followed by disease of the uterus and ovaries. Sterility almost always results, and peritonitis may occur secondarily. The symptoms are those of chronic pelvic inflammatory disease. Diagnosis should be based on examination of tissue from the endometrium and from lesions visible through the laparoscope and cultures of the menstrual fluid or vaginal discharge. As with renal tuberculosis, drug therapy usually is successful, but excisional surgery may be indicated for residual lesions or persistently draining sinuses.

SKELETAL TUBERCULOSIS. The presence of a gibbus or hunchback deformity of the thoracic spine (Pott's disease) has served as a marker of tuberculosis since prehistoric times. *Tuberculous spondylitis* is still the most common manifestation of bone and joint infection. At present, it is mainly a disease of adults that arises by reactivation of dormant foci. The common areas of involvement are thoracic and lumbar; the cervical spine may be involved in 2 to 3 per cent of cases. The destructive process usually begins in the intervertebral discs, where it first produces narrowing of the disc space, then destruction of the two adjacent vertebral bodies through the bony end plates. Sometimes, however, the anterior portion of the vertebral body is destroyed first. Inflammation often extends into the soft tissues surrounding the spine, either in the form of a spreading, phlegmonous reaction or as a cold abscess that may be paravertebral, in and around the psoas muscle, or retropharyngeal, depending upon the site of disease. The symptoms are usually dominated by back pain, sometimes followed by the neurologic manifestations of compression of the spinal cord and nerve roots. There may be fever. Active tuberculosis of the lungs may be absent, although some evidence of past disease usually is seen.

Radiographic examination of the spine shows destructive lesions in the commonly involved sites. The paraspinal involvement appears as widening of the mediastinum or an oval-shaped density behind the heart. It may be manifested as a psoas abscess, a retropharyngeal abscess, or a mass in the groin or in the supraclavicular area. A similar radiographic appearance may occur in pyogenic infection of the spine. A needle biopsy sample usually is necessary to establish the proper diagnosis. Even when a pyogenic organism such as *Staphylococcus aureus* is isolated, caseating granulomas and a culture positive for *M. tuberculosis* sometimes can be found by biopsy. Occasionally open biopsy of the vertebral body may be necessary.

The disease has a natural tendency to heal by spontaneous fusion of the vertebral bodies. Treatment consists of antituberculosis chemotherapy according to the modern regimens described under Treatment. Preliminary results with short-course treatment are encouraging, but they cannot be recommended for routine use until further experience has accumulated. Published studies of the British Medical Research Council Working Party on Tuberculosis of the Spine have suggested that prolonged bed rest, immobilization of the spine, and spinal fusion operations are no longer necessary, although some indications still exist for surgical procedures: decompression of the spinal cord if there has been no neurologic improvement after several weeks of drug treatment and debridement and anterior spinal fusion for dangerous instability of the spine. The inflammatory reaction with or without pus around the spine often improves with drug treatment so that drainage is not always necessary.

Tuberculous arthritis occurs mainly in hips and knees but also may involve many other joints including elbows, shoulders, and the joints of the hands and feet. The patient usually has chronic monoarticular arthritis. Diagnosis is made by synovial biopsy and bacteriologic study of tissues and pus. The process usually responds to antituberculosis chemotherapy without the necessity for operative procedures, but occasionally excision of extensively destroyed synovium and temporary immobilization may be beneficial.

Tuberculous tenosynovitis is usually secondary to involvement of adjacent bone. At least two distinctive processes may result from involvement of the hand: carpal tunnel syndrome, and compound palmar ganglion, a distinctive bilobed swelling on either side of the volar carpal ligament. Chemotherapy often needs to be supplemented by debridement and evacuation of fibrinous material.

ABDOMINAL TUBERCULOSIS. *Intestinal tuberculosis* secondary to chronic pulmonary disease once was so common that patients were routinely screened by radiography of the small bowel upon admission to the sanatorium. This situation continued long after the ingestion of *M. bovis* was brought under control by the pasteurization of milk. Lately, the emphasis has been on primary intestinal disease in the absence of recognizable pulmonary lesions. The route of infection in these cases remains unknown. Tuberculosis may involve all parts of the alimentary canal from top to bottom, but by far the most common location is in the ileocecal area. The predominant tissue reaction may be either ulcerative or hyperplastic, with accompanying bleeding, perforation, fistula formation, obstruction, or combinations of two or more of these processes. The early symptoms are nonspecific, consisting mainly of anorexia, loss of weight, abdominal pain, and alternating periods of diarrhea and constipation. The clinical picture is not unlike that of Crohn's disease. Indeed, the differential diagnosis of these two conditions may not be possible, even on the basis of intestinal radiography. Tuberculosis of the colon also may occur and needs to be distinguished from carcinoma, diverticulitis, and inflammatory bowel disease of nonspecific nature. Perirectal abscess and fistula formation may result from lower colon lesions. The disease usually responds well to antituberculosis chemotherapy, but surgical correction may be necessary for the complications described earlier. The diagnosis often is made unexpectedly at surgery or autopsy.

Tuberculous peritonitis may result from bloodborne infection or by extension of disease from the intestine, mesenteric lymph nodes, or fallopian tubes. The classic form is that of a chronic adhesive peritonitis that produces a doughy, tender abdomen, abdominal masses, low grade fever, anorexia, and weight loss. A much more common manifestation is painless ascites. When this occurs in adults with alcoholic cirrhosis and ascites, it makes for a difficult differential diagnosis. Tuberculosis should be suspected when the combination of fever, ascites, and a positive tuberculin skin test reaction are found. Examination of the fluid is helpful. A high total protein concentration with a moderate number of leukocytes, mostly lymphocytes, is suggestive of tuberculosis. A more definitive diagnosis may be obtained by laparoscopy or laparotomy. Usually the entire peritoneal surface is studded with tubercles that are easily differentiated from carcinomatosis histologically. The fluid is rarely positive for AFB by stained smear and even by culture test is positive in somewhat less than 50 per cent of cases. Response to antituberculosis chemotherapy is good.

Isolated tuberculosis of the liver or spleen occasionally has been described. These organs are usually involved in disseminated or miliary tuberculosis, but occasionally a liver biopsy done in an attempt to explain enlargement of the liver, jaundice, or abnormal liver function studies leads to a diagnosis of tuberculosis when there is apparently no disease elsewhere.

Central Nervous System. In the past, *tuberculous meningitis* was one of the most dreaded complications of primary tuberculosis in young children, appearing in about one in a thousand cases and almost always resulting in fatality. It usually occurred two to six months after the primary infection in infants and was commonly associated with miliary tuberculosis. In this country it is now more likely to be seen in adults than in children. Invasion of the meninges occurs by direct extension from subjacent caseous foci in the cerebral cortex, cerebellum, choroid plexus, middle ear, or spine. Brain infarcts secondary to tuberculous arteritis sometimes occur. The syndrome of inappropriate secretion of antidiuretic hormone may accompany the meningitis.

The inflammatory reaction is concentrated around the base of the brain where the thick exudate may eventually obstruct the basal foramina to produce hydrocephalus. Examination of the spinal fluid reveals a characteristic pattern of high protein, low sugar, and a moderate number (up to a few hundred) of leukocytes, most of which are lymphocytes. However, early in the course of the disease neutrophils may predominate; the shift to a lymphocytic exudate rarely does not occur; the sugar level may be normal or only slightly decreased; and the number of leukocytes may reach several thousand. Occasionally the protein content is high enough that a thin web or pellicle appears in undisturbed refrigerated fluid. Acid-fast bacilli may be seen in this web, although they are not visible in the sedimented fluid. Stained smears of the fluid are usually positive in no more than 25 per cent of samples, but there are a few colonies of tubercle bacilli in cultures in about 75 per cent of cases. The larger the sample of spinal fluid submitted, the greater the chance of finding the organism. The tuberculin skin test should be positive in approximately 75 per cent of cases, provided that those nonrective to 5 TU are retested immediately with 250 TU. A careful search reveals evidence of tuberculosis elsewhere in the majority of cases, although the disease in the lungs may appear to be inactive.

The onset is usually insidious, extending over a period of many weeks. Occasionally, however, there is a much more acute onset that resembles pyogenic or aseptic meningitis. The most common symptoms are headache, fever, lethargy, and confusion. Later, focal neurologic signs appear in the form of ocular palsies, other cranial nerve palsies, and increasing stupor progressing to coma. Stiffness of the neck is common. The outcome of therapy depends mainly on the stage of disease at the time treatment is instituted. Treatment should start immediately when tuberculous meningitis is suspected, without waiting for confirmation of diagnosis. A triple-drug regimen including INH and RMP is recommended. Ethionamide and PZA achieve therapeutic concentrations in spinal fluid even in the absence of an inflammatory reaction. Ethambutol penetrates reasonably well through inflamed meninges. It should be remembered that SM does not appear in therapeutic concentrations and that infections with INH-resistant organisms occur more often in children than in adults. It has been recommended that the third drug should be either ethionamide or PZA. Treatment should be continued for at least one year, although administration of the third drug may be discontinued after two or three months once it has been determined that drug resistance is not a problem. The use of corticosteroids is controversial. Intrathecal treatment is usually not necessary.

Tuberculomas of the brain may be seen at any age. Cases involving children still predominate in the developing countries, while in the United States they occur mainly in adults. The clinical presentation is that of a brain tumor with signs and symptoms of increased intracranial pressure, focal seizures, and focal neurologic defects. Indications of infection, such as fever, often are absent. Lesions may be single or multiple and must be differentiated from tumor and abscess of the brain. The spinal fluid may show slight lymphocytosis and elevated protein concentration, but often it is normal. The correct diagnosis may be suggested by radiographic scanning techniques, a positive tuberculin skin test reaction, and the presence of tuberculosis elsewhere, but the definitive procedures are needle aspiration through a burr hole and craniotomy for open biopsy. Drug treatment similar to that used for tuberculous meningitis should be used.

Miscellaneous. Almost every organ and tissue of the body can be involved in tuberculosis. In the upper respiratory tract and oral cavity, the larynx and the middle ear are most prone to infection. *Tuberculous laryngitis* used to be a rather common complication that was considered to be secondary to long-standing highly positive sputum associated with chronic cavitary disease. It was extremely painful and resulted in such difficulty in swallowing that severe inanition resulted. Response to drug treatment, even to administration of SM alone, was rapid and dramatic. The new face of tuberculous laryngitis is that of a primary laryngeal lesion that must be distinguished from carcinoma. Tuberculous middle ear disease, formerly common, is now rare. It was usually associated with advanced pulmonary or disseminated disease. Involvement of the eye is in the form of chronic uveitis, such as chorioretinitis, iridocyclitis, or iritis. Phlyctenular conjunctivitis produces small yellowish vesicles. Direct inoculation into the eye may produce conjunctivitis or keratitis. The specific origin of eye disease is difficult to prove. Cutaneous tuberculosis has all but disappeared, except for lesions associated with direct inoculation in laboratory workers and pathologists. Other manifestations include lesions like lupus vulgaris in which tubercle bacilli may be located and the tuberculids that are considered to be hypersensitivity reactions in which the organisms usually are not found. The larger blood vessels may harbor infections in their walls. Tuberculosis is a rare cause of aortic aneurysm. At one time tuberculosis of the adrenal gland was a common cause of adrenal insufficiency. Occasional cases of tuberculosis of the thyroid, breast, and soft tissues elsewhere than in the chest wall are still being reported.

DISSEMINATED AND MILIARY TUBERCULOSIS. These terms are used synonymously, although miliary tuberculosis is but one form of disseminated tuberculosis in which the widely dispersed small tubercles resemble millet seeds. During life these lesions usually are first recognized in the chest roentgenogram as very small nodules of uniform size that are evenly distributed throughout both lungs. The acute form was predominately an early complication of untreated primary tuberculosis, occurring mainly in young children and often associated with meningitis. During the past three decades the predominant age group has changed to the elderly, and the disease has become more subacute in its progression.

The diagnosis often is missed because it is difficult to distinguish the tuberculosis symptoms from those of the many underlying conditions that could be responsible for the weight loss, increasing fatigue, and low grade fever. Skin test anergy and frequent absence of chronic pulmonary tuberculosis may compound the difficulty. This sort of subacute disseminated tuberculosis has been called *cryptic* or *nonreactive tuberculosis*. The situation was admirably presented and analyzed by Slavin et al. in 1980. In their series of autopsied cases, only 15 per cent of patients admitted during the antibiotic era had the correct diagnosis made antemortem. A composite of such a case would be an elderly anergic patient without previously recognized tuberculosis who presented to the hospital with malignancy, renal failure, a renal transplant, or chronic alcoholism. Constitutional symptoms would be nonspecific, mainly fever, loss of weight, and increasing fatigue. Examinations would reveal no obvious tuberculosis in lungs or other organs, no hepatosplenomegaly, and no enlarged peripheral lymph nodes. There would be moderate anemia, a slight elevation of alkaline phosphatase, and a negative initial bacteriologic workup. The correct diagnosis depends upon a high index of suspicion and the demonstration of characteristic microscopic lesions and mycobacteria by biopsy. The most productive tissue is the liver, usually sampled by needle biopsy, with bone marrow next in line. Blood cultures should be obtained since they are sometimes positive at this stage of disease. At a later stage choroidal tubercles may be seen and radiographs of the lungs may show the typical miliary pattern.

Miliary tuberculosis almost always results from the discharge of infected caseous material into the bloodstream, usually from a well hidden lymph node in the mediastinum or the abdomen. When multiple bacteremic episodes occur, the process may be protracted. The patient may have serositis manifested by pleural effusion, pericardial effusion, or ascites. Hematologic abnormalities may be so prominent that a primary blood disease is suspected. The most common abnormality is a leukemoid reaction, although leukopenia, thrombocytopenia, and hemolytic anemia may occur. More commonly the primary disease is hematologic, complicated by a secondary tuberculosis dissemination, especially when large doses of corticosteroids have been given.

Treatment should consist of an intensive antituberculosis drug regimen using three drugs, including INH and RMP, plus EMB or PZA. After a few months, when a good response has occurred and after the drug susceptibility pattern of the infecting strain is known, the third drug can be discontinued. The total duration of therapy utilizing the suggested regimen has not been established, but it probably should be at least one year. Disseminated mycobacteriosis has been recognized as one of the common opportunistic infections in immunosuppressed and debilitated patients, including those with acquired immunodeficiency syndrome. Nontuberculous mycobacteria cause these infections even more often than does *M. tuberculosis*—a fact that should be considered in the choice of proper treatment.

Andrew OT, Schoenfeld PY, Hopewell PC, Humphreys MH: Tuberculosis in patients with end-stage renal disease. Am J Med 68:59, 1980. *A study of 10 patients with tuberculosis from a group of 172 undergoing dialysis in San Francisco gave a risk ratio of 12. The problems of diagnosis and treatment are admirably discussed.*

Anonymous: Is BCG vaccination effective? Tubercle 62:219, 1981. *The failure of the most recent large-scale trial in South India to demonstrate protection is brought into focus by this concise article.*

Canetti G: The Tubercle Bacillus in the Pulmonary Lesion of Man. New York, Springer Publishing Company, Inc., 1955. *A classic monograph detailing and integrating the pathogenesis of the disease in relation to histopathology, bacteriology, and immunology, as well as the influence of chemotherapy on the lesions.*

Centers for Disease Control: Primary resistance to antituberculosis drugs—United States. Morbid Mortal Wkly Rep 32:521, 1983. *The final report of a seven-year study in which 20 selected laboratories throughout the country submitted over 12,000 cultures to the CDC laboratory to be tested for drug susceptibility in a uniform manner.*

Clemens JD, Chuong JJH, Feinstein AR: The BCG controversy; a methodological and statistical reappraisal. JAMA 249:2362, 1983. *The authors reanalyzed the major BCG trial reports and concluded that vaccination was highly protective. Their appraisal was based on the superior study design and statistical precision of the more favorable trials.*

Costello HD, Caras GJ, Snider DE Jr: Drug resistance among previously treated tuberculosis patients: A brief report. Am Rev Respir Dis 121:313, 1980. *Among 4000 unsuccessfully treated patients in the United States, 41 per cent harbored drug-resistant strains.*

Daniel TM: The immunology of tuberculosis. Clin Chest Med 1:189, 1980. *A good summary of the immune spectrum exhibited by tuberculosis patients, the importance of further purification of mycobacterial antigens, and the mechanisms of immunoregulation.*

Daniel TM, Balestrino EA, Balestrino OC, Davidson PT, Debanne SM, Kataria S, Kataria YP, Scocozza JB: The tuberculin specificity in humans of *Mycobacterium tuberculosis* antigen 5. Am Rev Respir Dis 126:600, 1982. *Despite the fact that antigen 5 appeared to be limited to* M. tuberculosis *and* M. bovis, *it proved to be no more specific than tuberculin PPD when tested in the field. A good review of the previous attempts to produce specific skin test antigens to differentiate various mycobacterioses.*

Dannenberg AM Jr: Macrophages in inflammation and infection. N Engl J Med 293:489, 1975. *This study utilizing skin lesions in rabbits demonstrates the dynamic nature of mycobacterial lesions. Macrophages enter the arena as novices, become activated locally by interaction with immune lymphocytes, ingest bacilli, die, and are replaced by fresh cells recruited from the circulation.*

Farer LS, Lowell AM, Meador MP: Extrapulmonary tuberculosis in the United States. Am J Epidemiol 109:205, 1979. *An analysis of tuberculosis cases reported to the Centers for Disease Control reveals but little change in the number or rate of extrapulmonary disease from 1964 to 1976. Cases are analyzed according to age, anatomic site, sex, and race.*

Fox W: The chemotherapy of tuberculosis: A review. Chest 76S:785, 1979. *An excellent review of antituberculosis drug treatment up to 1979.*

Goodwin RA, Des Prez RM: Apical localization of pulmonary tuberculosis, chronic pulmonary histoplasmosis, and progressive massive fibrosis of the lung. Chest 83:801, 1983. *The higher oxygen tension at the apices of the lungs has been used as an explanation for the localization of adult-type tuberculosis. A more satisfactory theory based on diminished tissue clearance of antigens and lymph stasis is promulgated in this paper.*

Lichtenstein IH, MacGregor RR: Mycobacterial infections in renal transplant recipients: Report of 5 cases and review of the literature. Rev Infec Dis 5:216, 1983. *Among the cases were two that probably represented reactivation tuberculosis in the transplanted kidney. A survey of 26 transplantation centers revealed a tuberculosis rate of 480 cases per 100,000.*

Lincoln EM: Epidemics of tuberculosis. Arch Environ Health 14:473, 1967. *A review of 109 epidemics in 12 countries, the majority of them occurring in schools.*

Lorin MI, Hsu KHK, Jacob SC: Treatment of tuberculosis in children. Pediatr Clin North Am 30:333, 1983. *The latest recommendations for treatment of children, from a Houston group with long-standing interest in pediatric tuberculosis.*

Lurie MB: Resistance to Tuberculosis: Experimental Studies in Native and Acquired Defensive Mechanisms. Cambridge, Harvard University Press, 1964. *The role of native immunity in tuberculosis is well illustrated in this book, which summarizes the author's experiments using inbred rabbits.*

Sahn SA, Lakshminarayan S: Tuberculosis after corticosteroid therapy. Br J Dis Chest 70:195, 1976. *A recent review that emphasizes the usefulness of preventive therapy with isoniazid in patients already infected with* M. tuberculosis.

Slavin RE, Walsh TJ, Pollack AD: Late generalized tuberculosis: A clinical pathologic analysis and comparison of 100 cases in the preantibiotic and antibiotic eras. Medicine 59:352, 1980. *This study, from the Department of Pathology at Johns Hopkins University, consisted of an analysis of 200 autopsied cases. It contains a wealth of useful information on one form of disseminated tuberculosis.*

Snider DE Jr, Layde PM, Johnson NW, Lyle MA: Treatment of tuberculosis during pregnancy. Am Rev Respir Dis 122:65, 1980. *Presented are guidelines for the use of antituberculosis drugs in pregnant women.*

Stead WW: Control of tuberculosis in institutions. Chest 76 (Suppl):797, 1979. *Reviews recent outbreaks in nursing homes, prisons, schools, and hospitals, and suggests common-sense methods of control.*

Stead WW, Kerby GR, Schlueter DP, Jordahl CW: The clinical spectrum of primary tuberculosis in adults. Ann Intern Med 68:333, 1968. *Primary pulmonary disease was documented in 37 adults, of whom 9 had only minor symptoms, 11 developed pleural effusion, and 16 showed progression to adult-type chronic pulmonary disease.*

Youmans GP: Mechanisms of immunity in tuberculosis. Pathobiol Annu 9:137, 1979. *In this review article a former Department of Microbiology Chairman who published extensively in this field explains why he believes that "tuberculin sensitivity is an immune phenomenon that is quite distinct from the specific acquired immune response."*

299. OTHER MYCOBACTERIOSES

Emanuel Wolinsky

Organisms of the tuberculosis complex are not the only mycobacteria associated with human disease. The most popular label at present for these other mycobacteria is "nontuberculous." They have become more prominent in the total picture of mycobacterial disease because of the declining incidence of tuberculosis and a greater awareness and recognition of the other mycobacterioses. Indeed, there is evidence that the frequency of nontuberculous pulmonary disease may be increasing in certain areas of the country. In addition, disseminated mycobacterial infection is now recognized much more frequently as an opportunistic infection in immunosuppressed individuals, especially in those with the acquired immune deficiency syndrome (AIDS). Infection with other mycobacteria has been blamed, perhaps unfairly, for the apparent failure of bacille Calmette-Guérin (BCG) vaccination to protect adults in South India from subsequent tuberculosis. Leprosy, also a mycobacterial disease, is discussed in Ch. 300.

HISTORICAL PERSPECTIVE. The presence of many other species of *Mycobacterium* in the environment and in cold-blooded animals was recognized within a few years after the discovery of the tubercle bacillus. Scattered reports of the isolation of other mycobacteria from human secretions or pus date back to 1885. Several perceptive studies were published in the 1930's and the 1940's, but the realization that human disease surely was associated with nontuberculous mycobacteria did not occur until the mid 1950's. Since then, knowledge has been increasing at a rapid pace, although there are still many unanswered questions regarding the epidemiology, pathogenesis, and treatment of the other mycobacterioses.

MYCOBACTERIA. ***Mycobacterium avium-intracellulare (MAI).*** Mycobacteria of this species or complex constitute the most important agents of nontuberculous mycobacteriosis throughout the world. The organism known as the avian tubercle bacillus was described in 1890, although tuberculosis of chickens had been recognized for 22 years before that time. Supposedly quite resistant to infection with *M. avium,* people with documented *M. avium* disease were the subject of occasional literature reports. Recognition of the expanded role of these mycobacteria in pulmonary and disseminated disease occurred in the 1950's, when the organism was misnamed *Nocardia intracellularis* and given the common name of Battey bacillus. The official name of *Mycobacterium intracellulare* was assigned in the 1960's. The realization that *M. intracellulare* could not be distinguished from *M. avium* in most laboratories dictated another change to the presently used term MAI or *M. avium complex.* In this complex one can recognize 28 types by seroagglutination, of which types 1 to 3 represent the classic *M. avium* strains. Strains of MAI grow slowly; usually are nonpigmented or slightly yellow, becoming more highly pigmented with age but independently of light; are resistant to most antituberculosis drugs; and often produce colony variants of two or three types, including smooth translucent, smooth domed, and rough opaque. Of the three variants, the translucent colonies are usually most drug resistant and most virulent for experimental animals. Strains of MAI may be associated with all varieties of mycobacterial disease, especially pulmonary disease, childhood lymphadenitis, and opportunistic infection in patients who have AIDS.

Mycobacterium scrofulaceum. This is a scotochromogenic mycobacterium similar in many ways to MAI. The pigmentation varies from light yellow to dark orange. In some publications these organisms are lumped together with MAI, and the combination is called the *MAIS complex.* The name derives from the fact that the organism was recognized as the cause of scrofula in young children. Rarely, *M. scrofulaceum* may be associated with pulmonary disease in adults. Most of the disease-associated strains belong to one of three seroagglutination types, but it is not uncommon to see a strain of *M. scrofulaceum* agglutinate in one of the MAI serotypes.

Mycobacterium kansasii. The "yellow bacillus" was described in 1953 in Kansas City and was later given the official name of *M. kansasii.* It is responsible for a large number of pulmonary mycobacteriosis cases in some areas of the world. The organisms may be recognized in the initial sputum smears as large cross-barred acid-fast bacilli. Positive cultures may be identified by their distinctive photochromogenicity. The yellow color is light-dependent, developing within hours after the colonies have been exposed to light. Most strains are fully susceptible to rifampin and only slightly resistant to isoniazid, ethambutol, and streptomycin. *M. kansasii* is not found in nature except occasionally in samples of water.

Mycobacterium fortuitum-chelonei. Strains of this group grow rapidly, even on ordinary laboratory media. They are sometimes spoken of as the *M. fortuitum complex,* but it is better to retain at least two separate species because they can be distinguished from each other readily in the laboratory, and *M. chelonei* tends to be much more drug resistant than *M. fortuitum.* Both species are pathogenic for mice and resistant to the usual antituberculosis drugs. Long known for their ability to produce injection site abscesses and severe infections of traumatic wounds, strains of this group recently have become prominent as the cause of sternal osteomyelitis after cardiac surgery, of wound infection after implantation of silicone breast prostheses, of disseminated and localized infection in dialysis patients, of prosthetic valve endocarditis, and of disseminated infections with skin lesions in the immunosuppressed host.

Mycobacterium marinum. This organism is distinctive by virtue of its photochromogenicity and an optimal growth temperature of 30 to 33° C. It was named and recognized as a pathogen of fish in 1926. It is a common contaminant in fresh and salt water, accounting for the frequent occurrence of skin infection in individuals who work or play in a marine environment. Deep infections of the hand may also occur. Almost all strains are resistant to isoniazid but susceptible to rifampin and ethambutol. The organisms are also susceptible to tetracycline and sulfonamides.

Other Slow-Growing Species. *Mycobacterium xenopi* has an optimal growth temperature of 43° C and has been found as a contaminant in hot water generators and storage tanks. From these sites several outbreaks have occurred of respiratory tract colonization and pulmonary disease in the hospital environment. Other species that may cause disease are *M. simiae, M. szulgai,* and *M. malmoense.* Two species that may be associated with superficial soft tissue disease but not with pulmonary disease are *M. ulcerans* and *M. hemophilum.*

Species of Low Pathogenic Potential. A few cases have been reported in which strains of the *M. terrae* complex (including *M. triviale*) were the cause of pulmonary disease, arthritis, or tenosynovitis. Strains of this complex may be found in the soil. An organism long associated with water and considered to be saprophytic is *M. gordonae.* Documented infections with this organism now range from bursitis to widely disseminated disease. Cases of pulmonary disease and synovitis also have been ascribed to *M. flavescens,* an organism with an intermediate growth rate that was previously considered to be nonpathogenic for humans.

EPIDEMIOLOGY. In contrast to tuberculosis, the other mycobacterioses are not transmitted from person to person but are acquired from the environment by mechanisms that are not well understood. For *M. xenopi* and *M. kansasii* the evidence points to aerosols of infected water. Strains of MAI may be found in domestic animals, soil, dust, and water. There is evidence that infected droplet nuclei may be produced along coastlines. Still largely unexplained is the geographic variability in the incidence of other mycobacterioses and the relative proportion of these infections attributable to each of the two most important agents of disease, MAI and *M. kansasii.* In this country the highest rates of *M. kansasii* disease have been reported from New Orleans, Dallas, Houston, Kansas City, and Chicago, while Milwaukee and the states of Georgia and Florida have reported a predominance of MAI disease. From one institution in St. Louis, 27 per cent of newly diagnosed cases of mycobacterial pulmonary disease were associated with an equal proportion of MAI and *M. kansasii*. Australia, Israel, and Japan have reported an overwhelming predominance of MAI infections over those caused by *M. kansasii*. These figures refer to pulmonary disease; they do not reflect the distribution of disseminated infections. A recent increase in MAI and a concomitant decrease in *M. kansasii* disease has been reported from Virginia (Kim et al., 1984).

PATHOGENESIS. The localization of disease in the lungs suggests that the inhalation of infectious aerosols represents the primary route of infection. In many cases infection occurs by inoculation as a result of puncture wounds, lacerations, and foreign bodies. The question of whether the disease in adults usually represents primary infection or recrudescence of dormant foci cannot be answered at this time.

CLINICAL DESCRIPTION. ***Pulmonary Disease.*** The classic description is that of chronic cavitary disease resembling tuberculosis that occurs in a middle-aged rural man who has one or more of the following predisposing conditions: pneumoconiosis, healed tuberculosis, chronic bronchitis and emphysema, bullous disease, bronchiectasis, and malignant disease. However, there are many exceptions: the disease may be seen in all age groups except in children, in either sex, and in some individuals without any apparent predisposing factor. It sometimes appears as an acute condition in which there is an infected bulla or cyst or in a case resembling pneumonia. Solitary pulmonary nodules also have been described. The common etiologic agent is MAI, with *M. kansasii* second and *M. xenopi* a distant third.

The diagnosis may be suspected from the clinical appearance and the x-ray film, but it is the laboratory that must supply the correct identification of the mycobacterial agent. Skin tests are not helpful owing to a lack of adequately standardized antigens and the poor specificity of the presently available reagents. Pulmonary changes are characterized by one or more thin-walled cavities with little or no pleural disease or spread to the basal segments of the lungs. The sputum usually contains many acid-fast bacilli visible on smear and yields a heavy growth of the infecting agent. It may be possible to recognize the large banded forms of *M. kansasii* in the direct smear. A single positive culture test result in which there are only a few colonies usually represents environmental contamination. Repeatedly positive specimens may be indicative of transient or long-term colonization of the respiratory tract when they are not associated with new or enlarging cavities and a compatible clinical picture.

Treatment for *M. kansasii* disease usually is highly successful, provided that rifampin is included in the regimen. It is recommended that isoniazid, rifampin, and ethambutol be given for one year after the sputum becomes negative for the organism. Results of preliminary trials of short-course treatment have not been encouraging.

Therapy for MAI disease, on the other hand, has proved to be difficult. Most strains are resistant to the available antituberculosis drugs as well as the other anti-infectives, and the drug regimens recommended up to now have been chosen empirically. The necessity for treatment must first be established by an observation period to determine the stability of disease and the rate of progression if it is advancing. During this period the sputum should be examined at frequent intervals, and the patient should receive a comprehensive course of bronchial hygiene, including cessation of smoking, bronchodilator therapy, chest physiotherapy, and antibiotics if there are purulent secretions. These maneuvers have served to eliminate the organism from the secretions of some patients with chronic pulmonary disease. It may be necessary to initiate therapy immediately in certain cases of severe acute disease with a new cavitary lesion and no other apparent cause. Drug treatment may be considered at three levels. Level 1 is a triple-drug regimen consisting of isoniazid, rifampin, and ethambutol for a duration of at least two years provided there is some response within the first few months. This level would be suitable for a patient who had chronic stable disease with consistently positive sputum test results and in whom the mycobacterial infection was adding to the burden of pulmonary disease. Level 2 treatment consists of the same three drugs plus daily streptomycin administration for at least two years. Administration of streptomycin may be reduced to two or three times a week after an initial response has been demonstrated. This treatment level would be suitable for a patient who had slowly progressive disease, who had a poor response to level 1 treatment, or who had a relapse after discontinuation of level 1 drug therapy. Drug treatment at level 3 may be empiric combinations of five or six drugs or more reasonably, a regimen consisting of isoniazid, ethambutol, streptomycin, and ansamycin LM 427. The latter drug is an investigational rifamycin derivative that may be obtained at present from the tuberculosis control unit of the Centers for Disease Control. Most strains of MAI are susceptible to this ansamycin in vitro.

The response to drug treatment depends to a large extent on the underlying chronic lung disease and on the rate of progression of the mycobacterial infection. For those patients who have rapidly progressive infection in lungs that are already severely damaged, the prognosis is poor even with level 3 treatment. Some of these individuals have defects in cellular immune functions, especially those associated with T cells. Resectional surgery should be considered after a few months of treatment for those patients who have adequate pulmonary function and sufficiently localized mycobacterial disease. Treatment is not necessary for solitary pulmonary nodules that result from MAI infection, usually recognized after resection.

Disease caused by *M. xenopi* and *M. szulgai* usually is amenable to drug therapy. The exact combinations of drugs to be used depend on the drug susceptibility patterns in vitro. Suggested for *M. xenopi* disease is a regimen consisting of isoniazid, rifampin, and streptomycin and for *M. szulgai*, rifampin, ethambutol, and either ethionamide or streptomycin.

Infections associated with *M. scrofulaceum*, *M. simiae*, and *M. fortuitum-chelonei* are more difficult to control because of natural drug resistance. Strains of *M. simiae* usually are resistant to all of the antituberculosis drugs except cycloserine and ethionamide. Limited information on susceptibility of *M. scrofulaceum* suggests that ethionamide, rifampin, and ethambutol are most likely to be active in vitro. The same considerations as those described for MAI infection are applicable to these resistant infections. Although pulmonary infections with *M. fortuitum-chelonei* are quite rare, there is some information about the response to drug treatment from cases of extrapulmonary disease. Before sensitivity test results are available, full doses of amikacin should be given intramuscularly, together with one or more of the following drugs: doxycycline, erythromycin, cefoxitin, and a sulfonamide.

Lymphadenitis. Mycobacterial lymphadenitis is almost exclusively a disease of children of preschool age. Data from British Columbia published in 1974 indicated that the case rate for this new kind of scrofula was 0.37 per 100,000 persons per year, about ten times higher than for that caused by *M. tuberculosis*. Involved nodes may be found in the femoral, inguinal, epitrochlear, and axillary areas, although the most common location is around the angle of the jaw. The route of infection to the groin area is obvious after a penetrating injury or splinter entry into an extremity. The cervical nodes probably become infected by mucous membrane penetration in the mouth or pharynx. Examination shows a child who has had a painless localized swelling for several weeks and who is otherwise healthy. An unknown number of cases go on to suppuration and breakdown. Draining sinuses, whether spontaneous or following incision and drainage, may persist for many months. *M. scrofulaceum* was the most common cause of this infection, with MAI the second. However, there has been a recent reversal of this ratio so that strains of MAI now are the most common isolates from these infected nodes. Rare cases caused by several other species have been reported.

Correct diagnosis depends on the physician's familiarity with the disease, a positive tuberculin skin test result (sometimes requiring the use of second strength purified protein derivative), the absence of a history of contact with tuberculosis, absence of thoracic disease, and the location as well as the appearance of the involved nodes. Other conditions that need to be differentiated are tuberculosis, pyogenic lymphadenitis, cat scratch disease, congenital cyst, and lymphoma. The treatment of choice is excision of the involved nodes. In about 10 per cent of cases there is a recurrence of the infection in another group of nodes near the original site, occasionally on the other side. Rarely, there may be a third episode. Recurrences should be treated in the same manner as the original infection. There is no convincing evidence that drug treatment is beneficial. It should be remembered that as a result of this infection a child may have a positive tuberculin skin test reaction for many years.

Skin and Soft Tissue Infections. CUTANEOUS GRANULOMAS. Localized groups of papules have been called swimming pool granuloma or fish tank granuloma, depending on the source of infection. In another form of the disease there is a local abscess at the inoculation site, usually on the hand, followed by a series of secondary nodules that progress centrally along the lymphatics in a manner not unlike that seen in sporotrichosis. A few deep hand infections have also been described. The infection is not uncommon as an occupational or recreational illness in people who work or play in a marine environment. With few exceptions, the etiologic agent is *M. marinum.* Most superficial infections are self limited. When treatment is deemed necessary, the physician may use a combination of rifampin and ethambutol, rifampin alone, one of the tetracyclines, or trimethoprim-sulfamethoxazole. All of these regimens have been reported to be successful.

LOCAL ABSCESS. Many cases of local abscess following subcutaneous or intramuscular injection have been reported, some in outbreaks. The trouble usually is traced to a contaminated multiple injection vial, and the etiologic agent usually is *M. fortuitum-chelonei.* Incision and drainage usually will suffice to control the infection.

LOCAL TRAUMA. Most of these infections caused by *M. fortuitum-chelonei* occur as a result of penetrating or lacerating wounds contaminated with soil. Expert surgical handling is necessary, along with appropriate drug therapy as outlined under Pulmonary Disease.

DISSEMINATED NODULES. Multiple nodules and abscesses may be associated with widely disseminated mycobacterial disease, almost always in an immunocompromised host. The species most often isolated is *M. fortuitum-chelonei.* In addition, such nodules have been described in renal transplant patients as a result of infection with *M. hemophilum.*

BURULI ULCER. This deeply penetrating ulcer caused by *M. ulcerans* is confined mainly to Africa, Papua New Guinea, Malaysia, and Australia. The treatment is difficult and controversial.

Skeletal Infections. The synovia, tendon sheaths, and bursae are involved more often than other parts of the skeletal system in nontuberculous mycobacterial infections. A wide variety of species may be associated, including environmental strains with little pathogenicity for man, such as *M. terrae, M. gordonae,* and *M. flavescens.* Leading the list of etiologic agents is *M. kansasii,* with *M. fortuitum-chelonei* and MAI following in that order. Many of these infections follow trauma in which the wound is contaminated with soil or water. Others have occurred after injections of corticosteroids into arthritic joints; in these cases it is difficult to determine which condition was primary. The most common site is the hand, where the infection produces an indolent but persistent tenosynovitis, including the carpal tunnel syndrome. Osteomyelitis may occur in the form of multifocal lesions from hematogenous dissemination, often as a slowly progressive rather than a fulminant infection. The principal etiologic agent in these cases is MAI.

Treatment for skeletal infection usually demands close cooperation between a skilled surgeon and a physician specializing in infectious disease. Drug therapy depends on the etiologic agent (refer to earlier discussion).

Postsurgical Infections. Infections following surgery mainly are caused by *M. fortuitum-chelonei.* They include prosthetic valve endocarditis, sternal wound infection and osteomyelitis after open heart surgery, wound infection after augmentation mammoplasty, and infections associated with hemodialysis and peritoneal dialysis.

Disseminated Disease. Patients who acquire disseminated disease usually are severely immunocompromised from the standpoint of cellular immune functions. The recently recognized acquired immune deficiency syndrome has been associated with a dramatic increase in disseminated mycobacterial infections, since up to 50 per cent of such patients coming to autopsy in several cities have been found to have disseminated MAI infections. Prior to 1980 there were relatively few cases of disseminated mycobacterial disease reported throughout the world. Such cases usually involved patients who had underlying hematologic malignancies or who were under treatment with corticosteroids, or both. Both children and adults were affected, and the most common etiologic agents were *M. kansasii* and MAI. The case fatality rate was very high, even with the most intensive multiple-drug treatment. Diagnosis is most commonly made by biopsy and culture of liver, bone marrow, or lymph nodes. Cultures of the blood are often positive. Skin lesions or subcutaneous nodules or abscesses should be biopsied and examined for acid-fast bacilli. Strains of *M. fortuitum-chelonei* often are associated with these superficial lesions. The tissues may show a nonspecific necrotizing reaction in which macrophages are loaded with acid-fast bacilli, rather than a granulomatous reaction.

Treatment for disseminated disease is based on the same principles as those outlined for pulmonary disease. Infections caused by drug-sensitive organisms such as *M. kansasii* can usually be brought under at least temporary control provided that the human host is able to provide an adequate immune response. For infections related to MAI a multiple-drug regimen is usually chosen empirically, with a core of ansamycin* LM 427 and clofazimine.* Attempts to modify the host response by the use of transfer factor or prostaglandin inhibitors such as indomethacin have not yet been fully evaluated.

---

*Investigational drugs available from Centers for Disease Control, Atlanta, GA.

Bailey WC: Treatment of atypical mycobacterial disease. Chest 84:625, 1983. *In addition to a review of therapeutic regimens, the author proposes a new mycobacterial classification system based on responsiveness of associated diseases to treatment.*

Chapman JS: The Atypical Mycobacteria and Human Mycobacteriosis. New York, Plenum Medical Book Company, 1977. *A very informative monograph from one of the leaders in the field.*

Dixon JH: Nontuberculous mycobacterial infection of the tendon sheaths in the hand. J Bone Joint Surg 63B:543, 1981. *A report from a hospital in London of six cases caused by* M. kansasii. *The long delay in establishing the correct diagnosis is emphasized.*

Gribetz AR, Damsker B, Bottone EJ, Kirschner PA, Teirstein AS: Solitary pulmonary nodules due to nontuberculous mycobacterial infection. Am J Med 70:39, 1981. *This paper from New York's Mt. Sinai Medical Center describes the findings in 20 resected nodules positive for AFB during the period from 1969 to 1979. Twelve yielded* M. avium-intracellulare *on culture;* M. tuberculosis *was found in only one.*

Kim TC, Arora NS, Aldrich TK, Rochester DF: Atypical mycobacterial infections: A clinical study of 92 patients. South Med J 74:1304, 1981. *This is a study of pulmonary disease as seen in Charlottesville, Virginia, from 1970 to 1979. The majority of cases were attributed to* M. avium-intracellulare, *with a pronounced decrease of* M. kansasii *disease during the second five-year period.*

Macher AM, Kovacs JA, Gill V, Roberts GD, Ames J, Park CH, Straus S, Lane HC, Parillo JE, Fauci AS, Masur H: Bacteremia due to *Mycobacterium avium-intracellulare* in the acquired immunodeficiency syndrome. Ann Intern Med 99:782, 1983. *Eight patients had positive blood culture results on 1 to 14 occasions, requiring only 7 to 14 days with an automated radiometric technique.*

Marchevsky A, Damsker B, Gribetz A, Tepper S, Geller SA: The spectrum of pathology of nontuberculous mycobacterial infections in open-lung biopsy specimens. Am J Clin Pathol 78:695, 1982. *From 1969 to 1980 at New York's*

Mt. Sinai Medical Center, biopsy material from 40 patients revealed AFB. M. avium-intracellulare *accounted for 24 cases and* M. tuberculosis *for 6. A variety of histopathologic reactions are described in addition to the classic granulomas.*

Mason UG, Greenberg LE, Yen SS, Kirkpatrick CH: Indomethacin-responsive mononuclear cell dysfunction in "atypical" mycobacteriosis. Cell Immunol 71:54, 1982. *Cells from nine patients were studied. Seven had MAI infection. Evidence was found in favor of abnormal immunoregulation mediated by an imbalance of arachidonic acid metabolic products.*

Moran JF, Alexander LG, Staub EW, Young WG, Sealy WC: Long-term results of pulmonary resection for atypical mycobacterial disease. Ann Thorac Surg 35:597, 1983. *This report documents the good results of resectional surgery in 37 patients seen by the surgical group at Duke University from 1967 to 1981. All disease was attributed to* M. avium-intracellulare.

Sutker WL, Lankford LL, Tompsett R: Granulomatous synovitis: The role of atypical mycobacteria. Rev Infect Dis 1:729, 1979. *Presented are data from 25 adult patients observed from 1970 through 1977. Positive culture results were obtained in 15 cases: 4* M. tuberculosis, *6* M. kansasii, *2 MAI, and 1 each* M. marinum, M. gordonae, *and* M. chelonei. *There is also a good literature review.*

Wolinsky E: Nontuberculous mycobacteria and associated diseases. Am Rev Respir Dis 119:107, 1979. *A "state of the art" review of the entire subject.*

Woodley CL, Kilburn JO: In vitro susceptibility of *Mycobacterium avium* complex and *Mycobacterium tuberculosis* strains to a spiropiperidyl rifamycin. Am Rev Respir Dis 126:588, 1982. *Information from the laboratories of the Centers for Disease Control form the basis for the investigation of the use of ansamycin LM 427 in the treatment of MAI disease.*

300. LEPROSY (Hansen's Disease)

Ward E. Bullock

DEFINITION. Leprosy is a chronic granulomatous disease of man that is caused by *Mycobacterium leprae*. It is a disease of great chronicity, and the spectrum of its clinical manifestations is broad. At one end of the spectrum is tuberculoid (TT) leprosy, in which the clinical manifestations are localized to a single area of skin and the associated nerve supply. At the opposite end of the spectrum is lepromatous (LL) leprosy, in which there is massive infection of the dermis by *M. leprae* as well as involvement of the nerves, nasopharynx, testes, and lymphoreticular system. The intermediate forms of leprosy display mixtures of the clinical, histopathologic, and immunologic features typical of TT or LL disease. The intermediate forms are less stable clinically and often progress toward the lepromatous end of the spectrum; spontaneous improvement with a shift toward the tuberculoid spectrum occurs less frequently unless antimicrobial therapy has been instituted. These "upward" or "downward" shifts, as defined by gain or loss of host resistance, may be marked by inflammatory reactions within infected tissues, the immunologic mechanisms of which are poorly understood. Such reactions produce considerable functional impairment when they involve the peripheral nerve trunks. Reactions of this type occur in individuals with intermediate forms of leprosy but not in those with TT or LL disease. LL leprosy is associated with a different type of tissue reaction, erythema nodosum leprosum (ENL), that likewise may precipitate acute nerve dysfunction, presumably as a result of the humoral response to antigens of *M. leprae*.

EPIDEMIOLOGY. ***Incidence and Prevalence.*** The World Health Organization has estimated the total number of leprosy cases in the world to be approximately 11 million. However, valid statistics are not available from several countries with a high prevalence of leprosy including China. The actual number of cases probably exceeds 15 million. The highest prevalence rates are in Asia and Africa, followed by Central and South America and Oceania. Overall, the prevalence rate does not exceed 25 to 55 per 1000 in these areas, although it may be greater than 200 per 1000 within particular villages and surrounding areas.

The proportion of cases with lepromatous leprosy varies considerably from region to region; in Asia and the Americas it ranges from 25 to 65 per cent. In Africa the lepromatous forms of disease are distinctly less common, constituting from 6 to 20 per cent of the leprosy population. Roughly 20 per cent of the known cases of leprosy in India are of the lepromatous type. Although most cases of leprosy are found in the tropics, leprosy can flourish in colder climates, as for example in Korea, northern China, and Siberia. Within the United States, leprosy is endemic in Hawaii and in small areas of Texas, Louisiana, and Florida. Nevertheless, of the 1480 new cases reported to the U.S. Public Health Service from 1978 through 1982, 89 per cent occurred in foreign-born patients. This percentage represents a significant shift since the period from 1947 to 1966 when only 55 per cent of patients were foreign born. The largest number of patients with leprosy from 1978 through 1982 have come from Vietnam.

TRANSMISSION. The incubation period of leprosy is generally three to five years but may range from six months to decades. The precise modes of transmission have not been established. Traditionally, it had been thought that transmission involved prolonged close exposure of susceptible persons to the skin of an index case, especially one with lepromatous infection. In an endemic area, the risk of acquiring leprosy among household contacts of lepromatous cases is about eight times that in normal households; the risk of acquisition in households with tuberculoid leprosy is approximately four times normal (Doull et al., 1962). In fact, very few leprosy bacilli are shed from the intact skin of lepromatous patients; large numbers of organisms may be shed from skin ulcers, but these are relatively uncommon. By contrast, the nasal secretions of those with lepromatous disease contain up to 2×10^8 *M. leprae* in a single nose blow. Thus, a major portal of entry may be the respiratory tract. To date, however, there is little evidence to document primary respiratory tract infection *prior* to the onset of skin lesions. The granulomatous inflammation of leprosy does not caseate except occasionally within nerves. Since lesions heal without calcification, there are no residual tissue markers of primary infection equivalent to the Ghon complex of tuberculosis that might suggest the initial site of infection.

The gastrointestinal tract is a possible route for primary infection, since breast milk contains large numbers of *M. leprae*, but primary lesions have not been recognized within the gastrointestinal tract. Biting insects may provide still another means of transmission, since viable *M. leprae* can be isolated from the midguts of laboratory-bred arthropods for at least 48 hours after they have fed on lepromatous cases.

Although man has been thought to be the only natural host of *M. leprae*, a disease resembling lepromatous leprosy has been recognized in up to 10 per cent of feral armadillos from certain regions of Louisiana. The organism recovered from these animals is indistinguishable from *M. leprae* by available techniques. Leprosy has also been discovered in the sooty mangabey, a New World monkey. Thus, there may exist reservoirs of *M. leprae* other than man.

Susceptibility to Leprosy. The host factors that determine susceptibility to disease once an individual has been infected with *M. leprae* are poorly understood. The incidence of new cases usually is highest among older children and young adults. Although the cell-mediated immune responses of younger children may be relatively immature at the time of initial exposure to *M. leprae* and thereby predispose to increased disease incidence, environmental factors undoubtedly play a major role as well. The index case in childhood leprosy frequently is a parent with untreated disease with whom the child will have had prolonged and close contact.

Leprosy is diagnosed more frequently in males than in females, the ratio being 3:1 in some areas. The apparent predominance of leprosy in males probably is specious, since census figures in many regions are uncontrolled for sex selection.

Genetic factors long have been held to be important in determining susceptibility to leprosy, especially to the lepromatous type. Strong support for this concept is lacking. In a large study of monozygotic twins, it was found that 37 of 62 (60 per cent) of monozygotic twin pairs were concordant for leprosy of similar type, whereas in 25 pairs (40 per cent) only one member had leprosy. Others have failed to detect differences from normal in the segregation patterns of multiple genetic polymorphic systems among leprosy cases. Likewise, no consistent associations have been found between leprosy and HLA-A, B, or C antigens, although one group has found a statistically significant preferential inheritance of HLA-DR2 by siblings with tuberculoid leprosy but not by healthy siblings or by siblings afflicted with lepromatous disease. No associations between DR2 and nonfamilial cases of tuberculoid leprosy were detected.

ETIOLOGY. The causative agent of leprosy is a bacillus measuring 0.3 to 0.4 $\mu m \times$ 4 to 7 μm that is acid-alcohol fast when stained by the Ziehl-Neelsen method. Although the lepra bacillus was the first to be identified as the cause of human disease by Hansen in 1874, successful cultivation of this organism in vitro has not yet been achieved conclusively, and hence relatively little is known of its biology. A significant advance was made in 1960, when Shephard observed that a small inoculum (10^4) of *M. leprae* prepared from infected human tissues will multiply in the footpads of mice to a plateau level of 10^6. During multiplication, the doubling time of *M. leprae* is extraordinarily long, ranging from 10 to 13 days. The mouse footpad model has also made it possible to study the efficacy of many compounds against *M. leprae* in vivo.

Systemic infections with *M. leprae* can be achieved in mice and rats that are congenitally athymic or have been neonatally thymectomized. It is difficult to maintain immunodeficient animals for prolonged periods, and thus the utility of these models has been limited. Nine-banded armadillos and some species of monkeys are susceptible to infection with *M. leprae*. The former tend to develop an overwhelming infection that is analogous to lepromatous leprosy. The armadillo model will be more useful when these animals can be bred to produce pathogen-free animals. The need for specific pathogen-free animals is critical because wild armadillos may be infected with other noncultivatable mycobacteria.

PATHOGENESIS AND HISTOPATHOLOGY. Whatever the portal of entry for *M. leprae* may be, the first clinical manifestations of leprosy appear in the skin. The histopathology of an early lesion may be indeterminate and reveal only nonspecific inflammation composed of a scanty lymphocytic infiltrate around the dermal appendages and neurovascular bundles. Rarely, an acid-fast bacillus can be seen within small nerves of the dermis. In untreated cases, indeterminate lesions may resolve spontaneously or evolve until the histopathology becomes more characteristic of leprosy. It is then possible to classify a lesion within the leprosy spectrum based on the cell types and the number of bacilli observed within the areas of granulomatous inflammation. The best standardized classification of leprosy is that developed by Ridley and Jopling, in which the leprosy spectrum is divided into five groups as outlined in Table 300–1.

Tuberculoid (TT) Leprosy. The lesion of TT leprosy is characterized by well-developed granulomas composed of epithelioid cells with a uniform appearance and giant cells of the Langhans or foreign body type. Lymphocytes are abundant at the periphery of the granuloma, and acid-fast bacilli usually cannot be identified. Dermal nerves involved by the granulomatous inflammation are destroyed.

Borderline Tuberculoid (BT) Leprosy. The pathology of TT and BT leprosy is similar except that acid-fast bacilli are more readily seen in the latter, especially in dermal nerves, although the number is small.

TABLE 300–1. IMMUNOLOGIC MANIFESTATIONS WITHIN THE LEPROSY SPECTRUM*

Manifestation	TT	BT	BB	BL	LL
Lepromin reaction	3+	1+	±	–	–
ENL	–	–	–	±	2+
Bacilli in nose	–	–	–	1+	2+
Bacilli in granuloma	0	1–3+	3–4+	4–5+	5–6+
Epithelioid cells	1+	1+	1+	–	–
Langhans giant cells	1+	2+	–	–	–
Foam cells	–	–	–	1+	3+
Lymphocytes	3+	2+	1+	1+	±
Nerve destruction (skin)	2+	2+	1+	±	–

*Modified from Ridley DS: Int J Leprosy 40:102, 1972.

Borderline (BB) Leprosy. In BB leprosy, the histologic picture may vary considerably from lesion to lesion or even within the same lesion. Typically, the granuloma formation is less well developed. Epithelioid cells are spread more diffusely throughout the granuloma, giant cells are not present, and there are fewer lymphocytes within the infiltrate. The dermal nerves are less damaged, and therefore more easily visible. Acid-fast bacilli are numerous.

Borderline Lepromatous (BL) Leprosy. In this form, histiocytes are the predominant cell type with relatively few lymphocytes scattered among them, sometimes in aggregates. Epithelioid cells are absent. The damage within dermal nerves is less than that observed in BB disease, but there is increased perineural inflammation. This produces lamination of the perineurium that imparts an "onion skin" appearance to the nerve. Large numbers of acid-fast bacilli are present.

Lepromatous Leprosy (LL). The inflammatory infiltrate is composed almost exclusively of histiocytic cells that have a foamy appearance. Masses of bacilli are present intracellularly, many in large clumps called globi. Lymphocytes are very sparse. Characteristically, there is a "clear zone" beneath the epidermal basement membrane in which there is no inflammatory infiltrate, as contrasted with the tuberculoid forms of leprosy in which the granulomas extend to the dermal-epidermal junction.

Granulomas can be identified in the lymphoreticular organs of persons with tuberculoid leprosy. However, granulomatous pathology is far more extensive in BL and LL disease. For example, the paracortical regions of lymph nodes are heavily infiltrated by masses of histiocytes and literally are "choked" with acid-fast bacilli; T lymphocytes, normally abundant in this area, are largely displaced. The germinal centers, containing a predominance of B lymphocytes, are spared; they tend to be increased in both size and number. In the spleen, the white pulp is especially prone to invasion by histiocytic cells, although the red pulp also may be infiltrated. Aggregates of foamy histiocytes are present in the liver, most frequently around the portal tracts and scattered within the lobules. Patients suffering from LL disease manifest a continuous bacteremia with up to 1×10^5 bacilli per milliliter of blood, and the total body burden of *M. leprae* may approach 10^{12}.

IMMUNOPATHOLOGIC CONSIDERATIONS. Intracutaneous injection of healthy individuals and of patients with TT or BT leprosy with a heat-killed suspension of *M. leprae* (integral lepromin) prepared from skin lepromas will induce local granuloma formation within a three- to four-week period. Conversely, patients with LL disease are completely anergic to lepromin. Thus, the lepromin test provides a crude indication of an individual's capacity to mount a cell-mediated immune response against infection in *M. leprae*. If more purified preparations of *M. leprae* are employed to skin test for delayed-type hypersensitivity or to measure the proliferative responses of lymphocytes in vitro, the response to these antigens decreases progressively across the leprosy spectrum, i.e., they are greatest in TT leprosy and least in LL cases. Moreover, in a high percentage of the latter group, there is a generalized impairment of the delayed-type hypersensitivity response to a variety of "recall" antigens as measured by skin testing and lymphocyte proliferative responses. The anergy to antigens of *M. leprae* is very persistent despite long-term treatment, whereas the anergy to other antigens tends to be reversible.

Serum levels of the immunoglobulins generally are within the normal range in tuberculoid patients, whereas polyclonal hypergammaglobulinemia is a common feature of lepromatous leprosy. More than 90 per cent of lepromatous sera contain antibodies to *M. leprae* that cross-react with other mycobacteria; as antimicrobial therapy is continued, titers of these antibodies decline over a period of years. Ten per cent or more of patients with LL disease will have biologic false-positive reactions in tests for syphilis employing cardiolipin-type antigens, and more than 30 per cent will have cryoglobulinemia. Circulating immune complexes are present in a substantial but variable percentage of lepromatous cases, and in more than 50 per cent the serum contains elevated levels of amyloid-related serum protein component (SAA), an acute phase reactant. Although the relationship of SAA to tissue amyloid is unclear, secondary amyloidosis is not an uncommon complication of longstanding lepromatous leprosy. At least 50 per cent of cases have greatly elevated serum levels of C-reactive protein. Less frequently, antinuclear antibodies and rheumatoid factor are present, as well as low titers of antibody to thyroglobulin. In tuberculoid forms of leprosy, the prevalence of these serologic abnormalities is very low, presumably because the host immunoregulatory control mechanisms are less disordered.

CLINICAL MANIFESTATIONS. The variations of histopathology within the skin and peripheral nerves are reflected clinically by a wide range of skin lesions and peripheral neuropathies. The typical indeterminate lesion is usually, but not always, seen in children. It is a hypopigmented macule, of which there are rarely more than three or four. The macule measures 2 to 5 cm in diameter, and sensation may be impaired slightly within the macular area. In many cases the macules resolve spontaneously, whereas in others they evolve to become lesions more typical of tuberculoid or lepromatous disease.

TT leprosy generally presents as a single large plaque or macule that is very well defined. Occasionally, up to two or three lesions are present. Plaques are erythematous with sharply elevated outer borders that slope toward a flattened center, which is rough, dry, hairless, and anesthetic. Macules may be either erythematous or hypopigmented in the center. Enlarged dermal nerve twigs and related peripheral nerve trunks may be palpable or visible within the involved skin area. The most frequently enlarged nerves are the greater auricular, the ulnar above the elbow, the peroneal as it curves around the head of the fibula, and the posterior tibial. As with skin lesions, nerve damage is localized. Any area of the body may be affected, although the axillae, inguinal region, and perineal areas are spared, presumably because of the proclivity of *M. leprae* to grow in cooler areas of the body.

BT leprosy closely resembles TT disease; however, the plaques or macules tend to be more numerous, and satellite lesions sometimes are present near the larger lesions. The peripheral nerve trunks frequently are enlarged by granulomatous infiltrates. Some of the more common complications are (1) traumatic plantar ulcerations of the feet, (2) foot drop, (3) loss of hand function as a result of flexion contracture and repeated trauma to anesthetic digits, and (4) corneal abrasions if there is corneal nerve dysfunction.

The lesions of BB leprosy are polymorphic in appearance. Generally they are numerous and vary considerably in size. Unlike the tuberculoid forms of disease, in which lesions are localized to one side of the body, the lesions of BB leprosy are more symmetrical. In some cases they appear as large, erythematous bands with sharply demarcated centers and outer edges. Others appear as irregular erythematous plaques with poorly defined outer margins and hypopigmented centers that have a characteristic "punched-out" appearance. Not infrequently, both types are present simultaneously, and satellite lesions are common. The lesions tend not to be as anesthetic as those in TT or BT disease.

Skin manifestations of BL leprosy are perhaps the most heterogeneous of all. They are numerous, are distributed bilaterally, and can present as macules, plaques, papules, or nodules. BL skin lesions tend to include some nodules with a "dimpled" appearance in the center, and some plaques have centers that appear hypopigmented and "punched out." As a rule, the nasal structures are not involved, although the ear lobes may be thickened. Nerve thickening can be quite prominent near the site of cutaneous lesions, but anesthesia is less evident than in the forms described above.

During early stages of LL leprosy, the extensive inflammatory response within the dermis gives rise to widely distributed erythematous macules or papules. In dark-skinned individuals these are difficult to see unless viewed obliquely in good light. With progression, plaques and nodules become evident. In later stages they are the predominant types of lesions. The skin becomes progressively thickened with infiltrate to produce the classic leonine facies in association with thinning and loss of eyebrows. Occasionally, cases of LL leprosy can present without obvious localized lesions but instead have diffuse lepromatous infiltrates in the skin. This type of disease is observed most frequently in Central America. Those who suffer from it are prone to develop a distinctive vasculitis (the so-called "Lucio's phenomenon") involving the dermal vessels that results in ischemic necrosis of the epidermis. The lesions are stellate in appearance and heal with atrophic scar formation.

In LL leprosy, the eyes frequently are involved by keratitis and iritis; there is progressive destruction of the nasal cartilage and anterior maxillary spinous process, resulting in saddle nose deformity. Incisor teeth may be lost, and chronic inflammation of the larynx can lead to life-threatening stenosis. Extensive infection of the testes is common, leading to fibrosis and hyalinization of the seminiferous tubules and azoospermia; the testicular damage is reflected by elevated gonadotropin levels, reduced plasma testosterone levels, and gynecomastia. The ovaries are infected only rarely. Nerve involvement is more extensive in LL leprosy than in other forms, although functional deficits are less severe because the intensity of the intraneuronal inflammation is reduced consequent to poor cell-mediated immunity to *M. leprae*. The neurologic damage usually manifests as mononeuritis multiplex, i.e., an asymmetrical sensory polyneuropathy.

Reactional States. Although leprosy itself is an extremely torpid infection, the clinical course all too frequently is punctuated by acute and subacute reactional states that produce serious morbidity and even death. The most common of these reactional states is erythema nodosum leprosum (ENL), which occurs only in patients with high bacterial loads—namely, those with BL or LL disease. Occasionally, untreated patients experience ENL. Much more frequently, effective antileprosy treatment triggers the onset of ENL, which occurs in more than 50 per cent of patients within the first year. The onset of ENL is sudden over a 24- to 48-hour period with eruption of painful red papules or nodules over the face, trunk, arms, and thighs. Nodules may proceed to frank suppuration, requiring several weeks to heal, generally without scarring. Occasionally, ENL is chronic, lasting for several months. Histologically, early ENL nodules reveal polymorphonuclear infiltration within the lepromatous granulomas, and frequently there is panniculitis; a panvasculitis may involve both arteries and veins in the dermis. It is widely believed that ENL activated by antimycobacterial therapy is precipitated by degradation of *M. leprae* with release of antigenic material. Antibodies to *M. leprae* are presumed to complex with these antigens, thereby inducing a number of serious constitutional disturbances, including severe pyrexia, iridocyclitis, neuritis, orchitis, lymphadenitis, and polyarthritis. In addition, there is a high prevalence of glomerulonephritis in ENL. Acute proliferative glomerulonephritis and focal mesangial hypercellularity with thickening of the glomerular capillary loops are the most consistent findings. Deposits of subendothelial or subepithelial electron-dense material are seen by electron microscopy, and discontinuous linear deposits of IgG, IgM, and C3 have been demonstrated along the capillary membranes by fluorescence microscopy. To date, it has not been established that antigenic material derived from *M. leprae* is actually present within the glomeruli. Notwithstanding the severity of the inflammatory response in many cases of ENL, hypocomplementemia is unusual.

Reversal Reactions. Patients with BT, BB, or BL disease may experience a quite different type of tissue reaction after they have been treated for several months. As the clinical status of these patients improves, typically from a BL to a BB classification, some will develop induration and erythema within infected areas of the skin. Histologic examination reveals an influx of lymphocytes into areas of granulomatous inflammation, with concomitant reduction in the number of bacilli. Reversal reactions generally develop over days or weeks and last for weeks or months. Although these reactions are regarded as an "upgrading" of the host's cellular immune responses, the clinical consequences can be serious. For example, augmentation of the inflammatory response within peripheral nerves can irreversibly damage the already compromised fascicles. Reactions quite similar in appearance to reversal reactions but that signal a deterioration in the immune response may be experienced by patients whose compliance with therapy is poor or in whom the *M. leprae* has become drug resistant. These so-called "downgrading" reactions are associated with worsening of the clinical condition and an increased bacillary index within tissues.

DIAGNOSIS AND DIFFERENTIAL DIAGNOSIS. Isolation of a phenolic glycolipid I that appears unique to *M. leprae* (Brennan and Barrow, 1980) offers promise that serologic tests may be developed that will aid in the early diagnosis of leprosy. At present, however, the diagnosis must be established by clinical examination and histopathologic study. An anesthetic or hypoesthetic skin lesion immediately suggests the diagnosis of leprosy; associated nerve thickening further supports the diagnosis. A skin biopsy is essential for confirmation and accurate classification of the disease. An adequate biopsy specimen must include both central and peripheral areas of a lesion and should be deep enough to remove subcutaneous fatty tissue en bloc. Elliptical excision biopsy 12 to 15 mm long is preferred to punch biopsy. When lesions of varying types are present, it is advisable to obtain biopsies from two different sites.

M. leprae in paraffinized tissues is poorly stained by the Ziehl-Neelsen method. A much better stain is obtained by the Wade-Fite method, or its equivalent, which restores the acid-fast property of *M. leprae* by impregnating the tissue section with an oily substance such as turpentine or peanut oil. Control sections known to contain acid-fast staining organisms should be prepared simultaneously. In patients with paucibacillary disease (i.e., TT or BT), serial histologic sections may have to be searched for hours to identify one or two bacilli; these most frequently will be located within dermal nerve twigs. The Ziehl-Neelsen stain is adequate for smear preparations as from nasal scrapings and the buffy coat of blood. Acid-fast staining bacilli are readily visualized in both types of smears in BL or LL disease. In buffy coat smears, mononuclear cells contain bacilli, as do occasional polymorphonuclear leukocytes.

Some clinical signs and symptoms that may be helpful in establishing the diagnosis of lepromatous leprosy include the following: (1) The ear lobes are thickened and have a "succulent" appearance. (2) The patient complains of a chronically stuffy nose with discharge that sometimes is bloody; frequently the examiner will note a fetid odor. (3) There may be ENL lesions scattered widely over the body, including the face. Erythema nodosum that is associated with other conditions usually is localized to the pretibial regions of the lower extremities. ENL is not seen in tuberculoid leprosy. (4) Not infrequently there is a brawny type of edema involving the lower extremities and the hands. Fusiform swelling of the digits that extends to the dorsum of the hands is seen, mimicking scleroderma.

Certain types of nerve deficits or deformities should suggest the possibility of leprosy in any form. These include (1) plantar ulcerations in a person who is neither diabetic nor tabetic; (2) footdrop without a history of poliomyelitis or heavy metal exposure; and (3) a characteristic claw deformity of the hands, with digital damage resulting from motor and sensory dysfunction of the ulnar nerve and other nerve supply to the hand. Occasionally, leprosy will be misdiagnosed as lupus erythematosus; fluorescent antibody staining of a skin biopsy may reveal immunoglobulin deposits resembling those of lupus within the epidermal basement membrane. A Wade-Fite stain is most helpful in such situations.

TREATMENT—PRINCIPAL DRUGS. ***Dapsone.*** The standard drug for leprosy continues to be 4,4′-diaminodiphenylsulfone (dapsone, DDS). DDS is thought to block the p-aminobenzoic acid condensation reaction necessary for folate synthesis. The minimal inhibitory concentration (MIC) of DDS for *M. leprae* that are susceptible to the drug ranges between 0.01 and 0.001 μg per milliliter as determined by the mouse footpad assay. DDS is inexpensive, a factor of great economic significance in countries with high prevalence rates of leprosy. Its toxicity is low; however, adverse reactions to DDS occasionally occur. The most serious are hemolysis, agranulocytosis, hepatitis, exfoliative dermatitis, and, very rarely, severe hypoalbuminemia. A devastating combination of exfoliative dermatitis and hepatitis, known as the "DDS syndrome," has been observed in perhaps 1 per 1000 cases in the early stages of treatment (less than seven weeks). Immediate cessation of DDS, intensive care, and massive corticosteroid therapy (in excess of 100 mg per day of prednisone or its equivalent) may be lifesaving.

Twenty-four hours after ingestion of DDS, 100 mg, the plasma concentration in a 60-kg person ranges from approximately 0.12 to 0.4 μg per milliliter. This rather wide range is explained by large individual differences in rates of clearance from the body, resulting in part from genetic polymorphism in acetylation of the drug. Thus, the half-life in plasma varies from 10 to 50 hours, with an average of 28 hours. Regardless of an individual's acetylation status, however, the plasma levels of DDS under daily therapy with 50 to 100 mg will remain well in excess of the MIC for susceptible *M. leprae.*

Rifampin.* The MIC of rifampin against *M. leprae* is less than 1 μg per ml, and it provides a rapid bactericidal effect against organisms in tissues and nasal secretions. As little as 4 weeks of therapy with rifampin prevents multiplication in the mouse footpad of acid-fast bacilli harvested from tissue specimens or nasal secretions of patients with lepromatous leprosy. A comparable loss of infectivity cannot be achieved with DDS until 10 to 12 weeks of treatment. Rifampin therapy also rapidly reduces the morphologic index (MI) of *M. leprae.* The MI expresses a ratio of the number of bacilli, within tissues or secretions, that stain uniformly by acid-fast methods and that therefore are considered viable over the number of bacilli that strain irregularly and therefore are considered to be nonviable. The MI of *M. leprae* in lepromatous patients falls to nearly zero within four weeks after the start of rifampin therapy. By contrast, three to six months of DDS therapy may be required for comparable reduction of the MI.

Clofazimine. Clofazimine (B663) is a phenazine iminoquinone derivative that is effective in the treatment of leprosy, although its mechanism of action is not well understood. There is some evidence that it may act by inhibiting template formation of deoxyribonucleic acid. The compound is highly lipophilic and is deposited within fatty tissues, the skin, and the reticuloendothelial system, where it is taken up by macrophages. Clofazimine is a dye and therefore causes skin pigmentation over time, with a coloration varying from a reddish hue to a deep purple with prolonged high dosage therapy. After discontinuation of clofazimine therapy, the pigmentation clears gradually over a period of months to years. Clofazimine is eliminated very slowly with a half-life following oral administration of 70 days or more. Urinary excretion is negligible, whereas approximately 50 per cent of an administered dose may be recovered unchanged from the feces, possibly as a result of incomplete absorption from the gut and excretion via the bile, in which high concentrations have been found. Given in high concentrations (200 to 300 mg per day) for extended periods of time, the drug is deposited in the small intestinal wall and thereby causes segmental thickening that may be associated with mid-abdominal burning or cramping pain, diarrhea, and rarely partial small bowel obstruction. Clofazimine has not been approved by the Food and Drug Administration. It may be obtained under protocol from the National Hansen's Disease Center, Carville, Louisiana.

*This use is not listed in the manufacturer's directive.

TREATMENT—CURRENT RECOMMENDATIONS. Of great concern has been the emergence of both primary and secondary resistance to DDS as a consequence of its long-term use as the single therapeutic agent to treat leprosy. Worldwide, the prevalence of secondary resistance currently ranges from 20 to 190 per 1000, depending on locale. Primary resistance to DDS of varying prevalence and degree also has been reported worldwide. In view of these findings, it is essential that a variety of antibiotics be administered to all patients with leprosy.

The principal aims of multidrug therapy are to stem the increase in prevalence of primary and secondary resistance to DDS by *M. leprae* and to reduce the duration of treatment. For treatment of multibacillary forms of leprosy (BB, BL, and LL types), the following triple drug combination is suggested by the World Health Organization (WHO): (1) a self-administered oral dose of DDS, 50 to 100 mg daily; (2) a self-administered oral dose of clofazimine, 50 mg daily plus a 300-mg dose given once monthly under supervision; and (3) an oral dose of rifampin, 600 mg once monthly under supervision. When clofazimine is totally unacceptable, ethionamide* or prothionamide† should be considered in a self-administered oral dose of 250 to 375 mg daily. The case for use of the latter antibiotics is more compelling in patients harboring *M. leprae* that is resistant to DDS. Proof of resistance requires special procedures that are available at centers for the treatment of leprosy.

Combined therapy should be given for a minimum of two years. If possible, such therapy should be continued until all skin scrapings and biopsies become negative for acid-fast bacilli, a process that may require several years.

The WHO recommendation for intermittent rifampin treatment is made in part because of the heavy economic burden that the drug places upon nations with a high prevalence of leprosy. The scientific rationale is based on preliminary clinical trials and studies of intermittent chemotherapy in the mouse footpad infection model. Despite the early promise of intermittent rifampin therapy and the low incidence of reactions to the drug when it is given in this manner (influenza-like syndrome, thrombocytopenic purpura, and shock), the WHO recommendation is based on incomplete data. Some experienced physicians prefer to give 450 or 600 mg of rifampin* daily for two to three years when possible.

For treatment of paucibacillary disease (indeterminant, TT, and BT types), the WHO recommends administration of rifampin,* 600 mg orally once per month under supervision for a six-month period plus DDS, 100 mg orally daily for six months, self-administered. If relapse occurs, the treatment regimen should be repeated. The number of *M. leprae* in patients with paucibacillary disease rarely exceeds 10^6. Therefore, the risk of selecting drug-resistant mutants by treatment appears to be quite low. Moreover, the cell-mediated immune defense mechanisms of these patients are better able to deal with the leprosy bacillus than are those of patients with multibacillary disease. However, the long-term efficacy of intermittent rifampin therapy for paucibacillary disease has not been established. Thus some leprologists elect to treat such cases with DDS, 50 to 100 mg daily plus rifampin, 450 to 600 mg daily for six months with DDS therapy continued for two to five years.

In patients with multibacillary disease who are treated appropriately, clinical improvement generally can be detected after the third month of treatment and clearly is evident by the sixth month. Disappearance of recognizable bacillary forms usually requires three to five years even though viable bacilli rapidly become undetectable by currently available assay methods. Thus patients with lepromatous leprosy have difficulty not only in disposing of viable *M. leprae* but also in clearing nonviable organisms.

Patients with lepromatous leprosy who are under treatment with a drug regimen that includes rifampin can be regarded as noncontagious after a two- to three-week period. However, even the untreated patient represents only a very low risk of contagion and can be admitted to any general hospital in which ordinary procedures of barrier nursing are observed. Tuberculoid leprosy should be viewed as noncontagious.

*This use is not listed in the manufacturer's directive.
†Investigational drug.

Treatment of Reactions. ENL is by far the most common reaction in lepromatous leprosy. When mild, it can be managed with aspirin. Severe episodes are controlled rapidly by high dosages of prednisone (60 to 80 mg per day). However, as the dosage is tapered, a flare-up of ENL is encountered frequently. Thalidomide* is very effective in treating severe ENL. The initial dosage is usually 200 mg given twice daily with gradual tapering over several weeks to maintenance levels of 50 to 100 mg per day. This dosage can be continued for several months. Administration of both prednisone and thalidomide to patients with severe ENL brings about very prompt improvement by means of the steroid action and yet permits rapid steroid withdrawal within a few days as the thalidomide takes full effect. The use of thalidomide in women of childbearing age is hazardous because of its teratogenicity. Clofazimine is also effective in the management of ENL, although it requires from four to six weeks to exert its effect. ENL reactions in patients with BL leprosy are poorly controlled by thalidomide and are best managed by judicious use of steroids and/or clofazimine.

Reversal reactions associated with severe neuritis or in which there is a risk of skin ulceration should be treated with steroids in high dosage, followed by very gradual tapering. Alternatively, steroids plus clofazimine can be employed to attempt more rapid withdrawal of the steroid. Reversal reactions are far more chronic than the usual episodes of ENL and may require anti-inflammatory therapy for several months. Thalidomide is ineffective in treating these reactions.

Treatment of Other Complications. A cold abscess within a peripheral nerve requires surgical drainage. A sudden increase in the intensity of nerve pain and/or increase in the functional deficit of a nerve under full medical therapy may be helped in some cases by surgical decompression to relieve the intraneural edema. Excellent corrective surgical procedures are available for deformity of the hands secondary to permanent loss of motor innervation. The common problem of footdrop can be greatly improved by transfer of the tibialis posterior muscle so that it becomes a dorsiflexor. Plantar ulceration secondary to sensory loss responds well to appropriate medical and surgical management. Subsequently the patient should be fitted carefully with special footwear that will increase the area of load-bearing and reduce pressure at the ulcer-prone site. Madarosis (complete loss of eyebrows) can be corrected by swinging scalp flaps to the eyebrow area after infection has been arrested. This cosmetic procedure can make the difference between social acceptance or nonacceptance, since laymen in regions endemic for leprosy are well aware of the cause of eyebrow loss. Leprotic iridocyclitis is an insidious complication in lepromatous patients that may progress without pain. Treatment with mydriatrics and steroids is essential to prevent destruction of the ciliary body. Lagophthalmos secondary to involvement of the seventh cranial nerve also must be corrected to prevent exposure keratitis.

PROGNOSIS. Most cases of TT leprosy are self-curing, as are many of those with indeterminate disease. Some individuals with BT leprosy may self-cure with or without permanent nerve damage; however, there is a tendency for others to lose cell-mediated immune responsiveness to *M. leprae* and to drift toward the lepromatous end of the disease spectrum. Notwithstanding the more favorable prognosis in tuberculoid leprosy, all patients should be treated as detailed above.

Most cases of lepromatous leprosy can be brought to a state of arrest if not cure, provided that compliance is good and that appropriate therapy is continued for a prolonged period. Death caused by amyloidosis or inadequately treated ENL is relatively infrequent.

PREVENTION AND PROPHYLAXIS. The household contacts of leprosy patients, especially children, should be examined care-

*Investigational drug in leprosy.

fully for signs of leprosy, and suspicious skin lesions must be biopsied. Generally, household contacts of TT and BT patients should not be given prophylaxis, although it is advisable that they be examined annually. Children who have had extensive household contact with BL or LL patients who have been untreated should be considered for DDS prophylaxis; DDS has been shown to be of prophylactic value in children under the age of 16 when given according to recommended dosage schedules (Filice and Fraser). Adults appear to be less susceptible to leprosy; since the efficacy of DDS prophylaxis in this group has not been established, preventive treatment of older age groups usually is not recommended.

Three major trials to determine the preventive role of BCG vaccine against leprosy have yielded different results. At this time BCG is not recommended for prevention of leprosy.

Bullock WE: Immunology of leprosy. *In* Nahmias A, O'Reilly R (eds.): Immunology of Human Infection, Part I. New York, Plenum Publishing Corporation, 1981, p 369. *A thorough discussion of the immunologic disturbances associated with leprosy.*

Filice GA, Fraser DW: Management of household contacts of leprosy patients. Ann Intern Med 88:538, 1978. *Detailed recommendations.*

Ridley DS, Jopling WH: Classification of leprosy according to immunity. A five-group system. Int J Leprosy 34:255, 1966. *Most helpful for comprehending the spectrum of leprosy. Good illustrations.*

Serjeantson SW: HLA and susceptibility to leprosy. Immunol Rev 70:89, 1983. *A good review of the genetic aspects of leprosy.*

WHO Study Group Report: Chemotherapy of leprosy for control programmes. WHO Technical Report Series No. 675. Geneva, WHO, 1982. *A new report containing important recommendations for changes in the treatment of leprosy.*

Yawalkar SJ, Vischer W: Lamprene (Clofazimine) in Leprosy. Basel, Ciba-Geigy Limited, 1978, pp 1–15. *A concise summary of what is known about this important drug.*

Sexually Transmitted Diseases

P. Frederick Sparling

301. INTRODUCTION AND COMMON SYNDROMES

Sexually transmitted diseases (STDs) are a diverse group of infections, caused by biologically dissimilar microbial agents, which are grouped together because of certain common clinical and epidemiologic features. In recent years there has been a surge of interest by physicians, researchers, and the public in STDs. This interest in part is due to the prior lack of knowledge about these common diseases, to relaxation of former taboos about sexuality, and to recognition of the medical and economic importance of STD. This has resulted in a remarkable accumulation of information about "classic" venereal infections such as gonorrhea, as well as "new" sexually transmitted diseases such as hepatitis A and B, shigellosis, giardiasis, acquired immune deficiency syndrome (AIDS), and others. This chapter will discuss certain common features of some of these infections, as well as the differential diagnosis and management of several of the common syndromes of genital infections.

DEFINITIONS. Those infectious agents which are frequently transmitted by sexual contact, and for which sexual transmission is epidemiologically important, are considered sexually transmitted diseases. In some cases, such as gonorrhea and genital herpes simplex virus infection, sexual transmission is the only important mode of transmission, at least between adults. In others, such as the hepatitis viruses, giardiasis, shigellosis, and amebiasis, there are also important nonsexual means of acquiring infection. Table 301–1 lists the important infectious agents that are commonly transmitted sexually, as well as their known or probable disease syndromes. Other diseases, such as cervical carcinoma, for which there is strong epidemiologic evidence of association with sexual transmission but for which there still is not a known cause, will not be considered here. Diverse infections such as blastomycosis, histoplasmosis, and others for which sexual transmission has been documented generally will be considered. "Sexual" includes the full range of heterosexual or homosexual behavior, including genital, oral-genital, oral-anal, and genital-anal contact.

EPIDEMIOLOGIC CONSIDERATIONS. Sexually transmitted infections are prevalent in many segments of society, but, for obvious reasons, are most prevalent in the groups with the most promiscuous sexual activity. It is not sexual activity per se, but the number of different sexual partners that determines the risk of acquiring STD. The highest rates of gonorrhea are found in the young (15 to 30) and unmarried, and in groups of low educational and socioeconomic status. Rates of gonococcal infection may be 50-fold higher in young single inner-city persons than in married middle to upper-middle class persons. Decisions regarding the cost-effectiveness of screening for STD should be governed by these considerations; screening is most effective in high-risk groups.

Multiple infections are frequent in patients with sexually transmitted infection. In venereal disease clinics, about 20 per cent of men with gonorrhea also have urethral chlamydial infection, and 30 to 50 per cent of women with gonorrhea also have cervical chlamydial infection. In women with vaginitis, one study showed that 16 per cent of cases were caused by mixed infection with various combinations of *Candida, Trichomonas,* and *G. vaginalis*. However, there is no convincing evidence that one sexually transmitted infection directly increases the risk of acquiring others. Rather, the frequent coexistence of multiple sexually acquired infections probably reflects the frequency of these organisms and the multiplicity of sexual partners among patients who were the subjects of these studies.

Control of sexually transmitted infections is complicated by the frequent lack of significant symptoms. The majority of gonococcal and chlamydial infections in women probably are associated with few symptoms. From 10 to 50 per cent of urethral gonococcal infections in men are oligo- or asymptomatic. Urethral chlamydial infections of men are more common than gonococcal infections and frequently are asymptomatic. The importance of the asymptomatic male is underscored by the repeated observation that women with gonococcal pelvic inflammatory disease have male partners whose infection is asymptomatic. Thus, one of the crucial issues in management is proper diagnosis and treatment of the asymptomatically infected partner.

STD IN HOMOSEXUAL MALES. Homosexual males are recognized as a group at particularly high risk of acquiring sexually transmitted disease. The current epidemic of AIDS in homosexual men is a major concern. This subject is discussed in Ch. 430. AIDS is but one of many STD-related problems in homosexual males, however. Currently, approximately 50 per cent of all male patients in the United States with infectious (primary and secondary) syphilis name other males as their contacts. Some homosexual males are exceptionally promiscuous and are at high risk of acquiring not only syphilis but also gonococcal urethritis, proctitis, and pharyngitis; herpes genitalis and proctitis; hepatitis A and B; and a variety of enteric infections that are rarely transmitted in heterosexual sex, including giardiasis, amebiasis, and shigellosis. These enteric infections are probably transmitted by oral-anal or anal-penile-oral contact. Several cities in the United States with relatively large populations of homosexual males have had major increases in prevalence of giardiasis, amebiasis, and shigellosis. In some studies, the incidence of acute shigellosis and hepatitis A and B in men aged 20 to 39 was six to ten times that of any other age group of men or women. A study of a population of homosexual men

TABLE 301–1. SEXUALLY TRANSMITTED AGENTS AND THEIR SYNDROMES*

Microorganism	Syndromes
Bacteria	
Neisseria gonorrhoeae	Urethritis, cervicitis, bartholinitis, proctitis, pharyngitis, salpingitis, epididymitis, conjunctivitis, perihepatitis, arthritis, dermatitis, endocarditis, meningitis, amniotic infection syndrome
Gardnerella vaginalis	"Nonspecific" vaginosis (in association with anaerobic bacteria)
Treponema pallidum	Syphilis (multiple clinical syndromes)
Hemophilus ducreyi	Chancroid
Calymmatobacterium granulomatis	Granuloma inguinale
Shigella species	Enteritis in homosexual men
Campylobacter species	Enteritis in homosexual men
Group B *Streptococcus*	Neonatal sepsis and meningitis
Chlamydiae	
Chlamydia trachomatis	Nongonococcal urethritis, purulent hypertrophic cervicitis, epididymitis, salpingitis, conjunctivitis, trachoma, pneumonia, perihepatitis, lymphogranuloma venereum, ? Reiter's syndrome
Mycoplasmas	
Ureaplasma urealyticum	Nongonococcal urethritis, ? premature rupture of membranes and abortion
Mycoplasma hominis	Postpartum fever, ? pelvic inflammatory disease
Viruses	
Herpes simplex virus	Genital herpes, proctitis, meningitis, disseminated infection in neonates
Hepatitis A virus	Hepatitis in homosexual men
Hepatitis B virus	Hepatitis, ? periarteritis nodosa, hepatoma; especially prevalent in homosexual men
Cytomegalovirus	Congenital infection (birth defects, infant mortality, mental deficiency, hearing loss); mononucleosis syndrome
Genital wart virus	Condyloma acuminatum
Molluscum contagiosum virus	Molluscum contagiosum
Protozoa	
Trichomonas vaginalis	Trichomonal vaginitis, occasional urethritis
Entamoeba histolytica	Enteritis in homosexual men
Giardia lamblia	Enteritis in homosexual men
Fungi	
Candida albicans	Vaginitis, balanitis
Ectoparasites	
Phthirus pubis	Pubic lice infestation
Sarcoptes scabei	Scabies

*The relative importance of sexual transmission in the epidemiology of several of these agents remains to be defined; these include Group B streptococci, hepatitis A virus, cytomegalovirus, *Candida albicans*, and others.

in New York City showed that nearly 40 per cent had *E. histolytica, G. lamblia,* or both in their stool. It is not clear whether the apparent increase in STD in homosexual men is due to increased recognition and reporting of these diseases or to changing patterns of sexual behavior among certain groups of homosexual men. Homosexual women apparently do not have increased rates of STD.

INCIDENCE OF STDs. The true incidence of the STDs is not known in the United States because of serious problems of underreporting. Nevertheless, some estimates are available (Table 301–2). Gonorrhea is the most common of the reported infectious diseases in the United States, and infections by genital chlamydiae (which are not reportable at present) are probably of similar or greater magnitude. The relative incidence of STD is quite variable in different areas of the world. For instance, chancroid is presently quite uncommon in the United States, but is about as common as gonorrhea in certain areas of the Far East.

COMMON SYNDROMES. ***Urethritis in Males.*** Urethritis in males is a very common syndrome. It is ordinarily classified as either gonococcal or nongonococcal urethritis (NGU), depending on whether the presence of gonococci can be demonstrated by Gram stain or culture. In venereal disease clinics, the prevalence of gonococcal and nongonococcal urethritis is similar, but NGU is considerably more common in private practice and in college infirmaries. A recent study of asymptomatic sexually active military men found a 1 per cent prevalence of urethral gonorrhea but a 12 per cent prevalence of urethral chlamydial infection.

A large number of studies have established *Chlamydia trachomatis* as a cause of approximately 40 per cent of cases of NGU. Case-control studies have provided suggestive evidence that *Ureaplasma urealyticum* (formerly "T-strain" mycoplasma) is a significant factor in chlamydia-negative NGU. In addition, urethral inoculation of volunteers with pure cultures of *U. urealyticum* produced rather typical NGU. In practice, however, it is difficult to define the importance of *Ureaplasma* infection in patients with urethritis, because up to 50 per cent of asymptomatic sexually active persons are colonized by these organisms. A very small proportion of cases of male NGU is due to *Trichomonas vaginalis* or herpes simplex virus infection.

Diagnosis of urethritis requires demonstration of an inflammatory urethral exudate. A discharge may not be evident if the patient has recently voided, and patients preferably should be examined several hours after their last urination. The discharge may be present only in the morning, prior to urination. Demonstration of discharge often requires urethral "milking," and may require insertion of a small calcium-alginate or similar swab into the anterior urethra, with examination of a direct Gram-stained smear of the swab for leukocytes. Presence of an average of at least five polymorphonuclear leukocytes per high power (100×) field suggests the diagnosis of urethritis.

The patient should be questioned for past history of urethritis, and for symptoms suggestive of systemic diseases such as Reiter's syndrome or disseminated gonococcal infection. Examination should be made for signs of conjunctivitis, arthritis, dermatitis, and epididymitis. Prostatitis is rarely present unless there are symptoms of perineal, suprapubic, or rectal discomfort, and rectal examination is not routinely indicated. Rectal examination and urine culture are indicated in men with dysuria but without signs of anterior urethral discharge.

Laboratory studies are ordinarily limited to a Gram stain of urethral exudate. Demonstration of typical gram-negative diplococci, many of which are inside neutrophils, establishes the diagnosis of gonococcal urethritis. At least 90 per cent of men with symptomatic culture-proven urethral gonorrhea have a positive Gram stain. In occasional patients, especially those with equivocal Gram stain, it may be necessary to culture the anterior urethra or freshly voided urine sediment for gonococci. This is particularly important in asymptomatic male contacts of patients with disseminated gonococcal infection or gonococcal salpingitis, since Gram stain of urethral contents is positive in only about 60 per cent of men with asymptomatic urethral gonorrhea.

Diagnosis of NGU is made by exclusion of gonorrhea. Dem-

TABLE 301–2. INCIDENCE OF CERTAIN SEXUALLY TRANSMITTED DISEASES IN THE UNITED STATES, 1977*

Disease	Estimated Annual Incidence
Gonorrhea	2,000,000
Nongonococcal urethritis in men	1,000,000
Trichomoniasis	800,000
Condyloma acuminatum	300,000
Pelvic inflammatory disease	250,000
Genital herpes simplex virus	200,000
Pediculosis pubis	150,000
Syphilis (primary and secondary)	75,000

*Source: STD Fact Sheet, HEW Publication (CDC) 79–8195.

onstration of genital chlamydiae or ureaplasmas requires cultural methods that are not routinely available at present. Monoclonal antibodies recently were made available for diagnosis of chlamydiae in secretions; early results indicate a sensitivity of over 90 per cent compared with culture, with nearly 100 per cent specificity. There is no serologic test that is clinically useful to diagnose infection by either of these agents. Examination of a saline suspension of urethral exudate for motile trichomonads occasionally may be revealing in patients with recurrent urethritis who fail to respond to appropriate therapy. A serologic test for syphilis should be obtained, but the diagnostic yield is low.

Management is outlined in Figure 301–1 and is discussed further in Ch. 302. Sexual partners of men with gonococcal or nongonococcal urethritis should be treated both to prevent reinfection of the patient and to prevent development of complications in the partners.

The syndrome of *postgonococcal urethritis* (persistence or recrudescence of urethritis after administration of therapy that has eradicated gonococcal infection) is usually due to concomitant urethral chlamydial infection that was not eradicated by the original treatment. This syndrome is more common after therapy with intramuscular procaine penicillin or a single oral dose of ampicillin than after a five-day regimen of tetracycline, undoubtedly because of the greater efficacy of tetracycline for treating chlamydial infections. Accordingly, there is considerable merit to use of oral tetracycline for treatment of gonococcal urethritis, either as the sole therapy or to follow up penicillin or ampicillin therapy.

Genital Ulcer Syndrome. Genital skin lesions may be either ulcerative or nonulcerative. In patients seen in a venereal disease clinic, the most common sexually transmitted nonulcerative genital lesions are due to scabies, genital warts, molluscum contagiosum, or *Candida* species, but differential diagnosis includes a long list of dermatologic conditions.

The most common cause of ulcerative genital lesions in patients in the United States is herpes simplex virus, but differential diagnosis includes syphilis, chancroid, lymphogranuloma venereum (LGV), granuloma inguinale (GI), and trauma. Chancroid is uncommon in Western nations, and LGV and GI are rare. The most important distinction is between syphilis and genital herpes. Sometimes, the appearance is virtually diagnostic: grouped painful superficial vesicles are nearly diagnostic of herpes, whereas a single clean-based nonpainful ulcer with indurated margins suggests primary syphilis. In recent studies, only about 60 per cent of penile syphilitic chancres had this classic appearance. Painful ulcers suggest herpes, or possibly chancroid. Genital herpes may present as a single ulcer, particularly in patients with recurrent herpes, and syphilis may present with multiple ulcers. Secondarily infected lesions of primary syphilis may be painful.

It is a useful rule to obtain a serologic test for syphilis on all patients with genital ulcers, and, if the initial serology is negative and if the diagnosis remains uncertain, to obtain a second serology about two weeks later. A dark-field examination for syphilis should also be done, and it should be repeated twice on successive days if syphilis is seriously suspected and the initial examination is negative.

Infection by herpes simplex virus may be efficiently diagnosed by viral culture or by immunofluorescent methods, but these are frequently unavailable in practice. Papanicolaou smear is suggestive of herpes in about two thirds of culture-positive cases. Giemsa or Wright's stain of cells scraped from the base of a vesicle may reveal multinucleate giant cells (Tzanck test), but this test is particularly insensitive in herpetic lesions which have become ulcerated. Serologic tests for herpesvirus are not helpful. Referral of patients to centers with capability of viral culture may be indicated in diagnostically difficult patients.

In addition to herpesvirus infection, chancroid should be suspected in patients with painful genital ulcers. Chancroid is more likely if there has been recent sexual contact in Africa or the Far East. Attempts should be made to isolate the causative agent, *Hemophilus ducreyi;* selective culture media are an improvement over previously available methods. No serologic tests are available.

Therapy clearly depends on the correct diagnosis. Topical antibiotics are never indicated. Initial genital herpes (first infection) is best treated with topical or oral administration of acyclovir or intravenous administration for severe infections (see Ch. 28). Therapy of chancroid is with co-trimoxazole or erythromycin. Occasional empirical trials of oral co-trimoxazole or erythromycin are warranted in patients with persistent genital ulcers not readily attributable to herpesvirus or syphilis, but repeated attempts to isolate *H. ducreyi* should be made in such instances. It is not possible to arrive at an unequivocal diagnosis of the cause of genital ulcers in all patients.

Lower Genital Tract Infections in Women. Infections of the female genitourinary tract produce a variety of syndromes, often with overlapping symptoms (dysuria, vaginal discharge, vulvar irritation). These infections are very common, relatively poorly understood by most physicians, sometimes difficult to treat, and often frustrating for both doctor and patient. However, the various syndromes usually can be distinguished on relatively simple clinical and laboratory grounds, and a precise microbial etiology often can be established.

It is most helpful first to determine the primary anatomic site of infection: urethra or bladder, endocervix, or vagina. This can sometimes be accomplished by history; women with urinary tract infection (UTI) usually experience "internal" dysuria, whereas women with dysuria associated with vaginitis usually experience "external" dysuria owing to passage of urine over

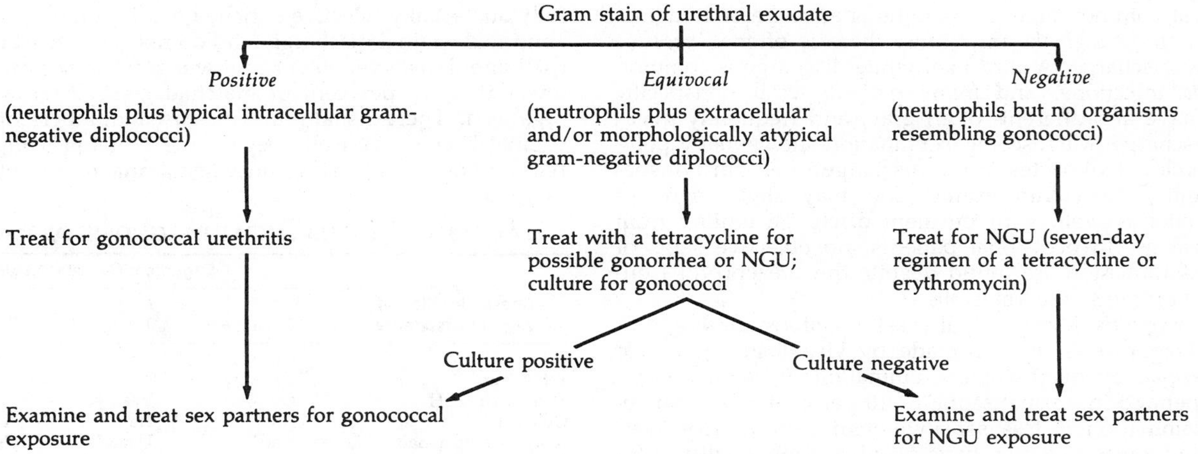

Figure 301–1. Management of male patients with urethritis.

inflamed labia. Cervicitis is diagnosed by physical examination; there are mucopurulent secretions emanating from the endocervical canal, and there is often a hypertrophic, mucoid, reddened "cobblestone" appearance to the cervical mucosa. Patients with cervicitis may also have urethritis or vaginitis. Vaginitis is associated with increased vaginal discharge of several types, as discussed below, and frequently there are associated signs and symptoms of vaginal, vulvar, and perineal irritation (dyspareunia, external dysuria, itching, pain). In patients with lower genitourinary infection, it is important to determine whether there is involvement of the upper genitourinary tract (pyelonephritis, salpingitis).

THE URETHRAL SYNDROME. Bacterial cystitis with or without pyelonephritis is usually diagnosed in women with dysuria, urinary frequency, and pyuria if they have colony counts of at least 10^5 bacteria per milliliter of urine. If similar symptoms are present but routine cultures grow less than 10^4 bacteria per milliliter of voided urine, the "urethral syndrome" is likely.

In a study of sexually active young women who presented to walk-in clinics with dysuria and urinary frequency, and who did not have vaginitis or active herpes simplex infection, 43 per cent had the urethral syndrome (urethritis). Among women with urethritis, 25 per cent had positive urethral cultures for *Chlamydia trachomatis.* Isolation of chlamydiae from the urethra was uncommon in women without urethritis. In other studies, gonococci also were shown to cause this syndrome. Thus, women as well as men may present with urethritis caused by gonococci and chlamydiae.

Management of patients with the urethral syndrome has not been carefully evaluated. Patients with symptoms of urinary tract infection who do not have bacteriuria should have urethral and cervical cultures for *N. gonorrhoeae.* If these cultures are also negative, a therapeutic trial may be made with a tetracycline or a sulfonamide for approximately seven days. There are no controlled trials of such therapy or of the management of sexual partners of women with the urethral syndrome.

VAGINITIS. In a large study of women in a primary care clinic who presented with lower genitourinary complaints, vaginitis was more than five times as common as urinary tract infections. In this and similar studies, there were three predominant types of vaginitis: yeast infection *(Candida albicans)*, trichomonas *(T. vaginalis)* infection, and "nonspecific" vaginitis caused by organisms other than *Candida* and *T. vaginalis.* The incidence of these types of vaginitis varies in different patient populations, but in general *Candida* and nonspecific vaginitis are more common than *T. vaginalis* vaginitis.

Symptoms of vaginitis include increased volume of vaginal discharge, which is often abnormally yellow or green in appearance, and may be malodorous. Vaginal and vulvar itching may be troublesome, especially in *Candida* infection. There may be vaginal tenderness and pain, dyspareunia, or dysuria.

The most common sign of vaginitis is an increased vaginal discharge. In *T. vaginalis* infections, there is often a profuse and frothy discharge. A curd-like, white discharge is common in *Candida* infections, and many patients with nonspecific vaginitis have an adherent, often gray, and frequently malodorous discharge. Microscopic examination shows many polymorphonuclear leukocytes in the discharge in all but nonspecific vaginitis. Speculum examination may show signs of endocervicitis as well, with purulent discharge issuing from the cervical os. In occasional patients, no objective signs of vaginal inflammation are found despite the presence of troublesome symptoms. See Table 301–3.

Candida Vaginitis. Most vaginal yeast infections are due to *C. albicans.* Diagnosis is usually made by visualizing yeasts or pseudohyphae by microscopic examination of vaginal secretions suspended in normal saline or 10 per cent KOH. Microscopic examination is less sensitive than culture. However, many asymptomatic women have positive vaginal cultures for *C. albicans,* and therefore some authorities advocate using microscopy in preference to culture. The discharge in *Candida* vaginitis is not malodorous and has a pH of less than 4.5 when a drop is applied to pH paper with a range of 4.0 to 5.5.

Therapy of *Candida* vaginitis is with intravaginal nystatin twice daily for seven days, or with one of the imidazole compounds (clotrimazole or miconazole) once each night for seven days. Several studies suggest that therapy with the imidazoles is more effective than with nystatin. There is no convincing evidence that attempts to eradicate yeast from the gastrointestinal tract by administration of oral nystatin have a significant effect on rates of cure or relapse of *Candida* vaginitis. There is no evidence to warrant therapy of sexual partners. Attempts should be made to correct ancillary conditions which increase susceptibility to vaginal candidiasis: antibiotic therapy, diabetes, or oral anovulatory steroids. Relapse is a significant problem in some patients. No therapy is indicated for asymptomatic vaginal carriers of *C. albicans.*

T. Vaginale Vaginitis. Diagnosis is made ordinarily by visualizing motile trichomonads in a normal saline suspension of vaginal secretions. The organisms are easily seen at high-dry (100×) magnification, and may usually be seen under low power magnification. The saline suspension should be examined promptly. Culture is more sensitive, but about 80 to 90 per cent of culture-positive cases are detected by microscopy. Addition of a drop of 10 per cent KOH to vaginal secretions usually results in liberation of a detectable fish-like odor, attributed to release of volatile amines. The pH of vaginal secretions is usually greater than 5.0. In these latter two respects, *T. vaginale* vaginitis is similar to nonspecific vaginitis.

Therapy of trichomoniasis is with one of the nitroimidazoles, either metronidazole or newer compounds such as tinidazole. The latter is extensively used in Europe but is not approved in the United States. A single 2.0-gram oral dose of metronidazole is as effective as multiple-day regimens. Metronidazole is mutagenic, and there is evidence that it is a weak carcinogen in certain animal systems (but, so far, not in humans). Accordingly, it should be used with caution; it has been advocated for women with asymptomatic trichomoniasis, but others would reserve its use for women with symptomatic infections because of possible adverse effects. Metronidazole should not be used in the first trimester of pregnancy. Since over one third of male sexual partners of women with trichomoniasis are asymptomatic urethral carriers of *T. vaginale,* the male partners should also be treated with a single 2.0-gram dose of metronidazole.

Although *T. vaginale* can be transmitted sexually, it probably is transmitted by other means as well. This conclusion is based on prevalence studies which show one peak in young, sexually active women and a second peak in older women who have no other evidence for sexually transmitted infection.

Nonspecific Vaginosis. Recent work has confirmed that this syndrome is probably due to infection by an organism formerly called either *Corynebacterium vaginale* or *Hemophilus vaginalis,* but now termed *Gardnerella vaginalis. G. vaginalis* is a small, gram-variable coccobacillus, which can be grown quite successfully on partially selective enriched media. Among women with abnormal vaginal discharge who do not have yeast infection or trichomoniasis, over 90 per cent will grow *G. vaginalis,* whereas fewer than 10 per cent of matched controls grow the same organism. There usually are increased numbers of anaerobic vaginal bacteria as well. Development of full symptoms may require both *G. vaginalis* and vaginal anaerobes, although the

TABLE 301–3. DIFFERENTIAL DIAGNOSIS OF VAGINITIS

Characteristics of Vaginal Discharge	Organism Causing Vaginitis		
	C. albicans	*T. vaginalis*	*G. vaginalis*
pH	4.5	>5.0	>5.0
White curd	Usually	No	No
Odor with KOH	No	Yes	Yes
Clue cells	No	No	Usually
Motile trichomonads	No	Usually	No
Yeast cells	Yes	No	No

precise pathophysiology of this syndrome is still under investigation.

Diagnosis of nonspecific vaginosis is by exclusion of trichomoniasis, candidiasis, and purulent cervicitis. Abnormal cells termed "clue cells" are often seen in a wet mount of vaginal secretions in normal saline; these are stippled, granular-appearing vaginal epithelial cells that contain large numbers of adherent *G. vaginalis*. Few polymorphonuclear leukocytes are present. Addition of a drop of 10 per cent KOH usually results in production of an unpleasant fishy odor. The pH of the vaginal secretions is nearly always greater than 5.0.

Optimal therapy is being investigated. Some but not all studies show that oral ampicillin (500 mg four times daily for seven days) is effective. Metronidazole has only borderline activity in vitro against *G. vaginalis*, but in a dose of 500 mg by mouth twice daily for seven days it was effective in eradicating both *G. vaginalis* and the symptoms of vaginitis from 80 of 81 patients in one trial; similar results have been obtained in other trials. This suggests that the principal cause of this syndrome is an anaerobe, since metronidazole is principally effective against anaerobes. Interest is now focused on curved gram-negative anaerobic rods that are often found in women with nonspecific vaginosis. Oral tetracycline and topical vaginal creams containing sulfonamides are usually ineffective. Over 90 per cent of male partners are urethral carriers of *G. vaginalis*, and therefore probably should be treated with the same regimen as the patient.

Mixed Vaginitis. In 2 to 16 per cent of patients, vaginitis may be due to polymicrobial infection with two or three of the organisms *C. albicans*, *T. vaginalis*, or *G. vaginalis*. Such mixed infection may account for some instances of treatment failure. Particular care should be given to identification of all causative organisms in patients who have recurrent or relapsing vaginitis.

CERVICITIS. Two organisms are recognized as probable causes of mucopurulent endocervicitis: *N. gonorrhoeae* and *C. trachomatis*. Women who are sexual partners of men with chlamydia-positive NGU have a much higher rate of isolation of chlamydiae from the cervix than do women who are partners of men with chlamydia-negative NGU, and they also have significantly higher rates of mucopurulent cervicitis. Herpes simplex virus can also cause cervicitis, especially in primary infection. However, the clinical appearance in herpetic cervicitis is different, with cervical vesicles and ulcers rather than mucopurulent cervicitis.

True cervicitis should not be confused with cervical ectopy, which is merely the appearance of endocervical columnar epithelium on the exposed, visible exocervix. This results in a red-appearing cervix and may result in increased production of a mucoid vaginal discharge, but does not require therapy.

Diagnosis of mucopurulent endocervicitis requires visualization of purulent discharge from the cervical os. There often is a roughened "cobblestone" appearance to the cervix. Gram stain is about 60 per cent sensitive and over 90 per cent specific for gonorrhea if typical intracellular gonococci are seen, but cultures for *N. gonorrhoeae* should be taken. Tissue culture methods for isolation of *C. trachomatis* are not widely available. Cytology is not sufficiently sensitive to warrant widespread use. New monoclonal antibodies against *C. trachomatis* may allow rapid, sensitive, specific immunofluorescent diagnosis from patient secretions.

Antibiotic therapy appears to result in clinical improvement in mucopurulent cervicitis. Patients with negative cultures for the gonococcus probably should be treated with tetracycline or erythromycin in a dose of 500 mg four times daily for at least seven days; their sexual partners probably should be treated similarly. One should recognize that only modest data support these recommendations. No other form of cervicitis has been shown to respond to antimicrobial therapy.

Upper Genital Tract Disease in Women: Salpingitis. Full coverage of this important topic is precluded by space considerations. This is a very important clinical problem, resulting in considerable morbidity in the estimated 250,000 to 500,000 women who are affected yearly in the United States.

ETIOLOGY. The gonococcus may account for as much as 50 per cent of cases in the United States. About 15 to 20 per cent of women with gonococcal cervicitis probably subsequently develop salpingitis. Increasingly strong evidence now implicates genital chlamydial infections as another significant cause of salpingitis; in Sweden, more cases of salpingitis are due to *C. trachomatis* than to *N. gonorrhoeae*. There is less convincing evidence that *Mycoplasma hominis* may occasionally cause a similar syndrome. Many cases of salpingitis are caused by mixed infection with microaerophilic streptococci and enteric bacilli, often including *Bacteroides* species. These polymicrobial infections appear to be more common in recurrent attacks of salpingitis.

DIAGNOSIS. Clinical diagnosis of salpingitis is inexact. Perhaps only 20 per cent of patients have the classic syndrome of lower abdominal pain and tenderness, cervical tenderness, fever, leukocytosis, and elevated sedimentation rate. The most common findings are lower abdominal tenderness, which is usually bilateral, and adnexal and cervical tenderness. Patients with gonococcal salpingitis are more likely to present with fever, and more commonly have onset near the menses, whereas patients with nongonococcal salpingitis more commonly present with adnexal masses. Laparoscopy is commonly used to diagnose salpingitis in certain countries, but is invasive and requires general anesthesia. In the United States, laparoscopy is usually used only in selected patients whose differential diagnosis includes ectopic pregnancy, appendicitis, ruptured abscess, or other potential emergencies.

COMPLICATIONS. Complications are primarily infertility and ectopic pregnancies. Rates of involuntary infertility are about 15 per cent after one attack of salpingitis and about 75 per cent after three or more attacks. Total hysterectomy may eventually be necessitated by symptoms of chronic salpingitis.

THERAPY. A controlled trial of outpatient therapy showed that ten-day regimens of either oral tetracycline or ampicillin were equally effective in both gonococcal and nongonococcal salpingitis. Recent recommendations from the Centers for Disease Control suggest initial therapy with cefoxitin 2.0 grams intramuscularly, or ampicillin 3.5 grams orally, or aqueous procaine penicillin G 4.8 mU intramuscularly, each along with probenecid 1.0 gram orally, followed by doxycycline 100 mg orally twice daily for 10 to 14 days. There are no controlled data on efficacy of various regimens used for hospitalized patients. Current recommendations call for doxycycline 100 mg intravenously twice daily plus cefoxitin 2.0 grams intravenously four times daily; or clindamycin 600 mg intravenously four times daily plus gentamicin or tobramycin 1.5 mg per kilogram intravenously three times daily; or doxycycline 100 mg intravenously twice daily plus metronidazole 1.0 gram intravenously twice daily in patients with normal renal function. Patients should usually be hospitalized if they are very ill, are pregnant, have significant adnexal masses, or have failed previous therapy, or if the differential diagnosis includes surgical emergencies such as appendicitis or ectopic pregnancy.

PREVENTION. Sexual partners of women with gonococcal salpingitis must be identified, examined, and treated to prevent subsequent reinfection of the patient. About one half of the infected male partners of women with gonococcal salpingitis are asymptomatic. Treatment of women with tetracycline (as compared with penicillin) to eradicate chlamydiae from the cervix reduced the incidence of posttherapy salpingitis in one recent study (Rees, 1980), which suggests that increased emphasis on treatment of chlamydiae in the male and female genital tract might reduce the incidence of salpingitis.

Baldson MJ, Pead L, Taylor GE, Maskell R: *Corynebacterium vaginale* and vaginitis: A controlled trial of treatment. Lancet 1:501, 1980. *A randomized trial of the therapy of nonspecific vaginitis. Tetracycline was ineffective, but metronidazole was effective.*

Bowie WR, Wang S-P, Alexander ER, Floyd J, Forsyth PS, Pollock HM, Lin J-SL, Buchanan TM, Holmes KK: Etiology of nongonococcal urethritis: Evidence for *Chlamydia trachomatis* and *Ureaplasma urealyticum*. J Clin Invest 59:735, 1977. *An excellent epidemiologic and clinical study of the etiology and therapy of nongonococcal urethritis in males.*

Centers for Disease Control: Sexually transmitted diseases treatment guidelines 1982. Morbid Mortal Wkly Rep (Suppl) 31(2S):33S, 1982. *The current United States Public Health Service treatment guidelines for all STDs.*

Chapel TA, Brown WJ, Jeffries C, Stewart JA: How reliable is the morphologic diagnosis of penile ulcerations? Sex Trans Dis 4:150, 1977. *Difficulties in clinical distinction among lesions caused by* T. pallidum, *herpesvirus hominis,* and Hemophilus ducreyi *are clearly elucidated.*

Cunningham FG, Hauth JC, Strong JD, Herbert WNP, Gilstrap LC, Wilson RH, Kappus SS: Evaluation of tetracycline or penicillin and ampicillin for treatment of acute pelvic inflammatory disease. N Engl J Med 296:1380, 1977. *The best available study of antibiotic therapy of mild to moderate pelvic inflammatory disease.*

Jacobs NF Jr, Kraus SJ: Gonococcal and nongonococcal urethritis in men: Clinical and laboratory differentiation. Ann Intern Med 82:7, 1975. *A study of clinical and laboratory features which allow distinction between gonococcal and nongonococcal urethritis.*

Mårdh P-A, Møller BR, Paavonen J: Chlamydial infection of the female genital tract with emphasis on pelvic inflammatory disease. A review of Scandinavian studies. Sex Transm Dis 8 (Suppl):140, 1981. *Review of the role of chlamydiae in pelvic inflammatory disease.*

McCue JD, Komaroff AL, Pass TM, Cohen AB, Friedland G: Strategies for diagnosing vaginitis. J Family Pract 9:395, 1979. *A study in a primary care clinic of simple methods for diagnosing the etiology of genitourinary symptoms in women.*

Pheifer TA, Forsyth PS, Durfee MA, Pollock HM, Holmes KK: Nonspecific vaginitis: Role of *Haemophilus vaginalis* and treatment with metronidazole. N Engl J Med 298:1429, 1978. *A clinical and therapeutic study of nonspecific vaginitis, showing that both* G. vaginalis *and vaginal anaerobes are probably important in causation of the syndrome, and also that metronidazole is effective therapy.*

Rees E: The treatment of pelvic inflammatory disease. Am J Obstet Gynecol 138:1042, 1980. *Treatment of women with chlamydial infection of the cervix with tetracycline as compared with penicillin reduced the incidence of subsequent salpingitis.*

Sohn N, Robilotti JG Jr: The gay bowel syndrome: A review of colonic and rectal conditions in 200 male homosexuals. Am J Gastroenterol 67:478, 1977. *A brief clinical review of the numerous kinds of venereal infections acquired by male homosexuals.*

Stamm WE, Koutsky LA, Benedetti JK, Jourden JL, Brunham RC, Holmes KK: *Chlamydia trachomatis* urethral infections in men: Prevalence, risk factors, and clinical manifestations. Ann Intern Med 100:47, 1984. *Asymptomatic male urethral carriers of chlamydiae are very common.*

Stamm WE, Wagner KF, Amsel R, Alexander ER, Turck M, Counts GW, Holmes KK: Causes of the acute urethral syndrome in women. N Engl J Med 303:409, 1980. *Females may also develop a form of nongonococcal urethritis resulting from infection with* Chlamydia trachomatis.

Tait IA, Rees E, Hobson D, Byng RE, Tweedie MCK: Chlamydial infection of the cervix in contacts of men with nongonococcal urethritis. Br J Vener Dis 56:37, 1980. Chlamydia trachomatis *is shown to cause mucopurulent cervicitis, and appropriate antibiotic therapy to result in clinical improvement.*

Taylor-Robinson D, Csonka GW, Prentice MJ: Human intraurethral inoculation of ureaplasmas. Q J Med 46:309, 1977. *Inoculation of the investigator's urethra with ureaplasmas resulted in nonspecific urethritis.*

302. GONOCOCCAL INFECTIONS

INTRODUCTION. *Neisseria gonorrhoeae* is a common sexually transmitted organism which causes anterior urethritis in males and endocervicitis and urethritis in females. Other types of primary infection include pharyngitis, proctitis, conjunctivitis, and vulvovaginitis; the last-named disorder occurs principally in prepubescent females. Complications may occur by direct extension of infection, including epididymitis, prostatitis, Bartholin gland abscess, salpingitis, and perihepatitis. Bacteremia may occur, with production of characteristic cutaneous lesions, arthritis, and tenosynovitis; rare complications include endocarditis and meningitis. Conjunctival infection formerly was a common cause of blindness in neonates.

Gonorrhea is the most common reportable infectious disease in the United States, with about 1 million reported cases annually. The true incidence is probably at least 2 million cases annually.

EPIDEMIOLOGY. The only natural hosts for *N. gonorrhoeae* are humans. The organism normally resides on the columnar epithelium of mucosal surfaces and is usually transmitted by intimate sexual contact.

The prevalence of gonorrhea varies greatly in different groups. As many as 5 per cent of persons in high-risk populations may be infected at any time. Surveys of private practices in the United States in the 1970's showed that about 2 per cent of sexually active young women had positive endocervical cultures for the gonococcus. Highest prevalence was found in young (15 to 30) single persons of low socioeconomic and educational status, probably because these factors correlate positively with sexual promiscuity.

The risk of acquiring infection depends on the type of contact with an infected person. About 60 to 80 per cent of females in contact with a male with urethral gonorrhea will develop gonococcal cervicitis. In contrast, it is estimated that only 20 to 30 per cent of males having sex with an infected female will develop gonorrhea. This difference may be due to exposure of females to a larger inoculum of gonococci. A person having oral sex with a male with gonococcal urethritis has considerable risk of acquiring pharyngeal gonorrhea. Transmission of infection by oral contact with the genitals of an infected female is rare. Infection is apparently efficiently spread by penile-rectal contact.

Gonococci die rapidly upon drying, and transmission by fomites is rare. Epidemics were reported in prepubertal females living in close proximity in orphanages, but such episodes are now very uncommon.

Control of gonorrhea is difficult because of the frequency of asymptomatic infection. Perhaps 50 per cent of infections in females are asymptomatic or only minimally symptomatic, and at least 10 per cent of infected males are asymptomatic.

In past years there was considerable emphasis on case finding by endocervical culture of young, sexually active females. The merit of this strategy depends on the prevalence of infection in the community and the life style of the patient. A more cost-effective method for finding infected patients is to culture patients about six weeks after treatment for gonorrhea; as many as 15 to 20 per cent of such persons will be culture positive, usually because of reinfection.

THE ORGANISM. *N. gonorrhoeae* is a gram-negative, aerobic diplococcus. Many strains require 3 to 10 per cent CO_2 for optimal growth. They are highly autolytic and die rapidly when outside their normal human environment. They are sensitive to fatty acids and grow best on media with added starch to inhibit fatty acids present in agar. Iron required for growth is usually provided by addition of hemoglobin (chocolate agar). Several partially selective media are available; most employ antibiotics such as trimethoprim, vancomycin, colistin, and nystatin to inhibit growth of other microorganisms. Replacement of vancomycin with lincomycin seems to improve the rate of isolation of gonococci.

Presumptive identification in vitro is made by colonial morphology, Gram stain, and a positive oxidase test. Differentiation from the closely related meningococcus and the various nonpathogenic *Neisseria* is ordinarily by patterns of utilization of various simple carbohydrates; gonococci use glucose but not maltose or sucrose.

Gonococci are highly variable and occur in a number of different colonial forms. Small colonial types are piliated and more virulent in humans than the larger, nonpiliated variants. Variation is also found in certain outer membrane proteins which affect colony opacity. Opaque colonies may attach to certain mucosal surfaces better than transparent colonies, whereas transparent colonies are more likely to invade and cause salpingitis or bacteremia and arthritis. All gonococci and meningococci are able to use transferrin as a source of iron, whereas nonpathogenic *Neisseria* organisms are rarely able to do so. The importance of other surface components of the gonococcus in pathogenesis of infection is under intense investigation. A surface capsule has been reported, but its composition and biologic importance, if any, are unknown.

Gonococci can be serotyped on the basis of antigenic differences in pili, outer membrane proteins, and other antigens. They also can be reliably biotyped by definition of their nutritional requirements on defined agar media ("auxotypes"). These tests are not routinely available at present.

PATHOGENESIS. The minimal infective dose of gonococci for establishment of urethritis in male volunteers is between 100 and 1000 colony-forming units. Surface pili undoubtedly help to attach the bacteria to the mucosal surface, and they also help prevent ingestion and killing by polymorphonuclear leukocytes. Typical urethral infections result in a moderately severe inflammatory response, which is probably due to release of toxic lipopolysaccharide from gonococci, and possibly to production of chemotactic factors which attract neutrophilic leukocytes. Certain strains, particularly those requiring arginine, hypoxanthine, and uracil for growth (Arg^- Hyx^- Ura^- auxotype) are likely to cause asymptomatic urethral infection for reasons not completely understood. These strains are usually penicillin sensitive, resistant to the bactericidal effects of normal human serum, and particularly likely to cause bacteremia and septic arthritis.

In the preantibiotic era, symptoms usually persisted for two to three months before host defenses finally succeeded in eradicating the infection. Host defenses include serum opsonic and bactericidal antibodies, as well as local (mucosal) antibodies of the IgG and IgA classes. All gonococci produce an enzyme, IgA protease, which cleaves the major class of secretory IgA, perhaps accounting in part for persistence of local gonococcal infections.

Serum bactericidal antibodies are undoubtedly important in prevention of bacteremic infection. The best evidence for this has been provided by patients who suffer from homozygous deficiency of one of the complement components C6, C7, or C8. This results in deficiency of serum bactericidal activity but no alteration of serum opsonic activity. Such individuals are particularly prone to recurrent bacteremic gonococcal infection, or to recurrent meningococcal meningitis or meningococcemia.

CLINICAL PATTERNS OF DISEASE. *Gonorrhea in Males.* Gonococcal urethritis in males ("the clap," or "the strain") is characterized by a yellowish purulent urethral discharge and dysuria. The usual incubation period is two to six days. The discharge of gonorrhea is slightly more copious and purulent than in nongonococcal urethritis (NGU). Symptoms are probably produced by 90 per cent of infections, although asymptomatic infections do occur and may persist for many months. Males with asymptomatic infection do not seek treatment, whereas those with symptomatic infection are usually promptly treated and cured. This is the probable explanation for prevalence studies which show that up to 50 per cent of infected males are asymptomatic. Asymptomatic infection in males and females is of great epidemiologic importance, since such carriers may continue to spread infection to new sexual partners for months if they are not properly diagnosed and treated.

Complications of gonococcal urethritis in males are now rare. Urethral stricture was formerly a common complication, but was probably due in part to the use of caustic treatment regimens. Epididymitis and prostatitis, relatively common complications in the past, are seen only occasionally today. The principal complication is disseminated gonococcal infection, which is estimated to affect about 1 per cent of men with gonorrhea. This entity is discussed below.

The differential diagnosis of gonococcal urethritis is discussed in Ch. 301.

Gonococcal infections of the pharynx and rectum are common problems in homosexual males. Most patients with pharyngeal infection are asymptomatic, but occasional patients have exudative pharyngitis with cervical adenopathy. Gonococcal infection of the rectum causes a wide spectrum of symptoms, ranging from asymptomatic carriers to severe proctitis with tenesmus and bloody mucopurulent discharge. Although approximately 40 per cent of females with cervical gonorrhea also have positive rectal cultures, symptoms of proctitis in females are unusual. This has suggested that the trauma of rectal intercourse may contribute to the proctitis observed in males. Sigmoidoscopy may be indicated to exclude ulcerative colitis, Crohn's colitis, rectal lacerations, or other infections such as shigellosis, amebiasis, or syphilis, all of which are common in male homosexuals.

Gonococcal epididymitis is usually unilateral. Both *Chlamydia trachomatis* and the gonococcus are significant causes of epididymitis in men under 35 years, whereas coliform bacteria are the usual cause in older males. The differential diagnosis includes trauma, tumor, and torsion of the testicle, the last of which is suggested by sudden onset and elevation of the testicle. If there is question of testicular torsion, consultation with a urologist is necessary. In epididymitis there is often a urethral exudate, which should be cultured for gonococci and other bacteria. Treatment of gonococcal epididymitis includes scrotal elevation and seven to ten days of appropriate antibiotics, as indicated in Table 302–1.

Gonorrhea in Females. In prevalence studies, approximately one half of women infected with the gonococcus are asymptomatic or have so few symptoms that they do not seek medical care. The most commonly involved site is the endocervix (80 to 90 per cent), followed by the urethra (80 per cent), rectum (40 per cent), and pharynx (10 to 20 per cent). Most pharyngeal, urethral, and rectal infections cause few or no symptoms. Cervical infection may result in vaginal discharge or abnormal menstrual bleeding. Neither of these symptoms is specific for gonococcal infection. Gonococcal urethritis may mimic cystitis caused by enteric bacilli, although standard urine cultures are negative because gonococci do not grow on culture media ordinarily used to diagnose urinary tract infection. Gonorrhea should be suspected in sexually active young women with urethral symptoms. A pelvic examination should be done, and cultures should be taken for the gonococcus from the endocervix and from the urethra if symptoms of urethritis are present. Culture methods are discussed below under Laboratory Diagnosis. The differential diagnosis of cervicitis, vaginitis, and the urethral syndrome is discussed in Ch. 301.

The most important complication of gonorrhea is salpingitis. The less precise term "pelvic inflammatory disease" (PID) is often used synonymously. Although many other organisms can cause a similar syndrome, the gonococcus accounts for about half of the estimated 500,000 annual cases of PID in the United States. About 15 per cent of women with gonococcal cervicitis develop PID, often in close proximity to a menstrual period. Symptoms usually include abdominal pain, and often there is fever. Physical examination usually discloses cervical motion tenderness and bilateral adnexal tenderness; in a small proportion of cases the disease may be unilateral, causing confusion with appendicitis or ectopic pregnancy. There may be signs of generalized peritonitis. Laboratory studies often show an elevation of the white blood cell count and sedimentation rate. The diagnosis of PID is inexact, as shown by laparoscopic examination; many patients with PID will be missed if undue reliance is placed on presence of fever or elevation of white blood cell count or sedimentation rate.

Although PID is uncommon in pregnancy, it may be particularly severe, and pregnant patients with PID should probably be hospitalized. The incidence of gonococcal PID is increased about three-fold in women using an intrauterine device (IUD) for contraception.

A single attack of gonococcal PID seems to increase two-fold the risk of developing another bout of PID with subsequent gonococcal cervicitis. About half of the male sexual partners of women with gonococcal PID are infected, and half of these infections are asymptomatic. Failure to diagnose and treat properly the male partners exposes the patient to the risk of further attacks of PID. After the patient has been effectively treated, it often is wise to refer her and her sexual partners to a public health clinic for follow-up.

The major complication of gonococcal PID is tubal scarring and infertility. The incidence of involuntary infertility is estimated as 15 per cent after one attack of PID and about 50 per cent after three attacks. The incidence of ectopic pregnancy is increased from seven- to ten-fold in women with previous salpingitis, with resultant increased fetal and maternal mortality. Treatment is indicated in Table 302–1.

Gonococci may spread upward to the liver, causing perihepatitis (Fitz-Hugh–Curtis syndrome). Gonococcal perihepatitis causes tenderness and pain in the region of the liver which mimics acute cholecystitis. However, it resolves promptly with appropriate antibiotic therapy. Peritoneoscopy may be indicated rarely for diagnostic purposes; "violin-string" adhesions between the liver capsule and the peritoneum are seen.

Gonorrhea in Children. Infants born to a mother with cervicovaginal gonorrhea may develop gonococcal conjunctivitis, although routine use of prophylactic 1 per cent silver nitrate eye drops (or, in some hospitals, topical erythromycin or tetracycline) has markedly reduced the incidence of this problem. Neonates may also acquire pharyngeal, respiratory, or rectal infection, and may develop gonococcal sepsis. Older children up to one year of age usually acquire conjunctival or vaginal infection by accidental contamination from an adult, whereas from one year to puberty most childhood gonorrhea is the result of purposeful sexual abuse by an adult.

TABLE 302–1. ANTIBIOTIC REGIMENS RECOMMENDED FOR GONOCOCCAL INFECTIONS

Diagnosis	Treatment
Uncomplicated genital infection, men and women	Aqueous procaine penicillin G (APPG), 4.8 million units IM in two divided doses, plus 1.0 gram of probenecid PO *or* Tetracycline, 0.5 gram PO four times daily for seven days *or* Ampicillin, 3.5 grams (or amoxicillin, 3.0 grams), in a single PO dose, plus 1.0 gram of probenecid PO *or* Spectinomycin, 2.0 grams IM
Anorectal infections in men	APPG, 4.8 million units IM, plus 1.0 gram of probenecid PO *or* Spectinomycin, 2.0 grams IM
Pharyngeal infection	APPG, 4.8 million units IM, plus 1.0 gram of probenecid PO *or* Tetracycline, 0.5 gram PO four times daily for seven days
Treatment failure (patients should be recultured and isolates tested for production of β-lactamase)	Spectinomycin, 2.0 grams IM
Penicillinase-producing *N. gonorrhoeae* or infection acquired in Africa or the Far East where PPNG are common	Spectinomycin, 2.0 grams IM *or* Ceftriaxone, 125 mg IM
Gonorrhea in pregnancy	APPG, 4.8 million units IM, plus 1.0 gram of probenecid *or* Spectinomycin, 2.0 grams IM
Salpingitis—outpatient	APPG, 4.8 million units IM, plus 1.0 gram of probenecid, or cefoxitin, 2.0 grams IM, followed by doxycycline, 100 mg PO two times daily for ten days *or* Doxycycline, 100 mg PO two times daily for ten days
Salpingitis—inpatient	Doxycycline, 100 mg IV twice daily plus cefoxitin, 2.0 grams IV four times daily until improved, followed by doxycycline, 100 mg PO twice daily to complete 14 days of therapy; alternative regimens include clindamycin plus an aminoglycoside, cefoxitin, or doxycycline, 100 mg IV twice daily plus metronidazole, 1.0 gram IV twice daily until improved, followed by same drugs, same dose PO to complete 14 days of therapy
Disseminated gonococcal infection	Penicillin G, 10 million units IV daily until improvement, followed by ampicillin, 0.5 gram PO four times daily to complete a minimum of seven days of therapy *or* Ampicillin, 3.5 grams PO, plus 1.0 gram of probenecid, followed by ampicillin, 0.5 gram PO four times daily for seven days *or* Tetracycline, 0.5 gram PO four times daily for seven days

Gonococcal Bacteremia. Approximately 1 per cent of adults with gonorrhea develop the syndrome of gonococcal bacteremia, dermatitis, and arthritis, or disseminated gonococcal infection (DGI). In most series, the majority of patients with DGI are women. The regional incidence of DGI probably varies because of geographic differences in prevalence of the antibiotic-sensitive, serum-bactericidal–resistant strains of *N. gonorrhoeae* which cause this syndrome. The severity of the syndrome is variable, from a slowly evolving mild illness with little or no fever, mild arthralgias, and few skin lesions to a fulminant illness with high fever and prostration. Most episodes of DGI are relatively mild in comparison with meningococcemia.

Many patients with DGI have no local symptoms of gonococcal infection. Initial manifestations are usually migratory asymmetrical polyarthralgias and skin lesions which are often accompanied by fever. Many patients have tenosynovitis, typically involving the flexor tendon sheaths of the wrist or the Achilles tendon (colloquially known as "lover's heels"). Skin lesions are few in number (less than 30 usually), are acral in distribution (fingers, toes, extremities), and may be painful before they are visible. The individual lesions may be papules, pustules, or bullae on an erythematous base; less commonly seen are petechiae or necrotic lesions. The rash is not pathognomonic, but is sufficiently typical that it should strongly suggest DGI when seen in young patients with polyarthralgias. Blood cultures are often positive at this stage, and circulating immune complexes may be present. Gram stain of the skin lesions is positive in only about 5 per cent of patients, but gonococcal antigens can be detected in these lesions in about two thirds of patients by use of immunofluorescent-labeled antigonococcal antibody.

The early stage of gonococcemia may subside spontaneously, or may merge indistinctly after about one week into a second stage of septic arthritis. Skin lesions have usually disappeared by this time, and blood cultures are nearly always negative. Septic arthritis may occur without preceding skin lesions or polyarthralgia. One large joint (elbow, wrist, hip, knee, ankle) is usually involved, although some series report involvement of two joints in a significant minority of patients. On infrequent occasions symmetrical involvement of the fingers may mimic acute rheumatoid arthritis. Physical examination typically discloses a swollen, warm joint with evident intra-articular fluid. Aspiration of the joint often reveals a marked neutrophilic leukocytosis (50,000 to 100,000 leukocytes per cubic millimeter), although early in the development of the septic joint the synovial leukocyte count may be much lower. Cultures of joint fluid are usually positive if the leukocyte count is 80,000 or greater, but are often negative when leukocyte counts are 20,000 or less.

Other complications of gonococcal bacteremia include mild hepatitis, myocarditis, the Fitz-Hugh–Curtis syndrome, meningitis, and endocarditis. In the preantibiotic era gonococcal infection accounted for up to 10 percent of all endocarditis, but it is now rare. Gonococcal endocarditis is often a rapidly progressive infection with severe valvular damage; it should be suspected in patients with a new murmur, severe prostrating illness, severe myocarditis, or evidence of renal failure, or in the presence of stigmata of peripheral embolization.

The differential diagnosis of the gonococcal bacteremia arthritis syndrome includes Reiter's syndrome, rheumatic fever, rheumatoid arthritis, systemic lupus erythematosus, other infectious or postinfectious arthritis, subacute bacterial endocarditis, meningococcemia, and viral hepatitis. In young males,

Reiter's syndrome is the principal consideration. Conjunctivitis is rarely seen in gonococcemia, but is common in Reiter's syndrome. In the absence of typical skin lesions, DGI may not be suspected until culture results are known.

Diagnosis of DGI is secure when gonococci are recovered from the blood, skin lesions, or synovial fluid. The diagnosis of DGI is probably correct in patients in whom the only positive cultures are from local mucosal surfaces, but in whom there are both typical skin lesions and a prompt response to antigonococcal therapy.

LABORATORY DIAGNOSIS. Gram's stain of urethral exudate in symptomatic males has a sensitivity of 90 to 98 per cent and a specificity of 95 to 98 per cent. Accordingly, urethral cultures are not ordinarily indicated in untreated symptomatic males. Since the sensitivity of the Gram stain is only about 60 per cent in asymptomatic male urethral infection, cultures of the anterior urethra or fresh urine sediment are recommended when epidemiologic evidence suggests possible asymptomatic urethral infection. Gram stain of the endocervix is about 50 to 60 per cent sensitive and about 82 to 97 per cent specific in women with positive cervical cultures for *N. gonorrhoeae.* Care must be taken to avoid mistaking normal endocervical flora and neutrophils for gonorrhea; only smears showing several neutrophils with multiple, typical intracellular gram-negative diplococci should be read as presumptively positive for gonorrhea. All women should be cultured for *N. gonorrhoeae,* even if the Gram stain appears positive.

Cultures should be plated immediately if possible onto chocolate agar or chocolate agar containing selective antibiotics (e.g., modified Thayer-Martin medium, MTM). Holding medium such as Amies' or Stuart's transport media may be used if necessary, but viability of gonococci drops after 12 to 24 hours in such media. In infected women, a single endocervical culture on MTM is about 80 to 90 per cent sensitive, as judged by yields obtained with multiple cultures from multiple sites. About 3 to 5 per cent of women will have their only positive culture at the pharyngeal, urethral, or rectal site. The yield from these sites is too low to warrant routine pharyngeal, urethral, or rectal cultures. Urethral cultures are indicated in women with the urethral syndrome. Both cervical and rectal cultures should be obtained as part of the test of cure in women after treatment, since inclusion of the rectal culture increases the diagnostic yield of treatment failures by as much as 50 per cent. Pharyngeal cultures should be obtained from patients with symptomatic pharyngitis, or from persons exposed by fellatio to infected males. Patients with possible disseminated gonococcal infection should have culture samples taken from all possible mucosal sites (pharynx, urethra, cervix, rectum), as well as blood and synovial fluid.

Cultures of the cervix should be taken under direct visualization during speculum examination, using a cotton-tipped swab. Lubricant jellies may be deleterious to gonococci and should be avoided. Cultures of tampons can be used if speculum examination is not possible. Cultures of the anterior urethra of males should be taken with calcium alginate swabs or a sterile wire loop.

Positive cultures from the pharynx or rectum should be carefully evaluated by the microbiology laboratory to avoid confusion between gonococci and meningococci. Meningococci are more common than gonococci in throat cultures. Male homosexuals apparently transmit meningococci sexually, and positive rectal cultures for meningococci are relatively common in this group.

A variety of inexpensive office kits is available for culturing gonococci. These offer the advantages of media with long shelf life. They are approximately equal to standard cultures when their use is limited to urethral or cervical samples; the presently available systems should not be used for pharyngeal or rectal cultures.

A variety of serologic tests for gonorrhea has been developed in the past, and more are being tested currently. No test available in 1984 is sufficiently sensitive and specific to merit use for screening purposes. Patients with complications of gonorrhea usually have detectable serum antibodies against crude or purified gonococcal antigens, but none of the tests is routinely available at present.

TREATMENT. Gonococci frequently have chromosomal mutations which result in relative resistance to penicillin, tetracycline, and other antibiotics. The resistance in these strains is usually low level and can be overcome by appropriate doses of penicillin or tetracycline.

Gonococci which carry a β-lactamase (penicillinase) plasmid recently emerged in the Far East and elsewhere, and have spread to much of the world. Penicillinase-producing gonococci (PPNG) account for about 30 per cent of all gonorrhea in certain cities in the Philippines, but are quite uncommon (less than 0.5 per cent) in the United States. The prevalence of PPNG is only about 1 per cent in northern Europe, but seems to be rising. There are two closely related gonococcal penicillinase plasmids of either 3.2 or 4.4×10^6 daltons; each encodes a typical enteric-type TEM β-lactamase. The gonococcal plasmids are similar to penicillinase plasmids found in *Hemophilus* species. PPNG are resistant to clinically attainable doses of penicillins, but are sensitive to spectinomycin, and to certain cephalosporins (cefuroxime, cefoxitin, ceftriaxone*). PPNG are known to cause DGI and salpingitis.

The antibiotic regimens recommended for gonorrhea in the United States are summarized in Table 302–1. Because gonococcal infections commonly are associated with genital chlamydial infection, most authorities now recommend a seven-day course of a tetracycline for all patients with gonorrhea, either as sole therapy or as follow-up to initial penicillin or ampicillin therapy.

Although the risk of anaphylaxis after penicillin is low (0.05 per cent if there is no history of penicillin allergy), up to 1 per cent of patients treated with 4.8 million units of procaine penicillin develop an acute neurotoxic syndrome caused by inadvertent intravenous administration of procaine, and up to 5 to 15 per cent develop rash caused by penicillin. The procaine penicillin regimen has the advantages of proven efficacy for incubating syphilis, and single-dose administration. The latter is of considerable theoretical advantage because of potential patient noncompliance with multidose oral regimens. The seven-day oral tetracycline regimen has little toxicity, but its principal merit is concomitant treatment of coexistent genital chlamydial or ureaplasmal infections. In men, this clearly results in reduced incidence of postgonococcal urethritis, which is usually due to chlamydial infection. Recent evidence suggests that generalized use of tetracyclines for gonorrhea in women would result in clinically significant benefits owing to simultaneous treatment of coexistent chlamydial infection.

In pharyngeal gonorrhea, the single-dose ampicillin and spectinomycin regimens result in about 50 per cent treatment failures. Consideration should be given to use of a pretreatment pharyngeal culture in patients treated with either of these regimens.

Each of the recommended regimens is highly effective for genital gonorrhea. If patients fail to respond to therapy, they should be cultured so that their isolates can be tested for production of penicillinase, and spectinomycin should be used for retreatment. However, most apparent failures are really reinfections. Some studies show that 15 per cent of patients are reinfected within six weeks of successful therapy. On this basis, many authorities recommend that patients should be recultured six weeks after treatment.

In the absence of an effective vaccine, control of this disease depends on proper diagnosis and treatment of patients' sexual contacts. If patients are given simple instructions, many will bring their contacts to the physician for examination. There are sound epidemiologic reasons for treating contacts immediately.

*Investigational drug.

Local health departments are not utilized sufficiently for help in examination and treatment of contacts.

Treatment of salpingitis (PID) has not been studied adequately. Two studies comparing ten-day oral ampicillin and tetracycline regimens found that they were equally effective in gonococcal and nongonococcal PID. Little is known about the relative merits of various regimens for hospitalized patients. Most authorities recommend removal of intrauterine devices in women with PID. It is crucial to examine and treat all sexual partners of women with gonococcal PID.

Therapy of gonococcal arthritis is ordinarily highly successful with each of the recommended regimens (Table 302–1). Failure to improve in three days suggests that the patient does not have DGI. Septic joints should be aspirated, both to make the initial diagnosis and to remove inflammatory exudate. Open drainage is rarely indicated, except in infection of the hip in childhood. Repeat closed aspiration may be necessary if joint fluid rapidly reaccumulates, but most patients require only one or a few joint aspirations. Antibiotics should not be injected into the joint space. Most patients with DGI should be hospitalized initially, but outpatient therapy may be used occasionally in carefully selected, compliant patients with a definite diagnosis and only mild infection.

Gonococcal conjunctivitis should be treated by immediate saline irrigation and intravenous penicillin G.

PREVENTION. Although vaccines are presently under intense study, an effective gonococcal vaccine is still only a hope. Condoms will prevent most infection, but those who need them most will often not use them. Certain contraceptive foams have antigonococcal activity but are of unproven efficacy clinically. Prophylaxis with a single dose of a tetracycline antibiotic was partially protective in a recent study, but failed in patients exposed to relatively resistant strains and therefore cannot be recommended. Prophylaxis with a five-day course of oral tetracycline has not been studied, but is undoubtedly effective and may be used in selected patients.

Barlow D, Phillips I: Gonorrhoea in women: Diagnostic, clinical, and laboratory aspects. Lancet 1:761, 1978. *A concise description of the clinical and laboratory findings in a large group of women.*

Brinton CC Jr, Wood SW, Brown A, Labik AM, Bryan JR, Lee SW, Polen SE, Tramont EC, Sadoff J, Zollinger W: The development of a neisserial pilus vaccine for gonorrhea and meningococcal meningitis. *In* Robbins JB, Hill JC, Sadoff JC (eds.): Seminars in Infectious Disease. Vol IV: Bacterial Vaccines. New York, Thieme-Stratton Inc., 1982, pp 140–159. *A gonococcal pilus vaccine protected human volunteers against experimental urethral infection. Unfortunately, this vaccine may not work for all strains.*

Brooks GF, Gotschlich EC, Holmes KK, Sawyer WD, Young FE (eds.): Immunobiology of *Neisseria gonorrhoeae.* Washington, D.C., American Society for Microbiology, 1978. *A comprehensive presentation of present research.*

Buchanan TM, Arko RJ: Immunity to gonococcal infection induced by vaccination with isolated outer membranes of *Neisseria gonorrhoeae* in guinea pigs. J Infect Dis 135:879, 1977. *This is one of several papers in the current literature which shows that it is possible to produce partial immunity to gonococcal infection with a vaccine. All studies to date show that the protection is only approximately 1000-fold, and there is little cross-protection against unrelated strains.*

Cunningham FG, Hauth JC, Strong JD, Herbert WNP, Gilstrap LC, Wilson RH, Kappus SS: Evaluation of tetracycline or penicillin and ampicillin for treatment of acute pelvic inflammatory disease. N Engl J Med 296:1380, 1977. *A prospective randomized comparison of outpatient therapy for pelvic inflammatory disease. Either tetracycline or ampicillin given for ten days is effective.*

Dans PE, Judson F: The establishment of a venereal disease clinic. II. An appraisal of current diagnostic methods in uncomplicated urogenital and rectal gonorrhea. J Am Vener Dis Assoc 1:107, 1975. *A critical examination of the utility of various diagnostic methods, including multiple cultures and Gram stains.*

Eisenstein BI, Sox T, Biswas G, Blackman E, Sparling PF: Conjugal transfer of the gonococcal penicillinase plasmid. Science 195:998, 1977. *Gonococci contain a conjugal plasmid which enables them to transfer sexually their penicillinase plasmid with efficiency.*

Handsfield HH, Hodson WA, Holmes KK: Neonatal gonococcal infection. I. Orogastric contamination with *Neisseria gonorrhoeae.* JAMA 225:697, 1973. *Maternal gonococcal infection is frequently associated with complications of delivery, and the neonate may develop systemic infection by gonococci.*

Handsfield HH, Lipman TO, Harnisch JP, Tronca E, Holmes KK: Asymptomatic gonorrhea in men: Diagnosis, natural course, prevalence and significance. N Engl J Med 290:117, 1974. *Asymptomatic infection of the male urethra by gonococci is carefully described, and is shown to be much more common than previously recognized.*

Handsfield HH, Murphy VL: Comparative study of ceftriaxone and spectinomycin for treatment of uncomplicated gonorrhoea in men. Lancet 2:67, 1983. *Among newer antibiotics, ceftriaxone appears most promising for single-dose therapy of penicillin-resistant gonorrhea.*

Handsfield HH, Wiesner PJ, Holmes KK: Treatment of the gonococcal arthritis-dermatitis syndrome. Ann Intern Med 84:661, 1976. *This is probably the best evaluation of the efficacy of various regimens for therapy of disseminated gonococcal infection.*

Kaufman RE, Johnson RE, Jaffe HW, Thornsberry C, Reynolds GH, Wiesner PJ, and The Cooperative Study Group: National gonorrhea therapy monitoring study: Treatment results. N Engl J Med 294:1, 1976. *The results of a large multiclinic evaluation of various regimens for outpatient therapy of gonorrhea.*

Lebedeff DA, Hochman EB: Rectal gonorrhea in men: Diagnosis and treatment. Ann Intern Med 92:463, 1980. *This paper briefly reviews the clinical findings, diagnostic methods, and efficacy of various methods of treatment for gonococcal proctitis in men.*

Luciano AA, Grubin L: Gonorrhea screening: Comparison of three techniques. JAMA 243:680, 1980. *Culture of the first voided urine in asymptomatic males is shown to be a highly reliable method for diagnosis.*

Mulks MH, Plaut AG: IgA protease production as a characteristic distinguishing pathogenic from harmless Neisseriaceae. N Engl J Med 299:973, 1978. *Gonococci and meningococci commonly produce an enzyme which cleaves immunoglobulin A1, and thereby probably increases the ability of the pathogenic* Neisseria *to escape local immune mechanisms.*

Peterson BH, Lee TJ, Snyderman R, Brooks GF: *Neisseria meningitidis* and *Neisseria gonorrhoeae* bacteremia associated with C6, C7, or C8 deficiency. Ann Intern Med 90:917, 1979. *A brief review of the clinical and laboratory findings in patients with homozygous complement deficiency and meningococcal or gonococcal bacteremia.*

Roberts RB (ed.): The Gonococcus. New York, John Wiley & Sons, 1977. *Contains comprehensive reviews of most clinical aspects of gonococcal infection.*

303. LYMPHOGRANULOMA VENEREUM

Lymphogranuloma venereum (LGV) is an acute to chronic sexually transmitted disease caused by strains of *Chlamydia trachomatis.* LGV typically produces transient genital lesions followed by significant regional lymphadenopathy, which may progress to late fibrosis and tissue destruction in untreated cases.

ETIOLOGY. The organisms causing LGV are closely related to the *C. trachomatis* strains which cause trachoma (serotypes A–C) or nongonococcal urethritis (serotypes D–K). By use of a microimmunofluorescent procedure the LGV strains have been grouped into three serotypes (L1, L2, and L3), of which L2 is apparently the most common. On one occasion the related organism *Chlamydia psittaci* caused a similar syndrome. All chlamydiae apparently contain a common group antigen, but recently an LGV-specific protein antigen has been partially characterized. As is the case with all chlamydiae, the LGV strains can be isolated only in tissue culture or in yolk sac culture.

EPIDEMIOLOGY. LGV is more common in tropical and subtropical climates but does occur in relatively low incidence throughout the western world. The true incidence is unknown. Screening of patients in venereal disease clinics with the LGV complement fixation test has sometimes shown 10 per cent with positive serologies; however, this may merely reflect cross-reactions between antibodies directed against the *Chlamydia trachomatis* serotypes D–K (the causes of nongonococcal urethritis and related syndromes) and the LGV serotypes L1, L2, and L3.

The disease is almost always transmitted by sexual contact. The site of primary infection is usually around the genitals but may be anal or oral, depending on the mode of sexual practice.

PATHOGENESIS AND PATHOLOGY. The incubation period is uncertain but has been estimated to be anywhere from a few days to several weeks. In approximately one fourth of patients a small evanescent primary vesicular or ulcerative lesion develops at the site of inoculation, but in the other three fourths of patients no primary lesion is clinically evident. Occasional patients may have symptoms of nonspecific urethritis, presumably owing to intraurethral infection. Approximately two to six weeks after sexual contact most patients develop significant regional lymphadenopathy. Primary infection of the anterior vulva or penis results in inguinal adenopathy, whereas primary infection of the vagina or posterior vulva or rectum results in primary perirectal or pelvic adenopathy. Most patients seen in venereal disease clinics are males with inguinal adenopathy. In about one third of patients the adenopathy is bilateral. Involvement of lymphatic tissue may result in significant lymphedema and, if untreated, may lead to elephantiasis of the external genitalia. Chronic infection of the perirectal tissues may lead to rectal strictures. The histologic appearance of involved tissues is nonspecific with acute and chronic inflammation.

CLINICAL MANIFESTATIONS. The transient primary lesion usually appears as an infiltrated papule or small erosion. It may mimic herpes but is frequently unnoticed or not present. In its earlier stages the adenopathy syndrome is manifested by discrete tender movable nodes. After several days the nodes become matted, with an ovoid firm lobulated swelling with adherent erythematous overlying skin. In about 10 to 20 per cent of patients, nodes are involved above and below the inguinal ligament, and fibrosis may result in the so-called "groove sign" (linear depressions parallel to the inguinal ligament). The nodes may undergo necrosis, and, if not aspirated, spontaneous fistula tracts may develop. Lymphatic obstruction may result in vulvar edema or polypoid masses around the anal orifice. In early stages anal masses may resemble hemorrhoids. There may be fever, chills, and headache, associated with other nonspecific systemic symptoms such as nausea and weight loss. Infrequently, there is generalized rash, polyarthralgia, splenomegaly, generalized lymphadenopathy, or meningismus. Cutaneous manifestations may include erythema nodosum, erythema multiforme, urticaria, or a scarlatiniform eruption.

Late complications are usually limited to strictures or scarring of the rectum. This complication is more common in women, but is now fortunately rare. There is often no preceding adenopathy syndrome. The strictures may be bandlike or may involve extensive areas of the lower large bowel.

DIAGNOSIS. LGV must be considered in patients with enlarged inguinal lymph nodes, draining inguinal fistulas, and rectal strictures. Differential diagnosis includes reactive nodes secondary to distal sites of pyogenic infection on the extremities (which may be small and not noticed unless careful examination is performed), chancroid, granuloma inguinale, syphilis, and a variety of other diseases associated with adenopathy or adenitis. Diagnosis is made by one of two methods: either by direct demonstration of LGV organisms in lesion material or by appropriate serologic tests. Material may be obtained for culture from affected lymph nodes by inserting a needle into the area of fluctuance, being careful to insert the needle through normal skin. The aspirated pus is characteristically extremely viscous. Organisms may sometimes be directly demonstrated in this material by immunofluorescence, although this test is not routinely available. Culture may be performed in yolk sacs or in tissue cell culture. A complement fixation test, using group-specific antigen, is widely available for serologic diagnosis. In the presence of a compatible clinical syndrome a titer of greater than or equal to 1:16 is strongly suggestive of LGV. Serial samples frequently show a four-fold or greater rise in titer in the acute stage of the disease. Most patients with LGV develop peak titers of at least 1:64. Other serologic tests are under development, including indirect immunofluorescence and counterimmunoelectrophoresis; each of these tests uses antigens specific for LGV, but neither is widely available at present. A recently developed direct immunofluorescence test employing monoclonal antibodies against *C. trachomatis* serotypes L1, L2, and L3 offers promise for rapid specific diagnosis, but it is not yet widely available.

Other laboratory tests are of little help. Many patients have a modest elevation in total leukocyte count with predominance of lymphocytes. There may be a reversal of the albumin globulin ratio, and some patients have elevated cryoglobulins or rheumatoid factor.

TREATMENT. Both tetracycline and sulfonamide drugs are effective. Usual therapy for adults is tetracycline, 500 mg four times daily for at least three weeks. When tetracycline is contraindicated as in pregnancy, sulfisoxazole may be given in a dose of 500 mg four times daily for at least three weeks. Tense nodes should be aspirated through normal skin to prevent formation of fistulous tracts. Patients with early stages of the disease respond well to therapy, but those with late complications, including chronic lymphatic obstruction and rectal stricture, respond poorly or not at all to antibiotic therapy. Surgery may be needed to correct rectal stricture. After an initial course of treatment, patients should be seen at least every three months for one year, and the titer of the LGV complement fixation test should be followed. Retreatment should be given if there is a four-fold increase in serologic titer or if there is clinical evidence of relapse. Sexual contacts should be treated similarly.

PREVENTION. There are no specific data regarding modes of prevention. Presumably, use of condoms would help to prevent transmission. An effective vaccine is not available.

Caldwell HD, Kuo CC: Serologic diagnosis of lymphogranuloma venereum by counterimmunoelectrophoresis with a *Chlamydia trachomatis* protein antigen. J Immunol 118:442, 1977. *A specific test for LGV is under development.*

Klotz SA, Drutz DJ, Tam MR, Reed KH: Hemorrhagic proctitis due to lymphogranuloma venereum serogroup L2: Diagnosis by fluorescent monoclonal antibody. N Engl J Med 308:1563, 1983. *LGV may cause hemorrhagic proctitis that mimics ulcerative colitis in homosexual males; monoclonal antibodies provide rapid diagnosis.*

Schachter J: Lymphogranuloma venereum and other nonocular *Chlamydia trachomatis* infections. *In* Hobson D, Holmes KK (eds.): Nongonococcal Urethritis and Related Infections. Washington, D.C., American Society for Microbiology, 1977, pp 91–97. *An excellent short review of the biology of the organism and the clinical manifestations of the disease.*

Sowmini CN, Gopalan KN, Chandrasekhara Rao G: Minocycline in the treatment of lymphogranuloma venereum. J Am Vener Dis Assoc 2:19, 1976. *Tetracyclines were effective in infected military personnel in Vietnam.*

304. GRANULOMA INGUINALE (Donovanosis)

Granuloma inguinale, also known as donovanosis, is a slowly progressive ulcerative disease involving principally the skin and subcutaneous tissues of the genital, inguinal, and anal regions. It is primarily transmitted sexually, but probably can be transmitted by nonsexual contact as well. Multiple sexual contacts with an infected partner seem necessary for transmission of infection. The disease is uncommon in the United States, with less than 100 recorded cases annually. It is quite common, however, in certain other areas of the world, especially Papua New Guinea.

ETIOLOGY. The causative organism is *Calymmatobacterium granulomatis*, a gram-negative bacterium which is immunologically related to certain *Klebsiella* strains. Current evidence suggests that *C. granulomatis* is not a member of the *Klebsiella-Enterobacter-Serratia* family; its exact taxonomic status is uncertain. The organism can be grown in yolk sacs, but only with great difficulty on artificial medium. It is apparently a facultative intracellular parasite, since in infected lesions it is found primarily in histiocytes or other mononuclear cells.

CLINICAL MANIFESTATIONS. The initial lesion usually appears as a subcutaneous nodule which erodes through the surface and develops into a beefy, elevated granulomatous lesion. This usually is painless and unassociated with systemic symptoms. Secondary bacterial infection may cause a necrotic painful ulcerative lesion which may be rapidly destructive. A cicatricial form may also occur with a depigmented elevated area of keloid-like scar containing scattered islands of granulomatous tissue. Lesions in the genital area are commonly associated with pseudobuboes in the inguinal region; these swellings are usually not due to involvement of the inguinal lymph nodes but rather to granulomatous involvement of the subcutaneous tissues. Metastatic infection of bones or other viscera is occasionally seen. Clinical experience suggests that secondary carcinomas may be a complication of granuloma inguinale.

DIFFERENTIAL DIAGNOSIS. The differential diagnosis includes tumor, lymphogranuloma venereum, chancroid, syphilis, and other ulcerative granulomatous diseases. Chancroid is usually differentiated by its irregular undermined borders, which are not seen in the usual cases of granuloma inguinale. Dark-field examination and serologic tests should help to distinguish syphilis. Biopsies may be necessary to distinguish granuloma inguinale from certain tumors.

DIAGNOSIS. Diagnosis is made by demonstrating intracellular "Donovan bodies" in histiocytes or other mononuclear cells from lesion scrapings or biopsies. Wright's stain or Giemsa stain of fresh impression smears or unfixed biopsies will usually demonstrate the bacilli relatively easily, although multiple biopsies may be necessary in chronic cases. Culture is not practical at present. A serologic test has been devised but is not clinically available. Histologic examination of biopsies shows mononuclear cells with some infiltration by polymorphonuclear leukocytes but no giant cells.

TREATMENT. Treatment consists of tetracycline or sulfisoxazole in a dose of 0.5 gram four times daily for at least three weeks. Other regimens which have proved effective include ampicillin, chloramphenicol, gentamicin, or co-trimoxazole. Limited experience suggests that lincomycin may be used successfully. Patients should be followed for at least several weeks after discontinuation of treatment because of the possibility of relapse. Although the risk of communicability appears to be low, sexual contacts should also be examined; at present, treatment of contacts is not indicated in the absence of clinically evident disease.

PREVENTION. No effective prevention is known.

Breschi LC, Goldman G, Shapiro SR: Granuloma inguinale in Vietnam: Successful therapy with ampicillin and lincomycin. J Am Vener Dis Assoc 1:118, 1975. *Ampicillin was frequently effective in patients previously unresponsive to tetracycline.*

Garg BR, Lal S, Sivamani S: Efficacy of co-trimoxazole in donovanosis. A preliminary report. Br J Vener Dis 54:348, 1978. *Trimethoprim and sulfamethoxazole were effective.*

Kuberski T: Granuloma inguinale (donovanosis). Sex Trans Dis 7:29, 1980. *An excellent short review.*

Maddocks I, Anders EM, Dennis E: Donovanosis in Papua New Guinea. Br J Vener Dis 52:190, 1976. *A description of the epidemiology and clinical manifestations in an endemic area of granuloma inguinale.*

305. CHANCROID

Chancroid is a sexually transmitted infection caused by the gram-negative bacillus *Hemophilus ducreyi.*

EPIDEMIOLOGY. On a worldwide basis chancroid is considerably more common than syphilis, and in parts of Africa and in Southeast Asia is nearly as great a problem as gonorrhea. In the United States it is an uncommon disease, but the incidence is rising. Epidemics have been documented in several cities in North America in recent years. About 90 per cent of reported cases occur in males. An outbreak in Greenland was exceptional in that about 40 per cent of cases were noted in women. It is quite likely that there has been significant underdiagnosis in women in the past.

CLINICAL MANIFESTATIONS. The usual incubation period is two to five days, but may be up to 14 days. In the Greenland outbreak the incubation period averaged nearly two weeks in women. The initial clinical manifestation is an inflammatory macule that then becomes a vesicle-pustule and finally a sharply circumscribed, somewhat ragged, and undermined painful ulcer. The base is moist and may be covered with a grayish necrotic exudate. Removal of the exudate reveals purulent granulation tissue. There is usually surrounding cutaneous erythema. Lesions typically are single but may be multiple, possibly owing to autoinoculation of nearby tissues. There are rarely systemic symptoms. Inguinal adenopathy is noted in half of patients, approximately two thirds of whom have unilateral adenopathy. Lesions are usually noted on the shaft or glans of the penis or around the anal orifice in males. In females lesions may occur on the cervix, vagina, vulva, or perianal area. Lesions may occasionally occur primarily on or spread to the abdomen, thigh, breast, fingers, or lips. Intraoral lesions are quite uncommon.

There are reports of a transient genital ulcer, followed by significant inguinal adenopathy. This may be difficult to distinguish from lymphogranuloma venereum. Other uncommon clinical variants include the *phagedenic type* of ulcer with secondary suprainfection and rapid tissue destruction; *giant chancroid,* which is characterized by a very large single ulcer; *serpiginous ulcer,* which is characterized by rapidly spreading indolent shallow ulcers on the groin or the thigh; and a *follicular* type with multiple small ulcers in a perifollicular distribution.

DIFFERENTIAL DIAGNOSIS. The differential diagnosis includes syphilis, herpes genitalis, lymphogranuloma venereum, traumatic ulcers, and granuloma inguinale. Of these the most commonly confused are syphilis and herpes genitalis. Multiple infections are relatively common. Outpatients with suspected chancroid should have a serologic test for syphilis and preferably a dark-field examination as well.

DIAGNOSIS. The diagnosis of chancroid is made on the basis of the clinical appearance of the lesions plus either morphologic demonstration of typical organisms in the lesions or recovery of *H. ducreyi* by culture. Culture is the preferred method. Positive cultures can be obtained in over 80 per cent of cases. Best culture results seem to be obtained with a chocolate agar medium containing 3 μg per milliliter of vancomycin. Necrotic debris should be removed from the ulcer with physiologic saline. The base and edges of the ulcer should be swabbed with a cotton-tipped swab and inoculated directly onto the culture plate if possible; swabs may be put into Amies transport medium if culture plates are not immediately available. Smears obtained from the undermined edges should be gently rolled onto a slide. *H. ducreyi* is a small gram-negative bacillus with rounded ends, which typically forms chains or parallel aggregates in lesions. Typical organisms are seen in 50 to 80 per cent of cases. Organisms may also be obtained by aspiration of inguinal nodes. Nodes should be aspirated by placing the needle through normal skin to avoid formation of fistulous tracts. Nodes should not be incised. There is no serologic test for chancroid.

TREATMENT. The drug of choice is probably erythromycin, in a dose of 500 mg orally four times daily for ten days. Combinations of trimethoprim and sulfamethoxazole (co-trimoxazole) are highly effective. Ampicillin should not be used, since some strains of *H. ducreyi* produce a typical TEM-type β-lactamase and are quite ampicillin resistant. Interestingly, the plasmid containing the gene for production of β-lactamase is very closely related to the penicillinase plasmids found recently in *H. influenzae* and *Neisseria gonorrhoeae.* All regular sexual partners should be examined and epidemiologically treated with a similar regimen.

PREVENTION. No vaccine is available. Use of a condom is presumably helpful. There are no data regarding efficacy of antibiotic prophylaxis.

Hammond GW, Lian CJ, Wilt JC, Ronald AR: Comparison of specimen collection and laboratory techniques for isolation of *Haemophilus ducreyi.* J Clin Microbiol 7:39, 1978. *Use of selective media improves rates of cultural isolation.*

Hammond GW, Slutchuk M, Scatliff J, Sherman E, Wilt JC, Ronald AR: Epidemiologic, clinical, laboratory, and therapeutic features of an urban outbreak of chancroid in North America. Rev Infect Dis 2:867, 1980. *An excellent summary of a recent epidemic in Winnipeg.*

Lykke-Olesen L, Larsen L, Pedersen TG, Gaarslev K: Epidemic of chancroid in Greenland 1977–78. Lancet 1:654, 1979. *A remarkable epidemic, affecting 3 per cent of the adult population. Tropical climates are not necessary to disease transmission or expression.*

Plummer FA, D'Costa LJ, Nsanze H, Maclean IW, Karasira P, Piot P, Fast MV, Ronald AR: Antimicrobial therapy of chancroid: Effectiveness of erythromycin. J Infect Dis 148:726, 1983. *Documents the efficacy of erythromycin.*

306. SYPHILIS

DEFINITION. Syphilis is a subacute to chronic infectious disease caused by the bacterium *Treponema pallidum.* It is usually acquired by sexual contact with another infected individual. Syphilis is remarkable among infectious diseases in its large variety of clinical presentations. It progresses, if untreated, through primary, secondary, and tertiary stages. The early stages (primary and secondary) are infectious. Spontaneous healing of early lesions occurs, followed by a long latent period. In about 30 per cent of untreated patients, late disease of the heart, central nervous system, or other organs ultimately develops. At one time this disease was termed "the great imitator." Although the disease is less common now than previously, it remains a great challenge to the clinician because of its protean manifestations, and is of great interest to biologists as well because of the long and tenuous balance between the host and the invading spirochete.

ETIOLOGY. The etiology of syphilis was discovered in 1905 by Schaudinn and Hoffman when they visualized spirochetal organisms in early infectious lesions. The causative agent of syphilis, *Treponema pallidum,* is closely related to other pathogenic spirochetes, including those causing yaws *(Treponema pertenue)* and pinta *(Treponema carateum). T. pallidum* is also related in a more distant manner to other pathogenic spirochetes, including *Leptospira* (cause of leptospirosis) and *Borrelia* (cause of relapsing fever).

T. pallidum is a thin, helical cell approximately 0.15 μ wide and 6 to 50 μ long. Ordinarily there are approximately 6 to 14 spirals. The organism is tapered on either end. It is too thin to be seen by ordinary Gram stain but can be visualized in wet mounts by dark-field microscopy (see below), or by silver stains or fluorescent antibody methods.

The organism bears considerable structural resemblance to gram-negative bacteria. A superficial hyaluronic acid slime layer is formed around the organism, and may contribute to virulence. Beneath the slime layer is the outer membrane, or outer envelope, which is structurally similar to the outer membrane of gram-negative bacteria. Between the outer membrane and the peptidoglycan cell wall are six axial fibrils. The axial fibrils are attached three at each end and overlap in the center of the organism. They are structurally and biochemically similar to flagellae, and may be in part responsible for the motility of the organism.

It has not been possible to culture *T. pallidum* in vitro. Motility is prolonged under microaerophilic to anaerobic conditions. *T. pallidum* was formerly considered a strict anaerobe, but recent evidence shows that it is a microaerophilic to aerophilic organism. It can be maintained by serial passage in rabbits without loss of virulence. Only a few strains of *T. pallidum* have been isolated in rabbits and carefully studied, and little evidence is available regarding the genetic diversity of the organism. All studied isolates have been susceptible to penicillin and are similar antigenically. Immunity to the homologous strain develops after prolonged infection in rabbits. The only known natural hosts for *T. pallidum* are man and certain monkeys and higher apes.

HISTORY. A great epidemic of syphilis occurred throughout Europe in the late fifteenth century. Because of the severity of the infection it was termed the "great pox" in contrast to another prevalent infection, smallpox. The pandemic started soon after Columbus returned from the West Indies, and one school holds that the disease was imported into a nonimmune population by the returning sailors. However, there is evidence in the Old Testament and also in ancient Chinese writings of similar diseases, and there are other reasons for disbelieving the Columbian origin of syphilis. It seems more likely that syphilis was endemic in Europe, but rose to particular prominence in the late fifteenth century because of wartime conditions.

The disease was recognized to be sexually transmitted in the early sixteenth century. Its name is derived from the sixteenth century poem by Fracastorius about the mythical shepherd, Syphilis, who was afflicted with the disease. The major cardiovascular and neurologic complications were recognized in the eighteenth and nineteenth centuries. Many great figures of Western civilization had syphilis of the central nervous system, with untold effects on the course of history. The disease was confused with gonorrhea for some time. A clear distinction between syphilis and gonorrhea was finally made by Ricord in the mid 1800's.

Syphilis was treated for centuries with various heavy metal preparations. Until 1910, inunctions of mercury were the mainstay of therapy, which was apparently moderately effective, although extremely toxic. In 1910, Ehrlich introduced arsphenamine, the "magic bullet." This and subsequent arsenical compounds were more effective and less toxic than mercurial compounds and were revolutionary at the time. They had to be administered for periods of up to two years to be effective. Bismuth salts also were effective and were frequently used in combination with arsenicals between World War I and World War II. The final revolution occurred in 1943, when penicillin was introduced for therapy of syphilis. It was so effective and exhibited so little toxicity that many thought that this ancient disease would soon be eradicated. Although syphilis did decline rapidly in incidence after World War II, it has proved to be a resilient foe and continues to be a significant problem.

PATHOGENESIS AND HOST RESPONSE. *T. pallidum* may penetrate through normal mucosal membranes and also may penetrate through minor abrasions of epithelial surfaces. In experimental rabbit syphilis, spirochetes can be found in the lymphatic system within 30 minutes of inoculation and are found in blood shortly thereafter. There have been occasional instances in man of transfusion syphilis resulting from use of blood from a donor who was in the incubation stage of his disease. Therefore it seems clear that syphilis is a systemic disease from the onset in man as well. However, the first lesions appear at the site of primary inoculation, presumably because of the large numbers of treponemes implanted at this site. In laboratory animals, there is an inverse relationship between numbers of treponemes inoculated and time required for development of the primary cutaneous lesion. The minimal number of treponemes required to establish infection is not known, but may be as low as one treponeme. Multiplication of organisms is very slow, with a division time in rabbits of approximately 33 hours. Similarly slow growth of treponemes in man probably accounts in part for the protracted nature of the illness, and for the relatively long incubation period.

T. pallidum is not known to produce any toxins. Although the outer membrane structurally resembles those of gram-negative bacteria, there is no biologically active endotoxin in *T. pallidum.* Treponemes are capable of specific attachment to host cells, but it is not known whether attachment results in damage to host cells. Most treponemes are found in intercellular spaces, but occasional treponemes can be seen within phagocytic cells. However, there is no evidence for intracellular survival of treponemes.

The primary pathologic lesion of syphilis is a focal endarteritis. There is an increase in adventitial cells, endothelial proliferation, and presence of an inflammatory cuff around affected vessels. Lymphocytes, plasma cells, and monocytes predominate in the inflammatory lesion, and in some cases polymorphonuclear cells are seen as well. The vessel lumen is frequently obliterated. With healing there is considerable fibrosis. Treponemes may be seen in most early lesions of syphilis, and in some of the late lesions such as the meningoencephalitis of general paresis.

Granulomatous reaction is also frequent in secondary syphilis and in late syphilis. The granuloma is histologically nonspecific, and cases of syphilis have been incorrectly diagnosed as sarcoidosis or other granulomatous diseases. Human inoculation studies suggest that the pathogenesis of the gumma, which is a granulomatous lesion, involves hypersensitivity to small numbers of virulent treponemes introduced into a previously sensitized host.

Intracutaneous inoculation of patients with syphilis in various stages with partially purified antigens of *T. pallidum* showed that delayed cellular hypersensitivity developed only in late secondary syphilis but was uniformly present in latent syphilis. There may be temporary hyporesponsiveness of lymphocytes from patients with primary and secondary syphilis to treponemal antigens. It is possible but not yet proved that the unusual waxing and waning of lesions in early syphilis depend on the balance between development of effective cellular immunity and suppression of thymus-derived lymphocyte function.

The host also responds to infection with production of numerous antibodies, and in some instances circulating immune complexes may be formed. The nephrotic syndrome has been recognized occasionally in secondary syphilis, and renal biopsies from such cases have shown membranous glomerulonephritis characterized by focal subepithelial basement membrane deposits. The deposits contain both IgG and C3, and treponemal antibody.

Rarely patients may develop paroxysmal cold hemoglobinuria. This is due to production of an IgG antibody that binds to the red cell at 4° C and, upon rewarming of the blood in the presence of complement, results in hemolysis. Thus patients may develop massive hemolysis and hemoglobinuria after cold exposure. This was formerly usually due to congenital syphilis but is now almost always due to other infections. Treatment with penicillin usually stops the attacks.

Antibodies useful in diagnosis are discussed under Serologic Tests, below.

EPIDEMIOLOGY. Syphilis, with the exception of congenital syphilis, is acquired almost exclusively by intimate contact with the infectious lesions of primary or secondary syphilis (chancre, mucous patches, condylomata lata). This is usually through sexual intercourse, including anogenital and orogenital intercourse. Health workers have sometimes been infected during unsuspecting examination of patients with infectious lesions. Infection by contact with fomites is extremely uncommon.

Syphilis is most common in large cities, and in young sexually active individuals. The highest rate in both men and women occurs at ages 20 to 24, followed by ages 25 to 29 and 15 to 19 years. Among predominantly rural areas in the United States the disease is most prevalent in the southeast.

Syphilis spares no class, race, or group, but is more prevalent in the United States among the poorly educated and economically deprived than among more prosperous groups. Increased numbers of different sexual partners and perhaps indiscriminate choice of partner increase the risk of acquiring sexually transmitted disease. Patients with primary and secondary syphilis name on the average nearly three different sexual contacts within the previous 90 days. A cornerstone of syphilis control is epidemiologic investigation of sexual contacts of patients with primary or secondary lesions, and of patients with early latent disease.

In recent years male homosexuals have apparently accounted for an increasing proportion of the total cases of infectious syphilis. The ratio of male:female cases of primary and secondary syphilis in the United States rose from 1.6:1.0 in 1965 to 2.5:1.0 in 1975, and is now about 3:1. In many large cities over 50 per cent of all infectious syphilis occurs in male homosexuals. Currently, more than half of all white males with infectious syphilis name at least one male sexual partner during the recent past. In contrast only 2 per cent of primary and secondary syphilis in females occurs in women who name a female sexual contact. Similar trends have been noted in other countries.

Another important method of case detection is routine serologic testing. Of the approximately 38 million blood specimens examined annually in the United States, approximately 1 million are reactive. Approximately 35 per cent of primary and secondary syphilis and 75 per cent of early latent syphilis are detected annually by either serologic screening or contact treating.

The annual incidence of syphilis has generally declined worldwide for approximately 100 years with the exception of periods of extensive war. Reported cases of infectious primary and secondary syphilis in the United States peaked in 1947 at approximately 73 cases per 100,000 population. With introduction of penicillin there was a rapid decline in primary and secondary syphilis after World War II, to annual rates of approximately 4 cases per 100,000 in 1957. This resulted in declining federal expenditure for syphilis control, however, and there was a subsequent resurgence in infectious primary and secondary syphilis in the United States, reaching peaks of over 12 cases per 100,000 several times in the period 1965–1983. Total reported cases of primary and secondary syphilis in 1983 were 33,613. Since many cases of syphilis are not reported, the true incidence is much higher, perhaps 75,000 to 100,000 annually.

Reported deaths from syphilis declined from 2434 in 1965 to 200 in 1976. Infant deaths from syphilis and first admissions for syphilitic psychoses have fallen by 98 to 99 per cent since 1940. Patients with clinically manifest late syphilis, particularly gummas, are becoming less common, perhaps as a result of the effectiveness of penicillin therapy for early syphilis. However, surveys indicate that there still are significant numbers of patients with untreated cardiovascular and neurologic syphilis, especially among older age groups. There is suggestive evidence that neurosyphilis may be presenting with atypical clinical manifestations and therefore may not be easily recognized.

NATURAL COURSE OF UNTREATED SYPHILIS. The incubation period from time of exposure to development of the primary lesion at the place of initial inoculation of treponemes averages approximately 21 days, but ranges from 10 to 90 days. A painless papule develops, and gradually breaks down to form a clean-based ulcer with raised indurated margins. This persists for two to six weeks and then heals spontaneously. Several weeks later the patient characteristically develops a secondary stage characterized by low grade fever, headache, malaise, generalized lymphadenopathy, and a mucocutaneous rash. There may be involvement of visceral organs. The secondary eruption may occur while the primary chancre is still healing or several months after the disappearance of the chancre. The secondary lesions heal spontaneously within two to six weeks, and the infection then enters latency. Some patients may later develop relapsing lesions similar to those of the secondary stage; rarely the relapse will take the form of recurrence of the primary chancre. About one third of untreated patients eventually develop late destructive tertiary lesions involving one or more of the eyes, central nervous system, heart, or other organs, including skin. These may occur at any time from a few years to as late as 25 years following infection.

The course of untreated syphilis has been extensively studied in two large groups of patients. In the Oslo Study (1891–1951), over 2000 untreated patients diagnosed clinically (without serologic tests or lumbar punctures) were followed for the ultimate course of the disease. None of these patients received treatment with arsenicals or other compounds. A smaller prospective study was also done in the United States among black American males in rural Alabama (the Tuskegee Study, 1932–1972). This study, which was initiated in the arsenical era because of uncertainty that the beneficial effects of treatment outweighed the toxicity of prolonged exposure to arsenical compounds, extended into the penicillin era. It has been subjected to much criticism because curative penicillin therapy was not given when it became available in the mid 1940's, although antimicrobial drugs given for other purposes may have influenced the course of the disease in some patients.

In the Oslo Study, relapsing secondary lesions developed in the first four years after infection in nearly 25 per cent of patients. Twenty-eight per cent eventually developed tertiary syphilis. The most common late lesions were benign tertiary gummas of the skin, mucous membranes, and skeleton. Cardiovascular syphilis was diagnosed in slightly over 10 per cent and symptomatic neurosyphilis in 6.5 per cent of patients. Syphilis was the primary cause of death in 50 per cent of males and 8 per cent of females. Pregnancy had a beneficial effect on the disease. Among autopsied patients cardiovascular syphilis was proved in 35 per cent of men and 22 per cent of women. Serious late complications were more common in men than in women.

The Tuskegee Study showed that among men age 25 to 50 years, death rates were 75 per cent greater in syphilitics than in appropriately matched noninfected control subjects. Cardiovascular or central nervous system syphilis was the primary cause of death in 30 per cent of syphilitic men. Among autopsied patients aortitis was found in about 50 per cent of syphilitics with a persistently positive serologic test. Central nervous system syphilis was found in only 4 per cent. There was no definite anatomic basis for some of the excess mortality among syphilitics noted in the Tuskegee Study. Thus the incidence of cardiovascular syphilis was higher but the incidence of neurologic syphilis was lower in the Tuskegee Study than in the Oslo Study. On the basis of these data, plus other uncontrolled clinical observations, it has been suggested that black patients are particularly prone to development of cardiovascular syphilis, and white patients to central nervous system syphilis, but the evidence is not definitive. The reasons for the possible racial differences are unknown.

The incidence of late complications of untreated syphilis is presently unknown, but seems less than noted previously. Cases of gumma are presently so rare as to be reportable.

CLINICAL MANIFESTATIONS. ***Primary Syphilis.*** The typical lesion of primary syphilis is the chancre, a painless, clean-based, indurated ulcer. The chancre starts as a papule, but then superficial erosion occurs, resulting in the typical ulcer. The borders of the ulcer are raised, firm, and indurated. Occasionally, secondary infections change the appearance, resulting in a painful lesion. Most chancres are single, but multiple ulcers are sometimes seen, particularly when skin folds are opposed ("kissing chancres"). The untreated chancre heals in several weeks, leaving a faint scar. The chancre is usually associated with regional adenopathy, which may be either unilateral or bilateral. The regional nodes are movable, discrete, and rubbery. If the chancre occurs in the cervix or in the rectum, the affected regional iliac nodes are not palpable. See Figure 306–1.

It was formerly taught that 90 per cent of chancres occurred in the genital region. Presently a much higher proportion of nongenital chancres is observed, particularly among male homosexuals, in whom chancres in or near the rectum are common. Rectal chancres may have an atypical appearance mimicking rectal fissures or other more benign lesions, and are frequently overlooked. Conversely, they have also been mistaken for malignant disease. In general it is reasonable to assume that any ulcer occurring in the genital area or, in male homosexuals, around the rectum is syphilitic until proved otherwise. Chancres may also be seen in the pharynx, on the tongue, around the lips, on the fingers, on the nipples, or in diverse other areas. The morphology depends in part on the area of the body in which they occur and also on the host immune response. Chancres in previously infected individuals may be small and may remain papular. Chancres of the finger may appear more erosive and may be quite painful.

The *differential diagnosis* of a genital ulcer should include lesions caused by herpesvirus hominis type II. Herpetic ulcers can usually be distinguished because they are multiple, superficial, and, if seen early, vesicular. They are often painful. Herpetic ulcers, unlike syphilitic ulcers, may have a positive Tzanck test—multinucleated giant cells in the base of the ulcer. The ulcers of chancroid are usually painful, often multiple, and frequently exudative and nonindurated. Lymphogranuloma venereum may produce a small papular lesion associated with a regional adenopathy. Other conditions which must be distinguished include granuloma inguinale, drug eruptions, carcinoma, superficial fungal infections, traumatic lesions, and lichen planus. Final distinction in most cases is made on the basis of dark-field examination, which is positive only in syphilis.

Secondary Syphilis. Approximately four to eight weeks following the appearance of the primary chancre, patients typically develop lesions of secondary syphilis. They may complain of *malaise, fever, headache, sore throat,* and other systemic symptoms. Most patients have generalized lymphadenopathy, including the epitrochlear nodes. Approximately 30 per cent of patients will have evidence of the healing chancre, although

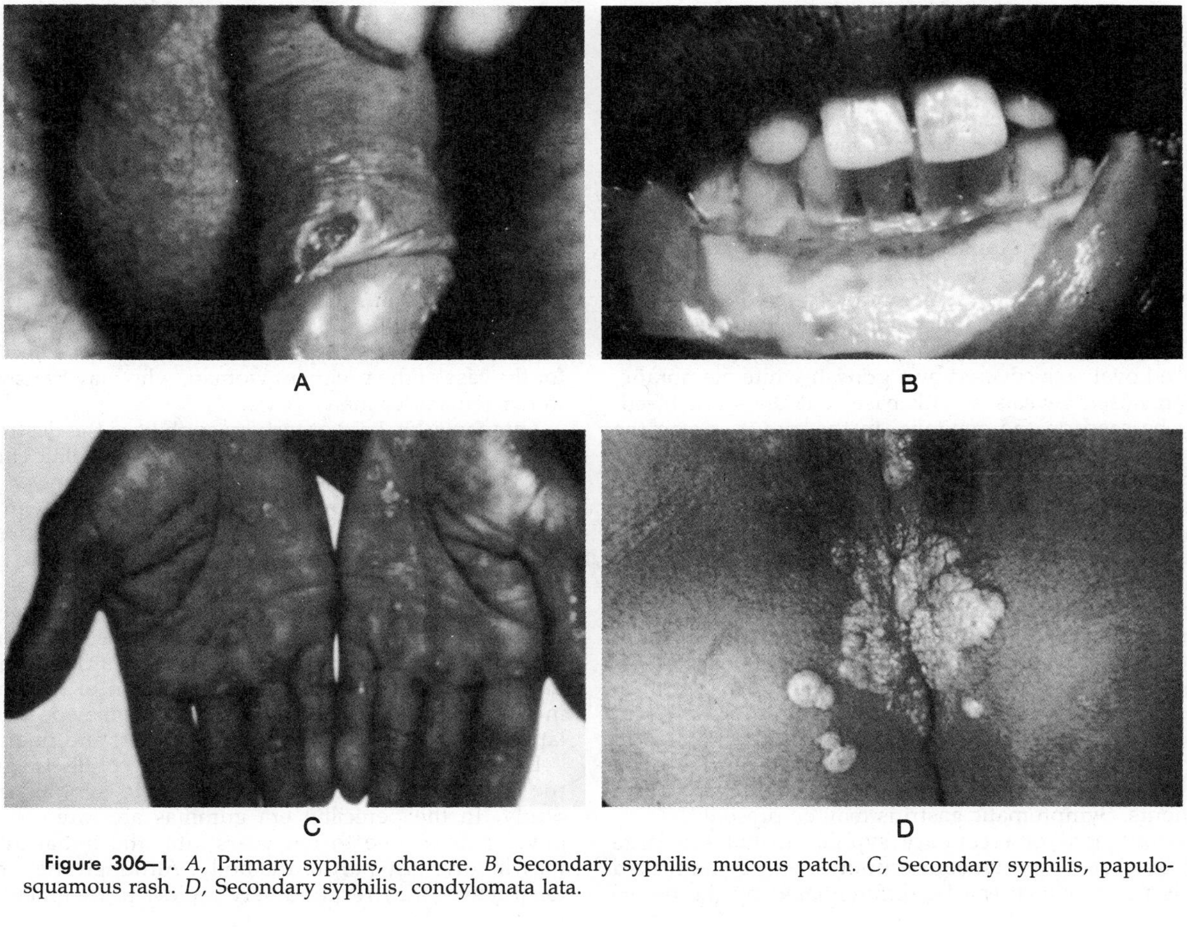

Figure 306–1. *A,* Primary syphilis, chancre. *B,* Secondary syphilis, mucous patch. *C,* Secondary syphilis, papulosquamous rash. *D,* Secondary syphilis, condylomata lata.

many patients, including male homosexuals and women, give no history of a primary lesion.

At least 80 per cent of patients with secondary syphilis have cutaneous lesions or lesions of the mucocutaneous junctions at some point in their illness. The diagnosis is usually first suspected on the basis of the cutaneous eruption. The rash is often minimally symptomatic, however, and many patients with late syphilis do not recall either primary or secondary lesions. The rashes are quite varied in their appearance, but have certain characteristic features. The lesions are usually widespread and are symmetrical in distribution. They often are pink, coppery, or dusky red, particularly the earliest macular lesions. They usually are nonpruritic, although occasional exceptions have been noted, and are almost never vesicular or bullous in adults. They are indurated except for the very earliest macular lesions and frequently have a superficial scale (papulosquamous lesions). They tend to be polymorphic and rounded, and on healing they may leave residual pigmentation or depigmentation. The lesions may be quite faint and difficult to visualize, particularly on dark-skinned individuals.

The earliest pink macular lesions are frequently seen on the margins of the ribs or the sides of the trunk with later spread to the rest of the body. The face is often spared except around the mouth. Subsequently a papular rash appears which is usually generalized but is *quite marked on the palms and soles.* These frequently are associated with a superficial scale and may be hyperpigmented. When the rash occurs on the face, it may be pustular, resembling acne vulgaris. On occasion the scale may be so great as to resemble psoriasis. Deep nodular lesions may cause confusion. Ulceration may occur, producing lesions resembling ecthyma. In malnourished or debilitated patients extensive destructive ulcerative lesions with a heaped-up crust may occur, the so-called rupial lesion. Lesions around the hair follicles may result in a patchy alopecia of the beard or of the scalp.

Ringed or annular lesions may occur, especially around the face, particularly on black individuals. Lesions at the angle of the mouth or the corner of the nose may have a central linear erosion (the so-called "split papule").

In warm, moist areas such as the perineum, large pale flat-topped papules may coalesce to form condylomata lata. These may also be seen in the axilla and rarely in a generalized form. They are extremely infectious. They are not to be confused with the common venereal warts (condylomata acuminata), which are small, often multiple, and more sharply raised than condylomata lata.

Other lesions of the mucous membranes are common. The palate and pharynx may be inflamed. Approximately 30 per cent of patients develop the so-called mucous patch. This is a slightly raised oval area covered by a grayish-white membrane, which when raised reveals a pink base that does not bleed. These may be seen on the genitalia, in the mouth, or on the tongue, and, like condylomata lata, are highly infectious.

Other manifestations of secondary syphilis include hepatitis, which has been reported in up to 10 per cent of patients in some series. Jaundice is rare, but an elevated alkaline phosphatase is common. Liver biopsy reveals small areas of focal necrosis and mononuclear infiltrate or periportal vasculitis. Spirochetes can often be visualized with silver stains. Periostitis with widespread lytic lesions of bone has been reported occasionally; use of bone scans appears to be a sensitive test for early syphilitic osteitis. An immune complex type of nephropathy with transient nephrotic syndrome has been rarely documented. There may be iritis or an anterior uveitis. From 10 to 30 per cent of patients have pleocytosis in the cerebrospinal fluid, but symptomatic meningitis is seen in less than 1 per cent of patients. Symptomatic gastritis may be present.

Differential diagnosis of secondary syphilis includes a large number of diseases. The cutaneous eruptions may be mimicked by pityriasis rosea, which can be differentiated by the occurrence of lesions along lines of skin cleavage and frequently by the presence of a herald patch in pityriasis rosea. Drug eruptions, acute febrile exanthems, psoriasis, lichen planus, scabies, and other diseases must also be considered in some cases. The mucous patch may superficially resemble oral candidiasis (thrush). Infectious mononucleosis may appear very similar to secondary syphilis, with sore throat, generalized adenopathy, hepatitis, and a generalized rash. Infectious hepatitis may also cause confusion. A high index of suspicion is required to make the diagnosis of syphilis in some cases. Unfortunately even classic cases with widespread, hyperpigmented, papulosquamous lesions involving the palms and the soles are not infrequently misdiagnosed in the current era. Fortunately, if the serologic tests for syphilis are obtained, they will be found to be positive in 99 per cent of patients. The condylomata lata and mucous patches contain large numbers of treponemes as seen on dark-field examination. Aspiration of lymph nodes may occasionally reveal motile *T. pallidum.*

Relapsing Syphilis. Condylomata lata are likely to recur. The skin manifestations tend to be unilateral, the eruptions more dense, marked, with fewer lesions, and sometimes solitary. They are also more infiltrated and of somewhat longer standing, and have some characteristics that resemble the skin lesions in late syphilis. This reflects the increasing immunity with the duration of the early disease. Neurorecurrences, as well as ophthalmic and other relapsing manifestations, may occur. If the patient has been inadequately treated, relapses may be delayed.

Latent Syphilis. By definition latent syphilis is that stage in which there are no clinical signs of syphilis and the cerebrospinal fluid is normal. Latency begins with the passing of the first attack of secondary syphilis and may last for a lifetime thereafter. It is usually detected by positive specific treponemal antibody tests for syphilis. The test must be shown to be reactive on more than one occasion to rule out technical errors. Diseases known to cause occasional false-positive treponemal reactions for syphilis, such as systemic lupus erythematosus, must be excluded. In addition, congenital syphilis must be excluded before the diagnosis of latent syphilis can be made. Patients may or may not have a history of earlier primary or secondary syphilis, although such history is obviously helpful in making a firm diagnosis of latent syphilis.

Latency has been divided into two stages: *early* and *late latency.* Early latency is ordinarily considered infection of less than four years' duration, based upon evidence in the Oslo Study that mucocutaneous relapse could occur at any time during the first four years. However, more recent evidence suggests that most relapses occur in the first year, and epidemiologic evidence shows that the most infectious spread of syphilis occurs during the first year of infection. *Therefore early latency in the United States is now defined as the first year after infection.* Late latent syphilis is ordinarily not infectious except for the case of the pregnant woman, who may transmit infection to her fetus after many years.

Late Syphilis. Late or tertiary syphilis is the destructive stage of the disease and can be crippling. Late syphilitic complications are still important medical problems, but newly recognized cases of late syphilis have been declining steadily in the United States since World War II. Although the incidence of late syphilis is unknown, the prevalence of various types of late syphilis has been approximated (Table 306–1).

Late syphilis is usually very slowly progressive, although certain neurologic syndromes may have sudden onset owing to endarteritis and thrombosis in the central nervous system. Late syphilis is noninfectious. Any organ of the body may be involved, but three main types of disease may be distinguished: late benign (gummatous), cardiovascular, and neurosyphilis.

LATE BENIGN SYPHILIS. Late benign syphilis or gumma was the most common complication of late syphilis in the Oslo Study. In the penicillin era gummas are rare. They typically develop from one to ten years after the initial infection and may involve any part of the body. Although they may be very destructive, they respond very rapidly to treatment and there-

TABLE 306–1. NEWLY DIAGNOSED TERTIARY SYPHILIS IN 105 PATIENTS IN DENMARK, 1961–1970

Type of Tertiary Syphilis	Number Observed*
Neurosyphilis	72
Asymptomatic	45
Tabes dorsalis	11
General paralysis	13
Meningovascular	1
Optic atrophy	2
Cardiovascular syphilis	44
Aortic insufficiency	16
Aortic aneurysm	13
Uncomplicated aortitis†	15
Late benign syphilis (gumma)	4

*Some patients had more than one form of late syphilis.
†Autopsy diagnoses only.

fore are relatively benign. Histologically the gumma is a granuloma. The histology is nonspecific and may be associated with central necrosis surrounded by epithelioid and fibroblastic cells and occasionally giant cells. There is sometimes vasculitis. *T. pallidum* is ordinarily not demonstrable by silver stains but can sometimes be recovered by inoculation of rabbits.

Gummas may be solitary or multiple. They are usually asymmetrical, and are often grouped. They may start as a superficial nodule or as a deeper lesion which breaks down to form punched-out ulcers. They are ordinarily indolent and slowly progressive with curving or polycyclic borders. They are indurated on palpation. There often is central healing with an atrophic scar surrounded by hyperpigmented borders. Cutaneous gummas may resemble other chronic granulomatous ulcerative lesions caused by tuberculosis, sarcoidosis, leprosy, and other deep fungal infections. Precise histologic diagnosis may not be possible. However, the syphilitic gumma is the only such lesion to heal dramatically with penicillin therapy. Another form of gumma is papulosquamous, and may mimic psoriasis.

Gummas may also involve deep visceral organs, of which the most common are the respiratory tract, the gastrointestinal tract, and bones. In earlier centuries gummas of the nose and palate commonly resulted in septal perforations and disfiguring facial lesions. Gummas may also involve the larynx or the pulmonary parenchyma. Gumma of the stomach may masquerade as carcinoma of the stomach or lymphoma. Gummas of the liver were once the most common form of visceral syphilis, presenting often with hepatosplenomegaly and anemia, occasionally with fever and jaundice. Skeletal gummas typically produce lesions in the long bones, skull, and clavicle. A characteristic symptom is nocturnal pain. Radiologic abnormalities when present include periostitis and either lytic or sclerotic destructive osteitis.

CARDIOVASCULAR SYPHILIS. The primary cardiovascular complications of syphilis are aortic insufficiency and aortic aneurysm, usually of the ascending aorta. Less commonly other large arteries may be involved, and rarely involvement of the coronary ostia results in coronary insufficiency. These complications in all cases are due to obliterative endarteritis of the vasa vasorum with resultant damage to the intima and media of the great vessels. This results in dilatation of the ascending aorta and eventually in stretching of the ring of the aortic valve, producing aortic insufficiency. The valve cusps remain normal. Death may eventually result from congestive heart failure. There has been some success with placing prosthetic heart valves in patients with syphilitic aortic insufficiency. Aneurysms occasionally present as a pulsating mass bulging through the anterior chest wall. Syphilitic aortitis may involve the descending aorta, but this is almost always proximal to the renal arteries, unlike atherosclerotic aneurysms, which typically involve the descending aorta below the renal arteries.

The disease usually begins within five to ten years after initial infection but may not become clinically manifest until 20 to 30 years after infection. Cardiovascular syphilis is thought to be more common in men than in women and possibly in blacks than in whites. The effects of genetic and nutritional factors on development of this and other complications of late syphilis are unclear. Cardiovascular syphilis does not occur after congenital infection—a phenomenon that remains unexplained.

Asymptomatic aortitis is best diagnosed by visualizing linear calcifications in the wall of the ascending aorta by x-ray. The signs of syphilitic aortic insufficiency are the same as for aortic insufficiency of other causes. In aortic insufficiency resulting from dilatation of the aortic ring, the decrescendo murmur is often loudest along the *right* sternal margin. Syphilitic aneurysms may be fusiform but are more typically saccular, and do not lead to aortic dissection. Approximately 10 to 25 per cent of patients with cardiovascular syphilis have coexistent neurosyphilis, and it is therefore mandatory to do a lumbar puncture in all patients with cardiovascular syphilis.

At present, syphilis is a relatively more common cause of aortic insufficiency among the elderly than among younger patients; this is due to the progressively decreasing incidence of new cases of late cardiovascular syphilis.

NEUROSYPHILIS. Neurosyphilis may be divided into four groups: asymptomatic, meningovascular, tabes dorsalis, and general paresis. Division is not absolute and there may be considerable overlap between syndromes. Current cases of neurosyphilis are more likely than heretofore to be variants of the classic syndromes, possibly as a result of use of antimicrobials for other diseases.

Asymptomatic Neurosyphilis. Asymptomatic neurosyphilis is diagnosed when there is a positive VDRL* in the cerebrospinal fluid (CSF) in the absence of signs and symptoms of neurologic disease. False-positive VDRL test results are very rare in CSF in the absence of a traumatic tap. The CSF usually shows an increased total protein and a lymphocytic pleocytosis, but these findings may be absent. If the CSF is normal two or more years after the initial infection, the patient is not likely to develop a positive CSF later. Athough up to 30 per cent of patients with untreated secondary syphilis have an abnormal CSF, penicillin therapy prevents progression to late symptomatic neurosyphilis. Because of this, routine lumbar punctures for examination of CSF are not indicated in early syphilis. Unfortunately, it has become common practice to avoid lumbar punctures in later stages of syphilis as well. Instead, patients are treated with doses of penicillin thought to be effective for neurosyphilis, if present. As a result, there are few data on the present frequency and course of asymptomatic neurosyphilis.

Some laboratories perform an FTA-ABS* test on spinal fluid. Interest in tests such as this has been prompted by good evidence that patients with untreated neurosyphilis may have a negative CSF-VDRL. There are published reports of positive FTA-ABS test results in the CSF of patients with otherwise normal spinal fluid, in whom there were clinical signs and symptoms compatible with neurosyphilis. However, the CSF FTA-ABS test has not been standardized, and there is some evidence that positive CSF test results are caused by passive transfer of serum antibody into spinal fluid. At present no diagnosis of asymptomatic (or symptomatic) neurosyphilis should be based solely on the CSF FTA-ABS* test.

Meningovascular Syphilis. An acute to subacute aseptic meningitis may occur at any time after the primary stage but usually within the first year of infection. It frequently involves the base of the brain and may result in unilateral or bilateral cranial nerve palsies. In about 10 per cent of cases, the onset of meningitis coincides with the rash of secondary syphilis. The spinal fluid shows a lymphocytic pleocytosis with increased protein and usually normal glucose concentration. The CSF-VDRL is nearly always positive. Rarely CSF glucose concentration is decreased. This syndrome can mimic tuberculous or fungal meningitis or nonpurulent meningitis of various causes.

*See Serologic Tests, below. Also refer to Table 306–2.

In other patients, the meningeal involvement may be less prominent but there is sufficient endarteritis and perivascular inflammation to result in cerebrovascular thrombosis and infarction, with signs and symptoms typical of those of cerebrovascular accidents of any cause. This usually occurs five to ten years after the initial infection and is more common in males. There often is an associated aseptic meningitis as well. Most cerebrovascular accidents are not due to syphilitic arteritis even in patients with a positive serologic test for syphilis. However, syphilis should be considered as the cause in young patients with a history of syphilis and without other causes for cerebrovascular accidents.

A variety of other meningeal syndromes may rarely be seen, including transverse myelitis and radiculitis. A rare syndrome of meningomyelitis may involve the lateral regions of the cord, resulting in anterior horn damage and paralysis of one or more extremities.

Tabes Dorsalis. Tabes dorsalis is a slowly progressive degenerative disease involving the posterior columns and posterior roots of the spinal cord, resulting in progressive loss of peripheral reflexes, impairment of vibration and position sense, and progressive ataxia. There may be chronic destructive changes in the large joints of the affected limbs in far advanced cases (Charcot's joints). Incontinence of the bladder and impotence are common. Sudden and severe painful crises of uncertain cause are a characteristic part of the syndrome. These may involve the larynx, vagina, rectum, or other organs. Not infrequently severe sharp abdominal pains lead to exploratory surgery. Lightning pains in the extremities may require opiates for relief. These may be triggered by exposure to cold or other stresses or may arise with no obvious precipitating cause.

The eyes are frequently involved as well. Optic atrophy is seen in 20 per cent of cases. The pupils are abnormal in 90 per cent of cases, with bilaterally small pupils which fail to constrict further in response to light but which do constrict normally to accommodation (Argyll Robertson pupils).

The cause of tabes dorsalis is unclear. Spirochetes cannot be demonstrated in the posterior column or dorsal root.

Onset of the disease is usually delayed, often 20 to 30 years after initial onset of infection. It is thought to be more common in whites and in males. Typical cases presenting with lightning pains, ataxia, Argyll Robertson pupils, absent deep tendon reflexes, and loss of posterior column function are easy to diagnose. Atypical cases may be more troublesome, particularly because the VDRL test result in the serum is normal in as many as 30 to 40 per cent of cases, and 10 to 20 per cent of cases (even before the advent of penicillin) have normal CSF-VDRL as well. The FTA-ABS test in serum is nearly always positive.

Treatment is unsatisfactory. Penicillin does not reverse the symptoms, although it does usually result in clearing of the abnormal spinal fluid. Carbamazepine in doses of 400 to 800 mg per day has been reported to be effective in treatment of the lightning pains.

Tabes dorsalis is now thought to be uncommon, although a survey of newly diagnosed late syphilis in Denmark in the decade 1961 to 1970 showed that in approximately 10 per cent of all persons with late syphilis and 40 per cent of all with clinical neurosyphilis there was evidence of tabes dorsalis.

General Paresis. This form of neurosyphilis is a chronic meningoencephalitis resulting in gradually progressive loss of cortical function. It typically occurs 10 to 20 years after the initial infection. Pathologically there is a perivascular and meningeal chronic inflammatory reaction with thickening of the meninges, a granular ependymitis, degeneration of the cortical parenchyma, and abundant spirochetes in the tissues.

The most devastating effect of general paresis is on the mind. With effective penicillin therapy this disease has become much less common; in the United States, first admissions to mental hospitals because of syphilitic psychosis have declined from 7694 in 1940 to 154 in 1968, the last year for which definite figures are available.

Symptomatically in its early stages general paresis results in nonspecific symptoms such as irritability, fatigability, headaches, forgetfulness, and personality changes. Later there is impaired memory, defective judgment, lack of insight, confusion, and often depression or marked elation. The patients may be delusional, and seizures are sometimes seen. There may also be loss of other cortical functions, including paralysis or aphasia.

Physical signs of the illness are primarily those of the altered mental status. Cranial nerve palsies are uncommon. Optic atrophy is rare. The complete Argyll Robertson pupil is also uncommon, but irregular or otherwise abnormal pupils are not infrequent. Peripheral reflexes are often somewhat increased.

The CSF is nearly always abnormal with lymphocytic pleocytosis and increased total protein. The VDRL is usually reactive in both spinal fluid and serum. The disease responds well to penicillin therapy if administered early, although as many as a third of treated patients may develop progressive neurologic decline in later years. Fever therapy induced with malaria was formerly an effective adjunct to treatment with arsenicals, but has now been abandoned.

Classic general paresis is now infrequently seen in the United States. However, it remains reasonable to suspect syphilis as the cause of undiagnosed neurologic illness. Since the VDRL may be negative in patients with late neurologic syphilis, the FTA-ABS test on serum must be performed before syphilis can be excluded.

Congenital Syphilis. Congenital syphilis results from transplacental hematogenous spread of syphilis from the mother to the fetus. The incidence of congenital syphilis among newborns or infants under one year of age in the United States rose from 180 cases in 1957 to 422 cases in 1972, but has since declined to about 100 cases annually. Each case of congenital syphilis represents a tragedy which possibly could have been prevented by better case reporting and by proper prenatal care. A VDRL should be obtained in all expectant mothers at the beginning and near the end of pregnancy.

It has generally been held that maternal syphilis cannot be transmitted to the fetus until the sixteenth to eighteenth week of pregnancy. However, spirochetes can be found in abortuses of as little as nine to ten weeks' gestation. The risk of fetal infection is greatest in the early stages of untreated maternal syphilis and declines slowly thereafter, but the mother may infect her fetus during at least the first five years of her infection. Adequate treatment of the mother prior to the sixteenth week will usually prevent manifest clinical illness in the neonate. Later treatment may not prevent late sequelae of the disease in the child. Untreated maternal infection may result in stillbirth, neonatal death, prematurity, or syndromes of early or late congenital syphilis among surviving infants.

Manifestations of early congenital syphilis are often seen in the perinatal period, but may not develop until the infant has been discharged from the hospital. The disease resembles secondary syphilis of the adult except that the rash may be vesicular or bullous, which is extremely rare in adults. There often is rhinitis, hepatosplenomegaly, hemolytic anemia, jaundice, and pseudoparalysis (immobility of one or more extremities) resulting from painful osteochondritis. There may be thrombocytopenia and leukocytosis. The early stages of congenital syphilis must be differentiated from rubella, cytomegalovirus infection, toxoplasmosis, bacterial sepsis, and other diseases.

Late congenital syphilis is defined as congenital syphilis of more than two years' duration. The disease may remain latent with no manifest late damage. Cardiovascular alterations have not been observed in congenital syphilis. Neurologic manifestations are common, and there may be eighth nerve deafness and interstitial keratitis. The latter occurs in over 10 per cent of patients but may not be manifest until the tenth year of life or later. Periostitis may result in prominent frontal bones, depression of the bridge of the nose ("saddle nose"), poor development of the maxilla, and anterior bowing of the tibias ("saber shins"). There may be late onset arthritis of the knees (Clutton's joints). The permanent dentition may show characteristic abnormalities known as Hutchinson's teeth; the upper central incisors are widely spaced, centrally notched, and tapered in the manner of a screwdriver. The molars may show multiple poorly developed cusps (mulberry molars). Some of the late manifestations such as interstitial keratitis and Clutton's joints may be due to hypersensitivity responses, and are benefited by corticosteroids in some cases.

DIAGNOSIS. ***Dark-Field Examination.*** The most definitive means of making a diagnosis is finding spirochetes of typical morphology and motility in lesions of early acquired or congenital syphilis. The dark-field examination is almost always positive in primary syphilis and in the moist mucosal lesions of secondary and congenital syphilis. It may occasionally be positive in aspirates of lymph nodes in secondary syphilis. Problems arise, however, because of false-negative results in primary syphilis owing to application by the patient of soaps or other toxic compounds to the lesions. A single negative result is therefore insufficient to exclude syphilis. Patients with suspicious lesions but with an initially negative dark-field examination should be instructed to avoid washing the lesion and to return daily for two successive examinations. Confusion may also arise because of presence of spirochetes which are morphologically indistinguishable from *T. pallidum* in the mouth, particularly around the gingival margins. For lesions in these areas, therefore, diagnosis often depends upon clinical appearance, history, and serologic testing.

To perform the dark-field examination, the surface of the suspected ulcerative lesion should be cleaned with saline solution and gauze without production of bleeding. Presence of red cells in the specimen makes it difficult to visualize small numbers of *T. pallidum.* Squeezing of the lesion (with gloves on) may help produce serous fluid, which is picked up on a glass slide, covered with a coverslip, and examined with the dark-field microscope. Living *T. pallidum* organisms demonstrate gradual motion to and fro, rotational movement around the long axis, and rather sudden 90 degree bending near the center of the organism. Since most physicians do not have the proper equipment and are not familiar with the techniques of dark-field microscopy, the state public health authorities can be called for assistance.

T. pallidum may also be demonstrated in biopsies or pathologic specimens by fluorescent antibody stains or by silver stains.

Serologic Tests. Two basic types of humoral antibody are stimulated by infection with *T. pallidum:* nonspecific antibody directed against diphosphatidyl glycerol (cardiolipin), which is a normal component of many tissues; and specific treponemal antibodies. Nonspecific antibodies against cardiolipin were formerly designated "reagin," a term which should be discarded to avoid confusion with another "reagin," IgE. The kinds of tests used in syphilis are summarized in Table 306–2.

TABLE 306–2. SEROLOGIC TESTS FOR SYPHILIS

Type	Use
Nonspecific (anticardiolipin) antibodies:	
VDRL (slide flocculation)	Screening, quantitation, following response to treatment
RPR (circle-card) (agglutination)	Screening
Kolmer (complement fixation)	Limited
Specific treponemal antibodies:	
FTA-ABS (immunofluorescence with absorbed serum)	Confirmatory, diagnostic, not for routine screening
MHA-TP (microhemagglutination)	Similar to FTA-ABS but can be quantitated and automated
TPI (immobilization)	Most specific but not generally available

VDRL = Venereal Disease Research Laboratories test.
RPR = Rapid plasma reagin test.
FTA-ABS = Fluorescent treponemal antibody absorption test.
TPI = *Treponema pallidum* immobilization test.
MHA-TP = Microhemagglutination assay for *T. pallidum.*

NONSPECIFIC TESTS. Anticardiolipin antibodies were first discovered by Wassermann in 1907, using extracts of congenitally syphilitic livers as the antigen for a complement fixation test. Subsequently it was shown that normal livers contained the same antigen as do many other tissues; the antigen for this class of test is now extracted from beef heart. As yet there is no convincing explanation for why patients infected with *T. pallidum* develop increasing titers of antibody against a normal tissue component.

The Wassermann test has now been replaced by related tests. The standard test in use today for detection of anticardiolipin antibody is the Venereal Disease Research Laboratories (VDRL) test, which is an easily quantitated slide flocculation test. Many similar tests, including the rapid plasma reagin (RPR) test and the unheated serum reagin (USR) test, are frequently used for screening for syphilis.

The VDRL and related tests are simple, well standardized, cheap, and easy to perform and are the screening tests of choice. The VDRL is the test of choice for following response of patients to treatment. Since the VDRL detects antibody against a normal tissue component, it may be falsely positive in a significant number of patients. The relative proportion of patients with a false-positive VDRL depends on the prevalence of syphilis in the community; the lower the prevalence of syphilis, the higher the proportion of positive VDRL tests which are due to nonsyphilitic causes.

The VDRL test begins to turn positive a week or two after the onset of the chancre. In large series of patients with primary syphilis, approximately two thirds have had a positive VDRL test. Obviously then a negative VDRL test does not exclude primary syphilis, particularly if the lesion is less than two weeks old. The VDRL is positive in 99 per cent of patients with secondary syphilis, the only exceptions being patients with such high titers of antibody that they are in antibody excess; dilution of the serum will then paradoxically result in conversion of a negative test to positive. VDRL reactivity tends to diminish in later stages of the disease, and only about 70 per cent of patients with cardiovascular or neurosyphilis have a positive VDRL test result.

The *quantitative titer* of the VDRL test is somewhat useful in diagnosis and quite useful in following therapeutic response. The titer is reported as the highest dilution which gives a positive response. Most patients with secondary syphilis have titers of at least 1:16. Most patients with false-positive VDRL tests have titers of less than 1:8. No single titer is in itself diagnostic. Significant rises (four-fold or greater) in paired sera, however, are strongly indicative of acute syphilis.

TREPONEMAL TESTS. There are many varieties of specific treponemal antibody tests. The first and still perhaps best test is the *Treponema pallidum* immobilization (TPI) test, which when properly performed is nearly completely specific for infection by *T. pallidum* or related pathogenic spirochetes. Unfortunately it is cumbersome and expensive and therefore is not routinely done in the United States at present. The most widely used treponemal antibody test is the fluorescent treponemal antibody absorption (FTA-ABS) test. Patient serum is absorbed with extracts of nonpathogenic cultivable treponemes to remove cross-reacting group treponemal antibody. The absorbed serum is reacted with dried *T. pallidum* on a glass slide, and specific antitreponemal antibodies are detected by subsequent addition of fluorescein-labeled anti-human gamma globulin. Other treponemal tests are based on agglutination of red cells to which *T. pallidum* antigens have been fixed, such as the microhemagglutination assay for *T. pallidum* (MHA-TP). Many other treponemal tests have been developed or are being investigated, but none is superior to the standard tests.

The precise nature of the antigens involved in these tests is not known. Characterization of the antigens of *T. pallidum* has been greatly hindered by inability to grow the organism in cell-free culture. Recent success in cloning *T. pallidum* antigens into

Escherichia coli may circumvent this problem. Antibodies reactive in the various tests are found in all major immunoglobulin classes (IgG, IgM, IgA). A modification of the FTA-ABS test has been developed using fluorescein-labeled anti-human IgM (IgM FTA-ABS). The IgM FTA-ABS test is of some use in diagnosis of early congenital syphilis but is of no use in distinguishing acute disease from old infections in adults.

The FTA-ABS test is best used as a confirmatory test. It is somewhat more difficult to perform than the VDRL test and cannot be easily quantitated. It is sensitive and has a high degree of specificity, being positive in only approximately 1 per cent of normal individuals. It is positive in 85 per cent of patients with primary syphilis, 99 per cent with secondary syphilis, and at least 95 per cent with late syphilis. It may therefore be the only test positive in patients with cardiovascular or neurologic syphilis. In late syphilis the FTA-ABS test usually remains positive for life despite adequate therapy. It (as well as the TPI and MHA-TP) is positive in other treponemal diseases such as pinta, yaws, and bejel.

The FTA-ABS test is reported in terms of relative brilliance of fluorescence, from borderline to 4+. Borderline reactivity has the same meaning as nonreactive for clinical purposes. Most laboratories report 1+ positive tests as reactive, but some studies have shown that such tests may be relatively difficult to reproduce. Occasional laboratories therefore only report as positive tests with 2+ or greater reactivity. In patients lacking historical or clinical evidence of syphilis but with a reactive FTA-ABS test, one should repeat the FTA-ABS test. Use of another treponemal test such as the MHA-TP may be helpful in certain problem cases.

The MHA-TP test is less sensitive than either the VDRL or the FTA-ABS test in primary syphilis. Its sensitivity and specificity otherwise are nearly identical to those of the FTA-ABS test, being positive in nearly all patients with secondary syphilis and in 95 per cent or more of patients with late syphilis. The reactivity of serologic tests for syphilis in various stages of disease is shown in Table 306–3.

False-Positive Serologic Test Results for Syphilis. The VDRL or RPR test may be positive in a variety of diseases other than syphilis. A false-positive result is defined as a reproducible positive test in a patient with no clinical or historical evidence of syphilis, and whose serum FTA-ABS or MHA-TP test is negative.

"Acute" (less than six months) false-positive VDRL test results occur with low frequency in atypical pneumonia, malaria, and other bacterial or viral infections, and may occur after smallpox or other vaccinations as well. *Chronic false-positive VDRL tests* (lasting longer than six months) are relatively common in autoimmune disorders such as systemic lupus erythematosus, in narcotic addicts, in leprosy, and in aged persons. From 8 to 20 per cent of patients with systemic lupus erythematosus have been reported as having a false-positive VDRL test, and the false-positive result may develop many years prior to the onset of other manifestations of the disease. A chronic false-positive VDRL test in females age 20 or younger carries a significant risk of future development of systemic lupus erythematosus, thyroiditis, or other autoimmune disorders, and such patients should be followed carefully for a considerable period of time. As many as one third of patients with narcotic addiction have a false-positive VDRL test. Over 1 per cent of patients aged 70 and 10 per cent of patients over age 80 have a low titer false-positive VDRL test. Most false-positive VDRL tests have a titer of 1:8 or less, although occasional patients with lymphoma and other diseases have been described with very high titer false-positive VDRL tests.

TABLE 306–3. FREQUENCY OF POSITIVE SEROLOGIC TESTS IN UNTREATED SYPHILIS

Stage	VDRL (%)	FTA-ABS (%)	MHA-TP (%)
Primary	70	85	50–60
Secondary	99	100	100
Latent or late	70	98	98

A positive FTA-ABS result is usually indicative of recent or past syphilis. However, there is an increased incidence of false-positive FTA-ABS results in systemic lupus erythematosus and in other chronic diseases associated with hyperglobulinemia, including rheumatoid arthritis, biliary cirrhosis, and others. False-positive results are of two kinds in systemic lupus erythematosus: the most common is one with a beaded pattern of fluorescence, which has been shown to be due to anti-DNA antibodies; there also may be homogeneous fluorescence of the treponeme indistinguishable from a true positive result in syphilis. Patients with systemic lupus who have a false-positive FTA-ABS result almost always have a negative VDRL result (and conversely, patients with SLE with a positive VDRL usually have a negative FTA-ABS).

Occasionally one encounters reproducible positive FTA-ABS results in patients with no clinical or historical evidence of syphilis and in whom there is no evidence of diseases associated with false-positive FTA-ABS results. It may be wise to obtain CSF for examination of total protein, cells, and VDRL reactivity in order to rule out neurosyphilis. If in doubt and if the patient is not allergic to penicillin, it is often wisest to treat such patients for possible syphilis.

IgM FTA-ABS Test for Congenital Syphilis. Mothers with a positive VDRL or FTA-ABS will deliver infants with a positive VDRL and FTA-ABS because of passive transfer of the IgG antibodies reactive in these tests. Since many infants with congenital syphilis are clinically normal at birth but develop serious symptomatic disease some weeks later, it is important to determine whether a newborn with a positive VDRL or FTA-ABS test has passively transferred maternal antibody or is actively infected. Since maternal IgM antibodies are not passively transferred to the fetus, an IgM FTA-ABS test has been developed to detect syphilis in the newborn. Unfortunately there is approximately a 35 per cent incidence of false-negative IgM FTA-ABS test results in delayed-onset congenital syphilis. There also is a false-positive rate of approximately 10 per cent. For these reasons the IgM FTA-ABS test is of limited use in diagnosis of neonatal syphilis.

If the mother has been adequately treated for syphilis during pregnancy and the infant is clinically normal at birth, one may elect to follow the infant carefully by serial examination and VDRL titers. If the positive VDRL in the infant is due to passively transferred maternal antibody, the titer of reactivity will fall markedly in the first two months of life. A rising titer indicates active disease and the need for treatment. Many physicians are unwilling to risk failure of proper follow-up of VDRL-positive but clinically normal neonates, and instead administer effective therapy immediately. The risk of penicillin allergy in neonates is very low.

TREATMENT. *T. pallidum* is highly susceptible to penicillin, being inhibited by less than 0.01 μg of penicillin G. Since treponemes divide slowly, and since penicillin acts only on dividing cells, it is necessary to maintain serum levels of penicillin for many days. Studies in animals and in man show that more therapy is required as the length of infection increases. Current recommendations for treatment of syphilis are summarized in Table 306–4.

Early (Less Than One Year) Infectious Syphilis. Early syphilis may be treated with a single injection of 2.4 million units of *benzathine penicillin G,* which provides low but effective serum levels for over two weeks. Extensive studies in the 1940's and 1950's with regimens which provided similar serum levels and duration of therapy showed that approximately 95 per cent of patients were cured by such treatment. Many of the remaining 5 per cent who had clinical or serologic evidence of relapse may actually have been reinfected. It is not necessary to examine the CSF at this stage, because penicillin prevents development of later neurosyphilis. Motile treponemes disappear from primary lesions in 24 hours.

TABLE 306-4. PENICILLIN TREATMENT PRACTICE IN SYPHILIS AS RECOMMENDED BY UNITED STATES PUBLIC HEALTH SERVICE

	Dosage and Administration*	
Indications for Syphilis Therapy†	*Benzathine Penicillin G*	*Aqueous Benzyl Penicillin G or Procaine Penicillin G*
Primary, secondary, and early latent syphilis (<1 year); epidemiologic treatment	Total of 2.4 million units; single IM dose of two injections of 1.2 million units in one session	Total of 4.8 million units IM in doses of 600,000 units daily for eight consecutive days
Late latent (>1 year) or when CSF was not examined in "latency"; asymptomatic neurosyphilis, symptomatic neurosyphilis, cardiovascular syphilis, late benign (cutaneous, osseous, visceral gumma)	Total of 7.2 million units IM in doses of 2.4 million units at seven-day intervals, over 21 days	Total of 9 million units IM in doses of 600,000 units daily over 15 days; in selected cases of symptomatic CNS syphilis, 2 to 4 million units of aqueous (crystalline) penicillin G intravenously every four hours for at least ten days
Congenital		
Early		
Up to two years of age	If CSF is normal: Total of 50,000 units per kilogram IM in a single or divided dose at one session	If CSF is abnormal: Total of 50,000 units per kilogram IM per day for ten consecutive days‡
Late		
Two to 12 years, weight 32 kg (71 lb) or less	Same as for early congenital syphilis	Same as for early congenital syphilis
Over 12 years, or over 32 kg	Same as for adult late latent syphilis	Same as for adult late latent syphilis

*Individual doses can be divided for injection in each buttock to minimize discomfort.

†In *pregnancy*, treatment is dependent on the stage of syphilis.

‡For aqueous penicillin, give in two divided doses per day; for procaine penicillin, give as one daily dose.

A single injection of 2.4 million units of *aqueous procaine penicillin*, which provides relatively high serum levels for a brief period, is ineffective in established early syphilis, but is curative if the disease is still in the incubating stage (e.g., in a patient who is being treated for gonorrhea and who happened to acquire syphilis simultaneously). Other regimens currently useful for gonorrhea have uncertain effects on incubating syphilis, and careful follow-up for syphilis is indicated in gonorrhea patients treated with regimens other than procaine penicillin. The incidence of incubating syphilis in gonorrhea patients is 2 per cent or more in several series.

For patients allergic to penicillin, tetracycline hydrochloride may be given in a total dose of 30 grams over 15 days, or erythromycin base may be given in a total dose of 30 grams over 15 days. Particularly careful follow-up is necessary in patients treated with drugs other than penicillin, because patients may not be fully compliant with these prolonged courses of oral therapy and these regimens have been less fully evaluated clinically. Cephaloridine or other cephalosporins may be effective but have not been well studied. Chloramphenicol is of equivocal efficacy and for this reason, as well as because of the risk of toxicity, should not be used. Spectinomycin has essentially no effect on syphilis.

Syphilis of More Than One Year's Duration. Larger doses of penicillin are needed for *neurosyphilis* (see Ch. 497) than for syphilis of less than one year's duration. In general, patients with general paresis respond better to treatment than do patients with tabes dorsalis, although patients with paresis should be expected to show residual effects of the infection. This is particularly true in advanced cases. Meningovascular syphilis usually responds well, except for residual damage to cranial nerves or cortical function resulting from ischemic infarcts. Published studies show that a total of 6.0 to 9.0 million units of penicillin G results in a satisfactory clinical response in approximately 90 per cent of patients with neurosyphilis.

Currently used benzathine penicillin regimens have received relatively little study in neurosyphilis. Benzathine penicillin G in a total dose of 7.2 million units given as 2.4 million units weekly for three successive weeks is effective in most patients. However, there are reports of patients who have failed standard penicillin therapy for neurosyphilis but who responded to intensive intravenous therapy which provided high serum levels of penicillin. Benzathine penicillin does not provide measurable levels of penicillin in the spinal fluid or aqueous humor of the eye. *Therefore in cases of symptomatic central nervous system syphilis, which is a serious disease, there is considerable rationale to treatment with intravenous penicillin G (20 million units per day for at least ten days in hospital).* Therapy of neurosyphilis not infrequently results in increased CSF pleocytosis for seven to ten days after starting treatment, and may transiently convert a normal CSF to abnormal.

Limited evidence suggests that treating *latent syphilis* with 7.2 million units total dose of benzathine penicillin is curative even if the patient has asymptomatic neurosyphilis. However, because of the possible lack of the efficacy of benzathine penicillin in some patients with central nervous system syphilis, it is desirable to examine CSF in all patients with latent syphilis to exclude asymptomatic neurosyphilis. Alternatively, one may reasonably elect to perform a lumbar puncture at the conclusion of the follow-up period (two years); if the CFS is normal, the patient can be reassured that neurosyphilis will not develop.

There is no evidence that therapy with antimicrobial drugs is clinically beneficial to patients with *cardiovascular syphilis*. Nevertheless, treatment of cardiovascular syphilis is recommended in order to prevent further progression of disease and because approximately 15 per cent of patients with cardiovascular syphilis have associated neurosyphilis.

There is no evidence as to the efficacy of other antimicrobials in treatment of later syphilis. Therefore if patients are allergic to penicillin, it is mandatory that the CSF be examined before therapy is undertaken. Either tetracycline, 2 grams daily for 30 days, or erythromycin, 2 grams daily for 30 days, is probably effective.

Syphilis in Pregnancy. All pregnant women should be examined with a VDRL or RPR test during pregnancy; if they are at high risk for syphilis, a second test should be obtained before delivery. Because of the risk to the fetus, evaluation and treatment of the VDRL-positive patient should be done as rapidly as possible, particularly for patients first seen in the later stages of pregnancy. If a confirmatory FTA-ABS is positive and the patient has not been treated, penicillin (or erythromycin for patients who are allergic to penicillin) should be administered in doses appropriate for early or late syphilis as outlined above. For patients who are VDRL positive but FTA-ABS negative and who have no clinical signs of syphilis, treatment may be withheld. In such patients a quantitative VDRL test and another FTA-ABS test should be repeated in four weeks. If the VDRL titer has risen by four-fold or more, or if clinical signs of syphilis have developed, the patient should be treated. If after repeat examination the diagnosis remains equivocal, the patient should be treated to prevent possible disease in the neonate. After treatment a quantitative VDRL titer should be followed monthly; if it rises four-fold, the patient should be treated a second time.

Congenital Syphilis. Proper treatment of the mother usually prevents active congenital syphilis in the neonate. However, infected infants may be clinically normal at birth, and the infant may be seronegative if the mother's infection was acquired late in pregnancy. The infant should be treated at birth if the mother has received no or inadequate treatment, or has been treated with drugs other than penicillin, or if the infant cannot be carefully followed up for several months after birth. CSF should be examined before treatment of the infant. If the CSF is normal, treatment may be with a single injection of 50,000 units per kilogram of benzathine penicillin G. If the CSF is abnormal, treatment should be with aqueous penicillin G, 50,000 units per kilogram intramuscularly or intravenously daily, given in two divided doses, for a minimum of ten days. Alternatively, a single daily intramuscular injection of procaine penicillin G, 50,000 units per kilogram, may be given for ten days. These recommendations are based upon the failure of benzathine penicillin to provide adequate treponemicidal levels in spinal fluid, and on evidence that aqueous or procaine penicillin does provide adequate CSF levels of penicillin.

Tetracycline should not be used to treat children of less than eight years of age. Antimicrobial agents other than penicillin are not recommended for treatment of congenital syphilis.

Follow-up Examinations. All patients with early syphilis or congenital syphilis should return for quantitative VDRL titers and clinical examination 3, 6, and 12 months after treatment. Patients with late latent syphilis should be examined also at 24 months after therapy; if CSF was not examined prior to therapy, a lumbar puncture should be done prior to discharge to rule out inadequately treated asymptomatic neurosyphilis.

The quantitative VDRL titer should return to normal within 12 months after therapy of primary syphilis or 24 months after therapy of secondary syphilis. In a small percentage of patients with early syphilis, the VDRL will remain reactive in low titer for long periods of time. Chronic low titer VDRL reactivity after therapy is much more common in late syphilis and should not be viewed with alarm. The FTA-ABS test usually remains positive for years, despite adequate therapy. The influence of therapy on serologic tests is shown in Table 306–5. A progressively rising VDRL titer after therapy (a four-fold or greater rise) is sufficient evidence for retreatment. Patients with treated early syphilis are fully susceptible to reinfection, and many clinical and serologic relapses after therapy are probably reinfections. As such they represent failures of proper epidemiologic case finding and preventive therapy of the patient's sexual contacts.

Patients with neurosyphilis should be followed with serologic tests for at least three years and with repeat examination of CSF at six-month intervals. The CSF pleocytosis is the first abnormality to disappear, but cell counts may not be normal for one to two years. The elevated CSF protein falls more slowly, followed by the positive CSF-VDRL test, which may take years to become negative. It is not known whether use of high-dose intravenous penicillin therapy will accelerate the return of CSF to normal. Rising CSF cell counts, protein, and VDRL titer obtained at follow-up are an indication for retreatment.

Epidemiologic Investigation and Treatment. All patients with syphilis should be reported to public health authorities. In the absence of an effective vaccine, control of syphilis depends on finding and treating persons with infectious lesions of primary and secondary syphilis before they can further transmit the disease, and on finding and treating persons with incubating syphilis before they have developed infectious lesions. All patients with early syphilis (less than one year) should be carefully interviewed by qualified persons to determine the nature of their recent sex contacts. Approximately 16 per cent of the named recent contacts of patients with early syphilis will be found to have active untreated syphilis on examination, and a similar proportion of individuals named as suspects or associates will also have active syphilis.

TABLE 306–5. EFFECT OF RECOMMENDED TREATMENT SCHEDULES ON SEROLOGIC TESTS FOR SYPHILIS

Stage of Disease When Treated	Time to Follow-up (Years)	Frequency of Positive Serologic Tests (%)	
		VDRL†	*FTA-ABS*
Primary (seropositive)*	2	0–3‡	>80
Secondary	2	0–24	>80
Late latent or tertiary	5–13	56–70	98

*Patients with primary syphilis and a positive VDRL test.

†Positive VDRL tests after treatment are almost always *low titer* unless reinfection or relapse has occurred.

‡The range of results reflects inclusion of data from several series, using different patient selection and treatment regimens.

Most authorities, particularly in the United States, recommend treatment of sexual contacts of patients with early syphilis even if the contacts are clinically and serologically normal on examination. This is justifiable, because 30 per cent of clinically normal individuals named as contacts of persons with infectious lesions of syphilis within the previous 30 days will go on to develop syphilis if untreated. In general, preventive treatment is given to all sexual contacts of the past 90 days, although nearly all cases of syphilis in contacts will have developed within 60 days of exposure.

Jarisch-Herxheimer Reaction. Up to 60 per cent of patients with early syphilis, and a significant proportion of patients with later stages of syphilis, experience a transient febrile reaction after therapy for syphilis. This usually occurs in the first few hours after therapy, peaks at six to eight hours, and disappears within 12 to 24 hours of therapy. Temperature elevation is usually low grade, and there is often associated myalgia, headache, and malaise. The skin lesions of secondary syphilis are often exacerbated during the Herxheimer reaction, and cutaneous lesions which were not visible may become visible. It is usually of no clinical significance and may be treated with salicylates in most cases. In patients with syphilis of the coronary ostia or of the optic nerve, there is a theoretical risk that local inflammation coincident with the Herxheimer reaction could precipitate serious damage. This is the subject of much discussion in the old literature, but there is little current evidence that "local Herxheimer reactions" constitute a significant risk to the patient. Corticosteroids have been used to prevent adverse effects of the Herxheimer reaction, but there is no evidence that they are clinically beneficial (other than reducing fever) or necessary. Institution of treatment with small doses of penicillin does not prevent the Herxheimer reaction.

The pathogenesis of the Herxheimer reaction is unclear. It may be due to liberation of antigens from the spirochetes. There is evidence of activation of the complement cascade, including transient consumption of C3, C4, C6, and C7, and of transient decrease in treponemal antibodies coincident with the Herxheimer reaction. There is also evidence for endotoxemia, obtained by positive limulus amebocyte gelation tests, at the time of the Herxheimer reaction, although *T. pallidum* does not contain biologically active endotoxin. These seemingly contradictory observations could be explained if the reaction resulted in release of endogenous endotoxin from the gut.

Persistence of Treponemes After Treatment. Studies in man and in rabbits have shown that spiral forms may be visualized by silver stains in lymph nodes after effective treatment. Living virulent treponemes have occasionally been recovered by rabbit inoculation from lymph nodes, CSF, or ocular fluids after effective treatment has been given. These documented cases of treponemal persistence are very rare, however. At present there is little reason to worry about persistence of virulent treponemes after therapy with penicillin, with the possible exception of central nervous system syphilis, which needs further evaluation. There is no evidence for selection of penicillin-resistant mutants of *T. pallidum* to date.

PROSPECTS FOR PREVENTION. Solid immunity develops in rabbits following prolonged infection with virulent *T. pallidum*. It has not yet been possible to transfer immunity passively in laboratory animals by either immune serum or immune lymphocytes alone, suggesting that both cellular and humoral systems are necessary for immunity. Rabbits have been effectively immunized with multiple injections of treponemes which have been rendered avirulent by irradiation or by exposure to cold. However, a very large number of injections and a large mass of treponemes are necessary to effect immunity in the laboratory animal. For this reason and since *T. pallidum* cannot yet be grown in a virulent state in cell-free medium, there is no immediate prospect for a vaccine. However, significant immunity does develop in man after prolonged infection. For the present, control depends entirely on clinical awareness on the part of physicians, adequate reporting to public health authorities, and vigorous application of epidemiologic investigation and preventive treatment of sexual contacts.

Drusin LM, Singer C, Valenti AJ, Armstrong D: Infectious syphilis mimicking neoplastic disease. Arch Intern Med 137:156, 1977. *A fascinating and frightening account of diagnostic problems caused by oral, rectal, or lymphatic syphilis, nearly leading to cancer surgery.*

Feher J, Somogyi T, Timmer M, Jozsa L: Early syphilitic hepatitis. Lancet 2:896, 1975. *A description of the frequency and histology of early syphilitic hepatitis.*

Fischer A, Kristensen JK, Husfelt V: Tertiary syphilis in Denmark 1961–1970. A description of 105 cases not previously diagnosed or specifically treated. Acta Dermatovener 56:485, 1976. *One of few studies of the prevalence of newly diagnosed late syphilis in the antibiotic era.*

Fulford KWM, Johnson N, Loveday C, Storey J, Tedder RS: Changes in intravascular complement and anti-treponemal antibody titres preceding the Jarisch-Herxheimer reaction in secondary syphilis. J Clin Exp Immunol 24:483, 1976. *A presentation of evidence that there may be an immunologic basis for the Jarisch-Herxheimer reaction.*

Gamble CN, Reardan JB: Immunopathogenesis of syphilitic glomerulonephritis: Elution of antitreponemal antibody from glomerular immune-complex deposits. N Engl J Med 292:449, 1975. *Clear evidence for an immune-complex etiology of syphilitic nephrosis.*

Gjestland T: The Oslo study of untreated syphilis: An epidemiologic investigation of the natural course of the syphilitic infection based upon a re-study of the Boeck-Bruusgaard material. Acta Derm Venereol 35:Suppl 34, 1955. *A medical classic, in which the long-term course of untreated syphilis is evaluated.*

Kaufman RE, Olansky DC, Wiesner PJ: The FTA-ABS (IgM) test for neonatal congenital syphilis: A critical review. J Am Vener Dis Assoc 1:79, 1974. *Unfortunately the initial hopes for the value of the FTA-ABS (IgM) test in congenital syphilis are dashed by experience.*

Lee TJ, Sparling PF: Syphilis. An algorithm. JAMA 242:1187, 1979. *An algorithm for management of patients who present with a positive VDRL or similar test.*

Lugar A, Schmidt B, Spendlingwimmer I, Horn F: Recent observations on the serology of syphilis. Br J Vener Dis 56:12, 1980. *A current evaluation of the merits of serologic tests for syphilis.*

Luxon L, Lees AJ, Greenwood RJ: Neurosyphilis today. Lancet 1:90, 1979. *A presentation of 17 cases, all of which were similar to types of neurosyphilis seen in the preantibiotic era.*

Magnuson HJ, Thomas EW, Olansky S, Kaplan BI, DeMello L, Cutler JC: Inoculation syphilis in human volunteers. Medicine 35:33, 1956. *A classic paper, in which prison volunteers were inoculated with virulent* T. pallidum. *Immunity to inoculation syphilis was observed only in individuals who had congenital or late syphilis.*

Musher DM, Schell RF, Jones RH, Jones AM: Lymphocyte transformation in syphilis: An in vitro correlate or immune suppression in vivo? Infect Immun 11:1261, 1975. *There is temporary T-lymphocyte hyporesponsiveness in secondary syphilis.*

Prewitt TA: Syphilitic aortic insufficiency. JAMA 211:637, 1970. *Observations on the epidemiology, serology, and clinical manifestations of syphilitic aortitis in the United States.*

Raskind MA, Eisdorfer C: Screening for syphilis in an aged psychiatrically impaired population. West J Med 125:361, 1976. *Syphilitic disease of the central nervous system may be more prevalent than hospital surveys suggest.*

Schroeter AL, Turner RH, Lucas JB, Brown WJ: Therapy for incubating syphilis: Effectiveness of gonorrhea treatment. JAMA 218:711, 1971. *A controlled study showing that single-dose procaine penicillin eradicates incubating syphilis.*

Sparling PF: Diagnosis and treatment of syphilis. N Engl J Med 284:642, 1971. *A critical review of syphilis serology.*

Syphilotherapy 1976: Position papers for the current USPHS recommendations. J Am Vener Dis Assoc 3:98, 1976. *Too many papers to be easily digested, but the definitive source for those who wish to have a summary of the available evidence.*

Tramont EC: Persistence of *Treponema pallidum* following penicillin G therapy: Report of two cases. JAMA 236:2206, 1976. *At least one of the cases of neurosyphilis probably was a true penicillin treatment failure.*

Turner TB: Syphilis and the treponematoses. *In* Mudd S (ed.): Infectious Agents and Host Reactions. Philadelphia, W. B. Saunders Company, 1970. *A scholarly review of the biology of the treponematoses.*

Wilner E, Brody JA: Prognosis of general paresis after treatment. Lancet 2:1370, 1968. *Neurosyphilis frequently shows clinical progression despite what is probably adequate therapy.*

Spirochetal Diseases Other Than Syphilis

307. NONSYPHILITIC TREPONEMATOSES*

Thomas Butler

DEFINITION. The nonsyphilitic treponematoses are the skin diseases called *yaws, bejel,* and *pinta.* They occur predominantly in tropical regions and are transmitted by skin contact with infected persons. Disfiguring ulcerations of the skin may be produced, and invasion of bone and other tissues has been described. Treatment with benzathine penicillin G is effective, and the World Health Organization has carried out extensive treatment campaigns in endemic areas.

ETIOLOGY. Yaws is caused by *Treponema pertenue;* pinta is caused by *T. carateum;* and bejel is caused by a treponeme that is indistinguishable from other species. Like *T. pallidum,* these treponemes are spirochetal bacteria with helical structures and measuring about 0.2 μ in diameter and 10 μ in length. They are visible by dark-field microscopy but cannot be cultivated in vitro.

DISTRIBUTION AND EPIDEMIOLOGY. Yaws is prevalent in rural areas of tropical Africa, the Americas, Southeast Asia, and Oceania. The highest incidence is in children between ages two and five years. Bejel occurs in Africa, in Eastern Mediterranean countries, on the Arabian peninsula, in Central Asia, and in Australia. It is most prevalent in arid regions. Pinta occurs in rural areas of tropical Central and South America. Pinta affects mostly older children and adolescents. Humans are the only known carriers of the nonsyphilitic treponematoses. The portal of entry is the skin, which must be broken, as by a scratch or insect bite, before the spirochete can enter. Transmission is believed to be by direct skin contact or indirectly by contaminated hands or fomites and is facilitated by conditions of poor personal hygiene and crowding.

CLINICAL FEATURES. *Yaws* produces a skin papule at the site of inoculation after an incubation period of three to four weeks. The most common sites are the legs and buttocks. The papule enlarges, ulcerates, and develops a serous crust from which treponemes can be recovered. Regional lymphadenitis may accompany the papule, which will heal spontaneously within six months. A generalized secondary rash will occur before or after healing of the initial lesion, and these rashes are also papular and often covered with brown crusts. Relapsing crops of lesions can occur. Papillomas may result, and the plantar surfaces of the feet are involved with hyperkeratotic lesions. Periostitis of long bones leads to tender bones, and fever may be present. Relapsing lesions may occur over several years, resulting in chronic ulcerations and destructive gummatous lesions affecting the skin and bones.

Bejel produces patches on the mucous membranes of the oral cavity and pharynx and can cause split papules at the mucocutaneous junction of the oral angles. Anal, genital, and other intertriginous skin areas can be affected by lesions that resemble secondary syphilis. Regional lymphadenitis is common, and generalized rashes are rare. Healing of these early lesions is followed by latency manifested by seropositivity or by late lesions that resemble tertiary syphilis. These include nodular ulcers of skin, deformities of bones, and gummatous lesions that can perforate the palate.

Pinta starts similarly as a cutaneous papule with regional lymphadenitis that is followed by a generalized maculopapular eruption. One to three years after healing of the initial lesion, large hyperpigmented macules that are brown or blue develop and subsequently lose their pigment and become white. The time required for lesions to pass through these stages varies, so that the same patient may have coexisting areas of increased pigment and loss of pigment.

DIAGNOSIS. By dark-field microscopy, the causative spirochetes from early skin lesions can be observed directly. Spirochetes have been demonstrated also in lymph node aspirates. Serologic tests for syphilis will detect cross-reacting antibodies in these diseases. The VDRL test, the serologic test for syphilis, and the fluorescent treponemal antibody absorption test will all give positive results if serum is taken at least two weeks after the appearance of initial lesions.

TREATMENT AND PROGNOSIS. Long-acting benzathine penicillin G given as 1.2 million units intramuscularly is the preferred treatment for patients with early lesions. For patients with late manifestations, this therapy should be repeated twice

*The author acknowledges the contribution of Dr. Thorstein Guthe on this subject in the 16th edition of *Cecil's Textbook of Medicine,* pages 1584–1589, and refers the interested reader to this more complete treatment of the subject, which includes photographs of skin lesions.

at approximately seven-day intervals. The early lesions will heal rapidly, and most seropositive patients will convert to seronegative status. Late destructive lesions take longer to show improvement.

PREVENTION. The prevalence of these diseases has been reduced in several areas of the world by mass treatment campaigns using penicillin. The World Health Organization has treated about 53 million cases of yaws and 350,000 cases of pinta in the field with good results. These campaigns, however, are not adequate to eradicate the disease. It has been suggested that reduction in transmission requires improvements in the sanitation and economic standards of people living in endemic areas.

Guthe T: Clinical serological and epidemiological features of framboesia tropica (yaws) and its control in rural communities. Acta Dermatovener 49:343, 1969.
Hackett CG, Guthe T: Some important aspects of yaws eradication. Bull WHO 15:869, 1956.
Hackett CJ, Lowenthal LJA: Differential Diagnosis of Yaws. WHO Monograph Series No. 45. Geneva, WHO, 1960.
Kantor I, Wilentz JM, Berger BB: Yaws. Arch Dermatol 103:546, 1971.

308. RELAPSING FEVER

Thomas Butler

DEFINITION. Relapsing fever is an acute febrile illness of humans that is caused by blood spirochetes belonging to *Borrelia* species. The two major kinds of relapsing fever are *louse-borne relapsing fever,* for which man is the reservoir and the body louse is the vector, and *tick-borne relapsing fever,* for which rodents and other animals are the predominant reservoirs and ticks are the vectors. The relapsing fevers are distributed worldwide in both tropical and temperate climates. The natural course of relapsing fever consists of one or more phases of fever and spirochetemia, which last for several days and are separated by afebrile intervals of several days without spirochetemia. Antiborrelial antibodies develop. Relapsing fever is usually a self-limited disease, but during epidemics of louse-borne relapsing fever high mortality rates have been recorded. The relapsing fevers are effectively treated with antibiotics, but after treatment patients will often experience a Jarisch-Herxheimer-like reaction that consists of a worsening of fever and signs of disease.

HISTORY. The term relapsing fever was coined by Craigie in Edinburgh in 1843. A year later in the same city, Henderson differentiated this disease from typhus fever. The etiologic agent of relapsing fever was first established in Berlin in 1873 by Obermeier, who used a microscope to observe spirochetes in the blood of patients. The transmission of *Borrelia* spirochetes by arthropod vectors was suggested in 1891 by Flugge, who postulated the body louse as a vector, and in 1905 by Dutton and Todd, who demonstrated the infection in the *Ornithodorus* ticks of Africa. The genus name *Borrelia* was proposed in 1907 in honor of the French bacteriologist A. Borrel.

Relapsing fever is certainly a disease of antiquity, and its known epidemic potential, particularly in times of war, migrations, and other conditions that favor human crowding and poor hygiene, suggests that relapsing fever has had a major impact on human history. Before the advent of microscopic diagnosis, however, it was not possible to distinguish relapsing fever from similar scourges of humankind such as malaria, typhoid fever, and typhus fever, and so the history of relapsing fever before 1873 is only speculative. Between 1910 and 1945, there have been at least seven epidemics of relapsing fever in North Africa, Sudan, Ethiopia, West Africa, Central Africa, Eastern Europe, and Russia. There were an estimated 15 million cases with over 5 million deaths and case fatality rates as high as 73 per cent.

ETIOLOGY. Relapsing fevers are caused by blood spirochetes of *Borrelia* species, which belong to the order of bacteria called Spirochaetales. *Borrelia* species differ from the other two genera of pathogenic spirochetes, *Leptospira* and *Treponema*, by structure, biochemical characteristics, and antigenic determinants. *Borrelia* spirochetes are spiral organisms that measure 5 to 40 μ in length and about 0.5 μ in diameter. They are too thin to be seen reliably by light microscopy of wet preparations, but they are easily visible when viewed by dark-field or phase contrast microscopy. They are stainable with aniline dyes, such as Wright or Giemsa stains, and can be visualized well in tissue by the application of silver stains, such as the Dieterle or Warthin-Starry stains. Like other bacteria, these spirochetes possess an outer cell wall (outer envelope) and an inner cytoplasmic membrane that contains muramic acid. Between the cell wall and the cytoplasmic membrane there are 15 to 20 flagella, which are anchored to the ends of the spirochete and wrap around its body until they meet at the middle region. In three dimensions the spirochetes have a helical configuration consisting of about four to ten coils with amplitudes of about 1 to 4 μ. Under dark-field or phase contrast microscopy, *Borrelia* spirochetes display an active corkscrew-like motility consisting of rotation and motion in helical waves to produce translational movement. *Borreliae* are microaerophilic and fermentative in their growth characteristics. They require long chain fatty acids for growth and are cultivable in Kelly's medium. *B. recurrentis,* the agent of louse-borne relapsing fever, is more fastidious than the tick-borne *Borreliae* and requires the further addition of asparagine and choline to Kelly's medium. The *Borreliae* grow slowly in Kelly's medium, with doubling times of 18 to 26 hours.

The species names of the tick-borne *Borrelia* are derived from the species names of *Ornithodorus* tick vectors that carry them. The more common ones in North America are *B. turicatae, B. hermsii,* and *B. parkeri* and in Africa *B. duttonii. Borrelia* spirochetes produce fever when injected into rabbits but do not possess endotoxin. In general, *Borrelia* spirochetes do not elicit acute inflammation, do not produce abscesses, and are confined predominantly to the plasma space of their mammalian hosts.

The relapsing feature of *Borrelia* infection has been attributed to antigenic variation in the infecting population of spirochetes. In experimental infections of rats with *B. hermsii,* three separate serotypes emerged sequentially during relapses, and specific antibody appeared in response to each of the antigenic variants.

DISTRIBUTION AND EPIDEMIOLOGY. The geographic distribution of the relapsing fevers is widespread, with occurrence in most continents of the world including the Americas, Europe, Africa, and Asia. Louse-borne relapsing fever has disappeared from the United States but still occurs in parts of South America, Europe, Africa, and Asia. From 1960 to 1979 louse-borne relapsing fever was documented in Ethiopia and Sudan. Although accurate statistics on the incidence of this disease are not available, Ethiopia appears to be the country with the highest incidence, estimated at approximately 10,000 or more cases a year. Tick-borne relapsing fever occurs in endemic foci in southern British Columbia, in the western United States, in the plateau regions of Mexico, and in Central and South America. This disease is present in all areas of Africa except for the Sahara Desert and the rain forest belt. It occurs also in Spain and Portugal. In Asia, tick-borne relapsing fever has been reported in Cyprus, Israel, Syria, Turkey, Iraq, Iran, southern Russia, China, Afghanistan, and India. Accurate statistics on tick-borne relapsing fever are not available, but the sporadic nature of human contact with rodent ticks and the small numbers of established diagnoses suggest that this form of relapsing fever occurs less frequently in humans than louse-borne relapsing fever.

The two types of relapsing fever, louse-borne and tick-borne, differ so much in their epidemiology that they must be considered separately. *Epidemic relapsing fever* refers to the louse-borne kind and *endemic* or *sporadic relapsing fever* to the tick-borne variety. The only species of *Borrelia* that causes louse-borne relapsing fever is *B. recurrentis.* Its vector is the human body louse, *Pediculus humanus humanus,* and the only known natural reservoir is humans. Thus, the cycle of infection is from person to person via the louse. Body lice acquire the infection by feeding on a spirochetemic person, and they remain infected for their entire life span, which is 10 to 61 days under laboratory conditions. The ingested spirochetes pass through the esophagus to the midgut, where they penetrate the gut epithelium to reach the hemolymph in which they will multiply. Spirochetes do not reach the salivary glands or ovaries of the lice. Therefore, infection is not transmitted to humans by bites of lice, and infection cannot be transmitted transovarially to offspring of infected lice. Infection is believed to be transmitted to humans by the crushing of lice on the skin, which allows liberated spirochetes to penetrate through a bite site or through intact skin. Body lice prefer the normal human body temperature of 37° C to higher temperatures; thus, lice are likely to leave the skin of a febrile patient to go to another person. This may explain, in part, the rapid transmission of infection during epidemics.

The persons at greatest risk for acquiring louse-borne relapsing fever are those living under crowded, unhygienic conditions that favor infestation with body lice. Migrant workers and soldiers in war are particularly prone to develop this infection. Males are at much greater risk than females, presumably because their lives more commonly expose them to infected lice. A strain-specific, short-lived acquired immunity develops following infection. This immunity helps to explain why migrant workers coming into an endemic area are more susceptible to infection than are the permanent inhabitants. In some endemic areas, such as Addis Ababa, Ethiopia, there is an increased incidence during the cool winter season when people wear heavier clothing that becomes louse-infested.

The species of *Borrelia* that cause tick-borne relapsing fever are numerous and include *B. duttoni* in East Africa, *B. hispanica* in Spain, *B. persica* in Asia, and *B. hermisii* and *B. turicatae* in North America. The vectors of these organisms are argasid ticks of the genus *Ornithodorus*. The major reservoirs of tick-borne relapsing fever are wild rodents, including squirrels, deer mice, rats, chipmunks, and rabbits, and occasionally lizards, toads, turtles, and owls. The infection is passed between the reservoir animals by tick bites, and humans are accidental hosts when they come into contact with infected animal ticks. The exception to the animal reservoirs may be *B. duttoni* in East Africa, which is carried by the domestic tick *Ornithodorus moubata*, for which humans appear to be the reservoir.

Ticks acquire the infection by biting and sucking blood from a spirochetemic animal. The spirochetes, after entering the hemocele, invade other tissues of the tick, including the salivary glands, the coxal glands on the legs, and the ovaries. Transmission of the infection to animals or to humans follows injection of infected saliva through the bite site or intact skin. Ticks are more durable vectors than body lice, being able to survive as long as 15 years between blood meals and to harbor viable spirochetes for years. In addition, female ticks can pass *Borrelia* spirochetes transovarially to their offspring, thus permitting ticks to be infective without having previously bitten an infected host.

Persons at greatest risk of infection are those who come in contact with infected ticks from wild rodents. In the United States the largest outbreak of tick-borne relapsing fever occurred in 62 campers and employees in the National Park at the Northern Rim of the Grand Canyon, Arizona, in 1973. They had all slept in log cabins that were inhabited by wild rodents. Another outbreak in Washington State affected 42 boy scouts who also camped in a log cabin. In tropical countries, people who live in dwellings that are not rodent proof are prone to infection.

PATHOGENESIS AND PATHOLOGY. After exposure to an infected louse or tick, spirochetes enter through the skin, and in the subcutaneous tissue they have access to the blood and lymphatic circulations. There are no symptoms during an incubation period estimated to last from 4 to 18 days after exposure while the spirochetes are dividing in the blood plasma. No local lesions develop at the skin site of entry, and there is no evidence for an intracellular phase of multiplication or sites of attachment of spirochetes to host cells. After the spirochetes have built up to a concentration of 10^6 to 10^8 per ml of blood, the symptoms of shaking chills, fever, headache, and fatigue begin suddenly. These symptoms may be continuous or intermittent and usually increase in intensity over several days. At this early stage of illness large numbers of spirochetes are regularly present in the plasma space and are easily visible on blood smears. A small number of the spirochetes are within circulating polymorphonuclear phagocytes, and some spirochetes have been phagocytosed by fixed macrophages of the reticuloendothelial system of the spleen, liver, and bone marrow. A decrease in blood platelets leads to diffuse petechial skin rashes. In some severely ill patients who have jaundice, liver function studies reveal intrahepatic obstruction of bile flow and hepatocellular inflammation.

There also is disseminated intravascular coagulation, which contributes to the decrease in platelets and produces prolonged prothrombin and partial thromboplastin times and elevated titers of fibrinogen-fibrin degradation products. During acute relapsing fever, there are decreased levels of serum complement, Hageman factor, and prekallikrein, suggesting that activation of certain plasma proteins contributes to the pathogenesis of features such as hypotension and disseminated intravascular coagulation.

In the hours after antibiotic treatment, most patients undergo a Jarisch-Herxheimer reaction characterized by rigor, rising temperature, and falling blood pressure. Disseminated intravascular coagulation is accelerated, and spirochetes are phagocytosed at increased rates while being cleared from the plasma. Some patients not receiving antibiotic treatment undergo a similar spontaneous crisis. It is during this crisis or Jarisch-Herxheimer reaction that patients are at the greatest risk of dying.

Autopsies performed in Ethiopia and Sudan in fatal cases of louse-borne relapsing fever showed characteristic disease most regularly in the spleen, liver, heart, and brain. The spleen is enlarged to as much as 900 grams, and the cut surface shows white microabscesses, which consist of necrosis and hemorrhage in the white pulp. Occasionally there are splenic infarcts and splenic rupture. The liver is also enlarged, often to over 2000 grams. The midzonal region shows scattered necrosis and hemorrhage, and Kupffer's cells are enlarged and numerous. The heart is normal in size but frequently shows evidence of myocarditis, consisting of interstitial edema and a cellular infiltrate of lymphocytes and plasma cells. Examination of the brain usually indicates cerebral edema, and in some cases there is hemorrhage into the subarachnoid space or cerebrum. Thus, the immediate causes of death in relapsing fever are varied and in any particular case may be liver failure, cerebral hemorrhage, or acute cardiac arrhythmia caused by myocarditis.

The majority of patients with relapsing fever recover from illness either with or without antibiotic treatment. Patients develop antiborrelial antibodies that can agglutinate, kill, or opsonize the spirochetes. In the absence of opsonizing antibody, spirochetes are rapidly phagocytosed and digested by polymorphonuclear leukocytes. These antibodies participate also in rendering patients immune to future infection with the same serotype of *Borrelia*.

CLINICAL SYNDROMES. The illness begins abruptly with shaking chills, fever, headache, and fatigue. Most patients have these symptoms almost continuously throughout the day, whereas some patients report the intermittent appearance of these symptoms several times a day. Patients complain frequently of myalgias, arthralgia, anorexia, dry cough, and abdominal pains. These symptoms are usually mild on the first day of illness and increase in intensity over a few days, until they result in prostration and a visit to a physician. The nonspecific nature of the symptoms leads the patient or the physician to believe the illness is flu-like.

The temperature is elevated in the range of 38.5° to 40° C, and the pulse rate is increased to about 115 beats per minute. The blood pressure is lowered to about 105/70 mm Hg. Patients appear lethargic or may be delirious. Common physicial signs are conjunctival injection, petechial skin rash that is more apparent on the trunk than on the extremities, and palpable liver and spleen. Jaundice is occasionally present. Generalized muscle weakness is common. Some patients have mental confusion or delirium or nuchal rigidity.

The laboratory results include a blood smear positive for spirochetes. The white blood cell count is usually normal, with increased band forms and decreased eosinophils. The platelet counts are often less than 50,000 per cubic millimeter, and there may be prolongation of prothrombin time and partial thromboplastin time. Liver function test results are frequently abnormal, with elevations in concentrations of serum alanine aminotransferase and bilirubin that are evenly divided between the conjugated and unconjugated fractions. Renal function studies often show mild abnormalities of the serum urea nitrogen and creatinine values, and patients may have proteinuria and microscopic hematuria.

DIAGNOSIS. The diagnosis of relapsing fever depends on the demonstration of spirochetemia. In most patients, this is readily accomplished by obtaining peripheral blood by either fingerstick or venipuncture methods and preparing a thin film on a microscope slide. *Borrelia* spirochetes are stained blue by aniline dyes. Thus a routine blood smear stained with Wright's or Giemsa stain is adequate. Blood smears, thin or thick, prepared for examination for malaria parasites, are also satisfactory. The spirochetes are 5 to 20 μ in length and lie in the plasma spaces between blood cells or may overlie the blood cells. Febrile patients with relapsing fever typically have large numbers of spirochetes in the blood, approximately 10^6 to 10^8 per ml, or several per high-power field. Patients who are afebrile in the interval between relapses will have smears negative for *Borrelia* and should be re-examined when the fever reappears. Spirochetemia also may be detected by dark-field or phase contrast microscopy. A drop of fresh blood is diluted with another drop of 0.9 per cent NaCl and overlaid with a coverslip. Spirochetes are readily identified by their characteristic rotational motility.

Serologic testing has been employed in endemic areas for seroepidemiology and examination of convalescent patients. Serum of convalescent patients contains antibodies that produce agglutination and immobilization of living spirochetes and that fix complement during reaction with spirochetal antigens. None of these tests, however, is standardized or commercially available for general use.

TREATMENT AND PROGNOSIS. The relapsing fevers are effectively treated with tetracycline and erythromycin. Tetracycline is the treatment of choice except in children less than seven years old and in pregnant women in whom tetracycline may stain developing fetal teeth. Recent studies in Ethiopia indicate that a single oral dose of tetracycline, 500 mg, is as effective in clearing spirochetemia and preventing relapse as a longer course of treatment. Erythromycin, 500 mg, given orally as a single dose, is equally effective and is a satisfactory alternative to tetracycline. For patients unable to take oral medication, intravenous injections of 250 mg of tetracycline or erythromycin are curative. For children weighing less than 30 kg, the dosage of tetracycline or erythromycin should be reduced to approximately 10 mg per kilogram. Penicillin G has been used to treat relapsing fever, but its use has been associated with slow clearance of spirochetes and relapses following treatment.

In most patients with louse-borne relapsing fever and in some with tick-borne relapsing fever, antibiotic treatment provokes a distressing Jarisch-Herxheimer-like reaction. During the reaction, the patient is extremely uncomfortable, feeling very cold with severe headache and myalgia. The blood leukocyte and platelet counts sharply decrease, and spirochetes disappear from the plasma. The patient may require intravenous infusions of 0.9 per cent NaCl to maintain adequate blood pressure. Over several hours, the temperature declines and the patient's condition improves. Attempts to ameliorate the severity of the reaction by giving antipyretic or anti-inflammatory drugs have not been entirely successful. The best approach is to anticipate reaction and to provide intensive nursing care and intravenous fluid support during the first day of treatment.

The prognosis is favorable for complete recovery in 95 per cent or more of treated cases of relapsing fever. Bad prognostic signs are the presence of jaundice, high spirochete counts in the blood, and hypotension. The prognosis of untreated disease is grave in the case of louse-borne relapsing fever, for which mortality rates of 40 per cent have been reported during recent epidemics. Untreated patients will also experience relapses. In louse-borne relapsing fever, the first attack lasts about six days and is followed by an afebrile period of about nine days. There usually is one relapse, which will last only about two days. In tick-borne relapsing fever, the first attack lasts about three days and is followed by an interval of about seven days, after which an average of three relapses occur, each lasting about two days. Relapses are usually milder in intensity than the first attacks.

PREVENTION. Available approaches for the control of relapsing fevers include the detection and treatment of human cases, vector control, rodent control, and public health education. Vaccines are not available for the prevention of relapsing fever. For louse-borne relapsing fever, the detection and treatment of cases has the effects of reducing the reservoir of infection and consequently of reducing transmission. More important is the control of louse infestation. Delousing of clothing and bodies with insecticides such as DDT can be employed, as can the application of insect repellents. In known epidemic situations, prophylactic antibiotics are a temporary measure to contain spread of infection to persons at high risk. The eventual control of this disease requires improvements in personal hygiene and housing conditions. For tick-borne relapsing fever, the treatment of human cases has no impact on the animal reservoirs. It is not possible to control this infection in wild rodents. Campers and hikers going into endemic areas should be advised to avoid cabins that are inhabited by rodents and ticks and to apply topical tick repellants to the skin.

Bryceson ADM, Parry EHO, Perine PL, Warrell DA, Vukotich D, Leithead CS: Louse-borne relapsing fever. A clinical and laboratory study of 62 cases in Ethiopia and a reconsideration of the literature. Q J Med 39:129, 1970.

Burgdorfer W: The epidemiology of the relapsing fevers. *In* Johnson RC (ed.): The Biology of Parasitic Spirochetes. New York, Academic Press, 1976, p 191.

Butler T, Hazen P, Wallace CK, Awoke S: *Borrelia recurrentis* infection: Pathogenesis of fever and petechiae. J Infect Dis 140:665, 1979.

Butler T, Jones PK, Wallace CK: *Borrelia recurrentis* infection: Single dose antibiotic regimens and management of Jarisch-Herxheimer reaction. J Infect Dis 137:573, 1978.

Warrell DA, Perine PL, Krause DW, Bing DH, MacDougal SJ: Pathophysiology and immunology of the Jarisch-Herxheimer–like reaction in louse-borne relapsing fever: Comparison of tetracycline and slow-release penicillin. J Infect Dis 147:898, 1983.

309. TROPICAL PHAGEDENIC ULCER

Anthony D. M. Bryceson

DEFINITION. Tropical phagedenic ulcer is an acute specific ulcer of skin and subcutaneous tissue, associated in its early stages with infection with *Borrelia vincentii* and anaerobic bacteria of the genus *Bacteroides*. The ulcer is usually situated below the knee, has certain typical characteristics, and commonly becomes chronic.

ETIOLOGY AND PATHOGENESIS. *B. vincentii* is a loosely coiled spirochete 5 to 10 μ long; it is a common oral commensal. *Bacteroides* is a curved, cigar-shaped rod 5 to 14 μ long, often beaded when stained; it, too, is an oral commensal and is common in moist soils. Either or both of these organisms are present in the acute stage of the ulcer. They gain entry through a tiny wound in the skin. Experimentally, they will cause ulcers only in malnourished subjects or animals. Other organisms, especially cocci, may also be found in established ulcers.

EPIDEMIOLOGY. The condition is common and widespread in the tropics and rare elsewhere. It may be found in all climates and at any altitude. In some countries hot wet areas are especially affected. In parts of some countries, active ulcers have a prevalence of 2 per cent and scars of 15 per cent. It is often the most common complaint of hospital outpatients, representing up to one third of new patients, and may be the most common cause of surgical admissions.

Tropical ulcer is typically a sporadic disease, especially affecting adolescent males. It is most common in the lower socioeconomic groups. Although the patient may not appear grossly malnourished, there is a clear clinical and experimental association with malnutrition. No specific nutritional deficiency has been identified, but tropical ulcer is rare in those who eat adequate animal protein and is especially common in labor gangs, ill-kept prisoners of war, and other physically deprived groups, among whom it can appear as an epidemic. This association with malnutrition and deprivation is also found in two other infections with the same organisms, cancrum oris (noma) and trench mouth (Vincent's angina).

PATHOGENESIS, CLINICAL MANIFESTATIONS, AND PROGNOSIS. The lesion starts at the site of a minor wound or insect bite, which the patient can usually recall. Often the site is neglected or treated with a native remedy, or sucked by mouth to clean it. A small blister appears, containing serosanguineous fluid, and ruptures, exposing an ash gray slough which has a characteristic foul smell. The ulcer spreads rapidly to involve subcutaneous tissue and often muscle and tendon down to bone. It reaches its final diameter of 1 to 40 cm in a few days. The central slough liquefies, exposing a gray-brown base. The ulcer is circular, with a raised edge and surrounding edema, and may encircle the limb. It is painful and bleeds easily. Regional lymph nodes may be enlarged and tender. The most common sites of tropical ulcers are over the bony parts of the leg at the level of, or just above, the ankle.

Histologic examination shows three layers: a superficial layer of coagulation necrosis in which organisms are abundant, a layer of granulation tissue, and a highly vascular base. The edge of the ulcer shows pseudoepitheliomatous hyperplasia.

Fifty per cent of ulcers heal spontaneously within three months, and 80 per cent within six months.

Chronic ulcers become less painful and lose their odor. They become irregular with a rigid base and edge and are filled with pink granulation tissue. Histologically there is much surrounding fibrosis. Squamous cell carcinoma develops in 9 per cent of chronic ulcers after a period of three months to 50 years. Tetanus and gangrene are rarer complications.

DIAGNOSIS. In the acute stage the appearances and smell are typical. The specific organisms can be demonstrated in a drop of fluid aspirated from the ulcer, either by dark-field microscopy or by Gram stain or staining with 1 per cent carbolfuchsin. Histologic examination is seldom needed. It is more difficult to identify the cause of chronic ulcers. The differential diagnosis includes yaws (serology and radiology), cutaneous diphtheria (climate, culture), Buruli ulcer (undermining, acid-fast bacilli), squamous cell carcinoma and melanoma (histology), and varicose ulcers (age group, venous abnormality).

TREATMENT. In the acute stage the patient is put to bed and the limb elevated. The ulcer is dressed with sterile saline or resorcinol monoacetate (Euresol). Hydrogen peroxide may be used for a few days to help slough out. Strong antiseptics are contraindicated. Penicillin is given by intramuscular injection for seven days; procaine penicillin, 600,000 units twice daily, or penicillin aluminium monostearate,* 1,200,000 units daily, is suitable. Metronidazole,† 200 mg thrice daily by mouth, is a suitable alternative to penicillin. The synergistic effect of the two drugs has not been tested.

This treatment controls the infection and cleans the ulcer. Ulcers under 5 cm in diameter should now heal satisfactorily. Ulcers over 5 cm should be grafted with split skin.

Chronic ulcers are treated initially in the same way and are then completely excised and grafted. A walking plaster may then be applied, and healing is complete within three weeks.

*No longer available in the United States.
†Investigational drug for this purpose.

PREVENTION. Good nutrition and physical health are the best preventives. Legs should be covered while walking in country where thorns or sharp grass may scratch them. Minor cuts and scratches should be washed and treated with local antiseptic.

Edington GM, Gillies HM: Tropical ulcers. *In* Pathology in the Tropics. London, Arnold, 1976, p 726. *Good pathologic account.*

Kuberski T, Koteka G: An epidemic of tropical ulcer in the Cook Islands. Am J Trop Med Hyg 29:291, 1980. *The little-known epidemic presentation.*

Lindler RR, Adeniyi-Jones C: The effect of metronidazole on tropical ulcers. Trans R Soc Trop Med Hyg 62:712, 1968. *One of the very few papers on chemotherapy.*

Lowenthal LJA: Tropical phagedenic ulcer: A review. *In* Lincicome DR (ed.): International Review of Tropical Medicine. New York, Academic Press, 1963, p 267. *Still the best major review.*

310. RAT BITE FEVERS

J. Bruce McClain

The term *rat-bite fevers* refers to illnesses caused by *Streptobacillus moniliformis* or *Spirillum minus*.

S. moniliformis previously has been called *Actinomyces muris, Streptothrix muris ratti,* or *Haverhilia multiformis.* It is an aerobic gram-negative branching rod in the same family as mycobacteria, 2 to 15 μ in length, and an inhabitant of the respiratory tracts of mice and rats.

Spirillum minus, sometimes called *Spirillum minor,* is a twisted gram-negative aerobic rod with bipolar tufts of flagella, which has not been grown on artificial media but which has been passed to animals. It is 2 to 5 μ in length and has been identified in the drainage from interstitial keratitis in rats.

EPIDEMIOLOGY. Neither streptobacillary nor spirillary rat-bite fevers are reportable diseases. The Centers for Disease Control receive two to three isolates annually. A survey from the 1940's of 400 rat bites reported 16 cases of clinical rat-bite fever, 8 of which had organisms identified. The highest reported rate of post–rat-bite fevers is 10 per cent. Many factors make the current prevalence in the United States difficult to determine: innate antibiotic responsiveness, the difficulty with which the causative organisms are isolated, and the lack of widely available serologic tests. The majority of recently reported cases are in laboratory workers with definite bite exposure, and these individuals constitute the population at highest risk. Other animals have been reported to transmit the disease, including weasels, dogs, cats, pigs, and mice. Streptobacillary fever may be transmitted by nonbite mechanisms, as demonstrated by an outbreak associated with consumption of unpasteurized milk in Haverhill, Massachusetts, and case reports of illness associated with trauma.

CLINICAL MANIFESTATIONS. ***Streptobacillary Fever (Haverhill Fever).*** The initial injury heals promptly in most cases. The incubation period from bite exposure is usually 3 to 4 days, with a range of 1 to 22 days. In the Haverhill outbreak most cases occurred within three days of exposure to contaminated milk. Ninety-five percent of patients will complain of fever, frequently in the 102° to 104° F range, usually with a sudden onset and a toxic effect on the patient. Bifrontal headache, nausea, vomiting, and myalgias usually accompany the fever initially. Occasionally there is a lessening of fever after a few days, with subsequent return of higher temperatures. A maculopapular rash develops within the first five days of illness in almost all patients. The rash is distributed distally and may involve the palms and soles of the feet. Occasionally the centers of the 0.3- to 1-cm lesions develop pustules. A fine desquamation occurs on healing in 20 per cent of patients. Arthritis occurs in 70 per cent of patients on the second through 14th days of illness and almost always involves more than one joint, especially the wrists and elbows. The arthritis is nondeforming, although in untreated cases it may persist for months and has been known to damage joints. Less frequently reported complications of streptobacillary fever are endocarditis, pericarditis, soft tissue abscesses, and amnionitis.

Spirillary Fever (Sodoku). The initial injury heals promptly in most cases, although induration, ulceration, or eschar may develop at the site of injury with the onset of illness. Regional adenopathy is frequently present. The incubation period is generally greater than 7 days, with a range of 1 to 36 days. The onset of sodoku is less abrupt than in streptobacillary fever, and temperatures are in the 102° F range. Fevers are recurrent with several days between episodes. Headaches, nausea, and vomiting are common, and a roseolar-urticarial rash is seen in half the patients. Arthritis is rare.

Spirilla are poorly characterized organisms. It seems that on occasion nonsodoku spirilla may cause illness in humans. These illnesses tend to be prolonged and to resemble endocarditis.

LABORATORY MANIFESTATIONS. Most patients with spirillary fever and less than 20 per cent with streptobacillary fever have false-positive results of serologic tests for syphilis. Leukocyte counts in both illnesses range from normal to 30,000 per cubic millimeter. Results of urinalysis usually are normal, although nephritic sediments have been seen in sodoku.

DIAGNOSIS. The diagnosis of streptobacillary rat-bite fever is made by culturing the organism from blood, joint fluid, or tissue or by demonstrating a four-fold rise in titer by an agglutination test that is available through the Centers for Disease Control. Titers may persist for two to four years. Streptobacilli from blood cultures will usually grow within a week. Their cultivation is complicated by requirements for animal serum in the medium and a CO_2 atmosphere as well as sensitivity to sodium polyanethol sulfonate (Liquoid, SPS), which is found in most automated blood culture systems at levels that are inhibitory (over 0.01 per cent). Specific measures to cultivate the organisms must be arranged with the laboratory.

Spirillary fever may be diagnosed by inoculation of mice with infected tissues or fluids and demonstration of morphologically compatible organisms in the peripheral blood by dark-field examination. Occasionally the diagnosis has been established by dark-field examination of peripheral blood or eschars in humans.

The differential diagnosis of rat-bite fever includes Still's disease, arthritis associated with hepatitis B, rubella, gonococcemia, meningococcemia, rickettsial disease, hypersensitivity vasculitis, and leptospirosis.

TREATMENT AND PROGNOSIS. Penicillin G, 1.2 million units per day in divided doses, is the treatment of choice for both types of rat-bite fever. Ampicillin or penicillin V, 2 grams per day is effective oral therapy. The duration of therapy should total ten days, and parenteral therapy may be followed with oral therapy. Higher doses have been used in endocarditis. The streptobacillary illness has responded to parenteral cephalosporin therapy. Oral cephalosporin therapy should not be substituted until more information is available. In the patient allergic to penicillin, both forms of the illness may be treated with tetracyclines, chloramphenicol, or streptomycin.

About 12 per cent of untreated patients with streptobacillary disease die, although in most cases the disease will run a course of 25 days with spontaneous resolution. Treatment with penicillin G will resolve most symptoms in one to four days, although patients who receive less than 400,000 units per day of penicillin have had illnesses persisting for several weeks. Penicillin resistance has been reported and should be kept in mind if treatment failure is suspected.

The mortality in untreated spirillary fever is 7 per cent. Without therapy the disease will last an average of 35 days. Spontaneous resolution is the rule. Penicillin therapy will cause resolution of symptoms in one or two days. A Herxheimer reaction is common.

Anderson LC, Leary SL, Manning PJ: Rat-bite fever in animal research laboratory personnel. Lab Anim Sci 33:292, 1983. *A case report and review of the clinical and epidemiologic characteristics of the group at risk for disease.*

Kowal J: Spirillum fever, report of a case and review of the literature. N Engl J Med 264:123, 1961. *An interesting review of nonsodoku spirillary illness.*

Roughgarden JW: Antimicrobial therapy of rat-bite fever. Arch Intern Med 116:39, 1965. *A comprehensive review of therapeutic results with various antimicrobials.*

Watkins CG: Ratbite fever. J Pediatr 28:429, 1946. *The best review of the clinical syndromes of rat-bite fever.*

311. LEPTOSPIROSIS

J. Bruce McClain

The term *leptospirosis* describes an infection with any serovar of *Leptospira interrogans*, regardless of the syndrome. Old names such as *canicola fever, Fort Bragg fever, Weil's disease,* or *peapicker's disease* are potentially confusing and should be avoided.

ETIOLOGY. *Leptospira* consists of two species: *interrogans,* which is pathogenic, and *biflexa,* which is saprophytic. Serotyping and serogrouping have established over 170 serovars in the species *L. interrogans*. The proper designation of a serovar is *L. interrogans* serovar pomona not *L.* pomona. The latter usage, although widespread, represents serovars as species and is incorrect.

The organism is a tightly coiled spirochete with one axial filament. With a diameter of about 0.15 μm, it is invisible on light microscopy and must be visualized by phase contrast or dark-field microscopy. It is easily cultured on Fletcher's medium and is an obligate aerobe.

EPIDEMIOLOGY. Leptospirosis is a ubiquitous enzootic disease. Reservoirs of infection include rodents, skunks, foxes, domestic livestock, and dogs. Many animals exhibit a prolonged urinary shedding of the organism without clinical illness. When humans contact infected tissues, fluids, or contaminated waters, they contract the illness. Transmission may occur through cuts, mucous membranes, and probably unabraded skin. In earlier series illness was reported associated with occupational exposure such as among sanitation, dairy, slaughter house, or fishing workers. The epidemiology has changed over the last 15 years, owing to the advent of multiuse land development with farmlands draining into recreational bodies of water. More recent reports indicate that at least half of cases result from nonvocational exposure. There has been a corresponding decrease in the age of persons infected, although males still comprise 80 per cent of cases. In the United States between 50 and 150 cases are reported annually. The national attack rate is 0.05 per 100,000, although rates as high as 1 per 100,000 occur in Hawaii. The disease is probably substantially underreported. Leptospirosis shows an annual peak in the summer months and has had a 4- to 5-year periodicity in attack rates over the last 25 years.

PATHOLOGY AND PATHOGENESIS. Gross anatomic findings in patients dying from leptospirosis are: (1) widespread hemorrhage in skin, mucosa, serosa, heart, lungs, spleen, liver, and kidneys; (2) hepatomegaly without prominent splenomegaly; (3) bile staining; and (4) enlargement of the heart and kidneys.

Histologic examination of the liver in autopsy material shows nonspecific inflammatory changes, bile stasis, and disruption of the limiting plate. Biopsy materials under light and electron microscopic examination show similar features with less destruction of architecture.

Kidneys in autopsy series show a spectrum of changes that reflect an initial tubular injury that is acellular. As the disease progresses and antibodies appear, inflammatory changes occur that result in an overt interstitial nephritis with disruption of the tubular architecture. Biopsy series show similar changes to a lesser degree. The glomeruli have foot-process fusion and mesangial hypertrophy but are otherwise spared. Leptospires are seen in most of the renal material.

Hemorrhagic manifestations are associated with areas of capillary wall damage and necrosis with perivascular round cell infiltration.

Striated muscle is frequently involved with degeneration of individual fibrils and loss of architecture associated with inflammation. This pattern is considered specific for leptospirosis. The myocardium is affected with similar changes. In one fourth of autopsy cases, myocarditis is listed as serious enough to be a contributing cause of death.

The mechanism by which *Leptospira* organisms cause damage to tissues is obscure. Toxic factors have been identified in culture supernatants, but organisms that do not produce some of these factors may cause serious disease. Early in the illness the evidence favors a direct leptospiral toxicity to certain tissues, while later in the illness damage secondary to inflammation is more pronounced.

CLINICAL FEATURES. Most natural infections appear 7 to 14 days after exposure, although the incubation period ranges from 2 to 20 days. The length of the incubation period has no prognostic significance. Clinical findings vary among reported series, but a general description includes: fever and headache, 95 per cent; myalgia and conjunctival suffusion, 80 per cent (in nonmilitary series suffusion is reported less often); gastrointestinal symptoms (nausea, vomiting, or abdominal pain), 60 per cent; cough or pharyngitis, 40 per cent; lymphadenopathy, 25 per cent; hepatomegaly, 15 per cent; rash, 10 per cent; and jaundice and gastrointestinal hemorrhage, 5 per cent each. Less commonly reported symptoms are splenomegaly, uveitis, and diarrhea. About one half of patients exhibit a "brutal beginning" with an abrupt onset of symptoms over a one- to two-hour period. The clinical picture that should bring leptospirosis to mind is a febrile patient with severe muscle aches and pain who is nauseated or vomiting. The presence of conjunctival suffusion may be very helpful in detecting the illness in military populations. It is not conjunctivitis as seen in allergic or viral conjunctivitis, but rather a *pericorneal reddening* or *hyperemia*.

The fever is high, usually above 102° C and frequently up to 104° C, and is accompanied by chills. Headache is severe and is characterized as retro-orbital or occipital. The presence of headache, high fever, and neck stiffness or pain due to profound myalgias suggests meningitis and may necessitate a lumbar puncture. Spinal fluid is usually acellular in the first five to seven days of illness, although leptospires may be seen. With the onset of antibody in the serum, an aseptic meningitis may occur in up to 90 per cent of patients, but only half will have meningeal symptoms. When a cutaneous hypesthesia is also present, patients may not tolerate the touch of a sheet. Other neurologic manifestations, such as changes in the level of consciousness, encephalitis, and cranial nerve palsies, have been reported less often. The muscle pains and tenderness are truly remarkable. The severity of myalgias may even prevent the patient from standing. The presence of nausea, vomiting, and anorexia with abdominal tenderness caused by muscle involvement can mimic pancreatitis. Acute dilatation of the gallbladder and cholecystitis can occur in leptospirosis and make the clinical evaluation of an ill patient very difficult, especially since there is already laboratory evidence of inflammation.

The illness usually lasts four to nine days. During that period all clinical findings resolve simultaneously, and both doctor and patients are surprised at how quickly the recovery has taken place and at how well the patient feels. In about 15 per cent of patients the illness persists beyond the ninth day. It rarely may last six to seven weeks.

Leptospirosis is generally a monophasic illness. In a minority of patients after an initial illness there will be a period of apparent recovery, after which symptoms worsen. This second phase is termed the *immune phase*. It lasts two to four days in most patients. It differs from initial illness in being more variable. Fever is not so high, myalgias and gastrointestinal symptoms are not so severe, but meningitis and abnormal spinal fluids and iridocyclitis are more common. The immune phase is so named because of its correlation with the onset of antibodies to leptospirosis in the blood, the disappearance of leptospiremia, and the onset of urine cultures positive for the germ.

The term *Weil's syndrome* is applied to one pole of a continuum of illness. It is not a specific subgroup of leptospirosis; it is simply severe leptospirosis. Any of the several manifestations of Weil's syndrome may occur alone. The clinical findings of intense jaundice, mental status changes, hemorrhage, purpura or petechiae, and renal insufficiency occurring in a previously normal patient are so memorable that it is not surprising that this was the syndrome that stimulated the search for leptospires. The first manifestation of severe illness is usually jaundice that develops between the fifth and ninth days. The intensity of jaundice has no prognostic significance. Renal insufficiency may develop concomitantly with jaundice. Oliguria is a grave prognostic sign. Hemorrhagic manifestations may develop: purpura and petechiae may appear on the oral, vaginal, or conjunctival mucosa. A biphasic pattern frequently may be seen, although the "stages" tend to merge into a single severe illness. Convalescence is rapid in most patients but may be delayed for up to ten weeks.

Childhood Disease. A recent report of nine pediatric cases reiterated the close contact of children to common reservoirs such as dogs. The pediatric syndrome shares many features of adult disease but is more intense, with several atypical features such as shock, hydrops of the gallbladder, skin desquamation, and chest x-ray abnormality.

LABORATORY FEATURES. Leukocyte counts are usually below 15,000 per cubic millimeter but may be as high as 50,000 per cubic millimeter. There is almost always neutrophilia. Hematocrit is normal in anicteric illness, but in prolonged illness anemia is common. The causes of anemia are many, with blood loss, microangiopathy, and leptospiral hemolysin all implicated in clinical cases. Thrombocytopenia is seen in severe cases. Coagulation studies occasionally demonstrate a vitamin K reversible prolongation of prothrombin time. However, this is not responsible for the hemorrhagic diathesis of severe leptospirosis. The sedimentation rate is elevated in half of cases.

Liver function tests reveal a mean SGOT/SGPT elevation of five times normal with occasional patients with elevations up to 20 times normal. The direct bilirubin concentration may rise as a manifestation of severe disease and may reach 64 mg per deciliter, but in most icteric cases it is below 20 mg per deciliter. The pattern is one of intrahepatic cholestasis.

Early in the illness 80 per cent of patients have abnormal urine findings. The most common abnormalities are microscopic hematuria, pyuria, and "2+" proteinuria. Gross hematuria rarely has been reported. One fourth of patients demonstrate elevations of the blood urea nitrogen between 20 and 100 mg per deciliter. The most common electrolyte abnormality is hyperkalemia, primarily in patients with renal failure.

The chest x-ray appears abnormal in one fourth of patients, including anicteric cases. The most common abnormality is patchy bronchopneumonia. A small pleural effusion is seen in 10 per cent of patients.

Electrocardiographic abnormalities occur in 10 to 40 per cent of patients, with bradycardia and low voltage accounting for one half of abnormalities. The remainder consists of nonspecific ST-T wave changes.

Cerebrospinal fluid may be abnormal in up to 90 per cent of patients. In 70 per cent of specimens the total cell count is below 500 per cubic millimeter, with frequent presence of neutrophils. Protein ranges from 50 to 110 mg per dl in 80 per cent of cases. The glucose concentration is usually normal.

IgM antibodies may be detected in blood by day four or five of illness in most patients.

DIAGNOSIS. A diagnosis of leptospirosis must be suspected in any patient with fever, myalgias, headache, and nausea or vomiting. The presence of conjunctival suffusion is an early and helpful sign. The most common misdiagnosis of a patient with leptospirosis is aseptic meningitis followed by viral hepatitis, viral syndrome, fever of unknown origin, bronchitis, influenza, nephritis, and rickettsiosis. The following differential points aid the clinician: (1) the myalgias of leptospirosis are not a prominent feature of viral hepatitis; (2) creatinine kinase is frequently elevated in leptospirosis, and this seldom occurs in viral hepatitis; (3) liver enzyme values in viral hepatitis may average 10 to 15 times higher than normal, but the average is five times higher in leptospirosis; (4) a conjunctival suffusion is very helpful in separating leptospirosis from other processes.

The diagnosis may be confirmed by culture (on Fletcher semisolid medium) of the blood in the first week of illness or of the urine thereafter. Cultures may take up to eight weeks to become positive. Since leptospires may be excreted in the urine for prolonged periods, the diagnosis may be established by urine culture in untreated patients even after clinical illness is over. Direct examination of the urine and blood are not sufficient to establish the diagnosis. There are many artifacts that may be mistaken for leptospires, especially by the inexperienced laboratory worker. When cultures are performed three to four times, organisms are recovered with regularity. The diagnosis may be established serologically by two methods. The macroagglutination is a screening test that uses pooled antigens from all of the serogroups of leptospirosis. Diagnosis is made by a four-fold rise in titer. This test is broadly available but will not detect infecting serovars that are not included in the pooled test antigens. The microagglutination requires a live pathogenic leptospiral culture and therefore is performed mainly in reference laboratories. Techniques for detecting genus-specific antibody or antigen using hemolytic assays and counterimmunoelectrophoresis have been published and are available as research tools. The most promising test for early diagnosis is a genus-specific antibody detection system.

PROGNOSIS. In most untreated cases this is a nonfatal, self-limited illness. The reported mortality of leptospirosis varies greatly among series. In military populations it is around 0.1 per cent. In civilian series it ranges from 5 to 10 per cent. In both military and civilian series mortality is related to age and presence of jaundice. Thirty per cent of patients over age 60 die. Jaundiced patients have a 15 per cent mortality. The differences in mortality may have to do with the underlying health of the host and the bias toward reporting of more serious cases. The military series involve large groups of well men in which high attack rates have been documented and physicians are sensitive to the diagnosis. If the patient lives, sequelae are uncommon even in severe cases. When sequelae occur, they consist of focal cerebral or peripheral nerve deficits or ocular problems caused by persistent uveitis. Several patients have been reported with persistent renal abnormalities.

THERAPY AND PREVENTION. Tetracycline or doxycycline (in controlled trials) are both effective in shortening the course of anicteric leptospirosis when they are given in the first two to four days of illness. Their efficacy in reducing symptoms if given later has not been established. Therapeutic trials were done in populations with no mortality in the placebo group, so the effect of these drugs on mortality is unknown. Doxycycline therapy prevents leptospiruria in infected patients. If leptospiruria is necessary for the mediation of renal damage, as some investigators have speculated, then doxycycline may affect the development of renal failure or Weil's syndrome. Although activities in vitro have been demonstrated for penicillins, aminoglycosides, and erythromycin, they have not been studied in a controlled trial. Uncontrolled experience suggests that penicillin is effective. The balance of therapy in leptospirosis consists of careful attention to the details of care in patients with renal, hepatic, hematologic, and central nervous system complications.

Doxycycline, 100 mg once a week, will prevent leptospirosis in high-risk groups for three weeks. Efficacy in longer periods of exposure has not been evaluated. There are no leptospiral vaccines for humans in use, although effective vaccines for animals are available.

Edwards GA, Domm BM: Human leptospirosis. Medicine 39:117, 1960. *An extensive analysis of the clinical and laboratory features of leptospirosis with a review of early papers.*

Feigin RD, Anderson DC: Human leptospirosis. CRC Crit Rev Clin Lab Sci 5:413, 1975. *The most comprehensive review of leptospirosis, including history, microbiology, pathogenesis, clinical findings, and therapy.*

McClain JBL, Ballou WR, Harrison SH, Steinweg DR: Doxycycline therapy of leptospirosis. Ann Intern Med 100:696, 1984. *A description of therapeutic effects of doxycycline in therapy of leptospirosis.*

Takafuji ET, Kirkpatrick JW, Miller RN, Karwacki JJ, Kelly PW, Gray MR, McNeil KM, Timboc HL, Kane RE, Sanchez JL: An efficacy trial of doxycycline chemoprophylaxis against leptospirosis. N Engl J Med 310:497, 1984. *Demonstrates efficacy in American soldiers with placebo controls.*

Diseases Caused by Chlamydiae

312. INTRODUCTION

Walter E. Stamm

Due to their obligate intracellular growth cycle, chlamydiae were originally considered large viruses and were variously called *Bedsonia* or *TRIC* (for *trachoma-inclusion conjunctivitis*) agents. These terms have been discarded, and chlamydiae now constitute a separate order (Chlamydiales), family (Chlamydiaceae), and genus *(Chlamydia).* All members of the genus are obligate intracellular pathogens, but they more closely resemble bacteria than viruses in that they possess both deoxyribonucleic acid (DNA) and ribonucleic acid (RNA), divide by binary fission, have bacterial ribosomes and a cell wall not unlike that of Enterobacteriaceae, and can be inhibited by antibiotics. Compared with other bacteria, they have a small genome of 6 to 8 $\times$ 10^5 base pairs. They also lack adenosine triphosphate (ATP)–generating enzymes and hence depend entirely upon host cell metabolism for energy production.

The genus *Chlamydia* contains two species, *C. psittaci* and *C. trachomatis.* The former is a ubiquitous cause of infection in birds and lower mammals, with humans being occasional accidental hosts, while *C. trachomatis* infects humans and has no apparent natural animal hosts. Characteristically, *C. psittici* produces long lived, persistent infections of birds and mammals. Persistent infections caused by *C. trachomatis* in humans may also be common but have not been well documented. The two species can be readily differentiated in the laboratory in that *C. psittaci* forms diffuse intracytoplasmic inclusions that do not contain glycogen and thus do not stain with iodine, while *C. trachomatis* forms compact glycogen containing inclusions that readily stain with iodine. Sulfonamides inhibit growth of *C. psittaci* but not of *C. trachomatis*.

All chlamydiae possess a genus-specific, heat-stable lipopolysaccharide antigen that serves as the basis for the widely available complement fixation serologic test. Species- and immunotype-specific antigens have also been described and serve as the basis for subdividing *C. trachomatis* into 15 immunotypes using the microimmunofluorescence test of Wang and Grayston. Specific immunotypes tend to cause particular clinical syndromes. Types A, B, Ba, and C produce endemic trachoma (see Ch. 313). Types D, E, F, G, H, I, J, and K cause genital infections in adults (see Ch. 301) and ocular and respiratory infections in infants (see Ch. 63). Types L1 to L3 produce lymphogranuloma venereum (LGV) (see Ch. 303) and proctocolitis (see Ch. 104). LGV strains of *C. trachomatis* possess properties that distinguish them from non-LGV strains biologically, including more efficient cell entry and cell-to-cell infectivity in tissue culture, as well as mouse lethality upon intracerebral injection. A subtyping system for *C. psittaci* has not been developed.

Chlamydiae replicate by means of a unique life cycle unlike that of other bacteria. The 300-nM elementary body (the infective and extracellular form of a chlamydiae) initiates infection by attachment to specific receptors in the susceptible host cell's outer membrane. Subsequently, the elementary body enters the host cell by endocytosis. Within the resulting phagosome, the elementary body reorganizes within six hours into the larger 800- to 1000-nM and more metabolically active reticulate body. These reticulate bodies undergo repeated binary division until a large inclusion occupying much of the cell's cytoplasm and containing many reticulate bodies is formed. Reticulate bodies possess many ribosomes and synthesize DNA, RNA, proteins, and other molecules but cannot generate ATP. After 24 hours, some of the reticulate bodies condense to form compact elementary bodies in the mature inclusion, and the latter are released into the extracellular environment to begin the cycle anew.

C. trachomatis preferentially infects columnar epithelial cells, while *C. psittaci* has a broader host cell range, including macrophages. In most patients, *C. trachomatis* infections remain superficial, involving mucosal surfaces of the eye, nasopharynx, cervix, urethra, and rectum. Many of these infections produce few or no symptoms and tend to be subacute in nature and mild in terms of the signs they produce. Ascending infection of the endometrium, fallopian tube, liver capsule, epididymis, or lung produce more severe symptoms and signs and can be regarded as more extensive or invasive infections. LGV strains of *C. trachomatis* cause the most invasive disease, manifested either by proctocolitis or painful inguinal adenopathy and fever. *C. trachomatis* occasionally causes nongenital systemic infection, including culture-negative endocarditis, peritonitis, and pneumonia in adults.

Since many chlamydial infections produce either no symptoms or nonspecific symptoms and signs, laboratory confirmation of infection often must be sought. Available techniques include direct microscopic examination of tissue scrapings for typical inclusions or specific antigen, isolation of the organism, and assessment of antichlamydial antibody in serum or secretions. Cell culture techniques for cultivation of *C. trachomatis* have replaced the much more cumbersome isolation method using embryonated yolk sac. Widespread adoption of McCoy and HeLa 229 cell lines for isolation of *C. trachomatis* from patient secretions or biopsies has been a major factor contributing to recognition of the wide spectrum of infections caused by *C. trachomatis.* These cell lines require pretreatment with cyclohexamide and centrifugation of the inoculum onto the monolayer for efficient isolation of *C. trachomatis.* Inclusions formed in the cell culture monolayers can be visualized using iodine, Giemsa, or immunofluorescent staining procedures. Despite widespread use in research laboratories, cell culture procedures for isolation of *C. trachomatis* have not been generally available to clinicians because of the expense and technical difficulty. Lack of an available confirmatory diagnostic test has been a major factor contributing to the increasing incidence of genital and neonatal *C. trachomatis* infections in this country. Newer immunodiagnostic procedures that detect chlamydial antigen in patients' secretions are now being developed and many prove more useful than chlamydial culture for routine diagnostic purposes.

Chlamydial infection stimulates both a humoral and a cellular immune response, but neither appears to be completely protective against subsequent infection with either homologous or heterologous strains. Both local and systemic antibody can be demonstrated after acute infection, and immunoglobulin G (IgG) antibody neutralizes infective elementary bodies. In ocular infection, it has been advocated by some that the immune response actually participates in the disease process by producing continued inflammation. Serodiagnosis of chlamydial infections has limited applicability except in specific circumstances. The complement fixation test, available in most health department laboratories, should be used for confirmation of suspected psittacosis or LGV (see Ch. 20). The microimmunofluorescence test may be useful in the diagnosis of infant pneumonia (see Ch. 63), pelvic inflammatory disease, or Fitz-Hugh-Curtis syndrome but is available only in research laboratories. Uncomplicated genital infections evoke only low titer antibody responses, and acute infections cannot be easily distinguished from pre-existing antibody in many patients.

C. trachomatis infections can be treated with a variety of antimicrobial agents. Those agents with greatest demonstrated inhibitory activity in cell culture assays and in clinical studies include the tetracyclines (tetracycline HCl, doxycycline, and minocycline), erythromycin, sulfonamides, sulfamethoxazole-trimethoprim, chloramphenicol, and rifampin. The β-lactam antibiotics produce abnormal inclusions in cell culture and inhibit replication but have been largely ineffective in clinical treatment trials. The aminoglycosides, vancomycin, and spectinomycin have no activity against chlamydiae. In general, antibiotic therapy of chlamydial infections require 7 to 21 days of treatment; single-day regimens have been largely ineffective. Treatment failure usually indicates noncompliance, reinfection, or inadequate duration of drug therapy. Resistance to tetracycline or erythromycin has not been described.

313. TRACHOMA

Walter E. Stamm

C. trachomatis causes two epidemiologically distinct patterns of ocular infection. In endemic parts of the world, *C. trachomatis* immunotypes A, B, Ba, and C cause trachoma, a chronic eye disease that may lead to severe visual impairment or blindness. In nonendemic areas, immunotypes D through K produce a milder, self-limited conjunctivitis in infants born to mothers with cervical infection or in adults who acquire ocular infection after secondary spread from genital sites (see Ch. 63).

Since antiquity, trachomatous infection has been recognized in the Mediterranean basin and in the Orient, and it remains prevalent in Africa and Asia. Although the incidence has been decreasing over the last 30 years, more than 500 million persons have eye infections with chlamydiae, with millions blinded as a result. Trachoma flourishes in hot dry areas that have a shortage of available water and poor hygienic customs. Initial infection usually occurs in early childhood, and in certain parts of the world virtually the entire population is infected with chlamydiae before reaching adulthood. Repeated exposure to chlamydiae and the high prevalence of bacterial superinfection with *Hemophilus spp.*, pneumococci, staphylococci, and Enterobacteriaceae in these populations contribute to the severity of the resulting eye disease. In the United States, trachoma is occasionally seen on Indian reservations in the southwestern United States, in Mexican-Americans, and in immigrants from endemic areas, but such cases rarely result in major visual impairment, perhaps because bacterial superinfection is infrequent.

Persons with active trachoma shed chlamydiae in desquamated conjunctival cells, in conjunctival exudate, and in tears, which then may be transmitted by fingers, fomites, and perhaps flies. In endemic areas, transmission by these routes occurs through close personal contact, especially within family units and in groups of young children. Patients with early active infection shed more infective chlamydiae than those with chronic infection. However, even patients with long-term eye disease unaccompanied by signs of current activity may shed chlamydiae and thus serve as a source of infection.

Typical trachoma in children begins insidiously at about age two as a follicular conjunctivitis, most noticeable in the conjunctiva of the upper lid and the tarsal plate. Histologically, inclusion bodies appear within the conjunctival epithelial cells, polymorphonuclear leukocytes infiltrate the epithelium, and subepithelial lymphoid follicles develop. Reinfection is common during this period. Next the cornea becomes involved, with epithelial keratitis and subepithelial corneal infiltration resulting in opacities. Blood vessels from the limbus, accompanied by fibroblasts, invade the cornea to form a pannus. Progression of the inflammatory response leads to necrosis and scarring of the conjunctiva and gradual corneal vascularization from the upper limbus downward. Eventually a dense fibrovascular pannus extends over part or all of the cornea to grossly impair vision. Linear or stellate scars appear on the conjunctiva. Progressive scarring of the subepithelial tissues leads to deformation of the tarsal plate that results in entropion, trichiasis, and further corneal damage. Destruction of the conjunctival goblet cells and lacrimal ducts and gland produces xerosis. The latter changes often follow secondary bacterial infection, which may also produce corneal ulceration and accelerate loss of vision. Typically there are no systemic symptoms or signs of infection. The disease process evolves over about ten years in endemic areas but may be milder and more slowly progressive in other cases.

Adult inclusion conjunctivitis usually appears as an acute follicular conjunctivitis with preauricular lymphadenopathy. Untreated, it regresses slowly, but keratitis with marginal infiltrates, subepithelial opacities, and corneal neovascularization may develop in the conjunctiva. Unlike trachoma, adult inclusion conjunctivitis rarely impairs vision permanently.

The traditional diagnostic criteria for trachoma include lymphoid follicles on the upper tarsal plate, limbal follicles, typical conjunctival scars, and vascular pannus. Early in the disease the latter two can be detected only by slit lamp examination. The presence of any two of these features confirms the diagnosis. Laboratory confirmation of trachoma is based on (1) identification of typical inclusions in epithelial cells from a conjunctival swab or scraping (usually done by Giemsa or immunofluorescence staining); (2) cultivation of chlamydiae from a conjunctival specimen in cell culture; or (3) microimmunofluorescent antibody in high titer in tears. Approximately 20 to 60 per cent of children with early inflammatory trachoma have Giemsa-positive scrapings; higher yields result from cultures of chlamydiae.

In the differential diagnosis of ocular chlamydial infection, epidemic keratoconjunctivitis (usually caused by adenovirus type 8 or type 19), herpetic keratoconjunctivitis, Newcastle disease virus conjunctivitis, acute hemorrhagic conjunctivitis caused by enterovirus type 70 or coxsackievirus, reactions to allergens and irritating chemicals, and other bacterial causes of conjunctivitis must be considered. Some of these entities may coexist with chlamydial infections, and repeated ophthalmologic examinations and extensive laboratory evaluation may be required to establish a correct diagnosis.

Control of chronic trachoma in endemic areas has been attempted using tetracycline or erythromycin ointment in the eyes of all affected children in the community for 21 to 60 days. Oral administration of erythromycin has been used as an alternative. Antibiotic therapy usually suppresses clinical activity and chlamydial as well as bacterial growth but may not eradicate chlamydiae permanently. However, in endemic areas, repeated courses of drug treatment are beneficial because they reduce severity of eye disease and thus avoid progression toward blindness. Even one dose per month of doxycycline, 300 mg (2.5 to 4 mg per kilogram), can provide clinical benefit by converting severe to mild eye disease. Drug therapy has no influence on scars or pannus. Surgical correction is required in serious entropion or trichiasis. Topical corticosteroids and caustic substances have no place in therapy. For acute adult inclusion conjunctivitis, tetracycline HCl, 1.0 to 2.0 grams given orally daily in divided doses, or erythromycin, 1.0 to 2.0 grams given daily for two weeks, will successfully treat genital tract as well as ocular involvement. Sulfisoxazole, 4 grams daily, may also be effective. Sexual partners must be treated simultaneously in order to avoid reinfection.

The potential measures to prevent trachoma include efforts to increase the supply of water, practices to maintain cleanliness such as frequent handwashing and avoidance of use of common towels, and measures to reduce flies. It is also important to detect mild early infection in young children in endemic areas and to apply effective drug treatment repeatedly to prevent the blinding progression of the disease. Detection and treatment of adults who already have visual impairment probably can reduce the source of infection for children. Entire family groups or communities should be treated simultaneously. Efforts to prevent trachoma with a vaccine have been unsuccessful.

314. NEONATAL CHLAMYDIAL INFECTIONS

Walter E. Stamm

Between 5 and 22 per cent of pregnant women have *C. trachomatis* infection of the cervix, with neonatal infection occurring when the infant passes through the infected birth canal. Ascending intrauterine infection of the fetus has not been demonstrated. Shortly after birth, 30 to 50 per cent of infants born to infected mothers have cultural evidence of infection, 25 per cent manifest clinically apparent conjunctivitis, and 10 to 15 per cent acquire nasopharyngeal infection, which in some cases progresses to chlamydial neonatal pneumonitis. Otitis media and symptomatic nasopharyngitis may be caused by *C. trachomatis* in some infants.

Neonatal *C. trachomatis* inclusion conjunctivitis begins 5 to 14 days after birth. The infection must be differentiated from gonococcal ophthalmia (which has a shorter incubation period of 1 to 3 days) and from other common causes of neonatal conjunctivitis (*S. pneumoniae, H. influenzae, S. aureus*, and group D streptococci). Typical manifestations include lid and conjunctival swelling, mucopurulent ocular discharge, conjunctival hyperemia, and membrane formation. Untreated, the disease persists 3 to 12 months but usually heals without sequelae. Rarely, conjunctival scarring and corneal neovascularization occur. Neonates with inclusion conjunctivitis frequently have concomitant chlamydial infection of the nasopharynx, rectum, urethra, and vagina, usually without associated clinical manifestations at these sites.

The diagnosis can be rapidly established by demonstration of chlamydial inclusions in conjunctival scrapings stained by Giemsa or immunofluorescence. Cultures for *C. trachomatis* can also be used if available and will be positive in some smear-negative cases. Tear antibody to *C. trachomatis* can be demonstrated in most cases, but the test is not readily available.

Silver nitrate drops instilled at birth do not prevent chlamydial inclusion conjunctivitis and in some instances cause chemical conjunctivitis. For this reason, many health departments now recommend prophylactic use of erythromycin ointment at birth. However, topical erythromycin prophylaxis does not cure concomitant nasopharyngeal or rectal infection. Perhaps a better preventive approach would be screening and treatment of pregnant women for *C. trachomatis* infection before term. This approach essentially appears to eliminate *C. trachomatis* infections in neonates and should be the strategy of choice when cultures are available.

Since many infants with inclusion conjunctivitis have concomitant nasopharyngeal, rectal, and vaginal *C. trachomatis* infection, systemic rather than topical therapy should be used. In addition, relapses often follow topical therapy. Erythromycin, 40 to 50 mg per kilogram per day in four divided doses for 14 to 21 days, cures more than 80 per cent of cases. Both parents should be examined for *C. trachomatis* infection and should be treated with tetracycline or erythromycin (for nursing mothers) if cultures are not available.

Approximately 10 per cent of infants born to infected mothers develop a distinctive subacute chlamydial pneumonia between the first and fourth months of life. Typically, tachypnea, a stacatto cough, inspiratory rales, elevated serum globulin concentrations, and eosinophilia are seen but fever is absent. Hyperinflated lungs with scattered interstitial infiltrates are evident on chest x-ray examination. The disease lasts for weeks to months but is mild in most infants and will resolve without specific therapy. However, marked hypoxemia and apnea have been reported in some cases. Lung biopsies have demonstrated chlamydial inclusions, alveoli with inflammatory exudate, and a lymphocytic interstitial infiltration of the bronchial submucosa. In some cases, *C. trachomatis* have been recovered from lung tissue. Diagnosis in most instances can be suspected on clinical grounds and confirmed by the demonstration of chlamydial inclusions on Giemsa or immunofluorescent stained smears of the conjunctivae or nasopharynx. If available, *C. trachomatis* should be sought by cell culture of eye scrapings, nasopharyngeal swabs, or rectal swabs. Rising high titer immunoglobulin M (IgM) microimmunofluorescent antibody to *C. trachomatis* can be demonstrated in the majority of infants with pneumonia. Erythromycin, 50 mg per kilogram per day in four divided doses for 14 to 21 days, has been recommended for treatment of infant pneumonia, although there are no control trials demonstrating the benefits of this regimen.

Holmes KK: The chlamydia epidemic. JAMA 245:1718, 1981.
Mardh PA, Holmes KK, Oriel JD, Piot P, Schachter J (eds.): Chlamydial Infections. New York, Elsevier Science Publishing Company, Inc., 1982.
Schachter J, Caldwell HD: Chlamydiae. Ann Rev Microbiol 34:285, 1980.

315. PSITTACOSIS (Ornithosis, Parrot Fever)

William Schaffner

DEFINITION. Psittacosis is an infection of birds that is produced by *Chlamydia psittaci*. When transmitted to man, this agent can produce asymptomatic infection, a transient influenza-like illness, or serious pneumonic disease characterized by high fever, headache, cough, myalgia, and pulmonary infiltrates.

HISTORY. In 1879, Ritter, a Swiss physician, described seven cases of an unusual pneumonia that occurred after contact with tropical birds. Morange, in 1894, established the parrot as a vector and termed the disease *psittacosis* after the Greek *psittakos* (the parrot). Bedson demonstrated the filterable agent in 1930. Over 90 species of birds can harbor the agent, and it has a worldwide distribution.

ETIOLOGY. *C. psittaci* is an obligate intracellular bacterium morphologically and serologically related to the agents of lymphogranuloma venereum and trachoma. Parrots and parakeets are common carriers and until recently represented the major source of human infection. With better control of psittacine disease in aviaries, other birds now contribute more human infections. Cases have resulted from contact with turkeys, pigeons, ducks, and other fowl. Persons working with birds are at greatest risk, notably pet shop employees, pigeon handlers, and poultry workers, especially in turkey processing plants. There is no risk associated with eating poultry products.

The agent is present in the blood, tissue, feathers, and discharges of infected birds. Although the avian disease can be fatal, infected birds frequently show only minimal evidence of illness, such as ruffled feathers, lethargy, diarrhea, and failure to eat. Birds having active infections are most likely to transmit the disease, but asymptomatic carriers are common, and birds can shed transmissible agent for months.

Psittacosis is generally acquired by the respiratory route through inhalation of infected dried bird excreta or by handling of infected birds. Mouth-to-beak intimacies have led to infection in humans. Cases have been reported after only brief exposure to birds, and 20 per cent of patients can show no history of exposure to birds. Person-to-person transmission of psittacosis is rare. These cases of "human strain" psittacosis have been severe, with high mortality.

PATHOLOGY. In birds, the principal sites of disease are the liver, spleen, and pericardium. In man, the lung is most commonly involved. The psittacosis agent gains access to the human body via the respiratory route, rapidly enters the blood, and reaches the reticuloendothelial cells of the liver and spleen. After replication in these sites, invasion of the lung is by hematogenous spread. The mature pulmonary lesion is a lobular pneumonitis. The process is initiated by inflammation and progressive edema of the alveoli. Exudation is often accompanied by small hemorrhages, accounting for clinical hemoptysis. Thick, gelatinous plugs of mucus may fill major and minor bronchi and account for the severe cyanosis and progressive anoxia seen in fatal cases. Foci of necrosis may occur in more severely affected areas of the lung and are sometimes associated with capillary thrombi. The process is generally most severe in dependent bronchopulmonary segments. Large monocytes and macrophages containing cytoplasmic inclusion bodies, which represent the agent (LCL bodies), are characteristic. Hyperplasia and monocytic infiltration of pulmonary and hilar lymph nodes and splenic enlargement with occasional areas of focal necrosis occurs. Rarely the liver shows intralobular focal necrosis and swollen Kupffer cells containing the psittacosis elementary bodies. Changes in the myocardium, heart valves, pericardium, meninges, brain, adrenal glands, pancreas, and kidneys have been reported.

CLINICAL MANIFESTATIONS. Wide variations can occur in the clinical picture. The incubation period ranges from 7 to 15 days but may be longer. Asymptomatic or mild influenza-like infections probably are the rule. Moderate or severe infections, although less frequent, are more commonly diagnosed. The onset of illness may be insidious, but it often starts with chills and a fever that rises slowly to 39 to 40.5° C during the first week of illness. As with some other instances of intracellular infection, the pulse may be slow relative to the level of the fever. Headache is severe. Malaise, anorexia, nausea, vomiting, severe myalgias, particularly in the neck and back, and arthralgias are common. Cough is generally prominent but may be delayed until late in the first week. Small amounts of mucoid sputum with occasional blood streaking are the rule. Changes in mentation are often seen. Delirium or stupor may occur in severe cases toward the end of the first week, and usually are associated with severe pulmonary involvement, cyanosis, and other evidences of anoxia. Other neurologic manifestations are uncommon. A macular rash (Horder's spots) resembling that seen in typhoid has occasionally been described. Jaundice and progressive nitrogen retention have been reported in severe cases. Severe dyspnea, tachypnea, tachycardia, cyanosis, jaundice, delirium, and stupor are all poor prognostic signs.

The physical findings of pneumonia are usually sparse. Chest roentgenograms often reveal infiltrates not detected at the bedside. Examination may reveal only fever, painful muscle groups, an elevated respiratory rate, and a relative bradycardia. Fine, crepitant rales may be heard in localized areas over the lungs, but true consolidation is less common. Pleurisy with effusion can occur but is unusual. Mild hepatomegaly is frequent. A palpable spleen has been noted in a substantial number of patients. Splenomegaly in a patient with undiagnosed acute pneumonitis should raise the consideration of psittacosis. An erythematous pharynx may be noted. In rare instances there may be signs of pericarditis or myocarditis. In prolonged, severe illness, thrombophlebitis and pulmonary infarction have been reported as late complications.

Patients with mild cases may recover in seven days. More severe infections may last 12 to 21 days without specific treatment. Fever is ordinarily sustained or remittent and, when accompanied by bradycardia, resembles the fever of untreated typhoid infections. Defervescence is generally slow, and a prolonged convalescence is common. Relapses have been reported even after appropriate treatment. Reinfections have been described. Occasional cases of endocarditis caused by *C. psittaci* in patients with sterile blood cultures have been described.

LABORATORY FINDINGS. Simple laboratory studies are not helpful in establishing a diagnosis. The leukocyte count is usually normal or slightly elevated. The erythrocyte sedimentation rate is generally elevated. Chest roentgenograms generally show soft patchy infiltrates radiating outward from the hilum, which tend to be more prominent in dependent lobes or segments. Occasionally diffuse miliary, nodular, or frank lobar distribution of infiltrates is seen.

A specific diagnosis can be made only by isolation of the agent or by serologic studies. The agent is present in the blood and sputum during the first two to three weeks, but isolation is hazardous and should not be attempted except in special laboratories. Diagnosis is generally made by a four-fold rise in complement-fixing antibodies. A significant change in antibody titers is generally present by the twelfth to fourteenth day of disease; the titers are usually maximal by 30 days, then slowly wane. Treatment can delay or suppress antibody response. A serum complement-fixation titer of 1:32 during the acute illness is presumptive evidence of psittacosis. There is considerable cross-reaction between antigens prepared from psittacosis and lymphogranuloma venereum agents. False-positive complement-fixation tests may occur with Q fever, brucellosis, or legionnaires' disease.

DIFFERENTIAL DIAGNOSIS. Specific diagnosis of psittacosis is of extreme importance because of its potential severity, its response to antimicrobials, and the public health significance of psittacosis infection. All cases should be reported to the local health department. The syndrome of viral pneumonia accompanied by protracted high fever, unusually severe headache, and relative bradycardia should suggest psittacosis. Often a history of contact with birds is the only clue to diagnosis and may be elicited only by repeated questioning of the patient and family. When pneumonic symptoms are prominent, psittacosis must be differentiated from legionnaires' disease, viral pneumonias, mycoplasmal pneumonia, influenza, Q fever, tularemia, tuberculosis, fungal infection, and bacterial pneumonia distal to an obstructed bronchus. If pneumonic symptoms are not prominent, psittacosis can be confused with other systemic febrile illnesses such as typhoid fever, brucellosis, infectious mononucleosis, infectious hepatitis, miliary tuberculosis, or the viral meningoencephalitides.

TREATMENT. The tetracyclines are the drugs of choice, and early diagnosis and initiation of treatment may be lifesaving. After institution of therapy with 2 to 3 grams daily, both fever and symptoms are generally controlled within 48 to 72 hours, although the response may be indolent. Although the disease apparently responds to penicillin in doses above 2 million units daily and to erythromycin, tetracycline remains the drug of choice. Treatment should be continued for at least 10 days after defervescence to prevent relapse. With treatment, mortality rates as low as 1 to 5 per cent can be achieved.

Byrom NP, Walls J, Mair HJ: Fulminant psittacosis. Lancet 1:353, 1979. *The difficulty in differentiating psittacosis and legionnaires' disease at the bedside is emphasized.*

Jariwalla AG, Davies BH, White J: Infective endocarditis complicating psittacosis: Response to rifampicin. Br Med J 1:155, 1980. *Endocarditis caused by psittacosis is reviewed concisely.*

Macfarlane JT, Macrae AD: Psittacosis. Br Med Bull 39:163, 1983. *A well written review.*

Schaffner W, Drutz DJ, Duncan GW, Koenig MG: The clinical spectrum of endemic psittacosis. Arch Intern Med 119:433, 1967. *Good descriptions of clinical presentations.*

Rickettsial Diseases

316. INTRODUCTION

Charles L. Wisseman, Jr.

The diseases commonly referred to as the rickettsial diseases of man consist of several clinical entities, usually acute, self-limited fevers, caused by bacteria of the family Rickettsiaceae. They fall naturally into the typhus-like diseases (typhus groups, spotted fever group, and scrub typhus group), Q fever, and trench fever. The typhus-like diseases are caused by organisms of the genus *Rickettsia;* Q fever by *Coxiella burnetii;* and trench fever by *Rochalimaea quintana.*

Organisms of the *Rickettsia, Coxiella,* and *Rochalimaea* genera, although very different in many respects, are very small bacteria with a gram-negative bacterium-like cell wall, bacterial type internal structure (typical prokaryotic DNA arrangement with a genome size roughly equivalent to that of *Neisseria;* ribosomes), often a slime layer or microcapsule, and a substantial independent metabolic activity. Organisms of the genus *Rickettsia* and *Coxiella burnetii* are obligate intracellular parasites, i.e., they are known to grow only within eukaryotic host cells. *Rochalimaea quintana* can be grown on cell-free medium and grows extracellularly in the louse gut. All organisms of the genus *Rickettsia* have the capacity to penetrate through the host cell plasma membrane into the cytoplasm, can cause host cell lysis from without, and multiply by binary fission free in the host cell cytoplasm not surrounded by a vacuolar membrane. Different species vary in their capacity to interact with other host cell membranes. Thus members of the spotted fever group can penetrate into the host cell nucleus, and these, as well as *R. mooseri,* can escape through the plasma membrane without requiring complete host cell destruction as does *R. prowazekii. Coxiella burnetii* enters host cells passively by endocytosis and grows within a membrane-bound vacuole. These differences in action on host cell membranes are probably related to differences in disease patterns (host response) and immune mechanisms. Active penetration of host cells appears to be correlated with mouse lethal toxic action, hemolytic properties, and phospholipase action. Members of the genus *Rickettsia* that have been studied and *Coxiella burnetii* also have endotoxins similar in physiologic action to those of gram-negative bacilli.

All rickettsioses are transmitted by arthropod vectors, although Q fever is usually acquired from domestic animals (Table 316–1). With the exception of louse-borne typhus and trench fevers, in which man is the key vertebrate host and reservoir, all the rickettsioses are zoonoses, existing in a natural cycle involving arthropods (vectors and in some cases reservoirs) and vertebrate (usually mammalian) hosts. In these, man acquires the disease by accidentally intruding into the natural cycle and is a "dead-end" host not sustaining the infection cycle. The reservoir mechanism varies considerably among the rickettsioses. The nonsterile immunity in the vertebrate host, with persisting infection and potential or proved capacity for recrudescence, appears to be important in louse-borne typhus and trench fever, in which the main reservoir is man. In these infections, the vector (the human body louse) does not transmit the organism transovarially to the next generation, and, in the case of louse-borne typhus, the infection in the louse vector is almost invariably fatal to the louse in a week or two. On the other hand, in tick-, mite-, and chigger-borne rickettsioses, the organism is efficiently transmitted transovarially to succeeding generations, a process which probably constitutes the main reservoir mechanism, whereas the vertebrate infection serves only an amplifying role in some instances. *Coxiella burnetii,* possibly originally tick-borne, is sustained by vertical passage in its vertebrate host (e.g., sheep, cattle) by virtue of its capacity to multiply to phenomenal levels in placental tissues and to be excreted in milk.

Thus, although they are commonly lumped together under the "rickettsial diseases of man," and possess some points in common, there are major differences in the biologic properties of the organisms involved, in their interactions with host cells, and in their natural infection cycles and reservoir mechanisms. However, some similarities in cell tropism and the restricted ways in which man responds to injury have conspired to produce a group of clinical entities with many to few common features.

PATHOGENESIS, PATHOLOGY, IMMUNITY. Since the human diseases caused by members of the genus *Rickettsia* share many common features, it is convenient to consider here pathogenesis and immunity in a generalized framework.

The route of infection is frequently through the skin, injected through the vector mouth parts in tick-, mite-, and chigger-

TABLE 316–1. SUMMARY OF SOME EPIDEMIOLOGIC FEATURES OF SELECTED RICKETTSIAL DISEASES OF MAN

Disease	Organism	Natural Cycle: Arthropod Vector	Natural Cycle: Reservoir/Mammalian Host	Usual Mode of Transmission to Man	Common Occupational or Environmental Association	Geographic Distribution
Typhus group						
Murine typhus	*Rickettsia mooseri (R. typhi)*	Flea	Rodents	Infected flea feces into broken skin or aerosol to mucous membranes	Rat-infected premises (shops, warehouses, grain elevators)	Scattered foci, worldwide
Epidemic typhus	*R. prowazekii*	Body louse	Man*	Infected crushed louse or feces into broken skin or aerosol to mucous membranes	Lousy human population with louse transfer	Worldwide
Brill-Zinsser disease	*R. prowazekii*	Recrudescence months to years after primary attack of louse-borne typhus			Unknown; ?stress	Worldwide
Spotted fever group (selected examples)						
Rocky Mountain spotted fever	*R. rickettsii*	Ixodid ticks	Ticks/small mammals	Tick bite, mechanical transfer to mucous membranes, ?airborne	Tick-infested terrain, houses, dogs	Western Hemisphere
Boutonneuse fever	*R. conorii*	Ixodid ticks	Ticks/rodents, dogs	Tick bite	Tick-infested terrain, houses, dogs	Mediterranean littoral, Africa, ?Indian subcontinent
Rickettsialpox	*R. akari*	Mouse mite	Mite/mice	Mouse mite bite	Unique mouse- and mite-infested premises (incinerators)	United States, U.S.S.R., Korea, ?Central Africa
Scrub typhus						
Tsutsugamushi disease	*R. tsutsugamushi* (multiple serotypes)	Chigger	Chigger/?rodents	Chigger bite	Chigger-infested terrain; secondary scrub, grass airfields, golf courses	Asia, Australia, New Guinea, Pacific islands
Q fever	*Coxiella burnetii*	?Ticks	Ticks/mammals	Inhalation of dried airborne infective material; ?tick bite	Domestic animals or products, dairies, lambing pens, slaughterhouses	Worldwide
Trench fever	*Rochalimaea quintana*	Body louse	Man	Infected crushed louse or feces into broken skin; ?aerosol to mucous membranes	Lousy human population with louse transfer	Africa, Mexico, ?South America, ?Eastern Europe

*Recent isolations of putative *R. prowazekii* from flying squirrels in the eastern United States have not been evaluated as reservoirs for human infection. Previous claims of involvement of domestic animals are now largely discounted.

borne rickettsioses and by contamination of broken skin by infected louse or flea feces in louse-borne typhus and murine typhus, respectively. Airborne rickettsiae in dried louse or flea feces may initiate airborne infection through the respiratory tract or conjunctiva. Aerosols of all rickettsiae are highly infectious via the respiratory tract.

Some local proliferation undoubtedly occurs at the inoculation site with all *Rickettsia* species. In some (e.g., scrub typhus, rickettsialpox, fièvre boutonneuse), a visible lesion (the *eschar*) develops at the inoculation site during the incubation period. Regional lymphadenopathy (as in scrub typhus) suggests lymphatic spread, whereas demonstration of rickettsiae in endothelial cells of small blood vessels at the inoculation site opens the possibility of early hematogenous dissemination. Patent rickettsemia probably appears only late in the incubation period, is regularly present at onset, and persists throughout the febrile period of disease despite the appearance of humoral antibodies by about the end of the first week of disease.

Disseminated focal infection of the small blood vessels (capillaries, arterioles, and venules) of the skin, and, to a lesser but significant extent, in other organs such as brain, lung, heart, and kidneys, is the single most important known pathophysiologic feature of these diseases. Thus, at focal points in the small blood vessels, rickettsiae infect, multiply in, and damage endothelial cells with cell necrosis, hypertrophy, and proliferation. Infection is limited to the endothelial cells in typhus and scrub typhus infections but may extend to all layers in Rocky Mountain spotted fever, causing necrosis of the media (Table 316–2). At the sites of endothelial damage, platelet-fibrin thrombi tend to form, which, along with endothelial hypertrophy and proliferation, partially or completely occlude vascular lumen. A typical perivascular inflammatory response develops, with polymorphonuclear and monocytic cells early and macrophages, lymphocytes, and occasional plasma cells later, coinciding approximately temporally with antibody response, suggesting the possibility of superimposition of a vascular immunopathologic component. This sequence suggests that a typical rickettsial infection evolves through an *early phase,* in which vascular damage is primarily the direct result of rickettsial infection, and a *late phase,* in which additional vascular damage is produced by immunologic mechanisms. The latter is unproved, but is consistent with the fact that in typhus and scrub typhus infections patients appear more "toxic" in this late phase and show greater vascular instability, and most deaths occur in the period *after* antibodies are demonstrable. On the other hand, the greater severity of vascular lesions and frequent deaths without detectable antibodies in early fatal cases of Rocky Mountain spotted fever suggest that direct rickettsia-induced vascular damage alone can initiate irreversible pathophysiologic changes.

The disseminated vascular lesions can account for many of the clinical and pathophysiologic abnormalities seen in these

TABLE 316–2. RICKETTSIA TARGET CELL RELATIONSHIPS, PATHOLOGIC LESIONS, AND CLINICAL MANIFESTATIONS OF HUMAN RICKETTSIOSES*

Disease	Target Cell	Host-Cell Association	Basic Lesion	Clinical Manifestations
Typhus-like fevers				
Typhus group	Endothelial	Free intracytoplasmic	Vasculitis	Acute self-limited fever
Scrub typhus	Endothelial	Free intracytoplasmic	Vasculitis	Acute self-limited fever
Spotted fever group	Endothelial, smooth muscle	Free intracytoplasmic and intranuclear	Vasculitis	Acute self-limited fever
Q fever	Reticuloendothelial	Intracytoplasmic vacuole	Granulomas	Acute self-limited fever, "atypical pneumonia," subacute hepatitis, subacute endocarditis
Trench fever	Unknown	Pericellular (in louse and cell culture)	Unknown	Recurring febrile episodes

*Adapted from Strickland (ed.): *Hunter's Tropical Medicine.* Philadelphia, W. B. Saunders Company, 1984.

infections, viz., rash, edema and increased extravascular fluid space, hypotension, and gangrene (in louse-borne typhus and Rocky Mountain spotted fever), as well as the clotting abnormalities (up to disseminated intravascular clotting), which have been recognized in several rickettsial diseases. The classic "typhus nodules" in the brain, most frequent in the midbrain and nuclear areas, are of the same vascular origin and help explain the mental changes and cranial nerve deficits. In Rocky Mountain spotted fever, discrete microinfarcts also may occur in the central nervous system with persisting electroencephalographic change. The heart often shows, in addition to the typical perivascular lesions, some edema, a diffuse mononuclear infiltrate of unknown origin, and a minor amount of muscle necrosis. Nonspecific electrocardiographic changes are common. Despite the dramatic histologic appearance of the heart, limited studies during World War II suggested that cardiac function was not impaired. This matter should be reinvestigated. Indeed, myocarditis has been suggested as a cause of death in Rocky Mountain spotted fever. Typical perivascular lesions occur in the portal areas of the liver, along with nonspecific focal areas of fatty degeneration in hepatocytes. However, the origin of abnormal blood transaminase levels remains unknown. The kidneys also show focal interstitial vascular lesions involving a few nephrons. The characteristic oliguria and azotemia of typhus have been attributed in the past to prerenal causes, e.g., hypotension, tissue catabolism, but evidence for transient immune complex disease should be sought by modern methods. The lungs show a variable degree of interstitial type pneumonitis on histologic examination and by x-ray regardless of route of infection. Cough is a common early clinical manifestation, but physical signs are scant.

Immunity to the infecting rickettsial strain following recovery from infection tends to be solid and longlasting but of a nonsterile type, i.e., the rickettsiae are not entirely eradicated and may remain "latent" for months to many years. The bases for immunity are not yet completely understood. An antibody response is detectable around the end of the first week of disease, but this does not cause an immediate control of rickettsemia. Cell-mediated immunity also develops, but the kinetics of its evolution in man have not yet been clearly documented. Laboratory studies suggest that both antibody-mediated and cell-mediated mechanisms contribute to immunity.

GENERAL CLINICAL DIAGNOSTIC CONSIDERATIONS. In classic form, the typhus-like rickettsial diseases (typhus group, spotted fever group, and scrub typhus group) display many common clinical features, which may vary in degree and in detail, e.g., fever, headache, cough, prostration, rash, altered mental state, hypotension, normal to low white blood count (Table 316–3). *Especially at the onset,* however, the signs and symptoms are those common to many acute infectious diseases, differential

TABLE 316–3. SOME CLINICAL FEATURES OF SELECTED RICKETTSIAL DISEASES

Disease	Usual Incubation Period (Days)	Eschar	Rash			Usual Duration of Disease* (Days)	Usual Severity†	Fever After Chemotherapy (Hours)
			Onset, Day of Disease	*Distribution*	*Type*			
Typhus group								
Murine typhus	12 (8–16)	None	5–7	Trunk → extremities	Macular, maculopapular	12 (8–16)	Moderate	48–72
Epidemic typhus	12 (10–14)	None	5–7	Trunk → extremities	Macular, maculopapular, petechial	14 (10–18)	Severe	48–72
Brill-Zinsser disease	—	None		Trunk → extremities	Macular	7–11	Relatively mild	48–72
Spotted fever group								
Rocky Mountain spotted fever	7 (3–12)	None	3–5	Extremities → trunk, face	Macular, maculopapular, petechial	16 (10–20)	Severe	72
Boutonneuse fever	5–7	Often present	3–4	Trunk, extremities, face, palms, soles	Macular, maculopapular, petechial	10 (7–14) 7	Moderate	—
Rickettsialpox	?9–17	Often present	1–3	Trunk → face, extremities	Papulovesicular	7 (3–11)	Relatively mild	—
Scrub typhus (tsutsugamushi disease)	1–12 (9–18)	Often present	4–6	Trunk → extremities	Macular, maculopapular	14 (10–20)	Mild to severe	24–36
Q fever	10–19	None		None		6 (2–21)	Relatively‡ mild	48 (occasionally slow)

*Untreated disease.
†Severity can vary greatly.
‡Occasional subacute infections occur (e.g., hepatitis, endocarditis).

clinical diagnosis is difficult, and specific laboratory diagnostic methods are limited. Sometimes an early sign, such as an eschar, which is variable even in the rickettsioses in which it occurs, is helpful. Later, rash, hypotension, changes in mental state, and the like may give clues. But rickettsioses vary in severity, and not all cases are classic. Moreover, in many areas, other infectious diseases exist which are confusing clinically, especially in that early period when the correct choice of chemotherapy may be lifesaving (as with Rocky Mountain spotted fever, meningococcemia, or cerebral malaria). Hence, one must be acutely sensitive to the different possibilities in one's area of practice and must devise a kind of strategy for the diagnosis and management, sometimes empirically on the basis of probabilities, of a rickettsia-like disease, using all available bits of epidemiologic, clinical, and laboratory information. Simple observation of the patient for the development of diagnostic clinical or laboratory features is a hazardous practice. In the United States, the single major factor contributory to the continuing 5 to 10 per cent mortality in Rocky Mountain spotted fever is delay in institution of specific chemotherapy. Listed below are some practical considerations that have emerged from analysis of experiences in several parts of the world.

The history of potential exposure (occupation, travel in endemic areas, recreational activities in wilderness areas), as well as of tick bite, is extremely important in alerting the physician to the possibility of a rickettsial disease. Modern air travel makes it possible to return from any part of the world within the incubation period of a rickettsial disease.

In a given area, certain diseases commonly cause difficult clinical differential diagnostic problems. For example, in the United States, the two diseases most commonly confused with Rocky Mountain spotted fever are measles and meningococcemia. In central and east Africa, two diseases which cause major differential diagnostic problems with louse-borne typhus are cerebral falciparum malaria and typhoid fever. Milder cases of typhus may be indistinguishable clinically from influenza. Patients with murine typhus fever commonly are found on enteric fever wards.

The most sophisticated modern laboratory diagnostic aids can sometimes help distinguish within hours between measles, meningococcemia, and Rocky Mountain spotted fever. Blood smears for malaria should be routine where malaria and rickettsial diseases coexist. Typhoid can be detected by cultures. Outside the United States and Europe, however, laboratory facilities may be unavailable, and an empirical therapeutic approach is often successful. For example, when it is not possible to distinguish between malaria, typhus, and typhoid, a combination of chloramphenicol and chloroquine, or other antimalarial appropriate for the resistance patterns of the area, often gives a satisfactory clinical response; or a "typhus suspect" not responding in 48 hours to a tetracycline drug can often be treated successfully with chloramphenicol.

Finally, outside the United States, a patient with a rickettsial infection may have another concurrent infection, e.g., typhus plus relapsing fever or trench fever; or typhus or scrub typhus plus malaria, bacterial pneumonia, or dysentery. These must also be diagnosed and treated specifically.

LABORATORY DIAGNOSIS. Methods for retrospective diagnoses (isolation of organism and serologic response) of rickettsial infections are reasonably well developed, although not universally available, but methods for specific diagnosis in the acute phase of disease, when crucial decisions about specific chemotherapy must be made, are generally unsatisfactory although improving. The following guidelines have been compiled especially for the practicing physician, beginning with methods applicable to the early, acute phase and proceeding to more specific methods, which sometimes tend to be only confirmatory or retrospective.

Exclusion of Diseases That Present Common Differential Diagnostic Problems in a Given Locality. Examples include malaria smear, skin lesion smear for meningococci, demonstration of measles antigen in respiratory epithelial cells by fluorescence microscopy, and cultures for typhoid and other enteric fevers.

Direct Demonstration of Rickettsiae in Tissues or Rickettsial Antigens in Urine in Acute Phase of Disease. Attempts to demonstrate rickettsiae directly in tissues or cells of patients and to demonstrate rickettsial antigens in body fluids, such as urine, have been explored for many years with variable degrees of success, although no method is yet available for routine diagnosis.

Direct Microscopic Demonstration of Rickettsiae in Tissues. For diagnostic purposes, rickettsiae have been demonstrated in endothelial cells of skin biopsies, blood leukocytes (with or without a short period of incubation in vitro), and bone marrow smears in typhus and spotted fever infections of man or animals. The use of fluorescein-conjugated antisera permits identification of the organisms, specific at least to group. Refinement and standardization of these methods promise to yield practical routine methods for the early specific diagnosis of rickettsial infections and should be pursued vigorously.

Demonstration of Rickettsial Antigens in Acute Phase Urine. Although theoretically feasible, reliable demonstration of rickettsial antigens in acute phase urine has been fraught with difficulty. Application of modern immunologic methods (radioimmunoassay, enzyme-linked immunosorbent assay [ELISA]) may improve sensitivity, specificity, and reliability and deserves concerted effort.

Isolation of Rickettsiae. The isolation of rickettsiae from the blood or tissues of a patient is hazardous, requires special laboratory facilities and trained personnel, usually does not yield results in time to influence patient management, and hence, was not encouraged as a routine procedure in the past. However, methods are improving, and moreover, it is now urgent to change this position because serologic retrospective diagnoses are ill equipped to identify new species or variants of rickettsiae. A growing diversity of rickettsial agents (e.g., the flying squirrel agent and *R. canada* in the typhus group, new members of the spotted fever group) is being recognized in the United States and elsewhere, whose importance as causes of human disease remains unknown; this is partly because conventional serologic tests for retrospective diagnosis are largely *group* specific, might not recognize variants at the species level, and would not detect infections with totally new agents. Isolation and characterization of the agent are the keystones of identification of new diseases.

Although isolation and identification of rickettsial agents are usually beyond the competence of the ordinary hospital laboratory, mechanisms do exist for accomplishing this. In the United States, properly collected and preserved specimens (frozen at $-70°$ C or lower) can be sent through state health departments to the Centers for Disease Control in Atlanta, Georgia, where trained personnel and facilities exist to handle and characterize such agents. Also, the World Health Organization has established a series of reference laboratories that are capable of handling such agents.

Serologic Diagnosis. Serologic methods remain the mainstay of routine laboratory diagnosis of rickettsial infections and for epidemiologic purposes. However, since an antibody response rarely occurs with any of the rickettsioses before the end of the first week of disease, and since a rise in antibody titer is more or less essential to a solid diagnosis, convincing serologic diagnosis may become available only *after* the critical point has been passed with respect to lifesaving decisions about chemotherapy. At present, serologic tests consist of (1) nonspecific (Weil-Felix) tests generally available to hospital laboratories through commercially produced antigens (a part of the "febrile agglutinin" package) and (2) more specific tests, generally available at state health departments, the Centers for Disease Control, and the WHO reference laboratories.

In those rickettsioses studied, antibody response following

primary infection consists of an early transient IgM response and a slower more persistent IgG response. Recrudescent typhus (Brill-Zinsser disease) is characterized by a brisk IgG response with low to negligible IgM response. Antibodies persist for many years following louse-borne and murine typhus but fall to low or negligible levels two to three years after scrub typhus and uncomplicated Q fever. Persistent high titers with Phase I *C. burnetii* antigen suggest subacute infection, e.g., hepatitis or endocarditis.

WEIL-FELIX REACTION. Based upon unique sharing of polysaccharide antigens between certain *Proteus* strains and some rickettsiae, this agglutination test performed with suspensions of rough *Proteus* OX-2, OX-19, and OX-K strains has an historical aura and the advantage of simplicity, ready availability of antigens, and sensitivity to early antibody response.

Proteus agglutinins tend to appear early (toward the end of the first week), attain peak titers between three and four weeks after onset, and then rapidly decline. The Weil-Felix test is not positive in all rickettsial infections (rickettsialpox and Q fever) and is variable in recrudescent typhus (Brill-Zinsser disease). It will not distinguish between typhus and spotted fever group infections (*Proteus* OX-2 and OX-190). *Proteus* OX-K agglutination is not positive in all scrub typhus infections (about 70 per cent positive in primary infections and fewer in secondary infections) but may yield false positive results in relapsing fever and leptospirosis. Nevertheless, properly applied and interpreted, the test can be useful. Until more specific tests are generally available to physicians within a time frame useful for patient management, the Weil-Felix test, despite its deficiencies, will not die.

INDIRECT FLUORESCENT ANTIBODY TESTS (IFA). IFA tests are now generally used for diagnostic and epidemiologic purposes. They are sensitive and useful with anticomplementary sera or blood collected on filter paper. IFA tests may be positive when blocking factors interfere with CF or MA tests. They can be made group specific. Methods for improved species differentiation are under study. IgG, IgM, and IgA antibody titers can be determined directly. The IFA test is currently the most sensitive and reliable test available for the diagnosis of scrub typhus.

OTHER TESTS. Complement fixation and microliter agglutination tests, formerly the mainstay of rickettsial serodiagnosis and still useful, have been displaced by the IFA test. Toxin neutralization tests, passive hemagglutination tests, and radioimmune precipitation tests have special uses. New tests, such as the ELISA type test and latex agglutination tests, are under development and evaluation.

TREATMENT OF RICKETTSIAL DISEASES. The general principles of therapy are similar for all the common rickettsial diseases. Optimal management includes (1) specific antimicrobial therapy directed against the offending rickettsial agent; (2) supportive measures to correct physiologic abnormalities; (3) good nursing care to prevent serious complications; and (4) prompt, appropriate therapy of complications. In mild cases, patients treated early may require little more than the specific antimicrobial therapy. Vigorous supportive measures and good nursing may be lifesaving in severe cases.

Antirickettsial Therapy. *Prompt adequate antirickettsial therapy is the single most important factor in shortening the disease, reducing mortality, and speeding convalescence.* In cooperative uncomplicated patients this may be the only medication required.

Antimicrobial drugs of the tetracycline series are the drugs of choice for treatment of all rickettsial diseases. Although also highly effective, chloramphenicol is not recommended, unless tetracyclines cannot be used, because of the occasional complication of aplastic anemia. These drugs shorten the course of disease dramatically and reduce fatality rates virtually to zero except in neglected, complicated, or fulminating cases. The patient often begins to respond by 24 hours and is afebrile in one to four days, usually two to three days, depending on the specific rickettsia and the stage of disease at the time therapy is begun.

Penicillin, streptomycin, and sulfonamides are clinically ineffective. Practical concentrations of a wide range of aminoglycosides, semisynthetic penicillins, and cephalosporins do not inhibit *R. prowazekii* growth in vitro in cell cultures. *Note: Except for chloramphenicol,* none of the drugs (ampicillin, amoxicillin, co-trimoxazole) used for the treatment of typhoid fever, a serious differential diagnostic problem in some areas, gives clinical and/or in vitro evidence of effectiveness in typhus fever.

Tetracycline HCl is given orally in a total daily dose of 25 to 50 mg per kilogram of body weight. Two grams per day in divided doses at 4- to 6- or even 12-hour intervals usually suffices for adult patients. Chloramphenicol is given orally in amounts of 50 and 75 mg per kilogram of body weight per day for adults and children, respectively, usually in divided doses at 4- to 6- or even 12-hour intervals. (*Caution:* Doses larger than 25 mg per kilogram of body weight may be severely toxic for *newborn infants.*) Intravenous tetracycline is given in a dosage of 0.5 gram every 6 to 12 hours, to a maximum of 2 grams per day for adults. Chloramphenicol succinate, appropriately diluted, is given intravenously to adults in a dose of 1.0 gram every 8 to 12 hours. Parenteral therapy should be replaced with oral therapy as soon as the patient can swallow. When parenteral preparations are unavailable or intravenous drip therapy is impractical, oral preparations suspended in fluid may be administered by stomach tube.

Since neither tetracycline HCl nor chloramphenicol is rickettsicidal under ordinary circumstances, and since neither eradicates the organism from the body, ultimate freedom from clinical relapse (i.e., "cure") is probably dependent on an adequate immune response by the patient. Duration of therapy is dependent on the pharmacology of the particular drug employed; the susceptibility of the organism to, and rate of recovery from, the inhibitory effects of the drug employed, which may vary from one species of organism to another; and the stage of the disease at the time therapy is begun. Although not necessarily the minimal effective regimen, a practical conservative guide to duration of tetracycline or chloramphenicol therapy is to administer the drug until the patient has been afebrile for 48 hours and for an additional period until the total time elapsed from onset of disease is 12 to 14 days. Relapses respond to retreatment with the same drug. The usual precautions are observed for administering antimicrobials, e.g., adjustment of dosage to compensate for problems of immaturity in infants and of renal or hepatic dysfunction of rickettsial or other origin, staining of developing teeth, changes in microbial flora and superinfection, pregnancy, drug susceptibilities, or blood dyscrasias.

The introduction of new lipotropic tetracycline derivatives which produce prolonged high blood and tissue levels after a single dose (viz., doxycycline and minocycline) has literally revolutionized the management of louse-borne typhus. A *single* 100-mg dose of doxycycline will *cure* most adults, and a *single* 50-mg dose will cure most children, with only an occasional transient relapse which does not require additional therapy. A single 200-mg dose is rarely followed by relapse. Under extreme circumstances, single-dose doxycycline therapy, requiring only a single contact between patient and medical personnel, has been applied successfully on an outpatient basis. Unless in extremis from typhus or suffering from some unrelated disease, almost all patients will survive whether hospitalized, at home, or transiently disoriented in the bush. Single-dose doxycycline is currently the treatment of choice for louse-borne typhus. Comparable results have been obtained with minocycline, but because of its tendency to cause otitic complications, it is not recommended as a first choice drug.

Experience with single-dose doxycycline treatment of other rickettsioses indicates that a single 200-mg dose of doxycycline will cure some, but not all, cases of scrub typhus. On the other hand, very limited and uncontrolled observations suggest that a single dose will not suffice for the treatment of murine typhus or Rocky Mountain spotted fever, although a daily dose of 100 to 200 mg on a schedule described for tetracycline HCl is highly effective.

Antimicrobial resistance has not yet been encountered in naturally occurring rickettsial disease.

Steroids. Although not rigorously controlled, studies have shown that corticosteroids given in conjunction with antimicrobial drugs may cause rapid defervescence, dramatic reversal of neurologic impairment (coma, difficulty in swallowing), and an apparent improvement in the general well-being of the patient without adversely affecting the infectious process. A comatose typhus patient given steroid therapy in the evening may be sitting up on the side of the bed in the morning, conversing with his fellow patients and able to take medication and fluids by mouth. Similar effects may be seen in patients unable to swallow. More limited observations with scrub typhus and Rocky Mountain spotted fever have shown similar apparently beneficial effects, although reversal of intravascular clotting in Rocky Mountain spotted fever will not be effected. This has been accomplished by giving 100 mg of hydrocortisone intravenously and 200 to 300 mg of cortisone acetate intramuscularly in addition to tetracycline or doxycycline upon admission. *(Falciparum malaria must be excluded by blood smear in patients at risk to both diseases.)* Often within 24 hours a typhus patient is able to swallow the final dose of antibiotic (100 mg of doxycycline), to take oral fluids, to attend to elimination, and to move spontaneously to reduce the chances of developing pressure necroses or thrombophlebitis. Usually no more therapy of any kind, antimicrobial or steroid, is required, and nutrition presents no problem. This therapy is reserved for seriously ill or "uncooperative" patients.

Fluid and Electrolyte Balance. Oral fluids sufficient to ensure a daily urine output of at least 1500 ml suffice for the conscious, cooperative patient. The comatose patient will require parenteral fluids to maintain an adequate urine output. Fluids should be given slowly so as not to tax the potentially labile cardiovascular system. Excess electrolytes contribute to the general edema and to cardiac load when the fluid re-enters the vascular compartment. Urine output, the presence of oliguria, and laboratory determinations will serve as guides to the proper volume and proportion of electrolytes, glucose, and water.

Hepatic and Renal Systems. The cause of the disturbed liver (abnormal test results, rarely jaundice) and kidney (azotemia, albuminuria, oliguria) functions remains controversial, but these abnormalities are usually transient and disappear with convalescence.

Cardiovascular System, Including Blood. The most prominent manifestations of the typhus, scrub typhus, and spotted fever groups of rickettsial diseases can be attributed to abnormalities of the cardiovascular system. Hypotension is common, and peripheral vascular collapse, frequently in the second week of disease, is a leading cause of death and has been difficult to manage. Its cause is only incompletely understood. However, the widespread focal lesions of the small vessels are assumed to be contributory.

Albumin may be used to combat hypoproteinemia. Red cells are preferred to correct significant anemia. Heparin has been described as treatment for rickettsia-associated intravascular clotting, but other reports have failed to record benefit.

The management of peripheral vascular collapse is empirical and largely of unproved benefit: (1) oxygen; (2) judicious use of salt-poor concentrated albumin as a plasma expander and to reduce edema; (3) vasopressor drugs, e.g., levarterenol bitartrate (Levophed); and (4) corticosteroids such as hydrocortisone.

Pulmonary edema and congestive heart failure, resulting from excessive intake of salt and water or from rapid resorption of edema fluid with vascular healing, are treated with digitalis. No guidelines are available for the use of diuretics, but if their use is contemplated, consideration should be given to the state of renal function.

Massive intravascular hemolysis, described in glucose-6-phosphate dehydrogenase deficient subjects with murine or scrub typhus, has been managed with dialysis.

Other Complications. Bacterial pneumonia, still frequent in epidemic typhus, or other bacterial infections are treated with appropriate antimicrobial agents according to the causative organisms and their sensitivity patterns. Gangrene, decubitus ulcers, and thrombophlebitis are treated by the usual surgical and medical methods. Unless caused by a large destructive process (hemorrhage or thrombosis of a large vessel), neurologic abnormalities usually resolve with convalescence, although personality changes, electroencephalographic abnormalities, and deafness have been known to persist in some patients for months.

Nursing Care. Patients may be irrational or agitated and may injure themselves or even attempt self-destruction. Close observation and restraint may be required. Comatose patients should be turned frequently to prevent pressure necrosis, thrombophlebitis, and hypostatic pneumonia. Special skin care and protection of bony prominences may be desirable in view of the vascular damage associated with these diseases. Good oral hygiene reduces the chances of suppurative parotitis.

Special Considerations. Although classic Q fever often responds promptly to chemotherapy with tetracycline drugs or chloramphenicol as outlined above, the response in some cases is slower and less dramatic. Treatment of chronic infection is less satisfactory. Chemotherapy of *C. burnetii* endocarditis is especially unsatisfactory, probably because of the fact that most antirickettsial drugs are primarily rickettsiostatic. There has been very limited success with combined chemotherapy administered over a period of many months. Surgical replacement of the affected heart valve has been successful in some cases, but colonization of the artificial valve may occur.

Trench fever has been reported to respond to tetracycline drugs, but no information is available concerning the effects of brief chemotherapy on the persistence of the organism in the blood or on subsequent relapse rates.

General

Horsfall FL Jr, Tamm I (eds.): Viral and Rickettsial Infections of Man. 4th ed. Philadelphia, J. B. Lippincott Company, 1965. *Although dated in many respects, the chapters on rickettsial diseases present much basic information and background and constitute the most recent authoritative and comprehensive general coverage.*

Weiss E: Growth and physiology of rickettsiae. Bacteriol Rev 37:259, 1973. *This is a good review up to the date of its publication. Although much has transpired since, no more recent review is available.*

Laboratory Diagnosis

Elisberg BL, Bozeman FL: Serologic diagnosis of rickettsial diseases by indirect immunofluorescence. Arch Inst Pasteur Tunis 43:193, 1966. Fiset P, Ormsbe RA, Silberman R, Peacock M, Spielman SH: A microagglutination technique for detection and measurement of rickettsial antibodies. Acta Virol (Praha) 13:60, 1969. Murray ES, O'Connor JM, Gaon JA: Differentiation of 19S and 7S complement-fixing antibodies in primary versus recrudescent typhus by either ethanethiol or heat. Proc Soc Exp Biol Med 119:291, 1965. Philip RN, Casper EA, MacCormack JN, Sexton DJ, Thomas LA, Anacker RL, Burgdorfer W, Vick S: A comparison of serological methods for diagnosis of Rocky Mountain spotted fever. Am J Epidemiol 105:56, 1977. *These four papers provide some introduction into serologic diagnostic methods.*

Woodward TE, Pederson CE Jr, Oster CN, Bagley LR, Romberg J, Snyder MJ: Prompt confirmation of Rocky Mountain spotted fever: Identification of rickettsiae in skin tissues. J Infect Dis 134:297, 1976. *This method is currently under evaluation for rapid diagnosis in the acutely ill patient.*

Pathology

Pinkerton H, Strano AJ: Diseases caused by rickettsiae. *In* Binford CH, Connor DH (eds.): Pathology of Tropical and Extraordinary Diseases, Vol 1. Washington, D.C., Armed Forces Institute of Pathology, pp 87-100. *This publication presents a well-illustrated comparison of the pathologies of common rickettsial diseases, along with some additional references.*

Chemotherapy

Woodward TE: Therapy of the rickettsial diseases with a discussion of chemoprophylaxis. Arch Inst Pasteur Tunis 35:507, 1959. *This review presents briefly the evolution of chemotherapy of rickettsial diseases through the introduction of chloramphenicol and the early tetracyclines. More recent tetracyclines are not included; their use is described in many scattered publications and from the author's personal experience.*

317. THE TYPHUS GROUP

Charles L. Wisseman, Jr.

Three clinical and epidemiologic entities comprise the established diseases of the typhus group: (1) primary louse-borne epidemic typhus *(Rickettsia prowazekii)*; (2) its recrudescent form, Brill-Zinsser disease *(R. prowazekii)*, and (3) flea-borne murine typhus *(R. mooseri [R. typhi])*. These diseases are similar clinically and pathologically but differ in intensity of certain symptoms and signs, severity, and case fatality rate. Tables 316–1 to 316–3 summarize selected features of the organisms, the diseases, and their epidemiologies. This conventional listing of typhus group diseases has been complicated in the United States in recent years by (1) the isolation of a new species, *R. canada*, from ticks in Canada and its implication on serologic grounds as the possible cause of a Rocky Mountain spotted fever–like disease in Georgia; (2) the isolation of a rickettsia indistinguishable from *R. prowazekii* from flying squirrels in the eastern United States, and the recent recognition of sporadic human cases serologically identified as *R. prowazekii* infection in houses harboring flying squirrels; and (3) the strong one-way serologic cross-reactions between *R. canada* and *R. prowazekii*. Much more information, especially isolation and characterization of the agents from human cases, is needed for clarification.

EPIDEMIC LOUSE-BORNE TYPHUS FEVER

SYNONYMS. Synonyms include *classic, historic, and European typhus; jail, war, camp, and ship fever; Fleckfieber* (German); *typhus exanthématique* (French); *tifus exantemático* and *tabardillo* (Spanish); and *dermotypho* (Italian).

DEFINITION. Classic typhus fever is an acute infectious disease transmitted by the human body louse *(Pediculus humanus humanus)* and characterized clinically by sudden onset, sustained high fever of about two weeks' duration, a macular rash, and altered mental state. Brill-Zinsser disease is a recrudescence of typhus occurring months to years after primary infection, caused by organisms persisting in tissues since the primary infection, and clinically resembling a mild form of classic typhus.

ETIOLOGY (see Ch. 316). *Rickettsia prowazekii* is the etiologic agent of both classic typhus fever and Brill-Zinsser disease. No evidence has been obtained for significant variations in antigenic composition or virulence for man in strains from different areas, but attenuation has been observed as a laboratory phenomenon.

TRANSMISSION AND EPIDEMIOLOGY. The "classic" infection cycle is restricted to man and the human body louse *(Pediculus humanus humanus)*, although the organism can also grow in the head louse *(Pediculus humanus capitis)*. The louse acquires the rickettsia by feeding on the blood of a typhus patient during the rickettsemic phase. The organism multiplies in and destroys cells of the louse midgut. Large numbers of rickettsiae are excreted in the feces. The organism is not transmitted by bite. Instead, crushed infective lice or louse feces contaminate bite sites or other breaks in the skin, or airborne infective louse feces gain access through the respiratory tract.

The louse regularly dies of *R. prowazekii* infection, does not transmit the organism transovarially to the next generation, and is not a reservoir of typhus. Putative domestic animal reservoirs have largely been discounted as laboratory artifacts. The origin and extent of the flying squirrel typhus phenomenon is unknown, and, hence, the importance of its role as a reservoir of classic epidemic typhus or any manifestation other than the known sporadic cases in the eastern United States is not yet known. In most other areas, man, through the phenomenon of persisting infection and subsequent recrudescence (Brill-Zinsser disease), is the only known interepidemic reservoir and the mechanism by which the rickettsiae are made available again to lice. Neither the factors that precipitate recrudescence nor the precise rate of recrudescence are known, although one estimate suggests a rate less than 10 per 100,000 cases of primary infection. The efficiency with which lice become infected with *R. prowazekii* is apparently less during feeding upon Brill-Zinsser disease patients than upon primary typhus patients. Nevertheless, this phenomenon is known to have initiated typhus outbreaks and probably also contributes to sustaining endemicity.

Typhus can occur anywhere when living conditions and political, socioeconomic, environmental, and cultural factors predispose to lousiness and the transfer of lice among people. These are currently supplied in mountainous parts of the Northern and Southern Hemispheres, as well as equatorial regions, in deserts (Sahara, Arabian deserts) where heavy clothing is worn continuously, and in tropical regions.

Louse-borne typhus can occur as a truly epidemic disease, as a prolonged endemoepidemic disease (as in Ethiopia today), or as a highly endemic infection with sporadic, often unrecognized infections in young age groups but with occasional sharp village outbreaks involving all ages (as in Andean countries today).

PATHOLOGY. The general pathology and pathophysiologic features are described in Ch. 316.

CLINICAL MANIFESTATIONS AND COURSE. The following description applies to untreated full-blown classic typhus fever in adults. The incubation period usually is from 8 to 12 days but may be as short as 6 or as long as 15 days.

Prodromes of vague malaise and headache are not uncommon. The early phase is usually ushered in by the abrupt onset of fever, severe headache, myalgia of the back and legs, and chills or chilly sensations. The headache is intense and intractable and persists day and night. Over the first two or three days the temperature attains a level of 39 to 41° C, where it remains with only slight fluctuations until death or recovery. The skin is usually hot and dry. The face is flushed or dusky; the conjunctivae are suffused; photophobia is frequent. Deafness, tinnitus, and sometimes vertigo are prominent features. The mental state is dull. Weakness and prostration may be mild early, but after two or three days may become profound. Unproductive cough with sparse physical findings occurs in about two thirds of the cases. Nausea, vomiting, and diarrhea occur but are uncommon. Constipation is usually present.

The characteristic rash appears between the fourth and seventh days. The lesions first appear on the trunk and axillary folds and spread to the extremities, sparing the face, palms, and soles, except in very severely ill patients. At first the lesions are pinkish red macules that blanch on pressure. The evolution of the rash depends on the severity of the illness. In mild cases it may fade completely in one or two days; in cases of greater severity it may become maculopapular, then petechial, changing to reddish brown and lasting for one to two weeks before fading; in very severe cases the lesions may be exceedingly numerous, almost confluent, quickly becoming hemorrhagic or even purpuric. The rash may be absent in 5 to 10 per cent of cases. With experience and proper lighting, it may be seen without too much difficulty in dark-skinned persons.

At first the pulse rate is slow in relation to the temperature, but by the end of the first week it becomes rapid (110 to 140), weak, and frequently undulating or irregular. The blood pressure is usually low, sometimes with a systolic pressure below 80 mm Hg, and there may be brief episodes of severe hypotension. Cyanosis may be present.

The mental state progresses from dullness to stupor or occasionally to coma. The stupor may be interrupted by brief periods of delirium. Cranial nerves are selectively and variably involved (deafness, dysphagia, dysphonia). Coarse tremors may appear. Incontinence of urine and feces is encountered in severely ill patients.

Oliguria, proteinuria, and azotemia are common. Jaundice is rare, but elevations in serum transaminases may appear early. The white blood count may show a leukopenia early. In the second and third weeks of the disease it is normal or only slightly elevated unless complications ensue. Anemia may develop in the second or third week.

Death from typhus usually occurs between the ninth and eighteenth day of illness. The terminal period is usually characterized by a profound stupor, peripheral vascular collapse, and severe renal failure. When recovery is the outcome, the temperature begins to decline after 14 to 18 days and reaches a normal level by lysis in two to four days. The mental and physical state of the patient improve strikingly as the temperature falls, but strength returns more slowly (two to three months).

Secondary bacterial bronchopneumonia, otitis media, and parotitis are common in untreated patients. Thrombosis may affect the large arteries with serious results (e.g., hemiplegia). Thrombosis of small vessels may lead to gangrene, particularly of the toes, fingers, or ear lobes. Necrosis of the skin may occur over the bony prominences, especially over the sacrum or greater trochanter.

Severity of disease and case fatality rate increase with age, being less severe and often uncharacteristic in younger children and increasing rapidly with age over 40 years. In persons who contract typhus after having received killed typhus vaccine, the disease is greatly modified, with negligible mortality.

Brill-Zinsser disease is similar to primary typhus but milder. The fever, on the average, is lower and of shorter duration, the rash is less intense and often absent, and the case fatality rate is low.

PROGNOSIS. Depending on host factors, such as age, stress, nutritional state, and other concurrent diseases, case fatality rate in untreated typhus may range from 10 per cent or less to 60 per cent. Deep coma and severe hypotension and tachycardia associated with falling body temperature are signs of poor prognosis. Even such cases, however, often respond dramatically to appropriate chemotherapy and supportive measures. Appropriate treatment reduces the mortality rate in ordinary severe typhus fever virtually to zero.

TREATMENT. Treatment is described in Ch. 316. A single 200-mg oral dose of the long-acting tetracycline doxycycline is the treatment of choice under ordinary circumstances. The response of uncomplicated typhus to specific antirickettsial chemotherapy, whether begun early or late, is highly predictable. The temperature returns to normal limits in 48 to 72 hours, averaging about 60 hours, accompanied by progressive lessening of headache and improvement of mental status. Occasionally, some manifestations, such as deafness, may appear during response to early therapy but subsequently subside.

PREVENTION AND CONTROL. Infected lice and louse feces on a typhus patient present a special hazard to all nonimmune contacts, including physicians and attendants among whom infection is a common occupational hazard. Decontamination and delousing of the typhus patient and his clothing (including blankets and hats) are performed immediately upon hospitalization. Clothing and bedding are best decontaminated by heat, because this will kill the lice as well as the rickettsiae. After the patient is decontaminated and deloused, isolation and quarantine are not necessary.

Control of louse-borne typhus currently depends heavily upon control of the louse vector. Application of insecticide dusts (10 per cent DDT, 1 per cent malathion, 1 per cent lindane, or newer carbamates, depending upon local louse-resistance patterns) to fully clothed persons is very effective for reducing louse populations and controlling disease in acute outbreaks. Insecticides alone are less effective for long-term louse control in areas where conditions conducive to lousiness persist and where louse strains resistant to insecticides can be, and are, selected. The older methods of subjecting clothes and bedding to heat or fumigants (e.g., methylbromide) are effective but cumbersome. It is possible but unproved that repellent-treated clothing (e.g., M-1960, diethyltoluamide) would reduce the chances of louse acquisition.

Conventional typhus vaccines composed of killed organisms are no longer available in the United States, pending development of improved vaccines of proven protective potency. The attenuated E strain of *R. prowazekii,* when used as a living vaccine, is protective but may produce a mildly symptomatic, self-limited infection in 10 to 15 per cent of recipients. It is not generally available in the United States.

Under current circumstances, ordinary tourists or resident expatriates are not very likely to be exposed to louse-borne typhus, in contrast to murine typhus, even in endemic areas if they maintain the usual separate households, pay attention to personal hygiene, and do not mix intimately with the affected local population. On the other hand, anyone who comes in contact with members of the affected population (in crowds, markets, buses, schools, or churches) is at risk. Depending upon the circumstances, the wearing of insecticide- or repellent-treated clothing and the overnight exposure of clothing to a dichlorvos strip (No-Pest) in an airtight bag may reduce exposure to lice. Under very special *short-term* circumstances, chemoprophylaxis with 100 mg of doxycycline once or twice a week might be effective, but this has not been formally tested with louse-borne typhus, and the disease might develop after the drug is discontinued. Prompt chemotherapy on the first or second day of disease reduces typhus to a relatively minor inconvenience.

MURINE OR FLEA-BORNE TYPHUS FEVER

DEFINITION. Murine typhus fever is an acute infectious disease communicable from rodent hosts to man sporadically by means of the rat flea *(Xenopsylla cheopis).* The disease is similar clinically to classic epidemic typhus except that it is milder.

ETIOLOGY (see Ch. 316). *Rickettsia mooseri (R. typhi)* shares some common antigens with *R. prowazekii* and *R. canada* but differs in specific antigens, host range, and certain other biologic properties. Significant cross-immunity between *R. mooseri* and *R. prowazekii* is produced by infection but not by killed vaccines. DNA homology studies show a difference between *R. mooseri* and *R. prowazekii* sufficiently large to preclude easy transition from one to the other by simple variation or mutation, except on an evolutionary scale. Thus, *R. mooseri* is an unlikely source of some contemporary outbreaks of classic louse-borne epidemic typhus, as has been suggested, although limited outbreaks of louse-borne *R. mooseri* infection may have occurred.

TRANSMISSION AND EPIDEMIOLOGY. Murine typhus is not communicable from man to man. It is a zoonosis maintained in nature in a cycle involving rats and certain other small mammals as amplifying hosts and reservoirs and fleas and rat lice as vectors. In the rat flea and perhaps the other fleas infected by feeding upon rickettsemic rats, the organism grows in cells of the gut without killing the flea and is shed in the feces for the life of the flea. There is no transovarial transmission. It is transmitted to man, not by bite of the flea, but rather by contamination of broken skin with infective feces or by inhalation of dried infective feces.

Murine typhus is widely distributed over the world in the areas penetrated by *Rattus rattus* and *Rattus norvegicus* and where the vector fleas coexist. In some areas under appropriate conditions there may be spillover of *R. mooseri* from *Rattus* into other spatially closely associated small mammals and to man. Seasonal incidence of human infections appears to correlate with the periods of abundance of vector fleas, which in the United States is in the summer months. Rats are commensal animals closely associated with buildings or structures containing food (such as warehouses, markets, grain elevators, and dwellings).

PATHOLOGY. Although because of the low death rate few postmortem studies have been made, it is assumed that the lesions in man, as is the case in experimental infection of laboratory animals, are similar to those in louse-born typhus.

CLINICAL MANIFESTATIONS AND COURSE. The incubation period of murine typhus lasts from 6 to 14 days. The symptoms are similar to those of louse-borne typhus, the principal differences being that murine typhus is a milder and shorter disease, the rash is less extensive and persists for shorter periods, there are fewer complications, and the case fatality rate is lower.

Although murine typhus is often referred to as mild, and truly mild cases do occur, this is mildness *relative* to louse-borne typhus. On an absolute scale it can be severe and debilitating and may require two to three months for convalescence in untreated patients.

DIAGNOSIS. ***Clinical Diagnosis.*** The diagnosis of murine typhus may be suspected when a patient has sustained fever of several days' duration accompanied by headache, generalized aches and pains, and a macular or maculopapular rash appearing on the trunk on the fifth or sixth day after onset of fever. The patient with murine typhus may give a history of activities that have brought him into contact with places where rats are numerous. However, there is often no definite recollection of a flea bite. It is impossible on clinical evidence alone to distinguish an ordinary case of murine typhus from a case of Brill-Zinsser disease or a mild case of louse-borne typhus.

In many areas of the world where typhoid or other enteric fevers are common, where specific laboratory diagnostic tests are not readily available, and where chloramphenicol is routinely employed to treat enteric fevers, significant occurrence of murine typhus and sporadic louse-borne typhus may be unsuspected or unrecognized, being hidden among the enteric fevers by virtue of some clinical similarity and response to chloramphenicol. However, when ampicillin or trimethoprim-sulfamethoxazole is used for the treatment of suspected typhoid fevers, the typhus fevers do not respond and their presence may then be unveiled.

Laboratory Diagnosis. Diagnosis can often be made by specific rickettsial serologic tests or by isolation of the agent. (See Laboratory Diagnosis in Ch. 316.)

PROGNOSIS. The case fatality rate is usually less than 5 per cent in untreated patients and is virtually zero with rapid convalescence in uncomplicated murine typhus treated with appropriate antirickettsial drugs.

TREATMENT. Treatment follows the guidelines given in Ch. 316 with respect to the *multiple* dose antimicrobial regimen.

PREVENTION AND CONTROL. Individual preventive measures include avoiding endemic foci where rats and their fleas abound (e.g., warehouses, storage areas, grain elevators) or wearing repellent-treated clothing to prevent acquisition of fleas. A vaccine is not available.

General control measures are directed at reducing rat and flea populations. Among others, these include rat proof construction and prevention of access of rats to food materials; reduction of rat populations by poison baits (e.g., warfarin, alphanaphthylthiourea), trapping, or poison gases into burrows; and reduction of the flea population through application of appropriate insecticides (such as DDT) to rat runs. When contemplating a rodent control program, it is important to plan insecticide application for flea control prior to, or simultaneously with, the rodent control measures to prevent increased exposure of man to fleas seeking alternative hosts.

Gaon JA, Murray ES: The natural history of recrudescent typhus (Brill-Zinsser disease) in Bosnia. Bull WHO 35:133, 1966. *This paper summarizes the definitive work that validated Zinsser's hypothesis about the nature of the disease described by Brill.*

Miller ES, Beeson PB: Murine typhus fever. Medicine 25:1, 1946. Stuart BM, Pullen RL: Endemic (murine) typhus fever: Clinical observations of 180 cases. Ann Intern Med 23:520, 1945. *These two papers record a wealth of clinical observations on murine typhus fever.*

Proceedings of the International Symposium on the Control of Lice and Louse-Borne Diseases, Washington, D.C., December 4–6, 1972. Pan-American Health Organization Scientific Publication No 263, 1973. *This is the most comprehensive modern consideration of the problems of lice and louse-borne diseases available today.*

Traub R, Wisseman CL Jr, Farhang-Azad A: The ecology of murine typhus—a critical review. Trop Dis Bull 75:237, 1978. *Although current work is introducing some additional concepts, this publication comprehensively covers most of the published work up to the time of its preparation.*

Wohlbach SB, Todd JL, Palfrey FW: The Etiology and Pathology of Typhus. Cambridge, Mass., Harvard University Press, 1922. *This is the classic, definitive work on the etiology and pathology of louse-borne typhus fever.*

Zarafonetis CJD: The typhus fevers. *In* Coates JB, Havens WP (eds.): Medical Department, United States Army. Internal Medicine in World War II, Vol II. Infectious Diseases. Washington, D.C., Office of the Surgeon General, Department of the Army, 1963, pp 143-223. *Clinical aspects of louse-borne typhus seen by Army physicians during World War II are summarized in this publication.*

318. ROCKY MOUNTAIN SPOTTED FEVER

Charles L. Wisseman, Jr.

SYNONYMS. This disease is also known as *spotted fever* and *tick typhus* (England), *fiebre manchada* (Mexico), *fiebre petequial* (Colombia), and *febre maculosa* or *São Paulo typhus* (Brazil).

DEFINITION. Rocky Mountain spotted fever is a mild to severe, sometimes fatal, acute infectious disease of the Western Hemisphere caused by *Rickettsia rickettsii* and transmitted to man by several species of ticks. The disease is characterized by sudden onset with chills and headache, by fever of about two to three weeks' duration, and by a rash on the extremities and trunk beginning about the fourth day of disease.

ETIOLOGY. The disease is caused by *Rickettsia rickettsii*, the prototype species of the spotted fever group of rickettsiae with members of which it shares group antigens but from which it can be differentiated by more specific tests (see Ch. 316). Both mild and highly virulent strains exist in many parts of the United States. Although several other species of the spotted fever group of rickettsiae have been isolated from ticks, to date only typical *R. rickettsii* has been *isolated* from infections of man. More intensive efforts to isolate and characterize rickettsiae from patients are needed to clarify the role of other spotted fever group agents as possible causes of human disease.

DISTRIBUTION AND INCIDENCE. Although originally encountered in Rocky Mountain states (Montana and Idaho), Rocky Mountain spotted fever has been recognized in at least 46 states and is actually more prevalent in the south Atlantic states than in the West. In the eastern United States it extends from Cape Cod and some adjacent islands, through a focus on Long Island, to Florida, with almost half the cases in the United States occurring in Maryland, Virginia, North Carolina, and Georgia. The number of cases per year in the United States has risen steadily over the past several years to more than 1000 since 1979. The reasons for this increase are not fully understood, but may include abundance of ticks, extension of suburbs into tick-infested rural areas, and increased recreational activities in wilderness areas. Rocky Mountain spotted fever has also been recognized in several provinces of Canada, in Mexico, in Central America (Panama, Costa Rica) and in South America (Colombia, Brazil).

TRANSMISSION AND EPIDEMIOLOGY. Rocky Mountain spotted fever is a zoonosis maintained in a natural cycle between certain tick species and small (rodents, rabbits) and perhaps larger mammals. Man, a dead-end host for *R. rickettsii*, becomes infected when he intrudes into this zoonotic cycle (as for recreational or occupational reasons) and is bitten by an infected tick. Rocky Mountain spotted fever is not communicable from man to man by ordinary contact.

Although multiple tick species (both hard and soft varieties) are known to become naturally infected and may play a role in transmission among animals, the main tick vectors for man are hard (Ixodid) ticks: the wood tick *Dermacentor andersoni*, in the western United States; the dog tick, *Dermacentor variabilis*, in the eastern United States; *Amblyomma americanum* in Texas and Oklahoma; the brown dog tick, *Rhipicephalus sanguineus*, in northern Mexico (and introduced into the United States); and *Amblyomma cajennense* in Brazil and Colombia.

PATHOLOGY. The pathology of Rocky Mountain spotted fever conforms in general to the description of the rickettsial diseases in Ch. 316. Of special note is the fact that the vasculitis in Rocky Mountain spotted fever is not limited to the endothelium and is more severe than in typhus or scrub typhus, causing more pronounced thrombotic occlusion and necrosis of the muscular layers. Microinfarcts are seen with some frequency in the central nervous system.

CLINICAL MANIFESTATIONS AND COURSE. A history of tick bite can be elicited in many, but not all, patients. Variations in incubation period (2 to 14, average 7 days) and severity of disease are seen in Rocky Mountain spotted fever, with a tendency for an inverse relationship between the two. Very severe disease often is preceded by a short (two- to five-day) incubation period. Prodromes, when present, consist of anorexia, irritability, malaise, feverishness, and chilly sensations. Attacks may be so mild that the patient remains ambulatory, or so severe that death may occur within three to six days of onset. The more typical infections are sudden in onset, with severe headache, chills, fever, prostration, myalgia (especially of the back and legs) nausea with occasional vomiting, conjunctival injections, and photophobia. There may be abdominal muscular pain, tenderness of muscles on palpation, and arthralgia.

Body temperature reaches 39 to 40° C in the first two days, is sustained at elevated levels for about two weeks, and declines by slow lysis over three or four days. Hyperthermia in the range of 41° C is a serious sign. Body temperature falling to near or below normal levels in the face of severe hypotension and tachycardia carries a grave prognosis.

The characteristic rash appears on about the fourth day (two to six days), first about the wrists and ankles, and then extends rapidly over all or most of the body, including palms, soles, face, and, occasionally, the mucous membranes of the mouth and throat. At first, the lesions are pink macules, 2 to 5 mm in diameter, which blanch on pressure. In two or three days, they become fixed, darker red, or purplish, maculopapular, and, about the fourth day, petechial. Hemorrhagic lesions may coalesce. The rash begins to disappear as the fever subsides but often remains as pigmented spots for weeks.

Early in the disease the pulse is full, regular, and elevated in proportion to fever. Later, it becomes more rapid and feeble, and some degree of hypotension develops. The electrocardiogram may show minor S-T deflections and prolonged P-R intervals. In some cases, hypotension may attain shock levels, and gangrene of fingers, toes, ears, nose, or genitalia may develop. Thrombosis of larger vessels may lead to a loss of a portion of a limb or hemiplegia. The skin may become necrotic over body prominences. Hemorrhage from the nose, gastrointestinal tract, or kidney may occur. Platelet counts are frequently low. Varying degrees of disseminated intravascular coagulation have been observed.

Central nervous system involvement is manifest by restlessness, insomnia, delirium, stupor, and, in severe cases, coma. Convulsions, muscular rigidity, tremors, and athetoid movements may occur. Cranial nerve involvement is variable. Transient deafness is common, but peripheral neuritis is uncommon. Electroencephalographic changes may persist for many months. Incontinence of urine and feces may be present in severe cases.

The liver may be enlarged and serum albumin depressed, but jaundice is not common. Oliguria and some azotemia are common in severe cases. Anuria and marked azotemia may be seen in critically ill patients. Complicating secondary bacterial infections (bronchopneumonia, otitis media, parotitis) occur but are uncommon.

Convalescence may take weeks to months. Death, when it occurs in the nonfulminant variety, usually occurs late in the second week of disease (range about 9 to 18 days after onset).

DIAGNOSIS. An acute febrile illness with or without rash, in a person with a history of tick-bite, exposure to ticks (either in a tick-infested rural or suburban area or contact with a tick-infested dog), or, equally important, recreational or occupational activities that might have brought the patient into a tick-infested area, should alert the physician to the possibility of Rocky Mountain spotted fever. Although other diseases, especially those with rash, may present transient early differential diagnostic problems, the two diseases that have consistently caused the greatest confusion are measles and meningococcemia. The most promising laboratory diagnostic method for providing a specific diagnosis early enough in the disease to permit effective specific therapeutic intervention is the demonstration by the fluorescent antibody technique of spotted fever group rickettsiae in skin biopsies. Isolation attempts and serologic methods (see Laboratory Diagnosis in Ch. 316) are useful and important but rarely yield results in time for most efficient management.

PROGNOSIS. Although mild cases occur, the rapid, severe course in some patients makes it imperative to regard any suspected case of Rocky Mountain spotted fever as a medical emergency. In untreated cases, the overall case fatality rate is about 20 per cent, with areas of low ($\leq$ 10 per cent) and high ($\geq$ 60 per cent) rates. Prognosis depends on severity of infection, host factors (such as age, presence of other disease), and *the time after onset at which specific antirickettsial chemotherapy is started.* Even with effective antirickettsial drugs available, the case fatality rate has remained at 5 to 10 per cent. Analysis of fatal cases has shown that the single most important factor was *delay in institution of antirickettsial therapy,* whatever the reason. With the time between onset and death as short as three to six days, the critical period when antimicrobial therapy can influence the outcome may be very short indeed and does not leave much latitude for correcting errors in clinical diagnosis.

TREATMENT. *Prompt* administration of a tetracycline antibiotic, including doxycycline, or chloramphenicol daily for about six days, is the single most important specific therapeutic measure (see Treatment of Rickettsial Diseases in Ch. 316). Because specific etiologic diagnosis may be impossible in the first few days of disease, any patient seriously considered to have Rocky Mountain spotted fever should be treated as such while other diagnostic procedures continue. Other antimicrobial agents, such as the penicillins, cephalosporins, aminoglycosides, and trimethoprim-sulfamethoxazole, which are commonly employed for other proven or suspected bacterial infections, *are without effect* on Rocky Mountain spotted fever at clinically permissible doses. Reliance upon them to gain time for a laboratory-confirmed diagnosis may be devastating.

Specific treatment of uncomplicated Rocky Mountain spotted fever on the first or second day of disease usually results in rapid defervescence, sometimes by 24 to 48 hours, with few residua. In sharp contrast, in the untreated severe cases, tissue damage caused by progressive infection may be accompanied by increasingly serious physiologic derangements, as in the cardiovascular and blood clotting systems, which do not respond directly to antimicrobial therapy and which often are poorly responsive to therapies specifically directed at the physiologic derangements. A patient may progress to this dangerous state, associated with high mortality rate, in five to seven days after onset of disease, and occasionally even more rapidly. It is not uncommon for a patient with an unsuspected case of Rocky Mountain spotted fever to enter the hospital after two to four days of fever and to enter the critical phase while routine diagnostic tests are still in progress, perhaps even under the misguided security of some combination of beta lactam and aminoglycoside antibiotics.

PREVENTION AND CONTROL. Individual preventive measures are directed primarily at prevention of tick bite. The chances of ticks attaching should be minimized by (1) avoiding places especially likely to harbor ticks (e.g., brush where livestock and game take refuge); (2) wearing protective clothing designed to exclude ticks (preferably impregnated with a tick repellent, such as N-N-butylacetanilide or high concentrations of diethyltoluamide, or sprayed with the acaricide 0.5 per cent permethrin); and (3) carefully inspecting the *entire* body once or twice daily to remove all ticks. Ticks usually crawl about on the body or in the clothing for some time prior to attaching. Thus frequent inspection usually discloses ticks before they attach. Moreover, since the chance of transmission of Rocky Mountain spotted fever appears to be a function of the duration of attachment, early removal of an attached tick probably reduces the chances of infection. Ticks should be removed (from man or dogs) with a pair of forceps, exerting gentle steady traction so that the mouth parts are released intact from the skin. Most other commonly recommended methods of tick removal are less satisfactory. Contact between tick and fingers should be avoided, because rickettsiae in tick feces or body fluids may enter a break in the skin or be transferred to mucous membranes and initiate infection.

For families living in tick-infested areas, an especially effective preventive measure is for parents to establish the routine of examining themselves and their children for ticks every evening at bath time during the tick season, and to teach the children to examine themselves as soon as they are old enough.

Dogs frequently bring ticks into houses. Ticks should be removed with the same care to avoid possible infection as described above. Acquisition of Rocky Mountain spotted fever by inhalation of airborne dried infected tick feces from the dog's coat is suspected but not proven. Commercial repellent-impregnated plastic collars may reduce, but not necessarily eliminate, ticks on dogs. *Rhipicephalus sanguineus* ticks may become established indoors.

If an attached tick is found, even if it is positive for *R. rickettsii* by the "hemolymph" test, it is best practice today to place a person from whom such a tick has been removed under close observation, recording morning and evening temperatures for two weeks, and instituting full antirickettsial chemotherapy only, but promptly, when a significant rise in temperature first appears. Attempts at chemoprophylaxis are likely only to delay onset of disease.

R. rickettsii vaccines have been removed from the market because of limited effectiveness.

Area control of ticks is still very difficult and is usually considered impractical. Ticks are unusually resistant to most insecticides. Yet, some measure of control may be achieved in time on small plots of ground, such as suburban lots, by intensive acaricidal treatment, the clearing of underbrush, intensive gardening or cultivation, and a reduction of the wild animal population. Changes in land use may affect tick populations. Some progress is being made toward identifying the specific habitat alterations that affect tick populations.

Note: In the last few years there has been a flood of publications on many aspects of the problems of Rocky Mountain spotted fever. No unifying reviews have yet appeared. The following references are limited to clinical aspects of Rocky Mountain spotted fever, because they, especially through the references that each cites, give a broad access to the rapidly evolving newer knowledge of the pathophysiologic manifestation of this disease.

Bradford WD, Croker BP, Tisher CC: Kidney lesions in Rocky Mountain spotted fever. A light-, immunofluorescence-, and electron-microscopic study. Am J Pathol 97:381, 1979.

Bradford WD, Hackel DB: Myocardial involvement in Rocky Mountain spotted fever. Arch Pathol Lab Med 102:357, 1978.

Fine D, Mosher D, Yamada T, Burke D, Kenyon R: Coagulation and complement studies in Rocky Mountain spotted fever. Arch Intern Med 138:735, 1978.

Harrell GT: Rocky Mountain spotted fever. Medicine 28:333, 1949. *A classic.*

Hatwick MAW, O'Brien RJ, Hanson BF: Rocky Mountain spotted fever: Epidemiology of an increasing problem. Ann Intern Med 84:732, 1976.

Linnemann CC Jr, Janson PF: The clinical presentations of Rocky Mountain spotted fever. Clin Pediat 17:673, 1978.

Walker DH, Crawford CG, Cain BG: Rickettsial infection of the pulmonary microcirculation: The basis for interstitial pneumonitis in Rocky Mountain spotted fever. Hum Pathol 11:263, 1980.

319. TICK-BORNE RICKETTSIOSES OF THE EASTERN HEMISPHERE

Charles L. Wisseman, Jr.

DEFINITION. Three diseases, caused by three different members of the spotted fever group of rickettsiae, are currently the best recognized tick-borne rickettsioses of the Eastern Hemisphere and occur over distinct broad geographic areas: (1) African tick typhus *(R. conorii),* (2) North Asian tick-borne rickettsiosis *(R. sibirica),* and (3) Queensland tick typhus *(R. australis).* Each is a zoonosis, with man an accidental, dead-end host, and is transmitted by the bite of one or more species of ixodid ticks. The three diseases, mild to moderate in severity, closely resemble one another with a short (average five- to seven-day) incubation period, a primary lesion (eschar, tache noire), a fever of a few days' to two weeks' duration, and a maculopapular to almost nodular rash which appears three to five days after onset.

HISTORY, ETIOLOGY, DISTRIBUTION, AND EPIDEMIOLOGY. The problem of the identity of the etiologic agents of the tick-borne rickettsial diseases of man in the Eastern Hemisphere is complex and poorly resolved. In addition to the three well-described agents, *R. conorii, R. sibirica* and *R. australis,* which have been isolated from human infections, a number of new spotted fever group rickettsiae have been isolated from ticks in different areas—e.g., Switzerland, Czechoslovakia, Israel, Pakistan, Thailand—but their capacity to cause human disease is still unknown. In Malaysia infections of man and small mammals have been identified by spotted fever group specific serologic tests, but the causative rickettsia(e) has not yet been isolated and identified. Reports of *R. conorii* infection in Indochina, based on inadequate serology, are likely to be erroneous. In contrast, a new spotted fever group rickettsia, tentatively designated *R. israeli,* has been isolated from human cases. Much remains to be done to clarify the tick-borne causes of human rickettsial infections of the Eastern Hemisphere. Accordingly, the descriptions included here will be confined to the three established entities.

Following the recognition of *boutonneuse fever* in Tunisia, similar tick-borne diseases with local names (e.g., Marseille fever, Kenya tick typhus, South African tick typhus, Indian tick typhus) were described over a wide area, which encompassed parts of Africa, southern Europe, the Middle East, and the Indo-Pakistan subcontinent. Serologic studies and some strain comparison suggested that all are caused by strains of *R. conorii* and that the unifying term *African tick typhus* should be applied to all. This probably is correct to a large degree. However, serologic methods employed have limitations.

The recent findings of a multiplicity of established and probable new species of spotted fever group rickettsiae along with *R. conorii* in some of the areas of presumed African tick typhus *(R. conorii)* distribution (e.g., Europe, Israel, Pakistan) suggest that considerable work must yet be done to clarify the question of distribution and nature of "African tick typhus." In the Mediterranean littoral, the main vector of fièvre boutonneuse is the dog tick, *Rhipicephalus sanguineus,* and the disease is often acquired in and around human habitations, i.e., a domestic or urban pattern. In other areas, the causative agent of the local disease is transmitted by ticks which are parasitic on wild animals, and hence the disease is acquired in rural areas, e.g., certain stretches of the South African veldt.

North Asian tick-borne rickettsiosis (Siberian tick typhus), now known to be caused by *R. sibirica,* is distributed from European Russia through Siberia to the Soviet Far East and possibly to the Indo-Pakistan subcontinent. Several species of ixodid ticks have been implicated as vectors in different geographic regions. Its acquisition is characteristically in a sylvan or rural setting.

Queensland tick typhus is usually acquired in rural areas heavily infested with the tick *Ixodes holocyclus* and a history of tick bite and an eschar are common. The agent, *R. australis,* has only been isolated from the blood of patients. Antibodies have been detected in the blood of some small marsupials and a rat, suggesting a natural sylvan small animal–tick cycle.

The identity of the strains causing disease in Southeast Asia is unknown.

PATHOLOGY. The findings are similar to those in Rocky Mountain spotted fever except for the presence of the tache noire, the black button–like necrotic primary lesion that is generally found on the surface areas of the body ordinarily covered by clothing. The basic pathologic changes are found in the small blood vessels (see Ch. 316).

SYMPTOMS, LABORATORY FINDINGS, AND DIAGNOSIS. The three tick-borne rickettsioses that occur in different parts of the Eastern Hemisphere resemble one another closely. After an incubation period of about five to seven days, the disease begins with fever, headache, malaise, myalgia, and conjunctival injection. The primary lesion, which is present in most cases at the onset of fever, consists of a small ulcer 2 to 5 mm in diameter with a black center and a red areola; the regional lymph nodes are enlarged. The generalized erythematous maculopapular rash appears about the fourth day and quickly involves most of the body, including the palms and soles and often the face. In severe cases the rash becomes hemorrhagic. Fever abates during the second week. The prognosis is good except in the aged and debilitated. Complications and sequelae are unusual.

North Asian tick-borne rickettsiosis has been the subject of considerable laboratory and clinical observation by Soviet investigators. Mild hypotension, electrocardiographic changes, a reversal of the A/G ratio in serum (depressed albumin, early increased alpha globulins, followed by increase in gamma globulins), and abnormal liver function test results are noteworthy.

Agglutinins against *Proteus* OX-19 develop during the second week, and complement-fixing antibodies appear shortly thereafter. Diagnosis is established by the clinical picture, including the tache noire, the geographic location, and positive serologic reactions.

TREATMENT. The broad-spectrum antimicrobial drugs are as effective in patients with African tick typhus and North Asian tick-borne rickettsiosis as in those with other rickettsioses (see Ch. 316 for details of therapy). Presumably, these measures are also applicable to the other tick-borne rickettsioses of the Eastern Hemisphere. All the newly recognized strains display susceptibility in vitro to doxcycline of the same order as *R. rickettsii* and presumably would respond to similar therapeutic regimens.

PROPHYLAXIS. Prevention of human disease is based on avoiding the bites of infected ticks. In Ch. 318 details are set forth regarding personal prophylaxis, including the use of protective clothing, chemical repellents, and reduction of tick population by measures involved in terrain control. Vaccines for human use are not available.

Campbell RW, Abeywickrema P, Fenton C: Queensland tick typhus in Sydney: A new endemic focus. Med J Aust 1:350, 1979. *An introduction to Queensland tick typhus.*

Goldwasser RA, Klingberg MA, Klingberg W, Steiman Y, Swartz TA: Laboratory and epidemiological studies of rickettsial spotted fever in Israel. *In* Frontiers of Internal Medicine, Proceedings of 12th International Congress of Internal Medicine, Tel Aviv, 1974. Basel, Karger, 1975, pp 270-275. *Identification of a new tick-borne spotted fever group rickettsial infection of man in an area of established* R. conorii *endemicity.*

Hoogstraal, H: Ticks in relation to human disease caused by *Rickettsia* species. Ann Rev Entomol 12:377, 1967. *An excellent means of access to literature on tick-borne rickettsioses up to 1967.*

Lyskovtsev MM: Tickborne rickettsiosis. (Translation from the Russian.) Misc Publ Entomol Soc Am 6:41, 1968. *Access to tick-borne rickettsioses of the Soviet Union.*

320. RICKETTSIALPOX

Charles L. Wisseman, Jr.

DEFINITION. Rickettsialpox is a mite-borne rickettsial disease, mild and self-limited, which is characterized by an initial eschar-like lesion and a fever of a week's duration accompanied by headache, backache, and a generalized papulovesicular rash.

ETIOLOGY. Rickettsialpox is caused by *Rickettsia akari,* a member of the spotted fever group on the basis of shared group antigens but with unique specific antigens and biologic properties.

DISTRIBUTION AND INCIDENCE. The disease has been reported from cities in the United States (New York, Boston, West Haven, Ct., Philadelphia, Pittsburgh, and Cleveland) and from the U.S.S.R. In the first three years after the disease was described in 1946, about 500 cases were reported in the United States, mostly from New York, but the number reported has since decreased markedly. Although the reasons for the decrease are not established, it may be due to under-reporting of disease or to control measures.

TRANSMISSION AND EPIDEMIOLOGY. Although detailed information is sparse, it is clear that rickettsialpox is a zoonosis which can involve house mice *(Mus musculus)* and mouse mites *(Allodermanyssus sanguineus). R. akari* has also been isolated from rats in the U.S.S.R. and from voles (small field "mice") in Korea. It is unknown whether the basic natural cycle involves field rodents and their ectoparasites with occasional spillover into the mouse-mite cycle or whether the latter is in fact the basic sustaining cycle. Regardless, in the United States the mouse-mite cycle, greatly amplified and concentrated in discrete foci artificially created by, and frequented by, man himself (e.g., improperly fired apartment house incinerators), was responsible for bringing *R. akari* and man into effective contact with one another. The unusually large mite population, which infested the walls and floors of the incinerator rooms, had access to people entering the foci with a frequency not usually encountered under natural circumstances. Transmission is presumably by bite of the mite.

PATHOLOGY. As no fatal cases have been encountered, studies of the pathology of rickettsialpox have been limited to an examination of skin biopsies. Histologically, the eschar of rickettsialpox resembles the eschars of scrub typhus and boutonneuse fever. The skin lesions composing the rash show a typical perivascular infiltration by monouclear cells. Later, necrosis of the superficial epithelium leads to intraepidermal vesicle formation.

CLINICAL MANIFESTATIONS AND COURSE. The incubation period varies from about ten days to three weeks. An initial lesion (the eschar) appears at the site of the mite bite about a week before onset of fever in about 90 per cent of the cases, gradually enlarging and progressing from a papular lesion through vesicle formation, finally to form a dark encrusted lesion 0.5 to 1.5 cm in diameter. The onset of an intermittent fever is sudden and is accompanied by chills or chilly sensations, drenching sweats, headache, anorexia, and photophobia. The temperature ranges from about 38 to 40° C, lasts for about a week, is accompanied by headache, lassitude, and myalgia, and then gradually subsides. A sparse eruption appears on the trunk, extremities, and mucous membranes between the first and fourth days of fever, beginning as discrete maculopapular lesions and evolving into a vesiculopapular rash. The vesicles are firm, are sometimes surrounded by erythema, and, on drying, form a dark crust that falls off without leaving a scar.

DIAGNOSIS. ***Clinical Diagnosis.*** The clinical characteristics of the disease are so distinctive that in most patients a presumptive diagnosis may be made on clinical grounds. Chickenpox in adults poses the most difficult diagnostic problem. Important points in differentiation are as follows: the vesicles in rickettsialpox arise from the center of discrete papules; the lesions tend to appear at the same time instead of in crops; on the average, the number of lesions is fewer than in chickenpox; and there often is an initial lesion at the site of the mite bite.

Laboratory Diagnosis. Laboratory diagnosis depends on isolation of the agent and on serologic response measured by rickettsial group and specific antigens. The Weil-Felix result is negative (see Ch. 316).

PROGNOSIS. Even without specific therapy, the course of the disease is benign, and the prognosis excellent.

TREATMENT. Response to tetracycline drugs, given as outlined in Ch. 316, is rapid without relapse.

PREVENTION AND CONTROL. The transient emergence of rickettsialpox from a silent zoonosis to a human disease problem was an artifact of urban living, and its apparent disappearance is probably a result of minor changes in human behavior. The prevention and control of rickettsialpox depend on rodent and mite control by (1) the elimination of mice and mouse harborages, which should include proper care and firing of incinerators in dwellings, and (2) the application of residual acaricides to walls and other mite-infested areas. No vaccines have been developed.

Greenberg M, Pelliteri O, Klein IF, Huebner RJ: Rickettsialpox—a newly recognized rickettsial disease. II. Clinical observations. JAMA 133:901, 1947. *Original clinical description of a newly recognized spotted fever group infection.*

Lackman DH: A review of information on rickettsialpox in the United States. Clin Pediat 2:296, 1963. *A resource for information on rickettsialpox in the United States.*

321. SCRUB TYPHUS

Charles L. Wisseman, Jr.

SYNONYMS. Scrub typhus is also known as *chigger-borne rickettsiosis.* It has many local names, including *tsutsugamushi disease, Japanese river* or *flood fever, mite-borne typhus, rural typhus, Mossman fever,* and others.

DEFINITION. Scrub typhus is an acute, febrile, typhus-like disease of rural Asia transmitted by the bite of larval trombiculid mites (chiggers). The site of infection is often marked by an eschar accompanied by regional lymphadenitis.

ETIOLOGY. The disease is caused by infection with *Rickettsia tsutsugamushi (R. orientalis).* The organism differs somewhat from other members of the genus *Rickettsia.* It shares an antigen with *Proteus* OX-K. Multiple serotypes exist that produce substantial homologous immunity but only transient cross-immunity in man. Hence multiple attacks of scrub typhus are possible. Virulence of strains for mice and man varies from low to very high.

DISTRIBUTION AND INCIDENCE. Scrub typhus is widely distributed in eastern and southern Asia and the islands of the western and southern Pacific. It is known as far north as the island of Hokkaido in Japan and the Primorye region of asiatic U.S.S.R., as far south as the northern tip of Australia, and as far west as Pakistan and Tadzhikistan. Endemic infection is unknown in the New World, Europe, Africa, and Western Asia; but cases imported during the incubation period following infection in an endemic area have been recognized in the United States.

Scrub typhus is best known from its occurrence in substantial numbers when large groups of nonimmune persons enter an endemic area, such as in military operations, road building, land clearing, and certain agricultural settings such as rubber plantations. Application of modern epidemiologic and laboratory methods is currently revealing, as expected, that scrub typhus is a major cause of febrile disease in rural populations indigenous to endemic areas.

TRANSMISSION AND EPIDEMIOLOGY. Scrub typhus is acquired from the bite of infected larval trombiculid mites (chiggers). Humans acquire the infection when they intrude into an enzootic focus. Four main elements are constant features of such foci: (1) *R. tsutsugamushi;* (2) chiggers of the *Leptotrombidium deliense* group (*L. deliense, L. akamushi, L. fletcheri, L. arenicola, L. pallidum, L. pavlovskyi,* others); (3) wild rats, especially of the subgenus *Rattus;* and (4) transitional vegetation. The mites, whose larval "chiggers" are the only stage to feed on man and rats, efficiently transmit the rickettsia from one generation to the next through the egg (transovarial passage) and probably constitute the main reservoir of *R. tsutsugamushi* as well as serving as vectors. Rats, especially wild rats of the subgenus *Rattus,* and other small mammals (field mice, voles, shrews) serve as hosts for the parasitic larval mites. Some kind of transitional or secondary vegetation provides the habitat for the chigger-mammal association—e.g., in cleared forest areas; the fringe vegetation along roads, forest trails, or streams; abandoned agricultural areas. Within such habitats, infected chiggers may occur in very circumscribed foci or "mite islands," accounting for the marked focal distribution of scrub typhus cases and sudden outbreaks in field personnel. Suitable habitats are widely distributed from tropical to temperate zones and occur in such extreme settings as semideserts, alpine meadow in the Himalayas, disturbed rain forests, and seashores. In temperate zones, the chiggers are usually active at some time during the warm months, although *L. scutellare*–transmitted *winter* scrub typhus occurs in the Izu Islands of Japan. In tropical or subtropical regions, the disease may be more prevalent at one time of the year than another, depending on rainfall, flooding, and other factors.

PATHOLOGY. The pathologic features of scrub typhus conform generally to those described in Ch. 316. Of special note in scrub typhus is the primary local ulcer with regional and, later, generalized lymphadenopathy. Vascular thrombosis is less frequent than in epidemic typhus and Rocky Mountain spotted fever.

CLINICAL MANIFESTATIONS AND COURSE. The spectrum of clinical severity of untreated scrub typhus ranges from inapparent or mild to severe or fatal in different places and outbreaks. The following description pertains to a classic, relatively severe untreated case of scrub typhus.

The bite of the infecting chigger, which may be on any part of the body, is usually unnoticed; but in roughly 60 to 70 per cent of the primary infections and substantially fewer in second infections, a small painless papule develops during the 6- to 18-day (usually 9- to 12-day) incubation period. It enlarges, undergoes central necrosis, and crusts to form the eschar or primary lesion, which is well developed at the onset of disease. The regional lymph nodes are enlarged and tender. Prodromes of headache, malaise, anorexia, and weakness may occur. The onset is usually acute. The fever rises progressively during the first few days, sometimes accompanied by chills after about the third day, to 39.5 to 40.5° C, accompanied by severe headache, ocular pain, conjunctival injection, anorexia, generalized aches, malaise, apathy, and cough. Interstitial pneumonitis is common. The pulse remains relatively slow. Toward the end of the first week, a macular rash, later sometimes papular, often appears, first on the trunk and then on the extremities. About this time there is generalized lymphadenopathy, soft splenic enlargement, and sometimes hepatomegaly.

During the second week of disease, the temperature remains elevated and signs of complex multiple organ system involvement appear. Apathy may give way to more pronounced signs of meningoencephalitis: delirium and restlessness, stupor, coma, convulsions, muscular weakness, hyperesthesias, and coarse intention tremors. Cranial nerves are selectively involved: varying degrees of nerve deafness and papilledema and congestion of retinal vessels are common; dysarthria and dysphagia are less frequent. Signs of diffuse and focal myocarditis may appear: soft first heart sound, systolic murmurs, ectopic beats, occasional cardiac enlargement, transient gallop rhythm, and minor abnormalities of the electrocardiogram (prolonged P–R interval, inverted T waves). Classic congestive failure is rare, but varying degrees of circulatory failure may appear: increasing pulse rate, falling blood pressure (commonly below 100 mm Hg systolic), rapid shallow respirations, cyanosis, sweating, and cold clammy skin. Gangrene is rare, but edema may be overt in severe cases. Clinical evidence for renal insufficiency is often absent, but oliguria or anuria occurs in some. Spontaneous diuresis is fairly common late in the febrile course or in early convalescence.

In untreated cases, defervescence is by lysis usually after about 10 to 14 days (21 or more days in severe cases). Convalescence is prolonged. All abnormalities appear to be completely reversible, although some, such as cardiovascular instability, personality changes, and deafness, may occasionally persist for weeks to months. Long-term (ten years or more) follow-up of United States servicemen who survived scrub typhus in World War II failed to reveal any significant residua.

An early leukopenia (1000 to 5000 white blood cells per cubic millimeter) gives way to slightly depressed or normal total white blood counts, which may become somewhat elevated late in the disease. Total serum proteins are usually normal or low, but the albumin/globulin (A/G) ratio is often reversed. Occasional clotting disturbances have been reported recently, including disseminated intravascular clotting syndrome. Jaundice is rare, but serum transaminase enzyme levels may be elevated. Albuminuria is common. Isosthenuria, oliguria, and azotemia may occur.

Second and subsequent attacks may be atypical (milder, without eschar, and with sparse or no rash).

DIAGNOSIS. A typhus-like illness with a history of possible exposure in endemic areas and an eschar (in only about 60 to 70 per cent) with regional lymphadenitis should alert the physician to the possibility of scrub typhus. Differential diagnosis may be difficult in some endemic regions where the clinical picture may suggest other rickettsial infections (especially tick-borne typhus, which may also have an eschar) and other nonrickettsial infections (see General Clinical Diagnostic Considerations in Ch. 316). The Weil-Felix test with *Proteus* OX-K, not positive in all cases, is useful because of general availability. The indirect fluorescent antibody test is currently the serodiagnostic method of choice (see Laboratory Diagnosis in Ch. 316). Isolation can be accomplished by inoculating blood or tissue homogenates intraperitoneally into white mice.

PROGNOSIS. Untreated, the mortality ranges from essentially zero to over 30 per cent in different foci. Prompt antibiotic therapy reduces mortality virtually to zero.

TREATMENT. Tetracycline drugs, given as recommended in Ch. 316, and appropriate supportive measures are recommended treatment. Concurrent malaria should not be overlooked.

PREVENTION AND CONTROL. Effective killed vaccines have not yet been developed to prevent scrub typhus. Chemoprophylaxis with weekly doses of doxycycline is feasible. But practically, preventive measures against scrub typhus are directed primarily against the chigger vector. Mite-infested terrain should be avoided whenever possible. Individual prophylaxis against attack by larval mites consists of wearing protective clothing, impregnated with a mite repellent (benzyl benzoate, M-1960), and applying diethyltoluamide to exposed skin areas. The vector population in and around camp sites in endemic zones can be reduced (1) by treating the area intensively with acaricides, (2) possibly by reducing the rodent population through intensive poison bait campaigns, and (3) by destroying vegetation (using bulldozers, power oil burners, herbicides). However, appropriate and relevant environmental, medical, and ecologic considerations must temper decisions on the use of persisting acaricides and herbicides.

Brown GW, Robinson DM, Huxsoll DL: Scrub typhus: A common cause of illness in indigenous populations. Trans R Soc Trop Med Hyg 70:444, 1976. *Illustrates previously unrecognized burden of scrub typhus on human populations indigenous to endemic zones.*

Deller JJ Jr, Russell PK: An analysis of fevers of unknown origin in American soldiers in Vietnam. Ann Intern Med 66:1129, 1967. *Description of recent experience with scrub typhus in military operations.*

Olson JG, Bourgeois AL, Fang RCY, Coolbaugh JC, Dennis DT: Prevention of scrub typhus: Prophylactic administration of doxycycline in a randomized double blind trial. Am J Trop Med Hyg 29:989, 1980. *Suggests feasibility of simple chemoprophylaxis. Unfortunately, bibliography to previous work is incomplete.*

Traub R, Wisseman CL Jr: The ecology of chigger-borne rickettsioses (scrub typhus) (review article). J Med Entomol 11:237, 1974. *Comprehensive review and reference to literature on ecology of scrub typhus up to time of writing.*

322. TRENCH FEVER

Theodore C. Eickhoff

SYNONYMS. Trench fever is also called *five-day* or *quintan fever, shin-bone fever,* and *Volhynia fever.*

DEFINITION. Trench fever is a self-limited febrile disease transmitted by the body louse, *Pediculus humanus corporis,* and characterized by headache, fever, and severe pain in the bones, joints, and muscles. Fatalities are rare, but the disease is characterized in most patients by a relapsing course.

ETIOLOGY AND EPIDEMIOLOGY. The etiologic agent, *Rochalimaea quintana,* is a rickettsia-like agent that grows extracellularly in the louse gut, and is excreted in louse feces. Human infection follows accidental inoculation of contaminated feces into abraded skin or conjunctivae. The etiologic agent is differentiated from other rickettsiae by its ability to grow on artificial media, true rickettsiae being obligate intracellular parasites.

The disease was a major military problem during World Wars I and II in Europe and occurs in endemic form in Mexico, parts of North Africa, and eastern Europe and Asia. Humans are generally considered to be the prinicipal reservoir, since the agent has been isolated from asymptomatic patients years after their initial infection. The louse then acquires its infection by ingesting the blood of an infected human. The recent finding that the so-called "vole agent" is in fact a strain of *Rochalimaea quintana* suggests that reservoirs may also exist in certain rodent populations.

PATHOLOGY AND CLINICAL MANIFESTATIONS. Histopathologic data are limited to skin biopsy studies that have revealed only nonspecific perivascular inflammation. Following an incubation period of 10 to 30 days, the presenting symptoms are fever, of either gradual or abrupt onset, severe weakness, headache, dizziness, and bone and body pain, frequently most dramatically severe in the shins. Physical and laboratory examination generally reveals only slight enlargement of the liver and spleen, pain and soreness in the muscles, and erythematous macules or papules which occur transiently in 70 to 80 per cent of patients. There may be a moderate leukocytosis. The initial febrile episode generally lasts three to five days but frequently recurs after a symptom-free interval of four to five days. Up to eight relapses of fever and symptoms similar to the initial episode have been described, but most patients fortunately experience only several such relapses. In some patients, the fever and symptoms are continuous for two to three weeks. In still others, the initial fever may decline, only to relapse without a true afebrile period, producing a typical "saddle-back" fever curve. Persistent rickettsemia is present during the initial attack, and continues during the relapses as well as the intervening asymptomatic periods; it may persist for months or sometimes years after apparent recovery.

DIAGNOSIS. A history of contact with lice within the appropriate incubation period is helpful. *R. quintana* can be cultivated on agar containing 10 per cent fresh defibrinated horse blood. Both a passive hemagglutination and an enzyme-linked immunosorbent assay test have proved useful in serologic diagnosis. During epidemics, typical cases may be diagnosed on clinical grounds alone. The differential diagnosis should include typhoid fever, typhus, dengue, relapsing fever, and leptospirosis.

TREATMENT AND PROGNOSIS. *Rochalimaea quintana* is highly sensitive in vitro to the tetracyclines and other broad-spectrum antimicrobials, and these may be expected to be as effective in the treatment of trench fever as in the treatment of other rickettsial diseases; there is, however, no direct information supporting their efficacy. Mortality is negligible, and the long-term prognosis is excellent. Approximately 85 per cent of patients recover fully within two months of onset; a few, however, continue to experience recurrences for months or years.

PREVENTION. Elimination of the louse vector by dusting clothing with residual insecticides should be as effective in controlling trench fever as in controlling epidemic typhus. Ten per cent DDT powders proved highly effective for louse control during World War II, but development of DDT resistance may require the use of lindane or malathion as a dusting powder.

Hurst A: Trench fever. Br Med J 2:318, 1942. *This is a lucid account of the clinical characteristics of trench fever in British troops in World War I.*

Vinson JW, Varela G, Molina-Pasquel C: Trench fever. III. Induction of clinical disease in volunteers inoculated with *Rickettsia quintana* propagated on blood agar. Am J Trop Med 18:713, 1969. *This study documents the isolation of the agent and induction of typical trench fever in volunteers.*

Weis E, Dasch GA, Woodman DR, Williams JC: Vole agent identified as a strain of the trench fever rickettsia, *Rochalimaea quintana*. Infect Immun 19:1013, 1978. *One of the few recent studies of trench fever, providing interesting, but speculative, epidemiologic insights.*

323. Q FEVER

Theodore C. Eickhoff

DEFINITION. Q fever is a self-limited rickettsial infection characterized by fever, chills, headache, and constitutional symptoms. In less than one half of patients, there may be an associated pneumonitis. It is unique among the rickettsial diseases of man in that infection is acquired by inhalation rather than by contact with an arthropod vector.

ETIOLOGY. The disease is caused by *Coxiella burnetii*, a rickettsial agent possessing a unique resistance to desiccation and to exposure in dusts and soils. The organism may be propagated in embryonated eggs and in mice, hamsters, and guinea pigs. Both patients and animals develop agglutinating and complement-fixing antibodies to the agents. *C. burnetii*, unlike other rickettsiae, does not stimulate the production of agglutinins to the X-strain of *Proteus vulgaris*.

EPIDEMIOLOGY. ***Incidence and Distribution.*** The true incidence of the disease in humans is impossible to determine because the majority of infections are undiagnosed. In the United States the disease, first found in Montana and California, is now recognized as prevalent in most of the states in which sheep and cattle are produced. Small numbers of cases have been reported from most of the remaining states. Serologic surveys have revealed that many persons exposed to infection in sheep and cattle ranches, abattoirs, meat packing plants or wool processing plants have serologic evidence of past infection. *C. burnetii* is now known to be distributed on a worldwide basis, except for Scandinavian countries.

TRANSMISSION. The epidemiology of Q fever is complex, involving two major patterns of transmission. The first pattern, described in Australia, is a disease cycle in wild animals with transmission of the agent from animal to animal by a tick vector. Such cycles involve up to 40 species of tick vectors. The agent can be transmitted indefinitely as an inapparent infection in the wild reservoir, such as kangaroos, by ticks, but it may also be transmitted laterally by arthropod vectors to a domestic animal in close contact with man. In these and similar cycles recognized in other parts of the world, *C. burnetii*, like the other rickettsial agents of human disease, is vector transmitted.

However, Q fever patients rarely give a history of tick bite. Human infection is now known to result almost exclusively from a second transmission cycle capable of sustaining itself independently of the wild animal cycle. The reservoirs of infection in the second pattern are domestic animals, principally cattle, sheep, and goats, in which *C. burnetii* produces an inapparent or at most mild infection. The organisms do, however, localize in placental tissue and mammary glands of pregnant animals. In sheep, *C. burnetii* is present in up to 10^{12} organisms per gram of placental tissue and to a lesser degree in amniotic fluid, milk, and feces. In the cow, and probably the goat, excretion occurs mainly through the placenta and milk. With all infected animals, the period of parturition is associated with the formation of a highly infectious aerosol. Such aerosols infect other cattle in the herd and also the human population in close contact with the animals. Further, because contaminated clothing, wool, hide, bedding, and soil may be the source of secondary aerosols, the infection may be transmitted by these vehicles at considerable distances from the infected cattle. The unique resistance of *C. burnetii* to prolonged exposure in nature contributes to the spread of the agent by such infectious microenvironments.

The domestic animal cycle has also resulted in several outbreaks of Q fever in personnel in United States medical schools carrying out research studies with pregnant ewes. In addition, Q fever is a recognized laboratory hazard; 50 cases were reported among personnel in one laboratory over a 15-year period. Only 21 of these personnel had been working directly with the organism. Rare reports of nosocomial transmission of Q fever suggest person-to-person transmission; this must be considered infrequent and unlikely.

C. burnetii is easily found in unpasteurized milk from infected cows. Several studies have reported serologic evidence of infection in raw milk drinkers, but there is no clear evidence of disease transmission via raw milk.

PATHOLOGY. Because the mortality rate is quite low, postmortem studies have been few. In patients with pneumonitis, the histopathology is similar to that seen in the viral pneumonias and psittacosis. During the acute phase of the disease, the systemic nature of Q fever is demonstrable both in biochemical abnormalities of liver function and in focal inflammation and noncaseating granulomas in hepatic biopsy specimens. Q fever endocarditis is the major serious complication of the disease, producing valvular vegetations from which rickettsiae may be isolated.

CLINICAL MANIFESTATIONS. After an incubation period of 10 to 28 days after exposure, most patients complain of an abrupt onset of high fever, rigors, headache, muscle pains, and severe malaise. The temperature may rise as high as 40° C and remain elevated, with considerable fluctuation, for one to two weeks. In contrast to all other rickettsial infections, there is no rash. In up to one half of patients there is roentgenographic evidence of pneumonitis, manifested clinically as a slight, nonproductive cough developing in the second week of fever.

Nevertheless, Q fever is more properly considered a severe systemic infection that infrequently causes significant pneumonitis. Hepatic involvement is common, manifested by hepatic enlargement, tenderness, or enzyme elevations; clinical jaundice is rare. Other complications of acute illness rarely reported include myocarditis, pericarditis, and encephalitis. The most serious late sequela, fortunately infrequent, is Q fever endocarditis, which may or may not be preceded by an illness compatible with the acute form of Q fever. Convalescence tends to be prolonged, lasting up to several months, even in uncomplicated cases.

DIAGNOSIS. Q fever should always be suspected in a patient having a severe febrile illness for which no obvious cause can be found. If the patient's vocation or avocation brings him into contact with sheep, cattle, or goats, or byproducts such as wool or hides, it should be particularly suspected.

The differential diagnosis of the acute systemic febrile illness includes influenza, infectious mononucleosis, brucellosis, typhoid fever, cytomegalovirus infection, leptospirosis, and toxoplasmosis. If pneumonitis is prominent, viral pneumonia, mycoplasma, psittacosis, and *Legionella pneumophila* must be considered as well. Evidence of hepatic involvement should suggest viral hepatitis or other intrahepatic processes in addition to those mentioned previously.

Diagnostic studies are usually limited to serologic studies. The complement-fixation test is the most generally available. Recent reports have emphasized the importance of phase variation in the selection of antigens for diagnostic use. Sixty-five per cent of patients will develop elevated titers against phase II antigen by the end of the second week of illness, and

90 per cent of patients will do so after four weeks. Elevated (≥1:200) antibody to phase I antigen is seen in patients with Q fever endocarditis, and the finding of such an elevated titer to phase I antigen during convalescence should raise the possibility of subacute or chronic infection.

TREATMENT AND PROGNOSIS. The tetracyclines and chloramphenicol are both effective in treatment of acute infections with *C. burnetii*, but owing to potential chloramphenicol toxicity, tetracycline is preferred, in a dose of 500 mg four times daily. The mortality is low (1 per cent or less) in untreated patients, and is lower still in those treated with antimicrobial drugs. Therapy should be continued for approximately one week, even though patients usually become afebrile within 48 to 72 hours. Patients occasionally may experience relapse after treatment, and when this occurs additional drug therapy should be administered.

Prognosis is less favorable for the rare patient in whom Q fever endocarditis develops. In some of these patients the disease has been reported to be unresponsive to antimicrobial therapy; long-term tetracycline therapy plus valve replacement as necessary is reported to reduce mortality in such patients to about 30 per cent.

PREVENTION. Experimental lots of yolk-sac vaccines have been effective in preventing clinical disease in volunteers experimentally infected via the respiratory route, and active immunization is still under study. Control measures are presently limited to minimizing exposure to the agents. This is generally not feasible for those occupationally exposed, save for those working in research or diagnostic laboratories. Milk from cattle, sheep, and goats in endemic areas should be pasteurized or boiled before use.

Ascher MS, Berman MA, Ruppanner R: Initial clinical and immunologic evaluation of a new phase I Q fever vaccine and skin test in humans. J Infect Dis 148:214, 1983. *Description of a promising vaccine.*

Baca OG, Paretsky D: Q fever and *Coxiella burnetii*: A model for host-parasite interactions. Microbiol Rev 47:127, 1983. *A current comprehensive exposition of the basic biology of* C. burnetii.

Clark WH, Lenette EH, Railsback OC, et al.: Q fever in California. VII. Clinical features in one hundred eighty cases. Arch Intern Med 88:155, 1951. *Well over thirty years old, but still among the best clinical studies of Q fever to be found.*

Kimbrough RC, Ormsbee RA, Peacock M, et al.: Q fever endocarditis in the United States. Ann Intern Med 91:400, 1979. *Illustrates the current management of Q fever endocarditis, and the use of phase I and II antigens in serodiagnosis.*

Meiklejohn G, Reimer EG, Graves PS, Helmick C: Cryptic epidemic of Q fever in a medical school. J Infect Dis 144:107, 1981. *Provides an insight into the potential Q fever problem in research settings.*

Tigertt WD, Benenson AR, Gochenour WJ: Airborne Q fever. Bact Rev 25:285, 1961. *A thorough review of the epidemiology of Q fever, emphasizing the extreme infectivity of this agent.*

Tobin MJ, Cahill N, Gearty G, et al.: Q Fever endocarditis. Am J Med 72:396, 1982. *Good discussion of the management of Q fever endocarditis.*

Section Three VIRAL DISEASES

324. INTRODUCTION TO VIRAL DISEASES

Edwin D. Kilbourne

Viruses are the most pervasive of infectious agents, infecting not only animals and plants but also bacteria, which are themselves agents of disease. Indeed, the ultimate causes of diphtheria and scarlet fever are the lysogenic viruses which infect the responsible bacteria. Viruses are the simplest and smallest of microorganisms. They are essentially transmissible genomes—life reduced to minimal complexity. The simpler viruses are protein-wrapped packages of nucleic acid carrying the blueprints for their own replication. Although simple, a virus is highly specialized. It functions not as a random source of genes, but as an exquisitely specialized package of information narrowly adapted by evolution to a way of life which not only permits its replication in the proper environment (i.e., in the proper cells of the proper host) but somehow programs for its exit from this environment and its attachment to and penetration of cells of the next host. Thus, the influenza virus mutant, so avirulent that it does not damage respiratory tract epithelial cells and thus provoke a cough and thereby effect the expulsion of its progeny, will have small chance for survival.

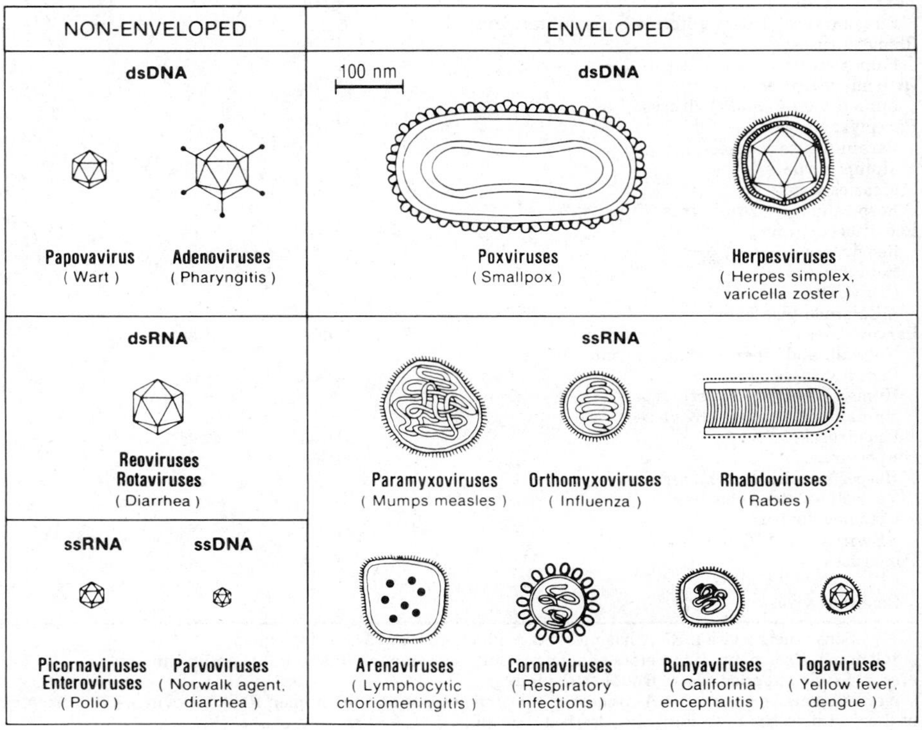

Figure 324–1. Families of known human viruses. (Modified from Matthews REF: Intervirology 12:158, 1979. By permission of S. Karger AG, Basel.)

Therefore, despite their utter dependence upon the cells of others and hence their formal lack of independence, viruses are most usefully considered as highly specialized organisms.

The dependence of viruses upon the host which they infect has favored the evolution of a temperate relationship for the most part of the viruses which are obligate and exclusive human parasites with man as their target and sustenance. Encountered early in life, sometimes damped by maternally transferred antibody, the obligate human viruses often cause asymptomatic infection and rarely kill. Paralysis in poliovirus infection is a rare event, measles encephalitis is uncommon, and fatal influenza usually occurs in previously damaged hosts.

But a large group of important and dangerous human viral infections are caused by viruses not specific for man. Such viruses as the agents of yellow fever and rabies cause primary infections of other hosts; they have not had to adapt to the human condition, and their ravages therefore are severe when human infection occurs as an accident of contact.

As shown in Figure 324–1, viruses come in a variety of shapes and sizes and vary widely in chemical composition (Table 324–1), from the simpler picornaviruses, which are composed only of RNA and protein, to the enveloped viruses, which contain glycoprotein spikes and lipid derived from the host cell membrane.

The relation of design and function of viruses is increasingly appreciated. Certain myxoviruses, including the influenza and parainfluenza viruses, possess a potent neuraminidase that probably abets their release from the mucin-coated cells of the respiratory tract. Most myxoviruses are fragile and unstable in the environment, whereas the enteroviruses, including poliovirus, can pass unscathed through the barrier of gastric acidity in their journey to the target cells of the small intestine.

Neither structural nor chemical similarity of viruses is any sure guide to the diseases that they may cause. Mumps and parainfluenza viruses are indistinguishable by electron microscopy and even share antigens in common, but one invades the salivary glands, pancreas, or meninges, whereas the other produces mild upper respiratory tract infection or infantile croup. Nor does viral dissimilarity predict dissimilar disease. The structurally variable, genetically plastic RNA virus of influenza and the geometrically precise DNA-containing adenovirus with its potential for latency both evoke similar clinical syndromes that may be difficult to differentiate.

BASIC CATEGORIES AND PROPERTIES OF HUMAN VIRUSES (VIRAL TAXONOMY). Is it important for the clinician to know that poliovirus is an enterovirus of the picornavirus family or that the agent of chickenpox is a herpesvirus? A physician who

TABLE 324–1. BASIC CATEGORIES AND PROPERTIES OF HUMAN VIRUSES

	Nucleic Acid			Virion		
Virus Families and Genera	*Type*	*Configuration*	*Sense**	*Size (nm)*	*Envelope*	**Obligate for Man**
Picornaviruses	RNA	ss	(+)	25	0	
Enteroviruses						
Poliovirus						Yes
Coxsackievirus						
Echovirus						
Rhinoviruses						
Togaviruses	RNA	ss	(+)			
Arbovirus A (alphavirus):				70	+	No
eastern, western, and Venezuelan encephalitis viruses						
Arbovirus B (flavivirus):				50	+	No
yellow fever, dengue viruses						
Rubella virus				60		Yes
Coronaviruses	RNA	ss	(+)	75–160	+	
Human coronavirus						Yes
Arenaviruses	RNA	ss	(−)†	50–300	+	No
Lymphocytic choriomeningitis virus; Lassa fever virus						
Bunyaviruses	RNA	ss	(−)†	90–100	+	No
Bunyamwera virus, California encephalitis virus						
Rhabdoviruses	RNA	ss	(−)	70 × 170	+	
Rabies virus						
Orthomyxoviruses	RNA	ss	(−)†	80–120	+	
Influenza A, B, and C viruses						†
Paramyxoviruses	RNA	ss	(−)	150 +	+	
Parainfluenza viruses						Yes (types 2 and 4)
Mumps virus						Yes
Measles virus						Yes
Respiratory syncytial virus						Yes
Reovirus subgroup	RNA	ds	(−)†	60–80	0	
Reoviruses						?
Rotaviruses						No
Orbiviruses:						No
Colorado tick fever						
Parvoviruses	DNA	ss		18–26	0	
Norwalk and other diarrheal agents						?
Papovaviruses	DNA	ds			0	
Human papilloma (wart) virus				52		Yes
Human polyoma JC, BK viruses				45		Yes
Adenoviruses	DNA	ds		70–90	0	Yes
Herpesviruses	DNA	ds		120–150	+	
Herpes simplex 1 and 2 viruses						Yes
Varicella-zoster virus						Yes
Cytomegalovirus						Yes
EB virus						Yes
Poxviruses	DNA	ds		170–260 × 300–450	+	
Smallpox virus						Yes

*(+) Sense means virion RNA has messenger function, i.e., RNA is infectious.
†Genome is segmented; therefore genetic reassortment among viruses of this group can occur.
ss = Single stranded. ds = Double stranded.
Not listed above are the DNA-containing hepatitis B virus and the human RNA retroviruses that have recently been associated with human T cell leukemia; neither of these viruses has been formally classified. Hepatitis A virus is an enterovirus.

possesses this information will not be surprised at the neurotropic potential of other enteroviruses, or at the reactivation of varicella virus as herpes zoster years after primary infection. If he appreciates the nuances of viral taxonomy he will know that it is a jungle of acronyms, sigla, neologisms, Greco-Latin hybrids, and morphologic descriptions. He will not be much aided by knowing that the togaviruses are cloaked (toga) with a host-derived envelope, because other enveloped viruses (Fig. 324–1, Table 324–1) are not so designated. However, the arbovirus designation of some members of the togavirus family will indicate to him that they are *ar*thropod *bo*rne. The term echovirus—*e*nteric *c*ytopathogenic *h*uman *o*rphan viruses—reminds him that these enteroviruses were recognized first as cytopathic agents in tissue culture and only later were associated with specific human diseases. In any case, it is the function of Table 324–1 to show where measles, mumps, and influenza viruses fit into the scheme of things and also to define the nature of their genomes as central to their replicative strategy and potential. Certain generalizations can be inferred on the basis of the nature of the viral nucleic acid. RNA viruses infrequently participate in true intrachromosomal genetic recombination with other viruses, and except for RNA tumor viruses (only recently found in humans) lack the capacity to integrate their genomes with that of the host—a capacity now proven for the DNA herpesviruses. On the other hand, certain of these viruses bear their RNA in pieces that can be readily reassorted during dual infection to create new viruses combining genes from both parents. Viruses as different as influenza and reoviruses share this property, which obviously enhances their adaptability and evolutionary potential. Viral nucleic acid may be double (ds) or single stranded (ss) in configuration, and RNA viruses contain either messenger RNA (mRNA) available for direct translation in the manufacture of viral proteins or RNA of nonmessage sense, which must be transcribed by a virion transcriptase to mRNA. Enveloped viruses (except for the poxviruses) emerge from infected cells by a budding process, incorporating host cell membrane lipids.

A CLASSIFICATION OF VIRUS INFECTIONS ACCORDING TO MECHANISM OF PATHOGENESIS. All viruses have in common the following replicative steps in the initial stage of pathogenesis: (1) *adsorption* through specific viral receptors to specific receptors on susceptible host cells; (2) *penetration* of the cell membrane; (3) *uncoating* of viral nucleic acid to permit expression of the viral genes (this step is usually carried out by host cell enzymes and coincides with the *eclipse period,* during which time infective virus cannot be found in the cell); (4) *macromolecular synthesis* of nucleic acid and protein; (5) *assembly* of virion components; and (6) *release* of infective virus from the cell. These events may occur in association with severe disruption of host cell function and rapid cytonecrosis, or host cell function may be virtually unaffected, depending on the nature of the invading virus. The damage to primary target cells may in itself directly cause the disease state, or characteristic symptoms may reflect involvement of secondary or even tertiary target cells in organs remote from the initial site of invasion (Fig. 324–2). Cellular damage may be the direct result of viral replication or may be indirectly mediated through the cellular immune response.

As illustrated in Table 324–2, initial and primary invasion of

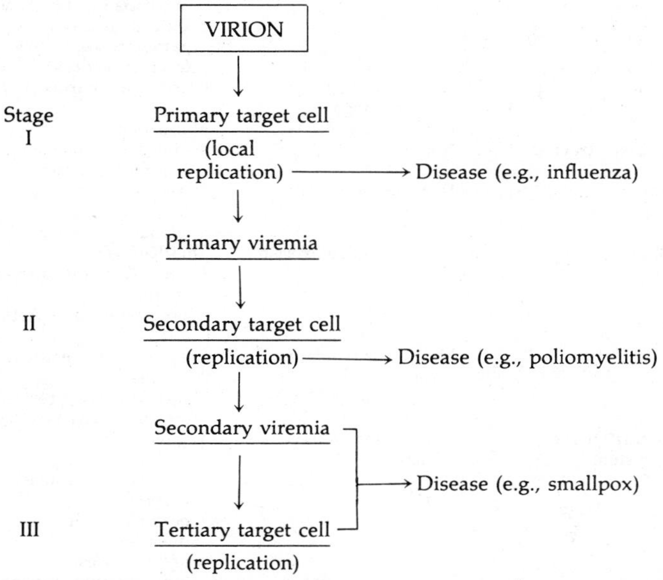

Figure 324–2. Stages of viral pathogenesis. Initial invasion may involve only primary target cells (influenza) or may lead to secondary or tertiary target cell invasion (poliomyelitis and smallpox), which results in the characteristic disease.

TABLE 324–2. PATHOGENETIC CLASSIFICATION OF HUMAN VIRAL INFECTIONS

I. Primary and definitive infection of the respiratory tract
 A. Orthomyxoviruses (influenza A, B, and C viruses)—influenza
 B. Paramyxoviruses
  1. (Parainfluenza viruses 1–4)—rhinitis, laryngotracheitis "croup"
  2. Respiratory syncytial (RS) virus—croup, infantile pneumonia
 C. Rhinoviruses (1–89 +)—"common cold," rhinitis
 D. Coronaviruses—mild upper respiratory tract infection
II. Primary respiratory tract infection with secondary infection elsewhere
 A. Adenoviruses (types 1–28)—febrile pharyngitis, ocular involvement with some types (especially, type 8); viruses can multiply in the small intestine
 B. Paramyxoviruses
  1. Mumps virus—parotitis, orchitis, oophoritis, pancreatitis, meningoencephalitis, viremia
  2. Measles virus—conjunctivitis, rhinitis, pharyngitis, bronchitis, pneumonia, viremia, exanthem, encephalitis
 C. Rubella virus (German measles)—mild upper respiratory infection, viremia, exanthem, encephalitis
 D. Poxvirus (smallpox virus)—respiratory tract symptoms, exanthem (see Fig. 324–3)
 E. Herpesviruses
  1. (Varicella-zoster virus)—chickenpox; herpes zoster—extremely mild respiratory symptoms → pneumonia in adults, exanthem
  2. Cytomegalovirus (cytomegalic inclusion disease)—mild or absent respiratory symptoms, pneumonia, hepatitis, viremia (congenital transplacental infection may occur)
  3. EB virus—lymphoproliferative disease, infectious mononucleosis
III. Primary and definitive enteric infections
 Reoviruses, rotaviruses, and parvoviruses have recently been implicated in diarrheal disease of man on the basis of demonstration of their presence in high concentration by electron microscopy of fecal specimens and by specific immune response
 Although the enteroviruses and the hepatitis viruses multiply initially and principally in the gut, multiplication is not restricted to this site, and viremia and secondary manifestations occur
IV. Primary enteric infection with secondary infection elsewhere (all picornaviruses except rhinoviruses)
 A. Polioviruses (types 1–3)—pharyngitis, meningoencephalitis, poliomyelitis, viremia
 B. Coxsackievirus: group A (types 1–24); group B (types 1–6)—vesicular pharyngitis (herpangina), aseptic meningitis, exanthem (macular or vesicular), epidemic pleurodynia and myalgia, myocarditis, viremia
 C. Echoviruses (*e*nteric *c*ytopathogenic *h*uman *o*rphan viruses) (types 1–30 +)—upper respiratory infection, aseptic meningitis, gastroenteritis, exanthem (macular), viremia
 D. Herpesviruses (herpes simplex)—primary oral or genital infection
 E. Hepatitis virus A—virus not yet cultivable in cell culture systems, viremia
V. Percutaneous (parenteral) infections by viruses nonobligate for man
 A. Togaviruses (200 + viruses in 20 different antigenic groups)—all multiply in hematophagous (bloodsucking) vectors—mosquitoes, ticks, sandflies, or gnats—and in avian or nonhuman mammalian hosts; diverse systemic disease (see clinical classification, Table 324–3) and viremia
 B. Rhabdovirus—(rabies) encephalitis
 C. Arenaviruses—Lassa fever
 D. Bunyaviruses—California encephalitis
VI. Percutaneously acquired obligate human viruses
 A. Herpesvirus
  1. Herpes simplex type 2 virus—genital, venereal infection
  2. Hepatitis virus B (serum hepatitis) or hepatitis virus A (infectious hepatitis) when administered via hypodermic needle
VII. Transplacentally acquired (congenital or vertical) human viral infections (all characterized by maternal viremia)
 A. Rubella
 B. Cytomegalic inclusion disease
 C. Others on occasion

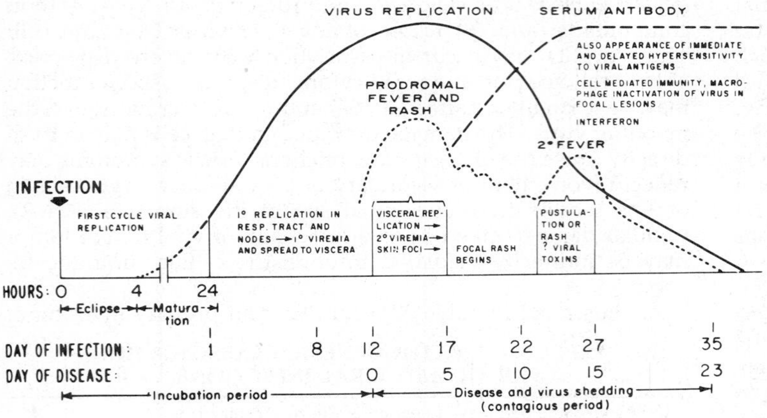

Figure 324–3. Pathogenesis of smallpox (based in part on inferences from animal models).

cells occurs with contagious viral infections (those spread from man to man) at respiratory or enteric portals. If replication is confined to these primary sites, as with rhinovirus and influenza virus infections in the respiratory tract, and rotavirus infection of the gut, then symptomatology similarly reflects this focal organ involvement. Viremia rarely occurs with these infections, and the malaise, myalgia, and other systemic signs of toxicity remain unexplained.

In other cases, the respiratory or intestinal tract, although the site of initial invasion, is not the definitive site of infection and disease. Measles and poliomyelitis viruses, although they first infect cells, respectively, of the respiratory tract or intestine, are spread through a viremic stage to other organs in which the characteristic disease is expressed. The transient involvement of the primary target cells may or may not be attended by minor or prodromal symptoms. It can be assumed that all virus diseases with rash, as well as those parenterally transmitted, must have a viremic stage. Furthermore, all viremic infections have the potential for congenital transplacental transmission. In fact, only rubella and cytomegaloviruses seem to be important causes of congenital disease.

The temporal aspects of viral pathogenesis are important to comprehend. A schematic profile of the pathogenic sequence in smallpox as a prototype is presented in Figure 324–3. Infection, probably initiated by one or very few viral particles, occurs in a cell or cells of the respiratory tract, in which the first cycle of viral replication takes place in a matter of hours. During the subsequent ten or eleven days of the *incubation period,* cell-to-cell spread locally in the respiratory tract and to regional nodes occurs by contiguity, associated with a transient primary viremia in which virus is disseminated to other viscera, including the liver and spleen. Symptoms of the disease begin about the twelfth day of infection in association with extensive visceral replication of virus, secondary viremia, and the establishment of skin foci. A prodromal fever and rash are associated with these events. On about the fifth day of disease (seventeenth day of infection) specific neutralizing antibody is first detectable in the serum. Thereafter it increases rapidly in titer coincidentally with the decline in fever, which occurs with appearance of the characteristic focal skin lesions.

Pustulation of the rash occurs between the ninth and fourteenth days as the result of cytonecrosis, from either viral toxins or perhaps immunopathologic reactions. This pustulation is associated with a secondary increase in fever and is not the result of secondary bacterial invasion.

Other events associated with the host's response which are difficult to indicate on a specific timetable are the appearance of both immediate and delayed hypersensitivity to viral antigens, the occurrence of cell-mediated immunity, and the inactivation of virus in focal lesions by macrophages. As with other viral infections, interferon probably plays a role in recovery, but the nature and extent of this role have not yet been defined.

A CLINICAL CLASSIFICATION OF VIRAL INFECTIONS. Finally, the physician must confront the end result of virus replication and the final stage of pathogenesis, which is clinical disease. Although certain viruses such as mumps, measles, and polioviruses are pathognomonic in their effects, clinical distinction among many virus infections is difficult. Indeed, fever and myalgia in the absence of obvious focal signs are generally regarded by physicians and laymen alike as manifestations of "a virus." Although the definitive diagnosis of viral infection

TABLE 324–3. CLINICAL CLASSIFICATION OF HUMAN VIRAL INFECTIONS (ACCORDING TO SITE OF CARDINAL SYMPTOMATOLOGY)

Site of Cardinal Symptoms	Presenting Disease	Causative Viruses
Upper respiratory tract	Rhinitis, pharyngitis, "common cold"	Rhinovirus, enterovirus, adenovirus, parainfluenza virus, coronavirus
Middle and lower respiratory tract	Tracheitis, bronchitis, pneumonia	Parainfluenza virus, RS virus, influenza viruses
Mouth	Gingivostomatitis, pharyngitis	Herpes simplex (type 1) virus
Genitalia	Vesicular or ulcerative lesions, orchitis, oophoritis	Herpes simplex (type 2) virus, mumps virus
Gastrointestinal	Gastroenteritis, hepatitis	Reoviruses, echoviruses, hepatitis viruses (A & B), rotaviruses, parvoviruses, yellow fever (arbovirus)
	Gastrointestinal hemorrhage	(Certain arboviruses)
	Pancreatitis	Mumps virus
Urinary tract	Nephritis	Yellow fever and some other arboviruses
Eye	Keratoconjunctivitis	Herpes simplex, herpes zoster, adenovirus type 8
Skin	Papular-vesicular rash	Smallpox virus, varicella-zoster, herpes simplex, coxsackieviruses A-16, 5, 10
	Macular-erythematous rash	Certain enteroviruses, rubella
	Macular-hemorrhagic rash	Measles, dengue, certain other arboviruses
Central nervous system	Encephalomyelitis, meningitis	Togaviruses, enteroviruses, rhabdovirus (rabies), herpesviruses, paramyxovirus (measles), arenaviruses, bunyaviruses, mumps
Peripheral lymph nodes	Lymphadenopathy	EB herpes virus
Salivary glands	Parotitis	Mumps virus

depends on isolation and identification of the virus and a study of specific immunologic response, consideration of the site of cardinal symptomatology is often helpful in reducing the range of etiologic possibilities (Table 324–3).

But as with other diseases, the clinical diagnosis of viral infections is aided by the context and circumstances in which infections occur. Acute pharyngitis in summer is usually caused by enteroviruses; in winter adenoviruses and rhinoviruses prevail. The individual case of influenza is easily confused with a number of other prostrating viral infections, but when the disease occurs in a sudden community-wide epidemic, it is readily diagnosed.

Viral infections are more frequent in childhood, at which time they are, in general, better tolerated. Except for the neonatal period, the severity of virus diseases increases with age *if such infection represents initial or primary contact with the virus.* On the other hand, reinfections of the adult (as with parainfluenza or adenoviruses) may be so modified by prior immune response that they are very mild or even asymptomatic. Needless to say, the severity of viral disease is often unfavorably influenced in chronically ill or immunologically compromised patients. In leukemic children with impaired cell-mediated immunity, varicella, among the mildest of viruses, can produce fatal illness; the rare paralytic complications of live poliovirus vaccines occur most commonly in children with immune deficiency states.

In summary, the clinical expression of disease in any given viral infection is a spectrum of response related to the virulence of the infecting virus (which tends to be relatively fixed), the infecting dose, the age and prior immunizing experience of the patient, and the integrity of his immune system and his general physiologic state, as well as host genetic factors which still remain to be defined.

These generalizations will gain substance in the separate consideration of individual virus infections in the chapters which follow.

Baltimore D: Expression of animal virus genomes. Bacteriol Rev 35:235, 1971. *Classic analysis of the differing replication strategies of viruses.*

Dulbecco R, Ginsberg HS: Virology. Harper & Row, 1980. *Excerpted from the classic* Microbiology *text. Good discussion of pathogenesis.*

Evans AS (ed.): Viral Infections of Humans—Epidemiology and Control. 2nd ed. New York, Plenum Medical Book Company, 1982. *Solid work with emphasis on viral epidemiology in general and particular.*

Fenner FJ, White DO: Medical Virology. 2nd ed. New York, Academic Press, 1976. *Dated but admirably succinct and well organized consideration of all aspects of human viral infections.*

Joklik WK: Principles of Animal Virology. New York, Appleton-Century-Crofts, 1980. *Strong basic text on virology and human virus diseases.*

Kilbourne ED: Segmented genome viruses and the evolutionary potential of asymmetrical sex. Perspect Biol Med 25:66, 1981. *Discussion of the potential evolutionary advantage of the several groups of viruses with segmented genomes, as well as practical applications of viral genetic reassortment.*

Luria SE, Darnell JE Jr, Baltimore D, Campbell A: General Virology. 3rd ed. New York, John Wiley & Sons, 1978. *Holistic consideration of general principles of virology, as well as a limited specific examination of prototype viruses of animals, plants, and bacteria.*

Reitz MS Jr, Kalyanaraman VS, Robert-Guroff M, Popovic M, Sarngadharan MG, Sarin PS, Gallo RC: Human T-cell leukemia/lymphoma virus: The retrovirus of adult T-cell leukemia/lymphoma. J Infect Dis 147:399, 1983. *Basic information about the first human leukemia virus to be isolated, written by the discoverer (R. C. Gallo) and his colleagues.*

Viral Infections of the Respiratory Tract

325/326. THE COMMON COLD*

Albert Z. Kapikian

DEFINITION. Although the term "common cold" does not denote a precisely defined disease, it has an almost universally comprehended meaning of an acute self-limited common illness of all age groups, in which the major clinical manifestations involve the upper respiratory tract, with nasal discharge (coryza) or nasal obstruction as the predominant symptom.

HISTORY. Although it was known since 1914 that bacteria-free filtrates of nasal secretions from patients with common cold could induce similar illnesses in volunteers inoculated intranasally, the discovery of etiologic agents from common colds eluded scientists for many years. Despite the isolation of numerous viruses that were associated etiologically with acute respiratory illnesses, such as influenza virus in 1933, and the adeno-, parainfluenza, and respiratory syncytial viruses in the 1950's, it soon became clear that the major etiologic agent(s) of the common cold had not yet been discovered. However, beginning gradually in the 1950's and escalating rapidly in the 1960's, largely because of the development of human diploid cell cultures (which were extremely sensitive for the propagation of certain viral agents), over 100 distinct common cold viruses were discovered and shown to be the major causative agents of the common cold. These heretofore fastidious agents were named rhinoviruses (rhin- is Greek for nose), since they caused predominantly nasal symptoms. Shortly thereafter, in the mid 1960's, another group of fastidious viruses, the coronaviruses, were discovered with the use of tissue and organ cultures and shown to be the second most important etiologic agents of the common cold and related diseases.

ETIOLOGY. Rhinoviruses have emerged as the major known causative agents of adult upper respiratory illnesses such as common colds. They have been isolated from approximately 15 to 40 per cent of adults with these illnesses (Table 325/326–1). The isolation rate is lower in children with upper respiratory tract illness, since only 4 to 5 per cent are rhinovirus positive. Rhinoviruses are classified as a subgroup of the picornavirus family and possess certain common characteristics, including small size (15 to 30 nm), ribonucleic acid (RNA) core, ether resistance, and complete or almost complete inactivation at pH 3. The latter property is a major characteristic distinguishing rhinoviruses from the other major subgroup of the picornaviruses, the enteroviruses (poliovirus, coxsackievirus, and echovirus), which are stable at pH 3. There are 89 officially designated rhinovirus serotypes, but the number will exceed 100 when the numbering system is extended further.

The second most important etiologic agents of common colds are the coronaviruses, which are associated with 10 to 20 per cent of common colds in adults. Their importance as etiologic agents of common colds in infants and young children has not been determined. These viruses possess certain common characteristics, including (a) a unique electron microscopic appearance characterized by pleomorphic 80 to 200 nm enveloped particles possessing relatively widely spaced club- or pear-shaped surface projections (reminiscent of the solar corona, from which the name coronavirus is derived); (b) an RNA genome; and (c) ether and acid lability. There are at least three distinct human coronavirus serotypes, designated B814, 229E, and OC43. Owing to difficulties in propagating these fastidious agents, fewer than 50 isolates have been recovered since their discovery; most epidemiologic studies have thus relied on serologic studies with the 229E and OC43 viruses for which suitable antigens could be prepared. As shown in Table 325/326–1, many other viruses such as influenza, parainfluenza, respiratory syncytial, adeno-, echo- and coxsackieviruses can also cause common-cold–like symptoms. These other agents are described in other sections of this text. A diagnosis of the etiology of a common cold cannot be made clinically, since the

*In the interests of an organized and coherent treatment of the topic, the originally planned chapters on The Common Cold and Rhinoviral Respiratory Disease have been combined into this single chapter.

TABLE 325/326–1. PERCENTAGE OF COMMON COLDS ASSOCIATED WITH SPECIFIC ETIOLOGIC AGENTS IN ADULTS*

Rhinoviruses (over 100 serotypes)	15–40%
Coronaviruses (at least 3 serotypes)	10–20%
Influenza viruses A, B, C, Parainfluenza viruses (4 serotypes) Respiratory syncytial virus (1 serotype) Adenoviruses (various serotypes)	5–10%
Coxsackieviruses (various serotypes) Echoviruses (various serotypes)	1–2%
Group A beta-hemolytic streptococci	2–10%
No specific agent known but presumed to be viral	30–50%

*Each of these agents can also cause common colds in the pediatric age group, but their relative roles are not clearly defined. Viruses associated with specific syndromes such as rubeola, rubella, and varicella have also been associated with common-cold–like symptoms in children.

agents causing the syndrome are so numerous. In addition, about one third to one half of common colds have yet to be associated with an etiologic agent.

INCIDENCE AND PREVALENCE. The common cold is probably the most frequently occurring illness in humans worldwide. The National Center for Health Statistics estimated that in the United States in 1981 the population experienced more than 93 million common colds for an incidence of 41.4 per 100 persons per year. Common colds represented 19.5 per cent of all acute conditions and were estimated to cause over 261 million days of restricted activity.

In the Cleveland Family Study, which spanned a period of about 10 years and included over 25,000 illnesses, common respiratory diseases accounted for 60 per cent of all illnesses. The overall incidence of common respiratory diseases (which included illnesses diagnosed as the common cold, rhinitis, laryngitis, bronchitis, and other undifferentiated acute respiratory illnesses) was 5.6 per person per year. Children under one year of age experienced about seven respiratory illnesses per year; the highest incidence occurred in the one-year age group (8.3 cases per year) and the incidence remained rather high through age five (7.4 cases per year). A progressive decrease was observed beginning at age six. As expected, adults had relatively fewer common respiratory illnesses than children (adults averaged over four per year). The average incidence was slightly greater in boys than in girls, whereas in adults, mothers experienced higher rates than fathers. In addition, the incidence of common respiratory diseases was greater in young children attending school than in those of the same age who were not in school; also, preschool siblings of school children had more respiratory illnesses than preschool siblings without brothers or sisters attending school. The incidence of common respiratory diseases increased progressively as family size increased from three to seven members. Such illnesses were introduced into the home most frequently by school children under six years of age, followed in order of decreasing frequency by preschool children, school children six years of age and over, mothers, and fathers. Analysis of secondary attack rates in families revealed that on the average 25 per cent of all exposures in the home were followed by illness; one- and two-year-olds experienced the highest secondary attack rates (about twice the average).

In a more recent survey of acute respiratory illnesses over a six-year period in Tecumseh, Michigan, the mean incidence of respiratory illnesses per person per year was 3. The highest incidence was in the one-year age group (6.1) and the next highest in the one- to two-year age group (5.7). A viral or potentially pathogenic bacterial agent was isolated from about 25 per cent of the specimens collected, with rhinoviruses accounting for 38.5 per cent of the total number of isolates, a figure representing more than twice the number of isolates of the next most frequently detected group, the parainfluenza viruses.

Studies of the prevalence of neutralizing antibodies in serum against various rhinovirus serotypes have revealed a gradual acquisition of antibody beginning early in childhood and reaching a maximum of at least 50 per cent in the fifth decade, thus providing further evidence that rhinovirus infections occur throughout early life and into adulthood. The prevalence of serum antibody to specific serotypes was not consistent. Although all individuals studied had neutralizing antibodies to each of the 55 serotypes tested, the prevalence of antibody to each serotype varied from about 10 to 80 per cent. Limited surveys of the prevalence of neutralizing antibody to rhinoviruses in various developed and developing countries including several tropical areas indicate a generally worldwide presence of rhinovirus antibody.

The prevalence of coronavirus serum antibody has been difficult to ascertain since only two serotypes, 229E and OC43, can be studied in cell cultures and, in addition, results have been variable in different locations with these two viruses. For example, in one study, 29 per cent of children and 69 per cent of adults had serum complement-fixing (CF) antibody to OC43 virus. Such antibody to 229E virus was present very infrequently in children, whereas about one third of adults were antibody positive. However, in the United Kingdom, about 25 per cent of children and 41 per cent of adults had neutralizing antibody to 229E virus. In United States marine recruits, over 80 per cent had serum hemagglutination inhibition antibody to OC43 virus and 12 per cent had CF antibody to 229E virus. A true evaluation of the prevalence of antibody to the coronavirus group must await the development of serologic assays for other members of this fastidious group of agents.

EPIDEMIOLOGY. In the temperate climates common colds occur most frequently in the colder months of the year. For example, in the Cleveland family study a consistent pattern of a low summer and high winter incidence of common respiratory diseases was documented. In September, a rise in respiratory illnesses to about six cases per person-year from a summer low of three cases per person-year was observed. After a slight dip in October an average rate of about seven cases per person-year was observed for each month from November through March. Some of the factors influencing the spread of common colds have already been described. However, with the discovery of rhinoviruses as the major etiologic agent of common colds, important questions relating to the epidemiology of these specific agents finally could be addressed.

Rhinoviruses are spread from person to person by direct contact, usually with transmission by infected droplets. In early volunteer studies, rhinoviruses induced common colds when administered in nasal drops or by swabbing the nasal mucosa or conjunctiva but not by swabbing the throat. More recent volunteer studies have highlighted a heretofore unrecognized mode of transmission that involves self-inoculation of the conjunctival or nasal mucosa with a rhinovirus-contaminated finger. Virus was recovered in 15 of 16 trials from fingers that were rubbed on plastic surfaces contaminated with rhinovirus one to three hours previously. In addition, rhinovirus was recovered from three of five subject pairs after exposures of uninfected skin to infected skin. The efficiency of transmission of infection from experimentally infected volunteers to susceptible volunteers by hand-to-hand contact followed by self-inoculation was compared with that of transmission by large- and small-particle aerosols. It was striking that 11 of 15 hand-to-hand exposures initiated infection, whereas only 1 of 12 large-particle exposures (donor and contact in social setting) and none of 10 small-particle exposures (donor and contact separated by double mesh barrier) induced such infection.

Rhinovirus communicability was evaluated in childless married couples in a study in which both lacked serum antibody. The overall transmission of a rhinovirus-related cold between partners was 38 per cent, which is similar to the secondary attack rate in the Cleveland Family Study or to those in epidemiologic studies of naturally occurring rhinovirus infections. Transmission rarely occurred unless (1) at least 1000 $TCID_{50}$ of virus was present in the donor's nasal washing, (2) the donor's hands and anterior nares were rhinovirus positive, (3) the donor had at least moderate symptoms, and (4) the partners spent many hours together (at least 122 hours during a seven-day period). Virus in saliva was not strongly associated with transmission.

The effect of exposure to cold temperatures on the course of common colds was evaluated in volunteers who were challenged with rhinovirus by small-particle aerosol or intranasal installation. Exposure to the cold environment did not have a significant effect on host resistance to rhinovirus infection and illness. Exposure to cold temperature did not induce a common cold in uninoculated volunteers. This finding is consistent with results of early studies on the epidemiology of common colds on the island of Spitzbergen. These early studies demonstrated that very few colds occurred during the bitter Arctic winter, but sharp outbreaks began shortly after the first ship arrived at the end of May. Thus, cold weather by itself did not induce common colds; the ingredient needed to initiate the outbreak was exposure to infected individuals. In early volunteer studies using common cold agents, fatigue and sleep deprivation caused an insignificant increase in the frequency with which colds occurred; however, in females, susceptibility was related to the menstrual cycle, with attempts to infect during menstruation being relatively unsuccessful.

The incubation period of rhinovirus-related common colds is quite short, ranging from one to five days with a mean of two days. Virus shedding generally begins with the onset of symptoms and continues for one week or even longer. Although there are over 100 distinct rhinovirus serotypes, no one serotype has assumed special importance because numerous serotypes usually circulate at the same time. Rhinoviruses can be detected during most months of the year but reach peak prevalence during the fall season. They are least prevalent during the cold winter months of December, January, and February when common colds still occur frequently. However, coronavirus infections have been found to be prevalent during the late fall, winter, and early spring, when rhinovirus infections occur infrequently. Thus, coronaviruses can be considered to be the major known etiologic agents of the common cold in the winter.

A cyclic pattern in infection rates of coronaviruses 229E and OC43 has been described. With the 229E virus, infections appear to occur in the same years in various locations, including Chicago, Maryland, Virginia, and Michigan; a two-year cycle of activity has been suggested. For OC43 virus, a two- to four-year cycle was found that did not coincide in all locations. The 229E virus was shed in nasal washings of volunteers for one to at least four days after challenge; the peak frequency of virus excretion generally coincided with the peak of clinical symptoms. Virus shedding was also detected in certain volunteers who did not develop colds after challenge. Reinfections have also been observed frequently with coronaviruses under natural conditions; recently, however, volunteers inoculated with the same coronavirus strain 8 to 12 months after initial challenge failed to develop illness on rechallenge. It appears that serum antibody to a specific rhinovirus serotype correlates with protection against natural or experimental challenge with that serotype. However, serum antibody may not in itself be responsible for protection but may be a reflection of the level of specific nasal secretory antibodies. In one volunteer study in which the protective effects of neutralizing antibody in serum and in nasal secretions were compared, it was found that only nasal secretory antibody was associated with resistance to rhinovirus infection and illness.

PATHOLOGY. The pathologic mechanisms whereby a common cold is induced by a virus are not known. However, the pathology of viral rhinitis in general has been described. In the initial acute period of viral rhinitis the nasal mucosa is thickened and edematous and depending on the degree of hyperemia is pale gray to red in color and covered by a thin watery mucoid discharge. The nasal cavities are narrowed by the enlargement of the turbinates. Histologically, there is extreme edema of the mucosal tissue, which is also infiltrated sparsely with neutrophils, lymphocytes, plasma cells, and eosinophils. Secretory hyperactivity of the mucus-secreting submucosal glands is also observed. The edematous nasal mucosa can cause obstruction of the orifices of the accessory air sinuses and lead to sinusitis. Bacterial superinfections can result in serious sequelae including osteomyelitis, cavernous sinus thrombophlebitis, epidural or subdural abscess, meningitis, or brain abscess. Nevertheless, such complications are exceedingly rare.

Information on the pathologic findings in acute rhinovirus infections is extremely limited. Biopsies of nasal epithelium were obtained from volunteers prior to and after rhinovirus inoculation and from volunteer controls who were not inoculated. Fixed smears prepared with Papanicolaou's stain demonstrated that most of the cells were ciliated columnar epithelial cells. Smaller numbers of nonciliated epithelial cells, goblet cells, and mononuclear and polymorphonuclear cells were also observed. However, consistent histologic changes were not observed in specimens obtained during infection or illness.

CLINICAL MANIFESTATIONS. The major clinical manifestation of common colds occurring under natural or experimental conditions is coryza or nasal congestion. The most common complaints in rhinovirus-positive respiratory illnesses in 139 civilian adults were rhinorrhea and sneezing, which were recorded in one half to two thirds of the cases. The next most frequent complaint was sore throat, which occurred in nearly one half, while hoarseness and cough were less common, being present in one quarter to one half of the cases. Temperature elevation was unusual. An oral temperature of 99.6° F (37.6° C) or greater at the time of study was documented in less than 1 per cent of the cases. Nonrespiratory complaints were not common except for headache, which occurred in approximately one quarter of the cases. The mean duration of symptoms was about 9 days with a median of 7.4 days and a mode of 4 days.

The clinical manifestations of coronavirus-229E–like infections under natural conditions in adults are quite similar. Of nine patients who shed this agent, all had coryza, eight had nasal congestion, seven had sneezing, and five had sore throat at the time of study. Less common manifestations were headache (in four), cough (in three), muscular or general aches (in three), and chills and fever (in two). Coryza or nasal congestion was the chief complaint in eight of the nine patients.

Administration of rhinoviruses or coronaviruses to volunteers has provided an opportunity to define the clinical manifestations associated with these agents under carefully controlled conditions (Table 325/326–2). The mean incubation period of colds induced by coronaviruses was significantly longer (about one day), the duration of the illness somewhat shorter, and the mean maximum number of paper tissues used per day (for nasal discharge) greater than in rhinovirus-induced illnesses. In later studies, each of six other coronavirus strains was also administered by the nasal route to volunteers: cumulatively, 35 of 49 volunteers developed common-cold–like illnesses. Thus, the ability to induce common colds in adults under experimental conditions is now as firmly established for the coronaviruses as for the rhinoviruses.

Rhinoviruses also cause common colds in children. The role of rhinoviruses as etiologic agents of bronchitis, bronchiolitis, bronchopneumonia, pneumonia, and croup is unclear. However, it appears certain that rhinoviruses are not important causes of these syndromes, even though administration of a rhinovirus by small-particle aerosol induces a tracheobronchitis in volunteers. Coronaviruses can also cause common-cold–like illnesses in children. In one study, coronavirus 229E was recovered from two infants with pneumonia, and serologic evidence of coronavirus infection was demonstrated in 8.2 per cent of pediatric patients hospitalized with lower respiratory tract disease. However, in other studies such an association was not found. Coronavirus OC43 infections also were observed in four military recruits with pneumonia with pleural

TABLE 325/326–2. COMPARISON OF THE CLINICAL FEATURES OF COLDS PRODUCED BY INTRANASAL ADMINISTRATION OF CORONAVIRUSES OR RHINOVIRUSES

	Coronaviruses		Rhinoviruses	
	229E	*B814*	*Type 2 (HGP or PK)*	*DC*
Number of volunteers inoculated	26	75	213	251
Number getting colds	13 (50%)	34 (45%)	78 (37%)	77 (31%)
Incubation period (days)				
Mean	3.3	3.2	2.1	2.1
Range	2–4	2–5	1–5	1–4
Duration (days)				
Mean	7	6	9	10
Range	3–18	2–17	3–19	2–26
Maximum number of tissues used daily				
Mean	23	21	14	18
Range	8–105	8–120	3–38	3–60
Malaise	46%	47%	28%	25%
Headache	85%	53%	56%	56%
Chill	31%	18%	28%	15%
Pyrexia	23%*	21%*	14%	18%
Mucopurulent nasal discharge	0	62%	83%	80%
Sore throat	54%	79%	87%	73%
Cough	31%	44%	68%	56%
Number of volunteers with colds of indicated severity				
Mild	10 (77%)	24 (71%)	63 (80%)	36 (47%)
Moderate	2 (15%)	7 (20%)	12 (15%)	28 (36%)
Severe	1 (8%)	3 (9%)	4 (5%)	13 (17%)

*Between 99.2° F (37.3° C) and 100.4° F (38° C). After Bradburne, Bynoe, Tyrrell: Br Med J 3:767, 1967.

reaction. The etiologic significance of such associations is not known. Rhinovirus and coronavirus infections have been associated with exacerbations of chronic bronchitis in adults. The association of rhinovirus infections with exacerbations of chronic lung disease has been reported in several studies; rhinoviruses have characteristically been the single most frequently detected agents (14 to 43 per cent). A transient decrease in pulmonary function has also been observed in volunteers infected with rhinovirus.

Complications of common colds include sinusitis, otitis media, acute infectious exacerbations in patients with chronic bronchitis, precipitation of asthma, and extensions of infections into the central nervous or cardiovascular systems, as noted in the pathology section. The role of bacteria acting in concert with the virus infection in certain of these complications must be kept in mind in establishing therapeutic regimens.

DIAGNOSIS. Since most respiratory viruses can induce common colds, an etiologic diagnosis cannot be made on clinical grounds. Specific viral diagnosis of the common cold is essentially a research procedure that requires tissue or organ cultures for virus isolation or antigens for certain serologic studies. Complement fixation (229E, OC43), hemagglutination-inhibition (OC43), enzyme-linked immunosorbent assay (229E), or radioimmunoassay (OC43) can be performed in order to demonstrate serologic evidence of infection with certain coronaviruses. However, antigens for such tests are not generally available. The most important test for a patient with a common-cold–like illness is a throat culture for group A beta-hemolytic streptococci because symptoms of illnesses associated with the common cold viruses and the streptoccoccus may overlap. Appropriate antibiotic therapy is available for treatment of this bacterial infection.

TREATMENT AND PREVENTION. There is no specific treatment for patients with the common cold. Only symptomatic treatment measures should be employed. The use of acetyl salicylic acid (aspirin) for children with colds should be approached with caution because of the epidemiologic association of this drug with Reye's syndrome when the drug is administered during a viral illness, usually influenza or varicella—both of which can cause symptoms resembling those of the common cold (Table 325/326–1). The Committee on Infectious Diseases of the American Academy of Pediatrics stated in a special report, "In balancing this probability (the risk) with the benefits of aspirin, it is the opinion of the Committee that aspirin should not be prescribed under usual circumstances for children with varicella or those suspected of having influenza on the basis of clinical or epidemiologic evidence."

Antibiotics have no value in the therapy of the uncomplicated common cold. Previous tonsillectomy did not significantly affect the number of common respiratory illnesses or the induction of experimental colds in volunteers in the Cleveland Family Study. The use of vitamin C for the treatment or prevention of common colds has aroused great interest and much controversy. Available evidence indicates that its use does not reduce the number of episodes of respiratory illness but does decrease somewhat the total number of days of disability. The routine use of large doses of vitamin C for preventive treatment of common colds does not appear to be warranted from evidence available at this time.

Although there was great enthusiasm for producing a vaccine against common colds in the 1960's, when the rhinoviruses were finally cultivated in tissue cultures with ease, this enthusiasm rapidly waned when the number of distinct serotypes gradually increased to 89. Currently over 100 serotypes are known to exist, and no one serotype or group of serotypes appears to be consistently more important than others. Experimental rhinovirus vaccines against single serotypes have been made and shown to be effective in preventing or modifying illnesses induced by the serotype present in the vaccine. Although some heterotypic antibody responses have been observed with decavalent rhinovirus vaccines, the production of a rhinovirus vaccine appears to be impractical because of the multiplicity of serotypes. Until the number of serotypes of coronaviruses can be elucidated and the role of antibody in preventing or modifying illnesses can be established, consideration of a coronavirus vaccine is premature. Antiviral drugs or compounds may hold promise as specific treatment measures. Interferon inducers or interferon itself applied topically in the nose have been shown to be effective in reducing symptomatic illness induced by a rhinovirus under experimental conditions.

One method available for preventing rhinovirus colds may

be the application of rigid personal hygienic measures when a family member has a common cold. This would entail hand washing and avoidance of finger-eye and finger-nose contact.

Committee on Infectious Diseases of the American Academy of Pediatrics (Fulginiti VA, Brunell PA, Cherry JD, Ector WL, Gershon AA, Gotoff SP, Hughes WT, Mortimer EA Jr, Peter G): Special report. Aspirin and Reye syndrome. Pediatrics 69:810, 1982. *After weighing the available evidence, this Committee has made a strong recommendation against the use of aspirin under usual circumstances in children with varicella or influenza (both of which can cause common-cold–like symptoms).*

D'Alessio DJ, Peterson JA, Dick CR, Dick EC: Transmission of experimental rhinovirus colds in volunteer married couples. J Infect Dis 133:28, 1976. *A carefully conducted study describing the communicability of rhinoviruses in married couples. Conditions for transmissibility of infection are elucidated.*

Dingle JH, Badger GF, Jordan WS: Illness in the home. A study of 25,000 illnesses in a group of Cleveland families. Cleveland, The Press of Western Reserve University, 1964. *A classic study of illnesses experienced by a group of families over an almost ten-year period. Detailed epidemiologic data are given on the patterns of illnesses, including common respiratory diseases.*

Douglas RG Jr, Lindgren KM, Couch RB: Exposure to cold environment and rhinovirus common cold. Failure to demonstrate effect. New Engl J Med 279:743, 1968. *This classic study examines the role of cold temperatures on host resistance to rhinovirus infection and illness.*

Dykes MHM, Meier P: Ascorbic acid and the common cold. JAMA 231:1073, 1975. *A thoughtful and careful analysis of numerous studies on the efficacy and safety of ascorbic acid in the prevention and treatment of the common cold. The authors conclude that "the unrestrictive use of ascorbic acid for these purposes cannot be advocated on the basis of the evidence currently available."*

Editorial: Cold comfort for hot children. Br. Med J 286:1163, 1983. *Reviews some of differential diagnoses when a child has a fever. Also examines the role of aspirin in Reye's syndrome and concludes that ". . . aspirin should be avoided in children with fever, especially during epidemics of influenza or chickenpox."*

Gwaltney JM Jr: Rhinoviruses. *In* Evans AS (ed.): Viral infections of humans. Epidemiology and control. New York, Plenum Medical Book Company, 1982, pp 491–517. *An up-to-date review of rhinoviruses from the epidemiologic perspective by a major contributor to this field (178 references).*

Gwaltney JM, Moskalski PB, Hendley JO: Hand-to-hand transmission of rhinovirus colds. Ann Intern Med 88:463, 1978. *An important paper by a pioneer group in rhinovirus research describing the efficient transmission of rhinovirus in common colds by hand exposure followed by self-inoculation. This route was more efficient for transmission than large- or small-particle aerosols.*

Jackson GG, Dowling HF, Anderson TO, Riff L, Saporta J, Turck M: Susceptibility and immunity to common upper respiratory viral infections—the common cold. Ann Intern Med 53:719, 1960. *The authors examine clinical aspects of experimentally induced common colds in volunteers. They also study environmental and physiologic factors in relation to susceptibility to common colds.*

Larson HE, Reed SE, Tyrrell DAJ: Isolation of rhinoviruses and coronaviruses from 38 colds in adults. J Med Virol 5:221, 1980. *This study demonstrates that the isolation rate of fastidious viruses from common colds can be enhanced substantially with the use of organ cultures and volunteers. This type of carefully executed study may also eventually lead to the discovery of new etiologic agents of common colds.*

Monto AS: Coronaviruses. *In* Evans AS (ed.): Viral infections of humans. Epidemiology and control. New York, Plenum Medical Book Company, 1982, pp 151–165. *An up-to-date review of the coronaviruses from the epidemiologic perspective (65 references).*

Reed SE: The behavior of recent isolates of human respiratory coronavirus in vitro and in volunteers: Evidence of heterogeneity among 299E related strains. J Med Virol 13:179, 1984. *Studies at the Common Cold Unit in Salisbury continue to expand our knowledge of the immunologic relationships among various strains of coronaviruses. Such studies may have an important bearing on vaccine approaches.*

Robbins SL, Cotran RS: Pathological Basis of Disease. 2nd ed. Philadelphia, W.B. Saunders Company, 1979, pp 881–882. *In a chapter on nasal cavities and accessory air sinuses, the authors describe the pathologic changes in viral rhinitis and also discuss bacterial complications.*

327. VIRAL PHARYNGITIS, LARYNGITIS, CROUP, AND BRONCHITIS

Maurice A. Mufson

DEFINITION. Viral infections that localize to the upper and middle respiratory passages produce an acute inflammatory response and depending upon the anatomic site involved, evoke the clinical manifestations of pharyngitis, laryngitis, croup (laryngotracheobronchitis), and bronchitis. These infections do not ordinarily involve the pulmonary alveoli. Pharyngitis, laryngitis, and bronchitis can occur in persons of any age. Croup occurs exclusively in children and mainly during the second year of life. The illnesses often begin abruptly with predominant upper respiratory tract signs and symptoms and limited systemic findings, and the uncomplicated illness abates after five to ten days. However, croup can be a life-threatening illness; the most common complications include respiratory failure and pneumonia.

ETIOLOGY. Many viruses that primarily infect the upper and middle respiratory passages can cause pharyngitis, laryngitis, croup, and bronchitis (see Table 327–1). The main viral pathogens of pharyngitis and laryngitis include rhinoviruses, coronaviruses, influenza A and B viruses, adenoviruses, parainfluenza viruses, enteroviruses, and respiratory syncytial virus. The principal viral pathogens of croup are the parainfluenza viruses types 1, 3, and 2 (in decreasing frequency). Influenza A and B viruses and respiratory syncytial virus are uncommon causes of croup. Acute viral bronchitis has been associated with influenza A and B virus, coronavirus, adenovirus, respiratory syncytial virus, and rhinovirus infections. In any individual case, the etiology of pharyngitis, laryngitis, croup, and bronchitis cannot be determined on the basis of the clinical characteristics of the illness. A definitive etiologic diagnosis can be made only by application of diagnostic virology tests.

Pharyngitis also can occur as part of systemic viral illnesses associated with *Epstein-Barr virus* (see Ch. 338) or *cytomegalovirus* (see Ch. 337) infection, and laryngitis and bronchitis occur in *measles* virus infection (see Ch. 332). When coryza represents the main feature of an upper respiratory infection, the term *common cold* (see Ch. 325) prevails. When the infecting virus is an influenza virus, the designation *influenza* describes an acute respiratory tract infection with fever and prostration (see Ch. 330). Since many viruses can cause either pharyngitis, laryngitis, croup, or bronchitis, and since the anatomic site of infection underlies the basis for the clinical manifestations, it seems preferable to retain these terms and modify them by adding the name of the infecting virus when it has been identified.

INCIDENCE AND PREVALENCE. Viral pharyngitis, laryngitis, and bronchitis occur commonly. Most children and adults experience three to five viral infections of the upper respiratory tract each year. Since croup is a serious illness of infants and children immediately recognizable by a distinctive complex of symptoms and signs (see later discussion), estimates of its incidence have been calculated among two populations studied during several years (Denny, 1983). The incidence of croup reached a peak during the second year of life, at 14.9 and 47.0 cases per 1000 children per year, and by age four to five it declined to 3.1 and 14.5 cases, respectively, in the two different populations.

EPIDEMIOLOGY. Viral pharyngitis, laryngitis, croup, and bronchitis occur during all months of the year, with peaks of occurrence paralleling epidemics of individual viruses. Respiratory syncytial virus, influenza A and B viruses, coronaviruses, parainfluenza virus type 1, and to a lesser extent type 2, occur in epidemics, mainly in the late fall, winter, and spring. The other viral pathogens occur endemically, although they may exhibit some seasonal variation from year to year. Virus infections of the respiratory tract spread by direct person-to-person contact, by infectious aerosols, or by fomites.

CLINICAL MANIFESTATIONS. ***Viral Pharyngitis.*** Acute viral pharyngitis is usually characterized by a scratchy and sore throat, but pain upon swallowing is not a prominent or constant feature. When dysphagia is present, it suggests a streptococcal infection. Cough is not a feature of acute viral pharyngitis. Fever and malaise accompany influenza and adenovirus infections, but these findings are infrequent with the other respiratory viral pathogens. Pharyngeal erythema and edema and enlarged and tender lymph nodes may be the only physical findings. Adenovirus pharyngitis may be associated with conjunctivitis. Exudative tonsillitis occurs in adenovirus infections, infectious mononucleosis associated with Epstein-Barr virus infection, herpetic pharyngitis (with or without vesicles or small ulcers), as well as streptococcal pharyngitis. Exudative tonsillitis alone does not serve to distinguish these infections. An attempt

TABLE 327–1. ETIOLOGY OF VIRAL PHARYNGITIS, LARYNGITIS, CROUP, AND BRONCHITIS

Virus	Serotype	Occurrence in Indicated Illness			
		Pharyngitis	*Laryngitis*	*Croup*	*Bronchitis*
Respiratory syncytial		+		+	+ + +
Parainfluenza	1	+ +	+ +	+ + + +	+ +
	2	+	+	+ + +	+
	3	+ +	+ +	+ + + +	+ +
Influenza	A	+ + +	+ + +	+	+ + +
	B	+ +	+		+
Adenovirus	1–7	+ + + +	+ +	+	+ +
Coronavirus	Few	+ +	+		+ + +
Rhinovirus	Many	+ + + +	+ + +		+ +
Enterovirus	Many	+ +			
Herpes simplex	1	+ +			

Frequency and importance of virus occurrence are graded from minimal importance (+) to major importance (+ + + +). Blank = uncommon occurrence.

must be made to estabish the cause in these cases and should include appropriate diagnostic laboratory tests.

Viral Laryngitis. In acute viral laryngitis, hoarseness predominates, associated with difficulty in talking, pain on clearing respiratory secretions, and often fever, depending upon the infecting virus. Cough and pharyngitis may be present. The larynx is erythematous and edematous, and the regional lymph nodes are slightly enlarged and tender. Wheezes may be audible upon auscultation.

Viral Croup. The clinical picture of croup characteristically includes inspiratory stridor, hoarseness, and a brassy cough. This distinctive triad of symptoms reflects the acute and intense edema and mucoid exudative secretions of the larynx and associated obstruction of the subglottic portion of the upper airway. These symptoms develop acutely, accompanied by fever, cough, tachypnea, and wheezing. Retractions of the chest wall occur. Hemoptysis does not occur. Rhonchi, rales, or wheezes, alone or in combination, may be audible upon auscultation of the lungs. Radiographic examination of the neck can demonstrate subglottic narrowing, and a chest roentgenogram may show hyperinflation of the lungs. In the uncomplicated case, the findings resolve in several days, but some children develop respiratory failure and pneumonia. Children who previously experienced multiple episodes of croup manifest hyperreactive airways several years later.

Viral Bronchitis. In acute viral bronchitis, cough, with or without sputum production, and fever are the main features. The sputum is slightly mucoid or watery and white. Other common symptoms include hoarseness, nonpleuritic substernal chest pain, and malaise. Rhonchi or rales may be heard upon auscultation of the chest. The chest roentgenogram may show increased intensity of the vascular pattern, but pulmonary infiltrates do not occur. Acute bronchitis associated with influenza or coronavirus infection occurs often as an exacerbation of chronic bronchitis.

TREATMENT AND PROGNOSIS. The treatment of pharyngitis, laryngitis, and bronchitis associated with virus infections of the upper respiratory tract aims at the relief of distressing local and systemic symptoms. These illnesses are self-limited and not severe. Antibiotics are not indicated, except when secondary bacterial infection occurs. In pharyngitis, pharyngeal pain or dysphagia should be treated with analgesics and fluids. The treatment of laryngitis and bronchitis also requires analgesics, fluids, and rest. Cough in adults and older children that is relentless and causes fatigue should be treated with cough suppressant preparations.

The less serious cases of croup can be managed by having the child rest in bed at home. Vaporizers that produce a mist of moist air may be beneficial. Children with severe croup require hospitalization, supportive treatment, and constant monitoring for the development of respiratory distress. If hypoxemia develops, oxygen therapy is essential; hypoxemia requiring oxygen can develop even before cyanosis becomes evident. Subglottic edema may be reduced by the administration of racemic epinephrine. Administration of corticosteroids in the treatment of croup may have limited benefit.

Buscho RO, Saxtan D, Shultz PS, Finch E, Mufson MA: Viruses and *Mycoplasma pneumoniae* infections in exacerbations of chronic bronchitis. J Infect Dis 137:377, 1978. *A longitudinal study of acute viral exacerbations among a group of adult men with chronic bronchitis, employing virus isolation and serodiagnosis. Exacerbations were significantly associated with influenza and coronavirus infections compared with periods of remission.*

Denny FW, Murphy TF, Clyde WA Jr, Collier AM, Henderson FW: Croup: An 11-year study in a pediatric practice. Pediatrics 71:871, 1983. *A comprehensive investigation of the viral etiology and epidemiology of croup among a large population of ambulatory children. Viral infections were identified by virus isolation attempts on oropharyngeal cultures.*

Gwaltney JM Jr, Hendley JO: Transmission of experimental rhinovirus infection by contaminated surfaces. Am J Epidemiol 116:828, 1982. *The first demonstration that environmental surfaces contaminated with rhinovirus-containing secretions could serve as a reservoir for the spread of these viruses to susceptible persons.*

Koren G, Frand M, Barzilay Z, MacLeod SM: Corticosteroid treatment of laryngotracheitis *v* spasmodic croup in children. Am J Dis Child 137:941, 1983. *Recent re-evaluation of the effectiveness of corticosteroid therapy for croup. Double-blind random design was employed in the treatment of two categories of croup using a single high dose of dexamethasone. Six hours after the start of corticosteroid therapy, the respiratory rate of patients classified as having spasmodic croup had decreased significantly compared with the placebo group, but no change in respiratory rate was detected among patients classified as having laryngotracheitis.*

Sherter CB, Polnitsky CA: The relationship of viral infections to subsequent asthma. Clin Chest Med 2:67, 1981. *Review of the evidence for a causal relationship between virus infections of the respiratory tract during childhood and subsequent asthma.*

328. RESPIRATORY SYNCYTIAL VIRUS

Robert M. Chanock

DEFINITION. Respiratory syncytial virus (RSV) is the most important cause of viral lower respiratory tract disease in infants and children. This ubiquitous virus causes an extensive epidemic every year during fall, winter, or early spring. During these epidemics there is a dramatic increase in admission to hospitals of infants and young children with severe lower respiratory tract disease. Older children and adults commonly undergo reinfection, but disease is usually milder than that experienced during infancy and early childhood.

ETIOLOGY. The virus was first isolated in 1956 from a symptomatic laboratory chimpanzee during an outbreak of illness resembling the common cold. Shortly thereafter, a similar virus was recovered from children with pneumonia or croup, and its characteristic syncytial (giant cell) cytopathic effect in tissue culture was noted. RSV is an enveloped virus that belongs to the family Paramyxoviridae, genus *Pneumovirus*. It resembles the parainfluenza viruses of the genus *Paramyxovirus* but differs from them in morphology of its nucleocapsid, in failure to agglutinate erythrocytes (hemagglutination), and in absence of a neuraminidase enzyme. The viral genome consists of a single negative (−) strand of ribonucleic acid (RNA) approximately 15,000 bases in length. The genetic information of RSV is expressed as a series of viral messenger RNAs (mRNAs) transcribed from the viral genome that code for ten viral-specific proteins. One of these proteins, nucleocapsid protein, coats the viral RNA to form a helical nucleocapsid. This structure is enclosed within a bilayer lipid membrane that is studded with two different viral glycoproteins. One of these, the fusion protein, lyses the host cell membrane, permitting entry of virus into the cell. This protein is also responsible for fusion of infected cells to neighboring cells, a process that results in syncytium formation, a prominent feature of the virus during its growth in tissue culture.

Although antigenic variation among strains has been noted, it does not have epidemiologic significance. A related RSV is a common cause of respiratory disease in calves, but this virus does not appear to infect humans.

EPIDEMIOLOGY. RSV has a worldwide distribution. Whenever appropriate studies have been performed, RSV has been found to be the major pediatric respiratory tract pathogen. The highest incidence of severe lower respiratory tract disease is observed in infants between one and six months of age, with a peak incidence at two months. Serious lower respiratory tract disease occurs more commonly in males than in females and in nonblack than in black infants. Approximately 50 per cent of infants who live through a single RSV epidemic become infected. In certain settings, such as day care centers, the attack rate approaches 100 per cent during an outbreak.

Reinfection occurs with high frequency during childhood. Adults are also reinfected frequently, particularly when there is exposure to a large amount of virus. For example, during annual RSV epidemics, 25 to 50 per cent of the staff of pediatric wards undergo reinfection. In families into which virus is introduced, spread of RSV among older siblings also occurs with high frequency (40 per cent). In individuals of all ages, reinfection is usually symptomatic, and adults exposed to a large amount of virus may develop an influenza-like disease.

Most individuals infected with RSV have upper respiratory illness. However, a surprisingly large proportion of infants (25 to 40 per cent) also develop lower respiratory tract disease. Hospitalization of infants for RSV disease varies with environmental and socioeconomic conditions. Overall, 1 in 120 to 1 in 200 infants requires hospital care for RSV pneumonia or bronchiolitis during the first year of life. RSV is responsible for approximately 50 to 75 per cent of bronchiolitis and for 20 to 25 per cent of pneumonia that necessitate admission of infants and young children to hospital.

In developed countries, severe RSV lower respiratory tract disease is usually nonfatal (0.5 to 2.5 per cent). Fatal RSV disease occurs most often in infants with other underlying illnesses, particularly congenital heart disease (37 per cent), bronchopulmonary dysplasia, serious renal disease, and diseases such as cancer that are treated with immunosuppressive drugs. In a British study of 46 infants and children who died with lower respiratory tract disease, 13 were infected with RSV. In addition, a number of babies dying from sudden infant death syndrome are infected with RSV.

RSV has a clear seasonality in temperate zones of the world. In urban centers, epidemics occur yearly in the late fall, winter, or spring but not during the summer. In the northern hemisphere, the virus is rarely isolated during August or September. Each RSV epidemic lasts approximately five months, with 40 per cent of infections occurring during the peak month in the temporal center of the outbreak. In the northern hemisphere, most outbreaks peak in February or March, but the peak may occur as early as December or as late as June. RSV is spread by infected respiratory secretions in the form of large droplets or through fomite contamination.

During epidemic intervals, RSV is one of the commonest causes of hospital-acquired infection on pediatric wards. The risk of infection increases as hospital stay is extended beyond one week. The mortality in such hospital-acquired infections is considerably higher than in community-acquired infetions because the patients involved are frequently at high risk because of other diseases, malnourishment, or immunosuppressive drugs.

Since reinfection with RSV is common and often associated with disease, it is clear that immunity is neither permanent nor complete. However, multiple reinfections induce temporary immunity to infection, and their cumulative effect prevents severe lower respiratory tract disease. Studies in adult volunteers indicate that immunity to induced infection correlates better with the level of nasal neutralizing immunoglobulin A (IgA) antibody than with serum antibody. On the other hand, there is some evidence that maternally transmitted antibody in small infants offers some protection from serious lower respiratory tract disease. Nonetheless, a considerable amount of severe RSV disease occurs in young infants who possess a moderate level of maternally derived serum neutralizing antibody.

CLINICAL MANIFESTATIONS. During infancy, RSV infection usually causes upper respiratory symptoms. In 25 to 40 per cent of infections the respiratory tract below the larynx is also involved. Lower respiratory tract signs are preceded by a prodromal phase of rhinorrhea that is sometimes accompanied by a decrease in appetite. Low grade fever is common. Cough is often accompanied by wheezing, and if disease is mild, symptoms may not progress beyond this stage. Examination usually reveals moderate tachypnea, diffuse rhonci, fine rales and wheezes, as well as profuse rhinorrhea and intermittent fever. Otitis media is also common. The chest x-ray usually appears normal. In most instances, uneventful recovery occurs after 7 to 12 days.

In more severe cases, coughing and wheezing progress and the child becomes dyspneic and refuses feedings. Hyperexpansion of the chest is evident, and there may be intercostal and subcostal retractions. Severe tachypnea is common even in the absence of visible cyanosis, and in advanced disease as the child tires and hypoxia becomes more extreme, listlessness and apnea occur. The chest may appear normal on x-ray examination, but often there is a combination of air trapping (hyperexpansion) and peribronchial thickening or interstitial pneumonia. Segmental or lobar consolidation is also occasionally seen, usually involving the right upper lobe. Pleural effusion is rare. In infants with underlying cardiac or respiratory disease, the progression of symptoms may be rapid. In these instances, respiratory failure requiring intubation and ventilation may appear on the second or third day of illness.

Almost all infants who require hospitalization are hypoxemic on admission and remain so for a prolonged period—up to several weeks—although recovery has ensued. The hypoxemia reflects an abnormally low ventilation-perfusion ratio. Hypercarbia may also be present.

In infants who were born prematurely, and sometimes in normal infants under six weeks of age, apneic spells may develop during RSV infection. This often occurs in the absence of significant respiratory signs and may be the predominant symptom bringing the infant to medical attention. Such apneic spells, while often recurrent during acute infection, are usually self-limited and rarely cause neurologic or systemic damage. However, exceptions to this pattern occur, and such episodes are an indication for hospitalization and careful medical supervision. Apnea at the peak of severe illness is a poor prognostic sign.

In the newborn infant, most RSV infections produce only

upper respiratory symptoms. Bronchiolitis is rare, and severe infection is more often characterized by lethargy, irritability, and fever or unstable body temperature than by specific respiratory signs.

Children who have apparently recovered completely from RSV bronchiolitis or pneumonia may still retain both measurable and symptomatic respiratory abnormalities for many years. A study of 23 children examined ten years after an episode of bronchiolitis found that although all were symptom free (a criterion for admission to the study), 20 had some measurable physiologic abnormality of lung function or arterial blood gases.

Acute RSV infections are common in adults, particularly in medical personnel or in those caring for small children. These infections are occasionally asymptomatic but usually are associated with rhinorrhea, pharyngitis, cough, constitutional symptoms of headache and fatigue, and fever. Disease usually lasts about five days but may be more prolonged, particularly in hospital staff. Alterations in pulmonary function, such as elevated total respiratory resistance and increased airway reactivity, often last for eight weeks. There is some evidence that RSV infection in the elderly is a cause of febrile bronchitis and severe or even fatal pneumonia.

DIAGNOSIS. Presumptive diagnosis of RSV infection can often be made on the basis of the clinical syndrome in relation to the time of year and other epidemiologic features. Definitive diagnosis depends upon the laboratory. In older children and adults, an increase in serum RSV antibody concentration, either complement fixing (CF) or neutralizing, is a fairly sensitive index of reinfection with RSV. Serologic tests in infants are less sensitive, particularly in patients under four months of age. In young infants, only 2 to 15 per cent of RSV infections are detectable by CF and 2 to 20 per cent by neutralization assay. Antibody measurement by solid-phase immunoassay (enzyme-linked immunosorbent assay; ELISA) recently has been shown to be a more sensitive indicator of infection in small infants than CF or neutralization. At all ages, however, isolation of virus or detection of antigen in respiratory secretions is the procedure of choice. Specimens are best obtained by aspiration or gentle washing out of nasopharyngeal secretions. These may be examined by inoculation of tissue culture, immunofluorescence, or ELISA. Infectivity of RSV in secretions is labile; hence samples should be placed on wet ice while being transported to a tissue culture laboratory.

TREATMENT AND PREVENTION. Treatment of RSV infections of the lower respiratory tract consists primarily of supportive care: mechanical removal of secretions, proper positioning of the infant, administration of humidified oxygen, and in severe cases respiratory assistance. When wheezing is an important symptom, some infants, particularly those over a year of age, will benefit from the use of theophylline or adrenergic drugs.

Ribavirin (1-b-D-ribofuranosyl-1,2,4-triazole-3-carboxamide), delivered by small-particle aerosol, shows some promise for treatment of severe RSV disease in young infants. In one study, the drug hastened recovery and diminished virus shedding.

Because immunity to RSV is neither permanent nor complete, the goal of immunoprophylaxis is prevention of severe lower respiratory tract disease. It should be possible to achieve this through the cumulative effect of repeated vaccination. Efforts to develop an effective vaccine have been frustrated by the ineffectiveness of formalin-inactivated virus and by the genetic instability of satisfactorily attenuated temperature-sensitive mutants that initially showed promise as live virus vaccine strains. Perhaps recent success in cloning complementary deoxyribonucleic acid (cDNA) copies of RSV genes in *E. coli* may open the way to the preparation of immunogenic viral surface glycoprotein antigens, or alternatively, recombinant DNA techniques may prove useful in constructing stable attenuated mutants that can be used in a live vaccine.

Chanock RM, Kim HW, Brandt CD, Parrott RH: Respiratory syncytial virus. *In* Evans AS (ed.): Viral Infections of Humans: Epidemiology and Control. New York, Plenum Publishing Corp., 1982, pp 471–489. *A summary of biologic properties of RSV as well as its epidemiology and the pathogenesis of the disease.*

Hall CBH, Geiman JM, Biggar R, Kotok DI, Hogan PM, Douglas RG Jr.: Respiratory syncytial virus infections within families. N Engl J Med 294:414, 1976. *Longitudinal surveillance of RSV infections in families. During an epidemic, infection occurred in 44 per cent of families; within these families the infection rate was 62 per cent in infants and 43 per cent in adults, the latter rate representing reinfection.*

Hall CBH, McBride JT, Walsh EE, Bell DM, Gala CL, Hildreth S, Ten Eyck LG, Hall WJ: Aerosolized ribavirin treatment of infants with respiratory syncytial viral infection. N Engl J Med 308:1443, 1983. *Administration of ribivirin by small-particle aerosol hastened recovery of infants with severe RSV lower respiratory tract disease.*

Henderson FW, Collier AM, Clyde WA Jr., Denny FW: Respiratory-syncytial-virus infections, reinfections and immunity. N Engl J Med 300:530, 1979. *Longitudinal surveillance of children in a day care center demonstated high frequency of reinfection; also, after several reinfections partial immunity developed to RSV.*

Henderson FW, Collier AM, Sanyal MA, Watkins JM, Fairclough DL, Clyde WA Jr., Denny FW: A longitudinal study of respiratory viruses and bacteria in the etiology of acute otitis media with effusion. N Engl J Med 306:1377, 1982. *Important role of RSV infection in initiating acute otitis media with effusion.*

329. PARAINFLUENZA VIRAL DISEASES

Robert M. Chanock

DEFINITION. Infection with parainfluenza viruses occurs early in life and is an important cause of *pediatric respiratory tract disease.* The spectrum of illness varies from mild upper respiratory disease to severe croup, pneumonia, or bronchiolitis. Reinfection is common in later life and is associated with mild respiratory tract disease.

ETIOLOGY. The parainfluenza viruses are enveloped viruses that belong to the family Paramyxoviridae, genus *Paramyxovirus.* The single stranded ribonucleic acid (RNA) viral genome has negative polarity (antimessenger sense) and is approximately 15,000 bases in length. Its genetic information is expressed as a series of messenger RNAs (mRNAs) transcribed from the viral genome that code for seven viral-specific proteins. One of these proteins, nucleocapsid protein, coats the viral RNA to form a helical nucleocapsid. This structure is enclosed within a lipid bilayer envelope that is studded with the two viral glycoprotein surface antigens, the hemagglutinin-neuraminidase, and the fusion protein. Parainfluenza viruses share many properties with the influenza viruses, but they differ from these agents in their wider RNA nucleocapsid (18 nm as compared with 9 nm) and in the distribution of hemagglutination and neuraminidase functions on their surface glycoproteins. Both parainfluenza hemagglutinin and neuraminidase are located on the same surface glycoprotein, whereas these functions reside on separate surface glycoproteins of the influenza viruses. The parainfluenza viruses have common antigens that are not shared by the influenza viruses. Mumps virus shares the foregoing properties, as well as related antigens, with the parainfluenza viruses.

There are four antigenically distinct serotypes of human parainfluenza virus. These viruses were first recognized by cytopathic effects that developed in infected tissue cultures (type 2) or by the hemadsorption reaction in which guinea pig erythrocytes become adsorbed to an infected tissue culture monolayer (types 1, 3, and 4). Initially, these viruses were designated *hemadsorption viruses,* but later they were classified as parainfluenza viruses. Related parainfluenza viruses cause respiratory disease in mice (Sendai virus, a subtype of type 1), dogs (SV5, a subtype of type 2), calves (bovine shipping fever virus, a subtype of type 3), and birds (seven distinct serotypes not closely related to human parainfluenza viruses). Animal and avian parainfluenza viruses are distinct antigenically from human parainfluenza viruses and do not appear to infect humans.

EPIDEMIOLOGY. The four parainfluenza virus types have wide geographic distribution. The first three types have been identified in most areas where appropriate tissue culture and hemadsorption techniques have been applied to the study of childhood respiratory tract diseases. So far, type 4 viruses (subtypes 4A and 4B), which are more difficult to recover in tissue culture, have been isolated in fewer areas, but serologic studies suggest that they are also relatively ubiquitous. Each of the four parainfluenza virus types causes acute respiratory tract disease in humans.

The parainfluenza viruses are exceeded only by *respiratory syncytial virus (RSV)* as an important cause of lower respiratory tract disease in young children. These viruses, particularly type 3, commonly reinfect older children and adults to produce upper respiratory tract disease. Illness usually occurs less often and is less severe during reinfection than during primary infection.

There is considerable diversity in both epidemiologic and clinical manifestations of infections caused by the parainfluenza viruses. Parainfluenza virus type 1 is the principal cause of croup (laryngotracheobronchitis) in children, and parainfluenza virus type 3 is second only to RSV as a cause of pneumonia and bronchiolitis in infants less than six months of age. Parainfluenza virus type 2 resembles type 1 virus in clinical manifestations but causes serious illness less frequently. Infections with parainfluenza virus type 4 are detected infrequently, and associated illnesses are usually mild.

The parainfluenza viruses are most important as respiratory tract pathogens during infancy and childhood, when they (types 1 through 3) cause a spectrum of effects ranging from inapparent infection to life-threatening lower respiratory tract disease. Studies in different parts of the world indicate that types 1, 2, and 3 are associated with approximately 40 to 70 per cent of severe croup. In addition to croup, these three viruses are also responsible for a smaller but appreciable percentage of other acute respiratory tract diseases of infancy and early childhood. Eighty per cent of individuals undergoing primary infection with type 3 virus develop a febrile illness, and in one third there is involvement of the lower respiratory tract. Approximately one half of initial type 1 virus infections and two thirds of initial type 2 virus infections produce a febrile illness. Severe croup, although the most dramatic and serious manifestation of initial parainfluenza virus infection, is noted in only 2 to 3 per cent of primary type 1 or type 2 virus infections.

Primary parainfluenza virus infection generally occurs early in life. Type 3 virus often causes illness during the first months of life while infants still possess circulating neutralizing antibody derived from their mothers. In contrast, in young infants, maternally derived antibody appears to prevent both infection and severe disease caused by type 1 and type 2 viruses. After age four months, there is an increase in the number of cases of croup and other lower respiratory tract diseases caused by type 1 and type 2 viruses. This high incidence continues until approximately six years of age, after which age there is a much lower incidence. It is unusual for type 1 or type 2 virus to cause lower respiratory tract illness during adolescence or adult life, although this does occur on occasion.

At present, type 1 and type 2 virus epidemics are synchronous, occurring during the autumn of odd-numbered years. For many years, type 3 virus exhibited an endemic pattern, with infection occurring during all seasons of the year. Within this endemic pattern, small outbreaks occurred, but there was no predictable periodicity. Within the past five years, there has been a shift toward yearly spring epidemics of type 3 virus infection. Nosocomial infection with the parainfluenza viruses, particularly type 3 virus, is common and often leads to serious lower respiratory tract disease.

Transmission of parainfluenza viruses is by direct person-to-person contact or large droplet spread. The high rate of infection early in life, coupled with the high frequency of reinfection, suggests that these viruses spread readily from person to person. Reinfected individuals appear to be infectious, and a relatively small inoculum is able to initiate infection. Type 3 virus appears to be the most transmissible of the parainfluenza viruses.

In experimental infection of adult volunteers, the interval between administration of type 1, 2, or 3 virus and onset of upper respiratory tract symptoms ranged from three to six days. The incubation period in pediatric infections has not been defined; however, the interval between exposure to type 3 virus and the subsequent initial shedding of this virus is two to four days. Resistance to type 1 or type 2 parainfluenza virus infection and associated upper respiratory disease appears to be a function of local respiratory tract, secretory, immunoglobulin A (IgA)-neutralizing antibodies. Infants may also be partially protected from infection and disease by serum antibodies. This protective relationship is suggested by the relative sparing of young infants from type 1 and type 2 virus infection and associated disease at a time when they possess serum antibodies passively acquired from their mother. Also, the risk of infection with type 3 virus during the first four months of life is inversely related to the level of neutralizing antibody present in cord serum at birth. However, the protective effect of passive immunity is less than that observed for type 1 and type 2 viruses, since a significant number of infants with moderately high levels of maternally derived serum antibody become infected with type 3 virus and develop severe illness.

CLINICAL MANIFESTATIONS. In children, the most common type of illness consists of rhinitis, pharyngitis, and bronchitis, usually with fever. The most common initial symptoms are cough, hoarseness, and fever. The cough may be croupy, but respiratory distress is not present. Approximately three fourths of such ill children have temperatures above 37.8° C; fever usually lasts two to three days. Coarse breath sounds, rhonchi, erythema of the pharyngeal mucous membranes, and rhinitis are characteristic physical findings. Cervical adenopathy is uncommon.

When croup develops, the initial symptoms of rhinitis, pharyngitis, fever, and cough progress. After several days, the cough worsens and becomes brassy, seal-like, or barking and stridor ensues. At this stage, most children recover uneventfully after 24 to 48 hours, but in some air hunger develops, with cyanosis, sternal and intercostal retractions, and progressive airway obstruction. The lateral x-ray of the neck (which should be obtained only under carefully controlled medical supervision, if at all) shows glottic and subglottic narrowing (the "steeple sign") and differentiates this disease from epiglottitis.

When bronchiolitis or pneumonia develops, fever persists and the cough progresses and becomes somewhat productive. It is accompanied by wheezing, tachypnea, and retractions and in severe cases by cyanosis. The x-ray shows interstitial or perihilar infiltrates and air trapping. In some patients a combined bronchopneumonia-croup syndrome occurs.

DIAGNOSIS. Presumptive diagnosis of parainfluenza virus infection can be made on the basis of age, history, clinical findings, and relation to known or characteristic prevalence of virus in the community. Definitive diagnosis, however, requires recovery of the virus from appropriate specimens taken from the respiratory tract or identification of viral antigens in respiratory tract secretions by immunofluorescence or another form of immunoassay. Serodiagnosis by hemagglutination inhibition, complement fixation, or neutralization can establish that infection with a member of the parainfluenza virus group has occurred, but frequent heterotypic responses make type-specific diagnosis by serology extremely difficult.

TREATMENT. Symptomatic treatment of croup usually includes humidification of air by ultrasonic nebulizer and periodic inhalation of racemic epinephrine. Antibiotics are usually contraindicated. The use of corticosteroids is controversial, but many physicians prescribe high doses of dexamethasone if croup is severe. Specific antiviral treatment or effective vaccines for prevention of parainfluenza virus disease are not available.

Chanock RM, Parrott RH, Johnson KM, Kapikian AZ, Bell JA: Myxoviruses: Parainfluenza. Am Rev Respir Dis 88:152, 1963. *A discussion of the importance of parainfluenza viruses in pediatric respiratory tract disease and the first description of pattern of spread and reinfection.*

Denny FW, Murphy TF, Clyde WA, Jr, Collier AM, Henderson FW: Croup: An 11-year study in a pediatric practice. Pediatrics 71:871, 1983. *Eleven-year evaluation of the role of parainfluenza viruses in croup. These viruses accounted for 74 per cent of all virus isolates from croup patients.*

Fox JP, Hall CE: Infections with other respiratory pathogens: Influenza, mumps, and respiratory syncytial viruses; *Mycoplasma pneumoniae. In* Fox JP (ed.): Viruses in Families. Littleton, John Wright/PSG Inc, 1980, pp 335–381. *Longitudinal surveillance of families for parainfluenza virus infection and illness. Infection rate was 44 per 100 person years for all ages, while attack rate for illness associated with parainfluenza virus infection was 76 per cent for babies under age 2 years and 25 per cent for adults.*

Glezen WP, Denny FW: Epidemiology of acute lower respiratory disease in children. N Engl J Med 288:498, 1973. *Excellent summary of contribution of parainfluenza viruses to pediatric respiratory disease.*

Glezen WP, Loda FA, Denny FW: Parainfluenza viruses. *In* Evans AS (ed.): Viral Infections of Humans: Epidemiology and Control. New York, Plenum Publishing Company, Inc., 1982, pp 441–454. *Summary of natural history of parainfluenza virus infection and pathogenesis of disease.*

330. INFLUENZA

R. Gordon Douglas, Jr.

DEFINITION. Influenza is an acute, usually self-limited febrile illness that occurs in outbreaks of varying severity almost every winter. Although the causative virus is transmitted by the respiratory route, systemic symptoms are out of proportion to those in the respiratory tract. Infection with influenza virus can produce several other clinical syndromes common with infection with respiratory viruses, such as common colds, pharyngitis, croup, tracheobronchitis, bronchiolitis, or pneumonia. Conversely, infections with other respiratory viruses, such as respiratory syncytial virus, rhinovirus, or adenovirus, may produce sporadic cases indistinguishable from those of typical influenza. In addition to enormous morbidity and loss of time from school and work, influenza epidemics are associated with substantial mortality caused in large part by pulmonary complications.

HISTORY. Epidemics of respiratory disease similar to modern influenza have been recorded through the centuries. Since the year 1510, 31 pandemics have been described, 5 of which have occurred in the 20th century (1900, 1918, 1957, 1968, and 1977). Of these, the pandemic of 1918 was the most severe, accounting for at least 21 million deaths. Influenza A virus was first isolated in 1933 and influenza B virus in 1936. Effective inactivated viral vaccines were first produced in the 1940's, and antiviral chemotherapy became available in the late 1960's. Since 1968, over 200,000 deaths have occurred in the United States from epidemic influenza.

ETIOLOGY. Influenza viruses belong to the family Orthomyxoviridae. Influenza A virus constitutes one genus and influenza B virus another. The virion is a medium-sized (80 to 100 nm in diameter) enveloped sphericle or elongated particle covered with surface projections that are glycoproteins possessing either hemagglutinin (H) or neuraminidase (N) activity (Fig. 330–1). The envelope is composed of a lipid bilayer, on the inner surface of which is the matrix (M) protein. Within the envelope are eight segmented pieces of nucleocapsid, formed by a single species of protein, the nucleoprotein (NP), and by pieces of segmented single stranded ribonucleic acid (RNA). Three polymerase (P) proteins and two nonstructural (NS) proteins of unknown function are found within the envelope. The H is responsible for binding of the virus to the cell. Antibody to this protein neutralizes viral infectivity, and thus is the major determinant of immunity. The viral N is instrumental in release of virus from cells. Antineuraminidase antibody is not neutralizing but limits viral replication and therefore the severity of infection. The M protein plays a role in stability of the membrane and in organization of the virion during assembly. The three polymerases are important in viral replication. The internal M, NP, and P proteins are antigenically indistinguishable in all influenza A viruses but vary for influenza B and C viruses. Thus, type-specific (A, B, or C) distinction of influenza viruses depends on serologic reactions mediated by these internal antigens. However, the surface proteins (H and N) do vary, not only among influenza virus types but also among subtypes of influenza A.

The viral genome comprises eight segments of RNA, seven of which code for a single viral protein each. The eighth codes for the two nonstructural proteins. Reassortment of gene segments occurs frequently during infection to provide an unusually high frequency of genetic recombination. Influenza B and C viruses have been studied much less but appear to be structurally similar to influenza A virus. Antigenic variation is much less frequent with influenza B, and it may not occur with influenza C.

EPIDEMIOLOGY. ***Antigenic Variation.*** One of the unique and most remarkable features of influenza virus is the frequency with which changes in antigenicity occur. Such changes help

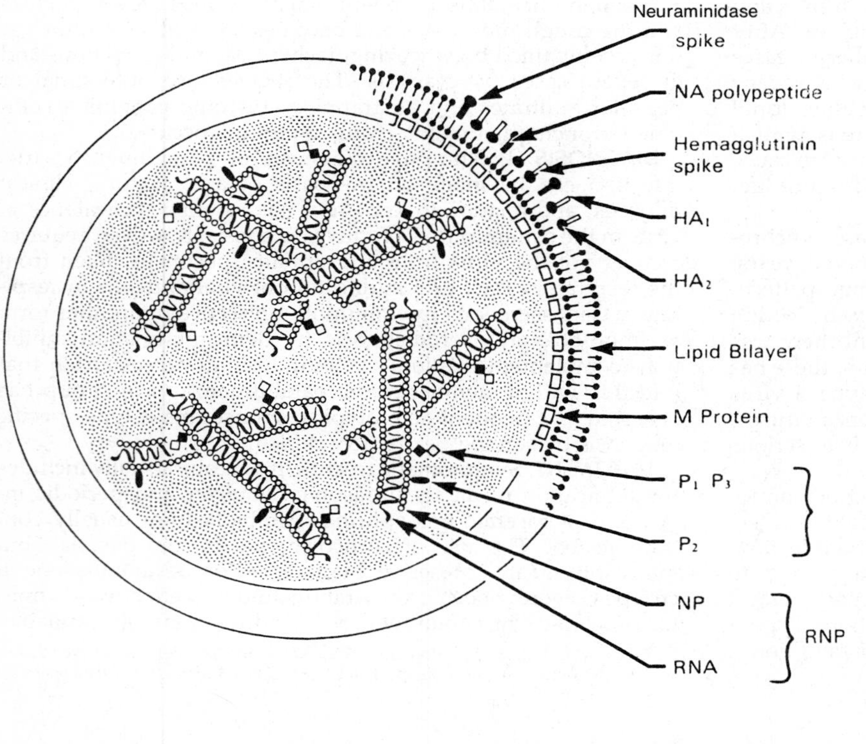

Figure 330–1. Schematic model for influenza virus virions. (Modified from Ginsberg HS: Orthomyxoviruses. *In* Davis BD, Dulbecco R, Eisen HN, Ginsburg HS (eds.): Microbiology, 3rd ed. Hagerstown, MD, Harper & Row, Publishers, 1980, p. 1119.)

explain why influenza continues to be a major epidemic disease in humans. As noted previously, antigenic variation involves only the H and N proteins among the proteins of influenza virus. The H is the most important since it is more frequently involved in antigenic variation than the N protein and since antibody to this protein neutralizes infection. Antigenic variation is referred to as *antigenic drift* or *antigenic shift*, depending on whether the variation is great or small.

Antigenic Drift. Antigenic drift refers to relatively minor changes that occur frequently (every year or every few years) within an influenza A subtype. Each subtype is named by its hemagglutinin and neuraminidase. To date, three hemagglutinins (H1, H2, and H3) and two neuraminidases (N1 and N2) have been recognized. The former designations, HO and HSW1, are now classified as variants of H1. Each strain within the subtype is identified by site and year of isolation. Thus, influenza A/Bangkok/79/H3N2 indicates an influenza virus of type A and subtype H3N2 that was isolated in 1979 in Bangkok. The original H3N2 variant, A/Aichi/68/H3N2, was isolated in Aichi, Japan, in 1968. All isolates worldwide for the next three years were serologically identical. Subsequent antigenic drifts resulted in recovery of variants possessing minor differences: A/England/72/H3N2, A/Port Chalmers/73/H3N2, A/Scotland/74/H3N2, A/Georgia/74/H3N2, A/Victoria/75/H3N2, A/Texas/77/H3N2, A/Bangkok/79/H3N2, A/Philippines/2/82/H3N2, and so on. Antigenic drift results from point mutations that usually affect the RNA segment coding for the hemagglutinin. Complete nucleotide sequencing of hemagglutinins of several H3 strains has been determined, in support of this hypothesis. As a result, there is an alteration in protein structure that involves one or a few amino acids and results in minor changes in antigenicity. There is immunologic selection in which a new virus is favored over the old for person-to-person transmission because of the less frequent presence of antibody in the population.

Antigenic Shift. Major antigenic shifts result from genetic reassortment when two influenza viruses simultaneously infect a single cell. Such an event results in a hemagglutinin or neuraminidase, or both, that is completely new in comparison with the previously circulating strain. Because of the high level of immunity to the old strain and lack of immunity to the new strain within the human population, the new strain, provided that it possesses intrinsic viral properties such as virulence and transmissibility, can readily cause a major outbreak of influenza.

Epidemic Influenza. An epidemic is an outbreak of influenza confined to one location such as a city, town, or country. In a given community, epidemics of influenza A virus infection have a characteristic pattern. A graphic description of an epidemic due to an A/Victoria/75/H3N2 like virus, which occurred in 1976 in Houston, Texas, is shown in Figure 330–2. Such localized epidemics begin rather abruptly, reach a sharp peak in two to three weeks, and last five to six weeks. Reports of increased numbers of children with febrile respiratory illness are often the first indication of influenza in a community. This is usually soon followed by the occurrence of influenza-like illnesses among adults. The next event is increased hospital admissions of patients with pneumonia, exacerbation of chronic obstructive pulmonary disease, croup, and congestive heart failure. There are increases in school and industrial absenteeism and in the number of deaths caused by pneumonia and influenza. Although the latter finding is a highly specific indicator of influenza, it invariably lags behind the others. Viral isolation studies show a peak that parallels that of acute febrile respiratory illness. Year-round studies indicate that almost all isolates are obtained during the epidemic period. It is rare to recover influenza virus during other periods of the year, although occasionally there is serologic evidence of infection during other months.

Epidemics occur almost exclusively during the winter months—October through April in the northern hemisphere and May through September in the southern hemisphere. When observed in large countries such as the United States or

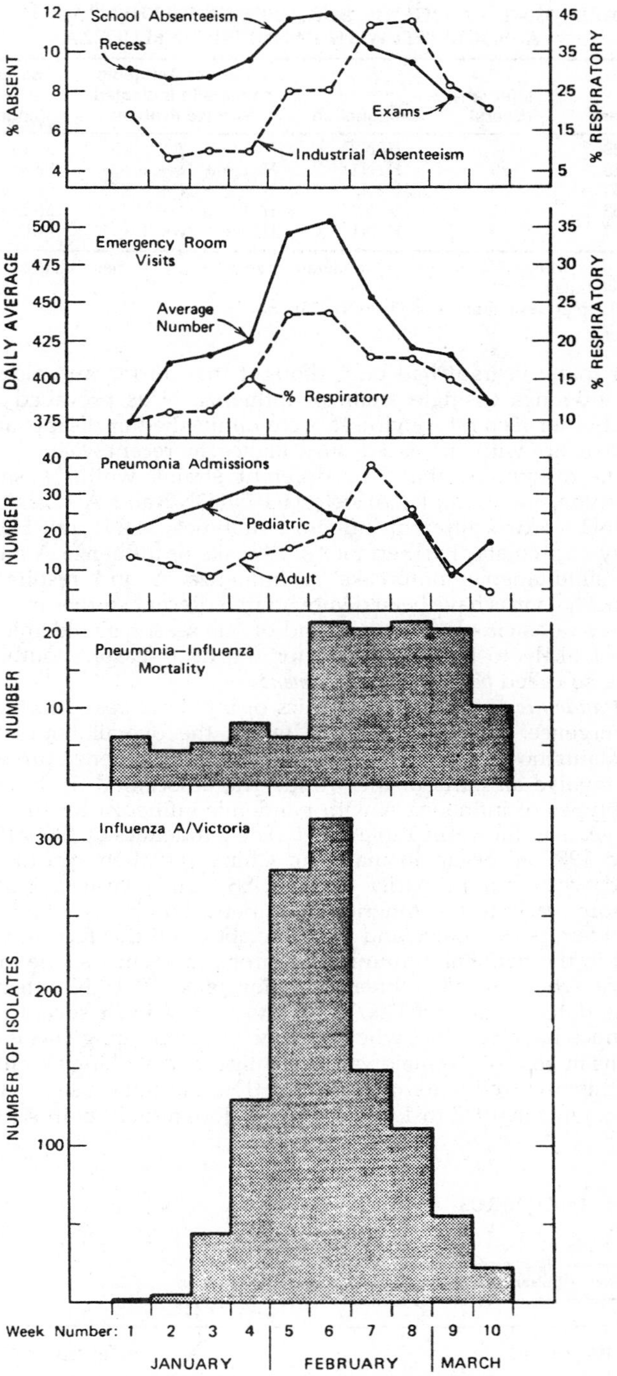

Figure 330–2. Correlation of the nonvirologic indexes of epidemiologic influenza with the number of isolates of influenza A/Victoria virus according to week, Houston, 1976 (industrial absenteeism is indicated by percentage with respiratory complaints). (From Glezen WP, Couch RB, Six HR: N Engl J Med 298:589, 1978.)

Australia, regional differences in the time of occurrence of influenza outbreaks are apparent. It is not uncommon to have major outbreaks occurring in some communities or regions while others are experiencing no activity whatsoever. Often those so spared will experience similar outbreaks at a later time, particularly if the prevalent virus demonstrates significant antigenic variation compared with previously prevalent viruses. During epidemics, the average overall attack rates are estimated to be 10 to 20 per cent; however, in selected populations or age groups, attack rates of 40 to 50 per cent are not uncommon.

TABLE 330–1. ANTIGENIC SUBTYPES OF INFLUENZA A VIRUS ASSOCIATED WITH PANDEMIC INFLUENZA

Year	Interval (Years)	Designation	Extent of Antigenic Change in Indicated Surface Protein*	Severity of Pandemic
1889	—	H3N2	?	Moderate
1918	29	H1N1†	H + + + N + + +	Severe
1957	39	H2N2	H + + + N + + +	Severe
1968	11	H3N2	H + + + N –	Moderate
1977	9	H1N1	H + + + N + + +	Mild

*+ = Minor change; + + = moderate change; + + + = major change; – = no change.

†Former designation was Hsw1N1 (35).

For many years it had been thought that during an epidemic of influenza a single strain of influenza virus prevailed and that other respiratory viruses were diminished or disappeared. However, with increased surveillance in recent years it has been recognized that two different strains within a single subtype, for example, A/Victoria/3/75/H3N2 and A/Texas/1/77/H3N2, or two different influenza subtypes, H1N1 and H3N2, may cocirculate. Furthermore, outbreaks of influenza A and B or simultaneous outbreaks of influenza A and respiratory syncytial virus have been demonstrated. Recent studies indicate that strains circulating at the end of one season's epidemic are most likely to be responsible for the next season's outbreak (the so-called *herald wave phenomenon*).

Pandemic Influenza. Pandemics of influenza result from the emergence of a new virus to which the overall population contains no immunity, so that epidemics of influenza progress to involve all parts of the world. The association of different subtypes of influenza A with pandemic influenza for the past 80 years is shown in Table 330–1. The pandemics of 1957, 1968, and 1977 all began in mainland China and then spread east and west, but primarily to the USSR and Western Europe before reaching the American continent. The interval between pandemics is variable and unpredictable, and this fact, in part, led to the national immunization program against swine influenza, when a small outbreak of A/New Jersey/76/H1N1 infection was detected at Fort Dix, New Jersey. The most severe pandemics have resulted when there were major antigenic alterations in both of the major surface antigens. A striking exception to this occurred when A/USSR/77/H1N1 did not cause a severe pandemic in 1977 to 1978, despite major shifts in both surface glycoproteins. This discrepancy may be due to the fact that much of the world's population of 1977 to 1978 had been alive during the previous H1N1 era, from 1947 to 1957, and thus possessed protective immunity. Furthermore, it appears that transmissibility from person to person and intrinsic virulence (severity of disease) are virus-coded functions that vary much as does antigenicity. Intrinsic virulence with H1N1 viruses appears to be milder than with H3N2 viruses.

Proposed Mechanism of Epidemic Behavior. The scheme shown in Figure 330–3 ties together the concepts of antigenic shifts and antigenic drifts in relation to population immunity. When a new virus, here called A HXNX, is introduced into a population lacking appropriate antibody, pandemic influenza results. After one or more waves of pandemic influenza, the level of immunity in the population increases. Such a chain of events provides a setting for emergence of a variant showing antigenic drift, since the level of immunity to it will be less than that to the original strain. Repeated epidemics caused by strains showing antigenic drift within the HXNX subtype occur in subsequent years. After 10 to 30 years of circulation of variants within this given subtype, the population's immunity to all variants within the subtype is very high, and the conditions for the spread of a new virus are favorable. Such a virus originates by genetic reassortment. Thus, it possesses an H or N protein, or both, that is markedly different with respect to the A HXNX subtype. When such a virus circulates, the next pandemic occurs. While the concepts of immunity of the population and antigenic variation are important in understanding the epidemiology of influenza, they do not provide the entire explanation. It is apparent that virus factors must contribute to virulence and transmissibility. Furthermore, it should be emphasized that other than the association of influenza outbreaks with colder seasons, the factors that allow an epidemic to develop remain unexplained. The factors responsible for the tapering off of an epidemic after five or six weeks, when only a portion of susceptible persons are infected, are also unknown. Finally, the host or medium where the virus has been between epidemics is not understood.

Mortality. In addition to the substantial morbidity associated with epidemic or pandemic influenza, mortality is also associated with such outbreaks. Pneumonia and influenza deaths fluctuate annually in predictable fashion, with peaks in the winter and troughs in the summer. When pneumonia and influenza deaths exceed the epidemic threshold, this is almost always due to influenza A virus activity or occasionally to influenza B virus activity.

PATHOLOGY AND PATHOGENESIS. Influenza virus infection

INFLUENZA VIRUS

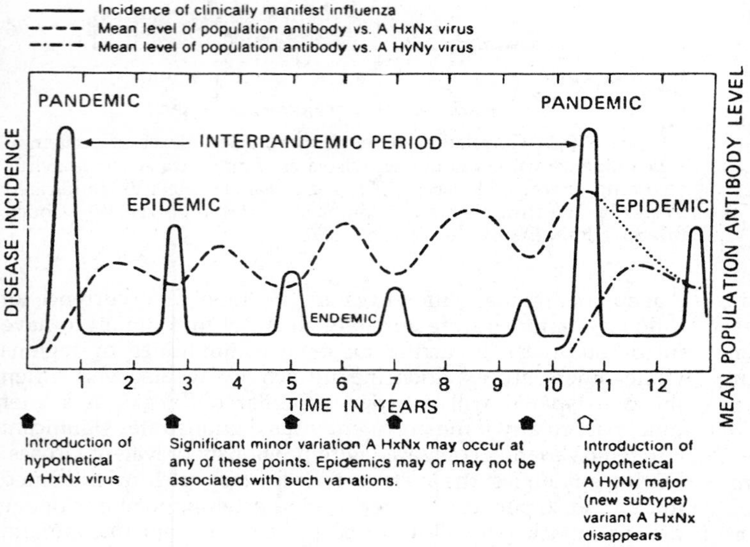

Figure 330–3. Schema of occurrence of influenza pandemics and epidemics in relation to the level of immunity in the population. AHxNx and AHyNy represent influenza viruses with completely different hemagglutinins and neuraminidases. (From Douglas RG Jr: *In* Galasso GJ, Merigan TC, Buchanan RA (eds.): Antiviral Agents and Viral Diseases of Man. New York, Raven Press, 1979.)

is acquired by transfer of virus-containing respiratory secretions from an infected to a susceptible person. Small-particle aerosols (less than 10 μ mass medium diameter) may be most significant in such person-to-person transmission. Once the virus has been deposited in the respiratory tract epithelium, unless it is prevented by specific secretory antibody, nonspecific mucoproteins, or mechanical actions of the mucociliary blanket, it attaches to and penetrates columnar epithelial cells. After absorption has taken place, the virion initiates its replication cycle. This cycle lasts four to six hours, and virus release continues for several hours before cell death ensues. Infection of adjacent and nearby cells follows, so that within a few replication cycles large numbers of cells in the respiratory tract are infected. The duration of the incubation period until onset of illness and virus shedding, which occur in close proximity, varies from 18 to 72 hours, depending in part on the inoculum size. Quantitation of virus in respiratory tract specimens reveals a characteristic pattern that correlates with severity of illness. This correlation suggests that a major mechanism in the production of illness is cell death resulting from viral replication. Serum or secretory antibody or cell-mediated immune mechanisms are not detectable at this time, indicating that immunologic mechanisms are probably not involved in production of illness. The occurrence of systemic illness and fever suggests hematogenous dissemination of virus or release of cellular products into the blood, but infectious virus only rarely has been detected in the blood.

Interferon is frequently detected in respiratory tract and serum specimens. Shedding of virus precedes by one to two days the appearance of interferon, which is correlated with improvements of signs and symptoms and decrease of virus titer and thus suggests that interferon is active in the recovery process. Nasal and bronchial biopsy specimens from persons with uncomplicated influenza reveal desquamation of the ciliated columnar epithelium. Individual cells show shrinkage, pyknotic nuclei, and loss of cilia. In addition, the lungs in fatal influenza show extensive hemorrhage, hyaline membrane formation, and paucity of polymorphonuclear cell infiltration. Patients with secondary bacterial pneumonia have the changes characteristic of bacterial pneumonia in addition to the tracheobronchial findings of influenza in the tracheobronchial tree.

Neutralizing, hemagglutination-inhibiting, antineuraminidase, complement-fixing, enzyme-linked immunosorbent assay (ELISA), and immunofluorescent antibodies begin to develop in the sera of persons with primary influenza virus infection during the second week after exposure to antigen and reach a peak by four weeks. Secretory antibodies develop in the respiratory tract after influenza infection and consist predominantly of immunoglobulin A (IgA) antibodies that reach peak titers in 14 days. Protection against infection is afforded by serum HAI titers of 1:40 or greater, serum-neutralizing titers of 1:8 or greater, or nasal-neutralizing antibody titers 1:4 or greater.

CLINICAL FINDINGS. Many patients can pinpoint the hour of onset. Initially, systemic systems predominate, and symptoms include feverishness, chilliness or frank shaking chills, headache, myalgias, malaise, and anorexia. In more severe cases, prostration is observed. Usually myalgias or headache are the most troublesome symptoms, and their severity is related to the level of the fever. Arthralgias are commonly observed. Ocular symptoms, although less commonly present, are helpful diagnostically and include photophobia, tearing, burning, and pain on moving the eyes. Respiratory symptoms, particularly dry cough and nasal discharge, are usually also present at the onset but are overshadowed by the systemic symptoms. Nasal obstruction, hoarseness, and dry sore throat may also be present.

Fever is the most important physical finding. The temperature usually rises rapidly to a peak of 38 to 40° C and occasionally to 41° C within 12 hours of onset, concurrently with the development of systemic symptoms. Fever is usually continuous but may be intermittent, especially if antipyretics are administered. On the second and third days of illness, the temperature elevation is usually less than on the first day. As fever subsides, the systemic symptoms diminish. Typically, the duration of fever is three days, but it may last from one to five or more days. In a few cases, a second fluctuation in fever occurs on the third or fourth day, resulting in a biphasic fever curve. Early in the course of illness, the patient appears toxic, the face is flushed, and the skin is hot and moist. The eyes are watery and reddened. Clear nasal discharge is common, but nasal obstruction is uncommon. The mucous membranes of the nose and throat are hyperemic, but exudate is not observed. Small tender cervical lymph nodes are often present, and transient scattered rhonchi or localized areas of rales are found in less than 20 per cent of cases.

As systemic signs and symptoms diminish, respiratory complaints and findings become more apparent. Cough is the most frequent and troublesome of these symptoms and may be accompanied by substernal discomfort or burning. Nasal obstruction, discharge, pharyngeal pain, and injection are also common. Such symptoms and signs usually persist three to four days after fever subsides; however, cough, lassitude, and malaise may persist for one, two, or more weeks before full recovery.

This pattern of illness just described occurs with any type or subtype of influenza A or B virus. Attack rates are higher in children than in adults, although the incidence of pulmonary complications is lower in children. Maximum temperatures are higher in children, cervical adenopathy may be more frequent, and croup occurs only among children.

PULMONARY COMPLICATIONS. Three kinds of pulmonary complications are well recognized: *primary influenza viral pneumonia, secondary bacterial pneumonia,* and *mixed viral and bacterial pneumonia.* In addition, during an outbreak of influenza, less distinct and milder pulmonic syndromes often occur that may represent viral tracheobronchitis, localized viral pneumonia, or possibly mixed viral and bacterial infection.

Primary Influenza Viral Pneumonia. This syndrome first became well documented in the pandemic of 1957 to 1958. However, it is clear that many of the deaths in the 1918 to 1919 outbreak were due to this syndrome in healthy young adults. Primary influenzal viral pneumonia has occurred predominantly among persons with cardiovascular disease, especially rheumatic heart disease with mitral stenosis. Although this syndrome occurs in healthy young adults in every large outbreak, other chronic disorders and pregnancy have been implicated as risk factors in some epidemics. Following a typical onset of influenza, there is rapid progression of fever, cough, dyspnea, and cyanosis. Physical examination and chest roentgenograms reveal bilateral findings consistent with the adult respiratory distress syndrome. Blood gas studies show marked hypoxia. Gram stain of the sputum fails to reveal significant bacteria, and bacterial culture yields sparse growth of normal flora. Viral cultures of sputum or tracheal aspirates yield high titers of influenza virus. Such patients do not respond to antibiotics, and mortality is high.

Secondary Bacterial Pneumonia. Bacterial superinfection is often clinically distinguishable from primary viral pneumonia. The patients are most often elderly or have chronic pulmonary, cardiac, metabolic, or other diseases. Following a typical influenza illness, a period of improvement lasting from one to four days may occur. Recrudescence of fever is associated with symptoms and signs of bacterial pneumonia, such as cough, sputum production, and a localized area of consolidation apparent on physical and chest roentgenogram examination. Gram stain and culture sputum reveal predominance of a bacterial pathogen, most often *S. pneumoniae, S. aureus,* or *H. influenzae.* Such patients will usually respond to specific antibiotic therapy.

Mixed Viral and Bacterial Pneumonia. During an outbreak of influenza, many cases are observed that do not clearly fit into either of the categories just described. The disease is not relentlessly progressive, and yet the fever pattern may be persistent and not biphasic. These patients may have a milder form of primary viral, secondary bacterial, or mixed viral and bacterial infection. Many will respond to antibiotics. Milder forms of primary viral pneumonia involving only one lobe or segment have been described that do not invariably lead to death. Such cases are more likely to be confused with a pneumonia due to *M. pneumoniae* than to that produced by bacterial infection. In children, pneumonia may occur but is less common than in adults. In addition, bronchiolitis and croup may be caused by influenza A or B virus infection.

Exacerbation of Chronic Obstructive Pulmonary Disease. In adults with chronic obstructive pulmonary disease, influenza A or B virus infection may lead not only to pneumonia but also to acute exacerbation of chronic bronchitis, a syndrome that is associated with other respiratory viruses and bacteria as well.

NONPULMONIC COMPLICATIONS. ***Reye's Syndrome.*** Reye's syndrome is a frequently recognized hepatic and central nervous system complication of influenza A and B infection as well as varicella-zoster virus infection. The syndrome occurs exclusively in children, most often between the ages of 2 and 16 years. Because of the epidemic nature of the occurrence of influenza A and B virus infections, Reye's syndrome also has an epidemic occurrence. Large outbreaks have occurred in the United States since 1967 in association with influenza A and B outbreaks. Reye's syndrome occurs several days after a typical upper respiratory, gastrointestinal, or chickenpox infection. The most significant manifestation is change in mental status, ranging from lethargy to delirium, obtundation, seizures, and respiratory arrest. In 75 per cent of the cases, central nervous system manifestations are preceded by nausea and vomiting, lasting one to two days. The children are usually afebrile and have hepatomegaly but are not jaundiced. Mortality is related to the stage of coma on admission and has decreased from approximately 40 per cent when the syndrome was first described to 10 per cent today. Lumbar puncture reveals normal protein values and cell counts confirming the presence of encephalopathy rather than encephalitis or meningoencephalitis. The most frequent laboratory abnormality is elevation of the blood ammonia value, which occurs in almost all patients. Hypoglycemia is present more often in patients with antecedent varicella-zoster or gastrointestinal illness, as compared with upper respiratory illness. Serum glutamic oxaloacetic transaminase (SGOT), serum glutamic pyruvic transaminase (SGPT), and bilirubin values are commonly elevated, as are creatine kinase (CK) and lactic dehydrogenase (LDH) levels. The prothrombin time is usually increased. Stage 4 or 5 coma on admission, evidence of increased intracranial pressure, and blood ammonia level greater than 300 μg per deciliter are all associated with mortality. Among survivors, 30 per cent of those who develop either decerebrate posturing or seizures during hospitalization have serious neurologic sequelae. Pathologically, the striking feature is absence of inflammatory changes. Liver biopsy specimens are usually pale yellow. Microscopic examination shows fatty infiltration of the hepatocytes with numerous small droplets of lipid uniformly distributed. The main ultrastructural finding is alteration of the hepatocyte mitochondria, including swelling and pleomorphism. Pathologic findings most often detected in the brain are cerebral edema, anoxia, and anoxic neuronal degeneration, but there is no inflammation. The pathophysiologic mechanism is unknown. Recently, an association with aspirin therapy during the antecedent illness has been indicated, but this finding has also been challenged.

Other Complications. Myositis and myoglobinuria with tender leg muscles and elevated serum CK levels have been reported, mostly occurring in children. Myocarditis, pericarditis, and myocardial infarction rarely have been associated with influenza A and B virus infection. Guillian-Barré syndrome has been reported to occur after influenza A, but no definite causal relationship has been established. Transverse myelitis and encephalitis have also been reported rarely.

DIAGNOSIS. In an individual case, influenza often cannot be distinguished from infection with a number of other viruses and bacteria that produce headache, muscle aches, fever, and cough. On occasion, other respiratory viruses can produce an influenza-like illness, as can streptococcal pharyngitis. In the summer months, enteroviruses produce a clinically indistinguishable picture, and the acute manifestations of many other infections, such as dengue, may mimic influenza. On the other hand, in the context of an epidemic, influenza may be readily distinguished from other acute infections. When the local, state, or national health authorities report the occurrence of an epidemic of influenza A or B virus infection in a given community, and a patient is seen with the acute onset of fever, headache, muscle aches, and cough, it is highly likely that these symptoms are caused by an influenza virus infection.

Definitive diagnosis depends on detection of infectious virus or viral antigen in secretions from patients or the detection of a serum antibody response. Influenza virus is readily isolated from throat or nasal swab specimens, sputum, or tracheal secretion specimens in the first two or three days of illness. Usually infectivity is detected within 48 to 72 hours in monkey kidney cell cultures. Viral antigen may be detected more rapidly in such specimens by use of immunofluorescence or ELISA, but these techniques are not widely available. Serologic methods are less useful clinically because they require a convalescent sera obtained 10 to 14 days after the onset of infection. However, they are of great use in epidemiologic studies and to document the occurrence of an outbreak. A four-fold increase in antibody titer comparing an acute to convalescent phase is diagnostic. The complement fixation antibody test is most useful for diagnosis because it is not dependent on strain or subtype variation, as is hemagglutination inhibition.

TREATMENT. Amantadine shortens the duration of fever and of systemic and respiratory symptoms by about 50 per cent. The dose is 100 to 200 mg per day orally for three to five days. Rimantadine, although not yet licensed, has a similar effect and reduces the likelihood of the mild transient central nervous system side effects that occur with amantadine. Other symptomatic measures include antipyretics and cough suppressants. Many authorities consider that aspirin should not be used, especially for persons under 16 years of age, because of its possible association with the occurrence of Reye's syndrome. There is no evidence that amantadine or rimantadine is effective in treatment of pulmonary complications of influenza.

Currently, primary influenza viral pneumonia in its severe stages is best managed in an intensive care unit with supportive measures such as respiratory therapy, supplemental oxygen, and fluids. Secondary bacterial pneumonia should be treated with appropriate antibiotics. When from studies of the sputum it is not clear which bacterium may be infecting the patient, coverage should include antibiotics that are effective against *S. aureus*, *S. pneumoniae*, and *H. influenzae*.

PREVENTION. The mainstay of prevention is the use of inactivated influenza virus vaccines. These vaccines provide about 80 per cent protective efficacy. The antigenic composition is reviewed annually so that the vaccine contains the most recently circulating strains. Usually the vaccine is a trivalent product containing one or more subtypes of influenza A and influenza B. The recent vaccines have been purified by density gradient centrifugation or chromatography and have very low reaction rates. One to two per cent of persons vaccinated will have fever and systemic symptoms peaking at 8 to 12 hours after vaccination, and up to 25 per cent may have mild local reactions at the site of vaccination. "Split" virus (subvirion) vaccines contain antigens with disrupted virus and may be less reactigenic than "whole" virus vaccines. The highest priority for vaccination should be given to persons with cardiac or pulmonary conditions requiring ongoing medical care and to residents of nursing homes and other chronic care facilities. Physicians, nurses and other personnel who have extensive contact with high-risk patients constitute the next priority for vaccination. Finally, persons over age 65 and persons with other chronic disease of any age should be vaccinated. Vaccine may also be given to well persons under age 65 who wish to reduce the likelihood of acquiring influenza.

Amantadine and rimantadine are also effective in preventing influenza A and should be used to supplement vaccine programs. Persons who are not vaccinated in the fall should be placed on amantadine when an outbreak occurs or throughout the influenza season for the highest risk group. If vaccine is available, persons may be vaccinated simultaneously, and amantadine therapy should be stopped after 14 days. Alternatively, if vaccine is not available, amantadine administration may be continued for the duration of the outbreak, the dose being 100 to 200 mg per day orally.

A Consensus Development Conference: Diagnosis and treatment of Reye's syndrome. JAMA 246:21, 1982. *Up-to-date summary of Reye's syndrome with description of staging.*

Barker WH, Mulloohy JP: Pneumonia and influenza deaths during epidemics: Implications for prevention. Arch Intern Med 142:85, 1982. *Rationale for influenza vaccination.*

Center for Disease Control: Prevention and Control of Influenza. Morbidity and Mortality Weekly Report 33:253–266, 1984. *Rationale and details of extensive revisions of recommendations for use of influenza vaccine.*

Dolin R, Reichman RC, Madore HP, Maynard R, Linton PN, Webber-Jones J: A controlled trial of amantadine and rimantadine in the prophylaxis of influenza A infection. N Engl J Med 307:580, 1982. *Definitive study comparing prophylactic efficacy of amantadine and rimantadine.*

Glezen WP, Couch RB, Six HR: The influenza herald wave. Am J Epidemiol 116:4, 1982. *Prediction of epidemic influenza from previous year's outbreak.*

Hauptmann R, Clarke LD, Mountford RC, Bachmayer H, Almond JW: Nucleotide sequence of the hemagglutinin gene of influenza virus A/England/321/77. J Gen Virol 64:215, 1983. *Studies on the molecular mechanism of antigenic drift.*

Younkin SW, Betts RF, Roth FK, Douglas RG: Reduction in fever and symptoms in young adults with aspirin or amantadine. Antimicrob Agents Chemother 23:577, 1983. *Recent study comparing therapeutic effects of amantadine and aspirin.*

331. ADENOVIRUS DISEASES

Stephen G. Baum

The clinically most significant diseases caused by adenoviruses are infections of the respiratory system and the eye. Recently, adenoviruses have been shown to play a major role in causing diarrheal disease in children and respiratory and urinary tract infections in immunocompromised patients. Adenoviruses are the object of intensive research efforts because they possess several fascinating and important biologic capabilities. Today they are perhaps the best characterized human virus group.

HISTORY. The term adenovirus derives from the fact that Rowe and colleagues first isolated these agents in 1953 from surgically removed adenoids that had been placed in tissue culture. The adenoidal cells underwent spontaneous cytopathic effects (CPE), and the virus could be passed serially in epithelial cells with reproducible characteristic CPE. In the past 30 years, 41 serotypes of human adenovirus have been identified (types 1 to 41). These have been isolated from adenoidal tissue, respiratory secretions, conjunctival exudate, urine, and stool samples. Many of the serotypes have been associated with specific syndromes, but over half the adenovirus types have not been shown to cause disease.

ETIOLOGIC AGENT. Adenoviruses are double-stranded DNA viruses that average 70 nm in diameter and have a unique outer structure, which permits their morphologic identification by electron microscopic examination. The virus is icosahedral with 20 equilateral triangular faces and 12 vertices. The faces are made up of hexon subunits, and the vertices each contain a penton subunit. From each vertex, an antenna-like structure, the fiber, projects with a knob at the end. Each class of these surface subunits differs antigenically from the others. The hexon contains group-specific and type-specific antigens. The 41 serotypes of adenovirus have been divided into four groups according to ability to agglutinate different erythrocytes. This artifactual grouping correlates well with the ability of different serotypes to cause specific syndromes and to induce tumors in animals.

In acute infections, adenoviruses cause cell death and lysis with release of new progeny virions. The mechanisms of latency and animal oncogenesis are not completely understood, although many of the functions of adenovirus have been accurately mapped on the deoxyribonucleic acid (DNA) genome. Adenoviruses can form a family of hybrid viruses with an unrelated DNA virus, SV40. Portions of the DNA of adenovirus and SV40 are covalently linked within an adenovirus outer coat. The hybrid virus has unique biologic and oncogenic capabilities in vitro and in animals in vivo. Neither adenovirus alone nor the hybrid viruses have been shown to cause cancer in humans.

A small defective DNA parvovirus has been isolated from some adenovirus preparations and from some patients with adenovirus infection. This *adeno-associated virus (AAV)* requires adenovirus for its replication. It is not known to cause disease by itself and does not appear to contribute to adenovirus pathogenesis.

EPIDEMIOLOGY. Most people experience an adenovirus infection during the first decade of life. The initial infecting serotype and the syndrome it causes are a function of the age of the patient and the route of infection. Studies of large populations show that adenoviruses cause 3 to 5 per cent of all clinically apparent infections in children. Adenoviruses are the most common viral isolates in this age group, and at least half of these isolations are associated with subclinical infections. Respiratory infection is transmitted by person-to-person contact or through contaminated swimming water.

Conjunctival infection may be transmitted directly, through water, or by fomites such as towels or ophthalmologic equipment and solutions. Pneumonia and urinary tract infection in immunocompromised patients may be acquired exogenously or may represent reactivation of latent infection. There are many adenoviruses that infect other animals and birds, but these play no known role in human disease.

CLINICAL PRESENTATIONS OCCURRING MOSTLY IN CHILDREN. ***Respiratory Infection.*** Infants most commonly manifest adenovirus infections as coryzal symptoms, but occasionally adenovirus type 7 causes fulminant bronchiolitis and pneumonia in this age group. In older children, pharyngitis and tracheobronchitis are most prevalent. Adenoviruses are the most common viral isolate from children with the whooping cough syndrome. It is not known whether this virus contributes to the pathogenesis of *Bordetella pertussis* infection or whether adenovirus alone can cause the syndrome.

Pharyngoconjunctival Fever. This syndrome occurs in small epidemics in summer camps where it is probably spread in swimming water. Adenovirus type 3 has been the most common isolate. The incubation period is three to five days, and symptoms, which are acute, include pharyngitis, rhinitis, conjunctivitis, cervical adenitis, and elevation in temperature to about 38° C. The bulbar and palpebral conjunctivae have a granular appearance. The symptoms last one to two weeks. Permanent sequelae are rare, and there is no specific therapy.

Intestinal Disease. Immunoelectron microscopy has revealed viruses in the stool in many cases of infantile diarrhea. The most common viruses visualized are rotaviruses and adenoviruses. These adenoviruses appear to be defective in their replication and require special cells for isolation in tissue culture. Two new serotypes, types 40 and 41, have been found most often in this situation. Intussusception in children has also been linked to adenovirus types 1, 2, 3, and 5, although a causal role is unproven. Many of the children with this syndrome have intercurrent adenoviral respiratory infection.

Hemorrhagic Cystitis. Adenovirus types 11 and 21 have been associated with hemorrhagic cystitis in American and Japanese children. Boys are affected more often than girls, in contrast to the situation with bacterial cystitis. Gross hematuria may persist for one to two weeks.

CLINICAL PRESENTATIONS OCCURRING MOSTLY IN ADULTS. ***Respiratory Infection.*** The first isolation of adenoviruses directly from sick patients occurred during an epidemic of acute respiratory disease in military recruits. This population seems extremely susceptible to infection with types 4 and 7, as it is to infection with *Mycoplasma pneumoniae* and the meningococci. In general, the manifestations are those of atypical pneumonia, of which up to 40 per cent of cases are caused by adenovirus. Fever to 39° C, cough, pharyngitis, rhinorrhea, and pulmonary rales are the most common signs and symptoms. Radiographic examination of the chest shows patchy interstitial infiltrates that are unilateral in most cases. Small pleural effusions can occur.

In nonepidemic situations, it is impossible to make a definitive clinical diagnosis of adenoviral pneumonia. Some factors useful in comparing adenoviral with mycoplasmal pneumonia are: lower incidence of cold agglutinins, shorter incubation period, and better correlation of x-ray and physical findings in the chest in adenovirus infection. Influenza and parainfluenza viruses produce similar syndromes. Adenoviral pneumonia usually lasts one to two weeks. There is no specific therapy, and bacterial superinfection and death are rare.

Adenoviruses have been isolated from the lungs of immunocompromised patients with pneumonia and from the urine of renal transplant recipients and patients with acquired immune deficiency syndrome (AIDS). Many of the higher serotypes were first isolated from such patients. In some of these instances, adenovirus operates as an opportunistic agent; in others it may play a primary role in causing disease.

Neurologic disease, most often appearing as meningoencephalitis, has been attributed to adenovirus. It sometimes occurs in minor epidemic form and is frequently associated with recent respiratory infection. The clinical presentation is that of encephalitis or aseptic meningitis. There are no pathognomonic findings.

Epidemic Keratoconjunctivitis. The initial epidemic of adenoviral keratoconjunctivitis involved shipyard workers who sustained minor eye trauma from paint and rust fragments. Adenovirus type 8 was isolated in this and many other epidemics. Serotypes 19 and 37 have caused keratoconjunctivitis that was spread by fomites such as roller towels. The incubation period is from 3 to 24 days. The onset is insidious, and both eyes often are affected. Eye irritation and exudation may last one to four weeks. Preauricular adenopathy often occurs early. Corneal involvement is a late complication and may persist for a month or more with blurring of vision. Residual blindness is unusual. There is no specific antiviral therapy as there is for herpes keratitis. Secondary spread to household contacts occurs in about 10 per cent of cases, varying with the duration of the index case.

TREATMENT AND PREVENTION. There is no effective antiviral chemotherapy for human adenoviral infections. Live, enteric coated oral adenovirus vaccines of types 4 and 7 have been effective in immunizing military populations. In epidemic situations, mass immunization with the live virus vaccine promptly interrupts the epidemic. The vaccine is not recommended or available for civilians because of the low incidence and sporadic occurrence of infection with adenovirus types 4 and 7.

Baum SG: Adenovirus. *In* Mandell A, Douglas RA, Bennet JE (eds.): Principles and Practice of Infectious Diseases. 2nd ed. New York, John Wiley & Sons, 1984. *An expanded version of the material in this chapter, containing correlative tables, fully referenced.*

Horwitz MS: Adenoviruses. *In* Fields BN, Melnick JL, Chanock R, Roizman B, Shope RE (eds.): Human Viral Diseases. New York, Raven Press (in press), 1984. *An encyclopedic chapter on the molecular biology of the adenoviruses.*

RNA Viral Infections Characterized by Cutaneous Lesions

332. MEASLES (Morbilli, Rubeola)

Samuel L. Katz

DEFINITION. Measles is an acute, highly contagious disease characterized by fever, coryza, cough, conjunctivitis, enanthem, and exanthem. Its morbidity and mortality vary greatly with host and environmental factors, and its epidemiology has been altered strikingly in the past 22 years in those nations where vaccine has been utilized widely.

ETIOLOGY. The virus is an enveloped, RNA paramyxovirus (genus morbillivirus) measuring 120 to 250 nm in diameter, similar to other members of the paramyxovirus family but lacking a neuraminidase. Its single antigenic serotype has been remarkably stable throughout the world for many years with no variation noted. Related animal morbilliviruses are canine distemper and bovine rinderpest, which show some cross-reactivity with measles. The virus contains six major polypeptides, which are responsible for a number of structural and functional properties, including hemagglutination (of primate erythrocytes), hemolysis, cell fusion, viral assembly, and virus penetration. Isolation of virus from clinical specimens is most successful with primary kidney cell cultures of human or simian origin. Laboratory passage has selected variants which grow well in other primary and continuous cell lines of mammalian and avian origin.

Certain simian species provide a reliable animal model of measles after respiratory tract or parenteral inoculation of human isolates. Some virus strains have been adapted to produce central nervous system infection in rodents.

EPIDEMIOLOGY. Classic descriptions of measles epidemiology are no longer applicable to those many areas of the world where measles vaccination is widely practiced. Instead of an inevitable childhood illness, the disease has become an unusual one. The age pattern has shifted to a greater proportion of cases among adolescents and young adults who remain susceptible because of lack of either childhood immunization or exposure to natural infection. In contrast, the epidemiology has been unaltered in developing nations where vaccine programs have been sporadic, incomplete, or totally lacking. Isolated communities such as the Faröe Islands (Panum) are infrequently attacked by measles, at which time manifest illness appears in virtually all persons not previously infected.

Throughout most of the world, measles was a disease of children; most adults acquired active immunity in childhood. Beyond the age of ten more than 90 per cent of the population had specific antibody. Although the peak attack rate coincided with the beginning of school (age six) in technologically advanced societies, it occurs much younger in most developing countries. Morbidity and mortality rates do not appear to be influenced by sex or race. Case fatality rates are highest in children less than five years of age, and are also relatively high in the aged. Congenital infection has occurred but intrauterine infection is more apt to produce a stillborn or premature infant.

There is no evidence that the virus may vary in virulence in nature. The excess morbidity and mortality of the disease in developing, isolated, or crowded populations may be explained as a corollary of (1) more prevalent infection of infants under one year of age, (2) poor environmental conditions, (3) inadequate medical care, and (4) secondary bacterial infections. A strikingly increased mortality rate is observed in areas where protein-calorie malnutrition is prevalent.

Communicability. Measles is one of the most highly contagious infections. Demonstration of virus in nasopharyngeal secretions during the prodromal, pre-eruptive phase and in the first days of rash is in accord with epidemiologic evidence that infection is disseminated and acquired by the respiratory tract. Close physical proximity or direct person-to-person contact is the usual requisite for infection.

Immunity. An unmodified attack of measles is usually followed by lifelong immunity. This observation is in accord with the observed enduring persistence of antibodies after infection. The mechanism of lifelong immunity after measles is undefined. Although persistence of infective virus seems not to occur, defective virus is demonstrable years after infection in the brain and peripheral lymph nodes of those rare individuals afflicted with subacute sclerosing panencephalitis (SSPE) (see Ch. 504).

Careful studies of isolated or closed populations after administration of live virus vaccine have demonstrated a lower level of antibody titer than in populations in which measles virus is circulating. Anamnestic antibody response in the absence of disease has been shown in immune contacts of patients with measles. However, studies of children in protected environments have demonstrated that re-exposure or reinfection is not necessary for maintenance of enduring immunity. Passively transferred maternal antibody protects the young infant for the first four to eight months of life.

PATHOLOGY AND PHYSIOLOGIC RESPONSES. Pathologic changes in fatal measles usually represent the compound effect of viral and secondary bacterial infection. Pneumonia is almost invariably present; it is most frequently interstitial. More representative are changes of the uncomplicated viral disease within the tonsillar, nasopharyngeal, and appendiceal tissue removed during the prodrome. These changes consist of round cell infiltration and the presence of multinucleated giant cells. Similar cells are commonly observed in tissue cultures infected with measles virus. Cytoplasmic and nuclear inclusions may be seen in epithelial cells. Koplik's spots show inflammatory mononuclear cell infiltration of buccal submucous glands and necrosis of focal vesicular lesions of the mucosa. Rash is the result of proliferation of capillary endothelial cells in the corium and the coincident exudation of serum, and occasionally erythrocytes, into the epidermis. Viral microtubular aggregates are found in the endothelium of dermal capillaries, but not in the epidermal layer. Simultaneous with the onset of rash, measles-specific antibodies are detectable in serum and, by immunofluorescence, in areas of rash. A marked leukopenia is frequently observed throughout the febrile period. Initially, the leukopenia is occasioned by a decline in lymphocytes on the first day of fever; subsequently, granulocytopenia ensues as well. Measles virus replicates in lymphoid tissues (spleen, thymus, lymph nodes), can multiply in vitro in peripheral blood T and B lymphocytes and monocytes, and can be isolated from blood leukocytes during the course of the disease. The virus is propagable in suspensions of leukocytes in vitro.

Immunosuppressive Effects of Measles. It has long been known that cell-mediated immunity is impaired during measles. There is transient suppression of the tuberculin reaction (observed also with measles vaccines), improvement in eczema and allergic asthma, delay in wound healing, and the induction of remissions in nephrosis. Actual infection of activated lymphocytes may explain the depression of cell-mediated immunity during the acute disease. In severe disease, the magnitude of depression of the total lymphocytes has been positively correlated with a lessened chance of recovery.

CLINICAL MANIFESTATIONS. After an incubation period that averages 11 days, measles becomes clinically manifest with symptoms of fever, malaise, myalgia, and headache. Within hours *ocular symptoms* of photophobia and burning pain are manifested by conjunctival injection, tearing, and exudate in the conjunctival sac. Concomitantly, or soon thereafter, *catarrhal inflammation of the respiratory tract* leads to sneezing, coughing, and nasal discharge. Less commonly, hoarseness and aphonia may reflect laryngeal involvement. In this prodromal stage of one to four days' duration, petechial lesions of the palate and pharynx or tiny white spots on the buccal mucosa *(Koplik's spots)* may herald the appearance of skin rash. The white lesions described by Koplik characteristically occur lateral to the molar teeth, and typically are mounted on red areolae of injected mucosa, which may coalesce to form a diffuse red background. They constitute a valuable, if not pathognomonic, diagnostic sign. The enanthem may involve other mucous membranes such as the palpebral conjunctiva and vaginal lining. It may "overlap" the subsequent appearance of the cutaneous rash by one to three days. See Figure 332–1.

The *rash* of measles follows the prodromal symptoms by two to four days, occasionally as late as seven days. It first appears behind the ears or on the face and neck as a blotchy erythema, spreads downward to cover the trunk, and finally is manifest on the extremities. The hands and feet may escape involvement. Initially, the eruption consists of discrete, reddish-brown macules that blanch with pressure. Subsequently, these lesions become papular, tend to coalesce, and may develop a hemorrhagic, nonblanching component. Rash is sometimes very extensive in children with protein-calorie malnutrition, and skin lesions associated with kwashiorkor may develop at the site of the exanthem. The rash fades in the order of its appearance; its disappearance about five days after onset is attended by a fine, powdery desquamation that spares the hands and feet. At its maximum the exanthem usually marks the termination of malaise and fever in the uncomplicated illness.

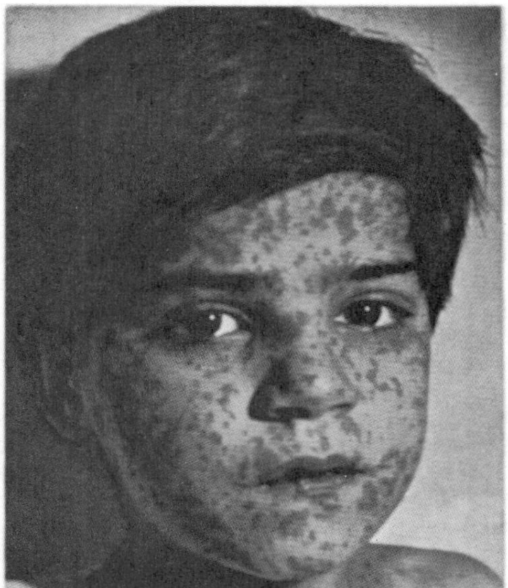

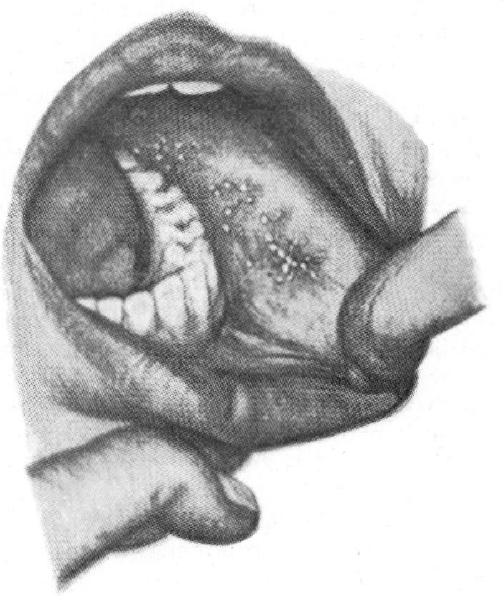

Figure 332–1. *Upper:* Early measles eruption. (Reproduction from Therapeutic Notes, by courtesy of Parke, Davis & Company.) *Lower:* Koplik's spots in measles (Hecker, Trumpp, and Abt).

The *fever* of measles is commonly of the typhoidal, progressively rising type, and falls by lysis. It persists for about six days, and frequently reaches 40 or 41° C. Throughout the febrile period, productive *cough* and auscultatory evidence of bronchiolitis may be evident. These manifestations may persist after defervescence, and cough is often the last symptom to disappear. Bronchopulmonary symptomatology is an integral part of the primary viral infection; roentgenographic evidence of pulmonary involvement is frequently seen in the uncomplicated disease in the absence of leukocytosis and obvious bacterial infection. Generalized lymphadenopathy accompanies the acute febrile illness and may persist for several weeks thereafter.

COMPLICATIONS. It is difficult to distinguish between those complications directly attributable to the virus of measles and those resulting from secondary bacterial infections. The persistence or recurrence of fever and the development of leukocytosis are presumptive evidence of the usual bacterial sequelae of *otitis media* or *pneumonia*. Superimposed bacterial infection is common, and pneumonia accounts for most of the severe or fatal cases. Pneumococcus, *Streptococcus hemolyticus*, *Staphylococcus aureus*, and *Hemophilus influenzae* are the usual secondary invaders.

Serious complications directly related to the measles virus are rare. *Laryngitis* of sufficient severity to embarrass respiration has been observed, and may warrant tracheostomy. Keratoconjunctivitis is part of the acute phase but rarely progresses to actual corneal ulceration. *Electrocardiographic abnormalities* may be found in as many as 30 per cent of children, but clinical evidence of cardiac disease is absent. *Abdominal pain* or *diarrhea* may be related to invasion of lymphoid tissue of the appendix or Peyer's patches. These symptoms may lead to unnecessary surgery before the appearance of the typical rash. The frequency of stomatitis and gastrointestinal symptoms is greater in malnourished children in tropical areas and may reflect coincident bacterial and parasitic infection. They may result in severe dehydration and acidosis as fluid and electrolyte losses rise in the face of diminished oral intake.

Encephalomyelitis. A rare (0.1 per cent) but serious consequence of measles is a demyelinating encephalomyelitis that may appear from 1 to 14 days after the onset of infection. This complication is associated with a recurrence of fever, and headache, vomiting, and stiff neck. Stupor and convulsions usually follow. Localizing neurologic symptoms may be present. Death ensues in about 10 per cent of patients; more than half of survivors suffer permanent residuals of varying severity. Abnormal electroencephalograms were recorded in 51 per cent of children with measles *without clinical signs of encephalitis*. In some of the children the abnormal encephalographic findings were persistent. As noted above, the presence of virus has been demonstrated in patients with subacute sclerosing panencephalitis. Infection of brain cells results in an incomplete viral replicative cycle with production of defective virions lacking one ("M") of the measles-virus proteins. Studies of patients with acute measles encephalomyelitis and of those with late onset subacute sclerosing panencephalitis show high titers in serum and cerebrospinal fluid of antibodies to all the measles virus proteins except M. This protein is an internal membrane protein crucial to viral assembly.

Other late sequelae of measles are thrombocytopenic purpura and exacerbation or activation of pre-existing pulmonary tuberculosis. The late complication of subacute sclerosing panencephalitis (see Immunity, above) is discussed in Ch. 504.

Giant-Cell Pneumonia. In children with severe disease compromising normal cellular and humoral immune mechanisms, measles virus may induce an interstitial pneumonia characterized by giant cells and intracellular inclusion bodies. The disease is usually fatal; if the patient survives, persistence of virus and poor or absent antibody formation are evident in convalescence. The pneumonia may occur in the absence of rash so that its etiologic relation to measles may be unsuspected.

Measles Modified by Antibody Administration. Attenuation of the natural disease by antibody prophylaxis may result in an illness of lessened severity comparable with the milder infection of the maternally immunized newborn. Fever alone may be observed, but some degree of exanthem is usually apparent. Koplik's spots may not appear. In general, the course is truncated and relatively uncomplicated. Lasting immunity is uncertain and serologic studies should be obtained to check for measles-specific antibodies after modified illness.

Atypical Measles—A New Disease. From 1963 to 1967, two types of measles vaccine, one live attenuated, the other inactivated or "killed," were available in the United States. The live attenuated vaccine has since 1967 been the sole product licensed and utilized in this country. From 1965 to 1968 a series of reports was published describing a severe, atypical form of disease occurring after exposure to natural measles of children who had previously received the inactivated vaccine. These patients had high fever, pneumonia, pleural effusion, obtundation, and an unusual rash. The exanthem frequently was initially urticarial and rapidly progressive to maculopapular, petechial, and sometimes vesicular lesions. It was most striking, and often began, on the extremities and was sometimes accompanied by edema of hands and feet. Concomitantly these patients' sera revealed extraordinarily high titers of measles-specific antibodies (25,000 to 200,000 by hemagglutination-inhibition testing).

Subsequent investigations showed that patients who had received inactivated measles vaccines failed to develop antibodies to the "F" protein of the virus. This polypeptide is responsible for cell fusion, viral penetration, and hemolysis. Lack of antibodies to the cell fusion factor permitted these patients to support measles infection in superficial respiratory mucosal cells by cell-to-cell spread. The other measles virus antigens released by these infected cells stimulated a hyperimmune response to those polypeptides that had been present in the inactivated vaccines. Thus the atypical measles syndrome is an imbalance of immune response.

In addition to the rash and pulmonary findings, these patients may have elevated liver enzymes, disseminated intravascular coagulation, and marked myalgia. The pulmonary changes have persisted for longer than 18 months in patients followed with serial chest films. Initial diagnoses on presentation have included Rocky Mountain spotted fever and meningococcemia because of the similarities of rash and toxicity. Since inactivated vaccines were available only from 1963 through 1967, the past recipients are now in adolescence or young adulthood. This atypical measles syndrome is of increasing importance to the internist.

DIAGNOSIS. The experienced layman can diagnose typical measles. The querulous, bleary-eyed child, his face blotched and his nose crusted with exudate, presents a characteristic, if miserable, picture as he breathes open-mouthed between paroxysms of sneezing and coughing. The severity of the catarrhal symptoms distinguishes the disease from other eruptive fevers. In the prodromal period the diagnosis should be suggested by (1) fever higher than that of the usual respiratory virus infection, (2) known measles in the community, and (3) Koplik's spots on the buccal mucosa.

Differential diagnosis (see Table 332–1) includes consideration of rubella, scarlet fever, exanthem subitum, infectious mononucleosis, secondary syphilis, drug eruptions, and infection with certain coxsackie- and echoviruses. Of value in excluding these possibilities are the milder course, postauricular nodes, and pinker rash of rubella; the sore throat, eventual desquamation, strawberry tongue, and leukocytosis of scarlet fever; and serologic tests for infectious mononucleosis and syphilis. The rash of exanthem subitum does not appear until the termination of fever. Fever, enanthem, and catarrh are uncommon with the cutaneous manifestations of drug hypersensitivity. Erythema infectiosum is an afebrile illness with rash on the cheeks, arms, and legs. There is no prodrome or accompanying respiratory tract involvement.

Specific Diagnosis. Specific diagnosis depends on the isolation of measles virus from throat washings, blood, or urine by inoculation of tissue culture with materials obtained optimally during the prodrome or first days of rash. Increase in specific antibody may be detected as early as the first or second day of rash by the complement fixation test. Antibody is also demonstrated by neutralization and hemagglutination-inhibition

TABLE 332–1. A GUIDE TO THE DIFFERENTIAL DIAGNOSIS OF MEASLES

	Conjunctivitis	Rhinitis	Sore Throat	Enanthem	Leukocytosis	Specific Laboratory Tests Available
Measles	+ +	+ +	0	+	0	+
Rubella	±	±	±	±	0	+
Exanthem subitum	±	±	0	0	0	0
Enterovirus infection	0	±	±	0	0	+
Scarlet fever	±	±	+ +	0	+	+
Infectious mononucleosis	0	0	+ +	±	±	+
Drug rash	0	0	0	0	0	0

0 Not usually present; no test available.
± Variable in occurrence.
+ Present; test available (virus or bacterial culture, serology).
+ + Present and severe.

procedures. The latter is generally employed because of rapidity and reliability.

Presumptive diagnosis may be made if giant cells are detected in stained smears of nasal exudate in the pre-eruptive period.

PROGNOSIS. Uncomplicated measles is rarely fatal, and complete recovery is the rule. Fatalities are almost always the result of pneumonia, occurring principally in children below the age of two years. Mortality in economically underdeveloped countries may be 250 times that observed in the United States or northern Europe. Case fatality rates are also high in elderly and tuberculous patients. Congestive cardiac failure is a common cause of death in patients over 50 years old.

Antimicrobial drugs effective against the usual secondary invaders have reduced the case fatality rate of measles sharply. They have not proved effective in prophylaxis of bacterial complications, but in therapy.

Encephalitis occurs as frequently in mild as in severe measles (i.e., about one in a thousand cases). However, the incidence of neurologic sequelae after administration of attenuated live virus vaccine is only one in a million.

TREATMENT. There is no specific antiviral therapy for measles.

Symptomatic Therapy. In the absence of complications, bed rest is the essence of treatment in this usually benign, self-limited disease. Codeine sulfate may be useful in the amelioration of headache and myalgia and is effective in the management of cough. Aspirin may be employed for its analgesic and antipyretic actions. Fluids should be encouraged. Bright light is not an ocular hazard, but photophobia may require darkening of the patient's room.

Antimicrobial Prophylaxis. The course of uncomplicated measles is not influenced by antimicrobial drugs, and their use during the acute illness has resulted in no decrease of secondary bacterial complications (otitis, sinusitis, pneumonia). Instead, the same rates of complications (about 10 to 15 per cent) have been observed, but with organisms resistant to the antibiotics used during the viral illness. If careful observation of the patient is possible, rational therapy is based on the prompt recognition and etiologic definition of complications, followed by initiation of the appropriate antimicrobial drug in proper dosage.

PREVENTION. ***Vaccination.*** A highly effective vaccine available for the prevention of measles is derived from the Edmonston strain of virus isolated originally in the laboratory of Dr. John Enders. This live virus vaccine produces immunity by infection and therefore needs to be given only as a single injection. It induces antibody response of somewhat lesser magnitude than that following natural infection. In children over one year of age, seroconversion after vaccination is 90 to 97 per cent. Although a gradual fall in antibody titer occurs in the absence of exposure to wild type virus (see Epidemiology: Immunity), serum antibody is demonstrable in most individuals more than 15 years after a single administration of vaccine. The occasional failure of live virus vaccine to protect has recently been related to vaccination at less than 12 months of age, at which time maternal antibody may inhibit replication of the vaccine virus. It is now recommended that measles immunization be deferred until 15 months of age in technologically advanced countries in which infantile infection is uncommon. Reimmunization is not harmful and is recommended for those who have received vaccine before age one year. The current vaccine is fully effective and safe in susceptible adults also.

Contraindications to live virus vaccine include pregnancy, immunodeficiency, leukemia, and other systemic malignant diseases, active tuberculosis, and administration of resistance-depressing drugs such as corticosteroids and antimetabolites.

Eradication of measles through administration of live virus vaccines is a scientifically reasonable possibility. The introduction of immunization in the United States in 1963 has led to a decrease in incidence from about 500,000 cases annually to fewer than 1500 cases in 1983. Although it may be possible to eliminate indigenous measles in the United States, the problem of "imported infection" has arisen with the influx of susceptible children from Southeast Asia and certain Latin American nations.

Annunziato D, Kaplan MH, Hall WW, Ichinose H, Linn JH, Balsam D, Paladino VS: Atypical measles syndrome: Pathologic and serologic findings. Pediatrics 70:203, 1982. *Excellent clinical description and explanation of a syndrome now seen in young adults.*

Choppin PW, Richardson CD, Merz DC, Hall WW, Scheid A: The functions and inhibition of the membrane glycoproteins of paramyxoviruses and myxoviruses and the role of measles virus M protein in subacute sclerosing panencephalitis. J Infect Dis 143:352, 1981. *The ultimate correlation of molecular virology and clinical expression of measles and related viruses.*

Hinman AR, Brandling-Bennett AD, Bernier RH, Kirby CD, Eddins DL: Current features of measles in the United States: Feasibility of measles elimination. Epidem Rev 2:153, 1980. *A "state-of-the-art" review of measles surveillance, immunization, and plans for eradication of indigenous disease in the United States.*

Johnson RT, Griffin DE, Hirsch RL, Wolinsky JS, Roedenbeck S, deSoriano IL, Vaisberg A: Measles encephalomyelitis—clinical and immunologic studies. N Engl J Med 310:137, 1984. *Pathogenesis of central nervous system complications studied by modern immunologic approaches.*

Katz SL, Krugman S, Quinn TC (eds.): International symposium on measles immunization. Rev Infect Dis 5:389, 1983. *An all-inclusive presentation of measles and its prevention throughout the world.*

Panum PL: Observations Made During the Epidemic of Measles on the Faröe Islands. Delta Omega Society, 1940. *A classic clinical epidemiologic description of measles introduced into an isolated population with disease among all susceptibles born since the previous epidemic 65 years earlier.*

Sabin AB, Arechiga AF, deCastro JF, Sever JL, Madden DL, Shekarchi I, Albrecht P: Successful immunization of children with and without maternal antibody by aerosolized measles vaccine. JAMA 249:2651, 1983. *A new approach to vaccine administration, with promise of great benefit for developing nations.*

333. RUBELLA (German Measles)

Samuel L. Katz

DEFINITION. Rubella is an acute, usually benign infectious disease characterized by a three-day rash, generalized lymphadenopathy, and minimal or absent prodromal symptoms. Since 1941, it has been known to cause congenital malformations when infection occurs during the early months of pregnancy.

Rubella was recognized as a distinct clinical entity by German physicians in the mid-eighteenth century; it continued to be the subject of moderate interest through the next two centuries until 1941, when the Australian ophthalmologist Gregg called attention to its role as a teratogen. Over the next 20 years the association of rubella in early pregnancy with fetal defects (cataracts, heart disease, and deafness) was corroborated by a number of clinical epidemiologic studies. In 1962, techniques for viral culture and serologic confirmation became available.

ETIOLOGY. Rubella virus is a pleomorphic agent when viewed by electron microscopy, usually spherical, with a central nucleoid 30 nm in diameter contained within an outer envelope 60 to 70 nm wide. Its genome is RNA, and the virus is classified as a special member (genus rubivirus) of the togavirus group on the basis of its biochemical, biophysical, and ultrastructural properties. Unlike most of the togaviruses it does not utilize an arthropod vector in its natural cycle. In the human, its natural host, the virus behaves like a paramyxovirus, and many of its laboratory characteristics are like those of that group. It will multiply in a variety of primary cell culture systems and in some continuous cell lines, usually without detectable cytopathic effects. Hemagglutination of avian erythrocytes provides a convenient method for virus assay, and by inhibition of this hemagglutination the presence and titer of antibody are readily measured. By polyacrylamide-gel electrophoresis eight distinct viral polypeptides have been identified.

EPIDEMIOLOGY. Prior to the availability of rubella vaccines, the disease was worldwide in distribution, produced major epidemics at six- to nine-year intervals, and occurred mainly in school-age children, but also produced outbreaks in settings such as military recruit bases and college campuses where large numbers of susceptible young adults gathered in relatively crowded conditions. The use, since licensure in 1969, of more than 125 million doses of rubella vaccine in the United States has strikingly altered the epidemiology. There has been no major epidemic since 1964–1965, and the age-specific attack rate has altered with a significant increase in the proportion of cases reported in adolescents and young adults who failed to be immunized in childhood. In other nations, where rubella vaccine has not been widely utilized, the epidemiology has remained unchanged and epidemics were observed in 1971–1972 and in 1978–1979. Because the usual disease may be quite nonspecific clinically, with evidence that nearly one third of adults may undergo infection without rash, epidemiologic reporting has been variable. Since 1966, congenital rubella has been a reportable disease. It is probable that rubella is spread by the respiratory route by close and sustained personal contact. The usual infection is contagious during the period of prodromal symptoms and for as long as seven days after the appearance of rash. However, the infant with congenitally acquired infection may excrete virus in respiratory secretions and in urine for months after birth and is contagious during this time. In hospital environments, especially in nurseries, the congenital rubella baby has been a source of nosocomial infection of personnel involved in his care.

Immunity is lifelong in duration after initial infection. Authenticated second attacks are exceedingly rare, and require serologic documentation because of the nebulous nature of the clinical syndrome. *Subclinical* reinfection demonstrated by increase in IgG serum antibody has been documented with increasing frequency as better serologic methods and increased surveillance have become available. Reinfection occurs most commonly in crowded populations in which the density of infection and probability of spread are high. Such reinfections are not associated with viremia and thus pose little threat in pregnant women. IgM response serves to distinguish primary infection from reinfection. Immunity that follows artificial immunization with live virus vaccine is apparently of equal duration even though the antibody titers induced may be somewhat lower. (See Prevention, below.)

PATHOLOGY. Death from postnatal rubella is an almost unheard-of event, so the histology has not been studied. Since 1962, it has been possible to investigate the pathogenesis and to correlate clinical findings with virologic events. After initial invasion of the upper respiratory tract, virus spreads to local lymphoid tissue where it multiplies and starts a viremia of approximately seven days' duration. Respiratory tract shedding of virus and the viremia rise to peak levels until the onset of rash, at which time the latter becomes undetectable, whereas respiratory secretions contain diminishing quantities of virus over the succeeding 5 to 15 days. Specific antibodies can be demonstrated with the onset of rash, and circulating immune complexes are detectable soon thereafter.

Congenital Rubella. Necropsies of fetal and neonatal victims of intrauterine infection have shown a variety of embryonal defects related to developmental arrest involving all three germ layers.

The virus establishes chronic persistent infection of many tissues, with inhibition of mitosis and a resultant intrauterine growth retardation. Delayed and disordered organogenesis produces embryopathic structural defects (eye, brain, heart, large arteries), and continued viral infection in fetal and postnatal cells causes organ and tissue damage (hepatitis, nephritis, myocarditis, pneumonia, osteitis, meningitis, cochlear degeneration, pancreatitis).

CLINICAL MANIFESTATIONS. ***Postnatally Acquired Rubella.*** Fourteen to 21 days after exposure, the onset of rubella is manifested by the appearance of a rash with mild accompanying constitutional symptoms of malaise and occasional sore throat. Palpable, tender, and occasionally visible lymphadenopathy involves postauricular and suboccipital nodes. Moderate fever, coryza, and faint conjunctivitis may accompany the rash. Generalized peripheral lymphadenopathy and, more rarely, splenomegaly may occur.

The exanthem of rubella is usually apparent within 24 hours of the first symptoms as a faint macular erythema that first involves the face and neck. Characterized by its brevity and evanescence, it spreads rapidly to the trunk and extremities, sometimes leaving one site even as it appears at the next. The pink macules that constitute the rash blanch with pressure and rarely stain the skin. Rubella virus has been isolated from the skin lesions as well as from uninvolved sites. The truncal rash may coalesce, but the lesions on the extremities remain discrete. The eruption vanishes by the third day. Rubella may occur without rash. An enanthem has been described that is inconstant in form and occurrence. The lesions consist of red macules that usually involve the soft palate. Infections with adenoviruses, enteroviruses, and Epstein-Barr virus can mimic rubella with rash, fever, and lymphadenopathy. In the absence of an epidemic and of serologic (or virologic) confirmation, the clinical diagnosis of rubella is not reliable.

COMPLICATIONS. Recovery is almost always prompt and uneventful. In contrast to measles, secondary bacterial infections are not encountered in rubella. Arthritis is more common among adolescents and adults with rubella, particularly females. It appears three or more days after onset of rash and may last five to ten days. Large joints (knees, elbows, ankles) are most often involved, but small and medium-sized joints may also be affected. Surveys during urban epidemics have revealed rates of 5 to 15 per cent in males and 10 to 35 per cent in females. There appears to be no association with later rheumatoid arthritis or other joint disease.

Thrombocytopenia, when sought by serial platelet counts, is a common complication but rarely of clinical significance. The unusual patient who develops purpuric manifestations may also have evidence of increased capillary fragility and a prolonged bleeding time. A meningoencephalitis of short duration may occur one to six days after the appearance of rash. Its incidence is estimated at 1 in 6000 cases, and it is fatal in approximately 20 per cent of those afflicted. Rubella encephalopathy is not associated with demyelinization (in contrast to other postviral encephalitides). Survivors may have electroencephalographic abnormalities, but intellectual function seems to be preserved.

Congenital Rubella. Congenital transplacental infection of the fetus occurs as a consequence of maternal infection (which may or may not be clinically evident), usually in the first four months of pregnancy. Virus is demonstrable in placental and fetal tissues obtained by therapeutic abortion at that time. If pregnancy is not interrupted, fetal infection persists, and upon delivery of the infant, virus is recoverable from the throat, urine, conjunctivae, bone marrow, and cerebrospinal fluid of the living infant and from most organs at autopsy. From 20 to 80 per cent of infants born to mothers infected in the first trimester of pregnancy have stigmata of infection readily recognizable in the first year of life. These include *cardiac lesions* and *eye defects* (cataracts, glaucoma, retinitis, microphthalmia). Most infants in whom virus is detectable do not have evidence of disease at birth or may simply have intrauterine growth retardation. In others, disease of intermediate severity occurs. Most prominent of these manifestations is *thrombocytopenic purpura*, which disappears soon after birth. *Hepatosplenomegaly* with active hepatitis may persist for months. Other involvement includes *interstitial pneumonia, meningoencephalitis, hearing loss* of varying extent, and *lesions of the long bones*. A chronic recurrent erythematous rash associated with the presence of rubella virus in the skin has been reported in some patients. Recently, a progressive panencephalitis simulating subacute sclerosing panencephalitis has been observed in the second decade following congenital infection. The long-term sequelae for most congenital rubella infants include psychomotor retardation, hearing loss, and retinopathy.

A striking finding has been the persistence of virus in the pharynx, urine, and cerebrospinal fluid for as long as one year after birth (9 per cent). Infective virus was present in a congenital cataract after three years, and in the urine of a victim of congenital rubella 29 years after her birth. This evidence of continuing viral synthesis occurs coincidentally with circulating antibody (initially of maternal origin). The character of the antibody changes during the first months from IgG (presumably maternal) to IgM, indicating a primary response of the infant to the persisting viral antigen. Studies of older infants and children with stigmata of congenital rubella show them to be free of demonstrable virus and to possess the IgG immunoglobulins that characteristically persist after other viral infections. The defect in host response that is responsible for viral persistence has not yet been defined fully, but there is depressed T cell response to rubella virus antigens in some congenitally infected infants.

DIAGNOSIS. Rubella may be diagnosed clinically with assurance only during an epidemic. Distinction from measles may be made on the basis of fainter, nonstaining rash, the milder course, and the minimal or absent systemic complaints. Sore throat is a more prominent complaint in scarlet fever; the course of infectious mononucleosis is often more protracted, and splenomegaly is more frequent than in rubella. Specific diagnosis of rubella is made by isolation of the virus in any of several cell culture systems, or by demonstration of neutralizing, hemagglutination-inhibiting (HI), or complement-fixing antibody response during infection. HI antibodies are most rapidly and reproducibly available in diagnostic laboratories throughout the nation. A simple, ten-minute latex-agglutination card assay for antibodies enables the physician to determine rubella susceptibility or immunity within the time of an office or clinic visit.

PROGNOSIS. Complete recovery from postnatally acquired rubella is almost invariable. The rare deaths attributable to rubella follow the infrequent complication of meningoencephalitis. Infection in pregnancy constitutes a grave hazard to the fetus but not to the mother.

TREATMENT. There is no specific antiviral therapy. Few patients suffer discomfort severe enough to warrant symptomatic medication. Headache and myalgia may be controlled by aspirin.

PREVENTION. ***Passive Immunization.*** *Administration of gamma globulin to the pregnant woman may only mask her symptoms of infection yet not protect the fetus from viral invasion.* Its use may thus only obscure the picture and confound decision about the need for therapeutic abortion.

Active Immunization. Rubella may be prevented in children and adults by the parenteral administration of attenuated live virus vaccines produced in cell cultures. Seroconversion rates after immunization are at least 95 per cent. As with other live virus vaccines, serum antibody titers are somewhat lower than those that follow natural infection. However, antibody persists for at least 15 years after vaccination. Natural reinfection of individuals immunized with vaccine is not uncommon, although such infection is asymptomatic and without viremia. In children, vaccination is attended by little or no reaction; but in women, malaise, arthralgia, and mild, acute arthritis occur frequently, the incidence being directly related to age. It was initially recommended in the United States that immunization be carried out principally in childhood. The success of these efforts, with reduction of rubella cases to fewer than 1000 in 1983, has encouraged a more aggressive attempt to immunize susceptible women and adolescent girls. Current policy recommends vaccination of all such persons who have no history of previous rubella immunization. Of this population, only nonpregnant individuals should be immunized, and contraception (when appropriate) should be carried out for at least three months after vaccination. The inadvertent administration of vaccine to pregnant women has demonstrated that attenuated vaccine viruses can reach the products of conception; but in 143 such cases studied, no infant has been observed with congenital malformations as a result. The use of vaccine in the United States prevented a large epidemic of rubella expected in the early 1970's and has reduced the reported annual occurrence from more than 50,000 cases annually (with epidemic peaks of 200,000 to 500,000) to an all-time low of 953 in 1983, with only 20 cases of congenital rubella.

Centers for Disease Control: Rubella and congenital rubella—United States, 1980–83. Morbid Mortal Wkly Rep 32:505, 1983. *Fourteen years since licensure of rubella vaccine, a statement of achievements and the need for a focus on unimmunized adults and hospital personnel.*

Clarke M, Schild GC, Miller C, Seagroatt V, Pollock TM, Finlay S, Barbara JAJ: Surveys of rubella antibodies in young adults and children. Lancet 1:667, 1983. *The English approach to prevention of congenital rubella, very different from that in the United States and with persistence of congenital rubella 13 years after its initiation.*

Gregg NM: Congenital cataract following German measles in the mother. Trans Ophthal Soc Aust 3:35, 1941. *The original "classic" associating rubella in pregnancy with congenital malformations.*

Hanshaw JB, Dudgeon JA: Rubella. *In* Viral Diseases of the Fetus and Newborn. Philadelphia, W. B. Saunders Company, 1978. *For the interested scholar, an all-inclusive presentation with nine pages of references.*

Herrmann KL: Rubella virus. *In* Lennette EH, Schmidt NJ (eds.): Diagnostic Procedures for Viral, Rickettsial and Chlamydial Infections. 5th ed. Washington, D.C., American Public Health Association, 1979. *Excellent presentation of the laboratory support for confirmation of the clinical diagnosis.*

Hinman AR, Orenstein WA, Bart KJ, Preblud SR: Rational strategy for rubella vaccination. Lancet 1:39, 1983. *The architects of United States rubella eradication re-examine the problem.*

Tingle AJ, Yang T, Allen M, Kettyls GD, Larke RPB, Schulzer M: Prospective immunological assessment of arthritis induced by rubella vaccine. Infect Immunol 40:22, 1983. *The unresolved issue of rubella's relationship to rheumatoid arthritis and other disorders.*

334. FOOT AND MOUTH DISEASE (Aphthous Fever, Epizootic Stomatitis)

Catherine M. Wilfert

Foot and mouth disease (FMD) is a highly contagious illness of cloven-hoofed animals, especially cattle, sheep, goats, and pigs. The etiology was first ascribed to a filterable agent in 1898 by Loeffler and Frosch. The virus is now known to be a member of the picornavirus family. It belongs to the aphthovirus genus, which is composed of small (diameter of 25 to 30 nm) acid-labile RNA viruses containing naked icosahedral nucleocapsids. The disease in animals is characterized by fever and increased salivation, with the appearance of vesicular lesions on the mucous membranes of the mouth, tongue, and lips, between the paws, and on the teats and udder. Vesicular fluid is highly infectious. There are seven different serotypes of FMD which tend to be found in localized geographic areas. This virus is highly communicable among animals, and the epidemic spread of this agent among domestic animals can result in tremendous loss of livestock. The rigid quarantine regulations of the Bureau of Animal Diseases, U.S. Department of Agriculture, in the United States has freed this country of FMD. Indeed, public law prevents importation of the virus into the mainland of the United States even for experimental purposes. An inactivated vaccine for use in animals utilized polyvalent, cell culture–grown FMD virus. More recently, DNA recombinant technology and chemically synthesized peptides corresponding to specific regions of a capsid polypeptide have been successfully used as immunogens in animals.

FMD in its natural hosts is clinically indistinguishable from two other diseases which do occur in the United States. These are vesicular stomatitis virus of horses, cattle, and occasionally humans, and vesicular exanthema of swine. The rapid diagnosis of FMD in cattle is important to allow its differentiation from the other two diseases. This is accomplished by a qualified laboratory with the use of differential inoculations of infectious material into appropriate hosts.

Man is an extremely rare incidental host of FMD. The illness is usually self-limited, febrile, and characterized by excessive salivation and vesicular lesions on the buccal or lingual epithelium, and possibly the skin of the hands, feet, and other parts of the body. Humans apparently carry the virus for at least 24 hours in their nasopharynx and can transmit it to other humans or susceptible animals via infectious droplets. For diagnostic purposes vesicular fluid can be used as antigen in a serotype specific complement fixation test. Antibody assessment can be accomplished by hemagglutination inhibition assays and tissue culture neutralization assays. This illness has no relationship to hand-foot-and-mouth disease caused by coxsackieviruses.

Bittle JL, Houghten RA, Alexander H, Shinnick TM, Sutcliffe JG, Lerner RA, Rowlands DJ, Brown F: Protection against foot-and-mouth disease by immunization with a chemically synthesized peptide predicted from the viral nucleotide sequence. Nature 298:30, 1982.

Kleid DG, Yansura D, Small B, Dowbenk T, Moore DM, Grubman MJ, McKercher PD, Morgan DO, Robertson BH, Bachrach HL: Cloned viral protein vaccine for foot and mouth disease: Responses in cattle and swine. Science 214:1125, 1981. *Description of recombinant DNA technology applied to development of specific polypeptide antigen.*

335. MUMPS (Epidemic Parotitis)

Catherine M. Wilfert

DEFINITION. Mumps or epidemic parotitis is an acute communicable viral infection. The characteristic clinical manifestations were described in the fifth century B.C. by Hippocrates.

ETIOLOGY. Mumps virus is placed in the Paramyxovirus genus of the paramyxoviridiae family. The diameter of the virus particle is approximately 150 nm, and it has enveloped helical nucleocapsids. It is an RNA virus with a nonsegmented single stranded genome that apparently codes for six polypeptides, three of which are nucleocapsid proteins and three of which are envelope proteins. One of the surface glycoproteins is the spike containing the hemagglutinin and neuraminidase (HN). The hemagglutinin causes the agglutination of erythrocytes of several species. The second surface glycoprotein spike (F) is responsible for the cell fusing and hemolyzing activities of the virus. The remarkable feature of the two paramyxovirus glycoproteins F and HN is that they must be cleaved once by a cellular protease for the virus particles to become infectious. If the cells lack the protease, only noninfectious virus particles are produced. The paramyxoviruses enter cells by fusing with cell membranes and liberating their nucleocapsids into the cytoplasm of the host cell. Mumps virus replication occurs in a variety of cell cultures and is infective for monkeys and chick embryos. It is relatively heat labile, with loss of infectivity resulting from heating to 55 to 60° C for 20 minutes.

EPIDEMIOLOGY. Mumps virus infection is endemic in all areas of the world and occurs throughout the year. Mumps is predominantly a disease of childhood, and prior to the advent of vaccine the majority of clinically evident infections were seen in children between the ages of five and ten years. Serologic evidence suggested that approximately 85 per cent of mumps infections occurred in those under 15 years of age.

Infection is transmitted via respiratory droplets, but mumps virus is less communicable than measles or varicella. Epidemiologic evidence suggests that the period of infectivity is from several days before onset of symptoms until the subsidence of the salivary gland swelling. Prolonged or recurrent excretion of virus is unknown. As many as 25 to 40 per cent of mumps infections are entirely asymptomatic. For these reasons attempts to control the spread of mumps infection by isolation of a patient are usually futile. The asymptomatic patients excrete virus, may transmit infection, and have a self-limited infection. The resulting immunity is comparable to that following symptomatic infection. There are no known animal reservoirs for mumps.

PATHOGENESIS AND PATHOLOGY. The portal of entry of the virus is thought to be the upper respiratory tract. The time interval after exposure to virus before the appearance of the clinical symptoms ranges from 14 to 21 days, with the usual incubation period being 16 to 18 days. After entering the host, the virus replicates and viremia occurs, which may result in secondary invasion of several organ systems. Tissues such as the salivary glands (predominantly the parotids), meninges, testes, pancreas, ovaries, thyroid, and heart may show evidence of infection. Virus is also excreted in the urine, and transient abnormalities in renal function have been found.

Pathologic examination of involved tissues has been infrequent because of the usually benign nature of the illness. Available studies of salivary glands indicate that there is no disruption of the general architecture of the gland. The involved salivary ducts may demonstrate changes in the epithelial lining cells, ranging from edema to complete desquamation. The ducts are dilated, and the lumen may be filled with cellular debris and polymorphonuclear cells. There may be a moderate amount of periductal edema around the involved ducts. Mononuclear inflammatory cells predominate in the interstitium. The pathology of other involved tissues is similar, and no specific hallmarks allow the diagnosis of mumps infection to be made solely on the basis of the observed pathology.

CLINICAL MANIFESTATIONS. Salivary gland involvement usually precedes other clinical symptoms, lasts for two to seven days, and may be unilateral or bilateral. Infection of the salivary glands is manifested by pain, and the characteristic swelling of the parotid gland provides the diagnosis of mumps. The infection less frequently involves the submandibular or sublingual salivary glands. Although other manifestations of mumps most often coincide with the parotid swelling, they may precede or occur in the absence of salivary gland involvement.

Meningitis. Central nervous system involvement with mumps virus occurs frequently. Viral meningitis has been said to occur in 65 per cent of hospitalized persons with parotid swelling when lumbar puncture is done. The cerebrospinal fluid (CSF) shows a predominantly lymphocytic pleocytosis in affected individuals, although only one half of them will display clinical signs of meningitis. The signs of meningeal involvement are most often manifest two to ten days after the onset of parotitis and last three to five days. Illness is characterized by fever, headache, nausea, vomiting, nuchal rigidity, is self limited, and clears with minimal (if any) sequelae.

Encephalitis. A more serious and much less frequent central nervous system manifestation is encephalitis or encephalomyelitis. The onset is usually later than the transient meningitis and occurs 10 to 14 days after the clinical salivary gland involvement. The patient appears severely ill, is deeply obtunded, and may have seizures or die. Although occurring much less often than the encephalitis associated with measles or varicella, mumps encephalitis is clinically and pathologically indistinguishable from them.

In 1967 suckling hamsters inoculated intracerebrally with the virus developed hydrocephalus. Virus replication occurred within ependymal cells of the ventricles and choroid plexus. Two to six weeks after infection, as inflammation resolved, aqueductal stenosis and hydrocephalus developed at a time when viral antigens and infectious virus were no longer demonstrable. The clinical application of such observations remains to be established, but recognition that sequelae of a virus infection can occur when the virus is no longer detectable is a useful concept.

Epididymo-orchitis. The complication of mumps infection best known by nonmedical persons is the involvement of the testes. This manifestation occurs predominantly in postpubertal males with 20 to 30 per cent manifesting orchitis during the course of mumps infection. Bilateral testicular involvement occurs in 2 to 6 per cent of patients with orchitis. Orchitis usually begins abruptly with fever, chills, headache, and lower abdominal pain. The systemic reaction ordinarily parallels the extent of gonadal involvement. The testis swells rapidly and becomes very painful and tender. The pain and swelling disappear as fever subsides, usually within five days of onset. Testicular tenderness may persist for a longer period. There is no theoretical or factual basis for the fear of sexual impotence following mumps orchitis. In the vast majority of instances the disease is unilateral. At least one half of those patients who have unilateral disease have completely normal testes after the acute infection; the remainder may have some degree of unilateral testicular atrophy, which does not result in sterility.

Pancreatitis. Pancreatitis may occur in association with mumps infection, with typical symptoms of abdominal pain, fever, and vomiting. Symptoms gradually subside over a period of three to seven days, and the patient usually recovers completely. Studies in vitro have demonstrated that mumps virus can replicate in human pancreatic beta cells and pancreatic epithelial cells. There is no firm epidemiologic or clinical evidence linking mumps virus infection to subsequent development of diabetes mellitus.

Other Clinical Manifestations. Especially in adults, infection of other tissues may rarely occur. Oophoritis has been described in adult females. The characteristic lower quadrant or back pain suggests the clinical diagnosis, but involvement of the ovaries may occur in the absence of recognizable symptoms. Sterility is not a known consequence of mumps oophoritis. Extremely rare manifestations of infection include polyarthritis, mastitis, myocarditis, thyroiditis, dacryoadenitis, and bartholinitis.

HOST RESPONSE. In the normal individual a single infection with mumps virus confers permanent immunity against clinically evident infection. It is probable that reinfection, defined as an antibody rise after exposure to the virus, may occur, but neither virus shedding nor clinical illness has been demonstrated with such reinfection. Although second attacks of parotitis have been observed, there are other possible causes, including coxsackievirus or lymphocytic choriomeningitis virus infections, starch ingestion, sarcoidosis, iodine sensitivity, and thiazide therapy. At present there is no documentation by culture or serology of two clinical attacks of mumps virus infection in the same individual.

Mumps virus infection induces the formation of specific humoral antibodies. Initially antibody of the IgM class and subsequently antibody of the IgG class are formed. Neutralization of infectivity, inhibition of hemagglutination, and the inhibition of neuraminidase activity are functions attributable to antibody to the HN protein. Specific neutralizing antibodies can be detected during the first week of symptoms and ordinarily persist for a lifetime. Hemagglutinating inhibiting and complement-fixing antibodies become detectable from one to three weeks after onset and usually reach peak titers within three to six weeks.

In vitro, mumps virus replicates in human lymphoblastoid cell lines with T cell characteristics and in peripheral blood mononuclear cells. Pokeweed mitogen enhances replication that occurs primarily in T lymphocytes, suggesting that these cells might be infected during natural infection.

DIAGNOSIS. The clinical diagnosis is strongly suggested when a known exposure to mumps is followed in two to three weeks by an illness with compatible clinical findings such as parotitis. In the absence of parotitis or if parotitis has occurred previously, specific laboratory studies are necessary to confirm the diagnosis.

Johnson and Goodpasture established that mumps was caused by a filterable virus. Successful propagation of virus in chick embryos preceded the now generally employed standard tissue culture techniques. Virus has been isolated from such varied sources as blood, CSF, urine, saliva, salivary gland tissue, and human milk. Viral diagnostic laboratories are available in many academic and large hospital settings for unusual or complicated situations.

Many diagnostic laboratories are better able to offer serologic diagnosis than viral isolation. Evaluation of sera for antibodies to mumps virus is readily accomplished. With acute serum one can determine if a person has ever had mumps infection. An increase in antibody titer on convalescent serum is indicative of recent mumps virus infection. Complement-fixation (CF) tests are most commonly employed by diagnostic laboratories for this purpose. Occasionally it is useful to obtain additional information about the temporal relationship of an illness to the antibody response. Two complement-fixing antigens, the nucleoprotein or soluble (S) antigen and the viral surface antigen (V), have been recognized for years. CF antibodies against the S antigen are detectable within two to three days of onset, peak at about ten days, and disappear in eight to nine months. CF antibodies against the V antigen, which includes the HN and F proteins, are not detectable until approximately the tenth day of infection and persist for years. Comparison of the transient nature of the S antibodies with the delayed appearance of the V antibodies may assist in defining recent infection.

PROGNOSIS. In general the prognosis of infection with mumps virus is excellent. Fatalities have been associated with encephalitis, myocarditis, and nephritis but are extremely rare. An occasional sequel to mumps virus infection is deafness, which may occur even in the absence of other evidence of central nervous system involvement. The loss of hearing may be preceded by tinnitus and a sense of fullness of the ear. Deafness is relatively uncommon but occurs suddenly during the period of parotid swelling. It is usually unilateral, but an estimated 20 per cent of those affected may have bilateral disease. Once deafness has occurred, the damage is irreversible.

TREATMENT. Mumps is a self-limited infection, and there is no specific therapy available.

PREVENTIVE MEASURES. *Passive Protection.* A common question concerns what to do when a susceptible person is exposed to mumps infection. Administration of hyperimmune globulin or pooled serum IgG after such exposure has not decreased the number of patients acquiring illness nor has it lessened the severity of illness. There is a single controlled study reporting that administration of hyperimmune globulin after the appearance of parotitis can decrease the incidence and severity of orchitis. Other studies under epidemic conditions failed to demonstrate any alteration in the attack rate or in the subsequent development of orchitis or meningoencephalitis. Therefore, the use of hyperimmune globulin is of dubious value.

Immunization. Live attenuated mumps virus vaccine is available for prophylactic use. The attenuated virus vaccine is produced in tissue cultures of chick embryo fibroblasts and is administered parenterally. Virus is not shed by the vaccinee, and immunization does not cause any side effects. The vaccine produces 95 to 100 per cent serologic conversion from antibody negative to positive in vaccinated susceptibles. Although the antibody levels are considerably lower, they parallel those produced by natural infection and have persisted for the 14 to 16 years that the vaccine has been available for study. The presence of detectable mumps antibody correlates with protection against clinical illness. Immunized children in contact with naturally occurring mumps have been protected against clinical illness. It is recommended for administration to children more than one year of age and to adolescents and adults for induction of immunity. Live attenuated mumps vaccine has been combined with measles and rubella virus vaccines.

There is only a single serologic strain of mumps virus; hence a single infection with either natural or attenuated virus confers immunity. Approximately 40 million doses of mumps vaccine have been distributed since 1968, and this increasing use of mumps vaccination has resulted in a marked decline in the incidence of reported disease in the United States.

The vaccine will not offer protection against mumps if someone has already been exposed to natural infection and is in the incubation period of illness. On the other hand, no harmful effects have been noted after administration of vaccine to an exposed susceptible. If the original exposure is not followed by mumps infection, the vaccine would then induce protection against subsequent exposures.

Fleischer B, Kneth HW: Mumps virus replication in human lymphoid cell lines and in peripheral blood lymphocytes: Preference for T cells. Infect Immun 35:25, 1982. *In vitro studies suggesting that activated T lymphocytes are the major site of replication of mumps virus in peripheral white blood cells.*

Gordon JE, Kilham L: Ten years in the epidemiology of mumps. Am J Med Sci 218:358, 1949. *A general, thorough description of mumps prior to the advent of vaccine.*

Jensik SC, Silver S: Polypeptides of mumps virus. J Virol 17:363, 1976. *Viral glycoprotein containing neuraminidase and hemagglutinating activity corresponds to V antigen of mumps virus.*

Kilham L, Margolis G: Induction of congenital hydrocephalus in hamsters with attenuated and natural strains of mumps virus. J Infect Dis 132:462, 1975. *Experimental induction of intrauterine infection with attenuated and wild type mumps virus resulting in central nervous system infection.*

Koplan JP, Preblud SR: A benefit-cost analysis of mumps vaccine. Am J Dis Child 36:362, 1982. *Statistical demonstration of the reduction in morbidity, mortality, and costs associated with a mumps vaccination program.*

Orvel C: Structural polypeptides of mumps virus. J Gen Virol 41:527, 1978. *The experimental definition of mumps virus polypeptides is described.*

Prince GA, Jenson AB, Billups LC, Notkins AL: Infection of human pancreatic beta cell cultures with mumps virus. Nature 271:158, 1978. *The demonstration by immunofluorescence of mumps antigen in human beta cells.*

Westmore GA, Pickard BH, Stern H: Isolation of mumps virus from the inner ear after sudden deafness. Br Med J 1:14, 1979. *A case report documenting mumps virus in the inner ear in association with subsequent deafness.*

Diseases Caused by Herpes-Type Viruses

336. HERPES SIMPLEX VIRUS INFECTIONS

R. Gordon Douglas, Jr.

Herpes simplex virus produces diseases ranging from inapparent infections and fever blisters to fatal encephalitis. The word herpes is derived from the Greek word "herpein," meaning "to creep," in reference to the skin manifestations.

ETIOLOGY. Herpes simplex virus (herpesvirus hominis, HSV) is a member of the Herpetoviridae family, which consists of a group of large enveloped DNA-containing viruses, belonging to two genera: herpesvirus and cytomegalovirus. Members of the herpesvirus genus that infect man include herpes simplex virus types 1 and 2, varicella-zoster virus, and Epstein-Barr virus. Only a single member of the cytomegalovirus genus, human cytomegalovirus, causes disease in man. Herpes simplex virus has an internal core containing double-stranded DNA, which is surrounded by an electron dense capsid, an icosahedron of 162 hollow capsomeres surrounded by a lipid-containing laminated envelope studded with glycoprotein projections. Because of the variable size of the envelope, the overall diameter of the virus ranges from 150 to 200 nm.

Viral replication occurs primarily within the cell nucleus, and viral envelopes are derived, at least in part, from the nuclear membrane. Complete replication is associated with lysis of the infected cell.

Herpes simplex viruses differ in host range from other members of the Herpetoviridae family. For example, herpes simplex types 1 and 2 grow well in a variety of human and animal cell lines, in embryonated hens' eggs, and in laboratory animals. Varicella-zoster virus is more restricted, not replicating in embryonated hens' eggs or in experimental animals, and only replicating in a few cell lines. Human cytomegalovirus is further restricted in host range to human fibroblast cell lines, and Epstein-Barr virus will not yield productive infection in any animal, egg, or conventional cell culture system, but viral replication occurs in continuous human lymphoblastoid cell cultures.

HSV types 1 and 2 share common antigens so that cross-reacting antibodies are induced following infection with either virus. They can be differentiated by monoclonal antibody and restriction enzyme techniques. As shown in Table 336–1, they differ also by route of transmission, by usual site of disease, by type of complications, by differences in physical properties, and by biologic characteristics.

EPIDEMIOLOGY. Herpes simplex viruses are distributed worldwide. There are no known seasonal patterns of infection. Since infection with virus is followed by development of antibody that persists for life, incidence of infection can be determined by antibody studies. The prevalence of antibody is inversely related to socioeconomic status. In lower socioeconomic groups, almost 100 per cent of adults have antibody to HSV, whereas in higher socioeconomic groups, this proportion falls to 30 to 50 per cent. The time of maximal acquisition of infection varies with the two types. The prevalence of antibody to HSV type 1 rises during childhood, whereas the major period of infection with HSV type 2 follows puberty.

Transmission apparently occurs by direct contact from person to person, and there is no animal reservoir. HSV type 1 is transmitted primarily by contact with oral secretions, and HSV type 2 by contact with genital secretions. A small percentage of adults may be excreting HSV type 1 or type 2 at any time, and this may occur in the absence of active lesions. Apparently, transmission can occur both from overtly infected persons and from asymptomatic excretors. The portal of entry is most commonly the oral cavity for HSV type 1 and the genital tract for HSV type 2. However, either type of HSV may be intro-

TABLE 336–1. COMPARISON OF PREDOMINANT CHARACTERISTICS OF HSV TYPE 1 AND TYPE 2

Characteristics	HSV-1	HSV-2
Transmission	Oral route	Genital route
Usual site of lesions	Skin of face and mouth, upper trunk	Genitals, skin of thighs, buttocks
Complications		
Keratitis	+	−
Encephalitis (adults)	+	−
Neonatal infection	−	+
Physical characteristics		
Temperature sensitivity (40° C)	−	+
Heparin sensitivity	+	−
Biologic characteristics		
Pock size on chorioallantoic membranes	Small	Large
Plaques in cell cultures	Small	Large
Syncytial formation in human embryonic kidney cells	Small	Large
Experimental infection in mice	Less neurotropic	More neurotropic

duced directly into the eye, a skin site, or the oral cavity or genital area. Transmission of HSV type 2 to skin sites other than those in the genital area can occur to infants born to mothers with genital infections. Also, anal and perianal infections of HSV type 2 are common among homosexual populations. Autoinoculation from either oral or genital sites to hands, thighs, or buttocks is not unusual. Extraoral acquisition of HSV is a hazard in certain occupations, and persons such as dentists, respiratory care unit personnel, and wrestlers are at higher risk. Laboratory-acquired infection and nosocomial outbreaks in hospital personnel or in neonatal nurseries have been reported.

Recurrent infections are one of the hallmarks of the Herpetoviridae family, and they occur frequently with both HSV type 1 and type 2. Recurrent infections of the lips or perioral area with HSV type 1 occur in 20 to 40 per cent of the population, and some data suggest that this rate may be increased among persons with the major histocompatibility type, HLA-A1. Recurrences may occur as frequently as once every several weeks or as infrequently as once or twice per year. They usually occur at the same site and occur despite the presence of circulating or local antibodies. They may be triggered by sunlight, fever, local trauma, menstruation, emotional stress, or other factors. Recurrent HSV type 2 usually occurs as lesions on the external genitalia, and with either type recurrences may appear at other sites, e.g., the eye.

Genital recurrences occur in up to 60 per cent of those with initial episodes. This frequency depends on sex, HSV type, and presence and titer of neutralizing antibody. Although most recurrences are due to reactivation of latent virus, exogenous reinfection accounts for some cases.

PATHOGENESIS AND PATHOLOGY. Following spread of virus from one person to another, the virus replicates locally in peribasal and intermediate epithelial cells, resulting in lysis of cells and initiation of a local inflammatory response. This results in a characteristic thin-walled vesicle on an inflammatory base. Histologic study reveals multinucleated cells with ballooning degeneration, marked edema, and the characteristic Cowdry type A intranuclear inclusions which are indistinguishable from those caused by varicella-zoster virus. Lymphatics and regional lymph nodes may become infected, and in neonates or compromised hosts viremia and visceral dissemination may occur. In most persons, however, infection is controlled at the local site by host defense mechanisms. Although neutralizing antibody may contribute, cellular immune mechanisms, such as the production of interferon and induction of T cell reactivity and development of both natural killer cell and antibody-dependent lymphocyte cytotoxicity, are thought to have the major function in controlling HSV infections. Adults and children with depressed cell-mediated immune mechanisms appear to be more susceptible to severe disseminated HSV infections than those with depressed humoral immunity. Disease resulting from primary infection with HSV type 2 is more severe in those who have not experienced HSV type 1 infection previously than in those who have and who consequently possess immunity to HSV type 1. This suggests that heterotypic protective immunity is present.

Following primary infection, HSV becomes latent in the ganglia of the nerves supplying the infected areas; for HSV type 1 the trigeminal ganglion and for HSV type 2 the lumbosacral ganglia are most frequently involved. The virus does not remain latent at the skin or mucous membrane site. While the virus is latent, infectious virus is no longer detectable in specimens from patients and lesions do not occur. Viral DNA, but not intact virus, can be demonstrated in the ganglia. Methylation of viral DNA may play an important role in the maintenance of HSV latency. Productive infection in epithelial cells with cell lysis follows reactivation. In contrast, neurons do not undergo cell lysis during recurrences. Infectious virus appears to spread peripherally along sensory nerves to skin sites where productive infection leads to cell lysis, an inflammatory response, and development of the characteristic lesions.

CLINICAL MANIFESTATIONS. ***Primary Infection.*** Most commonly, primary infection with HSV type 1 is asymptomatic, but *gingivostomatitis* will occur in a small number, usually children one to three years of age. It can also occur in older children and adults. Following an incubation period of 2 to 12 days, prodromal symptoms of low grade fever and cervical adenopathy may occur. As the oral lesions appear, the temperature rises to 38.3 to 38.9° C, and there is intense oral pain, increased salivation, and foul breath. The oral lesions begin on the buccal and gingival mucosa and tongue and appear as multiple vesicles on an erythematous base. The vesicles coalesce and rupture, and ulcerative lesions appear with an erythematous margin covered with a yellowish, necrotic membrane. Leukocytosis is common. The disease varies considerably in severity and duration; however, it is self-limited and usually disappears by 14 days. The lesions heal without scar formation. In children, dehydration may occur because of poor fluid intake, drooling, and fever.

In adolescents, symptomatic primary infection with HSV type 1 more commonly takes the form of *pharyngitis* rather than gingivostomatitis, although the two may occur in combination. Pharyngitis alone also may be seen in younger children. Pharyngitis caused by HSV is characterized by sore throat, cervical adenopathy, exudate, fever, and headache in about two thirds of cases. It also may be associated with leukocytosis, dysphagia, chills, and myalgia. Submaxillary adenopathy is usually absent. Autoinoculation of other skin sites by the hands, with development of characteristic lesions, can occur in persons with either gingivostomatitis or pharyngitis.

Herpes simplex virus infections of the eye are usually caused by HSV type 1. Primary infection is an acute *keratoconjunctivitis* with or without skin involvement. If the lids are uninvolved, acute conjunctival follicular disease with nonsuppurative preauricular adenopathy is present. The presence of vesicles on the lid margins, which may require a magnifying lens or a slit lamp to see, is helpful in diagnosis. Overt involvement of the lids with multiple vesicles and lid edema may occur. Corneal involvement most characteristically takes the form of a branching (dendritic) ulcer. However, corneal manifestations may be atypical, especially early in illness, and consist of diffuse punctate lesions or wandering serpiginous ulcers without clear-cut branching. The disease is self-limited and resolves entirely without scarring in many cases. However, corneal involvement may lead to permanent scarring.

Primary *genital infection* is most common in adolescents and in young adults and is usually caused by HSV type 2. In the male, characteristic vesicular lesions on an erythematous base usually appear on the glans penis or the penile shaft. In the female, lesions may involve the vulva, perineum, buttocks, cervix, and vagina and are frequently accompanied by vaginal discharge. Primary infection in both sexes may be associated with fever, malaise, anorexia, and tender bilateral inguinal adenopathy. Although vesicular lesions may persist for several days, they usually ulcerate rapidly and become covered with a grayish-white exudate. These lesions are often exquisitely tender, and in the female urethral involvement may result in dysuria or urinary retention. Lesions of primary genital herpes may persist for several weeks before healing is complete. Herpetic sacral radiculomyelitis may rarely accompany genital infection.

Although manifestations of primary infection are generally oral or genital with either type of HSV, primary infection may involve other skin sites. When it involves the fingers, it is referred to as herpetic whitlow.

Primary perianal and rectal HSV infections are being recognized more frequently, particularly in male homosexuals. Pain, tenesmus, discharge, difficulty in urinating, and sacral paresthesias, as well as fever, chills, malaise, and headache occur commonly. Examination reveals vesicles and ulcerations. The disease is usually self-limited except in the setting of acquired immune deficiency syndrome (AIDS), in which proctitis may be progressive.

Recurrent Infections. The most common manifestation of recurrent infection with HSV type 1 is herpes labialis (fever blister, herpes simplex). The lesions of recurrent labial herpes are localized to the mucocutaneous junction of the lips or adjacent skin. The lower lip is more frequently involved than the upper lip, and in an individual patient lesions tend to occur at the same site. It is notable that although primary infections commonly occur within the mouth, recurrent oral herpes infections rarely involve mucous membranes. They are frequently heralded by prodromal symptoms, such as tingling or itching, which last for a few hours. Vesicles then appear and are often associated with considerable pain. The lesions progress from vesicle to ulcer to crust within 48 hours. Pain is most severe in the first 24 hours, and healing is complete within eight to ten days.

Recurrent ocular infection may take the form of epithelial infections or trophic ulcers, stromal disease (interstitial or disciform keratitis), iridocyclitis, or combinations of these. It is usually unilateral. Often the characteristic branching (dendritic) ulcers that stain with fluorescein are observed, and these are virtually diagnostic of HSV infection. Stromal disease is manifested by various forms of infiltrates underlying the ulcers, which result in opacification. Superficial keratitis usually heals, but recurrent infection with deep stromal involvement and uveitis may persist. Gradual diminution in visual acuity takes place with recurrent attacks, and permanent visual loss may result.

Recurrent genital lesions in both sexes are associated with less severe systemic symptoms and less extensive local involvement than primary attacks. They are often preceded by a prodrome of tenderness, itching, burning, or tingling. However, in occasional individuals, severe recurrent attacks may occur over a period of one or more years.

Other Manifestations. ENCEPHALITIS. Herpes simplex encephalitis is a rare complication of herpes virus infection. It is thought to be the most common sporadic viral encephalitis in the United States and is fully described in Ch. 499. The virus is believed to spread by neural routes into the brain, most often during recurrent infection, but also during primary infection. Almost all isolates from brain tissue of adults with encephalitis are HSV type 1. Encephalitis may also occur as part of disseminated neonatal infection with HSV type 2.

ASEPTIC MENINGITIS. Infrequently, in association with HSV type 2 genital infection, the clinical syndrome of aseptic meningitis, including fever, headache, stiff neck, and cerebrospinal fluid (CSF) pleocytosis, may occur. HSV type 2 has been isolated from the spinal fluid and blood in such cases. Isolation from the CSF, however, is rare.

CONGENITAL INFECTIONS. Congenital infection is very rare and probably results from retrograde spread of HSV type 2 from maternal genital infection to the placenta. Such infection may be recognized at birth by central nervous system manifestations such as microcephaly, intracranial calcifications, microphthalmia, seizures, and chorioretinitis, which are common to a number of chronic intrauterine infections.

NEONATAL INFECTIONS. Neonatal infections result from passage of the infant through an infected maternal genital tract or retrograde ascending infection if the membranes have ruptured. The overall risk of neonatal infection is low in women with primary or recurrent HSV type 2 infection after 32 weeks' gestation, but is higher if lesions are present at delivery. Infants born to mothers with primary infection during pregnancy are at greater risk of developing severe infection than are those whose mothers have recurrent genital herpes. Disease may range from mild self-limited skin infection to fatal disseminated infection with or without encephalitis. Localized skin disease occurs in 10 per cent of cases and is self-limited. Isolated involvement of the central nervous system (encephalitis) and eye (chorioretinitis) may lead to death or serious sequelae.

Disseminated neonatal infection usually appears a few days after birth, and vesicles may or may not be present. Vesicles eventually occur in 50 per cent of the infants, but may be absent early in infection. Patients may show constitutional signs and symptoms, irritability, seizures, respiratory distress, jaundice, petechiae, ecchymosis, and shock-like syndrome. Neurologic signs occur in 50 per cent of cases and include seizures, cranial nerve palsies, lethargy, and coma. CSF pleocytosis with increased protein and normal glucose also is commonly observed. Many of these patients will develop destructive encephalitis, disseminated intravascular coagulation, or hepatic and adrenal necrosis. About 75 per cent of patients die, and few recover without sequelae.

COMPROMISED HOSTS. Patients compromised by immunodeficiency or immunosuppression, by malnutrition, or by disorders of skin integrity such as burns or eczema are at greater risk of developing severe herpes simplex viral infections. Frequently the cardiac transplant recipient, and less so the renal transplant recipient, excretes HSV in throat washings for the first few months following grafting. Although some such patients may not have overt disease, some develop lesions which can be severe and persist for many weeks to months. Lesions may spread down the respiratory or gastrointestinal tracts and result in tracheobronchitis, pneumonia, or esophagitis. Patients with hematologic and lymphoreticular neoplasms and children with congenital thymic disorders may develop severe, chronic, progressive mucocutaneous HSV infection or disseminated disease. Disseminated disease has also been observed in pregnancy and in geriatric populations. Herpetic esophagitis may be related to nasogastric intubation and results in dysphasia and substernal pain. Burn wound infections with HSV are becoming increasingly well recognized, as are HSV infections in patients with a variety of other skin disorders.

Severe herpes infections, particularly progressive perianal ulcers, colitis, esophagitis, and pneumonia, are prominent features of AIDS.

ERYTHEMA MULTIFORME. About 5 to 15 per cent of all cases of erythema multiforme are regularly preceded by an attack of herpes simplex. Either HSV type 1 or HSV type 2 infections may be involved, and the cutaneous manifestations may range from mild to severe (Stevens-Johnson syndrome) and may be recurrent.

OTHER SYNDROMES. Attempts have been made to relate HSV infections to a variety of neurologic syndromes such as multiple sclerosis, Bell's palsy, some atypical pain syndromes, ascending myelitis, trigeminal neuralgia, temporal lobe epilepsy, and others, but there is no definitive proof of a causal relationship for any of these associations. However, there is evidence of infectious virus (HSV type 2), viral antigens, and viral DNA sequences in cervical carcinoma cells, but the exact role of HSV type 2 in the production of cervical cancer is not clear.

DIAGNOSIS. In most minor infections, diagnosis is dependent on clinical recognition. Gingivostomatitis must be differentiated from aphthous stomatitis, Stevens-Johnson syndrome, Vincent's infection, infectious mononucleosis, herpangina, and streptococcal or diphtheritic pharyngitis. Pharyngitis caused by HSV infection must be differentiated from that caused by streptococci, EB virus, and other viruses. Cervical adenopathy, exudate, and fever are more common in HSV than in other kinds of viral pharyngitis. If dendritic ulcers are present in patients with keratitis, they are virtually diagnostic of HSV infection; however, these ulcers have also been observed in varicella-zoster virus infections, and corneal abrasions are occasionally mistaken for HSV infection. The presence of multiple vesicular genital lesions or ulcerative lesions associated with pain helps differentiate herpes simplex genital infections from other forms of venereal disease such as syphilis and chancroid. Infections of other skin sites, particularly if they have a dermatomal distribution, must be distinguished from varicella-zoster virus infection. Severe anorectal pain, difficulty in urination, and sacral paresthesias are more common in HSV perianal and rectal disease than in other forms of proctitis. Recurrent herpes labialis is easily recognized clinically. Recurrent intraoral lesions are usually not herpes simplex but rather aphthous stomatitis or some other malady, but intraoral lesions may occur with HSV infections in the immunocompromised or immunosuppressed patient. Recurrent eye and genital infections commonly can be recognized by their characteristic clinical manifestations. Congenital infections may be difficult to distinguish from similar syndromes caused by rubella virus, cytomegalovirus, or *Toxoplasma gondii.* Neonatal infection with HSV may be mistaken for neonatal sepsis, erythema toxicum, streptococcal infection, and enteroviral infection. In more severe infections viral isolation attempts are helpful. Severe skin infection in older patients and disseminated infection in immunocompromised patients may also be diagnosed by recovery of virus. Burn wound infections, unless there are typical vesicular areas, usually must be diagnosed by viral isolation or biopsy for intranuclear inclusions.

Definitive diagnosis can be made by isolation of HSV from lesions. However, 1 to 15 per cent of asymptomatic normals will shed HSV in oral secretions and presumably a similar number in genital secretions. Therefore, isolation of virus from these sites may not be related to active disease. HSV types 1 and 2 replicate in a variety of cell lines, and cytopathic effects appear rapidly, usually within 24 to 48 hours. Specimens should be collected early by aspiration of vesicles or swabbing the open lesions, and promptly inoculated into cell cultures. If transportation to the laboratory must be delayed, specimens can be stored at 4° C for a few hours, or, if storage is longer than 24 hours, they should be stored at −70° C.

Histologic diagnosis is based on the presence of giant cells, intranuclear inclusions, or both in scrapings of lesions or biopsies of tissue. Scrapings may be smeared, fixed with ethanol or methanol, and stained with Giemsa, Wright, or Papanicolaou (preferred) stain. Usually only giant cells are seen on scrapings and smears, and intranuclear inclusions in HSV infection cannot be distinguished from those of varicella-zoster virus infection.

Development of serum antibodies when none existed previously is often helpful in recognizing primary infection but is of little value in recurrent infections. Measurement of IgM antibodies to HSV may be helpful in the diagnosis of neonatal infection. Such antibodies usually appear within the first four weeks of life in infected infants and persist for many months. Unfortunately, measurement of IgM antibodies in older persons has not proved useful in separating primary from recurrent infection.

TREATMENT. Specific antiviral chemotherapy is now available for some HSV infections. Vidarabine (adenine arabinoside, ara-A), has been shown to be effective and is licensed in the United States. Ophthalmic ointment (3 per cent) is administered as one half inch of ointment into the lower conjunctival sac five times a day at three-hour intervals. Intravenous vidarabine is effective in patients with HSV encephalitis. It is administered to patients with proven or suspected HSV encephalitis in a dose of 15 mg per kilogram per day for ten days. This drug is somewhat insoluble (maximum 0.75 mg per milliliter with warming) and thus requires substantial amounts of fluid, and patients may experience difficulties with fluid overload. Intravenous vidarabine has also been shown to be effective in neonatal disseminated herpes simplex infections. It is not effective topically against herpes labialis or other skin or genital infections.

Idoxuridine (IDU or 2′-deoxy-5-iodouridine) and trifluorothymidine have also been shown to be effective in the treatment of HSV keratitis, and are licensed for this purpose in the United States.

Acyclovir is effective for treatment of primary herpes genitalis, progressive mucocutaneous disease in immunosuppressed patients, and herpes keratitis. It is available as a topical 5 per cent ointment and as an intravenous form. An oral form is under study. Topical therapy is effective in primary but not in recurrent genital infections. Intravenous and oral acyclovir

are more effective in recurrent and may be effective in primary genital infections. Topical acyclovir therapy is not recommended for recurrent herpes labialis.

As one might expect, immune serum globulin is not effective for treatment, since recurrent infections develop in the presence of high titers of circulating antibodies.

PROPHYLAXIS. Medical and dental personnel should be strongly encouraged to avoid direct contact with potential infectious lesions by wearing gloves. Patients with extensive herpetic lesions should be isolated. Either temporary abstinence or at least the use of condoms has been recommended to prevent genital spread when one sexual partner has active lesions. Continued use of condoms may be useful if there is a history of recurrent genital infections.

Prevention of neonatal disease in offspring of mothers with genital infection presents special problems in which considerable controversy exists. If there is clinically apparent cervical infection or genital virus excretion is detected at parturition before membranes rupture, a cesarean section is recommended. If rupture of the membranes has occurred, it is uncertain whether cesarean section will be effective in preventing infection, although rapid delivery by either route is clearly indicated to lessen exposure to the infant. If no lesions are obvious at delivery, only rarely is virus recoverable and vaginal delivery appears safe.

Corey L, Adams HG, Brown ZA, Holmes KK: Genital herpes simplex virus infections: Clinical manifestations, course and complications. Ann Intern Med 98:958, 1983. *Recent, well referenced review of genital HSV.*

Goodell SE, Quinn TC, Mkrtichian E, Schuffler MD, Holmes KK, Corey L: Herpes simplex virus proctitis in homosexual men. Clinical, sigmoidoscopic and histopathological features. N Engl J Med 308:868, 1983.

Hirsch MS, Schooley RT: Treatment of herpes virus infections. N Engl J Med 309:963, 1983. *An up-to-date, well referenced review of acyclovir, vidarabine, and other therapeutic agents in HSV infections.*

Whitley RH, Soong SJ, Hirsch MS, Karchmer AW, Dolin R, Galasso G, Dunnick JK, Alford CA, the NIAID Collaborative Antiviral Study Group: Herpes simplex encephalitis. Vidarabine therapy and diagnostic problems. N Engl J Med 304:313, 1981. *Follow-up of original controlled study with emphasis on diagnosis and prognosis.*

Wong KK, Hirsch MS: Herpes virus infections in patients with neoplastic disease. Ann Intern Med 76:464, 1984. *Well referenced summary of diagnosis and therapy with vidarabine, acyclovir, and alpha interferon.*

337. CYTOMEGALOVIRUS INFECTION

David J. Lang

DEFINITION. Infections caused by cytomegalovirus (CMV) may be asymptomatic or may cause disseminated and even fatal multisystem disease, depending upon the mode and timing of virus acquisition and the immune competence of the host. CMV infections occur commonly, although with variable severity, in the fetus and in immunocompromised individuals.

ETIOLOGY. CMV is a species-specific member of the herpesvirus group. Like other herpesviruses, CMV has the capacity to replicate persistently in the face of normal host immunity and to establish latent infections subject to reactivation. CMV cytopathology is focal in vitro, and replication of the virus is largely limited to cell cultures of species-specific fibroblasts. In vivo, however, CMV replicates in epithelial as well as fibroblastic elements. Subtypes of CMV can be distinguished, although the variants are without apparent clinical significance.

EPIDEMIOLOGY. CMV is worldwide in distribution, and the incidence of infection lacks consistent seasonality. Persistence, latency, and reactivation of CMV have made it difficult to interpret the etiologic significance of the recovery of the virus.

The age of acquisition of CMV is variable. In less developed parts of the world, CMV infection is acquired universally in infancy, probably at or shortly after parturition. Where interpersonal contact is reduced and sanitation is more universal, the acquisition of CMV infection is delayed and occurs gradually through infancy, childhood, and even adulthood. No specific genetic factors have as yet been identified that contribute to CMV colonization, infection, or persistence. Transmission of CMV is associated with close interpersonal (including sexual) contact or with direct introduction of cells or body fluids. CMV virus has been recovered from virtually all organs and tissues and can be found in urine, saliva, blood, semen, milk, secretions of the uterine cervix, and stool. This very prevalent virus is opportunistic; it reactivates in, is transmitted to, and spreads from hosts whose defenses are compromised. Since these patients are often found in hospital settings, this virus can provide a troublesome nosocomial problem, although spread occurs infrequently.

Prenatal CMV infection is the most common known congenital infection of humans. It occurs in about 1 per cent of infants born in the United States (0.5 to 8 per cent depending upon the population studied). Most of these infections reflect prenatal transmission of CMV reactivated during pregnancy in otherwise healthy immune women. As many as 30 per cent of pregnant women may shed CMV at some time and from some site during pregnancy. Active CMV shedding and perinatal transmission occur more frequently in young women.

PATHOGENESIS AND PATHOLOGY. CMV replicates slowly in vitro. Infected cells swell and develop characteristic intranuclear and paranuclear inclusions. In vitro CMV infections are accompanied by some changes associated with morphologic transformation. It has been possible to transform cells permanently by infecting with irradiated virus and in this way interfering selectively with the full cycle of virus replication and cytopathology. These CMV-transformed cells have malignant potential in certain animals. Whether CMV plays a role in the pathogenesis of malignancy in humans is unresolved.

CMV can and frequently does reactivate in immune hosts. When immune function is immature or compromised, reactivated virus can spread, causing significant injury and functional impairment. The pathogenesis of transplacental spread in the presence of intact maternal immunity remains unclear.

That CMV is carried in circulating cells of healthy individuals appears certain on the basis of epidemiologic observations. It is estimated that approximately 5 per cent of donor units of blood can transmit CMV. Nevertheless, it has been difficult to recover this virus from the circulating cells of healthy individuals.

Latent CMV may also be transmitted with transplanted organs. The superimposition of iatrogenic immunosuppression then further encourages CMV spread. Transmission of CMV with blood products has provided a particularly difficult problem for blood banks. The use of CMV antibody-negative units has been recommended for high-risk groups such as selected newborns or allograft recipients.

CLINICAL MANIFESTATIONS. ***Postnatal CMV Infection in Normal Hosts.*** In healthy individuals CMV infection is usually asymptomatic or unrecognized. Occasionally primary CMV infection is accompanied by a self-limited mononucleosis-like syndrome characterized by fever, splenomegaly, mild hepatocellular dysfunction, lymphoid hyperplasia including the presence of atypical lymphocytes, occasional thrombocytopenia, hemolysis, and inconsistent skin rash. Pharyngitis is not prominent. The fever may range from 39° to over 40° C (103 to 105° F) and in some instances is accompanied by night sweats and chills. Between febrile episodes the patient, although tired, does not feel very ill.

Some cases of mild to moderate hepatitis have been associated with CMV infection, and infrequently a normal host will experience an interstitial pneumonitis caused by this virus. There have been reports associating prior CMV infection with the Guillian-Barré syndrome. CMV infections have also been associated with isolated thrombocytopenia, hemolytic anemia, and ulcerative gastrointestinal disease.

Postnatal CMV Infection in Abnormal Hosts. Individuals undergoing open-heart surgery requiring perfusion and others receiving multiple units of blood may experience a mononucleosis-like illness about three to six weeks later. The illness can be mistaken for bacterial sepsis or endocarditis, a particularly important distinction in recipients of cardiac prostheses.

CMV infections have been a major problem for allograft recipients. Latent virus may be reactivated by immune suppression. Alternatively, the response to the allograft or, in the case of marrow transplantation, a graft versus host reaction, may stimulate virus reactivation. Immune suppression limits the ability of the host to restrict virus spread. Infection with this virus can be associated with significant and even fatal interstitial pneumonitis, hepatitis, encephalitis, and diffuse cytomegalic inclusion disease.

CMV infections have been found prominently in the acquired immune deficiency syndrome (AIDS). There has been speculation concerning the etiologic relevance of CMV to AIDS and to Kaposi's sarcoma. However, CMV (and other) infections associated with AIDS are more likely to be opportunistic, since immunologic impairment is prominent in this condition. Nevertheless, since CMV infections are often associated with some depression of the helper-suppressor T cell ratio, the differentiation between cause and effect, opportunism and pathogenesis, remains unclear.

Prenatal and Perinatal CMV Infection. Prenatal CMV infections were first appreciated through retrospective pathologic studies. Since the recognition of the infection depended on post-mortem examinations, it was initially concluded that prenatal CMV infection was rare and always fatal. The severe disseminated infection was termed *cytomegalic inclusion disease.* Subsequently, cytologic techniques identified CMV infection in living infants by the presence of large nuclear-inclusion–bearing cells in urinary sediment. The isolation of virus in vitro proved to be an even more sensitive technique. It became apparent that infants congenitally infected with CMV could survive and that manifestations of these infections resembled those associated with other prenatal infections. The CMV-infected infants were often small for gestational age and microcephalic. In some cases they exhibited intracerebral calcifications, hepatosplenomegaly, chorioretinitis, thrombocytopenia with purpura, macular rash, hemolytic anemia, and a variety of structural and functional organ impairments.

Prospective studies determined that congenital infections with CMV were not unusual or rare. Overall, about 1 per cent of babies were found to be prenatally infected with CMV. Prenatal CMV infection is particularly prevalent among infants of primiparous, young, unmarried, and promiscuous women. Most CMV-infected infants appear normal at birth, but as many as 10 to 20 per cent of such apparently symptomless congenital CMV infections are associated with learning disabilities, hearing impairment, or evidence of cognitive dysfunction.

Women who are immune prior to conception may give birth to CMV-infected infants. The birth to one woman of more than one CMV-infected infant with identical viral strains has been documented. It seems certain that at least some prenatal CMV infections are acquired from previously latent maternal virus reactivated during gestation.

Perinatal acquisition of CMV infection (from infected cervix, breast milk, or saliva) is usually asymptomatic. However, an infant born to a CMV-seronegative woman may develop significant postnatal pneumonia or hepatitis if infected with CMV via transfusions.

DIAGNOSIS. The laboratory isolation of CMV is accomplished in tissue culture and requires the prompt transportation of refrigerated specimens to a prepared virus laboratory. Up to five weeks can be required for recovery and identification of virus. Occasional prolonged shedding of virus and the intermittent reactivation of latent CMV may confuse the interpretation of virus recovery. The isolation of CMV at certain times (from urine taken during the first days of life) or from unusual sites (blood, spinal fluid, or tissues specifically involved in the disease process) makes the etiologic association of virus and clinical condition more likely. Demonstration of simultaneous seroconversion or significant (four-fold or greater) serologic change further strengthens the association. CMV serology may be assessed by complement-fixation, immunofluorescence, enzyme-linked immunosorbent assay (ELISA) procedures, and indirect hemagglutination. The use of CMV-specific IgM serology to identify recent infections may be rendered less useful by the presence of rheumatoid factor (false positives) and by the tendency of CMV IgM to persist in some instances and to reappear when latent virus is reactivated.

DIFFERENTIAL DIAGNOSIS. Congenital infections caused by toxoplasmosis, rubella, syphilis, and herpes simplex virus may be difficult to distinguish from those caused by CMV. All may be associated with intrauterine growth retardation, hepatic and splenic enlargement, purpura, thrombocytopenia, and hemolysis. Congenital toxoplasmosis can be associated as well with chorioretinitis and intracerebral calcifications.

Congenital rubella is associated with glaucoma, microphthalmia, cataracts, and cardiac malformations more frequently than is congenital CMV infection. The retinitis of congenital rubella, unlike that of CMV, is often marked by punctate retinal pigmentation.

Herpes simplex virus can be transmitted transplacentally, although usually neonatal herpes infection reflects the perinatal acquisition of the virus. Herpes infections are often associated with vesicular skin lesions, although systemic visceral and central nervous system infection may occur without rash.

In all of these instances the distinctions are made ultimately by laboratory studies. Specific IgM determinations are available for CMV, toxoplasmosis, rubella, and herpes simplex. The presence of a positive test for specific IgM to only one of these agents is usually diagnostic. The recovery of the specific agent in the case of CMV, rubella, or herpes simplex is also a rigorous means of identification. Differentiation of all of these conditions is important, since specific treatment is available for herpes simplex and for toxoplasmosis. The distinction of congenital syphilis or of bacterial sepsis, other potentially confusing entities in the neonate, is also important to facilitate specific therapy.

Postnatally acquired CMV infections may be difficult to distinguish from those caused by Epstein-Barr virus (EBV). EBV mononucleosis is often associated with a positive heterophil-agglutination reaction. CMV mononucleosis is always heterophil-negative. Hepatitis associated with CMV infection is generally milder than that associated with hepatitis A, B, or non-A, non-B viruses. The ultimate distinction between these conditions is dependent upon the results of virus-specific tests.

CMV interstitial pneumonitis cannot be identified on clinical grounds alone but requires the use of virologic studies applied to clinical samples, especially those from lung biopsies and needle aspirations.

PROGNOSIS. The outlook for normal development is poor in infants who are infected prenatally with CMV. Even among those with the apparently symptomless congenital CMV infections, as many as 20 per cent by school age may manifest significant sensorineural dysfunction.

Among individuals with acquired CMV infections, the prognosis is dependent upon the immune status of the host. In otherwise healthy persons, acquired CMV infections are self-limited and generally not associated with late complications. Among immunocompromised individuals, including transplant recipients, the outlook may vary from those who recover, maintain (allograft) function, and are without sequelae, to those who die with progressive interstitial pneumonitis. Disseminated CMV may predispose to significant life-threatening bacterial infections.

TREATMENT. A variety of nucleoside analogs, other antiviral drugs, transfer factor, antiserum, and steroids have been administered in an effort to treat CMV infections. None of these has been conclusively successful. Some drugs such as cytosine and adenine arabinoside have been associated with transient depression of virus titers. None has altered the clinical condition, nor has any of these agents curtailed the ultimate course of the virus infection. The intensive use of interferon in renal transplant recipients has reduced the shedding of virus and apparently improved the associated clinical conditions. Withdrawal of immunosuppression has been used as a means to control CMV infections in allograft recipients.

PREVENTION. "Attenuated" CMV vaccine strains have been produced in England and the United States. These candidate vaccine strains have been administered to volunteers, including health care workers, and to some individuals awaiting an allograft. The vaccines proved to be immunogenic and have not thus far been associated with detectable virus shedding or reactivation. Inoculated individuals who later received transplants and were immunosuppressed nevertheless did experience CMV reinfection and associated virus shedding.

Because of the questions associated with the production and use of attenuated CMV strains coupled with the evidence that immunity does ameliorate if not prevent prenatal and postnatal CMV infections, attention is also being directed to the development of subunit and peptide immunogens.

Adler SP: Transfusion-associated cytomegalovirus infections. Rev Infect Dis 5:977, 1983. *Comprehensive up-to-date review of transfusion-associated CMV infections with discussion of mechanisms as well as straightforward clinical issues.*

Betts RF: Cytomegalovirus infection in transplant patients. Prog Med Virol 23:44, 1982. *A very good discussion of the reciprocal impact of CMV upon all varieties of allograft. Contains an excellent summary of epidemiologic factors.*

Ho M: Cytomegalovirus, Biology and Infection. New York, Plenum Publishing Corp., 1982. *Treatise covering all aspects of CMV infection in humans. Small but thorough section pertinent to murine CMV. Very comprehensive bibliography.*

Mintz L, Drew WL, Miner RC, Braff EH: Cytomegalovirus infections in homosexual men. Ann Intern Med 99:326, 1983. *Prospective study covering aspects of sexual transmission of CMV in a homosexual population, with implications for AIDS.*

Zaia JA, Lang DJ: Cytomegalovirus infection of the fetus and neonate. Neurol Clin 2:387, 1984. *Recent review covering all aspects of pre- and perinatal CMV infection with discussion of some current hypotheses as well as comprehensive data review.*

338. INFECTIOUS MONONUCLEOSIS

*John A. Zaia**

DEFINITION. Infectious mononucleosis is an acute infection caused by Epstein-Barr virus (EBV). Symptomatic disease includes fever, sore throat, lymphadenopathy, and lymphocytosis with splenomegaly.

ETIOLOGY. EBV is a member of the herpesvirus group and was first isolated in tissue culture cell lines derived from Burkitt's lymphoma. Observation of EBV antibody seroconversion in a laboratory technician with infectious mononucleosis led to the etiologic connection of EBV with infectious mononucleosis. EBV has been isolated from cultures of peripheral blood, nasopharynx, and lymph nodes of persons with acute infectious mononucleosis.

Attempts to transmit infectious mononucleosis experimentally to volunteers by means of blood, throat washings, or stool suspensions from patients in the acute phase of infectious mononucleosis have been inconclusive or negative, probably because of the inclusion of seropositive nonsusceptible persons in the volunteer group. Infectious mononucleosis can be transmitted by blood transfusion. Seropositive college students with antibody to the viral capsid antigen (VCA) do not develop acute infectious mononucleosis. The disease is seen only in seronegative individuals.

INCIDENCE AND PREVALENCE. As in the other human herpesvirus infections, the incidence and prevalence of EBV infection are functions of socioeconomic factors that determine crowding and hygienic conditions. Infection occurs early in life in the less developed countries and is usually inapparent. In the more developed nations, EBV infection occurs later in life, usually in older children and adolescents. The ratio of asymptomatic to symptomatic disease in the middle class college population is approximately 2:1.

---

*With the assistance of David J. Lang.

EPIDEMIOLOGY. The source of EBV infection is contaminated body fluid(s), usually oropharyngeal secretions. EBV is readily demonstrated in the saliva of patients with infectious mononucleosis and also occurs late after infection in persons who have periodic reactivation of this virus. Antibody-positive individuals have been shown to be permanent carriers and to become intermittent excretors of EBV. Contact with infected saliva during intimate oral contact or from contaminated eating and drinking utensils provides the usual means of infection. Infections are transmitted by extracellular virus and occasionally by infected cells, as during blood transfusions. The incubation period is estimated to be between five and seven weeks when the disease occurs in young adults.

PATHOLOGY AND PATHOGENESIS. The pathology of EBV infection is confined to the lymphoid tissues. There is extensive hyperplasia of the lymph nodes, with partial obliteration and distention of lymphoid sinuses by macrophages, atypical lymphocytes, and plasma cells. Lymphoid follicular structure is maintained with occasional areas of focal necrosis and perivascular infiltration by atypical mononuclear cells. In the liver, patchy mononuclear cell infiltrates occur in the portal areas and in the lobular sinusoids. The bone marrow may contain granulomas.

The lymphoproliferative manifestations are related to two pathogenetic aspects of EBV infection: an initial virus infection with virus-induced proliferation of B lymphocytes and a secondary reaction of T lymphocytes to control the infection. The resultant immunopathologic events lead to the clinical syndrome of infectious mononucleosis. The peripheral blood contains large atypical lymphocytes (Downey cells), which consist of both transformed B cells and reactive T cells. Although these cells can be seen in other viral infections, they are most pronounced in infectious mononucleosis.

CLINICAL MANIFESTATIONS. Following a prodromal period lasting four to five days in which malaise, fatigue, and headache can occur, the principal clinical features of fever, sore throat, and cervical lymphadenopathy appear. Signs and symptoms can be quite variable and atypical, especially in children and the elderly. In the usual case of mononucleosis, fever persists for seven to ten days and may be greater than 39.5° C. Concomitantly, sore throat develops during the first week of disease, with inflammation and edema of the pharynx and exudative tonsillitis. A palatal enanthem can occur, consisting of petechiae on the palate, which cannot be distinguished from streptococcal pharyngitis. Lymph node enlargement is especially prominent in the anterior and posterior cervical nodes, but generalized adenopathy is often present. The lymph nodes are readily palpable and can be exquisitely tender. The lymphadenopathy persists for several weeks.

Splenomegaly occurs in approximately 50 per cent of patients and is greatest during the second and third weeks of illness. A rare complication of infectious mononucleosis is splenic rupture, which can be life-threatening. Although hepatosplenomegaly occurs in only 10 per cent of patients, liver function test results are frequently abnormal and clinical jaundice may develop during the first two weeks of illness. Elevated serum enzyme levels can persist for several weeks. During the first week as many as 10 per cent of patients develop a skin rash consisting of transient erythematous maculopapular eruptions on the trunk and proximal extremities. Although usually rubelliform in nature, the rash occasionally can be scarlatiniform, urticarial, or even hemorrhagic. Use of ampicillin and other antibiotics is frequently associated with skin rash. Bilateral supraorbital edema has been described as an early clinical finding.

Complications involving the central nervous system include Guillain-Barré syndrome, Bell's palsy, transverse myelitis, and meningoencephalitis. In addition, pneumonitis, myocarditis, pericarditis, nephritis, acquired hemolytic anemia, thrombocytopenic purpura, agranulocytosis, and aplastic anemia have been described during EBV infection.

The X-linked lymphoproliferative syndrome is a genetically inherited disease in which EBV infection can result in a lethal outcome. Susceptible individuals have been described with overwhelming EBV infection and fatal hepatitis, lymphoma, or agammaglobulinemia following EBV infection.

DIAGNOSIS. Infectious mononucleosis is diagnosed on the basis of clinical manifestations, characteristic blood abnormalities, and heterophile and EBV antibody titers. The white blood cell count may be normal or slightly low during the first week of infectious mononucleosis, but during the second and third weeks the white blood cell count is elevated to between 10,000 and 20,000 per square millimeter. The white blood cell differential count generally shows more than 50 per cent mononuclear cells, of which at least 10 per cent are atypical, with considerable pleomorphism. The atypical lymphocytosis may persist for several months. Occasionally, the total white blood cell count in the second and third weeks of illness is markedly elevated and can be as high as 50,000 per square millimeter. The Downey cells appear as large variably shaped cells with round, indented, or lobulated nuclei and with basophilic vacuolated cytoplasm.

Heterophile antibodies, mostly of the IgM class, develop transiently during the course of infectious mononucleosis and can be directed against sheep, horse, and bovine erythrocytes and also against such factors as I/i blood groups, immunoglobulin, nuclear factors, and Proteus OX19. The most frequent and useful heterophile antibodies in infectious mononucleosis are the agglutinins for sheep or horse erythrocytes and the hemolysins of bovine red blood cells. The development of antibody to sheep erythrocyte agglutinins in infectious mononucleosis was first described in 1932 by Paul and Bunnell. These antibodies were subsequently shown to be adsorbed by guinea pig kidney cell suspensions but not by bovine erythrocytes. The antibodies are referred to as the *heterophile agglutinins of Paul-Bunnell-Davidson (PBD).* The heterophile agglutinins are, with very rare exceptions, specific for infectious mononucleosis and form the basis for the currently available slide agglutination tests. These commercially available test kits give quick results and are generally specific for infectious mononucleosis, although false negative results can be observed when heterophile antibody titers are low, and false positive results occasionally can be seen. The PBD heterophile agglutinins are usually detectable during the first week of illness, but approximately 10 per cent of adolescent patients and a larger percentage of children fail to develop heterophile antibodies.

The EBV-specific serologic tests consist of the viral capsid antigen (VCA), the viral membrane antigen, the viral early antigens (EA), and the viral nuclear antigens (EBNA). Diagnostically significant increments in titer of antibody to VCA from acute to convalescent phases are observed in no more than 10 to 20 per cent of infectious mononucleosis patients. This is because VCA antibody is usually produced prior to clinical symptoms that are mediated by early immunopathologic events. IgM antibody to VCA is frequently present and is of proven value in the serodiagnosis of primary EBV infection. Antibody to EA is observed in 70 to 85 per cent of patients in the acute phase of infectious mononucleosis. This test is interpreted in two ways: diffuse staining of the nucleus and cytoplasm is seen during the acute phase of infectious mononucleosis, and a restricted staining of the cytoplasm is seen in prolonged cases of EBV infection. Antibody to EBNA appears only weeks or months after onset of illness and can be utilized to document EBV infection when early sera are not available. The EBV-specific antibody assays are not essential for the diagnosis of infectious mononucleosis when the heterophile antibody test result is positive. These tests should be reserved for heterophile-antibody–negative cases of mononucleosis-like illnesses and for evaluation of syndromes suggestive of EBV complications.

DIFFERENTIAL DIAGNOSIS. Infectious mononucleosis resembles several disorders associated with the nonspecific findings of fever, exudative tonsillitis, lymphadenopathy, and splenomegaly. Adenoviral pharyngitis and tonsillitis, streptococcal pharyngotonsillitis, diphtheria, and Vincent's angina can have oropharyngeal pathology similar to that associated with EBV infection. Mononucleosis syndromes are associated with cytomegalovirus infection, toxoplasmosis, hepatitis A, and hepatitis B and cannot be readily distinguished from infectious mononucleosis. Appropriate serologic tests should be used to exclude these entities. The heterophile agglutination tests specific for infectious mononucleosis are never positive in these conditions.

Blood dyscrasia, especially acute lymphocytic leukemia, can be similar to changes associated with infectious mononucleosis. Bone marrow examination should be performed in those individuals having a lymphoproliferative disease that lacks the diagnostic criteria of infectious mononucleosis.

TREATMENT. Infectious mononucleosis can be treated with corticosteroids when life-threatening complications are present. A ten-day course of prednisone is used starting with 60 mg per square meter on the first day and gradually decreasing this dosage by 5 mg per square meter per day. This is indicated for such complications as airway obstruction, neurologic complications, thrombocytopenia purpura, hemolytic anemia, and myocarditis.

The possible use of corticosteroid therapy for the treatment of uncomplicated infectious mononucleosis remains controversial. A well controlled study of steroid therapy demonstrated a decrease in the number of days of fever in the steroid-treated group. There is no clear evidence that this treatment increases the risk of other complications or the long-term potential risks of EBV infection such as lymphoproliferative disease and malignancy. At present, because of the known increased risks of lymphoproliferative neoplasm occurring in immunosuppressed allograft recipients with EBV infection, it would appear prudent to use steroid therapy only for severe complications of EBV infection.

PROGNOSIS. Infectious mononucleosis is generally a self-limited disease in which the acute symptoms subside within four to six weeks. Marked fatigue usually accompanies the convalescent period, and the patient should anticipate certain limitations to normal activity. Occasionally, these symptoms of fatigue persist for several months with or without abnormal liver function tests or other laboratory abnormalities. There is no explanation for the prolonged period of convalescence, which can last for many months in certain persons.

Andiman WA: The Epstein-Barr virus and EB virus infections in childhood. J Pediatr 95:171, 1979. *A review of EBV infection in the pediatric patient.*

Epstein MA, Achong BG: The Epstein-Barr Virus. New York, Springer-Verlag, 1979. *A complete review of laboratory and clinical aspects of EBV infection.*

Fleisher GR, Collins M, Fager S: Limitations of available tests for diagnosis of infectious mononucleosis. J Clin Microbiol 17:619, 1983. *Description of specificity and sensitivity of diagnostic tests for EBV.*

Hoagland RJ: The transmission of infectious mononucleosis. Am J Med Sci 229:262, 1955. *A classic description of EBV epidemiology.*

Horowitz CA, Henle W, Henle G, Schapiro R, Borken S, Bundtzen R: Infectious mononucleosis in patients aged 40 to 72 years: Report of 27 cases, including 3 without heterophil-antibody responses. Medicine 62:256, 1983. *A description of clinical EBV infection in older persons.*

Purtilo DT, Sakamoto K, Saemundsen AK, Sullivan JL, Synnerholm AC, Anvret M, Pritchard J, Sloper C, Sieff C, Pincott J, Pachman L, Rich K, Cruzi F, Cornet JA, Collins R, Barnes N, Knight J, Sandstedt B, Klein G: Documentation of Epstein-Barr virus infection in immunodeficient patients with life-threatening lymphoproliferative diseases by clinical, virological, and immunopathological studies. Cancer Res 41:4226, 1981. *Review of X-linked lymphoproliferative syndrome.*

339. VARICELLA AND HERPES ZOSTER

Sidney Kibrick

DEFINITION. Varicella (chickenpox) is an acute infectious disease, characterized by a generalized vesicular eruption which appears in crops over several days. It is most common in childhood.

Herpes zoster (shingles) is an acute infectious disease involving sensory ganglia and their cutaneous areas of innervation. It is characterized by pain along the distribution of the affected nerve and crops of clustered vesicles over the corresponding dermatome. It is usually unilateral and involves a single or adjacent dermatomes. The disease represents reactivation of a latent varicella virus in individuals with partial immunity to this agent.

ETIOLOGY. The agent responsible for these disorders is the varicella-zoster virus (V-Z virus), a member of the herpesvirus group. Weller isolated etiologic agents from both diseases in 1953 and subsequently established their similarity. Only one serotype is recognized. The virion, which is about 200 nm in diameter, has a DNA core, an icosahedral capsid, and a lipid containing envelope. Man is the only known natural host. The virus is quite labile and loses its infectivity quickly (probably within hours) in the external environment.

VARICELLA

EPIDEMIOLOGY. The disease is spread by airborne droplets and by direct contact with infected lesions. It may also be spread from person to person by a third individual (i.e., by indirect contact) within a limited time and distance, as on a hospital ward. Varicella is communicable from one to two days before onset of the rash until all the vesicles have crusted—five or six days after the rash appears in the average case, somewhat longer in more severe cases. The prodrome and early stages of eruption represent the periods of greatest communicability.

Although V-Z virus may be spread by respiratory secretions, it has rarely been possible to isolate this agent from nasal or pharyngeal secretions. By contrast, infectious virus is easily recovered from vesicle fluid.

Incidence and Prevalence. Varicella is primarily a disease of childhood. In temperate zones it is most common between two and eight years, with a peak on beginning school. Cases occur throughout the year but predominate in winter and spring. Inapparent infections are rare. Newborns of mothers who have had the disease are protected by maternal antibodies for up to about six months, but the degree of protection varies. Varicella is one of the most contagious of infectious diseases. Susceptible children exposed to cases in the same household had a secondary attack rate of 87 per cent. Histories of this disease in adults are often unreliable; in one study only 8 per cent of adults with supposedly negative histories acquired varicella from household contacts. Individuals with varicella usually develop lifelong immunity (but may subsequently develop zoster).

PATHOGENESIS AND PATHOLOGY. It is assumed that the virus enters and initially replicates in the respiratory tract. A viremia follows that disseminates virus throughout the body. Focal lesions then appear in the skin and occasionally in the viscera and enlarge by virus spread from infected to contiguous cells. The occurrence of the lesions in crops is consistent with an intermittent viremia. With appearance of circulating antibody (about one to four days after onset of the rash) the viremia ceases and symptoms begin to subside.

The histopathology of the skin lesions in varicella, herpes zoster, and herpes simplex is identical. Cells in the basal and prickle layers undergo ballooning degeneration, and edema fluid quickly accumulates, elevating the stratum corneum to form a clear vesicle containing large amounts of infective virus. The adjacent infected cells develop an eosinophilic inclusion in each nucleus. In addition, multinucleated giant cells containing such inclusions begin to form at the edges and base of the lesion. As the vesicles begin to dry, they become cloudy with accumulated inflammatory cells and desquamated epidermal cells, and the viral content declines. Finally the lesions crust, the epithelial cells at their base regenerate, and the crusts are shed. In fatal cases, areas of focal necrosis associated with cells showing characteristic intranuclear inclusions may be found throughout the respiratory tract, kidneys, adrenals, liver, and other organs.

The pathologic changes associated with varicella encephalitis are nonspecific and are similar to those seen in the other viral postinfectious encephalitides (see Ch. 506).

CLINICAL MANIFESTATIONS. After an incubation period of 14 to 16 days (range, 10 to 23 days), the disease is usually manifested in young children by low grade fever, malaise, and rash. In older patients, the eruption may be preceded by a one- or two-day prodrome consisting of fever and constitutional signs such as malaise, myalgia, and headache. The lesions, which first appear on the trunk and scalp, begin as small red macules and progress rapidly over 12 to 24 hours through stages to papules, vesicles, pustules, and crust formation. Pruritus is associated with the vesicular stage and may be quite marked. The vesicles are thin walled, superficial, and surrounded by prominent red areolae, which fade as the lesions dry. The crusts may fall off in a week or persist for several weeks, especially in lesions that become secondarily infected. Underlying areas generally heal completely over weeks to months; occasionally a pit or scar may persist.

The exanthem appears in successive crops over a one- to six-day period. Thus, as the disease progresses, a characteristic feature is the presence of lesions in various stages of development in the same anatomic area. Those in the final crop may regress after reaching the maculopapular stage.

The varicella rash has a centripetal distribution, being most abundant on the trunk and face and relatively sparse on the extremities, especially the distal extremities. It is usually increased, however, in areas of irritated, damaged, or inflamed skin.

Vesicles may also occur on the mucous membranes, especially in the mouth. Other sites which may be involved include the vaginal mucosa, conjunctiva, and pharynx. Lesions on mucous membranes break down to form shallow, generally painful white ulcers, which heal without crusting.

Fever parallels the severity of the rash and persists while new lesions continue to appear. Prolongation or recurrence of fever is associated either with bacterial superinfections, most commonly involving the skin lesions, or with some other complication of the disease. As with many other viral infections, varicella is usually more severe in adults than in children, with higher fever, more marked rash, and more frequent complications.

About 16 to 33 per cent of adults, and uncommonly children, develop clinical or radiologic evidence of pneumonitis during the disease. Chest films show diffuse nodular densities throughout both lung fields with a tendency to concentrate at the bases and hilum. The changes may persist for several months in severe cases. In some patients, fibrotic scars remain and gradually calcify, resembling the radiologic changes in healed miliary tuberculosis.

Encephalitis may occur with both mild and severe cases of varicella and is responsible for 90 per cent of the neurologic complications of this disease. Its incidence is estimated at less than one per 1000 cases. The manifestations are similar to those associated with measles or vaccinial encephalitis and may be quite severe with coma, seizures, appreciable mortality, and permanent sequelae. In about one third of patients with encephalitis, especially in children, cerebellar dysfunction with ataxia is the most prominent feature, and such patients generally do well, recovering completely within one to three weeks. Transverse myelitis, neuritis, and aseptic meningitis have also been observed.

Patients who are susceptible to varicella and who have leukemia, lymphoma, or congenital or acquired immunodeficiency or are on immunosuppressive medication represent a high-risk group for development of more severe disease, progressive varicella. Newborns of mothers who have onset of varicella less than five days before delivery or within 48 hours after delivery also fall into this category, presumably because they have received no maternal antibodies against this disease. This condition is characterized by continued eruption of lesions and high fever. In addition, pneumonia, disseminated visceral disease, secondary bacterial infection, central nervous system involvement, and hemorrhagic phenomena are more common, and mortality is significantly increased.

Additional manifestations that have been noted in varicella include *bullous rash, hepatitis, carditis, nephritis, orchitis, thrombocytopenia, and arthritis.* About 10 per cent of cases of Reye's syndrome (acute encephalopathy and fatty degeneration of the viscera) have been associated with an immediately preceding varicella (see Ch. 507).

Maternal infection with V-Z virus during the first four months of pregnancy has been reported to result occasionally in a syndrome of severe congenital malformation characterized by low birth weight for age, atrophy of a limb, scarring of the skin of that extremity, neurologic deficits, and eye abnormalities. The incidence of such cases appears to be quite low.

DIAGNOSIS. The typical case of varicella can be easily recognized on the basis of its characteristic clinical features. A history of exposure within the preceding several weeks is helpful. The demonstration of multinucleated giant cells in Wright- or Giemsa-stained scrapings of young vesicles (Tzanck smear) or in biopsies of affected tissues establishes the lesions as due to either V-Z or herpes simplex virus. Further differentiation among varicella, herpes zoster, and herpes simplex can then generally be made on the basis of associated clinical findings.

Viral isolation and/or serologic tests are generally necessary only to confirm unusual cases. Sera for testing should be collected within the first week after onset of illness and two to four weeks later. The virus can be readily isolated from vesicle fluid and identified in appropriate tissue cultures, or the presence of viral antigen can be confirmed by immunofluorescence. The demonstration of a rising titer of complement-fixing antibodies to V-Z antigen is also useful but must be interpreted with care, as this virus shares some antigenic components with herpes simplex virus. Complement-fixing antibodies decline rapidly and may not be detectable after six to twelve months. Neutralizing antibodies persist, but their determination is technically difficult. Immune status may be determined by an indirect fluorescent test with the patient's serum for antibody against V-Z virus-induced membrane antigen in infected cells (FAMA test). The presence of such antibody indicates immunity.

Other entities with a generalized vesicular eruption include smallpox (now extinct), eczema vaccinatum, eczema herpeticum, rickettsialpox, disease caused by certain coxsackieviruses, and some allergic rashes. None of these meet the criteria for diagnosis of varicella, and their differentiation from this disorder should present little difficulty.

TREATMENT. There is no specific therapy for varicella. Treatment is symptomatic and directed at relief of local discomfort and control of secondary infection. Supportive therapy includes acetaminophen (Tylenol) for high fever and constitutional symptoms and lukewarm starch baths, calamine lotion, and/or antihistamines for pruritus. The Centers for Disease Control recommend that salicylates not be used pending clarification of their possible causative role in Reye's syndrome. Nails should be kept clean and short to minimize skin infection from scratching. Patients with varicella pneumonia or encephalitis may need ventilatory support and attention to hydration, electrolyte balance, and nutrition. Bacterial or fungal superinfection may be important in the compromised host. Patients who develop varicella while on immunosuppressive doses of steroids should have the dose of such medication reduced to one to one and a half times physiologic levels (0.7 to 1.0 mg of cortisone per kilogram per day or its equivalent) as rapidly as is consistent with safety, and should be maintained at this level until the disease has subsided. Patients receiving other immunosuppressive therapy should also have the dose of their medication reduced.

Treatment with adenine arabinoside* (Ara-A, vidarabine), a DNA inhibitor, is of value for reducing the incidence of complications in immunocompromised patients with varicella. Early treatment is most effective. A dose of 10 mg per kilogram intravenously every 24 hours in a 12-hour infusion for five to seven days has been used. Acyclovir, another DNA inhibitor presently undergoing clinical trials, is less toxic and appears to be equally effective.

PREVENTION. Human immune serum globulin given to normal children within three days of exposure to varicella does not prevent but will attenuate the disease. V-Z immune globulin (VZIG), a more potent preparation, prepared from outdated normal blood with high antibody titers for V-Z virus, prevents varicella in normal hosts and reduces morbidity and mortality in susceptible high-risk hosts. VZIG is intended primarily for susceptible pediatric patients who meet high-risk criteria, for high-risk newborns, and on an individual basis for susceptible older compromised hosts. It is also available for prophylaxis for the patient with a history of chickenpox who has subsequently received a bone marrow transplant. Since such subjects are at high risk for severe disseminated disease, VZIG should be administered within 96 hours after exposure. It may be obtained by calling the local regional American Red Cross Office. Exposed patients on immunosuppressive therapy should not only receive VZIG but also have the dose of their medication reduced until the risk of varicella is past.

An attenuated live virus vaccine is currently being tested. It appears to be effective even in compromised hosts. Field trials in this country have been limited, however, by controversies regarding the long-term consequences and safety of a vaccine prepared with a virus that may establish a latent infection. It is presently being used in controlled studies on children with leukemia and other malignant diseases in whom the potential benefits outweigh the possible risks.

HERPES ZOSTER

EPIDEMIOLOGY. Herpes zoster represents a reactivation of a latent varicella infection; this disease may occur, therefore, in any subject who has had a prior infection with V-Z virus. Although shingles has been reported following contact with either varicella or herpes zoster, such cases most probably represent a coincidental reactivation of V-Z virus. The sporadic occurrence of herpes zoster as compared with the seasonal prevalence of varicella indicates that herpes zoster does not usually result from exogenous infection.

Susceptible persons may acquire varicella by close contact with patients with herpes zoster, but the estimated attack rate, 15 per cent or less, is considerably lower than that following similar exposure to varicella. This probably reflects the more limited skin and mucosal involvement, the presence of preexisting antibodies, and the decreased role of respiratory spread in patients with herpes zoster. Although the patient with herpes zoster does not disseminate virus so readily as the patient with varicella, vesicles yielding virus can persist longer than in varicella—for four to seven days after onset of the rash, longer in compromised hosts. As in varicella, the crusts in herpes zoster are not infectious.

Incidence and Prevalence. Herpes zoster may occur at any age but is uncommon in young hosts. The attack rate increases with age, with the peak incidence occurring in those over 50 years. In infancy or childhood the disease generally results from reactivation of an infection with V-Z virus acquired either in utero or in early infancy while protected by maternal antibodies. Although multiple episodes may occur, they are uncommon in the normal host. Data on age incidence suggest that 50 per cent of individuals will have had one episode by the age of 85 and 1 per cent will have had two attacks. The disease is more common in hosts with impaired cellular immunity, e.g., patients receiving immunosuppressive drugs and those with certain malignancies, especially Hodgkin's disease and lymphomas.

PATHOGENESIS AND PATHOLOGY. The exact pathogenesis of herpes zoster is not known. It is hypothesized that the V-Z virus enters the cutaneous endings of sensory nerves during varicella and travels centripetally along the nerve fibers to the sensory ganglia, where it becomes latent within the neurons. Although latency of V-Z virus in sensory ganglia remains to be proved, the virus has been demonstrated in ganglia of affected dermatomes obtained at autopsy from patients with active herpes zoster. Subsequently, in association with a variety of conditions, including development of malignancy, local x-irradiation, immunosuppressive therapy, tumor involvement of the dorsal root ganglion or adjacent structures, and treatment with certain drugs such as arsenicals, reactivation of the virus occurs. In many patients no obvious association or stimulus is apparent, and reactivation has been attributed to a decrease in host resistance with age. Virus replicates in the affected ganglia, producing an active ganglionitis causing pain along its sensory distribution. Virus is then believed to pass down the nerve and multiply again in the skin, where it produces the characteristic segmental, clustered, vesicular lesions of herpes zoster. A transitory viremia may also occur, as indicated by the appearance of a disseminated, generally sparse, varicella-like rash, usually several days after the dermatomal lesions, in up to one third of the patients. Rarely, spread to the viscera may also occur. The attack of herpes zoster is presumably terminated by the reactivated defense mechanisms of the host. Resolution and limitation of the rash correlate poorly with the antibody response. An impaired cellular immunity probably plays an important role in the pathogenesis of this disease.

Pathologic studies of involved sensory ganglia in herpes zoster reveal extensive lymphocytic infiltration, focal hemorrhage, and nerve cell destruction, followed in weeks to months by fibrosis. In addition, there is inflammation in the adjacent segments of the cord or brain stem. There may also be a localized leptomeningitis involving the affected segments; this process may occasionally spread to the anterior horn, resulting in motor paralysis, a rare complication of this disease.

The pathologic changes of zoster encephalitis are similar to those seen in varicella. The histopathology of the cutaneous lesions and the disseminated visceral lesions in herpes zoster is identical with that of varicella.

CLINICAL MANIFESTATIONS. Segmental or cutaneous paresthesias and pain of a burning or stabbing nature are characteristic of herpes zoster. These symptoms may be intermittent or constant and generally accompany the rash. Occasionally they may precede it by four or five days, presenting a prodromal picture easily confused with a variety of other illnesses characterized by localized pain. Malaise and fever may be present. The cutaneous lesions of zoster, like those of varicella, begin as erythematous maculopapules that progress over the next several days to form single or confluent clumps of vesicles, pustules, and crusts. Regional adenopathy generally accompanies the rash. New lesions continue to appear in crops for several days or longer, progressing to crusts which may persist for several weeks or more. Deep-seated lesions may result in scarring, and severe involvement may lead to gangrene. Typically, the rash appears in a unilateral, dermatomal distribution corresponding to the innervation of the affected sensory nerves. Occasionally the lesions may overlap onto adjacent dermatomes. Rarely, affected dermatomes may be separated or on opposite sides of the body.

The lesions of herpes zoster occur with the greatest frequency in those dermatomes in which the rash of varicella is most commonly found, i.e., the trunk in over 50 per cent of patients and, less often, the cervical and lumbar regions. The cranial nerve most commonly affected is the trigeminal, especially the ophthalmic branch. Ophthalmic zoster may be associated with a keratoconjunctivitis and impairment of oculomotor function

---

*Investigational drug for this purpose.

manifested by extraocular muscle weakness, ptosis, and mydriasis. Adjacent nerve roots may also be involved. Herpes zoster oticus (Ramsay Hunt syndrome) results from involvement of the facial and auditory nerves. Presenting features include vesicles in the external ear and ipsilateral facial paralysis, which is usually transitory. This localization of zoster may be accompanied by hearing loss, vertigo, loss of taste, tongue vesicles, and other signs consistent with involvement of additional cranial ganglia, especially those of the ninth and tenth cranial nerves.

Since the primary lesion of herpes zoster is in the nervous system, the cerebrospinal fluid may show a pleocytosis and elevation of protein. This is most frequent in patients with involvement of the cervical ganglia. Symptoms referable to meningeal involvement are minimal or absent. Although the cerebrospinal fluid changes may last for several weeks, recovery is usually complete.

Motor paralysis occasionally accompanies herpes zoster but is not common. It usually occurs within the first few weeks after onset of the rash, attains peak severity within days, and may persist for weeks or more. The paralysis almost always involves muscle groups innervated by nerves arising from the same spinal segment as that associated with the rash. About 75 per cent of such patients show complete or functional recovery. Major central nervous system infections with herpes zoster are rare, but cases of transverse myelitis, disseminated encephalitis, and acute cerebellar ataxia have been described.

The occurrence of segmental neuralgic pain without accompanying vesicles (zoster sine herpete) in serologically confirmed cases of V-Z infection has suggested that this virus may occasionally be activated in sensory ganglia without spread to the skin. Evidence in support of this hypothesis is limited.

Generalized herpes zoster occurs in 2 to 5 per cent of patients, most commonly in compromised hosts. It usually begins within a week or two of the localized rash, and is manifested as a varicella-like rash of varying severity, occasionally with widespread visceral involvement and fatal termination.

The neuralgia associated with herpes zoster generally subsides with recovery from the illness. It is rarely present in pediatric patients with this disease. In about 50 per cent of patients over 60 years it may persist for up to several months, and in a small percentage it may continue for a year or more.

Herpes zoster in pregnancy has not been shown to cause adverse effects in either the mother or the fetus.

DIAGNOSIS. Herpes zoster can generally be recognized by the characteristic development of pain and clustered vesicles in a unilateral, segmental distribution. Herpes simplex virus may occasionally produce a similar-appearing eruption, zosteriform simplex. Multiple recurrences are common with herpes simplex but uncommon in herpes zoster. Support for the diagnosis of herpes zoster may be obtained by the demonstration of multinucleated giant cells and intranuclear inclusions in stained scrapings of vesicular lesions (Tzanck smear) or in biopsies of affected tissues, but this does not differentiate between lesions of herpes zoster and herpes simplex. Such differentiation may be made by fluorescent antibody staining of cells in scrapings from vesicles. Specific diagnosis can also be made by isolation of the virus from vesicle fluid (and occasionally from cerebrospinal fluid with pleocytosis) in appropriate tissue culture systems. The virus may then be identified by standard serologic procedures, using specific antisera.

Methods for serologic diagnosis of herpes zoster are available but are not commonly employed. The complement fixation test, which is useful for confirmation of varicella, is less satisfactory for herpes zoster, since some patients show an elevated antibody titer in the acute phase serum with little subsequent rise. In addition, cross reactions occur with herpes simplex virus, so that simultaneous serologic tests must be carried out against both viruses before an antibody rise against V-Z virus may be considered as diagnostic.

TREATMENT. Uncomplicated herpes zoster requires only symptomatic and supportive therapy: analgesics such as aspirin or codeine for the neuralgia, and antihistamines and drying lotion for the pruritus. Ophthalmic zoster should be treated promptly by an ophthalmologist. Severe, prolonged postherpetic neuralgia presents a problem in management, since it is refractory to the usual analgesics and often leads to depression and occasionally to addiction in the search for relief. The combined use of analgesics, tranquilizers, and soporifics to break the pain cycle, followed by more limited use of such medication may be helpful. Treatment with prednisone is of questionable value.

Immunocompromised patients on immunosuppressive therapy who develop herpes zoster should have the medication dosage reduced as far as is practical. Treatment of such patients with adenine arabinoside early in the course of the infection (≤ 72 hours) has been shown to reduce systemic spread of virus as indicated by decreases in cutaneous spread of lesions and visceral disease. Controlled studies with acyclovir in such patients have given similar results.

Dissemination of herpes zoster lesions has been shown to occur in the presence of high levels of antibody. Administration of V-Z antibody preparations, therefore, would not be expected to affect the course of this illness.

PREVENTION. At present no effective means for prevention of herpes zoster is available.

Balfour HH Jr, Bean B, Laskin OL, Ambinder RF, Meyers JD, Wade JC, Zaia JA, Aeppli D, Kirk LE, Segreti AC, Keeney RE, the Burroughs Wellcome Collaborative Acyclovir Study Group: Acyclovir halts progression of herpes zoster in immunocompromised patients. N Engl J Med 308:1448, 1983. *Detailed double-blind collaborative evaluation of acyclovir.*

Herrmann KL: Congenital and perinatal varicella. Clin Obstet Gynecol 25:605, 1982. *A review with comments on management.*

Marcy SM, Kibrick S: Varicella and herpes zoster. *In* Hoeprich PD (ed.): Infectious Diseases. 3rd ed. New York, Harper & Row, 1982, pp 876–891. *Includes detailed accounts of less common complications of these disorders.*

Reichman RC, Mazur MH, Whitley RJ: *In* Dolin R (moderator): Herpes zoster–varicella infections in immunosuppressed patients. Ann Intern Med 89:375, 1978. *An edited transcription of a Combined Clinical Staff Conference at the Clinical Center, Bethesda, Md. (113 references).*

Weller TH: Varicella and herpes zoster. *In* Lennette EH, Schmidt NJ (eds.): Diagnostic Procedures for Viral, Rickettsial and Chlamydial Infections. Washington, D.C., American Public Health Association, 1979, pp 375-398. *A summary of procedures for isolation and study of varicella–herpes zoster virus in the laboratory. Includes data on interpretation of results.*

Weller TH: Varicella-herpes zoster virus. *In* Evans AS (ed.): Viral Infections of Humans, Epidemiology and Control. 2nd ed. New York, Plenum Publishing Corporation, 1982, pp 569–595. *The epidemiology and clinical features of varicella and herpes zoster are reviewed. Vaccine studies are summarized. Up-to-date, clearly written, and heavily referenced.*

Weller TH: Varicella and herpes zoster. Medical progress. N Engl J Med 309:1362, 1434, 1983. *A review of recent advances in knowledge about varicella and herpes zoster. Heavily referenced.*

Whitley RJ, Soong SJ, Dolin R, Betts R, Linneman C Jr, Alford CA Jr, the NIAID Collaborative Antiviral Study Group: Early vidarabine therapy to control the complications of herpes zoster in immunosuppressed patients. N Engl J Med 307:971, 1982. *Detailed double-blind collaborative evaluation of vidarabine.*

340. VARIOLA AND VACCINIA

Donald A. Henderson

The Thirty-third World Health Assembly "declares solemnly that the world and all its peoples have won freedom from smallpox . . . an unprecedented achievement in the history of public health. . . ." (Resolution 33.3, May 8, 1980, Geneva, Switzerland.)

This announcement was made some 30 months after the last known endemic case—a 23-year-old Somali cook who developed smallpox on October 26, 1977. In 1978, two additional cases of smallpox occurred in Birmingham, England, following a laboratory accident, but except for these cases no others have been found.

To confirm that eradication had been achieved, each country where smallpox had been endemic since 1967 and those at risk of importations conducted a search for cases for at least two years after the last known case. At the end of this period, World Health Organization (WHO)-appointed International Commissions reviewed the records of work and conducted extensive field visits to confirm the results. Between 1973 and 1979, 21 different commissions visited and certified eradication in 49 countries.

Finally, a Global Commission for the Certification of Smallpox Eradication reviewed the findings of each of the International Commissions and made special field visits. After satisfying itself that eradication had been achieved, the Commission reported its findings to the World Health Assembly. The Assembly members concurred and recommended that "smallpox vaccination be discontinued in every country except for investigators at special risk," and advised that "an international certificate of vaccination against smallpox should no longer be required of any traveller."

Thus concluded the first successful global program to eradicate a disease—one whose origins antedate written history and which over the centuries had proved to be one of the most devastating diseases known to man (McNeill).

HISTORY. Because of the need for variola virus to spread continually from person to person to survive, historians speculate that it emerged at some time after the first agricultural settlements, about 10,000 B.C. The presence of the distinctive smallpox rash on the mummy of Pharaoh Ramses V (1160 B.C.) documents its existence more than 3000 years ago (Dixon). In ancient times, only a few populated areas, probably in India, could have sustained its transmission. In the early Christian era descriptions suggestive of smallpox appear in historical accounts of western Asia, and by the eighth century it had established itself in Europe. Central and southern Africa were probably infected sometime later. In 1520, Spanish conquistadors brought the disease to the Americas.

Case-fatality rates of 20 per cent and greater were characteristic, and where population densities permitted the disease to become endemic virtually all persons eventually contracted smallpox. Deities to smallpox became a part of the culture in India, China, and a number of African countries. At the end of the eighteenth century, it was killing an estimated 400,000 Europeans each year and was responsible for one third of all cases of blindness.

VACCINATION. Edward Jenner's discovery in 1796 that smallpox could be prevented by "vaccination" with material from a cowpox lesion was widely acclaimed. Before his discovery, the only defense against smallpox was to deliberately inoculate (variolate) scabs or pustular material from smallpox patients into the skin of susceptibles. The resulting infection was usually less severe than infection acquired naturally by inhalation. Although case-fatality rates among those with induced infection were "only" 1 to 2 per cent, they readily transmitted infection to others. Within three years after Jenner first published his findings, more than 100,000 had been vaccinated in England. By 1803, the new vaccine had been transported to the Americas, Asia, and Africa, often by means of children who were vaccinated arm-to-arm in succession during the voyages.

During the nineteenth century, vaccination was increasingly widely practiced in temperate-climate countries, but the difficulties of sustaining the virus through arm-to-arm inoculation resulted in an uncertain supply. The discovery, late in the nineteenth century, that vaccinia virus could be propagated on the flank of a calf was an important advance. However, such vaccine remained viable for only a few days at ambient temperature. Finally, in the 1950's a commercially feasible technique was developed for producing a dried heat-resistant vaccine.

In the industrialized countries, smallpox incidence declined steadily, and Europe and North America succeeded in interrupting smallpox transmission after World War II. In these areas, the impetus for vaccination had diminished early in the century when a less virulent strain, variola minor, replaced variola major. Variola minor, with a case-fatality rate of about 1 per cent, was a less significant problem than variola major. In most of Africa, however, 5 to 15 per cent died of smallpox, and in Asia the virulent variola major prevailed. Neither in Africa nor in Asia was vaccination widely practiced.

ERADICATION OF SMALLPOX. Each year since 1948, the World Health Assembly had encouraged its member countries to take more vigorous control measures. It was a problem to all countries. Even those without disease feared importations and conducted vaccination programs to prevent epidemics should cases be imported. Although the global control of smallpox was in everyone's best interests, progress was slow. Finally, in 1959, the Assembly decided that a global eradication program should be undertaken. During the succeeding seven years, a number of countries undertook campaigns, but few succeeded in interrupting smallpox transmission. The few countries that were successful were plagued by importations from neighbors. Serious setbacks in WHO's other eradication program, the malaria program, caused the concept of eradication itself to be viewed with skepticism.

In 1966, the Assembly decided that one further effort should be made. It voted to allot $2.5 million annually for an intensified eradication program. A ten-year goal was proposed. The program commenced on January 1, 1967 (Henderson). In 1967, smallpox was endemic in 33 countries, and 14 additional countries reported importations. Although 131,000 cases were officially reported, later studies showed the true number to be about 10 to 15 million. Four geographic reservoirs of smallpox were identified: (1) Africa south of the Sahara; (2) a group of Southeast Asian countries, extending from Bangladesh through India, Nepal, Pakistan, and Afghanistan; (3) Indonesia; and (4) Brazil. The estimated population of these countries was more than 1.2 billion.

WHO's strategy called for each country to undertake a program of vaccination with the objective of reaching at least 80 per cent of the population during a two- to three-year period. During this time, a reliable reporting system was to be developed to identify foci of smallpox that would be eliminated by isolation of patients and vaccination of contacts. Extensive vaccination was believed necessary to increase population immunity and so reduce the number of cases to permit disease surveillance and containment activities to be effective.

Experience soon showed that the surveillance-containment strategy was more effective than had been thought, and, in fact, this proved to be the key to the program's success. In part, this was due to the unique characteristics of smallpox. An infected patient was able to transmit infection only from the time of first appearance of rash until the last scabs had separated. There were no chronic carriers or individuals with latent infection and no animal reservoir. The rash was sufficiently characteristic to be diagnosed with a high degree of accuracy by clinicians and villagers alike. The presence or absence of smallpox in an area could thus be reliably determined without laboratory studies. Moreover, approximately two thirds of recovered patients had characteristic residual facial scars. Thus, it was possible to determine both the present status of smallpox and its past history in an area.

To persist, smallpox virus had to be transmitted in a continuing chain of infection from patient to susceptible contact. By isolation of the patient and by vaccination of contacts, a barrier to transmission was created and a chain of infection interrupted. In small villages and in scattered populations, chains of transmission often terminated without intervention. Because smallpox did not spread rapidly, and then only to those in face-to-face contact, secondary cases usually were found among neighbors and relatives, and cases tended to cluster within parts of a town and in localized geographic regions. A patient rarely infected more than two or three others, and, even in infected households, three and sometimes four generations of cases occurred. Because of these factors, early detection of outbreaks and their containment proved effective in stopping transmission, even when there was a low level of population immunity (Foege et al.).

Smallpox vaccine that conferred excellent and durable immunity was an important factor in the program's success. Studies during the program revealed vaccine efficacy ratios of more than 90 per cent after 20 years. Because the lyophilized vaccine retained its potency after incubation at 37° C for at least one month, the logistics of vaccine storage and distribution were greatly simplified. The vaccination technique was greatly facilitated by the inexpensive newly developed bifurcated needle, a device best described as a large sewing needle with part of the eye ground off to leave two small prongs. Vaccine was held between the tines by capillarity. Fifteen rapid punctures were made with the needle held perpendicular to the skin. The technique was learned quickly and produced a high proportion of successful vaccinations.

PROGRESS IN THE PROGRAM. By 1969, eradication programs were in progress in all of the infected and immediately adjacent countries except for Ethiopia, whose program began in 1971. By 1970, the number of endemic countries had decreased from 33 to 18. Eleven of the 15 that became smallpox free were in western and central Africa. Brazil registered its last case in 1971 and Indonesia and Afghanistan in 1972. By 1973, all of Africa had become smallpox free except for Ethiopia and Botswana. In Asia, there remained only four smallpox-endemic countries: India, Pakistan, Nepal, and Bangladesh. However, the population of these four was over 700 million, and the techniques of surveillance and containment which had been applied in other areas had been less successful.

A new strategy in India began in the autumn of 1973 (Basu et al.). Far more rapid case detection and more effective containment of outbreaks were required. Accordingly, for one week each month more than 100,000 health workers were mobilized to search house by house, to detect cases. Hundreds of special surveillance-containment teams contained the outbreaks which were found. Between searches, the teams asked questions at markets and in schools to uncover rumors of cases. A similar strategy was adopted in the neighboring countries. By the summer of 1974, new cases began to decline, and a cash reward was offered to anyone who reported a case. In May 1975 the last case was detected in India, and on October 16, 1975, the last case in Asia.

The only remaining endemic country was Ethiopia. More than half of its population of 25 million lived more than a day's walk from any road, and its health structure was all but nonexistent. With the end of smallpox in Asia, resources were shifted to Ethiopia. In August 1976, the last case was isolated. Unfortunately, Somalian guerrilla forces had meanwhile introduced the disease into neighboring Somalia, and yet another year was to elapse before finally, on October 26, 1977, the last case occurred.

POSSIBLE SOURCES FOR A RETURN OF SMALLPOX. As of June, 1984, variola virus was known to exist in only two laboratories, each of which had been inspected by international teams. The risk of accidental escape is extremely small.

Extensive studies had been conducted since 1967 to discover a possible animal or other natural reservoir of the virus. None was found. The best evidence that such a reservoir does not exist is that all smallpox outbreaks detected in otherwise smallpox-free areas since 1967 were traced to known human cases.

Almost 200 cases of a newly recognized disease that is clinically indistinguishable from smallpox but caused by the related monkey pox virus occurred in six central and west African countries between 1970 and 1984. Almost all of the patients lived in small villages in the tropical rain forest. Person-to-person transmission occurred in several instances, but it is apparent that the virus is transmitted only with difficulty. Genome maps of this and other animal poxviruses reveal many differences between them and variola, suggesting that mutation to variola would be highly unlikely.

The recurrence of smallpox resulting from a deliberate release of variola virus cannot be ruled out. However, the potential damage of such an act should not be exaggerated. Smallpox does not spread rapidly as does influenza or measles, and an outbreak caused in this manner should be able to be contained within three to four weeks. Moreover, if someone were to decide to employ biologic weapons, there are other agents whose virulence and characteristics of spread are superior to those of variola virus.

As insurance against unforeseen events, WHO has established vaccine storage reserves of some 200 million doses of vaccine. Additional stocks are being retained by a number of governments.

Barring improbable circumstances, a human case of smallpox will never again be seen. However, the problem of mistaken diagnosis is a real one. For this reason, WHO medical officers with expertise in diagnosis remain on call to investigate rumors, and an expertise in laboratory diagnosis will be maintained by WHO Diagnostic Reference Laboratories (Centers for Disease Control, Atlanta, and the Institute for Virus Preparations, Moscow).

VARIOLA (Smallpox)

ETIOLOGY. Variola virus is one of a group of orthopoxviruses which includes vaccinia, monkey pox, rabbit pox, cowpox, camel pox, buffalo pox, and ectromelia (Nakano). The poxviruses are the largest viruses so recognized. The virions are brick-shaped structures with a diameter of about 200 mμ. The genome consists of a single molecule of a double-stranded DNA.

INCIDENCE AND PREVALENCE. The disease was declared to be eradicated on May 8, 1980.

PATHOLOGY AND PATHOGENESIS. The site of entry of the smallpox virus was probably the respiratory tract. In the 12-day incubation period the virus multiplied in the regional lymphoid tissues. Viremia occurred at the onset of fever and continued during the first two or three days of the pre-eruptive phase. During this time, the virus localized in mucous membranes, skin, and internal tissues. Antibodies appeared as early as the fourth day of disease. The virus multiplied in the epithelial cells of the skin and mucous membranes, causing pustulation. Patients became infectious at the time of onset of rash. Scabs separated during the third to fourth week of illness and, although virus could be detected in scabs, they were less infectious than vesicular or pustular secretions.

CLINICAL MANIFESTATIONS. The incubation period of smallpox was about 12 days with a range of 7 to 17 days. The illness began with severe malaise, prostration, head- and backache, and high fever lasting two to five days (Rao). Following the initial febrile period, a macular rash developed, which quickly became papular, and within two days the papules developed into vesicles and then pustules. On the eighth or ninth day of rash, crusting began. The scabs separated over the succeeding two to three weeks, leaving pigment-free skin. Subsequently, scarring or pitting developed. An important diagnostic feature of variola was the fact that lesions in any one area were all at the same stage of development, whereas in varicella they are in all stages. The eruption was characteristically more severe on the face and the distal parts of the arms and legs, and less severe over the trunk and abdomen. This centrifugal distribution was distinct from the rash of varicella, which tends to be centripetal. Lesions were often found on the palms of the hands and the soles of the feet, a finding uncommon in childhood varicella, although not unusual in the adult form. The characteristic pustular lesions of smallpox were round, raised, and tense, with a tendency to central depression as they began to dry. The majority of deaths occurred during the second week of rash.

VARIOLA MINOR AND INTERMEDIATE FORMS. In the early twentieth century, a milder clinical form of smallpox (variola minor, alastrim) became prevalent in the Americas, Europe, and parts of southern and eastern Africa. Case-fatality rates were 1 per cent or less. Variola major and minor were distinct although at times coexisting. Each of the two types gave rise to illnesses with a spectrum of severity ranging from fatal hemorrhagic cases to mild cases with only a few lesions. In outbreaks of variola major the severe cases predominated, whereas in variola minor most cases were mild. There was cross-protection between each of these forms and vaccinia.

DIFFERENTIAL DIAGNOSIS. Most cases of smallpox could readily be identified by the typical deep-seated rash, the centrifugal distribution of lesions, and the fact that in any area on the body all lesions were at the same stage of development. The infrequent severe hemorrhagic cases were frequently mistakenly diagnosed as meningococcemia, acute leukemia, or drug toxicity. Mild cases with few lesions were confused with varicella. Most problematic were severe cases of chickenpox in adults, which often were misdiagnosed as smallpox. Of help in diagnosis, however, was the fact that in any outbreak 80 per cent or more of the cases were clinically typical.

LABORATORY TESTS. Diagnosis of a poxvirus infection can be rapidly established by electron microscope identification of virus particles in vesicular or pustular fluid or scabs. Differentiation as to which poxvirus may be causing illness requires that the virus be isolated on chick chorioallantoic membrane and its properties characterized by specific biologic tests. WHO Reference Laboratories are prepared to undertake necessary diagnostic studies. For patients who have recovered, neutralizing antibody in serum specimens serves to identify which poxvirus was responsible for the illness.

TREATMENT. No specific treatment is available.

IDENTIFICATION OF A SUSPECT CASE OF SMALLPOX. Because smallpox has been eradicated, the occurrence of a single case has profound international implications. Should a suspect case be identified, *immediate notification of local, state, and national health officials is essential.* From time to time clinicians may suspect smallpox in a severely ill patient with fever and rash. Most suspected cases in recent years have been cases of varicella in adults. Visualization of varicella particles in vesicular, pustular, or scab material by electron microscopy will confirm the diagnosis. Under the electron microscope, orthopoxviruses such as vaccinia, monkey pox, and smallpox appear alike and must be further characterized by other biologic tests. Should a case prove to be smallpox, the source of virus must be assumed to be inadvertent or deliberate release from a laboratory.

A suspect patient should be placed under strict isolation and the diagnosis determined as an emergency measure. Additional measures will be dictated by epidemiologic circumstances.

VACCINIA (Vaccination)

No countries now require international certificates of vaccination and none conduct vaccination programs. Vaccination is recommended only for investigators who are working with poxviruses in the laboratory or who are engaged in field studies of monkey pox virus.

THE VACCINE. Vaccinia virus is believed to have derived from cowpox virus, although comparisons of contemporary strains of cowpox virus and vaccinia virus show them to have different biologic characteristics. Vaccinia virus is grown on the scarified flank of a calf or sheep. After purification and the addition of stabilizing agents, the suspension is freeze dried. Inoculated intradermally, vaccinia virus induces a mild infection and confers protection against all orthopoxviruses known to infect man—monkey pox, variola, and cowpox.

VACCINE PROTECTION. Following successful vaccination, protection against variola is virtually complete for five years, but effectiveness wanes over time. In poxvirus laboratories, vaccination at least every three years has been customary, and none so vaccinated has developed disease.

RISKS OF VACCINATION. Those who are candidates for vaccination are adults, a diminishing proportion of whom have received primary vaccinations as children. Although the risk of complications following revaccination is very low, primary vaccination of adults has been thought to be associated with a high incidence of serious complications, especially postvaccinial encephalitis. Most of the studies that document this are from Europe, where especially pathogenic strains had been used. Studies in the United States, where the New York Board of Health strain was used, reveal a much lower incidence of complications. A special study of vaccination complications among military recruits failed to document any cases of postvaccinial encephalitis among an estimated 2 million primary vaccinees.

FIRST VACCINATION (PRIMARY TAKE). Three days after vaccination a papule appears at the vaccination site. The papule is small, round, bright red, and hard but superficial. The papule changes to a vesicle, and by the seventh day is fully developed. It is whitish, umbilicated, and multilocular and contains clear lymph. An erythematous areola expands to reach a maximal diameter about nine days after vaccination. Crusting begins at the center, and the dry brownish crust falls off about three weeks after vaccination, leaving a scar.

REVACCINATION. When vaccination is performed on persons who possess some immunity, a gradation of cutaneous responses is observed. Individuals who have not been vaccinated for several decades may develop what appears to be a primary take. In persons with an intermediate level of immunity, the course of development of the lesion is more rapid and the maximal diameter of erythema is reached in from three to seven days. In the highly immune person, virus multiplication may not occur. However, in such persons, a hypersensitivity response to vaccinial protein may occur. A papule and sometimes a vesicle with erythema may develop. The reaction reaches its peak in the first 48 hours, but by the sixth day, there is no evidence of an inflammatory process. This reaction was formerly termed a "reaction of immunity," implying that the individual was immune to smallpox. However, experiments have shown that vaccine that has been inactivated by heat may induce a similar response.

To distinguish the hypersensitivity type of reaction from one in which virus multiplication has taken place, the site of inoculation is examined between the sixth and eighth days. If there is evidence of induration or congestion, virus multiplication may be assumed. If there is no evidence of induration or congestion, virus multiplication may or may not have taken place, and repeat vaccination is advised.

CONTRAINDICATIONS. Four groups of persons are at special risk of complications: (1) persons with eczema or other forms of chronic dermatitis; (2) pregnant women; (3) patients with leukemia, lymphoma, and other reticuloendothelial malignancies; and (4) those receiving immunosuppressive drugs, especially glucocorticosteroids. Vaccinees in close contact with persons with eczema may infect them, sometimes with serious consequences. If vaccination is required for persons at special risk, vaccinia immune globulin (0.3 ml per kilogram intramuscularly) should be administered simultaneously.

COMPLICATIONS. ***Postvaccinal Encephalitis.*** Encephalitis following vaccination is a rare event and occurs between the eighth and fifteenth days. The disease may be associated with fever, headache, vomiting, drowsiness, and sometimes paralysis, meningitic signs, coma, and convulsions. The cerebrospinal fluid usually shows an increase in cells. Paralysis, when it occurs, is generally spastic in type. Recovery may be complete, or residual paralysis and other central nervous system symptoms may persist. There is no treatment. Studies conducted in the United States in 1963 and 1968 (Neff et al., Lane et al.) revealed 28 cases, 9 fatal, among 11.3 million primary vaccinees. No cases occurred among 16.3 million revaccinees.

Progressive Vaccinia (Vaccinia Gangrenosa). Progressive vaccinia is an exceedingly rare but often fatal complication among vaccinated persons who have deficient immune responses. The initial vaccinial lesion fails to heal and progresses to involve adjacent skin with necrosis of tissue. Dissemination of virus may result in metastatic vaccinial lesions in other parts of the skin, bones, or viscera. In the United States studies, 12 cases, including 2 deaths, occurred among 11.3 million primary vaccinees and 8 cases, including 2 deaths, among 16.3 million revaccinees. Treatment with vaccinia immune globulin and thiosemicarbazone* is beneficial.

Eczema Vaccinatum. Eczema vaccinatum is sometimes a serious complication, which may occur in persons with either active or healed eczema. It may occur among eczematous subjects who are in contact with recent vaccinees. The disease tends to localize at sites where eczematous lesions are or have been present.

*Available for experimental use only.

Vaccinia immune globulin and the thiosemicarbazone* drugs are of help in therapy.

Generalized Vaccinia. Generalized vaccinia represents a secondary eruption resulting from bloodborne dissemination of vaccinia virus. Almost all cases occur after primary vaccination. The lesions become evident between six and nine days after vaccination. The number of lesions may range from a few to a generalized involvement of the skin. It is a self-limited illness, and complete recovery occurs without specific therapy.

Fetal Vaccinia. Fetal vaccinia results from a bloodborne dissemination of vaccinia virus in the pregnant woman given primary vaccination. It may occur during any trimester of pregnancy and frequently results in death of the fetus.

Miscellaneous Complications. A great variety of rashes has been reported to be caused by vaccination. Most common are erythema multiforme and variously disturbed urticarial, maculopapular, blotchy erythematous eruptions.

Basu RN, Jerek Z, Ward NA: The Eradication of Smallpox from India. New Delhi, India, World Health Organization, 1979. *A well-written, detailed, profusely illustrated book describing the epidemiologic and operational aspects of the program in India.*

*Available for experimental use only.

Dixon CW: Smallpox. London, J & A Churchill, Ltd., 1962. *A 500-page, well-illustrated book, which presents a comprehensive historical account of smallpox and vaccination as well as the clinical features, pathogenesis, and epidemiology of the disease and laboratory characteristics of the virus.*

Foege WH, Miller JD, Lane JM: Selective epidemiologic control in smallpox eradication. Am J Epidemiol 94:311, 1971. *A description of the surveillance-containment methodology in West Africa and its implications for the global program.*

Henderson DA: Smallpox: Eradication of a killer. *In* Medical and Health Annual. Chicago, Encyclopaedia Britannica, 1979, pp 125–141. *An illustrated account of the global eradication program.*

Lane JM, Ruben FL, Neff JM, Miller JD: Complications of smallpox vaccination, 1968. N Engl J Med 281:138, 1969. *With the paper by Neff et al., one of the few detailed studies of the frequency of complications following smallpox vaccination.*

McNeill WH: Plagues and People. Garden City, N.Y., Anchor Press/Doubleday, 1976. *An historian's account of the impact on history of a number of pestilential diseases, among which smallpox is prominently featured. Although some of the interpretations are subject to dispute, the book provides an unusual perspective.*

Nakano JH: Poxviruses. *In* Lennette EH, Schmidt NJ (eds.): Diagnostic Procedures for Viral, Rickettsial and Chlamydial Infections. New York, Americn Public Health Association, 1979, pp 257–308. *An exhaustive description of the virologic characteristics and diagnostic methods for the poxviruses.*

Neff J, Lane JM, Pert JH, Moore R, Miller JD, Henderson DA: Complications of smallpox vaccination. N Engl J Med 276:1, 1967. *With the paper by Lane et al., one of the few detailed studies of the frequency of complications following smallpox vaccination.*

Rao AR: Smallpox. Bombay, India, Kothari Book Depot, 1972. *Written by a clinician who treated more than 3000 cases, this book is an excellent reference on the clinical aspects of variola major.*

World Health Organization, Final Report of the Global Commission for the Certification of Smallpox Eradication. Geneva, WHO, 1979. *A comprehensive report of the eradication program, the activities which were conducted to certify eradication, and much useful statistical data about the program and its progress.*

Enteroviral Diseases

Raphael Dolin

341. INTRODUCTION

Enteroviruses cause a wide variety of diseases in humans and other mammals. These viral agents comprise a separate genus (enterovirus) within the Picornavirus (*pico*, small; *rna*, ribonucleic acid) family, and share the following common properties: (1) size of 17 to 30 nm, (2) capsids with cubic symmetry, (3) RNA genome, and (4) four major and one minor structural polypeptides. The virion lacks a lipid envelope, which renders the viruses resistant to lipid solvents.

Enteroviruses have been historically subdivided into *polioviruses, groups A* and *B coxsackieviruses,* and *echoviruses.* These divisions were based on antigenic relationships and differences in host range. Sixty-seven distinct immunotypes (species) were originally identified, although these have been reduced to 63 because of reclassification and redundancy in numbering (Table 341–1). However, this classification is not entirely satisfactory, since several enteroviruses have properties which overlap groups defined by the criteria cited above. Therefore, newly recognized enteroviruses are no longer classified as echoviruses or coxsackieviruses, but are simply designated "enterovirus," and are numbered sequentially beginning with enterovirus 68. To avoid confusion within the older literature, the previous classification (coxsackievirus groups A and B, and echovirus) has been retained for the 63 original immunotypes (Table 341–1).

Since infections with polioviruses are presented in Ch. 502, this discussion will be limited to consideration of nonpolio enteroviruses.

CHARACTERISTICS OF NONPOLIO ENTEROVIRUSES

COXSACKIEVIRUSES. Coxsackieviruses were originally isolated from stools of children who were suffering from paralytic poliomyelitis in Coxsackie, New York. Unlike polioviruses, these viruses cause disease in suckling mice and were therefore presumed to be distinct from polioviruses (see Table 341–1). Subsequently, additional coxsackievirus immunotypes have been isolated from widespread geographic locations. These viruses are divided into two groups, A and B, depending on the histopathology of lesions induced in mice. Group A coxsackieviruses produce a generalized myositis of skeletal muscle, which results in flaccid paralysis. Group B coxsackieviruses produce a focal myositis and a generalized infection of brown fat, myocardium, pancreas, and central nervous system, which results in spastic paralysis. Group B coxsackieviruses can be readily cultivated in primate tissue culture, whereas group A coxsackieviruses grow inconsistently or not at all in tissue culture. Twenty-three immunotypes of group A and six of group B have been identified.

ECHOVIRUSES. Echoviruses were first isolated from the stools of healthy children, but were not pathogenic for primates or suckling mice. They were given the acronym echo (*e*nteric

TABLE 341–1. CHARACTERISTICS OF HUMAN ENTEROVIRUSES

Virus	Number of Immunotypes	Numerical Designation	Isolated in Tissue Culture	Pathogenic for Suckling Mice	Pathogenic for Primates
Polioviruses	3	1–3	Yes	No	Yes
Coxsackieviruses A	23	A1–A24*	Occasionally†	Yes	No‡
Coxsackieviruses B	6	B1–B6	Yes	Yes	No
Echoviruses	31	1–34§	Yes	No	No
Enteroviruses**	4	68–71	Yes	Variable	No¶

*A23 has been reclassified as echovirus 9.
†Primary isolation in tissue culture is difficult for most immunotypes except A7, 11, 13, 15, 16, 18, 20, and 21.
‡Coxsackie A7 is neuropathogenic for monkeys.
§Echovirus 10 is reovirus 1; echovirus 28 is rhinovirus 1A; echovirus 34 is a variant of coxsackievirus A24.
¶Enterovirus 70 is neuropathogenic for monkeys.
**Hepatitis A virus will likely be classified as an enterovirus in the future.

TABLE 341–2. ILLNESSES ASSOCIATED WITH NONPOLIO ENTEROVIRUSES*

Coxsackieviruses Group A	Coxsackieviruses Group B	Echoviruses	Enteroviruses
Asymptomatic infection	Asymptomatic infection	Asymptomatic infection	Asymptomatic infection
Undifferentiated febrile illness with or without respiratory symptoms; common cold (21, 24); pneumonitis of infants (9, 16)	Undifferentiated febrile illness with or without respiratory symptoms; URI and pneumonia (4, 5)	Undifferentiated febrile illness with or without respiratory symptoms (4, 9, 11, 20, 25)	Undifferentiated febrile illness with or without respiratory symptoms; pneumonia, bronchiolitis (68)
Aseptic meningitis (1-14, 16, 17, 21, 22, 24); rare paralysis or encephalitis (4-7, 9, 10, 16)	Aseptic meningitis (1-6); rare paralysis or encephalitis (2-5)	Aseptic meningitis (all); rare paralysis or encephalitis (all except 23, 26, 28, 29, 32)	Aseptic meningitis (70, 71); paralysis (70)
Mucocutaneous infection: herpangina (2-6, 8, 10, 22); lymphonodular pharyngitis (10); hand-foot-and-mouth disease (5, 9, 10, 16); exanthem (4, 5, 6, 9, 16)	Myocarditis (1-5)†	Exanthem (2, 4, 6, 9, 11, 16, 18)	Acute hemorrhagic conjunctivitis (70)
Acute hemorrhagic conjunctivitis (24)	Pericarditis (1-5)†	Neonatal diarrhea (18)	Hand-foot-and-mouth disease (71)
	Pleurodynia (1-6)		Exanthem (71)
	Generalized disease of newborn (1-5)		
	Exanthem (1-5)		

*Immunotypes with strongest association are in parentheses.
†Myopericarditis has less frequently been associated with coxsackieviruses A1, 4, 9, and 16 and echoviruses 1, 3, 6 to 9, 11, 14, 19, 22, and 30.

cytopathic *h*uman *o*rphan), indicating that they were not associated with disease. Subsequently, a variety of diseases have been associated with echoviruses, and 31 immunotypes have been recognized. Most echoviruses can be readily cultivated in tissue culture (see Table 341–1).

NEWLY RECOGNIZED ENTEROVIRUSES. Four newly recognized enteroviruses, immunotypes 68 to 71, have been reported since the adoption of the new classification schema. Illnesses produced by enteroviruses 68 and 71 are similar to those produced by coxsackieviruses and echoviruses (Table 341–2). Enterovirus 70 causes acute hemorrhagic conjunctivitis and is discussed in Ch. 94. Enterovirus 69 has not as yet been associated with illness. In addition, hepatitis A virus is now known to have the biophysical properties of enteroviruses and will likely be classified within the enterovirus genus in the future. Hepatitis A infections are discussed in Ch. 120.

GENERAL FEATURES OF NONPOLIO ENTEROVIRAL INFECTIONS

EPIDEMIOLOGY. Enteroviruses have a worldwide distribution. In temperate climates, the incidence of infection and illness is markedly increased in the summer and early fall, although enterovirus-associated disease has been reported at other times as well. In tropical climates, enterovirus infections occur throughout the year. The prevalence of individual immunotypes varies widely according to geographic locale and year. Generally, one or two immunotypes account for the bulk of enterovirus-induced disease during any given season, but occasionally multiple immunotypes may be equally prevalent. Because of the prolonged shedding of virus from the gastrointestinal tract (see below), the presence of enteroviruses in surface waters and in sewage is a good indicator of the prevalence of infection in the community.

Transmission of enteroviruses is primarily by the fecal-oral route, and the frequency of infection is increased by factors that promote such transmission, e.g., poor hygiene and low socioeconomic status. Young children have the highest attack rates and serve as the vehicles for spread within communities. Once infection occurs within a family, susceptible (nonimmune) family members are rapidly infected. Coxsackievirus infections appear to be somewhat more communicable than echovirus infections.

PATHOGENESIS AND CLINICAL MANIFESTATIONS. Models of the pathogenesis of enteroviral infection are based largely on studies with polioviruses. However, the pathogenesis of nonpolio enteroviral infection appears to be similar, except for the major organs that are affected. Initial replication of the virus takes place in the oropharynx or in the gastrointestinal tract. Viral infection may be limited to the mucosa, or may proceed deeper into lymphoid tissue. The latter may be followed by viremia and dissemination of virus to distant organs, such as the heart or the central nervous system. The marked variation in clinical manifestations associated with nonpolio enteroviral infections reflects the relative involvement of different target organs (Table 341–2).

The bulk of enteroviral infections (50 to 80 per cent) are asymptomatic, and many of the remainder consist of "undifferentiated febrile illnesses," often with respiratory symptoms. The latter illnesses are generally mild and last a few days. The enterovirus infections most frequently coming to the attention of a physician are those resulting in central nervous system, heart, or skin involvement. Enteroviruses have been associated with a wide variety of clinical syndromes referable to those organ systems (Table 341–2), the most important of which are discussed below. As with "undifferentiated febrile illnesses," these syndromes are rarely sufficiently distinctive to permit diagnosis of infection with a particular immunotype. Immunotypes from different groups can produce similar syndromes, and alternatively a single immunotype can produce clinically diverse illnesses. Thus, coxsackievirus B1 can induce aseptic meningitis in one patient and pericarditis in another, even during the same outbreak. The factors that determine which clinical manifestation will be expressed in any individual infection are poorly understood.

LABORATORY DIAGNOSIS. Laboratory diagnosis is based on virus isolation and/or immunotype-specific antibody rises in acute and convalescent serum specimens. Enteroviruses can frequently be isolated from throat secretions and stools obtained from patients with enteroviral infections. Such isolations are most frequent in younger children, particularly in lower socioeconomic groups. However, interpretation of the significance of such isolates in individual cases is difficult. Intercurrent subclinical infections or prolonged fecal shedding of virus (up to three months) may occur, so that an etiologic association between an isolate and a current disease episode cannot be made with certainty. A rising titer of immunotype-specific antibodies in acute and convalescent sera indicates that a recent infection has taken place, but similarly does not assign an etiologic role to the virus in question. The strongest evidence for enteroviruses as etiologic agents of a variety of diseases originates from two sources: (1) large scale studies in which isolation rates from cases are matched with controls and (2) isolation of virus from sites from which asymptomatic shedding of virus does not occur, e.g., cerebrospinal fluid, myocardium, or pericardial fluid. In this regard, virus culture of blood has been reported to be useful in infants with enterovirus-related illness.

Serologic diagnosis of enteroviral infections is particularly difficult because group specific tests, such as complement fixation, do not exist, and thus immunotype-specific neutralization tests must be carried out. Since there are 67 currently recognized immunotypes, neutralization tests against all potential agents cannot be performed. Of necessity, neutralization tests must be limited to those directed against the patient's isolate (if one is present), or perhaps against isolates prevalent in the community. A possible exception is the case in which only a few immunotypes are likely to be present (e.g., hand-foot-and-mouth disease—coxsackievirus A16; myocarditis—coxsackieviruses B1 to 6). In addition, patients may be seen late in the course of illness, at which time high, stable antibody titers are present, which further reduces the utility of serologic tests.

PREVENTION AND TREATMENT. Highly successful live and inactivated virus vaccines directed against poliovirus infections have been developed (see Ch. 502). Immunity to nonpolio enteroviruses has been less well studied, but appears to be similarly dependent on the presence of immunotype-specific local and humoral antibodies. Thus, the development of vaccines against these agents is theoretically possible. However, the large number of immunotypes among nonpolio enteroviruses (67), as compared to polioviruses (3), and the benign nature of most enteroviral-induced disease have precluded the development of such vaccines.

Specific antiviral chemotherapy or chemoprophylaxis directed at enteroviral infection is not currently available. Treatment consists of symptomatic or supportive therapy for severe illness, particularly that involving the central nervous system or the heart (see below). However, the vast majority of enteroviral illnesses are self-limited and require no therapy. Appropriate control measures include maintenance of good hygienic practices such as hand washing, and proper disposal of potentially infectious stools. Isolation of patients is impractical and rarely indicated.

Grist NR, Bell EJ, Assad F: Enteroviruses in human disease. Prog Med Virol 24:114, 1978. *An excellent review with a comprehensive bibliography. Emphasis is on recent developments in the field.*

Moore M: Enteroviral disease in the United States, 1970–1979. J Infect Dis 146:103, 1982. *A summary of the most recent ten-year experience of surveillance data from the Centers for Disease Control. Provides an excellent epidemiologic overview.*

Young NA: Picornaviridae. *In* Mandell GL, Douglas RG, Bennett JE (eds.): Principles and Practice of Infectious Diseases. New York, John Wiley & Sons, 1979, p 1083. *The best single work which covers the molecular biology, epidemiology, and clinical manifestations of enteroviral diseases. Contains an exhaustive bibliography.*

POLIOMYELITIS AND ASEPTIC MENINGITIS

The most important enteroviral infections are poliomyelitis, discussed in Ch. 502, and aseptic meningitis caused by coxsackieviruses and enteroviruses, discussed in Ch. 499.

342. PARALYSIS AND OTHER NEUROLOGIC COMPLICATIONS OF NONPOLIO ENTEROVIRUSES

Paralysis has been rarely associated with nonpolio enteroviral infections. The majority of reported cases have been diagnosed on the basis of isolation of echoviruses and coxsackieviruses from stool, with relatively few isolations from central nervous system tissue or cerebrospinal fluid. Generally, muscle weakness rather than paralysis has been observed in these patients. When present, paralysis and weakness are generally less extensive than in poliomyelitis, and tend to resolve over a variable period of time. Cranial nerve and severe bulbar involvement have also been reported. Coxsackievirus A7 has been the immunotype most commonly implicated in paralytic disease, and small outbreaks have been recognized in the USSR and Scotland. A poliomyelitis-like syndrome has also been reported to accompany acute hemorrhagic conjunctivitis caused by enterovirus 70 (see Ch. 94). Other neurologic complications include transverse myelitis and the Guillain-Barré syndrome, although the precise relationship of these illnesses to enteroviral infection is unclear.

Infants, children, and occasionally young adults infected with nonpolio enteroviruses have developed encephalitis as manifested by seizures, coma, cerebellar ataxia, hemiplegia, or extrapyramidal movements. Up to 10 per cent of children who acquired enteroviral meningitis during the first year of life have developed mild mental retardation and spasticity, suggesting that involvement of central nervous system parenchyma may be more frequent than has previously been suspected. Echovirus infection of the central nervous system in agammaglobulinemic patients has resulted in a chronic meningoencephalitis associated with a dermatomyositis-like syndrome.

Grist NR, Bell EJ: Enteroviral etiology of the paralytic poliomyelitis syndrome. Arch Environ Health 21:382, 1970. *A good review of the uncommon association of nonpolio enteroviruses with paralytic disease.*

Wilfert CM, Buckley RH, Mohanakumarz T, Griffith JF, Katz SL, Whisnant JK, Eggleston PA, Moore M, Treadwell E, Oxman MN, Rosen FS: Persistent and fatal central nervous system echovirus infections in patients with agammaglobulinemia. N Engl J Med 26:1485, 1977. *A description of the syndrome of chronic echovirus central nervous system infection and dermatomyositis in patients with abnormal B cell function.*

343. EPIDEMIC PLEURODYNIA (Bornholm Disease, Epidemic Myalgia, Devil's Grip, Sylvest's Disease)

DEFINITION. Epidemic pleurodynia (*pleura*, side; *odyne*, pain) is an acute febrile disease characterized by sudden, sharp chest (intercostal) or abdominal pain. Pain is paroxysmal in nature, and relapses frequently occur after periods of well-being.

ETIOLOGY. Group B coxsackieviruses (1 to 6) are the major causes of pleurodynia. Outbreaks have also been associated with echovirus 1, and sporadic cases with coxsackieviruses A4, A6, and A10 and echoviruses 1, 6, 9, and 19.

EPIDEMIOLOGY. Epidemic pleurodynia was first described in the mid-nineteenth century in Iceland and Norway. In 1933, Sylvest published a classic monograph describing the illness on the Danish island of Bornholm. Subsequently, outbreaks and sporadic cases have been described in many parts of the world. In contrast to the annual occurrence of aseptic meningitis, epidemics of pleurodynia occur much less frequently, often 10 to 20 years apart. As with other enteroviral infections, illness is most common in summer and early fall. Person-to-person transmission occurs, particularly within families, with incubation periods of two to five days. Attack rates are highest in children, but the peak incidence is at a somewhat older age (5 to 15 years) than with other enteroviral infections.

PATHOGENESIS. Although detailed studies of the histopathology of pleurodynia are not available, the infection appears to involve skeletal muscle rather than pleura or peritoneum. Often muscle tenderness and occasionally swelling can be noted at the site of pain. Hyperesthesia can be elicited over affected muscles as well. In contrast, pleural rubs have been infrequently and inconstantly noted, and peritonitis has not been present in cases that have come to laparotomy. However, coxsackievirus B has not been unequivocally isolated from affected muscle.

CLINICAL MANIFESTATIONS. Characteristically, pleurodynia begins as an abrupt paroxysm of pain, located over the lateral chest (ribs) or upper abdomen. The pain is of variable intensity, but can be severe, and is often described as "catching," "stabbing," "crushing," or "vise-like." Acute shortness of breath is also frequently present. Adults most commonly have chest pain, whereas children more frequently have abdominal pain, generally in the epigastrium and upper abdomen. Patients have been described with pain primarily in the lower abdomen, as well as in the extremities. Prodromal symptoms are not present in the majority of cases, although up to 25 per cent of individuals report headache, malaise, myalgia, and sore throat prior to the onset of pain. Fever of 37.8 to 40.0° C is present at the onset of pain, but resolves between paroxysms. Multiple paroxysms of pain occur and last from two to ten hours, during which time the patient may appear diaphoretic and acutely ill. The initial paroxysm of pain is most severe, and subsequent ones are generally milder. Splinting of the chest or guarding of the abdomen is usually observed, so that in one outbreak 9 of 49 patients underwent laparotomy before the disease was recognized. Tenderness or swelling of the affected muscles, or both, has been noted in up to 25 per cent of cases. During paroxysms, patients tend to lie quietly in bed and try to avoid any motion which may aggravate the pain. The patient may appear relatively well between bouts of pain.

Acute illness generally lasts one to six days, but a range of up to three weeks has been reported. Approximately 10 per cent of the patients experience at least one recurrence of pain within one or more months after the last paroxysm. Such recurrences often develop at the same site as the initial paroxysm of pain.

LABORATORY DIAGNOSIS. Specific diagnosis is made by isolation of coxsackie B virus from the throat or stools of acutely ill patients, along with rises in immunotype-specific neutralizing antibody titers in acute and convalescent sera. Detection of virus is most frequent in samples taken early in illness. Other laboratory tests are not helpful in making the diagnosis. White blood cell and differential counts are generally normal, although mild leukopenia has been reported in approximately 25 per cent of cases.

DIFFERENTIAL DIAGNOSIS. Because of the location of the pain, Bornholm disease can be confused with a variety of acute chest diseases, including pneumonia, pulmonary infarction, and myocardial ischemia. The absence of physical and roentgenographic signs of pulmonary infiltrates, the lack of sputum production, and a normal ECG help exclude these diagnoses. When the pain is primarily abdominal, differentiation from other causes of an acute abdominal pain can be difficult. The absence of signs of peritonitis and a normal white cell count may be helpful. The most useful distinguishing clinical feature of Bornholm disease is the paroxysmal nature of the pain. Epidemiologic information, such as the occurrence of a cluster of cases in the late summer, may also suggest the diagnosis.

PROGNOSIS AND TREATMENT. Patients with epidemic pleurodynia will eventually recover fully, although relapses are common (see above). Occasionally, malaise or asthenia may persist for months after the acute illness. Complications are uncommon, but may include aseptic meningitis (3 to 7 per cent of cases), orchitis (less than 5 per cent) and rarely pericarditis.

Treatment is entirely supportive and symptomatic. Episodes of acute pain can usually be controlled by salicylates or other mild analgesics. Occasionally, narcotic analgesics may be required for relief.

Finn JJ Jr, Weller TH, Morgan HR: Epidemic pleurodynia: Clinical and etiologic studies based on one hundred and fourteen cases. Arch Intern Med 83:305, 1949. *An excellent clinical review of the subject.*

Huebner RJ, Risser JA, Bell JA, Beeman EA, Biegelman PM, Strong JC: Epidemic pleurodynia in Texas: A study of 22 cases. N Engl J Med 248:267, 1953. *Demonstration of the viral etiology of an outbreak of pleurodynia.*

Pickles NW: Sylvest's disease (Bornholm disease). N Engl J Med 250:1033, 1954. *A vivid and dramatic discussion of the clinical presentation.*

Sylvest E: Epidemic Myalgia: Bornholm Disease. London, Oxford University Press, 1934, pp 1-155. *The classic monograph in the field.*

344. MYOCARDITIS AND PERICARDITIS CAUSED BY ENTEROVIRUSES

Enteroviruses are well recognized causes of myocarditis and pericarditis, with clinical manifestations that appear to be age dependent. Neonatal infection is a severe illness in which extensive involvement of the myocardium, widespread dissemination to other organs, and high fatality rates are seen. In older children and adults, pericarditis is most prominent, and the disease is generally self-limited.

ETIOLOGY. The group B coxsackieviruses, immunotypes 1 to 5, are the enteroviruses most frequently implicated in pericarditis and myocarditis. Depending on the study, group B coxsackieviruses have been reported to cause from 3 to 44 per cent of cases of acute pericarditis and approximately 33 per cent of cases of acute myocarditis. Group A coxsackieviruses (1, 4, 9, and 16) and echoviruses (1, 3, 6 to 9, 19, and 22) have also been implicated, but considerably less frequently. Since routine serologic testing is available for group B but not for group A coxsackieviruses or echoviruses, it is conceivable that the proportion of cases caused by the latter groups may be higher. The etiology of the majority of cases of "idiopathic" pericarditis and myocarditis remains unknown.

EPIDEMIOLOGY. Enteroviral myopericarditis occurs most frequently during the summer and early fall, and both epidemics and sporadic cases are seen. Neonatal myocarditis was first recognized in outbreaks in nurseries for the newborn in South Africa, Rhodesia, and the Netherlands in the mid-1950's. Subsequent reports have been largely confined to sporadic cases. Illness in nursery outbreaks appears to be postnatally acquired, presumably by the fecal-oral route. However, cases in which infection was acquired at birth and even in utero have been described. In the latter cases, infection of mothers appeared to take place within two weeks of delivery.

Among older children and adults, myopericardial involvement with enteroviral infection is sporadic, and even in the presence of outbreaks of enteroviral infection myopericardial involvement in this age group is uncommon. Despite the likely overreporting of serious infections, only 3 per cent of group B coxsackievirus infections reported to the World Health Organization involved the myocardium predominantly.

PATHOGENESIS. Infection of the heart by enteroviruses is most likely a result of viremia after initial replication of virus in the gastrointestinal tract. Histopathology of acute enteroviral myocarditis consists of a mixed polymorphonuclear leukocytic and lymphocytic infiltrate, which can be either diffuse or focal. Focal myocardial muscle degeneration and necrosis are also seen. The histopathology of enterovirus-induced pericarditis is similar, and is frequently accompanied by focal areas of subepicardial myocarditis. For this reason, some authors prefer the term "myopericarditis" rather than simply "pericarditis."

During acute illness, virus may be isolated from myocardium, pericardium, or pericardial fluid, and therefore the pathogenesis appears to be direct viral invasion of myopericardium. However, chronic inflammatory lesions from which infectious virus cannot be isolated have been described in humans and in experimental myocarditis. Chronic lesions, and perhaps clinically apparent relapses, may have an immunopathologic basis. Direct evidence is lacking in humans, but in weanling mice the severity of coxsackie B3 myocarditis is increased by intact T-lymphocyte functions.

CLINICAL MANIFESTATIONS. ***Neonatal Myocarditis.*** Myocarditis of the newborn presents from two days to three weeks after birth (mean of seven days) with the acute onset of fever and listlessness, often accompanied by coryza and/or diarrhea. When congestive heart failure is present, respiratory distress and tachycardia are prominent. In approximately one third of patients, a biphasic illness is seen. The first phase consists of a febrile prodrome followed by a period of well-being lasting one to seven days, after which the phase of clinically evident cardiac involvement appears. The latter is predominantly myocarditis with little or no pericarditis. Circulatory failure can develop rapidly and be profound, as manifested by cyanosis, abdominal distention, and edema. In addition, viral infection may be disseminated widely, with involvement of the central nervous system, lungs, liver, pancreas, spleen, and kidney. In cases of fulminant disease, death may ensue within 24 hours, although the majority of fatalities occur two to seven days after the onset of illness. Among survivors, cardiac function and general well-being improve rapidly once the fever and acute illness have resolved.

Myopericarditis of Older Children and Adults. In older children and adults, the clinical features of enteroviral infection of the heart are those of acute pericarditis. Sixty to 90 per cent of patients present with fever and chest pain, preceded by an upper respiratory tract illness in approximately two thirds of cases. The chest pain is most frequently precordial and dull, but can on occasion be sharp with pleuritic and positional components. Dyspnea, malaise, myalgias, and arthralgias are frequently seen. Physical examination reveals a pericardial friction rub, often transient, in 36 to 76 per cent of cases. Pericardial effusions have been reported in 0 to 45 per cent of cases, but acute cardiac tamponade is rare. Increased areas of cardiac dullness and gallop rhythms have been reported in up to 25 per cent of patients in some series, but are ordinarily not observed. Despite histopathologic evidence of subepicardial myocarditis accompanying pericarditis, clinically apparent congestive heart failure is unusual. When present, the latter indicates widespread myocardial involvement. Serologic evidence for enteroviral infection in cases clinically diagnosed as acute myocardial infarctions has been reported, but the etiologic role, if any, of viruses in that setting is unknown. Pleural effusions, particularly left-sided, have been reported in 20 to 50 per cent of cases of enterovirus-associated myopericarditis.

LABORATORY DIAGNOSIS. The etiology of illness is established by isolation of enterovirus from the myocardium, pericardium, or pericardial fluid. Specimens from these sites should be submitted for virus isolation whenever available. However, only throat and/or stool cultures are obtained in the majority of cases. Isolation of virus from these latter sites, along with rises in immunotype-specific serum antibodies, provides circumstantial evidence for the diagnosis of enteroviral myopericarditis. Diagnosis is made more difficult by the fact that many patients present late in the course of illness, when virus shedding has ceased, and when high, stable titers of antibodies are already present. In the latter case, detection of immunotype-specific IgM antibodies indicates recent infection.

The laboratory hallmark of myopericarditis is an abnormal ECG, seen in virtually all cases. Changes in pericarditis or mild myopericarditis are S-T segment elevation and T wave flattening or inversion. In severe myocarditis, Q waves, conduction disturbances, and arrhythmias can be seen. In the latter cases, elevations of myocardial enzymes have been noted. Chest x-ray reveals enlargement of the cardiac silhouette in 50 to 75 per cent of cases, which may reflect either cardiac dilatation or pericardial effusion. To determine the presence and location of effusions, echocardiograms can be very helpful. Analyses of pericardial fluid in documented viral myopericarditis have been infrequent, but the characteristics of the fluid are generally those of an exudate, with a predominantly polymorphonuclear leukocytic content. Considerable overlap exists between the cell counts, differentials, and protein content of pericardial fluid in cases of viral pericarditis and fluid from cases of pericarditis of other etiologies.

Other laboratory tests are generally not helpful in establishing the diagnosis. A moderate polymorphonuclear leukocytosis may be present, and elevated erythrocyte sedimentation rates have been reported in 70 to 90 per cent of patients.

DIFFERENTIAL DIAGNOSIS. Neonatal myocarditis can mimic pneumonia, bacterial sepsis, or other disseminated viral infections such as those caused by herpes simplex and cytomegalovirus. The prominent ECG changes, evidence of congestive heart failure, and absence of skin lesions may be helpful in suggesting the diagnosis of neonatal myocarditis. The differential diagnosis of myopericarditis in older patients is discussed in Ch. 51 and 52.

PROGNOSIS. Neonatal myocarditis was initially reported to have an extremely high case-fatality rate; however, recent experience suggests that with aggressive supportive therapy, mortality is less than 50 per cent. Long-term follow-up of survivors is not available.

The majority of older children and adults with enteroviral myopericarditis recover without clinically apparent sequelae. The duration of illness is highly variable (days to weeks), and up to 20 per cent of patients experience one or more episodes of recurrent myopericarditis within one year of the initial illness. Electrocardiographic abnormalities may persist in 10 to 20 per cent of patients, and long-term cardiomegaly has been described in 5 to 10 per cent. Constrictive pericarditis is an extremely rare complication. Chronic congestive heart failure also appears to be an unusual sequel of illness, although in one series 5 of 22 patients were reported to have this complication. The role of enterovirus-induced myocarditis in chronic cardiomyopathies of unknown etiology remains controversial.

TREATMENT. Specific antiviral chemotherapy for enteroviral infections is not available. Management of patients with enteroviral myopericarditis consists primarily of control of pain with analgesics and treatment of arrhythmias or congestive heart failure as they appear (see Ch. 42 and 50). In experimentally induced myocarditis in mice, vigorous exercise is deleterious, and therefore bed rest or restriction of activity is frequently recommended to patients. Corticosteroids also increase the severity of infection in the same animal model, but anecdotal reports of corticosteroid treatment of cases in humans have claimed either benefit or lack of harm. Controlled studies of corticosteroid therapy of enteroviral myopericarditis are not available.

PREVENTION. Specific preventive measures have not been developed. In neonatal myocarditis, patients and mothers should be isolated as a unit, and women at term should subsequently be admitted to a separate facility. Isolation of cases of myopericarditis in older children and adults is not indicated (see Ch. 89).

Grist NR, Bell EJ: A six-year study of coxsackievirus B infections in heart disease. J Hyg 73:165, 1974. *A solid, laboratory based investigation of the problem.*

Lansdown ABG: Viral infections and diseases of the heart. Prog Med Virol 24:70, 1978. *A comprehensive review of infections with all known virus groups, as well as with enteroviruses.*

Lerner MA: Myocarditis and pericarditis. *In* Mandell GL, Douglas RG, Bennett DE (eds.): Principles and Practice of Infectious Diseases. New York, John Wiley & Sons, 1979, p 711. *A thoughtful review of the subject, with a good presentation of the evidence for a viral etiology. Mechanisms of pathogenesis are also discussed.*

Sainani GS, Krompotic E, Slodki SJ: Adult heart disease due to coxsackievirus B infection. Medicine 47:133, 1968. *A study of 22 adult patients which illustrates the clinical presentations and difficulty in establishing an etiologic diagnosis.*

Woodruff J: Viral myocarditis: A review. Am J Pathol 101:425, 1980. *A good general review of the subject.*

345. MUCOCUTANEOUS INFECTIONS CAUSED BY ENTEROVIRUSES

ENANTHEMS

Herpangina (*herpes*, vesicular eruption; *angina*, inflammation of the throat) is a vesicular eruption of the posterior pharynx which is most frequently caused by coxsackievirus A (1 to 6, 8, 10, 16, and 22), although other enteroviruses have also been implicated. Lesions most commonly occur on the soft palate and anterior pillars of the tonsils, and less commonly on the posterior pharyngeal wall or buccal mucosa. Illness begins abruptly with fever ranging from 37.8 to 40.5° C, sore throat, and dysphagia. The pharynx appears mildly injected, with little or no tonsillar exudate. Discrete oropharyngeal lesions can be seen, which begin as macules, progress to gray papules, and eventually become erythematous-based vesicles, 2 to 5 mm in diameter. Lesions progress from macules to papules over a period of one to two days, and may evolve into ulcers that can last up to one week. The lesions are usually less than six in number, occasionally up to twelve, and are only moderately painful. Malaise, myalgia, and headache frequently accompany the fever at the onset of illness, but resolve over two to four days as the fever abates. Abdominal pain and vomiting have also been noted during acute illness.

Acute lymphonodular pharyngitis is a syndrome in which lesions occur with a distribution similar to that seen in herpangina. However, the lesions consist of small nodules of lymphocytes on an erythematous base, rather than vesicles or ulcers. Mild to moderate fever, headache, and sore throat are present as in herpangina, and symptoms last 4 to 14 days. Coxsackievirus A10 has been isolated from patients with this syndrome.

Hand-foot-and-mouth disease (vesicular stomatitis with exanthem) is a mucocutaneous infection with both an enanthem and an exanthem. The enanthem consists of vesicles and/or ulcers in the anterior pharynx, most commonly on the anterior buccal mucosa, tongue, lips, and hard palate. The oral lesions are accompanied in 75 per cent of cases by vesicular or papulovesicular lesions on the palms, soles, or extensor surfaces of the hands and feet. Occasionally, lesions are seen on the buttocks or genitalia. Lesions are surrounded by erythema and are usually tender. Initially, patients complain of sore throat or refuse to eat, and manifest a low grade fever (38 to 39° C) for 24 to 48 hours. Illness is generally mild and lasts less than one week. This syndrome is caused most frequently by coxsackievirus A16, less frequently by A5, A9, and A10, and occasionally by B2 or B5 or enterovirus 71.

EPIDEMIOLOGY. As with other enteroviral infections, the enanthems are seen most frequently during the summer and early fall. Attack rates are highest in younger children, but cases occur in adolescents and young adults as well. Both sporadic cases and outbreaks have been described. Several children within a family unit can become infected sequentially, with an incubation period of two to ten days. Less frequently, illness can spread to adults. Asymptomatic infection of contacts is common.

DIFFERENTIAL DIAGNOSIS. Herpangina and acute lymphonodular pharyngitis involve the posterior pharynx, whereas hand-foot-and-mouth disease involves the anterior pharynx. The latter is associated with cutaneous lesions which are absent in herpangina. Primary herpes simplex stomatitis is also an anterior stomatitis, but often has gingivitis and more prominent systemic signs and symptoms, including cervical lymphadenitis. Chickenpox occasionally has an enanthem, but cutaneous lesions are more numerous and widely distributed than in hand-foot-and-mouth disease. Bacterial pharyngitis or tonsillitis is generally manifested by more systemic signs of illness, as well as by the presence of more extensive pharyngeal exudate. However, individual cases of bacterial infection may be difficult to distinguish from those caused by enteroviruses. Bacterial pharyngitis, as well as pharyngitis caused by viruses other than enteroviruses, generally does not produce vesicular lesions.

LABORATORY DIAGNOSIS. The principles of diagnosis are the same as those discussed in Ch. 89. Virus is frequently isolated from throat, stool, or vesicular lesions.

TREATMENT. The enteroviral enanthems are benign, self-limited illnesses which ordinarily require only symptomatic therapy for sore throat and headache.

EXANTHEMS

Nonpolio enteroviruses cause a variety of exanthems that accompany "undifferentiated febrile illness" or specific disease syndromes such as aseptic meningitis, or that occur independently. The rate of exanthems associated with enteroviral infection is highest in young children, and the pathogenesis of the majority of these exanthems has not been clearly established. Virus has been isolated from the vesicular exanthem associated with hand-foot-and-mouth disease, and it is likely that these lesions are the result of viremia. Virus isolation has not been reported from enteroviral maculopapular exanthems, and some authors have suggested that an immunopathologic component may be present.

The characteristics of the enterovirus exanthems are not sufficiently distinctive for establishment of an etiologic diagnosis on clinical grounds alone. Multiple immunotypes of echoviruses, coxsackieviruses, and enterovirus 71 cause exanthems. The most common clinical presentation is that of a *morbilliform* exanthem which is caused most frequently by echovirus 9. The rash consists of fine, discrete macules and/or papules, and occurs primarily on the face, neck, and, to a lesser extent, chest and extremities. It is most commonly confused with rubella, although posterior cervical and auricular lymphadenopathy are generally not present. Occasionally, rashes may have petechial components and even frank purpura, which may lead to confusion with meningococcemia. Fever is generally low grade and is present at the time that the rash develops. The rash and fever last for three to seven days. Both outbreaks and sporadic cases have been described.

Roseoliform exanthems have been caused most commonly by echovirus 16 ("the Boston exanthem"). Typically, fever (38 to 39.5° C) appears first, and the rash develops as the fever subsides. The rash consists of salmon pink macules and papules on the face and chest, but may involve the extremities on occasion. Fever lasts for 24 to 36 hours, and the rash persists for one to five days. The rashes in roseoliform as well as rubelliform exanthems are usually not pruritic or painful, and complete resolution is the rule. As with other enteroviral-induced illnesses, exanthems are seen most frequently in the summer and early fall. Attack rates are highest in very young children, and both epidemic and sporadic cases are seen.

Diagnosis of enteroviral exanthems depends on laboratory demonstration of viral infection, as discussed in Ch. 89. In general, patients with enteroviral exanthems are only mildly ill, although occasionally infants may be more severely affected. Since little morbidity is associated with enteroviral exanthems, supportive or symptomatic therapy is rarely required. However, the presence of enteroviral exanthems should alert physicians to the potential development of other types of enteroviral illness in the community.

Adler JL, Mostow SR, Mellin H, Janney JH, Joseph JM: Epidemiologic investigation of hand-foot-and-mouth disease. Am J Dis Child 120:309, 1970. *A detailed investigation of an outbreak due to coxsackievirus A16.*

Horstmann DM: Viral exanthems and enanthems. Pediatrics 41:867, 1968. *A concise review of the subject.*

Huebner RJ, Cole RM, Beeman EA, Bell JA, Peers JH: Herpangina. Etiologic studies of a specific infectious disease. JAMA 145:628, 1951. *Demonstration of association of herpangina with coxsackievirus A infection.*

Neva FA, Feemster RF, Gorbach IJ: Clinical and epidemiological features of an unusual epidemic exanthem. JAMA 155:544, 1954. *The original description of the Boston exanthem.*

Sabin AB, Krumbiegel ER, Wigand R: ECHO type 9 virus disease. J Dis Child 96:197, 1958. *A detailed review of the spectrum of disease associated with an epidemic of this immunotype and the types of rashes which were present.*

346. ACUTE HEMORRHAGIC CONJUNCTIVITIS

DEFINITION. Acute hemorrhagic conjunctivitis (AHC) is an acute viral infection of the eye characterized by painful conjunctival inflammation, subconjunctival hemorrhages, and swelling of the eyelids. AHC has occurred in explosive epidemics in Africa, India, and Asia.

ETIOLOGY. Epidemic AHC has been caused primarily by enterovirus 70. A smaller number of cases have been caused by coxsackievirus A24 and by adenovirus 11.

EPIDEMIOLOGY. Epidemics of AHC caused by enterovirus 70 first appeared almost simultaneously in Ghana and Indonesia in 1969. Extensive outbreaks were subsequently observed in northern and southeastern Africa, as well as in India, Southeast Asia, and other areas of the Far East. Localized outbreaks have occurred in the United Kingdom, continental Europe, and the USSR. The USSR outbreaks have been most often related to index cases in travelers and subsequent spread at eye clinics. Cases in the United States had been reported only in Southeast Asian refugees until 1981, when cases originating in the Western hemisphere with subsequent spread to the southern United States were first noted.

Patterns of antibody prevalence to enterovirus 70 suggest

that AHC has emerged as a relatively new disease. In endemic areas, antibody studies of serum specimens obtained prior to 1969 revealed low or absent levels of neutralizing antibody to enterovirus 70 in the population. After the occurrence of epidemics in 1969–72, antibody prevalence rates of 40 to 50 per cent were noted, indicating that widespread subclinical as well as clinical infection had taken place. Attack rates for clinical illness are highest among young adults, but infection is most common in young children. It is estimated that tens of millions of cases of AHC caused by enterovirus 70 have occurred since 1969. Simultaneously, a variant of coxsackievirus A24 has been implicated in several hundred thousand cases of AHC, including cases in mixed outbreaks.

PATHOGENESIS. In contrast to other enteroviral infections, AHC is spread by fomites and by direct inoculation of conjunctiva from contaminated fingers. Incubation periods are relatively short (12 to 72 hours), and likely reflect the large inoculum transmitted by these means. Transmission rates are increased by crowding and by poor hygiene. Enterovirus 70 appears to replicate preferentially at 33 to 35° C, which may represent an adaptation to conjunctival temperatures, rather than to the higher temperatures of the gut.

CLINICAL MANIFESTATIONS. AHC begins abruptly with pain, photophobia, swelling of the eyelids, and serous or seromucous conjunctival discharge. Involvement is initially unilateral but rapidly spreads to the other eye. Subconjunctival hemorrhages are present in up to 90 per cent of patients with disease caused by enterovirus 70, but are less frequent in disease caused by coxsackievirus A24. Lesions vary in size from petechiae to hemorrhages that cover the entire bulbar conjunctiva. Conjunctival folliculitis and preauricular lymphadenopathy are also frequently present. Slit lamp examination often reveals corneal erosions or punctate epithelial keratitis. Low grade fever, headache, coryza, and malaise may be present in up to 20 per cent of cases.

LABORATORY DIAGNOSIS. Virus can be recovered from conjunctival scrapings in a high proportion of cases. Unlike other enteroviral infections, virus is rarely isolated from the throat or stool. The diagnosis is supported by immunotype-specific antibody rises in acute and convalescent sera.

PROGNOSIS. Signs and symptoms peak on the first day of illness, abate over the next 48 hours, and resolve within ten days. Permanent sequelae are rare, although discoloration from hemorrhages can persist for days. Keratitis rarely leads to permanent corneal damage. Occasionally, secondary bacterial infection may follow the acute viral conjunctivitis. In adults, a rare aseptic meningitis accompanied by a poliomyelitis-like motor paralysis has been reported usually in association with enterovirus 70 infection. Paralysis develops 5 to 42 days after acute illness and has been observed almost exclusively in adults with an increased prevalence in men. The pathogenesis of the neurologic syndrome is unclear, although enterovirus 70 has been reported to be neuropathogenic in monkeys.

TREATMENT AND PREVENTION. Treatment is entirely symptomatic. If bacterial conjunctivitis develops, topical application of antibacterial ophthalmic ointment is indicated. Prevention of spread of AHC depends on careful handwashing, avoidance of contaminated towels or clothing, and sterilization of ophthalmologic instruments.

Arnow JC, Hierholzer JC, Higbee J, Harris DH: Acute hemorrhagic conjunctivitis: A mixed virus outbreak among Vietnamese refugees on Guam. Am J Epidemiol 105:68, 1977. *Description of an outbreak caused by enterovirus 70 and adenovirus 11.*

Christopher S, Theogaraj S, Godbole S, John TS: An epidemic of acute hemorrhagic conjunctivitis due to coxsackievirus A24. J Infect Dis 146:16, 1982. *Report of a large outbreak of AHC in India with good clinical descriptions and virologic studies.*

Hierholzer JC, Hilliard KA, Esposito JJ: Serosurvey for "acute hemorrhagic conjunctivitis" virus (enterovirus 70) antibodies in the southeastern United States, with review of the literature and some epidemiologic implications. Am J Epidemiol 102:533, 1975. *A detailed review of the seroepidemiology and spread of this agent.*

347. RESPIRATORY TRACT ILLNESS ASSOCIATED WITH ENTEROVIRUSES

Enteroviruses have been associated with upper respiratory tract illness, primarily the "common cold syndrome," in both children and adults. Lower respiratory tract illness, including bronchitis, tracheitis, bronchiolitis, croup, and pneumonia, has been induced by enteroviruses in children, but infrequently in adults. The majority of respiratory tract symptoms have presented as part of the "undifferentiated febrile illness" or "summer grippe" associated with enteroviral infections (see Table 341–2). Coxsackievirus A21 has caused outbreaks of pharyngitis in military recruits and has induced respiratory tract disease in normal adult volunteers. Group B coxsackieviruses, enterovirus 68, and several echoviruses (chiefly echovirus 11) have also been implicated as causes of respiratory tract illness. Respiratory illness induced by enteroviruses cannot be differentiated on clinical grounds from that caused by respiratory tract viruses, such as rhinoviruses, parainfluenza viruses, respiratory syncytial virus, or adenoviruses. However, infection with the latter groups of viruses occurs most frequently during the winter months, whereas enterovirus infection is seen most frequently in the summer and early fall. Viral respiratory tract infections are discussed in Ch. 73 to 78.

Viral Disease of the Gastrointestinal Tract

348. VIRAL GASTROENTERITIS (Acute Infectious Nonbacterial Gastroenteritis, Epidemic Diarrhea, Winter Vomiting Disease)

Raphael Dolin

DEFINITION. The term "nonbacterial gastroenteritis," along with the descriptive phrases cited above, refers to a group of acute, common, self-limited illnesses characterized chiefly by vomiting and/or diarrhea. An infectious etiology for these diseases had been previously suspected, but it has only been recently that specific viral agents that cause at least a portion of such illnesses have been detected.

ETIOLOGY. Two groups of viral agents that induce acute gastroenteritis have been described. The first is the Norwalk-like agents, generally named after the location of the outbreak from which they have been derived (Norwalk, Hawaii, Montgomery County, Marin County, Snow Mountain, "W," Ditchling, Cockle, and Parramatta agents). These agents have not been cultivated in vitro and have been only partly characterized. They are small (approximately 25 to 32 nm in diameter), nonenveloped viral agents found in the stools of acutely ill patients. Since the Norwalk-like agents have been only partly characterized biochemically, definitive classification within virus families is not possible at this time. Preliminary analysis of the Norwalk-like agents has detected at least five antigenic types.

The second group is the rotaviruses, which have been classified within the family of Reoviridae. They are 66 to 70 nm in diameter, contain double-stranded RNA in 11 discrete segments, and have a characteristic double shell appearance. Although strain differences have not been fully analyzed, human rotaviruses appear to be of two subgroups and at least four neutralization serotypes. Human rotaviruses have recently been grown efficiently in vitro by employing rhesus monkey kidney cells in roller tubes to which trypsin has been added. Rotaviruses can be detected directly in stool by a variety of techniques (see later discussion).

In addition, other groups of viruses have been implicated in outbreaks of gastroenteritis. These include noncultivatable adenoviruses, astroviruses, caliciviruses, and coronaviruses. The etiologic association of these agents with human gastroenteritis is less well established than that for rotaviruses and Norwalk-like agents. Additional studies are required to determine the relative importance of those virus groups.

The enteroviruses (coxsackieviruses, echoviruses), discussed in Ch. 89 to 95, commonly infect the gastrointestinal tract but do not appear to be major causes of acute gastroenteritis. Echovirus 18 has been implicated in an outbreak of diarrhea in a nursery for newborns.

EPIDEMIOLOGY. Because of the lack of suitable detection methods, seroepidemiologic studies have been carried out only with the Norwalk and Snow Mountain agents within the Norwalk-like group. Naturally occurring illness with these agents appears to be exceedingly common and widespread, and to involve all age groups. In one study, evidence of infection with the Norwalk agent was found in 34 per cent of 70 outbreaks of acute nonbacterial gastroenteritis. Infection with the Norwalk or Snow Mountain agent generally occurs late in childhood, so that antibody prevalence rates rise from less than 20 per cent by age 5 to 50 per cent or greater by age 19. Illness occurs most frequently during the winter months, but outbreaks in other seasons have been reported. Both sporadic cases and explosive outbreaks have been noted, including several common source outbreaks, which have involved shellfish, drinking water, and swimming pools.

In contrast to the Norwalk-like agents, illness associated with rotaviruses has a striking predilection for the very young. Rotavirus-induced gastroenteritis occurs most frequently between 6 and 24 months of age, and occasionally up to four years of age. Widespread infection occurs, so that 52 to 90 per cent of individuals above two years of age have serum antibody against rotavirus. Illness in neonates, older children, and adults is infrequent but can occur. Asymptomatic reinfection in older age groups is common.

Rotavirus infections are worldwide in distribution, and are seen primarily during the winter months in both Northern and Southern Hemispheres. Cases occur both sporadically and in distinct outbreaks. Rotavirus infections have accounted for 42 to 55 per cent of infants and young children hospitalized with gastroenteritis in studies carried out throughout the world.

PATHOGENESIS. Acute infection with Norwalk and Hawaii agents results in reversible histopathologic lesions, which primarily involve the upper jejunum, with relative sparing of the stomach and rectum. The jejunal mucosa remains intact, but there is marked blunting of villi and shortening of microvilli. The lamina propria is infiltrated with both polymorphonuclear and mononuclear cells. Acute illness is also accompanied by malabsorption of d-xylose and fat. Rotavirus infections induce a similar pathology in the duodenum and jejunum, although inflammatory changes can on occasion be seen in the stomach and rectum.

In human volunteer studies, resistance to rotaviral infection correlated with the presence of circulating antibody, while the relationship to local antibody was less clear-cut. Resistance to infection with the Norwalk-like agents appears to be unrelated to serum antibody titers, but other determinants of immunity are not well understood.

CLINICAL MANIFESTATIONS. Illness induced by the Norwalk-like agents consists of nausea, abdominal cramps, vomiting and/or diarrhea, often accompanied by headache and myalgias. Onset of illness is often abrupt, and both vomiting and diarrhea usually occur, although either can be present alone. Low grade fever (38.9° C) can be found in approximately 50 to 60 per cent of patients. The incubation period for illness is generally from 18 to 48 hours, and disease manifestations last from 48 to 72 hours. Disease remits spontaneously and without known sequelae. Rotavirus infections have clinical features similar to those described for the Norwalk-like agents. Incubation periods range from 24 to 96 hours, and among hospitalized children illness lasts for five to eight days. Even in the latter cases, illness appears to be generally mild, although occasionally more severe and rarely fatal cases have been reported.

DIAGNOSIS. Infection with Norwalk-like agents currently can be detected only by immune electron microscopy or by radioimmunoassay, which are specialized techniques not widely available. Norwalk agent is found in stools during the first four to five days of illness, and serum antibody rises are noted two to six weeks later. Rotaviruses are easily detected in stools by a variety of techniques, including complement fixation (CF), immunofluorescence, conventional electron microscopy, and enzyme-linked immunosorbent assays (ELISA). Virus can be found in stools for up to eight days and occasionally longer after onset of illness, and serum antibody rises are seen by two weeks after illness.

Infection with Norwalk-like agents or rotaviruses can be suspected on the basis of epidemiologic information (age, time of year, secondary cases). Although illness is generally milder than that observed with several bacterial pathogens, individual cases cannot be differentiated from other causes of acute gastroenteritis on clinical grounds alone. Fecal leukocytes are absent in Norwalk-induced disease, and are usually absent in rotavirus infections, which may prove helpful for early differentiation from *Shigella* or *Salmonella* enteritis (see Ch. 173 and 179).

TREATMENT. Acute viral gastroenteritis is generally a benign, self-limited illness which requires no specific therapy. In some cases, particularly in the very young or debilitated, fluid replacement may be necessary; this can generally be provided in the form of clear liquids by mouth. With severe fluid loss, intravenous fluid and electrolyte replacement should be administered promptly. Occasionally, symptomatic treatment of headache or nausea may be required. Administration of bismuth subsalicylate has resulted in a mild reduction in symptoms in Norwalk-induced illness, but the effect of administration of inhibitors of intestinal motility in viral gastroenteritis has not been studied. Restriction of activity during acute illness according to the patient's own symptoms appears to be prudent.

PREVENTION. There are currently no available methods for prevention of viral gastroenteritis, which represents a major uncontrolled public health problem. Considerable interest exists in the development of live attenuated vaccines directed against rotaviruses. Candidate vaccines would have to be safe and effective in very young age groups.

Dolin R, Blacklow R, Chanock RM: Biological properties of Norwalk agent of acute infectious nonbacterial gastroenteritis. Proc Soc Exp Biol Med 140:578, 1972. *The initial description of experimentally induced illness associated with the Norwalk agent and the biologic properties of the infectious agent.*

Dolin R, Reichman RC, Roessner KD, Tralka TS, Schooley RT, Gary W, Morens D: Detection by immune electron microscopy of the Snow Mountain agent of acute viral gastroenteritis. J Infect Dis 146:184, 1982. *Description of the use of immune electron microscopy for detection of the Snow Mountain agent, as well as the humoral immune response to infection.*

Greenberg HB, Wyatt RG, Kalica AR, Yolken RH, Black R, Kapikian AZ, Chanock RM: New insights in viral gastroenteritis. *In* Perspectives in Virology. Vol XI. New York, John Wiley & Sons, 1981, p 163. *Current review of Norwalk and rotavirus infections, with an extensive bibliography.*

Kapikian AZ, Kim HW, Wyatt RG, Cline WL, Arrobio JO, Brandt CO, Rodriguez WJ, Sack DA, Chanock RM, Parrot RH: Human reovirus-like agent as the major pathogen associated with winter gastroenteritis in hospitalized infants and young children. N Engl J Med 294:965, 1976. *A prospective study demonstrating the importance of rotavirus infection in very young children.*

Sato K, Inaba Y, Shinozaki T, Fujii R, Matumoto M: Isolation of human rotavirus in cell cultures. Arch Virol 69:155, 1981. *Description of the technique employed to cultivate human rotavirus efficiently in vitro.*

Tyrrell DAJ, Kapikian AZ: Virus Infections of the Gastrointestinal Tract. New York, Marcel Dekker, Inc., 1982. *An entire volume devoted to viral infections of the gastrointestinal tract, with chapters on virology, pathophysiology, and immune response. An excellent reference source for in-depth reading.*

Arthropod-Borne Viral Fevers

349. INTRODUCTION

Karl M. Johnson

Arthropod-borne viruses (arboviruses) and the diseases they produce in man can be defined in a variety of ways. In biologic terms, any virus which multiplies in one or more arthropods and is therafter transmitted to a vertebrate such that this mechanism is significant in the natural maintenance of the agent is an arbovirus. More than 400 distinguishable viruses have been tentatively so classified, and about 100 of these are known to infect man. Arboviruses also can be organized into virologic families based on morphologic, biophysical, and biochemical properties. Most of those which cause human disease belong to one of two such families: the Togaviridae and the Bunyaviridae, which in turn have been subdivided into genera such as alphaviruses, flaviviruses, phleboviruses, bunyaviruses, and nairoviruses. Within these genera, in turn, agents have been clustered immunologically on the basis of shared antigens. For example, most mosquito-borne flaviviruses can be readily distinguished from tick-borne members of this genus by this means (see Table 349–1).

Finally, arboviruses can be separated by the clinical syndromes they produce in man. Although mild undifferentiated fever is the most common consequence of infection, more serious illness can sometimes be induced by certain of these viruses. These individual descriptions are placed in one of the following groups: (1) *fevers of undifferentiated type,* with or without rash; (2) *encephalitides,* often severe and with significant case-fatality rates; and (3) *hemorrhagic fevers,* also frequently severe and fatal. Some of the variables used to classify arboviruses and the diseases they produce are illustrated in the accompanying table. All of the agents contain RNA, and all except the reoviruses have lipid-containing envelopes.

The largest number of viruses has been associated exclusively with mild, undifferentiated disease, and most of these are encountered in tropical and semitropical countries (see Table 350–1). Those to be described represent but a small sample that has caused many human illnesses in either endemic or significant epidemic patterns.

All arboviruses conspicuously associated with encephalitis are included. Similarly, viruses causing hemorrhagic fever are described. All are zoonotic agents, but not all are vector-borne arboviruses. Except for the nairovirus *Congo-CHF* and the unclassified Bunyavirus, *Hantaan,* which causes hemorrhagic fever with renal syndrome, arboviruses causing hemorrhagic fever are flaviviruses. Other zoonotic viruses causing hemorrhagic fever include three Arenaviruses, *Junin, Machupo,* and *Lassa,* and the as yet unclassified agents, *Marburg* and *Ebola.*

Arenaviruses are fundamentally parasites of wild rodents and display a high order of host specificity, characterized by chronic infection with persistent viremia and shedding of virus in urine. Lymphocytic choriomeningitis virus (see Ch. 499) is the prototype of the family and is associated with the common house mouse, *Mus musculus.* Other Arenaviruses are usually restricted to a single rodent species in nature and are thus sharply circumscribed as geographic pathogens by the distribution and ecology of the specific rodent host.

All of the agents considered in these chapters are zoonotic viruses, and infection in man produced by them is determined by geographic and ecologic features peculiar to a given agent. All of these viruses most often produce clinically undifferentiated febrile disease in man. Thus, the most important elements in differential diagnosis of possible zoonotic viral disease are a *carefully taken history* emphasizing geography and exposure, and the use of *specific diagnostic tests.* In many parts of the world, malaria is the most likely cause of acute febrile disease in adults. The finding of malaria parasites in blood, however, may not solve the clinical problem; it should be remembered that either a simultaneous zoonotic viral infection or a drug-resistant parasite may account for the lack of response to supposed specific chemotherapy.

Virus isolation, together with an antibody rise to that agent in sequentially obtained sera from the patient, provides strong evidence for an etiologic association between virus and the observed illness. *Whole blood* is the best source of virus for nearly all of the disease here described, and it *should be obtained on the very first day the patient is seen,* because viremia often disappears rapidly during clinical illness, especially in the case

TABLE 349–1. CLASSIFICATION PARAMETERS FOR ARBOVIRUSES AND CERTAIN OTHER ZOONOTIC VIRUSES CAUSING ACUTE HUMAN DISEASE

Virus Family	Virus Properties	Vector	Human Disease	Examples
Togaviridae	Spherical, 50–70 nm (alpha), 40–50 nm (flavi); single-stranded infectious RNA			
Alphaviruses		Mosquitoes	Undifferentiated fever, encephalitis	Mayaro, Ross River, eastern equine encephalitis
Flaviviruses		Mosquitoes, ticks	Undifferentiated fever, encephalitis, hemorrhagic fever	Dengue, West Nile, St. Louis encephalitis, yellow fever
Bunyaviridae	Spherical, 90–100 nm; RNA segmented, circular, noninfectious			
Bunyaviruses		Mosquitoes	Undifferentiated fever, encephalitis	California encephalitis
Phleboviruses		Mosquitoes, phlebotomine flies	Undifferentiated fever	Sandfly, Rift Valley fevers
Nairoviruses		Ticks	Hemorrhagic fever	Congo-CHF
Hantaan virus		Rodents	Hemorrhagic fever	Hemorrhagic fever, renal syndrome
Arenaviridae	Spherical or pleomorphic, 50–300 nm; segmented, circular, noninfectious RNA	Rodents	Hemorrhagic fever	Junin, Machupo, Lassa
Reoviridae, arboviruses	Spherical, isometric, nonenveloped, 65-80 nm; RNA is 10 linear segments	Ticks	Undifferentiated fever	Colorado tick fever
Marburg-Ebola viruses	90 × 700-800 nm rods; single-stranded RNA	Unknown	Hemorrhagic fever	

of the encephalitides. An acute-phase serum sample for antibody studies should be collected at this same time, and a convalescent specimen gotten 7 to 30 days later usually discloses an increase in specific antibodies when measured by the complement-fixation (CF), hemagglutination-inhibition (HI), immunofluorescent (IF), or neutralization (N) method. Binding assays for antibodies, particularly of immunoglobulin M (IgM) subclass, may often provide specific diagnosis during the acute phase of illness.

Fenner F: Classification and nomenclature of viruses. Intervirology 7:1, 1976. *Definitive exposition of internationally accepted game rules by the chairman of the committee in charge.*

Shope RE, Sather GE: Arboviruses. *In* Lennette EH, Schmidt NJ (eds.): Diagnostic Procedures for Viral, Rickettsial and Chlamydia Infections. 5th ed. Washington, D.C. American Public Health Association, 1979, pp 767–814. *Carefully detailed explanation of current technology, with an excellent discussion of indications and limitations of various diagnostic procedures.*

Undifferentiated Fevers

350. DENGUE

Robert B. Tesh

DEFINITION. "Classic" dengue is an acute, self-limited illness characterized by fever, prostration, headache, myalgia, rash, lymphadenopathy, and leukopenia. It is caused by a mosquito-borne flavivirus. Typically the disease lasts five to seven days and is followed by one or more weeks of depression and weakness.

ETIOLOGY. Four antigenically related but distinct subtypes of dengue virus have been recovered from patients. Infection with each of these agents results in long-lasting immunity against the homologous virus and partial immunity, which persists only for about six months, against the other three heterologous subtypes.

EPIDEMIOLOGY. Dengue fever affects millions of people annually; in terms of human morbidity, it is by far the most important arthropod-transmitted viral illness. Dengue is mainly a disease of the tropics and subtropics, although it can also occur in temperate areas during warm weather. In fact, the first accurate clinical description of the disease was provided by Benjamin Rush during an epidemic in Philadelphia in the summer of 1780. However, the inability of *Aedes aegypti,* the principal mosquito vector, to survive prolonged winter weather has prevented the disease from becoming permanently established in temperate regions of the world.

The basic cycle of dengue virus involves man and certain *Aedes* mosquitoes. The character of dengue outbreaks often varies from one locality to another, depending on climatic conditions, the size and age of the susceptible human population, and the abundance and vector competence of the local mosquitoes. Thus dengue may appear as a nearly silent continuously endemic infection, as repeated seasonal epidemics, or as massive outbreaks affecting populations previously free of the disease for many years. Classic dengue is generally a much milder disease in children than in adults.

When a dengue-infected mosquito feeds or probes, it usually introduces virus-contaminated saliva into its host. If the person is susceptible (nonimmune), the virus multiplies, and within five to seven days viremia follows. This viremic period usually corresponds with the acute phase of the illness and lasts about six days. During this time, the patient is infectious to mosquitoes. After ingestion of infected human blood by a susceptible mosquito, eight to ten days is required at warm temperatures for the virus to multiply in the insect's body and to infect its salivary glands. The mosquito is then infectious for life.

Aedes aegypti is by far the most important vector. It breeds, rests, and feeds in or near human habitations. It is strongly attracted to man, biting in daylight or twilight. These attributes make it an ideal virus vector and explain why dengue is principally an urban disease. In rural areas other *Aedes* species such as *Ae. albopictus* transmit infection, but their habits and smaller human populations make explosive epidemics uncommon.

PATHOLOGY. Dengue virus infection occasionally produces hemorrhagic fever and shock. This syndrome is discussed in Ch. 359. Since classic dengue is rarely fatal, the only information available about its pathology is from biopsies of the skin rash. Such lesions consist of endothelial swelling, perivascular edema, and mononuclear infiltration of small vessels. Petechiae are characterized by extravasation of blood without significant inflammatory reaction.

CLINICAL MANIFESTATIONS. The incubation period of dengue fever is five to eight days. The onset in adults is sudden; during the first 12 to 24 hours the patient develops progressively severe malaise, fever, chills, headache, backache, and generalized myalgia. By the second day the patient is usually acutely ill and prostrate with fever up to 40° C, severe headache, retro-orbital pain, photophobia, generalized muscle aches, and joint stiffness. Other frequent symptoms include anorexia, altered taste sensations, nausea, vomiting, abdominal tenderness, sore throat, and depression. During this early phase, a flush or fleeting erythematous eruption may appear on the face, neck, and chest. The lymph nodes usually become enlarged and palpable, but the liver and spleen do not. The fever generally lasts five to seven days. Occasionally the temperature briefly falls on the third or fourth day, giving a "saddleback" fever curve.

About the third or fourth day of illness, a maculopapular or scarlatiniform rash appears, beginning on the trunk and spreading in centripetal fashion. This lasts several days, becomes itchy as it fades, but rarely desquamates. Initially, the leukocyte count may be normal; but by the third or fourth day of illness, a generalized leukopenia develops. Toward the end of the febrile period, small clusters of petechiae may appear, especially on the lower extremities, but the thrombocyte count and clotting time are normal in classic dengue. Convalescence begins on the sixth or seventh day when the fever ends, but full recovery often takes several weeks because of lingering weakness and depression.

DIAGNOSIS. During epidemics of dengue fever, when a large number of cases occurs within a short time, the diagnosis is relatively easy. Isolated cases of the disease are more difficult to recognize, because influenza, rubella, and a number of other arbovirus diseases may be mistaken for dengue. Thus laboratory confirmation of a *few* cases during an epidemic and of *every* case when the pattern is sporadic is important. Dengue is endemic in a number of countries in the Caribbean, South and Central America, Africa, and Southern Asia; thus a history of travel during the previous ten days is essential whenever dealing with a suspect case in areas where the disease is rare.

Isolation of the virus is the preferred method of diagnosis. Dengue virus can frequently be recovered from the blood or serum of patients during the febrile stage of their illness. Inoculation of specimens into live mosquitoes or mosquito cell cultures is the most sensitive culture technique. Serologic diagnosis, using acute and convalescent specimens drawn 14 to 21 days apart, is the alternative. However, interpretation of serologic results may be difficult if the patient has been infected before with another flavivirus. An anamnestic immune response generally develops after a second flavivirus infection, making identification of the specific infecting agent difficult or impossible.

TREATMENT AND PROGNOSIS. There is no specific therapy. Bed rest is indicated, as well as the usual supportive measures to maintain fluid and electrolyte balance, particularly if repeated vomiting occurs. Secondary bacterial infection is uncommon but should be anticipated and treated appropriately. Aspirin should be avoided in dengue patients to prevent exacerbation of the thrombocytopenia and hemorrhagic manifestations which occasionally develop. The prognosis in patients with classic dengue is excellent, although convalescence may be prolonged.

PREVENTION. No vaccines for dengue viruses are yet available. Individual protection is difficult, because the mosquito vectors bite during the day, and continuous use of repellents is not practical. Community protection is possible through effective control or eradication of the *Aedes* vectors. Dengue patients should be protected from mosquitoes during the first five or six days of their illness in order to prevent further virus transmission, and space-spraying of buildings frequented by patients should be done to eliminate mosquitoes possibly infected prior to the diagnosis of the disease.

Halstead SB: Dengue and dengue hemorrhagic fever. *In* Steele JH (ed.): CRC Handbook Series in Zoonoses, Sect. B: Viral Zoonoses. Vol. 1. Boca Raton, CRC Press, 1981, pp 421–435. *A good review of the disease and its epidemiology.*

Kuberski TT, Rosen L, Reed D, Mataika J: Clinical and laboratory observations on patients with primary and secondary dengue type 1 infections with hemorrhagic manifestations in Fiji. Am J Trop Med Hyg 26:775, 1977. *A comparison of symptoms in patients with primary and secondary dengue infections. Hematologic and serologic results as well as the level and duration of viremia are reported.*

Schlesinger RW: Dengue Viruses. Vol 16. New York, Springer-Verlag, 1977. *This monograph covers all aspects of dengue viruses. The clinical picture of classic and hemorrhagic dengue fever is described in detail.*

351. WEST NILE FEVER

Robert B. Tesh

DEFINITION. West Nile fever is an acute, febrile, mosquito-borne viral illness marked by headache, myalgia, lymphadenopathy, and rash. It is generally self-limited, although occasional deaths resulting from encephalitis occur in aged persons.

ETIOLOGY. The disease is caused by a small ribonucleic acid–containing virus (family Togaviridae, genus *Flavivirus*), which is closely related antigenically to Japanese B, Murray Valley, St. Louis, and Rocio encephalitis viruses. West Nile virus also is related to dengue and yellow fever viruses.

EPIDEMIOLOGY. Millions of people have been infected with West Nile virus, which occurs in many rural areas of Africa, the Middle East, southwest Asia, and southern Europe. The disease occurs in both endemic and epidemic forms. In areas where West Nile virus is highly endemic, infection occurs early in childhood and most of the adult population is immune. In regions where the virus is less active, sporadic epidemics of West Nile fever occur among persons of all ages. Epidemics usually occur during the summer months and are correlated with seasonal peaks in populations of culicine mosquitoes. The virus is thought to be maintained in nature by a cycle involving *Culex* mosquitoes and birds, with man serving as only an incidental host.

CLINICAL MANIFESTATIONS. The disease begins suddenly after an incubation period of three to six days. The character of clinical illness produced by West Nile virus infection is largely age dependent. Infants and young children generally experience a mild, nonspecific febrile illness. Adolescents and adults usually develop a dengue-like disease, characterized by fever, rash, severe frontal headache, orbital pain, backache, generalized myalgia, anorexia, lymphadenopathy, and leukopenia. The rash is nonpruritic and maculopapular in type, occurs mainly on the trunk, and clears without desquamation. Other, less frequent symptoms include sore throat, nausea, vomiting, and diarrhea. A few patients in this age group also develop signs of meningeal involvement (stiff neck, Kernig's sign) during the acute phase of their illness. The cerebrospinal fluid in these cases usually shows a slight increase in cells and protein. In elderly and debilitated patients, West Nile virus infection sometimes produces meningoencephalitis and occasionally causes death. Neurologic symptoms in the latter patients may include depressed sensorium, somnolence, involuntary twitches, and coma.

West Nile fever is generally a self-limited disease, lasting three to six days, although general weakness and fatigue may persist for one or two weeks after the illness. In patients who develop neurologic involvement, the encephalitic signs do not usually appear until the fourth or fifth day of illness, and after the temperature has returned to normal.

DIAGNOSIS. Clinically this disease is so similar to dengue and phlebotomus fever that laboratory diagnosis is essential in all cases. Virus isolation is by far the best method, and blood specimens obtained as late as the fourth symptomatic day yield a reasonably high percentage of strains when inoculated into newborn mice or a variety of cell cultures. Serologic diagnosis may also be attempted with acute and convalescent serum samples, but previous infection with related flaviviruses, such as the 17D yellow fever vaccine strain, may render interpretation of results extremely difficult owing to the heterologous immune response that develops after a second flavivirus infection.

TREATMENT AND PREVENTION. Management of patients is completely symptomatic. Complications are uncommon. Since there is no vaccine available, the only effective prevention of West Nile fever is to avoid mosquito bites. Mosquito control programs can reduce the vector population and thus the incidence of the disease. Visitors to areas where West Nile virus is endemic should use mosquito netting, screens, and insect repellent.

Goldblum N: West Nile fever in the Middle East. Proc 6th Int Congr Trop Med Malar 5:112, 1959. *A review of the clinical picture and epidemiology of West Nile fever in Israel.*

Southam CM, Moore AE: Induced virus infections in man by the Egypt isolates of West Nile virus. Am J Trop Med Hyg 3:19, 1954. *This paper reports in great detail the clinical course of terminal cancer patients inoculated with West Nile virus. Encephalitic symptoms were common in this group of patients.*

Taylor RM, Work TH, Hurlbut HS, Rizk F: A study of the ecology of West Nile virus in Egypt. Am J Trop Med Hyg 5:579, 1956. *This paper describes results of field and laboratory studies to identify the mosquito vectors and vertebrate reservoirs of West Nile virus. It is a classic work in arbovirology.*

352. PHLEBOTOMUS FEVER

Robert B. Tesh

DEFINITION. Phlebotomus fever, also referred to as sandfly or pappataci fever, is an acute, self-limited, flu-like illness of two to four days' duration, which is transmitted by the bite of infected phlebotomine sandflies. The disease occurs annually during the warm season in the Mediterranean littoral and central Asia. Sporadic cases have also been recognized in tropical America.

ETIOLOGY. The phlebotomus fever group of arboviruses (family Bunyaviridae, genus *Phlebovirus*) currently consists of 36 antigenically distinct and geographically dispersed virus serotypes. Although many of these agents are capable of producing "classic" phlebotomus fever, most cases of the disease are due to the Naples and Sicilian serotypes.

EPIDEMIOLOGY. Phlebotomus fever is a public health problem mainly in the Old World where it occurs in both endemic and epidemic forms. The occurrence of the disease in this region closely parallels the geographic distribution and abundance of *Phlebotomus papatasi*, its principal vector. In areas where the disease is endemic, most of the indigenous population is infected and thereby acquires immunity early in life. The disease in children is a relatively benign, nonspecific febrile illness. However, when nonimmune adults enter an endemic area and are bitten by infected sandflies, they develop "classic" phlebotomus fever. For this reason, historically the disease has been of some military importance.

The principal vector, *Phlebotomus papatasi*, is a tiny (2 to 3 mm) sand-colored midge. Because of their small size, they can readily pass through ordinary screens and mosquito netting. Sandflies usually move in short hops and rarely travel more than a few hundred meters from their resting and breeding sites. The larvae develop in loose soil and organic debris in stone walls, wells, gardens, animal shelters, and privies, usually near human dwellings. *P. papatasi* is active mainly at night and readily feeds on humans. Available evidence suggests that many viruses in the phlebotomus fever group are maintained in the sandfly population by transovarial (hereditary) transmission. This mechanism ensures survival of the viruses during winter months when the vector is inactive and during periods when susceptible vertebrate hosts are not available.

Phlebotomus fever also occurs in tropical America; however, in this region the important vectors are sylvan species belonging to the genus *Lutzomyia*. Therefore cases of the disease in the New World are sporadic in occurrence and found mainly in persons who enter the tropical forests for work and recreation.

PATHOGENESIS. Since there are no fatalities, the pathology of this disease in humans is unknown. Experimental studies in man, however, indicate that after intracutaneous inoculation the incubation period is three to six days. Viremia is brief and lasts only one or two days, usually being confined to the day prior to and that of the onset of symptoms. Postinfection immunity is type specific and probably lifelong.

CLINICAL MANIFESTATIONS. The disease is sudden in onset and is characterized by fever, headache, myalgia, photophobia, retro-orbital pain, and marked conjunctival injection. The face often has an erythematous flush, but a true rash is absent. Nausea and vomiting sometimes occur, but other gastrointestinal and respiratory symptoms are uncommon. Most patients with phlebotomus fever develop a marked leukopenia, consisting of an initial lymphopenia followed by a protracted neutropenia. The acute symptoms last only two to four days; however, a general feeling of weakness and depression often persists for a week or more.

DIAGNOSIS AND TREATMENT. Epidemiologic or travel history represents the best clue to diagnosis. Virus isolation is difficult. Serologic procedures may be carried out but serve principally to exclude other possible causes such as dengue, West Nile fever, and influenza. Management of patients is symptomatic. No vaccine is available, but insecticides are highly effective in controlling the peridomestic sandfly vectors.

Bartelloni PJ, Tesh RB: Clinical and serologic responses of volunteers infected with phlebotomus fever virus (Sicilian type). Am J Trop Med Hyg 25:456, 1976. *A description of the clinical, hematologic, and serologic responses of volunteers infected with sandfly fever. References are given to other similar studies.*

Sabin AB, Philip CB, Paul JR: Phlebotomus (pappataci or sandfly) fever. JAMA 125:693, 1944. *A report of research on sandfly fever among American troops during World War II. It presents a detailed clinical description of the disease.*

Tesh RB, Saidi S, Gajdamovic SJ, Rodhain F, Vesenjak-Hirjan J: Serological studies on the epidemiology of sandfly fever in the Old World. Bull WHO 54:663, 1976. *A review of the epidemiology of phlebotomus fever in the Old World. It includes a map showing the geographic distribution of the principal vector,* Phlebotomus papatasi.

353. RIFT VALLEY FEVER

Robert B. Tesh

DEFINITION. Rift Valley fever is an acute viral illness, usually of short duration, which is characterized by high fever, headache, retro-orbital pain, myalgia, prostration, photophobia, and conjunctival injection. A small percentage of patients with this disease develop hemorrhagic and encephalitic complications which are sometimes fatal. Humans generally acquire the disease by contact with infected domestic animals, although the virus may also be mosquito borne.

ETIOLOGY. The causative agent is a 90-nm, ribonucleic acid–containing virus that is antigenically related to a number of viruses in the phlebotomus fever group (family Bunyaviridae, genus *Phlebovirus*). However, because of the virulence of Rift Valley fever virus for animals and humans, the disease that it causes is considered separately.

EPIDEMIOLOGY. The known geographic distribution of the virus includes most of the eastern half of Africa. Rift Valley fever is primarily a disease of domestic ruminants. Epizootics produce heavy mortality among lambs and calves and cause increased rates of abortion among ewes and cows. Outbreaks of the disease in domestic animals are sporadic; the virus is presumed to be transmitted from animal to animal by infected mosquitoes. The maintenance mechanism of the virus between epizootics is unknown.

Humans usually acquire the virus by aerosol transmission or by direct contact with blood or tissues of infected animals. Veterinarians, ranchers, herdsmen, slaughterhouse employees, and persons working in animal disease diagnostic laboratories are all at special risk during epizootics. Rift Valley fever virus is highly infectious to humans; cases of the disease have occurred in persons who have only been present in a room where a sick animal has been slaughtered or autopsied. It is uncertain what role, if any, mosquitoes play in the transmission of Rift Valley fever to man. During an extensive Rift Valley fever epizootic in Egypt during 1977 and 1978, many thousands of people became ill with the disease and more than 600 deaths were recorded. Because of the value of domestic animals in many economically depressed regions of Africa, animals are often housed within family compounds. Furthermore, sick or dying animals are usually killed to salvage their meat. Both of these practices greatly increase the risk of virus transmission to humans.

CLINICAL MANIFESTATIONS. The incubation period is three to six days. Uncomplicated Rift Valley fever in man is similar to phlebotomus fever. The disease begins suddenly with fever up to 40° C, chills, severe headache, retro-orbital pain, photophobia, generalized myalgia, and prostration. Patients with this disease appear acutely ill, with flushed faces and marked conjunctival injection. Occasionally nausea, vomiting, and diarrhea occur. Physical examination early in the disease is unremarkable. The white blood count may be decreased, normal, or elevated. In most cases the illness lasts two to four days, although sometimes a brief recrudescence of fever occurs, giving a biphasic temperature curve. Recovery in uncomplicated cases is complete.

A few patients with Rift Valley fever develop serious complications. One is loss of central visual acuity and occasionally blindness. The eye symptoms do not usually become apparent until several days or weeks after the febrile illness has ended. Funduscopic examination in these cases shows white macular exudates and occasionally retinal hemorrhages. In some patients, vision gradually improves; in others, it does not.

A second complication is hemorrhagic manifestations. These usually appear between the second and fourth days of illness, about the time that the patient becomes afebrile. The patient becomes progressively jaundiced and drowsy and manifests petechiae, purpura, bleeding gums, hematemesis, and melena. Liver function test results, including bilirubin, serum transaminases, alkaline phosphatase, and prothrombin time, are abnormal. The prognosis in these cases is poor; death often occurs within a week and is due to shock and hepatic failure.

A third complication is meningoencephalitis. Neurologic symptoms appear several days after the febrile period ends and may include mental confusion, hallucinations, vertigo, meningismus, paresis, convulsions, and coma. The cerebrospinal fluid shows increased protein and pleocytosis. The outcome is gradual recovery or death.

PATHOGENESIS. At autopsy, patients with hemorrhagic complications have petechiae and hemorrhages throughout the gastrointestinal tract. The most characteristic lesion is in the liver and consists of diffuse central necrosis and hemorrhage. Affected hepatic cells show eosinophilic cytoplasmic degeneration similar to that seen in yellow fever. The brain in fatal cases of encephalitis shows focal necrosis and perivascular infiltration with macrophages and lymphocytes.

DIAGNOSIS. Rift Valley fever is primarily a disease of place and particular human activity. A history is more valuable than any other procedure. Blood obtained during the febrile period almost always contains virus. Serologic diagnosis is also fairly specific, although low level cross-reactions may occur with some heterologous antigens in the phlebotomus fever group.

TREATMENT AND PREVENTION. Management of patients with this disease is entirely symptomatic. Those with hemorrhage and shock obviously need blood replacement.

Live attenuated and formalin-killed vaccines are available in limited quantities for certain high-risk groups such as veterinarians and laboratory workers. These are protective for at least two years. Individual antimosquito measures would also seem prudent during epizootics.

Peters CJ, Meegan JM: Rift Valley fever. *In* Steele JH (ed.): CRC Handbook Series in Zoonoses, Section B: Viral Zoonoses. Vol. 1. Boca Raton, CRC Press, 1981, pp 403–420. *A complete review of all aspects of the disease.*

354. FEVERS CAUSED BY ALPHAVIRUSES: CHIKUNGUNYA, O'NYONG-NYONG, MAYARO, ROSS RIVER, AND OCKELBO

Robert B. Tesh

DEFINITION. Chikungunya, o'nyong-nyong, Mayaro, Ross River, and Ockelbo virus infections are acute nonfatal illnesses that usually include fever, arthralgia, and rash. They are caused by a group of antigenically related, geographically diverse, mosquito-borne viruses.

EPIDEMIOLOGY. These five diseases affect persons of all ages, although they are generally milder in children. Clinically, they are practically indistinguishable, but their epidemiology is quite different. Chikungunya is the most widely distributed of the five diseases and occurs in sub-Sahara Africa, India, Southeast Asia, and the Philippines. Epidemics are sporadic in occurrence and usually appear during warm rainy months. In rural Africa, the virus is maintained in a cycle involving wild primates and forest mosquitoes *(Aedes africanus* and *Ae. furcifer).* Urban outbreaks of chikungunya are usually associated with *Aedes aegypti.* In this situation the virus is probably transmitted from man to mosquito to man.

Little is known about the epidemiology of o'nyong-nyong fever. It has occurred in Uganda, Kenya, Tanzania, Malawi, and Senegal. Between 1959 and 1962, a major epidemic of this disease swept across East Africa, affecting millions of people. The suspected vectors are *Anopheles funestus* and *An. gambiae.*

Mayaro virus has been isolated in Trinidad, Surinam, Brazil, Colombia, and Bolivia. Cases of this disease have been associated mainly with persons who live or work in tropical forests, mostly males. Sylvan mosquitoes of the genus *Haemagogus* are thought to be the principal vectors. Wild animals probably serve as the virus reservoir.

Ross River fever, also known as "epidemic polyarthritis," has occurred in Australia, New Guinea, the Solomon islands, Fiji, American Samoa, and a number of other South Pacific islands. In southern Australia, sporadic cases of the disease usually occur during warm weather among vacationers traveling in rural areas. There the virus is thought to be maintained in a wild vertebrate-mosquito cycle, with *Culex annulirostris* and *Aedes vigilax* serving as principal vectors. However, explosive epidemics of this disease have also occurred on several South Pacific islands where the virus appeared to be transmitted from man to mosquito to man, analogous to urban outbreaks of chikungunya. In the latter epidemics, *Aedes polynesiensis* was the presumed vector.

Less is known about the epidemiology of Ockelbo fever. The disease was first recognized in Sweden. A similar illness has also been reported in Finland and adjacent regions of the Soviet Union, where it is referred to as "Pogasta disease" and "Karelian fever," respectively. In all three countries, the disease typically occurs in late summer among picnickers, berry collectors, and other persons entering wooded areas. A single recovery of the virus has been made from *Culiseta* mosquitoes.

CLINICAL MANIFESTATIONS. The usual incubation period for this group of illnesses is three to five days. Typically, the onset is abrupt with fever, headache, myalgia, and weakness. In Mayaro and chikungunya infections, the fever may reach 39 to 40° C. A saddleback or biphasic temperature curve sometimes occurs with chikungunya. In Ross River, Ockelbo, and o'nyong-nyong infections, the fever is generally lower and constitutional symptoms are milder. Arthralgia and rash may appear with the initial symptoms or develop several days later. Arthralgia is the most striking feature of these illnesses. It is usually bilateral and mainly affects joints in the extremities. Symptoms vary from excruciating pain to vague joint stiffness. Affected joints are often swollen and tender, but other signs of inflammation are absent. Previously injured joints are particularly susceptible. The rash is maculopapular in type and occurs mainly on the trunk and extremities, although the palms and soles may also be affected. The rash clears in four or five days without desquamation, leaving a brownish stain to the skin. Lymphadenopathy is also common. Many patients have a leukopenia with relative lymphocytosis during the first week of illness. One serious but rare complication of chikungunya virus infection is hemorrhagic manifestations. Epistaxis, hematemesis, melena, petechiae, and purpura have all been reported occasionally.

DIAGNOSIS. These viruses can usually be recovered from the blood or serum of patients during the first few days of illness by inoculation of newborn mice or various cell cultures. Standard serologic techniques are also highly reliable in making a specific diagnosis, provided that a first serum specimen is collected early in the disease and a second is obtained 10 to 14 days later. Diagnosis during epidemics is relatively easy; the occasional or isolated case is more difficult to recognize. The differential diagnosis includes other diseases producing fever, arthralgia, and rash.

TREATMENT AND PROGNOSIS. Treatment is symptomatic, and the prognosis is excellent. In general, these illnesses last only about one week, although the arthralgia sometimes persists for several weeks or months. In such a case, recurrent attacks of joint pain and swelling are common. The pathogenesis of the joint disease is unknown.

Skogh M, Espmark A: Ockelbo disease: Epidemic arthritis—exanthema syndrome in Sweden caused by Sindbis-virus like agent. Lancet 1:795, 1982. *Brief description of Ockelbo disease.*

Tesh RB: Arthritides caused by mosquito-borne viruses. Ann Rev Med 33:31, 1982. *A review of the clinical manifestations and epidemiology of diseases caused by five alphaviruses. Many references are given.*

355. COLORADO TICK FEVER

Theodore C. Eickhoff

DEFINITION. Colorado tick fever (CTF) is an acute, benign, tick-transmitted viral infection that occurs throughout the Rocky Mountain area, and is characterized by headache, back pain, a biphasic febrile course lasting about one week, and leukopenia.

ETIOLOGY. CTF virus is an arbovirus that is transmitted to humans by the bite of the hard-shelled wood tick, *Dermacentor andersoni.* Human cases appear to be limited to the combined geographic distribution of the vector, and the major mammalian reservoirs, ground squirrels and chipmunks. CTF virus is in the orbivirus genus of the reoviruses and is unrelated to other arbovirus groups.

EPIDEMIOLOGY. The disease occurs during the spring and summer months, when tick exposure in the mountains is common. Disease activity appears to follow springtime in the mountains, for cases occur at lower altitudes during April and May, and at higher altitudes during June and July, presumably reflecting the slower emergence of ticks at higher altitudes. Most patients give a history of having found attached ticks, but others will not be aware of the tick attachment and bite, even though they may have seen ticks on their body or clothing. Cases may occasionally be encountered in other areas of the country as a result of travel outside the endemic area during the incubation period, or accidental transportation of infected adult ticks in clothing or bedding.

The virus has been recovered from as many as 14 per cent of *Dermacentor andersoni* collected in endemic areas. Replication of the virus within these ticks has been documented. It is not clear whether the virus is passed transovarially within the vector species. The reservoir of the virus probably resides in numerous small mammals, particularly golden mantled ground squirrels and chipmunks, which have a prolonged viremia and infect nymphal ticks. Overwintering may thus occur in either nymphal ticks or hibernating small mammals. Adult ticks then transmit the virus to other small animals, with humans being accidental hosts.

INCIDENCE AND PREVALENCE. The disease has been reported from most states in the Rocky Mountain area and from western Canadian provinces, but the largest number of cases has generally been reported in Colorado. Several hundred cases are diagnosed annually in the endemic area, but it is likely that this represents only a fraction of the total. Mild or wholly subclinical infections do occur, but their frequency has not been systematically evaluated.

The virus has been isolated from other species of ticks and from numerous species of small mammals, suggesting that the disease may occur over a wider geographic area than is presently appreciated.

PATHOGENESIS. There is no unusual local reaction at the site of the tick bite inoculation, and the site of initial localization and replication of the virus is unknown. The onset of symptoms occurs three to seven days after tick exposure. Viremia can be demonstrated at the time of onset of fever, not only persisting during the febrile illness itself, but remarkably persisting in red blood cells long after the virus has disappeared from serum and neutralizing antibody has appeared. The virus can be demonstrated within erythrocytes by fluorescent antibody staining for up to 120 days, and has been grown from washed erythrocytes 100 days after the original infection.

Few pathologic data in man are available, since only one fatal case has been recorded. In experimental animals, the heart, lungs, spleen, bone marrow, and lymph nodes are important sites of viral replication. Occasional patients have clinical evidence of central nervous system or meningeal involvement, and CTF virus has been recovered from cerebrospinal fluid.

CLINICAL MANIFESTATIONS. The disease begins abruptly, with chilly sensations, fever of 38 to 40° C, myalgias most prominent in the back and legs, headache, retro-orbital pain, and photophobia. Malaise and nausea may occur, but vomiting is uncommon. Physical findings during the first two to three days of illness are nonspecific. The patient may be flushed, with conjunctival and pharyngeal erythema. Lymphadenopathy is not prominent, although mild splenomegaly is sometimes present. Rashes have been reported in up to 12 per cent of patients, commonly macular or maculopapular and distributed over the entire body, sometimes petechial and involving primarily the extremities. Tachycardia is in proportion to the temperature elevation.

In approximately half of the cases, a distinctly biphasic illness occurs, the so-called "saddleback" fever. Symptoms abate after two to three days, temperature becomes normal or nearly so, and the patient feels relatively well for one or two days, following which there is an abrupt return of fever, headache, and back pain, often more intense than in the first phase. The second phase lasts two to four days and then subsides, leaving the patient with weakness and lassitude that disappear entirely during the succeeding week or two. Some patients do not exhibit the typical biphasic course, and experience only one bout of fever, or have a typical illness but with a third phase of fever, or have a single prolonged febrile illness lasting five to eight days.

Central nervous system involvement has occurred in a few patients, invariably children. The presenting findings have been those of aseptic meningitis with nuchal rigidity and mononuclear pleocytosis, or encephalitis with a depressed sensorium or stupor. Hemorrhagic manifestations have been described in a few children with encephalitis.

Laboratory findings very early in the illness are generally not helpful, but leukopenia is usually present by the third day of illness, and becomes even more pronounced during the second phase, reaching levels as low as 2000 per cubic millimeter. The most striking decrease is in the granulocyte series, with a relative lymphocytosis, and there is frequently an accompanying thrombocytopenia. Atypical, vacuolated lymphocytes are frequently observed. Bone marrow examination reveals a maturation arrest in the granulocyte series. The white blood count returns to normal during convalescence.

DIAGNOSIS. The diagnosis should be suspected in any person with a history of tick exposure in the endemic area three to seven days prior to the onset of a febrile illness. Findings during the first phase, however, cannot be differentiated from many other acute febrile illnesses. A brief symptom-free interval followed by a second febrile illness should strongly suggest CTF. Profound leukopenia is usually present by that time, and lends support to the diagnosis.

The diagnosis is confirmed by isolation of the virus from serum or whole blood, via inoculation of suckling mice. More rapid diagnosis is possible by direct immunofluorescent staining of virus in the patient's erythrocytes. A diagnostic rise in both neutralizing and complement-fixing antibodies can generally be detected by examination of acute and convalescent sera.

The differential diagnosis can be troublesome, inasmuch as Rocky Mountain spotted fever is transmitted in the tick fever endemic area by the same vector, *Dermacentor andersoni.* Paradoxically, Rocky Mountain spotted fever has become an unusual disease in the state of Colorado and is outnumbered by CTF in Colorado by 20-fold. Nevertheless, differential diagnosis may be impossible early in the course of disease, before the characteristic rash of Rocky Mountain spotted fever appears. A relatively symptom-free interval after two or three days would be most unusual in Rocky Mountain spotted fever, and strongly favors the diagnosis of CTF.

TREATMENT. Therapy is entirely supportive, there being no specific therapy. Salicylates may be necessary to minimize headache and myalgias, but are neither required nor advisable in most patients.

PROGNOSIS. The disease is almost invariably benign, and the prognosis is excellent. Severe illness, complicated by central nervous system involvement, is seen infrequently and only in children.

PREVENTION. Both inactivated and live attenuated vaccines have been studied, but the modest number of cases and the benign nature of the disease suggest little need for active immunization.

The most effective means of preventing the disease is the use of protective clothing or repellents by people outdoors in endemic areas during the spring and summer months, together with frequent body inspection and prompt removal of ticks. Transfusion-associated disease can be prevented by exclusion of convalescent donors for a minimum of six months.

Goodpasture HC, Poland JD, Francy DB, Bowen GS, Horn KA: Colorado tick fever: Clinical, epidemiologic and laboratory aspects of 228 cases in Colorado in 1973–1974. Ann Intern Med 88:303, 1978. *A recent, thorough clinical study.*

Oshiro LS, Dondero DV, Emmons RW, Lennette EH: The development of Colorado tick fever virus within cells of the haematopoietic system. J Gen Virol 39:73, 1978. *Recommended for those interested in the unusual host-parasite relationship in CTF.*

356. ARTHROPOD-BORNE VIRAL ENCEPHALITIDES

Thomas P. Monath

Of the more than 450 arboviruses presently registered, 13 are important causes of encephalitis, some responsible for intermittent epidemics, and 14 are occasionally associated with encephalitis (see Table 356–1). Arboviral encephalitis is a significant health problem in Europe and the Soviet Union (tick-borne encephalitis), parts of Asia (Japanese encephalitis), and in the New World where the disease assumes great importance, owing to a proliferation of etiologic agents, widespread occurrence, potential for epidemic spread, and concurrent affliction of domestic animals and man. Only the African continent is spared from epidemiologically important arboviral encephalitides. The physician faced with a case should attempt to establish an early specific diagnosis, because it provides information about the occurrence of a potentially epidemic disease and directs investigative, preventive, and control measures by the responsible public health authority.

The viruses under consideration are transmitted between wild or domestic animals by the agency of blood-feeding mosquitoes or ticks (see Fig. 356–1). Vertebrate hosts circulate virus in their blood at titers sufficiently high to infect a specific arthropod vector(s). After ingestion of an infectious blood meal, a temperature-dependent delay (extrinsic incubation period) of a week or more is required for replication in salivary gland tissue before transmission by bite can occur; thereafter arthropods remain infective for life. Man is not an essential host in the transmission cycles of the arboviral encephalitides. Human infection is most often abortive or subclinical, and the severe manifestations of central nervous system inflammation occur in only a small fraction of persons infected. The ratio of inapparent to clinically overt infections is a distinctive, age-dependent quality of each disease.

CLINICAL FEATURES. In encephalitis, the brain parenchyma itself is affected, resulting in diffuse or localizing signs of cerebral dysfunction. Signs of meningeal irritation are also nearly always present *(meningoencephalitis)*, but may be masked in the very young, the elderly, or the comatose patient. In some patients, inflammation of the leptomeninges may occur without evidence for disturbance of brain function (aseptic meningitis). A still milder form of arboviral central nervous system infection is manifested by fever and headache only; in such cases, however, cerebrospinal fluid pleocytosis may be present, indicating a forme fruste of meningitis.

The neurologic disease usually begins after a variable period of nonspecific, grippe-like symptoms. The clinical features and rate of evolution of encephalitis are quite variable. A degree of alteration of the state of consciousness is a universal finding in encephalitis. Convulsions, more often generalized than focal, may occur. Paresis, paralyses, hyperactive reflexes, and plantar extensor responses reflect damage to corticospinal tracts. A prominent feature of some infections (especially St. Louis and

TABLE 356–1. ARTHROPOD-BORNE VIRUSES WHICH CAUSE ACUTE CENTRAL NERVOUS SYSTEM INFECTION AND ENCEPHALITIS

Virus	Taxonomic Group	Mode of Transmission	Geographic Distribution	Disease in Domestic Livestock
I. Viruses Principally Associated with the Encephalitis Syndrome; Epidemic and Endemic				
Eastern equine encephalitis	Togaviridae, alphavirus	Mosquito	Eastern North America, Caribbean, South America	Equines, penned pheasants
Western equine encephalitis	Togaviridae, alphavirus	Mosquito	Western North America, South America	Equines
Venezuelan equine encephalitis	Togaviridae, alphavirus	Mosquito, possibly other modes (see text)	Florida, Central and South America	Equines
St. Louis encephalitis	Togaviridae, flavivirus	Mosquito	North America, Caribbean, Central and South America	None
Japanese encephalitis	Togaviridae, flavivirus	Mosquito	East, Southeast Asia; India	Equines, swine
Rocio encephalitis	Togaviridae, flavivirus	Mosquito	Brazil	None
Murray Valley encephalitis	Togaviridae, flavivirus	Mosquito	Australia	(Equines)*
California encephalitis and La Crosse	Bunyaviridae, California serogroup	Mosquito	North America	None
Tick-borne encephalitides: Russian spring-summer and Central European encephalitis	Togaviridae, flavivirus	Tick, ingestion of milk	Europe, USSR	None
Louping ill	Togaviridae, flavivirus	Tick	British Isles	Sheep, equines, cows
Powassan	Togaviridae, flavivirus	Tick	North America	None
II. Viruses Principally Associated with Other Syndromes, but Occasionally Causing Encephalitis; Epidemic and Endemic				
Sindbis (febrile illness with rash)	Togaviridae, alphavirus	Mosquito	Africa, Europe	None
West Nile (febrile illness with rash)	Togaviridae, flavivirus	Mosquito	Africa, Middle East	(Equines)*
Yellow fever (hemorrhagic fever)	Togaviridae, flavivirus	Mosquito	Africa, tropical America	None
Rift Valley fever (febrile illness, hemorrhagic fever)	Bunyaviridae, phlebotomus fever group	Mosquito, direct contact	Africa	Sheep, cows, goats
Colorado tick fever (febrile illness)	Reoviridae, orbivirus	Tick	Western North America	None
Tick-borne hemorrhagic fevers:				
Kyasanur Forest disease	Togaviridae, flavivirus	Tick	India	None
Omsk hemorrhagic fever	Togaviridae, flavivirus	Tick	Central Asia	None
Crimean hemorrhagic fever-Congo	Bunyaviridae, nairovirus	Tick	Eastern Europe, USSR, Africa	None
III. Rare and Sporadic Infections Associated with Encephalitis				
Semliki Forest†	Togaviridae, alphavirus	Mosquito	Africa, Southeast Asia	(Equines)*
Ilheus	Togaviridae, flavivirus	Mosquito	South America	None
Negishi	Togaviridae, flavivirus	Tick	Japan	None
Langat†	Togaviridae, flavivirus	Tick	Asia	None
Thogoto	Orthomyxovirus	Tick	Africa	None

*Disease suspected but not well documented.
†Encephalitis recorded in laboratory infections or experimental infections of cancer patients only; significance in naturally acquired infections unknown.

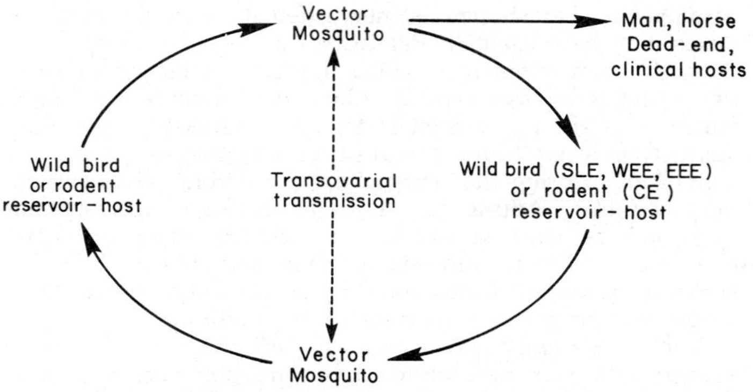

Figure 356–1. Generalized transmission cycle of the mosquito-borne encephalitides in North America.

Japanese encephalitis) is involvement of extrapyramidal structures, with tremor and muscular rigidity. Cerebellar dysfunction is manifested by muscular incoordination, dysmetria, and ataxic speech. Cranial nerve palsies are not uncommon and reflect damage to brainstem nuclei or supranuclear tracts. Autonomic disturbances (sialorrhea, cardiovascular irregularity, urinary retention) may be present. Infection of the cerebral cortex or hypothalamic–thalamic–temporal lobe regions produces confusion; defective memory; changes in speech, personality, and behavior; and the appearance of pathologic reflexes (e.g., suck, snout). Hyperthermia and the syndrome of inappropriate antidiuretic hormone secretion indicate disturbance of the pituitary-hypothalamic axis. Spinal cord involvement may be manifested by lower motor neuron and sensory deficits, hyperreflexia, and bladder paralysis. Interference with respiratory function, laryngeal paralysis, cardiac arrhythmia, and cerebral edema are potentially life-threatening complications. Surviving patients may be left with permanent neuropsychiatric sequelae. In the pregnant female, infection of the developing fetus may result in central nervous system damage or fetal death.

Clinical laboratory findings are relatively nonspecific. A modest peripheral leukocytosis is usual. The cerebrospinal fluid is under increased pressure and contains white blood cells (predominantly polymorphonuclear cells early and lymphocytes later). The cell count is generally less than 500 per cubic millimeter. Cerebrospinal fluid protein may be moderately elevated; glucose and lactate concentrations are normal. Changes in serum enzyme levels have been reported, reflecting myocarditis or damage to skeletal muscle or liver.

PATHOLOGY AND PATHOGENESIS. Two basic pathologic processes are common to the arboviral encephalitides; (1) neuronal and glial damage mediated by intracellular viral infection, and (2) an inflammatory response involving migration of immunologically active cells (lymphocytes, microglia, macrophages) into the perivascular space and brain parenchyma. Endothelial cell swelling and proliferation, vasculitic changes, and destruction of myelin sheaths in deep white matter areas are present in some of the arboviral encephalitides. Since the immune mechanism is responsible for the inflammatory response, an immunopathologic component has been postulated to occur in arboviral encephalitis. A balance apparently occurs between dual roles of the immune response in (1) viral clearance and recovery from infection and (2) enhancement of pathologic processes and acceleration of death.

After inoculation of virus by the bite of an infected arthropod, primary replication occurs in local tissues and in regional lymph nodes. Virus is carried by efferent lymphatics to the thoracic duct and into the bloodstream. This primary viremia seeds extraneural tissues, which in turn support further replication and release into the circulation. Viremia is modulated by replication in extraneural sites, by the rate of viral clearance by the reticuloendothelial system, and by the appearance of humoral antibodies. If viremia is prolonged and intense enough, the neural parenchyma is invaded, with or without ensuing clinical disease. The sites of extraneural infection vary from virus to virus. In the case of many alpha- and flaviviruses, experimental studies have shown that striated muscle and vascular endothelium are important sites of replication; in the case of Venezuelan encephalitis virus, myeloid and lymphoid tissue tropism has been emphasized. The mode of penetration of virus across the blood-brain junction is incompletely understood, but it is likely that passive movement of virus across cerebral capillaries plays a role. Factors that increase vascular permeability (heavy metal poisons, CO_2 inhalation, vasoactive amines) promote viral neuroinvasion. In experimental animals infected with flaviviruses, virus enters the central nervous system by way of the olfactory neuroepithelium. Olfactory neurons are infected by blood-borne virus, and the infection spreads by axonal transport to the brain.

The immature brain is more susceptible to damage by some arboviruses (e.g., western and Venezuelan equine and California encephalitis), accounting for the predominance of encephalitis in the younger age groups. But other central nervous system infections principally affect the elderly (e.g., St. Louis encephalitis), or have a bimodal incidence, striking both children and the very old. In endemic areas, accumulated immunity with increasing age may reduce the incidence of disease in the elderly. The reasons for the increased incidence and severity of some diseases in old persons are poorly understood; underlying hypertensive and arteriosclerotic cerebrovascular disease is suspected to play a role in viral neuroinvasion.

DIFFERENTIAL DIAGNOSIS. The primary task is to differentiate viral encephalitis from acute central nervous system infection by organisms which may respond to antibiotic therapy. Early clinical manifestations of bacterial meningitis (especially if partially treated), brain abscess, subdural empyema, and cerebral thrombophlebitis may mimic viral encephalitis, and cerebrospinal fluid changes are sometimes similar. Culture and repeated examination of the cerebrospinal fluid will help clarify the etiology in cases of bacterial meningitis. Diagnostic tests (computed tomography [CT], electroencephalography, brain scan) help define localized lesions, such as abscess. Subacute bacterial endocarditis may present with meningoencephalitis. Tuberculosis and fungal meningitis cause a mononuclear pleocytosis but reduced glucose values in the cerebrospinal fluid. Other infections that occasionally cause meningoencephalitis include Rocky Mountain spotted fever, leptospirosis, falciparum malaria, trichinosis, *Naegleria*, typhoid, and *Mycoplasma pneumoniae*.

Acute infection with viral agents other than arboviruses is associated with meningoencephalitis, including herpesviruses, mumps virus, enteroviruses, lymphocytic choriomeningitis virus, rabies, influenza, adenoviruses, respiratory syncytial virus, and encephalomyocarditis virus. Principal clues to an arboviral etiology are the history, presence of an outbreak of similar disease in the community, summer-fall occurrence, and the probable geographic locality in which infection was acquired. Echo- and coxsackieviruses cause summer-fall outbreaks in arbovirus epidemic areas, but the predominant syndrome produced is aseptic meningitis, and there may be clinical clues to the diagnosis (e.g., presence of rash, pleurodynia). In the individual case, herpes encephalitis presents the most important diagnostic challenge, since chemotherapy may be indicated. The presence of localizing neurologic signs, other clinical features (previous herpetic infection, subacute onset, predominant behavioral or confusional disturbance), and tests (e.g., CT scan) to detect a mass-like lesion are clues to the clinical diagnosis of herpes encephalitis. If brain biopsy is performed, fluorescent antibody tests and virus isolation attempts may be performed for both herpes and, if suspected, the arthropod-borne encephalitides.

Acute encephalitis may occur following exanthematous viral infections of childhood or administration of rabies or smallpox vaccines. The history of antecedent illness or vaccination and the prominence of myelitis in many cases are clues to the diagnosis.

Cerebrovascular accident may be confused with viral encephalitis. St. Louis encephalitis, a disease of the elderly, has been misdiagnosed as stroke. Subarachnoid hemorrhage produces meningismus, fever, headache, and neurologic signs that mimic an infectious etiology; CT scanning and lumbar puncture clearly distinguish these etiologies.

Metabolic (toxic) encephalopathies (caused by hypoxia, hypoglycemia, diabetic ketoacidosis, hepatic and renal failure, remote carcinoma, intoxications, and addisonian crisis) may present features suggesting infectious encephalitis. Careful history and physical, neurologic, and cerebrospinal fluid examination usually differentiate these conditions.

Neoplastic or *granulomatous diseases* involving the central nervous system and a variety of diseases of uncertain etiology (cat scratch disease, Behçet's disease, Reye's syndrome, acute multiple sclerosis, Lyme arthritis, and systemic lupus erythematosus) must occasionally be considered in the differential diagnosis.

Western Equine Encephalitis (WEE)

ETIOLOGIC AGENT. WEE virus, a member of the family Togaviridae, alphavirus genus, was first isolated in 1930 from a horse with encephalitis in California. A relative of WEE virus (Highlands J virus) present in the eastern United States is not associated with human (and rarely with equine) disease. WEE virus is pathogenic for a wide range of laboratory animals, embryonated eggs, and cell cultures. Isolation and viral assays are generally performed in infant mice inoculated intracranially or by plaque formation in primary avian cell cultures.

EPIDEMIOLOGY. ***Incidence and Prevalence.*** Between 1955 and 1981, 963 cases of WEE were reported in the United States. The annual incidence has varied from less than 10 cases to over 170 cases in epidemic years. Although classically an important disease on the west coast, the area most affected in recent years has been the central tier of states from the Mississippi River west to the Rocky Mountains, including adjacent parts of Canada. In Argentina and Uruguay, equine epizootics occur with little involvement of humans.

Epidemics generally occur in early or mid-summer, and may be precipitated by heavy snow melt or flooding, which produces conditions favorable for breeding of mosquito vectors. Cases of encephalitis in equines frequently precede the appearance of human disease by several weeks. The disease principally affects residents of rural agricultural communities. The incidence is higher in males than in females because of increased exposure to the vector during farming and recreational pursuits. WEE is most severe in infants and young children; these age groups also represent the immunologically most susceptible population in endemic areas. The case-fatality rate is between 3 and 7 per cent. In the western United States, mixed outbreaks of WEE and St. Louis encephalitis are the rule.

Transmission. The virus circulates between wild birds and *Culex tarsalis* mosquitoes. *Culex tarsalis*, an abundant breeder in irrigated areas and flooded pastures, is responsible for infection of man and equines, which develop low or undetectable viremias and do not perpetuate the chain of transmission. In temperate areas, transmission ceases during the winter months; the mechanism(s) whereby WEE virus persists in local winter reservoirs or is reintroduced in the spring is unknown.

CLINICAL FEATURES AND PATHOLOGY. The disease usually begins with generalized and nonspecific symptoms of fever, headache, malaise, and aches, lasting one to four days. Somnolence and lethargy, photophobia, vomiting, and neck stiffness signal the neurologic infection and progress, often quite rapidly, to stupor, coma, and, in a high proportion of children, convulsions. Paresis, cranial nerve deficits, and abnormal reflexes may be present. In fatal cases patients die one to two days after development of coma. Recovery often begins suddenly and progresses rapidly. About half of surviving infants suffer retardation, cerebellar damage, choreoathetosis, and spastic paralysis. Young age at onset, duration of illness, and convulsions during the acute phase are harbingers of permanent sequelae. Adults may have a prolonged convalescent syndrome of asthenia and neuropsychiatric complaints, but objective residua are rare and parkinsonism is extremely uncommon. Congenital infections are documented and result in severe and progressive neurologic deterioration.

A moderate leukocytosis and left shift are usual. The cerebrospinal fluid contains white cells (at first polymorphonuclear, then mononuclear), rarely in excess of 500 per cubic millimeter, and elevated protein concentration (usually 90 to 110 mg per deciliter).

Pathologic examination of the brains of infants reveals massive neuroparenchymal destruction; children dying months or years after the acute insult often have large cystic lesions in many areas of the brain. In older children and adults, acute WEE is characterized by focal necrosis and perivascular cuffing, predominantly in the basal ganglia and thalamic nuclei, but also in deep cerebral white matter. The highest titers of virus and interferon have also been found in basal ganglia and thalamus.

DIAGNOSIS. Viral isolation from blood or cerebrospinal fluid is almost never successful; a postmortem diagnosis may sometimes be achieved by isolation of the virus from brain tissue. Diagnosis is usually achieved by demonstration of a rise in hemagglutination-inhibiting (HI), fluorescent, complement-fixing (CF), or neutralizing (N) antibody titers in appropriately timed paired sera. An acute phase serum is obtained as early as possible in the illness, and a second serum a minimum of 10 to 14 days later.

TREATMENT. No specific chemotherapeutic agent is known. Supportive and good nursing care is essential and may reduce mortality. Control of high fever by sponging or ice packs and administration of antipyretics orally or rectally is recommended. Prompt administration of anticonvulsants (intravenous diazepam for acute control and phenytoin for more prolonged control) should be used to prevent protracted seizures and attendant hypoxia. Dehydration caused by fever, vomiting, and insufficient oral intake may be prominent, especially in children, and fluid and electrolyte balance must be restored and maintained by intravenous infusions. Management of airways in semicomatose and comatose patients is essential. Arterial blood gases should be monitored and respiratory assistance provided if hypoxia occurs. Prevention and treatment of secondary bacterial infections may be required; good pulmonary toilet and care of urinary catheters are essential. If clinical signs suggest cerebral edema or if the cerebrospinal fluid pressure is very high (>400 mm H_2O), measures to reduce brain swelling are indicated. Clinical signs that suggest progressive intracranial hypertension include deepening obtundation; prolonged delerium; respiratory, ocular, and motor signs of diencephalic deterioration; and loss of brainstem reflexes. Treatment consists of intracranial pressure monitoring, osmotic agents (mannitol), neuromuscular blocking agents, and/or hyperventilation.

PREVENTION AND CONTROL. An experimental formalin-inactivated vaccine grown in chick embryo cell cultures has been used exclusively for protection of laboratory workers. A commercial vaccine is available for horses; since equines are dead-end hosts, vaccination plays no role in preventing human disease. A high level of vaccine immunity in equines reduces their value as sentinels of WEE activity (see Epidemiology). In threatened or ongoing epidemics, residents should be advised to avoid mosquito bite by use of protective clothing, repellents, window screens, and restricted outdoor activity in the early morning, late afternoon, and evening. Public health measures include spray application of insecticides aimed at the adult *Culex tarsalis* vector.

EASTERN EQUINE ENCEPHALITIS (EEE)

ETIOLOGIC AGENT. EEE virus, first isolated in 1933, is an alphavirus. Two antigenic subtypes (North and South American) are distinguishable by special serologic tests. Methods for viral isolation and assay are as described for WEE.

EPIDEMIOLOGY. ***Incidence and Prevalence.*** The disease in man is relatively rare; 147 recognized cases were reported in the United States between 1955 and 1981. The largest outbreak occurred in 1959 in New Jersey (32 cases), but the usual pattern is one of a predominant equine epizootic involving 100 to 300 animals and associated with several human cases. The Atlantic and Gulf coastal areas are prone to recrudescent viral activity. Enzootic transmission and sporadic cases occur in inland fresh-water swamp areas of the United States east of the Mississippi River. Outbreaks also occur in eastern Canada and in the Caribbean area (Jamaica, Hispaniola, Cuba) caused by the North American viral subtype. Equine epizootics have appeared in Panama, Brazil, Guyana, Venezuela, and Argentina, but human disease is rare or unrecognized.

Despite the small size of EEE epidemics, their cost in terms of severity is high. The case-fatality rate is 60 to 70 per cent. The incidence and mortality are highest in children under 15 and in persons over 55 years, with no sex predilection. A risk of human disease may be predicted by the occurrence of equine cases or outbreaks of fatal encephalitis in penned exotic birds (pheasants, chukar partridges), which precede the appearance of human cases by several weeks or more. Vaccination of horses and birds or inadequate surveillance may abrogate their usefulness as sentinels. Outbreaks occur during the late summer and early fall.

Transmission. In temperate areas, EEE virus circulates between wild birds and *Culiseta melanura* mosquitoes in fresh water swamp habitat. Transmission is favored by excessive rainfall during the autumn of the preceding year and the summer of the current year. Sporadic infections may be acquired in or near fresh water swamps by the bite of the primary enzootic vector, which is principally attracted to birds and rarely feeds on horses and man. Other species, in particular *Aedes sollicitans* and *Coquillettidia perturbans*, are implicated in epidemic-epizootic spread and extension of viral activity from swamp to salt marsh and woodland habitat. Transmission between penned pheasants and chukars is by contact, through pecking and cannibalism. The overwintering cycle is presently unknown.

CLINICAL FEATURES AND PATHOLOGY. The disease is more acute and rapidly progressive than the other arboviral encephalitides. The onset is abrupt, with high fever, vomiting, somnolence, stupor, coma, myoclonus, and generalized convulsions appearing within 24 to 48 hours. Autonomic disturbances (sialorrhea) may be prominent, and respiratory difficulty and cyanosis are frequent. A curious feature of the disease in children is facial, periorbital, or generalized edema. Death usually occurs during the first week after onset; in surviving patients, recovery begins during the second week and may progress rapidly. Residual damage, in 30 to 50 per cent of the patients, is often severe, especially in children, and is characterized by retardation, spastic paralyses, and atrophy of brain substance.

Examination of the cerebrospinal fluid provides a clue to the diagnosis. Early in infection, EEE is characterized by high cell counts (500 to 2000 per cubic millimeter) and a predominance of polymorphonuclear cells. The total cell count falls after day three or four, but polymorphonuclear cells persist as a significant fraction. Red blood cells may be present, the protein elevated, and glucose normal. A striking peripheral leukocytosis and left shift are frequent findings.

In contrast to St. Louis and western equine encephalitis, the brain is grossly edematous and congested, and the inflammatory response is predominantly polymorphonuclear rather than mononuclear. Focal vasculitic lesions, endothelial cell swelling, and intravenous and arteriolar thrombus formation are present. Demyelination, necrosis, neuronolysis, and neuronophagia are prominent. The areas most affected are basal ganglia, thalamus, hippocampus, and frontal and occipital cortex.

SPECIFIC DIAGNOSIS. Isolation of virus from blood and spinal fluid is rarely successful. A postmortem diagnosis can be achieved by virus isolation from brain in approximately 75 per cent of fatal cases. Serologic diagnosis is as described for WEE virus; because of the rapid course of the clinical disease, sera should be obtained at two- to three-day intervals during the acute phase of illness. An early serologic diagnosis can often be made by this means.

TREATMENT. Treatment is supportive (see previous discussion of WEE).

PREVENTION AND CONTROL. An experimental formalin-inactivated chick embryo cell culture vaccine is used to protect laboratory and field workers. Vaccination prevents disease in equines but does not interrupt transmission or prevent human infection. Reduction of mosquito populations by appropriate use of insecticides may be effective in threatened or established outbreaks.

VENEZUELAN EQUINE ENCEPHALITIS (VEE)

ETIOLOGY. The causative agent is an alphavirus first isolated in 1938 from a sick horse in Venezuela. Five antigenic subtypes (I to V) are separable by serologic tests; multiple antigenic variants of subtypes I and III are also recognized. Subtypes IAB and IC are responsible for epidemics involving man and equines. In Florida, subtype II is enzootic and produces sporadic human disease. Definition of the antigenic subtype and variant responsible for infection requires isolation of the virus and characterization by a specialty laboratory.

EPIDEMIOLOGY. ***Incidence and Prevalence.*** Large equine epizootics occur at five- to ten-year intervals in Venezuela, Colombia, Ecuador, and Peru. The capacity of VEE virus to invade new territory was demonstrated in 1969, when subtype IAB virus appeared in Guatemala and spread in waves throughout Central America, Mexico, and south Texas. Individual epizootics have involved many thousands (sometimes more than 100,000) of animals, with up to 40 per cent mortality rates. Associated human morbidity has also been great (up to 30,000 clinical cases). Truly subclinical infections are rare. The predominant syndrome is a self-limited grippe-like illness, and only about 4 per cent of infected persons, principally children under 15 years, develop encephalitis. The case-fatality rate in children up to five years old with encephalitis is approximately 35 per cent, but in older persons it is less than 10 per cent. Laboratory infections are common in unvaccinated persons working with the virus or infected animals.

Transmission. Transmission of subtypes IAB and IC viruses during epizootic-epidemics is effected by a large variety of mosquito vectors, including species of the genera *Aedes*, *Psorophora*, and *Mansonia*; equines are the principal viremic hosts. Viremia in man is of sufficient magnitude to infect mosquitoes, but man-mosquito-man transmission is of minor importance in the generation and maintenance of an outbreak. Virus may be present in pharyngeal excretions of human patients; contact or aerosol person-to-person spread, although possible, is not epidemiologically important. Aerosol transmission in the laboratory is nevertheless well documented. The interepidemic maintenance transmission cycle of these viral subtypes is unknown.

The other members of the VEE viral complex, including subtype II in Florida, have enzootic transmission cycles involving *Culex (Melanoconion)* species mosquitoes and small forest rodents and marsupials. Equines are not involved in transmission; human disease is sporadic and relatively uncommon, but may be clinically severe.

CLINICAL FEATURES AND PATHOLOGY. The incubation period is two to five days. Onset is sudden, with fever, chills, generalized malaise, and headache; these symptoms are followed by myalgia (especially in the lumbar region), nausea, vomiting, and occasionally diarrhea. Physical examination reveals fever, tachycardia, conjunctival injection, and, in some cases, nonexudative pharyngitis. Acute symptoms generally subside in four to six days; a convalescent fatigue syndrome may follow, lasting up to three weeks. A biphasic course has sometimes been noted; acute symptoms reappear after a brief remission, within a week after the initial onset.

Evidence of mild central nervous system involvement (photophobia, somnolence, confusion) may be present in cases of the typical, grippe-like illness described above. Severe encephalitis develops in a small proportion of those infected, principally children, and is characterized by meningeal signs, convulsions, tremor, stupor, coma, spastic paralysis, abnormal reflexes, cranial nerve palsies, and central respiratory failure. Residual neurologic damage occurs in severe cases. Congenital infections acquired during the first and second trimesters result in fetal encephalitis and death.

In the first few days of illness, the peripheral leukocyte count may be depressed, with decrease in both lymphocytes and neutrophils, or normal, with a relative lymphopenia. Eosinopenia and vacuolization of monocytes have been described. In cases with central nervous system signs, the cerebrospinal fluid contains up to 500 cells per cubic millimeter, predominantly lymphocytes. The serum lactic dehydrogenase and glutamic-oxaloacetic transaminase levels may be elevated. Impaired glucose tolerance and insulin release were found in experimental animals after VEE infection, but there are no reports of a diabetogenic effect in man.

The neuropathologic features of the disease in man have not been clearly documented. In the congenitally infected fetus there is massive and widespread necrosis of brain tissue, hemorrhages, and resorption of brain material, resulting in hydranencephaly.

DIAGNOSIS. Virus can be isolated from the blood during the first three or four days after onset, with peak titers on day two. Isolation from throat swabs or washings may also be successful. HI and N antibodies appear in the first week and CF antibodies in the second week after onset; serodiagnosis is achieved by testing appropriately timed paired sera.

TREATMENT. No specific therapy is available, and treatment of encephalitis cases is supportive (see earlier discussion of WEE).

PREVENTION AND CONTROL. An experimental live, attenuated vaccine (TC-83) is used in adult laboratory personnel and provides solid immunity to the immunizing subtype (IAB) and its closest relative (IC), but incomplete protection against infection with some heterologous VEE viruses. Epidemics and epizootics can be prevented by effective vaccination of equines (the principal viremic hosts), using live, attenuated, or inactivated TC-83 vaccines. In the face of an ongoing epidemic, spraying of insecticides to reduce the adult (infective) mosquito populations is the only means of immediate control; vaccination of equines at the periphery of the outbreak prevents spread.

ST. LOUIS ENCEPHALITIS (SLE)

ETIOLOGY. St. Louis encephalitis virus, a member of the flavivirus genus of the family Togaviridae, shares close antigenic relationships with Japanese encephalitis, Murray Valley encephalitis, and West Nile viruses. The virus is pathogenic for infant and adult mice inoculated intracerebrally and may also be assayed in a variety of avian and mammalian cell cultures. Strain differences in pathogenicity and genome composition are recognized and provide a geographic and epidemiologic classification. Strains associated with *Culex pipiens*-borne epidemics in the eastern United States are distinct from endemic strains transmitted by *Culex tarsalis* in the western states.

EPIDEMIOLOGY. ***Incidence and Prevalence.*** The virus is present in all parts of the Western Hemisphere, but causes epidemics only in North America and some Caribbean islands. During epidemic years, the virus has been responsible for up to 80 per cent of all reported cases of encephalitis of known etiology in the United States. A total of 4965 cases were reported between 1955 and 1981. In recent years, epidemics have occurred mainly in urban-suburban localities of the Ohio–Mississippi River basin, in eastern and central Texas, and in Florida. Small outbreaks have also occurred in rural areas of the western United States. Epidemics generally occur between July and September, with a peak in August, but may arise later in the year in warm areas such as Florida. No racial difference in disease susceptibility exists, but, owing to socioeconomic factors, attack rates have been higher in the black than in the white population of some cities. Prior exposure and immunity to dengue may provide a degree of cross-protection against clinical SLE.

The overall case-fatality rate is approximately 9 per cent; mortality is negligible in persons under 20 years, and it rises steeply after age 55 to approximately 30 per cent in patients over 65 years of age. The inapparent:apparent infection ratio is 800:1 in children up to nine years, 400:1 in persons 10 to 49 years, and 85:1 in persons over 60 years.

In tropical America, a high prevalence of antibody in many areas indicates widespread transmission; disease is sporadic and rarely recognized.

Transmission. In most of the eastern United States, SLE virus circulates between wild birds and *Culex pipiens* mosquitoes. *Culex pipiens* breeds in polluted water and achieves high densities in urban-suburban areas with poor sanitation. In Florida and in parts of the Caribbean, *Culex nigripalpus* is the principal vector. The cycle in the western United States also involves wild birds, but the vector is *Culex tarsalis.* The ecology of SLE and WEE viruses in the west is thus similar, and transmission occurs in rural, agricultural areas. Horses develop antibodies but not overt disease or significant viremia. The primary vectors *(C. pipiens, nigripalpus, tarsalis)* are responsible for transmission to man.

Above-average summer temperatures and deficient rainfall (which creates stagnant pools suitable for *Culex pipiens* breeding) are associated with epidemics in the eastern United States. *Culex tarsalis*–borne SLE in the western states is favored by warm spring temperatures, heavy winter-spring precipitation, high river runoff, and flood conditions.

During the winter, the virus is probably maintained locally in infected hibernating adult female *Culex.*

CLINICAL FEATURES AND PATHOLOGY. Three clinical syndromes are recognized: febrile headache, aseptic meningitis, and encephalitis. As discussed above, encephalitis is a more frequent presentation in the elderly and the milder syndromes in young patients. The incubation period is 4 to 21 days. Onset is characterized by a variable period of nonspecific symptoms, including fever, headache, generalized malaise, drowsiness, myalgias, and sore throat, followed by the acute or subacute onset of meningeal or encephalitic signs or both. Fever ranges from 38.3 to 41° C; poor prognosis is associated with persistent high temperatures of 40 to 41° C. Nausea and vomiting and photophobia are common. Neurologic abnormalities include altered sensorium, meningismus, cranial nerve deficits (principally lower motor neuron N. VII), abnormal reflexes, and tremors. Signs of thalamic, brainstem, and cerebellar dysfunction include myoclonic twitching, nystagmus, and ataxia in up to 25 per cent of patients. Motor abnormalities are infrequent and sensory changes extremely uncommon. Convulsions occur in 10 per cent of patients and are a poor prognostic sign. In general, extrapyramidal abnormalities (tremor of tongue, face, and limbs) and the altered state of consciousness are the most significant findings. Signs of markedly increased intracranial pressure are very unusual. Acute inflammatory polyradiculoneuropathy (Guillain-Barré syndrome) has occasionally been associated with SLE, both as an acute presentation and during the convalescent period. Approximately half of the patients with fatal outcome succumb during the first week and 80 per cent within two weeks after onset. Complications of the neurologic disease include pneumonia, bacterial septicemia, pulmonary embolism, and gastrointestinal hemorrhage. Underlying conditions, especially hypertensive and arteriosclerotic disease, chronic brain syndromes, diabetes mellitus, and chronic bronchopulmonary disease, appear to play a role in determining severity and outcome, and may relate to the virulence of the disease process in older persons.

In uncomplicated cases of SLE, there is a moderate peripheral neutrophilic leukocytosis and left shift. Cerebrospinal fluid is under increased pressure and contains up to 500 cells per cubic millimeter, with polymorphonuclear predominance early, changing to lymphocyte predominance within several days. Spinal fluid protein is mildly elevated and glucose usually normal; in one series, however, cerebrospinal fluid glucose was less than 50 per cent of the blood level in 5 of 23 adult patients. Elevations of serum enzymes (creatine phosphokinase and glutamic-oxaloacetic transaminase) are frequently found. Serum aldolase levels may be elevated, but muscle biopsies have shown no changes. The electroencephalogram typically shows amorphous delta wave activity and diffuse generalized slowing most prominent in the frontal and temporal regions. The brain scan is normal. Disproportionately high cerebral blood flow in relation to metabolic demands has been documented, indicating a disturbance in cerebrovascular autoregulation. Mild hyponatremia and fluid overload in about one third of patients with encephalitis are due to the syndrome of inappropriate secretion of antidiuretic hormone.

Genitourinary tract symptoms (urgency, frequency, incontinence, and retention), microscopic hematuria, pyuria, and proteinuria, and elevated blood urea nitrogen are frequent. SLE viral antigen in cells of the urinary sediment has been detected by fluorescent techniques and virus-like particles in urine by immunoelectronmicroscopy. The possibility that the kidney is a site of SLE replication and injury remains problematic.

A convalescent fatigue syndrome characterized by weakness, fatigue, nervousness, tremulousness, sleeplessness, irritability, depression, difficulty in concentrating, and headaches occurs in 30 to 50 per cent of older persons and clears in 80 per cent of these within three years.

Pathologic changes in fatal cases are limited to microscopic examination. Leptomeningitis is characterized by lymphocytic inflammation. Parenchymal changes consist of lymphocytic perivascular cuffing, cellular nodule formation, and neuronal degeneration. Changes are most pronounced in substantia nigra, thalamus and hypothalamus, cerebellar cortex, cerebral cortex, and basal ganglia.

DIAGNOSIS. In approximately half of the fatal cases, a diagnosis may be made by virus isolation from brain tissue or immunofluorescent staining of frozen sections of brain. The virus is rarely isolated from blood or spinal fluid obtained during the acute phase of illness. Serologic diagnosis is achieved by demonstration of changing antibody titers; the HI, immunoassay, and N tests demonstrate antibody within the first week after onset, and titers rise during the ensuing two weeks. CF antibodies appear 10 to 20 days after onset. Rapid early diagnosis is possible by measurement of IgM antibodies by enzyme-linked immunosorbent assay (ELISA) and serum and cerebrospinal fluid. Specific serologic diagnosis may be complicated by cross-reactions in persons with prior exposures to dengue and other related flaviviruses.

TREATMENT. Treatment is supportive (see earlier discussion of WEE). Hyponatremia and clinical signs of water intoxication are generally of mild to moderate severity and are managed by restricting fluid intake.

PREVENTION AND CONTROL. No vaccine is available. Surveillance of vectors, antibody prevalence in wild birds, or serologic conversions in sentinel fowl are used to detect viral transmission before the occurrence of human infections. The information may be used to initiate vector control efforts. Source reduction and larviciding of vector breeding sites are useful preventive measures. In the case of an established outbreak, avoidance of mosquito bites and spraying to reduce infected adult mosquitoes are the only effective means of control.

CALIFORNIA ENCEPHALITIS

ETIOLOGY. Four members of the California serogroup of the Bunyavirus genus, LaCrosse, California encephalitis, Jamestown Canyon, and snowshoe hare viruses, cause encephalitis. California encephalitis virus occurs in the western United States (California, New Mexico, Utah, Texas) and has been implicated in only three human cases. In contrast, LaCrosse virus, distributed more widely in the eastern half of the United States and southern Canada, is a major human pathogen. It was first isolated from the brain of a child who died of encephalitis in 1964 at LaCrosse, Wisconsin. Recently Jamestown Canyon and snowshoe hare viruses have been implicated in sporadic human encephalitis cases in the north central United States and in Canada. Mice and a variety of cell cultures are useful for virus isolation and assay.

EPIDEMIOLOGY. ***Incidence and Prevalence.*** Between its recognition as a nosologic entity in 1964 and 1981, a total of 1310 cases of LaCrosse viral encephalitis have been reported in the United States, with an annual incidence of 50 to 150 cases. Undoubtedly far underreported, it occurs as an endemic rather than an epidemic disease, with individual or small clusters of cases scattered across the affected areas. It is most prevalent in the north central states, where it is responsible for as many as 20 per cent of cases of acute central nervous system infection in children. It primarily affects persons less than 15 years of age living in rural and suburban areas characterized by deciduous hardwood forests. Focal "hot spots" (communities, even backyards) of recurrent summertime viral activity are recognized. Cases occur between July and September, with peak incidence in August. The case-fatality rate is low (less than 1 per cent).

TRANSMISSION. The vectors of LaCrosse virus are *Aedes* mosquitoes (principally *Ae. triseriatus*), which breed both in forest tree-holes and in peridomestic artificial containers. The vector serves as a reservoir of LaCrosse virus, which is efficiently passed transovarially from female mosquitoes to progeny. The virus survives the winter months in infected eggs of *Aedes triseriatus*. In the summer months, wild rodents (squirrels, chipmunks) contribute to a cycle of transmission as viremic hosts. Man becomes infected by the bite of an infected mosquito but does not play a role in transmission.

CLINICAL FEATURES. The true clinical spectrum of California virus infection is not known, but undoubtedly includes nonspecific febrile illness, aseptic meningitis, and meningoencephalitis. Encephalitis may be quite severe in the acute stage, but the disease is almost always self-limited and death is extremely uncommon. The disease begins with a nonspecific syndrome of fever, headache, sore throat, and gastrointestinal symptoms, with appearance of the neurotropic disorder within one to three days. In mild cases of encephalitis, central nervous system signs appear on the third day after onset and subside within seven to eight days. In the more severe form, neurologic signs appear earlier (within 24 to 48 hours of onset), usually in the form of generalized seizures and altered consciousness, and are more prolonged. Papilledema or abnormal optic disc margins have been noted, but signs of progressive intracranial hypertension are rare. Intensive care and respiratory support are frequently required in severe cases. The question of permanent sequelae is unsettled. Although there are conflicting reports, many workers believe LaCrosse virus infection is responsible for residual psychologic problems, emotional lability, hyperkinesis, infantilism, compulsive behavior, and auditory and visual perceptual problems. There are case reports of hemiparesis and persistent seizure disorders.

The peripheral white cell count is often moderately elevated, with a predominance of granulocytes and band forms. The cerebrospinal fluid shows up to 500 lymphocytes per cubic millimeter, normal or mildly elevated protein, and normal glucose concentrations. The abnormalities on the electroencephalogram include generalized slowing in the delta and theta range, indicating diffuse cortical dysfunction. Focal delta wave activity related to cortical destruction or focal seizures is also a common finding.

DIAGNOSIS. The virus has been recovered from the brain in fatal cases, but not from blood or spinal fluid obtained during the acute phase. Diagnosis is best achieved by tests for antibody in paired acute and convalescent sera. The counterimmunoelectrophoresis, HI, CF, FA, ELISA, and N tests are applicable. However, the most practical, sensitive, and reliable methods are the HI test using the LaCrosse viral antigen and the IgM antibody capture ELISA.

TREATMENT. Treatment is supportive.

PREVENTION AND CONTROL. There is no vaccine. Vector control methods are of uncertain usefulness in this disease because of the multifocal, endemic pattern of disease incidence and the inherited nature of infection in mosquito vectors. In defined "hot spots" of recurrent viral activity, efforts to eliminate breeding sites for *Aedes triseriatus* should be made. Avoidance of mosquito bites and protection of children by limiting exposure and use of repellents are reasonable suggestions to parents.

JAPANESE ENCEPHALITIS

ETIOLOGY. Japanese encephalitis is caused by a flavivirus first isolated in 1934 from the brain of a fatal human case in Japan. Unlike SLE, it causes epizootics of clinical encephalitis in equines. The virus also produces abortion and stillbirth in swine, an important economic problem in parts of Asia. Serologic cross-reactivity with other flaviviruses may lead to confusion in diagnostic tests.

EPIDEMIOLOGY. ***Prevalence and Incidence.*** The disease is endemic and epidemic in Asia, including Japan, Korea, Taiwan, China, Okinawa, Vietnam, the Philippines, Burma, Malaysia, Bangladesh, east and south India, Thailand, and Indonesia. Morbidity in some outbreaks is high (thousands of cases); case-fatality rates of 50 per cent or more have been reported but reflect underrecognition of nonfatal cases. In hyperendemic areas, over 70 per cent of adult populations surveyed have antibodies, and children under 15 years old are principally affected by the disease. In areas without a high prevalence of background immunity (e.g., northern India), however, all age groups are affected; and in Japan, where school children have been protected by vaccination campaigns targeted at this age group, occurrence of encephalitis in the elderly has become evident. The inapparent:apparent infection ratio is over 500:1 in children and decreases with age; in Korea, the ratio among American servicemen was estimated at 25:1. In temperate areas, JE is a summertime disease; in the tropics, it occurs year-round as a sporadic infection. Epidemics have been most frequent at the northern fringe of the tropical zone. JE is predominantly a rural disease, and the incidence in males is often higher than in females.

Transmission. The natural cycle involves *Culex* mosquito vectors and vertebrates susceptible to viremic infection, including wild birds and swine. Man and equines are incidental (dead-end) hosts. The vector species varies with geographic area; *Culex tritaeniorhyncus*, a rice-paddy breeder, is the most widespread and important. Overwinter survival and springtime recrudescence in temperate areas are unexplained, but evidence suggests that transovarial viral transmission in mosquitoes may play a role.

CLINICAL FEATURES AND PATHOLOGY. The spectrum of illness includes febrile headache, aseptic meningitis, and meningoencephalitis. The disease is more severe than St. Louis encephalitis. Onset is abrupt, with fever, headache, and gastrointestinal symptoms. Meningeal irritation develops within 24 hours and is followed on the second or third day by the appearance of irritability, impaired consciousness, convulsions (especially in children), muscular rigidity, mask-like facies, ataxia, coarse tremor, involuntary movements, cranial nerve deficits, paresis, hyperactive deep tendon reflexes, and pathologic reflexes. Weight loss and dehydration are often striking findings. In patients with mild involvement, fever subsides on the sixth or seventh day and neurologic signs resolve by the end of the second week after onset. In severe cases, hyperpyrexia and progressive neurologic dysfunction and coma result in death between the seventh and tenth days, or the patient undergoes a prolonged recovery, often leaving permanent sequelae. Cardiorespiratory complications are frequent during the acute stage in these patients. Atypical forms with predominance of bulbar or myelitic signs have been described. A poor prognosis is associated with prolonged high fever, frequent or prolonged seizures, high protein content in the cerebrospinal fluid, Babinski signs, and early appearance of respiratory depression.

The occurrence of sequelae correlates with severity of the acute stage of illness; young children are most susceptible, and sequelae, including mental impairment, emotional lability, choreoathetosis, tremor, parkinsonism, autonomic disturbances, motor paralysis, and pathopsychologic syndromes, including schizophrenia, have been reported in up to 75 per cent of patients.

Transplacental infection, resulting in fetal death and abortion, has been reported.

Clinical laboratory tests show a moderate peripheral leukocytosis early in the disease (usually characterized by neutrophilia) and cerebrospinal fluid pleocytosis, polymorphonuclear early but predominantly mononuclear later in the disease. Spinal fluid protein is mildly elevated and glucose concentration normal.

Neuropathologic changes and distribution of lesions are similar to those described for St. Louis encephalitis (see earlier discussion of SLE).

DIAGNOSIS. In many patients dying during the first week after onset, the virus may be isolated from brain or viral antigen demonstrated by immunofluorescence. Isolations from blood or spinal fluid are uncommon, and diagnosis is best achieved by serologic tests. HI and N antibodies appear during the first and CF antibodies during the second week after onset. In areas where other flaviviral infections are common, cross-reactions make serodiagnosis difficult; increased precision may be obtained by measuring early, specific IgM antibodies by immunoassays on serum or cerebrospinal fluid.

TREATMENT. Treatment is supportive (see earlier discussion of WEE).

PREVENTION AND CONTROL. Inactivated, partially purified mouse brain vaccines produced in Asia are used principally in preschool- and school-age children. Although not yet licensed for use in the United States, a vaccine produced in Japan is available on a limited scale to United States citizens traveling to high-risk areas. Information should be sought from state health departments or the Centers for Disease Control. Since three doses of the inactivated vaccine are used, and approximately one month is required to confer protection, vaccination is not a practical measure in the face of an ongoing epidemic. Reduction of vector mosquito populations by ultra-low volume application of insecticides may be used to abort outbreaks.

MURRAY VALLEY ENCEPHALITIS AND ROCIO ENCEPHALITIS

Murray Valley encephalitis and Rocio encephalitis are similar to Japanese encephalitis in pathogenesis and clinical features and are caused by closely related flaviviruses.

Murray Valley encephalitis has occurred in small epidemics in the Murray and Darling River valleys of Victoria and New South Wales, Australia. The virus is endemic in Northern Australia and New Guinea, where it is maintained in a bird-mosquito cycle. It has been postulated that the virus is intermittently brought south by migratory birds; in southern Australia, transmission involves water birds, domestic fowl, and *Culex annulirostris* mosquitoes. Diagnosis requires laboratory studies similar to those for other flaviviruses. No vaccine is available.

Rocio encephalitis was first described in 1975, when a new flavivirus by the same name was isolated from the brains of patients with fatal encephalitis during an epidemic in São Paulo State, Brazil. In several discrete outbreaks in 1975–1976, over 1000 cases occurred in this region, but the disease has not been recognized elsewhere. The transmission cycle is poorly understood, but probably involves wild birds and mosquitoes. An inactivated suckling mouse brain vaccine has been prepared but has been found to be of low potency.

TICK-BORNE ENCEPHALITIS

ETIOLOGIC AGENTS. A complex of six antigenically related tick-borne flaviviruses consists of Powassan, tick-borne encephalitis virus (TBE), louping ill, Kyasanur Forest disease (KFD), Omsk hemorrhagic fever (OHF), and Langat viruses. The predominant syndrome in KFD and OHF is hemorrhagic fever (see earlier discussion of VEE),but meningoencephalitis may be a component of the disease spectrum. Two subtypes of TBE virus (Central European encephalitis and Russian spring-summer encephalitis) are distinguished by special serologic tests, are ecologically distinct, and differ in virulence for man. Powassan and louping ill viruses are rare causes of encephalitis in North America and the British Isles, respectively. These viruses are serologically easily distinguished from mosquito-borne flaviviruses, but induce cross-reactions within the complex. The viruses may be isolated and assayed in infant mice and a variety of cell cultures.

EPIDEMIOLOGY. ***Incidence and Prevalence.*** TBE occurs in Europe (including European Russia), southern Scandinavia, and the far eastern USSR. Several hundred to 2000 cases are reported annually, with morbidity rates of up to 20 per 100,000 inhabitants. Inapparent infections are common. The disease is seasonal, corresponding to peak summertime tick vector populations. Adults over 20 years are principally affected, and persons frequenting tick-infested foci (e.g., forestry workers, shepherds, campers) are at highest risk. Family outbreaks are caused by drinking infected milk (see Transmission, below). In Europe, the disease is relatively mild (case-fatality rate 1 to 2 per cent); but in the Far East, it is severe (20 to 25 per cent). In the United States, the disease should be considered in persons with a history of travel to endemic areas.

Louping ill causes encephalitis in sheep and cattle in Scotland and in northern England and Ireland. Sporadic human cases have been recognized in veterinarians, butchers, and laboratory workers. Serologic surveys indicate that natural infections are uncommon. Powassan virus encephalitis has been documented in a total of 15 cases in the northeastern United States and eastern Canada. The case-fatality rate is 50 per cent. The virus is not associated with animal disease. Serosurveys indicate that human infections in the endemic area are rare (prevalence rates less than 1 per cent).

Transmission. In Europe, the vector of TBE is *Ixodes ricinus*, and in the Far East, *I. persulcatus*. The tick vector also serves as a reservoir of the virus, which is transmitted both transovarially and from one stage (instar) to the next. Larval ticks parasitize small rodents, which serve as amplifying viremic hosts during the spring and summer; hibernating rodents may also harbor the virus during the winter. Man is a dead-end host, incidental to the transmission cycle. Large vertebrates (goats, sheep, cattle) are hosts for nymphal and adult ticks and may become infected and shed virus in the milk. Outbreaks have occurred in families or groups of individuals ingesting unpasteurized goat or sheep milk or cheese.

Louping ill virus is maintained in nature by *Ixodes ricinus* ticks and a variety of hosts, including small mammals, ground-dwelling birds (grouse), and, probably, sheep. Humans become infected by direct contact with infected sheep, or by tick bite. The transmission cycle of Powassan virus involves *Ixodes cookei*, *I. marxi* (and possibly other tick species), and mammals, particularly rodents and carnivores. Human infection is acquired by tick bite; because of the small size of the vector, a history of bite is infrequently obtained.

CLINICAL FEATURES. TBE in Europe typically (but not invariably) has a diphasic course, beginning 7 to 14 days after exposure with an influenza-like syndrome lasting one week, followed by a period of clinical remission for several days, and then abrupt onset of aseptic meningitis or meningoencephalitis. The latter is usually benign, although severe paralytic illness, myelitis, myeloradiculitis, and bulbar forms may occur. Convalescence is often prolonged, and residual paralysis may follow in severe cases. In the Far East, TBE begins suddenly with fever, headache, and gastrointestinal symptoms, followed rapidly by appearance of depressed sensorium, coma, convulsions, and paralysis. Bulbar paralysis and cervical myelitis are frequent findings. In fatal cases, death occurs in the first week after onset. Survivors have a high incidence of residual paralyses, especially lower motor neuron paralysis of upper extremities or shoulder girdle. Aseptic meningitis and milder forms of encephalitis also occur. Chronic forms of TBE have been described, with active clinical and pathologic abnormalities a year or more after onset.

The clinical features of louping ill resemble the European form of TBE. Powassan encephalitis is characterized by a variable period of fever and nonspecific symptoms, followed by the development of encephalitic signs, which are frequently severe. Residual paralysis may occur.

Peripheral blood and cerebrospinal fluid changes are similar to those described in other forms of flaviviral encephalitis.

DIAGNOSIS. The virus may be isolated from brain tissue. In TBE, virus isolation from blood is also possible during the early phase of illness. Serologic diagnosis is achieved by the HI, CF, N, or ELISA techniques.

TREATMENT. Treatment is supportive (see earlier discussion of WEE).

CONTROL. In eastern Europe and the USSR, TBE vaccines are used in high-risk groups (forestry and agricultural workers, military personnel). Avoidance of tick exposure by use of protective clothing and repellents may be recommended to visitors in areas of high TBE activity. Surveillance of viral transmission and use of insecticides to control ticks have met with variable success. In years of high rodent population density, rodent control in natural foci has also been recommended.

Bennett NM: Murray Valley encephalitis, 1974. Clinical features. Med J Aust 2:446, 1976. *A useful guide to the clinical aspects of this rare infection.*

Blaškovič D, Nosek J: The ecological approach to the study of tick-borne encephalitis. Prog Med Virol 14:275, 1972. *Comprehensive review of the ecology, epidemiology, prevention, and control of tick-borne encephalitis; exhaustively referenced.*

Calisher CH, Thompson WH (eds.): California Serogroup Viruses. New York, Alan R. Liss, Inc., 1983. *Symposium covering all aspects of this virus group.*

Grabow JD, Matthews CG, Chun RWM, Thompson WH: The electroencephalogram and clinical sequelae of California arbovirus encephalitis. Neurology 19:394, 1969. *Clear descriptions of clinical course and residual damage in children with California encephalitis; should be consulted together with reference by Matthews et al.*

Hilty MD, Haynes RE, Azimi PH, Cramblett HG: California encephalitis in children. Am J Dis Child 124:530, 1972. *Useful clinical descriptions of this infection.*

Johnson KM, Martin DH: Venezuelan equine encephalitis. Adv Vet Sci Comp Med 18:79, 1974. *A superbly written, detailed, and well-referenced review of the clinical, virologic, and epidemiologic aspects of this disease.*

Leon CA, Jaramillo R, Martinez S, Fernandez F, Tellez H, Lasso B, Guzman R de: Sequelae of Venezuelan equine encephalitis in humans: A four-year follow-up. Int J Epidemiol 4:131, 1975. *The only well-documented study of neurologic residua of this infection.*

Lincoln AF, Sivertson SE: Acute phase of Japanese B encephalitis. Two hundred and one cases in American soldiers, Korea, 1950. JAMA 150:268, 1952. *The leading reference in English to the clinical features of Japanese encephalitis.*

Lopes O de S, Sachetta L de A, Coimbra TLM, Pinto GH, Glasser CM: Emergence of a new arbovirus disease in Brazil [Rocio]. II. Epidemiologic studies on 1975 epidemic. Am J Epidemiol 108:394, 1978. *First description of this newly recognized disease; contains only epidemiologic information.*

Matthews CG, Chun RWM, Grabow JD, Thompson, WH: Psychological sequelae in children following California arbovirus encephalitis. Neurology 18:1023, 1968. *Useful to the physician facing questions from patients about sequelae in children recovering from this infection.*

Monath TP (ed.): Saint Louis Encephalitis. Washington, D.C., American Public Health Association, 1980. *Encyclopedic coverage of all aspects of St. Louis encephalitis, including clinical features and differential and definitive laboratory diagnosis. Contains references to all previously published studies.*

Venezuelan Encephalitis. Washington, D.C., Pan-American Health Organization Publication No. 243, 1972. *Proceedings of a symposium containing a wealth of published and unpublished information; all aspects of the disease are covered, but emphasis is on virology and ecology-epidemiology.*

Wallis RC: Recent advances in research on the eastern encephalitis virus. Yale J Biol Med 37:413, 1965. *A review; emphasizes epidemiologic and ecologic aspects.*

Viral Hemorrhagic Fevers

357. INTRODUCTION*

Karl M. Johnson

The viral hemorrhagic fevers form a group of acute diseases in which bleeding is a prominent clinical manifestation. These diseases occur in different parts of the world, are caused by ribonucleic acid (RNA)–containing viruses, and may be transmitted to man by mosquitoes, by ticks, or by direct contact with excreta of virus-infected rodents (see Table 358–1). Despite its longstanding fame as a cause of acute hepatocellular necrosis, *yellow fever* is included under this heading because of its recognized ability to induce gastrointestinal hemorrhage and a shock syndrome similar to that seen with other viruses of the group.

After a variable period of a few days to one to three weeks, during which the virus multiplies in lymphoid cells and produces a viremia, hemorrhagic fever patients experience fever, myalgia, and other nonspecific symptoms. Bleeding ensues, generally near the end of the febrile period, and although usually not sufficient per se to account for it, such hemorrhage is the harbinger of a clinical crisis dominated by hypovolemic shock. In at least two conditions, hemorrhagic fever with renal syndrome and dengue hemorrhagic fever, there is evidence that shock is caused by a widespread capillary vascular lesion in which plasma protein escapes the circulation much faster than erythrocytes. Thrombocytopenia and deficits in various circulating hemostatic factors are frequently present, but it is not clear whether they are etiologically related to this condition.

How the hemorrhagic syndrome is produced thus remains a mystery. No evidence for a direct virus-induced lesion of capillary endothelium has been obtained to date. Disseminated intravascular coagulation (DIC) has been shown in a few instances and postulated in others. Nevertheless, we have no clear idea about the important pathophysiologic events that induce hemorrhage and shock. Acute hepatocellular damage is present in many of these diseases and may play some role. Altered immunologic function also may be important; inflammatory reaction to tissue injury is notably absent in most hemorrhagic fevers, B cell lymphocyte suppression is suggested by high incidence of secondary bacterial infection and delay in antibody formation in Junin, Machupo, and Congo-CHF infections, and antigen-antibody complexes may prove to be important in dengue, Lassa, and Hantaan virus disease. Elucidation of the operative variables is important because case management and development of effective vaccines appear to offer more hope of averting fatal infection than interruption of nonhuman natural virus cycles.

358. YELLOW FEVER

Thomas P. Monath

DEFINITION. Yellow fever is an acute mosquito-borne viral infection characterized, in its severe form, by fever, jaundice, hemorrhage, and albuminuria. The disease is endemic-epidemic in tropical regions of the Americas and Africa (see Fig. 358–1), where it remains a major public health problem, but it does not occur in Asia.

*The views of the author in this and subsequent chapters do not purport to reflect the positions of the Department of the Army or the Department of Defense (Para. 4-3, AR 360-5).

ETIOLOGY. Yellow fever virus is the prototype of the flavivirus taxonomic group, which is composed of a variety of other medically important, antigenically related viruses, including several which also cause hemorrhagic fevers (see Table 358–1). Yellow fever virus and other flaviviruses are spherical, enveloped, RNA-containing particles of approximately 38 mμ in size; virions develop by budding from intracytoplasmic membranes of infected cells and accumulate in cisternae of the endoplasmic reticulum. Since the virus shares antigenic determinants with many other flaviviruses, serologic responses to infection are often nonspecific or difficult to interpret. Strains of yellow fever virus from Africa and South America are distinguishable in special serologic tests; strain variation in virulence markers for laboratory animals also occurs. However, no clear geographic differences have been shown in the clinical features of the human disease. Yellow fever virus is pathogenic for a variety of cell cultures, newborn mice, adult mice (when injected intracerebrally), and some monkey species. Rhesus monkeys have been used as an experimental model of the human disease.

EPIDEMIOLOGY. Two epidemiologic forms of yellow fever are classically distinguished on the basis of different mosquito vectors and vertebrate hosts involved in the cycle of virus transmission. These forms are clinically and pathoanatomically identical. In the *urban* form, yellow fever virus is passed from a viremic person to another, nonimmune individual by the peridomestic mosquito, *Aedes aegypti.* As with other arboviruses, a period of extrinsic incubation in the vector is required before virus can be transmitted. *Jungle* (or sylvan) yellow fever is a zoonotic infection, acquired through the bite of forest mosquito vector species, which maintain the virus in a monkey-mosquito-monkey cycle. The epidemiology of the disease in the Americas and in Africa differs and must be considered separately.

Between 50 and 300 cases of *jungle yellow fever* are recognized annually in South America. The virus is active primarily in Brazil, Peru, Bolivia, and Colombia in forested and sparsely populated areas under limited cultivation, drained by tributar-

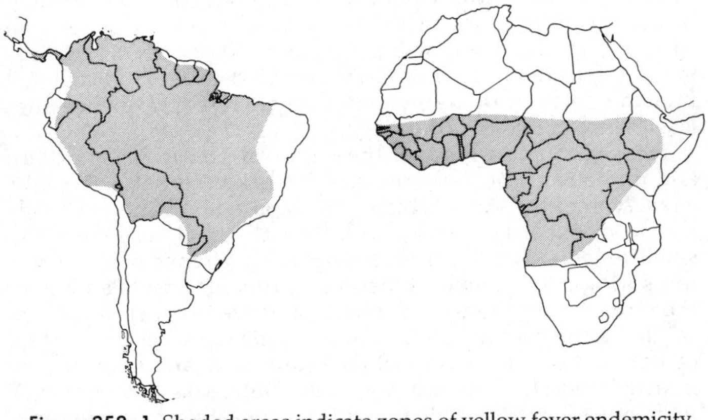

Figure 358–1. Shaded areas indicate zones of yellow fever endemicity. Some countries do not require certificate of yellow fever vaccination from travelers; nevertheless, vaccination is recommended for travel outside the urban areas of countries in the endemic zones. Yellow fever should be suspected in unvaccinated persons with fever and jaundice acquired in these areas.

TABLE 358–1. VIRAL HEMORRHAGIC FEVERS: ETIOLOGIC AND EPIDEMIOLOGIC CONSIDERATIONS

	Causative Agent	Vector(s)	Vertebrate Host(s)	Geographical Distribution	Epidemiologic Features of Involvement of Man	Control	Remarks
Yellow fever (urban)	YF virus—a flavivirus	*Aedes aegypti* in cities	Man	Human populations (usually urban) in tropics of South and Central America and Africa	Person-to-person passage by *Aedes aegypti*	*Aedes aegypti* control; vaccination	Sylvan YF can spread to cities
Yellow fever (sylvan)	YF virus—a flavivirus	*Haemagogus* mosquitoes in New World; *Aedes* species in Africa	Monkeys of several genera and species	Forests and jungles of South and Central America and West, Central, and East Africa	Man infected by exposure in jungle (e.g., woodcutters, hunters)	Vaccination	Human cases sporadic and unpredictable; disease often a "silent" epizootic in forests
Dengue hemorrhagic fever	Dengue viruses of four types; flaviviruses	*Aedes aegypti*	Man (involvement of other primates has been postulated)	Tropical and subtropical cities of Southeast Asia and Philippines; Caribbean	Small children usually involved in cities where *Aedes aegypti* densities ae high	*Aedes aegypti* control; mosquito repellent, screens, etc.	Disease may represent an immunologic over-response to a sequential infection with a different dengue strain
Omsk hemorrhagic fever	OHF virus—a flavivirus	Ticks of genus *Dermacentor*	Small rodents and muskrats	Omsk region of USSR; northern Rumania	People exposed in fields and wooded lands	Tick repellents and protective clothing	
Kyasanur Forest disease	KFD virus—a flavivirus	Ticks of several species in genus *Haemaphysalis*	Monkeys (rhesus and langur) and small rodents and birds	Mysore State, India	People exposed in fields and wooded lands	Tick control; tick repellents and protective clothing	Monkey mortality signals epidemic activity
Argentine hemorrhagic fever	Junin virus, an arenavirus	None recognized	Small rodents; *Akodon; Calomys laucha, musculinus*	Argentina: NW of Buenos Aires extending west to Province of Cordoba	Field workers at harvest time are particularly at risk	None practical	Infected rodents contaminate environment with urine
Bolivian hemorrhagic fever	Machupo virus—an arenavirus	None recognized	Small rodent, *Calomys callosus*	Beni Province of Bolivia	Residents of small rodent-infested villages and homes; 1971 nosocomial outbreak in Cochabamba, Bolivia	Rodent control in villages	High mortality in man
Lassa fever	Lassa virus, an arenavirus LCM-related	None required	Small rodent, *Mastomys natalensis*	West Africa; Nigeria, Liberia, Sierra Leone	Residents of small, rodent-infested villages; dramatic nosocomial outbreaks	None known; possibly rodent control	High mortality in man
Crimean hemorrhagic fever	Congo-CHF virus—a nairovirus	Ticks of several genera	Larger domestic animals implicated; also African hedgehog	Southern USSR, Bulgaria, East and West Africa	Cowhands and field workers in USSR; nosocomial outbreaks reported	Tick control relating to livestock; full isolation in patient care	Human disease important in USSR; importance to man in Africa not known
Korean hemorrhagic fever (hemor. nephroso-nephritis)	Hantaan virus—a bunyavirus	None recognized	Small rodents: *Apodemus, Clethrionomys*	Korea; northern Eurasia to and including Scandinavia	Rural or sylvan exposure (military, forest occupations farmers, laboratory workers)		Urban rats may be reservoirs Related viruses present in North and South America, Africa, without recognized human disease

ies of the Amazon, Orinoco, and Magdalena rivers. Human cases reach a peak during the rainy months. Human cases are often sporadic, but small epidemics (involving 20 to 50 cases) are not uncommon. In the past, large outbreaks have been associated with monkey epizootics which appear at 5- to 40-year intervals and spread through natural corridors into forested areas, such as Central America, normally outside the enzootic zone. In the forest canopy, the virus circulates in a primary cycle involving monkeys and marmosets and mosquitoes of the genus *Haemagogus.* The exact location of virus activity in the vast tropical forests of South America is difficult or impossible to ascertain at any time, and indeed the virus is constantly moving, thus assuring a supply of susceptible hosts adequate for maintenance of the cycle. Presence of the virus is, however, sometimes evident on the basis of monkey deaths, because some New World species succumb to the infection. Humans may acquire the disease during activities, such as woodcutting, which bring them into contact with *Haemagogus* mosquitoes. Dramatic outbreaks have occurred when groups of unvaccinated laborers have penetrated jungle areas.

In the Americas, *urban yellow fever* has not occurred since 1954 (in Trinidad), largely because of the eradication of *Aedes aegypti* mosquitoes from population centers of South America. Nonetheless, some *aegypti*-infested areas of northern South America remain in juxtaposition to the jungle cycle, and the risk of a viremic individual traveling to receptive regions of the Caribbean and southern United States is recognized. The recent occurrence of dengue epidemics in the Caribbean is prima facie evidence that this region is receptive to yellow fever.

The situation in Africa is considerably more complex. Relatively few sporadic cases are recognized annually, but this reflects inadequate surveillance and diagnostic facilities. Large epidemics, which occur at irregular intervals in areas of West, Central, and East Africa between 0 and 15 degrees N, have involved as many as 100,000 cases, with 30,000 deaths. Epidemics sustained by the peridomestic *Ae. aegypti* vector have occurred in both the urban and rural environments of West Africa. Epidemic yellow fever in savannah and forest-savannah transition areas of West Africa has been transmitted by tree-hole breeding *Aedes,* including *furcifer-taylori, africanus,* and *luteocephalus,* with both monkeys and man as intermediate hosts. During the long dry season adult mosquitoes disappear, and the virus may survive in transovarially infected eggs of *Aedes* vectors.

In the more extensive forests of Central and East Africa, a jungle cycle analogous to that in the Americas operates, with *Aedes africanus* as the principal vector. Sporadic cases and epidemics in persons entering the forest or living at the forest fringe have resulted from exposure to this mosquito. In some areas, another vector, *Ae. simpsoni,* links the jungle cycle with human populations and has been responsible for intensive interhuman transmission.

All races are equally susceptible to yellow fever infection. The disease in native populations of Africa is thought to be milder than in whites, but this is probably a reflection of background immunity and cross-protection by related endemic flaviviruses; some outbreaks of yellow fever involving Africans have been severe, with high death rates. Nonimmune persons of all ages and both sexes are equally susceptible. The age and sex distribution is, however, determined by natural immunization and vaccination, and by occupational exposures. Adult males employed in woodcutting or agricultural pursuits are primarily affected by jungle yellow fever.

PATHOLOGY AND PATHOGENESIS. Gross pathologic lesions include icterus; hemorrhages or petechiae of the mucous membranes, stomach, duodenum, renal capsule, and urinary bladder; and small amounts of pleural and peritoneal fluid. Histopathologic changes of the liver may be characteristic, but even experienced pathologists may not be able to make an unequivocal diagnosis in atypical cases. Conditions with which yellow fever has been confused on the basis of liver pathology include Lassa fever, African (Marburg-Ebola virus) hemorrhagic fever, viral hepatitis, and leptospirosis. The typical yellow fever lesion is marked by cloudy swelling, then by coagulative necrosis of hepatocytes in the midzone of the liver lobule, sparing cells bordering the central vein. Eosinophilic degeneration of hepatocytes results in the formation of *Councilman bodies;* intranuclear eosinophilic granular inclusions (Torres bodies) have also been described. Multi- and microvacuolar fatty change is nearly always present, especially after the eighth day of illness. An inflammatory response is absent or mild. The reticulin framework is preserved. Characteristic changes have been seen in biopsy specimens taken as early as the third day of illness; interpretation of biopsy or necropsy material obtained after the tenth day is often difficult. Renal glomerular changes are relatively insignificant compared to acute tubular necrosis and fatty metamorphosis, which may be marked. The myocardial fibers show cloudy swelling, degeneration, and fatty infiltration. Lymphocytic elements in the spleen and nodes are depleted, and large mononuclear or histiocytic cells accumulate in the splenic follicles. The brain may show edema and petechial hemorrhages.

The *pathologic physiology* of yellow fever is poorly understood. Direct viral injury to the cells of major target organs such as the liver undoubtedly underlies the pathogenic process. Hepatic coma has not been clinically or electroencephalographically defined, and the role of hepatic failure in the disease is uncertain. Some patients have prominent signs of acute renal failure, and deaths have been attributed to uremia. It is not known whether acute tubular necrosis is due to direct viral injury or is secondary to hemodynamic causes or hepatocellular necrosis. Deaths (especially late in the disease) have occurred because of cardiac failure or arrhythmia, but are rare. Hemorrhage undoubtedly exacerbates hypotension and oliguria and may precipitate vascular collapse and death. Evidence for disseminated intravascular coagulation as the basis for the hemorrhagic diathesis is conflicting. Acidosis and hyperkalemia are probable terminal events. At present, the complex pathophysiologic interrelationships of yellow fever cannot be specified, and directions for specific therapeutic interventions are consequently undetermined.

CLINICAL MANIFESTATIONS. Yellow fever infection produces a clinical spectrum from very mild, nonspecific, febrile illness to a malignant, sometimes fatal form with pathognomonic features. The precise frequency with which the various clinical forms occur is uncertain; however, abortive infections are the rule, and the classic symptoms of severe yellow fever are found in only 10 to 20 per cent of cases. The incubation period (interval between bite of infected mosquito and onset of symptoms) is generally three to six days.

The mild case will not be suspected or clinically diagnosed except in the setting of an epidemic. In its mildest form it is characterized by sudden onset of fever and headache, without other symptoms, lasting 48 hours or less. In other patients, the fever is higher, the headache more distressing, and the illness accompanied by a grippe-like syndrome with nausea, myalgia, slight albuminuria, and bradycardia in relation to the presence of fever (Faget's sign). The illness lasts several days, with uneventful recovery.

The severe forms of yellow fever begin abruptly with fever to 40° C, chills or chilliness, severe headache, and generalized myalgia often most acute in the lower back. The patient appears distressed and anxious, the conjunctiva congested, the face and neck flushed, the tongue reddened at the tip and edges, the breath foul smelling. Anorexia, nausea, and vomiting are present, and minor gingival hemorrhages or epistaxis may occur. Despite a persistent or rising temperature, the pulse may fall. This syndrome, persisting for approximately three days, corresponds to the "period of infection," during which yellow fever virus is present in the blood. It may be followed by a "period of remission," with partial or complete defervescence and mitigation of symptoms, usually lasting several to 24 hours. The fever and systemic symptoms then reappear with more *frequent vomiting, epigastric pain, prostration,* and the *appearance of jaundice* ("period of intoxication"). Viremia is generally absent, and antibodies appear during this phase. Hematemesis, coffee grounds–appearing or black vomit (vomito negro), is a characteristic and frightening sign. Other hemorrhagic manifestations include melena, metrorrhagia, petechiae, ecchymoses, and diffuse oozing from the mucous membranes. Dehydration resulting from vomiting and increased insensible losses is frequent. Renal damage is marked by the sudden appearance of albuminuria, which may rapidly increase, and by diminishing urine output. The pulse remains dissociated from fever, but may weaken as the blood and pulse pressures decrease. The patient recovers either rapidly after a period of intoxication of three to four days or over a protracted course of up to two weeks. Fatalities (occurring in up to 50 per cent of severe yellow fever cases) generally occur on the seventh to tenth day of illness, and are preceded by increasing albuminuria, hemorrhages, rising pulse, hypotension, oliguria, and azotemia. Hypothermia, a severe agitated delirium, intractable hiccup, stupor, and coma are terminal signs.

In individual cases hepatic, renal, or myocardial involvement predominates, with clinical signs of relatively pure hepatitis, acute renal failure, or hypotension and hypokinetic heart failure. Pre-eminent central nervous system involvement, producing meningoencephalitic signs, has also been described. Atypical, fulminant cases occur, with death on the second or third day in the absence of hepatic or renal signs.

Physical findings during the period of intoxication include scleral and dermal icterus, hemorrhagic manifestations, epigastric (rarely hepatic) tenderness without organomegaly, and the changes already noted in vital signs.

The convalescent stage is sometimes prolonged, with profound asthenia lasting one to two weeks. Late death, occurring at the end of convalescence or even weeks after complete recovery from the acute illness, is a rare phenomenon attributed to yellow fever myocardial damage, cardiac arrhythmia, or failure. Suppurative parotitis (resulting from dehydration) and secondary bacterial pneumonia are recognized complications.

CLINICAL LABORATORY FINDINGS. Leukopenia (neutropenia) occurs most often during the early phase of illness; the white blood count is, however, often normal or elevated. Prolongation of the clotting, prothrombin, and partial thromboplastin times is marked in cases with jaundice. The platelet count may be decreased, and fibrin split products may be present in serum. The total and conjugated serum bilirubin rise together and may reach levels of 15 to 20 mg per deciliter in severe cases. Serum glutamic oxaloacetic transaminase and serum glutamic pyruvic transaminase levels are markedly elevated in all icteric (but inconstantly and to lower levels in anicteric) patients, with peak values between days five and ten of the illness, and return to normal by days ten to twenty. The alkaline phosphatase is generally normal. In patients with severe hepatic damage, hypoglycemia has been noted.

During the period of infection, the urine may contain a small amount of albumin, which then increases suddenly on the fourth or fifth day, reaching levels of 3 to 5 (rarely as high as 40) grams per liter. The urine contains bile; the cell sediment may be abnormal but is not diagnostically helpful. The cerebrospinal fluid is clear, without cells, but it is often under increased pressure, and contains a mildly raised concentration of protein. ST-T wave electrocardiographic abnormalities have been described.

DIAGNOSIS. In endemic areas, recognition and diagnosis of a case are of great importance because it may indicate the presence of an epidemic and stimulate preventive or control measures. Because the incubation period is sufficient to permit an infected person to travel a long distance, the diagnosis should be suspected in all patients with fever and jaundice coming from tropical America or Africa. Specific diagnosis depends upon histopathologic study, isolation of the virus, or demonstration of a specific antibody response. The hemorrhagic diathesis renders liver biopsy hazardous, and pathologic diagnosis is thus a postmortem procedure. The virus is most readily isolated (by inoculation of mice or cell cultures) from serum obtained during the first three or four days of illness (period of infection), but it may be recovered from serum up to the twelfth day and occasionally from liver at death. Rapid early diagnosis may be possible by direct detection of yellow fever antigen in serum by means of enzyme immunoassay.

Serologic methods useful in the diagnosis of yellow fever include hemagglutination-inhibition (HI), complement-fixation (CF), neutralization (N), fluorescence, and immunoassay tests. The HI and N antibodies appear within a week of onset; the CF antibodies appear later. Paired, acute, and convalescent phase specimens are usually required to establish the diagnosis by rise in antibody titer. Cross-reactions with other flaviviruses and the high prevalence of background immunity to flaviviruses in tropical populations make serodiagnosis difficult. Determination of immunoglobulin (IgM) antibody titers by fluorescent assay or immunoassay may provide a more precise diagnosis.

Virus isolation and serologic tests are applicable to the diagnosis of all clinical forms of yellow fever and are the only means available of establishing the cause of abortive and mild infections.

DIFFERENTIAL DIAGNOSIS. Mild yellow fever cannot be clinically distinguished from a wide array of other infections. In the presence of jaundice and the other signs of severe yellow fever, conditions that must be differentiated include viral hepatitis, falciparum malaria, spirochetal infections (tick-borne relapsing fever and Weil's disease), Rift Valley fever, typhoid, Q fever, typhus, and surgical, drug-induced, and toxic causes. Other diseases (usually without jaundice) that may be confused with yellow fever include Lassa, African (Marburg-Ebola virus), Bolivian, and Argentine hemorrhagic fevers.

PROGNOSIS. Up to 50 per cent of patients with severe forms of yellow fever die; unfortunately, patients in most reported series have been cared for under primitive conditions. The fatality rate of *all* patients with clinical illness is much lower (2 to 5 per cent). The prognosis should be guarded for the patient who, after a brief remission, enters a period of intoxication with rising fever, jaundice, and albuminuria. Features which correlate with a poor prognosis include early onset of bilirubinemia and albuminuria rising to high levels; prolongation of the prothrombin time below 25 per cent of normal; a rising and weakening pulse during the period of intoxication; severe hemorrhage; and the appearance of shock, coma, hypothermia, and intractable hiccup.

Relapses have not been described. The possibility of late death from myocardial or renal injury must be considered.

TREATMENT. No specific therapy exists. Complete bed rest, supportive care, and close monitoring of vital functions are essential. During the period of infection, mild sedatives, analgesics, and antiemetics may be indicated, and attention should be given to fluid and electrolyte balance. Aspirin is contraindicated because of the bleeding diathesis. Supportive measures are of critical importance during the period of intoxication if vomiting is severe, if hemorrhage appears, or if hypertension, hypokinetic heart failure, oliguria, azotemia, and electrolyte and acid-base imbalance become evident. In theory, these consequences of severe yellow fever might be lessened by intensive counter-regulation. In patients with evidence of acute tubular necrosis, dialysis may be indicated. Cautious consideration may be given to early heparin treatment of disseminated intravascular coagulation if laboratory tests indicate its occurrence.

Secondary bacterial infections or concurrent infections (in particular, malaria) should be treated by the usual appropriate means.

Return to activity should be gradual.

PREVENTION AND CONTROL. The patient with yellow fever should be isolated from possible contact with mosquitoes under netting or in a screened room. Yellow fever 17D is one of the safest live, attenuated vaccines available and provides effective, long-lasting immunity. For purposes of international certification, vaccination is considered valid for ten years, but immunity has been documented to last more than thirty years and may be lifelong. Since yellow fever exists as a silent enzoosis over wide areas of the tropics (see Fig. 358–1) and appears in epidemic form with little warning and without early recognition, vaccination of travelers is imperative. Immunity can be demonstrated within ten days after vaccination. Mild vaccine reactions occur rarely, and serious complications have been exceedingly uncommon. No untoward consequences for the fetus have been recorded, but on theoretical grounds, pregnant women should not be vaccinated unless the risk of acquiring yellow fever is considered great. The vaccine is prepared in chicken embryos and should not be used in persons hypersensitive to egg proteins. The French neurotropic viral vaccine produced in mouse brain is no longer manufactured; remaining stocks are used to a limited extent in parts of Africa.

In the event of an epidemic, the disease may be controlled by mass vaccination and the use of insecticides to reduce infected vector populations.

359. HEMORRHAGIC FEVER CAUSED BY DENGUE VIRUSES (DHF)

Karl M. Johnson

DEFINITION. Dengue hemorrhagic fever is an acute, infectious, urban mosquito-borne disease. Endoepidemic in pattern, it is clinically defined as a dengue disease that worsens two or more days after onset and is characterized by hypoproteinemia and one or more hemostatic abnormalities such as thrombocytopenia, prolonged bleeding time, or elevated prothrombin time. The *dengue shock syndrome* consists of hemorrhagic fever plus shock (hypotension or a pulse pressure of 20 mm Hg or less) and hemoconcentration (hematocrit at least 20 per cent greater than convalescent value).

ETIOLOGY. All evidence suggests that dengue hemorrhagic fever is caused by each of the four recognized dengue virus types. How they produce such disease is still not clear. A current hypothesis is that severe dengue disease is produced by an immunologic reaction that occurs in some individuals experiencing a second dengue infection. However, hemorrhagic fever has been unequivocally caused by primary dengue infection.

EPIDEMIOLOGY. Dengue hemorrhagic fever was first seen in epidemic proportions in Manila and Bangkok (1954) and in Singapore (1960). Other outbreaks have been reported from Malaysia, South Vietnam, India, Indonesia, Oceania, and recently in Cuba. In Bangkok age-specific rates in children have reached 7 to 8 per 1000. In most outbreaks cases occur only in children, principally below the age of eight years; otherwise, the epidemiology of infection leading to dengue hemorrhagic fever is basically similar to that associated with ordinary dengue fever.

PATHOLOGY. Autopsy data are scant. The chief abnormalities include generalized vascular congestion and dilatation with edema and multiple focal hemorrhages in most organs, mild to moderate pleural effusion and ascites, mononuclear cell infiltration of interstitial tissues and alveolar walls of lungs, focal myocardial congestion, and a decrease in mature lymphocytes with proliferation of mononuclear forms in the germinal centers of lymph follicles.

Tissue necrosis is unusual. Perivascular mononuclear cell infiltration is common, but there is no evidence for direct damage to vessels or intravascular thrombosis. Globulin deposition on endothelial surfaces of arterioles has been noted in some cases. The marrow may exhibit megakaryocyte maturation arrest and generalized transitory hypoplasia.

Focal necrosis, usually mild, is observed in the liver, and Councilman bodies similar to those seen in yellow fever may be present.

PATHOGENESIS OR MECHANISM OF DISEASE. Vascular congestion, dilatation, and increased permeability lead to the extensive edema and hemorrhage observed in the gastrointestinal tract, the skin, and other tissues. The cause of these vascular changes is unknown, but they result in loss of plasma volume and associated electrolyte disturbances. Platelet deficiency probably plays a role in the hemorrhages. Bleeding time is usually prolonged, prothrombin times are somewhat prolonged, clot retraction is poor, and the blood fibrinogen is slightly reduced. Depression of C3 and C4 proactivation levels indicates activation of both arms of the complement system. None of these changes is very profound. The circulatory collapse and shock observed appear to be far in excess of what might be expected from the extent of loss of edema fluid and blood. The adrenal changes suggest exhaustion of steroid reserve. Death in some cases has been accompanied by severe hyperkalemia.

CLINICAL MANIFESTATIONS. The onset is that of a dengue infection, usually abrupt, with fever. Nausea and vomiting are common. The throat appears injected, and there may be a dry cough. About the second or third day petechiae appear, usually first on the face or distal portions of the extremities but sparing the axillae and chest. The tourniquet test may be conspicuously positive before petechiae appear. Purpura and large ecchymoses as well as other manifestations of bleeding tendency are occasionally prominent. There may be severe abdominal pain and tenderness. About the third or fourth day, vomiting may produce copious coffee-ground-like material. Melena also is not uncommon, but gross bleeding from the intestines is rare. Shock is likely to occur in severe cases about the fourth day, and this critical state lasts about 12 to 24 hours. At this time the temperature falls to normal, the blood pressure and pulse pressure are low or unmeasurable, and the limbs are cool and present a purple or brownish mottled appearance. Perspiration is frequently profuse. The face and hands appear edematous. Restlessness and apprehension are conspicuous as the patient enters shock. Thrombocytopenia is noted during this period, and bleeding time is prolonged. Leukocytes remain at approximately normal levels, but are elevated in number in serious cases more frequently than they are depressed. The total and differential leukocyte counts are not those observed in dengue. Although the numbers of both immature and mature polymorphonuclear cells are decreased, there is an increase in lymphocytes and sometimes in monocytes.

DIAGNOSIS. Hemorrhagic fever begins as an extension of a classic dengue infection, and the early dengue syndrome intergrades into the milder and atypical manifestations of the later hemorrhagic syndrome. The diagnosis in a febrile child acutely ill for only two or three days is rendered highly probable by the presentation of petechiae, purpuric lesions, and unusual ecchymosis of the skin with most prominent distribution on the extremities and face, together with melena, thrombocytopenia, and a relatively normal leukocyte count. In a milder case or at an earlier stage, the tourniquet test may be of great assistance in detecting unusual capillary fragility. The rapid development of circulatory collapse and shock during the fourth to sixth day, associated with the aforementioned findings, differentiates this from most other exanthematous diseases. Meningococcemia and the Waterhouse-Friderichsen syndrome need careful consideration. Thrombocytopenic purpura can be expected to have an entirely different onset and is usually not associated with fever. Laboratory methods available for diagnosis are those described for dengue fever.

TREATMENT. There is no specific therapy, but case-fatality rates can be greatly reduced by skillful management directed toward combating shock. Close monitoring of pulse, respiration, and blood pressure during the course of treatment is essential for at least 48 hours, because shock can occur and recur. Oxygen should be administered if there is cyanosis or labored breathing. Hypovolemia should be treated by administration of lactated Ringer's solution or 5 per cent glucose in normal saline, on the basis of 20 ml per kilogram of body weight, administered rapidly. In profound or unresponsive shock, plasma or a plasma expander (dextran in normal saline) can be given at the rate of 20 ml per kilogram of body weight. When signs improve, 5 per cent glucose in normal saline or in lactate-supplemented Ringer's solution should be given at the rate of 10 ml per kilogram per hour, and continued until vital signs are normal. Acidosis should be corrected with sodium bicarbonate as necessary.

Whole blood should be given only if blood loss is known to be large. Administration of whole blood to a patient with elevated hematocrit may result in heart failure. Paraldehyde or chloral hydrate may be required for children who are markedly agitated. Salicylates administered during the febrile period may cause bleeding and acidosis, and they should not be given to febrile patients during a hemorrhagic fever outbreak. Pressor amines, alpha-adrenergic blocking agents, and steroids have not been demonstrated to be of value in treatment.

PROGNOSIS. Death is almost always associated with shock, and ranges from 5 to 50 per cent, depending to a large extent upon the condition of patients on admission and the facilities available for treatment. Residual effects have not been observed, and, in contrast to primary dengue, recovery is usually prompt and complete seven to ten days after onset.

PREVENTION. Prevention is similar to that for dengue fever.

360. TICK-BORNE FLAVIVIRUS DISEASES: KYASANUR FOREST DISEASE AND OMSK HEMORRHAGIC FEVER

Karl M. Johnson

DEFINITION. Kyasanur Forest disease (KFD) and Omsk hemorrhagic fever (OHF) produce acute febrile illness with hemorrhagic manifestations and/or mild encephalitis in India and western Siberia, respectively.

ETIOLOGY. These diseases are produced by antigenically related flaviviruses which also share antigens with other tick-borne flaviviruses causing encephalitis (see Ch. 358). Neutralizing antibody measurement is required to distinguish OHF infection from that of tick-borne encephalitis (RSSE), which also occurs in western Siberia. The OHF agent produces hemorrhagic pneumonia in inoculated muskrats, and KFD virus induces encephalitis and hemorrhage in langur and bonnet monkeys.

EPIDEMIOLOGY. These viruses are maintained in discrete geographic foci by circulation between wild and domestic vertebrates and ixodid ticks of the genera *Ixodes, Dermacentor,* and *Haemaphysalis.* Rodents, birds, bats, sheep, goats, and cattle experience clinically silent, viremic infection; in addition, these agents are transmitted transovarially in ticks, thus providing a mechanism for winter or dry season virus survival. Viremia with overt fatal infection occurs naturally in muskrats and monkeys, and major epizootics among these mammals often precede or accompany epidemics.

Residents of rural forested areas are at highest risk of infection, and seasonal patterns of disease transmission are determined by the influence of temperature or moisture on tick activity. Winter outbreaks of OHF occur among trappers and skinners of muskrats, and both viruses have induced aerosol-transmitted infection in laboratory workers.

CLINICAL MANIFESTATIONS AND PATHOLOGY. The incubation period ranges from 3 to 12 days and is terminated by the abrupt onset of fever, headache, myalgia, and gastrointestinal disturbances. There is leukopenia and, after four to five days, the onset of mildly hemorrhagic bronchopneumonia, petechiae, and mild bleeding from the intestines. Epistaxis may occur. Pneumonia and clinical shock are the most serious clinical signs, but occur in a minority of infections. KFD patients, in addition, frequently exhibit recurrent fever with signs of meningitis or encephalitis during the second week of illness.

Pathologic lesions noted at autopsy include scattered necrotic foci in liver and gastrointestinal mucosa, hemorrhagic bronchopneumonia, capillary hemorrhages without inflammation in many tissues, and, in the case of KFD, occasional inflammatory vascular lesions in the brain.

DIAGNOSIS AND TREATMENT. Isolation of virus from blood or brain tissue or serologic diagnosis by standard methods is possible. Treatment is symptomatic.

PROGNOSIS AND PREVENTION. Mortality ranges from 0.5 to 5 per cent. There are no definitive methods for prevention.

361. CRIMEAN HEMORRHAGIC FEVER

Karl M. Johnson

DEFINITION. Crimean hemorrhagic fever (CHF) is an acute febrile disease, often marked by severe hemorrhage, high mortality, and nosocomial transmission, occurring in the Soviet Union, Bulgaria, the Middle East, and Pakistan.

ETIOLOGY. The CHF agent is a nairovirus first isolated from human blood specimens in 1967. It is pathogenic for suckling mice and grows in several types of cultured cells. This virus is indistinguishable from Congo virus of Africa in complement fixation and neutralization tests. Strains from Eurasia and Africa are thus referred to as Congo-CHF virus.

EPIDEMIOLOGY. Congo-CHF virus is naturally transmitted by several species of hard ticks belonging to the genera *Hyalomma, Rhipicephalus, Amblyomma,* and *Boophilus.*

Active foci of infection exist in the lower Don and Volga river basins and in Kazakhstan, Uzbekistan, Iran, Iraq, Dubai, western China, and northwest Pakistan. Few human cases have been reported from Africa. This is a disease of adults tending domestic animals. Cases appear in April and peak during early summer. Vertebrate hosts for the virus include cattle, goats, hares, and hedgehogs. Transovarial tick transmission has been demonstrated. The incubation period is about one week, and nosocomial human infections have occurred repeatedly.

CLINICAL MANIFESTATIONS. Onset is typically abrupt with high, unremittent fever, chills, headache, and myalgia. There may be hyperemia of the upper trunk and neck, conjunctival effusion, vomiting, and diarrhea. Hepatomegaly is noted in about half the cases; splenomegaly is uncommon. Pronounced panleukopenia is almost invariably present, as is thrombocytopenia. Bleeding begins on about the fourth day of illness. Petechiae appear in the oral mucosa and skin, at times presenting as frank *purpura hemorrhagica.* Nose, gums, and intestinal tract are the most common sites of bleeding, and in this disease above all other viral hemorrhagic fevers, blood loss per se may be life threatening. Stiff neck, hyperexcitability, or coma occurs in about 10 per cent of cases, and these are grave prognostic signs. The cerebrospinal fluid, however, contains no leukocytes or increased protein. There may be proteinuria and microscopic hematuria, but renal function is rarely compromised. The fever and bleeding generally resolve by lysis at about the eighth day. Hypovolemic shock with a paradoxical rising hematocrit may appear just prior to the end of fever and is the most common cause of death.

DIAGNOSIS. Virus can be easily obtained from blood of patients during the first few days of illness. Specific complement fixation and neutralizing antibodies appear in the sera of most patients 30 to 60 days after onset of symptoms.

TREATMENT AND PROGNOSIS. Therapy is symptomatic. Management of fluid, electrolyte, and erythrocyte balance forms the continuous clinical challenge. Shock is a grave problem and should be anticipated and treated as outlined in Ch. 43 and 362. Whole blood transfusion may be necessary. Intercurrent bacterial infection is very common, especially pneumonia. Mortality in the Soviet Union ranges from 20 to 50 per cent. Patients surviving the acute illness generally recover completely, albeit quite slowly. Several instances of mono- or polyneuritis persisting for several months have been recorded.

PREVENTION. There is no vaccine yet available; thus avoidance of the disease in endemic foci depends on personal measures designed to prevent tick bites. Several nosocomial infections have occurred in the Soviet Union and Pakistan. Thus strict isolation of patients and use of protective clothing and respirators by medical personnel are indicated.

362. HEMORRHAGIC DISEASES CAUSED BY ARENAVIRUSES: ARGENTINE AND BOLIVIAN HEMORRHAGIC FEVERS AND LASSA FEVER*

Karl M. Johnson

DEFINITION. Argentine and Bolivian hemorrhagic fevers and Lassa fever are acute diseases caused respectively by Junin, Machupo, and Lassa viruses. Clinically, the diseases share the common features of fever, severe myalgia, leukopenia, hemorrhagic manifestations, shock, and neurologic abnormalities.

ETIOLOGY. The three viruses are serologically and morphologically related, and belong to the family Arenaviridae.

GEOGRAPHICAL DISTRIBUTION, INCIDENCE, AND PREVALENCE. Argentine hemorrhagic fever is localized to the provinces of Córdoba and Buenos Aires in northern Argentina, where several hundred to several thousand cases occur annually, principally among workers harvesting maize. Bolivian hemorrhagic fever has been reported only from Beni province of Bolivia, between the rivers Mamore and Branco. Infections are seen in inhabitants of certain of the small towns, as well as in rural populations. Lassa fever occurs in West Africa, notably Nigeria, Liberia, and Sierra Leone. Fatality rates in hospitalized cases of all three diseases range from 10 to 20 per cent.

EPIDEMIOLOGY AND PROBABLE MODE OF TRANSMISSION. The viruses have been isolated from wild rodents: Junin, most commonly from *Calomys musculinus, Calomys laucha,* and also *Akodon arenicola;* Machupo, from *Calomys callosus;* and Lassa, from *Mastomys natalensis*. An attractive current hypothesis is that infection is acquired by direct human contact (ingestion, inhalation, or entrance through mucous membranes or skin breaks) with virus-containing rodent excreta. For all three agents, persistent infection in rodents has been demonstrated, with viruria readily detectable for months. A similar pattern of chronic virus infection in rodents has been described for lymphocytic choriomeningitis virus.

PATHOLOGY. Few cases have received full study. Findings include irregularly focal diapedesis and capillary hemorrhage without much evidence of inflammatory reaction. Gross hemorrhages may be seen in the mucosa of the stomach and intestines and in the brain. Pulmonary infection, probably intercurrent, is frequently seen. Focal liver necrosis is prominent in Lassa fever.

CLINICAL MANIFESTATIONS. Although as many as half of all etiologically confirmed cases appear as acute undifferentiated fevers, the findings and clinical course of "full-blown" Argentine and Bolivian infections are so nearly identical as to justify joint description. The same holds for Lassa fever. Onset is usually gradual, with increasing fever, headache, diffuse myalgia, and anorexia. By the third day the temperature may be 39.5 to 40.5° C, with severe myalgia, particularly in the lumbar regions (or legs in Lassa fever). Conjunctival injection is present, a flush involving the upper trunk and face is frequently observed, and there may be a relative bradycardia. Beginning about the fourth day, scattered fine petechiae may appear on the face and neck, about the pectoral girdle, and/or in the buccal mucosa or palate. Aphthous ulcers of the oral mucosa and exudative pharyngitis have been a noteworthy feature of Lassa infections. The Rumpel-Leede test is frequently positive. Frank hemorrhages from one or more sites, including the stomach, intestines, nose, gums, and uterus, accompanied by microscopic hematuria, may occur. Hemorrhagic phenomena are not a common feature of Lassa infections. Although hemorrhage per se is rarely the precipitating cause, a hypotensive crisis frequently develops between the sixth and eighth days, coincident with a rapid return of temperature to normal after five or more days of sustained fever. Patients surviving this stress for 48 hours generally make a slow but complete recovery.

Perhaps a fifth of the patients with the Bolivian or Argentine disease develop neurologic signs. These are quite characteristic, and begin on about the fifth or sixth day with a fine intention tremor of the tongue. This may become so severe as to render speech unintelligible and to preclude oral ingestion of solid or even liquid food. If so, gross intention tremors of the extremities usually appear, occasionally accompanied by an intermittent nystagmus. Such patients often become delirious, and may experience generalized clonic and tonic convulsions. The cerebrospinal fluid appears normal, however, and contains neither leukocytes nor virus. Convalescence is marked by weakness and signs of autonomic nervous system lability such as postural hypotension, spontaneous flushing and blanching of the skin, and episodes of diaphoresis.

In addition to delirium and occasional coma, 5 to 10 per cent of Lassa fever patients suffer significant permanent damage to one or both eighth cranial nerves. Some Lassa fever patients have shown electrocardiographic evidence of myocardial involvement.

Transient loss of scalp hair and typical Beau's lines in the nails, particularly those of the fingers, are observed in a majority of cases several weeks after subsidence of the high sustained fever. Many patients are not able to resume full activity for at least one month after illness.

Leukopenia is almost invariably present, and cell counts may be as low as 1000 per cubic millimeter by the fourth or fifth day. All elements are reduced nearly equally, and there is often a mild to moderate thrombocytopenia during the first week. Usually the peripheral blood picture returns to normal rapidly after defervescence, although there may be transient relative lymphocytosis and mild anemia. During the latter portion of the febrile period, progressive increase in hematocrit similar to, but usually milder than, that of hemorrhagic nephrosonephritis (q.v.) is frequently observed. At about the same time, moderate proteinuria is common, although renal function is rarely compromised seriously, and frank azotemia and hyperkalemia are almost never present.

DIAGNOSIS. Fever, myalgia, and leukopenia in a patient having a history of rural contact in endemic areas should be interpreted as arenaviral disease until proven otherwise. Laboratory procedures are necessary. Virus can be recovered from blood of patients with Argentine hemorrhagic fever or Lassa fever. Specific antibodies appear within the first month of illness in Lassa fever. Diagnosis of Bolivian hemorrhagic fever may be difficult because virus is infrequently detectable in blood or other secretions and antibodies do not appear during the acute phase of illness.

These three agents have been responsible for several fatal laboratory infections, and work with the viruses should be carried out only with strictest precautionary measures, and complete isolation from other activities, in special high-risk laboratories.

TREATMENT. Careful measurement of fluid and electrolyte balance is mandatory. Frequent measurements of hematocrit and urinary protein excretion are crucial for recognition of incipient hypovolemic shock. Plasma expanders may be used to treat this condition, but often provoke intractable pulmonary

*The author wishes to express his thanks to Dr. Wilbur G. Downs for his considerable assistance in the preparation of this chapter, particularly with reference to the material on Lassa fever.

edema if treatment is delayed until frank clinical shock develops. Secondary bacterial infections must be recognized and promptly treated. Passive anti-Junin antibodies have been proved to reduce mortality in Argentine hemorrhagic fever if administered during the first eight days of illness, but are not of proven value in Lassa fever or the Bolivian disease.

PROGNOSIS. Although case mortality may reach 20 per cent in Argentine and Bolivian hemorrhagic fever, there are no early findings which aid prognosis. The onset of shock or neurologic abnormalities is an ominous sign, and at least half of such patients succumb. In Lassa fever admission levels of virus and glutamic oxalic transaminase in serum are highly and directly correlated with outcome of infection.

PREVENTION. Effective elimination of intimate human contact with certain wild rodents represents the only proven method for prevention of disease. This may be achieved by maintaining sound standards of personal and environmental hygiene. Campaigns to eliminate rodents, repair buildings, and clean rubbish near dwellings are highly successful when the disease is acquired mainly from peridomestic animals.

Hospital outbreaks involving medical staff have occurred several times with Lassa virus. Current evidence suggests that these are usually due to direct contact with blood and excreta rather than to infectious aerosols.

363. AFRICAN HEMORRHAGIC FEVER (Marburg-Ebola Disease)

Karl M. Johnson

DEFINITION. African hemorrhagic fever is an acute, highly fatal disease characterized by fever, prostration, rash, proteinuria, major hemorrhagic manifestations, pancreatitis, and hepatitis.

HISTORY. The disease was first described in Germany in 1967 and named Marburg disease. It was acquired through contact with green monkeys, *Cercopithecus aethiops*, imported from Uganda. Secondary nosocomial cases occurred. A few further cases occurred in South Africa (1975) and Kenya (1980). Major outbreaks with several hundred cases were recorded in Sudan (1976 and 1979) and Zaire (1976).

ETIOLOGY. This syndrome is caused by morphologically identical viruses, Marburg and Ebola, which are immunologically distinct.

EPIDEMIOLOGY. The ecology of Marburg and Ebola viruses is presently unknown. No evidence for Marburg infection was detected in green monkeys captured in Uganda subsequent to the original outbreak. The source of the index infection in the other outbreaks remains a mystery. Transmission is person-to-person, associated with close contact with patients. In Zaire contaminated needles were the source of many infections. Incubation period is about one week.

PATHOLOGY. These viruses attack the lymphoreticular system, the liver, and possibly the pancreas. Prominent hepatocellular necrosis without inflammatory reaction is a hallmark of infection. Large eosinophilic inclusions are found in liver cells, but the overall pattern of destruction is diffuse, rather than strongly mid-zonal as in yellow fever.

CLINICAL MANIFESTATIONS AND PATHOLOGIC PHYSIOLOGY. Onset is abrupt or insidious with headache and progressive fever. There is severe myalgia, and often vomiting and/or diarrhea occur. About the fourth day of illness sore throat and abdominal pain appear, and a day or so later many patients develop a fine maculopapular rash over the trunk and back which spreads to the limbs and may fade in two or three days. Bleeding, principally gastrointestinal, begins on the fifth to seventh day and is associated with rapid decompensation, ending in shock and death. Leukopenia, thrombocytopenia, and proteinuria are almost invariably present. There are extreme elevations of plasma transaminases and of amylase. In the few cases studied, definitive evidence for disseminated intravascular coagulation was found.

DIAGNOSIS. High persistent viremia is the basis for establishment of the diagnosis in acute cases. Virus is recovered by inoculation of blood into Vero cell cultures or guinea pigs that undergo a febrile infection. Immunofluorescent antibodies appear during the second week after onset and persist for several years. This method is more sensitive than the complement-fixation technique, which also has been used.

PROGNOSIS AND TREATMENT. With sophisticated medical management, mortality in Marburg infection is 25 to 30 per cent. Ebola virus infections treated in rural hospitals were 50 to 90 per cent fatal, the worst prognosis of any viral disease other than rabies. In addition to intensive supportive care, which should include continuous nasogastric aspiration to combat pancreatitis, intravenous heparin therapy may be of value to combat incipient intravascular coagulation.

PREVENTION. The secondary attack rate in African hemorrhagic fever rarely exceeds 10 per cent. Transmission can be interrupted by scrupulous isolation of patients, careful disposal of virus-contaminated excreta and fomites, and use of protective clothing and full-face respirators by medical personnel.

364. HEMORRHAGIC FEVER WITH RENAL SYNDROME (HFRS)

Karl M. Johnson

DEFINITION. Hemorrhagic fever with renal syndrome is an acute disease that occurs in northeastern Asia and, in milder form, in northern European USSR, Scandinavia, Czechoslovakia, Rumania, and Bulgaria. It is characterized by fever, prostration, vomiting, proteinuria, hemorrhagic manifestations, shock, and renal failure.

HISTORY. The disease was first described in the far east of the Soviet Union in the 1930's, with suggestive history as far back as 1913. An epidemic in United Nations troops in Korea, beginning in 1951, attracted much attention.

ETIOLOGY. The disease is caused by Hantaan virus, first recovered from the striped field mouse, *Apodemus agrarius*, in Korea. Strains also have been recovered from patients.

EPIDEMIOLOGY. The disease is rural, characterized by isolated cases widely separated in place. Environmental exposure in forests or fields near forests is invariably noted. Person-to-person transmission does not occur. Soviet workers believe that the disease is transmitted directly from asymptomatically infected rodents to man by means of virus-contaminated rodent excreta. Some outbreaks in Europe have coincided with population "explosions" of the redbacked vole *(Clethrionomys glareolus)*, involving invasion by rodents of fields, barns, and even houses. An urban form of the disease was recognized in Osaka, Japan, and several recent outbreaks in Japanese medical centers were traced to virus-infected colonized Wistar rats. Hantaan-related agents have been isolated from wild rats and voles, *Microtus*, in North America.

PATHOLOGY. Profound, protein-rich retroperitoneal edema is characteristic of early death in shock, but not of later deaths. Changes in various organs apparently have a similar pathogenesis and consist of widespread, often focal, congestion and hemorrhage, sometimes accompanied by necrosis, without significant inflammatory response. The "pathognomonic" lesion is found in the kidneys, which appear swollen and, when incised, exhibit extreme hemorrhagic congestion sharply localized to the medulla. Gross congestion or hemorrhage derived from dilated, congested small blood vessels is also found frequently in the right atrium, the pituitary, and the stomach, and less often in intestines, adrenals, lungs, and central nervous system. Liver and spleen are usually not grossly involved. Petechial hemorrhages may occur in the skin, heart, adrenals, brain, and serous surfaces.

CLINICAL MANIFESTATIONS AND PATHOLOGIC PHYSIOLOGY. Most patients exhibit fever, variable proteinuria, and isohyposthenuria. Only a minority of infections result in the severe clinically classic and highly unique hemorrhagic syndrome. This is initiated by a *febrile phase* lasting three to eight days, marked by severe myalgia and malaise, a flush over the face and neck, and conjunctival and palatine injection. Toward the end of this phase, thrombocytopenia, proteinuria, and petechiae appear and hematocrit increases, heralding a *hypotensive phase,* which develops rapidly and lasts one to three days. Effective blood volume decreases; hematocrit values may reach 70 per cent; nausea, vomiting, and abdominal or lumbar pain appear and have occasioned ill-advised laparotomy in misdiagnosed cases. Heavy proteinuria and oliguria occur, and clinical shock is an ever-present danger. Capillary hemorrhages are most common during this phase, and blood leukocytes now show a mild leukemoid reaction.

Patients surviving this acute clinical crisis proceed to an *oliguric phase,* with renal shutdown, hyperkalemia, secondary pulmonary infection, and, in some cases, pulmonary edema. There are biochemical changes associated with renal failure, and some patients exhibit a reactive hypertension related to functional hypervolemia which responds to phlebotomy. Patients who survive this phase must still endure a *diuretic phase,* which lasts for days to weeks. Management of fluid and electrolytes during this interval often proves extremely difficult, and bacterial pulmonary infections also are common. Nearly one third of all deaths occur during this period, and survivors often require one to three months for return of strength and normal urinary concentrating function.

DIAGNOSIS. Specific diagnosis is made by immunofluorescent technique, using cell cultures infected by Hantaan virus as source of antigen. Most patients already have low titers of antibody in acute phase sera, but diagnostic increases in titer regularly occur by the end of the second week of symptoms. The antibodies persist at least ten years. Retrospective serodiagnosis has now been confirmed in patients from the Soviet Union, China, Finland, and Japan, as well as Korea. Asymptomatic infections are unusual, but mild clinically apparent cases have been documented.

PROGNOSIS AND TREATMENT. Treatment is supportive and complex. Fluid management is critical. Plasma expanders are important in shock therapy. Hemodialysis may be required to cope with azotemia and hyperkalemia during the oligemic phase, and electrolyte balance requires delicate and precise handling during diuresis. Under optimal conditions mortality should not exceed 6 per cent.

PREVENTION. Avoidance of contact with rodent excreta is the only available method of prevention.

Barnes WJS, Rosen L: Fatal hemorrhagic disease and shock associated with primary dengue infection on a Pacific island. Am J Trop Med Hyg 23:495, 1974. *Clear evidence that severe hemorrhagic disease can result from first dengue virus infection. Whether host factors or a particular virus strain is responsible is not clear.*

Casals J, Henderson BE, Hoogstraal H, Johnson KM, Shelokov A: A review of Soviet viral hemorrhagic fevers, 1969. J Infect Dis 122:437, 1970. *A clinical, virologic, and epidemiologic report based on extensive travel of authors in Soviet Union. Data on hemorrhagic fever with renal syndrome (Korean) and Crimean hemorrhagic fever are of special value.*

Halstead SB, et al.: Observations related to pathogenesis of dengue hemorrhagic fever. Yale J Biol Med 42:261, 1970. *Epidemiologic case for secondary dengue infection as trigger for hemorrhagic fever.*

Halstead SB: In vivo enhancement of dengue virus infection in rhesus monkeys by passively transferred antibody. J Infect Dis 140:527, 1979. *Experimental data making secondary infection concept highly plausible.*

International symposium on arenaviral infections of public health importance. Bull WHO, 52:381, 1975. *Best single collection of articles on Lassa fever.*

Johnson KM, Halstead SB, Cohen SN: Hemorrhagic fevers of Southeast Asia and South America: A comparative appraisal. Prog Med Virol 9:105, 1967. *Extensive comparative review of dengue and South American arenavirus hemorrhagic fevers.*

Johnson KM, Webb PA, Lange JV, Murphy FA: Isolation and partial characterization of a new virus causing haemorrhagic fever in Zaire. Lancet 1:569, 1977. *Describes circumstances of initial recognition and depicts unique morphology of Ebola virus.*

Lee HW, Lee PW, Johnson KM: Isolation of the etiologic agent of Korean hemorrhagic fever. J Infect Dis 137:298, 1978. *Classic report of initial isolation of Hantaan virus, using convalescent human sera for immunofluorescent detection of agent in tissues of single wild rodent species.*

Mertens P, Patton R, Baum JJ, Monath PP: Clinical presentation of Lassa fever cases during the hospital epidemic at Zorzar, Liberia, March–April 1972. Am J Trop Med Hyg 22:780, 1973. *Excellent description of the most severe form of Lassa fever.*

Pantier R: Yellow fever. *In* Debré T, Celers J (eds.): Clinical Virology. Philadelphia, W. B. Saunders Company, 1970, pp 299–315. *A good review with summary of the clinical features of, and diagnostic procedures for, this disease.*

Pattyn SR (ed.): Ebola Virus Haemorrhagic Fever. Amsterdam–New York, Elsevier/North-Holland, 1978. *Proceedings of a symposium documenting events surrounding initial recognition of this disease in Sudan and Zaire.*

Sabattini M, Maiztegui JI: Fiebre hemorrágica argentina. Medicina (Buenos Aires) 30:Suppl 1, 111, 1970. *Definitive review of epidemiology of Argentine hemorrhagic fever. In Spanish.*

Simpson DIH, Knight EM, et al.: Congo virus: A hitherto undescribed virus occurring in Africa. Part I. Human isolation clinical notes. East Afr Med J 44:87, 1967. *First description of the agent indistinguishable from virus causing Crimean hemorrhagic fever. Hemorrhage was not a prominent feature of the cases reported here.*

Smorodintsev AA, Kazbintsev LI, Chudakov VG: Virus Haemorrhagic Fevers (Y Halperin, translator). Washington, D.C., Office of Technical Services, U.S. Department of Commerce, 1964. *Still the most comprehensive description of viral hemorrhagic fevers occurring in the Soviet Union.*

Strode GK: Yellow Fever. New York, McGraw-Hill Book Company, 1951. *A landmark volume documenting the work of the Rockefeller Foundation at home and abroad during the dawn of modern virology, the 1920's through 1940's.*

Symposium on epidemic hemorrhagic fever. Am J Med 16:617, 1954. *The definitive review on clinical pathophysiology of Korean hemorrhagic fever.*

WHO Expert Committee on Yellow Fever: Third report. WHO Tech Rep Ser No 479, 1971. *Thorough summary of continuing trends in patterns of occurrence of sylvan yellow fever worldwide. Recommendations for diagnostic approach to outbreaks and for use of yellow fever vaccines.*

Section Four THE MYCOSES

David J. Drutz

365. INTRODUCTION

Fungi differ from bacteria in three major respects:

1. Like mammalian cells, they are *eukaryotes.* That is, they possess a discrete nucleus bounded by a membrane containing several chromosomes. Bacteria are *prokaryotes,* possessing a single continuous chromosome and no true nucleus or nuclear membrane.

2. Fungi may reproduce sexually or asexually. When mating has taken place, the "sexual state" or *"perfect state"* is said to be present. Spores formed by the perfect state are of major importance in taxonomy. When the perfect form of fungi has not been identified, they are referred to as *deuteromycetes* or *fungi imperfecti* (e.g., *Coccidioides immitis, Candida albicans*).

3. Fungi may be *biphasic,* with one form in nature and a different form in the infected host. For example, *C. immitis, Histoplasma capsulatum, Blastomyces dermatitidis,* and *Sporothrix schenckii* are mycelia (molds) in the environment, but yeasts *(H. capsulatum, B. dermatitidis, S. schenckii)* or endosporulating spherules *(C. immitis)* in man. Because these fungi are basically soil saprophytes and do not appear to require mammalian hosts, it is not clear what benefit accrues to them by attacking man.

Fungal diseases are referred to as *mycoses.* Some mycoses are *endemic.* That is, susceptibility is conferred by living in a geographic area constituting the natural habitat of that fungus (e.g., coccidioidomycosis in California, Arizona, and Texas; paracoccidioidomycosis in South America). Most endemic mycoses (coccidioidomycosis, paracoccidioidomycosis, histoplasmosis, blastomycosis) are acquired by the respiratory route, are minimally symptomatic, and are recognized in retrospect by skin tests or serology. Occasionally pulmonary disease may be progressive, or systemic infection may occur. Race and hormonal factors appear to play some role (e.g., chronic pulmonary histoplasmosis is especially common in middle-aged white men with emphysema; disseminated coccidioidomycosis is most common in black or Filipino men, and in pregnant women regardless of race).

Some mycoses are chiefly opportunistic, occurring in a setting of immunosuppression (candidiasis, cryptococcosis, aspergillosis, mucormycosis) or diabetic ketoacidosis (mucormycosis). Certain other fungi may behave as opportunists in patients with depressed cell-mediated immunity (CMI) (*H. capsulatum, C. immitis,* and perhaps *Paracoccidioides brasiliensis* and *B. dermatitidis*). A separate phenomenon is the occurrence of anergy and depressed correlates of CMI in vitro that are seen in some patients with disseminated histoplasmosis, coccidioidomycosis, sporotrichosis, and paracoccidioidomycosis. Such defects may be associated with excessive suppressor T cell activity and are reversible with elimination of the pathogen.

Diagnosis of the mycoses is usually dependent on morphologic and cultural criteria. *Serologic tests* show cross-reactions and are often more confusing than helpful. However, there are outstanding exceptions: coccidioidomycosis complement-fixing (CF) antibody in the cerebrospinal fluid (CSF) is diagnostic of coccidioidal meningitis; detection of cryptococcal polysaccharide antigen in the blood or CSF is virtually diagnostic of systemic cryptococcosis. *Skin tests* are more useful in epidemiologic surveys than in diagnosis of individual infections. A positive skin test result indicates merely that infection has taken place in the past. Many skin tests are poorly standardized; some (e.g., blastomycin) are valueless for any purpose. The histoplasmin skin test stimulates antibody formation, thereby canceling the limited capabilities of histoplasma serology. Neither of the skin tests available for coccidioidomycosis (coccidioidin, spherulin) has an effect on coccidioidomycosis serology. Further, in a patient with known disseminated coccidioidomycosis a negative skin test result suggests a poor prognosis (especially if associated with a high CF titer), and return to positivity is a clue to therapeutic response.

Effective antifungal chemotherapy is limited. Amphotericin B has been in use for nearly three decades and remains the treatment of choice for most mycoses. Only *Petriellidium (Pseudoallescheria) boydii* is routinely resistant to amphotericin B. Dosage regimens are based more on clinical experience than on objective criteria, and therapy is limited by toxic side effects, principally azotemia. Flucytosine is an orally absorbed drug that serves as an adjunct to amphotericin B in cryptococcal meningitis and in some forms of candidiasis. Its therapeutic efficacy is limited by rapid development of resistance by fungi, and by bone marrow toxicity that appears at least partially related to its conversion to 5-fluorouracil in vivo. Miconazole is a parenteral imidazole with efficacy in coccidioidomycosis and several other mycoses. Its side effects include hyperlipidemia, hyponatremia, and pruritus. It is currently secondary in importance to amphotericin B, except in the treatment of *Pseudoallescheria* infection. Ketoconazole, an orally administered, broad-spectrum imidazole, has shown efficacy in chronic mucocutaneous candidiasis, *Candida* esophagitis, histoplasmosis, blastomycosis, paracoccidioidomycosis, and some forms of coccidioidomycosis. It covers essentially the same spectrum of mycoses as miconazole and can be administered on a long-term basis with minimal side effects (gastrointestinal distress; hepatitis; and interference with endogenous steroid synthesis, especially testosterone).

Dismukes WE, Stamm AM, Graybill JR, Craven PC, Stevens DA, Stiller RL, Sarosi GA, Medoff G, Gregg CR, Gallis HA, Fields BT Jr, Marrier RL, Kerkering TA, Kaplowitz LG, Cloud G, Bowles C, Shadomy S: Treatment of systemic mycoses with ketoconazole: Emphasis on toxicity and clinical response in 52 patients. Ann Intern Med 98:13, 1983. *The ease of ketoconazole administration and its low toxicity relative to that of amphotericin B has stirred major clinical interest in its use for diverse mycoses. This important paper provides a perspective for the likely efficacy of ketoconazole in a variety of mycoses. Additional data from this National Institute of Allergy and Infectious Disease collaborative study are eagerly anticipated.*

Drutz DJ: Newer antifungal agents and their use, including an update on amphotericin B and flucytosine. *In* Remington JS, Swartz MN (eds.): Current Clinical Topics in Infectious Diseases, 3. New York, McGraw-Hill Book Company, 1982, pp 97–135. *The clinical roles of amphotericin B, flucytosine, and miconazole are discussed in detail.*

366. HISTOPLASMOSIS

DEFINITION. Histoplasmosis is the most common endemic respiratory mycosis in the United States. The disease is noncommunicable and ordinarily self-limited, but reinfection, chronic pulmonary infection, and disseminated infection all may occur.

ETIOLOGY. *Histoplasma capsulatum* (perfect form: *Emmonsiella capsulata*) is a biphasic fungus, occurring in the mycelial phase in the environment, and in the yeast phase at 37° C and in infected hosts. The mycelial form produces two types of spores: tuberculate macroconidia (8 to 16 μm), and microconidia of a size (2 to 5 μm) more appropriate to be inhaled. The yeasts are ovoid (2 to 3 × 3 to 4 μm) and unencapsulated, bud singly from a narrow neck, and occur intracellularly in macrophages.

INCIDENCE AND PREVALENCE. Histoplasmosis occurs worldwide. Over 40 million people have been infected in the United States, and about 500,000 develop skin test positivity each year. Eighty to 95 per cent of persons in the Mississippi, Missouri, and Ohio River valleys are histoplasmin positive. *H. capsulatum var. duboisii* produces a disease restricted largely to central Africa ("African histoplasmosis") with slightly different clinical and histopathologic features.

EPIDEMIOLOGY. *H. capsulatum* is a soil saprophyte that prefers moderate temperatures and moist environments. Droppings from chickens, pigeons, starlings, blackbirds, and bats support its growth. Birds are not infected, but carry the fungi on their feathers. Bats are infected and excrete yeasts from an ulcerated intestinal mucosa. Histoplasmosis ("cave disease") may follow exploration of bat-infested caves. Although the fungus is found in greatest abundance in bat or bird-related microenvironments, microconidia are commonly present as "air pollutants" in endemic areas and probably account for the majority of sporadic infections. Focal outbreaks occur with disturbances that raise dust (e.g., demolition of old buildings where birds or bats have roosted), especially on the edge of an endemic zone where histoplasmin skin test reactivity is not universally present. Because histoplasmin reactivity may wane, persons who live in highly endemic areas are subject to reinfection.

PATHOGENESIS AND PATHOLOGY. Following the inhalation of microconidia, fungi replicate locally and disseminate hematogenously to the mononuclear phagocyte system. With the development of cell-mediated immunity, granuloma formation occurs, often with caseation necrosis, and the histoplasmin skin test becomes positive. Healing may be marked by exuberant calcification at pulmonary parenchymal and hilar loci (Ghon complex) and in the spleen. An exaggerated fibrotic response may lead to *fibrosing mediastinitis* with bronchial or vascular occlusion (e.g., superior vena caval obstruction). Layers of collagen may be deposited at the site of pulmonary coin lesions *(histoplasmomas),* their growth leading to thoracotomy for suspected malignancy.

H. capsulatum stains poorly with hematoxylin-eosin, but well with periodic acid–Schiff, Giemsa, or Gomori methenamine silver stains. Organisms are ordinarily found in macrophages, but large bizarre extracellular forms may be seen in endocarditis lesions or necrotic loci. The spectrum of host response is related directly to the effectiveness of cell-mediated immune mechanisms. With optimal immunity, fungi are rare, granuloma formation is well developed, and the disease is restricted in extent. With deficient immunity, macrophages, including those in circulating blood, are packed with intracellular yeasts, granuloma formation is poor, and disease is extensive. Granulocytes and serum factors play a secondary role in host defense.

In patients with centrilobular or bullous emphysema, histoplasmosis is opportunistic. Subintimal arterial proliferation leads to infarct-like pulmonary necrosis. In infants and older adults without obvious host defense defects, and in patients with chronic lymphocytic leukemia, Hodgkin's disease, steroid therapy, or other defects of cell-mediated immunity, progressive hematogenous dissemination may occur. Some of the manifestations (meningitis, adrenal insufficiency, intestinal ulceration) are attributable to an accompanying perivasculitis.

CLINICAL MANIFESTATIONS. ***Primary Histoplasmosis.*** At least 90 per cent of all respiratory encounters with *H. capsulatum* pass unnoticed or are attributed to "the flu." Manifestations include cough, fever, headache, myalgias, stomach cramps, and pleuritic pain. With heavier exposure, there may be dyspnea, cyanosis, deep chest pain, and pericarditis. Occasionally, there may be erythema nodosum, erythema multiforme, diffuse rash, or arthralgias—especially in white women. The chest roentgenogram may show patchy infiltrates; hilar lymphadenopathy is common, especially in children. Cavitation and pleural effusion may occur. Ghon complexes tend to be more highly calcified than in tuberculosis. Multifocal pulmonary lesions may heal with diffuse "buckshot" calcifications. These may erode into bronchi and be expectorated later as broncholiths.

Reinfection Histoplasmosis. The potential for re-exposure to microconidia is constantly present in endemic areas. Reinfection is characterized by a shorter incubation period (three to seven versus ten to eighteen days), miliary nodulation (rather than patchy bronchopneumonia), lack of hilar adenopathy, and a shorter and less severe disease course. However, very severe pulmonary disease with cyanosis and respiratory distress may also be seen.

Chronic Pulmonary Histoplasmosis. This disease occurs most commonly in middle-aged white men with pre-existing chronic obstructive pulmonary disease and centrilobular or bullous emphysema. Multiplication of inhaled *H. capsulatum* in an emphysematous bleb (characteristically in an apical-posterior location) results in antigenic spillage to contiguous lung areas and an acute segmental interstitial pneumonitis. Symptoms include cough, fever, and malaise. Microorganisms are sparse, and in 80 per cent of cases the disease resolves over two to three months with infarct-like necrosis, contraction of damaged tissue, and a fibrous residual. There may be later recurrences. In 20 per cent of patients, persistent infection leads to chronic cavitary disease. Thick-walled cavities expand by contiguity into the surrounding lung ("marching cavity"), and bronchogenic spread of their contents results in pneumonitis and fibrosis in dependent lung areas. Patients may have fever and a productive cough; one third have hemoptysis. Sputum cultures are positive in only 50 to 70 per cent. The patients usually pursue a declining course, less from actual infection than from progressive loss of functioning lung.

Disseminated Histoplasmosis. One third of cases occur in infants, the remainder predominantly in men over age 40. A clinically apparent pulmonary infection may precede dissemination in infants, but is less likely to do so in adults. Dissemination in adults may follow immunosuppression, with arousal of disease from latency. Infants have the poorest host response to infection, and the most fulminating course; disease in adults is usually subacute or chronic.

Clinical manifestations include weight loss, fever, weakness and malaise, hepatosplenomegaly, lymphadenopathy, and impaired bone marrow function (anemia, leukopenia, and thrombocytopenia). Oropharyngeal, nasopharyngeal, and laryngeal ulcerations, usually painful and often associated with dysphagia or hoarseness, constitute a major clue to the diagnosis. Gastrointestinal tract ulcerations (especially common in the ileocecal area) may present with bleeding, obstruction, perforation, or malabsorption. Adrenal insufficiency is common and may occur years after successful eradication of fungi. Chest roentgenograms may show evidence of primary or hematogenous infection. Endocarditis (aortic more than mitral or tricuspid valves) may present with emboli to large blood vessels. Central nervous system histoplasmosis may present with focal cerebritis or diffuse chronic meningitis with hypoglycorrhachia. The kidneys, prostate, and skin may also be involved, but osteomyelitis and arthritis are rare.

Ocular Histoplasmosis. Presumed ocular histoplasmosis syndrome (POHS) refers to a focal chorioretinitis in the macular area that is thought to be related to a hypersensitivity response to products of *H. capsulatum*. No direct relationship to fungal infection has been proved.

DIAGNOSIS. Histoplasmosis is as clinically diverse as tuberculosis. Particularly suggestive features include mucous membrane ulcerations, leukopenia, thrombocytopenia, adrenal insufficiency, buckshot pulmonary calcifications, and splenic calcifications. The diagnosis depends on demonstrating or culturing *H. capsulatum* from involved tissues, seldom a simple task. The roles of skin and serologic tests are limited. The *histoplasmin skin test* is seldom useful diagnostically because positive results are common in the endemic area. Conversely, disseminated disease is not necessarily associated with a negative result (unlike the situation with coccidioidomycosis). A positive skin test result also elevates titers of serum antibodies. The skin test should therefore be restricted to use in epidemiologic investigations. The *complement fixation test* (using mycelial or yeast phase antigen) may show cross-reactions with blastomycosis or coccidioidomycosis. Low level antibody titers may persist for years following primary histoplasmosis. A titer $\geq$1:32, or a four-fold titer rise, suggests but does not prove active histoplasmosis; nor does a negative titer rule out the disease. Titers do not parallel disease activity and are of little value in following therapy or estimating prognosis. Tests for antibody by the *immunodiffusion* method produce two bands (m, h) of potential diagnostic value. The occurrence of both bands in the serum of a patient who has not been skin tested with histoplasmin is highly suggestive of histoplasmosis. If only an m band is observed, early histoplasmosis may be present because the m band usually precedes the h band. The *latex agglutination test* with histoplasmin-sensitized latex particles is a useful aid to diagnosis of acute histoplasmosis, especially in titers $\geq$1:16. False positive and negative results may occur, and confirmatory diagnostic tests are required.

Primary pulmonary histoplasmosis is rarely diagnosed in the absence of a suggestive epidemiologic history or the investigation of a common-source outbreak. Most cases are probably overlooked or misdiagnosed as bacterial or viral processes. Sputum cultures are positive in only 20 per cent of cases. Skin test conversion is diagnostic, but seldom documented. Serologic tests may be helpful in diagnosis, as noted above.

Chronic pulmonary histoplasmosis is diagnosed on the basis of suggestive roentgenographic changes and positive sputum smears or cultures. Less than one third of cultures are positive in early, self-limited disease, whereas 70 per cent are positive in patients with marching cavities. Multiple cultures may be required before the fungus is found.

Disseminated histoplasmosis in one large series demonstrated positive cultures in the following distribution: oral lesions (91 per cent), lymph node (72 per cent), bone marrow (70 per cent), sputum (60 per cent), liver biopsy (57 per cent), blood (54 per cent), CSF (45 per cent), and urine (43 per cent). Organisms have also been cultured from the stool, prostatic secretions, and skin lesions. Fungi may be demonstrated directly by Wright, Giemsa, or methenamine silver stains of the buffy coat of blood, ulcer swabs or scrapings, sputum, or other infected materials.

TREATMENT. Primary pulmonary infection rarely requires treatment. Those with acute respiratory insufficiency following massive spore exposure may require a brief course of corticosteroid therapy, with or without accompanying antifungal therapy. Chronic pulmonary histoplasmosis resolves spontaneously in 80 per cent of cases, but resolution may be assisted by restriction of activity or bed rest. Progressive cavitary pulmonary histoplasmosis generally requires therapy with amphotericin B (approximately 2 grams over ten weeks), but repeated courses of treatment may be required. If pulmonary function permits, surgical resection of marching cavities should be considered. Patients with progressive disseminated infection should receive approximately 2 grams of amphotericin B over ten weeks (for infants, the dosage is 1 mg per kilogram per day for six weeks), although lower total dosages may be curative in some patients. Relapses can occur. Endocarditis may be more difficult to cure. Adrenal function should be evaluated at the time of diagnosis and monitored indefinitely thereafter. Adrenal insufficiency may occur years later, and patients should be warned of this possibility. Fibrosing mediastinitis is a manifestation of excessive host response rather than progressive infection. Antifungal chemotherapy is not necessarily indicated.

The role of the imidazoles (miconazole, ketoconazole) in histoplasmosis is currently unsettled. Recently studies suggest efficacy of ketoconazole in both pulmonary and disseminated histoplasmosis. However, caution is warranted in using this oral agent for immunocompromised patients with severe disease. In such patients, amphotericin B is clearly the drug of choice. Sulfonamides are of historical interest only.

PROGNOSIS. Chronic cavitary pulmonary histoplasmosis usually results in death from respiratory insufficiency. Progressive disseminated histoplasmosis (once uniformly fatal in those with poor host defenses) is curable, although relapses may occur.

PREVENTION. A 3 per cent solution of formalin sprayed on *H. capsulatum*–containing soil will destroy the fungi and control common-source outbreaks.

Goodwin RA Jr, Loyd JE, Des Prez RM: Histoplasmosis in normal hosts. Medicine 60:231, 1981. *When learning about histoplasmosis, this is the paper with which to begin.*

Goodwin RA Jr, Owens FT, Snell JD, Hubbard WW, Buchanan RD, Terry RT, Des Prez RM: Chronic pulmonary histoplasmosis. Medicine 55:413, 1976. *The definitive article on the subject by the group with the greatest clinical experience with this disease. There is a strong emphasis on immunopathogenesis.*

Goodwin RA Jr, Shapiro JL, Thurman GH, Thurman SS, Des Prez RM: Disseminated histoplasmosis: Clinical and pathologic correlations. Medicine 59:1, 1980. *An extensive review of experience with this disease in middle Tennessee. Immunopathogenesis is emphasized, but this paper is also an outstanding clinical contribution. Amphotericin B was usually curative.*

Wheat J, French MLV, Kohler RB, Zimmerman SE, Smith WR, Norton JA, Eitzen HE, Smith CD, Slama TG: The diagnostic laboratory tests for histoplasmosis: Analysis of experience in a large urban outbreak. Ann Intern Med 97:680, 1982. *This paper discusses the diagnostic usefulness of the complement fixation and immunodiffusion tests for histoplasmosis. Antibody responses differed among clinical syndromes, and titers were not necessarily elevated in patients with disseminated infection.*

367. COCCIDIOIDOMYCOSIS

DEFINITION. Coccidioidomycosis is a noncontagious respiratory mycosis of the southwest, and the second most common endemic mycosis in the United States, after histoplasmosis. It is usually self-limited, but may lead to chronic pulmonary infection or hematogenous dissemination.

ETIOLOGY. *Coccidioides immitis* is a biphasic fungus. The mycelial phase, a soil saprophyte of semiarid regions, fragments to release box-like arthroconidia (arthrospores) of a size suitable to be inhaled (2 to 5 μm). In the infected host, the fungus grows as large spherules, 10 to 80 μm in diameter, the cytoplasm of which segments to produce hundreds of endospores (2 to 5 μm diameter). Spherule rupture results in dispersal of endospores to surrounding tissues, where they mature to spherules, repeating the growth cycle.

INCIDENCE AND PREVALENCE. Coccidioidomycosis occurs in the southwestern United States and neighboring Mexico (the "Lower Sonoran life zone"), and in parts of Central and South America. Approximately 100,000 cases occur yearly. The *spherulin* (spherule-endospore) and coccidioidin (mycelial) skin tests detect approximately equal numbers of *C. immitis*-exposed patients. Each test misses 12 to 15 per cent of patients that the other test detects. Eighty to 95 per cent of the population is skin test positive in parts of California and Arizona. Infection is more common in those with outdoor activities. Extrapulmonary dissemination occurs in 1 of 2000 to 3500 white women, 1 of 500 white men, and 1 of 50 black men. The risk may be even greater in Filipinos. Pregnancy, depressed cell-mediated immunity, and corticosteroid therapy increase the risk of dissemination.

EPIDEMIOLOGY. *C. immitis* is distributed sporadically within the endemic zone. Arthroconidia are spread on the wind by any activity that raises dust; fomites may carry the spores outside the endemic area. Risk of infectivity drops dramatically once land is cultivated. Animals are commonly infected but pose no hazard for man. Newcomers to the southwest are at high risk for infection. A World War II study documented a 50 per cent skin test conversion rate within six months in airmen stationed in the Phoenix area. Skin test reactivity is associated with solid immunity; reinfection is almost unknown.

PATHOGENESIS AND PATHOLOGY. Coccidioidomycosis is characterized by suppuration (endospore response) and granuloma formation (spherule response). Cell-mediated immunity is the major host defense mechanism. In patients with extrapulmonary dissemination or chronic progressive pulmonary coccidioidomycosis, *C. immitis* skin test reactivity may never develop or may wane, and there is nonspecific suppression of reactivity to recall-type skin tests and tests of cell-mediated immunity in vitro. Most defects are reversible with therapy. Granuloma formation may be deficient, and suppuration may dominate. Antibody plays no apparent role in host defense.

CLINICAL MANIFESTATIONS. ***Primary Coccidioidomycosis.*** Sixty per cent of primary infections are asymptomatic. Symptoms in the other 40 per cent include cough, fever, headache, and pleuritic pain. Up to 5 per cent (predominantly white women) present with erythema nodosum or erythema multiforme and arthralgias ("valley fever"). Others may have "toxic erythema" resembling measles. Eosinophilia is common. The chest roentgenogram may show segmental or lobar infiltrates, often with hilar adenopathy. Pleural fluid is present in 5 to 20 per cent of cases, and fungi may be demonstrable by pleural biopsy. Cavitation may occur, usually without specific symptoms. Thin-walled cavities may persist and be discovered later on a routine roentgenogram. They are usually single, less than 4 cm in diameter, and seldom symptomatic, although the sputum may contain *C. immitis*. Up to one half of cavities will close spontaneously in two to four years. Rarely, they may lead to hemoptysis, become secondarily infected, or enlarge to encroach on normal surrounding lung.

Persistent coccidioidal pneumonia is manifested by persistence of the primary infection for six to eight weeks, with worsening pulmonary infiltrates, fever, chest pain, prostration, and productive cough. Resolution is slow; healing may result in fibrosis, bronchiectasis, and calcification. Fatality is especially common in immunosuppressed patients.

Chronic progressive coccidioidal pneumonia is an indolent disease process with weight loss, fever, hemoptysis, chest pain, and dyspnea. It is characterized by chronicity and biapical fibronodular lesions and cavities that resemble tuberculosis or histoplasmosis.

Pulmonary nodules (coccidioidomas) result from resolution of earlier infiltrative disease. Most are 1 to 4 cm in size and have semisolid centers that contain *C. immitis*. The lesions may cavitate, resulting in an "abscessing nodule."

Disseminated Coccidioidomycosis. Extrapulmonary dissemination usually occurs soon after primary infection, but diagnosis may be delayed, depending on the pace and sites of dissemination. The chest roentgenogram may or may not be abnormal. Dissemination may be unifocal or multifocal. The *skin and subcutaneous tissues* are the most common sites involved. Lesions are papular, verrucous, or ulcerative; subcutaneous abscesses may occur. *Osteomyelitis* occurs in 10 to 50 per cent of cases, involves single or multiple bones, and is most common in the vertebrae, tibia, skull, metatarsals, and metacarpals, especially at sites of tendon or ligament insertion. Complications include muscle abscesses or draining cutaneous fistulas. *Joints* may be involved by penetration from contiguous osteomyelitis or by hematogenous infection of the synovium. Large weight-bearing joints such as the knee and ankle are most commonly involved. There may be rapid joint destruction, or chronic nonerosive synovitis with progressive villous hypertrophy and pannus formation resembling rheumatoid arthritis. *Meningitis* occurs in 30 to 50 per cent of patients, often as the sole site of involvement. Most cases are hematogenous in origin; some reflect direct spread from skull or vertebral osteomyelitis. The disease process is subtle, with headache, lethargy, personality changes, and diverse neurologic abnormalities. The meningitis is predominantly basilar in location; intracerebral infection may be demonstrable by CT scan; hydrocephalus is common. Other manifestations of disseminated disease include *thyroiditis, tenosynovitis,* and *prostatitis.* Liver, spleen, lymph node, and kidney involvement is common but often clinically silent. Adrenal insufficiency may occur. Gastrointestinal tract involvement is rare.

DIAGNOSIS. Coccidioidomycosis may be confused with a variety of infections, including tuberculosis and other mycoses. Joint involvement may mimic primary rheumatologic disorders. Diagnosis is readily achieved by demonstrating endosporulating spherules in 10 per cent KOH wet mounts of sputum or inflammatory exudates. Biopsy specimens stained with hematoxylin-eosin, Gridley, periodic acid–Schiff or Gomori methenamine silver stains may demonstrate the fungi in diverse tissues. Cerebrospinal fluid (CSF) findings include pleocytosis, elevated protein, and hypoglycorrhachia; when present, eosinophils are a valuable clue to the diagnosis. *C. immitis* is not fastidious and can be recovered on most standard media. However, the mycelial phase is biohazardous and demands great care in laboratory handling. Fungi can be cultured from the CSF in only 20 to 40 per cent of instances. Urine cultures may disclose *C. immitis* in the absence of any abnormality of renal function or urinalysis. Bone marrow cultures may be positive, but blood cultures are rarely positive until disease is nearly terminal.

Serologic tests are extremely important in diagnosis and prognosis, and are uninfluenced by skin testing. Patients with symptomatic disease generally manifest an IgM antibody response that peaks by the second to third week of illness, and is replaced by an IgG response. The IgM antibody is demonstrable by tube precipitin, latex particle agglutination, or immunodiffusion (ID) techniques. The IgG response is detectable by complement fixation (CF) or ID methods. CF titers seldom exceed 1:8 to 1:16 in uncomplicated primary infection. Persistent elevations at 1:16 to 1:32 or more raise the likelihood of dissemination, particularly if associated with loss or absence of skin test reactivity. Minimal work-up for suspected dissemination includes wet mounts, biopsies and cultures from any suspicious lesions, lumbar puncture, bone scans, and cultures of concentrated morning urine. Patients with unifocal dissemination (particulary meningitis) may not show elevated CF titers in the serum or loss of skin test reactivity. CF antibody is present in the CSF in 75 to 95 per cent of cases of meningitis, however, and is diagnostic.

TREATMENT. Primary pulmonary infection seldom requires treatment, although a "prophylactic" course of 1 gram of amphotericin B may be given to patients at particular risk of dissemination (blacks, immunosuppressed patients). Isolated thin-walled cavities are usually asymptomatic, although surgical resection may be required for life-threatening hemoptysis or threatened rupture into the pleural space. Progressive pulmonary infection may benefit from a total course of 1 to 2 grams of amphotericin B; fungi are difficult to eradicate once significant destruction of pulmonary parenchyma has occurred. Disseminated coccidioidomycosis is characterized by spontaneous exacerbations and remissions, making therapeutic response difficult to interpret. Amphotericin B is often more likely to be ameliorative than curative. A total dose of 2 grams constitutes a minimal course of therapy; the goal is to produce clear clinical improvement and a persistent fourfold fall in the serum CF titer. Relapse is typical and necessitates retreatment. Meningitis must be treated by the intrathecal or intraventricular route; cure is elusive. Synovitis may require synovectomy or arthrodesis for cure.

Miconazole lacks nephrotoxicity, but is not clearly superior to amphotericin B in any other sense, and must also be given intrathecally for meningitis. Daily dosage ranges from 1800 to 3600 mg; treatment should be continued for two to three months. Major side effects include symptomatic hyponatremia, hyperlipidemia, and itching. The role of ketoconazole in therapy of coccidioidomycosis is controversial. It appears to be most useful in maintaining remissions induced by amphotericin B. However, it occasionally shows benefit in the primary management of infection that has disseminated to the skin and soft tissues. Optimal dosage and duration of therapy remain uncertain.

PROGNOSIS. Meningitis is usually fatal within two years without therapy. Even with therapy, mental deterioration or fatality may occur from hydrocephalus unless the complication is anticipated and managed by CSF shunting. Other forms of coccidioidomycosis tend to be more debilitating than lethal, although fulminating pulmonary infection may be fatal in the severely immunosuppressed.

PREVENTION. Partial control of *C. immitis* at dusty sites can be achieved by saturating the soil with 1-chloro-2-nitropropane. Patients from nonendemic areas who have risk factors for coccidioidal dissemination should be warned of the danger in working or residing in highly endemic areas.

Bouza E, Dryer JS, Hewitt WL, Meyer RD: Coccidioidal meningitis: An analysis of thirty-one cases and review of the literature. Medicine 60:139, 1981. *Coccidioidal meningitis is difficult to diagnose, harder to manage, and refractory to cure. This paper recounts the experience of UCLA-affiliated hospitals with coccidioidal meningitis between 1964 and 1976 and provides a valuable literature review.*

DeFelice R, Galgiani JN, Campbell SC, Palpant SD, Friedman BA, Dodge RR, Weinberg MG, Lincoln LJ, Tennican PO, Barbee RA: Ketoconazole treatment of nonprimary coccidioidomycosis: Evaluation of 60 patients during three years of study. Am J Med 72:681, 1982. *Although ketoconazole may produce clinical improvement in patients with various forms of coccidioidomycosis, relapse is not uncommon. Similar results are reported in a series of 29 patients (Catanzaro A, Einstein H, Levine B, Ross JR, Schillaci R, Fierer J, Friedman PJ: Ketoconazole for treatment of disseminated coccidioidomycosis. Ann Intern Med 96:436, 1982).*

Drutz DJ: Coccidioidal pneumonia. *In* Pennington JE (ed.): Respiratory Infections: Diagnosis and Management. New York, Raven Press, 1983, pp 353–373. *A thorough review of all aspects of pulmonary coccidioidal infection, including medical and surgical management.*

Drutz DJ, Catanzaro A: Coccidioidomycosis. State of the art. Am Rev Respir Dis 117:559, 727, 1978. *A review of all aspects of coccidioidomycosis and its treatment.*

Stevens DA (ed.): Coccidioidomycosis. A Text. New York, Plenum Medical Book Company, 1980, p 279. *An up-to-date compendium of the microbiology, epidemiology, immunology, serology, pathology, and clinical manifestations of coccidioidomycosis.*

368. BLASTOMYCOSIS (North American Blastomycosis, Gilchrist's Disease)

DEFINITION. Blastomycosis is a noncontagious, subacute or chronic endemic mycosis that follows inhalation of the conidia of *Blastomyces dermatitidis.* The organs most commonly affected are the lungs, skin, bones, and male genitourinary system.

ETIOLOGY. *B. dermatitidis* (perfect form: *Ajellomyces dermatitidis*) is a dimorphic fungus, occurring in the mycelial phase at ambient temperatures and as yeasts at 37° C or in the infected host. The yeast phase is characterized by cells of 8 to 15 (or more) μm in diameter that reproduce by single budding. Daughter cells are attached at a very broad (4 to 5 μm) base, and may reach the size of the mother cells before separating.

INCIDENCE AND PREVALENCE. Blastomycosis is encountered far less commonly than histoplasmosis and coccidioidomycosis. There is no diagnostic skin test or serologic test. Hence, the extent to which subclinical disease occurs is largely unknown, and endemic areas are defined in terms of clinical cases.

EPIDEMIOLOGY. Blastomycosis occurs most commonly in the southeastern United States, especially in the Ohio and Mississippi River valleys, and in areas of the United States and Canada adjacent to the Great Lakes. However, the disease is also encountered in Africa, Mexico, and Central and South America, so that "North American blastomycosis" is a misnomer. The ecologic niche for the fungus appears to be the soil, but its recovery has been sporadic and uncommon, and the factors governing its distribution are unknown. Persons at risk often have outdoor vocations or avocations. Clinical illness is most common in middle-aged men. However, studies during common-source outbreaks indicate that self-limited infection is independent of sex, age, or race. Dogs and horses are highly susceptible to blastomycosis, and the occurrence of veterinary cases helps to define endemic areas. In some instances hunters and their dogs have acquired blastomycosis simultaneously. Percutaneous inoculation of fungi has been documented in laboratory accidents, but in virtually all other circumstances cutaneous lesions result from hematogenous spread of apparent or inapparent pulmonary disease.

PATHOGENESIS AND PATHOLOGY. The factors governing host defense against *B. dermatitidis* are poorly understood. Human granulocytes kill yeast-phase organisms ineffectively in vitro; animal studies suggest that cell-mediated immunity contributes significantly to host defense. The serum of patients with blastomycosis contains an acquired heat-stable factor that impairs the locomotion of polymorphonuclear leukocytes, and may help to potentiate the disease. Disseminated disease may occur with greater frequency in the presence of immunosuppression.

Histopathologically, blastomycosis is marked by the simultaneous presence of suppurative and granulomatous foci. In fulminating infections, the suppurative component may predominate. Caseation necrosis is uncommon. Cutaneous and mucous membrane lesions are characterized by the presence of pseudoepitheliomatous hyperplasia. Identification of microabscesses and single budding yeasts helps in establishing the diagnosis.

CLINICAL MANIFESTATIONS. ***Pulmonary Blastomycosis.*** In most cases, respiratory infection is probably asymptomatic. In some cases, pleuritic chest pain, nonspecific "flu-like" symptoms, or arthralgias and erythema nodosum may mark the occurrence of acute infection. The correct diagnosis is probably seldom made in the absence of a specific search for a fungal etiology, as during a suspected common-source outbreak. Clinically apparent pulmonary blastomycosis has no distinguishing clinical or radiographic characteristics. Bronchitis is present in up to one third of cases and may contribute to rapid endobronchial spread. Cavitation, hilar adenopathy, and pleural involvement are all well documented. Fibrosis is common, but residual calcification is rare. Expanding mass-like lesions may be confused with malignancies. Miliary pulmonary lesions may be present in cases with fulminating hematogenous dissemination.

Disseminated Blastomycosis. Extrapulmonary disease may occur in the presence or absence of obvious lung disease, either during or after the initial pulmonary infection. Some cases may reflect late endogenous reactivation. The frequency of multisystem involvement is directly related to the thoroughness of diagnostic studies. The most common site of extrapulmonary dissemination is the skin, and skin lesions are often the presenting feature of blastomycosis. Lesions begin as papules, pustules, or subcutaneous nodules, and may involve exposed or unexposed areas. Some become verrucous and progress over weeks or months to produce an elevated, warty, crusted lesion with a serpiginous, indurated, dusky red or violaceous, abruptly sloping outer border. Prominent "black dots" at the surface mark the location of necrotic papillary blood vessels. Removal of crusts reveals a granulomatous base with numerous ulcers exuding bloody purulent material. Central healing and scarring may occur, with disease activity most prominent at the advancing borders. In some patients superficial ulcerative lesions may predominate. Disseminated papulopustular skin lesions have followed incision of pulmonary blastomycotic mass lesions at exploratory thoracotomy for suspected malignancy.

Bone lesions are encountered in 25 to 60 per cent of cases. They are most common in the axial skeleton (especially the vertebrae) and long bones, but may be detectable only by bone scan or radiographic bone survey. Lytic lesions with or without sclerotic margins may be seen. Draining sinuses without a verrucous appearance may mark underlying osteomyelitic foci. An acute arthritis, usually monarticular, occurs in three to five per cent of cases, either hematogenously or by direct bony spread. Involvement of the prostate, testis, and epididymis may be signaled by dysuria, pyuria, hematuria, urinary hesitancy, and tender intrascrotal mass lesions. Renal, hepatic, and splenic infections are common but usually clinically inapparent. Adrenal involvement may rarely cause Addison's disease. Central nervous system invasion occurs in about 5 per cent of cases, and may present as an intracranial mass, isolated meningitis, or spinal epidural granulomas or abscesses. Gastrointestinal involvement is rare.

DIAGNOSIS. Pulmonary blastomycosis may be confused with tuberculosis, other mycoses, bacterial pneumonia, or malignancy. Cutaneous blastomycosis is highly characteristic in appearance, but may be confused with chromomycosis, coccidioidomycosis, or some cutaneous malignancies. Diagnosis may be reached most quickly by direct microscopic examination of biologic specimens digested in 10 per cent KOH. Under these circumstances, characteristic single-budding yeasts may be seen in sputum, prostatic fluid, and other biologic specimens. Stains are not necessary. *B. dermatitidis* will grow on most standard culture media, but specimens should be held for at least one month. The mycelial phase is not sufficiently distinctive to permit a precise identification, so that conversion in vitro to the diagnostic yeast phase is required. Animal inoculation is not necessary. In fixed tissue specimens, hematoxylin-eosin staining reveals characteristic yeast cells with a doubly refractile cell wall, often accentuated by retraction of the protoplast from the outer cell wall. The periodic acid–Schiff stain preserves intracellular detail and helps differentiate *B. dermatitidis* (multinucleated) from *C. neoformans* and *H. capsulatum* (single nuclei). Fungi are easily seen with Gomori methenamine silver stain, but internal detail is lost.

Patients with blastomycosis should have complete evaluation for skin, bone, and genitourinary lesions, as the response to therapy may be monitored by observing the progress of disease in these sites. Adrenal function should also be evaluated as a few patients may go on to develop adrenal insufficiency.

The blastomycin skin test is valueless as a diagnostic or prognostic tool, and should not be used. The blastomycosis complement fixation test shows cross-reactivity with *H. capsulatum* and *C. immitis*, and is almost never clinically useful. An immunodiffusion test has shown more promising results.

TREATMENT. Most acute pulmonary infections are probably self-limited. In patients with progressive lung disease, extrapulmonary lesions, or immunosuppression, systemic antifungal therapy is indicated.

Amphotericin B and 2-hydroxystilbamidine reportedly provide similar rates of improvement in patients with noncavitary pulmonary disease or disseminated disease involving only the skin. However, amphotericin B (given in a total dose of at least 2 grams) is associated with fewer relapses, and is probably the choice for all forms of the disease. 2-Hydroxystilbamidine is given in a total dose of 4 to 15 grams (225 mg per day). Its side effects include nausea, vomiting, chills, fever, elevation of hepatic transaminase levels, and rare hypotensive or idiosyncratic reactions. Ketoconazole has shown promise in clinical trials, but treatment failures have occasionally been reported and experience is insufficient to warrant its recommendation as a drug of first choice, especially in severely ill patients.

PROGNOSIS. The natural history of extrapulmonary blastomycosis is that of a slowly progressive disease with a 20 to 90 per cent mortality, and severe disfigurement, depending upon the series reported. Case mortality with either amphotericin B or 2-hydroxystilbamidine is about 8 per cent. Most relapses occur within one year of treatment, but have been documented after as long as nine years. All patients with untreated pulmonary disease should be carefully observed for later evidence of disease activity.

Parker JD, Doto IL, Tosh FE: A decade of experience with blastomycosis and its treatment with amphotericin B. Am Rev Respir Dis 99:895, 1969. *The only published study comparing therapeutic effectiveness of amphotericin B and 2-hydroxystilbamidine. Except for noncavitary pulmonary disease and isolated cutaneous dissemination, amphotericin B was superior.*

Sarosi GA, Davies SF: Blastomycosis. State of the art. Am Rev Respir Dis 120:911, 1979. *A valuable review paper with a particular emphasis on pulmonary blastomycosis. An excellent companion piece to the Witorsch and Utz reference.*

Witorsch P, Utz JP: North American blastomycosis: A study of 40 patients. Medicine 47:169, 1968. *This paper contains a wealth of information concerning both pulmonary and systemic blastomycosis.*

369. PARACOCCIDIOIDOMYCOSIS

DEFINITION. Paracoccidioidomycosis (South American blastomycosis) is a noncontagious respiratory mycosis that may be acute and self-limited, or may produce progressive pulmonary disease or extrapulmonary dissemination. It is the most common systemic mycosis in South America.

ETIOLOGY. *Paracoccidioides brasiliensis* is a dimorphic fungus which in its mycelial phase is probably a soil saprophyte. In tissues or at 37° C the fungus is a spherical double-walled yeast cell, 6 to 60 μm in diameter, that has multiple buds on narrow necks, producing the appearance of "ship's wheels," "crown of buds," or "Mickey Mouse" figures.

INCIDENCE AND PREVALENCE. Paracoccidioidomycosis is limited to an area 20° N in Mexico to 34° S in Argentina. Brazil accounts for 70 per cent of the 5000 to 6000 reported cases, followed by Venezuela and Colombia. Natural infection in animals has not been documented, and common-source outbreaks in humans have not been reported.

EPIDEMIOLOGY. Equal numbers of men and women have positive paracoccidioidin skin tests, but clinical disease is 15 times more prevalent in men. Only 4 per cent of cases have been reported in children. Hormonal or occupational factors (especially agricultural work) may influence susceptibility. Asian and European immigrants often have more severe illness than patients who are native born. Whether this indicates a racial predisposition or merely exposure of a population with a lack of prior disease experience is uncertain.

Prominent oropharyngeal ulcerations in disseminated paracoccidioidomycosis led to the assumption that infection was acquired from contaminated vegetation introduced into the mouth. It is now clear that virtually all cases are acquired by the respiratory route. The vast majority of cases are probably self-limited, manifesting themselves by positive skin tests and minimal abnormalities of the chest roentgenogram.

PATHOGENESIS AND PATHOLOGY. The host response consists of a combination of suppuration and granulomas. In patients with impaired host defense, the suppurative response may dominate. The disease process is limited to the lungs in most cases, but lymphohematogenous dissemination may occur, especially in males beyond puberty and in immunosuppressed patients.

The spectrum of disease encountered clinically is a function of the integrity of cell-mediated host defense responses. In patients with progressive disease, there is secondary suppression of immunity with impaired skin test reactivity to paracoccidioidin and other recall-type skin test preparations. There is also an impairment of correlates of cell-mediated immunity in vitro (migration inhibition factor, lymphocyte blastogenesis). All these parameters commonly improve with treatment.

CLINICAL MANIFESTATIONS. Pulmonary paracoccidioidomycosis may be symptomatic or asymptomatic and may or may not be apparent when extrapulmonary disease is discovered. There is nothing distinctive about the acute pulmonary process. Progressive pulmonary lesions may be unilateral or bilateral, with or without hilar adenopathy. Chest roentgenograms may reveal cavitation (20 to 33 per cent of cases), infiltration, nodules, tumor-like masses, or fibrosis. Pulmonary paracoccidioidomycosis is commonly confused with tuberculosis but less often leads to residual calcification.

Extrapulmonary dissemination may occur acutely, especially in young persons, under which circumstance the disease process is dominated by lymphadenopathy, hepatosplenomegaly, and a miliary pattern on the chest roentgenogram. The disease may also disseminate after a period of years to decades. Many cases have been documented in persons who have long since emigrated from endemic areas so that continued exposure to the fungus is not an important predisposing factor. The clinical presentation is variable, depending on the sites of involvement. Oropharyngeal mucosal invasion is characteristic. Ulcerating lesions involve the gums, lips, tongue, palate, uvula, pharynx, tonsillar areas, or floor of the mouth. Lesions eventually become so painful that eating is extremely difficult. Gingival destruction may result in loss of teeth. Involvement of the epiglottis and larynx results in dysphonia. Ulcers of the nasal, conjunctival, and perianal mucous membranes may be encountered. There may be massive cervical and abdominal lymphadenopathy. Lymph nodes may break down to produce draining fistulas. A wide variety of crusted ulcerative, verrucous, and granulomatous skin lesions have been described, often on the face or at mucocutaneous borders. Ulcerating lesions of the intestinal tract may be encountered; the stomach is usually spared. Complications include malabsorption, protein-losing enteropathy, or intestinal perforation. There may be signs of adrenal insufficiency and involvement of the bones, testes, epididymis, heart, and pancreas. Central nervous system disease may present as a space-occupying lesion or meningitis. Hepatic, splenic, and renal involvement is common but usually clinically silent.

DIAGNOSIS. Paracoccidioidomycosis must be differentiated from tuberculosis, histoplasmosis, sporotrichosis, leishmaniasis, yaws, and syphilis.

Multiple-budding *P. brasiliensis* can usually be demonstrated in wet mounts or 10 per cent KOH preparations from sputum or infective foci. Characteristic fungus cells can also be seen in hematoxylin-eosin stained slides from biopsy material, but special stains (e.g., periodic acid–Schiff, Gridley, and Gomori methenamine silver) demonstrate the cells much more effectively. Fungi can be recovered in two to four weeks on blood agar at 37° C (tissue phase) or on Sabouraud's agar at 30° C (saprobic phase). Cultures of blood, urine, bone marrow, spinal fluid, and biopsy specimens (liver, lymph node, intestine) may be helpful in appropriate instances. In one study of 39 cases, diagnosis could be made from direct examination of biopsy material in 95 per cent and by culture of these materials or sputum in 85 per cent. Animal inoculation is not necessary for diagnosis.

Serologic tests are useful in following the course of established disease. Precipitins are the first antibodies to appear, and the first to disappear with successful therapy. Complement-fixing (CF) antibodies appear later in a titer proportional to the severity of infection. Sera from 85 to 95 per cent of patients with active disease demonstrate CF titers ≥1:32. Numbers of precipitin bands formed in the immunodiffusion (ID) test rather than the actual antibody titer indicate the degree of disease activity. (ID and CF tests are available at the Centers for Disease Control in Atlanta.)

There is still a need for a specific paracoccidioidin skin test. The present preparations appear to share antigens with *H. capsulatum* and *S. schenckii*. There is no commercially available paracoccidioidin skin test reagent in the United States.

TREATMENT. The largest therapeutic experience is with sulfonamides. Their low cost, relatively low toxicity, and good gastrointestinal absorption are partially offset by slow response, a 40 per cent failure and relapse rate, and the occurrence of sulfonamide resistance. The recommended dose of sulfadiazine for adults is 4 to 6 grams per day. Once clinical improvement has occurred (a matter of weeks to months), dosage is reduced by half and continued for three to five years. Amphotericin B produces a higher response rate and is considered the drug of choice for disseminated disease. However, relapses occur even after total doses of 2 grams, whether or not sulfonamides are added to the regimen. Therapy should be continued until CF titers stabilize at a low level and the number of precipitin bands is reduced. *P. brasiliensis* is extraordinarily susceptible to miconazole in vitro (MIC ≤0.001 per milliliter), and there is a good clinical response. Ketoconazole and trimethoprim-sulfamethoxazole also appear highly promising and have the advantage of oral administration. Iodides, flucytosine, and 2-hydroxystilbamidine are without benefit.

PROGNOSIS. Disseminated paracoccidioidomycosis is generally fatal in the absence of therapy, with death occurring from extensive pulmonary disease, central nervous system lesions, intestinal perforation, or adrenal insufficiency.

Londero AT, Ramos CF, Lopes JOS: Progressive pulmonary paracoccidioidomycosis. A study of 34 cases observed in Rio Grande do Sul (Brazil). Mycopathologia 63:53, 1978. *Emphasizes the pulmonary aspects of this respiratory mycosis.*

Restrepo A, Gomez I, Cano LE, Arango MD, Gutierrez F, Sanin A, Robledo MA: Post-therapy status of paracoccidioidomycosis treated with ketoconazole. *In* Graybill JR (ed.): Proceedings of a Symposium on New Developments in Therapy for the Mycoses. Am J Med 74 (#1B):53–57, 1983. *The promise of ketoconazole is emphasized in this paper as well as in the following reference, which is somewhat more difficult to obtain: Del Negro G: Ketoconazole in paracoccidioidomycosis. A long-term study with prolonged follow-up. Rev Inst Med Trop Sao Paulo 24:27, 1982.*

Restrepo A, Greer DL, Vasconcellos M: Paracoccidioidomycosis: A review. Rev Med Vet Mycol 8:97, 1973. *A thorough review of the disease; a classic article.*

Restrepo A, Robledo M, Giraldo R, Hernandez H, Sierra F, Guiterrez L, Londono M, Lopez R, Calle G: The gamut of paracoccidioidomycosis. Am J Med 61:33, 1976. *An excellent review with an emphasis on pulmonary and extrapulmonary clinical manifestations, and helpful photographs.*

370. CRYPTOCOCCOSIS

DEFINITION. Cryptococcosis is a noncontagious, often opportunistic mycosis characterized by respiratory tract colonization, acute or chronic pulmonary infection, or hematogenous dissemination, often with meningitis.

ETIOLOGY. Pathogenic cryptococci are budding yeasts, 4 to 20 μm in diameter with a characteristic polysaccharide capsule. Buds are usually single and narrow-necked. Serotypes A and D, and B and C, respectively, show mating compatibility, and their respective perfect forms are *Filobasidiella neoformans* and *F. bacillispora*. Pathogenic cryptococci produce characteristic pigmentation on agar containing phenolic substrates or extracted birdseed (niger seed: *Guizotia abyssinica*), and progressive neurologic infection when injected intracerebrally into mice. They are not found as laboratory contaminants.

INCIDENCE AND PREVALENCE. Because there is no skin test or epidemiologically useful serologic test, the incidence and prevalence of cryptococcosis are unknown. However, the disease occurs worldwide, with several hundred new cases yearly in the United States. Most pulmonary infections are probably overlooked. Cryptococcal meningitis, which accounts for some 90 per cent of reported disease, is dramatic and seldom overlooked. Cryptococcosis has increased in incidence as immunosuppression has become more common and diagnostic techniques have improved and has emerged as a particular problem in patients with acquired immune deficiency syndrome (AIDS).

EPIDEMIOLOGY. Serotype A causes most disease in the United States, serotype D in Europe. Disease caused by serotypes B and C is largely restricted to southern California. Serotypes A and D are most commonly found in avian habitats, especially in pigeon dung. Up to 5×10^7 viable *C. neoformans* per gram of pigeon feces has been recovered from urban environments. Although the feet, beaks, crops, and gut contents of pigeons may harbor cryptococci, the birds are not infected. High humidity and protection from weathering or soil contact promote survival of *C. neoformans* in the environment. Indoor sites may harbor cryptococci more frequently than outdoor sites. Serotypes B and C are rarely recoverable from the environment, suggesting that *C. bacillispora* occupies a unique ecologic niche.

Because most patients give no history of contact with pigeons, infection probably results from inhalation of airborne organisms. A few infections have been traced to air conditioners in which birds have nested. Ocular cryptococcosis has been transmitted by corneal transplantation. Many animals are infected with cryptococci, but pose no threat to man.

PATHOGENESIS AND PATHOLOGY. Cryptococci in the environment are unencapsulated. Either these forms or the basidiospores of *Filobasidiella* are small enough to be inhaled. Encapsulation takes place in the lung, and virulence is related to the presence, but not the amount, of encapsulation. (Occasional infections with unencapsulated cryptococci occur.) Phagocytes can kill unencapsulated cryptococci, but phagocytosis of capsulated fungi is impaired, apparently because attached opsonic antibody is masked from phagocytes by capsular material. Studies in athymic nude mice suggest that cell-mediated immunity (CMI) is crucial to host defense. Patients with defective CMI (Hodgkin's disease and other lymphoreticular malignancies, corticosteroid therapy) are especially susceptible to cryptococcal dissemination. Neutropenia appears to confer no additional risk.

The histopathology of cryptococcosis varies from a foamy, gelatinous process to a more granulomatous response. Caseation, calcification, and fibrosis are rare. Cryptococci are fragile and may collapse during fixation, leading to a crescentic appearance. They stain poorly with hematoxylin-eosin, but well with methenamine silver and periodic acid–Schiff. Mucicarmine specifically stains capsular mucopolysaccharide.

CLINICAL MANIFESTATIONS. Respiratory tract colonization usually occurs in patients with underlying lung disease and may be transient or persistent.

Pulmonary Cryptococcosis. Manifestations include fever, malaise, pleuritic pain, cough, scanty sputum, and hemoptysis. A pleural effusion or friction rub may be present. Solitary or multiple nodules or nodular-confluent infiltrates, tumor-like masses, or miliary densities may be found on chest roentgenograms; any lobe may be involved. Cavitation is present in 10 to 16 per cent of cases. Hilar adenopathy may occur with advanced disease. Chronic infection is common; slowly progressive pulmonary involvement over four to nineteen years has been documented. Many such cases are diagnosed at thoracotomy for suspected malignancy. Although some cases are associated with alveolar proteinosis, only 10 per cent of all patients with pulmonary cryptococcosis have evidence of immunologic deficiency.

Disseminated Cryptococcosis. Manifestations of central nervous system cryptococcosis reflect exudate over the base of the brain (meningitis and hydrocephalus), extension of infection along perivascular spaces with involvement of the gray matter (encephalitis), direct invasion of the optic pathways (visual impairment), focal ischemic damage related to brain stem vasculitis, and cryptococcomas in the brain or spinal cord. Meningitis is the most common manifestation of systemic cryptococcosis, and its principal symptom is headache. Associated findings include mental changes (confusion, lethargy, personality alteration, defective memory, agitation, or frank psychosis); ocular symptoms (blurred vision, retrobulbar pain, diplopia, and photophobia); stiffness of the neck and back; nausea and vomiting; and fever, nystagmus, ataxia, aphasia, hearing deficits, cranial nerve palsies, seizures, and paresthesias. Up to 50 per cent of patients have papilledema or optic neuritis. Deterioration of mentation may reflect the development of hydrocephalus. Cryptococcal meningitis may be quite chronic, with disease presenting over weeks to months, or very rarely even years. *Skin and mucous membrane* involvement is seen in 10 to 15 per cent of cases and can take the form of papules, pustules, abscesses, chancres, nodules, or cellulitis followed by vesiculation and ulceration. *Bone* involvement occurs in 5 to 10 per cent of cases and may be mistaken for malignancy. Joint involvement is extremely rare. Other sites of invasion may include the *liver* (hepatitis, hepatic necrosis), *kidneys* (urinary tract symptoms, pyelonephritis, papillary necrosis), *prostate* (prostatism), *adrenals* (adrenal insufficiency), spleen, lymph nodes, and testes.

DIAGNOSIS. The differential diagnosis of pulmonary cryptococcosis includes diverse infections and malignancies. Cryptococcal meningitis may be confused with various hypoglycorrhachic syndromes, including tuberculosis and coccidioidomycosis. A primary psychiatric disorder is often suspected.

Sputum cultures are positive in only 20 per cent of pulmonary infections. Sixty per cent of cases have been diagnosed by exploratory thoracotomy for suspected malignancy in older series. Patients with positive sputum cultures should be evaluated for systemic infection, with cultures of blood and urine; biopsy and culture of skin lesions; and a lumbar puncture, whether or not central nervous system disease is apparent. Bone marrow aspiration, liver biopsy, and prostatic massage may also be indicated. In a recent series of patients with cancer and disseminated cryptococcosis, 15 per cent of blood cultures and 27 per cent of urine cultures were positive. Positive blood cultures do not routinely predict a poor therapeutic outcome.

In patients presenting with meningitis, the chest roentgenogram may or may not be abnormal. Sputum cultures should be obtained along with a careful baseline evaluation for other foci of infection. Characteristic cerebrospinal fluid (CSF) findings include elevated pressure (90 per cent of cases); pleocytosis (usually lymphocytic, sometimes polymorphonuclear) with a total white blood cell concentration generally below 500 per cubic millimeter; and hypoglycorrhachia (CSF glucose level less than 50 per cent of a simultaneously obtained blood glucose) (55 per cent of cases). When spun CSF sediment (or other body fluid) is mixed with a drop of India ink or nigrosin and examined under high dry magnification, cryptococci stand out against the darkened background by their halo-like capsules. The India ink preparation is positive in only about 50 per cent of cases of cryptococcal meningitis, whereas CSF cultures are eventually positive in about 95 per cent. Diagnostic yield is improved by examining CSF by cytologic techniques, looking carefully for extracranial sites of infection, obtaining large volumes of CSF exclusively for culture (~10 ml, provided that there are no contraindications to removal of this volume), repeated lumbar punctures, and, in particularly refractory diagnostic situations, tapping the cisterna magna or lateral ventricles. Reports of elevated CSF alcohol concentrations reflect detection of the alcohol used to prepare the skin for lumbar puncture.

The latex cryptococcal agglutination test (LCAT) is based upon the agglutination of latex spheres coated with anticryptococcal antibody in the presence of capsular antigen. Cryptococcal antigen is found in the CSF in up to 93 per cent of proven cases of cryptococcal meningitis, and may also be found in the blood. Patients with AIDS tend to have particularly high blood lecithin:cholesterol acyltransferase titers. In some cases, the LCAT is positive when all other tests of CSF are nondiagnostic. Serum or pleural fluid LCAT determinations may be helpful in the differential diagnosis of pneumonia in immunosuppressed patients. Tests for cryptococcal antibody are seldom of diagnostic value.

TREATMENT. Patients with respiratory tract colonization or resolving pulmonary infection and intact immunity seldom require therapy. Patients whose pulmonary cryptococcosis is diagnosed at thoracotomy should have careful postoperative evaluation for extrapulmonary disease, including a lumbar puncture. If none is found, therapy may be safely withheld in those with intact host defenses, provided that there is careful follow-up evaluation. If long-term follow-up is unlikely, antifungal therapy should be administered because there may be a 3 to 10 per cent risk of meningitis occurring up to three years following surgery. Patients with progressive pulmonary infection, especially if immunosuppressed, and all patients with extrapulmonary infection require systemic antifungal therapy.

Therapy for pulmonary cryptococcosis is poorly defined, but an arbitrary total dose of 1 gram of amphotericin B delivered intravenously over five to six weeks (up to 50 mg on alternate days) would be expected to control most cases. Immunosuppressed patients may require more aggressive therapy.

Therapeutic guidelines for cryptococcal meningitis are more clearly defined. Combination therapy with amphotericin B and flucytosine is currently favored on three bases: (1) the two drugs are synergistic against cryptococci in vitro; (2) flucytosine reliably crosses the blood-brain barrier, whereas amphotericin B does not; and (3) a national cooperative study has demonstrated that a six-week treatment course with intravenous amphotericin B (0.3 mg per kilogram per day) plus oral flucytosine (150 mg per kilogram per day) cured or improved more patients, produced fewer failures or relapses, and was associated with less nephrotoxicity than amphotericin B given alone for ten weeks in a dose of 0.4 mg per kilogram per day. Potential problems relate to the added toxicity of flucytosine (bone marrow suppression, liver function abnormalities, diarrhea, and rash). Flucytosine induced marrow suppression is usually reversible.

In patients who fail to show clinical improvement with combination chemotherapy, or those whose CSF cultures remain persistently positive, consideration must be given to delivery of amphotericin B into the lumbar sac, cisterna magna, or a lateral ventricle via an Ommaya reservoir or similar device. Complications related to amphotericin B irritability or catheter placement are common. Patients must also be carefully evaluated for hydrocephalus, since therapeutic CSF shunting may be required.

Too few clinical data are available to warrant the use of miconazole except in unusual circumstances. Ketoconazole may have some value in the management of extrameningeal infection, but its penetration of the blood-brain barrier is insufficient to permit its use in cryptococcal meningitis. Flucytosine should never be used alone because of a high risk of acquired drug resistance by the fungi.

PROGNOSIS. Prior to the amphotericin B era, 80 per cent of cryptococcal meningitis patients died within two years. With current therapeutic regimens, 80 to 90 per cent of patients can be cured, although more than one treatment course may be required. Adverse prognostic factors include lymphoreticular malignancy or corticosteroid therapy; cerebrospinal fluid with high opening pressure, a low glucose level, less than 20 leukocytes per cubic millimeter, and positive India ink preparations; cryptococci isolated from the blood or extraneural sites; and high titers of cryptococcal antigen in CSF and serum. Treated patients with persistently elevated titers of cryptococcal antigen have a tendency to relapse. Elevated CSF protein concentrations and positive India ink preparations may persist for years following curative therapy, and have no apparent prognostic significance.

PREVENTION. Hydrated lime and sodium hydroxide may be used to control cryptococcal growth in droppings of pet pigeons, but are otherwise impractical. Control of pigeon populations in urban areas might be expected to reduce the risk of acquiring cryptococcosis in this setting.

Bennett JE, Dismukes WE, Duma RJ, Medoff G, Sande MA, Gallis H, Leonard J, Fields BT Jr, Bradshaw M, Haywood H, McGee ZA, Cate TR, Cobbs CG, Warner JF, Alling DW: A comparison of amphotericin B alone and combined with flucytosine in the treatment of cryptococcal meningitis. N Engl J Med 301:126, 1979. *This important paper provides the rationale for the combined therapeutic approach to cryptococcal meningitis used in the United States at this time.*

Diamond RD, Bennett JE: Prognostic factors in cryptococcal meningitis a study in 111 cases. Ann Intern Med 80:176, 1974. *An excellent review of the factors predictive of early death in cryptococcal meningitis, as well as those factors that influence response to therapy.*

Hermann KJ, Powell KE, Christianson CS, Huggins PM, Larsh HW, Vivas JR,

Tosh FE: Pulmonary cryptococcosis: Clinical forms and treatment. A Center for Disease Control Cooperative Mycoses Study. Am Rev Respir Dis 108:1116, 1973. *This interesting paper compares the presentation of pulmonary cryptococcosis in patients in chronic chest hospitals with that of patients in other settings. Colonization, infection, and treatment are discussed.*

Perfect JR, Durack DT, Gallis HA: Cryptococcemia. Medicine 62:98, 1983. *Cryptococcemia identifies patients with poor prognoses, largely because of underlying disease. However, some patients will respond to aggressive therapy with amphotericin B and flucytosine.*

371. SPOROTRICHOSIS

DEFINITION. Sporotrichosis is a subacute or chronic noncontagious mycosis of the skin and regional lymphatics that results from the percutaneous introduction of *Sporothrix schenckii*. In some cases, pulmonary disease results from inhalation of spores. Rarely, there is lymphohematogenous dissemination to joints, bones, and skin.

ETIOLOGY. *Sporothrix (Sporotrichum) schenckii* is a dimorphic fungus. In tissues and at 37° C in vitro it is yeast-like, appearing as spherical or cigar-shaped budding cells. In nature (25° C), the fungus exists as sporulating hyphae that produce conidia of a size (2 to 3 μm) suitable to be inhaled. *S. schenckii* is commonly found on vegetation or wood, or in the soil; it is related to *Ceratocystis stenoceras*, a plant pathogen.

INCIDENCE AND PREVALENCE. Sporotrichosis is especially common in Mexico, Central America, and Brazil, and occurs more frequently in the United States than in Europe. Susceptibility is less related to sex, age, or race than to opportunities for environmental exposure. Skin test data suggest that sporotrichosis may occur as a subclinical infection, especially in nursery workers.

EPIDEMIOLOGY. *S. schenckii* is a potential cause of infection in anyone who has frequent contact with vegetation (e.g., sphagnum moss, timber, hay, thorn bushes). Thus, it is an occupational hazard for farmers, gardeners, florists, greenhouse workers, timber cutters, and others. Some cases may be transmitted by insect or animal bite. The source of infection may be obscure in those with pulmonary or visceral involvement. In the most famous outbreak of sporotrichosis, nearly 3000 otherwise healthy South African gold miners acquired lymphocutaneous sporotrichosis from brushing past contaminated mine timbers. Spread from patient to patient, pulmonary disease and disseminated disease were notable by their absence. Epidemiologic proof that alcoholism predisposes to sporotrichosis ("syndrome of the alcoholic rose gardener") is lacking.

PATHOGENESIS AND PATHOLOGY. *S. schenckii* enters the skin through apparent or inapparent trauma. Strains that multiply well at 35° C but poorly at 37° C can produce cutaneous lesions, but not lymphatic spread or systemic involvement. Strains that multiply well at 35 or 37° C are capable of producing lymphocutaneous or visceral disease. Cell-mediated immunity is important in determining the extent of disease, and immunosuppressed patients appear more likely to develop multifocal systemic spread of infection. Patients with disseminated but not localized lymphocutaneous sporotrichosis show evidence of depressed cell-mediated immunity (delayed-type hypersensitivity and lymphocyte transformation) that reverses with treatment.

The basic histopathologic pattern is a combination of suppuration and granulomas, occasionally with caseation necrosis. Chronic cutaneous lesions demonstrate prominent pseudoepitheliomatous hyperplasia and may be confused with malignancies.

CLINICAL MANIFESTATIONS. In lymphocutaneous sporotrichosis, which accounts for 75 per cent of cases, a single lesion usually develops on an exposed skin surface, commonly following trauma. The pimple, wart, pustule, ulcer, abscess, or chancre fails to heal and typically spreads up the extremity over days to weeks, evoking a series of subcutaneous nontender nodular lesions along the thickened lymphatics. The nodules may ulcerate, releasing thin pus. Systemic signs and symptoms of infection are notably absent. Incision and drainage and

antibacterial drugs are without benefit. The disease may slowly progress over months or even years; a few cases heal spontaneously.

In 20 per cent of cases, the process is strictly limited to the site of introduction in the skin ("fixed"). It is likely that this disease pattern is produced by *S. schenckii* strains that grow poorly at 37° C (see above). Lacking the diagnostic appearance of nodules following lymphatics, this form of sporotrichosis may be quite difficult to diagnose.

About 50 cases of pulmonary sporotrichosis have been reported. Disease may occur acutely, but more frequently presents as a chronic (thin-walled) cavitary process involving upper lobes and apices, and accurately mimicking pulmonary tuberculosis. Extracutaneous sporotrichosis is very rare. It may result from direct, deep implantation of fungi; from direct contiguous spread of lymphocutaneous disease; or by hematogenous spread from apparent or inapparent cutaneous or pulmonary loci. Common sites of dissemination include joints (especially knees, ankles, wrists, and small joints of the hands and feet) and bones (especially the tibia), sometimes with pathologic fractures. When joint disease occurs in the absence of a primary lymphocutaneous focus (as it does in more than 80 per cent of cases), it is classically confused with rheumatoid arthritis, sarcoidosis, villonodular synovitis, or gout. In immunocompromised patients with multifocal disease, there is often abrupt development of widespread subcutaneous nodules in a hematogenous distribution. Multiarticular joint disease may be present, and multifocal osteolytic foci may be visible roentgenographically. Cultures of the urine, bone marrow, and rarely even the blood may be positive. There are a few recorded cases of central nervous system sporotrichosis; chronic meningitis may be present.

DIAGNOSIS. The differential diagnosis of lymphocutaneous sporotrichosis includes sporotrichoid granulomas caused by atypical mycobacterial infections, other cutaneous mycoses, leishmaniasis, syphilis, anthrax, tularemia, cat scratch disease, and even furunculosis. Pulmonary sporotrichosis resembles pulmonary tuberculosis; sometimes the diseases coexist.

The diagnosis of lymphocutaneous sporotrichosis on histopathologic grounds is very difficult, as the fungi may not be easily demonstrable. Direct immunofluorescence or immunoperoxidase staining may be helpful, but is not generally available. *S. schenckii* is also difficult to identify directly in the sputum. In deep lesions, fungi may be demonstrable with special stains (e.g., methenamine silver, periodic acid–Schiff). Regardless of the locus of infection, diagnosis is made most accurately by recovering *S. schenckii* in culture. These fungi grow well on most standard media; cultures should be held at least four weeks before being discarded as negative. Conversion to yeast form in vitro or animal inoculation may assist in identification. Rarely, *S. schenckii* may be recovered from the sputum in the absence of any demonstrable disease process, thus reflecting the possibility of asymptomatic colonization.

Serologic tests are useful in establishing the diagnosis of extracutaneous or systemic forms of sporotrichosis when distinct clinical features are lacking. The yeast cell and latex particle agglutination tests are more sensitive than immunodiffusion or complement fixation techniques. In general, patients with extracutaneous disease have higher titers than those with lymphocutaneous involvement. A slide latex agglutination titer of 1:8 or above is considered presumptive evidence of sporotrichosis by the Centers for Disease Control, Atlanta. The test has limited prognostic value, since antibody levels may show little change during or after convalescence.

A sporotrichosis skin test is not commercially available.

TREATMENT. The treatment of choice for lymphocutaneous sporotrichosis is saturated solution of potassium iodide (SSKI). Its mechanism of action is unclear. Daily dosage is increased in dropwise fashion (usually 50 mg per drop) in a palatable vehicle until 3 to 5 grams or more is being administered each day. If signs of toxicity ensue (e.g., indigestion, rash, lacrimation, parotid swelling), dosage may have to be reduced. Amphotericin B is indicated when SSKI fails.

SSKI may be efficacious for noncavitary pulmonary sporotrichosis, but neither SSKI nor amphotericin B shows clear therapeutic superiority in cavitary infection. Resectional surgery may be indicated. Disseminated sporotrichosis is generally treated with intravenous amphotericin B (minimal dose, 2 grams), together with local intralesional therapy, arthrotomy, and other indicated drainage procedures. Amphotericin B appears substantially superior to SSKI in disseminated infection. Flucytosine, miconazole, and ketoconazole are poorly effective in any form of the disease.

PROGNOSIS. Cutaneous, lymphocutaneous, and mucocutaneous sporotrichosis commonly remit and relapse for years without therapy. Spontaneous cures are unknown in disseminated disease. The natural history and, indeed, the incidence and prevalence of pulmonary sporotrichosis are unknown. Cavitary pulmonary disease may be curable medically, but more often requires surgery. Untreated chronic pulmonary sporotrichosis is usually fatal.

Jung JY, Almond CH, Elkadi A, Tenorio A: Role of surgery in the management of pulmonary sporotrichosis. J Thorac Cardiovasc Surg 77:234, 1979. *A discussion of the disease process and the limitations of medical and surgical management.*

Kwon-Chung KJ: Comparison of isolates of *Sporothrix schenckii* obtained from fixed cutaneous lesions with isolates from other types of lesions. J Infect Dis 139:424, 1979. *Provides important information relating patterns of clinical disease with temperature optima for* S. schenckii.

Wilson DE, Mann JJ, Bennett JE, Utz P: Clinical features of extracutaneous sporotrichosis. Medicine 46:265, 1967. *Still the best reference concerning extracutaneous sporotrichosis.*

372. CANDIDIASIS (Candidosis)

DEFINITION. Candidiasis is a general term for a variety of local and systemic processes sharing in common colonization or infection by *Candida* species.

ETIOLOGY. The most common etiologic agent is *Candida albicans*. Others include *C. tropicalis, parapsilosis, stellatoidea, krusei, parakrusei, pseudotropicalis,* and *guilliermondi. Torulopsis glabrata* may be reclassified as *Candida glabrata. Candida* species are biphasic, but not in the usual sense (i.e., temperature or host dependent). Instead, yeasts (the usual colonizing form) may assume a pseudomycelial configuration, especially during tissue invasion. (*T. glabrata* remains yeastlike). Pseudomycelia result from the sequential budding of yeasts (blastospores), with resultant branching chains of elongated organisms, clearly delineated by constrictions. *C. albicans* can be readily identified in vitro by the production of unconstricted germ tubes within two to four hours of exposure to serum.

INCIDENCE AND PREVALENCE. Candidiasis occurs worldwide. Superficial infections such as thrush, paronychia, and intertrigo are universal. Invasive candidiasis has become a problem with the advent of antibiotics (destruction of normal inhibitory bacterial flora) and the use of myelotoxic or immunosuppressive agents, especially corticosteroids. Candidiasis is the most common opportunistic mycosis in the world.

EPIDEMIOLOGY. *Candida* species can be found in nature, but more commonly originate with man. *C. albicans* is found in the oropharynx, gastrointestinal tract, and vagina of a variable proportion of normal persons, but only rarely on the skin. Non-*albicans* species frequently colonize the skin. Vaginal colonization is increased by diabetes, pregnancy, and oral contraceptive agents. Carriage at all sites is increased by antibiotics. Unlike most other fungi, *C. albicans* is transmissible (e.g., from colonized birth canal to neonatal oropharynx, between sexual partners, by hands of medical attendants). Cutaneous infection generally requires skin trauma, maceration, and persistent moisture. Systemic candidiasis occurs most frequently in a hospital setting, among severely ill, antibiotic-treated patients with breaches of normal mucocutaneous barriers (e.g., indwelling intravascular lines or Foley catheters; gastrointestinal ulcerations from chemotherapeutic agents; burns or gastrointestinal surgery). Endocarditis may follow intravenous drug abuse, prolonged intravenous therapy, or placement of a prosthetic heart valve.

PATHOGENESIS AND PATHOLOGY. Candidiasis is a suppurative infection that sometimes has a granulomatous component. Both granulocytes and cell-mediated immunity are important in host defense. Polymorphonuclear leukocytes (PMNs) kill ingested yeasts by oxidative and nonoxidative mechanisms. *C. albicans* sometimes escapes the PMNs by germ tube penetration of the leukocyte wall. Pseudomycelia are attacked by apposition of PMNs, with exocytosis of lysosomal enzymes. Serum factors serve as opsonins and cause *Candida* clumping, assisting in bloodstream clearance. Neutropenia is a major risk factor for *Candida* dissemination. Patients with defective cell-mediated immune mechanisms (AIDS, the syndrome of chronic mucocutaneous candidiasis) are more susceptible to thrush and esophagitis than to hematogenous *Candida* dissemination.

CLINICAL MANIFESTATIONS. ***Mucocutaneous Infection.*** *Thrush* is characterized by a creamy to gray pseudomembrane, patchy or confluent, that covers the tongue, buccal mucosa, or other oropharyngeal surfaces. Ulceration and necrosis may be present. Membrane removal leaves a red, oozing base. Laryngeal involvement results in hoarseness. *Esophagitis* is often an extension of oropharyngeal disease, may be manifested by retrosternal pain and dysphagia, and has a highly suggestive appearance on barium swallow. *Intestinal candidiasis* is commonly asymptomatic, but is a major source of hematogenous invasion in the immunosuppressed. *Perianal* candidal overgrowth may follow antibiotic therapy, and produces or aggravates pruritus ani. *Intertrigo* involves the axillae, groins, inframammary folds, and other warm, moist areas. Lesions may be red and oozing or dry and scaly, with sharp scalloped borders and satellite vesicles, pustules, or bullae. *Paronychia* often follows chronic exposure of the hands or feet to moisture. The nails may become hardened, thickened, grooved, and discolored *(onychomycosis). Vulvovaginitis* is characterized by a variable discharge and pruritus. *Balanitis* is manifested by superficial penile erosions and pustules.

Chronic mucocutaneous candidiasis is a rare syndrome based upon limited T cell immunodeficiency. One fifth of patients show a familial tendency. In about half the cases, there is associated endocrinopathy (especially hypoparathyroidism, hypoadrenalism, hypothyroidism, or diabetes mellitus). Clinical features include persistent superficial *Candida* infection of the skin, scalp, nails, and mucous membranes, often in association with a dermatophyte infection. Disease may begin at any age and be extensive or very limited. Associated findings include alopecia, depigmentation, cheilosis, blepharitis, keratoconjunctivitis, and corneal ulcers. In the most severe cases, there is horn formation with thick, plaque-like, hyperkeratotic scales (*Candida* granuloma) involving the skin or nails. Immunologic abnormalities include decreased or absent response to *Candida* antigens by skin test or by tests of cell-mediated immunity in vitro.

Systemic Candidiasis. Most cases of systemic candidiasis are due to *C. albicans* and *C. tropicalis,* with an increasing number attributable to *C. glabrata.* Clinical manifestations of *C. albicans* and *C. tropicalis* infection tend to be apparent in three specific "target organs":

Eyes: A variable proportion of patients has *Candida* endophthalmitis, with single or multiple raised, white, fluffy chorioretinal lesions, in the presence or absence of overlying vitreous haze. Lesions are usually in the macular area within easy range of the ophthalmoscope and extend forward into the vitreous. They serve as a major clue to diagnosis and are a potential cause of blindness.

Kidneys: Renal involvement is attributable to the ability of bloodborne *Candida* to invade the renal tubules directly. Manifestations include diffuse renal abscesses, papillary necrosis, obstruction of the ureters by sloughed papillae or *Candida* balls (bezoars), and progressive renal insufficiency with flank pain and dysuria. *Candida* pyelonephritis must be differentiated from *Candida* cystitis, a benign infection often associated with prolonged catheterization or vaginitis.

Skin: Maculonodular skin lesions on an erythematous base may mark the occurrence of hematogenous *Candida* infection, sometimes with accompanying arthralgias or myalgias. The temptation to disregard these lesions as "pimples" must be overcome, lest a major clue to a lethal disease be overlooked.

Other manifestations of systemic candidiasis may include osteomyelitis (especially vertebral), arthritis, meningitis, and cerebral, myocardial, hepatic, splenic, and thyroid abscesses. Abscesses at the latter sites are seldom appreciated clinically. *Candida* pneumonia is rare. Although hematogenous involvement of the lungs is common, the miliary pulmonary lesions are usually too small to be seen on a chest roentgenogram.

Endocarditis. *C. albicans* endocarditis is most common in a setting of prolonged intravenous therapy, hyperalimentation, or a cardiac valve prosthesis. Non-*albicans* species are most frequent with intravenous narcotics abuse. Fungal valvular lesions are large and friable. Embolization and occlusion of large blood vessels are more common than in bacterial endocarditis; intracerebral lesions are common.

DIAGNOSIS. Superficial infections are diagnosed by examination of scrapings or swabs of infected lesions in the presence of 10 per cent KOH. *Candida* organisms can also be demonstrated by Gram stain. Endocarditis is diagnosed by blood cultures, echocardiographic demonstration of bulky valvular vegetations, or demonstration of fungi in an excised embolus. Systemic candidiasis may be difficult to diagnose. The presence of heavy colonization at usual carriage sites sets the stage for systemic disease, but does not prove that dissemination has occurred. The most reliable evidence of systemic candidiasis is biopsy demonstration of tissue invasion (hematoxylin-eosin or special fungal stains) or recovery of fungi from fluid in a closed body cavity (e.g., CSF, pleural or peritoneal fluid). Blood cultures are most likely to be positive when vented bottles and biphasic media are used. However, positive blood cultures or cultures from the tips of an intravenous line do not necessarily establish the diagnosis of systemic candidiasis, because fungemia may clear spontaneously with the removal of an intravascular focus of infection. Positive urine cultures may indicate cystitis or invasive upper urinary tract disease. The differentiation is not assisted by quantitative urine cultures (even 10^3 *Candida* per milliliter may be associated with pyelonephritis), fluorescent antibody coating studies, or the presence of pseudomycelia in the urine. Declining renal function and evidence of renal destruction (papillary necrosis), urinary tract fungal bezoars, and fungi from catheterized renal pelvis urine suggest that invasive disease is present. Positive sputum cultures usually indicate respiratory tract colonization; pneumonia is relatively rare and must be documented by invasive means. Meningitis is usually manifested by PMN pleocytosis, hypoglycorrhachia, and a positive CSF culture in 40 to 45 per cent of cases.

Skin testing is not helpful in diagnosing candidiasis, because delayed type hypersensitivity to *Candida* antigens is so common among normal persons that the test is used to screen for cutaneous anergy. *Serologic* studies based upon detection of antibodies (precipitins or agglutinins) may be falsely positive or negative, and do not clearly differentiate heavy colonization from systemic infection, although rising titers must be considered compatible with dissemination. Tests for specific cell wall carbohydrates (mannose or arabitol by gas liquid chromatography; mannan by various immunoassays) show great promise in the early diagnosis of invasive disease, and have the advantage of not relying on an immune response by an immunocompromised host.

TREATMENT. Topical preparations (nystatin, amphotericin B, clotrimazole, miconazole, haloprogin, gentian violet) may be used in the treatment of mucocutaneous infections. Chronic mucocutaneous candidiasis syndrome may respond to topical or systemic therapeutic agents (in particular, amphotericin B), but often relapses when medication is discontinued. Ketoconazole is particularly useful in this disease because it can be given indefinitely with relatively few adverse effects. Transfer factor and other immunologically active reagents have been used with variable success.

Systemic candidiasis should be treated with amphotericin B. The removal of precipitating factors (especially intravenous lines) is very important. Because removal of an intravascular focus does not guarantee that fungemia will be self-limited, treatment should be instituted in immunocompromised patients. In acutely ill patients, dosage should be raised quickly to 0.5 to 1.0 mg per kilogram of body weight per day, as tolerated. Alternate-day therapy can be employed and the dosage lowered once clinical improvement is apparent. The usual total dosage recommendation is 1.5 to 2.0 grams, but higher dosage or prolonged therapy may be required in refractory cases. Flucytosine may be added, using the same rationale as that employed for cryptococcosis (see Ch. 370). There are too few clinical data with either miconazole or ketoconazole to judge their value in systemic candidiasis; thus, amphotericin B remains the drug of choice.

Candida cystitis is often cured by Foley catheter removal and the substitution of intermittent ("straight") catheterization. Eradication of infection in those who must have an indwelling catheter, or those with non-catheter-related infection, may be attempted with amphotericin B bladder rinses; with low dose short-course intravenous therapy (amphotericin is excreted in the urine at a therapeutic level for days following intravenous dosing); or even with oral flucytosine, provided no catheter is in place. This is one of the few situations in which flucytosine may be used alone. Ketoconazole is largely metabolized by the liver; therefore, little active ketoconazole reaches the kidneys. There is an approximate 50 per cent failure rate when ketoconazole is used to treat candiduria.

Endocarditis is essentially incurable without valve replacement. Surgical treatment should be accompanied by a six- to ten-week course of amphotericin B and flucytosine, but cure is elusive. Endophthalmitis generally responds to amphotericin B and flucytosine. Local (sub-Tenon) treatment is employed in addition by many ophthalmologists.

PROGNOSIS. Chronic mucocutaneous candidiasis can be ameliorated, but rarely cured. Endocarditis patients often show evidence of disease activity after having been declared cured. Systemic candidiasis is curable, especially in those with intact immune mechanisms. Systemic candidiasis is common but difficult to document in febrile neutropenic patients. Empiric therapy with amphotericin B has led to an improved prognosis for recovery in these patients.

PREVENTION. Systemic candidiasis is avoided by adherence to sound principles of antibiotic use (avoidance of excessive dosage, duration, or breadth of antimicrobial spectrum) and avoidance of indwelling intravascular devices in favor of steel needles. If plastic cannulas are used, they must be changed at least every three days. In immunosuppressed patients, lowering colonization of the gastrointestinal tract with nystatin or ketoconazole is widely practiced, although its efficacy in preventing systemic spread has been questioned. Foley catheters should be avoided whenever possible.

Edwards JE Jr (moderator): Severe candidal infections. Clinical perspective, immune defense mechanisms, and current concepts of therapy. Ann Intern Med 89:91, 1978. *An up-to-date review of systemic candidiasis and chronic mucocutaneous candidiasis in the format of an Interdepartmental Clinical Case Conference from UCLA.*

Edwards JE Jr: Candida endophthalmitis. *In* Remington JS, Swartz MN (eds.): Current Clinical Topics in Infectious Diseases. Vol. 3. New York, McGraw-Hill Book Co., 1982, pp 381–397. *A timely review of this extremely important manifestation of hematogenous* Candida *dissemination.*

Edwards JE Jr, Foos RY, Montgomerie JZ, Guze LB: Ocular manifestations of *Candida* septicemia: Review of seventy-six cases of hematogenous *Candida* endophthalmitis. Medicine 53:47, 1974. *A review of this important complication of* Candida *septicemia.*

Eras P, Goldstein MJ, Sherlock P: *Candida* infection of the gastrointestinal tract.

Medicine 51:367, 1972. *An important paper that describes the types of lesions that occur in this frequent source of* Candida *sepsis.*

Fisher JF, Chew WH, Shadomy S, Duma RJ, Mayhall CG, House WC: Urinary tract infections due to Candida albicans. Rev Infect Dis 4:1107, 1982. *This paper provides valuable guidelines for the differentiation of renal and bladder* Candida *infection and recommends appropriate therapy for each.*

Kirkpatrick CH, Rich RR, Bennett JE: Chronic mucocutaneous candidiasis: Model-building in cellular immunity. Ann Intern Med 74:955, 1972. *A definitive review of this unique disease.*

Meunier-Carpentier F, Kiehn TE, Armstrong D: Fungemia in the immunocompromised host: Changing patterns, antigenemia, high mortality. Am J Med 71:363, 1981. *This paper documents the increasing importance of* C. tropicalis *as an opportunistic pathogen in immunocompromised patients.*

Pizzo P, Robichaud K, Gill F, Witebsky F: Empiric antibiotic and antifungal therapy for cancer patients with prolonged fever and granulocytopenia. Am J Med 72:101, 1982. *Premortem diagnosis of candidiasis in immunocompromised patients is accomplished in fewer than 40 per cent of cases. Hence, empiric antifungal therapy has become important in the management of persistently febrile leukopenic patients. This important paper explores the rationale and approach to therapy.*

373. ASPERGILLOSIS

DEFINITION. Aspergillosis is a poorly descriptive term encompassing a variety of disease processes that share an etiologic relationship with *Aspergillus* species. The dominant element may be any of the following:

1. *Colonization* of previously damaged respiratory tissues (aspergillary bronchitis, aspergilloma).
2. *Allergy* to inhaled spores or to fungi colonizing the bronchial tree (atopic asthma, allergic bronchopulmonary aspergillosis, extrinsic allergic alveolitis).
3. *Invasion* of (a) the lung, especially in immunocompromised hosts, with or without systemic spread, or (b) other loci, e.g. eyes, external ear canals, paranasal sinuses, burn wounds, prosthetic heart valves.
4. *Intoxication and/or neoplasm,* especially with ingestion of aflatoxin.

ETIOLOGY. *Aspergillus* species are ubiquitous and can be isolated from numerous sources (e.g., grains, leaves, grasses, soil, refrigerator walls, wet paint, construction and fireproofing materials). Their spores are frequently isolated from the air and are constantly being inhaled. The rarity of disease attests to the potency of normal host defenses. Although more than 300 *Aspergillus* species are known, only a few thermotolerant species are ordinarily pathogenic for man: *A. fumigatus* (the most common overall), *A. flavus* (especially in upper airway disease and sinusitis), *A. niger* (especially in external otitis), *A. nidulans, A. terreus, A. sydowi, A. clavatus,* and *A. glaucus*. In the tissues, *Aspergillus* hyphae are uniform, 2 to 7 μm in diameter, septate, and dichotomously branched with angles of ~ 45 degrees. These features are not diagnostic. There may be confusion with *Candida* pseudomycelia, *Pseudoallescheria* hyphae, or other fungi. *Aspergillus* species grow rapidly on most media and can be differentiated by their pattern of sporulation. They are rarely found in normal sputum or gastrointestinal contents.

INCIDENCE AND PREVALENCE. Aspergillosis is increasing in prevalence, particularly in patients with chronic respiratory disease or immunosuppression. Among the immunosuppressed, aspergillosis is second only to candidiasis as an opportunistic mycosis, and both are increasing in frequency because of better methods of controlling bacterial infection.

EPIDEMIOLOGY. *Aspergillus* infections occur worldwide, with no regard to age, sex, race, or occupation. Allergic bronchopulmonary aspergillosis is more common in the United Kingdom than in the United States, but is increasing in frequency in this country. Outbreaks of invasive aspergillosis in burned or immunosuppressed patients have followed exposure to spores released by hospital construction, contaminated air conditioning ducts and filters, and fireproofing materials above false ceilings. Filtration of hospital air results in lowered spore counts. Aflatoxin-related hepatotoxicity and malignancies have been documented in African tribes among whom spoiled peanuts are a major dietary component. *Aspergillus* infections are not considered transmissible from animals to man or from man to man.

SPECIFIC SYNDROMES (INCLUDING PATHOGENESIS, PATHOLOGY, CLINICAL MANIFESTATIONS, DIAGNOSIS, TREATMENT, AND PROGNOSIS). ***Colonization.*** *Aspergillary bronchitis* is characterized by the growth of sporulating mycelia on the surface of the bronchial mucosa, without tissue invasion. The mucosa shows only a mild inflammatory response. Bronchial casts containing mucus and mycelia may be expectorated.

Aspergillomas are fungal balls composed of tangled degenerating hyphae and amorphous debris that lie free in pulmonary cavities lined partially by modified bronchial epithelium. There is little surrounding inflammation. The cavities have generally been produced by other disease processes (tuberculosis, sarcoidosis, bronchiectasis, bullae, infarcts, necrotic neoplasms) and are particularly common in the upper lobes. The typical radiographic appearance is that of a freely movable intracavitary mass surrounded on its superior surface by a crescent of air (crescent sign, Monod's sign). This sign is not pathognomonic and may be mimicked by necrotizing tumors or pulmonary infarcts, echinococcal cysts, or other fungal balls. The natural history of aspergillomas is unknown, but some may undergo spontaneous liquefaction and absorption. Invasiveness is extremely rare, but may occur. Hemoptysis is encountered in 60 to 75 per cent of cases and is sometimes life threatening. Sputum cultures are often negative. Diagnosis may be established by bronchoscopy, bronchial brushing, or percutaneous transthoracic needle aspiration. Diagnosis may be assisted by the finding of elevated *Aspergillus* precipitins in the serum. Systemic antifungal therapy has been valueless. Intrabronchial amphotericin B therapy may occasionally be successful. Treatment is probably not indicated except with life-threatening hemoptysis. Under these circumstances, segmental resection or lobectomy is the treatment of choice. Selective bronchial artery embolization has been used in nonsurgical candidates.

Allergy. *Allergic bronchopulmonary aspergillosis* (ABPA) occurs in up to 20 per cent of patients with asthma and is related to the development of tissue hypersensitivity to antigens of *Aspergillus* species (usually *A. fumigatus*) that colonize the bronchial mucous membranes. Its immunopathogenesis includes type I hypersensitivity (IgE-mediated) with bronchospasm and type III (immune complex) and perhaps type IV (cell-mediated) hypersensitivity with permanent bronchial damage. The *Aspergillus* skin test is characterized by an early wheal and flare response (type I) and sometimes by a more delayed (four to six hours) Arthus (type III) reaction. Serum levels of IgE (both *Aspergillus*-specific and nonspecific) are significantly raised, and precipitating antibodies (involved in the type III response) are usually demonstrable in the serum. Clinical features include episodic bronchospasm, peripheral blood eosinophilia, history of transient or fixed pulmonary infiltrates (especially upper lobes), and central saccular bronchiectasis. Additional, less constant features include *Aspergillus* species in smears or cultures of sputum, eosinophils in the sputum, history of expectoration of brown plugs or flecks, and fever. Mucous impactions may result in segmental atelectasis or more generalized lung collapse. Irreversible complications of ABPA include pulmonary fibrosis, lung retraction, and bronchiectasis. In rare instances, aspergillomas may mimic some of the immunologic features of ABPA, and aspergilloma is a rare but recognized complication of the saccular bronchiectasis of ABPA.

Patients with a history of asthma and pulmonary infiltrates should be skin tested with *Aspergillus* antigen. If positive, serum should be obtained for determination of IgE and *Aspergillus* precipitins. The treatment of choice is prednisone in a dose of 0.5 mg per kilogram of body weight per day for two weeks, followed by the same dose on alternate days until the IgE serum level drops to a stable titer. At this point, steroid therapy is gradually withdrawn. The steroids appear to change the bronchial milieu to one unfavorable for colonization by *Aspergillus* species, as well as interfering with pulmonary hypersensitivity reactions. Some patients require no further therapy. Others will have recurrent attacks of ABPA (characteristically preceded by a jump in the IgE titer). These patients may require prednisone indefinitely.

In patients with *atopic asthma*, the inhalation of *Aspergillus* spores results in immediate bronchospasm based upon a type I immune response. There is no spore germination in bronchial passageways.

Extrinsic allergic alveolitis occurs predominantly in nonatopic patients who inhale *Aspergillus* spores, and is characterized by dyspnea, dry cough, malaise, myalgias, rales, diffuse micronodular infiltrates, and serum precipitins to *Aspergillus*. The skin test shows an Arthus response, with or without the preceding wheal and flare reaction. Similar processes include farmer's lung, maple bark stripper's disease, pigeon breeder's disease, and bagassosis.

Invasion. *Chronic necrotizing pulmonary aspergillosis* is an indolent cavitary process, often with mycetoma formation, that occurs predominantly in middle-aged patients with underlying pulmonary parenchymal disease. It is distinct from aspergilloma in that invasion of pulmonary tissue is clearly present. However, it is only semi-invasive when compared with the opportunistic form of infection described later. Patients have fever, productive cough, and pulmonary infiltrates with cavities. Demonstration of lung invasion by *Aspergillus* species and response to amphotericin B support the diagnosis, as does an elevated *Aspergillus* precipitin titer.

Opportunistic pulmonary aspergillosis occurs characteristically in patients with hematologic and lymphoreticular malignancy or organ transplants, generally in the face of intense immunosuppression, and often following the use of various antibacterial drug regimens for septic episodes. The basis whereby immunosuppression sets the stage for invasive pulmonary aspergillosis is unclear, since normal host defenses against this fungus are not fully understood. Apparently macrophages are responsible primarily for the killing of conidia, whereas neutrophils attack mycelia. Full-blown invasive disease occurs in settings in which there is damage to both arms of the immune system. However, even isolated neutrophil defects such as chronic granulomatous disease are characterized by an increased incidence of pulmonary infection and osteomyelitis caused by *Aspergillus* species.

Opportunistic pulmonary aspergillosis is characterized by widespread bronchial erosion and ulceration, followed by invasion of the pulmonary vasculature with thrombosis, embolization, and infarction. Clinical manifestations include a necrotizing patchy bronchopneumonia with or without signs and symptoms of accompanying hemorrhagic pulmonary infarction. The disease process may evolve slowly or rapidly, and abscesses may appear at the site of an apparently resolving pneumonia. In many instances, the abscesses have "crescent signs" and have been referred to as aspergillomas. However, they contain sequestra of infarcted lung tissue and invasive *Aspergillus* infection, and are thus distinct from the benign aspergillomas described earlier. In about 60 per cent of cases, the disease process remains confined to the lungs. In the others, there is hematogenous spread to the brain, liver, kidneys, gastrointestinal tract, thyroid, heart, skin, and other sites. Sometimes the pulmonary process itself is inapparent. In all infected loci, the disease is characterized by vascular invasion and tissue infarction and necrosis. Suppuration predominates; granulomatous response is rare. The differential diagnosis includes mucormycosis, nocardiosis, and necrotizing bacterial pneumonia. Any of these processes may also coexist with aspergillosis.

Invasive aspergillosis is commonly fatal. For patient survival, an aggressive approach to diagnosis and treatment is required. Patients whose therapy begins more than three to four days after the initiation of the infection seldom survive. Even with aggressive culturing, only one tenth to one third of patients have positive sputum cultures for *Aspergillus*. Recovery of *Aspergillus* species from the nasal mucous membrane may signal that deeper respiratory infection is taking place. If other conditions permit, diagnostic maneuvers should include transtracheal aspiration, fiberoptic bronchoscopy with brushing and transbronchial biopsy, percutaneous transthoracic pulmonary aspiration, or open lung biopsy. Fungi can be seen in impression smears and biopsies by Gomori methenamine silver or periodic acid–Schiff stains, but are also visible with hematoxylin-eosin. Identification may be hastened by immunofluorescent staining. Blood, urine, and CSF cultures are rarely positive. Skin tests and precipitin tests are of no value in diagnosis. Experiences with detection of circulating *Aspergillus* antigen by radioimmunoassay techniques provide hope that serologic methods may play a more useful role in diagnosis.

The treatment of choice is amphotericin B. The dosage should be raised rapidly to 0.5 to 1.0 mg per kilogram of body weight per day, as tolerated. Treatment may be given on alternate days once improvement is underway. Optimal total dosage is unsettled, but should probably be no less than 2 grams. Although some patients have received flucytosine or rifampin in combination with amphotericin B, proof of the superiority of such regimens is not available. The efficacy of granulocyte transfusions in leukopenic patients is unproven. Miconazole and ketoconazole are not useful in the management of aspergillosis.

Other loci: Aspergillosis is the most common fungal infection of the paranasal sinuses in otherwise healthy patients. Roentgenograms show opacification, with or without bony erosion. Surgery is usually sufficient for cure. Immunosuppressed patients may exhibit facial cellulitis and palatal necrosis reminiscent of mucormycosis. Aspergillosis is a rare but devastating complication of burn wounds. Antibiotics and local debridement are seldom effective. Amputation is often required for cure. *Aspergillus* infection of prosthetic cardiac valves is a rare but devastating complication of cardiac surgery. Blood cultures are virtually never positive. Antifungal antibiotics are ineffective, and valve replacement is necessary if there is to be any possibility of cure. Invasive cutaneous aspergillosis has occurred at the site of taping of extremities to boards used to stabilize intravenous infusions. Invasive eye disease may follow local trauma, surgery, or hematogenous spread of infection from other sites.

Binder RE, Faling LJ, Pugatch RD, Mahasaen C, Snider GL: Chronic necrotizing pulmonary aspergillosis: A discrete clinical entity. Medicine 61:109, 1982. *This paper calls attention to the fact that a form of limited invasive aspergillosis can occur in patients with underlying pulmonary parenchymal disease but little immunosuppression.*

Rinaldi MG: Invasive aspergillosis. Rev Infect Dis 5:1061, 1983. *A current review of the pathogenesis and pathologic and clinical features of this increasingly common infectious disease.*

Rosenberg M, Patterson R, Mintzer R, Cooper BJ, Roberts M, Harris KE: Clinical and immunologic criteria for the diagnosis of allergic bronchopulmonary aspergillosis. Ann Intern Med 86:405, 1977. *The best reference concerning allergic bronchopulmonary aspergillosis. Authors from the same group define aspects of management of this syndrome in Ann Intern Med 96:286, 1982.*

Weiner MH, Talbot GH, Gerson SL, Filice G, Cassileth PA: Antigen detection in diagnosis of invasive aspergillosis: Utility in controlled, blinded trials. Ann Intern Med 99:777, 1983. *This study indicates that radioimmunoassay for* A. fumigatus *antigen is a highly specific and moderately sensitive serodiagnostic test for invasive pulmonary aspergillosis.*

Young RC, Bennett JE, Vogel CL, Carbonne PP, DeVita VT: Aspergillosis. The spectrum of the disease in 98 patients. Medicine 49:147, 1970. Meyer RD, Young LS, Armstrong D, Yu B: Aspergillosis complicating neoplastic disease. Am J Med 56:6, 1973. *The best two references concerning invasive pulmonary and systemic aspergillosis.*

374. MUCORMYCOSIS (Phycomycosis, Zygomycosis)

DEFINITION. Mucormycosis is an acute suppurative opportunistic mycosis that produces predominantly rhinocerebral disease in patients with diabetic ketoacidosis; rhinocerebral, pulmonary, or disseminated disease in immunosuppressed patients; local or disseminated disease in patients with burns or open wounds; and gastrointestinal disease in patients with malnutrition or pre-existing intestinal disorders.

ETIOLOGY. "Phycomycosis" is an extremely broad term that includes mycoses attributable to fungi in the class Zygomycetes (zygomycosis). "Zygomycosis" includes diseases produced by fungi in the orders Mucorales (mucormycosis) and Entomophthorales (entomophthoromycosis). Entomophthoromycosis is due to infection with *Basidiobolus* and *Conidiobolus* species; occurs as a subcutaneous infection of normal young people, generally in the tropics; and is clinically and histologically distinct from mucormycosis. Mucorales known to produce mucormycosis include *Rhizopus, Mucor, Absidia, Mortierella, Cunninghamella, and Saksenaea* species. In the tissues, all these fungi appear as broad (6 to 50 μm), wavy, nonseptate (coenocytic), thick-walled hyphae with right-angle branching at haphazard intervals. They can be distinguished from one another only in vitro.

INCIDENCE AND PREVALENCE. Mucorales occur worldwide in soil and on decaying organic debris, and are economically important as food spoilage agents. Airborne spores may contaminate bacteriologic media. Colonization and infection are uncommon in normal persons. Mucormycosis is increasing in incidence because of expanding numbers of susceptible, immunosuppressed patients.

EPIDEMIOLOGY. Mucormycosis is acquired sporadically, by inhalation, by ingestion, or by contamination of wounds with spores. It is not communicable. Infection is unrelated to age, sex, race, or climate. Diabetics usually acquire their infections in the community; immunosuppressed patients, within the hospital. A recent outbreak of *Rhizopus* wound infections was related to the use of elasticized adhesive tape (Elastoplast, a nonsterile product), in direct contiguity with open wounds. The tape was found to be contaminated with spores of *R. oryzae* and *R. rhizopodoformis.* Mucormycosis of burn wounds may follow the use of topical mafenide, which suppresses other etiologic agents of burn wound infection.

PATHOGENESIS AND PATHOLOGY. Mechanisms of immunity are poorly understood. Evidence from various experimental models suggests roles for serum factors, polymorphonuclear leukocytes, and cell-mediated immunity, but in no consistent pattern. Acidosis appears more important than hyperglycemia in the susceptibility of experimental animals to rhinocerebral disease. This may relate to the acidic growth optima of the causative fungi, and the delay in polymorphonuclear leukocyte chemotaxis engendered by diabetic ketoacidosis.

The pathologic process in humans is characterized by suppuration with little granulomatous response. Invasion of blood vessels is characteristic, resulting in thrombosis, infarction, and embolization. Disease spreads by both direct and hematogenous extension, but the fungi are almost never recovered from the blood. Agents of mucormycosis stain readily with hematoxylin-eosin (eosinophilic hyphae). The Gomori methenamine silver stain is also useful, but results with the periodic acid–Schiff and Gridley stains are poor. Hyphae are generally surrounded by an acute inflammatory cell infiltrate, but sections with marked hyphal invasion sometimes show little or no cellular response.

CLINICAL MANIFESTATIONS. *Rhinocerebral mucormycosis* accounts for about half of all cases of mucormycosis. More than 75 per cent of cases of rhinocerebral mucormycosis occur in patients with acidosis, especially diabetic ketoacidosis. However, increasing numbers of cases are being seen in neutropenic patients with hematologic malignancies. It is one of the most rapidly fatal fungus diseases of man, death occurring within two to ten days of onset in untreated patients. Infection is presumably initiated by the germination of spores deposited on the nasopharyngeal mucous membranes. Early clinical manifestations include nasal stuffiness, blood-tinged nasal discharge, facial swelling, and facial or orbital pain. Examination of the nasal mucosa reveals dirty red or black necrotic turbinates—an appearance commonly mistaken for dried blood, and a major clue to the diagnosis. Facial cellulitis, palatal or nasal septal perforation, and signs of sinusitis may be present. Radiographs of the sinuses reveal nodular thickening of the mucous membranes, spotty destruction of the bony walls, and the absence of air-fluid levels. Spread of infection to the orbit results in orbital cellulitis, proptosis, and failing vision. Ultimately, there is a full-blown orbital apex syndrome reflecting the destruction of cranial nerves (III, IV, VI, and the ophthalmic branch of V) and blood vessels traversing the optic foramen and superior orbital fissure. Manifestations include complete ophthalmoplegia; a fixed, dilated pupil; corneal and upper facial anesthesia; chemosis and conjunctival hemorrhage; and blindness resulting from obstruction of the central artery of the retina. The disease commonly spreads to involve the internal carotid artery, and sometimes the cavernous sinus, cribriform plate, meninges, brain, and bones of the skull. Cerebral infarction caused by vascular compromise is common. The cerebrospinal fluid may disclose pleocytosis (≥50 per cent polymorphonuclear leukocytes) and elevated protein concentration, but hypoglycorrhachia is rare, and fungi are virtually never seen or cultured.

Pulmonary mucormycosis is nearly as common as rhinocerebral disease, and typically occurs as a complication of hematologic malignancy and cytotoxic or immunosuppressive therapy. Infection presumably follows inhalation of fungal spores. There are no characteristic clinical or roentgenographic findings, but the pattern of infarction and cavitation may resemble that of invasive pulmonary aspergillosis. Sputum cultures are rarely positive, and successful diagnosis usually requires invasive techniques such as open lung biopsy.

Gastrointestinal mucormycosis may result from the ingestion of fungal spores in patients with pre-existing gastrointestinal abnormalities or malnutrition. It is seldom suspected prior to laparotomy or autopsy.

Cutaneous mucormycosis: Local cutaneous infection may follow deep burns, application of contaminated wound dressings, or injections at contaminated skin sites.

Disseminated mucormycosis may follow pulmonary or burn wound infection. Cerebral involvement is common, but no organ is spared.

DIAGNOSIS. Rhinocerebral mucormycosis may be confused with midline granuloma, rhinoscleroma, thyroid disease, syphilis, tuberculosis, or nasal and orbital tumors. Pulmonary mucormycosis may be confused with a variety of opportunistic pulmonary infections in the immunosuppressed host, or with bland pulmonary embolization and infarction. The diagnosis of all forms of mucormycosis depends upon the *direct demonstration* of the characteristic hyphae in the tissues. Diagnosis is urgent and may be achieved by crushing fresh biopsy material between two slides, clearing with 10 to 20 per cent KOH, and examining for hyphae. Smears and swabs of sputum or wound exudate rarely disclose the fungus. Cultures are positive in less than 20 per cent of cases, and even positive cultures from superficial tissues might reflect the presence of fungal contaminants. No skin test is available, and there are no reliable serologic tests. Neither a negative tissue examination nor a negative culture rules out mucormycosis in the presence of a suggestive clinical picture, and collection of additional tissue specimens is indicated along with appropriate, aggressive therapy.

TREATMENT. Amphotericin B is the only drug with proven efficacy, and results of therapy do not necessarily correlate with results of tests of susceptibility to the drug in vitro. Successful therapy requires early diagnosis, control of the underlying disease process, aggressive debridement, and aggressive use of amphotericin B. Control of burn infection may necessitate amputation. The dose of amphotericin B should be rapidly increased to 0.5 to 1.0 mg per kilogram per day, in accordance with the patient's ability to tolerate the drug. Consideration should be given to local administration of drug into infected paranasal sinuses. With clinical improvement, amphotericin B can be given in an alternate-day regimen. A total dose of 2 to 4 grams is commonly suggested.

PROGNOSIS. The prognosis of mucormycosis is directly related to the rapidity of diagnosis and the aggressiveness of therapy. Prior to the advent of amphotericin B, rhinocerebral disease was fatal in 80 to 90 per cent of instances. Current data indicate that 75 per cent of patients with no systemic disease, 60 per cent of diabetics, and 20 per cent of patients with other underlying disorders survive rhinocerebral disease. Prognosis is poor in patients with hemiplegia, facial necrosis, or nasal deformity. Only about 15 patients have been reported to have recovered from pulmonary infection.

Blitzer A, Lawson W, Meyers BR, Biller HF: Patient survival factors in paranasal sinus mucormycosis. Laryngoscope 90:635, 1980. *An analysis of 179 cases of rhinocerebral infection with emphasis on significant prognostic factors.*

Lehrer RI (moderator): UCLA Conference Mucormycosis (part I). Ann Intern Med 93:93, 1980. *A thorough and up-to-date review of clinical, mycologic, and immunologic aspects of mucormycosis. The best reference on the subject.*

Meyer RD, Rosen P, Armstrong P: Phycomycosis complicating leukemia and lymphoma. Ann Intern Med 77:781, 1972. *The best reference available for pulmonary mucormycosis.*

375. MYCETOMA (Maduromycosis)

DEFINITION. A mycetoma is a localized lesion, usually of an exposed area such as the unshod foot (Madura foot), characterized by swelling and deep sinuses that discharge pus and grains (microbial colonies embedded in a host-derived proteinaceous matrix).

ETIOLOGY. Half of all mycetomas are produced by fungi (eumycetoma); the other half by actinomycetes (actinomycetoma). They resemble a syndrome produced by certain bacteria (botryomycosis). The etiologic agents originate in plant debris and soil, and are introduced by trauma. Etiologic agents of eumycetoma include (1) white to yellow grains—*Petriellidium (Pseudoallescheria) boydii* and *Acremonium (Cephalosporium), Trichophyton,* and *Microsporum* species; (2) yellow to brown grains—*Neotestudina (Zophia) rosatii;* and (3) black grains—*Madurella mycetomi* and *grisea (Pyrenochaeta romeroi), Phialophora (Exophiala) jeanselmei,* and *Leptosphaeria senegalensis* and *thompkinsii.* Etiologic agents of actinomycetoma include (1) white to yellow grains—*Nocardia asteroides, brasiliensis,* and *cavae* (tiny grains) and *Actinomadura madurae* (extremely large grains); (2) yellow to brown grains—*Streptomyces somaliensis;* (3) red grains—*Actinomadura pelletierii;* and (4) black grains—*Streptomyces paraguayensis.*

EPIDEMIOLOGY. Mycetomas are encountered worldwide, but especially in semitropical zones such as Sudan and Mexico. *P. boydii* is the most common cause of mycetoma in Europe and the United States, *N. brasiliensis* in Mexico.

The mycetomas occur most frequently in adult males from rural areas who work out of doors, experience repeated trauma, and care poorly for local wounds. The disease is not contagious, occurs in sporadic fashion, and is unrelated to animal contact. Mycetomas usually involve the feet or legs, but may involve the back, neck, or shoulders (in bearers of burdens), or the head (where *Trichophyton* and *Microsporum* eumycetomas are especially likely to occur).

PATHOGENESIS AND PATHOLOGY. The host-parasite interactions that foster the development of grains instead of free filaments by the weakly pathogenic organisms responsible for mycetomas are unknown.

Typical mycetomas consist of large granulomatous areas with a purulent center surrounded by a thick, fibrous capsule. Fistulous tracts that contain grains pass deep into underlying tissues, usually along fascial planes, and also drain at the skin surface. Focal areas of subcutaneous necrosis and intense fibrosis result in typical tumefaction. Tracts open and close over long periods of time. In actinomycetomas, the suppurative response tends to persist indefinitely, and there is a tendency to invade bones and muscles. Eumycetomas take on the character of foreign body granulomas.

CLINICAL MANIFESTATIONS. Mycetomas usually begin as a painless draining nodule at a site of trauma. Multiple secondary nodules develop over years and drain through sinus tracts. Lesions extend deeply into subcutaneous tissues, under the cover of thick fibrosclerous tissue. A common complaint is a sensation of deep itching. Disease may spread to bone (including medullary canal and epiphyses), joints, muscles, tendons,

and nerves. When extensive bony remodeling occurs, the process becomes painful. Blood and lymphatic vessels are damaged or interrupted, but regional lymphadenopathy is rare. In the typical "Madura foot," the destruction of tarsal bones, nonimpairment of the tendons, and widespread plantar fibrosis give the foot a characteristic shortened and raised appearance. The sole is typically convex. The general health of the patient remains little affected. Rapid local or lymphohematogenous spread may occur when mycetomas involve the buttocks, chest, or trunk.

DIAGNOSIS. Mycetomas can be diagnosed by the presence of characteristic sinuses and grains. Collection of grains may be facilitated by gentle abrasion of lesions or overnight occlusion with saline-saturated gauze. Grains should be crushed, and wet mounts prepared in 10 to 20 per cent KOH. Examination of grains permits the broad differentiation of actinomycetoma (fine filaments), eumycetoma (broad hyphae), and botryomycosis (cocci or rods without filaments). Culture is necessary for etiologic diagnosis. Serologic tests are not routinely available.

TREATMENT. Treatment for actinomycetomas depends upon identification of the infecting agent and determination of its in vitro antibiotic susceptibility. Therapeutic responses have followed high dose penicillin regimens (e.g., 10 million units per day), with or without probenecid, 1 gram per day; sulfadiazine, 3 to 10 grams per day; or minocycline, 150 mg twice daily. *Nocardia brasiliensis* infections are especially likely to respond, perhaps because the smaller grains pose a less formidable barrier to drug penetration. Other useful drugs include diaminodiphenylsulfone (dapsone), 50 to 200 mg daily by mouth; co-trimoxazole (160 mg trimethoprim plus 800 mg sulfamethoxazole daily, by mouth); or streptomycin (3 grams intramuscularly per day for three weeks, then 2 grams daily for three weeks, then 1 gram daily). Prolonged streptomycin regimens carry the danger of vestibulotoxicity. Limb perfusion therapy and topical antimicrobial agents have also been used, together with judicious resectional surgery. Eumycetoma is considerably more difficult to treat. Amphotericin B given intravenously or locally has produced equivocal results. *P. boydii* may respond to miconazole, ketoconazole, or even thiabendazole. Unfortunately, eumycetoma often requires amputation.

PROGNOSIS. The mycetomas are often brought to medical attention late in the course of illness. Reasons include the absence of pain, the remote living conditions of patients, and the fear of amputation. In general, the prognosis for life is good, but the disease may be incapacitating.

Mariat F, Destombes P, Segretain G: The mycetomas: Clinical features, pathology, etiology and epidemiology. *In* Contributions to Microbiology, Vol 4, Host-Parasite Relationships in Systemic Mycoses; Part II, Specific Diseases and Therapy. Basel, Karger, 1977, pp 1-39. *A masterful, easily readable, and up-to-date review article with an emphasis on pathophysiology.*

Smego RA Jr, Gallis HA: The clinical spectrum of *Nocardia brasiliensis* infection in the United States. Rev Infect Dis 6:164, 1984. Nocardia brasiliensis *is a common cause of mycetoma throughout the world. It can also produce a variety of other skin, soft tissue, and systemic manifestations. This is an important review of the pathogenesis, diagnosis, and therapy of the gamut of* N. brasiliensis *infections.*

Tight RR, Bartlett MS: Actinomycetoma in the United States. Rev Infect Dis 3:1139, 1981. *A case report and review of 28 cases of actinomycetoma in the United States that emphasizes the importance of etiologic diagnosis, antibiotic susceptibility testing in vitro, identification of osteomyelitis, and protracted therapy in disease management.*

376. CHROMOMYCOSIS

Chromomycosis (dermatomycosis) is a general term for mycotic infections produced by dematiacious (brown-pigmented) fungi. There are three clinical forms: cutaneous, cystic, and cerebral.

CUTANEOUS CHROMOMYCOSIS

DEFINITION. Cutaneous chromomycosis (chromoblastomycosis, verrucous dermatitis), the classic form of chromomycosis, is a noncontagious chronic granulomatous infection, usually of exposed areas such as the extremities, and characterized by warty plaques, nodules, and cauliflower-like excrescences.

ETIOLOGY. Chromomycosis is produced by a variety of brown-pigmented saprophytic soil fungi that are genetically related, morphologically identical, and distinguishable only in vitro. They include principally members of the genera *Phialophora (Exophiala), Fonsecaea,* and *Cladosporium. Fonsecaea pedrosoi* is the most common etiologic agent.

INCIDENCE AND PREVALENCE. Cutaneous chromomycosis occurs worldwide, but is most common in tropical and subtropical areas, especially Brazil and Costa Rica. The first case report was from New England in 1915, and numerous cases have been documented in Texas and Louisiana.

EPIDEMIOLOGY. The etiologic agents reside in soil, decaying wood, or rotting vegetation. They are usually introduced by trauma, especially in barefoot persons. Cutaneous chromomycosis is most common in adult males who work out of doors, especially those with suboptimal nutritional or hygienic status.

PATHOGENESIS AND PATHOLOGY. There is pseudoepitheliomatous hyperplasia of the surface epithelium, and microabscesses with epithelioid and giant cell granulomas in the underlying dermis. Eventually, a chronic fibrosing inflammatory reaction supervenes. The characteristic tissue fungi develop as large, thick-walled, dark-colored rounded cells (4 to 12 μm in diameter), the so-called "sclerotic bodies." They multiply by septation and not by budding, and frequently remain attached to one another in clusters of two or more.

CLINICAL MANIFESTATIONS. Cutaneous chromomycosis starts as a small pink scaly papule, and slowly enlarges to a warty tumor that may spread to form a plaque. Mucous membranes are not often involved. Plaques may be verrucous with central scarring, extensively scarred with a serpiginous border, scaly, or indurated with fistulas. Some patients develop a papillomatous tumor reminiscent of a cauliflower. Ulceration may follow trauma or secondary infection, and local spread may occur by direct or lymphatic extension, or by autoinoculation through scratching. Regional lymphadenopathy is not common. It may take ten to fifteen years for a whole limb to be involved. Lymphedema and elephantiasis may result. Rarely the disease may be complicated by an epithelioid carcinoma. In some patients, widespread hematogenous dissemination occurs. Lesions have been documented in the pancreas, liver, bowel, lymph nodes, brain, and meninges. The organs may contain sclerotic bodies and/or hyphae.

DIAGNOSIS. Early lesions may be confused with malignancy, mycetoma, other mycoses, cutaneous tuberculosis, leishmaniasis, yaws, and "mossy foot" (lymphostatis verrucosis). Laboratory diagnosis is relatively easy. Although superficial crusts digested in 10 to 20 percent KOH may contain long brown branching hyphae, the diagnostic sclerotic bodies are more likely to be found intracellularly or extracellularly in pus, in granulation tissue obtained by curettage, or in biopsy specimens. The brown pigmentation of the fungi serves to identify them; special stains are seldom needed. Cultures may grow slowly and should be kept at least eight weeks. Serologic or skin tests are not available.

TREATMENT. Treatment is successful in inverse relation to the duration and extent of infection. Except when the lesions are small and early, surgery is nearly always followed by recurrence. Systemic amphotericin B may not produce fungistatic concentrations at the lesions. Intralesional amphotericin B has been tried with variable success, but is painful. Flucytosine* (150 mg per kilogram of body weight per day by mouth) cured 16 of 23 patients in a recent series. The other seven developed flucytosine-resistant fungi. Amphotericin B given simultaneously with flucytosine might retard emergence of flucytosine-resistant fungi. Thiabendazole (2 grams per day, orally), an anthelmintic, has given promising results, but is not approved for this use in the United States. Unpublished results suggest that ketoconazole, an orally administered imidazole, may be efficacious.

Response to therapy may be monitored by serial biopsies and cultures.

PROGNOSIS. Cutaneous chromomycosis usually remains localized and will not debilitate the patient if left untreated. Secondary infection resulting in lymphostasis and elephantiasis is disabling. There is a slight risk of hematogenous dissemination, probably increased by immunosuppression.

CYSTIC CHROMOMYCOSIS

Cystic chromomycosis (phaeosporotrichosis, phaeomycotic cyst, phaeohyphomycosis, hypodermomycosis) is characterized by the formation of a granulomatous cyst-like lesion, usually deep in subcutaneous or muscle tissue. The lesion, which is usually encapsulated, becomes necrotic and may ulcerate. The principal etiologic agent is *Exophiala jeanselmei.* Pigmented hyphae are present in exudate and in the abscess wall; sclerotic bodies are not seen. However, "yeast-like" cells of odd shapes and sizes have been reported.

Cystic chromomycosis must be differentiated from sebaceous cysts, tendon sheath granulomas, foreign body granulomas, or gummas. Hematogenous spread is rare. Treatment consists of surgical excision.

CEREBRAL CHROMOMYCOSIS

Cerebral chromomycosis (cerebral dermatomycosis, cladosporiosis, encephalomycosis) is a general term for any cerebral mycosis caused by a dematiacious fungus. The most important form, caused by *Cladosporium trichoides,* is characterized by the formation of abscesses containing pus, giant cells, and pigmented hyphae. Sclerotic bodies are not seen. Blood vessel invasion by hyphae occurs (reminiscent of aspergillosis or phycomycosis). Meningitis is present in about half the cases, sometimes as an isolated occurrence. The cerebrospinal fluid usually shows a polymorphonuclear leukocyte response; hypoglycorrhachia has not been reported. The site of primary infection may be the lung, but there is seldom evidence of pulmonary involvement. Cerebral chromomycosis is rarely diagnosed early enough to permit the evaluation of therapeutic regimens. Optimal management would seem to require surgical debridement and the use of flucytosine* or an imidazole, with or without amphotericin B.

---

*Investigational drug for this purpose.

Bennett JE, Bonner H, Jennings AE, Lopez RI: Chronic meningitis caused by *Cladosporium trichoides.* Am J Clin Pathol 59:398, 1973. *Comprehensive discussion of cerebral infection with dematiaceous fungi.*

Carrion AL: Chromoblastomycosis and related infections: New concepts, differential diagnosis, and nomenclatorial implications. Int J Dermatol 14:27, 1975.

Vollum DI: Chromomycosis: A review. Br J Dermatol 96:454, 1977. *Two brief, excellent reviews of the spectrum of disease produced by dematiaceous fungi.*

Part XX
DISEASES CAUSED BY PROTOZOA AND METAZOA

377. INTRODUCTION TO PROTOZOAN AND HELMINTHIC DISEASES

Adel A. F. Mahmoud

Human infections with parasitic protozoa and helminths account for a major proportion of the diseases caused by infectious agents. In spite of some worldwide efforts to control the spread and consequences of these infections, the associated morbidity and mortality have not been appreciably reduced. Furthermore, in the developed countries infection with protozoa and helminths is being seen with increasing frequency in immigrants and is also among the more important causes of disease in the growing number of patients with depressed immune responses.

The biology of the interaction between protozoa and helminths and their host is less well understood than that of other infectious agents. Most of these infections are prevalent in the developing countries in which limited attention has been paid to studies on pathogenesis, chemotherapy, or control. There are no reliable data on prevalence and morbidity caused by human protozoan and helminthic infections. Nevertheless, their magnitude is staggering; malaria infects 600 million, and ascariasis and trichuriasis one billion each, and 600 million are estimated to be infected with either schistosomiasis or filariases. Other infectious protozoa and helminths such as *Toxoplasma gondii, Entamoeba histolytica, Giardia lamblia, Pneumocystis carinii,* and *Strongyloides stercoralis* occur worldwide. Although the major burden of disease due to protozoan and helminthic infections falls on the developing world, some of these infections are becoming clinically recognized pathogens in the more developed countries. An additional dimension of the problem of protozoan and helminthic infections concerns the lack of effective chemotherapeutic agents in some instances and the excessive toxicity of these agents or the development of resistance to them in other instances.

BIOLOGY OF PARASITIC PROTOZOA AND HELMINTHS

This group of infectious agents belongs to the animal kingdom, unlike bacteria, viruses, or fungi. Such distinction led to restricting the term "parasite" to include only protozoa and helminths, and may have hampered our clinical as well as basic understanding of the mechanisms by which they cause disease and how to enhance host resistance effectively. The host-parasite relationship in protozoan and helminthic infections is complex because of the distinctive biological features of the organisms. Although protozoa are unicellular pathogens and are mainly microscopic in size, they are far larger than viruses and bacteria. A major biological feature of protozoa is their ability to multiply within mammalian hosts as do viruses, bacteria, and fungi. Protozoan infection, therefore, can be initiated by a relatively small inoculum of organisms, which then multiply within the host and reach the numbers that cause disease. A single infected mosquito bite, for example, can deliver enough malaria sporozoites to establish infection in the liver, where the organisms multiply and cause clinical disease upon invasion of red cells.

In contrast, helminths are multicellular organisms with well developed organ system structures. They vary in size from 1 cm to approximately 10 meters. Unlike other infectious agents, helminths do not multiply within mammalian hosts. Re-exposure is, therefore, necessary to increase the number of helminths in a host. This distinguishing feature has important clinical significance, as disease in most helminthiasis is closely related to intensity of infection. For example, anemia results from hookworm infection only if the individual is harboring a significant worm load or there are other reasons for nutritional deficiencies. In rare circumstances such as strongyloidiasis in the immunosuppressed, the worm can increase its population through an autoinfection cycle. This leads to life-threatening infection that necessitates aggressive medical attention.

Parasitic protozoa and helminths have developed elaborate mechanisms for evasion of host protective responses. One of the best studied is antigenic variation noted in African trypanosomiasis. Parasitemia in infected individuals declines with the development of a protective antibody response but is followed by the emergence of a new parasite variable antigen and an increase in their numbers. These organisms are capable of expressing at least 100 different variable antigens allowing a long chronic course of infection. The phenomenon of antigenic variation in trypanosomiasis is expressed through a surface glycoprotein of a molecular weight 65,000. The trypanosomes contain individual genes for all the different variable glycoproteins but only one is expressed at a time. The multiplicity of trypanosome variable glycoprotein genes and mechanisms for introducing mutations into them illustrate the degree of complexity and sophistication of these human pathogens.

The constantly changing nature of infectious disease is best illustrated in some parasitic protozoan and helminthic infections. For example, relatively unsuspected pathogens such as *Giardia lamblia* are now being recognized as the major identifiable cause of water-borne diarrhea in North America and several parts of the world. New human pathogens such as *Isospora* and *Cryptosporidium* species have been appreciated only recently as causes of diarrheal illness, particularly in the immunosuppressed. This group of patients, including those with acquired immune deficiency syndrome (AIDS), is particularly susceptible to several opportunistic Protozoan infections such as *Pneumocystitis carinii, Toxoplasma gondii,* and the coccidia. These new developments add to the difficulties experienced in the treatment and control of parasitic protozoa and helminths. For several, effective and safe chemotherapeutic agents are lacking (e.g., onchocerciasis and South American trypanosomiasis). In some circumstances the pathogen (e.g., *Plasmodium falciparum)* is rapidly developing resistance to the available drugs; insecticide resistance is also complicating vector control attempts. On the other hand, malaria vaccine may be a reality soon and new chemotherapeutic agents for onchocerciasis are to be introduced in the near future.

APPROACH TO THE PATIENT WITH PROTOZOAN OR HELMINTHIC INFECTION

Since most of the clinical manifestations of protozoan and helminthic diseases are not specific or pathognomonic, a high degree of suspicion is essential. The simple question "Where have you been?" and knowledge of the general geographic distribution of parasitic protozoa and helminth will often save exhaustive and costly diagnostic workups and may spare human lives.

The next phase in attempting to reach correct diagnosis

involves interpretation of the presenting symptoms and signs. Definitive diagnosis in most cases requires isolation and identification of the specific pathogen. Since the number of cases seen by any single laboratory in North America is limited, certain expertise is required for correct identification that may not be available to many practicing physicians. Consultations with the Centers for Disease Control are, therefore, helpful.

Schmidt GD, Roberts LS, eds.: Foundations of Parasitology, 2nd edition. C. V. Mosby Company, St. Louis, 1981. *A concise text for basic information on morphology and biology of protozoa and helminths.*

Warren KS, Mahmoud AAF, eds.: Tropical and Geographical Medicine. McGraw-Hill Book Company, New York, 1984. *Detailed description of the biology and molecular understanding of protozoa and helminths and the diseases they cause in individuals and in populations.*

Section One PROTOZOAN DISEASES

378. MALARIA

Louis H. Miller

DEFINITION. Malaria remains today one of the major health problems in the tropics. It is caused by four species of *Plasmodium, P. falciparum, P. vivax, P. ovale* and *P. malariae,* each of which produces disease with its own morphology and clinical characteristic (Table 378–1). The asexual erythrocytic parasite is the stage in the life cycle that causes disease, including the characteristic malarial paroxysm (fever, chills, and sweats). *P. falciparum* malaria causes the most morbidity and mortality and presents the therapeutic problem of chloroquine resistance. Since effective therapy is available for *P. falciparum* malaria, high mortality usually results from failure of the physician to include malaria in the differential diagnosis of a febrile patient who has traveled in the tropics or received a blood transfusion.

ETIOLOGY. Malaria parasites undergo a developmental cycle in female anopheline mosquitoes, the vector, and in humans. Mosquitoes, during a blood meal, inoculate *sporozoites* that rapidly enter liver parenchymal cells. The sporozoite surface is covered by a membrane protein with a multiply repeated epitope. Sporozoites may develop immediately in liver cells into thousands of individual merozoites (all types of malaria) or remain dormant as uninucleate hypnozoites for months to years before undergoing proliferation (the relapsing malarias, caused by *P. vivax* and *P. ovale*). Different strains of *P. vivax* produce their own characteristic timing patterns of relapse in patients who contract the disease. Some strains (e.g., from New Guinea) cause relapse monthly after the primary attack. Others cause relapse six months or longer after the primary attack or may not produce a primary attack.

Merozoites rupture from liver cells and pour into the bloodstream to invade erythrocytes. Development of the intraerythrocytic parasite follows one of the two pathways: asexual proliferation or differentiation into sexual parasites, the gametocytes, which await ingestion by the mosquito. In the mosquito they ultimately develop into infectious *sporozoites.* Asexual erythrocytic parasites develop from young ring forms through *trophozoites* to the dividing form, the *schizont.* Each mature schizont contains 6 to 24 merozoites, the number varying with the particular species. Merozoites, on rupture of infected erythrocytes, are released to invade other erythrocytes and thus continue the cycle.

Merozoites attach to erythrocytes by specific receptors. Erythrocytic determinants required for *P. vivax* and *P. falciparum* invasion are the Duffy blood group system and glycophorin, respectively. Blacks who are Duffy blood group negative *(FyFy)* are completely refractory to erythrocytic infection by *P. vivax.* En(a-) erythrocytes that completely lack glycophorin A have reduced susceptibility to invasion by *P. falciparum.*

The agents producing the three types of malaria, *P. vivax, P. ovale,* and *P. falciparum,* invade reticulocytes preferentially. *P. falciparum,* however, can infect erythrocytes of all ages and produces high parasitemias with resultant morbidity and mortality. *P. malariae* infects mature erythrocytes.

Each type of malaria induces characteristic morphologic changes on the infected erythrocyte membrane: knobs by asexual parasites of *P. falciparum;* knobs by sexual and asexual parasites of *P. malariae;* and *Schuffner's dots,* pink stippling of the infected erythrocyte, by sexual and asexual parasites of *P. vivax* and *P. ovale.* A histidine-rich parasite protein forms the knobs on the membrane of *P. falciparum*–infected erythrocytes, which mediate attachment to venular endothelium (sequestration) and may be a factor in obstruction of cerebral vessels leading to cerebral malaria. This sequestration explains the predominance of young parasites, ring forms, in the peripheral blood.

The asexual erythrocytic parasite has a haploid genome. Cloned populations of asexual parasites can change their expression of antigens on the erythrocyte surface (antigenic variation) in order to evade the host immune response.

EPIDEMIOLOGY. Most malaria patients seen in Europe and in the United States are infected in Africa, Asia, and Latin America (imported cases). Mosquito vectors capable of transmitting malaria still exist in countries where malaria has been eradicated (e.g., *Anopheles freeborni* in the Western United States). In these areas, rare episodes of transmission have occurred following infection of local mosquitoes by individuals infected in the tropics (introduced cases). Congenital infections occur; the clinical symptoms are not evident until weeks to months after delivery. Other causes of infection in nonendemic areas include blood transfusion and communal use of syringes by drug addicts. The single most important factor in preventing transfusion malaria is the exclusion of donors who have lived or traveled in endemic areas until their risk of infection is negligible, because chronic infections are often asymptomatic. Most

TABLE 378–1. CLINICAL AND DIAGNOSTIC DIFFERENCES AMONG THE FOUR SPECIES OF MALARIA

	P. falciparum	*P. vivax*	*P. ovale*	*P. malariae*
Clinical features	High parasitemia, severe anemia, renal failure, cerebral malaria, pulmonary edema, death	Splenic rupture, anemia		RBC infection persists for years; nephritis
Chloroquine resistance	Yes	No	No	No
Asexual cycle	48 hours	48 hours	48 hours	72 hours
Relapse	No	Yes	Yes	No
Characteristic on thin blood film	Rings predominate; multiply infected RBCs, rings with thread-like cytoplasm, double nuclei, banana-shaped gametocytes	Enlarged RBC with Schuffner's dots; trophozoite cytoplasm amoeboid; 12 to 24 merozoites in mature schizont	Oval RBC with fringed edges; Schuffner's dots; trophozoite cytoplasm compact; 6 to 16 merozoites in mature schizont	Trophozoite cytoplasm compact (band forms); 6 to 12 merozoites in mature schizont; RBC unchanged

P. falciparum–infected individuals undergo self-cure in three years; a rare case may persist for four years. Disease caused by *P. vivax* and *P. ovale* may last for three to five years. That from *P. malariae* may persist as an asymptomatic, erythrocytic infection for decades. Since infection by *P. falciparum* and *P. vivax* is most serious, blood donation should be excluded for four years after the traveler's return from the tropics.

The endemicity of malaria in the tropics is determined by vector capacity, host factors such as immunity, political stability and the commitment to malaria control, and the character of the parasite. The central concept in understanding malarial transmission in any part of the world is *vector capacity,* which is defined as the expected number of new infections produced per infective case per day. Vector capacity is determined by the interaction of the vector mosquito and its biology with the environment and the parasite.

INNATE RESISTANCE. Genetically determined host factors influence susceptibility to malaria. Certain polymorphisms have been associated with the distribution of *P. falciparum* in the world (e.g., hemoglobin S, thalassemia, and glucose-6-phosphate dehydrogenase [G-6-PD] deficiency). The evidence for a selective advantage of polymorphisms in malarious areas is most convincing for sickle trait (HB SA). Children who die of malaria in West Africa rarely have sickle trait, although the frequency of this phenotype is high in this region. In areas where the heterozygote has an advantage over either homozygote, a balanced polymorphism results. The mechanism of protection at the cellular level appears to be inhibition of growth in HB SA erythrocytes because *P. falciparum*–infected erythrocytes sequester along venules where O_2 tension is low.

Black Africans who have the Duffy blood group–negative genotype *(FyFy)* are resistant to infection by *P. vivax.* Elliptocytosis, a skeletal abnormality of erythrocytes, occurs throughout lowland tropical areas of Southeast Asia and Melanesia that are endemic for malaria; the erythrocytes are partially resistant to invasion by all types of malaria.

IMMUNITY. Immunity to malaria is primarily directed against the asexual erythrocytic parasite. Immunity to sporozoites occurs in adult populations of Africa but probably is of little importance in host survival. Immunity to the asexual erythrocytic parasite develops only after prolonged or repeated infection. Immunity usually does not prevent reinfection but reduces the severity of the disease or leads to an asymptomatic infection. The asymptomatic person, however, can infect mosquitoes and can transmit the infection directly to others through blood transfusion. Immunity wanes in a few years when the person is unexposed to reinfection. Recurrence of disease may occur in an immune person immediately after surgery or during pregnancy.

Immunity is species-specific (e.g., immunity to *P. falciparum* does not protect against *P. vivax*). Further, the immunity against *P. falciparum* is strain-specific, indicating variant antigens among strains. Passive transfer of antibody from hyperimmune adult West Africans to East or West African children reduced parasitemia.

The spleen is of primary importance in host survival against malaria. One mechanism may involve antibody and cells within the spleen. Alternatively, parasites may be killed by natural killer (NK) cells or other antibody-independent mechanisms.

PATHOGENESIS AND PATHOLOGY. The asexual erythrocytic cycle causes the symptoms and pathology. Fever and the associated symptoms of headache, nausea, and muscular pain occur at the time that schizont-infected erythrocytes rupture and new ring forms appear. Although pyrogens and other toxins may be released from ruptured schizonts to cause fever and symptoms of malaria, none has been identified to date.

Anemia is caused by hemolysis of infected erythrocytes and dyserythropoiesis. Coombs-positive hemolytic anemia occurs rarely and usually results from quinine sensitivity. Severe acute hemolytic anemia results in patients who are heavily infected with *P. falciparum.* African children with chronic low-grade *P. falciparum* parasitemia have severe anemia associated with dyserythropoiesis and a low reticulocyte count. Reticulocytosis occurs after antimalarial therapy. Drugs administered to patients with G-6-PD deficiency may cause severe hemolysis. Thrombocytopenia results from binding of malaria-specific IgG to malaria antigen adsorbed on platelets.

Renal failure and cerebral malaria occur in *P. falciparum* malaria. Mechanisms for renal failure include severe hemolytic anemia, hemoglobinuria, hypovolemia, and possibly splanchnic vasoconstriction.

Blackwater fever is severe hemolytic anemia and hemoglobinuria in a falciparum malaria patient; it may cause renal failure. Prior to the introduction of chloroquine in the 1940's, quinine was used for prevention and treatment of malaria. Because of this, Coombs-positive hemolytic anemia following quinine administration was the most common cause of blackwater fever. Today, blackwater fever results from high parasitemia.

P. falciparum malaria causes diffuse cerebral disease. The decreased deformability of infected erythrocytes and their tendency to adhere by knobs to vascular endothelium probably cause the plugging of capillaries in the brain. Ring hemorrhages develop around obstructed capillaries. The brain may become edematous, although usually the cerebrospinal fluid pressure is normal.

Unusual complications of severe falciparum malaria include centrilobular necrosis of the liver and pulmonary edema. The lungs have microvascular congestion, interstitual edema, and hyaline membrane formation as evidence of increased capillary permeability.

P. malariae produces chronic progressive nephritis. Immune complexes are deposited in the glomerular capillary wall. Antibody in the complexes is specific for *P. malariae.* The majority of kidneys with immune complexes contain the C3 component of complement; 25 per cent have *P. malariae* antigen.

CLINICAL MANIFESTATIONS. No sign or symptom is pathognomonic of malaria. *Fever* need not be accompanied by the characteristic *malarial paroxysm.* The paroxysm begins with a chilly feeling, bedshaking chills, and a rise in temperature. The skin appears pale, with cyanosis of the lips and nail beds. The patient experiences *headache* and *nausea,* and may vomit. Within one to two hours the temperature rises toward 39 to 40.5° C, the patient feels hot, and the skin is warm and dry. As the temperature falls, *sweating* begins and drenches clothing. The patient feels fatigued and weak and often sleeps. This description is most typical of benign malarias; fever may persist and symptoms are prolonged in *malignant falciparum malaria.* Fever is usually not periodic in malignant falciparum malaria, and during the initial attack of *P. vivax* malaria, when the infection is asynchronous. Periodicity of fever occurs only in synchronized infections when the majority of infected erythrocytes containing mature schizonts rupture at the same time. This occurs at intervals determined by the length of the asexual erythrocytic cycle. The cycle in *P. vivax* and *P. ovale* malaria takes 48 hours and thus the fever occurs every other day. *P. malariae* matures in 72 hours and causes fever every third day.

The pulse rate is elevated but not commensurate with the fever. A nonproductive cough may occur during fever. Orthostatic hypotension is common in falciparum malaria, and weakness may persist for weeks. Splenomegaly occurs frequently and hepatomegaly less frequently. Tenderness on palpation of liver and spleen may be due to sudden stretching of their capsules; splenic rupture, a potentially fatal complication, should be considered. The absence of hepatosplenomegaly does not exclude the diagnosis of malaria. Labial herpes simplex lesions are often present. Rashes and lymphadenopathy are uncommon and point to a diagnosis other than malaria.

Abnormalities in routine laboratory test results in uncomplicated malaria may include evidence of a hemolytic anemia, leukopenia caused by a decrease in granulocytes and lymphocytes, thrombocytopenia, and minimal albuminuria. The thrombocyte count returns rapidly to normal on treatment. Hyponatremia, which is seen frequently in *P. falciparum* malaria, is caused by salt depletion and water retention.

Asymptomatic Infection and Recrudescence. Partial therapy or immunity reduces parasitemia and symptoms may disappear. Despite persistent erythrocytic infection during these asymptomatic periods, parasites are difficult to locate on blood films. Periodic rises in parasitemia cause recurrent clinical attacks (recrudescence). The total duration of erythrocytic infection varies for each type of malaria. Most falciparum infections are eliminated in one year; a few persist for up to three years. *P. malariae* infection may persist as an asymptomatic infection for the life of the patient. How *P. malariae* evades the immune response for years while infecting new erythrocytes every 72 hours remains a mystery. The asymptomatic erythrocytic infection poses two potential risks to other individuals: first, donated blood induces malaria in the recipient; second, the asymptomatic patient can infect vector mosquitoes.

Relapse differs from recrudescence in that the infection that induces the relapse persists as a latent form in hepatic parenchymal cells. Relapses occur only in *P. vivax* and *P. ovale* malaria.

COMPLICATIONS. High parasitemia in *P. falciparum* infection accounts for the severe morbidity and mortality. When the parasitemia rises above 100,000 infected erythrocytes per cu mm and the hematocrit falls below 30 per cent, the patient may develop serious complications, which most commonly include severe hemolytic anemia, renal failure, and coma. Acute renal failure can be associated with hemolytic anemia and hemoglobinuria (blackwater fever). The hemolytic anemia may be caused by high parasitemia, quinine sensitivity, or oxidant drugs in patients with G-6-PD deficiency. Renal failure may occur in the absence of severe hemolysis and may be associated with hypovolemia. It may occur with normal urine volume. Blood urea nitrogen may rise rapidly in renal failure because of an increased catabolic rate.

Cerebral malaria presents as disturbances in consciousness ranging from somnolence to coma, major motor seizures, and organic psychosis. Since the signs and symptoms are not pathognomonic of malaria, other diseases should be excluded, even in patients with circulating malaria parasites. Marked hypoglycemia, especially during infusion of quinine and in pregnancy, may cause lapses in consciousness. Febrile seizures in young children are impossible to distinguish from seizures of malaria. Neurologic examination may reveal hyper-reflexion and bilateral Babinski's signs. Focal neurologic findings occur rarely. The cerebrospinal fluid pressure may be elevated and the concentration of protein increased. Pleocytosis is rare.

Greatly elevated bilirubin and transaminase occur rarely. Another unusual complication, pulmonary edema, may be associated with fluid overload. Since it is caused by increased capillary permeability, it is difficult to reverse and the outcome is often fatal.

Splenic rupture, a rare and serious complication, occurs most commonly in *P. vivax* infections.

Chronic infection with *P. malariae* in children may produce progressive nephritis that responds poorly to treatment with antimalarials or steroids.

Falciparum Malaria During Pregnancy in the Semi-immune. Parasites sequester in the vascular beds of the placenta. The primigravida, although previously immune, may have severe attacks of malaria and marked anemia. Consequently, chemoprophylaxis is indicated throughout the first pregnancy in the semi-immune. Malaria causes stillbirths and underweight newborns, especially in the primigravida.

Tropical Splenomegaly Syndrome. Patients living in regions of Africa and New Guinea endemic for falciparum malaria develop massive splenic enlargement, hepatic sinusoidal lymphocytic infiltrates, and elevated levels of serum IgM. They respond to chronic antimalarial chemoprophylaxis with decrease in spleen size and reversal of liver pathology. Mortality is high in patients who do not receive antimalarial therapy. Splenectomy is contraindicated because severe malaria may occur following splenectomy, even in a previously immune individual.

Burkitt's Lymphoma. This tumor occurs in areas of Africa hyperendemic for *P. falciparum* and is believed to be an atypical response to Epstein-Barr virus infection.

DIAGNOSIS. The high mortality from falciparum malaria in nonendemic areas results from the failure of clinicians to consider the diagnosis and to obtain malaria blood films. The diagnosis of malaria should be suspected in a febrile patient who has traveled in the tropics or who has received a blood transfusion. The incubation period—the time from inoculation of sporozoites by mosquito to the first symptoms—is about 10 to 16 days. Drug prophylaxis may suppress the initial attack of *P. falciparum* malaria for weeks to months and of the relapsing malarias caused by *P. vivax* and *P. ovale* for months to years. The definitive diagnosis is made from identification of malarial parasites on a Giemsa-stained thick and thin blood film. Blood examinations should be obtained immediately and repeated at 12-hour intervals, because the parasitemia may fluctuate. Parasites may be undetectable during the first few days of the initial attack and in asymptomatic, semi-immune persons. The clinician should not wait for a paroxysm to obtain a blood film, since delay in diagnosis and treatment of *P. falciparum* malaria increases the risk to the patient. If malaria is strongly suspected on clinical grounds in a patient with repeatedly negative blood films, a therapeutic trial may be instituted.

Well-prepared and properly stained thick and thin blood films simplify diagnosis. A cleaned slide should be labeled with the patient's name, the date, and the time. For the thick film, one drop of blood at one end of the slide should be evenly spread in a circular motion to a diameter of 2 cm with the edge of another slide. A second drop of blood should be spread on the slide for the thin film as for a routine blood cell examination. After the blood films are dry, the thick film should be lysed in water and the thin film should be fixed with absolute methanol. Both should be stained with Giemsa at pH 7.0 to 7.2.

Once malaria parasites are identified on the blood film, the most important distinction is whether the patient has *P. falciparum* malaria, because this will influence the initial therapy. Criteria suggestive of *P. falciparum* include predominant small ring forms and multiply infected erythrocytes, rings with double nuclei, rings as applique forms, and the diagnostic crescent-shaped gametocytes. Except during high parasitemia, trophozoites and schizonts are rarely seen; infected erythrocytes adhere to venular endothelium. *P. falciparum* does not cause enlargement or pink stippling (Schuffner's dots) of infected erythrocytes. If more than 5 per cent of the erythrocytes are infected, *P. falciparum* should be suspected. Diagnosis of a malaria other than that caused by *P. falciparum* does not exclude the diagnosis of *P. falciparum* malaria, since mixed infections may occur. Slides should be saved for evaluation by an expert. Inclusions in erythrocytes (e.g., Howell-Jolly bodies and siderocytes) and artifacts (e.g., platelets on erythrocytes, precipitated stain and dirt) may be confused with malarial parasites. *Babesia microti* resembles *P. falciparum* rings but can be differentiated by an experienced microscopist.

Serologic tests have no place in the diagnosis of the acutely ill patient. The indirect fluorescent antibody test is useful in identifying infected donors in cases of transfusion malaria.

THERAPY. ***P. falciparum.*** Prompt diagnosis and early treatment are essential. Delay in chemotherapy increases morbidity and mortality. All patients should be hospitalized and treated as a medical emergency. Patients whose condition appears stable on admission may have rapid worsening.

The decision on drug regimen will depend on the origin of the infection. Chloroquine resistance is widespread and will continue to appear in new areas. Therefore, every falciparum malaria case should be considered potentially chloroquine resistant. Resistance extends today from India through Southeast Asia to New Guinea and Vanuatu in the Pacific Islands, from

Panama to South America, and from East Africa to Zambia, Madagascar and the Comoros. *P. falciparum* malaria in patients from Central and West Africa should be treated with chloroquine and the response followed closely. Because partial resistance to quinine (i.e., response followed by recrudescence) occurs in Southeast Asia and other areas, quinine is usually not used alone in treatment. Resistance to Fansidar, a fixed-drug combination of pyrimethamine and sulfadoxine, has been reported in Southeast Asia and South America.

Since treatment failure may occur with any drug regimen, the course of parasitemia must be followed at 12-hour intervals. Failure to reduce parasitemia in the first 24 to 48 hours of treatment should raise the possibility of parasite resistance to that treatment. No asexual parasites should be detectable on smears four to five days after a course of chloroquine is completed; persistence after the fifth day indicates drug failure. A simple method for estimating parasitemia from the thin blood film is as follows: at low parasite densities, the number of infected erythrocytes in 25 oil emersion fields is counted; at high parasite densities, the number of infected erythrocytes per 500 erythrocytes is counted.

Gametocytes may persist in the blood for weeks after asexual forms have been successfully eliminated. Gametocytes do not cause disease and their presence does not indicate treatment failure.

Partially resistant parasites recrudesce up to two months after treatment in the nonimmune. The patient should be warned that any febrile episode weeks to months after treatment may indicate drug failure and requires evaluation for malaria.

Symptomatic and Supportive Measures. Treatment includes aspirin, sponging with tepid water, and fanning to increase evaporation. Orthostatic hypotension, usually observed early in infection, is an indication for complete bed rest.

Packed erythrocytes or whole blood should be infused slowly in severe anemia. Platelet transfusions are generally not indicated for thrombocytopenia, as the platelets rapidly return toward normal during specific chemotherapy. Uremia may progress rapidly because of the high catabolic rate and is an indication for early hemodialysis. Administration of excessive fluids may aggravate cerebral symptoms or precipitate pulmonary edema. Pulmonary edema is usually not associated with a rise in central venous pressure during intravenous fluid administration and often results in death despite treatment.

Although splenic tenderness is common in acute malaria, evidence of peritoneal and diaphragmatic irritation may indicate splenic rupture. This life-threatening complication is more common in *P. vivax* malaria.

Treatment of Chloroquine-Sensitive *P. falciparum*. Chloroquine-sensitive strains occur in Western India, Pakistan, West and Central Africa, and Central America (except Panama). These patients should be treated with chloroquine or amodiaquine unless they have high parasitemia, in which case they should be treated as described in the section on severe and complicated malaria. The recommended therapy for adults is either chloroquine phosphate, 1000 mg initially, 500 mg six hours later, and 500 mg on each of two succeeding days; or amodiaquine hydrochloride, 780 mg initially and 520 mg on each of the two succeeding days. The major acute toxicity occurs in Africans who experience severe itching of the palms of the hands and soles of the feet without any obvious skin abnormalities, but this is not an indication for discontinuing choloroquine unless the symptoms are severe.

Because of the possibility of chloroquine resistance, the parasitemia should be followed closely during treatment (see above) and alternative drugs instituted if indicated. Fever occurring weeks after therapy may indicate a recrudescence.

Treatment of Chloroquine-Resistant *P. falciparum*. The regimen combines three drugs given orally: quinine sulfate, 650 mg every eight hours for ten days; pyrimethamine, 25 mg twice daily for three days; and a sulfonamide (sulfisoxazole or sulfadiazine), 0.5 grams every six hours for five days. Occasionally, after treatment with this regimen, the patient may suffer a subsequent recrudescence. Recrudescent attacks may be treated either with a second course of quinine, pyrimethamine, and sulfonamide, or, alternatively, with the following regimen: quinine sulfate, 650 mg every eight hours for three days, plus tetracycline hydrochloride, 250 mg every six hours for ten days.

Cinchonism (nausea, vomiting, tinnitus, and vertigo) commonly results from treatment with quinine and is not an indication to alter or discontinue therapy. A rare complication of quinine therapy, Coombs-positive hemolytic anemia, is an indication for immediate withdrawal of the drug.

Mefloquine, a new experimental antimalarial drug, is highly effective against chloroquine-resistant *P. falciparum*. As more data become available on its relative safety, it may become the treatment of choice for *P. falciparum* malaria. Mefloquine alone or in combination with pyrimethamine and sulfadoxine is now undergoing extensive clinical trials. Mefloquine rarely causes disorientation, hallucinations, and lapses of consciousness two to three weeks after drug administration.

Treatment of Severe and Complicated Malaria. Patients with *P. falciparum* malaria who have parasitemia greater than 100,000 per cu mm, marked anemia, cerebral complications, or are vomiting repeatedly should be treated with intravenous quinine dihydrochloride. Quinine dihydrochloride, 600 mg dissolved in 250 ml of 5 per cent glucose in 0.075 M sodium chloride should be infused slowly over eight hours. This should be repeated every eight hours until oral medication is tolerated, at which time a combination of quinine, sulfonamide, and pyrimethamine should be administered orally. Since quinine is excreted by the kidneys and metabolized by the liver, the dosage in patients with renal failure and hepatic disease should be decreased by at least half.

Hypoglycemia is a life-threatening complication of severe malaria and occurs most commonly during intravenous quinine therapy and in pregnant women. Blood glucose should be monitored closely, especially in patients who have a change in the level of consciousness.

If quinine is not immediately available from the Centers for Disease Control and the patient is severely ill with high parasitemia, intravenous quinidine should be considered until quinine can be obtained. Although there is limited experience with intravenous quinidine in malaria, oral quinidine has been shown to be as effective as oral quinine against chloroquine-resistant *P. falciparum*. Quinidine does not have FDA approval for use in malaria; therefore, the physician should obtain informed consent. Quinidine gluconate (10 mg per kilogram maximum of 600 mg) should be infused slowly over four to six hours followed by a continuous infusion of quinidine gluconate (5 mg per kilogram over six hours maximum of 300 mg) until intravenous quinine becomes available. Quinidine is contraindicated in patients who have conduction disturbances, untreated cardiac failure, and hypotension. The patient should be monitored closely, although lengthening of the $Q\text{-}T_C$ interval is to be expected.

Exchange transfusions may improve survival in patients who have parasitemia greater than 15 per cent, although controlled studies have not been performed. Glucosteroids are contraindicated because they increase morbidity and mortality. Heparin is contraindicated even in patients with disseminated intravascular coagulation because of the risk of hemorrhage.

P. vivax, P. ovale, and P. malariae. Acute attacks with any of these species should be treated with chloroquine or amodiaquine (see regimen under treatment of chloroquine-sensitive *P. falciparum*).

P. vivax and *P. ovale* infections acquired by mosquito bites may have persistent hepatic forms and these must be eliminated to prevent relapses. After completion of chloroquine treatment, primaquine phosphate, 26.6 mg daily for 14 days, is administered. Primaquine causes hemolysis in patients with G-6-PD deficiency. Patients who have a mild G-6-PD deficiency may be treated under close supervision because the hemolysis is self-limited. Severe G-6-PD deficiency is a contraindication to the use of primaquine, each relapse requiring retreatment with chloroquine. Primaquine is not indicated in the treatment of transfusion malaria because erythrocytic parasites of blood-induced infections do not infect the liver.

Sites of Action of Antimalarial Drugs. Only the sites of action of pyrimethamine and sulfonamide are known. Pyrimethamine has a greater affinity for parasite than host dihydrofolate reductase and blocks folate metabolism. Pyrimethamine-resistant parasites have either a higher concentration of dihydrofolate reductase or an enzyme with a lower affinity for pyrimethamine. Sulfonamides block utilization of para-aminobenzoic acid (pABA). It has been suggested that chloroquine interferes with enzymatic digestion in the parasite's food vacuole or the processing of ferriprotoporphyrin into hemozoin pigment. It is proposed that unprocessed ferriprotoporphyrin is toxic to the parasite.

PREVENTION. ***Protection for the Individual.*** Ideal chemoprophylaxis is not available because of chloroquine-resistant *P. falciparum* in many areas of the world. In addition, chloroquine eliminates only the primary attack of *P. vivax* and *P. ovale* but has no effect on relapses that may occur months to years later. Therefore the patient should be warned that fever during or after travel in endemic areas may be caused by malaria, even though the patient was on drug suppression.

Prevention of malaria can usually be accomplished in adults by chloroquine phosphate, 500 mg orally once weekly, or amodiaquine hydrochloride, 520 mg orally once weekly. Long term use of chloroquine at recommended doses for malaria prophylaxis does not cause eye disease. The drug should be continued for six weeks after leaving an endemic area. Travelers who were heavily exposed to malaria and are not G-6-PD deficient should receive primaquine phosphate, 26.6 mg daily for 14 days, on return from an endemic area to eliminate hepatic forms of *P. vivax* and *P. ovale*.

Fansidar, each tablet of which contains pyrimethamine, 25 mg, and sulfadoxine, a long-acting sulfonamide, 500 mg, is effective for prevention of chloroquine-resistant *P. falciparum*, although Fansidar resistance occurs in Southeast Asia and Brazil. The dose is one tablet weekly. Long-acting sulfonamides, but not sulfadoxine, have been rarely associated with Stevens-Johnson syndrome. Chloroquine weekly prophylaxis should be taken with Fansidar because of strains of *P. vivax* resistant to this medication.

Because drug prophylaxis is not ideal, the traveler should be advised to prevent contact with night-biting *Anopheles*. The traveler should use netting over the bed, insecticides, and mosquito repellents such as Off (N,N-diethyltoluamide).

Chemoprophylaxis in Pregnancy and for Nursing Mothers. Drugs in pregnancy always present a potential risk to the fetus, especially for prolonged use as in chemoprophylaxis. Chloroquine is considered generally safe when used at the recommended dosage. Chemoprophylaxis in areas of chloroquine-resistant *P. falciparum* presents a more difficult problem. Fansidar, the drug of choice, contains pyrimethamine, which has exhibited teratogenicity in some animal experiments. Although there are no documented cases of fetal abnormalities during human pregnancy (e.g., during the treatment of toxoplasmosis in pregnant women), a low frequency of congenital defects could have been missed. In addition, sulfonamides may increase the risk of kernicterus in hyperbilirubinemic neonates, because sulfonamides displace unconjugated bilirubin from albumin. Therefore, short-acting sulfonamides should be used close to term, should be discontinued as soon as labor begins, and should not be given to a mother nursing a newborn.

Acute malaria because of its risk to mother and child should be treated according to the regimens outlined under Therapy. Primaquine should not be used during pregnancy for the treatment or prevention of relapsing malarias (*P. vivax* and *P. ovale*).

Eradication and Control in Endemic Areas. The major tools for the control of malaria have been directed against the vector. Antimalarial drugs, especially chloroquine, are used primarily to reduce morbidity and mortality. When malaria eradication was first instituted as a program of WHO in the 1950's, the program mainly emphasized spraying walls with residual insecticides, detecting malaria cases, and treating patients with antimalarial drugs. Insecticide resistance, avoidance by mosquitoes of sprayed surfaces, and outdoor feeding of mosquitoes have created major problems and led to the failure of malaria eradication in many areas. In addition, the spread of multidrug-resistant *P. falciparum* will probably increase morbidity and mortality in regions of resurgent malaria. There is no question that new tools such as vaccines and novel approaches to vector control will be sorely needed in the decades ahead.

Boyd MF (ed.): Malariology. Philadelphia, W. B. Saunders Company, 1949. *The best description of the course of each of the four human malarias in the nonimmune.*

Brown HW, Neva FA: Basic Clinical Parasitology. 5th ed. Norwalk, Appleton-Century-Crofts, 1983. *Color plates of malaria parasites for the inexperienced microscopist.*

Miller LH: Malaria. *In* Warren KW and Mahmoud AAF (eds.): Tropical and Geographical Medicine. New York, McGraw-Hill Book Company, 1983. *A general review of malariology with references.*

White NJ, Warrell DA, Chanthavanich P, Looareesurvan S, Warrell MJ, Krishna S, Williamson DH, Turner RC: Severe hypoglycemia and hyperinsulinemia in falciparum malaria. N Engl J Med 309:61, 1983. *A new complication of falciparum malaria.*

Udeinya IJ, Miller LH, McGregor IA, Jensen JB: *Plasmodium falciparum* strain-specific antibody blocks binding of infected erythrocytes to amelanotic melanoma cells. Nature 303:429, 1983. *An example of variant antigens in falciparum malaria.*

Development of mefloquine as an antimalaria drug. Bull WHO 61:169, 1983. *Review of data on an important, experimental antimalarial drug for chloroquine-resistant P. falciparum.*

379. AFRICAN TRYPANOSOMIASIS (Sleeping Sickness)

B. M. Greenwood

DEFINITION AND ETIOLOGY. Sleeping sickness, an infection caused by *Trypanosoma brucei*, occurs in two forms—West African or Gambian sleeping sickness and East African or Rhodesian sleeping sickness. Trypanosomes causing these diseases cannot be distinguished morphologically, but differentiation of isolates that are pathogenic for man from those that are not is often important. In general, nonpathogenic strains (*T. b. brucei*) lose their infectivity for laboratory animals when incubated in human serum, whereas strains pathogenic for humans (*T. b. gambiense* and *T. b. rhodesiense*) do not. These two subspecies can be differentiated by the electrophoretic pattern of their component enzymes.

On light microscopy *T. brucei* is seen to be an elongated trypanosome with a prominent nucleus, kinetoplast, and flagellum. Its length varies from 10 to 40 μ, slender and stumpy forms being found in the patient at the same time. Electron microscopy has revealed the detailed structure of the trypanosome. It is coated with an amorphous material which contains the variant antigens that are of vital importance to its survival.

EPIDEMIOLOGY. ***Distribution and Prevalence of Sleeping Sickness.*** Sleeping sickness is restricted to tropical Africa, where it has been recognized since the fourteenth century. Major epidemics, affecting several million people, occurred throughout the first half of the twentieth century. Sleeping sickness is now a less serious health problem, but many cases still occur in Zaire and in Uganda. Smaller foci persist in other countries such as the Ivory Coast.

Pathway of Infection. Tsetse flies are the natural vector of African trypanosomiasis. Intrauterine transmission has been recorded but is rare. Infections have followed accidental inoculation with trypanosomes in the laboratory.

When a tsetse fly bites an infected host, trypanosomes are sucked into the midgut with the blood meal. Here they pass around or through the peritrophic membrane, migrate forward between it and the gut wall, penetrate the gut wall, and reach the salivary glands, where development into new infective forms occurs. When a new host is bitten, trypanosomes pass down the proboscis with the saliva to start a new infection. Development within the fly takes two to five weeks.

Epidemiology of Gambian Sleeping Sickness. Humans are the main host of *T. b. gambiense,* but there is increasing evidence that animals such as the pig and sheep form an important reservoir of the infection. Gambian sleeping sickness is spread mainly by two species of tsetse fly, *Glossina palpalis* and *G. tachinoides*. These flies inhabit the shaded areas alongside rivers and streams, areas where their human victims can often be found. In some areas flies also rest and bite within a village. Thus, contact between humans and these tsetse flies is often very close, providing ideal conditions for transmission of the infection.

Epidemiology of Rhodesian Sleeping Sickness. *T. b. rhodesiense* differs from *T. b. gambiense* in being primarily a parasite of wild game, man acting only as an occasional and accidental host. Rhodesian sleeping sickness is spread by tsetse flies of the *G. morsitans* group, flies that can survive in open savanna. Rhodesian sleeping sickness is primarily an occupational disease, occurring mainly in those whose work takes them into areas of bush where wild game, especially the bushbuck, survives. Hunters, fishermen, honey-gatherers, and tourists are all at risk. This form of trypanosomiasis is usually a sporadic infection, but epidemics can occur. In the epidemic situation direct person-to-person transmission probably takes place.

PATHOLOGY. In the early stage of the disease the lymph nodes and spleen are enlarged and infiltrated with plasma cells and macrophages. Later, lymph nodes shrink and patchy fibrosis occurs. Lymphocytic infiltration of the pericardium and myocardium may be found, especially in the Rhodesian form of the disease. Characteristic changes are found in the brain and meninges once invasion of the central nervous system has occurred. These changes are most marked in long-standing cases of Gambian sleeping sickness. The meninges are thickened and infiltrated with lymphocytes, plasma cells, and morular cells. Morular cells are large cells with an eccentric nucleus displaced by numerous cytoplasmic vesicles which contain IgM. As the disease progresses, chronic inflammatory changes extend along the perivascular spaces to produce prominent perivascular cuffing. Finally, infiltration of the brain substance with lymphocytes, plasma cells, and morular cells takes place with accompanying neuronal degeneration and microglial proliferation.

PATHOGENESIS AND IMMUNITY. The immune response of the host plays an important part in the pathogenesis of sleeping sickness, but the nature of the immunopathologic reactions occurring in this infection has not been defined clearly. Patients

TABLE 379–1. SOME CONTRASTING FEATURES OF GAMBIAN AND RHODESIAN SLEEPING SICKNESS

	Gambian Sleeping Sickness	Rhodesian Sleeping Sickness
Causative organism	*Trypanosoma brucei gambiense*	*Trypanosoma brucei rhodesiense*
Distribution	West and Central Africa	East Africa
Source of infection	Humans (domestic animals)	Wild game (man)
Vector	*Glossina palpalis* or *tachinoides* (riverine tsetse)	*Glossina morsitans* (savanna tsetse)
Clinical features		
Lymphadenopathy	+ +	+
Heart failure	0	+ +
Neurologic	+ +	+
Disseminated intravascular coagulation	0	+
Diagnosis	Trypanosomes in lymph node juice or CSF	Trypanosomes in blood or CSF
Course of infection	Slow	Rapid

with sleeping sickness have high serum immune complex levels and show laboratory abnormalities indicating activation of the complement and kinin systems. However, it is uncertain whether these immune complexes cause tissue damage; glomerulonephritis and arthritis are not usual features of the disease. Stimulation of the reticuloendothelial and B lymphoid systems may contribute to the lymphadenopathy and splenomegaly of the early phase of the infection. Large amounts of IgM are present in the serum and in the cerebrospinal fluid of patients with the infection. Only a small proportion of this immunoglobulin is parasite-specific antibody; the rest contains antibodies with a wide variety of specificities, including autoantibodies. Several aspects of lymphocyte function are impaired in patients with sleeping sickness. The resulting suppression of cellular and humoral immunity may contribute to the increased susceptibility of patients with sleeping sickness to other infections.

African trypanosomes possess surface and core antigens, both of which can induce an antibody response. Little is known about the role of cell-mediated immunity in this infection. In the presence of antibody to surface antigens, trypanosomes are lysed or taken up by cells of the reticuloendothelial system. However, successful eradication of the parasite is prevented by the process of antigenic variation. By progressive alteration of its surface antigens, the trypanosome is able to keep one step ahead of the host's immune response and thus to persist until the host eventually dies. The possible mechanisms of antigenic variation are of great interest to biologists. It is probable that each trypanosome possesses the necessary genetic information to synthesize several surface antigens, antigenic change being initiated by environmental factors such as contact with antibody.

CLINICAL FEATURES. Sleeping sickness passes through three pathologic and clinical phases: an initial phase in which trypanosomes are localized to the site of the tsetse fly bite; an early or systemic phase in which trypanosomes are widely distributed throughout the body; and a neurologic or advanced stage in which trypanosomes are largely restricted to the central nervous system. Rhodesian sleeping sickness is usually a much more rapidly progressive illness than Gambian sleeping sickness with less distinction between systemic and neurologic stages. However, this distinction is not an absolute one; in some outbreaks Gambian sleeping sickness has progressed rapidly, whereas occasionally Rhodesian sleeping sickness follows a more benign course.

Gambian Sleeping Sickness. Ten days after a bite by an infected tsetse fly, a small nodular lesion, a chancre, may develop at the site of the bite and persist for two to three weeks. This lesion, if it occurs, frequently passes unnoticed.

Months or even years after an infected bite, clinical features of systemic invasion with trypanosomes occur. Fever and lymphadenopathy are the main features of this early stage of the infection. Fever is usually intermittent and may be mild. Lymphadenopathy may be general, but the posterior cervical nodes are nearly always involved. Enlarged nodes are firm but not usually tender. Moderate splenomegaly may occur. Urticarial rashes, erythematous rashes, and localized edema may be seen. A variety of eye lesions have been recorded, but these are rare. Electrocardiograms are often abnormal, but clinical signs of heart disease are unusual. Mild normocytic anemia and mild thrombocytopenia are common. The serum IgM level is nearly always raised.

Months or years after the first appearance of symptoms, the clinical features of the early phase of the disease regress to be replaced by new symptoms and signs indicating invasion of the nervous system. Mild behavioral and personality changes are often the first signs of central nervous system involvement. Later, more florid psychologic changes may occur with hallucinations and delusions. Headache and backache are common complaints. Drowsiness during the day, the feature from which the disease takes its name, may occur but is not invariable, and some patients are manic. If no treatment is given, the patient's level of consciousness progressively deteriorates until finally he lapses into stupor. Convulsions occasionally occur. Chorea and athetosis are the most frequently encountered localizing neurologic signs. Pyramidal tract involvement is less frequent and cranial nerve lesions are rare. Obesity and impotence or amenorrhea frequently occur and perhaps follow from damage to the hypothalamus. Severe itching is an unexplained symptom that may lead to skin changes. The cerebrospinal fluid shows an increase in cells and protein, much of which is IgM. Free immunoglobulin light chains may be present. Most of the cells are lymphocytes, but a few are plasma cells and morular cells. Trypanosomes may be present.

Rhodesian Sleeping Sickness. The clinical picture of Rhodesian sleeping sickness is similar to that described above, but on presentation the patient is usually more acutely ill than a patient with Gambian sleeping sickness, and the disease progresses more rapidly. Heart failure and jaundice occur more frequently than in Gambian sleeping sickness, but lymphadenopathy is usually less prominent. Neurologic features similar to those described above may be present, but sometimes death occurs before these have had time to develop. Anemia and thrombocytopenia are usual, and disseminated intravascular coagulation may occur. Liver function test results are often abnormal, and an abnormal electrocardiogram is usually obtained. Cerebrospinal fluid changes are the same as those described above.

DIAGNOSIS. The chancre of trypanosomiasis has no special features and is unlikely to be recognized unless there is a strong reason for suspecting trypanosomiasis. It must be differentiated from an allergic reaction to a tsetse fly bite. Trypanosomes are present in juice obtained from the lesion.

The clinical features of the early phase of sleeping sickness are similar to those of many infectious, neoplastic, and connective tissue diseases. Trypanosomiasis must be considered in the differential diagnosis of unexplained pyrexia or lymphadenopathy in any patient who has visited an endemic area, even if only for a short holiday. Diagnosis of Rhodesian sleeping sickness can usually be made by the demonstration of trypanosomes in a thick blood film. However, trypanosomes are found less frequently in the blood of patients with Gambian sleeping sickness even when concentration methods such as ion-exchange chromatography, culture, or animal inoculation are used. Diagnosis is made most readily in the early stage of Gambian sleeping sickness by the detection of trypanosomes in the juice obtained on puncturing an enlarged lymph node with a venipuncture needle.

Once invasion of the central nervous system has occurred, clinical diagnosis of sleeping sickness is usually not difficult. However, tragic misdiagnoses have been made in patients with predominantly psychologic features. Chorea may be so marked as to suggest Sydenham's chorea, and confusion with other extrapyramidal syndromes may occur occasionally. Diagnosis of the advanced stage of sleeping sickness is confirmed by examination of the cerebrospinal fluid. Trypanosomes can be found in most patients, provided both that the cerebrospinal fluid is examined immediately after collection and that scrupulously clean glassware is used. Measurement of the cerebrospinal fluid IgM level is often of great diagnostic help in patients in whom trypanosomes cannot be found. A high cerebrospinal fluid IgM in the presence of a modest increase in total protein is almost pathognomonic of sleeping sickness.

Many different serologic tests have been used to diagnose sleeping sickness. These tests have proved of great value in survey work but are of less value in the investigation of individual patients, as false-positive and false-negative reactions can occur.

TREATMENT. *General Measures.* Whenever possible, a patient with sleeping sickness should be treated in hospital. Lumbar puncture to determine the stage of the disease must be carried out before treatment is started. If abnormalities are found (a raised cell count or protein), the patient must be treated as having advanced disease, even if there are no clinical signs of central nervous system involvement. Poorly nourished patients may require dietary supplements. A search should be made for any associated infections, and these should be treated appropriately.

Many different drugs and dosage regimens have been used in the treatment of sleeping sickness, but few controlled trials have been undertaken and the treatment schedules currently in use were established empirically. All the drugs used in the treatment of sleeping sickness were developed many years ago, and all are toxic; there is still a great need for safer effective drugs.

Chemotherapy of Early Disease. Suramin is an effective treatment for early Gambian and Rhodesian sleeping sickness, but it is ineffective in advanced disease, since it penetrates poorly into the cerebrospinal fluid. Suramin* is a white powder that is made up in an aqueous solution immediately before use and given intravenously in a dose of 20 mg per kilogram of body weight. Occasionally it causes vomiting and collapse, so it is customary to start with a test dose of one fifth of this amount. A course comprises five to ten injections given at two- to five-day intervals. The drug can cause renal damage; because of this, the urine should be tested for protein and casts before each injection. Mild proteinuria can be ignored; but if heavy proteinuria develops or if casts are found, treatment should be stopped. Three injections of melarsoprol (see below) is an effective alternative form of treatment of early disease. Berenil is also effective but has been used less widely.

Chemotherapy of Advanced Disease. Melarsoprol (Mel B) is the treatment of choice for both Gambian and Rhodesian sleeping sickness once involvement of the central nervous system has occurred, even though the drug is very toxic. It is possible that toxicity is reduced by prior treatment with one or two injections of suramin, but melarsoprol should be started right away in patients who are very sick. Mel B is dispensed as a 3.6 per cent solution in propylene glycol. This is very irritating and is liable to produce thrombophlebitis. The full dosage of Mel B* is 3.6 mg (0.1 ml) per kilogram of body weight given intravenously up to a maximum of 5.0 ml. The following is an effective schedule of treatment for an adult: 2.5 ml on days 1 and 3, followed by 5.0 ml on day 5; rest for one week; 5.0 ml on days 15, 17, and 19; rest for a further week; and then 5.0 ml on days 29, 31, and 33 (total dose, 40.0 ml). Other schedules employ a more gradual build-up to full dosage. Treatment schedules should be kept flexible and slowed down if reactions occur. Febrile reactions are common after the first injection of Mel B, especially if suramin has not been given. Mel B can produce rashes, marrow depression, and renal damage, but its most serious side effect is an encephalopathy which occurs in about 5 per cent of patients. Encephalopathy occurs most frequently at the time of the third or fourth injection; it may develop very rapidly and has a mortality of about 50 per cent. It is uncertain whether it is due to arsenic poisoning or to an immunopathologic reaction. Dimercaprol (BAL) has been used to treat this complication of Mel B treatment, but its value has not been clearly established. It has been suggested that corticosteroids protect patients from Mel B encephalopathy, but this assertion has never been clearly documented.

Follow-up and Treatment of Relapses. The results of treatment of patients with early disease with suramin or melarsoprol are excellent, but occasional patients subsequently develop neurologic disease and require treatment with a full course of Mel B. Regular follow-up with clinical examination and lumbar puncture is therefore necessary for at least one year after treatment and preferably for longer.

---

*Available from the Centers for Disease Control (404–329–3670); (404–329–2888) evenings, weekends, and holidays.

Patients with neurologic disease also require regular follow-up, for treatment failures and relapses occasionally occur. Patients with a relapse of advanced disease should receive another full course of Mel B* (total dosage, 40.0 ml for an adult) together with nitrofurazone, for, despite the toxicity of this drug, there is an impression that relapsed patients treated with melarsoprol and nitrofurazone do better than those receiving melarsoprol alone. The adult dosage of nitrofurazone* is 0.5 gram given by mouth every six hours for five days, this course being repeated on two or three occasions. Nitrofurazone is a toxic drug causing peripheral neuropathy and hemolytic anemia, especially in those with glucose-6-phosphatase deficiency.

PROGNOSIS. Many patients with early Gambian sleeping sickness remain relatively well for months or years without treatment, and it is possible that a few recover spontaneously. Once central nervous system involvement has occurred, death is inevitable unless treatment is given. Death frequently follows a secondary infection, often pneumonia, in a stuporous and malnourished patient. Patients with Rhodesian sleeping sickness may die from heart failure.

The results of treatment of patients in the early phase of sleeping sickness are excellent, over 90 per cent making a complete recovery. However, a few patients subsequently develop central nervous system involvement and require further treatment. Mel B achieves a parasitologic "cure" in at least 90 per cent of cases of advanced disease, and many patients make a complete recovery. Unfortunately some patients are left with irreversible neurologic damage. These patients must be differentiated from those who have had a true relapse and require further treatment. About 5 per cent of patients die during the course of Mel B treatment.

An attack of sleeping sickness does not induce protective immunity, and reinfection may occur.

CONTROL AND PROPHYLAXIS. Many different approaches have been made to the control of sleeping sickness. In West Africa, survey teams have been used extensively to detect and treat asymptomatic patients early in the course of their disease, thus reducing the reservoir of infection. In East Africa, attempts have been made to reduce the reservoir of infection in wild game. A wide variety of techniques has been used to destroy tsetse flies, ranging from hand trapping to aerial spraying with insecticides. Currently, the potential control value of traps baited with animal odors is being evaluated.

Pentamidine* has been successfully used as a chemoprophylactic in Gambian sleeping sickness when given by a single intramuscular injection of 4 mg per kilogram every three to six months. However, its use carries the risk of producing cryptic infections, and the drug can cause diabetes. It should therefore be used only in those who are at considerable risk of being infected.

The occurrence of antigenic variation has been a major obstacle to the development of a successful vaccine. However, progress in culture of *T. brucei* in vitro and in analysis of the chemical structure of its variant antigens and the mechanisms underlying their expression holds out some hope for the future.

---

*Available from the Centers for Disease Control (404–329–3670); (404–329–2888) evenings, weekends, and holidays.

Apted FIC: Clinical manifestations and diagnosis of sleeping sickness. *In* Mulligan HW (ed.): The African Trypanosomiases. London, George Allen and Unwin, 1970, pp 661–683. *A comprehensive review of the clinical features of sleeping sickness.*

Ford J: The role of African Trypanosomiases in African Ecology. Oxford, Clarendon Press, 1971. *A very readable account of the social impact of human and cattle trypanosomiasis in Africa.*

Greenwood BM, Whittle HC: The pathogenesis of sleeping sickness. Trans Roy Soc Trop Med Hyg 74:716, 1980. *A review of the ways in which the immune response of the host may contribute to the pathology and clinical features of sleeping sickness.*

Lambert PH, Berney M, Kazyumba G: Immune complexes in serum and in cerebrospinal fluid in African trypanosomiasis: Correlation with polyclonal B cell activation and with intracerebral immunoglobulin synthesis. J Clin Invest 67:77, 1981. *An account of the possible role of immune complexes in the pathogenesis of sleeping sickness.*

Vickerman K: Antigenic variation in trypanosomes. Nature 273:613, 1978. *A concise and lucid review of this complex but very interesting biologic phenomenon.*

WHO and FAO: The African Trypanosomiases. Technical report series 635. Geneva, World Health Organization, 1979. *A short report covering various aspects of African trypanosomiasis in man and in cattle. Contains several tables with epidemiologic information.*

380. CHAGAS' DISEASE (American Trypanosomiasis)

Vanize Macedo

DEFINITION. Chagas' disease, an infection caused by *Trypanosoma cruzi* and named after its Brazilian discoverer, Carlos Chagas, is found only in the Western Hemisphere. A distinction must be made between infection and disease. The majority of infected patients develop no signs of clinically detectable disease. Chagas himself described the two main disease forms occurring years after the initial infection: a chronic cardiomyopathy often with intracardiac conduction defects, and dilatation of the esophagus or colon (the mega syndromes).

ETIOLOGY. The trypanomastigote is visible in peripheral blood films of man and the multitude of naturally or experimentally infected animals studied in the early or acute phase of the disease. It is polymorphic, 15 to 25 μ long, and has a large subterminal kinetoplast. Multiplication takes place only in an amastigote phase in host cells. The trypanomastigote penetrates a host cell (frequently a cardiac or smooth muscle cell), rounds up, and commences to replicate by binary fission every 12 hours. The time of rupture of this host cell will depend on its size. The amastigotes change into trypanomastigotes, which are released to circulate in the peripheral blood and penetrate new cells. After a period of weeks, the host immune response suppresses the trypanomastigote parasitemia to subpatent levels. Small numbers continue to circulate for years.

EVOLUTIONARY CYCLE. The insect vector of *T. cruzi* is a hemipteran, a reduviid bug of the subfamily Triatominae, of which about 100 species have been described. They are obligate blood suckers and withdraw a large blood meal rapidly by directly tapping a subcutaneous capillary with their stylet mouth parts. The great majority of these are sylvatic and maintain cycles among wild animals. Such bugs are found from within 200 miles of New York to the south of Argentina. For reasons that are unclear, a small number of species have become highly domesticated, and those cohabiting with man are the transmitters of Chagas' disease. The most important species in this respect are *Triatoma infestans, Panstrongylus megistus,* and *Rhodnius prolixus.*

EPIDEMIOLOGY. Transmission is usually at night, when the bugs are active. They feed mainly on the face and arms, the uncovered parts of sleeping man. As they engorge with blood, the rise in intra-abdominal pressure promotes defecation, and the trypanomastigotes in the feces can penetrate mucous membranes or small skin abrasions. The three main species of transmitting bugs all tend to defecate soon after feeding.

Congenital transmission and infection by blood transfusion can occur. More rarely, transmission may occur as a result of a laboratory accident. There exists the possibility of contamination by the digestive tract.

Chagas' disease has been described in all the countries of South America and Central America with the exception of Guyana and Surinam. In Mexico it is rare. Two autochthonous acute cases have been reported in Texas. The high standard of housing and the discrete nature of the sylvatic cycles makes transmission to man a very rare event in North America. Chagas' disease is a serious public health problem in South America, principally in Argentina, Brazil, Chile, Uruguay, and Venezuela. There are geographic differences in the disease; for example, cardiomyopathy is rare in Chile, and the mega syndromes are unknown in Venezuela. From some countries (e.g.,

Bolivia) there is little information on the status of Chagas' disease.

It is estimated that the prevalence of trypanosomiasis may reach 20 per cent in the rural zones of the countries where it is endemic. Socioeconomic conditions are bad in these areas and dwellings are of poor construction with mud and sticks, building materials which favor bug colonization. Chagas' disease is intimately linked with economic underdevelopment.

The medicosocial importance of the disease has not been determined, and we do not know for certain the role American trypanosomiasis plays in the economy of countries where it is endemic. Cardiopathy is the most important form of the disease, causing a significant mortality and inability to work in the most productive phase of life. Many employers in Brazil will not hire a worker with positive serology.

PATHOGENESIS. The local tissue inflammation promoted by rupture of nests of amastigotes of *T. cruzi* was the first interpretation of the pathology of the disease. This view explains the alterations that occur in the acute phase but not all those that occur in the chronic phase. In this phase amastigotes are rarely found.

There is evidence suggesting that an autoimmune process is at work in the chronic cardiomyopathy of Chagas' disease. Santos, Buch, and Teixeira have demonstrated that sensitized lymphocytes from rabbits chronically infected with *T. cruzi* are cytotoxic to normal cardiac cells. Cossio and colleagues have identified circulating autoantibodies to heart tissue in patients with chronic cardiomyopathy.

The importance of strains of the parasite or reinfection in the pathogenesis of Chagas' disease is still not clear.

PATHOLOGY. In the acute phase the infection is generalized, and amastigotes of *T. cruzi* can be found in cells of the reticuloendothelial system. Initially reticular cells are parasitized, and in a short time smooth and striated muscle cells, including cardiac muscle, glial and nerve cells, and fat cells, are invaded.

The inoculation lesion shows inflammation with infiltration of lymphocytes and plasma cells and fibroblastic proliferation. The heart is enlarged and flabby, with predominance of dilatation over hypertrophy. Hemorrhagic foci may be seen on the endocardium. Microscopically there is diffuse edema, both intestinal and interfibrillar congestion, and the presence of amastigotes in the cardiac fibers. The cardiac fibers show hyaline necrosis and degeneration (lesions of Margarino Torres). In the central nervous system there is mononuclear infiltration of the leptomeninges, congestive perivascular inflammation, and hemorrhage with glial proliferation and neurophagia. Amastigotes may be encountered in the cells of the central nervous system.

In the chronic cardiac form the heart is enlarged with both hypertrophy and dilatation, so that the apex is formed by the terminations of both ventricles. The epicardium is congested, and there may be a small pericardial effusion. There are no organic valvular lesions. The thinned myocardium of the apex may distend to form an apical aneurysm, a characteristic lesion of Chagas' disease. Mural thrombosis is frequent on the endocardium, particularly in the right atrium and the apex of the left ventricle. Thrombosis at the apex is an important finding in Chagas' myocarditis. These intracardiac thrombi are the source of emboli principally to the lungs, kidneys, cerebrum, and spleen. There is chronic passive congestion of the organs.

Microscopy demonstrates an intense diffuse myocarditis with focal areas of cellular infiltration containing mononuclear cells, lymphocytes, and plasma cells. There is hypertrophy of the cardiac fibers with small areas of focal necrosis, hemorrhage, and granular degeneration. A variable degree of fibrosis is associated with edema and vascular dilatation and congestion. Tissue amastigotes are rarely seen in chronic cases.

Andrade has shown that these inflammatory changes directly involve the conducting system of the heart, particularly the sinoatrial node, the inferior third of the atrioventricular node, the right half of the main bundle, the right bundle branch, and the anterior ramification of the left bundle branch. He established a good correlation between the electrocardiogram in life and these pathologic changes.

In the indeterminate form of Chagas' disease, active myocarditis with granuloma formation and neuronal destruction of Auerbach's plexus has been found, but in lesser degree than established cardiomyopathy. In megaesophagus and megacolon the organ is dilated with focal myositis associated with a diminution in the number of nerve cells in Auerbach's plexus.

In the congenital form a chronic placentitis with ischemia of the chorionic villi occurs. Edema and a histiocytic inflammatory infiltrate are present with small foci of necrosis in these villi. Amastigotes are visible in the cytoplasm of macrophages.

CLINICAL PRESENTATION. Chagas' disease has an acute and chronic phase. In endemic areas discrepancies exist between the prevalence of the chronic phase and the small number of cases diagnosed as acute disease.

Acute Phase. In areas endemic for Chagas' disease, the acute phase is diagnosed in about 1 per cent of patients. Probably in the majority of individuals the initial phase of the infection is not apparent. Seventy per cent of patients in this phase are children under ten years of age. Acute Chagas' disease is rare in adults.

The incubation period is 4 to 12 days. The signs at the portal of entry often call the attention of the physician to the possible diagnosis of the disease. Romaña's sign is present in half the patients in the acute phase. This is a unilateral, bipalpebral, firm, violaceous edema, frequently with conjunctivitis and enlargement of the preauricular gland. An inoculation chagoma may occur in exposed areas, such as the face or arms, where the bug has an opportunity of biting. This also is characterized by erythema and infiltrative tumefaction of the skin with satellite ganglion reaction, which, when it disappears, leaves hyperpigmentation. It is found in 25 per cent of patients in the acute phase. A minority of patients do not present signs of a portal of entry.

The disease is characterized by prolonged fever, asthenia, enlargement of lymphatic glands, edema of the face and legs, and hepatosplenomegaly. Tachycardia is frequently present even in the absence of fever. This is a sign of myocarditis, which is benign in the majority of cases and diagnosed only on electrocardiogram.

The signs of the acute phase disappear in two to four months. The so-called schizotrypanides are skin rashes that rarely occur in the acute phase. They may take the form of erythematous indurated plaques or may be morbilliform or urticarial in type, suggesting an allergic nature. Meningoencephalitis is also a rare complication, often occurring in children under one year of age and usually fatal. Clinical evidence of encephalitis may be complicated by convulsions.

Congenital Disease. Since this is rarely diagnosed, its prevalence in endemic areas cannot be estimated. Such newborns are underweight and afebrile, and have hepatosplenomegaly and often edema. Petechiae, bruising, and frank hemorrhage may be noted. Meningoencephalitis may produce convulsions and tremors of the face and limbs. If jaundice is present, it disappears in the third week. Metastatic chagomas have been described, with skin infiltration, infection, and even necrosis.

The Chronic Phase. INDETERMINATE FORM. After the acute phase, individuals can stay for many years or all their lives in a latent or indeterminate phase. These subjects do not have clinical, radiologic, or electrocardiographic signs. In endemic areas, approximately half of those infected show this form. It is probable that this number will diminish as more sophisticated methods for detecting disease are developed.

CARDIAC FORM. This is the most important clinical form of the chronic phase, and its prevalence can reach 30 per cent of individuals in an endemic area. The majority of patients have no cardiac symptoms or signs but only electrocardiographic evidence of disease.

Palpitations, usually the result of extrasystoles, are a frequent initial symptom. They may be accompanied by dizziness and precordial pain. Right-sided ventricular failure predominates, and dyspnea is infrequent.

Physical examination shows an irregular pulse and distant heart sounds, fixed splitting of the pulmonary second sound, gallop rhythm, and a functional regurgitant murmur in the mitral area. In advanced cases, tricuspid regurgitation can occur and cyanosis is present. Thromboembolic phenomena are very frequent and may precede symptoms of cardiac insufficiency. Total atrioventricular block is rare but is frequently accompanied by Stokes-Adams attacks.

Digestive Form. The digestive form is characterized by dilatation and alteration in motility of the esophagus or colon. Rarely the stomach or small intestine shows similar changes.

In megaesophagus the principal symptom is long-standing dysphagia, which begins with difficulty with solid food and progresses until the patient can swallow only soft foods with the aid of frequent sips of water. In advanced cases, patients have pain on swallowing, regurgitation, and pyrosis with a sensation of suffocation. Hiccup, sialorrhea, and nocturnal cough are associated symptoms. Hypersalivation is accompanied by parotid gland enlargement. Marked weight loss is present, and aspiration pneumonias may occur in advanced cases.

Megacolon is manifested by retention of feces and gas and often progresses to fecaloma formation. Volvulus and intestinal obstruction are frequent complications. The majority of cases of megacolon are associated with megaesophagus. Half of the patients with digestive forms of Chagas' disease have abnormal electrocardiograms.

Other Clinical Forms. Rare complications are megaureter, megabladder, megagallbladder, and bronchiectasis. The forms of central nervous system involvement in chronic infection, described by Chagas himself, are still debatable. The denervation process has been implicated in the dysfunction of various exocrine and endocrine glands.

DIAGNOSIS. ***Acute Phase.*** The acute phase is usually diagnosed by finding the trypanomastigote in the peripheral blood on direct examination of thick films. This is the best criterion for diagnosing the acute phase. Should this fail, simple concentration methods are usually positive, such as examination of the leukocyte cream after centrifugation or allowing the blood to clot and examining the supernatant (Strout's method). Biopsy of the calf muscle shows myositis and frequently nests of amastigotes.

The *xenodiagnostic test* is often positive before 30 days owing to the high number of circulating trypanosomes. Similarly, cultures (NNN) and subinoculation of mice recover the organism. The serologic reactions, usually positive in this early stage, are precipitins and agglutinins. There is a raised IgM. The complement fixation test result becomes positive four to six weeks after infection. The indirect immunofluorescent test becomes positive earlier than the hemagglutination and complement fixation tests. The white cell count shows leukocytosis caused by an intense lymphocytosis with atypical lymphocytes. The erythrocyte sedimentation rate is increased, as are the mucoproteins. Heterophil antibodies may appear in the serum, and the Paul Bunnell reaction may be positive. Protein electrophoresis reveals a slight hypoalbuminemia with a rise in gamma and alpha 2 globulins. The transaminases are slightly elevated. The electrocardiogram may show sinus tachycardia, low voltage complexes, first degree atrioventricular block, increased QT space, primary alterations in ventricular repolarization, and sometimes subepicardial ischemia. Alterations in cardiac rhythm are rare at this stage and a bad prognostic sign.

On x-ray examination, there may be enlargement of the cardiac shadow, which may be transitory. At times such enlargement is due to a pericardial effusion. Marked cardiomegaly indicates a bad prognosis.

Chronic Phase. Evidence of infection is established mainly by serologic tests such as complement fixation, hemagglutination, and immunofluorescence. Xenodiagnosis, using 40 bugs, will isolate an organism in about 50 per cent of cases. In the indeterminate phase, only these investigations will be positive.

A chest x-ray may be normal, but frequently a degree of cardiomegaly is seen progressing to marked global enlargement of the heart. The electrocardiogram is valuable, as conduction defects are common. In the endemic area of São Felipe, Brazil, the following abnormalities were present in a frequency of 15 to 20 per cent: complete right bundle branch block with anterior hemiblock, ventricular extrasystoles, first degree atrioventricular block, and alterations in ventricular repolarization. Total atrioventricular block or complete left bundle branch block occurred in only 0.2 per cent. There may be evidence of septal fibrosis. Digestive tract involvement is revealed by radiologic studies in a patient with a suggestive history. Both the esophagus and colon are dilated, with abnormal peristalsis and evidence of retained food residues.

DIFFERENTIAL DIAGNOSIS. Romaña's sign must be distinguished from conjunctivitis, orbital cellulitis, cavernous sinus thrombosis, insect bites, and trauma, all of which produce unilateral orbital edema. Clinically the acute phase may resemble typhoid fever, infectious mononucleosis, kala-azar, brucellosis, toxoplasmosis, and acute glomerulonephritis. Other types of acute myocarditis must be considered.

Congenital infections must be distinguished from syphilis, toxoplasmosis, and cytomegalic inclusion disease.

Chronic cardiomyopathy involves a differential diagnosis from the cardiomyopathies associated with alcohol, pregnancy, idiopathic cardiomyopathy, endomyocardial fibrosis, and ischemic heart disease. The absence of organic valvular lesions usually permits a distinction from rheumatic valvular disease. Carcinoma of the esophagus may mimic megaesophagus. The presence of positive serology and electrocardiographic changes assist in the differential diagnosis from megaesophagus and megacolon not caused by Chagas' disease.

EVOLUTION AND PROGNOSIS. Chagas' cardiomyopathy is variable in its course and of uncertain prognosis. In the acute phase 10 per cent of patients die of myocarditis or acute meningoencephalitis. The latter condition usually occurs in children under one year of age. The indeterminate phase can last a lifetime. The factors influencing the evolution of the disease are not clear. There is some evidence that reinfections could play a role in an endemic area. The strain of parasite and the host's response to it could be important. Cardiomyopathy begins in the second to fifth decade. Heart failure in these age groups leads to death one to five years after its initial appearance. The prognosis is poor if cardiac failure appears before 30 years of age.

A longitudinal study in São Felipe, Brazil, showed that each year the disease made a detectable progression in 5.5 per cent of patients. The mortality was 0.7 per cent per year. The principal cause of death was cardiac failure in 58.3 per cent. Sudden death from conduction defects occurred in 37.5 per cent. The following electrocardiographic changes were associated with a 50 per cent mortality in five years: total atrioventricular block, atrial fibrillation, left bundle branch block, multifocal extrasystoles, and septal fibrosis.

TREATMENT. Two drugs appear to kill circulating trypanosomes and may have value in the specific treatment of Chagas' disease. These are nifurtimox, a nitrofuran derivative (Bayer 2502 [Lampit]), and benznidazole, a nitroimidazole (RO7–1051 Rochagan).

Nifurtimox* is used in a dose of 8 mg per kilogram of body weight per day for a period of 120 days. With regard to eradicating parasitemia, it has given good results in patients in the acute and chronic phases in Chile, Argentina, and southern Brazil. In other areas of Brazil, such as Bahia, Goiás, and Minas

*Available from Centers for Disease Control (404–329–3670); (404–329–2888) evenings, weekends, and holidays.

Gerais, the results have been less satisfactory, only 40 per cent of individuals being uniformly negative on repeated xenodiagnosis after treatment. Experiments in animals infected with different strains of *T. cruzi* demonstrated different susceptibilities to nifurtimox. This reinforces the hypothesis that different strains of *T. cruzi* may be responsible for these variations in response to treatment. Benznidazole* is used in a dose of 5 mg per kilogram per day for 60 days and also eradicates parasitemia in a proportion of patients. Both these drugs have serious side effects and should be used only under direct medical supervision. The side effects include polyneuritis, dizziness, loss of weight, nausea, and insomnia. With use of benznidazole, exfoliative dermatitis and thrombocytopenic purpura have also been seen.

It is not known how important such specific treatment is in arresting the disease. If parasitemia is an important factor in the evolution of the disease, then certainly the acute phase should be treated. In the acute phase, both serologic tests and xenodiagnosis may remain negative after treatment. In the chronic phase, those in whom xenodiagnosis becomes negative remain positive serologically. It is still not clear whether such treatment is of value in the chronic phase.

When chronic myocarditis is associated with heart failure, the treatment is symptomatic. Digitalis must be used with care because of sensitivity of the damaged cardiac fiber, and the response is poor in relation to other cardiomyopathies. Extrasystoles, the most frequent arrhythmia, may be helped by procainamide. In ventricular tachycardia, procainamide and lidocaine are the drugs indicated. Beta-adrenergic blocking agents are dangerous in acute arrhythmias in Chagas' myocarditis, as they may produce bradycardia and shock. Deaths have been reported after the use of propranolol. In Stokes-Adams crises, isopropyl norepinephrine is useful. In patients with total atrioventricular block and a normal or slightly enlarged heart, implantation of a pacemaker is indicated. Marked cardiac enlargement carries a poor prognosis, because either the weak cardiac muscle cannot support the new rhythm or an intramural clot may become dislodged.

Initially megaesophagus is treated by balloon dilatation; in more advanced cases cardiotomy is often successful. Operations consisting of excision of the aperistaltic esophagus and replacement with a segment of colon or small intestine have been developed. In megacolon, evacuation of a fecaloma may be an emergency procedure. It has to be carried out with care, for rupture of the colon and septicemia can follow the procedure. Resection of the aperistaltic segment may relieve persistent constipation.

PROPHYLAXIS. The important prophylactic measures in the control of Chagas' disease are better housing, public health education, and application of insecticides in the house and its environs. Benzene hexachloride (BHC), the insecticide of choice, is applied in a suspension of 500 mg of the gamma isomer per square meter every six months.

In blood banks in endemic areas of Chagas' disease, 1:4000 gentian violet is added to stored blood 24 hours before use in order to kill the trypanosomes. To date, no results that can be applied to humans have been obtained with immunoprotection for Chagas' disease.

---

*Available from Centers for Disease Control (404–329–3670); (404–329–2888) evenings, weekends, and holidays.

American Trypanosomiasis Research. PAHO Scientific Publication 318, 1975. *A monograph with extensive reviews of many aspects of research.*

Andrade Z, Andrade SG: Chagas' disease (American trypanosomiasis). *In* Marcial-Rojas RA (ed.): Pathology of Protozoal and Helminthic Disease. Baltimore, Williams & Wilkins Company, 1971. *An account of the pathology of Chagas' disease.*

Chagas C: Processos patojênicos da tripanosomiase americana. Memórias do Instituto Oswaldo Cruz 8:5, 1916. *A classic account demonstrating Carlos Chagas' remarkable insight into the disease he discovered.*

Köberle F: Patologia y anatomia patológica de la enfermedad de Chagas. Bol Sanit Panam 51:404, 1961. *A paper examining the role of parasympathetic denervation in the pathogenesis of megasyndromes and cardiopathy.*

Laranja FS, Dias E, Nóbrega G, Miranda A: Chagas' disease—a clinical epidemiologic and pathologic study. Circulation 14:1035, 1956. *One of the first satisfactory accounts of the clinical cardiology.*

Prata A, Andrade Z, Guimarães A: Chagas' heart disease. *In* Shaper AG, Hutt MSR, Fejfar Z (eds.): Cardiovascular Disease in the Tropics. London, British Medical Association, 1974. *A review of Chagas' heart disease.*

World Health Organization: Chagas' Disease: Report of a Study Group. Technical Report Series No 202, 1960. *The first report published before the current wave of interest.*

381. LEISHMANIASIS

Franklin A. Neva

DEFINITION. Leishmaniasis is a protozoan infection caused by various species of the genus *Leishmania*. Paradoxically, the host cells for these intracellular parasites are macrophages, the very cells normally involved in defense mechanisms. The natural cycle of infection is usually a zoonosis, with phlebotomine sandflies as vectors transmitting the parasite among wild or domestic animals, especially rodents and canines. Humans are generally incidental hosts.

The traditional view that all human leishmanial infections result in either visceral or cutaneous involvement needs modification. Visceral involvement when it happens represents a severe systemic disease with parasites invading the reticuloendothelial system, and is characterized by hepatosplenomegaly, fever, weight loss, leukopenia, and ultimately death. The cutaneous disease is manifested by one or more indolent, ulcerative lesions that can heal spontaneously, but sometimes the disease later produces metastatic destructive lesions of the oronasopharynx—i.e., mucocutaneous leishmaniasis. While these concepts of visceral and cutaneous prototypes are useful, it is now apparent that clinical leishmaniasis is a spectrum of manifestations, especially as it involves the skin. There is increasing evidence that the clinical outcome of leishmanial infection is determined by the interaction of intrinsic characteristics of the infecting organism with immune response of the host. Unfortunately, nomenclature and speciation of *Leishmania* are still uncertain because of development of new technologies for classification.

ETIOLOGY. *Leishmania* exist in two morphologic forms, a motile flagellate or *promastigote*, and a smaller, nonmotile intracellular form, the *amastigote*. Promastigotes are found in the sandfly vector as well as in artificial cultures, both habitats requiring temperatures of about 22 to 26° C. Amastigotes, the form of the parasite in humans and other vertebrate hosts, are round or oval bodies of about 2 × 5 μ, without a free flagellum. Also called *Leishman-Donovan* or *LD bodies* after their describers, amastigotes contain a nucleus and a characteristic rodlike structure of extranuclear DNA, the *kinetoplast*. When stained by Giemsa or Wright's, the nucleus is reddish, the kinetoplast purple, and the cytoplasm a pale blue.

In the infected animal, leishmania are found only in macrophages where they multiply by binary fission, rupture out, and infect new cells. An appropriate sandfly vector becomes infected by ingesting infected cells from the skin or blood during a blood meal. In the gut of the sandfly, the parasites transform to promastigotes and multiply as spindle-shaped flagellates of 15 to 25 μ length and 2 to 3 μ width. In vectors ultimately capable of transmitting the parasite, promastigotes tend to migrate to a higher level in the gut of the fly, even into the pharynx and buccal cavity. At least seven days are needed before the sandfly becomes infective. The actual mechanism by which infective promastigotes are transferred to a new vertebrate host is not clear—possibly by regurgitation into the bite wound during a blood meal or perhaps even being rubbed into abrasions after a successful swat. Once inoculated, the promastigotes are taken up by macrophages; they are transformed into amastigotes and begin to multiply. Amastigotes that rupture from infected macrophages are taken up by adjacent cells; some infected cells may be transported to distant sites via the blood or lymphatics.

Classification of *Leishmania* was previously determined mainly by geographic origin of the parasite, and the nature of disease produced in the hamster. *L. donovani* was associated with visceral disease and produced fatal hepatosplenic disease in hamsters. This behavior in the hamster was consistent, even with isolates from different regions of the world. Strains causing cutaneous disease in the Old World produced only modest cutaneous lesions in the hamster and were called *L. tropica*. The situation with cutaneous strains from the Americas was more complicated, with isolates broadly separable into two groups, the *L. mexicana* and *L. braziliensis* complexes. Rapidity of growth in culture was considered an additional criterion for these two groups. In recent years, biochemical taxonomy based upon isoenzyme patterns and DNA peptide mapping has permitted a more detailed grouping of strains. In addition, immunologic reactivity to monoclonal antibodies and to membrane shed antigens (EF factors) is being used. In the final analysis, the most meaningful taxonomy of leishmania will probably come from correlating these biochemical and immunologic findings with biologic characteristics of the organisms. For example, the course of infection in genetically defined mice and sensitivity to heat appear to be two very useful biologic criteria.

PARASITE-HOST INTERACTION. Studies of leishmania with host cells under various conditions *in vitro* have illuminated clinically relevant issues in the host-parasite interaction. First, promastigotes are rapidly lysed by fresh serum, by activating the classical complement pathway. They are also destroyed by polymorphonuclear leukocytes. Since promastigotes often meet the same fate when ingested by macrophages, infection would seemingly be difficult or impossible to initiate. This paradox now appears to be explained by the recent finding that stationary phase leishmania are more infective than log phase organisms, from cultures as well as in the sandfly. Interestingly, the intracellular amastigotes are more resistant than promastigotes to the oxidative response of macrophages. However, if macrophages are activated by exposure to specific or nonspecific lymphokines, they are then capable of destroying most species of amastigotes.

When leishmania are ingested by macrophages they are enclosed in a phagocytic vacuole, whose membranes subsequently fuse with lysosomal vacuoles. Presence of acid hydrolases on the amastigote surface membrane is one of the features that protects the parasite from being destroyed.

Variation in temperature sensitivity of various species of leishmania is another critical factor that determines clinical expression of the disease. For example, *L. donovani* can survive and multiply in macrophages at higher temperatures than cutaneous strains. Among isolates causing cutaneous disease in the Americas, some members of the *L. mexicana* complex are inhibited to a greater extent at 37° C than are strains of the *L. braziliensis* complex. These differences in temperature tolerance probably explain why some varieties of cutaneous leishmaniasis can be treated successfully by local heat.

IMMUNOLOGY. The pattern of humoral and cell-mediated immune responses that normally develops during or after leishmanial infection varies with the clinical form of disease. Serum antibody can be demonstrated by a variety of tests, usually indirect immunofluorescence (IFA) or enzyme-linked immunosorbent assay (ELISA) in patients with established visceral or cutaneous leishmaniasis. Cell-mediated immunity in leishmaniasis can be evaluated by a delayed hypersensitivity skin test (leishmanin test, or Montenegro test) or by lymphocyte proliferation to leishmanial antigen. Positive skin test results and lymphocyte proliferation are normally present in patients with cutaneous disease, but only after recovery or effective treatment in patients with visceral disease. Cell-mediated immunity is absent or suppressed during active visceral infections.

Resistance to leishmaniasis is best correlated with presence of cell-mediated immunity. Its absence in visceral disease has already been noted, and it is dramatically demonstrated in a rare form of disease called *diffuse cutaneous leishmaniasis* (DCL). In patients with DCL, not only is there specific anergy to the skin test but parasites are very abundant in lesions, whereas lymphocytes are scanty, lesions do not ulcerate, and response to chemotherapy is poor. Antigen specific suppressor cells have been demonstrated in DCL. In contrast, a normal immune response in cutaneous leishmaniasis is generally associated with lesions that ulcerate and show relatively few parasites and abundant lymphocytes and even giant cells, plus a positive skin test. Thus, it is helpful to compare the clinical forms of leishmaniasis with the spectrum of disease response in leprosy.

Jaffe CL, McMahon-Pratt D: Monoclonal antibodies specific for *Leishmania tropica*. J Immunol 131:1987, 1983. *One of a series of papers on monoclonals for differentiating species.*

Kreutzer RD: Identification of *Leishmania* spp. by multiple isozyme analysis. Am J Trop Med Hyg 32:703, 1983. *One of the other main techniques being used in biochemical taxonomy.*

Neal RA, Hale C: A comparative study of susceptibility of inbred and outbred mouse strains compared with hamsters to infection with New World cutaneous leishmaniasis. Parasitology 87:7, 1983. *This provides comparative information on mouse vs. hamster susceptibility to leishmanial species, and also recent references to the extensive literature on inbred mice in leishmanial work.*

Sacks DL, Perkins PV: Identification of an infective stage of leishmania promastigotes. Science 223:1417, 1984. *Clarifies a previously suspected critical issue—that the parasite is infective for cells in stationary but not in log phase of growth, in the fly as well as in culture.*

Turk JL, Bryceson ADM: Immunological phenomena in leprosy and related diseases. Adv Immunol 13:209, 1971. *Provides the clinical and experimental bases for regarding leishmaniasis as a disease spectrum.*

VISCERAL LEISHMANIASIS (Kala Azar)

EPIDEMIOLOGY. The visceral form of leishmaniasis, caused by *L. donovani* and related organisms, has a worldwide distribution. Certain regions continue to be endemic areas of this disease. These include the following: northeast India, especially Assam and Bihar states; Kenya, Sudan, and Ethiopia in east Africa; northeast China; the shores of the Caspian Sea and Iran in south Asia; the countries of Europe, North Africa, and the Middle East surrounding the Mediterranean; and northeast Brazil. In addition to these macrofoci, smaller foci outside these extensions occur. In the western hemisphere, for example, visceral leishmaniasis is sporadically seen in southern Brazil, Paraguay, and northern Argentina, as well as in the vicinity of Belem at the mouth of the Amazon. Additionally, there are foci of transmission in Venezuela and Colombia, and extending north into Central America with isolated cases reported from El Salvador, Guatemala, Honduras, and even from Mexico.

With such a wide geographic distribution of the disease, it is not surprising that different species of phlebotomine flies are involved in the various regions. What is surprising is that the causative organisms from these widely separated regions are relatively uniform in their properties. Yet some investigators prefer to assign separate species designations to the parasites from certain geographic foci, such as *L. infantum* for the Mediterranean variety and *L. chagasii* for that from Brazil. While up to now such species designations have been based partly upon epidemiologic grounds, they are likely to be upheld by more discriminating analyses in current use of isoenzyme patterns and DNA characteristics.

FACTORS AFFECTING TRANSMISSION. Since *L. donovani* is usually transmitted as a zoonosis, consideration must be given to the various factors favoring natural transmission, and the manner in which humans become involved in the cycle. Since phlebotomine sandflies have a limited flight range, humans must come into their habitat to become infected, or the vector and reservoir host must both live close to people. The latter condition is fulfilled when dogs are reservoir hosts. The domestic dog, as well as wild canines such as the fox, develop a chronic systemic disease very similar to that of humans when infected with *L. donovani*. But an additional unique feature of leishmanial infection in canines is the frequent presence of organisms in the skin, including the nose and ears, which are favorite feeding sites of sandflies. An epidemiologic cycle of the parasite involving wild foxes, domestic dogs, and humans via the vector *Lutzomyia longipalpis* has been documented in northeast Brazil. The domestic dog has also been incriminated as an important reservoir host for visceral leishmaniasis of the Mediterranean region and in certain areas of China.

Rodents such as the Nile rat (*Arvicanthus niloticus*) are the likely reservoir in the Sudan, and the activity of the vector, *P. orientalis,* is high in clumps of acacia woodland near villages. In Kenya transmission of disease is associated with termite hills, which serve as resting places for the vector, *P. martini,* and around which village men gather in the evening. However, the animal reservoir in Kenya has not been identified. In some regions such as in northeast India, humans appear to be their own reservoir, and several factors serve to facilitate person-to-person transmission. The vector, *P. argentipes,* has a preference for human blood. The parasite is found in circulating monocytes in Indian cases of kala azar more frequently than usual. An additional source of parasites for the vector are dermal lesions containing large numbers of parasites that develop after the initial disease in Indian patients.

The last few decades have seen a resurgence of visceral leishmaniasis in regions where it had disappeared after the widespread use of DDT for malaria control. Phlebotomine populations were greatly reduced around houses, but zoonotic transmission was not affected. When use of residual insecticides was discontinued, transmission to people was re-established. This has occurred in the countries around the Mediterranean, with an epidemic reported in western Italy.

Outbreaks of visceral leishmaniasis have often followed famine, wars, and civil or political disturbances resulting in malnutrition and mass migration of people. It is not known whether this is due to greater exposure to infected vectors, defective immune response, reactivation of latent infection, or a combination of these and other factors.

PATHOLOGY. The organs mainly affected are the liver, spleen, bone marrow, and elements of the reticuloendothelial system in diverse sites. These organs and tissues hypertrophy, with the increased cells made up of parasitized macrophages and histiocytes, but little or no lymphocytic response. Generalized enlargement of lymph nodes is not a consistent finding (see below), but hyperplasia of lymphoid tissue in the nasopharynx and in the Peyer's patches of the gut is common. Endothelial proliferation occurs in certain organs such as within septae of pulmonary alveoli and in renal glomeruli.

The spleen is enlarged, sometimes to tremendous size, but is firm and has a thick capsule. While the splenic pulp is friable and there may be infarcts, the nature and chronic course of the enlargement make the spleen relatively resistant to tears from an aspirating needle. Enlargement of the liver is due to hyperplasia of the Kupffer cells, which are packed with amastigotes. Only rarely are parenchymal cells of the liver parasitized. There may be focal granulomas in the liver, with some fibrosis in chronic untreated cases.

The bone marrow is infiltrated with parasitized macrophages. Red cell and white cell production are normal initially but may be impaired late in the disease as the bone marrow is replaced by parasitized macrophages. Even in early disease, however, the peripheral blood shows leukopenia and anemia. Both of these are due to pooling and destruction of cellular elements in the enlarged spleen. There is a striking polyclonal B cell activation that results in high IgG and total serum protein values.

Some organs, most notably the kidneys, may show pathologic changes secondary to deposition of immune complexes. Connective tissues of various organs exhibit deposition of hyaline substance, probably related to elevated serum protein levels, with a distribution similar to that of secondary amyloidosis.

In the early stages of visceral leishmaniasis small nodules in the skin containing parasites have been described at or near the site of inoculation. There are scattered reports of parasites being demonstrated even in apparently normal skin. A more obvious type of skin involvement, although variable by geographic location, is post–kala azar dermal leishmaniasis. This is the development in some patients after recovery from disease of subcutaneous nodules of varying size that contain large numbers of parasites. For unknown reasons the lesions do not ulcerate in spite of their heavy load of organisms; thus they resemble the entity of diffuse cutaneous leishmaniasis (see below).

CLINICAL FEATURES. The incubation period is long, generally one to three months, but it may be as short as 10 to 14 days. There are well documented instances of activation of latent infection several years after exposure to the parasite, under conditions of immunosuppression. The onset is usually insidious and difficult to date, especially among people who regard intermittent fevers and lassitude as normal. The course may continue gradually, with intermittent fevers becoming noticeable, accompanied by sweats, weakness, and weight loss. These symptoms, perhaps including nonproductive cough and abdominal discomfort produced by an enlarging liver and spleen, may continue for months with the patient still up and about. In some patients the course of disease is more rapid, with high fever and chills, simulating typhoid fever or acute brucellosis. The most prominent physical findings are fever, splenomegaly, and cachexia, which is especially evident in the thorax and shoulder girdle. While the fever pattern can be variable, ultimately it often exhibits characteristic twice daily elevations to 38 to 40° C for some time. Generalized adenopathy is common in patients in some geographic areas, but it is seldom striking. In light-skinned patients hyperpigmentation of the abdomen and extremities may be noted; the term *kala azar* is Hindi for "black sickness." Splenic enlargement can be extreme in this disease, often reaching the iliac fossa, and the organ is firm and nontender. Some otherwise typical cases may involve only modest splenomegaly. The liver is also firm and nontender but not invariably palpable or enlarged.

COURSE AND COMPLICATIONS. Although there is strong indirect evidence from skin tests and serologic results that spontaneous recovery from visceral leishmaniasis can occur, it probably happens only early in the course of infection. As the disease progresses, weight loss, anemia, and other signs become clinically more apparent. Subcutaneous edema, ascites, and other evidences of hypoalbuminemia may develop. Bleeding from the nose or gums can occur. Finally, after a illness that may be as short as a few months or as long as a year, the patient becomes emaciated and exhausted. In the great majority of instances death is due to intercurrent infections such as pneumonia, tuberculosis, dysentery, and gangrenous stomatitis. Advanced cases are particularly susceptible because of leukopenia and undoubted impairment of cell-mediated immunologic function, although specific mechanisms have not been defined. Another cause of death is massive gastrointestinal bleeding.

Post–Kala Azar Dermal Leishmaniasis. As noted earlier, a small percentage of patients, after treatment or spontaneous recovery, develop skin lesions containing parasites. This is fairly common in India, less common in Africa, and quite rare in Brazil. The lesions begin as a hypopigmented or erythematous macular rash soon or late after treatment and are often located on the face. When the dermal lesions persist they are likely to become papular or nodular, especially on the forehead, cheeks, and earlobes, and closely resemble lepromatous leprosy. This syndrome combines clinical and parasitologic features of relapse of the visceral infection and a type of skin involvement seen in diffuse cutaneous leishmaniasis. Unfortunately, detailed assessment of immune response is not yet available in post–kala azar dermal leishmaniasis.

SPECIFIC LABORATORY DIAGNOSIS. Since other clinical states may mimic certain features of visceral leishmaniasis, demonstration of the parasite, preferably by culture, is essential before treatment is undertaken. In addition, presence or absence of the parasite can be used to monitor response to treatment. Organisms are most readily recovered by aspiration from bone marrow, spleen, liver, lymph nodes, or blood. Material obtained is:

1. Used to make thin smears on a slide, dried, fixed and stained with Giemsa or some other Romanovsky stain for examination under oil immersion for amastigotes. Parasitized macrophages often rupture on smearing so free parasites usually are present. Bone marrow aspiration is the method of choice because adequate material can be obtained. Splenic puncture in this disease is safe if the spleen is readily palpable below the costal margin, if prothrombin and bleeding times are normal, and if proper technique is used. A 21-gauge needle on a 10-ml syringe is inserted quickly; suction is applied and withdrawn in less than a second. The main disadvantage of splenic puncture is the small amount of material obtained, which must be kept sterile for dilution and culture after a few smears are made. Aspirates of lymph nodes are done similarly, but yield of positive results is much less than with bone marrow or spleen. Biopsies of either liver or lymph nodes could provide more material for culture. Buffy coat preparations of peripheral blood are seldom positive except in India.
2. Inoculated into NNN (Novy-MacNeal-Nicolle) medium, a blood agar slant made with 30 per cent defibrinated rabbit blood and overlaid with a liquid phase of balanced salt solution containing antibiotics (not amphotericin or Mycostatin). Schneider's insect culture medium containing 30 per cent fetal bovine serum (FBS) may be just as effective as NNN but can vary with strains and lots of FBS. Cultures are incubated at 22 to 25° C (not 37° C) and a few drops of material can be removed and examined fresh for motile promastigotes at intervals. A positive culture will usually show organisms within 10 to 14 days, but this may require up to 30 days.
3. Hamsters are very susceptible to *L. donovani* and can be inoculated. However, it may require three or four months before organisms are demonstrable in their liver or spleen, so this method is not very practical.

IMMUNOLOGIC TESTS. By the time patients with visceral leishmaniasis come to clinical attention they invariably have readily demonstrable antileishmanial serum antibodies. Although the IFA test with amastigotes as antigen has had the longest use, it now appears that ELISA using promastigotes for antigen is just as reliable and more practical. The ELISA test can be read visually if necessary, and has advantages for testing large numbers of sera, including eluted blood specimens collected in the field onto filter paper. Direct agglutination of fixed promastigotes is another test that can be used, but it requires treatment of serum samples to eliminate cross-reacting IgM and is not as specific as other tests. Serum from individuals infected with *Trypanosoma cruzi* will cross-react with leishmanial antigens; this is a problem only in certain areas of Latin America. The leishmanin skin test for delayed hypersensitivity is negative in cases of active visceral leishmaniasis but becomes positive after recovery. A low frequency of positive leishmanin reactors among certain populations residing in endemic areas but without a history of visceral leishmaniasis is generally interpreted as evidence for inapparent infections or spontaneous cures of the disease. Some investigators attribute otherwise unexplained positive leishmanin skin tests to human infections with nonpathogenic species of leishmania.

LABORATORY FINDINGS. Most of the laboratory abnormalities involve the hematopoietic system. Leukopenia, with absolute reductions in neutrophils and eosinophils and a relative increase in lymphocytes and monocytes, is characteristic. In one series the total white cell count was below 4000 in 90 per cent of cases by one month after onset of symptoms, and it frequently may be around 2000 or less per cu mm. Thrombocytopenia is also present, and the sedimentation rate is increased. A moderately severe normocytic and normochromic anemia, unless complicated by blood loss or deficiency states, is very common, caused by increased red cell destruction. In late stages of the disease prothrombin, bleeding, and clotting times are prolonged.

Total serum proteins are increased to levels of 9 to 10 grams per deciliter, virtually all IgG, because of polyclonal B cell activation. Serum albumin levels, especially in advanced cases, are normal or low. The striking hyperglobulinemia is the basis for the old recommended diagnostic tests, such as the formol-gel and Chopra reaction, before specific serodiagnosis was available. Evidence for circulating immune complexes, based upon C1q binding in the serum, is readily demonstrable. Liver function tests show only mild abnormalities, if any.

DIFFERENTIAL DIAGNOSIS. Chronic malaria in endemic regions may present some problems in differential diagnosis. In malaria-immune individuals the presence of malaria parasites in the blood does not rule out the additional diagnosis of leishmaniasis. Conversely, an enlarged spleen is hardly enough on which to base the diagnosis. Tropical splenomegaly syndrome (an exaggerated immune response to malaria) easily could be confused with the clinical picture of visceral leishmaniasis. Several different forms of schistosomiasis may also mimic visceral leishmaniasis; the acute disease with fever and hepatosplenomegaly, the severe chronic variety with Symmers' fibrosis and portal hypertension, and chronic relapsing enteric fever that can be a complication of schistosomiasis. Other diseases that may resemble kala azar include lymphoma, cirrhosis of the liver with hypersplenism, miliary tuberculosis, brucellosis, typhoid fever, and subacute bacterial endocarditis.

TREATMENT. The drug of choice for treatment has been and remains pentavalent antimony, even with novel approaches to possible use of other drugs. The antimony preparation available in the United States (from Centers for Disease Control, 404-329-3670, 8:00 A.M. to 4:30 P.M. EST Monday through Friday; 404-329-2888, evenings, weekends, and holidays) and some European countries is sodium stibogluconate (Pentostam), a preparation containing 100 mg antimony (Sb) per ml. The dose is 0.1 to 0.2 ml per kilogram of body weight, given daily by intramuscular or intravenous injection, not exceeding 1000 mg Sb per day. Another pentavalent antimony preparation used in Latin America, meglumine antimonate (Glucantime), is virtually identical but contains 85 mg Sb per ml. Children with this disease require more Sb than adults, and the total dosage required for cure varies in different parts of the world. In India ten daily doses are usually adequate, while the disease in Kenya requires 30 injections, and up to 30 per cent of cases may still relapse within six months. Pentavalent antimony is relatively nontoxic in comparison to the trivalent Sb, except for local pain at the injection site when given intramuscularly. Other side effects are cumulative with dose and include nausea, vomiting, slight elevation of liver enzyme values, and nonspecific T wave changes if electrocardiograms are taken.

Response to treatment is not dramatic and may not be apparent for several weeks. Useful indicators to follow are temperature, spleen size, hemoglobin, and white blood count. Weekly splenic aspirates were used by one group, with "cure" defined as two successively negative aspirates a week apart. Since relapse may occur up to a year after apparent cure, monthly follow-up for six months and then after a year is recommended.

Primary unresponsiveness to Sb, that is, little or no improvement during or after the first course, occurs in up to 10 per cent of cases. Resistance of *L. donovani* to Sb can be induced experimentally but has not been documented to occur in humans. Second-line drugs for unresponsive or relapsed patients are pentamidine or amphotericin B. The dose of pentamidine* is 4 mg per kilogram given intramuscularly three times weekly for ten doses, but severe pain at the injection site is common and sterile abscess formation can occur. Additional systemic side effects of anorexia, nausea, abdominal pain, hypotension, and development of diabetes in 10 per cent make the decision to use pentamidine a difficult one. The other second-line drug, amphotericin B, must be given intravenously on alternate days at 1 mg per kilogram each time over many weeks in order to achieve the recommended 1.5 to 2.0 gram total dosage. This drug regularly produces chills, fever, and nausea with each dose and a cumulative reduction of hemoglobin and renal function. New approaches to treatment include use of allopurinol or its derivatives and incorporation of drugs

*Available from Centers for Disease Control, Atlanta, GA.

in liposomes for more efficient and prolonged uptake by macrophages.

Supportive treatment can be very important, especially in the malnourished and debilitated. These patients are prone to develop complicating bacterial infections for which proper treatment must be instituted. Fluid and electrolyte balance must be corrected, and hemorrhagic complications may require blood transfusion. Good nursing care, attention to oral hygiene, adequate diet and correction of nutritional deficiencies are, of course, desirable.

PREVENTION. Since the epidemiology of kala azar varies between different geographic areas, the local conditions responsible for transmission must be understood in order to implement preventive measures. Where sandflies are in or around houses, vector control with insecticides is appropriate. If an animal reservoir such as the domestic dog is involved, destruction of infected dogs, especially strays, can be instituted. If focal sites of infected flies are known, they can be destroyed or avoided. Personal protection by wearing protective clothing in the evenings, use of insect repellents, and sleeping under fine mesh netting is applicable under some circumstances.

Chulay JD, Bhatt SM: A comparison of three dosage regimens of sodium stibogluconate in the treatment of visceral leishmaniasis in Kenya. J Infect Dis 148:148, 1983. *Report by a group with extensive experience in use of Pentostam. They used it in much larger doses than did others.*

Kager PA, Rees PH: Splenic aspiration; experience in Kenya. Trop Georg Med 35:125, 1983. *Report on large experience with this procedure in diagnosis of kala azar and response to treatment. Same tissue has review of literature on same topic.*

Most H, Lavietes PK: Kala azar in American military personnel. Medicine 26:221, 1947. *A classic paper, still one of the best on clinical aspects.*

CUTANEOUS LEISHMANIASIS OF THE OLD WORLD (ORIENTAL SORE) AND NEW WORLD INCLUDING MUCOCUTANEOUS OR ESPUNDIA

EPIDEMIOLOGY. Although basically the same disease, there are differences in epidemiology and clinical course in cutaneous leishmaniasis of the Old and New Worlds. In the Mediterranean basin, Middle East, and Southern Asia the disease tends to be clinically more benign and occurs in semiarid and desert climates; transmission can become established in villages and cities. Cutaneous leishmaniasis in the Americas is acquired by workers in the jungle or by farmers and their families living at its edges. The New World disease sometimes produces later metastatic and destructive lesions of the mucous membranes.

The epidemiology of cutaneous leishmaniasis is best understood in South Russia, Iran, and Middle Eastern countries where infected desert rodents (*Rhombomys opimus* and *Psammomys obesus*) live in burrows with phlebotomine vectors (often *P. papatasi*). People are infected with *L. tropica major* when they invade this environment to establish settlements, exacavate archaeologic ruins, or make war. If settlements are established, the parasite is likely to become involved in a new transmission cycle with dogs and humans as reservoirs and an urban sandfly such as *P. sergenti* as vector. Parasite species from such locations are often identified as *L. tropica*. The commonness of typical facial scars in adults in Iran, Afghanistan, Syria, and Iraq indicates the high frequency of cutaneous leishmaniasis in these countries.

The epidemiology of cutaneous leishmaniasis in West Africa and the sub-Sahara belt is less clear. Human cases are sporadic, with a rural transmission cycle, and the parasite species is often *L. tropica major*. In Ethiopia and Kenya, however, the animal reservoir is often the hyrax (*Procavia*), the vector is *P. longipes*, and the parasite species is *L. aethiopica*.

In the Americas cutaneous leishmaniasis occurs from Texas to northern Argentina, with only Chile free of the disease. Except for some areas of Peru, where the domestic dog is a reservoir, New World cutaneous leishmaniasis is a forest or jungle zoonosis with forest rodents or sloths serving as animal reservoirs. Western hemisphere sandfly vectors are now classified as members of the genus *Lutzomyia*.

The organism in Mexico and northern central America is classified as *L. mexicana mexicana*, an organism that does not produce mucocutaneous disease. The predominant organisms in the remainder of Central America, Panama, and northern South America are members of the *L. braziliensis* complex. These are considered capable of causing late mucous membrane involvement. Mucocutaneous leishmaniasis is generally believed to be associated with *L. braziliensis braziliensis*, occurring commonly in central Brazil, Bolivia, and tropical regions of Peru. However, this association of leishmanial species with clinical types of disease and with geographic distribution is still provisional. For example, a number of isolates of *L. b. braziliensis* have recently been reported from Belize, where *L. mexicana* was supposed to predominate, and members of the *L. mexicana* complex (*L. m. amazonensis*) have been recovered from classic mucous membrane lesions. It is likely that additional members of the two major complexes will be described as the newer methods of taxonomy are applied.

PATHOLOGY. The earliest changes at the site of inoculation have not been described. Established lesions show a large accumulation of macrophages containing amastigotes, with variable numbers of lymphocytes and plasma cells. There may be focal accumulations of polymorphonuclear cells, especially in areas of necrosis, but the exact mechanism for ulceration of the epithelium is not clear. With time, numbers of parasites diminish and the lesion heals. In other instances the lesion persists and a tuberculoid histologic reaction is seen with granulomas including multinucleated giant cells. This is the type of pathology seen in *chronic relapsing cutaneous leishmaniasis*, also known as the *lupoid* or *recidiva* form. Delayed skin test reactivity to leishmanial antigen is present in normally healing and recidiva leishmaniasis.

The unusual complication known as diffuse cutaneous leishmaniasis (DCL), associated with anergy to leishmanial antigen, has a different histologic picture. DCL lesions show a heavy infiltrate of foamy or vacuolated macrophages containing large numbers of amastigotes with only scant numbers of lymphocytes. Moreover, the overlying epithelium is not ulcerated.

The lesions of mucocutaneous leishmaniasis represent metastatic spread of organisms via the bloodstream to mucous membranes of the nose, mouth, and upper pharyngeal tissues. The histology is a confusing mixture of granulomatous inflammatory cell reaction with necrosis, fibrosis, and often response to secondary bacterial infection. Organisms are usually scanty. Tissue destruction involves cartilage with perforation of the nasal septum, loss of much of the nose and palate, and even involvement of the larynx.

CLINICAL MANIFESTATIONS. The lesion begins as a small erythematous papule on exposed areas, often the face or extremities, within two to eight weeks after infection. The papule may develop a tiny vesicle that opens and oozes some serous fluid and enlarges to several centimeters, with firm, raised, and reddened edges. The ulcer can remain relatively dry with a central crust (dry form) or may ooze (wet form). Lesions can be single or multiple; small satellite papules may occur at the edge of a larger lesion. Subcutaneous nodules in a centripetal alignment from an ulcer may develop (sporotrichoid form). Cutaneous leishmanial lesions will generally heal spontaneously, but the process can take a few months to a year or more. The result is a depressed, depigmented scar. *Recidiva* or *lupoid leishmaniasis* may sometimes develop, persisting for years. This lesion exhibits central healing with papules developing in the periphery or center of the scar. Regional adenopathy may or may not occur with cutaneous leishmaniasis; this finding is not helpful in differential diagnosis.

COMPLICATIONS. Metastatic spread of parasites and development of destructive naso-oropharyngeal lesions is a serious later sequel to cutaneous disease. This mucous membrane involvement occurs almost exclusively in the western hemisphere and is said to be associated primarily with *L. braziliensis*

braziliensis infections. Mucocutaneous disease due to *L. mexicana amazonensis* does occur, so until more data correlating parasite type with clinical disease are available, this complication can be equated with geographic region rather than parasite species. Thus, mucocutaneous leishmaniasis is most common in central Brazil and adjacent portions of Bolivia, Peru, and Ecuador, and relatively uncommon in Panama and Central America, for example. Mucosal involvement generally does not become manifest until the initial skin lesion has healed, even many years later, and presumably is more likely to occur if there has been no or inadequate treatment of the original ulcer.

Earliest signs and symptoms of mucosal disease commonly involve the nose, with epistaxis and obstruction. Perforation of the nasal septum is common, or the upper lip may be involved. The process can destroy cartilaginous structures of the nose and palate and extend to the larynx. Death may result from aspiration pneumonia or suffocation. Distinction should be made between the mucous membrane involvement that occurs as direct extension from a facial lesion, as in Ethiopia, and the late metastatic form seen in South America.

Diffuse cutaneous leishmaniasis (DCL) is a rare complication that offers insight into immunity to leishmaniasis because it features antigen-specific anergy and cell-mediated immunosuppression. DCL seems to occur more commonly in certain countries (Dominican Republic, Venezuela, and Ethiopia), and in the Americas is caused by organisms belonging to the *L. mexicana* complex. The disease begins with one or only a few nodular lesions that do not ulcerate but go on to metastasize to other cutaneous sites, primarily the face and extensor surfaces of the limbs. The subcutaneous nonulcerative nodular lesions are not associated with fever or other systemic symptoms and do not involve visceral organs. The appearance, distribution, and chronic nature of DCL has often led to the erroneous diagnosis of lepromatous leprosy. There is no mortality associated with DCL, but disfigurement and ulceration secondary to trauma at pressure points lead to morbidity, since this disease is notoriously unresponsive to the usual antileishmanial drugs.

DIAGNOSIS. Leishmaniasis can be suspected in anyone who develops one or more chronic ulcers on exposed areas of skin after recently visiting or working at archaeologic sites in the Middle East, at Mayan ruins, or in jungle or rural areas of Latin America. Ideally, diagnosis should be confirmed by culture of the organism in NNN or other appropriate media from a biopsy or aspirated specimen obtained from the edge of the lesion. Culture is the most sensitive method for detection of organisms. Excisional or punch biopsy offers an additional advantage of providing a portion of the specimen for histopathologic examination and routine bacteriologic, fungal, and acid-fast cultures in cases in which a wider differential diagnosis is required. Appropriate impression smears can also be made and stained from biopsied material, whether culture is possible or not. If biopsy is not possible because of circumstances or location of the lesion, scrapings from a slit made in involved skin or from the debrided base of an ulcer can be cultured or stained for organisms. The characteristic amastigotes in lesions appear larger and are more easily recognized in smears than in tissue sections. A recent technique that may permit direct and rapid species differentiation of leishmania, as well as diagnosis, is blotting with radiolabeled DNA probes. Numbers of parasites present and ease of culture vary with the strain, but the concentration of parasites in lesions tends to diminish with time as healing occurs, and they are also reduced if the ulcer is secondarily infected with bacteria. It is also usually difficult to culture or demonstrate organisms in the late lesions of mucocutaneous disease.

A positive leishmanin skin test and serum antibody can usually be demonstrated in patients by the time a cutaneous lesion has ulcerated. These tests remain positive in mucocutaneous disease. The most reliable serologic tests are the ELISA with promastigote antigen and indirect immunofluorescence with amastigote antigen. Cross-reactions with leishmanial antigens do occur in individuals with *Trypanosoma cruzi* infection and previous kala azar. It must also be remembered that positive skin and serologic tests can reflect a previous rather than a current leishmanial infection.

Cutaneous leishmaniasis must be differentiated from the following conditions, with decreasing likelihood of occurrence: nonspecific tropical or traumatic ulcers due to bacterial infection or stasis; fungal infections, especially sporotrichosis and blastomycosis; mycobacterial infections such as *M. marinum* and tuberculosis; syphilis and other treponematoses of the skin; sarcoidosis and neoplastic ulcers. Mucocutaneous leishmaniasis is especially likely to mimic infection with *Paracoccidiodes brasiliensis*, histoplasmosis, Wegener's mid line granuloma, or rhinoscleroma.

TREATMENT. As described earlier for visceral leishmaniasis, the standard and recommended treatment for cutaneous leishmaniasis is pentavalent antimony, available in the U.S. as Pentostam.* The dose is 0.1 to 0.2 ml per kilogram by intramuscular or slow intravenous injection, not exceeding 10 ml per dose. The drug is given daily for 10 to 15 days. Modest elevation of liver enzymes and/or mild nonspecific ST or T wave electrocardiographic changes may occur during therapy, especially after six or eight doses. These changes are generally not associated with symptoms, but it may be prudent to monitor them.

Old World cutaneous leishmaniasis, especially in patients from the Middle East, will often heal spontaneously within six months. Since leishmaniasis in this region does not metastasize to mucosal tissues, treatment may justifiably be withheld if the lesion is not extensive and appears to be healing.

In contrast, if the infection is known or suspected to originate from an endemic area of mucocutaneous disease, some authorities recommend that three courses of pentavalent antimony treatment be given for a cutaneous lesion. The possibility of later mucous membrane involvement, usually manifested by nasal obstruction and/or epistaxis, should be explained to the patient so that medical attention will be sought.

Regardless of the infecting species of parasite, it is not unusual for cutaneous leishmanial lesions to require a second course of antimony treatment. Two weeks of rest are generally allowed between courses of treatment. Although different strains of leishmania can vary in their susceptibility to antimony, naturally occurring resistance is very unusual. Yet the circumstances required to eliminate the organisms from a lesion are not fully understood, and probably a normal immunologic response on the part of the host is required.

Amphotericin B is indicated in cases in which antimonials have failed to control the disease. Side effects are severe and common. The effective total dose is lower than for many systemic mycoses, with a total dose of 1.5 to 2.0 grams for a 60 kilogram adult often being sufficient.

A number of other drugs with varying degrees of antileishmanial activity may be useful in treatment under certain circumstances. Cycloguanil pamoate,† an injectable repository, is moderately effective and popular among workers in camps who cannot afford to spend 10 to 15 days away from a distant workplace. Orally administered drugs such as rifampin, metronidazole, and ketoconazole have been touted on the basis of uncontrolled trials in a few patients, but they are clearly inferior to antimony. Innovative new approaches to therapy are under way with allopurinol analogues, liposome-encapsulated compounds, and even topically applied drugs; their ultimate usefulness remains to be established. The application of local heat (40 to 41° C) for 25 hours or more over a period of four or five days may be effective for lesions caused by the *L. mexicana* complex organisms.

PREVENTION. Transmission of leishmaniasis in cities can be prevented by control of sandfly populations with insecticides

---

*Available from Centers for Disease Control, Atlanta, GA.
†Investigational drug in the United States.

or destruction of breeding sites. Where reservoirs and vectors are sylvatic, other measures must be employed, such as insect repellents and use of protective clothing over exposed parts of the body. Vaccines should theoretically be effective since there is immunity to second episodes of cutaneous disease. However, the effectiveness of immunization with either viable or killed organisms has been difficult to evaluate.

Lainson R: The American leishmaniasis: Some observations on their ecology and epidemiology. Trans Roy Soc Trop Med Hyg. 77:569, 1983. *Perhaps heavier on taxonomy of parasites than justified, but excellent overview by a world's expert in ecology of this disease.*

Marsden PD, Nonata RR: Mucocutaneous leishmaniasis: A review of clinical aspects. Rev Soc Bras Med Trop 9:309, 1975. *This is a very good article, in English, with emphasis on Brazilian experience.*

Neva FA: Diagnosis and treatment of cutaneous leishmaniasis. *In* Remington JS and Swartz MN (eds.): Current Clinical Topics in Infectious Diseases. Vol. 3. New York, McGraw-Hill Book Company, 1982, p 364. *More detailed account of these aspects of the subject.*

Petersen EA, Neva FA: Specific inhibition of lymphocyte proliferation responses by adherent suppressor cells in diffuse cutaneous leishmaniasis. N Engl J Med 306:387, 1982. *Documentation of a basic immunologic defect in the diffuse cutaneous disease.*

382. TOXOPLASMOSIS

Henry Masur

Toxoplasmosis is a common disease of birds and mammals caused by the protozoon *Toxoplasma gondii.* The name *T. gondii* is descriptive of this arc-shaped protozoon, being derived from the Greek word *toxon,* meaning arc, and from the name of the North African rodent *gondi,* in which the organism was first recognized. *T. gondii* currently infects over 500 million humans around the world. This obligate intracellular organism can proliferate readily and cause clinically important disease in individuals with normal or abnormal immune function. A clear distinction must be kept in mind between *T. gondii* infection, which is defined by the presence of viable organisms in a patient, and toxoplasmosis, a relatively uncommon occurrence that indicates an active disease process.

HISTORY. In 1907 Nicolle and Manceaux first recognized this organism in the gondi. The first human case of congenital infection was described by Janku in Prague. The parasite was initially isolated from a case of congenital disease by Wolf, Cowen, and Paige in 1938. Three years later Pinkerton and Henderson recognized the first case of disease in adults. Frenkel subsequently suggested that retinochoroiditis might be caused by *Toxoplasma;* Wilder confirmed such an association in 1952. Epidemiologic studies over the last 40 years by Feldman, Jacobs, Thalhammer, and Desmonts led to the recognition that the infection is very common in most parts of the world including the United States. In 1967 Hutchison suggested that the cat played an important role in the life cycle of *T. gondii.* Subsequently, Wallace proved that there is a sexual cycle in the cat intestine that produces a newly recognized form, the *oocyst.* This provides an important link that explains the frequency of this infection in certain populations.

THE PROTOZOAN. Three forms exist in the life cycle of *T. gondii:* the *cyst,* the *trophozoite,* and the *oocyst.* The trophozoite has an arc or oval form and is about 3 to 4 μ in diameter and 6 to 7 μ in length. It is an obligate intracellular form that proliferates in acute infection. Trophozoites can enter vacuoles in any nucleated mammalian cell. They divide by endodyogeny, an asexual process whereby two daughter cells are formed within one parent cell. Division continues until the cell ruptures, releasing trophozoites to infect adjacent cells. As the host develops immunity, trophozoite proliferation slows.

Toxoplasma cysts are 10 to 200 μ forms that contain several thousand 'very slowly dividing organisms; these appear to develop within host cells. Cysts can be seen in any tissue, but they are most commonly found in brain, skeletal muscle, and cardiac muscle. Cysts are more resistant to environmental conditions than are trophozoites, and are able to remain viable after exposure to digestive enzymes.

Oocysts are 10 to 12 μ oval forms that exist uniquely in the intestinal mucosa of cats. Toxoplasma released from cysts or oocysts in the cat intestine enter epithelial cells where they proliferate and then mature by gametogony into micro- or macrogametocytes. A zygote is formed by the union of the gametocytes; this zygote matures in one to four days into an oocyst. Large quantities of oocysts (up to 10 million per day) are excreted by the cat for one to three weeks beginning three to five days after ingestion of the *Toxoplasma*-containing tissue. Cats also get a concurrent systemic infection. Oocysts are not infectious until they undergo sporogony outside the body, a process that requires 1 to 21 days depending on environmental conditions. Oocysts are quite hardy: they can exist outside the body for at least a year in warm moist soil. *Toxoplasma*-infected cats will probably excrete oocysts for a brief period when they are rechallenged orally with *Toxoplasma.*

EPIDEMIOLOGY. *Toxoplasma* infection is a world-wide zoonosis. Natural infection occurs by ingestion of cysts or oocysts and by transplacental transmission. In nature the cycle of infection is probably maintained by cats and birds and small mammals. Primary human infection usually occurs by accidental ingestion of infected cat feces or by consumption of inadequately cooked meat. The relative importance of these primary routes probably depends on the amounts of rare meat consumed, hygienic practices, and the proximity of a feline population. When cats consume infected animals or inadequately cooked meat scraps they become infected and excrete oocysts. Children are particularly likely to come into contact with contaminated cat feces when playing in sand, or to inhale aerosolized dried feces under dusty conditions. Cockroaches and flies have also been shown to transfer oocysts to uncovered food.

In North America and Western Europe where many cats are confined to the home and eat only processed foods, and where food is usually covered and refrigerated, the consumption of rare meat is probably of greater epidemiologic importance than contact with cats or insects. Pork and lamb are more likely to contain cysts than is beef. If meat is not cooked to 60° C, or frozen to -20° C (a temperature not reliably reached by most commercial freezers), the cysts will be infective.

Toxoplasma has been transmitted rarely by needle stick accidents involving laboratory workers, by accidental inoculation during autopsy procedures, and by transplantation of an infected heart or kidney. Since some immunodeficient patients (particularly those with chronic myelogenous leukemia) have parasitemia, and since persistent parasitemia for a year has been described in an apparently healthy individual, blood products could be a source of infection. However, a healthy blood donor has never been documented to transmit *Toxoplasma* infection and in general blood product transmission seems to be a very rare event.

Secondary *Toxoplasma* infection can occur by transplacental transmission. Such transmission occurs only if the mother acquires *Toxoplasma* infection during the pregnancy or perhaps during the few months prior to conception. The frequency of congenital toxoplasmosis is thus dependent on the frequency with which women of childbearing age acquire *Toxoplasma* infection. In the United States and Europe 0.5 to 1 per cent of women show high or rising antitoxoplasma titers during pregnancy. About 40 per cent of these infections are transmitted to the fetus, the likelihood of transmission increasing progressively during successive trimesters of pregnancy from 17 to 65 per cent.

The frequency of *Toxoplasma* infection in any population depends on a variety of sociologic, economic, and environmental factors. Among both men and women there is increasing prevalence of positive serologic results with increasing age. In the United States less than 1 per cent of infants have congenital *Toxoplasma* infection; there is an abrupt rise in prevalence during teenage years; and from age 15 to 50 years there is an increase of approximately 1 per cent per year. Thus, about 20 to 70 per cent of adults in this country have positive serologic tests for *Toxoplasma* infection, the precise number depending on the specific population studied. Individuals in cold, arid, or mountainous regions tend to have a lower frequency than those in tropical areas. There are isolated communities that have little or no *Toxoplasma* infection. The regional variations cannot all be explained on the basis of meat eating habits, the presence of felines, or climatic extremes.

PATHOGENESIS AND PATHOLOGY. *Toxoplasma* are liberated from cysts or oocysts in the gastrointestinal tract where they multiply in the mucosal cells. Trophozoites then disseminate via the bloodstream or lymphatics to infect any nucleated host cell. Multiplication of the trophozoites within host cell vacuoles does not appear to disturb host cell function until the dividing organisms cause the cell to rupture. As adjacent cells are infected and they are themselves ruptured, progressive tissue necrosis occurs and an inflammatory response is elicited. The inflammatory response typically consists of mononuclear cells, a few polymorphonuclear cells, and edema. How extensive the tissue necrosis and dissemination become depends on the effectiveness of both humoral and cellular immune mechanisms. Although any organ can be involved, small foci of infection are most often established in lymph nodes, skeletal muscle, myocardium, and brain. Even after effective immunologic response the organisms are not eradicated: a few cysts form in these organs as early as the first week of infection and remain dormant for the lifetime of the host unless host immunity is diminished, in which case active proliferation of the organisms can again cause substantial local disease and dissemination. In some patients primary infection can be associated with widely disseminated disease: most of these patients have defects in cell-mediated immune mechanisms.

Histopathologically the changes in lymph nodes are so characteristic of toxoplasmosis that they are virtually diagnostic even in the absence of a visualized or cultivated organism. The lymph node shows reactive follicular hyperplasia with irregular clusters of epithelioid histiocytes. These histiocytes have vesicular nuclei and abundant eosinophilic cytoplasm; they encroach upon the germinal centers and obscure their margins. The germinal centers have many mitoses and many necrotic cells. Monocytoid cells produce focal distention of subcapsular and trabecular sinuses. Trophozoites or cysts are rarely seen in lymph nodes, although promptly performed cultures will grow the organism in many cases.

When other organs are involved, the pathologic findings can vary from a few isolated cysts to a marked inflammatory response associated with extensive necrosis. In skeletal muscle or brain an isolated cyst can be found unassociated with any inflammatory response or with any clinical manifestations of organ dysfunction. In patients with disseminated disease, however, the heart, brain, liver, spleen, kidney, pancreas, or other organs can manifest an intense inflammatory response surrounding areas of necrosis that can vary greatly in size. The inflammatory response consists of lymphocytes, plasma cells, and monocytes in association with edema. Perivascular mononuclear inflammatory changes are often seen contiguous to the necrotic areas. Intracellular and extracellular trophozoites are usually found in the periphery of the lesion rather than in the necrotic center.

In the central nervous system the necrotic lesions with margins of mononuclear cell infiltrate may be single or multiple. Periaqueductal and periventricular necrosis in congenital infection may lead to obstruction of the aqueduct of Sylvius or the foramen of Monro, resulting in obstructive hydrocephalus. The necrotic areas may ultimately calcify. In the eye, single or multiple necrotic lesions in the retina are the first manifestations of *Toxoplasma* infection. Mononuclear cell infiltrates are seen in association with cysts or trophozoites. Granulomatous inflammation occurs secondary to the necrotizing retinitis. The disease involves the posterior chamber almost exclusively and may be complicated by iridocyclitis, glaucoma, or cataracts.

In immunocompetent patients primary *Toxoplasma* infection is associated with both a humoral and cellular immune response. Antibodies against various *Toxoplasma* antigens can be detected in the blood. Subsequently, lymphocytes become responsive to *Toxoplasma* antigens and produce lymphokines. These lymphokines enable mononuclear phagocytes to inhibit *Toxoplasma* replication and to kill the intracellular organisms. Even immunocompetent individuals are not able to eliminate all *Toxoplasma* organisms from the body: cysts characteristically form in brain and muscle and remain viable for the lifetime of the host. Outside of the retina these cysts do not cause disease unless host immune function is altered.

CLINICAL MANIFESTATIONS. ***Acquired Toxoplasmosis in the Immunocompetent Individual.*** The vast majority of individuals who are infected with *T. gondii* after birth have no apparent clinical symptoms. In the small number of individuals with a symptomatic illness lymphadenopathy (90 per cent), fever (40 per cent), and malaise (40 per cent) are the common manifestations. The lymphadenopathy classically occurs symmetrically in the posterior auricular, anterior cervical, or posterior cervical chains. Generalized lymphadenopathy or localized unilateral enlargement or enlargement of a solitary node can also be seen. The nodes are characteristically rubbery and nontender. Splenomegaly occurs in about 30 per cent of patients. The fever is usually low grade but on occasion can be high, rapidly fluctuating, and prolonged. Fatigue can be a prominent feature. A minority of patients has a sore throat, maculopapular rash, myalgias, arthralgias, urticaria, or headache. The sore throat presents as hyperemia rather than as an exudative pharyngitis. Thus, for most patients with clinically apparent disease toxoplasmosis manifests as either asymptomatic lymphadenopathy or as a mild disorder associated with malaise, fever, and lymphadenopathy, which is self-limiting over a period of several weeks. Toxoplasmosis can, however, be a prolonged, severely debilitating disorder that may prevent the patient from working for many weeks or months. The lymph nodes may fluctuate in size during the recovery period.

In immunocompetent individuals specific organ involvement can lead to clinically significant disease involving the lungs, myocardium, pericardium, liver, skin, brain, and skeletal muscle. These manifestations may dominate the clinical picture. Glomerulonephritis has been reported. Death due to toxoplasmosis in immunocompetent individuals is an extremely unusual event.

Laboratory evaluation reveals a normal leukocyte count with a slight lymphocytosis or monocytosis. When atypical lymphocytes are present they are found only in small numbers. The hemoglobin is usually normal, although a Coombs-negative hemolytic anemia has occasionally been reported. Serum transaminases are rarely elevated to more than twice normal. The chest radiograph is usually normal; hilar adenopathy is unusual. On the electrocardiogram ST and T wave abnormalities may be seen if myocarditis is present.

Ocular Involvement in the Immunocompetent Individual. *Toxoplasma* has been estimated to cause 20 to 35 per cent of cases of retinochoroiditis in children and adults. This ocular disease is almost always a consequence of congenital infection: there are very few well documented cases of eye disease caused by infection acquired by adults.

Symptoms of retinochoroiditis are usually noted initially during the second or third decade of life. Symptoms and the degree of visual loss depend on the location and the extent of retinal involvement. Patients may complain of blurred vision, scotomas, pain, or epiphora. Strabismus may be an early sign in children. The lesions appear acutely as white or yellow cotton-like patches that have indistinct, elevated margins. Inflammatory exudate in the vitreous may obscure visualization of the fundus. As the lesions age they become atrophic with whitish-gray plaques, more distinct borders, and black spots of choroidal pigment. Lesions may be peripheral, but characteristically they occur near the posterior pole of the retina. They are usually multiple and vary in age, but single lesions do occur. Panuveitis and papillitis with optic atrophy can occur, especially in association with central nervous system disease.

Exclusively anterior uveitis has never been proven to be caused by toxoplasma.

Patients with *Toxoplasma* retinochoroiditis have an unpredictable clinical course. Episodes of active disease may occur once or many times but usually stop after the age of 40. Recurrent episodes are often associated with progressive loss of vision.

Toxoplasmosis in the Immunodeficient Patient. Toxoplasmosis can occur as a disseminated disease in patients with immunodeficiencies, particularly those with defects in cell-mediated immunity. The majority of patients are those with hematologic malignancies (particularly Hodgkin's disease), organ transplants, and the acquired immune deficiency syndrome (AIDS). The clinical manifestations are variable. Fever, hepatosplenomegaly, pneumonitis, maculopapular rash, myositis, myocarditis, meningoencephalitis, and central nervous system mass lesions may be seen. The lymphadenopathy characteristic of acquired disease in the immunocompetent patient is often absent. This syndrome is usually fulminant and rapidly fatal. It is very difficult to distinguish from numerous other infectious and noninfectious processes that can present in a similar fashion. The most common presentation includes central nervous system involvement in which fever, headache, confusion progressing to coma, and focal neurologic signs occur. Seizures and signs of increased intracranial pressure may be present. The cerebrospinal fluid shows nonspecific changes that usually include pleocytosis and moderately elevated protein, and normal glucose content. Computerized tomography usually shows one or more lesions that are contrast-enhancing in a ring or nodular pattern.

Toxoplasmosis has been serologically associated with progressive polymyositis. It is unclear whether the association reflects the etiology of the muscular disorder or whether the disorder activates *Toxoplasma* infection. A few patients with polymyositis and high antitoxoplasma antibody titers have responded symptomatically to antitoxoplasma therapy.

Congenital Disease. Congenital toxoplasmosis is the result of acute infection acquired by the mother just before or during gestation. These *Toxoplasma* infections acquired by the mother are usually asymptomatic, as is *Toxoplasma* infection acquired by other immunocompetent hosts, and thus there is nothing to make the mother or her physician suspicious unless serologic testing is routinely performed. The likelihood that the fetus will become infected and the severity of the congenital infection are largely dependent on when during the gestation the infection is acquired. In cases in which the infection occurs late during gestation or involves very few organisms, the infant will probably have no clinical manifestations but will have positive humoral and cellular immune responses to *Toxoplasma*. Although the infant is asymptomatic, *Toxoplasma* trophozoites may continue to replicate after birth, causing more damage. Cysts of *Toxoplasma* will persist in the retina, brain, myocardium, and/or skeletal muscle for the infant's lifetime. If the infant remains immunocompetent during its lifetime, the only subsequent clinical manifestations that might occur are retinochoroiditis, which usually flares during the second or third decade of life; seizures; and mild retardation. In infants who are infected early during gestation or with large inocula, the clinical sequelae can be severe. Spontaneous abortion, stillbirth, and prematurity may result. The infant may be born with microophthalmia, microcephaly, seizures, cerebral calcifications, bilateral retinochoroiditis, rash, lymphadenopathy, pneumonitis, fever, or hepatosplenomegaly, which can result in severe incapacity. If the cerebral inflammatory response involves the aqueduct of Sylvius, hydrocephalus may result. Clinical manifestions of these complications may be apparent at birth or may become obvious several months later when the infant fails to reach normal milestones.

DIAGNOSIS. The diagnosis of toxoplasmosis can be based on serologic tests, lymph node histology, the demonstration of trophozoites in body tissues or fluids, or isolation of *T. gondii* from certain sites. Which diagnostic test is most appropriate depends on the clinical situation.

Serology. Measurement of antitoxoplasma antibody titers is the most commonly employed mechanism for diagnosing toxoplasmosis. The *Sabin-Feldman dye test* is a highly sensitive and highly specific dye exclusion test that uses live *T. gondii.* This test is the reference procedure with which other tests must be compared. The Sabin-Feldman dye test and the indirect fluorescent antibody (IFA) test give comparable titers: titers begin to rise one to two weeks after infection and reach a peak after two to eight weeks that is almost always ≥ 1:1000. Titers drift down slowly over several years and persist at low levels (1:16–1:64) for the patient's lifetime. The height of the initial peak does not correlate with severity of clinical disease. Sabin-Feldman dye test titers are positive at stable low levels in adults with reactivated ocular disease and in most immunoincompetent patients with disseminated toxoplasmosis. Titers in infants may be elevated because of passively transferred maternal antibodies. Sequential studies over four to six months must be performed to determine if the infant's titers are rising, suggesting that the infected infant is producing antibody, or if they are falling (usually by 50 per cent per month) and attributable to passively transferred maternal antibodies.

The IgM-fluorescent antibody (IgM-IFA) test is particularly useful for establishing recent *Toxoplasma* infection because titers appear early (as early as five days after infection) and disappear within several months. IgM-IFA tests have not been carefully standardized: the significance of specific titers needs to be evaluated by the laboratory performing the test. Detection of IgM antibodies by the double sandwich ELISA is more sensitive and specific than the IgM-IFA test but also has not been carefully standardized. The IgM-IFA titers are elevated in acute disease in immunocompetent individuals and in infants with congenital disease but are not elevated in adults with reactivated ocular disease or in most immunoincompetent individuals with disseminated toxoplasmosis.

The complement fixation test using soluble *Toxoplasma* antigen becomes positive three to six weeks after infection, rises for the succeeding two to eight months and falls to very low levels after one to two years. This test can be useful for documenting a titer rise in someone whose Sabin-Feldman dye test titer has already peaked and whose IgM-IFA or IgM-ELISA peak has already occurred, i.e., a patient whose infection occurred more than two to four months previously but less than six to eight months previously. Titers are often elevated in infants with congenital disease and in some immunologically abnormal patients with disseminated disease. Titers are not elevated in adults with reactivated ocular disease.

The indirect hemagglutination (IHA) test as performed in most laboratories measures antibodies that rise very late in the course of infection and persist for years. Titer rises occur so late that the test has very little clinical utility and is particularly poor for use as a screening device to identify pregnant women who have acquired *Toxoplasma* infection early during gestation and who might therefore elect abortion if still medically feasible. The indirect hemagglutination tests that are available in commercial kits are often poorly standardized and are therefore difficult to interpret.

False positive results are not known to occur with the Sabin-Feldman dye test. The IFA and IgM-IFA tests may produce false positive results if antinuclear antibody is present. Rheumatoid factor can also cause false positive IgM-IFA titers.

In summary, acute acquired toxoplasmosis is suggested serologically by Sabin-Feldman dye test or IFA titers ≥ 1:1000 and proven convincingly by the documentation of elevated IgM-IFA or IgM-ELISA titers, or the documentation of a two tube (or greater) titer rise in the Sabin-Feldman dye test, IFA test, complement fixation test, and perhaps the indirect hemagglutination test. Congenital toxoplasmosis in infants is documented by demonstrating elevated complement fixation or IgM-IFA titers, or by showing that Sabin-Feldman dye test or IFA titers are stable or rising over four to six months. Ocular toxoplasmosis or toxoplasmosis in the immunoincompetent host cannot be diagnosed with certainty by antibody testing: a negative Sabin-Feldman dye test or IFA test titer excludes *Toxoplasma* as a cause of the ocular disease.

Isolation of the Organism. *T. gondii* can be isolated from leukocytes, body fluids, or tissue by direct inoculation of the specimens subcutaneously or intraperitoneally into mice. The mice are then examined periodically for the presence of antibody to *Toxoplasma;* for the presence of trophozoites in the peritoneum; or for the presence of cysts in the brain. The isolation of *Toxoplasma* from leukocytes or body fluids is convincing evidence of acute infection, although parasitemia persisting for a year has been described. The isolation of *Toxoplasma* from tissue does not provide convincing evidence of acute infection because a tissue cyst may have been present for many years and may thus be irrelevant to the disease process active at the time of biopsy. *Toxoplasma* isolation requires several weeks to perform and is not a rapid diagnostic technique.

Histologic Diagnosis. The histologic findings in the lymph nodes of patients with acute toxoplasmosis, described earlier, are so characteristic as to be diagnostic. The inflammatory reaction in other tissues is much less specific diagnostically. In these other tissues free or intracellular trophozoites must be demonstrated for the diagnosis of toxoplasmosis to be established. The demonstration of *Toxoplasma* cysts proves that the patient was infected by *T. gondii* at some time in the past but does not document that the current clinical disease is related.

DIFFERENTIAL DIAGNOSIS. The differential diagnosis of a patient with lymphadenopathy includes lymphoma, Hodgkin's disease, acquired immune deficiency syndrome (AIDS), sarcoidosis, mycobacterial disease, cytomegalovirus disease, mononucleosis, brucellosis, tularemia, cat scratch disease, and many other infectious processes. Toxoplasmosis can be distinguished from mononucleosis by the absence of atypical lymphocytosis, exudative pharyngitis, elevated serum transaminases, and heterophile antibodies. Appropriate serologies, cultures, and lymph node biopsies are necessary to distinguish the other processes. Toxoplasmosis in immunosuppressed patients may mimic other disseminated infections: the central nervous system mass lesions need to be distinguished by biopsy from *Herpes simplex* infection, bacterial abscesses, fungal processes, and neoplasms.

Toxoplasma retinochoroiditis needs to be distinguished on the basis of lesion morphology, serology, and appropriate cultures from cytomegalovirus, herpes, tuberculosis, histoplasmosis, syphilis, and sarcoidosis. Congenital toxoplasmosis must be distinguished from cytomegalovirus disease, syphilis, *Herpes simplex* infection, rubella, erythroblastosis fetalis, and bacterial sepsis.

THERAPY. The need and duration of therapy depends on the clinical setting. Most immunocompetent adults with lymphadenopathic disease do not need specific antitoxoplasma therapy. Patients with severe or prolonged constitutional symptoms, patients with specific organ dysfunction, immunoincompetent patients, and probably patients infected by direct inoculation (laboratory workers and transfusion recipients) merit treatment. Treatment for patients with retinochoroiditis or for pregnant patients is more controversial.

A combination of pyrimethamine (Daraprim) and sulfadiazine has been shown to be effective in inhibiting the replication of trophozoites. There are no drugs that will kill trophozoites or eradicate the cyst form. Pyrimethamine can only be given orally: in adults an initial dose of 75 mg is given, followed by 25 mg daily. Infants should be given 1 mg per kilogram for three days followed by 0.5 mg per kilogram per day. Sulfadiazine 1 gram orally every six hours is the adult dose. Infants should receive 100 mg per kilogram per day. Triple sulfonamides can be substituted for sulfadiazine, but sulfisoxazole (Gantrisin) is ineffective. Good urine flow should be maintained by adequate fluid intake to prevent crystalluria. Since sulfa drugs and pyrimethamine inhibit folate synthesis, folinic acid (leucovorin) 3 to 9 mg should be administered two to three times weekly to prevent bone marrow toxicity. Platelet counts and white blood cell counts should be monitored at least twice weekly during therapy. Pyrimethamine is a potential teratogen and should not be used in pregnant women.

Evaluation of the effectiveness of sulfadiazine and pyrimethamine therapy has been limited by the marked variability in clinical course and the frequency of spontaneous improvement. There is considerable anecdotal experience, however, that specific therapy can shorten the symptomatic period of fever and fatigue (although not the lymphadenopathy) in immunocompetent patients with acquired disease and is probably effective in hastening the resolution of serious organ dysfunction. Often a four- to six-week course of therapy is given and then the clinical situation re-evaluated. In *Toxoplasma* retinochoroiditis primary therapy should be directed at controlling the hypersensitivity response with anti-inflammatory drugs such as corticosteroids if the lesions are extensive or central. Pyrimethamine and sulfadiazine should be used to prevent local proliferation of the organisms and potential dissemination during the period of drug-induced immunosuppression.

Sulfadiazine and pyrimethamine have been effective in a number of immunosuppressed patients in controlling systemic symptoms and specific organ dysfunction. Long-term therapy should be strongly considered for the duration of immunosuppression. Bone marrow toxicity is a major management problem in many of these patients, particularly those with AIDS or those treated with antineoplastic chemotherapy.

In pregnant women who plan to complete their pregnancy despite the acquisition of *Toxoplasma* infection during gestation, pyrimethamine is dangerous to give because of its teratogenic potential. There is some evidence that sulfadiazine alone may be effective therapy. In Europe spiramycin (not available in the United States) has been used but its efficacy has not been clearly established. Congenital toxoplasmosis should be treated aggressively whether or not the infant is symptomatic, because organism proliferation can continue after birth. Antitoxoplasma therapy will not reverse damage that has already occurred.

For patients who cannot tolerate sulfadiazine and pyrimethamine, there are no clearly effective alternatives. Studies in vitro and animal data suggest that trimethoprim, either alone or in combination with sulfa drugs, has some antitoxoplasma activity, although less than pyrimethamine. Clindamycin and spiramycin do not have an established role in the treatment of systemic human disease. There is some evidence suggesting that clindamycin may be useful for treating retinochoroiditis.

PREVENTION. Toxoplasmosis is usually transmitted by the consumption of undercooked meat or exposure to oocyst-infected cat feces, so effective prevention should be directed against minimizing exposure to these two sources. Meat should be cooked as mentioned earlier. Pet cats should be kept in the house and they should not be fed raw meat or have access to wild rodents or birds. Particularly susceptible individuals should avoid sandboxes or moist soil where outdoor cats may defecate.

Congenital toxoplasmosis can be largely avoided if pregnant women follow the aforementioned precautions carefully. Serologic testing at the time of the mother's first prenatal examination and again at 16 to 18 weeks of gestation permits recognition of mothers who have acquired toxoplasmosis early in pregnancy and allows consideration of therapeutic abortion.

There are no current guidelines for preventing *Toxoplasma* infection related to blood transfusions or organ transplantation, nor is it clear how reactivated disease can be prevented in immunodeficient patients.

Desmonts G, Couvreur J: Congenital toxoplasmosis. A prospective study of 378 pregnancies. N Engl J Med 290:110, 1974. *The risk of congenital toxoplasmosis is documented in this prospective study.*

Dorfman RF, Remington JS: Value of lymph node biopsy in the diagnosis of acute acquired toxoplasmosis. N Engl J Med 289:878, 1973. *The specific histologic characteristics of toxoplasma lymphadenitis are documented.*

Ruskin J, Remington J: Toxoplasmosis in the compromised host. Ann Intern Med 84:193, 1976. *The clinical manifestations in immunosuppressed patients are described.*

Schlaegel TF Jr: Ocular Toxoplasmosis and Pars Planitis. New York, Grune & Stratton, 1978. *This detailed volume comprehensively covers ocular toxoplasmosis.*

Wallace GD: The role of the cat in the natural history of *Toxoplasma gondii.* Am J Trop Med Hyg 22:313, 1973. *The sexual cycle of* T. gondii *in the cat is described.*

Welch PC, Masur H, Jones TC, Remington JS: Serologic diagnosis of acute lymphadenopathic toxoplasmosis. J Infect Dis 142:256, 1980. *The usefulness of different serologic techniques is assessed for diagnosing acute lymphadenopathic toxoplasmosis.*

Wilson CB, Remington JS, Stagno S, Reynolds DW: Development of adverse sequelae in children born with subclinical congenital *Toxoplasma* infection. Pediatrics 66:767, 1980. *An analysis of the sequelae that congenital* Toxoplasma *infection produced in 24 children.*

383. PNEUMOCYSTOSIS

Henry Masur

Pneumocystosis is a pulmonary disease characterized by dyspnea, tachypnea, and hypoxemia that occurs in immunodeficient patients and in malnourished or premature infants. It is caused by species of the genus *Pneumocystis*, organisms that are probably protozoa. *Pneumocystis* cause asymptomatic infection in healthy mammalian hosts and are seen extracellulary in the pulmonary alveoli.

HISTORY. In 1909, while studying the lungs of guinea pigs experimentally infected with *Trypanosoma cruzi*, Carlos Chagas described what he thought was a new sporogony stage of the trypanosome. In 1910, Carini noted an identical form in the lungs of rats infected with *T. lewisi.* Two years later, Delanoe and Delanoe recognized that this lung cyst of Carini was in fact a distinct organism. Numerous workers then identified *Pneumocystis* in the lungs of mice, rats, guinea pigs, rabbits, dogs, monkeys, and horses that had not been infected with trypanosomes. Subsequently, epidemics of interstitial plasma cell pneumonia of unknown cause were described in Europe. Although Chagas had recognized his sporogony stage in a human lung in 1911, it was not until 1953 that Vanek, Jirovec, and Lukes recognized the association between interstitial plasma cell pneumonia and *Pneumocystis*. Since that time, *Pneumocystis* pneumonia has been recognized with increasing frequency, particularly as the use of immunosuppressive therapies for malignant neoplasms and organ transplantation has increased, and as the life span of individuals with congenital immunodeficiencies has improved.

ORGANISM. The life cycle of *Pneumocystis carinii* is not known with certainty. Morphologic data suggest that a thick-walled cyst and a thinner-walled trophozoite are the major stages in the life cycle of this extracellular organism. The cyst is 5 to 6 μ in diameter, and usually contains a cluster of six to eight round sporozoites (1 to 2 μ in diameter). When the sporozoites are released by the cyst, they develop into the trophozoites (1 to 5 μ in diameter). Under certain conditions, the trophozoites undergo a series of changes, including loss of internal structure, appearance of villous projections on the outer membrane, and development of an unusual trilaminar membrane, changes which transform the trophozoite into the cyst stage. A trophozoite-to-trophozoite cycle may also occur. The intra-alveolar exudate contains a mixture of cysts and trophozoites, as well as cellular and microbial debris and plasma proteins. The cyst is the stage of the organism usually identified in clinical specimens by means of the characteristic outer membrane staining with methenamine silver nitrate (Color plate 5G), Gram-Weigert, or toluidine blue O stains. With Giemsa stain, sporozoites can be identified within the cyst, as can the trophozoites, especially in touch preparations of fresh lung tissue or in bronchial secretions.

EPIDEMIOLOGY. *Pneumocystis* species are widely distributed, infecting rodents, rabbits, dogs, goats, horses, sheep, and other mammals, including humans. There is no evidence that animals serve as a reservoir for infection of humans. Experimental animal models and epidemiologic investigations of human disease best support the theory that transmission is by a respiratory route via droplet spray. In a few cases, congenital transmission has appeared to be the most likely route of infection.

Epidemiologic data suggest that *Pneumocystis* is infectious, that healthy or diseased individuals can transmit the infection, and that infection is usually persistent and asymptomatic. Nude mice or cortisone-treated germ-free rats will not develop pneumocystosis unless they have respiratory contact with communally raised non-germ-free rats. Epidemics of human disease among institutionalized malnourished infants, outbreaks of pneumocystosis among hospitalized immunodeficient patients, family clusters of pneumocystosis, and the increased prevalence of antipneumocystis antibody among healthy medical personnel further support these concepts.

Pneumocystosis occurs most commonly in malnourished infants (especially in the second to fourth months of life when passively transferred maternal antibodies first reach low levels), patients with deficiency of immunoglobulins G or M, and patients with deficiencies in cell-mediated immune mechanisms. The vast majority of adult patients have either the acquired immune deficiency syndrome (AIDS) or have received chemotherapy for hematologic malignancies or organ transplantation.

PATHOLOGY AND PATHOGENESIS. In latent *Pneumocystis* infection, rare clusters of cysts unassociated with marked cellular response or alveolar exudate can be seen. In the rat model, latent *Pneumocystis* infection can develop into active pulmonary disease after corticosteroid or cyclophosphamide therapy, but not after irradiation, splenectomy, or neonatal thymectomy. In humans, the relative importance of specific predisposing factors is less clear. When the *Pneumocystis* organisms are able to multiply, the inflammatory response includes transudation of fluid into the alveoli and a mononuclear cell infiltrate of interstitial spaces. The alveoli become filled with a foamy, proteinaceous material that contains clumps of both trophozoites and cysts. In malnourished or premature infants with pneumocystosis, the interstitial spaces contain predominantly plasma cells and alveolar epithelial cells—hence the pathologic description, interstitial plasma cell pneumonia. In immunodeficient children and adults, however, the inflammatory response consists of lymphocytes, macrophages, and occasionally eosinophils. Polymorphonuclear leukocytes are not seen, even in patients with normal white blood cell counts. The lung is usually involved diffusely, although localized disease has occasionally been described. The lung is usually firm and rubbery in consistency. Other infections can be found in association with pneumocystosis, including generalized infections as well as viral or fungal or bacterial pneumonias. Rarely, *Pneumocystis* may occur outside the lungs, involving lymph nodes, spleen, or bone marrow.

CLINICAL MANIFESTATIONS. The major symptoms of pneumocystosis are dyspnea, tachypnea, and a nonproductive cough. Fever and cyanosis are often present. The clinical syndrome can progress rapidly over several days or can appear insidiously over weeks or months. The rapidly progressive form is characteristic of patients with malignant neoplasms, especially during corticosteroid withdrawal. The insidious form is typically seen in children with congenital immunodeficiencies and in adults with AIDS.

On physical examination, the patient usually shows signs of respiratory distress (tachypnea, dyspnea, and cyanosis) associated with fever, but some patients, particularly those with AIDS, may have a paucity of signs. Auscultation of the lungs usually reveals no abnormalities, although scattered rales and rhonchi may be heard.

Routine laboratory tests are not generally helpful in distinguishing pneumocystosis from other pulmonary processes that are common in immunodeficient patients. Leukocytosis can be seen, but most often the white blood cell count reflects the underlying disease or the effects of chemotherapy. Eosinophilia has been reported, especially in children with humoral immune deficiencies. The arterial blood gases will demonstrate decreased oxygen saturation and hyperventilation despite continuous oxygen therapy, consistent with alveolar capillary block. A mild respiratory acidosis may be seen. Early in the course of the disease the chest radiograph usually shows a perihilar interstitial or patchy reticulogranular infiltrate with peripheral sparing. At the time of presentation some patients, particularly those with AIDS, may have normal arterial blood gases and/or normal chest x-rays. As pneumocystosis progresses, diffuse alveolar infiltrates with air bronchograms usually involve the entire lung fields. Pleural reaction, pleural effusion, asymmetry of infiltrates, or nodular infiltrates are unusual manifestations of pneumocystosis alone, but can be seen in up to half of the cases, since more than one disease process is often present in the lungs.

COURSE. The course of untreated pneumocystosis is one of progressive pulmonary consolidation, hypoxemia, and death. After institution of appropriate specific therapy, improvement usually occurs in five to ten days. The radiologic findings may become transiently worse after institution of therapy, but will then improve over one to three weeks. An association of pneumocystosis with interstitial fibrosis or emphysema has been reported, but the etiologic role of pneumocystosis has been difficult to document in view of the many factors that could lead to pulmonary changes in these patients.

DIAGNOSIS. Once the suspicion of pneumocystosis is raised by the clinical setting of immune deficiency and progressive pulmonary symptoms, pulmonary secretions or lung tissue should be examined by methenamine silver, Gram-Weigert, Giemsa, or toluidine blue O stains. Sputum smears and transtracheal aspirates demonstrate the organism in fewer than 15 per cent of patients. Bronchoscopy can be diagnostic in the majority of patients if products of lavage and brushings are examined carefully. Percutaneous needle biopsy of the lung and transbronchial biopsy of the lung are also diagnostic in most patients, although sufficient lung tissue for satisfactory pathologic evaluation is not always obtained. Open lung biopsy provides the optimal chance for complete and accurate diagnosis. For most patients, the operative risk is justified by the need to distinguish *Pneumocystis* from other, clinically similar pulmonary processes that may be caused by viruses, fungi, bacteria; neoplastic disease, hemorrhage, or drugs. Definitive lung biopsy results permit specific therapy, thus avoiding the complications of prolonged broad-spectrum antimicrobials. If the biopsy must be delayed, or if surgery is contraindicated, a therapeutic trial with specific drugs against *Pneumocystis* should be instituted.

Reliable serologic techniques have not yet been developed for diagnostic purposes. Immunofluorescent antibody titers are significantly elevated in only about 30 per cent of patients with pneumocystosis, but are also elevated in some immunosuppressed patients without apparent pneumocystosis, and in some healthy contacts. These titers may be useful in the epidemic infantile form of pneumocystosis, and in epidemiologic investigations.

TREATMENT. If started early in the course of the disease, therapy for pneumocystosis is quite successful. Pentamidine isethionate was used to treat pneumocystosis in the United States for over a decade; its use decreased mortality from nearly 100 per cent to less than 50 per cent, particularly if the patient survived long enough to receive the drug for nine or more days. Pentamidine has now been supplanted by co-trimoxazole as the therapy of choice for pneumocystosis. Co-trimoxazole, the fixed combination of trimethoprim and sulfamethoxazole, appears to be as effective as pentamidine and less toxic. This drug combination interferes with the synthesis of folinic acid. Adults should be given at least a 14-day course of 20 mg per kilogram per day of trimethoprim and 100 mg per kilogram per day of sulfamethoxazole in four equal oral or intravenous doses. Serum concentrations should be monitored because critically ill patients may not absorb orally administered drugs optimally, and because factors such as abnormal renal function or unusual volumes of distribution may make levels unpredictable even after intravenous administration. Peak serum levels of 5 to 10 μg per ml trimethoprim and 100 to 150 μg per ml sulfamethoxazole, drawn 90 minutes after drug administration, have been documented in some successfully treated patients. Folinic acid can be administered orally or intravenously to prevent or to treat folate deficiency; the dose is 10 mg two to three times weekly. Hypersensitivity rashes and leukopenia are uncommon adverse effects in patients with malignant neoplasms but occur with unusually high frequency in AIDS patients.

If the patient is unable to tolerate co-trimoxazole because of hypersensitivity or an adverse reaction, or if the patient has not responded to seven to ten days of co-trimoxazole therapy, then the use of pentamidine should be considered. Pentamidine is available in the United States only from the Parasitic Drug Service, U.S. Public Health Service (404–329–3670, days; 404–329–2888, nights). The mechanism of action of pentamidine on *Pneumocystis* is unknown, but the drug inhibits incorporation of nucleotides into DNA and RNA, inhibits oxidative phosphorylation, and causes megaloblastic cell changes. Pentamidine is administered in one single daily intramuscular dose for 10 to 14 days. Pentamidine isethionate, the drug available from the Parasitic Drug Service in the United States, should be given at a dose of 4 mg per kg per day. In Canada and certain other countries the methylsulfonate salt of pentamidine is available; the dose is calculated differently since the product is labelled with the amount of pentamidine base present, rather than the amount of pentamidine salt: the dose is 2.3 mg of base per kg per day. In over 40 per cent of patients, pentamidine causes adverse effects, including renal insufficiency, abnormal liver function, and disturbances in bone marrow function or glucose metabolism (hypoglycemia or hyperglycemia). These adverse effects are usually reversible. Intramuscular administration often results in large and painful sterile abscesses. Intravenous administration has been associated with significant hypotension in the past and has thus been avoided. Recent experience suggests that slow infusion over 60 to 90 minutes of pentamidine diluted in 100 to 150 ml of fluid may be safe. Such an infusion must be considered experimental, however.

Repeat episodes of pneumocystosis have been documented after pentamidine and after co-trimoxazole therapy, particularly in patients with AIDS.

PREVENTION. Since the diseased patient may be able to spread the organism to other patients, to healthy medical personnel, and to family members, respiratory precautions should be maintained when the diagnosis is suspected. Such precautions may prevent hospital clusters of pneumocystosis. For certain highly susceptible patient populations such as children with acute lymphoblastic leukemia at institutions with high attack rates, and perhaps for patients with AIDS, continuous prophylactic treatment with co-trimoxazole is beneficial. The daily preventive dose is trimethoprim, 5 mg per kilogram per day, and sulfamethoxazole, 25 mg per kilogram per day, in two equally divided doses.

Burke BA, Good RA: *Pneumocystis carinii* infection. Medicine 52:23, 1973. *This thoroughly referenced review summarizes a large clinical experience as well as the literature to date, covering the biology, the clinical and pathologic aspects, and the epidemiology of pneumocystosis.*

Hughes WT, Kuhn S, Chaudhary S, Feldman S, Verzosa M, Aur RJA, Pratt C, George SL: Successful chemoprophylaxis for *Pneumocystis carinii* pneumonitis. N Engl J Med 297:1419, 1977. *This randomized, double blind study demonstrates the efficacy of co-trimoxazole for the prevention of pneumocystosis in a high risk pediatric population.*

Kovacs JA, Hiemenz JW, Macher AM, Stover D, Murray HW, Shelhamer J, Lane HC, Ormacher C, Hoenig C, Longo DL, Parker MM, Natanson C, Panillo JE, Fauci AS, Pizzo PA, Masur H: *Pneumocystis carinii* pneumonia: A comparison between patients with the acquired immunodeficiency syndrome and patients with other immunodeficiencies. Ann Intern Med 100:663, 1984. *The clinical presentation of pneumocystis pneumonia in AIDS is demonstrated to be more subtle than in other disease states, but response to therapy does not differ dramatically between the two groups.*

Singer C, Armstrong D, Rosen PP, Schottenfeld D: *Pneumocystis carinii* pneumonia: A cluster of eleven cases. Ann Intern Med 82:772, 1975. *An epidemiologic investigation of an outbreak of pneumocystosis. This article provides documentation about probable routes of transmission, with important implications for disease prevention.*

Walzer PD, Perl DP, Krogstad DJ, Rawson PG, Schultz MG: *Pneumocystis carinii* pneumonia in the United States. Epidemiologic, diagnostic, and clinical features. Ann Intern Med 80:83, 1974. *This article summarizes 194 confirmed cases of pneumocystosis in terms of information supplied to the Centers for Disease Control. Its data are useful and well organized.*

Winston DJ, Lau WK, Gale RP, Young LS: Trimethoprim-sulfamethoxazole for the treatment of *Pneumocystis carinii* pneumonia. Ann Intern Med 92:762, 1980. *The efficacy of intravenous co-trimoxazole in 11 adults with confirmed pneumocystosis is documented. Pharmacologic guidelines for therapy are provided.*

384. BABESIOSIS (Piroplasmosis)

Morton N. Swartz

DEFINITION. Babesiosis is a tick-borne malaria-like acute febrile illness caused by protozoa of the genus *Babesia* and usually occurring in sharply circumscribed endemic areas. Infection with *Babesia* was first recognized in animals, in which primary symptomatic illness (babesiosis) may be followed by persistent low-grade infection manifested only by the presence in blood of the parasites (babesiasis). Only recently has transmission of infection to humans been recorded—usually by ticks, rarely by transfusion of blood from an asymptomatic carrier.

HISTORY. Babès, in Romania in 1888, described an intraerythrocytic organism in cattle with fever and hemolytic anemia. Five years later, Theobold Smith identified a similar organism as a protozoan and the cause of Texas cattle fever, a disease that he went on to show was transmitted by ticks. The first human case of babesiosis, one which ended fatally, occurred in 1956 in a farmer in Yugoslavia who was exposed to tick infested cattle and who had undergone splenectomy 11 years earlier following an accident. However, babesiosis in humans may have been identified as early as 1904 when Wilson and Chowning noted organisms resembling those in piroplasmosis of cattle in the blood of several patients in Montana. Since these cases occurred in the endemic area of Rocky Mountain spotted fever, the findings were attributed to the latter disease. In the past 17 years 118 additional cases of infection with *Babesia* have been reported, a few from Europe but most from the northeastern United States.

PROTOZOAN AND VECTOR. Babesia is a protozoan that in mammalian hosts propagates only in erythrocytes and by a process of nonsynchronous budding. Different species of *Babesia* have been described in specific vertebrate hosts: e.g., *B. canis* (dogs); *B. bovis* (cattle); *B. equi* (horses); *B. microti* (rodents). The latter has been the etiology of most reported human cases, particularly those recently observed in the northeastern United States; rare cases in Europe have been due to *B. bovis* and *B. divergens*.

Ixodes dammini (northern deer tick) is responsible for the spread of babesiosis from rodents to humans. In development through its three stages (larva, nymph, adult) the tick requires three animal hosts (of the same or different species), each as a source of a blood meal. Deer are the usual hosts for the adult tick. The initial step in the cycle of transmission occurs when larvae feed on rodents (white-footed mice in endemic areas of Massachusetts and New York) and acquire *B. microti* in the process. Infection in this rodent population can be extensive in endemic areas (60 per cent of white-footed mice on Nantucket Island harbor this protozoan). Infection in the larvae ultimately involves the salivary glands. Nymphs, the next stage, are the most abundant ticks on rodent reservoir hosts and usually feed from May through September. When the nymph takes its blood meal from rodents or man (requiring a period of at least 48 hours of feeding during which sporozoites replicate, mature, and become infectious), human infection ensues. Although transovarial transmission of other babesial species in other tick hosts occurs, there is no evidence as yet that *B. microti* is transmitted in this way in *I. dammini*.

EPIDEMIOLOGY. Seven cases of babesiosis have been reported from Europe and over 100 additional human infections have been documented in the United States. The European cases have been caused by bovine *Babesia* (primarily *B. divergens*), have all occurred in splenectomized individuals, and have represented serious illness (57 per cent mortality). With the exception of two splenectomized patients in California who had infections thought to have been caused by equine *Babesia* and a patient in Georgia who harbored *Babesia* that were not defined as to species but were morphologically distinct from *B. microti*, the infections in the United States have all been caused by *B. microti*. The endemic area for human infection during the summer months includes circumscribed adjoining areas of Massachusetts (Nantucket Island, Martha's Vineyard, Cape Cod) and New York (Shelter Island, Fire Island, eastern Long Island).

Only about 5 per cent of nymphal *I. dammini* on Nantucket were found to be infected with *B. microti*. This finding, plus the fact that at least 48 hours of attachment and feeding are needed for transmission of infection, may account for the fact that infection is not more prevalent in endemic areas. However, the very high current frequency of parasitemia in white-footed mice in the offshore islands and the replacement of other rodent ticks by the newly dominant *I. dammini* may account for the increasing occurrence of human babesiosis (15 clinical infections in 1980) in the endemic areas of the Northeast.

Subclinical infection occurs in humans: 4 to 7 per cent of asymptomatic individuals spending time outdoors in endemic areas during the summer months had significant IFA antibody titers to *B. microti*, and seroconversion had occurred in most. This appreciable rate assumes importance in view of the occurrence of transfusion-induced babesiosis in four patients. In several instances asymptomatic blood donors had been in endemic areas and had significant IFA titers against *B. microti; B. microti* was isolated on intraperitoneal inoculation of hamsters with blood from one such donor.

CLINICAL MANIFESTATIONS. The incubation period following a tick bite is one to six weeks. However, since the engorged nymph is only 2 mm in diameter, its presence may be easily overlooked. The incubation period for blood (or platelet) transfusion-induced babesiosis has been long (six to nine weeks) in three cases. Unlike the European cases, which were very severe and uniformly occurred in splenectomized patients, 80 per cent of clinical cases from the United States have occurred in patients with intact spleens. Most patients have been over 50 years of age and, with two exceptions, all recovered.

The initial symptoms are nonspecific: malaise, fatigue, anorexia, headache, weakness. Fever (39 to 40° C), drenching sweats, chills, myalgias, and arthralgias then develop. Nausea and vomiting may occur; mental depression, mood lability, photophobia have been noted in some patients but meningeal signs have been absent. The onset may occur acutely over a period of a few days or may be more protracted over several weeks. Lymphadenopathy is absent, but splenomegaly is detected in some patients. Rash is not observed. However, simultaneous infection with Lyme disease (vector also *I. dammini*) has occurred.

More severe disease occurs in splenectomized patients. Of the 22 patients with reported cases, six died (including five Europeans with cases due to bovine strains) with prominent hemolytic anemia, hemoglobinuria, jaundice, and renal insufficiency.

Occasional asymptomatic cases of human babesiosis have been described (Mexico, Georgia, Massachusetts) in which the protozoan has been identified on blood smear or on animal inoculation of the individual's blood.

Hematologic changes consist of a hemolytic anemia with reticulocytosis, reduced serum haptoglobin level, normal or slightly reduced leukocyte count, and mild to moderate thrombocytopenia. Rarely, disseminated intravascular coagulation has developed in severe cases. In some patients with clinical babesiosis direct antiglobulin tests are positive on their red blood cells as in patients with malaria. Usually, from 1 to 10 per cent of erythrocytes on peripheral blood smears contain the parasite. Parasitemias well below 1 per cent and as high as 85 per cent have been reported in patients with clinical illness. Mild elevations of serum bilirubin, SGOT, and alkaline phosphatase are common. Urinalysis shows proteinuria and hemoglobinuria.

IMMUNITY. Babesiosis in humans caused by *B. microti* is a self-limited disease in most instances, presumably because of control exercised by the host immune defenses. IgM and IgG antibodies are detectable within a few days of the initial clinical manifestations, probably reflecting the relatively long prepatent period. However, parasitemia continues in the presence of such antibodies during the course of the clinical illness and after subsidence of symptoms. Considerable evidence indicates a role for the spleen in the host defense against *Babesia:* (1) increased severity of illness in asplenic humans, (2) increased level of parasitemia in experimental animals splenectomized before or during infection, and (3) recrudescent parasitemia following recovery from babesiosis in hamsters subsequently splenectomized.

The cellular immune response plays an important role in protection. Administration of antilymphocyte serum (ALS) to hamsters prior to infection with *B. microti* results in failure to induce specific antibody, exaggerated parasitemia, and death; in animals that have successfully handled infection, later administration of ALS results in recrudescent parasitemia and some mortality despite high serum antibody levels. Also, athymic mice are more susceptible to babesial parasitemia than normal mice. In humans with acute babesiosis T and B cell function is often suppressed on assay in vitro.

DIAGNOSIS. The diagnosis of babesiosis should be considered in a febrile patient from an endemic area in the tick season or who has received a blood transfusion (including platelet infusions or transfusions of frozen-thawed blood). The diagnosis is established by finding characteristic intraerythrocytic forms (pyriform, ring, tetrad) on thin or thick Giemsa-stained blood smears. Ring forms of *Babesia* (often several in a single red cell) may be mistaken for *Plasmodium falciparum* but can be distinguished by the presence of pigment in erythrocytes parasitized by older forms of the latter. Also, schizonts and gametocytes are absent in *Babesia* infection but may be present in blood smears of patients with malaria. Tetrad (maltese cross) forms are uncommonly present in human blood smears but are sufficiently distinctive when present to indicate babesiosis. With intense parasitemia extraerythrocytic parasites (merozoites) in clusters may be seen occasionally in blood smears. Since parasitemia may vary, smears should be repeated over several days in suspected cases. Confirmation of diagnosis can be made by demonstration of IFA antibody (Centers for Disease Control) to *B. microti* in sera of patients; titers rise to ≥ 1:1024 within the first few weeks of illness and then fall gradually over the next six months. Confirmation of the diagnosis can also be made by demonstration of parasitemia in blood smears of hamsters inoculated intraperitoneally with a patient's blood.

THERAPY. Patients with intact spleens, low level parasitemia, and mild symptomatology often recover without specific treatment. An effective treatment for this infection has not yet been established. Although chloroquine may produce symptomatic improvement, it has little activity against the parasite itself. The combination of quinine (650 mg orally every six hours) and clindamycin (300 mg intravenously every 6 hours) has been used successfully in treating two markedly symptomatic adults with prominent parasitemia. Pentamidine isethionate* (4 mg per kg intramuscularly daily) has been used in treatment but is of questionable benefit in eliminating parasitemia. Other antimalarial drugs (pyrimethamine-sulfadoxine, primaquine) have no effect on parasitemia in animals. Exchange transfusions have been very helpful in several severely ill patients with intense degrees (40 to 60 per cent) of parasitemia and hemolysis.

PREVENTION. Prevention consists of avoiding contact with nymphal *I. dammini* in endemic areas during May through September. If tick infested areas are to be entered, use of repellents containing diethyltoluamide is advisable. Also, careful daily examination for ticks should be performed, and any found to be attached should be removed by fine forceps placed close to the site of attachment. Asplenic patients particularly should avoid endemic areas where they might come in contact with ticks.

In view of the cases of transfusion-induced babesiosis, current policy is not to accept as blood donors anyone with a history of babesiosis or any permanent residents of endemic areas (Shelter Island, Nantucket, etc.).

*Available from Centers for Disease Control, Atlanta, GA.

Dammin GJ: Babesiosis. *In* Weinstein L, Fields BN (eds.): Seminars in Infectious Disease. New York, Stratton Intercontinental Book Corporation, 1978, p 169. *Comprehensive review of important aspects of babesiosis as a zoonosis and a disease of humans.*

Jacoby GA, Hunt JV, Kosinski KS, Demirjian ZN, Huggins C, Etkind P, Marcus LC, Spielman A: Treatment of transfusion-transmitted babesiosis by exchange transfusion. N Engl J Med 303:1098, 1980. *The role of exchange transfusion in the treatment of intense* B. microti *parasitemia.*

Rosner F, Zarrabi MH, Benach JL, Habicht GS: Babesiosis in splenectomized adults. Am J Med 76:696, 1984. *Helpful summary of the 22 reported cases of human babesiosis that have occurred in splenectomized patients.*

Ruebush TK II, Cassaday PB, Marsh HJ, Lisker SA, Voorhees DB, Mahoney EB, Healy GR: Human babesiosis on Nantucket Island. Ann Intern Med 86:6, 1977. *Good description of the clinical illness.*

Ruebush TK II, Juranek DD, Spielman A, Piesman J, Healy GR: Epidemiology of human babesiosis on Nantucket Island. Am J Trop Med Hyg 30:937, 1981. *Good overview of the epidemiology of babesiosis in a major endemic area.*

Sun T, Tenenbaum MJ, Greenspan J, Teichberg S, Wang RT, Degnan T, Kaplan MH: Morphologic and clinical observations in human infection with *Babesia microti*. J Infect Dis 148:239, 1983. *Detailed electron and light microscopic studies of* Babesia *infection in a patient with 85 per cent parasitemia.*

Wittner M, Rowin KS, Tanowitz HB, Hobbs JF, Saltzman S, Wenz B, Hirsch R, Chisholm E, Healy GR: Successful chemotherapy of transfusion babesiosis. Ann Intern Med 96:601, 1982. *An important paper describing a case of transfusion-induced babesiosis successfully treated with the combination of quinine and clindamycin.*

385. AMEBIASIS AND AMEBIC MENINGOENCEPHALITIS

Donald J. Krogstad

AMEBIASIS

DEFINITION. Amebiasis is defined as infection with the protozoan parasite *Entamoeba histolytica*.

ETIOLOGY. *E. histolytica* exists in both cyst and trophozoite forms. Motile trophozoites (12 to 50 μm) are typically found in the bloody and mucoid stools of patients with active disease. Cysts are smaller (10 to 20 μm) and nonmotile. They are the infectious form of the parasite and are characteristically found in the formed stools of asymptomatic patients and those with minimal disease. Their double cyst membrane is an adaptation that presumably protects them from desiccation and from gastric juice after ingestion. In contrast, trophozoites (which do not have this protective double membrane) disintegrate rapidly after excretion into the external environment and are not infectious on oral ingestion.

PREVALENCE. Available data suggest that less than 1 per cent of the United States population is infected with this organism (by stool examination) or has serologic evidence of previous infection (a positive antibody titer). The 5 to 10 per cent prevalence estimates of 50 to 70 years ago are no longer valid, although they may still be applicable in some developing countries.

EPIDEMIOLOGY. The epidemiology of amebiasis in most developed countries is a mixture of indigenous and imported disease. Because the organism does not require a soil phase in its life cycle, it is not restricted to warmer climates. Thus, it may be transmitted by the fecal-oral route in areas far from the tropics. For example, there have been well-described outbreaks of disease in the northern United States and Europe, including a recent outbreak that was transmitted by the practice of colonic irrigation. Amebiasis may also be transmitted by sexual activity and is an important public health problem among homosexual populations.

Imported disease may result from the immigration of infected persons or from foreign travel by tourists. Although many refugees who come to the United States are screened for amebiasis, most returning tourists and their physicians are unaware of this risk. Thus, these patients may be mistakenly diagnosed as having ulcerative colitis and inappropriately treated with steroids.

In developing countries, the lack of sanitation and the high prevalence of infection combine to produce a greater risk of transmission than in developed countries. In both developing and developed countries, patients severely ill with amebiasis are less likely to transmit the infection than relatively well or asymptomatic patients, because they excrete the more fragile trophozoite form in their stool. Thus, the epidemiology of amebiasis is complicated by the fact that the persons most important for transmission are minimally symptomatic or asymptomatic, and are thus less likely to seek medical help.

PATHOGENESIS AND MECHANISMS OF DISEASE. *Entamoeba histolytica* directly invades the intestinal mucosa to cause amebic colitis and may also travel via the bloodstream to produce metastatic infections in the liver and at other sites. Although the mechanism(s) by which *E. histolytica* produces disease is incompletely defined, contact-dependent killing of target cells may be an important pathogenetic factor. Ravdin and his colleagues have found that direct contact (between the parasite and the target cell) is necessary for the killing of mammalian target cells by amebae.

PATHOLOGY. Amebic colitis is characterized by flask-shaped ulcers that contain pus and amebic trophozoites. On histologic examination, trophozoites are usually identifiable with routine hematoxylin and eosin staining at the periphery of these ulcers. Except for the presence of *E. histolytica* and their characteristic flask shape, these lesions may be mistaken for the colitis of inflammatory bowel disease. In contrast, amebic abscesses in the liver and elsewhere usually contain few identifiable amebae, which tend to be at the border between the abscess and normal tissue.

CLINICAL MANIFESTATIONS. The vast majority of patients infected with *E. histolytica* have few or no detectable symptoms. In a minority of patients, this commensal relationship breaks down for unknown reasons and the organism becomes a pathogen. The manifestations of amebic colitis may be subtle or severe, and range from mild watery diarrhea to explosive, bloody dysentery with a fulminant course. In addition, it is not uncommon for the disease to wax and wane. The same patient may experience both exacerbations and remissions over a period of months to years without treatment.

Outside the gastrointestinal tract, amebic disease typically presents as a slowly expanding mass lesion. Abscesses are most frequently found in the liver, where right-sided lesions are much more common than left-sided ones (presumably owing to the vascular supply of the liver). For reasons that are not clear, amebic liver abscesses are much more common in males than females (6 to 7:1). Important clues to the presence of an amebic liver abscess include elevation of the right hemidiaphragm and right upper quadrant pain.

Although amebic abscesses are most common in the liver, the infection may also extend to the lung or pericardium and metastasize to other sites, including the central nervous system. Less frequently, lesions may present in the anogenital area. These have been confused with squamous cell carcinoma of the rectum, penis, and cervix on the basis of their macroscopic appearance, although histologic examination typically reveals *E. histolytica* trophozoites.

DIAGNOSIS. ***Stool Examination.*** Stool examination for *E. histolytica* is one of the most difficult tests to perform correctly in the clinical laboratory. False negatives are common because morphology is insensitive. In addition, false-positive results have been reported by inexperienced observers who have confused both white blood cells and other amebae with *E. histolytica*. *Entamoeba hartmanni* is a particular problem, because the only criterion by which it can be distinguished from *E. histolytica* is size. It tends to be smaller in diameter (cyst 5 to 8 μm, trophozoites 6 to 10 μm) than *E. histolytica*. This distinction is difficult for even experienced observers and is impossible without the use of an ocular micrometer to measure parasite size accurately.

In patients with severe intestinal disease, *E. histolytica* trophozoites tend to be large (25 to 50 μm in diameter) and actively motile. Another useful clue is the presence of ingested red blood cells, which are characteristic of *E. histolytica* but not the nonpathogenic protozoa. However, ingested red blood cells are not diagnostic of amebiasis. Macrophages may ingest red blood cells and have often been misdiagnosed as amebae on this basis in both shigellosis and salmonellosis. Although material should be preserved in polyvinyl alcohol fixative for a permanent record, the use of supravital stains such as methylene blue may be invaluable in defining the nuclear morphology of the parasite to distinguish it from white cells and other actively motile cells in the stool at the time of the initial stool examination.

The most important cause of false-negative stool examinations for *E. histolytica* is the presence of substances that interfere with the stool examination for parasites. These include particulate material that obscures the presence of the parasite (barium sulfate, bismuth, and kaolin compounds), agents that lyse trophozoites (soap and tap water enemas), and antimicrobials that decrease the number of parasites excreted in the stool (tetracycline, sulfonamides, antiprotozoal agents). After excluding the presence of these substances (for seven to ten days prior to stool examination), there are several additional procedures worth considering in patients with negative stool examinations who are suspected of having amebiasis. Because long delays in transporting specimens to the laboratory may produce false-negative results, the next step should be to obtain fresh material from the patient and to examine it directly. If these examinations are negative, one may often increase the yield by examining pus or exudate taken at proctoscopy or sigmoidoscopy. This material should be taken with a glass rod or metal spatula, because parasites tend to adhere to cotton swabs. If these results are negative, biopsy of a rectal valve is frequently diagnostic. Even if all efforts to make a morphologic diagnosis are unsuccessful, serology is often positive.

Serology. Because most patients develop symptomatic amebiasis over months to years, the usual two- to four-week delay for the development of antibodies is not a significant problem. In areas such as the United States where amebiasis is rare, a positive antibody titer is strong suggestive evidence for amebiasis. Most patients ($\geq$ 80 per cent) with active intestinal disease have a positive indirect hemagglutination (IHA) test. The sensitivity of this test is even greater in extraintestinal (metastatic) disease, and 96 to 100 per cent of patients with liver abscess have a positive titer ($\geq$ 1:128). Conversely, in areas where amebic infection is common, a positive titer is less useful because titers may remain elevated for years after resolution of the acute infection.

Recent studies by Pillai and colleagues suggest that many patients with active amebic disease have circulating immune complexes which contain amebic antigen, and that the titers of these immune complexes may decrease rapidly with treatment—in contrast to the IHA.

Radiology. Radiologic examination is often positive in amebic colitis. It may reveal mass lesions (ameboma), ulcerations, pseudomembranes, or toxic megacolon. These lesions are nonspecific and may readily be confused with either cancer or inflammatory bowel disease. Their lack of specificity emphasizes the need for a more specific diagnosis based on morphology or a positive serology.

A number of radiologic techniques have been used to demonstrate extraintestinal amebic disease. The most frequently used technique is the technetium 99 scan, which characteristically reveals an area of decreased uptake in amebic liver abscess. However, amebic liver abscesses have also been visualized by ultrasonography, gallium scan, and computed tomography. In selecting a radiologic technique, observer experience is a more important variable with ultrasonography than with the other techniques. We recommend the technetium scan as the initial radiologic test for liver abscess and computed tomography or ultrasonography if the technetium scan is negative, and for disease outside the liver.

TREATMENT. The treatment of amebiasis remains unsatisfactory. It is complicated because different forms of the infection require different treatment regimens (Table 385–1), and because several antiamebic drugs have significant toxicity. Emetine and dehydroemetine are cardiotoxic; metronidazole is mutagenic in bacteria and produces tumors in rodents.

Although susceptibility testing is not yet practical for individual patients, it is nevertheless important to individualize the treatment of patients with amebiasis. For instance, metronidazole penetrates the blood-brain barrier well, and is an excellent

TABLE 385–1. TREATMENT OF PATIENTS WITH AMEBIASIS*

Intestinal infection:	
Cysts on stool examination (patients with few or no symptoms):	
Diloxanide furoate (Furamide)†	500 mg three times a day for ten days
Diiodohydroxyquin‡	650 mg three times a day for twenty days
Metronidazole (Flagyl)	750 mg three times a day for five to ten days
Trophozoites on stool examination (patients with symptomatic disease):	
Metronidazole (Flagyl)	750 mg three times a day for five to ten days
Dehydroemetine†	1.0 to 1.5 mg per kilogram per day for ten days intramuscularly or subcutaneously
Extraintestinal infection:	
Metronidazole (Flagyl)	750 mg three times a day for five to ten days
Chloroquine plus diiodohydroxyquin‡	500 mg a day for ten weeks, plus 650 mg three times a day for twenty days
Dehydroemetine† plus chloroquine	As above, plus 500 mg a day for two to three weeks
Dehydroemetine†	As above

*Doses suggested are for adults: Unless otherwise noted, doses are for oral administration.

†Available from the Parasitic Disease Drug Service, Centers for Disease Control, Atlanta, Ga 30333 (404–329–3670; nights and weekends, 329–2888).

‡Now used less frequently because a close congener (iodochlorhydroxyquin-Enterovioform) has been associated with subacute myelo-optic neuropathy. Available from Panray Division of Orment Drug and Chemical, Englewood, NJ 07631, and Glenwood Laboratories, Tenafly, NJ 07670.

Reproduced with permission of The New England Journal of Medicine (from Krogstad et al., 1978).

choice for patients with suspected central nervous system involvement. Conversely, diloxanide furoate is the preferred agent for patients with minimal or no symptoms who are passing cysts in stool.

PROGNOSIS. The prognosis of amebic infection is usually excellent if it is recognized before the patient is critically ill. However, steroids have been shown to enhance the pathogenicity of *E. histolytica* in animals and may also interfere with the response to therapy in humans. In addition, peritonitis may result from colonic perforation in amebic colitis, or from rupture of an amebic liver abscess, and clearly results in a worse prognosis.

Although high IHA antibody titers are associated with active disease, patients whose titers fall more slowly after therapy do not necessarily have persistent disease. Therefore, we recommend that patients should be followed clinically and that those with persistently high titers should not be re-treated on this basis alone.

PREVENTION. Amebiasis can be prevented by careful hygiene. Because amebic cysts are killed by cooking, only uncooked foods such as salads or those contaminated after cooking can transmit the infection. In endemic areas, it is best to avoid fresh uncooked vegetables and fruits that cannot be peeled. The concentration of chlorine necessary to kill amebic cysts ($\geq$ 10 ppm) is substantially greater than the levels used for water purification (1 to 2 ppm) and is unpalatable. Therefore, most water systems depend on sedimentation and filtration to remove amebic cysts.

Adams EB, MacLeod IN: Invasive amebiasis. I. Amebic dysentery and its complications. Medicine 56:315, 325, 1977. *The extensive experience of these investigators with over 7000 cases documents the favorable outcome of uncomplicated amebic colitis and liver abscess (case-fatality rates of < 1 per cent) and the unfavorable outcomes associated with complications such as peritonitis and pericardial extension (case-fatality rates of 30 to 40 per cent).*

Cedeno JR, Krogstad DJ: Susceptibility testing of *Entamoeba histolytica.* J Infect Dis 148:1090, 1983. *With methods such as this one, it may ultimately be possible to perform susceptibility testing on isolates obtained from individual patients.*

Healy GR, Kraft SC: The indirect hemagglutination test for amebiasis in patients with inflammatory bowel disease. Am J Dig Dis 17:97, 1972. *Indirect hemagglutination antibody titers to* E. histolytica *are a reliable method of screening patients with inflammatory bowel disease for amebiasis.*

Istre GR, Kreiss K, Hopkins RS, et al.: Outbreak of amebiasis spread by colonic irrigation at a chiropractic clinic. N Engl J Med 307:339, 1982. *This outbreak demonstrates the potential danger of such practices (presumably including penile-rectal intercourse), which transfer colonic contents from one person to another.*

Krogstad DJ, Spencer HC Jr, Healy GR, Gleason NN, Sexton DJ, Herron CA: Amebiasis: Epidemiologic studies in the United States, 1971–1974. Ann Intern Med 88:89, 1978. *This study demonstrates that lack of diagnostic skill in the United States produces both false-positive and false-negative laboratory results that lead to inappropriate therapy and increased morbidity and mortality. It also emphasizes the difficulty of distinguishing clinically between inflammatory bowel disease and amebic colitis.*

Pillai S, Mohimen A: A solid-phase sandwich radioimmunoassay for *Entamoeba histolytica* proteins and the detection of circulating antigens in amebiasis. Gastroenterology 83:1210, 1982. *This report suggests that the disappearance of circulating immune complexes from the serum may be a clinically useful indicator of successful treatment.*

Ravdin JI, Croft BY, Guerrant RL: Cytopathogenic mechanisms of *Entamoeba histolytica.* J Exp Med 152:377, 1980. *These studies demonstrate that cell-to-cell contact is necessary for the killing of target cells by the parasite.*

AMEBIC MENINGOENCEPHALITIS

Amebic meningoencephalitis is an infection of the brain and meninges caused by free-living amebae. It has been associated with *Naegleria, Acanthamoeba, Hartmanella,* and other free-living amebae. (*Acanthamoeba* may also cause a keratitis that is similarly resistant to treatment.)

This is a rare disease; only 100 to 200 cases have been reported. However, its prevalence has probably been underestimated because of difficulty in making the diagnosis. There are two different forms of primary amebic meningoencephalitis. One occurs primarily in young, healthy individuals who have been swimming in artificial fresh water lakes and is typically caused by one of the free-living *Naegleria* species. The other is more subacute and is associated with immunocompromised hosts. It is usually due to *Acanthamoeba, Hartmannella,* or other free-living amebae, but not *Naegleria.*

In both of these infections, the morbidity and mortality are caused by meningitis and a hemorrhagic encephalitis. In disease caused by *Naegleria,* inflammatory and hemorrhagic changes along the olfactory tract are often prominent. This infection is thought to gain access to the central nervous system by crossing the cribriform plate from the nose during swimming exposure in fresh water. The pathogenesis of disease caused by *Acanthamoeba* and the other organisms not associated with fresh water exposure is less clear. However, several investigators have described other amebic infections at distant sites in these patients and have postulated hematogenous spread to the central nervous system.

Both types of amebic meningoencephalitis are characterized by fever, meningismus, and obtundation. The major distinctions between them are in the epidemiologic history and in the tempo of the disease. Infections caused by *Naegleria* tend to be more fulminant with a course of several days to a week and a half. In contrast, disease among immunosuppressed hosts tends to be more subacute.

The diagnosis of amebic meningoencephalitis is often missed because the organisms are mistaken for lymphocytes in the cerebrospinal fluid. In previously healthy young patients, the disease is also confused with viral infection. In compromised hosts, it may be confused with toxoplasmosis, cytomegalovirus infection, and other opportunistic pathogens. The diagnosis is best made by careful examination of spinal fluid wet mounts for motile trophozoites, 8 to 15 μm in size.

The outlook for patients with this infection is grim. There are only four known survivors. The limited data available suggest that intravenous and intrathecal amphotericin B and miconazole, plus oral rifampin, may be effective. However, serologic studies in areas with known cases suggest that subclinical illness and spontaneous recoveries do occur with this infection. Although the only preventive measure is to avoid swimming in lakes epidemiologically associated with this infection, the risk is low (probably less than one in a million).

Carter RF: Primary amebic meningoencephalitis—clinical, pathological and epidemiological features of six cases. J Pathol Bacteriol 96:1, 1968. *This early report describes cases associated with swimming exposure in Australia and identifies* Naegleria *as the responsible pathogen.*

Duma RF, Helwig WB, Martinez AJ: Meningoencephalitis and brain abscess due to a free-living ameba. Ann Intern Med 88:468, 1978. *This report documents a fatal case of amebic meningoencephalitis caused by a free-living ameba that could not be identified. It raises the possibility that an unknown number of the free-living amebae may be capable of causing this disease.*

Key SN III, Green WR, Willaert E, Stevens AR, Key SN Jr: Keratitis due to *Acanthamoeba castellani*: A clinicopathologic case report. Arch Ophthalmol 98:475, 1980. *This newly recognized entity* may *be amenable to treatment with topical polyenes such as pimaricin.*

Seidel JS, Harimatz P, Visvesvara VS, Cohen A, Edwards J, Turner J: Successful treatment of primary amebic meningoencephalitis. N Engl J Med 306:346, 1982. *The* in vitro *susceptibility studies in this report suggest that the combination of amphotericin B plus miconazole may be synergistic against* Naegleria.

386. OTHER PROTOZOAN DISEASES

David P. Stevens

The human host provides an ever-changing environment for protozoan infections. With the increasing prevalence of acquired immune deficiency, caused by either immunosuppressant drugs or the acquired immune deficiency syndrome (AIDS), protozoan infections that were previously considered rare or exotic are now observed more frequently. Notable examples are *Cryptosporidium* and *Giardia* infections in the presence of AIDS. With this changing epidemiologic setting, it will not be surprising in the future to find additional protozoa that play the opportunist's role as pathogenic agents.

These infections should be distinguished, however, from the numerous nonpathogenic protozoa that may be found in the stool of apparently healthy persons. Notable among them are *Entamoeba coli, Endolimax nana, Iodamoeba butschlii, Dientamoeba fragilis, Trichomonas hominis,* and *Chilomastix mesnili*. The clinician must rely on a skilled laboratory technician to differentiate these agents from pathogenic species such as *Entamoeba histolytica* and the organisms discussed in the following chapters.

GIARDIASIS

DEFINITION. Giardiasis is an infection of the small intestine caused by the flagellated protozoan *Giardia lamblia.* When symptomatic, it results in diarrhea, malabsorption, and weight loss.

INCIDENCE AND PREVALENCE. Giardiasis is present in all climates from the equator to the poles. Its prevalence is greater where community water supplies are chronically contaminated by human sewage. It is particularly prevalent in developing regions of the world where water supplies are not formally treated or where they overlap with sewage disposal systems such as local streams. Endemic giardiasis, however, is also found in certain areas of industrialized countries. Unexpected examples of the latter include the municipal water supply of Leningrad and many of the pristine streams of the Rocky Mountains. The prevalence of giardiasis in the United States was estimated from 24 published surveys to be 7.4 per cent. It is the most commonly identified cause of water-borne infectious diarrhea and the most frequently isolated stool parasite in the United States.

ETIOLOGY. Although van Leeuwenhoek was the first to observe *G. lamblia* when he peered at his own stool with his primitive microscope in 1681, several centuries elapsed before the pathogenicity of this small intestinal flagellate was appreciated. It was long thought to be a commensal. Only in the last several decades was its role as a cause of infectious diarrhea and malabsorption recognized.

The organism exists either as the motile, flagellated, pear-shaped trophozoite, 12 to 15 μm in length, or as the somewhat smaller, tough-walled oval cyst. Infection occurs in the small intestine of the host. Trophozoites either attach to the microvilli of the intestinal epithelium with single ventral foot-like sucking discs or move about in the unstirred layer of mucus just above the epithelial surface. The trophozoites, carried caudally by peristalsis, eventually encyst and are passed out into the environment. The cyst is resistant to many environmental stresses, including concentrations of chlorine normally found in treated municipal water supplies. It is ingested eventually by a subsequent host. Excystation occurs in the acid environment of the stomach, and infection is again established in the small intestine.

EPIDEMIOLOGY. *Giardia* spreads by two routes: water-borne infection, particularly in contaminated community water supplies, and direct person-to-person transmission. Over two dozen epidemics have been described in the United States consequent to breakdown of community water filtration systems. Epidemics in day-care centers for children and among promiscuous male homosexuals indicate that direct person-to-person spread can occur.

A possible role for animal reservoirs of infection has been suggested by the demonstration of *Giardia*-infected beaver upstream from communities where outbreaks of human infection have occurred. Although controversy remains about the possibility of cross-species transmission of human *Giardia,* it is now suspected that both beaver and dogs may carry *Giardia* species infectious for humans.

Giardia is a frequent source of diarrhea in travelers returning from endemic areas. Twenty-three per cent of North American travelers returning from Leningrad have been shown to have giardiasis. Typically, the infected traveler develops symptoms several weeks after returning home, and on this basis the infection may be distinguished from that caused by toxigenic *E. coli* and other forms of infectious traveler's diarrhea with shorter incubation periods.

Its presence in persons with humoral immune deficiency syndromes has long been recognized. It has been estimated that 80 per cent of persons with common variable immune deficiency and diarrhea—so-called immunodeficient sprue—improve when treated with anti-*Giardia* drugs.

PATHOGENICITY. Jejunal mucosal biopsies from infected persons range in appearance from normal to marked subtotal mucosal atrophy with submucosal inflammatory cell infiltration, reduced villous height, and elongated crypts. Electron microscopic observation of epithelial cells beneath overlying adherent trophozoites show deformation and blunting of the individual microvilli. The mechanisms for these changes remain unknown. Possible hypotheses include mechanical interference by *Giardia* overlying the epithelium, elaboration by the parasite of an unidentifiable soluble toxin, competition between the parasite and host for nutrients, direct damage of the epithelium by adherent trophozoites, concurrent abnormal small intestinal bacterial overgrowth, invasion of submucosa by *Giardia* trophozoites with consequent elicitation of cellular inflammation, and immunopathogenic mechanisms mediated by the host's immune system.

CLINICAL MANIFESTATIONS. The majority of infections with *Giardia* are asymptomatic. In those persons who are ill, disease ranges from mild diarrhea to severe debilitating malabsorption and weight loss. Reversible lactase deficiency as well as malabsorption of fat and vitamin B_{12} has been documented. The majority of symptoms result from malabsorption and include abdominal distention, cramps, nausea, flatulence, borborygmi, and frequent loose, bulky, foul, and urgent stools. Although some persons have a self-limited infection of several weeks' duration, many have a prolonged indolent illness with waxing and waning symptoms and progressive weight loss.

DIAGNOSIS. The diagnosis is established in the suspected patient by demonstration of cysts or trophozoites in stools, or trophozoites in small bowel contents. Because excretion of the organism in stool is episodic and its demonstration elusive, at least three stool specimens should be examined before a negative conclusion is drawn. If no organisms are seen, the small bowel contents should be sampled. This can be achieved by aspiration or passage of a string which will absorb sufficient jejunal fluid for examination. Microscopic examination of a wet preparation of jejunal contents will usually reveal motile organisms in the infected person. Small bowel biopsy may be reserved for situations when these measures are unsuccessful. The small bowel roentgenogram will usually show an edematous mucosa, but this finding is nonspecific. Hematologic studies are normal. Eosinophilia should not be expected, since this is a finding associated with infections by worms, not protozoa.

TREATMENT. All infected persons should be treated. Moreover, there is occasional justification for a trial of therapy in the rare patient with typical signs and symptoms of giardiasis but in whom exhaustive efforts to demonstrate the organism fail. Therapy is achieved with quinacrine hydrochloride, 100 mg three times daily for ten days. When this drug is contraindicated, metronidazole,* 250 mg three times daily for seven days, is an alternative. Treatment with either drug may be unsuccessful in 5 to 20 per cent of patients, requiring a second course of therapy. Resolution of symptoms is often slow, in spite of effective therapy.

Hoskins LC, Winawer SJ, Bortman SA, Gottlieb LS, Zamcheck N: Clinical giardiasis and intestinal malabsorption. Gastroenterology 53:265, 1967. *Virtually every aspect of the clinical presentation of giardiasis is described in this series of case reports.*

Mahmoud AAF, Warren KS: Algorithms in the diagnosis and management of exotic diseases. II. Giardiasis. J Infect Dis 131:621, 1975. *A succinct and critical outline for the process of evaluation and treatment of the patient with giardiasis. The bibliography is highly selective.*

Stevens DP: Giardiasis: Host-pathogen biology. Rev Inf Dis 4:851, 1982. *A detailed review of the sparse knowledge available on the pathogenesis of this infection.*

TRICHOMONIASIS

Trichomonas vaginalis is probably the only species of the trichomonads that is pathogenic for humans. It is a 10 to 20 μ motile flagellated organism that ordinarily inhabits the urethra, urinary bladder, vagina, and prostate. Nearly half of infections are asymptomatic. Recognized symptoms, however, include a yellow creamy vaginal discharge associated with itching and burning. Dysuria may be prominent. Infection in the male is almost always asymptomatic.

Diagnosis is made microscopically by identification of the organism in a wet preparation of the exudate. While long-term complications are unrecognized in otherwise healthy persons, treatment of both partners is required for cessation of symptoms of this sexually transmitted disease. Treatment is accomplished with a single 1 to 2 gram dose of metronidazole, although this is frequently associated with side effects of nausea, a metallic taste, or alcohol intolerance.

Fouts AC, Krause SJ: Trichomonas vaginalis: Re-evaluation of its clinical presentation and laboratory diagnosis. J Infect Dis 141:137, 1980. *An authoritative clinical report for further detailed study.*

BALANTIDIASIS

Balantidium coli is a large, motile, oval ciliate, some five to ten times the size of an erythrocyte. The trophozoite form resides as a facultative anaerobe in the colon. The great majority of infections in humans are noninvasive, asymptomatic, and self-limited. Infrequently a cause of disease, this protozoan can penetrate the colonic mucosa with formation of deep ulcers. Illness consists of dysentery, usually bloody, often with resulting dehydration and prostration. Complications include colonic perforation at the site of the ulcers. Infection may extend to mesenteric lymph nodes and, less commonly, the appendix and terminal ileum. Isolated reports of infection of vagina, liver, lung, and pleura have documented that extraintestinal migration of the organism is rare.

Balantidia infect numerous nonhuman reservoirs, particularly swine. It is said that 80 per cent of pigs in England carry this organism. The relevance of various other animal reservoirs, such as rats, to human infection is debated. The importance of porcine infections to human disease is borne out, however, by the documented high prevalence of balantidiasis in communities where swine and humans live together closely, e.g., in New Guinea, Micronesia, Peru, and southern Russia. Poor nutrition and debilitating illness seem to predispose to symptomatic balantidiasis. Person-to-person spread probably occurs in settings where crowding and poor hygiene exist.

Ingestion of *Balantidium* cysts leads to infection in the susceptible host. Excystation occurs at an unknown location in the gastrointestinal tract, and multiplication occurs in the colon. An immune response develops in humans when tissue invasion occurs and is demonstrated by the presence of circulating immunofluorescent antibodies. Encystation occurs in the distal colon or after expulsion into the environment. The cyst, resistant to drying and other environmental stresses, becomes again the infectious form for the subsequent host.

The diagnosis is confirmed in the suspected patient by microscopic demonstration of trophozoites in fresh wet preparations of liquid stool or scrapings of colonic ulcers. Cysts are less frequently observed in stool, and concentration techniques are usually required. Differentiation from amebiasis and idiopathic ulcerative colitis must always be considered.

Therapy is reserved for the patient with symptomatic infection and consists of tetracycline, 500 mg four times daily for ten days. Metronidazole, 250 mg four times daily for seven days, is probably effective and may serve as alternative therapy when tetracycline is not tolerated.

Knight R: Giardiasis, isosporiasis, and balantidiasis. Clin Gastroenterol 7:31, 1978. *There are few timely clinical reviews on balantidiasis; this is the best of the lot.*

COCCIDIOSIS (Cryptosporidiosis, Isosporiasis)

Coccidia may infect humans, usually with a short-lived infection characterized by diarrhea, malaise, and weight loss. Increasingly, these organisms have been found to cause chronic debilitating infections in human hosts suffering from immune deficiency states such as acquired immune deficiency syndrome.

The 4 to 6 μ oocysts of *Cryptosporidium*, a protozoa previously recognized exclusively as an animal parasite, have been found in stools of immune-compromised human hosts by the use of modified acid-fast staining techniques. The clinical presentation includes prolonged and debilitating diarrhea, weight loss, fever, and abdominal pain. Spread to the trachea and bronchial tree has been reported. Therapy including metronidazole, quinacrine, or antibiotics has been generally disappointing.

Infection with *Isospora belli*, the oocysts of which are 23 to 33 μ long and 12 to 14 μ wide, is often asymptomatic. Nevertheless, *I. belli* may result in malabsorption, diarrhea, weight loss, and even death. It is usually found in the tropics, often where uncooked meats are consumed. It is also spread directly by fecal-oral transmission. Consequently its presence in institutions where hygienic practices are poor should be suspected when the appropriate clinical presentation is observed. Microscopic examination of small bowel biopsy specimens show flattened mucosal villi accompanied by inflammatory cell infiltration. Several case reports describing *I. belli* infection in association with lymphoma suggest that it, too, should be suspected in immunosuppressed patients with diarrhea.

Pitlik SD, Fainstein V, Garza D, Guarda L, Bolivar R, Rios A, Hopfer RL, Mansell PA: Human cryptosporidiosis: Spectrum of disease. Report of six cases and review of the literature. Arch Intern Med 143:2269, 1983. *A detailed study of the clinical picture and timely review of available references.*

Treatment of cryptosporidiosis in patients with acquired immunodeficiency syndrome (AIDS). Morbid Mortal Wkly Rep 33:117, 1984. *A compendium of therapy administered to a total of 112 patients. The results were dismal.*

SARCOSPORIDIOSIS

Infections with *Sarcocystis hominis* (previously designated *Isospora hominis*) may be associated with abdominal pain, diarrhea,

*This use is not listed in the manufacturer's directive, but is recommended by the Centers for Disease Control.

and nausea. The human is the definitive host with sexual reproduction taking place in the small intestine; cattle are the intermediate host where the sarcocyst resides in the skeletal or cardiac muscle with little or no reaction. While infection in humans is relatively common in areas of the world where undercooked beef is ingested because of local custom, the definition of the precise role of this agent in human disease remains clouded by its frequent coincidence with other pathogenic agents.

Beaver PC, Gadgil RK, Morera P: Sarcocysts in man: A review and report of five cases. Am J Trop Med Hyg 28:810, 1979. *This reference provides a good starting point into the available clinical literature.*

Section Two HELMINTHIC DISEASES

387. INTRODUCTION

Adel A. F. Mahmoud

"Parasite" is an all-embracing definition for infectious causes of human disease and should include viruses, bacteria, protozoa, fungi, and helminths. Within this definition, a useful distinction between microparasites and macroparasites has been suggested. The former refers to all infectious agents that directly reproduce within the definitive or mammalian host (Ch. 377). On the other hand, macroparasites that include most helminthic infections have certain biologic characteristics that set them apart from other pathogens; these features are essential in understanding host-parasite relationship. Helminths or worms have no direct reproductive capabilities within their definitive host. Therefore, an increase in worm numbers in a particular host necessitates repeated exposures to the infective stage of the pathogen. Furthermore, worm infections are usually of long duration (mean life span varies from several months to several decades), and in most circumstances reinfection potential is abundant in endemic areas. In helminthiases, a majority of infected individuals harbor few worms; the resultant morbidity is therefore generally mild. In a minority of infected individuals, worm loads are high (infection is characteristically aggregated and not normally distributed in human populations); these subjects are at higher risk of developing significant pathologic sequelae. The multicellular nature of worms, their complex antigenic structures and their elaborate evasive mechanisms add to the complexity of host-parasite relationship. Unfortunately, there are as yet no clear approaches to induction of protective immunity in humans against worm infections.

Helminthiases are prevalent in many parts of the developing and developed countries. For example, *Ascaris lumbricoides* infects approximately one fourth of the world's population while *Enterobius vermicularis* is estimated to infect 40 million people in the United States. Some worm infections such as *Strongyloides stercoralis* are particularly important in the immunosuppressed host since hyperinfection may lead to grave morbidity and considerable mortality. A systematic clinical approach to individuals with suspected worm infections should include knowledge of the geographic distribution, mode of infection, and specific symptoms and signs, if any. Diagnosis is usually dependent on obtaining and handling appropriate samples to be examined by experienced laboratory personnel. Serologic tests may be of help in some specific circumstances, such as toxocariasis, when obtaining a definitive parasitologic diagnosis may be impossible or may expose the infected subject to unnecessary and potentially hazardous procedures.

Eosinophilia, when present, is a useful clinical manifestation of worm infections that migrate in host tissues. Worms that reside exclusively in body cavities such as adult *Ascaris lumbricoides* in the lumen of small intestines are not associated with eosinophilia. Increased eosinophil counts may be observed in peripheral blood or affected tissues of infected individuals. Specific chemotherapy is usually followed by an increase of cell count before it subsides to normal levels. Eosinophilia in helminthic infections results from a combination of specific worm components that are either chemotactic or that induce other host cells to release chemotactic, eosinophilopoietic, or activating factors. The cells obtained from individuals with helminthiases and eosinophilia exhibit more Fc and complement receptors on their surface, are metabolically activated, and may be more efficient than those from uninfected subjects in killing invading stages of worms. Because of the large size of most invading stages of worms, killing of these targets by eosinophils occurs extracellularly and is mediated by a combination of oxidative and nonoxidative mechanisms.

Chemotherapy of helminthic infections has changed drastically over the last few years. Currently, there are effective, safe, and orally administered chemotherapeutic agents for most worm infections. These agents are of great help to the clinician in treating individual cases and to the public health authorities in planning control programs.

Mahmoud AAF, Austen KF (eds.): The Eosinophil in Health and Disease. Grune & Stratton, New York, 1980, p 364.
Schmidt GD, Roberts LS (eds.): Foundations of Parasitology, 2nd ed. C. V. Mosby Company, St. Louis, 1981, p 795.
Warren KS, Mahmoud AAF (eds.): Tropical and Geographical Medicine, McGraw-Hill Book Company, New York, 1984, pp 345–541.

The Cestodes

Martin S. Wolfe

388. INTRODUCTION

More than 30 species of tapeworms, or cestodes, may infect man. They are dorsoventrally flattened and creamy white, and their habitat is the intestinal tract of vertebrates. With the exception of *Hymenolepis nana*, which can be passed directly from person to person, all the species that parasitize man require at least one intermediate host to complete their life cycle.

Adult cestodes range in size from the smallest, *Echinococcus* species of 2 to 9 mm long, to the largest, *Diphyllobothrium latum*, which ranges in size from 3 to 10 meters long. They all have characteristic morphologic and biologic features that differentiate them from other helminths and from each other. Most adult tapeworms consist of a head or scolex for attachment to the intestinal wall of the host. Behind this is an unsegmented narrow neck from which immature segments or proglottides develop progressively to fully developed mature proglottides. Most distal are the oldest and gravid segments, which are essentially a sac of eggs. The entire worm, from the scolex to and including the distal gravid proglottides, is called the strobila. Each mature proglottid has both sets of sex organs, nerve trunks, and an excretory canal. There is no alimentary canal in tapeworms, and food is absorbed directly from the cuticle, which has a microvillus surface similar to intestinal mucosa of vertebrates. Diagnosis of certain species can be made from the gravid segments, which may have particular branchings and shape of the uterus or position of the genital pore.

Eggs are passed from the bowel either in the segment or free in the stool, and contain a form infective for an intermediate host. Eggs may be operculate, an adaptation for hatching in water, or nonoperculate, which usually develop in soil. Operculate eggs, exemplified by *Diphyllobothrium latum*, are undeveloped when passed, and a free-swimming larva or coracidium hatches in 9 to 12 days. This is ingested by a copepod, in which further development takes place to a procercoid larva; this in turn is ingested by an appropriate fish, in whose flesh the infective or plerocercoid larva is found. When man ingests fish with a plerocercoid larva, the larva adheres to the small intestinal wall, where it develops. When nonoperculate eggs of other species are ingested by an appropriate intermediate host, an embryo or oncosphere is released, which has the capability of penetrating the intestinal mucosa. Oncospheres of *Taenia* species penetrate the intestinal wall of the intermediate host and develop into small fluid-filled structures called cysticerci, which are distributed in various tissues and cause the disease cysticercosis. *Hymenolepis nana* oncospheres penetrate only into the villi of the small intestine and develop into cysticercoids, which eventually break out into the lumen of the intestine and attach and develop into adults. With *Echinococcus granulosus* usually only one oncosphere develops into a cyst in the intermediate host, but this hydatid or echinococcal cyst is capable of producing daughter cysts, each containing many scoleces, from an internal germinating membrane.

Pathogenesis and symptomatology are determined by the various forms of development. Humans are the definitive host of adult *D. latum* and *Taenia* worms, but the most serious effects occur when man becomes an accidental intermediate host of *Taenia solium* and cysticerci lead to many small lesions in the muscle and brain. The cysticercoids and adults of *H. nana* and adults of *Taenia* species may cause irritation of the small intestine. *Echinococcus* and *Multiceps* species produce large space-occupying cysts with symptoms depending on their location.

In the following chapters, geographic distribution, essential biology, epidemiology, pathogenesis, symptomatology, diagnosis, and prevention will be described for each of the common and some less common related cestode species which parasitize man. A final chapter will deal with the treatment of tapeworms.

Beaver PC, Jung RC, Cupp EW: Clinical Parasitology, 9th Ed. Philadelphia, Lea & Febiger, 1984, Ch 25. *An encyclopedic review of both common and very rare tapeworms of man.*

Marcial-Rojas RA (ed.): Pathology of Protozoal and Helminthic Diseases with Clinical Correlations. Baltimore, Williams & Wilkins Company, 1971, pp 585–657. *A well-illustrated and very complete discussion of pathologic and clinical aspects of the major tapeworms.*

389. DIPHYLLOBOTHRIUM LATUM (The Fish Tapeworm)

This parasite is most prevalent in parts of the northern and southern temperate zones where fresh water fish are commonly eaten. The highest incidence of infection of humans is in the countries bordering the Baltic Sea, particularly Finland and Sweden. In North America, a high incidence of *D. latum* infection occurs in Alaska, Canada, and the smaller lake areas of northern Michigan and Minnesota. A related species carried by marine fishes, *Diphyllobothrium pacificum*, has recently been described from coastal Peru.

D. latum adults are the largest tapeworms of man and may reach 10 meters in length with up to 4000 proglottides. The scolex has two deep sulci or bothria, one dorsal and one ventral, for attachment to the wall of the ileum. The last four fifths of the worm consists of maturing and gravid proglottides. The mature proglottid is broader than it is long, and in its middle is a dark, rosette-shaped, coiled uterus, which is of diagnostic value. The distalmost proglottides gradually disintegrate and release eggs in the bowel lumen, rather than separating from the parent worm like *Taenia* segments. Eggs are yellowish-brown, ovoid, and operculated and measure 56 to 76 μ long by 40 to 56 μ wide. They contain immature embryos when discharged into the feces, and under favorable conditions they mature and hatch into a ciliated coracidium in 9 to 12 days. This is ingested by the first intermediate host, a freshwater copepod of the genus *Cyclops* or *Diaptomus*, wherein it develops into a procercoid larva. The copepod is in turn ingested by the second intermediate host, certain freshwater fish species, including pike, perch, and salmon. The procercoid larva develops into a plerocercoid larva (sparganum) within the muscle and viscera of the fish in 7 to 30 days. Man becomes infected by eating raw or insufficiently cooked fish. The sparganum adheres to the wall of the small intestine and reaches maturity in three to six weeks, and eggs begin to appear in the feces. Inadequate sewage disposal allows pollution by human feces of fresh water containing suitable intermediate hosts. The fishes of small lakes are more important sources of infection than those of the Great Lakes, since the cold deep waters of the latter inhibit the hatching of eggs. Women of particular ethnic groups, such as Jews, Russians, and Scandinavians, are more frequently infected, by eating raw or undercooked fish in the preparation of ethnic foods such as gefilte fish. *D. latum* may live for up to 20 years.

The great majority of infections are with a single worm in the ileum. Most infected persons are asymptomatic, but some may experience intestinal symptoms from mucosal irritation. A moderate eosinophilia may be present. The most harmful effect of the fish tapeworm is vitamin B_{12} malabsorption and, rarely, a megaloblastic anemia. The exact mechanism is not certain, but it is related to the absorption of vitamin B_{12} by the worm. This is reported primarily in Scandinavians.

Diagnosis can be made by recovering characteristic eggs in the feces, or from the typical proglottides which are broader than long and have a characteristic rosette-shaped uterus. There is no satisfactory serologic method of diagnosis.

Prevention is with adequate disposal of raw sewage. Fish from known or suspected infected lakes must be thoroughly cooked at 56° C for at least five minutes or frozen at −10° C for 72 hours to ensure destruction of the infective larvae.

SPARGANOSIS

Sparganosis is an uncommon infection of man with larval diphyllobothroid tapeworms closely related to *D. latum*. It is caused by the sparganum or plerocercoid larva of the genus *Spirometra*, which measures up to several centimeters in length. Most human infections have been encountered in the Orient and are caused by *S. mansonoides*. Very rarely, infection is with a budding larval tapeworm, *S. proliferum*. The life cycle is similar to that of *D. latum*. Adult worms are found in dogs and cats, and in man only the larval form occurs. Eggs hatch in water and develop into procercoid larvae in *Cyclops* species, which are swallowed by the secondary intermediate host—a frog, snake, bird, or mammal. A plerocercoid larva develops in the muscle and is finally ingested by the definitive host. Humans usually become infected by ingesting infected copepods containing the procercoid larvae. Infections in the Far East may occur from the ingestion of infected raw flesh of amphibians and reptiles or by the use of these animals' flesh for medicinal skin or eye poultices. After penetrating the intestinal wall, the larvae usually migrate through the tissues and localize in the subcutaneous or muscular tissues. When infected poultices are applied to the eye, localization and edema may occur around the eye. A slowly growing, pruritic nodule develops over a three- to ten-month period, eventually measuring up to 3 cm. Local indurations, periodic urticaria, edema, erythema, chills, fever, and marked peripheral eosinophilia may occur. The parasite should be considered in anyone with a localized subcutaneous swelling and a possible exposure history. Diagnosis is by finding the characteristic larvae in the removed nodules. Infection can be prevented by avoiding untreated drinking water in endemic areas and avoiding the ingestion of uncooked flesh of amphibians and reptiles or the use of this flesh for poultices in the Far East.

Editorial: Pathogenesis of tapeworm anemia. Br Med J 2:1028, 1976. *A brief update on this most intriguing aspect of fish tapeworm infection.*
Swartzwelder JC, Beaver PC, Hood MW: Sparganosis in southern United States. Am J Trop Med Hyg 13:43, 1964. *A number of interesting case reports.*
Von Bonsdorff B: Diphyllobothriasis in Man. London, Academic Press, 1977. *Written from a medical rather than parasitologic viewpoint. A useful reference book which covers developments in diphyllobothriasis since Birkeland's monograph of 1932.*
Weinstein P, Krawczyk HG, Peers JH: Sparganosis in Korea. Am J Trop Med Hyg 3:112, 1954. *Three case reports and discussion of snake eating among Koreans and its possible relationship to sparganosis.*

390. TAENIA SAGINATA (The Beef Tapeworm)

Cattle are the most important intermediate hosts. In Africa cattle are frequently and heavily infected, and human infection rates may exceed 10 per cent in some areas. The parasite occurs throughout Asia, there is a low level of endemicity in Latin America and Europe, and rare cases are indigenously acquired in the United States. *Taenia saginata* is one of the most frequently diagnosed tapeworms in the United States, usually being acquired abroad.

The adult worm ranges from 4 to 10 meters in length and consists of 1000 to 2000 proglottides. The scolex has four prominent muscular suckers for attachment to the small intestinal wall. Proglottides are usually detached singly and have muscular power that allows them to move through the anal sphincter, or they may be carried out with the feces. The eggs are liberated from the proglottid. They are yellow-brown and cannot be morphologically differentiated from those of *Taenia solium*. Eggs become mature in approximately two weeks, and are then infective to the intermediate hosts, primarily cattle. After hatching in the intestine, the oncospheres penetrate the intestinal wall and eventually localize in the skeletal muscles of cattle, where they develop in 60 to 75 days into small cysticerci having an opaque invaginated neck and a scolex with four suckers. In about 12 months the cysticercus degenerates and calcifies. Humans are the only definitive host and become infected by ingesting raw or undercooked beef containing cysticerci. The scolex evaginates and attaches to the jejunal mucosa, where in 8 to 12 weeks it develops into an adult worm. *Taenia* worms may live up to 25 years in man. Human infection is favored by the ingestion of meat in the form of beef tartare, rare steak, and undercooked shashlik or kabobs.

Usually only one worm is present, but multiple infections can occur rarely. In most cases the adult worms are in the upper jejunum and cause no damage or symptoms. Irritation, however, may cause flatulence, cramps, or diarrhea. Eosinophilia occurs in almost half of those infected and is usually less than 10 per cent. Infection is usually recognized by the spontaneous passage of gravid proglottides out of the anus or in the feces.

Diagnosis is made by pressing the passed proglottid between two large glass slides and counting the number of lateral uterine segments. *T. saginata* usually has 15 to 30 of these uterine segments, whereas the only other similar-appearing segment, that of *T. solium*, usually has less than 13 and an average of 9 uterine segments. Identification of lateral uterine segments can be made only on mature proglottides. In doubtful cases, diagnosis may require fixation and staining of the segments. Typical *Taenia* ova may be found on stool examination, but differentiation between *T. saginata* and *T. solium* cannot be made on egg morphology alone. Eggs may also be recovered from the perianal region with use of a scotch tape swab. Serologic tests have not proved useful in the diagnosis of *T. saginata*.

Infection can best be prevented by avoiding rare or raw beef in highly endemic areas such as Africa. Thorough cooking of beef at 56° C for five minutes or freezing at −10° C for ten days will kill cysticerci.

Pawlowski Z, Schultz MG: Taeniasis and cysticercosis (*Taenia saginata*). Adv Parasitol 10:269, 1972. *Detailed coverage of all aspects of this parasite.*
Penfold HB: The signs and symptoms of *Taenia saginata* infestation. Med J Aust 1:531, 1937. *Common and uncommon findings in 100 patients.*

391. TAENIA SOLIUM (The Pork Tapeworm; Human Cysticercosis)

Human infection is cosmopolitan but is especially prevalent where man commonly consumes raw or insufficiently cooked pork. Infections with both adult worms and tissue larvae are particularly common in India, Africa, Mexico, and Latin America, but are rare in the United States and western Europe where most recognized cases are imported.

The adult worm is smaller than *T. saginata*, measuring 2 to 4 meters long, and contains 800 to 1000 segments. The scolex has four cup-shaped suckers and differs from *T. saginata* in having a double crown of between 25 and 30 hooks on a low rounded rostellum. Mature proglottides are flabby, have less muscular action than those of *T. saginata*, and have 7 to 12 lateral branches. The ova are morphologically identical to *T. saginata* ova. Gravid proglottides or eggs are ingested by the usual intermediate host, the hog, and less frequently by other intermediate hosts, including wild boars, sheep, camels, and humans. Eggs must first be digested by gastric juice before they hatch and liberate oncospheres, which then penetrate the intestinal wall and are carried throughout the body. They typically are filtered out in the muscles but can also reach other organs. In 60 to 70 days cysticerci develop that contain an invaginated scolex with hooks and suckers. Cysticerci may remain viable in the hog for three to six years or, rarely, longer. Man is the only natural definitive host and becomes infected by eating raw or undercooked pork. The cysticerci are dissolved by gastric juices, and the larval worm attaches to the upper jejunum by its evaginated scolex. In 5 to 12 weeks it develops into an adult worm. Human infection with *Cysticercus cellulosae* occurs when people ingest eggs in contaminated food or water or eggs transferred from the anus to the mouth, or, rarely, by the regurgitation of ova into the stomach by reverse peristalsis associated with vomiting in the presence of an adult worm. Human infection is most common in populations with a preference for pork, thus being rare in Moslems and Jews. Infection is also related to general poor hygienic conditions in which hogs are allowed to have frequent contact with infected feces. As it often takes some years for cysticerci to develop, die, and lead to overt symptoms, most cases are recognized in adulthood.

Intestinal infection is usually with one adult worm, and this seldom causes anything more than local irritation and mild eosinophilia. Cysticerci may develop in any tissue or organ of the body. The cysticercus matures in man in a few months and forms a translucent cyst, which gradually becomes surrounded by a fibrous capsule. Eventually the larvae die and calcify. No serious effects result from cysticerci in their most frequent locations, the subcutaneous tissue and skeletal muscles, although palpable or visible subcutaneous nodules can be recognized in approximately half of those with established infections. These are more frequently felt in the pectoral and abdominal superficial tissues than in the limbs and may simulate neurofibromatosis. The invasive stage often causes no symptoms, but fever, eosinophilia, muscle aches, and fatigue have been described. In the brain cysticerci may be present in the cortex, meninges, ventricles, or substance of the cerebrum. Cysts in the ventricle may cause hydrocephalus. When parasites die in the brain, they provoke a severe inflammatory reaction that can lead to increased pressure symptoms. Calcification occurs after the parasite has been dead for some years.

Cerebrospinal changes occur more often in the presence of cysts in contact with the subarachnoid space rather than with parenchymatous cysts, and include pleocytosis, eosinophilia, increased protein, and decreased sugar. Patients with larvae in the brain may present with epilepsy, intracranial hypertension, and motor or sensory or personality changes many years after initial infection. *Cysticercus* is the most common larval tapeworm to invade the eye, which it reaches through the retinal artery. The unencapsulated larva is 6 to 14 mm in size and sausage shaped. It may lodge anywhere in the orbit, conjunctiva, or anterior chamber, but most commonly is subretinal in the vitreous. Reactions to live larvae are usually minimal, but dead parasites produce iridocyclitis, clouding of the vitreous, and severe retinal inflammation or detachment. Patients may present with intraorbital pain, light flashes, and blurred or absent vision. Cysts may rarely localize in all layers of the heart tissue and may produce myocarditis or congestive heart failure.

Diagnosis of adult worms can be made by finding *Taenia* eggs or characteristic segments in the stool. Cysticercosis is suggested by a history of infection with an adult worm, the presence of multiple subcutaneous nodules, typical symptoms, earlier residence in a highly endemic area where undercooked pork may have been eaten, and a moderate eosinophilia. Definitive diagnosis is by removal of subcutaneous nodules or brain cysts. After calcification of larvae, roentgenologic diagnosis from typical lesions may be made, but this is usually not possible until after five years of muscle infection or until after ten years of brain infection. Brain scan, EEG, and CT scan can confirm space-occupying lesions. With CT scan, different stages of development of the cysticerci may be seen in an individual patient. Cerebral cysticercosis must be differentiated from hydatid or coenurus cyst, brain tumors, and cerebral lues. An indirect hemagglutination test is presently the best available serologic test and is positive in a significant number of cases. However, a negative result cannot rule out cysticercosis. A complement fixation test may be positive on cerebrospinal fluid, particularly when inflammatory changes are present in the CSF.

Infection with adult worms can be prevented by heating pork from 49 to 53° C for at least a half hour, or freezing at −10° C for four days, which kills larvae. Pickling and smoking are usually not sufficient to destroy cysticerci. Proper hygienic measures and disposal of human excrement can prevent human cysticercosis.

Bickerstaff ER: Cerebral cysticercosis. Common but unfamiliar manifestations. Br Med J 1:1055, 1955. *Illustrative case reports and good discussion.*

Byrd SE, Locke GE, Biggers S, Percy AK: The computed tomographic appearance of cerebral cysticercosis in adults and children. Radiology 144:819, 1982. *The best available method for diagnosis of brain cysts.*

Dixon HBF, Lipscomb FM: Cysticercosis: An Analysis and Followup of 450 Cases. London Privy Council, Med Res Special Rept Ser No 299, 1961. *A classic review of 450 cases in British troops returned from India.*

Powell SJ, Proctor EM, Wilmot AJ, MacLeod IN: Cysticercosis and epilepsy in Africans: A clinical and serological study. Ann Trop Med Parasitol 60:152, 1966. *Clinical descriptions and value of hemagglutination test in diagnosis.*

Reddy PS, Satyendran DM: Ocular cysticercosis. Am J Ophthalmol 57:665, 1964. *Ten cases and general review of subject.*

392. HYMENOLEPIS NANA (The Dwarf Tapeworm)

Hymenolepis nana has a worldwide distribution but is most prevalent in warm, dry climates. It is common in southern and eastern Europe, the Middle East, Africa, and Latin America. In the United States it is particularly common in the southeastern and southwestern states and in institutional populations.

This parasite takes its name of the dwarf tapeworm from the very small size of the adult worm, which measures 25 to 40 mm long by 1 mm wide. It has a minute scolex with four cup-shaped suckers and a short rostellum armed with 20 to 30 small hooks. Individual segments are not seen in the stool, and mature proglottides are approximately 0.85 mm long by 0.22 mm wide. Eggs are set free by gradual disintegration of the distalmost proglottides. Eggs are characteristic in having a clear area between the shell and an inner envelope, and four to eight threadlike filaments arising from each of two polar thickenings of the inner envelope. They measure 45 by 35 μ. Eggs are immediately infective when passed in the feces. No intermediate host is required, and upon ingestion of the eggs by the definitive host (man, mouse, or rat) oncospheres hatch in the small intestine and penetrate into the villi, where they develop into cysticercoid larvae. In about four days these break out into the intestinal lumen and attach to villi in the upper two thirds of the ileum, where they become adults in 10 to 12 days. Internal autoinfection may lead to continued heavy infection. The life duration of the worm is only a few months. Infection is transmitted directly from hand to mouth and also by contaminated food and water. Children are infected more often than adults, as resistance increases with age.

Infections in man with over 1000 worms can occur. In most light infections no injury is caused to the mucosa and there are no symptoms, but mucosal irritation from heavy worm loads may lead to anorexia, abdominal pain, and diarrhea. Mild eosinophilia is often present.

Diagnosis is by the recovery of characteristic double membrane eggs in the stool. Personal hygiene, particularly in families and institutions, is the most effective method of prevention.

Otto GF: Human infestation with the dwarf tapeworm (*Hymenolepis nana*) in the southern United States. Am J Hyg 23:25, 1936. *Clinical aspects as seen in an earlier time in the United States.*

393. ECHINOCOCCOSIS (Hydatid Disease)

Three main species of *Echinococcus* infect man. *Echinococcus granulosus* is by far the most common with a worldwide distribution, especially in sheep-raising areas. Sheep are the main intermediate hosts, with dogs being the definitive host. Human infection rates are highest in southern Europe, the Mediterranean littoral, the Middle East, eastern Africa, Australia and New Zealand, and Latin America. The majority of cases in the United States are found in immigrants from endemic areas, but autochthonous cases are found in sheep-raising areas of western states. Another strain variant, *Echinococcus granulosus var. canadensis,* has a sylvatic cycle with wild animals as the main hosts and occurs in Alaska and Canada. Alveolar hydatid disease, caused by *Echinococcus multilocularis,* is restricted to the Northern Hemisphere, occurring in Europe, northcentral United States, Canada, and Alaska, with foxes as definitive hosts and rodents as intermediate hosts. A related species, *Echinococcus oligarthus,* with cats as normal hosts and small rodents as the main intermediate hosts, has been described in a few human cases in Panama and Colombia. The following discussion will refer primarily to *E. granulosus.*

Adult worms of the three species can be differentiated morphologically and are the smallest of the tapeworms, measuring from 2 to 9 mm long and consisting of a scolex, a neck, and usually three segments, the last of which is gravid. Adult worms inhabit the upper jejunum of the definitive host, principally dogs, wolves, coyotes, foxes, and cats. In dogs, their life span is three to six months. Ova, similar to those of *Taenia* species, are evacuated in the feces of the definitive host and are ingested by the intermediate host, primarily sheep and rodents, and less commonly by man. Eggs can live for some months in moist, shady soil. The shell is digested in the duodenum, and the freed embryo penetrates into the intestinal mucosa and is carried by the bloodstream until it is filtered out in a small capillary. This usually occurs in the liver, the first capillary filter; next most commonly in the lung; and less frequently in other tissues and organs of the body. The parasite then develops into a bladderlike cyst, which increases at a rate of approximately 1 cm per year. As the cyst grows, a fibrous connective tissue cyst wall is formed by reaction of the host. Inside this is a germinal layer from which budding secondary daughter cysts develop. Hydatid fluid fills the cyst, which in the case of *E. granulosus* is unilocular. With *E. multilocularis,* multilocular or alveolar cysts occur, owing to the very thin laminated membrane, which is not sharply separated from the surrounding tissue and allows for exogenous budding and malignant-like growth. Metastases may occur via the circulation. *E. oligarthus* cysts also tend to be multilocular. When dogs or other definitive hosts eat the infected flesh or offal of intermediate hosts, embryonic tapeworms within developed cysts are freed in the duodenum and attach by their scoleces to the intestinal wall, becoming adult worms.

Man is infected only by the larval or hydatid cyst stage through intimate contact with infected dogs or other definitive hosts. Infection of dogs and other reservoir hosts depends upon the dog-sheep (or rarely cattle), or wild animal-moose or rodent relationship, whereby reservoir hosts are infected by consuming infected carcasses or offal. Most *E. granulosus* infections occur in childhood by hand-to-mouth transmission of eggs picked up from the fur of dogs.

Pathology in man depends upon the location of the cyst. About 65 per cent of unilocular and 90 per cent of multilocular cysts occur in the liver, usually in the right lobe. *E. granulosus* cysts are multiple in about one quarter of patients. Lung cysts account for approximately 20 per cent of total *E. granulosus* infections, whereas the remaining 15 per cent may involve almost any other body organ or tissue. Physical signs and symptoms do not usually occur until cysts are at least 10 to 20 cm in diameter, about 10 to 20 years after initial infection. Rupture or leakage of viable cysts may lead to secondary multiple implantations of the peritoneum or other organs. Cysts may lead to compression or atrophy of surrounding tissue. Cysts may become inactive and calcify without ever causing symptoms, although there may still be some viability in a calcified cyst. There is less resistance to spherical growth in the lung than in the liver, and lung cysts may attain greater size more rapidly and rarely calcify. Brain cysts usually present at a younger age because of increased intracranial pressure, and they rarely calcify.

As many as 20 per cent of *E. granulosus* cysts may never cause symptoms. Symptoms related to liver cysts include right upper quadrant pain, hepatomegaly, and jaundice. Approximately half of patients with pulmonary cysts are asymptomatic, but cysts may cause chest pain, cough, and hemoptysis. Brain cysts may give signs of increased intracranial pressure and convulsions. With slow leakage of a cyst, urticaria and other allergic symptoms may occur, whereas rupture or needle puncture of a cyst may lead to anaphylaxis, which is often fatal. When eosinophilia is present, it is usually related to some leakage of fluid.

Echinococcosis must be suspected in anyone with a history of a slowly growing cystic tumor, particularly in the liver or lung, who has lived in an endemic area. A characteristic physical sign over a hepatic cyst on ballottement is the hydatid thrill. Liver function tests are usually normal with hepatic cysts except for a frequent elevation of alkaline phosphatase. Radiography may show older calcified lesions in the liver, spleen, or kidney. Echinococcal cyst is the leading cause of a round, reticulated calcified lesion in the liver, but the differential diagnosis includes calcified hemangiomas, metastases, and old amebic or bacterial abscesses. Radioactive or CT scans or sonography are useful in localizing noncalcified cysts. Invasive angiographic techniques are rarely required. Pulmonary cysts present as regular, well-defined, round shadows, which cannot be differentiated from a tumor. If a pulmonary cyst becomes detached from the adventitia, the so-called *water lily sign* is produced. Immunologic techniques are quite valuable and should always be employed preoperatively to alert the surgeon to the likely presence of a hydatid cyst. When the Casoni skin test, using an antigen with an appropriate nitrogen content, shows an immediate negative reaction, this is good but not absolute evidence of the absence of hydatid disease. False-positive test results may occur. Serologic procedures include indirect hemagglutination, bentonite flocculation, latex or complement fixation, and immunoelectrophoresis. Immunoelectrophoresis is the only one absolutely specific for hydatid disease, but it is presently not readily available. The diagnosis is confirmed by the finding at surgery of daughter cysts and scoleces in the cyst fluid. Closed needle aspiration of a lesion with any possibility of its being a hydatid cyst should never be performed before radiologic and immunologic studies have been done.

In endemic areas, infected dogs should be treated with a taeniafuge such as arecoline or niclosamide, and stray dogs should be destroyed. Dogs should be kept from eating uncooked carcasses or offal.

Gamble WG, Segal M, Schantz PM, Rausch RL: Alveolar hydatid disease in Minnesota. First human case acquired in the contiguous United States. JAMA 241:904, 1979. *Case report and literature review with particular reference to the disease in North America.*

Katz AM, Pan CT: *Echinococcus* disease in the United States. Am J Med 25:759, 1958. *A very thorough review of 556 cases diagnosed in the United States, the great majority of which were imported from highly endemic areas.*

Thatcher VE: Neotropical echinococcosis in Colombia. Ann Trop Med Parasitol 66:99, 1972. *A discussion of 11 cases from Colombia with this rare form of multilocular hydatid disease, which is also found in Panama.*

Wolcott MW, Harris SH, Briggs JN, Dobell ARC, Brown RK: Hydatid disease of the lung. J Thorac Cardiovasc Surg 62:465, 1971. *A series of 37 Tunisian cases treated by Hope Ship physicians. Emphasizes the need for surgery in diagnosis and treatment.*

394. OTHER, RARER TAPEWORMS

Hymenolepis diminuta, a common tapeworm of rats and mice, infrequently infects man. It has a cosmopolitan distribution worldwide, and the few cases reported in the United States have mostly been from the South. Various species of larval and adult insects are intermediary hosts and become infected by taking in eggs deposited in rodent stool. Man and dog are incidental hosts, becoming infected by ingesting one of the insects containing a cysticercoid larva, usually by eating stale grains or cereals infested with insects. The majority of human infections are in young children. Adult worms are 20 to 60 cm long and reside in the small intestine. No pathologic changes are recognized, but bowel irritation may cause minor gastrointestinal symptoms. The eggs resemble those of *H. nana,* differing in having no filaments at the pointed poles of the inner membrane. Diagnosis is by finding typical eggs in the stool.

Dipylidium caninum is the most common tapeworm of dogs and cats worldwide. Adult worms measure 15 to 80 cm in length and reside in the small intestine. Eggs, passed onto the ground in packets or in proglottides by infected animals or man, are ingested by larval fleas in which they hatch and develop into cysticercoid larvae. Humans having close contact with dogs or cats are infected by ingesting an infected flea. Human infection is infrequent, and small children are usually infected. The majority of cases are asymptomatic, but diarrhea, abdominal pain, restlessness, and eosinophilia have been reported. Diagnosis is by finding characteristic cucumber seed-shaped proglottides or characteristic eggs singly or in packets in the stool. Proglottides are motile and may migrate from the anus and can be mistaken for pinworms by history.

Coenurosis is a well-recognized disease of the central nervous system of animals. Humans are rarely infected. The adult tapeworm of the genus *Multiceps* is a common parasite of dogs and wolves. *Taenia*-like eggs are passed in the host's feces and are ingested by an intermediate host, a sheep or other ruminant, and occasionally by people. After hatching, larvae lodge primarily in the brain and central nervous system, but may also involve the eye or subcutaneous tissue, where they metamorphose into a coenurus, a bladder worm with multiple scoleces. Infections in temperate climates are probably due to *Multiceps multiceps,* usually involve the central nervous system, and may lead to increased intracranial pressure. The majority of subcutaneous cysts have been described from East Africa where the prevalent species is *Multiceps (Taenia) brauni*, and are manifested by a solitary tender subcutaneous nodule on the trunk or rarely by an eye cyst within the vitreous chamber, attached to the retina or choroid. Diagnosis is possible only with surgery. Both clinically and microscopically it is often difficult to distinguish coenurosis of the central nervous system from hydatid cyst or cysticercosis.

Cohen R, Mackey K: *Hymenolepsis diminuta* unresponsive to quinacrine. West J Med 127:340, 1977. *Case report of a symptomatic Mexican-American child.*

Hermos JA, Healy GR, Schultz MG, Barlow J, Church WG: Fatal human cerebral coenurosis. JAMA 213:1461, 1970. *The cerebral form of this disease seems to occur only in temperate climates and must be differentiated from hydatid cyst and cysticercosis.*

Templeton AC: Anatomical and geographical location of coenurus infection. Trop Geogr Med 23:105, 1971. *Review of 14 cases from Uganda involving subcutaneous nodules.*

Turner JA: Human dipylidiasis (dog tapeworm infection) in the United States. J Pediatr 61:763, 1962. *This tends to be primarily a disease of childhood but may not be as rare as earlier supposed.*

395. TREATMENT OF TAPEWORM INFECTIONS

The present drug of choice for *D. latum*, *Taenia* species, *Hymenolepis* species, and *D. caninum* is niclosamide (Niclocide). For *D. latum*, *T. saginata*, *T. solium*, and *D. caninum*, adults are given a single 2-gram dose. The tablets are chewed thoroughly in the morning and followed by water. No fasting or purging is necessary. The head and much of the worm disintegrate so that proof of cure depends on a negative stool examination for eggs at three months. For *H. nana* and *H. diminuta* the adult dose is 2 grams daily for five to seven days. Side effects are rare. Another effective drug against *D. latum*, *Taenia* species, and *H. nana* is paromomycin (Humatin), a poorly absorbed antibiotic that is considered an investigational drug for tapeworms in the United States. For *H. nana*, the adult dose is 45 mg per kilogram once a day for five to seven days, while for the other worms 1 gram every 15 minutes for four doses is administered. Quinacrine hydrochloride had formerly been used for these parasites but is most effective when administered through a duodenal tube, and cure rates are lower than with niclosamide. The anthelmintic drug mebendazole (Vermox) is effective against *Taenia* species in a dose of 300 mg twice daily for three days, but is not yet approved for this indication in the United States. Praziquantel, in a single dose treatment is very effective against intestinal *Taenia*, *Hymenolepsis*, and *Diphyllobothrium* infections in humans but is also not yet approved for cestode infections in the United States.

Praziquantel has also been shown to be effective against human cysticercosis of the brain and subcutaneous and muscle tissue. This has greatly improved the prognosis for this infection, formerly treated only surgically, with many cases being inoperable. To prevent potential immunologic reactions in the brain tissue caused by death of parasites, steroids are administred concurrently. Calcified cysticerci do not respond to this treatment, and when they cause seizures, anticonvulsants must be used for control. Successful treatment of neurocysticercosis in Mexico has been obtained by means of specific internal radiation with anti-*Cysticercus* antibodies labeled with iodine 131. Ocular cysticerci must be removed surgically; praziquantel is not recommended for treatment of ocular cysticercosis because of concern about ocular damage after parasite destruction in the eye.

Surgery is recommended for accessible symptomatic *E. granulosis* cysts. Sterilization of cysts should be performed at surgery by scolecidal solutions, such as hypertonic saline or a 10 per cent formaldehyde solution. Cysts may also be marsupialized, or cryosurgery may be used. For multiple cysts, poor surgical risk patients, and inaccessible cysts, mebendazole in large doses for several months has led to subjective improvement in most cases of *E. granulosis* and evidence of regression of cysts in some; in other patients, cysts continued to grow or were proved viable even after lengthy treatment. Hepatic lobectomy is the only operation for *E. multilocularis*, but complete removal is usually difficult. In patients with inoperable *E. multilocularis* cysts, the progressive course of the disease can be arrested by mebendazole, but treatment apparently has not killed the parasite. Related benzimidazole drugs, flubendazole, fenbendazole, and albendazole, also appear to be promising in inoperable hydatid infections.

Symptomatic coenurosis must be managed surgically. Complete surgical excision is the treatment of choice for sparganosis; if it is inoperable, injections of alcohol into the lesion will kill the parasite.

Groll E: Praziquantel for cestode infections in man. Acta Tropica 37:293, 1980. *Single-dose treatment of intestinal cestodes.*

Jones WE: Niclosamide as a treatment for *Hymenolepsis diminuta* and *Dipylidium caninum* infection in man. Am J Trop Med Hyg 28:300, 1979. *Effective treatment of these uncommon cestodes.*

Peña Chavarria A, Villaraejos VM, Zeledon R: Mebendazole in the treatment of *Taeniasis solium* and *Taeniasis saginata*. Am J Trop Med Hyg 26:118, 1977. *An alternative treatment for the commoner intestinal cestodes; not yet an approved indication in the USA.*

Perera DR, Western KA, Schultz MG: Niclosamide treatment of cestodiasis. Clinical trials in the United States. Am J Trop Med Hyg 19:610, 1970. *An early review of this drug, which has been further substantiated, showing it to be safe, simple, and effective.*

Sayek I, Yalin R, Savac Y: Surgical treatment of hydatid disease of the liver. Arch Surg 115:847, 1980. *A review of 100 surgically treated cases in Turkey.*

Schantz PM, Van den Bossche H, Eckert J: Chemotherapy for larval echinococcis in animals and humans: Report of a workshop. Z Parasitenkd 67:5, 1982. *Review of published literature and proceedings of a workshop on use of benzimidazoles against larval echinococcosis.*

Skromne-Kadlubik G, Celis C: Cysticercosis of the nervous system: Treatment by means of specific internal radiation. Arch Neurol 38:388, 1981. *Encouraging results in 500 patients in Mexico.*

Sotelo J, Escobedo F, Rodriguez-Carbajal J, Torres B, Rubro-Donnadieu F: Therapy of parenchymal brain cysticercosis with praziquantel. N Engl J Med 310:1001, 1984. *Promising new drug treatment of neurocysticercosis.*

Wittner M, Tanowitz H: Paromomycin therapy of human cestodiasis with special reference to hymenolepiasis. Am J Trop Med Hyg 20:433, 1971. *Successful treatment of various common cestodes with an alternative to niclosamide.*

The Trematodes

396. SCHISTOSOMIASIS (Bilharziasis)

Adel A. F. Mahmoud

DEFINITION. Schistosomiasis, a chronic worm infection, affects more than 200 million people in the world; several hundred million more live in endemic areas and are at risk of exposure to the parasites. In view of its prevalence and the morbidity it causes, schistosomiasis ranks among the most important public health problems of tropical and subtropical areas. The schistosomes are blood flukes that parasitize the venous channels of the definitive human host; infection is transmitted via freshwater snails. Man may be infected by one of three species: *Schistosoma haematobium*, *S. mansoni*, or *S. japonicum*. Each species is endemic in specific geographic areas of the world and results in defined clinical syndromes which, if left undiagnosed and untreated, may cause major morbidity or mortality. Other species that occasionally infect man include *S. intercalatum*, *S. mekongi*, *S. bovis*, *S. matthei*, and some avian schistosomes. In many parts of the world, enhancing agricultural productivity by developing and expanding water conservation schemes is an economic necessity. Inadvertently, these projects create ideal breeding places for the snail intermediate host, thus increasing prevalence of schistosomiasis in the population and possibly causing its spread to new areas. Currently, schistosomiasis is endemic in various areas of Africa, Asia, South America, and the Caribbean islands. In the United States, there are approximately 400,000 cases; these usually occur in Puerto Rican immigrants or travelers who have been infected while in endemic areas. Because of the absence of susceptible snails, the life cycle of the schistosomes cannot be established in this country.

Schistosomiasis has been the subject of much scientific and public health investigation, particularly over the past two decades. This has resulted in better understanding of the pathogenesis of disease syndromes and the development of new effective chemotherapeutic antischistosomal agents. Furthermore, a global strategy for schistosomiasis control is now emerging that could bring about its containment.

ETIOLOGY. The schistosomes are the most significant trematode parasites of man. Moreover, ancient Egyptian records and the presence of calcified *S. haematobium* eggs in mummies indicate that schistosomiasis existed as a human infection for several thousand years. The schistosomes differ from other trematode infections of humans in having separate sexes. The species of schistosomes that infect humans share some common features, although they are morphologically distinctive. Each worm has two suckers (anterior and ventral), and the bifurcate intestinal ceca unite posteriorly. The larger male (0.6 to 2.2 cm × 2 to 4 mm) has a ventral gynecophoric canal in which the female is held during copulation. The slender female worm (1.2 to 2.6 cm × 1 to 2 mm) has a rounded body with pointed ends.

The schistosome worms parasitize defined sites of the venous vasculature of humans. *Schistosoma haematobium* worms inhabit the venous plexus around the lower end of the ureters and the urinary bladder, whereas *S. mansoni* and *S. japonicum* are respectively located in the inferior and the superior mesenteric veins. Sexual maturity of female worms requires the presence of living mature males; when ready to deposit eggs, the worms move against the bloodstream toward the small venous radicles. The female schistosomes deposit ova singly or in bunches, depending on the species of the parasite, and retreat in the direction of blood flow. Egg deposition has been estimated at 300 per day for female *S. haematobium* and *S. mansoni* worms and 3000 per day for those of *S. japonicum*. The ova of each species have characteristic morphologic features, which are of diagnostic importance. Once deposited in the host, the eggs attempt to penetrate the venous capillaries and escape to the bladder or intestinal lumen; enzymatic secretions are thought to aid egg migration. The proportion of ova escaping from infected individuals varies in each species, and also may depend on the extent of pathology and state of resistance in the host. Eggs that fail to reach the lumen of urinary tract or gut are trapped in these organs or may be carried by portal blood to the liver; these ova result in inflammatory and immunopathologic changes which are a major cause of disease in schistosomiasis.

The schistosome eggs, upon deposition by female worms, contain immature miracidia; they take approximately 10 to 12 days to develop while migrating through the host tissues. Once mature, miracidia have a mean life span of 11 to 12 days, during which they must reach, via the bladder or intestinal lumen, the snail intermediate host. Promiscuous urination and defecation by infected individuals result in dissemination of the parasite eggs in the environment. In fresh water the schistosome ova hatch within a few hours. Miracidia escape head first and swim, usually near the surface of water; they remain infective to the snail intermediate host for approximately eight hours. On encountering the specific snail, the miracidia penetrate its tissues and undergo tremendous asexual multiplication and transformation into hundreds of cercariae. Schistosome infection of snails causes varying degrees of pathology in their liver and sexual organs and reduces their life span. Development of schistosomes inside the snail takes approximately four to six weeks, but it varies with the species of the parasite and mollusc and with changes in environmental conditions. Cercariae, the infective forms to man, emerge from the snails under specific conditions of light and temperature; they are elongate with a pear-shaped body and a long forked tail, and measure approximately 400 to 600 μm in length. They can survive in fresh water for almost 72 hours, but lose their infectivity considerably within the first 24 hours. Cercariae attach to skin of mammalian hosts by their oral or ventral suckers. Burrowing of the skin is helped by vertical vibratory movements of their bodies and secretions of the cephalic penetration glands; the process is usually completed within a few minutes. During penetration, the cercariae shake off their tails and change into the next stage of life cycle, the schistosomula, which lie in tunnels in the stratum corneum parallel to the skin surface. Schistosomula are anaerobic organisms with heptalaminar membrane (instead of the trilaminar cercarial membrane) and can no longer survive fresh water. They are thought to remain in the skin for one to three days before migrating to the lungs, finally reaching the liver in two to four weeks. The pathway of migration of the schistosomula inside the host is still controversial. They migrate via the venous circulation to the lungs, but how they reach the liver and their final habitat is still unclear. In the intrahepatic portal system the worms complete the major digestive and sexual stages of their development. Adult worms start their migration to their final habitat in two weeks and mate; viable eggs can be seen in the excreta five to nine weeks after cercarial penetration.

The mean life span of adult schistosome worms inside the human host is not exactly known. Several individual case reports indicate that worms may live 20 to 30 years. This, however, represents extreme cases, as examination of infected individuals who migrated to nonendemic areas and mathematic calculations indicate that the mean life span of the worms is much shorter, in the range of three to ten years. Such a mean duration of survival is still considerable in view of the capability of the worm to produce eggs continually and cause pathologic changes in the host.

EPIDEMIOLOGY. The endemicity of schistosomiasis in any specific area is dependent upon the unsanitary disposal of urine and feces, the presence of suitable snail hosts, and human exposure to cercariae-infected water bodies. Furthermore, the epidemiology of schistosomiasis is complex because of the existence of several stages of the life cycle of the parasite and the multitude of factors affecting each. These worms reach sexual maturity but do not multiply in the definitive host (man) whereas asexual division and extensive multiplication occur inside the snail intermediate host. Since adult schistosomes, like many parasitic worms and contrary to all other infectious agents, do not multiply in the human body, close correlation between worm load and fecal or urinary egg counts has been shown; estimates of intensity of infection can therefore be obtained by ova-enumerating procedures. Quantifying worm loads is important epidemiologically as well as for the individual patient, as it determines the extent of participation in transmission of schistosomiasis and predicts, to a large extent, the risk of morbidity and pathologic outcome.

In endemic areas, schistosomiasis prevalence and intensity show characteristic association with age and sex; infection is more common in the young and in males. Schistosomiasis is acquired early in childhood; prevalence and intensity gradually increase to a peak in the second decade of life. In older individuals, a modest reduction of prevalence may be seen in contrast to a sharp fall in intensity of infection. As schistosomiasis is acquired through contact with infected water bodies, the marked drop in intensity in adults may be due to a decrease in their water-related activities. Development of immunity may also explain age-related decrease in intensity, although there is not yet convincing evidence for acquisition of resistance against schistosomiasis in man. Intensity of infection in endemic communities shows another characteristic feature: most infected individuals harbor low worm loads, and only a small proportion acquire heavy infection. The underlying mechanism of this clustering of heavy infection in schistosomiasis is not known, but may be due to varying degrees of susceptibility and/or response of man to the parasites.

Determination of the incidence and rate of acquisition of schistosomiasis in the population of endemic areas is important for risk assessment and planning control strategies. The prevalence and intensity of infection peak in the age group 10 to 20 years in spite of the presumed multiple reexposures to the parasite. These observations suggest that the schistosomiasis transmission rate in endemic areas is slow. Several ecologic as well as host factors help maintain these features. For example, the prevalence of schistosomal infection in the snail intermediate host is usually low, ranging between 0.6 and 2 per cent. Cercarial dispersion in water bodies is considerable; they appear in significant numbers only during certain hours of the day and lose their infectivity shortly thereafter. Once on its way to invade a certain host, no more than 40 per cent of cercariae mature into adult worms. In addition, attempts to measure incidence rates in endemic areas confirmed the relatively slow rate of transmission, ranging from 2 to 4 per cent per year.

In some areas, the endemicity of schistosomiasis may be maintained by animal reservoirs; this is especially the case with *S. japonicum,* which infects dogs and cows. Although both *S. haematobium* and *S. mansoni* can infect primates and rodents, the role of these animals as reservoirs does not seem to be epidemiologically important.

PATHOGENESIS. Schistosomiasis is initiated by cercarial penetration of skin; inside the host three maturational forms of the parasite evolve: schistosomula, adults, and eggs. These stages are associated with morphologic, biochemical, and antigenic changes of the worm, which add to the complexity of host-parasite relationship. Disease caused by schistosomiasis occurs in only a small percentage of infected individuals, mainly those with high eggs counts. This relationship, however, is not exact, as the roles of other factors such as genetic background and immunologic modulatory mechanisms are now being elucidated.

Three distinct disease syndromes caused by schistosomiasis have been described; each corresponds roughly to a stage in the parasite development in the host. Cercarial dermatitis or swimmer's itch may be seen in infections with human schistosomes but more commonly when avian or other nonhuman cercariae penetrate the skin. Swimmer's itch caused by nonhuman schistosomes is commonly seen in the north central United States where some lakes are infected. The condition has also been reported in subjects exposed to *S. mansoni* or *S. haematobium* but rarely after exposure to *S. japonicum.* Primary exposure to these larvae results in either no reaction or immediate pruritic macular rash. On repeated exposures, sensitization occurs, and a more pronounced papular eruption develops with erythema, edema, and pruritus. Histopathologically, edema, round cell infiltrate, and eosinophila can be seen in the dermis and epidermis. Although the mechanism of this reaction is not known, it is probably due to host response to dying larvae and the subsequent development of humoral and cellular immunity.

Acute schistosomiasis or Katayama fever is a serum sickness–like syndrome which occurs three to nine weeks after infection. This period coincides with the onset of egg production and its associated increase in antigenic challenge to the host. Clinically significant acute schistosomiasis occurs more often with *S. japonicum* infections but has also been reported with the other two species. It is seen in previously unexposed individuals; the severity of symptoms and signs correlates with intensity of infection. There is very little known of the mechanism of this syndrome; it manifests itself as fever, abdominal pain, and headache with hepatosplenomegaly and eosinophilia. Elevations of serum IgG, IgM, IgE, and specific antischistosomal antibodies have also been observed, leading to the suggestion that the syndrome is a form of immune complex disease.

The basic pathologic lesion in chronic schistosomiasis is the egg granuloma. Although the schistosomes do not multiply in the definitive host, they continually produce eggs; some of these are trapped in the tissues. Enzymes and antigens are subsequently released from the eggs to facilitate their migration out of the body. These parasite products sensitize the host lymphocytes, which migrate to areas of egg deposition and recruit other cells through the secretion of lymphokines, and a compact cellular infiltrate "granuloma" is formed. Several cell types are prominent in the schistosome egg granuloma: lymphocytes, macrophages, eosinophils, and fibroblasts. Granuloma formation around the schistosome eggs leads to the development of lesions far bigger than the parasite ova. The extent of these granulomas along with the ultimate deposition of collagen results in most of the chronic fibro-obstructive lesions in schistosomiasis. In *S. haematobium* infection, granulomas at the lower end of the ureters impede urine flow and cause hydroureter and hydronephrosis. In *S. mansoni* infection, granulomas in the intestinal wall are associated with the abdominal manifestations of the disease, and those in the liver result in presinusoidal obstruction of portal blood flow, portal hypertension, splenomegaly, and esophageal varices. Similar lesions are seen in schistosomiasis japonica. Less commonly, eggs may be carried to almost any organ or tissue in the body eliciting granuloma formation and its pathologic sequelae. The mechanisms and control of granuloma formation and its modulation in schistosomiasis have been extensively studied; in *S. mansoni* and *S. haematobium,* cell-mediated immunologic reactions play a key role in granuloma production, whereas the etiology of *S. japonicum* granuloma is not yet clear. Furthermore, the size of the granulomatous response represents a delicate balance between sensitizing and modulating mechanisms. In chronic schistosomiasis, granulomas spontaneously modulate, i.e., their size decreases significantly, and may result in slow progression of disease manifestations. Modulation has been shown to be mediated by several arms of the host's immune system, including serum antibodies, immune complexes, suppressor lymphocytes, and macrophages. Functionally, granulomas serve to destroy the parasite eggs. Recent observations indicate that among the cells constituting the granulomatous response, eosinophils play a key role in egg destruction. The pathologic lesions seen in individuals infected with *S. intercolatum* are similar to those produced by *S. haematobium,* whereas infection with *S. mekongi* clinically closely resembles that with *S. japonicum.*

The immune response of individuals with schistosomiasis includes humoral as well as cellular components. The degree and extent of these responses provide the balance that may result in either asymptomatic infection or disease manifestations. Furthermore, mechanisms which control the host immune response such as genetic background have been demonstrated to influence the extent of granuloma formation and consequently disease. Recently, it has also been demonstrated that the host immune response to schistosome antigens also is inversely related to intensity of infection; impaired responses are seen only in those with heavy worm loads. These observations are similar to what has been demonstrated in other overwhelming mycobacterial or fungal infections. Whether the defect in immunity is a cause or consequence of infection is not yet clear. Another aspect of the host's immune response in schistosomiasis relates to the development of peripheral blood as well as tissue eosinophilia. Schistosomiasis, similar to other worm infections with tissue phases, results in significant increase of peripheral blood eosinophils; this is especially seen during the acute phase of infection. Later, in the chronic stage, eosinophil count may not be significantly elevated. Eosinophils are seen in subcutaneous tissues around the entry points of cercariae, and they constitute approximately 50 per cent of the cells in egg granulomas. The eosinophils have been shown to play a central role in host defenses against the invading stage of the parasite (schistosomula) and the phase (ova) retained in the tissues.

The occurrence of immunity to schistosomiasis in humans

has not convincingly been shown, as noted above. Although the drop of intensity and prevalence of infection in older individuals in endemic areas may reflect the development of resistance, these phenomena may be explained equally by the differences in patterns of contact with infected waters, or by changes in the rate of egg production by adult worms. Studies in vitro have demonstrated that several human cells—eosinophils, neutrophils, basophils, monocytes, and cytotoxic T lymphocytes—may alone or in combination with complement components or antischistosomal antibodies damage the larval stage of the parasite. The biologic relevance of these observations in man is not yet clear.

MANAGEMENT. Diagnosis of schistosomiasis must be based on the clinical presentation, positive geographic history, and finding the parasite eggs in the excreta or biopsy material. Quantification of infection and assessing viability of the eggs are important procedures not only for planning therapy but also for prognostic evaluation. Although tremendous advances have been made in serologic tests for schistosomiasis over the past decade, their diagnostic and prognostic value is not yet at the stage at which they can be used on a routine basis. Safe chemotherapeutic antischistosomal agents are now available and provide high cure rates. None of these drugs have any effect on cercarial penetration, on swimmer's itch, on the course of acute schistosomiasis, or as a prophylactic measure. Their major action is on the adult egg-producing worms. Appropriate management of patients with schistosomiasis must take into consideration the extent of disease and intensity of infection; measures directed against the parasite and those needed to alleviate the clinical, chronic manifestations of disease must be considered. Antischistosomal therapy, if given early enough during the course of disease, may lead to reversal of pathologic lesions. In late cases, chemotherapeutic measures may be useful only in preventing further damage resulting from the presence of the parasite.

CONTROL. The intimate relationship between humans and bodies of water in their environment leads to schistosomiasis endemicity. In addition, the lack of precise knowledge of the epidemiology of infection and disease in schistosomiasis has hampered efforts for its control. Recently, several developments such as single oral dose chemotherapeutic agents and better appreciation of transmission dynamics have led to clearer definition of strategies for control of schistosomiasis. Ideally, eradication of infection should be the target, but this is impossible to achieve with the currently available tools and the economic and social structure of the endemic areas. A more realistic approach, based on control of disease and reduction of transmission, may contain the infection and reduce its pathologic sequelae. The most cost-effective measure currently advocated is targeted mass chemotherapy, combined with focal mollusciciding if needed. Because of the specific features of infection dynamics, treated individuals remain with low egg counts for a few years. In addition, health education, attempts at raising socioeconomic standards, providing privies, and abandoning obsolete agricultural practices offer additional means for achieving progress in containing this infection.

Those traveling to endemic areas should be given proper advice. There are virtually no safe freshwater bodies in most of the areas endemic for schistosomiasis. Avoiding contact with these water sources is to be strongly recommended.

Butterworth AE, Vadas MA, David JR: Mechanisms of eosinosphil mediated helminthotoxicity. *In* Mahmoud AAF, Austen KF (eds.): The Eosinophil in Health and Disease. New York, Grune & Stratton, 1980, pp 253–273. *Description of how human eosinophils destroy the schistosomula stage of the parasite.*

Ellner JJ, Olds GR, Osman GO, El Kholy A, Mahmoud AAF: Dichotomies in the reactivity to worm antigen in human schistosomiasis mansoni. J Immunol 126:309, 1981. *Demonstration of an inverse relationship between intensity of infection and immune response to schistosome antigens.*

Hofstetter M, Nash TE, Cheever AW, dos Santos JG, Ottesen EA: Infection with *Schistosoma mekongi* in Southeast Asian refugees. J Infect Dis 144:420, 1981. *Description of clinical and parasitological features of schistosomiasis mekongi.*

Iarotski LS, Davis A: The schistosomiasis problem in the world. Bull WHO 59:115, 1981. *An attempt to determine the global prevalence of schistosomiasis.*

Mahmoud AAF, Arap Siongok TK, Ouma J, Houser HB, Warren KS: Effect of targeted mass treatment on intensity of infection and morbidity in schistosomiasis mansoni. Lancet 1:849, 1983. *Evaluation of the clinical and parasitologic effects of targeting chemotherapy to those with hepatosplenomegaly and heavy infection.*

Mahmoud AAF, Warren KS, Peters PA: A role for the eosinophil in acquired resistance to *Schistosoma mansoni* infection as determined by anti-eosinophil serum. J Exp Med 142:805, 1975. *Demonstration of the in vivo protective function of eosinophils in animals with schistosomiasis.*

Olds GR, Mahmoud AAF: Role of host granulomatous response in murine schistosomiasis mansoni: Eosinophil-mediated destruction of eggs. J Clin Invest 66:1191, 1980. *Granuloma formation in schistosomiasis is a protective mechanism aimed at egg destruction. Ablation of eosinophils in the host leads to delay in egg destruction and exacerbation of disease.*

Warren KS: The immunopathogenesis of schistosomiasis: A multidisciplinary approach. Trans R Soc Trop Med Hyg 66:417, 1972. *Review of the sequence of events leading to disease in schistosomiasis.*

Warren KS: Regulation of the prevalence and intensity of schistosomiasis in man: Immunology or ecology? J Infect Dis 127:595, 1973. *A lucid discussion of the factors controlling transmission and regulation of infection in schistosomiasis.*

World Health Organization: Epidemiology and control of schistosomiasis. Technical report series 643, 1980. *Review of epidemiology, progress in some national control programs, and the different control strategies.*

SCHISTOSOMIASIS HAEMATOBIA
(Urinary Bilharziasis)

Schistosomiasis haematobia is due to human infection with the trematode *S. haematobium;* adult worms reside in the venous plexus around the urinary bladder, and their eggs are mainly found in urine of infected individuals. *S. haematobium* infection is endemic in Africa and some parts of the Middle East; it is highly prevalent in the Nile valley and extends along the Mediterranean coast of the continent. In West Africa it is more widely disseminated than *S. mansoni;* its distribution in East and South Africa is patchy. The parasite is endemic also on the islands of the Malagasy Republic. In southwest Asia, the endemic area includes most countries of the Middle East and Arabian peninsula. Clinically, infection with *S. haematobium* is the most significant of human schistosomes. Symptoms and signs of disease occur in over half of the infected individuals, including those with light worm loads. Because of the anatomic location of the pathologic lesions, gross urinary tract disease can result from a few granulomas at the lower end of ureters. In endemic areas, extensive hydroureters and hydronephrosis can be demonstrated in a considerable proportion of infected children; the natural history of these lesions and the course of disease in adults have not been clearly defined.

The adult male *S. haematobium* worms are distinguished by their finely tuberculate surface and by the presence of four to five large testes. The ovaries are found in the posterior half of the female body and contain 20 to 30 eggs. Mature *S. haematobium* eggs measure approximately 143×50 μm and are spindle shaped with a rounded anterior end and a conical posterior end which tapers to a terminal delicate spine. Eggs are mainly found in urine of infected individuals but may occasionally be seen in stools or rectal biopsies. The main intermediate hosts of *S. haematobium* in North Africa and the Middle East are freshwater snails of the genus *Bulinus;* in Africa south of the Sahara they belong to the subgenus *Physopsis.*

PATHOLOGY AND CLINICAL MANIFESTATIONS. The ova of *S. haematobium* pass from the venules of the vesical plexus into the bladder wall and the lower end of ureters, where most of the pathologic changes in infected individuals are seen. In the urinary bladder, the formation of egg granulomas leads to hyperemia, tubercles, ulcers, and polyps; as healing proceeds, sandy patches and scarring may be seen. Obstructive uropathy is the main functional disturbance caused by schistosomiasis haematobia. Other urinary tract lesions such as bacteriuria, calculi, and bladder cancer have been epidemiologically associated with *S. haematobium* infection, but no causal relationship has yet been confirmed. Ova of *S. haematobium* have occasionally been found in the lungs with subsequent focal pulmonary arteritis and diffuse hypertensive arteriolar changes; chronic cor pulmonale may occur in these patients.

Swimmer's itch and acute schistosomiasis have rarely been

described in *S. haematobium* infection. In contrast, symptoms caused by egg deposition in the urinary tract occur in a large proportion of infected individuals. In endemic areas, 50 to 90 per cent of infected subjects complain of dysuria, hematuria, or frequency. Hematuria is characteristically terminal, but with extensive ulceration the whole stream of urine may be bloody along with passage of clots. In late cases, symptoms related to secondary infection of the urinary tract, severe obstructive uropathy, or neoplasia may appear. Urine examination reveals proteinuria and hematuria; both signs are closely related to intensity of infection. An association between *S. haematobium* infection and bacteremia, mainly caused by *Salmonella* organisms, has been reported. Renal function may be compromised in patients with obstructive uropathy; both minimum urine osmolality and the ability to excrete an ingested water load are reduced, but there are nonspecific changes. Cytoscopic examination shows some degree of pathology in almost all infected individuals, the most common being hyperemia near the ureteral openings and the bladder trigone. Sandy patches, tubercles, ulcers, and polyps are less frequently seen. Radiographically, bladder calcification is a characteristic feature of urinary schistosomiasis; it is found in approximately 50 to 80 per cent of infected individuals. Other pathologic lesions are also frequently seen in 40 to 60 per cent of patients, including obstructive uropathy, hydroureters, hydronephrosis, and filling defects in the bladder and ureters. The severity of most of these symptoms and signs of schistosomiasis haematobia correlates with intensity of infection; however, in individuals with light infection, considerable pathologic changes can still be demonstrated.

DIAGNOSIS. Urine examination for *S. haematobium* eggs can be performed by direct or concentration methods. Excretion of the parasite eggs is maximal around midday, when samples should optimally be obtained. Diagnosis and quantification of infection can be achieved by filtering 10 ml of urine through Nucleopore membranes. Examination of more than one urine sample may be necessary to establish the diagnosis; rectal biopsy may alternatively be obtained in suspected cases with negative urine results. Once *S. haematobium* infection is diagnosed, assessment of urinary tract pathology by cystoscopy and intravenous pyelography is recommended. In addition, care must be taken in some endemic areas for early detection of bladder cancer by appropriate cytologic and histologic examinations.

TREATMENT. The drug of choice is metrifonate, an organophosphorus anticholinesterase compound that is highly effective against *S. haematobium* infections. Metrifonate is administered orally (7.5 mg per kilogram of body weight); the dose is repeated twice at weekly intervals. Cure rates are in the range of 60 to 90, with a more than 90 per cent drop in egg counts. Trials with a single oral dose of 10 mg per kilogram of body weight have shown high efficacy for field use; the percentage of reduction of egg counts was 96. No major side effects or contraindications to metrifonate use have been demonstrated. Following drug administration a few patients may complain of abdominal pain, nausea, or diarrhea. The main laboratory side effect is decrease of serum and red blood cell cholinesterase; however, it returns to normal within two to eight weeks. Praziquantel, a new broad-spectrum antischistosomal drug, is equally effective against *S. haematobium* infection. Antischistosomal therapy in schistosomiasis haematobia eliminates the parasites and reduces the extent of pathologic lesions. Residual urinary tract defects are treated medically; in rare cases surgical correction may be needed.

Davis A, Baily DR: Metrifonate in urinary schistosomiasis. Bull WHO 41:209, 1969. *A review of the therapeutic effect of metrifonate against* S. haematobium *infection.*

Lehman JS Jr, Farid Z, Smith JH, Basily S, El Masry NA: Urinary schistosomiasis in Egypt: Clinical, radiological, bacteriological and parasitological correlations. Trans R Soc Trop Med Hyg 67:384, 1973. *A complete clinical description of 200 individuals infected with* S. haematobium.

Mott KE, Dixon H, Osei-Tutu E, England EC: Relation between intensity of *Schistosoma haematobium* infection and clinical haematuria and proteinuria. Lancet 1:1005, 1983. *Correlation of proteinuria and hematuria to counts of* S. haematobium *eggs in urine.*

Peters PA, Mahmoud AAF, Warren KS, Ouma JH, Siongok TKA: Field studies of a rapid, accurate means of quantifying *Schistosoma haematobium* eggs in urine samples. Bull WHO 54:159, 1976. *Simple quantitative technique for urine examination.*

Smith JH, Kamel IA, Elwi A, von Lichtenberg F: A quantitative post mortem analysis of urinary schistosomiasis in Egypt. I. Pathology and pathogenesis. Am J Trop Med Hyg 23:1054, 1974. *Description of the pathology of schistosomiasis haematobia as it relates to egg counts and parasite load.*

Warren KS, Mahmound AAF, Muruka JF, Wittaker LR, Ouma JH, Siongok TKA: Schistosomiasis haematobia in Coast Province, Kenya. Am J Trop Med Hyg 28:864, 1979. *Correlation of morbidity with egg counts in schistosomiasis haematobia; even in lightly infected children disease manifestations are significant.*

SCHISTOSOMIASIS MANSONI
(Intestinal or Hepatosplenic Bilharziasis)

Schistosomiasis mansoni is due to human infection with the blood fluke *S. mansoni*, which parasitizes the inferior mesenteric venous channels. Parasite eggs are detected in stools of infected individuals, and far less commonly in their urine. Infection with *S. mansoni* is endemic in Africa, the Middle East, South America, and some Caribbean islands. The distribution of schistosomiasis mansoni in Africa overlaps with that of schistosomiasis haematobia; it is prevalent in the Nile delta in Egypt, in the Sudan, in Ethiopia, and in a broad belt across central Africa. In southwest Asia, it occurs in Yemen and Saudi Arabia. *S. mansoni* is sporadically distributed all over the northern part of South America and is endemic in several Caribbean countries and islands and in many parts of Puerto Rico.

Adult male *S. mansoni* worms have a grossly tuberculate surface and usually contain seven small testes. In the female, the ovary occupies the anterior half of its body, with a short uterus containing one to four ova. Mature eggs measure 155 $\times$ 66 μm, and are oval in shape with a lateral, long spine. *Schistosoma mansoni* infects man and primates and is found also in rodents such as mice and hamsters, but none of these animals play an important role as reservoirs for the infection. The intermediate snail hosts of *S. mansoni* are species of the genus *Biomphalaria* in Africa and *Australorbis tropicorbis* in the Americas.

PATHOLOGY AND CLINICAL MANIFESTATIONS. Cercarial dermatitis may occur following skin penetration by these larvae but is remarkably uncommon. Acute schistosomiasis mansoni appears between three and seven weeks after exposure; the presenting symptoms, in their order of occurrence, are fever, anorexia, abdominal pain, and headache. Less often, diarrhea, nausea, and vomiting may occur. Hepatosplenomegaly, eosinophilia, and elevated serum immunoglobulins are the main clinical signs. In a recent study, most of these manifestations correlated significantly with intensity of infection as evaluated by stool egg counts.

Schistosoma mansoni eggs are primarily deposited in the small veins around the large intestine of infected individuals; some of the eggs may be trapped in the gut wall or break loose into the portal circulation to be carried to the small intrahepatic portal venules. In patients with schistosomal hepatosplenomegaly, adult worms apparently move up to the veins surrounding the small intestine. On examination of the intestinal mucosa of infected subjects, it appears red and granular with pinpoint elevations surrounded by hyperemic zones. There may be minute hemorrhages and ulcerations. Sessile and pedunculated polyps, mainly in the rectosigmoid area, have been reported in Egyptians infected with *S. mansoni*, but not from other endemic areas. Pathologic examination of the liver in lightly infected individuals shows schistosome eggs with and without granulomas and mild portal inflammation. In advanced cases, the typical picture of Symmers' fibrosis is seen; the eggs are concentrated in and around large portal tracts with marked fibrosis and obstructive portal venous lesions. The lobular arrangement of liver parenchyma and its function are usually maintained. However, these structural changes lead to marked alteration of hepatic hemodynamics such as obstruction of portal blood flow through the liver and increase in number and size of intrahepatic arterial branches, thus shifting the blood flow through the liver from mainly portal to arterial sources. Portal hypertension leads to congestive splenomegaly and the formation of portosystemic venous shunts at the lower end of the esophagus and other sites. In these patients, the schistosome eggs may find their way to the pulmonary circulation, bypassing the obstructed portal blood flow. In the lungs, granulomas form around the trapped eggs, leading to arteriolar fibrosis and pulmonary hypertension.

Nervous system involvement in schistosomiasis mansoni is rare; the main clinical presentation, as in schistosomiasis haematobia, is transverse myelitis. The preferential involvement of the spinal cord may be due to the anatomic location of adult worms; both species rarely produce cerebral lesions. The underlying pathologic lesions are usually granulomas forming around eggs in the spinal cord.

Infection with *S. mansoni* does not have characteristic or specific symptomatology, in contrast to schistosomiasis haematobia. In several recent studies, infected individuals had a slightly higher incidence of crampy abdominal pain (21 to 48 per cent) and bloody diarrhea (4 to 28 per cent) than matched uninfected controls from the same endemic area. Examination of stools demonstrates an association between intensity of infection and the amount of blood detected. Other frequently mentioned nonspecific symptoms and signs, such as weakness, inability to work, or diarrhea, have not been convincingly demonstrated in any controlled studies. Significant enlargement of the liver is seen in 4 to 11 per cent of infected subjects, and splenomegaly occurs in 3 to 7 per cent. Patients with schistosomal hepatosplenomegaly present with a unique form of liver disease. The pathophysiologic changes are based on alteration of hemodynamics, fibrosis of large portal tracts, and very little derangement of liver function. Enlargement of the liver usually occurs in the left lobe, but later, in the course of infection and particularly in adults, uniform hepatomegaly may be seen. Simultaneously, gross enlargement of the spleen may occur; the organ is characteristically rubbery hard. Laboratory examination may show indications of anemia and a low degree of eosinophilia but no changes in liver function tests until late in the course of disease. Total serum proteins are usually normal, but gamma globulin elevations are common. An association between schistosomal hepatosplenomegaly and hepatitis B antigen and antibody presence has been described, but its pathophysiologic significance is not clear. Although hepatosplenomegaly usually occurs in heavily infected individuals, other underlying mechanisms may be involved. Recently, an association between HLA haplotypes and schistosomal hepatosplenomegaly has been demonstrated. In patients with pure schistosomal fibrosis uncomplicated by cirrhosis or viral hepatitis, liver function is preserved for a long time. These individuals often present clinically with an episode of hematemesis caused by rupture of esophageal varices without prior complaints. Bleeding may recur several times while the liver parenchyma maintains its normal functions. Finally, however, symptoms and signs of liver cell failure ensue, along with the development of stigmata of chronic liver disease and ascites.

Several less defined clinical syndromes have been associated with schistosomiasis mansoni. Formation of antigen-antibody complexes and their deposition in the kidney glomeruli have been demonstrated in infected laboratory animals as well as in individuals with chronic schistosomiasis mansoni. However, the prevalence of this syndrome and the rate at which it occurs in schistosomiasis are unknown, since proteinuria and nephrotic syndrome are not particularly prevalent in schistosomiasis-endemic areas. Schistosomiasis cor pulmonale is a better defined disease entity, although its incidence is not known. It usually occurs in patients with advanced hepatosplenic schistosomiasis mansoni or japonica because of the development of collateral circulation. In *S. haematobium*–infected individuals, the anatomic location of adult worms may help eggs reach the systemic circulation directly and become trapped in the pulmonary arterioles. Patients with schistosomal pulmonary hypertension present clinically with symptoms and signs similar to those in cor pulmonale of other causes. Aneurysmal dilation of the pulmonary artery and its branches, along with right ventricular hypertrophy, may occur. Other signs and symptoms of chronic schistosomiasis are usually detected, as well as parasite eggs in excreta or tissue sections.

DIAGNOSIS. Stool examination for the characteristic *S. mansoni* eggs is the definitive diagnostic procedure. Since assessing intensity of infection is essential, quantitative techniques are recommended. The Kato thick smear method involves examination of sieved 50-mg stool samples placed on glass slides and spread under a cellophane cover slip pre-soaked in 50 per cent glycerol. The slides should be left at least 24 hours to allow for clearing of fecal material; the embryo within the ova also clears, but the characteristic shape of the egg shell is retained. Rectal biopsy may be used for diagnosis of stool-negative cases, particularly in lightly infected individuals.

TREATMENT. The current drug of choice for treatment of schistosomiasis mansoni is oxamniquine. It is administered as a single oral dose of 15 to 20 mg per kilogram of body weight. In *S. mansoni* infections acquired in South America, this dose results in 70 to 100 per cent cure rates and a drop of 95 to 97 per cent in egg counts. If the patient to be treated was infected in Africa, higher doses are needed (60 mg per kilogram).* The drug is safe, and is associated with a few side effects such as dizziness and drowsiness. They occur in no more than 30 per cent of treated patients and disappear within six hours. Praziquantel, a new broad-spectrum antischistosomal drug, is equally effective against *S. mansoni.* In patients with advanced hepatosplenomegaly, antischistosomal chemotherapy may halt the advance of the disease process, but other medical measures are usually needed. Hematemesis and ascites should be treated medically; these patients do not require shunting surgery after their first bleeding episode. Although they are good surgical risks, postoperatively the incidence of portal encephalopathy is considerable.

Abdel Salam E, Ishaac S, Mahmoud AAF: Histocompatibility-linked susceptibility for hepatosplenomegaly in human schistosomiasis mansoni. J Immunol 123:1829, 1979. *The first demonstration of a relationship between defined HLA haplotypes (HLA-A1 and B5) and schistosomal hepatosplenomegaly.*

Cheever AW: A quantitative post mortem study of schistosomiasis mansoni in man. Am J Trop Med Hyg 17:38, 1968. *Correlation of worms loads with egg counts in tissues and feces, and detailed description of pathology of* S. mansoni *infection.*

Omer AHS: Oxamniquine for treating *Schistosoma mansoni* infection in man. Br Med J 2:163, 1978.

Peters PA, El Alamy M, Warren KS, Mahmoud AAF: Quick Kato smear for field quantification of *Schistosoma mansoni* eggs. Am J Trop Med Hyg 29:217, 1980. *Detailed description of the Kato thick smear technique for quantification of* S. mansoni *eggs.*

Siongok TKA, Mahmoud AAF, Ouma JH, Warren KS, Muller AS, Handa AK, Houser HB: Morbidity in schistosomiasis mansoni in relation to intensity of infection: Study of a community in Machakos, Kenya. Am J Trop Med Hyg 25:273, 1976. *Correlation of symptoms and signs of* S. mansoni *with fecal egg counts.*

SCHISTOSOMIASIS JAPONICA

Schistosomiasis japonica or Oriental schistosomiasis is due to human infection with the fluke *S. japonicum.* This schistosome species characteristically infects humans and domestic animals such as cats, dogs, and cattle, thus providing reservoir hosts which may contribute to its endemicity in certain areas of the Far East. On the main Asian continent, schistosomiasis japonica is prevalent in some parts of China, Thailand, Laos, Cambodia, and Malaysia. It is also endemic in Taiwan, Japan, the Philippines, and Celebes.

Adult *S. japonicum* male worms have a nontuberculate surface and seven medium-sized testes. The ovary occupies the middle part of the body of female worms and contains 50 to 100 ova. *S. japonicum* eggs are found in stools of infected individuals; they measure 89 × 67 μm and are oval or rounded with a lateral short, sometimes curved spine. The intermediate hosts

*This dose exceeds the manufacturer's recommended dosage.

for *S. japonicum* are snails of the genus *Onchomelania*. They are amphibious and have separate sexes, and each infected snail sheds an average of two cercariae daily. These organisms emerge in the evening and lie very close to the surface film of water; they can penetrate mammalian skin within a minute.

PATHOLOGY AND CLINICAL MANIFESTATIONS. *S. japonicum* infection results in pathologic lesions in the human definitive host which generally follow the same time course as described for schistosomiasis mansoni. Cercarial dermatitis is not a prominent feature of schistosomiasis japonica. Katayama fever, or acute schistosomiasis, was named after the district in Japan endemic for *S. japonicum* infections. Symptoms usually begin five to seven weeks after infection and are similar to those associated with schistosomiasis mansoni. The clinical features usually subside in a few days but may last for several months, and fatalities have been reported. The chronic manifestations of schistosomiasis japonica are related to ova deposited in the intestines and liver; adult worms produce ten times more eggs than those of *S. mansoni*. These ova are laid in aggregates and remain so in the intestinal wall or when carried to the liver by the portal blood flow. In addition, *S. japonicum* eggs differ from *S. mansoni* in their tendency to calcify in tissues. Schistosomiasis japonica granulomas vary in size tremendously and tend to show signs of necrosis.

The major pathologic lesions in schistosomiasis japonica are seen in the intestines, liver, lungs, and occasionally brain of infected individuals. Morphologically these lesions are initiated by the presence of eggs and proceed to granuloma formation and fibrosis as in schistosomiasis mansoni. Although it has always been assumed that, because of the ten-fold difference in egg productivity, disease in schistosomiasis japonica is more severe, there are no studies to confirm this suggestion. Individuals with chronic schistosomiasis japonica may present with no symptoms or several nonspecific complaints. Controlled surveys performed recently in endemic areas have shown no particular increase in complaints of weakness, abdominal pain, or diarrhea in infected individuals. Clinical signs of hepatosplenomegaly are more frequently seen in infected rather than uninfected individuals, but they were not uniformly correlated with intensity of infection. Severe hepatosplenic disease caused by schistosomiasis japonica may be seen in endemic areas, but its prevalence and relationship to intensity of infection and other complicating factors are unknown.

Cerebral schistosomiasis japonica is a unique syndrome reportedly occurring in 2 to 4 per cent of infected individuals in the endemic countries. *Schistosoma japonicum* infection of the central nervous system preferentially affects the brain. The lesions consist of large aggregates of eggs in the cerebral venous system, but adult worms have never been found in the brain. Cerebral schistosomiasis japonica presents clinically early in the course of the infection; the most frequent manifestation is focal jacksonian epilepsy; less commonly, generalized encephalitis may be the presenting feature.

DIAGNOSIS. Stool examination for *S. japonicum* eggs is the only reliable diagnostic procedure. The Kato thick smear technique provides both diagnosis and quantitative assessment of infection. Rectal biopsy may be used in individuals with light infections, particularly when a less common manifestation, such as cerebral schistosomiasis, is encountered.

TREATMENT. Currently, the drug of choice for treating schistosomiasis japonica is praziquantel. It is given orally as three doses of 20 mg per kilogram body weight. This dose of praziquantel has been shown to result in parasitologic cure in 70 to 80 per cent and to reduce fecal egg excretion by approximately 95 per cent. Praziquantel administration is associated with slight and clinically insignificant side effects such as abdominal pain. The same general medical recommendations outlined for advanced *S. mansoni* hepatosplenomegaly may be used in patients with late manifestations of schistosomiasis japonica.

Domingo EO, Tiu E, Peters PA, Warren KS, Mahmoud AAF, Houser HB: Morbidity in schistosomiasis japonica in relation to intensity of infection: Study of a community in Leyte, Philippines. Am J Trop Med Hyg 29:858, 1980. *A controlled study of the correlation between symptoms and signs of schistosomiasis japonica and fecal egg counts.*

Santos AT: Current chemotherapy of schistosomiasis japonica in the Philippines. SE Asian J Trop Med Public Health 7:306, 1976. *A review of the efficacy of niridazole and other schistosomal agents in schistosomiasis japonica.*

Santos AT, Blas BL, Nosenas JS, Portillo GP, Ortega OM, Hiyashi M, Boehme K: Preliminary clinical trials with praziquantel in *Schistosoma japonicum* infections in the Philippines. Bull WHO 57:793, 1979.

Warren KS, Su DL, Xu CY, Yuan HC, Peters PA, Cook JA, Mott KE, Houser HB: Morbidity in schistosomiasis japonica in relation to intensity of infection; study of 2 royal brigades in Anhui Province, China. N Engl J Med, 309:1533, 1983.

397. HERMAPHRODITIC FLUKES

S. K. K. Seah

The hermaphroditic flukes, unlike *Schistosoma* flukes, have male and female sex organs in the same worm, and self-fertilize. Those of medical importance are (1) flukes that parasitize the biliary tract, i.e., *Clonorchis sinensis, Opisthorchis* spp., *Fasciola hepatica, Dicrocoelium dendriticum*, and *Metorchis conjunctus;* (2) flukes that parasitize the intestinal lumen, i.e., *Fasciolopsis buski, Heterophyes heterophyes, Echinostoma ilocanum, Gastrodiscoides hominis*, and *Metagonimus yokogawai;* (3) flukes that parasitize the lung, i.e., *Paragonimus westermani* and other species; and (4) the mesocercarial stage of *Alaria americana*, which causes generalized systemic infection.

All of these flukes parasitize other mammals, and some of them, such as *Fasciola hepatica*, are of major importance in veterinary medicine. Most of these flukes have limited geographical distribution. However, with the migration of people around the world, human infections are often seen in nonendemic areas.

The hermaphroditic flukes are leaf-like, nonsegmented, and bilaterally symmetrical, ranging in size from a few millimeters to several centimeters. On one end is the anterior or oral sucker and just behind it the ventral sucker or acetabulum. The acetabulum acts as a holdfast to the epithelial tissue of the final host.

Eggs appear in bile and stool and, in the case of the lung fluke, in sputum and stool. The eggs are operculated. Some are fully embryonated when passed; others may require time for embryonation. The embryonated egg contains the first stage larva or miracidium. After hatching in fresh water the miracidium penetrates, or is ingested by, a suitable first intermediate host, a snail. In the snail the miracidium develops into thousands of cercariae, which are released into the water. The cercariae attach themselves to or penetrate into the second intermediate hosts, which, depending on the flukes, may be freshwater fish, crustaceans, frogs, or aquatic plants. The final definitive hosts (man or animals) acquire the infection by ingesting encysted metacercariae.

The treatment of digenetic trematodes is by the broad-spectrum anthelminthic praziquantel. Personal prevention of infection includes eating only well-cooked fish or crustaceans and avoiding raw watercress in endemic areas. Community prevention consists of cleaning up the environment and preventing infection of the intermediate hosts.

Seah SKK: Digenetic trematodes. Clin Gastroenterol 7:87, 1978. *A good review of all the hermaphroditic flukes; up to date and well referenced.*

HEPATIC HERMAPHRODITIC FLUKES

Clonorchiasis (Clonorchis Sinensis)

This infection is common in the Far East, especially southern China, Hong Kong, Taiwan, Japan, and Korea, where raw or undercooked fish have long been considered a delicacy. More than 40 species of freshwater fish, mainly the carp and salmon group, harbor metacercariae.

Clonorchis sinensis has a very long life span (probably up to 50 years), and this parasitic infection will likely be important in these areas for many years. Clonorchiasis occurs in all parts of the world where there are Asian immigrants from endemic areas.

After ingestion of the contaminated fish, the metacercariae excyst in the duodenum. Most of the larval flukes ascend the biliary tree directly, but some may pass via the portal circulation to the liver. During maturation of the fluke there is marked desquamation of biliary epithelium. The fluke matures in two to three weeks and begins to lay eggs. Flukes prefer to reside in the second order bile ducts, but in heavy infection they are found throughout the biliary system, including the gallbladder, and sometimes in the pancreatic duct. Adult flukes are grayish-brown, 15 × 3 mm. They feed on secretions from the bile duct mucosa. They cause low grade inflammatory changes of the biliary tree, proliferation of the biliary epithelium, and progressive portal fibrosis. As a rule there is no parenchymal damage and cirrhosis does not result from uncomplicated clonorchiasis.

CLINICAL MANIFESTATIONS. *Acute clonorchiasis* occurs one to three weeks after the ingestion of encysted metacercariae. There may be fever, chills, abdominal pain, diarrhea, tender hepatomegaly, and mild jaundice. The white blood cell count is raised with marked eosinophilia, and serum alkaline phosphatase, SGOT, SGPT, and bilirubin levels are elevated. The clinical presentation is often confused with acute viral hepatitis and seldom recognized. The ova of *C. sinensis* appear in the stool or bile three or four weeks after ingestion of the metacercariae. The history of eating raw fish in the endemic area and the eosinophilia should suggest the diagnosis.

The majority of people with ova of *C. sinensis* in their stools have no symptoms even when heavily infected. It is impossible to predict who will develop the complications of chronic clonorchiasis. *Acute suppurative cholangitis* is a severe febrile illness often associated with hypoglycemia and *Escherichia coli* bacteremia. The biliary system is blocked by numerous flukes and becomes secondarily infected. This condition carries a very high mortality rate. *Recurrent pyogenic cholangitis* is a recurrent febrile illness associated with clonorchiasis and intrahepatic bile duct calculi. During surgical operation or autopsy, *Clonorchis* flukes are not consistently found as in the case of acute suppurative cholangitis. With recurrent pyogenic cholangitis cirrhosis may eventually develop. The flukes occasionally block the pancreatic ducts and induce pancreatitis. Cholangiocarcinoma is a late complication of chronic clonorchiasis. Clonorchiasis has no causal relationship with hepatocellular cancer.

DIAGNOSIS. The diagnosis is made by finding the small operculated eggs in the stool or duodenal aspirate. The eggs average 29 × 16 μ; they are light brown and ovoid. Unfortunately the *C. sinensis* egg is almost identical to those of *Opisthorchis, Heterophyes,* and *Metagonimus.* To be absolutely certain of the diagnosis one must examine the adult fluke. However, geographic distribution may help in separating *Clonorchis* from *Opisthorchis.* Expulsion and eradication of the flukes by a course of bephenium hydroxynaphthoate will indicate whether the ova are *Heterophyes* or *Metagonimus.* In a patient with abdominal or other symptoms and *C. sinensis* eggs in the stool, it is often difficult to decide if the complaints are due to clonorchiasis. It is often necessary to eliminate other current illnesses before attributing the symptoms to clonorchiasis. As a rule in uncomplicated established clonorchiasis, there is no eosinophilia, elevation of sedimentation rate, anemia, or abnormal liver function test results, and radioisotope scan and ultrasound (B scan) of the liver are normal.

In acute clonorchiasis, leukocytosis, marked eosinophilia, and abnormal liver function test results are present. This condition must be distinguished from hepatic amebiasis and visceral larva migrans. In the former, eosinophilia is absent and serology for amebiasis is positive. In the latter, the serology for toxocariasis is positive. The presence of the flukes in the liver provokes irregular antibody response, and a large variety of serologic and skin tests is available in some centers. However, these are not sufficiently specific and sensitive for clinical use.

TREATMENT. Until recently there was no satisfactory treatment for clonorchiasis, but praziquantel has revolutionized the treatment of this condition. The recommended dosage is 75 mg per kilogram of body weight, divided into three doses on the same day. Praziquantel is well tolerated and no long-term toxicity has been shown. At the dose recommended there may be some gastrointestinal disturbance and transient headaches. Because this drug is safe, it is recommended that all cases of clonorchiasis whether symptomatic or not be treated. The cost of this drug may limit its use in mass chemotherapy in the endemic area.

The treatment of complications such as calculi, suppurative cholangitis, recurrent pyogenic cholangitis, and pancreatitis is both medical and surgical. Conservative treatment consists of broad-spectrum antibiotics and intravenous fluids. If this is not effective, a permanent and adequate drainage procedure, such as choledochoduodenostomy, is required. Suppuration usually kills many flukes, and medical treatment is not urgent. At surgery as many flukes as possible should be removed from the biliary tree.

PREVENTION. In the endemic areas, freshwater fish must be well cooked before eating.

Opisthorchiasis
(Opisthorchis Viverrini and Felineus)

Opisthorchis felineus is common in eastern Europe, the USSR, India, Japan, the Philippines, and Vietnam. *Opisthorchis viverrini* is common in northern Thailand and Laos. In northeast Thailand 90 per cent of the people over the age of ten have *O. viverrini* infection. The life cycles of these flukes are similar to those of *C. sinensis.* Infection is acquired by eating undercooked freshwater fish. Many animals, especially the cat, are natural reservoirs.

The pathology, clinical manifestations, and complications of opisthorchiasis are similar to those of clonorchiasis. Cholangiocarcinoma can also result from chronic opisthorchiasis. The eggs of *Opisthorchis* are almost identical to those of *Clonorchis.* This emphasizes the importance of geographic history, for the only other way of distinguishing the parasites would be by examination of the adult flukes. The treatment is the same as for clonorchiasis.

Dicroceliasis

Dicrocoelium dendriticum is a lancet-shaped fluke, measuring 10 × 2 mm, that normally inhabits the biliary tract of sheep and cattle. Man is occasionally infected by ingesting ants that have eaten slime balls containing cercariae secreted by the snail. This occurs in Europe, in Asia, and around the Mediterranean basin. Infection is usually asymptomatic, and there is little information on the pathologic changes in man. It is important for the physician to recognize the small (40 × 25 μ), fully embryonated, thick-shelled operculated eggs for what they are. This infection requires no treatment.

Fascioliasis (Fasciola Hepatica)

This is a common parasite in the biliary tract of sheep and cattle, but it may also infect all types of mammals, including man. Worldwide in distribution in sheep, it is prevalent in low wet pastures where suitable species of snails are present. The cercariae, discharged from the snails, attach themselves to the water plants and encyst as metacercariae. Man is infected mainly as a result of eating watercress and other aquatic plants gathered in these pastures. In the duodenum the immature fluke penetrates the mucosa, enters the abdominal cavity, and through some unexplained hepatotropism penetrates Glisson's capsule. The immature flukes migrate throughout the liver for some weeks until they reach the biliary tract, where they mature in about two months. The fluke measures 3 × 1.3 cm, and the eggs are large, ovoid, and operculated, measuring 140 × 75 μ.

CLINICAL MANIFESTATIONS. ***Acute Fascioliasis.*** Invasion and maturation occur during the first three months after ingestion of the metacercariae. The immature flukes produce small necrotic foci along the migration paths. There may be no significant symptoms, or there may be abdominal pain, hepatomegaly, fever, vomiting, and jaundice. Leukocytosis and marked eosinophilia are present, but *F. hepatica* eggs are not found in the stool at this stage.

Established Infection. The mature flukes now produce metabolites that irritate the biliary passages, resulting in hyperplasia. Obstruction and dilation of the biliary passage and cholecystitis may occur. There may be abdominal pain, hepatomegaly, recurrent urticaria, jaundice, irregular fever, diarrhea, and weight loss. Anemia from blood loss can be severe. The obstruction and irritation may produce thickening of the biliary tree, atrophy of the hepatic cells, and biliary cirrhosis. Cholelithiasis is common. The relationship of fascioliasis and biliary cancers is not proved.

Extrabiliary Fascioliasis. Ingestion of raw sheep and goat liver containing young flukes causes the condition called "halzoun" (suffocation). This pharyngeal fascioliasis is due to lodgment of flukes in the upper respiratory and digestive tracts. Inflammation and edema may lead to dysphagia, dyspnea, and even asphyxiation. Cutaneous fascioliasis, usually in the upper abdomen, presents as migratory nodules which are pruritic, painful, and inflamed, and vary in size from 2 to 5 cm. Rarely, the flukes may be found in the lung, peritoneum, muscles, eye, and brain.

DIAGNOSIS. In acute infection the diagnosis is made in an endemic area by a high index of suspicion and the clinical triad of fever, hepatomegaly, and marked eosinophilia. A history of ingestion of wild watercress supports the diagnosis. At this stage the stool does not contain eggs. Serologic tests, such as the complement fixation test, are helpful. In chronic infection the stool contains the characteristic large operculated eggs (140 × 75 μ). Duodenal and biliary aspirate will provide a higher yield than fecal examination. Liver function test results reflect the degree of hepatic cellular damage and biliary obstruction. Intravenous or percutaneous cholangiography may show abnormalities and filling defects. The diagnosis is often made during surgical operation for biliary disease. The diagnosis of halzoun in an endemic area is made by the history of ingestion of raw liver and the finding of a pharyngeal mass.

TREATMENT. In the past, bithionol, emetine, dehydroemetine, and chloroquine were used with some success in this condition. Praziquantel is now the drug of choice in fascioliasis. The recommended dosage is 75 mg per kilogram of body weight divided into three doses per day for two days. Ectopic flukes are removed surgically. Prevention consists of not eating raw watercress and raw sheep and goat liver in the endemic areas.

Fasciola Gigantica

This large fluke is a liver parasite of herbivorous animals and occasionally of man in Asia and Africa. The life cycle, mode of infection, clinical manifestations, and treatment are similar to those of *F. hepatica.*

Clonorchiasis

Flavell, DJ: Liver fluke infection as an aetiological factor in bile duct carcinoma of man. Trans Roy Soc Trop Med Hyg 75:814, 1981. *Reviews the evidence of liver flukes as factors in causing bile duct cancer.*

Gibson JB, Sun T: Clonorchiasis. *In* Marcial-Rojas RA (ed.): Pathology of Protozoal and Helminthic Diseases. Baltimore, Williams & Wilkins Company, 1971, pp 546-566. *Profusely illustrated; very good on all aspects, especially on epidemiology and pathology as seen in Hong Kong.*

Liu YH, Qiu ZD, Wang WG, Wang QN, Qu ZQ, Chen RX, Liu JB, Zhang CD, Qin SA: Praziquantel in clonorchiasis: A further evaluation of 100 cases. Chin Med J 95:89, 1982. *Describes the evaluation of this drug in China.*

Pearson RD, Guerrant RL: Praziquantel: A major advance in anthelminthic therapy. Ann Intern Med 99:195, 1983. *A good review of the pharmacology, toxicity, and usefulness of this drug in schistosoma, trematode, and cestode infections.*

Praziquantel—a new antiparasitic drug. Med Lett Drugs Ther 24:108, 1982. *A very good summary of this wonder drug.*

Rim HJ, Lyu KS, Lee JS, Joo, KH: Clinical evaluation of the therapeutic efficacy of praziquantel (Embay 8440) against Clonorchis sinensis infection in man. Ann Trop Med Para 75:27, 1981. *Describes the early use of this drug in large number of patients in Korea.*

Xu Z, Zhong H, Cao W: Acute clonorchiasis. Chinese Med J (Peking) 92:423, 1979. *Good description and documentation of the clinical course of the seldom recognized acute clonorchiasis.*

Opisthorchiasis

Viranuvatti V: Liver fluke infection and infestation in Southeast Asia. Progr Liver Dis 4:537, 1972. *Concise review of liver flukes, especially* Opisthorchis.

Fascioliasis

Jones EA, Kay JM, Milligan HP, Owens D: Massive infection with *Fasciola hepatica* in man. Am J Med 63:836, 1977. *Report of an unusual case with a prolonged course of illness. Illustrates many of the complications of this disease.*

Marcial-Rojas RA: Fascioliasis. *In* Marcial-Rojas RA (ed.): Pathology of Protozoal and Helminthic Disease. Baltimore, Williams & Wilkins Company, 1971, pp 490-497. *Good on the epidemiology and pathology of this disease.*

LUNG HERMAPHRODITIC FLUKES
(Paragonimiasis)

Paragonimiasis is due to infection with the adult *Paragonimus westermani* and other species. As a rule the infection is in the lung, where the flukes are encapsulated in the parenchyma. The disease is also called pulmonary distomiasis, endemic hemoptysis, and Oriental lung fluke disease. Human paragonimiasis occurs most commonly in the Far East, especially central China, Japan, Korea, Vietnam, Laos, Thailand, and the Philippines. It also occurs in the Indian subcontinent, Central and South America, and West Africa. In addition to *P. westermani,* over 30 species may affect man. Most of these flukes are parasites of mammals, especially of the cat family (cat, tiger, leopard), foxes, dogs, cattle, and pigs. *P. westermani* was first discovered in 1877 by Westerman in a tiger in the Amsterdam zoo.

The adult flukes live singly or in pairs encapsulated in the cystic spaces of the lung. They are ovoid, plump, and leaf-like, and measure about 1 × 0.5 × 0.4 cm. Oval yellowish-brown operculated ova (90 × 55 μ) are coughed up and expelled in the sputum or are swallowed and passed in the feces. The flukes have a life span of five to six years. In fresh water the miracidia escape from the ova and penetrate the first intermediate host, a suitable snail. After several weeks the cercariae emerge and penetrate the second intermediate host, the crayfish or crab. Man or animal acquires the infection by eating raw meat or viscera of the freshwater crustacean. In Korea and West Africa, fresh crab juice is used as a home remedy in the treatment of measles. In the duodenum the metacercariae excyst, enter the abdominal cavity, migrate through the diaphragm into the pleural space, and end up in the lung parenchyma, where they mature and begin to lay eggs about two months after ingestion of the crayfish. This circuitous route of migration explains the extrapulmonary cysts of *Paragonimus.*

PATHOLOGY. The migratory larval flukes tunnel into the lung at the periphery. This is accompanied by inflammatory reaction with many eosinophils. They finally encyst with a fibrous tissue wall. The cyst may communicate with a bronchus and may often be secondarily infected with abscess formation. The death of the fluke is followed by calcification. Flukes in the abdominal cavity may cause abscess and adhesion and intestinal ulceration, resulting in bloody diarrhea with mucus and ova. In the brain the temporal and occipital lobes are the favored sites of eosinophilic granulomas containing the flukes or ova. Lodgment of the flukes in the spinal cord causes transverse myelitis. Adult flukes have been found in other organs, including the genitalia and muscle. Some species are prone to cause ectopic paragonimiasis. Thus the characteristic feature of *P. skrjabini* is migratory subcutaneous nodules containing active flukes.

CLINICAL MANIFESTATIONS. In the rare case of acute paragonimiasis there may be fever, chills, and chest pain. The symptoms and physical findings are indistinguishable from those of bronchopneumonia. As a rule the onset is insidious and the symptoms are those of chronic bronchitis and bronchiectasis. Cough, especially in the morning, productive of thick, gelatinous, blood-tinged sputum, is the most prominent symptom. Exertional dyspnea and night sweats are common. Frank hemoptysis often occurs after a paroxysm of coughing. Chest pain and pleural effusion may be present, and clubbing of fingers may occur. The most characteristic physical finding is persistent moist, coarse rales over the area of involvement. Chest x-rays early in the disease show patchy, cloudy infiltrations, but later dense nodular opacities or ring shadows indicate the site of the cysts. Pleural thickening and calcification may be seen late in the disease.

Abdominal paragonimiasis occurs when the flukes localize in the abdomen. The symptoms are nonspecific dull ache, tenderness, and diarrhea, which may be bloody and accompanied by mucus. An abdominal mass with lung disease in a patient from an endemic area should raise this suspicion. On rare occasions the fluke localizes in the brain, resulting in a seizure disorder similar to cysticercosis. There may be pareses of varying degrees and optic atrophy with papilledema. The cerebrospinal fluid shows a raised protein concentration, and eosinophils are present. Children with cerebral paragonimiasis are usually mentally retarded. Subcutaneous localization of the fluke results in abscess formation.

DIAGNOSIS. This rests mainly on finding ova in the sputum. In more than half of the cases stools will also reveal the ova, especially after concentration. The main differential diagnoses in the chest x-rays are bronchopneumonia, bronchiectasis, tuberculosis, tumor, and the rarer fungal infections. In practice the most important differential diagnosis is tuberculosis. Active tuberculosis and paragonimiasis often are present in the same individual from the endemic area.

Abdominal paragonimiasis must be differentiated from intestinal parasitic and nonparasitic infections and other intra-abdominal disorders. The finding of the ova in the stool does not necessarily indicate abdominal paragonimiasis. The cerebral presentation must be differentiated from other causes of seizure disorder, space-occupying lesions, cysticercosis, hydatid disease, and meningoencephalitides.

Moderate eosinophilia is usual in the early cases, but in established cases there may be no abnormal hematologic findings. Serology, as a rule, is not useful in helminthic infections, and this is also true in paragonimiasis. The complement fixation test, using extract of the adult fluke as antigen, is positive when the fluke is alive, but the skin test may remain positive long after the fluke is dead.

TREATMENT. Praziquantel, because of its safety, ease of use, and high degree of efficacy, is replacing bithionol and niclofolan as the treatment of choice in pulmonary paragonimiasis. The recommended dosage of praziquantel in this infection is 75 mg per kilogram of body weight divided into three doses daily for two days.

Paragonimiasis of the central nervous system requires surgery. Praziquantel should be given before the operation. Subcutaneous flukes should also be surgically removed.

PREVENTION. In theory prevention is simple. Freshwater crustaceans must be well cooked before eating, and hands and utensils should be thoroughly washed after contact with raw crabs and crayfish. However, in endemic areas it is difficult to persuade people to relinquish long-established cooking and eating habits and the use of raw crab juice for medicinal purposes.

Chung CH: Human paragonimiasis. *In* Marcial-Rojas RA (ed.): Pathology of Protozoal and Helminthic Diseases. Baltimore, Williams & Wilkins Company, 1971, pp 504-535. *Very detailed description of the pathologic changes of this disease. Well illustrated.*

Monson MH, Koenig JW, Sach R: Successful treatment with praziquantel of six patients infected with the African lung fluke *Paragonimus uterobilateralis.* Am J Trop Med Hyg 32:371, 1983. *Describes the usefulness of this drug in the common Western African species of Paragonimus.*

Spitalny KC, Senft AW, Meglio FD, Moran J, Peter G: Treatment of pulmonary paragonimiasis with a new broad-spectrum antihelminthic, praziquantel. J Pediatr 101:144, 1982. *Report of an Indochinese refugee to America with pulmonary paragonimiasis successfully treated with this drug.*

Yokogawa M: *Paragonimus* and paragonimiasis. Adv Parasitol 7:375, 1969. *Good review of the finer parasitologic points on this fluke.*

INTESTINAL HERMAPHRODITIC FLUKES

Fasciolopsiasis (Fasciolopsis Buski)

Fasciolopsis buski is the largest intestinal fluke and is normally a parasite of pigs. Human infection is widespread in Southern China, Southeast Asia, and the Indian subcontinent. The eggs are passed in the feces, and the miracidia are released to penetrate a snail. The cercariae encyst as metacercariae on edible water plants. Often the infected plants are peeled by using the teeth to remove the "skin," and the metacercariae are swallowed in the process. The larvae attach themselves to the upper small intestine, where they mature in about four weeks. The adult fluke has an average size of 3 × 1.2 cm.

CLINICAL MANIFESTATIONS. Many light infections are asymptomatic, but heavy loads of flukes produce symptoms, especially in children. The worm load may be up to several thousand. The flukes attach themselves to the duodenal and jejunal mucosa and produce symptoms by trauma, obstruction, and toxin production. There may be abdominal pain, gastrointestinal hemorrhage, diarrhea, and intestinal obstruction. In severe cases there may be edema of the face, trunk, and legs, as well as ascites.

DIAGNOSIS. This rests on finding the large ova (135 × 80 μ), or recovery of characteristic adult flukes in the stool. Difficulty may be encountered in distinguishing the ova of *F. hepatica* and *F. buski*. Eosinophilia is common and may exceed 50 per cent of the white cell count. Serologic tests, such as the indirect fluorescent antibody test, are available in some centers. The specificity of serologic tests is unproved, and definitive diagnosis cannot be based on serologic tests alone. This is also true of skin tests. Facial edema may require differentiation of fasciolopsiasis from trichinosis or the nephrotic syndrome.

TREATMENT. In the past the drug of choice in endemic areas has been hexylresorcinol (Crystoid anthelmintic), given in a single dose of 1.0 gram by mouth. Tetrachloroethylene in a dose of 0.1 ml per kilogram is equally effective. These two inexpensive medications are not available in North America. Piperazine or bephenium hydroxynaphthoate can be used. Not all the flukes are eradicated in one treatment, but it may be repeated in one week. Praziquantel will probably emerge as the drug of choice in this condition. The dosage is 75 mg per kilogram of body weight divided into three doses per day for one or two days. Personal prevention consists of cooking aquatic plants before eating. Community prevention entails eradication of the snails with molluscacides, public education, and prevention of fecal contamination of ponds.

Other Intestinal Hermaphroditic Flukes

Heterophyes heterophyes and *Metagonimus yokogawai* are small flukes that are acquired by eating raw or undercooked fish that contain the metacercariae. The former is found in Egypt, Tunisia, south China, India, and the Philippines, and the latter in the Far East and Indonesia. The adult flukes are 2 to 3 mm long and attach themselves to the intestinal mucosa. Usually the infection is light and there are few symptoms. Very rarely the eggs gain access to the circulation and may be found in the organs. As a rule the eggs are passed in the stool; they closely resemble *Clonorchis* eggs. Both flukes can be treated with tetrachloroethylene as used for hookworm. Differentiation of the two species requires examination of the adult flukes by experts. Many species of the genus *Echinostoma* infect man in the Far East, but they rarely produce symptoms. *Gastrocoides hominis* occurs in India and Malaysia, and may cause diarrhea. In Western Canada the eggs of *Metorchis conjunctus*, which are somewhat similar to those of *Clonorchis*, are occasionally found in the stools of humans who eat raw fish. If treatment is called for, praziquantel (75 mg per kilogram of body weight in three divided doses for one day) is the treatment of choice.

Alaria americana is an intestinal trematode of carnivores, such as the fox, wolf, lynx, or skunk. Two cases of human infection by the mesocercariae of this fluke have been reported in Ontario. Mesocercaria is a stage of development between the cercaria and the metacercaria. The cercariae emerging from the snail penetrate tadpoles. As the tadpole grows into a frog the mesocercariae tend to concentrate in the hind legs. When the frog is eaten by a carnivore, the mesocercariae develop into metacercariae and adult flukes in the lung and the gut, respectively. When man, who is not the normal host, eats the frog the mesocercariae migrate all over the body. In the first reported case the mesocercaria was surgically removed from the retina

of the eye. The second case was a fatal systemic infection manifested by severe respiratory distress, coma, a coagulation abnormality, and vasculitis. At autopsy mesocercariae were found in all organs. The diagnosis is by biopsy of affected organs. There is no known treatment, although praziquantel may be useful.

Faust EC, Beaver PC, Jung RC: Intestinal flukes. *In* Faust EC, Beaver PC, Jung RC: Animal Agents and Vectors of Human Disease. 4th ed. Philadelphia, Lea & Febiger, 1975, pp 134-141. *Emphasis is on the parasitology, life cycles, and morphology. A good reference for the lesser important parasites.*

Fernandes BJ, Cooper JD, Cullen JB, Freeman RS, Ritchie AC, Scott AA, Stuart PF: Systemic infection with *Alaria americana* (Trematoda). Can Med Assoc J 115:1111, 1976. *This is the first report of generalized infection with mesocercariae of this fluke. Good description of the clinical course and autopsy findings.*

The Nematodes

398. INTRODUCTION

Daniel S. Blumenthal

Nematodes are primitive, elongated, unsegmented worms, with a body cavity that is not lined with a peritoneum of mesodermal origin as is the body cavity of higher animals. The sexes are separate, but parthenogenesis occurs in some parasitic forms. The class includes half a million species; some are free-living, while others are parasitic for plants, invertebrates, and both wild and domestic vertebrates.

Eleven species are important parasites of humans. These may be classified as intestinal parasites or tissue parasites. The former include the hookworms *Ancylostoma duodenale* and *Necator americanus*, the large roundworm *Ascaris lumbricoides*, the whipworm *Trichuris trichiura*, the pinworm *Enterobius vermicularis*, and *Strongyloides stercoralis*. The adult *Trichinella spiralis* also inhabits the human intestine, but it is classified as a tissue nematode because its clinical manifestations are produced by larvae invading the tissues. The filariae are also tissue parasites; species commonly causing serious disease in humans include *Onchocerca volvulus*, the agent of river blindness; *Dracunculus medinensis*, the Guinea worm; *Loa loa;* and *Wuchereria bancrofti*. Several other nematodes are human parasites of lesser importance, and a variety of nematodes that ordinarily infect non-human species may occasionally infect people, sometimes causing serious disease.

The parasitic nematodes have evolved a great variety of mechanisms by which they are transmitted from one definitive host to another. Some (such as *Enterobius*) produce ova that may be passed from person to person, while the eggs of others (for instance, *Ascaris* and hookworm) must incubate in the soil before they become infective. Some, such as *Trichinella*, require an intermediate host that is eaten by the definitive host, whereas the intermediate hosts of some nematode parasites of animals release infective larvae. The filariae are transmitted by insect vectors.

Of the major nematode parasites of man, only *Strongyloides stercoralis* is capable of reproducing in the definitive host. This is true of most other helminthic infections as well, and distinguishes them from infections with viruses, bacteria, and protozoa. As a consequence, it is not usually necessary to seek total elimination of the parasite in a patient (or a community), since a light infection is not generally clinically significant. An exception is ascariasis, in which a single worm can cause serious morbidity or mortality.

It is hard to overestimate the amount of worldwide morbidity that is caused by parasitic nematodes. There are an estimated one billion cases each of *Ascaris* and *Trichuris*, a number equal to a quarter of the world's population. Approximately 600 million persons are infected with hookworm and 300 million with filariae. Nematode infections are still common in many communities in the United States. There are perhaps 4 million persons infected with *Ascaris* in this country; 2.2 million with *Trichuris*, 700,000 with hookworm, and 400,000 with *Strongyloides*.

In areas where soil and climatic conditions are suitable, nematode infections may be considered a marker of rural poverty. Only when this poverty, with its accompanying inadequate levels of sanitation and education, has been alleviated, will the prevalence of these parasites be reduced to unimportant levels.

Major nematode infections; other nematode infections. *In* Intestinal Protozoan and Helminthic Infections. Report of a WHO Scientific Group. Technical Report Series 666. Geneva, World Health Organization, 1981. *A comprehensive public health approach.*

Schultz MG: Parasitic diseases. N Engl J Med 297:1259, 1977. *Schultz discusses all parasitic disease, not just nematode infections, but speaks eloquently of the magnitude of the problem.*

Warren KS: The control of helminths: Nonreplicating infectious agents of man. Ann Rev Public Health 2:101, 1981. *A thoughtful commentary on efforts to control nematode and other helminth infections in developing countries.*

399. STRONGYLOIDIASIS

Daniel S. Blumenthal

DEFINITION. Strongyloidiasis is infection with the parasitic phase of *Strongyloides stercoralis*. Clinical manifestations may be caused by the adult worms in the small intestine or by the migrating filariform larvae.

ETIOLOGY AND LIFE CYCLE. The adult female *Strongyloides* is about 2 mm long and lives in the mucosal epithelium of the duodenum and jejunum, extending above or below this in the gastrointestinal tract in heavy infections. There is no parasitic male; reproduction in the parasitic phase is parthenogenic.

The life cycle of this parasite is complex and proceeds by several alternative pathways. Each worm produces fewer than 100 eggs daily. They hatch in the intestine of the host, and rhabditiform larvae are passed in the stool. These may metamorphose in the soil into infective filariform larvae or may mature into free-living adults that reproduce bisexually. They may then give rise to infective larvae in a later generation. The infective larvae invade the human host by penetrating the skin, travel through the venous circulation to the lungs, migrate through the alveolar capillary walls, ascend the respiratory tree to the epiglottis, and are swallowed to reach the small intestine, where they mature.

Alternatively, *Strongyloides* larvae may develop to the infective stage in the intestine, penetrate the intestinal wall to reach the circulation, and enter the cycle of infection. This process of *internal autoinfection* is unique to this species among nematodes. Infective larvae may also penetrate the perianal skin after being passed with the stool to enter the host by *external autoinfection*. These processes may enable an infection to persist 30 to 40 years in the absence of re-exposure of the host.

In immunosuppressed or malnourished patients, internal autoinfection may assume massive proportions with ectopic migration of the larvae, resulting in the *hyperinfection syndrome.*

EPIDEMIOLOGY. *Strongyloides* is found in warm climates throughout the world, but, except in institutions for the retarded, high community prevalence rates have not been reported. In the United States, strongyloidiasis is most common in Southern Appalachia, but occasional autochthonous cases have been found in northern cities. There is at least one report of transmission from dog to man. *Strongyloides fulbornii,* a parasite of monkeys, has been reported to infect people in Africa.

PATHOLOGY. As the larvae migrate through the lungs, they sometimes cause a pneumonic process similar to Löffler's syndrome in ascariasis.

In the small intestine, microscopic abnormalities include stunted, swollen, or fused villi; eosinophilic infiltration of the lamina propria; and mononuclear infiltration of the mucosa.

In the hyperinfection syndrome and in other severe cases of strongyloidiasis, intestinal changes are more pronounced. Parasites may be found in all layers of the intestinal wall, which is thickened by edema and fibrosis. An inflammatory response is seen, but without eosinophilia, and there may be micro- and macroscopic ulcerations. Pulmonary involvement in the hyperinfection syndrome is characterized by extensive larval migration and hemorrhagic pneumonia. Larvae may be found throughout the body, especially in the kidneys, brain, and heart.

CLINICAL MANIFESTATIONS. As the larvae penetrate the skin, particularly in cases of external autoinfection, they may cause a migratory pruritic eruption known as *larva currens.* Larvae migrating through the lung may cause pneumonia, with cough, dyspnea, and hemoptysis, but this is not common.

Mild intestinal infections are often asymptomatic. Moderate infections generally result in epigastric pain and intermittent diarrhea, whereas heavy infections may cause significant malabsorption with bulky, foul-smelling stools, abdominal distention, and hypoproteinemia with edema. In patients who are malnourished, the malabsorption may persist even after the infection is adequately treated.

COMPLICATIONS. The hyperinfection syndrome has been increasingly recognized in recent years in hosts with altered immune status, those with malignancies or malnutrition, and rarely those who are otherwise normal. The onset of symptoms in this complication is characteristically relatively abrupt, with fever and severe abdominal pain and distention, often accompanied by shock. Gram-negative sepsis frequently ensues; intestinal ulcerations caused by the parasite are thought to permit the entry of enteric pathogens into the circulation. When larval invasion of the lungs is severe, dyspnea and cough productive of blood-tinged sputum may be prominent.

DIAGNOSIS. *Strongyloides* ova do not appear in the stool; diagnosis is dependent on the identification of larvae. Multiple stool examinations, using concentration techniques, are generally necessary in light or moderate infections. Larvae may be identified in duodenal fluid when they cannot be found in stool specimens; the string test (Enterotest) is useful for obtaining samples of duodenal fluid for this purpose. In cases of hyperinfection, larvae may often be found in the sputum.

Eosinophilia is often present, but may be absent in cases of hyperinfection. Contrast media examination of the small bowel often demonstrates thickening and edema of the mucosal folds. Chest x-ray in patients with hyperinfection may show patchy infiltrates.

TREATMENT. The drug of choice, in both ordinary intestinal strongyloidiasis and hyperinfection, is thiabendazole, 25 mg per kilogram twice a day for two to five days. Nausea, vomiting, drowsiness, and vertigo are common side effects. Other drugs that have been used include pyrvinium pamoate, mebendazole, diethylcarbamazine,* and levamisole (not available in the United States). None of these drugs is recommended for pregnant women. A follow-up stool examination should be obtained two to six weeks following treatment, and stool examinations should also be obtained on other family members.

PREVENTION. This parasite, like the other soil-transmitted nematodes, is associated with rural poverty and its attendant conditions of poor sanitation and inadequate education. Alleviation of these conditions interrupts transmission. The wearing of shoes protects against infection.

Secondary prevention of the hyperinfection syndrome is important in persons from endemic areas who have altered immune status. Such patients should have studies appropriate to rule out *Strongyloides* infection, particularly when they exhibit suggestive gastrointestinal symptoms and/or eosinophilia.

Burke JA: Strongyloidiasis in childhood. Am J Dis Child 132:1130, 1978. *A comprehensive survey of this infection and review of the literature, complete with case studies.*

Igra-Siegman Y, Kapila R, Sen P, et al.: Syndrome of hyperinfection with *Strongyloides stercoralis.* Rev Infec Dis 3:397, 1981. *Reviews 103 cases of hyperinfection syndrome reported in the English language literature since 1964.*

Walzer PD, Milder JE, Banwell JG, Kilgore G, Klein M, Parker R: Epidemiologic features of *Strongyloides stercoralis* infection in an endemic area of the United States. Am J Trop Med Hyg 31:313, 1982. *Southeastern Kentucky is an area of particularly high prevalence of this parasite. This paper defines the epidemiology of* Strongyloides *in this area and points out that the infection is more common in geriatric patients than are other parasitic infections.*

400. CAPILLARIASIS

Daniel S. Blumenthal

Capillaria philippinensis infection was first observed in the north Philippines in 1963. Since then, it has also been found in Thailand. At least 1500 cases have been reported, with a case-fatality rate of about 10 per cent. This nematode is thought to parasitize birds, with fish and crustaceans serving as intermediate hosts. Humans are infected by eating the raw intermediate hosts. The ingested larvae mature and live in the crypts of the small intestine, where they reproduce. (*Strongyloides* is the only other nematode that reproduces in man.) The result is often a heavy infection; up to 40,000 adult worms have been recovered at one autopsy. The clinical syndrome is one of severe malabsorption and protein-losing enteropathy. The diagnosis is made by finding eggs or larvae in the stool; the eggs resemble those of *Trichuris.* An intradermal test is also available. The treatment of choice is mebendazole, 200 mg twice a day for 20 days; an alternative is thiabendazole, 25 mg per kilogram daily for 30 days. Fluid and electrolyte replacement and a high protein diet are also important.

Capillaria hepatica is a parasite of rats that occasionally infects the liver of man. The result is an acute or subacute hepatitis with eosinophilia. Diagnosis is made on liver biopsy; there is no known treatment.

Singson CN, Banzon TC, Cross JH: Mebendazole in the treatment of intestinal capillariasis. Am J Trop Med Hyg 24:932, 1975. *Little has been written about this parasite in the last 10 years. This study documents the value of mebendazole in treatment.*

401. HOOKWORM DISEASE

Daniel S. Blumenthal

DEFINITION. Two species of hookworm infect man: *Ancylostoma duodenale,* the so-called Old World hookworm, and *Necator americanus,* the so-called New World hookworm. Both species attach themselves to the mucosa of the small intestine and ingest blood. When this results in anemia, hypoproteinemia, and clinical symptoms, the condition is termed hookworm disease. If these findings are lacking, the host is said merely to have hookworm infection.

ETIOLOGY AND LIFE CYCLE. Hookworms are about 1 cm long; the female is slightly larger than the male, and *Ancylostoma* is

*Production of this drug in the United States has been discontinued.

slightly larger than *Necator*. *Ancylostoma* bears two pairs of upper teeth in its mouth, whereas *Necator* has a pair of upper and a pair of lower cutting plates.

The female *Ancylostoma* produces about 25,000 eggs per day; *Necator*, about 7000. These eggs are passed in the stool of the host and hatch in the soil within 48 hours. The emerging rhabditiform larvae molt twice within five to ten days and become infective filariform larvae. These may survive for several months in the soil.

Upon coming in contact with the skin of man, the filariform larvae penetrate, enter the venous circulation, and are carried into the lungs. There they migrate across the alveolar capillary walls, ascend the respiratory tree, and are swallowed to reach the small intestine. Infection with *Ancylostoma* may also be acquired by ingesting the filariform larvae; *Necator* is not infective by this route. The life span of *Necator* in the human host is two to six years; that of *Ancylostoma* is probably less.

EPIDEMIOLOGY. *Necator americanus* was once endemic throughout the southeastern United States, where it caused considerable disability among the rural poor. Its prevalence was greatly reduced by the work of the Rockefeller Sanitary Commission from 1910 to 1920, and has since continued to decline. *Necator* was originally imported to the New World from sub-Sahara Africa and has, in the past, been described as the predominant species in that part of the world, as well as in most of South and Central America. *Ancylostoma* was previously found exclusively in the Mediterranean basin, Asia, and parts of coastal South America. In more recent years, this distribution has become blurred.

In endemic areas, the highest prevalence rates are found in school-age children. During the time when hookworm was widespread in the southeastern United States, whites were noted to be more susceptible than blacks.

PATHOLOGY. A local inflammatory response occurs at the site of skin penetration by the filariform larvae, and as the larvae migrate through the lungs, an eosinophilic and mononuclear infiltration takes place along with local hemorrhages. A heavy passage of larvae through the lungs may cause a pneumonic process similar to Löffler's syndrome in ascariasis.

In the intestine, the adults attach themselves to the mucosa and actively suck blood. *Ancylostoma* ingests more blood (0.15 ml per worm per day) than *Necator* (0.03 ml per worm per day). The worms change sites of attachment at frequent intervals, leaving bleeding lacerations at their previous sites. The wall of the intestine becomes edematous, and a mononuclear and eosinophilic infiltrate surrounds each parasite.

CLINICAL MANIFESTATIONS AND COMPLICATIONS. Light infections, such as those generally found in the United States, are usually asymptomatic. In tropical countries, where worm burdens are often in the thousands, clinical manifestations of hookworm disease are frequent.

A pruritic vesicular or papular eruption, known as ground itch, may develop at the site of larval invasion. This is particularly pronounced after multiple exposures to the parasite. The passage of larvae through the lungs is sometimes associated with wheezing, dyspnea, and cough productive of blood-streaked sputum.

Abdominal pain and diarrhea may be caused by the adult worms in the intestine, particularly as the parasites attach themselves to the mucosa. The most important clinical manifestations, however, are those of anemia and hypoalbuminemia resulting from chronic blood loss. Weakness, fatigue, lassitude, and growth retardation are characteristic findings in patients with hookworm disease. Signs and symptoms of high-output congestive heart failure may be present, and peripheral edema may occur as a result of both the heart failure and hypoalbuminemia. The severity of anemia developed by the patient depends on the adequacy of dietary iron intake. Residents of communities endemic for hookworm often have inadequate diets and may be anemic independent of hookworm infection. On the other hand, an adequate diet may prevent anemia and hypoproteinemia despite significant infection.

DIAGNOSIS. The diagnosis of hookworm infection is made

by the finding of characteristic ova in the stool. The ova of *Necator* and *Ancylostoma* are identical, but species differentiation is not necessary for appropriate treatment and follow-up.

Quantitation of hookworm ova by either the Stoll or Kato thick smear technique may be performed as an aid in estimating the intensity of infection. Egg counts greater than 2000 per milliliter of feces in women and children or greater than 5000 per milliliter of feces in men are considered clinically significant in infections with *Necator*.

Other laboratory findings associated with hookworm infection include eosinophilia, Charcot-Leyden crystals in the stool, and, in heavy infections, hypoalbuminemia and anemia as low as 2 grams of hemoglobin per 100 ml of blood.

TREATMENT. In holoendemic areas in the tropics, where resources are limited, it has generally been the practice to treat only moderate or heavy infections. In the United States, however, light infections should also be treated when discovered, and measures should be taken to prevent reinfection.

The drug of choice is pyrantel pamoate, which is given in a single dose of 11 mg per kilogram of body weight (maximum, 1 gram). Mebendazole, 100 mg twice a day for three days, is equally effective. Neither drug should be used in pregnant women; mebendazole should be used with caution in children less than two years old. The anemia should be treated with oral iron supplementation; in cases of severe anemia with hypoalbuminemia, transfusion may be necessary.

A follow-up stool examination should be performed two to six weeks after treatment; stool examinations should also be performed on other family members.

PREVENTION. Hookworm, like the other soil-transmitted nematodes, is prevented by alleviating the conditions of rural poverty with which it is associated. The most important factors in this regard are the construction of sanitary facilities for the disposal of human wastes and community education regarding the etiology of the infection. The wearing of shoes is also important. Iron supplementation of the diet in endemic areas will prevent most cases of anemia.

Gilman RH: Hookworm Disease: Host-pathogen biology. Rev Infec Dis 4:824, 1982. *A concise review of the topic.*

402. CUTANEOUS LARVA MIGRANS

Daniel S. Blumenthal

DEFINITION. Cutaneous larva migrans (creeping eruption) is infection with a larval nematode that wanders in the subcutaneous tissues. The most common agent is *Ancylostoma braziliense*, a hookworm of dogs and cats.

ETIOLOGY AND EPIDEMIOLOGY. In addition to *A. braziliense*, the larvae of several other nematodes can cause cutaneous larva migrans. These include *Ancylostoma caninum* (a dog hookworm) and several other species of hookworm and *Strongyloides* that oridinarily infect nonhuman hosts. The larvae of these species penetrate human skin if it is exposed to soil contaminated with the feces of infected animals. Rather than complete their life cycle, however, the larvae continue to migrate in the subcutaneous tissues.

The infection is most common in tropical and subtropical areas, particularly on beaches frequented by dogs. The coasts of the Gulf of Mexico and Florida are common locales in the United States. Children, farmers, plumbers (working under beach houses) and sunbathers are most often affected.

The larvae of *A. braziliense* tunnel in the epidermis just above the basal layer, rarely penetrating into the dermis. The tunnel is surrounded by eosinophil and round cell infiltration.

CLINICAL MANIFESTATIONS. An erythematous pruritic papule or nonspecific dermatitis occurs at the site of skin contact with the contaminated soil. In two or three days (occasionally weeks or months), this becomes a 2 to 3 mm wide, slightly elevated, serpiginous track or burrow. The patient experiences intense itching.

DIAGNOSIS AND TREATMENT. The diagnosis is clinical. There are no diagnostic tests and usually no eosinophilia.

Topical application, four times a day, of the commercially available 10 per cent suspension of thiabendazole appears to work as well as giving the drug orally. If the oral route is elected, the dosage is 25 mg per kilogram in two divided doses for two to five days.

Edelglass JW, Douglass CM, Stiefler R, Tessler M: Cutaneous larva migrans in northern climates. A souvenir of your dream vacation. J Am Acad Dermatol 7:353, 1982. *A good review with typical case presentations in United States tourists. The literature on topical and oral therapy is discussed.*

403. TRICHOSTRONGYLIASIS

Daniel S. Blumenthal

Several species of the genus *Trichostrongylus* infect both man and domestic ruminants. The infection is found widely in the Middle and Far East and Australia. Particularly high prevalence rates have been reported from Iran.

Ova are passed in the stool and hatch in the soil; larvae are ingested with leafy vegetables. The adult worms live in the intestines and suck small amounts of blood; heavy infections result in anemia. Diagnosis is made by identifying ova, which resemble those of hookworm, in the stool.

Treatment is with thiabendazole, 25 mg per kilogram twice a day for two days, or with pyrantel pamoate in a single dose of 11 mg per kilogram.

Ghadirian E, Arfaa F: Present status of *Trichostrongylus* in Iran. Am J Trop Med Hyg 24:935, 1975. *Documents the high prevalence of this parasite in Iran and discusses the reasons for this.*

404. GNATHOSTOMIASIS

Daniel S. Blumenthal

Gnathostomiasis is infection with the larvae of *Gnathostoma spinigerum*, an intestinal nematode of dogs and cats for which fish serve as an intermediate host. Infective larvae are ingested when raw or undercooked fish is consumed. The larvae do not complete their life cycle in humans but migrate through the body.

The infection is found throughout the Far East; the greatest number of cases has been reported from Thailand.

The larvae most often migrate to the subcutaneous tissues, where they are found in eosinophilic granulomata. In central nervous system gnathostomiasis, hemorrhagic tracks may be found in the brain. Fever, vomiting, and abdominal pain occur a few days after ingestion of the infective fish. A few weeks later, skin lesions appear; these consist of subcutaneous nodules or swellings that may be either pruritic or painful and are often migratory. Abscesses may form. In the CNS variety, there is paralysis of the extremities, encephalitis, and subarachnoid hemorrhage. Eye involvement with uveitis and orbital cellulitis represents a third variety. Gnathostome larvae have also been reported from many other parts of the body.

Peripheral eosinophilia is usual in cutaneous gnathostomiasis; the diagnosis is usually established by biopsy. In central nervous system infection, peripheral eosinophilia is an inconstant feature, but there are many eosinophils in the cerebrospinal fluid. This must be distinguished from the eosinophilic meningitis caused by *Angiostrongylus*, which is usually less severe. Diagnosis may be assisted by an enzyme-linked immunosorbent assay (ELISA), and an intradermal test has been described. Treatment of subcutaneous lesions consists of surgical removal. For central nervous system infection, mebendazole* 200 mg every three hours for six days may be given. The infection may be prevented by cooking fish thoroughly before eating.

*This use is not listed in the manufacturer's directive.

Boogird P, Phuapradit P, Siridej N, Chirachariyavej T, Chuahiran S, Vejjajiva A: Neurological manifestations of gnathostomiasis. J Neurol Sci 31:279, 1977. *A clinical and epidemiologic description of a series of 24 cases of CNS gnathostomiasis.*
Stowens D, Simon G: Gnathostomiasis in Oneida County. NY State J Med 81:409, 1981. *A typical case of cutaneous gnathostomiasis, with discussion.*
Daengsvang S: Gnathostomiasis in Southeast Asia. Southeast Asian J Trop Med Public Health 12:319, 1981. *A review of the literature on both human and animal gnathostomiasis.*

405. PRIMATE NEMATODIASES

Daniel S. Blumenthal

Several nematodes that ordinarily parasitize the intestine of monkeys occasionally infect man. *Oesophagostomum* sp. has been reported from Africa, Asia, and Brazil; it is responsible for the formation of granulomas in the intestinal wall. *Ternides deminutus* is sometimes found in the human colon in Africa and Asia; a heavy infection may cause anemia. *Physaloptera mordens,* also reported from Africa, may attach itself to the esophagus, stomach, or small intestine of humans.

Barrowclough H, Crome L: Oesophagostomiasis in man. Trop Geogr Med 31:183, 1979. *Presents a case, discusses the difficulties in diagnosis, and reviews the literature.*

406. ASCARIASIS

Daniel S. Blumenthal

DEFINITION. Ascariasis is infection with the large roundworm, *Ascaris lumbricoides.* Clinical manifestations may result from the migration of the larvae through the lungs, from the presence of the adult worms in the lumen of the small intestine, or from extraintestinal migration of the adults.

ETIOLOGY AND LIFE CYCLE. *Ascaris* is the largest of the intestinal nematodes. Adult females measure 20 to 45 cm in length; adult males are about three fourths as large. Worm loads in the intestine may range from only one or two to hundreds; the life span of the parasite averages about 18 months.

The female produces about 200,000 ova per day. These are passed by the host in the stool and become infective after an obligate period in the soil of about ten days. The eggs are killed by direct sunlight and temperatures above 45° C, but under proper soil and climatic conditions they may remain viable for years.

After ingestion by the host, the eggs hatch in the duodenum, and the larvae penetrate the intestinal wall, enter the venous circulation, and are carried to the lungs, where they migrate across the alveolar capillary walls. They then travel up the respiratory tree to the epiglottis and are swallowed, returning to the small intestine, where they mature. The worms reach maturity and begin producing eggs in about two months.

EPIDEMIOLOGY. It is estimated that a quarter of the world's population is infected with *Ascaris.* The parasite occurs throughout the world but is most common in warm climates. In the United States, ascariasis is common in many rural parts of the southeast. The prevalence of the infection is greatest in children 1 to 13 years of age.

PATHOLOGY. As the larvae pass through the lungs, they may cause an eosinophilic pneumonitis known as *Löffler's syndrome.* The pathologic process appears to be a combination of physical damage to the alveoli caused by the migrating larvae and an exudative interstitial pneumonia. The large numbers of eosinophils (and the scarcity of neutrophils) in the exudate suggest a hypersensitivity reaction, and previous exposure to the parasite may be important in the development of this response.

The adult worms in the small intestine do not invade the mucosa, but maintain their position by bridging across the lumen. Nonetheless, they may cause mucosal damage demonstrable on barium-contrast examination of the upper gastrointestinal tract. Microscopically, this damage is seen as broadening and shortening of villi, elongation of crypts, and round cell infiltration of the lamina propria. Mucosal disaccharidase deficiency has been described.

The adult worms may migrate to extraintestinal sites in response to drug administration, intercurrent illness in the host, or unknown causes, and in so doing may cause considerable damage.

CLINICAL MANIFESTATIONS AND COMPLICATIONS. The *Ascaris* pneumonia caused by the migration of the larvae through the lungs is characterized by cough, fever, and malaise and, in severe cases, by chest pain, dyspnea, and hemoptysis. Patchy pulmonary infiltrates are seen on chest x-ray.

Various nonspecific gastrointestinal symptoms have been described in association with the worms in the intestine. These include abdominal pain, diarrhea, vomiting, irritability, and anorexia.

Malnutrition in children has been associated with ascariasis, but the amount of malnutrition caused by the infection is controversial. Lowered serum vitamin A and C and protein values have been reported in infected children. Improvement in growth rates have also been reported following de-worming. The nutritional effects of ascariasis seem to stem more from the malabsorption of fats, protein, and carbohydrate caused by mucosal damage than from the ingestion of host nutrients by the parasite.

Serious and life-threatening complications of ascariasis include intestinal obstruction by a bolus of worms, intussusception, volvulus, appendicitis, intestinal perforation, hepatic abscess, aspiration of a worm, cholangitis secondary to bile duct obstruction, and pancreatitis secondary to pancreatic duct obstruction. Of these, intestinal obstruction is the most common; it occurs particularly in children under age six.

DIAGNOSIS. Infection is diagnosed by the finding of ova on microscopic examination of the stool. Often the patient will describe a typical worm passed in the stool; in endemic areas, this is sufficient evidence of ascariasis to warrant treatment.

Eosinophilia is an inconstant feature of intestinal ascariasis. Serologic tests are available, but do not reliably distinguish current from past infection, or *Ascaris lumbricoides* infection from visceral larva migrans.

Ascaris pneumonia is not associated with eggs in the stool unless adult worms are simultaneously present in the host intestine. A marked peripheral eosinophilia provides evidence for the etiology of the pneumonia, but may not be present until late in the course of the illness. Larvae may sometimes be identified in the sputum.

TREATMENT. Pyrantel pamoate is the drug of choice; it is administered in a single dose of 11 mg per kilogram (maximal dose, 1 gram). Mebendazole is equally effective and is particularly useful in mixed *Ascaris-Trichuris* infections; the dose is 100 mg twice a day for three days. It should be used with caution in children less than two years old. Piperazine citrate, in a dose of 75 mg per kilogram daily for two days (maximal daily dose, 3.5 grams), is another effective drug; it is contraindicated in persons with seizure disorders or impaired renal or hepatic function. Levamisole is also effective but is not available in the United States.

Because the goal in treatment of ascariasis is complete elimination of the parasite, a follow-up stool examination should always be obtained two to six weeks after treatment. Stool examinations should also be performed on other members of the patient's household.

No specific treatment is available for *Ascaris* pneumonia. Oxygen and steroids may be indicated in severe cases.

Intestinal obstruction caused by ascariasis should be treated conservatively with nasogastric suction, intravenous fluids, and the instillation of an anthelmintic via the nasogastric tube. Surgery is indicated only in the event of failure of medical management.

PREVENTION. *Ascaris,* like the other soil-transmitted nematodes, is a marker of rural poverty in areas of suitable soil and climatic conditions. Primary prevention is largely dependent on the alleviation of poverty with its accompanying inadequate levels of education and sanitation.

Secondary prevention is possible through the periodic mass treatment of all children or all persons in an endemic community. Such a program may result in the near-eradication of the infection; but in the absence of improved hygiene and education, it is likely that the parasite will eventually become reestablished.

Pawlowski ZS: Ascariasis: Host-pathogen biology. Rev Infec Dis 4:806, 1982. Schultz MG: Ascariasis: Nutritional implications. Rev Infec Dis 4:815, 1982. *Two companion papers that together constitute a comprehensive review of the topic.*

Stephenson, LS: The contribution of *Ascaris lumbricoides* to malnutrition in children. Parasitology 81:221, 1980. *Argues that ascariasis negatively affects growth in children and that mass treatment of children should be undertaken in endemic areas.*

407. TOXOCARIASIS

Daniel S. Blumenthal

DEFINITION. Toxocariasis is infection with larvae of the dog ascarid, *Toxocara canis,* or less often, the cat ascarid, *Toxocara cati.* The larvae do not complete their life cycle in humans but migrate through the body, invading various organs and producing a syndrome known as *visceral larva migrans.* When the eye is involved, other organs are usually spared; this is known as *ocular larva migrans.*

ETIOLOGY. Humans become infected by ingesting soil contaminated with the feces of infected dogs or cats. Children with geophagia are at highest risk. Swallowed ova hatch in the small intestines and the larvae penetrate the intestinal wall to enter the circulation. When they reach a blood vessel with a diameter smaller than their own, they bore into the surrounding tissue. Larvae have been found in the liver, lungs, heart, and brain, as well as the eye.

EPIDEMIOLOGY. Toxocariasis is predominantly a childhood infection; fewer than 20 per cent of cases occur in adults. Visceral larva migrans tends to occur in younger children, while the ocular form of the infection tends to occur in older children. When both syndromes coexist, however, the patient is usually very young (under five years of age). Most cases are reported from the southern states. There is a strong association with the presence of a dog (especially a puppy) in the household. Serosurveys in the United States demonstrate a prevalence of antibodies to *Toxocara* of 15 to 25 per cent in black children age 1 to 11; white children have a prevalance of 4 to 5 per cent. This suggests that the vast majority of infections are asymptomatic.

PATHOLOGY. Migrating larvae leave tracks of hemorrhage, necrosis, and inflammatory cells. Eosinophilic granulomas or abscesses remain at the site of destruction of larvae; other larvae are walled off and may resume their migration up to years later.

CLINICAL MANIFESTATIONS. Common symptoms of visceral larva migrans are fever, coughing, wheezing, malaise, and weight loss. Physical findings commonly include wheezes, rales, and hepatosplenomegaly. Occasionally the central nervous system is involved, resulting in seizures or behavior disturbances. The white count may be greatly elevated (30,000 to 100,000) with 50 to 90 per cent eosinophils. Serum IgG, IgM, and IgE are usually elevated, as are isohemagglutinins.

In ocular larva migrans, the presentation may be one of visual loss, strabismus, or less often, eye pain. Funduscopic findings may range from a retinal granuloma to severe exudative endophthalmitis with retinal detachment. The condition often mimics retinoblastoma and must be distinguished by serologic testing to avoid needless enucleation.

DIAGNOSIS. Visceral larva migrans should be considered in any child with a persistent eosinophilia, especially if there is a history of pica and/or a household dog. Diagnosis may be confirmed by enzyme-linked immunosorbent assay (ELISA), which has a sensitivity of about 80 per cent and a specificity of about 90 per cent.

TREATMENT AND PREVENTION. Most cases of visceral larva migrans are mild and self-limited, and no treatment is indicated. In severe cases, thiabendazole in a dose of 25 mg per kilogram twice a day for five days may be given, although its benefits remain controversial. Corticosteroids should also be given in severe cases to alleviate symptoms and to limit eye damage in ocular larva migrans.

Household dogs should be examined by a veterinarian for intestinal nematodes and treated as necessary. Leash laws and control of stray dogs may reduce fecal contamination of public parks and playgrounds.

Glockman LT, Schantz PM: Epidemiology and pathogenesis of zoonotic toxocariasis. Epidemiol Rev 3:230, 1981. *An extensive review with emphasis on the seroepidemiology of toxocariasis.*

408. ANISAKIASIS

Daniel S. Blumenthal

Anisakiasis is infection with the larvae of an intestinal nematode of marine mammals. Several species of fish, including herring, serve as intermediate hosts, and human infection may be acquired when raw fish is eaten. The larvae of both *Anisakis* sp. and *Phocanema decipiens* have been implicated. Most cases have occurred in Japan or western Europe, particularly Scandinavia and the Netherlands. Fewer than 30 cases have been reported from the Western Hemisphere.

The larvae invade the wall of the small intestine, where they produce eosinophilic granulomata; intestinal obstruction or perforation may result. Living larvae are sometimes regurgitated. Serologic and intradermal diagnostic tests have been studied, but the diagnosis is generally made at laparotomy. Thiabendazole, 25 mg per kilogram twice a day for three days, may be given if surgical intervention is not required. The disease may be prevented by cooking or freezing fish prior to eating.

Smith JW, Wootten R: Anisakis and anisakiasis. Adv Parasitol 16:93, 1978. *An exceptionally complete review.*

409. TRICHURIASIS

Daniel S. Blumenthal

DEFINITION. Trichuriasis is infection with the whipworm, *Trichuris trichiura.* Clinical manifestations are caused by parasites in the cecum and large intestine; migration of larvae or adults elsewhere in the body has not been reported.

ETIOLOGY AND LIFE CYCLE. Both male and female adult *Trichuris* are about 30 to 50 mm long and have an elongated whiplike anterior portion which is embedded in the submucosa of the host's colon. The female produces 5000 to 10,000 eggs per day; these are passed in the stool and must incubate in the soil for at least three weeks. Embryonated eggs can survive in the soil for years.

Upon ingestion, the ova hatch in the small intestine, and the larvae proceed to the cecum and colon, where they mature. Egg production begins in two to three months. Adult worms survive for three to ten years in the host. Worm loads may number in the thousands.

EPIDEMIOLOGY. Trichuris is found in warm climates throughout the world. In the United States, it is estimated that 2.2 million persons are infected; over 40 per cent of children and adolescents in some rural communities in the southeastern United States harbor the parasite. Soil and climatic requirements for this parasite are similar to those for *Ascaris,* and infections with both worms often coexist in the same host.

PATHOLOGY. Pathologic findings are limited to the large intestine. Light infections cause little tissue reaction. Heavier infections cause edema and hyperemia of the mucosa; microscopically, there is a plasma cell, eosinophil, and polymorphonuclear infiltrate.

CLINICAL MANIFESTATIONS AND COMPLICATIONS. Light infections are often asymptomatic. Heavy infections are accompanied by abdominal pain and diarrhea, which may be severe and prolonged. Since the infection is limited to the large intestine, however, true malabsorption does not occur.

Rectal prolapse is a not infrequent complication of heavy infection. The visible white worms on the edematous mucosa have given the condition the name "coconut cake" prolapse. Worms have also been reported to obstruct the appendix and cause acute appendicitis. The question of whether trichuriasis causes intestinal bleeding is unresolved. Two studies using similar techniques have reached differing conclusions.

DIAGNOSIS. Characteristic eggs, with a mucous plug in each end, may be found on direct fecal smear. In light infections, stool concentration techniques are helpful in making the diagnosis.

Worms may be observed directly on proctosigmoidoscopy. An eosinophilia frequently accompanies infection.

TREATMENT. The drug of choice is mebendazole, 100 mg twice a day for three days regardless of body weight. Since side effects with this drug are very uncommon, even light asymptomatic infections may be treated. However, mebendazole should be used with caution in children under two years, and it should not be given to pregnant women. Oxantel is also effective; it is not available in the United States. A follow-up stool examination should be performed following treatment, and stool examinations should be obtained on other family members.

Reduction of rectal prolapse may be accomplished with a tissue-paper–covered finger; the tissue paper, which facilitates withdrawal of the finger, remains in the rectum and is later expelled. The buttocks may be taped together for a day or two after the prolapse is reduced.

PREVENTION. As with the other soil-transmitted nematodes, this parasite is associated with rural poverty. The provision of sanitary means for the disposal of human feces, combined with community education regarding the transmission of worms, is essential in prevention.

Chanco PP, Vidad JY: A review of trichuriasis, its incidence, pathogenicity and treatment. Drugs 15 (Suppl. 1):87, 1978. *A historical review.*

Greenberg ER, Cline BL: Is trichuriasis associated with iron-deficiency anemia? Am J Trop Med Hyg 284:770, 1979. *A slight reduction in hemoglobin levels was found in* Trichuris-*infected children compared to controls. Reviews the articles relevant to the controversy concerning trichuriasis and gastrointestinal blood loss.*

410. ENTEROBIASIS

Daniel S. Blumenthal

DEFINITION. Enterobiasis is infection with the pinworm, *Enterobius (Oxyuris) vermicularis.* This is a generally benign, although often symptomatic, parasitosis.

ETIOLOGY AND LIFE CYCLE. The adult female pinworm is about 1 cm long, the male, one fourth to one third as large. The parasites inhabit the cecum and colon. Gravid females emerge from the anus while the host sleeps, each female depositing several thousand eggs on the perianal skin. These are transmitted by person-to-person contact via the host's hands. Alternatively, they may be transmitted by bedclothes or become airborne. They remain viable in the environment only a few days. Swallowed eggs release larvae in the small intestine; these pass directly to the colon, where they mature.

EPIDEMIOLOGY. Pinworms are common throughout the world, in urban as well as rural populations and in the affluent as well as the poor. They are particularly common in group living situations, and their prevalence in institutions for the mentally retarded often exceeds 50 per cent. Adults are affected less often than children.

PATHOLOGY. The parasites in the intestine provoke little or no inflammatory response. Worms sometimes migrate into the appendix or fallopian tubes or escape into the peritoneum or elsewhere in the body, where they cause an inflammatory or granulomatous reaction.

CLINICAL MANIFESTATIONS. Many infections—perhaps the majority—are asymptomatic. The characteristic manifestation of symptomatic infections is pruritus ani caused by the deposited ova. This itch may result in restlessness or insomnia.

Nocturnal enuresis has been attributed to enterobiasis, and there are documented cases of bedwetting which resolved promptly upon treatment of concurrent pinworm infection. Most cases of enuresis are not associated with enterobiasis, however.

Numerous other symptoms in children have been attributed to this parasitosis, but no cause-and-effect relationship has been demonstrated. These include tooth-grinding, nose-picking, sleeping in the knee-chest position, anorexia, and abdominal pain.

COMPLICATIONS. Perianal scratching may result in excoriations or impetigo. Young girls may suffer bouts of cystitis or vaginitis caused by pinworms which enter the urethra or vagina during their nocturnal wanderings, carrying enteric bacteria. Thus, it is worthwhile to perform cellophane tape tests on girls with urinary tract infections. Pinworms have also been found in inflamed appendices. Rare manifestations of migrating pinworms include salpingitis, pelvic granulomas, and intestinal perforation. Syndromes resembling regional enteritis or carcinoma have been reported as resulting from enterobiasis.

DIAGNOSIS. Pinworm ova are usually not found in the stool but may be identified with a cellophane tape test. This test is performed by pressing the gummed side of a piece of cellophane tape to the perianal area, and then sticking the tape to a glass slide. The preparation is then examined microscopically for ova. At least three tests, performed on three different mornings before bathing, are necessary to attain a sensitivity of 90 per cent. On occasion, the worms may be seen if the suspected host's perianal area is inspected during sleep. Eosinophilia is not commonly associated with enterobiasis.

TREATMENT. A single-dose treatment with any of three drugs is effective in enterobiasis: pyrantel pamoate, 11 mg per kilogram (maximum, 1 gram); pyrvinium pamoate, 5 mg per kilogram (maximum, 350 mg); or mebendazole, 100 mg regardless of body weight. Patients should be warned that pyrvinium stains stools red. Mebendazole should be used with caution in children less than two years of age; none of these drugs should be given to pregnant women.

Treatment should be repeated in two weeks. Since this parasite is readily transmitted from person to person, it is best to treat the entire household in which a single case is identified. Treatment should be accompanied by the washing of bedclothes, but further environmental measures, such as the scrubbing of floors and toilet seats, should be discouraged. Parents should be reassured about the relative harmlessness of this infection.

PREVENTION. Residents of institutions should be examined periodically for this and other intestinal parasitoses. However, no effective measures for preventing enterobiasis in the general population have been described.

Sachdev YV, Howards SS: *Enterobius vermicularis* infestation and secondary enuresis. J Urol 113:143, 1975. *Describes several cases of nocturnal enuresis which resolved after treatment of pinworm infections.*

Simon RD: Pinworm infestation and urinary tract infection in young girls. Am J Dis Child 128:21, 1974. Kropp KA, Cichocki GA, Bansal NK: *Enterobius vermicularis* (pinworms), introital bacteriology and recurrent urinary tract infection in children. J Urol 120:480, 1978. *Two papers which provide evidence that pinworms play a role in causing urinary tract infections in girls.*

411. TRICHINELLOSIS (Trichinosis)

Donald W. Hoskins

DEFINITION AND ETIOLOGY. Trichinellosis is an intestinal and tissue nematode disease resulting from the ingestion of inadequately cooked meat containing larvae of *Trichinella spiralis*. The chief sources are pork, pork products, and bear or walrus meat.

The enteral phase of the infection is largely unnoticed. Diffuse tissue invasion by *Trichinella* larvae, the result of the intestinal union of the adult worms, produces the trichinellotic syndrome of muscle pain and tenderness, fever, periorbital edema, and petechiae. The severity of an infection is directly related to the number and strain of *T. spiralis* larvae ingested, the duration of larval production, and poorly defined host factors.

The ingested larvae, resistant to acid-pepsin digestion, penetrate the villi of the small intestine, molt, and develop into mature adults within 48 hours. After fertilization, the gravid female burrows deep into the mucosa, discharging larvae (500 to 1500 per female) beginning 5 to 46 days after infection and continuing for two to four weeks or occasionally longer. Widely disseminated via lymphatics and bloodstream, *Trichinella* larvae (0.1 mm) enter most organs, but persist only in individual skeletal muscle fibers. Increasing almost ten-fold in size (to 1.0 mm) over succeeding weeks, larvae gradually become surrounded by a cyst wall of muscle origin. Although the capsules calcify within six months to two years, the larvae within remain viable for months to years, rarely for decades.

The adult worms are usually expelled from the intestinal tract after the third or fourth week of infection, the result of immunologic mechanisms, including mast cell degranulation and B and T lymphocyte activity.

The definitive hosts of this infection include numerous carnivorous and omnivorous mammals, although the hog remains the single most important source of human infection.

EPIDEMIOLOGY. Approximately 28 million people worldwide are infected with this parasite, close to 75 per cent of whom reside in the United States. The disease is most prevalent in the temperate zones. Most infections are mild and go unrecognized or misdiagnosed. At present, approximately 100 cases are reported annually in the United States; this represents a significant decrease (except for occasional outbreaks—Louisiana, 44 cases 1979–80) from earlier decades.

From 1940 to 1970, autopsy studies of human diaphragm revealed a drop in the prevalence (16.1 to 4.2 per cent) and severity of infection. The current infection rate is 1.6 to 2.2 per cent. This decline is largely attributable to laws prohibiting the feeding of raw garbage to swine. Currently, more than 98.5 per cent of swine in the United States are grain fed, and only 0.1 per cent are infected with *Trichinella;* garbage-fed swine have an infection rate of 0.5 per cent, down from 10 per cent in 1940.

Pork and pork products, especially sausage, account for 75 per cent of all human *Trichinella* infection; nonpork products account for 13 per cent, and in 12 per cent the source is undetermined. Ground beef contaminated by pork (e.g., in the meatgrinder) is a common source of nonpork-induced disease. Bear and walrus meat account for less than 6 per cent of the reported cases of trichinellosis in this country.

PATHOLOGY AND PATHOGENESIS. Microscopic ulceration, mucosal hyperemia, localized edema, punctate hemorrhages, and intestinal inflammation may result from the penetration of the adult *Trichinella* into the mucosa of the small intestine.

The larvae produce basophilic granular alteration of muscle fibers within 48 hours of invasion. The fibers enlarge, and edema, nuclear proliferation, and interstitial inflammation ensue. Later, fatty metamorphosis is followed by atrophy and fibrosis. Larvae may produce a severe myocarditis with focal necrosis and eosinophilic infiltration, but encystment does not occur in cardiac muscle. Eosinophilic infiltration of the endocardium with fibrosis has been reported in fatal trichinellosis. Nonpurulent encephalomeningitis with larvae in the cerebrospinal fluid, choroid, and retina may also occur.

CLINICAL MANIFESTATIONS. The vast majority of persons infected with *T. spiralis* exhibit few or no symptoms. Less than 12 per cent have gastrointestinal symptoms. Heavy infection may produce an acute enteritis (abdominal discomfort, diarrhea) one to two days following ingestion, with systemic symptoms occurring five to seven days later. The usual incubation period is seven to fourteen days, extending to three weeks or more in mild infections.

The onset of the trichinellótic syndrome is often acute with fever, muscle pain and tenderness, weakness, malaise, bilateral periorbital edema, and headache. Subungual, retinal, and subconjunctival petechiae and hemorrhage may be present, and a macular, petechial, or urticarial rash is not uncommon. Within the first two weeks of severe systemic disease, allergic phenomena such as edema, pneumonitis, and pleural transudate may occur.

Mild infection is characterized by fever of less than 38° C and symptoms of less than three weeks' duration; *moderate* infection persists for more than four weeks, and fever is usually greater than 38° C for one to two weeks. *Severe* infection persists for six weeks or more, fever is greater than 39° C for two weeks or more and serum albumin is usually less than 2.5 grams per deciliter.

Serious complications, including myocarditis, pneumonitis, and meningoencephalitis, occur most often in the third to ninth week of the disease. Mortality is less than 1.5 per cent and is almost always related to complications.

DIAGNOSIS AND DIFFERENTIAL DIAGNOSIS. Once considered, the diagnosis is not difficult. The trichinellotic syndrome coupled with marked peripheral blood eosinophilia (20 to 70 per cent), elevation of muscle enzymes (CPK, LDH, aldolase, and transaminases), and normal sedimentation rate should strongly suggest the diagnosis. Finding encysted larvae in any remaining suspected food source would be additional evidence.

Confirmation of the diagnosis is often accomplished by serologic testing, skin test, or muscle biopsy. Serologic testing is simple, highly sensitive, and specific. Antibodies are not detected, however, until three weeks or more after the onset of infection. Available tests include rapid screening counterimmunoelectrophoresis (CIE) and enzyme-linked immunosorbent assay (ELISA), passive hemagglutination (PHA), and indirect immunofluorescence (IF). The bentonite flocculation test is the most widely used; a titer of one to five or greater is considered positive, although a four-fold rise in the titer is more convincing. False positives do occur; 13.5 per cent of typhoid-paratyphoid sera may react positively. Two independent methods are often required to establish serodiagnosis of trichinellosis. Skin testing does not distinguish between past and present infection and therefore does not prove active disease.

Muscle biopsy may be positive as early as the second week of infection but is often not required. A small amount of muscle is excised under local anesthesia from a tender, painful, swollen muscle, a portion sent for routine pathologic examination, and a small amount crushed between glass slides and examined directly under a scanning or low power objective for motile larvae. Pepsin–hydrochloric acid digestion of 1.0 gram of muscle may also be performed and larvae sought microscopically.

The differential diagnosis in a disease with multisystem involvement is extensive. Common misdiagnoses include viral syndromes (influenza, gastroenteritis, various exanthems), collagen disease (periarteritis, dermatomyositis), sepsis (typhoid, pneumonitis, meningitis), allergic phenomena, and polymyositis.

TREATMENT. Rarely, infection with *T. spiralis* is suspected within hours or days of ingestion of infected meat. Treatment of the immature worms in the small intestine is usually successful and will abort or markedly inhibit systemic disease. Furthermore, given the relationship of the severity of infection to continued larval production by the adult female *T. spiralis* and the unknown duration of its fecundity, treatment of the intestinal phase in all cases up to six weeks after infection is advisable. Thiabendazole (Mintezol) 25 mg per kilogram twice daily (maximum 3.0 grams per day) for one week has been replaced by another benzimidazole, mebendazole (Vermox) 200 mg daily for four days, largely for improved patient tolerance. Alternatively, pyrantel pamoate (Antiminth) 10 mg per kilogram (maximum 1.0 gram per day) for four days has been used with similar results. Although none of these drugs is advocated during pregnancy, mebendazole is specifically contraindicated.

Mild to moderate systemic infection is treated with rest and analgesics; recovery may take weeks and complications are rare. All patients must be carefully observed, especially in the first two weeks following onset of systemic symptoms, for progression to a more acute and severe form of trichinellosis.

Acute severe trichinellosis will require corticosteroids in high doses (prednisone, 60 mg daily) for two or more weeks, primarily for inhibition of host response. Since the enteral phase of *T. spiralis* may be prolonged (and larval production extended) with the use of corticosteroids, the concomitant administration of a benzimidazole (mebendazole, 5 mg per kilogram daily for five to ten days) is advisable. The benzimidazoles (thiabendazole, mebendazole) have been used singly in the treatment of moderate to severe trichinellosis with improvement in well-being and defervescence of fever; the analgesic and anti-inflammatory properties of the drugs may account for the improvement seen rather than any tissue larvicidal properties in man. The risk of a hypersensitivity (Jarisch-Herxheimer) reaction on day three or four of treatment with benzimidazole therapy favors the combined corticosteroid-benzimidazole regimen in acute severe trichinellosis. Adverse effects of the benzimidazoles include headache, nausea, vomiting, dizziness, rash, and agitation.

PREVENTION. Thorough cooking of infected meat kills larvae; a temperature of 58.3° C throughout the meat is adequate. Freezing meat at −32° C for 24 hours or at −15° C (home freezer) for three weeks is also effective. Government inspection of meat in the United States does not exclude *Trichinella* infection, nor does the smoking, salting, or drying of meat.

The application of an enzyme-linked immunosorbent assay (ELISA) for the detection of antibody to *T. spiralis* in pooled hog sera at slaughter may be practical in the detection of infected sources.

Campbell WC (ed.): *Trichinella* and Trichinosis. New York, Plenum Press, 1983. *An expensive but highly valuable update on all aspects of parasite and pathogen. The practicing physician will especially appreciate the chapters on chemotherapy, clinical aspects, and immunodiagnosis. Extensively referenced work.*

Kim CW, Pawlowski ZS (eds.): Proceedings of the Fourth International Conference on Trichinellosis. University Press of New England, 1978. *This volume is strong in the clinical, pathologic, and therapeutic areas. Report of a symposium in Poland in 1976.*

Most H: Current concepts in parasitology. Trichinosis—preventable yet still with us. N Engl J Med 298:1178, 1978.

412. ANGIOSTRONGYLIASIS

Daniel S. Blumenthal

The larvae of two rodent parasites, *Angiostrongylus cantonensis* and *A. costaricensis*, may infect man. The pathology and clinical findings caused by the two species are quite different. The genus is also known as *Morerastrongylus*.

ANGIOSTRONGYLUS CANTONENSIS. Eosinophilic meningitis caused by larvae of the rat lungworm occurs in southeast Asia and many Pacific islands. The first cases in the Western Hemisphere were reported in 1981 from Cuba.

Humans are infected by ingesting, in an uncooked state, the snails, slugs, and crustaceans that serve as intermediate hosts. The infective larvae migrate to the capillaries of the meninges, where they cause an eosinophilic inflammatory response with granuloma formation. Clinically, there are signs of meningeal irritation, and there may be localizing neurologic findings, including paresthesias and cranial nerve palsies. There is a peripheral and cerebrospinal fluid eosinophilia. The eosinophilic meningitis of angiostrongyliasis must be differentiated from that caused by gnathostomiasis, cysticercosis, and other parasitoses. Most cases resolve uneventfully, but some result in permanent sequelae or death. There are no specific diagnostic tests available. Thiabendazole has been given for this infection, but there is no convincing evidence that it is effective. Steroids may control symptoms.

ANGIOSTRONGYLUS COSTARICENSIS. Human larval infection with this species has been reported in children in Central America, Mexico, and Venezuela. Adult *A. costaricensis* live in the mesenteric arteries of rats and other rodents; a slug serves as intermediate host. Larvae are shed in the slime of the slug, and children may become infected by handling slugs and then putting their hands in their mouths. Vegetables on which slugs have crawled may also be infective. Once ingested, the larvae travel to the mesenteric arterioles, where they cause edema of the wall of the cecum, appendix, and ascending colon. Yellow granulations of the subserosa and eosinophilic infiltrates are common pathologic findings. There may be ulcerations, peritonitis, and fistula formation. The clinical picture is similar to that of acute appendicitis, with fever and right lower quadrant pain and tenderness. A tumor-like mass may often be palpated in the right lower quadrant. There is usually marked eosinophilia. Contrast studies of the gastrointestinal tract may show abnormalities of the cecum, ascending colon, and terminal ileum. The diagnosis is usually established at surgery. If surgery is not required, thiabendazole may be tried, but its efficacy is in doubt.

Prevention of both types of infection is dependent on education and rodent control.

Chin-Yun Y: Clinical observations on eosinophilic meningitis and meningoencephalitis caused by angiostrongylus cantonensis on Taiwan. Am J Trop Med Hyg 25:233, 1976. *A series of 125 cases of this infection, including four deaths and three with permanent sequelae.*

Loria-Cortes R, Lobo-Sanahuja JF: Clinical abdominal angiostrongylosis. Am J Trop Med Hyg 29:538, 1980. *The largest series of* A. costaricensis *infection to date (116 children), with clinical and epidemiologic findings.*

Filariasis

413. INTRODUCTION

Eric A. Ottesen

Eight filarial parasites commonly infect humans (Table 413–1), but three are responsible for most of the pathology associated with these infections. There are the lymphatic dwelling filariae *Wuchereria bancrofti* and *Brugia malayi* and the subcutaneous filarid *Onchocerca volvulus*.

All eight species are transmitted by biting arthropods (Table 413–1) and go through complex life cycles that include a slow maturation phase of 3 to 18 months from the time infective larvae are introduced by the vector until the adult worms mature and reside in the lymph nodes, subcutaneous tissue, or body cavities. The offspring of these adults (microfilariae) are 200 to 250 μm long and 5 to 7 μm wide. They either circulate in the blood or migrate through the skin, awaiting ingestion by the appropriate arthropod in which they develop over one to two weeks to infective forms capable of initiating this life cycle again. Adult worms are long lived (probably 8 to 15 years), while microfilariae probably live about 6 months. Patent infection is generally not established unless exposure to infective larvae is intense and prolonged, and manifestations of disease usually develop slowly.

Diagnosis can be extremely difficult because it relies almost exclusively on parasitologic techniques to demonstrate microfilariae in the blood or tissue. At present, there are no completely satisfactory methods for making a definitive diagnosis in states of "amicrofilaremic filariasis" (before or after the microfilaremic state). When microfilariae circulate in the blood, they do so with or without a distinct periodicity (Table 413–1). Some are garbed in sheaths while others are sheathless. These two features, as well as other more subtle morphologic distinctions, are helpful diagnostically. Microfilariae can be identified either by direct observation of Giemsa-stained blood smears or, more sensitively, by concentration techniques using Knott's method (examination of centrifuged sediment after mixing 1 ml of blood with 9 ml of 2 per cent formalin) or membrane filtration of one or more ml of blood through a 3 μm- or 5 μm-pore Nucleopore membrane filter. Skin microfilariae are best sought by performing skin snips either as described in Ch. 422 or using a corneal-scleral (Holth) biopsy punch. Antibody detection, although helpful in certain situations, is generally nondiagnostic because it cannot differentiate current from past infection or exposure and because of antigenic cross reactivity between the filariae and other helminth parasites.

Diethylcarbamazine (DEC)* has been the single mainstay of treatment for all filarial infections since the late 1940's; however, it shows variable effectiveness for the different conditions. Suramin,† although extremely toxic, is also used for onchocerciasis. While little advance in the chemotherapy of these diseases has been made until recently, current prospects for more effective, less toxic drugs for filarial infection appear hopeful.

*Not commercially available in the United States but may be obtained in special circumstances from Lederle Laboratories.

†Available from the Centers for Disease Control, Parasitic Disease Drug Service, Atlanta, GA.

Hawking F: Diethylcarbamazine and new compounds for the treatment of filariasis. Adv Pharm Chemother 16:129, 1979. *A complete account of the most important drugs currently used to treat filarial infections.*

Ottesen EA: Filariasis and tropical eosinophilia. *In* Warren KS and Mahmond AA

TABLE 413–1. THE COMMON FILARIAL PARASITES OF MAN

				Microfilariae		
Species	**Distribution**	**Vector**	**Primary Pathology**	*Primary Location*	*Periodicity*	*Presence of Sheath*
Wuchereria bancrofti	Tropics worldwide	Mosquitoes	Lymphatic, pulmonary	Blood, hydrocele fluid	Nocturnal, subperiodic	+
Brugia malayi	Southeast Asia	Mosquitoes	Lymphatic, pulmonary	Blood	Nocturnal, subperiodic	+
Brugia timori	Indonesia	Mosquitoes	Lymphatic	Blood	Nocturnal	+
Onchocerca volvulus	Africa; Central and South America	Black fly	Skin, eye, lymphatic	Skin	None or minimal	–
Loa loa	Africa	Horse fly	Allergic	Blood	Diurnal	+
Mansonella perstans	Africa; South America	Midge	? Allergic	Blood	None	–
Mansonella streptocerca	Africa	Midge	Dermal	Skin	None	–
Mansonella ozzardi	Central and South America	Midge	Vague	Blood	None	–

(eds.): Tropical and Geographical Medicine. McGraw-Hill Book Co., 1983, pp 390–412. *Detailed clinical, parasitologic and epidemiologic discussions of filarial diseases.*

Sasa M: Human Filariasis. Baltimore, University Park Press, 1976, pp 819. *A book giving a global view of the epidemiology of filariasis.*

414. DRACUNCULIASIS

Donald R. Hopkins

Dracunculiasis, or guinea worm disease, is caused by infection with the parasite *Dracunculus medinensis.* It occurs mainly in the Indian subcontinent and West Africa, where up to about 10 million persons living in rural areas are thought to be affected.

Diagnosis of patent infections is easy. The thin white female worms, each up to 1 meter long, emerge directly through the skin, usually of the lower leg, ankle, or foot. The adult worms emerge 10 to 14 months after victims have drunk water containing infected *Cyclops,* a barely visible crustacean that serves as the parasite's intermediate host. When persons harboring such emerging worms enter a stagnant source of drinking water such as a step well or pond, larvae are released into the water. Some such larvae are ingested by *Cyclops,* where they undergo two molts before becoming infective to humans. When humans drink water containing *Cyclops* with infective larvae, the larvae penetrate the intestinal or stomach wall, mature, and mate, after which the male worms die.

The adult female worms emerge very slowly, over a period of weeks or months. Emergence may be preceded by generalized allergic symptoms and is usually accompanied by a burning sensation, then a blister that ruptures to form an ulcer at the site of emergence. Some worms present first as a serpentine cord just beneath the skin or at the center of an abscess. No immunity develops, so persons in endemic areas are infected year after year.

The great social and economic significance of dracunculiasis, which rarely is fatal, derives from the fact that emergence of the worm is very painful and is often associated with swelling, local arthritis, and secondary infection. Thus, victims are often unable to farm or sometimes even walk for weeks or months. Over half of the adults in a village may be crippled at the same time, and because the infection tends to be seasonal, these effects appear precisely when villagers need to harvest or plant their crops. School attendance is also affected.

Treatment is difficult because anthelmintics such as thiabendazole or metronidazole only marginally reduce the duration of emergence and associated pain. Aspirin can help relieve the pain. Emerging worms are best rolled around a small stick as their predecessors have been for centuries, care being taken not to break the worm (which would exacerbate the inflammation). Some worms can be removed surgically. Victims should be immunized against tetanus, which is an all too frequent complication caused by secondary infection of the ulcer around the emerging worm. Persons at risk should be taught to boil their drinking water or filter it through a piece of cloth, and to avoid entering sources of drinking water when the infection is patent.

Since the most effective intervention against this infection is to provide safe sources of drinking water, efforts are under way to take advantage of the International Drinking Water Supply and Sanitation Decade (1981–1990) to provide safe water to dracunculiasis-endemic areas as a priority, and thereby control or eliminate the disease.

Hopkins DR: Dracunculiasis: An eradicable scourge. *In* Epidemiologic Reviews. Vol 5. Baltimore, The Johns Hopkins School of Hygiene and Public Health, 1983, pp 208–219. *A recent review of all aspects pertaining to control and eradication of dracunculariasis.*

Muller R: *Dracunculus* and dracunculiasis. *In* Dawes B (ed.): Advances in Parasitology. Vol 9. New York, Academic Press, 1971, pp 73–151. *A thorough consideration of the parasite's biology, life cycle, and the disease it produces.*

415. LYMPHATIC FILARIASIS (Wuchereria bancrofti, Brugia malayi, and Brugia timori)

Eric A. Ottesen

ETIOLOGY. There are three lymphatic-dwelling filarial parasites of man, *Wuchereria bancrofti, Brugia malayi,* and *Brugia timori.* Adult worms are thread-like in form (2 to 10 cm long by less than 0.4 mm wide) and usually reside in the lymph nodes or afferent lymphatic channels. The female worms produce large numbers of microfilariae (175 to 300 μ long), which circulate in the peripheral blood awaiting ingestion by mosquito intermediate hosts, which are necessary to continue the parasite's life cycle. After about two weeks in these mosquitoes, the microfilariae develop into infective third stage larvae (L_3's). When infected mosquitoes feed, these L_3's leave the mosquito mouth parts and come to rest on the surface of the host's skin. If they then manage to penetrate the skin through the puncture wound at the site of the bite, transmission is successful; after a further developmental period lasting as long as 4 to 12 months, adult worms can again be found in the lymphatic tissues, where they mate and produce another generation of microfilariae. The adult parasites may remain viable in the human host for decades.

EPIDEMIOLOGY. For *W. bancrofti* man is the only definitive host and, thus, the natural reservoir for infection. Indeed, considerable experimental effort to establish the parasite in a wide variety of potential mammalian hosts has met with little success. *W. bancrofti* is found throughout the tropics and subtropics, including areas of South America and the Caribbean, Africa, Asia, and the Pacific. Two forms of the parasite are distinguished by the periodicity of their circulating microfilariae. Nocturnally periodic forms have microfilariae detectable in peripheral blood primarily at night, whereas in the subperiodic forms the microfilariae are usually present in the blood at all hours but with maximal levels often in the late afternoon. Generally, subperiodic bancroftian filariasis is found only in the Pacific islands east of 160° E longitude (including New Caledonia, Fiji, Samoa, Ellis and Cook Islands, Society Islands, and the Marquesas); elsewhere *W. bancrofti* is nocturnally periodic. The natural vectors are *Culex fatigans* in urban settings and usually anopheline or aedean mosquitoes in rural areas.

The distribution of brugian filariasis is much more restricted, being limited primarily to Malaysia, Indonesia, India, China, Korea, the Philippines, and Japan. Again, there are both nocturnally periodic and subperiodic forms of the parasite. The former is more common and is transmitted in coastal rice fields primarily by mansonian and anopheline mosquitoes; mansonian mosquitoes, found in swamp forests, are the major vectors of the subperiodic form. Unlike *W. bancrofti, B. malayi* can be a natural infection of cats and can be established in a number of laboratory animals. *B. timori* has been described only from two Indonesian islands.

PATHOLOGY. Most of the pathology of bancroftian and brugian filariasis is initiated in the lymphatics. Although details of the pathogenesis are lacking, the progression of pathologic changes is clear. Damaged lymphatics lead first to reversible lymphedema and then to chronic obstructive changes (elephantiasis) in the limbs, breasts, or genitalia, or to chyluria. The location of lymphatic damage determines the site and type of pathology expressed.

Adult worms, residing in the afferent approaches or cortical sinuses of the lymph nodes, incite local inflammatory reactions by undefined (probably immunologic) mechanisms. These reactions result in dilatation of the lymphatics and hypertrophy of the vessel walls. Endothelial and connective tissue proliferation leads to polypoid growths that protrude into the lymphatic lumen; but so long as the worm remains alive, the vessel appears to stay patent. Patency, however, does not assure normal lymphatic function, as lymphangiographic studies have clearly documented the development of a characteristic tortuosity of the lymph vessels with loss of valvular function and backflow of lymph leading to lymph stasis and lymphedema even during this "preobliterative phase."

Death of adult worms is accompanied by local necrosis and granulomatous reaction around the parasite with infiltration of plasma cells, eosinophils, and giant cells. Fibrosis occurs and the fragmented parasites are either completely resorbed or partially calcified. Lymphatic obstruction develops and associated endophlebitis may further complicate the lymphatic obstruction. Although there is subsequent formation of collateral lymphatics and some recanalization of obstructed vessels, lymphatic function remains compromised. Repeated infection with increasing host response to the parasite leads to the chronic changes of advanced elephantiasis.

CLINICAL MANIFESTATIONS. The three most common clinical presentations of the lymphatic filariases are asymptomatic microfilaremia, "filarial fever," and lymphatic obstruction. A fourth presentation, the tropical eosinophilia syndrome, is considered in Ch. 416.

Patients with asymptomatic microfilaremia rarely come to the physician's attention except through an incidental finding of microfilariae in the peripheral blood smear during mass surveys in endemic regions, or when blood eosinophilia leads to a diagnostic evaluation for filariasis. Such asymptomatic persons appear to be clinically unaffected by the parasites. It is likely that in some of these individuals the infections clear spontaneously, whereas the infections of others subsequently progress and become symptomatic, but what determines such clinical changes is unclear.

"Filarial fevers" are acute febrile episodes characterized by high fever (often with shaking chills), lymphatic inflammation (i.e., lymphadenitis and lymphangitis), and transient local edema. They occur as often as six to ten times per year in affected persons and usually last three to seven days before subsiding spontaneously. The factors that initiate these episodes are unknown, but they are definitely parasite related. The lymphangitis characteristically develops in a retrograde fashion, extending peripherally *from* the draining node where the adult parasites reside. Regional nodes are enlarged and painful, and the entire lymphatic tract often becomes indurated and inflamed. Concomitant local thrombophlebitis is common. In brugian filariasis especially, a single local abscess may form along the inflamed lymphatic and subsequently rupture to the surface, leaving a characteristic scar whose presence has been used epidemiologically as an indication of the clinical "activity" of filarial infection in *Brugia* endemic regions. Neither the lymphatic inflammation nor the characteristic abscesses appear to be bacterially induced. Such lymphadenitis and lymphangitis occur in the upper and lower extremities with both bancroftian and brugian filariasis, but involvement of the genital lymphatics is almost exclusively a feature of *W. bancrofti* infection. Thus, acute *bancrofti* episodes may also involve funiculitis, epididymitis, scrotal pain, and tenderness. Patients with filarial fevers may be microfilaremic but more often are not.

As lymphatic damage progresses, the edema and anatomic distortion that were initially transient develop into the permanent changes of elephantiasis. Pitting edema yields to brawny edema, and there is both thickening of subcutaneous tissue and hyperkeratosis. Fissuring of the skin develops along with nodular and papillomatous hyperplastic changes. Superinfection of these poorly vascularized tissues becomes a problem. In addition, in bancroftian filariasis, obstructed genital lymphatics may lead to scrotal lymphedema or hydrocele, whereas obstruction of the retroperitoneal lymphatics can increase hydrostatic pressure in the renal lymphatics, causing their rupture into the renal pelvis or tubules and leading to chyluria. Characteristically chyluria is intermittent, sometimes lasting for days or weeks before abating spontaneously and then recurring; often it is most prominent in the morning after the patient first arises.

DIAGNOSIS. Definitive diagnosis of filariasis can be made only by the demonstration of parasites, either adult worms associated with the lymphatics (rarely observed) or microfilariae in the blood, hydrocele fluid, or chylous urine. These fluids can be examined directly (20 cu mm on a slide with or without red blood cell lysis), after concentration of the parasites by centifugation in 2 per cent formalin (Knott's technique), or after filtration through a membrane (3- to 5-μm Nuclepore) filter. The time of blood collection should take into account the parasite's possible nocturnal periodicity.

Because many persons with filariasis (especially those with chronic pathology) are not microfilaremic, diagnosis must often be made clinically. The differential diagnosis is broad but in the acute episodes primarily includes thrombophlebitis, infection, and trauma. The edema and other lymphatic obstructive changes associated with chronic filariasis must be distinguished from the manifestations of congestive heart failure, malignancy, trauma, postsurgical scarring, and a number of less common congenital and idiopathic abnormalities of the lymphatic system. The many disorders associated with serum IgE and blood eosinophil elevations must be considered in evaluating asymptomatic filarial infections. Several specific points may help in this differential diagnosis: (1) Exposure to filariae must be prolonged or intense (for at least several months) before persons become infected; (2) the physical finding or history of *retrograde* lymphangitis can often aid in distinguishing filarial from bacterial lymphangitis; (3) although lymphadenopathy is characteristic of filariasis, alone it is never diagnostic; (4) lymphangiographic patterns of elephantiasis and chyluria are well defined so that, even though not always diagnostic, lymphangiography is sometimes useful in distinguishing filarial from congenital or neoplastic lymphatic abnormalities; (5) although total serum IgE and blood eosinophil levels are elevated in all filarial infections, they cannot distinguish filarial from other helminth infections except in the case of the tropical eosinophilia syndrome (see Ch. 416); and (6) because most residents of endemic regions have been immunologically "sensitized" to filarial antigens through years of bites by infected mosquitoes and because filarial antigens cross-react extensively with those of other nematode parasites, positive results in the numerous serologic and skin tests that have been developed are of little diagnostic value *except* in those who are not native to endemic areas.

TREATMENT. Available chemotherapy for lymphatic filariasis is both limited and inadequate. Diethylcarbamazine* (DEC, 5 mg per kilogram per day given in single or divided doses for two to three weeks) rapidly kills microfilariae in vivo, but its effect on adult parasites is not so clearly defined. Thus, following treatment with DEC, although the blood is temporarily free of microfilariae, the infection itself has often not been terminated, and several courses of DEC or long-term intermittent treatment with low doses of DEC are often required to kill the adult parasites. There are no other clinically useful drugs available for eradicating the infection.

Side effects of DEC treatment, although not so frequent or severe as those seen in onchocerciasis, can be troublesome, especially in brugian filariasis. These include fever, chills, headache, dizziness, nausea, vomiting, and arthralgias, all usually occurring in the first 24 to 36 hours. Both the likelihood of developing such reactions and the degree of their severity are directly related to the number of circulating microfilariae. Thus, the side effects of DEC administration at these dosage levels are due not to direct drug toxicity but to allergic or immunologic responses of the host to dying parasites. To avoid these reactions in highly parasitemic persons, one can initiate treatment with very small doses of DEC or premedicate the patients with steroids, as suggested for onchocerciasis (see Ch. 422). A very few patients may also develop filarial fever episodes with lymphangitis and lymphadenitis in the first days after DEC treatment. All of these side effects occur early in

*Production of this drug has been discontinued in the United States.

treatment and generally subside even with continued administration of the drug.

The results of severe chronic lymphatic damage generally are not reversible, but long-term low dose DEC has been shown to reverse early lymphedematous changes and careful attention to the management of lymphedema can minimize the development of further damage. Limb elevation, elastic stockings, and perhaps even diuretics are important, as well as local foot care to prevent damaging bacterial and fungal infection in these already compromised tissues. In the most extreme cases, surgical excision of redundant tissue can be performed. Hydroceles can be repeatedly drained or managed surgically. Chyluria also can sometimes be corrected surgically, but, interestingly, many cases have been reported in which diagnostic lymphangiography itself appears to have terminated the leak of chyle into the urine, probably as a result of its sclerosing effects.

PREVENTION. Because DEC kills developing preadult forms of many filarial species, it is used in veterinary practice as a prophylactic agent to prevent filarial infection of dogs. Its potential for prophylaxis in man, however, has not been evaluated. In public health programs DEC has been used successfully as a protective measure to reduce infection rates in selected populations. Because of its microfilaricidal effects, small doses administered intermittently to all residents of an endemic region (e.g., 3 mg per kilogram monthly) reduce the number of blood-borne microfilariae in the community to levels so low that successful transmission of the infection by mosquitoes cannot occur. Other approaches to filariasis control designed to eradicate the mosquito vectors have also proved effective.

Gooneratne BWN: Lymphangiography—Clinical and Experimental. London, Butterworths, 1974. *General description of lymphangiographic techniques, edited by a physician with great personal experience in the lymphangiography of filarial lymphatic obstruction. Three chapters are devoted exclusively to the lymphatic lesions seen in filariasis.*

Hawking F: Diethylcarbamazine and new compounds for the treatment of filariasis. Adv Pharmacol Chemother 16:129, 1979. *A thorough review of the pharmacology and clinical effects of the major chemotherapeutic agent used for treating filariasis. An evaluation of alternative drugs is also given.*

Ottesen EA: Immunopathology of lymphatic filariasis in man. Springer Semin Immunopathol 2:373, 1980. *Reviews the major immunologic findings in lymphatic filariasis and attempts to relate these findings to the pathogenesis of the various clinical syndromes associated with the infection.*

Sasa M: Human Filariasis: A Global Survey of Epidemiology and Control. Baltimore, University Park Press, 1976. *A fine compendium of epidemiologic observations, taxonomic detail, and host, parasite, and vector interactions. Techniques for detection of microfilariae in clinical specimens are described in detail.*

416. TROPICAL EOSINOPHILIA

Eric A. Ottesen

Tropical eosinophilia is a syndrome of acute and chronic lung disease first defined in the 1940's but not generally recognized as being of filarial etiology until the 1960's. Its main clinical features are a history of residence in a filaria-endemic region; paroxysmal cough and wheezing, which generally occur at night; scanty sputum production; occasional weight loss, low-grade fever, and adenopathy; and extreme blood eosinophilia (>3000 per microliter). It appears to be more common in Indians than in persons of other nationalities and more common in men than in women. Chest x-rays can be normal but generally show increased bronchovascular markings, diffuse miliary lesions, or mottled opacities primarily involving the mid and lower lung fields. Tests of pulmonary function almost always indicate restrictive abnormalities and often show obstructive defects as well. The association of the syndrome with filarial infection was first recognized by finding very high levels of antifilarial antibody in these patients and by noting the favorable response to treatment with antifilarial drugs (now diethylcarbamazine [DEC]* in doses of 5 to 6 mg per kilogram per day for two to three weeks). Later, several reports described microfilariae or their degenerating remnants in lung biopsy specimens. Most recently, extremely high levels of total serum IgE (usually 10,000 to 100,000 ng per milliliter) have been found in these patients, and an appreciable fraction of this IgE has been shown to be directed against filarial antigens.

*Production of this drug has been discontinued in the United States.

Because of these and other findings, tropical eosinophilia is now considered to be a form of "occult filariasis" in which host immunologic hyperresponsiveness to the parasite results in such rapid clearance of microfilariae from the blood that this stage of the parasite is essentially never detectable. Generally this microfilarial clearance takes place in the lungs, and the clinical symptoms appear to result largely from the allergic and inflammatory reactions elicited by the cleared parasites. In some subjects, however, trapping of the microfilariae occurs predominantly in other organs of the reticuloendothelial system (liver, spleen, lymph nodes), and in these persons the major clinical manifestations are those resulting from hepatomegaly, splenomegaly, or lymphadenopathy. It has been postulated that infection with nonhuman filarial parasites is the major cause of tropical eosinophilia. More likely, however, the syndrome is caused not by an "abnormal parasite" but rather by an abnormal host response to those same parasites (*Wuchereria bancrofti* and *Brugia malayi*) that commonly cause lymphatic filariasis (see Ch. 415). In this respect, tropical eosinophilia is likely quite similar to another pulmonary eosinophilic disorder, allergic bronchopulmonary aspergillosis, both in its clinical expression and in its pathogenesis (see Ch. 373).

Diagnosis depends primarily on distinguishing tropical eosinophilia from the other important eosinophilic syndromes with pulmonary involvement, namely, Löffler's syndrome, chronic eosinophilic pneumonia, allergic aspergillosis, certain vasculitic syndromes, the idiopathic hypereosinophilia syndrome, drug allergies, and some helminth infections. Although there is no one clinical or laboratory criterion that will distinguish tropical eosinophilia from these other conditions, a history of residence in the tropics along with the presence of specific filarial antibodies and the response to DEC therapy are the most helpful differential points. Within three to seven days following administration of DEC, there is almost always marked improvement or disappearance of symptoms. Relapse may occur, however, months to years later and require retreatment. DEC will not, of course, reverse permanent pulmonary damage (primarily an interstitial fibrosis), which frequently develops prior to successful diagnosis and treatment of the disorder.

Neva FA, Ottesen EA: Tropical (filarial) eosinophilia. N Engl J Med 298:1129, 1978. *Concise review of historical, clinical, and pathogenetic aspects of the tropical eosinophilia syndrome.*

Udwadia FE: Pulmonary Eosinophilia. Progress in Respiration Research, Vol 7. Basel, S Karger, 1975. *Extensive review of tropical eosinophilia by a physician operating a chest clinic in Bombay, India, who has followed and studied over 450 patients with this disease. Rich in clinical detail and perspective.*

417. LOIASIS

Eric A. Ottesen

Loa loa is indigenous only to the rain forest belt of western and central Africa. Mature female parasites, about twice the size of the males, are 50 to 70 mm long and 0.5 mm wide. They live wandering through the subcutaneous tissue in humans, usually attracting attention only when they cross the eye subconjunctivally. The sheathed microfilariae produced by these females circulate with a diurnal periodicity that peaks about noon.

Clinical loiasis presents in two primary forms, one more common among individuals native to endemic regions and the other more common in visitors to these areas who acquire infection. Among the natives loiasis is often entirely asymptomatic until an adult worm appears moving across the eye or blood examination reveals microfilaremia. Such individuals may also have occasional episodes of "Calabar swellings." These are characteristic localized areas of erythema and angioedema (up to 5 to 10 cm in diameter) that occur primarily on the extremities and last one to three days before regressing spontaneously. These swellings appear to be a hypersensitivity reaction to the adult worm, whose presence can also be detected in some patients by either a subcutaneous crawling sensation or the appearance of a fine vermiform hive in the skin. When the inflammation extends to nearby joints or peripheral nerves, corresponding symptoms may develop. Rarely, nephropathy (probably immune complex mediated) and encephalopathy have been reported.

The major difference between this presentation and that seen in outsiders who acquire infection is the greater predominance of allergic or hyper-reactive symptoms in the latter. Episodes of angioedema are likely to be more frequent and debilitating, and patients are much less likely to have microfilariae in the blood. In addition, they often present with extensive blood eosinophilia (30 to 60 per cent of an elevated total leukocyte count) much like patients with tropical eosinophilia (Ch. 416). Diagnosis in these patients often cannot be made parasitologically and must be based on the characteristic history, clinical presentation, blood eosinophilia, and elevated filarial antibody titers. If untreated, a small (but undefined) percentage of such patients develops severe cardiomyopathy presumably secondary to the hypereosinophilia elicited by the infection.

Treatment is with diethylcarbamazine (DEC)* (6 to 10 mg per kilogram per day) for two to three weeks. The drug is extremely effective against microfilariae but less so against adult worms, so that multiple courses of treatment are often necessary before there is complete resolution of signs and symptoms. In cases of heavy microfilaremia (greater than several hundred microfilariae per ml of blood) allergic and other inflammatory side effects of treatment may be so severe that a regimen of 0.5–1 mg per kilogram DEC per dose (with or without simultaneous steroids) is safer for initiating treatment. Some evidence exists that DEC is effective in preventing loiasis when taken in doses of 5 mg kilogram per day for three days each month, but large trials of this prophylactic regimen have yet to be carried out.

Brockington IF, Olsen EGJ, Goodwin JF: Endomyocardial fibrosis in European residents in tropical Africa. Lancet i:583, 1967. *Description of the cardiomyopathy believed to result from the hypereosinophilia induced in some patients by loiasis.*

Duke BOL: Studies on the chemoprophylaxis of loiasis. II. Observations on diethylcarbamazine citrate (Banocide) as a prophylactic in man. Ann Trop Med Parasitol 57:82, 1963. *The only published experience on the potential chemoprophylactic effects of diethylcarbamazine in human loiasis.*

418. *MANSONELLA OZZARDI* INFECTION

Eric A. Ottesen

M. ozzardi is restricted in distribution to Central and South America and certain islands of the Caribbean. Adult worms have been recovered in humans only twice, both times from the peritoneal cavity. *Unsheated* microfilariae circulate in the blood with little or no periodicity.

Many investigators consider these parasites to be non pathogenic, but in one of the fullest clinical studies of an affected population it was asserted that the major clinical presentation is severe articular pain or dysfunction, especially in the arms and shoulders. Headache, fever, pulmonary symptoms, adenopathy, hepatomegaly, and pruritic skin eruptions also occurred in a small number of patients with a frequency greater than that in nonparasitized individuals in the same population. Diethylcarbamazine* has little or no effect on this infection.

Marinkelle CJ, German E: Mansonelliasis in the comisaria del Vaupes of Columbia. Trop Geogr Med 22:101, 1970. *A very complete and interesting account of clinical manifestations ascribed to* M. ozzardi *infections in South American Indians.*

Weller PF, Simon HB, Parkhurst BH, Medrek FF: Tourism acquired *Mansonella ozzardi* microfilaremia in a regular blood donor. JAMA 240:858, 1978. *Evidence for the ineffectiveness of diethylcarbamazine in* M. ozzardi *infections.*

419. PERSTANS FILARIASIS

Eric A. Ottesen

Mansonella perstans (formerly *Dipetalonema perstans*, *Acanthocheilonema perstans*) is distributed in a broad belt across the center of Africa and in northeast South America. Adult worms, up to 70 to 80 mm long, reside in the body cavities (pleural, peritoneal, and pericardial) and in the mesentery, perirenal, and retroperitoneal tissues. Microfilariae are liberated *unsheathed* from the females and circulate in the blood without regular periodicity.

M. perstans infection was long thought to be asymptomatic, because up to 90 per cent of individuals with the parasite appeared to have no difficulty with it. Subsequent studies, however, indicate clearly that *M. perstans* is capable of inducing a variety of symptoms including angioedematous swellings much like the Calabar swellings of loiasis; fever; headache; pain in bursae and/or joint synovia, in serous cavities, or over the liver; neurologic or psychologic symptoms, and extreme exhaustion. There is some evidence that symptoms are more prominent in "outsiders" coming to endemic regions, but in all series at least a quarter of the patients were asymptomatic despite persistent microfilaremia.

Treatment with diethylcarbamazine* (5-6 mg per kilogram per day for two to three weeks) is often ineffective, with multiple courses usually necessary to achieve cure. When the parasites are eliminated, however, patients characteristically lose their symptoms (no matter how vague), lose their eosinophilia, and regain a sense of well-being.

Adolph PE, Kagan IG, McQuay RM: Diagnosis and treatment of *Acanthocheilonema perstans* filariasis. Am J Trop Med Hyg 11:76, 1962. *Results from a series of patients evaluated in the United States after returning from doing missionary work in Africa.*

Clarke V deV, Harwin RM, MacDonald DF, Green CA, Rittey DAW: Filariasis: *Dipetalonemia perstans* infections in Rhodesia. Cent Afr J Med 17:1, 1971. *Discussion of the clinical expression of* M. perstans *filariasis in Africans and Europeans living in East Africa.*

420. DIROFILARIASIS

Eric A. Ottesen

Dirofilaria species are filarial parasites mostly of dogs, cats, and raccoons that sometimes infect man but almost never fully develop to complete their life cycles in this abnormal host. The distribution of cases is worldwide and reflects the distribution of the parasites in animals.

Two general types of clinical presentation predominate. Pulmonary dirofilariasis, caused by the dog heartworm *D. imitis*, usually presents as an asymptomatic solitary pulmonary nodule ("coin lesion") but occasionally with chest pain, cough, or hemoptysis. Microscopically there is local eosinophilia and granuloma formation accompanied by infarction and thrombosis around an impacted, immature worm. The second common clinical presentation is that of a subcutaneous nodule found anywhere on the body (or within the eye) that results usually from infection with the subcutaneous dwelling filarids of dogs (*D. repens*) or raccoons (*D. tenuis*) but occasionally from infection with *D. immitis.* Local lesions again are granulomatous and eosinophilic and are sometimes accompanied by bacterial superinfection.

Definitive diagnosis and treatment most often result from the same surgical (excisional) procedure. Blood eosinophilia is not a regular finding in these patients nor are detectable antifilarial antibodies. Furthermore, since the worms are usually incompletely developed, microfilaremia occurs only in the rarest of circumstances. These "abnormal" parasite infections do not respond to diethylcarbamazine and their treatment is primarily surgical.

Dissanaike AS: Zoonotic aspects of filarial infections in man. Bull WHO 57:349, 1979. *A scholarly, readable discussion of man's interaction with zoonotic filarial infections.*

Gershwin LJ, Gershwin E, Kritzman J: Human pulmonary dirofilariasis. Chest 66:92, 1974. *Description of the 35th of the more than 100 cases now reported, with a good discussion.*

*Not commercially available in the United States but available in special circumstances from Lederle Laboratories.

*Not commercially available in the United States but available in special circumstances from Lederle Laboratories.

421. POSSIBLE HUMAN MENINGONEMIASIS

Eric A. Ottesen

According to Orihel, microfilariae recovered from patients with neurologic disorders in Rhodesia (now Zimbabwe) resemble *Meningonema peruzzii* (which inhabit the leptomeninges of the brainstem in African monkeys) more closely than *Dipetalonema perstans*.

Orihel TC: Cerebral filariasis in Rhodesia—a zoonotic infection. Am J Trop Med Hyg 22:596, 1973. *Evidence that microfilariae recovered from the cerebrospinal fluid are* M. peruzzii.

422. ONCHOCERCIASIS (River Blindness)

Brian O. L. Duke

Onchocerciasis is a disease of the skin and eye which follows infection with the filarial worm *Onchocerca volvulus*.

ETIOLOGY. Infection comes from the bites of female blackflies (buffalo gnats) of the genus *Simulium*, which transmit the infective larvae of the parasite. Over some 10 to 20 months these larvae grow to threadlike adult worms (males 5 cm; females, 50 cm), which live for up to 15 years tangled together in fibrous nodules under the skin, in the intermuscular fascial planes, and against the capsules of joints or the shafts of long bones. The adult females produce a continuous supply of live embryos or microfilariae, which have a life span of 12 to 24 months in the subepidermal layer of the skin and which may invade the eye, lymph glands, or other organs. Skin microfilariae ingested by biting *Simulium* develop in seven to ten days to infective larvae and can be transmitted to a new host.

PREVALENCE AND EPIDEMIOLOGY. Some 20 to 40 million people are infected with *O. volvulus*, mostly in tropical Africa south of the Sahara; there are also foci in Yemen, Guatemala, Mexico, Venezuela, Ecuador, Colombia, and Brazil.

Infections are mostly found in communities located within 10 to 20 km of fast-flowing water courses in which *Simulium* flies breed. The main vectors are *S. damnosum* s.l. and *S. neavi* s.l. in Africa, and *S. ochraceum* in Guatemala and Mexico. In many communities almost all the people are infected, and in some West African savanna villages 10 to 15 per cent of the whole population may be blind from onchocerciasis.

PATHOGENESIS AND PATHOLOGY. The nodules arise from a granulomatous and fibrous reaction in the host's tissues produced in response to the adult worms. Apart from being unsightly or inconvenient, they seldom cause clinical manifestations. Dead microfilariae in the tissues produce small granulomas infiltrated with eosinophils and leading to fibrosis. In the skin in acute cases this produces an itchy papular rash. Prolonged heavy infection leads to fibrosis, scarring of the papillae, replacement of dermal collagen by hyalinized scar tissue, and atrophic changes. In the eye similar reactions around microfilariae give rise to the inflammatory and scarring lesions in the cornea, anterior uvea, chorioretinal tissues, and optic nerve head, any of which can lead to blindness.

Onchocerciasis is a cumulative infection. Repeated inocula of infective larvae lead to intense infections both in terms of adult worms and microfilariae. The more intense the infection, the greater is the risk of severe lesions. The host's immune response to the parasite also influences the clinical picture.

CLINICAL MANIFESTATIONS. Cases presenting in temperate climates are likely to be light infections, probably newly acquired, in persons who have recently resided in an endemic area. Commonly there is an adult worm(s) near the limb girdle on one side. The microfilariae from this invade the skin locally, giving rise to a persistent itchy rash, which typically has a lopsided distribution (e.g., one leg and buttock, or one arm and shoulder). The rash is composed of discrete red papules 1 to 3 mm in diameter, but wheals, vesicles, scratch marks, and secondary infection may be superimposed. The skin fold on the affected side is thickened, the draining lymph glands are slightly enlarged, and there may be deep aches and pains in the limb concerned. Seldom can a nodule be palpated. Sometimes there is no rash, but the skin is thickened and lichenified and may itch. Such patients are unlikely to have more eye involvement than a few fluffy opacities (punctate keratitis) around microfilariae dying in the cornea.

Heavy and chronic onchocercal infection is likely only among natives of the endemic area. Palpable nodules may be abundant over bony prominences. In the skin gross lichenification and hyperpigmentation occur, giving way later to atrophy, "lizard skin," and mottled depigmentation (especially over the shins). The femoral and inguinal lymph glands enlarge. They may come to lie in pockets of loose skin (known as "hanging groins"), which predispose to hernia. In the eyes severe visual loss or blindness can result from (1) sclerosing keratitis; (2) chronic iridocyclitis with acute exacerbations, leading to secondary glaucoma; (3) chorioretinal lesions (typically the Hissette-Ridley fundus); or (4) postneuritic optic atrophy.

DIAGNOSIS. Definitive diagnosis depends on finding an adult worm in an excised nodule, or microfilariae in a skin snip, which should be taken from an area of affected skin or, failing that, from the iliac crest or calf (in Africa) or from the scapula (in America). A cone-shaped fold of skin is raised with a needle point and sliced off with a razor blade to give a bloodless piece of skin 2 to 3 mm in diameter. This is placed in normal saline and examined under the microscope, at 20- to 100-fold magnification, for microfilariae, which usually emerge within a few minutes to a few hours. Microfilariae may also be seen in the cornea or anterior chamber with a slit lamp. In lightly infected cases in which no microfilariae can be detected, a presumptive diagnosis often has to be made on clinical grounds, and the Mazzotti test (50 mg of diethylcarbamazine citrate* by mouth produces an exacerbation of itching and rash in the affected parts within 24 hours) is very useful. Eosinophilia and a positive filarial indirect fluorescent antibody or skin test are suggestive but not specific.

Differential diagnosis includes scabies, prickly heat, insect bites (especially *Culicoides*), contact dermatitis, and, rarely, streptocerciasis (see Ch. 423).

TREATMENT. Nodules on the head should always be removed because of extra danger to the eye, but removal of all palpable nodules will not result in cure. Treatment depends on chemotherapy with diethylcarbamazine citrate (DEC-C)* to kill the microfilariae, followed by suramin† to kill the adult worms, and then more DEC-C to mop up the residual microfilariae. The full course of treatment lasts two to three months and requires regular knowledgeable medical supervision on account of (1) the severe systemic and local reactions (in skin and eye) which may supervene as the microfilariae are killed by DEC-C and (2) the intrinsic toxicity of suramin.†

In all but the lightest cases DEC-C* should be given under corticosteroid "cover" (betamethazone 1 to 2 mg t.d.s. started two days before the DEC-C)* since there is always a danger of doing damage to the posterior segment of the eye in infected persons. DEC-C* may be started at 50 mg for an adult on the first day and increased to 100 mg on the second day and then to 200 mg daily for one week. Suramin† is best given weekly by intravenous injection according to the schedule 0.2 gram, 0.4 gram, 0.6 gram, 0.8 gram, 1.0 gram, 1.0 gram for a 60-kilogram adult.

PROGNOSIS. In the absence of reinfection the parasites will die out within 15 years, but signs and symptoms of disease will persist and may get worse during this period.

PREVENTION. There is no chemoprophylaxis. Personal prophylaxis consists of avoiding the haunts of *Simulium* and of wearing clothing that reduces the area of skin exposed to bites.

The larvae of *Simulium* are highly susceptible to regular

---

*Production of this drug in the United States has been discontinued.

†Available from Centers for Disease Control (404–329–3670 8:00 A.M. to 4:30 P.M. Monday through Friday; 404–329–2888 evenings, weekends, and holidays).

intermittent application of insecticides (currently Abate is used) to their aquatic breeding sites. Control of transmission of *O. volvulus* has been achieved in this way in the Volta River Basin in West Africa.

Buck AA (ed.): Onchocerciasis: Symptomatology, Pathology and Diagnosis. Geneva, World Health Organization, 1974. *Provides excellent photographs of skin and eye lesions.*

Epidemiology of Onchocerciasis. Report of a WHO Expert Committee. Geneva, World Health Organization, Technical Report Series NO 597, 1976. *Full account of epidemiology and diagnostic methods.*

Ledingham JGG, Warrell DA, Wetherall JJ (eds.): The Oxford Textbook of Medicine. 13th ed. Oxford, Oxford University Press, 1981. *Section on onchocerciasis gives detailed, up-to-date account of treatment.*

423. STREPTOCERCIASIS

Brian O. L. Duke

Mansonella streptocerca is transmitted by midges, especially *Culicoides grahamii*. It occurs in the tropical forest belt of Africa from Ghana to Zaire. The adult worms are subcutaneous,

especially over the torso; and the microfilariae, which have shepherd's-crook tails, are found in the skin (see Ch. 422 for skin-snipping technique).

Infection is usually symptomless, but the adult worms may produce hypopigmented macules (to be distinguished from leprosy), and the microfilariae occasionally cause itching papular rashes similar to those of onchocerciasis. Both adult worms and microfilariae are killed by diethylcarbamazine citrate* (e.g., seven to ten days of treatment at 2 mg per kilogram three times daily for an adult).

Meyers WM, Connor DH, et al.: Human streptocerciasis: A clinicopathologic study of 40 Africans (Zairians) including identification of the adult filaria. Am J Trop Med Hyg 21:528, 1972. *Covers the clinical aspects and gives references to other aspects.*

*Production of this drug in the United States has been discontinued.

Section 3 ARTHROPODS AND ANIMAL POISONS

424. ARTHROPODS AND LEECHES

William L. Krinsky

ARTHROPODS AS AGENTS OF DISEASE

Disease associated directly with arthropods results from toxic or allergic responses to the organisms or their products when humans are exposed by bites or stings, simple contact, or invasion through the skin or natural orifices. Arthropods most often involved in these types of exposure are listed in Table 424–1.

Physicians usually become aware of insects and their relatives (spiders, mites, ticks, scorpions, millipedes, and centipedes) when patients present with skin lesions caused by arthropods, when infestations of the creatures themselves are seen, when foreign bodies extracted from skin or sense organs are identified as arthropods, or when respiratory symptoms develop in response to arthropods or their products. Dermatoses associated with arthropods and human infestations with arthropods (e.g., lice, mites, fly larvae) are discussed in detail in this chapter. Arthropods as vectors are mentioned here; detailed discussions of arthropod-borne pathogens may be found elsewhere in this book. Arthropods as sources of respiratory and skin allergens are discussed in Ch. 434.

TABLE 424–1. ARTHROPODS CAUSING HUMAN PATHOLOGY

Human Exposure	Arthropod	Antigens or Toxins
Bites	Insects (lice, bed bugs and other true bugs; fleas; flies including mosquitoes, black flies, biting midges, sand flies, horse and deer flies, stable flies, tsetse flies, keds; ants)	Salivary secretions, venoms
	Arachnids (chigger and other rodent and bird mites; ticks; spiders)	
	Centipedes	
Stings	Insects (some ants, wasps, and bees)	Venoms
	Arachnids (scorpions)	
Invasion	Insects (fly larvae, *Tunga* fleas)	Salivary secretions, excretions
	Arachnids (scabies mites)	
Simple contact	Insects (caterpillars, pupae or adults of moths and butterflies; blister and some rove beetles)	Setae, spines, secretions (venoms) and excretions
	Arachnids (stored product mites)	
	Millipedes	

Disease associated with fear of insects (entomophobia) or a preoccupation with an imagined infestation (delusory parasitosis) falls within the realm of psychiatry. However, diagnosis of the latter requires careful, repeated examinations by a physician in consultation with an entomologist to rule out an unusual infestation or the presence of microscopic arthropods or their products.

Canizares O: Clinical Tropical Dermatology. Oxford, Blackwell Scientific, 1975. *This text includes detailed clinical information about cutaneous lesions caused by arthropods.*

Harwood RF, James MT: Entomology in Human and Animal Health. 7th ed. New York, The Macmillan Company, 1979. *This is a comprehensive textbook that provides detailed references to the diverse arthropod-associated problems discussed here.*

Biting Arthropods

Louse Infestations (Pediculosis)

Pediculosis is infestation of the body with lice (small wingless, dorsoventrally flattened insects in the order Anoplura). Pruritus is the primary symptom of pediculosis, although some infestations are asymptomatic. Infested persons may be irritable and restless as a consequence of physical discomfort and lack of sleep. Louse eggs (nits) seen cemented to hairs of the scalp or the observation of lice themselves confirms the diagnosis of head lice (*Pediculus capitis*). Nits (or lice) attached to the seams of clothing (often in undergarments) indicate the presence of body lice (*Pediculus humanus*), and nits or lice attached to pubic hairs indicate a pubic (crab) louse (*Phthirus pubis*) infestation.

The eggs are pearly yellow-white and opaque, elongate-oval, about 0.8 mm long and 0.3 mm wide and are attached singly to each hair or clothing fiber. After hatching, the nits appear translucent and opalescent. Although nits may be numerous, usually not more than 10 to 20 lice are found on or associated with most infested persons. The head louse egg is cemented on a hair about 1 mm above the scalp surface. Because hair grows 0.4 to 0.6 mm a day and most eggs hatch within five to ten days after deposition, generally it can be assumed that nits attached over 7 mm from the surface are nonviable. Pseudopediculosis is a condition in which other materials such as dandruff, hair casts, dried sebaceous secretions, or solidified hair spray droplets mimic head louse infestation.

Head and body lice are very similar in appearance. Adult head lice are 2.5 to 3.5 mm long and adult body lice are 3 to 4.5 mm long. Immature and adult head and body lice each have three pairs of about equal-sized legs bearing claws for gripping hairs or fibers. Adult pubic lice, somewhat crablike in appearance, are 1 to 2 mm long, about as broad, grayish-white or yellowish-brown, and have forelegs narrower than the other pairs; all pairs have strong claws for gripping coarse hairs. All louse immatures (three stages in each species) resemble their respective adults except in size, and all immatures and adults are obligate bloodsucking ectoparasites. The body louse is the only known natural vector of the pathogens of louse-borne typhus, trench fever, and louse-borne relapsing fever.

Head lice and their nits are found most frequently in the hair over the postauricular and occipital regions. Body lice, although occasionally found on the body, are usually seen in clothing with nits in the seams and creases in areas that contact the body. Crab lice and nits are found on hairs in the pubic and perianal regions, sometimes on hairs on the thighs and abdomen, less commonly on axillary hairs, beard, mustache, eyebrows, eyelashes, and rarely on the margin of the scalp. Pubic infestations are found only in postpubertal individuals.

The skin lesions produced by the bites of lice are erythematous papules that may be accompanied by urticaria or lymphadenopathy. Extensive erythema and pruritus result from hypersensitivity to louse saliva that develops after repeated feedings. Crab lice typically induce nonpruritic small gray-blue macules (0.3 to 1 cm diameter) with irregular borders (maculae ceruleae) that may persist for months. The lesions produced by any of the species may be covered with hair matted with eggs, dried serous secretions, and dark louse excrement. The latter, seen on the body or in underclothing, should trigger a physician's search for lice. Excoriations from scratching further disguise original bite lesions and may lead to impetigo, furuncular, or eczematous lesions. The possibility of louse infestation should be considered when pyoderma is seen. The lichenification and pigmentation seen in chronically infested individuals is called vagabond's disease (*morbus vagabondus*). A nondescript macular or papular erythematous rash on the trunk may be the presenting sign for an undiscovered head louse infestation. Similarly, postauricular and posterior cervical lymphadenopathy in the absence of other node enlargement should be suspected as a sign of head lice. Body louse infestation may be differentiated from scabies (see later discussion) by the absence of lesions on the hands and feet and the common occurrence of lesions in the intrascapular region. The differential diagnosis of louse-induced dermatitis from various mite-induced lesions or nonarthropod-associated dermatoses is made by finding nits or lice.

Treatment for lice includes shampoos, creams, and lotions containing insecticides. The most often used preparations contain lindane (gamma benzene hexachloride) or pyrethrins with piperonyl butoxide. Malathion lotion has recently been approved for use in the United States. One effective treatment for head lice is a four-minute shampoo with about 25 ml of 1 per cent lindane shampoo. This may not be ovicidal; therefore, to ensure that subsequently emerging lice are killed, the treatment may be repeated seven to ten days later, or only if lice are seen. Patients infested with body lice or pubic lice may apply lindane (1 per cent) lotion or cream to affected areas. This should be thoroughly washed off six to eight hours later. A repeat application may be necessary. Infested clothing and linen should be washed in hot water (60° C) for 20 minutes or dry cleaned.

After being treated, lice and nits can be removed with a metal comb with teeth 0.1 mm apart. Moisture or oil rinses may make removal easier. Mechanical removal is recommended for facial pubic lice infestations. Lice and nits may be removed from eyelashes with a trachoma (roller) forceps. This may be followed by treatment with one of various pediculicide ointments, such as yellow oxide of mercury (1 to 2 per cent), pyrethrin in Vaseline (1:8), or petrolatum, applied twice a day for seven to ten days. Blepharitis and other secondary infections associated with lice may require specific antibiotic therapy.

Prevention of recurrence involves treatment of infested human contacts and materials (fomites). Pillow cases, hats, scarves, and other items with which a person with head lice had contact should be washed or cleaned as recommended for clothing. Infested combs and brushes should be cleaned and boiled or soaked for one hour in lindane shampoo or Lysol (2 per cent). Head and body lice will survive only about three days (ten days maximum) away from the body. Sexual partners of persons with pubic lice should be treated, and bedding, towels, and clothing contacted should be washed or dry cleaned. Pubic lice will not survive longer than 24 hours away from a body; transmission via toilet seats is unlikely. Fumigation after any louse infestation is unnecessary, but vacuuming is helpful to remove stray lice and shed hairs with affixed nits.

Domonkos AN, Arnold HL, Odom RB: Andrews' Diseases of the Skin. 7th ed. Philadelphia, W. B. Saunders Company, 1982, pp 554–557. *This text has excellent photographs of nits, lice, and skin lesions seen in pediculosis.*

Raber IM: Pediculosis ciliaris. *In* Parish LC, Nutting WB, Schwartzman RM (eds.): Cutaneous Infestations of Man and Animal. New York, Praeger, 1983, pp 138–143. *This is a lucid description of the clinical aspects and treatment of pubic louse infestation of the eyelashes.*

Witkowski JA, Parish LC: Pediculosis. *In* Parish LC, Nutting WB, Schwartzman RM (eds.): Cutaneous Infestations of Man and Animal. New York, Praeger, 1983, pp 125–137. *A concise, well-documented discussion of clinical louse infestations.*

Flea Bites

Most fleas, unlike lice, do not infest the body. The common flea species that suck blood from humans visit the body for a few minutes to hours, during which time feeding occurs. As in louse infestations, flea bites generally cause pruritus, although some bites are asymptomatic. Each bite lesion is an erythematous papule with a hemorrhagic punctum. Sensitization of an individual to flea saliva may result in papular urticaria (common in affected children), bullous eruptions, or erythema multiforme–type lesions. Bites are usually multiple and irregularly grouped. Commonly seen bites in adults appear as widespread papules that become lichenified, or as grouped papules overlying erythema or edema. Persons entering a previously infested room that has been vacant for weeks or months often suffer from multiple bites on the ankles and legs as hungry fleas, stimulated by a warm-blooded host, emerge from pupal cocoons that have laid dormant in floor crevices, debris, or carpeting. As with louse bites, excoriated lesions may become infected and furuncular.

Fleas are small (about 1.5 to 4 mm long), wingless, laterally flattened, brown to black, obligate bloodsucking, temporary ectoparasitic insects (order Siphonaptera). The eggs are usually laid off the host, and larvae (resembling some fly larvae) live off the host, feeding on organic debris. Adults reach their hosts by jumping. Flea species that most often bite humans are the cat flea (*Ctenocephalides felis*), the dog flea (*C. canis*), and somewhat less commonly the so-called human flea (*Pulex irritans*). Occasional household infestations with these and other fleas may arise from abandoned wild animal nests built near houses.

Treatment of flea bites is usually symptomatic and involves the use of antipruritic and anti-inflammatory creams or lotions, or oral antihistamines. Secondary infections may require antibiotic therapy. Infested pets should be treated with specific insecticide powders, sprays, mists, or dips. Floors, carpets, upholstered furnishings, and pets' sleeping quarters should be sprayed or dusted with insecticides to kill larval, pupal, and adult fleas. Thorough cleaning, including vacuuming, of infested premises should eliminate the insects. Because fleas at all stages can live for weeks or months, a repeat insecticide application may be necessary.

Persons may protect themselves from fleas with repellents containing dimethyl phthalate or diethyl metatoluamide. Wild animal (especially rodent) fleas that may feed on humans present the greatest health risks because of their potential to transmit the bacilli of plague or tularemia, as well as the less virulent rickettsia of murine (flea-borne) typhus. Less commonly seen pathogens that are transmitted by accidental ingestion of fleas (mostly by children) are the dwarf tapeworm *Hymenolepis diminuta* and the dog tapeworm *Dipylidium caninum*.

Bagnall B, Rook A: Arthropods and the skin. *In* Rook A (ed.): Recent Advances in Dermatology. No. 4. Edinburgh, Churchill Livingstone, 1977. *This review includes information about the ecology of fleas and pathogenesis and clinical features of infestations.*

Smit FGAM: Siphonaptera (Fleas). *In* Smith KGV (ed.): Insects and Other Arthropods of Medical Importance. London, British Museum (Natural History), 1973. *This is a careful overview of the medical importance of fleas.*

Bed Bugs and Kissing Bugs

Bed bugs (Cimicidae) are flat, mahogany brown, wingless insects (5 to 7 mm long). Most of the species are bloodsucking ectoparasites of birds and bats. Two species (*Cimex lectularius* and *C. hemipterus*) feed almost exclusively on humans; the former is cosmopolitan, the latter has a tropical distribution. Both species may cause irritating, pruritic bite lesions in sensitized individuals. The bugs become engorged with blood in 3 to 15 minutes and feed only at night or in subdued light. They hide in crevices of bedding, beds, floors, and furnishings and in wood and paper trash accumulations during the day. The bites are often seen in short linear groups and vary from small urticarial lesions to large erythematous papules or bullae. The lesions are often excoriated, and eczematous reactions and pyoderma may be seen. Hypersensitivity reactions may include asthma, generalized urticaria, and arthralgia. While some affected persons complain of being awakened at night, most are troubled by the lesions on arising in the morning. Treatment is symptomatic. Prevention includes removal of debris that harbors the bugs, use of insecticides in crevices and hiding places, and cleaning of bedding and infested furnishings.

Triatomine kissing bugs (Reduviidae) that suck blood from a diversity of hosts are found in the New World subtropics and tropics and in Asia. Most of these cone-nosed bugs (8 to 38 mm long) are tan, brown, or black, with yellow or red spots around the dorsal edge of the abdomen. The bugs feed rapidly at night and, like bed bugs, these insects and their bites often go unnoticed. Sensitive individuals may develop papular lesions, small vesicles or, in the extreme, large urticarial or hemorrhagic nodular to bullous lesions. Generalized anaphylactoid reactions including shock and angioneurotic and laryngeal edema have occurrred. Despite the name, kissing bugs may feed not only near the lips but anywhere on the body. Domesticated species in the tropics are found most often in thatched houses or those with mud floors. In the southwestern United States, a species (*Triatoma protracta*) living in wood rat nests in desert areas occasionally invades homes. Unlike bed bug-infested dwellings, those affected premises harbor only one or a few bugs. Treatment of bites or severe allergic reactions is symptomatic. The major medical problems associated with triatomine bugs occur in Central and South America, where these insects are vectors of Chagas' disease trypanosomes.

Crissey JT: Bedbugs—an old problem with a new dimension. Int J Dermatol 20:411, 1981. *This review article discusses bed bug biology and the possible role of these bugs in human disease.*
Ryckman RE: Host reactions to bug bites (Hemiptera, Homoptera): A literature review and annotated bibliography. Parts I, II. Calif Vector Views 26:Nos. 1–2, 1979. *This is an excellent source of specific references about all bugs that prey on humans.*

Mosquitoes and Other Bloodsucking Flies

Mosquitoes (Culicidae) are found throughout the world, breeding wherever there is stagnant water. While biting, a female mosquito (3 to 6 mm long) induces a pruritic wheal that becomes an erythematous papule within 24 hours of the bite. In very sensitive persons, bullous lesions, cellulitis, or hemorrhagic necrotic reactions may follow the bites. Systemic anaphylactic reactions are rare. The most serious medical problems associated with mosquitoes relate to their transmission of the agents of yellow fever, dengue, arboviral encephalitides, malaria, and filariasis.

Biting midges (Ceratopogonidae), also called punkies or no-see-ums because of their minute size (most are 0.6 to 2 mm long), give a painful bite that feels like an ember on the skin. The resulting erythematous punctiform lesions may become papular and pruritic. Vesicles may develop that ooze fluid for days. These midges, especially *Culicoides* species, bite mostly on exposed parts of the body and may be pestiferous in sandy seashore or marshy areas where they breed. Biting occurs mostly at dawn or dusk.

Black flies (Simuliidae), also called buffalo gnats, are small (1 to 5 mm long), humpbacked, tan to black insects that breed only in running water. They are troublesome bloodsuckers in northern temperate regions where they harass woodland visitors. The bites may become hemorrhagic papules that ooze blood for hours. These lesions may be painful and cause recurrent pruritus as well. Lymphadenopathy is common in sensitive individuals, who may develop localized edema. Cephalalgia, fever, and nausea have occurred in persons receiving large numbers of bites. Black fly species found at high elevations in Central and South America and along rivers in Africa are of greatest medical importance because they transmit *Onchocerca volvulus*, the etiologic agent of river blindness.

Phlebotomine sand flies (Psychodidae) are delicate, small (2 to 3 mm long), hairy flies that are found mainly in subtropical and tropical areas. Various species are abundant in rain forests in the New World and in arid areas in the Mediterranean region and Asia. Biting occurs at night or in subdued light. The bites, which may be painful, occur usually on the extremities and cause pruritus and elevated pale urticarial lesions that become papular. Vesicular or bullous lesions may occur. Phlebotomine flies are of major medical importance as vectors of the pathogens of sand fly (pappataci) fever, bartonellosis, and leishmaniasis.

Other flies that may attack man and cause painful bites are the robust horse and deer flies (Tabanidae), stable flies, and tsetse flies. Tsetse flies, found only in Africa, should be avoided because they transmit the trypanosomes of African sleeping sickness. Sheep keds (wingless flies) that infest the wool of sheep occasionally bite sheep farmers and handlers of fresh wool.

Treatment of any of these fly bites is symptomatic and often includes the use of topical corticosteroids and oral antihistamines to reduce itching. Personal protection from biting flies mostly involves avoidance of the insects by use of screen enclosures, headnets, and insect repellents. Protective clothing and open mesh jackets impregnated with repellents are effective.

Allen JR: Mosquitoes and other biting flies. *In* Parish LC, Nutting WB, Schwartzman RM (eds.): Cutaneous Infestations of Man and Animal. New York, Praeger, 1983, pp 344–355. *This is a concise, clearly presented review of pathogenesis and clinical aspects of fly bites.*

Chiggers and Other Biting Mites

Chiggers are the larvae (six-legged stage) of trombiculid (itch or harvest) mites. These larvae (0.15 to 0.40 mm long), which are white to yellow or orange-red, are found on a diversity of vertebrates. Human infestation occurs following contact with grassy or shrubby vegetation inhabited by the mites. First exposure may not produce dermatitis or may produce only slightly irritating, transient erythematous macules or papules (1 to 2 mm). The more commonly seen skin reactions to chigger feeding are extremely pruritic, papular, papulovesicular or papulourticarial lesions (4 to 20 mm) that may persist with burning and itching for days to weeks. The lesions may fade and flatten or become hemorrhagic, purpuric, or vesicular. Diagnosis is dependent upon morphology and distribution of lesions, exposure history, and observation of the mites. Engorging chiggers may be apparent as minute reddish blebs embedded in hair follicles. The mites most often attach to skin covered by clothing, especially near belts, straps, or elastic bindings. Scrub itch (a misnomer) mites of Asia and South Pacific Islands usually do not cause dermatitis, but they are of major medical concern as vectors of scrub typhus rickettsiae.

Other mites that bite man but that are rarely recovered from the lesions they cause are pyemotid (straw, hay, or grain itch) mites, cheyletiellid (cat and dog fur) mites, and dermanyssoid (chicken, red, house mouse, tropical rat, fowl, and rodent) mites. All of these mites are extremely small (about 0.4 to 1 mm long) and, depending on the species, the six-legged larvae or eight-legged nymphs and adults may attack man. The resulting skin lesions may be extremely variable.

Differential diagnosis of mite-induced dermatitis from other forms of pruritic eruptions usually depends on associating the patient with a source of mites. Sources include wild and domestic animals, agricultural commodities, infested furniture, and, in chigger-associated cases, particular outdoor activities or habitats.

Treatment of dermatitis associated with biting mites is symptomatic. Antipruritic topical lotions and creams or oral antihistamines are useful. Secondary infections caused by excoriations may require antibiotic therapy. Rare allergic reactions, including edema and asthma, require emergency treatment (see Ch. 434).

Prevention of recurrences is dependent on destruction or fumigation of the mite source. Personal repellents (containing sulfur or diethyl toluamide) are helpful in preventing chigger infestation, although avoidance of infested areas is the best prevention. *Rickettsia tsutsugamushi* is the only pathogen of major medical importance specifically associated with mite transmission. *R. akari*, the etiologic agent of rickettsialpox, is transmitted by the house mouse mite.

Krinsky WL: Dermatoses associated with the bites of mites and ticks (Arthropoda: Acari). Int J Dermatol 22:75, 1983. *This review includes a list of mites causing human dermatitis and discusses clinical findings.*

Parkhurst HJ: Trombidiosis (infestation with chiggers). Arch Dermatol Syphilol 35:1011, 1937. *This is an extensive review of the biology and clinical importance of chiggers.*

Tick Bites and Tick Paralysis

Ticks, like mites, are arachnids that have six-legged larvae and eight-legged nymphs and adults. Ticks, found worldwide, are grouped in two major families, soft ticks (Argasidae) and hard ticks (Ixodidae). The former, which have rugose integuments, are associated with restricted habitats, such as rodent burrows and bird nests, and rarely feed on humans. When they do, most attach for only a matter of minutes and produce maculate, erythematous lesions (6 to 30 mm in diameter). Some species in Africa cause extensive ecchymosis; pain, pruritus, edema, ulceration, and necrotic lesions have also been observed. The pajaroello (talaja) tick (*Ornithodoros coriaceus*), found in Mexico, California, and Oregon, is known to produce hemorrhagic, painful lesions. In Europe, bites of the pigeon tick (*Argas reflexus*) have caused dyspnea, nausea, and loss of consciousness. Soft ticks are of primary medical importance as vectors of the borreliae of relapsing fevers.

Hard ticks have smooth, hard, shiny integuments and are found on a diversity of animals and in tall grass and forests. Ticks carried on dogs, cats, or other animals sometimes drop off and attach to man. Hard ticks remain embedded in the skin for days while becoming engorged with blood, and usually do not cause pain or discomfort. Engorging ticks, mistakenly identified as pedunculated moles or warts, are usually noticed only by chance observation. Typical tick bite lesions are small indurations with peripheral erythema. Unusual manifestations of hard tick bites include various forms of nonspecific dermatitis, acrodermatitis chronica atrophicans, necrotic ulcers, and alopecia. Most hard ticks attach, feed, drop off, and are never noticed. Nodular lesions that may persist for years at the sites of bites must be differentiated from malignancies, such as lymphomas. Hard ticks are of major medical concern as vectors of the etiologic agents of various arboviral hemorrhagic fevers and encephalitides, several kinds of tick-borne typhus (including Rocky Mountain spotted fever), tularemia, babesiosis, and Lyme disease. An engorging tick itself may induce tick paralysis (discussed below).

Attached soft ticks may be easily removed by gentle traction with a forceps. Hard ticks, usually more deeply embedded, require strong constant traction. Use of heat, flames, or caustic substances is ill-advised and may cause unnecessary damage to the patient. Hard ticks embedded in sensitive sites, such as the ear canal or genitals, may be covered with petrolatum. The ticks then detach within about two hours and can be gently removed. Complete extraction of the mouthparts lessens the chance of secondary infection. Persistent nodules that cause discomfort should be surgically excised.

Tick paralysis is an unusual form of ascending flaccid paralysis that may occur while a tick is attached to the body. Mostly children (especially girls) are affected. Tick paralysis in humans has been associated with only a small number of hard tick species but has been observed in North America, Europe, South Africa, and Australia. Most cases have been caused by female wood ticks, the Rocky Mountain wood tick (*Dermacentor andersoni*) in western North America, and the common dog tick (*D. variabilis*) in eastern North America, but only rare individuals, which are indistinguishable from other ticks of the same species, induce paralysis. Although nonspecific numbness or irritability may occur before the onset of paralysis, the initial consistent sign is *weakness in the legs*. Leg tendon reflexes are reduced or absent and Romberg's sign is often present. Sensory changes are rarely noted. Blood counts and lumbar puncture usually give no indication of the disease. Complete paralysis of the extremities may occur within a few days after a tick attaches. If the cause is unrecognized, paralysis usually progesses causing speech dysfunction, dysphagia, and ultimately death from aspiration or respiratory paralysis. If a tick is found, removal usually results in reversal of paralysis with a return to normal function in hours to weeks, depending on the severity of the neurologic deficit. The patient should be examined for other ticks, with special attention to concealed areas such as the scalp, ear canals, axillae, popliteal fossae, anus, and genitals. Even after all ticks are removed, death may occur in patients who exhibit bulbar or respiratory paralysis. A different form of paralysis is seen in Australia, where severe paralysis occurs about two days after the causative tick, *Ixodes holocyclus*, is removed. Supportive therapy usually leads to recovery after days to weeks.

The clinical presentation of tick paralysis may suggest poliomyelitis, Guillain-Barré syndrome, diphtheritic polyneuropathy, transverse myelitis, botulism, or other acutely developing neuropathies. The specific etiologic agent and mechanisms for the reduction in maximal motor nerve conduction velocities and decreased nerve action potentials seen in *Dermacentor* tick paralyses are unknown. A toxin isolated from *I. holocyclus* causes paralysis in dogs that is reversible with antiserum, but no substance or pathogen has been found in other tick species that induces paralysis in experimental animals or that is associated with human tick paralysis.

Prevention of tick bites and tick paralysis includes avoidance of tick-infested habitats. Individuals and their pets who enter such habitats should be thoroughly examined for crawling or attached ticks. Personal measures that may prevent ticks from reaching the skin include wearing long-sleeved shirts and long pants, tucking pants legs into socks, and using chemical repellents.

Gothe R, Kunze K, Hoogstraal H: The mechanisms of pathogenicity in the tick paralyses. J Med Entomol 16:357, 1979. *This review lists the tick species that have been associated with paralysis, general clinical aspects and experimental observations.*

Krinsky WL: Dermatoses Associated with the Bites of Mites and Ticks (Arthropoda: Acari). Int J Dermatol 22:75, 1983. *This is a review of skin lesions caused by acarines and epidemiologic and clinical factors helpful in diagnosis.*

Spider Bites

All spiders are eight-legged arachnids that use venom to immobilize their prey. Relatively few species have mouthparts (chelicerae) large and strong enough to inject venom into human skin. Among the better known spiders that cause moderate to severe reactions in man are the widows (*Latrodectus* species) of the Old and New Worlds, brown spiders (*Loxosceles* species) of the Americas, wandering spiders (*Phoneutria* species) and wolf spiders (*Lycosa* species) in South America, species of *Chiracanthium* in both hemispheres, funnel web spiders (*Atrax* species) in Australia, and *Harpactirella* species in South Africa.

The black widow (shoe button) spider (*Latrodectus mactans*) female may bite if it or its web is disturbed. Its abdomen is 6 mm wide and 9 to 13 mm long and is shiny black with a reddish hourglass marking or less well-defined markings on the underside. The spider lives in sheltered, dark, dry places such as corners of garages and in old stone walls and outhouses. The bite, which may not be felt, may become slightly swollen and appear as two erythematous puncture marks. Within a few hours, a bitten person develops intense muscle pains and commonly a tightening feeling in the chest. Abdominal (board-like) rigidity and waves of excruciating cramping pain are characteristic. Respiratory distress, nausea, vomiting, profuse perspiration, headache, vertigo, paresthesias of the extremities, and hyperactive reflexes are common. Speech difficulty and visual dysfunction may occur. The clinical presentation reflects the generalized neurotoxic effects of the venom that stimulates central, peripheral, and autonomic nerve activity. In untreated adults, the pathologic effects of the venom usually disappear within two to three days. Death from cardiac or respiratory arrest occurs mostly in very young children and elderly or hypertensive persons.

Differential diagnosis requires consideration of various abdominal and cardiovascular crises, such as perforated ulcer, acute appendicitis or pancreatitis, cholelithiasis, nephrolithiasis, splenic, renal, or mesenteric embolism, volvulus, porphyria, tetanus, and strychnine and lead poisoning. The generalized muscle pain, lack of abdominal tenderness, and the peripheral sensory changes help to differentiate widow spider bite from these other diseases.

Treatment with muscle relaxants, such as intravenous injection of 10 ml of 10 per cent calcium gluconate, temporarily relieves muscle pains. A specific antivenin available from Merck, Sharp and Dohme is effective against all *Latrodectus* venom and neutralizes the effects of the venom. Because the antivenin is derived from horses, horse serum sensitivity testing is required before the antivenin is administered.

The brown (violin or fiddleback) spiders, including *Loxosceles reclusa* (brown recluse) and *L. laeta* of the western hemisphere, are also secretive, living in secluded places in houses and nesting in clothing, and may bite when disturbed. They are 10 to 15 mm long and have a dark violin-shaped mark on the brown to gray cephalothorax. Their bites may cause only mild skin reactions but are most often recognized when a more serious condition, *necrotic arachnidism,* is the result. The sometimes painful lesion that develops two to six hours after a bite is a bulla or pustule surrounded by concentric rings of ischemia and erythema. Within 24 to 48 hours the lesion becomes cyanotic, and a central necrotic area begins to form. This area may slowly expand (up to 20 cm) over days to weeks. The resulting ulcer may not heal for weeks or months. Tissue destruction is thought to result from the enzyme activity of the venom and, possibly, venom activation of complement. Systemic reactions to the bite include fever, chills, edema, nausea, vomiting, dizziness, myalgias, and arthralgias; morbilliform and petechial eruptions may occur within 48 hours of the bite. A fatal complication, most often seen in children, is *intravascular hemolysis,* followed by hemoglobinuria and acute renal failure.

Treatment of necrotizing lesions is mainly symptomatic and may include surgical debridement and antibiotic therapy for secondary infection. Systemic corticosteroid therapy has been successful in reducing symptoms and skin destruction. Skin grafts may be needed to promote healing of chronic lesions.

Phoneutria (wandering) spiders often enter houses and may bite, causing intense pain, visual disturbance, tremors, profuse sweating, convulsions, priapism, tachycardia, and respiratory distress. Wolf spiders (*Lycosa* species) may produce painful but localized bite reactions. Specific treatment for *Phoneutria* and *Lycosa* bites is administration of antivenins available from the Butantan Institute, Sao Paulo, Brazil.

Chiracanthium species may bite producing erythema, edema, and pruritus. Necrotic lesions thought to be caused by these spiders may be confused with those of *Loxosceles* species. The mygalomorph funnel-web spiders (*Atrax* species) and *Harpactirella* spiders are aggressive and produce painful bites that have resulted in death.

Maretic Z, Lebez D: Araneism with Special Reference to Europe. Belgrade, Yugoslavia, Nolit Publishing House, 1979. *This book has extensive clinical information about* Latrodectus *envenomation and biological and clinical discussions relevant to other spider bites.*

Millikan LE: Loxoscelism and other arachnid problems. *In* Parish LC, Nutting WB, Schwartzman RM (eds.): Cutaneous Infestations of Man and Animal. New York, Praeger, 1983, pp 284–295. *This chapter includes excellent photographs of the necrotic lesions caused by recluse spider bites and a discussion of pathophysiology and treatment.*

Southcott RV: Arachnidism and Allied Syndromes in the Australian Region. Rec Adelaide Child Hosp 1:99, 1976. *This detailed review treats basic biology and clinical aspects of arachnid bites and infestations and is relevant to much of the world's fauna.*

Centipede Bites

Centipedes are multi-legged, elongated (up to 30 cm) arthropods with one pair of legs on each body segment. The first pair of legs is modified as poison claws that are used to inject venom into prey. Centipedes shun the light and are found under rocks and forest litter. The characteristic lesion resulting from a bite has two punctate hemorrhages in the center of an erythematous swelling. Centipede bites may cause severe (fiery) local pain that may be followed by inflammation, edema, and superficial necrosis. Systemic reactions may include headache, dizziness, and vomiting. The transient effects of a bite may be accompanied by irregular pulse, muscle spasm, or lymphadenopathy. There are a few reports of children dying from the bites of large tropical species, but their reliability has been questioned. Treatment is symptomatic and despite the venomous nature of these creatures, they rarely bite because of their nocturnal habits and tendency to escape when uncovered or disturbed during the day. In general, centipede bites cause few or no long-term pathologic effects.

Southcott RV: Arachnidism and allied syndromes in the Australian region. Rec Adelaide Child Hosp 1:99, 1976. *This includes a careful review (pp 174–177) of clinical aspects of centipede bites and some case histories.*

Stinging Arthropods

Bee, Wasp, and Ant Stings

Bees, wasps, and ants (order Hymenoptera) are insects that include solitary and social species that have females in which the egglaying tube (ovipositor) has been modified as a sting that secretes venom from abdominal glands. Solitary species rarely sting humans and their stings usually cause only minor pain or discomfort. The social bees that include honeybees and bumblebees all have two pairs of membranous wings, are stocky, hairy, and often colored with yellow and black or brown. The honeybee (*Apis mellifera*) and its various racial forms and close relatives are found worldwide and often are responsible for human sting reactions. Unlike other Hymenoptera, the honeybee has a barbed sting that becomes embedded in skin and, as the bee tries to escape, it leaves its venom apparatus and other abdominal organs and soon perishes. Social wasps include vespid wasps (yellowjackets, hornets, paper wasps) that are smooth insects sleeker than bees and often colored yellow and black, or with combinations of yellow, red, brown, or black. These wasps make the paper nests often found in trees, under eaves of houses, or underground. Honeybees and bumblebees may sting when accidentally disturbed while seeking nectar or pollen at flowers. Vespid wasps may become pestiferous around foodstuffs, being especially attracted to sweet or fermented liquids, fruit, and meats. Mutillid wasps (velvet ants, cow killers), which are hairy and wingless, sometimes sting persons in sandy, arid environments.

Human reactions to stings usually include intense local pain, followed by the appearance of a red punctum surrounded by a blanched area and erythema. A wheal forms and the swelling and erythema, accompanied by pruritus, may last for a few hours. Multiple stings, especially on the face, may cause more extensive edema, severe skin lesions such as multiple vesicles or bullae, or purpura that results from the hemolytic and anticoagulant properties of wasp venoms. Treatment includes gentle removal of the sting by scraping with a sharp blade (in cases of honeybee envenomation), application of ice, and topical hydrocortisone or oral antihistamines. Severe and sometimes fatal allergic reactions to stings of bees and wasps that occur in sensitized individuals are discussed in Ch. 434.

Ants (Formicidae) of some species can sting, causing severe pain. Two notable groups of New World stinging ants are the fire ants (*Solenopsis* species) and harvester ants (*Pogonomyrmex* species). Fire ants build ground nests that protrude as large mounds. Persons that encounter the ants are readily stung. Each ant grips the skin with its mandibles and then inserts its sting. The ant may pivot and sting many times. This behavior, compounded by the common occurrence of mass attacks, leads to a clustering of lesions. The usual reaction to the sting is fiery, sharp pain, followed by a wheal and flare response. Within hours, a clear vesicle appears that becomes pustular after about 24 hours. This sterile pustule may persist for three to ten days and dry as a crust that sloughs, leaving a macule, scar, or fibrous nodule. Systemic reactions such as dizziness, nausea, vomiting, profuse perspiration, cyanosis, and asthma usually occur in allergic individuals, but may also be seen in cases of multiple stings. Harvester ants also make mound nests and cause similar local sting reactions. Symptomatic treatment of local reactions is similar to that for bee and wasp stings. Treatment of allergic reactions is discussed in Ch. 434.

Harwood RF, James MT: Venoms, defense secretions, and allergens of arthropods. *In* Entomology in Human and Animal Health. 7th ed. New York, The Macmillan Company, 1979. *This is a review of the biology and clinical importance of stinging Hymenoptera.*

Rhoades RB, Schafer WL, Schmid WH, et al.: Hypersensitivity to the imported fire ant. A report of 49 cases. J Allergy Clin Immunol 56:84, 1975. *This is a detailed review of clinical data and treatment of fire ant stings.*

Scorpion Stings

Scorpions are mostly subtropical and tropical arachnids that have a pair of lobster-like claws (pedipalps) anteriorly and a curved spine posteriorly that is an outlet for the proteinaceous venom produced by a pair of venom glands. Scorpions are nocturnal predators and will sting man quickly and repeatedly when disturbed in their hiding places under rocks, lumber, vegetation or in materials such as shoes, bedding, or clothing left on the ground. In the United States only one scorpion species, *Centruroides sculpturatus*, of about 40 native species causes severe pathologic effects in humans. This small (about 6 cm long), straw-colored species is found only in Arizona. In Mexico, six species of *Centruroides* sting humans and cause serious envenomation. In Trinidad, *Tityus trinitatis* is of medical importance. In South America, this species and five others in the genus as well as one *Centruroides* species cause severe sting reactions. The arid regions that extend from North Africa to India are inhabited by the most abundant and dangerous scorpions.

The nature and severity of human reactions to scorpion stings are not consistent with the size, appearance, or aggressiveness of different species, so that closely related scorpion species may elicit disparate pathologic reactions. Intense and immediate pain at the site of a sting is common to all cases. When a mildly toxic scorpion such as *C. vittatus*, a common southern United States species, is involved, the pain may be followed by local swelling and perhaps skin discoloration, regional lymphadenopathy, pruritus, or paresthesias, and less commonly by nausea and vomiting. These reactions are transient, lasting for only minutes to as long as 24 hours. The more toxic species cause similar local pain but little or no skin response, and systemic effects are usually noted within a few minutes to 24 hours after the sting. The neurotoxic venoms of these species have cholinergic and adrenergic effects and may be hemolytic. Symptoms may include anxiety, drowsiness, syncope, increased salivation, lacrimation, and perspiration, diminished vision, photophobia, numbness and sluggishness of the tongue, vomiting, diarrhea or involuntary defecation and micturation, priapism, muscular fibrillations or spasms, and convulsions. Clinical signs may include hypotension or hypertension, irregular pulse, tachycardia and arrythmias, irregular respiration, rapid shifts in body temperature, oliguria or polyuria, and hemiplegia. Laboratory tests may reveal hyperglycemia, glycosuria, SGOT elevation, hematuria, and melena. Severe pathologic changes that may lead to death include myocarditis, pulmonary edema, and shock. Respiratory paralysis is the usual immediate cause of death. In the most toxic cases, death may occur within minutes of the sting or not for over 40 hours later, but most deaths occur in 2 to 20 hours after the sting. The mortality rate is highest in children. Close monitoring of affected patients is important because sudden relapses, often involving acute respiratory distress, may occur after a patient's condition seems to have stabilized.

Treatment of the least toxic stings is symptomatic and often includes application of ice and a local anesthetic to the sting site. The most important treatment for moderate to very toxic stings is administration of an antivenin. Antivenin to *C. sculpturatus* is available in Arizona from the Antivenom Production Laboratory, Arizona State University, Tempe, Arizona 85281 (602-965-3116; outside of business hours 602-965-3456; ask for Dr. William Northey). Antivenins against other species are available from laboratories in Mexico, Brazil, Turkey, Algeria, Egypt, and South Africa (addresses listed in Keegan, 1980).

Early treatment of these stings should include cooling of the sting site for up to two hours and, if the sting is on an extremity, use of a tourniquet for five to ten minutes. Oxygen administration or artificial respiration, sodium phenobarbitol injection, and parenteral solutions, including blood plasma, may be needed to treat respiratory distress, convulsions, and shock, respectively. Calcium gluconate (10 ml of 10 per cent solution) given as a slow intravenous injection will reduce muscle spasms. In the United States, morphine and meperidine are contraindicated because they enhance the toxic effects of *C. sculpturatus* venom. Morphine and barbiturates are not recommended for treatment of any scorpion stings because these drugs inhibit the bulbar respiratory centers.

Personal prevention against stings includes wearing heavy gloves and boots when reaching into hidden areas or when moving materials in which scorpions may hide. Shaking out shoes and other materials left on the ground before using them is essential. Removal of litter from around houses, sealing cracks in foundations, and selective use of pesticides are helpful means of preventing scorpions from inhabiting houses and gardens.

Keegan HL: Scorpions of Medical Importance. Jackson, University of Mississippi Press, 1980. *This book reviews scorpion morphology, taxonomy, biology, and geographic distribution, and clinical aspects and prevention of scorpion envenomation.*

Invasive Arthropods

Scabies

The scabies mite (*Sarcoptes scabiei*), unlike the other mites discussed, burrows into the skin and, because it reproduces on humans, can maintain a continuous infestation. Fertile female mites burrow into the skin and lay their eggs as they tunnel. Individuals of the resulting immature stages (larvae and nymphs) move out to the surface and rapidly enter hair follicles. Further development and mating takes place near the skin surface. The mite burrows are slightly raised, curved, or tortuous gray lines, 5 to 15 mm long, and at the end of each is a female, a minute pearly bleb. The burrows are restricted to the horny layer of the skin and occur most often in the sides of the fingers, the interdigital webs, flexor surfaces of the wrists, elbows, skin around the nipples, and penis. Other lesions, including erythematous papules, lichenified patches, and pustules, which occur in sites other than the burrows, may be seen on the abdomen, thighs, and buttocks. In infants and young children, burrows may occur in the palms and soles, and papular lesions may be seen on the scalp, face, and neck.

Intense pruritus that begins from two to six weeks after first exposure to the mite is presumably an allergic response to the mite or its products. Definitive diagnosis of the lesions is often difficult because of excoriations. In very clean individuals, few lesions may be present and burrows may not be clearly visible. Generalized urticarial papules may result from previous treatment with fluorinated corticosteroids. Some patients have pruritic inflammatory nodules (≤ 12 mm in diameter) that occur on covered skin, especially the axillae, abdomen, scrotum, and penis. A severe form of scabies most often seen in immunologically compromised persons is called *crusted scabies* (originally called Norwegian scabies). As the name implies, warty plaques occur frequently on the hands and feet and extensive scaling covers the scalp to the trunk or below. Horny debris collects under the fingernails, which are usually distorted and thickened. Pruritus, erythema, and lymphadenopathy may occur to varying degrees.

Diagnosis of any scabies infestation depends on observation of a mite in skin scrapings of a burrow or in situ, by gently raising the top of a burrow with a sterile needle and looking with a magnifier. In most scabies cases, only 10 to 15 mites are present on the body. In crusted scabies, large numbers of mites (possibly more than a million) are present. To obtain a scraping of a burrow, an area suspected of infestation is scraped with a scalpel blade. The scraped material is examined at 50 to 100 times magnification. The movements of a living mite may be observed if the material is placed on a slide without any mounting media. Otherwise, the scraping may be cleared in a drop of potassium hydroxide (20 per cent) or suspended in mineral oil under a coverslip on the slide. The adult female mite is about 300 to 400 μm long, oval, with the dorsum convex and venter flattened. It has four pairs of legs, two pairs directed anteriorly and two posteriorly. Each anterior leg ends in an unjointed stalk with a distensible thin-walled sac at its tip; each posterior leg ends in a long, thick bristle. The size of the mite egg is about 100 × 150 μm.

Scabies lesions initially may be diagnosed as those of other skin conditions, e.g., neurodermatitis, dermatitis herpetiformis, lichen planus, and various other kinds of mite-associated dermatitis, such as that caused by *Cheyletiella* fur mites. The distribution of lesions and finally the observation of the mite will rule out these other diagnoses. Secondary infections appearing as pyoderma are common and nephrogenic strains of streptococci infecting the lesions may cause acute glomerulonephritis.

Treatment of uncomplicated scabies involves application of one of various acaricide lotions or creams. Lindane (1 per cent) is often used in a manner similar to that suggested for pediculosis; namely, a 6- to 12-hour treatment for adults and a 6-hour application for children, followed by thorough washing. The treatment should not be repeated more than once in seven days. Pruritus and dermatitis may persist for days after adequate treatment. Antipruritic medications such as antihistamines and Schamberg's lotion are often prescribed. Topical corticosteroids are contraindicated because of the urticarial reaction they sometimes cause.

Transmission occurs during contact with infested persons or with clothing recently worn by such persons. Transmission between bed partners is common and does not require bodily contact. All household and intimate contacts should be treated to prevent recurrence or continued transmission. The female mite will survive for only two to three days away from a host; therefore, as with louse infestations, fumigation of premises is unnecessary. Clothing, especially undergarments, bedding, and towels, should be laundered in hot water.

Scabies mites infesting domestic animals, including dogs and cats, occasionally cause dermatitis in man, but the lesions are usually limited to the areas that contact the animals. These mites are usually not recovered from humans.

Mellanby K: Scabies. Middlesex, England, E. W. Classey (1943), 1972. *This classic work available in this reprinted form is a comprehensive review of the basic biology, clinical evolution, and treatment of scabies.*

Parish LC, Nutting WB, Schwartzman RM (eds.): Scabies—Part II. *In* Cutaneous Infestations of Man and Animal. New York, Praeger, 1983, pp 53–109. *Several concise chapters give a clear and thorough review of the biology and clinical aspects of scabies.*

Myiasis and Tungiasis

Myiasis is the infestation of living vertebrate tissue by fly larvae. Many flies (order Diptera) that normally deposit eggs or larvae on carrion, manure, or decaying organic matter sometimes deposit their immature stages in open wounds or infected human tissues. These include blow flies, also called greenbottle or bluebottle flies (Calliphoridae), flesh flies (Sarcophagidae), and house flies (Muscidae). The larvae of some of these flies are attracted to draining infections, or clothing stained with urine or feces. The larvae crawl into lesions or natural orifices when an infected person sleeps on the ground or is otherwise exposed to flies. Individuals immobilized because of physical illness or old age who have such open lesions or infections, and especially those who are living in poor sanitary conditions, are particularly susceptible. Urogenital myiasis may cause dysuria, hematuria, and pyuria.

The sheep bot fly (*Oestrus ovis*) sometimes larviposits in the nose, ears, or eyes of sheep herders, who may develop external ophthalmitis from the migration of the larvae over the conjunctival surfaces. Other flies always oviposit in wounds. The screw worm fly (*Cochliomyia hominivorax*) of cattle in the southern United States and Mexico may oviposit on humans and is such a species. Other fly larvae always invade intact skin of domestic animals or man; species in this group include the human bot fly (*Dermatobia hominis*) found in Central and South America, the African Tumbu fly *Cordylobia anthropophaga,* and some species of *Wohlfahrtia* that have a predilection for the tender skin of infants. Larvae of cattle warble flies (*Hypoderma* species) and horse stomach bot flies (*Gasterophilus* species) may accidentally infest man and crawl about subcutaneously causing a creeping eruption that appears as erythematous, serpentine lesions or painful swellings.

Fly larvae that live in foodstuffs or organic detritus, e.g., vinegar flies (Drosophilidae) and cheese skippers (Piophilidae), are sometimes accidentally ingested and may cause gastrointestinal discomfort.

Wound or dermal myiasis often results in furuncular lesions, and an infested individual notices a swelling and feels pain or movement under the skin where the larvae are feeding on tissue fluids. Careful observation of the top of a lesion enables one to see two dark respiratory openings (spiracles) through which the larva breathes. Treatment consists of removal of the larvae by gentle compression of the swelling and pulling a larva out with a forceps. A local anesthetic may be helpful because the recurved spines that hold many larvae tightly under the skin may make removal difficult and painful. Topical antibiotics are used to control or prevent secondary infections. Removal of larvae that crawl into sensory openings or urogenital and anal orifices may require irrigation or surgical intervention, as may treatment of ophthalmomyiasis. Intestinal myiasis is usually self-limited, ceasing when the larvae are passed in the stool. Dermal myiasis of most kinds, if untreated, progresses until the mature larvae back out of the skin and drop to the ground to pupate. The physical and emotional distress caused by the presence of living larvae can be prevented if a physician considers the possibility of such an infestation and removes the larvae early in the infestation. Warble fly larvae, which normally migrate from the legs of cattle through the body to the back, in human infestations will also migrate dorsally and, unless they reach a cutaneous exit site, may cause extensive tissue damage that leads to chronic illness or death.

Prevention of myiasis requires use of frequently changed dressings on wounds and infections, and personal protection from flies such as screening or changes in behavior related to outdoor activities and eating habits. Use of eye protection in sheep bot fly areas is advisable.

Tungiasis is the infestation of vertebrate, including human, skin by the female flea *Tunga penetrans* (chigoe, jigger, or sand flea). This flea occurs in sandy soil in subtropical and tropical regions of the Americas, the West Indies, and Africa. It usually feeds between the toes, under a toenail, or in the sole of the foot, and becomes embedded as it gorges on blood. By eight to ten days after the flea begins feeding, it has grown to ≥5 mm from its original 1 mm size and it begins to release eggs through the skin opening. The flea, which remains embedded permanently, may cause irritation, pain, or pruritus, and the resulting swelling is often pustular. Secondary infections, including cellulitis and tetanus, are complications of infestations, and autoamputation of digits in Africans is apparently caused by inflammatory reactions to the flea.

Treatment of tungiasis includes removal of the flea with a sterile needle or pointed blade, tetanus vaccination, and application of topical antibiotics. Sometimes curettage is required to remove the flea, feces, or eggs retained in the skin. Personal protection against *T. penetrans* includes wearing footwear and using insect repellent. Because the flea is a poor jumper, sleeping above the ground surface usually prevents the flea from reaching the body.

Brothers W, Heckmann R: Tungiasis (*Tunga penetrans*) in Utah. J Parasitol 65:782, 1979. *This note succinctly describes the clinical problem and gives references to recent cases.*

Harwood RB, James MT: Myiasis. *In* Entomology in Human and Animal Health. New York, The Macmillan Company, 1979. *This is a thorough review of different clinical forms of myiasis.*

Arthropods and Contact Dermatitis

Various species of nonbiting mites found in stored products may cause dermatitis when they contact human skin. These microscopic foodstuff mites (Acaridae, Glycyphagidae) are found in various commodities including grains, cereals, seeds, bulbs, dried herbs, copra, dried vegetables, cured meats, mushrooms, humus, cheese, and animal and plant material used for stuffing furniture, pillows, and mattresses. Dried fruit mites (Carpoglyphidae) are found not only in various dried fruits but also in jams, jellies, spoiled fruit, wine, caramel, flour, and dried milk products. The skin reactions to these mites vary with the extent of exposure and host differences, but pruritic diffuse erythema with urticarial wheals or erythematous papular eruptions with each papule surmounted by a small vesicle are common. Laborers in granaries, food processing plants, and commercial kitchens and dockworkers are most susceptible.

Another form of pruritic dermatitis is caused by contact with various caterpillars, pupae, adults, and less often egg masses of moths and butterflies (order Lepidoptera). Urticating setae and spines on these life stages may cause mechanical irritation of the skin or may have toxic effects. Venomous materials are sometimes extruded from setae and spines connected to poison glands. Some of these toxins contain histamine and proteolytic enzymes. Mechanical or chemical irritation is often enhanced by barbs on the setae, which cause these structures to become tightly embedded in the skin. Dermatitis may result when setae or spines are touched or when people contact those that have become airborne around large infestations of the insects. Contact with setae, spines, or hairs from these caterpillars may cause intense stinging or fiery pain, followed by the formation of wheals, local edema, erythema, and pruritus. Less common reactions include lymphadenopathy, cephalalgia, shocklike symptoms, or convulsions.

Treatment of dermatitis caused by foodstuff and dried fruit mites or lepidopteran spines or setae is mainly symptomatic. Antipruritic substances including antihistamines, corticosteroids, and anesthetics have been used. Calcium gluconate (10 ml of a 10 per cent solution) given intravenously provides relief from the intense pain following contact with puss caterpillars (Megalopygidae). Specific treatment involves removal of the source of irritants. Commodities containing mites must be fumigated or destroyed. Spines or setae of lepidopterans may be removed from the skin with fine forceps. Use of protective clothing and thorough washing of exposed materials will help prevent continuation of these forms of dermatitis.

A third form of contact dermatitis results from vesicants produced by blister beetles (Meloidae) and some rove beetles (Staphylinidae). Cantharidin, first isolated from the meloid called the Spanish fly, is found in all species of blister beetles. This substance causes the mild to severe vesicular dermatitis that results when these beetles or their secretions are touched. The worldwide staphylinid genus *Paederus* contains more than 30 species that cause vesication.

Similar lesions, which usually follow a burning sensation and tanning of the skin, result from contact with defensive secretions of millipedes. Some species of these otherwise harmless herbivorous myriapods exude a fluid from pores along the length of the body. Secretions from the aforementioned beetles or millipedes will cause burning pain and conjunctivitis if they are rubbed into the eyes.

Treatment of toxic dermatitis associated with beetles or millipedes includes rapid washing of the skin or eyes, if affected, and use of local anesthetics. The dermal reactions caused by contact with mites, lepidopterans, beetles, and millipedes are usually transitory and do not have long-lasting effects.

Harwood RB, James MT: Vesicating Coleoptera. *In* Entomology in Human and Animal Health. New York, The Macmillan Company, 1979, pp 441–443. *This section discusses the nature of vesicant chemicals from beetles and reviews clinical cases.*

Radford AJ: Millipede burns in man. Trop Geogr Med 27:279, 1975. *Geographical distribution, toxicology, pathogenesis, clinical features, and treatment of millipede envenomation are carefully reviewed.*

Southcott RV: Lepidoptera and Skin Infestation. *In* Parish LC, Nutting WB, Schwartzman RM (eds.): Cutaneous Infestations of Man and Animal. New York, Praeger, 1983, pp 304–343. *This chapter gives a comprehensive review of worldwide lepidopterism, including pathogenesis and clinical presentations.*

PENTASTOMIASIS (Linguatuliasis)

Pentastomiasis is infestation with pentastomes, little-known invertebrates called tongue worms, which have been variously classified as arthropods or helminths. These bloodsucking endoparasites are found as adults in the lungs of reptiles and birds, or in the nasal cavity of carnivores, especially cats and dogs. Herbivores are normal intermediate hosts, but humans and other mammals can be dead-end aberrant hosts for the larvae. Ingested eggs hatch and the larvae burrow through the intestine and migrate to diverse tissues where they molt several times and become encysted as third stage larvae.

Human infestations have occurred in Europe, Africa, and North, Central, and South America. Two species account for most cases, *Armillifer armillatus,* found in pythons and other vipers in tropical Africa, and *Linguatula serrata,* found in canids in Europe and the Near and Middle East.

Infection occurs by accidental ingestion of tongue worm eggs contaminating food or drink, by ingestion of eggs picked up on fingers from handling infected snakes or lizards, or by ingestion of improperly cooked or raw reptiles. The third stage larvae (20 to 25 mm long) encysted in fibrous capsules occur most often in the liver and are rarely noted except incidentally at autopsy or as calcified cysts (3 to 6 mm in diameter) on x-ray examination. Rarely, a mass of cysts in the intestinal wall may cause obstruction. Cysts compressing vital structures such as bile ducts or bronchi may lead to infections or obstructions.

Linguatuliasis, the direct infection of humans with third stage larvae of *Linguatula* species, occurs most often in Lebanese people who eat raw or inadequately cooked liver or lymph nodes of goats and sheep. The ingested larvae migrate to the nasopharynx from the stomach. These larvae (5 to 10 mm long) cause Halzoun's syndrome, characterized by paroxysmal coughing, sneezing, nasal and lacrimal discharge, accompanied by pain and itching in the throat. Other symptoms may include hoarseness, dyspnea, dysphagia, and vomiting. Submaxillary and cervical lymph nodes may be enlarged. Recovery in most cases is spontaneous and occurs in seven to ten days; however, death from asphyxiation caused by tonsillar edema has been reported. A similar syndrome seen in Sudan, Turkey, and Greece is called Marrara's syndrome.

Prevention of pentastomiasis includes proper cooking of

exotic foods such as herbivore organs and reptiles, as well as improved hygiene of persons handling reptiles.

Hopps HC, Keegan HL, Price DL, Self JT: Pentastomiasis. *In* Marcial-Rojas RA (ed.): Pathology of Protozoal and Helminthic Diseases. Baltimore, Williams & Wilkins Company, 1971, pp 970–989. *This is a comprehensive review that includes basic biological and clinical information.*

LEECHES AS AGENTS OF DISEASE (Hirudiniasis)

Leeches of medical importance are bloodsucking annelid worms. Each has a ventral anterior or posterior sucker enclosing teeth that cut through the skin after the leech attaches. Feeding occurs within a half hour or more.

The leeches most often feeding on humans are aquatic (fresh water) species of *Hirudo,* the cosmopolitan medicinal leeches, *Limnatis,* the nasal leeches found from the Canary Islands east through Europe, Africa, and Asia, *Dinobdella,* found in Asia, and terrestrial species of *Haemadipsa,* found in Asia, Indonesia, Australia, Pacific Islands, and Central and South America. Humans are subject to attack by large leeches in tropical rain forests or infestation with aquatic species while wading or swimming.

Wounds produced by leeches are often painless and go unnoticed, except for the oozing blood or prolonged bleeding caused by an anticoagulant, hirudin. Pruritus is common at bite sites and although leeches are not known to transmit any human pathogens, secondary infections may occur. Immature aquatic leeches may be ingested with water and infest the upper respiratory and digestive tracts, or may invade the mouth, nose, eyes, vagina, urethra, or anus of swimmers.

Attachment of leeches to the nasal passages may cause epistaxis. Attachment to the larynx may cause hoarseness, dyspnea, and hemoptysis, and attachment to the pharynx or esophagus may cause dysphagia and hematemesis. Hemorrhaging from leech infestations may be so severe, especially in children, that anemia occurs that leads to death.

Techniques used for removing leeches from the respiratory and digestive tracts include a steady pull on the specimen with a forceps or hemostat, or narcotizing the leech with a spray of 5 per cent cocaine hydrochloride before removal. In genitourinary infestations, irrigation with a strong salt solution may cause the leeches to detach. A leech attached to skin, respiratory, or digestive tract surfaces may be induced to release its grip by holding it in a hemostat and touching the exposed part of the worm with a small flame or other cauterant.

Prevention of attack by aquatic and land leeches includes use of protective clothing and of insect repellents. Repellents applied to boots, trouser legs, and exposed skin are quite effective, but, because they are water soluble, must be reapplied every few hours in wet tropical regions where leeches are commonly found.

Keegan HL, Radke MG, Murphy DA: Nasal leech infestation in man. Am J Trop Med Hyg 19:1029, 1970. *This paper discusses two cases and reviews other clinical reports and treatment.*

425. SNAKE BITES

Jay P. Sanford

EPIDEMIOLOGY. Of the nearly 3500 species of snakes, fewer than one tenth are venomous. The poisonous varieties belong to five families (Table 425–1). Throughout the world, snake bites are estimated to account for 30,000 to 40,000 deaths annually. The largest number occur in Burma and Brazil. In the United States, the number of snakes bites is estimated at 8000 per year. Some 20 to 30 per cent of the bites by venomous snakes in the United States do not result in envenomation (poisoning). Most bites occur in the states bordering on the Gulf of Mexico. Despite the large number of bites with envenomation, fewer than 15 deaths occur and almost all of these are due to rattlesnake bites. This low case fatality ratio reflects the virtual absence of members of the species Elapidae and Hydrophidae in the United States.

Coral snakes, eastern and western varieties, are found in southern and western states (North Carolina, South Carolina, Georgia, Florida, Alabama, Mississippi, Louisiana, Arkansas, Texas, New Mexico, Arizona). Their fangs are short and permanently erect. They envenomate through chewing movements. Since they are nocturnal and shy, they rarely bite humans.

TABLE 425–1. VENOMOUS SNAKES OF THE WORLD

Family	Common Varieties	Geographic Distribution
Crotalidae	Pit vipers (rattlesnakes, water moccasins, copperheads), fer-de-lance, bushmaster	Americas, Asia
Elapidae	Cobras, kraits, mambas, coral snakes, death adder	Worldwide except Europe
Colubridae	Boomslangs, bird snakes	Africa
Hydrophidae	Sea snakes	Indo-Pacific waters
Viperidae	True vipers, puff adder	Worldwide except Americas

The pit vipers (Crotalidae) are identified by a small depression between the eyes and nostrils. Their fangs are long and hinged, folding back when the mouth is closed and erect when open. Upon contact, venom is expressed by muscular contraction. The pit vipers are generally aggressive. The eastern (*Crotalus adamanteus*) and western (*C. atrox*) diamondback rattlesnakes are the largest and most dangerous in the United States. Their distribution includes the aforementioned states plus California, Nevada, and Oklahoma. Cottonmouths (*Agkistrodon piscivorus*), or water moccasins, are found along streams in the southern and southeastern states. They may inflict facial bites when disturbed while resting on tree branches. Contrary to lore, they can bite under water. Copperheads (*A. contortrix*), or highland moccasins, have a geographic distribution similar to the cottonmouths. Their bite is painful but rarely fatal.

PATHOGENESIS. Snake venoms are probably the most complex of all poisons. Due to the heterogenous composition and multiplicity of effects, snake venoms cannot be classified simply as neurotoxic, cardiotoxic, or hematotoxic on the basis of the snake family (Table 425–2).

Venoms from Elapidae and Hydrophidae contain basic polypeptides that produce a nondepolarizing neuromuscular block with resultant flaccid paralysis including respiratory paralysis. Cobra cardiotoxin, an additional basic polypeptide, depolarizes cell membranes of skeletal, cardiac, and smooth muscles, thus contributing to paralysis. Venom of the South American rattlesnake contains an acidic protein with nondepolarizing curare-like neuromuscular blocking effects. Viperatoxin isolated from the Palestine viper causes a peripheral nerve conduction block. A variety of enzymes, mostly hydrolases and phospholipase A, are present in most venoms. Bradykinin is released from bradykininogen by most crotalid and viperid venoms but not by Elapidae except the king cobra (*Ophiophagus hannah*). The venom of a single snake seldom contains all of the toxins. The composition and potency of venom is highly variable and differs not only among species but even among individual snakes.

SYMPTOMS AND SIGNS. ***Pit Viper Envenomation.*** In the United States, most patients reach a physician within 15 minutes to 3 hours. At that time it is essential to determine whether or not envenomation has occurred and, if it has occurred, to determine the severity; this has important therapeutic implications. The clinical effects are summarized in Table 425–3. The most important early findings of envenomation are swelling at the bite, usually occurring within ten minutes, and pain, although pain may be absent. Mild envenomation is characterized by local edema (one to five inches in diameter) and pain without systemic symptoms or signs. With moderate enven-

TABLE 425–2. BIOCHEMISTRY OF SNAKE VENOMS

Toxins	Family	Mechanism of Injury-Death
Neurotoxin (basic polypeptide)	Elapidae, Hydrophidae, South American rattlesnake *(Crotalus durissus terrificus)*, Palestine viper *(Vipera palestinae)*	Respiratory paralysis
Cardiotoxin	Elapidae	Cardiovascular depression
Enzymes	Elapidae, Hydrophidae, Crotalidae, Viperidae	Hemolysis
Phospholipase A		
5-Nucleotidase		
Phosphodiesterase		
Deoxyribonuclease II		
Ribonuclease		
Adenosine-triphosphatase		
Nucleotide pyrophosphatase		
Exopeptidase		
Hyaluronidase	(Absent in spitting cobra)	
l Amino acidoxidase		
Proteases	Crotalidae, Viperidae	Hypotension due to release
Acetylcholinesterase	Elapidae (absent in spitting cobra, mamba, coral)	
Alkaline phosphatase		
Acid phosphatase		

omation, local findings are more extensive—edema of 6 to 12 inches in diameter. Systemic findings occur: weakness, sweating, nausea, faintness, dizziness, ecchymoses, and tender regional lymph nodes. With severe envenomation systemic involvement includes tachycardia; tachypnea; hypothermia; hypotension; ecchymoses; paresthesias of the scalp, finger and toe tips; and muscle fasciculations. With very severe envenomations, gingival bleeding, hematemesis, hematuria, melena, oliguria, and coma occur.

Over the first 12 hours, the skin develops a tense discolored appearance and bullae, which may be either serous or hemorrhagic.

Coral Snake Envenomation. The bite wound usually resembles scratch marks and is somewhat painful, but there is little or no edema. The onset of systemic manifestations is usually delayed one to six hours. Paresthesias around the bite may occur within several hours. Systemic symptoms may include weakness, apprehension, giddiness, nausea, vomiting, excess salivation, and even a sense of euphoria. Bulbar and cranial nerve paralysis may develop with ptosis, diplopia, papillary dilatation, excess salivation, dysphagia, dysphonation, and respiratory failure.

LABORATORY FINDINGS. Proteolytic enzymes in venoms produce not only tissue damage but have a marked effect on coagulation, thrombin-like activity being most prominent. Within the first few hours there is a drop in platelets due to local consumption (occasionally to less than 10,000 per cu ml), a decrease in fibrinogen, and an increase in fibrin degradation products. Striking increases in prothrombin time and partial thromboplastin time occur with severe envenomation. Erythrocytes show a peculiar "burring" indicating membrane damage, and drops in hematocrit and hemoglobin concentration occur.

With pit viper envenomation, baseline laboratory tests should include complete blood count, platelet count, prothrombin time, partial thromboplastin time, bleeding time, urinalysis, and serum electrolytes. Blood should be obtained for typing and cross matching. In patients with envenomation of moderate or greater severity arterial blood gas determinations and an electrocardiogram are indicated. Hematologic studies should be repeated every four to six hours for the first day or until the coagulopathy has stabilized. With coral snake envenomation, repetitive coagulation studies are not indicated.

TREATMENT. ***First Aid.*** In general, too much emphasis has been placed on first aid at the expense of delay in definitive hospital care. The snake should be killed if this can be done quickly and safely and taken along with the patient to allow accurate identification; this may obviate unnecessary therapy. The dead snake must be handled with care since the head of an apparently dead snake can deliver a venomous bite for up to an hour after being severed. The value of incision and suction (I and S) has been questioned. It has been stated that if I and S is begun within three minutes after subcutaneous envenomation, 22 to 50 per cent of injected venom can be removed. Recovery is much less after intramuscular envenomation and if I and S is delayed. As a practical matter, if the patient cannot reach definitive care (antivenin) within one and one-half hours, prompt I and S is appropriate. If more than 15 minutes have elapsed since a bite, I and S should not be performed. Mouth suction should be used only if no other method is available. In the absence of oral lesions, mouth suction poses no risk to the first aider because ingestion of venom is harmless; however, mouth suction does result in the equivalent of a human bite to the victim. If a constricting band (not a tourniquet) is used, it should be placed immediately proximal to the wound. Linear incisions, 1 cm long and no deeper than 3 mm, should be made over each fang mark. If I and S is not to be used, the Australian Serum Institute recommends application of a broad firm constrictive bandage immediately over the bite, then bandaging of as much of the limb as possible. The affected part should be immobilized (splinted) promptly and the patient transported to the nearest medical treatment facility. The affected area should not be placed on ice. Cryotherapy results in greater tissue damage with the potential for necessitating amputation.

Hospital Care. On admission it is important to determine, if possible, if the bite was inflicted by a pit viper or a coral snake and whether envenomation has occurred. The mainstay of therapy is antivenom (antivenin), which is a horse serum product; hence it has a high potential of causing serum sickness later. There are two antivenoms: one polyvalent for North American pit vipers and another for eastern coral snakes. For minor envenomation, antivenin is not indicated. For more serious envenomation, antivenin should be administered. For mild pit viper envenomation, three to five ampules of antivenin should be diluted (10 ml each), then added to 500 ml of

TABLE 425–3. PIT VIPER ENVENOMATION: SYMPTOMS AND SIGNS (PERCENTAGE)

Local		Systemic: *Generalized*		*Hematologic*		*Neuromuscular*	
Fang marks	100	Weakness	70	Thrombocytopenia	42	Paresthesia scalp, fingertips	63
Edema	74	Tachycardia	60	Increased clotting time	37	Faintness, dizziness	57
Pain	65	Hypotension	54	Decreased hemoglobin	37	Paresthesias of affected part	57
Vesicles	40	Sweating	43	Burring of RBC	18	Fasciculations	41
Necrosis	27	Nausea/vomiting	42	Thrombocytosis	16		
		Hypothermia	42	Bleeding	15		
		Tachypnea	40				
		Regional adenopathy	40				

Adapted from Russell, FE: Ann Rev Med 31:247, 1980.

intravenous fluid. The patient should be skin tested for horse serum hypersensitivity. If the skin test is negative, the 500 ml should be given intravenously over 60 minutes. If the amount is adequate, the swelling will not progress and paresthesias will decrease. If progression occurs, the dose should be repeated. For moderate envenomation 5 to 10 vials, for severe envenomation 10 to 20 vials, and for very severe envenomation up to 40 vials (400 ml) may be required. In one series, the average dose required for adults with severe bites was 16 vials. Larger doses are required for bites in children and for those involving the fingers. Antivenin neutralizes both the local and systemic effects of the venom.

In coral snake bites, if any symptoms or signs develop within the first several hours, 3 to 5 vials of antivenin (Micrurus fulvius) should be given intravenously. Even in the absence of symptoms, patients should be observed in the hospital for approximately 48 hours because onset of symptoms may be delayed and insidious.

Antibiotics are usually recommended. Bacteriologic cultures of rattlesnake venom and fangs show growth from over 90 per cent. Aerobic gram-negative bacilli (*Enterobacter* sp., *Pseudomonas* sp., and *Citrobacter* sp.) and histotoxic clostridia (*C. perfringens*) are the predominant isolates. On the basis of the microbiologic results, administration of one of the newer beta-lactam antibiotics, piperacillin or azlocillin, is most appropriate. Such agents would also be effective against the human bite wound. Although *Clostridium tetani* were not isolated and there are only one or two reports of tetanus following snake bite, a tetanus toxoid booster is recommended.

In the severely envenomated patient, concurrent supportive measures include the management of shock and respiratory and renal failure. Pharmacologic doses of glucocorticords comparable with those used in "endotoxic shock" have been recommended, but benefits have not been demonstrated. Despite the hypofibrinogenemia and elevation of fibrin degradation products, heparin is not of benefit. Attention to early recognition and management of anaphylaxis is essential.

Decompressive fasciotomy is indicated if edema within closed muscular compartments is inadequately controlled and arterial blood supply is compromised. From the end of the first to the third week the majority of patients will develop serum sickness, the prevalence approximating 1 per cent per milliliter of horse serum administered.

PROGNOSIS. If adequate antivenom was administered intravenously, mortality is virtually nil. If cryotherapy was avoided, amputation or serious resultant deformities are uncommon.

Jimenez-Porras JM: Biochemistry of snake venoms. Clin Toxicol 3:389, 1970. *A detailed review of the enzymatic and toxic properties of snake venoms with an extensive bibliography.*

Ledbetter EO, Kutscher AE: Aerobic and anaerobic flora of rattlesnake fangs and venom. Arch Environ Health 19:770, 1969. *This is the only study available that addresses the potential microbiologic contaminants in snake bite wounds. It provides a reasonable basis for antibiotic selection.*

Medical Letter: Treatment of snake bite in the USA. The Medical Letter 24:87, 1982. *The process utilized by the Medical Letter results in a consensus among consultants. This provides a necessary balanced view in light of the facts that differences of opinion exist as to ideal management and that the number of annual cases is too few and dispersed to allow a prospective therapy trial.*

Russell FE: Snake venom poisoning in the United States. Ann Rev Med 31:247, 1980. *An excellent general review by one of the foremost authorities on the subject in the United States. An excellent source of clinical features.*

Simon TL, Grace TG: Envenomation coagulopathy in wounds from pit vipers. N Engl J Med 305:443, 1981. *This study on experimental envenomation in rabbits enables a sequential assessment of the clotting abnormalities that occur.*

Walt CH Jr: Poisonous snakebite treatment in the United States. JAMA 240:654, 1978. *A report on an extensive personal clinical experience utilizing the treatment approaches recommended by the Medical Letter.*

426. VENOMOUS AND POISONOUS* MARINE ANIMALS

John Williamson

The world's seas contain a formidable array of venomous and poisonous marine creatures capable of harming or even

killing the human intruder. The story of their relationship to humankind dates from antiquity but their scientific study remains relatively neglected; for example, about 95 per cent of known marine biotoxins have scarcely been examined for their biological activity. The animals are found in greatest variety and profusion in warmer tropical and subtropical waters—the very seas that attract human activities. Communities dependent on the seas as a food source or as a tourist attraction are typically foremost in studying the subject. Current research is being conducted in Australia, French Polynesia, Japan, and the United States (including Hawaii). Although the subject has now emerged from the realm of folklore, lack of objectivity still causes misconceptions. Human injury by venomous marine creatures results from accidental or intentional human interference with the animal or its territory.

Taxonomic Classification

Taxonomic classification is customary but is of limited practical value to those responsible for treatment and prevention of marine envenomation. The animals listed in Table 426–1 have accounted for the majority of human deaths and a significant number of the poisonings and injuries that are documented to date.

Animals Causing Human Fatalities

Table 426–1 lists invertebrates and vertebrates that cause fatalities by envenomation, and those animals responsible for fatal poisonings in humans.

BOX JELLYFISH. The box jellyfish (*Chironex fleckeri*), the world's only coelenterate known to be lethal to humans, has been responsible for 71 documented human deaths since 1884; many more reports remain unconfirmed. Found only in tropical West Indo-Pacific waters, it is a true jellyfish, carrying up to 60 extendable tentacles. These tentacles bear a vast number of nematocysts (stinging capsules, microbasic mastigophores) that discharge massively when a person blunders into them and becomes entangled. The animal is almost impossible to see under natural conditions. This massive envenomation produces rapid systemic absorption that is enhanced by struggling, and collapse occurs within minutes in serious cases. Seventy per cent of fatalities occur in women and children (small body mass and hairless skin). The venom is a high molecular weight protein mixture containing "lethal" and dermatonecrotic factors. The densely adherent tentacles produce whip wheals with a diagnostic ladder pattern on the envenomated skin. Treatment is immediate resuscitation on the beach, vinegar dousing, compressive bandaging, and injection of the specific antivenom, intravenously if possible, in a dosage large enough to be effective. The antivenom is sheep antiserum; therefore, appropriate precautions are necessary.

BLUE-RINGED OCTOPUS. At least two species (*Hapalochlaena maculosa* and *H. lunulata*) have produced morbidity and mortality. The venom is located in the salivary glands and is

TABLE 426–1. MARINE ANIMALS CAUSING HUMAN FATALITIES

I. From Envenomation
   A. Invertebrates
      1. Box jellyfish (*Chironex fleckeri*)
      2. Blue-ringed octopuses (Family *Octopodidae*)
      3. Venomous cone shells (Family *Conidae*)
   B. Vertebrates
      1. Venomous sea snakes (Family *Hydrophiidae*)
      2. Scorpionfishes, including stonefishes (Family *Scorpaenidae*)
      3. Catfish (Suborder *Siluroidei*)
      4. Stingrays (Order *Rajiformes*)
II. From Poisoning
   A. Ciguatoxic fishes
   B. Tetrodotoxic fishes
   C. Shellfish
   D. Sea turtles
   E. Viscera of whales, porpoises, polar bears, walruses, seals

*The currently held view is that the administration of venoms requires mechanical penetration, whereas the term poison implies oral ingestion. The term toxins (here marine zootoxins) refers to both venoms and poisons.

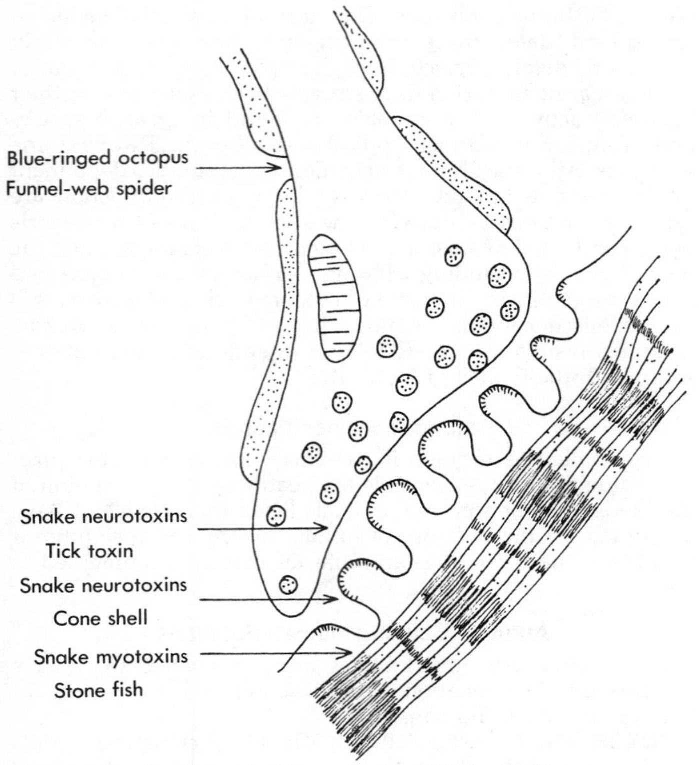

Figure 426–1. Scheme of a somatic neuromuscular junction, showing sites of action of a number of animal toxins (Courtesy of Dr. V. Callanan, Townsville).

injected by a bite that may be painless. The salivary toxin contains tetrodotoxin (M.W. 319), a unique biological material also found in the flesh of puffer fish (see below). It inhibits action potentials (Fig. 426–1) by specific blockade of sodium ion transport, and is thus in addition a valuable physiologic research tool. Clinically the danger is respiratory failure and hypoxia. Airway protection and expired air resuscitation will be life saving. There is no antivenom. First aid is as for snakebite (see Ch. 425).

VENOMOUS CONE SHELLS. There are 37 cases of cone shell envenomation in the literature, eight of them fatalities. Seven species of cone shells are considered dangerous. The injected venom produces postsynaptic neuromuscular blockade (Fig. 426–1) and thus death from hypoxia (respiratory failure). On-the-spot airway protection and expired air resuscitation will be life saving. No antivenom presently exists, but research is promising. First aid is identical to that for snakebite (see Ch. 425).

VENOMOUS SEA SNAKES. Apart from their predominance in warmer waters, the proven lethality of several species, and the availability of a specific antivenom (*Enhydrina schistosa* antivenom), the subject of sea snakebite can be considered in the same manner as land snakebite (see Ch. 425).

SCORPIONFISHES AND STONEFISHES. Deaths from zebrafish stings have been documented. No firm record of a fatality caused by stonefish (*Synanceja*) stings has been located from Australia, where these stings are not uncommon. In this group of animals dorsal spines inject the venom. The ensuing pain is a devastating experience, with intense local tissue swelling and discoloration. Immersion of the envenomated part in hot water offers partial pain relief. Medical management is concerned with pain relief (conduction anesthesia), prevention of wound infection, and in the case of stonefish stings specific antivenom injection with appropriate precautions. Tourniquets or compressive bandages should not be used.

CATFISH AND STINGRAYS. Despite their ubiquity, these animals rarely cause human death. A full account of their injuring and envenomating capabilities is given by Halstead (1978). Pieces of the brittle stingray spines not infrequently break off in wounds, necessitating careful exploration under anesthesia.

CIGUATERA (POISONING BY FISH IN THE TROPICS). This occurs in all tropical and subtropical seas and is a major public health and economic problem in the Pacific. About 1500 cases of ciguatera poisoning occur annually in the South Pacific alone. Deaths have been reported. The hoped-for simple chemical test of fish flesh to reveal the presence of ciguatoxin has not yet been developed. The most common symptoms are gastrointestinal (nausea, abdominal pain, vomiting, and diarrhea) and peripheral neurologic (paresthesiae, especially circumoral and intraoral, dental discomfort, and a classic reversal of peripheral temperature sense; that is, hot feels cold and vice versa). Ciguatoxin is believed to be passed along in the food chain, and at least one source has been traced to a dinoflagellate, *Gambierdiscus toxicus*. There is no antidote and treatment is symptomatic. Symptoms can persist for months. The chemical structure of ciguatoxin remains to be elucidated.

TETRODOTOXIC FISHES. These include toad fish and puffer fish. Ingestion of the toxin in the fish flesh produces symptoms and signs characteristic of tetrodotoxin's action potential blockade (Fig. 426–1), viz.: numbness, motor weakness, ataxia, and respiratory failure. Tetrodotoxin is one of the most toxic of known poisons and is the active component in blue-ringed octopus envenomation (see above). There is no specific antidote, so management of a patient is symptomatic.

SHELLFISH POISONING. Paralytic shellfish poisoning is due to the ingestion of saxitoxin and is associated with a fatality rate of about 8.5 per cent. This condition should be distinguished from the gastrointestinal and the allergic types of shellfish poisoning. Like ciguatoxin (see above), saxitoxin is thought to originate in dinoflagellate organisms, at the beginning of the marine food chain. Treatment is symptomatic. No specific antidote is known.

WHALES, PORPOISES, POLAR BEARS, WALRUSES, AND SEALS. Poisoning results from the ingestion of the viscera of these animals, notably liver or kidneys. The intoxication from such organs of polar bears, walruses, and seals is believed to be due to hypervitaminosis A.

Some Nonfatal Envenomations (Table 426–1)

These have occurred from true jellyfish (Class *Scyphozoa*), including *Carybdeid medusae* and the "hydroids" (Class *Hydrozoa*), including *Physalia* species (bluebottle, Portuguese man o'war), sea nettle (*Chrysaora quinquecirrha*), and mauve stinger (*Pelagia noctiluca*). Others have included corals and anemones (Class *Anthozoa*), and toxic sponges (Class *Demospongiae*).

A vast array of marine animals continues to be involved in less serious human envenomations, ranging from mild local itching to serious allergic manifestations. Certain treatment principles are becoming established.

1. Household vinegar inactivates undischarged nematocysts of several species of jellyfish (*Physalia, "Irukandji," Carybdia tamoya*, and *Cyanea*). Vinegar does nothing for the pain of the sting.

2. In general, ethyl alcohol should not be applied to marine stings.

3. Allergic phenomena can play a significant role in some marine envenomations such as jellyfish stings and toxic sponge contacts.

4. Immediate pain relief continues to be a problem. Local cooling (ice) helps in some jellyfish stings.

Bowerman M: Joint research on ciguatera. South Pacif Undw Med Soc J July to September: 24, 1980. *A useful summary of current research findings from the major centers in the Pacific.*

Burnett JW, Cobbs CS, Kelman SN, Calton GJ: Studies on the serologic response to jellyfish envenomation. J Am Acad Dermatol 9:229, 1983. *A controlled investigation of allergic reactions to sea nettle and Portuguese man-of-war stings.*

Edmonds C: Dangerous Marine Animals of the Indo-Pacific Region. Newport, New South Wales, Wedneil Publications, 1975. *A readable and well-illustrated overview of the subject.*

Halstead BW: Paralytic shellfish poisoning guide. Geneva, WHO Publication, 1982. *A good review of the subject.*

Halstead BW: Poisonous and Venomous Marine Animals of the World; Revised Edition. Princeton, Darwin Press, 1978. *The classic and encyclopedic reference text on the subject; an essential starting point.*

Hartwick R, Callanan V, Williamson J: Disarming the box jellyfish. Nematocyst inhibition in *Chironex fleckeri*. Med J Aust 1:15, 1980. *Demonstrates the value of vinegar and the problems of alcohol application in the first aid treatment of box jellyfish stings.*

Sutherland SK: Australian Animal Toxins. Melbourne, Australia, Oxford University Press, 1983. *This detailed and profusely illustrated work is the most recent hallmark in the subject of animal envenomation and poisoning, both marine and terrestrial. Destined to become a classic work. The definitive work on snake and spider bite management.*

Torda TA: Tetrodotoxic fish—clinical management. *In* Sutherland SK: Australian Animal Toxins. Cambridge, Oxford University Press, 1983, pp 458–459. *A recent update on a potentially dangerous clinical situation.*

Williamson J: Some Australian Marine Stings, Envenomations and Poisonings. 3nd ed., Brisbane, Surf Life Saving Association of Australia, Queensland State Centre, 1984. *A concise illustrated account at the level of first aiders and paramedics.*

Williamson JA, Callanan VI, Hartwick RF: Serious envenomation by the Northern Australian box jellyfish (*Chironex fleckeri*). Med J Aust 1:13, 1980. *A fully documented account of a near fatal sting that deals with all aspects of management.*

Part XXI
DISEASES OF THE IMMUNE SYSTEM

427. INTRODUCTION: THE IMMUNE SYSTEM

William E. Paul

The immune system consists of the recirculating pool of *lymphocytes* and *monocytes* and of cells in the bone marrow and in the organized lymphoid tissues, including the *lymph nodes, spleen, Peyer's patches,* and the *thymus*. The principal cells that comprise this system are the *B* and *T lymphocytes* and cells of the *monocyte-macrophage* lineage. These cells and their products, most notably *antibodies* and *lymphokines,* are responsible for the protective immunity that is so critical for survival of humans in the sea of potentially pathogenic microorganisms in which we live. The consequences of the failure to make an immune response or of major dysfunction in the immune system is graphically and tragically demonstrated by the fate of infants with severe combined immunodeficiency disease or of adults with acquired immune deficiency syndrome.

The immune response is initiated by introduction of an immunogenic substance into an immunocompetent individual. Such immunization results in activation and proliferation of T and B lymphocytes, which bear membrane receptors specific for antigenic determinants (epitopes) on the immunogen. This leads to the selective expansion of clones of specific lymphocytes that initially represented a very small fraction of the total lymphocyte population.

Stimulated B lymphocytes differentiate into antibody-secreting cells, of which plasma cells are a major morphologic type. Antibody-secreting cells produce *immunoglobulin* (Ig) molecules with antigen-combining sites that are identical to the antigen-combining sites of the membrane receptors expressed on their B lymphocyte progenitors. Ig's exist in a series of structurally distinct classes, including IgM, IgD, IgG, IgA, and IgE. Each of these types of Ig molecules has a distinctive function.

Stimulated T lymphocytes may differentiate into effector cells, such as specific cytotoxic T lymphocytes. Other members of the T cell population play critical roles in regulation of the immune system. Among these regulatory cells are *helper* T lymphocytes, which interact with B lymphocytes and aid them to develop into antibody-secreting cells, and *suppressor* T cells, which inhibit immune responses, principally by diminishing the action of helper T cells.

The negative regulatory aspects of the immune system, as exemplified by suppressor cells, are necessary to prevent the uncontrolled growth of individual B or T cells that might result as a consequence of continued antigenic stimulation. An equally critical need of the immune system is to limit the production of antibodies specific for *self* antigenic determinants and the appearance of effector T lymphocytes with self-specificity. Lymphocytes potentially capable of such self-specific responses are eliminated or their activation inhibited by the establishment of immunologic tolerance. Disorders in immunoregulation or of tolerance induction are a major feature of autoimmune diseases, such as systemic lupus erythematosus.

This Introduction will serve to describe briefly the principal cell types that participate in the immune response, the means through which these cells are activated, how they communicate with one another, the nature of the antibodies and other soluble products that they secrete, and how these cells mediate their immunologic functions.

B LYMPHOCYTES

B lymphocytes are precursors of antibody-secreting cells. They are found in all of the peripheral lymphoid tissues and in the recirculating pool of lymphocytes. In lymph nodes, B cells are mainly located in primary follicles within the subcapsular cortex. B cells bear membrane receptors through which they recognize foreign antigens. These receptors are Ig molecules, mainly of the IgM and IgD classes, that are specialized for expression within membranes. All of the membrane receptors of any individual B cell have the same binding specificity. When these cells differentiate into antibody-secreting cells, they produce antibodies with specificity identical to that of the membrane Ig (mIg) of the B cells. Thus, the extremely large number of distinct antibodies that may be produced in the course of immune responses represents the existence of a correspondingly large number of antibody-secreting cells, each of which produces antibody of only a single specificity.

ONTOGENY, MOLECULAR GENETICS, AND DIVERSITY OF B LYMPHOCYTES. B lymphocytes are derived from hematopoietic stem cells. These cells are found in embryonic life within the blood islands of the yolk sac, later in gestation within the liver, and in postnatal life principally within the bone marrow. The earliest identifiable member of the B lymphocyte lineage is the *pre-B* cell. This cell lacks mIg, but expresses in its cytoplasm one of the two constituent polypeptide chains of IgM molecules, the μ heavy (H) chain. Early pre-B cells rapidly cycle, but more mature pre-B cells are small and quiescent.

Within pre-B cells a series of remarkable genetic translocations occur, involving the genes coding for both of the polypeptide chains of Ig's (H and light [L] chains). Both H and L chains consist of amino-terminal regions, which are highly variable and which form the walls of the antigen-combining sites of Ig's, and of carboxy-terminal regions, which, for a given H chain class or L chain type, are essentially constant, except for allotypic variation (Fig. 427–1). These regions are designated the variable (V) and constant (C) regions of the H and L chains respectively. The H chain V region is encoded by three distinct genes, the *V, D,* and *J* genes (Fig. 427–2). In the germline DNA and in DNA of nonlymphoid cells, the H chain *V, D,* and *J* genes, which are on chromosome 14, are widely separated from one another, but in the course of pre-B cell development, two separate translocation events occur that bring these genes together to produce a single *VDJ* gene. This *VDJ* gene specifies an individual H chain V region. Germline DNA contains a large number (~300) of distinct V genes, a large but not yet determined number of *D* genes, and four functional *J* genes. It appears that these genes can be randomly combined, making possible the formation of a large number, probably more than 10,000, *VDJ* genes simply by combinatorial association. Furthermore, there are opportunities for somatic genetic changes, both in the translocation process and due to mutation and gene conversion events, so that the actual number of distinct *VDJ* genes that may be formed is much greater. Within any individual cell, only one functional set of *VDJ* translocation events appears to occur. The *VDJ* gene is initially assembled near the gene encoding the μ constant region (*Igh-C*μ gene). This leads to the expression within pre-B cells of μ H chains.

The L chain V region is also constructed by the translocation of distinct genes. L chain V regions are encoded by *V* and *J* genes, which are brought into apposition with one another; no *D* gene exists for L chains. L chains are of two different types, κ and λ. The *V* and *J* genes for κ (V_κ and J_κ) as well as the gene for the κ constant region (C_κ) are found on chromosome 2. The comparable λ genes (V_λ, J_λ, and C_λ) are on chromosome 22.

Translocation of H chain *V, D,* and *J* genes appears to precede translocation of L chain *V* and *J* genes; V_κ, J_κ translocation appears to precede translocation of V_λ, J_λ. In general, if V_κ and J_κ translocation events are successful and lead to an active κ gene, λ gene translocation events are not observed. Thus, an individual cell expresses only κ or λ chains but not both. Furthermore, a set of translocation events leading to the formation of active H or L chain genes generally occurs on only one of the two allelic chromosomes that specify H or L chains.

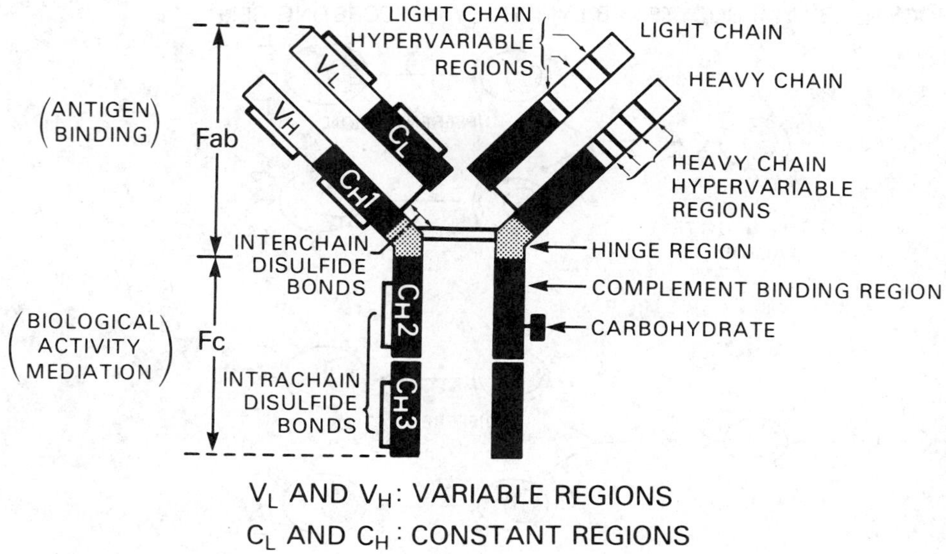

Figure 427–1. Structure of an Ig molecule. A schematic representation of an IgG molecule indicating the chain and domain structure of the molecule and the existence of hypervariable regions within variable regions of both H and L chains. *Fab* and *Fc* refer to fragments of the IgG molecule formed by papain cleavage. The former contains the V_H and C_{HI} H chain regions and an intact L chain; the latter consists of C_{H2} and C_{H3} region of two H chains, linked to one another by disulfide bonds. (From Wasserman RL, Capra JD: Immunoglobulins. *In* Horowitz MI, Pigman W (eds.): The Glycoconjugates. New York, Academic Press, 1977, pp 323–348.)

Thus, Ig H and L chains produced by any individual cell are derived from only one of the allelic chromosomes, resulting in the phenomenon of *allelic exclusion*.

The completion of functional H and L chain genetic translocation within a pre-B cell is associated with the appearance of mIg on the surface of the cell and thus with the differentiation of the pre-B cell into a B cell. Immature B cells express mIg only of the IgM class. As these cells mature further, they also express mIgD. This expression of mIgD, in addition to mIgM, by developing B cells appears to be associated with acquisition of new immune functions, such as resistance to tolerance induction and responsiveness to polysaccharide antigens.

Mature B cells express a series of other markers that have potential functional significance. These include receptors for the Fc portions of Ig's (*Fc receptors*), receptors for complement components (i.e., for the C3b and C3d fragments of C3), and class II *major histocompatibility complex* (MHC) molecules. (A complete discussion of the MHC is found in Ch. 436.) Although the precise physiologic roles of Fc and C3 receptors are still uncertain, class II MHC molecules on B cells are involved in the process by which helper T cells recognize and interact with B cells in the course of B cell responses to antigenic stimulation.

The events in pre-B cell and B cell development described thus far are antigen independent. Subsequent events in B cell development appear to require antigenic stimulation or stimulation by soluble factors made by antigen–activated T cells.

CONTROL OF B CELL RESPONSES. Resting, mature B cells can be activated as a result of cross-linkage of their membrane receptors by antigen or by anti-Ig antibodies (Fig. 427–3). B cells may also be activated by mitogenic agents such as the Cowan I strain of *Staphylococcus aureus*, bacterial lipopolysaccharide, and dextran sulfate. Responses to anti-Ig antibodies and to other mitogens are often used to assess B cell function. B cells activated by cross-linkage of their receptors enter the S phase of the cell cycle and then divide upon stimulation by a T cell-derived–B cell growth factor, now designated B cell stimulatory factor (BSF)-p1. This process also depends upon the presence of a macrophage-derived factor, *interleukin-1* (IL-1). B cells that are activated by receptor cross-linkage and that then proliferate following the action of BSF-p1 and IL-1 develop

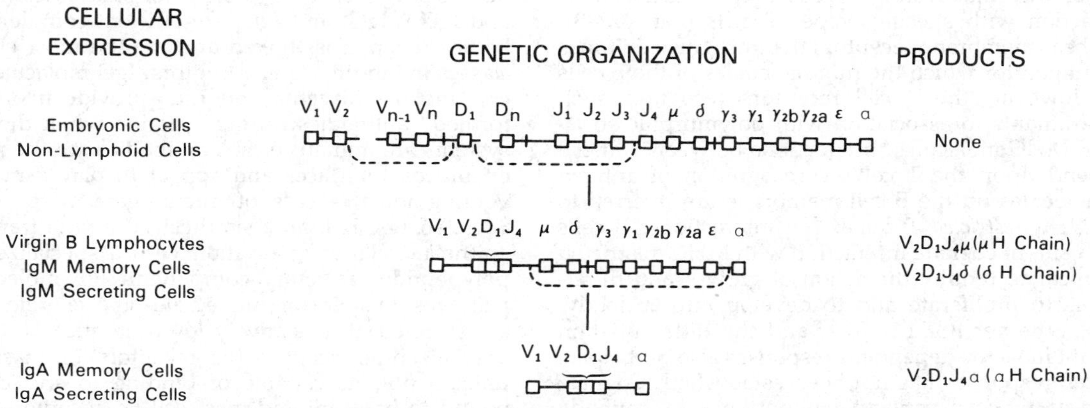

Figure 427–2. Organization and translocation of Ig genes. Immunoglobulin H chains are encoded by four distinct genetic elements: *Igh-V(V)*, *Igh-D(D)*, *Igh-J(J)*, and *Igh-C* genes. The *V*, *D*, and *J* genes together specify the variable region of the H chain. The Igh-C gene specifies the C region. The same V region can be found in association with each of the C regions (e.g., in the mouse, μ, δ, γ3, γ1, γ2b, γ2a, ε, and α). A generally similar situation exists for human C region genes, but these genes have not been precisely ordered. In the germline genome, the *V*, *D*, and *J* genes are far apart, and there are multiple forms of each of these genes. In the course of lymphocyte development, a *VDJ* gene complex is found by translocation of individual *V* and *D* genes so that they lie next to one of the *J* genes, with the excision of intervening genes. This *VDJ* complex is initially expressed with μ and δ C genes, but may be subsequently translocated so that it lies near one of the other C genes (e.g., α) and in that case leads to the expression of a VDJα chain. (From Paul WE: The immune system: An introduction. *In* Paul WE (ed): Fundamental Immunology. New York, Raven Press, 1984, p 8.)

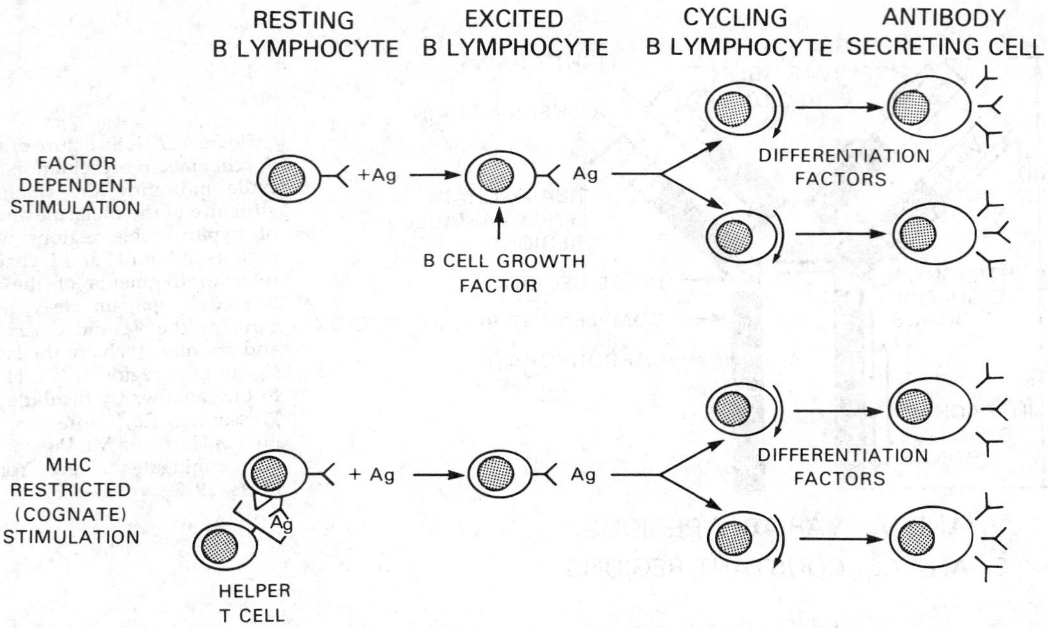

Figure 427–3. B cell stimulation. Resting B cells may be stimulated to proliferate and then to differentiate by two distinct mechanisms. One mechanism is designated factor-dependent activation. In this pathway, resting B cells are activated to an excited, or G_1, state by the action of agents that appropriately cross-link their receptors. Excited cells are acted upon by soluble factors, including B cell growth factor, and enter the S phase. Differentiation factors act upon these cells to cause them to synthesize and secrete Ig. The second major pathway involves the interaction of "histocompatibility-restricted" helper T cells with resting B cells. These T cells recognize antigen and class II molecules on the B cell surface and stimulate the cell to enter an excited state. This activation pathway is often designated cognate activation. The subsequent progress of the excited B cell may depend upon further interaction with helper T cells or soluble factors. Differentiation factors are probably necessary for differentiation of these into cells secreting Ig.

into antibody-secreting cells as a result of the action of B cell differentiation factors. This pathway of B cell responsiveness, which is controlled by the sequential action of a series of soluble T cell and macrophage products (lymphokines), is sometimes referred to as *factor-dependent* stimulation. Although detailed studies of the physiologic significance of factor-dependent activation in in vivo immune responses of humans have not yet been carried out, it seems most likely that it is mainly responsible for antibody responses to polysaccharides and to a related set of antigens designated type II antigens. Factor-dependent B cell stimulation would thus be critical to the development of immunity to the capsular polysaccharides of many pyogenic microorganisms, such as *Streptococcus pneumoniae*.

An additional way that resting B cells may be activated is through interaction with specific helper T cells (Fig. 427–3). Helper T cells bear membrane receptors that recognize epitopes on the same antigen for which the mIg molecules of the B cells are specific. However, the T cell receptors recognize such antigenic determinants in association with polymorphic structures of class II MHC molecules. Interactions between T and B cells that depend upon the T cell's corecognition of antigen and class II molecules on the B cell membrane are referred to as *cognate* or *MHC restricted* T cell–B cell interactions. B cells activated as a result of cognate interaction with MHC–restricted T cells also appear to require the action of growth and differentiation factors to proliferate and to develop into antibody-secreting cells. Whether BSF-p1, IL-1, and the differentiation factors important in factor-dependent responses also participate in cognate B cell responses has not been established. Cognate responses appear to be of principal importance in antibody responses to protein antigens.

IMMUNOGLOBULINS. Antibodies are Ig molecules. They exist in a series of classes that, as already noted, have distinct functions. Ig's are composed of one or more units, each of which consists of two identical H and two identical L chains. Both H chain and L chain polypeptides are divisible into a series of regions of 100 to 110 amino acids in length (Fig. 427–1). L chains consist of two such regions, an amino-terminal V region and a single carboxy-terminal C region. H chains consist of a V region and three or four C regions (C_{H1}, C_{H2}, . . .), depending on H chain class. Some classes of Ig's also have a hinge region, imparting segmental flexibility to the molecule. Hinge regions are located between C_{H1} and C_{H2} regions. The Ig's that consist of more than one unit of 2H and 2L chains (pentameric IgM and polymeric IgA) also contain one J chain per polymeric Ig molecule; the J chain is critical to maintaining such Ig's in their polymer form.

The various Ig classes have distinct functional properties (Table 427–1). IgM, in its membrane form, is one of the principal membrane receptors of B cells. In its secreted form and when cross-linked by antigen, IgM activates complement and thus is important in lysis and opsonization of bacteria and other foreign particles. IgG exists in a series of subclasses (IgG_1, IgG_2, IgG_3, and IgG_4). IgG_3 and IgG_1 are efficient complement-fixing antibodies when cross-linked and are the most efficient IgG subclasses in binding to Fc receptors. IgG molecules are capable of crossing the placenta and thus provide neonates with "preformed" antibodies during a period when their own immune systems are immature. IgA antibodies are the major Ig's found on mucosal surfaces and appear to play a major role in preventing initial access of microorganism to portals of entry. Secreted IgA is locally synthesized and is tranported through epithelial cells in association with a specialized 70,000-dalton polypeptide, secretory component. IgE molecules are principally responsible for immediate-type allergic reactions. They are secreted at a relatively low rate and are tightly bound to specialized Fc receptors (Fc_ϵ receptors) on mast cells and basophils. Antigens capable of binding to and cross-linking IgE bound to basophil and mast cell Fc_ϵ receptors cause the rapid release of vasoactive amines and other mediators from such cells; this mediator release is responsible for allergic and *anaphylactic* responses. IgD, as already mentioned, functions almost exclusively as a membrane receptor. Although it is secreted in small amounts, no specific function has been identified for IgD as a secretory Ig.

The initial Ig's expressed by any cell are mIgM and mIgD. The descendants of such cells may secrete antibody of any of

TABLE 427–1. PROPERTIES OF HUMAN IMMUNOGLOBULINS

	IgG	IgA	IgM	IgD	IgE
H chain class	γ	α	μ	δ	ε
H chain subclass	γ1,γ2,γ3,γ4	α1,α2	μ1,μ2		
L chain type	κ and λ	κ and λ	κ and λ	κ and λ	κ and λ
Molecular formula	γ_2L_2	α_2L_2* or $(\mu_2L_2)_2$SC†J‡	$(\mu_2L_2)_5$J‡	δ_2L_2	ϵ_2L_2
Molecular weight (approximate)	150,000	160,000 400,000§	900,000	180,000	190,000
Complement fixation (classic)	+	0	+ +	0	0
Serum concentration (approximate; mg/dl)	1,000	200	120	3	0.05
Serum half-life (days)	23	6	5	2–8	1–5
Placental transfer	+	0	0	0	0
Reaginic activity	?	0	0	0	+ +

*Monomeric serum IgA; † secretory component; ‡ J chain; § secretory IgA.
Adapted from Goodman JW: Immunoglobulins, I. *In* Stites DP, Stobo JD, Fudenberg HHY, Wells JV (eds.): Basic and Clinical Immunology. Los Altos, Lange Medical Publications, 1982, p 34.

the other Ig classes. Such Ig possesses the same V region as did the mIg of the progenitor B cell. The change in Ig class expression that occurs during B cell differentiation is known as "switching" and is dependent on a genetic translocation event, in which the chromosomal segment containing the assembled *VDJ* gene is moved from its location proximal to the C_μ gene into a new position proximal to the *C* gene for the Ig H chain constant region that will be expressed by the cell (i.e., $C_{\gamma1}$, $C_{\gamma2}$, $C_{\gamma3}$, $C_{\gamma4}$, C_α, C_ϵ) (Fig. 427–2).

T LYMPHOCYTES

T cells mediate both effector and regulatory functions. In general, these distinct functions are mediated by separate subpopulations of T cells. The principal T cell effector functions are the destruction of antigen-bearing target cells by specific "killer" T cells and the production of potent mediators. These mediators are responsible for induction of a variety of inflammatory phenomena, such as delayed-type hypersensitivity that is associated with activation of macrophages and with the chemotaxis of granulocytes and monocytes.

As regulatory cells, T cells function in a variety of distinct ways. They produce *interleukin-2* (IL-2), the T cell growth factor, which is critical to the development of cytotoxic T cell responses. They act as helper cells, collaborating with B cells and enabling them to produce antibodies to thymus-dependent antigens. Helper T cells play an important role in determining the class and idiotype of antibody produced in an immune response. A separate set of regulatory T cells, the suppressor T cells, inhibits both antibody synthesis and cell-mediated immune responses, including delayed-type hypersensitivity.

T lymphocytes can be identified and quantitated because they bear specific membrane molecules that can be detected with *monoclonal antibodies.* (Monoclonal antibodies are homogeneous populations of antibody molecules, generally produced by somatic cell hybrids between activated normal B cells and a plasmacytoma cell line. Such hybrids are referred to as hybridomas.) All peripheral human T cells bear a determinant recognized by the monoclonal antibodies OKT3 and Leu 4. This determinant is borne on a membrane molecule that appears to play an important role in the process through which T cells are activated. Mature T cells may be subdivided into two major groups, recognized by distinct monoclonal antibodies, OKT4 and OKT8. T4-positive cells generally include helper T cells, and T8-positive cells include cytotoxic and suppressor T cells, although exceptions to this generalization exist. Measurement of the numbers of T cells in each of these subpopulations and their responsiveness to several mitogenic lectins, such as phytohemagglutinin (PHA), concanavalin A (con A), and pokeweed mitogen (PWM), provides a convenient *initial* means to assess certain aspects of T cell function. More specific and complex in vitro assays can be performed to measure helper and suppressor function.

T CELL DEVELOPMENT. T cells originate from hematopoietic stem cells. In contrast to B cells, T cell precursors undergo critical aspects of their differentiation in a specific central lymphoid organ, the thymus (Fig. 427–4). T cell precursors enter the thymus where an extensive series of proliferative events occurs and in which these cells develop into mature, antigen-reactive T cells that are seeded into the peripheral lymphoid tissue. Much of the functional repertoire of possible T cell responses seems to be formed within the thymus. T cell receptors have a complex specificity pattern. Their receptors corecognize epitopes of foreign antigens in association with structures on class I or class II MHC molecules. These structures on MHC molecules are designated *histotopes.* A single T cell receptor molecule recognizes an epitope-histotope complex.

The mature T cells of an individual are principally specific for antigenic epitopes in association with the histotopes expressed on the individual's own class I or class II MHC molecules. This corecognition of antigen with *self*-MHC molecules is often referred to as *histocompatibility restriction* (Fig. 427–5). It appears that the intrathymic selection events that shape the T cell repertoire are based on the capacity of developing thymocytes to recognize histotopes of self-class I or class II MHC molecules on thymic epithelial cells or thymic macrophages. Such events lead to the development of mature populations of T cells that have partial specificity for self-MHC molecules. It also appears that tolerance to many self-antigens may be established within the thymus.

Upon leaving the thymus, T cells are found in all the peripheral lymphoid tissues and in the blood and lymph.

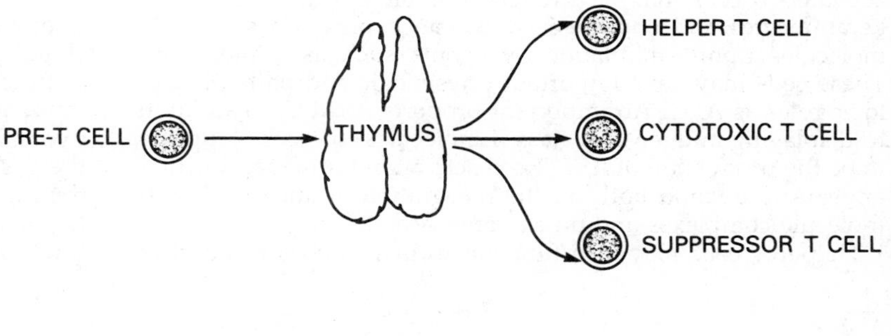

Figure 427–4. T cell differentiation. Precursors of T cells found in the hematopoietic tissue enter the thymus where they undergo differentiation and emerge into the periphery as cells of distinct function, bearing markers that allow their characterization. Whether a single pre-T cell can develop into each of the three T cell lines illustrated here or whether there are distinct sets of pre-T cells has not yet been elucidated.

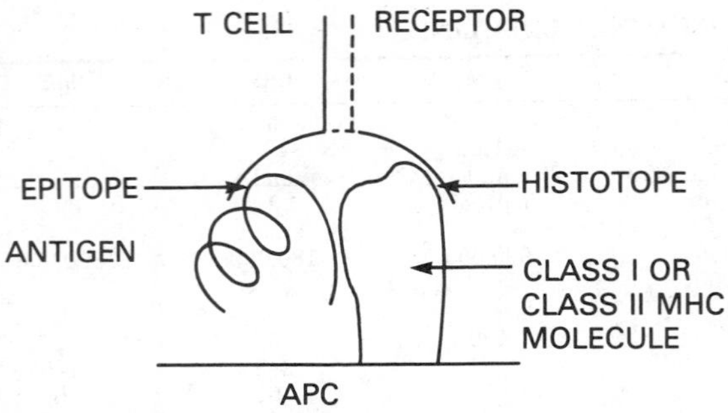

Figure 427–5. Corecognition of epitopes and histotopes by "MHC-restricted" T cell receptors. T cells that express histocompatibility-restriction in their interactions with B cells and macrophages have a complex antigen recognition system. These cells corecognize an antigenic determinant on a foreign molecule (an epitope) and a site on a self-MHC molecule (a histotope). Helper T cells generally corecognize epitopes with histotopes of class II MHC molecules. Cytotoxic T cells and their precursors generally corecognize epitopes with histopes of class I MHC molecules. The antigen recognition element of the T cell may be a single receptor with specificity for both the epitope and the histotope, or it may be two linked receptors, one specific for the epitope, the other for the histotope.

Within lymph nodes they tend to be principally found in the paracortex.

ANTIGEN-RECOGNITION BY T CELLS. Identification and characterization of the nature of the T cell receptor for antigen have been major goals of modern immunology. Recent work has provided very substantial insights into the nature of the T cell receptor. Monoclonal antibodies specific for unique structures on T cell clones block T cell activation by antigen. These antibodies, when polymerized onto polyacrylamide beads, can stimulate responses by the T cell clones for which they are specific. Such antibodies, designated *clonotypic* antibodies, appear to recognize epitopes on the antigen-binding receptors of T cells. The receptor molecule is a disulfide-linked heterodimer, consisting of two distinct chains (α chains and β chains), each of ~40,000 daltons. Both the α and β chains contain constant and variable peptides, suggesting that they may have a structure generally similar to immunoglobulins. A recently obtained complementary DNA clone appears to specify one of the two constituent polypeptide chains of the receptor. Detailed knowledge of the structure of the T cell receptor and of the genetic basis of antigen-binding repertoire of T cells will probably become available during the next several years.

HELPER T CELLS. Helper T cells play a critical role in antibody responses to many antigens. They provide B cells with critical signals enabling them to respond to typical protein antigens. As discussed in Control of B Cell Responses, T cells may help B cell responses in several ways. Cognate T cell help depends upon the corecognition by T cells of antigen bound to the B cell as a result of interaction with its receptor, and of histotopes of class II MHC molecules. The activation of helper T cells for this purpose is most efficiently achieved by their interaction with specialized *antigen-presenting cells* (APC), which take up antigen nonspecifically and which express class II molecules. Macrophages, epidermal Langerhan's cells, and dendritic cells appear to be important APC, but evidence is growing that activated B cells may also function as effective APC. Indeed, keratinocytes and endothelial cells can express class II MHC molecules upon stimulation by agents such as γ-interferon. These cells may have important physiologic and pathophysiologic roles as APC. An important property of APC, in addition to displaying antigen and class II molecules to T cells, appears to be the production of IL-1. T cell activation for helper function appears to depend both on the recognition of antigen-class II molecule complexes and on the presence of IL-1.

Helper T cells may also function to help B cells respond to antigen by producing BSF-p1, which is important in B cell proliferation, and by secreting a series of B cell differentiation factors.

Stimulated T cells produce IL-2 and thus play a critical role in proliferation of cytotoxic T cells. Recently the existence of T cell factors responsible for differentiation of precursors of cytotoxic T cells into active killer cells has been reported.

Whether the same T cells act as "cognate" helpers, as producers of B cell growth and differentiation factors, and as producers of IL-2 and cytotoxic differentiation factors is under current investigation. The means by which the production of these factors is regulated is poorly understood.

T cells also play an important role in regulating the class of Ig synthesized and in the selective expansion of clones of B cells that express certain unique antigenic determinants (*idiotopes*) on their receptors and on the antibodies that their descendants secrete. Such T cells appear to function by recognizing Ig determinants on the B cell rather than by recognizing antigen. Our understanding of the physiology and relative importance of "receptor-specific" helper T cells is much less complete than is that of cognate and factor-producing helper cells (see Idiotypic Networks).

SUPPRESSOR T CELLS. Suppressor T cells play important roles in the immune system both by inhibiting immune responses against self-components and by regulating responses to conventional antigens. The suppressor system is highly complex, consisting of a series of cell types that act sequentially. Several distinct suppressor systems have been described by investigators working with different experimental models and a consensus suppressor pathway has not yet been agreed upon. The sequential action of the cells that are members of suppressor pathways appears to have an important amplification effect; the final cell in the pathway inhibits the function of helper T cells. The action of such *suppressor-effector* cells on antibody-secreting cells and on cytotoxic T cells, or their precursors, has been less intensively studied, but evidence exists to suggest that these cells are also important sites of suppressor action.

CYTOTOXIC T CELLS. Cytotoxic T cells recognize, interact with, and destroy cells bearing specific foreign antigens. Cytotoxic T cells play a major role in the destruction of virally infected cells, which bear viral glycoproteins on their membranes. In addition, they may be very important in destroying tumor cells, which display unique tumor-associated antigens on their surfaces. Cytotoxic T cells generally corecognize foreign antigens together with histotopes on class I MHC molecules. Since essentially all cells express class I MHC molecules, cytotoxic T cells are capable of destroying cells of any type that express appropriate foreign antigens. The bulk of cytotoxic T cells are recognized by the OKT8 monoclonal antibody.

Cytotoxic T cells appear to lyse their target cells through a series of steps, including recognition and binding to the target cell and subsequent formation of "holes" in the membrane of the target cell. After this has been accomplished, the cytotoxic T cell may detach from its target and is free to attack other antigen-bearing cells. The cell in which membrane lesions have been induced will then undergo osmotic lysis (Fig. 427–6).

IDIOTYPIC NETWORKS

Since distinct antibodies have variable regions of different structure, it is hardly surprising that the antibodies themselves express unique antigenic determinants on their variable regions against which specific antibodies may be produced. These determinants are designated *idiotopes,* and the complement of idiotopes expressed by an individual Ig is its *idiotype.* The clonotypic antigenic determinants of T cells should be regarded as functionally equivalent to idiotopes of Ig. A provocative and influential theory holds that the immune system exists in a dynamic equilibrium in which members of each clone within the system are recognized by members of other clones (or by their products) through idiotope-antiidiotope interactions. A key postulate of this theory is that there is considerable structural similarity between many of the epitopes on exogenous

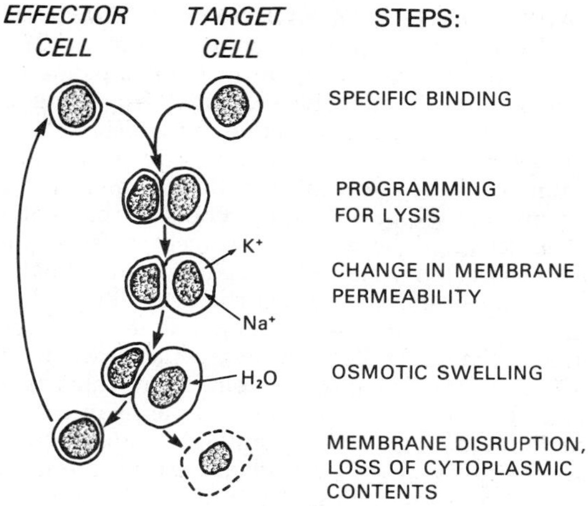

Figure 427–6. Stages in T cell-mediated lysis. (From Henry CS, Gillis S: Cell-mediated cytotoxicity. *In* Paul WE (ed.): Fundamental Immunology. New York, Raven Press, 1984, p 676.)

antigens and the idiotopes of Ig's or T cell receptors. Such idiotopes have sometimes been designated internal images of antigen. Thus, individual B cells and T cells may recognize internal images of antigen and may themselves be recognized by antibodies and T cells specific for the idiotopes they express. Such an interrelated system can allow an immune regulation based on recognition of receptors, without need for exogenous antigen, and can lead to dominance of a given immune response by cell types expressing particular idiotopes because of the action of idiotope-specific T cells or antibodies. Idiotopes that are dominantly expressed in immune responses because of such regulatory action have been designated *regulatory idiotopes.* The idiotope regulatory mechanism may offer opportunities for manipulation of the immune system to either enhance or suppress specific response. Furthermore, these idiotopes, as unique clonal markers, may also have value as specific markers of clonal malignant lymphoid disease. Therapy of human and experimental malignant lymphoid disease with idiotope-specific reagents appears to offer an exciting potential application of idiotypic network concepts.

MACROPHAGES

Cells of the monocyte-macrophage lineage play an important role in several aspects of the immune response. They have a critical function in (1) degrading complex structures, such as intact microorganisms, (2) processing the resulting antigens, and (3) presenting these antigens, in association with class II MHC molecules, to T cells that act as helper cells and that participate in cellular immune responses such as delayed hypersensitivity. This function depends upon the expression of class II MHC molecules on the macrophage. γ-Interferon, which is a product of activated T cells, can induce class II MHC molecules in macrophages. Thus, interactions between antigen-presenting macrophages and specific T lymphocytes are dynamic processes in which an initial activation step leads to the production of soluble factors capable of rendering many other macrophages competent to act as APC. A second important element in antigen presentation and T cell activation appears to be the production by macrophages of IL-1, a substance that has effects in many systems but that appears critical to activation of resting T cells.

Macrophages also function as phagocytic cells. They recognize and ingest foreign particles that are coated by antibodies or complement components (Ch. 148). Macrophages possess membrane Fc receptors, which bind avidly to the aggregated Ig found in antigen-antibody complexes; they also bear receptors for fragments of the third component of complement. These complement fragments are generated in the course of the activation of the complement cascade and are found on opsonized microorganisms and in association with immune complexes.

Whether phagocytosed microorganisms and tumor cells are destroyed depends on both the nature of the ingested particle and the state of activation of the macrophage. Phagocytosis itself appears to be associated with a respiratory burst that enhances the bactericidal activity of the macrophage. Furthermore, T cell products, such as macrophage-activating factor, increase the capacity of macrophages to destroy ingested microorganisms and cells.

NATURAL KILLER CELLS AND ANTIBODY-DEPENDENT CELLULAR CYTOTOXICITY

Natural killer (NK) cells are lymphoid cells from normal individuals that can lyse certain cell types, particularly members of certain long-term tumor cell lines. The NK cells in human peripheral blood are large lymphoid cells with prominent granules and are referred to as large granulocytic lymphocytes. However, their precise cellular lineage remains uncertain; they may be members of the T cell lineage, of the monocyte-macrophage lineage, or of an independent lymphoid lineage. Some patients with severe combined immunodeficiency have depressed NK activity while others display normal NK activity.

The cytotoxic mechanism employed by NK cells is probably very similar to that of specific cytotoxic T lymphocytes. It has been proposed that NK cells play an important role in surveillance mechanisms postulated to destroy emerging clones of malignant cells, but firm evidence for this view is still lacking.

Antibody–dependent cellular cytotoxicity (ADCC) is the destruction of antibody-coated cells by cytotoxic cells that possess Fc receptors. Evidence suggests that NK cells, or closely related cells, mediate ADCC. In general, the ADCC effector cells recognize the Fc region of IgG (Fc_γ) on the target cell, but Fc_μ- and Fc_ϵ-specific ADCC has been described.

ADCC almost certainly has immunopathologic significance. It appears to be important in autoimmune states in causing lysis of autoantibody-coated cells, in destruction of antibody-coated tumor cells, and in destruction of antibody-coated parasites.

CONCLUSIONS

The basic elements of the immune system, working together in a regulated manner, allow a rapid, specific and highly protective response against foreign substances such as those associated with pathogenic microorganisms and against neoantigens expressed by tumor cells. Disorders, both qualitative and quantitative, in this system can have profound effects. It is clear that deficient immune responses may expose the individual to potentially devastating consequences. Furthermore, much of the tissue damage that occurs in a wide range of diseases is due to abnormal action of immune mechanisms. The subsequent chapters of this part, Diseases of the Immune System, outline in detail the pathophysiology of the immune system itself, describing disorders that directly relate to its function. Chapters in Part XXII, Connective Tissue Diseases, describe many key examples in which disordered immune responses or, perhaps, normal responses to abnormal stimuli lead to profound disruption of normal function. Furthermore, immunologically mediated inflammation and tissue damage are key features of many diseases, affecting virtually every organ system. Progress in preventing and treating these disorders will require clear understanding of the nature of the immunologic abnormalities in each case. In turn, this will require a much deeper understanding of the normal physiology of the immune system than is now available to us.

Annual Review of Immunology, 1983–1984, Vol 1 & 2. *A yearly series of reviews on topics in fundamental and clinical immunology aimed at providing a means of keeping up with this rapidly developing field.*

Parker CW (ed.): Clinical Immunology. Philadelphia, W. B. Saunders Company, 1980. *A detailed discussion of the application of immunologic mechanisms in pathophysiologic situations and a discussion of immunologic aspects of many disease states.*
Paul WE (ed.): Fundamental Immunology. New York, Raven Press, 1984. *A general textbook of basic immunologic mechanisms.*
Samter MD (ed.): Immunologic Diseases. 3rd ed. Boston, Little, Brown & Company, 1979. *An extended discussion of immunologic diseases and the mechanisms that underlie them.*
Stites DP, Stobo JD, Fudenberg HH, Wells JV (eds.): Basic and Clinical Immunology. 4th ed. Los Altos, Lange Medical Publications, 1982. *A good introductory text.*

428. COMPLEMENT

Douglas T. Fearon

GENERAL CONSIDERATIONS. Complement functions as part of the immune system to protect the individual from microbial infection by mediating a variety of biologic reactions: opsonization, chemotaxis of leukocytes, increased vascular permeability, and cytolysis of target organisms. These activities of complement that promote an inflammatory reaction also carry the potential for damaging the host. Human disease related to complement may manifest either as defective resistance to infection secondary to impaired activation of the system or as hypersensitivity states caused by excessive complement activation.

The complement system consists of 18 proteins (Table 428–1) found in highest concentrations in plasma. These proteins are said to be in the "classic pathway" or "alternative pathway," names which arose from common usage rather than considerations of relative importance or phylogenetic priorities. The proteins of the classic pathway are designated by letter C and a number: C1 (which comprises three distinct proteins, C1q, C1r, and C1s, that are held together by calcium), C4, C2, C3, and C5 to C9. Proteins of the alternative pathway are designated by capital letters: B, D, P, H, and I. Although C3 has been found to be an essential constituent of the alternative pathway, it has retained its classic pathway nomenclature. Cleavage fragments of components are denoted by lower case letters, as in C3a, C3b, Ba, and Bb, and inactive components are signified by the letter i, as in C3bi and Bbi. An overbar, as in $\overline{C1}$, indicates that a component has been converted to its enzymatically active form.

TABLE 428–1. PROTEINS OF THE COMPLEMENT SYSTEM

Name*	Former Designation	Molecular Weight	Serum Concentration (μg/per Milliliter)
C1q	—	400,000	70
C1r	—	95,000	35
C1s	—	85,000	35
C4	—	209,000	400
C2	—	117,000	25
C3	—	185,000	1500
C5	—	200,000	85
C6	—	128,000	75
C7	—	121,000	55
C8	—	153,000	55
C9	—	80,000	200
B	C3 proactivator, glycine-rich β glycoprotein	95,000	250
D	C3 proactivator convertase	25,000	2
P	Properdin	160,000	25
$\overline{C1}$ inhibitor	—	105,000	180
C4-binding protein	—	$1.2-1.5 \times 10^6$	250
H	β1H	150,000	400
I	KAF, C3b inactivator	90,000	50

*This nomenclature for the alternative pathway proteins has been submitted by the Nomenclature Committee of the International Union of Immunology Societies to the World Health Organization for final approval and adoption.

ACTIVATING AND EFFECTOR PATHWAYS OF COMPLEMENT. The cleavage of C3 by complement enzymes, termed "C3 convertases," is the most critical reaction in the complement system for the elaboration of its biologic activities. There are two pathways, the classic and alternative, by which C3 convertase enzymes may be formed. The classic pathway is initiated by certain antigen-antibody complexes which confer immunologic specificity on this system. The phylogenetically older alternative pathway is activated by a variety of cell surfaces (including those of some bacteria, parasites, fungi, and mammalian cells) which possess certain biochemical characteristics. The alternative pathway is not necessarily dependent on antibody for recognition of the target. Both pathways may efficiently activate C3 and C5–C9 of the "effector" proteins from which are derived the biologically active peptides and complexes of complement.

Classic Pathway (Fig. 428–1). Only IgM and IgG can activate the classic pathway, as other antibody classes are not capable of binding C1 and converting it to its active form, $\overline{C1}$. Binding of the C1q subcomponent of C1 to the Fc regions of one IgM or of at least two adjacent IgG molecules within an antigen-antibody complex induces a conformational change in C1q that leads to conversion of C1r to active $\overline{C1r}$. This subcomponent then proteolytically activates C1s to $\overline{C1s}$. The $\overline{C1s}$ subcomponent of $\overline{C1}$ sequentially cleaves C4, whose major C4b fragment covalently binds to the immune complex, and C2 to generate C2a, which is taken up by C4b to form C4b,2a, the classic pathway C3 convertase. The site for proteolysis of C3 resides in C2a, which also acquires C5-cleaving activity after the major cleavage fragment of C3, C3b, covalently binds to adjacent sites on the target. The C4b,2a enzyme undergoes spontaneous decay of C3- and C5-cleaving activities by release of C2a, which immediately becomes inactive C2ai.

Three plasma proteins regulate activation of the classic pathway. The $\overline{C1}$ inhibitor ($\overline{C1}$INH) irreversibly binds to and blocks the enzymatic sites on $\overline{C1r}$ and $\overline{C1s}$, which prevents activation of C1s by the former and cleavage of C4 and C2 by the latter. $\overline{C1}$INH also retards spontaneous activation of C1. The C4 binding protein (C4bp) binds to C4b to prevent uptake of C2 or to dissociate C2a that is already complexed to C4b. Binding of C4bp also makes C4b susceptible to proteolytic inactivation by C3b/C4b inactivator (I), which yields two degradation fragments, C4c and C4d.

Alternative Pathway (Fig. 428-2). The alternative pathway is more complex than the classic pathway, since two C3 convertases are formed. The *"priming" C3 convertase*, C3,Bb, is assembled by the slow interaction in the fluid phase of C3 (in which the internal thiol ester has been hydrolyzed), B, D, and properdin regardless of the presence of activating substances, and

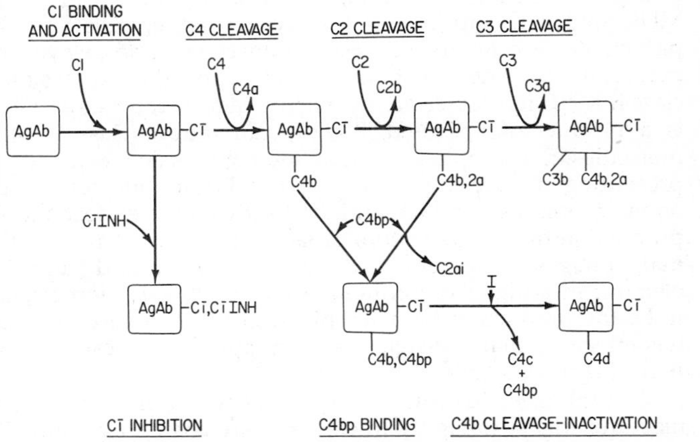

Figure 428–1. The classic pathway of complement activation. An antigen-antibody complex (AgAb) initiates the reaction by binding C1, which then self-activates. The $\overline{C1}$ cleaves C4 and C2, whose major fragments form a bimolecular complex, C4b,2a, the classic pathway C3 convertase. Formation of the C3 convertase is regulated by the control proteins $\overline{C1}$INH, C4bp, and I.

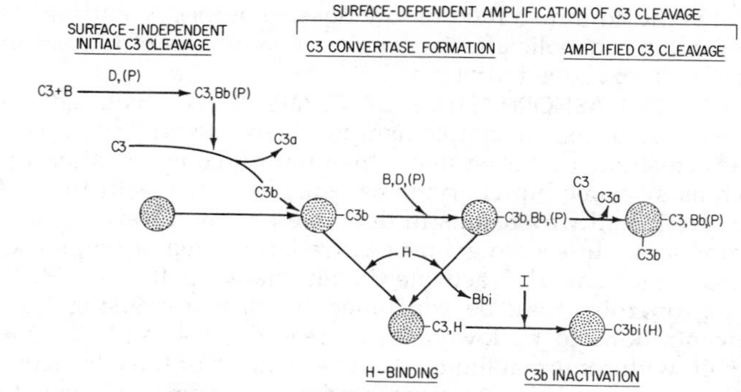

Figure 428–2. The alternative pathway of complement activation. C3b, which is slowly and continuously generated by a "priming" C3 convertase, C3b,Bb(P), may attach to bystander cells. If the cell is an activator of the pathway, the amplification C3 convertase, C3b,Bb(P), is formed and catalyzes cleavage and deposition of additional molecules of C3b. In contrast, C3b bound to a nonactivator binds the regulatory protein, H, and is converted to inactive C3bi by I. P is shown in parentheses to indicate that it augments C3 convertase activity but is not required for alternative pathway activation.

it continuously provides small amounts of C3b that can initiate formation of the *"amplification" C3 convertase*, C3b,Bb. This amplification C3 convertase is responsible for effective C3 cleavage by the alternative pathway, and the adjective "amplification" is used because C3b is both a subunit and a product of this enzyme. C3b that has attached covalently to cell surfaces binds B, and the latter is cleaved by D to uncover the C3 cleaving site on the Bb fragment. C3b,Bb rapidly loses activity by spontaneous dissociation of the catalytic Bb subunit, which becomes inactive Bbi. Properdin serves to stabilize C3 convertase activity by binding to the C3b subunit and retarding dissociation of Bb. C3b,Bb acquires C5 convertase activity after cleavage of additional C3 and deposition of C3b at an adjacent site on the activating target. Regulation of the amplification C3 convertase is essential because of its positive feedback potential and is effected by two control proteins, H and I. The capacity of H to bind to C3b endows it with three inhibitory effects: blocking formation of C3b,Bb, dissociation of Bb that is already bound to C3b, and increasing the susceptibility of C3b to proteolysis by I which yields C3bi, an inactive form of the protein.

The outcome of the competition between B and H for uptake by C3b on a cell membrane determines whether that cell activates the alternative pathway. C3b that is in the fluid phase or affixed to the surface of a nonactivator of the pathway binds H with almost 100-fold greater affinity than that with which it binds B, whereas C3b on the surface of an activator binds H less effectively, and uptake of the control protein is not favored relative to uptake of B. The latter circumstance results in formation of C3b,Bb on the surface of the activating cell and amplifies the reaction by cleavage of additional C3.

A biochemical characteristic of cell membranes that influences the affinity of cell-bound C3b for H is the relative amount of sialic acid that is present in membrane-associated glycoproteins and glycolipids. This carbohydrate increases the affinity of C3b for H but not for B so that its presence on a cell membrane prevents alternative pathway activation. Conversely, the absence of cell surface sialic acid permits activation to occur on a membrane.

The capacity of the alternative pathway to respond to cells that are deficient in sialic acid residues may be relevant to its role in natural resistance to infection, since most bacteria, some parasites, and all plants lack this carbohydrate. Moreover, some of the bacterial species having capsular sialic acid, such as Type III Group B *Streptococcus*, Groups B and C *Neisseria meningitidis*, and K1 *Escherichia coli*, are pathogenetic for man, suggesting that capsular sialic acid facilitates evasion of host defense. The capacity of antibody to enhance activation of the alternative pathway by bacteria and mammalian cells without involvement of classic activating components also has been demonstrated and may be related to alteration of the distribution of membrane structures capable of regulating the uptake and function of cell-bound C3b.

Effector Sequence (Fig. 428–3). Assembly of C5 convertases by the two activating pathways provides the enzyme specificity that is necessary to continue the complement reaction through the effector sequence. Proteolytic cleavage of C5 liberates the C5a peptide that has anaphylatoxic and chemotactic activities and yields the major C5b fragment that initiates assembly of the membrane attack complex of C5b–9. C6 and C7 bind to C5b to form a trimolecular complex with exposed hydrophobic regions that inserts partially into the membrane of the target cell bearing the C5 convertase. The uptake by membrane-associated C5b–7 of C8 and as many as five C9 molecules leads to further insertion of the complex into the membrane; formation of a transmembrane channel through which water, salt, and small molecules can pass; swelling of the cell; and, eventually, lysis.

Although the cytolytic function of complement may protect the host against certain organisms, many pathogenetic bacteria are resistant to the action of C5b–9. In these instances, the most critical reactions for host defense would be the proteolytic cleavages of C3 and C5, which generate activities that can recruit leukocytes to the extravascular focus of complement activation and enhance the capability of the cells for phagocytosis of the target. The C3a and C5a peptides release histamine from mast cells, increasing local vascular permeability. Another peptide derived from C3, C3e, promotes leukocytosis by releasing neutrophils from the bone marrow. C5a also causes accumulation of inflammatory cells at the site of complement activation by inducing adherence of neutrophils to endothelial cells and chemotaxis of polymorphonuclear leukocytes and monocytes. In addition, C5a increases the number of C3b receptors on neutrophils and monocytes. Once these cells have arrived, their capacity to ingest and kill the target organism is greatly enhanced by the presence of C3b on the complement-activating particle, as this opsonin attaches the target to the phagocyte via C3b receptors on the latter's plasma membrane. The functions of C3b receptors on B lymphocytes have not been entirely defined, although uptake of antigen, generation of B memory cells, and enhanced responses to pokeweed mitogen have been described. Thus, complement may kill cells directly by cytolysis or indirectly by recruitment of certain leukocyte functions.

INHERITED ABNORMALITIES OF COMPLEMENT (Table 428-2). ***Association with Increased Susceptibility to Infection.*** An increased incidence of bacterial infections in patients with homozygous deficiencies of C3, I, H, C5, C6, C7, or C8 has been

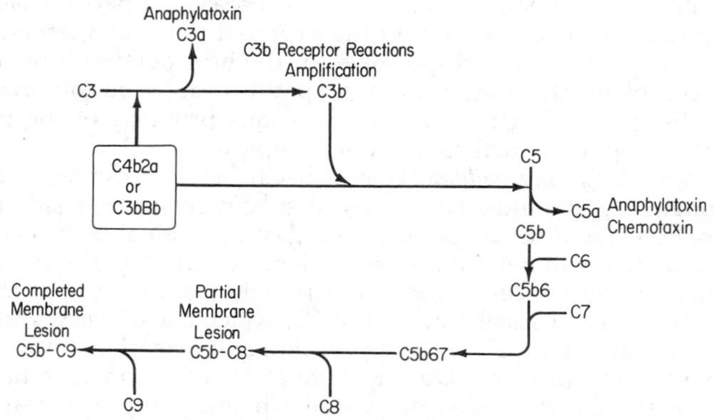

Figure 428–3. The effector sequence of complement, which is activated by the C3/C5 convertases of the classic and alternative pathways. Some of the prominent biologic activities associated with cleavage fragments and multimolecular complexes are shown.

TABLE 428–2. DISEASES ASSOCIATED WITH DEFICIENCIES OF COMPLEMENT

Deficient Component	Disease
Clq	SLE, vasculitis
Clr	Glomerulonephritis, SLE*
Cls	SLE
C̄1INH	HAE†, discoid LE, SLE
C4	SLE
C2	Glomerulonephritis, SLE, discoid LE, purpura, dermatomyositis, hemolytic anemia, JRA‡
C3	Pyogenic infections
I	Pyogenic infections
H	Pyogenic infections
C5	Neisserial infections, SLE
C6	Neisserial infections, Raynaud's phenomenon
C7	Neisserial infections, Raynaud's phenomenon
C8	Neisserial infections
C9	None
P	Neisserial infections

*Systemic lupus erythematosus.
†Hereditary angioedema.
‡Juvenile rheumatoid arthritis.

noted. Absence of C3 abolishes the capacity of serum to opsonize some pathogenetic bacteria, and prevents activation of C5–C9, from which are derived the chemotactic and cytolytic activities of complement. Thus, individuals with this deficiency have had multiple serious pyogenic infections. Two patients with homozygous deficiency of I or H and secondarily depressed serum concentrations of C3 and B also have increased susceptibility to bacterial infections. Absence of C5, which would impair both chemotactic and cytolytic activities of complement, was found in a patient with recurrent bacterial infections who also had systemic lupus erythematosus. Individuals with deficiency of C5, C6, C7, or C8 appear to have a selective propensity for developing disseminated neisserial infections without experiencing an increased incidence of infections with other pyogenic organisms, suggesting that cytolysis rather than phagocytosis is the primary host mechanism for defense against gonococci and meningococci.

Associations with Immunologic Disease. A variety of diseases with immunologic bases have been found in association with inherited deficiencies of C1q, C1r, C1s, C4, C2, and C3 components of the classic activating pathway. Also, patients with systemic lupus erythematosus have an inherited partial deficiency of C3b receptors on erythrocytes. Possible consequences of these deficiencies that may predispose to diseases associated with elevated levels of circulating immune complexes include impaired solubilization of immune complexes, impaired clearance of immune complexes, and lack of generation of peptide fragments of C3 that have immunoregulatory functions. The relatively low frequency of infectious diseases in persons lacking C1, C4, or C2 has led to the proposal that the alternative pathway is primarily responsible for the host defense function of complement, while the classic pathway may be important for the processing of potentially noxious products of the immune response, such as immune complexes.

Hereditary Angioedema (see also Ch. 431). Episodic, occasionally trauma-induced attacks of subcutaneous and submucosal edema of the respiratory and gastrointestinal tracts occur in patients with heterozygous deficiency of C̄1INH. The diminished plasma concentration of this protein results in the continual presence of small amounts of C̄1, which consumes C4 and, to a lesser extent, C2, causing secondary depressions of these complement proteins. During acute attacks the concentrations of C4 and C2 are further depressed. The mediator of increased vascular permeability is not known. As C̄1INH inhibits not only C̄1r and C̄1s of complement but also activated Hageman factor and kallikrein, regulation of several plasma protein enzyme systems is impaired in those patients. Current treatment is the administration of low doses of impeded androgens with potent anabolic effects to increase synthesis of C̄1INH in these heterozygous individuals.

ACQUIRED ABNORMALITIES OF COMPLEMENT. Acquired abnormalities of serum complement levels usually indicate excessive activation of the system. In immune complex diseases, such as systemic lupus erythematosus, excessive activation of the classic pathway results in depressed serum levels of these components. In severe gram-negative bacteremia or cryptococcemia, organisms that activate the alternative pathway, C3, B, and properdin, may be consumed in plasma, causing their concentrations to be lowered, whereas C1, C4, and C2 may remain within normal limits. Acute activation of the alternative pathway occurs also in patients undergoing hemodialysis with cellulosic membranes. The C5a that is generated during this procedure causes aggregation of neutrophils and their sequestration within the pulmonary vasculature. Some studies suggest this effect of C5a may have a role in the adult respiratory distress syndrome.

An unusual mechanism for alternative pathway activation occurs in some patients with membranoproliferative glomerulonephritis and in most patients with partial lipodystrophy with or without glomerulonephritis. Their sera have low levels of C3, normal concentrations of C1, C4, and C2, and an IgG autoantibody, termed C3 nephritic factor, which is specific for antigenic determinants on the amplification C3 convertase. Binding of this autoantibody to C3b,Bb creates a stable trimolecular complex that is resistant to dissociation of its catalytic Bb subunit by H, causing deregulated consumption of C3 by the alternative pathway. An IgG autoantibody to the classic pathway C3 convertase with analogous stabilizing activity has been described in a few patients with systemic lupus erythematosus.

CLINICAL MEASUREMENTS OF COMPLEMENT. Activation of a complement protein results in loss of its precursor, native activity, and in its accelerated clearance from plasma. If hypercatabolism is not compensated for by increased synthesis, the determination of depressed levels of complement protein in plasma or other body fluids may provide evidence for activation of the system. Complement can be measured by assaying the function of its components, by utilizing hemolytic assays which detect only native, unaltered proteins, or by immunochemical assessment of the protein concentration of individual components, usually by immunoprecipitation assays which do not discriminate between native and altered components. The most frequently employed functional assay of complement activity is the determination of the amount of serum or other body fluid required to lyse 50 per cent of a sample of sheep erythrocytes that has been sensitized with rabbit antibody, and is reported as CH50 units. The test measures the overall activity of C1–C9; is not influenced by the alternative pathway proteins B, D, or properdin; and is relatively insensitive to a modest decrease in the activity of a single component. However, the CH50 is useful as an initial screen to detect marked consumption of complement proteins or homozygous deficiencies of individual components. Specific functional assays for all components of both pathways require specialized reagents that are not available in most clinical laboratories, and individual components are usually measured by immunoprecipitation. For the evaluation of patients with hypocomplementemia, determination of the C4 and C3 protein concentrations is most informative. Low concentrations of C4 indicate that classic pathway activation has occurred, since C4 is extremely sensitive to C̄1. Depressed levels of C3 suggest that rather intense activation of either pathway is occurring, and, if found to be associated with normal levels of C4, indicate that exclusive activation of the alternative pathway is occurring. Recently developed radioimmunoassays for the peptide activation fragments of C4 and C3, C4a and C3a, may also be useful for determination of complement activation. Finally, the involvement of complement in a pathologic process is most directly assessed by immunofluorescent staining of individual complement proteins in the involved tissue.

Alper CA, Rosen FS: Inherited deficiencies of complement proteins in man. Springer Semin Immunopathol. In press. *Discussion of the clinical pathologic correlations of complement deficiency states.*

Fearon DT, Wong WW: Complement ligand receptor interactions that mediate biological responses. Ann Rev Immunol 1:243, 1983. *Review of cellular receptors for complement proteins, an aspect of complement that is the basis for many of the biologic effects of this system.*

Lachmann PJ, Peters DK: Complement. *In* Lachmann PJ, Peters DK (eds.): Clinical Aspects of Immunology. Boston, Blackwell Scientific Publications, Ltd., 1982, pp 18–49. *An excellent review of the basic biochemistry, biology, and clinical aspects of complement.*

429. PRIMARY IMMUNODEFICIENCY DISEASES

Rebecca H. Buckley

The first example of human immunodeficiency was described in 1952. Similar or related syndromes have subsequently been reported with increasing frequency. Immunodeficiency diseases may involve all components of the immune system, including lymphocytes, phagocytic cells, and the complement proteins. This chapter will focus on abnormalities of lymphocytes. Deficiencies of the complement system (see Ch. 428) are mentioned briefly. A review of the syndromes associated with neutrophil dysfunction is presented in Ch. 149 and an overall review of the compromised host is given in Ch. 257. The acquired immunodeficiency syndrome (AIDS) is described in Ch. 430.

Despite the large body of knowledge gained regarding functional derangements and cellular abnormalities in the various primary disorders of lymphocytes, the fundamental biologic errors for most of them remain unknown. Exceptions include two defects accompanied by purine salvage pathway enzyme deficiencies—adenosine deaminase in some cases of autosomal recessive severe combined immunodeficiency and purine nucleoside phosphorylase in some patients with Nezelof's syndrome. The genetic error in many other immunodeficiencies must, by definition, be located on the X chromosome. None of the primary defects studied have been found to have associated deficiencies of particular HLA antigens; thus they are unlikely to represent defects involving HLA-linked immune response genes on chromosome 6. Since trace amounts of immunoglobulins of all five isotypes can usually be found in the serum of even the most severely agammaglobulinemic patient, it is also unlikely that immunoglobulin deficiency states are due to deletions of genes encoding for immunoglobulin heavy chains. This does not, however, exclude the possibility of regulatory gene defects.

Various classifications of immunodeficiency disorders involving lymphocytes have attempted to postulate the cellular levels at which the defects occur. Cells with mature differentiation markers of both T and B lymphocytes, however, have been found in most of the known defects. In many cases, normal numbers of such cells have been found despite profound absences of T or B cell function or both. Thus, in most cases the suspect cell lineage is not missing but malfunctional. Table 429–1 lists the current state of knowledge of the most prominent functional deficits and the presumed cellular level of the defect in 18 primary immunodeficiency syndromes.

In contrast to the acquired immune deficiency syndrome (AIDS), which has a new case acquisition rate of 50 per week, primary immunodeficiency diseases are rare. The incidence of agammaglobulinemia is estimated at 1 in 50,000. Selective absence of serum and secretory IgA, the most common, has a reported prevalence of 0.03 to 0.97 per cent.

ANTIBODY DEFICIENCY DISORDERS

Antibody deficiency may occur either as an apparent congenital disorder or as an "acquired" abnormality. Most patients are recognized because they have recurrent infections, but some individuals with selective IgA deficiency or infants with transient hypogammaglobulinemia may have few or no infections. Table 429–2 lists some of the general features of these disorders.

X-LINKED AGAMMAGLOBULINEMIA. A majority of boys afflicted with this malady remain well during the first six to nine months of life, presumably by virtue of maternally transmitted immunoglobulin. Thereafter they repeatedly acquire infections with high-grade extracellular pyogenic organisms such as pneumococci, streptococci, and *Hemophilus* unless given prophylactic antibiotics or gamma globulin therapy. The most common types of infections include sinusitis, pneumonia, otitis, furunculosis, meningitis, and septicemia. Chronic fungal infections are usually not present, and *Pneumocystis carinii* pneumonia rarely occurs unless there is an associated neutropenia. Viral infections and live virus vaccines are also usually handled normally, with the notable exceptions of hepatitis and enterovirus infections. Several examples of paralysis after polio vaccine administration have occurred, presumably because of mutation of persistent vaccine virus to a more neurotropic form. In addition,

TABLE 429–1. CLASSIFICATION OF PRIMARY IMMUNODEFICIENCY DISORDERS*

Disorder	Functional Deficiencies	Presumed Cellular Level of Defect
X-linked agammaglobulinemia	Antibody	Pre-B cell
Common variable (B lymphocyte) hypogammaglobulinemia	Antibody	B lymphocyte
Selective IgA deficiency	IgA antibody	IgA B lymphocyte
Secretory component deficiency	Secretory IgA	Mucosal epithelium
Selective IgM deficiency	IgM antibody	T helper cells
Immunodeficiency with elevated IgM	IgG and IgA antibodies	IgG, IgA B lymphocytes
Transient hypogammaglobulinemia of infancy	None; immunoglobulins low, but antibodies present	Unknown
Antibody deficiency with near-normal immunoglobulins	Antibody	Unknown; ?B cell
X-linked lymphoproliferative disease	Anti–EBV nuclear antigen antibody	B cell; ?also T cell
DiGeorge's syndrome	T cellular; some antibody	Dysmorphogenesis of 3rd & 4th branchial pouches
Nezelof's syndrome (including with PNP deficiency)	T cellular; some antibody	Unknown; ?thymus; ?T cell; metabolic defects
Severe combined immunodeficiency syndromes (autosomal recessive; ADA deficiency; X-linked recessive; bare lymphocyte syndrome; reticular dysgenesis)	Antibody and T cellular; phagocytic in reticular dysgenesis	Unknown; metabolic defect(s); ?T cell; ?stem cell; ?thymus
Wiskott-Aldrich syndrome	Antibody; T cellular	Unknown
Ataxia-telangiectasia	Antibody; T cellular	B lymphocyte; helper T lymphocyte
Immunodeficiency with short-limbed dwarfism	T cellular	G1 cycle of many cells
Immunodeficiency with thymoma	Antibody; some T cellular	B lymphocyte; excessive T suppressor cells
Hyperimmunoglobulinemia E	Specific immune responses; excessive IgE	Unknown
Chronic mucocutaneous candidiasis	Variable cellular	?Antigen overload

*From Buckley RH: Immunodeficiency. J Allergy Clin Immunol 72:627–641, 1983.

TABLE 429–2. CLINICAL CHARACTERISTICS OF ANTIBODY DEFICIENCY DISORDERS

1. Recurrent infections with high grade extracellular encapsulated pathogens
2. Few problems with fungal or viral (except enterovirus) infections
3. Chronic sinopulmonary disease
4. Growth retardation not striking
5. Antibody deficiency in serum and secretions
6. May or may not lack B lymphocytes with surface immunoglobulins or complement receptors
7. Absence of cortical follicles in lymph node and spleen in X-linked agammaglobulinemia
8. Paucity of palpable lymphoid and nasopharyngeal tissue in X-linked agammaglobulinemia
9. Compatible with survival to adulthood or for several years after onset except for those with persistent enterovirus infections, autoimmune disorders, or malignancy

a dermatomyositis-like syndrome accompanied by chronic, eventually fatal central nervous system disease caused by various echoviruses has occurred in more than 20 patients. Approximately 20 per cent of patients have an arthritis resembling juvenile rheumatoid arthritis.

The diagnosis of X-linked agammaglobulinemia is suspected if serum concentrations of IgG, IgA, and IgM are below the 95 per cent confidence limits for appropriate age and race-matched controls (usually there is <100 mg per deciliter total immunoglobulin). The demonstration of antibody deficiency in serum and in external secretions is of great importance in distinguishing this disorder from transient hypogammaglobulinemia of infancy. Tests for natural antibodies to blood group substances, for antibodies to antigens given during standard courses of immunization, e.g., diphtheria, tetanus, or pneumococcus, and for antibodies to and ability to clear bacteriophage $\phi \times 174$ are markedly abnormal. Polymorphonuclear functions are usually normal, but some patients with this condition have had transient, persistent, or cyclic neutropenia.

Lymphopenia is uncommon, and the percentages of T cells and T cell subsets have been found to be normal or elevated in most instances. In contrast, blood lymphocytes bearing surface immunoglobulin, "Ia-like" antigens or the EBV receptor, or reacting with a specific anti-B cell serum are absent or present in very low number. Hypoplasia of adenoids, tonsils, and peripheral lymph nodes is the rule; germinal centers are not present, and plasma cells are rarely found (Fig. 429–1). Conversely, normal numbers of pre-B cells are found in the bone marrow. Mixed lymphocyte responsiveness and lymphocyte responses to antigens and mitogens are normal. Cell–mediated immune responses can be detected in vivo, and the capacity to reject allografts is intact. The thymus has appeared normal in all autopsied cases, and lymphoid cells are abundant in thymus-dependent areas of peripheral lymphoid tissues.

Except in those unfortunate patients who develop polio, persistent echovirus infection, or lymphoreticular malignancy (an incidence as high as 6 per cent has been reported), the overall prognosis is reasonably good if humoral replacement therapy is instituted early. Systemic infection can be prevented by administration of immune serum globulin (ISG; primarily IgG) by the intramuscular or intravenous route. Use of the traditional loading dose of 200 mg per kilogram and maintenance dose of 100 mg per kilogram every three to four weeks is currently under review; it is likely that higher or individualized doses, or both, will be recommended. Thus far, there have been no reports of the transmission of AIDS with ISG, and such preparations are also known to be free of hepatitis antigens. Use of random donor plasma as a source of Ig carries the risk of transmission of both of these, although plasma from a known safe donor is a valuable source (10 ml per kilogram will provide approximately 100 mg IgG per kilogram). Many patients go on to develop crippling sinopulmonary disease despite this therapy, since no effective means now exists for replacing secretory IgA at the mucosal surface. Intermittent or chronic antibiotic therapy is often necessary in addition for the management of such patients.

AGAMMAGLOBULINEMIA WITH IMMUNOGLOBULIN-BEARING B LYMPHOCYTES. This condition, also known as common variable agammaglobulinemia (CVAγ), may appear similar clinically in many respects to X-linked agammaglobulinemia. Although this disorder may occur in infants and young children, most patients present with a history of recurrent infection beginning several years after birth. This disorder is distinguished from X-linked agammaglobulinemia by later age of onset, somewhat less severe susceptibility to infections, and almost equal sex distribution. In contrast to patients with the X-linked form, patients with CVAγ may have normal-sized or enlarged tonsils and lymph nodes, and the latter may have cortical follicles. Additionally, such patients often have normal or near-normal numbers of circulating immunoglobulin-bearing B lymphocytes. Nevertheless, the serum immunoglobulin and antibody deficiencies are usually just as profound by measurement, and the bacterial etiologic agents are the same as in the X-linked disorder. Thus far no documented examples of fatal

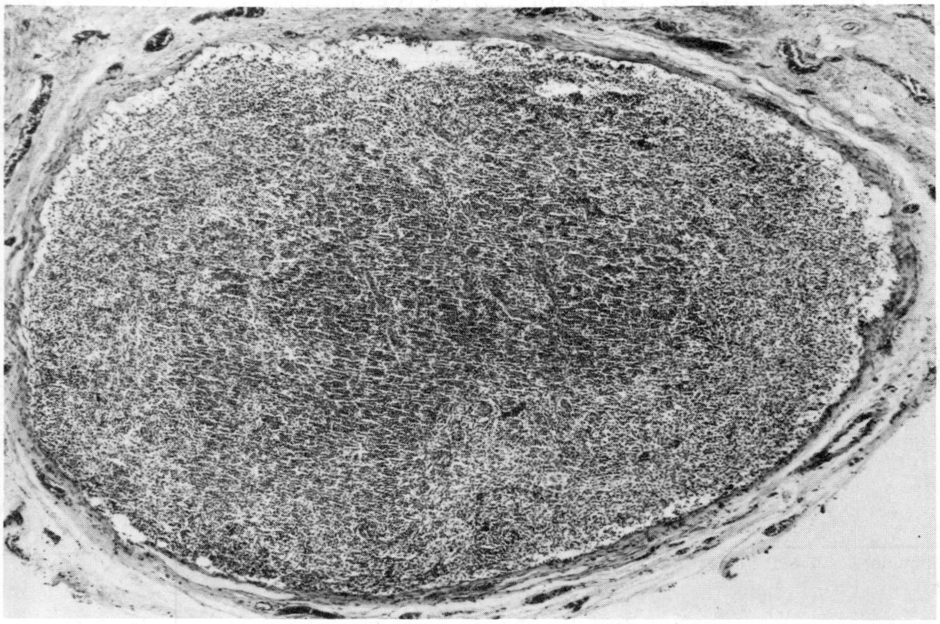

Figure 429–1. Section of lymph node from boy with infantile X-linked agammaglobulinemia, a classic example of an antibody deficiency disorder. Note absence of cortical follicles but relatively dense paracortical area. (From Buckley RH: *In* Middleton E, Reed CE, Ellis EF [eds.]: Allergy: Principles and Practice. St. Louis, C. V. Mosby Company, 1978, p 200.)

echovirus meningoencephalitis have occurred in patients with CVAγ.

This condition has been variably associated with a sprue-like syndrome, with or without nodular follicular lymphoid hyperplasia of the intestine; thymoma; alopecia areata; and autoantibody formation leading to hemolytic anemia, gastric atrophy, achlorhydria, and pernicious anemia. Frequent complications include giardiasis (seen far more often here than in X-linked agammaglobulinemia), bronchiectasis, gastric carcinoma, lymphoreticular malignancy, and cholelithiasis. Lymphoid interstitial pneumonia, pseudolymphoma, amyloidosis, and noncaseating granulomas of the lungs, spleen, skin, and liver have also been seen.

Despite normal numbers of circulating immunoglobulin-bearing B lymphocytes and the presence of lymphoid cortical follicles, the lymphocytes do not differentiate in vivo or in vitro into immunoglobulin-producing plasma cells, even in the presence of the polyclonal B cell activator, pokeweed mitogen. Although the primary biologic error responsible for this defect is unknown, in most patients it appears to be due to abnormal terminal differentiation of the B cell line. Because this disorder occurs in first-degree relatives of patients with selective IgA deficiency, and some patients with hyper-IgM have later become panhypogammaglobulinemic (or vice versa), it is possible that these diseases all belong to the same spectrum of B cell maturation arrests. The inconstancy of excessive suppressor T cell activity suggests that this mechanism is not etiologic for these disorders as a whole. The treatment of CVAγ is the same as for the X-linked disorder.

SELECTIVE IgA DEFICIENCY. An isolated near-absence (i.e., <10 mg per deciliter) of serum and secretory IgA is the most common immunodeficiency disorder so far detected, a frequency of 1:886 being reported among blood donors. Although IgA deficiency has been observed in apparently healthy individuals, it is commonly associated with ill health. The kinds of health problems experienced often reflect the type of clinic from which the patients are drawn. Among 75 from an allergy-immunology clinic, there were high frequencies of chronic or recurrent respiratory tract infection and atopic diseases. In contrast, 30 IgA-deficient patients drawn from a rheumatology clinic had a high frequency of autoimmune and/or collagen vascular disease.

IgA is the major immunoglobulin of external secretions. As would be expected, its deficiency is associated with infections occurring predominantly in the respiratory, gastrointestinal, and urogenital tracts. Bacterial agents responsible are essentially the same as in other types of antibody deficiency syndromes. A high incidence of viral hepatitis was noted in one group of IgA-deficient patients, but there is no clear evidence that patients with this disorder have an undue susceptibility to other viral agents. Children with IgA deficiency produce local IgM and IgG antipolio antibodies to killed vaccine given intranasally and IgM and IgG antirubella antibodies during convalescence from natural rubella. The compensating IgM seems to be locally synthesized and capable of combining with secretory piece for local secretion similar to IgA. Serum concentrations of other immunoglobulins are usually normal in patients with selective IgA deficiency, although an IgG_2 subclass deficiency has been reported in some, and IgM (usually increased) may be of the low molecular weight variety.

In addition to limiting the attachment of infectious agents to mucosal surfaces, secretory IgA antibodies probably act to prevent absorption of other foreign antigens, such as those in the diet. There is a high incidence of allergy and of IgG antibodies against cow's milk and ruminant serum proteins in patients with IgA deficiency. The antiruminant antibodies often present technical problems in immunoassays of IgA which employ goat (but not rabbit) antisera. Intestinal nodular hyperplasia has been seen in a few such patients. A sprue-like syndrome may occur in adults with selective IgA deficiency and sometimes responds to a gluten-free diet.

The basic defect leading to selective IgA deficiency is unknown. IgA–bearing blood B cells from most such patients also coexpress surface IgM and IgD, similar to cord blood B cells, suggesting maturation arrest. In addition, the B lymphocytes fail to secrete IgA in vitro. Some have exhibited excessive isotype-specific T suppressor cells. Studies of T cell function have been normal in most patients. The defect may not always be permanent. The author, in following over 150 such patients, has seen the spontaneous development of normal serum IgA concentrations in ten children documented for several years to have absence of or extremely low concentrations of IgA. The occurrence of IgA deficiency in both males and females and in families suggests autosomal inheritance.

Serum antibodies to IgA are found in as many as 44 per cent of such patients. This observation is of possible etiologic and great clinical significance. At least seven IgA-deficient patients have had severe or fatal anaphylactic reactions after intravenous administration of blood products. For this reason, only multiply washed erythrocytes or blood products from other IgA-deficient individuals should be administered to these patients; ISG (which contains a small amount of IgA) is contraindicated.

Currently the only treatment for IgA deficiency is vigorous treatment of specific infections with appropriate antimicrobial agents. Even if serum IgA could be replaced (in the face of anti-IgA antibodies), it would not be transported into the external secretions, since the latter is an active process involving only locally produced IgA.

SECRETORY COMPONENT DEFICIENCY. A patient with chronic intestinal candidiasis and diarrhea was found to lack IgA in his external secretions, despite having a normal concentration of serum IgA. This was traced to a lack of secretory piece, which prevented the normal secretion of locally produced IgA.

SELECTIVE IgM DEFICIENCY. If one uses a strict definition of a serum IgM concentration less than 10 mg per deciliter, there are very few well-documented cases of this entity. Fatal septicemia caused by meningococci and other gram-negative organisms has been noted in some such patients. Others have experienced bacterial infections of other types, including pneumococcal meningitis, tuberculosis, recurrent staphylococcal pyoderma, periorbital cellulitis, bronchiectasis, and recurrent otitis. There is no specific therapy; early and vigorous treatment with antibiotics is recommended to avoid the fatal septicemia that has occurred in some patients.

IMMUNODEFICIENCY WITH ELEVATED IgM. This disorder is characterized by very low serum concentrations of IgG and IgA but a markedly elevated concentration of polyclonal IgM. Some patients have low molecular weight IgM molecules. Similar to patients with X-linked agammaglobulinemia, those with this defect commonly become symptomatic during infancy with recurrent pyogenic infections, including otitis media, sinusitis, pneumonia, and tonsillitis. In contrast to patients with X-linked agammaglobulinemia, however, the frequent presence of lymphoid hyperplasia often leads away from a diagnosis of immunodeficiency. There is an increased frequency of autoimmune disorders, such as hemolytic anemia and thrombocytopenia, and transient, persistent, or cyclic neutropenia is common. Thymic-dependent lymphoid tissues and T cell functions are usually normal, but several have had partial T cell deficiencies. A sex-linked mode of inheritance has been proposed, but several examples of the disorder in females now seem to make this less certain.

The pathogenesis of the hyper-IgM syndrome has yet to be elucidated. Normal or only slightly reduced numbers of Ig-bearing B lymphocytes have been found in the blood; however, cultured B cell lines from such patients have shown the capacity to synthesize only IgM, suggesting a B cell maturation defect that prevents isotype switching. Plasma cells in lymph nodes contain only IgM.

Because these patients are unable to make IgG antibodies, the treatment is the same as for agammaglobulinemia.

TRANSIENT HYPOGAMMAGLOBULINEMIA OF INFANCY. This condition has been described as a prolongation and accentuation of the "physiologic" decline in serum immunoglobulin concentrations normally seen during the first three to seven months of life. Unlike patients with X-linked or common variable agammaglobulinemia, those with transient hypogammaglobulinemia can synthesize antibodies to human type A and B erythrocytes and to diphtheria and tetanus toxoids, usually by six to eleven months of age, well before immunoglobulin concentrations become normal. The finding of only eleven cases of transient hypogammaglobulinemia of infancy among over 10,000 sera tested by the author over a twelve-year period suggests that, contrary to popular opinion, this is not a common entity.

Gamma globulin replacement therapy is not indicated in this condition. In addition to the known risks of inducing anti-IgG allotype antibodies, passively administered antibodies could block endogenous primary antibody formation in the same manner that RhoGAM suppresses anti-D antibodies in Rh-negative mothers delivering Rh-positive infants.

ANTIBODY DEFICIENCY WITH NEAR-NORMAL IMMUNOGLOBULINS. Only scattered reports have appeared in the literature describing patients with deficient antibody responses despite apparently normal T cell function and normal or near-normal immunoglobulin concentrations. The author and her associates have studied the antibody-forming capacities of twelve such patients. Blood group antibody titers were absent in all but two, diphtheria titers were low in all, and tetanus titers were low in ten. Geometric mean antibody titers to thirteen pneumococcal serotypes were significantly lower than those of normal controls before and after immunization with tridecavalent pneumococcal polysaccharide vaccine. All patients cleared bacteriophage $\phi \times 174$ normally, but all primary immune responses were far below the normal range. Secondary responses to $\phi \times 174$ were also below the normal range in all but two, but, in both cases, most of the secondary response was IgM rather than IgG. This type of immune problem would not be detected unless functional tests of antibody-forming capacity are regularly conducted in the assessment of humoral immunity. Patients with this disorder are candidates for immunoglobulin replacement therapy.

X-LINKED LYMPHOPROLIFERATIVE DISEASE. This disorder, also referred to as *Duncan's disease* (after the original kindred in which it was described), is characterized by an impaired immune response to Epstein-Barr virus (EBV). Males affected with this condition are apparently healthy until they experience infectious mononucleosis. Two thirds of the 100 patients studied thus far died of overwhelming EBV–induced B cell proliferation during mononucleosis. A majority of the survivors developed hypogammaglobulinemia or B cell lymphomas or both. Such individuals have marked impairment in production of antibodies to the EBV nuclear antigen, whereas titers of antibodies to the viral capsid antigen have ranged from zero to markedly elevated. Antibody-dependent cell-mediated cytotoxicity against EBV-infected cells and natural killer function are depressed, and there is a deficiency in long-lived T cell immunity to EBV. Despite normal numbers of B and T cells, there is an elevated percentage of lymphocytes of the suppressor (T8) phenotype. In addition, lymphocyte immunoglobulin synthesis in response to polyclonal B cell mitogen stimulation in vitro is markedly depressed. Thus, both EBV-specific and nonspecific immunologic abnormalities occur in these patients.

CELLULAR IMMUNODEFICIENCY DISORDERS

Some important clinical characteristics of cellular immunodeficiency disorders are listed in Table 429–3. In general, patients with partial or absolute defects in T cell function have infections or other clinical problems for which there is no effective treatment or which are often of a more severe nature than in those with antibody deficiency disorders. It is therefore rare that such individuals survive beyond infancy or childhood.

TABLE 429–3. CLINICAL CHARACTERISTICS OF CELLULAR IMMUNODEFICIENCY DISORDERS

1. Recurrent infections with low grade or opportunistic infectious agents such as fungi, viruses, or *Pneumocystis carinii*
2. Delayed cutaneous anergy
3. Accompanied by growth retardation, short life span, wasting, and diarrhea
4. Susceptible to graft-versus-host (GVH) disease if given fresh blood, plasma, or unmatched allogeneic bone marrow
5. Fatal reactions from live virus or BCG vaccination
6. High incidence of malignancy

THYMIC HYPOPLASIA (DIGEORGE'S SYNDROME). This condition results from dysmorphogenesis of the third and fourth pharyngeal pouches, leading to hypoplasia or aplasia of the thymus and parathyroid glands. Other structures forming at the same age are also frequently affected, resulting in anomalies of the great vessels (right-sided aortic arch), esophageal atresia, bifid uvula, congenital heart disease (atrial and ventricular septal defects), a short philtrum of the upper lip, hypertelorism, an antimongoloid slant to the eyes, mandibular hypoplasia, and low-set (often notched) ears. The diagnosis is usually first suggested by the presence of hypocalcemic seizures during the neonatal period. DiGeorge's syndrome has occurred in both males and females, and there is little evidence that it is heritable.

A variable degree of hypoplasia is more frequent than total aplasia of the thymus and parathyroid glands. Some children with the features of this syndrome have little trouble with infections and show evidence of some cell-mediated immunity. They are often referred to as having partial DiGeorge's syndrome. Those with marked thymic hypoplasia may resemble infants with severe combined immunodeficiency in their susceptibility to infection with low-grade or opportunistic pathogens (i.e., fungi, viruses, and *Pneumocystis carinii*) and to graft-versus-host (GVH) disease from nonirradiated blood transfusions.

Serum immunoglobulins are usually normal for age, but some fractions, particularly IgA, may be diminished and IgE may be elevated. T cell numbers are decreased, and there is an increased number of B cells. Responses of peripheral blood lymphocytes following mitogen stimulation, like the intradermal delayed hypersensitivity response, have been absent, reduced, or normal. Careful postmortem studies have sometimes revealed tiny nests of thymic tissue containing Hassall's corpuscles and a normal density of thymocytes. Lymphoid follicles usually appear normal, but lymph node paracortical areas and thymus-dependent regions of the spleen show variable degrees of depletion, depending upon the degree of thymic hypoplasia. Because of variability in the severity of the immunodeficiency, it is difficult to evaluate claimed benefits of fetal thymus transplantation.

CELLULAR IMMUNODEFICIENCY WITH IMMUNOGLOBULINS (NEZELOF'S SYNDROME). This syndrome is characterized by lymphopenia, diminished lymphoid tissue, abnormal thymus architecture, and the presence of normal or increased levels of most of the five immunoglobulin classes. Children with this condition may have recurrent or chronic pulmonary infections, failure to thrive, oral or cutaneous candidiasis, chronic diarrhea, recurrent skin infections, gram-negative sepsis, urinary tract infections, severe varicella, progressive vaccinia, or combinations of these. An autosomal recessive pattern of inheritance has been suggested in some cases, but an X-linked mode seemed more likely in others. Other findings include neutropenia and eosinophilia. Serum immunoglobulins may be normal or elevated for all classes, but selective IgA deficiency and marked elevation of IgE occur not infrequently.

Studies of cellular immune function have shown delayed cutaneous anergy to ubiquitous antigens and low to absent in vitro lymphocyte responses to mitogens and allogeneic cells.

Such patients have profound deficiencies of total T cells and T cell subsets, with usually a normal helper (T4+) to suppressor (T8+) cell ratio, in contrast to patients with AIDS who characteristically have marked inversion of the T4:T8 ratio due to selective deficiency of T4+ cells. Peripheral lymphoid tissues demonstrate paracortical lymphocyte depletion. The thymuses are very small and have a paucity of thymocytes and usually no Hassell's corpuscles; however, again in contrast to AIDS, thymic epithelium is present. These could all be useful in distinguishing Nezelof's syndrome from AIDS in the pediatric age group, since it is the primary immunodeficiency disorder most likely to be confused with it. Fatal or serious infections have included varicella, vaccinia, *Pneumocystis carinii*, cytomegalovirus, rubeola, *Pseudomonas*, and *Mycobacterium kansasii*. Antibody-forming capacity has been apparently normal in roughly one third of the reported cases. Plasma cells are usually abundant in the lamina propria and lymph nodes. Although in one patient with this disorder reconstitution was successful by means of a matched sibling bone marrow transplant, most other forms of therapy have been unsuccessful.

With Purine Nucleoside Phosphorylase Deficiency. More than a dozen patients with Nezelof's syndrome have been found to have purine nucleoside phosphorylase (PNP) deficiency. In contrast to patients with adenosine deaminase (ADA) deficiency, serum and urinary uric acid are markedly deficient, and no characteristic physical or skeletal abnormalities have been noted. Three patients have suffered from a progressive neurologic disorder with spastic tetraplegia, two developed an autoimmune hemolytic anemia, and one has idiopathic thrombocytopenic purpura. Deaths have occurred from generalized vaccinia, varicella, lymphosarcoma, and GVH disease following a blood transfusion. In contrast to a majority of patients with Nezelof's syndrome, the thymuses of PNP-deficient patients have had some Hassall's corpuscles, reminiscent of some patients with ADA deficiency. Analyses of lymphocyte subpopulations with monoclonal antibodies in two such patients revealed marked deficiency of T cells and T cell subsets but increased numbers of cells with natural killer (NK) phenotype and function. Attempts to correct the immunologic and enzymatic deficiencies of PNP-deficient patients by enzyme replacement therapy, using normal erythrocyte transfusions or deoxycytidine, have not been very successful.

SEVERE COMBINED IMMUNODEFICIENCY (SCID) DISORDERS

The syndromes of SCID are distinguished by their apparent congenital absence of all adaptive immune function. Unless immunologic reconstitution can be achieved through immunocompetent tissue transplants or enzyme replacement therapy or unless gnotobiotic isolation can be carried out, death usually occurs before the patient's first birthday. For some time it has been assumed that an absence or a failure of proliferation and/or differentiation of the "primordial" stem cell was the basis of these syndromes. Unfortunately, this theory does not explain the great diversity of genetic, enzymatic, hematologic, and immunologic features observed. The major subcategories of this disorder are discussed below.

AUTOSOMAL RECESSIVE SEVERE COMBINED IMMUNODEFICIENCY DISEASE. Within the first few months of life, infants affected with this first-described SCID syndrome have frequent episodes of otitis, pneumonia, sepsis, diarrhea, and cutaneous infections. Growth may appear normal initially, but extreme wasting soon develops. Infections with opportunistic organisms such as *Candida albicans*, *Pneumocystis carinii*, vaccinia, varicella, measles, cytomegalovirus, and BCG frequently lead to death caused either by difficulties encountered in diagnosis or by a lack of effective treatment. These infants also lack the ability to reject foreign tissue and are therefore at risk for GVH disease. GVH reactions can result from maternal immunocompetent cells crossing the placenta or from the administration of blood products containing viable histoincompatible lymphocytes.

Immunologic evaluation reveals serum immunoglobulin concentrations to be diminished or absent, and no antibody formation occurs following immunization. There is a near-total lack of cellular immune function, with lymphopenia and absence of or extremely low lymphocyte responses to mitogens or allogeneic cells, delayed cutaneous anergy, and inability to reject foreign tissues. Marked heterogeneity of lymphocyte subpopulations exists among SCID patients, even among those with similar inheritance patterns. Despite the uniformly profound lack of T or B cell function, some patients have had low numbers of both B and T lymphocytes, whereas others have had elevated numbers of B cells; occasionally even normal numbers of both T and B cells have been found. Cytofluorographic studies with monoclonal antibodies to mature T cells and subsets have generally revealed some, albeit low, percentages of cells reacting with all such reagents; however, there is no increase in cells bearing the T6 antigen present on immature cortical thymocytes. Thus the lymphocytes present appear to have acquired surface markers characteristic of mature T cells. In contrast to similarly lymphopenic patients with AIDS, SCID patients rarely have an inverted ratio of helper (T4+) to suppressor (T8+) cells. Recently a new phenotype of SCID was characterized by the author in which virtually all of the lymphocytes of two infants with SCID were large granular lymphocytes with NK cell phenotype and function. NK function has been totally lacking in other SCID patients, again illustrating the striking heterogeneity at a cellular level. Typically, these patients have very small thymuses (less than 2 grams), which usually fail to descend from the neck, contain few thymic lymphocytes, lack corticomedullary distinction, and usually lack Hassall's corpuscles (see exception below). Despite the profound thymocyte depletion in SCID patients, thymic epithelium is present—in contrast to the situations in AIDS in which there is marked epithelial atrophy. Both the follicular and paracortical areas of the peripheral lymph nodes are depleted of lymphocytes. Tonsils, adenoids, and Peyer's patches are absent or extremely underdeveloped.

ISG fails to halt the progressively downhill course of SCID. Transplantation of bone marrow cells from HLA genotypically identical or D locus compatible donors has resulted in apparent complete correction of the immunologic defect in a number of these patients, with some 40 known long-term survivors. Fetal tissue transplants have been much less effective. Recently a major advance has allowed the use of haploidentical (half-matched) bone marrow cells for correction of the immunologic defect in SCID. In this technique, which takes advantage of the affinity of human T cells for soybean lectin and for sheep erythrocytes, post-thymic T cells are selectively and completely removed, leaving the stem cells intact for transplantation. To date, over 30 infants with SCID who would have otherwise died because of lack of an HLA-identical donor have been treated successfully with this approach, with virtually no signs of GVH reaction.

With Adenosine Deaminase (ADA) Deficiency. Absence of the enzyme ADA has been observed in some but not all patients with the autosomal recessive form of SCID; approximately 30 families have been identified in which ADA deficiency was associated with severe immunodeficiency. A marked accumulation of deoxyadenosine and its triphosphate may provide the biochemical mechanisms responsible for the immunodeficiency. Deoxyadenosine is an apparent suicide inactivator of the enzyme S-adenosylhomocysteine (SAH) hydrolase and could alter methylation in a manner which would lead to cell death. Although most such patients have had profound lymphopenia from the earliest age studied, a few have had early normal or fluctuating lymphocyte counts that declined by six weeks to two years of life. In marked contrast to "classic" SCID, some ADA-deficient patients have been found to have a few Hassall's corpuscles in their thymuses and changes suggestive of early differentiation. Other distinguishing features of ADA-deficient SCID disorders have included the presence of rib cage abnormalities similar to a rachitic rosary and multiple skeletal abnormalities of chondro-osseous dysplasia on radiographic examination.

Both matched sibling and haploidentical post-thymic T cell–depleted bone marrow transplants have resulted in lymphocyte chimerism and partial or complete correction of the immunologic defect in ADA-deficient SCID. Enzyme replacement therapy, consisting of the administration of 15 ml per kilogram of glycerol-frozen, irradiated, packed normal erythrocytes every two to four weeks, has resulted in temporary immunologic or clinical improvement or both in some such patients.

X-LINKED RECESSIVE SEVERE COMBINED IMMUNODEFICIENCY DISEASE. This is thought to be the most common form of SCID in the United States. There have been no examples of deficiencies of the purine salvage pathway enzymes ADA or PNP in association with SCID in pedigrees in which there has been proven X-linked inheritance. Clinically, immunologically, and histopathologically, these patients appear similar to those with the autosomal recessive form.

BARE LYMPHOCYTE SYNDROME. In this form of combined immunodeficiency there is a lack of expression of HLA antigens and the absence of B_2 microglobulin on lymphocytes. Nine examples of this defect have now been reported, all from the Mediterranean area. The associated defects of immunity and of HLA expression support the concept of a biologic role of HLA determinants in the development of functional T lymphocytes.

SEVERE COMBINED IMMUNODEFICIENCY WITH LEUKOPENIA (RETICULAR DYSGENESIS). In 1959, identical twin male infants were described who exhibited a total lack of both lymphocytes and granulocytes in their peripheral blood and bone marrow. Seven of eight infants reported died between 3 and 119 days of age from overwhelming infections; the eighth underwent complete immunologic reconstitution from a bone marrow transplant. The organisms responsible have been both bacterial and viral, including cytomegalovirus, *Pseudomonas, Klebsiella,* and pyogenic cocci. A genetic, probably autosomal, influence seems likely from reports of familial occurrences.

Serum immunoglobulins were very low and no lymphocyte responses to mitogens occurred in the four patients in whom immunologic evaluations were conducted. The thymus glands all weighed less than 1 gram, and no Hassall's corpuscles and few or no thymocytes were seen.

PARTIAL COMBINED IMMUNODEFICIENCY DISORDERS

IMMUNODEFICIENCY WITH THROMBOCYTOPENIA AND ECZEMA (WISKOTT-ALDRICH SYNDROME). This X-linked recessive syndrome is characterized clinically by the triad of eczema, megakaryocytic thrombocytopenic purpura, and undue susceptibility to infection. Often there is prolonged oozing from the circumcision site or bloody diarrhea during infancy. Atopic dermatitis and recurrent infections usually develop during the first year of life. Infections are caused by pneumococci and other bacteria with polysaccharide capsules, resulting in episodes of otitis media, pneumonia, meningitis, and sepsis. Later, as cellular immunity wanes, infections with *Pneumocystis carinii* and the herpesviruses become more frequent. Survival beyond the teens is rare; major causes of death are infections or bleeding, but a 12 per cent incidence of fatal malignancy also occurs in this condition. A papovavirus has been recovered from a reticulum cell sarcoma of the brain and from the urine of patients with this syndrome.

The earliest evidence of immunodeficiency is an impaired humoral immune response to polysaccharide antigens. Absent or markedly diminished isohemagglutinin titers are uniformly found, and poor or no responses are seen following immunization with polysaccharide antigens. Antibody titers to protein antigens also fall with time, and anamnestic responses are often poor or absent. Studies of immunoglobulin metabolism have shown an accelerated rate of synthesis, as well as hypercatabolism, of albumin, IgG, IgA, and IgM, resulting in highly variable immunoglobulin concentrations. The predominant dysgammaglobulinemia is a low IgM, an elevated IgA and IgE, and a normal or slightly low IgG concentration. Lymphocyte responses are moderately depressed, and cutaneous anergy is a frequent finding. Analyses of blood lymphocytes with monoclonal reagents have revealed low percentages of cells reacting with antibodies to all T cells and to the helper (T4+) and suppressor (T8+) subsets. However, as with the other primary cellular immunodeficiencies, there is usually no imbalance in the T4:T8 ratio.

The thrombocytopenia appears to be due to an intrinsic platelet abnormality, since antiplatelet antibodies are not usually demonstrated and survival times of homologous but not autologous ^{51}Cr-labeled platelets have been normal in these patients.

Treatment has been directed primarily toward control of bleeding with platelet transfusions, splenectomy, or both and of infections by intravenous administration of ISG. Several patients have had complete corrections of both the platelet and immunologic abnormalities by HLA-matched sibling bone marrow transplants after being conditioned with irradiation or busulfan and cyclophosphamide.

ATAXIA-TELANGIECTASIA. This is a complex syndrome with neurologic, immunologic, endocrinologic, hepatic, and cutaneous abnormalities. The most prominent clinical features are progressive cerebellar ataxia, oculocutaneous telangiectasia, chronic sinopulmonary disease, a high incidence of malignancy, and variable humoral and cellular immunodeficiency. Ataxia typically becomes evident soon after the child begins to walk and progresses until he or she is confined to a wheelchair, usually by ten to twelve years of age. Telangiectasias usually develop by three to six years of age. Recurrent, usually bacterial, sinopulmonary infections occur in roughly 80 per cent of these patients; common viral exanthems and smallpox vaccination have not usually resulted in untoward sequelae. However, varicella was fatal in one of the author's patients.

The malignant tumors reported have usually been of the lymphoreticular type, but others have been seen. Cells from such patients, as well as those from heterozygous carriers, have been reported to have increased sensitivity to ionizing radiation, defective DNA repair, and frequent chromosomal abnormalities. An autosomal recessive mode of inheritance seems operative.

The most frequent immunologic abnormality is selective absence of IgA, found in from 50 to 80 per cent of these patients. IgE concentrations are usually low, and the IgM may be of the low molecular weight variety. Specific antibody levels may be decreased or normal. In vivo, there is impaired but not absent cell-mediated immunity, as evidenced by delayed cutaneous anergy and prolonged allograft survival. Death from GVH disease has not been reported. Enumeration of blood T cells and subsets in five patients with this disorder revealed reduced percentages of total T cells and T cells of the helper (T4) phenotype, with normal or increased percentages of cells of the suppressor (T8) phenotype. In vitro studies of lymphocyte function have shown moderately depressed proliferative responses to mitogens, decreased T helper cell function, and an intrinsic defect in B cell IgA synthesis. The thymus is very hypoplastic and lacks Hassall's corpuscles. No satisfactory treatment has been found.

IMMUNODEFICIENCY WITH SHORT-LIMBED DWARFISM. An unusual form of short-limbed dwarfism with frequent and severe infections has been reported among the Amish; some affected individuals also had cartilage-hair hypoplasia. Features include short and pudgy hands; redundant skin; hyperextensible joints of hands and feet but an inability to completely extend the elbows; and fine, sparse light hair and eyebrows. Severe and often fatal varicella infections appear to be a particular hazard.

Progressive vaccinia and vaccine-associated poliomyelitis have also been observed.

The severity of the immunodeficiency varies; in one series, 11 of 77 patients died before age 20 but two were still alive at age 76. Three patterns of immune dysfunction have emerged: defective antibody-mediated immunity, defective cellular immunity, and severe combined immunodeficiency. The most striking abnormality appears to be one of defective cell proliferation due to an intrinsic defect related to the G1 phase, resulting in a longer cell cycle for individual cells. The trait appears to be autosomal recessive with variable penetrance.

IMMUNODEFICIENCY WITH THYMOMA. These patients are adults who almost simultaneously develop hypogammaglobulinemia, deficits in cell-mediated immunity, and benign thymoma (see Ch. 439). The thymomas are predominantly of the spindle cell variety. Eosinophilia or eosinopenia, aregenerative or hemolytic anemia, thrombocytopenia, or pancytopenia may also occur. Antibody formation is poor, although percentages of immunoglobulin-bearing B lymphocytes are normal, and progressive lymphopenia develops. Several patients with this disorder have been shown to have excessive suppressor T cell activity.

HYPERIMMUNOGLOBULINEMIA E SYNDROME. The hyper-IgE syndrome is a primary immunodeficiency characterized by recurrent staphylococcal abscesses and markedly elevated serum IgE concentrations. The disorder was first reported by the author and her coworkers in two young boys in 1972. These patients all have lifelong histories of severe recurrent staphylococcal abscesses involving the skin, lungs, joints, and other sites. Persistent pneumatoceles develop as result of their recurrent pneumonias. The pruritic dermatitis that occurs is not typical atopic eczema and does not always persist; respiratory allergic symptoms are usually absent. An autosomal dominant form of inheritance with incomplete penetrance seems possible. Laboratory features include exceptionally high serum IgE concentrations but usually normal IgG, IgA, and IgM concentrations; pronounced blood and sputum eosinophilia; abnormally low anamnestic antibody responses; and poor antibody and cell-mediated responses to neoantigens. In vitro studies have shown normal percentages of E rosette-forming, T3-, T4-, and T8-positive lymphocytes, and there is no increase in the percentage of IgE–bearing B lymphocytes. Lymphocyte responses to mitogens are normal, but responses to antigens or to related allogeneic cells have been absent or very low. Histologic sections of lymph nodes, spleen, and lung cysts show striking eosinophilia.

Phagocytic cell ingestion, metabolism, and killing mechanisms and total hemolytic complement have been normal in all patients. Defects of mononuclear and/or polymorphonuclear chemotaxis are present in some but not all patients, and thus are not the basic problem in this syndrome.

The most effective therapy is long-term administration of a penicillinase resistant penicillin, with the addition of other antibiotic or antifungal agents as required for specific infections.

CHRONIC MUCOCUTANEOUS CANDIDIASIS. This clinical syndrome, probably of multiple causes, is associated with chronic candidal infection of the skin and mucous membranes but only rarely life-threatening systemic infections of the types seen in patients with severe T cell dysfunction. Some patients have endocrinopathies involving the parathyroid, thyroid, adrenal, and/or pancreatic glands (see Ch. 240); however, many do not have either associated endocrinopathy or any demonstrable immunologic abnormality. Serum immunoglobulins are generally normal or increased, but IgA deficiency has been reported. Precipitating or agglutinating antibodies to *Candida* are usually present. Even in those patients who have had in vivo and/or in vitro evidence of deficient cell-mediated immunity, it is not clear whether it was primary or secondary to extensive fungal disease (e.g., an antigen overload mechanism). Ketaconazole (Nizoral) has been found to be the single most effective form of therapy. Nephrotoxicity prohibits continuous therapy with amphotericin B.

PRIMARY DEFICIENCIES OF THE COMPLEMENT SYSTEM

In addition to congenital or hereditary disorders of lymphoid cells, there are several well-defined primary immune defects involving the complement system. Genetically determined deficiencies have been described for all of the components of complement, and undue susceptibility to infection is a characteristic of certain of these, particularly for deficiencies of C2, C3, C5, C6, and C7. The types of infections experienced in C2, C3 and in some with C5 deficiency are generally similar to those of patients with antibody deficiency syndrome, whereas those in patients with deficiencies of the terminal components are usually of meningococcal or gonococcal causes. A normal CH50 would exclude all heritable complement deficiencies. The complement system is discussed in detail in Chapter 428.

Buckley RH: Normal and abnormal development of the immune system. *In* Joklik WK, Willett HP, Amos DB (eds.): Zinsser Textbook of Microbiology and Immunology. 18th ed. New York, Appleton-Century-Crofts, 1984, pp 317–340. *A concise review of ontogeny of the normal human immune system as well as the primary immunodeficiency disorders.*

Buckley RH: Immunodeficiency diseases. *In* Kelley WN, et al. (eds.): Textbook of Rheumatology. Philadelphia, W. B. Saunders Company, 1981, pp 1351–1377. *A comprehensive, extensively referenced chapter on primary immunodeficiency, with particular emphasis on the occurrence of collagen vascular and autoimmune diseases in certain of these disorders.*

Buckley RH, Sampson HA: The hyperimmunoglobulinemia E syndrome. *In* Franklin EC (ed.): Clinical Immunology Update. New York, Elsevier North Holland, 1980, pp 147–167. *A review of the clinical and immunologic features of 21 well-studied patients with the hyper-IgE syndrome.*

Purtilo DT, Sakamoto K, Barnabei V, et al.: Epstein-Barr virus–induced diseases in boys with the X-linked lymphoproliferative syndrome (XLP): Update on studies of the Registry. Am J Med 73:49, 1982.

Reisner Y, Kapoor N, Kirkpatrick D, Pollack MS, Cunningham-Rundles S, Dupont B, Hodes MZ, Good RA, O'Reilly RJ: Transplantation for severe combined immunodeficiency with HLA-A, B, D, DR incompatible parental marrow cells fractionated with soybean agglutinin and sheep red blood cells. Blood 61:341, 1983.

Rosen FS, Cooper MD, Wedgewood RJP: The primary immunodeficiencies. N Engl J Med 311:235, 300, 1984. *An excellent recent Medical Progress article which presents an overview of the basic biology and the clinical manifestations of these disorders. 260 references*

Stiehm ER, Fulginiti VA (eds.): Immunologic Disorders in Infants and Children. Philadelphia, W. B. Saunders Company, 1980. *The second edition of the only comprehensive textbook on pediatric immunology. Well referenced.*

Wedgwood R, Rosen FS, Paul NW (eds.): Primary Immunodeficiency Diseases. New York, Alan R. Liss Publishers, 1983. *Proceedings of the Fourth International Symposium on Immunodeficiency Diseases. Contributions by most authorities in the field. It is comprehensive and presents the state of the art as of 1982.*

430. ACQUIRED IMMUNODEFICIENCY SYNDROME (AIDS)

Anthony S. Fauci

DEFINITION. The acquired immunodeficiency syndrome (AIDS) has been defined by the Centers for Disease Control (CDC) as the presence of a reliably diagnosed disease that is at least moderately indicative of an underlying defect in cell-mediated immunity, for example, Kaposi's sarcoma in an individual who is less than 60 years of age, *Pneumocystis carinii* pneumonia, or other life-threatening opportunistic infections. Critical to the case definition is the absence of known causes of underlying immune deficiency and of any other host defense defects reported to be associated with the disease, such as immunosuppressive therapy or malignant lymphoreticular disease.

ETIOLOGY. AIDS is clearly caused by a transmissible agent. Although its precise etiology has not yet been conclusively proven, recent viral isolation and sero-epidemiologic studies have provided compelling evidence that the etiologic agent is a retrovirus of the human T cell leukemia/lymphoma virus (HTLV) family, which has been designated HTLV-III. This virus is lymphocytotropic, with a selective affinity for thymus-derived (T) lymphocytes that are of the inducer/helper subset defined by the T4 or Leu 3 phenotypic markers. Although other viruses such as the Epstein-Barr virus (EBV) and the cytomegalovirus (CMV) have been implicated by some investigators as being causal to the syndrome, it is now clear that they are either secondary infections or cofactors that result in immunosuppression and/or activation of lymphocytes, rendering them susceptible to infection with the primary etiologic agent.

INCIDENCE AND PREVALENCE. AIDS is either an entirely new disease or it existed in an epidemiologic setting whereby its incidence was low enough to remain unnoticed. The medical community first became aware of the syndrome in June and July, 1981, when CDC announced the unexplained occurrence of *Pneumocystis carinii* pneumonia in five previously well homosexual men in Los Angeles and Kaposi's sarcoma in 26 previously well homosexual men in New York and Los Angeles. By September, 1984, more than 5785 cases had been reported from at least 45 states and hundreds of additional cases worldwide. Since the incubation period is believed to be approximately one year, and in occasional cases it is felt to have been as long as four years, the full scope of the syndrome has not been realized, and it is difficult to project accurately the full impact and ultimate prevalence of AIDS. The epidemiologic pattern strongly suggests that sexual contact is the major means of transmission. The second most common mode of transmission appears to be via blood or blood products, as in individuals sharing needles for intravenous drug abuse or receiving a large number of transfusions of blood products. Thus the disease up to this point has remained largely confined within certain well-defined risk groups.

Clearly, homosexual or bisexual men constitute the largest risk group, accounting for over 70 per cent of all cases reported in the United States. Almost half of the reported cases in the world are from the New York City area, which has the largest concentration of male homosexuals in the United States. The next largest groups of patients are found in San Francisco and Los Angeles, cities that also have large concentrations of male homosexuals. Intravenous drug abusers with no history of homosexuality comprise the next largest group, with 17 per cent of the total patients. Haitian immigrants to the United States with no admitted history of homosexuality or intravenous drug abuse compose 5 per cent of cases. Recently it has become apparent that the disease is indeed seen in Haitians living in Haiti. However, it is unclear at this point what proportion of these fall into the first two risk groups of homosexuality and intravenous drug abuse. Lastly, hemophiliacs with no history of other risk factors compose almost 1 per cent of patients. Hemophiliacs are probably exposed to the transmissible agent of AIDS through the large numbers of transfusions of plasma products required for replacement of deficient clotting factors. This is especially true of individuals who receive large amounts of factor VIII concentrates. Almost 6 per cent of patients fall into none of the above categories. Within this group are several transfusion-related cases, infants born of mothers at risk for AIDS, and small numbers of women who are the heterosexual partners of individuals who either have AIDS or are at risk for AIDS. Others within this group with no known risk factors are a few patients who died before adequate information could be obtained and a very few others who truly have no apparent risk.

Physicians, nurses, and other health care or laboratory workers who deal with AIDS patients have not contracted AIDS unless they themselves fell into one of the recognized risk groups. This observation strongly suggests that casual or even close nonsexual contact will not transmit AIDS. Although AIDS is clearly epidemic in the risk groups mentioned, it seems likely to remain largely confined to these risk groups unless individuals in non-risk groups either have sexual contact with or are exposed to blood-borne transmission from someone with AIDS or incubating AIDS.

PATHOGENESIS AND IMMUNE DEFECT. The common denominator of AIDS is a profound acquired defect in cell-mediated immunity. Patients are anergic with a defect that is remarkably selective for the T lymphocyte. Most patients are lymphopenic with selective quantitative diminution in the inducer/helper T cell subset that is defined by the T4 or Leu 3 phenotypic markers. The suppressor/cytotoxic subset of T cell defined by the T8 or Leu 2 phenotypic marker is generally normal in number or only slightly increased or decreased, thereby resulting in marked decrease in the T4-T8 ratio within the peripheral blood. The T4 cells are not only quantitatively decreased but are also qualitatively defective in their functional capability. The selective defect in the T4 lymphocyte subset likely reflects the fact that HTLV-III is T4 lymphocytotropic. Natural killer cell and virus-specific T cell cytotoxicity are also defective in AIDS. This defect may well be due to the lack of induction of cytotoxic cells by the T4 cell or its soluble products. Finally, patients manifest hypergammaglobulinemia that reflects polyclonal hyperactivity of B lymphocytes. This B cell hyperactivity results in an actual B cell defect, as patients do not respond with an appropriate humoral response to in vivo antigen exposure as with immunizations.

The underlying defect in cell-mediated immunity leads to a dramatic decrease in host defenses, in turn leading to extraordinary susceptibility to recurrent opportunistic infections, one of the hallmarks of the syndrome. Patients are also susceptible to the development of Kaposi's sarcoma and, to a much lesser extent, of Burkitt-like lymphomas. It is unclear why patients develop Kaposi's sarcoma; furthermore, Kaposi's sarcoma is found to a much higher proportion in homosexuals with AIDS than in individuals in the other risk groups. AIDS patients who develop Kaposi's sarcoma have a significantly higher incidence of the HLA-DR5 haplotype.

Thus, the underlying pathogenesis of the syndrome itself relates to a profound defect in T-cell–mediated immunity caused by infection with a T lymphocytotropic virus. The subsequent manifestations of the syndrome result from this remarkable immune defect.

CLINICAL MANIFESTATIONS. Patients with AIDS exhibit a number of disease patterns. By strict definition, they must have either an opportunistic infection or Kaposi's sarcoma. In this regard, 50 per cent of patients have *Pneumocystis carinii* pneumonia without Kaposi's sarcoma, and approximately 26 per cent develop Kaposi's sarcoma without *Pneumocystis carinii* pneumonia. Smaller percentages of patients have both Kaposi's sarcoma and *Pneumocystis carinii* pneumonia or other opportunistic infections without Kaposi's sarcoma or *Pneumocystis carinii* pneumonia. The clinical manifestations reflect the particular opportunistic infection or the distribution of the neoplastic process. It is not uncommon for a given patient to have more than one opportunistic infection simultaneously.

Patients who develop *Pneumocystis carinii* pneumonia have the typical findings of this disease, with dyspnea and hypoxemia (see Ch. 383). The pneumonia may be abrupt and fulminant or insidious, with symptoms accelerating over weeks before the diagnosis is realized. CMV infections are manifest by fever and disseminated organ system involvement. Of particular importance is the chorioretinitis that often relentlessly progresses to total blindness. Herpes simplex virus may manifest as fulminant and life-threatening mucocutaneous dissemination. *Candida albicans* is commonly seen as oral thrush or esophagitis. *Cryptococcus neoformans* infections occur as meningitis or disseminated disease. Of particular interest are the disseminated infections with *Mycobacterium avium-intracellulare*. This infection is very rarely seen in individuals with iatrogenic immunosuppression or immunosuppression due to congenital cellular immunodeficiencies or spontaneous neoplasms. Yet this infection is relatively common in patients with AIDS. Disseminated *Mycobacterium tuberculosis* infection is seen to a lesser extent in AIDS, except in Haitian patients in whom it is relatively common. *Toxoplasma gondii* infections occur as intracerebral mass lesions or as chorioretinitis. Finally, a peculiar diarrheal syndrome has been linked to infection with the coccidial protozoa *Cryptosporium*. Many patients with AIDS have or develop intractable diarrhea for which no offending agent can be identified.

Another peculiar clinical syndrome associated with AIDS is a neurologic disorder that is characterized by progressive dementia with or without localizing signs. The etiology of this syndrome is unclear at present, and no etiologic agent has been identified, although biopsy specimens have revealed nonspecific inflammation, cerebral atrophy, or multifocal leukoencephalopathy.

Certain patients develop an unexplained syndrome of fever, weight loss, and wasting that is seemingly unrelated to the other manifestations of their disease, i.e., obvious opportunistic infections or Kaposi's sarcoma. However, in several patients these findings were ultimately explained by disseminated CMV or unrecognized *Mycobacterium avium-intracellulare* infections.

Kaposi's sarcoma in AIDS patients follows a significantly different pattern from Kaposi's sarcoma in nonepidemic groups, such as elderly men in the United States and Europe and organ transplant recipients. In these latter groups, the disease is generally indolent and confined to the skin, with only a 10 per cent incidence of extracutaneous organ involvement. In the Kaposi's sarcoma seen in children and young adults in certain areas of Africa, the incidence of extracutaneous involvement is 20 per cent, whereas in AIDS patients it is over 70 per cent. The most commonly involved organs are the lymph nodes, gastrointestinal tract, and lungs; however, virtually any organ system can be involved in this disseminated form.

Finally, a large number of male homosexuals have an unexplained lymphadenopathy syndrome that has been defined by the CDC as the presence for three months or longer of extrainguinal sites of lymphadenopathy with no recognizable cause for it. Biopsy, when available, reveals nonspecific lymphoid hyperplasia. Other individuals may have a wasting syndrome described above with or without lymphadenopathy. This constellation of signs and symptoms has been termed AIDS-related complex and even "pre-AIDS" by some. However, this terminology is not entirely appropriate, since it is unclear what proportion of these individuals will progress to full-blown AIDS. In this regard, HTLV-III has been isolated from over 80 per cent of such individuals.

DIAGNOSIS. The diagnosis of AIDS is made on the basis of the clinical criteria listed above. There are no laboratory tests that are diagnostic of the syndrome, although the selective diminution of the T4 lymphocyte subset in an otherwise well individual is strongly suggestive of the underlying immune defect. The presence of opportunistic infections or Kaposi's sarcoma in this setting confirms the diagnosis. It is of importance to realize that a mere reversal of the T4-T8 ratio of lymphocyte subsets does not of itself indicate that an individual is at risk to develop the full-blown syndrome. A number of common and relatively benign viral infections cause an increase in the T8 subset without substantially lowering the T4 subset, yet this will also result in inversion of the T4-T8 ratio. Since many homosexual males who do not have AIDS are frequently infected with viruses such as CMV and EBV, which cause reversals of T cell subset ratios, it would be inappropriate at this point to designate them as having a pre-AIDS condition.

TREATMENT AND PROGNOSIS. There is no known treatment for the underlying immune defects in AIDS, and there has been no report of spontaneous reversal of this defect. A number of attempts at immune reconstitution have been undertaken, including bone marrow transplantation, infusion of histocompatible lymphocytes, and administration of alpha interferon, gamma interferon, and interleukin 2. Despite the fact that some beneficial effects on the viral infections and Kaposi's sarcoma have been noted, there has thus far been no impressive and long-lasting reconstitution of immune function. However, extensive trials with these agents have not yet been completed. Kaposi's sarcoma has been treated with irradiation, chemotherapy, and certain of the immune reconstitutions mentioned above. Again, although partial and complete remissions of Kaposi's sarcoma have been effected in some patients, the underlying immune defect persists, and patients remain susceptible to repeated bouts of opportunistic infections or return of Kaposi's sarcoma or both. Several of the opportunistic infections such as *Pneumocystis carinii*, candidiasis, toxoplasmosis, cryptococcosis, typical tuberculosis, and herpes simplex can be effectively treated to a greater or lesser degree with antimicrobial agents, but there is no effective treatment for *Mycobacterium avium-intracellulare*, CMV and EBV infections, and cryptosporidosis.

The typical clinical course of the syndrome is one of repetitive and relentless attacks of a variety of opportunistic infections with or without Kaposi's sarcoma, ultimately leading to the death of the patient. The overall mortality of the syndrome is approximately 40 per cent. However, there are very few survivors among those who have had the disease since 1981, and given the fact that there are no reported cures, the true mortality of AIDS, at this point, may approach 100 per cent.

Fauci AS: The syndrome of Kaposi's sarcoma and opportunistic infections: An epidemiologically restricted disorder of immunoregulation. Ann Intern Med 96:77, 1982. *Description of the syndrome and discussion of potential scope and pathophysiologic mechanisms.*

Fauci AS, Macher AM, Longo DL, Lane HC, Rook AH, Masur H, Gelman EP: Acquired immune deficiency syndrome (AIDS). Ann Intern Med 100:92, 1984. *Detailed updated review and discussion of the epidemiology, clinical and pathologic manifestations, immune defect, potential etiologic factors, and currently utilized therapeutic approaches to AIDS.*

Gottlieb MS, Groopman JE, Weinstein WM, Fahey JL, Detels R: The acquired immunodeficiency syndrome. Ann Intern Med 99:208, 1983. *Extensive review of the syndrome with focus on the UCLA clinical experience.*

Murray JF, Felton CP, Garay SM, Gottlieb MS, Hopewell PC, Stover DE, Teirstein AS: Pulmonary complications of the acquired immunodeficiency syndrome: Report of a National Heart, Lung, and Blood Institute workshop. N Engl J Med 310:1682, 1984. *An excellent, recent, concise overview.*

Popovic M, Sarngadharan MG, Read E, Gallo RC: Detection, isolation, and continuous production of cytopathic retroviruses (HTLV-III) from patients with AIDS and pre-AIDS. Science 224:497, 1984. *Classic report providing compelling evidence that a retrovirus of the HTLV family (HTLV-III) is in fact the etiologic agent of AIDS.*

431. URTICARIA AND ANGIOEDEMA

Nicholas A. Soter

DEFINITION. Urticaria and angioedema are commonly encountered clinical entities that occur as evanescent areas of cutaneous edema. Urticaria appears as circumscribed elevated erythematous and usually pruritic areas of edema involving the superficial portions of the dermis. When the edema extends into the deep portions of the dermis or subcutaneous and submucosal tissues or both, it is designated angioedema and appears as large erythematous areas with diffuse borders. In addition to the skin, the respiratory and gastrointestinal tracts as well as the cardiovascular system may be involved singly or in any combination. The etiology of urticaria-angioedema is frequently unknown; however, its pathogenesis in many instances is believed to be related to activation of mast cells and/or basophils and release of their products, termed mediators of immediate hypersensitivity. Similar symptoms and signs may occur in association with activation of other inflammatory systems, such as the arachidonic acid metabolic pathways, the complement system (see Ch. 428), and the Hageman factor–dependent pathways of coagulation, fibrinolysis, and kinin generation with or without the participation of mast cells.

INCIDENCE AND PREVALENCE. Urticaria-angioedema may develop at any age. The highest incidence is in young adults, in whom it occurs in approximately 15 to 20 per cent. In patients with urticaria-angioedema, about 50 per cent will have both, 40 per cent urticaria alone, and 10 per cent angioedema alone. Approximately 50 per cent of patients with urticaria alone are free of lesions within one year, but 20 per cent continue to experience lesions for more than twenty years. Of patients with both urticaria and angioedema, 75 per cent experience symptoms for more than one year, 50 per cent for more than five years, and 20 per cent for more than twenty years. Age, race, sex, occupation, geographic location, and season of the year are involved as factors only insofar as they may contribute to exposure to an eliciting cause.

PATHOGENESIS AND PATHOLOGY. Urticaria-angioedema is often attributed to an immediate-type immunologic reaction (Type I, anaphylactic, or IgE-mediated hypersensitivity) produced by the antigen-induced release of biologically active materials from mast cells sensitized with specific IgE. Antigen-dependent activation and secretion in mast cells is initiated by bridging of pairs of adjacent IgE molecules and is dependent upon several subsequent intracellular events, including the activation of adenylate cyclase, membrane phospholipid methylation, and calcium flux (see Fig. 59–3). Urticaria-angioedema may also occur after mast cell degranulation induced by complement factors C3a and C5a, kinins, insect venoms, highly charged polyanions, or certain therapeutic and diagnostic agents. Physical stimuli such as trauma, pressure, cold, light, and heat may affect the mast cell via IgE or by unknown mechanisms.

The skin is rich in mast cells; the mean number is 7000 to 12,000 per cubic millimeter (see Fig. 438–1). The biologic effects of mast cells (described more fully in Ch. 438) are produced by the release of mediators, which alter venular permeability, contract smooth muscles, influence the motility of leukocytes, affect the generation and release of biologically active materials from other cell types, and enzymatically degrade complex substrates such as proteoglycans and collagen (see table in Ch. 438).

Urticaria-angioedema occurring after mast cell–mediated reactions is attributed primarily to the release of *histamine*, although other mediators, such as prostaglandin D_2, may play a role. Two tissue receptors, classified as H_1 and H_2, mediate the biologic activities of histamine. H_1-mediated effects include smooth muscle contraction, alterations in venular permeability, increases in airway resistance, and augmentation of motility of certain leukocytes. H_2-mediated effects include alterations in venular permeability, inhibition of T-lymphocyte function, depression of motility of certain leukocytes, suppression of basophil mediator release, increases in cardiac rate and force of contraction, and augmentation of gastric acid secretion. Inasmuch as the human skin vasculature contains both H_1 and H_2 receptors, vascular permeability may depend on the effect of histamine on both.

Skin biopsy specimens show edema involving the superficial portion of the dermis in the case of urticaria and the deeper dermis and subcutaneous tissue in the case of angioedema. Both urticaria and angioedema are associated with dilation of the venules with or without tissue infiltration by various numbers of lymphocytes and/or eosinophils and neutrophils. In some instances, necrotizing vasculitis with fibrinoid necrosis of the venule is present. In individuals with hereditary angioedema, examination of biopsy specimens from skin, larynx, and jejunum has shown subcutaneous or submucosal edema without infiltrating inflammatory cells.

CLINICAL MANIFESTATIONS. Urticaria and angioedema may occur together or individually in any location; however, angioedema most commonly affects the face. Episodes of urticaria-angioedema appear suddenly, usually persist fewer than 24 hours, and may recur. Recurrent episodes of fewer than four to six weeks' duration are considered acute, whereas those persisting longer are chronic.

Urticaria-angioedema can be classified into five groups that include those types which are IgE dependent or complement dependent, those which are due to a direct action on mast cells, those which occur after presumed alterations of the arachidonic acid metabolic pathways, and those which are idiopathic (see Table 431–1).

Idiopathic Urticaria-Angioedema. In at least 70 per cent of individuals with chronic episodes of urticaria-angioedema, the cause is unknown. Since this clinical condition is common, is easily recognized, and manifests a capricious course, it is often associated with concomitant events. Such attributions must be interpreted with caution. Although viral, fungal, bacterial, and helminthic infections, foods, medications, diagnostic agents, metabolic and hormonal abnormalities, malignant conditions, and emotional factors are frequently claimed as causes, proof of their etiologic relation often is lacking. Although idiopathic urticaria-angioedema is the most prevalent form, the diagnosis is one of exclusion and can be made only after the other types of urticaria-angioedema, discussed below, are eliminated. The laboratory studies to be considered in patients with urticaria-angioedema are noted under Laboratory Findings, below.

IgE-Dependent Urticaria-Angioedema. ATOPIC DIATHESIS. A history of acute episodes of urticaria-angioedema may be elicited in individuals with a personal or family history of asthma, rhinitis, or eczema. The prevalence of chronic urticaria, however, is not increased in atopic individuals. Moreover, in atopic persons urticaria-angioedema should not be too readily attributed to the atopic diathesis without a search for other causes.

SPECIFIC ANTIGENS. IgE-mediated urticaria-angioedema occurs after exposure to agents that include foods, diagnostic and therapeutic agents, pollens, and Hymenoptera venoms. In some instances, vasoactive substances or chemical additives may be responsible factors.

PHYSICAL STIMULI. Physical urticaria-angioedema occurs after a variety of stimuli, some of which are IgE dependent as demonstrated by passive transfer with serum of the cutaneous response to normal individuals (Prausnitz-Küstner reaction).

Dermographism. Dermographism occurs in 1.5 to 4.2 per cent of the normal population. It is usually recognized as a linear wheal appearing after the skin is briskly stroked with a firm object; however, its configuration depends on the eliciting stimulus. The transient pruritic wheal appears rapidly and fades within 30 minutes. Dermographism has been passively transferred to the skin of normal persons with both serum and its IgE fraction. Elevations in blood histamine levels have been detected after experimental scratching.

Pressure Urticaria-Angioedema. Pressure urticaria appears as erythematous, deep, often painful swelling that arises within minutes or up to six hours after sustained pressure, such as occurs under shoulder straps and belts, on the soles of the feet after running, and on the palms after manual labor. Although pressure urticaria-angioedema often occurs in individuals with dermographism or chronic idiopathic urticaria, an IgE-dependent mechanism has not been documented.

Vibratory Angioedema. Angioedema occurring after a vibratory stimulus has been reported with an autosomal dominant pat-

TABLE 431–1. CLASSIFICATION OF URTICARIA-ANGIOEDEMA

I. Idiopathic urticaria-angioedema
II. IgE-dependent urticaria-angioedema
  A. Atopic diathesis
  B. Specific antigen sensitivity
  C. Physical stimuli
  D. Contact urticaria
III. Complement-mediated urticaria-angioedema
  A. Hereditary angioedema
  B. Acquired C1 inhibitor abnormalities associated with angioedema
  C. Necrotizing venulitis
  D. Serum sickness
  E. Reactions to the administration of blood products
IV. Urticaria-angioedema due to agents with a direct action on mast cells
V. Urticaria-angioedema dependent on agents that alter the arachidonic acid metabolic pathways

tern of inheritance. It occurs also in association with cholinergic urticaria and after several years of occupational exposure to vibration. In the heritable form, the swelling appears rapidly, is transient, and is accompanied by facial flushing. A transient rise in plasma histamine was noted during experimental induction of vibratory angioedema both in the hereditary form and in those patients with acquired disease.

Cold-Induced Urticaria-Angioedema. There are both inherited and acquired forms of cold-induced urticaria-angioedema. The acquired form is more common. After exposure to changes in ambient temperature or direct contact with cold objects, patients experience a pruritic, urticarial eruption that may evolve into angioedema. Headaches, syncope, or wheezing may accompany an attack. If the entire body is cooled, as in swimming, hypotension and collapse, a potentially lethal event, may occur. Passive transfer with serum and its IgE fraction to the skin of a normal recipient has been documented, and the release into the serum of histamine and factors chemotactic for eosinophils and neutrophils has been detected after experimental challenge. Also, successful passive transfer with serum containing IgM antibody has been accomplished. In rare instances, acquired cold urticaria has been associated with underlying cryoproteins, notably cryoglobulins, cryofibrinogens, or cold hemolysins. The mechanism by which cryoproteins induce cold urticaria may be activation of the complement system.

Dominantly inherited cold urticaria has been described in immediate and delayed forms. In the immediate type, the eruption appears as erythematous macules or papules which manifest a burning sensation and which are accompanied by pyrexia, arthralgias, and a neutrophilic leukocytosis. In the delayed form, erythematous deep swellings develop 9 to 18 hours after cold challenge. This disorder is infrequently recognized, and its pathogenesis is unknown.

Light Urticaria. Idiopathic light or solar urticaria is a rare condition manifested by pruritus and urticaria-angioedema developing within minutes after exposure to the sun or to artificial light sources. Light urticaria also occasionally occurs in patients with systemic lupus erythematosus and erythropoietic protoporphyria. Classification of the urticarial response into subtypes is based on the reaction to specific portions of the light spectrum; however, individuals may respond to more than one portion of the spectrum. Histamine and factors chemotactic for eosinophils and neutrophils have been detected in serum after experimental exposure to UVB (290 to 320 nm), UVA (320 to 400 nm), or visible (400 to 700 nm) light. In some individuals the response has been passively transferred; in other subjects a serum factor induced by irradiation has been implicated in the development of the lesions.

Cholinergic Urticaria. Cholinergic urticaria is a distinctive eruption that develops after stimuli that allegedly raise core body temperature, such as a hot shower, exercise, or episodes of pyrexia. After an initial sensation of warmth, pruritic wheals 1 to 2 mm in size appear, surrounded by extensive areas of erythema. Wheezing has been noted, and obstructive alterations in pulmonary function have been documented during experimental induction of the clinical syndrome by exercise. Elevations in serum histamine and the appearance of factors chemotactic for eosinophils and neutrophils have been noted. Although injection of cholinergic agents such as methacholine into the skin has been employed as a diagnostic test, in only one third of individuals with cholinergic urticaria does this maneuver reproduce the skin lesions.

Heat Urticaria. Heat urticaria is a rare disorder in which urticaria-angioedema develops within minutes after exposure to locally applied heat. Elevations in plasma histamine levels have been noted after experimental challenge.

Aquagenic Urticaria and Aquagenic Pruritus. Contact of the skin with water of any temperature may result in pruritus alone or, more rarely, urticaria. The eruption consists of small wheals reminiscent of cholinergic urticaria. After experimental challenge, elevations of blood histamine have been noted in both aquagenic urticaria and aquagenic pruritus.

Contact Urticaria. Urticaria may occur after direct local contact with a variety of chemical substances. The eruption appears within minutes, is transient, and usually disappears within hours. Occasionally, systemic manifestations have been noted. Although passive transfer has been documented in some instances, agents such as stinging nettles, arthropod hairs, and chemicals may directly release histamine from mast cells.

Complement-Mediated Urticaria-Angioedema. Hereditary Angioedema. Hereditary angioedema (HAE) occurs as episodes of edema of the skin and of the upper respiratory and gastrointestinal tracts. Episodes of swelling are self-limited, subside within 72 hours, and may occur over any area of the body, particularly on the face or an extremity. Urticaria alone is not a manifestation of HAE. Swelling of the face or buccal mucosa may progress to involve the larynx, with the danger of death by asphyxiation. The severity of the abdominal pain mimics surgical abdominal conditions.

HAE is transmitted as an autosomal dominant trait, and afflicted individuals are heterozygotes; however, the absence of a family history does not exclude the diagnosis. There are two forms of this inherited disease, each of which is characterized by the absence of function of the inhibitor ($C\bar{1}INH$) of the activated form of the first complement protein ($C\bar{1}$) of the classic activating pathway (see Ch. 428). Either the $C\bar{1}INH$ protein and its function are lacking or normal levels of $C\bar{1}INH$ protein without function are present. The absence of $C\bar{1}INH$ provides a genetic marker for HAE and introduces the possibility that the lack of function of this complement factor is involved in pathogenesis of the clinical attacks. Levels of the fourth complement protein (C4) are also low, and levels of C4 and of the second complement protein (C2) diminish during clinical attacks. With the possible exception of post-traumatic attacks, the reasons for the episodic activation of C1 are unknown. In the absence of the $C\bar{1}INH$, the activation of Hageman factor after tissue trauma may lead to the conversion of plasminogen to plasmin, which subsequently activates C1. It is speculated that the angioedema is a result of a smooth muscle–contracting, heat-stable polypeptide derived by the action of plasmin on a complement fragment produced by the action of $C\bar{1}$ on C4 and C2. Urinary histamine levels are increased during attacks, presumably reflecting the degranulation of mast cells by C3a anaphylatoxin. Kallikrein has been found in the fluid of blisters induced over areas of edema, and increased bradykinin has been detected in plasma during attacks.

Acquired $C\bar{1}INH$ Deficiency. The acquired depletion of the $C\bar{1}INH$ sometimes associated with angioedema has been observed in patients with different types of lymphoproliferative disorders, in a patient with a rectal adenocarcinoma, and in some individuals with lupus erythematosus. In addition to low serum levels of $C\bar{1}INH$ and C4, C1 and C1q levels are also reduced, thus permitting its differentiation from HAE. Abnormalities of complement in family members have not been reported.

Necrotizing Venulitis. Recurrent episodes of urticaria-angioedema may be manifestations of cutaneous necrotizing venulitis. An idiopathic clinical syndrome occurs primarily in women with associated transient arthralgia. The episodes of urticaria are chronic; individual lesions are transient, lasting fewer than 24 hours in many instances but occasionally up to three to five days. Most patients experience transient arthralgias of the peripheral joints. In some instances, diffuse glomerulonephritis has been noted as well as pyrexia, lymphadenopathy, obstructive pulmonary disease, and benign intracranial hypertension. These cases have been described under the terms erythema multiforme, lupus erythematosus–like syndrome, and hypocomplementemia-vasculitis-urticaria syndrome. Although some patients manifest serum hypocomplementemia with circulating C1q precipitins, many do not. Some patients with systemic lupus erythematosus or Sjögren's syndrome also manifest an urticarial form of cutaneous necrotizing venulitis.

SERUM SICKNESS. Serum sickness is a clinical symptom complex occurring after the administration of serum or drugs and lasting four to five days. The clinical manifestations include pyrexia, urticaria, lymphadenopathy, myalgia, and arthralgia. Urticaria is seen in over 70 per cent of patients with serum sickness, and often occurs at the site of injection.

REACTIONS TO BLOOD PRODUCTS. Urticaria-angioedema frequently occurs after the administration of blood products. Both the urticarial and the anaphylactic reactions noted after the transfusion of blood, serum, or IgG fractions are usually the result of immune complex formation with complement activation. Such immune complex reactions are especially prevalent in patients with IgA deficiency, in whom antibodies against IgA are present. Occasionally the urticaria may be due to the transfusion of IgE directed toward an antigen to which the recipient is subsequently exposed or to the transfusion of an antigen into a sensitized recipient. Activated Hageman factor has also been implicated in urticarial transfusion reactions.

Urticaria-Angioedema Due to Agents with a Direct Action on Mast Cells. The administration of opiates, polymyxin B, curare and tubocurarine, or radiocontrast media may be associated with the idiosyncratic release of histamine from mast cells. Between 5 and 8 per cent of individuals receiving radiocontrast media experience urticarial reactions, especially following intravenous administration.

Agents Which Presumably Alter Arachidonic Acid Metabolism. Urticaria-angioedema in response to administration of aspirin or nonsteroidal anti-inflammatory agents occurs commonly. Aspirin intolerance in patients with chronic urticaria is reported to be as high as 20 to 50 per cent. Patients intolerant to aspirin also react to indomethacin and to azo dyes, notably tartrazine, as well as to benzoates used as preservatives. Such reactions are often unrecognized, may serve to aggravate preexisting urticaria, and may occur from 15 minutes to 20 hours after ingestion. In patients intolerant to aspirin, reactions do not occur after exposure to structurally related compounds such as sodium or choline salicylate, whereas structurally unrelated agents such as indomethacin may precipitate the response.

LABORATORY FINDINGS. Laboratory evaluation is usually not helpful in patients with acute episodes of urticaria-angioedema. Historical information and physical findings offer better diagnostic clues. Acute urticaria may present as a manifestation of hepatitis B viral disease or serum sickness. In those patients whose acute urticaria-angioedema suggests an IgE-mediated allergic process, prick skin testing or assessment in vitro by radioallergosorbent test (RAST) of specific IgE antibody may be indicated; however, the likelihood of obtaining diagnostically relevant information from unselected prick skin tests or RAST is minimal. Prick skin testing is unreliable in the presence of dermographism.

Evaluation of chronic episodes of urticaria-angioedema requires more extensive laboratory analysis. The RAST has allowed the diagnosis of sensitivity to a variety of antigens, including foods, pollens, insect venom, and animal danders. Eosinophilia, when present, is a helpful feature in implicating a drug reaction or parasitic infestation as a cause of urticaria. Anti–hepatitis B surface antibody has been noted in some patients. Antinuclear antibody is helpful in detecting associated lupus erythematosus. Total serum concentrations of IgE in the absence of atopy are normal in patients with chronic urticaria-angioedema.

Assessment of the serum complement system is of value in detecting patients with hereditary and acquired forms of angioedema. In patients with HAE, immunochemical measurements of both $C\overline{1}INH$ and C4 are low with normal levels of C1 and C3. If the $C\overline{1}INH$ protein level is normal and the C4 low, functional assessment of $C\overline{1}INH$ may be performed to confirm the diagnosis.

In patients with chronic idiopathic urticaria-angioedema the finding of an elevated erythrocyte sedimentation rate should prompt a biopsy of an urticarial lesion to search for underlying cutaneous necrotizing venulitis. In some patients with necrotizing venulitis hypocomplementemia may be detected. As not all patients with necrotizing venulitis manifest hypocomplementemia, the sedimentation rate has proved to be a more sensitive screening test than serum complement analysis.

DIAGNOSIS AND DIFFERENTIAL DIAGNOSIS. Urticaria and angioedema are easily recognizable. Urticarial eruptions are episodic and evanescent, with multiple lesions occurring in various stages of evolution and resolution. The differential diagnosis of urticaria includes papular urticaria, which consists of small wheals occurring after insect bites; the eruption of erythema multiforme that includes iris or target lesions; the early urticarial stages of the Henoch-Schönlein syndrome that evolve into palpable purpura; urticaria pigmentosa, which is a generalized, pigmented, papular or even nodular mast cell infiltration in which the skin lesions become urticarial upon rubbing (see Fig. 438–2); and the syndrome of perceptive deafness, fever with urticaria, and renal insufficiency consequent to amyloidosis.

Disorders included in the differential diagnosis of angioedema are contact dermatitis appearing as recurrent episodes of eyelid and facial swelling; cellulitis and erysipelas, which may at times resemble angioedema; lymphedema occurring after cutaneous pyoderma or surgery; and congestive heart failure, renal insufficiency, obstruction of the superior vena cava, myxedema, thrombophlebitis, and stasis, which may produce recurrent swelling. The Melkersson-Rosenthal syndrome consists of swelling of the lips, facial paralysis, and a fissured tongue.

TREATMENT AND PREVENTION. When urticaria-angioedema is due to a known agent, avoidance is the therapeutic choice. Since patients may respond to the administration of placebos and the disease tends to spontaneously remit, evaluation of therapeutic intervention is difficult. Avoidance of aspirin or food additives has been claimed to improve many patients. Recurrent episodes of idiopathic urticaria-angioedema are most effectively treated by the prophylactic administration of H_1 antihistaminic agents. A variety of H_1-type antihistamine preparations exist, which are used empirically. These agents are administered in divided doses; representative examples are chlorpheniramine maleate, 4 to 8 mg, or diphenhydramine hydrochloride, 25 to 50 mg, every four to six hours. The combination of H_2 antihistamines in combination with H_1 agents is of value in a small number of individuals. Epinephrine is rarely required, and the chronic systemic administration of corticosteroid preparations creates risks out of proportion to the therapeutic benefits. The treatment of physical urticaria includes avoidance of the precipitating stimulus and the empiric administration of antihistamines.

The treatment of HAE can be divided into management of the acute episode, preoperative prophylaxis, and long-term prevention of spontaneous attacks. Specific therapeutic measures to interrupt spontaneous attacks are not available. The primary maneuver is to maintain the airway. Preoperative preparation of patients with antifibrinolytic agents suppresses attacks of angioedema. Nonandrogenic or impeded anabolic steroids, such as oxymetholone, danazol, and stanozolol, are effective in prevention of spontaneous attacks. Toxicity caused by attenuated androgens is dose related; however, the adverse effects that occur with daily therapy subside with alternate-day therapy. Although statistically significant mean increases in the serum levels of $C\overline{1}INH$ occur with both daily and alternate-day therapy, a significant mean rise in C4 levels occurs only on daily therapy. Thus clinical control can be achieved with therapeutic regimens of attenuated androgens that are not accompanied by immunochemical correction. Impeded androgens have also been used to treat acquired $C\overline{1}INH$ deficiency with recurrent angioedema. There is no proven effective treatment for the urticaria-angioedema that occurs as a manifestation of underlying necrotizing venulitis although some patients benefit from the administration of prednisone or nonsteroidal anti-inflammatory agents.

Gigli I: Hereditary angioneurotic edema (hereditary angioedema). *In* Franklin EC (ed.): Clinical Immunology Update: Reviews for Physicians. New York, Elsevier Biomedical, 1983, pp 317–335. *A current review of hereditary angioedema, its pathogenesis, and treatment.*

Juhlin L: Recurrent urticaria: Clinical investigation of 330 patients. Br J Dermatol 104:369, 1981. *A recent epidemiologic study of a large number of patients with urticaria-angioedema.*

Monroe EW: Urticarial vasculitis: An updated review. J Am Acad Dermatol 5:88, 1981. *A review of patients with chronic urticaria-angioedema as a manifestation of necrotizing venulitis.*

Soter NA: Physical urticaria/angioedema as an experimental model of acute and chronic inflammation in human skin. Springer Semin Immunopathol 4:73, 1981. *A review of the types of physical urticaria and the use of such disorders to study mast cell participation in human cutaneous disease.*

Warin RP, Champion RH: Urticaria. London, W. B. Saunders Company, 1974. *The definitive monograph considering the entity urticaria-angioedema.*

432. ALLERGIC RHINITIS

John E. Salvaggio

DEFINITION. Allergic rhinitis is an IgE-mediated, inflammatory disease of the nasal mucous membranes, characterized by paroxysms of sneezing, itching of the nose, eyes, palate, pharynx, and conjunctivae, nasal stuffiness with partial or total obstruction of airflow, and mucous secretion often accompanied by postnasal drainage. The disease is often seasonal, depending on the pollination patterns of inhalant allergens that have direct impact on the respiratory mucosa. The condition may be perennial when due to nonseasonal allergens, such as dust, animal danders, some plant products, and molds.

ETIOLOGY. The most apparent seasonal allergens acting as etiologic agents in allergic rhinitis are pollens, such as ragweed, and mold spores. Tree pollens are usually released during the spring, and, in most parts of the country the height of the grass pollen season is late spring to midsummer. Much of the nasal symptoms caused by airborne weed pollens occur in late summer and the early fall months. Ragweed pollen is by far the worst offender in the eastern, midwestern, and southern United States. Many individuals with allergic rhinitis have an IgE-mediated response to crude house-dust antigen, which is a mixture of lint, danders, insect parts, fibers, and other particulate matter. In many geographic areas and household situations, mites, including *Dermatophagoides farinae* and *D. pteronyssimus,* appear to be the primary sources of antigen in house dusts. Animal danders, particularly cat dander, may be especially potent in inducing sudden, violent nasal symptoms, even when there is contact only with the dander, saliva, or urine of the animal. In certain patients, other inhalant allergens, including cottonseed and flaxseed, which may be constituents of animals feeds, fertilizers, and inexpensive upholstery, may cause perennial or sporadic symptoms. Mold spores may be very important perennial allergens, since they are found in both outdoor and indoor environments.

INCIDENCE AND PREVALENCE. Approximately 9 per cent of all patients seeking care at a physician's office do so for one of the common allergic diseases. It is estimated that 35 million Americans have allergic diseases: An estimated 8.9 million suffer from asthma with or without allergic rhinitis, 14.7 million have allergic rhinitis alone, and 11.8 million have other allergic manifestations, such as urticaria, angioedema, eczema, or food, drug, or insect hypersensitivity. Stated in another way, 17 per cent of all Americans have at least one common allergic disease, and 7 per cent of all Americans have allergic rhinitis alone. These incidence figures are deceptively low, since they approximate only the number of patients who, at the time of the particular study, are actually afflicted with the condition, and they do not include the large numbers of individuals who have had diseases such as allergic rhinitis in the past, but have since "recovered."

PATHOGENESIS AND MECHANISMS. Airborne particles (allergens) initially impact on the upper respiratory tract mucosa during inhalation. Many of the relevant allergens, which are water soluble, diffuse onto the respiratory epithelium, and a host IgE antibody response ensues with subsequent sensitization of respiratory tissues. Continued exposure of the appropriately sensitized upper respiratory tract mucous membranes to aeroallergens results in antigen-antibody interactions on the surface of submucosally located mast cells, with release of mediators of acute inflammation and production of clinical symptoms.

Both tissue mast cells and circulating basophils concentrate IgE on their surfaces, which may have up to 500,000 IgE molecules per cell. The IgE fixes to a glycoprotein receptor site on the membrane by its Fc fragment, resulting in an arrangement that permits exposure of the antibody combining sites (or Fab) to the surrounding milieu. Cross-linking of two IgE antibody molecules by specific antigen aggregates the corresponding receptor sites and results in initiation of a series of cellular biochemical events, culminating in the expulsion of secretory granule contents (Fig. 432–1). Among the important mast cell–derived mediators are histamine; bradykinin; thromboxanes; leukotrienes C, D, and E, which are derived from arachidonic acid released during the allergic reaction; eosinophil chemotactic factors of anaphylaxis (ECF-A), which are derived from the mast cell granule; heparin, which makes up 30 per cent of the dry weight of mast cell granules; superoxide dismutase (SOD), which is formed by the univalent reduction of oxygen; prostaglandins, which are C_{20} unsaturated fatty acid derivatives of arachidonic acid; platelet activating factor (PAF), a small phospholipid derivative of phosphoryl choline released from rabbit basophils; neutrophil chemotactic factor of anaphylaxis (NCF-A); inflammatory factors of anaphylaxis, which are constituents of the mast cell granules that induce a late–phase allergic inflammatory reaction; and a number of enzymes that are found in mast cell granules, such as chymotrypsin and trypsin. These enzymes may contribute to the tissue destruction accompanying various late–phase allergic reactions. There are immunologic as well as nonimmunologic triggers of this mast cell degranulation process. It is not uncommon for patients to note associations between symptoms and exposure to certain nonspecific irritants, such as strong odors, insecticides, and cigarette smoke.

CLINICAL MANIFESTATIONS. Common symptoms include *nasal stuffiness*, paroxysms of *sneezing*, profuse *mucous secretion*, and frequent *itching* of the nose, eyes, posterior pharynx, or conjunctivae. Soreness or inflammation of the conjunctivae, with excessive *tearing* and mucoid conjunctival discharge may be present in severe cases, and it is not uncommon for patients with recurrent symptoms to note a certain degree of fatigue, malaise, anorexia, and irritability. Many offending plants pollinate during the early morning hours. Thus, morning symptoms may be followed by improvement during the day, with a lessened degree of exposure. Repeated rubbing of the nose upward to relieve itching may cause a crease to develop across the nose, especially in children. Mouth breathing is common, as are typical dark, discolored infraorbital "shiners" (Fig. 432–2).

Examination of the nasal mucous membranes characteristically reveals bluish, edematous, boggy, pale nasal turbinates, often coated with clear secretion; but many persons with allergic rhinitis have an erythematous, boggy nasal mucosa, which can easily be confused with that seen in infectious rhinitis. At times the nasal airways may be completely obstructed, as a result of accumulation of mucus and turbinate swelling. Scleral and conjunctival injection and edema, plus periorbital swelling and tearing, may be noted. Nasal polyps are relatively uncommonly associated with uncomplicated rhinitis. They may, however, be associated with aspirin intolerance. Since asthmatics with aspirin intolerance often have severe disease, visualization of even small polyps in patients with rhinitis and asthma may provide important diagnostic leads.

In *seasonal rhinitis*, symptoms recur each year with regularity during the pollination season characteristic for a given area. IgE–mediated perennial rhinitis presents with a continuance of low-grade symptoms, which may improve only with removal

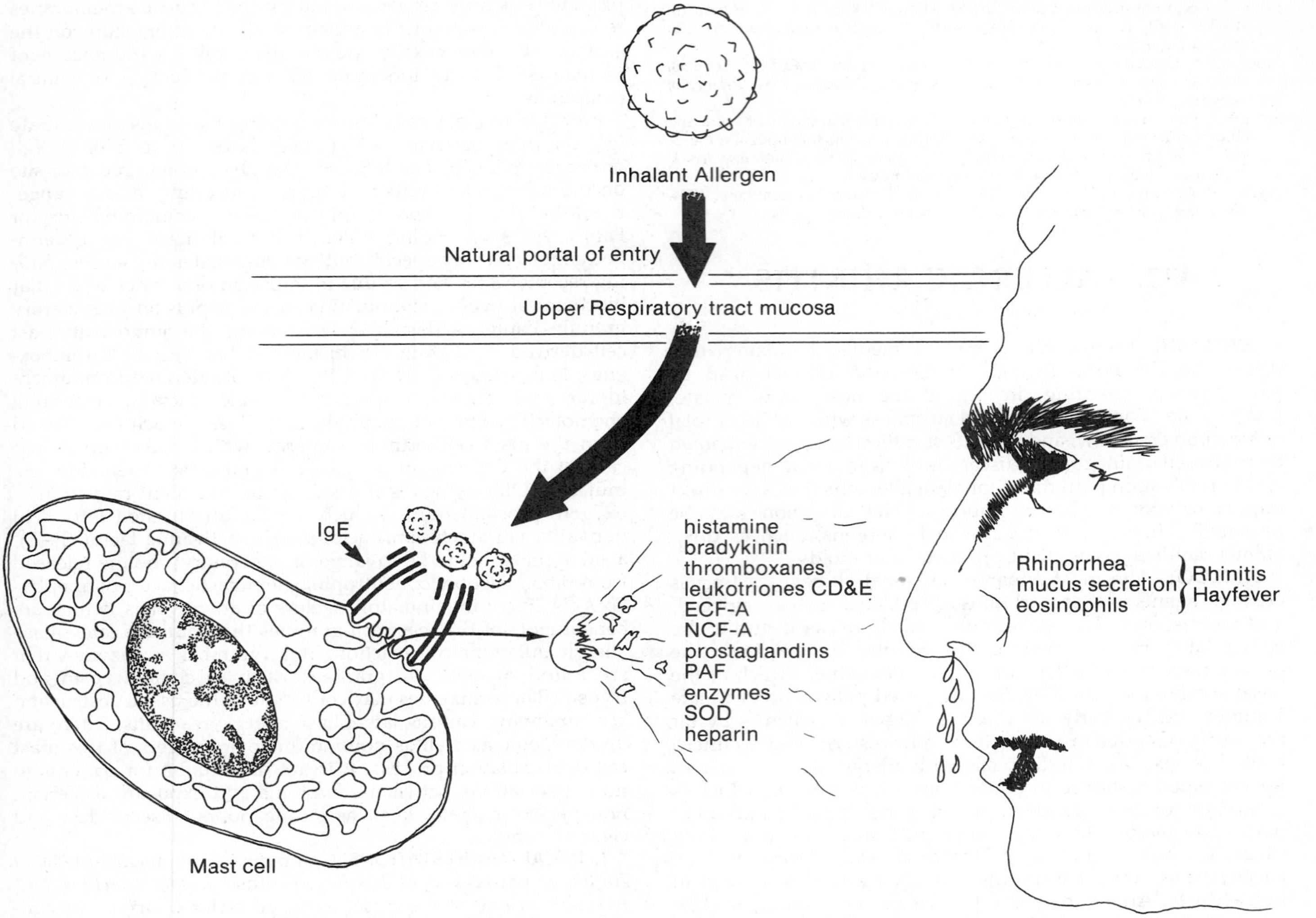

Figure 432–1. Pathogenesis of allergic rhinitis; antigen-antibody interaction and mediator release.

from the inciting causes. *Perennial rhinitis* of unknown cause (also called vasomotor rhinitis) also produces persistent symptoms without correlation to any specific allergen exposure. This type of perennial rhinitis is often worsened by changes in temperature or humidity or with exposure to irritants or other types of air pollutants. It is also often associated with profuse nasal discharge after the patient eats chilled, highly spiced, or heated foods, and such symptoms may be erroneously attributed to food allergy.

Serous otitis media may be superimposed upon the symptoms of seasonal or perennial allergic rhinitis. In many instances of serous otitis media, allergic factors cannot, however, be identified. Serous otitis can be an important complication in children, and may result from nasal obstruction or obstructive dysfunction of the eustachian tube as a result of mucosal edema and secretions. It can also lead to hearing loss with adverse effects on cognition or speech development in the young child. The diagnosis of serous otitis media is suggested by a history of symptoms such as delayed speech development or decreased auditory perception. The tympanic membrane on physical examination is frequently amber-colored and retracted, with decrease in motion if there is negative middle ear pressure, or no motion at all if there is a serous effusion.

Chronic sinusitis may be another complication, often manifested by the presence of chronic nasal discharge, nocturnal cough associated with postnasal discharge, pain, fever, headache, and recurrent otitis media. In adults, however, pain, headache, and low-grade fever are the most frequently recognized signs. Chronic sinusitis as a complication of seasonal allergic rhinitis should be considered whenever symptoms of allergic rhinitis are more protracted than expected, when the patient has severe dull-to-intense throbbing pain over the involved sinus area, or when prolonged or persistent cough develops that is suggestive of bronchitis that has failed to respond to appropriate therapy.

DIAGNOSIS (WITH DIFFERENTIAL DIAGNOSIS). A good history is most important in correctly diagnosing rhinitis. In addition to the history of classic physical signs and symptoms, careful skin testing with common inhalant preparations together with positive and negative control substances is a mandatory procedure in diagnosing specific allergic factors associated with rhinitis. Direct skin tests of the scratch, prick, and intradermal variety are the least expensive and time consuming. The intradermal test should never be performed without prior performance of negative scratch or prick tests. In general, negative skin test responses with common inhalant allergens indicate that rhinitis is of nonallergic origin. In vitro methods of detecting IgE antibodies have now been available for several years. In patients who are receiving medications that might prevent skin reactivity, or in those with extensive eczema or dermatographia that negate the use of skin tests, these in vitro assays for serum IgE antibodies can be of diagnostic aid. Total serum IgE levels

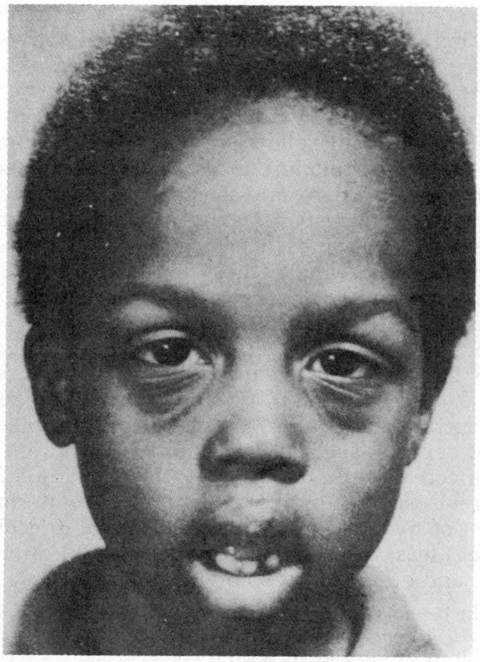

Figure 432–2. Typical appearance of highly allergic 6-year-old child. Note dark circles under eyes ("allergic shiners") and mouth breathing. Allergic nasal crease from constant "saluting" was also present. (Reprinted with permission from Mathews KP: Respiratory atopic disease. JAMA 248:2588, 1982.)

are elevated in only 30 to 40 per cent of patients with allergic rhinitis. They may also be elevated in many nonallergic conditions. Although frequently elevated in allergic rhinitis, the peripheral blood eosinophil count may be normal. A high peripheral eosinophil count may also be seen in nonallergic perennial rhinitis associated with nasal polyps, hyperplastic sinusitis, and idiopathic asthma. Of more significance is a smear of nasal secretions for eosinophils.

Clear-cut seasonal allergic rhinitis due to inhalant allergens seldom presents a differential diagnostic problem. Symptoms of the common cold may, however, be quite similar, although they usually last less than one week and are often associated with fever, pain, and the presence of considerable neutrophils in nasal secretions. Symptoms associated with structural abnormalities of the nasal area, such as polyps, deviated nasal septum, enlarged tonsils, or foreign bodies, are relatively constant rather than episodic as in classic seasonal allergic rhinitis. A suspected diagnosis of so-called rhinitis medicamentosa due to the rebound effects of nose drops, sprays, ovarian hormonal agents (such as oral contraceptives), reserpine derivatives, or hydralazine can often be confirmed when symptoms gradually improve following avoidance of the suspected agent. Nasal symptoms may accompany metabolic disorders such as hyperthyroidism or emotional states, but the relationship is unclear. During pregnancy and premenstrually, hormonally related rhinitis may occur. A condition known as nasal mastocytosis is associated with symptoms of perennial allergic rhinitis; the diagnosis can be made by nasal mucosal biopsy.

TREATMENT. Three basic principles are important in the treatment of rhinitis: avoidance of offending allergens of allergic rhinitis; use of symptomatic treatment, such as antihistamines, sympathomimetic drugs, and topical steroids; and allergenic extract immunotherapy.

Avoidance. When practical, avoidance of aeroallergens is the treatment of choice, since it removes the cause of difficulty and prevents symptoms. When a specific food, drug, occupational allergen, or animal dander is involved, it is the only measure that serves to both prevent and treat disease. All physicians should be familiar, for example, with standard antidust regimens for use in home environments. Although avoidance of outdoor exposure to ubiquitous seasonal and perennial pollens is virtually impossible, commonsense measures to avoid heavy exposure often help to prevent severe exacerbations of symptoms. For example, mold-sensitive patients should avoid barns, working with hay, raking leaves, or mowing grass. Simply keeping doors and windows closed significantly decreases indoor pollen and mold spore concentrations, and air conditioning makes a closed environment more tolerable. Although electrostatic air-purifying devices do not provide cooling or dehumidification, they are quite efficient in removing pollen grains and other large mold spores. In certain cases a patient may choose to leave an area of exposure during a particularly symptomatic season. Such measures may be applicable when well-defined seasons, such as the late-summer-and-early-fall ragweed season, are involved. Only rarely should consideration be given to making a permanent move from an area of exposure to particularly aggravating allergens, since, with time, allergic individuals generally tend to acquire new sensitivities to allergens in their adopted environment.

Symptomatic Treatment. Although, in general, antihistamines are only partially effective and are often associated with a side effect of drowsiness, they are often used alone or in combination with oral sympathomimetic agents, anticholinergics, cromolyn sodium, and topical corticosteroids. The H_1 antihistaminics often control symptoms of profuse nasal itching and sneezing. They act as competitive inhibitors for histamine at its H_1 receptor site. Since receptor sites can be effectively blocked prior to histamine release, better results are often obtained when these drugs are administered on a regular basis rather than intermittently. Antihistamines have been classified into six groups on the basis of chemical structure. These include the ethanolamines, such as diphenhydramine (Benadryl); the ethylenediamines, such as tripelennamine (Pyribenzamine); the alkylamines, such as brompheniramine (Dimetane); and chlorpheniramine (Chlor-Trimeton); the piperazines, such as hydroxyzine (Atarax, Vistaril); the phenothiazines, such as promethazine (Phenergan); and a miscellaneous group including cyproheptadine (Periactin), and azatadine (Optimine). In a typical case, one might start with one of the alkylamines such as chlorpheniramine maleate or brompheniramine maleate 4 mg three or four times a day in the adult (0.4 mg per kilogram per day in three or four divided doses in children). Both of these compounds are also available in long-acting preparations that can be given in 8- to 12-mg quantities two times a day.

The most commonly employed sympathomimetic nasal sprays and drops that contain alpha-adrenergic agonists are phenylephrine hydrochloride, a short-acting agent, and longer-acting preparations, such as oxymetazoline hydrochloride. In most cases, use of these compounds for more than a few days will result in progressively severe nasal obstruction secondary to rebound swelling of the nasal mucosa that may be a self-perpetuating process (known as rhinitis medicamentosa). Thus these agents are not recommended for long-term use in allergic rhinitis. Sympathomimetic agents administered orally, such as pseudoephedrine and phenylpropanolamine, may also reduce nasal congestion, although when used alone they may have significant CNS stimulatory effects, often leading to insomnia and nervousness. A 4 per cent solution of cromolyn sodium applied topically can also be of some benefit in the treatment of allergic rhinitis or conjunctivitis, or both, if administered frequently on a regular basis.

Topical corticosteroids are now widely used and highly successful in the symptomatic treatment and prevention of allergic rhinitis. These usually include the highly potent and rapidly metabolized corticosteroids such as beclomethasone dipropionate, flunisolide acetate, budesonide, and triamcinolone acetonide. These agents act primarily topically, and have a relative lack of systemic effects, which is most advantageous. Although of substantial value in treating seasonal allergic rhinitis, these agents may not work well in acute, severe cases associated with considerable nasal mucosal edema and obstruction. They also do not relieve ocular symptoms. If used intermittently on a regular basis, they can help in perennial allergic rhinitis and vasomotor rhinitis. In addition, they may be of some help in weaning patients from excessive use of vasoconstrictor nasal sprays. The rule for use of corticosteroids is "as much as necessary but as little as possible."

Dose response investigations in hay fever patients have shown total control of nasal symptoms in about 30 per cent of patients treated with 200 or 300 μg of beclomethasone dipropionate per day. This percentage is increased to 60 per cent when 400 μg per day are employed. Seasonal treatment on a daily basis with 400 μg per day is recommended and is considered to be quite harmless. (Each puff of beclomethasone dipropionate from a nasal inhaler is equal to approximately 42 μg of beclomethasone dipropionate, USP). Thus, one puff per nostril four times per day from the nasal inhaler would be a typical dose. Some attention should be paid to the frequency of prescription; for example, when 400 μg is recommended, one aerosol container will last approximately four weeks. In all cases, clinical improvement is usually apparent within several days, but symptomatic relief may not occur in some patients for as long as two weeks. In adults and children, the inhalation of 400 μg daily is without risk of systemic steroid side effects. There is also substantial evidence that this is the case in adults who use up to 800 μg daily (approximately 16 inhalations). In addition, cushingoid changes probably do not occur until the very large dose of approximately 1 mg (20 inhalations or more) is reached. When this drug is used it should be remembered that, in regard to therapeutic potency, eight inhalations is roughly equivalent to 7.5 mg of oral prednisone. These drugs should be used with caution in the presence of viral and fungal nasal diseases, such as ocular herpes or related diseases, in which there appears to be an associated defect in cell-mediated immunity.

Inhalant Allergen Immunotherapy (Desensitization or Hyposensitization). With this form of therapy, one attempts to alter the immunologic reactivity of an allergic inidividual so that there is less response upon natural reexposure to the offending allergen. The clinical decision to use immunotherapy in the patient with allergic rhinitis depends on several factors: (1) the existence of clinically important rhinitis should be confirmed; (2) maximum environmental control procedures should be utilized; and (3) the response to medication should be well defined. Immunotherapy is usually employed in patients who have substantial allergic components to their illness and who are not attaining satisfactory clinical improvement with environmental control and symptomatic treatment. The technique involves injecting increasing amounts of allergen subcutaneously, usually at weekly intervals, starting with a very low dose with gradual increases (usually a doubling of dosage) at each subsequent injection. One should always carefully monitor for the development of any untoward reactions. After incremental increases in the amount of allergen injected, a maintenance dose is achieved, the interval between subsequent maintenance injections varying from two to six weeks, depending upon individual patient reactivity and requirements. In most cases, a decrease in nasal symptoms following immunotherapy is usually obvious during the first six months to one year, and is maximum by three years of therapy. There are no universally accepted guidelines for the duration of therapy, and many physicians attempt trials of discontinuation after approximately four years of a successful program.

Symptomatic improvement with immunotherapy has been clearly shown in hayfever due to ragweed, grass, mountain cedar pollen, or birch pollen and asthma due to house dust mite, ragweed pollen, grass pollen, and cat dander. Beneficial results depend on an adequately high dosage of antigen; relapse may occur once continuing maintenance injections are abandoned. Results are specific for particular allergens employed. A variety of immunologic changes have been demonstrated following immunotherapy, but it is not known which are responsible for clinical improvement. Among these changes are a rise in serum IgG-blocking antibodies against the allergens employed; suppression in the usual seasonal rise in IgE antibodies, which normally follows environmental seasonal exposure; increase of blocking IgA and IgG antibodies in secretions; reduced basophil reactivity and sensitivity to allergens; reduced in vitro lymphocyte responsiveness to allergens; and an increase in specific T suppressor cells following immunotherapy.

New experimental approaches to the therapy of allergic rhinitis include the use of altered antigens (such as allergoids and polymerized forms of antigen) that ultimately result in a heightened degree of immunization, with considerably less chance to trigger sensitized mast cells and produce local or systemic reactions. The use of other routes of antigen administration (such as intranasally) has also been attempted, as have efforts to depress specific IgE antibody synthesis with or without effects on suppressor T cells, by linking allergens to certain agents such as polyethylene glycol, with subsequent production of tolerance. Still other efforts are directed toward such novel ideas as inhibition of IgE receptors on mast cells, basophils, and other IgE receptor–bearing cells.

Bellanti J (ed.): Immunology II. Philadelphia, W. B. Saunders Company, 1978. *A concise, well-illustrated text stressing simple fundamentals of clinical immunology.*

Middleton E Jr, Reed CE, Ellis EF: Allergy: Principles and Practice. 2nd ed. St. Louis, C. V. Mosby Company, 1983. *A multi-authored, two-volume reference work stressing immunologic, pharmacologic and clinical aspects of the common allergic diseases.*

Patterson R (ed.): Allergic Diseases. 2nd ed. Philadelphia, J. B. Lippincott Company, 1980. *A concise volume devoted to practical clinical aspects of the common atopic diseases.*

Parker C (ed.): Clinical Immunology. Philadelphia, W. B. Saunders Company, 1980. *A comprehensive two-volume text (basic and clinical) concentrating on experimental and clinical aspects of human diseases with strong immunologic overtones.*

Salvaggio J (ed.): Primer on allergic and immunologic diseases. JAMA 248:2579, 1982. *Compact article on the essentials of respiratory atopic disease, in a setting of other articles that stress the clinical implications of immunology for the medical student and resident.*

Stites D, Stobo J, Fudenberg H, Wells V (eds.): Basic and Clinical Immunology. 4th ed. Los Altos, Lange Medical Publishers, 1982. *A text outlining relevant features of basic immunology, immunologic laboratory tests, and clinical immunology. Clinical chapters focus on primary immunologic diseases and disorders with important immunopathologic characteristics.*

433. ANAPHYLAXIS*

Lawrence M. Lichtenstein†

Systemic anaphylaxis is the most dramatic example of an immediate hypersensitivity reaction. The first known report of this syndrome describes the sudden death of King Menes of Egypt, from the sting of a wasp, during the twenty-sixth century B.C. The experiments of Richet and Portier in the early 1900's, which gained them the Nobel Prize, showed that dogs who survived a large dose of sea anemone toxin died within a few minutes when given a minute dose some weeks later. They coined the term "anaphylaxis" to describe how this type of immunization led to a lack of protection rather than the expected immunity (i.e., prophylaxis).

Human anaphylactic reactions are uncommon, but have always received considerable medical attention because of their unexpected nature and occasionally fatal outcome. They occur in previously sensitized individuals after re-exposure to foreign antigens or low molecular weight substances that act as haptens. These reactions are mediated by IgE antibody, begin a few minutes after antigen exposure, and result from the release of basophil and mast cell mediators. Other "anaphylactoid" reactions probably involve the nonimmunologic release of the same chemical mediators. Systemic anaphylactic reactions involve the cutaneous, respiratory, circulatory, gastrointestinal, and hematologic systems. They range in severity from distress-

*Supported by Grant AI 08270 from the National Institute of Allergy and Infectious Diseases, National Institutes of Health.

†I would like to thank my colleague, Eugene R. Bleecker, M.D., for his aid in the preparation and writing of this chapter.

TABLE 433–1. AGENTS CAUSING ANAPHYLAXIS

Type	Common	Rare
Proteins	Venoms (Hymenoptera)	Hormones (insulin, ACTH, vasopressin, parathormone)
	Pollens (ragweed, grass, etc.)	Enzymes (trypsin, penicillinase)
	Foods (eggs, seafood, nuts, grains, beans, cottonseed oil, chocolate)	Human proteins (serum proteins, seminal fluid)
	Horse and rabbit serum (antilymphocyte globulin)	
Haptens and other low molecular weight substances	Antibiotics (penicillins, cephalosporins, tetracyclines, amphotericin B, nitrofurantoin, aminoglycosides)	Vitamins (thiamine, folic acid)
	Local anesthetics (lidocaine, procaine, etc.)	
Polysaccharides		Dextrans, iron-dextran

ing but self-limited, generalized urticarial reactions to sudden death.

ETIOLOGY. During the early part of this century, anaphylaxis was most often seen as a reaction to the proteins of horse serum, which was used in the preparation of diphtheria and tetanus antitoxins. Table 433–1 lists the inciting agents that are now most common. Proteins likely to cause these reactions are those in horse serum (now used to make antihuman lymphocyte globulin), hormones, enzymes, Hymenoptera venoms (in insect stings as described in Ch. 434), pollen extracts, and various foods (seafood, eggs, wheat products, nuts). Polysaccharides such as dextran are rarer causes of anaphylaxis. The most common etiologic agents are drugs, low molecular weight substances that are not antigenic in themselves but act as haptens, combining with native proteins to form an antigen. Antibiotics (penicillin, cephalosporins, tetracycline, nitrofurantoin), local anesthetics, vitamins, and some diagnostic agents are thought to act by this mechanism. Some substances (Table 433–2) that are administered by intravenous injection (iodinated radiopaque dyes or hypertonic solutions [mannitol]) as well as some nonsteroidal anti-inflammatory agents (acetylsalicylic acid, aminopyrine, indomethacin) may induce mediator release by nonimmunologic mechanisms that are poorly understood, or vascular shock by direct systemic vasodilatation. Although the parenteral administration of these agents is the cause of most reactions, oral and topical exposure can also cause systemic anaphylactic reactions in highly sensitive individuals.

In the two best-studied situations, penicillin and insect sting anaphylaxis, the incidence of sensitivity (e.g., a positive skin test) is not greater in patients with a familial or personal history of atopy. However, not all individuals with a positive skin test, indicating the presence of specific IgE antibody, are at risk of an anaphylactic reaction. Although the degree of risk in skin test–positive patients is very much higher than in skin test–negative patients, not all will react to any particular challenge.

PATHOGENESIS. In a susceptible individual, exposure to an antigenic agent causes the production of IgE antibodies. With repeat exposure, the antigen combines with IgE antibodies on the surface of basophils and mast cells to initiate a sequence of biochemical reactions that result in the active secretion of mediators such as histamine, arachidonic acid metabolites, and factors that attract and activate platelets, eosinophils, and neutrophils (see table in Ch. 438). These mediators constrict bronchial smooth muscle, increase vascular permeability, affect systemic and pulmonary vascular muscle tone, induce platelet aggregation and degranulation, attract inflammatory cells to the reaction site, and, in general, are responsible for the manifestations of anaphylaxis. Elevated levels of histamine have been measured during human anaphylactic shock and the intravenous injection of this mediator causes urticaria, bronchospasm, vasodilation, hypotension, and vomiting. It seems likely that other mediators are also involved. It is not yet possible, however, to describe the mechanisms involved in anaphylaxis in detail. The alterations in coagulability which have been reported, for example, may be due to platelet activating factors or to an enzymatic mediator which activates Hageman factor.

TABLE 433–2. AGENTS CAUSING ANAPHYLACTOID REACTIONS*

Curare
Hypertonic solutions (mannitol)
Nonsteroidal anti-inflammatory agents (acetylsalicylic acid, aminopyrine, indomethacin)
Radiopaque contrast material

*Reactions to these small molecular weight compounds may not be due to IgE-mediated immunologic mechanisms (see text).

CLINICAL FEATURES. The onset and clinical manifestations of systemic anaphylaxis vary, depending on the route of administration of the antigen or hapten. The physiologic features are also determined by the type, quantities, and sites of release of pharmacologic mediators, by factors that control releasability, and by differing sensitivity of the organs to the released mediators.

There is no universal response pattern or "shock" organ that is always involved in man. Individuals do, however, have a characteristic pattern of response which tends to repeat. This pattern is often preceded by an aura that is also characteristic and well recognized by the patient. Attention to these subjective symptoms, which precede the physiologic events by one to two minutes, may be valuable. The most common manifestations of systemic reactions are *cutaneous*: erythema, pruritus, urticaria, and angioedema, often of the eyes, lips, or tongue. In adults, the cutaneous symptoms are usually accompanied by one or more other features. There are two patterns of respiratory failure. The first is *upper airway obstruction* owing to edema of the larynx and/or epiglottis, which can cause acute distress and death by suffocation. The second involves *diffuse lower airway bronchoconstriction* similar to the respiratory abnormalities observed in status asthmaticus. Such airflow limitation is not relieved by endotracheal intubation and may lead to abnormalities of pulmonary gas exchange with subsequent hypoxemia and hypercarbia.

Perhaps the most severe clinical manifestation of anaphylaxis is *hypotensive shock*, which can develop with or without other symptoms. The cause is thought to be either peripheral vascular pooling of blood resulting from vasodilation or increased capillary permeability with functional loss of intravascular blood volume into the interstitial spaces. Electrocardiographic abnormalities, including conduction disturbances, arrhythmias, and ischemic or infarction patterns, have been noted during anaphylactic shock. These changes may reflect myocardial ischemia and arrhythmias caused by decreased coronary perfusion and oxygenation.

Rarely, other symptoms are associated with systemic anaphylactic reactions. These include gastrointestinal (vomiting, nausea, and diarrhea) and central nervous system symptoms. Prolonged hypotension or anoxia can, of course, cause a variety of secondary, more permanent changes.

Metabolic abnormalities in severe human anaphylactic shock include increased blood histamine levels, which correlate with the duration and severity of shock. There is also depletion of clotting factors V, VIII, and fibrinogen, activation of complement, and loss of high molecular weight kininogen. The utilization of these coagulation factors is consistent with acute intravascular coagulation and may account for clotting defects observed in clinical anaphylactic syndromes.

DIFFERENTIAL DIAGNOSIS. The diagnosis of systemic anaphylaxis is generally easy with a characteristic history of immediately antecedent exposure to foreign antigenic material and appropriate evidence of systemic involvement on physical examination. The presentation may, however, involve a patient unable to provide a history and suffering the secondary effects of shock, e.g., a myocardial infarction or an arrhythmia. Occasionally, this syndrome must be distinguished from other related clinical conditions, i.e., sudden acute bronchospasm in an asthmatic, vasovagal syncope, acute drug toxicity, hereditary angioedema, cold or idiopathic urticaria. Nonimmunologic "anaphylactoid" reactions to radiopaque dyes, hypertonic solutions, and nonsteroidal anti-inflammatory agents (indomethacin, aminopyrine, acetylsalicylic acid) have a similar clinical presentation and require an identical therapeutic approach, even though they may not be mediated by IgE antibody.

Because of the rapid onset of these reactions, initial laboratory testing is not helpful in making a diagnosis. The retrospective diagnosis of specific allergic sensitivity is by skin testing, or the measurement of specific IgE antibody by the radioallergosorbent test.

PREVENTION AND TREATMENT. The sudden, usually unexpected onset of human anaphylaxis with a rapid clinical course that leads to either swift recovery or death has provided little opportunity for prospective, controlled, therapeutic studies. Even when anaphylaxis is treated in an intensive care unit by trained personnel and a well-planned therapeutic approach, severe systemic reactions often do not respond to medical treatment. Therefore, every attempt must be made to prevent these reactions. A careful medical history should include inquiry about any previous allergic drug reactions. Patients who have previously experienced anaphylactic episodes should wear a Medic-Alert bracelet and be instructed in the importance of relating details of their specific drug allergies before taking medications; their medical records should prominently state the patient's allergic history. The physician should be aware of which medications, proprietaries, and foods contain allergens or cross-reacting antigens. Sensitization may occur in the absence of clinical symptoms; previous tolerance of a substance provides no guarantee that an anaphylactic reaction will not occur.

If diagnostic tests are not available, as with most drugs, it is appropriate to substitute another therapeutic agent for the treatment of a patient with a history of sensitivity to a particular drug. Again, knowledge of cross-reactivity is necessary. If, for example, cephalosporins are substituted for penicillin, there is a significant risk of reaction, since these agents share a common β-lactam ring. Penicillin causes more anaphylactic reactions than any other drug, but at least 80 per cent of patients with a history of a previous reaction will have negative skin tests (to penicilloyl-polylysine and a mixture of haptens [MDM]) and can tolerate the drug with impunity. This is an important consideration, since penicillin is a relatively nontoxic drug and most antibiotics that would be substituted have a significant incidence of side effects. (See Ch. 437 for a further discussion of penicillin allergy.) When penicillin or other allergens must be used in a sensitive patient, an effort can be made to desensitize the patient by the use of sequential low doses, initially intradermally, then subcutaneously, and finally intramuscularly into the peripheral part of an extremity. Such a procedure should be carried out by experienced personnel, and potentially allergenic substances should be administered in a setting where anaphylactic reactions can be effectively treated.

Early recognition of anaphylaxis is critical, since death or irreversible anoxic organ damage can occur rapidly. When an anaphylactic reaction is initiated by an injection into the arm or leg, a tourniquet should be placed around that extremity to stop antigen absorption. The initial pharmacologic treatment is the subcutaneous administration of 0.2 to 0.5 ml of a 1:1000 solution of epinephrine. This is the agent of choice. Antihistamines and corticosteroids play *no* role in the treatment of an acute reaction, although some physicians believe they limit late or recurrent cutaneous manifestations. Extrathoracic upper airway obstruction must be differentiated from diffuse bronchospasm, since severe laryngeal and epiglottic edema may require careful endotracheal intubation or an emergency tracheostomy to facilitate ventilation. Bronchospasm can be handled in a manner similar to the therapy for status asthmaticus, by the administration of inhaled B-2 sympathomimetics or by intravenous aminophylline (see Ch. 59). Hypoxemia should be treated with supplemental oxygen. Hypervolemic shock requires rapid intravenous fluid administration (normal saline and colloid) to maintain blood pressure. Additionally, epinephrine can be given intravenously in severe shock, and, if it is ineffective, an alpha-adrenergic vasoconstrictor (norepinephrine) should be tried. If severe vascular anaphylactic shock does not respond immediately to these measures, supportive treatment should be continued, preferably in an intensive care unit setting where vascular monitoring is available to guide additional therapy. Any patient who has had significant shock or airway obstruction should be hospitalized for at least 24 hours after the acute episode is handled, since these symptoms may recur many hours after an initial favorable response.

Bleecker ER, Lichtenstein LM: Systemic anaphylaxis. *In* Lichtenstein LM, Fauci AS (eds.): Current Therapy in Allergy and Immunology, 1983–1984. St. Louis, C. V. Mosby Company, 1983, pp 78–83. *A detailed description of how to treat this serious disorder.*

Parker CW: Systemic anaphylaxis. *In* Parker CW (ed.): Clinical Immunology. Philadelphia, W. B. Saunders Company, 1980, pp 1208-1218. *An up-to-date textbook review of what is known about etiology, pathogenesis and treatment.*

Smith PL, Sobotka AK, Bleecker ER, Traystman R, Kaplan AP, Gralnick H, Valentine MD, Permutt S, Lichtenstein LM: Physiologic manifestations of human anaphylaxis. J Clin Invest 66:1072, 1980. *Physiologic and biochemical changes monitored in human anaphylaxis occurring during a trial of therapy for insect allergy. Includes comments on therapy.*

434. INSECT STING ALLERGY*

Lawrence M. Lichtenstein†

The stings of insects of the order Hymenoptera have long been recognized as a potential cause of severe, often life-threatening reactions in susceptible individuals. These reactions are unrelated to the toxic chemicals in the venoms, being due to allergic sensitization. Insect sting allergy has recently become the most intensely studied model of anaphylaxis in man, resulting in important advances that have had rapid clinical application.

EPIDEMIOLOGY. The incidence of immediate hypersensitivity to insect stings based on history is 4 per cent; more than 20 per cent of the population, however, has positive skin test reactions to insect venoms without having had a reaction. Other allergies do not seem to predispose to insect sting sensitivity. The frequency varies with exposure and is therefore greater in children and males as well as those inclined to outdoor activities or beekeeping. Insect stings cause few fatalities, but the morbidity, fear, and change in life style caused by these reactions is significant. A large number of people suffer prolonged and unusually large local inflammatory reactions to insect stings, which are allergic in nature. As with other allergies, there appears to be an inherited predisposition, since multiple family members are often affected.

ETIOLOGY. The only insects possessing true stingers are those of the order Hymenoptera. There are two families of importance, the bees (honeybees, bumblebees) and the vespids (yellow jackets, hornets, wasps). The bees have barbed stingers which remain in the skin after a sting. Yellow jackets are the most common culprits, but honeybees are more commonly implicated in the western United States. Wasps are more common in the south central United States (especially Texas). The fire ant, common in the South and the Caribbean, is a

*Supported by Grant AI 08270 from the National Institute of Allergy and Infectious Diseases.

†I would like to express my thanks to my colleague, David B. K. Golden, M.D., for his aid in the preparation and writing of this chapter.

hymenopteran whose sting can also cause anaphylaxis. Sensitivity develops to antigens in the insect venom, most of which have enzymatic activity. A major allergen in both insect families is phospholipase, but they do not cross-react with one another.

PATHOGENESIS. The injection of foreign proteins commonly causes the production of specific antibodies of the IgE and IgG classes. Individuals may develop venom-specific IgE antibodies after any sting, this response persisting for less than three months to more than 25 years. Tissue mast cells and circulating basophils are sensitized by bound IgE, and a repeat encounter with the offending allergen will trigger release of the mediators of anaphylaxis (see Fig. 59–3). The initiation and persistence of this sensitization are related to inheritable and other unknown determinants. Sensitization may occur at any time in life, even after many uneventful stings. The sensitizing sting itself causes no unusual reaction, and is often so remote as to evade recollection.

Generalized mediator release from sensitized basophils and mast cells causes the many manifestations of anaphylaxis (see table in Ch. 438). Localization of symptoms to specific target tissues is not well understood. The pathology observed in fatal cases includes upper airway edema and obstruction, the visceral consequences of hypotension, or occasionally no discernible abnormality (see Ch. 433 for a discussion of anaphylaxis).

Large local reactions most often appear to be IgE dependent, but their prolonged time-course is not typical of immediate hypersensitivity. These reactions may involve a cascade of events beginning with mediator release from mast cells and culminating with local inflammation involving many cell types and numerous mechanisms. The potential roles of eosinophils, neutrophils, basophils, lymphocytes and lymphokines, complement, and mediators with prolonged release or activity have not been elucidated.

The venom-specific IgG antibody response to a sting is usually short lived, lasting only a few months. Repeated stings (as in beekeepers) are associated with high titers of IgG antibodies, which protect against allergic sting reactions. Beekeepers who do not have anaphylactic reactions have high IgG titers, as do affected individuals immunized with venoms. Passive transfer of these IgG antibodies protects sensitive patients from a sting. These protective antibodies are thought to block the allergic reaction by competing with IgE for the allergenic venom proteins and have therefore been termed "blocking" antibodies.

CLINICAL MANIFESTATIONS. Allergic reactions to insect stings are either generalized (systemic) or large local reactions. *Systemic sting reactions* present the classic manifestations of anaphylaxis described in Ch. 433. The observed frequency of the most common symptoms in adult patients is presented in Table 434–1. The risk of a fatal outcome increases, as might be expected, with age. Fatal anaphylaxis may occur without a past history of sting allergy.

The onset of systemic symptoms is rapid, within two to three minutes, and uncommonly occurs more than 30 minutes after a sting. Symptoms presenting hours later (except large local reactions) are not usually associated with immediate hypersensitivity or IgE antibodies. Unusual reactions such as vasculitis, nephropathies, encephalitis, and other neurologic manifestations have been reported, but no causal relationship has been established. Allergic respiratory symptoms may occur in beekeepers and their families owing to sensitization to the dust in the hives that contains bee body proteins. This sensitivity is unrelated to sting reactions.

Large local reactions are slow in onset and occur with or without concomitant early systemic reaction. The area of induration increases in size progressively for the first 24 to 48 hours, and then resolves gradually over several days. These reactions may be so large as to immobilize an entire limb, and are a significant cause of morbidity in sensitive individuals. Red streaks resembling lymphangitis may be observed and are often treated with antibiotics despite a lack of evidence for true cellulitis. Some individuals develop large local sting reactions in the absence of allergic sensitivity. These are exaggerated reactions to the toxic and inflammatory venom components, and often occur in persons who report similar large swellings to mosquito or fly bites, or who have cutaneous sensitivity to many irritants.

TABLE 434–1. SYMPTOMS REPORTED BY 245 PATIENTS

Symptom	%
Cutaneous only	14
Urticaria-angioedema	78
Dizziness-hypotension	61
Dyspnea-wheezing	53
Throat tightness-hoarseness	40
Loss of consciousness	33

NATURAL HISTORY. The natural history of insect sting allergy has been incompletely documented. The incidence of venom sensitization in the general population was noted above, but the actual risk of reaction associated with sensitization is unknown. There is considerable variability in the reaction to a sting among those who are clearly allergic as demonstrated by positive skin tests and a history of previous reaction. In a small study 60 per cent of adults had a systemic reaction when stung by the appropriate insect. In children a repeat sting causes a reaction in only 8 per cent. The incidence in adolescents and young adults must lie between these extremes. This variability confounds the prediction of risk associated with sensitization.

Many patients and physicians believe that allergic sting reactions become progressively more severe with every sting. Although some patients progress from large local through mild systemic reactions to life-threatening anaphylaxis, most of those affected maintain a similar pattern of symptoms with every sting. Less than 10 per cent of those experiencing large local reactions will subsequently have systemic reactions. Factors favoring a systemic reaction include multiple stings, or stings in close temporal proximity (only weeks apart).

Sensitization may decrease or disappear in time, more commonly in children. However, resensitization has been observed upon resting.

DIAGNOSIS. The acute presentation of anaphylaxis may be easily diagnosed in the presence of classic symptoms and signs. The insect sting may be inapparent. Differential diagnosis is more difficult in localized reactions such as acute chest pain and dyspnea or syncope without urticaria or recognition of the sting.

The diagnosis of insect sting allergy currently rests on a convincing history and positive skin tests. Demonstration in vitro of venom-specific IgE by the radioallergosorbent test (RAST) is less sensitive than skin tests, but may be useful in equivocal cases.

Skin tests are performed intradermally with venoms diluted to concentrations in the range of 1 to 1000 ng per milliliter. Five venoms are used: honeybee (HB), yellow jacket (YJ), yellow hornet (YH), white-faced hornet (WH), and *Polistes* wasp (POL). Positive intradermal skin tests develop, within 20 minutes, a wheal greater than 5 mm in diameter with at least 20 mm of erythema. The degree of skin test sensitivity does not correlate with clinical sensitivity. Within a few months after a systemic sting reaction, skin tests are almost uniformly positive. Stings more remote in time are more commonly associated with an apparent loss of sensitivity (similar to the situation in penicillin-related anaphylaxis).

Honeybee venom sensitivity occurs independent of other venom allergies, but about 10 per cent of patients are sensitive to both bee and vespid venoms. The vespid venoms are highly cross-reactive, so that almost all vespid sensitive patients have positive YJ, YH, and WH skin tests even though most have been stung only by YJs. Half of these patients are also sensitive to POL venom. A few individuals are allergic to only one or two of the vespid venoms. In vitro RAST inhibition techniques are useful to distinguish cross-reactivity from specific sensitivity.

TREATMENT. The treatment of choice for anaphylactic reactions is subcutaneous epinephrine 1:1000, 0.5 ml initially and repeated twice at ten-minute intervals, if necessary, to reverse the progression of symptoms. Sublingual isoproterenol is probably ineffective. Antihistamines and glucocorticoids do not contribute to the management of life-threatening symptoms, but may reduce the duration and severity of cutaneous manifestations. Their use should not be considered until the termination of the acute episode. Intravenous volume expansion or airway maintenance may be necessary. In a few individuals, the process is resistant to epinephrine; in such instances an α-adrenergic agent (i.e., norepinephrine) may be tried. Affected persons not yet protected by immunotherapy are advised to carry, and are instructed in the use of, a kit containing a syringe device preloaded with one or two recommended doses of epinephrine.

Venom immunotherapy is successful in virtually all patients. Less than 3 per cent of those immunized have any systemic symptoms after a challenge sting, and these are uniformly less severe than their previous reactions. The indications for venom immunotherapy are currently based on an incomplete understanding of the natural history of the disease. Those with a history of life-threatening reactions should be treated. The risk of progression from strictly cutaneous to life-threatening respiratory or vascular reactions is uncertain. Cutaneous reactors who are more likely to be stung in their daily activities or who can, for a variety of reasons (location, age, cardiovascular disease), ill afford a more severe reaction should be treated. The cost and inconvenience of treatment may deter other cutaneous reactors from undergoing immunotherapy. Children, much more commonly than adults, have cutaneous symptoms only. These children may be left untreated. Venom immunotherapy is contraindicated in the absence of positive skin tests. Treatment is currently recommended using all venoms causing a positive skin test. While other mechanisms may contribute, the induction of increased serum levels of venom-specific IgG antibodies is the most apparent mechanism of protection for venom immunotherapy; about 5 μg per milliliter is required.

Rapid immunization in six to eight weekly visits is recommended, since it is associated with a significantly greater and more rapid immune response, and with fewer adverse reactions than a slower (more than 20 weeks) regimen. The maintenance dose of 100 μg of each venom is repeated monthly for at least six months, and is then continued at six- to eight-week intervals for an indefinite time. If treatment is interrupted for more than three months, it is likely that protection will diminish to inadequate levels. Although unusual in adults, loss of sensitivity during maintenance immunotherapy may occur. Skin tests should, therefore, be repeated every two years.

Adverse reactions to venom immunotherapy may be early or late. Immediate reactions include all the manifestations of anaphylaxis. During the initial course of treatment, 10 to 15 per cent of patients report systemic complaints, only half of which require epinephrine. At maintenance doses, systemic reactions occur rarely. After a systemic reaction, the dose should be reduced by up to 50 per cent on the subsequent visit, and then increased gradually toward 100 μg again.

Large local reactions occur frequently. Fifty per cent of treated patients experience at least one such reaction. These occur after 10 out of every 100 injections in the induction phase, most commonly in the midrange of doses (10 to 50 μg) and much less often at maintenance doses. Large local reactions do not presage systemic reactions and require a reduction of dose only for the most severe reactions. Long-term side effects have not been observed with venom immunotherapy or in beekeepers stung frequently for over 30 years.

Hunt KJ, Valentine MD, Sobotka AK, et al.: A controlled trial of immunotherapy in insect hypersensitivity. N Engl J Med 299:157, 1978. *A comparison of venom immunotherapy with whole body extract and placebo. Demonstrates efficacy of venom therapy and the clinical consequences of challenge stings.*

Lichtenstein LM, Valentine MD, Sobotka AK: Insect allergy: The state of the art. J Allerg Clin Immunol 64:5, 1979. *A review of diagnostic and therapeutic problems in insect allergy. Details the parameters which dictate the choice of patients for treatment.*

Schuberth KC, Lichtenstein LM, Kagey-Sobotka A, et al.: Epidemiologic study of insect allergy in children. II. Effect of accidental stings in allergic children. J Pediatr 102:361, 1983. *A prospective epidemiology study of repeat stings in children. Has implications for young adults.*

435. IMMUNE COMPLEX DISEASES

Charles G. Cochrane

DEFINITION. Immune complex diseases are caused by the deposition or formation of antigen-antibody complexes in tissues. Inflammation results and leads to acute or chronic disease of the organ system in which the immune complexes have been deposited. The antigen-antibody complex localizes in a particular organ by two major mechanisms: (1) when antigens of that organ are exposed to antibodies entering from the circulation; and (2) antigen-antibody complexes may form in the circulation, to be subsequently deposited in renal glomeruli, arteries, or venules, inducing inflammatory disease of each structure. Thus immune complexes are capable of causing severe inflammation in many organs of the body. For example, immune complexes may contribute to the pathogenesis of systemic lupus erythematosus, serum sickness, acute and chronic glomerulonephritis, rheumatoid arthritis, arteritis, vasculitis, and tissue injury associated with a wide spectrum of infectious agents. This chapter will examine the mechanisms by which the interaction of antigens and antibodies may form immune complexes and how this process may be injurious to the host.

PATHOGENESIS. The pathogenesis of immune complex diseases is best understood by examining several well-studied experimental models that closely mimic human diseases.

Immune Complex Disease with Tissue-Fixed Antigen. When the antigen is bound in an organ or is released locally from a tissue, the antibodies react with antigen at that locus to induce local inflammatory injury. As an example, antibodies in the circulation may react with antigens in the glomerular basement membrane of the kidney and result in inflammation of the glomerulus (glomerulitis) with acute or chronic injury. In human beings this takes the form of Goodpasture's disease. Similarly, when antigen-antibody complexes form in a joint space, synovitis results. This may play an important role in the pathogenesis of rheumatoid arthritis, in which antibodies have been found in the joint fluid complexed with many host proteins, especially IgG itself.

Immune Complex Disease Caused by the Deposition of Circulating Immune Complexes in Tissues. Acute immune complex disease, or serum sickness, can be produced in experimental animals by injection of serum protein antigens. The associated lesions are generally those of arteritis, glomerulonephritis, endocarditis, cutaneous rash, and synovitis. A mechanism for the production of immune complex disease is given in Figure 435–1. A chronic disease follows injections of the serum protein antigens for 30 days. In this form of the disease, chronic glomerulonephritis most characteristically results, often without the other lesions of the acute disease. In cases in which a large antibody response occurs, pulmonary inflammation and fibrosis of the lung result. The glomerular lesions of chronic immune complex disease contain lumpy deposits rich in antigen, immunoglobulin, and complement along the outer edge of the basement membrane (Figs. 435–2 to 435–4). These morphologic characteristics have formed the diagnostic features of immune complex glomerulonephritis of human beings. However, in contrast to the lesions of chronic serum sickness of experimental animals, the amount of the inducing antigen (when known, such as in poststreptococcal glomerulonephritis) is vanishingly small in concentration. By contrast, the IgG–

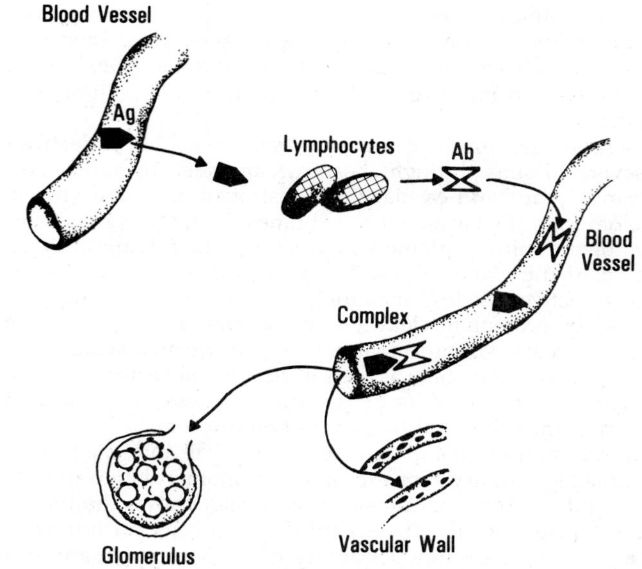

Figure 435–1. Schematic mechanism of the production of antibody by an antigen, the formation of antibody-antigen complexes in the circulation, and the localization of the complexes in tissues where inflammatory injury develops. Ag = antigen; Ab = antibody.

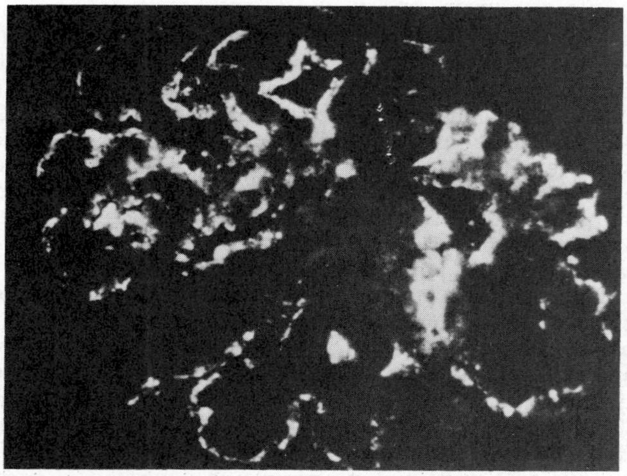

Figure 435–3. Fluorescent photomicrograph of a glomerulus similar to that in Figure 435–2, showing the presence of rabbit immunoglobulin along the glomerular basement membrane. The specific antigen and the third component of complement were localized in the same pattern.

anti-IgG complexes and cryoglobulins may dominate, suggesting that a nonspecific stimulation of the immune system followed the initial exposure to antigen. Possibly a polyclonal stimulation of B lymphocytes and diminished activity of immune-suppressor systems are important pathogenic mechanisms in these human autoimmune diseases. Some antibodies to IgG proteins are anti-idiotypic; they form complexes with the immunoglobulin of the appropriate idiotype.

The Mechanism of Deposition of Circulating Immune Complexes. Several factors determine the ability of circulating complexes to localize in the vessel walls of a particular organ. Important among these factors are the quantity of complexes and the size of the complex. No definite minimal concentration of the complexes in the circulation has been established, but there seems to be a requirement for the complex to be of a particular size (19S or greater) for its deposition in blood vessel walls. The size of the three-dimensional lattice of antigen-antibody complexes depends largely upon the affinity of the antibody for the antigen. For example, in experimental animals complexes of intermediate size circulate and cause tissue injury, whereas larger complexes are insoluble and are rapidly cleared from circulation by the reticuloendothelial system. Smaller complexes may fail to activate the mediator systems or be too small to be trapped in vessel walls. The small complexes may therefore circulate for long periods. Another factor that may play a role in the deposition of immune complexes is charge. By virtue of the overall anionic charge of the glomerular basement membrane, cationic immune complexes or free antigens possess an affinity for glomeruli and are retained longer than neutral or anionic molecules. Whether this plays a role in the development of glomerulonephritis, however, is unclear.

An increase in vascular permeability is required for circulating immune complexes to deposit in tissues and to initiate acute injury. The local release of vasoactive amines appears responsible for this increased permeability. Circulating antigen reacts with specific surface IgE on sensitized basophils to release an array of constituents, including histamine and a platelet acti-

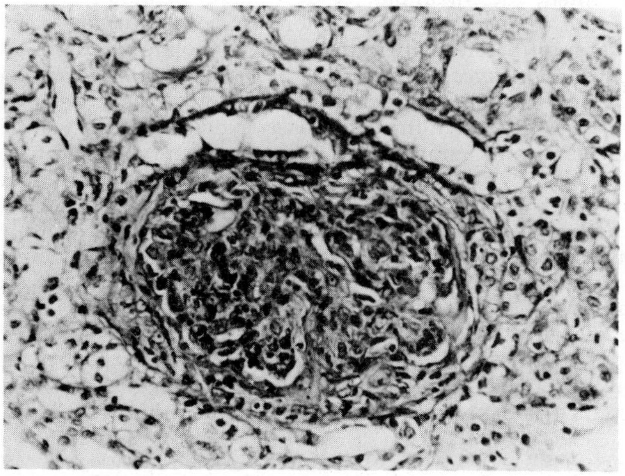

Figure 435–2. Glomerulus of a rabbit with subacute immune complex-induced glomerulonephritis. Inflammatory cells have accumulated, and injury of the glomerular basement membrane was evidenced by marked proteinuria. (× 150.)

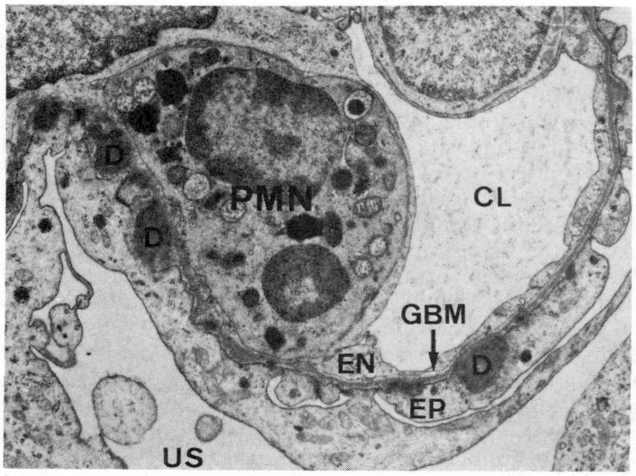

Figure 435–4. A polymorphonuclear leukocyte (PMN) is seen closely approximated along the glomerular basement membrane (GBM) in proximity to subepithelial (EP) electron dense deposits (D) in a rabbit with chronic serum sickness glomerulonephritis. The deposits are rich in antibody, complement, and, to a lesser extent, antigen by fluorescent antibody microscopy. Similar or identical deposits are observed in human immune complex glomerulonephritis. The endothelial cell (EN) has been displaced. Other abbreviations: CL = capillary lumen; US = urinary space.

vating factor (PAF). This latter factor causes clumping and degranulation of platelets and release of platelet histamine and serotonin. Thus an allergic reaction induces deposition of the circulating complexes in blood vessel walls. The anaphylatoxins C3a and C5a, generated by complement activation (see Ch. 428), also degranulate basophils and mast cells to liberate vasoactive amines and other substances. These may augment the increase in vascular permeability and facilitate the deposition of immune complexes along vascular basement membranes. In immune complex disease of man, the role of increased vascular permeability in the local deposition of circulating immune complexes has been documented in cutaneous vasculitis. In addition, in patients with active systemic lupus erythematosus, the circulating basophils undergo loss of granules and contain diminished levels of PAF. Basophils from patients with quiescent systemic lupus degranulate and release PAF upon exposure to DNA.

Host Factors Responsible for the Inflammation Caused by Immune Complexes. Immune complexes deposited in tissues activate mediator systems. These mediators are the cellular and humoral effectors of inflammatory injury—activated enzymes, biologically active peptides, oxidizing substances, polyamines, and prostaglandins—that are released in the tissues as a consequence of antigen-antibody complex deposition. The classic and, to a lesser extent, the alternative pathways of the complement system are activated by the complexed Ig molecule to initiate the complement cascade. This leads to the limited proteolytic cleavage of C3 and C5 to liberate small peptides, C3a and C5a and the fragment C3b, which rapidly bind to tissue structures such as vascular basement membrane. As noted, the peptides also degranulate basophils and mast cells releasing histamine, slow-reacting substance, and other substances that cause increased vascular permeability, smooth muscle contraction, and hypotension (see Table 438–1). C5a is also a potent chemoattractant for leukocytes. The remaining portion of the C3 molecule, C3b, binds white blood cells through the process of immune adherence, thus facilitating phagocytosis and discharge of lysosomal granules. Short-lived oxidants (usually free radicals of oxygen) are generated in vivo in inflammatory foci and produce injury through mechanisms that have not been clarified. Of particular interest, antioxidants have a profound therapeutic effect in experimental inflammatory disease.

White blood cells, platelets, and macrophages specifically bind the Fc portion of the antigen-antibody complex and in the process are stimulated to generate injurious oxidizing radicals (e.g., superoxide anion and H_2O_2) and to release their lysosomal granules containing proteolytic enzymes, peptides, and vasoactive amines into the surrounding fluid. The C5a peptide has a similar effect on leukocytes. The discharge of these effector molecules results in the inflammatory tissue injury characteristic of immune complex disease.

Acute immune complex–mediated injury depends, therefore, upon an interaction of the complement system and neutrophils at the local site. This has been clearly demonstrated in experimental studies of the Arthus reaction, pneumonitis, and arteritis in serum sickness; of immunologic synovitis; and of at least one form of experimental glomerulonephritis. In each reaction, an antigen-antibody complex is formed in the tissues, complement is rapidly activated, and neutrophils accumulate at the site. Inhibition of complement activation prevents the accumulation of neutrophils and prevents injury, suggesting that immune adherence by tissue-fixed C3b and stimulation of neutrophil chemotaxis by C5a are important functions in the genesis of these lesions. Production of neutropenia with specific antibody or by the use of nitrogen mustard also prevents the development of experimental immune complex injury even though complement is present. The release of mediators of inflammatory injury by neutrophils at the site of antigen-antibody complex deposition has been described above. Mononuclear leukocytes are also capable of generating oxidizing radicals and of releasing lysosomal constituents. C3e, a fragment derived from further degradation of C3b, stimulates leukocytosis.

Experimental immune complex disease is capable of destroying several tissues through these mechanisms. In joints, glycosaminoglycans and cartilage are destroyed; in blood vessels and glomeruli, the basement membranes are hydrolyzed. Fragments of the injured glomerular basement membrane may be excreted in the urine. Elastic fibers of arteries are destroyed, and connective tissues, including collagen in the lung, are damaged by proteolytic cleavage. In man the histologic features of arteritis, acute streptococcal glomerulonephritis, acute homograft rejection, and some aspects of rheumatoid arthritis imply a similar mechanism of tissue destruction. Loss of elastin and collagen in the lungs is a hallmark of emphysema.

Chronic immune complex disease may call into play other mechanisms of injury. For example, the glomerulonephritis of experimental chronic serum sickness, which shows the typical lumpy appearance of antigen-antibody deposits on immunofluorescence, occurs independently of both complement and neutrophils. Macrophages, which may be attracted by chemotactic factors from neutrophils and by other substances, probably play an important role in this lesion. Macrophages cause tissue injury by mechanisms similar to those described for neutrophils. They may also be stimulated to divide at the site of tissue injury by macrophage growth factors present in the inflammatory exudate. There is increasing evidence for an important role for the macrophage in both experimental models of chronic immunologic diseases and in immunologic lung disease in man. In a model of chronic membranous nephritis, marked by immune complex formation along the epithelial side of the glomerular basement membrane, complement appears to play an essential role in the development of proteinuria independently of leukocytes. In this lesion, which closely resembles membranous nephritis of humans, the immune complexes and activated complement components lie on or adjacent to the delicate slit-pore diaphragm that bridges the space between epithelial foot processes. This diaphragm may be an essential barrier to the passage of protein molecules, and its disruption by the membrane attack complex of complement may constitute a major cause of the glomerular dysfunction in chronic membranous nephritis.

Experimental myasthenia gravis is another interesting example of the role of mediators in the pathogenesis of diseases caused by antigen-antibody complexes. In this disease, antibodies react with motor end-plates (acetylcholine receptors); this reaction activates complement and stimulates the local accumulation of monocytes. If the activation of complement is prevented, the inflammatory destruction of motor end-plates and the loss of muscle function do not occur, despite the reaction of the antibody with the acetylcholine receptors.

The Significance of Circulating Immune Complexes in Human Disease. Circulating immune complexes have been detected in a wide variety of human diseases. Nevertheless, in diseases such as chronic glomerulonephritis, which is most probably caused by immune complexes, circulating complexes frequently cannot be detected. In other diseases in which immune complexes do not appear to play a role in pathogenesis, complexes may be readily measured in plasma. Thus the mere detection of circulating immune complexes does not necessarily imply that they play a role in the pathogenesis of the disease. Nevertheless, since the potential of immune complexes to deposit and establish inflammatory injury is established, their detection in the circulation should alert the physician to seek evidence of their pathogenicity in the individual patient.

Lambert PH, et al.: A WHO collaborative study for the evaluation of eighteen methods for the detection of immune complexes in serum. J Clin Lab Immunol 1:1, 1978. Theofilopoulos AN, Dixon FJ: The biology and detection of immune complexes. Adv Immunol 28:89, 1979. *These two references cover the mechanisms available for detecting immune complexes in the circulation of patients with a wide variety of disorders. The latter reference offers, in addition, useful information on the effects of immune complexes on the host's response.*

Salant DS, Belok S, Madaio MP, Couser WG: A new role for complement in experimental nephropathy in rats. J Clin Invest 66:1339, 1980. *This article reviews the finding that immune complexes can form on the epithelial side of the glomerular basement membrane and, through the activation of complement, produce injury.*

Schraufstatter IU, Revak SD, Cochrane CG: Proteases and oxidants in experimental pulmonary inflammatory injury. J Clin Invest 73:1175, 1984. *This article provides evidence that oxidants are generated in situ in inflammation, and reviews the available data on oxidants and proteases in human pulmonary inflammatory disease.*

436. THE MAJOR HISTOCOMPATIBILITY COMPLEX AND DISEASE SUSCEPTIBILITY

Hugh O. McDevitt

The major histocompatibility complex (MHC) in mouse and man was originally defined as a linked cluster of genes on one chromosome that determines the structure of a group of cell surface molecules that are the strongest antigenic barrier to tissue transplantation between two unrelated individuals of the same species. This genetic region was first identified by tumor graft and skin graft rejection experiments. Subsequently serologic analysis became feasible with antisera produced in one individual by application of skin grafts or injection of lymphocytes from another individual of the same species. With the development of sophisticated skin grafting techniques following World War II, and the advent of kidney transplants, interest in detailed analysis of the major histocompatibility system increased. Great progress was made in our knowledge of the structure of the human MHC, of the number of alleles at each locus in the system (genetic polymorphism), and of the structure of the gene products themselves.

All of this knowledge developed directly out of research in transplantation immunology, although a moment's reflection will make it obvious that this system could not have evolved to frustrate the transplant surgeon. Tissue compatibility systems are well described in plants and in invertebrates. These systems may have evolved in the transition from unicellular to multicellular organisms so that these gene products play a major role in the discrimination of self from nonself. The MHC regulates the recognition of antigenic foreignness at several levels by several different effector components of the immune system. This phenomenon has been amply documented and carefully analyzed at the cellular level, although the molecular mechanisms are not yet clear.

The genotype of several MHC gene products (MHC antigens) shows a striking association with susceptibility to a wide variety of human diseases as well as to a number of animal disease models. This presumably results from their role in regulating specific immune responses. A wide variety of diseases in almost every subspecialty of internal medicine, many of them autoimmune in nature, shows strong associations with particular alleles (alternate forms) of particular loci in the human MHC, as determined by typing MHC molecules on peripheral blood lymphocytes (human leukocyte antigens—HLA). An understanding of the MHC and of the functions of the MHC genes is therefore important in understanding the association with disease susceptibility, and may be vital in understanding the pathogenesis of these diseases.

This chapter will describe the genetic structure of the murine and human MHC, the biochemistry and molecular genetics of the MHC gene products, and the function of these genes at the cellular level. The chapter will conclude with a brief discussion of (1) the possible mechanisms of action of these gene products at the molecular level and (2) an attempt to relate these functions to regulation of the immune response and to the determination of susceptibility to particular diseases. Some or all of the MHC antigens are expressed on all cell types. They clearly play a major role at the cell surface in recognition of antigenic foreignness. This may be only one of several regulatory functions of a group of cell surface molecules whose evolutionary origins may extend much farther back than the appearance of vertebrates in evolution.

THE MAJOR HISTOCOMPATIBILITY COMPLEX IN THE MOUSE

Analysis of the major histocompatibility complex is most advanced in the mouse and in man. MHC genes, gene products, and the functions of the complex in these two species share extensive homology. The genetic organization of the MHC differs slightly in the two species. Unfortunately the nomenclature differs radically. Since the genetic analysis of the murine MHC is farther advanced, this system will be presented first, followed by a discussion of the corresponding genes in the human MHC. In this textbook of medicine, discussion of important and fundamental work in the mouse must of necessity be curtailed. The reader is referred to a more extensive discussion of this topic in the articles cited at the end of this chapter.

The mouse MHC was the second histocompatibility-determining locus described in the mouse, and therefore has been designated H-2.

Figure 436–1 is a linkage map of the seventeenth mouse chromosome. The histocompatibility-2 (H-2) region is approximately 15 centimorgans (cM) to the right of the centromere. (Genetic map units or distances are expressed as crossover frequencies. Two loci on the same chromosome that show genetic recombination, resulting from crossing over, 15 times in 100 matings are said to be 15 map units, or crossover units, or centimorgans, apart.) The H-2 complex is a small portion of the seventeenth mouse chromosome, and spans a genetic distance of 1.0 cM. Although this is small in terms of the size of the seventeenth chromosome, it is sufficient to encode for over 200 structural genes for polypeptides of approximately 20,000 daltons. The exact number of genes in the H-2 complex is not known. To date, over 50 genes have been mapped in the H-2 complex.

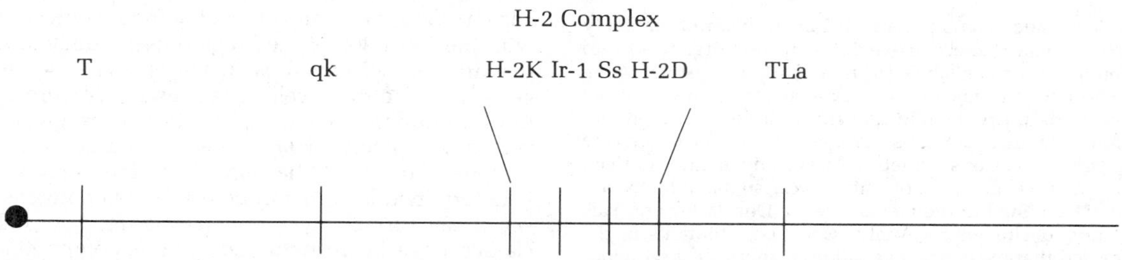

Figure 436–1. A schematic diagram of some of the genes on the seventeenth mouse chromosome. T is the short tail or brachyury locus. qk is the quaking locus. The H-2 complex is explained in detail in the text. TLa is the thymus leukemia antigen locus. (From McDevitt HO: *In* McCarty DJ [ed.]: Arthritis and Allied Conditions. 9th ed. Philadelphia, Lea & Febiger, 1979.)

The MHC includes three major classes of genes and gene products that are also found in man (cf. Fig. 436–1). They will be discussed as a background for understanding the corresponding systems in man.

THE CLASS I GENE PRODUCTS ENCODED BY H-2K AND H-2D. ***Genetics and Biochemistry.*** The class I gene products are cell surface glycoproteins, molecular weight 45,000 daltons, that are present in the membranes of all nucleated cells as well as on red cells and platelets. These antigens were originally detected by isoimmunization to produce isoantisera. The presence or absence of H-2 incompatibility in a donor-recipient pair of mice is correlated with rapid versus subacute or chronic graft rejection. The structure of the class I histocompatibility antigens is determined by several genes, H-2K, H-2D, H-2L, and H-2R, and consists of a two-chain molecule in which each H-2K or H-2D polypeptide chain is tightly bound to a 12,000-dalton polypeptide known as β_2-microglobulin (Fig. 436–2). The β_2-microglobulin molecule is under the control of a structural gene on a separate chromosome. This two-chain structure, with a heavy and light chain, is reminiscent of the structure of immunoglobulins. In fact, β_2-microglobulin has a very marked amino acid sequence homology with a portion of the constant region of the IgG immunoglobulin heavy chain. In addition, H-2K and H-2D gene products also have partial amino acid sequence homology with some immunoglobulin molecules. This finding has led to speculation that immunoglobulins may have evolved from a primitive recognition system represented by the transplantation antigen system.

There is also marked amino acid sequence homology between the K and D gene products. This indicates that the two gene products probably arose by a process of tandem duplication from a single ancestral gene. The serologically different forms (alleles) of the K and D genes show multiple differences in amino acid sequence primarily in the first and second domains. As would be expected, the K and D gene products show remarkable amino acid sequence homology with their counterparts in the human MHC. The major characteristics of the H-2K and H-2D gene products are presented in Table 436–1.

The major histocompatibility antigens are unique among

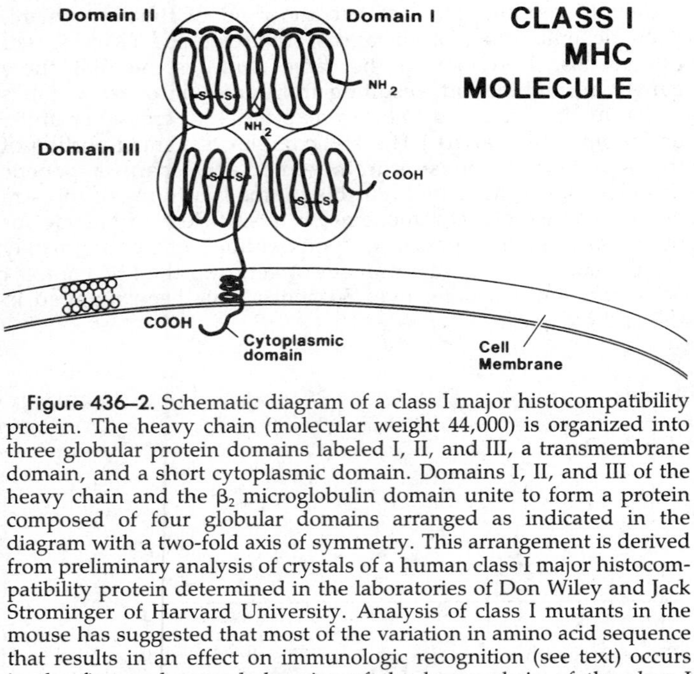

Figure 436–2. Schematic diagram of a class I major histocompatibility protein. The heavy chain (molecular weight 44,000) is organized into three globular protein domains labeled I, II, and III, a transmembrane domain, and a short cytoplasmic domain. Domains I, II, and III of the heavy chain and the β_2 microglobulin domain unite to form a protein composed of four globular domains arranged as indicated in the diagram with a two-fold axis of symmetry. This arrangement is derived from preliminary analysis of crystals of a human class I major histocompatibility protein determined in the laboratories of Don Wiley and Jack Strominger of Harvard University. Analysis of class I mutants in the mouse has suggested that most of the variation in amino acid sequence that results in an effect on immunologic recognition (see text) occurs in the first and second domains of the heavy chain of the class I histocompatibility protein. The sites of these variations are indicated by arcs, but their true position in space is unknown.

TABLE 436–1. MAJOR PROPERTIES OF THE CLASS I (H-2K AND H-2D) GENE PRODUCTS OF THE MOUSE

Molecular weight:	45,000 dalton glycoprotein
Tissue distribution:	Found on all nucleated cells, but especially on lymphocyte plasma membranes; constitutes 1 to 2 per cent of membrane protein of the lymphocyte
Polymorphism:	Extremely high degree of genetic polymorphism
Biologic properties:	Incompatibility of *H-2K* and/or *D* elicits rapid graft rejection, *strong* cytotoxic T cell reponse, *weak* mixed lymphocyte reaction, and production of IgG isoantibody

mammalian isoantigenic systems in their high degree of stable polymorphism. (Polymorphism is said to exist in a population when two or more different forms of the same gene and gene product are found in the population, both of which are present in more than 1 per cent of the individuals.) One of the most striking characteristics of the MHC is the enormous degree of genetic polymorphism for the class I genes. Each new population of wild mouse isolates from different geographic regions has shown at least one or two previously undetected H-2K or H-2D antigenic specificities. In man, a very high degree of polymorphism for the homologous loci is also seen.

Function of the H-2K and H-2D Genes. The major biologic properties that can be attributed to the H-2K and D gene products are listed in Table 436–1. These gene products elicit a very strong cytotoxic T cell response, and a very weak or minimal mixed lymphocyte culture reaction. They are in some way involved in or influence the specificity of cytotoxic T cells for foreign antigenic molecules. The experimental findings are as follows. Following immunization with viruses, minor histocompatibility antigens, or haptens complexed to cell surface antigens, the cytotoxic T cells that subsequently develop are capable of killing target cells *only* when the target has on its surface both the foreign antigenic determinant (virus, minor histocompatibility antigen, or hapten) *and* molecules of the same H-2K or D gene products that were present on the immunizing cells originally injected. Two possible explanations for these findings have been considered: (1) cytotoxic T cells are differentiated to recognize only "altered self," and therefore recognize a foreign antigenic determinant on the cell surface only in combination with H-2K or D or both; or (2) the cytotoxic T cell carries two receptors, one of which is specific for self H-2K and D, and the other of which is specific for foreign antigens, the two receptors being in some way closely linked on the cytotoxic T cell surface.

The evidence presently available indicates that the T cell receptor is a single immunoglobulin-like molecule of 80,000 daltons, which is made up of two 40,000-dalton chains. This receptor "sees" a compound antigenic determinant created by the association of self H-2K or D with the foreign antigen on the cell surface.

THE CLASS II GENE PRODUCTS ENCODED BY THE H-2I REGION. ***Genetics and Biochemistry.*** The I region was initially identified because it was possible to show that genetic control of the immune response to a series of related synthetic polypeptide antigens was localized to a gene or genes mapping between the H-2K and S regions (Fig. 436–3). In closely related inbred strains of mice that were genetically identical for the other 19 chromosome pairs, and at most of the seventeenth chromosome with the exception of the I region itself, antisera were produced that reacted selectively with lymphocyte cell surface alloantigens. Because these cell surface antigens were associated with the I immune response region, they were given the name of I region associated, or Ia antigens. To date, Ia antigens are the only gene products that have been identified whose structure is determined by I region genes. The Ia antigens are a discrete set of cell surface glycoproteins. So far, two molecular weight classes have been identified—one a polypeptide of 33,000 to 34,000 daltons and the second a polypeptide of 28,000 to 29,000 daltons. These two chains form a heterodimer of 62,000 molecular weight (Fig. 436–4). The major characteristics of the Ia antigens are listed in Table 436–2. In the mouse there are only

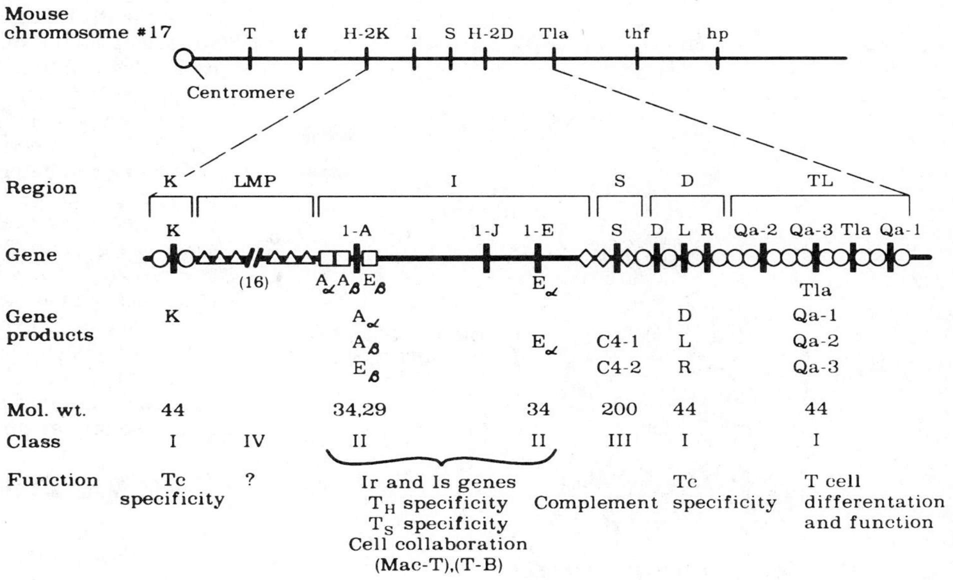

Figure 436–3. Schematic diagram of the genes of the murine major histocompatibility system. These genes are located on the seventeenth chromosome in the mouse, which is shown at the top of the diagram. The major histocompatibility system is shown in an expanded version in the second tier of the diagram in which it is broken up into subregions. Class I major histocompatibility genes are found in the K, D, and TL regions, while class II major histocompatibility genes (defined in the text) are found in the I region. Class III genes encoding several of the components of the complement system are found in the S region, and a set of 16 polypeptides is encoded by genes in the LMP region. The function of class I and class II genes is described in the text, and the function of class IV genes is unknown. ○ = class I genes; □ = class II genes; ◇ = class III genes; △ = class IV genes.

two class II molecules, I-A and I-E, encoded by four genes—A_α, A_β, E_α, and E_β.

The antigens eliciting the mixed lymphocyte culture reaction were also mapped to the I region. The mixed lymphocyte culture reaction is a proliferative response that occurs when lymphocytes from two unrelated individuals of the same species are cocultured together. T cell recognition of the allogeneic lymphocyte cell surface class II antigens results in rapid proliferation of a subpopulation of the T lymphocyte population from each donor.

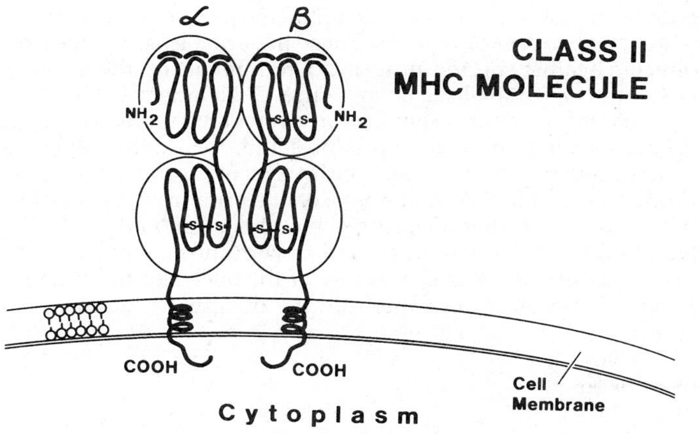

Figure 436–4. Schematic diagram of a class II major histocompatibility protein. This protein is composed of two polypeptide chains, an α chain of 34,000 molecular weight and a β chain of 29,000 molecular weight. As indicated in the diagram, three of these domains have intrachain disulfide loops with spacing reminiscent of immunoglobulin domains. Analysis of nucleotide sequence of complementary DNA clones of several different genetic forms (alleles) of the α chain by Mathis and Benoist in the author's laboratory, and of the β chains in John Seidman's laboratory at Harvard University, S. Tonegawa's laboratory at Massachusetts Institute of Technology, and the author's laboratory have shown that the major sequence differences between different alleles of the α and β chains occur in the first domain and that within the first domain, they occur in three "allelic hypervariable" regions that are positioned similarly to the hypervariable regions seen in immunoglobulin molecules. The position of these allelic hypervariable regions in space is as yet unknown but in the diagram is indicated as occurring at one end of the molecule (indicated by arcs) open to the aqueous environment in a manner similar to that seen in the three-dimensional folding of the antibody molecule.

The Functions of the I Region. The I-immune response region is defined primarily by the Ir genes—specific immune response genes that determine the ability of the individual's immune system to recognize an antigen as foreign and to mount an effective immune response, or to fail to recognize the antigen as foreign, in which case the animal is classified as a nonresponder to the antigen in question. More than 30 antigens have been shown to be under the control of Ir genes. Most of these antigens possess a restricted range of antigenic determinants available for recognition by the animal being immunized. For example, some of the antigens under Ir gene control are (1) simple synthetic polypeptides made up of two or three amino acids and therefore presenting a restricted range of antigenic determinants; (2) minor histocompatibility antigens, which presumably differ from the structure of the same antigen in the recipient by only a few amino acid residues; or (3) complex proteins for which Ir gene control operates only at a very low dose of antigen in which presumably one or a few antigenic determinants are "dominant." Although only 30 to 40 antigens have been shown to be under H-2 linked Ir gene control, it is likely that this control operates for most if not all foreign antigens.

I region genes appear to regulate immune reactivity by influencing the manner in which foreign antigens are seen by, or "presented to," T lymphocytes. One of the best examples of this comes from an analysis of the immune response of inbred guinea pigs to bovine insulin. Strain 2 guinea pigs respond primarily to antigenic determinants on the A chain of insulin, whereas strain 13 guinea pigs fail to recognize antigenic differences in the A chain of insulin but recognize antigenic differences in the insulin B chain. These two strains can then be crossed to produce an F_1 hybrid. When these hybrid animals

TABLE 436–2. MAJOR PROPERTIES OF THE CLASS II (I REGION) PRODUCTS (Ia ANTIGENS) OF THE MOUSE

Molecular weight: 34,000 and 29,000 dalton glycoprotein
Present in the cell membrane as a dimer between 34,000 and 29,000 dalton polypeptides
Tissue distribution: B lymphocytes, macrophages, some T cells, and epidermal cells
Polymorphism: High degree of polymorphism, not as great as *H-2K* and *D*
Biologic properties: Incompatibility at the *I* region elicits rapid rejection of bone marrow (lymphocyte), skin, and cardiac muscle grafts; *weak* cytotoxic T cell immune response; *strong* mixed lymphocyte culture reaction; and production of IgG isoantibody

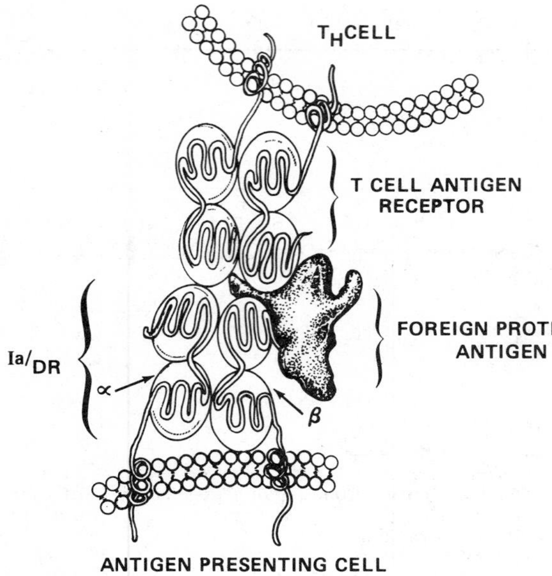

Figure 436–5. Schematic diagram of the interaction between the T helper lymphocyte (which is responsible for triggering proliferation and differentiation of B lymphocytes to produce antibody) and the foreign antigen on the surface of an antigen presenting adherent cell, or macrophage. The T lymphocyte is "restricted" in its ability to recognize a foreign antigen on the surface of the antigen presenting cell by the genotype of the class II histocompatibility protein on the antigen presenting cell. The T helper lymphocyte can recognize foreign antigen only if it is in association with a class II molecule of the same genotype as that present on the initial antigen presenting cell that induced the initial proliferation and differentiation of the T helper lymphocyte. This phenomenon of specificity of the T cell for both foreign antigen and class II histocompatibility antigen was initially described by Alan Rosenthal, Ethan Shevach, William Paul, and Ira Green at the National Institutes of Health.

are immunized to bovine insulin, their T lymphocytes will recognize antigenic differences in *either* the A chain or the B chain, when the insulin molecule is "presented" to the F_1 lymphocytes bound to the surface of F_1 macrophages. However, when the insulin molecule is presented to F_1 T lymphocytes on strain 2 macrophages, only A chain specific immune responses are elicited. When the insulin molecule is presented on strain 13 macrophages, only B chain antigenic differences are recognized. These findings are compatible with the possibility that class II determinants on the macrophages interact with foreign antigens. This interaction would influence the availability of particular foreign antigenic determinants for interaction with the helper T cell (T_H) receptor. This model postulates that Ia antigens engage in a wide variety of "specific" protein interactions with foreign antigens present on the macrophage cell surface. This interaction is similar to the interaction of class I molecules with foreign antigen that is the target of the cytotoxic T cell receptor. The only distinction is that helper T cells "see" foreign antigen in association with class II MHC molecules. This is diagrammed in Figure 436–5.

The I region determines the development of specific immune suppression as well as specific immune responsiveness. However, the effector cells mediating specific immune suppression express a genetically and functionally distinct Ia antigen that is the product of a gene mapping in a separate subregion (I-J). One class of Ia antigen determined by the I-J subregion appears to be selectively expressed on suppressor T cells.

I region genes also affect the efficiency of cell-cell interaction. Thus, the ability of T cells and macrophages, and T cells and B cells, to interact appears to require identity at the I region, or in one subregion (I-A or I-E) of the I region.

THE MAJOR HISTOCOMPATIBILITY COMPLEX IN HUMANS

The human MHC has been designated the *h*uman *l*eukocyte *a*ntigen or HLA system. The HLA system is found on the short arm of human chromosome 6 and spans a genetic distance of about 4.0 cM. A schematic diagram of the HLA system is presented in Figure 436–6.

HLA-A, B, AND C REGIONS. The HLA-A and B gene products of humans are homologous with the H-2K and D gene products of the mouse. The HLA-C gene product may be a tandem duplication of the HLA-B gene product. HLA-A, B, and C are the 44,000–dalton cell surface glycoproteins that are found on the surface of all nucleated cells in association with a 12,000–dalton β_2-microglobulin chain. Maternal isoantisera are routinely used to type for HLA-A, B, and C antigens. During the course of pregnancy, sufficient fetal lymphocytes leak into the maternal circulation to induce a significant titer of anti-HLA antibodies in the weeks following delivery in approximately 30 per cent of women. These maternal isoantibodies are directed against specific antigenic determinants on the HLA-A, B, C and (as we shall see below) HLA-D isoantigens. Thus any one maternal isoantiserum has a number of antibodies in it directed against these gene products and, in addition, appears to have several different antibodies specific for any one gene product, e.g., HLA-A. Maternal isoantiserum from a primipara will react with the offspring's lymphocytes, and with the lymphocytes of the father, as well as with those of anyone else in the population who shares any of the alleles of the HLA-A, B, and C loci with the father and the offspring. The maternal

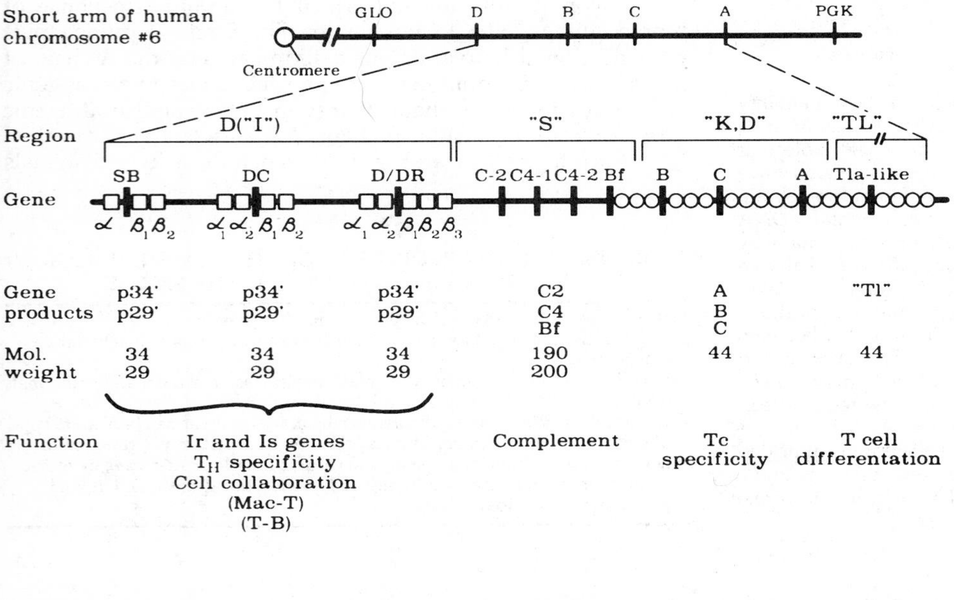

Figure 436–6. Schematic diagram of the human major histocompatibility complex on the sixth human chromosome. Aside from the difference in *position* and *number* of class II genes, the human and mouse systems are strikingly homologous. The symbols are the same as those given in Figure 436–3.

isoantiserum can thus be used to define the presence of these antigens in other members of the population.

By using a large number of different maternal sera, and a large panel of normal donor lymphocytes, combined with computer analysis of associations of reactions of paired sera with particular lymphocytes, many allelic antigenic specificities at the HLA-A, B, and C loci have been defined. There are approximately 20 different allelic antigenic specificities at the HLA-A locus, over 40 allelic antigenic specificities at the HLA-B locus, nearly 6 distinct antigenic specificities at the HLA-C locus. These allelic antigenic specificities have been assigned numbers; i.e., HLA-A1, A2, A3; HLA-B12, B16, B17, B27; and HLA-C1, C2, C3.

HLA-D REGION. The major difference in the genetic organization of the HLA system relative to the murine H-2 system is that the genes for determining the structure of the cell surface molecules eliciting the mixed lymphocyte culture reaction (MLR) map at a position *outside* of the region bounded by the two genes determining the class I histocompatibility antigens (HLA-A, B). The genetic region determining the structure of the antigens eliciting the MLR in the HLA system has been termed HLA-D. The HLA-D gene products in man were initially typed by using the mixed lymphocyte culture reaction. (By x-irradiating the lymphocytes of one of the two donors to a mixed lymphocyte culture reaction, it is possible to eliminate the responsiveness of that lymphocyte population. The mixed lymphocyte culture in this situation is termed a one-way mixed lymphocyte culture reaction, and measures only the ability of the responder lymphocytes to recognize alloantigens on the surface of the irradiated stimulator cells.) If stimulator cells are used that are homozygous at the HLA-D locus, then nonresponsiveness in the MLR in this situation is said to give a "typing reaction," and the responder lymphocyte population can be identified as possessing that particular HLA-D allele. Such homozygous typing cells (HTCs) were originally identified in the population, and at the Sixth and Seventh International Histocompatibility Testing Workshops were given provisional "workshop" or "w" designations as HLA-Dw1, Dw2, Dw3, and so forth. A total of ten HLA-D locus types or alleles have been identified by this method. Utilizing these homozygous typing cells, it is possible to identify somewhat more than 50 per cent, but less than 75 per cent, of the HLA-D genes (two genes for each individual) present in a normal population.

Differences at the HLA-D locus also elicit the production of isoantibodies in maternal sera, antibodies that are specific for B cell alloantigens whose structure is determined by HLA-D–linked genes. These sera show a distinct correlation with HLA-D locus types as determined by homozygous typing cells in the mixed lymphocyte culture reaction. These B cell alloantigens identified by maternal isoantisera have been provisionally identified as HLA-DR (for D-related) antigens. Since the HLA-D locus is analogous to the I region locus in terms of function in eliciting the mixed lymphocyte culture reaction, it is not surprising that HLA-D gene products are analogous to the I region polypeptides in the mouse. Indeed, HLA-D gene products are composed of two classes of polypeptide chains of 34,000 and 29,000 daltons displayed on macrophages, B cells, some T cells, and endothelial cells. The amino acid sequence of the human p34 polypeptide is homologous with the 34,000-dalton polypeptide of the I-E/C segment (E_α) of the I region of the mouse.

Murine Ia and human HLA-DR determinants are similar with regard to their ability to stimulate in a mixed lymphocyte reaction and in their tissue localization and structure. These genes also appear to function as immune response genes in man.

Despite these biochemical, structural, and functional similarities, there are marked differences in the genetic organization of the HLA-D genetic region when compared to the murine H-2I region. There are many more Class II MHC genes and gene products in man than in the mouse. There are three separate *types* of class II molecules in man, designated DR, DC, and SB (compared to two types, I-A and I-E, in the mouse). For each

type there are multiple genes. In terms of genes expressed by gene products at the cell surface (in contrast to pseudogenes) there are: $1DR_\alpha$, $3DR_\beta$, $2DC_\alpha$, $2DC_\beta$, $2SB_\alpha$, and $2SB_\beta$ chains. This is a striking contrast with the mouse, and presumably results in much greater complexity in regulation of the immune response by class II molecules in man.

Population Genetics and Disease Associations

Specific combinations of particular alleles at the HLA-A, B, C, and D loci tend to occur together on the same chromosome in a particular combination more often than would be expected by chance. This phenomenon, known as *linkage disequilibrium*, is the opposite of linkage equilibrium. Equilibrium can be said to exist when any given allele of one gene is found on the same chromosome in combination with any specified allele of a second linked gene in a frequency determined by the product of the gene frequencies of the two specified alleles at the two loci. This linkage equilibrium develops because genetic crossing over will occur between the two loci and scramble any particular combination of specified alleles at the two loci. For a newly introduced (mutant) allele of one of the two genes, genetic equilibrium will develop more rapidly for genes that are farther apart. Even for closely linked genes, genetic equilibrium will ultimately develop, given sufficient numbers of generations and a random choice of breeding partners.

The HLA system constitutes one of the most remarkable examples of linkage disequilibrium in the human genome. There are several chromosomal combinations or haplotypes (a set of particular alleles of linked genes on one chromosome, the haploid number, is designated as a haplotype) that occur in a particular population at a frequency much higher than would be predicted by chance. Thus, in Caucasian populations, the A1,B8,Dw3 combination occurs much more frequently than would be predicted by the product of the gene frequencies of these three alleles in the population. The same is true for the A3,B7,Dw2 haplotype and for several other haplotypes. These alleles are thus said to be in linkage disequilibrium.

Linkage disequilibrium may reflect a selective survival advantage of a particular combination of alleles at linked loci. In most systems the precise mechanism of selective survival advantage is unclear. The same is true for the HLA system. There is clear evidence that HLA-A and B can influence cytotoxic T cell specificity, and presumptive evidence indicates that genes in the HLA-D region can dictate immune reactivity to a given antigenic determinant. This suggests at least one mechanism of selective advantage. Particular combinations of HLA-A, B, and D alleles might confer a very strong selective survival advantage in a population exposed to a particular selective force, such as a viral or bacterial infection. This would presumably vary with climate and environment, and similar variation in the occurrence of linkage disequilibrium has also been observed. Thus, the HLA-A3,B7,Dw2 haplotype is much more prevalent in Scandinavian countries and in temperate European areas than in Caucasian populations of European origin in Mediterranean countries and countries closer to the equator.

It must be kept in mind that an alternative mechanism may be operative in some cases, and has been documented in the mouse. This mechanism is suppression of crossing over due to an inversion in gene order on the chromosome exhibiting linkage disequilibrium.

Associations of the HLA Systems with Disease Susceptibility

Figure 436–7 indicates some of the more than 40 diseases for which it has been shown that susceptibility is associated with a particular HLA-A, B, or D locus type. Only a few diseases show primary association with an HLA-A or B type. Susceptibility to idiopathic hemochromatosis is associated with HLA-A3 in some populations, but is due to a linked gene influencing iron metabolism. Susceptibility to a wide variety of rheumatic

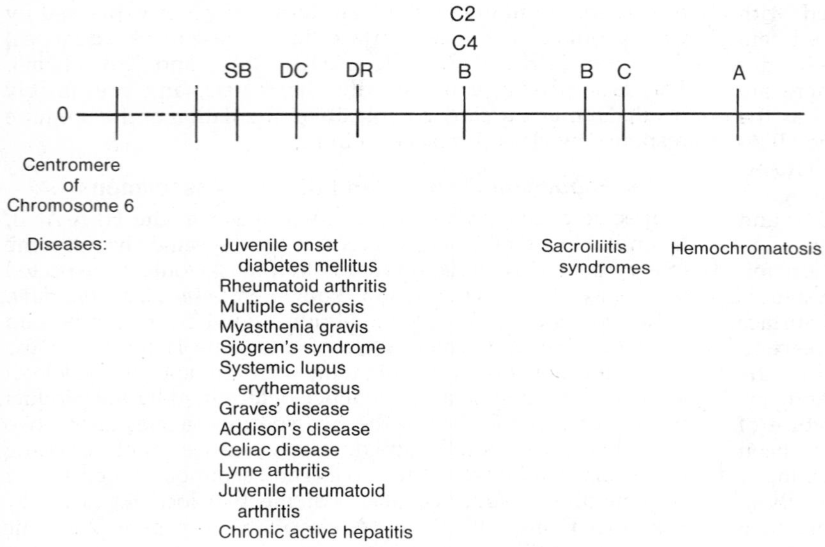

Figure 436–7. The HLA system and HLA-associated diseases.

diseases in which sacroiliitis and spondylitis are prominent features is associated with HLA-B27—one of the strongest associations between HLA and disease susceptibility. HLA-B27 occurs in approximately 5 per cent of the normal Caucasian population and in more than 90 per cent of patients with ankylosing spondylitis, more than 75 per cent of patients with Reiter's disease, and a majority of patients with psoriatic arthritis and inflammatory bowel disease in whom sacroiliitis occurs as a complication of their illness.

By far the largest category of HLA-associated diseases consists of those in which the primary association is with a particular HLA-DR or Dw type. Many of these diseases were originally reported to be associated with a particular HLA-B locus type, but subsequent studies have revealed that this is due to preferential combination of particular alleles of HLA-A, B, and D occurring together on the same chromosome more often than would be expected by chance owing to linkage disequilibrium.

The list of HLA-D locus–associated diseases is extensive and ranges from examples such as celiac disease, in which almost 100 per cent of the patients are HLA-Dw3, to thyrotoxicosis, in which slightly more than half of the patients are HLA-Dw3 (Dw3 occurring in the normal population in approximately 20 per cent of individuals).

In Caucasians the HLA-A1,B3,Dw3 haplotype is associated with a number of autoimmune diseases, including myasthenia gravis, thyrotoxicosis, Addison's disease, juvenile–onset diabetes mellitus, Sjögren's syndrome, and chronic active hepatitis. The A3,B7,Dw2 haplotype is associated with susceptibility to multiple sclerosis. A particularly intriguing example of this type is the frequent occurrence of the HLA-A10,B18,Dw2 haplotype with a deficiency in the structural gene for the second component of complement. Most of the cases of absolute deficiency of the second component of complement (a recessive defect) carry at least one dose of this haplotype. In addition, the A10,B18,Dw2 C2 deficiency haplotype in the heterozygote appears to be associated with a markedly increased incidence of autoimmune syndromes resembling systemic lupus erythematosus. This is one of several examples in which the C4,C2, properdin factor B genes of the HLA system may be playing a role in disease susceptibility.

The mechanism of the association of HLA-D type with susceptibility to this wide variety of diseases is unknown. However, four generalizations can be made from the available data: (1) Most of these diseases have a definite or suspected autoimmune pathogenesis. Examples of diseases in which an autoimmune pathogenesis is clearly established include myasthenia gravis, thyrotoxicosis, and systemic lupus erythematosus. Diseases in which an autoimmune pathogenesis is suspected but not yet clearly established include rheumatoid arthritis, multiple sclerosis, and juvenile–onset diabetes mellitus, as well as chronic active hepatitis, celiac disease, Sjögren's syndrome, and nontuberculous Addison's disease. (2) Susceptibility is a dominant trait, as is Ir gene–controlled immune responsiveness. (3) Only a minority of those carrying a susceptibility allele ever develop the disease, suggesting that environmental factors also play a role. (4) Not all individuals with a particular disease possess the allele associated with susceptibility, suggesting that other genes may influence disease occurrence, as has been shown for MHC-determined thyroiditis in chickens and myasthenia gravis in humans.

These four generalizations have a very major bearing on our attempts to understand the mechanism underlying the association between the HLA system and susceptibility to disease. Since the pathogenesis of these diseases is for the most part a mystery, any attempt to explain the mechanism of association with HLA must be, in part, speculative. Thus, the association of ankylosing spondylitis and Reiter's disease with HLA-B27 might be due to a direct effect of the B27 allele on the development of cytotoxic T cell responsiveness to an exogenous antigen that triggers an immune response to a cross-reacting self antigen. Alternatively, the association could reflect the effect of a gene closely linked to HLA-B27 and in very strong linkage disequilibrium with it. Definitive family studies to settle this point have not yet been carried out.

Similarly the association of a wide variety of autoimmune diseases, including rheumatoid arthritis, with the HLA-D locus raises the speculation that a hypernormal or hyponormal immune response to an exogenous antigen or to a self antigen might underlie the association. For example, the association of Graves' disease and myasthenia gravis with HLA-Dw3 might be due to a hypernormal immune response to an environmental agent that cross-reacts with either the thyrotropin receptor or the acetylcholine receptor, or alternatively might be due to a deficit in suppressor T cells that normally suppress what might otherwise be a damaging autoimmune response to the thyrotropin receptor or the acetylcholine receptor. Some of these possibilities are susceptible to experimental tests, but evidence is as yet lacking.

The existence of linkage disequilibrium in the HLA system, which has been referred to above, raises the possibility that none of the measured genes are responsible for the observed associations. The associations might in fact be due to other linked genes that are in linkage disequilibrium with the measured genes, including the DC and SB class II molecules. Our methods of genotyping for these molecules are at present imperfect. For example, the association of Graves' disease and juvenile–onset diabetes mellitus (as well as a number of other autoimmune diseases in Caucasians) with HLA-Dw3 might be due to a strong linkage disequilibrium between HLA-Dw3 and other genes predisposing to these diseases. In this situation none of the HLA-A, B, C, or D genes would be the true disease susceptibility genes.

It is clear that the HLA-D region is subdivided into several loci (at least 5_{α} and 7_{β} chain genes). Some of these loci might be of major importance in determining disease susceptibility. Typing methods specific for these additional D region subloci may reveal very strong disease associations, whereas current typing methods reveal only partial or weak association with DR type.

The possibility of gene complementation in disease susceptibility must also be taken into account. The relative risk of juvenile-onset diabetes in individuals who are HLA-DR3/DR3 or HLA-DR4/DR4 is very much less than that of individuals who are HLA-DR3/DR4. This is the first example suggesting gene complementation for susceptibility to a disease, and appears to be analogous to complementing Ir genes and Ia molecules described in the mouse. As our knowledge of the HLA-D region advances, our understanding and identification of the susceptible genotypes and of the mechanisms at work may well advance in parallel. Studies utilizing cDNA probes for the various class II α and β chain genes reveal a striking degree of genomic DNA restriction endonuclease fragment length polymorphism. Analysis of these polymorphisms, as well as DNA sequence analysis of class II α and β chain genes, will almost certainly refine and subdivide current HLA-DR haplotypes, and can be expected to refine and sharpen association of particular DR, DC, and SB genotypes with particular diseases. Application of these findings will undoubtedly have major impact on diagnostic approaches, prognosis, and ultimately on therapy.

Hood L, Steinmetz M, Malissen B: Genes of the major histocompatibility complex. Ann Rev Immunol 1:529, 1983.

Kaufman JA, Auffray C, Korman AJ, Shackleford DA, Strominger J: The class II molecules of the human and murine major histocompatibility complex. Cell 36:1, 1984.

Klein J: The Major Histocompatibility Complex. Chapter 8. *In* Immunology: The Science Of Self–Non Self Discrimination. New York, John Wiley & Sons, 1982.

Ryder LP, Svejgaard A, Dausset J: Genetics of HLA disease association. Annu Rev Genet 15:169, 1981.

437. DRUG ALLERGY

Charles E. Reed

An allergic cause of a drug reaction is suspected when an inflammatory lesion characteristic of those provoked by immunologic mechanisms follows administration of the drug. The variety of drug allergies gives the initial impression that any drug can cause any reaction; in fact, distinct patterns are the rule. Any particular drug tends to cause a similar reaction in different subjects. Typical examples include urticaria after penicillin G injection, lymphocytic pneumonitis after nitrofurantoin, or contact dermatitis from an ointment containing ethylenediamine. Allergic drug reactions need to be distinguished from expected side effects, idiosyncratic reactions of unknown cause, toxic reactions, psychophysiologic reactions, and also from immunologic manifestations of the underlying disease. A further distinction is made between allergic inflammation initiated by a ligand reacting with an antibody or a specifically reacting lymphocyte and similar inflammation initiated by some other chemical reaction. Unfortunately these distinctions are not always easy at the bedside, and there are few reliable clinical or laboratory tests.

Many patients relate a history of allergy to one or more drugs, often without an objective basis. Usually this history can be accepted and serves as a deterrent to excessive drug therapy. Sometimes, however, it is important to evaluate the possibility of allergy to a potentially lifesaving drug for which

there is no substitute, since many patients with a history of a reaction will tolerate the drug, particularly if several years have passed. If the allergy is still present, taking the drug can be disastrous with fatality from anaphylaxis, Steven-Johnson's syndrome, exfoliative dermatitis, interstitial pneumonitis, or vasculitis. A decision for a particular course of action often rests on judicious weighing of the potential benefits and risks rather than on a definitive diagnosis.

INCIDENCE AND PREDISPOSING FACTORS. Allergic reactions constituted only about 6 per cent of all adverse drug reactions in a 1968 study. The frequency is thought to be less today, except for reactions to radiographic contrast agents, which now account for about 60 per cent of drug-induced anaphylaxis and about 20 per cent of all cases of anaphylaxis. Radiographic contrast dyes do not cause anaphylaxis as a result of specific antibodies (see below). In one large study of drug reactions, which may have underestimated reactions in organs other than skin, the following distribution was found: erythematous and maculopapular rashes, 46 per cent; urticaria, 23 per cent; fixed eruptions, 10 per cent; erythema multiforme, 5 per cent; exfoliative dermatitis, 4 per cent; purpura, 2 per cent; anaphylaxis, 1 per cent; and vasculitis, 0.5 per cent.

Several predisposing factors exist. Previous drug allergy to the same or a related drug is most important, and the frequency of allergy is increased by multiple courses of treatment. Topical administration is the route most likely to sensitize, oral administration least, and parenteral intermediate. Parenteral administration provokes more severe reactions, especially anaphylaxis. Children are less likely than adults to react, and men less than women. Persons with history of atopic allergy may be at increased risk of anaphylaxis or urticaria but not of other kinds of allergic drug reactions. Indeed, subjects with atopic dermatitis are less easily sensitized than normal persons to antigens that cause contact dermatitis. The antigenic determinant in drug allergy is usually a metabolite rather than the drug itself; genetic differences in drug metabolism therefore influence allergic reactions. For example, persons with reduced acetyltransferase activity are more likely to develop drug-induced systemic lupus erythematosus from hydralazine.

MECHANISMS. Foreign macromolecules acting as complete antigens are the most likely to sensitize, eliciting an IgE or IgG antibody response that on a subsequent administration causes anaphylaxis, serum sickness, or vasculitis. Classic serum sickness that occurs after injections of large amounts of rabbit or horse serum requires large amounts of antigen and relatively high concentrations of circulating immune complexes. Most episodes of urticaria, fever, and arthralgia after the relatively small doses of macromolecules in current use probably involve a combination of IgE- and IgG-initiated events.

Low molecular weight drugs and diagnostic agents elicit an immune response only after reacting covalently with proteins. The hapten may be the drug itself, but is more often a drug metabolite. The hapten-protein carrier then functions as the complete antigen, both initiating sensitization and eliciting the reaction. An allergic reaction requires a multivalent ligand to cross-link antibody molecules either in fluid phase or bound to cell surface receptors. Univalent haptens actually inhibit cross-linking by occupying the antigen-binding sites. Some chemicals may react with host proteins in such a way that their tertiary structure is altered and the new antigenic determinant is not the hapten itself but the altered structure of the host protein. The allergic reaction may take any of the forms of allergic reaction described in Part XXI. The mechanisms of immune defense and hypersensitivity, like many other biologic functions, exhibit redundancy such that a drug reaction may involve more than one allergic mechanism at the same time. The fact that the hapten so often is a drug metabolite may explain the characteristic involvement of some particular organ where the metabolism occurs; alternatively, the hapten may react with a specific organ protein to account for the location of the reaction.

TABLE 437–1. ALLERGIC DRUG REACTIONS

- I. Systemic
  - A. Anaphylaxis
    - 1. Macromolecules
      - Allergenic extracts
      - Dextrans (including iron dextran)
      - Enzymes
        - Asparaginase
        - Chymopapain
        - Chymotrypsin
        - Trypsin
      - Heparin
      - Hormones (ACTH, insulin, etc.)
      - Human gamma globulin
      - Organ extracts
      - Protamine
      - Vaccines
      - Xenogenic sera
    - 2. Diagnostic agents
      - Fluorescein
      - Iodinated contrast media
    - 3. Antimicrobials
      - Aminosalicylic acid
      - Amphotericin B
      - Cephalosporins
      - Clindamycin
      - Ethambutol
      - Kanamycin
      - Lincomycin
      - Penicillins
      - Streptomycin
      - Sulfonamides
      - Tetracyclines
      - Vancomycin
    - 4. Other drugs
      - Aspirin
      - Bleomycin
      - Cisplatin
      - Colchicine
      - Cromolyn
      - Cytarabine
      - Dantrolene
      - Ethylenediamine
      - Indomethacin
      - Local anesthetics
      - Mephyton
      - Meprobamate
      - Organic mercurials
      - Niacin
      - Opiates
      - Pentamidine and stilbamidine
      - Probenecid
      - Sulfite
      - Tolmetin
      - Triamterene
      - Tubocurarine and other muscle-relaxing agents
      - Vitamin B_{12}
  - B. Serum Sickness
    - 1. Macromolecules
      - Dextrans
      - Heparin
      - Hormones (insulin, ACTH)
      - Vaccines
      - Xenogenic sera
    - 2. Antimicrobials
      - Cephalosporins
      - Griseofulvin
      - Lincomycin
      - Penicillins
      - Streptomycin
      - Sulfonamides
    - 3. Other Drugs
      - Barbiturates
      - Cholecystographic dyes
      - Hydantoins
      - Hydralazine
      - Mercurial diuretics
      - Phenylbutazone
      - Procarbazine
      - Thiouracils

- I. Systemic (*Continued*)
  - C. Drug Fever
    - 1. Antimicrobials
      - Aminosalicylic acid
      - Cephalosporins
      - Chloramphenicol
      - Erythromycin
      - Isoniazid-kanamycin
      - Nitrofurantoin
      - Penicillins
      - Pyrazinamide
      - Quinine
      - Streptomycin
      - Sulfonamides
      - Tetracyclines
    - 2. Other drugs
      - Allopurinol
      - Heparin
      - Hydantoins
      - Hydralazine
      - Iodides
      - Mercurial diuretics
      - Methyldopa
      - Penicillamine
      - Phenobarbital
      - Pneumococcal vaccine
      - Procainamide
      - Propylthiouracil
      - Quinidine
  - D. Vasculitis
    - Allopurinol
    - Busulfan
    - Colchicine
    - Diphenhydramine
    - Ethionamide
    - Furosemide
    - Hydantoins
    - Indomethacin
    - Iodides
    - Isoniazid
    - Meprobamate
    - Methamphetamine
    - Penicillins
    - Phenothiazines
    - Phenylbutazone
    - Propranolol
    - Propylthiouracil
    - Sulfonamides
    - Tetracyclines
    - Thiazide diuretics
    - Vaccines
  - E. Systemic lupus erythematosus syndrome
    - Chloroquine
    - Griseofulvin
    - Hydralazine
    - Isoniazid
    - Methyldopa
    - Oral contraceptives
    - Phenytoin
    - Procainamide
    - Tetracycline
    - Thiouracil
- II. Skin
  - A. Urticaria and angioedema
    - 1. Antimicrobials
      - Aminoglycosides
      - Cephalosporins
      - Isoniazid
      - Metronidazole
      - Miconazole
      - Nalidixic acid
      - Penicillin
      - Quinine
      - Rifampin
      - Spectinomycin
      - Sulfonamides
      - Suramin
    - 2. Other drugs
      - Aspirin and other nonsteroidal anti-inflammatory drugs
      - Calcitonin
      - Chloral hydrate

- II. Skin (*Continued*)
  - Cyclophosphamide
  - Doxorubicin
  - Ergotamine
  - Ethchlorvynol
  - Ethosuximide
  - Ethylenediamine
  - Methaqualone
  - Penicillamine
  - Phenothiazines
  - Procainamide
  - Quinidine
  - Tragacanth
  - B. Morbilliform-maculopapular rash
    - 1. Antimicrobials
      - Aminosalicylic acid
      - Ampicillin
      - Erythromycin
      - Gentamicin
      - Penicillin
      - Sulfonamides
    - 2. Other drugs
      - Allopurinol
      - Barbiturates
      - Gold salts
      - Hydantoins
  - C. Erythroderma and exfoliative dermatitis
    - Allopurinol
    - Carbamazepine
    - Chloral hydrate
    - Chlorpromazine
    - Ethylenediamine
    - Glutethimide
    - Gold salts
    - Hydantoins
    - Iodides
    - Penicillin
    - Phenobarbital
    - Sulfonamides
    - Trimethadione
  - D. Erythema multiforme
    - Acetaminophen-phenacetin
    - Ampicillin
    - Barbiturates
    - Chloroquine
    - Chlorpropamide
    - Clindamycin
    - Ethosuximide
    - Gold salts
    - Hydantoins
    - Hydralazine
    - Penicillins
    - Phenolphthalein
    - Phenylbutazone
    - Rifampin
    - Streptomycin
    - Sulfapyridine
    - Sulfonamides
    - Sulfonylureas
    - Trimethoprim-sulfamethoxazole
    - Vaccines
  - E. Photosensitive
    - 1. Topical
      - Fluorouracil
      - Halogenated salicylanilides
      - Hexachlorophene
      - Para-aminobenzoic acid esters
      - Promethazine
      - Sulfanilamide
    - 2. Systemic
      - Carbamazepine
      - Chlorpromazine
      - Griseofulvin
      - Imipramine
      - Lincomycin
      - Nalidixic acid
      - Phenothiazines
      - Quinethazone

- II. Skin (*Continued*)
  - Sulfonamides
  - Sulfonylureas
  - Thiazide diuretics
  - F. Fixed drug eruptions
    - Aspirin
    - Barbiturates
    - Gold salts
    - Iodides
    - Meprobamate
    - Penicillins
    - Phenacetin
    - Phenolphthalein
    - Phenylbutazone
    - Quinine
    - Sulfonamides
    - Tetracyclines
  - G. Erythema Nodosum
    - Bromides
    - Iodides
    - Oral contraceptives
    - Penicillin
    - Sulfonamides
  - H. Contact dermatitis
    - Ammoniated mercury
    - Ampicillin
    - Antihistamines
    - Bacitracin
    - Benzalkonium chloride
    - Benzocaine
    - Chlorpromazine
    - Ethylenediamine
    - Fluorouracil
    - Formaldehyde
    - Glucocorticoids
    - Glutaraldehyde
    - Hexachlorophene
    - Idoxuridine
    - Iodochlorhydroxyquin
    - Lanolin
    - Local anesthetics
    - Neomycin
    - Opiates
    - Para-aminobenzoic acid
    - Parabens
    - Penicillin
    - Phenothiazines
    - Propylene glycol
    - Streptomycin
    - Sulfonamides
    - Thimerosal
- III. Lung
  - A. Asthma
    - Aspirin and other nonsteroidal anti-inflammatory drugs
    - Cromolyn
    - Pituitary snuff
    - Sodium glutamate
    - Sulfite
    - Occupational exposures to:
      - Cephalosporins
      - Glutaraldehyde
      - Pancreatic enzymes
      - Papain
      - Penicillin
      - Phenylmercurials
      - Psyllium
      - Spiromycin
  - B. Eosinophilic pneumonitis
    - Aminosalicylic acid
    - Azathioprine
    - Carbamazepine
    - Chlorpropamide
    - Cromolyn
    - Gold salts
    - Mephenesin
    - Nitrofurantoin
    - Penicillin
    - Sulfonamides
  - C. Fibrotic and pleural reactions
    - Bleomycin
    - Busulfan

(*Table continues on facing page*)

TABLE 437–1. ALLERGIC DRUG REACTIONS (*Continued*)

- III. Lung (*Continued*)
    - Cyclophosphamide
    - Ganglionic-blocking drugs
    - Gold salts
    - Hydrochlorothiazide
    - Melphalan
    - Methotrexate
    - Methysergide
    - Mitomycin
    - Nitrofurantoin
    - Procarbazine
- IV. Liver
    - A. Cholestatic
        - Chlorzoxazone
        - Erythromycin estiolate
        - Ethchlorvynol
        - Imipramine
        - Nalidixic acid
        - Nitrofurantoin
        - Phenothiazines
        - Sulfamethoxazole
        - Sulfonylureas
        - Troleandomycin
    - B. Hepatocellular
        - Aminosalicylic acid
        - Amphotericin B
        - Ethacrynic acid
        - Furosemide
        - Gold salts
        - Griseofulvin
        - Halothane
        - Hydantoins
        - Isoniazid
        - Methyldopa
        - Monoamine oxidase inhibitors
- IV. Liver (*Continued*)
    - Nitrofurantoin
    - Oxyphenisatin
    - Propylbutazone
    - Propylthiouracil
    - Pyrazinamide
    - Quinidine
    - Rifampin
    - Sulfonamides
    - Trimethadione
    - C. Chronic Active Hepatitis
        - Methyldopa
        - Nitrofurantoin
        - Oxyphenisatin
- V. Kidney
    - A. Glomerulonephritis. See *Vasculitis*
    - B. Interstitial nephritis
        - Cephalosporins
        - Diuretics
        - Furosemide
        - Nonsteroidal anti-inflammatory drugs
        - Penicillins, especially methicillin
        - Phenytoin
        - Rifampin
        - Sulfonamides
        - Thiazide
- VI. Bone Marrow and Blood Cells
    - A. Bone Marrow Aplasia
        - Chloramphenicol
        - Gold salts
        - Mephenytoin
        - Penicillamine
        - Phenylbutazone
        - Trimethadione
- VI. Bone Marrow and Blood Cells (*Continued*)
    - B. Anemia
        - Cephalosporins
        - Cisplatin
        - Penicillin
        - Acetaminophen
        - Aminosalicylic acid
        - Chlorpromazine
        - Insulin
        - Isoniazid
        - Melphalan
        - Phenacetin
        - Quinidine
        - Quinine
        - Rifampin
        - Stibophen
        - Sulfonamides
        - Sulfonylureas
        - Chlorpromazine
        - Hydantoins
        - Ibuprofen
        - Levodopa
        - Mefenamic acid
        - Methyldopa
        - Methysergide
    - C. Thrombocytopenia
        - Acetaminophen
        - Acetazolamide
        - Acetylsalicylic acid
        - Aminosalicylic acid
        - Carbamazepine
        - Cephalothin
        - Chloramphenicol
        - Chlorpheniramine
        - Digitoxin
        - Ethchlorvynol
        - Gold salts
- VI. Bone Marrow and Blood Cells (*Continued*)
    - Heparin
    - Hydantoins
    - Isoniazid
    - Levodopa
    - Meprobamate
    - Methyldopa
    - Penicillamine
    - Phenacetin
    - Phenylbutazone
    - Procainamide
    - Quinidine
    - Quinine
    - Rauwolfia alkaloids
    - Rifampin
    - Stibophen
    - Sulfonamides
    - Sulfonylureas
    - Thiazide diuretics
    - D. Granulocytopenia
        - Chloral hydrate
        - Chlorpropamide
        - Dipyrone
        - Mercurial diuretics
        - Methimazole
        - Penicillins (Semisynthetic)
        - Phenothiazines
        - Phenylbutazone
        - Phenytoin
        - Procainamide
        - Propranolol
        - Sulfamethoxypyridazine
        - Sulfapyridine
        - Tolbutamide
    - E. Lymphoid hyperplasia
        - Phenytoin
        - Mephenytoin

PREVENTION. The likelihood of serious drug allergy can be reduced by avoiding drugs with high sensitivity potential whenever possible. For this reason only a few macromolecules capable of acting as complete antigens remain in current use. Passive immunization with horse serum has been replaced with human serum except for anti-snake venoms. Egg-containing vaccines have either been replaced by tissue culture vaccines or are highly purified to remove most of the contaminating proteins. Reactions to highly purified vaccines like tetanus and diphtheria toxoids do occur occasionally, however. ACTH has been largely supplanted by glucocorticoids, and human insulin is available for the occasional patient who becomes allergic to beef or pork insulin. A few enzymes are still used, particularly asparaginase and chymopapain. Occasional reactions follow use of heparin and protamine. Dextran is avoided whenever possible because of its potential for causing anaphylaxis. Allergenic extracts are a special class of diagnostic and therapeutic materials carefully prepared to elicit allergy, and an excessive dose naturally can cause serious anaphylactic reactions.

The likelihood of serious drug allergy can be reduced by taking a careful history of drug allergy, by a high index of suspicion when fever, rash, or organ damage occurs during treatment, by careful recording of manifestation of drug reactions and diagnosis in the chart when they do occur and by proper instruction of the patient.

DIAGNOSIS. The history and physical examination provide the essential information for pattern recognition. A key point of the history is the time course of the reaction as well as the identity of the drug. Anaphylactic reactions follow within minutes, drug fever within an hour or two, contact dermatitis in a day or two, but cholestatic jaundice requires several days or a week. The character of the lesion is also important. Ampicillin characteristically causes a morbilliform rash that may be delayed for two days after the drug is stopped. All penicillins may cause urticaria within ten minutes, but the urticaria may not occur for several days. This distinction is important because the immediate reactions are more likely to be associated with anaphylaxis. A physician observing a drug reaction should record the physical findings for future use. For example, by history alone it is difficult to distinguish between laryngeal edema from anaphylaxis and the hyperventilation syndrome, but the presence of stridor and swelling of pharyngeal or laryngeal mucosa makes the distinction clear. Distinction between a drug reaction and an immunologic event from the underlying disease is important. For instance, many children with viral respiratory infections have transient urticaria that can be mistaken for a penicillin rash. Or, on the first or second day of penicillin treatment a patient with endocarditis may have a macular hemorrhagic rash and fever, reflecting a reaction to antigens released by antibiotic lysis of the bacteria rather than drug allergy.

Some of the most important patterns of drug reactions are summarized in Table 437–1.

Skin tests may be helpful in predicting anaphylaxis from macromolecules and are usually positive in patients with allergy to foreign sera, insulin, vaccines, and similar complex materials. With the important exception of penicillin, skin or in vitro allergy tests with low molecular weight drugs are not reliable for detecting anaphylactic (IgE-mediated) drug allergy, although positive skin tests have occasionally been reported after anaphylaxis from local anesthetics, cisplatin, and a few other drugs. Patch tests with single components are useful for identifying contact allergens. Ethylenediamine, one of the ingredients of many creams and ointments, is currently the most frequently encountered contactant. Attempts to adapt lymphocyte transformation tests for diagnosis of drug allergy have been unsuccessful. Deliberate trial of small doses of the drug strictly for diagnostic purposes is unwise and unnecessary, though it may be indicated as a precaution in situations in which the diagnosis of drug allergy is uncertain and no chemically unrelated substitute is available for an urgently needed drug.

MANAGEMENT. In addition to stopping use of the offending drug, the reaction itself may need symptomatic or supportive treatment appropriate to the specific situation. As a rule it is unwise to attempt to continue using the offending drug under a protective umbrella of antihistamines or glucocorticoids, although occasional desperate situations may justify an exception. The emergency treatment of anaphylaxis is described in Ch. 433.

SPECIFIC DRUG ALLERGIES. ***Penicillin.*** Penicillin is one of the most common drugs causing allergy, and as the most fully understood, it serves as a model for other drugs. Penicillin reactions include anaphylaxis, urticaria, vasculitis, dermatomyositis, maculopapular rashes, hemolytic anemia, drug fever, interstitial nephritis, pneumonitis, and contact dermatitis. Airborne penicillin can cause asthma in workers who produce or use it. The nature of the reaction is determined not only by the specific metabolite that becomes the hapten but also by the carrier molecule. For example, the penicilloyl determinant commonly evokes IgE antibody in cases of urticaria, but it also evokes IgG, and if it is combined with red cell membrane protein, it may be responsible for hemolytic anemia during the course of intravenous penicillin treatment. Many patients who claim to be allergic to penicillin tolerate it without adverse effect. In such patients, treatment with more expensive or toxic antibiotics would be unnecessary. Reliable tests are available for predicting which patients with a history of penicillin reactions will have a reaction. Cautious skin testing with dilute solutions of the antibiotic itself and with commercially available benzylpenicilloyl-polylysine (Pre-Pen) will provide guidance. If skin test reactions are negative to these reagents and to the "minor" determinants (the plain drug, penicilloate and penilloate), the probability of an allergic reaction is very low, no higher than in subjects receiving penicillin for the first time. The minor determinants are as yet available only in research settings, but only about 10 to 15 per cent of patients react to this reagent alone. Therefore, tests with the available reagents interpreted in the light of the history will usually allow appropriate treatment to proceed. The skin test with penicilloyl-polylysine begins with a prick of the 6.0×10^{-5} M solution, and if negative in 20 minutes, one proceeds to intradermal testing. Skin testing with the penicillin solution starts with a prick test with a solution containing 6000 units per milliliter of penicillin G or 4 mg per milliliter of other penicillins.

TABLE 437–2. ORAL DESENSITIZATION PROTOCOL FOR PENICILLIN

Dose*	Units	Route†
1	100	P.O.
2	200	P.O.
3	400	P.O.
4	800	P.O.
5	1,600	P.O.
6	3,200	P.O.
7	6,400	P.O.
8	12,800	P.O.
9	25,000	P.O.
10	50,000	P.O.
11	100,000	P.O.
12	200,000	P.O.
13	400,000	P.O.
14	200,000	S.C.
15	400,000	S.C.
16	800,000	S.C.
17	1,000,000	I.M.

*Interval between doses, 15 min.
†P.O. = oral; S.C. = subcutaneous; I.M. = intramuscular.
From Sullivan TJ, Yecies LD, Shaty GS, et al.: Desensitization of patients allergic to penicillin using orally administered β lactam antibiotics. J Allergy Clin Immunol 69:276, 1982.

Desensitization can be undertaken when skin test reactions are positive or when there are other reasons for suspecting an appreciable risk of anaphylaxis, but the patient has life-threatening infection with an organism for which no alternative antibiotics are available. Oral desensitization is preferred (Table 437–2).

Radiographic Contrast Agents. Iodinated contrast agents injected for radiographic examinations are now the most common cause of anaphylactic drug reactions. These reactions are not truly anaphylactic, for these materials do not combine with proteins to act as haptens but rather appear to act pharmacologically. As yet these reactions are not fully understood, but it is known that these drugs activate complement and release anaphylotoxin. Skin tests or small test doses do not predict reactivity. Persons who have had a previous reaction are at increased risk of a similar reaction from a subsequent injection. When a second examination is necessary, the patient should be given prednisone 50 mg every six hours for three doses, ending one hour before the procedure, and also an antihistamine shortly before.

Local Anesthetics. Most adverse reactions to local anesthetics are either toxic or psychophysiologic, but allergic reactions can occur. The most frequent is contact dermatitis; anaphylaxis is more serious though not as common. It has not yet been determined that skin testing with local anesthetics is useful in predicting anaphylaxis in patients with a history of reactions to local anesthetic. When local anesthesia is needed, an anesthetic as unrelated as possible to the one suspected of causing the reaction should be chosen, and a small test dose should be given first. Lidocaine seems to carry a low risk of allergy.

Aspirin and Other Nonsteroidal Anti-inflammatory Drugs. Shortly after its introduction in the late nineteenth century, aspirin was observed to provoke severe reactions in some patients with asthma. Such patients react in the same way to other nonsteroidal anti-inflammatory agents that inhibit cyclooxygenase, the key enzyme in the generating of prostaglandins from arachidonic acid. The typical reaction consists of acute bronchospasm, rhinorrhea, and occasionally urticaria. Most of the asthmatic patients who react to these agents also have nasal polyps and lack IgE-mediated allergy to common airborne allergens. In some patients with chronic urticaria but no respiratory disease, urticaria is the only manifestation of the reaction. The mechanism of this adverse response to aspirin is not allergic; extensive search for IgE antibodies has been unrewarding. Rather, it is presumably due to the inhibition of cyclooxygenase, but the precise mechanism is still undefined. Patients who have reacted to aspirin need not avoid other salicylates (except methylsalicylate), and salicylate-free diets are unnecessary. Five to ten per cent of aspirin-reactive subjects react similarly to tartrazine (FD&C yellow no. 5) added to foods or drugs. Skin tests to aspirin and similar agents are not useful and may be dangerous. No biochemical tests are available for diagnosis.

Sulfite. Sulfites, metabisulfites, and sulfur dioxide are added to foods to prevent discoloration and spoilage. Some asthmatic subjects develop acute severe reactions a few minutes after ingesting 10 to 100 mg. Though these reactions resemble those provoked by aspirin, they occur in different persons, and the biochemical pathway involved is presumably different. Lettuce and other salad ingredients prepared in restaurants in advance are often sprayed with sulfites to preserve freshness. This is perhaps the most common exposure. Other food sources include dried fruits, wine, some beers, and some soft drinks. Sulfites added as antioxidants to some medications for parenteral injection or aerosol administration can provoke similar reactions. No tests are available.

Parker CW: Drug allergy. N Engl J Med 292:511, 732, 957, 1975. *A masterful discussion of the principles of drug allergy that stresses immunologic mechanisms.*

Van Arsdel PW: Adverse drug reactions. *In* Middleton EJ, Ellis FF, Reed CE (eds.): Allergy Principles and Practice. 2nd ed. St. Louis, C. V. Mosby Company, 1983. *A detailed review and extensive listing of agents and reactions.*

438. MASTOCYTOSIS

Robert A. Lewis

DEFINITION. Mastocytosis is a rare disease of mast cell proliferation, which occurs in both cutaneous and systemic forms. The mast cell is a connective tissue cell normally found in most organs. It is not surprising, therefore, that systemic mastocytosis has been reported to involve virtually all tissues except the central nervous system, most commonly the skin, bones, gastrointestinal tract, liver, spleen, and lymph nodes. Mast cell leukemia and malignant transformation of solid tumors have been described in a few cases.

Mast cells are generally identifiable by their metachromatic granules (Fig. 438–1), which contain histamine, heparin, a tryptic protease, and a number of acid hydrolases, the last of which defines the granules as modified lysosomes. Mast cells, activated by either immunologic or nonimmunologic stimuli, secrete their lysosomal contents into the microenvironment and additionally liberate arachidonic acid from their membrane phospholipid stores, metabolizing it selectively to prostaglandin D_2 (PGD_2), and the sulfidopeptide leukotriene, LTC_4. LTC_4 is then further metabolized to its peptide cleavage products, LTD_4 and LTE_4, extracellularly. (A discussion of arachidonic acid metabolism is presented in Ch. 233.) Several of the clinical manifestations of mastocytosis as well as the choice of some therapeutic agents are based on the pathophysiologic actions of these substances, termed "mediators of immediate hypersensitivity," owing to their suspected roles in allergic disease (Table 438–1).

INCIDENCE AND PREVALENCE. Fewer than 1000 cases of mastocytosis have been reported, with equal occurrence in men and women. As the hallmark of this disease is based on cutaneous manifestations, mastocytosis is said to involve the skin in over 95 per cent of patients. The actual frequency with

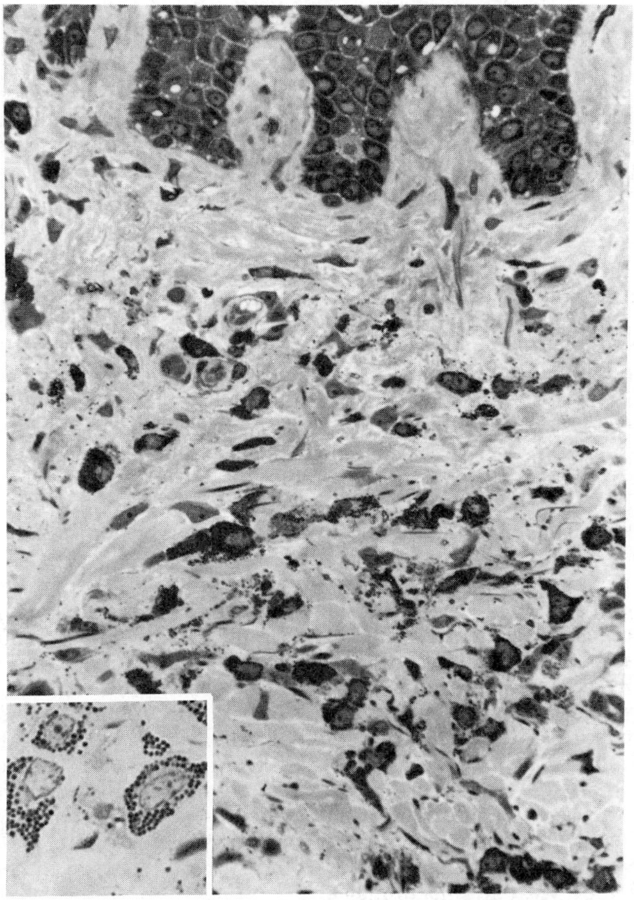

Figure 438–1. Mast cell proliferation in the dermis (Giemsa-stained lesional skin biopsy; × 520). Inset of dermal mast cells (× 1310). (Courtesy of J. Caulfield and A. Hein.)

TABLE 438–1. HUMAN MAST CELL–DERIVED PRODUCTS

Mediator	Function
Histamine	Increased vasopermeability; nonvascular smooth muscle contraction
Heparin	Anticoagulation; inhibition of complement activation
Prostaglandin D_2	Vasodilation; nonvascular smooth muscle contraction
Eosinophil and neutrophil chemotactic factors*	Eosinophil and neutrophil chemotaxis
Tryptase, arylsulfatase, N-acetyl-β-D-glucosaminidase, β-glucuronidase	Enzymatic degradation of proteoglycans and glycoproteins
Sulfidopeptide leukotrienes	Vasoconstriction; increased vasopermeability; nonvascular smooth muscle contraction (LTC_4)
	Vasodilation; increased vasopermeability; nonvascular smooth muscle contraction (LTD_4 and LTE_4)

*Evidence for association with human mast cell granule is indirect.

which mastocytosis involves other organs with sparing of the skin may thus be underestimated because of the bias of ascertainment. Cutaneous lesions begin more frequently in early childhood than after maturity. Visceral disease is not commonly associated with single isolated skin lesions, especially those arising in infancy or early childhood. However, approximately one quarter of adults with cutaneous lesions have visceral involvement.

CLINICAL MANIFESTATIONS. Involvement of the skin in mastocytosis is termed *urticaria pigmentosa.* The lesions may be isolated mastocytomas or generalized and multiple (Fig. 438–2); they are usually reddish-brown and plaque-like or nodular. More rarely, telangiectatic or doughy-feeling erythrodermic forms of the skin lesions occur. When a cutaneous lesion is stroked firmly, it becomes pruritic and raised with surrounding erythema (Darier's sign). In many patients, stroking of seemingly uninvolved skin produces a wheal of dermographism, owing to microscopic dermal mastocytosis. Generalized pruritus and flushing may occur with or without cutaneous lesions.

Acute symptomatic episodes may occur, marked by systemic vasodilation with headache, dizziness, tachycardia, hypotension, syncope, and even frank shock. Rarely, such attacks may be fatal. These acute symptoms do not necessarily indicate systemic mastocytosis, since extensive cutaneous lesions are capable of releasing large amounts of the potent mediators

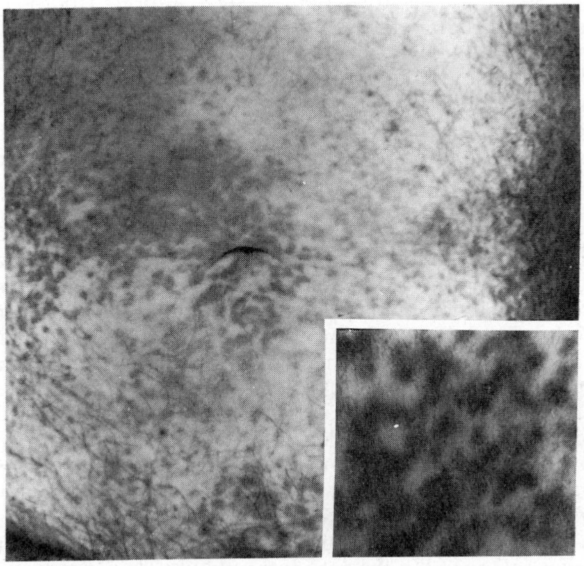

Figure 438–2. Skin lesions of mastocytosis (urticaria pigmentosa). Inset showing close-up view. (Courtesy of N. Soter.)

summarized in the table. Even the diagnostic test of stroking a cutaneous lesion to whealing may provoke systemic symptoms, especially those of flushing and colic in affected infants. Ingestion of alcohol may degranulate mast cells and set off acute symptoms.

Gastrointestinal symptoms may dominate the clinical picture. Anorexia, nausea, vomiting, diarrhea, and a possible predilection for peptic ulceration with or without hyperchlorhydria may complicate mastocytosis whether or not mast cells have proliferated in the gastrointestinal tract. Some patients have developed the malabsorption syndrome (see Ch. 103), which may be due to the release of mediators from mast cells infiltrating the small bowel mucosa and lamina propria. Hepatomegaly or hepatosplenomegaly may result from mast cell infiltration. The liver in mastocytosis may also be fibrotic and sometimes exhibits piecemeal inflammation. Rarely there is associated portal hypertension and gastroesophageal varices.

Osseous lesions occur in approximately 10 per cent of all patients with mastocytosis, or two thirds of those with systemic disease. These lesions, most commonly found in the pelvis, ribs, vertebrae, skull, and proximal long bones, may occasionally resemble Paget's disease radiologically. Bone pain may occur with or without pathologic fractures.

Occasionally rhinorrhea and rarely audible wheezing occur, reminiscent of the signs of allergic rhinitis and asthma, respectively. Ill-defined neuropsychiatric symptoms, ranging from malaise to decreased attention span and irritability, have been described. Anemia, leukopenia, thrombocytopenia, and even mast cell leukemia have been rarely reported in association with severe bone marrow infiltration by mast cells. Modest blood eosinophilia occurs occasionally, and the coagulation abnormalities of prolonged prothrombin and bleeding times related to heparin release, although uncommon, have also been reported.

DIAGNOSIS. The cutaneous lesions of urticaria pigmentosa in conjunction with Darier's sign are pathognomonic for mastocytosis. In their absence, additional criteria are necessary for the diagnosis. Osseous infiltration by mast cells may be suspected from radiologic lesions with adjacent areas of osteoporosis and mottled osteosclerosis. Bone marrow biopsy of involved areas demonstrates abnormally high numbers of mast cells and rarefaction of the spongiosa or, alternatively, myelofibrosis and sclerosis. In the absence of radiologic abnormalities, ^{99}Tc bone scans may define areas of increased radionuclide uptake to guide the site of the biopsy. Histaminuria two to three times greater than normal 24-hour levels (36 ± 14 μg) is common among patients with extensive cutaneous and/or visceral disease and useful when present, although both normal values and striking elevations up to 1300 μg per 24 hours have been reported. Two unique PGD_2 metabolites, which are, respectively, minimally present and undetectable in normal urine, have recently been described in urine specimens from patients with systemic mastocytosis. This observation, if confirmed and extended, may provide another sensitive diagnostic test.

For the patient with flushing, intermittent hypotension, diarrhea, tachycardia, and possibly hepatomegaly and peptic ulceration, the main differential diagnosis is with the carcinoid syndrome. The most direct criterion is a biopsy demonstrating mast cell proliferation as opposed to argentaffin cell infiltration in an involved organ. Failing this, the measurement of grossly elevated levels of histamine and its metabolites in the urine favors mastocytosis, whereas elevated urinary levels of 5-hydroxyindoleacetic acid (5-HIAA) are noted in the carcinoid syndrome. It must be recalled, however, that marked increases of urinary histamine may occur in gastric carcinoid (see Ch. 242), and elevated urinary excretion of serotonin metabolites may rarely occur in mastocytosis.

In addition to other clinical and laboratory manifestations, histopathology will differentiate the skin lesions of mastocytosis from those of histiocytosis X, myelomonocytic leukemia, cutaneous myelosarcoma, granular cell tumor, and dermatofibroma.

PATHOPHYSIOLOGY AND TREATMENT. When mast cells degranulate, they release their preformed granule-associated mediators and also generate newly formed PGD_2 and LTC_4. The mast cell in mastocytosis releases normal mediators in approximately normal amounts per cell. The most striking abnormalities seem to lie in the sensitivity of the degranulation response of the neoplastic cell to numerous physical stimuli, including not only gentle stroking (Darier's sign) but usually also moderate heat or cold. Once a skin lesion urticates, it requires up to three days to regenerate adequate granule histamine to form a second wheal.

In the past, the majority of the symptoms and signs of mastocytosis were ascribed to the effects of released histamine. Histamine is probably the major cause of local cutaneous whealing and pruritus as well as rhinitis. Vasodilation and gastrointestinal symptoms in this disease probably have a more complex pathogenesis. The combined use of antihistamines of both the H_1 antagonist group, such as chlorpheniramine maleate, and the H_2 antagonists, exemplified by cimetidine, has failed to control either the gastrointestinal symptoms or the hypotension in some patients with mastocytosis.

The identification of a vasodilating prostaglandin (PGD_2) formed by mast cells may therefore be relevant both to the pathophysiology of mastocytosis and to the development of effective therapy. Aspirin and other nonsteroidal anti-inflammatory compounds inhibit prostaglandin synthesis. It is therefore reasonable to try the use of such agents in mastocytosis. Aspirin therapy should be started in very small initial doses of 16 mg four times daily, with the dose doubled on each subsequent day for one week until either symptomatic relief is achieved or the side effects of salicylism supervene. The minimal therapeutic aspirin dose should then be maintained indefinitely. Aspirin should be given only after first initiating treatment with oral therapeutic doses of H_1 and H_2 antihistamines, such as 8 mg of chlorpheniramine maleate and 300 mg of cimetidine four times daily for an adult patient. The caution employed in initiating aspirin therapy follows from reports of a few patients with mastocytosis who have sustained precipitous hypotension after aspirin ingestion, suggesting the possibility that massive release of mediators may occur, including enhanced LTC_4 synthesis when nonsteroidal anti-inflammatory agents inhibit the cyclooxygenase pathway of arachidonate metabolism to prostaglandins.

The heparin released from islands of mast cells has been implicated in the prolonged local bleeding time at the sites of excised lesions, the occasionally reported purpura underlying cutaneous mastocytomas, and the rare incidence of significant gastrointestinal bleeding related to local mast cell infiltration. The development of osseous lesions that are both porotic and sclerotic may relate to the combined capacities of mast cell acid hydrolases and tryptase(s) for proteoglycan degradation which precedes collagenolysis, followed by tissue repair. Heparin has also been reported to cause osteopenia. Hepatic fibrosis when documented may also be a product of altered tissue repair in the presence of these enzymes. Therefore, drugs known to cause mast cell degranulation, such as alcohol, morphine, and codeine, are to be prohibited.

Disodium cromoglycate (cromolyn),* given as 100 mg orally four times daily, has been used successfully, particularly for the gastrointestinal symptoms. Cromolyn is thought to reduce mast cell degranulation by interfering with cellular calcium uptake. As little or none of the drug is absorbed, its local action on the gastrointestinal mast cells probably occurs without preventing histamine release from other mast cell infiltrated organs. Histaminuria is not modified by successful therapy with cromolyn. Less easily explained are the therapeutic effects of this agent in decreasing cutaneous symptoms of pruritus, whealing and flushing, as well as in relieving some of the neuropsychiatric complaints. Cromolyn may be given in combination with antihistamines and aspirin.

PROGNOSIS. Isolated cutaneous mastocytomas of infancy

*Approved for investigational use only.

commonly involute spontaneously. If this does not occur, the single lesions may be excised surgically. None of the suggested medical therapies reduce the number of mast cells in either cutaneous or visceral lesions.

Malignant mastocytosis is a very rare disorder with high mortality within two years of diagnosis. It may occur as either a cutaneous or a systemic disease and reportedly may appear by malignant transformation of a small minority of the clinically benign mastocytomas, especially of the systemic variety. Special histopathologic techniques may be necessary to detect the immature granules of malignant cells. Leukemia is associated with mastocytosis in fewer than 5 per cent of cases and may be monocytic, mastocytic, or myeloid, in approximately equal frequencies.

Lewis RA, Austen KF: Mediation of local homeostasis and inflammation by leukotrienes and other mast cell-dependent compounds. Nature 293:103, 1981. *A review of the biology of mast cell-derived mediators, including the leukotrienes.*

Parker CW, Cryer PE, Kissane JM: Clinicopathologic conference: Systemic mastocytosis. Am J Med 61:671, 1976. *An excellent review of the signs and symptoms of mastocytosis.*

Roberts LJ II, Sweetman BJ, Lewis RA, Folarin VF, Austen KF, Oates JA: Increased production of prostaglandin D_2 in patients with systemic mastocytosis. N Engl J Med 303:1400, 1980. *Important for future diagnostic and therapeutic considerations.*

Soter NA, Austen KF, Wasserman SI: Oral disodium cromoglycate in the treatment of systemic mastocytosis. N Engl J Med 301:465, 1979. *A prospective evaluation of cromolyn therapy for mastocytosis.*

439. DISEASES OF THE THYMUS

Daniel P. Stites

DEVELOPMENT, STRUCTURE, AND FUNCTION. The thymus is a central lymphoid organ which functions in the development and maintenance of immunologic competence. It arises embryologically from the third and fourth branchial clefts and then migrates caudad, as a bilobed organ, to the anterior mediastinum. Ectopic thoracic and cervical thymic rests are present in 30 per cent of normal individuals. The thymus enlarges until late puberty and then involutes, the lymphocytes and epithelial cells being nearly completely replaced with fat by the fifth or sixth decade. The normal thymus varies greatly in size. It is uniquely susceptible to marked involution within hours owing to the stress of serious illness or to treatment with glucocorticoids. The thymus is composed primarily of lymphocytes encased in a lattice of epithelial cells. It also contains a few myoid cells, macrophages, and plasma cells. The thymus is arranged into discrete lobules containing a cortex and medulla. Hassall's corpuscles are specialized aggregates of epithelial cells whose function is unknown.

The thymus begins to function by about ten to twelve weeks of gestation when immunocompetent T cells can first be detected. Undifferentiated stem cells migrate to the thymus from fetal liver and bone marrow prenatally and from the bone marrow postnatally. Local influences, probably from epithelial cells, induce maturation of thymic lymphocytes, which then divide in the cortex, migrate to the medulla, and emigrate to the peripheral lymphoid tissue as mature T cells. The cortex is also the site of intense lymphopoiesis. The thymus secretes a variety of incompletely defined hormones which maintain T cell competence in peripheral lymphoid organs. These substances are variously known as thymopoietin, thymin, and thymosin. The immunosuppressive effects of thymectomy vary with age, being most pronounced at younger ages (see below). The thymus also appears to play an important role in maintenance of tolerance to various antigens, in immune surveillance, and possibly in leukemogenesis (as judged by animal experiments).

THYMIC HYPOPLASIA. Hypoplastic thymus may be either congenital or acquired. In neonates and infants, *congenital thymic hypoplasia* is expressed as marked T cell and variable B cell immunodeficiency. Resulting diseases include reticular dysgenesis, severe combined immunodeficiency disease, DiGeorge's and Nezelof's syndromes, and ataxia-telangiectasia (see Ch. 429). Essentially all of these patients are diagnosed in childhood; the severity of the thymic lesion, if untreated, rarely allows survival beyond age ten to twelve years. Congenital thymic hypoplasia has been treated by thymic or bone marrow transplantation and by thymic hormone injections with variable success. *Acquired hypoplasia* or thymic involution occurs normally with age or results from stress (within hours or days), malnutrition, pregnancy, x-rays, glucocorticoids, or cytotoxic drugs. Acquired involution may be reversible after withdrawal of the offending cause.

THYMIC HYPERPLASIA. An enlarged thymus is very difficult to evaluate accurately because of its large normal variability in size. In the past, so-called status thymolymphaticus, a condition diagnosed with respiratory distress, and large thymic shadow on chest roentgenogram frequently led to unnecessary removal or radiation of normal thymuses. The concept of status thymolymphaticus has been abandoned. The thymus may rarely enlarge in thyrotoxicosis, Addison's disease, anencephaly, acromegaly, castration, cysts, or tumors (see below).

THYMUS AND MYASTHENIA GRAVIS. Myasthenia gravis is an autoimmune disease caused by the presence of antiacetylcholine receptor (AchR) antibodies (see Ch. 539). In myasthenia gravis there is a 10 per cent incidence of thymoma. In fact detectable enlargement of the thymus in myasthenia gravis usually heralds the presence of a thymoma. In 65 per cent of cases, the thymus is hyperplastic with increased numbers of germinal centers but not clinically enlarged. In the remaining 25 per cent of patients the thymus is normal. In large series of thymomas, 30 to 60 per cent of patients have myasthenia gravis. Rarely myasthenia gravis develops years after total thymectomy for thymoma, which militates against an absolute requirement for thymoma in the pathogenesis of this disorder. Neonatal myasthenia gravis occurs without any thymic abnormality, presumably owing to transplacental transfer of maternal antibody. There is little correlation with serum levels of anti-AchR antibody and clinical improvement in myasthenia following thymectomy. Damage to AchR antigen shared between muscles and thymic epithelial or myoid cells may explain the rather obscure relationship of the thymus to this autoantibody disorder.

EFFECTS OF THYMECTOMY. Total removal of the thymus during the neonatal period in rodents results in severe immunodeficiency, loss of T cells, and a wasting disease, a result of chronic unopposed infection. Thymectomy in adult animals, however, is associated with much subtler changes in T cell function. What is the effect of thymectomy in man? Because of the high incidence of extramediastinal thymic rests (30 per cent), thymectomy can rarely be considered total. Total thymectomy intentionally done during cardiothoracic surgery in children does not appear to result in compromised transplantation immunity. In patients with thymoma, a transient decrease in circulating lymphocytes and T cell functions is noted. Following thymectomy for myasthenia gravis, functional loss in some T cell populations occurs. However, the long-term effects of thymectomy either in immunologically normal patients during cardiac surgery or in cancer patients with thymomas is not known. These individuals should be carefully observed for development of autoimmune disease, infection, certain malignancies, or other signs of T cell deficiency.

THYMOMA. ***Definition.*** A thymoma is a neoplasm of thymic epithelial cells. This definition excludes other tumors that may affect the thymus such as lymphoma, germ cell tumors, and carcinoid. Thymomas are rare; fewer than 1000 cases have been reported. Nevertheless, it is the most common tumor of the anterior superior mediastinum (see Ch. 69).

Pathology. Thymomas contain various proportions of epithelial cells and lymphocytes. The latter are T cells and may constitute a large proportion of cellular content of the tumor; hence the term *lymphoepithelioma.* Although their significance is

TABLE 439–1. DISEASES ASSOCIATED WITH THYMIC TUMOR

Thymoma
Myasthenia gravis
Red cell aplasia
Hemolytic anemia
Neutrophil agranulocytosis
Hypogammaglobulinemia (Good's syndrome)
Systemic lupus erythematosus
Polymyositis
Pemphigus vulgaris
Chronic mucocutaneous candidiasis
Carcinoid
Cushing's syndrome
Multiple endocrine neoplasia syndromes (see Ch. 240)

unknown, the activated appearance of these lymphocytes suggests a host reaction to neoplastic epithelial cells. These T cells all have the surface characteristics of thymocytes rather than peripheral blood T cells. Various histologic degrees of malignancy from minimal cytologic atypia to undifferentiated carcinoma exist. However, correlation of microscopic appearance with clinical malignancy is notoriously poor. In fact, local invasion of pleura, pericardium, vessels, and nerves is the major criterion for determining clinical malignancy of the tumor.

Clinical Manifestations. Median age of patients with thymoma is about 50 years, and no sex predominance is noted. About 30 per cent of patients present with myasthenia gravis; another 30 per cent are asymptomatic, and the diagnosis is suggested by an anterior mediastinal mass on chest roentgenogram. The remaining 30 to 40 per cent of patients have a variety of symptoms and medical syndromes associated with the tumor (Table 439–1). Symptoms and signs include cough, chest pain, dysphagia, dyspnea, hoarseness, neck mass, and superior vena cava syndrome.

A few patients with spindle cell thymomas have marked *hypogammaglobulinemia.* Whether the relationship is causal is not established. The rare occurrence of red cell aplasia with or without immunodeficiency and thymoma raises the possibility of T cell-mediated suppression of erythropoiesis or immunoglobulin synthesis. Direct evidence to support these notions is only fragmentary.

Diagnosis. The presence of a round or oval anterior mediastinal mass visualized in posteroanterior and lateral chest roentgenograms in the presence of myasthenia gravis or of some other known systemic manifestations is suggestive of thymoma. Computed tomographic (CT) imaging is useful in defining the size and location of thymomas and is occasionally useful in differentiating various thymic lesions. Thymic biopsy has no place in evaluation of anterior mediastinal masses, and mediastinoscopy is of little or no value. Some centers claim success with fine needle aspiration and cytology. Thoracotomy with adequate exposure to determine whether capsular invasion has occurred is needed for diagnosis of any thymic tumor. Differential diagnosis includes other primary or secondary thymic tumors (see below), cysts, post-traumatic hemorrhage, aneurysm or other abnormalities of the anterior mediastinal contents including metastatic tumors, giant lymph node hyperplasia, mesothelioma, thyroid and parathyroid tumors, and paragangliomas (see Ch. 69).

Treatment. Surgical removal of tumor followed by local irradiation if extracapsular extension has occurred is the treatment of choice. Distant metastases are rare; the tumor spreads mainly by local invasion of adjacent structures.

Prognosis. The prognosis is nearly entirely dependent on presence of local invasion and cannot be predicted by histologic appearance of the tumor. Noninvasive thymomas are usually cured by excision. Patients with invasive thymoma have about 50 per cent five-year survival.

OTHER TUMORS OF THE THYMUS. *Thymolipoma* probably represents a lipoma arising within normal thymus. This tumor is usually radiolucent and asymptomatic and has not been associated with myasthenia gravis. *Carcinoid tumor* of the thymus arises from neuroendocrine cells within the thymus (see Ch. 242). Fifty per cent produce ACTH-like molecules and cause Cushing's syndrome or hyperparathyroidism, or are associated with multiple endocrine adenomatosis; 30 per cent are malignant and metastasize. Surgery and radiotherapy are indicated. *Carcinomas,* particularly squamous cell types, may rarely occur. *Germ cell tumors* rarely occur: seminoma, teratoma, teratocarcinoma, choriocarcinoma, embryonal cell carcinoma, and yolk sac tumors. The thymus may be involved by *malignant lymphomas.* T cell lymphomas with acute lymphoblastic leukemia occur in the second decade. Cells from these tumors may have C receptors and are positive for terminal deoxynucleotidyl transferase. Hodgkin's disease usually is of nodular sclerosing type (see Ch. 158 and 160).

Baron RL, Lee JKT, Sagel SS, Levitt RG: Computed tomography of the abnormal thymus. Radiology 142:127, 1982. *This article delineates indications for CT scans in patients with clinical, surgical, and pathologic evidence of thymic diseases. It indicates that, on occasion, CT may suggest the specific nature of a thymic lesion.*

Namba T, Brunner NG, Grob D: Myasthenia gravis in patients with thymoma with particular reference to onset after thymectomy. Medicine 57:411, 1978. *Excellent review of literature on relationship of thymoma to myasthenia gravis with 72 locally studied cases.*

Pahwa R, Ikehara S, Pahwa SG, Good RA: Thymic function in man. Thymus 1:27, 1979. *Careful description of thymic physiology, with emphasis on role of thymic hormones.*

Salyer W, Eggleston JC: Thymoma. A clinical and pathological study of 65 cases. Cancer 37:229, 1976. *Clinicopathologic description of a large series of thymoma patients, annotating association with other medical syndromes.*

Part XXII
MUSCULOSKELETAL AND CONNECTIVE TISSUE DISEASES

440. APPROACH TO THE PATIENT WITH MUSCULOSKELETAL DISEASE*

James F. Fries

The rheumatic diseases present a major challenge to clinical judgment. The chronicity, variability, tendency to exacerbate and remit, biochemical and immunologic complexity, unknown pathogenesis, variable response to specific treatment, and myriad ways in which these diseases affect the patient's lifestyle, family relationships, self-image, and employability all combine to complicate the therapeutic equation. Difficult therapeutic decisions must be made for the most part without adequate experimental justification and evaluated against a poorly understood natural history.

Balanced against these tremendous uncertainties, contemporary management is relatively straightforward but has changed substantially. Present therapeutic strategy has shifted from dogma to flexibility. Good management now requires that therapeutic decisions be based upon individual circumstances rather than upon diagnosis per se. Further, treatment decisions are never final but are modified in a continuing feedback between application of treatment and observation of response. Decisions evolve and change over time as appropriate to the trends, tempo, and previous response of the particular patient. Clinical judgment is essential to good outcome. It is more than a truism to note that the art of medicine is reborn in the approach to a patient with a chronic disease. The broad principles underlying contemporary management strategy are set forth in this chapter and are divided into six major facets. The medical history, the physical examination, and the laboratory data, which are discussed in following chapters, are integrated into decisions regarding these six areas.

DETERMINING THE PATHOPHYSIOLOGY

Modern management individualizes therapy within diagnostic categories, based upon subgroups of patients with differing prognoses and different therapeutic requirements. Patients with the same diagnosis often should be managed very differently. Rheumatic disease patients frequently have features of several diagnostic entities at the same time.

Diagnosis is *not* the most important factor in selecting management in rheumatic disease. Management in musculoskeletal disease is more closely linked to the underlying pathophysiologic process than to the disease entity. Reversal of the pathophysiologic process (or negation of its impact) requires a clear visualization of that process. Even such a basic pathophysiologic concept as "inflammation" has different therapeutic implications. The inflamed synovial membrane (synovitis) typical of rheumatoid arthritis responds to a different spectrum of anti-inflammatory agents than does the inflammation of ligamentous insertions (enthesitis) typical of ankylosing spondylitis or the inflammation within the joint space induced by microscopic crystals.

Eight specific types of musculoskeletal pathology are readily distinguished by history and physical examination in most patients and provide a framework for pathophysiologic categorization. These categories are not mutually exclusive, but categorization of the predominant pathophysiology in a given patient is usually straightforward. The eight categories are discussed in the following paragraphs and are listed in Table 440–1 together with the prototype disease of the category, examples of the most useful laboratory tests for that category, and the typical treatments required. Management implications for each category are surprisingly distinct and provide guidelines for the ordering of laboratory investigations and the selection of initial treatment.

SYNOVITIS. Inflammation of the synovial membrane, with eventual damage to surrounding joint structures, is most strikingly manifested in the disease "rheumatoid arthritis." The synovium is tender, thickened, and palpable and may demonstrate warmth and, less often, redness. Joint destruction is caused by the enzymatic products of inflammation and develops slowly over many years. Management is based upon reducing the *rate* of damage to joint structures. The sedimentation rate is consistently elevated with significant synovitis, and the latex fixation or other tests for rheumatoid arthritis are often useful for further categorization. A wide range of pharmacologic and other treatments may be required, and many patients require sequential trials with a variety of agents. Some useful drugs, such as gold, penicillamine, and hydroxychloroquine, are not proven therapeutically effective in any other category, and others, such as aspirin, find their greatest use here.

ENTHESOPATHY. Inflammation in certain diseases is most marked at the enthesis, that transition region where ligament attaches to bone. Such inflammation is the hallmark of a family of rheumatic diseases of which the most common is ankylosing spondylitis. The distribution of musculoskeletal involvement in these diseases thus follows the location of regions of enthesis throughout the body. The marked predilection for the sacroiliac joints, heels, and spine identifies a process affecting areas characterized by ligament and tendon attachment. This specific pathophysiology has been recognized only in the last several years and provides a unifying basis for the observed clinical features of the diseases and their typical response to specific therapy. The HLA-B27 gene is usually present, and rheumatoid factor is predictably absent from the serum. Nonsteroidal anti-inflammatory agents, in particular indomethacin, phenylbutazone, and naproxen, are therapeutically effective and usually

*Adapted with permission from Kelley WN, Harris ED Jr, Ruddy S, Sledge CB: Textbook of Rheumatology. Philadelphia, W. B. Saunders Company, 1981, pp 353–358.

TABLE 440–1. CATEGORIES OF RHEUMATIC DISEASE

Pathology	Prototype	Most Useful Tests	Typical Treatment
Synovitis	Rheumatoid arthritis	Latex, erythrocyte sedimentation rate	Acetylsalicylic acid, gold
Enthesopathy	Ankylosing spondylitis	Sacroiliac radiographs, HLA-B27	Indomethacin
Cartilage degeneration	Osteoarthritis	Radiographs of affected area	Analgesic
Crystal-induced synovitis	Gout	Joint fluid crystal examination	Colchicine
Joint infection	Staphylococcal	Joint fluid culture	Antibiotics
Myositis	Dermatomyositis	Muscle enzymes, muscle biopsy	Corticosteroids
Focal conditions	Tennis elbow	None, radiographs of affected area	Localized
Generalized conditions	Fibrositis	Erythrocyte sedimentation rate	Conservative

are well tolerated over the long term. The spectrum of effective anti-inflammatory drugs used for enthesopathy is different from the spectrum effective in synovitis. Prednisone, for example, is neither indicated nor effective in most patients.

CARTILAGE DEGENERATION. Degenerative and other processes can cause fraying and destruction of the articular cartilage, with subsequent injury to the underlying subchondral bone. This occurrence is usually termed osteoarthritis (or osteoarthrosis), and a group of specific syndromes is recognized within this category. Narrowing of the apparent joint space and development of bony spurs make radiography the most useful investigative procedure; other ancillary tests are usually negative. Few patients have significant inflammation, and it is not surprising that anti-inflammatory treatment is not frequently useful. The analgesic effects of aspirin or nonsteroidal anti-inflammatory agents may be helpful; doses required for optimal effect are often considerably less than doses required for anti-inflammatory effects with the same compound. Treatment is symptomatic and is seldom dramatically effective.

CRYSTAL-INDUCED SYNOVITIS. Microcrystalline arthritis occurs when crystals forming in the synovial fluid (or injected therein) induce an acute inflammatory reaction in the joint fluid and the surrounding synovium. Gout is the prototype disease, with the inflammation in gout induced by crystals of monosodium urate. Similar syndromes may occur with crystals of several other types. The inflammatory response develops with a rather sudden clinical onset, increases to very intense inflammation within a period of hours, and spontaneously resolves without treatment over a period of a few days to a few weeks; this resolution is markedly accelerated with treatment. The physical factors underlying crystal formation determine that only one or, at most, a few joints are involved at a time. The crucial laboratory observation is inspection of the aspirated joint fluid for crystals under polarized light microscopy. Drugs inhibiting polymorphonuclear leukocytes are particularly effective, as exemplified by colchicine, a drug with little effect in any other rheumatic disease category.

JOINT INFECTION. The synovium encloses a body space that can be the site of direct infection by microorganisms. Critical to investigation of the patient with suspected joint infection is aspiration and culture of the joint fluid and, in many instances, culture of other body fluids as well. Treatment consists principally of prescribing an antibiotic specific for the microorganism involved. Drainage may be required.

MYOSITIS. Inflammation of muscle occurs in two closely related diseases, dermatomyositis and polymyositis, and in a distant relative, polymyalgia rheumatica. Determination of muscle enzyme levels and histologic examination of involved muscle may be the critical laboratory observations. In polymyalgia, the sedimentation rate is greatly elevated and is often the sole objective finding. Temporal artery biopsy may be useful when giant cell arteritis is demonstrated. Corticosteroids are almost always required in inflammatory muscle disease and, in contrast to every other rheumatic disease category, are usually required from the outset.

FOCAL CONDITIONS. A wide variety of conditions affecting the musculoskeletal system do not truly warrant the term "disease." Tendinitis, bursitis, low back strain, calcific tendinitis, and a variety of other entities can affect almost any area of the body and are among the most common of all medical problems. Laboratory aids are few, although radiography occasionally may be useful in locating calcium deposits or spurs or in ruling out fracture. The therapeutic imperative in localized problems (unfortunately often neglected) is to emphasize localized rather than general treatment measures. Treatment of the entire organism for a problem in one local area is seldom rewarding. Splints, slings, heat, and local injection are usually the most reasonable initial approach.

GENERALIZED CONDITIONS. A variety of ambiguous entities fall into this poorly defined category. Terms such as "fibrositis" or the "chronic muscle contraction syndrome" are sometimes used to indicate the likelihood of organic disease. The terms "psychogenic rheumatism," "nonarticular rheumatism," or "depressive equivalent" are frequently used to suggest an emotional component to such complaints. These patients are rich in symptoms but poor in objective evidence of pathology. The conditions may be extremely troublesome for the individual but are not progressive and do not result in physical crippling. Laboratory test results, such as the sedimentation rate, are normal and are employed only to rule out other categories of illness. Treatment is best termed "conservative." The therapeutic approaches listed for other categories are unlikely to be beneficial, and the physician who attempts pharmacologic intervention rather than reassurance, lifestyle counseling, and support often ends with a drug-dependent patient who gets no better.

These eight categories and the brief descriptions presented are supported by generalizations to which there are some exceptions. However, Table 440–1 suggests quite specific directions in which laboratory investigation and the therapeutic approach should begin. The experienced physician soon moves far beyond this table, but it provides a particularly useful framework upon which to place the more detailed clinical knowledge of following chapters.

USING THE LABORATORY SELECTIVELY

Laboratory tests in the rheumatic diseases usually provide confirmatory data rather than conclusive evidence. After the three exceptions of (1) the sacroiliac radiograph in ankylosing spondylitis, (2) the identification of specific crystals within the joint fluid, or (3) a positive bacteriologic culture from joint fluid, laboratory tests have varying degrees of lack of sensitivity and lack of specificity and, except in the unusual case, add relatively little to clinical assessment. As a result, the majority of patients presenting with musculoskeletal problems do not require any laboratory evaluation whatsoever. The key to appropriate use of the laboratory is selective use. Every test should have a specific indication, and blind "surveys" or "panels" should not be used.

One in six visits by a patient to a health professional is for a musculoskeletal complaint. The great majority of such physician visits occur for the common "focal conditions" of life. Low back pain, sprained ankles, tennis elbows, and other common musculoskeletal complaints account for most initial visits. The overwhelming majority of such problems are easily identified as self-limited. Optimal management includes ruling out more significant illness, advice about activity or rest, reassurance, occasionally symptomatic medication, and transmission of the expectation that the natural healing process will resolve the difficulty. The usual healing period for local musculoskeletal problems ranges from two to six weeks, depending upon the magnitude of the often inapparent injury, with the healing process beginning again from the start if there is reinjury during this period. Healing cannot be pharmacologically accelerated. Thus, optimal treatment usually requires "masterly inactivity," with confident reliance upon the natural healing process. Inappropriate rigor with test or treatment can lead to investigative mishaps, therapeutic side reactions, and an intensity of focus upon the problem entirely inappropriate to its magnitude. The careful rheumatic disease clinician uses time to establish the trends and tempo of the condition in the individual; time is used to remove the self-limited condition from the hazards of inappropriate response.

The critical initial decision, therefore, is whether the problem requires immediate action or whether the decision to investigate or treat can be postponed until the course of the disease and the magnitude of the appropriate response may be better estimated. A six-week "rule of thumb" is appropriate. In the absence of specific indication or immediate threat, a waiting period of six weeks from onset of symptoms serves to minimize inappropriate use of laboratory tests or treatment. Four major exceptions to the six-week rule obtain. First, a condition that is severe and involves a single joint (or, at most, a few joints) is much more likely, paradoxically, to require immediate attention than is a widespread polyarthritis. Acute gouty arthritis and infections, the usual causes of the "single hot joint," require immediate attention. In contrast, in rheumatoid arthritis, a period of six weeks is required even before the criteria for diagnosis can be met, and management in the first days of disease is most appropriately conservative. Many "possible rheumatoid arthritis" patients have minor problems that disappear as the viral or minor hypersensitivity reaction subsides. They need not be given the emotional burden of a "serious" diagnosis.

Secondly, a patient who is febrile, systemically ill, and otherwise showing signs of major disease deserves immediate attention. Endocarditis, neoplasm, tuberculosis, and other illnesses are frequently identified through musculoskeletal clues, and a connective tissue disease with systemic manifestations deserves immediate attention.

Third, if the problem is associated with significant trauma, the possible need for immediate orthopedic management should be considered. Fourth, an associated neurologic problem such as carpal tunnel syndrome, sciatic nerve compression, or cervical nerve root compression may be benefited by immediate attention. In practice, these four indications for action are relatively unusual. The large majority of patients with initial complaints of the musculoskeletal system are not found to have conditions requiring either intensive efforts at diagnosis or employment of hazardous therapy.

ESTABLISHING MANAGEMENT GOALS

Following current biomedical training, disease impact has often been defined in terms of numerically expressed test results. The level of autoantibodies, titer of rheumatoid factor, number of radiographic erosions, and sedimentation rate too often become the criteria for therapeutic success. The patient (and the patient's family) is much more directly interested in quite a different list of disease endpoints: in survival, in normal mobility and function, in absence from pain and other symptoms, and in the ability to remain solvent through the duration of a chronic illness. These five "D's" (death, disability, discomfort, drug toxicity, and dollar cost) are the major dimensions of patient outcome in the patient's own terms.

In some disease areas, such as oncology, consideration of the single outcome dimension of death suffices to dominate most clinical decisions. In contrast, in the rheumatic diseases value "trade-offs" among several outcome dimensions must be based upon the values of the particular patient, since different treatments may have contrasting effects on different outcome dimensions. For example, pain may be reduced by narcotics but disability increased; disability may be reduced by cyclophosphamide but a risk of death incurred; or short-term symptomatic relief by plasmapheresis may be obtained at very high cost.

Careful establishment of management goals must precede development of the individual management strategy. In some instances, a limited goal, such as regaining the ability to walk, may be dramatically useful to the patient and far more valuable to him or her than a modest reduction in the general severity of the disease. Some very worthy goals may not be achievable in the particular instance, and their pursuit may only increase the dimension of therapeutic toxicity. The question of what is desirable is usually subordinate to the question of what is achievable.

PLANNING FOR OPTIMAL LONG-TERM OUTCOME

Hospital-based training tends to focus attention on improving the patient's status at admission by the time of discharge. In chronic illness, such short-term benefits may be desirable but illusory. Corticosteroids, narcotic analgesics, and intra-articular injections often provide obvious short-term benefit. Unfortunately, the agent that provides the best initial response may lead to iatrogenic disaster over the longer term.

The basic therapeutic strategy holds that simple and nontoxic measures should be used first, and hazardous medications withheld unless the simpler approaches fail. But the individual patient frequently has special considerations requiring modification of such progressions. Thus, the tempo of disease may be such that joint destuction is developing over a short period of months; the therapeutic progression then requires acceleration. Or a major therapeutic attempt with gold, penicillamine, or an immunosuppressant agent may require months until the expected date of response. Meanwhile, the patient may have exhausted sick leave prior to forced retirement because of disability. Addition of a generally contraindicated agent, such as prednisone, might, under such circumstances, provide temporary support for the individual while more definitive therapy is taking hold. In a patient of advanced age, concern about the eventual hazard of malignancy secondary to a drug might well be small. In a vigorous and active male patient, there may be little concern about corticosteroid osteopenia. For a young patient, the expectation for patient outcome should perhaps be integrated over twenty to thirty years. In the older patient, both the risks and the benefits of treatment might be reduced, but not by the same amount. Again, the necessity for the individual program is seen.

The inexperienced clinician is often trapped by taking the short view of a chronic illness. The quack practitioner more intentionally follows the same strategy, that is, attempting to maximize immediate benefits while disregarding future problems. A chronic disease cannot be managed by short-term tactics; it requires a long-term strategy, shared and negotiated with the patient.

Such a strategy, it must be admitted, requires tactical modification at nearly every physician-patient encounter. At each visit, new information is always present, even if it is only the information about what has transpired in response to the last set of decisions. A decision is thus followed by observation, then by further decision, then by another period of observation. The decision strategy is flexible and, in the final analysis, frequently empiric.

USING A COMPLETE CLINICAL REPERTOIRE

Treatment of musculoskeletal disease is frequently discussed in terms of the available pharmacologic agents. This myopic view neglects the dominant contributions often afforded by reconstructive surgical procedures, by the use of appliances and devices to allow handicapped individuals to function more normally, by exercise to strengthen bones and tissues, or by personal interaction to increase the motivation and self-image of the patient.

A drug-based strategy tends to find its greatest use in early, systemic, inflammatory disease processes. Orthopedic approaches tend to have the greatest utility if the number of joints or regions involved is small, if major problems are concentrated in a single anatomic region, or after an inflammatory process has "burned out." Improvement after occupational therapy is often seen in patients with moderate to major disability who require adaptive devices to render the environment more friendly. The will to live a normal life sometimes can be more important to outcome than any specific therapy, and patient confidence (personal efficacy) is a useful therapeutic adjunct. Medical therapy that interferes with mental or emotional adaptation frequently appears to make things worse.

The novice at managing rheumatic diseases employs only a limited therapeutic repertoire. Typically, the patient requires a diverse program individualized to specific needs and frequently making use of a variety of individuals from different disciplines. Development of rational strategies requires intimate knowledge of the strengths and weaknesses of all available therapeutic modalities. The physician cannot manage chronic musculoskeletal diseases effectively without detailed knowledge of the techniques of complementary disciplines or a good working relationship with individuals who possess these skills.

ACHIEVING PATIENT UNDERSTANDING

The informed patient is the physician's greatest single asset in managing chronic illness. Consider even the recommendation that a patient should take aspirin. The lay media describe the hazards of aspirin, colloquialisms associate aspirin with physician neglect, and the over-the-counter availability suggests that aspirin is a minor remedy. Yet, for anti-inflammatory treatment with aspirin, the physician may aim for a narrow therapeutic range just below toxicity and far above the dose the patient expects. While establishing dosage, the patient is almost certain to encounter one or another side effect, even though the aspirin later may be well tolerated. The informed patient must know that anti-inflammatory and analgesic activities of aspirin are different, that a particular therapeutic range is important, that the drug is active against the inflammatory process itself, and that several weeks may be required to see the full effects of the drug. In the absence of such understanding, it is extremely unusual for a patient to do well on aspirin; patient education is a prerequisite for therapeutic success.

Most clinicians believe that patients with positive expectations have better outcomes. While causality is not established from this observation, it is reasonable to assume that restoration of hope and a positive self-image are beneficial parts of the treatment program. The patient with arthritis is under intense psychologic pressures. Self-image is threatened by diseases that may cripple and prevent remunerative employment. The possibility of dependence upon others is often present. Yet prognosis is generally better than that anticipated by the patient. The physician who is unaware that every patient with arthritis has significant fears may do great harm by inadvertently increasing those fears.

Additional considerations mandate careful patient education. The informed patient is more likely to comply with a particular therapeutic regimen. The patient's report of success or failure with previous recommendations is essential for the next clinical decision and must be as accurate as possible, again emphasizing the need for direct patient-physician communication. Unrealistic expectations followed by perceived therapeutic failures are a major cause of the burgeoning business in quack treatment of arthritis. The patient must be educated to recognize the falsity of overstated claims and the losses in courage, independence, and money that may result. The obscenity of the quack practitioner who makes a living by defrauding patients with arthritis focuses the attention of most physicians upon the outrage. At the more important level, however, the patient susceptible to the claims of the quack does not have a confident and informed relationship with his or her personal physician.

The management of musculoskeletal disease is directed in large part at maintenance of the independence of the individual. Most persons with arthritis can be independent and healthy individuals despite their musculoskeletal condition. This independence is the final goal of the individualized management strategy.

Fries JF: Education for outcome. J Rheum 5:1, 1978.
Fries JF, Holman HR: Systemic Lupus Erythematosus: A Clinical Analysis. Philadelphia, W. B. Saunders Company, 1975.
Fries JF, Mitchell DM: Joint pain or arthritis. JAMA 235:199, 1976.
Rodnan GP, Schumacher HR (eds.): Primer on the Rheumatic Diseases. Atlanta, Georgia, Arthritis Foundation, 1983.
Urowitz MB: SLE subsets—divide and conquer. J Rheum 4:332, 1977.

441. CONNECTIVE TISSUE STRUCTURE AND FUNCTION

Stephen M. Krane

Connective tissues are responsible for the form and shape of the animal body and, in addition, provide protection for vital organs and facilitate locomotion. The term connective tissue is also applied in a more restricted sense to structures such as dermis, tendons, fascia, bone, cartilage, and the capsules of the joint. All cells, however, make contacts with surrounding structures which involve connective tissues as components of the extracellular matrix. The matrix possesses chemical, physical, and mechanical properties uniquely suited to the function of tissues and organs of which the cells are a part. The extracellular matrix may be rigid (e.g., bone), elastic (e.g., blood vessel walls), compressible (e.g., cartilage), or liquid (e.g., synovial fluid). Most connective tissue matrices derive these properties by virtue of the content of fibrillar proteins, nonfibrillar macromolecules, and low molecular weight proteins and electrolytes. The properties of the matrix are therefore determined predominantly by the function of cells, specific for each tissue, which are responsible for synthesis of the matrix components. Many of the functions of the component cells, in turn, are influenced by the character of the extracellular matrix. The properties of connective tissues are also influenced by their relationships to the vascular system from which critical components are derived, such as water, electrolytes, and proteins. Indeed, the walls of blood vessels may themselves be considered as connective tissues. However, although some connective tissues are highly vascular (e.g., bone), others are essentially avascular (e.g., cartilage).

COMPOSITION OF EXTRACELLULAR MATRICES. The major components of the extracellular matrix are fibrillar proteins (collagens and elastin), globular proteins, complex carbohydrates, and, in the case of bone, the inorganic mineral phase. In most connective tissues the fibrillar proteins make up the bulk of the organic material. The *elastic fibers* consist of two distinct protein components. The most abundant is an amorphous protein (elastin) with no distinct periodicity by electron microscopy. The minor component associated with the elastin is a microfibrillar glycoprotein. Elastic fibers are most abundant in walls of large arteries and in some tendons and ligaments. In joints, however, collagens are the major fibrillar proteins. Collagens belong to a family of proteins which have similar chemical and structural properties. The term "collagen" is also used to refer to fibers or fiber bundles observed in tissue sections. The form of collagens in tissues is determined by the type of molecule that predominates and by interactions with other components of the matrix. Collagen fibers usually have diameters of 0.1 μm to 10 to 15 μm. The most abundant species, the interstitial collagens, such as those which predominate in tissues such as dermis, tendons, bone, and cartilage, have a characteristic banding pattern seen on electron microscopy with major periods of approximately 64 to 70 nm (Fig. 441–1). Some collagens such as those comprising basement membranes or others which are deposited pericellularly, appear amorphous and do not have a banded structure detected by electron microscopy. The collagen molecules of most collagens consist of three polypeptides (α chains) which have a characteristic and unique helical structure determined by the amino acid sequence. The collagen molecules of the interstitial collagens can be solubilized from some tissues. In solution these molecules behave as long, rigid rods with dimensions of approximately 300 $\times$ 1.5 nm. Each of the collagen polypeptide chains contains a glycine residue at every third position and is rich in amino acids such as alanine and proline. Collagens contain little phenylalanine and tyrosine and essentially no tryptophan, and, with the exception of type III collagen and the basement membrane collagens, usually lack cysteine in the body of the helical portion.

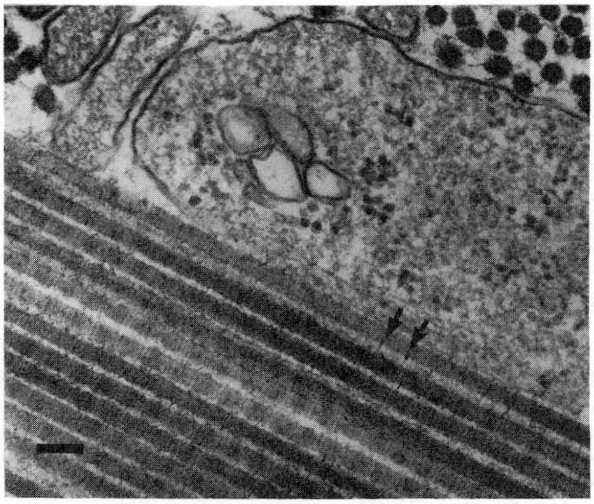

Figure 441–1. Electron micrograph of sections of 17-day-old chick Achilles tendon. Collagen fibrils are seen in longitudinal section in the lower left portion of the figure. These fibrils have a period of ~67 nm, as indicated by the distance between the two arrows. Fibrils seen in cross section at the upper portion of the figure have an average diameter of ~50 nm. Collagen fibers, which are made up of many fibrils, have diameters which range from 0.1 to 15 μm. Bar = 100 nm. (Courtesy of Dr. Romaine Bruns.)

Collagen chains in the course of synthesis also undergo unique post-translational modifications of several component amino acids. The most important of these modifications involves the introduction of a hydroxyl group in the 4 position of specific prolyl residues. The 4-hydroxyproline residues are considered to be responsible for stabilization of the collagen helix. In addition, there is a small amount of 3-hydroxyproline in most collagens, whose function is not known. Specific lysyl residues also are modified by hydroxylation in the 5 position to form hydroxylysine. The hydroxyproline and hydroxylysine of collagens liberated by proteolytic cleavage of the polypeptide chains in the course of physiologic remodeling or pathologic degradation are not reutilized for collagen biosynthesis. Quantitation of the urinary excretion of these amino acids therefore provides some index of collagen turnover. Certain ε-amino groups of lysines as well as hydroxylysines are oxidized to their respective aldehydes to form derivatives known as allysines and hydroxyallysines, respectively. Lysine, hyroxylysine, and their derivatives are involved in crosslinking between the chains that constitute the collagen molecules (intramolecular) as well as crosslinking one collagen molecule to another (intermolecular).

In the case of the interstitial collagens the characteristic banding pattern is accounted for by an ordered staggered arrangement of the collagen molecules within the collagen fibrils and the collagen fibers. The manner of molecular packing within the fibril in turn is determined by the amino acid sequence. The way the molecules are staggered in the fibril, however, gives rise to regions in which the molecules overlap and others in which there is no overlap (Fig. 441–2). It is probable that the mineral phase of bone is deposited predominantly within the voids or holes of the nonoverlap region. The

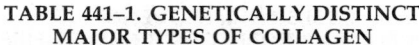

TABLE 441–1. GENETICALLY DISTINCT MAJOR TYPES OF COLLAGEN

Type	Chains	Form	Major Tissues
I	α1, α2	$[\alpha 1(I)]_2 2$	Bone, dermis, tendon fascia, arteries, parenchyma
I	α1	$[\alpha 1(I)]_3$	Embryo tendons
II	α1	$[\alpha 1(II)]_3$	Hyaline cartilage
III	α1	$[\alpha 1(III)]_3$	Dermis, arteries, uterus, parenchyma
IV	α1, α2	?	Basement membranes
V	α1, α2, α3 (A, B, C)	?	Basement membranes, pericellular, placenta, muscle

macromolecular structure of type IV collagen, the major fibrillar component of basement membranes, is very different from that of the interstitial collagens. Type IV collagen structure consists of a network of individual 390 nm-long molecules that are aggregated and crosslinked via identical ends to form a distinctive lattice.

These proteins with structural homologies make up the collagen family. The different homologous species are referred to as types, with each type the product of a different (nonallelic) genetic locus. The five most common and best characterized collagen types are listed in Table 441–1. These types do not have a unique tissue distribution, although some tissues are characterized by a marked predominance of one type—e.g., type II collagen in cartilage and type I collagen in bone. It is likely that each of these collagen types is largely responsible for the functional and morphologic properties of each connective tissue, although it has not yet been possible to relate function to a particular chemical modification. In addition to those types listed in Table 441–1, there are other less abundant collagens (at least five more types) described and partially characterized, each the product of a different gene. These include intima, long chain, endothelial cell, high molecular weight, and short chain collagens.

There is considerable information concerning the pathways of synthesis of various collagens. Even the genes from several animal species for the component polypeptide chains of several collagen types have been partially characterized, illustrating the enormous progress that has been made in the study of these molecules. Although the chains of the interstitial collagen molecules contain approximately 1000 amino acids, and the procollagen precursor contains additional polypeptide sequences at either end which would require a messenger RNA of approximately 4500 bases, the genes coding for each of the proα1 and proα2 chains have a length of approximately 38,000 bases. The enormous size of the genes is due to the presence of approximately 50 intervening DNA sequences (introns), which do not code for amino acid sequences of the mature collagen chains. A possible sequence of events in the course of synthesis of the collagen molecule is shown in Table 441–2. Further complexities are illustrated by the finding that, in the case of type I collagen, the genes coding for the constituent chains are not even on the same chromosome. In humans, the gene for the α1 chain is on chromosome 17 and that for the α2 chain on chromosome 7.

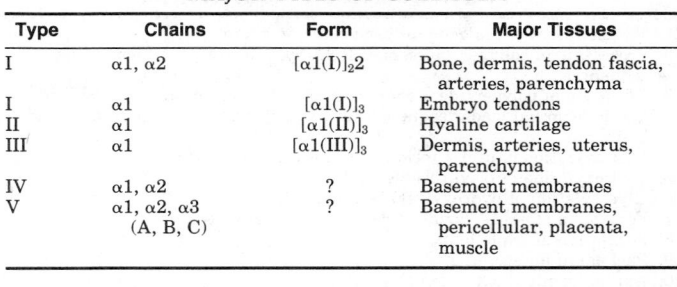

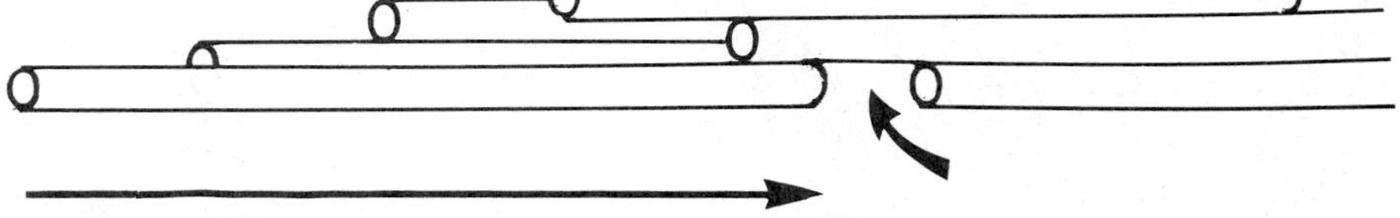

Figure 441–2. A model of the packing of the collagen molecules within the collagen fibril. The molecules, each consisting of three helical polypeptide chains, are depicted as long rigid rods and represented here by the cylinders. The length of the molecules is indicated by the long arrow. The structure gives rise to regions where adjacent molecules are in contact and others in which there are holes, indicated by the short arrow. It is suggested that the inorganic crystals of bone are located predominantly in these holes.

TABLE 441–2. SEQUENCE OF CELLULAR COLLAGEN BIOSYNTHESIS

1. Transcription of the gene for each collagen chain
2. Processing of collagen messenger RNA by removing ~ 50 noncoding sequences
3. Initiation of polypeptide α chain synthesis by formation of hydrophobic amino terminal leader sequence, followed by assembly of proregion and helix
4. Hydroxylation of prolyl residues begins on nascent chains
5. Hydroxylation of lysyl residues
6. Glycosylation of hydroxylysyl residues
7. Formation of –S–S– bonds at carboxyterminal extension
8. Formation of triple helix
9. Packaging for secretion
10. Amino terminal extension cleavage
11. Carboxyterminal extension cleavage
12. Formation of microfibril
13. Lysyl and hydroxylysyl oxidation
14. Formation of reducible crosslinks
15. Maturation and growth
16. Further crosslinking and interaction with other components

Despite the complexity of this synthetic process, there are several heritable disorders of connective tissue in which it is possible to demonstrate abnormalities in biosynthesis. Defects in synthesis of a particular type of collagen, type III collagen, have been demonstrated in a form of the Ehlers-Danlos syndrome (type IV), characterized by tissue friability and rupture of viscera and major blood vessels. Defects in hydroxylation of lysine have also been noted, which gives rise to another clinical form (type VI) of the Ehlers-Danlos syndrome. In addition, defects in processing of the procollagens have been demonstrated (Ehlers-Danlos syndrome type VII) as well as problems with crosslinking accounted for by failure to oxidize critical lysine and hydroxylysine residues (certain forms of cutis laxa). Insufficient synthesis of type I collagen has also been found in certain forms of osteogenesis imperfecta, particularly the classic dominant variety of moderate severity, associated with deafness and blue sclerae. In other cases of osteogenesis imperfecta, which fall into a different clinical and genetic grouping, additions or deletions of portions of the coding region for the procollagen extensions or the helical portions have been described. In one extraordinary case, no α2 chains are present in skin and bone nor are such chains secreted by fibroblasts. The defect lies in a portion of the extension peptides that does not permit normal assembly of the procollagen trimer. Thus, absence of α2 chains is not lethal; trimers of α1 chains can be formed.

Other major components of connective tissues include the *high molecular weight carbohydrates* that make up the so-called ground substance of the interfibrillar matrix. These macromolecules, formerly known as mucopolysaccharides, are composed of a glycosaminoglycan portion (the complex carbohydrate itself) linked to a core protein. The core protein with the glycosaminoglycans attached is termed the proteoglycan subunit. In articular cartilage, proteoglycans constitute approximately half the dry weight of the tissue. Another abundant complex carbohydrate present in many tissues and the major polysaccharide of synovial fluid is hyaluronic acid. The complex carbohydrates of cartilage are composed of high molecular weight polymers of the proteoglycan subunits, with the polysaccharide side chains of chondroitin sulfate and keratan sulfate linked to serine residues of the core protein. The polymeric components consist of these proteoglycan subunits bound to high molecular weight hyaluronic acid chains through interactions with another glycoprotein, called link protein. These proteoglycan aggregates are envisioned as occupying the spaces in cartilage surrounded by the collagen fibers and other components of the matrix. Both the proteoglycans and the collagens are synthesized by the articular chondrocytes.

In general, the cells of the connective tissues interact with the complex carbohydrates and the collagen fibers through glycoproteins, which are probably specific for each type of connective tissue. For example, the cell membranes of epithelial cells interact with a glycoprotein known as laminin, which by interacting with type IV collagen, a unique heparan sulfate glycoprotein, and another protein, nidinogen, together make up the structure of the basement membrane. Many connective tissue and other cells interact with collagens through the protein fibronectin. A protein similar to cellular fibronectin also circulates in plasma where it is known as cold insoluble globulin. Chondrocytes interact with their extracellular matrix through another glycoprotein called chondronectin.

STRUCTURE AND FUNCTION OF JOINTS. The structure and characteristics of the diarthrodial joints are determined by the

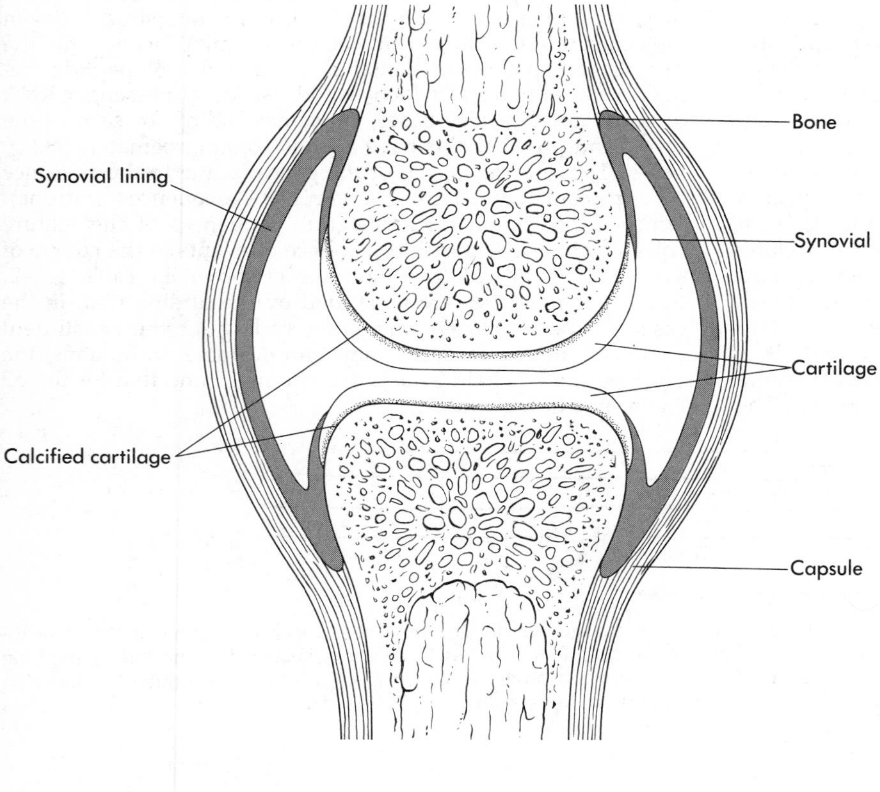

Figure 441–3. A schematic view of a diarthrodial joint.

function of specific cells which produce unique extracellular matrices. A typical joint such as that depicted schematically in Figure 441–3 has its characteristic components. The joint is ideally suited for the demands of weight bearing and motion, which must be operational with a minimum of wear over the lifetime of the individual. The functional properties of the joint are dependent upon a compressible, deformable cartilaginous surface which is properly lubricated and supported by relatively rigid subchondral bone. The stability of the joint, in turn, is determined by the connective tissue structure of the joint capsule, tendons, and ligaments, and is influenced by function of muscles concerned with movement or support of that joint. The joint cavity is lined by a synovial membrane, which normally consists of one or two layers of cells. Some tendency to piling up of the cells is observed at the margins of the joint where the synovium is reflected. The synovial lining cells are derived from connective tissue (they are not epithelial) and do not rest on a continuous basement membrane. In the normal synovium, at least two types of cells have been recognized. The type A cell is a phagocytic cell possibly related to macrophages; the type B cell is fibroblast-like.

The joint cavity contains a characteristic synovial fluid. Its high viscosity is due to the presence of hyaluronic acid, which is probably synthesized by the synovial lining B cells. Water, electrolytes, and some low molecular weight serum proteins such as albumin are derived by filtration from the subsynovial capillaries. Glucose and electrolytes are present in normal synovial fluid at concentrations similar to those in plasma. In inflammation of the synovium, glucose entry is impaired and utilization increased to account for the lower synovial fluid glucose concentrations in some forms of arthritis, such as rheumatoid and septic arthritis. The concentration of proteins in normal synovial fluid is inversely proportional to their molecular weights. Albumin is therefore the most abundant protein. Plasma α_2-macroglobulin, IgM, and fibrinogen are essentially excluded from normal fluids, possibly owing to molecular sieving effects of the hyaluronic acid in the interstitial regions of the synovium and the synovial fluid. In joint inflammation, there is increased entry of the high molecular weight proteins into the synovial fluid. These pathologic fluids may thus form a *fibrin* clot, whereas normal fluids do not. This is to be distinguished from the so-called *mucin* clot, which is composed of a protein–hyaluronic acid complex, which can be produced by the addition of dilute acetic acid to synovial fluid. A tight, ropy mucin clot is characteristic of normal or traumatic fluids, whereas inflammatory fluids tend to produce a fragmented clot or a dispersed sediment upon addition of acetic acid. The clinical diagnostic usefulness of the mucin clot test is not uniformly accepted, however.

The cartilage of the diarthrodial joint is avascular, and the chondrocytes must receive their nourishment from the synovial fluid; products of their metabolism are in turn disposed of through the synovial fluid. The function of the articular cartilage is critically dependent upon the interaction of the fibrillar collagenous matrix and the proteoglycans. By virtue of the highly negative charge on the proteoglycans, these molecules occupy a large domain. The extent to which articular cartilage is deformed on compression and the ability of the cartilage to regain its shape following release from compression is determined by interactions of the proteoglycan aggregates with the fibrillar matrix. It is envisioned that alternate compression and relaxation of the cartilage during motion and weight bearing are responsible for movement of fluid and electrolytes in and out of the cartilage interstitium and provide a mechanism for the nutrition of the chondrocytes. The properties of articular cartilage with its surface in contact with synovial fluid account for the extraordinarily low coefficient of friction upon movement of the joint. The viscous hyaluronic acid which serves a lubricating function for the synovial membrane is probably not responsible for lubrication of the articular cartilage itself. Other components such as lubricating glycoproteins interact with components on the surface of the articular cartilage, providing a so-called boundary type of lubrication. The very fact that the cartilage is capable of deforming under load and regaining its shape following release of the load also contributes to the low coefficient of friction of moving joints. This elastic, spongy nature of cartilage allows it to weep fluid when squeezed under high loads, which, in part, creates a film of lubrication at the head of the moving surfaces. It is also postulated that the highly ordered structure of the cancellous bone supporting the articular cartilage dissipates the shock of impact under loading and permits some of the mechanical forces to be dispersed away from the articular cartilage.

ALTERATION OF STRUCTURE AND FUNCTION OF JOINTS IN DISEASE. When joints are subjected to mechanical or chemical trauma, there are several predictable responses that occur in the articular cartilage and surrounding structures. Repeated mechanical trauma is associated with loss or decrease of the proteoglycan of the cartilage matrix, which can be appreciated histologically as a loss of the staining properties (e.g., metachromasia) attributed to this component. The mechanism for the proteoglycan loss probably involves the secretion of proteolytic enzymes, by the chondrocytes or by cells in the synovial fluid or the synovial lining, which, at neutral pH, cleave the core protein of the proteoglycans near the linkage region with the hyaluronic acid. Following cleavage of the core protein, the partially degraded proteoglycan is leached from the matrix. Alterations of this type have been observed following arthrotomy or bleeding into the joint. Since the articular chondrocytes have the capacity to resynthesize proteoglycans, if the mechanical injury is only temporary, some structure of the matrix can be restored. However, persistent deficiency of cartilage proteoglycan is accompanied by alteration in mechanical properties of the matrix manifested by an increased tendency of the cartilage to deform under load and a decreased ability to regain form following removal of the load. Only late in the course of injury is the collagenous component of the matrix affected. Although articular chondrocytes have retained the capacity for replication and to increase, often in clusters, in response to chronic injury, these cells have a limited capacity to resynthesize type II collagen and reconstitute the normal fibrillar matrix. The proliferation of cartilage cells in response to trauma and mechanical stress may also be followed by vascularization and activation of the endochondral sequence, resulting in formation of osteophytes, usually at the margin of joints. Trauma may also produce reactions in the synovium, probably mediated by altered vascularization in addition to increased numbers and activity of the synovial lining cells. These synovial reactions may in turn result in the formation of increased synovial fluid, manifested clinically as effusions. The composition of these synovial fluids closely resembles that of normal synovial fluid with respect to viscosity (the concentration of hyaluronic acid) and the type and relative concentration of the protein components (predominance of albumin and absence of high molecular weight plasma proteins such as fibrinogen, IgM, and α_2-macroglobulin). Thus, a mild degree of "synovitis" may be a component of either acute or chronic injury. Under these circumstances, however, few cells (100 to 500 per cubic millimeter) are present in the synovial fluid; lymphocytes and monocytes predominate, whereas polymorphonuclear leukocytes are scarce.

In almost all types of joint inflammation, however, whether acute, as in urate gout or pseudogout (calcium pyrophosphate deposition disease), or chronic, as in typical rheumatoid arthritis, there is an exudation of cells, particularly polymorphonulear leukocytes, into the synovial cavity. In these inflammatory joint diseases, the synovial fluid usually is characterized by a decreased viscosity, an inability to form a normal tight mucin clot, and an increased concentration relative to normal of macromolecules such as immunoglobulin, α_2-macroglobulin, and fibrinogen. Enzymes released from the inflammatory cells have the capacity to degrade the proteoglycan core protein and collagen of the articular cartilage and surrounding structures if their concentrations (activities) exceed those of inhibitors present in synovial fluid and synovial tissues.

The synovitis seen, for example, in rheumatoid arthritis may be particularly intense with chronic inflammatory cells present, especially at the margins of the joint where the synovial membrane is reflected. With persistent synovial inflammation, a mass of proliferating cells (pannus) may burrow beneath the articular cartilage and subchondral bone or appear to work its way over the surface of the articular cartilage, degrading matrix structures in its wake. These degradative processes are probably mediated by enzymes such as specific collagenases and elastase-like proteases capable of attacking matrix components. Alterations also occur in the subchondral bone in joint disease. In the noninflammatory forms, the subchondral bone may increase in mass by new bone formation (sclerosis). In contrast, in inflammatory joint disease, subchondral bone is frequently resorbed, producing the typical radiologic appearance of juxta-articular osteoporosis. Diaphyseal cortical bone is usually not thinned until late in rheumatoid disease; in some subjects, it may even be increased in thickness owing to periosteal new bone formation. When the inflammation subsides, bony erosions may heal, and some restoration of the diffuse juxta-articular bone loss may also occur. Defects or clefts in articular cartilage, on the other hand, generally do not heal with restoration of the original form because of the limited capacity of chondrocytes to resynthesize the specific collagenous fibrillar component of extracellular matrix.

Each of the extracellular components of the matrix of the joint structures has its unique pattern of composition with respect to the collagen type, proteoglycan, and glycoprotein component. The composition of these matrices must in turn determine their function. Return of function with healing of disease therefore requires restoration of the original composition, which, in turn, is dependent upon the ability of the tissue to undergo remodeling. The limited capacity for remodeling of some tissues, such as articular cartilage, therefore accounts for disability in several of the rheumatic diseases. Thus, in instances in which structure is sufficiently distorted and return of function impossible, the only alternative may be to use the artificial surfaces of joint prostheses to permit or regain motion and weight-bearing capacity and to alleviate pain.

Bornstein P, Sage H: Structurally distinct collagen types. Ann Rev Biochem 49:957, 1980. *The material discussed in this review complements that considered by Eyre and by Prockop et al.*

Brandt KD: Glycosaminoglycans. *In* Kelley WN, Harris ED Jr, Ruddy S, Sledge CB (eds.): Textbook of Rheumatology. Philadelphia, W. B. Saunders Company, 1981, pp 239–254. *This review on glycosaminoglycans extends and updates that of Lindahl and Höök.*

Eyre DR: Collagen: Molecular diversity in the body's protein scaffold. Science 207:1315, 1980. *An updated review of collagen structure and biosynthesis.*

Harris ED Jr: Biology of the joint. *In* Kelley WN, Harris ED Jr, Ruddy S, Sledge CB (eds.): Textbook of Rheumatology. Philadelphia, W. B. Saunders Company, 1981, pp 255–276. *A consideration of joint development, structure, and function as well as mechanisms proposed to account for the lubricating properties of joints. The formation of synovial fluid and its functions are also described.*

Hollister DW, Byers PH, Holbrook KA: Genetic disorders of collagen metabolism. Adv Human Genet 12:1, 1982. *A complete review of heritable disorders of collagen metabolism.*

Krane SM: Mechanisms of tissue destruction in rheumatoid arthritis. *In* McCarty DJ (ed.): Arthritis and Allied Conditions. A Textbook of Rheumatology. Philadelphia, Lea and Febiger, 1984. *A discussion relating the histologic features to the connective tissue degradation in rheumatoid arthritis.*

Kühn K: Chemical properties of collagen. *In* Furthmayr H (ed.): Immunochemistry of the Extracellular Matrix. Vol I. Methods. Boca Raton, CRC Press, 1982, pp 1–28. *Concepts of collagen composition as it relates to organization of the molecules in tissues are well-documented.*

Lindahl U, Höök M: Glycosaminoglycans and their binding to biological macromolecules. Ann Rev Biochem 47:385, 1978. *A review of the structure of the complex carbohydrates and their interactions with intracellular and extracellular macromolecules.*

Merlino GT, McKeon C, de Crombrugghe B, Pastan I: Regulation of the expression of genes encoding types I, II, and III collagen during chick embryonic development. J Biol Chem 258:10041, 1983. *A modern study of the regulation of collagen gene expression in which references to other applications are also given.*

Nimni M: Collagen: Structure, function and metabolism in normal and fibrotic tissues. Semin Arthritis Rheum 13:1, 1983. *A well-referenced review of collagen structure with particular attention to abnormalities in disease.*

Piez K, Reddi AH: Extracellular Matrix Biochemistry. New York, Elsevier-North Holland, 1984. *A comprehensive treatise on collagen biochemistry and metabolism as well as discussions of alterations in heritable and acquired diseases.*

Prockop DJ, Kivirikko KI, Tuderman L, Guzman N: The biosynthesis of collagen and its disorders. N Engl J Med 301:13,77, 1979. *A good review of what is known about the details of collagen biosynthesis and how this is disordered in certain diseases.*

Tsipouras P, Myers JC, Ramirez F, Prockop DJ: Restriction fragment length polymorphism associated with the proα2 (I) gene of human type I procollagen. J Clin Invest 72:1262, 1983. *An example of the kind of investigations that are currently being conducted in human beings using probes for the collagen genes.*

Wuepper KD, Holbrook KA, Pinnell SR, Vitto J: Supplemental issue: Structural elements of the dermis. J Invest Derm 79(Suppl 1):1, 1982. *Short reviews on most aspects of connective tissue function including adherence glycoproteins, elastic fibers, and proteoglycans.*

Yamada KM: Cell surface interactions with extracellular materials. Ann Rev Biochem 52:761, 1983. *Detailed discussion of how cells interact with the matrices in their environment with particular emphasis on fibronectin and laminin.*

442. MECHANISMS OF INFLAMMATION AND TISSUE DESTRUCTION IN THE RHEUMATIC DISEASES

Ralph Snyderman

Immunologic processes mediate the localization and rapid destruction of substances which, if disseminated, could disrupt the host's complex internal milieu. The immune system has several unique features which permit it to combat microbial invasion and provide resistance against the development and spread of cancer. Unlike other tissues, it consists not only of fixed structures (i.e., thymus, spleen, and lymph nodes) but also of motile cells which wander throughout the body, performing surveillance. It is also the only tissue which is able to destroy other components of the host. Both the protective and destructive abilities of immunologic processes relate largely to their inflammatory potential. Understanding how inflammation is initiated is thus essential for understanding the mechanisms of immunologically mediated resistance and for comprehending how tissue destruction occurs in the rheumatic disorders.

To fulfill its function of host defense, the immune system must differentiate self from nonself and then rapidly destroy substances recognized as nonself. An orderly progression of immunologic recognition, amplification of the immune reaction, accumulation of inflammatory cells, and finally destruction of the inciting agent is ordinarily an ongoing subclinical process. Inflammatory reactions can be initiated by either specific or nonspecific means (Table 442–1). Recognition of unique determinants (epitopes) on antigens by antibodies or by receptors on small lymphocytes initiates immunologically mediated in-

TABLE 442–1. COMPONENTS OF THE INFLAMMATORY RESPONSE

Function	Mediator
Recognition	
Specific	Immunoglobulins
	Lymphocytes
Nonspecific	Macrophages*
	Polymorphonuclear leukocytes
	Alternative complement pathway
	Hageman factor
Amplification	Complement
	Cytokines—lymphokines, monokines
	Kinin-forming system
	Arachidonic acid metabolites
	Mast cell products
Destruction of antigen	Macrophages
	Polymorphonuclear leukocytes
	Lymphocytes

*Macrophages are also involved in specific recognition since they are required for antigen presentation to lymphocytes.

flammation. Nonspecific recognition can be initiated by components of the immune system which bind to materials based on their charge, hydrophobicity, or lectin composition. Nonspecific recognition is mediated in part by phagocytic cells, such as polymorphonuclear leukocytes and macrophages, as well as by C3b, an initiator of the alternative pathway of the complement system (see Ch. 428), and by Hageman factor.

Following recognition of nonself, amplification systems are activitated and lead to the production of mediators of inflammation. The type of amplifier involved depends upon the recognition component and the nature and location of the inciting material. Amplification components of the immune system such as complement cleavage products, cytokines, and other phlogistic factors magnify the initial response to nonself. Inflammatory reactions can also be initiated by nonimmunologic means. For example, inflammation following tissue necrosis results from the direct cleavage of complement components by lysosomal proteases released by injured cells. This phenomenon may play a role in extending cardiac tissue damage following myocardial infarction. In gout or pseudogout, inflammation follows the phagocytosis, by polymorphonuclear leukocytes, of monosodium urate or calcium pyrophosphate dihydrate crystals. Ingestion of these agents by leukocytes leads to the release of lysosomal hydrolases as well as the synthesis of chemotactic factors, which attract other inflammatory cells into the joint.

Regardless of the type of inflammatory response, the accumulation of granulocytes and macrophages can result in the phagocytosis and degradation of the material that initiated the inflammatory event. The factors which determine whether an inflammatory response will be protective or destructive are poorly understood. They depend in part upon the nature and location of the inciting agent as well as its quantity and digestibility. The genetic makeup and the immunoregulatory competency of the host are also important. In general, when the antigen or other inciting agent is rapidly disposed of, the inflammatory process is protective and self-limited. When antigen persists or is excessive in amount, the inflammatory response can be locally destructive and become clinically apparent.

RHEUMATOID SYNOVITIS AS A MODEL OF INFLAMMATORY-MEDIATED TISSUE DESTRUCTION

A chronic, locally destructive inflammatory reaction in humans is exemplified by the synovitis present in some connective tissue disorders. The prototype disease is rheumatoid arthritis. The diarthrodial joint has several features that influence inflammatory processes which occur there. The synovial membrane is highly vascular and lines all intra-articular structures, except for cartilage. The synovial lining is devoid of a basement membrane and thus permits relatively free diffusion of soluble substances. Moreover, the synovium lines a closed cavity, the joint space; therefore any reactive materials gaining entrance to the joint space are difficult to remove.

Normal synovium is a thin layer of tissue whose lining is composed of two principal cell types supported by a loose connective tissue stroma (Fig. 442–1*A*). The Type A cell is rich in surface pseudopodia, and its cytoplasm has many lysosomes and prominent Golgi complexes but little rough endoplasmic reticulum. Type A synoviocytes have many characteristics of macrophages and are phagocytic, but ultrastructural studies have implied a secretory role for these cells as well. The Type B synoviocyte exhibits prominent rough endoplasmic reticulum, but few vacuoles, lysosomes, or cell processes. This cell is primarily a secretory cell, hyaluronic acid being an important product. Synoviocytes may, however, be multipotential, with their morphology reflecting the net result of stimuli present in the local milieu. Beneath the synovial membrane there are collagen fibrils, fatty tissue, and an extensive capillary network. Fibroblasts in this area produce Types I and III collagen. Lastly, the dense fibrous joint capsule provides a support for the

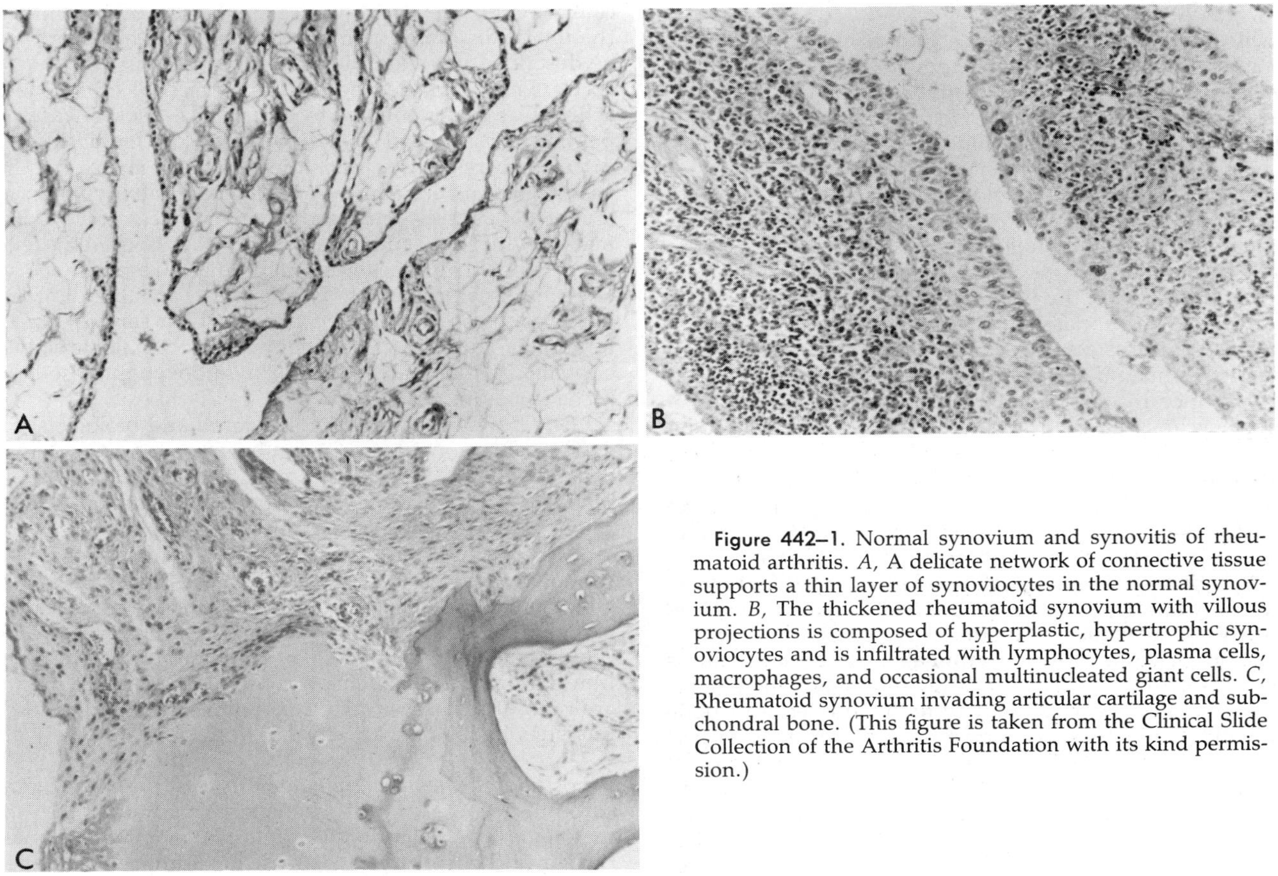

Figure 442–1. Normal synovium and synovitis of rheumatoid arthritis. *A,* A delicate network of connective tissue supports a thin layer of synoviocytes in the normal synovium. *B,* The thickened rheumatoid synovium with villous projections is composed of hyperplastic, hypertrophic synoviocytes and is infiltrated with lymphocytes, plasma cells, macrophages, and occasional multinucleated giant cells. *C,* Rheumatoid synovium invading articular cartilage and subchondral bone. (This figure is taken from the Clinical Slide Collection of the Arthritis Foundation with its kind permission.)

synovial lining membrane and separates the articular space from surrounding structures.

Rheumatoid synovitis exhibits three main components: inflammation, proliferation, and infiltration. In early stages, both Types A and B cells proliferate and increase in size. Fibrin deposits are frequently present on the inner synovial lining. Polymorphonuclear leukocytes predominate in the synovial fluid exudate, but cells are seen as infiltrates only in the superficial synovial layer. The supporting stroma beneath the lining cell layer becomes edematous and develops an increase in the number of small blood vessels. Concurrently, there are focal accumulations of inflammatory cells consisting of lymphocytes, plasma cells, macrophages, and occasionally mast cells. If the inflammatory synovitis persists, a proliferative lesion develops, characterized by synovial membrane thickening and projection of villous formations into the articular cavity (Fig. 442–1*B*). There is a concomitant increase in supporting connective tissue, small blood vessels, mononuclear cell infiltrates, and occasional multinucleated giant cells, as well as increased numbers of undifferentiated mesenchyme-like cells which have both phagocytic and synthetic potential. As the proliferative lesions progress, infiltration of surrounding structures develop as the fibrous-mesenchymal tissue (pannus) begins to invade and replace cartilage and bone at the periphery of the synovial reflection (Fig. 442–1*C*). The invasion of cartilage, subchondral bone, and tendon by inflammatory synovial tissue results in collagen destruction, degradation of proteoglycans in the cartilage matrix, and bony resorption.

MEDIATORS OF INFLAMMATION THAT PARTICIPATE IN THE RHEUMATIC DISEASES

Inflammatory reactions result from the local production of a number of mediators derived from humoral or cellular sources. A complex interplay of activation and suppression mechanisms modulates the type and magnitude of the inflammatory response which develops.

ARACHIDONIC ACID METABOLITES. Phospholipids are major constituents of cell membranes, including those of leukocytes and platelets, and are subject to degradation by cellular phospholipases under certain conditions such as exposure of cells to inflammatory or noxious stimuli. Cleavage of phospholipids results in the release of arachidonic acid, which can be further metabolized into a number of biologically potent mediators and modulators of inflammation. Prostaglandins (PG) are synthesized from arachidonic acid following the action of the enzyme cyclo-oxygenase, which forms PGG_2, which is then reduced to PGH_2. Depending upon the isomerase enzymes present in the particular tissue, the classic prostaglandins (PGE_2, $PGF_{2\alpha}$), thromboxanes, or prostacyclins will be formed. Leukocytes and explants of rheumatoid synovia produce predominantly PGE_2, platelets produce thromboxane A_2, and endothelial cells produce prostacyclin. Thromboxanes are potent vasoconstrictors, whereas prostacyclins are potent vasodilators. PGE_2 appears to modulate a number of inflammatory events. It enhances vascular permeability, is pyrogenic, and increases sensitivity to pain. PGE_2 also stimulates the formation of cAMP in many types of inflammatory cells and thereby suppresses a number of immunologic responses, including release of mediators from mast cells, lymphocyte blastogenesis, and lymphocyte-mediated cytotoxic reactions. An important source of PGE_2 in immunologic reactions is the macrophage. Supernatant fluids from explants of rheumatoid synovium stimulate bone resorption by enhancing osteoclast activity and the release of bone calcium. This phenomenon is probably mediated in large part by PG since it is inhibitable by indomethacin, an inhibitor of their formation.

Arachidonic acid can also be metabolized into another class of biologically active derivatives by the enzyme lipoxygenase. The hydroxy-eicosatetraenoic acids (HETEs) and the derivatives of 5-hydroperoxy-eicosatetraenoic acid (termed leukotrienes) are examples of these arachidonic acid metabolites and are synthesized by granulocytes, macrophages, and basophils. 5,12-HETE, also termed leukotriene B_4 (LTB_4), is a potent chemotactic factor, whereas leukotrienes C and D stimulate bronchoconstriction. LTB_4 has been identified in the synovial effusions of patients with rheumatoid arthritis and ankylosing spondylitis. Large amounts of LTB_4 are produced when granulocytes phagocytize monosidium urate crystals. This chemoattractant may, therefore, be important in the pathogenesis of gouty inflammation.

BIOLOGICALLY ACTIVE AMINES, HISTAMINE, AND SEROTONIN. Histamine is derived from the decarboxylation of histidine by the enzyme L-histidine decarboxylase. The majority of histamine is stored in mast cells and basophils and is complexed with mucopolysaccharides such as heparin. Stimulation of mast cells and basophils by a number of mechanisms causes secretion of histamine. This agent has diverse biologic activities, including constricting smooth muscle, enhancing vascular permeability, depressing leukocyte chemotaxis, blocking T lymphocyte function, and depressing further histamine release from mast cells and basophils. Histamine thus may modulate both acute and chronic inflammatory responses. Serotonin (5-hydroxytryptamine) is produced by the decarboxylation of 5-hydroxytryptophan. More than 90 per cent of body stores of serotonin are found in the gastrointestinal tract and the central nervous system; the remainder is present in the dense granules of platelets. The biologic role of serotonin in inflammation is not well understood, but it enhances the chemotactic responses of leukocytes and increases fibroblast growth in vitro. It also stimulates collagen formation.

BIOLOGICALLY ACTIVE PEPTIDES. ***Complement Cleavage Products.*** The complement (C) system functions as an important amplifier of inflammatory events initiated by immunoglobulins IgG and IgM as well as inflammatory reactions initiated by release of hydrolytic enzymes from traumatized cells or by leukocytes. The biology and biochemistry of this complex series of proteins are described in Ch. 428. Two complement cleavage products, C3a and C5a, derived from the third and fifth C components, respectively, are mediators of inflammation in rheumatic disorders such as rheumatoid arthritis and will thus be described in greater detail here.

C3a: Enzymatic cleavage of the α chain of C3 by the earlier-acting C components or by other proteases releases C3a, a peptide consisting of 77 amino acids. C3a mediates a number of biologic responses, including smooth muscle contraction, vasodilatation, enhanced vascular permeability, the degranulation of mast cells and basophils, and the secretion of lysosomal enzymes by leukocytes. C3a also has immunoregulatory effects and suppresses humoral immune responses in vitro by affecting T lymphocytes. C3a is the most abundant of the C peptides released upon activation of C in serum. The COOH-terminal arginine of C3a is required for its biologic activity, and cleavage of this amino acid by a carboxypeptidase-B–like enzyme in serum renders the peptide inactive.

C5a: C5a has a number of structural and biologic similarities to C3a. C5a consists of 74 amino acids, the COOH-terminal constituent also being arginine. C5a is derived from cleavage of the α chain of C5. In addition to having all the biologic activities of C3a, C5a is also an extremely potent chemoattractant for polymorphonuclear leukocytes, monocytes, and macrophages. C5a is the major source of chemotactic activity generated in serum treated with immune complexes or endotoxin and is also an important source of chemotactic activity in rheumatoid synovial fluids. In contrast to C3a, C5a potentiates humoral immune responses in vitro. Cleavage of the terminal arginine of C5a by a serum carboxypeptidase-B markedly diminishes its biologic activity but does not completely abrogate it.

Eosinophil Chemotactic Factors of Anaphylaxis (ECF-A). Eosinophil accumulation is characteristic of a number of rheumatologic and allergic disorders. Basophils and mast cells contain inflammatory mediators, including two tetrapeptides,

Val-Gly-Ser-Glu and Ala-Gly-Ser-Glu. Both of these substances are chemoattractants for eosinophils and to a lesser degree for neutrophils.

Crystal-Induced Chemotactic Factors. Leukocytes accumulate in the synovial fluid of individuals with gout or pseudogout following the ingestion by neutrophils of monosodium urate or calcium pyrophosphate dihydrate crystals, respectively. Incubation of neutrophils with these crystals in vitro results in the production by the cells of LTB_4 and a polypeptide chemoattractant with a molecular weight of 8400. The production of these chemoattractants are blocked by colchicine. A mechanism by which colchicine abrogates acute gouty arthritis may be its ability to inhibit the synthesis of chemoattractants by neutrophils.

Kinin-Forming System. An intimate association exists between the activation and regulation of the intrinsic clotting, fibrinolytic, and kinin-forming systems. Hageman factor (HF), factor XII of the clotting system, is central to the activation of all three systems. HF is activated nonspecifically by a number of agents, including exposure to crude preparations of collagen, vascular basement membranes, monosodium urate crystals, calcium pyrophosphate crystals, and endotoxin. Negatively charged surfaces also activate HF. Upon activation, HF (an 80,000 dalton β globulin) is cleaved, and its active form HF_A initiates the conversion of factor XI of the clotting pathway to XIa, and the conversion of prekallikrein to kallikrein. Kallikrein in turn activates plasminogen forming plasmin, an enzyme important in fibrinolysis. Kallikrein also cleaves a serum protein termed high molecular weight kininogen to form bradykinin, a nonapeptide with potent biologic activities. Interestingly, C1 esterase inhibitor (C1INH), a protein which functions as an inhibitor of activated C1, is also an important inhibitor of HF_A and kallikrein. Bradykinin and two other kinins produced by tissue kallikreins from kininogen induce smooth muscle contraction, increase vascular permeability, and induce pain. Cleavage of fibrinogen by plasmin results in the production of a number of products, including fibrinopeptide B, an agent which potentiates the action of bradykinin and has chemotactic activity for neutrophils in vitro.

Interleukins. Interleukins are immunoregulatory molecules synthesized by mononuclear leukocytes. Stimulation of macrophages by antigens as well as by factors from lymphocytes initiates the secretion of interleukin I (IL-1), a 15,000-dalton peptide with diverse biologic activities. Macrophages are required for many of the activities of lymphocytes, and certain of the "helper" functions of macrophages are mediated by IL-1. IL-1 may be identical to a factor termed mononuclear cell factor (MCF) which stimulates synovial cells to produce collagenase. IL-1 may also be identical to leukocytic pyrogen.

Interleukin 2 (IL-2), previously termed T-cell growth factor, is a 15,000-dalton polypeptide produced by T lymphocytes and stimulates the continuous proliferation of activated T lymphocytes in culture. Another class of mediators produced by stimulated lymphocytes is the lymphokines. These are discussed later in this chapter under the heading Inflammatory Reactions Initiated by Mononuclear Leukocytes.

LYSOSOMAL ENZYMES. Lysosomal enzymes are contained in a class of subcellular organelles termed lysosomal granules. One function of these enzymes is digestive in that they break down complex macromolecules. Lysosomal granules also contain antimicrobial constituents such as myeloperoxidase and lactoferrin. Leukocytes contain two types of lysosomal granules based on staining characteristics. These are termed the azurophilic and specific granules. Lysosomal enzymes play an important role in the digestion of antigens following phagocytosis. However, since these enzymes may also be released during phagocytosis or upon cell death, they can cause tissue destruction which sometimes accompanies inflammatory reactions. Lysosomal proteases found in leukocytes include collagenase, elastase, cathepsin D, and cathepsin G. These enzymes are capable of destroying extracellular structures and may thus participate in mediating tissue injury in the rheumatic diseases. Cathepsin D cleaves cartilage proteoglycan, whereas granulocyte collagenase is active in cleaving Type I and, to a lesser degree, Type III collagen substrates found in bone, cartilage, and tendon. The substrates of granulocyte elastase include collagen crosslinkages and proteoglycans, as well as the elastin components of blood vessels, ligaments, and cartilage. Lysosomal hydrolyases are also capable of producing mediators of inflammation through their direct action on C components such as C5, thereby producing C5a. Leukocytic hydrolyases can liberate kinin from kininogen. Plasminogen activator, an enzyme that converts plasminogen to plasmin (which stimulates fibrinolysis) is found in both granulocyte and macrophage lysosomes. Rheumatoid synovial collagenase is usually present as an inactive lysosomal proenzyme which requires plasminogen activator for conversion to its active form.

Regulation of the potent tissue destructive potential of the lysosomal proteases is mediated by protease inhibitors such as α_2 macroglobulin and α_1 antiprotease. These antiproteases are present in serum and in synovial fluids and inhibit protease enzymes by binding to them and covering their active sites.

PHYSIOLOGIC MECHANISMS OF INFLAMMATORY CELL ACCUMULATION

The accumulation of inflammatory cells at sites of antigen is central to the inflammatory process. Polymorphonuclear leukocytes and macrophages are motile cells which have many common physiologic characteristics. Both can perceive gradients of chemoattractant molecules and migrate directionally along such gradients. They also perform endocytosis (ingestion), secrete lysosomal enzymes, and generate superoxide anions (see Ch. 148). Polymorphonuclear leukocytes and macrophages perceive chemotactic factors by means of specific surface receptors. These cells have receptors for synthetic polypeptide chemotactic factors which may be analogous to bacterial products, as well as for C5a, CCF and LTB_4. Binding of chemoattractants to the surface of phagocytes results in orientation of the cells toward the source of the chemotactic gradient. Upon orientation, the cells lose their round configuration and become polarized in shape. The configuration of motile cells is triangular, with the base of the triangle facing toward the chemoattractant gradient (Fig. 442–2). This change in cell shape requires rearrangement of intracellular cytoskeletal elements. Microtubules provide a front-to-back polarization, whereas actin filaments accumulate at the front and back of the cells and provide the contractile forces required for movement. Chemotactic factors can also initiate other cellular responses by leukocytes, such as superoxide anion production and lysosomal enzyme secretion. The concentration of chemotactic factors required to initiate these latter processes approximately ten fold is greater than that required for the induction of chemotaxis. This phenomenon may prevent the release of potentially toxic products from the cells until they arrive at the inflammatory site where the concentration of chemoattractants is the greatest.

The mechanism by which chemotactic factors initiate their biologic responses in phagocytes is not entirely clear at present, but it is known that these factors induce transmembrane fluxes of calcium, sodium, and potassium which alter cellular transmembrane potential. Following exposure to chemotactic factors, there is a transient elevation of cAMP. Arachidonic acid is released from phospholipids in the phagocytic cell membrane through activation of phospholipases. Metabolism of arachidonic acid via enzymatic pathways involving cyclooxygenase and lipoxygenase results in the production of prostaglandins and leukotrienes. Transmethylation reactions mediated by S-adenosylmethionine are required for chemotaxis but methylation of phosphatidylethanolamine is inhibited by chemotactic factors in macrophages. This results in changes in the composition of newly synthesized phospholipids in cells exposed to chemoattractants. Alterations in the phospholipid composition

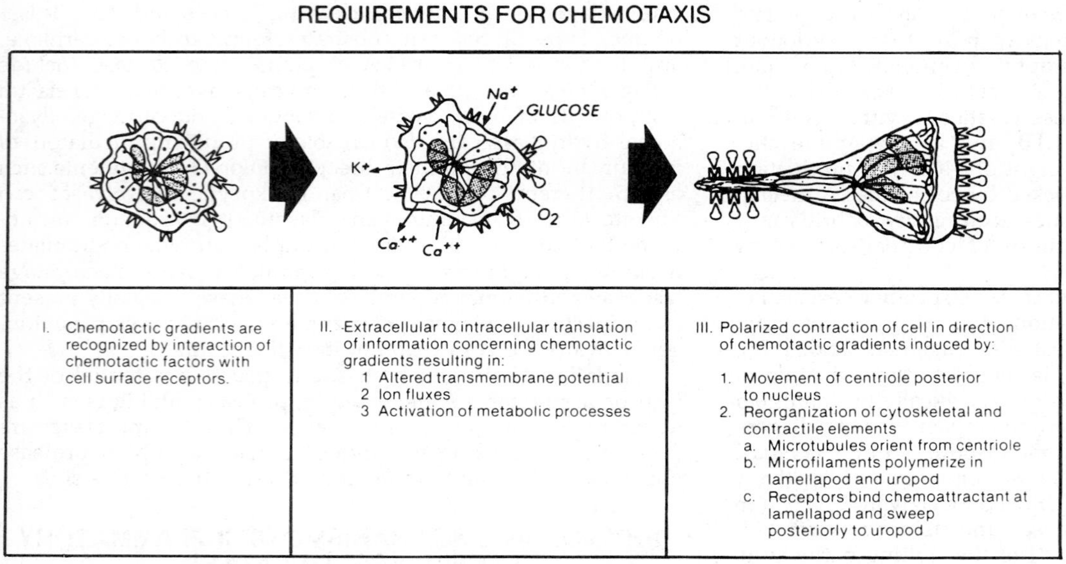

REQUIREMENTS FOR CHEMOTAXIS
Na^+
GLUCOSE
K^+
O_2
Ca^{++} Ca^{++}
I. Chemotactic gradients are recognized by interaction of chemotactic factors with cell surface receptors.
II. Extracellular to intracellular translation of information concerning chemotactic gradients resulting in:
1 Altered transmembrane potential
2 Ion fluxes
3 Activation of metabolic processes
III. Polarized contraction of cell in direction of chemotactic gradients induced by:
1. Movement of centriole posterior to nucleus
2. Reorganization of cytoskeletal and contractile elements
a. Microtubules orient from centriole
b. Microfilaments polymerize in lamellapod and uropod
c. Receptors bind chemoattractant at lamellapod and sweep posteriorly to uropod

Figure 442–2. The interaction of chemotactic factor receptors with chemotactic factors triggers the indicated cellular responses.

of the membrane at the leading edge of the chemotactically stimulated cells may be important for motility and for the activation of membrane associated enzymes such as protein kinase C. Lymphocytes are also highly motile cells but do not respond to the same chemotactic factors as do polymorphonuclear leukocytes and macrophages. The migration of lymphocytes is stimulated by specific antigens, mitogens, and by as yet undefined factors produced by lymphocytes.

Phagocytosis is initiated by binding of a particle to the surface of phagocytic cells. Particles carrying bound immunoglobulin or the complement fragments C3b or C3bi are more readily phagocytosed since they bind to Fc and C3b receptors on both polymorphonuclear leukocytes and macrophages. However, phagocytosis can occur in the absence of receptor involvement. Particle ingestion results from the envelopment and fusion of phagocytic cell membrane around the foreign material (Fig. 442–3). Intracellular lysosomes migrate to the phagocytic vesicle, fuse with it, and empty their contents, thus forming a phagolysosome. Within the phagolysosome, antigenic digestion and microbial killing generally occur. During the process of phagocytosis, lysosomal hydrolases and toxic oxygen radicals may be released.

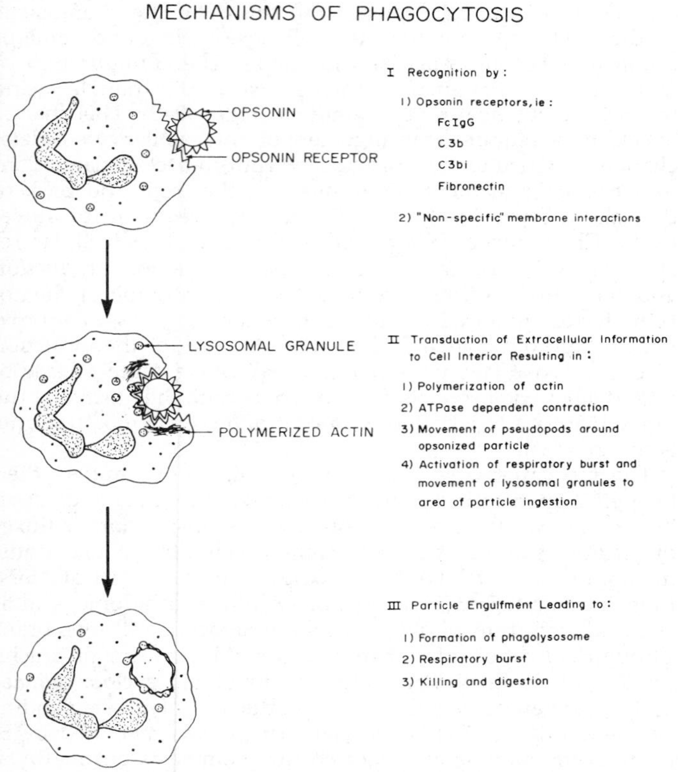

MECHANISMS OF PHAGOCYTOSIS
OPSONIN
OPSONIN RECEPTOR
I Recognition by:
1) Opsonin receptors, ie:
FcIgG
C3b
C3bi
Fibronectin
2) "Non-specific" membrane interactions
LYSOSOMAL GRANULE
POLYMERIZED ACTIN
II Transduction of Extracellular Information to Cell Interior Resulting in:
1) Polymerization of actin
2) ATPase dependent contraction
3) Movement of pseudopods around opsonized particle
4) Activation of respiratory burst and movement of lysosomal granules to area of particle ingestion
III Particle Engulfment Leading to:
1) Formation of phagolysosome
2) Respiratory burst
3) Killing and digestion

Figure 442–3. Requirements for phagocytosis. Particulate antigen binding to the membrane of phagocytic cells initiates cellular responses which lead to envelopment of the antigen. The process is enhanced when the antigens have bound opsonins.

IMMUNOLOGICALLY MEDIATED TISSUE INJURY

Inflammatory responses can produce adverse reactions in the host, ranging from minor local tissue irritation to selective destruction of organs or even sudden death. The nature of immunologically mediated inflammatory responses depends upon the immunologic recognition component which identifies the antigen. Four general types of immunologically mediated inflammatory reactions have been defined (Table 442–2). In clinical and experimental situations it is not infrequent to have more than one, and even all types, of these immune reactions operative simultaneously.

TYPE I REACTIONS: INFLAMMATION INITIATED BY REAGENIC (IgE) ANTIBODIES. IgE antibodies bind to mast cells and basophils by means of their Fc portion, which allows the Fab portion of the molecule to be available for binding to specific antigen. Shortly after the appropriate antigen binds, the cells degranulate and secrete their intracellular products, which include histamine, ECF-A, and heparin. Release of mediators from basophils or mast cells causes an increase in local vascular permeability within seconds and produces vascular stasis and smooth muscle contraction. Type I reactions are responsible for such allergic phenomena as urticaria, seasonal rhinitis, asthma, and systemic anaphylaxis (see Ch. 431 to 434).

TYPE II REACTIONS: TISSUE DESTRUCTION MEDIATED BY CYTOTOXIC ANTIBODY. The development of antibody to antigens on the surface of a host's own cells can lead to tissue destruction. Injury results from the binding of C-fixing antibodies to host tissue cells. Activation of the C cascade leads to the release of inflammatory mediators and the accumulation of inflammatory cells. Release of lysosomal enzymes and toxic oxygen radicals by inflammatory cells and direct cytolysis of target cells through C action contribute to tissue destruction. An example of a human disease resulting from the development of antibody directed toward self tissues is Goodpasture's syndrome (see Ch. 62). The result of antibody deposition is the explosive

TABLE 442–2. TYPES OF IMMUNOLOGICALLY MEDIATED INFLAMMATION

Type of Inflammation	Recognition Component	Soluble Mediator	Inflammatory Response	Disease Example
I. Reagenic, allergic	IgE	Basophil and mast cell products (i.e., histamine, SRS, ECF)	Immediate flare and wheal, smooth muscle constriction	Atopy, anaphylaxis
II. Cytotoxic antibody	IgG, IgM	Complement	Lysis or phagocytosis of circulating antigens, acute inflammation in tissues	Autoimmune hemolytic anemia, thrombocytopenia associated with systemic lupus erythematosus
III. Immune complex	IgG, IgM	Complement	Accumulation of polymorphonuclear leukocytes and macrophages	Rheumatoid arthritis, lupus erythematosus
IV. Delayed hypersensitivity	T lymphocytes	Cytokines	Mononuclear cell infiltrate	Tuberculosis, sarcoidosis, polymyositis, granulomatosis, vasculitis

onset of hemorrhagic pneumonitis and rapidly progressive glomerulonephritis. Spontaneous development of antibody to tissues is frequently seen in certain rheumatologic disorders, particularly systemic lupus erythematosus. Autoimmune hemolytic anemia occurs following the deposition of C-fixing antibodies plus C3 cleavage products on circulating red blood cells. As a consequence of this, the cells are rapidly destroyed either by macrophages in the reticuloendothelial system (particularly in the spleen) or, less commonly, by intravascular hemolysis mediated by C. Also common in individuals with systemic lupus erythematosus is idiopathic thrombocytopenic purpura, in which antibody develops against platelet antigens. This leads to thrombocytopenia owing to the rapid clearance of platelets by the reticuloendothelial system.

TYPE III REACTIONS: INFLAMMATION INITIATED BY IMMUNE COMPLEXES. The formation or deposition of certain types of immune complexes in local tissues produces an inflammatory response characterized by the accumulation of polymorphonuclear leukocytes within hours, followed by the influx of macrophages. Several mechanisms exist by which immune complexes initiate this reaction. The combination of IgM or IgG (subclasses 1, 2 or 3) antibodies with antigen leads to the binding and activation of the first component of C. As a result of this activation, C4 and C2 are cleaved and activated, and then C3 is cleaved into two fragments. The large fragment (C3b) binds to the immune complex; the small fragment (C3a) diffuses away from the immune reaction. C3a enhances vascular permeability, contracts venular smooth muscle, and degranulates mast cells and basophils. Diffusion of C3a from the site of the immunologic reaction toward nearby blood vessels initiates early events of the acute inflammatory response. Cleavage of the next component of complement, C5, releases the extremely potent inflammatory polypeptide C5a. Diffusion of C5a from the site of immunologic reactions establishes a gradient of this chemoattractant, the highest concentrations being at the site of the immune complex deposition itself. Polymorphonuclear leukocytes and macrophages detect this gradient by means of receptors for C5a and migrate to the site of immune complex deposition. Upon arrival at the site of immune complex formation, Fc and C3b receptors enhance complex binding to the phagocytic cells, and phagocytosis ensues (see Fig. 442–3).

If the amount of immune complex deposited locally is not great, the material can be phagocytized and digested by polymorphonuclear leukocytes and macrophages without tissue destruction. If the amount of immune complex formation is large or if a significant portion of the immune complexes is lodged in vessel walls, permanent tissue destruction can ensue. Polymorphonuclear leukocytes and macrophages contain abundant lysosomal enzymes and are capable of producing toxic oxygen radicals. In the process of phagocytizing immune complexes, particularly when these complexes are not easily internalized, the cells release their lysosomal enzymes and oxygen radicals externally. Cell death also results in enzyme release. The lysosomal enzymes are than capable of cleaving additional C5, thereby producing more C5a. These processes, when occurring within vessel walls, produce vasculitis and can lead to hemorrhagic necrosis and local tissue destruction.

Tissue damage initiated by C-fixing immune complexes can occur following the formation of antigen-antibody complexes in local tissue sites (an Arthus-type reaction) or in the circulation (a serum sickness reaction).

Serum sickness reactions occur when an individual develops C-fixing antibody to a circulating antigen. As antibody is produced, antigen-antibody complexes form in the circulation. During the early phase of antibody synthesis, the amount of antibody available for binding is small so that the complexes are formed in a setting of great antigen excess. Such complexes are not pathogenic. As antibody production increases, usually by seven days after antigenic exposure, the immune complexes become larger and the ratio of antigen to antibody decreases. When the complexes are in slight antigen excess, they tend to be deposited in the walls of small blood vessels, where they initiate inflammatory lesions. Palpable purpuric skin lesions (leukocytoclastic vasculitis), arthritis, glomerulitis, and fever, as well as depressed serum C levels, are common clinical manifestations. As antibody production continues, the remaining immune complexes in the circulation increase in size and are rapidly cleared by the reticuloendothelial organs. If the exposure to antigen ceases, the illness resolves. Examples of both types of inflammation initiated by immune complexes are common in rheumatic diseases such as rheumatoid arthritis and systemic lupus erythematosus (SLE).

Certain animals develop spontaneous immune complex diseases that bear striking similarities to human SLE. By studying such animals, a great deal has been learned about the immunopathology of human autoimmune diseases. The F_1 hybrid cross between New Zealand Black (NZB) and New Zealand White (NZW) mice (NZB/W F_1) develops an immunologic disorder characterized by the development of circulating antibody to nuclear proteins, glomerulonephritis, autoimmune hemolytic anemia, and vasculitis. In contrast to the NZB/W F_1 hybrids, NZB mice develop severe autoimmune hemolytic anemia but insignificant glomerulonephritis. NZW mice do not develop spontaneous autoimmune disease.

NZB/W disease illustrates the contribution of genetic, immunologic, and infectious factors to the production of a spontaneous immune complex disease. Genetically, multiple autosomal genes appear to be involved. Immunologically, the animals have heightened B cell responsiveness and depressed T cell suppressor function. The mice produce excessive levels of antibody to many experimental antigens and have a depressed ability to reject skin grafts. The disease itself appears to occur when the NZB/W mice begin to produce unusually large amounts of antibody to Gross leukemia virus, an agent that infects many normal mouse strains but usually produces no disease. In the NZB/W mice, however, antigen-antibody complexes develop and deposit in a granular "lumpy-bumpy" immunofluorescent pattern in the renal glomerulus, leading to immune complex–induced glomerulonephritis. The formation of circulating immune complexes causes a fall in the serum C titer, and a systemic vasculitis occurs.

Recently, mice with genetic backgrounds quite different from those of NZB/W have also been shown to develop spontaneous immune complex disease. MRL and BXSB animals develop an illness characterized by circulating immune complexes, depressed serum C, and immune complex nephritis. A single mutant gene termed lpr found in these mice appears to be responsible for autoimmune disease. As in the NZB/W mice, one of the antigens appears to be an oncornavirus protein. Interestingly, mice of the MRL strain differ from the NZB/W F_1 in that they produce antibody to a nuclear antigen termed Sm. This type of antibody has been previously found only in humans with SLE. The immune defect in MRL mice is associated with increased helper T cell activity and elaboration of a T cell factor that stimulates B cells.

The requirement for a genetic predisposition along with exposure to the appropriate infectious agent or other environmental factor is also likely in human SLE. Recent studies have demonstrated that humans with SLE usually share similar histocompatibility antigens at the DR locus. Moreover, abnormal T cell suppressor function is seen not only in patients with this disease but also in family members. There are numerous other examples of human illnesses that appear to occur secondary to the development of either circulating or localized immune complexes. These include certain adverse reactions to drugs, hypersensitivity pneumonitis, and reactions to viruses such as hepatitis B virus.

TYPE IV REACTIONS: INFLAMMATORY REACTIONS INITIATED BY MONONUCLEAR LEUKOCYTES. Recognition of antigen by lymphocytes initiates a different type of inflammatory reaction than does antibody, manifested in the kinetics of inflammation and in the types of cells that accumulate. Lymphocyte-initiated inflammatory reactions are termed "delayed hypersensitivity" because maximal inflammatory cell accumulation does not appear for 48 to 72 hours after secondary antigenic exposure. For example, if an individual previously sensitized to the tubercle bacillus is injected locally with antigen from this organism, a delayed type of inflammatory response ensues. The foreign material is encountered first by macrophages, which partially digest and alter the antigen. This altered form of antigen is recognized by small lymphocytes that contain specific surface receptors for the antigen. Exposure to the antigen initiates synthesis and release of cytokines (Table 442–3). Lymphokines diffuse from the lymphocytes to areas of the vessel wall closest to the immunologic event. Increased vascular permeability ensues; chemotactic gradients that attract macrophages and other lymphocytes result in inflammatory cell accumulation. Small numbers of granulocytes precede the mononuclear cell influx, but the number of these cells is far less than that seen in the inflammatory response mediated by immune complexes. Lymphokines also activate the macrophages, which become more metabolically active, develop higher levels of hydrolytic enzymes, and are better able to bind to and destroy tumor cells or many intracellular parasites.

TABLE 442–3. EFFECTOR MOLECULES (CYTOKINES) RELEASED BY MONONUCLEAR LEUKOCYTES

Lymphocyte Products (Lymphokines)	Function
Macrophage activating factor (MAF)*	Macrophage activation
Lymphocyte-derived chemotactic factors (LDCF)	Chemotactic factors for monocytes, granulocytes, and fibroblasts
Lymphotoxin	Target cell lysis
Interferon-δ	Antiviral activity, immunoregulation
Connective tissue activating peptide I (CTAP-I)	Enhances glycosaminoglycan synthesis by synovial cells
Osteoclast activating factor (OAF)	Bone resorption
Interleukin II (IL-II, T cell growth factor)	T lymphocyte replication
Monocyte Products (Monokines)	**Function**
Lymphocyte activating factor (LAF, interleukin I (IL-I)	Lymphocyte activation for blastogenesis, leukocytic pyrogen
Mononuclear cell factor (MCF), probably identical to IL-I	Stimulates synovial dendritic cells to produce collagenase
Monocyte-derived chemotactic factor	Leukocyte accumulation
Prostaglandins	Immunoregulation, bone resorption, enhances vascular permeability
Lysosomal hydrolases	Proteolytic functions
Complement components	Inflammatory mediators

*MAF is probably identical to interferon-δ.

Lymphocytes at the inflammatory site undergo blastogenesis and release lymphokines which recruit other nonsensitized lymphocytes, thus expanding the clones of cells capable of recognizing and responding to the specific antigen. If successful in complete destruction of the antigen, the inflammatory response resolves and produces no tissue necrosis. The inflammatory process continues, however, if the antigen is large in quantity or is difficult to digest, as are the waxes of the tubercle bacillus, or if the antigen is an organism resistant to phagocytic destruction. New cells arrive to replace the dying cells already present at the site, resulting in the release of proteolytic enzymes and toxic oxygen radicals. Lesions typical of delayed hypersensitivity reactions are seen in mycobacterial and fungal diseases, sarcoidosis, and a number of rheumatologic disorders, including polymyositis and the granulomatous vasculitides.

MECHANISM OF TISSUE DESTRUCTION IN RHEUMATOID ARTHRITIS

One can construct models which describe how the joint and its surrounding structures are injured by immunologic reactions in rheumatoid arthritis. Similar models can be devised for other rheumatic diseases, the differences largely relating to the location and type of the inflammatory reactions. In most instances a combination of types of immune reactions contributes to the tissue destruction.

The characteristic tissue reaction in rheumatoid arthritis is the development of synovitis, in which the normally thin, loose connective tissue is replaced by a rich infiltrate of lymphocytes, macrophages, and plasma cells (see Fig. 442–1*B*). In the synovial fluid, the predominant inflammatory cells are the polymorphonuclear leukocytes. The cells which have infiltrated the synovia are metabolically active; the plasma cells produce rheumatoid factors, and the mononuclear cells produce cytokines. Rheumatoid factors are immunoglobulins of the IgM, IgG, or, rarely, IgA class. These factors bind to the Fc portion of IgG antibodies, which either have combined with antigen or have been aggregated or denatured. Polymorphonuclear leukocytes taken from synovial fluids contain inclusions of immune complexes, many of which contain rheumatoid factors. Synovial fluid C levels are depressed in relation to the serum C level. The turnover of C components, particularly components of the classic pathway, is markedly enhanced in rheumatoid synovial fluid. Cleavage products such as C5a are present in rheumatoid synovial fluid, as are hydrolytic enzymes derived from inflammatory cells, kinins and LTB_4.

The sequence of events leading to the development of synovitis and destruction of surrounding structures in rheumatoid arthritis can be envisioned as follows: some as yet undefined antigen localizes in the synovium and is phagocytized by the Type A synovial cells. One can assume that the antigen is not completely destroyed, so that a partially digested form persists and diffuses into the synovial fluid. Binding of the processed antigen to B lymphocytes induces their differentiation to plasma cells, which then produce antibodies and rheumatoid factors upon chronic stimulation. Antigen activation of T lymphocytes triggers lymphokine synthesis followed by blastogenesis. The role of viruses as stimulators of the immune response in rheumatoid arthritis must be considered. Rheumatoid synovial explant cells established in permanent lines exhibit many characteristics of virally transformed lymphocytes. Cell lines of the

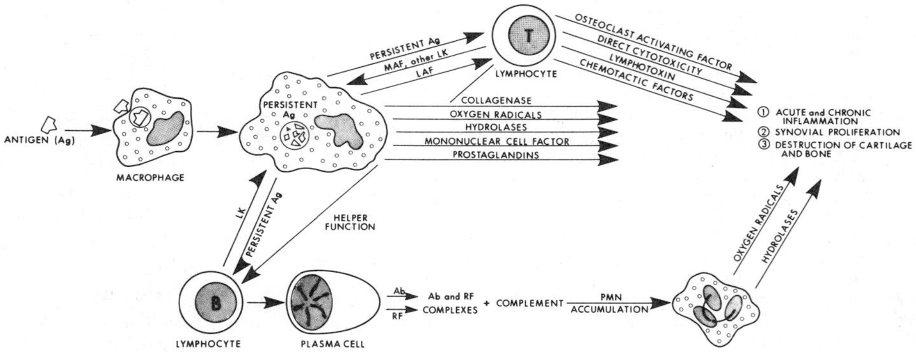

Figure 442–4. Model for the pathogenesis of articular inflammation in rheumatoid arthritis. Ab = antibody, LAF = lymphocyte activating factor, LK = lymphokines, MAF = macrophage activating factor, RF = rheumatoid factor.

B lymphocyte variety frequently contain antigens of the Epstein-Barr virus (EBV). This finding is interesting in that sera from approximately 65 per cent of patients with rheumatoid arthritis contain antibody, called a rheumatoid arthritis precipitin (RAP), which is directed at certain nuclear antigens present in human lymphoblastoid cell lines infected with EBV. The antigens have been termed rheumatoid arthritis nuclear antigens (RANAs). RANAs are found only in B lymphoblastoid cell lines, whose genomes contain the EBV genome, but no infectious viral particles are produced. RAPs are commonly present in the sera of patients who are rheumatoid factor positive but are also found in the sera of patients who are rheumatoid factor negative. The specificity of RAPs for rheumatoid arthritis has been questioned, as RAPs can be present in up to 20 per cent of normal individuals. In rheumatoid arthritis, there is no firm evidence to relate EBV causally to the disease, and serum antibody levels to EBV are not increased in the sera of rheumatoid arthritis patients. However, EBV does act as a polyclonal stimulator of antibody production and increases the mitogenic activity of lymphocytes. Regardless of the initiating agent, combination of antibody with antigen, as well as combination of antigen-antibody complexes with rheumatoid factors, or self-association of rheumatoid factors, activates C as well as the kinin-forming system by means of activating Hageman factor. This results in the production of inflammatory products such as C5a, arachidonic acid metabolites, kinins, and fibrinopeptides, which diffuse into the synovial fluid and to synovial blood vessels. These phlogistic agents enhance vascular permeability and attract polymorphonuclear leukocytes and macrophages. Polymorphonuclear leukocytes ingest the abundant immune complexes in the fluid, release lysosomal enzymes, and generate superoxide anions. This causes destruction of hyaluronate polymers in the joint fluid, as well as injury to cartilage. Cytokine production in the synovium leads to the further accumulation of macrophages, fibroblasts, and additional lymphocytes.

The unique structure of the joint space is important, as enzymes present in synovial fluid or released and synthesized locally by the cells constituting the proliferative synovial lesion contribute to the pathology evident in articular structures. The cartilage-degrading lysosomal enzymes collagenase and elastase are primarily derived from inflammatory cells. Proteinases released by dying cells may aid in superficial cartilage destruction by virtue of their role in uncrosslinking collagen fibrils, thus increasing their susceptibility to enzymatic degradation. Macrophages in the synovium produce prostaglandins, hydrolytic enzymes, collagenase, plasminogen activator, and IL-1. The synovial cell that is the most abundant source of collagenase in the rheumatoid synovium is one which has an unusual dendritic appearance and is adherent to glass but is nonphagocytic. Collagenase synthesis by this cell is greatly enhanced in the presence of IL-1 (mononuclear cell factor). With ongoing synovitis, early changes in cartilage involve the loss of proteoglycan content, often manifested microscopically as diminished metachromatic staining. In addition to collagenases, lysosomal proteinases can degrade aggregates of proteoglycans, and, once released from cartilage, these solubilized components are then sensitive to further enzymatic attack.

The final stage of the destructive process, demineralization of bone, may result from combined elements present initially in the inflammatory and later in the proliferative responses. Demineralization must occur in bone before this tissue is susceptible to collagenolytic enzymes. In rheumatoid synovitis, prostaglandins stimulate calcium release from bone matrix; other arachidonic acid metabolites are responsible for long-term leaching of mineral from bony matrix. In addition, bone demineralization is enhanced by heparin, which is released upon the degranulation of mast cells. Cellular mechanisms may also be operative in demineralization in that lymphocytes produce an osteoclast activating factor (OAF). In addition, connective tissue activating peptides (CTAPs) and specific lymphokines such as lymphocyte-derived chemotactic factor for fibroblasts (LDCF-F) attract and stimulate fibroblasts to produce collagen and may contribute to the ultimate fibrosis evident in the destroyed ankylosed joint.

The net effect, resulting from either persistence of antigen or disordered regulation of T and B cell activation, is a chronic inflammatory response in the synovium (Fig. 442–4). Continued cellular proliferation and influx lead to synovial proliferation and its invasion into surrounding structures. Diffusion of collagenase, PGEs, hydrolytic enzymes, and lymphokines into cartilage and bone results in erosion of these tissues. Rheumatoid arthritis thus illustrates the devastating local tissue destruction that results from chronic inflammatory reactions produced by the immune complex and delayed hypersensitivity types of immune responses.

Alspaugh MA, Tan EM: Serum antibody in rheumatoid arthritis reactive with a cell associated antigen. Demonstration by precipitation and immunofluorescence. Arthritis Rheum 19:711, 1976. *The initial description of rheumatoid arthritis precipitins.*

Bomalaski JS, Williamson PK, Zurier RB: Prostaglandins and the inflammatory response. Clin Lab Med 3(4):695, 1983. A detailed review of the role of prostaglandins in inflammation.

Dayer JM, Krane SM: The interaction of immunocompetent cells and chronic inflammation as exemplified by rheumatoid arthritis. Clin Rheum Dis 4:517, 1978. *An overview of cellular interactions in the generation of destructive rheumatoid synovitis.*

Kaplan AP: The intrinsic coagulation, fibrinolytic, and kinin-forming pathways of man. *In* Kelley WN, Harris ED, Ruddy S, Sledge CB (eds.): Textbook of Rheumatology, Vol. 1. Philadelphia, W. B. Saunders Co., 1981, pp 97–119. *A complete review of the Hageman factor–dependent pathways, including those that lead to kinin generation.*

McPhail LC, Snyderman R: Oxygen-dependent microbicidal activity of leukocytes. *In* Snyderman R (ed): Contemporary Topics in Immunobiology, Vol. 14. "Regulation of Leukocyte Function." New York, Plenum Press, 1984, pp 247–281. *A comprehensive overview of oxygen metabolism in phagocytes.*

Pisetsky DS, Caster SA, Roths JB, Murphy ED: *lpr* gene control of the anti-DNA antibody response. J Immunol 128:2322, 1982. *Evidence concerning the genetic regulation of anti DNA-antibody production and an autoimmune disease is presented.*

Samuelsson B: The leukotrienes: An introduction. *In* Samuelsson B, Paoletti R (eds.): Leukotrienes and Other Lipoxygenase Products. New York, Raven Press, 1982, pp 1–27. *An excellent review of the biochemistry of the leukotrienes and their potential biological roles.*

Smith HR, Steinberg AD: Autoimmunity—a perspective. *In* Paul WE, Fathman EG, Metzgar H (eds.): Annual Review of Immunology, Vol. 1. Palo Alto,

Annual Reviews Inc., 1983, pp 175–210. *A very readable review of human and animal autoimmune disease mechanisms. Many references.*

Snyderman R, Goetzl EJ: Molecular and cellular mechanisms of leukocyte chemotaxis. Science 213:830, 1981. *A thorough review of the mechanisms of leukocyte responses to chemotactic factors.*

Snyderman R, Pike MC: Transductional mechanisms of chemoattractant receptors on leukocytes. *In* Snyderman R (ed.): Contemporary Topics in Immunobiology, Vol. 14. "Regulation of Leukocyte Function." New York, Plenum Press, 1984, pp 1–28. *An up-to-date review of the biochemistry and biology of chemotactic factors and their receptors on leukocytes. Many references on inflammatory mechanisms.*

Theofilopoulos AN, Dixon FJ: Etiopathogenesis of murine SLE. Immunol Rev 55:179, 1981. *Interesting concepts and a good review of animal models of systemic lupus erythematosus.*

Theofilopoulos AN, Dixon FJ: Immune complexes in human diseases. Am J Pathol 100:531, 1980. *A comprehensive review of the role of immune complexes in human diseases.*

Wasserman SI: Mediators of immediate hypersensitivity. J Allergy Clin Immunol 72(2):101, 1983. *An exposition of the physiologic aspects of immediate types of hypersensitivity reactions.*

Weissmann G: Pathways of arachidonate oxidation to prostaglandins and leukotrienes. Sem Arth Rheu 13:123, 1983. *A recent review of arachidonate metabolism and its relevance to inflammation.*

Weissmann G, Smolen JE, Korchak HM: Release of inflammatory mediators from stimulated neutrophils. N Engl J Med 303:27, 1980. *A good update on the mechanisms of secretion by leukocytes.*

Wooley DE, Harris ED Jr, Mainardi CL, Brinckerhoff CE: Collagenase immunolocalization in cultures of rheumatoid synovial cells. Science 200:773, 1978. *This article stresses the importance of the dendritic cell as a source of collagenase in rheumatoid synovium.*

Ziff M: Pathophysiology of rheumatoid arthritis. Fed Proc 32:131, 1973. *A classic review of the pioneering work dealing with the immunology of rheumatoid arthritis.*

Zvaifler NJ: Pathogenesis of the joint disease of rheumatoid arthritis. Am. J. Med. 75:3, 1983. *A review of the role of various components of the immune response in rheumatoid arthritis.*

443. SPECIALIZED DIAGNOSTIC PROCEDURES IN THE RHEUMATIC DISEASES

Alan S. Cohen

An increasing number of specialized procedures are available for evaluation of patients with articular disease. Although many are useful, very few are diagnostic of a specific disorder. Laboratory data must be combined with clinical evaluation in order to arrive at a working diagnosis.

SYNOVIAL FLUID. In the patient with undiagnosed articular disease and an associated joint effusion, examination of the synovial fluid is mandatory. The preferred method of joint aspiration (most frequently the knee) is through the extensor surface, where major blood vessels and nerves are sparse and the synovial pouch is more superficial. If the synovial fluid sugar is to be measured, the patient should have fasted for at least six hours if possible. Careful sterile technique virtually precludes infection, the one very rare complication of arthrocentesis. The needle should be at least 19 gauge. After appropriate draping and intracutaneous instillation of 1 to 2 per cent procaine or Xylocaine, the needle is inserted through skin and subcutaneous tissue. It meets a small amount of resistance when it reaches the capsule and finally passes easily into the joint cavity. Although minimal amounts of fluid will suffice for basic studies, as a rule 10 to 15 ml will allow the necessary laboratory testing.

The synovial fluid is then ideally allocated as follows: (1) an aliquot (1 to 3 ml) in a sterile tube with heparin—for bacteriologic studies (cultures and Gram stain); (2) an aliquot (1 ml) in a clean nonsterile tube with heparin—for routine cytology, white cell count, and differential (can also be used for mucin test and crystal examination); (3) an aliquot (2 to 3 ml) without anticoagulant in a clean nonsterile tube—for color, viscosity, clot turbidity, mucin clot test, crystals, and inclusions (as well as proteins, rheumatoid factors, and complement if indicated); and (4) an aliquot (2 ml) in a clean nonsterile tube with preservative—for glucose analysis with parallel determination of serum glucose.

Cultures must be obtained on all synovial fluids, since indolent infections (bacterial, tuberculous) can mimic or be superimposed on well defined articular disease. Blood agar medium should be used; but if gonococcal infection is suspected, chocolate agar or its equivalent should be inoculated at the bedside. Appropriate cultures should be obtained if tuberculosis is suspected. A direct Gram stain should be performed on a concentrated specimen from the first tube, spun for 20 minutes in a clinical centrifuge.

Normal synovial fluid is a clear pale yellow viscous liquid that does not clot. It was appropriately named by Paracelsus because of its viscosity and physical resemblance to egg white. The few cells normally present (less than 200) are mononuclear. Although serous cavity fluids are plasma ultrafiltrates, synovial fluid is unique owing to the presence of hyaluronic acid (about 0.3 gram per deciliter) produced by the synovial lining cells. This large asymmetric molecule further influences the composition of synovial fluid, for because of its steric structure, some solute passage through the water surrounding the molecules may be hindered. Thus, according to the concept of excluded volume, the size and shape of the molecule plays a large role; i.e., large molecules such as fibrinogen and macroglobulin would be excluded, and small molecules would more easily enter the compartment. The state of hyaluronate (as roughly determined by the mucin clot test) may be a primary determinant of the nature of the synovial fluid in various pathologic conditions.

When a synovial membrane is inflamed for any reason, the white cell count in the synovial fluid increases. In a rough fashion one can classify such fluids into four groups (Table 443–1). Noninflammatory effusions (Group I) occur when the white cell count is normal or minimally increased, as in traumatic arthritis or degenerative joint disease. Only rarely will such fluid have white cell counts of over 2000 cells per cubic millimeter. Noninfectious mildly inflammatory effusions (Group II) with white cell counts rarely over 5000 occur in systemic lupus erythematosus and scleroderma. In noninfectious acute inflammatory effusions (Group III) characteristic of classic rheumatoid arthritis, gout, pseudogout, and rheumatic fever, the white cell count varies from 5000 to 25,000 but may exceed 50,000 or even 100,000 cells per cubic millimeter. Finally, in inflammatory effusions caused by infection (Group IV) the white cell count commonly varies from 25,000 to over 100,000 cells per cubic millimeter and in some instances resembles frank pus. As the white cell count becomes elevated, the percentage of polymorphonuclear leukocytes generally increases, the hyaluronate becomes degraded, and the synovial fluid sugar falls.

Normal synovial fluid does not clot owing to the absence of several clotting factors, including fibrinogen. Pathologic fluids do contain clots, and their size is roughly proportional to the degree of inflammation. Hyaluronate degradation can be roughly assessed by diluting 1 ml of joint fluid with 4 ml of 2 per cent acetic acid solution. When the mucin is normal, a tight ropy mass forms in a clear solution. This is termed a "good" mucin. A softer mass with shreds is a "fair" mucin, whereas a "poor" mucin shows shreds and soft small masses in a turbid solution.

Under normal conditions, the total synovial fluid protein is about one quarter that of the blood. Multiple studies have been performed to assess whether specific fractions might be related to specific disease states, but findings in general are nonspecific. One may conclude that if the synovial fluid total protein is over 2.5 grams per deciliter, the fluid is not normal, and that if it is over 4.5 grams per deciliter, there is significant inflammation.

Rheumatoid factors (antigamma globulins) are also found in the synovial fluid, occasionally when they are absent from the serum. Their presence and presumed local manufacture in the synovial membrane may be of diagnostic value. Antinuclear antibodies have been found not only in the synovial fluids of patients with systemic lupus erythematosus but also in those

TABLE 443–1. SYNOVIAL FLUID ANALYSIS

Diagnosis	Appearance	Total White Cell Count per Cubic Millimeter*	Polymorphonuclear Cells	Mucin Clot Test	Synovial Fluid-Blood Glucose Difference (Mean Milligrams per Deciliter)	Miscellaneous (Crystals, Organisms)
Normal	Clear, pale yellow	0–200 (200)	<10%	Good	No significant difference†	—
Group I (noninflammatory effusions)						
Degenerative joint disease; traumatic arthritis	Clear to slightly turbid	50–4000 (600)	<30%	Good	No significant difference	—
Group II (noninfectious, mildly inflammatory)						
Systemic lupus erythematosus; scleroderma	Clear to slightly turbid	0–9000 (3000)	<20%	Good (occasionally fair)	No significant difference	Occasional LE cell; decreased complement
Group III (noninfectious severe inflammatory effusions)						
Gout	Turbid	100–160,000 (21,000)	~70%	Poor	10	Monosodium urate crystals
Pseudogout	Turbid	50–75,000 (14,000)	~70%	Fair-poor	Not enough data	Calcium pyrophosphate dihydrate crystals
Rheumatoid arthritis	Turbid	250–80,000 (19,000)	~70%	Poor	30	Decreased complement
Group IV (infectious inflammatory effusions)						
Acute bacterial	Very turbid	150–250,000 (80,000)	~90%	Poor	90	Culture positive for gram-positive or gram-negative bacteria
Tuberculosis	Turbid	2500–100,000 (20,000)	~60%	Poor	70	Culture positive for *M. tuberculosis*

*Averages in parentheses.
†Less than 10 mg per deciliter difference.

of patients with rheumatoid arthritis and several other connective tissue diseases. Since DNA, especially in the native form, can be found free in synovial fluids from individuals with a variety of disorders, it is probable that its presence may reflect nonspecific tissue damage.

Complement levels in the synovial fluid depend upon rates of synthesis, catabolism, and local consumption. Analysis of complement components has been utilized not only for diagnosis but for evaluation of prognosis and for determination of the potential for immunologically related factors in the pathogenesis of the synovitis. The most severe depressions in complement factors have occurred in seropositive rheumatoid arthritis patients and in those with systemic lupus erythematosus (SLE). In rheumatoid arthritis the *serum* complement is not depressed, whereas in SLE it is low, in a fashion comparable to that of the synovial fluid. Although C4, C2, and C3 may be depressed in rheumatoid arthritis (when corrected for globulin in synovial fluid), and C3 particularly depressed in SLE, the fact that some persons with gout and bacterial arthritis also have depressed levels makes these determinations less specific. Elevated complement levels have been reported in Reiter's syndrome, gout, and ankylosing spondylitis. Cryoproteins, predominantly of fibrinogen but including cryoglobulins with DNA and IgG, are also found in synovial fluids of patients with rheumatoid arthritis and other types of synovitis, and rheumatoid fluids may contain complexes with Igs, rheumatoid factors, complement, and DNA.

The intense inflammatory activity of various synovial diseases is associated with the presence of a variety of enzymes in the synovial fluid. Some, but not all, investigators have implicated lysosomal enzymes (e.g., myeloperoxidase, lactoferrin, lysozyme, chymotryptic cationic protein) in the process of joint destruction. Collagenase, collagen, and antibodies to collagen have also been extensively studied. Such investigations have advanced our concepts of the pathogenesis of synovitis (especially rheumatoid), but generally measurements of these substances have not reached the routine clinical domain. Other proteins and peptides (C-reactive protein, plasminogen, vasoactive peptides, and oxygen-derived free radicals) have also been measured in synovial fluid, but their precise role in diagnosis is not clear.

Synovial fluid normally contains little lipid, but it demonstrates increased lipid content in rheumatoid effusions. Prostaglandin E_2 appears to be elevated in the fluid of patients with inflammatory synovitis. The glucose content of synovial fluid, which normally approximates that of serum, is markedly diminished in the presence of infection and may show a modest decrease (10 to 30 mg per deciliter) in other inflammatory effusions. Several of these nonspecific parameters are collectively useful in evaluating the degree and type of inflammatory synovitis (Table 443–1).

Several types of crystals have been found in synovial fluids. The two most important are monosodium urate, characteristic of gouty effusions, and calcium pyrophosphate dihydrate (CPPD), characteristic of the effusions of pseudogout (crystal deposition disease). Crystals that cause inflammation are usually 0.5 to 20 μm in length, sparingly soluble in water, and capable of being phagocytized. At the peak of inflammation most are intracellular. Other crystals such as calcium hydroxyapatite, calcium oxalate, cholesterol, and corticosteroid esters may also be associated with inflammatory effusions.

Crystals are demonstrated in synovial fluid (collected without oxalate) by examining a drop of synovial fluid placed on a slide and covered with a thin glass coverslip for examination in the polarizing microscope. Birefringent materials demonstrate two refractive indices when plane polarized light passes through them. The birefringence is termed positive when the crystals (which then appear blue) are aligned parallel to the slow rays of the retardation plate (first-order red plate compensator) and negative when the crystals appear yellow when in parallel alignment (blue when perpendicular). On polarization microscopy the monosodium urate crystals demonstrate strong negative birefringence and are usually long (8 to 10 μm) and needle-like in appearance. They may occur extracellularly or within polymorphonuclear or mononuclear cells. They are almost invariably in effusions associated with acute gout and are virtually diagnostic. They may, however, be present in gouty fluids between attacks. The CPPD crystals are often broader than urate crystals, may show a faint "line" down their center, appear parallelopiped, and in the polarizing microscope exhibit a weak positive birefringence. They have a significant association with acute attacks of arthritis in patients with chondrocalcinosis (articular cartilage calcification).

Under certain circumstances joint fluids, when nontraumatically aspirated, may demonstrate gross blood. One must consider bleeding disorders such as hemophilia, overdosage with anticoagulants, rare lesions such as pigmented villonodular synovitis and joint tumor, as well as neuropathic and traumatic forms of arthritis.

SYNOVIAL MEMBRANE HISTOPATHOLOGY. Synovial membrane is a non–basement membrane–lined, highly vascular structure consisting of several cell types (macrophages, fibroblasts, and possibly intermediate cells). It proliferates extensively during inflammation, such that synovial biopsy is often useful in establishing a diagnosis. The procedure is simple and may be an extension of the synovial fluid aspiration technique, using a wider bore Parker-Pearson needle. A specimen can also be obtained by arthroscopy or open surgical biopsy.

Although in the common rheumatic diseases (rheumatoid arthritis, degenerative joint disease, systemic lupus erythematosus) there are no common pathognomonic synovial membrane findings, the patterns of histologic involvement may be diagnostically useful. For example, severe synovial lining proliferation and especially the presence of lymphoid follicles are characteristic of rheumatoid arthritis, whereas the SLE membrane shows only minimal hyperplasia but may show dense surface fibrin and perivascular mononuclear infiltrates; rarely a pathognomonic hematoxylin body will be seen.

The procedure is very useful in the diagnosis of tuberculosis; the demonstration of an organism in section (or in culture) or a caseating granuloma with giant cells virtually establishes the diagnosis. Other instances in which the synovial biopsy could be helpful include hemochromatosis (in which iron is seen in the synovial lining cell), pigmented villonodular synovitis (villous hypertrophy, hemosiderin deposits with numerous giant cells), tumors (malignant cells in synovium), and ochronosis (fragments of pigmented cartilage in synovium). Although in properly fixed tissue (use of absolute alcohol) one can observe the crystals associated with gout on histologic examination, the procedure is not necessary to establish this diagnosis, since examination of synovial fluid so commonly demonstrates the crystals.

ACUTE PHASE PHENOMENA. The ancient Greeks observed the sedimentation of blood following venesection and used it as a basic diagnostic tool. It was reintroduced by Fahraeus and refined by Westergren, whose method is in common use today. The sedimentation rate is only one, albeit the most popular, of the acute phase phenomena utilized by rheumatologists to follow inflammation in their patients. Acute phase reactions refer to the increases in certain plasma proteins that occur after an extraordinary variety of tissue damage, i.e., toxic, chemical, infectious, inflammatory, or malignant. The functions of most of these proteins are not known, although presumably the damage led to increased protein synthesis in some cases. Only the sedimentation rate and C-reactive protein (CRP) will be briefly discussed here.

The basic measurement in the Westergren sedimentation rate is the rate of fall of erythrocytes in plasma; when rouleaux formation occurs owing primarily to increases in asymmetric proteins such as fibrinogen or macroglobulins (that alter the red cell zeta potential), the red cells sediment more rapidly. The original normal values are a 1 to 3 mm fall in one hour for men and a 4 to 7 mm fall in one hour for women. These levels may be elevated during menses or by certain drugs and appear to increase with aging. The cause of the last-named phenomenon is not clear despite several reports that seem to document it well. Many now accept sedimentation rates of 0 to 10 mm per hour for men and 0 to 15 mm per hour for women and suggest that the values may be as much as 10 mm per hour higher at age 50. Whether these represent changes in serum proteins with aging or undetected disease in the normal person is not yet clear. In the rheumatic diseases, however, the value of this determination is that when elevated (and it is often in the 30 to 100 mm per hour range), it can be an index for following the severity of inflammation and, when falling, for following the response to therapy. In addition, disorders such as temporal arteritis are characteristically associated with sedimentation rates of over 100 mm per hour.

One must be constantly aware, however, of the lack of specificity of this determination and that in selected series highly elevated sedimentation rates (over 100 mg per hour) are more commonly due to infections or malignancies. It is also documented that a small number of patients can have an active rheumatic disease (i.e., rheumatoid arthritis) with a normal sedimentation rate.

The CRP until recently has played little role in the evaluation of rheumatic diseases, although it has been the prototype acute phase reactant—virtually absent in normal conditions and appearing in large quantities in inflammation. It was named for its property of precipitating with pneumococcal cell wall polysaccharide. In recent years it has been isolated and characterized as a pentameric structure, and its molecular weight and primary structure have been determined. It has many homologies with a protein (AP) found uniquely in amyloid disease but is immunologically distinct. The existence and identification of these substances in phylogenetically distinct species add fascination to their role in man and their relation to one another. CRP rises under circumstances (infection, inflammation) similar to those that elevate the erythrocyte sedimentation rate.

The major differences between CRP and erythrocyte sedimentation rate are that CRP rises earlier (in hours), is a rapid indicator of tissue injury or infection, and tends to fall and reflect potential recovery faster. In addition, in uncomplicated systemic lupus erythematosus the CRP generally is only minimally elevated but becomes more clearly elevated in the presence of infection.

RHEUMATOID FACTORS. Fifty years ago, when Cecil and coworkers found high titers of "streptococcal agglutinators" in the sera of some rheumatoid patients, they were actually alluding to rheumatoid factors. Such factors are now defined as antibodies (present largely in the IgM fraction, but in other Ig fractions as well) to determinants of the Fc fragment of numerous animal (especially human and rabbit) IgGs. As antibodies they possess the characteristics of such proteins. They were named when their frequency in the sera of patients with rheumatoid arthritis (about 70 per cent) was observed. They lack both sensitivity and specificity in the detection of rheumatoid syndromes.

Most clinical tests depend upon the detection of IgM antibodies. In such assays particles (red blood cells or latex or bentonite particles) are coated with immunoglobulin G, mixed with the test serum, and observed for appropriate agglutination or flocculation. Various standardization procedures exist as well as different tube dilutions that are interpreted as positive. Internal standardization as well as the use of cross-reference laboratories is important.

The IgM antibody reacts with IgG to form a soluble complex which sediments in the ultracentrifuge with a coefficient of 22. In addition, IgG-IgG complexes sedimenting at an intermediate range can also occur, as well as larger, insoluble IgM-IgG complexes. In some instances the IgM rheumatoid factor is firmly bound to autologous IgG such that it is not detected on routine agglutination tests. Gel filtration under mildly acid conditions dissociates these IgG and IgM fractions. When the rheumatoid factor activity is found in such instances, the term "hidden rheumatoid factor" is sometimes applied.

Rheumatoid factors are uncommon in children with chronic arthritis. High titers have been correlated with severe progressive rheumatoid arthritis in patients with multiple rheumatoid nodules, vasculitis, skin ulcers, and other visceral manifestations. Rheumatoid factors are found in many diseases other than rheumatoid arthritis (other connective tissue diseases, leprosy, leishmaniasis, liver disease, tuberculosis). In some series of subacute bacterial endocarditis 50 per cent of the patients will transiently show rheumatoid factors in their sera. Although family studies of seropositive propositi suggest that there is a higher incidence in its members, epidemiologic use of rheumatoid factors has been of little help in determining the incidence of rheumatoid arthritis, since it may so often mark parasitic or infectious disease.

Since rheumatoid factors have been induced experimentally with bacterial antigens and since they are so commonly associated with chronic infectious diseases, the concept that an as yet unknown infectious agent or agents may play a pathogenetic role in rheumatoid disease is still under active investigation. Data thus far suggest that rheumatoid factor is an epiphenomenon and not a direct cause of rheumatoid arthritis.

The absence of rheumatoid factors in well defined groups of rheumatoid variants has led to the classification of seronegative spondyloarthritis for disorders such as psoriatic arthritis, ankylosing spondylitis, forms of juvenile chronic polyarthritis, and Reiter's syndrome.

ANTINUCLEAR ANTIBODIES AND THE LE CELL. The discovery of the LE cell by Hargraves in 1948 and subsequent studies demonstrating a lupus factor that reacted with nuclear material opened the door to a series of immunologic investigations that have led to new concepts of pathogenesis, diagnosis, and clinical course of systemic lupus erythematosus (SLE) and related disorders. The LE factor was initially regarded as a 7S immunoglobulin, but it is now known that this is only one of many autoantibodies in lupus sera, and that these occur in all immunoglobulin classes, although most are IgG's.

The evolution of this field is such that contradictory statements often appear concerning the role of autoantibodies in the immunopathogenesis of the disease, their diagnostic value, and clinical relevance in patient follow-up. The list of reported nuclear, cytoplasmic, and cell membrane antigens is long and somewhat confused by different methods of testing. We are concerned here only with those that are generally accepted and will take note of several new developments.

The prototype LE cell is a phagocytic polymorphonuclear cell containing (on Wright's stain) a homogeneous purple nuclear inclusion surrounded by a rim of cytoplasm and a compressed nucleus. It is produced in vitro from blood samples but can be found on direct examination of synovial, pleural, peritoneal, and pericardial fluid. It represents phagocytized deoxyribonucleoprotein (DNA-histone complex) and has as its tissue equivalent the isolated hematoxylin body. It has a high association with SLE. The LE cell can be present in other connective tissue diseases. However, it has a low sensitivity, is technically a time-consuming test and has been largely replaced by other immunologic procedures.

The next developments in the identification of antigen-antibody complexes involved complement fixation and precipitation tests, or particles (latex, bentonite, or red blood cells) coated with antigen which agglutinated on exposure to antibody. However, the fluorescence of isolated nuclear constituents or cells (especially the nuclei) on tissue slides after exposure to test sera was found to provide the most practical method for defining these antigen-antibody interactions (antinuclear antibodies) in a simple and reproducible fashion (Table 443–2). A homogeneous pattern of nuclear fluorescence indicates the presence of an antideoxyribonucleoprotein (LE cell factor), a peripheral (rim) pattern suggests the presence of anti-DNA antibody, and the speckled pattern reflects a variety of anti-acidic nuclear proteins. By appropriate dilution of sera, titers

TABLE 443–2. AUTOANTIBODIES TO DNA AND HISTONES

Antibody Reactive with	Clinical Association
Double-strand DNA only	SLE. Rare cases reported.
Double/single-strand DNA with reaction of immunologic identity	SLE (60–70%). Rarely in other diseases where it is usually in low titer
Single-strand DNA only. Antigenic determinants related to exposed purines and pyrimidines	SLE, other rheumatic diseases, and certain nonrheumatic diseases
Histones (H1, H2A, H2B, H3, H4)	Drug-induced LE (95–100%), rheumatoid arthritis (15–20%), and SLE (30%)

Reprinted with permission from: Tan EM: Autoantibodies to nuclear antigens (ANA): Their immunobiology and medicine. Adv Immunol 33:172, 1982.

of antibody can be determined. Unfortunately the use of a variety of kits and of various substrates (mouse liver cells, buccal cells, tissue culture cells) has prohibited further standardization. Despite this, certain generalizations can be made, although the correlations are not absolute and exceptions occur. Indeed, there are patients with SLE in whose sera antinuclear antibodies cannot be identified. In addition to fluorescent methodology DNA binding assays, the *Crithidia* (a hemoflagellate with apparent specificity for nDNA antibody) assay, or commercial kits are increasingly employed.

From a pathogenetic point of view it is likely that multiple immunologic aberrations, seen particularly in SLE, do mediate certain aspects of the disease and may be responsible for renal and other tissue damage. However, in tissue culture, such antinuclear antibodies have been shown not to cause cell damage, and the IgG antibodies passed transplacentally have not been shown to cause permanent fetal damage. The closest association has been the presence of anti-nDNA antibodies in patients with SLE and active renal disease. These preparations usually contain some ssDNA antibody as well, but these are not highly specific and have been observed in a number of nonrheumatologic conditions associated with tissue damage, i.e., infection.

Antibodies to deoxyribonucleoprotein are present in many patients with SLE, but they also occur in other connective tissue diseases and in unaffected relatives and may be present in moderate titers for years in asymptomatic SLE patients.

The study of the extractable nuclear antigen (ENA), an acidic component, has led to the discovery that it contains several constituents. Antibodies against one, termed Sm antigen, are specifically associated with SLE but are found in only 20 to 30 per cent of such patients. Another, antiribonucleoprotein (anti-RNP), has led to the identification of mixed connective tissue disease—MCTD—either as a separate entity or a milder subset of lupus or scleroderma. Anti-RNP is found in SLE, scleroderma, and polymyositis, as well as in MCTD (Table 443–3). Even more recently, antigens associated with the sicca syndrome, SS-B, an acidic nuclear antigen (cross-reactive with Ro antigen of cytoplasmic extracts), and SS-A antigen, a similar antigen (cross-reactive with La cytoplasmic antigen), have been described. These antibodies and others appear to identify certain connective tissue diseases (i.e., anti-Scl-70 in scleroderma; anti-Jo-1 in polymyositis) but often have a low sensitivity. The accepted antigens and antibodies and an estimate of their incidence in disease are listed in Tables 443–2 and 443–3.

In addition to these, another nuclear antigen, termed RANA, has been found to have a close association with the Epstein-Barr (EB) virus and also a high association with rheumatoid arthritis. Whether this simply represents a marker for rheumatoid arthritis or implicates the EB virus in the pathogenesis of the disease remains to be seen.

Tests for cell-mediated immunity and for immune complexes are of interest, but currently their significance in the rheumatic diseases is not well defined.

RADIOGRAPHIC TECHNIQUES IN THE DIAGNOSIS OF ARTICULAR DISEASES. ***Clinical Radiology of Joints.*** Skeletal radiographs

TABLE 443–3. AUTOANTIBODIES TO NONHISTONE NUCLEAR PROTEINS AND RNA-PROTEIN COMPLEXES

Antibody Reactive with	Clinical Association
Sm antigen	SLE (30–40%). Marker antibody
Nuclear ribonucleoprotein (nRNP) or U1-RNP	MCTD (95–100%). Lower frequency in SLE, discoid LE, and scleroderma
SS-A/Ro antigen	Sjögren's syndrome (60–70%), SLE (30–40%)
SS-B/La antigen	Sjögren's syndrome (50–60%), SLE (10–15%)
Scl-70	Scleroderma (15–20%). Marker antibody
Centromere/kinetochore	CREST (70–90%). Marker antibody
RANA (rheumatoid arthritis associated nuclear antigen)	RA (90–95%)
Ma antigen	SLE (20%)
PCNA (proliferating cell nuclear antigen)	SLE (5–10%)
PM-1	Polymyositis/scleroderma overlap (87%) Dermatomyositis (17%)
Mi-1	Dermatomyositis (11%)
Jo-1	Polymyositis (31%)
Ku	Polymyositis/scleroderma overlap (55%)

Reprinted with permission from: Tan EM: Autoantibodies to nuclear antigens (ANA): Their immunobiology and medicine. Adv Immunol 33:173, 1982.

can contribute to the diagnosis of articular diseases because the bone and joint changes reflect the basic pathology. Proper integration depends upon an understanding of the pathophysiology of the various diseases and an appreciation of the typically affected areas. This discussion will highlight general patterns and differential diagnostic aspects of major diseases. The simplest classification is that used in assessing synovial fluid, i.e., inflammatory and noninflammatory articular disease.

General radiologic features of noninflammatory disease (such as degenerative disease) include uneven narrowing of the joint space, sclerosis of juxta-articular bone, and the presence of bone spurs and cysts. Target areas include the distal interphalangeal and first carpometacarpal joints, acromioclavicular joint, vertebral column, hip, and knee, with the appearance of genu varum.

Inflammatory joint disease (such as rheumatoid arthritis) is generally characterized by local bony demineralization, erosions, and narrowing of the joint space. The pattern includes bilateral symmetry with involvement of the metacarpophalangeal joints, ulnar styloid area, and glenohumeral and atlantoaxial joints, as well as metatarsophalangeal joints. Involvement of the knees leads to genu valgum.

In addition there are patterns of change that assist in the differentiation of several types of inflammatory articular disease. For example, in tophaceous gouty arthritis the eroded joint may demonstrate an "overhanging ledge," as opposed to the erosion of rheumatoid arthritis. It may show asymmetric intra- and extra-articular erosions, as opposed to the marginal intra-articular erosions of rheumatoid arthritis. Gout does not lead to osteopenia, and joint space narrowing will be a late phenomenon rather than an early manifestation as it is in rheumatoid arthritis.

In the seronegative spondyloarthropathies (e.g., psoriatic arthritis) the articular involvement is less likely to be symmetrical, the interphalangeal joints of the feet may be more involved than the metatarsophalangeals, osteopenia is uncommon, and periosteal new bone formation may be seen as well as bony ankylosis. Finally, evidence of sacroiliitis with narrowing, erosions, sclerosis, and obliteration of the sacroiliac joint, is common. Descriptions of specific changes, such as calcinosis in scleroderma and polymyositis and aseptic necrosis (osteonecrosis) associated with systemic lupus erythematosus, are detailed in the chapters devoted to the individual disease entities.

Several additional principles should be stressed in the radiographic examination of joints. First, films are of little value if they are not of good technical quality. Occasionally, for fine points, microradiography (high resolution magnification radiography) can clarify whether or not an erosion or lesion is present. Second, the use of radiography must be selective and usually can be limited both for safety and cost effectiveness. For example, in evaluating rheumatoid arthritis: (1) in the upper extremities the key films are those of the hands (including the wrists) in posteroanterior and 15 degree oblique views; (2) in the neck, a lateral view in flexion alone will give sufficient data; and (3) in the feet, posteroanterior and lateral views without the oblique will often suffice. To assess degenerative joint disease of the knee, it is vital to include a standing anteroposterior view of both knees in one frame. For examination of the patient with seronegative spondyloarthropathy, limited views of the spine—i.e., a posteroanterior view of the pelvis to visualize the sacroiliac joints, anteroposterior and lateral views of the lumbosacral spine, and a lateral view of the neck in flexion—may suffice.

Joint Scintigraphy—Radioisotopes in the Evaluation of Articular Disease. The use of labeled isotopes in tracer amounts to measure their accumulation over normal and pathologic joints for the assessment of articular disease was introduced in the 1960's. The isotope evaluated first was technetium-99m (^{99m}Tc) pertechnetate, which largely binds to serum protein and is localized in areas of increased tissue vascularity. These scans correlate well with clinical assessment of joints and routine radiography, and on occasion allow the earlier detection of inflammation (increased blood flow). However, they are nonspecific, usually do not add significantly to routine radiography, and add (albeit a small amount) to the total body exposure.

The introduction of the bone seeking isotope ^{99m}Tc-diphosphonate added a new dimension to scintigraphy, since this allowed better evaluation of the axial skeleton. In many centers this has become the scan of choice. It can on occasion localize early sacroiliac inflammation prior to routine radiography since new bone is laid down in the involved sacroiliac joint. However, it, too, gives nonspecific results (the lesions of degenerative joint disease are often not distinguishable from those of rheumatoid arthritis), and the other problems noted above pertain. A negative scintigram is believed to be predictive of the absence of serious articular disease. However, in assessments of normal individuals an occasional joint has appeared positive.

The routine history, physical examination, selected laboratory studies, and selected routine radiographs make the use of joint scintigraphy a procedure to be chosen by experts for a specific purpose rather than a routine part of the workup of a patient with arthritis.

Arthrography (Synoviography). The injection of a contrast medium, often together with air or carbon dioxide, to visualize a joint space has become an accepted diagnostic procedure. Its value lies in the assessment of internal derangements of a joint space (usually a knee or shoulder) rather than in diagnosing inflammatory disease. The usual contraindications are infection or a bleeding diathesis. The radiopaque dye is introduced and the radiograph obtained promptly to determine its dispersion.

Orthopedists use the technique widely (as well as arthroscopy) in the diagnosis of cartilage tears in the knee and rotator cuff injuries of the shoulder. It is of great value medically in assessing masses in the popliteal area. When the differential diagnosis of deep venous thrombosis versus a ruptured popliteal cyst arises, venography is almost always indicated as a prior procedure.

Synovial cysts in rheumatoid disease, e.g., popliteal (Baker's) cysts, may rupture and lead to pain and discomfort about the knee and in the gastrocnemius area. Often the differential diagnosis is between acute thrombophlebitis and ruptured synovial cyst. When thrombophlebitis has been excluded, arthrography can often define the medical problem. On occasion, large synovial cysts can be instrumental in the development of thrombophlebitis caused by the pressure effect. Synovial cysts can occur about other joints but usually are asymptomatic.

Arthroscopy. Arthroscopy is an endoscopic procedure that has widespread orthopedic use. Its major application is in injuries about the knee joint, especially meniscal tears. With advancing technology the procedure has also been utilized in other articular spaces.

It is occasionally used by the rheumatologist in undiagnosed monarticular knee disease as a method of obtaining a selective biopsy from a local area of the joint under direct observation. It is not, however, a routine procedure and should only be performed by those with appropriate expertise.

Miscellaneous. Other technologies have been applied to the diagnostic evaluation of articular disease. These include angiography (useful in defining synovial tumors), ultrasonic scanning (increasingly helpful in the assessment of intact popliteal cysts), and, most recently, computed tomography of the joint space. All these procedures have limited utility.

Allen JC, Kunkel HG: Hidden rheumatoid factors with specificity for native gamma globulin. Arthritis Rheum 9:758, 1966. *Early studies of rheumatoid factors (RFs) showed that IgM RFs existed in the serum complexed with autologous IgG for which they were specific. When the binding was strong, these RFs could go undetected in certain systems.*

Bartfield H, Epstein WV: Rheumatoid factors and their biological significance. Ann NY Acad Sci 168:1, 1969. *A volume devoted to clinical and investigative aspects of the nature of rheumatoid factors and their relevance to disease.*

Cohen AS (ed.): Laboratory Diagnostic Procedures in the Rheumatic Diseases. 2nd ed. Boston, Little, Brown & Company, 1975. *A definitive review of the methodology and interpretation of laboratory tests in rheumatology. Not included are radiologic aspects.*

Dixon AS, Rasker JJ: Synoviography. Clin Rheum Dis 2:129, 1976. *A fine exposition of synoviography (arthrography) of various joints and the information to be gleaned from these procedures.*

Goldenberg DL, Cohen AS: Synovial membrane histopathology in the differential diagnosis of rheumatoid arthritis, gout, pseudogout, systemic lupus erythematosus, infectious arthritis and degenerative joint disease. Medicine 57:239, 1978. *An analysis of synovial membrane histopathology in the common inflammatory articular diseases, pointing out patterns that are diagnostically useful even though individual pathognomonic findings are rare.*

Griffiths ID, Dick WC: Antibodies to DNA antigens: Their specificity and clinical relevance. Eur J Clin Invest 9:239, 1979. *An editorial that focuses on the many ways of determining anti-DNA antibodies. It stresses the current multiple sources of DNA used (12 different sources in a recent multicenter study) and points out that in using radiolabeled nuclear antigens the present binding activity is linearly dependent upon the DNA molecular weight.*

Hadler NM, Spitznagel JK, Quinet RJ: Lysosomal enzymes in inflammatory synovial effusions. J Immunol 123:572, 1979. *A useful study of lysosomal enzymes of synovial fluid that discusses both sides of the question as to whether these enzymes are major causes of articular tissue destruction.*

Harris ED Jr, Krane SM: Collagenases. N Engl J Med 291:557, 605, 652, 1974. *A scholarly review of an increasingly important enzyme (collagenase) that might itself (or through its inhibitor) play a role in cartilage destruction.*

Jackson RW, Dandy DJ: Arthroscopy of the Knee. New York, Grune & Stratton, 1976. *A simple text that outlines the advantages and hazards of arthroscopy.*

Kushner I, Volanakis JE, Gewurtz H: C-Reactive protein and the plasma protein response to tissue injury. Ann NY Acad Sci 389:1–482, 1982. *The latest update of the chemistry and significance of C-reactive protein.*

Ng KC, Brown KA, Perry JD, Holborow EJ: Anti RANA antibody: A marker for seronegative and seropositive rheumatoid arthritis. Lancet 1:447, 1980. *A new and interesting test for rheumatoid arthritis that may have pathogenetic significance.*

Resnick D, Niwayam G: Diagnosis of Bone and Joint Disorders with Emphasis on Articular Abnormalities, Vols 1–3. Philadelphia, W. B. Saunders Co., 1981. *An extensive review of the radiologic findings in articular diseases.*

Ropes MW, Bauer W: Synovial Fluid Change in Joint Disease. Cambridge, Mass., Harvard University Press, 1953. *The definitive work on synovial fluid analysis in various articular diseases. The data on synovial fluid white counts, differentials, mucin, clot, etc., of 30 years ago are still valid and represent the basis for most subsequent joint fluid analyses.*

Rosenspire KC, Kennedy AC, Russomanno L, Steinbach J, Blau M, Green FA: Comparisons of four methods of analysis of ^{99m}Tc pyrophosphate uptake in RA joints. J Rheumatol 7:461,1980. *One of the first critical comparisons of the value and limitations of various methods of joint scintigraphy.*

Sokoloff L (ed.): The Joints and Synovial Fluid I. New York, Academic Press, 1978. *A modern treatise on the development, ultrastructure, immunobiology, and macromolecules of joints.*

Tan E: Autoantibodies to nuclear antigens (ANA): Their immunobiology and medicine. Adv Immunol 33:167, 1982. *An authoritative review of antinuclear antibodies and their clinical significance by a major contributor.*

444. RHEUMATOID ARTHRITIS

J. Claude Bennett

Rheumatoid arthritis (RA) is a systemic inflammatory disorder of a chronic nature that is characterized primarily by the pattern of involvement of synovial joints. The inflammatory process may involve soft tissue such as tendons, ligaments, fascia, and muscle and may extend into bone. By virtue of the mediators of inflammation that are involved in the rheumatoid process, systemic involvement of a generalized inflammatory nature affecting many different organ structures may also be seen.

For purposes of classification of rheumatoid arthritis, for usefulness in the uniformity of diagnosis, and for adherence to investigative protocols, the American Rheumatism Association (ARA) has developed 11 criteria for the diagnosis of RA. Of these 11 criteria, 7 are needed for diagnosis of *classic RA,* 5 for diagnosis of *definite RA,* and 3 for diagnosis of *probable RA.* Also required is that criteria 1 through 5 be fulfilled by observation of the continuous presence of the signs or symptoms for at least 6 weeks. The following criteria have been developed: (1) morning stiffness; (2) pain on motion or tenderness in at least one joint (observed by a physician); (3) swelling in at least one joint (observed by a physician); (4) swelling (observed by a physician) of at least one other joint (any interval free of joint symptoms between the two joint involvements may not be more than three months); (5) symmetric joint swelling (observed by a physician) with simultaneous involvement of the same joint on both sides of the body; (6) subcutaneous nodules (observed by a physician) on bony prominences, extensor surfaces, or in juxta-articular regions; (7) roentgenographic changes typical of rheumatoid arthritis; (8) a positive agglutination test result to demonstrate the presence of rheumatoid factor; (9) a poor mucin precipitate from synovial fluid (with shreds and cloudy solution) obtained on adding synovial fluid to dilute acetic acid; (10) characteristic histologic changes in the synovium; (11) characteristic histologic changes in the nodules.

The ARA criteria also incorporate 20 exclusions that were developed in order to rule out the many other forms of rheumatic disease that might in their early stages mimic rheumatoid arthritis. It is not surprising, with the rheumatoid factor assay as the only quantitative criterion, that the ARA set of diagnostic criteria is somewhat cumbersome to use for diagnosis on a broad basis. A more rigorous set of criteria proposed at the Third International Symposium of Population Studies of the Rheumatic Diseases in New York City in 1966 tends to exclude the probable cases as defined by ARA criteria but still suffers from the same absence of a quantitative basis on which to make the diagnosis. Nevertheless, the ARA criteria have been extremely useful in terms of description of the disease, anticipation of its clinical course, and for allowing physicians to talk with each other in commonly agreed-upon terms regarding patients with this disorder. Rheumatoid arthritis has a worldwide distribution and seems to affect all racial and ethnic groups. There is a female to male preponderance of approximately 2:1 to 3:1. However, if one focuses on the more specific findings of the disease, such as the positive serologic test for rheumatoid factor and erosive changes on roentgenograms, the striking female preponderance becomes less obvious. Although the peak incidence of onset is between the fourth and sixth decades, there is an increasing prevalence with advancing age up to the seventh decade. There have been many determinations of prevalence in a number of different populations, and in general it varies from 0.3 to 1.5 per cent. For convenience it is acceptable to consider a frequency of rheumatoid arthritis of about 1 per cent in the general adult population.

ETIOLOGY

The etiology of rheumatoid arthritis remains elusive even after many years of intensive investigation along various lines of study. These avenues of research have involved studies of metabolic, endocrine, and nutritional factors, as well as those defined by family studies, geographic locations, occupation, and psychosocial variables. Currently the most promising approaches lie along two major avenues of research: (1) studies of abnormalities in the immune system and its regulation; and (2) a search for some infectious agent or agents.

The discovery of rheumatoid factors in the synovial inflammatory process has focused attention on the immune system for the past 30 years. There is clear evidence that rheumatoid arthritis is an autoimmune disorder in the sense that it involves antibodies against autologous immunoglobulin G (IgG). On the other hand, there is no compelling reason to believe that this has occurred de novo; rather, it may be a response to some specific initiating external agent. The immunologic factors that might play a role in the etiology are discussed in subsequent paragraphs.

For many years investigators have found evidence for the occurrence of polyarthritis in association with microbial organisms, including bacteria. These have included the streptococci, clostridia, diphtheroids, and mycoplasmas. The association of several viral diseases with inflammatory rheumatic syndromes has provoked the possibility that rheumatoid arthritis itself is caused by a virus. The striking synovitis sometimes seen following rubella infections and the arthritis that may precede the onset of jaundice in infectious hepatitis are interesting examples of viral associations with rheumatic syndromes. In addition, the Ross River virus can produce an epidemic syndrome that in many clinical respects resembles the systemic-onset form of juvenile chronic arthritis. The arboviruses, particularly those of the togavirus family, can cause profound joint manifestations (e.g., Chikungunya and O'nyong-nyong fever). However, direct experimental evidence for viral infection in RA has not been forthcoming in spite of extensive searches. Interestingly, Lyme arthritis, which is caused by a spirochete, has some features of chronic rheumatoid disease but is clearly separable from the usual form of RA. Perhaps the strongest reason investigators have pursued microbial organisms as primary inciting agents in RA is that a large number of animal models of RA exist that are caused by microorganisms or their products. These include particularly mycoplasma infections in rats, pigs, mice, and poultry and also *Erysipelothrix* infections in pigs. Other animal models involve the immunologic reactivity against adjuvant or against bacterial cell wall peptidoglycans. Both of these processes produce an erosive, destructive, and fibrosing picture of joint pathology.

Nevertheless, in spite of numerous investigations for an initiating event, there are no generally accepted scientific data for a causative organism in adult rheumatoid disease. There are, however, a number of immunologic abnormalities that develop in parallel with the inflammatory process and that will be described in the paragraphs that follow.

PATHOLOGY

It appears that the earliest events in the rheumatoid synovium involve microvascular injury and edema of the subsynovial tissues, leading to a mild synovial lining cell proliferation. However, there are some who believe that the first visible event is synovial cell proliferation followed by injury and inflammation. Polymorphonuclear leukocytes (PMNs) may develop in the superficial synovium, the small blood vessels may be involved by inflammatory cells, and tiny thrombi may often be seen. Phagocytic events occur in proliferating synovial tissues and involve large mononuclear cells. In established RA the synovium develops slender villous projections and appears edematous and proliferative as it protrudes into the joint cavity. At this time one may see hyperplasia and hypertrophy of the synovial lining cells, which increase in thickness two- to threefold in terms of cell layers. At this stage of synovial proliferation, segmental vascular changes may be seen, and there may also be venous distention and infiltration of the arterial walls by PMNs together with areas of thrombosis and perivascular hemorrhage. The subsynovial stroma, which in the normal state is acellular, becomes packed with inflammatory cells, largely mononuclear, which may collect into aggregates or follicles. Rarely one actually sees true germinal centers. Lymphocytes usually predominate in the follicles with a layer of plasma cells around the periphery. Although immunofluorescence demonstrates large numbers of immunoglobulin-producing cells (B-lymphocytes), the majority of lymphocytes in the rheumatoid synovium are T cells. Progression to chronicity is associated with an expansion of the synovial surface area. This growing synovium actually erodes into bone, causing roentgenographic changes, and into soft tissue (such as tendons and fascia), which ultimately give rise to the deforming qualities of the clinical picture of RA.

PATHOGENESIS AND IMMUNOLOGIC FEATURES

Researchers in the rheumatic diseases have generally tended to develop hypotheses of pathogenesis along one of two lines. One involves extravascular immune complex formation, which sets into process the inflammatory response. The other is that the disease itself may result from a cellular hypersensitivity. Proponents of the latter hypothesis would say that an accumulation of activated T-lymphocytes in the synovium is associated with the production of soluble factors (lymphokines) and that this stimulates the dramatic synovial proliferation and general inflammatory response. The observation of a rheumatoid-like arthritis in some agammaglobulinemic children may be cited as possible evidence for an important role of the cellular immune reaction in rheumatoid synovitis.

Nevertheless, the first concept, based on the formation of immune complexes, is the one currently adhered to by the greatest number of investigators. It implies that the immune response is triggered in a sufficient, and perhaps specific, way against some foreign antigen. Clearly the genetic makeup of the individual would be a determinant of this host response. Hence, one might expect to see characteristic association with histocompatibility markers as has been noted in seropositive RA with HLA-D4 and HLA-DR4. A local reaction ensues within the joint itself. RA seems to involve a multicentric immune response, that is, each synovial tissue reacts in its own way, and therefore one might see a different B-lymphocyte clonal reactivity in different locations within the same individual. Antigen-antibody complexes thus formed from this reaction within the joint cavity would then become trapped in hyaline cartilage and fibrocartilage and produce changes in matrix macromolecules. In addition, within the synovial fluid the immune response activates the complement system, kinins, phagocytic cells, and lysosomal enzyme release. Mediators produced through this mechanism would cause synovial cells to proliferate and to produce proteinases and prostaglandins. These products cause dissolution of the connective tissue macromolecules within the associated connective tissue and the articular cartilage. Mediators also activate fibroblasts to produce a denser, richer connective tissue matrix and further synovial proliferation.

The rheumatoid factors produced by subsynovial lymphocytes are perhaps a reaction to IgG that has become immunogenic because of its combination with an antigen or because of its alteration in some fashion. These complexes in the synovial fluid can fix and activate complement and perpetuate the inflammatory process. Finally, in order for progressive destruction of joint tissue to occur, the usual control mechanisms that inhibit inflammation, i.e., inhibit the degradative enzymes and their activators, must be overwhelmed. Presumably this occurs through saturation of the synovial fluid and the tissue inhibitors of specific enzyme systems. The evolution of these processes gives rise to a continuing and perpetuating proliferation of cells, stimulation of enzyme systems, and destruction of normal tissue matrices.

Much is now known about the ability of rheumatoid synovial tissue to produce large quantities of collagenase, elastase, cathepsins, and prostaglandins. Collagenase production seems to be markedly stimulated in synovial sites when they are exposed to interleukin I, derived from mononuclear cells and blood macrophages. This enzyme is generally inactive when released from synovial cells but may be activated by appropriate proteolytic enzymes. The important activator may be plasmin. Synovial cells produce a plasminogen activator that attacks plasminogen in the circulation and converts it to plasmin. Plasmin then activates the latent collagenase bound to collagen fibrils. This allows rapid destruction of collagen-containing tissues. These pathogenetic events may stop at any stage, but over the long, chronic evolution of the disease, it is their summation in conjunction with the mechanical forces of weight bearing that give rise to the clinical picture of arthritis and the production of the characteristic deformities.

Rheumatoid factors are specific antiglobulins that react against the Fc portion of IgG molecules. They are produced by B-lymphocytes in the blood and other tissues, including synovial tissue. Their presence has turned out to be a useful clinical test for RA, as they occur in the circulating blood in approximately 80 per cent of patients, the so-called seropositive group. It must be emphasized that a positive test result is not diagnostic and that it does occur in 1 to 5 per cent of normal subjects with an increasing incidence in older individuals. It also occurs in a variety of other diseases usually associated with hyperglobulinemic states such as cirrhosis, leprosy, schistosomiasis, and sarcoidosis.

High titers of rheumatoid factors generally are associated with more severe and active joint disease and more frequently are found in the presence of rheumatoid nodules. A variety of rheumatoid factor activities may be discerned. They may react only with autologous IgGs or with isologous ones and sometimes even with the IgG of other species (heterologous). IgM rheumatoid factor can react with five IgG molecules and produce very large components with sedimentation constants of 22S. Intermediate-size complexes (between 7S and 19S) containing only IgG molecules, some of which have rheumatoid activity against self and usually consist of three molecules, can be discerned. There is some evidence that these complexes occur to a greater extent in those individuals with widespread systemic disease and vasculitis.

The question arises as to why rheumatoid factors should be produced. It appears that they are in fact reacting to altered autologous IgG. The alteration in the IgG could be the result of its having bound to a specific antigen molecule. There is some evidence for this concept, primarily from the finding of rheumatoid factors in bacterial endocarditis and in other diseases associated with chronic antigenic stimulation. Associations have been made between RA and the Epstein-Barr virus, which is a polyclonal stimulator of B cells. It has been suggested that certain individuals may be stimulated to produce rheumatoid factor molecules because of their special host response to this virus. Although the association of rheumatoid factors with RA is overwhelming, they clearly do not cause the disease, since the transfusion of rheumatoid factors into normal volunteers does not initiate an inflammatory process. Nonetheless, this association bespeaks some fundamental process that must be taking place within the synovial tissues. The recent concept of multicentric immunoreactivity within various synovial tissues is of great importance to our understanding of the total clonal repertoires that might be involved. Perhaps the B-lymphocytes of individuals who are susceptible to RA react in special ways against a variety of antigens and subsequently stimulate the production of rheumatoid factors.

CLINICAL FEATURES

Rheumatoid arthritis has a highly variable clinical course. It could in fact be an expression of a heterogeneous group of diseases of diverse etiologies. The course may range from a mild disease of brief duration to a progressive, destructive, and crippling arthritis. Although there is no direct correlation among the extent of articular manifestations, joint destruction, and systemic manifestations, individuals who have very high titers of rheumatoid factors tend to have a more generalized

systemic disease and a more erosive, destructive arthritic process.

Onset of Symptoms

The majority of patients, perhaps two thirds, have an insidious onset of their disease over weeks to months. During this period of time, malaise, fatigue, and perhaps diffuse musculoskeletal pain may be the predominant complaints. Only later do specific joints become involved with swelling, redness, pain, and tenderness. Frequently the onset of disease is symmetrical, involving especially the small joints of the hands, but also the elbows, the wrists, and the shoulders. As noted in the ARA diagnostic criteria, the symmetrical pattern is particularly useful in early disease in helping to differentiate RA from other forms of inflammatory arthritis. During this period of time, a frequent complaint is that of stiffness following inactivity. It can occur in the morning upon arising or following prolonged sitting. It is described by some as a "gelling" process and seems to be associated with edema within the inflamed tissues. So characteristic is this symptom that the duration of morning stiffness has been taken as a guide to the severity of the inflammatory process. In most clinical studies of RA, it is a useful bit of quantitative data that may be used to follow the activity of the disease. As the process evolves, the patient may have increasing difficulty with pain and stiffness. This limits the ability to move about, climb stairs, open doors, open jars, or to do detailed small movements, such as sewing. The patient may develop an associated psychologic depression and weight loss, and sometimes a low-grade fever may occur in association with the systemic manifestations of the disease.

An acute onset of disease is seen in about 20 per cent of patients. "Acute" refers to the rapid buildup of symptoms usually over a period of a few days. Occasionally an individual retires in the evening with no symptoms and wakes up the next morning with acute generalized RA. Such rapid onset of pain involving joints and surrounding soft tissues, as well as muscles, can present a difficult diagnostic picture. Such an acute onset of RA may be confused with acute myositis, viral syndromes, or, if focal, even septic arthritis.

Joint Manifestations

RA can affect any diarthrodial joint, and those most commonly involved are the small joints of the hands, wrists, knees, and feet. As the disease spreads, it may involve elbows, shoulders, sternoclavicular joints, hips, ankles, and, less commonly, the temporomandibular and cricoarytenoid joints. Spinal involvement in RA is generally limited to the upper cervical articulations, at least from the standpoint of clinically significant lesions.

Because of the synovial proliferation and inflammatory destruction of soft tissues, a laxity of ligaments and tendons develops, which, in conjunction with mechanical pressures and regular use, gives rise to typical deformities.

HANDS. One of the most common early signs of disease is swelling of the proximal interphalangeal (PIP) joints, giving the fingers a fusiform or spindle-shaped appearance. This is generally associated with bilateral and symmetrical swelling of the metacarpophalangeal (MCP) joints (Fig. 444–1). Although the distal interphalangeal (DIP) joints can be involved, they generally are not, and this is important in the differential diagnosis of RA and osteoarthritis. Soft tissue laxity gives rise to the appearance of an ulnar deviation of the fingers (Fig. 444–2*A*) that is frequently accompanied by palmar subluxation of the proximal phalanges. Swan neck deformities develop owing to hyperextension of the PIP joints in conjunction with flexion of the DIP joints (Fig. 444–2*B*). Flexion deformity of the PIP joints and extension of the DIP joints give rise to the boutonniere deformity. These changes are associated with loss of strength in the hands and frequently loss of the ability to maintain a

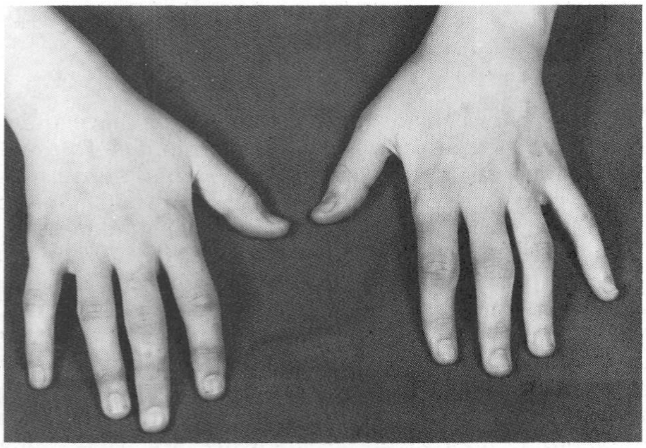

Figure 444–1. Early rheumatoid arthritis manifest as symmetrical swelling and slight flexion deformities of proximal interphalangeal joints of the hands. Roentgenograms were normal except for evidence of soft tissue swelling.

good pinch. Synovial erosions of tendons may lead to their rupture and sudden loss of the ability to extend the fingers.

WRISTS. The wrists are almost invariably involved in RA and frequently demonstrate easily palpable, boggy synovium. Such synovial proliferation on the volar aspect may compress the median nerve and produce the carpal tunnel syndrome. This consists of paresthesia and dysesthesia of the thumb and the second and third digits and the radial aspect of the fourth digit. It may also be accompanied by atrophy of the thenar eminence. Frequently, one of the first losses of motion in rheumatoid arthritis is the inability to dorsiflex the wrist fully. Normally the wrist should be able to move through nearly 180 degrees in its extremes of palmar and dorsiflexion.

KNEES. Synovial hypertrophy and effusion in this weight-bearing joint places it among the more frequently affected joints in RA. Effusions may be detected by ballotting the patella or by demonstrating a "bulge sign" along the patella when fluid is pushed into the suprapatellar pouch and then expressed back into the joint. One may expect to see quadriceps atrophy in association with chronic knee arthritis. Baker's cysts may form owing to enlargement of the semimembranous bursa into the popliteal space. Such synovial cysts may occasionally dissect and rupture and can give rise to symptoms mimicking acute thrombophlebitis. Sonargrams and arthrograms may be useful for confirmation of the diagnosis. Destruction of soft tissue about the knee can also give rise to marked joint instability.

FEET AND ANKLES. Arthritis is frequently present in the feet and may involve changes analogous to those described in the hands. Cock-up of the toes may produce subluxation of the metatarsal heads and finally a clawlike appearance.

NECK. Symptoms of neck pain are frequent in rheumatoid arthritis and may be associated with significant bony erosions because of involvement of the rheumatoid process in the cervical vertebrae. Although rare, continuous erosion may produce atlantoaxial subluxation, which can give rise to cervical dislocation and spinal cord compression, producing neurologic manifestations.

Extra-articular Manifestations

The occurrence of constitutional symptoms, occasionally a low-grade fever and minimal lymphadenopathy, are to be expected in RA. As the disease progresses, muscle atrophy, weakness, and sometimes the development of tremor can be seen. The latter is presumably caused by muscle fatigue and is usually associated with more severe disease and a poor prognosis.

SKIN. Subcutaneous nodules may develop at some time in approximately 20 to 25 per cent of patients. They are nearly always associated with seropositive disease and are found most frequently in the rapidly progressive and destructive form of the disease. Periarticular structures and areas subject to pressure, such as the elbows, the occiput, or the sacrum, tend to be the primary sites for subcutaneous nodules. They may occasionally break down or become infected but generally are asymptomatic. Another common skin manifestation in RA is the result of vasculitis. In the skin the vasculitic process often produces small brown spots, frequently in the nail folds or in the digital pulp. Larger areas of ischemic involvement may occur in the lower extremities with infarction of a toe or the development of skin sloughs over the malleoli. Histologic examination of the vasculitis may show only a mild venulitis with a relatively bland proliferation of affected digital vessels, or it may be a severe and widespread necrotizing vasculitis of the small and medium-size arteries, indistinguishable from polyarteritis nodosa. Rheumatoid vasculitis is frequently associated with high fever and other manifestations of systemic disease, including a depression of serum complement.

Another common skin manifestation is that of a tendency to easy bruisability and production of ecchymotic lesions. This seems to be caused by the general fragility of the skin in rheumatoid disease and is possibly associated with the systemic manifestations of the inflammatory process.

CARDIAC MANIFESTATIONS. Although symptomatic cardiac disease is not common in RA, a relatively frequent symptomatic lesion is acute pericarditis. It is unrelated to the duration of the arthritis and seems to appear most often in seropositive disease. The pericardial fluid characteristics include a low glucose concentration, increased lactic dehydrogenase (LDH) level, elevated immunoglobulin levels, and low complement activity. Pericardial disease may vary from a mild, fleeting process to a sizable effusion to cardiac tamponade and death. Some evidence of pericardial involvement with old fibrinous adhesions is found in about 40 per cent of RA patients at autopsy.

Lesions similar to rheumatoid nodules may be found involving the myocardium and the valves. Sometimes a focal inter-

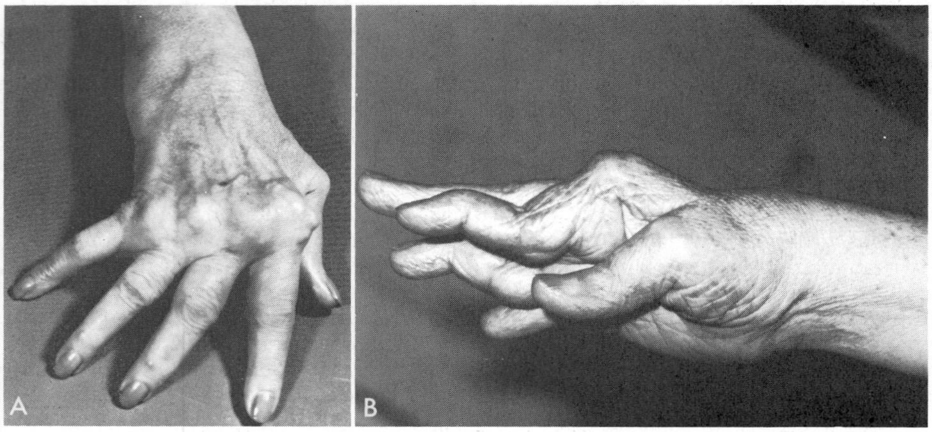

Figure 444–2. Hand deformities characteristic of chronic rheumatoid arthritis. *A*, Subluxation of metacarpophalangeal joints with ulnar deviation of digits. *B*, Hyperextension ("swan neck") deformities of proximal interphalangeal joints.

stitial myocarditis and arteritis of coronary vessels may be recognized. Occasionally valvular insufficiency, conduction abnormalities, and myocardial infarction secondary to these inflammatory lesions may be seen as clinical manifestations of rheumatoid heart disease.

PULMONARY MANIFESTATIONS. Rheumatoid pleural disease, though frequently found at autopsy, is most commonly asymptomatic. Occasionally a pleural effusion may be of sufficient size to cause respiratory limitation. Typically the pleural fluid is exudative, and white cell counts vary greatly but generally are less than 5000 per cu mm. Glucose levels tend to be low, and the LDH enzyme level is high. Total hemolytic complement, C3, and C4 levels are low. Immune complexes and rheumatoid factors are frequently found in the pleural fluid.

Intrapulmonary nodules may also be seen. Although they are usually asymptomatic, they may become infected and may cavitate or rupture into the pleural space with the production of a pneumothorax. Similar but distinct nodular infiltrates may also be seen in rheumatoid lungs in association with pneumoconiosis (Caplan's syndrome). Finally one may see a diffuse interstitial fibrosis and pneumonitis. This may progress to a honeycomb appearance on the roentgenogram, bronchiectasis, chronic cough, and progressive dyspnea. Pulmonary function tests show a diminished compliance and a restrictive ventilatory pattern.

NEUROLOGIC MANIFESTATIONS. Rheumatoid vasculitis is frequently associated with a mononeuritis multiplex syndrome in which there is patchy sensory loss in one or more of the extremities, frequently in association with foot drop or wrist drop. Biopsy of the sural nerve (when there is an abnormal conduction time) can confirm the diagnosis of vasculitis. As mentioned previously, neurologic complaints can also be produced in association with proliferating synovium, causing compression of nerves. This can result in conditions such as a median neuropathy (carpal tunnel syndrome) or a tarsal tunnel syndrome caused by an anterior tibial nerve palsy (resulting in foot drop). Although the central nervous system is usually spared, rheumatoid vasculitis and rheumatoid nodule-like granulomas have been known to occur in the meninges.

OPHTHALMOLOGIC MANIFESTATIONS. Episcleritis is a self-limited condition and may develop in association with mild pain and discomfort. Sjögren's syndrome can occur and cause corneal and conjunctival lesions associated with dryness of the eyes. Scleritis can be accompanied by severe pain and occasional visual impairment. Lesions may be found in the superior sclera as raised yellow nodules surrounded by hyperemia of the deep scleral vessels. If this progresses over a period of time, allowing the dark blue color of the choroid beneath to show through, it is termed scleromalasia perforans. The histologic picture is similar to that of the rheumatoid nodule.

FELTY'S SYNDROME. This syndrome is found in chronic RA associated with splenomegaly, lymphadenopathy, anemia, thrombocytopenia, and a selective leukopenia involving only the neutrophils. Although hypersplenism is proposed as one cause of the leukopenia, splenectomy fails to correct the abnormality in many patients. Gram-positive infections are common and frequently fail to respond to antibiotics. Interestingly, the incidence of infection may decline after splenectomy even when the neutropenia remains unaltered.

Clinical Laboratory Findings

A mild anemia, usually of the normocytic normochromic or hypochromic type, may be found. Sometimes there is a low serum iron level and normal or low iron binding capacity. The anemia, however, is generally resistant to iron therapy. The erythrocyte sedimentation rate tends to be elevated in most patients but only roughly parallels the disease activity. Although the white cell count and differential are usually normal, there may be a significant eosinophilia in association with systemic rheumatoid disease, especially vasculitis. The presence of rheumatoid factor by agglutination test is helpful in the clinical diagnosis of rheumatoid disease, and other serologic abnormalities, including antibodies against DNA and nuclear antigens in low titer, occur in a small percentage of patients. Although the finding of HLA-DR4 positivity by B cell typing is important for investigational purposes, it is not generally useful in the diagnosis of RA. Evidence now suggests that it is associated with a more aggressive disease, especially striking when found among seronegative RA patients.

Synovial fluid analysis generally shows white cell counts in the range of 5000 to 20,000 per cu mm with approximately 50 to 70 per cent as polymorphonuclear leukocytes. Synovial fluid complement is usually low, rheumatoid factors are usually present, and there is evidence of hyaluronate degradation, as shown by a poor mucin clot test.

Differential Diagnosis

The differential considerations in the diagnosis of RA are numerous. Although there is seldom confusion in classic rheumatoid arthritis, diagnosis can be more difficult in patients with early acute polyarthritis or those with involvement of only a few joints. One must consider osteoarthritis, gout, chondrocalcinosis, systemic lupus erythematosus (SLE), and progressive systemic sclerosis (PSS) as the more common diseases that might be confused with RA. In addition, a variety of systemic diseases, including sarcoidosis, inflammatory bowel disease, Whipple's disease, amyloidosis, chronic infection, and malignancies, can all present with arthritic syndromes mimicking RA. Therefore, a complete medical evaluation is indicated on all patients with joint manifestations. One must assess the patient for general systemic diseases and also for curable causes, such as bacterial infections. The careful analysis of synovial fluid is critical to differentiate rheumatoid arthritis from chronic gout and chondrocalcinosis. Critical evaluation of inflammatory joint effusions is useful not only for diagnosis but also as a guide for therapeutic responses.

COURSE AND PROGNOSIS

Although rheumatoid arthritis can follow several possible courses, most commonly the disease is initially intermittent but becomes more sustained with the passage of time. However, the course cannot be predicted, and although some patients show an unrelenting progression to deformity and occasionally even death, most patients will have episodes of relative or complete remission. An ARA committee has proposed criteria for clinical remission of rheumatoid arthritis in which five or more of the following requirements must be fulfilled for at least two consecutive months: (1) duration of morning stiffness not exceeding 15 minutes; (2) no fatigue; (3) no joint pain (by history); (4) no joint tenderness or pain on motion; (5) no soft tissue swelling in joints or tendon sheaths; and (6) erythrocyte sedimentation rate (Westergren method) less than 30 mm per hr for females or 20 mm per hr for males.

Remissions may be more frequent than generally appreciated, but a spontaneous remission is not likely beyond the first two years of the disease. It is usually helpful in chronic arthritis to establish an evaluation of functional capacity. Although there have been a number of suggested systems, a rough division would be the following:

Class I—No restriction of ability to perform normal activities.

Class II—Moderate restriction but adequate for normal activities.

Class III—Marked restriction, inability to perform most duties of the patient's usual occupation or self-care.

Class IV—Incapacitation or confinement to a bed or wheelchair.

THERAPEUTIC MANAGEMENT

The physician should recognize that RA is a chronic systemic disease that may be expected to have a prolonged course and an uncertain outcome. Therefore, one must remember that the majority of patients can continue to lead active lives with varying degrees of restrictions. In this setting of chronic disease, undue or excessive drug therapy, especially adrenocorticosteroids and immunosuppressive agents, can cause greater morbidity than the underlying disease itself. Objectives of management should include (1) relief of pain, (2) reduction of inflammation, (3) minimizing undesirable side effects, (4) preservation of muscle strength and joint function, and (5) as rapid a return to a normal lifestyle as possible. All patients with rheumatoid arthritis should begin with a basic program that includes (1) adequate rest, (2) adequate salicylate therapy, and (3) maintenance of joint function by physical measures.

Neither the patient nor the physician should be confused by the dual goals of balanced rest and exercise in rheumatoid disease. As has been noted for many years, it is only a rare patient with RA who does not improve significantly upon being hospitalized. From this we have learned that bed rest tends to decrease the general systemic inflammatory response. Most patients will soon learn that their fatigue, which occurs in the mid-afternoon, can be significantly reduced by a period of rest. This tends to give them a "second wind" for handling their functional requirements during the remainder of the day. Therefore, a regularly disciplined rest period in the mid-afternoon is most effective in maintaining the patient's overall sense of well-being. In acute exacerbations of disease, longer rest periods and perhaps even bed restriction are required to assist in suppression of the inflammatory process. Although it is clear that physical overexertion will increase synovitis and inflammation in the rheumatoid joint, it is also important that full range of motion be maintained. This can usually be accomplished by graded exercise programs for the patient. However, during acute phases, passive range of motion exercises by a physical therapist or an instructed lay person may be indicated.

Salicylate therapy is critical to this basic program. Salicylates are cheap, generally well-tolerated, and have a good track record of control of inflammation in RA. The patient needs to understand that salicylates should be taken in a continual daily dosage that provides a constant blood level of 20 to 30 mg per dl. For most people this will require between 3 and 6 grams of aspirin per day. If one expects to obtain anything more than analgesia from aspirin, this dose level must be reached. All patients should be monitored for toxicity, as indicated by blood tests, ototoxicity (deafness or ringing in the ears), or gastrointestinal intolerance. Because of the availability of buffered aspirin and coated aspirin, one can usually find a salicylate preparation for almost any patient.

Physical measures and various heat modalities such as shower, bath, warm pool, paraffin baths, hot packs, and so forth, should be employed to loosen the joints and to relieve stiffness. Exercise following these applications is designed to maintain motion of affected joints and to prevent muscle atrophy. These goals can generally be achieved without aggressive overactivity and can usually keep a patient fully mobile during the course of the disease. Acutely inflamed joints may need to be rested with either total body rest or splinting.

Drug Therapy

Even though the appropriate approach to aspirin therapy has been discussed previously, it should be pointed out that many salicylate preparations cause silent gastrointestinal bleeding. Fortunately, this is usually minimal and may not require a change of therapy. Overt gastrointestinal tract hemorrhage caused by aspirin is rare, but if gastrointestinal bleeding is contributing to a constant anemia, modification of the therapeutic regimen should be instituted.

Several nonsteroidal anti-inflammatory drugs (NSAIDs) are available, and many of them have effective analgesic, antipyretic, and anti-inflammatory activity in patients with rheumatoid arthritis. Indomethacin and phenylbutazone have been available for some time. Although they are more frequently used in osteoarthritis, they are also effective in some patients with RA. Newer nonsteroidals have recently been introduced in this country. They include the derivatives of phenylacetic acid (ibuprofen, fenoprofen), naphthalene acetic acids (naproxen), pyrrolealkanoic acid (tolmetin), indoleacetic acids (sulindac), a halogenated anthranilic acid (meclofenamate sodium), and, even more recently, piroxicam, zomepirac, and diflunisal. Most of these drugs are beneficial in patients with rheumatoid arthritis. They are generally no more effective than aspirin but may be better tolerated. Their major current disadvantage is their expense. The experience of physicians dealing with rheumatoid arthritis generally is that they will have to shift drugs occasionally in order to lessen side effects or to adjust to the needs of a given patient.

If the nonsteroidal anti-inflammatory drugs fail to control the disease, then one must consider the more slowly acting drugs, including antimalarials, gold, and penicillamine. Antimalarials are usually given as hydroxychloroquine 200 mg twice daily. This drug and chloroquine may cause retinal lesions and loss of vision; therefore the patient should be checked by an ophthalmologist at least twice a year. Gold salts are widely used and can produce remission in many cases. Because of the potential of gold toxicity on the kidney and bone marrow, frequent urinalysis and routine blood work (CBC) must be done, especially during the early phases of the therapeutic program. Treatment with gold is usually begun with a 10 mg test injection (Myochrysine or Solganal) for idiosyncrasy, then a 25 mg dose the second week, and a 50 mg injection weekly up to a total of about 1 gram. Usually during this period of time a therapeutic response occurs, and at that point the dose can be cut to alternate weeks and subsequently to every third or fourth week. Many patients have been on prolonged gold therapy for a number of years. However, side effects are common, with as many as 30 per cent of patients having to discontinue therapy because of them. The most common and the most annoying to the patient are pruritic skin rashes. More painful are mouth ulcers. Severe manifestations include bone marrow suppression, usually leukopenia or thrombocytopenia, and renal damage with proteinuria and rarely the nephrotic syndrome. Penicillamine is now available for the treatment of rheumatoid arthritis and is also quite effective in inducing improvements in the disease and sometimes even in inducing remissions. It suffers from some of the same problems as gold in that it affects both the bone marrow and the kidney. Therefore, patients must be carefully monitored for toxicity. Immunosuppressive agents such as azathioprine, cyclophosphamide, chlorambucil, and methotrexate have been used to treat especially severe and unremitting RA. Azathioprine has been given FDA approval for the treatment of rheumatoid arthritis, and large-scale cooperative studies are now under way to evaluate methotrexate therapy in specific cases of rheumatoid disease.

Other experimental approaches to the treatment of drug-resistant patients include plasmapheresis, leukapheresis, and total nodal irradiation. All of these procedures are experimental, and long-term effects are unknown.

One cannot ignore corticosteroids when considering the therapy of RA. Because of their side effects they are generally discouraged by most rheumatologists. Patients with active rheumatoid disease do not tolerate alternate-day steroids well, and therefore one quickly gets into a pattern of daily therapy. Although they can be useful in those patients who have neuropathy, vasculitis, pleuritis, pericarditis, scleritis, and related conditions, for the usual patient with only joint disease it is wise to avoid them. Local steroid injections can sometimes be helpful for the relief of persistent effusions or to get patients more mobile in preparation for appropriate physical therapy.

Finally, one must not overlook the very great importance of reconstructive orthopedic surgery. Perhaps the greatest contribution to the management of rheumatoid arthritis in the last 10 years has been the development of superb techniques for joint replacement therapy. The use of prosthetic devices for the patient with hip and knee disease has given excellent results, and the results for ankle, elbow, and shoulder replacement are improving rapidly. Reconstructive orthopedic surgery in patients who have had long-term destructive disease is a very major part of our total therapeutic armamentarium.

JUVENILE CHRONIC ARTHRITIS

Rheumatic diseases are not rare in children, but they differ somewhat from those in adults, and that difference is worth noting. Although the various subclasses of chronic arthritis in children have not yet been fully defined and although some still prefer the use of the term "juvenile rheumatoid arthritis," it is becoming increasingly popular to use the term "juvenile chronic arthritis." Currently, the disease is further subdivided into the following: systemic onset disease, polyarticular onset disease, and pauciarticular onset disease.

The first, systemic onset (Still's disease), accounts for about 20 per cent of patients. The disease can begin at any age. The rheumatoid factor and antinuclear antibody test results are generally negative. Clinical characteristics include a high intermittent fever, maculopapular rash, polyserositis, lymphadenopathy, hepatosplenomegaly, leukocytosis, and anemia. Although the disease is rarely life-threatening, it can be confused initially with leukemia or infection. A chronic polyarthritis usually develops in these patients within the first few months of the disease but sometimes not until years later.

Polyarticular onset disease without any extra-articular manifestations occurs in approximately 40 per cent of patients, and there is a female preponderance. The majority of these children are seronegative for rheumatoid factors. Those who are seropositive are generally older than eight years of age when the disease begins. Positive test results for antinuclear antibodies are often found. These patients may have malaise, low-grade fever, adenopathy, anemia, and growth retardation. With polyarticular disease one commonly sees cervical spine involvement, most typically at the C2-C3 apophyseal joints.

Pauciarticular onset disease affects another 40 per cent of children with juvenile arthritis, and there are several subgroups of this pattern. At least two can be identified. One subgroup is characterized by early onset with a female preponderance. The serum of these patients often is positive for antinuclear antibodies but negative for rheumatoid factors. Some tend to develop inflammation of the anterior uveal tract (iridocyclitis). This occasionally can be the major manifestation and can progress to blindness. Therefore, evaluation of these children for progressive ophthalmologic manifestations is important. The second subgroup of pauciarticular onset has a strong male preponderance, and many of these individuals are HLA-B27 positive, so they appear as young children with spondyloarthropathy.

Treatment is usually helpful for these children. Aspirin is a basic standby for therapy, and physical and psychosocial support are indicated. Although these subsets have many properties in common with adult rheumatoid disease, there are many distinctions, and one must be aware that there may be several different diseases with different etiologies grouped within this general category.

ADULT-ONSET STILL'S DISEASE

As indicated in the previous section, one of the subsets of juvenile chronic arthritis is the systemic onset form, which is Still's disease There have been several cases, now up to a total of 70 or more, of adult-onset Still's disease in which the clinical features are almost identical to those occurring in children. These patients exhibit high fevers, polyarthritis, tenosynovitis, and a salmon-colored maculopapular measles-like rash, particularly over the trunk and along pressure lines. Nodules sometimes occur in these patients, but the fever and rash are the most characteristic of the initial signs of disease and help to point toward the adult-onset form of Still's disease. Pericarditis and pleural effusions have been reported but are generally mild. Other systemic manifestations do occur. Acute symptoms

generally respond to an adequate dose of salicylates, but occasionally nonsteroidal anti-inflammatory drugs or even prednisone may be necessary for short periods of time.

Alarcón GS, Koopman WJ, Acton RT, Barger BO: Seronegative rheumatoid arthritis: A distinct immunogenetic disease? Arth Rheum 25:502, 1982. *An interesting study of the association of histocompatibility markers and immunogenetic epidemiology in seronegative rheumatoid arthritis.*

Ansell B: Diagnostic criteria, nomenclature, classification. *In* Munthe E (ed.): The Care of Rheumatoid Children. Basel, EULAR, 1978, p 42. *A succinct description of the basis for diagnosis and classification of the juvenile chronic arthritides.*

Aptekar RG, Decker JL, Bujak JS, Wolff SE: Adult onset juvenile rheumatoid arthritis. Arth Rheum 16:715, 1973. *An excellent clinical discussion of the adult onset form of Still's disease.*

Bennett JC: The infectious etiology of rheumatoid arthritis. Arth Rheum 21:531, 1978. *A discussion of the various possibilities for the role of infectious agents in rheumatic diseases.*

Blumberg B, Bunim JJ, Calkins E, Pirani CL, Zvaifler NJ: ARA nomenclature and classification of arthritis and rheumatism. Arth Rheum 7:93, 1964. *The general outline of the ARA Diagnostic Criteria*

Hollingsworth JW: Local and Systemic Complications of Rheumatoid Arthritis. Philadelphia, W. B. Saunders Co., 1968. *An excellent and comprehensive discussion of the nonarticular complications of rheumatoid disease.*

Kotzin BL, Strober S, Engleman EG, Calin A, Hoppe RT, Kansas GS, Terrell CP, Kaplan HS: Treatment of intractable rheumatoid arthritis with lymphoid irradiation. N Engl J Med 305:969, 1981. *An interesting description of a current investigative approach to the treatment of rheumatoid arthritis.*

Krane SM: Aspects of the cell biology of the rheumatoid synovial lesion. Ann Rheum Dis 40:433, 1981. *Description of the biology of tissue destruction in the rheumatoid process dealing with both the enzymes involved and their regulation.*

Lewis JR: New antirheumatic agents. JAMA 237:1260, 1977. *A succinct description of the nonsteroidal anti-inflammatory agents.*

Pinals RS, Masi AT, Larsen RA: Preliminary criteria for clinical remission in rheumatoid arthritis. Arth Rheum 24:1308, 1981.

Schumacher HR: Synovial membrane and fluid morphologic alterations in early rheumatoid arthritis: Microvascular injury and virus-like particles. Ann NY Acad Sci 256:39, 1975. *An excellent description of the pathology of rheumatoid synovial tissue and synovial fluid.*

Short CL, Bauer W, Reynolds WS: Rheumatoid Arthritis. Cambridge-Harvard University Press, 1957. *A superb documentation of modes of onset and clinical features of rheumatoid arthritis throughout its entire natural history.*

Steinbrocker O, Traeger CH, Batterman RC: Therapeutic criteria in rheumatoid arthritis. JAMA 140:659, 1949.

Wees SJ, Sunwoo IN, Oh SJ: Sural nerve biopsy in systemic necrotizing vasculitis. Am J Med 71:525, 1981. *Description of a useful diagnostic procedure for vasculitis and peripheral neuropathy.*

Ziff M: Systemic rheumatoid disease: Immunological aspects. Adv Inflam Res 3:123, 1982. *A comprehensive review of the immunological mechanisms involving the pathogenesis of rheumatoid arthritis.*

445. THE SPONDYLARTHROPATHIES

Andrei Calin

The seronegative spondylarthritides are characterized by involvement of the sacroiliac joints, by peripheral inflammatory arthropathy, and by the absence of rheumatoid factor. Other features include (1) pathologic changes concentrated around the enthesis (i.e., the site of ligamentous insertion into bone) rather than the synovium. Nonenthesopathic changes may also develop in the eye, the aortic valve, the lung parenchyma, and the skin. (2) Clinical evidence of overlap among the various seronegative spondylarthritides. Thus, a patient with psoriatic arthropathy may well develop uveitis or sacroiliitis; a patient with inflammatory bowel disease may develop ankylosing spondylitis or mouth ulcers. (3) A tendency toward familial aggregation, with the suggestion that these entities "breed true" within families.

TYPES

The spondylarthropathies include the prototype disorder ankylosing spondylitis, as well as Reiter's syndrome (both the postvenereal, or endemic, and the postinfective, or epidemic, forms), the reactive arthritides (caused by infections with Yersinia and Salmonella), certain subsets of juvenile arthropathy (juvenile ankylosing spondylitis and the seronegative enthesopathic arthropathy syndrome), enteropathic sacroiliitis (ul-

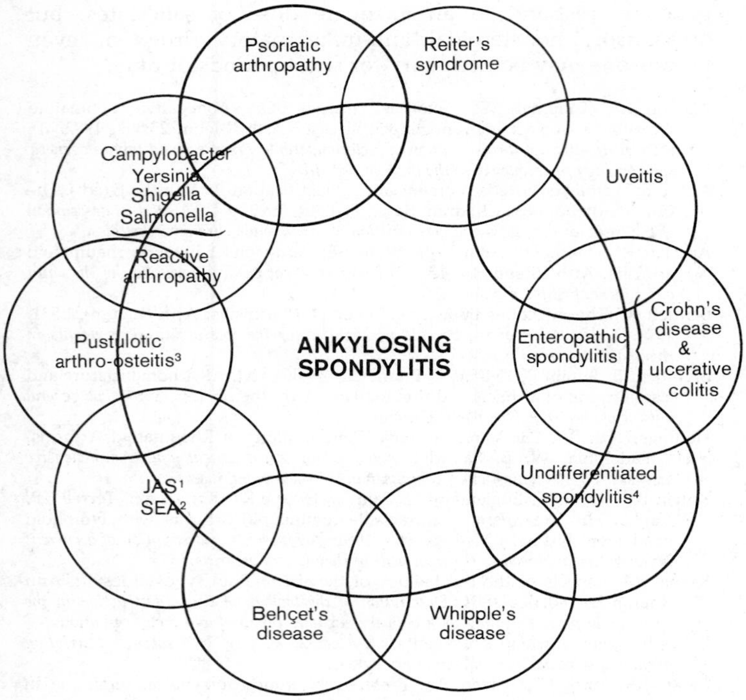

Figure 445–1. Individual conditions that overlap to form the spondyloarthritides. (1) Juvenile ankylosing spondylitis. (2) Seronegative enthesopathic arthropathy syndrome. (3) Considered by Japanese to be part of spondyloarthropathy spectrum (rare in United States and Europe). (4) Undifferentiated spondylitis (i.e., subset of patients who have spondyloarthropathic features but who fail to meet criteria for ankylosing spondylitis, Reiter's syndrome, or other condition, e.g., dactylitis, uveitis, plus unilateral sacroiliitis).

cerative colitis and Crohn's disease), psoriatic arthropathy, and perhaps a group of rarer disorders (Behçet's syndrome, Whipple's disease, and pustulotic arthro-osteitis) (see Fig. 445–1).

These disorders can be categorized according to the specific periarticular or articular involvement. The various spondylarthropathies can be distinguished from one another according to the particular peripheral joints involved, the associated clinical features (i.e., urethritis, conjunctivitis, skin involvement), and the manner in which the disease progresses (i.e., remission or relapse) (see Table 445–1).

HEREDITARY FACTORS

Hereditary factors play an important role in the development of the spondylarthropathies. Approximately 20 per cent of HLA-B27–positive individuals develop ankylosing spondylitis following an unknown environmental event or develop Reiter's syndrome after exposure to Shigella or other environmental agents. The offspring of an individual with HLA-B27 have a 50 per cent chance of carrying the same antigen and, thus, an overall 10 per cent chance of developing ankylosing spondylitis or Reiter's syndrome if exposed to a specific arthritogenic trigger.

The explanation for the link between HLA-B27 and the spondylarthropathies remains unknown. Hypotheses include (1) B27 acts as a receptor site for an infective agent; (2) B27 is a marker for an immune response gene that determines susceptibility to an environmental trigger; or (3) B27 may induce tolerance to foreign antigens with which it cross-reacts.

Patients with ankylosing spondylitis or Reiter's syndrome who lack HLA-B27 may be more likely to have a cross-reacting antigen such as B7, Bw22, or Bw42. We now know that the

TABLE 445–1. COMPARISON OF SERONEGATIVE SPONDYLOARTHROPATHIES

	Ankylosing Spondylitis	Reiter's Syndrome	Psoriatic Arthropathy	Enteropathic Spondylitis	Juvenile Arthropathy (JAS* subset)	Reactive Arthropathy
Sex	Male ≥ Female	Male ≥ Female	Female ≥ Male	Female = Male	Male > Female	Male = Female
Age at onset	20	Any age	Any age	Any age	<16	Any age
Uveitis	+	+ +	+	+	+	+
Conjunctivitis	−	+	−	−	−	+
Peripheral joints	Lower > Upper: often	Lower usually	Upper > Lower	Lower > Upper	Lower > Upper	Lower > Upper
Sacroiliitis	Always	Often	Often	Often	Often	Often
HLA-B27	95%	80%	20% (50% with sacroiliitis)	50%	90%	80%
Enthesopathy	+	+	+	?	+	?
Aortic regurgitation	+	+	?+	?	?	+
Familial aggregation	+	+	+	+	+	+
Risk for HLA-B27–positive individual	±20%	20%	?	?	?	20%
Onset	Gradual	Sudden	Variable	Gradual	Variable	Sudden
Urethritis	−	+	−	−	−	+/−
Skin involvement	−	+	+ +	−	−	−
Mucous membrane involvement	−	+	−	+	−	+
Symmetry (spinal)	+	−	−	+	+	−
Self-limiting	−	+/−	+/−	+/−	+/−	+/−
Remission, relapses	−	+/−	+/−	−	+/−	+/−

*JAS = Juvenile ankylosing spondylitis.

risk of developing ankylosing spondylitis for a B27-positive relative of a B27-positive patient is 25 to 50 per cent compared with about 5 per cent for a B27-positive subject. This argues for genetic differences between the two B27 groups.

ANKYLOSING SPONDYLITIS

Criteria for Diagnosis

The criteria for diagnosing ankylosing spondylitis have been evolving in recent years. The New York criteria have limitations. For example, precisely what constitutes reduced spinal mobility has not been adequately defined. Also, the criterion based on limitation of chest expansion is somewhat imprecise: it is difficult to measure chest expansion accurately, and the reduction below 2.5 cm occurs late in the course of the disease. A simpler approach defines ankylosing spondylitis as the presence of symptomatic sacroiliitis. A patient with back discomfort and radiologic evidence of sacroiliitis would be diagnosed as having ankylosing spondylitis. Symptomatic sacroiliitis is usually associated with a decreased range of spinal mobility.

Prevalence

Once considered a rare disease, the illness is now known to have a prevalence comparable to that of rheumatoid arthritis. Twenty per cent of HLA-B27–positive individuals have symptomatic sacroiliitis. Because the B27 antigen occurs in six to 14 per cent of white individuals, approximately 1 to 1.5 per cent of whites have ankylosing spondylitis. The distribution of this disease follows the population frequency of HLA-B27, and it is more common in whites than in blacks.

Ankylosing spondylitis has often gone undiagnosed; inappropriate diagnostic procedures lead to erroneous diagnoses (i.e., mechanical back disease). Such patients often receive incorrect therapy.

Although ankylosing spondylitis was formerly considered a predominantly male disease, several studies now suggest that there may be a more uniform sex distribution. Female patients are less frequently diagnosed, perhaps because physicians and radiologists may be reluctant to diagnose a disease that they consider to be rare in females. The disease may be milder in females and present with a greater number of peripheral joint manifestations. In the past, many women with ankylosing spondylitis were inappropriately diagnosed as having seronegative rheumatoid arthritis.

Clinical Presentation

A history of several of the following five features is suggestive of inflammatory spinal disease: insidious onset of discomfort, age less than 40 years, persistence for more than three months, association with morning stiffness, and improvement with exercise.

If this simple screening test is positive, radiologic evidence of sacroiliitis confirms ankylosing spondylitis. Many radiologists have been unfamiliar with rheumatologic joint disease and have diagnosed ankylosing spondylitis only when there was evidence of major ankylosis of the sacroiliac joints and spine. Ankylosing spondylitis can be diagnosed, however, in the presence of only minimal sacroiliitis. The severity of sacroiliitis is graded from 0 to IV, based on the amount of radiographically observed joint distortion. In many patients, the disease does not progress beyond Grade II or III.

Early change in the lumbar spine is manifested as squaring of the superior and inferior margins of the vertebral body. This phenomenon is caused by inflammatory disease at the site of insertion of the outer fibers of the anulus fibrosus (i.e., enthesopathy). Later changes result in the classic, though rare, bamboo spine. Comparable spinal changes are seen in primary ankylosing spondylitis and in the spondylitis associated with inflammatory bowel disease. In spondylitis associated with Reiter's syndrome and psoriatic arthropathy, however, the changes tend to be asymmetric and random.

Radionuclide scans, computed tomography, and other advanced radiologic techniques have been suggested to evaluate the condition of the sacroiliac joints, but a simple anteroposterior radiograph usually suffices.

Physical Examination

Examination of the spine may reveal muscle spasm and loss of the normal lordosis. In contradistinction to mechanical spinal disease, mobility is decreased symmetrically in both anterior and lateral planes. The degree of restriction of forward flexion can be documented by measuring the distraction, on flexion, of two points—the lower point at the level of the lumbosacral junction and the upper point 10 cm above this level. In a normal individual, the distraction of this 10-cm line is 5 to 12 cm, compared with 0 to 7 cm in an untreated spondylitis patient. Lateral spinal flexion is measured by the distraction, on contralateral flexion, of a 20-cm line drawn in the midaxillary plane. In this case, normal distraction varies from 5 to 12 cm, compared with 0 to 7 cm in spondylitis patients.

Peripheral joint involvement, especially in the lower limb, occurs at some stage in approximately 20 to 30 per cent of cases; the frequency increases with the severity of the disease. Inflammatory disease of the hip and shoulder may produce progressive disability. Enthesopathic features may include plantar fasciitis, costochondritis, and Achilles tendinitis.

Laboratory Findings

HLA-B27 testing should not be used as a routine screening procedure; it is expensive and usually unnecessary. A diagnosis of ankylosing spondylitis does require radiologic evidence of disease. B27 is present in over 95 per cent of white patients.

Other laboratory changes are less striking. Elevation of the erythrocyte sedimentation rate occurs in most patients but may be normal despite severe disease. Elevation of IgA levels and the presence of immune complexes suggest aberrant immunity. Serum creatine kinase and alkaline phosphatase activities may be elevated. Lymphocytes predominate in the synovial fluid, and synovial histologic findings are nonspecific.

Pathology

The synovial lesions of ankylosing spondylitis and rheumatoid arthritis share identical histopathologic characteristics: intimal cell hyperplasia; a diffuse lymphocyte and plasma cell infiltrate; formation of lymphoid follicles; and plasma containing IgG, IgA, and IgM. IgM is found less frequently in ankylosing spondylitis than in rheumatoid disease. Synovitis per se, however, does not explain the propensity toward ligamentous ossification and widespread new bone formation observed in ankylosing spondylitis. Inflammation at the enthesis accounts for the unique pathology, or enthesopathy, of ankylosing spondylitis; new bone formation appears to be a specific reparative process occurring at the enthesopathic site. Complications of severe spinal disease include fractures and spondylodiskitis after minimal trauma.

Extraskeletal Involvement

Extra-articular features include fatigue, weight loss, and low-grade fever. Cord compression resulting from spinal fractures or the cauda equina syndrome may cause neurologic symptoms. The negative effects of systemic involvement and of radiotherapy on the survival of patients with ankylosing spondylitis are well recognized.

EYE INVOLVEMENT. Uveitis develops in up to 25 per cent of patients during their illness. It occurs most often in HLA-B27–positive patients with peripheral joint disease but shows no correlation with the severity of the spondylitis. The visual episodes are usually self-limiting but may require local steroid therapy. Progressive visual impairment is more common in Reiter's syndrome than in ankylosing spondylitis.

PULMONARY DISEASE. Patients with severe disease may exhibit chronic infiltrative and fibrotic changes in the upper lung fields that mimic tuberculosis. Pulmonary ventilation is usually well maintained by the diaphragm, despite the chest wall rigidity. The pulmonary fibrosis is occasionally clinically silent, but most affected patients present with cough, sputum, and dyspnea. Cyst formation and subsequent *Aspergillus* invasion may cause hemoptysis.

CARDIOVASCULAR DISEASE. Aortic incompetence, cardiomegaly, and persistent conduction defects occur in 3.5 to 10.0 per cent of patients with severe spondylitic disease. Cardiac involvement may be clinically silent or may dominate the clinical picture. Thickened aortic valve cusps and scar tissue in the root of the aorta represent the major histologic changes.

AMYLOIDOSIS. Amyloid deposition is an occasional complication of ankylosing spondylitis, particularly in Europe. It may be present in up to 10 per cent of patients, although it appears to be of little clinical significance in most cases.

KIDNEY. In contrast with patients with rheumatoid arthritis who may show renal impairment as an expression of disease, renal glomerular function is apparently unimpaired in ankylosing spondylitis, despite recognized pathologic changes. An IgA nephropathy, however, has been described in patients with seronegative spondylarthropathy.

Treatment and Prognosis

Ankylosing spondylitis is a gratifying condition to recognize and treat early: much can be accomplished toward ameliorating symptoms and, perhaps, preventing spinal deformity. The primary objectives are to relieve pain, decrease inflammation, begin remedial strengthening exercises, and maintain good posture and function.

Anti-inflammatory agents relieve inflammation, pain, and spasm and permit patients to follow an adequate exercise program. There is some evidence that phenylbutazone decreases the rate of spinal fusion. Nevertheless, indomethacin is the drug of choice. Phenylbutazone, although more efficacious, may be more toxic. Indomethacin, started at a dosage of 25 mg three times a day, may be increased to a maximum of 150 mg daily. The dose should be titrated against response and side effects. Possible side effects include headache, vertigo, and depression, especially in older patients, and nausea, gastric discomfort, and diarrhea in all age groups. Phenylbutazone (100 mg t.i.d. or q.i.d.) is remarkably effective but must be used with caution. Dangerous side effects include agranulocytosis and aplastic anemia. Agranulocytosis is an idiosyncratic response, developing chiefly in young individuals within three to six weeks of the start of therapy. Aplastic anemia appears to be dose-related and occurs primarily in individuals more than 60 years of age.

Nonsteroidal anti-inflammatory drugs (NSAIDs) include ibuprofen (Motrin), naproxen (Naprosyn), fenoprofen (Nalfon), tolmetin (Tolectin), sulindac (Clinoril), meclofenamate sodium (Meclomen), and piroxicam (Feldene). If indomethacin is efficacious but not tolerated, one of these NSAIDs may be given. In general, these agents play a minor role in the management of the spondylarthritides. Phenylbutazone should be tried when indomethacin is ineffective.

Gold and penicillamine have not been adequately studied; radiotherapy, once the treatment of choice, is no longer practiced in view of the high risk of inducing leukemia.

The patient also needs remedial strengthening exercises and postural training. A firm mattress and small pillow are ideal when resting; attention to posture at work and at rest must be stressed. The best exercise regimen includes extension exercises and hydrotherapy; swimming is highly recommended.

In those few patients who, despite optimal management, develop an irreversible deformity, wedge osteotomy may be indicated. For those with destructive arthropathy of the hip, arthroplasty is useful despite the risk of postoperative reankylosis.

REITER'S SYNDROME

The most common cause of an inflammatory oligoarthropathy in a young male is Reiter's syndrome. This classic triad of urethritis, conjunctivitis, and arthritis represents the one chronic rheumatic disorder related to both a specific genetic background (HLA-B27) and a specific infection. Reiter's syndrome is often not self-limiting. Progressive disease may result in major disability. The disease may be defined as "an episode of arthropathy within one month of urethritis or cervicitis."

Whether a dysenteric (epidemic) or a venereal (endemic) infection is the most common precipitating event remains a matter of controversy. In young children, however, the former is the rule. In many cases, the distinction between urethritis as a precipitating factor and urethritis as an integral manifestation of the syndrome remains unclear; the association with venereal disease, however, creates a sense of guilt for the patient. In postvenereal Reiter's syndrome both *Chlamydia* and *Mycoplasma* have been implicated. In a patient with a specific predisposing genetic background, a variety of different organisms may be responsible.

Prevalence

The prevalence of Reiter's syndrome remains unknown. The disorder develops in at least one per cent of patients with nonspecific urethritis. *Shigella* dysentery is followed by Reiter's syndrome in one to two per cent of cases (i.e., 20 per cent of B27-positive patients).

The sex distribution of Reiter's syndrome is difficult to define because the syndrome is diagnosed only with difficulty in females, in whom urethritis is often clinically inapparent. Formes frustes of the syndrome are now being recognized. A woman presenting with uveitis and an inflammatory arthropathy of the knee in association with the HLA-B27 antigen may have Reiter's syndrome. Similarly, the disorder is difficult to recognize in children; a diagnosis is usually made only if an epidemic of dysentery is present and Reiter's syndrome has been recognized in other family members. Postdysenteric Reiter's syndrome almost certainly has an equal sex distribution.

Clinical Picture

Reiter's syndrome should be considered a symptom complex rather than the association of three specific features. The syndrome may present as a tetrad (i.e., with the addition of buccal ulceration or balanitis to the classic triad); alternatively, only two of the three cardinal features may be present. Several of the classic features may appear insignificant and be overlooked. For example, the urethritis may be mild, perhaps forgotten; the discharge may be minimal and remembered by the patient only after direct questioning. Balanitis may not be evident unless the prepuce is retracted and the glans penis closely inspected. Buccal ulceration is usually painless and apparent only after close inspection. A red eye may be forgotten or considered irrelevant, and the various skin lesions typified by keratoderma blennorrhagicum may be misdiagnosed.

Rheumatologic features include arthralgias, tenosynovitic episodes, plantar fasciitis, and other enthesopathies, as well as frank arthritis. The typical sausage-shaped digit is a frequent occurrence related to the disorder's enthesopathic nature.

Some 20 per cent of patients with Reiter's syndrome develop sacroiliitis and ascending spinal disease. Whether spondylitis should be considered a complication of the Reiter's syndrome or a manifestation of B27 disease remains unclear. Other radiologic evidence of Reiter's syndrome includes plantar spurs and periosteal new bone formation. Cardiac complications similar to those in ankylosing spondylitis occur late in Reiter's syndrome.

The hyperkeratotic skin lesions seen in Reiter's syndrome cannot be distinguished from those in psoriasis.

Formerly considered a self-limited process, Reiter's syndrome is now known to be a more or less persistent disease in many patients. About 80 per cent of patients have evidence of disease activity when they are re-examined after a five-year period.

Laboratory Evaluation

It is unclear whether the presence of HLA-B27 correlates with increased severity of Reiter's syndrome. A patient with severe Reiter's syndrome may have an erythrocyte sedimentation rate in the normal range or one as high as 100 mm per hour or more. Synovial fluid analysis is rarely diagnostic, apart from the fact that it reveals a relatively high complement level (reflecting a nonspecific inflammatory reaction), rather than the low level seen in rheumatoid arthritis (reflecting immune complex disease).

Occasionally, the diagnoses of ankylosing spondylitis and Reiter's syndrome may prove difficult to disentangle. Some patients who are diagnosed as having ankylosing spondylitis may have presented originally with Reiter's syndrome, but the episodes of urethritis have subsequently been forgotten by the physician and patient. Similarly, patients dignosed as having Reiter's syndrome may actually have ankylosing spondylitis with peripheral joint disease and a chance occurrence of urethritis.

Management

There is no cure for Reiter's syndrome. The patient's feelings of guilt and anxiety about sexual misconduct must be allayed. Although anecdotal evidence suggests that individuals with postvenereal Reiter's syndrome may develop a relapse following sexual activity, many individuals have spontaneous exacerbations. An explanation of allergic response may help the patient: asthma may develop on exposure to a known or unknown allergen in sensitive individuals; in the same way, Reiter's syndrome may flare up following an unknown allergic event.

Symptomatic management includes the use of indomethacin or phenylbutazone. Antibiotic therapy is controversial and probably unnecessary. Patients with severe recurrent uveitis may require steroid eye drops or subconjunctival preparations. The syndrome may remit, recur, or continue unabated despite steroid or even cytotoxic therapy.

THE REACTIVE ARTHROPATHIES

Reactive arthropathy refers to an inflammatory arthritis that follows an infection in which there is no microbial invasion of the synovial space. The B27-linked arthropathies following *Shigella, Salmonella, Yersinia,* and *Campylobacter jejuni* infection are in this group. Why some patients develop only an arthropathy whereas others have the full spectrum of Reiter's disease after exposure to one of these agents is unknown.

Yersinia Infection

Yersinia enterocolitica infection may produce the following: fever, mild gastrointestinal illness, and, after a latent period, polyarthropathy and erythema nodosum, especially in B27-positive individuals. The symptom complex may mimic acute rheumatic fever. The arthropathy may last for weeks or months, and in HLA-B27–positive individuals, sacroiliitis may occur.

Salmonellosis

An arthropathy associated with *Salmonella* infection mimics that caused by *Yersinia.*

Treatment of these disorders is the same as that of Reiter's syndrome.

JUVENILE CHRONIC ARTHROPATHY

Chronic arthritis in a child or teenager often persists into adulthood; therefore, an awareness of juvenile chronic arthropathy is relevant when attending adult patients. Until recently, the term juvenile rheumatoid arthritis was used, inappropriately, to describe all forms of childhood arthritis. As in adults, arthritis in children may be associated with psoriasis, inflammatory bowel disease, and other conditions. The acute systemic form, Still's disease, presents with fever, rash, and toxicity in young children who are negative for B27 and rheumatoid factor (IgM-anti-IgG). Still's disease is also recognized in adults. Another subset (in the spondylarthropathy group) consists largely of adolescent males who predominantly exhibit oligoarthropathy affecting the large joints of the lower limbs: such individuals are frequently positive for HLA-B27. This group may develop sacroiliitis or ankylosing spondylitis; the presence of B27 is associated with spinal disease involvement. Another group includes B27-negative individuals (usually females less than five years of age) presenting with an oligoarthropathy characterized by a positive fluorescent antinuclear antibody (FANA) test. These subjects are at risk for developing asymptomatic chronic iridocyclitis, in contrast with FANA-negative and B27-positive patients, who develop clinically obvious acute uveitis. A few older children (preponderantly females) develop a seropositive, nodular, and erosive disease that resembles adult rheumatoid arthritis. A B-27–related syndrome known as seronegative enthesopathy and arthropathy (SEA syndrome) is now also recognized in children.

THE ENTEROPATHIC ARTHROPATHIES

Two major clinical patterns of arthropathy associated with inflammatory bowel disease (ulcerative colitis and Crohn's disease) are peripheral arthropathy and spondylarthropathy.

Peripheral Arthropathy

Approximately 20 per cent of individuals with severe Crohn's disease or ulcerative colitis develop an acute migratory inflammatory polyarthritis, often of abrupt onset and involving the larger joints of the lower extremities. The arthritis resolves in weeks or months. Arthritis flare-ups usually parallel exacerbations of the underlying disorder. The pathogenesis of the joint complication is unknown. B27 antigen is not present. Treatment is directed at the primary disorder and is more effective in ulcerative colitis than in Crohn's disease.

Spondylarthritis

About one patient in five with inflammatory bowel disease develops sacroiliitis and, occasionally, severe ankylosing spondylitis. The spinal disease may precede the bowel disease or follow it. There is no correlation between the severity of the bowel disorder and the spondylitis, which mimics primary ankylosing spondylitis rather than the spondylitis associated with psoriasis or Reiter's syndrome. Therapy is the same as for classic ankylosing spondylitis. Despite the bowel disease, the nonsteroidal anti-inflammatory drugs are usually well tolerated.

About 50 per cent of individuals with both inflammatory bowel disease and ankylosing spondylitis are B27-positive, a percentage lower than that found in patients with primary ankylosing spondylitis.

A post–intestinal-bypass syndrome consisting of arthropathy and occasionally dermatitis is well recognized. Immune alterations have been described in these patients, and B27 is occasionally associated with this syndrome.

PSORIATIC ARTHROPATHY

Different subsets of psoriatic arthropathy are recognized, several forms of which appear to be enthesopathic rather than purely synovitic. Uveitis, sacroiliitis, and ascending spinal disease occur in up to 20 per cent of cases. Patients are seronegative for rheumatoid factor and exhibit sausage digits and characteristic radiologic changes. The disease may be markedly destructive.

Psoriasis itself is a genetically determined disease, associated with HLA-B13, HLA-Bw17, and HLA-Cw6. Moreover, HLA-B27 is present in approximately 20 per cent of individuals with psoriatic arthropathy even in the absence of sacroiliitis. HLA-Bw38, HLA-DR4, and HLA-DR7 appear to be genetic markers for patients with peripheral arthropathy. About 50 per cent of psoriatic spondylitis patients are B27-negative; thus, as with inflammatory bowel disease, other genetic or environmental factors are relevant.

Psoriatic arthropathy is a common disease, occurring in about 20 per cent of individuals with psoriasis, particularly in those patients with psoriatic nail disease. Women are affected only slightly more commonly than men, in contrast to the more marked sex distribution in rheumatoid disease. Several forms of psoriatic arthropathy, separated by indistinct boundaries, have been described.

1. Asymmetric oligoarthropathy. In general, there is little relationship between joint and skin activity. Patients with this common form of psoriatic arthropathy remain seronegative for rheumatoid factor. Asymmetric involvement of both large and small joints is seen; the sausage-shaped digit is common. A disparity is often observed between the clinical appearance and subjective symptoms. Any patient presenting with this form of arthropathy should be carefully examined for signs of psoriasis (scalp, umbilicus, gluteal region, and nails). In the past, many such individuals were considered to have seronegative rheumatoid arthritis.

2. Symmetric polyarthropathy resembling rheumatoid arthritis. Rarely, the pattern of arthritis may be indistinguishable from that seen in rheumatoid disease. This form may represent coincidental rheumatoid arthritis in a patient with psoriasis.

3. Arthritis mutilans. A resorptive arthropathy, arthritis mutilans is the severest form of destructive arthritis. The telescoping digits appear as the so-called opera-glass hand.

4. Psoriatic spondylitis. Approximately 20 per cent of subjects with psoriatic arthropathy have radiologic sacroiliitis (ankylosing spondylitis).

5. Psoriatic nail disease and distal interphalangeal joint involvement. Nail pitting, transverse depressions, and subungual hyperkeratosis often occur in association with distal interphalangeal joint disease. The relationship between the psoriasis and the arthritis remains unclear.

Laboratory Features

An elevated erythrocyte sedimentation rate, anemia, and rarely, hyperuricemia may occur. The frequency of positive tests for rheumatoid factor is the same as that found in the general population. The synovial tissue and fluid changes are nonspecific.

Radiologic Findings

Characteristic changes in this sometimes highly destructive disease include whittling of the distal ends of the phalanges, giving the joints a "pencil-and-cup" appearance; extensive bone resorption can result in an opera-glass hand. Erosions, ankylosis, periostitis, sacroiliitis, and ankylosing spondylitis are other typical radiologic findings.

Therapy

The skin and joints are treated separately. Improvement of the skin disease may be associated with amelioration of the joint inflammation. For mild arthropathy, indomethacin (25 to 50 mg t.i.d.) is the drug of choice. If this fails, phenylbutazone may be given. Gold and penicillamine may be useful, but few controlled studies have been done. Methotrexate is helpful in resistant cases.

Calin A (ed.): Spondylarthropathy. New York, Grune and Stratton, 1984, pp 1–427. *A multiauthored international text on spondylarthropathy including discussions on immunogenetics, the environment, and ethnic differences.*

Calin A, Marder A, Becks E, Burns T: Genetic difference between B27 positive patients with ankylosing spondylitis and B27 positive healthy controls. Arthritis Rheum 26:1460–1464, 1983. *An up-to-date analysis of the genetics of B27-associated disorders.*

Fox R, Calin A, Gerber R, and Gibson D: The chronicity of symptoms and disability in Reiter's syndrome: An analysis of 131 consecutive patients. Ann Intern Med 91:190–193, 1979. *A detailed evaluation of 131 consecutive patients with Reiter's syndrome.*

Wright V, Moll JMH: Seronegative Polyarthritis. Amsterdam, North Holland Publishing Company, 1976. *The best introduction to the concept of the spondylarthropathies.*

446. INFECTIOUS ARTHRITIS

Stephen E. Malawista

BACTERIAL ARTHRITIS

Bacterial arthritis usually results from bloodborne infection and much less commonly from direct penetration (e.g., needle aspiration) or contiguous osteomyelitis. Acute bacterial joint infections may be divided into two general groups, nongonococcal and gonococcal, based on their typically differing target populations, clinical characteristics, and ease of treatment. (This chapter emphasizes principles of diagnosis and management. Other areas of the text contain more detailed accounts of the problems and management of sepsis caused by specific bacteria.)

Nongonococcal Arthritis

Staphylococcus aureus heads the list of common infecting organisms in this group, followed by other gram-positive cocci (*Streptococcus pyrogenes, pneumoniae, viridans*) and gram-negative bacilli (*Escherichia coli, Salmonella* sp., *Pseudomonas*, etc.); *Hemophilus influenzae* is unusual except in children under four years of age, before protective immunity develops. Patients are often either very young or very old. Risk factors for bacterial arthritis during septicemia include debilitating chronic disease, immunosuppressive therapy, previous joint damage (e.g., rheumatoid arthritis, neuropathic arthropathy, joint surgery), sickle cell anemia, hypogammaglobulinemia, and intraarticular corticosteroid injections. After prosthetic joint replacement, an increasing problem has been late infection by organisms of low virulence, such as *Staphylococcus epidermidis*.

CLINICAL MANIFESTATIONS. A patient may present typically with the abrupt onset of a single severely tender red hot swollen joint, especially the knee or another weight-bearing joint; shaking chills and fever may occur. However, signs of inflammation may be masked in severely debilitated patients or in those given adenocorticosteroids or immunosuppressive agents. Bacterial arthritis superimposed on a noninfectious inflammatory joint disease may also be easily overlooked. For example, infection in one or a few joints of a patient with rheumatoid arthritis may be mistaken for a flare in the chronic disease. An infected joint in a gouty individual may go unrecognized for too long, even when the patient does not respond to his usual regimen for acute gouty arthritis (a good clue that something else is going on). A high index of suspicion is essential in these circumstances, because delay can lead rapidly to destruction of cartilage and bone and eventual fibrous or bony ankylosis.

DIAGNOSIS. When bacterial arthritis is suspected, prompt joint aspiration and both Gram stain and culture of synovial fluid are imperative; most nongonococcal bacterial will be recovered. Cultures for both aerobic and anaerobic organisms should be made. Synovial fluid leukocyte counts are frequently greater than 50,000 per cubic millimeter, and the glucose level low and lactate level high compared to those of serum, but these findings are not specific for infection. Bacteriologic studies should of course be extended to blood and other material (sputum, urine, etc.) from which the infection may have disseminated. On x-ray, only soft-tissue swelling is likely to be seen during the first week, but evidence of loss of articular cartilage and erosion of bone may appear rather soon thereafter in untreated patients.

MANAGEMENT. Successful management of bacterial arthritis depends primarily on early institution of appropriate antimicrobial therapy and effective drainage of the joint space. The selection of antimicrobial agents and recommendations regarding dose and duration of therapy are discussed in other areas of the text (Part XIX). Antibiotics are given parenterally, often in high doses, for two to four weeks, depending on the clinical situation and the patient's response. They generally attain adequate levels in joint fluid and need not be given intraarticularly; indeed, the latter procedure may induce a chemical synovitis. For drainage, daily (or even more frequent) closed joint aspiration through a large-bore needle is carried out until fluid no longer accumulates. Open surgical drainage usually can be avoided except when the hip or the shoulder is infected (difficult to evacuate completely by needle), when tissue debris or fibrin interfere with closed aspiration, or when loculations, gross joint destruction, or contiguous osteomyelitis is present. The affected joint should be at rest while inflamed, and mobilized to prevent atrophy when signs of acute inflammation have subsided.

Gonococcal Arthritis

Gonococcal infection is discussed in Ch. 302. The associated arthritis is by far the most common bacterial joint problem in generally healthy, sexually active teenagers and young adults, especially in urban populations. Gonorrhea is more likely to disseminate in women and in homosexual men, whose infections are often asymptomatic and therefore untreated. The risk of dissemination is particularly high during menses and pregnancy, in the post-partum period, and in individuals with genetic deficiency in the terminal components of serum complement (C5, C6, C7, or C8). Additional features that help to distinguish gonococcal from other bacterial arthritides include a high frequency of associated tenosynovitis and rash and of multiple joint involvement, especially in the wrists and hands. Diagnosis is frequently presumptive because synovial fluid smear and culture—which requires special media—are often negative, and corroborating cultural evidence from urethra, cervix, throat, rectum, blood, or skin may be lacking. Highly suggestive diagnostically is a history of fever and migratory polyarthralgias that progress to frank oligoarticular arthritis and are associated with tenosynovitis and skin lesions. The latter are either vesiculopustular on an erythematous base, often with necrotic centers, or hemorrhagic. Similar lesions are seen with arthritis caused by the meningococcus. Response to (even oral) antibiotic therapy (Ch. 302) and drainage is usually dramatic. Resistance to penicillin of gonococci that disseminate is known but is uncommon.

Tuberculous Arthritis

The general decline in the frequency of pulmonary tuberculosis in the western world is reflected in the relative rarity of tuberculous bone and joint disease. Infection usually reaches the joint from hematogenous dissemination to bone and direct extension from an osteomyelitic focus. Formerly, the classic presentation was chronic low back pain in a child because of involvement of lower thoracic or lumbar vertebrae, leading to collapse and sharp-angle kyphosis (Pott's disease). Currently, the typical target is a tuberculin-positive adult, often without evidence of pulmonary disease, who presents with chronic, insidious pain and swelling, usually in a single joint, especially the hip, knee, or wrist; this presentation is often mistaken for monoarticular rheumatoid arthritis. Tenosynovitis is common. Diagnosis depends upon culture of *Mycobacterium tuberculosis* from synovial fluid (positive in 80 per cent) or synovial biopsy (positive in 90 per cent). Sensitivities to chemotherapeutic agents must be determined; caseating granulomata and acid-fast bacilli are sometimes due to atypical mycobacteria resistant to the usual antituberculous drugs. Usual therapy for uncomplicated infections consists of long-term isoniazid and ethambutol or rifampin.

Masi AT, Eisenstein BI: Disseminated gonococcal infection (DGI) and gonococcal arthritis (GCA). Clinical manifestations, diagnosis, complications, treatment, and prevention. Semin Arthritis Rheum 70:173, 1981. *A careful review that satisfies its subtitle.*

Rosenthal J, Bole G, Robinson WD: Acute non-gonococcal infectious arthritis. Evaluation of risk factors, therapy and outcome. Arthritis Rheum 23:889, 1980. *Presentation of experience with 63 patients and general review.*

VIRAL ARTHRITIS

Many specific viral infections are associated with polyarthritis, notably hepatitis B and rubella, but also mumps and vaccinia (and formerly, smallpox) and occasionally adenovirus type 7, EB virus (in infectious mononucleosis) and other herpes viruses, and certain enteroviruses. Polyarthritis may dominate the picture of various mosquito-transmitted arbovirus infections, especially epidemic polyarthritis of Australia (Ross River virus) and the dengue-like illnesses, chikungunya and o'nyong-nyong.

In general, diagnosis is suggested by the exposure history (drug abuse for hepatitis B, immunization for rubella, epidemiologic considerations for arbo- or enteroviruses); recognition of the associated viral syndrome, which often includes fever, rash, and regional lymphadenopathy; brevity of the joint involvement (days to weeks); and changing antibody titers against specific antigens. Routine laboratory tests are nonspecific, and except for rubella, virus has rarely been recovered from synovial fluid. Little is known about pathogenesis, but studies of hepatitis B and rubella provide some clues.

Transient, often symmetrical polyarthritis or arthralgias resembling acute rheumatoid arthritis may be associated with both hepatitis B and rubella infections. In the case of *hepatitis B*, 10 to 30 per cent of patients have arthritis, often accompanied by urticaria, fever, and lymphadenopathy, all occurring days to weeks before the onset of frank hepatitis. This prodromal syndrome typically occurs when hepatitis B surface antigen (HBsAg) is in excess over antibody, hypocomplementemia is present, and serum contains immune complexes composed of HBsAg and anti-HB, other immunoglobulins, and complement components. Similar material has been found in affected dermal blood vessels, and the antigen has been seen in synovial tissue. With the development of antibody excess, complexes disappear, the arthritis and rash resolve, and frank hepatitis may supervene. The process resembles experimental serum sickness, and suggests an inflammatory pathogenetic mechanism driven by deposition of immune complexes. Joint symptoms may respond dramatically to salicylates.

Rubella arthritis is primarily a disease of adult women. It usually follows onset of the characteristic rash by a few days, but the rash may be absent and rheumatoid factor present, inviting diagnostic confusion. Arthritis is usually sudden in onset, symmetrical and polyarticular in distribution (fingers, knees, wrists), brief in duration (less than a month), and without residua. Salicylates are useful for pain and stiffness.

Arthritis may also occur within a few weeks of vaccination by attenuated rubella virus. Again, attacks are brief but may recur periodically for a few years without permanent joint damage. Rubella virus has been recovered from synovial fluid in both the natural and vaccine-induced disease and more recently in a few patients with various chronic joint syndromes. It seems capable of replicating in synovium; whether its new association with chronic disease is critical or coincidental remains to be determined.

Steere AC, Malawista SE: Viral arthritis. *In* McCarty D J (ed.): Arthritis and Allied Conditions. 10th ed. Philadelphia, Lea & Febiger (in press). *Survey of common and uncommon arthritides associated with specific viral illnesses.*

Wands JR, Mann E, Alpert E, Isselbacher KJ: The pathogenesis of arthritis associated with acute hepatitis B surface antigen-positive hepatitis. Complement activation and characterization of circulating immune complexes. J Clin Invest 55:930, 1975. *Clinical description and characterization of immunologic aspects of the syndrome.*

LYME DISEASE

Lyme disease (formerly Lyme arthritis) was recognized in 1975 because of unusual geographic clustering of children with inflammatory arthropathy in the region of Lyme, Connecticut. It is now known to be a complex immune-mediated multisystem disorder occurring at any age, in either sex, whose clinical hallmark is an early expanding skin lesion, *erythema chronicum migrans* (ECM), which may be followed weeks to months later by neurologic, cardiac, or joint abnormalities. Symptoms may refer to any one of these systems alone. Foci of Lyme disease have been found elsewhere along the northeastern coast of the United States, in many other states, in Europe, and in Australia. The disease is caused by a newly recognized spirochete, and transmitted by the minute tick *Ixodes dammini* or by related ixodid ticks.

In summer or early fall, days to weeks after a tick bite that may have gone unnoticed, a typical patient may present with ECM at the site and perhaps with systemic symptoms: chills and fever, malaise and fatigue, headache or stiff neck. Most such patients have circulating immune complexes. Those who also have elevated levels of serum IgM and cryoglobulins containing IgM are at high risk for subsequent organ involvement. This high-risk group tends to have the histocompatibility antigen DR2, which in turn correlates with the development of severe disease (but not with ECM alone). Within weeks, typical ECM expands to several inches in diameter with central clearing, then fades; secondary annular non–tick-associated lesions may occur.

Within weeks to months of ECM, there may be neurologic abnormalities (15 per cent of patients)—especially lymphocytic meningitis, cranial neuritis (including bilateral Bell's palsy), and motor and sensory radiculoneuritis—and cardiac abnormalities (8 per cent)—fluctuating degrees of A-V block and myopericarditis (but *not* valvulitis; cf. rheumatic fever). Early rheumatic complaints include migratory polyarthritis and arthralgias and tendinitis. Later (weeks to years), frank arthritis (without morning stiffness) may occur (60 per cent of patients) in a few large joints, especially knees, persist for weeks to months, and recur for years. Chronic joint disease, with erosion of cartilage and bone, is much less common.

Changes in synovium and synovial fluid resemble those in rheumatoid arthritis. Immune complexes are present, even when absent from blood. However, rheumatoid factor and antinuclear antibodies are lacking. Spirochetes have been isolated from blood (early), skin (ECM), and cerebrospinal fluid, but not yet from joints. Diagnosis, when ECM is lacking or missed, is facilitated by high or changing antibody titers against the *I. dammini* spirochete.

Oral tetracycline (or penicillin) eradicates ECM and usually prevents major complications. High-dose intravenous penicillin cures the meningitis and is currently used for complete heart block (with high-dose prednisone, when failure is present). The high-dose penicillin regimen has recently been shown to cure established arthritis in the majority of patients.

Steere AC, Malawista SE: Lyme disease. *In* Kelly WN, Harris ED Jr, Ruddy S, Sledge CB (eds.): Textbook of Rheumatology. 2nd ed. Philadelphia, W. B. Saunders Company (in press). *In depth presentation of the epidemiology, pathogenesis, natural history, immunology, diagnosis, and treatment of Lyme disease.*

Steere AC, Pachner AR, Malawista SE: Successful treatment of neurologic abnormalities of Lyme disease with high-dose intravenous penicillin. Ann Intern Med 99:767, 1983. *Meningitis, formerly treated with high-dose prednisone tapered over months, responds to penicillin in days.*

OTHER FORMS OF INFECTIOUS ARTHRITIS

Syphilitic Arthritis

Syphilis is discussed in Ch. 306. Joint disease associated with congenital and acquired syphilitic infections is now rare. In infants with congenital disease, musculoskeletal complaints are related to periostitis and osteochondritis. About the time of puberty, painless knee effusions (Clutton's joints) may be confused with rheumatoid or pyogenic arthritis. With acquired infection, arthralgias, arthritis, or tenosynovitis may accompany classic signs of secondary syphilis: rash, mucous plaques, alopecia, or lymphadenopathy. In tertiary lues, gummatous arthritis or periostitis (tibia, clavicles) may occur. Neuropathic arthropathy (Charcot joint) is reviewed in Ch. 497.

Fungal Arthritis

Any of the invasive mycoses can affect joints, usually by direct extension from bone. Frequent infectious agents include coccidioidomycosis and histoplasmosis—both of which may also be accompanied by erythema nodosum with joint involvement—sporotrichosis (often by direct penetration: rose thorns), blastomycosis, actinomycosis, and candidiasis. Clinically, the affected joint or joints resemble those in other forms of granulomatous arthritis (e.g., tuberculous). For diagnosis, the causative agent must be seen in appropriately stained synovial biopsy material or grown from synovial tissue or fluid.

447. SYSTEMIC LUPUS ERYTHEMATOSUS

Alfred D. Steinberg

Systemic lupus erythematosus (SLE) is a disease of unknown etiology characterized by inflammation in many different organ systems associated with the production of antibodies reactive with nuclear, cytoplasmic, and cell membrane antigens. Individual patients may have some, but not necessarily all, of the following: fatigue, anemia, fever, rashes, sun sensitivity, alopecia, arthritis, pericarditis, pleurisy, vasculitis, nephritis, and central nervous system disease. The course is often unpredictable with variable periods of exacerbations and remissions. There is no one clinical abnormality that definitely establishes the diagnosis, nor is there a single test for the disorder. As a result, criteria have been developed and modified in an attempt to include patients with SLE and to exclude patients with other disorders (see Table 447–1). Although these criteria have been developed for epidemiologic and research purposes, they are helpful in diagnosis as well. Nevertheless, it is possible to fulfill these criteria and not have SLE, and it is possible to fail to fulfill the criteria and still have SLE. Thus, a teen-age girl with a "butterfly" rash of the face, pleurisy, and large amounts of serum antibodies reactive with native DNA undoubtedly has SLE even if she does not yet manifest any other criteria. The disease derives its name (lupus = wolf) from the facial rash, which resembles the malar erythema of a wolf.

INCIDENCE. Although SLE can occur at any age (it has been diagnosed at birth and in individuals in the tenth decade of life), more than 70 per cent of patients experience the onset of disease between ages 13 and 40 years. Among children, SLE occurs three times as commonly in females as in males. In patients in their teens, twenties, and thirties, 90 to 95 per cent are female. Thereafter, the female predominance again falls to that observed before puberty.

The disorder is approximately three times more common among American blacks than American caucasians. Certain North American indian tribes (Sioux, Crow, Arapahoe) have an even greater predisposition toward SLE. Orientals have been less well studied; however, the data suggest that they are affected to approximately the same extent as American blacks. The overall annual incidence of SLE is about 6 new cases per 100,000 population per year for relatively low-risk populations and approximately 35 per 100,000 for relatively high-risk populations. The chance of a black female developing SLE in her lifetime is approximately 1 in 250.

These data suggest that both genetic factors and sex hormones may affect the probability of developing SLE. If a family member has SLE, the likelihood of SLE increases (approximately 70 per cent for identical twins and 5 per cent for other first degree relatives). Although males develop SLE less frequently than do females, their illness is not milder.

ETIOLOGY. The etiology of SLE is unknown. The signs and symptoms are thought to be due to the autoantibodies that react with self constituents and initiate inflammatory responses. The initiation of this process may be multifactorial (Fig. 447–1). Moreover, the factors may be different in different individuals with SLE. These factors are currently poorly understood. One or more genetic factors appear to be important in many individuals. These may be genes that allow augmented antibody responses following a variety of stimuli as well as genes that predispose to particular autoantibody responses. In addition, hormonal, metabolic, and environmental factors appear to act

TABLE 447–1. THE 1982 REVISED CRITERIA FOR CLASSIFICATION OF SYSTEMIC LUPUS ERYTHEMATOSUS*

Criterion		Definition
1. Malar rash		Fixed erythema, flat or raised, over the malar eminences, tending to spare the nasolabial folds
2. Discoid rash		Erythematous raised patches with adherent keratotic scaling and follicular plugging; atrophic scarring may occur in older lesions
3. Photosensitivity		Skin rash as a result of unusual reaction to sunlight, by patient history or physician observation
4. Oral ulcers		Oral or nasopharyngeal ulceration, usually painless, observed by a physician
5. Arthritis		Nonerosive arthritis involving two or more peripheral joints, characterized by tenderness, swelling, or effusion
6. Serositis	a)	Pleuritis—convincing history of pleuritic pain or rub heard by a physician or evidence of pleural effusion *OR*
	b)	Pericarditis—documented by ECG or rub or evidence of pericardial effusion
7. Renal disorder	a)	Persistent proteinuria greater than 0.5 grams per day or greater than 3+ if quantitation not performed *OR*
	b)	Cellular casts—may be red cell, hemoglobin, granular, tubular, or mixed
8. Neurologic disorder	a)	Seizures—in the absence of offending drugs or known metabolic derangements; e.g., uremia, ketoacidosis, or electrolyte imbalance *OR*
	b)	Psychosis—in the absence of offending drugs or known metabolic derangements, e.g., uremia, ketoacidosis, or electrolyte imbalance
9. Hematologic disorder	a)	Hemolytic anemia—with reticulocytosis *OR*
	b)	Leukopenia—less than 4000/mm^3 total on two or more occasions *OR*
	c)	Lymphopenia—less than 1500/mm^3 on two or more occasions *OR*
	d)	Thrombocytopenia—less than 100,000/mm^3 in the absence of offending drugs
10. Immunologic disorder	a)	Positive LE cell preparation *OR*
	b)	Anti-DNA: antibody to native DNA in abnormal titer *OR*
	c)	Anti-Sm: presence of antibody to Sm nuclear antigen *OR*
	d)	False positive serologic test for syphilis known to be positive for at least 6 months and confirmed by *Treponema pallidum* immobilization or fluorescent treponemal antibody absorption test
11. Antinuclear antibody		An abnormal titer of antinuclear antibody by immunofluorescence or an equivalent assay at any point in time and in the absence of drugs known to be associated with "drug-induced lupus" syndrome

*The proposed classification is based on 11 criteria. For the purpose of identifying patients in clinical studies, a person shall be said to have systemic lupus erythematosus if any 4 or more of the 11 criteria are present, serially or simultaneously, during any interval of observation.

on the genetically conditioned immune substratum to predispose to or protect against disease expression. Androgens appear to protect against the development of SLE except in a subgroup of males who inherit a Y chromosome accelerating factor from their fathers. Estrogens probably predispose to SLE to a lesser extent than androgens protect against the expression of the illness. In general, factors that augment immunity favor disease expression whereas those that retard immunity, especially antibody production, tend to protect. Any of a variety of bacterial or viral infections may stimulate the immune system as may drugs or food additives.

The central role of immune regulations in the expression of illness has led to the concept that some patients may have a primary abnormality in the ability of their immune systems to perform normal self-regulatory functions. It is probably best to consider abnormal immune regulation as one of several factors that may contribute to illness. If any one is very abnormal, disease may occur. Under most circumstances, several defects probably combine to incite disease. However, once the process is initiated, impaired self-regulation would favor perpetuation of the disease-inducing abnormalities.

It has long been known that some individuals with SLE have disease exacerbations following exposure to ultraviolet light. Several different mechanisms are likely: UV light induces keratinocytes to secrete interleukin 1, which, in turn, stimulates B cells and induces T cells to produce growth factors (interleukin 2, B cell growth factors, B cell differentiation factors, interferon), which stimulate the immune system; UV light impairs processing of antigen and immune complexes, thereby increasing the load of pathogenic complexes on target organs; UV light induces cytosine and thymine dimer formation, which stimulates immune responses.

Certain drugs can cause an SLE-like illness in apparently healthy individuals. The drugs (Table 447–2) do not share common structural or chemical properties. The mechanisms of disease induction probably vary depending upon the structure of the drug. Even chemicals in foods may induce SLE. For example, alfalfa sprouts contain L-canavanine, which can induce an SLE-like illness. The extent to which "idiopathic" SLE is triggered by such specific environmental factors is unknown.

A variety of complement deficiencies have been associated with SLE. The most common is C2 deficiency. It is not clear whether the association is one of genetic linkage or predisposition because of the deficiency itself. The latter might occur if the deficiency led to increased susceptibility to infections that trigger illness.

For many years it has been thought that there might be a "lupus virus," a particular virus that induces disease. Patients with SLE have, in the endothelial cells of their kidneys and in their lymphocytes, structures that resemble viral nucleocapsids. In addition, retroviruses have been implicated in the immune-complex renal disease of animals with SLE-like disorders. Nevertheless, the evidence suggests that even if such a virus is important, it is only one of many factors critical to the development of disease.

AUTOIMMUNITY AND DISEASE IN SLE. In prior years it was believed that an anti-self response was harmful and that such responses did not occur normally. More recently it has become appreciated that normal immune responses involve self-self recognition. Moreover, many individuals produce nonpathogenic antibodies reactive with self antigens. As a result, disease occurs only when anti-self reactions are either excessive or productive of especially injurious immune responses. SLE is characterized by the production of large amounts of antibodies reactive with a great variety of different antigenic specificities. Some individual antibody molecules have been shown to cross-react with more than one antigen (DNA and cardiolipin or IgG and nucleoprotein). As a result, the true range of antibody molecules reactive with self-determinants may be less than the number of specificities as measured by the reactive antigens. Nevertheless, the range of determinants against which SLE antibodies may react is impressive (Table 447–3).

How could such self reactivity come about? It is believed that self-tolerance is a complex state brought about and maintained by several mechanisms. Very early in life, exposure to antigens tends to produce tolerance rather than immunity. Subsequently, several immune mechanisms tend to maintain self-tolerance. Although B lymphocytes and their progeny are

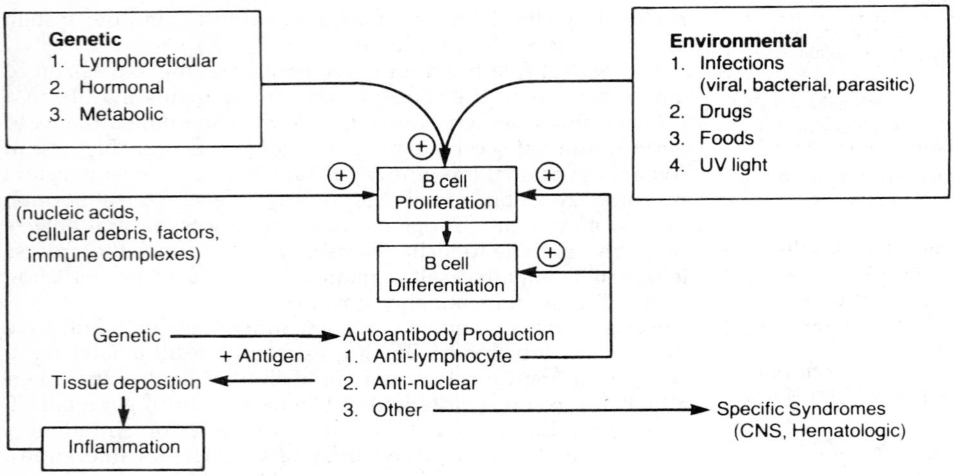

Figure 447–1. Initiation and perpetuation of systemic lupus erythematosus.

responsible for antibody production, under most circumstances they require helper T lymphocytes for activation, proliferation, and differentiation into antibody secreting cells. Moreover, specialized T cells (suppressor cells) appear capable of down-regulating immune responses. If the T cell population is self-tolerant, it may prevent B cells capable of differentiating into autoantibody producing cells from proliferating and differentiating. A defect in self-tolerance mechanisms could occur at any of several steps in the immune pathway. In addition, strong immune stimulation can overwhelm normal regulatory mechanisms rendering them incapable of function adequate to regulate the immune stimuli. Such strong immune stimuli as graft-versus-host disease (as after allogeneic bone marrow transplantation) or stimulation by any of a variety of powerful polyclonal immune activators (endotoxin) or even viruses that stimulate B cells (Ebstein-Barr virus) may drive B cells to produce antibodies and autoantibodies without the usual requirements for or regulation by T cells. Individuals with B cells capable of producing pathogenic autoantibodies that had been previously held in check by T cells may, under such circumstances, be driven to produce large amounts of injurious antibodies. Since it is often the quantity of autoantibody that determines whether or not disease occurs, quantitative aspects of immune regulation and immune stimulation may be critical to the balance between disease development versus relative health with minor immune abnormalities.

PATHOGENESIS. Systemic lupus is often classified as an immune complex type disorder. This designation is, at best, an oversimplification. SLE is a disease primarily mediated by antibodies; however, the details of pathogenesis are not proven for many of the clinical and pathologic findings. It is clear that patients with SLE produce autoantibodies and that many of these are injurious. This has been well demonstrated for the

TABLE 447–2. SOME DRUGS ABLE TO INDUCE FEATURES OF SLE

Related to Dose-Time Administration	More Idiosyncratic
Hydralazine	Aminosalicylic acid
Procainamide	D-Penicillamine
Alpha-methyldopa	Griseofulvin
Isoniazid	Penicillin
Chlorpromazine	Ampicillin
Chlorthalidone	Streptomycin
Phenytoin	Sulfonamides
Mephenytoin	Tetracycline
Trimethadione	Methylthiouracil
Primidone	Propythiouracil
Ethosuximide	Phenylbutazone
Carbamazepine	Oxyphenisatin
Phenylethylacetylurea	Practolol
	Tolazamide
	Methysergide
	Reserpine
	Quinidine
	Isoquinazepan
	Guanoxan

TABLE 447–3. AUTOANTIBODIES FOUND IN PATIENTS WITH SLE

Specificity	Comments
Nuclear	Present in most but not all patients
Native DNA	Essentially restricted to SLE
Denatured (single-stranded) DNA	May also cross-react with double-stranded DNA. High titers in SLE; lower titers in other diseases
Histones H1, H3-H4	SLE
Histones H2A-H2B	More common in drug-induced SLE
Sm	In a minority of SLE patients, but not found in other diseases.
Nuclear ribonucleoprotein	Found in SLE, but highest titers in "mixed connective tissue disease." Multiple small proteins and combined RNA have been discovered.
Nucleolar antigens	Scleroderma, SLE, Sjögren's Syndrome
SS-B (La, Ha)	Sjögren's Syndrome, SLE
SS-A (Ro)	Sjögren's Syndrome, SLE
Proliferating cell nuclear antigen	SLE
RANA	Especially in rheumatoid arthritis (Ebstein-Barr virus)
DNA-RNA hybrids, double-stranded RNA	SLE
Cytoplasmic	Less information available on these
Ribosomal ribonucleoprotein	SLE
Mitochondria	Primary biliary cirrhosis, SLE
Microsomal antigens	Chronic active hepatitis, malignancies
Lysosomes	SLE
Single-stranded RNA, tRNA	SLE
SS-B and SS-A	Sjögren's Syndrome, SLE
Cell membrane determinants	Common in SLE
Red cells	May occur without important hemolysis
White cells	Granulocytes, T cells, B cells
Platelets	Common without thrombocytopenia
Lipomodulin	SLE, RA, others ?
Receptors	Insulin, IL 2, others
Ia	Interferes with immune functions
Others	
Mitotic spindle and intracellular supporting proteins	SLE and other rheumatic diseases
Immunoglobulins	JRA, RA, SLE, Sjögren's Syndrome, others
Clotting factors	SLE and other diseases
Cardiolipin	May cross react with DNA
Thyroid antigens	Thyroid diseases, SLE, Sjögren's Syndrome

renal disease associated with SLE. Antibody reacts with antigen either in the circulation or in the glomerulus and complement is fixed, leading to release of chemotactic factors, attraction of leukocytes, and release of their injurious mediators of inflammation. The degree of pathology is determined, to a large extent, by the magnitude of the antibody deposition and the magnitude of the inflammatory process initiated. Continued deposition of antibody and continued induction of inflammation ultimately leads to irreversible renal damage. Similar processes occur in other organs. However, antibody and complement may be deposited in the skin or in the choroid plexus with or without an attendant inflammatory response. It must be presumed that the qualitative character of the antibody molecules (affinity, isotype, charge), the nature of the antigen or their combined properties (size, molecular configuration), or additional factors may be critical to pathogenesis.

It has long been taught that immunopathology of SLE results from the deposition of DNA–anti-DNA immune complexes. Although immune complexes may contribute to the immunopathology, it is likely that uncomplexed antibody may reach an organ where antigen is already present and there bind to antigen and initiate the inflammatory process. This idea is supported by demonstrations of DNA binding to basement membranes without antibody. Moreover, antibodies of other specificities appear to contribute to disease.

Antibody plays a role in SLE not only by depositing in vessels, but by binding to the surfaces of cells. Patients with SLE produce antibodies to erythrocytes, granulocytes, lymphocytes, and macrophages. These antibodies can cause such cells to be removed from the circulation by the reticuloendothelial system, killed by complement-mediated cytotoxicity, or more likely, by the mechanism of antibody-dependent cellular cytotoxicity (ADCC). In this non–complement-mediated killing, leukocytes recognize antibody-coated target cells and kill them. It is possible that ADCC may be responsible for some of the pathology initiated in the kidneys and other organs by other antibody-mediated mechanisms. In addition, antibody directed against renal antigens, for example renal tubular or glomerular basement membrane, may be generated as a result of immunization by fragments released from the inflammatory process. Such antibody induces additional renal pathology and may account for much of the disease in some patients.

It appears that many of the inflammatory lesions that occur in SLE are initiated by antibody and that the injury occurs in small vessels. Thus, any organ so affected could be a site of inflammation with the possibility of scarring, dysfunction, or both. Many of the central nervous system problems of patients (seizures, psychoses) as well as hematologic (anemia, thrombocytopenia, leukopenia), cardiac (coronary artery disease), dermal (alopecia, sun sensitivity), and other clinical and laboratory abnormalities have additional pathogenetic mechanisms. The hematologic abnormalities could all be explained by antibodies specifically reactive with the formed elements of the blood; however, many relate to suppression at the level of the bone marrow. The central nervous system disorders are multiple, and each may have its own pathogenetic mechanism. Because central nervous system involvement in SLE is not a single entity, individual patients may require different approaches to understanding and therapy.

PATHOLOGY. The pathologic abnormalities of SLE follow directly from the pathogenetic mechanisms; moreover, the same degree of variability is encountered. In organs affected by small vessel vasculitis, the first lesions are usually characterized by granulocytic infiltration and periarteriolar edema. This is usually (except in some cases of leukocytoclastic involvement of the skin) followed by round cell infiltration and ultimately a relatively acellular eosinophilic material composed of fibrin, immunoglobulins, and complement (fibrinoid) containing scattered hematoxylin bodies. These basophilic-staining bodies are nuclear debris, often associated with anti-nuclear antibody, and represent a correlate of the LE cell in vivo. Immunofluorescence analysis of affected areas demonstrates immunoglobulin and complement in the vessels in the affected areas. Arterioles, venules, and sometimes arteries and veins are involved.

Individual organs often have their peculiar abnormalities. The spleen has "onion skin lesions," concentric fibrosis of the walls and surrounding tissues of the central and penicilliary arteries. These lesions are thought to be diagnostic of SLE in patients with "idiopathic" thrombocytopenia. Nonbacterial verrucous endocarditis (Libman-Sacks) consists of vegetations on the heart valves or chordae tendineae; they can extend along the endocardium and become quite large.

The renal pathology varies from mild to severe glomerular inflammation and variable interstitial involvement. Most patients have relatively normal kidneys or a renal lesion consisting of minimal focal hypercellularity, thickening of the capillary basement membrane, and fibrinoid change. In clinically important glomerulonephritis, these lesions are more generalized and are usually a mixture of proliferative and membranous changes with increases in endothelial, mesangial, epithelial, and inflammatory cells, capsular inflammation leading to crescent formation, and focal thickening of the basement membrane and mesangial hypercellularity. Some kidneys are found to have membranous glomerulonephritis with considerable thickening of the basement membrane. Basement membrane thickening, when associated with fibrinoid changes, results in the so-called "wire loop" lesions. There may also be hyaline thrombi in glomeruli, focal necrosis, hematoxylin bodies, and sclerosis in healed lesions. Tubular degenerative changes and mixed inflammatory interstitial inflammation are common. Some patients have primarily mesangial disease; this carries a better prognosis than does capillary loop involvement. Extensive crescent formation and substantial glomerular or interstitial scarring are bad prognostic signs.

CLINICAL MANIFESTATIONS. SLE is a highly variable disease in terms of onset and course. A young woman may present with a butterfly rash, a history of recent sun sensitivity, pleuropericarditis, arthritis, fever, extreme fatigue, seizures, and nephrotic syndrome. This "typical" presentation, which is easily recognized as SLE, occurs in only a minority of patients. More commonly, patients may have only one or two signs or symptoms of SLE for a period of time, such as arthritis and fatigue. Only later do additional features of SLE occur. As a result, the initial presentation may not allow a definitive diagnosis nor insight into the organ systems that may become involved in the future. Many patients never develop major organ involvement. Some have kidney but not central nervous system involvement or vice versa. Thus, the clinical manifestations of one patient may be very different from those of another. Nevertheless, some associations between serologic findings and clinical features are valid on a statistical basis but may not hold for a given individual. Thus, patients with large amounts of anti-DNA, especially precipitating antibodies, are more likely to have renal disease. Those with antibodies to Ro (SS-A) and La (SS-B, Ha) are most likely to have sicca syndrome, muscle disease, lung disease, and inconsequential or no renal disease. In the paragraphs that follow, individual clinical features of patients with SLE are described (see also Table 447–4). Patients vary greatly in terms of organ system involvement and also in terms of the severity of disease when a given organ system is affected. Thus, most patients do not have many of the abnormalities described. In addition, SLE is characterized by periods of active disease followed by periods of less intense disease or even remission. In rare cases the patient has a rapidly progressive disease, but the majority can look forward to the time when the disease no longer interferes with their lives.

Constitutional Problems. The majority of patients have fatigue, fever, and weight loss at the time of diagnosis. However, before attributing these to SLE, a diligent search for other causes is necessary to rule out the concurrent presence of serious infection. Later in the illness, the recurrence of one or

TABLE 447–4. COMMON CLINICAL ABNORMALITIES IN PATIENTS WITH SLE

Abnormality	Approximate Frequency (%)*
Constitutional	
Fatigue	90
Fever	80
Weight loss, anorexia	60
Musculoskeletal	
Arthritis, arthralgia	90
Myalgia, myositis	30
Skin and mucous membranes	
Butterfly rash	60
Alopecia	50
Photosensitivity	40
Raynaud's phenomenon	30
Mucosal ulcers	30
Discoid lupus	20
Urticaria	10
Edema or bullae	10
Eye (conjunctivitis/episcleritis/sicca syndrome)	20
Gastrointestinal	30
Serosal (pleurisy, pericarditis, peritonitis)	50
Lymphoreticular	
Lymphadenopathy	50
Splenomegaly	30
Hepatomegaly	30
Hypertension	30
Bacterial infections	40
Pneumonitis (all)	30
"lupus"	10
Renal (all)	50
severe	20
Central nervous system	
Personality disorders	50
Seizures	20
Psychoses	20
Stroke or long tract signs	10
Migraine headaches	10
Cardiac	
Myocarditis	30
Murmurs and valvular disease	30
Coronary artery disease	20
Hematologic	
Anemia (all)	70
Hemolytic	10
Purpura (all)	50
Thrombocytopenia	10
Peripheral neuropathy	10

*Frequencies are compiled from a number of series and are rounded off to the nearest 10 per cent. There was some variation from series to series depending upon patient population, non-SLE therapy, and therapy for SLE. Some abnormalities are more common in younger patients than in older patients (e.g., splenomegaly and lymphadenopathy) and vice versa (e.g., muscle disease and sicca syndrome).

more of these findings often indicates an increase in disease activity. Fatigue, difficult as it may be to evaluate, often is the first sign that a flare is imminent.

Musculoskeletal Problems. Arthralgias are the single most common manifestation in SLE. They characteristically are much more transitory than in patients with rheumatoid arthritis (RA), lasting minutes to days in a given joint. With more longstanding or more severe disease, the pain may be constant and frank arthritis is observed. It is often symmetrical, the proximal interphalangeal joints of the hands, metacarpophalangeal joints, wrists, and knees being most commonly affected. Morning stiffness is reported by many patients with SLE and joint disease. Although the bony erosions characteristic of RA do not occur, deformities similar to those in RA develop in 10 to 15 per cent of patients and are thought to result from tendon disease. Occasionally patients experience rupture of the Achilles or quadriceps tendons. Myalgias occur in approximately 30 per cent of patients; only a portion of these have muscle tenderness. Many patients with SLE and muscle disease do not have elevations of creatine kinase activity; some of these have an elevated aldolase value. Muscle samples from such patients may be normal or show perivascular infiltration or atrophy. Some patients have a vacuolar myopathy that is also observed in corticosteroid-treated individuals.

Skin and Mucous Membranes. The typical butterfly rash varies from a slight blush to a clear-cut and somewhat edematous nonpapular erythematous covering of both cheeks and the bridge of the nose. Patients with a butterfly rash often look as though they have healthy rosy cheeks or have applied too much rouge. This lesion may occur in the absence of sun exposure, but is often exacerbated by the sun. It often precedes other manifestations of disease. A maculopapular erythematous eruption is also common. Indistinguishable from a drug eruption, it is often induced or exacerbated by sunlight and sometimes by a drug (Gantrisin and ampicillin are common offenders). The palms and soles are not always spared. Healing usually occurs without scarring. Urticaria and angioedema are more common than subepidermal bullae, which occur in only a few per cent of patients. Discoid lupus in SLE is indistinguishable from discoid lupus without systemic involvement; however, systemic disease may develop in patients with longstanding discoid lesions. In this rash, central atrophy, hyper- and hypopigmentation, telangiectasia, and follicular plugging accompany the usual stages of erythema followed by hyperkeratosis and then by atrophy. The hypopigmentation may be extensive and particularly disturbing to blacks.

Livedo reticularis occurs commonly in patients with SLE, but only rarely is it severe. Splinter hemorrhages, tender fingertip pulp lesions, and palmar erythema are sometimes remarkable. Purpura is more often secondary to vasculitis or capillary fragility (corticosteroid therapy is often responsible) than to thrombocytopenia.

Lupus profundus (relapsing nodular nonsuppurative panniculitis) occurs rarely in SLE patients. It may be limited to superficial panniculitis or may extend deeply into the thighs or buttocks. The overlying skin may ulcerate, and the deeper lesions often calcify.

One fifth of patients demonstrate vasculitic lesions of the skin. These can occur on the fingertips, forearms, lips, or lower leg (these latter may ulcerate). Although they are signs of disease activity, they do not usually imply impending disaster. The related mucosal ulcers are often painless and occur on the hard and soft palate, the nasal septum, other parts of the upper respiratory tract, and even the vagina. They are usually harmless, but occasional patients with involvement of the upper airway may require emergency tracheotomy.

Alopecia is usually diffuse; patients report increased hair on comb or brush or pillow. The hair will regrow in areas not scarred by discoid lesions.

Raynaud's phenomenon may be severe enough to cause digital gangrene and spontaneous amputation of the distal parts of the digits. More often it follows a more benign and variable course. Thrombophlebitis occurs in approximately 10 per cent of patients and may be accompanied by pulmonary emboli.

Eyes. Conjunctivitis or episcleritis or both are usually observed in younger patients at times of disease activity. Cytoid bodies (white exudates next to retinal vessels) are associated with active central nervous system involvement. Spasm of the retinal vessels may lead to transient or permanent blindness. Keratoconjunctivitis sicca occurs in 10 per cent of patients and is usually slowly progressive, but it often improves temporarily with therapy for other symptoms.

Gastrointestinal System. Anorexia, nausea, vomiting, and abdominal pain are observed in a minority of patients. Diffuse abdominal pain with or without rebound tenderness may be a manifestation of serositis or mesenteric arteritis. The latter can be complicated by intestinal infarct, which may lead to perforation and death. Corticosteroid therapy often improves symptoms in both situations; however, if perforation has already occurred, the symptoms may be blunted and therapy inappropriately delayed. Pancreatitis is occasionally due to SLE.

Dysphagia may be associated with reduced peristalsis, ulcerations of the esophagus caused by arteritis, or, more commonly, *Candida albicans* infection.

Liver. Liver enlargement occurs in about 30 per cent of patients with SLE. This is usually inconsequential. Fatty infiltration of the liver is common and rarely may be associated with hepatic insufficiency. Liver enzyme elevations often occur early in the illness in the absence of therapy. Aspirin treatment may induce such enzyme elevations. Chronic hepatitis is only occasionally observed in patients with SLE.

Heart. Pericarditis is usually symptomatic but without consequence; however, an occasional patient may experience tamponade. The most common EKG abnormality is nonspecific T wave changes. A prolonged P-R interval or evidence of ischemia or infarction may be found. Myocarditis may be manifested by unexplained tachycardia or mild dyspnea on exertion. More severe involvement is associated with frank heart failure. Coronary artery disease, most often atherosclerotic but occasionally arteritic, can lead to myocardial infarction, even in women in their early twenties.

Lung. Pleuritic chest pain occurs more commonly than x-ray evidence of effusion; however, massive effusions may occur. Pneumonitis in patients with SLE is often infectious; however a noninfectious syndrome occurs in SLE patients that varies from fleeting infiltrates (usually hemorrhagic) to marked consolidation and hypoxia. Diffuse interstitial pneumonitis also has been found in SLE.

Hematologic and Lymphoreticular Problems. Lymphadenopathy and splenomegaly may be sufficiently marked that it suggests a lymphoproliferative disorder. Moreover, polyclonal immune hyperactivity in the lymph node may be mistaken for giant follicular or other lymphomas. Hematologic abnormalities are almost invariably present in patients with active disease. The most common is the anemia of chronic disease—a normocytic anemia caused by impaired erythropoiesis. Hemolysis may occur in patients with or without a positive Coombs' test result, but significant hemolysis occurs in less than 10 per cent of patients. Iron deficiency often contributes to anemia. Many patients with lupus bruise easily; therapy and capillary fragility are more often the cause than a bleeding disorder. Mild thrombocytopenia occurs in a substantial proportion of patients with active disease; however, serious thrombocytopenia occurs in less than 10 per cent of patients. Two types of "anticoagulants" occur. One is a laboratory artifact caused by antibodies reactive with the phospholipids used in the partial thromboplastin time (PTT) test. This abnormality is not associated with prolonged bleeding and is not a cause of concern with regard to surgery or biopsies. Other antibodies may react with clotting factors (VIII, IX, XII, and others) and may be responsible for clinically important bleeding.

Nervous System. Peripheral neuropathies have been observed in about 15 per cent of patients with SLE, sometimes in the absence of other nervous system involvement. In addition to a sensory neuropathy, a mononeuritis multiplex picture (e.g., footdrop) is notable. Central nervous system involvement is quite variable. Psychological problems include personality disorders of every variety and numerous forms of frank psychosis (depression, paranoia, mania, schizophrenia). Differentiating that caused by lupus and that caused by corticosteroids is often a challenge.

Seizures, often grand mal, are common, especially in younger patients. Migraine headaches and cytoid bodies may be indications of disease activity. An organic brain syndrome with impaired mentation can progress to coma. Recovery may be complete, or there may be residual impairment. Movement disorders are more common in younger patients: chorea, athetosis, and hemiballismus are observed. Cerebellar abnormalities may occur independently or with other defects.

Transverse myelitis occurs in patients with SLE. Paralysis may also occur following intracerebral hemorrhage or thrombosis. Sterile meningitis may be observed. Despite the large variety of lupus-related nervous system problems, bacterial and other non-lupus causes must be sought and treated.

Kidney Disease. The great majority of patients have some degree of renal involvement. In many, the degree of abnormality is mild enough to escape clinical detection. In others, it is clinically detectable, but does not progress to functional impairment. Only a minority of patients have renal involvement that is threatening to the function of the organ. Hypertension and lupus renal involvement synergize in bringing about destructive changes. As a result, the presence of untreated hypertension poses a threat in patients with renal abnormalities.

Involvement in the kidney represents a multidimensional spectrum: rapidly progressive disease (a subacute glomerulonephritis picture), membranous involvement (usually with some mesangial hypertrophy) with nephrotic syndrome, a nephritic picture (mild to severe), and minimal abnormalities. Most patients have mesangial involvement. The progression to capillary loop pathology carries a worse prognosis. The biopsy picture can change from one form to another; as a result, the degree of active disease (e.g., necrosis) and scarring (glomerular hyalinization, interstitial) offers a much more useful measure than precise histologic classifications. The less scarring, the more there is to treat and preserve. If progression to renal failure occurs, chronic dialysis and renal transplantation are well tolerated. Most patients can be maintained with adequate renal function by modern therapy. Low-grade activity may be associated with slow progression to renal failure. Complete remissions of renal disease occur.

Menses and Pregnancy. Disease activity in menstruating women tends to be greatest in the period between ovulation and menses. Flares generally occur or worsen in this period. Menses are frequently irregular during active disease. Bleeding may be increased in patients with antibodies to clotting factors or with thrombocytopenia. Repeated spontaneous abortions are common in some women. Others, especially when in remission, carry to term without difficulty. Patients in remission at the time of conception tend to have relatively normal pregnancies. Advanced cardiac, central nervous system, or renal disease is a contraindication to pregnancy. The risk of a disease flare after induced abortion is the same as after delivery. Patients with active renal disease often experience exacerbation during pregnancy and may develop pre-eclampsia. Patients without renal involvement tend to have calmer pregnancies, but the disease often flares postpartum or postabortion. Increased dosage of corticosteroids during the time of delivery and for several weeks thereafter tends to reduce the likelihood of a disease flare. Babies of mothers with antibodies to SS-A may have congenital cardiac problems, including heart block.

LABORATORY FINDINGS. Specific tests for SLE are not available. The presence of large amounts of antibodies to native DNA is the single most useful diagnostic laboratory finding. A variety of abnormalities depend in large measure upon the organs involved. The lupus band test consists of a biopsy of nonlesional skin and staining for the presence of immunoglobulin and complement. This test is positive in about three fourths of patients with active SLE and one third of patients with inactive SLE; however, positive tests also occur in patients with rheumatoid arthritis, non-SLE renal disease, and certain dermatologic disorders. Many regard the test as not very helpful.

The LE cell consists of a nucleus that has been phagocytized. The phagocytosis requires antibodies reactive with DNA-histone and complement. In patients with extremely low complement, LE material that has not been phagocytized may be noted. About 80 per cent of patients with SLE are positive for LE cells. A small percentage of patients with related disorders are also positive: rheumatoid arthritis, especially with Felty's syndrome; Sjögren's syndrome; polymyositis-dermatomyositis. The fluorescent antinuclear antibody test (FANA or ANA) has been used as a screening test; however, many patients with related and unrelated diseases may also have positive tests. It is now possible to measure antibodies specifically reactive with various antigens (native DNA, Sm, various low molecular weight RNA species, SS-A, SS-B, etc.). These are much more informative than the FANA despite the improvement in usefulness of the FANA by virtue of analysis of patterns of staining.

Most patients with active SLE have impaired skin tests. Especially important is the common failure to respond to tuberculin in inactive patients as well.

Hematologic. Anemia usually is present in patients with active disease. Although leukopenia occurs in half of the patients, others may manifest leukocytosis. Corticosteroids may increase the white count. Infection in patients with SLE is to be suspected if there is an increase in percentages of granulocytes or immature granulocytes or both even in the absence of leukocytosis. Thrombocytopenia may precede other features of SLE. Antibodies to coagulation factors may be measured in coagulation abnormalities. Antibodies to phospholipids, which prolong the PTT, do not cause bleeding. A false-positive serologic test for syphilis is also observed in 15 per cent of patients.

Immune. The erythrocyte sedimentation rate (ESR) is usually elevated in patients with active disease; however, a minority of patients have normal ESR during periods of disease. Serum albumin levels are usually near normal except in patients with renal disease. Hypergammaglobulinemia may be marked in an untreated patient. Cryoglobulins may be increased in quantity. Rheumatoid factor occurs in low titer in patients with SLE. Reduced hemolytic complement levels (CH_{50}) are common in active disease, especially with renal involvement. Some patients have selected congenital complement deficiencies. Immune complexes may be found in the serum or plasma. Antibodies reactive with leukocytes (granulocytes, B cells, T cells) are found in the majority of patients. Platelet-bound immunoglobulin often occurs in the absence of thrombocytopenia as does a positive Coombs' test result in the absence of hemolysis. Antibodies are found that react with DNA, RNA, histones, nuclear ribonucleoprotein, and cytoplasmic antigenic determinants (see Table 447–3). Rarely, unusual antibodies have been found to react with histamine (inducing acquired Type I hyperlipoproteinemia), insulin receptors (exacerbating difficulties in sugar regulation), and other substances.

Renal. Proteinuria, granular or cellular casts, and cells (RBC, WBC) are found in the urine of patients with active kidney disease. Elevated serum creatinine levels may be reversible or fixed. Hypertension is common, even in the absence of renal failure. Renal biopsies are best used to determine therapy rather than to confirm the diagnosis.

Cardiac. Abnormal T waves are the most common EKG abnormality; evidence of coronary artery or hypertensive disease may be noted. Valvular abnormalities and pericardial fluid may be detected with echocardiograms.

Pulmonary. Pleural fluid may be seen on the x-ray. It is usually an exudate; however, the protein content may not be very high in patients with hypoalbuminemia. The glucose level is usually much higher than is observed in rheumatoid effusions. LE cells may be seen in the fluid. Pleural biopsies can show varying degrees of fibrosis and infiltration. Lung biopsies may show alveolar hemorrhage only; alveolar damage with interstitial edema and hyaline membranes; hypertrophy with or without vasculitis; or acute alveolitis. There is mild to severe hypoxemia. Patients with interstitial fibrosis show decreased vital capacity; others have disproportionately impaired diffusing capacities.

Nervous System. The EEG most commonly shows diffuse slowing. Seizures often occur in the absence of the typical patterns observed in patients with foci. The cerebrospinal fluid may be normal or have moderately elevated protein levels. The gammaglobulin levels are not increased. Granulocytes are indicative of infection; some patients have small numbers of round cells. Aseptic meningitis is occasionally found. A loss of brain substance may be noted in patients with chronic disease. Isolated loss of cortical or cerebellar neurones occurs.

DIAGNOSIS. SLE should be suspected in any person with a multisystem disease including joint pain. For epidemiologic and study purposes, four of the 11 criteria listed in Table 447–1 are required; however, the diagnosis may be made for other purposes with fewer criteria. SLE should be suspected if any of the criteria shown in Table 447–1 are present and unexplained. The disorder should be considered if any of the following are present: unexplained fever, purpura, splenomegaly, adenopathy, pneumonitis, myocarditis, or aseptic meningitis. The presence of a single symptom, such as serositis, and antibodies to native DNA in a young woman is highly suggestive of SLE.

Children are frequently misdiagnosed as having rheumatic fever or juvenile rheumatoid arthritis. Adults most commonly are misdiagnosed as having rheumatoid arthritis. Other diagnoses often applied to patients with SLE include Raynaud's disease, hemolytic anemia, idiopathic thrombocytopenia, thrombotic thrombocytopenic purpura, psychosis, vasculitis, progressive systemic sclerosis, lymphoma, autoimmune neutropenia, secondary syphilis, drug reaction, porphyria, multiple sclerosis, myasthenia gravis, polymyositis, glomerulonephritis, Henoch-Schönlein purpura, personality disorder, stroke, and seizure disorder.

In addition to those just listed, other diseases should be considered in patients suspected of having SLE: subacute bacterial endocarditis, bacterial peritonitis, gonococcal septicemia, meningococcal septicemia, tuberculosis, sarcoidosis, serum sickness, leukemia, leprosy, angioimmunoblastic lymphadenopathy, Wegener's granulomatosis, leptospirosis, Lyme arthritis, Rocky Mountain spotted fever, and acquired immune deficiency syndrome (AIDS).

Overlaps occur between SLE and other diseases such as progressive systemic sclerosis and Sjögren's syndrome. Some have defined these as "mixed connective tissue disease" or the "overlap syndrome;" others prefer less rigid categorizations.

THERAPY. The diagnosis of SLE often induces an emotional reaction. In addition, many patients with SLE have psychological problems that may be a result of the disease. Therefore it is necessary to provide effective emotional support. This includes an honest but optimistic assessment. Most patients with SLE can look forward to a normal lifespan, but with the requirement for periodic visits to the physician and treatment with various drugs. Many of the more serious problems do not affect most people. Renal failure can be handled by dialysis. Thus, although the patient must realize the presence of a serious and chronic disease, a dire prognosis should not be issued. Early involvement in educational programs and with physical therapists, dieticians, and occupational therapists may be helpful.

Patients with SLE usually need more than normal rest. Ten hours of sleep at night plus an afternoon nap would not be inappropriate. The more active the disease, the more rest needed. Ultraviolet light should be avoided: outdoor swimming should be limited to periods of reduced exposure (not at 1:00 PM $\pm$ 4 hours) and sunscreen should be used even for trips to the store. Drugs that augment the effects of UV light, such as tetracyclines and psoralens should be avoided. The same is true of foods containing large amounts of psoralens (celery, parsnips, figs, and parsley). Exercise should be appropriate to the clinical situation; however, exercise to the point of exhaustion should be discouraged. Stresses, including surgery, infections, childbirth, abortions, and psychological pressures may exacerbate the process and dictate additional treatment.

Although certain drugs can induce a lupus-like syndrome, there is little evidence that those drugs are detrimental to patients with SLE. Therefore, such drugs as alphamethyldopa and dilantin may be used without undue concern. However, sulfonamides are poorly tolerated by many patients; patients with active disease experience a rash up to one half of the time. Estrogens may worsen disease; therefore, birth control pills with minimum amounts of estrogens are preferred. Since hypertension is synergistic with immune-complex disease in bringing about pathology, the blood pressure should be kept in the middle of the normal range for age and sex.

Corticosteroids are frequently given. Short-acting drugs such as prednisone or methylprednisolone are preferred so that every other day therapy can be attempted and the hypothalamic-pituitary-adrenal axis not disrupted. The side effects of every other day steroids are much less than those of daily therapy. Low doses are less than 30 mg per 1.7 square meters per day of prednisone, and every attempt should be made to maintain patients on less than 25 mg per 1.7 square meters every other day. Moderate doses are 30–50 mg per 1.7 square meters per day. Higher doses may be necessary. Patients with marked multisystem involvement may temporarily require corticosteroids in divided doses. Heroic and experimental therapy includes boluses of very large doses of corticosteroids (1 gram or more of methylprednisolone) or of cyclophosphamide (0.5–0.75 grams per square meter) and plasmapheresis.

The role of prophylactic vigorous therapy has not been established for non–life-threatening situations. Total nodal irradiation may induce long-term suppression of disease as may monthly boluses of cyclophosphamide; however, these experimental procedures require further study. Azathioprine has long been used to treat patients with SLE; its usefulness may be limited to a subset of patients with moderate kidney disease or those with intractable skin disease or arthritis.

A major problem in the management of patients with SLE is not the acute treatment but the long-term management. The clinical picture (history plus physical exam) is usually a very good guide to the therapy of nonrenal and nonhematologic problems. In the latter two situations, the laboratory measures are helpful. Anemia, fatigue, and hypergammaglobulinemia tend to weigh in favor of more therapy. The long-term toxicities of corticosteroids (cataracts, asceptic necrosis of bone, infections) must always be balanced against the benefits of continued vigorous therapy. In tapering corticosteroids, it is generally advisable to drop rapidly to 30 mg per 1.7 square meters per day and then to reduce dosage more slowly. The lower the dose, the slower the tapering process should be. Rapid tapering can cause a disease flare, which requires re-institution of high doses.

The variable severity and extent of involvement in SLE dictate individualized treatment. It is helpful to divide problems into those of major organs, which therefore are life threatening, and those which are unpleasant but not life threatening (Table 447–5). The major exception to this division is a syndrome of acute toxic lupus observed primarily in pre-corticosteroid times: a young woman with high fever, serositis, rash, and arthritis might succumb to SLE in the absence of major organ involvement. This syndrome appears to be quite susceptible to therapy with corticosteroids in modest doses.

TABLE 447–5. MAJOR VERSUS NON-MAJOR ORGAN INVOLVEMENT IN SLE

Non-Major Organ SLE*	Major Organ SLE†
Alopecia	Glomerulonephritis
Fever	Central nervous system disease
Fatigue	Myocarditis
Anorexia	Pneumonitis
Arthritis	Thrombocytopenic purpura
Myalgia	Hemolytic anemia (marked)
Pleurisy	Severe granulocytopenia (rare)
Pericarditis	Mesenteric vasculitis
Peritonitis	
Rash	
Skin vasculitis	
Raynaud's phenomenon	
Mucosal ulcers	
Splenomegaly	
Lymphadenopathy	
Peripheral neuropathy	
Episcleritis	
Hepatitis	

*Usually does not require high-dose corticosteroids or other vigorous treatment. In all cases, a careful search for infection is carried out.

†Usually requires high-dose corticosteroids or other vigorous treatment. Individual patients vary greatly and some do not require vigorous therapy.

Non–major-organ involvements are best handled with symptomatic therapy: the less medicine the better. Hydroxychloroquine (200 mg–600 mg/d) is effective for skin involvement; it also may help treat arthritis and other manifestations. Nonsteroidal anti-inflammatory drugs (NSAIDs) such as aspirin and ibuprofen are useful for arthritis, serositis, and fever. Some patients tolerate one NSAID better than another—bizarre neurologic reactions may occur in SLE patients receiving ibuprofen; liver enzyme abnormalities may follow aspirin treatment; gastrointestinal tolerance varies. The combination of hydroxychloroquine + NSAID may be sufficient. The addition of low doses of corticosteroids may be necessary. Initial every other day therapy may not be possible; however, a subsequent switch to alternate day treatment reduces steroid-induced side effects. In patients with continued disease activity, symptoms may be prominent every other day, necessitating return to daily steroids. Even in the face of corticosteroid therapy, NSAID and hydroxychloroquine may add substantial benefit and allow a lower steroid dosage. Fevers occurring in spite of daily corticosteroids may respond to NSAIDs. Indomethacin may be especially effective in pericarditis.

The management of major organ involvement is usually directed at preservation of function and prevention of organ failure and disability or death. Myocarditis usually responds to the symptomatic treatment of SLE, but occasional patients may require specific treatment; moderate doses of corticosteroids are usually adequate. Thrombocytopenia and hemolytic anemia are treated more or less as they are in the absence of SLE. The hematologic parameters are followed. High-dose corticosteroids are instituted; if inadequate or they cannot be tapered to a reasonable dose, immunosuppressive drugs or splenectomy may be necessary. Plasmapheresis may be of temporary benefit. Plasma exchange may be helpful in patients with features of thrombotic thrombocytopenia (look for fragmented RBC on the peripheral smear). Patients with factor VIII deficiency caused by specific antibodies should be treated with plasmapheresis and immunosuppression. Mild pneumonitis usually responds to moderate doses of corticosteroids; severe disease requires heroic measures. Central nervous system involvement may require moderate to high corticosteroid therapy; in patients with severe involvement, intravenous cyclophosphamide (0.75–1.0 gram per 1.7 square meters) can be lifesaving. Seizures require treatment with both corticosteroids and anticonvulsants.

The most studied and controversial area is the treatment of SLE kidney disease. If there is active disease on biopsy and little scarring, high-dose corticosteroids or corticosteroids plus an oral immunosuppressive drug (azathioprine for example) may be sufficient. If there is active disease and more scarring, vigorous therapy may be considered. This includes the following choices: intravenous corticosteroids in large doses, intravenous cyclophosphamide, or plasmapheresis + cyclophosphamide. Randomized trials to determine the relative efficacy of these therapies are in progress. In the face of little disease activity and moderate scarring, aggressive therapy is usually not indicated.

Am J Kidney Dis 11(Suppl 1) (July, 1982). *Devoted to a symposium on SLE.*

Decker JL: Systemic lupus erythematosus: Evolving concepts. Ann Intern Med 91:587, 1979. *The experiences of a leading center for SLE research and patient care.*

DuBois EL: Lupus Erythematosus. Los Angeles, University of Southern California Press, 1978. *A lengthy monograph citing many case reports. Extensively referenced.*

Koffler D: Current perspectives on the immunology of systemic lupus erythematosus. Arthritis Rheum 25:721, 1982. *Devoted to a symposium on SLE.*

Ropes MW: Systemic Lupus Erythematosus. Cambridge, Harvard University Press, 1976. *Observations of a physician with over 40 years' experience with SLE patients.*

Rothfield NF: Systemic lupus erythematosus. Clin Rheum Dis Vol 1, Dec 1975. *Thirteen chapters dealing with systemic lupus.*

Smith HR, Steinberg AD: Autoimmunity—A perspective. Ann Rev Immunol 1:175–210, 1983.

Steinberg AD: Systemic lupus erythematosus. Insights from animal models. Ann Intern Med 100:714, 1984. *Up-to-date discussion of pathogenetic mechanisms of disease.*

Winchester RJ: New directions for research in systemic lupus erythematosus. Arthritis Rheum (Supplement to June 1978 issue). *Proceedings of a multicenter conference on systemic lupus.*

448. SYSTEMIC SCLEROSIS (Scleroderma)

Edward D. Harris, Jr.

Systemic sclerosis (Scl) is a generalized disorder of connective tissue characterized by thickening and fibrosis of the skin (scleroderma), prominent abormalities of the small arteries and microvasculature, and by distinctive patterns of involvement of internal organs including the gastrointestinal tract, heart, lungs, and kidneys. The initial manifestation of Scl is typically Raynaud's phenomenon which is eventually present in over 95 per cent of cases. Although Raynaud's phenomenon may be the only complaint for decades, skin involvement usually begins within two years, initially on the fingers and hands (acrosclerosis) but with variable extent and progression and in many cases involving the face, arms, legs, and trunk (diffuse or generalized scleroderma). Localized scleroderma, a term which includes morphea and linear scleroderma, involves the skin exclusively.

The diagnosis of Scl is most often made in patients between the ages of 35 and 55, yet all age groups may be affected. The disease is four times more common in females than in males and is found in all racial groups and geographic areas. The incidence of Scl remains uncertain with estimates of 4 to 12 cases per million population per year reported. Some observers feel many people are misdiagnosed as having Raynaud's syndrome alone or as having a related connective tissue disease. Although the cutaneous manifestations are clinically prominent, morbidity and mortality are related to the extent and severity of internal organ involvement.

PATHOGENESIS. The etiology and pathogenesis of Scl are unknown. Familial aggregation has been reported but is uncommon. Studies of HLA phenotypes have failed to reveal any consistent associations. Any hypothesis concerning the pathogenesis of Scl must explain a diverse body of findings including the heterogeneous patterns of disease; its progression and internal organ involvement; the high frequency of abnormal serologic and cellular immune reactions; the activated state of connective tissue; and the prominent vascular abnormalities.

Raynaud's phenomenon is the initial complaint in 70 per cent of patients with Scl. Histopathologically, the digital arteries reveal a distinctive accumulation of collagen and ground substance along with endothelial cell proliferation in the intima that leads to severe attenuation (greater than 75 per cent) of the arterial lumen in the majority of cases. Similar findings are evident in the small arteries of the heart, lung, kidney, and gastrointestinal tract. Nailfold capillaroscopy reveals distinctive abnormalities of enlarged, tortuous capillary loops interspersed with areas of capillary loss. While it is not clear whether these capillary abnormalities precede or develop concurrently with Raynaud's phenomenon in systemic sclerosis, the derangement of the capillary bed has been found to correlate with the degree and extent of internal organ involvement and is also felt to be a differentiating feature between Raynaud's disease and Raynaud's phenomenon as a manifestation of systemic sclerosis. Similar capillary lesions are evident in clinically unaffected muscle tissue and in the tissues of affected internal organs.

The factor or factors responsible for initiation of these vascular lesions is unknown. Patients with Scl sometimes have high levels of circulating immune complexes, yet there is little evidence of deposition of immunoglobulin and complement in involved tissues. A trypsin-like endothelial cytotoxic factor in serum has been reported, yet a similar activity has been found in other connective tissue diseases and its specificity for endothelium remains in doubt. The finding of increased von Willebrand factor activity and factor VIII/von Willebrand factor antigen in patients with Scl suggests that endothelial injury and repair are ongoing processes. Signs of platelet activation in vivo in Scl include moderate thrombocytosis, elevated plasma β-thromboglobulin levels, and increased numbers of circulating platelet aggregates.

The role of this platelet-endothelial interaction in the pathogenesis of the proliferative vasculopathy of Scl is unclear. The digital arteries of Scl have abnormal reactivity to cold and to serotonin but not to catecholamines. Recent studies have demonstrated cold-induced vasospasm in the circulation of the heart, lungs, and kidneys, suggesting that internal organ "Raynaud equivalents" may play a role in the visceral abnormalities of Scl as well.

Skin biopsies reveal dermal thickening secondary to increased collagen deposition and variable degrees of T lymphocyte accumulation. Although areas of recent fibrosis may have a higher ratio of Type III to Type I collagen, no significant abnormalities of physical properties, amino acid analysis, cross-linking, or solubility of collagen have been reported. Dermal collagenase activity appears normal.

Dermal fibroblasts from Scl cultured in vitro produce collagen and glycosaminoglycan at increased rates. This abnormality can be sustained for several generations of tissue culture. The cause of the increased collagen and matrix synthesis is unknown, but in vivo may be related to stimulation by monokines, lymphokines, or substances such as platelet-derived growth factor. The finding of dermal thickening and fibrosis in chronic graft-versus-host disease similar to Scl suggests that cellular immune factors may be fundamental elements in this process. Many patients with Scl have evidence of humoral immune abnormalities including serum antinuclear antibodies, rheumatoid factor, and hypergammaglobulinemia.

PATHOLOGY. Systemic involvement is characterized by sclerosis. Early findings in the *skin* in active scleroderma have revealed edema, plasma cell and/or lymphocyte infiltrates around eccrine sweat glands, loss of capillaries, and endothelial proliferation. Larger vessels may show fibromucinous accumulations in the intima. The *reticular dermis* is usually thickened. It may have a normal collagen-bundle pattern or may show broad, homogeneous, acellular deposits of collagen with indistinct bundle patterns. Other findings include atrophy of the rete pegs of the epidermis, atrophy of the hair follicles and sweat glands, perivascular lymphocytic infiltration, and hyalinization of arterioles. The subcutaneous tissue is replaced by thick collagen bundles which bind the dermis to deeper structures. Pathologic changes in the musculoskeletal system include acute and chronic inflammation in the *synovium* with no pannus formation but with more sclerosis than is found in rheumatoid synovium with an equivalent inflammatory response. Fibrin deposits are laid down around *tendons*, and *muscles* show a variety of abnormalities, the most common being fibrosis of the perimysium and epimysium, scattered cellular infiltrates, and atrophy and necrosis of muscle fibers similar to that seen in polymyositis.

In the internal organs, microvascular abnormalities (see Pathogenesis), mild inflammation, and edema in connective tissue are followed by increased deposition of fibrous tissue in both appropriate and inappropriate loci. This leads to distortion of the architecture of the tissues affected. In the *lungs*, a relatively low-grade interstitial pneumonitis is followed by interstitial fibrosis, most marked in lower lobes. After this, cyst formation and bronchiectasis may develop. Arteriolar thickening (concentric intimal proliferation or medial hypertrophy) is seen, particularly in those patients with clinical evidence of pulmonary hypertension. In the gastrointestinal tract, atrophy of the muscularis is more prominent than fibrotic replacement. The lower two thirds of the *esophagus* frequently is involved with muscle atrophy and fibrosis. Lesions secondary to reflux of gastric contents are present in 20 per cent of cases. Involvement of the *small bowel* begins with patchy subserosal fibrosis and may progress to almost complete replacement of smooth muscle with fibrous tissue. The small bowel may develop multiple sacculations, presumably at sites of weakness in the continuity of the wall. Dilation, muscle atrophy, and fibrosis are seen in the *colon;* the fibrosis is irregular, leading to the characteristic sacculations and diverticula. The *heart* is frequently enlarged and may be the only organ weighing more than predicted for the subject's body weight. Small patches of interstitial myocardial fibrosis commonly are found. In very severe cases, as much as 60 per cent of cardiac muscle is replaced by dense, relatively acellular and avascular fibrous tissue. Endocardial or valvular thickening is unusual and is rarely of hemodynamic significance. Fibrinous pericarditis is found quite often, even in the absence of uremia. *Kidneys* in Scl are normal in size when renal involvement has not been present clinically. In patients dying with uremia they may be small and frequently have small cortical infarcts. Histologically, fibromucinous intimal proliferation in the interlobular arteries, fibrinoid necrosis of small arteries and arterioles (including the glomerular tufts), and thickening of the basement membrane (the "wire-loop" lesions) may all be present. These changes are similar to those seen in kidneys from patients with malignant hypertension.

CLINICAL MANIFESTATIONS AND DIAGNOSIS. Paroxysmal vasospasm of the fingers with the characteristic sequential color changes of Raynaud's phenomenon is the typical initial manifestation of Scl. In individuals destined to develop generalized or *diffuse Scl,* Raynaud's phenomenon may be preceded by finger and hand edema, polyarthralgia or polyarthritis, or both, weakness, weight loss, or signs of specific internal organ involvement. Patients destined to develop more limited Scl may have Raynaud's phenomenon alone for many years prior to the development of other manifestations of disease. Confident diagnosis of early Scl is frequently confounded by the clinical resemblance to other connective tissue diseases or to idiopathic Raynaud's phenomenon alone.

Classification. Scl is variable in extent and progression but can be grouped into two principal syndromes of important prognostic and therapeutic implications. Individuals with *diffuse scleroderma* are at risk for rapidly progressive and generalized skin involvement and the full spectrum of visceral abnormalities. A nearly equal number of patients are characterized by slowly progressive and restricted skin changes—confined to the fingers, hands, and face—that have been termed the *CREST syndrome variant* (subcutaneous calcinosis, Raynaud's phenomenon, esophageal dysmotility, sclerodactyly, and telangiectasia). Patients with the CREST syndrome have a relatively benign and protracted course of disease and are at far less risk of involvement of the skeletal muscles, joints, heart, and kidneys.

Calcinosis, Raynaud's phenomenon, and telangiectasia are seen in both syndromes; thus accurate classification depends upon assessment of the extent of skin involvement, although other clinical and laboratory features should be considered (Table 448–1). Less commonly, patients may present with typical internal organ manifestations of Scl but without skin changes (systemic sclerosis sine scleroderma).

TABLE 448–1. CLINICAL CLASSIFICATION OF SYSTEMIC SCLEROSIS

	Diffuse Scleroderma	CREST Syndrome
Onset of Raynaud's phenomenon	Within 2 yrs	May be present alone for decades
Skin involvement	Acral and Trunk	Acral Only
Tendon friction rubs	60%	< 1%
Arthritis	40%	20%
Myositis	20%	< 5%
Interstitial pulmonary fibrosis	75%	Rare
Pulmonary hypertension	Rare	10%
Myocardial involvement	15–50%	5%
Renal involvement	25%	Rare
Esophageal dysmotility	90%	90%
Anti-centromere antibody	5–10%	50–70%
Anti-Scl 70 antibody	30–40%	Rare

Cutaneous System. The earliest change is painless pitting edema of the hands and fingers and occasionally more proximal locations. There may be symptoms of hand stiffness or of carpal tunnel syndrome. As the edema lessens, gradual tightening and thickening of the skin develop. The skin may appear shiny and taut with loss of normal skin folds. Joints become immobilized from tight encasement in thickened skin as well as from contractures of muscles, tendons, and palmar fascia. Generalized hyperpigmentation or spotty hypopigmentation may ensue. Recurrent traumatic ulcerations occur over the proximal interphalangeal joints. Chronic ischemic ulcerations may develop at the tips of the digits and the fingers themselves may shorten through progressive resorption of the terminal phalanges. Telangiectasia and subcutaneous calcinosis are common later findings. The skin of the face may appear smooth and waxy with a pinched immobile facies. Narrowing of the oral aperture may ensue, restricting lip movement and preventing adequate dental hygiene. Pruritus is uncommon, but scaling and erythema can be seen. Late in the course of illness, the skin tends to soften and atrophy.

The extent and severity of skin thickening typically worsen in the first several years of disease and thereafter many patients enjoy spontaneous improvement, an observation that complicates interpretation of long-term therapeutic trials. An individual patient with diffuse scleroderma may manifest rapidly progressive skin involvement or may have long intervals of stable or even spontaneously improving skin thickening, some of which may be due to waxing and waning of skin edema.

Musculoskeletal System. Almost half of patients with Scl present with joint pain or develop it during the first year of illness. Small joints are involved more often than large ones. Although an erosive synovitis can be seen, most joint deformity and immobility are best explained by periarticular soft tissue thickening and fibrosis. Tendons are frequently involved in *diffuse scleroderma,* mimicking arthritis. A leathery friction rub can be felt on active and passive motion of involved tendons. Muscle atrophy is often severe in areas such as the hands. Proximal muscle weakness indistinguishable from idiopathic polymyositis may be seen but is more typically a chronic and insidious process.

Gastrointestinal Tract. Of the internal organ systems, the gastrointestinal tract is the one most often involved in Scl. Oral symptoms include xerostomia and a progressive decrease in the size of the mouth. Sjögren's syndrome is seen often, and the frequency of its association with systemic sclerosis is probably underestimated. Symptoms referable to the esophagus, ranging from simple dysphagia to heartburn, nausea, and substernal fullness, are found in 45 to 60 per cent of cases. The dysphagia is related to absence of coordinated peristalsis, followed by loss of amplitude of esophageal body waves and incompetence of the lower esophageal sphincter. If reflex esophagitis becomes a persistent complication, stricture may develop. Vomiting, abdominal distention, and pain or diarrhea may indicate involvement of the small intestine. As in the esophagus, motility of the small bowel is decreased, and there may be malabsorption secondary to intraluminal stagnation with concomitant bacterial overgrowth. Functional bowel complaints secondary to pathologic changes in the colon are common. Disease of both large and small bowel may produce a clinical picture identical to paralytic ileus with incomplete obstruction at any level. An association between primary biliary cirrhosis and scleroderma with CREST syndrome is now recognized.

Heart and Lungs. Dyspnea is the most common cardiorespiratory symptom in Scl and is present in more than 50 per cent of patients. Fine, dry crackles at the bases of the lung are the first abnormality found on physical examination. In some patients, progression to respiratory insufficiency and death from hypoxemia are related to progressive pulmonary fibrosis. The earliest abnormality of pulmonary function is a decrease in pulmonary diffusion capacity. Those exposed in their occupation to silicate dust have a predilection to develop this form of the disease. Restriction of chest wall expansion by dermal fibrosis around the thorax rarely affects respiratory function. A few patients with severe cystic and fibrotic changes in the lungs have developed multifocal alveolar cell carcinomas.

Increasingly recognized as a prominent cause of late morbidity and a principal cause of mortality in patients with CREST syndrome is progressive pulmonary hypertension in the absence of significant pulmonary interstitial fibrosis. Rales are frequently absent but an increased pulmonic heart sound or signs of right ventricular failure may be seen. Pulmonary hypertension should be suspected if a severely reduced diffusion capacity is present.

Replacement of myocardium with fibrous tissue ("scleroderma heart disease") is an occasional primary cause of heart failure. In addition, impaired cardiac function can be attributed to right ventricular failure secondary to pulmonary hypertension. Fibrosis of the conducting system may lead to atrioventricular conduction defects and arrhythmias. The occurrence of angina-like pain and sudden death in patients with Scl associated with pathology showing ischemic reperfusion has suggested that a Raynaud's phenomenon in the heart is probably a true clinical event.

Kidneys. The sudden development of malignant hypertension resistant to therapy and uremia progressing rapidly to death is a dreaded complication of Scl. Most patients have had skin changes before development of abnormal renal function. Careful monitoring of blood pressure by the patient at home and search of peripheral blood smears for evidence of microangiopathic hemolyis may occasionally give warning that accelerated hypertension is developing. Progression to renal failure and death may follow quickly unless treatment is vigorous. Renal complications of Scl develop more often in cold months of the year.

Nervous System. Involvement of the nervous system is rare. Facial pain, questionably related to a trigeminal neuropathy, is seen occasionally and may be disabling. Significant reduction in mean conduction velocity of peripheral nerves has been reported.

LABORATORY FINDINGS. The erythrocyte sedimentation rate is elevated in most patients with Scl, and a mild anemia of chronic disease may be present. In addition, iron deficiency anemia may result from bleeding from esophagitis, and vitamin B_{12} and/or folic acid deficiency from overgrowth of organisms in an atonic bowel. Hemolysis is unusual, except for microangiopathic hemolytic anemia, which heralds severe accelerated hypertension. A number of serologic abnormalities link Scl to other connective tissue diseases. Mild hypergammaglobulinemia is present in 30 to 50 per cent of patients, rheumatoid factor in 25 to 35 per cent, antinuclear antibodies (often with a speckled or a nucleolar pattern) in sera of 40 to 80 per cent, depending on the assay used, and LE cells in less than 10 per cent of patients. Antinuclear antibody is directed against a soluble nuclear antigen, Scl-70 (particularly in patients with diffuse disease), nucleolar RNA, and the centromere of chromosomes (particularly in patients with CREST variant). DNA-binding activity in serum is absent.

The electrocardiogram shows nonspecific abnormalities in almost 50 per cent of patients. The pattern of conduction defects with very low voltage is seen only in those uncommon patients with marked myocardial replacement by fibrous tissue. Echocardiogram in these cases will reveal reduced ventricular wall motion. This technique is also useful in documenting small pericardial effusions. In general the electromyogram is normal; most patients have polyphasic waves of normal duration and size. Denervation potentials are seen only rarely.

Roentgenography. Roentgenograms are important for diagnosis and follow-up evaluation. The findings of soft tissue atrophy, subcutaneous calcinosis, and resorption of the tufts of the terminal phalanges without loss of apparent joint spaces between phalanges are virtually pathognomonic of Scl when seen on hand films. Upper gastrointestinal films reveal a dilated, atonic esophagus in about 60 per cent of patients. Small bowel studies may demonstrate segmental atony, dilation, and sacculation in the duodenum and jejunum. Linear or cystic pneumatosis (air in the wall of the gut) is occasionally seen in flat plates of the abdomen of patients with severe small bowel involvement. Barium studies of the colon reveal wide-mouth, asymmetrical diverticula in 20 to 40 per cent of patients; progression to a dilated, atonic megacolon rarely occurs. In patients with pulmonary involvement, chest roentgenograms reveal a diffuse reticular pattern with a honeycomb appearance in the lower lung fields. Serial films may document progression to dense interstitial fibrosis amid radiolucent cystic areas.

DIFFERENTIAL DIAGNOSIS. When Scl presents as persistent symmetrical polyarthritis involving the hands, as edematous puffy hands, or as Raynaud's phenomenon, a specific diagnosis may be impossible to make. Rheumatoid arthritis, systemic sclerosis, SLE, and dermatomyositis-polymyositis can all present in this fashion. If symptoms persist and the skin begins to appear thickened or bound down to underlying fascia, the physician should look for one or more of the following, which would help consolidate a diagnosis of Scl: (1) diminished numbers and dilation or tortuosity of nail-bed capillaries; (2) pitting scars in the distal digits below the nails; and (3) signs of systemic fibrosis such as bibasilar pulmonary fibrosis or disturbances of gastrointestinal (especially esophageal) motility. In a large multicenter study, *proximal* scleroderma itself was identified as the sole criterion necessary to make the diagnosis. The differential diagnosis of varied manifestations of Scl is listed in Table 448–2.

TREATMENT. Because so little is known about the pathogenesis of Scl, no specific treatment is available. Innumerable therapies have been attempted, but controlled trials have been few and outcome measures seldom uniformly applied. The inflammatory symptoms wax and wane as is characteristic of the connective tissue diseases. The tendency for skin involvement to improve spontaneously in late disease and the variability in progression of skin changes in early Scl confound the interpretation of uncontrolled trials and of long-term therapies.

TABLE 448–2. DIFFERENTIAL DIAGNOSIS OF SYSTEMIC SCLEROSIS

Raynaud's phenomenon
- Raynaud's disease
- Occupational trauma
- Shoulder-hand syndrome
- Heavy metal or ergot poisoning
- Vascular disease (including SLE and polymyositis)
- Hematologic abnormalities
  - Polycythemia vera
  - Cryoglobulinemia
- Vinyl chloride toxicity

Skin changes
- Werner's syndrome
- Progeria
- Chronic hypostatic edema
- Lichen sclerosus et atrophicus
- Porphyria cutanea tarda
- Scleredema
- Chronic graft-versus-host reactions
- Bleomycin therapy
- Fasciitis with eosinophilia
- Carcinoid syndrome
- Chronic insulin-dependent diabetes mellitus

Telangiectasia
- Hereditary telangiectasia
- Cirrhosis of the liver

Visceral disease
- Idiopathic pulmonary fibrosis
- Rheumatoid arthritis
- Sarcoidosis
- Infiltrative cardiomyopathies
- Intestinal obstruction

In view of the prominent immunologic abnormalities of Scl, corticosteroids and immunosuppressants have been employed, but the consensus of this experience has been that neither affect significantly the natural history of Scl. Corticosteroids have been implicated in provoking Scl renal involvement, and their use should be reserved for patients with inflammatory muscle disease and some patients with rapidly progressive interstitial lung disease. Anti-platelet and vasodilator therapies including aspirin, dipyridamole, and calcium channel blockers have attracted recent interest, but results of preliminary trials have been disappointing. D-Penicillamine has been investigated in a number of trials for its known effect in inhibiting inter- and intramolecular cross-linkages of mature collagen. A recent large retrospective study suggested that patients receiving high doses ($\geq$ 750 mg per day) for prolonged periods of time (18 months) enjoyed lessening of skin thickening and a decreased incidence of new internal organ involvement, resulting in an improved survival when compared to a well-matched population not receiving this treatment. D-Penicillamine therapy was not associated with improvement of previously existing internal organ involvement nor with improvement in the vascular or immunologic aspects of Scl, and the rationale for such therapy in CREST syndrome remains unclear.

Previously refractory to all but the most desperate therapies (bilateral nephrectomy, renal transplantation), the accelerated hypertension, rapidly progressive renal insufficiency, and hyperreninemia of Scl renal crisis are now felt to respond to aggressive antihypertensive treatment. Dramatic successes have been reported with both captopril and minoxidil in which hypertension was controlled and renal damage reversible if treatment was begun at early stages (serum creatinine less than 4.0 mg/dl). Intriguingly, many of these patients have experienced reversal of skin involvement in a time course similar to that associated with D-penicillamine treatment, lending support to the concept of a vascular pathogenesis of Scl.

The mainstay of treatment of Scl is supportive. Many patients lead productive and useful lives. An important goal of therapy is to preserve function in and prevent injury to the hands. Vocational and occupational therapy can be important in maintenance of hand function. Digital ulcerations must be treated immediately with wound care, topical or systemic antibiotics, and vasodilators before they progress to substantial tissue damage. Antacids, cimetidine, and simpler maneuvers such as elevation of the head of the bed and avoidance of postprandial recumbency and tight clothing can lessen the symptoms of reflux esophagitis and delay or prevent secondary lower esophageal stricture. Esophageal dilatation is of help in certain patients but frequently must be repeated at regular intervals. Malabsorption and crampy diarrhea sometimes respond to broad-spectrum antimicrobials (e.g., tetracycline 0.25 gm twice daily) for presumed bacterial overgrowth. Constipation responds to agents that soften and increase the bulk of stool.

Symptomatic management of the vasospastic phenomena of Scl includes avoidance of cold, attention to proper dress, including both warm mittens and layered clothing for the trunk, and avoidance of emotional stress, nicotine, and caffeine. No drug therapy of Raynaud's phenomenon in Scl is universally effective or tolerated, but direct vasodilators such as nitroglycerin, calcium channel blockers, and prazosin appear better choices than sympatholytic drugs.

EOSINOPHILIC FASCIITIS. Eosinophilic fasciitis (EF) is a disorder characterized by rapidly developing symmetrical inflammation and scleroderma-like sclerosis of the deep fascia, lower subcutis, and dermis. Chiefly affected are the extremities and in many instances the face and trunk as well. In contrast to Scl, the fingers, hands and feet are typically spared; Raynaud's phenomenon, nailfold capillary abnormalities, and internal organ involvement are rarely present. Although the etiology of EF is unknown, some cases, especially in men, appear to have been precipitated by strenuous physical activity such as rapid assumption of physical fitness programs. All age groups are affected, but the majority of patients are between 30 and 60 years. Clinically, one finds erythema, edema, and severe induration of the skin and subcutaneous tissues. The overlying skin typically has an "orange-peel" appearance and exaggerated furrowing over the course of superficial veins is noted in anti-dependent postures. Arthritis is uncommon, but carpal tunnel syndrome is frequent and virtually all patients develop joint contractures. Muscle weakness secondary to disuse atrophy and occasionally occurring as an extension of inflammation deep to the fascia are seen.

Laboratory abnormalities include elevation of erythrocyte sedimentation rate, hypergammaglobulinemia, circulating immune complexes, and striking peripheral eosinophilia (typically over 2000/mm^3). Biopsy specimens should include skin to skeletal muscle; they reveal edema of the deep fascia and subcutis and infiltration with eosinophils, lymphocytes, and histiocytes in early disease. Later, tissue eosinophils are less conspicuous or are absent, and the predominant feature is fibrosis and thickening of the deep fascia, which can extend to the dermis.

Moderate corticosteroids (prednisone $\leq$ 20 mg/day) provide rapid symptomatic relief and readily obliterate the tissue and peripheral eosinophilia, although they have not been demonstrated to speed the resolution of tissue fibrosis. The majority of patients experience clinical and biopsy resolution within three to five years, yet others have recurrences or persistent disease. The precise relationship of EF to Scl remains speculative. Many observers are struck by the clinical and laboratory resemblance of EF to acute generalized subcutaneous morphea.

OVERLAP SYNDROMES. Some patients with Scl present with simultaneous clinical and laboratory features of SLE, rheumatoid arthritis, polymyositis, or all three. The term "overlap syndrome" has replaced such colorful names as lupoderma and sclerodermatomyositis to describe patients with features of two or more connective tissue diseases. In general, patients with overlap syndromes tend to have less extensive Scl skin involvement, milder signs of digital ischemia, and less renal disease from either Scl or SLE.

Mixed connective tissue disease (MCTD) is recognized as a distinct overlap syndrome and describes patients with a positive antinuclear antibody test result with a speckled pattern and a high titer of serum antibody to extractable nuclear protein antigen (RNP) in a clinical setting of features of Scl, SLE, and polymyositis. Diffuse hand swelling, fever, and lymphadenopathy are frequent as well. Low levels of anti-DNA antibodies are sometimes found but antibody to Sm antigen is uncommon. Involvement of the kidneys and central nervous system occurs less frequently than in SLE, and the polymyositis responds to corticosteroids. In long-term follow-up of patients originally said to have MCTD, the majority were found to evolve toward more classic Scl, yet others had protracted clinical courses dominated by the features of SLE or polymyositis. Not all patients with clinical MCTD have antibody to RNP, and many patients with antibody to RNP have clinical manifestations consistent with diagnoses of SLE, Scl, or polymyositis alone. MCTD illustrates the ambiguities and the idiosyncratic nature of the clinical expressions of connective tissue diseases. Proper management requires close assessment of the features present in the individual patient. All patients presenting with an overlap syndrome should have tests of the presence and extent of muscle, renal, hematologic, and pulmonary involvement. A screening serologic profile, including serum rheumatoid factor, sedimentation rate, antinuclear antibody, anti-DNA antibody, and serum complement levels is appropriate. A high titer of speckled antinuclear antibody suggests that antibody to extractable nuclear antigen, either RNP or Sm, may be present, and in such instances these should be measured as well.

Follansbee WP, Curtiss EI, Medsger TA Jr, Steen VD, Mretsky BF, Owens GR, Rodnan GP: Physiologic abnormalities of cardiac function in progressive systemic sclerosis with diffuse scleroderma. N Engl J Med 310:142, 1984. *Abnormalities of myocardial perfusion are common in PSS and appear to be due to a disturbance of myocardial microcirculation of both ventricles.*

Fritzler MJ, Kinsella TD, Garbutt E: The CREST syndrome: A distinct serologic entity with anticentromere antibodies. Am J Med 69:520, 1980. *Anticentromere antibody was found in 26 of 27 CREST patients but only 8 of 115 with diffuse Scl and related connective tissue diseases.*

Haynes DC, Gershwin ME: The immunopathology of progressive systemic sclerosis (PSS). Sem Arthritis Rheum 11:331, 1982. *An extensively referenced review of the various immunologic aspects of Scl.*

Moore TL, Zuckner J: Eosinophilic fasciitis. Sem Arthritis Rheum 9:228, 1980. *A detailed literature review of 53 patients with illustrative case material.*

Nimelstein SH, Brody S, McShane D, Holman HR: Mixed connective tissue disease: A subsequent evaluation of the original 25 patients. Medicine 59:239, 1980. *In surviving patients, inflammatory disease manifestations (arthritis, serositis, fever, myositis) responded to steroid therapy and became less severe. Sclerodermatous manifestations (sclerodactyly, esophageal disease) persisted. There was a general evolution away from an MCTD picture toward Scl. Renal disease remained infrequent.*

Rodnan GP, Myerowitz RL, Justh GO: Morphologic changes in the digital arteries of patients with progressive systemic sclerosis (scleroderma) and Raynaud's phenomenon. Medicine 59:393, 1980. *This paper provides good examples of the histopathology of the arterial lesion of Scl as well as an excellent discussion of Raynaud's phenomenon in Scl versus Raynaud's disease.*

Steen VD, Medsger TA, Rodnan GP: D-Penicillamine therapy in progressive systemic sclerosis (scleroderma). Ann Rheum Dis 97:652, 1982. *A large and long-term retrospective experience with D-penicillamine treatment. Includes good clinical detail and a discussion of the difficulties inherent in treatment of Scl.*

Subcommittee for Scleroderma Criteria: Preliminary criteria for the classification of systemic sclerosis (scleroderma). Arthritis Rheum 23:587, 1980. *This large multicenter study has compiled the clinical and laboratory features of scleroderma and developed criteria for diagnosis of this disease.*

Traub YM, Shapiro AP, Rodnan GP, Medsger TA, McDonald RH Jr, Steen VD, Osial TA Jr, Tolchin SF: Hypertension and renal failure (scleroderma renal crisis) in progressive systemic sclerosis. Review of a 25-year experience with 68 cases. Medicine 62:335, 1983. *With renal dialysis and more effective treatment of severe hypertension, together with bilateral nephrectomy in selected patients, survivals of greater than one year were achieved in 11 patients treated in the past few years.*

Whitman HH, Case OB, Larugh JH, Christian LL, Botstein G, Maricq H, LeRoy EC: Variable response to oral angiotensin-converting-enzyme blockage in hypertensive scleroderma patients. Arthritis Rheum 25:241, 1982. *Experience with 12 patients emphasizing the need for early, aggressive intervention in Scl renal crisis.*

449. SJÖGREN'S SYNDROME

Norman Talal

DEFINITION. Sjögren's syndrome is a chronic inflammatory and autoimmune disease in which the salivary and lacrimal glands undergo progressive destruction by lymphocytes and plasma cells resulting in decreased production of saliva and tears. The term autoimmune exocrinopathy has been introduced. The spectrum of this illness includes a primary form (sicca complex), a secondary form accompanying rheumatoid arthritis (or occasionally another connective tissue disease), and a form characterized mainly by lymphoproliferation of either a benign infiltrative or a malignant nature. Females are involved ten times more commonly than males.

PATHOGENESIS. The several factors involved in the etiology of autoimmune diseases such as Sjögren's syndrome include genetic, immunologic, hormonal, and probably infectious (? viral). The discovery of the immune response (IR) genes, which exist in linkage disequilibrium with other genes in the major histocompatibility complex, has helped distinguish primary from secondary Sjögren's syndrome. The former is associated with HLA B8 DR3, whereas the latter is associated with DR4 (when rheumatoid arthritis is the accompanying illness). The Ia cell surface antigens, the presumed products of the IR genes, mediate the lymphocyte-lymphocyte and lymphocyte-macrophage interactions necessary for proper immune regulation. Autoimmune diseases probably arise as a consequence of disordered immunologic regulation. Although just how immune regulation becomes disturbed is not yet known, it seems likely that internal factors (such as sex hormones and latent viruses) as well as external factors (drugs or infectious agents) play a role. For example, the predominant female incidence of Sjögren's syndrome may relate to an ability of androgen to suppress and estrogens to accelerate autoimmune disease, as in the NZB/NZW F_1 mouse model.

CLINICAL MANIFESTATIONS. The symptoms of Sjögren's syndrome may be subtle and brought out only by careful and persistent questioning.

Ophthalmologic (Keratoconjunctivitis Sicca). The patient may notice accumulation of thick ropy secretions along the inner canthus owing to a decreased tear film and an abnormal mucus component. Related complaints include erythema, photosensitivity, eye fatigue, decreased visual acuity, and the sensation of a "film" across the field of vision. Desiccation can cause small superficial erosions of the corneal epithelium. Slit lamp examination may reveal filamentary keratitis (filaments of corneal epithelium and debris) in severe cases. Conjunctivitis caused by *Staphylococcus aureus* is a complication.

Salivary. Complaints resulting from dryness of the mouth are varied. The "cracker sign" describes the difficulties encountered in trying to eat dry foods without sufficient lubrication. Many subjects require frequent ingestion of liquids. They may resort to carrying water bottles or candy in purse or pocket. Additional features include oral soreness, adherence of food to buccal surfaces, fissuring of the tongue, and dysphagia. Angular cheilitis resulting from superimposed candidiasis may occur. Patients may lose the ability to discriminate foods on the basis of taste and smell. Dental caries are accelerated. The parotid gland enlarges in many patients secondary to cellular infiltration and ductal obstruction. Usually asymptomatic and self-limited, the enlargement can be recurrent and associated with pain or erythema. Focal infiltrates of lymphocytes are also found in the minor salivary glands of the lower lip. When biopsied, these lesions provide histologic confirmation and quantification of the degree of infiltration.

Other Symptoms. Dryness may also involve the nasal mucosa, leading to recurrent epistaxis, and may extend throughout the upper respiratory tract, causing hoarseness, recurrent bronchitis, and pneumonitis. Eustachian tube blockage can result in conduction deafness and chronic otitis. Dysphagia may be ascribed to several causes: decreased saliva, infiltration of the glands of the esophageal mucosa, esophageal webbing, and abnormal motility. Other exocrine gland functions may be affected, leading to loss of pancreatic secretions, hypo- or achlorhydria, dermal dryness, and lack of vaginal secretions.

Extraglandular Involvement. Extraglandular involvement occurs more frequently in patients with primary than secondary Sjögren's syndrome. Dependent nonthrombocytopenic purpura is generally associated with hyperglobulinemia. Raynaud's phenomenon is present in 20 per cent of patients. A diffuse interstitial pneumonitis resulting from lymphocytic infiltration may cause dyspnea. Obstructive disease (in the absence of smoking) may result from lymphocytic infiltration surrounding small airways. The most common renal abnormalities involve the tubules, particularly overt or latent renal tubular acidosis and hyposthenuria. The presence of glomerulonephritis should suggest coexisting systemic lupus erythematosus, cryoglobulinemia, or immune complex deposition. Peripheral and cranial neuropathy has been associated with vasculitis involving the vasa nervorum.

Lymphoproliferation and Lymphoma. The incidence of lymphoma is increased 44-fold in Sjögren's syndrome. Pseudomalignant or malignant lymphoproliferation may be present initially or may develop later in the illness. Most lymphomas belong to the B cell lineage, although the histologic appearance is variable. Many cases previously described as histiocytic lymphoma represent B cell lymphomas and remain sufficiently differentiated to synthesize monoclonal immunoglobulins. Other monoclonal immunoglobulin B cell proliferations in Sjögren's syndrome patients include Waldenström's macroglobulinemia, light chain myeloma, and non-IgM monoclonal gammopathies (IgG κ and IgA λ). A diminution of a previously elevated Ig class may signify malignant transformation. Pseudolymphoma is an intermediate stage in this transition from benign to malignant lymphoproliferation.

Other clinical indications of an increased risk of malignancy include persistent or greatly increased parotid swelling, generalized lymphadenopathy, and splenomegaly. Serial measurement of serum β-2 microglobulin offers another clue as to the clinical subset or course. β-2 microglobulin is elevated in the saliva of Sjögren's syndrome patients and in the synovial fluid of patients with rheumatoid arthritis. Salivary levels correspond with the degree of lymphocytic infiltration, and serum levels may be elevated in patients with renal and lymphoproliferative complications.

DIAGNOSIS. ***Clinical.*** The presence of dry eyes is suggested by a positive Schirmer test (less than 5 mm of wetting per five minutes, unanesthetized), but the frequency of both false-negative and false-positive results is high. The pattern and intensity of staining with rose bengal dye and slit lamp examination are more reliable in diagnosis. The presence of filamentary keratitis and corneal ulcerations indicates advanced keratoconjunctivitis sicca.

Diminution in stimulated parotid flow rate (PFR) (<5 ml per gland in ten minutes) is a sensitive indicator of xerostomia. Salivary scintigraphy, which measures the uptake, concentration, and excretion of ^{99m}Tc-pertechnetate by the major salivary glands, is a sensitive index of glandular function. Scintigraphy is expensive, however, and offers no advantage in diagnostic sensitivity over minor salivary gland biopsy. Lip biopsy is a sensitive and specific diagnostic procedure, is well tolerated by the patient, and causes no disfigurement. Further, biopsy offers more information; in addition to confirming the diagnosis, it allows quantification of the degree of lymphocytic infiltration and tissue damage. Aggregates of lymphocytes within the acinar tissue are scored, each aggregate of 50 or more cells representing a focus. The number of foci within 4 sq mm of glandular tissue is determined and constitutes the focus score. A focus score of more than 1 is characteristic of Sjögren's syndrome and is seen in less than 1 per cent of both normal and autopsy controls. The diagnosis of Sjögren's syndrome is based upon the presence of two of the following three criteria: (1) focus score of more than 1 in the labial salivary gland biopsy, (2) keratoconjunctivitis sicca, and (3) an associated connective tissue or lymphoproliferative disorder.

Clinically, a "sicca-like" syndrome may be caused by a number of other disease processes, including hyperlipoproteinemias IV and V, hemochromatosis, sarcoidosis, and amyloidosis. Use of anticholinergic drugs as well as a number of other medications may be the single most frequent cause of xerostomia. Thus, it is essential to establish the presence of focal lymphoid infiltrates and autoimmunity in a patient suspected of having Sjögren's syndrome.

Laboratory. Autoantibodies are common in Sjögren's syndrome. Rheumatoid factor may be found in 75 to 90 per cent; antinuclear antibodies may be positive in 50 to 80 per cent. Multiple organ-specific antibodies are noted, including antibodies directed against gastric parietal, thyroid microsomal, thyroglobulin, mitochondrial, smooth muscle, and salivary duct antigens.

An autoantibody to a nucleoprotein antigen called SS-B (also termed La) occurs in approximately 50–70 per cent of patients with primary Sjögren's syndrome and to a lesser extent in Sjögren's syndrome accompanied by SLE. Antibodies to a related nucleoprotein SS-A (also termed Ro) are less specific for Sjögren's syndrome, also occur in SLE, and are associated with vasculitis. An antibody (RAP) to an EB virus-related nuclear antigen (RANA) occurs in secondary Sjögren's syndrome with RA.

Antibodies to SS-A are less specifically associated with any one disease. A recent report identifies antibodies to SS-A in as few as 13 per cent of Sjögren's syndrome patients and as many as 46 per cent of systemic lupus erythematosus patients without Sjögren's syndrome.

Persons with Sjögren's syndrome manifest B cell hyperactivity. Evidence for this includes the polyclonal hyperglobulinemia seen in over 50 per cent of patients and the presence of numerous autoantibodies and circulating immune complexes. The lymphoid infiltrates in the salivary glands synthesize immunoglobulins locally. Serum hyperviscosity may result from either macroglobulinemia or polymerizing IgG with rheumatoid factor activity which forms intermediate complexes.

Cryoglobulinemia may be present, as well as vasculitis and glomerulonephritis. A high proportion of patients with Sjögren's syndrome have circulating immune complexes as measured by C1q binding and Raji cell assays. Serum levels of complement are only infrequently low.

Peripheral blood T lymphocytes are decreased in about one third of patients. Immunoglobulin-positive lymphocytes in peripheral blood may be increased slightly. Abnormalities in T cell function may be present, particularly in patients with lymphoproliferative or other systemic features. These patients tend to have alterations in T cell subsets and decreased autologous mixed lymphocyte responses. Natural killer (NK) cell activity is also diminished as a consequence of immunoregulatory abnormalities rather than intrinsic deficits.

There is also a defect in reticuloendothelial clearance in patients with Sjögren's syndrome. In 12 of 19 patients, labeled IgG sensitized autologous red cells, which are usually cleared rapidly by splenic macrophages via surface membrane Fc receptor binding, persisted in the circulation for an abnormally long period. Eleven of the 12 patients had either extraglandular manifestations of Sjögren's syndrome or secondary Sjögren's syndrome.

TREATMENT. Treatment of Sjögren's syndrome is aimed at symptomatic relief and limiting the damaging local effects of chronic xerophthalmia and xerostomia. Ocular dryness responds to the use of artificial tears containing methylcellulose. Since staphylococcal blepharitis occurs in two thirds of patients, the lids should be cultured and infection eradicated. Soft contact lenses may be used to protect the cornea; this is controversial. Moisture may be maintained with frequent use of saline drops. Saran wrap occlusion or diving goggles may be worn at night in an attempt to prevent tear evaporation. Topical steroid use should be avoided unless specifically indicated, because corneal thinning and subsequent perforation may occur. The use of diuretics, many antihypertensive drugs, and antidepressants may further diminish lacrimal and salivary gland function. Xerostomia may respond to an increased fluid intake, use of a 2 per cent solution of methylcellulose, and sour sugar-free candies given as sialagogues. Scrupulous care of teeth is imperative; patients should avoid a high sucrose intake or the frequent use of sugar-containing candies to decrease oral dryness. Vigorous dental plaque control and topical application of fluoride should be used regularly. Oral candidiasis may be treated with mycostatin tablets for a prolonged course, with separate treatment of dentures. Vaginal dryness can be treated with propionic acid gels.

Only those patients with severe functional disability or life-threatening complications warrant corticosteroid or immunosuppressive therapy. Prednisone may suppress parotid swelling and improve the restrictive component of pulmonary disease. Immunosuppressive agents have decreased extraglandular lymphoid infiltrates and improved exocrine gland function in some individuals. Their use has been restricted to those patients with severe renal and pulmonary manifestations.

Strand V, Talal N: Advances in the diagnosis and concept of Sjögren's syndrome (autoimmune exocrinopathy). Bull Rheum Dis 30:1046, 1980. *This is an up-to-date and comprehensive review of clinical, laboratory, and pathogenetic features of Sjögren's syndrome.*

Talal N: Sjögren's syndrome and connective tissue disease with other immunologic disorders. *In* McCarty D (ed.): Arthritis and Allied Conditions. 10th ed. Philadelphia, Lea & Febiger, in press.

450. THE VASCULITIC SYNDROMES

Anthony S. Fauci

Vasculitis is a clinicopathologic process characterized by an inflammatory response within the blood vessel itself. Associated with this inflammation is a compromise of the vessel lumen with resulting ischemic changes in the tissues supplied by the vessel. Any size, location, and type of blood vessel may be involved, including large muscular arteries, medium-sized and small arteries, arterioles, capillaries, postcapillary venules, and veins. This heterogeneous category of diseases comprises unique syndromes as well as diseases with overlapping clinical and pathologic features. The vasculitis may be the primary process, or it may be a component of another underlying disease. Furthermore, vasculitis varies considerably in its clinicopathologic manifestations. Certain of the vasculitic disorders are rarely life threatening, e.g., the hypersensitivity vasculitic syndromes in which cutaneous involvement usually predominates. Other vasculitic syndromes may be fulminant and, if untreated, rapidly fatal diseases, e.g., Wegener's granulomatosis and polyarteritis nodosa.

The vasculitic syndromes are generally thought to result from immunopathogenic mechanisms; however, the evidence for this varies among the different syndromes. Among these mechanisms, the deposition of circulating immune complexes with subsequent vessel damage has emerged as the major immunopathologic event associated with most of the vasculitic syndromes. However, many individual patients with active vasculitis have not shown circulating or deposited immune complexes. This result could reflect an insensitivity of techniques in detecting certain types of immune complexes. In addition, complexes could be cleared at such a rapid rate as to preclude their detection. On the other hand, the presence of circulating immune complexes does not prove that the associated vasculitis is caused by them, since many nonvasculitic diseases are also associated with circulating immune complexes, and complexes per se need not result in vasculitis, even in diseases in which vasculitis is present.

In only a few diseases has the actual antigen involved in the immune complex been identified. The most noted of these is the hepatitis B surface antigen that has been demonstrated in the circulating immune complexes, cryoprecipitable serum components, and involved tissues of certain patients with hepatitis B antigenemia–associated vasculitis.

The mechanism of tissue damage from immune complexes is thought to be similar to serum sickness. In this model, soluble immune complexes are formed in antigen excess and deposited in blood vessel walls in areas of increased vascular permeability. The increased permeability is attributed to release of vasoactive amines from platelets or mast cells under the influence of specific IgE. Following deposition of complexes, various components of complement are activated, particularly C5a, which is strongly chemotactic for neutrophils. The neutrophils infiltrate the vessel wall at the site of immune complex deposition and release intracytoplasmic enzymes such as collagenase and elastase that directly damage the vessel wall. Compromise of the lumen occurs with resulting ischemic changes.

Certain of the vasculitides are characterized by granulomatous inflammation in and around the blood vessels. Although granulomatous responses are generally of the delayed hypersensitivity type, immune complexes themselves can trigger granuloma formation and thereby produce granulomatous vasculitis.

Why certain persons develop vasculitis and others do not is an extraordinarily complex issue and likely involves a number of host factors such as genetic predisposition, immunoregulatory mechanisms, and the integrity of the reticuloendothelial system, which clears the complexes from the circulation. In addition, the reasons why certain complexes cause vasculitis and why certain types of vessels and not others are involved probably relate to the size and physicochemical properties of the immune complex and to other physical factors such as turbulence of blood flow, hydrostatic pressure within vessels, and previously damaged vessel endothelium.

CLASSIFICATION OF THE VASCULITIC SYNDROMES

The remarkable heterogeneity and the obvious overlap among the vasculitic syndromes have led to difficulties in classification of this group of diseases. The first complete report of a vasculitic syndrome was in 1866 by Kussmaul and Maier who elegantly described the clinicopathologic features in a patient with what is now recognized as classic polyarteritis nodosa. Following this publication polyarteritis nodosa was the reference for all subsequently described vasculitides. It soon became evident that there were numerous vasculitis syndromes with diverse clinical and pathologic manifestations, but diagnostic criteria were controversial. More precise and accurate classification schemes now have emerged, based upon reexamination of clinical, pathologic, and immunologic features, as well as responses to certain therapeutic regimens. Table 450–1 illustrates one such classification scheme.

The first major group is the systemic necrotizing vasculitides. Within this group falls classic polyarteritis nodosa. This syndrome is described in detail in Ch. 451. It is the prototype of serious systemic necrotizing vasculitis and manifests certain features such as small and medium-sized muscular artery involvement, hypertension, visceral vessel involvement, and a noticeable lack of lung involvement. In the classic syndrome, eosinophilia, granulomatous reactions, and an allergic diathesis are not characteristic. Soon after the original description physicians recognized a systemic vasculitis which resembled classic polyarteritis nodosa except that lung involvement was a prominent feature. These patients generally manifested eosinophilia, granulomatous reactions, and a strong allergic diathesis, usually severe asthma. Most of these patients had what is now referred to as the allergic angiitis and granulomatosis of Churg-Strauss. This disease is quite similar to classic polyarteritis nodosa except for the divergent features mentioned above. Many systemic necrotizing vasculitides manifest clinicopathologic characteristics which overlap these two syndromes as well as the hypersensitivity group of vasculitis (discussed below). This subgroup has been referred to as the "polyangiitis overlap syndrome" of systemic necrotizing vasculitis, and is probably more common than either classic polyarteritis nodosa or Churg-Strauss disease.

In addition to the polyarteritis nodosa group of systemic necrotizing vasculitides, certain other vasculitides are systemic and involve multiple organ systems. However, they are referred to by different names, since they possess characteristic clinical and/or pathologic features. This is true of diseases such as Wegener's granulomatosis (see Ch. 452) and the giant cell arteritides. In the latter group, the two major subcategories—i.e., cranial or temporal arteritis (see Ch. 453) and Takayasu's

TABLE 450–1. THE CLINICAL SPECTRUM OF VASCULITIS

1. Systemic necrotizing vasculitis (polyarteritis nodosa group)
    - Classic polyarteritis nodosa
    - Allergic angiitis and granulomatosis (Churg-Strauss disease)
    - Polyangiitis overlap syndrome
2. Hypersensitivity vasculitis
    - Henoch-Schönlein purpura
    - Serum sickness and serum sickness–like reactions
    - Other drug-related vasculitides
    - Vasculitis associated with infectious diseases
    - Vasculitis associated with neoplasms (most lymphoid)
    - Vasculitis associated with connective tissue diseases
    - Vasculitis associated with other underlying diseases
    - Congenital deficiencies of the complement system
    - Erythema elevatum diutinum
3. Wegener's granulomatosis
4. Giant cell arteritides
    - Cranial or temporal arteritis
    - Takayasu's arteritis
5. Other vasculitic syndromes
    - Mucocutaneous lymph node syndrome (Kawasaki's disease)
    - Behçet's disease
    - Vasculitis isolated to the central nervous system
    - Thromboangiitis obliterans (Buerger's disease)
    - Miscellaneous vasculitides

arteritis (see Ch. 53) are systemic diseases involving large muscular arteries with mononuclear cell and often giant cell infiltration within the walls of the involved arteries. Despite the predisposition for certain vessels in these diseases (temporal artery in cranial arteritis and subclavian artery in Takayasu's arteritis), these are systemic diseases which involve multiple arteries. Lymphomatoid granulomatosis (see Ch. 452) is generally considered in the differential diagnosis of systemic necrotizing vasculitis with lung involvement such as Wegener's granulomatosis. However, it is not strictly speaking an inflammatory response in vessels, but an infiltration of blood vessel walls with atypical and often neoplastic appearing lymphoid cells.

The hypersensitivity vasculitides include a broad and heterogeneous group of disorders which have often caused confusion in categorization. These are discussed in detail in this chapter.

Other vasculitic syndromes can be considered under the category of "miscellaneous" for want of a better term. These include Behçet's disease, the major pathologic feature of which is a true vasculitis (see Ch. 464), and thromboangiitis obliterans, which is an inflammatory and occlusive disease of arteries and veins, although its true vasculitic character has been questioned. In addition to the granulomatous vasculitis of the central nervous system, which is seen in association with certain lymphoproliferative malignancies, there is also an uncommon syndrome of isolated vasculitis of the central nervous system that occurs in the apparent absence of systemic vasculitis or other systemic disease.

Finally, the coronary arteritis and myocardial disease of the mucocutaneous lymph node syndrome (Kawasaki's disease) will be discussed below.

HYPERSENSITIVITY VASCULITIS

Hypersensitivity vasculitis is a term applied to a heterogeneous group of disorders that are thought to represent a hypersensitivity reaction to an identifiable antigenic stimulus such as a drug or an infectious agent; hence the word "hypersensitivity." This immediately becomes a source of confusion, since many, or even all, of the vasculitic syndromes represent hypersensitivity reactions of one form or another. Although the antigenic stimuli associated with this group are heterogeneous, these disorders generally share the characteristic of involvement of small vessels. They can be subdivided into two basic groups. The vast majority of the patients manifest involvement of the postcapillary venules, and hence have a venulitis. A smaller group of patients falls into the second category, in which arterioles are predominantly involved (arteriolitis). Most importantly, there is a predominant and often exclusive involvement of the vessels of the skin. Confusion in the literature generally resulted from grouping this category of vasculitis with the more serious systemic varieties such as classic polyarteritis nodosa and related diseases. It is true that the hypersensitivity vasculitides may have variable degrees of organ system involvement other than of the skin. However, this is usually less severe than that of typical systemic vasculitis of polyarteritis nodosa and Wegener's granulomatosis. Most frequently, the skin is exclusively involved or, if other organ systems are involved, the cutaneous disease still dominates the clinical picture.

ETIOLOGY. As indicated by the terminology, the etiology is usually a recognizable antigenic stimulus such as a drug, microbe, toxin, or foreign or endogenous protein. From an etiologic standpoint the hypersensitivity vasculitides segregate into two distinct groups, depending on the source of the sensitizing antigen. In the classic original group, the antigen is foreign to the host. In the second group the antigen is endogenous. For example, certain connective tissue diseases may manifest a typical hypersensitivity small vessel vasculitis. These diseases are generally characterized by circulating immune complexes in which one of the components is an endogenous protein to which antibody is directed. This is true of patients with systemic lupus erythematosus who develop immune complexes composed of endogenous DNA and anti-DNA antibodies; in addition, patients with rheumatoid arthritis may develop immune complexes of rheumatoid factor with antibody activity against endogenous immunoglobulin. Thus, in most of the hypersensitivity vasculitides, the identity of the etiologic agent which triggers the formation of immune complexes is at least strongly suspected.

INCIDENCE AND PREVALENCE. It is difficult to determine an accurate incidence for the hypersensitivity group of vasculitides owing to the marked heterogeneity among these diverse syndromes. However, the hypersensitivity group of vasculitides is much more common than the group of systemic necrotizing vasculitides and other syndromes such as Wegener's granulomatosis and Takayasu's arteritis. The disease can be seen at any age and in both sexes; however, this varies considerably with the particular subgroup in question.

PATHOLOGY AND PATHOGENESIS. The histopathologic hallmark of the hypersensitivity vasculitides is a leukocytoclastic venulitis. The term leukocytoclasis refers to nuclear debris derived from the neutrophils that have infiltrated in and around the involved vessels. In skin biopsies, this type of involvement is most common in the postcapillary venules just beneath the epidermis. When biopsies are obtained in the acute phase of active disease, the typical pattern of neutrophil infiltration is readily observed. In the subacute or chronic stages, biopsies often reveal mononuclear cell infiltration. In certain of the subgroups, eosinophilic infiltration predominates. In the second and smaller category of hypersensitivity vasculitis, arterioles and capillaries are predominantly involved. In the typical case of hypersensitivity vasculitis with a predominance of cutaneous involvement, the lesions are usually found in the lower extremities or in the dependent areas such as the sacrum in supine patients. This is most likely due to the increase in hydrostatic pressure within the postcapillary venules in these areas.

Although immune complex deposition is widely considered to be the pathogenic mechanism of this group of vasculitis, not every case of hypersensitivity vasculitis has had immune complexes demonstrated, even when, carefully sought, as mentioned above.

CLINICAL MANIFESTATIONS. Just as this broad group is etiologically heterogeneous, so too are the clinical manifestations. However, the hallmark of the group is the predominance of cutaneous involvement. The skin lesions may appear as the classic palpable purpura which results from the extravasation of erythrocytes into the tissue surrounding the involved venules. In addition, one may see macules, papules, vesicles, bullae, subcutaneous nodules, ulcers, and even recurrent or chronic urticaria.

Even though skin lesions generally dominate, various organ system involvements can be seen. Certain constellations of clinicopathologic findings define relatively distinct syndromes. For example, in *Henoch-Schönlein purpura* the typical syndrome consists of palpable purpura (usually over the buttocks), arthralgias, gastrointestinal symptoms, and glomerulonephritis. Henoch-Schönlein purpura is usually seen in children; however, adults of any age may be affected. The disease usually remits spontaneously after one week. However, the disease is remarkable for its tendency to recur a number of times over weeks to months before remission is complete. The characteristic skin lesions are present in virtually all patients. The majority of patients also have arthralgias involving multiple joints, but frank arthritis is rare. The gastrointestinal involvement is usually manifested as colicky abdominal pain which may mimic an acute surgical abdomen. Patients may experience nausea, vomiting, diarrhea, constipation, and occasionally the passage of blood and mucus per rectum. In the more severe and rare case, bowel intussusception may occur. Renal disease is a glomerulitis (see Ch. 80), which is usually expressed as a microscopic hematuria without significant renal functional impairment. However, in rare cases renal failure can occur. Most frequently, patients recover spontaneously and completely.

Other groups within the hypersensitivity category include *serum sickness and serum sickness–like reactions*. The classic manifestations are fever, urticaria, arthralgias, and lymphadenopathy occurring seven to ten days after primary exposure to the antigen in question, which for serum sickness is usually a heterologous serum protein and for serum sickness–like reactions is usually a drug such as penicillin. Most of the manifestations of this disorder are not due to a vasculitis. However, in rare cases cutaneous vasculitis typical of the hypersensitivity group is documented. In addition, patients may rarely progress to a typical systemic necrotizing vasculitis involving multiple organ systems.

A number of disorders have vasculitis as a manifestation of an underlying primary disease. Included in these diseases are *systemic lupus erythematosus, rheumatoid arthritis, mixed cryoglobulinemia*, and *other connective tissue diseases*. In these disorders, the manifestations of the underlying disease usually predominate. When vasculitis is observed, it is generally of the small vessel cutaneous type, which is virtually indistinguishable from the vasculitis seen in the hypersensitivity group with recognized exogenous antigens. However, patients with these disorders, particularly systemic lupus erythematosus and rheumatoid arthritis, may also develop a systemic necrotizing vasculitis which closely resembles the polyarteritis nodosa group in manifestations and severity. Nevertheless, in the typical case, the cutaneous vasculitis usually dominates the clinical picture with respect to the vasculitic process.

Other diseases which may fall into this category of small vessel hypersensitivity vasculitis are the *vasculitis associated with congenital deficiencies of various complement components* such as C1r, C1s, and C2; *erythema elevatum diutinum; hypocomplementemic vasculitis;* the *vasculitis associated with certain neoplasms, particularly of the lymphoid type;* and the *vasculitis associated with other primary disorders such as ulcerative colitis, Crohn's disease, biliary cirrhosis, and retroperitoneal fibrosis.*

DIAGNOSIS. The diagnosis of hypersensitivity vasculitis rests on the demonstration of vasculitis on biopsy. Since the predominant organ involved is the skin, histopathologic material is usually readily available. Since cutaneous involvement is often present in severe systemic vasculitides, one should undertake a systematic workup of other organ systems in patients who present with apparently isolated cutaneous vasculitis.

TREATMENT AND PROGNOSIS. Therapy of the hypersensitivity group of vasculitides has in general been unsatisfactory. Since most cases resolve spontaneously, the lack of response to therapeutic regimens is of less importance. However, in those patients who go on to develop persistent cutaneous disease or serious organ system involvement, several regimens have been tried with variable results. In cases in which a recognized antigenic stimulus is present, the first order of therapy is to remove the antigen; e.g., to remove sensitizing drugs or responsible organisms by appropriate antibiotic therapy when possible. In situations in which disease appears to be self-limited, no specific therapy is indicated. However, when disease persists or results in organ system dysfunction, a glucocorticosteroid is the drug of choice. Prednisone is usually administered in doses of 1 mg per kilogram per day with rapid tapering when possible, in some instances directly to discontinuation or initially to an alternate-day regimen followed by ultimate discontinuation (see Ch. 29). In cases which prove refractory to corticosteroid therapy, cytotoxic agents such as cyclophosphamide have been used, as has plasmapheresis with or without cytotoxic drugs. The efficacy of these regimens has not yet been fully evaluated in hypersensitivity vasculitis. Thus, one should be reluctant to institute cytotoxic agents in persons with disease limited to the skin, particularly since the response of the cutaneous variety of hypersensitivity vasculitis to cytotoxic agents has not been as dramatic as the response of the systemic vasculitides such as Wegener's granulomatosis (see Ch. 452) and the polyarteritis nodosa group.

The prognosis of most of the diseases in this category is generally excellent, with spontaneous and complete remissions in most patients. However, certain patients may develop persistent and debilitating cutaneous disease, and others may evolve a typical systemic vasculitis with a serious prognosis.

MUCOCUTANEOUS LYMPH NODE SYNDROME
(Kawasaki's Disease)

The mucocutaneous lymph node syndrome is an acute febrile illness of infants and young children.

Patients manifest characteristic changes in the skin and mucous membranes with nonsuppurative lymphadenopathy. This disease is also discussed in Ch. 557. Although the course is generally benign and self-limited, a small percentage of patients (approximately 1 to 2 per cent) develop fatal complications. These complications almost invariably result from a vasculitic involvement of the coronary arteries. In fact, it is now generally agreed that many cases of "polyarteritis nodosa in children" were in fact the arteritic complications of unrecognized mucocutaneous lymph node syndrome.

The disease has occurred in almost epidemic proportions in Japan. Although the etiology is unknown, an infective agent is suspected. Clusters of cases have appeared throughout the United States.

Most fatalities occur as sudden deaths in infants and children in the convalescent stage of the disease (usually between the third and fourth week of illness). In virtually all autopsied cases, the coronary arteries manifested arteritis. Typically, bead-like aneurysms with thrombosis are noted along the main trunk and branches of the coronary artery. There is a typical vasculitic picture with intimal proliferation and infiltration of the vessel wall with mononuclear cells. Other manifestations include myocarditis, pericarditis, myocardial infarctions, and cardiomegaly.

One of the difficult questions is the extent to which one should examine a child with the syndrome for cardiac involvement. Since the coronary arteritis occurs in such a small percentage of patients, invasive cardiovascular procedures do not seem warranted. Noninvasive procedures such as echocardiograms and scanning techniques are currently being employed to detect incipient cardiac involvement.

The prognosis of Kawasaki's disease on the whole is excellent, and the vast majority of patients recover uneventfully. However, the consequences for those who develop coronary arteritis are often devastating, with sudden death the rule. Preliminary studies indicate that treatment with aspirin (30 mg per kilogram per day) has resulted in a lessening of the incidence of cardiac complications. There is some unconfirmed evidence that corticosteroids are not effective and may increase the incidence of cardiac complications. At present, it is recommended that children be treated with aspirin during the acute and convalescent phases of the disease.

Alarcon-Segovia D: The necrotizing vasculitides. Med Clin North Am 61:240, 1977. *A brief though rather complete coverage of a classification scheme of the necrotizing vasculitides. One of the latest well-organized attempts to categorize these syndromes appropriately.*

Christian CL, Sergent JS: Vasculitic syndromes: Clinical and experimental models. Am J Med 61:385, 1976. *Excellent review of the vasculitis syndromes with emphasis on the pathophysiologic mechanisms in several of the human diseases as well as in animal models of vasculitis.*

Cupps TR, Fauci AS: The Vasculitides. Philadelphia, W. B. Saunders Company, 1981, pp 1–211. *Comprehensive treatise on the entire spectrum of the vasculitic syndromes. Pathogenesis, clinicopathologic manifestations, and updated therapeutic approaches are discussed in detail.*

Fauci AS, Haynes BF, Katz P: The spectrum of vasculitis. Clinical, pathologic, immunologic, and therapeutic considerations. Ann Intern Med 89:660, 1978. *Review article which introduced an updated classification scheme of the vasculitis syndromes and which has employed this scheme to develop guidelines for an approach to a patient with vasculitis.*

Fauci AS: Systemic vasculitis. In: Current Therapy in Allergy and Immunology

1983–1984. Lichtenstein LM, Fauci AS (Editors), Philadelphia, B. C. Decker, Inc, 1983, pp 130–136. Detailed description of the various therapeutic modalities currently employed for the spectrum of systemic vasculitis with a practical guide for the use of these regimens.

Zeek PM: Periarteritis nodosa and other forms of necrotizing angiitis. N Engl J Med 18:764, 1953. *Classic article which represents the first well-organized approach to the rational classification of the vasculitic syndromes. It is still employed as the backbone of most classification schemes.*

451. POLYARTERITIS NODOSA GROUP

K. Frank Austen

DEFINITION. Kussmaul and Maier introduced the term periarteritis nodosa in 1866 to designate a morbid process manifested by numerous grossly visible or palpable nodules along the course of medium-sized muscular arteries. The lesions are segmental in distribution, have a predilection for the crotch of bifurcations and branchings, and involve all but the pulmonary arteries. The clinical manifestations are disparate and polymorphic, and result from partial or complete arterial occlusion, hemorrhage, and glomerulitis. In view of the necrotizing nature of the process, involving the entire arterial wall, Ferrari in 1903 suggested the alternative name of polyarteritis acuta nodosa; this entity is now termed *classic polyarteritis nodosa* to distinguish it from other entities falling within the polyarteritis nodosa group or syndrome (Table 450–1).

Pulmonary lesions, parenchymal and pulmonary arterial, are absent in classic polyarteritis but almost always precede the onset of polyarteritic lesions in other organs in the entity termed *allergic angiitis and granulomatosis* by Churg and Strauss. Such patients typically present with bronchitis, bronchial asthma, or pulmonary infiltration. The polyarteritic process in other organs is indistinguishable from that of classic polyarteritis nodosa, and thus Rose and Spencer have preferred the term *polyarteritis with pulmonary involvement* for this entity.

A polyarteritic process associated with hepatitis B antigenemia and extending from the medium-sized muscular arteries to arterioles and venules was recognized in 1970 by Gocke and colleagues and is now termed *polyangiitis* or *generalized necrotizing angiitis* to emphasize that the presentation of this polyarteritic process may include venulitis manifested in skin as palpable purpura or urticaria. Serous otitis media and amphetamine abuse are major associated events in the hepatitis B negative group with generalized necrotizing angiitis. On clinical grounds no criteria have been identified to distinguish between the hepatitis B positive and negative patients except that all positive hepatitis B antigenemia patients had abnormal liver chemistries. These were, however, occasionally minimal and then not different from those of the hepatitis B negative group.

Polyarteritis nodosa of childhood has a predilection for the coronary arteries and represents a fourth subgroup of the polyarteritis group or syndrome. In view of the recent evidence that approximately 1 to 2 per cent of children with the mucocutaneous lymph node syndrome (Kawasaki's disease) develop coronary arteritis, it may be that Kawasaki's disease or similar entities are the source of polyarteritis of childhood.

The incidence, age distribution, and male-to-female ratio of polyarteritis nodosa are difficult to determine because a diagnostic serologic procedure is lacking, and the spotty distribution of lesions makes biopsy uncertain. Nonetheless, the condition occurs from infancy to old age, with a peak incidence in the fifth and sixth decades of life, and the male to female ratio has been estimated at from 2 to 3:1.

PATHOLOGY. The lesions of polyarteritis involve arteries of medium and small caliber, especially at bifurcations and branchings. The segmental process involves the media, with edema, fibrinous exudation, fibrinoid necrosis, and infiltration of polymorphonuclear neutrophils and varying numbers of eosinophils, and extends to the adventitia and intima. Thrombosis and infarction or hemorrhage occur at this stage. Subsequently, the regions of fibrinoid necrosis are replaced by cellular granulation tissue, and the intima proliferates. Finally the involved segment is replaced by scar tissue with associated intimal thickening and periarterial fibrosis. These changes produce partial occlusion, thrombosis and infarction, and palpable or visible aneurysms with occasional rupture.

The glomerulitis is characterized by capillary microthrombi, focal fibrinoid necrosis, polymorphonuclear neutrophil infiltration, and capsular proliferation. With progression, the necrotizing feature of the glomerulitis is less apparent, and the process is difficult to distinguish from glomerulonephritis of other causes.

In allergic angiitis and granulomatosis and in polyangiitis, the acute fibrinoid necrosis with cellular infiltration involves arterioles and venules as well as medium-sized muscular arteries, whereas in classic polyarteritis such vessels are spared except in areas contiguous to involved medium-sized muscular arteries. It is characteristic of the polyarteritis nodosa group for the vascular lesions to be in different stages of evolution, i.e., acute, subacute, and healed. In allergic angiitis and granulomatosis the pulmonary granulomatous lesions in vascular and extravascular sites are accompanied by an intense eosinophilic infiltration. The granulomas often include an eosinophilic core of altered collagen and necrotic eosinophils surrounded by radially arranged macrophages, lymphocytes, plasma cells, and varying numbers of polymorphonuclear leukocytes, both neutrophilic and eosinophilic.

In patients with polyangiitis associated with hepatitis B antigenemia, the specific antigen has been recognized in immune complexes present in the circulation and deposited in affected vessels along with complement proteins. It is presumed that this pathogenetic mechanism prevails in the entire polyarteritis nodosa group, but the basis for arterial deposition is unknown. The deposition of immune complexes in venules and glomeruli is attributed to changes in permeability and to physical trapping.

CLINICAL MANIFESTATIONS AND DIAGNOSIS. The widespread distribution of the arterial lesions produces diverse clinical manifestations, which reflect the particular organ systems in which the arterial supply has been impaired. Among the early general symptoms and signs of polyarteritis nodosa are tachycardia, fever, weight loss, and pain in viscera and/or the musculoskeletal system so that the differential diagnosis is of fever of unknown origin. Striking and specific presenting signs may relate to abdominal pain, acute glomerulitis, polyneuritis, or myocardial infarction. Pulmonary manifestations, especially intractable bronchial asthma, would indicate allergic angiitis and granulomatosis rather than classic polyarteritis nodosa.

Renal. Renal involvement in two forms, renal polyarteritis and a glomerulitis, may occur separately or together. Renal polyarteritis is the most common lesion at postmortem examination (Table 451–1). Manifestations of the renal involvement include intermittent proteinuria and microscopic hematuria with occasional hyaline and granular casts. The glomerulitis is manifested by marked microscopic and even macroscopic hematuria, proteinuria, cellular casts, and progressive renal failure; survival of the acute phase is followed by progressive hypertension. Hypertension reflects healing renal polyarteritis, progressive glomerulitis, or both. Renal involvement is the cause of death in about two thirds of patients with classic polyarteritis nodosa and about one third of those with allergic angiitis and granulomatosis.

Gastrointestinal. Arterial lesions are commonly found in one or more abdominal viscera. The principal manifestation is pain, especially in the umbilical region or right upper quadrant; anorexia, nausea, and vomiting are less prominent. Impaired arterial supply to the bowel can produce mucosal ulcerations, perforation, or infarction with melena or bloody diarrhea. Involvement of appendix, gallbladder, or pancreas can stimulate appendicitis, cholecystitis, or hemorrhagic pancreatitis. Liver involvement can range from hepatomegaly with or without jaundice to the signs of extensive hepatic necrosis. Sple-

TABLE 451–1. INCIDENCE OF NECROTIZING ANGIITIS IN VARIOUS ORGANS AT NECROPSY*

	Polyarteritis Nodosa (Classic) (Per Cent)	Allergic Angiitis and Granulomatosis ("Polyarteritis with Pulmonary Involvement") (Per Cent)
Lungs (pulmonary arteries)	0	47
Heart	35	60
Kidneys: Glomerulitis	30	57
Renal polyarteritis	65	60
Stomach and intestines	30	40
Liver	54	37
Pancreas	39	17
Spleen	35	43
Brain	4	3
Periadrenal connective tissue	41	40
Voluntary muscle	20	33

*Reproduced in modified form from Rose GA, Spencer H: Quart J Med 26:43, 1957. There were 54 cases in the periarteritis group and 30 with the diagnosis of allergic angiitis and granulomatosis.

nomegaly is uncommon. There has been no consistent relationship between the development of necrotizing angiitis and the appearance of liver disease in patients with hepatitis B antigenemia. Some of the observed combinations include necrotizing angiitis as the initial clinical finding, superimposed upon chronic active hepatitis, or appearing simultaneously with an acute hepatitis. Death in this group can occur from liver failure but is more commonly due to the generalized necrotizing angiitis.

Central and Peripheral Nervous System. Neurologic manifestations are generally late occurrences in the course of polyarteritis nodosa, and their particular presentation reflects the specific brain area compromised. Headache, convulsive seizures, papillitis, and retinal hemorrhages and exudates occur with or without localizing signs referable to the cerebrum, cerebellum, or brainstem; meningeal irritation may occur as a result of subarachnoid hemorrhage. Multiple mononeuropathy, i.e., involvement of several or even many individual nerves at the same or different times, is a common finding and is attributed to arteritis of the vasa nervorum. The peripheral neuropathy is usually asymmetrical with both sensory and motor distribution. The former can be extremely painful, but the latter, with attendant muscular degeneration, has on occasion been so severe as to dominate the clinical presentation.

Articular and Muscular. Arthralgia and myalgia are frequent in polyarteritis nodosa. Arthralgia is migratory, generally without swelling, and apparently due to small localized arterial lesions rather than extensive synovitis. The interpretation of those rare instances of synovitis with deformity and arterial changes of periarteritis nodosa is difficult, but it seems preferable to consider such cases as rheumatoid arthritis. Muscle pain or weakness reflects either direct involvement of the arterial supply or a peripheral neuropathy from involvement of the vasa nervorum.

Cardiac. Polyarteritis of the coronary arteries and their branches has a frequency approaching that of renal polyarteritis, and heart failure is responsible for or contributes to death in one sixth to one half of the cases. An infantile form of polyarteritis nodosa, affecting children mainly under ten months of age, is manifested primarily by involvement of the coronary arteries. The clinical manifestations of cardiac involvement are those of partial or complete arterial occlusion as modified by the superimposition of renal hypertension and an appreciable incidence of acute pericarditis without effusion. Whereas the combination of infarction and hypertension commonly leads to left-sided failure, an occasional patient with allergic angiitis and granulomatosis will present with predominantly right-sided decompensation.

Genitourinary. Involvement of the ovaries, testes, and epididymis is frequent, though usually asymptomatic. Mucosal ulceration in the bladder can occasionally precipitate gross hematuria with dysuria.

Cutaneous. Cutaneous involvement of some form is believed to occur in over 25 per cent of those affected with polyarteritis nodosa. The acute cutaneous manifestations include polymorphic exanthemata—purpuric, urticarial, and multiform in character—and severe subcutaneous hemorrhage, resulting from necrotizing arteritis, with secondary gangrene. Ulcerations and a persistent livedo reticularis are associated with the more chronic stage of the disease. A most characteristic but uncommon finding is cutaneous and subcutaneous nodules; these occur at any time in the disease course. The nodules tend to group, appear in crops, are usually movable, may regress in days or persist for months, range in size from a pea to a walnut, and may cause the overlying skin to become reddened or to ulcerate.

Pulmonary. Although the bronchial arteries can be involved in classic polyarteritis, only allergic angiitis and granulomatosis which involves the pulmonary arteries and parenchyma with granulomatous lesions gives rise to clinical manifestations. Asthma, when present, is intractable and associated with a marked peripheral eosinophilia. Pneumonic episodes are transient or progressive and may be accompanied by hemoptysis and/or pleuritic pain. Respiratory involvement accounts for about one half of the mortality, with the remainder being due to the polyarteritic process in other organs.

COURSE UNTREATED. The course of polyarteritis nodosa is progressive with destruction of vital organs. Intermittent acute episodes resulting from thrombosis of vital or nonvital structures are prominent. Death is most frequently attributed to renal involvement in cases of classic periarteritis nodosa and to pulmonary lesions in those cases classified as allergic angiitis with granulomatosis. Cardiac failure caused by a combination of infarction and renal hypertension is an additional frequent cause of death in both groups, and acute vascular accidents in the gastrointestinal tract or central nervous system account for much of the remaining mortality. In the retrospective postmortem study of Rose and Spencer, the five-year survival rate was about 10 per cent in classic periarteritis nodosa, and about 25 per cent in allergic angiitis and granulomatosis if onset was dated from the start of respiratory symptoms. The more recent report of the British Medical Research Council in 1960 placed the 54 months' survival rate in polyarteritis nodosa at nearly 50 per cent. Rare patients with polyarteritis limited to nonvital sites have been reported to experience an unusually long course or even a lasting remission.

LABORATORY FINDINGS. Leukocytosis, predominantly polymorphonuclear, is apparent in over 75 per cent of the cases of polyarteritis nodosa or allergic angiitis and granulomatosis, eosinophilia often being marked in the latter group. The association of hepatitis B antigenemia with generalized necrotizing angiitis may be as high as one third of the cases, but probably this figure will prove to be smaller as experience widens. Hypocomplementemia, which has not been observed in classic periarteritis nodosa, has been present in patients with generalized necrotizing angiitis with or without hepatitis B antigenemia. The erythrocyte sedimentation rate is customarily elevated with or without some increase of the globulins. Abnormalities in the urine sediment, especially hematuria and proteinuria, reflect renal involvement. Abnormalities of the electrocardiogram and electroencephalogram are those expected on the basis of arterial occlusive disease or those secondary to the metabolic disturbances of uremia. Lesions apparent on chest roentgenograms are the rule in patients with allergic angiitis and granulomatosis. The findings range from transient or progressive infiltration to consolidation, cavitation, or scarring; upper and lower lobes are involved with equal frequency. As none of these findings is specific, antemortem diagnosis of polyarteritis depends upon biopsy. Since the arterial involvement is segmental and spotty in distribution, it is advisable to obtain tissue from a symptomatic site, and it is essential to section completely the entire specimen. A deep, open surgical biopsy, including subcutaneous tissue and underlying muscle, should be obtained whenever possible from a skeletal muscle exhibiting pain and tenderness. Involvement of the epididymis and testes is sufficiently common to make this a useful biopsy site if palpation reveals the typical nodularity of segmental vascular lesions. Needle and surgical biopsies of internal organs with clinical involvement, such as liver or kidney, are gaining in favor. As an alternative or additional procedure, angiography to detect aneurysms of medium-sized muscular arteries in renal, hepatic, or intestinal sites may be helpful.

DIFFERENTIAL DIAGNOSIS. The differential diagnosis of the polyarteritis group includes not only the constituent syndromes but also all those conditions associated with necrotizing angiitis. The key differences between classic polyarteritis nodosa and other causes of necrotizing angiitis include the absence of extravascular granulomas, sparing of the pulmonary arteries, failure of venous involvement except by contiguous spread, and predilection for medium-sized arteries. For allergic angiitis and granulomatosis the striking granulomatous response excludes all but Wegener's granulomatosis. The prominence of bronchial asthma, peripheral eosinophilia, and the usual absence of necrotizing lesions in the upper respiratory tract permit a tentative clinical distinction between allergic angiitis and granulomatosis and Wegener's granulomatosis. The relative absence of venular involvement, with or without hepatitis B antigenemia, separates classic periarteritis nodosa from the more common polyangiitis. The hypocomplementemia in some patients with polyangiitis is more characteristic of certain patients with hypersensitivity angiitis than of polyarteritis nodosa. Underlying connective tissue diseases are still recognized by their clinical characteristics even when necrotizing arteritis becomes prominent. For example, cases of rheumatoid arthritis with ulcerating cutaneous lesions and peripheral neuropathy often exhibit prominent rheumatoid nodules and a high titer of rheumatoid factor. The specificities of the immunoglobulins which accompany active systemic lupus erythematosus or mixed cryoglobulinemia are distinctive; in addition, in the presence of active renal disease both entities manifest a reduced serum complement level not generally observed in classic polyarteritis nodosa. Giant cell arteritis, in its limited form, cranial (especially temporal) or aortic arch (Takayasu's) arteritis, or in its disseminated state lacks the glomerulitis, peripheral neuropathy, and cutaneous manifestations notable in polyarteritis nodosa. The combination of progressive nephritis and pulmonary hemorrhage seen in Goodpasture's syndrome is unlike polyarteritis nodosa. The drug-induced hypersensitivity angiitis group may be difficult to separate on purely clinical grounds, although the history of antecedent drug administration, the frequency of pulmonary involvement, infrequency of gastrointestinal manifestations, and absence of nodules along arteries are useful points. The clinical presentation in Henoch-Schönlein purpura, mostly in children and with a relatively good prognosis, is distinctive. Necrotizing vasculitis with or without renal disease in C2 deficiency, hypergammaglobulinemic purpura, and other syndromes listed under hypersensitivity angiitis are differentiated by the unique features responsible for designating the entity.

Additional entities to be considered in the differential diagnosis are certain microbial and occlusive diseases with diverse manifestations, notably chronic meningococcemia, subacute infective endocarditis, trichinosis, and certain rickettsial diseases. A few vascular occlusive diseases, including Degos' disease and thrombotic thrombocytopenic purpura, must also be considered. Necrotizing papulosis of Degos, with its occlusive arterial lesions of the skin, gastrointestinal tract, and brain, is best characterized by the cutaneous manifestations. These lesions typically involve the trunk and extremities, begin as pink to gray papules, undergo central umbilication, and persist for variable periods with depressed (porcelain-like) centers covered with a removable scale and surrounded by a red elevated margin. The absence of both thrombocytopenia and intravascular hemolysis distinguishes periarteritis nodosa from thrombotic thrombocytopenic purpura. Additional points of help in the differential diagnosis of periarteritis nodosa in general are the rarity of Raynaud's phenomenon, the absence of the nephrotic syndrome, and the lack of lymphadenopathy.

TREATMENT. The commonly employed anti-inflammatory agents such as salicylates or phenylbutazone have little or no clear effect on the polyarteritis group, and thus corticosteroids have been employed most widely. Large doses, in the range of 40 to 60 mg of prednisone per day, afford symptomatic relief and apparently do improve the one-year survival statistics. On the other hand, the study by the Medical Research Council of England did not reveal a better 54 months' survival period in a steroid-treated group as compared with a control series, whereas early steroid treatment was considered efficacious in the Mayo Clinic series. In a series of 17 patients falling within the polyarteritis group, including two with allergic angiitis and granulomatosis and six with hepatitis B–associated polyangiitis, 14 experienced dramatic remission with the introduction of cyclophosphamide at a dose of 2 mg per kilogram per day. It was subsequently possible to reduce the cyclophosphamide and to taper the steroids to every other day and yet maintain a remission state by clinical criteria and in some instances by resolution of microaneurysms on repeat celiac axis angiography. Although this experience is uncontrolled, the historical outcome and time course of response to the addition of a cytotoxic agent justify the approach.

Churg J, Strauss L: Allergic granulomatosis, allergic angiitis, and periarteritis nodosa. Am J Pathol 27:277, 1951. *This is the classic reference to the polyarteritis nodosa subgroup termed allergic angiitis and granulomatosis, and describes the cardinal clinical and pathologic manifestations.*

Collagen Diseases and Hypersensitivity Panel: Report to Medical Research Council. Br Med J 1:1399, 1960. *This is the classic reference on the natural history of the polyarteritis nodosa group, untreated and with steroid intervention.*

Cupps TR, Fauci AS: The Vasculitides. Philadelphia, W. B. Saunders Company, 1981. *An excellent and up-to-date general review of differential diagnosis, classification, and treatment.*

Fauci AS, Katz P, Haynes BF, Wolff SM: Cyclophosphamide therapy of severe systemic necrotizing vasculitis. N Engl J Med 301:235, 1979. *A most important contribution dealing with the effectiveness of cyclophosphamide therapy in the management of a series of patients falling within the polyarteritis group and including such subgroups as allergic angiitis and granulomatosis and hepatitis B–associated polyangiitis.*

Moore PM, Fauci AS: Neurologic manifestations of systemic vasculitis. A retrospective and prospective study of the clinicopathologic features and responses to therapy in 25 patients. Am J Med 71:517, 1981. *An up-to-date analysis of the beneficial effects of therapy.*

Mowrey FH, Lundberg RA: The clinical manifestations of essential polyangiitis (periarteritis nodosa) with emphasis on the hepatic manifestations. Ann Intern Med 40:1145, 1954. *A useful description of the gastrointestinal manifestations observed in patients with the polyarteritis nodosa group.*

Reza JJ, Dornfeld L, Goldberg LS, Bluestone R, Pearson CM: Wegener's granulomatosis. Long-term follow-up of patients treated with cyclophosphamide. Arthritis Rheum 18:501, 1975. *The introduction of cyclophosphamide therapy altered the natural history not only of Wegener's granulomatosis but subsequently also of the polyarteritis nodosa group, and thus this is an important reference article.*

Rose GA, Spencer H: Polyarteritis nodosa. Quart J Med 26:43, 1957. *This classic article argued most effectivly that allergic angiitis and granulomatosis was not a distinct entity from classic polyarteritis nodosa but could most easily be considered polyarteritis nodosa with pulmonary involvement. This is the current interpretation, and from a clinical point of view nothing need be added to the clinical and pathologic material contained herein.*

Sergent JS, Lockshin MD, Christian CL, Gocke DJ: Vasculitis with hepatitis B antigenemia. Long-term observations in nine patients. Medicine 55:1, 1976. *This represents the five-year experience of the group which originally described the association of hepatitis B antigenemia with necrotizing vasculitis and contains important information with regard to the natural history and clinical course of the disease.*

452. WEGENER'S GRANULOMATOSIS AND MIDLINE GRANULOMA

Anthony S. Fauci

WEGENER'S GRANULOMATOSIS

DEFINITION. Wegener's granulomatosis is characterized by the classic clinicopathologic features of necrotizing granulomatous vasculitis involving the upper and lower respiratory tracts, glomerulonephritis, and variable degrees of systemic, small vessel vasculitis.

ETIOLOGY. The cause is unknown, although it is generally considered to represent an aberrant hypersensitivity reaction to an unknown antigen. There have been no associations with allergic diatheses, geographic location, travel, or domestic or occupational exposure.

INCIDENCE AND PREVALENCE. Although an uncommon disease, Wegener's granulomatosis is no longer thought of as being extremely rare, as it is now recognized earlier and more frequently in clinical practice. The male:female ratio is approximately 1.3:1. The disease can be seen in any age group from infancy to old age. The mean age of onset is 40.6 years.

PATHOLOGY AND PATHOGENESIS. The characteristic histopathologic feature of this disease is necrotizing vasculitis of small arteries and veins together with granuloma formation.

The upper airway disease most often involves the paranasal sinuses and nasopharynx with necrotizing granuloma, with or without demonstrable vasculitis. Pansinusitis with erosion of adjacent bone may occur, as well as nasal septal perforation and saddle nose deformity.

Almost all patients have lung involvement (see Ch. 62). The infiltrates are usually multiple, bilateral, and nodular, with a tendency to cavitate. Endobronchial disease may result in airways obstruction and atelectasis.

Histopathologically, the renal lesion begins as a focal and segmental necrotizing glomerulitis which may lead to rapidly progressive glomerulonephritis and renal failure (see Ch. 80).

In addition to these classic features, virtually any organ can be involved with granuloma, vasculitis, or both.

The immunopathogenesis of the disease remains an enigma. Circulating immune complexes and immune complex–like renal deposits have been demonstrated in some patients. In contradistinction, the extensive granuloma formation in various organs is suggestive of delayed type hypersensitivity or cellular immune mechanisms. It is possible that there is an overlap of more than one type of immunologic mechanism, or that there is a granulomatous response to a particular type of immune complex in this disease.

CLINICAL MANIFESTATIONS. Wegener's granulomatosis is a multisystem disease manifesting a variety of signs and symptoms. However, in most patients the upper airway and, less frequently, the pulmonary symptoms dominate the presenting clinical picture.

Patients usually complain of severe upper respiratory symptoms and signs such as paranasal sinus pain, drainage, and purulent or bloody nasal discharge. Nasal mucosal ulceration and septal perforation may occur, as well as the classic saddle nose deformity. Serous otitis media commonly results from eustachian tube blockage, and variable degrees of hearing impairment may occur.

Eye involvement occurs in up to 60 per cent of patients and may range from mild conjunctivitis to severe episcleritis, granulomatous sclerouveitis, ciliary vessel vasculitis, and proptosis.

Pulmonary manifestations may include cough, hemoptysis, chest discomfort, and shortness of breath. However, it is not uncommon that asymptomatic pulmonary infiltrates are discovered on chest x-ray during workup for other problems.

Nonspecific symptoms such as weakness, malaise, arthralgia, anorexia, and weight loss are common. Fever may result from the underlying disease, but often reflects secondary infection in paranasal sinuses.

Skin disease resulting from vasculitis with or without granuloma is seen in 45 per cent of patients. Heart involvement is infrequent and usually appears as pericarditis or coronary vasculitis. Nervous system involvement, seen in up to 20 per cent of patients, may be exhibited as cranial neuritis, mononeuritis multiplex, or cerebral vasculitis and/or granuloma.

Renal disease usually determines the course and ultimate outcome of generalized Wegener's granulomatosis. Proteinuria with variable degrees of hematuria, red blood cell casts, and other sediment abnormalities may indicate smoldering disease activity. However, once renal function abnormalities appear, evidence of rapidly progressive glomerulonephritis usually ensues, leading to renal failure if appropriate therapy is not instituted. A limited form of Wegener's granulomatosis without renal involvement has been described. However, it most likely constitutes part of the spectrum of the generalized disease.

There are no diagnostic laboratory findings in this disease. The erythrocyte sedimentation rate is invariably markedly elevated. Mild anemia and leukocytosis may be seen, but eosinophilia is not characteristic. Mildly elevated rheumatoid factor titers are common, as is mild hypergammaglobulinemia, particularly of IgA.

DIAGNOSIS. The diagnosis can be strongly suspected when the classic picture of upper and lower airway disease together with renal involvement is present. It is confirmed by the histopathologic demonstration of necrotizing granulomatous vasculitis in appropriate tissues such as nasal or sinus mucosa. The pulmonary infiltrates are the source of tissue with the highest diagnostic yield. Percutaneous renal biopsy is extremely important in documenting glomerulonephritis, particularly in early disease or when the diagnosis is unclear.

Recognition of the classic clinicopathologic complex of Wegener's granulomatosis should make differentiation from other similar disorders relatively easy. However, differential diagnosis should include the vasculitides, connective tissue diseases, infectious and noninfectious granulomatous diseases, and tumors of the upper airway or lung. Goodpasture's syndrome is differentiated by the demonstration of antiglomerular basement membrane antibody. Idiopathic midline granuloma (see below) is a localized destructive disease which mutilates the upper airway and facial tissues. Wegener's granulomatosis does not erode through facial tissue, and idiopathic midline granuloma does not include lung or renal disease. Of particular interest in the differential diagnosis is a disease called *lymphomatoid granulomatosis*. It involves predominantly lungs, skin, central nervous system, and kidney. It is clearly different from Wegener's granulomatosis. It is not a classic inflammatory vasculitis, but an invasion and destruction of vessels by atypical lymphocytoid and plasmacytoid cells resembling a lymphoma; the renal disease is not a glomerulonephritis but a nodular infiltration of the kidney by these bizarre lymphoid cells; and upper airway disease is quite uncommon. Up to 40 per cent of cases of lymphomatoid granulomatosis may evolve into a frank lymphoma.

TREATMENT AND PROGNOSIS. The treatment of choice in this disease is cytotoxic agents, and of the cytotoxic agents cyclophosphamide* is clearly the most effective. It should be given in daily oral doses of 1 to 2 mg per kilogram per day. In initiation of treatment in fulminant cases, the drug may be given intravenously in doses of 4 to 5 mg per kilogram per day for a few days with subsequent change to the lower oral dosage regimen. A therapeutic response can usually be induced and maintained without causing severe leukopenia. Leukocyte counts should be closely monitored during therapy, and dosages of cyclophosphamide should be adjusted to maintain the leukocyte count above 3000 per cubic millimeter and the neutrophil count no less than 1000 to 1500 per cubic millimeter in order to avoid risk of infection. Cyclophosphamide should be continued for 1 full year following remission. In patients who cannot tolerate cyclophosphamide, azathioprine* in similar doses may be used.

Corticosteroids should be used initially, together with cyclophosphamide. Prednisone, 60 mg per day for a brief period of time, is recommended until the cyclophosphamide becomes effective (usually within 2 to 3 weeks). The prednisone should then be converted to an alternate-day regimen, tapered, and discontinued after approximately 6 months.

The disease was formerly universally fatal, usually within months after onset of renal disease. With cyclophosphamide

*Investigational drug for this purpose.

use, the prognosis is quite good, and long-term remissions have been achieved in over 90 per cent of patients. Several patients have maintained remission for years following discontinuation of cyclophosphamide. Several patients in drug-induced remissions, but with residual irreversible renal failure, have undergone successful renal transplantation.

Fauci AS: Granulomatous vasculitides: Distinct but related. Ann Intern Med 87:782, 1977. *An editorial which outlines the distinctions and overlaps among the various granulomatous vasculitides.*

Fauci AS, Haynes BF, Katz P: The spectrum of vasculitis. Clinical, pathologic, immunologic, and therapeutic considerations. Ann Intern Med 89:660, 1978. *Comprehensive review article which describes the entire spectrum of the vasculitides and places Wegener's granulomatosis in perspective in relation to the other systemic vasculitides.*

Fauci AS, Haynes BF, Katz P, Wolff SM: Wegener's granulomatosis: Prospective clinical and therapeutic experience with 85 patients for 21 years. Ann Intern Med 98:76, 1983. *Clinicopathologic features of the disease are discussed and detailed information on use of the combined cyclophosphamide-alternate day prednisone regimen is provided. Complete remissions were achieved in 93 per cent of patients.*

Liebow AA, Carrington CRB, Friedman PJ: Lymphomatoid granulomatosis. Hum Pathol 3:457, 1972. *Original description of the newly recognized entity of lymphomatoid granulomatosis. Extensively details the cases from a restrospective standpoint. An important paper, but overly long and cumbersome to read.*

Steinman TI, Jaffe BF, Monaco AP, Wolff SM, Fauci AS: Recurrence of Wegener's granulomatosis after kidney transplantation. Successful re-induction of remission with cyclophosphamide. Am J Med 68:458, 1980. *Wegener's granulomatosis recurred four years after renal transplantation and responded to cyclophosphamide after failing to respond to azathioprine.*

MIDLINE GRANULOMA

DEFINITION. Midline granuloma is a rare disease manifested by a relentlessly progressive, localized destructive process that predominantly involves the nose, paranasal sinuses, and palate, with erosion through contiguous structures such as the orbit and face. It is characterized by nonspecific acute and chronic inflammation and necrosis with or without granuloma formation.

ETIOLOGY. The cause of midline granuloma is unknown. Since the tissue reaction is suggestive of a hypersensitivity or immunologically mediated process, a localized fulminant response to an unidentified antigen has been proposed. No etiologic connections have been made with prior allergic rhinitis, chronic sinusitis, or infection. Certain upper airway tumors can result in inflammatory and granulomatous responses with necrosis. The underlying histopathology of the neoplasm is masked and the process closely resembles midline granuloma. However, true midline granuloma is a distinct entity in which no identifiable cause can be found despite multiple deep biopsies, long-term follow-up, and postmortem examination. This entity should appropriately be referred to as idiopathic midline granuloma, as opposed to the inflammatory and granulomatous responses associated with upper airway neoplasms.

PATHOLOGY. The typical histopathologic features are nonspecific acute and chronic inflammation with necrosis. The tissue is infiltrated with neutrophils, monocytes, lymphocytes, plasma cells, and, in some cases, eosinophils. True granuloma formation with or without typical Langhans giant cells may not be present in every case. Thrombosis of small vessels, perivascular cellular infiltration, and secondary involvement of vessels resulting from the inflammatory process may occur, but true primary vasculitis is rarely seen. If neoplastic cells are identified, the process can no longer be considered idiopathic midline granuloma. Secondary pyogenic infection of the involved tissue with its added inflammatory response is frequent.

CLINICAL MANIFESTATIONS. The disease can occur in all age groups, but most patients are in the fifth and sixth decades. It is slightly more common in women than men and occurs in all races.

The clinical presentation can vary, but in most cases symptoms are first related to the nose and paranasal sinuses with rhinorrhea and nasal stuffiness, followed by purulent nasal discharge resulting from superimposed infection. Nonhealing ulcerations of the nasal mucosa occur, and perforation of the nasal septum is frequent. Some patients present with disease in the oral cavity with or without nasal and paranasal sinus involvement. This usually occurs as ulcerations of the buccal mucosa, gums, or hard and soft palate. Some patients present with relatively painless perforation of the palate noted by the regurgitation of food or saliva into the nasal cavity. Occasionally, patients initially complain of symptoms related to the eye. The disease may be relatively indolent or fulminant, but it is always progressive. Relentless destruction of soft tissue, cartilage, and bone occur. Erosion of paranasal sinus walls occurs, with spread into contiguous structures such as the orbit. Destruction of the soft and hard palate, the nasal septum, and even the entire nose occurs. The destructive process may erode through the skin, resulting in dramatic mutilation of facial structures. The necrotic tissue and paranasal sinus cavities frequently becomes infected, usually with *Staphylococcus aureus*. The necrotic tissue can be quite malodorous, although the patients themselves frequently lose their sense of smell. Local lymphadenopathy occurs rarely and is suggestive of an underlying malignancy.

There are no characteristic laboratory findings except those related to the inflammatory process such as leukocytosis, elevated erythrocyte sedimentation rate, mild anemia of chronic disease, and hyperglobulinemia. Roentgenographic studies reveal pansinusitis with destruction of various cartilaginous and bony structures of the upper airways. Since this is a localized disease, laboratory abnormalities related to other organ systems should prompt one to investigate other possible causes.

Surgical procedures in the involved areas can lead to rapid acceleration of the disease, although, following appropriate treatment, debridement may benefit healing. Death usually occurs from secondary systemic infection or from inanition. Other causes are erosion into a major blood vessel with exsanguination or erosion into the central nervous system and subsequent meningitis.

DIAGNOSIS. The diagnosis of midline granuloma is made by the characteristic clinical presentation together with characteristically nonspecific histopathologic findings, but, most important, after other diseases with similar findings have been ruled out.

Midline granuloma is sometimes confused with Wegener's granulomatosis. They are clearly distinct entities. Wegener's granulomatosis is a systemic disease characterized by necrotizing granulomatous vasculitis of the upper and lower respiratory tracts with glomerulonephritis (in the generalized form). Midline granuloma rarely manifests true primary vasculitis in the lesions and by definition is a localized disease without pulmonary or renal involvement. Furthermore, Wegener's granulomatosis rarely if ever causes palatal perforation and does not erode facial tissues.

The greatest difficulty arises in distinguishing true idiopathic midline granuloma from neoplasms of the upper airways, particularly midline malignant reticulosis and certain lymphomas, whose malignant histopathology can be masked by the intense inflammatory reaction. Careful search for disseminated malignancy as well as complete examination of multiple adequate biopsy specimens often either reveal the neoplastic disorder or confirm midline granuloma.

Other diseases which must be ruled out are infectious diseases such as tuberculosis, syphilis, lepromatous leprosy, histoplasmosis, blastomycosis, coccidioidomycosis, mucocutaneous leishmaniasis, and rhinoscleroma (caused by a *Klebsiella* species). Pseudotumor of the orbit must also be ruled out.

TREATMENT. Corticosteroid therapy is ineffective and can worsen infection. Cytotoxic agents have been used with variable results, most of which were ultimately failures.

The treatment of choice is local radiation therapy. High dose (5000 rads) radiotherapy to the involved areas results in a high percentage of remissions.

PROGNOSIS. If untreated, the disease is uniformly fatal. Since the use of high dose local radiotherapy, the prognosis for survival is excellent, with greater than 70 per cent remission rate and even cures after up to 15 years of follow-up. Hence the disease should no longer be referred to as "lethal" midline granuloma. High dose radiotherapy is associated in some cases with serious complications and side effects. However, the risk is outweighed by the fatal alternative. The mutilation and disfigurement that result from far advanced disease are often a source of great psychologic difficulty. Reconstructive plastic surgery and prostheses have resulted in dramatic functional and cosmetic improvements in some patients.

Fauci AS, Johnson RE, Wolff SM: Radiation therapy of midline granuloma. Ann Intern Med 84:140, 1976. *Prospective, 15-year study of ten patients with idiopathic midline granuloma which establishes the efficacy of high dose local irradiation therapy. Discusses differential diagnosis as well as the salient features that distinguish midline granuloma from Wegener's granulomatosis.*

Fechner RE, Lamppin DW: Midline malignant reticulosis. A clinicopathologic entity. Arch Otolaryngol 95:467, 1972. *Important paper pointing out that certain types of destructive upper airway neoplasms can closely mimic midline granuloma.*

Friedmann I: Midline granuloma. Proc R Soc Med 57:289, 1964. *Classic description of many of the clinicopathologic features of midline granuloma.*

Stewart JP: Progressive lethal granulomatous ulceration of the nose. J Laryngol 48:657, 1933. *Original complete description of midline granuloma with firm establishment of the disease as a distinct clinicopathologic entity.*

Tsokos M, Fauci AS, Costa J: Idiopathic midline destructive disease (IMDD). A subgroup of patients with the "midline granuloma" syndrome. Am J Clin Pathol 77:162, 1982.

453. POLYMYALGIA RHEUMATICA AND GIANT CELL ARTERITIS

Louis A. Healey

POLYMYALGIA RHEUMATICA

Polymyalgia rheumatica is a syndrome consisting of pain and stiffness in pelvic and shoulder girdles, very rapid erythrocyte sedimentation rate, and a prompt response to a small dose of corticosteroid. For reasons unknown, it is a disease of older patients. The diagnosis is made with reluctance in anyone less than 50 years old, and most patients are over age 60. It is seen more often in women than in men (2.5:1). Almost all patients affected are Caucasian. Both polymyaligia and giant cell arteritis show statistical association with HLA determinants CW_3, DR_3, and DR_4.

Patients experience pain in the neck, back, shoulders, upper arms, and thighs. The onset may be gradual but at other times is so abrupt that patients go to bed well and awaken in the morning stiff and sore as if they had chopped wood or shoveled snow. Morning stiffness and jelling after prolonged sitting are essential features of the history. Patients graphically describe how a spouse has to pull them out of bed or, if they are alone, how it is necessary for them to wiggle like a snake and then push themselves up from a kneeling position. Although such a story may initially suggest weakness, the limitation is actually due to pain and stiffness rather than lack of strength. Some patients experience widespread symptoms and complain that they hurt all over. In others the pain and stiffness is in either shoulders or hips, but in all it is symmetrical. Low grade fever, malaise, apathy, and weight loss are sometimes present. Carpal tunnel syndrome has been noted.

Despite the severity of complaints, the physical examination of these patients is surprisingly normal. Tenderness or limitation of shoulder and hip motion may be detected; effusions are present in the knees at times. Muscle strength is normal when tested. Radiographs are unremarkable. The clue to the diagnosis is the erythrocyte sedimentation rate, which is always elevated, usually very high, and may exceed 100 mm per hour (Westergren method). Unless this test is performed, the diagnosis is easily missed. Fibrinogen and alpha II globulins are both high. Slight anemia may be present. Rheumatoid factor and antinuclear antibodies are not present, serum complement is normal, and circulating immune complexes have not been consistently detected. Serum levels of muscle enzymes, electromyograms, and muscle biopsies are normal. Evidence from scans, biopsies, arthroscopy, and synovial fluid cell counts suggests that the symptoms of pain and stiffness may stem from synovitis.

Although polymyalgia rheumatica appears to be a distinct clinical entity, it is obvious from this description that it is not a specific one, and as such it is often necessary to exclude other diseases in order to make the diagnosis. The sedimentation rate indicates that this is an inflammatory disease and serves to separate it from osteoarthritis or the functional musculoskeletal pain of fibrositis. Difficulty in getting out of bed or rising from a chair may suggest the weakness of polymyositis, but, as mentioned, muscles are normal. The common diagnostic problem is to differentiate polymyalgia rheumatica from the onset of rheumatoid arthritis. Patients with rheumatoid arthritis tend to have synovitis of the distal joints—wrists, metacarpophalangeal, and metatarsophalangeal. When present, the rheumatoid factor is helpful, but at times, the diagnosis only becomes evident with follow-up visits.

The response of the pain and stiffness of polymyalgia rheumatica to 10 to 20 mg of prednisone may truly be described as dramatic. Many patients are well by the next day; improvement is so invariable that if it does not appear within one week, the original diagnosis should be questioned. After two to four weeks, the dose can be tapered and patients remain free of symptoms on 5 to 7.5 mg of prednisone daily, without risk of steroid side effects. The duration that therapy will be required is uncertain. Some patients can stop after one year, but others will have to continue. The duration can be determined only by attempting to withdraw the drug and observing for a recurrence of stiffness and pain. Aspirin and other nonsteroidal anti-inflammatory drugs provide partial relief but are not so effective as even small doses of steroid.

GIANT CELL ARTERITIS

Since the recognition that any of the larger arteries may be involved, the term *giant cell arteritis* has been preferred to the original names *temporal* or *cranial arteritis*. In contrast to polyarteritis, smaller arterioles are not affected; thus pulmonary and renal complications are not seen, and stroke or myocardial infarction does not occur more frequently than would be expected in this age group.

Clinical manifestations may conveniently be divided into localized or systemic. Local manifestations depend on the artery involved. Inflammation of the temporal artery produces severe headache, most often in one temple. The artery may be tender and swollen. Sudden unilateral blindness is due to occlusion of the terminal branches of the ophthalmic artery. Since blindness is irreversible, this is the most dreaded complication of the disease. Pain in the masseter muscles with chewing is attributed to involvement of the facial artery. This "jaw claudication" is a pathognomonic symptom of giant cell arteritis. Transient diplopia from ischemia of extraocular muscles is important to recognize, since it may lead to early diagnosis, steroid treatment, and preservation of vision. Arteritic involvement of the aorta can cause aortic arch syndromes with claudication in the arms and unequal pulses or, rarely, aneurysm formation. Systemic manifestations include fever, anemia, weight loss, malaise, and polymyalgia rheumatica. Some or all of these may be present in varying degree. If headache and other cranial symptoms are either not present or minimal and systemic symptoms predominate, the patients may present such diagnostic problems as fever of unknown origin, unexplained anemia, or possible occult carcinoma.

As with polymyalgia rheumatica, the only laboratory abnormality is the rapid erythrocyte sedimentation rate. Anemia is usually mild but can be more significant with hematocrit as low as 28 per cent. Red blood cell indices are normal, and there is a failure to utilize iron despite the presence of normal stores in the marrow. Tests of liver function, particularly the alkaline phosphatase, may show slight to moderate abnormalities, but biopsy of the liver shows normal tissue or slight fatty changes.

The diagnosis is established by biopsy of the temporal artery, which is safe and convenient to perform as an office procedure. The characteristic histologic picture shows zones of inflammatory infiltrate composed of histiocytes, lymphocytes, and giant cells surrounding markedly fragmented internal elastic lamina with intervening segments of normal artery. When headache, visual symptoms, or other signs of cranial artery involvement are present, the diagnosis may be suspected and the biopsy is usually positive. However, the characteristic arteritis has also been found in some patients with polymyalgia rheumatica, fever, or other systemic symptoms even when the temporal artery appears clinically normal.

Giant cell arteritis responds well to steroid treatment, but higher doses are needed to suppress the inflammation. When cranial arteritis is diagnosed or even suspected, treatment should be started immediately with at least 50 mg of prednisone in order to preserve vision. If the diagnosis is proved by biopsy, this dose should be continued for four weeks before gradual reduction is instituted with the aim of achieving the same maintenance dose and duration of therapy as described for polymyalgia rheumatica. Such a program carries a risk of steroid toxicity, particularly osteoporosis and vertebral collapse, which must be balanced against the risk of blindness. Symptoms are a better guide to titrating the steroid dose than the sedimentation rate. If the patient has been treated with high-dose steroid for one month, it is preferable to follow the clinical response as the dose is tapered. The risk of steroid toxicity from treating the sedimentation rate is greater than the risk of a complication of arteritis in a patient whose sedimentation rate increases somewhat as the steroid dose is lowered.

The exact nature of the relation between polymyalgia rheumatica and giant cell arteritis is uncertain, in large part because the etiology of both diseases is not known. Both are diseases of older patients, the vast majority of whom are Caucasian. Both frequently are seen in the same patient. Sixty per cent of patients with giant cell arteritis experience polymyalgia rheumatica either as a prodrome or at some time during their illness. Conversely, of patients with polymyalgia rheumatica and normal-appearing temporal arteries, only 10 per cent show arteritis on biopsy. The majority of polymyalgia patients respond well to low-dose prednisone and never develop clinical evidence of arteritis.

Chuang T-Y, Hunder GG, Ilstrup DM, Kurland LT: Polymyallgia rheumatica. A 10-year epidemiologic and clinical study. Ann. Intern Med 97:672, 1982. *Based on an entire county population, this study gives the best information on incidence. The 10-year follow-up provides a look at the course of the disease, response to treatment, outcome, and complications.*

Healey LA, Wilske KR: The Systemic Manifestations of Temporal Arteritis. New York, Grune & Stratton, 1978. *This 140-page monograph describes clinical manifestations, histology, and treatment. English language references are critically reviewed. Research and possible etiology are discussed.*

454. DERMATOMYOSITIS AND POLYMYOSITIS

Ronald P. Messner

DEFINITION. Polymyositis is an inflammatory disease of skeletal muscle of unknown etiology, characterized by symmetrical weakness of the limb girdles, neck, and pharynx. Patients with this illness can be divided into five clinical categories:

Type I —Adult polymyositis
Type II —Dermatomyositis
Type III—Myositis with malignancy
Type IV—Childhood myositis
Type V —Myositis associated with other connective tissue diseases (overlap syndromes)

In this chapter the term polymyositis is used to characterize the whole group of patients, while adult polymyositis is used to denote Type I patients.

Proposed criteria for diagnosis of polymyositis are (1) symmetrical proximal muscle weakness, (2) elevation of muscle enzyme activities in serum, (3) typical EMG abnormalities, (4) positive muscle biopsy, and (5) typical rash of dermatomyositis. Patients are classified as having definite disease with four, probable disease with three, and possible disease with two criteria. The use of this system has helped to standardize the diagnosis and has greatly facilitated comparision of different reported series of patients.

INCIDENCE. Polymyositis has an annual incidence of approximately 7 cases per 1 million population. There is no relationship to birth order, family size, socioeconomic level, or geographic location. Familial cases are unusual. Age distribution is bimodal, with a small peak between ages 10 and 14 and a larger peak around age 50. Patients with myositis associated with malignancy have a mean age just over 60, whereas those with overlap syndrome have a mean age around 35. In adult and childhood polymyositis, females outnumber males by two to one. In cases associated with overlap syndromes the female dominance is even more pronounced. The sex ratio is nearly equal in dermatomyositis and myositis associated with malignancy.

PATHOLOGY AND PATHOGENESIS. The characteristic features of polymyositis on muscle biopsy include (1) degeneration of individual fibers, sometimes with vacuolation; (2) regeneration indicated by sarcoplasmic basophilia, large vesicular nuclei, and prominent nucleoli; (3) necrosis of part or all of a muscle fiber (moth-eaten fibers) and phagocytosis of the debris by macrophages; (4) increased variation in fiber size without hypertrophy of individual fibers; (5) interstitial and/or perivascular mononuclear cell infiltrate; (6) perifascicular atrophy; and (7) interstitial fibrosis. These findings may vary from patient to patient and even on multiple biopsies of a single patient. Approximately 15 per cent of initial muscle biopsies are normal, and the full picture of typical changes can be expected in about 50 per cent. Biopsy should be performed on a muscle that is involved but not totally weakened. Electromyography may aid in localizing an involved area, but the biopsy should not include the exact site of the electromyograph needle puncture, for these areas may show focal fiber destruction.

Skin biopsy should be done in an area of clinical dermatitis rather than relying on that obtained at muscle biopsy without regard for the condition of the skin. Marked dermal edema, basal vacuolation, and colloid bodies occur in the skin in both dermatomyositis and systemic lupus erythematosus, but in dermatomyositis the basement membrane is normal in thickness and does not stain for immunoglobulin or complement in indirect immunofluorescence studies.

One leading theory of the pathogenesis of polymyositis attributes muscle damage to cell-mediated autoimmunity. Evidence that supports this hypothesis includes the presence of lymphocytes and macrophages in the inflammatory infiltrate, sensitivity of lymphocytes to muscle antigens in vitro, and direct cytotoxicity of lymphocytes to cultured muscle cells. Recent information has, however, cast doubt on the ability of polymyositis lymphocytes to kill muscle cells. Although cell-mediated immune damage remains an attractive explanation, the exact mechanisms responsible for muscle injury are unknown.

There is little evidence to support the idea that antibodies participate in the pathogenesis of polymyositis. Antibodies to crude muscle extracts or myosin are no more frequent in polymyositis than in muscular dystrophy. Antibodies reactive with intact muscle are absent. Antimyoglobin antibodies occur in about two thirds of patients, but it is unclear whether they are primary or secondary factors in the disease process. A subset of children with polymyositis experiences cutaneous ulceration and intestinal infarction suggestive of necrotizing vasculitis, but examination of tissue reveals primarily noninflammatory endarteropathy and lymphocytic perivasculitis. Direct evidence of immune complex deposition is lacking in these children and in most adults, but a growing body of evidence suggests that ischemic damage caused by capillary abnormalities may be important in the pathogenesis. Replication of the capillary basement membrane and alterations in endothelial cells are frequent findings on electron microscopy, and the area of muscle served per capillary is increased. Loss of capillaries characteristically starts in the periphery of the fascicles and is more pronounced in children than in adults. These changes are probably not due to muscle atrophy, because the ratio of capillary lumina to muscle cell area does not change in Duchenne dystrophy and increases in denervation atrophy.

Infection caused by a virus or an organism such as *Toxoplasma gondii* has also been postulated as a cause of polymyositis. The incidence of IgM *anti-Toxoplasma* antibodies is increased in patients with polymyositis, and *Toxoplasma* organisms have been identified in a few cases of adult polymyositis, but treatment for toxoplasmosis has had little effect on the muscle disease. Whether these cases represent secondary infection with *Toxoplasma* or true toxoplasmic myositis is unclear. Coxsackievirus has been isolated from a few cases of polymyositis, and the incidence of antibodies to coxsackie B virus is increased in children with dermatomyositis. A good animal model has not been available for study of this disease. The recently described myositis that occurs in newborn mice after injection with coxsackie B1 virus might provide a system to study both the role of infection and the role of cell-mediated immunity in muscle damage.

CLINICAL MANIFESTATIONS. Weakness of the proximal muscles occurs in nearly all patients and is the presenting complaint in 70 per cent. The typical case begins with gradual onset of weakness in the hip girdle and proximal leg muscles. Muscle pain and tenderness are absent or mild. Weakness of the shoulders, proximal arm muscles, and neck flexors follows. Involvement of the pharyngeal muscles may occur with dysphagia, dysphonia, and dysarthria. Early symptoms include inability to rise from a low chair, climb stairs without the use of a railing, or raise the arms above the head to comb the hair. In advanced cases, the patient may be unable to lift the limbs against gravity. Muscular wasting is variable and frequently minimal until late in the disease. Contractures are almost exclusively associated with longstanding disease. The ocular muscles are almost never involved, and weakness of distal muscles occurs in less than 20 per cent of cases. Asymmetric weakness, weakness of isolated muscle groups, and acute onset with global weakness are unusual. Deep tendon reflexes are normal or slightly reduced. Muscle symptoms of childhood polymyositis are similar to those of the adult form, but fever, weight loss, rash, contractures, and subcutaneous calcification are more common.

Arthralgias occur in about one quarter of patients with adult polymyositis or dermatomyositis. True arthritis is usually mild; begins prior to or coincident with weakness; involves the hands, wrists, and knees; and responds quickly to steroid treatment. Synovial fluid has good viscosity and mononuclear cells. Synovial biopsy reveals fibrin deposition, focal loss of lining cells without proliferation, and mild inflammation. Patients with myositis and overlap syndromes may have joint involvement typical of rheumatoid arthritis or systemic lupus erythematosus. A peculiar arthritis of the hands with erosions, periosteal calcification, and instability of the interphalangeal joints of the thumb has also been described.

An erythematous skin rash occurs on the forehead, neck, shoulders, trunk, and arms of about one third of the patients with polymyositis. A lilac or heliotrope rash occurs on the upper eyelids and face in 15 per cent and is highly suggestive of the diagnosis of dermatomyositis. The rash may be associated with edema. Reddened, elevated, scaly patches are characteristically seen over the extensor surfaces of the small joints of the hands, the elbows, the knees, and the medial malleoli. Nailfolds may show periungual telangiectasia, dilated and distorted nailfold capillary loops alternating with avascular areas, or thickening and roughening without redness. In some patients, the finger pads become shiny and atrophic with constant peeling. Patients with myositis and overlap syndromes may display the whole spectrum of dermatologic changes associated with connective tissue diseases. Raynaud's syndrome occurs in one half of the patients with overlap syndrome and one fifth of those with adult polymyositis and dermatomyositis. It is less common in children and in patients with malignancy.

Dysphagia in polymyositis is primarily due to weakness of the striated musculature of the posterior pharynx. Dysfunction of the esophagus occurs, but is usually overshadowed by pharyngeal dysfunction. Hypomobility and poor absorption in the small intestine have been seen in a few patients without symptoms of frank scleroderma. Vasculitis associated with the childhood form of the disease may lead to mesenteric thrombosis.

Asymptomatic electrocardiographic abnormalities are common in polymyositis, but cardiac involvement manifested by congestive heart failure or heart block occurs in only 5 per cent of patients. Inflammatory cardiomyopathy, fibrosis, and small vessel disease have been found in some of these patients at autopsy. Interstitial pneumonitis occurs in 5 to 10 per cent of the patients. Cough and dyspnea precede muscle weakness in one half of the cases of interstitial pneumonitis. No relationship is apparent between the severity of the lung and muscle involvement. Vasculitis is not characteristic of this lesion, and pleurisy is uncommon. The presence of active inflammation on lung biopsy correlates well with steroid responsiveness. Renal involvement is rare. When renal failure occurs, it is most often attributable to myoglobulinuria. A few renal biopsies have revealed mesangial proliferation, suggesting that immune complexes may play a role in some cases.

About 10 per cent of patients with polymyositis have coexistent malignancy. The incidence of tumors is highest, 15 per cent, in dermatomyositis. It is also increased in adult polymyositis, but not in childhood polymyositis. Females are affected as frequently as males. Patients with associated malignancy are older than the average patient with polymyositis. Myositis precedes or occurs simultaneously with the diagnosis of malignancy in two thirds of patients, and in most instances the two diagnoses are made within the span of a year. Tumors of the breast and lung are the most common. Those of the ovary and stomach occur more frequently than in the general population, whereas tumors of the colon and rectum are less frequent. Polymyositis associated with malignancy has no clinical features that differentiate it from polymyositis alone. Extensive undirected radiographic screening of these patients for cancer has proved unrewarding. Clues to the coexistence of a malignancy are almost always present on history, physical examination, or routine laboratory tests.

CLINICAL COURSE AND PROGNOSIS. The five-year survival rate of patients followed over the last 20 years is approximately 80 per cent. The best survival rate occurs in children, and the worst in adults with malignancies. Death within the first year is usually due to pneumonia associated with dysphagia and aspiration. The leading causes of death are malignancy, infection, and cardiovascular disease. Deaths from muscular weakness are relatively rare. About half of the surviving patients will attain almost complete recovery of muscle strength.

LABORATORY DATA. Serum levels of muscle-derived enzymes, principally creatine kinase (CK), transaminases (SGOT, SGPT), lactate dehydrogenase (LDH), and aldolase, are elevated at some time during the course of the disease in 99 per cent of the patients and will be normal at any one time in about 10 per cent. The CK may be normal in as many as 36 per cent of cases at the time of presentation. Diagnostic accuracy can be improved by obtaining a battery of enzyme assays. The levels of these enzymes correlate reasonably well with disease activity and can be used as guides to therapy. Serum levels of myoglobin are elevated in approximately half of the patients and also correlate with clinical activity.

The incidence of rheumatoid factors and fluorescent antinuclear antibodies is remarkable only in patients in the overlap category. Antibodies to the Sm antigen are absent, but anti-RNP antibodies have been reported. Polymyositis patients have a number of antibodies directed against antigens present in calf thymus nuclear extracts that are separate from the Sm, nRNP, SS-A, and SS-B systems found in other autoimmune disorders. The JO-1 system occurs exclusively in polymyositis and defines a subset of patients with a high incidence of pulmonary fibrosis. The JO-1 antigen has been identified as histidine tRNA synthetase. Children with polymyositis have an increased incidence of HLA-B8 and DR3.

Anemia may be present but is rarely severe. The erythrocyte sedimentation rate is abnormal on initial evaluation in only half of the patients and cannot be relied upon as an index of disease activity. Gamma globulins are normal or elevated. With few exceptions total hemolytic complement and C3 are normal. Radionuclide scanning with ^{99m}Tc-polyphosphate may reveal increased uptake in areas of active myositis.

The electromyogram (EMG) is abnormal in almost all patients. The most common abnormalities, reduction in amplitude and duration of motor unit potentials, occur in 90 per cent of cases but are not specific for polymyositis. Evidence of membrane irritability, including fibrillation, positive sharp waves, and increased insertional activity, occur in half to three quarters of the EMGs. Spontaneous bizarre high frequency discharges are also characteristic. Electromyographic patterns do not differ among the clinical types of disease. In some patients the characteristic pattern is present only in certain muscle groups. The paravertebral musculature is frequently involved and should be included in diagnostic electromyography.

DIAGNOSIS AND DIFFERENTIAL DIAGNOSIS. Polymyositis is but one of a variety of diseases that may be present with muscle weakness and pain.

Neurologic disease is a primary concern in the evaluation of these patients. The history and physical examination will usually establish the neurologic origin, and EMG will show neuropathic changes. In muscular dystrophy a family history is often present and the symptoms progress over years rather than months. The CK may be elevated and may decrease on treatment with corticosteroids, but clinical improvement does not occur. The early involvement of the ocular and facial muscles helps differentiate myasthenia gravis.

Steroid myopathy begins insidiously in the proximal leg and hip muscles and spreads to involve the shoulders and arms. Other signs of glucocorticosteroid excess are usually present, but there is a poor correlation between the actual dose of corticosteroids and this syndrome. Raising the dose over a previously tolerated level may induce myopathy, and decreasing it to the previous level may relieve the symptoms. Muscle biopsy is normal. The combination of elevated urinary creatine and normal serum enzyme activities has been suggested as a useful differential point in favor of steroid myopathy. Other drugs that may cause myopathy include alcohol, clofibrate, penicillamine, azathioprine, phenytoin, polymyxin, chloroquine, and emetine.

Both hyper- and hypothyroidism may cause proximal muscle weakness. Thyrotoxic myopathy is usually insidious in onset and occurs most often in men. Muscle biopsy shows mild atrophy without inflammation. The electromyogram is nonspecific, and muscle enzymes are not elevated. In hypothyroidism, however, serum creatine phosphokinase may reach exceptionally high levels, and the electromyogram may be identical to that in polymyositis. Hyperparathyroidism may also cause proximal muscle weakness, an abnormal electromyogram, and muscle atrophy without an inflammatory infiltrate.

Weakness and myalgia may occur after exercise in McArdle's syndrome, carnitine palmityltransferase deficiency, myoadenylate deaminase deficiency, or renal tubular acidosis. A syndrome closely mimicking polymyositis may be seen in phosphate depletion, which is most often due to the use of nonabsorbable antacids. Muscle enzymes are not elevated. The electromyogram may be normal or show a pattern of denervation. Weakness disappears upon restoration of body phosphorus.

Direct invasion of muscle by an infectious agent may also mimic polymyositis. Trichinosis is characterized by a history of an antecedent gastrointestinal infection and coexisting symptoms of fever, edema of the eyelids, an urticarial rash, and eosinophilia. Muscle biopsy and positive serologic tests for trichinosis will confirm the diagnosis. Tropical pyomyositis is caused by *Staphylococcus aureus* in 90 per cent of patients. The onset is usually subacute with pain in the gluteal, quadriceps, or trunk muscles. Abscesses develop deep within the muscle and result in an initial hard woody swelling. Serum muscle enzymes are normal, and blood cultures are usually negative. Treatment requires antibiotics and surgical drainage.

Acute exertional rhabdomyolysis is characterized by muscular pain, swelling, induration, and weakness. It occurs after strenuous exercise in apparently healthy individuals. The urine contains heme pigment but not erythrocytes. Serum levels of muscle enzymes are elevated.

Patients with hypereosinophilic syndrome may have proximal muscle weakness, muscle tenderness, elevated serum enzymes, and a myopathic electromyogram, but muscle biopsy shows striking eosinophilic infiltrate. Eosinophilia is also present in the blood, and systemic features such as congestive heart failure and peripheral neuropathy are prominent. Eosinophilia also occurs in diffuse fasciitis with eosinophilia. These patients have sore and tender muscles and a peculiar puckering and thickening of the skin, and may develop contractures over a few weeks' time. They can be identified by the characteristic thickening of the fascia between the subcutaneous fat and muscle on biopsy.

Microemboli from atheromatous plaques in the aorta, or from nonbacterial endocarditis associated with carcinoma may produce a syndrome described as monomyositis multiplex. Pain usually involves the legs. It is sudden in onset and lasts for a short time, only to recur in a different site. Serum levels of muscle-derived enzymes and the erythrocyte sedimentation rate may be elevated and a myopathic pattern is present on electromyography, but the muscle biopsy is diagnostic. Diabetic amyotrophy may cause asymmetrical pain, weakness, and wasting in the proximal lower limbs, but the electromyogram and muscle biopsy are those of a neuropathy rather than a myopathy.

Polymyalgia rheumatica occurs in the elderly and is characterized by proximal muscle pain and stiffness without weakness. The only laboratory abnormality is a striking elevation of the erythrocyte sedimentation rate. Prompt relief after treatment with a small dose of corticosteroid is a helpful differentiating point. Other rheumatic connective tissue diseases may have myositis as part of the symptom complex. These patients should be labeled as having polymyositis only if they meet the independent criteria for the diagnosis.

TREATMENT. Bed rest is necessary during the active stage of the disease. Active physical therapy should be reserved until the inflammation has subsided.

In spite of a lack of adequately controlled therapeutic trials, corticosteroids are generally accepted as the drug of choice. Prednisone, 50 to 100 mg, is given daily in divided doses, and continued until definite improvement occurs. Serum enzymes typically decrease to half their pretreatment values one month after initiation of therapy, and reach normal values in two to three months. Muscle strength usually shows definite improvement in two months. Attempts to decrease steroid dosage rapidly or discontinue treatment prematurely may lead to a recurrence of the disease. A single daily dose or alternate-day steroid therapy may be tried in order to decrease the side effects, but should be attempted only when the disease is in good control. Maintenance therapy will be necessary for years in many cases. Failure to respond to steroids occurs in about 20 per cent of the patients. Immunosuppressive drugs such as methotrexate or cyclophosphamide or plasma exchange may be beneficial in these instances, but controlled studies to substantiate their efficacy are not available. Combined therapy with azathioprine and prednisone has been shown to reduce steroid requirements and improve function in long-term treatment compared to steroid alone. Polymyositis associated with malignancy may occasionally undergo a dramatic remission when the tumor is removed.

Bohan A, Peter JB, Bowman RL, Parson CM: A computer-assisted analysis of 153 patients with polymyositis and dermatomyositis. Medicine 56:255, 1977. *Presents data on which the classification and diagnostic criteria recommended in this chapter are based.*

Bunch TW: Prednisone and azathioprine for polymyositis. Arthritis Rheum 24:45, 1981. *A three-year controlled study suggesting the addition of azathioprine to conventional treatment with prednisone may have long-term benefits.*

Callen JP: Dermatomyositis and malignancy. Clin Rheum Dis 8:369, 1982. *Contains practical advice on the question of how extensively polymyositis patients should be investigated for malignancy.*

Crowe WE, Bove KE, Levinson JE, Hilton PK: Clinical and pathogenetic implications of histopathology in childhood polydermatomyositis. Arthritis Rheum 25:126, 1982. *Contains a clear description of the vascular lesions present in biopsies of the childhood form of polymyositis.*

Kagen LJ: Approach to the patient with myopathy. Bull Rheum Dis 33:2, 1983. *A concise discussion of the use of various tests and grading systems in diagnosis of muscle disease.*

455. CALCIUM CRYSTAL DEPOSITION ARTHROPATHIES

H. Ralph Schumacher, Jr.

At least three different calcium-containing crystals are now known to deposit in joints and to be associated with a variety of patterns of arthritis in much the same way as urate crystals cause the various features of gouty arthritis. Calcium pyrophosphate and occasionally calcium oxalate crystals produce linear or punctate calcifications in menisci and articular cartilage that can be readily seen on roentgenograms. These calcifications are termed chondrocalcinosis. Both these crystals and calcium apatite can also deposit diffusely in synovium and periarticular tissues, giving a soft tissue pattern on roentgenograms. X-rays may not show obvious calcifications when crystals are relatively few. Definitive diagnosis is only made by aspiration of synovial fluid for identification of the crystal type.

CALCIUM PYROPHOSPHATE DIHYDRATE (CPPD) CRYSTAL DEPOSITION DISEASE (Pseudogout Syndrome)

This is defined by the identification of rod or rhomboid-shaped weakly positively birefringent crystals (2 to 25 μ long) in synovial fluid or articular tissue. This is a common cause of arthritis; it is most frequent in the elderly. Up to 27 per cent of nursing home patients in their 80's have x-ray evidence of chondrocalcinosis on this basis. Familial cases have been described in populations of various ethnic origins. Both sexes are affected.

The cause of CPPD crystal deposition is not established, but deficiency of phosphatases and local connective tissue changes are probably important. CPPD crystals deposit only in joints and adjacent tendons or bursas, where they produce hematoxyphilic clumps replacing the normal tissue. Virtually any joint can be involved, but knees, wrists, and second and third metacarpophalangeal joints are the ones most commonly involved, so that chronic cases can be confused with rheumatoid arthritis. Acute bouts of crystal-induced arthritis in one or more joints can mimic gout, which led to the early term "pseudogout." CPPD crystal deposition often complicates osteoarthritis; crystals were seen in 42 per cent of osteoarthritic knee effusions in one series. Whether crystals contribute to cartilage degeneration in osteoarthritis is not yet clear. Occasionally, severe arthritis mimics the destruction seen in neuropathic joints. Radiographic evidence of calcification can be present in some patients for years without producing any symptoms.

Synovial effusions are generally inflammatory with leukocyte counts up to 100,000 per cu mm and contain 80 to 90 per cent neutrophils during acute attacks. Between attacks crystals can be seen in clear, noninflammatory joint effusions.

CPPD deposition can be an important clue to a number of associated diseases, many of which have specific treatments that can control systemic features if not the arthropathy. Diseases seen in association with CPPD include hyperparathyroidism, hemochromatosis, myxedema, ochronosis, hypophosphatasia, hypomagnesemia, and perhaps acromegaly and Wilson's disease. CPPD deposition frequently is seen as a complication of other advanced arthritides such as gout and rheumatoid arthritis. Septic arthritis can complicate CPPD deposition.

Treatment of inflammatory episodes with thorough aspiration and use of nonsteroidal anti-inflammatory agents is generally successful. Intra-articular steroid injections may provide relief for refractory involvement of individual joints. Intravenous colchicine may also be helpful. No long-term preventive measures are known, and the prognosis is slow progression punctuated by inflammatory bouts. Chronic use of nonsteroidal agents can be tried in patients with chronic or recurrent inflammation.

McCarty DJ: Proceedings of a conference on pseudogout and pyrophosphate metabolism. Arthritis Rheum 19(Suppl), 1975 (275 pages). *Multiple authors discuss clinical picture, pathogenesis, and management.*

Schumacher HR, Gibilisco P, Reginato A, et al.: Implications of crystal deposition in osteoarthritis. J Rheum (Suppl 9), 40, 1983. *The association of crystals with osteoarthritis is reviewed.*

APATITE CRYSTAL DEPOSITION DISEASE

Individual apatite crystals can be seen only by electron microscopy (EM), but clumps of these crystals appear as shiny (but not generally birefringent) globules 2 to 15 μ in size that can suggest the diagnosis. Apatite crystal deposition and crystal-induced inflammation are common findings in bursitis and periarthritis. Apatite also occurs in some otherwise unexplained acute arthritides and like CPPD is common in osteoarthritic joint effusions. Most joints or bursas can be involved, but the more common sites include shoulders, hips, knees, and digits. X-rays can show soft-tissue calcifications with or without bony erosions and occasionally with severe destruction. Calcium stains such as Alizarin red can help suggest the presence of apatite. Definitive diagnosis of the crystal type can only be made by EM with electron probe elemental analysis, x-ray diffraction, or infrared spectroscopy. Synovial or bursal effusions can have many or only a few leukocytes. Serum studies are generally normal, except that phosphate levels are often elevated in renal dialysis patients, who are at high risk of apatite deposition.

Apatite deposition can also be associated with scleroderma and the other connective tissue diseases. In most instances the cause of soft-tissue apatite deposition is not known. Treatment for acute arthritis or periarthritis is with nonsteroidal anti-inflammatory agents or colchicine. Aspiration of crystals and local injection with depot corticosteroids can also be effective.

Paul H, Reginato AJ, Schumacher HR: Alizarin red S staining as a screening test to detect calcium compounds in synovial fluid. Arthritis Rheum 26:191, 1983. *This describes a simple office screening test for apatite and other calcium-containing crystals.*

Pinals RS, Short CL: Calcific periarthritis involving multiple sites. Arthritis Rheum 9:566, 1966. *This recurrent calcific periarthritis is related to apatite crystals.*

Schumacher HR, Somlyo AP, Tse RP, et al.: Arthritis associated with apatite crystals. Ann Intern Med 87:411, 1977. *Clinical picture, diagnostic evaluation, and review.*

OTHER CALCIUM-CONTAINING CRYSTALS

Calcium oxalate deposition can occur in joints of renal failure patients on chronic hemodialysis, producing x-ray evidence of soft tissue calcification and chondrocalcinosis. Acute or chronic joint effusions can be seen. Diagnosis is made by identification of typical bipyramidal crystals. When less characteristic crystals are seen, other techniques as described under apatite deposition can be used. Calcium hydrogen phosphate dihydrate (brushite) and octacalcium phosphate have also been described in synovial fluids and tissues; their relationship to joint disease is not yet defined.

Hoffman EC, Schumacher HR, Paul H, et al.: Calcium oxalate microcrystalline-associated arthritis in end stage renal disease. Ann Intern Med 97:36, 1982. *Three cases with oxalosis and arthritis are described. Methods to identify oxalate crystals are included.*

456. RELAPSING POLYCHONDRITIS

H. Ralph Schumacher, Jr.

This uncommon disease is characterized by recurrent inflammation and destruction of cartilaginous and other connective tissue structures. Commonly involved cartilages are the pinnae of the ears, nasal cartilages, and tracheal rings. Polychondritis occurs nearly equally in both sexes and at any age but with a peak of onset between the ages of 30 and 50.

The pathologic lesion seen by light microscopy consists of loss of matrix staining, predominantly superficial infiltration with polymorphonuclear neutrophils or lymphocytes, and eventual destruction of normal structures followed by fibrosis. Electron microscopy in addition shows alterations of superficial chondrocytes, matrix, and elastic fibers. The cause of polychondritis is unknown, but the location of lesions and the frequency of associated systemic diseases suggest the importance of systemic factors. Antibodies to type II collagen and the presence of cell-mediated immunity to proteoglycan are evidences of immunologic aberrations.

The most common initial clue to the diagnosis is inflammation of the cartilaginous structures of the ears. There is generally rather acute onset of pain and tenderness with erythema and swelling of one or both helices. The lobe is spared. Inner and middle ear involvement can occur, causing hearing loss or vertigo. Nasal cartilage involvement can produce a saddle nose. Laryngeal and tracheal disease can cause hoarseness or life-threatening upper respiratory obstruction. Ocular manifestations are common and include conjunctivitis, episcleritis, iritis, and rarely other problems such as optic neuritis. Antigens in the eye that are cross-reactive with cartilage proteoglycans and their link protein have been identified.

Cardiac involvement, especially of the aortic root with aortic insufficiency, is seen in up to one fourth of cases. There may also be aortic aneurisms. Arthritis is reported in about three fourths of cases. This is nondestructive. It is not clear whether articular cartilage is involved in the same way that other cartilages are or whether other factors account for the arthritis. Fever, rashes, and neurologic and renal disease can occur.

There are no diagnostic laboratory tests for relapsing polychondritis, although the erythrocyte sedimentation rate is often elevated. There may be anemia and leukocytosis. Roentgenograms can detect the tracheal narrowing.

Relapsing polychondritis is associated with other diseases in one third or more of cases. These include rheumatoid arthritis, systemic lupus erythematosus, Sjögren's syndrome, thyroid disease, ulcerative colitis, vasculitis of various types, cryoglobulinemia, diabetes mellitus, biliary cirrhosis, malignancies, sinusitis, mastoiditis, and occasionally other diseases.

In mild cases, nonsteroidal anti-inflammatory agents can be used for symptomatic treatment, although adrenocorticosteroids are generally needed for acute inflammatory episodes and severe respiratory involvement. There is no evidence that steroids alter the long-term course of the disease. Immunosuppressives have been used with apparent benefit. Dapsone has recently been used with success in several series.

The course is unpredictable. Deaths have occurred from cardiac or respiratory involvement, and aortic valve disease has required surgery. Remissions do occur; some patients have chronic or relapsing disease over many years.

Conn DL, Dickson ER, Carpenter HA: The association of Churg-Strauss vasculitis with temporal artery involvement, primary biliary cirrhosis and polychondritis in a single patient. J Rheum 9:744, 1982. *Vasculitis and other associated diseases are common.*

Ebringer B, Rook G, Swana T, Bottazzo GF, Doniach D: Autoantibodies to cartilage and type II collagen in relapsing polychondritis and other rheumatic diseases. Ann Rheum Dis 40:473, 1981. *Immune mechanisms are described and discussed.*

Martin J, Roenigk HH Jr, Lynch W, et al.: Relapsing polychondritis treated with dapsone. Arch Dermatol 112:1272, 1976. *The interesting beneficial effects of dapsone.*

McAdam LP, O'Hanlan MA, Bluestone R, et al.: Relapsing polychondritis: Prospective study of 23 patients and a review of the literature. Medicine 55:193, 1976. *The best general review.*

Ruhlen JL, Huston KA, Wood WG: Relapsing polychondritis with glomerulonephritis: Improvement with prednisone and cyclophosphamide. JAMA 245:847, 1981. *Renal involvement can occur. Drug therapy can include immunosuppressives.*

Shaul SR, Schumacher HR: Relapsing polychondritis. Electron microscopic studies of ear cartilage. Arthritis Rheum 18:617, 1975. *Pathologic findings and their implications are described and reviewed.*

457. OSTEOARTHRITIS (Degenerative Joint Disease)

David S. Howell

Osteoarthritis (OA) is a complex response of joint tissues to aging and to genetic and environmental factors, characterized by degeneration of cartilage, bony remodelling, and overgrowth of bone. Idiopathic osteoarthritis refers to the common variety encountered during aging that is unrelated to known systemic or local diseases and includes certain hereditary and erosive subsets. *Secondary* osteoarthritis refers to the form indistinguishable from the idiopathic (primary) type on a pathologic basis but clearly provoked by antecedent events, such as an inflammatory, metabolic, endocrine, developmental, or heritable connective tissue disorder (Table 457–1). Effects of a macrotrauma, repeated microtrauma, or prolonged immobilization

TABLE 457–1. ETIOLOGIC CLASSIFICATION OF OSTEOARTHRITIS*

- Idiopathic (primary)
  - Localized
    - Hands: Heberden's nodes, erosive interphalangeal arthropathy
    - Feet: hallux valgus, hammer toes; talonavicular osteoarthritis
    - Knees: medial, lateral, patellofemoral compartments
    - Hips: sites of cartilage loss—eccentric (superior), concentric (axial, medial), diffuse
    - Spine: zygoapophyseal joints, osteophytes, intervertebral discs (spondylosis); ligaments, e.g., disseminated idiopathic skeletal hyperostosis
    - Other single sites: shoulder, temporomandibular, carpometacarpal joints
  - Generalized—Includes three or more areas listed above (described by Kellgren and Moore)
  - Mineral deposition diseases
    - Calcium pyrophosphate deposition disease
    - Hydroxyapatite arthropathy
    - Destructive disease (e.g., Milwaukee shoulder)
- Secondary
  - Post-traumatic
  - Congenital or developmental
    - Legg-Calvé-Perthes hip dislocation
    - Epiphyseal dysplasias
  - Disturbed local tissue structure by primary disease, e.g., ischemic necrosis, tophaceous gout, hyperparathyroid cysts, Paget's disease, rheumatoid arthritis, osteopetrosis, osteochondritis
  - Miscellaneous additional diseases
    - Endocrine: diabetes mellitus, acromegaly, hypothyroidism
    - Metabolic: hemochromatosis, ochronosis, Gaucher's disease
    - Neuropathic arthropathies
    - Miscellaneous: frostbite, Kashin-Beck disease, caisson's disease
    - Mechanical: obesity, unequal lower extremity length; valgus/varus deformities, ligamentous laxity

*Compiled by Osteoarthritis Diagnostic Criteria Committee. American Rheumatism Association, 1983.

on normal joints may dispose the joints to secondary osteoarthritis.

When bony hypertrophy estimated by roentgenographic changes is used as a criterion, the majority of the population over 50 years of age is afflicted with osteoarthritis. By the eighth decade there is evidence of disease in 90 per cent of persons. It is the leading cause of joint pain and related disablements in middle-aged and elderly patients.

PATHOLOGY. Minor cartilage softening in non–weight-bearing sites and hypertrophic bony changes may persist a lifetime without producing symptoms. Osteoarthritis depends on development of progressively deepening clefts and erosions typically in weight-bearing sites. The disease advances over a period of years but rarely reaches the level of severity seen in rheumatoid arthritis, i.e., there is rarely joint fusion or pannus formation, and major subluxations are uncommon.

The earliest histologic changes may be documented in the surface, subsurface, and deep zones of articular cartilage. These changes include loss of staining reactions for proteoglycans, with areas of cell injury, or loss followed by proliferation. On electron microscopic views, lipid accumulations, reduced cartilage collagen fibril size, edema, and surface irregularities are found. Clefts, microcysts, and erosions arise at the site of these changes. Aggressive lesions consist usually of vertical clefts in cartilage, which progress to deep erosions and exposure of subchondral bone. Bony thickening, eburnation, cysts, and bone-on-bone contact across the joint surface typifies end-stage disease.

ETIOLOGY. The most accepted premise is that primary changes in articular cartilage underlie development of osteoarthritis. Nevertheless, in a substantial subset of patients, biomechanical deficiencies arising from dysplasias of major or minor nature are causative. Similar biomechanical deficiencies may arise related to adolescent and adult remodelling of bones and abnormal distribution of weight-bearing forces (Table 457–1).

Repeated industrial or sports-invoked macro- and microtraumatic events may produce excessive wear and hypertrophic remodelling responses. Evidence has been obtained for reduced biomaterial properties of cartilage as a function of aging and for possible metabolic disturbances in cartilage metabolism, as in diabetes mellitus, acromegaly, and ochronosis.

The subchondral bone table is disturbed by tissue remodelling early in the disease or by such afflictions as Paget's disease or hyperparathyroidism with subchondral cysts. Hyperlaxity of ligaments per se or as part of certain overt (heritable) disorders of connective tissue can lead to osteoarthritis.

PATHOGENESIS. As a result of a multiplicity of etiologic factors, an apparent final common pathway of disease expression involves breakdown of cartilage both by direct physical injury and enzymatic degradation resulting from injury to chondrocytes and indirectly by subchondral bone stiffening from remodelling. Most important in this context is injury of the collagen network or framework that holds together articular cartilage. This network retains in a semi-dehydrated conformed state the abundant, intensely hydrophobic, charged, proteoglycan macromolecules. The latter exert an osmotic pressure of several atmospheres against the network. Ungluing or cleavage of the collagen network by maldistributed or excessive weight-bearing forces, or degradation of the network by enzymes elaborated by injured cartilage cells may occur. This response to various precipitating events leads to loss of essential elastic properties.

In early osteoarthritis, repair responses by local chondrocytes are usually of a poor quality, leading to almost no replacement of lost tissue. From advanced erosions penetrating the marrow, tissue repair is more effective and consists of mixtures of fibro- and hyaline cartilage. Normal rugged biomaterial properties are never recovered by the repair cartilage. As degeneration proceeds, wear particles break off from both original and repair cartilages. These fragments are carried to the synovial lining membrane where a phagocytic response engenders low-grade inflammation and synovial effusion, proliferation of synovial cells, and thickening of the synovial membranes. In some cases, it is speculated that membrane-engendered inflammatory factors may then amplify cartilage breakdown.

Several biochemical abnormalities have been noted in osteoarthritic cartilage: increased water content, decreased aggregation and content of proteoglycans, decreased chain length and altered profiles of glycosaminoglycans, and increased proteolytic enzyme levels.

CLINICAL MANIFESTATIONS. The clinical presentation may be divided into early and late stages. Throughout these stages, there is deep, aching pain in the afflicted joints, morning stiffness of short duration, and variable joint thickening and effusion. Early stages are dominated by pain on motion with stiffness, night pain, and responsiveness to anti-inflammatory medication. The late stages are dominated by joint instability, predominance of pain at rest accentuated on weight-bearing, and failure of responsiveness to anti-inflammatory agents. The present description of clinical features is developed largely on an anatomic basis inasmuch as signs and symptoms reflect regional patterns of involvement. Roentgenographic and laboratory workup and treatment are discussed later.

Hands. Heberden's nodes refer to the osteoarthritic disfigurements of distal interphalangeal joints, and Bouchard's nodes signify equivalent lesions of the proximal interphalangeal joints of the hands (Fig. 457–1). Early Heberden's nodes have a soft consistency and may be associated with prominent inflammatory signs. In the chronic stage, they are characterized by bony enlargement and angular deformities with variable symptom-

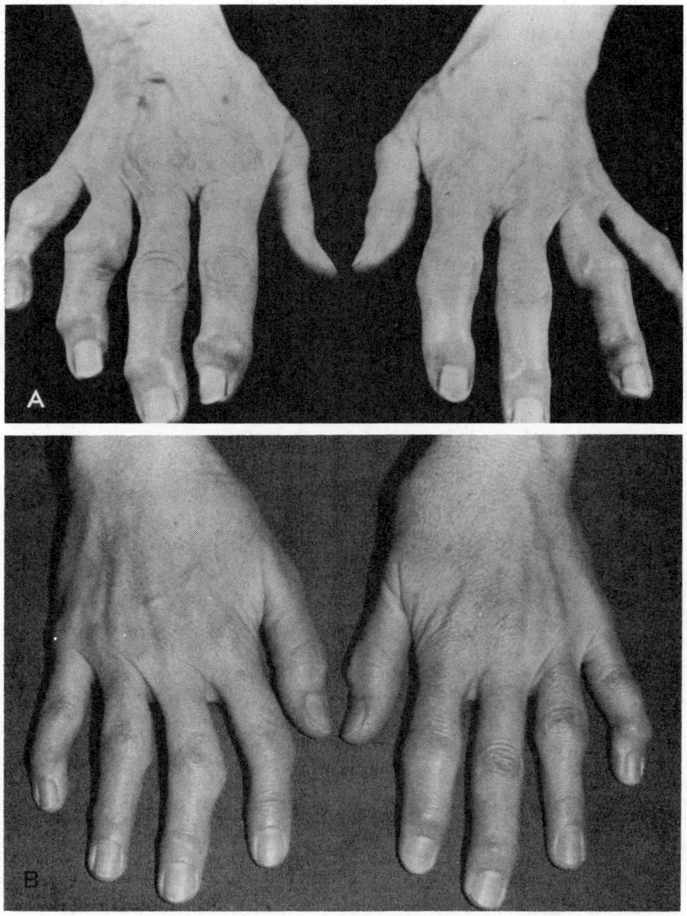

Figure 457–1. Typical hand deformities in osteoarthritis. *A,* Typical Heberden's and Bouchard's nodes comprise hypertrophic joint capsular and bony enlargement of the distal and proximal interphalangeal joints, respectively. *B,* Prominent Bouchard's nodes and minor subluxations may cause misdiagnosis of rheumatoid arthritis.

atology. Heredity and sex, in addition to microtrauma, are prominently involved in the development of Heberden's nodes, which are more common in women at menopause or late middle age. The only other common hand lesion involves the first carpometacarpal joint. Such lesions are associated with pain in the radial side of the wrist, intensified by physical activities such as golf, tennis, and knitting.

Knees. The commonest source of major disability in osteoarthritis is from knee involvement. At any one time, heat, synovial thickening, or effusions have been documented in at least 50 per cent of cases. Elicitation of crepitus, which persists on repeated flexion and extension of the knee, bony marginal overgrowth, mediolateral instability (in the late stages), and synovial effusion are important diagnostic aids. Degenerative changes are usually more prominent in the medial compartment of the knee, leading to varus (bowleg) deformities. Developmental defects, i.e., knock knee or bowleg deformity, predispose to OA.

Degenerative alteration of the patellofemoral joint is termed chondromalacia patellae. This syndrome of mild effusion and knee pain is usually associated with trauma and occurs predominantly in young adults. It is usually preceded by developmental biomechanical disturbances influencing knee flexion. There is often spontaneous remission of symptoms, but some cases progress to irreversible patellofemoral osteoarthritis.

Malum Coxae Senilis (Coxarthrosis). Clinical manifestations of primary hip joint disease appear usually in late middle or old age. Perhaps one third or more of cases arise from acetabular dysplasia, as well as growth or maturational disturbances in the femoral neck and head. Altered bone growth as well as developmental thickening at the zenith of the acetabulum may be causative in less than 5 per cent of cases. Beyond these factors, there is a background of adult bone remodelling and altered joint incongruity, which may further compromise normal weight-bearing patterns and chondrocyte nutrition. In addition, a variety of acquired disorders such as rheumatoid arthritis and ischemic necrosis of the femoral head are important etiologically.

Groin pain on weight-bearing or motion is a dominant symptom and is usually referred to the anterior aspect of the thigh above the knee. Over a period of months or a few years, invalidism from severely restricted mobility and pain is a common outcome of untreated disease.

Spinal Osteoarthritis (Including Herniated Disc Syndrome). Throughout the spine, weight-bearing compressive forces are largely supported by one set of articulations—the intervertebral discs. These are elastic organs similar to articular cartilage in respect to the fact that they depend on properties of the semidehydrated proteoglycan molecules. A high osmotic pressure at rest results from proteoglycan confinement by cartilage endplates in two dimensions and the annulus fibrosis in the third. An additional important elastic component is provided by the annulus fibrosis. Rotary motions in the back and neck depend upon the zygoapophyseal joints. All of these joints undergo osteoarthritic changes almost identical in nature to those of the peripheral joints (see Ch. 459 for specific clinical features). Ordinarily, the former joints protect the latter against severe torsional trauma; under certain conditions, especially flexion of the lumbosacral spine, the rotary joints are of much less protectional value, and annular tears may occur under these (and several other) conditions. Resultant displacement of discal products into the spinal foramen adjacent to nerve rootlets and/or spinal canal occurs, depending on the conditions of damage. Injury of these structures both by mechanical trauma and activated inflammatory pathways comprises one of several causes of neural dysfunction leading to symptoms. The relationship of the posterior zygoapophyseal joints in the cervical, thoracic, and lumbar spines to their respective nerve roots as they traverse the intervertebral foramina, and the proximity of an additional set of *joints of Luschka* in the cervical spine (segment C2 to C7) have similar importance because of potential damage to nerves by inflammation secondary to mechanical irritation.

Notably, symptoms of osteoarthritis in the cervical spine depend upon the neural segment involved. Pain, aggravated by motion, often radiates into the supraclavicular and upper trapezius regions, as well as the occiput and distal upper extremities. Overgrowth of bone in either the cervical or lumbar spine can cause narrowing of the spinal canal and encroachment on the spinal cord rather than the nerve roots. In the neck, a myelopathy of a painless nature may result. Constriction of the spinal cord by surrounding bone, disc, or ligamentous thickening, leads to the syndrome of spinal stenosis most common in the lumbosacral spine. Neurogenic claudication pain (resembling vascular claudication) is an important symptom in this condition and must be differentiated from vascular insufficiency (see Ch. 459 for management of discogenic claudication).

Diffuse Idiopathic Skeletal Hyperostosis. This is characterized by a flowing ligamentous calcification along the anterolateral aspects of vertebral bodies. There is usually only minor symptomatology, and the thoracic spine is most often affected without intervertebral disc narrowing.

LABORATORY FINDINGS. There are no specific abnormalities in osteoarthritis. The sedimentation rate is usually within normal limits, synovial fluid is clear and exhibits a normal range of viscosity, and there is a negative mucin clot test result. Leukocyte counts in synovial fluid generally vary from 150 to 1500 per cu mm; wear particles including whole fragments containing proteoglycans and collagen fibers as well as mineral particles are often identified in the fluid.

ROENTGENOGRAPHIC FEATURES. There is usually narrowing of the radiolucent interosseous joint space resulting from destruction of articular cartilage. Bony cysts varying in size may be seen in subchondral or denuded bone, which may be densely sclerotic. Osteophyte formation at the margins of affected joints is the basis for the most striking roentgenographic findings. Degeneration of lumbar and cervical intervertebral discs results in narrowing of the interspaces. A vacuum sign or marked translucency in the disc may be seen. Evidence for disc degeneration is usually documented in anteroposterior and lateral roentgenograms. For visualization of osteophytes blocking foramina, particularly in the cervical spine, oblique views are mandatory. Oblique views are also valuable for defining bony sclerosis and joint-space narrowing of the zygoapophyseal joints of the lumbar spine.

DIFFERENTIAL DIAGNOSIS. Osteoarthritis and rheumatoid arthritis are readily distinguished in terms of their usual clinical presentation. The latter is generally associated with prominent signs of joint inflammation, characteristically afflicting the hands and wrists symmetrically, especially the metacarpophalangeal joints. These joints almost never are affected in osteoarthritis.

Differentiation of these disorders is more complicated when seronegative rheumatoid arthritis involves only (or predominantly) the lower extremities. The presence of a normal erythrocyte sedimentation rate, negative serum rheumatoid factor test result, and minimal synovial fluid change support the diagnosis of osteoarthritis. Despite severe deformities, occasionally seen with Heberden's and Bouchard's nodes, the lack of ulnar drift and metacarpophalangeal and diffuse wrist involvement help to rule out rheumatoid arthritis. Erosive osteoarthritis characteristically shows bony destruction and inflammatory changes in the proximal and distal interphalangeal joints but not in the metacarpophalangeal joints.

Secondary osteoarthritis must be considered in the presence of joint hypermobility, chondrocalcinosis, heritable disorders such as the Ehlers-Danlos syndrome, mechanical derangements of the joints, metabolic bone disorders, ochronosis, neuropathies, and hemochromatosis. Spinal involvement in osteoarthritis is distinctly different from that in ankylosing spondylitis; the latter predominantly afflicts young men and has characteristic and distinctive roentgenographic features involving sacroiliac sclerosis and fusion, calcification and ossification of the annulus fibrosus and adjacent paravertebral ligaments, and formation of bridging syndesmophytes (bamboo spine).

TREATMENT. Although treatment depends in large measure on the site and severity of joint involvement, the outlook with a multidisciplinary long-term management program is relatively optimistic for functional restoration and symptomatic improvement.

Early disease with signs of mild to moderate inflammation but without joint instability can usually be managed successfully with a combination of measures: (1) Relief of pain with mild analgesics (e.g., acetaminophen 500 mg three or four times a day) or nonsteroidal anti-inflammatory agents (e.g., aspirin 2400 to 3600 mg daily) or both. Indomethacin, ibuprofen, naproxen, fenoprofen, and tolmetin are alternative agents, advantageous as substitutes for aspirin. Where possible, intermittent rather than continuous usage is encouraged to avoid gastrointestinal side effects, especially acid peptic disease; (2) Revision of daily schedule of activities, increased joint rest, and selected avoidance of activities unfavorable to the symptomatic joints; (3) Protection of joints with relevant devices, i.e., splints, crutches, walkers, canes, etc.; (4) Use of weight-reducing diets; (5) Diazepam, 5 mg three to four times daily or another suitable agent may be used sparingly for acute episodes of muscle spasm; (6) Application of moist heat or cold packs may help; (7) Symptomatic response, in refractory cases, to intra-articular or para-articular injections of small amounts of corticosteroid at infrequent intervals is useful; (8) Once pain and muscle spasm have been relieved, a formalized program of physical therapy followed by a prolonged home exercise program is often recommended in the hope of retarding further joint deterioration.

In the case of cervical osteoarthritis, hyperextension and hyperflexion should be avoided. The patient should sleep flat on one pillow and employ intermittent traction devices available for home use. A cervical collar restricts motion and minimizes pain (see Ch. 459 for treatment of osteoarthritis in the lumbar spine).

The principal anatomic regions that are most benefited by orthopedic surgery are the knee, hip, and spine. Several surgical procedures are appropriate for patients with severe hip involvement, including osteotomy, mold arthroplasty, total joint replacement, and arthrodesis. For the knee, debridement, either through an arthroscope or via open surgery, osteotomy, and a variety of partial or complete arthroplasties are used for treatment. Tibial or femoral osteotomies may be of long-term benefit by realigning weight-bearing forces, but considerable follow-up rehabilitation is required. Otherwise, joint replacement is the treatment of choice for many cases of advanced osteoarthritis of the knees characterized by intractable pain, loss of function, instability, or all three. Some indications for spinal surgery are: (1) advancing intractable nerve deficits, (2) spinal instability, and (3) spinal stenosis affecting bladder or rectal function because of autonomic nerve involvement.

Bland JH, Cooper S: Osteoarthritis: A review of the cell biology involved and evidence for reversibility; management rationally related to known genesis and pathophysiology. Semin Arthritis Rheum. In press. *Emphasis is on practical management as influenced by cell biology, physiology, and what is known concerning etiology and pathogenesis.*

Howell DS, Talbott JH: Osteoarthritis symposium. Semin Arthritis Rheum 11:1, 1981. *Studies of fundamental and clinical nature relating to inflammatory components of osteoarthritis. For those not daunted by scientific data.*

McCarty DJ (ed.): Arthritis and Allied Disorders. Osteoarthritis, Section IX. Philadelphia, Lea and Febiger, 1979, pp 1135–1189. *A useful reference with chapters amplifying all topics discussed in this chapter, but not at a level too burdensome for the internist.*

458. THE PAINFUL SHOULDER

David S. Howell

Shoulder pain is a common source of incapacitation and can result from numerous causes. Intrathoracic, diaphragmatic, and cervical pathologic lesions all can cause pain referred to the shoulder, a fact that deserves early consideration and strong emphasis. A characteristic of intrinsic painful disorders is that they often originate in periarticular soft structures—synovial membranes, tendons, and associated muscles. These structures have a unique role in joint stabilization. Loading forces are attenuated by the action of muscles across the coordinated bearings—glenohumeral, acromioclavicular, and sternoclavicular joints—as well as across the scapulothoracic surfaces. Multiple bursae and tendons near their attachment sites, particularly the rotator cuff tendons, are subject to microinjury and inflammation. Secondary recurrent pain and muscle spasm occur, followed by atrophic or reflex dystrophic responses or both. The most common disorders afflicting these structures are briefly reviewed in this chapter.

CALCIFIC TENDINITIS. A frequently encountered cause of painful shoulder is focal injury or degeneration of the rotator cuff tendons. Roentgenograms reveal calcium-containing minerals in the tendons of the rotator cuff in roughly 3 per cent of middle-aged persons, usually from prior insults. Mineral deposits in tendinous sites may engender bursal inflammation of variable intensity. Acute shoulder pain with radiation into the upper arm and neck is common. Associated muscle hypertonicity with limitation of shoulder motion and guarding, exquisite local tenderness over the inflamed site, and pain on motion or during prolonged rest are prominent. Most often roentgenograms show linear densities in the supraspinatus, infraspinatus, or subscapularis tendons. Occasionally, a diffuse calcific pattern in the subacromial bursa is seen. Evidence of acute inflammation usually subsides within one week, but subacute rotator cuff tendinitis may persist or recur for months to years.

Management is conditioned by the duration and intensity of attacks. Adequate early pain relief is of paramount importance and is usually attainable by use of moist heat or ice compresses, rest, including arm support, analgesics, and a nonsteroidal anti-inflammatory agent. Newer agents are discussed in Ch. 444. In most patients, pain and muscle spasm subside with variable reduction of mineral deposits. Injection of an adrenocorticosteroid derivative commonly hastens symptomatic recovery.

Follow-up evaluation is important to assess completeness of recovery. Residual loss of strength or joint motion or chronic pain deserves a conscientious program of active exercises, including both supervised therapy in a physical medicine facility and a home program of daily exercise. Long-term physical therapy or surgical excision of mineral deposits is seldom necessary.

BICIPITAL TENDINITIS. Inflammation of this tendon and synovial sheath is a frequent cause of shoulder pain. The tendon through attrition may subluxate from the bicipital groove or rupture. Localized tenderness on palpation with accentuation of pain by flexion or extension of the elbow against resistance or by internal rotation and abduction distinguishes the diagnosis clinically.

Treatment includes moist heat or ice compresses, rest, and nonsteroidal anti-inflammatory agents in the acute stages, and frequently the instillation of corticosteroids. Chronic recurrent disease is suggestive of the aforementioned mechanical derangements or an additional rotator cuff tear. Surgical transfer of the tendon may lead to satisfactory recovery.

ROTATOR CUFF TEARS. After heavy work, sports, or accidental injury, degenerative lesions in the rotator cuff often engender breakdown with moderate to major tendinous and ligamentous tears, predominantly in middle-aged persons. Complete rupture of the rotator cuff renders the arm incapable of abduction to 90 degrees. With mild tears, there is pain between 60 and 90 degrees abduction. Either preceding or following these tears, an impingement syndrome frequently occurs at the coracoacromial arch. Often this is associated radiographically with cysts or sclerosis of the greater tuberosity of the humerus, osteophytes at the anterior margin of the acromion, and narrowing of the distance between the humeral head and acromion. These changes are related to trauma from impingement of the aforementioned bones. Since the rotator cuff forms, in part, the roof of the glenohumeral joint and floor of the subacromial and subdeltoid bursae, tears in the cuff permit synovial joint fluid extrusion into these bursae—demonstrable by arthrogram.

Primary treatment of rotator cuff tears consists of heat and aspirin, 2.4 to 3.6 gm per day, or other nonsteroidal anti-inflammatory agents such as ibuprofen, 1200 to 2400 mg per day. Partial immobilization and exercise programs are indicated for incomplete tears. When these measures fail, surgical repair is often required.

ADHESIVE CAPSULITIS. This (frozen shoulder) disability of middle-aged persons develops more commonly in women than in men and is of unknown etiology. The diagnosis is suspected when persons with no primary shoulder disease develop active and passive restricted motion of the glenohumeral joint attended by increasing pain in the shoulder over a period of weeks to months, and it is more certain when an arthrogram shows a contracted joint capsule. Fibrosis is seen on pathologic study. Rotator cuff tears, hemarthroses, anterior shoulder capsule tear, psychophysiologic shoulder dysfunction, and shoulder-hand syndrome can all cause immobile painful shoulders and may be confused with adhesive capsulitis.

The key feature of management is prevention of severe pain through early use of heat, analgesics, range of motion exercises, and, if these are unsuccessful, the judicious use of intra-articular or systemic corticosteroids.

Manipulation mobilization under general anesthesia followed by a course of intensive physical therapy rarely is required for advanced disease.

SHOULDER-HAND SYNDROME. Shoulder pain and stiffness concurrent with pain, swelling, and vasomotor changes in the hands, wrists, and arms of various intensity and duration characterize this syndrome. Thickening of the skin and edema may follow, resembling Sudeck's atrophy. A small per cent of cases eventually develop adhesive capsulitis and sclerodactyly. This syndrome, which affects patients over age 50 years and follows acute severe illness such as cerebral vascular accident, myocardial infarction, and trauma to the distal upper extremity, is believed to be caused by reflex sympathetic stimulation. Associated changes of cervical osteoarthritis probably have a minor role if any. When the disease is bilateral, the differentiation from acute rheumatoid arthritis or polymyalgia rheumatica may be difficult. The most important feature of treatment is aggressive physical therapy assisted by analgesics and prednisone in a short moderate dosage trial of 20 to 30 mg per day for three weeks, tapered at the end of the course. Stellate ganglion blocks and local corticosteroid injections are sometimes employed.

AMYLOID ARTHROPATHY. In two thirds of patients, there is shoulder involvement usually secondary to myeloma. There is para-articular infiltration with amorphous amyloid fibers causing the "shoulder pad sign." Acute inflammatory signs are usually absent (see Ch. 210).

ISCHEMIC NECROSIS. This disease is half as common in the humeral head as in the hip. Diffuse shoulder pain precedes conventional radiologic changes, the most helpful of which is an irregular translucent band localized in subchondral bone.

POLYMYALGIA RHEUMATICA. This syndrome is often characterized by severely painful shoulders and upper arms in aged persons with anemia, high sedimentation rates, and negative rheumatoid factor test, and in a small percentage of cases temporal arteritis and retinal ischemia threatening to vision (see Ch. 548). Dramatic response of shoulder pain to low-dose corticosteroid administration (prednisone 10 mg per day) is characteristic.

MILWAUKEE SHOULDER. This syndrome consists of a painful, destructive, bilateral arthropathy in middle-aged and elderly patients with capsular calcification, joint effusions, and a high frequency of eroded rotator cuff tendons. Synovial fluids are virtually free of inflammatory cells despite a reported high collagenase activity.

Kozin F: Painful shoulder and the reflex sympathetic dystrophy syndrome. *In* McCarty DJ (ed.): Arthritis and Allied Conditions. Philadelphia, Lea and Febiger, 1979, pp 1091–1120. *An extremely concentrated and detailed coverage, especially useful as a reference for differential diagnosis.*

Post M: The painful shoulder. Clin Orthop 173:2, 1983. *A symposium by multiple authors on various clinically important syndromes and discussion of current management.*

459. THE PAINFUL BACK

David S. Howell

Among degenerative disease, low back pain is the leading cause of industrial absenteeism and chronic disablement in some studies. The back is a complex structure serving weight-bearing and locomotor functions. It provides for major support of body structures and transmission of loading forces through the sacroiliac joints to the lower limbs. The fundamental functioning unit is an articular triad composed of two zygoapophyseal joints posteriorly and the intervertebral disc anteriorly. The disc is comprised of a nucleus pulposus encompassed by the annulus fibrosis. These structures are arranged in a series and stabilized throughout the spine by ligaments. The spinal bones also encase the spinal cord and the cauda equina, and through successive foramina rootlets connect the spinal cord with peripheral neural pathways (see Ch. 457 for detailed discussion of the cervical spine and Ch. 445 for the Spondyloarthropathies).

ETIOLOGY OF BACK PAIN. In Table 459–1, the numerous causes of back pain are displayed according to disease subgroups. Although all vertebral levels can be affected, pain

TABLE 459–1. ETIOLOGY OF BACK PAIN

Mechanical or Traumatic
Paraspinal ligaments and musculature
Myofascial syndrome, sacroiliac strain
Spondylogenic
Osteoarthritis-related lesions-zygoapophyseal joints
Degenerative lesions—intervertebral discs
Mechanical insufficiency, congenital and acquired, of ligaments and bones
Spondylolisthesis
Spinal stenosis
Fractures
Metabolic
Vertebral bodies, partial collapse and distortion—osteoporosis; osteomalacia—Paget's disease—often with secondary osteoarthritis
Tumors
Neural tumors, osteosarcoma, metastatic tumors, e.g., from breast, thyroid, kidney
Myeloma, lymphoma, leukemia
Systemic Inflammatory Disease
Spondylitis (ankylosing)—Reiter's disease; psoriatic or enteropathic arthropathy
Disseminated ankylosing skeletal hyperostosis
Infections
Pyogenic, fungal, tuberculous disc infection, *Herpes zoster* infection, paraspinal abscesses
Referred Pain
Vascular—aneurysms, sclerosis of aorta and branches
Tumors or inflammation of pleural, pulmonary, pericardial, cardiac, or neck origin
Viscerogenic disease of gallbladder, pancreas, stomach, intestines, kidneys, ureters, bladder, prostate, uterus
Pelvis or retroperitoneal tumors or inflammation
Non-Organic Components
Hysterical conversion
Learned painful behavior
Psychosis
Litigation neurosis, malingering
Chronic pain syndrome
Substance abuse

in the low back is most prevalent. The majority of patients present with problems relating to functional or mechanical disturbances, and these must be distinguished from a wide variety of diseases either of focal origin or referred from multiple organ systems.

MEDICAL HISTORY. *Sex.* Compression vertebral fractures from osteoporosis have their highest prevalence in postmenopausal women. Gynecologic pathology such as endometriosis is the basis for some referred patterns of back pain. Reiter's disease, ankylosing spondylitis, and back injuries are found more commonly in males.

Age. Young people with back pain most commonly suffer with congenital abnormalities, injury, spondyloarthropathies, and herniated disc syndromes. In middle and old age, osteoporosis, vertebral collapse, degenerative states, including spinal stenosis, and malignant lesions are common.

Family History. Familial patterns of segregation are often detected in respect to spondyloarthropathies and uncommonly in respect to spinal degenerative conditions.

Nature of Pain. A review of events or conditions that accelerate or retard symptoms should be gathered. The chronic inflammatory diseases (spondyloarthropathies) are associated with increased pain and stiffness on inactivity. Patients with lumbar disc protrusion and radicular pain generally are relieved by lying flat with the knees flexed and are uncomfortable sitting. Sudden or acute onset of symptoms is suggestive of a mechanical or infectious origin of symptoms respectively. Constitutional symptoms such as fever, weight loss, and fatigue are important clues to infectious, inflammatory, or neoplastic disorders.

In regard to localization, the dorsal segment suggests osteoarthritis, vertebral fracture, neoplasm, herpetic radiculitis, or referred pain from the viscera (see later paragraph). Localization of pain in the low back is usually of little help in regard to differential diagnosis.

Claudication-type pain, with onset after sustained walking, suggests either spinal stenosis or arterial insufficiency. The former condition often refers pain to the thigh and is poorly relieved by standing still. Usually neurogenic claudication is relieved by sitting, whereas vascular claudication is reduced by standing.

Referred Pain. A deep aching pain referred to various sites in the upper and midback may be engendered by lesions in the upper gastrointestinal tract. Pain of malignancy (whether local or referred) is typically severe and unrelieved by change of position or mild analgesics.

In respect to neuropathic symptoms, alteration of the structure of the vertebral foramina may lead to radicular dissemination of pain. In such instances, compression or traction of nerve rootlets or extension of inflammation to them can lead to sensory and motor nerve symptoms and signs, i.e., paresthesias, hypoesthesias, and muscle weakness.

Symptomatology. Discogenic pain is characteristically aggravated by cough or sneeze. Rarely, loss of bowel or urinary sphincter function can result from cord compression or bilateral involvement of sacral nerve roots from spinal stenosis, tumors, or infectious lesions.

PHYSICAL EXAMINATION. General examination of the back is discussed in Ch. 440. Descriptions here are confined to vertebral compression fractures, degenerative disc disease, and lumbosacral strains and sprains.

Lumbosacral Strain. This and related myofascial syndromes are the most common ailment seen in office practice. A history of injury is often followed by prompt or delayed low-back pain. Transient disc prolapse, subluxation of facet joints, and injury to muscles or ligaments are diagnostic considerations. Physical signs are usually limited to paravertebral muscle spasm, tenderness, and restricted lower back motion without evidence of nerve root involvement.

Vertebral Compression Fractures. These are the most common complication of osteoporosis with resultant traction or compression of rootlets adjacent to collapsed vertebrae. Sudden onset of severe pain associated with the postural strain of lifting heavy objects or hyperflexing the trunk is found. Major physical findings consist of localized tenderness and muscle spasm related to the level of the nerve roots affected. Poorly localized back pain may be associated with osteoporosis in the absence of vertebral collapse. Metastatic tumor, myeloma, and metabolic bone disease, especially osteopenia of aging, are common underlying conditions.

Discogenic Disease. The commonest form of low back pain with radiculitis is associated with prolapse, protrusion, or extrusion of intervertebral disc substance. Usually the onset of acute symptoms is preceded by chronic intermittent low-back pain, although a discrete injury may precipitate an attack. Ninety per cent of disc herniations are localized at L4–L5 or L5–S1 levels. A proprioceptive neuromuscular disturbance may engender a fixed forward flexion or lateral list of the spine. Discs involving the L4 nerve root or above may cause pain referred along the course of the femoral nerve with hip extension and knee flexion. Knee extension may be weak and the patellar reflex reduced or absent. Patients with L5 nerve root disturbance complain of classic sciatic distribution of pain, i.e., radiating to the posterior thigh and the anteromedial leg and foot, in association with weakness of the toe extensors. First sacral radiculopathy is associated with pain over the posterior thigh, calf, and heel, weakness of the ankle and toe flexors, and reduced or absent achilles tendon reflex. Frequently, loss of neurologic function is subtle and requires repeated testing to document. A positive response to straight leg-raising is most frequently indicative of L4–L5 or L5–S1 disc protrusion. Usually there is elicitation of pain on hip flexion with the knee extended and absence of pain on repetition of hip flexion with the knee flexed (positive Lasègue's sign). The cauda equina syndrome is a form of spinal stenosis and is an uncommon but an important complication of massive disc prolapse. In the cauda equina syndrome, central midline disc displacement causes paralysis of the sacral root with bladder and bowel dysfunction. It is characterized by severe bilateral leg pain, urinary retention, weakness of the anal sphincter, and bilateral nerve root abnormalities. Once complete neurologic block has occurred, deceptively pain is often alleviated, and the patient will require a neurologic examination to verify the need for emergency surgery.

Spondylolisthesis. This term, which refers to forward displacement of one vertebra on another, commonly involves the L4–L5 and L5–S1 levels. Bursts of segmental severe girdle pain are typical, often worse on activity and relieved by rest.

LABORATORY PROCEDURES. Tests performed are dictated by the results of medical history and physical examination. Simple x-rays of the back may suffice if a traumatic injury is causative. In instances of suspected metabolic disturbance, appropriate screening tests such as serum calcium, phosphorus, and alkaline phosphatase measurements should be obtained. Complete blood counts, sedimentation rate, urinalysis, and automated serum chemical profiles are sometimes justified to clarify the diagnosis. Anemia and an elevated sedimentation rate should prompt a more extensive search for infectious, inflammatory, and neoplastic diseases.

X-RAY STUDIES. *Routine X-ray Studies.* These include frontal, lateral, and oblique films of the lumbosacral spine, which can demonstrate foraminal encroachment, compression fractures, degenerative changes, and subluxation of zygoapophyseal joints, as well as interspace narrowing (see Ch. 457). There may be severe degenerative changes by x-rays with few or no relevant symptoms, and severe back pain may occur in the absence of significant radiographic signs and be of discogenic origin.

Additional Imaging Procedures. When surgical intervention is planned or a diagnosis remains questionable and requires an imperative answer and high resolution, cat scans (noninvasive) are increasingly preferred to myelography, although the latter may be necessary. It is not usually necessary to perform a discogram (injection of radiopaque dye directly into the disc). When osteomyelitis or neoplastic involvement is likely, radionuclide bone scans are helpful. A percutaneous vertebral biopsy under fluoroscopic guidance may be performed to establish histopathologic diagnosis or bacteriologic diagnosis at highly suspicious sites obvious from scans or x-rays. Epidural venography scans have become an additional useful tool in precisely delineating sites of discogenic disease. Electromyography can confirm the presence of nerve root deficits.

MANAGEMENT. Conservative therapy for mechanical disorders of the spine and disc herniation focuses on bedrest, analgesics, muscle relaxants, and anti-inflammatory medication. Pelvic traction is also of benefit in some patients. Application of moist heat, e.g., hydrocollator packs wrapped with a wet towel, may relieve pain and muscle spasm. Cyclobenzaprine (10 mg) or diazepam (5 mg) three to four times daily serves as a useful muscle relaxant. The amount of bedrest is dependent on the severity of symptoms. After enforced bedrest for about a two-week period, gradual ambulation and a program of exercises together with back protection including a lumbosacral support are recommended. Most cases of disc herniation respond to conservative therapy; those unresponsive require further measures, including intrathecal and epidural steroids, nerve root or sleeve infiltrations with steroids, and injections of chymopapain into the disc space. This latter treatment is now approved for general use by the FDA. Before surgery is indicated, a psychological assessment, a thorough program of muscle relaxants, and exercises emphasizing back stretching and abdominal strengthening should be attempted.

Progressive muscular weakness and progressive neurologic deficit despite bedrest and other aforementioned measures, as well as the cauda equina syndrome, are indications for surgery. Relative indications for laminectomy are severe pain, unrelieved by bedrest, and recurrent episodes of incapacitating pain. Ninety to ninety-five per cent improvement following surgery is anticipated, although 70 per cent of patients experience relief of pain whether or not the disc is removed.

Following either conservative therapy or laminectomy, a program of prophylactic management thereafter includes postural education, performance of daily exercise program to strengthen the lumbar and abdominal muscles, and avoidance of lower spine stress. Besides laminectomy, joint fusion for spondylolisthesis and discogenic disease or unroofing procedures for spinal stenosis are sometimes necessary. Myelography or cat scans are indicated preoperatively to establish definitively the nature and extent of disease as well as the level of vertebral involvement.

Acute symptoms from compression fractures require appropriate rest and relief of pain with analgesics. Activities must be selected to avoid additional compression fractures. (See Ch. 249 for management of osteoporosis.)

Brown MD (ed.): Intradiscal Therapy: Chymopapain or Collagenase. Chicago, Year Book Medical Publishers, Inc, 1983. *Clinical research results on an important alternative procedure to laminectomy. Results are cautiously interpreted.*

Lipson SJ: Low back pain. *In* Kelley WN, Harris ED Jr, Ruddy S, Sledge CB (eds.): Textbook of Rheumatology. Philadelphia, W. B. Saunders Company, 1981, pp 451–471. *A useful reference; concisely written orthopedic diagnostic and therapeutic steps.*

MacNab I: Backache. Baltimore, Williams & Wilkins Company, 1977. *This monograph reviews practical aspects of diagnosis and management of backache. Excellent philosophic concepts and relevant classification of backache by a pioneer innovator in orthopedic surgery.*

Quinet RJ, Hadler NM: Diagnosis and treatment of backache. Semin Arthritis Rheum 8:261, 1979. *Detailed exposition of diagnosis and management tailored for the internist.*

460. DISEASES WITH WHICH ARTHRITIS IS FREQUENTLY ASSOCIATED

Giles G. Bole

Arthritis can be a significant feature of each of the diseases discussed in this chapter. Description of the disorder is brief and limited to the rheumatic manifestations of the disease. More detailed discussion of each entity is found in other chapters devoted to these diseases.

SARCOIDOSIS

The most common rheumatic manifestation of sarcoidosis is an acute, symmetric polyarthritis associated with erythema nodosum and hilar adenopathy (Löfgren's syndrome). The ankles are most frequently involved, followed by the wrists, the proximal interphalangeal joints, and the elbows. Arthritis and the other acute manifestations usually resolve spontaneously within a few weeks without sequelae. Circulating immune complexes and an increased frequency of HLA-B8 are found in these patients. Treatment with salicylates, oral colchicine, or corticosteroids has been symptomatically beneficial in individual cases. Chronic granulomatous sarcoid synovitis is an uncommon form of oligoarthritis that can cause joint destruction. It is less responsive to drug treatment and follows a variable clinical course.

HEMOCHROMATOSIS

Joint involvement has been observed in approximately half of the patients with idiopathic hemochromatosis. Joint swelling with bony enlargement is particularly common in the small joints of the hands, but the wrists, hips, and knees may be affected. The clinical and roentgenographic features resemble osteoarthritis more than they do inflammatory joint disease. There is roentgenographic evidence of narrowing of the joint space with subchondral erosions and sclerosis. Chondrocalcinosis is present in about 50 per cent of patients with arthropathy and may lead to acute episodes of crystal-induced synovitis (see Ch. 485). Management of this arthropathy includes the use of a nonsteroidal anti-inflammatory drug and prosthetic weight-bearing joint replacements in advanced disease.

SICKLE CELL DISEASE AND OTHER HEMOGLOBINOPATHIES

Severe polyarthralgia is a frequent manifestation of the crises of sickle cell disease. Occasionally the pain is accompanied by transient joint effusions. Skeletal abnormalities result from widening of bone marrow spaces and focal sickle cell thrombosis in bone. The most common bony lesion is avascular osteonecrosis of the femoral head; less commonly the humerus and vertebral bodies are involved. This complication is also associated with sickle cell trait, hemoglobin C disease, sickle cell disease, and sickle cell–thalassemia disease. In children, periostitis may result in transient diffuse swelling of the hands and feet (dactylitis). Sickle cell disease is associated with an increased incidence of bacterial arthritis and osteomyelitis, especially those caused by gram-negative organisms. Arthropathy in patients with the thalassemia syndromes is attributed to stress fractures of weakened subchondral bone.

HYPERLIPOPROTEINEMIA

In familial hypercholesterolemia (Type II hyperlipoproteinemia) recurrent episodes of acute migratory polyarthritis occur in homozygous cases. In heterozygous patients achilles tendonitis, monoarthritis, or polyarthritis of brief duration and variable severity can involve both large and small joints. Tendinous xanthomas appear in late stages of this disease. In some individuals with hypertriglyceridemia (Type IV hyperlipoproteinemia) a mild asymmetric oligoarthritis of chronic or recurrent type has been observed. Several of these patients have had periarticular bone cysts identified in joint radiographs. Certain of the reported cases may have occurred in association with familial combined hyperlipidemia, which includes individuals with both of these plasma lipoprotein profiles. Several authors have reported gradual reduction in the severity and frequency of articular symptoms after correction of the plasma lipid abnormalities by appropriate dietary and drug therapy.

HYPOGAMMAGLOBULINEMIA

A polyarthritis, rarely deforming in character, has been observed in as many as one third of patients with congenital or acquired hypogammaglobulinemia. The pattern of joint involvement resembles that of rheumatoid arthritis; in addition, other connective tissue diseases such as systemic lupus erythematosus, systemic sclerosis, and dermatomyositis have been associated with immune deficiency states. A variety of autoimmune phenomena and connective tissue syndromes, including juvenile arthritis, have been observed in patients with selective IgA deficiency. Regression of arthritis has been observed following institution of gamma globulin therapy. (See Ch. 429.)

HYPERPARATHYROIDISM

Patients with hyperparathyroidism are subject to a variety of associated rheumatic disorders that may occur singly or in combination. These include hyperuricemia and gouty arthritis, chondrocalcinosis with episodes of calcium pyrophosphate dihydrate crystal-induced synovitis (CPPD disease), and osteoarthritis resulting from deformation of atrophic subchondral bone. Rheumatic symptoms, particularly those associated with CPPD disease, may be the first manifestations of hyperparathyroidism.

ACROMEGALY

The majority of patients with acromegaly develop an atypical form of osteoarthritis. Increased levels of growth hormone result in hypertrophy of articular cartilage, subchondral bone, and periarticular tissues. Hypermobility of joints, a common manifestation, may contribute to degenerative change. The fingers and knees are most frequently affected. Pathognomonic radiographic features include overgrowth of bone and cartilage. Median nerve entrapment (carpal tunnel syndrome) secondary to wrist synovitis is common.

FAMILIAL MEDITERRANEAN FEVER

Joint involvement is second only to peritonitis as the most common manifestation in this disease. The arthritis is usually monoarticular and acute in onset and most commonly affects the large weight-bearing joints. The articular attacks remit in a few days, and only in a few cases do joint symptoms persist for weeks to months. Arthritis, like other manifestations of this syndrome, is recurrent, but permanent damage to joints other than the hip is rare. (For a more complete discussion, see Ch. 209.)

WHIPPLE'S DISEASE

This disease is now recognized as an unusual host response to a bacterial infection. It is characterized by diarrhea, malabsorption, fever, anemia, increased skin pigmentation, and migratory polyarthralgia or polyarthritis. Permanent joint damage is rare, and the disease is suppressed by chronic antibiotic therapy (see Ch. 103).

461. MISCELLANEOUS FORMS OF ARTHRITIS

Giles G. Bole

NEUROPATHIC JOINT DISEASE (Charcot Joints)

This chronic progressive degenerative arthropathy can be a complication of a variety of neurologic disorders. Impairment of proprioceptive and pain sensations deprives the affected joint of the normal protective reactions that ordinarily modulate the forces of weight bearing and motion. Diabetic neuropathy is now the most common and syphilitic tabes dorsalis the second most common cause of this joint disorder. Syringomyelia, myelomeningocele, and congenital indifference to pain are less frequent causes of neuropathic arthropathy. The basic neurologic lesion determines the distribution of the affected joints. In tabes dorsalis, the knees, hips, ankles, and vertebrae are frequently involved. In diabetic neuropathy, the changes are limited to the distal lower extremities, and in syringomyelia the shoulder and elbow joints are most commonly affected.

Although pain is generally present, discomfort tends to be disproportionately mild relative to the degree of joint destruction. Clinical, pathologic, and roentgenographic features of chronic neuropathic joint disease reflect severe degrees of destruction and disorganization of the involved joints. Synovial fluid is usually noninflammatory, but it can be hemorrhagic and contain destructive debris (fragments of cartilage or bone). In the early stages, the differentiation from other causes of joint derangement depends upon the demonstration of a sensory neuropathy.

Management includes immobilization of affected joints and restriction of weight-bearing activities with crutches, splints, and braces. Surgical arthrodesis, although frequently unsuccessful, is indicated in selected individuals. Total joint replacement has been attempted, but success has been severely limited and most consider this approach contraindicated at the present time.

HEMARTHROSIS

Recurrent or chronic hemarthrosis is the most common complication of a group of heritable disorders of blood coagulation (see Ch. 167). Hemarthrosis can be a complication of anticoagulant therapy or severe trauma to a normal joint.

In hemophilia, joint bleeding usually begins before the age of five and tends to recur repeatedly during childhood in response to even minor injury. The most common sites are the knees, elbows, and ankles, but any joint can be involved.

Acute hemarthrosis usually results in marked local inflammation and joint symptoms that can last for days to weeks. Approximately half of the patients with hemophilia develop chronic deformities in one or more joints. Some of them develop a chronic progressive synovitis, restricted to one or a few joints, which clinically and roentgenographically resembles rheumatoid arthritis. In chronic cases there is marked synovial membrane hyperplasia, destruction of articular cartilage, and erosions of subchondral bone. This chronic progressive pattern probably results from a low level of continuous or intermittent bleeding into involved joints. Joint fluid, in chronic cases, usually contains blood and very high levels of leukocyte-derived proteases. Other musculoskeletal manifestations of hemophilia include bleeding into muscle and bone. The resolution of large hematomas can produce chronic cysts within these tissues.

The first principle in management is to prevent trauma, a goal not easily achieved in children. Acute hemarthrosis should be managed by immobilization, analgesic therapy, and the administration of appropriate plasma concentrates that contain the required coagulation factor. Aspirin and other nonsteroidal analgesics that alter platelet function should be avoided. If there is marked distention of a joint or bursa, aspiration can be accomplished after the defect in coagulation has been corrected. When pain and acute inflammation have subsided, an exercise program to restore joint range of motion should be initiated. For the patient with severe chronic deforming joint disease, the availability of potent plasma concentrates has made it possible to perform synovectomy and arthroplasty in selected instances.

HENOCH-SCHÖNLEIN PURPURA

Polyarthralgia and a nondeforming arthritis, most frequently affecting knees and ankles, are common manifestations of this disorder. Other features include nonthrombocytopenic purpura, abdominal pain, and glomerulonephritis. The syndrome is rare in adults. (For a more detailed discussion see Ch. 166.)

MULTICENTRIC RETICULOHISTIOCYTOSIS (Lipoid Dermatoarthritis)

This rare disorder usually begins in the middle decades of life and affects females three times more frequently than males. It is characterized by the development of multiple histiocytic nodules in the skin and severe polyarthritis that may simulate rheumatoid arthritis. The firm reddish-brown or yellow papular nodules are most commonly found on hands, forearms, head, neck, and chest. Mutilating joint destruction, especially in the interphalangeal joints, occurs in approximately half of the patients with this syndrome. Diagnosis is made by demonstration of histiocytes and multinucleated giant cells, containing PAS-positive material, in skin or synovium. Similar infiltrates have been observed in other organs. Reports of apparent benefit from adrenocorticosteroid or immunosuppressive therapy are difficult to interpret because of the tendency for spontaneous remission in this disorder.

HYPERTROPHIC OSTEOARTHROPATHY

This term refers to a syndrome that includes clubbing of fingers and toes, periostitis at the ends of long bones, arthritis, and in some cases signs of autonomic dysfunction such as flushing, blanching, and profuse sweating of the extremities. The syndrome occurs with a wide variety of underlying disease states. There is a rare hereditary and idiopathic (pachydermoperiostosis) form of this disorder. The fully expressed pattern is usually associated with intrathoracic disease: lung carcinoma, lung abscess, emphysema, bronchiectasis, chronic interstitial pneumonitis, or mesothelioma. Clubbing, usually without periostitis, can be seen with cyanotic heart disease, cystic fibrosis, bacterial endocarditis, biliary cirrhosis, ulcerative colitis, regional enteritis, or thyroid disease.

The distal joints (wrist, elbows, ankles) and long bones of the forearms and legs are most frequently affected. There are inflammatory changes in the periosteum, synovial membrane, and periarticular structures. The periosteum is "lifted" by the deposition of new bone matrix and subsequent mineralization. Clubbing results from edema, cellular infiltration, and connective tissue proliferation in the nailbeds.

Pain, tenderness, and enlargement of the distal portions of extremities may be accompanied by an acute polyarthritis that superficially resembles rheumatoid arthritis. Correct diagnosis of the acute polyarthritis syndrome is established by the recognition of digital clubbing and roentgenographic evidence of periostitis and intrathoracic disease.

The production of a humoral substance that mediates increased vascularity or connective tissue proliferation or both has long been suspected as the pathogenic factor in hypertrophic osteoarthropathy, but no such factor has been demonstrated. Evidence that neural factors are involved is derived from observations of striking resolution of signs and symptoms after denervation of the hilum or vagotomy on the same side as the thoracic lesion. Regression of osteoarthropathy has also been observed after resection of pulmonary neoplasms.

Aside from therapy directed at the associated disease, there is no effective treatment of hypertrophic osteoarthropathy. Symptomatic benefit may be obtained from salicylates, other analgesics, or adrenocorticosteroids.

PALINDROMIC RHEUMATISM AND INTERMITTENT HYDRARTHROSIS

These terms describe two different constellations of clinical findings in which no pathogenic mechanism or mechanisms have been defined and in which the symptoms are often the prodrome of another rheumatic disease. *Palindromic rheumatism* is a term applied to a recurrent pattern of polyarthritis that in

individual cases is quite constant. The episodes are usually of brief duration. Many patients eventually develop typical features of rheumatoid arthritis. *Intermittent hydrarthrosis* is typified by recurrent joint effusions usually occurring in young females at menstruation and involving the knee. Like palindromic rheumatism, there is a strong tendency for cases to evolve into rheumatoid arthritis. Diagnostic arthrocentesis is justified in each condition based upon the local joint findings during an acute attack. Since each of the disorders remits spontaneously for variable periods of time, there is no uniform opinion regarding treatment, which is strictly symptomatic.

462. NONARTICULAR RHEUMATISM

Giles G. Bole

This term designates a group of painful disorders resulting from involvement of tendons, bursae, and other periarticular structures. Conditions causing shoulder pain are considered separately in Ch. 458.

BURSITIS

Bursae are closed synovial spaces located at sites of friction between skin, ligaments, tendons, muscles, and bones. Trauma is the most common cause of acute bursitis, but almost any illness characterized by joint synovitis can be associated with inflammation in the lining of bursae. Bursae commonly involved include the following: subdeltoid, trochanteric, olecranon, and prepatellar. Septic or gouty bursitis can be documented by appropriate studies of aspirated fluid. Protection of an inflamed bursa from friction and trauma is the most important aspect of treatment, but moderate doses of salicylates or other nonsteroidal anti-inflammatory drugs can be helpful. Local injection with an adrenocorticosteroid preparation is indicated if symptoms are severe or refractory to other treatment.

TENOSYNOVITIS

Tendon sheaths, like bursae, have synovial linings and can be involved by any process capable of inducing joint synovitis. Transient tenosynovitis in the hand or foot is a frequent manifestation of gonococcemia. Calcific tendinitis, a common source of shoulder pain (see Ch. 458), can be associated with severe inflammation and simulate acute gout. Focal thickening of a tendon sheath and adjacent tendon can result in "locking or trigger" phenomena. This problem, termed stenosing tenosynovitis, is most common in the flexor tendons of the fingers. Involvement of the abductor pollicis longus and extensor pollicis brevis tendons of the thumb (De Quervain's syndrome) produces pain and tenderness at the radial aspect of the wrist. There are few generalizations regarding management, since tenosynovitis can be a manifestation of various disease states, including rheumatoid arthritis and other connective tissue syndromes, infection, crystalline synovitis, or hyperlipidemia. The most common form of tenosynovitis, unassociated with systemic disease, often subsides with rest of the part. If symptoms are severe or recurrent, local injections of adrenocorticosteroid preparations are usually effective. Surgical excision of the affected tendon sheath is indicated for those patients with persistent disability.

TENNIS ELBOW (Epicondylitis)

This common disorder is characterized by pain over the lateral aspect of the elbow. Tenderness is localized at the site of origin of the extensor communis apparatus at the lateral epicondyle. The problem, most common in middle-aged males, is related to sports activities or occupations that involve repetitive wrist extension or pronation-supination. Pain is accentuated by resisted wrist extension. If symptoms fail to respond to rest, local injection of an adrenocorticosteroid preparation is usually successful. An exercise program designed to stretch and strengthen the forearm extensor muscles may also be required.

Medial epicondylitis, sometimes referred to as golfer's elbow, is associated with pain and tenderness over the medial aspect of the elbow, at the site or origin of the wrist flexors. Therapy is similar to that for tennis elbow.

CARPAL TUNNEL SYNDROME

This problem results from entrapment of the median nerve as it passes deep to the transverse carpal ligament at the wrist. Inflammation of the adjacent flexor tendons and their sheaths, the most common basis for median nerve entrapment, can be a feature of rheumatoid or other forms of arthritis; but in most patients the tenosynovitis is localized and unassociated with systemic disease. The syndrome can be seen in endocrine disorders, granulomatous infections, amyloidosis, and pregnancy. The most consistent symptoms are dysesthesia, paresthesia, and hypesthesia in the middle three digits of the hand. Referred pain to the more proximal upper extremity is common. Symptoms are usually intermittent, occurring most frequently during the night. Forced flexion of the wrist or nerve compression locally (Tinel's sign) can induce characteristic symptoms. In a minority of patients, there is progressive wasting of the muscles of the thenar eminence. Conservative management consists of fitting a removable wrist splint and the local injection of an adrenocorticosteroid preparation. Surgical release of the transverse carpal ligament is indicated for patients with persistent disability.

TIETZE'S SYNDROME

This anterior chest wall disorder is characterized by painful enlargement of the upper costal cartilages. It is usually unilateral and limited to a single costochondral juncture. Occasionally the manubriosternal and sternoclavicular joints are affected. The disease may be recurrent, but remission is the rule. If discomfort is severe or recurrent, analgesics, heat, or local infiltration (adrenocorticosteroid or local anesthetic agents) may be beneficial. The condition is distinct from costochondritis, which occurs at multiple sites lower in the anterior rib cage and is unattended by local palpable swelling of a costochondral junction.

FIBROSITIS

This term has been applied to a poorly defined symptom complex that is characterized by pain and stiffness in varying areas, most commonly in the neck, shoulder girdle, and posterior aspect of the trunk. Physical signs except for questionable nodules or thickening of the deep fasciae are lacking, and results of laboratory and roentgenographic studies are normal. Localized areas of tenderness, commonly in the paravertebral areas medial to the scapula, have been termed tender or "trigger points." The syndrome usually begins in the middle years of life and is most common in females. Because the majority of patients appear tense and anxious and have no recognizable objective basis for their symptoms, the syndrome is often considered psychogenic. Patients with fibrositis frequently report difficulty with sleep, and electroencephalographic studies have demonstrated disturbances in slow wave non-REM sleep in some cases. Since pain and stiffness can be manifestations of a variety of musculoskeletal, neurologic, and systemic disorders, the diagnosis of fibrositis requires the exclusion of more specific disease entities. Patient and physician tend to share an unhappy experience in efforts to control symptoms. The results of strong reassurance that serious disease is lacking are variable, as are the results of therapy with salicylates, sedatives, tranquilizers, and muscle relaxants. Some authors favor the use of moderate doses of one of the tricyclic antidepressants to control the patient's reported sleep disturbance and other symptoms.

463. SYNOVIAL TUMORS

Giles G. Bole

Primary malignant tumors of joints are rare. Synovioma is a highly malignant fibroblastic sarcoma which usually originates in the knee or periarticular structures of the thigh. This neoplasm is most common in late childhood or early adult life. The recommended therapy is wide excision (frequently requiring amputation), irradiation, or systemic chemotherapy or all three. Synovial chondrosarcoma is a rare neoplasm that may simulate synovial chondromatosis. It most frequently involves the knee and is slow in producing distant metastases. Radical excision or amputation is the treatment of choice.

Benign tumors arising within joints include lipoma, chondroma, hemangioma, and xanthoma. These neoplasms are rather uncommon and are most frequently found in or about the knee.

Synovial chondromatosis is uncommon. It is characterized by multiple foci or cartilage metaplasia in the synovial tissues. The metaplastic growths form nodules and can detach and grow as loose bodies in the joint space. The lesions can also undergo ossification. The latter condition is referred to as synovial osteochondromatosis. The knee is the most common site of involvement; the disease is rarely polyarticular. Symptoms include crepitation, swelling, limitation of motion, and intermittent locking of the affected joint. Treatment is surgical synovectomy.

Pigmented villonodular synovitis is the most common term applied to a disorder characterized by villous or nodular growths that invade the synovial lining of joints, bursae, or tendons. It has a characteristic histopathologic picture, i.e., presence of inflammatory granulomas that contain hemosiderin, cholesterol crystals, and multinucleated giant cells. Authorities disagree about whether the condition should be classified as a form of chronic synovitis or as a true neoplasm. The knee is most frequently involved, but it can occur in the hip, elbow, ankle, or foot. Synovial fluid is usually hemorrhagic or xanthochromic. The inflammatory granuloma frequently invades the cartilage, subchondral bone, and periarticular structures. Localized pigmented villonodular synovitis can affect extra-articular bursae or tendon sheaths or occur as a solitary nodule in a single joint. The treatment of choice for each of these conditions is synovectomy or local excision of the tumor masses. Recurrence is uncommon.

464. BEHÇET'S DISEASE

Ralph Snyderman

DEFINITION. Behçet's disease is an inflammatory disorder of unknown etiology characterized by recurrent oral and genital aphthous ulcers, ocular inflammation, and skin lesions of erythema nodosum and acneiform eruptions. Behçet's disease also frequently involves the joints, the central nervous system, and the gastrointestinal tract.

INCIDENCE AND PREVALENCE. Behçet's disease is common in northern Japan, Turkey, and Israel. In Japan the current prevalence is 1 per 10,000. The frequency in the United States is far less. An annual incidence of 1 per 300,000 was determined for Olmstead County, Minnesota. The disease does not occur frequently in Japanese-Americans, perhaps suggesting environmental factors in addition to genetic predisposition in the etiology of this illness.

ETIOLOGY AND PATHOGENESIS. No infectious agent has been consistently isolated. Sera frequently contain circulating immune complexes of the IgA and IgG variety, as well as elevated levels of chemotactic activity for leukocytes. Antibodies reactive against oral mucosal cells have been found, and factors produced by patients' lymphocytes are toxic for oral mucosal cells. However, these findings are also present in individuals with recurrent aphthous stomatitis alone. Serum complement levels in Behçet's disease are usually elevated, particularly levels of C9. Most patients with neurologic involvement have demyelinating antibodies in their sera. There is a strong association of HLA-B5 with Behçet's disease in Japan and in the Mediterranean area. Heavy metal exposure, certain foods (particularly English walnuts), and toxic factors such as organophosphates have initiated attacks in some individuals.

PATHOLOGY. Behçet's disease is primarily an inflammatory disorder involving small blood vessels, particularly venules. Areas of ulceration initially show an intense mononuclear cell infiltration around blood vessels. As the lesion evolves, polymorphonuclear leukocytes and plasma cells predominate. The early lesions resemble a delayed hypersensitivity reaction, the later lesions an immune complex–Arthus-type reaction. The role of immune complexes in causing the venulitis is, however, questionable, since immunoglobulins are not routinely found in vessel walls.

CLINICAL MANIFESTATIONS. Behçet's disease can occur in many forms, but recurrent oral aphthous ulcers are present in 99 per cent of patients, and in almost 70 per cent these are the initial symptoms. Ocular symptoms occur in 90 per cent, skin lesions in 85 per cent, and genital ulcerations in nearly 70 per cent. Arthritis is present in approximately half of the patients with Behçet's disease. The onset is usually in the third or fourth decade. Behçet's disease affects men and women approximately equally. Indicators of poor prognosis include neurologic and posterior uveal tract involvement. In the absence of these, the disease tends to be unpredictable and remitting. In Japan, the mortality is approximately 4 per cent, with blindness occurring in as many as 65 per cent of untreated individuals. Young males have the worst prognosis.

The diagnosis of Behçet's disease is based upon the criteria listed in Table 464–1. Complete Behçet's syndrome is associated with all four major criteria. Persons with three major sites of involvement, or ocular lesions plus one other major site, have incomplete Behçet's disease. The diagnosis should be suspected when two major sites are affected. Since all manifestations need not appear, some investigators have grouped this illness into subtypes based upon the primary tissue involvement (i.e., neuro-Behçet's, oculo-Behçet's).

The oral aphthous ulcers are painful, unlike those of Reiter's syndrome, and occur singly or multiply on the lingual, gingival, buccal, or labial mucosal membranes. In Reiter's and Stevens-Johnson syndromes, the ulcers occur on the palate, pharynx, and tonsils, structures rarely involved in Behçet's disease. The aphthae of Behçet's disease usually last for approximately a week and may heal with or without scarring. Ulcers can also appear on the scrotum, vulva, penis, vaginal mucosa, or perianal areas. These lesions may be painless in women. Their gross appearance is similar to that of the oral aphthous ulcers. Vulvar lesions frequently occur premenstrually. Other types of cutaneous involvement are common. Painful, recurrent lesions of erythema nodosum may appear in crops over the tibia. Superficial thrombophlebitis can occur in the upper or lower extremities. Skin eruptions resembling acne vulgaris frequently appear on the upper thorax and face.

TABLE 464–1. DIAGNOSTIC CRITERIA OF BEHÇET'S DISEASE (SYNDROME)*

Major criteria
1. Recurrent oral aphthous ulcers
2. Eye lesions
   a. Recurrent hypopyon, iritis, or iridocyclitis
   b. Chorioretinitis
3. Genital ulcerations
4. Skin lesions
   a. Erythema nodosum-like eruptions
   b. Superficial thrombophlebitis
   c. Pustular skin lesions
   d. Hyperirritability of the skin (pathergy)

Minor criteria
5. Arthritis
6. Gastrointestinal lesions
7. Epididymitis
8. Vascular lesions (occlusion of blood vessels, aneurysms)
9. Central nervous system involvement
   a. Brainstem syndrome
   b. Meningoencephalomyelitic syndrome
   c. Organic confusional states

*Modified from the recommendations by the Behçet's Syndrome Research Committee of Japan (1972).

Approximately 40 per cent of patients with Behçet's disease exhibit a cutaneous phenomenon termed "pathergy." Venipuncture or injection of sterile saline into the skin of these patients results in the formation of a pustule. This phenomenon is not pathognomonic for Behçet's disease.

Ocular lesions may consist of anterior or posterior uveitis. Anterior uveitis frequently produces hazy vision as an initial manifestation. The development of a hypopyon is not unusual. Recurrent posterior uveitis is an ominous expression of Behçet's disease which, if untreated, frequently leads to bilateral blindness. Choroidal exudates and bleeding may be seen.

Articular manifestations consist of arthralgias and arthritis. The involvement is usually asymmetrical, affects one to several large joints such as the knees, ankles, elbows, and wrists, and resolves during remissions. Permanent joint damage is rare.

Gastrointestinal involvement during acute attacks, present in approximately 50 per cent of patients, is most commonly manifested by vomiting, abdominal pain, diarrhea, flatulence, or constipation. More specific for Behçet's disease are erosions or superficial ulcers in the terminal ileum or colon. Intestinal ulcers occasionally perforate. Differentiation of Behçet's disease from ulcerative colitis or regional enteritis may be difficult.

Nervous system involvement occurs in approximately 10 per cent of patients and can be extremely severe, explosive, and associated with a poor prognosis. Manifestations include hemiplegia, paraplegia, cerebellar dysfunction, and psychologic changes.

Superficial venous occlusions, perhaps related to abnormalities in the blood fibrinolytic system, occur in up to 40 per cent of patients. Inferior or superior vena caval obstructions can lead to death. Occlusive lesions have also occurred in the aorta and other large arteries. Epididymitis occurs in approximately 6 per cent of male patients.

TREATMENT. No therapy has been proved uniformly effective. Since the illness is unpredictable and frequently remitting, long-term continuous therapy with potentially dangerous drugs is not justified except in specific situations. Chlorambucil (0.1 to 0.2 mg per kilogram per day) has been reported to prevent blindness in patients with posterior retinal involvement. Other immunosuppressive agents such as azathioprine, cyclophosphamide, and 6-mercaptopurine have also been used. Since neuro-Behçet's syndrome is life-threatening, immunosuppressive agents are frequently used for this manifestation. Corticosteroids are strictly palliative for the inflammatory lesions (i.e., anterior uveitis) and should not be used except during acute flares of the disease. Avoidance of factors known to precipitate attacks (i.e., particular foods or toxic materials) should be encouraged. Colchicine (0.6 mg orally twice a day) is sometimes effective in treating the mucocutaneous and cutaneous lesions. Transfer factor has not been effective in double-blind clinical trials. In patients with gastrointestinal manifestations, a trial of sulfasalazine (2 to 4 gm per day) is warranted. Sulfasalazine may also be useful in patients without obvious gastrointestinal complaints. Fibrinolytic agents have been recommended for patients with occlusive vascular disease. Because the disease is remitting in nature, the efficacy of therapy is difficult to evaluate.

Chajek T, Fainaru M: Behçet's disease. Report of 41 cases and a review of the literature. Medicine 54:179, 1975. *Concise but thorough review of clinical features in a large number of patients with Behçet's disease.*
Lehner T, Barnes CG: Behçet's Syndrome. London, Academic Press, 1979. *Book devoted to Behçet's disease. Good review of the immunologic findings and clinical manifestations of the illness.*
Marquardt JL, Snyderman R, Oppenheim JJ: Depression of transformation and exacerbation of Behçet's syndrome by ingestion of English walnuts. Cell Immunol 9:263, 1973. *An immunologic study of Behçet's disease with a potential clue for pathogenesis.*
Michelson JB, Chisari FV: Behçet's disease. Surv Ophthalmol 26:190, 1982. *An up-to-date review of Behçet's disease, particularly good for ocular manifestations.*
Shimizu T, Ehrlich GE, Inaba G, Hayashi K: Behçet disease (Behçet syndrome). Semin Arthritis Rheum 8:223, 1979. *Comprehensive review of clinical features, pathology and potential pathogenic mechanisms of Behçet's disease.*

465. PANNICULITIS AND DISORDERS OF THE SUBCUTANEOUS FAT

Gerald S. Lazarus

INTRODUCTION. The subcutaneous tissue is a fibrofatty layer spread between the flexible skin and the rigid muscles. It functions not only as a thermal and mechanical insulator but also as an active metabolic organ. The mature lipocyte contains an eccentric nucleus and a single large vacuole. The characteristic signet ring lipocytes are organized into lobules by fibrous septa, which are continuous with the dermis and contain the blood and lymph vessels and reticuloendothelial cells.

The diagnosis of panniculitis frequently requires skin biopsy. The most important histologic characteristic of the deep skin biopsy is the location of the inflammatory process. Inflammation primarily in the septa is designated *septal panniculitis,* whereas the presence of inflammatory cells primarily in the fat lobules is designated *lobular panniculitis.* The presence or absence of vasculitis further differentiates panniculitis into the four major groups.

LOBULAR PANNICULITIS WITHOUT VASCULITIS. ***Nodular Panniculitis—Weber-Christian Disease.*** Nodular panniculitis describes a group of syndromes or diseases characterized by subcutaneous nodules and inflammatory cells in the fat lobules. The term Weber-Christian disease is applied when cutaneous lesions are associated with systemic complaints.

The etiology of this group of diseases is unknown. In the early stages the fat lobules are infiltrated with polymorphonuclear leukocytes. Later, macrophages appear and ingest fat, producing the characteristic lipophagic granuloma. The lesions heal with lobular fibrosis. Uncommonly, minimal septal vasculitis may be observed.

Lobular panniculitis most commonly presents in females between the ages of 30 and 60, although cases have been reported in all age groups. The lesions begin as red, slightly tender nodules deep in the skin. They appear more or less in symmetrical crops on thighs and lower legs, but lesions may also occur on arms, trunk, and face. The number of lesions may vary enormously. The lesions become firmer, less red, and less tender over a period of weeks. They heal, leaving a depressed hyperpigmented scar. *Liquefying panniculitis* is a variant in which the lesions become necrotic and drain an oily, yellow-brown fluid. *Rothmann-Makai syndrome* is a very rare variant of lobular panniculitis, affecting children with numerous large lesions; the lesions do not liquefy, and healing usually occurs within 12 months.

Systemic nodular panniculitis or *Weber-Christian disease* is a widespread process affecting cutaneous and visceral fat. Patients usually present with unequivocal cutaneous nodules and arthralgias, malaise, fatigue, weight loss, and abdominal pain. Involvement of the bone marrow may produce anemia, leukocytosis or leukopenia, and bone pain. Hepatomegaly, steatorrhea, and intestinal perforation have also been reported. Inflammation may occur in other internal organs such as lungs, pleura, pericardium, spleen, kidney, and adrenal glands. Visceral involvement may be confined to the retroperitoneal space, producing abdominal pain, nausea, and vomiting. Alpha$_1$-antitrypsin deficiency and lymphoma have occasionally been reported in association with nodular panniculitis.

The prognosis of nodular panniculitis is good in patients with only cutaneous involvement. There are frequent remissions and exacerbations of the lesions. Some cases recover after a few months, and permanent remission is usual after several years. On rare occasions visceral involvement may be fatal.

There is no specific therapy for this disease. Saturated potassium iodide, increasing from 5 drops three times daily by 1 drop per day to 30 drops three times daily, has been suggested. Hydroxychloroquine, 200 mg twice per day, has also been advocated as treatment. High dose prednisone, 40 to 60 mg for one to two weeks with gradual tapering over six to eight weeks, has also been reported to be of value in patients with severe disease; steroids should be used only for acute attacks and for limited periods of time.

Lobular Panniculitis Associated with Pancreatic Disease. The diagnosis is made by skin biopsy, which reveals acute fat necrosis with characteristic ghost cells. These patients often have associated arthritis, ascites, and eosinophilia. Acute pancreatitis, trauma to the pancreas, chronic pancreatitis, pancreatic cysts, and pancreatic carcinoma have been reported to be associated with this syndrome. Diagnosis depends upon the histologic findings at skin biopsy and documentation of a specific pancreatic abnormality. Therapy is directed at the underlying pancreatic disease.

Poststeroid Lobular Panniculitis. Children who receive large doses of steroid for a short period of time, followed by abrupt discontinuance, may develop lobular panniculitis. Lesions may occur in the viscera, and a fatal case has been reported.

Physical Lobular Panniculitis. Physical trauma of any kind and cold injury, especially in children, can produce lobular panniculitis. A unique traumatic panniculitis occurs in the obese breasts of women in their 50's. Injection of silicones or other foreign materials into female breasts or buttocks and into the male genitalia may induce a granulomatous foreign body nodular panniculitis. Similar inflammatory lesions may be seen following injections of Talwin.

Lobular Panniculitis Associated with Systemic Disease. Lupus erythematosus, sarcoidosis, granuloma annulare, and infections including deep fungi and pyogens may present as lobular panniculitis. Lymphoma or leukemia may also present as panniculitis; histologically, these lesions demonstrate malignant cells in the fat lobules. Lupus erythematosus confined primarily to the fat is known as lupus profundus. The skin may be exclusively involved, or the panniculitis may be associated with systemic disease. Granuloma annulare, a disease characterized by ring-shaped lesions of the skin, may also involve the fat.

LOBULAR PANNICULITIS WITH VASCULITIS. This category of disease includes *nodular vasculitis* and *erythema induratum.* The eruption consists of recurring, tender, painful nodules on the calves, which often ulcerate and heal with scarring. It is much more common in females than in males. Increased erythrocyte sedimentation rate and hypertension have been associated with this syndrome. Bazin gave the name erythema induratum to this disease when histologic examination revealed caseation necrosis and the lesions were associated with tuberculosis.

There is no specific therapy for this syndrome. Most patients have remission of lesions with bed rest. Severe cases have been successfully treated with nonsteroidal anti-inflammatory drugs, dapsone, and prednisone. In the very rare case of nodular vasculitis associated with tuberculosis, appropriate antituberculous therapy is indicated.

SEPTAL PANNICULITIS WITHOUT VASCULITIS. This histology in a patient with nodular, painful, tender lesions, especially on the anterior leg, is diagnostic of *erythema nodosum,* which is discussed in Ch. 556. A chronic disease similar to erythema nodosum clinically and histologically except that the lesions spread peripherally over months, forming rings, is called *sub-*

acute migratory panniculitis. This disease responds to therapy with increasing doses of saturated potassium iodide as described for nodular panniculitis. Septal panniculitis without vasculitis can also be seen in scleroderma, eosinophilic fasciitis, and necrobiosis lipoidica diabeticorum.

SEPTAL PANNICULITIS WITH VASCULITIS. *Thrombophlebitis* may present with subcutaneous nodules. Histology reveals inflammation of veins with adjacent panniculitis (see Ch. 54).

Cutaneous polyarteritis is a chronic and recurring, painful nodular eruption, primarily of the legs. There is often an associated mottled livedo vascular pattern. Cutaneous polyarteritis is associated with myalgias, arthralgias, and increased erythrocyte sedimentation rate. Histologic examination demonstrates leukocytoclastic vasculitis of medium-sized arterioles. This disease is usually not associated with systemic involvement. It has a benign course, but lesions may recur for years.

Therapy includes nonsteroidal anti-inflammatory agents and short courses of corticosteroids. Cutaneous polyarteritis associated with granulomatous bowel disease has responded to short courses of Cytoxan.

LIPOATROPHY. Loss of subcutaneous tissue can occur as a consequence of healing in almost any of the panniculitides described previously. The most common diagnosable cause of lipoatrophy is recurrent insulin injection. Insulin lipoatrophy is usually associated with repetitive injections of high doses of insulin in exactly the same location in females. Talwin injections may also produce panniculitis and severe lipoatrophy.

Total lipoatrophy associated with diabetes may occur in children and adults. The clinical picture is dramatic, and there is almost complete loss of subcutaneous fat. Partial lipoatrophy usually begins in children or young adults. It is five times more common in females than in males. Patients often lose the fat in the face and the upper half of the body. In some cases, there is hypertrophy of the fat on the lower half of the body. Patients with partial lipodystrophy often develop progressive mesangiocapillary glomerulonephritis and hypocomplementemia. Diabetes develops in one third of these patients. Retinitis pigmentosum has also been reported with this disease. The prognosis depends upon the severity of the renal disease.

Ackerman AB: Panniculitis. *In* Ackerman AB: Histologic Diagnosis of Inflammatory Skin Diseases. Philadelphia, Lea & Febiger, 1978, pp 779-826. *An outstanding review of the classification and histopathology of panniculitis.*

Bennett WM, Bardana EJ, Wuepper K, Houghton D, Border WA, Gotze O, Schreiber R: Partial lipodystrophy, C3 nephritic factor and clinically inapparent mesangiocapillary glomerulonephritis. Am J Med 62:757, 1976. *Description of the association of lipodystrophy with glomerulonephritis.*

Bondi EE, Lazarus GS: Panniculitis. *In* Fitzpatrick TB, Eisen AZ, Wolff K, Freedberg IM, Austen KF (eds.): Dermatology in General Medicine. 3rd ed. New York, McGraw-Hill Book Company, In press. *A complete overview of panniculitis, emphasizing clinical description, mechanisms, and treatment.*

Epstein EH Jr: Lipodystrophy. *In* Fitzpatrick TB, Eisen AZ, Wolff K, Freedberg IM, Austen KF (eds.): Dermatology in General Medicine. New York, McGraw-Hill Book Company, 1979, pp 795-797. *Concise review of the lipodystrophy syndromes with appropriate pertinent references.*

Parks DL, Perry HO, Muller SA: Cutaneous complications of pentazocine injections. Arch Dermatol 104:231, 1971. *Good discussion of the cutaneous complications of pentazocine injections.*

Winkelman RK, Bowie BM: Hemorrhagic diathesis associated with benign and systemic histiocytosis. Arch Intern Med 140:1460, 1980. *A review of severe systemic lobular panniculitis.*

466. MULTIFOCAL FIBROSCLEROSIS (Multicentric Fibrosclerosis, Fibrosing Syndromes)

H. Ralph Schumacher, Jr.

In rare instances the delicate fibrous areolar tissue in a certain anatomic region becomes the site of a chronic low-grade inflammatory process, leading to deposition of dense sclerotic plaques, which may obstruct or limit the movement of adjacent viscera. When the process is in the active phase, there are characteristic findings of chronic or granulomatous inflammation, with mononuclear cell infiltration and occasional giant cells. In the end-stages the pathologic lesion is simply that of scar tissue, so that by the time this process causes clinical manifestations there may be little evidence of the initial inflammatory reaction. In at least some cases there is an accompanying vasculitis. As a general rule the process tends to originate in the midline, around the great vessels, then spreads laterally. In most cases a clue to the inciting mechanism is lacking; hence the frequent use of the term "idiopathic" in describing the various syndromes.

Syndromes that have been considered as manifestations of multifocal fibrosclerosis include retroperitoneal fibrosis, mediastinal fibrosis, sclerosing cholangitis (see Ch. 129), Riedel's thyroiditis (see Ch. 228), pseudotumor of the orbit, Peyronie's disease (a sclerotic induration of the corpora cavernosa of the penis), and practolol peritonitis. Other sites of a similar fibrosis, such as the testes, vagina, and suprasellar area, have also rarely been reported. A case of retroperitoneal fibrosis occurring with scleroderma has been described. The toxic syndrome following ingestion of adulterated rapeseed oil in Spain exhibits vascular disease and multiple areas of fibrosis but apparently does not include the sites seen with multifocal fibrosclerosis. Pulmonary and myocardial fibrosis syndromes have generally not been seen as related to multifocal fibrosclerosis.

The fibrosing pattern of response in multifocal fibrosclerosis may follow different kinds of injury. For example, there is an association between therapy with methysergide and some cases of retroperitoneal fibrosis, and the suggestion has been made that fibrosing mediastinitis can occur as a sequel to infection with *Histoplasma capsulatum.* In a number of instances the disease has developed concurrently with a neoplastic process such as reticulum cell sarcoma or carcinoid tumor. Sclerosing cholangitis is sometimes associated with ulcerative colitis or with Crohn's disease. Other associated factors have been retroperitoneal or intraabdominal surgery, several infectious agents, drugs, and systemic vasculitis.

Although most of these syndromes have been described as separate entities, depending on the clinical manifestations and the interests of the writers who have reported them, it should be emphasized that several anatomic areas may become affected in one person. For example, retroperitoneal fibrosis and sclerosing mediastinitis may be present at the same time. Even more interesting is the report by Comings and his associates of two brothers, offspring of a consanguineous marriage, who exhibited varying combinations of retroperitoneal fibrosis, mediastinal fibrosis, sclerosing cholangitis, Riedel's thyroiditis, and pseudotumor of the orbit. This brings up the possibility of a genetic predisposition to disease of this character, but of course does not exclude other precipitating factors, e.g., common exposure to some chemical. The former possibility is given support by the description of an association between the occurrence of fibrosing syndromes and alpha$_1$-antitrypsin deficiency. Some reports also have described an association of familial mediastinal or retroperitoneal fibrosis with seronegative spondyloarthropathies.

Comings DE, Skubi KB, Van Eyes J, Motulsky AG: Familial multifocal sclerosis. Ann Intern Med 66:884, 1967. *Description of multiple sites of fibrosis in two brothers.*

Goldbach P, Mohsenifar Z, Salick AI: Familial mediastinal fibrosis associated with seronegative spondyloarthropathy. Arthritis Rheum 26:221, 1983. *Two siblings with both diseases but HLA-B27 negative.*

RETROPERITONEAL FIBROSIS

In retroperitoneal fibrosis the process usually begins over the promontory of the sacrum and extends laterally across the ureters and up as high as the level of the second or third lumbar vertebra. Less commonly the lesion develops in other extraperitoneal areas, for example, contiguous with the kidneys, duodenum, descending colon, or urinary bladder. In some cases there has been an associated vasculitis in the skin and subcutaneous tissue, manifested by the formation of nodules, erythematous discolorations, and ulcerations. Similarly, inflammatory changes in small vessels at the sites of the sclerosis have been noted. Glomerulonephritis has been seen in a few patients.

The occurrence of retroperitoneal fibrosis in patients taking methysergide for migraine has been reported with greater frequency than could be due to chance. Occasional cases have been reported in association with use of various beta-adrenergic blocking agents, hydralazine, or methyldopa.

The disorder is about twice as common in males, and the peak age incidence is in the fifth and sixth decades. Cases have been reported in children. The manifestations are variable, depending on the anatomic location of the process. Pain is the most common symptom; it is vague, tends to be located in the low back, and may be accompanied by symptoms referable to the gastrointestinal tract. The patient is likely to lose weight and have low-grade fever. There may be some anemia and elevation of the erythrocyte sedimentation rate. Although the ureter is the structure most often affected, symptoms referable to the urinary tract are uncommon until obstructive uropathy has led to azotemia and other clinical manifestations of renal insufficiency. The fibrosing process may surround the inferior vena cava, but signs of obstruction of that vessel are relatively uncommon. Thromboembolism and hypertension can be complications. Arterial invasion has been described. Retroperitoneal fibrosis occasionally develops in association with abdominal aortic aneurysm.

Diagnosis of retroperitoneal fibrosis is difficult because of the lack of localizing manifestations. It is most often suggested by the findings at intravenous pyelography: displacement of the ureters toward the midline and evidence of obstruction, usually at the level of the pelvic brim. One or both ureters may be affected. In rare instances a mass can be palpated in the pelvis or on the posterior abdominal wall. Ultrasound, computed tomography (CT) scans, and nuclear magnetic resonance (NMR) imaging can also identify the fibrosing masses. Once the presence of a mass has been disclosed, the main problem in differential diagnosis lies in distinguishing retroperitoneal fibrosis from retroperitoneal tumor. For that reason multiple deep biopsies should be made at the time of laparotomy.

Surgical treatment, if employed before there has been severe renal damage, is often highly successful. Inasmuch as the fibrosing process is seldom invasive, the constricted organ can usually be freed by blunt dissection so that normal movement or flow is restored. Relief of ureteral obstruction is usually achieved simply by dissecting this structure free of its fibrous encasement and bringing it out on the anterior surface of the sclerotic mass. Occasionally, however, the obstruction recurs months or years after such treatment. Some surgeons wrap the ureters in omentum to try to decrease recurrent obstruction. Steroid therapy may be helpful, but the evidence for this is limited, and prompt surgical relief should usually be attempted whenever significant obstruction is present. Steroid treatment may be employed as an adjunct to surgical measures. When the inferior vena cava is obstructed, surgical relief is technically difficult and risky; here it may be preferable to temporize, in the hope that development of collateral pathways may alleviate the circulatory block.

The long-term outlook is fairly good if the disease is recognized and if its obstructive consequences can be treated suitably by surgical means. The disease often tends to run its course and subside. Most deaths have been caused by renal failure.

Hricak H, Higgins CB, Williams RD: Nuclear magnetic resonance imaging in retroperitoneal fibrosis. Am J Radiol 141:35, 1983. *Documentation of the increasing value of CT scans and NMR in diagnosis.*

Littlejohn GO, Keystone E: The association of retroperitoneal fibrosis with systemic vasculitis and HLA-B27: A case report and review of the literature. J Rheum 8:665, 1981. *Vasculitis has been documented histologically in 37 of 500 cases reviewed and may be much more common. An association with HLA-B27 and sacroiliitis is seen in this case.*

MEDIASTINAL FIBROSIS

Taut bundles of collagenous tissue form in the superior and anterior mediastinum with impingement on the aorta, trachea, esophagus, and pericardium, but the predominant manifestations are those caused by obstruction of the superior vena cava: puffy, suffused appearance of the face and conjunctivae; nonpitting edema of the face, neck, and upper extremities; and distended veins in the neck and upper extremities. Rarely the principal vessels affected are the pulmonary arteries, causing pulmonary hypertension. More frequently the pulmonary veins are involved, and here severe hemoptysis may be the most prominent manifestation. The main task in differential diagnosis is to distinguish this relatively benign condition from obstruction caused by tumor. Roentgenographic examination of the chest may reveal little or no abnormality, but angiographic studies show obstruction of the affected vessels. Thoracotomy may be required for histologic diagnosis.

As already mentioned, histoplasmosis, and possibly tuberculosis too, may be a cause of mediastinal fibrosis; therefore these should be considered. Some patients with this syndrome have shown gradual improvement over months or years, presumably because of development of collateral circulation. Successful superior vena cava bypass surgery has been described.

Doty DB: Bypass of superior vena cava: Six years experience with spiral vein graft for obstruction of superior vena cava due to benign and malignant disease. J Thorac Cardiovasc Surg 83:326, 1982. *Superior vena cava syndrome relieved for up to six years. Four patients had fibrosing mediastinitis.*

Dye TE, Saab SB, Almond MD, Watson L: Sclerosing mediastinitis with occlusion of pulmonary veins. J Thorac Cardiovasc Surg 74:137, 1977. *An unusual and serious but treatable cause of hemoptysis.*

Goodwin RA, Nickell JA, Dez Prez RM: Mediastinal fibrosis complicating healed primary histoplasmosis and tuberculosis. Medicine 51:227, 1972. *Excellent review, certainly implicating histoplasmosis.*

PRACTOLOL PERITONITIS

An unusual fibrotic syndrome has been observed in patients treated with the beta-adrenergic blocking drug practolol. This drug closely resembles propranolol in chemical structure, but the risk of fibrotic reaction in the peritoneum is far smaller, perhaps nonexistent, with propranolol.

Practolol peritonitis seldom manifests itself in less than 12 months after beginning treatment. Some cases have developed a year or longer after cessation of therapy. Thus, although practolol has been withdrawn from use, occasional late occurring cases might still be seen. The peritonitis consists of a thick fibrous encasement of the small intestine, and the symptoms are those of subacute obstruction. It has usually been possible to relieve the symptoms by surgery, with blunt dissection to peel away the fibrous tissue. Some improvement occurs with time. A few patients have developed apparently related respiratory disease.

Part XXIII
NEUROLOGIC AND BEHAVIORAL DISEASES
Section One CLINICAL STUDY OF THE PATIENT WITH NEUROLOGIC SYMPTOMS

467. APPROACH TO THE PATIENT, INCLUDING GENERAL MANAGEMENT

Fred Plum

Patients with symptoms and signs referable to the nervous system place special requirements on the physician's clinical approach. The most immediate task is to consider whether the symptoms are merely the nonspecific signals of a systemic disorder or reflect intrinsic neurologic disease. Pain, headache, nausea, dizziness, fatigue, and weakness all lack specificity until taken in context with the rest of the history and physical findings; as often as not, such symptoms can reflect the emotional ravages of disturbed psychologic adjustment. To understand and treat human beings requires that the doctor know *who* is sick as much as or more often than *what* is sick. Put in Peabody's words, "The secret of the care of the patient is caring for the patient."

A second major consideration is to realize that although all patients are to some degree frightened of illness, concern over the possibility of paralysis, severe pain, or mental impairment instills an especial terror which requires the doctor's attention and reassurance. When examining such patients, if at all possible follow Osler's dictum: "Do the kind thing and do it first."

The third major consideration stems from the nervous system's vulnerability to damage and its inability to repair itself. In a broad sense, the purpose of the practice of medicine is to protect the brain. Man's brain makes him human. Damage it and life loses its meaning in direct proportion, no matter what other physiologic benefits may accrue in the process. The brain cannot be regenerated, repaired, or homotransplanted. It accumulates no metabolic debts, and, unless supplied continuously by an effective circulation carrying a large volume of oxygen and substrates, it digests itself promptly and irreparably. The doctor's mandate is clear: in seriously and acutely ill patients with neurologic abnormalities, life- or brain-threatening complications must be treated even while proceeding with diagnostic procedures which may take several more minutes, hours, or days to complete.

Wise and sensitive management of the neurologic patient requires attention to both disease and humane need. In general, the more specific and acute the illness, the less immediately important become the broad concerns of the patient. By contrast, patients whose diseases lack quick and specific remedies (e.g., most degenerative diseases, most residua of severe trauma) usually need far more from the doctor than the local pharmacy can supply. Three important maxims apply to all treatment situations: protect the brain first, no matter what successive steps must follow; relieve pain even while proceeding with diagnosis; and give reassurance, hope, and explanation at every step along the way. To plan long-term management effectively and economically, try to construct an accurate prognosis as early as possible. In acute, self-limited illnesses, such as meningococcal meningitis or most acute inflammatory polyneuritis, for example, one knows the probable outcome within a few days of onset. One even knows for most such patients the difference in convalescent time required before they will return to their former occupations. However, with diseases with intermediate outcomes such as multiple sclerosis, full recovery is less certain and the risk of relapse or chronic disability may require the physician to appraise all aspects of the patient's life in order to give proper guidance. At the third extreme are patients who become severely aphasic and hemiplegic from stroke or demented from Alzheimer's disease. They may never recover independence, and their proper early management requires that one guide whole families through major social and financial readjustments in planning for the future. How the doctor manages such complexities determines to a considerable degree his effectiveness as a physician.

Bennett AE: Communication Between Doctors and Patients. London, Oxford University Press, 1976. *A series of essays with a particularly good chapter by Maguire and Rutter on interviewing techniques for medical students.*

DeJong RN: The Neurological Examination. 4th ed. Hagerstown, MD, Harper & Row, 1979. *A comprehensive and detailed explanation of the technique and physiology of the examination.*

Elstein AS, Shulman LS, Sprafka SA: Medical Problem Solving. An Analysis of Clinical Reasoning. Cambridge, MA, Harvard University Press, 1978. *An excellent description of how clinical problems are solved.*

Emerson CP: Reminiscences of Sir William Osler. Int Assoc Med Museums Bull 1926, p 294. *A volume of gems on teaching, care, and scholarship by America's greatest clinician.*

Mayo Clinic and Foundation: Clinical Examinations in Neurology. Philadelphia, W.B. Saunders Company, 1981. *A useful compendium of clinical and electrophysiologic approaches to neurologic diagnosis.*

Peabody FW: The care of the patient. JAMA 88:877, 1927. *A thoughtful and compassionate statement about the doctor-patient relationship.*

468. PRINCIPLES OF DIAGNOSIS

Fred Plum

Two major, alternative strategies underlie the way that most physicians approach the process of diagnosis. One, *pattern recognition,* is the classic technique of putting together the symptoms and signs into a syndrome and determining that the result conforms to a condition that the doctor has read about, has previously observed, or can ferret from the medical literature. The method profits by experience and specialization and relies relatively less on an analytic consideration of basic mechanisms in disease. The other, *logic and probability,* consists of analyzing signs and symptoms as manifestations of disordered physiology and deducing their meaning in terms of the anatomic structures involved and the way diseases affect these structures. The reliability of the resulting diagnostic hypothesis is tested by estimating the probability that certain abnormalities in bodily mechanisms will accompany one another and by the knowledge of the frequency with which such involvements occur. History, physical examination, and laboratory tests serve as constant back-checks and extensions of the deductive process. Skillful physicians utilize both pattern recognition and logic-probability in varying measure. The pattern-recognizing qualities of astute clinicians can reach legendary quality, but even the most experienced doctors usually mentally test their diagnostic impressions against a physiologic benchmark to see if the implied pathophysiology "makes sense" (i.e., fulfills physiologic probabilities). For the young physician, especially as scientific knowledge grows in medicine, a logical approach based on deductions from pathophysiology is imperative, for it focuses attention on the patient's main problem and avoids the pitfall of treating minor symptoms or laboratory perturbations that provide no threat to the patient's health. Particularly in neurologic diagnosis the strong communicative power of the nervous system and its reflections of the patient's inner self mean that information derived from the history and neurologic examination usually lends itself to logical analysis and probability testing (e.g., is it likely that *this* patient would have *this* disorder at *this* time with *this* combination of symptoms?).

Armed with a provisional diagnostic formulation in anatomic and physiologic terms, the physician then should require only a limited number of laboratory tests to establish the precise mechanism of disease or to rule out the presence of some other, unsuspected condition or illness. One should recall, however, that the complexity of disease is such that even the most exhaustive efforts accurately diagnose only about 85 per cent of first time admissions to major medical centers. The number of relatively trivial uncertainties and errors probably rises higher in ambulatory patients with self-limited problems which inherently receive less attention or disappear without causing serious disability.

The first step in neurologic diagnosis is anatomic. To arrive at a regional diagnosis one asks: Does the patient have a structural disease (i.e., is the process organic, physiologic-functional, or psychiatric)? If a disease is present, is it monofocal or diffuse? Given the likelihood that a neurologic disorder is present, one asks in succession: Are the lesions peripheral (i.e., at the receptor, muscle effector, synapse, or nerve) or central (i.e., in the spinal cord or brain)? If central, does the disease affect structures above or below the foramen magnum, above or below the tentorium, on the right or the left side? Is the process static, worsening, or improving? Given the answer or answers to these questions, one can then formulate a patho-logic-etiologic diagnosis according to whether the evidence suggests a disorder that is genetic, developmental, traumatic, environmental-toxic, infectious, immunologic, degenerative, neoplastic, metabolic, nutritional, physiologic (e.g., epilepsy, migraine), or psychophysiologic (e.g., tension backache, vasodepressor syncope). One then proceeds to nonspecific and specific laboratory tests in order to confirm the clinical diagnostic hypotheses.

469. THE NEUROLOGIC HISTORY

Jerome B. Posner

In most respects, the neurologic history is similar to the general medical history. The purpose (to supply diagnostic information that will direct the physical and laboratory examinations and lead to an appropriate diagnosis) and the format (e.g., chief complaint, present illness, past history, social history, review of systems) are the same. However, the neurologic history usually supplies a greater proportion of the diagnostically relevant information than does a medical history; many neurologic diseases are not accompanied by abnormal physical or laboratory findings, and in these instances the physician must depend solely on the history to reach an appropriate diagnosis. Even when the patient suffers from a neurologic disease marked by physical signs and/or laboratory abnormalities, the history usually supplies about 80 per cent of the total diagnostic information. Furthermore, because neurologic abnormalities affect such important functions as thinking, moving, and feeling, it is unusual for patients to have significant abnormal signs which have not been perceived as symptoms by the patient. (Exceptions occur in demented patients and those with lesions of the nondominant parietal lobe, characterized by denial of disability. In these instances, abnormal behavior is recognized by family and friends.) Thus, findings on examination not recognized by the patient (or his family) are likely to be irrelevant or even misleading. By contrast, symptoms complained of by the patient, such as mild weakness or alterations of sensation, are probably significant even if too subtle to be detected by the most meticulous neurologic examination. (For example, a patient who complains of horizontal diplopia on extreme left lateral gaze is probably suffering from weakness of the left lateral rectus even if the finding is absent at the time of examination, e.g., myasthenia gravis, or too subtle for the physician to detect. On the other hand, the physician's finding by "red glass test" of horizontal diplopia in extreme lateral gaze in a patient who does not complain of diplopia probably represents congenital weakness of the muscle and is of no consequence.) Finally, because neurologic symptoms are so keenly appreciated by the patient, a meticulous history often allows a physician to localize the disease anatomically and to understand its pathophysiology even before he begins the physical examination.

Taking the neurologic history does (or should) occupy the majority of time spent with a patient suffering a neurologic disorder. At the completion of the history, the physician should be able either to make a definite diagnosis or to formulate three or four hypotheses which can be tested by the physical and laboratory examinations. Because there are an almost infinite number of potential questions which might be asked of a patient with a neurologic disorder, the physician must develop a strategy that allows him to achieve the maximal useful information in a reasonable period of time. Elements of that strategy are listed below. (Specific questions which might elicit useful diagnostic information in patients suffering from neurologic disease may be found in standard texts on the neurologic history and evaluation and, in this textbook, under the descriptions of specific diseases.) In taking a neurologic history, the physician must observe the following guidelines:

BE INTERESTED AND SUPPORTIVE. The purpose of the neurologic history is not only to gain diagnostic information but also to learn enough about the patient's psychologic and social background to establish a satisfactory doctor-patient relationship, and thus to be able to manage the patient's illness satisfactorily. Diagnostic information is often lost when the patient does not volunteer symptoms that he believes would not interest the physician or that are too intimate or embarrassing to tell to an "unsympathetic stranger." Such information will be volunteered to the physician who demonstrates by his attitude his interest, reassurance, and support.

BE ALERT TO NONVERBAL CUES. What the patient does is often as important as what he says. The patient's overall appearance and demeanor, his tone of voice, or a sigh or a tear in discussing what appear to be relatively trivial symptoms may be important clues to an underlying depression or severe anxiety over those symptoms.

REQUIRE PRECISION. Interviewers should not accept jargon or names of diseases from the patient. Jargon terms such as "dizziness" or diagnostic appellations such as "sinus headache" require a thorough exploration of the exact nature of the symptom and its effect on the patient. For example, a patient who complains of dizziness may mean vertigo (a vestibular symptom), lightheadedness (potentially caused by cardiovascular disease), syncope, ataxia, diplopia, or psychogenic dissociation—all symptoms which have very different physiologic meanings. "Sinus headache" is a diagnostic term often given to or used by patients to describe headaches which in fact are rarely caused by sinusitis but are usually migraine or tension headache.

MAINTAIN A BALANCE BETWEEN LISTENING AND ASKING. Physicians should elicit the history in the patient's own words and, whenever possible, should allow the patient to tell the story without interruption. Excessive interruptions indicate to the patient that the physician is in a hurry or disinterested, and may lead the patient to exclude vital information. By hearing the patient out, the physician often gains important information concerning the patient's fears and anxieties. However, the physician must ask direct questions to encourage relevance, achieve precision, and place each symptom in its correct context. If the patient does not volunteer it, the physician must ask about the intensity and frequency of the complained symptoms, their duration, events and factors that precipitate or relieve them, and any other symptoms associated in time with the patient's major complaint. For example, a patient with "cluster headaches" (see Ch. 477) may complain only of severe, disabling headache, but careful questioning may reveal that the headaches occur in two- to three-month clusters once or twice a year, characteristically appear three times a day, are always localized in and around the left eye, last no more than 30 to 40 minutes, are the most intense pain the patient has ever experienced, frequently awaken him at night, and can always be precipitated by alcohol intake during the cluster period. Such a precise history allows no other diagnosis.

FORM HYPOTHESES. The physician cannot be a passive recipient of the patient's story. The patient supplies too much information, much of it not diagnostically relevant, for the physician to recall at a later time, even with notes. Thus, the physician, while taking the history, must sift and distill the information as he receives it in order to retain what is relevant and be allowed to forget irrelevant information. Concurrently, he must form hypotheses about the nature of the patient's symptoms as they are presented, and test those hypotheses by asking pertinent questions. Hypotheses are tested and refined during the course of taking the history, so that by the end of the history the physician has three or four potential diagnoses to guide his physical and laboratory examinations. The best hypotheses are broad explanations of the patient's symptoms in anatomic and/or pathophysiologic terms, which are gradually refined into etiologic terms as the history develops. (For example, in a patient complaining of weakness of the right arm and leg, the hypotheses might include a left hemispheral structural lesion or a cervical cord lesion. As the physician elicits a history of weakness in the face and difficulty with language, the cervical cord hypothesis can be discarded and the left hemispheral lesion accepted. Additional history of slowly progressive weakness accompanied by headache and lethargy will lead the physician to hypothesize a mass lesion of the left hemisphere, possibly hematoma, tumor, or abscess, and a history of heavy smoking with recent cough could lead him to consider a metastatic lung tumor. At the end of the history, the physician has arrived at the conclusion that the patient has a mass lesion in the left hemisphere and has hypothesized several etiologic entities.) Hypotheses should give preference to those illnesses that are probable (i.e., common diseases are more likely than rare diseases), serious (e.g., brain tumors should be considered before tension headache), treatable (e.g., combined systems disease and spinal cord meningioma should be ruled out before making a diagnosis of multiple sclerosis), and novel (some patients do indeed have rare diseases, and these should not be forgotten in taking the history).

ALWAYS TAKE A COMPLETE HISTORY. Even if the diagnosis seems clear from the chief complaint and the present illness, other aspects of the patient's history must be elicited to ensure that other physical or psychologic disabilities are not playing a role in the patient's discomfort. In particular, inquiry must be made about the patient's mood (e.g., is he depressed or suicidal?), his usual daily activities (and whether the illness interferes with them), his sexual activities, the nature of psychologic and physical support at home, and his view of the illness and how it affects him.

END BY SUMMARIZING. At the end of the history it is useful to summarize the history as the physician understands it, asking the patient if the summary is correct and if anything has been missed. Such a summary gives the patient a chance to supply information which may have been left out in the initial history and to correct any misunderstandings. It also allows the patient to present new data on areas concerning him.

OBTAIN FURTHER HISTORY FROM THE PATIENT'S FAMILY AND FRIENDS. If the history appears incomplete, and particularly if part of the patient's illness involves changes in mental state or episodic unconsciousness, the patient's family, friends, and colleagues should be asked to corroborate the history and to supply missing elements, giving their views on how the signs and symptoms affect the patient's daily life.

GEAR THE NEUROLOGIC EXAMINATION TO THE HYPOTHESES. It is neither possible nor desirable to perform all elements of the neurologic examination on every patient. Thus, the hypotheses generated during the course of the history determine which of the nonroutine neurologic maneuvers the physician will carry out during the course of his examination. For example, olfactory sensation need not be tested routinely, but if the physician has hypothesized a frontal lobe tumor, significant head injury, or pernicious anemia, all of which may affect olfactory sensation, then this function must be tested. A complaint of intermittent numbness in an upper extremity should lead the physician to test for compromise of the thoracic outlet, even though that is not part of the routine neurologic examination. In similar fashion, hypotheses generated during the history direct the laboratory examination even in the presence of a normal neurologic examination. For example, if the history gives strong evidence of a left hemispheral mass lesion, failure to find a hemiparesis on examination does not rule out a brain tumor, and a computed tomographic scan must be performed. Even if the tests are initially uninformative, a strongly suggestive history requires that the doctor follow the patient closely.

470. THE NEUROLOGIC EXAMINATION

Fred Plum

Several texts can be consulted for the detailed techniques of bedside neurologic examinations. The necessary length of the complete examination and the potentially bewildering complexity of detailed neuroanatomy sometimes intimidate students and general physicians. This is unfortunate, because an understanding of a few fundamental principles about the nervous system plus the mastering of a relatively brief but systematically thorough approach to the examination can give a working knowledge that allows for the reliable and effective practice of medicine. The secret is to learn a relatively rapidly applied approach that covers the main elements of nervous system function and to be familiar with how to apply more exhaustive evaluations to selective functions if and when material in the history or the baseline examination suggests abnormalities in special parts.

An effective neurologic examination proceeds from general to specific in its principles and rostral to caudal in its anatomy. Such an examination checks on the integrity of major functions and yet avoids bogging down in details which do not relate to the complaints of most patients. In awake and talking patients, listen to them as they give their histories. Begin at that point to evaluate mental status and language (inconsistencies? vagueness on important points? word-blocking? circumlocutions? paraphasias? agrammaticisms?). Apply at least a brief mental examination on everyone, but be gentle and understanding: "How has your memory been? Can I just check a couple of points with you?" Check orientation. Examine memory for recent events, for public figures, and for three unrelated words at five minutes. Review the capacity to handle abstractions (boy—dwarf, small tree—bush, proverbs). Provide a problem in simple arithmetic (nickels in $1.35). Check serial sevens. Have the patient repeat five numbers backwards or the spelling of "world." But be patient and remember that anxiety can occlude the performance of even a normally good mind. Have the patient stand and walk; remember that the nervous system is the organ of communication and behavior, and that one learns most about man while watching him attempt natural tasks. Watch the patient at least partially dress and undress (apraxia); remark on alertness-dullness; hyperactivity-apathy; adventitious movement–akinesia; visible deformities, asymmetries, or weaknesses in functional tasks; hypertrophies-atrophies; cutaneous abnormalities (pox, birthmarks, café au lait spots, pigmented or hair spots over spinal defects); a straight, flat, or crooked spine. In other words, learn to observe constantly and closely, comparing always what you see with what you already have seen in thousands of people living everyday lives.

Examine cranial functions, screening certain structures and

innervations in every patient. Palpate the skull and test the neck gently for suppleness and length. Then examine in everyone vision (rough fields and acuity), the optic fundi, pupillary activity, ocular movements, corneal reflexes, jaw movement, facial movement, bilateral hearing, swallowing, speaking, and breathing. One can omit or defer from most routine examinations such tests as those of smell, taste, facial sensation, labyrinthine-vestibular activity, sternocleidomastoid function, or the integrity of detailed tongue movements unless symptoms suggest the involvement of these bodily areas. Examine in everyone the extremities and trunk for symmetry (hypertrophy or atrophy), size, at least grossly for strength, muscle tonus, adventitious movements (e.g., tremors, fasciculations, tics), coordination (rhythmic movements and point-to-point tests), and reflexes. If the patient has no sensory symptoms, he is unlikely to have abnormal sensory signs. Nevertheless, make a brief check of the distal extremities for the threshold perception of vibration and pin prick before deciding that things are normal. Examine the plantar responses. Evaluate autonomic and sphincter functions as part of the general medical examination. Get in the habit of examining the neck over the carotid arteries for bruits that may herald partial stenoses. Above all, be systematic and consistent in the approach and *do not jump at diagnosis until all the evidence is in.* Doctors often make diagnoses too quickly and surrender wrong ones reluctantly. By contrast, they view even partial unknowns as challenging problems. Try to choose the latter approach until matters become certain.

USE OF LABORATORY TESTS. Advances in laboratory methods during recent years have remarkably increased the accuracy of diagnosis and physiologic evaluations. At the same time, excessive technology raises the costs of medical care unnecessarily. More than anything else, the physician's ordering practices influence this aspect of health care costs. The doctor must recognize the precise advantages for both positive and negative knowledge that derive from each test, and order only those which add substantially to the patient's evaluation and treatment. To give an example: when managing an adult with recent onset of headache, the results of a computed tomographic scan, whether normal or abnormal, commonly help the doctor's management and provide the patient with great reassurance. However, to repeat the scan just to intensify reassurance for a querulous patient or an insecure physician wastes the time and resources of all concerned.

471. NEUROLOGIC DIAGNOSTIC PROCEDURES

Samuel Rapoport

LUMBAR PUNCTURE

With the advent of modern brain imaging devices, lumbar puncture is performed far less often currently than in the past. Nevertheless, sampling the cerebrospinal fluid (CSF) remains an indispensable step in diagnosing several infectious diseases and is an emergency procedure in cases of suspected bacterial meningitis. Table 471–1 gives other indications and contradications. Other considerations of when and when not to do lumbar puncture can be found in Ch. 476. Postlumbar puncture headache is discussed in Ch. 475.

TABLE 471–1. INDICATIONS AND CONTRAINDICATIONS FOR LUMBAR PUNCTURE

Diagnostic:	Known or suspected meningitis-encephalitis Acute: Bacterial, viral Subacute: Tuberculous, syphilitic, fungal, neoplastic Chronic: Syphilitic, granulomatous, neoplastic Intracranial-intraspinal hemorrhage (when no CT is available)
Useful:	Multiple sclerosis Acute polyneuropathy Suspected benign intracranial hypertension (CT negative)
Contraindicated:	Noninfectious states of undiagnosed increased intracranial pressure Thrombocytopenia or anticoagulated states Local skin or epidural infections
Therapeutic:	Antimicrobial or anticancer therapy

IMAGING TECHNIQUES

Brain, Dura, and Skull

COMPUTERIZED TOMOGRAPHY. Computerized tomography (CT) is performed by measuring transmission of an x-ray beam across the brain and computing density differences in two dimensions based on the amount of radiation that is transmitted across a tomographic slice of variable thickness. The resulting image displays density of tissue on a black and white scale. Water produces the least dense reference and is portrayed as black. Relatively more dense tissue appears progressively whiter, with bone and metallic objects being the whitest. A typical scan depicts the spinal fluid in the cerebral ventricles and subarachnoid spaces as black, the calvarium as dense white, the cortical gray matter as light gray, and the cortical white matter as a darker gray. Masses of blood within brain tissue appear as circumscribed white or gray-white images, while areas of encephalomalacia, such as result from cerebral infarcts, emerge as dark gray. Resolution with current instruments yields excellent images of the cerebrum, differentiating among cortical mantle, white matter tracts, deep nuclei, and cerebral ventricles. Shifts of intracranial structures caused by mass lesions are readily detectable. CT is currently the most accessible way of accurately and safely evaluating structural lesions of the brain and surrounding dural and osseous structures. The 5 mm spatial resolution of present techniques, as well as the ability of many machines to calculate the volume of a desired brain area, makes it easy to determine changes in the size of lesions as a function of time or treatment. Intravenously administered iodinated x-ray contrast agents leak across the abnormally permeable capillary beds of certain intraparenchymal brain lesions, providing an increase in the scan density of the desired areas. Such enhancement becomes particularly useful in detecting lesions that are isodense with normal surrounding brain on routine CT scans, as well as lesions whose small size falls below the spatial resolution of the instument.

Advantages. The general availability of CT scans, as well as the short time required for a complete examination, renders it a most valuable emergency diagnostic procedure. In victims of head trauma with neurologic abnormalities, CT scanning allows immediate determination of whether hemorrhage has occurred intraparenchymally or in one of the dural compartments, thus guiding therapy. In patients with acute stroke, CT readily distinguishes hemorrhage from ischemia, guiding decisions for anticoagulant therapy. Brain tumors usually can be differentiated from their surrounding edema, and the response of intracranial abscesses to antimicrobial therapy can be monitored. The degree of cerebral atrophy can be assessed. The ratio of ventricular size to the size of the cortical subarachnoid spaces provides a useful index of hydrocephalus, and the density of the white matter surrounding the ventricies often gives an indication of how recently the process has arisen. Most abnormalities of the skull, orbits, neural foramina, and cranial sinuses can be detected, making obsolete most skull x-rays and almost all nuclide brain scans.

Disadvantages. CT scans cannot detect lesions smaller than 5 mm in diameter, and they often visualize posterior fossa structures poorly because of artifacts generated by surrounding bone. Subacute subdural hematomas sometimes generate an image isodense with surrounding brain, rendering them undetectable. Small brain tumors located superficially on the cortex are often difficult to detect, even after contrast injections, because of averaging artifact from the surrounding bone. Small, low-grade infiltrating brain tumors may have a density very close to that of surrounding brain tissue and possess too little blood-brain barrier permeability to be detected. Almost no nonstructural brain diseases disfigure the CT scan. The technique often cannot differentiate between tumor and infarct, or among metastatic tumor, primary tumor, and brain abscess. The resolution of CT is insufficient to detect any but giant cerebral aneurysms. Assessment of the cerebral vasculature requires angiography.

NUCLEAR MAGNETIC RESONANCE (NMR). NMR measures the energy required to align the nuclear dipoles of hydrogen protons so that they point in the same direction when tissue is placed in a magnetic field. The technique provides a density map of hydrogen protons that can be processed to generate a video image that reproduces the cross-sectional anatomy of the brain with very high spatial detail and contrast resolution.

Indications. NMR, unlike CT, is unaffected by the artifact of x-rays reflected from bone, so that it generates better images of the structures of the posterior fossa. For similar reasons, better assessment of the intrasellar contents can be achieved. NMR has the unique ability to image the longitudinal axis of the brain and cervical spine, and it depicts both the normal and abnormal anatomy of the craniocervical and spinomedullary junctions more clearly than does any other diagnostic procedure. Owing to substantially better resolution powers, down to a millimeter or less with powerful magnets, NMR can detect plaques of multiple sclerosis and post-traumatic contusions far better than can CT. NMR is clearly superior to CT scanning in detecting intra-axial brainstem tumors. It is not yet fully established whether one technique is more sensitive than the other for detection of the majority of brain tumors, strokes, and other structural lesions. Instrumentation of NMR is advancing so rapidly that any conclusions at this juncture would be premature.

Disadvantages. NMR is not suitable for emergency situations, since life-support equipment can be drawn vigorously and violently into the magnet. Similarly, patients with surgical clips or metallic prostheses cannot be introduced into the magnetic field. The procedure currently requires 45 minutes to complete fully satisfactory images. The long-term risks of exposure to a large magnetic field are believed to be negligible; the technique is totally noninvasive and free of exposure to x-rays.

Spine, Spinal Cord, and Cauda Equina

Bony abnormalities of the spine, including primary or metastatic tumors and vertebral collapses, usually can be detected by conventional x-rays. Radiographs of the cervical spine are indispensable for evaluating abnormalities of the foramen magnum and displacement of the odontoid due to fractures. Demonstration that such abnormalities are impinging on neural tissue requires myelography. When one suspects root compression alone, such as with herniated discs, myelography performed with water-based contrast agents provides superior resolution to other agents, especially in the region of the cauda equina, and outlines the configuration of individual roots. Water-based agents, however, frequently cause nausea, vomiting, headache, and transient encephalopathy; since these agents are absorbed from the spinal fluid into the systemic circulation and excreted through the kidney, they can trigger allergic reactions in susceptible individuals. Rarely, they may cause renal insufficiency. These side effects are seldom observed with oil-based myelographic dyes such as Pantopaque. In patients with metastatic cancer it is advisable to perform myelography with Pantopaque so that the effects of treatment can be evaluated later by flouroscopy. NMR can provide longitudinal views of the spine, epidural space, and neural tissue, outlining bony abnormalities and intervertebral discs as they impinge on neural tissue.

Myelography demonstrates intrinsic spinal cord abnormalities such as tumors or syrinxes as circumscribed narrowings of the contrast column in the subarachnoid space. CT scanning through areas of such abnormalities reveals their tissue density, differentiating solid tumor from cyst. Longitudinal images of the spinal cord on NMR permit one to visualize the total length of the tumor or syrinx as well as cross-sectional views through the abnormality. Conventional CT scanning fails to provide longitudinal views of the spine and spinal cord, and to be certain of the total length and of the level of the spinal abnormality one must perform multiple transverse CT cuts. The spinal cord is not well visualized by CT scan, which must be enhanced with subarachnoid contrast material for adequate evaluation of intraspinal lesions. Intervertebral disc protrusion can be confirmed with conventional transverse CT scans, but clear definition of impingement on spinal roots or cord similarly requires the injection of subarachnoid contrast material.

NEURAL PLEXUS. In patients in whom soft tissue masses are suspected of impinging on the brachial or the lumbosacral plexus, CT scanning through the area provides the most valuable available technique for delineating the lesion and the local extent of its spread.

ELECTRODIAGNOSTIC STUDIES

Electroencephalography (EEG)

The electroencephalogram is a record of the electronically amplified dendritic activity of the superficial layers of the cerebral cortex. The instrument is indispensable for documenting the presence and type of epileptiform discharges, aiding the diagnosis of seizure disorders. In patients with altered states of consciousness, EEG helps differentiate seizures from metabllic encephalopathy and aids in distinguishing between organic and psychogenic causes of unresponsiveness. When seizures develop in comatose or theraputically paralyzed patients, the EEG can delineate the response to treatment, making it possible to titrate anticonvulsant dosage against cessation of epileptiform discharges. Absence of EEG activity supports the diagnosis of brain death.

Sensory Evoked Potentials

Measurement of the EEG time-locked to a visual, auditory, or somatosensory stimulus generates modality-specific potentials that are highly reporducible and provide information on the integrity of the pathway carrying the signal.

VISUAL EVOKED POTENTIALS (VEP). VEP usually are performed by haveing the subject fixate on a reversing black-white checkerboard pattern. Electrodes placed over the scalp record a positive potential, the latency of which is related to conduction in the optic nerve and central visual pathways. The method is

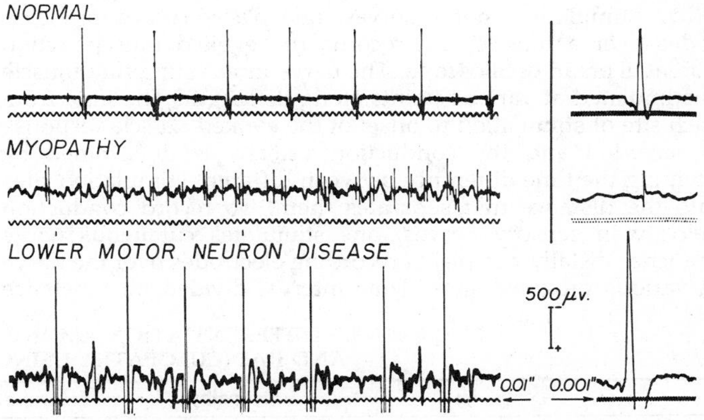

Figure 471–1. Diagram of muscle electrical activity showing motor action potentials during weak voluntary contraction of the biceps brachii. Note the normal amplitude and duration of the potentials on the top line compared to small, short duration potentials in muscular dystrophy and the enlarged amplitude and duration in amyotrophic lateral sclerosis. (From Aronson AE, Anger RG, et al.: Clinical Examinations in Neurology, 5th ed. Mayo Clinic and Mayo Foundation, 1981.)

TABLE 471–2. PATTERN OF EMG AND NERVE CONDUCTION ABNORMALITIES IN MONONEUROPATHY, POLYNEUROPATHY, RADICULOPATHY, AXONOPATHY, AND MOTONEURON DISEASE

	EMG Abnormality	Nerve Conduction Abnormality
Mononeuropathy	Limited to muscles innervated by damaged nerve	Limited to damaged nerve
Polyneuropathy	Diffuse	Diffuse
Radiculopathy	Limited to muscles innervated by damaged root	Usually none
Axonopathy/Motoneuron Disease	Diffuse	None

highly sensitive for detecting demyelination of the optic nerve, whether produced by compression, toxic agents, metabolic abnormalities, or multiple sclerosis.

BRAINSTEM AUDITORY EVOKED POTENTIALS (BAEP). Presentation of a white noise click stimulus to the ear generates a series of potentials from the brainstem auditory relay pathway, which can be recorded over the scalp at the vertex. The clinically relevant potentials occur within the first 10 milliseconds following the stimulus. The first potential recorded is generated by the auditory nerve, and subsequent potentials are generated, respectively, in the superior olive, lateral lemniscus, and inferior colliculus. Thus, a measure of conduction between various points along the auditory pathway between eighth nerve and inferior colliculus is provided. BAEPs detect abnormalities due to demyelinative, destructive, or compressive lesions affecting brainstem auditory pathways.

SOMATOSENSORY EVOKED POTENTIALS (SEP). Stimulation of a peripheral nerve by pulse of constant voltage or constant current gives rise to potentials that can be recorded over the spine and scalp. The median or peroneal nerves are most often stimulated. Stimulation of a lower extremity nerve, such as the peroneal, gives rise to a volley whose transit can be recorded at all levels of the spine. If bipolar electrode arrays are placed over the spine, the latency of the recorded potential increases progressively from lumbar to cervical spine and brain. Measurement permits calculation of a conduction velocity that is thought to reflect conduction in the posterior columns of the spinal cord. The time interval between the potential recorded at the cauda equina and over the scalp measures total conduction time in the somatosensory pathway. Any lesion, whether demyelinative, nutritional, compressive, or destructive, that affects this ascending pathway in spinal cord or brainstem can delay the total conduction time.

Electromyography and Nerve Conduction Studies

Appropriate percutaneous electrical stimulation of a peripheral nerve excites the nerve to generate an action potential. When stimulating motor nerves, one places recording elelctrodes over a muscle and records the evoked muscle action potential on an oscilloscope. The nerve innervating that muscle is stimulated at various points along its length. The time from each site of stimulation to onset of the evoked muscle response is recorded and the conduction velocity is determined by dividing the time difference between different stimulation sites into the distance that separates them. To record conduction velocity in sensory nerves, one stimulates cutaneous nerve branches distally and places recording electrodes over the nerve at various proximal sites. Time interval divided into distance again provides the conduction velocity. The *F-response* gives an indication of conduction in motor nerves from the site of stimulation antidromically to the motoneuron and orthodromically back to the site of recording; when analyzed in conjunction with the conduction velocity of the more distal portions of the nerve, it provides a measure of conduction in the proximal portions of a motor nerve and ventral root. The *H-reflex* provides the electrical equivalent of the stretch reflex by stimulating sensory fibers of the posterior tibial nerve in the popliteal fossa at low intesnsities and recording the muscle evoked action potential from the soleus muscle. These peripheral nerve and muscle electrophysiologic studies assist in determining whether disease involves nerve, muscle, or both and in determining the distribution of abnormality. They facilitate the differentiation of demyelinating neuropathy from axonal neuropathy, neuropathy from radiculopathy, and primary muscle disease from disease of the motor unit. Demyelinating neuropathies affect mainly large fibers and slow the conduction velocity. When disease damages axons in addition to myelin, there is a decrease in the number of axons that can be electrically activated, resulting in a diminution in the size of the compound action potential.

Electromyography (EMG) is performed by inserting a needle electrode into the muscle to record the structure's electrical activity (Fig. 471–1). Under normal circumstances muscle at rest is silent, but in denervated or diseased states muscle membranes become spontaneously excitable, generating fibrillation potentials of small amplitude. When the nerve itself is diseased, entire motor units may become spontaneously active. The resulting fasciculations are often visible percutaneously and can be detected by the electrode. Furthermore, when damaged axons cease to innervate muscle fibers, remaining axons gradually sprout collaterals that reinnervate the denervated fibers; consequently, the size of the few remaining motor units increases. As a result, in partially denervated muscles one records during voluntary contraction a decrease in the number and an increase in the size of the electrical potentials generated by the activated motor units. By contrast, as muscle fibers degenerate in primary disease of muscle, the size of motor units decreases, since each nerve now innervates fewer fibers: during voluntary contration the number of activated units is normal but their amplitude is smaller. The anatomic distribution of abnormalities helps differentiate a mononeuropathy from a generalized neuropathy and a radiculopathy from a neuropathy. In primary myopathies, the distribution of abnormality helps in characterizing the myopathy itself. Tables 471–2 and 471–3 provide guides to the usefulness and pertinent changes in electrophysiologic tests in various neuromuscular disorders.

TABLE 471–3. DIFFERENTIATION AMONG MYOPATHY, AXONOPATHY, MYELINOPATHY, AND RADICULOPATHY USING ELECTROPHYSIOLOGIC STUDIES

	Myopathy	Axonopathy	Myelinopathy	Radiculopathy
Nerve conduction velocity	Normal	Normal	Slow	Normal
F-response	Normal	Normal	Delayed/absent	Delayed/absent
H-reflex*	Normal	Normal	Delayed/absent	Delayed/absent
EMG				
Voluntary contraction	Predominance of small motor units	Predominance of large motor units	Normal	Normal/some large motor units
Spontaneous activity	Fibrillations	Fibrillations, fasciculations	Normal	Fibrillations, fasciculations

*Usually studied with posterior tibial nerve stimulation, recording the soleus contraction, thus providing an index of S1 root function only.

NEUROMUSCULAR TRANSMISSION STUDIES

Diseases of the neuromuscular junction (myasthenia gravis, Eaton-Lambert myasthenic syndrome, botulism) are characterized by normal nerve conduction velocity and usually a normal EMG. Repetitive electrical activation of the neuromuscular junction, however, will produce either an abnormal diminution or an abnormal facilitation of the evoked muscle action potential. In myasthenia gravis repetitive stimulation of a peripheral nerve most often causes a rapid progressive decrement of the amplitude of the muscle evoked action potential owing to rapid saturation of the small number of post-synaptic receptors by the released acetylcholine. In botulism and Eaton-Lambert myasthenic syndrome, where the defect is on the presynaptic membrane, repetitive stimulation of the nerve overcomes the presynaptic blockade of acetylcholine release and usually elicits an increase in the size of the muscle evoked action potentials.

Bradbury M, Radda GK, Allen PS: Nuclear magnetic resonance techniques in medicine. Ann Intern Med 98:514, 1983. *A well-written summary of this rapidly advancing field.*

Chiappa KH: Evoked Potentials in Clinical Medicine. New York, Raven Press, 1983. *This and the below-mentioned three texts provide excellent summaries and current references for the field.*

Goodgold J, Eberstein A: Electrodiagnosis of Neuromuscular Disease. Baltimore, William and Wilkins, 1983.

Johnson EW: Practical Electromyography. Baltimore, Williams and Wilkins, 1983.

Mayo Clinic: Clinical Examinations in Neurology. 5th ed. Philadelphia, W. B. Saunders Company, 1981.

Spehlmann R: EEG Primer. New York, Elsevier, 1981. *An excellent general reference on electroencephalography.*

Weisberg LA: Computed tomography in the diagnosis of intracranial disease. Ann Intern Med 91:87, 1979. *A useful summary article.*

Section Two DISORDERS OF CEREBRAL FUNCTION

472. DISTURBANCES OF CONSCIOUSNESS AND AROUSAL

472.1 Sustained Impairment of Consciousness

Jerome B. Posner

PATHOGENESIS

DEFINITIONS. From the medical standpoint, consciousness include two interdependent but separate functions: wakefulness and psychologically recognizable mental activity. Its antithesis, *coma*, is a state of complete mental unresponsiveness with eyes closed and no evidence of psychologically or physiologically appropriate responses to stimulation. Between these antipodes lie a series of abnormal states of mentation and arousal that reflect the effects of different degrees, loci, and acuteness of brain dysfunction damage. *Obtundation* and *drowsiness* describe states of impaired alertness or wakefulness wherein patients continue to respond to verbal stimuli. *Stupor* is a state wherein subjects arouse when vigorously stimulated but immediately sink back to unresponsiveness as soon as external stimuli are withdrawn. Amnesia, asphasia, and dementia are conditions in which the content of consciousness is reduced but relatively normal arousal and sleep-wake cycles remain. The *vegetative state* describes a usually chronic or semichronic condition wherein patients with severe forms of brain damage sleep and awaken but have no recognizable psychological functions. Brainstem and autonomic functions are retained. Vegetative states may follow severe acute brain injuries caused by head trauma or cardiac arrest, for example. Chronic vegetative states also comprise the terminal stages of progressive organic dementias such as Alzheimer's or Huntington's disease. The *locked-in state* describes patients who are awake and retain mental content but owing to paralysis of descending motor pathways, cannot express themselves because of paralysis of the muscles that control speach or facial expression or move the limbs. The site of the lesion usually involves motor pathways in the base of the pons or, less often, midbrain. Sparing of the brainstem tegmentum in these structures explains why consciousness is retained.

MECHANISMS OF CONSCIOUSNESS AND UNCONSCIOUSNESS. The physiologic basis of consciousness depends on close interaction between the intact cerebral hemispheres and activating mechanisms located in the central gray matter of the upper brainstem. The cerebral hemisphere contribute the substrate for most of the specific psychologic components, including language, memory, intellect, and learned responses to sensory stimuli. However, in order for the cerebrum to function and to integrate its component psychologic activities, the hemispheres must be aroused or activated by structures that originate in the thalamus, hypothalamus, midbrain, and tegmentum of the upper pons. An important component of this arousal mechanism is located within what Magoun, Morruzzi, and their colleagues called the ascending reticular activating system; other brainstem systems lying along the deep central gray matter core of the brainstem also influence cerebral cortical activity and the state of consciousness. In addition, conscious behavior is heavily influenced by the activity of intra- and interhemipsheric interconnecting neural pathways.

The relation of the cerebral cortex to consciousness is both quantitative and qualitative. All hemispheric lesions of any great size interfere with both specific somatosensory areas (e.g., vision, cutaneous sensation, movement control) and association cortex. Lesions of the latter alter the integrative aspects of consciousness, and the sudden total loss of the cortex or its connections to the deeper nuclei causes several days or weeks of coma even if the brainstem remains intact. Between the extremes of alert, intelligent consciousness and a state of unresponsive coma lies a continuum along which the size and location of the lesion and the impairment of mind, memory, wit, and personality are roughly proportional to one another.

GENERAL CAUSES AND MANIFESTATIONS OF DELIRIUM, STUPOR, AND COMA

As indicated above, to produce an alteration of consciousness, disease or dysfunction must damage or depress either the two cerebral hemispheres or the upper brainstem or both.

TABLE 472–1. THE COMMON CAUSES OF STUPOR AND COMA

Supratentorial lesions (causing upper brainstem dysfunction)
Cerebral hemorrhage
Large cerebral infarction
Subdural hematoma
Epidural hematoma
Brain tumor
Brain abscess (rare)
Subtentorial lesions (compressing or destroying the reticular formation)
Pontine or cerebellar hemorrhage
Infarction
Tumor
Cerebellar abscess
Metabolic and diffuse lesions (see also Table 472–2)
Anoxia or ischemia
Hypoglycemia
Nutritional deficiency
Endogenous organ failure or deficiency
Exogenous poison
Infections
Meningitis
Encephalitis
Ionic and electrolyte disorders
Concussion and postictal states
Psychogenic unresponsiveness

A potentially bewildering series of individual disorders can have one or both of these effects, as may be seen in Table 472–1. However, if one examines the mechanisms by which neurologic diseases cause coma, real or apparent, these maladies fall into four categories that can be distinguished by their anatomic distribution and the resulting signs and symptoms they produce. These are (1) supratentorial mass lesions, (2) subtentorial compressive or destructive lesions, (3) metabolic brain diseases, and (4) psychogenic unresponsiveness.

Supratentorial Mass Lesions

Supratentorial masses impair consciousness because as they expand they shift and squeeze the contents of the supratentorial compartment and, in so doing, compress the diencephalon. The expanding process can originate anywhere in the hemisphere and ultimately produces this reaction because the fibrous tentorium and the bones of the base of the skull resist movement except toward the tentorial opening. As a result, the diencephalic tectum and adjacent midbrain become compressed, and the diencephalon may be displaced downward through the tentorial notch (transtentorial herniation).

How do supratentorial masses progress so that these reactions occur? The brain has certain common responses to injury, including edema, vascular dilatation, and the invasion of leukocytes and proliferation of glial cells. The intensity and tempo of these individual pathologic responses vary according to the nature of the original lesion and the rate at which it appears, but the end result of neoplasms, infection, and infarcts is often the same: the original lesion gradually enlarges and, ripple-like, its effects expand outward to impair structures ever more remote from itself in the inexpansible intracranial cavity. Effects that lie remote from the primary lesion are due partly to edema spreading away from its edges and partly to an actual shift of the brain within the skull, compressing normal tissues and blood vessels against rigid structures such as the falx cerebri and the tentorium. At this stage, clinical signs of increased intracranial pressure are common and imply that an intracranial lesion is already exerting generalized deleterious effects.

The clinical picture of supratentorial mass lesions producing stupor or coma has several distinctive features. Localizing symptoms such as frontal headache, focal seizures, or other changes consistent with hemispheric disease almost always precede the development of unconsciousness. Physically, most patients demonstrate a combination of *focal* hemispheral signs, e.g., sensorimotor defect, aphasia, and visual field defect, reflecting the site of the original pathologic process, plus *diffuse* signs of supratentorial dysfunction, indicating that the lesion is exerting remote effects on the opposite hemisphere and the deep-lying diencephalon. An important negative finding is that, unless the patient is in the terminal stages of illness, no evidence of direct subtentorial brainstem dysfunction can be found: pupillary and oculovestibular reflexes remain intact. As a supratentorial lesion progresses, the neurologic signs and symptoms evolve in a characteristic, orderly, rostral-caudal pattern. The more rostrally located neurologic functions disappear first, followed by more caudal impairment, first in the diencephalon and then down the brainstem almost as if the structures were being progressively transected from above downward, each plane of function being removed before the next becomes greatly impaired.

The aforementioned description needs amplification to be complete. Some supratentorial masses that begin and enlarge in neurologically silent areas such as the frontal lobes or the subdural space can lack a focal signature. Lesions of this type may be revealed only when the patient develops signs of diffuse forebrain dysfunction plus, perhaps, headache and evidence of increased intracranial pressure.

Stupor or coma with supratentorial lesions is ominous because it implies that the deeply located upper brain stem is already compressed or distorted and that the much more serious complication of herniation of the forebrain into the tentorial notch threatens to occur. Such herniation begins either with direct downward displacement of the diencephalon (central herniation) or with the uncus of the temporal lobe squeezing into the tentorial notch and against the midbrain (uncal herniation). Either way, if the hernia develops fully, it usually impacts itself upon the midbrain and nearly always results in permanent brain damage or death. A characteristic constellation of symptoms heralds each of these patterns of transtentorial herniation. With impending *central* herniation, stupor becomes gradually deeper, and the subjects sigh, yawn, or develop periodic respirations. The pupils shrink to 1 to 2 mm in diameter, but retain their light reflexes. Oculocephalic reflexes (doll's eye maneuver) are brisk and oculovestibular responses (cold caloric test) are marked by tonic deviation of the eyes toward the stimulated side rather than by physiologic nystagmus. The extremities stiffen into bilateral rigidity or spasticity, combined with extensor plantar responses. With *uncal* herniation, signs are in many ways similar to the above except that as the uncus slides over the tentorial edge, it often compresses the third nerve ahead of it, even before the diencephalon is squeezed. The result is that the pupil on the side of the herniation begins to dilate more than its fellow. Eventually, the pupil dilates widely and becomes light-fixed, and the patient declines into stupor. Shortly afterward, oculomotor functions of the third nerve are usually impaired, and the involved eye turns outward. If the herniating process continues, the opposite third nerve becomes involved, and then the brainstem. To initiate effective treatment one must recognize the process before this advanced stage and halt it with osmotic jecompressing agents or surgical treatment. Otherwise, when conditions progress this far, few subjects recover without residual neurologic injury.

Subtentorial Mass or Destructive Lesions

The subtentorial regions critical to consciousness extend along the paramedian tegmentum from the level of the rostral midbrain down to roughly the middle of the pons. Destruction or compression of this critical area causes stupor or coma, and partial damage to it impairs cognition. Expanding lesions of the posterior fossa produce a similar effect if they compress the upper brainstem. Compression of the medulla oblongata by the cerebellar tonsils causes stiff neck, along with irregularities of respiratory and cardiac rhythm, but does not directly impair consciousness.

The characteristic clinical feature of subtentorial destruction or compression causing coma is evidence of focal brainstem dysfunction, usually asymmetrical, which frequently can be anatomically pinpointed by the clinical findings. The pupils are almost always abnormal, because either pontine or medullary sympathetic pathways or third nerve nuclei or fibers are destroyed. Dysconjugate eye movement are common, and bizarrely or independently moving eyes, ocular bobbing, or rotating ocular deviation usually means primary brainstem dysfunction. Unilateral facial anesthesia involving both the brow and lower face, absent caloric responses to one side, and eye deviation toward the paralyzed arm and leg all suggest a subtentorial lesion. The combination of flaccidity in the arms and flexor responses in the legs signifies pontine-midbrain damage. Seldom do the signs indicate complete brainstem transection. This restricted, discrete localization is unlike metabolic lesions causing coma in which the signs commonly indicate incomplete dysfunction at several different levels of the brain, and also is unlike the secondary brainstem dysfunction and coma that follow supratentorial herniation, in which *all* function at any given level tends to be lost as the process progressess from rostral to caudal along the neuraxis.

Purely compressive lesions of the posterior fossa rarely cause coma until late in their course when the patient is near death. The pathologic process involved is usually a hemorrhage, abscess, or tumor of the cerebellum or fourth ventricle. In such instances, occipital haadache, nystagmus, diplopia, nausea, vomiting, cranial nerve signs, and ataxia usually precede unconsciousness. Important points in distinguishing destructive and compressive posterior fossa lesions from metabolic depression of the brainstem are that in metabolic depression, other than that caused by sedative drugs, oculovestibular responses are generally preserved until the advanced stages, and pupillary light reflexes are nearly always preserved with both endogenous and exogenous metabolic depression. By contrast, structural brainstem lesions causing coma always disrupt the oculovestibular responses, and those involving the midbrain also interrupt the pupillary reflexes.

Delirium and Exogenous Metabolic Brain Disease

DEFINITIONS. Metabolic encephalopathy is a term applied to the behavioral changes which result from diffuse or wide spread multifocal failure of cerebral metabolism. The disorder usually begins acutely or subacutely and often subsides with time and/or treatment. The clinical picture is one in which confusion, thinking errors, behavioral abnormalities, disorders of consciousness, and abnormal motor activity predominate. In some instances (e.g., vitamin B_{12} deficiency or hypothyroidism) metabolic encephalopathy is more insidious in onset. The usual clinical findings then resemble dementia (see definition below) rather than delirium. However, the brain disorder remains reversible by appropriate treatment. Some causes of metabolic encephalopathy are listed in Table 472–2. The table also includes some primary disorders of the central nervous system such as encephalitis, meningitis, concussion, and seizures disorders, because these develop acutely, are reversible with appropriate treatment, and clinically resemble acute metabolic brain disease.

Metabolic brain disease is common and often misdiagnosed. When mild, it produces intellectual dullness, social indifference, and vague perplexity easily mistaken by observers for psychogenic depression or simply low intelligence. More severe

TABLE 472–2. SOME CAUSES OF METABOLIC BRAIN DISEASE

- I. Deprivation of oxygen, substrate, or metabolic cofactors
  - *A. Hypoxia (interference with oxygen supply to the entire brain—cerebral blood flow normal)
    - 1. Decreased oxygen tension and content of blood
      - Pulmonary disease
      - Alveolar hypoventilation
      - Decreased atmospheric oxygen tension (e.g., high altitude)
    - 2. Decreased oxygen content of blood—normal tension
      - Anemia
      - Carbon monoxide poisoning
      - Methemoglobinemia
  - *B. Ischemia (diffuse or widespread multifocal interference with blood supply to brain)
    - 1. Decreased cerebral blood flow resulting from decreased cardiac output
      - Stokes-Adams syndrome, cardiac arrest, cardiac arrhythmias
      - Myocardial infarction
      - Congestive heart failure
      - Aortic stenosis
      - Pulmonary embolism
    - 2. Decreased cerebral blood flow resulting from decreased peripheral resistance in the systemic circulation
      - Syncope: orthostatic, vasovagal
      - Carotid sinus hypersensitivity
      - Low blood volume
    - 3. Decreased cerebral blood flow due to generalized or multifocal increase in cerebrovascular resistance
      - Hyperventilation syndrome
      - Increased blood viscosity (polycythemia, cryo- and macroglobinemia, sickle cell anemia)
      - Bacterial meningitis and encephalitis
      - Subarachnoid hemorrhage
    - 4. Decreased local cerebral blood flow due to widespread small vessel occlusion or tissue necrosis
      - Disseminated intravascular coagulation
      - Systemic lupus erythematosus
      - Subacute bacterial endocarditis
      - Cardiopulmonary bypass
      - Small emboli (fat, fibrin, platelets)
      - Acute viral encephalitis
    - 5. Alterations of blood flow due to failure of autoregulation
      - Hypertensive encephalopathy
  - *C. Hypoglycemia
    - Resulting from exogenous insulin
    - Spontaneous (endogenous insulin, liver disease, etc.)
  - D. Cofactor deficiency
    - Thiamine (Wernicke's encephalopathy)
    - Niacin
    - Pyridoxine
    - B_{12}
    - Folate
- II. Diseases of organs other than brain
  - *A. Diseases of nonendocrine organs
    - Liver (hepatic coma)
    - Kidney (uremic coma)
    - Lung (CO_2 narcosis)
    - Pancreas (exocrine pancreatic encephalopathy)

- II. Diseases of organs other than brain (*Continued*)
  - *B. Hyper- and/or hypofunction of endocrine organs
    - Pituitary
    - Thyroid (myxedema-thyrotoxicosis)
    - Parathyroid (hyper- and hypoparathyroidism)
    - Adrenal (Addison's disease, Cushing's disease, pheochromocytoma)
    - Pancreas (diabetes, hypoglycemia)
  - C. Other systemic diseases
    - Diabetes
    - Cancer
    - Porphyria
    - Sepsis
- III. Exogenous poisons (see also Ch. 25)
  - *A. Sedative drugs
  - B. Acid poisons or poisons with acidic breakdown products
    - Paraldehyde
    - Methyl alcohol
    - Ethylene glycol
  - C. Psychotropic drugs
    - Tricyclic antidepressants and anticholinergic drugs
    - Amphetamines
    - Lithium
    - Phenothiazines
    - LSD-mescaline
    - Monoamine oxidase inhibitors
  - D. Others
    - Penicillin
    - Anticonvulsants
    - Steroids
    - Cardiac glycosides
    - Cimetidine
    - Heavy metals
    - Organic phosphates
    - Cyanide
    - Salicylates
- IV. Abnormalities of fluid, ionic, or acid-base environment of CNS
  - A. Water and sodium (hyper- and hyponatremia) (hypo- and hyperosmolality)
  - B. Acidosis (metabolic and respiratory)
  - C. Alkalosis (metabolic and respiratory)
  - D. Magnesium (hyper- and hypomagnesemia)
  - E. Calcium (hyper- and hypocalcemia)
  - F. Phosphorus (hyper- and hypophosphatemia)
  - G. ? Trace metal deficiency or excess
- V. Disordered temperature regulation
  - A. Hypothermia
  - B. Heat stroke, fever
- VI. Infections or inflammation of CNS
  - A. Leptomeningitis
  - B. Encephalitis
  - C. Acute "toxic" encephalopathy
  - D. Parainfectious encephalomyelitis
  - E. Cerebral vasculitis
  - F. Subarachnoid hemorrhage
- VII. Miscellaneous diseases of unknown cause
  - A. Seizures and postictal states
  - *B. "Postoperative" delirum
  - C. Concussion
  - *D. Acute delirious states
    - Sedative drug withdrawal
    - "Postoperative" delirium
    - Intensive care unit delirium
    - Drug intoxications

*Alone or in combination, the most common causes of delirium seen on medical or surgical wards.

encephalopathy elicits either a florid picture of tremulous agitation, rich and frightening hallucinations, and periods of seemingly complete loss of contact with the environment, or a more quiet, withdrawn, akinetic state which may fade into stupor or coma. The former, often called *delirium* or *toxic psychosis*, may be confused with a functional psychosis, and the latter, often called *acute* or *subacute confusional state*, is likely to be mistaken for structural brain disease or psychological depression. Although certain specific systemic disorders characteristically cause one or another of the aforementioned syndromes, each can occur with any of the metabolic brain diseases; thus the terms "delirium," "toxic psychosis," and "confusional state" are used interchangeably in this chapter to describe the wakeful stage of metabolic encephalopathy.

The term *dementia* is used operationally to describe an irreversible loss of memory and cognitive functions, usually insidious in onset, irreversible, and often, but not always, resulting from intrinsic disease of the brain. Demented patients usually do not have the clouding of consciousness associated with deliriuim. However, an insidiously developing, quiet delirium may be clinically indistinguishable from the early stages of dementia.

CLINICAL FEATURES OF METABOLIC BRAIN DISEASE. The purpose of the physical and laboratory examination in a patient with suspected metabolic brain disease is two-fold: first to determine if the observed changes in consciousness are due to metabolic brain disease (i.e., to rule out structural brain disease or psychiatric dysfunction); and second, to determine exactly the type of metabolic defect causing the delirium. In general, evaluation of the state of consciousness, motor activity, and autonomic acitivity, as detailed below, helps answer the first question, whereas the general physical examination, examination of ventilation, and laboratory examination (the latter two detailed below) help answer the second question. It cannot, however, be overemphasized that, despite the difficulties of examining a delirious patient, a thorough and systematic general physical, neurologic, and laboratory examination *must* be undertaken if a definitive diagnosis is to be established and definitive treatment to be applied. Some principles of the examination are outlined in Table 472–3.

State of Consciousness and Mental Content. Disorders of attention are the earliest sign and the hallmark of metabolic brain disease. The patient may appear quietly perplexed or preoccupied and be unable to concentrate sufficiently to deal with significant stimuli in the environment. Conversely, he may appear hypervigilant and distractible, attending briefly to each new environmental stimulus no matter how trivial or irrelevant. Attentional defects may be subtle at onset and are easily mistaken for normal if slightly odd behavior. At about the same time, restlessness or lethargy, emotional lability, insomnia or drowsiness, and vivid nightmares may appear. Patients often appear fearful and anxious, or depressed, and may express the fear that they are "going crazy." They may be restless, irritable, and easily distracted. Conversely, they may lie quietly or sleep when left alone, and rarely read or attend to the world around them. With more severe metabolic disturbances, patients become drowsy and finally stuporous or comatose. The particular affect that prevails in patients with metabolic encephalopathy depends partly on the nature of the illness and partly on the rapidity of its development; previous personality often has suprisingly little influence. Thus, barbiturate- or alcohol-withdrawal syndromes, acute liver necrosis, and porphyria often cause an agitated delirium, whereas uremia, pulmonary encephalopathy, and anoxia usually produce a more quit illness. Rapijly developing metabolic abnormalities are more likely to produce agitated delirium than those that develop more slowly.

TABLE 472–3. PHYSICAL EXAMINATION OF PATIENTS WITH SUSPECTED METABOLIC BRAIN DISEASE

- History (from relatives or friends)
  - Previous medical illness (diabetes, uremia, heart disease)
  - Previous psychiatric history
  - Access to drugs (sedative, psychotropic drugs)
  - Recent complaints (headache, depression)
- General physical examination
  - Evidence of trauma
  - Evidence of chronic or acute systemic illness
- Neurologic examination
  - Mental status
    - Affect (agitated, depressed, apathetic)
    - Alertness (delirium, obtundation, stupor, coma)
    - Memory (recent events, recall of objects)
    - Orientation (time, place, person)
    - Perceptual abnormalities (illusions, delusions, hallucinations)
    - Psychomotor activity
  - Motor examination
    - Focal weakness
    - Tremor
    - Asterixis
    - Myoclonus
    - Seizures
  - Autonomic examination
    - Pupillary size and responses
    - Temperature
    - Heart rate and rhythm
    - Diaphoresis
    - Ventilation

Disturbances in cognition appear along with altered alertness and awareness and are characterized by difficulties with immediate recall and the ability to abstract. Normal subjects readily recall and repeat 6 or 7 digits forward and 5 or 6 backward and can identify the common denominator between such pairs as an apple and an orange or a fly and a tree, but delirious patients cannot. However, innate intelligence and education also determine cognitive abilities and, unless the physician has examined the patient previously, it is difficult to attribute mild disturbances to a metabolic defect. An early sign of delirium, although usually not as early as altered alertness and cognition, is impairment of memory and orientation. Loss of memory for recent events is a hallmark of metabolic and other organic brain disease and is tested by asking the patient about the names of his doctors, some important current events, and his recent activities. Orientation to place and time should be specifically tested by asking the date and year, the day of the week, and the present location. Orientation for time, particularly the year, is lost early in patients with delirium and orientation for place a little later.

Perceptual errors, e.g., mistaking the physician for an old friend or family member, illusions and hallucinations are common accompaniements of delirium. They frighten and agitate some patients, but are quietly tolerated by others. The nature of the illusions and hallucinations seems to reflect the individual's personality, and often the same hallucinations accompany separate episodes of delirium. A quiet, withdrawn patient must be specifically asked about hallucinations, because he often fails either to volunteer the information or to behave as if he were hallucinating. Hallucinations of metabolic origin may be visual, auditory, tactile, or a combination, contrasting with those of schizophrenia, which are usually auditory only.

Fluctuations of the mental status are common in metabolic encephalopathy. Patients may be totally out of contact one moment and lucid the next. Lucid intervals appear unpredictably and last for minutes or hours. Some of the fluctuation is environmentally related. Thus delirious patients characteristically become more disoriented at night, in unfamiliar surroundings, and in situations in which restraints and background noise and unfamiliar activity replace familiar sensory stimuli. One study demonstrated a higher incidence of postoperative delirium in patients treated in a windowless intensive care unit than in those treated in a similar one with windows.

Motor Activity. Tremor, asterixis, and multifocal myoclonus are characteristic of metabolic brain disease, and the specificity of the latter two makes them the most important physical signs that distinguish metabolic encephalopathy from psychiatric illness or from structural brain disease.

The *tremor* of delirious patients is coarse and irregular at a rate of about eight to ten per second. It is usually absent at complete rest. It is best seen in the fingers of the outstretched hands. It is less specific than asterixis and multifocal myoclonus, and may affect patients with psychiatric disease as well as those with systemic illness not associated with delirium.

Asterixis is an abnormal, involuntary jerking movement elicited in the hands by asking patients to dorsiflex the wrist and spread the extended fingers. Its mildest form involves irregular random lateral jerking movements of the fingers at the metacarpophalangeal joints. With fully developed asterixis there is sudden palmar flexion of the fingers at the metacarpophalangeal joints and of the wrist. The movements are asynchronous in the two hands and nonrhythmic. They occur every 2 to 30 seconds, recover quickly, and cannot be controlled by the patient, even when he is aware of their presence. Asterixis may also involve the feet and tongue. In the obtunded patient the same movement can sometimes by evoked by passively dorsiflexing the wrist or the ankles. Bilateral asterixis almost universally accompanies metabolic encephalopathy at some stage of the illness. It is absent in patients with spychiatric disorders unless they are taking large amounts of drugs, and is encountered rarely, and then unilaterally, in patients with structural brain disease such as decompensating subdural hematomas or deep hemispheral infarcts, especially involving the basal ganglia.

Multifocal myoclonus consists of sudden nonrhythmic, nonpatterned gross muscle contractions in a resting person. The movements are most common in the face and shoulders but occur anywhere in the body. Multifocal myoclonus can often be elicited, if not present at rest, by passive movements of the shoulder and upper arm. It occurs in a later and more severe stage of metabolic illness than does asterixis, and may physiologically represent a more intense and widespread manifestation of that abnormal movement. Multifocal myoclonus makes its most frequent appearance in uremia, hypercarbic-anoxic encephalopathy, and penicillin overdose, but can occur in virtually all metabolic encephalopathies.

Psychomotor activity ranges from extreme hyperactivity to total immobility. Delirious patients may be unwilling or unable to stay in bed, pacing the halls, in constant movement, with outbursts of aggressiveness which may culminate in attacks on others. With more severe delirium, there may be groping movements, picking at the bedclothes, and constant tossing and turning. Such patients may fall out of bed and injure themselves. Increased psychomotor activity is typically observed in acute deliria such as delirium tremens and drug withdrawal states. More commonly, delirium is manifested by reduced activity, with the patient lethargic, drowsy, and generally bradykinetic. The same patient may run the gamut from psychomotor overactivity to reduced activity during the course of the delirium. *Speech* is often abnormal. Patients with increased psychomotor behavior often speak rapidly, with a muttering or slurred speech which, because of its speed, is incomprehensible. Patients with reduced psychomotor activity may speak slowly, monotonously, and so softly as not to be clearly heard.

Seizures, hyperactive stretch reflexes, and *focal signs* frequently accompany severe metabolic brain disease. The seizures are usually generalized and the motor abnormalities usually symmetrical. However, focal paresis and focal seizures are not rare, especially with anoxia, hypoglycemia, or hyperosmolality. Signs of focal disturbance make it more difficult to distinguish between metabolic and structural brain disease. However, in metabolic brain disease the focal signs are usually mild and fleeting, and they are accompanied by more widespread neurologic dysfunction than occurs with gross structural disease.

Autonomic Activity. *Pupillary light reactions are always preserved in metabolic coma with the few exceptions to be mentioned, and absence of the pupillary light reaction strongly suggests a structural lesion.* The exceptions are glutethimide intoxication, which may produce mid-position or slightly dilated fixed pupils; anticholinergic drug administration, which produces fixed, dilated pupils; and exposure to severe anoxia, or asphyxia, which produces fixed dilated pupils and, if sustained, probably implies irreversible brain damage. The pupils, whatever their size and reaction to light, are usually symmetrical in patients comatose from metabolic brain disease, but often asymmetrical in patients comatose from structural brain disease.

TABLE 472–4. LABORATORY EVALUATION OF METABOLIC BRAIN DISEASE

Test	Reason for Test
Immediate:	
Glucose	Hypoglycemia, hyperosmolar coma
Na^+	Osmolar abnormalities
Ca^{++}	Hyper- or hypocalcemia
BUN	Uremia
Arterial blood pH, Pco_2, Po_2	Acidosis, alkalosis, hypoxia
Lumbar puncture	Infection, hemorrhage
Later:	
Liver function tests	Hepatic coma
Sedative drug levels	Overdose
Blood and CSF culture	Sepsis, encephalitis, meningitis
Full electrolytes, including Mg^{++}	Electrolyte imbalance
Coagulation profile	Intravascular coagulation
EEG	

Hypothermia is common in delirious patients with myxedema, hypoglycemia, and barbiturate intoxication. Hyperthermia with profuse perspiration and tachycardia accompanies most agitated deliria and is especially common with delirium tremens. Hyperthermia without perspiration suggests anticholinergic drug ingestion or infection. Hyperthermia also marks salicylate and occasionally phenothiazine overdosage.

LABORATORY TESTS. The causes of metabolic coma are legion, and a final diagnosis usually depends on extensive laboratory tests. The tests which should be performed immediately to establish the presence of life-threatening metabolic defects are listed in Table 472–4, along with those whose results are not available immediately but should be done as soon as possible if the diagnosis is unclear.

PSYCHIATRIC DISORDERS

Psychiatric dysfunction may mimic alterations in consciousness. Patients with psychiatric disorders may complain of memory loss, confusion, and/or hallucinations. Patients with psychiatic amnesia, unlike those with metabolic or structural brain disease, often claim disorientation for self (i.e., they deny that they know who they are), even though they may be oriented for place and time. Furthermore, if the patient's cooperation can be elicited, recent memory and cognitive functions are usually preserved. Hallucinations are auditory rather than visual or tacitile, and asterixis and multifocal myoclonus are never present. Patients with extreme anxiety may hyperventilate, producing respiratory alkalosis and a diffusely slow electroencphalogram. Except for that problem, however, the physical and laboratory evaluations are generally normal.

In patients with psychiatric unresponsiveness, the segmental neurologic examination is likewise normal. Breathing is eupneic or voluntarial hyperpneic. Such patients are quietly unresponsive, with all their limbs flaccid. Eye are usually closed and frequently resist eyelid opening. In some patients, the eyes may deviate toward the bed when the patient is turned on his side. The eyelids are incapable of the slow closure of the passively opened eyelids that accompanies true coma. Pupils are briskly responsive or, if psycho-plegics have been self-instilled, widely dilated. Oculocephalic responses are unpredictable, but if the diagnosis is doubtful, irrigating the tympanum with 50 ml of cold water produces physiologic nystagmus rather than the tonic eye deviaiton of the comatose patient with structural or metabolic disease. At times the diagnosis may be difficult because psychiatric delirium or unresponsiveness is superimposed on underlying physical illness (e.g., a patient hospitalized with a severe medical or neurologic illness may be so anxious that he is unable to cope with his environment and thus develops delirium or unresponsiveness). In instances in which there is serious doubt about the diagnosis, slow infusions of small amounts of sodium amobarbital (Amytal interview) may allow thucphysician to establish contact and rapport with the psychiatrically withdrawn patient. The drug may be similarly used to awaken patients rendered unconscious by continuous focal seizures.

GENERAL MANAGEMENT OF ALTERED CONSCIOUSNESS

HISTORY. Several questions must be asked and answered by the physician when he attempts to diagnose and manage the patient with severe brain dysfunction of unknown cause. First he must determine if the disease is focal (i.e., structural) or multifocal-diffuse. If focal, is it (1) supra- or subtentorial in distribution? (2) arrested, improving, or worsening? (3) best treated medically or surgically? If apparently multifocal-diffuse, is the disorder due to (1) exogenous drugs, (2) endogenous metabolic error, (3) CNS infection or hemorrhage, or (4) psychogenic unresponsiveness? Given the answers to these questions, what is the specific etiologic diagnosis? However, even before pursuing this logical approach, the physician must ensure that the brain and other vital organs receive no further injury while he obtains whatever history, examination, or laboratory data are required. This means that in critical situations, lifesaving measures should be underway while clinical and laboratory steps are undertaken to reach an accurate diagnosis and initiate definitive treatment.

It requires considerable restraint to approach a patient with altered consciuosness methodiccally, for the urge to act without delay is understandably strong but potentially dangerous. Inquiry into both the past medical history and the circumstances under which the patient lost ocnsciousness generally discloses more of diagnostic value than any other maneuver. Is there any suggestion that head trauma could have occurred recently? Is chronic renal, hepatic, or myocardial disease? Could a seizure have preceded the present unconsciousness? Has the subject been taking insulin? Have there been recent changes in mood, behavior, or neurologic function to suggest an evolving intracranial process? Was the subject "blue," depressed, or moody, and did he have access to depressant drugs? Is he a "spree" drinker? These and other questions must be covered comprehensively with relatives, past physicians, friends, police, or ambulance personnel. One should always remember that most cases of "coma of unknown cause," whether found at home or in the emergency room of a busy hospital, are due to self-induced drug intoxication.

PHYSICAL FINDINGS. One must perform both a meticulous neurologic examination and a thoughtful physical review of every body system, because disease in remote organs often causes or accentuates dysfunction in the brain.

Fever implies infection, inflammation, or neoplasm. On the other hand, hypothermia, (30 to 36° C) in a patient not severely exposed to cold suggests depressant drug poisoning, hypoglycemia, or severe lower brainstem injury, as by infarction. Hypertension may be the cause of hypertensive encephalopathy or the underlying cause of cerebral hemorrhage. Conversely, an elevated blood pressure can be a symptom of subarachnoid hemorrhage in a subject not previously hypertensive. Hypotension in a supine patient implies low blood volume (hemorrhagic or traumatic shock, severe nutritional and fluid depletion), low cardiac output (myocardial infarction), or low peripheral resistance (depressant drug poisoning). Extreme tachycardia (over 180 per minute) can mean that unconsciousness is the result of lowered cardiac output from a supraventricular cardiac arrhythmia. Bradycardia suggests heart block and the Adams-Stokes syndrome or a myocardial infarct.

The pattern and depth of respiration are often informative in evaluating both neurologic function and acid-base balance. A rapid evaluation of the patient's ventilatory status, coupled with an estimate of blood acid-base balance, frequently narrows the range of possible causes of metabolic coma. A careful clinical examination of the respiratory rate and depth usually allows the physician to estimate whether his patient is hyperventilating, eupneic, or hypoventilating. Caution must be excerised in evaluating patients with severe emphysema whose respiratory effort is increased and who may be tachypneic but nevertheless hypoventilating because of ineffective lungs. Caution must also be used in evluating patients poisoned with depressant drugs who appear to be hypoventilating but are actually eupneic because their metabolic needs are so low. Unexplained abnormalities in the respiratory pattern demand rapid determination of blood gas and acid-base status. A delirious and clinically *hyperventilating* adult with a low serum pH probably has diabetic ketosis, uremia, lactic acidosis, or poisoning with an acidic product. Severe metabolic acidosis, if not treated, is rapidly lethal. Uremia, diagetes, and Addison's disease can be treated specifically (see Ch. 78, 230, and 229), and the others often respond to prompt and urgent treatment of the acidosis by infusion of bicarbonate. If, however, the serum pH is elevated in the delirious and hyperventilating adult, pulmonary disease, cardiac disease, hepatic coma, or neurogenic hyperventilation probable cause. Pneumonia is probably the most common cause of mild respiratory alkalosis in unconscious patients; the others can be evaluated by appropriate laboratory tests. When the serum pH is elevated and the bicarbonate is between 10 and 15 mEq per liter (mixed respiratory alkalosis and metabolic acidosis), sepsis, especially with Gram-negative organisms, salicylism severe hepatic coma are the probable causes.

A similar analysis can be applied to *hypoventilating* patients. In these, the severe problems are depressant drug poisoning, which produces a low serum pH with a normal bicarbonate, and chronic pulmonary failure, which produces a low serum pH and usually a high serum bicarbonate. (The serum bicarbonate level indicates the duration of hypoventialtion.) Both situations demand ventilatory support.

The skin should be searched for petechiae (thrombocytopenic or nonthrombocytopenic purpura, meningococcemia, and bacterial endocarditis), bruises, evidence of nutritional deficiency, icterus, angiomatous spiders, and the bright pinkness of carbon monoxide poisoning. Fleshy or clubbed fingertips suggest carcinoma of the lung, or less often, lung abscess or congenital heart disease (with brain embolism or abscess). A meticulous examination of the optic fundi is imperative but should be completed without cycloplegics, the use of which destroys the potential diagnostic value of pupillary reactions in coma. In the fundus oculi, the pathologic changes of many diseases causing coma can be viewed directly: increased intracranial pressure, hypertensive vascular diase, diabetes, blood dyscrasias, tuberculosis, sarcoidosis, bacterial endocarditis, cryptococcosis, collagen vascular disease, and even subarachnoid hemorrhage producing subhyaloid bleeding.

Chest examination has two potentially rewarding findings: cardiac murmurs suggest bacterial endocarditis with consequent focal, embolic encephalitis; the wheezes and obstructive sounds of the pulmonary cripple suggest CO_2 retention causing narcosis. In the abdominal examination, the presence of masses suggesting polycystic kidneys increases the chances that subarachnoid hemorrhage has occurred, whereas liver enlargement (hepatic coma is common with hepatomas) or splenic enlargement (both blood dyscrasias and infectious mononucleosis can cause encephalitis-like illness) can provide valuable leads.

During the neurologic examination, certain potentially informative steps are sometimes overlooked. The skull should always be palpated and isnpected meticulously. Edema of the scalp commonly overlies fresh fracture lines, and basal skull fractures predispose to blood pigment stains behind the ear (Battle's sign) and about the orbit (raccoon eyes). Blood also may escape from basal fractures into the ear canals, the middle ears, or the nostrils. The skull should be percussed, because focal or unilateral skull tenderness, manifested by grimacing or withdrawal in a stuporous subject, often overlies an intracranial mass lesion. The neck should be tested carefully: stiff neck can reflect meningitis, cerebellar tonsillar herniation, or, occasionally, simply skeletal muscle spasticity. The stiff neck of acute bacterial meningitis is rarely equivocal; that of impending herniation is commonly less severe and lacks accompanying signs of infection or a prominent Kernig sign. It usually requires several hours or a day or more for stiff neck to develop after subarachnoid bleeding.

Table 472–5 gives a profile of neurologic functions useful for evaluating patients with acute brain dysfunction. As the table indicates, certain signs discriminate among normal, impaired, or absent cerebral hemispheric functions, whereas others point toward the presence of moderate or severe brainstem dysfunction. This fundamental examination is easily completed within a few minutes in most patients and can be employed both for immediate anatomic diagnosis and for indicating whether the patienimproving or worsening as time and treatment transpire.

Laboratory Tests. A *CT scan* often resolves much of the issue of the diagnosis of impaired consciousness, particularly in potentially lethal but surgically treatable diseases. If the diagnosis is in doubt, an emergency CT scan should be obtained whenever possible. An abnormal CT scan which identifies supratentorial or subtentorial mass lesions indicates that urgent treatment must be applied. A negative CT scan reassures the physician that he can safely perform a lumbar puncture and informs him that no mass lesion exists, greatly narrowing the choices and suggesting metabolic brain disease.

When to do a lumbar punture is always a serious question. All physicians are aware that in patients with increased intracranial pressure the procedure sometimes induces fatal herniation of the brain through the tentorium or foramen magnum. For this reason, lumbar puncture is best avoided if the physician strongly suspects his patient of having an expanding intracranial mass, particularly in the posterior fossa. Such forbearance is particularly advisable when CT scanning is immediately available. There are certain treatable diseases such as meningitis, however, that can be diagnosed only by lumbar puncture, and many others such as encephalitis or subarachnoid hemorrhage in which the procedure yields valuable preliminary diagnostic informaiton. When the advice of neurologic specialists is unavaialble, the doctor has no choice but to proceed with lumbar puncture if the diagnosis is in doubt and he believes the procedure has a reasonable chance of offering valuable information. Certain steps minimize the risk. One is to use a small (No. 20 or 22) needle. Another is to attach the manometer to the needle before releasing fluid, a technique that prevents sudden subarachnoid pressure shifts. Jugular manometrics should *never* be performed, for they offer little useful data and increase the risk of impacting potential intracranial herniations.

The *electroencephalogram* (EEG) is moderatley useful in evaluating patients with alterations in consciousness. In patients with metabolic brain disease, the EEG is usually slow but symmetrical, and bilateral synchronous paraxysmal bursts of 1 to 3 per second (Hz) activity are frequently superimposed upon the slow background. The degree of slowing roughly parallels the severity of the encephalopathy. Patients with agitated delirium are often exceptions and particularly those suffering from drug withdrawal may have rapid rather than slow EEGs. Normal 8 to 13 Hz activity, however, is usually absent. In patients with supratentorial structural disease, the slow activity is usually more prominent on the side of the lesion. In some patients, alteration of consciousness is caused by a continuosly discharging focal lesion (focal status epilepticus), and such abnormalities may be detected by the presence of focal spikes or sharp waves.

TABLE 472–5. THE NEUROLOGIC EXAMINATION OF THE PATIENT WITH ACUTELY ALTERED OR CHANGING CONSCIOUSNESS*

Verbal function—oriented, syntactically normal; confused; aphasic; incomprehensible sounds only; mute
Spontaneous eye movements—conjugate pursuit; roving conjugate; dysconjugate; none
Eye opening—spontaneous; in response to verbal stimuli; in response to noxious stimuli; none
Corneal response to stimulation—present; *absent*
Pupillary (note size) response to light stimulation—brisk; *unequal* (test directly and consensually); *sluggish; absent*
Oculocephalic-oculovestibular responses—quick phase nystagmus present; tonic conjugate; *dysconjugate; absent*
Motor response to noxious stimulation—appropriate; stereotyped withdrawal; asymmetrical; abnormal flexor ("decorticate"); abnormal extensor ("decerebrate"); *flaccid*
Breathing pattern—eupneic; rhythmic hyperpnea or hypopnea; regularly irregular (Cheyne-Stokes); *ataxic or bizarrely irregular; absent*

*Each function is subdivided in best-worse order and roughly indicates the rostral-caudal level of impairment. Signs of impaired or absent brainstem function are italicized. (For details consult Plum F, Posner JB: Diagnosis of Stupor and Coma. 3rd ed. Philadelphia, F. A. Davis Company, 1980.)

†Note that eye opening reflects only the state of arousal and not necessarily the presence of psychologic awareness or interaction.

EMERGENCY MANAGEMENT OF COMA

The definitive treatment of altered states of consciousness requires removing, correcting, or halting the specific process responsible to whatever degree possible. Often, however, accurate diagnosis and specific therapy require time to carry out and become effective. In the meantime one must move immediately to protect the brain against permanent damage.

Certain general therapeutic measures apply to the care of all patients:

1. *Assure an adequate airway and oxygenation.* Immediately check and clean out the upper airway. If the patient is entirely unresponsive, arragne for the skillful insertion of an endotracheal airway, but first give 1 mg of atropine intravenously to guard against hypoxigenic vagal cardiac arrest. Be sure that no neck fracture exists before extending the head for intubation. Ausculate both lung bases after inserting the tube to assure that lower airway is open. If a ventilator is used, a rate less than 16 per minute and adjust the volume to give arterial blood gases of Pa_{O_2} >80 mm Hg and Pa_{CO_2} 30 to 35 mm Hg. It is difficult to avoid leaving the patient supine while diagnosis is pursued; but once the diagnosis of metabolic encephalopathy is made, place the patient in mild Trendelenburg position and turn from side to side each hour.
2. *Maintain circulation.* Check the blood pressure and pulse frequently (insert a venous line immediately to replace volume loss), and infuse vasoactive agents to keep mean blood pressure at 80 to 90 mm Hg or more.
3. *Give glucose.* Draw bloods for emergency blood gas and chemical determinations (see Table 472–4) and, if hypoglycemia is a possible diagnosis, immediately give 50 ml of 50 per cent glucose. The glucose will not appreciably intensify hyperosmolality, but there is evidence that hyperglycemia may enhance ischemic brain disease, and thus glucose should be given with caution. However, it is potentially too dangerous to the brain to wait. (Bloods are drawn first in order not to lose evidence for the diagnosis.)
4. *Stop generalized seizures.* Repetitive convulsions can result from either intracranial mass lesions or metabolic-diffuse encephalopathies. In either event, status epilepticus can cause coma and within a short period of time produces irreversible brain damage as well. Start treatment with intravenous diazepam, 10 mg, keeping ventilator available to treat depressed breathing. As soon as convulsions stop, give between 500 and 1000 mg of phenytoin intravenously at a rate of less than 50

TABLE 472–6. COMMON DRUG POISONINGS, SIGNS OF TOXICITY, AND TREATMENT

Drug	Signs and Symptoms: *Mild*	Signs and Symptoms: *Severe*	Diagnostic Test	Treatment
Opiates				
Heroin Morphine Meperidine Methadone Hydromorphone Oxycodone Levorphanol	"Nodding" drowsiness, small pupils, urinary retention, slow and shallow breathing; skin scars and subcutaneous abscesses; duration 4–6 hours; with methadone, duration to 24 hours	Coma; pinpoint pupils, slow irregular respiration or apnea, hypotension, hypothermia, pulmonary edema	Response to naloxone Urine	Naloxone, 0.4 mg intravenously or intramuscularly; repeat at 15-minute intervals not more than twice; repeat in 3 hours if necessary; if no response by second dose, suspect another cause; treat shock; find and detect infection
Depressants				
Alcohol Barbiturates Chloral hydrate Glutethimide (Doriden) Meprobamate (Equanil)	Confusion, rousable drowsiness, delirium, ataxia, nystagmus, dysarthria, analgesia to stimuli	Stupor to coma; pupils reactive, usually constricted; oculovestibular response absent; motor tonus initially briefly hyperactive, then flaccid; respiration and blood pressure depressed; hypothermia; with glutethimide, pupils moderately dilated, can be fixed; with meprobamate, withdrawal seizures common; with methaqualone, coma, occasional convulsions, tachycardia, cardiac failure, bleeding tendency	Blood, urine, breath Blood Blood Blood	Intubate, ventilate, gavage; drainage position; antimicrobials; keep mean blood pressure above 90 mm Hg and urine output > 300 ml per hour; avoid analeptics; hemodialyze severe phenobarbital poisoning
Methaqualone (Quaalude, Sopor, Mandrax)	Hallucinations, agitation, motor hyperactivity, myoclonus, tonic spasms		Blood	
Benzodiazepines (Librium, Valium, Tranxene, Ativan, Dalmane, etc.)	Usually taken with another sedative if poisoning is attempted		Blood	As above; diuresis of little help
Ethchlorvynol (Placidyl)				
Stimulants				
Amphetamines Methylphenidate	Hyperactive, aggressive, sometimes paranoid, repetitive behavior; dilated pupils, tremor, hyperactive reflexes; hyperthermia, tachycardia, arrhythmia Acute torsion dystonia	Agitated, assaultive and paranoid excitement; occasionally convulsions; hypothermia; circulatory collapse	Blood	Chlorpromazine
Cocaine	Similar but less prominent than above; less paranoid, often euphoric	Twitching, irregular breathing, tachycardia, occasionally convulsions	None: clinical appraisal only	Sedation
Psychedelics (LSD), mescaline, psilocybin, phencyclidine, STP)	Confused, disoriented, perceptual distortions, distractable, withdrawn or eruptive, leading to accidents or violence; wide-eyed, dilated pupils; restless, hyperreflexic; less often, hypertension or tachycardia	Panic		Reassure; diazepam satisfactory; avoid phenothiazines
Scopolamine-atropine (knockout drops, Transderm delirium)	Agitated or confused, visual hallucinations, dilated pupils, flushed and dry skin	Florid toxic disoriented delirium, visual hallucination; later, amnesia, fever, dilated fixed pupils, hot flushed dry skin, urinary retention		Reassure; sedate lightly; (1) avoid phenothiazines; (2) do not leave alone
Antidepressants				
Tricyclics (Tofranil, Elavil, Desipramine, etc.)	Restlessness, drowsiness, tachycardia, ataxia, sweating	Agitation, vomiting, hyperpyrexia, sweating, muscle dystonia, convulsions, tachycardia or arrhythmia	Clinical	Symptomatic; gastric lavage; inject physostigmine for coma or arrhythmia. Intensive care, anticonvulsants, and antiarrhythmics for severe cases
MAO inhibitors (Parnate, Nardil, Eutonyl, etc.)	Hypertensive crises, agitation, drowsiness, ataxia	Hypotension; headache; chest pain; agitation; coma, seizures and shock	Clinical	Symptomatic; gastric lavage

Table continued on opposite page

TABLE 472–6. COMMON DRUG POISONINGS, SIGNS OF TOXICITY, AND TREATMENT (*Continued*)

Drug	Signs and Symptoms: *Mild*	Signs and Symptoms: *Severe*	Diagnostic Test	Treatment
Phenothiazines	Acute dystonia, somnolence, hypotension	Coma; convulsions (rare); arrhythmias; hypotension	Clinical	Symptomatic; gastric lavage
Lithium	Mild lethargy	Lethargy; muteness with appearance of distraction; coma; multifocal seizures; slow or fluctuating course	Blood	Hydrate if mild; hemodialyze for coma or convulsions
Acid-forming intoxicants				
Methanol (formic); ethylene glycol (oxalic and hippuric); other organic alcohols	Inebriation with hyperpnea	All produce progressive hyperventilation, drunkenness, stupor, eventually convulsions and death. Early blindness with methanol	Blood shows increasingly severe anion-gap acidosis	Inhibit hepatic alcohol dehydrogenase by giving alcohol until acidosis controlled, Treat acidosis vigorously
Salicylate				
Aspirin	Tinnitus, dyspnea	Older persons: confusional state or toxic delirium leading to stupor, convulsions, coma	Blood salicylate > 60 mg/dl	Alkaline diuresis

mg per minute. IF seizures continue, give more diazepam or resort to barbiturate general anesthesia. Repetitive focal seizures and myoclonus are potentially less damaging to brain, and their continuation does not require that one resort to anesthesia.

5. *Restore blood acid-base and osmolar balance.* Extremes of either acidosis or alkalosis usually reflect profound metabolic problems, severe circulatory insufficiency, the postictal state (muscular lactic acidosis), or hyperadrenocorticism. Since secver metabolic acidosis can precipitate cardiovascular irregulalarity and alkalosis depresses breathing, they should be corrected. Extreme hypo- and hyperosmolality are equally dangerous to brain and should be corrected, the first with hypertonic saline and the second with fluids (and insulin for hyperglycemia). Beware of too rapid reversal, however, because osmotic delays across the blood-brain barrier during treatment can lead to large fluid shifts in or out of brain. A reasonable goal is to correct blood by about 15 to 20 mOsm in 24 hours.

6. *Treat infection.* Several kinds of infection cause or intensify delirium and coma. Obtain nose, throat, blood, and would cultures, and perform lumbar puncture if indicated. With any sign of infection, begin antimicrobial treatment after obtaining the cultures cited above, based on either the results of smears or the most probable organism.

7. *Treat extreme body temperatures.* Hyperthermia above 40° C or hypothermia below 34° C should be brought to within 2° C of normal.

8. *Give thiamine, 50 to 100 mg intravenously.* Many patients admitted to emergency rooms in stupor or coma are malnourished and therefore vulnerable to Wernicke's encephalopathy if loaded with glucose.

9. *Consider specific antidotes.* Most patients admitted to emergency rooms in coma have taken an overdose of drugs, often in combination. For narcotic overdose, give 0.4 mg of naloxone intravenously every five minutes until the subject awakens. If the subject may be an addict, dilute the dose in 10 ml of saline and give slowly, trying to avoid withdrawal phenomena. Remember that naloxone's duration of action of two to three hours is shorter than that of several narcotics, and the dose may require repeating.

10. *Control agitation,* avoiding barbiturates but employing diazepam or haloperidol as necessary.

11. *Protect the corneas against abrasions,* using ophthalmic ointment and, if necessary, taping the lids shut.

472.2 Acute Central Nervous System Poisoning

Fred Plum

This portion of the chapter briefly discusses the diagnosis and treatment of the most frequent forms of self-induced and accidental poisoning that produce acute severe neurologic dysfunction. At one time sedative drugs, especially the barbiturates, were the chief offenders, but patients and industry recently have become more imaginative in their choices and the list of common agents has lengthened. To find descriptions of poisons not included in this section, especially chronic neurotoxic agents, the reader should consult the textbooks listed in the references.

Table 472–6 lists the most common acute neurotoxic poisonings in the United States, gives their principal signs of toxicity, and outlines their treatment. Antidepressants, benzodiazepines, phenothiazines, barbiturates, opiates, and alcohol either alone or in combination cause the great majority of coma-inducing poisonings. Clinical appraisal must be used to diagnose the agent causing several of these reaction patterns, specific chemical tests being either unavailable or impractically slow. Nevertheless, when any doubt exists, one should keep admission serum samples for possible later analysis. Blood levels or size of the dose are unreliable guides to the potential depth of coma or other risks with most of the drugs because tolerance develops to chronic ingestion, making individuals react differently to similar doses. The mixing of drugs and alcohol adds to the unreliability. Only the opiates and some of the sedatives create an immediate risk of death; concurrent alcohol ingestion enhances both these risks. Opiate poisoning is discussed in more detail in Ch. 481.

PATHOGENESIS. All sedative drugs depress the central nervous system, although not equally on a gram-molecular weight basis, and not to the same degree so far as different central structures are concerned. The duration of action varies widely and depends largely on how the particular drug is detoxified or eliminated. The short-acting barbiturates, pentobarbital, secobarbital, and amobarbital, are detoxified by the liver, as is methaqualone. They exert their maximal effects promptly after being absorbed and, even in huge doses, seldom cause neurologic depression lasting longer than three to five days. Barbital and phenobarbital are partially detoxified by the liver and partially excreted in the urine. Severe poisoning with the latter agent can cause coma lasting 10 to 14 days. Glutethimide has a short duration of action comparable to that of secobarbital, but it is poorly absorbed from the gut and may generate more long-lasting neurotoxic metabolites. Meprobamate has an intermediate duration of effect lasting for days. Bromide rarely causes full coma, but, once it reaches high levels, it replaces chloride in the blood and tissues and persists for weeks to cause symtoms without further ingestion.

Although the sedatives have few important effects outside the nervous system, barbiturates, glutethimide, and meprobamate in toxic doses tend to produce hypotension. Also, glutethimide possesses anticholinergic properties and is the only sedative that predictably produces lightfixed pupils in anesthetic doses.

A withdrawal syndrome consisting of tremulousness, agitation, and sometimes delirium, and convulsions can develop after prompt withdrawal of any of the hypnotic sedatives. Convulsions are a particular problem after withdrawal from meprobamate and methaqualone.

CLINICAL MANIFESTATIONS. Stupor or coma caused by depressant drug poisoning presents the characteristic picture of severe metabolic brain disease. The depression of the central nervous system tends to be bilateral and symmetrical, and the drug affects simultaneously many levels, including the spinal cord. Respiratory and circulatory controlling mechanisms in the lower brainstem are affected only with very high doses or not at all, and, except with glutethimide or extremely large, smooth muscle-paralyzing doses of the barbiturates, the pupillary light reflexes are preserved. Early in the course of acute poisoning, patients can demonstrate muscular hypertonus or even spasticity as the result of uneven depression of different neurologic levels. Within a short time, usually an hour or less, flaccidity supervenes, and the stretch reflexes tend to disappear. Even moderate degrees of drug depression can depress or block the oculovestibular reflexes.

As mentioned, blood levels are a poor index to the depth of coma. Generally speaking, however, blood levels of short-acting barbiturates of more than 2.5 mg per deciliter and phenobarbital blood levels of more than 12 mg per deciliter are associated with very deep coma to the level at which apnea and hypotension become management problems. Apnea rarely supervenes with the benzodiazepines.

DIAGNOSIS. The combination of unresponsiveness, preserved or sluggish pupillary reactions, absent oculovestibular reactions, motor areflexia, hypothermia, and depression of respiration and circulation is clinically diagnostic of sedative-anesthetic drug poisoning. Only infarction or hemorrhage of the pons resembles this clinical state, and with lesions of the pons the pupils are usually small or pinpoint, the stretch reflexes are generally preserved or hyperactive, and the plantar responses are extensor. Specific chemical tests will detect barbiturates, glutethimide, meprobamate, methaqualone, and bromides in blood or urine, and can be done as emergency measures.

MANAGEMENT OF COMA. Treat the patient first, not the drug. First comes general physiologic support. There are no specific antidotes, but certain precautions must be taken. Patients with drug overdose can sink rapidly and unexpectedly to deeper levels of anesthesia and should never be left alone with unskilled attendants.

Assure the Airway First and Throughout. Depressant drugs suppress the cough reflex and the ciliary action of the tracheal and bronchial mucosa. Give atropine, 1 mg intravenously, and place a cuffed endotracheal tube fefore attempting gastric lavage. Subsequently, deflate the endotracheal cuff hourly, replace the tube at 48 hours, and consider tracheostomy at 96 hours if no signs of awakening have occurred.

To empty the stomach in still arousable subjects, give apomorphine subcutaneously, 6 mg for adults and 1 to 2 mg for children. If not available, ipecac 20 ml may be given orally, followed with glasses of water to induce vomiting. Place vomiting subjects prone to avoid aspiration. For patients already in coma once the endotracheal tube is in place, gavage the stomach until clear, using a large double-barreled tube and plain water or half-normal saline for the irrigating solution. To absorb remaining drug in the gut, instill 2 tablespoons of activated charcoal before withdrawing the tube. Repetitive dosing with charcoal may accelerate phenobarbital elimination if coma lasts longer than 12 hours.

Start moistened oxygen 25 per cent via a suitable nonobstructing airway connector. Treat any evidence of hypoventilation immediately with an automatic ventilator. Shallow breathing in a deeply comatose patient frequently reflects no more than the subject's depressed metabolism; if the rate falls below 12 per minute or the physician entertains serious doubts as to the adequacy of ventilation, artificial respiration is indicated. Measure arterial blood gases and initiate artificial respiration in any case if the arterial Po_2 falls below 100 mm Hg on 25 per cent oxygen or if the Pco_2 climbs above 45 mm Hg. High concentrations (greater than 30 per cent) of oxygen therapy should be confined to patients receiving artificial respiration, for such treatment increases the risk of CO_2 retention in nonventilated subjects.

Treat the Circulation. Maintain the blood pressure, but avoid overhydration. Shock is rare with depressant posioning, but the action of the drugs on smooth muscle commonly produces moderate hypotension, which in turn impairs glomerular infiltration and renal clearance of drugs. Beware of patients with tricyclic antidepressant poisoning. These drugs cause bizarre and sometimes fatal arrhythmias whose treatment may require an experienced cardiologist. A widened QRS or QT interval may particularly predispose to ventricular tachycardia.

For all patients with depressant poisoning give fluids and pressor agents so as to maintain mean blood pressure at 80 to 90 mm Hg and a urine flow approaching 300 ml or more per hour. Dopamine will be sufficient to attain perfusion in many patients. Norepinephrine can be used cautiously if less vigorous pressor agents fail to maintain ideal systemic pressures. Judge fluid intake by urine output, after first inserting a catheter for accurate collections. If hour-by-hour fluid excretion does not match intake by the third hour of treatment, try raising the blood pressure rather than first loading in more fluids. Oliguric renal failure almost never occurs except in patients who have been in profound shock. Remember, however, that patients who have been in coma for several hours before reaching hospital may have shifted enought of their blood volume into extravascular compartments to be seriously hypovolemic. Nevertheless, avoid fluid overload. Check electrolytes at intervals of 12 hours; once diuresis is attained, replace sodium with half-normal saline and potassium at a rate of 80 to 120 mEq or more per day. Digitalis or other cardiac drugs are useful only for patients with heart disease.

Monitor blood pressure, pulse, and respiration every half hour. In the unventilated patient, the presence of a respiration rate above approximately 20 implies either pneumonitis or, less often, incipient pulmonary edema. Most patients with drug poisoning are hypothermic, and body temperatures above 37.5° C generally imply infection. Hypothermia above 33° C requires no special treatment.

Prevent Complications. Keep unconscious patients semi-prone in the drainage position and change their position from side to side, but never place them fully supine. Treat potential pulmonary infection with a broad-spectrum antibiotic. These patients will be unconscious for only a few days, and the risk of emergence of drug-resistant bacterial infections is of less concern than is pneumonia caused by already aspirated material.

Hemodialysis is not necessary to treat poisoning with the short-acting hypnotics. However, hemodialysis may shorten the duration of coma for patients who have ingested large amounts of long-acting barbiturates such as barbital or phenobarbital, or who are in very deep coma from glutethimide overdose. Dialysis also is indicated for severe lithium or bromide poisoning.

Analeptics and pharmacologic stimulants are contraindicated for coma caused by depressant drug poisoning. Most carry the risk of overstimulating or producing convulsions in lightly poisoned patients.

RECOVERY AND PROGNOSIS. Patients recovering from coma require close medical supervision. Severe pneumonitis can develop as late as three to four days after recovery. If antimicrobial drugs were started during coma, they are best continued for at least 48 hours after it ends. Permanent physical sequelae are rare. Among 356 of our own such cases, residual brain injury was observed only once (in a patient who suffered an acute cardiac arrest). Peripheral nerve injuries from pressure developed in 6 subjects, and 14 subjects had pressure skin lesions leaving scars. Thre were no other physical residua.

Later management varies according to the patient's underlying psychiatric disorder and his attitudes upon recovery. Serious suicide attempts are never accidents, and reports of near-fatal ingestion caused by misunderstanding the dose or forgetting previous doses carry little validity. The expert opinion of a psychiatrist should be sought before deciding whether to release or to institutionalize a patient. The immediate prognosis is good, but there is a high incidence of recurrent attempts over the years.

Gilman AG, Goodman LS, Gilman A (eds.): The Pharmacological Basis of Therapeutics. 6th ed. New York, Macmillan, 1980. *The bible of its field.*

Hulten BA, Heath A: Clinical aspects of tricyclic antidepressant poisoning. Acta Med Scand 213:275, 1983 *A study of laboratory findings, complications, and treatment of 225 severely ill patients with a 2 per cent mortality.*

Spencer PS, Schaumberg HH: Experimental and Clinical Neurotoxicology. Baltimore, Williams and Wilkins, 1980. *A valuable compendium to nervous system poisons, mostly of the chronic variety.*

472.3. Prognosis in Severe Brain Damage and Diagnosis of Brain Death

Fred Plum

An important part of the physician's responsibility includes forecasting the outcome of illness. Modern medical advances save many lives that only a few years ago would have been lost to severe disease or trauma. Unfortunately, however, when severe brain dysfunction accompanies acute illness, it creates the risk that if the brain does not recover, vigorous treatment may be followed by an unwanted outcome. Several surveys conducted among both laymen and professionals have indicated that most persons would prefer death over a life of overwhelming and permanent neurologic disability. These considerations have resulted in the development of several empirically based guidelines to help the physician predict between possibly good and almost certainly very poor neurologic outcomes following severe illnesses causing severe brain damage or coma.

Nontraumatic Coma

The outcome from severe medical coma depends upon its cause and, with the exception of depressant drug poisoning, upon the initial severity and extent of neurologic damage as revealed by certain clinical neurologic signs obtainable at onset and within the first few days of illness.

At the onset it must be emphasized that depressant drug poisoning, no matter how deep the coma, reflects a state of general anesthesia; barring severe complications, almost all such patients who survive to reach medical attention can recover physically unscathed. This favorable prognosis applies even when coma is so profound that normal brainstem reflexes and the EEG temporarily disappear. Since most coma of unknown origin leading to emergency house calls or emergency room visits will be due to drug ingestion, such initially undiagnosed patients should receive maximal treatment unless direct evidence points to severe structural brain damage or systemic disease and the use of drugs by ingestion or for therapy has been ruled out.

TABLE 472–7. NEUROLOGIC TESTS THAT BEST INDICATE THE COURSE OF COMA AND ITS PROGNOSIS

Verbal responses	Ocular movements
Eye opening	a. Spontaneous
Pupillary reactions	b. Vestibular reflex
Corneal responses	Motor responses to noxious stimulation

Aside from drug poisoning, the acute or subacute development in the course of medical illness of loss of consicousness lasting more than a very few hours carries a poor prognosis in which only about 15 per cent of patients are likely to make a good recovery. The major problem in making early treatment decisions lies in attempting to discriminate between patients who have a chance of reaching a good outcome and those whose chances of a self-rewarding neurologic recovery are extremely small. In making such early decisions, clinical signs of abnormal foregrain and/or upper brainstem function have been found to be the most powerful available prognostic indicators. The nature of the underlying illness has secondary influence on whether or not a good outcome occurs but does not modify the accuracy of predictions between the extremes of good and bad prognosis as indicated by early signs. No laboratory determinants have been found accurately to predict outcome, nor does age significantly influence the quality of survival of adults in medical coma.

The clinical tests most valuable for estimating the capacity for recovery after medical coma are identical with those used in making the initial diagnosis and in following the later course of the patient in coma (Table 472–7). Verbal responses and eye opeining reflect mainly forebrain functions whereas tests of pupils, corneals, eye movements, and motor activity reflect the state of brainstem activity. In most instances, one cannot reliably estimate the outcome of coma immediately after the event, a time when rapid improvement often occurs. After about six hours, however, so long as the patient has not received heavy doses of sedative drugs or alcohol, certain neurologic findings begin to correlate increasingly strongly with teh potential for neurologic recovery and also confidently predict the outcome of about one third of those patients who ultimately will do badly. By the end of the first day, clinical signs accurately predict about two thirds of the patients who actually will do well. With each successive day, the signs develop greater predictive power. When considered appropriate, treatment can be adjusted accordingly.

Figure 472–1 provides a series of algorithms that describe the actural outcome of 500 patients in medical comas as related to their neurologic findings at 6 hours and on days one, three, and seven following onset. Reference to the charts discloses that signs of brainstem dysfunction (absent pupillary or corneal responses, imperfect or absent oculocephalic responses, or abnormal motor responses to stimulation) worsened the prognosis and, in combination, made it essentially hopeless when they persisted beyond the third day.

A few patients following an acute diffuse brain injury such as follows cardiac arrest, become immediately vegetative following the ictus and remain so as the days pass into weeks. Most who regain verbal abilities later than the end of the second week are left with prominent intellectual defects, especially in recent and anterograde memory, even if sensorimotor activities return to normal. No recorded example exists of an adult who has regained independent recovery after spending more than three weeks either in coma or a vegetative state. Care must be taken in such instances, however, to rule out a locked-in state (Ch. 472.1).

Traumatic Coma

Coma following head injury enjoys a somewhat more favorable outcome than that associated with medical illness. About

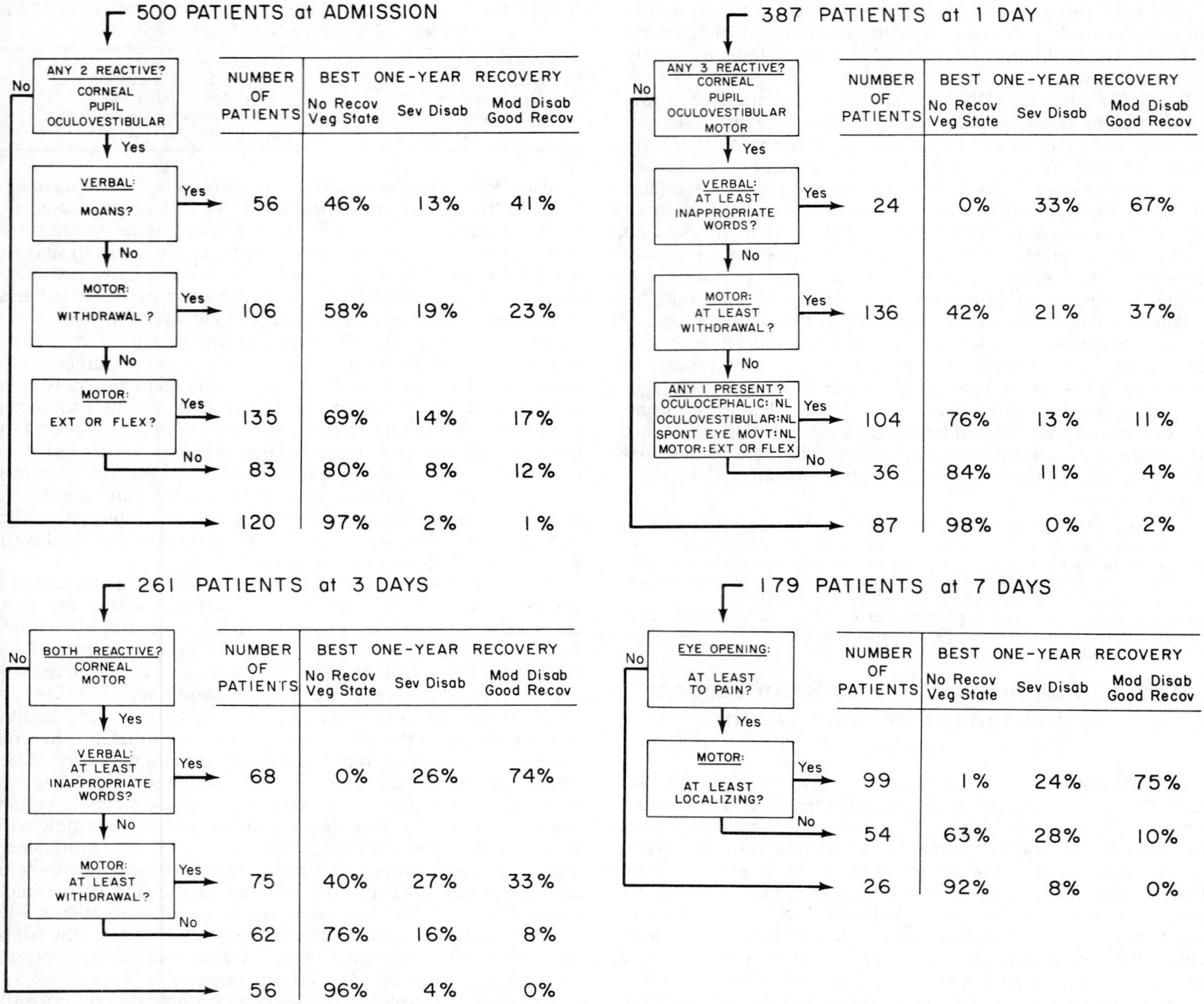

Figure 472–1. The best one-year outcome for 500 optimally treated patients in coma from nontraumatic causes. For each time period following onset, the diagram correlates the degree of recovery with clinical signs observed at that point. Although the diagrams describe actual events in a specific population, the numbers in most instances are sufficiently large to provide a basis for estimating prognosis among similarly affected patients in the future. (From Levy DE, Bates D, Caronna JJ, Cartlidge NEF, Knill-Jones RP, Lapinski RH, Singer BH, Shaw DA, Plum F: Prognosis in nontraumatic coma. Ann Intern Med 94:293, 1981, with permission.)

50 per cent of patients in coma from head injury die, and neurosurgeons debate whether treatment greatly affects that figure. Recovery is closely linked to age: the younger the better. As with medical coma, abnormal neuro-ophthalmologic signs reflecting brainstem dysfunction carry from the start a prognosis for death or disability with approximately 90 per cent of such patients either dying or remaining in near-vegetative states.

Brain Death

Modern resuscitative devices can maintain the functions of the heart, lungs, and visceral organs for hours or days after the life-maintaining brainstem dies. The modern emergence of this hopeless condition has led countries worldwide to adopt the principle that death of the person occurs whenever either the brain or the heart irreversibly fails in its functions. In the United States the time of brain death has been accepted as the time of the person's death in all instances in which the matter has been brought to judicial attention. Many states accept the brain death concept by statute, and in none has judicial review overturned it. The advantages to making the diagnosis and acting upon it are several. Proper medical preparations in such instances may preserve vital organs for transplantation so that other may live. Furthermore, the highly expensive hospital care of an artifically maintained corpse both offends humanity and adds to already burdensome medical costs. The Presidential Commission sets as the criterion for brain death the "irreversible cessation of all functions of the entire brain, including the brainstem." Criteria for the practical application of these principles are listed in Table 472–8.

Certain points in the diagnosis of brain death must be emphasized. *Recoverable drug depressant poisoning can in all ways resemble brain death and must be explicitly ruled out.* In any doubtful case, any evidence of EEG activity or of reflex activity of the

TABLE 472–8. CRITERIA FOR DIAGNOSIS OF BRAIN DEATH

1. Nature and duration of coma is known
   a. Known structural disease or irreversible systemic metabolic cause
   b. No chance of drug intoxication or hypothermia; no paralyzing or sedative drugs recently given for treatment
   c. Six-hour observation of no brain function is sufficient in cases of known structural cause when no drug or alcohol is involved in cause or treatment; otherwise, 12 to 24 hours plus negative drug screen required
2. Absence of cerebral and brainstem function
   a. No behavioral or reflex response to noxious stimuli above foramen magnum level
   b. Fixed pupils
   c. No oculovestibular responses to 50 ml ice water calories
   d. Apneic during oxygenation for ten minutes
   e. Systemic circulation may be intact
   f. Purely spinal reflexes may be retained
3. Supplementary (optional) criteria
   a. EEG isoelectric for 30 minutes at maximal gain
   b. Brainstem-evoked responses reflect absent function in vital brainstem structures
   c. No cerebral circulation present on angiographic examination

brainstem means that the brain is not dead and contravenes immediate discontinuation of life support. However, purely spinal reflex activity can persist after brain death, including reflexes of the limbs and even some upper cervical-controlled trunk movements.

In these controversy-laden and litigious times, it is recommended that physicians faced with applying and acting upon the diagnosis of brain death familiarize themselves with the additional pertinent material listed in the references.

Abrams MB, et al: Deciding to Forego Life-Sustaining Treatment. A Report on the Ethical, Medical, and Legal Issues in Treatment Decisions. President's Commission for the Study of Ethical Problems in Medicine and Biomedical and Behavioral Research. Washington, D.C., United States Government Printing office, March, 1983. *A long and thoughtful report on the problems associated with the terminally ill and the neurologically hopelessly damaged patient.*

Arena JM: Poisoning: Toxicology, Symptoms, Treatment. 4th ed. Springfield, IL, Charles C Thomas, 1979. *A detailed, classic text on all aspects of poisoning.*

Barber J, et al.: Guidelines for the determination of death: Report of the medical consultants on the diagnosis of death to the President's Commission for the Study of Ethical Problems in Medicine and Biomedical and Behavioral Research. Neurology 32:395, 1982. *The detailed report describing that cardiac death and brain death are equivalent and giving criteria for each.*

Driesbach RH: Handbook of Poisoning. 10th ed. Los Altos, CA. Lange Medical Publishers, 1980. *Succinct and handy, an excellent and up-to-date quick source to consult in emergencies.*

Levy DE, Bates D, Caronna JJ, Cartlidge NEF, Knill-Jones RP, Lapinski RH, S.INGER BH, Shaw DA, Plum F: Prognosis in nontraumatic coma. Ann Intern Med 94:293, 1981. *Provides detailed information correlating nature of illness and early clinical neurologic signs with best one-year outcome in 500 patients with loss of consciousness due to medical illness.*

Plum F, Posner JB: Diagnosis of Stupor and Coma. 3rd ed, revised printing. Philadelia, F. A. Davis Company, 1982. *Comprehensively discusses pathogenesis, diagnosis, prognosis, and emergency management of patients with acute severe brain dysfunction. Extensive references, especially to mechanisms and metabolic-diffuse brain diseases.*

472.4. Brief Loss of Consciousness

Fred Plum

Brief, not immediately explained loss of consciousness is a frequent complaint of patients entering any hospital emergency room. The cause of most such attacks, if diagnosable at all, can be determined on the basis of an accurate history alone. Routine physical and simple laboratory procedures, including blood work and ECG, are the most important additional diagnostic measures. Vasovagal reflex syncope is by far the most frequent cause of brief loss of consciousness (Table 472–9). Among patients with unwitnessed attacks, however, the cause of as many as one third eludes exact diagnosis even after comprehensive laboratory evaluation and a year or more of follow-up.

TABLE 472–9. PRINCIPAL CAUSES AND APPROXIMATE FREQUENCIES OF BRIEF LOSS OF CONSCIOUSNESS

Syncope	
Vasovagal/psychophysiologic	55%
Cardiovascular	10%
Central nervous system	
First seizure	10%
Other	5%
Drug-metabolic	5%
Undiagnosed, including hysteria	15%

Certain immediate guidelines aid empirically in differential diagnosis and prove valuable in deciding whether and to what extent further laboratory investigations will be necessary or fruitful. Among patients younger than age 40 years, brief loss of consciousness is almost always either vasodepressor syncope or undiagnosable unless the history or physical findings explicitly indicate the presence of severe heart disease, systemic illness, a seizure disorder or epileptiform movements during the attack, or alcohol-drug abuse. Among patients older than age 40 years, cardiac causes of syncope increase in frequency; but even among older patients, if the history, physical, and standard laboratory evaluation disclose no evidence of severe cardiac, systemic, or neurologic illness, the symptom most often has benign implications. Cryptic thrombophlebitis producing pulmonary infarction is a threat at any age; hypoglycemia or other metabolic perturbations are rare causes of brief loss of consciousness in the absence of strongly suggestive associated symptoms.

Neurologic causes of brief loss of consciousness other than syncope are comparatively few and are usually diagnosable by history: CT scans and EEGs almost never provide the diagnosis in patients unsuspected of neurologic disease. Drugs contribute importantly to loss of consciousness, producing hypotension in cardiacs and other older persons and predisposing to withdrawal seizures at any age over about 25 years. Head injury, while a common cause of brief concussion-amnesia, seldom represents a diagnostic problem unless neither witnesses nor evidence of surface trauma are present. Malingering-hysteria is a possible explanation for unexplained loss of consciousness, but the diagnosis should be considered only when social circumstances are appropriate, when history reveals evidence of previous similar difficulties, or when the examiner witnesses an obviously factitious attack. Even then, underlying associated physical disease should be ruled out.

SYNCOPE

Syncope is the commonest cause of brief unconsciousness and results, by definition, from an acute, global reduction in cerebral blood flow (CBF) sufficient to deprive cerebral-reticular neurons of substrate. Among otherwise healthy young persons syncope almost always carries a benign prognosis except for the associated inconvenience or specific attack-related dangers that future episodes may carry. Among persons in older age groups, cardiac causes for syncope become more common and must be meticulously searched for, as studies in some groups of patients with cardiogenic syncope show a one-year mortality as high as 30 per cent. Syncope rarely results from focal cerebral vascular disease, the only exception to this maxim being in patients in whom more than one of the four internal carotid-vertebral arteries are occluded so that any further arterial flow reduction globally affects brain perfusion.

With any cause of syncope, the degree of impaired unconsciousness depends upon (1) the severity of reduction of CBF and (2) its duration. Table 472–10 lists the major causes and the following paragraphs discuss the principal mechanisms and disorders following the order of the table.

SYNCOPE DUE PRIMARILY TO IMPAIRED RIGHT HEART FILLING (Mainly Reflex Syncope). Most examples of syncope resulting from a failure of right heart filling are associated with abnormalities in the neural feedback loop that reflexly controls the systemic circulation. The normal heart rate and blood pressure are regulated by efferent parasympathetic and sympathetic projections that originate from nuclei in the lower pons and medulla. Limbic forebrain and hypothalamic influences modulate cardiac action and the circulation mainly by acting on these medullary areas. Parasympathetic influences act predom-

TABLE 472–10. PRINCIPAL MECHANISMS OF SYNCOPE

I. Impaired right heart filling, cardiac rate slow and abnormal (mainly reflex)
  A. Vasodepressor syncope (vasovagal)
    1. Psychophysiologic (including hyperventilation)
    2. Visceral reflex (micturition, pain, gastrointestinal dilatation, acute vertigo)
    3. Carotid sinus, type 2
  B. Orthostatic hypotension
    1. Reduced blood volume (hemorrhage, acute salt and water loss, protein loss, enteropathy, burns)
    2. Hypotensive drugs
    3. Neurogenic and idiopathic
  C. Mechanically impaired right heart venous return (cough syncope, acute pulmonary infarction, fainting lark, near-term pregnancy, pericardial tamponade)
II. Impaired cardiac output
  A. Vagovagal attacks (transient sinus arrest)
    1. Psychophysiologic (uncommon)
    2. Visceral trauma (glossopharyngeal neuralgia, swallow syncope, tracheal stimulation, dilatation of hollow viscus)
    3. Carotid sinus, type 1
  B. Cardiac arrhythmia or asystole
    1. Extreme tachycardia > 160–180/minute
    2. Severe bradycardia < 30–40/minute
    3. Heart block: Morgagni-Adams-Stokes syndrome
    4. Ventricular fibrillation
III. Cerebral ischemia (rare)
  A. Severe cervical arterial obstructive disease plus transient ischemic attack (TIA) in remaining single carotid or vertebral artery
  B. Transient acutely increased intracranial pressure (plateau waves)
  C. Basilar migraine

inantly to slow the heart; they exert a minimal influence on the blood vessels. Postganglionic sympathetic fibers originate in the paravertebral cervical and thoracic sympathetic ganglia. They innervate the heart as well as both the arterial (resistance) and venous (capacitance) vascular beds of the viscera, trunk, and extremities. Closing the peripheral sympathetic reflex loop on the afferent side are fibers that arise in the baroreceptors of the aortic arch, other arteries, and, especially, the carotid sinus: their stimulation reduces the descending sympathetic outflow of the medullary pressor area.

Syncope resulting from failure of right heart filling nearly always reflects pooling of blood in the venous, capacitance vessels of the lower extremities or the splanchnic abdominal circulation. Relaxation of arterial resistance vessels plays a lesser role. Since gravitational factors contribute importantly to the impaired venous return, fainting caused by impaired right heart filling almost always occurs in the erect or, occasionally, sitting positions.

Acute Vasodepressor (Vasovagal) Syncope. This is the most common cause of fainting and typically is marked by a diphasic course. During an initial brief period of apprehension and anxiety, heart rate, blood pressure, total systemic resistance, and cardiac output all may increase. *This initial sequence*, however, often is *lacking*. The vasodepressor phase follows, during which heart rate and blood pressure fall, cardiac output declines, and the CBF eventually drops. Both sympathetic and parasympathetic abnormalities are involved, since atropine prevents the bradycardia but not the depressor response. Symptoms of palpitation, salivation, and anxiety characteristically mark the first phase, whereas progressive sensations of lightheadedness, giddiness, abdominal sinking sensations, nausea, urinary urgency, and finally "gray-out" or faintness accompany the vasodepressor component. Occasionally the reflex suppression of sympathetic tone comes so rapidly that the affected subject topples like a log. Rarely, with a severe attack of vasodepressor syncope, as with other forms of profound reduction of cardiac output and cerebral ischemia, brief tonic convulsive movements result.

Vasodepressor syncope most often is precipitated by conscious or unrecognized feelings of fear, disgust, and especially anxiety that precipitate discharges from the forebrain limbic system to activate medullary vasodepressor centers. During the course of the faint, such subjects appear pale rather than cyanotic, and the accompanying parasympathetic hyperactivity characteristically induces piloerection and sweating. Awareness and normal cardiovascular reflexes usually return promptly once the subject becomes supine. Occasionally dysautonomic influences on the heart are so profound as to induce arrhythmia. Engel and others have speculated that this is one mechanism causing sudden death, associated with sudden grief or fright.

Fainting is more likely in hungry subjects, in a warm moist environment, and after prolonged standing. A few individuals give a history of lifelong susceptibility to fainting attacks, and rarely one gets a history of multiple family members in several generations who have been susceptible to recurrent vasodepressor syndope.

Visceral reflex syncope acts via the same medullospinal pathways as the examples cited above. Afferent small myelinated pain fibers project directly on depressor and parasympathetic centers in the medulla. Thus a sense of faintness or even complete syncope can follow immediately after any of the following: emptying a full bladder from the standing position (micturition syncope), acute visceral pain (as occurs with a suddenly distended gut or an abrupt joint or ligament injury), or an attack of severe vertigo (as occurs with Menière's disease).

Carotid Sinus Syncope Type 2 describes a severe vasodepressor response to carotid sinus massage. The condition is rare and seldom a practical consideration except with neoplasms of the neck that directly irritate afferent glossopharyngeal fibers.

The diagnosis of vasodepressor syncope is made largely by history; rarely are the events medically witnessed. Among young persons who lack histories of neurologic or cardiovascular disease and have normal physical examinations, laboratory examinations beyond routine blood work and an ECG are almost always uninformative and therefore unnecessary. Treatment is symptomatic. Impending sensations of faintness should be treated promptly by placing the subject supine. Placing the head far forward in a sitting position is customary but less effective, because it fails to drain the enlarged pool of blood located in the muscles and veins of the lower extremities. If the heart rhythm is regular, no further resuscitative measures are needed. With severe irregularities or asystole, cardiopulmonary resuscitation is in order, but this is a rare requirement. Subjects who have fainted should be mobilized slowly, because the reflex abnormality occasionally can persist for as long as two hours. Prophylactic treatment has little value except when fainting occurs in response to disease or injury which requires attention.

Orthostatic Hypotension. Acute orthostatic hypotension occasionally can occur in normal persons after acute blood loss or following prolonged standing; affected subjects undergo a sudden collapse of sympathetic reflex tone, e.g., as with soldiers at parade rest in a hot sun. Recurrent symptoms of syncope or faintness accompanying the erect position, however, usually can be traced to the presence of the chronic use of vasodepressor drugs or to neurologic disorders involving the peripheral or central nervous system. Increased age tends to intensify the effects of the neurologic disorder; in a few instances, autonomic failure appears to be attributable entirely to blunting of central autonomic reflex control. Many drugs accentuate tendencies to orthostatic hypotension, including almost all of the antihypertensive agents and a large proportion of the antidepressants, phenothiazines, and sedatives. Bed rest deconditions sympathetic vasomotor reflexes and predisposes to orthostatic hypotension. Any tendency to impaired sympathetic reflex control is accentuated by a reduced blood volume such as is caused by Addison's disease, protein loss, or enteropathy. The combination of chromic diuretic use and vasodepressant medication outnumbers all other causes combined.

Orthostatic hypotension sufficient to cause cerebral symptoms can occur either rapidly upon standing or develop insidiously over seconds or minutes. Although symptoms of faintness and giddiness predominate in some patients, others lack such warnings, presumably because of the absence of strong efferent parasympathetic activity. When patients in this latter group sit for long periods or stand, they may become confused or tremulous without the usual sensations of faintness. Mental cloudiness, staggering, or falling is more common than complete unconsciousness. Diagnosis comes from observing an acute or progressive decline in the mean blood pressure of more than 10 to 15 torr in the erect position. Autonomic insufficiency can be inferred by observing an unchanging pulse rate despite the hypotension, and confirmed by establishing other evidence of autonomic impairment. The simplest way to evaluate sympathetic tone at the bedside is to take the pulse while the supine patient performs a vigorous Valsalva maneuver; the normal response consists of a palpable post-Valsalva slowing of pulse and a 10 to 30 torr rise in mean blood pressure. Other autonomic changes are discussed in Ch. 478 on Autonomic Disufficiency.

Treatment of orthostatic hypotension depends upon the cause. Symptomatic treatment requires eliminating drugs that cause hypotension, searching for and correcting causes of blood volume depletion, and applying elastic stockings to the lower extremities. When other measures fail, an increased salt intake and, subsequently, administering the salt-retaining steroid fludrocortisone, 0.3 to 0.8 mg per day in divided doses, can be cautiously initiated. The chronic use of vasopressor agents seldom helps. Just as vasomotor reflexes can be deconditioned by excess bed rest, they can be at least partially reconditioned by erect activity. Every effort should be made to keep affected patients up and walking.

Most other instances of syncope caused by *mechanical impairment of right heart filling* result from conditions in which the diagnosis and mechanism are fairly self-evident, as noted in Table 472–10. Treatment is directed at the underlying cause.

SYNCOPE DUE PRIMARILY TO IMPAIRED LEFT HEART OUTPUT (Mainly Cardiac Syncope). *Vagovagal attacks* consist of reflexly induced changes in the cardiac rhythm, including nodal or sinus arrest, atrioventricular asystole, atrioventricular block, sinoatrial block, and ventricular arrhythmias. Usually these are accompanied by relatively minor vasodepressor changes in the peripheral vasculature, implying a lesser sympathetic component. Most but not all patients with vagovagal attacks belong to the older population and have associated heart disease. Most vagally induced cardiac arrhythmia or arrest represents an abnormally intense cardiac response to a relatively normal degree of increased parasympathetic stimulatioc or sympathetic inhibtion. Vagal bradycardia or arrest occasionally is induced by sudden emotional stimuli, but more commonly follows acute noxious or abnormal visceral stimulation. Severe bradycardia or arrest especially accompanies glossopharyngeal neuralgia, swallowing in patients with mechanical esophageal lesions, sudden painful dilatations of a hollow viscus, prostatic manipulation, tracheal stimulation, or visceral wounds. *Carotid sinus syncope Type 1* is a rare phenomenon in which massage or pressure of the sinus induces transient asystole.

Cardiac-related syncope represents less than 10 per cent of all patients who present to emergency or outpatient facilities complainint of brief loss of consciousness. The symptom has medical importance far beyond that number, however, because of its implications of serious disease or sudden death if not effectively prevented or treated.

Cardiac syncope almost always reflects serious heart disease. Analyses of large series of patients show that serious associated risk factors include severe hypertension; a history of, respectively, myocardial infarction, congestive heart failure, or severe valvular disease (especially arotic stenosis); and electrocardiographic monitoring abnormalities on laboratory testing. With cardiac patients, even extensive laboratory studies often fail to disclose the specific reason for asystole-syncope, but major associated abnormalities on prolonged electrocardiographic monctoring include episodes of sinus pauses lasting more than 8 seconds, sinus bradycardia less than 40 per minute, atrial fibrillation with a slow ventricular rate, sustained supraventricular tachycardia, and Mobitz type II atrioventricular block. In the absence of specific predisposing abnormalities discovered by history, physical examination and ECG monitoring, direct electrophysiologic studies of the heart, cardiac catheterization, coronary or cerebral angiography, brain CT scanning, and electroencephalography seldom add diagnostically helpful information. Management of cardiac syncope depends upon the nature of the underlying heart disease, although affected persons should be considered for pacemaker insertion.

OTHER CAUSES OF BRIEF LOSS OF CONSCIOUSNESS

Hyperventilation is closely related to syncope in its mechanisms in that a globally reduced cerebral blood flow gives rise to sensations of giddiness, faintness, and other distress. Full unconsciousness rarely occurs without some additional abnormal maneuver. The abnormal state is most often part of an anxiety response, and often is accompanied by sensations of suffocation, pressure on the chest, and a sense of being unable to obtain the satisfaction of a lung-filling deep breath. Extreme or prolonged hyperventilation can produce feelings of unreality with anxiety bordering on panic.

In healthy subjects, only a modest increase in respiratory rate and depth is required to drop Pa_{CO_2} levels within a very few minutes to 25 mm Hg or less; once a new steady state develops, little more than the normal level of breathing is sufficient to match bodily CO_2 production and maintain hypocapnia. Accordingly, casual inspection may show no more than a respiratory rate of 16 to 18 per minute, interrupted perhaps by occasional sighs. Hypocapnia induces cerebral vasoconstriction, which reduces the amount of oxygen delivered to the brain and is the presumed basis of many of the accompanying sensations.

Symptoms and signs include feelings of unreality, difficulty in concentrating, and several hard-to-explain sensory complaints, such as unilateral or bilateral chest pain or paresthesias involving the body and extremities. Symptoms of facial twitching, carpal spasm, and perioral paresthesias are more easily understood as part of alkalotic tetany.

Diagnosis is easy when otherwise structurally healthy patients complain of the aforementioned symptoms in settings of anxiety dyspnea, but often is conjectural when made in retrospect. Some patients can reproduce their symptoms by voluntarily overbreathing, and insights gained from the maneuver can be helpful in guiding treatment. Most often the symptoms are observed as part of a larger pattern of anxiety and must be treated accordingly.

Hyperventilation occasionally precipitates syncope under special circumstances. Children sometimes voluntarily hyperventilate, then perform a vigorous Valsalve maneuver to induce syncope in the already partially oxygen-deprived brain (fainting lark). Athletes may unconsciously repeat a similar sequence when competing in contests such as weight lifting or squat jumps. More dangerous is a pattern wherein underwater swimmers hyperventilate before diving, then exhaust their oxygen reserves by exercise before producing sufficient carbon dioxide to result in dyspnea. The ensuing cerebral hypoxia can induce submersion syncope, which is sometimes fatal.

SEIZURE DISORDERS. Seizure disorders, discussed fully in Ch. 510, produce a diagnostic problem under four principal circumstances:

1. *Rapid, profound syncope* may induce a single brief tonic seizure or series of clonic twitches as a result of abrupt cerebral ischemia. The response is somewhat more frequent with severe episodes or when the subject has made maximal effort to stand or sit despite premonitory symptoms. Differential diagnosis rests on identifying the following as more consistent with syncope: the attendant psychologic circumstances and physical

appearance, the associated medical conditions and body position, the brief quality of the seizure, and the presence of a normal neurologic examination and interictal EEG.

2. *Akinetic seizures* in children consist of attacks of suddenly falling or pitching to the ground. Similar seizures occur in the supine position and are marked by psychologic unresponsiveness accompanied by generalized muscular hypotonia or brief body spasm. Diagnosis rests on the typical history, the absence of pallor during witnessed episodes, the age and frequency of onset, and the presence of an abnormal interictal EEG. *Absence (petit mal) seizures* rarely provide a diagnostic problem, since the child, although out of contact during the attacks, neither falls nor turns pale and usually has no memory of the episode. The EEG is abnormal.

3. *Partial complex (psychomotor) seizures* sometimes include brief behavioral automatisms in which the subject recalls only being out of contact and may retrospectively consider himself to have suffered a state of unconsciousness. Usually the presence of a characteristic, self-recognized aura or set of incipient symptoms indicates the diagnosis. Falling to the ground rarely occurs unless a generalized seizure develops. Witnessed attacks and the EEG usually are typical and, in any event, not syncopal in their appearance.

4. *Postictal unresponsiveness* from grand mal attacks produces unconsciousness for five to thirty minutes, the duration usually depending on the severity of the preceding convulsion. Diagnosis is a problem only if the seizure was unwitnessed, in which case the state may look like concussion or profound fainting. However, the postictal state is marked initially by flushing (cyanosis), giving way to pallor, hyperpnea, and deep unresponsiveness.

HYPOGLYCEMIA (see Ch. 231). Hypoglycemia, usually caused by excess exogenous insulin, less often by insulin secreted from endogenous tissues, can produce a variety of relatively brief episodes of neurologic dysfunction. These can consist, variably, of brief confusional episodes, seizures of a variety of types, narcoleptic-like syndromes, and focal or tetraparetic weakness with or without coma. The condition is rare except in insulin-receiving diabetics. Diagnosis depends on suspicion plus the detection of blood sugars of less than 30 to 40 mg per deciliter during an attack or following induced fasting.

DRUG OR ALCOHOL BLACKOUTS. Drug or alcohol blackouts consist of episodes of such severe intoxication that they anesthetize memory for the event, leaving the subject with an episode of focal amnesia. Many are accompanied by "passing out," a condition with a clinical appearance that differs in no way from deep, barely arousable sleep.

CONCUSSION-POSTCONCUSSION AMNESIA. Variable periods of memory loss for immediate sugsequent events can follow brief periods of concussive unconsciousness. The usual question is whether an intrinsic malady caused the fall or whether the fall represented the whole illness. Only diagnostic diligence can solve the issue.

ACUTE INTRACRANIAL HYPERTENSION. This condition occasionally produces brief episodes of loss of consciousness that may resemble syncope. The classic, but rare, example occurs with colloid cysts of the third ventricle which intermittently obstruct that cavity or produce plateau waves (Ch. 472.1). More frequently, brief unconsciousness may accompany the onset of acute subarachnoid hemorrhage. The unconscious episode, which is syncopal in its abruptness and often accompanied by either a tonic extensor spasm or brief clonic jerks, is most often due to an acute cardiac arrhythmia accompanying the onset of bleeding. Cerebral hemorrhage with intraventricular rupture can produce similar intracranial events.

CONDITIONS SOMETIMES RESEMBLING LOSS OF CONSCIOUSNESS

DROP SPELLS. These are poorly understood attacks affecting mainly women of middle age or older. The legs of affected subjects suddenly and unexplainedly give way, and the women fall, often injuring themselves but experiencing no observed interruption of consciousness. The cause is unknown, although basilar artery ischemia has been postulated. There is no known effective treatment.

TRANSIENT GLOBAL AMNESIA (see Ch. 493 to 495). This name is applied to attacks lasting usually one to six hours, rarely longer, wherein the subject loses knowledge of all immediate and many recent past events but retains knowledge of self, the distant past, and the maenities of behavior. The episodes affect the middle-aged or elderly, and are suspected but not proved to represent the effects of vascular disease. During the attack, patients have not associated neurologic deficits and recover spontaneously and completely, but with no memory for the content of the episode. Consciousness is not lost and only if the patient was entirely unattended during the episode would the diagnosis be in question.

CONVERSION REACTIONS OR MALINGERING. Hysterical or other psychogenic unresponsiveness is almost impossible to diagnose in retrospect from the history. If such a condition occurs during the physical examination, however, the diagnosis is based on the absence of physiologic abnormality and the presence of additional, often bizarre features. Most subjects awaken with gentle but firm confrontation. A few do so only when advised that psychiatric admission lies in store. Mutilating stimuli are unjustified and often unsuccessful as ways to prove the diagnosis.

Day SC, Cook ET, Funkenstein H, Goldman L: Evaluation and outcome of emergency room patients with transient loss of consciousness. Am J Med 73:15, 1982. *An analysis of 198 patients, giving differential diagnosis, identifying low- and high-risk groups, and indicating relative value of laboratory tests.*

De Bono DP, Warlow CP, Hyman NM: Cardiac rhythm abnormalities in patients presenting with transient non-focal neurological symptoms: A diagnostic gray area? Br Med J 1:1437, 1982. *An evaluation of 89 patients versus controls. Only arrhythmias in young patients and bradyarrhythmia at any age were considered relevant. Monitoring contributed to diagnosis in less than one third.*

Engel GL: Psychological stress, vasodepressor (vasovagal) syncope and sudden death. Ann Intern Med 89:403, 1978. *Must reading for the internist by one of the pioneers in understanding of both the physiology and emotion of cardiovascular responses.*

Evans DW, Lum LC: Hyperventilation: An important cause of pseudoangina. Lancet 1:155, 1977. *A clinical article, emphasizing the often misleading symptoms of the disorder.*

Kapoor WN, Karpf M, Maher Y, Miller RA, Levey GS: Syncope of unknown origin. The need for a more effective approach to its diagnostic evaluation. JAMA 247:2687, 1982. *Among 121 older patients with syncope, cardiac monitoring, cardiac electrophysiologic studies, and cardiac catheterization provided diagnostic evidence in only 13. Glucose tolerance tests, head CT, brain scans, lumbar puncture, and skull x-ray aided diagnosis in none.*

Kapoor WN, Karpf M, Wieand S, Peterson PA, Levey GS: A prospective evaluation and follow-up of patients with syncope. N Engl J Med 309:197, 1983. *Among 204 mainly older patients with syncope, 40 per cent of whom were hospitalized from the start, diagnosis could be made in 53 per cent. Twenty-six per cent had a cardiovascular cause. At one year half the cardiovascular group had died, compared to 12 per cent with noncardiovascular causes and 6 per cent in the idiopathic group.*

472.5. Sleep and Its Disorders

J. Allan Hobson

Modern research supports three important changes in our common-sense orientation to sleep:

First, sleep is a complex biologic function with extremely variable length and depth. Individuals may vary in their baseline sleep need between four and ten hours. Short sleepers tend to be hyperactive but productive and well-adjusted, whereas long sleepers tend to be low-key, underachieving, and mildly depressed. Experiments in animals show marked differences in sleep length in genetically different strains; given the existence of a bell-shaped distribution of sleep length, the duration variable cannot, per se, be taken as an index of pathology, and the physician should beware of pushing patients against powerful biologic gradients.

Second, sleep is variable *within* individuals. Marked, built-in changes take place over the life span. The neonate sleeps two thirds of the time. At sexual maturity, this duration has fallen by half, but the capacity for deep, fulfilling sleep is still robust. By age 40 the sleep of fully productive humans is normally more shallow, and by age 60 sleep length may have decreased further. There is a linear positive correlation between age and the number of awakenings.

Third, sleep is also variable within individuals from one sleep-wake cycle to the next. There is a dynamic relationship between waking state variables and sleep characteristics over both the short and long term. Hence, during highly productive periods, sleep need may decrease; sleep length may also undergo unwanted but normal shortening during periods of anxiety and stress. Within limits—to be judged by the individual's adaptive responses—these should be regarded as signals to be heeded, understood, and dealt with during the awake state rather than symptoms of disease needing to be extinguished via the chemical manipulation of sleep.

Activity patterns also influence sleep variables. Few farmers complain of insomnia during the haying season, and animal experiments indicate that moderate exercise reduces sleep latency while also increasing sleep length and depth. These points should be brought home to the sedentary city dweller. Another point is that sleep is not only variable and responsive but carefully regulated. Thus good sleep can often be expected to follow poor. And, despite highly publicized initial results, sleep deprivation studies have not revealed specific or long-lasting ill effects, so that conservative management is not likely to be dangerous even to the patient who may ultimately need pharmacologic treatment.

PHYSIOLOGY AND PHARMACOLOGY OF SLEEP. The metabolism of all organisms is temporally ordered. Cosmic forces synchronize circadian rhythms, endogenous oscillations of slightly more than 24 hours in length, which are reset each day by light and other time cues. In all mammals, including man, the circadian oscillator appears to include the suprachiasmatic nucleus of the hypothalamus. The hypothalamus receives a direct input from the optic tract, which presumably delivers the light pulses that reset the rhythm each day. Lesions of the posterior hypothalamus produce hypersomnia, whereas lesions of the anterior hypothalamus produce insomnia.

As all who have crossed time zones in jet airplanes can testify, the circadian rhythm is a powerful, persistent, and plastic determinant of when we sleep and wake. Whether its action is mediated by the sleep-inducing peptides that have been isolated from the spinal fluid of sleep-deprived animals or by conventional neurotransmission is not yet clear, but it is certain that the EEG sleep cycle is under its control.

Each sleep period consists of a series of biphasic 90- to 100-minute cycles. The non–rapid eye movement (NREM) phase, which initiates sleep and each subsequent cycle is also called slow wave or synchronized sleep. It is characterized by progressive EEG slowing and by corresponding decreases in muscle tone, heart rate, respiratory rate, and blood pressure. When this deactivation process is maximal—at about mid-cycle—subjects are difficult to rouse and may be disoriented or even confabulate when asked to report their mental activity.

The rapid eye movement (REM) phase of the cycle, which follows NREM and ends each cycle, is also called fast wave or desynchronized sleep. It is characterized by progressive reactivation of the EEG and autonomic functions. Paradoxically, however, muscle tone is even further depressed in REM; this is caused by active inhibition which finally obliterates tonus and effectively paralyzes all but the ocular musculature. Silently signaling the intense internal activation of many neuronal systems of the brain, the eyes execute spectacular runs of nystagmiform movement behind the still-closed lids. Heart and respiratory rates quicken and blood pressure rises, especially during the clusters of REM. Upon awakening from REM sleep, subjects are easily aroused and often report detailed and vivid dreams.

This NREM-REM cycle repeats itself, usually without interruption, four or five times each night. Since the later cycles have shallower NREM troughs, relatively more time is devoted to REM toward morning. Major shifts in posture—of which the subject is generally unaware—occur at NREM-REM phase transitions, hence at least eight or ten times per night. The important point for the physician to grasp is that the physiologic systems underlying mentation, movement, and cardiorespiratory control are all undergoing dynamic and dramatic changes in their operating properties throughout the night.

Lesion and ablation studies in animals indicate that the system controlling the EEG sleep cycle is located in the pontine brainstem. Single cell recordings suggest that this pontine clock is composed of two interconnected neuronal populations whose activity levels fluctuate periodically and oppositely. Their out-of-phase oscillation appears to be due to the reciprocal interaction of their excitatory and inhibitory neurotransmitters.

During waking the resting activity level of aminergic inhibitory neurons is high. The nuclei containing these "waking" cells include the noradrenergic locus ceruleus and the serotonergic dorsal raphe, which have been implicated in control of sleep state, mood, and learning. As a consequence of aminergic inhibition, the resting activity level of cholinergic neurons in many brainstem reticular nuclei is actually low in waking. During the non-REM phase of the sleep cycle, aminergic inhibition gradually declines; simultaneously, cholinergic excitation gradually increases so that at mid-cycle the balance between aminergic inhibition and cholinergic excitation shifts. The REM period occurs when aminergic inhibition has fallen to its low point and cholinergic excitation becomes maximal. The microinjection of either cholinergic agonists *or* aminergic antagonists into the pontine brainstem is capable of converting an animal's state from awake to REM sleep. Unfortunately, the drugs used in clinical practice and in most research studies are administered by parenteral routes and may thus affect multiple peripheral and central systems with confusing, contradictory, and uninterpretable results.

A PATHOPHYSIOLOGIC APPROACH TO THE SLEEP DISORDERS. *A static shift* in net drive on one or both of the opposing brainstem populations will result in an increasing propensity for one state or the other to occur. Thus insomnia (or too much waking) will occur if there is either aminergic overactivity or cholinergic underactivity, or both. Examples are stress, anxiety, and amphetamine-induced insomnia; all are characterized by aminergic overactivity and all are countered by aminergic antagonists. Reciprocally, hypersomnia (or too little waking) will occur if there is either aminergic underactivity or cholinergic overactivity, or both. Examples are boredom, characterologic depression, and narcolepsy—all characterized by aminergic underactivity and all countered by aminergic agonists. The probability of waking or sleep is thus a function of the set-point of the controlling oscillator. Set-point level is susceptible to environmental influences: exogenous (e.g., noise) and endogenous (e.g., cortical or muscular) inputs both play their part.

The *dynamics* of the system are such that timing errors may occur, resulting in a temporal dissociation of sleep-wake state components. For example, if the subsystems controlling mentation and motor activity are not precisely coordinated, we may see hallucinosis (hypnagogic hallucinations) when falling asleep, or persistent immobility (sleep paralysis) when aroused from REM—as in narcolepsy; conversely, we may see motor activity emerge from deep NREM sleep—as in somnambulism, sleep talking, or enuresis.

The dynamic shifts in level of activity of the multiple neuronal subsystems that are integral to state regulation by reciprocal interaction also have predictable autonomic manifestations. Thus the decreasing aminergic drive on brainstem reticular neurons that is integral to sleep onset may be associated with cessation of breathing (as in central sleep apnea) if the set-point of the respiratory oscillator—which itself is a reticular system—is suddenly changed. Similarly, the deactivation (probably a disfacilitation) of motor systems that is integral to sleep onset may compromise a marginal airway via decreasing tonus of glossal and hypoglossal muscles (as in obstructive sleep apnea).

THE EVALUATION OF SLEEP COMPLAINTS. Until recently, sleep was neither directly observed nor measured, so that the physician was literally groping in the dark in his diagnostic efforts. Sleep laboratory studies indicate that there are two kinds of errors in subjective reporting: overestimation of time spent awake in insomnia, and underestimation of the physiologically important respiratory disturbances that occur in sleep. Thus an insomniac patient perceives his one or two hours of sleep loss as three or four, whereas a severely apneic patient can be unaware of the hundreds of arousals that occur causing recurrent cyanosis with oxygen saturations of 50 per cent or less! This irony is compounded by the fact that the anxious insomniac may put great pressure on the physician for a prompt, uncritical, and even potentially dangerous therapeutic program, whereas the apneic patient, urgently needing tracheostomy, remains lethargic and uncomplaining.

Objective observation can be accomplished in several direct and simple ways prior to referral for sleep laboratory evaluation. One is the sleep log, which should be kept for at least two and preferably for four weeks following an initial visit. On a single sheet, each line of which represents 24 hours, are recorded the times of retiring, falling asleep, arousals, awakening, and arising. Dated entries, corresponding to the lines, indicate subjective state and behavioral data for the intervening waking periods.

The sleep log can be more reliable if there is a cooperative bed partner or roommate. Since the bed partner is not only a potential investigative collaborator but often the plaintiff, it is important that he or she be invited to the follow-up visit, if not the intake. Because of the snoring (sleep apnea) or kicking (nocturnal myoclonus) of the patient, it may be the bed partner who is the more insomniac!

Obstructive apneic episodes can be documented by the bed partner, using an audio cassette recorder. The tape recorder is also useful in the characterization of sleep talking, sleep walking, bruxism, night terrors, and nightmares.

So sensitive is sleep to situational variables that even more vigorous efforts should be made to increase our capability of documenting both normal and abnormal sleep in its natural habitat. New techniques capable of clinical adaptations include actigraphic movement recording and visual monitoring by time-lapse photography or video of the posture shifts that normally accompany the NREM-REM stage shifts of the sleep cycle. These relatively simple, home-based recording techniques give values which correlate with subjective estimates of good and poor sleep and even provide measures of sleep latency, a critical variable in the documentation of insomnia and its therapeutic management.

At present, sleep laboratory studies provide the only definitive means of documenting the diagnostic signs of the specific sleep disorders. If narcolepsy, nocturnal myoclonus, or sleep apnea cannot be ruled out by the simple means described above, referral to a sleep laboratory is indicated.

CLASSIFICATION OF SLEEP DISORDERS. The balance of this chapter follows a simple, complaint-ordered scheme: too little sleep (insomnias), too much sleep (hypersomnias), or abnormal sleep behavior (parasomnias) (see Table 472–11).

The Insomnias. Sleep is so variable and complaints of insomnia are so common as to raise serious questions about the point at which complaints of too little sleep should be regarded as abnormal (in a statistical sense) or pathologic (in a medical sense). In the absence of objective data, considerable judgment is required in making these decisions. Current trends, spurred by the discovery of side effects of sedative medication, are toward a conservative, behaviorally oriented management approach of disorders of initiating and maintaining sleep. To be successful, this approach must first emphasize careful diagnostic study to determine specific underlying causes. In the most common, nonspecific cases, patients need education in the multifactorial determinants of sleep quality and duration, support in their behavioral and pharmacologic potentiation, and close follow-up monitoring of these interventions.

TABLE 472–11. CLASSIFICATION OF SLEEP DISORDERS BY COMPLAINT

- Too little sleep (the insomnias)
  - Specific
    - Circadian rhythm shifts
    - Nocturnal myoclonus
    - Sleep apnea syndromes (see below)
  - Secondary
    - Medical
      - Fever
      - Pain
      - Cardiopulmonary disease
    - Psychiatric
      - Anxiety, stress
      - Alcohol and drugs
      - Depression
      - Schizophrenia
- Too much sleep (the hypersomnias)
  - Specific
    - Narcolepsy
    - Kleine-Levin syndrome
    - Sleep apnea syndromes
  - Secondary
    - CNS lesions
    - Pickwickian syndrome
    - Depression
- Abnormal sleep behavior (the parasomnias)
  - Motor
    - Enuresis
    - Sleep walking
    - Sleep talking
    - Night terrors
    - Bruxism
  - Respiratory
    - Sleep apnea syndromes—central, peripheral, mixed types

Usually the primary care physician is the person who most possesses the proximity, continuity, and credibility necessary for success in this area in which time, knowledge, and care are the only effective substitutes for the illusion of magical cure. In addition to the conditions discussed here, it should be recognized that the sleep apnea syndrome is an important part of the differential diagnosis of insomnia.

Medical Insomnia. Specific and nonspecific effects on the sleep cycle oscillator are exerted by many medical conditions. These include diseases producing fever (which immediately suppresses REM sleep) and pain (which produces a general increase in arousal level). Sleep loss is common in hospital settings, where sleep-disruptive procedures combine with anxiety to make night life miserable for many patients. Patients with coronary or pulmonary insufficiencies may decompensate during the autonomic storm of REM sleep. The patient with congestive heart failure or emphysema may be aware or unaware of the frequent interruptions of sleep which are caused by anoxic stimulation of the reticular formation and which may be lifesaving. Before prescribing sedatives, specific treatment of the underlying medical disease and manipulation of environmental variables must be vigorously pursued.

Psychiatric Insomnia. A variety of neurotic and psychotic disorders, all known to be associated with disturbances in balance of central sympathetic and cholinergic activity, are characterized by difficulty falling asleep and staying asleep. Anxiety and obsessional neuroses, the schizophrenias, and the manic-depressive syndromes are now postulated to be mediated by abnormal neurotransmission in the same central adrenergic systems as those which regulate sleep.

The management of chronic anxiety, always notoriously difficult, is now further complicated by the discovery of three undesirable properties of the class of agents called benzodiazepines. One is a subtle but pernicious addiction syndrome, associated with the long-term use of diazepam. As in other cases of drug dependency, insomnia may be a presenting complaint and the physician must, by careful history-taking and restraint, avoid compounding or aggravating an already iatrogenic disorder of sleep. Another is rebound insomnia, a worsening of sleep following intermediate term use of nitrazepam, flunitrazepam, temazepam, and triazolam. The third is an interference with daytime functioning caused by the cumulative build-up of active metabolites of such "long-acting" agents as flurazepam, diazepam, and flunitrazepam, whose products have half-lives of 36 to 48 hours. Short-acting agents, with half-lives of ten to twelve hours, are less liable to suppress daytime effectiveness (lorazepam, triazolam, and temazepam).

GUIDELINES FOR PRESCRIBING SEDATIVES. A versatile and flexible approach to sedative prescription is needed to exploit the assets and minimize the liabilities of the medication used. For example, when the desired relief of acute anxiety and insomnia has been obtained from a diazepine such as diazepam (Valium), 2 to 5 mg at bedtime, patient and physician can expect some temporary worsening of sleep when the drug is withdrawn. One should not attempt to suppress this time-limited effect of the treatment itself by increasing drug administration. The other agents (e.g., triazolam [Halcion], 0.25 to 0.5 mg at bedtime) tend not to produce rebound and are effective hypnotics. They do not suppress REM, but, like their short-acting congeners, they do suppress Stages III and IV of NREM sleep. In cases of persistent or recurrent insomnia, intermittent and alternating drug use reduces the problems of habituation and withdrawal. Recent suggestions that barbiturates can be reconsidered seem ill advised in view of the low margin of safety and addictive potential of these agents.

Enthusiasm has been expressed for tryptophan sedation (1 to 5 grams at bedtime) but the efficacy of this naturally occurring amino acid has not been proved. The old standby chloral hydrate (0.5 to 1.0 gram at bedtime) still deserves consideration. Amitriptyline (50 mg at bedtime) has been reported to be sleep enhancing even in patients who are not depressed, and the tricyclic antidepressants also improve the sleep of severely depressed patients who may complain of sudden worsening of sleep when effective treatment is stopped. During such withdrawal, frightening hypnopompic hallucinations may mislead both patient and doctor into thinking that psychosis is recurrent when, in reality, a time-limited and transitory pharmacodynamic intensification of REM sleep is the cause. As with rebound insomnia, this complaint demands reassurance, not reinstitution of medication.

Alcohol is a self-administered CNS depressant with profound short- and long-term effects on sleep. The REM phase of the cycle is suppressed during the first part of the night when sleep may be unusually sound. An associated suppression of normal posture shifts may explain the Saturday night paralysis that results from nerve compression occurring in alcoholic sleep. Later in the night, when metabolic breakdown products accumulate, sleep is fitful and more REM deprivation is incurred. Hangover includes a feeling of sleepiness and fatigue which alcohol may temporarily reverse only to perpetuate and intensify. Long-term REM deprivation may be an intervening variable in the ultimate development of alcoholic hallucinoid syndromes; in fact, delirium tremens develops at the peak of REM rebound on about the third day of withdrawal.

NOCTURNAL MYOCLONUS. In late middle age and elderly patients, rhythmic muscle twitches may cause sleep-disturbing involuntary movements of the extremities. The benzodiazepine clonazepam (0.5 to 1.0 mg at bedtime) is reported effective, probably because of a combination of anticonvulsant, sedative, and muscle relaxant effects.

The Hypersomnias. The conditions to be considered as possibly responsible for the complaint of excessive sleep or sleepiness include sleep disorders (narcolepsy) and specific medical disorders (e.g., pickwickian syndrome, CNS lesions). They also include conditions in which the excessive sleepiness is secondary to the disturbed sleep of the parasomnias (sleep apnea syndromes) or a manifestation of underlying mood or personality disorder (depressive and passive dependent types).

NARCOLEPSY. Narcolepsy is a syndrome which is best understood as an increased excitability of the REM generator. Patients complain of persistent drowsiness and one or more of a tetrad of specific signs: (1) *Sleep attacks,* which occur suddenly, are often REM sleep attacks. (2) *Cataplexy* is an equally sudden muscle weakness akin to the atonia which normally occurs only in nocturnal REM. Cataplexy is often precipitated by surprise, mirth, or anger. (3) *Hypnagogic hallucinations* are the subjective accompaniment of sleep-onset REM periods. (4) *Sleep paralysis* is an abnormal extension of REM sleep atonia into the waking state. Thus the narcoleptic patient demonstrates both kinds of sleep pathophysiology: a low set-point level of the REM oscillator—which explains the direct precipitation of REM sleep from waking (the sleep attacks and the sleep onset REM periods); and a dissociation of the ascending (conscious state) and descending (muscle tone) components of REM sleep—which explains the sleep attacks without cataplexy, the cataplexy without sleep attacks, and the sleep paralysis.

Polygraphic studies of narcolepsy demonstrate increased sleepiness (multiple sleep latency test), identify the sleep attack as REM sleep, and disclose REM periods at nocturnal sleep onset. Since narcolepsy is vocationally disabling and sometimes life threatening, it is important that every effort be made to establish the diagnosis objectively. It is equally important not to label all patients who complain of drowsiness as narcoleptic, since many may have sleep apnea syndrome or a nonspecific sleep disorder. Because of stigmatization of affected individuals as "lazy" and because of the legal problems of long-term management with amphetamines, the existence of self-help groups is a welcome innovation.

The set-point of the pontine oscillator can be raised—and the narcolepsy syndrome prevented—by either decreasing cholinergic excitatory drive or increasing aminergic inhibitory drive, or both. The second mechanism best accounts for the traditional effectiveness of the amphetamines, which increase the efficacy of noradrenergic synapses by mimicry. The more recently described beneficial effects of the antidepressants, especially upon cataplexy, are probably due both to blockade of norepinephrine reuptake and/or monamine oxidase inhibition, both of which enhance noradrenergic inhibition by increasing the duration of physiologically released norepinephrine, and to the anticholinergic effects of these drugs. Because they produce fewer long-term problems, the amine reuptake blockers, if effective in a given patient, are the agents of choice.

KLEINE-LEVIN SNYDROME. This extremely rare disorder occurs primarily in adolescent males and is characterized by episodic periods of excessive sleep and overeating, lasting up to several weeks. The cause is unknown. There is no specific treatment, but the condition remits in adulthood.

DEPRESSION. Not only do asymptomatic long-sleepers tend to be depressed, some clinically depressed patients also tend to hypersomnolence (as well as to difficulty falling asleep). Markedly shortened REM latency, increased REM percentage, and increased REM density allow depressive sleep disturbance to be distinguished from that of the insomniac and of normal individuals. This depressive sleep disorder is best treated with amine reuptake blockers (which are also anticholinergic) and is aggravated by physostigmine.

PICKWICKIAN SYNDROME. Hypersomnia is integral to the pickwickian syndrome and a primary result of the anoxemia and hypercarbia consequent upon waking state hypoventilation. It should be emphasized that waking arterial oxygen levels are normal in the sleep apnea syndromes and that the hypersomnia seen in those conditions is, in part, secondary to the sleep disturbance.

The Parasomnias. All the parasomnias share the feature of loss of control of some neural subsystem during sleep. All appear to be age, sex, and sleep stage dependent.

ENURESIS. Bedwetting is a troublesome sleep disorder occurring predominantly in preadolescent males. (Roughly 10 per cent of boys aged four to fourteen are affected.) Because the full bladder does not trigger an awakening, enuresis has been conceived of as a disorder of arousal. The beneficial effects of imipramine (25 to 50 mg given at bedtime) have been attributed mainly to peripheral anticholinergic effects on the bladder. Because of the risks of using drugs and even behavioral treatment in children, only the most persistent and severe cases should be treated.

NIGHT TERRORS, NIGHTMARES, SLEEP WALKING, SLEEP TALKING, AND BRUXISM. Dissociation of sensory and motor integration during NREM sleep characterizes all of these conditions. In night terrors, there is a partial arousal, in panic, from Stages III and IV of NREM sleep, associated with tachycardia and tachypnea. Although capable of coordinated motor behavior and responsive to sensory input, the affected child may hallucinate and thus terrify his parents as much as himself. Fortunately night terrors are benign and short lived, so that reassurance is both appropriate and adequate. Nightmares also occur in older subjects. They can be precipitated from NREM sleep when they are characterized by pure fear (without visual hallucinoid imagery) or REM sleep (when vivid frightening dreams are reported). In both types, intense autonomic storm is measurable. Nightmares of the NREM type have been reported to respond to benzodiazepines with Stages III and IV suppressing properties (such as diazepam, 2 to 5 mg). Age is also helpful here, since Stage IV declines markedly in the fourth decade. The REM type of nightmare (or bad dream) may persist and may present as sleep interruption insomnia. No specific treatment has been reported.

In sleep talking and sleep walking, automatic motor activity begins in Stages III and IV of NREM sleep without full arousal and without accompanying mental activity; bruxism occurs in Stage I of NREM sleep. Sleep talking is entirely benign and should not be treated; disturbed roommates may have to make adjustments. Preventive measures are indicated in bruxism and sleep walking; a boxer's mouthpiece prevents enamel destruction by the persistent and automatic tooth grinding (in bruxism), and a child's stairway gate or other physical restraint may avoid embarrassment and injury to the sleep walker (in somnambulism). There is no evidence that any of these conditions are psychologically determined, and all are age related.

THE SLEEP APNEA SYNDROMES. The respiratory neurons of the brainstem constitute a reticular oscillator of similar design and close proximity to the sleep cycle clock. It is therefore little wonder that this system shows such dramatic state dependency. It may even turn out that some neurons, especially those of the so-called pneumotaxic center, are common to both systems.

At sleep onset and increasingly throughout the NREM phase of sleep, respiration slows and deepens as if the excitatory drive on the medullary respiratory oscillator were decreasing; in contrast, the advent of REM is associated with an increase in variability of both rate and depth of respiration. Hence, one may see a marked hyperpnea—a series of rapid short shallow breaths—or an apneic pause, or both, in association with the clusters of eye movement that punctuate REM and give this curious sleep phase its name.

The respiratory neural oscillator moves air through a complex peripheral system (the airway and lungs) and is influenced by a variety of feedback influences. All of these peripheral factors are also subject to the vicissitudes of the sleep-wake cycle via the autonomic and spinal pathways affecting smooth and skeletal muscle. Thus the decreases in muscle tone that are part of NREM sleep onset, and the further active inhibition of muscle tone that is an intrinsic part of REM, may render a marginal airway nonpatent, so that air cannot be moved even if the consequent changes in blood gases signal the sleep-depressed respiratory oscillation to increase its output. Upon such a background the terms central, peripheral, and mixed type of sleep apnea assume logical and lucid order. In fact, physiology suggests that all state-dependent respiratory changes, from the normal to the pathologic, must involve *both* central and peripheral factors.

Middle-aged male patients complaining of either excessive daytime sleepiness or incapability of staying asleep at night should be considered as possibly suffering from the sleep apnea syndrome. If they are obese and snore, then descriptions on tape recordings of their obstructive apneic spells—which occur on the order of 300 times per night—may be obtained from a bed partner. These peripherally mediated events are due to collapse of a fat-compromised airway by the negative intrathoracic pressure of inspiration; the situation is only made worse by the vigorous compensatory respiratory effects which ensue, accompanied by the strained grunting of the Müller maneuver, and which are often noted by the observant bed partner. Observable cyanosis may be a sign of the oxygen desaturation (50 per cent is not unusual). Recovery occurs only when arousal restores both the set-point of the respiratory oscillator and the tonus of the tongue and pharyngeal musculature. The frequent awakenings contribute to the excessive daytime sleepiness.

Even the peripheral obstructive type of apnea, which is often relieved by tracheostomy or a continuous positive-pressure nasally delivered airstream, probably has a central component because neither surgery nor weight loss eliminates the sleep apnea episodes. Furthermore, some men who are neither obese nor airway obstructed show only the apneas. These individuals may reflect most purely the CNS pathophysiology common to all the sleep apnea syndromes. Such cases are uncommon and difficult to diagnose—an important point, since sedative medication, prescribed as a well-intentioned response to the complaint of insomnia, may depress the sensitivity of the respiratory reticular formation which translates hypoxia into a life-saving arousal. Patients suspected of having sleep apnea syndrome are best referred for diagnosis and treatment to a sleep laboratory with pulmonary recording capability.

Cardiac abnormalities can complicate the pickwickian syndrome and the sleep apneas. Marked sinus arrhythmias may accompany the apneic spells, and extreme bradycardia, asystoles, second degree atrioventricular block, premature ventricular contractions, atrial flutter, and ventricular tachycardia have all been reported. The abnormalities clear if night-time apnea and its associated hypoxemia are prevented.

CONTRIBUTING FACTORS AND CLINICAL VARIANTS OF SLEEP APNEA SYNDROME. At all ages males are more prone than females to intrinsic sleep abnormalities. The tendency to snore, to stop breathing, and to collapse and/or obstruct the airway in sleep has a genetic component and is greater in men of the same family. The times in life at which pathologic consequences are most likely to emerge are infancy (sudden infant death syndrome), puberty (chubby puffer syndrome), and late middle age (sleep apnea syndrome).

Cardiorespiratory arrest is a likely cause of *sudden "crib" death* in infancy. In those infants who are "near-miss" for sudden infant death, apneas occur with increasing frequency at four and one half months of age, predominantly during NREM sleep. The period of greatest risk for fatal accidents is between birth and six months of age, and respiratory infection is thought to be a contributing factor. Home-monitoring systems have been developed to detect apneas and alert parents to the need for resuscitative maneuvers.

In the *chubby puffer syndrome,* obese prepubescent males may resemble adult pickwickians whose symptoms are ascribed to primary alveolar hypoventilation, and this sign may persist after temporary relief has been provided by adenotonsillectomy. These facts imply a central respiratory abnormality whose neural basis is as yet obscure. Treatments designed to increase central respiratory drive with aminophylline and progesterone have not been generally effective. Recent reports claim that the antidepressant tricyclic agent protriptyline has been effective.

Physiology and Pharmacology

Hobson JA, Brazier MAB (eds.): The Reticular Formation Revisited. New York, Raven Press, 1980. *This book covers the most recent basic research on the neurobiology of the reticular formation, including its role in control of respiration, muscle tone, and the states of consciousness.*

Hobson JA, Steriade M: Neuronal basis of behavioral state control. *In* Handbook of Physiology, Section on Neurophysiology, Volume on Intrinsic Regulatory

Systems of the Brain. American Physiological Society, 1984. *A comprehensive and critical review of cellular level studies of sleep phenomena and a detailed account of the neurophysiologic and neuropharmacologic basis of the reciprocal interaction model of sleep cycle control.*

Lader M (ed.): New perspectives in benzodiazepine therapy. Arz Forsch/Drug Res 30:851, 1980. *This set of papers provides an up-to-date survey of a rapidly developing area of neuropharmacologic research with important clinical applications.*

Sleep Disorders

Guilleminault C, Dement WC (eds.): Sleep Apnea Syndromes. New York, A. R. Liss, 1978. *A symposium addressing the clinical and physiologic aspects of the disorders.*

Hauri P: The Sleep Disorders. 2nd ed. Kalamazoo, MI, Upjohn, 1982. *A concise, complete, and sensible summary with excellent illustrations; for medical students, house officers, and practitioners.*

Hobson JA: Sleep: Order and disorder. Behav Biol Med Monogr 1:1, 1983. *A detailed and extensively referenced discussion of sleep pathophysiology.*

Roffwarg H: Diagnostic classification of sleep and arousal disorders. Sleep 2:1, 1979. *A comprehensive diagnostic inventory which constitutes an invaluable reference for the sleep disorders specialist.*

Sullivan CE, Issa EG, Berthon-Jones M, Eves L: Reversal of obstructive sleep apnea by continuous positive airway pressure applied through the nares. Lancet 1:862, 1981. *Description of a new, effective, nonsurgical treatment with a diagram of the effective nasal adapter.*

473. REGIONAL DIAGNOSIS OF CEREBRAL DISORDERS

Fred Plum

Localizing diagnosis is an important part of the evaluation of neurologic diseases. Although radiographic methods for examining the brain safely and painlessly have advanced a great deal during recent years, they commonly fail to detect the early stages of many tumors, some regional infections, and most degenerative diseases. The regional diagnosis of most epileptogenic foci also lies below the discriminatory powers of conventional radiography or imaging methods. Since therapy in epilepsy often depends on the anatomic locus of the seizure focus, clinical judgment becomes crucial. Regional diagnosis helps in differentiating neurologic from psychiatric disease and provides the additional reward that it tells the observer something about how the brain works, a philosophic interest that has increasingly drawn human inquiry for the past two centuries.

Several general principles influence the accuracy of regional clinical diagnosis. First, lesions that damage the corticospinal, somatosensory, or special sensory pathways generally can be localized earlier and more precisely than those that affect the brain's association cortex. Second, the rate at which a lesion appears and enlarges and the degree to which it irritates surrounding brain tissue influences not only how rapidly signs and symptoms develop but their severity as well. Slowly growing intracranial tumors, for example, sometimes can reach the size of small oranges before they produce notable signs and symptoms, even when they impinge on primary motor or sensory pathways. By contrast, pea-sized metastatic growths can in some instances produce incapacitating disabilities. Third, certain individual behavioral symptoms can reflect perturbed functions in any of several of the cerebral association areas; inattention, for example, can accompany disease in either the frontal or parietal lobe, and the distinction of its regional cause must be made by identifying additional signs that accompany it. Finally, by shifting soft tissues against the unyielding skull and dural meninges, large lesions of the brain sometimes produce functional changes in neural structures that lie at a distance from the lesion itself. Such remote effects especially accompany acutely arising lesions such as brain infarcts, hemorrhages, or malignant tumors. Sometimes, however, they can lead the unwary observer to errors of clinical localization even when slowly enlarging masses are at fault.

Frontal Lobes

The frontal lobes influence two principal functions, motor control and expressive behavior. The neurons constituting the primary motor area reside in the precentral gyrus and are arranged somatotopically along that structure in a manner that gives especially large representation to the fine movements regulating phonation and distal limb control, especially of the upper extremity. The adjacent, postcentral gyrus of the parietal lobe provides the cortical receiving area for sensory perceptions and is arranged with a similar somatotopic representation. The two cortical areas work interdependently, and the pre- and post-Rolandic banks often are described together as the primary sensorimotor cortex. Immediately anterior to the primary motor strip lies the premotor cortex on the lateral surface and the supplementary motor area on the medial frontal cortex. Cerebellar, basal ganglia, and cortical association projections feed into this premotor area, which provides prefinal integration of motor acts before the motor cortex synthesizes their final coordination and transmits the signal via the corticospinal tract. Within the prefrontal areas lie the principal zones influencing voluntary, saccadic control of eye movements. Broca's speech area is found along the inferior prefrontal region of the dominant hemisphere. The remainder of the lateral and medial surface, plus almost all of the inferior surface of the frontal lobes, contains neural mechanisms regulating behavior, emotion, and autonomic function, especially as these activities relate to motor expression.

Motor symptoms of frontal lobe disease (Table 473–1) are most prominent when lesions directly intrude on the Rolandic motor strip or its descending corticospinal pathways in the corona radiata or internal capsule. Selective premotor signs and symptoms occur when a lesion in that region either stimulates seizures or reaches a relatively large size.

Two major behavioral syndromes result from frontal lobe damage. Both usually reflect the presence of relatively large lesions directly or indirectly producing bilateral frontal lobe dysfunction; unilateral abnormalities, unless they produce seizures, often remain asymptomatic in their early stages. As an example, unilateral prefrontal lobe amputation can be carried out to remove localized tumors, often leaving no discernible change in personality or behavior. Similarly, minor effects have attended efforts to relieve or alter abnormal psychiatric traits by unilateral anterior frontal lobe removal. Such procedures, to cause a change in behavior, usually must interrupt limbic frontal pathways.

SYNDROME OF THE BASAL FOREBRAIN. This clinical constellation accompanies large, usually bilateral lesions involving the septal area and adjacent basal forebrain extending forward into the orbitofrontal cortex toward the frontal pole. Affective patients are apathetic, inattentive, hypokinetic, and hypophonic or mute. Many show an autonomic apraxia, being unable to initiate deep breathing or to micturate on command. There may

TABLE 473–1. MOTOR SYMPTOMS OF FRONTAL LOBE DISEASE*

	Paralysis	Seizure
Precentral gyrus	Focal distal weakness, maximal in lower face, hand, sometimes foot. Distribution occasionally resembles glove or stocking. Hyperactive reflexes, mild spasticity, Babinski if foot involved.	Jacksonian: focal onset of face, thumb, foot with "march" toward proximal limb and trunk.
Corona radiata or internal capsule	Increasingly spastic hemiplegia.	
Prefrontal area	Slow, hypokinetic, sometimes ataxic movements; ocular ipsiversion; paratonic resistance to passive stretch; palmar or plantar grasping; Broca's syntactic aphasia, occasionally mutism.	Adversive: ocular contraversion, elevated arm, body turning, speech arrest.

*All arise contralateral to the brain lesion.

be incontinence because of indifference. The lesions often displace more posteriorly located structures so as to produce corticospinal tract dysfunction with hyperactive deep tendon reflexes and extensor plantar responses on one or both sides of the body.

FRONTAL POLAR AND PREFRONTAL SYNDROMES. Small lesions often cause no measurable behavioral abnormalities. Large ones produce the frontal lobe syndrome of classic repute. Affected patients are distractible, euphoric, and facetious, and are unable appropriately to plan ahead or to judge the future implications of present acts or experiences. Lesions affecting the medial prefrontal cortex may result in urgency incontinence. Seizures, if they occur, include adversive or grand mal attacks. Enlarging lesions may eventually encroach upon premotor function to cause hypokinesia, contralateral inattention, paratonia, and grasp reflexes.

Parietal Lobe

The postcentral gyrus contains the neural mechanisms that abstract somatosensory stimuli into stereoperception and stereognosis. The more posteriorly located association cortex receives heavy afferent projections from somatosensory and visual receiving areas and progressively abstracts the information to create an internal map by which the subject gives attention to the spatial world of his body and the outer world that surrounds it. Several perceptual and cognitive functions of the parietal association cortex are predominantly lateralized to one or the other hemisphere. The nondominant hemisphere especially relates to recognition of external space, sometimes on both sides of the body, while the dominant parietal lobe abstracts right-sided body space but also influences the capacity for arithmetic calculation and for right-left orientation. Both hemispheres contribute importantly to the advanced programming of complex motor acts (praxis).

The *syndrome of the postcentral primary somatosensory cortex* includes impaired or absent capacities to recognize the form, texture, relative size, and weight of objects, especially of complex items producing multiple spatial-morphologic stimuli. The integration of morphologic perception into memory must also be coded in this area, since patients with only partial cortical sensory loss still have great difficulty in naming a palpated object even when they possess some residual capacity to describe its form. For example, one of our otherwise intelligent patients with a post-Rolandic parietal lesion was able to identify a block in her left hand as being "an edged, partly flat lump" but was unable to synthesize this into calling it either a block or a cube. Lesions confined to the primary cortical sensory area do not affect cutaneous thresholds for vibration, pain, temperature, or simple touch.

Small lesions affecting the posterior parietal areas produce few abnormal symptoms. Limited evidence from man plus physiologic analyses in the monkey suggests that the dorsal posterior region functions largely to make beginning abstractions of somatosensory perceptions and relate them to visual perception. The inferior parietal region, located where the parietal, occipital, and temporal lobes converge, serves a multimodal function in which somatosensory, spatial, visual, and auditory perceptions are integrated and related to the memory, limbic, and language functions of the temporal lobes. Most so-called parietal lobe syndromes reflect damage predominantly to this posterior inferior area.

Nondominant posteroinferior parietal lobe syndromes include symptoms whose severity and extent depend directly upon the size and acuteness of the lesion. Most frequent is constructional apraxia, really a spatial defect, reflected by difficulties in either drawing simple figures such as a clock face or in copying the outlines of a cube or intersecting hexagons. Selective spatial disorientation sometimes is striking. One of our patients, a milkman with a small neoplasm in this region, remained capable in all dimensions of his job except that he was no longer able to recall automatically the pattern of his delivery route. Dressing apraxia similarly may be a relatively isolated symptom of the nondominant parietal lobe. With larger lesions in this area, patients develop inattention to contralateral space, a phenomenon sometimes called neglect, which may extend to include the failure to perceive left-sided tactile or visual stimuli when such stimuli are presented to both sides of the body or visual field simultaneously (the phenomenon of extinction). With very large lesions extending deeply to involve the thalamus or forward to impair the descending corticospinal pathways, patients may fail to recognize the presence of the sensory defect and even deny that a hemiparesis exists (anosagnosia). Acutely, patients with such large lesions may suffer a protracted confusional delirium. Later or sometimes from the start some exhibit a remarkable emptiness of affect and a degree of inattentiveness that suggests that neither their bodies nor the world contralateral to the damaged hemisphere any longer exists in either their attention or their memory. Almost always the cause of such severe "parietal lobe" syndromes lies in cerebral infarcts that damage a substantial fraction of the territory of the middle cerebral artery, with the tissue injury extending well beyond the parietal lobe. Most specific agnosias or apraxias also can be traced to the presence of similarly large lesions or bilateral disturbances of the hemispheres.

Left-sided, dominant hemisphere parietal lesions produce symptoms somewhat different from the above. The effects of very large lesions usually cannot be judged because they nearly always are associated with severe aphasia. Constructional apraxia accompanies restricted left posterior inferior parietal lobe damage more frequently than right-sided damage. Patients with lesions in this area commonly have great difficulties making arithmetic calculations (acalculia) even of a simple nature. Some authorities attribute a combination of acalculia, right-left disorientation, agraphia, and finger agnosia (Gerstmann's syndrome) to damage of the left inferior parietal lobe, but it is doubtful that it occurs with lesions isolated to that area.

Temporal Lobes

The temporal lobes contain neural structures critical to auditory perception, memory, language, and emotion. Each auditory cortex receives projections from both ears so that hearing itself rarely is disrupted by cerebral lesions. The memory and language functions of the temporal lobes are discussed in Ch. 474. The inferior loop of the geniculocalcarine radiation passes through the temporal lobe, where its injury may give rise to characteristic visual field defects as described in Ch. 479.

The parahippocampal region and the hippocampus of the temporal lobe contribute to the phylogenetically ancient "limbic lobe" of the cerebral cortex, which rims the upper brainstem and together with certain subcortical nuclei makes up the *limbic system*. The limbic system integrates emotions and their expressions with memory and with the polymodal sensory input that converges upon the temporal lobe. The system projects to efferent motor and other areas of the cortex and via the hypothalamus to autonomic and reticular structures in the brainstem and spinal cord.

In monkeys, removal of the temporal lobes bilaterally gives

TABLE 473–2. ICTAL MANIFESTATIONS OF TEMPORAL LOBE EPILEPTIC FOCI

Medial Basal Structures	Lateral Cortical Structures
Uncus: Olfactory hallucinations Amygdala, Hippocampus: Memory disturbances (jamais or déjà vu); forced thinking, dreamy state	Language impairment; hissing, roaring, or clicking hallucinations; vertigo

↓ (both converge to)

Epigastric distress
Blank stare
Repetitive vegetative or somatic automatisms

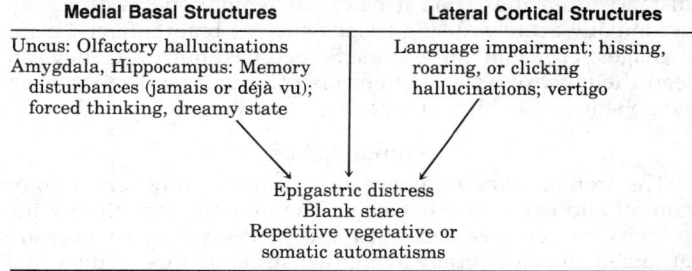

TABLE 473–3. COMMON INTERICTAL TRAITS OF PATIENTS WITH TEMPORAL LOBE EPILEPTIC FOCI

Humorless
Obsessional
Dependent
Philosophical
Sad
Hyposexual

rise to a remarkable behavioral disorder termed the Kluver-Bucy syndrome, marked by amnesia, excessive orality, distractibility, placidity, and indiscriminate sexuality. A somewhat similar constellation of symptoms, usually accompanied by more extensive behavioral changes, has been reported in humans, most often following diffuse brain injuries or in one of the degenerative dementias. More restrictive visceral and emotional aberrations mark the ictal and to some degree interictal behavior of patients with temporal lobe epilepsy (Ch. 510). Tables 473–2 and 473–3 list some of these major symptoms.

Controversy has surrounded the question of whether patients with temporal lobe or limbic system lesions or temporal lobe epilepsy are more given to violence or psychosis as a direct result of their lesions. Present evidence is inconclusive. If restrained during an attack, patients with temporal lobe epilepsy often will lash out physically. Unprovoked violence, however, probably is no more frequent among patients with temporal lobe epilepsy than among the remainder of the population. It seems doubtful that epilepsy or specific brain lesions can be regarded as a medically satisfactory explanation for aggressive crime.

Occipital lobe functions are discussed with disorders of the visual system (Ch. 479–2).

Baer D: Hemispheric specialization and the neurology of emotion. Arch Neurol 40:195, 1983. *Several studies are reviewed that suggest that the right hemisphere may be "dominant" for certain emotions.*

Baer DM, Fedio P: Quantitative analysis of interictal behavior in temporal lobe epilepsy. Arch Neurol 34:454, 1977. *An important effort to quantify differences in personality traits between epileptics and controls.*

Biemond A, Vinken PJ, Bruyn GW: Localization in Clinical Neurology. Handbook of Neurology. Vol 2. Amsterdam, North Holland, 1969. *A compendium of classic observations on the topic.*

Delgado-Escueta AV, Mattson RH, King L, et al.: The nature of aggression during epileptic sezures. N Engl J Med 305:711, 1981. *An NIH committee reports that the phenomenon is rare.*

Hier DB, Mondlock J, Caplan LR: Behavioral abnormalities after right hemisphere stroke. Neurology 33:337, 1983. *A careful analysis of large series of patients with damage to the right parietal lobe and more.*

Lilly R, Cummings JL, Benson DF, Frankel M: The human Klüver-Bucy syndrome. Neurology 33:1141, 1983. *Twelve patients with severe bilateral anterior temporal lobe damage are described with rather mixed syndromes.*

Mesulam M-M: A cortical network for directed attention and unilateral neglect. Ann Neurol 10:309, 1981. *A thoughtful synthesis of the sensory integrative functions of the parietal association areas.*

Pritchard PB, Lombroso CT, McIntyre M: Psychological complications of temporal lobe epilepsy. Neurology 30:227, 1980. *A confirmation of the high incidence of behavioral-personality difficulties in these patients.*

Roland PE: Astereognosis. Arch Neurol 33:543, 1976. *Empirical confirmation that stereognosis depends on mechanisms that arise in the immediate postcentral cortex.*

Roland PE, Larsen B, Lassen NA, Skinhøj E: Supplementary motor area and other cortical areas in organization of voluntary movements in man. J Neurophysiol 43:118, 1980. *Preprogramming of hand movement is associated with increased blood flow in supplementary motor areas, while during actual movement blood flow increased bilaterally in these areas as well as in the bilateral premotor and motor areas of the cortex. A classic in the physiologic substrate of behavior.*

Stevens JR, Hermann BP: Temporal lobe epilepsy, psychopathology, and violence: The state of evidence. Neurology 31:1127, 1981. *A vigorous defense against the view that psychopathology and temporal lobe epilepsy are directly linked.*

474. FOCAL DISTURBANCES OF HIGHER FUNCTION

Fred Plum

LANGUAGE AND APHASIA

Verbal language represents the process by which the forebrain applies symbolic terms to objects and concepts in order to formalize its knowledge of sensory perceptions, memories, emotional responses, and the stream of preverbal inner thoughts. The neuroanatomy of the mechanisms that accomplish language is known, albeit imprecisely, from three sources. One is the postmortem study of patients who have been carefully evaluated for language impairment. The second is the change produced in language by stimulating various regions of the cerebral cortex by skilled surgeons in the process of operating on appropriate patients. The third is radiography, including CT, NMR, and PET scans, which allow one to study the anatomy of language in the intact patient.

Although wide areas of both hemispheres contribute to language function, the critical regions are concentrated in two principal cortical zones, a posterior, predominantly receptor–integrative zone and an anterior region devoted predominantly to language expression. The principal posterior portion of the language cortex occupies the posterior superior temporal gyrus extending from approximately the transverse auditory gyrus back to the end of the Sylvian fissure. This, the Wernicke area, represents the region where sensory perceptions appear to be integrated with inner thought and memory so as to generate the fundamental abstractions of language. The region of the adjacent angular and supramarginal gyri, as well as of the superiorly adjacent parietal operculum and, perhaps, the pulvinar nucleus of the thalamus, contributes importantly but in a clinically less predictable manner to the fundamental synthesis of language. More anteriorly, *Broca's area,* lying in the inferolateral frontal lobe just anterior to the primary motor cortex and extending under the surface into the frontal operculum, is critical to the normal verbal or written expression of speech. Lesions surrounding the Wernicke area, interrupting pathways projecting into it but not the speech cortex itself, disrupt selective aspects of posterior language function, while peri-Brocal lesions somewhat similarly produce partial impairments in the expression of language. Evidence obtained by Penfield and others, who have removed tumors or epileptogenic lesions from Broca's area, indicates that in some of these patients most or all of verbal and written expression may return following damage to or even removal of parts of this region. Normal language function, however, rarely returns to the adult who suffers severe damage to the Wernicke area of the dominant hemisphere.

Language function is strongly lateralized in most human brains. Anatomically, the left hemisphere usually contains a longer Sylvian fissure than the right, and the planum of the left temporal lobe (the area lying in the Sylvian fissure in back of the posterior edge of the transverse (Heschl's) auditory gyrus) is larger than the right in two thirds of brains. The anatomic changes are found in infants and fetuses as well as in adult brains. Clinically, language laterality in patients can be estimated in two major ways: by correlating the side of temporofrontal brain lesions with the presence or absence of an aphasia and, in persons with normal speech, by observing the effect of injecting amobarbital sodium into the ispsilateral or contralateral carotid artery. The anesthetic briefly anesthetizes the ipsilateral hemisphere, including its language activities, and gives important preoperative knowledge of the risks of surgery to the particular area of brain. Both kinds of studies indicate that in almost all right-handed persons the left hemisphere is heavily dominant for speech and that aphasia resulting from damage to the left posterior language areas seldom fully recovers. Among the left-handed and the strongly ambidextrous, about 70 per cent show a left hemisphere language dominance or predominance. Of the remaining 30 per cent, about half show strong language representation in each hemisphere, while the remainder are right dominant. A feature of many left-handed and ambidextrous persons is that damage to the major language area on either side may produce acute symptoms of aphasia, but a higher percentage recover than do right-handed persons with comparable left hemispheric lesions.

Language function in children represents a special case. Most youngsters who suffer a severe hemispheric brain injury when less than six years of age recover normal or nearly normal language capabilities whether or not aphasia accompanies the early postinjury period. Even among such children, however, transient aphasia occurs nine times more often following damage to the left temporal frontal area than to the right.

Aphasia or dysphasia describes an impairment or loss of language function as a result of damage to the specific language areas of the cerebrum. The condition must be distinguished from *dysarthria,* a disturbance in the articulation of speech, as well as from defects in sensory systems that prevent perceptions from reaching the language cortex. Persons deaf and blind from peripheral causes can learn a language as long as the brain is intact, while disease of the motor system, the cerebellum, or the vocal apparatus can cripple or halt the outflow of words but does not produce aphasia.

The pattern of an aphasia depends on the part or parts of the speech brain that are damaged. Language represents the integration and expression of many aspects of brain function and injuries to its mechanisms can result in a number of somewhat varying symptom complexes. Among the properties of a language are (1) the comprehension of symbols, (2) the ability to transform perceptions or inner thoughts into words, and (3) the ability to express symbols. Geschwind (Table 474–1) has found that most aphasic disorders can be classified by testing comprehension of language, fluency of output, and ability to repeat phrases.

Lesions damaging the dominant posterior superior temporal gyrus and its adjacent area characteristically destroy the capacity to recognize the sensory symbols of language or to transform inner thoughts into meaningful words. The classic result is *Wernicke's aphasia.* Affected patients cannot recognize spoken, written, or symbolic instructions except, perhaps intermittently, the simplest verbal commands (e.g., "Stop!"). Despite the severe injury to comprehension, the brain preserves a memory storehouse of words so that expressed words often are chosen correctly. Patients with Wernicke's aphasia speak fluently with a natural rhythm, although the result possesses neither understandable syntax nor meaning. Insight is lost and prognosis for total recovery is poor. Posterior lesions outside the immediate Wernicke area tend to produce more restricted disturbances. Lesions of the parietal operculum may give rise to conduction aphasia, a disorder in which the patient speaks fluently but makes many errors similar to those of Wernicke's aphasia. However, comprehension is relatively normal.

Other strategically placed focal lesions of the posterior dominant hemisphere can destroy selectively one or another dimension of language perception. *Alexia* (inability to comprehend written language while retaining relatively good general vision, especially in the left visual field) without *agraphia* (the inability to write language despite the preservation of related motor function) results when a lesion destroys the left visual cortex and, in addition, extends to involve the splenium of the corpus callosum. The placement cuts off the projection that otherwise connects the unaffected right visual cortex to the language areas of the left. Such patients, despite their inability to comprehend the written word, can speak and write normally, in contrast to those with a combination of *alexia with agraphia,* in whom normal auditory comprehension, thought, and speech remain, but the comprehension of both visual and written language symbols is lost. The abnormality is rare and has been stated to follow lesions of the left angular gyrus. *Pure word deafness* describes the circumstance in which auditory language perception selectively is lost despite intact hearing and the preservation of other language capabilities. This rare phenomenon follows bilateral selective damage to the auditory cortex of the superior temporal gyrus or, reportedly, can accompany subcortical white matter damage in the left temporal lobe that injures the adjacent left auditory cortex and disconnects the transcallosal fibers from the right temporal lobe destined for Wernicke's area.

Broca's aphasia is characterized by severe disturbances in the output of either spontaneous or commanded speech and writing. Comprehension is relatively well preserved, although things spoken usually are understood better than things read. Largely because of vascular distributions, many patients with Broca's aphasia also have an associated right hemiparesis or hemiplegia, but this is the result of an independent internal capsular lesion. Enlargement of the lesion into the adjacent premotor cortex is believed to explain an associated motor apraxia observed in some such patients. A more restricted lesion may cause aphasia characterized by slow, effortful, dysarthric speech with normal syntax and preserved ability to write normally.

Global aphasia describes the combined severe loss of all major aspects of language function. Affected patients acutely are often mute and most have an accompanying right hemiplegia. Shortly thereafter it becomes apparent that they can neither comprehend nor express language except, perhaps, in the form of brief expletives or phrases. Insight, as judged from other behavior, is poor, as is prognosis for full recovery.

A group of aphasic disorders is characterized by the ability of the patient to repeat after the examiner phrases and often long sentences. Such ability to repeat implies that Wernicke's and Broca's areas as well as the primary connections between them must be intact and that the responsible lesions must be near to but not involving the primary speech areas. Geschwind has divided these aphasias with good repetition into those called (1) transcortical motor (similar to Broca's), (2) transcortical sensory (similar to Wernicke's), and (3) the isolation syndrome

TABLE 474–1. CLASSIFICATION OF APHASIAS

	Expression	Comprehension	Repetition	Other Signs	Localization
Broca's (expressive)	Nonfluent	+	–	Right hemiparesis worse in arm; mood depressed	Lower posterior frontal
Wernicke's (receptive)	Fluent	–	–	Often none; may be euphoric and/or paranoid	Posterior superior temporal area
Conduction	Fluent	+	–	Often none; cortical sensory loss in right arm; depressed	Usually parietal operculum
Global	Nonfluent	–	–	Right hemiparesis worse in arm; flat affect	Massive peri-Sylvian lesion
Transcortical motor	Nonfluent	+	+		Anterior to Broca's area or supplementary speech area
Transcortical sensory	Fluent	–	+		Surrounding Wernicke's area posteriorly
Transcortical mixed (isolation syndrome)	Nonfluent	–	+		Both of the above
Anomic	Fluent	+	+		Lesion of angular gyrus or second temporal gyrus

*After Geschwind, 1970.
+ = relatively or fully intact.
– = definitely impaired.

(caused by a large lesion producing a global type of aphasia except for normal repetition). Included in this group of disorders is *anomic aphasia,* associated with a lesion of the angular gyrus and characterized by rambling, lengthy, empty, and poorly focused speech, with transparent circumlocutions—talking around forgotten words. However, the diagnosis of anomic aphasia deserves a word of caution. Nonspecific difficulties in word-finding are common in the elderly and may accompany diffuse disorders of the brain that produce delirious or confusional states, only to disappear largely or entirely when the general illness subsides.

Mutism, the inability to speak, occurs in several forms. Acutely, it appears in association with vascular lesions of the left frontal lobe involving either part of Broca's area or its conducting pathways. Under such circumstances, mutism coupled with right hemiplegia, as indicated above, reflects the presence of a relatively large brain lesion and gives way to a less complete language disturbance within a few days. As an isolated symptom of a vascular lesion, however, acute mutism characteristically carries a benign prognosis and disappears within a few days to a week or so without leaving residual expressive symptoms. Acute mutism also occurs paroxysmally with epileptic attacks involving the left inferior premotor area, the commonest underlying cause being a neoplasm. More sustained mutism develops as a symptom of bilateral frontal lobe damage (Ch. 473) and is accompanied by apathy, inattention, and hypokinesia. Sustained mutism and behavioral withdrawal also can accompany severe psychiatric disorders. Such illnesses can be recognized by their lack of signs, symptoms, or laboratory findings of structural frontal lobe disease. *Anarthria,* the inability to speak because of abnormal innervation or mechanical disease of the vocal apparatus, differs from mutism in that affected patients make sounds and usually express vividly their frustration over being unable to speak. Occasionally, anarthria will reflect an hysterical disorder, in which case the alert, attentive subject usually displays insouciant indifference to the lack of vocal capacity. Neurogenic causes of anarthria include either severe bulbar or pseudobulbar palsy, conditions readily diagnosed by the presence of other signs and symptoms of nuclear or supranuclear paralysis.

Although brief disturbances in language function can result from seizures or transient attacks of vascular insufficiency, the development of a true aphasia, i.e., a selective disturbance in language function that is not part of a global decline in the intellect and lasting for more than a few hours, almost always reflects a focal structural lesion of the brain. The commonest cause is vascular damage, either from infarction or from hemorrhage, in the distribution of the middle cerebral artery or, less often, the posterior or anterior cerebral arteries. Occlusions of the latter may damage the pulvinar or disconnect right hemispheric sensory perceptions from the language areas in the left hemisphere. The second most frequent cause of aphasia is severe head trauma, neoplasms and other space-occupying lesions making up most of the remaining causes. None of these causes of aphasia typically produce very discrete brain lesions and several, such as vascular disease, are prone to generate either multifocal brain damage or large lesions whose effects extend considerably beyond the language zones. Language represents an exclusively human function, so that aphasia can be studied only in the damaged human brain. The anatomic variability of the lesions that cause aphasia necessarily leads to an equally inconsistent patterning of its major symptoms. The examiner must constantly recall these principles when trying to analyze a language defect in an effort to localize its anatomy and diagnose its cause.

APRAXIA

Apraxia refers to a disturbance of or an inability to perform learned motor acts despite retention of sufficient sensory and language function to understand the command and the motor capacity to carry it out (praxis). Students of brain function are inconsistent in their views about the mechanism of the phenomenon. Those disposed toward precise localizationist views of the brain postulate apraxia to occur under the following circumstances: (1) *Ideational apraxia.* Visual and receptive functions of the language areas of the left hemisphere are relatively preserved, but the propositional ideas of motor activity are lost, so that commands to carry out skilled acts cannot be executed. Imitation is also impaired and both sides of the body can be affected. Tools of daily living such as pencils, combs, and eating utensils can sometimes be recognized and even named by the affected subject but cannot accurately be utilized. The defect traditionally has been inferred to result from damage to the dominant posterior inferior parietal lobe area. (2) *Ideomotor apraxia.* Visual, receptive, and ideational functions of the dominant hemisphere are preserved, but the subject is unable to perform an act to command despite understanding the task, retention of the ability to move the involved body part, and ability to imitate the act. Affected patients tend to have insight into their motor incapacity and may shrug or smile hopelessly as their tentative efforts fail accurately to carry out the command. The condition is considered to reflect a conduction defect that interrupts commands that emanate from the posterior language area and are intended for Broca's area in the dominant hemisphere. We find the phenomenon rare except as an inconstant accompaniment to moderately severe posterior aphasias. (3) *Limb-kinetic, kinetic, or motor apraxia.* Patients with expressive aphasia may have great difficulty carrying out motor commands involving the face or hand of either side, despite their apparent ability to understand what is said. The defect is considered to reflect damage to a premotor area in the dominant hemisphere, which retains the command map (engram) for learned motor functions. Affected patients appear to understand instructions and may even haltingly repeat them verbally but are unable to imitate with either hand acts such as combing the hair, using a toothbrush, waving, and saluting. By contrast, some of these functions may be carried out in automatic settings, such as in performing the morning toilet. In our experience motor apraxia is uncommon except with frontal lobe lesions that are either large, bilateral, or only part of a more widespread forebrain dysfunction. (4) *Callosal apraxia.* Lesions producing destructive damage to the anterior portion of the corpus callosum or interrupting the transcallosal motor pathway that connects the left frontal lobe to the right can result in apraxia of the left hand to verbal but not to visually mediated commands. The disorder has been attributed to disconnection of the pathway that connects verbally released motor engrams putatively located in the left, dominant premotor area from reaching the premotor areas of the right hemisphere.

Except for the rare example of anterior callosal apraxia, we seldom have encountered motor apraxia as a distinct neuropsychologic deficit unaccompanied by wider functional impairments of aphasia or dementia, complications that make mechanistic interpretations difficult. The value of apraxia as a sign of specific physiologic impairment or anatomic localization has been commensurately small.

Constructional apraxia and *dressing apraxia* are disorders of skilled movements that relate more to damaged perceptual mechanisms than to motor impairments. Constructional apraxia describes difficulty in arranging or copying objects in accordance with their normal spatial relationships. Dressing apraxia refers to the inability properly to relate the shape and parts of garments to the appropriate part and form of the body so as to clothe oneself. In isolation, both constructional and dressing apraxia relate to large lesions that destroy or damage the spatial integrating functions of the posterior parietal lobe, especially the right, and its transcortical-subcortical connections. Alternatively, they tend to be prominent features of the bilateral temporoparietal abnormalities that accompany Alzheimer's disease. Constructional apraxia is the more common of the two defects and affects interpretations of material presented to either visual field or carried out by either side of the body. Dressing apraxia is less common and when associated with severe left somatosensory defects or denial tends more selectively to affect that side of the body. Both abnormalities tend to clear during convalescence. Their occurrence with acute damage to the parietal lobe suggests that they depend upon dysfunction in areas outside the immediate area of tissue destruction. We have observed a few instances of sustained bilateral dressing apraxia apparently related to single, focal, and only moderately large neoplasms involving the junctional area between the occipital and parietal cortex on the right side.

Several motor abnormalities sometimes have been called apraxia that are more appropriately considered to be combinations of pseudobulbar palsy and the effect of abnormal supranuclear reflexes. *Gait apraxia* due to a combination of bilateral pyramidal and extrapyramidal weakness of the lower extremities with paratonic rigidity and plantar grasping falls into this category (Ch. 480.2). Similarly, *oculomotor apraxia*, a term applied to complete or partial inability to look conjugately in particular directions on command is best understood as a bilateral interruption of the descending supranuclear oculomotor pathways from the frontal eye fields. The supranuclear defect of frontal pathways impairs but does not necessarily totally interrupt voluntary control of the direction of gaze and is enhanced by the sparing of an uninhibited, occipitally originating, visual fixation reflex. Characteristically, patients affected with the disorder must blink to block fixation before they can voluntarily redirect gaze toward the new point. They easily follow fixated objects.

AGNOSIA

Agnosia, at least as separated from a more global dementia with its attendant visual spatial defects, is an uncommon psychologic phenomenon characterized by the inability to recognize a complex sensory stimulus despite the preservation of elemental perceptions and the absence of a defect in language. The distinct existence and mechanisms of the disorder as an isolated neurologic event have been controversial, but all workers agree that agnosia requires bilateral impairment of the primary or association-cortical areas of the affected perception. The disorder is best considered as a form of monomodal amnesia or an interruption in the connection between the involved sensory area and the memory mechanisms of the hippocampal formation.

Visual agnosia is the most frequently encountered disturbance of this genre. It consists of the failure to recognize and name familiar objects, pictures, or faces despite, for example, the ability to describe or copy them. The phenomenon has been associated with bilateral posterior occipital-temporal-parietal lesions or with right-sided posterior parietal lesions plus dementia. Mechanistically, one can regard the disorder as a selective defect in the progressive abstraction of visual symbols into memory. Insight usually is lacking. *Auditory agnosia*, or pure word deafness, is extremely rare and has been described with the aphasias. The inability to recognize objects or events by the sounds they make also has been reported, but it too is rare except with direct damage to both transverse auditory gyri. *Tactile agnosia* exists only as a part of the astereognosis that results from damage to the primary postcentral sensory cortex.

MEMORY AND ITS IMPAIRMENT

Memory is the process by which the brain encodes, stores, and retrieves its sensory perceptions, ideas, and motor skills. The process is identical to learning. Disturbances of memory-learning include two dimensions: defects in past memory, called *retrograde amnesia*, and the inability to form new memories from ongoing events, called *anterograde amnesia*.

PATTERNS OF MEMORY FAILURE. The components of memory can be grouped into three major epochs—immediate, intermediate, and remote. *Immediate memory or recall* consists of holding in the mind material just heard or read with no necessary intervening process of memory storage. The capacity to register and repeat received stimuli lasts until the subject's mind is interrupted by some other stimulus and is reflected by such simple tests as repeating after the examiner a series of numbers. Except for grossly confused or delirious subjects, patients with organic brain disease usually show little or no defect in immediate memory.

Intermediate memory covers the time span beginning within a few seconds past and extending backward for 24 to 48 hours or more. It is tested by asking about knowledge of current events or the content of recent meals or asking the subject to repeat three unrelated words two to five minutes after having been given them. As with immediate memory, inattention may impair the answers. *Long-term memory* begins beyond that epoch, but this too has its gradations, for childhood memories tend to be singularly well recalled even as more recent ones begin to fade. As a result, standard I.Q. tests that examine primarily words and functions learned before the age of 14 years often give normal or nearly normal scores even in adults who have suffered from diseases that severely damage or destroy recent and anterograde memory.

MEMORY MECHANISMS. Memory has both nonspecific and specific substrates. Many regions of the cerebral hemispheres nonspecifically process the initial stages of learning about one's outer and inner world. Subcortical regions involved in translating events into memory are only partly known but relate closely to the limbic system. Structures located in the medial thalamic and probably hypothalamic regions as well as in the ascending brainstem reticular formation and basal forebrain activating systems are known to play an important role. Reflecting these widespread processings, at least some memory deficits accompany large lesions affecting any lobe of the brain.

Specific structures make especially important contributions to the anatomy of adult memory. In experimental primates, both the hippocampus and amygdala have been implicated in this regard. In humans, evidence suggests that at the cortical level, the hippocampus appears to play the major role in the retrieval of recent memories and the laying down of new ones. Unilateral damage to the human hippocampus results in relatively subtle defects, left hippocampal damage being followed by modest impairments in verbal memory while right hippocampal damage may produce difficulties in visual spatial memories and the recognition of musical tones. Occasional patients with inferomedial left temporal lobe damage develop transient, fairly severe amnesia for places, events, and verbal memories. If the opposite hemisphere is spared, this subsides in three to four days, leaving no clinically detectable residuals. In contrast to these mild or evanescent effects of unilateral injury, bilateral damage or surgical removal of the hippocampus in the adult is devastating and results in profound and usually permanent deficits in intermediate memory affecting especially the verbal-visual-spatial spheres. The degree of retrograde amnesia is proportional to the extent of hippocampal damage but rarely extends back beyond late adolescence. Proportional defects in anterograde learning accompany the retrograde loss. At the subcortical level, bilateral damage to the dorsal-medial nuclei of the thalamus and, less consistently, the ventral-medial hypothalamus, including the mammillary bodies, results in humans in a profound multidimensional disturbance of memory. The prominent memory loss that accompanies Huntington's disease suggests that striatal mechanisms may contribute to the normal memory process.

Understandings of the cellular physiology and molecular

biology of the memory-learning process are just beginning. Cerebral cortical memory mechanisms depend in an incompletely understood way on cholinergic projections that link the subcortical basal forebrain with the hippocampus and the association cortex of the temporal, parietal, and frontal lobes. Degeneration of these projections affects the memory functions of experimental animals and is a prominent accompaniment of the dementia of Alzheimer's disease. Anatomic studies have shown that an increase in neuronal connections in the hippocampus accompanies the learning process, while a reduction of dendritic synapses accompanies the memory failure of human dementia with Alzheimer's disease. Kandel, working with simple invertebrate nervous systems, has found that genetically regulated influences predispose to presynaptic increases in neurotransmitter output during the development of classic conditioning. These beginning steps may lead to better future understanding and treatment of the human amnesias.

CLINICAL MEMORY DISORDERS. Many middle-aged and elderly persons report an increasing but isolated difficulty in recalling proper names and recent events of minor importance. This "benign forgetfulness" bears no consistent relationship to the progressive dementias and is best treated with prompt and vigorous reassurance.

As discussed in Ch. 475, the most frequent causes of severe memory loss are the degenerative dementias, severe head trauma, brain anoxia or ischemia, nutritional impairment, encephalitis, and, less frequently, intracranial mass lesions.

Korsakoff's syndrome is a severe disturbance of recent memory that occurs most often as a sequel to acute and frequently repeated attacks of severe thiamine deficiency. The fully developed disorder includes profound recent memory loss, lack of insight, disorientation to time and place, and confabulation. In Western countries, nutritional Korsakoff's syndrome most frequently affects alcoholics and often accompanies or follows the florid signs and symptoms of acute Wernicke's encephalopathy (Ch. 482) or delirium tremens (Ch. 17). The condition, however, can follow any circumstance in which thiamine-free calories provide the major or only sustained source of nutrition. The memory failure in thiamine deficiency is accompanied consistently by bilateral damage to the dorsal medial nucleus of the thalamus. Other structural abnormalities affect the mammillary bodies as well as various areas of the cortex, including the hippocampus.

Severe retrograde and anterograde memory loss producing a Korsakoff syndrome can follow global cerebral anoxia-ischemia, status epilepticus, and subarachnoid hemorrhage. All of these conditions selectively damage vulnerable neurons in the hippocampus that normally relate to the functions of learning and memory. Even modest head trauma temporarily interrupts memory-mediating neural connections in the hippocampus and diencephalon: concussive injuries frequently produce an initially severe degree of retrograde and a lesser degree of anterograde amnesia; in most instances the retrograde memory loss almost fully disappears with time. Concurrently, anterograde learning increasingly improves. A less fortunate prognosis accompanies prolonged post-traumatic coma. When this lasts more than two to three weeks, most patients, particularly those over 25 years old, never fully recover from the memory loss.

Permanent or prolonged amnesia occasionally can follow bilateral cerebral infarction, large brain tumors, or surgical operations. Such cases have shown bilateral damage of either the hippocampus, the medial diencephalon, or both structures. Herpes simplex encephalitis characteristically leaves severe and often permanent amnesia in its wake. The disease has a predilection to produce necrotic-inflammatory lesions that destroy the limbic system lying along the medial surfaces of the temporal lobes.

Transient global amnesia (TGA) is a condition marked by fully alert periods lasting from several minutes to as long as 12 hours or so of acute confusion during which the affected person can identify himself but is severely disoriented for time and place. A severe deficit in retrograde memory accompanies the beginning of the attack and gradually disappears as it wears off. Status epilepticus with partial complex or nonconvulsive generalized (petit mal) seizures can produce a somewhat similar amnesic state. Attacks of such "minor status" are distinguished by dull, slow-witted, and inattentive behavior. Most TGA attacks come on in middle-aged or elderly persons and appear to reflect temporary vascular insufficiency affecting hippocampal memory areas or their immediate neural connections. Patients with TGA usually remain bright, attentive, and alert and are distressed by their acute confusion. They tend repeatedly to ask where they are and what is going on until, within a few hours, the disorientation gradually disappears. Most TGA attacks neither leave residual limitations nor carry a strong risk of recurrence.

Psychogenic memory impairment can affect either recent or remote recall, usually in clinically recognizable patterns. Preoccupation, forced inattention, or reduced arousal may result in inconsistent responses to testing, some answers to current events being given accurately and others not at all. Severe depressive illnesses may reduce language to near muteness or incomprehensible monosyllables. In general, organic disturbances in memory are marked by variability in what is remembered, emotionally reinforced material being recalled better than neutral events. With organic memory loss, disorientation is worst for time, less for place and persons, and never for self. In most instances, events of the recent past are unevenly forgotten more than remote memories, and the providing of cues often improves recall. By contrast, psychogenic amnesia tends to be greatest for emotionally important events, may elide from the patient's memory well-defined blocks of past events while leaving intact the recall of preceding or following material, may affect remote memories equally with recent ones, resists improvement with cues, and sometimes even includes disorientation to self. "Who am I? What's my name?", unless spoken during obvious delirium or a proved epileptic seizure, always reflects malingering.

TREATMENT. Patients with acute post-traumatic amnesia show a high rate of spontaneous recovery. Improvement of memory loss from other organic disorders is less predictable except when the amnesia can be traced to an excess use of medication or a temporary systemic disorder such as hepatic, renal, or pulmonary insufficiency. Memory loss with depression (pseudodementia) improves with the treatment of the psychiatric illness. A few patients with memory loss due to herpes simplex encephalitis enjoy a slow, spontaneous recovery, but most retain at least some permanent incapacity. Memory loss from thiamine deficiency or subarachnoid hemorrhage has an unpredictable prognosis; some patients improve, others do not, depending largely on the severity of the initial amnesia. Similar principles guide prognosis for recovery from postanoxic amnesia. In adults within these groups, whatever improvement occurs usually takes place within three to six months of onset. Permanent, incapacitating retrograde and anterograde amnesia affects patients with known bilateral destructive lesions of the hippocampus or the anterior-medial thalamic area. To date, neither neuroactive peptides, neurotransmitter precursors, neurotransmitters, nor dietary agents have achieved clinically useful benefits in the treatment of either the severe fixed amnesias or those that accompany the progressive dementias.

Beecher WB, Milner B: Loss of recent memory after bilateral hippocampal lesions. J Neurol Neurosurg Psychiatr 20:11, 1957. *Removal of the uncus and underlying amygdaloid complex in 31 patients resulted in little behavioral change beyond improved tractability, mentioned in several instances. When the hippocampus was bilaterally damaged as well, memory impairment resulted.*

Geschwind N: The apraxias. Neural disorders of learned movement. Am Sci 63:188, 1975. *A hard-line localizationist interpretation of the apraxias.*

Geschwind N: Disconnection syndromes in animals and man. Brain 88:237, 585, 1965. *A long and thoughtful review of the subject.*

Geschwind N: The organization of language and the brain. Science 170:940, 1970. *A summary of the organization of language areas and the syndromes that follow their damage.*
Guberman A, Stuss D: The syndrome of bilateral paramedian thalamic infarction. Neurology 33:540, 1983. *A review of vascular lesions in this area producing the amnesic syndrome.*
Heilman K, Valenstein E (eds.): Clinical Neuropsychology. Oxford, Oxford University Press, 1979. *A multiauthored collection of essays on major aspects of disorders of higher brain function.*
Kandel ER, Schwartz JH: Molecular biology of learning: Modulation of transmitter release. Science 218:433, 1982. *A well-written review of efforts to establish at the cellular level the fundamentals that underlie learning and memory.*
Penfield W, Roberts L: Speech and Brain Mechanisms. Princeton, Princeton University Press, 1959.
Victor M, Adams RD, Collins GH: The Wernicke-Korsakoff Syndrome. Philadelphia, FA Davis Co., 1971. *The classic monograph on the subject links the medial thalamus to memory.*
Woods BT, Schoene W, Kneisley L: Are hippocampal lesions sufficient to cause lasting amnesia? J Neurol Neurosurg Psychiatr 45:243, 1982. *The evidence from a well-studied case shows that they are.*

475. AMENTIA AND DEMENTIA

Fred Plum

GENERAL CONSIDERATIONS

DEFINITION AND PREVALENCE. Dementia is a clinical term describing a sustained or permanent decline in several dimensions of intellectual function so as to interfere with the individual's normal social or economic activity. The condition must be differentiated from *amentia,* or mental retardation, in which normal intellectual function fails to develop, and *delirium,* a reversible state of diffuse mental impairment usually unaccompanied by permanent neuropathologic abnormalities.

The symptom of a *static dementia* can follow any disease that permanently structurally damages large portions of the association areas of the cerebral hemispheres. Thus, for example, single episodes of severe head injury, global brain ischemia from cardiac arrest, large intracranial neoplasms or hemorrhages with their surgical removal, or infections such as severe encephalitis or meningitis each can injure the brain sufficiently to prevent intelligence from ever returning to a pre-illness level. Such conditions, however, represent but a fraction of the problem compared to the *progressive dementias* that affect increasing numbers of persons as the average life span grows longer. In the United States alone estimates indicate that close to a million persons are incapacitated by a fixed or progressive dementia. One can predict from present population age trends that this number will double or triple by the early twenty-first century unless scientific research slows or halts the epidemic.

Table 475–1 indicates the most common causes of the progressive dementias and provides rough estimates of their frequencies drawn from several sources. The figures emphasize the relatively greater problem of the progressive, "primary" dementias, especially of the Alzheimer type.

EARLY CLINICAL MANIFESTATIONS. The component symptoms of dementia vary as broadly as do the underlying components of the damaged mind whose worsening they reflect. The diagnosis of dementia implies the deterioration of several aspects of the intellect; monosymptomatic neuropsychologic defects such as aphasia or a circumscribed amnesia usually are classified separately. Acute, static dementia seldom provides a problem in diagnosis. Almost as soon as the acute illness passes, family, employers, and sometimes even the patient usually recognize that something is wrong, that things are different. Problems with social relationships or employment soon follow, and when no improvement takes place within weeks or months, the diagnostic problem becomes not whether a mental decline has occurred but to what degree and how the patient can restructure his world to his new, possibly permanent limitation.

TABLE 475–1. MAJOR CAUSES AND APPROXIMATE FREQUENCIES OF PROGRESSIVE DEMENTIA

1. Senile dementia, Alzheimer type	50%
2. Multi-infarct (arteriosclerotic) inflammatory	20%
3. Combination of 1 and 2	
4. Communicating hydrocephalus	5%
5. Alcoholic–post-traumatic	5%
6. Huntington's	5%
7. Intracranial mass lesions	5%
8. Uncommon or mixed with above: Chronic drug use; Creutzfeldt-Jacob; metabolic (thyroid, liver, nutritional); degenerative (spinocerebellar, amyotrophic lateral sclerosis, parkinsonism, multiple sclerosis, Pick's, Wilson's, epilepsy); static dementia	10%

Early diagnosis in the progressive dementias is less certain and more difficult. Initial symptoms especially involve deterioration in mood, personality, recent memory, judgment, and the capacity to form abstractions, none of which is easily quantified, especially in the elderly. In general, families or work associates notice a change before the patient does, and persons who live by intellectual efforts show their limitations earlier than do those with routine or manual jobs. Danger signals in mood and behavior consist of a loss of vitality, of curiosity, and of mental energy—of "sparkle." Some patients become so apathetic as to seem depressed, while in others great anxiety or increased irritability disrupts a once pleasant personality. Affective responses lose their depth; some early dements become paranoid. Loss of recent memory is a universal feature of the progressive dementias. One notes in affected patients an increasing tendency to make lists, then to forget where they left the lists. Appointments are missed, plans forgotten, stories of recent events become narrated repeatedly with no insight. Eventually orientation fails, first for days, then years, then months and finally for place but never for self. Interest lags—first in papers, books, and new challenges, later in work, and eventually in friends and family. Debts may be accumulated silently, property unwisely sold, accounts lost, meals cooked twice over or served half-cold. In a curious, even startling way mental capacities may fluctuate suddenly and widely without apparent relationship to external events. In Alzheimer's disease and some of the other primary progressive dementias social amenities tend to be retained until late in the course. Incontinence, soup on the shirt, and a disheveled appearance are more characteristic of frontal lobe disease and intracranial mass lesions than of the diffuse cortical and subcortical cellular diseases that produce progressive dementia.

DIAGNOSIS AND DIFFERENTIAL DIAGNOSIS. The three principal questions are (1) Does a true decline in intellect exist? (2) If so, what is its probable cause? (3) Can any aspect be treated effectively? Bedside testing answers the first, while the second and third require laboratory assistance.

The clinical examination of any patient with subacute or chronic central nervous system disease should include at least a brief evaluation of mental function. The test should be given gently and the results interpreted with due allowance for the patient's social background, schooling, innate capacities as judged by life attainments, and probable anxiety provoked by admission to hospital and fear of failure. The standard bedside examination measures orientation, language, and memory-retention by identifying recent major current events, the spelling of w-o-r-l-d backwards, and recalling three unrelated words at five minutes. Asking the subject to perform serial sevens backwards tests attention span, while proverbs and definitions (e.g., river from canal) give some idea of abstract capabilities.

As with other functions in medicine, quantitation of mental capacity is desirable and for this the Minimental Status examination (Table 475–2) provides valuable help. To obtain the evaluation usually requires considerably less than 10 minutes. Normals score 27 to 30, while clinically demented persons usually score less than 20. Psychologically depressed patients generally have intermediate scores.

When a quantitative baseline is desired against which to compare the effects of treatment or the rate of future deterioration, the Weksler Adult Intelligence Scale (WAIS) provides useful information but requires the assistance of a trained

TABLE 475–2. OUTLINE OF MINIMENTAL STATUS EXAMINATION

Test	Score
What is the *year, season, date, day, month*	5
Where are you: *state, county, town, place, floor*	5
Name three objects: State slowly and have patients repeat (Repeat until patient learns all three)	3
Do reverse serial 7's (five steps) or spell "WORLD" backwards	5
Ask for the three unrelated objects above	3
Name from inspection a pencil, a watch	2
Have patient repeat "No ifs, ands, or buts"	1
Follow a three-stage command (1 pt each) ("Take a paper in your hand, fold it, and put it on the floor.")	3
Read and obey, "Close your eyes"	1
Write a simple sentence	1
Copy intersecting pentagons	1

*From Folstein MF, Folstein SE, McHugh PR: Minimental state. A practical method for grading the cognitive state for the clinician. J Psychiatr Res 12:189, 1975. The authors found that out of a possible score of 30, mean score for dementia was 9.7, depression with cognitive impairment was 19.0, and uncomplicated affective depression was 27.6.

psychologist. In mild to moderate dementia the verbal score of the WAIS provides an index of learning capacity, while the performance part reflects current mental abilities. A discrepancy of more than 15 points between the two provides a strong indication of structural brain damage.

The laboratory evaluation of dementia depends on the combined results of the history, general physical and neurologic examinations, and preliminary laboratory results. In the absence of important leads from these sources (e.g., signs of chronic liver disease, uremia, severe vascular disease, bacterial endocarditis, a space-occupying intracranial lesion, etc.), the laboratory tests listed in Table 475–3 are in order and will detect nearly all of the treatable causes of dementia that would not quickly be suspected from the clinical examination. The yield will be low in suspected degenerative cases, but the seriousness of the problem deserves the dignity of careful evaluation.

Pseudodementia is a term applied to reversible states in which reduced cognitive functions appear to indicate progressive organic brain disease but instead are caused by chronic drug intoxication (usually prescribed) or depressive illness. The aging brain is especially susceptible to both conditions. Diagnosis in the first instance comes by taking a meticulous history of medications and reducing all potential offenders gradually so as to judge their effects on symptoms. Barbiturates, benzodiazepines, butyrophenones, tricyclic antidepressants, MAO inhibitors, anticholinergics, corticosteroids, and digitalis are most often responsible.

Psychologic depression (Ch. 476) is a common response to the physical and emotional deprivation of elderly life. The associated apathy, semi-mutism, akinesia, anxiety, and indifference often can suggest a mistaken diagnosis of dementia. Careful evaluation, however, quickly brings out differences. In contrast to demented patients, those with depression complain repeatedly of their poor memory. Patients with depression commonly eat little, often are severely constipated, sleep less than normal, and tend to behave best at night. They may answer questions slowly or reluctantly, but when they do, they respond to factual queries relatively well, revealing proper general orientation and understanding of commands. Errors occur because of indifference or obstinate refusal rather than poor comprehension. Depressed patients may stumble over tests requiring attention, but they rarely forget major recent events or political figures, and when they cooperate, they do not fail either simple tests of language or two- or even three-stage verbal commands. By contrast, patients with incapacitating dementia are disoriented, their nights are more agitated and confused than their days, they have difficulty following commands, both attention and recent memory are severely impaired, and many of them suffer difficulties in language and specific learned motor functions. Differences on mental status examinations usually are readily apparent. Laboratory tests add differentiating points. Brain imaging procedures show anatomic abnormalities in many of the dementias, and the EEG is slow in most of the dementias but not in depression.

TABLE 475–3. LABORATORY TESTS MOST USEFUL IN DEMENTIA OF UNKNOWN ORIGIN

Blood: CBC and ESR, serologic test for syphilis (STS)
Metabolic screen (SMA 12–16)
Serum thyroxine, B_{12} level
Chest x-ray and head CT scan
Lumbar puncture: cells (cytologic analysis if present), protein, STS

Depression sometimes accompanies dementia, especially that associated with multiple strokes, head trauma, and Huntington's disease, all conditions in which insight tends to be relatively preserved. One reaches the diagnosis of an associated psychologic problem by clinical sensitivity to the patient's mood and complaints and by observing behavior that is disproportionally withdrawn and mute for the degree of testable cognitive loss.

ALZHEIMER'S DISEASE

This commonest of the progressive dementias affects both men and women, beginning in rare instances as early as the late teens or 20's and increasing in frequency progressively with age to affect approximately 5 per cent of persons over age 65 years and over 20 per cent of those who reach 80 or more. In past years, patients younger than age 65 were classified as having Alzheimer's presenile dementia, while older ones were believed to have a different illness termed senile dementia. Clinical and biologic evidence, however, indicates that both terms describe the same disease, irrespective of age.

ETIOLOGY. The cause of Alzheimer's disease (AD) is unknown. The disease exists worldwide, and no evidence suggests a relationship to nutritional factors, infection, exposure to toxins, or other environmental factors. A history of affected family members occurs in about a quarter of cases. This plus the fact that patients with trisomy 21 (Down's syndrome) almost all develop Alzheimer's changes in the brain at about age 30 years suggests a genetic factor, with susceptibility transmitted perhaps as an autosomal dominant trait. Other influences, however, must be important, since identical twins show less than 50 per cent concordance for the illness, and when such cases have appeared, several years have separated their appearance within the affected pair.

PATHOLOGY AND PATHOPHYSIOLOGY. AD produces a progressive neuronal degeneration of selective cells in the association and memory areas of the cerebral cortex, combined with similar abnormalities in certain subcortical nuclei. Some of the latter, in turn, cause a secondary degeneration of the ascending cholinergic pathways that diffusely connect the basal forebrain with the cerebral hemispheres. The locus ceruleus degenerates in many, but not all, cases, reducing noradrenergic influences on the forebrain and brainstem.

When viewed at autopsy examination, the temporal lobe in AD is usually smaller than in brains of similarly aged normals. Gross, more generalized atrophy sometimes is seen in younger, chronic victims of the disease. Histologic examination usually discloses characteristic abnormalities. Neuronal loss affects especially the large pyramidal cells of the parietal and frontal association areas, the hippocampus, and the amygdala. This change may account for the decline in somatostatin found in most areas of the cortex. The basal forebrain nucleus of Meynert, which gives rise to the major cholinergic projection to the cortex, suffers severe degeneration. Silver-staining plaques containing degenerating neuronal products are scattered prominently in the cortex and subcortex. Many of the degenerating nerve cells contain tangles of twisted intracellular fibrils of a unique protein configuration.

The pathologic changes of AD are more quantitatively than

qualitatively different from other brains. Somewhat similar abnormalities occur in other disorders, and neuronal loss, plaques, and tangles can be found in the brains of many intellectually intact old persons, although in substantially lesser concentrations than in most AD victims. The reduction in cholinergic innervation appears to be a more specific alteration, although its functional impact remains unclear. Cell loss in the hippocampus and amygdala correlates with the prominent amnesia of the disease. The pyramidal cell dropout in areas of association cortex explains many of the early psychologic symptoms and correlates with recent research studies that show that brain metabolism is moderately reduced in early cases of AD, with the temporal-parietal-occipital association areas suffering the greatest decline.

SIGNS AND SYMPTOMS. Failure of recent memory is the earliest prominent symptom. Amnesia is followed in frequency by disturbances in emotional behavior consisting most often of either a reduction in affect or an increase in anxiety. Focal psychologic deficits are prominent, demonstrated by difficulty in managing spatial relationships or in initiating motor skills, and by a nominal memory loss that may become so severe as to resemble a specific aphasia. Disorders of descending motor pathways almost never occur, so that strength and reflexes remain unscathed. No defects arise in somatosensory or special sensory functions. Social amenities are preserved until very late; even with moderately advanced, incapacitating dementia almost all AD patients continue to dress well, to maintain neat appearances, and to avoid incontinence. Only in very rare instances do either myoclonic or generalized convulsions mark either the early or intermediate stages of the illness.

The onset of AD usually is insidious, although hints of abnormal behavior sometimes appear several years before sustained clinical changes allow a firm diagnosis. Among older victims a suddenly unexpected delirious or paranoid reaction associated with a minor febrile illness or an operation such as cataract extraction may be the first harbinger. The early progressive loss of recent memory can be difficult to distinguish from the "benign forgetfulness" for names and trivial events that affects many older persons in their sixth or seventh decade. When the defect extends to a failure to keep appointments, to initiate or keep track of important business or domestic matters, or becomes coupled with a progressive loss of interest, early AD should be suspected. Less frequently, isolated psychologic deficits producing spatial disorientation, apraxia, syntactic aphasia, or acalculia may be prominent. The time course of evolution varies widely from patient to patient. In younger individuals a period of years sometimes separates the first suggestions of "peculiar" behavior from the advent of a readily diagnosed dementia.

Except for the signs of abnormal mental status, the physical and neurologic examinations remain normal in early or intermediate stage AD. Laboratory tests are not helpful except in a negative sense. CT scans of the brain may or may not show moderate cortical atrophy but are otherwise unremarkable; blood and CSF studies are uninformative. The EEG usually is moderately but nonspecifically slow.

DIFFERENTIAL DIAGNOSIS. Diagnosis in AD is made by exclusion and largely on clinical grounds. No specific laboratory determinants exist, and brain biopsy is unjustified. The main problem occurs when laboratory tests show no abnormality. Early multi-infarct dementia, psychologic depression, drug intoxication, some of the diffuse angiopathies, metabolic deficiency, chronic meningitis, Pick's disease, or diffuse primary or metastatic brain tumor sometimes may create diagnostic errors. Within a matter of weeks to a very few months, however, clinical diagnosis proves accurate in about 80 per cent of cases, the exceptions being mainly neuropathologic rarities or another form of primary degenerative dementia such as the rare Pick's disease or an unclassifiable neuropathologic change.

MANAGEMENT. There is no specific treatment of AD. Dietary efforts aimed at increasing acetylcholine levels in the brain have resulted in no discernible benefit. Research workers have given prostigmine orally or by injection, but any ensuing mental-behavioral changes have been too small to suggest this as a practical approach.

The brunt of the care usually falls on family or social agencies during the early and intermediate stages of illness. Institutionalization often is required in the late stages when patients may sink to a purely vegetative level. Occasionally depression is a prominent early symptom; it responds to small doses of the usual antidepressants. Sedatives or tranquilizers tend only to make matters worse. With restless, agitated patients, tasteless liquid haloperidol can be given in doses of 0.5 to 1 mg two to three times daily as needed. The Alzheimer's Disease Foundation can provide the family with useful advice. Mace and Rabin's valuable guide is listed in the references.

OTHER PRINCIPAL DEMENTIAS

MULTI-INFARCT DEMENTIA (MD). This term describes diffuse mental impairment resulting from cerebral vascular disease. The condition is much less common than Alzheimer's disease and usually is readily distinguishable clinically. A general decline in intellectual function results from multifocal occlusion of cerebral arteries and arterioles either from remotely arising emboli or from intrinsic cerebral arteriolar occlusive disease. The condition appears most often in association with diabetic or hypertensive vascular disease, producing infarcts large and small that involve specific sensorimotor areas as well as areas of association cortex dealing with specific and nonspecific cognitive functions. As a result, disturbances in gait, station, and skeletal motor function accompany abnormalities in language, praxis, gnosis, mood, abstract thinking, and attention. Lesions can affect any area of the brain but are most frequent in the distribution of the middle and anterior cerebral arteries. Pseudobulbar palsy is common, as is pathologic crying and laughing and abnormal motor reflexes. A high incidence of frontal lobe infarction is accompanied by a reduction in attention as well as emotional lability, often coupled with a disregard for neatness and social niceties. Insight often is retained and accompanied by depression of mood. Many patients develop urinary incontinence. Multi-infarct dementia characteristically progresses in steps, with each new bite out of the brain accompanied by an abrupt minor or major worsening, sometimes with modest improvement between. Occasionally, the individual infarcts of hypertensive arteriolar disease may be so small (lacunae) that the effect of their successive appearance gives the impression of an insidiously developing and gradually progressing process. Nevertheless, the presence of prominent motor changes and abnormal motor reflexes almost always differentiates the process from Alzheimer's disease; radiographic studies rule out a space-occupying lesion or communicating hydrocephalus and CSF analysis eliminates infection as the mechanism of the mental decline. Signs of systemic vascular disease are almost invariably present.

HYDROCEPHALIC DEMENTIA. Chronic communicating hydrocephalus, sometimes called normal pressure hydrocephalus, occasionally produces an insidiously beginning and gradually progressive dementia, with forebrain functions becoming especially impaired by the abnormal hydrodynamic process. Affected persons may give a history of remote subarachnoid hemorrhage, recurrent head trauma, or meningeal infection, but the cause of the hydrocephalus often lies in the remote past and remains unknown. The condition is most frequent in late middle-aged or elderly men. In hydrocephalic dementia, CT scans or other imaging studies show marked enlargement of the cerebral ventricular system, especially the lateral and third ventricles. Sometimes one finds narrowing of the aqueduct of Sylvius, but more frequently there is dilatation of all of the ventricles with reduced or absent sulcal markings over the surface of the brain, especially at the vertex. The periventricular white matter often appears abnormally lucent owing to increased water content. The cerebrospinal fluid pressure usually lies in the range of 180 to 220 mm H_2O, but lower levels often are found. CSF contents are normal and the presence of an elevation of cell count or protein immediately suggests a more active meningeal abnormality. With such chronic obstructive hydrocephalus, the periventricular white matter of the cerebral hemispheres, especially of the frontal lobes, undergoes gradual atrophy, resulting in progressive signs and symptoms of frontal lobe dysfunction.

The typical signs and symptoms of hydrocephalic dementia comprise a triad of frontal-type dementia, broad-based ataxia, and urinary incontinence. Attention declines, abstract reasoning and the capacity to anticipate future events decays in parallel, and patients become careless in appearance and attire. Motor dysfunction is prominent and consists of a rigid-spastic increased resistance to passive movement of the extremities, especially the lower, coupled with a stiff, broad-based, hesitating, small-stepped, tottering gait, often accompanied by palmar and plantar grasp reflexes. Diagnosis depends principally on the clinical picture and the characteristic CT scan. Surgical CSF-shunting procedures are followed by intellectual and motor improvement in about half the cases. The operation is more often successful when the cause of the meningeal obstruction is evident or improvement follows a brief trial of spinal drainage by lumbar puncture.

HUNTINGTON'S DISEASE. Huntington's disease (HD), an inherited disorder transmitted as an autosomal dominant trait with close to complete penetrance, produces a combination of a choreiform movement disorder and dementia, as discussed in Ch. 485. The brain at autopsy shows prominent gross atrophy of the caudate, putamen, and, to a lesser degree, globus pallidus, with loss of the small neurons of the caudate and putamen being the most prominent cellular change. Studies of brain oxidative metabolism of asymptomatic family members at risk for HD have shown selective hypofunction in the region of the caudate possibly heralding onset of the disease. Early symptomatic patients show hypometabolism in both caudate and putamen but not at the cortical level. Postmortem pharmacologic studies of the striatum and its connections in HD have shown prominent decreases in the content of the synthesizing enzymes for GABA and acetylcholine, as well as decreases in the peptide neurotransmitters, substance P, enkephalin, and cholecystokinin. These changes relate more firmly to our understanding of the pathophysiology of the movement disorder than to the dementia, which currently lacks a satisfactory mechanistic explanation. The recent apparent identification of the locus of the Huntington gene suggests that preclinical diagnosis and genetic counseling may soon be a 100 per cent accurate opportunity for family members.

The earliest certain abnormalities in HD are usually those of the movement disorder. Early cognitive changes consist of a difficulty in anticipating and planning the future combined with a patchy memory loss, especially for serial tasks or memorization. Word memory and language functions are relatively well retained, as is spatial recognition. Later, the dementia takes on a more general quality. Prominent psychiatric symptoms mark the early stages in about two thirds of cases. Depression or schizophreniform behavior is common, and approximately 10 per cent of patients with HD commit suicide.

CREUTZFELDT-JAKOB DISEASE. Creutzfeldt-Jakob disease (CJD) is an infrequent disorder transmitted by a submicroscopic agent of unknown type ("slow virus") (Ch. 504). The brain is marked by a diffuse involvement of gray matter, with all affected areas showing neuronal loss, astrocytic proliferation, and a spongy appearance on histologic examination. The cardinal clinical features are the early appearance and rapid progression over several months of signs of upper motor neuron dysfunction coupled with increasing dementia, focal motor or myoclonic convulsions, and prominent changes in the EEG. CT scans are normal. These features distinguish CJD from the other dementias described in this chapter.

PICK'S DISEASE. This is a rare cortical atrophy of unknown cause with an age incidence that overlaps that of AD. The illness usually develops insidiously and progresses slowly for a period of three to ten years or more. Severe atrophy affects the cortical mantle, especially in the frontal and temporal regions, including the hippocampus. Microscopic examination shows neuronal loss, extensive gliosis, and characteristic swollen, pear-shaped "Pick cells." Plaques and tangles are unusual. The caudate, globus pallidus, and thalamus show less consistent cellular losses. Physiologic studies during life disclose a reduction in cerebral blood flow and, by implication, metabolism in the frontotemporal areas, maximally frontally. CT scans reveal frontotemporal atrophy. In keeping with the pathologic findings, early clinical signs and symptoms include prominent disturbances in memory and in the anticipation and regulation of planned activities. Affected patients are apathetic, slovenly, and hypoactive and tend to forget the purpose of their acts, yet they retain spatial orientation and direction. Incontinence develops early and vocal productivity declines, often to the level of mutism. Signs of extrapyramidal and corticospinal motor dysfunction develop late, adding further distinction from the clinical picture of AD, the alternate diagnosis most likely to be considered. There is no treatment.

Blackwood W, Corsellis JAN: Greenfield's Neuropathology. Chicago, Arnold-Yearbook, 1976. *The standard reference for the classic morphology of the dementias.*

Chase TN, Foster NL, Fedio P, Brooks R, Mansi L, DiChiro G: Regional cortical dysfunction in Alzheimer's disease as determined by positron emission tomography. Ann Neurol 15:S170, 1984. *The greatest reduction in metabolism affected posterior association cortex.*

Coyle JT, Price DL, DeLong MR: Alzheimer's disease: A disorder of cortical cholinergic innervation. Science 219:1184, 1983. *Construction of the cholinergic hypothesis of AD by the group that discovered the abnormality of the basal forebrain projection to the cortex.*

Cummings JL, Benson DF: Dementia: A clinical approach. Boston, Butterworths, 1983. *The best current monograph on the subject.*

Hachinski VC, Iliff LD, Zilhka E, DuBoulay GH, McAllister VL, Marshall J, Ross RW, Symon L: Cerebral blood flow in dementia. Arch Neurol 32:632, 1975. *A validation of the vascular defect in multi-infarct dementia, together with helpful scales aimed at defining the presence of dementia and the criteria for suspecting stroke as its cause.*

Katzman R, Terry R: The Neurology of Aging. Philadelphia, FA Davis, 1983. *This recent monograph discusses many aspects of the needs of the aging patient, including conditions that must be differentiated from dementia.*

Kuhl DE, Phelps ME, Markham CH, Metter EJ, Riege WH, Winter J: Cerebral metabolism and atrophy in Huntington's disease determined by ^{18}FDG and computerized tomographic scan. Ann Neurol 12:425, 1982. *Caudate metabolism is shown to be reduced both in patients with HD and in some at-risk offspring.*

Mace NL, Rabin PV: The 36-hour Day. A family guide to caring for persons with Alzheimer's disease, related dementing illnesses, and memory loss in later life. Baltimore, Johns Hopkins University Press, 1981. *An invaluable book for families and friends of the affected.*

Sulkava R, Haltia M, Paetau A, Wikstrom J, Palo J: Accuracy of clinical diagnosis in primary degenerative dementia: Correlation with neuropathological findings. J Neurol Neurosurg Psychiatr 46:9, 1983. *Clinical criteria accurately predicted autopsy findings in 22 of 27 patients, two of whom showed no diagnosable morphologic abnormality.*

Terry RD, Katzman R: Senile dementia of the Alzheimer type. Ann Neurol 14:497, 1983. *A summary of the most recent scientific information about the disorder.*

476. PSYCHOLOGIC ILLNESS IN MEDICAL PRACTICE

Paul R. McHugh

FUNCTIONAL PSYCHOSES

The psychoses gather together several different clinical entities. To be placed within the category an entity must produce disturbances in thinking and perception that are inexplicable solely as responses to experience and are severe enough to distort the patient's appreciation of the world and the relationship of events within it. The category psychosis has no uniform foundation as in somatic pathology nor any more objective aspect of psychopathology to mark its distinction from other collections of psychiatric symptoms. It is thus a term difficult to use with precision. Sometimes psychosis is used as a euphemism for insanity, sometimes as a synonym for schizophrenia, one of the entities within the category, and sometimes to draw an elusive distinction as between neurotic and psychotic depression.

The unmodified term can be qualified by a differentiation into organic and functional psychoses. Here the term psychosis means only severe mental illness. The organic psychoses, delirium, dementia, and Korsakoff's syndrome, are produced by a variety of cerebral pathologies. The functional psychoses, schizophrenia and manic-depressive disorder, lack a recognizable neuropathology.

This differentiation is practical. It draws a distinction in kind that affects treatment and prognosis, and it indicates the character of the clinical problem. For the organic psychoses the central problem is the cause of the pathologic changes. For the functional psychoses the central problem is consistent diagnosis.

Schizophrenia and manic-depressive disorder are clinical disease entities. The criteria for their diagnosis are their symptoms alone. There are no objective tests verifying a diagnosis. Only the natural history or response to empirically discovered treatments can confirm a diagnostic opinion. Since they lack a recognized neuropathology and are by definition inexplicable as responses to experience, there are no comprehensive etiologic explanations for these disorders. Treatment therefore is symptomatic rather than fundamental. Both prevention and radical cure await a chance discovery or a major scientific advance in understanding the biologic foundations of human behavior.

McHugh PR, Slavney PR: The Perspectives of Psychiatry. Baltimore, The Johns Hopkins University Press, 1983. *The authors discuss theconcept of disease as it arises in psychiatric thinking and address the methodologic problems of psychiatry as a medical discipline.*

Schizophrenia

Schizophrenia is a devastating disturbance of mind and personality appearing in clear consciousness and characterized by several distinctive alterations in mental experiences, modes of thinking, and mood that are seldom completely resolved. The most characteristic features occur during the active phases of the disturbance, and take the form of hallucinations, delusions, and altered behavior toward others. Specific intellectual and affective disabilities varying from minimal to severe can develop insidiously or remain after an attack. A crucial element of the definition is that all these symptoms occur in a patient free of any relevant and discernible pathologic change in his nervous system.

CLINICAL MANIFESTATIONS. The symptoms of schizophrenia can begin at almost any stage in life, but most commonly occur during adolescence and early adulthood and then either insidiously or as an acute attack followed by a series of attacks, each leaving behind personality defects of increasing severity.

In some patients it is possible to recognize a particular premorbid personality. They may have seemed more timid or seclusive than others. They may have been bookish, unsociable, and preoccupied with philosophic and religious ideas to the exclusion of friendships and community experiences. But this so-called *schizoid personality* is not found in most patients who develop schizophrenia. *At least half of schizophrenic patients had premorbid personalities indistinguishable from normal.*

Among the mental changes that mark the onset of a schizophrenic illness, only some are specific to this disorder. Emotional unrest, uncertainty, perplexity, and confusion can be found in many disorders other than schizophrenia, and therefore a diagnosis of schizophrenia cannot rest on them. There are, however, a number of mental changes that are more or less diagnostic. These can be usefully divided into abnormal mental experiences and disturbed modes of expression. The abnormal mental experiences seem somewhat more reliable evidence of the illness simply because they are easier to elicit with confidence and less dependent upon interpretation than disturbances in expression.

Hallucinations and delusions are the outstanding schizophrenic mental experiences. Although hallucinations can occur in many disorders such as delirium, dementia, and occasionally manic-depressive disorder, certain forms of hallucinations are more specific for schizophrenia. Thus auditory hallucinations are the most common hallucinations in schizophrenia, and certain kinds of auditory hallucinations are almost diagnostic. Thus hearing one's thoughts aloud or hearing voices commenting about one's every action or several voices engaged in a conversation in which derogatory and praising remarks are passed with the patient discussed in the third person are the most typical schizophrenic hallucinations.

Although delusions, i.e., false beliefs that are incorrigible, idiosyncratic, and preoccupying, also can be found in many disorders other than schizophrenia, in this illness delusional experiences are dramatic and well developed. They can begin as vague, fearful interpretations and "half-beliefs" and develop into firm incorrigible convictions. A delusion coming on suddenly, not prompted by any hallucination or previous delusion, nor related in any obvious way to the patient's mood, is called a "primary delusion" and is highly suggestive of schizophrenia. Many other schizophrenic experiences are of delusional form, but have such individual characteristics that they have been named for themselves.

Commonly schizophrenics have delusions about bodily control, the so-called passivity experiences. The patient feels as though he were under the control of some outside force or power making him behave as an automaton without a will of his own. He may feel hypnotized and feel forced to make particular movements, speak with a special voice, or walk to certain areas. The patient may believe these feelings come to him as penetrating waves from electronic or telephonic equipment.

The schizophrenic patient may experience changes in his thinking. Particularly he may feel that his thoughts are disrupted by some outside agency, that his thoughts are withdrawn from his mind, or that other thoughts are inserted into it. He may believe that people can hear his thoughts, which are leaving his mind as waves broadcast to others.

In contrast to these abnormalities of experience are the disturbances in the patient's mode of expression. Particularly noticeable is his abnormal language. Characteristically, he is difficult to understand. His thinking is expressed in a vague and awkward fashion with words poorly chosen and ideas poorly related to one another. Strikingly, the patient makes no effort to correct the vagueness of this thinking or to improve the clarity of his talk. Often, asking a question of the patient, the examiner receives a reply that is off the point and that goes into unnecessary details. Although the questions of the interview seem to start the patient toward a particular answer, it is never reached, but the patient takes up abstract and unnecessary ideas and must be redirected toward his goal. The examiner, laying the responsibility for the confusion on himself, may work to express himself more clearly, and only after considerable effort recognize that the difficulty in communication rests with the odd replies from the patient.

Another prominent disturbance is emotional expression of these patients. They seem distant, unresponsive, and cold. On some occasions the patient's emotional attitude seems incongruous, particularly for the thoughts he is expressing. Thus he may laugh while saying that he is in mortal danger. This cold or incongruous attitude and manner give the schizophrenic patient his most striking features, and even when at their mildest can be baffling and distressing symptoms to his family.

Other abnormal modes of expression of the schizophrenic patient are disturbances in stance and mobility called catatonic symptoms. Gestures may seem stiff, slow, and mannered. Some schizophrenic patients make repetitive movements or facial grimaces. Others may become totally immobile and mute. Still others may assume unnatural postures and hold them for long periods.

During the active phases of the schizophrenic illness the flamboyant subjective experiences are most prominent. During the chronic phase of schizophrenic illness expressive disturbances in thought and emotion are more evident, varying from mild to severe. Although at times some patients seem free of symptoms, whether a careful examination does reveal mild residual disturbances in thinking and emotional responsiveness is debated and difficult to disprove.

DIAGNOSIS. The diagnosis of schizophrenia rests on recognition of the distinctive clinical symptoms of this disorder and the exclusion of other conditions which may produce similar symptoms.

Many disorders of brain function can imitate schizophrenic symptoms; but with the exception of the three schizophrenia-like disorders to be discussed, patients with the other brain disturbances also manifest disturbed consciousness, disorientation, and disruption of cognitive abilities, particularly recent memory function, that are not found in schizophrenia.

Mania or depression can be confused with schizophrenia (to the considerable embarrassment of the diagnostician when the patient recovers completely on receiving treatment appropriate for these conditions). A source of difficulty is the occurrence of delusions, which are common enough in mania and depression but usually spring directly from the mood and the attitudes of self-confidence or self-blame that are so prominent in those disorders.

In schizophrenia disturbances in experience, including the auditory hallucinations and delusions just described, form the most secure basis for diagnosis. Thus, in a person free of brain disease or drug intoxication, recognition of auditory hallucinations with voices commenting on the patient in the third person, primary delusional experiences, passivity experiences, or disturbances in "thought control" permit the diagnosis of schizophrenia to be made with some confidence. In fact, Kurt Schneider has referred to these as "first rank symptoms" of schizophrenia because of the diagnostic confidence their discovery brings.

If these symptoms cannot be found, then diagnosis must rest upon recognition of manifest disturbances in thought and emotional expression. It should be pointed out, however, that opinion holding a person's thought to be illogical and vague, or his affective responses to be inadequate or incongruous, is an evaluative judgment and must be held with somewhat less confidence, if the difficulties are minimal or inconstant, than opinion resting on recognition of delusions and hallucinations.

Catatonic symptoms of immobility, posturing, and grimacing, along with the disturbances in behavior described as negativism or reluctance to cooperate, must be carefully interpreted. Only in those patients in whom no evidence of a prominent mood change can be found should a diagnosis of schizophrenia be made. Motility changes in the direction of psychomotor retardation are prominent features of depressive disorder, a condition as common as schizophrenia and more common than the catatonic variety of schizophrenia.

Symptoms of emotional unrest, anxiety, withdrawal, and hostility can be found in schizophrenic patients, but these are common to many other psychiatric disorders, and therefore can never form the basis for a secure diagnosis of schizophrenia. However, that diagnosis is rendered more likely if it can be established that the patient was developing normally without an apparently vulnerable personality, and if these symptoms appeared without a change in the patient's mood or the pattern of his life. Since these more general symptoms can be found in both schizophrenia and many other psychiatric disturbances, it is important to search carefully for the more basic symptoms of hallucinations and delusions from which emotional unrest and unpredictable behavior may stem. Often repeated efforts are required to gain cooperation of the patient so that he will divulge the existence of those basic symptoms that make a diagnosis of schizophrenia certain.

ETIOLOGY. There is no neuropathology or consistent pathophysiology that can be observed to develop with progression of the disorder and that might give some hint of causation. An approach to a consideration of etiology has to be more circuitous and the opinions derived held with somewhat less assurance than is true of other clinical entities. Two aspects of etiology can be conveniently separated for the purpose of organizing the information we have. One aspect is "cause," that is, any prerequisite element needed to set in motion a train of events leading to the entity. The other is "mechanism," that is, the particular nature of the train of events, be they psychologic, neurologic, or biochemical, that produce the symptoms. For schizophrenia there is some information relating to "cause" and also to "mechanism," but it is far from conclusive.

"Cause" or Prerequisite Elements in Schizophrenia. The genetic constitution has been decisively demonstrated to be one of the "causes" of schizophrenia. The risk of schizophrenia increases with the closeness of genetic relationship to a schizophrenic patient. Thus only 1 per cent of very distant relatives of a schizophrenic patient will themselves suffer from the disorder. This is no higher than the risk in the general population. But 5 to 6 per cent of siblings and 40 to 50 per cent of monozygotic twins of schizophrenic patients will have schizophrenia.

The possible objection that these data merely reflect the increasingly common environment of progressively closer relatives has been refuted by observations on monozygotic twins brought up apart who continue to show an identical high risk. Heston made the same point in a different fashion by studying a group of offspring of schizophrenic mothers. These particular children were raised from earliest infancy in foster homes by normal, nonschizophrenic mothers and fathers. The incidence of schizophrenia in these children was exactly the same as that reported for children raised by a schizophrenic parent. They thus resembled their biologic mother although reared apart from her.

It has nevertheless been impossible to fit schizophrenia into a clear mendelian pattern of dominant or recessive inheritance. Some students of the disease would describe the hereditary contribution to schizophrenia as polygenic, i.e., the sum of a number of contributions from the genes no one of which is solely responsible. The polygenic concept might permit environmental factors to play a large role in causation. Thus a mild genetic vulnerability might express itself in a schizophrenic phenotype only in those who face injurious environments, whereas those carrying a more severe genetic vulnerability might show the disorder in any environment. It is difficult at the moment to propose a test that would exclude the polygenic hypothesis as a possibility.

The same studies that have established a genetic contribution to the etiology of schizophrenia have also given evidence of the inadequacy of genetics as a sufficient cause for the disorder. That 50 per cent of monozygotic twins of schizophrenic patients are free of this illness means one of the following: (1) Although the genetic constitution is necessary and sufficient to produce schizophrenia, the symptoms employed to define a case fail to provide an adequate means of recognizing all examples of the disorder, and 50 per cent are mistakenly called normal. (2) The defining symptoms encompass a mixed group of disorders, and in only 50 per cent of these disorders are genetic features necessary. (3) A genetic vulnerability for schizophrenia is necessary but not sufficient. It must be combined with certain life experiences that need not be common for genetically identical individuals.

The present inadequacy of the genetic hypothesis to provide a complete description of the "cause" for schizophrenia reinforces a search for environmental and experiential causes. It has proved just as difficult to determine an environmental contribution as to define the genetic contribution. Thus the experiences of being raised by a cold and distant mother, or of receiving insistent, simultaneous, but incompatible directions from the parents, or of simply living in a disharmonious family incapable of providing a healthy environment for psychologic growth have all been considered causes of schizophrenia.

Such disturbed experiences have been found in the lives of some schizophrenic patients when viewed retrospectively after the onset of the illness. But none has proved to be a common experience in all schizophrenic people. Nor has it been possible to predict an increased incidence of schizophrenia among individuals living in comparably disturbed situations. At present the most economical view of the role of life experiences in the "cause" of schizophrenia holds that *any* adversity, be it a psychologic shock, abnormality in critical relationships, or physical injury (particularly brain injury) may provide a partial contribution in causing schizophrenia, but that most of these adversities are exerting their causal effects upon a genetically vulnerable individual.

"Mechanism" of the Schizophrenic Syndrome. This is the other aspect of etiology. Given that some combination of genetic and environmental attributes is probably prerequisite for the illness, by what derangements are the symptoms produced? Are they produced by some change in a psychologic function that might have been learned or developed through experience, or are they produced by some morbid change in the nervous system that alters the normal capacity to perceive, integrate, and respond? There have been proposals for each of these "mechanisms."

It has been proposed that the mechanism of the disturbance has been through the production of a particular psychologic change fundamental to the whole syndrome and from which all the symptoms can be explained. Thus Federn has proposed a "loosening of ego boundaries" as the essential feature mediating this illness, whereas Bleuler proposed a basic disturbance in associational thinking. A crisis of identity has been proposed by proponents of existential psychiatry. These views have a ring of plausibility perhaps derived from their resemblance to experiences common to all people, part of which can seem to be reflected in the behavior of schizophrenic patients. But they depend on concepts that are difficult to define except in terms of what they purport to explain.

Other studies have attempted to demonstrate the possibility that the mechanism is a change in the central nervous system. No such change has been demonstrated in schizophrenia as yet, so supporters of this possibility have had to reason by analogy.

Three well-documented conditions affecting the brain can give rise to a mental disturbance resembling schizophrenia. The most familiar is the syndrome found with *chronic amphetamine intoxication.* In this condition the patient is alert and oriented but preoccupied by auditory hallucinations and delusional ideas indistinguishable from those seen in schizophrenia. The disturbance may last from several days to a few weeks, but disappears eventually after the withdrawal of the stimulant.

Slater, Beard, and Glithero have demonstrated that among patients suffering from *psychomotor epilepsy,* caused by an irritative lesion in the limbic portions of the temporal lobe, a certain number develop a paranoid schizophrenia-like syndrome after 10 to 15 years of epilepsy. This condition displays all the classic delusional and hallucinatory symptoms of schizophrenia, but there is less tendency toward deterioration of thinking and personality.

Finally, certain patients, *withdrawing from excessive alcohol ingestion,* suffer from a period of auditory hallucinations. Although in most of these patients the hallucinatory experience clears within 24 to 48 hours, in a small proportion a chronic condition of persisting auditory hallucinations associated with delusional beliefs, incongruous affect, and disturbed thought develops. This chronic condition may be indistinguishable from the schizophrenic syndrome, and may persist for many years.

For all these schizophrenia-like conditions the possibility exists that the pertinent features might be the expression of a latent predisposition for schizophrenia in the affected individuals. But there is no evidence of a predisposition. The relatives of these patients do not have an increased incidence of schizophrenia, and the patients themselves do not have schizoid traits in their premorbid personalities.

The existence of these conditions demonstrates that the symptoms of schizophrenia are capacities of the damaged human brain. Yet we are ignorant of any common pathologic feature of these brain disorders that could by implication be the fundamental mechanism for schizophrenia. One possibility is that each of these disorders represents an extraexcitatory arousal of the brain, particularly of the reticular formation and limbic system, either directly via amphetamine or epileptic discharge or in rebound from long-continuing action of the depressant ethanol. It may be that the condition of schizophrenia itself is thus produced by some excessive activity in these or related brain regions evoked by the genetic-environmental "causes" discussed above. Mednick and Schulzinger have also found some evidence suggestive of hyperarousal in children of schizophrenic mothers who go on to develop the disease themselves.

Another proposed mechanism for producing schizophrenia is through some change in body metabolism or chemistry that could itself alter cerebral and psychologic functions. In fact the difficulties in establishing a role for biochemistry in the etiology of schizophrenia rest not with chemical methodology but with such issues as defining the group being studied, avoiding chemical artifacts related to dietary habits or medications given chronically hospitalized people, and deciding what biochemical change to look for. The papers of Kety should be consulted for a more thorough discussion of these difficulties.

New methods for imaging the brain are being employed in an effort to discern a neuropathology of schizophrenia. Computer axial tomography (CAT) has demonstrated that some patients with schizophrenia have enlarged ventricles and an apparent loss of brain tissue. This change may be more obvious in patients with prominent expressive changes as defined above, rather than those with the acute symptoms of hallucinations and delusions.

Any brain change in schizophrenia will likely be chemotransmitter specific. The most likely candidate for this transmitter problem is dopamine. The hypothesis that some functional excess of dopamine is present in schizophrenia was proposed by Snyder from observations that the therapeutic potency of phenothiazines parallels their capacity to block dopamine receptors. This hypothesis has provoked postmortem chemical studies of the brains of schizophrenics and the employment of positron emission tomography (PET). Both methods have provided suggestive, but as yet inconclusive evidence for an increase in dopamine receptors in schizophrenia. Complications of diagnosis, drug treatment, and age effects remain to be sorted out. However, we seem closer to defining a pathologic basis and mechanism for at least some forms of this disease.

Thus our knowledge of "mechanism," as much as our knowledge of "cause," is still fragmentary and provisional. But on the bits of evidence at hand, the view that seems easiest to defend is that schizophrenia will prove to be due to some deranged neural mechanism that can occasionally be produced by brain disease but more often is the outcome of an anomaly of the genetic constitution.

TREATMENT. The treatment for any schizophrenic patient is complex and should not be attempted by the inexperienced. A period of hospitalization will usually be required. There a program to include drug therapy, psychologic treatment, and social evaluation can be planned.

The sheet anchor of treatment now for schizophrenia is the *phenothiazine* drugs, discovered in the 1950's almost by accident. To date there is no secure explanation for their effectiveness. Clearly they are not simply acting by virtue of their sedative effect, since their remarkable action is not mimicked by other sedatives. They can remove the symptoms of schizophrenia, including the delusions, hallucinations, and disordered thought, and are not restricted to relieving excitement or anxiety as the term tranquilizer might imply.

The most versatile phenothiazine preparation is the original: chlorpromazine. The dose required to treat acute symptoms varies widely from patient to patient, and amounts from 200 to 2000 mg per day may be necessary. Maintenance dosage is similarly an individual matter, but 100 to 200 mg per day is usually an effective range. Since cessation of treatment results in the reappearance of symptoms in 60 to 70 per cent of patients within six months, drug therapy is often given over years. This practice, however, must be evaluated in light of a movement disorder (tardive dyskinesia) that may appear with prolonged use of phenothiazines. Tardive dyskinesia is a chronic choreoathetotic disorder affecting primarily the faciobulbar musculature but in some examples the extremities as well. It is resistant to most pharmacologic treatment with the exception of giving larger doses of the phenothiazines that provoked it originally. Since it is a particular danger of chronic high dose phenothiazine treatment, the attempt should be to employ as small a dose as possible in chronic administration. The report of Crane gives details.

The *psychotherapy* suitable for the schizophrenic patient has been a subject of intense controversy. The more radical approaches based on psychologic and particularly psychoanalytic views of the genesis of schizophrenia have not achieved their optimistic goals of curing the patient by relieving some basic psychologic conflict. More modest psychotherapy is indispensable when it is intended to help the patient in his everyday affairs, taking advantage of those personal assets that persist despite his illness, and establishing a relationship of friendly rapport in order to guide him in his management of personal and social issues, which, if mishandled, can be demonstrated to provoke distress and further illness. In fact, Vaughn and Leff have shown that the social setting in which a schizophrenic patient is placed after hospitalization is as crucial for his outcome as is his medication. Placement in a household in which intense emotional engagement by some family member with the patient is the rule can be shown to provoke new symptoms regardless of the medication regimen. Thus his psychiatrist, usually at first with the help of a psychiatric social worker, must strive to find a domestic arrangement that is calm and supportive but not too emotionally demanding, and a daily routine that combats the tendency to withdraw from all social contacts into an isolated and perhaps fantasy-ridden existence. Efforts made to instruct the family members on the nature of the symptoms of schizophrenia and on the need to avoid an excess of expressed emotion over the patient have been usedful in reducing both medication requirements and relapses. To accomplish these goals is one of the most challenging exercises in medical treatment. The growth of "halfway houses" as residences for previously hospitalized schizophrenic patients has been prompted by recognition of the need for stable and structured social environments for schizophrenic patients once they have improved enough to leave the hospital.

PROGNOSIS. Prognosis for any patient diagnosed as schizophrenic is always guarded. Certain features carry a good prognosis: high intelligence, a normal premorbid personality, an acute onset, catatonic features in the illness, and a family history of affective disorder. Other features carry a poor prognosis: low intelligence, schizoid premorbid personality, insidious onset of the illness, symptoms of thought disorder, affective blunting in the illness, and a family history of schizophrenia.

The use of phenothiazines has considerably improved the prognosis of schizophrenia, 30 to 50 per cent of patients having complete remissions on follow-up over five years. Another 30 to 40 per cent show some residual symptoms but are able to live in the community, and only 10 to 20 per cent require further hospitalization if phenothiazine treatment is begun and maintained after their first attack of the illness.

Crane GE: Persistent dyskinesia. Br J Psychiatry 122:395, 1973. *Definitive study of the neuroleptic-induced movement disorder with epidemiologic and therapeutic implications.*

Fish FJ: Schizophrenia. Bristol, John Wright & Sons, 1976. *Still the best introduction to the clinical issues and methods of reasoning about this disorder.*

Heston LL: Psychiatric disorders in foster home reared children of schizophrenic mothers. Br J Psychiatry 112:918, 1966. *The original paper on the method of adoption study for discerning a genetic element in schizophrenia.*

Kety, SS: Biochemical theories of schizophrenia, I and II. Science 129:1528, 1590, 1969. *Still the best summary of the pitfalls and findings of biochemistry in the search for a mechanism and cause for schizophrenia.*

Slater E, Beard AW, Glithero E: The schizophrenia-like psychoses of epilepsy. Br J Psychiatry 109:95, 1963. *The classic demonstration of the important relationship between a schizophrenia syndrome and the brain.*

Snyder SN: The dopamine hypothesis of schizophrenia: Focus on the dopamine receptor. Am J Psychiatry 133:2, 1976. *The best described hypothesis offering some hope for the eventual comprehension of this condition.*

Tune LE, Creese I, DePaulo JR, Slavney PR, Coyle JT, Snyder SH: Clinical state and serum neuroleptic levels measured by radioreceptor assay in schizophrenia. Am J Psychiatry 137:2, 1980. *The demonstration that neuroleptic levels in blood have a clear relationship to their therapeutic effectiveness in schizophrenia. An indication that very soon such measurements will be standard for the proper care of these patients.*

Vaughn CE, Leff JP: The influence of family and social factors in the course of psychiatric illness. Br J Psychiatry 129:125, 1976. *An empirical demonstration with crucial therapeutic implications of the role of emotional and situational elements in provoking relapses in schizophrenia.*

Manic-Depressive Psychosis

The essential feature of this psychosis is an excessive disturbance of mood and self-appraisal from which its other mental symptoms seem to arise. This disturbance can be in the direction of elation and self-confidence or sadness and self-blame. The course tends to be episodic, even periodic, with attacks of elation (mania) or sadness (depression) interspersed with periods of apparent mental health varying in length from weeks to years. Individual patients may suffer attacks of only one kind throughout their lifetime. Single or repetitive attacks of depression seem to be the most common manifestation, but attacks alternately manic and then depressive or even repetitively manic are not unusual.

CLINICAL MANIFESTATIONS. *Depression.* During an attack of depression the patient complains of feeling miserable and uncertain of himself. He may give evidence of his sadness by a dejected appearance and by restlessness and distractibility. Some patients are slowed in their activity, and this can progress to a psychomotor retardation of such severity that the patient seems totally unresponsive.

Mental examination of the depressed patient usually brings to light not only his feelings of sadness or misery but also a lowered self-esteem that can vary in intensity from feelings of inadequacy and incompetence to convictions of personal worthlessness, blameworthiness, and evil. This combination of depressed mood with self-blame is the diagnostic sign of this condition. It will also explain most of the other symptoms, modes of behavior, and dangers faced by the depressed patient.

Other symptoms include delusional extrapolations of the attitudes of self-blame. These can increase to a belief that the patient's guilt is notorious, that he is to be arrested, and that he will be condemned to die or to suffer some extraordinary punishment either in this world or the next. Suspiciousness and fear of mistreatment based on these delusional beliefs may be difficult to distinguish from similar attitudes in the paranoid schizophrenic patient. A useful if not cast-iron distinction is the depressive's belief that the suspected ill treatment comes as a justified punishment and not, as with the schizophrenic, as an undeserved persecution.

In some severely depressed patients delusional ideas can become bizarre and even grandiose in concept. Thus they come to believe that they have been the cause of cosmic disasters, that the sun is darkened by them, that whole cities have been deserted because of their presence, or that they and their progeny are accursed in the sight of the Divinity. Delusions of bodily change may take the form that their brains are rotting, their bowels totally blocked, or their bones fractured and dislocated.

Delusional ideas may concern the relationship of the patient to the world and to others. He may believe that he has lost all his money, that he has become a burden to others, that he is universally despised, or even that he gives off such a bad odor that people cannot stand his presence. Again, these beliefs are usually reflective of the patient's inner attitude of self-blame, self-contempt, and hopelessness.

The point about these opinions is that they are delusional

and not just false. They are unshakable opinions held in the face of all contrary evidence. Only treatment of the depressive disorder will remove them.

The most worrisome symptom of the depressed patient is *inclination to suicide.* It is easily appreciated that attitudes of such hopelessness and despair as have been described could prompt self-destruction. But it is not necessary to have such exaggerated delusions for suicide to be a distinct risk. Vigilance for suicidal intentions must be maintained throughout the course of the depressive disturbance. The physician should ask any depressed patient about thoughts of self-injury. A series of questions useful in estimating suicidal risk is provided in the discussion of Depression (below). Often this simple action will reveal both the severity of the mood disturbance and the need to bring the patient into hospital for his own protection.

Homicide is also a possibility for the depressed patient, and is particularly likely in those who harbor beliefs that their family shares in their guilt and accursed characteristics. Any suggestions by the patient that he might prefer death should be most seriously believed.

Along with these psychologic symptoms the depressed patient will often suffer from disturbances in his sleep, particularly waking early in the morning and being unable to return to sleep. Other physical disturbances include bodily aches and pains, loss of appetite, constipation, and weight loss. These features may combine with the retardation to give the appearance of chronic physical ill health. In fact, many depressed patients will first consult internists complaining of such physical symptoms. Helpful to the differentiation of the patient whose somatic symptoms are part of a depressive illness is a discovery of the features of depressed mood, and attitudes of self-blame or hopelessness when these features are combined with complaints of poorly localized pains, with loss of appetite or weight loss, or even with preoccupations about the state of the inner organs.

Mania. Symptoms that are almost the exact opposite of those seen during an attack of depression appear during an attack of mania. Now the patient says that he is in excellent spirits, that he feels well, and in fact has never felt better. He is active and restless, and appears energetic, confident, and quick-witted. These characteristics tend to worsen, and it is in their more extreme form that they become recognized as symptoms. The restlessness and energy become overactivity, with the patient moving constantly and planning progressively less plausible projects. His speech becomes incessant, rapid, and disjointed, one idea following another with little connection between them. His attitude of confidence becomes grandiose self-satisfaction. He may be overbearing and pompous. He often will be irritated by his surroundings, easy to anger, and perhaps suspicious that the efforts being made to control him are unjust.

Although a manic patient can usually be recognized by his overactivity, ebullience, and great self-confidence, he can develop as well ideas of resentment and feelings that he is being in some way unfairly noticed or persecuted. These ideas, on investigation, are found to derive from his own delusional opinion that he is so important that he must be under scrutiny by forces such as foreign powers. Occasionally, these persecutory ideas are so prominent that a diagnosis of schizophrenia is entertained. It is, however, the direct connection of these ideas to the attitude of self-confidence that allows a diagnosis of mania to be made.

With the mental changes manic patients exhibit disturbed social behavior. They may have increased sexual interest and may become promiscuous. They tend to overspend and be reckless with money. They may insult their employers and so be fired from their jobs. In the first attack of mania and before the severe restlessness and disorganization of thought appear, these activities may not be recognized as the products of mental illness, but may be construed as actions for which the patient can be held accountable. Thus the patient can be subjected to severe losses, to legal actions, or to moral criticism that can hamper his life long after his manic attack is over. To protect him from these consequences hospitalization of the manic patient may be required.

ETIOLOGY. ***"Cause" or Prerequisite Elements in Manic-Depressive Disorder.*** As with schizophrenia, an important genetic contribution to the etiology of the manic-depressive disorder seems certain. There is a progressive frequency of incidence with increasing blood relatedness so that with monozygotic twins the concordance rate is over 50 per cent. It is likely that genetic constitution is a necessary but not sufficient cause for this disorder. Certain other features of the illness require consideration. First, the illness does appear in attacks interspersed with periods in which the person appears to be normal. Second, the attacks are somewhat seasonal, appearing more frequently in the spring and fall than in summer and winter. Third, although many attacks occur spontaneously, many seem to be precipitated by some disturbing event. Presumably some other elements must combine with the genetic vulnerability to explain these features. Again, the most easily defended position would hold that a necessary cause for manic-depressive disorder is the genetic constitution of the patient, but that any of a large number of environmental disturbances can bring out the disorder.

Mechanism in Manic-Depressive Disorder. As with schizophrenia, a pharmacologically induced disorder has enhanced confidence that, whatever the "cause," the mechanism for affective disorder is a neural one. Treatment with reserpine for hypertension produced depression in up to one of four patients, and this depression was accompanied by the typical delusional attitudes of the manic-depressive psychosis. The discovery that reserpine depleted brain neurons of biogenic amines, particularly norepinephrine and serotonin, has prompted a variety of hypotheses that propose some lack of norepinephrine, serotonin, or other biogenic amines at synaptic sites in the brain for emotional control. That many effective antidepressant agents also influence these same amines has been a further support to these hypotheses.

TREATMENT. The first rule in managing either manic or depressed patients is that most of them should be in a hospital. Their conditions can bring catastrophe to themselves and their families in the form of financial mismanagement in mania and suicide in depression. If these diagnoses are strongly suspected, then psychiatric opinion should be immediately sought so as to determine whether hospitalization should be imposed. It is critical to have expert help, because the patient can often hide the severity of the disorder in a mass of explanations which may appear quite plausible. In the hospital the suicidal patient must be closely supervised and definitive treatment should not be long deferred.

It is crucial to diagnose these patients and separate them from those with other conditions, because new drug treatments have proved effective for them and are specific to the affective disorders. Two classes of pharmacologic agents are effective in *depression.* Seemingly more effective are the so-called *tricyclic antidepressants,* the prototype of which is imipramine. This drug, given in doses of from 75 to 300 mg per day, will relieve a depressive attack in 50 per cent of patients. The recent development of the means for measuring plasma levels of tricyclic antidepressants has revealed a partial explanation for failures to respond. A narrow range (50 to 170 ng per milliliter) encloses therapeutic plasma nortriptyline levels. The failure to reach this level or the exceeding of it inhibits a full response. A rational pharmacology for these medications will soon require plasma measurements to be available as a routine. Maintenance therapy of 100 to 150 mg per day should be continued for six to eight months after recovery. If tricyclics are ineffective, the logical practice should be to switch to the other class, which includes the drugs that have as their primary action the capacity to inhibit the enzyme monoamine oxidase. These drugs, in doses of 45 to 75 mg per day, have also proved useful in depression.

If *monoamine oxidase inhibitors* are used, the patient must be warned to avoid foodstuffs such as cheese, broad beans, and some yeast extracts, which have pressor amines of the phenylethylamine group that includes tyramine. If absorbed by patients whose monoamine oxidase enzyme is depleted, they can cause sudden elevation of blood pressure with headache, blurred vision, and even cerebrovascular hemorrhage.

The mainstay of treatment for severe depression is *electroconvulsive treatment* (ECT). In contrast to the drugs which relieve the symptoms of depression, ECT will terminate an attack of depression usually in four to eight treatments. This treatment can produce the most dramatic and quick recovery from the depths of a life-threatening depression, and should not be withheld from a delusional patient or any seriously depressed patient who has failed to respond to drug treatment after three to four weeks. Maintenance with imipramine, 100 to 150 mg per day for six months, is recommended after ECT for the avoidance of relapse shortly after successful treatment.

The *treatment of mania* is often very difficult, particularly if the patient is suspicious about medicines. Haloperidol in doses of 2 to 10 mg thrice daily taken orally has proved effective. This compound is liable to produce severe extrapyramidal side effects which can be combated with antiparkinsonian drugs and with Benadryl. Chlorpromazine in doses of 300 to 1000 mg per day can also be tried.

An effective measure for controlling mania is the use of lithium ion in the form of lithium carbonate. This compound is available in 300 mg tablets, and daily intake of 900 to 2400 mg per day can relieve manic excitement. It is, however, essential to follow plasma lithium concentration in these patients, because toxic signs of disorientation, tremor, anorexia, and diarrhea can appear if plasma lithium concentration rises above 2 mEq per liter. The therapeutic level and the toxic level of lithium are close, and therefore the medication must be started when the patient can be carefully supervised in a hospital. Maintenance lithium treatment can be recommended, because there is fair clinical evidence that in this fashion some further attacks of mania may be avoided.

Maintenance lithium treatment is not without problems, however. It can produce several renal complications—in particular, nephrogenic diabetes insipidus and, rarely, a nephrotic syndrome secondary to an interstitial nephropathy.

These problems appear to increase with the duration as well as the dose of lithium given (DePaulo, 1980). No patients have had renal failure produced by lithium, but it would seem prudent to make some measure of glomerular filtration rate prior to beginning lithium treatment and annually as long as the treatment is maintained. A creatinine clearance test is an adequate screening test.

The diabetes insipidus, if severe, can be a serious problem if the patient being treated with lithium nonetheless falls ill with mania or depression and fails to sustain a fluid intake either because of the distractions of mania or the delusions and psychomotor retardation of depression. The patient in such circumstances can become dangerously dehydrated or can develop a severe lithium intoxication. The patient and family should be counseled about this problem and the need to maintain the fluid intake.

In the face of such complications, the decision on whether a given patient should be sustained on lithium is a judgment. The complications of the treatment must be weighed against the frequency and psychosocial impairments of subsequent attacks of affective disorder.

PROGNOSIS. The prognosis for a single attack of mania or depression is excellent. Even without treatment patients tend to recover completely within six months. With antidepressant treatment the medication can be withdrawn after six to eight months with fair assurance that symptoms will not recur at this time.

The longer-range prognosis is not so favorable. Eighty per cent of people who have suffered one attack of affective disturbance will have another at some time in their lives, but this may not be for many years. Some patients, however, will have recurrent attacks of mania or depression interrupted by only brief intervals of normal behavior.

The best advice to give patients who have suffered from their first affective attack is that they will very likely be quite well for years, but that they and their family should be aware that their mood changes are to be considered seriously, and they should seek psychiatric attention promptly if such a mood change tends to persist or worsen. Prien's work indicates that individuals who suffer recurrent attacks of any form of manic-depressive disorder are best maintained on lithium for an extended, even an indefinite, period.

Akiskal HS, McKinney WT: Overview of recent research in depression. Arch Gen Psychiatr 32:285, 1975. *A masterful consideration of ten possible models for the etiology of depression, ranging over psychoanalytic, behavioral, biologic, sociologic, and existential concepts. The authors attempt to be comprehensive, critical, but reconciling.*

Kragh-Sorensen P, Hasen CE, Asberg M: Plasma levels of nortriptyline in the treatment of endogenous depression. Acta Psychiatr Scand 49:444, 1973. *The definitive article indicating the need for plasma levels of antidepressants because it demonstrates an optimal level below which and above which the patients do not improve. A most clear demonstration of a therapeutic "window."*

Lewis A: Melancholia. J Ment Sci 80:1, 277, 1934; 82:488, 1936. *The classic triad of papers on the history, symptoms, and course of endogenous depression, written before the advent of effective physical treatments.*

Prien R, Klett J, Caffey E: Lithium prophylaxis in recurrent affective illness. Am J Psychiatry 131:198, 1974. *A clear indication of the utility of lithium in treatment.*

Winokur G, Clayton PJ, Reich T: Manic-Depressive Illness. St. Louis, C.V. Mosby Company, 1969. *This is the definitive monograph on the subject.*

PERSONALITY DISORDERS AND NEUROTIC SYMPTOMS

GENERAL CONSIDERATIONS. The concept of disease entities that supports our understanding of the functional psychoses does not suit all psychologic disturbances and particularly those that are described as personality disorders or neurotic symptoms. There is uncertainty both in terms and in concept here. For example, the designation neurosis is ambiguous in that it seems a name for a clinical entity with some sharp distinction from normal, but a cardinal symptom of one neurosis, *anxiety*, is an experience of all people at some time and is an appropriate mood in certain circumstances. What then is abnormal in *anxiety neurosis*? Is this abnormality of a quantitative or a qualitative nature? To what kind of patient can the term anxiety neurosis be applied? Should we use it only for patients in the emotional "state" of anxiety, or is it suitable regardless of the present state if a patient has "traits" that make him prone to this emotion?

The term *personality* and particularly its extension, *personality disorder*, can be just as troublesome. Personality seems a word similar to such terms as character or temperament, words intended to describe aspects of human psychologic variation distributed in a smoothly graded fashion in the population. But if that is true, then the distinction personality disorder can seem an arbitrary, socially contrived, or judgmental decision, since no sharp dividing line is to be expected in smoothly graded characteristics. In later sections of this chapter, an attempt is made to dispel some of these ambiguities while considering several emotional disturbances often called neurotic that occur in a general medical setting.

Although many mental changes and emotional disturbances in patients can be ascribed to known or presumed pathologic changes in brain function, certain varieties of human psychologic constitution and certain life experiences can themselves provoke emotional disturbance and disrupted behavior. The terms personality disorder and neurotic symptoms are intended to describe the disturbances that result from variation in human constitution and experience by invoking the concepts of potential and response. Personality always means *potential*. It encompasses and describes the abiding and distinctive traits or tendencies of an individual to react to circumstances in a particular fashion. Thus by "optimistic personality" is meant an individual who can be expected to respond with cheerfulness and optimism in situations in which others are less likely to do so. An individual's personality is the sum of numerous traits, and a comparison with others is implicit in the description of each trait. Thus every trait can be conceived as a dimension of variation along which people can be dispersed in a fashion similar to their dispersal along the dimensions of height, weight, or intelligence. Any definition of an individual's personality is an attempt to place him in relationship to others in respect to one or more traits. An individual can be said to have a disorder of personality if he deviates to such an extreme along the range of variation for some trait that either he or others complain of its effects.

Whereas personality and personality disorder indicate potential, the neurotic symptoms are emotional *responses* displayed when the individual is troubled by circumstances. For anyone certain environments and life events are conducive to anxiety, others to depression, and still others to suspiciousness. People with a disorder of personality have an increased potential for these responses and are provoked to them by less extreme circumstances and less specific stimuli. Thus paranoid personality disorder is a term used to describe an individual who tends to show attitudes of suspiciousness and feelings of persecution (the neurotic symptoms) in settings so minimally threatening that they will seldom provoke such attitudes in others. If, however, his life is relatively free of threatening features, these feelings will be diminished and, despite his personality traits, symptoms may be avoided.

Before such concepts can be used in the evaluation and management of a particular patient, that patient must be well known to the doctor, and the possibility of other conditions that could produce similar symptoms must be excluded. For this a detailed psychiatric history, mental status, and physical examination are needed. The latter two can be obtained during the first interview, but historical information about the patient's family background, developmental milestones, sexual adjustment, scholastic and occupational achievement, habits, and medical problems may require several hours of examination. Observations from his relatives improve the accuracy of such information, and their descriptions of his personality are indispensable. All these data, combined with the knowledge of the patient's present condition, form the basis for diagnosis, treatment, and prognosis, and to embark on such matters without this information is to commit a capital error. The result is often failure of treatment, because the patient has been misunderstood and emphasis given to minor rather than major features of his problem.

As it becomes clear that a given patient's disturbance is the outcome of the kind of person he is and the situations that he faces, the data of the psychiatric history and the mental status examination can usually be divided into three categories which, although closely related, are usefully distinguished: (1) the predisposing factors for the disturbance, including personality traits and formative life experiences; (2) the precipitating factors; and (3) the symptoms themselves and their effect on the patient.

PREDISPOSING FACTORS. Predisposing factors are those features special to an individual that make him vulnerable to emotional disturbance. The most critical factor is personality, the traits of which are distinguished in the patient's temperament, attitudes, and predictable responses. But personality is the outcome of genetic constitution, intellectual endowment, and lifetime experiences, and each of these is a predisposing factor in itself. Predisposing factors often overlooked are the patient's social status and cultural situation.

Finally, the state of health is an important predisposing feature, because physical illness, through the distress it produces or by direct effects on the central nervous system, interferes with a person's capacity to cope with circumstances and thus leads to psychologic symptoms.

PRECIPITATING FACTORS. The precipitating factors are events or experiences that have disrupted emotional equilibrium and bear a close temporal relationship to the disturbance for which the patient seeks help. The common-sense expectations that personal illness, or conflict produced by changes in family or occupational circumstances, could precipitate psychologic distress have been confirmed in studies reviewed recently by Wing. Holmes has attempted to grade life events in a hierarchy of emotional stressfulness, and many workers have found his scale useful for estimating the relative distress different patients have endured. Some psychologic precipitants are more recondite, because they depend on a special meaning an individual gives events, perhaps a symbolic meaning derived from the particular patient's early life experiences. Before emphasizing these more abstruse precipitants of a unique character, it is usually wise to consider the more immediate and obvious ones that may be present.

SYMPTOMS. Later in this chapter the symptoms of anxiety, depression, and hysterical reaction are discussed, because they are common in the general practice of medicine. These conditions do not exhaust the neurotic disorders, but are the most common seen in medical practice. For a comprehensive consideration of the neurotic reactions, reference can be made to the text by Goodwin and Guze.

All neurotic symptoms emerge as complaints either of the patient himself or of others who must deal with him. They are symptoms in the sense that they disturb the patient's sense of well-being or they interfere with his behavior and his adaptability to circumstances. They can vary from mild to severe, and they can be acute or chronic.

In the assessment of these symptoms the patient should be encouraged to describe how he feels, how the symptoms developed, what seems to make them worse or better, what they are like when compared with previous emotional reactions, and how they disturb him now. *The aim is to come to appreciate these symptoms as understandable responses of this particular person to his particular circumstances.* The overall principle is that we are considering here not classes of patients suffering from distinct disease entities, but individuals troubled by their special life circumstances and needing assistance tailored to their particular personal nature and situation. The specific symptoms, their characteristic predisposing and precipitating factors, their effects on behavior, and modes of treatment will be considered in the balance of this chapter.

A comprehensive consideration of the psychotherapy of neurotic reactions can be found in the monograph of Frank and his associates.

Frank, JD, Hoehn-Saric R, Imber SD, Liberman BL, Stone AR: Effective ingredients of successful psychotherapy. New York, Brunner/Mazel, 1978. *A thoughtful, practical, and scholarly approach to psychotherapy based on 25 years of painstaking empirical research. This book is the outstanding work in a field of many entries. Its documentation of (1) demoralization as the central issue for the patient, (2) those characteristics of patient and therapist conducive to successful treatment, and (3) the equal effectiveness of different therapeutic schools of thought is noteworthy.*

Goodwin DW, Guze SB: Psychiatric Diagnosis. 2nd ed. New York, Oxford University Press, 1979. *A brief but thorough text describing the psychiatric syndromes. A good introduction to the approach to psychiatry exemplified in the American classification of psychiatric disorder DSM III.*

Holmes TH, Rahe RJ: The social readjustment score. J Psychosomat Res 11:213, 1967. *The presentation of a scoreable approach to stressful life events that has helped take some of the subjectivity out of this awkward assessment.*

Wing JK: Innovations in social psychiatry. Psychol Med 10:219, 1980. *A thorough and up-to-date review of concepts and research into the precipitants of psychiatric disorders.*

Anxiety

DEFINITION. Anxiety is an unpleasant mood of tension and apprehension. It is fear's first cousin, and like fear it has prominent autonomic effects when severe, but fear is an emotion sharply focused on immediate dangers. Anxiety is usually imposed by the anticipation of future danger, distress, or difficulties. As an emotional response common to people, anxiety is useful. Activities that arouse it are avoided and those that diminish it are sustained. Although anxiety may spur people to perform difficult tasks skillfully and admirably, when excessive it is a hindrance, as some well-prepared students demonstrate when facing a critical examination. Anxiety is a medical problem when it is excessive, inappropriate, or without obvious cause.

FORMS OF ANXIETY AND THEIR PREDISPOSING AND PRECIPITATING FACTORS. Anxiety can occur (1) as an affective response of anyone under circumstances of threat or danger; (2) as a symptom of another psychiatric disorder, such as delirium, dementia, or schizophrenia; or (3) as a psychopathologic state in which excessive anxiety is the prominent feature.

It is not difficult to appreciate the predisposing and precipitating factors of anxiety as an affective response to danger. Anxiety is a psychologic reaction to anticipated troubles of all sorts. But people and troubles vary. Some—the timid, the inexperienced, the excessively conscientious—are frequently anxious in situations that seem not to affect others. Most people are at least mildly anxious whenever they seek medical advice; when threatening dangers are intense or prolonged as in chronic painful illness or in battle, even the most resistant individuals can develop an incapacitating anxiety. Resistance to anxiety varies with physical condition. When tired, sick, or injured, people are more easily threatened.

Common precipitants of anxiety in daily life are circumstances of conflict in which an action is demanded but the correct action may be difficult to discern. Thus, a person may be anxious over difficult decisions on which rest his economic and social future or because the decisions produce an unpredictable response in an inconsistent superior.

Laboratory models for this kind of conflict and its effects on the emotional state have been produced. Pavlov trained dogs to respond to the picture of a circle by rewarding such responses with food. He did not reward responses to an ellipse. Then by simply compressing the ellipse so that it gradually approached a circle in shape, he made a discrimination progressively more difficult. The emotional response of these dogs was remarkable. They became agitated when put into harness for the experiment. They tore at their restraints, barked, and refused to attempt the discrimination. In this state, they not only made many mistakes but they became unable to make discriminations that had previously been easy. It is not difficult to see analogies in both situation and behavior between these dogs and people in situations of conflict.

An emotional state of anxiety can, as mentioned, be a symptom of any of a number of neurologic and psychiatric disorders. The person with brain damage may become anxious in situations that do not seem immediately threatening, but appear so to him because of his disturbed capacity for analysis and discrimination. In fact, one of the first indications of a dementia can be an attack of severe anxiety without obvious provocation.

A prolonged, irritable anxiety state can follow a head injury, as one of the symptoms of the so-called postconcussional syndrome. Gronwall and Sampson demonstrate that it may be due to a mild disturbance in cognitive capacity subjectively evident to the patient but demonstrable objectively only with difficulty.

A mood of tension and agitation can occur in the delirious states, such as those that follow withdrawal from alcohol or barbiturates. It can also sometimes be produced by the hallucinogenic drugs such as LSD 25. In these situations it may be disturbed perceptions and misinterpretations that arouse anxiety, but occasionally the anxiety appears as one of the several symptoms of psychologic arousal and seems independent of anything that the patient experiences or understands.

The conditions in which anxiety can be recognized as a psychopathologic state are several. Included here are the phobic states in which the patient suffers an excessive fear of some object, animal, or situation such as the dark or thunder and lightning. These monosymptomatic phobias usually commence in childhood and are of less clinical importance because they are well encapsulated and seldom lead to medical attention.

It is the condition sometimes referred to as *agoraphobia with panic attacks* that should be distinguished from these other conditions. This disorder has carried many names, including neurasthenia, effort syndrome, neurocirculatory asthenia, and, most recently, *panic disorder*. The condition is a familial disorder, as first noted by Cohen and his associates. A careful family survey by Crowe et al. of first degree relatives of patients with panic disorder found a morbidity risk of 42 per cent among female relatives and 22 per cent among male relatives. In fact, familial morbidity risk for panic disorder is as high as any in the psychiatric genetics literature.

The precipitating event for panic attacks can be a calamitous emotional experience, such as a bereavement, separation, or injury, but it can be a more trivial distressing event superimposed upon a chronic state of some tension and uneasiness. The precipitating event then triggers off the panic attack, which will recur irregularly and unpredictably in the future.

These spontaneously occurring panic attacks that seem so inexplicable to the patient lead to the development of an anticipatory anxiety as the patient begins to fear the recurrence of another attack. In fact, this can lead to the phobic avoidance of any situation which can be thought to provoke these panic attacks, and this avoidance can grow to such an extreme that the patient is housebound; hence the term agoraphobia. But agoraphobia is probably a misnomer, in that what the patient is fearing is not open spaces but being away from familiar surroundings and entering settings where the inexplicable but very distressing panic attacks occur. The term panic disorder is preferable.

MANIFESTATIONS OF ANXIETY. Regardless of the cause of anxiety, its manifestations are divisible into three groups: (1) The inner feelings of tension, apprehension, and dread that form the anxious mood itself. (2) A disturbance of the intellectual power. The anxious patient is unable to think clearly and to use proper judgment, to learn efficiently, or to remember accurately. (3) The somatic and autonomic symptoms that accompany tension, anxiety, and fear. These include tension headache, tremor, giddiness, dyspnea, heart palpitation, gastric distress, urinary frequency, backache, and general feelings of weakness.

A model anxiety state is to be seen among combat soldiers. The infantryman is a prepared subject for anxiety. He is threatened with death or mutilation. He must go without sleep, remain exposed to the weather, and often be hungry. He is usually unable to understand all that is happening around him. He is repeatedly frightened by gunfire and distressed by the death of comrades. If he is exposed to such circumstances long enough, he develops a severe and persisting anxiety state, sometimes called combat exhaustion or battle fatigue. Swank, in his classic studies of combat exhaustion in the European campaign of World War II, described all the features. Soldiers complained of emotional tension and were easily startled, had difficulty sleeping, reported mental confusion and memory deficits, and complained of headache, back pain, palpitations, weakness, and fatigability. The complaint of persistent fatigue was found in all of the men.

Swank documented that this condition develops after severe or prolonged combat. The character of the individual symptoms and the sequence of the development were stereotyped but they appeared earliest among units with the highest casualty rates. All men apparently, though, will develop this condition if exposed to battle long enough. Wolff reported that the average man in the Army of the United States during the Korean conflict reached this point after 85 days of combat.

The symptoms of anxiety that physicians see in patients in circumstances that are threatening to them or as symptoms of other diseases are not different. The patients all have the same three groups of symptoms but may report that one is more prominent than the others, such as emphasizing the tension and fatigue, the intellectual difficulties, or the somatic and autonomic difficulties.

Panic attacks are distinct from the chronic tension and anxiety found in these circumstances and can be recognized by their characteristic features. They occur usually on a background of some persistent, generalized anxiety or apprehension, but the attacks occur at times when there appears to be no obvious threatening circumstance. Although the panic attack can occur at any time, a most favorite time is when the person is in a situation in which rapid exit would be difficult, such as traveling in a bus, train, or elevator; standing in a crowded store or restaurant; or waiting in a supermarket line.

The attacks are experienced as episodes of uneasiness that start without any identifiable precipitant and build up over ten to fifteen minutes to a level of severe panic, only to subside again by the end of an hour. As the feeling of anxiety increases, the patient may notice dyspnea, choking sensations, sweating, flushing, paresthesias, trembling or shaking, heart palpitations, weakness, or lightheadedness. A common complaint in an anxiety attack is the sensation of tightness in the chest, as though the lungs could not be adequately filled. The patient responds to this sensation by deep and sighing respirations, sometimes to the point of producing a respiratory alkalosis that adds to the feelings of giddiness with tingling of the fingertips and even tetany with carpopedal spasms. This is the *hyperventilation syndrome* that adds its symptoms to the panic feelings. The patient may act upon his symptoms by trying to flee from the situation and may in the future avoid the situations in which the panic attack appeared. This avoidance may get so extreme that the patient becomes essentially housebound.

A chronic anxiety may be provoked by a chronic situation of conflict and threat, or it may be the outcome of repeated panic attacks in which the anxiety is now focused particularly on the fear of further attack. With the chronic condition symptoms are less intense, although not different in quality from those of acute anxiety. The patient is tense and on edge. He may also report some feelings of sadness or hopelessness along with his anxiety. He will have a number of somatic complaints, particularly frontal or occipital headache, anorexia, and weight loss, and on examination he may have physical signs of tension, a fine tremor of the extended hands, brisk tendon reflexes, rapid heartbeat, and pupillary dilatation.

That there is a clear genetic vulnerability to panic disorder implies that there may be a biologic foundation to this condition distinguishing it from anxieties that can be understood as graded responses of an individual to varying threats. Certainly its stereotyped presentvation, its response to medication, and its tendency to remissions and exacerbations, as well as this genetic predisposition, encourage a search for a biologic system that can be provoked into action by some ordinarily nonthreatening event. The recent recognition that receptors for the benzodiazepine class of drugs are to be found naturally in the brain leads to proposals that there may be some natural "tranquilizer" ligand, with the implication that a pathophysiology of such a system of ligands and their receptors might prove to be a basis for this particular disorder. If such a system were discovered, it would also most likely illuminate the other anxieties generated by more obviously threatening circumstances and treatable with exogenous benzodiazepines.

DIAGNOSIS. Usually the recognition of anxiety is not difficult. The patient's voiced complaint is his distressing emotional state. His associated disturbances in thinking and autonomic functions serve to confirm the diagnostic impression. Most often the major issue is not the diagnosis of anxiety but rather the question of why the patient is anxious now. This question must be answered from knowledge of the circumstances of the onset of anxiety, the signs and symptoms that accompany it, and the personality of the patient. The decision as to whether this patient's anxiety is a response to circumstances, a symptom of some underlying psychiatric or neurologic disorder, or a psychopathologic state of its own can be made on the basis of this knowledge.

It is crucial, though, to recognize the panic disorder, since it will have a specific treatment. It can occasionally be presented by a patient who focuses his complaints on the physical symptoms that accompany the attacks, such as his cardiac palpitations or his giddiness and vertigo. Then the condition can be confused with episodic cardiac or neurologic conditions. Most helpful to the proper diagnosis is the discernment that the episodes are always accompanied by intense anxiety and by several autonomic reactions. A search for such particular symptoms as air hunger, tremulousness, and hyperventilation is diagnostically helpful. It is sometimes necessary to exclude other conditions with appropriate laboratory tests. As with all psychologically disturbed patients, laboratory studies should not be delayed or protracted, but should be decided upon, and this phase of the examination should be finished as promptly as possible. Knowledge of the existence of panic disorder as a specific condition is most helpful to its recognition.

TREATMENT. Treatment will vary with the cause and severity of the anxiety. Many mildly anxious patients whose anxiety is a response to threat or conflict can be helped by a physician who is willing to listen carefully to their difficulties and offer some support and occasional advice. These patients have disturbances that are transient and are based on some particular problem or self-doubt that can eventually be resolved.

Those with more severe anxiety but from the same source can be aided by a combination of pharmacologic treatment and repeated compassionate discussions of their difficulties. The pharmacologic agent to be recommended for this form of anxiety is chlordiazepoxide (Librium), which can be given in doses of 10 mg three to four times a day.

Only occasionally is it necessary to bring such patients into hospital. This is done in an effort to remove them from some pathogenic setting that has provoked a vicious circle of anxiety, decompensation, failure, and more anxiety. Yet such hospitalization is often remarkably effective in bringing such patients relief. Again some sedation as well as psychologic support can be given to them, and again chlordiazepoxide can be recommended in combination with a milieu of support and understanding that allows the patient to regain emotional balance.

Patients with chronic anxiety can be referred with confidence to specialists in psychotherapy. Jerome Frank and his associates have documented that certain personality features have prognostic significance in the psychotherapy of anxiety, and their monograph on the ingredients of successful psychotherapy can be consulted.

As emphasized, though, panic attacks must be specifically recognized. This is because (1) it is clear that they are distinct from other anxieties in family history, course, and phenomena, and (2) they do *not* respond to the sedatives such as chlordiazepoxide but do respond well to tricyclic antidepressants or monoamine oxidase inhibitors. The tricyclic antidepressant imipramine has proved particularly useful. Often patients respond at a relatively low dose of 25 to 50 mg per day, but it can be gradually raised until panic attacks abate. Doses that have been effective have ranged from 5 to 300 mg of imipramine. The monoamine oxidase inhibitor phenelzine in doses of 30 to 60 mg per day has also been demonstrated to be effective in this condition. These medications interrupt the panic attacks but may leave the patient with some continuing chronic tension. For this a small dose of chlordiazepoxide can be recommended. The medication for the panic attacks should be maintained until the patient is attack free for six to twelve months.

Psychologic management in the panic disorder does form a useful adjunctive treatment. It is particularly important to explain the nature of this condition to patients, because often they fear that the panic attacks indicate that they have some progressive mental disorder. Simply discovering that it is a recognized entity with an established treatment has been comforting to many patients through the period of adjusting medication and establishing a plan for managing the attacks. It is also helpful to remind the patient that recovery will not be immediate, that relapses can occur, and that, since it is the panic symptom that is being treated, panic will be experienced several times before it is controlled, but that in about 80 per cent of patients this control will ultimately be achieved.

The patient can aid in his own recovery if he tries not to flee from a situation in which he experiences a panic attack. To help the patient do this, he can be told truthfully that the panic will not lead to mental disruption or total loss of control but customarily will reach some peak intensity and then gradually abate over a period of ten to fifteen minutes. If the patient can simply sustain himself in the setting until some abatement occurs, the next occasion will often be less severe. Along with the medications that tend to suppress their occurrence, this behavioral management of the individual attacks gradually gives the patient a sense of control of the panic experience and with this a capacity to free himself from the constraints on his activity that he previously used to avoid panic.

Cohen ME, Badal DW, Kilpatrick A, Reed EW, White PD: The high familial prevalence of neurocirculatory asthenia (anxiety neurosis, effort syndrome). Am J Hum Genet 3:126, 1951. *The classic description of the panic attack syndrome and its familial occurrence. Most useful also for its consideration of differential diagnosis.*

Crowe RR, Pauls DL, Slymen DJ, Noyes R: A family study of anxiety neurosis. Arch Gen Psychiatry 37:77, 1980. *A recent confirmation of the familial prevalence of panic disorder.*

Gronwall DA, Sampson H: The Psychological Effects of Concussion. London, Oxford University Press, 1975. *An elegant demonstration of a deficit in information-processing capacity in patients after concussive injuries.This deficit is often inapparent to routine examination but can have profound effects on emotional reactivity. A model of neuropsychiatric research.*

Marks IM: Fears and Phobias. New York, Academic Press, 1969. *A readable and thorough discussion of various anxiety states, with particular consideration of treatment and prognosis.*

Rohs RG, Noyes R: Agoraphobia. Newer treatment approach. J Nerv Ment Dis 166:701, 1978. *A good review of psychologic and psychopharmacologic treatments of panic disorder.*

Swank RL: Combat exhaustion. J Nerv Ment Dis 109:475, 1949. *The classic description of the causes, symptoms, and signs of situation-specific anxiety. Still rewarding to study.*

Depression

DEFINITION. Depression is a term for a mood of sadness and gloom. It can be a symptom of manic-depressive psychosis (see above for a complete consideration of the subject). Here we are dealing with depression that occurs as a response to troubled life circumstances. Such depression can usually be given a more specific name, such as discouragement, demoralization, or grief—terms that carry specifically the connotation of an emotional reaction.

The troubled mood is usually not hard to recognize. The patient appears miserable, his face expressive of sadness and perhaps tension. He may move without confidence or purpose and report that his energy is decreased and his thinking slow and difficult. Appetite is usually lessened, often with weight loss, and sleep is restless and diminished. Sexual interest will be greatly reduced. The patient may also say that he is irritable and fearful. Depending on the severity of his depression, the patient will seem socially disorganized, proving inefficient in work, failing in duties, and neglectful of appearance. His acknowledged inadequacies in these respects may add to his sense of misery and may prompt thoughts of resigning from work, leaving his family, or even committing suicide.

Although various troubles can provoke depression, there is a specific response that illustrates features common to many depressive reactions. That response is *grief*, well studied by Dr. C. M. Parkes.

Grief is an experience in almost every lifetime and is the response that follows the loss, usually by death, of some relative or friend. The severity of the reaction and its duration depend upon many factors, but the most important is the closeness of the relationship and degree of dependence of the mourner on the lost individual.

Grief is a state that follows a pattern of development in which certain stages can be recognized even though the transition from one to the next is not possible to define exactly and features from one can persist in the others. The *first stage*, which lasts several days, begins upon learning of the death. The mourner feels stunned and appears bewildered, does not seem to grasp his loss fully or to relate its implications to his feelings coherently. He may appear irritable, tearful, or anxious, but can also seem calm and capable. Although his emotions and behavior may be unpredictable, they are often culturally modified as he carries out such customs as funeral rituals. He himself will usually report afterward that his emotions were blunted and his thinking uncertain, and that his depressed mood was not fully experienced. Parkes refers to this period as the stage of numbness, blunting, or shock.

This stage ends gradually but usually within one week of the bereavement, when there is an increase in the emotion of sadness and the appearance of an intense sense of loss that comes in waves, called pangs of yearning or pining by Parkes. In this *second stage*, between these surges of distressing feelings, which are so frequent at first as to be almost continuous, the patient is usually irritable and sad, with sleep and appetite diminished. Activity, which often takes the form of aimless moving about rather than productive work, may be increased, particularly so during a depressive surge, a point Parkes uses to support his analogy of this stage of grief to the searching behavior of animals separated from their mates. It is the phenomenon of *surges of misery*, however, that is most characteristic of grief and usually aids in its recognition. With time these occur less often, but it is common experience to have such a wave of depressive feelings sweep over a person following a reminder of the loss years after the bereavement.

The *third period of grief* appears with a diminution in the attacks of yearning and the anxious restlessness. This phase, usually entered into within several weeks of bereavement, customarily lasts the longest. It is a stage of depressed feelings with apathy and a disinclination to find purpose or interest in work. The patient is no longer restless, sleepless, or without appetite, but his emotional state is one of gloom and discouragement and his capacity for enjoyment or for physical or intellectual work is greatly reduced. Parkes refers to this as the stage of disorganization when the patient seems withdrawn, may complain of ill health, and fails to plan ahead. This state may last over a year and only gradually be replaced with more customary feelings. Recovery may be brought about in part by the natural but chance occurrence of new integrative activities and friendships, and can be facilitated by efforts of the mourner to expose himself to the opportunities for these restorative experiences.

Depressions that are responses to difficulties in life other than bereavement are very similar to this third stage. Symptoms like those in the first two stages of grief can appear briefly in distressing situations that have a sudden onset, such as being informed of an unexpected personal misfortune. But these are usually transient features and are soon replaced by a mood of sadness and discouragement very like that of the third stage.

PRECIPITATING FACTORS. In this form of depression it is usually not difficult to recognize the change as a response to some difficulty, for the patient is often preoccupied with the trouble itself and is ready to draw the link between it and his present mood. Precipitating situations can be of many kinds. They can be sudden and specific events in which something is lost, such as a relationship or a job. Other provocations are situations chronically thwarting to the sense of achievement and mastery, as in an education program in which students are confronted with their errors but given little effective teaching to overcome them. Moving away from home can provoke the very unpleasant depressive reaction, homesickness, especially in persons who depend a great deal on the support of friends and family. In general, circumstances that disturb a person's sense of stability, security, effectiveness, or worth provoke depressive responses.

The more such a precipitant is prolonged or accompanied by a growing realization of his difficulties, the more likely the person is to show a depressive response. A paradigm of these features for a precipitant is found in debilitating physical illnesses such as cancer. Here the protracted and continually worsening clinical situation provides constant reminders of losses suffered and brings more each day. That depression is a universal occurrence in such circumstances has been demonstrated by Hinton in his study of the dying.

For reasons not fully understood, there are some physiologic states and physical illnesses that commonly provoke depressive moods. Patients with hepatitis or any severe viral illness are particularly prone to report a depressive mood and to find reasons for it in trifles that did not trouble them when they were well. Endocrine alterations such as the postpartum state, Cushing's disease, or Addison's disease are also precipitants of depressive feelings that can be very distressing to the patient and of such profound degree as to occasionally promote a suicidal action. Certain brain diseases, particularly stroke, may also precipitate a prolonged and distressing depressive state. In all these circumstances the mood of depression may rest on some disturbed physiologic mechanism in the central nervous system as yet unknown. Their possible relationship to manic-depressive disorder is discussed above.

PREDISPOSING FACTORS. Given that situations of difficulty can lead to depression, there are features of personality that can make an individual more vulnerable to this response, perhaps by making him assess losses and difficulties more acutely and by inhibiting his power to resolve them. Especially vulnerable are those insecure and sensitive individuals who perceive criticism when none is intended and find a source of depressive feelings in their self-doubting.

Another depressive predisposition is that of the self-dramatizing and emotionally unstable and immature individual who tends to amplify emotional reactions of all sorts. When such an individual finds himself in situations of discomfort in which his feelings may be neglected, he seems more prone than others to develop a sense of dissatisfaction, distress, and depression. Slavney and McHugh present empirical evidence of this predisposition in their report of depressive symptoms in 80 per cent of patients hospitalized with the diagnosis of hysterical personality.

Finally, individuals limited in their capacity to cope with difficulties are predisposed to depressive responses. Particularly vulnerable for this reason are the mentally retarded. Even modest impairment in intellectual endowment will interfere with the person's ability to find solutions to situations that present him problems, and his failure and uncertainty tend to provoke a depressive mood. Borderline mental retardation is often overlooked in the search for predisposing factors, and a history of poor occupational and scholastic performance in a depressed patient warrants formal intelligence testing.

Social factors have been considered important in depression since Durkheim. Brown and Harris have documented in a careful epidemiologic study a group of predisposing features for depression among women in an urban setting. It was more frequent in working class than in middle class women and was highly related to threatening life events. Whether the woman suffered a depressive response to these events seemed to depend on four other vulnerability factors. These were the presence of three or more children under 14 at home; no employment for the woman outside the home; absence of a confiding, intimate relationship, as with the husband; and loss of the woman's mother before age 11. Such predisposing features emphasize the isolated life experience of young mothers and the importance of efforts to help them with these aspects as well as to aid them over more acute crises.

DIFFERENTIAL DIAGNOSIS. The differential diagnosis of depressive states can be difficult, particularly if it is not carried out methodically. The most important distinction to draw is that between depression as a response to troubled circumstances and depression as a symptom of manic-depressive disorder. This important discrimination rests on clinical grounds and cannot be made with certainty in all situations. Thus, although the depressions of the widow, the homesick, and the patient with a fatal illness can all be recognized as responses, the trap is in making this understandable connection with every depression and explaining it always as being due to some recent difficulty. If the family of the patient says he is more depressed than they would expect him to be under the circumstances, the diagnosis of a depressive response might be questioned. Also, the presence in the patient of remarkable changes in self-attitude such as the appearance of beliefs that he is a criminal or deserves punishment for minor transgressions, or that he is infectious and filled with physical corruption, are not seen in the usual depressive response and should lead to the consideration of manic-depressive psychosis. Finally, a previous history of mania or of depression, or a family history of affective disorder, should influence the interpretation of depression and sway the diagnosis away from the depressive response (see above).

TREATMENT. Although the depressive response is characteristic enough to be recognized easily again and again, the particular predispositions, precipitants, and interactions are never exactly the same from one patient to another. Treatment is based on these particulars and is thus unique to some extent to each occasion. It is therefore hard to describe the treatment of depression without some sense of dissatisfaction because, although the principles are simple, no list of them applies to every patient.

An important early decision in treatment is the need for hospitalization. This is usually determined by how severely the mood disturbance interferes with self-care, by the availability of a supportive and protective environment at home, and particularly by the presence of suicidal features. To assess the last, the patient must be asked if he has been considering self-injury. Although judgment is required in evaluating his answers, a sequence of questions probing for suicidal thoughts should be routine for every patient with depression. A proportion of the patients will deny all thought of self-injury and can be assumed to be of lesser suicidal risk. Those who admit to such thoughts should be asked if they have any means in mind. To that question still more patients will reassure the doctor that their thoughts on suicide have not reached so severe an intensity. Those patients, however, who admit to having considered a means (pill, gas, shooting) must be considered of higher risk, and thought must be given to protecting them, perhaps by hospitalization or by guaranteeing that they are under the supervision of friends or relatives. Finally, the patients should be asked if they have acquired any means or done anything to try them out. Again a proportion of patients will say that they have not been that despondent, but those who say that they have done such things are at very high risk and should in most cases be hospitalized.

Once a decision is made about the site of treatment, in a hospital or on an outpatient basis, the act of reaching a secure diagnosis of a depressive reaction in a patient is the first step in its treatment, because this judgment requires that the doctor has come to understand the patient and his predicament. To gain this understanding the doctor's first meetings should be devoted to listening to the patient's description of his circumstances, of his emotional changes, and of the connections he draws between his experiences and his depressive mood. If appropriate, other informants such as relatives can amplify on the patient's statements and give details of his past modes of coping with trouble. All these efforts are intended to bring the doctor an appreciation of this particular individual and the circumstances that he faces. Such knowledge, combined with the relationships of trust, respect, and empathy that develop naturally in its acquisition, provides the resources for treatment.

The therapeutic efforts from this foundation are directed toward re-engaging the patient in life experiences in which success can be found, replacements for losses enjoyed, and a sense of integrity and control regained. Usually the first need of the patient is some help in simple tactics for the management of his current troubles and for the avoidance of their repetition in the future.

At this stage a sense of helplessness often prompts the patient to abandon many of his activities and efforts, but if at all possible he must be encouraged not to give in to these promptings, because doing so tends to perpetuate the disturbed mood by holding him from opportunities to reassess his situation and to try out solutions. His daily work, even when less efficiently performed, is often helpful in directing his attention to matters other than his troubles.

With assistance in simple matters of personal management, the patient can be helped to some success in his circumstances, bringing him encouragement and promoting a willingness to maintain his efforts and to plan for the future. Educating the patient in how certain circumstances strike his particular vulnerabilities and so provoke depressive responses can be helpful.

The most useful ingredient of the treatment is the support and interest of the doctor. This is particularly true for those depressive feelings that emerge in the context of chronic or progressive medical illness. Patients report that the supportive information and sense of planning together provided by the physician managing such an illness are major sources of encouragement and relief. Such support encourages the patient to express his feelings and discuss his circumstances. In this way not only is the physician provided with more information about assets and vulnerabilities of the patient, but often there is spontaneous recognition by the patient of causal features for his difficulties that brings both relief to his mood and self-perceived tactics for their resolution. If this supportive relationship can be maintained and developed, improvement of depression can be expected. For the occasional patient with whom such a relationship fails or who succumbs frequently to depressive reactions because of some intractable predisposition, more prolonged treatment by specialists in psychotherapy can be recommended.

Finally, treatment with pharmaceutical agents may help. Chlordiazepoxide, 10 mg three times daily, may relieve agitation somewhat in the bereaved or otherwise reactively depressed. A sleeping medication, flurazepam hydrochloride (Dalmane), is helpful for the sleeplessness. The *antidepressant medications,* although most useful in the manic-depressive psychoses, can be tried in some patients with a prolonged depressive response. Imipramine in a dose of 150 to 250 mg a day or the monoamine oxidase inhibitor phenelzine, 15 mg three times daily, has helped individual patients, but this symptomatic relief should be considered a minor part of the treatment plan in patients with this form of depression.

Brown G, Harris T: Social Origins of Depression. London, Tavistock, 1978. *A readable account of several years of painstaking research on the psychosocial causes of depression in women.*

Durkheim E: Suicide: A Study in Sociology. (Translated by George Simpson.) Glencoe, IL, Free Press, 1951. *An excellent translation of this classic study by one of the fathers of sociology.*

Parkes CM: Bereavement: Studies of Grief in Adult Life. London, Tavistock, 1972. *A comprehensive and invaluable book for this universal human problem.*

Hysteria

DEFINITION. Hysteria is a disturbance of behavior in which symptoms and signs of physical ill health are imitated more or less unconsciously for some personal advantage. As the phrase "more or less unconsciously" implies, hysteria may be hard to distinguish from "malingering," in which the imitation of illness is a well-appreciated fraud. Frank malingering is rare, though, because the power of human self-deception is usually adequate to persuade a person of the validity of his own symptoms. The only ones who can be called malingerers with any confidence are some self-mutilating patients and the remarkable pathologic liars, picturesquely called examples of the *Munchausen syndrome,* who travel from hospital to hospital gaining admission by means of dramatic acts of illness.

PREDISPOSING AND PRECIPITATING FACTORS. Hysterical symptoms are to be seen as responses to distressing experiences. They can occur in almost any person facing danger or difficulty, especially if, as with soldiers in battle or prisoners, the distress is intense and prolonged and physical symptoms can provide a viable escape. Dull-witted or immature persons with inadequate powers of introspection and self-control may produce transparently hysterical symptoms in response to milder distress, such as school difficulties or family problems. Some of the exaggerations and elaborations of medical symptoms common in hospitalized patients may be similarly interpreted as responses to the distress of illness by persons whose capacity for self-control has been weakened by somatic illness. Hysterical symptoms can be the first manifestations of a dementing illness or of a depressive or schizophrenic psychosis, and these disorders must be considered when a previously well-balanced adult develops a suspiciously hysterical symptom.

Commonly, though, hysteria is a disturbance in the behavior of a person predisposed by an attention-seeking, emotionally unstable, and egocentric personality. In fact, these characteristics form what has become known as the "hysterical personality" even though hysteria can occur in other types of people, and these characteristics do not invariably produce hysterical symptoms. Most easily recognized in such people is their flair for the dramatic, and thus the recent term *histrionic personality* has been applied to them in the new American psychiatric classification (DSM III). They show this tendency in flamboyant dress and in exaggerated, even melodramatic, responses to questions about their symptoms. They are never so happy as when they are the center of attention. Karl Jaspers characterized the hysterical personalities as those who "crave to appear, both to themselves and others, as more than they are and to experience more than they are capable of." The zeal of these patients for exaggeration and drama renders them more liable to hysterical symptoms. But other kinds of people can have these symptoms. In all of them usually a discouraged, depressive mood has been prompted by difficulties in life, and the hysterical symptoms then emerge from this mood state.

As implied by the concept of gain from imitation of illness, there are social predisposing factors here. Perhaps most fundamental is the social advantages that derive in our society from what Parsons has called the "sick role." The sick are relieved of certain obligations such as working and self-sufficiency with the assumption that sickness is a state that is of itself unpleasant, that the patient is involuntarily victim to sickness, and that he will do all that is required to escape from it. For certain circumstances and certain people the "sick role" may offer such attractions that the illness-imitating behavior that we call hysterical appears. It is likely that the irritation some doctors feel for these patients derives from the belief that the patients are gaining unfair advantages and wasting resources needed by others. It is perhaps helpful to employ Pilowski's concept of "abnormal illness behavior" for these patients and so extricate ourselves from an inappropriate, judgmental, and ineffective approach toward them.

SYMPTOMS AND SIGNS. Many of the phenomena of somatic illness can be imitated by hysteria. The accuracy of the imitation depends on the medical sophistication of the patient. A doctor or nurse is more likely to produce a convincing imitation than is an unqualified person.

Common hysterical symptoms are vague subjective disorders, such as generalized weakness, dizziness, indigestion, or pain. Hysterical pain can occur in any part of the body, but the head and neck, the region over the heart, and the low back are particularly favored. Hysterical pain can be of any character, from dull aching to sharp and stabbing pain, but it is often described by the patient in vivid similes such as "like a bullet," "like a bolt of lightning," "aches like an abscessed tooth," or "sore as a hot boil." Usually, hysterical pain is not confined to a local area as around a pathologic lesion, nor is it referred into the distribution of a particular nerve or dermatome. Rather, hysterical pain is felt in a general region of the body and spreads, sometimes in bizarre ways, into contiguous areas without regard to neuroanatomic boundaries. Thus pain beginning in the face may spread along the side of the head and into the back, crossing from the region of the trigeminal nerve into the upper cervical nerve regions. Hysterical pain often varies in its character, intensity, and distribution, changing considerably with attention or suggestion. Occasionally it can be remarkably improved by a small amount of intravenous amobarbital sodium when analgesics do not help.

Although vague symptoms of a subjective kind such as pain or dizziness are the present vogue in hysteria, crude and gross symptoms are still seen. These may be psychologic, such as the amnesia or fugue states, in which memory is partially lost, often in situations in which the patient is depressed or anxious. Other psychologic symptoms shown occasionally include auditory and visual hallucinations and even flamboyant delusions. These must be carefully judged, but appear most commonly in young people who have read popular books on psychology and psychiatry and are apparently suggested into these symptoms by their reading at a time when they are distressed over other matters.

Motor disturbances in the form of abnormal movement, disturbed gaits, seizures, or paralyses are occasionally hysterical symptoms. Hysterical seizures can usually be distinguished from epileptic ones. The patients only rarely injure themselves, bite their tongues, or lose their urine. They do not have the typical tonic and then clonic phases of a seizure, but tend to show a dramatic flailing of the limbs. Consciousness is partially retained, and seizures hardly ever occur when the patient is alone. The EEG is normal.

Sensory disturbances are particularly favored hysterical symptoms. Thus, *blindness* or *deafness* is common, often developing dramatically at a time of emotional distress. Loss of sensation over one side of the body to pin prick or light touch is frequently found after a susceptible patient has been examined by a neurologist.

DIAGNOSIS. Diagnosis of hysteria is seldom easy and never popular. Ideally, it should rest on three supports: first, the *form* of the hysterical manifestation; second, the *personality* of the patient; and third, the *setting* in which the symptoms developed. Often it is not possible to find all three supports to a diagnosis, but all should be sought.

Commonly, hysterical symptoms are vague and variable. In fact, the more definite and consistent a patient's description of the onset, location, nature, and duration of his symptoms, the less likely the symptoms are to be hysterical. Hysterical symptoms and signs are also usually incompatible with what is known of anatomy and physiology. Thus sensory losses do not conform to patterns of nerve distribution; reflexes remain intact and unchanged in the palsies of arm and leg; seizures of the entire body do not disturb consciousness; total blindness appears without a disturbance of pupillary reflex or of opticokinetic nystagmus. The hysterically mute person can phonate on coughing. The hysterically deaf person speaks louder to be heard over increased ambient noises. Many other hysterical symptoms have been analyzed for such inconsistencies by Head.

Knowledge of the personality and past history of the patient is helpful to a diagnosis of hysteria. The recognition that the symptoms are occurring in an hysterical personality should prompt an observer to look very closely at the symptoms before embarking on extensive laboratory tests or upon surgery. Similarly, knowledge of a previous vague and poorly understood medical disturbance can lend weight to an opinion that a new symptom that has eluded diagnosis is occurring in an individual prone to hysteria. Conversely, hysteria can usually be eliminated as an explanation for symptoms in an emotionally stable, middle-aged person. People who have passed through adolescence and young adulthood without resorting to hysterical behavior are unlikely to employ it when older.

The setting in which the symptoms develop should be carefully scrutinized, and a search made for a distressing event that may have provoked an hysterical reaction or for any purpose that the hysterical symptoms may serve. Occasionally, a clear association between the symptoms chosen and a particular recent disturbance in the life of the subject can be found, such as an amnesia developing in a person who has done something shameful or criminal, or weakness and pain persisting in a person who is seeking financial compensation for an injury. Often, though, motivations behind hysterical symptoms are vague and uncertain. It is usual to find that the patient is unhappy or anxious about some aspect of his life circumstances and that the hysterical symptoms serve to call attention to his distress. Also, it may be possible to demonstrate that the development of particular symptoms has been prompted by suggestion: weakness of legs, for example, developing in a nurse caring for a paraplegic patient, or peculiar falling attacks after the patient has witnessed an epileptic seizure.

Guzé and his associates have pointed out a subgroup of patients with a chronic hysterical disorder who have had recurrent complaints of symptoms involving almost every bodily system. These patients, with what Guzé terms *Briquet's syndrome,* present diagnostic difficulties to many specialists as their complaints change, worsen, and improve in unpredictable ways. They usually have undergone multiple medical and surgical procedures. The same criteria that lead to the diagnosis of single hysterical symptoms can be applied to this group. Additionally they can be reliably differentiated from most medical patients by the sheer number of systems that have been involved in their past complaints.

A careful study of the symptoms, the personality, and the life setting of a patient usually allows a reasonably certain differentiation of hysterical symptoms from those of a medical illness. There are, however, certain medical problems that are notoriously easily confused with hysteria. These are the diseases that produce vague and changing symptoms that seem to vary with the patient's motivation and, at least in their early phases, lack convincing physical signs. If such an illness occurs in a patient who has features of the hysterical personality and who will therefore describe the symptoms in a dramatic and flamboyant fashion, physicians may be even more persuaded to believe that the illness is only deceptively physical. Examples of diseases frequently confused with hysteria because of their subtle clinical features are the first attack of multiple sclerosis, particularly if sensory changes alone are produced; the weakness of arms and legs seen early in acute idiopathic polyneuritis of the Guillain-Barré type; the difficulty in swallowing of bulbar myasthenia gravis; the attacks of muscular weakness in periodic paralysis; the tonic posturings and oculogyric crises of postencephalitic parkinsonism; the pain of a cauda equina tumor; and the abdominal pain of acute intermittent porphyria.

MANAGEMENT OF HYSTERIA. The management of hysterical patients is difficult. No one method can be recommended unqualifiedly. But there are certain principles that can be followed. To help hysterical patients it is essential to have sympathy for them. Many doctors find these patients irritating. It is just as possible to see them as individuals displaying an intriguing aspect of human behavior that has profound implications in their lives. It is pointless to argue with these patients about the validity of their symptoms. A useful approach is to agree that they have had an illness producing their symptoms, but that they are now improving even though total recovery has not arrived.

It is important to diagnose hysteria promptly. Hesitation in diagnosis leading to several hospital admissions for extensive laboratory investigations is a good way to solidify hysterical symptoms in a patient. Among other things, the uncertainty of doctors helps persuade a patient that the symptoms are real. Repeated examinations increase the consistency with which symptoms are reported. Long hospitalization, mounting bills, and the inconvenience caused to others make it difficult for a patient to abandon symptoms without embarrassment. The gratifying attention given to the patient in the hospital, perhaps as an example of an intriguing diagnostic problem, can feed the self-dramatizing tendencies and so encourage the behavior.

There is always a risk of error in any diagnosis, because diagnosis is only a weighing of probabilities. The diagnosis of hysteria, though, depends purely on a physician's judgment and, before relief of symptoms is accomplished, can be confirmed in the laboratory only by evidence of health. Physicians, for obvious reasons, fear more the error of calling a physically sick patient hysterical than the error of mishandling hysteria. They often prefer to exclude, by laboratory examination, progressively more unlikely diseases than to study carefully the symptoms and the individual who has produced them, even though this would lead more directly to a definite diagnosis as well as an understanding of the response. It may be unwise to counsel too strongly against this behavior because medical diagnosis is never easy. A compromise can be found in the admonition to perform immediately the laboratory tests that seem necessary for a patient but, when hysteria is suspected, to bring the period of investigation as quickly as possible to a close so that management of the specific symptom can be begun.

Treatment of the specific symptoms rests basically upon persuasion. The doctor is persuading the patient to perform the functions that the patient claims are disabled. Intravenous amobarbital sodium given to the point at which the patient is mildly intoxicated and his speech slurred is particularly helpful in making and establishing a persuasion. Usually, some ingenuity is required for success. The hysterically blind person can, for example, be persuaded first that he can distinguish light from dark and then gradually to distinguish forms, to read large print, and, finally, small newspaper type. The person who claims he cannot walk can be encouraged first to move his legs in bed, and then to stand, to make a few tentative shuffles, and finally to stride out. The hysterically deaf person can be persuaded to hear through a stethoscope and then gradually that he can hear without it. A dramatic show of some kind is often helpful in removing these symptoms. If a physician has success in partially removing hysterical symptoms, he should persist in his treatment without interruption in order to bring about as much improvement as possible and even to restore full function. When there is recovery of function, the patient should perform his recovered skills in public—before his family, other patients, and several doctors—to prevent his relapsing immediately into his former state.

The fear that sudden removal of hysterical symptoms will result in a disastrous psychologic collapse is exaggerated. Rarely, a depressed patient with hysterical symptoms has an increase in depression, but it is clear that in those situations a depression was overlooked and the more secondary hysterical symptoms were emphasized.

Some hysterical disorders are refractory to treatment. Among these are the disorders assumed for some material gain, such as compensation. They usually are not improved until some settlement is made. Episodic disorders such as hysterical seizures can be hard to control. Sometimes, however, a statement to the patient that they will not recur, given with full authority by a physician whom the patient trusts and respects, may eliminate these symptoms. The longer the patient has hysterical symptoms, the harder they are to remove. This is a corollary to the aforementioned observation that hysterical symptoms produced for transparent reasons and bordering on malingering are more difficult to eliminate than are the ones produced by an attention-seeking personality in some emotional distress.

Simultaneously with treatment of the specific symptoms, the emotional state and present life of the patient should be studied to discover any distress that may have precipitated the hysterical symptoms. Then advice, social assistance, or guidance can be offered to aid the patient in resolving these difficulties. This aspect of their psychologic treatment depends on developing a relationship of friendship and mutual respect identical to that found necessary in treating an anxious or depressed person.

Long-term management of hysterical patients is much more difficult than treatment of individual symptoms. It is not wise to have the average hysterical patient embark on depth psychotherapy, because he tends to produce more symptoms and to recount involved sexual and other fantasies in order to maintain the interest of his doctor. If possible, these patients should be followed by one physician who understands them and the behavior that they are liable to produce and is also competent to recognize physical illness should it arise. This physician can save these patients from needless surgery and long hospitalization. He can remove hysterical symptoms promptly by being alert to the diagnosis and providing help for the difficulties that precipitate them.

Guzé S: The validity and significance of the clinical diagnosis of hysteria (Briquet's syndrome). Am J Psychiatry 132:138, 1975. *This paper demonstrates the means and clinical utility of distinguishing patients with a chronic hysterical disorder.*

Head H: The diagnosis of hysteria. Br Med J 1:827, 1922. *A valuable description of a variety of hysterical manifestations that can be confused with neurologic disorders.*

Pilowski I: Abnormal illness behavior. Br J Med Psychol 42:347, 1969. *A most intriguing way of looking at hysteria as a socially provoked abnormal behavior.*

477. DRUG ABUSE AND DEPENDENCE

Robert B. Millman

Drug abuse results from the complex interaction of an individual, his social and cultural environment, and the pharmacology and availability of particular drugs. Frequently no sharp line distinguishes appropriate use from misuse of any drug. Drug abuse may therefore be defined as the use of any substance in a manner that deviates from the accepted medical, social, or legal patterns within a given society. These substances may be grouped into six major classes: (1) opiates; (2) central nervous system depressants, including alcohol, hypnotics, and tranquilizers; (3) central nervous system stimulants, including the amphetamine group and cocaine; (4) cannabis; (5) psychedelics; and (6) miscellaneous inhalants.

Abuse of some drugs may be intermittent and lead to little physical, psychologic, or social deterioration. In other cases, the user may become dependent on the drug in order to function at what he perceives to be a satisfactory level. This *psychologic dependence,* or habituation, varies in intensity and may culminate in *compulsive drug abuse,* in which the supply and use of particular drugs become primary concerns of living. In addition, certain drugs have the capacity to produce *physical dependence.* This is an altered physiologic state induced by the repeated administration of a drug that requires the continued administration of the drug to prevent the appearance of a syndrome characteristic for each drug, the *withdrawal,* or *abstinence, syndrome.* The term "*addiction*" should be reserved for a pattern of compulsive drug use that includes an overwhelming involvement with the acquisition and use of a drug, loss of control, and a tendency to relapse after withdrawal.

ETIOLOGY AND PATTERNS OF ABUSE. Initially, drugs may be taken to satisfy curiosity, to reduce pain, to influence mood, to change activity levels, to reduce tension and anxiety, to decrease fatigue and boredom, to facilitate social interaction, to heighten sensation and awareness, and for many other reasons. If caffeine, nicotine, alcohol, and prescription and over-the-counter depressants and stimulants are included, few people in the United States would be found who take no psychoactive drugs. Patterns of abuse vary from the experimental or intermittent use of a particular drug or combination under defined circumstances, such as the use of marijuana and alcohol at a party, to a compulsive "polydrug-abuse" pattern, in which a variety of drugs are taken in a disorganized and dangerous manner on a daily basis.

SOCIOLOGIC FACTORS AND EPIDEMIOLOGY. Social and cultural factors determine initial drug-experimentation patterns and define acceptable drug-abuse behaviors for a given group. The use of alcohol is condoned and even encouraged in many segments of society. Cocaine and depressant use have become an integral part of membership in some urban upper-middle-class groups. During the past several years, the use of heroin by the upper classes also has increased.

Drug-use trends may be broadly summarized. Large increases in the prevalence of marijuana use occurred in the mid-1960's among adolescents and young adults, particularly males and those living in metropolitan areas. This trend continued in the late 1960's, accompanied by increased involvement by other age groups, those living in rural areas, and females. Increased use of other drug classes occurred during this period as well. Currently (1984), the prevalence of marijuana and depressant use is remaining stable; heroin and cocaine use is increasing, and amphetamine and hallucinogen use has declined.

PSYCHOBIOLOGIC FACTORS. Personality and constitutional factors, in part, determine the individual's psychoactive responses and influence the choice of drugs and patterns of abuse. Amphetamines may produce tranquility in some people. Alcohol and barbiturates impair behavior control in others and may permit certain personality types to act in a hostile and violent manner. Genetic factors have been strongly implicated in the development of alcoholism.

No predictive test or system will determine whether or not a person will become a compulsive user, or which people will use which drugs. It is generally agreed that the experimental or intermittent abuse of drugs is not necessarily an indication of psychopathology. Compulsive drug use is frequently associated with psychopathology. In some people the drug use may be an attempt at *self-medication* of painful feelings of anxiety, shame, inadequacy, loneliness, guilt, and depression. Others may be seeking to allay unacceptable aggressive or sexual drives or to control psychotic symptoms. At the same time, some severely disturbed people have experimented with alcohol, opiates, and other drugs and have not become compulsive users.

Conditioned learning is an integral part of the development and maintenance of compulsive drug-abuse patterns. This may occur in the presence or absence of physical dependence. The drug-craving and withdrawal syndrome that long abstinent ex-addicts experience when they return to a site of former drug use is, in part, a reflection of this conditioning process. Learning also influences the nature of the subjective drug experience. The prolonged use of psychoactive drugs to treat medical illness sometimes induces addiction.

PHARMACOLOGIC FACTORS. *Tolerance* refers to the decreased effect obtained from repeated administration of a given dose of a drug or to the need for increased amounts to obtain the effects that occurred from the first dose. Tolerance may be either *drug disposition* (metabolic) in type, in which there is more rapid inactivation or excretion of a drug, or *pharmacodynamic* (cellular), in which cells in the nervous system adapt to drug concentrations. Both may occur with the same drug. The physical dependence that develops concurrently with tolerance to opiates, barbiturates, and alcohol is poorly understood and may be related to pharmacodynamic tolerance mechanisms. *Cross-dependence* refers to the ability of one drug to suppress abstinence symptoms produced by withdrawal of another. Cross-dependence may be complete or partial, as with alcohol and the barbiturates.

DIAGNOSIS. To provide adequate treatment, one must characterize the specific problems of drug abuse and dependence, the psychologic set, and the social situation. The nature and degree of drug-induced psychoactive effects and any abstinence symptoms and signs should be assessed. Drug abusers are often poor historians and may minimize or exaggerate the extent of their drug use, depending on their perception of the situation, their needs, and the attitude of the examiner. It is likely that an opiate user will exaggerate the extent of his use so as to obtain more opiates during the detoxification process and perhaps suffer decreased abstinence symptoms. A college student may minimize his diazepam dependence, since the extent of his use might be considered evidence of weakness or serious psychopathology.

Evaluation of the mode of administration and the adverse effects of the drugs is important in diagnosis. Signs of repeated intravenous injections ("tracks") suggest heroin, amphetamine, or cocaine abuse. These drugs are also "sniffed," whereby the material is inhaled and absorbed through the mucous membranes of the nasopharynx and respiratory tract, a route suggested by chronic sinusitis or perforation of the nasal septum.

Routine qualitative procedures for the detection in urine of morphine (the major metabolite of heroin), methadone, amphetamines, cocaine, marijuana, and the most frequently abused general depressants are currently available in many laboratories. Agents usually are detected if a dose sufficient to produce pharmacologic effects has been taken within 24 hours prior to the urine sample. Since results are not immediately available ordinarily and since false positives occur, these tests should be used to confirm the clinical impression. They are most useful as an adjunct to the continuing evaluation of patients already in treatment. In emergency situations, blood levels of suspected drugs can usually be obtained immediately.

TREATMENT AND PREVENTION. Treatment of specific addictions is given in subsequent sections. Drug abusers are often faced with prejudice and hostility on the part of treatment personnel; e.g., "They did it to themselves." Since many of their personality characteristics and behavior patterns occur in response to the attitudes of society, an inquiring, compassionate stance is crucial in the treatment of this group of patients.

Drug abusers often relapse after detoxification and varying periods of abstinence. This tends to frustrate the physician or the treatment team, who may give up on particular patients. The problem may be conceptual; physicians often regard substance abuse as an acute illness, not unlike pneumonia, and liable to complete cure after detoxification. This is an unrealistic assumption given the chronic nature of most psychologic and social difficulties. Then, too, the pharmacologic dependence may be more protracted than previously imagined. Patience and continuing enthusiasm are as essential as in most other branches of medicine.

Drug-abuse prevention programs have focused on educational efforts, in which the risks of drug abuse are publicized, and on legal sanctions. Both approaches have serious deficiencies. Perhaps more important than either of these would be the provision of reasonably attractive vocational, recreational, and educational alternatives to drug abuse in those most at risk, namely, the young and psychosocially disadvantaged. Physicians must be extremely prudent in prescribing potentially abusable drugs.

Jaffe J: Drug addiction and drug abuse. *In* Gilman AG, Goodman LS, Gilman A (eds.): The Pharmacological Basis of Therapeutics. 6th ed. New York, Macmillan, 1980, pp 535–584. *Overview of pharmacologic and clinical aspects of drug use and abuse.*

Lowinson JH, Ruiz P. (eds.): Substance Abuse: Clinical Problems and Perspectives. Baltimore, Williams and Wilkins, 1981. *Exhaustive compendium of substance abuse–related subjects considered from multiple perspectives.*

Pradhan SN, Dutta SN (eds.): Drug Abuse, Clinical and Basic Aspects. St. Louis, C. V. Mosby Company, 1977. *Comprehensive textbook on the pharmacology and clinical aspects of the drugs of abuse.*

OPIATES

Opiates or narcotic analgesics refer to natural or synthetic drugs that have pharmacologic actions similar to those of the derivatives of opium. Opium is obtained from the poppy plant *Papaver somniferum* and contains more than 20 alkaloids, of which morphine and codeine are relevant to this discussion. Heroin, the principal opiate of abuse in the United States, is converted from morphine by the addition of two acetyl groups (diacetyl-morphine). Meperidine and methadone are synthetic narcotic analgesics. Pentazocine is a synthetic analgesic compound that has actions similar to both the opiates and the narcotic antagonists.

INCIDENCE. People have used opium for medical, religious, or recreational purposes since ancient times. The use of patent medicines containing opiates was widespread in the United States during the period from 1850 to 1906, when the labeling requirements of the Pure Food and Drug Act caused many preparations to be withdrawn. The Harrison Narcotics Act of 1914 and Supreme Court decisions in the 1920's made possession of narcotics without a prescription a crime and created a climate in which addicts were considered to be criminals and in which physicians could not prescribe narcotics to addicts. The number of oral opiate users declined, and the primary remaining group were those who injected heroin or morphine. Illegal dealers became the only source of opiates. Prices rose precipitously, and addicts frequently resorted to criminal activity to finance their addiction. The growth of urban ghettos and the development of efficient production and delivery systems ushered in the present era of extensive heroin use associated with a pervasive street culture that supports the heroin-dependent life.

Heroin use reached epidemic proportions in the United States in the mid- to late 1960's. The majority of users were members of urban ethnic minority groups. Males predominated over females, and the population was quite young. After a decline in heroin use during the mid-1970's, there has been a resurgence of the problem. People of diverse socioeconomic and cultural groups are involved, including the urban affluent. A similar phenomenon is occurring in western Europe and appears to be related to increased supplies of more pure forms of heroin from southwest Asia and Iran. Estimates vary widely, although between 5 and 10 per cent of the youthful and young adult population in the United States are reported to have used the drug. Heroin addiction is a leading cause of death in urban males aged 15 to 35.

PATTERNS OF ABUSE. Street heroin ("smack," "scag," "junk," "dope") is adulterated ("cut") with quinine, lactose, mannitol, maltose, and other substances as it passes from the importer to the user. The purity of the final package varies enormously, from 4 to 70 per cent. Initial street use is generally by "sniffing." A user's first experience with the drug is often somewhat unpleasant because of nausea, vomiting, and anxiety; these symptoms abate with subsequent use. Effects may then be perceived as a sense of relaxation and peace with relief of worry and tension, a euphoric state in which all things are as they should be. At the outset, use may be intermittent and separated by weeks or months. It is not known how many people experiment with the drug and stop using it. Those who do continue to use heroin develop tolerance to its euphoric effects and begin to inject the drug subcutaneously and eventually intravenously ("mainlining"). Intravenous injection produces a warm flushing of the skin and pleasurable bodily sensations described as similar to sexual orgasm and called a "rush" or "kick." Chronic intravenous use of opiates and other drugs may occlude available veins, necessitating a return to subcutaneous injection.

As tolerance increases and physical dependence becomes manifest, more drug must be used more often; the street addict now devotes all his time and energy to supporting his addiction ("habit"). Involvement in the "junkie" subculture, with its own language and behavioral systems, ensures his supply of drug and provides the social structure that makes it possible to live as an addict. Any source of money is acceptable; males engage in theft and forgery, whereas females become prostitutes and shoplifters. Every user is a potential "dealer" of drugs, since this is the most efficient way of making money. Food, clothing, sexual desires, and dignity subordinate themselves to the ever-present need for opiates. In addition, an unknown number of heroin addicts are able to maintain employment and their families and avoid the behavior patterns of the street "junkie."

If heroin is not available or is in poor supply, addicts will use other opiates, particularly illicitly obtained ("street") methadone because of its long duration of action, to allay their withdrawal symptoms. Compulsive use of illicit methadone occurs, although usually after an initial period of heroin dependence. Most narcotic addicts also abuse alcohol, sedatives, stimulants, and marijuana, and mixed addictions are frequent.

Opiate addicts demonstrate appreciable psychopathology, including high levels of neurotic, personality, and psychotic characteristics, although no common pattern is apparent. Personality characteristics and behavior patterns result in part from the interaction of the addict and the drug in the sociocultural environment of addiction. Inner-city minority-group addicts are often remarkably stable given their difficult living situations and the high degree of personality integration and intelligence required to survive as a street addict. Middle-class people may be more severely disturbed, and the drug use may represent an attempt at self-medication for symptoms that reflect borderline or psychotic personality disorders.

PHARMACOLOGY. Morphine and heroin lose much of their analgesic potency when taken orally, whereas codeine and meperidine remain active, and methadone retains most of its analgesic efficacy after oral administration. Heroin is hydrolyzed to morphine in the body and, except for its greater potency and more rapid onset of action, has pharmacologic properties similar to those of morphine. Morphine is concentrated in parenchymatous tissues, skeletal muscle, and, to a lesser extent, brain. It is conjugated with glucuronic acid and excreted primarily in the urine and secondarily in the feces. Traces of morphine can be found in urine for 48 hours, although 90 per cent or more is excreted within the first 24 hours.

Administered subcutaneously, methadone and morphine exert approximately equal analgesic effects; heroin is three times stronger, whereas meperidine and codeine are approximately one tenth as potent. Morphine or heroin taken intravenously is effective almost immediately; duration of action varies from three to six hours. Oral administration prolongs the action of all the opiates, particularly that of methadone, in which the onset of effect occurs within 30 minutes and the duration of action in nontolerant individuals is four to ten hours.

Morphine or heroin administred to a nontolerant individual induces analgesia through a reduction in the anxiety and tension that result from the perception of pain. Related to this is a feeling of well-being or euphoria. Mental clouding, characterized by an inability to concentrate, sleepiness, or "nodding," also occurs. Opiates cause pupillary constriction, depression of respiration and body temperature, and stimulation of central nervous system centers to produce nausea and vomiting. Other acute effects include decreased motility of the stomach, diminished pancreatic and biliary secretions, decreased propulsive contractions of the small and large intestine, and increased tone of the anal sphincter, leading to constipation. Increased tone of the detrusor muscle leads to a sensation of urgency; increased tone of the vesical sphincter may result in urinary retention. Antidiuretic hormone release is stimulated while ACTH, corticotropin-releasing factor, and gonadotropin are inhibited. Peripheral vasodilatation produces pruritus and an increase in perspiration.

ADDICTION AND WITHDRAWAL PROCESSES. Repeated use of narcotic analgesics produces tolerance to most of the acute narcotic effects, and the lethal dose is markedly increased. Whereas a 10-mg dose of morphine may produce euphoria in a nontolerant individual, some addicts can consume as much as 5 grams daily. Tolerance to all the opiate effects does not occur equally; highly tolerant users will continue to demonstrate pupillary constriction and constipation. Cross-tolerance occurs with all narcotic analgesics. Tolerance to narcotics is primarily due to some form of cellular adaptation to the drug's action, with increased metabolism of lesser importance.

Physical dependence develops concurrently with tolerance and can emerge after only a few exposures on succeeding days. The syndrome varies according to the particular drug and its usage. With heroin, the first withdrawal signs are generally seen shortly before the next scheduled dose. They are purposive in nature and include feelings of anxiety, depression, restlessness, irritability, and drug craving. Lacrimation, rhinorrhea, yawning, and perspiration become apparent eight to fifteen hours after the last dose of narcotic. A restless sleep may intervene ("yen sleep") interrupted by more severe withdrawal symptoms and signs, including dilated pupils, sneezing, coryza, anorexia, nausea, vomiting, diarrhea, abdominal cramps, bone pains, myalgias, tremors, weakness, insomnia, goose flesh, and, very rarely, convulsions or cardiovascular collapse. With morphine and heroin, withdrawal symptoms peak at 36 to 48 hours, and most symptoms subside over the next five to ten days. With methadone, the onset of withdrawal symptoms is more gradual, the peak is less pronounced and later, and the duration may be more than two or three weeks. The abstinence syndrome may be precipitated within minutes in opiate-dependent persons by administration of a narcotic antagonist such as nalorphine, levallorphan, or naloxone, although there are no medical indications for this diagnostic procedure.

Pentazocine (Talwin), a drug with weak opiate-antagonist effects and moderate opiate-agonist effects, elicits morphine-like subjective effects in nontolerant individuals. Higher doses produce dysphoric effects, including nervousness, anxiety, and, infrequently, bizarre alterations in perception and behavior. To speed the onset of action of pentazocine and to lengthen the duration of psychoactive effects, pentazocine is frequently abused in combination with the antihistamine tripelennamine ("t's and blues"). Tolerance, physical dependence, and addiction can occur. Abrupt withdrawal of the drug from persons taking 500 to 700 mg daily results in irritability, abdominal cramps, nausea, vomiting, hyperthermia, lacrimation, and drug-seeking behavior. When pentazocine is administered to opiate-dependent patients, its antagonistic actions may precipitate withdrawal symptoms.

Subsequent to the termination of abstinence symptoms or after a course of detoxification, most addicts experience recurrent urges for narcotics and generally resume their use of these drugs. Psychologic factors play a role, however. Evidence is accumulating that metabolic and neurophysiologic changes persist long after the detoxification process is completed, as does some tolerance. Protracted abstinence signs, as indicated by alterations in blood pressure, pulse rate, body temperature, respiratory rate, and pupillary size, and symptoms, particularly depression and anxiety, have been documented for up to 30 weeks and may relate to the high incidence of relapse. The associations ex-addicts experience when they are exposed to their old neighborhoods and friends intensify the persistence of drug craving.

MECHANISM OF OPIATE ACTION. Structurally and sterically specific receptors for the opiates are located in areas of the nervous system associated with the integration of sensory information and emotion, particularly the limbic system. The presence of these receptors led to the discovery of naturally occurring morphine-like peptides in the brain and gastrointestinal tract (enkephalins) and pituitary gland (endorphins). The endogenous morphine-like compounds elicit analgesia, produce tolerance and physical dependence, and compete with radioactive opiates for the receptor. All the peptides so far identified except one have amino acid sequences present in the pituitary hormone, β-lipotropin. The enkephalins have been implicated in the control of pain, affective states, and appetitive drives. A model that includes a neurohumoral feedback mechanism has been postulated to play a part in the opiate addiction syndrome. If, under resting conditions, opiate receptors are exposed to a basal level of the morphine-like substances, when exogenous opiate is administered, the overloading of the receptors might suppress the synthesis or release of endogenous opioid. Termination of the exogenous opiate administration might deprive the receptor because of endogenous opioid deficiency, generating changes responsible for the immediate or protracted abstinence syndrome. The anxiety and panic of the opiate abstinence syndrome have been proposed to result from noradrenergic hyperactivity and have led to treatment of the state with adrenergic agonists (see below).

MEDICAL COMPLICATIONS. The patterns of use, unknown and markedly variable opiate dose, lack of hygienic administration techniques, and the variety of adulterants used to dilute the opiate produce an extensive morbidity and mortality (estimated to be about 1 to 3 per cent per year) associated with opiate abuse and dependence.

Acute heroin reactions secondary to the intravenous use of street drug are responsible for one half to four fifths of all fatalities from narcotics. Formerly thought of as true pharmacologic overdoses with respiratory depression, these reactions may also be due to opiate-induced cardiac arrhythmias or hypoxia by unexplained mechanisms. Acute reactions to adulterants, including quinine, allergic reactions, and synergistic effects from multiple-drug use, may also be implicated. The syndrome is marked clinically by the rapid development of cyanosis, pulmonary edema, respiratory distress, and varying levels of consciousness progressing to coma. Increased intracranial pressure and occasionally convulsive seizures are seen. Fever to 40° C may occur initially and may persist for 48 hours in association with leukocytosis. The pupils are usually pinpoint, although dilated, nonreactive pupils may occur with hypoxia or multiple-drug use. The pathologic picture includes pulmonary congestion and edema and frequently cerebral edema.

Skin abscesses, cellulitis, and *thrombophlebitis* are the most frequent complications of heroin addiction. Pentazocine injection causes characteristic chronic ulcers in areas of severe "woody" induration. *Septicemia* and *acute* and *subacute bacterial endocarditis* with involvement of either or both sides of the heart are seen. *Staphylococcus aureus* is frequently the causative organism in right-sided lesions. Peripheral and pulmonary embolic phenomena occur. Osteomyelitis occurs infrequently. The introduction of quinine as an adulterant and the eradication of malaria in this country have decreased the incidence of this complication.

Viral hepatitis transmitted by the communal use of contaminated needles is a frequent complication of intravenous drug use. Persistent abnormal liver function tests, hypergammaglobulinemia, and increased serum immunoglobulins are due in some cases to variants of chronic hepatitis, but may also be due to effects produced by alcohol, malnutrition, allergic phenomena, adulterants, and recurrent or chronic infections. False-positive serologic tests for syphilis and AIDS appear with appreciable incidence.

Pulmonary complications include pneumonia, abscess, infarction, and tuberculosis. Disseminated extrapulmonary tuberculosis has been reported. Angiothrombotic pulmonary hypertension and granulomatosis result from the intravenous injection of foreign bodies, including talc or cotton. Vascular lesions include local arterial occlusion, phlebitis, mycotic aneurysms, and necrotizing angiitis.

Neurologic complications of street heroin use include transverse myelitis, acute inflammatory polyneuropathy, peripheral nerve lesions, toxic amblyopia secondary to quinine, and muscle disorders, including acute rhabdomyolysis with myoglobinuria and a fibrosing chronic myopathy. Septic states may lead to bacterial meningitis and brain, subdural, and epidural abscesses. Narcotism is a leading cause of tetanus, particularly when the drugs are injected by the intramuscular route. Mortality rates lie in the 50 to 75 per cent range.

Pregnant addicts have a high incidence of toxemia and premature babies. Withdrawal symptoms are noted in a variable percentage of the newborns. Sexual difficulties, including decreased libido, impotence, and delayed ejaculation, are frequent in male heroin addicts.

Homicide, suicide, and *accidents* account for between 20 and 40 per cent of narcotic-related deaths. In any given case, it is often difficult to distinguish among the three.

TREATMENT. Methods of treatment of narcotic dependence vary, depending on the treatment goals, factors in the etiology of the addiction, and the characteristics of individual patients. The magnitude of the addict's desire to stop using opiates is an important factor in the selection of the appropriate treatment modality as well as in the outcome. These motivational factors are difficult to assess, since, within one or two years after the onset of the addiction, most addicts express the wish to terminate it. Nevertheless, many continue the compulsive use of heroin for many years and suffer repeated treatment failures. Approaches are primarily psychosocial, pharmacologic, or combinations of these. Since addiction has physical, psychologic, and social determinants, treatment is best provided by a well-organized team approach. Individual practitioners should be prepared to make an accurate diagnosis, treat the acute and chronic sequelae of the drug use, and effect the appropriate referral.

ACUTE OPIATE REACTIONS (OVERDOSE). If an acute opiate reaction is suspected, immediate nonspecific supportive, resuscitative measures should be instituted, and 0.4 mg of the narcotic antagonist naloxone should be given intravenously or intramuscularly. A positive response, consisting of pupillary dilatation, increased respiratory rate and minute volume, and increased alertness, should occur within one to two minutes after intravenous injection. If a positive response does not occur, a second 0.4-mg dose may be administered in five to ten minutes. If a positive response again fails to ensue, the existence of an acute opiate reaction is doubtful. If a response occurs, the patient's respiratory rate and volume and level of consciousness should be monitored for the next 24 hours, since the antagonistic actions of naloxone persist for only two to three hours, whereas the agonistic effects of large doses of heroin or morphine may last longer and the effects of methadone may persist for 24 to 36 hours. Naloxone administration may be repeated after two to three hours as necessary. If it is anticipated that the patient is physically dependent on narcotics, the initial intravenous injection of 0.4 mg of naloxone should be diluted to 0.1 mg per milliliter and given slowly and in the smallest amounts necessary, to minimize the precipitation of a violent abstinence syndrome. Evidence of infection or trauma should be sought and treated as necessary.

WITHDRAWAL TECHNIQUES. Withdrawal of narcotics is most effectively accomplished by inpatient or outpatient substitution of oral methadone for any of the natural or synthetic narcotic analgesics (detoxification). Doses ranging from 20 to 40 mg daily are instituted, followed by a gradual reduction of dosage over the course of 14 days or more. Detoxification with decreasing doses of propoxyphene napsylate, a mild analgesic, has been effective, particularly when the degree of dependence is minimal or methadone is not available. Clonidine,* an alpha-2-adrenergic agonist, has shown promise in suppressing the abstinence syndrome. After tapering and cessation of narcotic use, clonidine is given in divided doses of 0.1 to 0.2 mg. The dose is then increased over the course of the next four to ten days to a maximum of 1 to 1.5 mg daily in three divided doses. The clonidine is then tapered over a four- to five-day period. Clonidine can cause postural hypotension and sedation, necessitating close observation, frequent blood pressure checks, and dosage adjustment. Acupuncture has also been reported to be effective in reducing opiate withdrawal symptoms. As mentioned previously, however, whatever the treatment, the relapse rate remains high.

METHADONE MAINTENANCE. In the United States, methadone maintenance has been the most widely used approach in the treatment of opiate dependence. This mode of therapy emphasizes social and emotional rehabilitation rather than abstinence. The treatment is based on the two major properties that distinguish methadone from other narcotics: good oral efficacy and long duration of action. After oral ingestion in tolerant individuals, the duration of action of methadone is extended to 24 to 36 hours owing to a reservoir of drug in tissues. Initially, oral methadone is administered daily in doses that will allay symptoms of abstinence. The dose is gradually increased until a stabilization level is reached at which patients will be tolerant to the euphoric effects of the drug and will experience no persistent craving for opiates. If the stabilization level is high enough (60 to 100 mg), there is a good degree of cross-tolerance to the effects of other narcotics, such that the effects of even large doses of intravenous opiates will not be felt. Approximately 65 per cent of patients in well-run programs remain in treatment. Improvement has been noted in the work and school records of patients retained in the program, and their criminal activity has declined markedly. Long-term methadone maintenance has been shown to be medically safe, with no toxicity when properly administered. Performance and learning are normal in methadone-maintained subjects. Medication should be dispensed in a clinic situation that provides medical care and extensive rehabilitative services so as to facilitate satisfactory re-entry into non-drug-dominated ("straight") society. Late methadone detoxification is sometimes possible.

Many former addicts, although they may be heroin free, are unable to acquire the necessary skills and education to make a social adjustment. They continue to abuse alcohol and other drugs. Illicit diversion of methadone doses by clinic patients has led to the availability of the drug for the street-addict population.

NARCOTIC ANTAGONISTS. Naltrexone, a long-acting narcotic antagonist, should shortly become available for the treatment of detoxified addicts. This agent blocks the euphoriant effects of opiates and prevents the development of physical dependence in patients who continue to use opiates. Unfortunately, while naltrexone has proven to be effective in some patients when administered on a three-times-a-week basis, it does not relieve chronic opiate hunger, and patients tend to cease its use and relapse to heroin. Clinical trials are under way with buprenorphine, a drug that combines potent and long-term opiate agonist and antagonist properties. This promising new agent appears to suppress the opiate abstinence syndrome and blocks the effects of high doses of opiates. In contrast to methadone maintenance, abrupt termination of high-dose buprenorphine maintenance results in a mild, almost negligible withdrawal syndrome.

*This use is not listed in the manufacturer's directive.

PSYCHOSOCIAL APPROACHES—ABSTINENCE PROGRAMS. A number of programs exist that emphasize abstinence from opiates and other drugs as a primary component of treatment. These take the form of either voluntary groups or supervised institutionalization.

Voluntary groups are generally self-regulatory in nature and staffed predominantly by former drug users. The individual remains in a closed, drug-free environment for variable periods of time, frequently one to two years, and is encouraged to develop a new set of social and living skills that will enable him to remain drug free upon completion of the program. Outpatient programs are also under way. Some of the well-known therapeutic communities are Daytop Village, Phoenix House, and Project Return. Therapeutic communities are valuable for many people, although only a small percentage of heroin addicts are motivated to enter a community, and follow-up studies of individuals who have returned to society are disappointingly few.

Results of traditional psychotherapy has been disappointing for most compulsive opiate abusers. Specialized forms of group psychotherapy may help some patients. After variable and sometimes prolonged periods of addiction, an unknown number of addicts spontaneously cease opiate use. This "maturing-out" process may be related to advanced age and the difficulty of obtaining drugs, a decline of internal psychologic conflicts, and the cumulative effect of various treatment programs.

Dole VP, Nyswander M: A medical treatment for diacetyl morphine (heroin) addiction. JAMA 193:646, 1965. *First description of methadone maintenance treatment.*

Gold MS, Rea WS: The role of endorphins in opiate addiction, opiate withdrawal and recovery. Psychiatr Clin North Am 6(3):489, 1983. *Data and theoretical framework relative to the role of endogenous opioids in addiction, and treatment implications. Extensive references.*

Sternbach G, Moran J, Eliastam M: Heroin addiction: Acute presentation of medical complications. Ann Emerg Med 9(3):161, 1980. *Review of the acute presentation of medical sequelae of heroin abuse and treatments. Extensive references.*

Stimmel B: Heroin Dependency: Medical, Economic and Social Aspects. New York, Stratton Intercontinental Medical Book Corporation, 1975. *Comprehensive discussion of heroin dependency and treatment.*

CENTRAL NERVOUS SYSTEM DEPRESSANTS

All central nervous system depressants are subject to abuse. The most frequently abused drugs in this category are the benzodiazepines, particularly diazepam (Valium) and chlordiazepoxide (Librium); the short-acting barbiturates, particularly pentobarbital (Nembutal) and secobarbital (Seconal); assorted other hypnotics such as glutethimide (Doriden), methyprylon (Noludar), and methaqualone (Quāālude); and amitriptyline (Elavil), an antidepressant with sedative properties. Bromide abuse has become rare.

INCIDENCE AND PATTERNS OF ABUSE. A continuum of depressant use extends from appropriate use to compulsive abuse and addiction. Depressants in general and the benzodiazepines in particular have become the most widely prescribed drugs throughout the world. Currently in western society, about one in five adult females and one in ten adult males take benzodiazepines or other depressants in the course of one year. Approximately 30 per cent of general practitioners and internists prescribe these drugs. The pattern of abuse may begin intermittently at night to decrease anxiety and ensure sleep, progress to nightly use with increased doses, and culminate in prolonged daily use to maintain an adequate level of function. Whereas the risk of serious dependence on the benzodiazepines is lower than with the hypnotics, the prevalence of tranquilizer use has led to substantial drug dependence, particularly in women. An individual may obtain drugs from several physicians at one time, none of whom is aware of the magnitude of the patient's use. Alcohol is frequently used in association with the depressants.

Hypnotic and tranquilizer use also involves the drug subcultures.

Illicit sources of drugs are most often employed, and a wealth of street names have evolved, including "ludes" (methaqualone), "reds" (secobarbital), "yellows" (pentobarbital), and "double trouble" (amobarbital and secobarbital). Most use is oral, although some individuals inject the drugs intravenously or intramuscularly. The amounts taken vary, but some individuals ingest as much as 30 hypnotic doses of the short-acting barbiturates or benzodiazepines daily over many months.

Surveys suggest that 20 per cent of adolescents and young adults abuse depressants. Patterns and extent of use vary markedly, but generally depressants are taken in association with other drugs. Intermittent users may take several times the therapeutic dose, possibly in addition to marijuana, alcohol, and cocaine, to get "high" enough to enjoy a concert or party.

The "high" that the user obtains from abuse of depressant drugs has been characterized as the sense of tranquility or peace that occurs just prior to sleep in normal individuals. Inhibitions and anxiety are blunted, and there may be a feeling of aggressiveness, freedom, and pleasant numbness. Sexual pleasure and ability are said to be enhanced at low doses of these drugs; higher doses lead to a decreased ability to perform sexually. Violent and antisocial behavior frequently serves to isolate depressant abusers ("down heads") from other groups of drug abusers.

PHARMACOLOGY. Depressants are absorbed rapidly after oral administration and are distributed throughout the body. They are general depressants of nerves and of skeletal, smooth, and cardiac muscles, although at low doses the central nervous system is primarily affected. Central nervous system effects vary from mild sedation to coma, depending on the particular drug, the dose, the route of administration, the degree of excitability of the nervous system, and tolerance. In some individuals under certain circumstances, small doses produce an initial stimulation not unlike that produced by alcohol. Barbiturate-induced sleep is similar to physiologic sleep except for a reduction in the proportion of rapid eye movement (REM) sleeping time; benzodiazepines suppress REM sleep less. Duration of action varies with the particular depressants. After-effects, including drowsiness, depression, impairment of judgment and performance, and occasionally hyperexcitability, may persist for many hours.

Both drug-disposition and pharmacodynamic tolerance to the depressants develop rapidly with repeated administration. Drug-disposition tolerance in the short-acting barbiturates and some other depressants results from the activation of drug-metabolizing liver-enzyme systems and is characterized by the more rapid degradation of the drug and a decrease in sleeping time. The range of tolerance is narrow, and individuals tolerant to the sedating and intoxicating effects of 1 gram of pentobarbital may become intoxicated for prolonged periods upon the addition of 0.1 gram. Although the lethal dose of barbiturates varies in individuals, in distinction to the opiates, tolerance does not increase this dose significantly from that of nontolerant individuals. Severe poisoning is likely to occur when more than ten times the hypnotic dose is ingested at one time. Acute barbiturate poisoning may thus be superimposed on chronic intoxication at any time. The combination of sublethal doses of depressants with opiates or alcohol may also result in acute poisoning. Cross-tolerance develops to all barbiturates as well as to paraldehyde, meprobamate, and benzodiazepines. Partial cross-tolerance between alcohol and the depressants occurs.

CLINICAL MANIFESTATIONS. Acute depressant poisoning may occur either accidentally or incident to a suicide attempt. Approximately 25 per cent of all drug-related deaths are due to barbiturates and related hypnotics; few deaths have been ascribed to the benzodiazepines alone. Accidental overdoses may be due rarely to "drug automatism"; an individual may fail to fall asleep after several hypnotic doses, become confused, and ingest an overdose. Upon recovery, there may be no memory of the excessive drug ingestion. The clinical manifestations and treatment of severe poisoning are discussed in Ch. 472.2. The acute and chronic signs and symptoms of mild depressant intoxication resemble those of intoxication with alcohol. The individual shows general sluggishness, difficulty in thinking, slowness of speech and comprehension, poor memory, faulty judgment, emotional lability, and narrowed attention span. Neurologic signs include thick, slurred speech, nystagmus, diplopia, strabismus, vertigo, ataxic gait, hypotonia, dysmetria, and decreased superficial reflexes. Sensation, deep-tendon reflexes, and pupillary responses are unaltered. Skin rashes have been reported. Unexplained seizures in adults should always prompt one to consider chronic depressant drug abuse. Adverse effects of chronic depressant use include decreased psychomotor efficiency, anterograde amnesia, changes in interpersonal style, rebound insomnia, and drowsiness. Neurologic damage and permanent memory deficits have been reported but are poorly documented.

ABSTINENCE SYNDROME. A characteristic *general depressant withdrawal syndrome* occurs and is similar to the symptoms of withdrawal from alcohol. It varies in severity, depending on the drug, dose, and frequency of use. *In contrast to the opiate withdrawal syndrome, that from depressants may be life-threatening.* The first manifestation of this syndrome might be considered the rebound increase in nightly rapid eye movement sleep, associated with nightmares and a sense of having slept badly, that occurs after discontinuation of use of only therapeutic doses of barbiturates or benzodiazepines for several nights. In general, the time required to produce physical dependence is shorter with the short-acting depressants, and the withdrawal symptoms are more abrupt in onset and more severe than with the longer-acting sedatives.

When short-acting hypnotics are abruptly withdrawn, signs and symptoms of the intoxication clear over the initial 12 to 16 hours, and the patient appears to improve. Restlessness, anxiety, tremulousness, and weakness then occur, which may be accompanied by cramps, nausea, vomiting, and orthostatic hypotension. These symptoms progress, and coarse hand tremors, muscle twitching, hyperactive deep reflexes, and increased blink reflex appear within 24 hours. Symptoms generally attain their peak during the second and third days, and convulsions may occur then or before. Most patients who have seizures subsequently improve, but some develop typical delirium tremens, which potentially can lead to fatal cardiovascular collapse. The abstinence syndrome generally clears by about the eighth day, usually leaving no serious residua. Clearing is frequently preceded by a period of prolonged sleep. With longer-acting barbiturates and benzodiazepines, seizures may not occur until the seventh or eighth day. Irritability, anxiety, sleep disturbances, and severe psychiatric symptoms may persist for many months, but may be related to pre-existing psychopathology.

As with the opiates but not the barbiturates, specific receptors for the benzodiazepines have been found in all vertebrates studied. The binding sites are found in highest concentrations in the cortex, the cerebellum, and the amygdala and appear to relate to inhibition of central nervous system function.

TREATMENT. Treatment is composed of acute withdrawal procedures and long-term rehabilitation. Outreach and educational programs aimed at intermittent abusers of depressants before they become addicted may be important.

If physical dependence is determined or strongly suspected, hospitalization and close observation are indicated. A long-acting general depressant with which the physician is familiar should be administered after the intoxication clears but before major withdrawal symptoms have begun. Diazepam is widely used, since the agent produces measurable blood levels and protection against the development of either withdrawal symptoms or dangerous intoxication. Patients who are taking large amounts of lesser known sedatives should be withdrawn from the original drug of abuse. If the patient will not tolerate the oral administration of diazepam or more rapid sedation is required, intramuscular injections of the same doses may be used. Patients may usually be switched to oral drugs after a few intramuscular injections. With oral medications, an initial dose of 20 to 40 mg of diazepam should be administered and the patient carefully observed for signs of intoxication or withdrawal. Succeeding doses should be adjusted to provide a mild but manageable level of intoxication marked by inconstant, slow nystagmus on lateral gaze, slight dysarthria, and ataxia. A rough approximation of the dosage of depressant to be given daily is calculated by substituting 15 mg of diazepam for each 100 mg of the short-acting barbiturate the patient reports using. Most patients will require between 60 and 100 mg daily for stabilization, to be given in four divided doses; higher doses may be required in the case of severe tremulousness or hallucinations. This "stabilization dose" should be carefully controlled to prevent signs of increased intoxication. Patients should be maintained on this dose for 24 to 48 hours, after which the dose of diazepam can be reduced by 15 to 20 mg or less daily. The patient should be observed carefully for signs of insomnia, tremulousness, increased deep tendon reflexes, and orthostatic hypotension, at which point withdrawal should be suspended for one to two days. If severe symptoms emerge, diazepam should be administered parenterally. Delirium, convulsions, or fever should be treated as an emergency, with increased doses until the patient is able to sleep for eight to twelve hours, after which the stabilization dose is determined, as described above. Once a withdrawal delirium develops, increased doses of diazepam may only partially restore equilibrium; agitation and disorientation may persist for several days.

Satisfactory care requires that fluid and electrolyte losses be replaced and complicating medical and surgical conditions treated. Increasing fever without evidence of infection necessitates additional sedation, antipyretics, sponging, or cooling blankets. Phenothiazines, butyrophenones, and phenytoin are not indicated. In general, the substitution program may take from ten days to three weeks. It should not be hurried. During the process, patients should be as active as possible, eat regularly, and take part in group activities. Patients who are concurrently dependent on opiates should be withdrawn from the general depressant first, while being maintained on suitable doses of methadone. Opiate withdrawal procedures may then be effected.

Anxiety, irritability, depression, and insomnia often persist for weeks or months after withdrawal is completed and are associated with the danger of relapse or suicide. Provision must be made for inclusion of patients in well-structured, supportive, long-term therapeutic programs on either an inpatient or an outpatient basis.

Physicians must be cautious when prescribing depressants for the relief of anxiety and insomnia. Attempts should be made to diagnose and treat the source of these symptoms without medication. If necessary, benzodiazepine tranquilizers may be used in low doses for well-defined, short periods or on an intermittent basis.

BROMIDES. Chronic bromide intoxication (bromism) has become rare. However, the agent is still found in some proprietary headache remedies, and the daily ingestion of small doses can result in an accumulation of this long-acting drug to toxic levels over a period of weeks. Central nervous system symptoms and signs are variable and include drowsiness, impaired thought and memory, dizziness, and irritability, leading in severe cases to confusion, hallucinations, lethargy, and coma. Neurologic disturbances include tremors, thick speech, motor incoordination, and decreased superficial reflexes. Various types of skin eruptions, ranging from acneiform lesions to proliferative nodular lesions similar to those of tertiary syphilis, are found in 25 per cent of patients with mental symptoms. The diagnosis is established by serum bromide levels above 9 mEq per liter (75 mg per deciliter) in association with the aforementioned clinical picture.

Treatment consists of sedation when necessary and the daily administration of 200 mEq of either sodium or ammonium chloride, together with sufficient fluids to ensure a large urine output. This reduces the half-life of bromide to three or four days. Diuresis with chloruretic drugs may be useful if more rapid displacement of bromide is indicated. Hemodialysis rapidly clears bromides and may be indicated in treating comatose patients.

Tyrer P, Owen R, Dawling S: Gradual withdrawal of diazepam after longterm therapy. Lancet 1:1402, 1983. *A double-blind, placebo-controlled study of the incidence and characteristics of the diazepam withdrawal syndrome with relevant background and references.*

Wesson PR, Smith DE: Barbiturates: Their Use, Misuse and Abuse. New York, Human Science Press, 1977. *Comprehensive treatment of patterns of use, adverse consequences, and treatments.*

CENTRAL NERVOUS SYSTEM STIMULANTS

Central nervous system stimulants or sympathomimetics that are subject to abuse include cocaine, the amphetamines, methylphenidate (Ritalin), phenmetrazine (Preludin), and diethylpropion (Tepanil). This discussion will consider primarily cocaine, an alkaloid of the coca plant, which is indiginous to the mountain slopes of Central and South America, and the amphetamine group, including amphetamine, dextroamphetamine, and methamphetamine.

INCIDENCE AND PATTERNS OF ABUSE. Mountain-dwelling Indians in Bolivia and Peru have been chewing coca leaves to alleviate fatigue, suppress appetite, and increase productivity since pre-Incan times. The cocaine alkaloid was isolated in Europe in the mid-nineteenth century and was recommended briefly as a treatment for depression and other emotional disorders and even as a cure for morphine and alcohol addiction, before its usefulness as a local anesthetic was appreciated.

During the past 20 years, in association with the profound increases in other illicit drug use in American society, the prevalence of cocaine use has increased remarkably. Current estimates suggest that 25 to 30 per cent of youthful and young adult populations have used the drug, with about one-fourth of this number being current users. The affluent have been particularly at risk because of the expense of the drug, although users cut across all socioeconomic and demographic lines.

Cocaine is available through illicit channels as a variably adulterated white powder, with a "gram" costing between $100 and $125. The drug may be sniffed, ingested orally, smoked, administered intravenously or applied to mucous membranes. Upon insufflation, the primary mode of use in the United States, effects are perceived within minutes and persist for 20 to 40 minutes. Psychoactive effects include a feeling of increased energy, intensity, confidence, and alertness, coupled with irritability and often some anxiety. Increased activity, planning, and talking occur.

There is a continuum of abuse from the rare or occasional use of the drug to luxuriously punctuate a variety of occasions to a pattern of compulsive use in which it becomes the dominant concern of living. Regular users often use the drug continuously, and the higher the dose the more powerful is the compulsion to repeat the experience. During a "run" of varying duration, 1 to 10 grams of the drug or more may be used daily; at this stage the user is often irritable, nervous, and suspicious and unable to function. There may be intense involvement in complicated and often unnecessary tasks such as reorganizing a room or disassembling a television set. Alcohol, sedative-hypnotics, opiates, and marijuana are often taken concurrently to alleviate anxiety and irritability. When the supply of drugs is depleted or users become too disorganized or debilitated to continue, the "run" ends. Cessation of cocaine use is marked by apathy, fatigue, depressed mood, and often a period of deep sleep ("crashing"). Symptoms are reported to persist for days or weeks and serve as a powerful reinforcement to resumption of the drug use pattern.

Upon intravenous use, effects are perceived as a "rush" of intense euphoria and power, and the compulsion to repeat the experience is intense. Injections may be repeated at 10- to 20-minute intervals for many hours. A recent phenomenon is the marked increase in the smoking of "free base," an alkaline extraction of cocaine that is more volatile than the hydrochloride form and more rapidly absorbed in the lungs. Blood levels and psychoactive effects approach those of intravenous injection.

Most of the psychoactive effects of the *amphetamines* are similar to those of cocaine with regard to elevation of mood, decreased need for food and sleep, and hyperactivity. When amphetamines were prescribed by physicians for a variety of conditions, many people became dependent, finding that they had to continue to ingest the drug in order to prevent depression and maintain optimal levels of performance. The advent of tolerance necessitated increased doses, occasionally five to ten times the original 5- to 10-mg amount prescribed. A significant decline in use has occurred recently as a result of federal and state regulations that severely limit prescribing and manufacturing practices with respect to the amphetamines.

Patterns of use of amphetamines in chronic drug-abusing populations, particularly the young, resemble those of cocaine. Whereas any amphetamine or other sympathomimetic agent may be used, methamphetamine ("speed," "crystal," or "meth") is preferred because it has more pronounced central effects and fewer peripheral ones. The drugs are "sniffed," administered intravenously, and taken orally. Use may be intermittent and limited to special occasions such as a party or journey or may be continuous for several days or even longer. As tolerance develops, the dose is increased and the drug taken more frequently, such that 1 gram may be injected every two to four hours.

PHARMACOLOGY. Systemic effects of cocaine and amphetamines include increased cardiac contraction, increased blood pressure and heart rate, dilated pupils, constriction of peripheral blood vessels, rise in body temperature, relaxation of the bronchial musculature, increased contractility of the urinary bladder sphincter, and increased venous pressure, pulmonary arterial pressure, and renal blood flow. Central effects include stimulation of the cerebrospinal axis and the brainstem respiratory centers. In low doses these drugs increase alertness and physical and cognitive ability, particularly when performance has been compromised by lack of sleep. Appetite depression occurs and probably derives from a combination of factors, including an inhibitory effect on the lateral hypothalamus as well as the improvement in mood that occurs. Cocaine is an effective topical local anesthetic and vasoconstrictor of mucous membranes.

Tolerance develops to both the peripheral and central effects of the amphetamines. Tolerance to the psychoactive effects of cocaine does not occur; there may be some psychologic tolerance to the euphoric effects. Tolerance to the respiratory and cardiac stimulant effects of cocaine does occur. Cross-tolerance exists among the amphetamines, but no cross-tolerance has been demonstrated between the amphetamines and cocaine.

Cessation of cocaine or amphetamine use does not generally produce major physiologic symptoms. The depression, anxiety, increased appetite, lassitude, and prolonged sleep that ensue might be considered an abstinence syndrome and evidence of physical dependence. During the subsequent sleep, the EEG characteristically shows a marked increase in the percentage of REM sleep, and nightmares may occur. Rarely, withdrawal has been marked by headaches, profuse sweating, muscle cramps, disorientation, and confusion. Cocaine and the amphetamines are among the most powerful reinforcers of continued drug-taking behavior.

ADVERSE EFFECTS. The chronic intranasal administration of cocaine or amphetamines commonly causes irritation or ulceration of the nasal mucosa and may lead to perforation of the nasal septum. Corneal ulcers also occur. Chronic users may be debilitated and subject to infections as a result of lack of sleep and poor nutrition. A sensation of something crawling under the skin is described ("cocaine bugs") such that compulsive users will frequently have excoriations and open sores from constant scratching and pinching. The intravenous use of these drugs is associated with the expected complications that result from nonsterile conditions. A necrotizing cerebral angiitis with resulting stroke has been associated with methamphetamine abuse. *Acute cocaine toxicity* is dose related and is characterized by initial sympathomimetic effects including tachycardia, hypertension, hyperthermia, arrhythmias, and convulsions, followed by brainstem depression leading to respiratory failure and cardiovascular collapse. *Acute amphetamine toxicity* is also marked by extensions of the sympathomimetic effects. Stroke, coma, and sudden death remain rare but are increasing in association with the use of high doses of cocaine. Deaths have occurred as a result of the accidental breaking of bags containing large quantities of cocaine ingested in smuggling attempts. The lethal dose of cocaine is estimated to be about 1.2 grams; that of the amphetamines varies depending upon the extent of tolerance.

Compulsive cocaine and amphetamine abusers suffer from a variety of preexisting psychiatric problems and the abuse engenders even more. Depression, anxiety, irritability, insomnia, and decreased libido occur frequently. Paranoid ideation and stereotyped compulsive behavior are common. Chronic users are frequently aware of these characteristics of the drugs and will not act on ideas of persecution. Antisocial or violent behavior may occur when this insight is lacking. Continued use frequently leads to a well-described cocaine or amphetamine psychosis that is often indistinguishable from acute paranoid schizophrenia. The reactions appear to be inevitable if the dose and frequency of use are continually increased or high doses maintained. Psychotic episodes have been precipitated in some individuals after a single small dose. The syndrome is marked by paranoid ideation; stereotyped compulsive behavior; visual, auditory, and tactile hallucinations; and loosening of associations occurring in a setting of clear consciousness and correct orientation. The psychotic episodes invariably appear while the patients are under the influence of the drug and generally abate within a few days to several weeks after cessation of drug use. Subsequently, affected individuals have a lower threshold for precipitation of psychotic episodes even after long intervening periods. Prolonged psychotic episodes may relate to the premorbid personality of the user. A toxic hallucinatory state and dyskinetic and dystonic reactions occur rarely.

TREATMENT. Amphetamine and cocaine abusers demonstrate markedly diverse patterns of drug use. Accordingly, treatment must be flexible. Treatment of the medical complications is considered elsewhere in this textbook. Treatment of anxiety reactions marked by hypertension and tachycardia may be accomplished with benzodiazepines or similar agents. Withdrawal from these drugs requires a safe, supportive atmosphere, much reassurance, and benzodiazepines when necessary for extreme anxiety. Detoxification with decreasing doses of the sympathomimetics is not indicated, although many users will be addicted to alcohol or sedatives. Treatment of psychotic symptoms may require hospitalization. Phenothiazines or other major tranquilizers may be necessary for prolonged psychotic reactions. After recovery, depressive symptoms and the possibility of suicide must be considered.

Physicians should prescribe amphetamines and related drugs with great caution. Some authorities suggest that the childhood hyperkinetic disorders and narcolepsy are the only acceptable indications for their use.

Mule SJ (ed.): Cocaine: Chemical, Biological, Clinical, Social and Treatment Aspects. Cleveland, CRC Press, 1976. *Comprehensive review of the subject, with extensive bibliography.*

Wetli CV, Wright RK: Death caused by recreational cocaine use. JAMA 241:2519, 1979. *An analysis of deaths associated with cocaine use.*

CANNABIS (Marijuana and Hashish)

INCIDENCE AND PATTERNS OF ABUSE. Cannabis has been used extensively in many societies since antiquity as a form of folk medicine and for recreational purposes. The prevalence of cannabis use has increased explosively in the United States and Western Europe during the past 20 years. More than two thirds of people from 18 to 25 are estimated to have used the drug, with 35 per cent being current users. Increased use is being noted in younger and older age groups as well. Whereas geographic, social, and cultural considerations are determinants of whether a person will use cannabis, personality characteristics are important in determining the frequency and pattern of use.

The drug is peripheral to the life of the occasional user, and frequently there is no other drug use. Others demonstrate a compulsive abuse pattern, with lives dominated by the acquisition and use of cannabis and other drugs. Occasional users generally smoke in groups, where the ritual of preparation and sharing of the cigarette is an integral part of social interaction. Chronic smokers frequently smoke alone.

Marijuana is usually smoked in homemade cigarettes ("joints"). Hashish is smoked in a wide variety of small pipes. Both preparations may be ingested in combination with food or drink, although this is less common.

PHARMACOLOGY. Cannabis preparations are three to four times more potent when smoked than when taken orally. After inhalation, effects begin within minutes, peak within one hour, and are dissipated within three hours. After ingestion, effects begin in 30 minutes to two hours, peak at three hours, and persist for four to six hours. The effects of cannabis correlate with the appearance in plasma of active polar metabolites of delta-9-THC. Kinetic interactions have been described between several of the cannabinoids in marijuana, suggesting that, in accordance with popular belief, the pharmacologic and psychoactive effects of different strains may vary apart from the differences in delta-9-THC content.

The acute physiologic effects of cannabis are dose related and include an increase in heart rate, conjunctival vascular congestion, decreased intraocular pressure, bronchodilatation, increased airway conductance, and peripheral vasodilatation. Dryness of mouth and throat, fine tremors of fingers, ataxia, nystagmus, nausea, and vomiting have been noted. Orthostatic hypotension and loss of consciousness occur infrequently. Sleep patterns may be altered.

Psychoactive effects depend on the dose, the route of administration, the personality of the user, and the environmental and social setting in which the drug is used. Enhanced perception of colors, sounds, patterns, textures, and taste is reported. Mood changes are complex; a sense of increased well-being is frequently experienced, although anxiety and depression may be increased by the drug as well. Drowsiness or hyperactivity and hilarity may occur. Time seems to pass slowly, and short-term memory is impaired. Motor performance is variably impaired. It is probable that alterations in attention are responsible for some of the reported decrements in performance and cognitive function. *Driving performance is significantly impaired by marijuana intoxication.*

Inexperienced users of cannabis report fewer subjective effects than experienced users but demonstrate more decrement in perceptual and psychomotor performance. A social learning process may be involved in the initial perception of psychoactive effects. A varying degree of tolerance develops to some of the psychologic and physiologic effects of the drug, particularly the subjective "high" and the effects on heart rate. A mild withdrawal syndrome, marked by irritability, restlessness, sleep disturbances, sweating, tremor, nausea, and vomiting, occurs under experimental conditions of heavy use but has not been a clinical problem.

Cannabis preparations have been shown to reduce the nausea patients experience incident to cancer chemotherapy and to be effective in reducing intraocular pressure in glaucoma. Research continues on the therapeutic indications for the drug.

ADVERSE EFFECTS. There are no documented fatalities caused by an overdose of cannabis. The increased workload of the heart may pose a threat to patients with hypertension, cerebrovascular disease, and coronary atherosclerosis. Decreased pulmonary function, including vital capacity, has been reported in chronic users, with an increased incidence of bronchitis, sinusitis, and nose and throat inflammation. Marijuana smoke contains 50 to 100 per cent more benzopyrine and other hydrocarbons, as well as more tar, than cigarette smoke. Some of these compounds are considered to be carcinogenic, although an increased incidence of cancer in marijuana smokers has not been reported. The reported in vitro reduction in thymus-dependent lymphocytes and inhibition of DNA, RNA, and protein synthesis require clarification. Reduced gonadotropin and testosterone levels, altered characteristics and decreased production of sperm, compromised ovulation, decreased fertility, and increased fetal loss have been reported in animals, but the clinical significance of these findings is unclear.

Adverse reactions are generally psychologic in nature, infrequent, and dependent on the dose, the personality of the user, and the setting. The most common adverse effects are simple depression, acute panic reactions, and paranoid ideation. These symptoms usually abate in several hours. An acute toxic psychosis, transient in nature, with confusion, disorientation, and auditory and visual hallucinations, occurs infrequently. There is disagreement as to whether cannabis may precipitate a psychotic episode in a stable, well-structured personality, although prolonged psychotic episodes certainly arise in people with borderline psychologic adjustment.

The chronic, heavy use of marijuana may cause diminished goal-directed activity, apathy, and an inability to master new problems, particularly in workers who are engaged in complex tasks or for whom mental operations predominate —"amotivational syndrome." In populations involved in simpler tasks or with high motivation, work performance did not decline. There is no evidence that cannabis use leads to criminal activity.

TREATMENT. Treatment of the frequently seen depressive and panic reactions should be personal, supportive, and reassuring. The patient must be continually reminded of the drug-induced nature of his difficulty. Tranquilizers are sometimes indicated in violent or aggressive states. Psychotherapy and hospitalization may be indicated in more severe or chronic disorders.

Marijuana and Health. Report of a study by a Committee of the Institute of Medicine: Division of Health Sciences Policy. Washington DC, National Academy Press, 1982. *Comprehensive analysis of the impact of marijuana on health and behavior.*

Tashkin DP, Calvarese BM, Simmons MS, Shapiro BJ: Respiratory status of seventy-four habitual marijuana smokers. Chest 78(5):699, 1980. *Controlled study of the long-term effects of marijuana on respiratory status and lung function.*

PSYCHEDELICS

The psychedelic drugs characteristically produce distinctive alterations in perception, thought, feeling, and behavior. They are among the oldest known psychoactive drugs, having long been used as an adjunct to religious practices in some societies. They are sometimes classified as hallucinogens, psychotogens, or psychotomimetics. In this country, the most frequently abused drugs in this category are related either to the indolealkylamines such as the synthetic *lysergic acid diethylamide (LSD, "acid"), psilocybin* ("magic mushrooms"), *psilocin, dimethyltryptamine (DMT),* and *diethyltryptamine (DET),* or to the phenylethylamines such as *mescaline,* which is derived from the peyote cactus, and the substituted amphetamines such as 2,5-dimethoxy-4-methylamphetamine *(DOM, "STP").* Since the pattern of physiologic and psychologic effects produced by other agents is similar to that seen with LSD, this discussion will center on LSD. By virtue of their ability to produce bizarre alterations in behavior, anticholinergic compounds and the general anesthetics *phencyclidine* ("angel dust," PCP) and *ketamine* are included with the psychedelics.

PHARMACOLOGY. LSD is the most potent psychedelic known. It is more than 100 times more potent than psilocybin and 4000 times more potent than mescaline in producing psychologic effects. The usual illicit street dose is probably around 200 μg, but doses as low as 20 μg produce psychologic effects in susceptible individuals. The drug is generally taken orally, although it has been injected on occasion. Central sympathomimetic stimulation occurs within 20 minutes after ingestion, characterized by mydriasis, hyperthermia, tachycardia, elevated blood pressure, piloerection, increased alertness, and facilitation of monosynaptic reflexes. Nausea and occasionally vomiting occur.

Psychoactive effects are evident within one to two hours; these vary within and among subjects depending upon conditions of dose, mood, expectation, setting, and time. Perceptions are heightened and may become overwhelming. Afterimages are prolonged and overlap with ongoing perceptions. Objects may seem to move in a wavelike fashion or melt. Illusions and synesthesias, the overflow of one sense modality to another, are common. There may be a sense of unusual clarity, and one's thoughts may assume extraordinary importance. Time seems to pass slowly, and body distortions are commonly perceived. True hallucinations with loss of insight may occur in susceptible individuals. Mood is highly variable and labile, and may range from expansive reactions characterized by euphoria and self-confidence to a constricted reaction marked by depression and panic.

The syndrome begins to clear after 10 to 12 hours, and fatigue and tension may persist for an additional 24 hours. The duration of action of mescaline is about 12 hours, that of psilocybin is 4 to 6 hours, that of DOM is 6 to 8 hours, and that of phencyclidine is 4 to 6 hours. DMT must be injected or sniffed, and effects last less than 2 hours.

Tolerance to LSD develops rapidly. Repeated daily, doses become ineffective in three to four days. Recovery is equally rapid, so weekly use of the same dose is possible. Cross-tolerance has been demonstrated between LSD, mescaline, psilocybin, and the amphetamine-based psychedelics, but not between LSD and amphetamine. Some tolerance occurs with chronic PCP use. Physical dependence does not occur with LSD or any of the psychedelic drugs.

Mechanisms of action are unknown but may depend on a complex interaction of serotonin and norepinephrine systems in the central nervous system. LSD lowers the threshold for reticular arousal via sensory input and may influence the processes concerned with the filtration and integration of sensory information.

ADVERSE EFFECTS. Acute physiologic toxicity of the LSD-related psychedelic drugs is low at doses that produce marked psychologic effects. No deaths directly attributable to the use of these drugs have been reported. Evidence suggests that pregnant women exposed to illicit LSD have an elevated rate of spontaneous abortions. LSD may inhibit antibody formation and disrupt the body's immune system.

The acute panic reaction ("bad trip," "freak-out") is the most frequent complication of psychedelic use. These vary in intensity and rarely have led to suicide attempts and accidents. Fear of death or insanity and sensations of breathlessness or paralysis are common. In most cases, this acute reaction subsides as drug effects are dissipated. Other complications include prolonged psychotic disorders, acute and chronic paranoid reactions, and depressive states. Adverse psychologic reactions are most frequent in emotionally disturbed individuals in crisis situations or insecure environments who take the drug in unsupervised settings. High doses of psychedelic drugs lead to an increased incidence of these complications.

At low doses, the *acute toxic effects of phencyclidine* resemble those of LSD, although violent and psychotic reactions are reported more frequently. At higher doses, the drug produces severe physiologic toxicity, and deaths have been reported. Common features include emotional lability, excited intoxication, nystagmus, gross incoordination, elevated blood pressure, and increased deep-tendon reflexes which may progress to a state of extreme muscular rigidity. High doses may lead to arrhythmias, convulsions, and coma. A chronic dementia has been described in phencyclidine abusers, marked by memory gaps, disorientation, and visual and speech disturbances.

ANTICHOLINERGIC COMPOUNDS. Ingestion of the alkaloids *atropine, hyoscyamine,* and *scopolamine* in their natural plant forms occurs incident to the ingestion of "herbal teas" and a variety of proprietary medications, and several deaths have occurred. Excessive use of *antihistaminic* compounds with anticholinergic effects also occurs. Symptoms of the potent peripheral effects of intoxication include dilated, fixed pupils, dry skin and mouth, flushing, hyperthermia, and tachycardia. Psychoactive effects are those of an acute toxic delirium, with clouding of consciousness and loss of memory for the period of intoxication. Vivid sensory phenomena are not prominent, although hallucinations may occur.

TREATMENT. Treatment of the acute panic reaction may usually be accomplished by ensuring a supportive environment with someone in constant attendance and a minimum of other external stimuli. The user should be reminded continually that the effects he is experiencing are due to the drug and will pass in time. In particularly agitated patients, diazepam or haloperidol orally or intramuscularly may be used. In the event of precipitation of prolonged psychosis, hospitalization with supportive care may be required. Flashbacks are treated with reassurance and/or psychotherapy when these are severe. In general, the duration and severity of these decrease with time if psychedelic drug use ceases.

Treatment of the acute intoxication caused by low doses of phencyclidine is similar to that for the other psychedelics, particularly with respect to reduction of external stimuli and tranquilization. Toxic reactions from higher doses may require hospitalization and intensive supportive care.

Gastric lavage is indicated in the severely obtunded patient. To enhance the excretion of phencyclidine, acidification of the urine may be accomplished acutely by the intravenous administration of ammonium chloride, 75 mg per kilogram per day in four divided doses, or ascorbic acid, 500 mg every four hours, with repeated monitoring of blood pH, blood gases, BUN, blood ammonia levels, and electrolytes. If symptoms are mild, cranberry juice and 1 or 2 grams of ascorbic acid given orally four times daily may be sufficient.

Treatment of anticholinergic poisoning is symptomatic and consists of protecting the patient from self-injury, providing fluids, and reducing the fever. Administration of cholinesterase inhibitors and suitable tranquilizers may be indicated; phenothiazines are contraindicated because of their anticholinergic effects.

Arronow R, Done A: Phencyclidine overdose: An emerging concept of management. J Am Col Emerg Phys 7(2):56, 1978. *Summary of physical and psychologic symptoms of acute phencyclidine reactions and suggested treatment.*

Grinspoon L, Bakalar JB: Psychedelic Drugs Reconsidered. New York, Basic Books, 1979. *Comprehensive discussion of the use and abuse of psychedelics, with an extensive bibliography.*

INHALANTS

ORGANIC SOLVENTS. The inhalation of a wide range of organic solvents, particularly the toluene in glue, has become popular among young persons during the past 20 years. The drugs are easily available, inexpensive, and convenient to use. The material is usually squeezed into a plastic bag and the vapors inhaled. As used recreationally, these solvents produce intoxication and dizziness not unlike that experienced with alcohol. Few adverse effects have been reported, although suffocation caused by the plastic bag has apparently occurred. Prolonged exposure or overdose, as in the case of addicts or industrial workers, may have serious adverse effects on a variety of organ systems. Cerebral degeneration has been reported in sniffers, as have been deaths secondary to the inhalation of the anesthetic agent halothane, a halogenated hydrocarbon. The inhalation of aerosol sprays containing fluorocarbon propellants is also occurring. The rare occurrence of toxicity and death may be via the induction of cardiac arrhythmias or upper-airway obstruction and hypoxia.

AMYL NITRITE. Amyl nitrite ("amies," "poppers") inhalation has become quite prevalent in youthful and young adult populations, particularly as a sexual aid. A variety of other volatile nitrites, marketed as deodorizers or "aromas" under a variety of exotic brand names, are similarly used. Use is intermittent and characterized by an instantaneous feeling ("rush") of flushing, dizziness, hilarity, and activity. Effects persist for minutes. Adverse effects include palpitations, postural hypotension, and headache, occasionally progressing to loss of consciousness. Prolonged adverse effects have not been reported.

NITROUS OXIDE. Recreational inhalation of nitrous oxide alone or in combination with oxygen is a rarely reported phenomenon that occurs in some youthful populations. Psychoactive effects occur in 15 to 30 seconds and persist for less than five minutes. The experience is described as one of intoxication, euphoria, and hilarity. Adverse effects have not been reported.

TREATMENT. Since the effects of the inhalants are evanescent, specific acute treatments are generally not indicated. When inhalant use is chronic or associated with psychopathology, appropriate long-term treatments should be provided.

Lazar RB, Ho SU, Melen O, Daghestani AN: Multifocal nervous system damage caused by toluene abuse. Neurology 33:1337, 1983. *A recent description of cases, supplemented with a thorough bibliography.*

Sharp CW, Brehm ML (eds.): Review of Inhalants: Euphoria to Dysfunction. NIDA Research Monograph 15. US Department of Health, Education and Welfare, October 1977. *Comprehensive review of the preclinical and clinical data on the various inhalants.*

Section Three PATHOPHYSIOLOGY AND MANAGEMENT OF MAJOR NEUROLOGIC SYMPTOMS

478. AUTONOMIC DISORDERS AND THEIR MANAGEMENT

Fred Plum

THE NONENDOCRINE HYPOTHALAMUS

To survive in a constantly changing, often threatening environment, humans must continuously and automatically adjust the activity of both their internal organs and their outward behavior. The task of maintaining a stable internal environment in the face of minor potential perturbations falls largely to the autonomic nervous and endocrine systems. Major or more sustained challenges, however, must be met by emotional drives or reflex emergency motor acts, both mediated by the limbic system. The hypothalamus (HT) stands between these biologically comprehensive, internally and externally directed regulatory mechanisms, serving as a kind of command post that receives afferent signals of visceral, somatic, and emotional need or sufficiency, then integrates the sum and translates the message to coordinate internal homeostasis with outward behavior. Chapters 222, 224, and 226 further discuss the neuroendocrine role of the HT.

To accomplish its astonishingly complex functions, the hypothalamus has evolved into a neuroendocrine structure in which interneuronal connectivity, in addition to being mediated by conventional neurotransmitters, is modulated and sometimes mediated by endocrine-like peptides. Many of the latter substances spread diffusely from their secreting neurons, either through the HT itself or to remote points in the brain after entering the cerebral ventricles or blood. Anatomically the HT is tightly packed with fibers of passage interlaced among what, by conventional histologic stains, appears to be a diffuse reticulum of nerve cells. Only after applying modern immunocytochemical methods to discern specific nuclei and pathways does the remarkable anatomic richness of the structure and its connections emerge.

The tightly packed, interwoven contents of the hypothalamus make it difficult or impossible to assign specific signs and symptoms to any but a few local areas (Table 478–1). Ventromedial and posteriorly located lesions tend to produce greater functional abnormalities than those located elsewhere, because their position inevitably interrupts fibers leading to the endocrine and descending autonomic nervous systems, respectively. Except when they affect unilateral descending sympathetic projections, clinically detectable changes in autonomic function due to HT disorders always imply the presence of bilateral lesions. Table 478–2 lists the principal diseases that attack the structure.

COGNITIVE AND BEHAVIORAL ABNORMALITIES. Severe retrograde and anterograde memory loss and even a chronic delirium can accompany ventromedial hypothalamic destruction in man. Outbursts of fear and rage sometimes accompany lesions in this region, whereas lateral-posterior damage tends to be associated with apathetic hypoactivity. Disorders of specific neurotransmitter systems have not, as yet, been linked successfully to these functional changes. Loss of libido in the male frequently accompanies structural HT disease but usually reflects associated gonadotropic or autonomic deficiency.

DISTURBANCES OF SLEEP AND AROUSAL. In animals, stimulation of the anterior hypothalamus produces behavioral sleep, whereas destruction of that area results in chronic insomnia, findings consistent with the cholinergic-aminergic theory of sleeping-waking behavior (Ch. 472). Limited evidence suggests that similar effects apply in humans. Selective anterior HT destruction in man is too uncommon to permit conclusions, but posterior hypothalamic destruction or inflammation frequently produces sleep disorders, the most frequent causes being stroke, neoplasm, or encephalitis. Hypersomnolence and chronic sleeplike stupor or coma lasting longer than three to four weeks are pathognomonic for damage or dysfunction in this area. No evidence supports the suggestion that the *Kleine-Levin syndrome,* a condition marked by episodic hypersomnia and hyperphagia in young boys, reflects primary hypothalamic dysfunction (Ch. 472).

HEAT REGULATION. The preoptic anterior HT contains separate receptors for warmth and cold as well as for pyrogens. Diurnal changes in central excitability and in the level of circulating ovarian hormones provide additional nonspecific stimuli. In turn, the HT activates varying combinations of behavioral autonomic and endocrine responses that conserve or dissipate body heat. Diseases in the region can be responsible for hypothermia or, rarely, hyperthermia.

Hypothermia. RELATIVE POIKILOTHERMIA. Poikilothermia, defined as a fluctuation in body temperature of greater than 2° C with changes in ambient temperature, is the most common central abnormality of heat regulation in man. Most such cases are detected by a lowered body temperature. Poikilothermia results from damage to the posterior hypothalamus and rostral mesencephalon. Damage to this area impairs not only autonomic heat-regulating pathways but those that control the sense of thermal discomfort and the behavioral regulation of body temperature as well. As a result, many patients with poikilothermia are unaware of their condition and do little to avoid it. At ordinary ambient temperatures of 20 to 25° C, the degree of hypothermia tends to be proportional to the degree of functional hypothalamic impairment. Relative poikilothermia resulting from impaired hypothalamic-autonomic function frequently affects elderly persons (*senile hypothermia*), making them dangerously susceptible to lowered environmental temperatures. Chronic poikilothermia also accompanies several degenerative disorders that affect the HT in children and adults.

TABLE 478–1. REGIONAL SYNDROMES OF THE HYPOTHALAMUS*

	Preoptic Anterior Hypothalamus	Tuberal and Ventromedian Hypothalamus	Posterior Hypothalamus
Integrates	Endocrine, thermal, parasympathetic autonomic	Cognition; endocrine; sympathetic autonomic caloric balance; fluid balance	Consciousness; cognition; complex endocrine; autonomic; thermal
Contains	Sleep-inducing mechanism; forebrain parasympathetic paths; thermal sensing areas	Final common endocrine paths	Reticular activating system; regulatory and outflow autonomic effectors
Acute lesions	Insomnia; hyperthermia; diabetes insipidus; inappropriate ADH	Hyperthermia; diabetes insipidus; hypothalamic-endocrine disorders	Hypersomnia; poikilothermia; autonomic storm
Chronic lesions	Insomnia; complex endocrine changes (e.g., precocious puberty); endocrinotropic abnormalities; hypothermia; hypodipsia	Medial: memory loss; emotional disorders; hyperphagia and obesity; endocrinotropic abnormalities Lateral: emotional disorders; emaciation	Memory loss; apathy; hypersomnia; poikilothermia; autonomic incoordination; complex endocrine disorders (e.g., precocious puberty)

*As indicated in the text, functional localization is more precise for some activities than for others.

TABLE 478–2. PRINCIPAL CAUSES OF HYPOTHALAMIC DISEASES IN ADOLESCENTS AND ADULTS

Congenital midline brain defects, e.g., agenesis of corpus callosum
Stroke: Basilar artery occlusion, subarachnoid hemorrhage
Tumors: craniopharyngioma, glioma, hamartoma, dysgerminoma, dermoid, lipoma, lymphoma or leukemia, meningioma
Trauma
Encephalitis
Granulomas: sarcoid, tuberculosis, histiocytosis X
Wernicke's polioencephalopathy (thiamine deficiency)
Progressive idiopathic degeneration (rare, childhood)

Poikilothermia regularly follows extensive damage to the posterior hypothalamus or midbrain by stroke, trauma, neoplasm, encephalitis, or thiamine deficiency. Such central hypothermia must be differentiated from that caused by metabolic disorders such as acute or chronic sedative drug ingestion, hypoglycemia, and myxedema.

PAROXYSMAL HYPOTHERMIA. Sustained hypothermia (as opposed to relative poikilothermia) is rare in humans. Less uncommon is paroxysmal hypothermia consisting of attacks of lowered body temperature that vary widely in frequency from daily to more than a decade apart. Such attacks usually begin abruptly, last from minutes to days, and are characterized by sweating, flushing of the skin, and a fall in body temperature, usually to 32° C or lower. Fatigue, decreased mental responsiveness, hypoventilation, hypotension, cardiac arrhythmias, ataxia, lacrimation, and asterixis may accompany the temperature drop. The attacks subside either slowly (hours to days) or rapidly with shivering and peripheral vasoconstriction. During hypothermia, mechanisms for both heat production and heat dissipation respond normally, but around a lower temperature set-point. Most affected patients have had direct evidence for hypothalamic disease; several have suffered from congenital agenesis of the corpus callosum. In some instances anticonvulsant therapy stops the attacks.

Hyperthermia. Chronic fever never results from HT disease, and even acute neurogenic fever is rare. The most frequent causes of acute neurogenic hyperthermia include gross head injury, surgical trauma or spontaneous bleeding into the region of the anterior hypothalamus, and hemorrhage in the adjacent meninges or the third ventricle. With neurogenic hyperthermia, the body temperature can rise to potentially fatal levels of 42° C or higher as a result of active heat production unbalanced by heat dissipation. The cardiovascular changes that normally accompany fever are disproportionately lacking. If standard cooling measures fail, small (2 mg) doses of morphine can ameliorate dangerously high neurogenic fevers.

DISORDERS OF FEEDING BEHAVIOR AND CALORIC BALANCE. Influences generated by the forebrain, especially the limbic system, provide the major influences on feeding behavior in man; primary hypothalamic error accounts for no more than a tiny fraction of human obesity or emaciation, making it all the more important to recognize when it occurs.

In experimental animals, stimulation of the ventromedian region of the HT inhibits feeding, whereas lesions destroying this region produce hyperphagia and a weight gain that later stabilizes at a new elevated set-point. Evidence suggests that the changes are mediated by autonomic influences on the digestive tract and on insulin secretion to enhance appetite. Conversely, stimulation of the lateral hypothalamus induces feeding in excess of caloric requirement, whereas damage to the region results in a temporarily severe aphagia that slowly recovers to maintain a chronically lowered body weight. Both hyperphagia and hypophagia due to HT dysfunction occasionally can be observed in man.

Hypothalamic Obesity. Most patients with hypothalamic obesity have shown at autopsy diffuse or large lesions of the structure. A few, however, have suffered from precisely placed abnormalities of the ventromedian hypothalamus. Examples include leukemic infiltration, with the most severe damage localized in the ventromedian region; others have consisted of discrete tumors in this area. Affected patients have experienced remarkable combinations of food-seeking behavior, including ravenous hyperphagia, decreased motor activity, and sometimes enormous obesity.

The hypothalamus integrates a set-point that roughly regulates the individual's body weight. In patients who develop hypothalamic obesity, whether or not hyperphagia continues or disappears depends upon whether (a) the neurologic abnormality is fixed and (b) the new disease-related set-point for weight has been reached. Patients with obesity following surgical procedures or severe closed head trauma that affects the hypothalamus illustrate this principle. Characteristically, such persons eat ravenously and gain weight quickly following the injury until they reach their new set-point, at which point they become normophagic and stabilize at a new, higher weight.

Emaciation sometimes accompanies hypothalamic disease in man, but the associated lesions usually have been large and their specificity uncertain. Efforts to link hypothalamic disease and anorexia nervosa have been unsuccessful.

WATER BALANCE. The HT controls body water content and osmolality via coordinated mechanisms regulating affective thirst, drinking behavior, and the release of antidiuretic hormone (ADH) via the paraventricular (PV) and supraoptic (SO) nuclei. HT or limbic system disease can produce four principal disorders of water balance, including ADH deficiency (diabetes insipidus), inappropriate ADH secretion, neurogenic (essential) hypernatremia, and episodic hyperdipsia. Chapters 76 and 226 discuss much of the pathophysiology of these disorders. Important from the neural standpoint is to understand that osmoreceptors and volume receptors appear to reside in different areas of the hypothalamus. Osmoreceptors and central thirst receptors have been identified within the preoptic region. These respond to afferent stimulation from peripheral thirst receptors as well as to local sodium concentrations and circulating levels of the peptide angiotensin. Volume receptors appear to lie more laterally in the HT and project to the PV and SO nuclei by pathways different from those that carry osmoreceptor signals. Peripherally, thirst is stimulated or quenched by signals arising from receptors lying within the mouth and interstitial fluids, while different receptors arising from heart, large capacitance systemic veins, and carotid baroreceptors signal volume control needs. Differential peripheral stimulation of the two systems or selective damage to the central osmoreceptor-thirst area explains some examples of inappropriate ADH secretion and most if not all cases of neurogenic (essential) hypernatremia.

Neurogenic (Essential) Hypernatremia. This disorder is marked by four features: (1) elevated serum sodium unaccompanied by circulating volume deficiency, (2) a preserved renal tubular responsiveness to ADH, (3) an inadequate secretion of ADH in response to osmotic stimuli, and (4) the absence or deficiency of appropriate thirst (hypodipsia) despite otherwise relatively normal conscious behavior. True essential hypernatremia is rare; most cases of serum hyperosmolarity accompanying intracranial disease result from a nonspecific combination of dehydration and stupor-impaired drinking behavior.

Essential hypernatremia in its milder and more chronic forms often elevates the serum sodium only modestly, and such patients characteristically lack symptoms except for a remarkable lack of thirst. Close attention often discloses considerable fluctuation in daily serum sodium values above the 150 mmol per liter mark. When sodium levels climb to the 160 to 170 mmol per liter range, affected patients develop weakness and sometimes fever as well as muscle tenderness and cramping that may progress to fatigue, ataxia, and even myoglobinuria. Mental symptoms include lethargy, anorexia, depression, and irritability. With elevations of serum sodium above 180 mmol per liter, most patients become confused or stuporous, and some will die. Patients with essential hypernatremia fail to experience thirst, but many retain persistent habitual drinking, although at a volume insufficient to maintain a normal serum osmolality. They commonly lack clinical evidence of dehydration; only mild hypovolemia or even normovolemia can accompany serum sodium levels as high as 200 mmol per liter or more. An associated hypokalemia usually contributes to the muscular symptoms. Urine volumes may be low or normal but are always more dilute than appropriate for the serum hyperosmolality. The administration of exogenous ADH induces a more concentrated urine. Either an acute water load or a hypertonic saline load, however, can produce an increase in free water clearance, reflecting the failure of central osmoreceptors to respond to the latter stimulus.

The hypothalamic defect that produces essential hypernatremia is inexactly localized. Almost all affected patients have had associated neurologic or endocrine abnormalities, but many have lacked radiographic evidence of central nervous system abnormalities. Some give a history of diffuse head trauma, while in others space-occupying lesions destroy the entire hypothalamic region by the time of death. In a few patients, restricted tumors have involved the preoptic and tuberal region. The mechanisms of essential hypernatremia remain unsettled. The absence of thirst is critical, and this, along with direct measurements showing that serum vasopressin levels fail to increase when sodium levels rise but fall when blood volume increases, indicates either that osmoreceptor function is selectively uncoupled from the behavioral and hormonal control of water balance or that mechanisms that regulate natriuresis are distinct from ADH control.

Treatment consists of lowering the serum sodium and raising the potassium by manipulating the diet and conditioning the patient automatically to drink several liters of water each day regardless of thirst. Spironolactone, chlorpropamide, and the thiazide diuretics may help to achieve fluid balance. Treatment of hypernatremic crises must be initiated slowly: symptoms of water intoxication can develop if serum sodium is reduced by more than 20 mEq per deciliter per day.

Hyperdipsia and Self-induced Water Intoxication. Excessive water drinking in the absence of either hypovolemia or serum hyperosmolality is termed primary hyperdipsia and must be differentiated from the compensatory hyperdipsias of conditions such as diabetes insipidus, diabetes mellitus, or polyuric renal failure. In the absence of inappropriate ADH secretion, symptoms of severe hyperdipsia, i.e., hypervolemia, hyponatremia, and clinical water intoxication accompanied by stupor, delirium, and convulsions, are infrequent. The problem never arises, to our knowledge, as the result of primary central nervous system disease. Most severe hyperdipsia occurs in persons with acute psychiatric disorders who drink excessively to overcome delusional fears. Occasionally, acute water intoxication occurs in alcoholics with gastritis or in youngsters drinking huge amounts of fluids on a dare, e.g., during ritual hazing or tea-party games.

DISORDERS OF PERIPHERAL AND CENTRAL AUTONOMIC FUNCTION

Centripetal parasympathetic influences emanate largely from the anterior HT, whereas sympathetic descending pathways take their origin mainly in the posterolateral reticulum of the structure. Autonomic control extends to almost every organ of the body and perturbations in these regulatory systems probably take more American patients to doctors than all other conditions combined. The large number of autonomic drugs annually prescribed for cardiovascular, gastrointestinal, pulmonary, and genitourinary disorders affirms this premise.

Most *psychosomatic disorders* produce their symptoms at least partly and often predominantly through the limbic-autonomic system. As John Hunter said of his angina pectoris, "My life is in the hands of any rascal who chooses to annoy and tease me." (He subsequently died during an argument at a hospital board meeting.) Autonomic influences act in subtle ways, and abnormal responses to life stress are often highly individual matters, not easy to separate from the nervous system's routine adjustments to living. Clinical sensitivity to the possibility that the brain rather than the target organ sometimes causes the symptoms represents perhaps the most important first step in detecting pathologic autonomic adjustments to life stress.

Diffuse, moderate sympathetic-parasympathetic dysfunction can accompany occasional cases of otherwise typical parkinsonism and is seen as a component to several of the late-life cerebellar or olivopontocerebellar degenerative disorders. Similarly, many elderly patients gradually lose the briskness of their autonomic reflexes and suffer an insidious decline in orthostatic circulatory control, sexual function, heat regulation, urinary and rectal sphincter continence, and bowel motility, all of which must be treated symptomatically. More severe diffuse autonomic dysfunction occurs in two major forms: one is observed chiefly in association with chronic or acute disease of the peripheral nerves; the other consists of diffuse autonomic dysfunction accompanied by degeneration of corticospinal, extrapyramidal, or cerebellar pathways.

Peripheral Autonomic Insufficiency

Involvement of autonomic fibers is prominent in several axonal diseases and peripheral neuropathies, including, especially, acute poliomyelitis, acute inflammatory neuropathy, diabetic neuropathy, tabes dorsalis, and poisoning with the toxic chemical acrylamide. Autonomic impairment with predominantly sympathetic dysfunction accompanies the peripheral neuropathy of inherited amyloid disease.

A small number of patients have been recorded as suffering from a variably complete degree of acutely or subacutely developing failure of the major parts of peripheral sympathetic and parasympathetic function without accompanying somatomotor or sensory changes (*acute pandysautonomia*). Most cases have been in children, although the first reported example was in a middle-aged male. Recovery has been the rule, and the disorder generally is regarded as a selective variant of idiopathic inflammatory neuropathy, a condition in which more restricted autonomic signs and symptoms in the form of tachycardia, hypertension, sweating impairment, and gastrointestinal atony commonly accompany the more prominent motor and sensory changes. Similarly restricted adrenergic abnormalities also accompany the motor polyneuropathy of acute intermittent porphyria. The treatment in all instances is symptomatic.

FAMILIAL DYSAUTONOMIA. This disorder, also called Riley-Day syndrome, is a rare autosomal recessive disorder that predominantly affects Ashkenazi Jewish children and is characterized by several developmental defects, prominently including abnormalities in peripheral and probably central adrenergic and cholinergic neurotransmission.

Idiopathic Autonomic Insufficiency (Idiopathic Orthostatic Hypotension, Shy-Drager Syndrome)

This is a rare degenerative disorder of unknown etiology that strikes during middle age, causing progressive autonomic dysfunction; severe debility or death may occur within 5 to 15 years of onset. Associated extrapyramidal abnormalities and lesions of pigmented brain nuclei may play a prominent role in the genesis of symptoms.

Pathogenesis and Pathology. Histologic examination at autopsy has disclosed various changes, ranging from the severe to the barely detectable. Degenerative abnormalities may affect autonomic ganglia in the periphery, the preganglionic intermediolateral cell column in the spinal cord or autonomic centers in the hypothalamus, nigrostriatal system, pontine nuclei, and globus pallidus. Postmortem biochemical studies have revealed marked depression of dopamine-β-hydroxylase, which converts dopamine to norepinephrine, in sympathetic ganglia, whereas tyrosine hydroxylase, the rate-limiting enzyme in catecholamine biosynthesis, is decreased in locus ceruleus. In parkinsonian patients, tyrosine hydroxylase may be depressed in substantia nigra. The pathogenesis of the disease is unknown.

Several observers have suggested that at least two entities

may constitute idiopathic autonomic insufficiency. The first may consist of autonomic insufficiency alone, whereas the second may be characterized by autonomic insufficiency in association with a variety of neurologic signs, including movement disorders resembling Parkinson's disease. The degree of clinical overlap between these groups, however, is consistent with the existence of a broad continuum rather than distinct entities.

Clinical Manifestations. Symptoms of autonomic dysfunction predominate early in the course. Characteristically, initial difficulties consist of sexual impotence; urinary hesitancy, urgency, or incontinence; and/or anhidrosis. These early symptoms are frequently unrecognized and undiagnosed. Within months to years, the hallmark of the disorder, postural hypotension, appears. This may be manifested as dizziness, giddiness, or frank syncope upon standing. Less frequently, patients complain of generalized weakness, cervico-occipital discomfort, or leg weakness upon standing. Attendant autonomic symptoms include intermittent diplopia, dysphagia, and diarrhea, fecal incontinence, or constipation. A parkinsonian disorder, consisting of bradykinesia, coarse tremor, and rigidity, is common, and tends to progress inexorably. Myoclonus, gait disturbance, and signs of olivopontocerebellar dysfunction may also occur.

Physical signs of autonomic dysfunction parallel the aforementioned symptoms. Orthostatic hypotension, a greater than 30/20 mm Hg fall in blood pressure upon assumption of the erect position, constitutes the fundamental sign. Other signs include absence of sinus arrhythmia and absence of the normal overshoot in diastolic pressure during phase IV of the Valsalva maneuver. Autonomic dysfunction may express itself in Horner's syndrome, in parasympathetic pupillary changes, or as anhidrosis even with elevated ambient temperature. Muscle wasting, fasciculation, and extensor plantar responses occasionally have been observed.

A variety of clinical laboratory tests may be employed to evaluate autonomic function, and only the simplest will be delineated here. *Miosis* in response to ocular administration of dilute solutions of methacholine, or *mydriasis* after instillation of dilute epinephrine, suggests respectively parasympathetic or sympathetic denervation supersensitivity. On the other hand, absence of mydriasis after ocular instillation of cocaine or hydroxyamphetamine suggests that endogenous norepinephrine stores are defective. Absence of sweating with elevation of the ambient temperature and absence of the axon reflex after intradermal histamine suggest denervation of cutaneous structures. The presence of an abnormally accentuated blood pressure response to the intravenous infusion of norepinephrine is consistent with widespread denervation supersensitivity.

Differential Diagnosis. Orthostatic hypotension itself may accompany intravascular hypovolemia (as with massive hemorrhage or adrenal insufficiency), vasodepressor syncope, acute cardiac failure from a variety of causes, familial hyperbradykininism, and intracranial posterior fossa mass or vascular lesions. However, in these conditions other signs of autonomic dysfunction are absent. On the other hand, autonomic insufficiency, including orthostatic hypotension, may occur with any disease that alters peripheral or central autonomic pathways. Many disorders conform to this description. A variety of peripheral neuropathies may be accompanied by dysautonomia, including the acute Guillain-Barré syndrome; the chronic neuropathies of diabetes mellitus, amyloidosis, Wernicke's disease, and porphyria; and the congenital Riley-Day syndrome. Ganglion dysfunction may result from ingestion of ganglioplegic agents. Tabes dorsalis is commonly accompanied by autonomic signs. Autonomic dysfunction may result from interruption of descending pathways in the spinal cord, as observed with syringomyelia, trauma, or spinal tumor. Pontine hemorrhage may interrupt descending sympathetic pathways in the brainstem, thereby causing sympathetic dysfunction. Differentiation from these diseases is readily accomplished by suitable history, examination, and laboratory tests.

Course and Treatment. Although treatment does not alter the underlying pathologic process, it may allow an otherwise bedridden invalid to lead a considerably improved life. Orthostatic hypotension may be treated with a variety of measures, dictated by the severity of the problem. The first line of defense consists of antigravity stockings, which prevent pooling of blood in the lower extremities upon standing. In moderately severe cases, intravascular volume expansion may be achieved by using the mineralocorticoid desoxycorticosterone acetate or 9-α-fluorocortisone and sodium chloride, with potassium supplementation. In severe cases, oral sympathomimetic agents, including ephedrine or hydroxyamphetamine, may be added. Indomethacin may be effective in selected patients for the treatment of orthostatic hypotension. The use of monoamine oxidase inhibitors may be potentially hazardous in those patients who are subject to denervation suprasensitivity. Although the diet may be rigorously regulated in the hospital setting, this is rarely possible on an outpatient basis. For example, such foods as cheese, broad beans, Chianti, raisins, bananas, and aged or smoked meat contain significant quantities of vasoactive amines. Inadvertent ingestion of microgram quantities of vasoactive amines in the diet may result in alarming elevation of blood pressure in patients being treated with monoamine oxidase inhibitors for widespread sympathetic denervation.

Parkinsonian signs and symptoms may be successfully treated with L-dopa and the customary anticholinergic agents.

ABNORMALITIES OF SWEATING. *Anhidrosis,* a relatively uncommon complaint, occurs as part of a rare, probably autosomal recessive disorder in which it is associated with congenital insensitivity to pain. Anhidrosis due to congenital absence of the sweat glands is similarly rare. Anhidrosis also follows pre- or postganglionic sympathetic denervation produced by disease or surgical procedures and can occur in the appropriate territorial distribution of any diseased or damaged peripheral nerve.

Hyperhidrosis, defined as sweating in excess of apparent thermal requirements, is a common response to anxiety, especially among persons less than 30 years old. Longstanding severe hyperhidrosis causing constantly dripping hands and feet is an uncommon but socially troublesome disorder of unknown cause. Emotional factors seem to contribute little. Severe cases can be relieved by sympathectomy directed at the upper extremities. The procedure is best limited to either the upper or lower extremities, since compensatory accentuation of pre-existing sweating tends to affect nondenervated parts. Total sympathectomy produces too many undesirable side effects to be recommended. Hyperhidrosis localized to a particular body part occasionally occurs in association with irritation of the related preganglionic fibers or ganglia by an infection or neoplasm and deserves careful attention from that standpoint.

Urinary Bladder Control

Abnormalities in micturition, collectively termed *dysuria,* arise from four principal causes: local disease in the bladder and urethra, neurologic disorders, drug effects, and psychologic perturbation. Table 478–3 outlines a differential diagnosis of these conditions based on the predominant symptoms, while the following paragraphs briefly discuss neurogenic mechanisms.

The bladder is a hollow pelvic structure composed of the interlacing smooth muscle fibers of the detrusor covered by its internal mucous membrane and outer serosa. The bladder is smooth muscle and its resistance to stretch is determined predominantly by the viscoelastic properties of its wall rather than by direct neurogenic mechanisms. With progressive filling, the normal intravesical pressure rises slowly, remaining below about 15 cm of water until average capacities are reached, between 400 and 600 ml, at which point the intravesical pressure rises either abruptly owing to the onset of the micturition reflex or more gradually owing to reaching the elastic limits of the wall itself. Normal adult micturition volumes average between 200 and 400 ml, but with acute urinary retention the structure can stretch abnor-

TABLE 478–3. MECHANISMS OF DYSURIA

Painful Urination
- Cystourethral inflammation (Ch. 85)
- Urethral stricture
- Psychogenic

Increased Frequency-Urgency
- Increased fluid intake of any cause (e.g., diabetes, alcoholism)
- Cystourethral inflammation
- Psychogenic
- Partial outlet obstruction (e.g., prostatic hypertrophy)
- Neurogenic
  - Damage to prefrontal or spinal inhibitory pathways
  - Spinal reflex facilitation

Incontinence
- Stress: Small volumes, brief urgency, women more than men
  - Normal in 50 per cent of giggling girls
  - Multiparas with cystocele, other outflow damage
  - Increases with normal aging
- Retention-overflow: Dribbling or small volumes, pain in pelvis or flanks, palpable bladder
  - Causes as listed with retention
  - Severe cystitis (small bladder volume)
- Confusional: Small or large volumes, usually shameless
- "Spastic": Large volumes, sporadic occurrence, prominent urgency, emptying complete
  - Prefrontal lesions
  - Extramedullary advanced spinal compression
  - Occasionally partial outlet obstruction
  - Circumstance: bedridden or crippled elderly with facilities remote
- Spinal: Moderate volumes, brief urgency, frequent occurrence, high residual urine
  - Intramedullary cervical-thoracic-lumbar lesions (multiple sclerosis, neoplasms, etc.)
  - Occasionally with partial peripheral denervation

Retention
- Acute or chronic outflow obstruction
- Acute neurologic disease
  - Peripheral: Autonomic polyneuropathy, pelvic trauma, cauda equina compression, conus lesions
  - Central: Poliomyelitis, spinal transection
- Drugs (usually plus local structural problems)
  - Anticholinergics, antidepressants, opiates
- Psychogenic
- Postanesthetic

mally to accommodate one or more liters, while chronic infection and hypertrophy may contract it to a capacity of no more than 60 to 100 ml.

Urine enters the bladder from the paired ureters and normally leaves via the membranous urethra. In both sexes the lower detrusor musculature joins with elastic tissue to form an involuntary internal sphincter that normally can resist passively induced intra-abdominal–intravesical pressures as high as 150 mm Hg. The more distal urethra is encircled by voluntarily controlled striated muscle innervated by the somatomotor pudendal nerve. More competent in men than in women, this external sphincter can withstand briefly the intraurethral detrusor-induced pressure of normal micturition but is unnecessary to normal urinary continence.

The act of voiding represents a stretch-induced parasympathetic reflex of smooth muscle facilitated by brainstem and spinal mechanisms, normally inhibited or released by forebrain regulatory influences. The actual neuromuscular sequence consists of an initial voluntary relaxation of the skeletal muscle of the pelvic floor followed by the disinhibited reflex discharge, which contracts the detrusor, assimilates and relaxes the musculoelastic tissue of the internal sphincter, and empties the organ by a fusion of successive detrusor contractions.

The complete reflex mechanism for micturition exists within the spinal cord. The afferent route of the arc depends upon fibers that originate in stretch receptors in the bladder wall and travel centrally via sacral roots 2 to 4. Efferent preganglionic fibers arise in the lateral columns of the sacral segments of the conus medullaris, whence they travel in the cauda equina to and through the lower sacral foramina to synapse with their final ganglia over the outer surface of the bladder and the region of the proximal urethra. Centrally, afferent proprioceptive signals travel rostrally via the lemniscal system while descending inhibitory influences originate in the paramedian prefrontal cerebral cortex. These latter pathways are joined in the brainstem and upper spinal cord by reflex-facilitating fibers that enhance complete reflex bladder emptying. The pathway descends in the spinal cord within the lateral funiculus to synapse upon the sacral preganglionic neurons.

CEREBRAL DISTURBANCES IN MICTURITION. Damage to the bilateral prefrontal area lowers the micturition reflex threshold, resulting in a proportionately smaller bladder capacity. The chief symptoms are sudden, sometimes uncontrollable urgency with moderately large volumes, usually of less than 250 ml, but complete bladder emptying. The cystometrogram shows a normal bladder pressure-volume filling curve but a reduced micturition reflex threshold, with a comparably reduced threshold to filling sensation. Clinical evaluation or CT scanning of the head readily discloses evidence of structural frontal lobe disease.

Dementia leads to an incontinence of indifference (a loss of bladder training) in which visceral physiology remains intact but social restraints depart. Patients with severe physical disabilities such as hemiplegia, advanced arthritis, etc., may develop *pseudoincontinence* due to difficulty in reaching the toilet or, occasionally, as a depressed, angry, and frustrated response to the limitations of their condition.

SPINAL DISTURBANCES OF MICTURITION. Gradual *extramedullary* spinal cord compression produces few changes in bladder function until late in the course when the reflex is facilitated along with somatic motor reflex pathways. Urgency with moderately reduced voiding volumes results. Incontinence occurs only with advanced or sudden cord compression. *Intramedullary* spinal lesions can directly affect the descending parasympathetic pathways, releasing the reflex from higher inhibition and impairing brainstem-originating pathways that facilitate complete detrusor emptying. The reflex threshold drops and urgency-frequency with moderate volumes results, often leaving a high postvoiding residual volume. Sporadic reflex incontinence is common.

Acute spinal transection produces reflex inhibition in the distal segment ("spinal shock"), with loss of voiding reflexes as well as of somatomotor ones. Acute retention develops, stretching the smooth muscle wall and producing a flat pressure-volume curve with no reflex. Overflow dribbling incontinence ensues. Reflex recovery is marked by increasingly large, randomly spaced, reflex partial bladder emptyings that in many instances can be trained by skill and patience into complete self-stimulated reflex voidings.

PERIPHERAL (PREGANGLIONIC OR SOMATIC AFFERENT) DEFECTS IN VOIDING. These can result from disease of either efferent or afferent peripheral nerves (e.g., occasional inflammatory neuropathy, diabetic neuropathy, tabes dorsalis, pelvic carcinoma), of the cauda equina, or of the conus medullaris. Depending upon the rate of neuritic progression, the bladder gradually dilates, with sensations of fullness disappearing commensurately with the degree of mechanical stretching. Normal sensations of urgency disappear, and the reflex progressively loses its effectiveness. Residual urine volumes increase. Ultimately, moderate to severe retention occurs, with or without spontaneous dribbling or occasionally spurting, small-volume overflow incontinence. In the absence of cystitis, the cystometrogram shows a flat filling curve on which, in time, autonomous ganglion-induced local detrusor contractions increasingly become superimposed. Spontaneous parasympathetic activity eventually leads to nearly continuous autonomous local detrusor activity, producing a hypertrophied bladder wall with a decreased bladder capacity and a steep pressure-volume curve.

TREATMENT OF NEUROGENIC BLADDER DIFFICULTIES. This varies according to the anatomic distribution of the cause. Urinary tract infections intensify all neurogenic functional abnormalities and should be treated promptly and effectively. Urgency or urgency-incontinence due to cerebral lesions or spinal extramedullary compression sometimes is aided by antispasticity drugs such as baclofen or parasympathetic blocking agents such as oxybutynin chloride 5 mg bid or tid. Often such symptoms are relatively minor and can be treated by addressing the neurologic abnormality and forcing fluids in an attempt to stretch the bladder wall so as to raise the threshold for the voiding reflex. Urgency-retention-incontinence due to intramedullary spinal lesions can be difficult to manage, especially when a high residual urine volume leads to recurrent urinary tract infection. Many women and some men can be taught clean self-catheterization to assure complete bladder emptying every four to six hours, thereby minimizing infection. Effective control is more difficult to attain in persons who suffer damage to the conus or peripheral micturition pathways; they usually require the assistance of an experienced urologist to develop effective bladder care.

Male Sexual Function

Organic disturbances of male sexual function are limited almost entirely to loss of libido, failure to attain an erection of sufficient strength to carry out sexual intercourse (impotence), and failure to attain normal ejaculation-emission. Masters and Johnson define impotence somewhat generously as greater than a 25 per cent failure during attempted intercourse. Failure to reach orgasm or the presence of premature or delayed ejaculation with normal libido and erectile capacity almost always reflects a psychogenic rather than an organic problem.

Neural control over male sexual activities arises within forebrain limbic areas, generating sexual drives that, in turn, are chronically stimulated by the effects of circulating androgens. Descending pathways travel with the parasympathetic outflow. Parasympathetic sacral efferents control penile tumescence by inducing vascular engorgement and also stimulate a large proportion of the severally originating pelvic contractions that initiate ejaculation and lead to the sensation of orgasm. Sympathetic stimulation contracts the seminal vesicles and closes the bladder neck to prevent retrograde emission, thereby guaranteeing anterograde ejaculation. Genital sensory fibers reach the spinal cord via the S2 to S4 dorsal roots and thenceforth ascend in the lemniscal system. Considerable evidence gained from the study of sexual function in paraplegics with a lesion producing an isolated, distal thoracic and lumbosacral spinal cord indicates that the cord contains all the necessary reflexes to complete sensory-induced erection and ejaculation.

Male impotence is common and increases with age to affect at some time almost half the population over 55 years; at that age psychogenic causes appear to be primary in only about 25 per cent. Therapeutic drugs and alcohol excess represent the most frequent causes of male impotence. Aging itself, however, eventually becomes a cause, and about 25 per cent of males of 70 years or more have erection failure attributable to aging alone.

Impotence has several possible causes, as indicated in Table 478–4, and more than one can operate in a given patient. In perhaps 10 per cent of cases no satisfactory explanation can be found. Psychologic factors are always important. They account for as many as half of the overall cases and must be inquired into carefully even when adequate organic reasons appear to exist.

Differential diagnosis begins with a careful history. Does the patient's complaint reflect a recent change in libido and performance or a longstanding pattern that has finally proved more troublesome to a sexual partner than to self? Longstanding absence or low level of libido can reflect either psychologic factors, chronic temporal lobe disease, or primary or secondary androgenic failure. If the disease is recent in origin, does it relate entirely to a specific partner? Such instances are usually psychogenic and best managed by a sex therapist if a careful history, physical examination, and tumescence studies provide no suggestion of the organic disorders listed in Table 478–4. If recent in onset, did libido remain high as potency declined? The latter pattern is more common among drug-induced or neurologic disorders than among endocrine ones.

Specific drugs most often causing impotence are listed in Table 478–5. Among the endocrine disorders, most that are severe enough to cause impotence are readily recognized. Pituitary tumors and hypothalamic lesions impairing gonadotropic release usually give prominent additional symptoms (Ch. 225). Hypo- or hyperthyroidism similarly generates other systemic symptoms. In doubtful cases, measurement of serum prolactin, testosterone, thyroxin, and triiodothyronine should settle the question. Borderline changes of a single serum hormone value, however, seldom provide evidence for a disorder of potency that will be reversed by giving hormone therapy.

Neurologic disturbances cause only about 10 per cent of all cases of impotence, although the symptom affects patients with a number of neurologic diseases and deserves compassionate inquiry. Temporal lobe disease affecting limbic systems is associated with reduction in male libido, while structural lesions involving descending parasympathetic systems commonly interfere with the capacity to gain and maintain an erection. Peripheral neurologic disorders, as Table 478–4 indicates, are the commonest neurologic offenders and should be approached as indicated in Ch. 526 to 531.

Aside from a record of sexual inadequacy limited to a specific partner, little in the history alone guarantees psychogenic causes. Since patients with physical illness may suffer psychogenic impotence (e.g., postmyocardial infarction or post-stroke sexual failure) while others with prominent psychiatric disorders may have unsuspected physical illness (e.g., depressives with diabetic neuropathy), objective testing measures are valuable in differential diagnosis. Useful in this regard is the measurement of nocturnal penile tumescence (NPT), which, taken during sleep monitoring, records the frequency and intensity of the erections that normally accompany rapid eye movement sleep. When matched suitably for age with normal controls, the results correlate highly although not completely with psychogenic (no appreciable decline in NPT) versus organic (moderate to marked decline in NPT) impotence.

Treatment of male impotence depends upon the cause. Drug avoidance or readjustment can benefit many cases, as can substitution therapy when endocrine failure is demonstrated.

TABLE 478–4. PRINCIPAL ORGANIC CAUSES OF MALE SEXUAL FAILURE

Drugs
Endocrine
Secondary: pituitary adenoma; idiopathic or acquired hypogonadotropic hypogonadism; hyperprolactinemia
Primary gonadal failure
Advanced diabetes mellitus
Hypothyroidism, hyperthyroidism (rare)
Chronic Systemic Illnesses
Cirrhosis
Chronic renal failure
Disseminated malignancy, etc.
Neurogenic
Temporal lobe disorders: trauma, epilepsy, neoplasm, stroke
Intramedullary spinal lesions: paraplegia; demyelinating disorders; neoplasms; syrinx; Shy-Drager dysautonomia
Peripheral nerves. Somatic or autonomic neuropathies; pelvic neoplasms, granulomas, trauma; structural lesions of cauda equina or conus medullaris
Urologic
Complete prostatectomy; priapism; local trauma or neoplasms; Peyronie's disease; rectosigmoid "cleanouts"
Vascular
Severe aortic atherosclerosis; lower aortic bypass

TABLE 478–5. DRUGS OFTEN REPORTED TO INTERFERE WITH MALE POTENCY

Alcohol	Guanethidine
Anticancer chemotherapy	Immunosuppressives
Anticholinergics	Lithium
Antiparkinson agents	Opiates
Barbiturates and congeners	Phenothiazine
Benzodiazepines	Several antihypertensive ganglionic blockers
Bethanidine	Several diuretics
Cannabis	Tricyclic and MAO-inhibitor antidepressants
Cimetidine	

Local genital abnormalities should be approached surgically. A variety of surgically implantable prostheses to assist erection have become available in recent years to aid the patient affected with impotence caused by neurogenic or locally severe vascular disease. Thus far, attempts at revascularizing the penis have met with only limited success. Testosterone therapy given in the absence of a demonstrated androgen deficiency almost never provides more than placebo benefit and creates a carcinogenic risk as well.

Hypothalamus and Its Disorders

Greenberg HS, Rocher LL, Clavin DB, Ehren Kranz JRL: Episodic hyperhidrosis, hypothermia, and agenesis of the corpus callosum. Neurology 33:1122, 1983. *The most recent comprehensive review of this uncommon condition, with the addition of new material.*

Martin JB, Lourdis DMD: Potential implications of brain peptides in neurologic disease. *In* Martin JB, Reichlen S, Bick KL (eds.): Neurosecretion and Brain Peptides. New York, Raven Press, 1981. *Covers the known and possible associations of these newly identified neuromodulators with neurologic disease, some of the hypothalamus.*

Plum F, Van Uitert R: Non-endocrine diseases and disorders of the hypothalamus. Res Publ Assoc Res New Ment Dis 56:415, 1977. *A comprehensive review of the clinically important autonomic functions of the hypothalamus written at the dawn of the peptide era. Extensively referenced.*

Peripheral and Central Autonomic Functions

Appenzeller O: The Autonomic Nervous System. 2nd ed. New York, Elsevier, 1976. *The only available comprehensive monograph of recent origin.*

Bannister R, Oppenheimer DR: Degenerative diseases of the nervous system associated with autonomic failure. Brain 95:457, 1972. *A description of various autonomic syndromes associated with degenerative disease, with an attempt to classify the disorders tentatively.*

Black IB, Petito CK: Catecholamine enzymes in the degenerative neurological disease idiopathic orthostatic hypotension. Science 192:910, 1976. *An analysis of biochemical deficits in autonomic failure, with specific reference to catecholamine biosynthetic enzymes.*

Bradbury S, Eggleston C: Postural hypotension: A report of three cases. Am Heart J 1:73, 1925. *The first definitive report of idiopathic orthostatic hypotension.*

Hines S, Houston M, Robertson D: The clinical spectrum of autonomic dysfunction. Am J Med 70:1091, 1981. *An analysis of 297 patients with various forms of autonomic insufficiency of both secondary and primary causes.*

Kochar MS, Itskovitz HD: Treatment of idiopathic orthostatic hypotension with indomethacin. Lancet 1:1011, 1978. *The first report of the use of indomethacin, a potentially useful agent, in the treatment of postural hypotension.*

Nass R, Chutorian A: Dysesthesias and dysautonomia: A self limited syndrome of painful dysesthesias and autonomic dysfunction in childhood. J Neurol Neurosurg Psychiatr 45:162, 1982. *A description of three children with a self-limited selective sensory and autonomic neuropathy, presumably of the inflammatory type.*

Petito CK, Black IB: Ultrastructure and biochemistry of sympathetic ganglia in idiopathic orthostatic hypotension. Ann Neurol 4:6, 1978. *Correlation of ultrastructural and enzymatic deficits in one form of autonomic insufficiency.*

Shy GM, Drager GA: A neurological syndrome associated with orthostatic hypotension. Arch Neurol 2:511, 1960. *The definitive clinicopathologic analysis of autonomic insufficiency associated with generalized neurologic degeneration.*

Young R, Asbury A, Corbett J, Adams R: Pure pandysautonomia with recovery. Description and discussion of diagnostic criteria. Brain 98:613, 1975. *A detailed description of the entitled disorder.*

Ziegler MG, Lake CR, Kopin IJ: The sympathetic-nervous-system defect in primary orthostatic hypotension. N Engl J Med 296:293, 1977. *A clinical study using circulating catecholamines and metabolites to analyze the pathogenesis of idiopathic orthostatic hypotension.*

Urinary Bladder Control

Andersson K-E, Sjögren C: Aspects on the physiology and pharmacology of the bladder and urethra. Prog Neurobiol 19:71, 1982. *Describes bladder-urethral innervation and comprehensively lists drugs that have been used to treat bladder dysfunction.*

Boyarsky S, Labay P, Hanick P, Abramson AS, Boyarsky R: Care of the Patient with Neurogenic Bladder. Boston, Little, Brown and Company. 1979. *A well-balanced monograph describing all aspects of this difficult subject.*

Williams ME, Pannill FC: Urinary incontinence in the elderly. Physiology, pathophysiology, diagnosis and treatment. Ann Intern Med 97:895, 1982. *A thorough, highly practical guide with an extensive bibliography.*

Male Sexual Function

Bennett AH (ed.): Management of Male Impotence. Baltimore, Williams and Wilkins, 1982. *A useful multiauthored monograph that covers the organic causes of the problem.*

Kaplan HS: Disorders of Sexual Desire. New York, Bruner/Meizel, 1979. *A detailed review of the most frequent psychogenic sexual dysfunctions.*

Kolodny RC, Masters WH, Johnson VE: Textbook of Sexual Medicine. Boston, Little, Brown and Company, 1979. *A good textbook of sexual medicine designed for students and general physicians.*

Slag MF, Morley JE, Elson MK, et al.: Impotence in medical clinic outpatients. JAMA 249:1736, 1983. *Among 1181 men attendees at a VA Hospital, 34 per cent with a mean age of just over 60 years had erectile dysfunction.*

Spark RF, White RA, Connolly PB: Impotence is not always psychogenic. Newer insights into hypothalamic-pituitary-gonadal dysfunction. JAMA 234:750, 1980. *Thirty-seven of 105 consecutive patients evaluated for impotence in an endocrine clinic had previously unsuspected hypogonadism, hyperprolactinemia, or hyperthyroidism. Appropriate treatment restored potency in 33 cases.*

479. THE SPECIAL SENSES AND RELATED FUNCTIONS

479.1. Smell and Taste

Fred Plum

OLFACTION

The capacity to detect odor provides humans with both strong limbic system signals and potential safety warnings. Smell contributes importantly to the anticipation and ingestion of food, since much of what we "taste" derives from olfactory stimulation during the ingestion and chewing of food. Most humans can recognize and identify a thousand or more different odors; efforts to reduce this large repertory into the compoundings of a limited number of elemental aromas have been unsuccessful.

Olfactory receptors lie in a roughly dime-sized area of specialized pigment epithelium that archs along the superior aspect of each side of the nasal mucosa. Constantly regenerating bipolar sensory cells in this area thrust short receptor hairs into the overlying mucus to detect aromatic molecules as they dissolve. Central afferent fibrils traverse the cribriform plate to reach the olfactory bulb on the ventral surface of the frontal lobe whence second and third order neurons project directly and indirectly to the prepyriform cortex and parts of the amygdaloid complex of the same and opposite side of the brain, representing the primary olfactory cortex.

Olfactory sense can be reduced (hyposmia), absent (anosmia), or distorted (dysosmia). Dysosmia usually results from the products of local disease but occasionally represents a psychiatric symptom. Anosmia can be partial or complete, inherited or acquired. Thus, anosmia or hyposmia for specific selective odors occurs rarely an as autosomal or recessive inherited trait. Congenital anosmia accompanies certain autonomic and endocrinopathic disorders, notably hypogonadotropic hypogonadism (Kallman's syndrome).

Most acquired disturbances of smell result from transient or sustained disease of the nasal mucous membranes that deadens or dries out the receptor membrane. The disorder seldom is complete and commonly responds to local treatment. More severe and often permanent anosmia results from basal skull fractures, frontal fossa brain tumors affecting the olfactory pathways, and, much less often, herpes zoster, B_{12} deficiency, and multiple sclerosis. Sudden, idiopathic anosmia usually associated with loss of taste as well has been reported, possibly the result of a local neurotropic viral infection. No satisfactory treatment has been found for such neurogenic anosmias. Affected patients must be warned explicitly to avoid gas heating and to install smoke alarms to compensate for the life-threatening hazards of the defect. *Parosmia* is a distortion of olfactory perception (normal odors perceived as a foul smell) that may occur without prior anosmia or during recovery from anosmia.

Hallucinations of smell, usually of a foul quality, occur with epileptogenic lesions affecting the region of the amygdala and are termed uncinate fits.

GUSTATORY FUNCTION

Taste, like smell, has both vegetative and survival values, the latter perhaps more necessary among our primitive ancestors. The impairment or loss of taste is a serious complaint with a variety of illnesses, in some of which a concurrent olfactory loss is actually at fault.

The brain abstracts its specific sense of taste from signals fed from tastebuds and associated receptors that lie on the dorsal surface of the tongue and in the adjacent faucial areas. Fungiform papillary buds on the anterior tongue respond mainly to sweet and sour stimuli, while foliate and valate papillae located along the base of the tongue and adjacent areas detect predominantly bitter qualities. The distribution of selective taste receptors may vary from time to time within the individual so as partly to guide food selection according to nutritional need. The anterior two thirds of the tongue is innervated by branches of the chorda tympani division of the intermediate and facial nerves, making it especially susceptible to injuries or infections that affect the latter nerve on its route through the middle ear and petrous bone. Glossopharyngeal nerve fibers supply the taste receptors of the posterior two thirds of the tongue and fauces. Both innervations project to the nucleus tractus solitarius of the medulla and then via a series of relays to reach the postcentral somatosensory cerebral cortex. Taste receptors on the tongue have an innately relatively high threshold that increases further with age, often making specific testing difficult for diagnostic purposes.

Taste loss or reduction is termed *ageusia* or *hypogeusia*, distortion being *dysgeusia*. The reference by Schiffman provides a long list of specific disorders that sometimes can reduce or alter taste or smell sensations. Chief specific offenders from the neurologic standpoint are Bell's palsy, which reduces perception; epileptic aurae, which occasionally include gustatory sensations; and depressive or paranoid delusions, which more distort the sense of taste or smell than destroy them. Among systemic problems, aging, hepatitis, cancer, and various forms of drugs are the main causes of symptoms of taste reduction or distortion. Investigation for the symptom of taste loss or abnormal taste involves first a clinical search for local mucous membrane or neurologic disease, followed by a systematic review of medications being taken, possible exposure to toxic fumes, and, if still necessary, a more exacting inquiry into possibly hidden systemic illness.

As with defects in smell, there is no specific treatment for taste loss except giving attention to the underlying illness. Dietary zinc supplements provide no proven advantage. Nontoxic odorants and spices commonly increase the palatability of food, as does switching from one substance to another during meals.

Doty RL: A review of olfactory dysfunctions in man. Am J Otolaryngol 1:57, 1979. *A comprehensive basic review, extensively referenced.*

Howe JG, Gibson JD: Uncinate seizures and tumors, a myth re-examined. Ann Neurol 12:227, 1982. *Most patients with such seizures lack radiographic evidence of structural brain abnormalities.*

Schiffman SS: Taste and smell in disease. N Engl J Med 308:1275, 1337, 1983. *A two-part, well-referemced review of an often neglected medical problem.*

Smith M, Smith LG, Levinson B: The use of smell in differential diagnosis. Lancet 2:1452, 1982. *An amusing index to disease-produced odors useful to the clinician.*

479.2. Neuro-ophthalmology

Fred Plum

The mechanistic understanding of visual impairment, along with disturbances of pupillary and oculomotor control, lies close to the heart of diagnosing neurologic disorders. Diseases of the eye itself are further considered in Part XXIV.

ANATOMY OF THE VISUAL PATHWAYS

Light entering the eye falls on the retinal rods and cones, which transduce the stimulus into neural impulses to be transmitted to the brain. What each eye "sees" is termed its *visual field*. The geometry of the system dictates that the nasal side of the left eye and the temporal side of the right see the left side of the world and vice versa and, similarly, that the upper half of each retina sees the lower half of the world (Fig. 479–1) and vice versa.

Retinal sensitivity to light stimulation increases centrifugally toward the cones of the central macular area, which transmit a distinctive

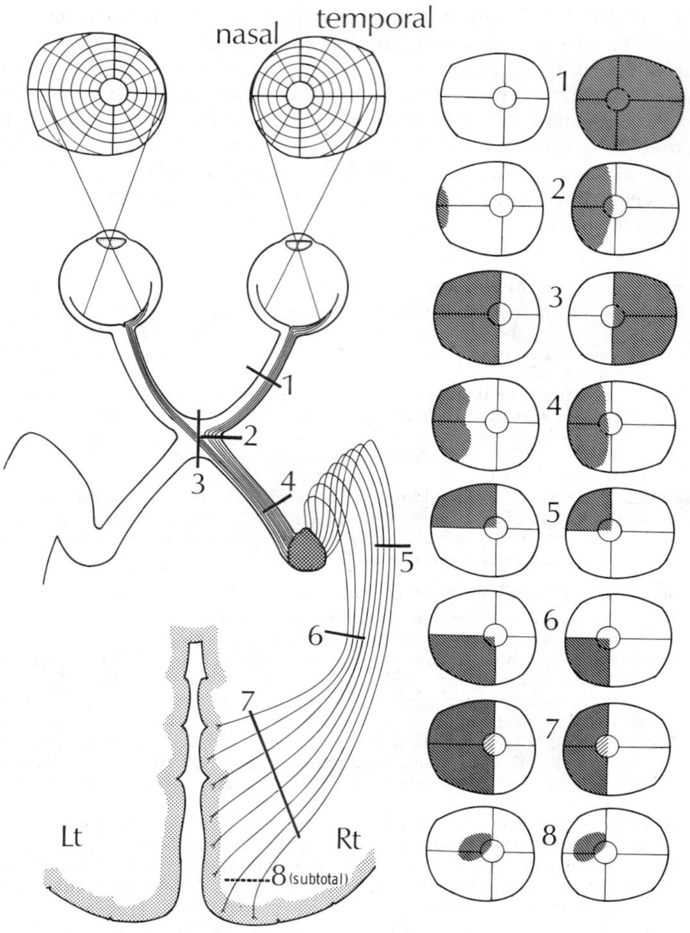

Figure 479–1. Visual fields that accompany damage to the visual pathways. 1. Optic nerve: Unilateral amaurosis. 2. Lateral optic chiasm: Grossly incongruous, incomplete (contralateral) homonymous hemianopia. 3. Central optic chiasm: Bitemporal hemianopia. 4. Optic tract: Incongruous, incomplete homonymous hemianopia. 5. Temporal (Meyer's) loop of optic radiation: Congruous partial or complete (contralateral) homonymous superior quadrantanopia. 6. Parietal (superior) projection of the optic radiation: Congruous partial or complete homonymous inferior quadrantanopia. 7. Complete parieto-occipital interruption of optic radiation. Complete congruous homonymous hemianopia with psychophysical shift of foveal point often sparing central vision, giving "macular sparing." 8. Incomplete damage to visual cortex: Congruous homonymous scotomas, usually encroaching at least acutely on central vision.

maculopapillary bundle that enters the temporal-lateral one third of the optic disc. Other nerve fibers from the retina lie axially within the optic nerve in a pattern that largely repeats their retinal distribution.

The arterial supply to the optic nerve and retina both derive from branches of the carotid-born ophthalmic artery. The *central retinal artery* approaches the eye along each optic nerve, and pierces the inferior aspect of the dural sheath about 1 cm behind the globe to enter the center of the nerve. The artery emerges in the fundus at the center of the nerve head whence it irrigates most of the retina by superior, medial, inferior, and lateral branches. Anastomotic branches derived from the choroidal and posterior ciliary arteries supply the nerve head itself and the macular region. Venous drainage from the retina and nerve head flows primarily via the central retinal vein, whose course of exit from the eye parallels that of the entry of the artery. The venous anatomy explains why inflammatory lesions of or adjacent to the optic nerve head cause venous distention and ipsilateral papilledema (optic neuritis), whereas inflammation lying posterior to the point where the vein leaves the nerve produces only visual loss without swelling of the nerve head (retrobulbar neuritis).

Behind the eye the optic nerve passes through the orbital foramen and sphenoid bone to reach the optic chiasm. In the chiasm, nerves from the nasal half of each retina decussate and join the fibers from the temporal half of the contralateral retina (see Fig. 479–1). From the chiasm, the *optic tracts* pass around the cerebral peduncles to reach the lateral geniculate ganglia of either side. At the level of the geniculate, fibers serving corresponding points in each retinal half visual field lie adjacent to each other, and this proximity is maintained in the subsequent relay to the calcarine cortex. The geniculocalcarine radiation initially fans out into superolateral and inferolateral projections, the latter passing around the lateral ventricle and for a short distance into the temporal lobe (Meyer's loop) before turning posteriorly to head for the striate cortex of the occipital lobe. At the occipital pole, the striate cortex (area 17) lies along the superior and inferior banks of the calcarine fissure, with macular fibers projecting most posteriorly to the occipital pole, and more peripheral retinal projections lying more anteriorly. Each occipital pole "sees" the opposite half world. Fibers serving the superior retinal quadrants project to the superior bank of the calcarine fissure, and those from the inferior quadrants project to the inferior bank. No satisfactory evidence indicates that the macula enjoys bilateral anatomic representations in the striate cortex.

DIAGNOSIS OF VISUAL IMPAIRMENT

DEFINITIONS. *Amblyopia* refers to dimness or partial loss of vision, *amaurosis* to blindness. *Scotomas* are errors of relative or complete visual loss circumscribed within a comparatively better total field of vision for the particular eye.

Abnormalities affecting structures lying anywhere from the retina to the occipital pole produce distinctive abnormalities in the visual field. Visual field defects impairing half or nearly half of a field are termed *hemianopic.* Those affecting less than this extent are termed partial field defects, often with the additional designation of *quadrantic* or *altitudinal* (superior or inferior), according to the abnormality. A visual defect that affects similar parts of the right or left half field in both eyes is called *homonymous;* identical errors of involvement from the two eyes are termed *congruent.* Scotomas may reflect abnormalities anywhere from the retina or its projecting pathways to the striate cortex. Most frequently they result either from prechiasmatic lesions of the optic nerve or retina, less often from partial lesions of the occipital cortex. Involvement of the macular area or its projections produces *central* scotomas. Scotomas that lie near the macular visual area are sometimes called *paracentral,* whereas those that extend into macular vision from the more peripheral field may be termed *cecocentral.* Central scotomas always interfere with visual acuity. An uncorrectable reduction in acuity below 20/50 indicates either a central scotoma or a diffuse impairment of the visual pathway of that eye.

Difficulty seeing may arise as a result of local disease in the eye as well as from neurologic disorders that affect tissues extending anywhere from the retina to the occipital cortex. Essential to understanding is a careful examination of the globes themselves, together with ophthalmoscopy and measurements of visual acuity and visual fields.

OPHTHALMOSCOPIC EXAMINATION. One should use bright tangential ophthalmoscopic light to detect any corneal, lenticular, or vitreous opacities. Ophthalmologists routinely dilate the pupil to examine the fundus, but this step should be avoided in acutely ill patients or those suspected of neurologic diseases until one is certain that intrinsic pupillary abnormalities will not be important in reaching a diagnosis or in following the patient's course.

VISUAL ACUITY. Visual function for neurologic purposes consists of the *best corrected visual acuity.* It is best tested quantitatively with refractive errors corrected and for each eye separately. The normal reference is a recognition of letters at an idealized 20 feet, and acuity charts are designed with ever larger letters that normally are recognized at proportionately greater distances. Thus if one reads at 20 feet letters no better than those normally perceived at 40 feet, vision is recorded as 20/40. Small visual charts that are easily carried in the physician's case permit quick and fairly accurate bedside appraisals of acuity.

Visual fields can be tested at the bedside by confrontation, and rough estimates of their integrity can be made even in patients with reduced alertness. With practice and a cooperative subject, accurate confrontation fields can be obtained that even outline scotomas. The examiner should place the test object, e.g., a red match head, midway between his eye and the patient's and test the patient's unilateral visual field against his own. The field should be tested individually for each eye, since the finding of an asymmetrical (incongruous) or symmetrical visual field change represents an important localizing sign.

PATHOLOGIC DIAGNOSIS OF VISUAL IMPAIRMENT

LESIONS OF THE EYE. Corneal, lenticular, or vitreous opacities large enough to produce visual symptoms almost always can be detected by inspection or funduscopic examination. Refractive errors can be distinguished from neurologic abnormalities by the pin hole test. Patients with uncorrected myopia or presbyopia will correct vision to normal by gazing at the test chart through a pin hole in a card held immediately over the eye. The tiny aperture overcomes any aberration created by the failure of the lens to accommodate.

Glaucoma caused by impaired absorption of the aqueous humor results in a high intraocular pressure that usually produces gradual visual loss with reduced night-time vision, "haloes" seen around illuminated lamps, and, often, pain in the affected eye. Uncommonly, rapid visual loss can occur with few premonitory symptoms. Diagnosis comes from the tonometric measurement of a high intraocular pressure and may be suspected by palpating an abnormally firm globe and observing a deep, pale optic cup and attenuated blood vessels.

Retinal tears and detachment give rise to unilateral distortions of the visual image, seen as sudden angulations or curves of objects containing straight lines *(metamorphopsia).* Hemorrhages into the vitreous humor or unilateral infectious or inflammatory lesions of the retina can produce scotomas that in all ways resemble those resulting from primary disease of the central visual pathway.

Serious visual losses due to abnormalities affecting the lower visual pathways tend to affect the two eyes asymmetrically or separately, produce non-homonymous visual field defects, and are prone to interfere with the pupillary light reflex.

Monocular visual loss is due to a lesion of one eye, its retina, or optic nerve. Ocular and retinal lesions can usually be detected with the ophthalmoscope. Most acute or subacute optic nerve disease is due to demyelinating-inflammatory illness, vascular obstruction, or neoplasm. Demyelinating disease of the nerve head (*optic neuritis* or "papillitis") produces papilledema along with loss of central vision only in the affected eye; subjectively unrecognized scotomas sometimes may be found in the other eye. Demyelination in the optic nerve behind where the retinal vein emerges (retrobulbar neuritis) initially leaves a normal-looking disc but a central or paracentral scotoma. Vascular lesions produce either total amaurosis or a sector field defect consistent with an intraocular arterial occlusion *(ischemic optic neuropathy).* Funduscopic appearances are characteristic. Tumors invading the nerve or space-occupying lesions compressing it anywhere between the orbit and the chiasm cause gradually declining unilateral impairment of either central vision (intrinsic or far advanced lesions), or a sector defect of the peripheral visual field. With such chronic lesions, the affected optic nerve becomes visibly atrophic. In doubtful cases, fluorescein ocular angiography, visual evoked responses, or electroretinography can assist in the localizing diagnosis of a prechiasmal or retinal lesion.

Binocular visual loss can result from disease located anywhere along the central visual pathways from the retinas to the occipital poles. Retinal, prechiasmatic optic nerve or chiasmatic lesions are the most common cause of bilateral global visual loss, i.e., amblyopia that involves both halves of the visual fields of each eye. Degenerative diseases of the postgeniculate radiations as well as traumatic, vascular, and rarely neoplastic disorders involving both occipital lobes serve as less frequent causes of such bilateral visual impairments. Most *bilateral retinal disease* producing visual failure in younger subjects is due to heredodegenerative conditions. Vascular diseases, diabetes, idiopathic (senile) macular degeneration, and bilateral retinal detachments are causes in older age groups. In the pigmentary retinal degenerations, visual loss begins peripherally and proceeds centrally and often very slowly before acuity (central vision) is impaired. By contrast, pigmentary macular degenerations affect mainly younger children and impair central vision early in their course. Most of the retinal degenerations produce characteristic and recognizable ophthalmoscopic appearances. With the pigmentary degenerations the visual fields shrink progressively in size. With the macular degenerations, on the other hand, the fields show noncongruent central scotomas.

Acute *bilateral optic nerve* disease with visual loss, although less common than unilateral disease, is caused most often by inflammatory-demyelinating illness, less frequently by optic nerve or retinal vascular disease, or by toxic or nutritional optic neuropathies. In younger persons and those lacking a clear history of toxic exposures, demyelinating lesions overwhelmingly predominate. Symptoms are of an abrupt or subacute onset with visual blurring or loss of acuity which may progress rapidly to blindness within hours or days. There may be pain about the eyes, particularly on eye movement.

Papilledema resulting from increased intracranial pressure occasionally causes visual loss under one of three circumstances: (1) Acute transient episodes of amaurosis lasting a few seconds and attributed to acute rises in intracranial pressure (plateau waves) that interfere with retinal venous drainage into the cavernous sinus or with vascular irrigation of the occipital lobe. (2) Acute bilateral sustained amaurosis following abrupt surgical relief of longstanding severely increased intracranial pressure. This is rare. (3) Progressive loss of peripheral vision with longstanding severe papilledema, presumably owing to pressure atrophy of the most peripherally lying fibers in the tightly sheathed optic nerve. Table 479–1 gives the main differential points between papilledema and optic neuritis.

Subacute or chronic optic nerve disease results mainly from toxic-nutritional causes and the inherited optic atrophies. The latter sometimes accompany spinocerebellar degeneration or selectively affect the optic nerves in both juvenile and adult (Leber's) forms. With either cause, visual loss is moderate or severe and affects primarily or initially central vision; ophthalmoscopy shows mild to moderate primary optic atrophy. (*Primary optic atrophy,* that caused by primary degeneration, retrobulbar compression or demyelination of the optic nerve, is characterized by a pale white optic disc, a reduced vascularity, and a sharply demarcated edge that separates the disc margin from the relatively normal-appearing surrounding retina. *Secondary optic atrophy* follows chronic papilledema and is characterized by pallor of the disc plus superimposed papilloretinal scarring: the disc looks atrophic but more gray, the vessels are attenuated, and the margin between the disc and the surrounding retina lacks clear demarcation.)

Lesions involving or compressing the *optic chiasm* produce nonhomonymous visual abnormalities that affect the unilateral visual fields incongruously (e.g., bitemporal hemianopia). Intrinsic or extrinsic neoplasms and parachiasmal arterial aneurysms are the common causes. Gliomas that arise in the chiasm are rare in adulthood but, when they occur, impair central vision early. Extrinsic space-occupying lesions compressing the chiasm can arise from its superior lateral or inferior aspect and include dysgerminomas, craniopharyngiomas, pituitary adenomas, meningiomas arising from the sphenoid bone, and large aneurysms of the carotid artery. Asymmetrical, lateral (bitemporal) inferior or superior visual field impairments combined with subtle primary optic atrophy are early signs. The patient often is unaware of visual impairment until the deficit encroaches on central vision in one or both eyes.

Optic tract abnormalities are comparatively rare but produce characteristic visual changes. The fibers serving identical points in the homonymous half fields do not fully commingle in the anterior optic tract so that lesions encroaching on this structure produce incongruous and usually incomplete homonymous hemianopias. Mild and sometimes subtle optic hemiatrophy accompanies longstanding tract lesions. Pupillary reactions usually appear normal by bedside testing.

LESIONS OF THE GENICULATE GANGLIA, VISUAL RADIATION, OR OCCIPITAL CORTEX. These most often result from vascular damage, traumatic injuries, neoplasms, or, rarely, inflammatory or degenerative disorders involving the cerebral white matter. Their localization can be deduced by the resulting visual field defects (see Fig. 479–1), most of which are fully congruent, occasional exceptions being observed in the horizontal margins of field defects occurring with temporal lobe lesions. Postgeniculate damage to the visual radiations can go long unrecognized unless hemianopia intrudes on macular vision. Even then, psychophysical adjustments shift the foveal point so that few patients with occipital lesions permanently split the visual image unless the adjacent parastriate cortex is involved.

Bilateral damage to the visual radiation or occipital cortex produces *cortical blindness.* Postgeniculate amaurosis can be differentiated from pregeniculate causes by (1) a normal funduscopic appearance, (2) intact direct and consensual pupillary light reflexes, and (3) the presence of anatomically appropriate lesions by CT scan. When the injury to the visual radiation concurrently involves the right parietal lobe, such patients may be unaware of or even deny the existence of visual loss. Visual evoked response studies will distinguish cortical visual loss from hysteria or malingering if any doubt exists following the CT scan.

Partial damage involving adjacent areas of the superior and inferior banks of the calcarine cortex is relatively rare, but occasionally can follow traumatic or ischemic injuries. Those at or near the occipital pole result in central or paracentral scotomas that are usually but not always hemianopic. Aside from the history and CT findings, differentiation from an optic nerve defect depends on the congruity of the resulting field defect, the absence of pupillary reflex abnormalities, and, often, the results of testing visual evoked responses.

PUPILLARY FUNCTIONS

Neural mechanisms controlling the pupil travel widely through the nervous system, making changes in pupillary activity a frequent clue to neurologic diagnosis.

ANATOMY AND DIAGNOSIS OF PUPILLOMOTOR ABNORMALITIES. The size of the pupil is governed by a tonic balance between sympathetic and parasympathetic innervation of the pupillodilator (sympathetic) and pupilloconstrictor (parasympathetic) muscles of the iris. Sympathetic stimulation widens the pupil *(mydriasis);* parasympathetic stimulation narrows it *(miosis).* Paralysis of either of the innervations results in a near maximal response in the unopposed direction. In the normal resting state, light entering the eye provides the major stimulus governing the size of the pupil; sympathetic mydriasis occurs characteristically as part of the more brief "fight or flight" defense reaction.

Retinal influences on the pupil take origin in the retinal rods and cones with maximal sensitivity in the macular area. The fibers follow the crossed and uncrossed visual pathways to the pregeniculate portion of the optic tracts where the light receptor fibers diverge to the pretectal area located at the midbrain diencephalic junction. Interneurons project from this region to the Edinger-Westphal nuclei atop the midbrain

TABLE 479–1. DIFFERENTIATION OF OPTIC NEURITIS FROM PAPILLEDEMA

	Optic Neuritis	Papilledema
Central-cecocentral visual loss	Present	Absent
Distribution	Usually unilateral	Usually bilateral
Ocular pain on movement	Present	Absent
Direct light reflex	± Reduced	Intact
CT scan of head	Normal	Often abnormal
Visual evoked responses	Abnormal	Normal
Lumbar puncture pressure	Normal	Elevated

third nerve complex of either side. From that point, paired parasympathetic efferents leave the midbrain with the third nerves to travel in the interpeduncular space across the petroclinoid ligament and edge of the tentorium whence, after traversing the cavernous sinus, they enter the superior orbital fissure. In the orbit, the parasympathetic efferents synapse in the ciliary ganglion from which short ciliary nerves enter the eye to reach the pupillary muscles.

The principal sympathetic control of the pupil originates in the ventrolateral hypothalamus (first order neuron), whence fibers descend ipsilaterally to the lower brainstem tegmentum and then the cervical cord, where they lie superficially and synapse with the preganglionic neurons in the intermediolateral cell column of the upper three thoracic segments. Preganglionic fibers (second order neurons) emerge with the ventral roots of C8, T1, and T2, and ascend in the neck to synapse in the superior cervical ganglion adjacent to the base of the skull. Postganglionic (third order neurons) pupillary fibers accompany the internal carotid artery through the skull, leaving it to follow the ophthalmic branch of the trigeminal nerve to reach the pupillodilator muscles of the eye.

Topologic diagnosis of pupillary abnormalities follows anatomic principles. Lesions of one retina or prechiasmatic optic nerve produce no pupillary abnormalities at rest, but light stimulation of the affected nerves evokes an impaired or absent pupillary constriction with an impaired consensual constriction in the opposite eye *(the afferent pupil).* The affected pupil may be slightly larger than its fellow. By contrast, stimulation of the opposite, normal eye elicits a brisk consensual response in the amaurotic eye. Chiasmal lesions produce pupillary defects proportional to the degree that they encroach on fibers of the maculopapillary bundles; pupillary changes are a late sign. Lesions compressing or damaging the tectal region interrupt the afferent light reflex bilaterally to produce midposition or moderately wide (greater than 5 mm) and light-fixed pupils. Pupillary constriction on accommodation is preserved until late stages. Damage to the midbrain tegmentum and third nerve nuclei destroys the preganglionic parasympathetic pupillary control but interrupts descending sympathetic pathways at the same time. The result is irregular, often unequal and fixed, midposition pupils of 3 to 5 mm diameter. Interruption of the emerging third nerve in the ventral midbrain or along the proximal part of its course produces a mid-dilated pupil 6 to 7 mm in diameter. For unclear reasons, injury to the third nerve in the cavernous sinus or anterior to it sometimes misleadingly spares the pupil.

Sympathetic paralysis of the eye with ptosis and miosis (Horner's syndrome) can result from lesions anywhere along the course of the pathway. Topical diagnosis is made best by identifying associated signs in the brainstem or neck or along the carotid artery. Failure of the affected eye to dilate after instilling hydroxyamphetamine 1 per cent indicates a postganglionic (third order neuron) lesion.

Certain pupillary problems may occur in relative isolation. These include *essential anisocoria,* a lifelong difference in the size of the two pupils with normal reflex reactions; the disparity remains constant during constriction and dilatation. *Adie's tonic pupil* is a medium to large (3 to 6 mm) pupil that constricts little or not at all to light and slowly to accommodation but constricts with the instillation of dilute pilocarpine (0.02 per cent) or mecholyl 2.5 per cent. The abnormal pupil is associated with diminished to absent deep tendon reflexes in the extremities. The condition usually affects one eye or occasionally both, is more frequent in women 25 to 45 years of age, and carries no serious implications. Its cause is unknown. *Argyll Robertson pupils* are small, 1 to 2 mm, unequal, irregular, and fixed to light, and constrict to accommodation.Their principal cause is tertiary neurosyphilis, although partial Argyll Robertson changes occur with diabetes and certain of the autonomic neuropathies. Unexplained unilaterally or bilaterally dilated pupils as an isolated finding can result from the accidental or intentional instillation of mydriatics. The recent widespread use of scopolamine skin pads has increased the problem. Failure of the pupil to constrict promptly with pilocarpine 1 per cent gives the diagnosis if the history is withheld.

DISTURBANCES OF OCULAR MOVEMENT

DEFINITIONS. Abnormal, disjunctive eye movements can result from disturbances at several levels. These include abnormalities in the action of the individual ocular muscles, the oculomotor myoneural junctions, the oculomotor nerves and their three paired nuclei in the brainstem, and the internuclear medial longitudinal fasciculus that yokes the eyes in parallel movements. The term strabismus describes an involuntary deviation of the eye from its normal physiological position. *Nonparalytic strabismus* is due to an intrinsic imbalance of ocular muscle tone and is usually congenital. *Paralytic strabismus* results from defects in ocular muscle innervation. Strabismus is called *comitant* when the relationship between the two ocular axes remains constant in all directions of gaze, *noncomitant* when they change, and *latent* when the imbalance is brought out only by covering one eye to prevent fixation. Latent strabismus can become manifest during great fatigue or in association with high fever and systemic illness. Congenital comitant strabismus present at birth or soon thereafter carries with it the strong risk that, if uncorrected, the subject will suppress vision in the nondominant eye during the developmental period when it usually forms its connections with the visual cortex. The result is unilateral, permanent reduction of vision in the nondominant eye *(amblyopia ex anopia).* Strabismus beginning after binocular fusion is developed produces sudden diplopia, which gradually disappears as the subject automatically suppresses the image from the misaligned eye. Postinfancy visual suppression does not lead to permanent visual loss.

Defects in ocular movement resulting from faulty action of the eye muscles or their peripheral innervation from the third (oculomotor), fourth (trochlear), or sixth (abducens) cranial nerves or their nuclei in the brainstem are called *ocular paralyses* or palsies. This contrasts with abnormalities in eye movement on conjugate gaze owing to abnormalities of the medial longitudinal fasciculus or supranuclear structures, which are called *gaze paralyses.*

OCULAR PARALYSES. The *abducens nerve* serves the external rectus muscle. Beyond the nucleus, selective involvement of the abducens nerve anywhere along its pathway inside or outside the brainstem leads to isolated weakness of abduction of the affected eye. Destruction of the specific area of the abducens nucleus in the brainstem damages not only the area that controls abduction in the ipsilateral eye but also the neurons that control lateral conjugate gaze to that side. The *trochlear nerve* serves the superior oblique muscle which intorts the eye and moves it down. Patients with superior oblique weakness often tilt the head in the opposite direction. One usually observes a slight upward deviation of the involved eye in vertical down gaze accentuated by adducting the affected globe. Involvement of the third nerve nucleus in the midbrain always produces at least some bilateral oculomotor weakness; either a nuclear or subnuclear lesion of the third nerve within the brainstem can be identified by the presence of other central neurologic defects that arise concomitantly. Peripheral third nerve paralysis can result from lesions damaging the structure anywhere from its origin from the ventral midbrain to where it enters the orbit via the superior orbital fissure. Depending upon its completeness, third nerve palsy produces a widely dilated pupil, severe ptosis, and an externally deviated eye held in position by the unopposed contraction of the external rectus muscle. In such conditions, the continued trochlear action reveals itself by intorsion of the eye as the subject fixes on an object brought from above to below the horizontal meridian.

ABNORMALITIES OF CONJUGATE GAZE. Conjugate movements of the eyes are regulated by supranuclear pathways that descend from the forebrain to reach the lower and upper ends of the medial longitudinal fasciculus (MLF) in the brainstem. The forebrain pathways direct gaze in response to voluntary action and visual reflex tracking, whereas the brainstem MLF yokes the two globes by reciprocal innervation and inhibition so as to assure normal fusion of the visual image.

Pathways descending from the frontal lobes regulate rapid voluntary and saccadic eye movements. *Saccades* are quick (up to 700° per second), ballistic movements that rapidly change fixation. Stimulation in humans of one frontal gaze area conjugately directs the eyes to the opposite side; acute damage to the same region (e.g., by hemorrhage or infarct) results in 24 to 72 hours of inability to direct the eyes contralaterally. Combined activity of both frontal lobes moves the eyes up or down. Bilateral damage to the gaze areas of both frontal lobes or their descending pathways may produce an inability to move the eyes voluntarily despite preserved visual reflex tracking movements, a condition termed oculomotor apraxia.

Pathways descending from the parieto-occipital region of the two hemispheres subserve slow visual tracking or *pursuit movements*. Visual pursuit movements cannot track faster than 50° per second (vestibulo-ocular reflex movements can track up to 400° per second). Loss of parieto-occipital function impairs smooth following movements reflected in a loss of opticokinetic nystagmus toward the diseased hemisphere.

Best present evidence indicates that pathways from the frontal eye fields descend initially in the ipsilateral internal capsule, then decussate to synapse in the para-abducens conjugate gaze area of the opposite side of the pons. Parieto-occipital eye fields send their impulses via the pretectal area to descend in the brainstem tegmentum and reach the pontine para-abducens region. Pathways from both cerebral areas that regulate vertical eye movements enter the MLF at both the lower pontine and the upper midbrain levels. In clinical situations, lesions at midbrain level more often affect vertical gaze than do those at the pontine level. This is especially seen in *Parinaud's syndrome,* in which lesions impinging on the pretectal area and the midbrain tegmentum interrupt incoming pathways from the light reflex and the cerebral eye fields. The result is wide, light-fixed pupils and a loss of upward gaze, which is at first voluntary and later reflex as well. Damage to either para-abducens area paralyzes lateral conjugate gaze to the side of the lesion. Thus with conjugate gaze paralysis of forebrain origin the eyes "look" toward the lesion, whereas with conjugate gaze paralysis of brainstem origin the eyes look away from the lesion.

The pathway for the MLF lies in the brainstem immediately ventral to the periaqueductal gray matter and decussates just rostral to the abducens nucleus. Lesions of the MLF characteristically produce an *internuclear ophthalmoplegia* (INO) with which the eyes in the primary position at rest may either be parallel or show a mild skew deviation, but move disjunctively in lateral gaze. (Skew results from any of a number of lesions involving the brainstem and has little localizing value.) Characteristic of a fully developed INO is that during lateral gaze toward the side of the interrupting lesion, the ipsilateral eye abducts and shows nystagmus, whereas the contralateral, adducting eye partially or completely fails to move nasally because of failure of ascending impulses to reach the opposite third nerve nucleus. Classically, adduction for near vision convergence is relatively well preserved. Internuclear ophthalmoplegia may be unilateral or bilateral, partial or complete, depending upon the location of the lesion and the degree of damage to the paired MLF structures. Demyelinating and small vascular lesions (e.g., systemic lupus erythematosus, hypertension) are the most common cause of a unilateral INO isolated from other ocular palsies or brainstem signs. Larger brainstem lesions that damage one or more oculomotor nuclei plus the MLF, often produce bizarre combinations of disjunctive eye movements coupled with nuclear oculomotor paralyses. Partial ophthalmoplegia from myasthenia gravis can sometimes resemble an inconstant INO and that disease should be tested for in doubtful cases.

NYSTAGMUS. Nystagmus, a rhythmic to-and-fro movement of the eyes, can be of two types. *Pendular nystagmus* oscillates at equal rates between the extremes of movement, whereas *jerk nystagmus* consists of a slow phase away from the visual object, followed by a quick saccade back toward the target. The two are not always easily differentiated, even with the aid of electronic recordings of eye movement. The deviation of jerk nystagmus is defined by the quick phase. Nystagmus should be described by its direction, relation to direction of gaze, and intensity (i.e., amplitude times frequency).

Nystagmus reflects a disorder or imbalance in a complex neural network that involves the visual pathways, the labyrinths, proprioceptive influences arising from neck muscles, the vestibular and cerebellar nuclei, the reticular formation of the pontine brainstem, and the oculomotor nuclei. The references at the end of this chapter give more detailed consideration. For most clinical purposes the discriminations to be made about nystagmus are whether it is congenital or acquired; if acquired, whether peripheral or central in origin; and if central, whether structural or metabolic in cause.

Congenital nystagmus is present by birth or early infancy and most often but not always relates to primary central visual loss. It may last into adult life, manifests itself equally in the two eyes, appears mainly pendular and horizontal, and produces a diagnostically characteristic wave form on ocular recordings. In most instances the head oscillates reciprocally with the eyes.

Acquired pendular nystagmus in adults most often reflects cerebellar or brainstem disease and frequently possesses a chaotic, multidirectional quality in which the eyes may move independently. Most jerk nystagmus in adults reflects dysfunction of the vestibular end-organ (the labyrinth), the vestibular nerve, or the vestibular nuclei in the brainstem.

Knowledge of the normal responses to *caloric irrigation* of the tympanum aids in understanding labyrinthine influences on eye movements. Warm water irrigation stimulates the ipsilateral labyrinth; cold water irrigation inhibits it (i.e., mimics disease or destruction). In the awake subject, cold water induces fast beating nystagmus away from the irrigation; in the subject with depressed forebrain but intact brainstem function, the eyes move slowly, tonically toward the irrigation but nystagmus is absent. Table 479–2 gives some criteria that help differentiate between nystagmus of peripheral and of central origin.

Purely horizontal fine nystagmus at the extremes of gaze is

TABLE 479–2. CLUES TO THE ORIGIN OF VESTIBULAR NYSTAGMUS*

Symptom or Sign	Peripheral (End-Organ)	Central (Nuclear)
Direction of nystagmus	Unidirectional, fast phase opposite lesion	Bidirectional or unidirectional
Purely horizontal nystagmus without rotary component	Uncommon	Common
Vertical or purely rotary nystagmus	Never present	May be present
Visual fixation	Inhibits nystagmus and vertigo	No inhibition
Severity of vertigo	Marked	Mild
Direction of environmental spin	Toward slow phase	Variable
Direction of past-pointing	Toward slow phase	Variable
Direction of Romberg fall	Toward slow phase	Variable
Effect of head turning	Changes Romberg fall	No effect
Duration of symptoms	Finite (minutes, days, weeks) but recurrent	May be chronic
Tinnitus and/or deafness	Often present	Usually absent
Common causes	Infectious (labyrinthitis), Ménière's disease, neuronitis, vascular, trauma, toxic	Vascular demyelinating, neoplastic

*Reprinted, with permission of the publisher and author, from Glaser JS: Neuro-ophthalmology. Hagerstown, MD, Harper & Row, 1977.

a common finding without pathologic significance. It is more common with fatigue or poor lighting. When bidirectional gaze-evoked nystagmus is prominent or involves vertical as well as horizontal movements to an equal degree, excessive sedative or anticonvulsant drug ingestion is probably the cause.

Several unusual forms of nystagmus have neurologic localizing qualities: *Dissociated nystagmus,* i.e., unequal in the two eyes, implies a brainstem lesion. *See-saw nystagmus* involves the eyes reciprocally rising and falling, then reversing their reciprocal directions. The phenomenon accompanies parasellar tumors or, less often, upper brainstem damage. *Convergence* or *retractory nystagmus* accompanies mesencephalic lesions. *Periodic alternating nystagmus* consists of a horizontal jerk nystagmus that changes its direction periodically. A typical sequence would be jerk nystagmus 90 seconds to the left, followed by a 10-second inert pause, followed by jerk nystagmus 90 seconds to the right, with the sequence then repeating itself. The finding has been associated with a variety of posterior fossa abnormalities, especially those involving the region of the craniocervical junction. *Down-beat* nystagmus produces downward jerks with the eyes in the primary gaze position; it often reflects a craniocervical abnormality such as the Arnold-Chiari malformation, but can occur with parenchymal lesions such as multiple sclerosis. Some subjects have the capacity to induce *voluntary nystagmus,* which is extremely rapid, occurs in short bursts of 10 to 15 seconds or so, is present on the extremes of gaze, and may be unequal in the two eyes. It is doubtful whether cervical disease produces clinically significant nystagmus.

Other abnormalities of conjugate eye movements include *ocular bobbing,* consisting of fast conjugate downward eye jerks followed by a slow return to the primary gaze position. The phenomenon accompanies severe displacement or destruction of the pons or, much less often, metabolic CNS depression. *Ocular myoclonus* consists of continuous rhythmic, pendular oscillations, most often vertical with a rate of two to five beats per second. Often it accompanies palatal myoclonus and has a similar pathogenesis. *Ocular flutter* consists of brief, intermittent, horizontal oscillations arising from the primary gaze position. It blends into *opsoclonus,* a pattern of rapid, chaotic, conjugate, repetitive saccadic eye movements ("dancing eyes"). Both of these disorders usually reflect cerebellar dysfunction, but can emerge as a remote effect of systemic neoplasm, especially neuroblastoma in children. *Ocular dysmetria* consists of saccadic overshoots or undershoots of conjugate eye movement during rapid following of a visual object. It reflects cerebellar dysfunction.

Glaser JS: Neuro-ophthalmology. Hagerstown, MD, Harper & Row, 1977. *An excellent one-volume didactic introductory text.*

L'Esperance FA (ed.): Current Diagnosis of Chorioretinal Disease. St. Louis, The C. V. Mosby Co., 1977. *A well-written and referenced text to diseases of the eye producing visual loss.*

Walsh FB, Hoyt WF: Clinical Neuro-ophthalmology, 3 vols. Baltimore, Williams & Wilkins Company, 1969. *An encyclopedic reference work. Although over a decade old, it provides the most comprehensive analysis to most aspects of the field.*

Zee DS, Leigh RJ: Disorders of Ocular Movement. Philadelphia, F. A. Davis Company, 1983. *An up-to-date monograph that gives the clinical and physiological details of modern investigations on ocular control.*

479.3. Hearing and Equilibrium

Jerome B. Posner

The neural pathways subserving hearing and those most important for equilibrium and spatial orientation are anatomically proximate through much of their course, from their end organs in the inner ear to their termination in the superior portion of the temporal lobe. Because of the close anatomic linkage, disorders that affect hearing often affect equilibrium as well, and vice versa. For this reason, they are considered together here. Despite their major anatomic similarities, there are substantial pathophysiologic differences that make clinical examination of the two systems quite different: (1) The auditory system is physiologically relatively isolated, so that its function and dysfunction can be tested independently of other neural systems. (2) The vestibular system, on the other hand, has many close physiologic linkages with the motor system (particularly the cerebellum, oculomotor system, and the autonomic nervous system) and can be tested only indirectly by noting secondary effects on oculomotor and cerebellar functions. (3) Abnormalities of the auditory system lead only to a few well-defined and unique symptoms, i.e., hearing loss or distortion and/or tinnitus. (4) Abnormalities of the vestibular system may cause symptoms that mimic disorders of other neural structures. Such symptoms include dizziness or vertigo, ocular abnormalities (nystagmus), motor abnormalities (including ataxia or sudden falls), and autonomic abnormalities (including nausea and vomiting and even syncope).

HEARING

Anatomy and Physiology of Hearing

In normal hearing, sound waves are transmitted from the tympanic membrane via the three ossicles of the air-filled middle ear (air conduction) to the oval window, to which is attached the basilar membrane of the fluid-filled cochlea. The ossicles serve to increase the gain from tympanum to oval window about 18-fold, compensating for the loss that sound waves moving from air to fluid would otherwise suffer. In the absence of this system, sound may reach the cochlea by vibration of the temporal bone (bone conduction) but with much less efficiency (approximately 60 db loss). Hair cells lying along the cochlear basilar membrane detect the vibratory movement of that membrane and transduce vibration into nerve impulses. The nerve impulses are relayed via nerve cells that synapse at the base of hair cells and have their bodies in the spiral ganglion to the cochlear nucleus of the ipsilateral pontine tegmentum. Auditory frequency receptors are distributed unevenly along the basilar membrane. Hair cells sensitive to higher frequencies (above 2000 to 4000 Hz) are localized along the basilar turn of the cochlea, while lower frequency receptors are distributed along the full length of the structure. For this reason, partial deafness characteristically affects the perception of higher more than lower frequencies. Within the brainstem, auditory signals ascend from the ventral and dorsal cochlear nuclei to reach the superior olivary nuclei of both sides. Thus, nervous system lesions central to the cochlear nucleus do not cause monaural hearing loss and, conversely, unilateral lesions do not cause deafness. From these structures, the pathway projects by way of the lateral lemnisci to the inferior colliculi. Each inferior colliculus transmits to the other and to its ipsilateral medial geniculate body which, in turn, sends the final projection to the transverse auditory gyrus lying in the superior portion of the ipsilateral temporal lobe.

The normal ear can detect sound frequencies ranging between about 20 and 20,000 Hz, with the upper range dropping off fairly rapidly with advancing age. The ear is most sensitive between 500 and 4000 Hz, in part because the middle ear has a resonant frequency of about 3000 Hz. Normal speech resonates at frequencies of 2000 Hz and below. Standard clinical audiograms test hearing frequencies only below 8000 Hz. The intensity of sound is quantified by decibels (db), a logarithmic abstraction calculated from the smallest perceptible difference in intensity that the normal ear can discriminate. A 30 to 40 db loss (about 100-fold decrease) impairs normal conversation; an 80 db loss is deafness.

Symptoms of Auditory Dysfunction

Only two symptoms result from disease of the auditory system: The first is hearing impairment, sometimes associated with a distortion as well as a decrease in the intensity of sound, and the second is tinnitus, a sound heard in the ear or head not arising from the external environment. Hearing loss is termed *conductive* (external and middle ear), *sensorineural* (cochlea and auditory nerve), or *central* (brainstem and cerebral hemispheres), according to the anatomic location of the abnormality. Most deafness is conductive or sensorineural.

Conductive hearing loss is characterized by equal loss of hearing at all frequencies and by well-preserved speech discrimination once the threshold for hearing is exceeded. With sensorineural hearing loss, the hearing levels for different frequencies are usually unequal, typically resulting in better hearing for low than for high frequency tones. Patients with sensorineural hearing loss often have difficulty hearing speech that is mixed with background noise and may be annoyed by loud speech.

Three important manifestations of sensorineural lesions are diplacusis, recruitment, and tone decay. Diplacusis and recruitment are common with cochlear lesions; tone decay usually accompanies eighth nerve involvement. With diplacusis the tonal quality of a pure tone is distorted so that it may sound like a complex mixture of tones. Binaural diplacusis occurs when the two ears are affected unequally so that the same frequency has a different pitch in each ear, i.e., the patient hears double. Monaural diplacusis occurs when two tones or a tone and noise are heard simultaneously in one ear. With recruitment there is an abnormally rapid growth in the sensation of loudness as the intensity of a sound is increased so that faint or moderate sounds cannot be heard, whereas there is little or no change in the loudness of intense sounds. The inability to maintain perception of a continuous tone presented above auditory threshold is called tone decay. Patients with conductive or cochlear lesions can usually hear a continuous tone for at least 60 seconds, whereas the perception of the tone rapidly decays in patients with eighth nerve lesions.

HEARING TESTS. Hearing may be examined either at the *bedside* or in the *laboratory*. The examiner can test for hearing loss in the speech frequencies by observing the patient's response to spoken commands at different intensities. Higher frequencies can be tested by noting the distance at which the patient can hear a watch tick. Loss of watch tick sound out of proportion to whisper or low speech suggests sensorineural hearing disorders, which often involve only higher frequencies. With the speech and watch tick tests the physician uses his own hearing level as a standard. With tuning forks, the physician can test hearing in each ear at different frequencies and distinguish conductive from sensorineural hearing loss. In the Rinne test, nerve conduction is compared to bone conduction by holding a tuning fork (256 or 512 Hz) against the mastoid process until the sound can no longer be heard. It is then placed one inch from the ear and, in normal subjects, can be heard about twice as long by air as by bone. If bone conduction is better than air conduction, the hearing loss is conductive, but care must be taken to assure that the bone conduction is not heard in the normal ear. In the Weber test, a 512 tuning fork is placed on the patient's forehead or upper teeth. Normally this sound is referred to the center of the head. If it is referred to the side of unilateral hearing loss, the hearing loss is conductive; if it is referred away from the side of unilateral hearing loss, the loss is sensorineural. The Weber test is often unreliable in conductive hearing loss because the patient cannot accept the fact that he hears better in what he knows to be the diseased ear. Hyperacusis and recruitment (see below), two components of sensorineural hearing loss, can often be tested for at the bedside by having the patient compare the pitch and intensity of the tuning fork tone in each ear as it is struck with progressively harder blows.

Although bedside tests are useful in screening hearing loss, more sophisticated audiometric hearing tests are necessary to localize the degree and site of hearing loss with certainty. These tests include audiometry, impedance measurement, and auditory evoked responses.

Pure Tone Audiometry. Pure tones at selected frequencies are presented via either earphones (air conduction) or a vibrator pressed against the mastoid portion of the temporal bone (bone conduction). The minimal level that the subject can hear is determined for each frequency. The *speech reception threshold* (SRT) is the intensity at which the patient can correctly repeat 50 per cent of the words presented. The SRT is a test of hearing sensitivity for speech and should reflect the hearing level for pure tones in the speech range. The *speech discrimination test* measures the ability to understand speech when it is presented at a level that is easily heard. In patients with eighth nerve lesions, speech discrimination can be severely reduced even when pure tone thresholds are normal or nearly normal, whereas in patients with cochlear lesions discrimination tends to be proportional to the magnitude of hearing loss.

Recruitment is usually measured by the alternate binaural loudness balance (ABLB) test (if the hearing loss is unilateral). This test compares the loudness for tones of varying intensity as perceived by the pathologic ear and the normal ear. Recruitment is present if smaller increases in stimulus intensity are required in the poorer ear than in the better ear to maintain equal loudness. *Tone decay* is usually tested by presenting a tone at a prescribed suprathreshold level and asking the patient to respond as long as he hears the tone. Special tests for central auditory lesions assess the patient's ability to understand *distorted speech* or speech that is presented to one ear with a *competing message* in the other ear.

Impedance Measurement. By inserting a probe in the external canal that both presents and measures the sound pressure level of a tone, the acoustic impedance of the middle ear can be assessed. Two types of impedance measurements are routinely used: *tympanometry* and *stapedius reflex measurement*. Tympanometry, the measurement of impedance as a function of ear canal air pressure, is primarily useful for detection of middle ear disorders; stapedius reflex measurements are particularly useful for identifying lesions of the eighth nerve and/or brainstem. The stapedius muscle contraction is measured indirectly by determining the impedance-change induced at the tympanic membrane when the muscle contracts. The reflex consists of (1) auditory nerve, (2) brainstem interneurons, and (3) facial nerve. If the middle ear structures are intact, loss of the stapedius reflex suggests a lesion in this reflex arc.

Auditory Evoked Responses. These can be recorded from scalp electrodes at 0 to 10 msec (early), 10 to 50 msec (middle), and 50 to 500 msec (late) following a click stimulus. The early potentials reflect electrical activity at the cochlea, eighth nerve, and brainstem, whereas the later potentials reflect cortical activity. Computer averaging of the responses to 1000 to 2000 clicks separates the evoked potential from background noise. Evoked responses may be used to estimate the magnitude of hearing loss and to differentiate among cochlear, eighth nerve, and brainstem lesions.

CAUSES OF HEARING LOSS

Conductive Hearing Loss

Conductive hearing loss arises from abnormalities of external or middle ear and can raise hearing threshold no more than 60 db, since bone conduction persists intact. Obstruction in the external auditory meatus (the most common cause of conductive hearing loss) impairs air transmission to the tympanum. This benign condition, caused by *impacted cerumen*, is usually first noticed after bathing or swimming, when a droplet of water closes the remaining tiny passageway. A *fluid-filled middle ear* reduces movement of the ossicles against the oval window. The most common serious cause of conductive hearing loss is inflammation of the middle ear, *otitis media*. Either infected (suppurative otitis) or noninfected (serous otitis) fluid accumulates in the middle ear, impairing the conduction of airborne sound. Since the air cavity of the middle ear is in direct connection with the mastoid air cells, infection can spread through the mastoid bone and occasionally into the intracranial cavity. Chronic otitis media with perforation of the tympanic membrane can result in an invasion of the middle ear and other pneumatized areas of the temporal bone by keratinizing squamous epithelium (cholesteatoma). Cholesteatomas can produce erosion of the ossicles and bony labyrinth, resulting in a mixed conductive-sensorineural hearing loss.

Otosclerosis is a process in which the annular ligament that attaches the stapes to the oval window overgrows and calcifies. It reduces ossicular transmission via the window to the cochlear basement membrane. Seventy per cent of patients with clinical otosclerosis notice hearing loss between the ages of 11 and 30, and there is a positive family history in approximately 50 per cent of cases. The hearing loss is typically conductive, although in some individuals the cochlea may be invaded by foci of otosclerotic bone, producing an additional sensorineural hearing loss. Otosclerosis usually stabilizes when the hearing level reaches 50 to 60 db and rarely progresses to deafness. Other common causes of conductive hearing loss include trauma, congenital malformations of the external and middle ear, and glomus body tumors.

Sensorineural Hearing Loss

Genetically determined deafness, usually from hair cell aplasia or deterioration, may be present at birth or develop in adulthood. The diagnosis of *hereditary deafness* rests on the finding of a positive family history. In many instances the inheritance is through a recessive gene or a dominant gene with low penetrance, making it difficult to determine the genetic nature of the disorder. *Intrauterine factors* resulting in congenital hearing loss include infection (especially rubella); toxic, metabolic, and endocrine disorders; and anoxia associated with Rh incompatibility and difficult deliveries.

Acute unilateral deafness usually has a cochlear basis. Bacterial or viral infections of the labyrinth, head trauma with fracture or hemorrhage into the cochlea, or vascular occlusion of a terminal branch of the anterior-inferior cerebellar artery all can damage extensively the cochlea and its hair cells. An acute, idiopathic, often reversible, unilateral hearing loss strikes young adults and is presumed to reflect either a viral infection or a vascular disorder of the cochlea. Sudden unilateral hearing loss, often associated with vertigo and tinnitus, can result from a perilymphatic fistula. Such fistulae may be congenital or may follow stapes surgery or severe or mild trauma to the inner ear.

Drugs cause sudden bilateral hearing impairment fairly often. Salicylates, furosemide, and ethacrynic acid potentially produce transient deafness when taken in high doses. More toxic to the cochlea are the aminoglycoside antibiotics (gentamicin, tobramycin, amikacin, kanamycin, streptomycin, and neomycin). These agents can destroy cochlear hair cells in direct relation to their serum concentrations and the cumulative duration of drug exposure, causing permanent hearing loss. Some anticancer chemotherapeutic agents, particularly cisplatin, cause severe ototoxicity.

Subacute, relapsing cochlear deafness occurs with *Ménière's syndrome*, a condition associated with fluctuating hearing loss and tinnitus, recurrent episodes of abrupt and often severe vertigo, and a sensation of fullness or pressure in the ear. Recurrent endolymphatic hypertension (hydrops) is believed to cause the episodes. Pathologically, the endolymphatic sac is dilated and the hair cells become atrophic. The resulting deafness is subtle and reversible in the early stages but subsequently becomes permanent and characterized by diplacusis and loudness recruitment. The disorder is usually unilateral. When bilateral (less than 20 per cent of cases), it begins in one ear before the other.

Gradually progressive hearing loss with age is known as *presbycusis*. Presbycusis reflects deterioration in the cochlear receptor system with degeneration of the hair cells, especially at the base. As a result, higher tones are lost early, with audiograms showing a characteristically sharp decline at each successive frequency above 2000 Hz. The recurrent trauma of noise-induced hearing loss affects approximately the same cochlear region and is almost as frequent, particularly among those with exposure to loud military or industrial noises. Loud, blaring modern music has become a recent offender. The increasing tone loss starts initially above a slightly higher threshold of about 4000 Hz but moves down toward speech frequencies with repeated exposure.

Hearing loss from direct damage to the acoustic nerve in the petrous canal occasionally results from abscesses within or trauma to the surrounding bone; severe, abruptly beginning deafness marks the event and is usually associated with acute vertigo due to concurrent vestibular nerve injury. Progressive unilateral hearing loss that arises insidiously and worsens by almost imperceptible degrees is characteristic of benign neoplasms of the cerebellopontine angle, such as acoustic neurinomas. Bilateral gradual eighth nerve deafness is uncommon, but when it occurs it suggests the angle tumors of neurofibromatosis.

Central Hearing Loss

Central hearing loss is unilateral only if it results from damage to the pontine cochlear nuclei on one side of the brainstem. Such can occur with ischemic infarction of the lateral brainstem, e.g., due to occlusion of the anterior-inferior cerebellar artery, a plaque of multiple sclerosis or, rarely, invasion or compression of the dorsal lateral pons by a neoplasm or hematoma. Bilateral degeneration of the cochlear nuclei accompanies some of the rare, recessively inherited disorders of childhood.

Because of the extensive cross innervation of the supranuclear auditory pathways, clinically important unilateral hearing loss never results from neurologic disease arising rostral to the cochlear nucleus. Bilateral hearing loss could in theory result from bilateral destruction of central hearing pathways anywhere along their course. In practice, involvement of neighboring structures in brainstem or hemisphere would usually lead to such severe neurologic disability that the hearing loss becomes an unimportant additional sign. Two exceptions occur: In rare instances, bilateral hearing loss has been reported as an early sign of pineal region tumors, presumably from compression of the inferior colliculi. Most affected patients also have other signs of brainstem tectal dysfunction, including loss of upward gaze. Bilateral infarctions of the anterior transverse gyrus of the temporal lobe may also cause central deafness, but usually it is accompanied by aphasia as well as some involvement of the nearby Wernicke's area in the dominant hemisphere. *Spatial orientation* for sound depends upon the integrity of several of the neural structures and pathways carrying auditory information in the brainstem to, as well as in, the auditory cortex itself. Lesions lying anywhere along this path can impair the function.

Diagnosis and Treatment of Hearing Loss

The physician should perform bedside tests of hearing in all patients, regardless of complaint. Many patients can gradually develop hearing loss in one ear without being aware of it. In others, hearing loss is detected only by some activity that requires a single ear, such as using the telephone. The tuning fork test can usually distinguish conductive from sensorineural hearing loss. Inspection of the external auditory canal and tympanic membrane can often identify the cause of conductive hearing loss. The presence of associated symptoms of vertigo, tinnitus, or pressure or fullness in the ear suggests cochlear damage, whereas those of ataxia and nystagmus may suggest eighth nerve or central damage. A complete evaluation of the patient's hearing loss requires testing by a skilled otolaryngologist using modern techniques of audiometry and evoked potential measurement. Such an evaluation should be carried out whenever the cause of hearing loss is not immediately apparent. The physician is likewise responsible for the monitoring of hearing in patients undergoing treatment with potentially ototoxic agents. Vestibular function should also be monitored, since many of the ototoxic agents damage the vestibular system before or in addition to the auditory system.

The treatment of most hearing loss is usually unsatisfactory and is best left to skilled specialists. If an underlying disorder has not yet destroyed the auditory system and can be ameliorated medically or surgically, hearing may be improved or preserved. Some patients with otosclerosis respond to stapedectomy. Closure of a perilymphatic fistula may improve hearing. Antibiotic and decongestive treatment of otitis media may be useful. The surgical treatment of Ménière's syndrome is still controversial. Some patients with nonreversible damage to their hearing can be assisted by hearing aids. Patients with conductive hearing loss require simple amplification, but those with sensorineural hearing loss often need frequency-selective amplification in order to make hearing aids useful.

TINNITUS

Tinnitus is the term applied generally to noises that arise spontaneously in one or both ears. Tinnitus may be classified as either *objective,* i.e., the patient is hearing a sound arising externally to the auditory system, a sound that can usually be heard by the examiner with a stethoscope, or *subjective,* i.e., the sound arises from an abnormal discharge of the auditory system and cannot be heard by the observer. *Objective tinnitus* usually has benign causes such as noise from temporomandibular joints, opening of eustachian tubes, or repetitive contraction of the stapedius muscle. Sometimes in a quiet room the patient can hear the pulsatile flow in the carotid artery or a continuous hum of normal venous outflow through the jugular bulb. The latter can easily be obliterated by gentle compression of the jugular vein. Pathologic objective tinnitus occurs when patients hear turbulent flow in arteriovenous anomalies or tumors (e.g., glomus jugulare tumor). Objective tinnitus may also be an early sign of increased intracranial pressure. Such tinnitus, which can be obliterated by pressure over the jugular vein, probably arises from turbulent flow of compressed venous structures at the base of the brain. The symptom is also transiently relieved by decreasing intracranial pressure, as for example by lumbar puncture.

Subjective tinnitus can arise from anywhere in the auditory system. The sounds most frequently complained of are metallic ringing, buzzing, blowing, roaring, or, less often, bizarre clangings, poppings, or nonrhythmic beatings. A degree of tinnitus, heard as a faint, moderately high-pitched metallic ring, can be observed by almost everyone if they concentrate their attention on auditory events in a quiet room. Sustained, louder tinnitus accompanied by audiometric evidence of deafness occurs in association with both conductive and sensorineural disease. The phenomenon can be a manifestation of salicylate, quinine, or quinidine toxicity. Tinnitus observed with otosclerosis tends to have a roaring or hissing quality, while that associated with Ménière's syndrome often produces sounds that vary widely in intensity with time and quality, sometimes including roarings or clangings. Tinnitus with other cochlear or auditory nerve lesions tends to be higher pitched and ringing in quality.

Tinnitus without observable deafness appears sporadically and for variable lengths of time in many persons without other evidence of an ongoing pathologic process. In many such instances, one suspects that the auditory experience is no more than an anxious preoccupation with normal auditory physiology. Beyond a careful audiologic examination, audiometric testing, and checking for a history of ingested medications, few diagnostic measures prove useful. Tinnitus may be a very distressing symptom to some patients. Masking sounds (white noise) delivered to the involved ear may give some patients relief, but no treatment removes the symptoms.

EQUILIBRIUM

Anatomy and Physiology of the Vestibular System

The paired vestibular end organs lie within the temporal bones proximate to the cochlea. Each end organ consists of three semicircular canals that detect angular acceleration and two otolithic structures, the utricle and saccule, that detect linear (gravitational) acceleration. Like the cochlea, these organs possess hair cells projecting into a fluid-filled (endolymph) membrane. The hair cells of the three semicircular canals, each of which is oriented at right angles to the others, are concentrated in the ampulla, where they are embedded in a gelatinous mass called the cupula. Movement of the head causes the endolymph to flow either toward or away from the cupula, distorting the hair cells and, depending on the direction of endolymphatic movement, either stimulating or inhibiting their firing. Since the hair cells of the semicircular canal are tonically active, both excitation and inhibition change the rate of discharge. Furthermore, the two sets of semicircular canals are approximately mirror images of each other, so that rotational movement of the head that excites one canal will inhibit the analogous canal on the opposite side. The hair cells of the otolith apparatus, the utricle and saccule, are concentrated in an area called the macula. The macula of the utricle lies approximately in the plane of the horizontal canal and the macula of the saccule is essentially vertical. The hair cells are imbedded in a membrane that also contains calcite masses or otoliths; the density of otoliths is considerably greater than that of the endolymph. As the head is moved, the force of gravity on the otoliths distorts the hair cells, producing firing of these organs.

A discharge of hair cells from either semicircular canals or otoliths is detected by nerve fibers at the base of the hair cells. These fibers have their cells of origin in Scarpa's ganglion. The nerve fibers travel in the vestibular portion of the eighth nerve contiguous with the acoustic nerve. The vestibular portion of the eighth nerve is divided into superior and inferior vestibular nerves. The fibers of the horizontal and vestibular canals as well as the utricle and anterior saccule compose the superior vestibular nerve, while those of the posterior canals compose the inferior vestibular nerve. Nerve fibers from various portions of the semicircular canal terminate in different vestibular nuclei at the pontomedullary junction. There are also direct connections between the semicircular canals and many portions of the cerebellum with the greatest representation in the floculonodular lobe, the so-called vestibulocerebellum. Efferent fibers from the brainstem travel through the vestibular nucleus to reach the hair cells of the semicircular canal and utricles. Efferent fibers are inhibitory in nature and may, like the efferent fibers of the cochlea, have as their function selecting input to which the brain will attend. From the vestibular nuclei, second order neurons make important connections to the vestibular nuclei of the other side, to the cerebellum, to motor neurons of the spinal cord, to autonomic nuclei in the brainstem, and, most importantly for the examining clinician, to the nuclei of the oculomotor system. Fibers from the vestibular nuclei also ascend through the brainstem and thalamus to reach the cerebral cortex, where the representation of the vestibular system is bilateral. The exact site of cortical representation is unclear. Clinical evidence points to both superior temporal and inferior parietal lobes as possible sites.

Symptoms and Signs of Vestibular Dysfunction

The vestibular system is a finely tuned tonically discharging system. Any imbalance in discharge between the paired peripheral vestibular end organs or their primary receiving areas in the vestibular nuclei, if not caused by a true movement of the head or body, produces a mismatch between vestibular input and other sense organs (such as the eyes and proprioceptive apparatus) and leads to an illusory sensation of movement in space called vertigo. Vertigo is the only direct symptom of a vestibular abnormality, but because the vestibular system influences other neural systems, vertigo may be accompanied by autonomic symptoms (nausea, vomiting, diaphoresis), motor symptoms (ataxia, past pointing, falling), or ocular symptoms (oscillopsia—a visual sensation that the environment is moving). Also because of the close interconnection among neural systems, the sensation of vertigo can be produced by abnormalities of the visual or somatosensory system as well as, much more commonly, the vestibular system.

Vertigo may be mild or severe, physiologic or pathologic. *Physiologic vertigo* occurs when there is a mismatch among the vestibular, visual, and somatosensory systems induced by an external stimulus. Common examples of physiologic vertigo include motion sickness, height vertigo (the sensation that occurs when one looks down from a great height), and visual vertigo (the sensation sometimes felt when one visualizes a motion picture of a roller coaster or other violent movement). *Pathologic vertigo* usually arises from an abnormality of the vestibular system but less commonly can be produced by visual or somatosensory disorders. *Severe vertigo* is a sensation usually well described by the patient and easily recognized by the physician. *Milder vertigo,* however, may easily be confused with the lightheadedness of syncope, the unsteadiness of ataxia, and the psychogenic symptoms of anxiety or dissociation.

The major clinical *sign* of a disordered vestibular system is *nystagmus*. Nystagmus, like vertigo, can be physiologic or pathologic. Examples of physiologic nystagmus include optokinetic nystagmus, which occurs when watching telephone poles from a moving train, and rotational nystagmus, such as occurs when one rotates himself in space. Like vertigo, nystagmus can originate from sites other than the vestibular system, particularly the visual or cerebellar systems, and may occur either with or without vertigo. Vestibular nystagmus arises when there is unbalanced input from the two vestibular systems. For example, stimulation of the horizontal canal on the left side increases the output from the left horizontal canal relative to the right and causes a reflex movement of the eyes toward the right. There is a rapid compensatory (non-vestibular) movement of the eyes back to the midline, so that in the awake patient the net movement of the eyes is only a few degrees. In the comatose patient, vestibular stimulation may produce full conjugate lateral deviation of the eyes with only slow return to the midline. Nystagmus is named for the direction of the rapid component. Thus, stimulation of the left horizontal canal which drives the eye slowly to the right with a compensatory movement to the left is called left beating nystagmus.

Tests of Vestibular Dysfunction

Most vestibular problems presenting to the physician are episodic, and there are neither symptoms nor signs when the physician examines the patient. The best test of vestibular dysfunction, therefore, is a careful *history*. The history should attempt to distinguish vertigo (the illusion of movement in space) from lightheadedness (syncope) and ataxia (dysequilibrium of the body without a true movement in space) and from psychogenic symptoms (the feeling of dissociation). If the history is not clear, bedside *provocative tests* to mimic the symptom may assist the physician in making a pathophysiologic diagnosis. *Hyperventilation,* which lowers the P_{CO_2} and decreases cerebral blood flow, causes a "light-headed" sensation associated with syncope. Ask the patient to *hyperventilate* maximally for three minutes to cause lightheadedness. If the episode exactly mimics the patient's symptoms, it suggests that anxiety and hyperventilation may be playing an important role. In addition, during the course of hyperventilation the patient may suffer dry mouth, chest tightness, and paresthesias, which he may then recognize are part of his spontaneous attacks, thus helping in the diagnosis. *Tandem walking* (heel to toe) with eyes opened or closed will reproduce the sensation of dysequilibrium. The *Bárány rotation maneuver* (rotating the patient about a vertical axis 10 times over 20 seconds), caloric tests (see below), and positional tests (see below) can reproduce the symptoms of vestibular vertigo. The physician should also examine the patient carefully for nystagmus. The patient should fix a light in both horizontal and vertical gaze and in both the erect and supine positions. Sustained nystagmus suggests pathology of the vestibular system, and vertical nystagmus suggests that it is central rather than peripheral. Nystagmus and vertigo can sometimes be precipitated by rapid movements of the head in space (*Nylen-Bárány test*). The examiner tilts the seated patient so that the head is hanging 45 degrees below horizontal, with first one ear and then the other dependent. He observes for nystagmus and vertigo. Bedside *caloric tests* in a patient without vertigo or nystagmus at the time of the examination can often reproduce the patient's symptoms and identify the site of the pathology. With the patient lying supine and the head elevated approximately 30 degrees, water 7° C above or below body temperature is douched against the tympanic membrane. In the normal situation, cold water produces nystagmus away from the side of stimulation (because of inhibition of the horizontal semicircular canal) and warm water nystagmus to the side of stimulation (because of stimulation of the semicircular canal). An astute patient suffering from labyrinthine vertigo can often tell which stimulation reproduces the symptoms, thus assisting in the localization of the lesion. Absence of response on one side suggests labyrinthine failure on that side. Because most peripheral nystagmus is partially inhibited by the visual fixation of the open eyes, accurate quantitative evaluation requires electrical recording of the eye movement with the eyes closed. *Electronystagmography* can be performed in the resting position, with the head rotated into various positions to provoke nystagmus, and before, during, and after caloric stimulation. Electronystagmography is often helpful in identifying the pathology of the vestibular system and localizing it when identified.

Causes of Vertigo

PHYSIOLOGIC VERTIGO. Table 479–3 lists some of the physiologic causes of vertigo. In almost all instances, the diagnosis is clear from the history. One exception may be head extension vertigo, a sensation of vertigo or postural imbalance induced with the head maximally extended while the patient is standing. This vertigo is abruptly terminated when the head is flexed to a neutral position. The symptoms may mistakenly be attributed to vertebral artery insufficiency. Physiologic head extension vertigo does not occur when the head is extended in the lying position and occurs only rarely when the patient is sitting. If physiologic vertigo becomes a clinical problem, it is best treated by supplying sensory cues that help to match the various sensory systems. Thus, motion sickness, which is often exacerbated by sitting in a closed space or reading, giving the visual system the miscue that the environment is stationary, may be relieved by looking out at the environment and watching it move. Height vertigo caused by a mismatch between sensation of normal body sway and lack of its visual detection can often be relieved by the patient's either sitting or visually fixing a nearby stationary object.

PATHOLOGIC VESTIBULAR VERTIGO. Vertigo can be caused by disease of either the peripheral or central vestibular apparatus (Table 479–4). In general, peripheral vertigo is more severe, is more likely to be associated with hearing loss and tinnitus, and often leads to nausea and vomiting. Nystagmus associated with peripheral vertigo is frequently inhibited by visual fixation. Central vertigo is generally less severe than peripheral vertigo and is often associated with other signs of central nervous system disease. The nystagmus of central vertigo is not inhibited by visual fixation and frequently is very prominent when vertigo is mild or absent.

PERIPHERAL VERTIGO. *Benign positional vertigo* is an extremely common disorder of middle age that accounts for at least 25 per cent of patients presenting to the physician complaining of vertigo. Typically, the patient first experiences severe whirling vertigo when turning over or first lying down in bed at night. Less commonly, the patient may experience similar symptoms when he sits up from a lying position or when he turns suddenly while standing or walking. Usually the symptoms are most severe when the patient lies on the side of the affected

TABLE 479–3. TYPES OF PHYSIOLOGIC VERTIGO

Motion sickness
Height vertigo
Visual vertigo (e.g., motion pictures)
Somatosensory vertigo
Auditory vertigo
Head extension vertigo
Bending vertigo
Space sickness

TABLE 479–4. CAUSES OF VESTIBULAR VERTIGO

Peripheral Causes	Central Causes
Peripheral vestibulopathy	Brainstem ischemia
Labyrinthitis and/or vestibular neuronitis	Cerebellopontine angle tumors
Acute and recurrent peripheral vestibulopathy	Demyelinating disease
"Benign" positional vertigo	Cranial neuropathy
Ménière's syndrome	Seizure disorders (rare)
Vestibulotoxic drugs	Heredofamilial disorders
Post-traumatic vertigo, metastatic tumor, etc.	Spinocerebellar degenerations
Other focal peripheral disease	Friedreich's ataxia
Infection	Olivopontocerebellar atrophy
Ischemia	Other central causes
Otosclerosis	Brainstem tumors
Perilymphatic fistula	Cerebellar degenerations
Cervical arthritis	Paraneoplastic syndromes

ear. The vertigo is sudden in onset, very severe, and may be accompanied by nausea or vomiting. The patient usually reports that the vertigo ceases when he moves out of the position that causes it, but in fact if he remains in that position, it rarely lasts more than a minute. About 15 per cent of patients with benign positional vertigo report that it followed a head injury, often mild; in most patients there is *no* pre-existing illness. The pathophysiology of the disorder is not established, but some investigators have postulated that debris from otoliths may enter the posterior canal and artificially stimulate that canal when it is in the dependent position. The diagnosis is made by the characteristic history and the reproduction of the attack by the Nylen-Bárány maneuver: With the affected ear dependent, there is a latent period of several seconds during which the patient has no abnormal sensation, followed by the sudden onset of severe vertigo accompanied by rotatory nystagmus when the patient looks toward the dependent ear, and vertical nystagmus when the patient looks away from that ear. The vertigo and nystagmus usually last 30 to 50 seconds and then cease. When the patient sits up there may be brief milder vertigo, with nystagmus in the opposite direction. If the maneuvers are repeated, each subsequent attack becomes less lengthy and less severe until attacks fatigue completely. The illness usually runs a course of several weeks and then resolves but may recur several times over many years. If the patient has the classic history and physical findings, no further evaluation is necessary. If the history or findings are atypical, the condition must be distinguished from other causes of vertigo and nystagmus (see below) and may occur with tumors or infarcts of the posterior fossa. Typical benign positional vertigo is very rarely associated with such conditions. The treatment for most patients is simple reassurance. Since the vertigo can be fatigued, many patients find that repetitively producing the vertigo each day gives them prolonged relief.

PERIPHERAL VESTIBULOPATHY. This disorder, also called acute labyrinthitis or vestibular neuronitis, may occur as a single bout or may recur repeatedly over months or years. Characteristically, the patient has the acute onset of severe vertigo, often associated with nausea and vomiting. This may follow a respiratory infection, but often there is no preceding illness. The vertigo may be so severe that the patient is unable to sit or stand without vomiting or ataxia and prefers to lie absolutely still in bed with the involved ear uppermost, often refusing to move. Nystagmus is invariably present, usually horizontal or rotatory, and directed away from the involved labyrinth. The severe symptoms usually improve substantially within 48 to 72 hours, allowing the patient to be up and about. However, the patient often notes for weeks or months following the episode that sudden movements of the head produce mild vertigo or nausea. The pathogenesis of the illness is not entirely known. Although the disorder is called *acute labyrinthitis,* suggesting a viral infection of the labyrinth, recent EEG and evoked potential studies suggest that in many patients there are accompanying eighth nerve or brainstem abnormalities, leading some to refer to the disorder as *vestibular neuronitis.*

In some patients, attacks (usually less severe) of acute vestibulopathy occur over many months or years. There is no way of predicting whether an individual with a first attack will have repetitive attacks. In the patient suffering from repetitive attacks, the differential diagnosis includes Ménière's syndrome (see above) and otosclerosis. At least 25 per cent of patients with otosclerosis suffer from vertigo. In both of these disorders, hearing tests will be abnormal as well. Labyrinthine fistulae have been reported to produce episodic vertigo. Fistula testing by a skilled otolaryngologist should establish that diagnosis.

MÉNIÈRE'S SYNDROME. Ménière's syndrome is also described on page 2039. The disorder accounts for about 10 per cent of all patients with vertigo. The diagnosis is established primarily on the basis of the hearing tests.

VESTIBULOTOXIC DRUG-INDUCED VERTIGO. Several drugs that damage the auditory system (see page 2039), such as the aminoglycosides, may also damage the labyrinth. The patient may suffer acute vertigo, either along with or independent of hearing loss and tinnitus. Unfortunately, many patients being treated with the drug are bedridden and are unaware of labyrinthine failure until they recover from their acute illness and attempt to ambulate. Then they discover that they are unsteady on their feet, the environment tends to jiggle in front of their eyes (oscillopsia), and they feel vertiginous. Younger patients adapt after weeks to the labyrinthine failure; older patients may be permanently disabled. Usually there is no nystagmus, but the patient is ataxic. Caloric tests may demonstrate absence or hypoactivity of the labyrinth, and the Bárány rotation test may fail to elicit either vertigo or nystagmus. The best treatment is prevention. If the drug is discontinued early during the course of symptoms, the disorder may stabilize or improve.

POST-TRAUMATIC VERTIGO. Head injury may lead to benign positional vertigo (see above) or may produce a more vaguely described, rather constant feeling of dizziness or vertigo, usually associated with anxiety, difficulty in concentrating, headache, and phonophobia. Vertigo in this complex of symptoms called the *post-traumatic syndrome* is probably peripheral in origin, but its exact pathogenesis is unknown. The post-traumatic syndrome often follows a mild head injury, and the vague vertiginous feelings may persist for weeks or months. Reassurance that the patient has no substantial brain damage may help. Vestibular suppressants (see page 2043) can diminish the symptoms.

OTHER PERIPHERAL CAUSES OF VERTIGO. Vertigo may be an additional symptom in patients suffering from *sudden hearing loss.* The pathogenesis of the disorder is unknown but may be vascular. Bacterial infection of the labyrinth or occasionally otitis media causes vertigo. Degenerative and genetic abnormalities of the labyrinthine system can cause vertigo. *Cervical vertigo* is the term given to the vertiginous feelings associated with head movement in patients with cervical osteoarthritis or spondylosis. The disorder probably is caused by unbalanced input from cervical muscles to the vestibular apparatus. Acute neck strain may occasionally be associated with vertigo. Local anesthetics injected into one side of the neck can produce vertigo and ataxia by a similar lack of balanced input. There is no nystagmus in these disorders.

Central Vertigo

Central causes of vertigo, less common than peripheral causes, are usually characterized by less severe vertigo than that resulting from peripheral lesions, no hearing loss or tinnitus, and concomitant neurologic signs of brainstem or cerebellar dysfunction. When central vertigo is usually accompanied by other neurologic signs or symptoms, the localization is strongly suggested by history and physical examination.

CEREBROVASCULAR DISEASE. If ischemia, infarction, or hemorrhage affects the brainstem or cerebellum, vertigo accompanied by nausea and vomiting is a relatively common symptom. Occipital headache usually accompanies the vertigo, and nystagmus as well as other neurologic signs suggesting brainstem or cerebellar dysfunction will be found. Rarely, vertigo is the sole symptom of *transient ischemic attacks* of the brainstem, but most patients suffering such attacks will, if carefully questioned, report headache, diplopia, facial or body numbness, and ataxia as well. However, even in the absence of other symptoms, elderly patients with risk factors for cerebrovascular disease, such as hypertension, diabetes, heart disease, or hyperlipidemia, should be evaluated for posterior fossa vascular disease: Caloric testing and auditory evoked potentials may provide evidence of central vestibular and auditory dysfunction. CT scans with fine cuts of the posterior fossa may reveal evidence of infarction, and digital venous angiography can rule out surgically correctable lesions of the posterior fossa vasculature. For further discussion of the diagnosis and treatment of cerebrovascular disease, see Ch. 494.

CEREBELLOPONTINE ANGLE TUMORS. Most tumors growing in the cerebellopontine angle (e.g., acoustic neuroma, meningioma) grow slowly, allowing the vestibular system to accommodate and thus usually producing a vague sensation of dysequilibrium rather than acute vertigo. Frequently the patient complains of tinnitus, hearing loss, and a sensation that he is being pulled or pushed when he walks. Occasionally episodic vertigo or positional vertigo will herald the presence of a cerebellopontine angle tumor. In virtually all of the patients, retrocochlear hearing loss is present, and responses to caloric tests are decreased or absent on the involved side. Careful CT scans through the temporal bone and posterior fossa usually reveal the tumor. Nuclear magnetic resonance may be an even more sensitive test in these disorders.

DEMYELINATING DISEASE. Acute vertigo may be the first symptom of *multiple sclerosis,* although only a small percentage of young patients with acute vertigo eventually develop multiple sclerosis. Such central vertigo is often accompanied by nystagmus and other signs of brainstem dysfunction. A past history of transient neurologic deficits suggests multiple sclerosis, and CT scan or, if available, nuclear magnetic resonance scan may reveal demyelinating plaques. Oligoclonal bands in the cerebrospinal fluid strongly suggest the diagnosis. Vertigo in multiple sclerosis is usually transient and often associated with other neurologic signs of brainstem disease, in particular internuclear ophthalmoplegia or cerebellar dysfunction. Vertigo may also be a symptom of *parainfectious encephalomyelitis* or, rarely, *parainfectious cranial polyneuritis.* In this instance, the accompanying neurologic signs establish the diagnosis.

CRANIAL NEUROPATHY. A variety of acute or subacute illnesses affecting the eighth cranial nerve may produce vertigo as an early or sole symptom. The most common such disorder is *herpes zoster.* The *Ramsay-Hunt syndrome (geniculate ganglion herpes)* is characterized by vertigo and hearing loss associated with facial paralysis and sometimes pain in the ear. The typical lesions of herpes zoster, which may follow the appearance of neurologic signs, are found in the external auditory canal and sometimes over the palate. Whether herpes zoster is ever responsible for vertigo in the absence of the full-blown syndrome is not certain. *Granulomatous meningitis* or *leptomeningeal metastases* and cerebral or systemic *vasculitis* may involve the eighth nerve, producing vertigo as an early symptom. In these disorders, cerebrospinal fluid analysis usually suggests the diagnosis.

SEIZURE DISORDERS. Patients suffering from temporal lobe epilepsy occasionally suffer vertigo as the aura. Vertigo in the absence of other neurologic signs or symptoms is never caused by epilepsy or other diseases of the cerebral hemispheres.

OTHER CENTRAL CAUSES. Many structural lesions of the brainstem or cerebellum, particularly if rapid in onset, may cause vertigo. In a few instances, *paraneoplastic brainstem or cerebellar degeneration* may present with vertigo, and, as with *brainstem tumors, cerebellar degenerative diseases,* and other structural disease of the brainstem and posterior fossa, there are usually other neurologic symptoms and there are almost always signs of brainstem or cerebellar dysfunction in addition to the vertigo and nystagmus.

Evaluation of the "Dizzy" Patient

1. Try to determine by history (see page 2040) whether the patient is suffering from vertigo or nonvestibular dizziness, e.g., syncope (Ch. 480), ataxia (Ch. 472), diplopia, or anxiety (Ch. 476).

2. Perform a standard physical and neurologic examination, with special attention to heart and blood pressure (orthostatic hypotension or cardiac arrhythmias) for suspected syncope, cerebellar or peripheral nerve dysfunction for ataxia, visual and oculomotor examination for visual vertigo, and nystagmus and past pointing for vestibular causes.

3. Try to elicit the symptoms by provocative tests (dizziness simulation battery).

4. Laboratory evaluation including routine blood studies and chemistries, 24-hour cardiac monitoring, electroencephalography, audiometry, and electronystagmography may be required to establish the cause of the dizziness.

5. If the symptoms are vestibular, decide by the above tests whether the abnormality is physiologic or pathologic. Physiologic abnormalities require little more than reassurance and the use of vestibulosuppressive drugs in appropriate circumstances (see below), whereas pathologic vertigo requires more careful vestibular evaluation.

6. The above examinations should also have indicated whether, if the vertigo is pathologic, it is peripheral or central. Peripheral vertigo that is not typically benign positional or Ménière's disease requires careful otolaryngologic examination, including hypocycloidal tomography and CT scanning of the temporal bones. A search for perilymphatic fistulae should be made. Most peripheral disorders are, however, benign and self-limited.

If the disorder is *central,* neuro-otologic evaluation should include CT scanning of the brain, with particular attention to the posterior fossa. It is likely that in the future nuclear magnetic resonance scanning will be superior to CT scanning in defining lesions of the posterior fossa. Spinal fluid evaluation may also be required. In most instances, careful attention to history, physical examination, and provocative tests will establish the diagnosis.

Treatment

The best treatment of symptomatic vertigo is successful treatment of the underlying disease. In many instances that is not possible and the physician can prescribe symptomatic treatment only. In acute vertigo, such as occurs with labyrinthitis, patients should be, and in fact will insist on being, at bedrest. Vestibulosedative drugs such as meclazine 25 mg 4 times daily or diazepam 5 mg 4 times daily may also be helpful. If the patient is vomiting, 25 mg prochlorperazine suppositories may be helpful. In more chronic vertiginous disorders, the vestibulosuppressive drugs such as meclazine are often helpful. Scopolamine 0.4 to 0.8 mg together with methylphenidate 5 mg orally may give relief of vertigo, particularly motion sickness. Recently transdermal scopolamine paste-on units placed behind the ear have been reported to be effective in the treatment of the vertigo of motion sickness for up to 72 hours. These, like all scopolamine products, may produce anticholinergic side effects. If head or neck movement precipitates vertigo, a cervical collar may relieve the symptoms.

Baloh WR: Dizziness, Hearing Loss and Tinnitus: The Essentials of Neurotology. Philadelphia, F. A. Davis Company, 1984. *A new monograph with sections on anatomy and physiology, clinical examination, and treatment.*

Brandt T, Daroff RB: The multisensory physiological and pathological vertigo syndromes. Ann Neurol 7:195, 1980. *An excellent clinical review of the pathophysiology of vertigo and the clinical findings in patients with that disorder.*

DeWeese DD, Saunders WH: Textbook of Otolaryngology. 6th ed. St. Louis, The C. V. Mosby Co., 1982. *A recent edition of an excellent text, with good chapters on hearing loss, tinnitus, dizziness, and vertigo. The bibliography is good.*

Rudge P: Clinical Neuro-Otology. Clinical Neurology and Neurosurgery Monographs, Vol. 4. Edinburgh, Livingstone, 1983. *A thorough and comprehensive discussion of the anatomy and physiology, clinical assessment, and specific diseases of the auditory and vestibular system.*

480. DISORDERS OF MOTOR FUNCTION

480.1. Asthenia, Fatigue, and Weakness

Fred Plum

The closely related symptoms of asthenia, fatigue, and weakness relate to motor activity in different ways. *Asthenia* is anticipatory, occurring in advance of the act. It consists of an inner sense of usually subacute or chronic lassitude in which persons feel weak before they start or expect that greater than normal effort will be required to perform tasks. Affected persons hesitate to undertake motor activity, fearing that strength or endurance may be insufficient to the requirement. Small reductions in motor power or impaired endurance can be difficult to measure, so that asthenia sometimes reflects the presence of clinically undetectable motor weakness as in mild myasthenia gravis or in the early course of acute polyneuropathy. Similarly, asthenia can be an early, prominent symptom of thyrotoxicosis. The symptom can accompany acute lateral cerebellar dysfunction, presumably due to impairment of neocortical long loop feedback control, and emerges with the complex difficulty in initiating movement that accompanies parkinsonism. Most asthenia, however, is non-neurogenic and accompanies several psychologic and systemic disorders.

Most organically based asthenia has a relatively recent onset and arises in association with other symptoms, signs, or laboratory findings of physical illness. Subacute or chronic asthenia (neurasthenia, formerly called "effort syndrome") contributes prominently to the symptoms of anxiety or depression. Its physiology is little understood. The symptom may be accompanied by signs of autonomic imbalance, including tachycardia, recurrent sighing, multifocal blushing, and inappropriate sweating. Neurasthenia is difficult to treat; affected patients often tenaciously regard their symptom and its accompaniments as expressions of some still-undiscovered organic disease rather than as a reflection of psychologic maladjustment.

Fatigue refers to an abnormal rate or degree of exhaustion during or following motor activity. Abnormal fatigue can be local or generalized and either acute, subacute, or chronic. Many systemic illnesses produce at least briefly a sense of generalized lassitude, purposelessness, and easy exhaustion, including bacterial and influenzal infections, hepatitis, infectious mononucleosis, myocardial infarction, endocrine disorders (e.g., Addison's disease, panhypopituitarism, and hypo- or hyperthyroidism), severe anemia, malnutrition, disseminated malignancy, and anticancer chemotherapy. Fatigue is a prominent symptom of certain chronic neurologic disorders such as parkinsonism and multiple sclerosis. A distressing sense of purposelessness, easy tiring, and lack of initiative characterize the postconcussion syndrome and states of chronic sedative drug ingestion. The managment of such complex mixtures of psychic and somatic reactions provides a major challenge for the physician. It is best to approach the matter directly, as the symptoms are common and easily self-reinforced if not managed effectively in their early stages. *Local* fatigability with a rapid decline in strength after repeated movement of a particular group of muscles is characteristic of myasthenia gravis. Less easily measurable feelings of muscle tiredness also accompany local peripheral motor neuropathy or radiculopathy. Chronic fatigue that remains unexplained by a careful search for systemic or neuromuscular causes often has a psychogenic basis.

Most acute fatigue states have a metabolic or musculoskeletal origin and can be related to a recent illness or to episodes of unusual exercise or muscular hyperactivity. Almost all kinds of muscular or neuromuscular weakness lower the threshold for the exercised part to tire, but persistent somatic fatigue rarely can be attributed to mere chronic overwork. Organically engendered fatigue states are worse in the evening than in the morning. They are accentuated by further activity and typically relieved by sleep. Psychogenic fatigue follows the opposite pattern, being maximal in the morning and declining in the evening as the social pace increases.

Weakness refers to a specific loss of strength in voluntary muscle movement, usually complained of as an inability to complete a specific and familiar act. The symptom can be subtle. Patients sometimes ignore even prominent degrees of weakness until noticed by friends or family ("your foot drags" or "why are you limping?") or brought out by the examiner's tests. The presence of weakness can reflect disease or dysfunction at any level of the nervous system: muscle, neuromuscular junction, peripheral nerve or root, anterior horn cell, descending motor systems, basal ganglia or cerebellum, and even hysteria or malingering. Muscular weakness can develop from locomotor indirect involvement with generalized metabolic dysfunction as with hyponatremia, hyper- or hypothyroidism, certain drug intoxications, and in the setting of starvation or cancer. Painful areas of bone and joint inflammation can induce local, non-neurogenic weakness as a protective response against the further discomfort of movement.

480.2. Ataxia and Related Gait Disorders

Fred Plum

Any neurologic illness that affects sensorimotor functions in the lower extremities can interfere with the coordinated act of walking. Accordingly, an introductory analysis of the differential features of certain gait abnormalities may prove helpful in diagnosis. Other chapters provide descriptions of the well-known abnormalities that characterize parkinsonism, chorea, athetosis, spastic paraparesis, and various forms of poly- and mononeuritic motor weakness.

ATAXIA. Ataxia is a failure of muscular coordination expressed as irregularity or awkwardness of movement. Common usage has applied the term most often to an unsteadiness of walking, but the same principles apply to disturbances in coordinated movements affecting the upper extremities, the speech mechanisms, or even the eye movements. In the literal sense, ataxia can result from any abnormality in motor function, whether induced by faulty peripheral sensory mechanisms or by disturbances of descending corticospinal, basal ganglion, or cerebellar control. Most often the analysis of ataxia as a diagnostic problem lies in distinguishing disturbances in proprioceptive control from those caused by weakness, cerebello-vestibular abnormalities, or the influence of toxic drugs.

PROPRIOCEPTIVE (SENSORY) ATAXIA. Proprioceptive ataxia can result from diseases of the large afferent fibers of the peripheral nerve, dorsal root, or the dorsal spinal funiculus, and less often from lesions of the brainstem lemniscal system or the sensory projection from the thalamus to the parietal lobe cortex. The functional defect results from a variable loss of knowledge of the location of the body part combined with relatively preserved strength in the member. Afferent peripheral nerve, dorsal root, and spinal lesions most often result from inflammatory-demyelinating neuropathy, diabetic neuropathy, syphilitic tabes dorsalis or meningomyelopathy, and any of several inherited forms of spinocerebellar degeneration. Cyanocobalamin (B_{12}) deficiency involves both the peripheral nerve and the dorsal column of the cord, whereas multiple sclerosis and allied demyelinating diseases affect the cord alone.

Nerve or root lesions cause a bilateral defect that characteristically (1) affects the lower more than the upper extremities; (2) involves position as much as or more than vibratory sensation but may sometimes be difficult to verify; (3) shows absent or greatly reduced deep tendon reflexes; and (4) produces a broad-based, weaving gait that with severe sensory loss becomes lurching, sometimes leg flinging, or pounding, and is worse in the dark (rombergism). Spinal dorsal column lesions produce similar symptoms except that position loss may be more profound, the signs may be less equally symmetrical, the tendon reflexes can be preserved, and pathologic reflexes may be present if the abnormality also involves the descending corticospinal tract. Brainstem lemniscal involvement resembles spinal impairment but is seldom bilateral. Position sense loss may outstrip vibratory impairment. Patients with peripheral or spinal sensory ataxia are subjectively well aware of their deficits. They are also aware that their lack of coordination is not due to "dizziness," which distinguishes them from patients with vestibular disorders. Parietal or thalamoparietal proprioceptive impairment produces an ataxia that is usually unilateral and (1) affects the contralateral upper extremity as severely as the lower, (2) disproportionately impairs position sense more than vibration, and (3) may go partially unrecognized or be denied by the patient (anosognosia).

CEREBELLAR ATAXIA. The motor abnormality associated with cerebellar lesions depends on the localization of the abnormality in the cerebellum and on whether or not adjacent or related neural structures are involved. Thus midline, lateral hemispheric, and cerebellar outflow lesions each tend to produce somewhat distinct syndromes. These differences become less typical and more individualized when cerebellar tumors compress the adjacent brainstem to produce additional dysfunction or when diseases such as disseminated sclerosis or spinocerebellar degeneration affect neurologic structures that lie remote from the cerebellum

Spinocerebellar disorders produce a predominantly sensory ataxia superimposed on which is a variable degree of cerebellar dyssynergia, depending on the extent to which specific cerebellar inflow and outflow pathways are affected in the particular disease in question.

Midline cerebellar dysfunction results principally from degenerative (nutritional-alcoholic, remote effects of carcinoma) or neoplastic (medulloblastoma, hemangioblastoma, metastasis) disease. The gait is characteristic with legs thrust widely apart and extended, the arms extended in compensatory balance, and walking accomplished by short steps. Affected patients usually look at the ground for additional sensory stabilization and turn en bloc. With extension into the anterior midline cerebellum, stretch reflexes become hyperactive. In the early stages of the illness, the upper extremities and cranial nerves can be affected little or not at all, even in the presence of substantial lower extremity ataxia. As the disorder advances, truncal titubation appears, as can difficulty in rhythmic movements of the upper extremities and, eventually, even nystagmus. Posterior midline space-occupying lesions may add retropulsion to this symptom complex. It is difficult to be sure whether this last-mentioned symptom emanates from cerebellar or underlying brainstem dysfunction.

Lateral cerebellar hemispheric abnormalities produce ipsilateral hypotonia and incoordination marked by an irregular swaying gait and a tendency to drift toward the side of the lesion. The feet are spread apart, although not so broadly as with midline lesions, and patients characteristically cannot manage close-footed tandem walking. Rombergism is absent, but, as with all ataxias, distorted vision or closing the eyes moderately accentuates the patient's unsteadiness. Rhythmic movements and point-to-point tests are impaired in both the upper and lower extremities. If classic intention tremor appears, it implies that the abnormality includes the outflow from the dentate nucleus or its projection through the superior cerebellar peduncle to the red nucleus of the midbrain.

DRUNKENNESS. Drunkenness, whether due to alcohol or depressant drug intoxication, results mainly from bilateral labyrinthine-vestibular dysfunction and is accompanied by sensations of both vertigo and dizziness. Few patients with cerebellar disease walk the streets with as much incapacity as a severe alcoholic. Severely intoxicated patients reel, lurch, twist, and fall. Lesser degrees of intoxication produce unsteadiness, a tottering, cautious gait with the feet placed moderately widely apart, clumsiness, dysarthria, and nystagmus in all directions.

VESTIBULAR ATAXIA. Chronic unilateral impairment of the vestibulosensory system can occur with lesions anywhere along the peripheral pathway, including labyrinthine destruction by disease or drugs, eighth nerve damage from cerebellopontine angle tumor, or compression, injury, inflammation, or neoplasms damaging the vestibular complex in the brainstem. Patients with such abnormalities tend to drift toward the side of impairment and then quickly correct the deviation in the opposite direction. Turning accentuates their unsteadiness and induces missteps. Bilateral damage to the vestibular nuclei in the brainstem results in a narrow-based ataxia with poor compensating movements in the limbs, drifting or falling to either side, and a tendency to retropulsion and falling backward. Patients with vestibular dysfunction depend heavily on visual proprioception so that closing the eyes accentuates the gait disorder.

SPASTIC ATAXIA. Combined abnormalities of the spinal dorsal columns and cortical spinal tracts produce a characteristic broad-based tottering and sometimes pounding gait with the knees held high but the legs moving stiffly. The condition occurs with demyelinating diseases and other intrinsic spinal disorders such as vascular malformations, cyanocobalamin deficiency, arachnoiditis, and, occasionally, neoplasms.

FRONTAL LOBE GAIT DISORDERS. Patients with frontal lobe disease can suffer any of several gait disorders, depending upon the anatomic distribution of the lesions. Unilateral injury to the foot-leg area of the somatosensory cortex produces a focal monoparesis, whereas bilateral motor-premotor damage results in a relatively narrow-based, stiff-legged impairment, sometimes with scissoring of the legs. More anteriorly placed premotor and prefrontal abnormalities arise in association with deep bilateral tumors, multiple cerebral infarctions, or communicating, "low pressure" hydrocephalus. The ensuing ataxia sometimes (and probably erroneously) is called "gait apraxia." It consists of a severe difficulty in walking or otherwise using the lower extremities so long as the patient is in the erect position. The feet appear glued to the floor (magnet reaction), and attempts to walk often consist of short shuffles or even hops, before the legs get moving. Walking, once (or if) it begins, proceeds as a halting and broad-based movement made easier by guidance or support. Advanced cases may be unable to get underway and, unless supported, increasingly tend to retropulse or fall backward, even from a sitting position. A degree of clinically obvious dementia accompanies the gait disorder.

Patients with frontal ataxia of this type show a greater ability to move their legs on command when lying supine than when standing. Examination of the lower extremities discloses an increased paratonic resistance to passive movements coupled with bilateral plantar grasp responses, extensor thrust responses, and usually accentuated tendon reflexes. These reflex abnormalities and physiologic dysfunctions, rather than the elusive mechanisms of an ill-defined apraxia, best explain the difficulty in movement.

HEMIPARESIS. Both pyramidal-corticospinal and extrapyramidal motor disorders sometimes have a hemiparetic pattern and in their early stages can be confused with one another clinically. Severe spastic hemiplegia from damage to the corticospinal tract or the full-blown stooped, festinating, semishuffling gait of parkinsonism is so well known and readily recognized as to require no discussion. More subtle hemiparesis, however, can easily be overlooked, especially when it reflects the akinesia of early parkinsonism. In their initial stages, both pyramidal and extrapyramidal disorders produce mild or inconstant weakness, a susceptibility to easy fatigue in the affected member, and a sense of stiffness. Both corticospinal and parkinsonian hemiparesis incipiently produce a gait disorder marked by a slack arm and a reduction of other automatic accessory movements on the affected side, a tendency to scuff the toe, and a measure of bodily akinesia. Both may result in an increase in muscular resistance to passive stretch on the involved side; in the early stages it may be difficult clinically to distinguish between pyramidal spasticity and extrapyramidal rigidity. The following points help in differential diagnosis. Patients with early pyramidal tract dysfunction tend to have unilaterally increased reflexes on the affected side. When walking, they flex the wrist and fingers, circumduct the lower extremity, and hold the foot in an equinovarus position. Patients with early hemiparetic parkinsonism, on the other hand, tend to have greater facial and bodily hypokinesia, to stoop, and to show at least some cogwheel resistance on rotary movements of the elbow or wrist. They extend the affected wrist and step the weak foot forward rather than circumducting it. The foot itself is held in simple varus position. The deep tendon reflexes may or may not be slightly asymmetrical.

GAIT DISTURBANCES IN THE ELDERLY. Any of several specific visual, somatosensory, or motor diseases may impair walking in elderly persons. Less easily classified but fairly typical walking difficulties include a tendency to walk with slow, short, mincing, and unsteady steps (marche à petits pas). Fairly common is a stooped position coupled with a moderately broad-based, unsteady gait, sometimes associated with CT evidence of a chronic communicating hydrocephalus (see Ch. 515).

RETROPULSION. A tendency to step backward from the standing position or to fall backward while sitting can be a symptom of several serious, acquired midline abnormalities of the brain. The physiology of the disorder is poorly understood. It accompanies midline tumors of the posterior cerebellum as well as degenerative disorders affecting the central vestibular mechanisms bilaterally, and has been reported in association with bilateral lesions affecting the sides of the third ventricle, the basal ganglia, and the frontal lobes. Occasionally the abnormality is associated with large, unilateral frontal lobe neoplasms that produce an increase in intracranial pressure and intracranial shift. Retropulsion of posterior fossa origin is especially dangerous, as it often comes on suddenly and is accompanied by a loss of the normal postural protective mechanisms that guard against injury during falling.

HYSTERICAL GAIT. Hysteria can mimic a variety of hemiparetic, steppage, or ataxic gait disorders. With a hemiparetic type, the pattern usually gives itself away by an atypical dragging behind of the affected leg during a series of hops or supported steps. The most obviously factitious hysterical disorder is a lurching, irregularly based, sometimes bent-forward walk in which the patient grasps any object in reach for support and reels from side to side inconsistently. Such patients may sink to the floor, but almost never endure an unsupported, self-injuring fall. Signs of altered muscular tonus or abnormal reflexes are absent, and the bizarre movements not only differ from the expected pattern of sensory or cerebellar dysfunction but often change from examination to examination.

De Jong RN, Magee KR: The Neurological Examination. 4th ed. Hagerstown, MD, Harper & Row, 1979. *A comprehensive text with detailed references.*

Garcin R: Coordination of voluntary movement and the ataxias. *In* Vinken PJ, Bruyn GW, Garcin R (eds.): Handbook of Clinical Neurology, Vol 1, Disturbances of Nervous Function. Amsterdam, North Holland, 1969, pp 293, 309. *A detailed and thoughtful exposition of clinical and physiologic principles.*

Kremer M: Sitting, standing and walking. Br Med J 2:63, 1958. *A succinct and readable analysis.*

480.3. Episodic Loss of Motor Function

Jerome B. Posner

Motor disorders cause paralysis, usually accompanied by alterations in muscle tone. In most instances, the weakness is either persistent or progressive. Sometimes, however, patients report episodic loss of motor function affecting one or more extremities which, although severe, is brief in duration and followed by a return to normal. Such episodic loss of motor function can be caused by a variety of pathophysiologic abnormalities. Because the symptoms are episodic, the patient is usually entirely normal when he presents to the physician; therefore, preliminary diagnosis depends on obtaining an accurate description of the event. The paragraphs below describe the potential causes of episodic loss of motor function. Individual disorders are described in detail under pertinent headings in other chapters.

Drop Attacks

PATHOPHYSIOLOGY. The most perplexing diagnostic problem associated with episodic loss of motor function is the so-called drop attack. A patient, usually in the later decades of life, who is standing or walking suddenly falls to the ground. In a classic drop attack, the patient does not lose consciousness, has not tripped or otherwise lost his balance, and is able to resume normal activity immediately or shortly following the fall. Affected persons suffer no accompanying neurologic signs but often fall with sufficient suddenness and force to cause injury.

Pathophysiologically, drop attacks without loss of consciousness occur when tonic, long loop, posture-controlling discharges from the central nervous system to extensor muscles of the leg transiently cease. The sudden loss of anterior horn or corticospinal tract function may result from direct damage to these structures, leading to transient paralysis, or from removal of tonic facilitation of these structures, leading to sudden failure of muscle tone. *Transient ischemia* can produce drop attacks when motor pathways are involved bilaterally. Such an event is likely only when the transient ischemia occurs in the distribution of either the anterior spinal or the vertebrobasilar arterial system. Episodic spinal cord ischemia is usually accompanied by sensory as well as motor changes, and the patient may be able to report a level of sensory change that localizes the dysfunction to the thoracic or lumbar spinal cord. Vertebrobasilar insufficiency may cause drop attacks as the only symptom, but more commonly the patient suffers other signs of brainstem ischemia (Ch. 494). The only detailed autopsy report of a patient with drop attacks shows infarction affecting the corticospinal tracts in the lower pons and upper medulla.

All drop attacks, however, do not have the implication of severe spinal or brainstem ischemia. *Cryptogenic drop attacks* occur in many middle-aged and elderly individuals whose evaluation reveals no evidence of either cardiac or central nervous system vascular disease. The attacks may occur episodically for months or years without the development of other nervous system disease. Although they are not rare, nothing is known of the pathophysiology of these drop attacks.

Cataplexy, the sudden loss of motor tone without paralysis or change in consciousness, is an occasional cause of drop attacks. The fall to the ground is usually slower than with the classic drop attack, and the patient rarely hurts himself. Cataplexy is thought to be a fragment of the loss of motor tone that occurs normally during REM sleep and usually occurs as a part of the narcolepsy syndrome (Ch. 472.5). Occasionally cataplexy occurs as an isolated symptom of the sudden rises of intracranial pressure (*plateau waves*) that sometimes accompany brain tumors or hydrocephalus (Ch. 515). Because there are important connections between the vestibular system and pathways controlling muscle tone, sudden *vestibular failure* can cause drop attacks. Such episodes are almost always accompanied by vertigo and usually by nausea and vomiting as well. *Akinetic* or *myoclonic seizures* causing drop attacks are common in childhood but rare in the adult. However, drop attacks occasionally have been reported in adults that appear to be epileptic in origin and respond to anticonvulsant drugs.

DIAGNOSIS. The first task for the physician in the differential diagnosis of drop attacks is to determine whether the patient was truly unconscious at any time throughout the episode. If unconsciousness is known or reasonably suspected, the first diagnosis should be syncope and the diagnostic evaluation directed toward that disorder (Ch. 472.4). If it is clear that the patient is conscious throughout the episodes and that the disorder cannot be attributed to tripping or loss of balance, the physician should probe carefully for accompanying symptoms or signs that may help to localize the cause. Back pain, lower extremity paresthesias or sensory loss, or sudden changes in bladder or bowel function accompanying the drop attacks suggest spinal cord dysfunction. Headache, diplopia, and dysarthria accompanying the attack suggest brainstem dysfunction, probably caused by vertebrobasilar arterial insufficiency. Tinnitus or vertigo suggests vestibular dysfunction. Severe headache, particularly if accompanied by nausea and vomiting, suggests plateau waves from increased intracranial pressure.

A CT scan will rule out a brain tumor or hydrocephalus leading to plateau waves. In the absence of demonstrated syncope or a cause of increased intracranial pressure, the most serious potential diagnosis is vertebrobasilar transient ischemic attacks. Patients in whom no other diagnosis can be made should be considered to have cerebral vascular disease and be so treated until proved otherwise (Ch. 493). In many patients, however, no diagnosis can be made and no definitive treatment prescribed. Elderly patients with drop attacks not due to cerebral vascular disease sometimes benefit by carrying a cane, which may prevent or lessen the force of the fall. Patients in whom no diagnosis can be made should probably be evaluated by electroencephalography and be considered for a trial of anticonvulsant agents.

Other Transient Paralyses

Episodic loss of motor function in one or more extremities can be a perplexing problem. Affected patients may complain of sudden or rapid loss of motor function involving an arm or a leg or both, with or without associated sensory symptoms, but without abnormal motor movements of either the arm or the leg. Several pathophysiologic abnormalities can cause such symptoms, and these abnormalities may be clinically indistinguishable from each other. The first and most common is a *transient ischemic attack* from vascular insufficiency in the distribution of the internal carotid artery. All patients suffering episodic loss of motor function on one side of the body should be considered to be suffering from transient ischemic attacks until proved otherwise. Other, less common, causes of transient loss of motor function include *plateau waves* associated with increased intracranial pressure, *nonconvulsive epileptic attacks,* and *late-life complicated migraine.* In transient ischemic attacks and plateau waves, there is usually sudden loss of motor function lasting 5 to 15 minutes and, in the instance of plateau waves, often an accompanying headache and sometimes some clouding of consciousness; with atonic seizures and migraine, the onset of motor dysfunction is usually but not always slower, but it too persists for 5 to 20 minutes. The motor weakness in late-life migraine may or may not be accompanied by a contralateral headache that appears as the motor change disappears. Patients with transient ischemic attacks or plateau waves also may have headaches at times indistinguishable from migraine.

Since the four entities may be clinically indistinguishable from each other, all must be considered in the differential diagnosis of episodic weakness. A CT scan establishes the presence and causes of increased intracranial pressure and plateau waves; digital venous angiography often establishes the initiating cause of transient ischemia as lying in the carotid or basilar artery distribution; electroencephalography may assist in the diagnosis of a seizure disorder, but the EEG is often normal between episodes. A past or family history of migraine assists in the diagnosis of late-life migraine but is not diagnostic. Therapeutic trials directed successively at treatment of the several causes of these episodic attacks sometimes help in reaching a definitive diagnosis.

481. DISORDERS OF SENSATION

Jerome B. Posner

MAJOR SENSORY PATHWAYS AND SYMPTOMS

An organism perceives its environment through its sensory systems. The sensory systems can be divided roughly into three physiologic entities: *special sensation,* including smell, vision, hearing, equilibrium, and taste (see Ch. 479); the *exteroceptive* or somatosensory system, which perceives environmental influences directly contacting the organism, including the sensations of pressure, touch, temperature, and pain; and the *enteroceptive* system, which senses the internal environment, including both consciously perceived pressure and pain sensation and unconsciously perceived alterations of osmolality, chemistry (aortic and carotid chemoreceptors, glycoreceptors, etc.), and pressure (cardiovascular baroreceptors). *Proprioception,* only some of which is perceived consciously, includes special sensation (vestibular system), exteroceptive receptors (joint position sense), and enteroceptive receptors (muscle sensation). When portions of the sensory system are diseased, the organism no longer accurately perceives its environment and thus cannot interact with it to full effect.

When the sensory system is disordered, sensation may be diminished, increased, or distorted. In the exteroceptive system, diminution or absence of function is called *hypesthesia* or *anesthesia*, respectively. Diminution or loss of pain sensation is called *hypalgesia* or *analgesia;* diminution or loss of temperature sensation, *thermhypesthesia* or *thermanesthesia,* etc. Hyperfunction of the exteroceptive sensory system is characterized either by a lowered threshold to stimulation (hyperesthesia), a phenomenon that occurs in some instances of physical (e.g., sunburn) or chemical abnormalities of cutaneous receptors, or by spontaneous discharge, leading to pins and needles or burning sensations that may or may not be painful (*paresthesias*). Distortion of sensory input leads to *dysesthesias,* usually an unpleasant or painful sensation produced by a stimulus that is ordinarily painless, or to hyperpathia. *Hyperpathia* follows damage to the sensory system that elevates the threshold of perception of noxious stimuli, but once that threshold is exceeded, a severely painful or unpleasant sensation is the response to what would normally be only a modestly unpleasant stimulus. *Causalgia* is a condition in which both painful paresthesias and hyperpathia exist and are characterized by a sense of burning pain.

Anatomy and Physiology of Sensory Pathways

Two major sensory pathways subserve both exteroception and conscious proprioception. The first pathway subserves the sensations of pain, temperature, and crude touch. It begins as free nerve endings of small myelinated and unmyelinated fibers. "Free nerve endings" have never been identified microscopically, nor is there complete agreement on the adequate stimulus for discharging these receptors, but current studies suggest that mechanical deformation and hot and cold are the important stimuli.

The receptors are connected to small (5 μ), thinly myelinated, "A delta" fibers, which conduct at about 35 meters per second, and to unmyelinated "C" fibers (1 to 2 μ), which conduct at about 0.5 meter per second. This dual set of fibers explains the phenomenon of "double pain." A noxious stimulus elicits first a sharp, pricking, well-localized pain mediated by the more rapidly conducting fibers, and the C fibers mediate a burning, poorly localized, exceedingly unpleasant "second pain."

All primary sensory afferents have their cell bodies in the dorsal root ganglion, but the small fibers of the first pathway enter the spinal cord via the dorsal root, lateral to the large myelinated (touch and proprioception) fibers, and then ascend or descend for one or two segments in the medial portion of Lissauer's tract to enter the more ventrally placed dorsal horn.

After synapsing in the dorsal horn, the ascending pain pathways in the spinal cord divide into two groups: the neospinothalamic tract, which is believed to subserve the perception of intensity and localization of pain, temperature, and crude touch, and the phylogenetically older paleospinothalamic tract, which is believed to subserve the arousal and emotional components of pain. The axons of the neospinothalamic tract arise from the dorsal horn, cross the anterior commissure, and ascend in the anterolateral quadrant of the spinal cord. The axons terminate in the ventral basal complex of the thalamus, principally within the ventral posterolateral nucleus (VPL) ipsilateral to the side of their ascent. The thalamic terminations of these fibers coincide to a large extent with those of the dorsal column, and the pathway shows somatotopic localization at the thalamic level, the face and upper body being represented most medially. Third order neurons from the thalamus project to somatosensory area 1 (sensorimotor cortex), with the same somatotopic localization as other sensory modalities. Lesions at the thalamic level often lead to chronic so-called "thalamic pain." The paleospinothalamic tract, whose cells of origin in the dorsal horn receive C fiber input, also crosses in the anterior commissure and ascends in the spinal cord closely applied to but more ventral than the neospinothalamic tract. Many of the fibers of the paleospinothalamic tract send collaterals to the reticular formation of the brainstem, but some reach the thalamus, terminating in several nuclei, particularly the nucleus centralis lateralis and the intralaminar nuclei.

The second system consists predominantly of larger myelinated fibers and subserves the functions of light touch, position sense, and tactile localization. The anatomy and physiology of the peripheral portion of this second pathway is described in Ch. 525. The central nervous system part begins where these large fibers enter the spinal cord via the dorsal root ganglion, lying in a position medial to the smaller fibers that subserve pain and temperature. Most of the large fibers ascend without synapsing in the posterior and to a lesser extent lateral columns of the spinal cord to reach the gracile and cuneate nuclei in the low brainstem. Second order neuron fibers then decussate and ascend in the medial lemniscus through the brainstem to reach the contralateral ventral posterior lateral nucleus of the thalamus. Third order neurons projected from the thalamus terminate in the cerebral cortex, prodominantly in the sensorimotor strip surrounding the Rolandic fissure. Lesions of this system lead to loss of sense of position of the limbs and body in space, inability to localize tactile stimuli or to distinguish between one and two closely placed stimuli (two-point discrimination), and inability to describe accurately the size, shape, and texture of objects (stereoanesthesia). Subcortical lesions of the system also cause loss of the ability to recognize vibratory sensation (pallesthesia).

The two major exteroceptive systems are anatomically separated through much of their course, particularly in the spinal cord, and they differ physiologically as a result of fiber size. Thus, lesions at different sites in the nervous system and lesions of different physiologic natures cause unique sensory syndromes that assist in localizing the site and nature of the disorder. Some of these syndromes are described in detail in other chapters. The paragraphs below describe the symptoms that help physicians localize sensory disorders, and the next section details the pathophysiology and clinical findings of common pain problems.

Localization of Sensory Disorders

PERIPHERAL NERVES. Sensory perception begins when a physical or chemical stimulus alters the activity of a *sensory receptor* in such a way that the stimulus is transduced into an electrical potential (receptor potential). If the potential is large enough, the nerve to which the receptor is connected will discharge and the stimulus will eventually reach the central nervous system. There are a wide variety of receptors, each of which transduces one of the physical and chemical stimuli that the organism is capable of perceiving. These receptors range from free nerve endings in the skin (touch, pressure, pain) to the highly specialized photoreceptors of the retina and the hair cells of the auditory and vestibular system. Certain degenerative diseases can affect the receptors in the eye or the ear, but no known disorders exist that affect receptors of the somatosensory system. Thus, the most peripheral disorders of the somatosensory system occur either in the axon itself (axonal neuropathy) or in the myelin sheath encasing the axon (Ch. 525). Many diseases of peripheral nerves affect both large and small fibers, leading to a diminution of all sensory modalities to approximately equal degree. In some disorders of peripheral nerves, however, small or large fibers can be involved preferentially, leading to a "dissociated sensory loss." When small fibers are predominantly affected, one finds pin and temperature sensation involved out of proportion to light touch, vibration, and position sense. Because autonomic fibers are also small, trophic changes in skin and joints may accompany such a small fiber peripheral neuropathy, but because motor fibers and the afferent portion of the stretch reflex are subserved by large fibers, these functions are relatively preserved despite sometimes profound loss of pain and temperature sensation. Such selective small fiber damage is sometimes encountered in diabetes and is common in some of the hereditary neuropathies as well as in toxic-nutritional neuropathies (Ch. 528 to 530). Large fiber loss is more common in demyelinating neuropathies and may lead to profound loss of localizing touch and proprioception, with relative preservation of crude touch, pin, and temperature sensation. Such disorders are commonly accompanied by paresthesias and sometimes spontaneous pain. The deep tendon reflexes are absent because of damage to large afferent fibers from muscle, and there is usually weakness as well. The diagnosis of a peripheral neuropathy involving sensory fibers is established by the distribution of the sensory loss, which may be in the distribution of a single nerve, multiple individual nerves (mononeuritis multiplex), or a symmetrical distal stocking-and-glove distribution (polyneuropathy). Polyneuropathies are distributed distally because longer axons are more vulnerable to disease than shorter ones. In general, mononeuropathies are caused by local disease (e.g., compression entrapment), mononeuritis multiplex by vascular disorders (e.g., polyarteritis), and polyneuropathies by immunologic or metabolic disorders (e.g., demyelination-inflammatory neuropathy, diabetes, uremia, nutritional neuropathy).

SPINAL CORD. True dissociation of sensory loss is more common in spinal cord disorders than in those originating in peripheral nerves or roots. Lesions of the posterolateral columns produce profound loss of position and vibration sense with normal crude touch, pin, and temperature sensation. Usually corticospinal tracts are involved as well as sensory pathways, and thus most such patients often have hyperactive reflexes and extensor plantar responses. Lesions of the spinothalamic tract or of crossing fibers from the posterior horn to the spinothalamic tract cause loss of pain and temperature sense with preservation of vibration, position, and localizing touch. Such dissociated sensory loss is common in syringomyelia and may occur with infarction of the anterior portion of the spinal cord from occlusion of the anterior spinal artery. In both of these disorders, motor function may be relatively well preserved. When only one side of the spinal cord is involved, one finds loss of proprioceptive sensation on the ipsilateral side and loss of pin and temperature sensation on the contralateral side, both below the level of the lesion. There is usually a small band of decreased sensation to all modalities resulting from damage to the posterior horn at the level of the lesion. This so-called Brown-Séquard syndrome is sometimes seen with tumors either compressing or invading the spinal cord and is a common presenting syndrome in radiation myelopathy. Lesions of the spinal cord are rarely confused with those of peripheral nerves, even when the latter show dissociated sensory loss, because the sensory loss in spinal cord lesions is usually proximal as well as distal and restricted to those segments below the spinal cord level damaged. Thus, by the time a polyneuropathy causes substantial sensory loss above the knees, nerve fibers supplying the fingertip are usually involved as well, whereas with a thoracic spinal cord lesion the arms are always spared. Furthermore, motor signs of upper motor neuron disease, particularly extensor plantar responses, usually correctly identify the central nature of a spinal cord disorder rather than pointing to a peripheral disturbance.

BRAINSTEM. In the lower brainstem, spinothalamic and proprioceptive pathways remain separated, lateral lesions of the medulla causing loss of pin and temperature sensation on the ipsilateral side of the face (a result of damage to the descending root of the trigeminal nerve) and the contralateral side of the body. This sensory abnormality is usually accompanied by other signs of lateral medullary damage (Wallenberg's syndrome) and spares proprioceptive pathways. Higher in the brainstem, as the two pathways converge in their route toward the thalamus, damage causes contralateral sensory loss to all modalities, usually accompanied by cranial nerve palsies, ataxia (from the cerebellar outflow), and motor weakness.

CEREBRUM. In the thalamus, damage to the ventral posterolateral nucleus causes decreased sensation of all modalities on the contralateral side of the body and face. Sensory loss is often accompanied by dysesthesias. A curious *thalamic syndrome* often appears four to six weeks after acute thalamic damage and has been attributed to denervation hypersensitivity of sensory neurons in the midbrain reticular formation. The patient develops spontaneous pain in the distribution of the sensory loss, usually associated with a dysesthetic response to touch and a hyperresponsiveness to pinprick once threshold is exceeded. The thalamic syndrome is rare but causes a particularly unpleasant pain intractable to most therapeutic endeavors. Conversely, surgical lesions of the intralaminar nuclei, which receive fibers from the paleospinothalamic tract, often decrease pain without affecting sensory thresholds.

Damage to the cerebral cortex causes sensory loss in which the synthetic qualities of sensation are involved out of proportion to crude sensation. Pain sensation is usually preserved, although the patient may describe a pin as feeling less sharp on the involved side. The distribution of sensory impairment follows the sensory homunculus. Depending on the cortical location of the lesion within that distribution, touch and vibration are usually relatively preserved as well. Position sense loss is often profound; the patient is unable to distinguish between one and two points touching the finger or foot, and cutaneous sensations, even though identified, may not be localized. Patients may be unable to identify the nature of an object placed in their hands, even though they are able to describe certain of its qualities (astereognosis). Patients with large cortical sensory lesions are often relatively inattentive to sensation from the contralateral side of the body, particularly if there is a distracting stimulus to the ipsilateral side. Thus, the patient presented with two symmetrical cutaneous sensory stimuli may fail to identify the one contralateral to the cortical lesion even though the strength of the stimulus exceeds threshold (extinction). With less severe damage, if two nonhomologous stimuli are presented (as, for example, to left hand and right face), the patient may perceive the stimulus on the involved side as occurring homologous to the stimulus on the uninvolved side ("You touched both sides of my face"). Such extinction phenomena are characteristic of parietal lobe lesions, particularly in the nondominant hemisphere. Smaller or more restricted lesions of the parietal lobe may lead to subtle changes in sensory function, with only synthetic modalities such as stereognosis, two-point discrimination, and graphesthesia (ability to identify numbers or letters traced on the palm or fingertip) involved.

PAIN

Pain is the most common symptom for which patients seek medical assistance, and chronic pain is among the most vexing problems which physicians face. Pain can have no precise definition because only the individual suffering it, not the observer, perceives it. Sir Thomas Lewis described the situation exactly when he said pain is "known to us by experience and described by illustration." Pain always has two aspects: the first is an emotionally neutral perception of a stimulus which is usually sufficiently strong to produce tissue damage; the second is an affective response to the perception of that stimulus. Pain implies damage to the organism, either physical or psychologic, and chronic pain, if untreated, will itself damage the organism. It is the physician's two-fold therapeutic task to discover and treat the cause of pain and also to treat the pain itself, whether or not the underlying cause is treatable.

Diagnosis of Painful Disorders

Pain is either "acute" or "chronic." The point at which acute pain becomes chronic pain varies, but pain of over six months' duration is usually considered chronic. Several clinical features differentiate acute from chronic pain. Patients suffering from severe acute pain can usually give a clear description of its location, character, and timing. Furthermore, objective signs, particularly of autonomic nervous system hyperactivity, with tachycardia, hypertension, diaphoresis, midriasis, and pallor, are present. Acute pain usually responds well to analgesic agents, and psychologic factors often play a minor role in its pathogenesis. By contrast, in patients suffering from chronic pain, the localization, character, and timing of the pain are more vague, and because the autonomic nervous system adapts, signs of autonomic hyperactivity disappear. Furthermore, chronic pain usually responds less well to analgesic agents, and psychologic factors are more important than in acute pain. All of these factors may lead the physician to believe that the patient's complaints are exaggerated. Since there are no reliable objective tests to assess chronic pain, the physician *must* believe the patient's report, taking into consideration his age, his cultural background, his environment, and other psychologic circumstances known to alter reaction to pain. *In general, the physician is wise to accept at face value the patient's report of the severity of his pain unless there is overwhelming evidence to the contrary.*

For purposes of classification by pathogenesis, chronic pain can be divided into three categories, although the physician should realize that there is much overlap among these categories. The first is chronic pain associated with structural disease. Such pain occurs with rheumatoid arthritis, metastatic cancer, or sickle cell anemia, and may be characterized by prolonged episodes of pain alternating with pain-free intervals, or by unremitting pain waxing and waning in severity. Psychologic factors may play an important role in exacerbating or relieving pain, but treatment of the pain by analgesics or therapy directed to the underlying disease is usually more helpful. The second group of patients suffers from psychophysiologic disorders causing pain. In these patients, structural disease such as a herniated disc or torn ligaments may once have been present, but psychologic factors have engendered chronic physiologic alterations such as muscle spasm, which produces pain long after the underlying deficit has healed. Such patients tend to respond poorly to analgesic drugs, but often respond well to combination therapy directed at the end-organ (e.g., injection of trigger points in muscles) and at psychologic factors which are disturbing them. The third group of patients complains of pain which appears to be caused by neither structural nor physiologic disorders. These patients are suffering from somatic delusions. Such patients usually have profound psychiatric disorders such as psychotic depression or schizophrenia, and the history of the pain is so vague and bizarre and its distribution so unanatomic as to suggest the diagnosis. These patients respond *only* to psychiatric therapy.

A thorough history, general physical examination, and careful neurologic examination are imperative in any patient complaining of pain. Often the description of the nature and distribution of the pain is so characteristic (e.g., trigeminal neuralgia or tabetic lightning pains) that it allows no other diagnosis. Inquiry should be made concerning (1) the temporal pattern of pain, (2) its distribution, (3) exacerbating factors, and (4) relieving factors.

For example, headache beginning early in the morning before arising suggests increased intracranial pressure, whereas headache occurring late in the day is more suggestive of tension. Back pain and sciatica made worse by sitting or walking suggest disc disease, whereas back pain and sciatica which are worse while in bed suggest intraspinal tumor. Back pain and sciatica exacerbated by cough or sneeze suggests intraspinal disease, whereas similar pain not exacerbated by cough or sneeze suggests disease in the pelvis. Pain in the back or legs exacerbated by straight leg raising suggests disease of the nervous system, whereas a similar pain exacerbated by rotating the hips suggests pelvic or hip disease. All pain is relieved to some extent by distraction and a pleasurable environment, and exacerbated by anxiety or psychologic stress.

A careful psychiatric history, looking particularly for signs and symptoms of depression, should be elicited from all patients. Specifically, physicians should inquire about the degree to which pain has interfered with the patient's activities, whether he is having difficulty sleeping, and whether there is a change in appetite or bowel habits. Early morning awakening, anorexia, and constipation are somatic manifestations of depression and may either be caused by chronic pain or exacerbate the effects of the pain.

A general physical examination must be performed. Both the physical and laboratory examination should begin with the assumption that the site of pathologic change is at the site of pain. The painful areas should be examined for swelling and redness as well as for any obvious deformity. (The pain of herpes zoster usually precedes the rash, and occasionally on examination one may note only the faintest reddening of the skin in a dermatomal distribution.) The areas reported as painful should be palpated, the temperature estimated, and points of tenderness sought. (If the site of pain is in a soft tissue, bone, or joint, it should be tender to palpation as well as spontaneously painful.) Joints should be taken through a full range of motion and the effect of movement on the pain assessed. Nerve trunks going to the extremities should be palpated and stretched by movement of that extremity (e.g., straight leg raising; abduction and extension of the arm). Inflamed and compressed nerve roots and nerve plexuses are more painful when stretched. A careful neurologic examination must also be performed. If there are neurologic abnormalities (e.g., weakness, sensory loss, reflex changes) in the painful part, one can infer that nervous system disease is responsible for the pain. The absence of specific neurologic abnormalities on first examination does not guarantee, however, that the nervous system is free of disease, because the process may simply not have advanced beyond the stage of selectively involving pain pathways. For example, a Pancoast tumor may produce pain in the shoulder and arm before other signs of neural involvement, such as Horner's syndrome or motor or sensory loss, appear.

Finally, laboratory examinations are performed. If the site of disease appears to be in bones or joints, x-rays of those structures or radioisotope scans may localize it. First attention should be paid to the local site of pain, but the physician should acquaint himself with the common referred patterns of pain (e.g., hip disease commonly causes knee pain, cardiac pain is frequently referred to the ulnar aspect of the arm and forearm, the pain of renal colic may be felt primarily in the groin and testicle, and pain resulting from disease of the throat may be referred to the ear).

Referred pain is pain perceived at a site remote from the source of the disturbance. Usually, referred pain is cutaneous and evoked by disease of deep structures innervated by the same dermatome. Referred pain may be associated with cutaneous hyperalgesia and even relieved by procaine injection into the area of referral. When pain is referred to the same dermatome or myotome as innervates the diseased structure (e.g., pain down the medial aspect of the arm [T1-T2] produced by myocardial infarction or angina pectoris), it is often helpful in diagnosis. However, pain is sometimes referred at a great distance from the primary site to segments not similarly innervated, and there the mechanism is perplexing (e.g., anginal pain referred to the jaw). Various theories have been suggested to account for referred pain. Such theories as division of the same nerve into deep and superficial branches, release of chemical mediators in the nervous system, and convergence of cutaneous and visceral nerves into common synaptic pools at the spinal cord all explain the dermatomal referral of pain but fail to explain pain at remote sites.

Management

In some patients, pain is best managed by treating the underlying disorder (e.g., steroids for giant cell arteritis relieve headache and muscle pain promptly; radiation therapy for bone pain caused by cancer is often helpful). In others, a particular kind of pain has a particular treatment (see Specific Pain Syndromes below), but in many patients the pain is chronic and the physician is able neither to treat the underlying disturbances nor to offer specific therapy for that type of pain. In treating this type of chronic and severe pain, certain general principles should be followed:

1. The pain should be treated by the simplest effective means, but all efforts should be made to relieve it. Pain, especially when chronic, is both physically debilitating and psychologically demoralizing. It should be considered by the physician as a serious symptom and treated to the extent that the patient is made comfortable.

2. Pain should be treated early. There is both clinical and experimental evidence that if pain goes untreated for an extended period of time, abnormal excitatory states arise in the central nervous system so that treatment directed toward peripheral structures which initially would have relieved the pain are no longer effective. In general, the earlier one undertakes to treat pain, the more successful one is.

3. Pain should be treated promptly. Clinical evidence suggests that if analgesic drug doses are spaced so far apart that severe pain recurs, the analgesic becomes less effective. Thus patients should be encouraged to take analgesic agents when the pain first reappears rather than wait until it becomes unbearable.

4. More than one treatment should be utilized. Various treatments of pain are additive and should be used together rather than separately. Combinations of narcotic and non-narcotic analgesics are often more effective than either alone and adjuvant analgesics such as the phenothiazines and butyrophenones (see Table 481–1) may enhance analgesic effect. Non-pharmacologic methods of pain control, including hypnosis, relaxation techniques, biofeedback, and "cognitive coping skills," can often help in selected patients with chronic pain.

5. Narcotic drugs should be used with discrimination, but they should not be withheld if no alternative therapy is effective. Long-term use of narcotics produces tolerance and physical dependence. These effects should not be confused with drug habituation or "addiction," which implies both a psychologic dependence and drug abuse for effects other than analgesia. The percentage of patients who actually become psychologically dependent on narcotics given to treat medical illness is unknown. Many physicians are impressed that narcotic psychologic dependence is unusual in patients treated for pain if the pain is later relieved by other means. The side effects of narcotic drugs include *tolerance,* which requires gradually increasing doses to maintain analgesia; *physical dependence,* which means that narcotics must be withdrawn gradually if they are to be discontinued after prolonged use; *constipation,* which requires careful attention to bowel function, including the use of stool softeners, laxatives, and enemas; and at times *somnolence.* All narcotic drugs produce some degree of somnolence; in individual patients, if somnolence is a problem, lower doses should be given more frequently, amphetamines added, or several different narcotics tried, because the patient may tolerate a particular drug better than another in comparable doses. Other than those mentioned, the side effects of narcotic drugs are few. Methadone maintenance programs as well as other long-term studies have proved that patients can take narcotics in large doses over long periods of time without physical damage and continue to function usefully in society. Rarely, multifocal myoclonus and seizures may occur following repetitive doses of meperidine from accumulation of the metabolite

normeperidine. Substitution of an alternative narcotic alleviates the seizures.

6. Psychogenic factors always play a role in chronic pain—the pain is more severe when the patient is anxious and stressed and less severe when he is relaxed. The physician must assess the psychologic factors in any patient with pain. However, no patient should be diagnosed as having "psychogenic pain" until an exhaustive examination has ruled out structural disease. Depression, whether endogenous or reactive, should be treated with antidepressant drugs. Tricyclic antidepressants have analgesic properties, and may be effective in relieving pain by themselves; more frequently they are effective as analgesic adjuvants. Psychiatric consultation is necessary if psychogenic factors are causing the pain.

7. Placebo effects are important. In most clinical studies, about one third of patients report relief of pain when given a placebo, although the extent of relief is rarely equal to that achieved by analgesic drugs. The physician can utilize a patient's desire to be free of pain by approaching the therapy in an enthusiastic and reassuring manner. It is less important whether it is the placebo or the drug which was effective than that the patient be relieved of his pain.

8. Multidisciplinary pain clinics which diagnose and treat intractable pain exist in many centers and should be utilized to evaluate and treat severe and chronic problems.

ANALGESIC AGENTS. Analgesics are drugs which decrease pain without causing loss of consciousness. Analgesics (see Table 481–1) can be divided clinically into those which are suitable for mild pain, generally non-narcotic agents; those suitable for moderate pain, usually narcotics or narcotic antagonists with low addiction potential; and those which are suitable for severe pain, generally narcotic agents except for methotrimeprazine, a phenothiazine. The mild analgesics appear to act peripherally by blocking the pain chemoreceptors and perhaps by relieving inflammation. There is also evidence for a central effect of some of these drugs as well.

The physician's strategy in treating chronic pain should begin with the mildest agents and add stronger agents or analgesic adjuvants only when mild agents fail to work. Drugs should always be given in sufficient amounts and at sufficiently short intervals to achieve relief of pain. Treatment should begin with aspirin or acetaminophen, 600 mg every three to four hours. If the pain is due to musculoskeletal spasm or if anxiety is prominent, one of the mild tranquilizers (diazepam or meprobamate) can be added. If the pain fails to respond to this mild regimen, one adds drugs used for the treatment of moderate pain (e.g., codeine, oxycodone). If the pain is still unrelieved

TABLE 481–1. ANALGESIC AGENTS

Type	Generic Name (Proprietary)	Usual Dose*: Oral (mg)	Usual Dose*: Subcutaneous or Intramuscular (mg)	Comment
Some agents used for mild to moderate pain	Aspirin	600 q 3–4 h		Side effects of dyspepsia and GI bleeding
	Acetaminophen (Tylenol)	650 q 3–4 h		Equal to aspirin but without GI side effects; less anti-inflammatory effect
	Dextropropoxyphene (Darvon)	65 q 3–4 h		Weak narcotic related to methadone
	Ibuprofen (Motrin)	200 q 6 h		Useful for pain associated with inflammation; less GI toxicity than aspirin
Some agents used for moderate to severe pain	Codeine	1 tab q 4–6 h	130 q 4–6 h	Narcotic with low addiction potential; additive effect if used with mild analgesics
	Oxycodone (with acetaminophen = Percocet)	5 q 4–6 h		Preferred over codeine by many patients
	Pentazocine (Talwin)	30–50 q 4–6 h	60 q 4 h	Narcotic antagonist (produces withdrawal in patients physically dependent on narcotics); hallucinations and dysphoria at higher doses; not recommended for general use
Some agents used for severe pain: narcotics and antagonists	Levorphanol (Levodromoran)	2 q 3–4 h	10 q 3–4 h	Potent oral narcotic; long plasma half-life†
	Morphine		2 q 3–4 h	The standard narcotic agent for treatment of pain
	Meperidine (Demerol)	50–100 q 3–4 h	75 q 2–4 h	More rapid onset and shorter duration of action than morphine; can cause CNS hyperirritability with chronic administration
	Methadone (Dolophine)	10–20 q 4 h	10–15 q 3–4 h	Potent oral narcotic; long plasma half-life
	Hydromorphone (Dilaudid)	7 q 3 h	1 q 3 h	Potent, short-acting
Non-narcotic agents	Methotrimeprazine (Levoprome)		20 q 4–6 h	Phenothiazine; no tolerance; produces sedation and postural hypotension
	Dextroamphetamine	10 q 6 h		Enhances narcotic effect and decreases somnolence in postoperative pain
Some agents used as analgesic adjuvants (probably little or no analgesic properties per se but used to relieve anxiety and/or depression)	Minor tranquilizers—muscle relaxants:			
	Diazepam (Valium)	5 qid		Useful with mild analgesics for acute or subacute pain associated with muscle spasm and/or anxiety
	Meprobamate (Miltown)	200–400 qid		
	Antidepressants:			Reported useful in pain associated with depressive symptoms (esp. atypical facial pain); may be useful when combined with analgesic agents for chronic pain of many kinds; may cause over-sedation or anticholinergic symptoms
	Amitriptyline (Elavil)	25–75 qd		
	Imipramine (Tofranil)	25 qid		
	Phenothiazines:			Reported useful in pain associated with anxiety or depression and in some specific pain syndromes (e.g., thalamic pain, postherpetic pain); these drugs may have analgesic properties or potentiate analgesics; fluphenazine and amitriptyline have been reported to relieve postherpetic pain; may cause oversedation, depression, Parkinson-like syndrome, hypotension, or urinary retention
	Chlorpromazine (Thorazine)	25–50 qid		
	Fluphenazine (Prolixin)	1–3 qd		
	Butyrophenones:			
	Haloperidol	2 mg tid		

*Intramuscular dose of narcotics is equivalent to 10 mg of morphine. Since tolerance develops to these drugs, doses must be increased with continued use. Oral doses are not equivalent to intramuscular doses but represent usual starting doses.

†Analgesic "half-life" differs from plasma half-life.

and the physician satisfies himself that psychogenic factors are not responsible, the agents used for moderate pain should be discontinued, and agents used for severe pain should be added to the mild analgesic. Levorphanol, 2 mg, methadone, 10 mg, or hydromorphone, 4 mg, every three to four hours, are the agents of choice if oral drugs are to be used, and morphine, 10 mg every three to four hours, if a subcutaneous or intramuscular agent is necessary. If the pain continues as a chronic and unremitting problem not relieved by these drugs, or if anxiety and depression appear to be the major contributors to the pain, a major tranquilizer (phenothiazine) or antidepressant agent, or both, may be added to the mild analgesics and narcotic agents. At times a satisfactory resolution of an intractable problem may be achieved by the combined use of a narcotic and non-narcotic analgesic with a tranquilizer or an antidepressant. The physician must be careful to adjust the doses of each so as to produce maximal pain relief with minimal sedation and unpleasant side effects. The physician should be prepared to increase the dose of those particular drugs to which tolerance develops as necessary to control pain. No tolerance develops to non-narcotic analgesics.

Non-Narcotic Mild Analgesics. Aspirin and acetaminophen (Tylenol, Tempra) are the most useful of the mild analgesics. However, acetaminophen differs from aspirin in that it does not have aspirin's anti-inflammatory properties. Either aspirin or acetaminophen may be given in doses of 600 mg every three to four hours, either alone for relief of mild pain or in conjunction with more potent drugs for relief of severe pain. Ceiling effects and unpleasant side effects prevent the use of increasing doses of these drugs to treat more severe pain. The side effects of aspirin (clotting disorders, dyspepsia, and gastrointestinal bleeding) make acetaminophen a safer drug and probably the drug of choice at usual therapeutic doses. However, acute overdose of acetaminophen can cause severe hepatotoxicity, and there is evidence that alcohol ingestion increases its toxic effects on the liver. Aspirin and acetaminophen taken together may be more effective than either one alone. Aspirin or acetaminophen plus codeine is more effective than codeine alone.

Narcotic Analgesics. Tolerance develops to all narcotics. Thus there is no set dose of these drugs, and with continued use dosage must increase. *The physician is wise to learn to handle two or three drugs and use those consistently rather than using all the drugs occasionally.* The physician must be prepared to use more than one, because some patients find that side effects of the drugs make one preferable to another. Morphine, 10 mg intramuscularly, is the standard by which other narcotic analgesics are judged. Intramuscular morphine has its maximal effect in 60 to 90 minutes and lasts between three and six hours. It requires 60 mg or more of morphine orally to give the same analgesic effect as 10 mg intramuscularly. Levorphanol has a relatively high oral/parenteral ratio for analgesia; 2 mg given intramuscularly is equal to 10 mg of morphine intramuscularly, and 4 mg given orally is equal in total effect to 10 mg of morphine given intramuscularly. Methadone also has a relatively high oral/intramuscular potency ratio; 10 mg intramuscularly or 20 mg orally equals 10 mg of morphine intramuscularly. Codeine and dihydrocodeine are also effective orally and are generally used in doses of 50 to 60 mg as a mild analgesic. They often cannot be used to relieve severe pain, because side effects preclude high doses. Pentazocine is a mild analgesic when given in doses of 30 mg and is equal to morphine if given in intramuscular doses of 60 mg. It is a mixed narcotic agonist-antagonist, and thus can produce withdrawal in a physically dependent patient. Pentazocine is not included in the Federal Controlled Substances Act. However, dysphoria, hallucinatory effects, and toxic psychoses are frequent side effects and limit its use. Like the other narcotics it can produce respiratory depression.

Other Agents. The phenothiazine methotrimeprazine (Levoprome) is a potent analgesic agent. Given intramuscularly in doses of 20 mg, it is equivalent to 10 mg of morphine intramuscularly. The drug is an effective antiemetic and does not suppress cough or respiration but does produce sedation and postural hypotension, making it useful only for hospitalized patients.

Anticonvulsant drugs are probably useful only in pain associated with spontaneous neuronal firing such as trigeminal neuralgia. Low doses of amitriptyline (25–75 mg daily) produce an analgesic effect independent of any antidepressant effect and the drug is useful in efforts to manage patients with chronic neurogenic pain syndromes.

Dextroamphetamine has been reported to enhance the effectiveness of narcotic agents in postoperative patients while counteracting the undesirable side effects of sedation and possibly respiratory depression. Whether the drug may also be an effective adjuvant for chronic pain remains to be established.

PHYSICAL METHODS OF PAIN RELIEF. There are a bewildering variety of physical methods designed to relieve pain. These vary from simply rubbing a partially denervated area with a soft towel to placing radiofrequency lesions stereotactically in the thalamic and hypothalamic reticular formations. The simpler procedures can be carried out by the general physician or even by the patient; the more complicated ones, depending on their nature, demand the expertise of a skilled anesthesiologist or neurosurgeon.

The physician's approach to the use of physical methods for intractable pain should embody certain general principles:

1. Nondestructive procedures should be tried first. Cutaneous stimulation, either by hand or by battery-driven electrodes, or local anesthetic blocks in conjunction with analgesic drugs may be effective in relieving pain. If these simple procedures fail, the services of an anesthesiologist or neurosurgeon should be procured and a treatment plan embodying the use of analgesics and physical procedures outlined.

2. The least destructive procedure should be tried first. In general, the procedure should be directed first at the peripheral nervous system, and only if this fails, at the spinal cord, brainstem, or cerebrum. Quantitative data on the incidence of pain relief and its duration are sketchy for most of these procedures and seem to vary from center to center, depending on the skill and enthusiasm of the investigator reporting.

3. Thus, the choice of a particular procedure often depends not only on the nature of the patient's disease but on the particular skills, experience, and bias of the physician.

4. If and only if a full trial of analgesic drugs has failed should destructive procedures for relieving pain be tried. These destructive procedures can and should be used in conjunction with analgesic drugs, because, even if the drugs have failed to relieve pain on their own, they may act synergistically with physical methods. Nerve blocks and surgical procedures often yield only temporary relief in patients with chronic pain. Thus many of the enthusiastic reports in the literature refer to patients followed for only a short period of time. When the patients are followed over months or years, the pain which was relieved shortly after the procedure often returns and is as bad as or worse than it was prior to the operation. For this reason, patients with cancer who are not expected to live a long time are often better candidates for surgical destructive procedures than are patients with pain originating from more benign conditions.

5. Patients with chronic pain being considered for destructive procedures must be thoroughly evaluated psychiatrically. If psychogenic factors play a major role in the genesis of pain, surgical procedures will not help, and often the pain will be exacerbated after surgical intervention.

Cutaneous Stimulation. Cutaneous stimulation of a painful area, particularly one which has been partly denervated, is often effective in relieving pain. This procedure, which probably has its greatest use in the treatment of postherpetic neuralgia, consists of rubbing the painful area with a soft cloth or terrycloth towel, almost constantly at first but then with gradually lengthening intervals of rest between rubbing periods. Often a period of rubbing will yield relief which long outlasts the stimulus, and continued intermittent rubbings may totally relieve the pain. The "gate theory" offers an explanation of the rubbing phenomenon, i.e., rubbing stimulates large fiber afferents which may close the gate against incoming pain fibers. Whatever the explanation, the procedure is often useful in the treatment of painful phantom limbs and in chronic cutaneous or extremity pain after surgery. Battery-powered electrical stimulators which give one control over the frequency and intensity of the cutaneous stimulation can also be used. The electrodes of the stimulator may be placed over the painful area or over the peripheral nerve supplying the painful area, and stimulation using an intensity and frequency which produces a vibratory sensation is applied.

Acupuncture Analgesia. Acupuncture analgesia has become increasingly popular in the past several years, but few carefully controlled studies attest to its usefulness. A needle is placed under the skin, often in a place remote from the painful site but at times into the painful site, and the area is stimulated either by twirling the needle or by electrically vibrating it. Recent experiments in animals and man suggest that the analgesic effect of acupuncture is partially reversed by naloxone, leading to the hypothesis that one mechanism of acupuncture analgesia is through release of endogenous analgesic substances. The usefulness of acupuncture in Western medicine is still not clear.

Nerve Blocks. Direct block of peripheral nerves, using either anesthetic agents (lidocaine) or neurolytic agents (phenol), has been popular in the treatment of thoracic and abdominal pain, particularly that pain which follows surgery. Blocks may be dangerous if used in the extremities, because they may paralyze as well as anesthetize; but in areas where they can be used, relief of pain sometimes long outlasts the period of anesthesia. The procedure is a simple one when performed by a skilled anesthesiologist.

Subarachnoid injection of anesthetics or neurolytics directed at nerve roots has been utilized in patients with widespread and intractable pain. Phenol can likewise be injected into the subarachnoid space and directed at particular nerve roots by positioning the patient. The mechanism of action is destruction of nerve fibers; if material spills into the cauda equina, bladder and bowel dysfunction are common. The relief of pain may be only transient. Spinal opiate administration with small doses (2 mg) of morphine given into the epidural or subarachnoid space may produce prolonged analgesia without substantial side effects. This technique is useful in the management of patients with postoperative pain. Continuous epidural infusions of opiates, using implantable infusion pumps, in cancer patients with chronic pain has been reported to be useful.

Other Procedures. Several nondestructive procedures directed at the affective component of pain are currently in use. These include not only psychotherapy and hypnotism but also more recently developed techniques of biofeedback, operant conditioning, relaxation techniques, and cognitive behavioral methods. These approaches have been gaining in popularity as our understanding of the psychologic components of chronic pain has improved. Preliminary studies suggest that stimulation of the medial thalamus following stereotactic placement of electrodes is effective in relieving some chronic neurogenic pain. Tolerance does not develop to this stimulation-produced analgesia.

Each nonsurgical procedure directed at the *peripheral nervous system* has its surgical counterpart. In patients with chronic pain such as that which follows herpes zoster, the skin has been undercut in an attempt to totally denervate it. Postoperative infection is a complication at times and the pain relief is transient, thus contraindicating this procedure. Peripheral nerves can be cut, particularly in the thorax and abdomen, but this should not be done unless prior nerve blocks have indicated that it will be effective and sustained. The peripheral nerves regenerate after a time, and often the pain returns. Dorsal root ganglia in the thorax and abdomen can be removed for chronic pain or the dorsal roots themselves cut. This procedure also should not be done unless nerve blocks have indicated that it will be effective. Several roots must be cut off either side of the painful area if one is to achieve long-term pain relief.

Surgery of the Central Nervous System. There are four kinds of surgical procedures directed at the central nervous system for the relief of pain. The *first type* involves the placement of electrodes on the skin, along peripheral nerves, and along spinal cord pathways. A few years ago there was some enthusiasm about electrodes surgically placed on the dorsal columns with a subcutaneous power pack which would allow the patient to control frequency and intensity of stimulation. Failure of this method to give prolonged relief and the morbidity of the procedure have led many neurosurgeons to abandon it. More recently, electrodes have been placed stereotactically in the periventricular gray matter, again using a power source controlled by the patient. Total body analgesia with increase in pain threshold has been observed for three to eight hours following stimulation, but tolerance develops to the analgesic effect. This procedure is still an experimental one, and its effectiveness requires further evaluation.

The *second type of procedure* destroys pain pathways in the spinal cord, brainstem, or brain. Spinothalamic tracts can be destroyed either surgically, after a laminectomy (open cordotomy), or by the placement of a radiofrequency lesion through a needle (percutaneous cordotomy). These procedures are particularly effective in relieving pain in the lower extremities and have the advantage that, although pain and temperature sensations are lost, cutaneous sensation and motor power remain intact. At times the level of anesthesia approaches within one or two cord segments of the level at which the destructive lesion is placed, but often there is a drop to about five segments below the placement of the lesion. Thus, the lesion must be placed considerably higher than the site of pain. If the lesion is placed unilaterally, pain often reappears on the other side of the body, necessitating another lesion. Bilateral lesions considerably enhance the risk of motor weakness and bladder and bowel dysfunction, but in skilled hands these risks are low. Occasionally patients with bilateral percutaneous lesions in the cervical cord suffer loss of automatic respiratory function (Ondine's curse). Percutaneous spinothalamic tract cordotomy, when done by a skilled technician, produces satisfactory pain relief in 70 to 90 per cent of patients, with a small mortality (1 to 5 per cent) and morbidity rate. The procedure is particularly useful in patients with terminal cancer, because the pain relief is usually sustained until death and the procedure does not require a major operation. An analogous lesion in the low brainstem placed in the descending tract of the trigeminal nerve has been reported useful in relieving facial pain. Pain and temperature sensation are lost, but cutaneous sensation remains intact. Lesions have been placed in the spinothalamic tract of the midbrain, so-called mesencephalic tractotomies. The dangers of this lesion are considerably greater than those of spinal cord lesions, and most centers have abandoned the procedure. Several neurosurgeons have placed lesions in the thalamus, both in the ventral-basal complex and in the interlaminar nuclei. Although good results are occasionally reported for both, the ventral-basal lesions appear only to produce transient relief of pain, whereas those placed in the intralaminar nuclei at the end-point of the paleospinothalamic tract appear to be more successful. There are rare reports of removal of sensory portions of the parietal lobe in relieving chronic pain, but the rarity of the reports implies the ineffectiveness of the treatment.

The *third surgical method* directed at pain relief is to place lesions in the frontal lobe, particularly the limbic projection to the frontal areas, in an attempt to alter the patient's psychologic response to pain rather than alter the pain pathways themselves. Several different surgical procedures, including frontal lobotomy, frontal leukotomy, and cingulotomy, have been tried with varied success. These procedures, which alter the patient's personality as well as his suffering, probably deserve trial only when all other procedures have failed.

The *fourth procedure* is directed at ablating the pituitary gland and is reported to be particularly effective in the treatment of pain from bony metastases from hormonally sensitive tumors such as those of breast or prostate. However, it has also been reported effective in pain caused by nonhormonally sensitive tumors. The pituitary may be ablated either surgically or by injection of destructive chemicals into the sella turcica (chemical hypophysectomy). In some series, 30 to 50 per cent of patients with pain from metastatic tumors have reported pain relief.

Good statistical data comparing the various surgical procedures for pain are difficult to come by. The best extant data indicate that initial relief of pain occurs with almost all procedures in 50 to 80 per cent of patients, with spinothalamic tract cordotomies yielding the best results. Longer-term follow-up suggests that considerably less than 50 per cent of patients achieve lasting relief, in many series the figure being as low as 20 per cent. Patients with malignant disease seem to have greater pain relief even initially than those with more benign conditions, probably because selection of patients with benign conditions often includes many with psychogenic pain.

Bonica JJ: The Management of Pain. Philadelphia, Lea & Febiger, 1953. *A classic monograph.*

Bonica JJ, Lindblom U, Iggo A (eds.): Proceedings of the Third World Congress on Pain, Edinburgh. Advances in Pain Research and Therapy. Vol 5. New York, Raven Press, 1983. *An up-to-date multi-authored monograph describing new developments in the physiology, pharmacology, and management of pain.*

Sternbach R: Pain Patients: Traits and Treatment. New York, Academic Press, 1974. *Important monograph on the psychology of chronic pain.*

Twycross RG, Lack SA: Symptom Control in Far Advanced Cancer: Pain Relief. London, Pitman Books Ltd., 1983. *An up-to-date monograph describing in detail the control of pain in patients with cancer. Many of the concepts are equally applicable to other chronic diseases causing pain.*

HEADACHE AND OTHER HEAD PAIN

Headache is one of man's most common afflictions. It ranks ninth among the causes of visits to physicians and is a major source both of time lost from work and of medical diagnostic procedures. The frequency of disabling headache is explained in part by the rich nerve supply to the head (including afferent nerve fibers from trigeminal, glossopharyngeal, vagus, and upper three cervical nerves) and in part by the psychologic significance of head pain, causing anxiety about even modest headache, whereas a pain of equal severity elsewhere in the body might be ignored. Head pain can result from distortion, stretching, inflammation, or destruction of pain-sensitive nerve endings as a result of intra- or extracranial disease in the distribution of any of the aforementioned nerves. However, most head pain arises from extracerebral structures and carries a benign prognosis. The physician's twofold task is first to distinguish the commoner, benign head pain from more serious causes and then to administer appropriate treatment. The diagnosis can usually be established by history and physical findings alone; skull x-rays, CT scans, and other diagnostic tests are seldom required. Table 481–2 is a simplified classification of the pathogenesis of head pain; the overwhelming majority of headaches are either muscle contraction or common migraine headaches, with both abnormalities frequently playing a role in a given individual. The other forms of headache are much less common.

Migraine and Other Vascular Headaches

The term *vascular headache* applies to a group of clinical syndromes of unknown etiology in which the final step in pathogenesis of the pain appears to be dilatation of one or more branches of the carotid artery, leading to stimulation of nerve endings supplying that artery. There may be a release of noxious substances by either the arterial wall or the nerve ending, causing a substantially lowered pain threshold. Such substances as serotonin, substance P, bradykinin, histamine, and prostaglandins alone or in combination have all been implicated in the pathogenesis of vascular headache. Most vascular headaches are unilateral in distribution and often but not always throbbing in quality, and they recur over months or years. Individual headaches are frequently precipitated by identifiable environmental or psychologic factors. During the course of a vascular headache, the involved arteries may be tender to the touch, and pain may be relieved temporarily by compression of the carotid artery, only to return with increased severity when compression is released. Most vascular headaches can be relieved by prompt administration of vasoconstrictive agents, and many recurrent headaches can be prevented by one of several vasoactive drugs. So-called "common migraine" may affect as many as 25 per cent of the population. Other vascular headache syndromes are less common, but each has distinctive clinical findings.

TABLE 481–2. PATHOPHYSIOLOGIC CLASSIFICATION OF HEADACHE

Vascular Headache
Migraine Headache
Classic migraine
Common migraine
Complicated migraine
Variant migraine
Cluster Headache
Episodic cluster
"Chronic" cluster
Chronic paroxysmal hemicrania
Miscellaneous Vascular Headaches
Carotidynia
Hypertension
Hangover
Toxins and drugs
Occlusive vascular disease
Muscle Contraction (Tension) Headache
Common tension headache
Depressive equivalent
Conversion reaction
Temporomandibular joint dysfunction
Atypical facial pain
Cervical osteoarthritis
Traction-Inflammation Headache
Cranial arteritis
Increased or decreased intracranial pressure
Extracranial structural lesions
Pituitary tumors
Cranial Neuralgias

Classic Migraine

Classic migraine is distinguished by well-defined symptoms of neurologic dysfunction that precede or less often accompany the headache. Neurologic symptoms are usually visual, consisting of bright flashing lights (scintillation or fortification scotomata) beginning in the center of a homonymous visual half-field and radiating over 10 to 30 minutes outward toward the periphery. Less commonly, the visual abnormalities are monocular (retinal) or consist of hemianoptic loss of vision in place of or following the scintillating scotomata. Other neurologic disturbances that can occur in classic migraine include unilateral paresthesias, usually involving the hand and perioral area, aphasia, hemiparesis, and hemisensory defects. An uncommon variant named *basilar artery migraine* occurs predominantly in children and adolescents and is characterized by vertigo, ataxia, and diplopia, along with hemiparesis or hemisensory changes. Rarely, confusion, stupor, or even coma may develop. Neurologic symptoms of classic migraine usually last no longer than 30 minutes and generally clear before the headache phase begins. However, in some instances neurologic signs may persist for hours or, rarely, for days, throughout and even beyond the headache phase of the illness.

The pathogenesis of the neurologic dysfunction is not fully understood. Measurements of regional cerebral blood flow during episodes of classic migraine have shown a wave of focal hyperemia followed by abnormally low flow (oligemia) spreading from posterior to anterior over the cerebral cortex. The degree of oligemia is not sufficient in and of itself to produce the neurologic symptoms, nor is it always accompanied by neurologic symptoms. One explanation is that there may be a wave of physiologic depression that spreads across the cortex, accounting for both the neurologic symptoms and the changes in blood flow. Changes in brain blood flow do not accompany common migraine, even though the headache phase of the illness is similar. Thus, it is likely that if "spreading depression" is the cause of the neurologic symptoms of migraine, it is only one of several precipitating factors that may produce the headache.

The syndrome of classic migraine has four parts: (1) The *prodromal phase* occurs in a minority of patients and consists of an alteration of mood, often occurring for 24 or more hours before the headache. Patients may complain of increased hunger or thirst, drowsiness, euphoria, or depression. In some patients, known precipitants such as red wine commonly induce an attack. (2) The second phase consists of the *neurologic symptoms* described above. The neurologic symptoms may occur without subsequent headache (termed migraine equivalent), particularly in older people. (3) The third phase usually begins as the neurologic symptoms clear and characteristically consists of a unilateral throbbing frontotemporal *headache* on the side opposite the neurologic symptoms. The headache is frequently accompanied by nausea, photophobia, vomiting, diarrhea, phonophobia (noise intolerance), and a general feeling of being unwell. The headache commonly lasts four to six hours but may persist for one or more days. If the headache is prolonged, it may change into a dull, aching, bilateral pain extending back into the neck and shoulders. The headache phase is often terminated either by vomiting or by a period of sleep. (4) The *post-headache* phase is characterized by a feeling of exhaustion, tenderness of the scalp at the site of the headache, and recurrence of headache on sudden head movement.

The diagnosis of classic migraine is made by history; physical findings are absent, and laboratory evaluation is not helpful. When the attacks are atypical, particularly when neurologic disability is severe or prolonged, CT scans or digital intravenous angiography (DIVA) may be required to rule out structural lesions of the brain or its vasculature (brain tumors, particularly meningiomas, or arteriovenous anomalies). However, such instances are rare. The treatment of classic migraine is similar to that of common migraine (see below), except that classic migraine attacks usually occur no more than four or five times a year and rarely more than once a month.

Common Migraine

Common migraine is similar to classic migraine except that neurologic symptoms are absent. Many patients with classic migraine also have episodes of common migraine. Common migraine is characterized by recurrent headaches, often severe, frequently beginning unilaterally, and usually associated with malaise, nausea and/or vomiting, and photophobia. The disorder often begins in childhood, affects women more often than men, and runs in families (70 per cent of patients give a family history). Characteristically, the headache affects individuals with perfectionistic and "driven" personalities. Identifiable factors that often precipitate individual headaches are holidays and weekends, menstrual periods, foods (especially red wine, chocolate, nuts, and aged cheese), environmental stimuli (such as bright sunlight, too much sleep, and undue emotional stress or resentment). Medical conditions and their treatment may also precipitate attacks. Vasodilators such as nitroglycerin and antihypertensives and serotonin releasers such as reserpine, as well as estrogens and oral contraceptives, have been reported to cause migraine attacks in susceptible individuals. The diagnosis of common migraine is usually made by the history. Important historical points that help distinguish migraine from the equally common tension headaches (see below) include their unilaterality, their association with nausea or vomiting, the tendency of migraine to awaken one from sleep, a positive family history, and a positive response to ergot preparations. When the diagnosis is in doubt, treatment of the patient for common migraine often clarifies the issue.

TREATMENT. The best treatment for migraine is prevention. Whenever possible, the patient should avoid precipitating factors. Medications known to cause migraine should be withdrawn if others can be substituted. Foods commonly implicated may also be withdrawn and, if withdrawal is effective, replaced one at a time to determine the specific precipitant. The patient should attempt to avoid undue stress or fatigue and not to sleep excessively on weekends. If these methods fail and severe headaches occur frequently (once a week or more), pharmacologic prophylaxis is indicated. Several agents have been reported effective in the prophylaxis of migraine, but not every patient responds to each agent. Perhaps the safest and most effective class of drugs are the beta-adrenergic blockers, particularly propranolol. The drug is begun at a dose of 80 mg a day in divided doses, and increased as tolerated until headaches are controlled. Recent reports suggest that calcium channel blockers such as verapamil* (80 mg three to four times daily) are also effective. Methysergide, a serotonin antagonist, is effective at a dose of 2 mg three to four times daily. Methysergide must be employed cautiously because it can cause serious side effects, including vascular insufficiency, retroperitoneal or pleural fibrosis, and fibrotic thickening of heart valves. The side effects can be minimized by gradually withdrawing the drug for one month after every four to six months of treatment. Amitriptyline in gradually increasing doses from 25 to 125 mg daily may be useful if the above drugs fail.

Acute attacks, if mild, often respond to analgesic agents and bedrest. More severe attacks are best treated by ergot preparations such as ergotamine tartrate. The drug, given parenterally, is sufficiently effective (85 to 90 per cent) to be useful as a diagnostic test. Oral ergot 1 to 2 mg given at the onset of a headache is effective in about 50 per cent of patients. However, during the headache, absorption of the oral form of the drug is often poor, and better results can be achieved with sublingual or rectal ergot preparations. The best nonparenteral results are generally achieved by the insertion of half of a 2-mg ergotamine rectal suppository. The side effect of *ergotism* makes it unwise to treat frequent migraine headaches in this way, and therefore one should switch to prophylaxis if the headaches occur more than once a week.

Migraine Variants

There are several migraine syndromes that differ sufficiently from classic and common migraine to earn separate names. *Ophthalmoplegic migraine* is the name given when an ocular motor palsy develops during the course of a severe migraine attack. Ophthalmoplegic migraine usually begins in childhood and is characterized by unilateral pupillary dilatation, ptosis, and paralysis of ocular muscles occurring 12 to 24 hours *after* the beginning of an attack of severe migraine. The ophthalmoplegia usually clears within hours to days but frequently recurs. Angiography (usually DIVA) may be required to rule out a carotid aneurysm. *Hemiplegic migraine* is a familial syndrome in which aphasia, confusion, and hemiparesis or hemiplegia precede or more often accompany the migraine attack. Repetitive episodes alternating from side to side may occur over many years. *Complicated migraine* is a term applied to attacks of migraine prodromes in which the focal neurologic defects may last for the entire headache attack and may even leave permanent residua. The few available anatomic studies of such patients have shown ischemic brain infarction involving the functionally impaired region.

Cluster Headache

Cluster headaches are short-lived attacks of severe, acute, and intense unilateral head pain that occur in clusters lasting

*This use is not listed in the manufacturer's directive.

several weeks, only to disappear for months or years on end. The disorder affects men much more than women and usually first begins between the third and sixth decades. Clusters characteristically occur in the spring and fall and last three to eight weeks. The individual headaches occur one to several times a day, particularly at night, and frequently with a predictability that allows one to set his clock by them. Each attack, which lasts 30 minutes to two hours, is characterized by rapid onset of a knife-like pain in the nostril or behind the eye which spreads to involve the forehead. During the attack, the ipsilateral nostril may be stuffy or water, and the eye may tear. In about 20 per cent of instances, a homolateral Horner's syndrome develops. During the course of the headache, the patient is usually unable to lie still (the opposite of the situation with migraine) and restlessly paces the floor. The pain may be so severe that the patient bangs his head against the wall or threatens suicide. The headache disappears as abruptly as it came, usually leaving no residua. Unlike the patient with migraine, the patient with cluster headaches does not feel systemically ill, and there is no nausea, vomiting, or feeling of exhaustion when the headache ceases. During the time when clusters are occurring, but not between such periods, alcohol will invariably induce an attack. When the headaches occur frequently, the Horner's syndrome may outlast the head pain.

The pathogenesis of cluster headache is unknown, although it is believed to be a vascular headache related to migraine. The diagnosis is established by the characteristic history. Treatment of an acute attack is usually not worthwhile, since by the time the patient absorbs the analgesic agents the attack is over. In some patients the headache rapidly responds to oxygen inhalation. Several drugs prevent attacks of cluster headache. Ergotamine tartrate given prophylactically in a dose of 1 mg four times a day, or 2 mg at bedtime if the attacks are all nocturnal, is often effective. The drug should be withdrawn every seventh day to prevent the symptoms of ergotism and to see if the cluster has ceased. Methysergide 2 mg three to four times daily is also often effective; since the cluster rarely lasts more than eight weeks, the drug can be discontinued and thereby is safe. Prednisone 40 mg daily in divided doses may also work and can be added to methysergide if the former is only partially effective. Lithium carbonate in daily doses of 0.9 to 1.5 grams sometimes works.

Cluster Variants

Several variants of cluster headache should be recognized by the physician, since their treatment may be different. The most striking is *chronic paroxysmal hemicrania,* a rare disorder consisting of painful episodes similar to cluster headaches that appear many times a day and recur unremittingly for years. There may be as many as 10 to 20 headaches daily, each lasting 10 to 30 minutes. Indomethacin orally in doses of 75 to 150 mg daily has relieved all subjects. A cluster variant characterized by daily cluster headache without remission, multiple brief jabs of pain in the head, and a background of continuous unilateral headache of variable severity exacerbated by exertion has recently been described and is said to respond to indomethacin in most instances. Patients who did not respond to indomethacin did so to tricyclic antidepressants.

Other Vascular Headaches

Several vascular headache variants deserve mention so that the physician may recognize them as benign and treat them appropriately. Included are *orgasmic headaches,* severe short-lived bilateral throbbing headaches occurring in either sex and appearing abruptly at orgasm. The attack can be differentiated from subarachnoid hemorrhage because the headache usually disappears within minutes to an hour or more and may recur repetitively. Usually the illness is self-limited, but if not it may respond to 1 mg of ergot given an hour before sexual activity. *Exertional headache* occurs, as the name implies, during active exercise. Like orgasmic headaches, these are usually bilateral and throbbing, and may last several hours. They respond well to indomethacin. Vascular headaches have been reported to follow minor *trauma* to the carotid artery in the neck and to *carotid endarterectomy*. These headaches are unilateral, recurrent, and severe and usually respond to prophylaxis with propranolol. *Carotidynia* is the name given to spontaneous vascular headaches associated with unilateral anterior neck pain and/or carotid tenderness. They usually respond to the same treatment as vascular headaches. When attacks of carotid pain and/or headache recur, the diagnosis is not difficult, but the first attack must be distinguished from a spontaneous dissection of the carotid artery and may require intravenous angiography for diagnosis.

Hangover headache is part of a larger syndrome, usually including premature awakening from an evening of overindulging and often accompanied by a fine tremor of the extremities and mild gastric distress or nausea, mental dulling, and mild incoordination. The pathogenesis is related to alcohol withdrawal, dehydration, and the toxic effect of various congeners found with different intoxicants. *Nitrites* can induce pulsating headache and, occasionally, facial flushing, most often after the ingestion of processed foods ("hot dog" headache). *Monosodium glutamate* has been blamed for the "Chinese restaurant syndrome," characterized by postprandial headache, tight sensations about the face and head, and, less often, giddiness and diarrhea.

Hypertensive headaches occur only in patients with very severe or episodic hypertension. They are characterized by early-morning, usually throbbing, occipital headache that responds to the treatment of the hypertension.

Muscle Contraction (Tension) Headache

Muscle contraction or tension headaches are characterized by a steady, non-pulsatile, unilateral or bilateral aching pain, usually beginning in the occipital regions but also often involving frontal or temporal regions as well. The headaches are so named because they are frequently accompanied by tight and tender muscles at the site of the most severe pain. They are probably the commonest cause of headache in the adult. In one clinic series of 726 consecutive headache patients, 279 were classified as due to tension and 181 as suffering from migraine; in 221 patients no exclusive diagnosis could be made. Tension headaches are recurrent, often present every day, and usually begin in early afternoon or evening, with a dull occipital or frontal pain that may spread to grip the entire head "in a vise." Unique among headaches, the pain may be constantly present for days, weeks, or months and is often associated with severe tenderness in the posterior cervical, temporalis, or masseter muscles. The pain may be quite severe, but patients rarely complain of nausea, vomiting, or malaise, although modest dizziness, blurring of vision, and sometimes tinnitus may occur. These headaches are more frequent in women, in individuals who are tense and anxious, and in those whose work or posture requires sustained contraction of posterior cervical, frontal, or temporal muscles. There is much overlap between the symptoms of common migraine and tension headaches, and many patients suffer from both. The distinguishing features favoring tension headaches include pressure or tightness, which is worst at the back of the neck, increased severity of pain as the day progresses, and pain that is preceded by or associated with clear anxiety-producing situations. Tension headaches are less commonly unilateral than migraine and less commonly associated with nausea and vomiting, do not usually awaken the patient from sleep, and do not respond to ergot preparations.

The pathogenesis of tension headaches is unclear. They are commonly accompanied by skeletal muscle contraction about the neck, face, and jaw, and palpation of those muscles may reveal sharply localized painful areas or nodules, injection of which with local anesthetics transiently relieves the headache. Sometimes massage has a similar effect. Patients are frequently aware that sustained contraction of muscles leads to headache. The contracting muscles or the nerves supplying them may release vasoactive substances such as lactate, serotonin, bradykinin, and prostaglandins, which lower pain threshold. Thus, some of the same substances implicated in migraine may also play a role in tension headache and explain the frequent overlap between the two syndromes. Muscle contraction headache may also be a result of sustained contraction of the head as a consequence of structural disease of the eye, ear, nose, paranasal sinuses, teeth, scalp, or intracranial contents.

TREATMENT. The first step in treatment is to identify causal factors. If these include abnormalities of posture leading to sustained muscle contraction, these should be corrected. Many patients with tension headache, particularly chronic ones, are depressed and respond to treatment with antidepressant agents such as amitriptyline. Others are tense and anxious and respond to anti-anxiety agents such as diazepam. This drug, in a dose of 15 to 20 mg a day for two to three weeks, is often effective as a diagnostic test. The relief of chronic headache establishes the diagnosis for the physician and helps to convince the patient that tension and anxiety are playing a major role in the headache, thus making the patient more amenable to psychotherapeutic endeavors. In addition, these drugs frequently break up a cycle of anxiety–muscle tension–anxiety, so that a short course may give prolonged relief.

An individual headache may be treated with aspirin. This drug is probably more useful for tension headaches than acetaminophen because of its anti-prostaglandin properties. Vasoactive agents used for the treatment of migraine have no role in this disorder unless vascular headaches are concomitantly present. Some clinics report that biofeedback treatments effectively relieve muscle contraction and thus the headache.

Tension Headache Variant

There are several rather characteristic headache syndromes of unknown cause that may have muscle contraction and psychologic tension as part of their pathogenesis. The syndrome most clearly related to muscle contraction headache is the so-called "temporomandibular joint syndrome." Patients complain of unilateral or bilateral head pain, usually in the temporal region and in the jaw, often radiating into the ear. The pain is often associated with tenderness of the masseter and temporalis muscles and may be exacerbated by chewing. Patients characteristically are tense and anxious individuals. Accompanying symptoms often include limitation of full movement at the temporomandibular joint when opening the jaw, bruxism, and malocclusion. The disorder sometimes responds to dental manipulation, particularly use of a mouth guard that prevents bruxism. However, for most patients analgesics and anti-anxiety manipulation effectively treat muscle contraction head pain. *Post-traumatic headaches* are dull, generalized, aching head pains that follow head injury. The injury is often mild, indeed sometimes trivial. The patient suffering the "post-traumatic syndrome" complains of headache often coupled with unsteadiness, giddiness, difficulty concentrating, insomnia, and fatigue. Contrary to popular belief, the syndrome is no more common in patients seeking compensation for the injury than not. It often persists for months or years. Treatment, like that of muscle contraction headaches, consists of psychologic support and reassurance and the use of mild analgesics and sometimes anti-anxiety agents. Patients should be encouraged to return to work as soon as possible and to try to live a normal life despite the symptoms. The disorder can blend into *depressive headache*, a chronic generalized headache, usually vaguely described, sometimes associated with giddiness and unsteadiness, that occurs as a frequent and sometimes predominant manifestation of depression. The headache may have muscle contraction and tension as its pathogenesis or may be a *somatic delusion* in a severely depressed patient. In either event, the treatment of choice is an antidepressant drug.

Atypical Facial Pain

Atypical facial pain or atypical facial neuralgia is a term used to describe a syndrome characterized by steady aching facial pain, usually unilateral, localized to the lower part of the orbit, maxillary area, and sometimes the jaw. The pain begins without a known precipitating episode and may last for hours to days. It may spread to involve the head or neck, and muscles of the jaw and neck are often tender. Sometimes autonomic symptoms including sweating, flushing, a nidus, and pallor are present. The disorder usually affects women, often in early middle age. Patients affected with the disorder are tense, anxious, and often chronically depressed. The pathogenesis of the illness is unknown. The autonomic changes have led some to suggest that the syndrome is a migraine variant, and the muscle tenderness and depression have led others to suggest that it be classified with musculoskeletal tension pain. Patients suffering from atypical facial pain should be examined carefully for local pathology of the eyes, nose, teeth, sinuses, and pharynx, but such is rarely found. Careful psychologic evaluation will often reveal a masked depression. Treatment is usually unsatisfactory. Analgesic agents are usually not helpful, and patients respond poorly to routine psychotherapy. In some patients, ergot preparations or propranolol appears to be effective, and others respond to physical methods such as massage and biofeedback. Antidepressants are sometimes helpful. It is important to recognize that the syndrome is not caused by structural disease and that patients require no invasive diagnostic or therapeutic procedures. Dental extraction does more harm than good.

Traction/Inflammation

Cranial Arteritis

This condition receives detailed consideration in Ch. 451 but deserves mention here as an important cause of headache in the elderly. The illness almost always appears after age 60 and usually later. The onset is usually with unilateral or bilateral temporal, occipital, or fronto-occipital head pain of variable intensity, often coupled with tenderness of the painful areas. Many patients have pain in the jaw muscles, making chewing uncomfortable. Nodules occasionally are palpable on affected vessels. The great risk is occlusion of retinal arteries secondary to untreated inflammation. Diagnosis depends on suspicion and usually on the presence of an elevated erythrocyte sedimentation rate. Diagnosis should be confirmed by arterial biopsy because definitive steroid treatment, once started, often must be maintained for many months. Since migraine-vascular headaches and depressive headaches also can have their onset in the elderly, a confirmed diagnosis is essential.

Meningitis and Subarachnoid Hemorrhage

Acute and subacute meningitis cause gradually developing headache resulting from inflammation of pain-sensitive structures surrounding the brain. The headache is usually generalized, throbbing, and very severe. It may be rapid or gradual in onset, and by the time it is fully developed is associated with nuchal rigidity. The diagnosis is established by lumbar puncture. In patients suspected of harboring an intracranial mass lesion, CT scan of the brain should be performed first and lumbar puncture deferred, unless the physician suspects that the patient is suffering from acute bacterial meningitis, in which case lumbar puncture must be done immediately. In *subarachnoid hemorrhage*, the initial sudden headache is caused by alteration of intracranial pressure. This headache is succeeded by a chronic persistent headache, often accompanied by nuchal rigidity that results from inflammation of the meninges caused by the blood. In a patient suspected of having suffered a subarachnoid hemorrhage, a CT scan should be performed first. The presence of extravascular blood establishes the diagnosis and obviates the need for lumbar puncture, which may exacerbate the bleeding by altering intracranial dynamics. The absence of identifiable hemorrhage on CT scan, however, does not rule out a small subarachnoid hemorrhage, and lumbar puncture then must be performed to establish or rule out the diagnosis definitively.

Alterations of Intracranial Pressure

Headache from altered intracranial pressure is caused by compression or traction of pain-sensitive vascular and neural structures over the apex and base of the brain. In the instance of *intracranial hypotension,* the loss of spinal fluid decreases the buoyancy of the brain so that the organ descends when the upright position is assumed, exerting traction on structures at its apex and compression on structures at its base. (In rare instances, the small bridging veins that enter the sagittal sinus may rupture and cause subdural hematomas.) In *intracranial hypertension,* the source of pain is probably compression of vascular and neural structures at the base of the brain by tumor or edematous brain.

INTRACRANIAL HYPERTENSION. Increased intracranial pressure per se does not lead to headache unless pain-sensitive structures are distorted. Many patients with high intracranial pressure from brain tumors, jugular venous obstruction, hydrocephalus, or pseudotumor cerebri do not suffer headache. If headache is present, it may be mild or severe, throbbing or steady, localized or generalized. When localized, it usually overlies the site of the lesion, but posterior fossa lesions may cause bifrontal headache. The headache is characteristically at its worst early in the morning, although it usually does not awaken the patient from sleep. It is exacerbated by stooping, coughing, moving the head suddenly, or straining at stool. Many patients prefer to sleep in the sitting position. The headache is rarely continuously intense. Reflecting transient rises of intracranial pressure, there are often waves of intense headache, sometimes accompanied by nausea, vomiting, or other neurologic signs. These "pressure or plateau waves," lasting 5 to 20 minutes, commonly are precipitated by assuming the upright posture.

The treatment of headache related to increased intracranial pressure is the treatment of the underlying disease (Ch. 513). Mild analgesics produce temporary relief; narcotic analgesics should not be used because of their tendency to produce respiratory depression and further raise the pressure in neurologically compromised individuals.

INTRACRANIAL HYPOTENSION (see Ch. 512). Intracranial hypotension usually follows a lumbar puncture and is due to continued leakage of cerebrospinal fluid through a rent in the dural sheath. (Rarely, a dural tear may occur spontaneously or follow mild trauma, producing the syndrome of *spontaneous* intracranial hypotension.) The syndrome develops 12 hours to several days after the lumbar puncture and is characterized by headache that occurs on assuming the upright position. There is no evidence that a period of recumbency after a lumbar puncture prevents subsequent development of the headache. The headache usually begins as a dull ache in the posterior cervical area, radiating laterally out toward the shoulders and cephalad toward the frontal area. It persists, often growing more severe, as long as the patient is in the upright position, and when most severe it may be associated with perspiration, nausea, and vomiting. Persistent headache of intracranial hypotension can lead to diplopia, probably a result of traction on the abducens nerves. The diagnosis of post–lumbar puncture headache is made by history; spontaneous intracranial hypotension is suspected by the history of positional headache and confirmed by low (<30 mm H_2O) or even negative CSF pressure on attempted lumbar puncture. The fluid is usually normal, but there may be an elevated protein concentration if the needle has entered a subdural or epidural fluid collection. Analgesics relieve the mildest headaches; the most severe ones can be controlled only by assuming the recumbent position. The headaches usually clear within a few days to a few weeks; in rare instances, surgical repair of the torn dura is necessary.

Extracranial Structural Lesions

Nasal and Sinus Headache

Although acute or chronic inflammation and neoplasms of the paranasal sinuses can cause headache, most patients who have been physician- or self-diagnosed as having sinus headaches are in fact suffering from either vascular or muscle contraction headache. Most true paranasal sinus headaches result from acute inflammation of the paranasal sinuses, which produces pain localized over the involved sinus and is associated with the stigmata of acute infection, including fever, swelling, and tenderness over the sinus and engorgement of the turbinates, ostia, nasofrontal ducts, and superior nasal spaces. Most of the discomfort comes from the ostia, which are many times more sensitive than the poorly innervated walls of the sinuses. Typically, "sinus" headache commences in the morning (frontal) or early afternoon (maxillary) and subsides in the early or late evening. The pain is dull and aching, is made worse by changing head position, and is seldom associated with nausea and vomiting. Sinus headache is best treated with decongestants and analgesics. Persistent purulent discharges should be cultured and appropriate antimicrobial drugs employed. Chronic suppurative disease in the frontal, ethmoid, and sphenoid sinuses, or in the mastoid air cells, may result in osteomyelitis and inflammation of adjacent cranial tissues. Headache persisting after surgical drainage of the diseased sinus is evidence for extradural and possibly subdural infection. More chronic inflammation and neoplasms, particularly when they occur in the sphenoid sinus, may not be accompanied by the usual physical signs of sinusitis. In such instances, sinus x-rays or CT scan may be required to establish the diagnosis.

Dental Pain

Noxious stimuli in a tooth usually evoke local toothache, but severe dental pain can be extremely difficult to localize. Afferent fibers for sensation in the teeth are contained in the second and third divisions of the trigeminal nerve. Headache in the areas supplied by the latter is, in rare instances, associated with prolonged, intense toothache or follows a tooth extraction. More commonly, in association with toothache, tooth extraction, or a tender, diseased tooth, distant tissues exhibit surface hyperalgesia, tenderness, and vasomotor reactions, such as tender eyeballs, reddening of the conjunctivae, and tenderness of the auricular and temporal tissues. Because of secondary muscle contraction, other sites of tenderness and pain may be noted behind the ears, behind the lower border of the mastoid process, and in the muscles of the occiput, neck, and shoulders. The upper teeth frequently hurt in association with disease of the nasal and paranasal structures. Occasionally, in coronary insufficiency, pain is experienced in the lower jaw. One should beware of ascribing bizarre pains in and around the jaws to a dental origin unless unequivocal acute inflammatory dental lesions are present. Dental extraction rarely ameliorates neuralgias or atypical facial pain. However, hysterical or delusional face pain is often attributed by the patient to prior dental work. Headache may not be attributed to a diseased tooth unless the injection of procaine into the tissues about the suspected tooth greatly reduces the intensity of, or eliminates, such headache.

Aural Pain

Severe pain in the vicinity of the ear can be caused by disease of the teeth, acute tonsillitis, inflammatory and neoplastic disease of the larynx and nasopharynx, temporomandibular joint disorders, tumors, inflammation in the posterior fossa, and disease of the cervical spine and its soft tissues. Pain in the ear is also associated with vascular headaches, atypical facial pain, and herpes zoster of the fifth and seventh cranial nerves and, rarely, the glossopharyngeal nerve. True glossopharyngeal neuralgia causes severe pain radiating from the tonsil into the ear. It has the usual timing feature of "tic."

Primary ear disease is relatively infrequent—but important—as a source of headache, because it almost always indicates inflammation or destructive disease. Acute otitis media (purulent or nonpurulent), furunculosis of the ear canal, traumatic rupture of the tympanum, and fracture of the anterior wall of the bony canal all cause pain in the ear associated with sustained tender contraction of adjacent skeletal muscles. Osteomyelitis of the mastoid bone may be associated with inflammation of the nearby periosteum as well as of dura and adjacent tissues (epidural abscess)—both sources of pain in or behind the ear. Pain in this region also accompanies tumors of the acoustic nerve and inflammation and thrombosis of the lateral sinus.

Eye Pain and Headache

Errors of refraction (hypermetropia, astigmatism, anomalies of accommodation), disturbances of ocular muscle equilibrium, and glaucoma are universally described as causing headache. Refractive errors are also said to give origin to such other symptoms as aching of the eyes, "sandy" feeling in the eyes, pulling sensations in and about the orbit, and conjunctival congestion. Headache is mild in degree and usually starts around and over the eyes and subsequently radiates to the occiput and back of the head.

The pain of glaucoma at first remains localized in the eyeball, then extends along the rim of the orbit and, finally, throughout most of the area supplied by the ophthalmic division of the trigeminal nerve. Nausea and vomiting sometimes accompany such headaches, which can become prostratingly severe if not treated promptly.

Simple myopia does not evoke headache because the myope, in attempting to improve his vision by the contraction of his eye muscles, actually makes his vision worse and soon abandons the attempt.

With inflammation of the iris and ciliary body, light may cause intense pain in the eye and adjacent areas because of movement of the inflamed iris. When the iris is immobilized, pain is allayed.

Pituitary Pain

Headache caused by pituitary tumors is the result of compression and distortion of pain-sensitive structures at the base of the skull, particularly the diaphragma sella. Pain is generally referred to the frontal or temporal regions bilaterally and may on occasion be referred to the vertex or occipital regions. Because the pain is not related to intracranial pressure, it does not have the same temporal characteristics of most brain tumor headaches and instead can occur at any time and is frequently chronic and unremitting. The headache is usually accompanied by evidence of endocrine failure, particularly loss of libido and impotence in the male. The combination of loss of libido and chronic headache may lead the physician to suspect depression rather than a pituitary lesion. The diagnosis can be established by endocrine examination and by CT scan of the pituitary fossa. Acute headache occurring with known pituitary lesions (*pituitary apoplexy*) usually results from infarction or hemorrhage into the tumor. Sudden expansion of the tumor may compromise the overlying optic chiasm, leading to visual loss, or invade the laterally lying cavernous sinus, producing ocular palsies. Pituitary apoplexy should be treated surgically by emergency drainage of the hemorrhagic or infarcted material.

Cranial Neuralgias

The term cranial neuralgias refers to several distinctive head pains that appear to result from sudden and excessive discharge from the involved nerve. The best-known cranial neuralgia is trigeminal neuralgia. The concept of cranial neuralgias has been expanded to include the chronic burning pain that frequently follows herpes zoster infection of the nerve. Some also include atypical facial pain and temporomandibular joint syndrome under the cranial neuralgias, but these probably have muscle contraction or vascular disturbances as their pathogenesis and in this chapter are included under those headings.

TRIGEMINAL NEURALGIA. Trigeminal neuralgia (tic douloureux) is a disease characterized by sudden, lightning-like paroxysms of pain in the distribution of one or more divisions of the trigeminal nerve. Most observers believe that most trigeminal neuralgia is caused by compression of the trigeminal nerve by arteries or veins of the posterior fossa. In some patients there is no identifiable structural disease. Occasionally trigeminal neuralgia may be a symptom of a gasserian ganglion tumor, of multiple sclerosis, or of a brainstem infarct involving the descending root of the trigeminal nerve.

The history is diagnostic. The pain occurs as brief, lightning-like stabs, frequently precipitated by touching a trigger zone around the lips or the buccal cavity. At times, talking, eating, or brushing the teeth serves as a trigger. The pains rarely last longer than seconds, and each burst is followed by a refractory period of several seconds to a minute in which no further pain can be precipitated. The pains, however, often occur in clusters so that the patient may report that each pain lasts for hours. The pain is limited to the distribution of the trigeminal nerve, usually affecting the second and third division or both. Spontaneous remissions and exacerbations are common, the exacerbations tending to occur in spring and fall. Between paroxysms of pain, the patient is asymptomatic. Tic pain rarely occurs at night. In idiopathic trigeminal neuralgia, the neurologic examination is entirely normal. In symptomatic trigeminal neuralgia, there may be sensory changes in the distribution of the trigeminal nerve, and such a finding should prompt a careful search for structural disease of the nervous system.

Carbamazepine is the drug of choice for the treatment of trigeminal neuralgia. The anticonvulsant drug is given in doses varying from 400 to 800 mg a day, but because of its sedative properties the initial dose is 100 mg twice daily, gradually increased to the required maintenance dose. No more than 1200 mg should be taken daily. The drug is not an analgesic and is only effective for specific kinds of pain such as trigeminal neuralgia, glossopharyngeal neuralgia, and the lightning pains of tabes dorsalis. Rarely, aplastic anemia has been reported, and complete blood counts are procured prior to the initiation of therapy and at intervals thereafter. Other side effects include dizziness and sedation. Phenytoin* in doses of 400 mg a day is also effective in trigeminal neuralgia but less so than carbamazepine. Occasionally the two drugs appear to be synergistic. Baclofen* 60 to 80 mg daily has also been found to be a useful agent. If medical treatment fails, surgical intervention is necessary. The most popular operations are radiofrequency lesions of the gasserian ganglion (radiofrequency gangliolysis) and posterior fossa craniotomy to relieve the trigeminal nerve of compression by vascular structures. The first operation can be done under local anesthesia and is generally effective initially, but has a high relapse rate. The second operation is as effective as the first, and appears to have a lower relapse rate. Both operations produce either mild or no loss of sensation in the face, and thus are preferable to such operations as section of the nerve root proximal to the ganglion, which, however, affords permanent relief. Local anesthesia of the ganglion or the peripheral branches of the nerve at some time prior to surgery is desirable because some patients find the anesthesia produced by nerve section less tolerable than the pain itself.

GLOSSOPHARYNGEAL NEURALGIA. Glossopharyngeal neuralgia is characterized by pain similar to that of trigeminal neuralgia but in the distribution of the glossopharyngeal and vagus nerves. The trigger zone is usually in the tonsil or posterior pharynx, and the pain spreads toward the angle of the jaw and the ear. Occasional patients suffer cardiac slowing or arrest during these attacks as a result of the intense afferent discharge over the glossopharyngeal nerve. Carbamazepine is often effective, but if it fails, glossopharyngeal nerve roots are sectioned in the posterior fossa. Symptomatic glossopharyngeal

*This use is not listed in the manufacturer's directive.

neuralgia is occasionally the presenting complaint in a patient with a tonsillar tumor, and careful examination of the pharynx and tonsillar fossa for mass lesions must be carried out.

OTHER NEURALGIAS. Similar but much rarer disorders than trigeminal or glossopharyngeal neuralgia have been reported to involve the greater occipital nerve and the nervus intermedius portion of the facial nerve. The clinical features and treatment of these rare disorders are similar to those for trigeminal neuralgia.

POSTHERPETIC NEURALGIA. Postherpetic neuralgia refers to severe and prolonged burning pain with occasional lightning-like stabs in the involved dermatome after an attack of herpes zoster. The disorder commonly affects the first division of the trigeminal nerve. Its treatment is discussed in Ch. 501.

Diagnostic Evaluation

Headache is an extremely common disorder, and the excessive application of expensive and highly technical laboratory procedures to the diagnosis and management of benign head pain has been a substantial cause of unnecessary medical costs. Set against this truism is the fact that in some instances a timely CT scan or lumbar puncture can give lifesaving information about an otherwise undiagnosable problem. Given these antitheses, the following principles may help in the management of the individual patient:

1. Patients with chronic classic or common migraine or with chronic tension headache rarely require more than a careful history and examination. Even when the unilateral prodromes and headache of longstanding, classic migraine consistently affect the same side, the incidence of associated intracranial lesions remains so low that CT scan is unnecessary and arteriography unjustified.
2. Headaches that are of recent origin or progression deserve investigation by CT scan. This principle especially applies to headaches that have a consistently focal distribution, follow trauma, or begin after the age of 30 years.
3. The EEG is almost never useful in the diagnosis of diseases causing headache and can be omitted. Skull x-rays are useful in diagnosing headache only (a) when searching for abnormalities involving the base of the brain such as sellar and suprasellar lesions or (b) immediately following head trauma. CT scans have superior discriminating capacities to plain x-rays and, when available, make x-rays unnecessary.
4. Diagnostic lumbar puncture should be performed with any acute headache that (a) is accompanied by fever or (b) is explosive or the most severe headache ever suffered (a history typical of acute subarachnoid hemorrhage). Lumbar puncture should, if possible, be deferred until after CT scanning with other forms of acute headache, especially if stiff neck but no fever is present. (This combination may indicate partial herniation of cerebellar tonsils into the foramen magnum secondary to an intracranial mass lesion.)
5. If CT scanning is available, radioisotopic brain scanning almost never adds useful information and is expensively superfluous.

Diamond S, Dalessio DJ: The Practicing Physician's Approach to Headache. 3rd ed. Baltimore, Williams & Wilkins, 1982. *This short, up-to-date monograph describes the practical approach to the management of headache. The book is beautifully illustrated.*

Headache and *Cephalgia. Two journals which publish original articles concerning new developments in the diagnosis and management of headaches and other types of head pain.*

Packard RC: Symposium on Headache. Neurol Clin Vol 1, No 2, May, 1983. Philadelphia, W. B. Saunders, 1983. *A comprehensive and up-to-date review of headache and its management.*

Saper JR: Headache Disorders. Current Concepts and Treatment Strategies. Boston, John Wright, PSG Inc., 1983.

NECK AND BACK PAIN

Neck and/or back pain, whether localized or radiating into the extremities, is one of man's most common afflictions. Low back pain is believed to affect about 80 per cent of all individuals at some time during their lives. Neck or back pain is a major cause of time lost from work. Most neck or back pain is transient and neither life-threatening nor associated with obvious pathologic abnormalities. Because the pathophysiology of most such pain is poorly understood, the physician often encounters patients for whom he can neither make a certain diagnosis nor prescribe rational therapy. Fortunately, most patients suffering neck or back pain recover within a few weeks no matter what the treatment. Estimates are that 70 per cent of patients recover within one month and 90 per cent within three months. Only 4 per cent of patients suffering neck or back pain are disabled longer than six months. In those patients who suffer transient episodes of neck or back pain, the cause is rarely established. Some authorities believe that the majority suffer from bulging or herniated intervertebral discs (see Ch. 519). Others believe that disc disease is a minor cause and that most neck and back pain is caused by lesions of other pain-sensitive structures in and around the spine, especially the facet joints, paravertebral musculature, sacroiliac joints, or vertebral bodies themselves.

A small number of patients develop chronic pain or neurologic dysfunction that portends serious disease. In this small number, meticulous diagnostic evaluation and vigorous therapy often prevent or reverse serious or potentially lethal neurologic sequelae. Most patients with chronic pain and neurologic dysfunction suffer from mechanical lesions compressing the nerve roots, paravertebral nerve plexuses, or spinal cord. The lesions are described in Ch. 518. The following provides a general discussion of the management of the patient who complains of acute or subacute neck or back pain.

ANATOMY AND PHYSIOLOGY OF THE SPINE. The functional unit of the spine is composed of two segments: The anterior segment contains two adjacent vertebral bodies separated by an intervertebral disc. The function of the anterior segment is to bear weight and cushion the shock to the spine from such activities as walking and running. The posterior segment is composed of the vertebral arches, the transverse processes, the posterior spinous processes, and the paired articulations known as "facets," with the facet joint between them. The posterior segment is a non–weight-bearing structure that has the function of protecting the contained spinal cord and nerves as well as allowing the spine to be mobile both in extension and in rotation. Not all of the structures of this unit are pain-sensitive. The vertebral body, at least its periosteum, is pain-sensitive (therefore, compression fractures are, at least initially, painful), whereas the intervertebral disc is not in itself pain-sensitive. However, if the intervertebral disc bulges and compresses the posterior longitudinal ligament, pain may result even if the nerve root itself is not involved. Posteriorly, the synovium-lined facet joints are pain-sensitive, although the intraspinal ligaments holding the posterior elements together are not. The paravertebral muscles surrounding and supporting the spine are pain-sensitive, particularly when they are overstretched or when they go into spasm. In the neutral position, the nerve root occupies only a small portion of the intervertebral foramen from which it exits the spinal canal. However, when the spine is extended, i.e., when it is in the hyperlordotic posture, the intervertebral foramen becomes smaller, potentially causing impingement on a nerve root and also leading to overlap of the facet joints, the latter allowing for irritation of the pain-sensitive synovial membranes. This is the reason that on examination of patients with intervertebral disc disease or with pain originating from the facet joints, the pain may be relieved somewhat by flexion of the spine and exacerbated by extension or lordosis. It is also the reason that hyperlordosis, a common postural abnormality, sometimes leads to chronic low back pain and why most back exercises have as their goal the production of a flat or slightly flexed but certainly not hyperlordotic lumbar spine.

Another anatomic finding of clinical importance in evaluating low back pain is that lumbar roots exit through that portion of the intervertebral foramen that is above the intervertebral disc. Thus, even though the L4 root exits between L4 and L5, a herniated disc between these vertebral bodies occurs just below the exit of the L4 root and thus will usually compress the L5 and not the L4 root. A herniated disc between the fifth lumbar and the first sacral vertebral body will usually compress the S1 root and not the L5 root. If, however, the disc protrudes more medially, an occurrence much less common than laterally protruding disc, an L4-L5 disc may involve the caudally directed sacral roots rather than the L5 lumbar root. Only if the disc completely extrudes into the vertebral canal will an L4-L5 disc compress the L4 root. In the cervical spine, the roots exit above a vertebral body with the same number (i.e., C4 root exits between C3 and C4). Thus, a herniated C4-C5 disc may compress the C6 or C5 root, but not the C4.

Neck or back pain may be severe and disabling and can originate from any of the pain-sensitive structures in the spine or surrounding muscles, the description giving no sure clue as to its etiology. Only if pain radiates in a clear dermatomal distribution can the physician infer that a nerve root has been damaged or compressed by the process.

EXAMINATION OF THE PATIENT. The task for the physician is to separate those patients with potentially serious disease who require extensive diagnostic evaluation from those with more common, if unknown, causes of neck and back pain who need only reassurance, sometimes coupled with bedrest, analgesics, and physical therapy.

The diagnostic evaluation begins with the history. Get a complete description of the pain. Most benign back pain is of acute or subacute onset, and frequently follows by minutes to hours some unaccustomed physical activity, particularly lifting or bending. Often patients awaken stiff and sore the morning after unusual exercise. Sometimes low back pain begins acutely, frequently on arising in the morning, without any obvious precipitating event. Most neck pain begins as a stiff neck, often on awakening in the morning, without a history of any unusual activity. In many patients neck or low back pain recurs episodically over many years. Most benign neck or back pain is dull and aching in quality, exacerbated by movement and relieved by rest. The majority of patients with benign neck or back pain are comfortable when they are recumbent and immobile, or are able to find at least one position that relieves the pain. Pain that is present when the patient is immobile and cannot be relieved by positional manipulation should lead the physician to search for a more serious disorder. Ask if the pain radiates from the neck or back, around the chest or abdomen, or into an extremity. If the radiation is in a dermatomal distribution, and particularly if it is accompanied by paresthesias or loss of sensation, there is probably mechanical compression of the root supplying that dermatome, and more likely than not the patient will have identifiable structural disease of the nervous system. However, radiating pain into an extremity may not follow a strict dermatomal distribution and may not be accompanied by paresthesias. Instead, there is diffuse aching often associated with muscle tenderness in a distribution different from and more widespread than a dermatome. The distribution labeled sclerotomal does not necessarily imply compression of a root. The pathogenesis of such sclerotomal pain is poorly understood, but has been produced by injection of noxious substances such as hypertonic saline into the posterior longitudinal ligament of the spinal canal, into facet joints, and into paravertebral muscles. Many believe the source of the pain is muscle spasm resulting from irritation of nerve endings in ligamentous and muscular structures.

Take additional history. A past history of serious systemic illness may suggest disease of vertebral bodies. For example, carcinoma of the breast or thyroid may cause back pain from bony metastases years after the primary tumor has been successfully treated. A previous systemic infection may lead to delayed onset of vertebral osteomyelitis or an epidural abscess. A family history may also give clues to the etiology of back pain. For example, neurofibromas causing neck or back pain by compressing nerve roots or the spinal cord may be associated with neurofibromatosis. Rheumatoid arthritis and ankylosing spondylitis are causes of familial back pain.

A careful general physical examination is mandatory. The examination may reveal evidence of systemic disease such as cancer or infection, indicating a similar process causing low back pain. Urinary tract infections, pelvic disease, abdominal aneurysms, and other intra-abdominal or intrathoracic processes may cause back pain by impinging on vertebral bodies or paravertebral structures. Peripheral nerves can be easily palpated at several sites (e.g., ulnar nerve at the elbow, peroneal nerve at the head of the fibula, sacral roots by pelvic or rectal examination). Palpable thickening may lead to a diagnosis of neurofibromatosis. Special attention should be paid to mobility of the spine and paravertebral structures. In most patients who complain of a stiff neck there is some limitation of movement of the cervical spine, but if gradual movement of the cervical spine causes intense pain, if pain on neck flexion is referred to the thoracic or lumbar area, or if neck flexion causes paresthesias radiating into the arms, legs or back (Lhermitte's sign), spinal cord compression should be suspected. Most low back pain not caused by a herniated disc is exacerbated by forward flexion and relieved by lying down. The paravertebral muscles are often in spasm, straightening the normally lordotic lumbar spine, and are often tender to palpation. Sometimes the palpating finger encounters nodule-like thickenings that, when pressed, produce pain radiating into an extremity in a sclerodermal distribution. In most people with severe low back pain, particularly if it radiates into a lower extremity, the pain increases when the extended leg is raised from the bed (straight leg raising sign). However, pain referred to the contralateral back or leg when the nonpainful leg is raised (crossed straight leg raising) implies root compression within the spinal canal. Point tenderness over a spinous process raises the suspicion of involvement of that vertebra by either tumor or infection.

The neurologic examination is important. Sensory loss, reflex diminution, and weakness all suggest serious structural disease and require further evaluation. The distribution of neurologic abnormalities localizes the lesion. Remember, however, that patients in severe pain are reluctant to move the painful part, particularly against resistance, and often appear to be weak when the neuromuscular structures are in fact normal. Likewise, guarding can affect deep tendon reflexes, either increasing or decreasing them with respect to the normal side. Such reflex alteration may mislead the observer into believing that the patient has nervous system disease. Repeating the neurologic examination after pain has been relieved by analgesics usually clarifies whether or not there is neurologic dysfunction. Clear and reproducible neurologic signs, particularly sensory loss in a dermatomal distribution or a diminished stretch reflex, imply root compression.

SIGNS AND SYMPTOMS OF NERVE ROOT AND SPINAL CORD COMPRESSION. The spinal cord and its attached motor, sensory, and autonomic nerve roots are the primary occupants of the spinal canal. The spinal cord itself extends in the adult from the first cervical to the first lumbar vertebral body, and the spinal roots continue in the subarachnoid space to the second sacral vertebra. The caudal portion of the spinal cord is called the conus medullaris, and the bunched roots below the cord the cauda equina. Within the spinal canal, the spinal cord and its roots can be subjected to mechanical compression and deformation by several processes. The resulting signs and symptoms depend on the location of the pathologic process, its speed of development, and whether it affects the nerve roots or the spinal cord alone.

Acute compression of nerve trunks and nerve roots is not generally painful. Pressing on the median nerve at the wrist or the ulnar nerve at the elbow is rarely painful. A sharp blow may cause the nerve to discharge, causing paresthesias in the distribution of that nerve but not severe pain. However, once a root or nerve is damaged, as when chronic compression produces edema, demyelination, and inflammation, the root becomes tender to compression or stretch. Then pain occurs, usually both at the site of compression and in part or all of the dermatomal distribution of that root (radicular pain). The symptoms of chronic compression of nerve roots are pain, paresthesias, sensory loss, weakness, atrophy, and hyporeflexia. These abnormalities are confined to the tissues supplied by the root(s) involved, thus localizing the lesion. Knowing the myotomal and dermatomal distribution of spinal roots (see Table 518–1) often allows one not only to localize the lesion but also to suggest its etiologic diagnosis, since involvement of a single root is more likely to occur with intervertebral disc herniation (see Ch. 519), whereas multiple root dysfunction is likely to be caused by tumor or chronic inflammation. However, myotomal and dermatomal localization must be utilized cautiously. In the first place, not everyone obeys the standard maps (e.g., in about 5 per cent of patients intrinsic muscles of the hand are supplied exclusively by the median or ulnar nerve rather than shared between the two). Also, there is much overlap between contiguous dermatomes and contiguous myotomes, and the apparent size of a dermatome may vary from day to day or even hour to hour, depending on the excitability of the central nervous system. Excepting these caveats, however, the localizing diagnosis of root lesions is usually quite accurate.

In most instances, pain is the prominent symptom of root compression. Pain is experienced in the overlying spine, deep in certain muscles supplied by the compressed root, and in the cutaneous distribution of the injured root. Pain is usually least severe when the patient is in a position that minimizes compression of the root and most severe in positions that compress or stretch the root. With intervertebral disc herniations, lying down may be very comfortable and sitting up uncomfortable, whereas with tumors within the spinal canal compressing nerve roots, the opposite may be true. With both disc herniation and tumor, pain is exacerbated by increasing intraspinal pressure, e.g., coughing, sneezing, and straining.

Pain, both local and radicular, is also an early complaint in patients with spinal cord compression. As with root disease, the pain of spinal cord compression is usually exacerbated by movements that stretch the cord (neck flexion, straight leg raising) or that increase intraspinal pressure (coughing, sneezing, straining). In addition, patients harboring compressive spinal cord lesions are often tender to percussion over the vertebral body at the site of compression. Other clinical signs of spinal cord compression depend on the speed with which the compression develops, the transverse and longitudinal site of the lesion, and the vulnerability of the individual spinal fibers. The spinal cord accommodates fairly well to gradually developing compression (as, for example, from meningiomas and neurofibromas), and these disorders may cause the gradual onset of painless paraparesis or paraplegia. Because the cord has accommodated to the evolution of a compressing lesion, subsequent decompression, even when patients are severely paraparetic, often leads to complete resolution of neurologic symptoms. On the other hand, rapidly developing lesions such as epidural hematomas, acute midline herniated discs, or epidural spinal cord compression from metastatic tumor cause rapidly developing neurologic signs that respond poorly to therapy once severe paraparesis has developed. The site of compression in the transverse plane also determines clinical signs, particularly when the compression develops slowly. For example, lateral lesions compressing one side of the spinal cord may cause Brown-Séquard's syndrome (ipsilateral hemiparesis and vibration and position sense loss, with contralateral pain and temperature loss); compression of the posterior portion of the cord may cause bilateral position and vibratory loss, with preservation of pin and temperature sensation and of motor power. However, because mass lesions twist the cord as they compress it and also interfere with the vascular supply to sites beyond the compression, one can depend only in a general way on the neurologic signs to evaluate the exact transverse site of spinal cord compression. The longitudinal location of the lesion is likewise important. Cervical lesions cause quadriplegia; thoracic lesions, paraplegia; and upper lumbar lesions, normal motor function with bowel and bladder dysfunction and extensor plantar responses (conus medullaris syndrome). Lesions below the first lumbar vertebral body compress the cauda equina, causing loss of bowel and bladder function with lower motor neuron leg weakness and normal plantar reflexes. Certain spinal tracts appear to be more vulnerable to compression than others. The corticospinal tracts and posterior columns appear particularly vulnerable, the spinothalamic tracts and descending autonomic fibers less so. As a result, weakness, spasticity, and reflex hyperactivity tend to be the earliest signs of spinal cord compression, with paresthesias and vibratory and position sense loss occurring soon thereafter. Loss of pain and temperature sensation and of bladder and bowel function usually occur late in the course of spinal cord compression. The spinocerebellar pathways are also sensitive to compression, and at times ataxia mimicking cerebellar disease may be the only sign of spinal cord compression.

LABORATORY AIDS TO INVESTIGATION. In most patients with benign neck or back pain no laboratory tests are required. However, if, after a careful history and examination, the physician suspects structural disease of the spine or root or spinal cord compression, laboratory tests will help confirm the clinical diagnosis and identify the site and nature of the disorder. Plain x-rays of the spine should be the first test in patients suspected of harboring structural disease. For suspected cervical lesions, frontal, lateral, oblique, and open-mouth odontoid views are required. If the patient has a short neck, the lower cervical area on lateral view may be obscured by the shoulders and require tomography. Flexion and extension views of the neck are often helpful to determine if subluxation is present. If the *patient* is allowed to control the degree of flexion and extension, these tests are not harmful. For the thoracic and lumbosacral spine, frontal and lateral views are usually sufficient. Flexion and extension views assess subluxation. Review the x-rays with the radiologist to assure that all potential lesions of the site in question have been assessed. Pay particular attention to the sagittal diameter of the cervical and lumbar canal (see Ch. 519), to the pedicles (see Ch. 520), and to the presence of osteophytes and loss of height in disc spaces (see Ch. 519). Congenital anomalies (see Ch. 523) should also be searched for, but the physician should recognize that congenital anomalies of the spine are common and most do not cause pain or other symptoms. Similarly, most patients of middle age or older have evidence of cervical and/or lumbar osteoarthritis. Such abnormalities do not prove that the radiologic defect is responsible for the symptoms. However, changes such as significant spondylolisthesis, marked multiple disc narrowings, stenosis of the lumbar canal, or vertebral destruction from tumor or infection are likely to be responsible for pain and often for neurologic disability. If back pain is referred to the lower extremities, x-rays of the pelvis and femora may reveal unsuspected abnormalities.

Computed tomography (CT scan) can detect erosion of vertebral bodies not identified on plain x-rays or bone scan, can identify paravertebral masses, dumbbell tumors growing through the intervertebral foramen, and herniated discs. With high resolution CT scanners, tumors and syrinxes within the cord can sometimes be identified. Thus, the CT scan is now the best radiologic test for the diagnosis of spine, nerve root, and spinal cord disease. Nuclear magnetic resonance (NMR) for scanning of the spinal cord and canal promises to identify intramedullary lesions such as tumor and syrinxes not currently seen by other techniques. NMR with or without CT may eventually replace more invasive diagnostic tests such as myelography.

X-ray tomography is useful in defining bony lesions in some areas of the spine, particularly at T1 and the sacrum where obscuration of the vertebral canal by overlying shadows makes plain films hard to interpret. Tomography is also useful in assessing minor degrees of bone destruction when plain x-rays are normal. It may sometimes be more sensitive than CT. A *radionuclide bone scan* is a more sensitive but less specific method of identifying lesions of the vertebrae. Destruction of bone by tumor may be identified by bone scan before plain x-rays become positive. Unfortunately, trivial traumatic, arthritic, and inflammatory lesions may also produce a positive bone scan. Occasionally the bone scan is normal even when plain x-rays reveal obvious bone destruction.

Myelography, using either lipid- or water-soluble radiopaque contrast material, will reliably outline compressive lesions. Myelograms must be viewed in both the frontal and lateral planes to determine if lesions are extradural, intradural, or intramedullary. If a complete block to the passage of the contrast material is encountered after lumbar injection, a cisternal or upper cervical injection of contrast material will determine the upper extent of the lesion. *Lumbar puncture* is useful to detect the presence of malignant cells or infecting organisms in the spinal fluid. When a mass lesion is suspected, a lumbar puncture should be performed only in conjunction with myelography. *Spinal angiography* is a specialized technique, sometimes essential for the detailed investigation of tumors and vascular malformations within the spinal cord. The technique is particularly useful to the surgeon who requires preoperative knowledge of the vascular supply. *Discography* is a controversial technique for identifying clinically important herniated discs. Under fluoroscopic control, less than 1 ml of contrast material is injected into the nucleus pulposus. Leakage of contrast material through the anulus fibrosis indicates disease of the disc space. More importantly, if the patient's spontaneous pain pattern is exactly reproduced, one can infer that it is that damaged disc which is producing the patient's symptoms. Unfortunately, at times asymptomatic discs may yield positive discograms.

Electromyography also helps in diagnosis. When the level of nerve root or spinal cord compression cannot be determined clinically, electromyographic evidence of lower motor neuron dysfunction restricted to a particular myotome strongly suggests root or anterior horn cell involvement at that level. Caution in evaluating lower motor neuron dysfunction in spinal cord compressive lesions is essential because tumors of the upper cervical spinal cord occasionally cause atrophy with fasciculations and fibrillations in the hand, probably from ischemia of anterior horns in the lower cervical cord. The paraspinous muscles are supplied by the posterior ramus of each emerging nerve root, and electromyographic evidence of denervation in those muscles implies a lesion close to the vertebral body before anterior and posterior rami diverge. In some patients with back pain but without clinically definable root symptoms, denervation of paraspinous muscles points to root involvement at the level of back pain. *Somatosensory evoked potentials* can be recorded along the spinal cord or in the brain after a peripheral nerve is stimulated. Abnormalities sometimes identify the site of a spinal cord lesion. Evoked potentials diminish or disappear with posterior column dysfunction. Their exact role in the diagnosis and prognosis of spinal cord lesions is still unresolved.

MANAGEMENT OF NECK AND BACK PAIN. If there are no clinical findings to suggest serious structural disease of the spine, nerve roots, or spinal cord, patients should be treated as if they suffered from an acute neck or back strain, without further diagnostic evaluation. Because most patients recover within a few weeks without specific therapy, it is difficult to assess various therapeutic regimens. For severe pain, the best treatment probably consists of bedrest on a firmly supported mattress in the position most comfortable for the patient. The best positioning for low back pain is usually semi-Fowler's position (head slightly elevated with pillows under the knees). Bedrest should be combined with analgesic agents (usually aspirin or acetaminophen) and with local heat. Patients should be encouraged to stay in bed except to go to the bathroom until they are free of pain. When the patient is free of pain, he should gradually ambulate and then start a program of strengthening exercises for the paravertebral muscles of the neck and back in order to prevent recurrence of the pain (see references). Other treatment modalities, including physical therapy, traction, procaine or saline injection into trigger points, and spinal manipulation, have not been shown to be more efficacious than the regimen described above. Manipulation of the neck is potentially dangerous because the vertebral arteries can be occluded as they enter the skull by excessive or unskilled manipulation. Using standard therapy, 70 to 80 per cent of patients will become free of pain within a four-week period and able to return to full activity. During the period of bedrest, repeated physical and neurologic examinations are unwise, since vigorous movement of the neck, back, and extremities often exacerbates the pain and delays improvement. A small minority of patients continue to have chronic pain, and these patients, along with those whose initial examination has suggested more serious disease, need further evaluation. For neck pain, a soft cervical collar often is as effective in immobilizing the neck as is bedrest.

The management of some specific causes of nerve root and spinal cord compression is considered in Ch. 519. Other causes of neck and low back pain, such as ankylosing spondylitis, rheumatoid arthritis, multiple myeloma, spinal tuberculosis, and Paget's disease, are discussed elsewhere in this text.

Cailliet R: Low Back Pain Syndrome. 3rd ed. Philadelphia, FA Davis, 1981. *A well-written monograph with schematic drawings illustrating the anatomy, physiology, causes, and treatment of low back pain.*

Cailliet R: Neck and Arm Pain. 2nd ed. Philadelphia, FA Davis, 1981. *This short monograph describes the clinical anatomy and physiology of the cervical spine and the causes of pain originating from disorders of that area.*

Keim HA, Kirkaldy-Willis WH: Low back pain. Clinical Symposia, Vol 32, No 6, 1980. Summit, NJ, Ciba-Geigy Corporation. *Beautifully illustrated monograph on the anatomy and pathophysiology of low back pain. Drawings demonstrate the physical examination of the back and therapeutic exercises.*

SOME SPECIFIC PAIN SYNDROMES

Some disorders causing pain produce a specific constellation of signs and symptoms that sets them apart from other and more common causes of pain. Moreover, many of these pain syndromes often respond completely to treatment with nonanalgesic medications. Thus, it behooves the physician to recognize these disorders and to prescribe appropriate treatment. Those disorders that particularly affect the head, neck or back are discussed above. Others are discussed in the paragraphs below.

LIGHTNING PAINS OF TABES. The lightning pains of tabes are acute, short-lived pains in the trunk or lower extremities which occur with structural lesions of the dorsal roots and particularly with tabes dorsalis. Lightning pains are analogous to trigeminal and glossopharyngeal neuralgia. Like those two disorders, the pain usually responds to carbamazepine. There is no surgical therapy.

"REFLEX SYMPATHETIC DYSTROPHIES." This is a term that applies to pain, hyperalgesia, hyperesthesia, and autonomic changes, usually after injury to an extremity. If the injury has involved a peripheral nerve, particularly the sciatic or median nerve, the syndrome is called *causalgia* (hot pain). If the injury has not involved a peripheral nerve, such terms as post-traumatic painful osteoporosis, Sudeck's atrophy, post-traumatic spreading neuralgia, minor causalgia, shoulder-hand syndrome, and reflex dystrophy have been applied, the particular term depending on the outstanding symptom. Whatever the term, the pathophysiology of all these disorders appears to be the same, as do their clinical manifestations and response to therapy.

The disorder may follow either a major or a minor injury to an extremity, after which severe pain, usually of a burning quality, develops in the extremity. The pain is continuous but exacerbated by emotional stress and is associated with severe hyperpathia, so that moving or touching the limb is often intolerable. At first the pain is localized to the site of the injury or the distribution of the nerve injured, but with time it spreads, often to involve the entire extremity. Along with the pain there are vasomotor changes, first of vasodilatation (warm and dry skin) but later a change to vasoconstriction (edema, cyanosis, cool skin). Other autonomic disturbances include either hyperhidrosis or hypohidrosis; trophic changes in the skin, subcutaneous tissue, and muscles; and osteoporosis. The entire symptom complex is rarely present in any one patient, and one sign or symptom usually predominates. Untreated, severe reflex sympathetic dystrophy leads to muscle atrophy, fixation of joints, osteoporosis, and a useless extremity. The exact mechanism of the pain and sympathetic changes is not understood.

Treatment should be undertaken as early as possible, because there is evidence that the earlier the treatment, the more effective it will be. Treatment begins with local anesthetic infiltration of the painful site, using 2 to 5 ml of 0.5 per cent lidocaine, repeated frequently enough to maintain relief of pain. When local measures fail, most patients are relieved by sympathetic block with lidocaine. This procedure often gives permanent relief, but if repeated local anesthetics produce only transient benefit, surgical sympathectomy should be considered.

POSTHERPETIC NEURALGIA. Postherpetic neuralgia refers to severe and prolonged burning pain with occasional lightning-like stabs in the involved dermatome after an attack of herpes zoster. Severe postherpetic neuralgia is usually a disease of elderly patients and, like most chronic pain, is exacerbated by emotional upset and relieved to some degree by distraction. Touching the involved area usually exacerbates the pain. Treatment of postherpetic neuralgia is not entirely satisfactory, but the initial treatment should be directed toward stimulating the painful area. Brisk rubbing for many hours a day with a terrycloth towel or stimulation of the dermatome with a cutaneous electrical stimulator often brings relief which long outlasts the stimulus. Initially, when therapy is undertaken, the hyperpathia may be so severe that the patient is unwilling to have the area stimulated. One can then spray the area with a local anesthetic (e.g., ethyl chloride) before stimulation is undertaken. During the first 48 to 72 hours, stimulation should be done as often as possible when the patient is awake and then decreased gradually. Care must be taken to keep the rubbing light so as not to excoriate friable skin. Relief of pain may take several weeks. Analgesic drugs are sometimes beneficial, and psychotropic drugs (amitriptyline, 75 mg daily, and fluphenazine, 1 to 3 mg daily) have been reported to be useful. The results of surgical therapy are usually poor. Recent evidence suggests that nerve blocks using agents injected paraspinally or epidurally may relieve postherpetic neuralgia if given early in its course. There is also some evidence that adrenocorticosteroids and interferon used for the treatment of acute herpes zoster may diminish the incidence of postherpetic neuralgia. In many patients the disease runs its course, and after a year or two the pain disappears spontaneously. Thus mutilating surgical procedures are probably not indicated.

PHANTOM LIMB PAIN. Phantom limb pain is a chronic and severe pain appearing to be localized in an amputated or totally denervated limb. All patients suffer phantom sensations after amputation, but in only about 10 per cent is it painful, usually when there has been severe pain prior to operation. The pain is frequently similar to that suffered before amputation, or at times it may resemble muscle pain with the phantom seeming to be in a cramped or uncomfortable position. In most instances, the pain lessens and disappears with time, but in occasional patients it is a chronic and severe problem. Therapy is difficult. A search should be made for painful neuromas, but these are an uncommon cause of phantom pain, and even if small neuromas are found and removed, the pain is not usually relieved. Surgical procedures directed at the central nervous system are often not helpful. The pain may be triggered by touching the amputation stump, but over the passage of time healthy areas of the body when touched may also trigger pain in the phantom. Phantom pain is sometimes permanently abolished by cutaneous stimulation, either rubbing or electrical stimulation, or by repeated anesthetic blocks of peripheral nerves proximal to the stump. Narcotic analgesics may be helpful; other analgesic agents are usually not helpful. Sympathetic blocks have been reported to relieve pain in some patients for prolonged periods, but sympathectomy rarely produces relief as lasting as with causalgia. The mechanism of phantom pain is unknown.

MYOFASCIAL PAIN SYNDROMES. Pain arising from skeletal muscle is common. Unaccustomed exercise causes soreness and tenderness in the involved muscles but is rarely a source of patient complaint. Prolonged tonic contraction of skeletal muscles, however, has an underlying pathogenesis of psychologic tension, resentment, and anxiety, and may produce pain in which the cause is not immediately apparent to the patient. Examples are tension headache arising from chronic contraction of paraspinous muscles at the base of the skull, anterior chest pain from contraction of pectoralis major, posterior thoracic or lumbar pain from paraspinous muscle contraction, and abdominal pain from rectus muscle retraction. The pain is initially localized over the area of muscle contraction but may spread widely into a distribution characteristic for the muscles involved. The muscles are usually tender to palpation, and there is often a particular tender area somewhere in the muscle, called a trigger area, which, when palpated, reproduces the entire distribution of the spontaneous pain. When the pain is acute, it may be treated with rest, local heat, and mild analgesic drugs, along with muscle relaxant drugs such as diazepam or meprobamate. When the pain is chronic or severe, particularly when a trigger area is found, local anesthesia with ethyl chloride spray or local injection of 0.2 per cent lidocaine or physiologic saline sometimes affords relief. At times, a single injection breaks the pain–muscle tension–pain cycle and permanent relief is achieved. At other times, repetitive injections with the addition of analgesic agents and muscle relaxants are required.

Section Four ALCOHOL-RELATED AND NUTRITIONAL DISORDERS OF THE NERVOUS SYSTEM

482. ALCOHOL-RELATED AND NUTRITIONAL DISORDERS OF THE NERVOUS SYSTEM

Ivan Diamond

Alcohol-related neurologic disorders usually occur in patients who have abused the agent for a long time on a regular basis. Such patients should be distinguished from "binge" drinkers, who resume adequate diets after brief bouts of drinking; instead they tend to be chronic alcoholics who often suffer poor nutrition over months to years. It is not known why some alcoholics develop neurologic complications while others do not. Genetic factors are suspected to play a role in alcoholism, and certain individuals within the susceptible population may carry an inherent risk for neurologic disease when nutrition is inadequate. The individual alcohol-related neurologic disorders described below often occur together in the same patient. The consequences of nonalcoholic malnutrition and specific vitamin deficiencies are discussed in Ch. 214 and 217.

WERNICKE'S ENCEPHALOPATHY

Wernicke's encephalopathy is an acute disorder that occurs most commonly in chronic alcoholics. It also develops in other

TABLE 482–1. CONDITIONS ASSOCIATED WITH WERNICKE'S ENCEPHALOPATHY

Chronic alcoholism
Starvation
Persistent vomiting
Hyperemesis gravidarum
Gastric malignancy
Gastritis
Intestinal obstruction
Digitalis intoxication
Systemic diseases
Malignancy
Hepatic failure
Disseminated tuberculosis
Uremia
Iatrogenic
Inadequate parenteral nutrition
Chronic hemodialysis

conditions listed in Table 482–1. This is the only alcohol-related neurologic disorder that can be corrected by a specific vitamin—thiamine.

CLINICAL MANIFESTATIONS. A clinical triad of ophthalmoplegia, ataxia, and global confusion is characteristic. Affected patients may complain of double vision or difficulty with balance. There is almost always horizontal nystagmus on lateral gaze. Vertical nystagmus, usually on upward gaze, occurs in about 50 per cent of cases. Bilateral, often asymmetric, lateral rectus palsies are characteristic and may develop rapidly. Defects in conjugate gaze are common. Bilateral ptosis and total external or an apparent internuclear ophthalmoplegia occurs rarely. Occasionally, one observes a diminished pupillary reaction to light, but light-fixed pupils should suggest an alternate or additional diagnosis.

Virtually all patients have an ataxic gait due to cerebellar involvement. This can be so mild that it is demonstrable only by tandem walking or rapid turning, or it can be so severe that the patient cannot stand. Peripheral neuropathy and vestibular dysfunction frequently complicate Wernicke's encephalopathy and contribute to the ataxia. Intention tremor is less common, and speech disturbances are rare.

Most patients have an acute confusional state characterized by inattention, disorientation, and sleepiness. Stupor or coma occurs but is rare. Sometimes patients may be hyperactive and agitated (alcohol withdrawal, see Ch. 17) but usually are apathetic, indifferent, and amnesic for new information.

Associated physical abnormalities related to chronic alcoholism or poor nutrition are often present. These include signs of liver disease and portal hypertension (see Ch. 121) as well as lesions of the skin and mucous membranes (see Ch. 552). Tachycardia and orthostatic hypotension are common. Hypothermia occurs less frequently; any fever should prompt a search for concomitant infection. Patients with Wernicke's encephalopathy do not develop beriberi heart disease (see Ch. 217).

PATHOLOGY. The distribution of lesions in the brain is unique and appears to account for the clinical findings. The major lesions occur in the periventricular regions of the diencephalon, mid-brain, and brain stem, and in the superior vermis of the cerebellum. The lesions of Wernicke's encephalopathy may vary in severity and age in the same patient. They consist of areas of demyelination and glial proliferation. Microglia are prominent in acute lesions and fibrous astrocytes in older ones. Acute lesions show capillary dilation with occasional petechial hemorrhages. In experimental animals, accompanying defects in serotonergic transmission can be demonstrated in affected areas.

TREATMENT. Thiamine is the only factor that produces sustained improvement in Wernicke's encephalopathy. Because intestinal absorption is impaired in malnourished alcoholics, thiamine (50 to 100 mg) is given parenterally before starting infusions. One must avoid administering glucose prior to giving thiamine, as it can precipitate or worsen the encephalopathy in thiamine-depleted patients. Recovery begins promptly. In most cases, ophthalmoplegia and gaze palsies begin to resolve rapidly during the first day; nystagmus, gait ataxia, and confusion may show improvement within days to weeks. After recovery from the acute encephalopathy, however, many patients are left with nystagmus and gait ataxia. This residual cerebellar disorder is clinically and pathologically identical to the sometimes independently arising syndrome of alcoholic cerebellar degeneration described below. Nearly all patients with Wernicke's encephalopathy recover from the global confusional state, but many are left with a residual, more circumscribed disorder of memory—Korsakoff's amnestic syndrome.

KORSAKOFF'S AMNESTIC SYNDROME

CLINICAL MANIFESTATIONS (see also Ch. 478). There is a characteristic defect in forming new memories (anterograde amnesia) and in summoning previously established memories (retrograde amnesia). Recent memories tend to be most severely affected. Patients are usually disoriented for place and time. Immediate recall is intact, but patients are unable to remember the same items several minutes later. Confabulation often occurs early in the course. Affected patients are usually unaware of their memory deficits and blissfully unconcerned. Other aspects of cognitive function, including arousal, language, praxis, and judgment, are spared.

PATHOLOGY. The pathologic findings of active or remote Wernicke's encephalopathy may be present. Consistent damage to the dorsal medial nucleus of the thalamus probably accounts for the memory deficits.

TREATMENT. Unlike the acute motor abnormalities of Wernicke's encephalopathy, Korsakoff's amnestic syndrome often does not improve after thiamine treatment. About 20 per cent of patients recover completely, but more than half show little or no change. If improvement occurs, it may take one to three months to be recognizable. All patients with Korsakoff's syndrome should be given thiamine to treat possible coexistent Wernicke's encephalopathy and to prevent progression of the amnesia.

METABOLIC CONSIDERATIONS. Thiamine (vitamin B_1) in human tissues is derived entirely from dietary sources and is absorbed in the small intestine (Ch. 217). A saturable, energy-dependent transport system regulates uptake of thiamine into the brain and CSF. A series of reactions produces phosphorylated thiamine derivatives, and thiamine pyrophosphate (TPP) is a required co-factor for certain enzymes in carbohydrate and amino acid metabolism. The four principal thiamine-dependent enzymes are pyruvate dehydrogenase, α-ketoglutarate dehydrogenase, transketolase, and branched-chain α-ketoacid dehydrogenase. A report that patients with the Wernicke-Korsakoff syndrome may have a genetic defect in transketolase activity awaits confirmation. In addition to its role as a co-factor, thiamine and thiamine triphosphate (TTP) may also be important in the electrical function of neural membranes. Defects in some of these thiamine-dependent activities may underlie the acute symptoms of Wernicke's encephalopathy or Korsakoff's syndrome. However, there is no proof that they are directly responsible for the findings in these disorders.

The confusional state and oculomotor disturbances seen in Wernicke's encephalopathy respond to thiamine treatment, and it is said that recovery may proceed during thiamine therapy whether or not alcohol consumption continues. However, calorie-containing ethanol appears to be an important contributing factor to the neurologic deficits. Malnourished prisoners of war who developed Wernicke's encephalopathy rarely exhibited the irreversible amnestic syndrome. Moreover, nystagmus, ataxia, and the memory deficits often fail to improve after thiamine therapy, indicating that some areas of the brain have become irreversibly damaged. The molecular metabolic defect that precedes tissue damage in Wernicke's encephalopathy and Korsakoff's amnestic syndrome is not known.

ALCOHOLIC CEREBRAL ATROPHY

Many chronic alcoholics develop cerebral atrophy that increases with age and that can be visualized on CT scans of the brain. There is usually symmetrical enlargement of the lateral ventricles and an increase in the size of cerebral sulci and the width of interhemispheric and sylvian fissures. The abnormalities may disappear if drinking is discontinued. Many chronic alcoholics also show deficiencies on psychometric examination. However, the CT scan abnormalities do not correlate well with such specific cognitive defects. The specific mechanisms of these cerebral abnormalities are not known.

ALCOHOLIC NEUROPATHY

CLINICAL MANIFESTATIONS. Polyneuropathy is common among alcoholic patients. The most typical complaints are weakness, pain, and paresthesias in the hands and especially the feet. Symptoms usually begin insidiously in the legs and progress proximally and symmetrically. Abnormal motor and sensory signs develop concomitantly. Patients may complain of burning pain and heat sensations on the plantar surfaces of the feet and aching pain in the calves. Dysesthesias can become so severe that light touch and deep pressure are intensely unpleasant. Burning pain made worse by contact can interfere with walking despite adequate strength.

On examination muscle weakness and wasting are usually more prominent distally, affecting legs more than arms and never the latter exclusively. The muscles may feel flabby and tender to pressure. Weakness can be so severe that contractures develop at the ankles and knees. Sensory abnormalities usually involve all modalities, but especially the pain and temperature modalities early in the course, and are more prominent distally. The deep tendon reflexes are usually absent to diminished in a distal to proximal distribution. Even asymptomatic patients often show mild sensory loss in the feet and absent Achilles tendon reflexes.

Involvement of the vagus nerve and thoracoabdominal sympathetic chain occurs rarely and can produce hoarseness, dysphagia, vocal cord paralysis, and hypotension. Cerebrospinal fluid protein levels are usually normal.

PATHOPHYSIOLOGY AND TREATMENT. The classic pathologic findings in alcoholic neuropathy are axonal degeneration and demyelination. Some investigators propose that alcoholic peripheral neuropathy, since it first affects smaller sensory fibers, is characterized by axonal degeneration with electromyographic signs of denervation and normal nerve conduction velocities being found at that stage. By contrast, superimposed nutritional neuropathies are prone to produce segmental demyelination of large fibers as well as axonal degeneration. This may result in slow nerve conduction velocities.

A specific vitamin deficiency has not been documented in alcoholic neuropathy. Treatment consists of a balanced diet with supplemental B vitamins. Recovery is always slow and often incomplete. Several weeks may be needed for motor improvement to begin, and it may take a year before patients with marked weakness begin to walk.

ACUTE AND CHRONIC ALCOHOLIC MYOPATHY

ACUTE MYOPATHY. This is a dramatic and life-threatening condition that develops in chronic alcoholics during prolonged heavy drinking. Symptoms begin abruptly with pain, cramps, tenderness, weakness, and swelling of the legs. Muscle involvement may be generalized or confined to one limb. Creatine phosphokinase activity in blood is elevated, and muscle biopsy shows acute rhabdomyolysis. Myoglobinuria often occurs and may lead to acute renal failure, hyperkalemia, and death. Electromyography usually shows evidence of a primary myopathy (Ch. 539). Recovery usually follows days to weeks of abstinence, occasionally leaving residual proximal muscle weakness in its wake.

CHRONIC MYOPATHY. This is a chronic, painless disorder of proximal muscle weakness and atrophy that occurs rarely in alcoholics. It can be mild or severe. Muscles of the pelvic girdle and thighs are involved most frequently; weakness of shoulder girdle muscles is less common. Improvement usually occurs within two to three months after ethanol withdrawal. A coexistent alcoholic peripheral neuropathy may contribute to the weakness.

ALCOHOLIC CEREBELLAR DEGENERATION

Cerebellar cortical degeneration occurs frequently in chronic alcoholics. About half the patients have an associated peripheral neuropathy. Men are affected more often than women. Most patients give a history of episodic binge drinking superimposed on heavy consumption extending back over many years. Some complain of progressive unsteadiness and difficulty in walking, but these more insidiously developing symptoms often reflect a superimposed peripheral neuropathy that may clear with treatment. Abnormalities of gait and station are the most common findings. Initially, unsteadiness is demonstrated when the patient turns rapidly, and tandem walking is difficult or impossible. Gradually, the feet become more widely based, walking becomes hesitant, and truncal ataxia is added. Ataxia of the legs may be demonstrable on heel to shin tests, but nystagmus, dysarthria, and tremor are rare. Often the cerebellar syndrome develops abruptly or rapidly over several weeks and then remains stable. Sometimes the disorder evolves more slowly, with exacerbation following a binge or during an intercurrent illness. The most prominent pathologic abnormality is degeneration of the neurons of the anterior and superior cerebellar vermis with loss of Purkinje cells. CT or NMR scans confirm cerebellar vermis atrophy. Abstinence and treatment with a balanced diet and supplemental B vitamins may produce moderate improvement in the gait ataxia as peripheral neuropathy recovers.

NUTRITIONAL AMBLYOPIA

This is a condition of retrobulbar neuritis involving the maculopapillary fibers. It is caused by a nutritional deficiency and is encountered primarily in alcoholics. The patient complains of dim or blurred vision that evolves gradually over weeks to months. Decreased visual acuity occurs in one or both eyes, accompanied by bilateral symmetrical central or centrocecal scotomas. Peripheral visual fields are usually unaffected, and funduscopic examination is usually normal. Treatment consists of abstinence and a balanced diet with supplemental B vitamins. The extent of recovery varies inversely with the severity of impairment before therapy.

CENTRAL PONTINE MYELINOLYSIS

Central pontine myelinolysis (CPM) is a rare disorder that affects alcoholics primarily but also occurs in children and adults with severe electrolyte disorders, liver disease, malnutrition, anorexia, burns, cancer, Addison's disease, sepsis, and Wilson's disease.

PATHOPHYSIOLOGY, SIGNS, AND SYMPTOMS. The signs and symptoms relate closely to the pathologic change, which consists of a varying extent of symmetrical focal myelin destruction involving the basal central pons, with similar lesions occasionally affecting extrapontine areas. There is no associated inflammation or nerve cell destruction, and the lesions appear to be reversible with time and proper nutritional and fluid balance.

Typically CPM evolves within days or weeks in severely ill patients, often in association with acute post-alcoholic complications. Almost always the condition follows by one to three days a period of profound hyponatremia followed by rapid osmolal correction of greater than 20 mEq per liter. Mental symptoms often are prominent and consist of clouded consciousness or an increase in a post-alcoholic delirious state. Reflecting interruption of corticospinal pathways in the pons, a flaccid or spastic quadriparesis ensues, accompanied in many instances by bulbar difficulties of speaking and swallowing. Some patients develop a supranuclear ophthalmoplegia and the mortality is high. Reflecting the sparing of the pontine tegmentum, sensory abnormalities usually fail to develop. Formerly, most cases were discovered at postmortem examination, but the characteristic story has recently led to many cases being diagnosed during life, confirmed by characteristic abnormalities on CT scan. Complete recovery can take place in patients whose underlying illness makes this possible. Treatment consists of meticulous maintenance of electrolytes, especially sodium balance and adequate nutrition. The exact pathogenesis is unknown but has been attributed to edema of the basis pontis associated with the rapid electrolyte changes.

MARCHIAFAVA-BIGNAMI DISEASE

This is a rare disorder consisting of symmetrical demyelination of the corpus callosum and adjacent white matter. Although at one time described in Italian men who drink red wine, the disorder affects mainly severely alcoholic middle-aged men addicted to various kinds of alcoholic beverages. The clinical features are variable, and diagnosis is seldom made before death. Patients may have a progressive dementia over several years accompanied by agitation or apathy, hallucinations, and emotional disorders until seizures, stupor, and coma supervene. Clinical findings such as rooting and sucking responses, grasp reflexes, paratonic rigidity, incontinence, and a slow hesitant gait suggest bilateral frontal lobe involvement. Recovery is rare. Symmetrical demyelination in the corpus callosum may be seen on CT scans. The specific etiology is unknown.

VITAMIN B_{12} DEFICIENCY

Vitamin B_{12} deficiency causes subacute degeneration of white matter in the dorsal and lateral columns of the spinal cord, peripheral nerves, optic discs, and cerebral hemispheres. The neurologic findings usually accompany a macrocytic (pernicious) anemia, but anemia need not be present. Hematologic and pathophysiologic considerations of vitamin B_{12} deficiency and details of treatment are discussed in Ch. 217.

CLINICAL MANIFESTATIONS. Neurologic symptoms develop in most patients with long untreated pernicious anemia, especially those in whom anemia has been masked by folate ingestion. Patients first complain of paresthesias in the hands or legs, such as tingling, numbness, and "pins and needles" sensations. Stiffness and weakness of the legs with unsteadiness in walking may be bothersome, particularly in the dark. Neurologic symptoms progress relentlessly if untreated; ataxia and stiffness eventually are followed by paraplegia and dysfunction of bowel and bladder. Psychologic symptoms are frequent and include apathy and depression, irritability and paranoid tendencies, nocturnal confusion, and dementia. Intellectual deterioration does not usually develop in the absence of other neurologic signs. Failing vision with central scotomas occurs rarely.

Initially one may find few objective changes despite complaints of paresthesias. Later, symmetrical distal impairment of vibratory sensation occurs, usually first in the legs but eventually reaching the trunk and arms. Position sense is affected less prominently, although Romberg's test may be positive. The earliest changes are those of a peripheral neuropathy. The patellar and Achilles tendon reflexes are diminished or absent, and there may be decreased perception of touch, pain, and temperature in the feet and ankles. In the intermediate advanced case, one finds symmetrical weakness in the legs associated with spasticity, clonus at the knees and ankles, increased or decreased deep tendon reflexes, and extensor plantar responses. Tingling distal paresthesias may follow flexion of the neck (Lhermitte's sign).

PATHOLOGY. The most prominent early findings are in the peripheral nerves and dorsal and lateral columns of the spinal cord. Fragmentation and spongy degeneration of myelin usually begin in the lower cervical and upper thoracic regions; in untreated patients the disease progresses up and down the spinal cord and reaches into the ventral columns. Myelin sheaths and axons are destroyed, and Wallerian degeneration is found in the spinal cord funiculi. Cerebral white matter is affected late. Peripheral nerves may show distal degeneration.

DIAGNOSIS. Serum vitamin B_{12} levels are low and appear to correlate with the severity of the neurologic findings. In pernicious anemia this is due to impaired absorption of vitamin B_{12}, which is the basis of the commonly used Schilling test. There is diminished or absent intrinsic factor, usually in association with gastric achlorhydria. Vitamin B_{12} deficiency can also result from intestinal malabsorption syndromes, gastrectomy, or inadequate diet. These are discussed in Ch. 217. Methylmalonic acid is increased in blood and CSF and its increased excretion in the urine is regarded as a sensitive and specific indicator of vitamin B_{12} deficiency. The CSF protein concentration may be increased slightly. Neurologic disorders that can be confused with vitamin B_{12} deficiency include multiple sclerosis, cervical spondylosis, spinal cord tumors, and syphilitic meningomyelitis. A virtually identical syndrome has been reported after chronic abuse of nitrous oxide (Ch. 481).

PATHOGENESIS. The molecular pathogenesis of the neurologic lesion in vitamin B_{12} deficiency is unknown. Vitamin B_{12} exists in different forms, some of which are required for at least two enzymes: N5-methyltetrahydrofolate homocysteine methyltransferase, which catalyzes the synthesis of methionine and regeneration of tetrahydrofolate, and methylmalonyl-CoA mutase, which generates succinyl-CoA. The activities of both enzymes are reduced in vitamin B_{12} deficiency. Methionine is a substrate for protein synthesis and is a precursor for transmethylation reactions in neurotransmitter, phospholipid, and protein metabolism. Prolonged exposure to nitrous oxide, which produces a neurologic disorder resembling combined system disease, also inhibits methionine synthesis. Reduced activity of methylmalonyl-CoA mutase probably accounts for the increased excretion of methylmalonic acid because methylmalonate is not converted to succinyl-CoA.

TREATMENT. Intramuscular administration of vitamin B_{12} is the only treatment for vitamin B_{12} deficiency due to pernicious anemia. Therapy should be started immediately and continued throughout the patient's lifetime as described in Ch. 217. Early neurologic changes can be rapidly and completely reversed if treatment with vitamin B_{12} is begun promptly within the first few weeks of the illness. If the neurologic manifestations have reached the stage of producing spinal cord dysfunction, therapy will halt progression of the disease but improvement cannot be guaranteed.

Charness ME, Diamond I: Alcohol and the nervous system. Current Neurology 5:383, 1984. *A discussion of recent advances in many alcohol-related neurologic disorders.*

Dreyfus PM, Geel SE: Vitamin and nutritional deficiencies. *In* Albers RW, Siegel GJ, Katzman R, Agranoff BW (eds.): Basic Neurochemistry. 3rd ed. Boston, Little, Brown and Company, 1981. *A clear discussion of the basic neurochemistry of the vitamins.*

Greenberg DA, Diamond I: Wernicke-Korsakoff syndrome. *In* Tartar RE, Van Thiel DH (eds.): Alcohol and the Brain: Chronic Effects. New York, Plenum Publishing Corp., 1984. *A discussion of recent advances.*

Norenberg MD, Leslie KO, Robertson AS: Association between rise in serum sodium and central pontine myelinolysis. Ann Neurol 11:128, 1982. *In 12 hyponatremic patients a rise in serum sodium of greater than 20 mEq per liter was followed by the disorder, which did not appear in other hyponatremic patients treated more cautiously. A good bibliography accompanies.*

Victor M, Adams RD, Collins GH: The Wernicke-Korsakoff Syndrome. Philadelphia, F. A. Davis Co., 1971. *A classic clinical-pathologic description of the disorder.*

Vinken PJ, Bruyn GW: Handbook of Clinical Neurology. Vol. 28, Metabolic and Deficiency Diseases of the Nervous System. Amsterdam, North Holland Publishing Co., 1976, Ch. 1–14. *A comprehensive review of nutritional diseases of the nervous system.*

Section Five THE EXTRAPYRAMIDAL DISORDERS

Stanley Fahn

Extrapyramidal disorders are associated with abnormalities of the basal ganglia and are characteristically manifested by a combination of abnormal involuntary movements, alterations in muscle tone, and disturbances in postural stability. Included are the syndromes of parkinsonism, tremor, chorea, athetosis, dystonia, and hemiballism, collectively referred to as *movement disorders,* a heading which also encompasses the syndromes of myoclonus and tics, maladies that probably arise from sites outside the basal ganglia. As a general rule, diagnosis of the particular abnormal involuntary movement depends more on careful clinical observation than on laboratory study. The age and mode of onset, genetic traits, exposure to drugs and toxins, progression of symptoms, and development of other neurologic features (e.g., dementia) usually provide the most important clues.

ANATOMIC, PHYSIOLOGIC, AND BIOCHEMICAL CORRELATES. The basal ganglia comprise five paired nuclei: caudate nucleus, putamen, globus pallidus (or pallidum), subthalamic nucleus, and substantia nigra (Fig. 1). The first three lie deep within the cerebral hemispheres and collectively are referred to as the corpus striatum. The subthalamic nucleus is in the diencephalon, and the substantia nigra is located in the midbrain.

Although separated by the internal capsule, the caudate and putamen are similar microscopically, chemically, and physiologically, and are considered collectively as the neostriatum or striatum. The striatum serves as the main site of neural input into the basal ganglia, receiving afferents from all parts of the cerebral cortex and from the nucleus centrum medianum of the thalamus. The major output of the striatum is to the pallidum and the zona reticulata portion of the substantia nigra. The pallidum and zona reticulata are also separated by the internal capsule, but are similar microscopically, chemically, and physiologically. These two regions serve as the major site of neural output from the basal ganglia, with the principal neural efferent pathway going to the ventral anterior (VA) nucleus of the thalamus and thence to the premotor cortex. The premotor cortex is one source of the corticospinal tract (pyramidal tract), the major descending cortical efferent pathway controlling motor function.

The subthalamic nucleus receives afferents from the pallidum and sends its efferents back to the pallidum. Thus, it can be considered to function as a modulator of the globus pallidus and probably regulates the basal ganglia output to the VA nucleus of the thalamus. In an analogous fashion, the substantia nigra can be considered to modulate the neostriatum. The dorsal part of the substantia nigra (zona compacta) sends efferents to the neostriatum (the dopaminergic nigrostriatal pathway), and the ventral part of the substantia nigra (zona reticulata) receives fibers from the neostriatum.

Considerable progress has been made in identifying and understanding the neurotransmitters of some of the neuronal pathways in the basal ganglia. The nigrostriatal pathway contains dopamine and may inhibit the striatum. The other inputs to the striatum (the thalamostriatal pathway and the glutamate-containing corticostriatal pathway) are excitatory. The GABA-containing efferents from the striatum to the pallidium and substantia nigra are inhibitory. Lesions of the substantia nigra with resulting loss of dopamine in the striatum result in the bradykinetic syndrome of parkinsonism. Drugs that deplete dopamine (e.g., reserpine) and drugs that block striatal dopamine receptors (e.g., phenothiazines) can also cause parkinsonism. By contrast, excessive dopamine activity (e.g., levodopa overdosage) produces the hyperkinetic state of chorea. A lesion of the subthalamic nucleus produces contralateral hemiballism. It is generally believed that such a lesion removes an inhibitory influence on the pallidum (disinhibition). Lesions in the corpus striatum produce inconsistent patterns of dyskinesias, depending on particular sites and mode of involvement. Athetosis and dystonia can follow trauma and vascular lesions of the striatum, whereas chorea accompanies degenerative loss of neurons in this structure (e.g., Huntington's chorea).

The basal ganglia serve as a major input to the pyramidal tract motor system. In fact, a lesion of the pyramidal tract sufficient to cause paralysis will eliminate existing dyskinesias, such as tremor and chorea. The term extrapyramidal system was originally coined to denote a motor system operating in parallel with and independent from the pyramidal tract. This is incorrect, but the long use of the term "extrapyramidal" in clinical medicine has embedded it as synonymous with the basal ganglia system.

Phylogenetically, the extrapyramidal system is ancient and serves as the predominant motor system for reptiles and birds. In higher animals it is believed to be involved in automatic movements (e.g., walking, swinging arms when walking, feed-

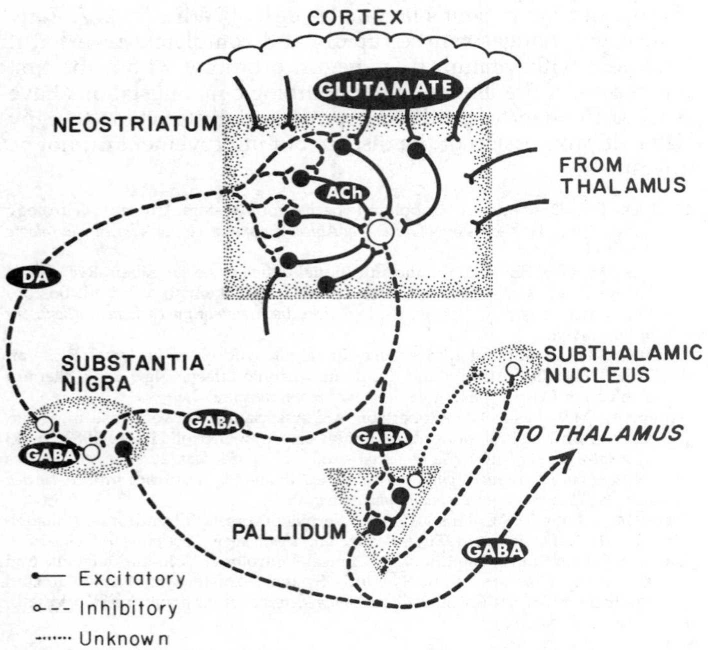

Figure 1. A simplified scheme of the neuronal pathways in the basal ganglia, depicting their function and suspected neurotransmitters. DA = dopamine; ACh = acetylcholine; GABA = gamma-aminobutyric acid.

ing), control of muscle tone, and maintenance of posture. Much of our knowledge of the function of the basal ganglia has been derived from clinicoanatomic correlations in humans.

ABNORMAL INVOLUNTARY MOVEMENTS. Movement disorders can be divided into *bradykinesia* (or *akinesia*), a paucity of automatic and spontaneous movement, and *hyperkinesia* (or *dyskinesia*), which is excessive or abnormal involuntary movements. Bradykinesia is a feature of parkinsonism and is virtually specific for that syndrome, whereas the dyskinesias are subdivided into specific types, depending on their rhythmicity, speed, duration, repetitiveness, and other characteristics. As a general rule, dyskinesias are absent during sleep, reduced with relaxation, and increased with stress.

Tremor refers to relatively rhythmic oscillatory movements. These can result from alternating contractions of opposing muscle groups (e.g., parkinsonian tremor) or from simultaneous contractions of agonist and antagonist muscles, with one group more forceful than the other (e.g., essential tremor). Clinical examination of tremor can aid in the etiologic diagnosis (Table 1). One should seek for (1) tremor at rest (hands in lap when patient is sitting or at side when patient is lying supine), (2) postural tremor (arms outstretched in front of body), (3) action tremor (when patient is moving arms or using hands to write or lift a cup of water to the mouth), and (4) intention tremor (finger-to-nose maneuver).

The classic parkinson tremor is present at rest. In the limbs, it is almost always distal, being present in the hands (pill-rolling) and feet. Tremor can also involve the tongue, lips, and chin, but rarely the head or neck. The rate of parkinsonian tremor is usually from 3 to 7 Hz. Characteristically, the tremor at rest transiently disappears when the patient initiates movement of the involved part. Some patients with parkinsonism may have an action tremor in addition to or instead of tremor at rest.

Postural and action tremors are more rapid than tremor at rest (rate between 7 and 11 Hz) and are also more severe distally than proximally. Drugs, metabolic illnesses, and essential tremor are common causes. These tremors can usually be suppressed by beta-adrenergic blockers such as propranolol and metoprolol. Intention tremor is a manifestation of cerebellar pathology, especially in the major outflow pathway, the superior cerebellar peduncle. The most common cause is multiple sclerosis; unfortunately, no effective drug is available for this problem. Thalamotomy may bring relief of all types of tremor.

Chorea refers to brief, irregular, nonrhythmic contractions that can involve any or all parts of the body. In disorders such as Huntington's disease and Sydenham's chorea, the choreic movements are not repetitive; instead, they flow from one muscle to another. This can be an important distinction from tardive dyskinesia, in which the brief movements are rhythmic and repetitive (stereotypic). In chorea, patients frequently try to mask the abnormal jerks by carrying out voluntary movements, so-called semipurposeful movements. Patients with chorea cannot maintain a sustained, even contraction, as manifested by "milkmaid" grips, inability to keep the tongue protruded, stuttering gait, and clumsiness with dropping of objects.

Ballism is a form of chorea in which the brisk, involuntary contractions affect proximal muscles and are of large amplitude, causing wild, flinging movements of the limbs. These movements usually occur unilaterally (hemiballism).

TABLE 1. A CLASSIFICATION OF COMMON ABNORMAL TREMORS

- I. Tremor at rest
  - A. Parkinsonism
- II. Postural and action tremor
  - A. Essential tremor
  - B. Accentuated physiologic tremor
    1. Epinephrine, amphetamines
    2. Thyrotoxicosis
    3. Anxiety, fatigue
    4. Lithium, tricyclics
    5. Alcohol withdrawal
- III. Intention tremor
  - A. Multiple sclerosis
  - B. Wilson's disease
  - C. Phenytoin toxicity

Athetosis refers to continual slow, writhing movements that can involve limbs (distal and proximal), trunk, head, face, and tongue. When the movements are brief, the term choreoathetosis is commonly applied; when sustained contractions occur at the end of an athetotic movement, the term athetotic dystonia can be used. It is common to see an increase of athetotic movements when the patient carries out voluntary movements or is speaking (overflow phenomenon).

Dystonia refers to involuntary movements with sustained contractions at the end of the movement. The positions can be prolonged (dystonic postures) but usually last only a second or less (dystonic movements). Dystonic movements are usually of a twisting nature; hence the term torsion dystonia. They may be brisk from the beginning to peak of the contraction, and a misdiagnosis of chorea is not uncommon. However, if a twisting aspect is present, a diagnosis of dystonia is appropriate even if sustained contractions are not obvious. Action dystonia refers to dystonic movements that occur only when the affected part of the body is in voluntary motion. For example, twisting movements of a leg or foot may appear only when the patient attempts to walk. As the dystonia becomes more severe, the involuntary contractions appear at rest as well. Another peculiar but characteristic feature of dystonia is the lessening of abnormal contractions by tactile or proprioceptive input. For example, patients with torticollis will frequently place a hand on the mandible to provide some relief from the involuntary muscular contractions. Dystonic movements may be generalized or limited to only one part of the body. The focal dystonias include spasmodic torticollis, writer's cramp, blepharospasm, and spastic dysphonia.

Myoclonus refers to shock-like or lightning-like movements due to muscular contractions or inhibitions (the latter is referred to as negative myoclonus). Myoclonic jerks can involve a single muscle or a group of muscles, with the amplitude ranging from a small muscular flicker to a large body-moving synchronous jerk. The myoclonus that accompanies the initial stage of sleep is an example of the latter and represents a normal physiologic form. Asterixis, which resembles a tremor, is an example of negative myoclonus. It occurs in metabolic encephalopathies and is due to brief periods of electrical silence in muscles.

Tics are complex coordinated movements that appear suddenly and transiently. Head shaking, eye blinking, shoulder shrugging, and complex facial contortions are examples. In addition to motor tics, vocal tics are common, and when present indicate a diagnosis of Tourette's syndrome (Ch. 486).

ALTERATIONS IN MUSCLE TONE. Increased muscle tone (rigidity) and decreased muscle tone (hypotonia) are common components of extrapyramidal disorders. Tone is determined by the examiner who manipulates the passive limb, neck, and trunk of the patient. Rigidity is most commonly encountered in parkinsonism, and must be differentiated from spasticity. The latter accompanies corticospinal tract lesions and is manifested by increased tone in either flexion or extension of a limb, with sudden relaxation as the muscle continues to be stretched (clasp knife phenomenon). Spasticity is also associated with weakness, increased tendon reflexes, and a Babinski sign. In contrast, rigidity is present in both flexion and extension and continues throughout the length of muscle stretch. Most often it is jerky (cogwheeling) owing to an underlying tremor rhythm, but it can be smooth (lead-pipe rigidity). Electromyographic recordings reveal that the agonist and antagonist muscles contract simultaneously, even when the patient attempts to relax. Hypotonia occurs characteristically in chorea and may also be present in patients with torsion dystonia at a time when the muscle is not involuntarily contracting.

DISTURBANCES OF POSTURAL REFLEXES. Normally, an individual can recover balance quickly if thrown off his center of gravity. However, such postural reflexes tend to be lost in parkinsonism, Huntington's disease, and Wilson's disease. The effect leads to falling when the patient attempts to walk or stand. Such reflexes can be tested by pulling the standing patient backward or forward toward the examiner with a quick tug on the shoulders. One must prepare to catch the patient should he not be able to recover owing to loss of postural reflexes.

Postural changes, such as stooping and kyphosis, are encountered in parkinsonism. Torsion dystonia can lead to postural deformities such as scoliosis, tortipelvis, and lordosis. Eventually, fixed postures develop as a result of contractures.

Carpenter MB: Anatomy of the corpus striatum and brain stem integrating systems. *In* Handbook of Physiology. The Nervous System II. 2nd ed. Bethesda, MD, American Physiological Society, 1982, pp 947–995. *A detailed review of basal ganglia anatomy.*

DeLong MR, Georgopoulos AP: Motor functions of the basal ganglia. *In* Handbook of Physiology. The Nervous System II. 2nd ed. Bethesda, MD, American Physiological Society, 1982, pp 1017–1061. *A review of basal ganglia physiology in terms of motor behavior.*

Jankovic J, Fahn S: Physiologic and pathologic tremors: Diagnosis, mechanism, and management. Ann Intern Med 93:460, 1980. *An etiologic classification of tremors and their mechanisms and treatment.*

Kita ST: Electrophysiology of the corpus striatum and brain stem integrating systems. *In* Handbook of Physiology. The Nervous System II. 2nd ed. Bethesda, MD, American Physiological Society, 1982, pp 997–1015. *A review of the physiology of the neuronal pathways within the basal ganglia.*

Martin JP: The Basal Ganglia and Posture. Philadelphia, J. B. Lippincott Company, 1967. *An outstanding discussion of the role of the basal ganglia in postural mechanisms in normal and disease states.*

Penney JB Jr, Young AB: Speculations on the functional anatomy of basal ganglia disorders. Ann Rev Neurosci 6:73, 1983. *A review of neurotransmitter pathways within the basal ganglia and speculations on their role in movement disorders.*

483. PARKINSONISM

Parkinsonism is a clinical syndrome consisting of four cardinal signs: tremor at rest, rigidity, bradykinesia, and loss of postural reflexes. Not all patients have all four cardinal signs. Bradykinesia refers to a paucity of automatic and spontaneous movements and difficulty in initiating voluntary movement. Bradykinesia is almost always present in parkinsonism and is virtually synonymous with this diagnosis. Bradykinesia accounts for the majority of parkinsonian symptoms and signs: a general slowing down of movement, masked face (hypomimia), decreased frequency of blinking with a staring expression, decreased swallowing resulting in drooling of saliva, soft voice (hypophonia), loss of speech modulation, impaired handwriting with micrographia, decreasing amplitude in performing rapid repetitive movements (such as opening and closing the hand or tapping the foot), difficulty in arising from a chair and turning in bed, loss of armswing on walking with a tendency to take short steps or shuffle, and loss of spontaneous gesturing when speaking.

Parkinsonism is the most common extrapyramidal disorder, and indeed is one of the most prevalent neurologic conditions, along with epilepsy, stroke, and dementia. Its prevalence has been placed at close to 1 million individuals in the United States, with the addition of 50,000 new cases each year. It is a prominent cause of disability.

Parkinsonism can be categorized into three etiologic groups (Table 483–1): (1) the primary or idiopathic disorder referred to as Parkinson's disease, (2) secondary or acquired parkinsonism, and (3) "parkinsonism-plus" syndromes, in which additional neurologic findings are present. A history of encephalitis, exposure to drugs or toxins, surgical removal of the parathyroid glands, or previous strokes suggests one of the secondary forms of parkinsonism. The presence of impaired ocular movements, orthostatic hypotension, cerebellar ataxia, or dementia suggests one of the "parkinsonism-plus" syndromes.

In parkinsonism, dopamine activity in the striatum is deficient. In Parkinson's disease, there is a loss of pigmented neurons in the substantia nigra and locus ceruleus with subsequent loss of their dopamine and norepinephrine neurotransmitters. In postencephalitic parkinsonism, the midbrain is particularly affected, with loss of substantia nigra neurons. In these two conditions degeneration of the dopaminergic nigrostriatal pathway leads to striatal dopamine deficiency. Reserpine depletes striatal dopamine, and antipsychotic drugs (e.g., phenothiazines and butyrophenones) block dopamine receptors. In other conditions (e.g., lacunar infarcts, hypoparathyroidism, striatonigral degeneration, and progressive supranuclear palsy), it is suspected that striatal dopamine receptors are directly affected. Involvement of the dopamine receptor renders treatment with levodopa or dopamine agonists ineffective.

TABLE 483–1. A CLASSIFICATION OF COMMON FORMS OF PARKINSONISM

I. Primary
    Idiopathic parkinsonism (Parkinson's disease)
II. Secondary
    A. Infectious: postencephalitic parkinsonism
    B. Toxins: manganese, carbon monoxide
    C. Drugs: antipsychotics, reserpine
    D. Hypoparathyroidism
    E. Vascular
III. Parkinsonism-plus
    A. Striatonigral degeneration
    B. Progressive supranuclear palsy
    C. Shy-Drager syndrome
    D. Normal pressure hydrocephalus
    E. Alzheimer's disease
    F. Wilson's disease
    G. Huntington's disease

PRIMARY PARKINSONISM (Parkinson's Disease)

The incidence of Parkinson's disease increases with age, but, because the population declines with age, the peak age at onset is in the sixth and seventh decades of life. Idiopathic parkinsonism can occur in younger adults and, rarely, in children. (Although juvenile parkinsonism can represent primary parkinsonism, it is often a feature of Wilson's disease, Huntington's disease, or rarer forms of pallidal degeneration.) Both sexes are affected, males more than females by a ratio of 3:2. Familial parkinsonism sometimes occurs.

Parkinson's disease begins insidiously, most commonly with tremor or bradykinesia in one limb. The symptoms then involve the other limb on the same side and tend to remain unilateral for several years before spreading to the opposite side. Rigidity, masked face, and soft voice appear early, and the patient reports a slowness in carrying out the day's activities. The gait becomes short stepped and shuffling. Loss of postural reflexes with unsteadiness on turning and festination (the need to walk faster and faster to avoid falling forward) appears as the disease progresses. Postural deformities appear: the head is flexed forward, the trunk is stooped and may be tilted to one side, the hands develop ulnar deviation with flexion at the metacarpophalangeal joints and extension at the interphalangeal joints, and the arms are adducted at the sides with elbows flexed. This characteristic posture plus masked face often allows first inspection to make the diagnosis even if tremor is not present.

As the disease progresses, patients develop gait hesitation ("freezing") on initiating gait (start-hesitation), when approaching a target (terminal-hesitation), and when trying to walk in a crowded area, as if the feet are glued to the ground. With progressive bradykinesia and loss of postural reflexes, the patient eventually becomes wheelchair bound. Swallowing difficulty with choking becomes a problem. Parkinson's disease is not lethal, but increased mortality occurs because of debility, aspiration pneumonia, urinary tract infections, and decubitus ulcers. The rate of progression varies. Disability seldom ensues until 10 to 15 years after onset.

Other symptoms include personality changes: the patient becomes less assertive and more passive, dependent, fearful, and indecisive, disabling qualities for persons in an executive position. Depression is common, and dementia may ensue as the disease progresses. Some patients complain of pain, tingling, numbness, and burning sensations, usually on the side of initial symptoms. These are frequently misdiagnosed as arthritis or bursitis. Primitive reflexes, such as Myerson's sign (repetitive blinking on repetitive tapping of the glabella), snout reflex, and palmomental reflex, are commonly found.

Pathologically, depigmentation of the normally pigmented brainstem nuclei is characteristic, and cytoplasmic eosinophilic inclusions (Lewy bodies) are seen microscopically in substantia nigra and locus ceruleus neurons. The cause of Parkinson's disease is unknown.

SECONDARY PARKINSONISM

This category comprises numerous disorders in which parkinsonism provides the predominant symptoms or in which it plays a smaller role in the clinical picture. The list includes poisonings with manganese, carbon monoxide and a synthetic opiate by-product (MPTP), brain tumors affecting basal ganglia function, cerebral trauma, intoxication with neuroleptic drugs, encephalitis, hypoparathyroidism and basal ganglia calcification, chronic hepatocerebral degeneration, and cerebrovascular disease. Most frequent are drug-induced parkinsonism, postencephalitic parkinsonism, and vascular parkinsonism.

DRUG-INDUCED PARKINSONISM. Drug-induced parkinsonism rivals idiopathic parkinsonism as the most common form of this syndrome. High dosages of both reserpine and the antipsychotic drugs (e.g., phenothiazines and butyrophenones) cause parkinsonism. Reserpine is now usually used only in low dosage to treat hypertension, making the antipsychotic agents the predominant offending agents. Reserpine depletes the storage of dopamine in the dopaminergic nerve terminals in the striatum; the antipsychotic agents block postsynaptic dopamine receptors in the striatum. The latter produce several extrapyramidal syndromes: (1) Acute *akathisia* (motor restlessness) can occur as the dosage is increased; sometimes anticholinergics relieve this symptom. (2) Acute *dystonic reactions* can appear with the initial doses, especially in children and young adults. These dystonic postures can be relieved with parenteral administration of anticholinergics (benztropine, 2 mg intramuscularly), antihistamines (diphenhydramine, 50 mg intravenously), or diazepam (5 to 7.5 mg intravenously). (3) *Oculogyric crisis,* in which the eyes are deviated in a fixed posture for minutes to hours, is a form of dystonia, but occurs in adults as well as children. It can be relieved by the drugs described above. (4) *Parkinsonism* can appear as a toxic reaction and resembles idiopathic parkinsonism in all the cardinal signs of the syndrome. Levodopa will not reverse this complication, probably because the dopamine receptors are blocked and occupied by the antipsychotic agent. Oral anticholinergic drugs are effective (e.g., trihexyphenidyl, 2 mg three times a day). If the antipsychotic drug is withdrawn, the symptoms will clear over several weeks to months. (5) *Tardive dyskinesia,* a chorea-like disorder presenting predominantly as an oral dyskinesia, can appear after long-term use of antipsychotic drugs. The condition may be irreversible and can worsen when the drugs are withdrawn.

POSTENCEPHALITIC PARKINSONISM. The pandemics of encephalitis lethargica (von Economo's encephalitis) that occurred between 1919 and 1926 left in their wake a variety of extrapyramidal disorders (chorea, dystonia, oculogyric crises, and parkinsonism). The onset of parkinsonism can occur years after the encephalitis and even after mild, subclinical cases. Although a viral etiology is suspected, the causative agent has never been established. An influenza strain is suspected, but serum antibody titers in patients with postencephalitic parkinsonism have been normal.

Clinically, postencephalitic parkinsonism is a more slowly progressive disorder than Parkinson's disease and may stabilize. Affected patients may have oculogyric crises and a variety of neurologic deficits, such as hemiplegia, ocular palsies, dystonia, chorea, tics, or behavioral disorders. Postencephalitic parkinsonism is more sensitive to levodopa therapy than is Parkinson's disease, and patients with the former may require approximately one half the usual dosage needed in the latter.

Rarely, other types of encephalitis may be followed by parkinsonism. The condition has been reported in association with coxsackieviruses, Japanese B encephalitis, and western equine encephalitis. In most cases, the parkinsonian syndrome either improves or remains stable.

VASCULAR PARKINSONISM. Most parkinsonism among persons over age 70 is of the idiopathic variety. However, vascular or arteriosclerotic parkinsonism does occur infrequently and can appear in middle life as well as in old age. Occasionally it follows a stroke, but more often it appears as a complication of multiple small infarctions involving the striatum. Gait disturbance is the most frequent complaint, with short steps, "freezing," and unsteadiness on turning common. Increased muscle tone and loss of postural reflexes are present, but tremor is rare, as are masked facies and classic bradykinesia. Dementia may be present, as well as hyperactive tendon reflexes and Babinski signs. Antiparkinson drugs have little benefit.

PARKINSONISM-PLUS (Multisystem Degenerations)

The clinical signs of parkinsonism can accompany other neurologic deficits in several multisystem degenerative diseases including striatonigral degeneration, olivopontocerebellar degeneration (with cerebellar ataxia), progressive supranuclear palsy (with ophthalmoplegia), and Shy-Drager syndrome (with orthostatic hypotension). Parkinsonism with profound dementia can occur in patients in whom cerebral pathology reveals features of both Alzheimer's disease and Parkinson's disease. The parkinsonism-dementia complex is also seen in some patients with normal pressure hydrocephalus, which typically presents as a triad of gait disturbance, dementia, and urinary incontinence. Rarely, parkinsonian features, with or without associated dementia, accompany otherwise typical amyotrophic lateral sclerosis.

STRIATONIGRAL DEGENERATION. First described in 1961, striatonigral degeneration presents clinically as Parkinson's disease. As the disease progresses, however, signs of cerebellar ataxia and laryngeal stridor may appear. Loss of neurons occurs predominantly in the substantia nigra and putamen, with additional degeneration in other basal ganglia and the cerebellum. This disorder may be one of the many types of the olivopontocerebellar degenerations (see Ch. 490). The diagnosis can be suspected clinically by its failure to respond to levodopa, explained by the loss of dopamine receptors with the neuronal loss in the striatum.

PROGRESSIVE SUPRANUCLEAR PALSY. Well delineated in 1964 by Steele, Richardson, and Olszewski, progressive supranuclear palsy can resemble Parkinson's disease, but tremor is rare. Additional distinguishing features are external ophthalmoplegia, nuchal dystonia (especially neck hyperextension), and a dystonic facial smile with deep nasolabial folds (rather than the flattened folds seen in Parkinson's disease). The presence of ophthalmoplegia is required for the diagnosis. Initially vertical eye movements are lost. Whereas upward gaze alone is limited in Parkinson's disease, downward gaze is also impaired in progressive supranuclear palsy. Eventually, horizontal eye movements become limited. The ophthalmoplegia is supranuclear, and a full range of reflex eye movements can be detected by the doll's eyes test. Pathologically, basal ganglia, brainstem, and cerebellum contain neuronal loss and neurofibrillary tangles. There is no effective treatment, but dopamine agonists help some patients.

MANAGEMENT OF PARKINSONISM

GENERAL PRINCIPLES. The overall goals of therapy should be directed toward keeping the patient functioning independently as long as possible. Athough symptoms can often be suppressed, at least for a short period of time, the consequences of chronic drug administration must be considered, since long-term levodopa use may be accompanied by disabling adverse effects. It is best to individualize therapy in such matters as when to start drugs, which ones to utilize, and regulation of medications. The last-named point is a continual process in treating parkinsonism; one must constantly adjust drug dosage and timing to achieve the optimal balance between amelioration of symptoms and avoidance of unacceptable adverse reactions.

Parkinsonism is frequently accompanied by fearfulness, passivity, dependence, and depression, and affected patients need repeated encouragement and reassurance in meeting the stresses of everyday life and their all-too-realistic fears of the future.

PHYSICAL THERAPY. Parkinsonism inherently produces immobility. Patients must be encouraged to be as active as possible; the family must participate in this as well. Maintaining employment as long as feasible, taking long walks, gardening, and becoming active in hobbies are among the possibilities. As the disease advances, more formal home exercise programs with a physiotherapist can be arranged. Appropriately placed hand bars enable patients to get up unassisted from toilet seats or beds. Patients should be encouraged to carry out activities of daily living as independently as possible. For gait difficulty and unsteadiness, a cane is not useful but may serve as a warning that the patient is handicapped, thereby avoiding unnecessary jostling and preventing falls and fractures, a common complication. Pain from rigid cervical muscles may be relieved by heat and massage.

DRUG THERAPY. When the disease is mild and symptoms not troublesome, drugs are not necessary. The physician can explain that the symptoms may progress very slowly in the first few years, that drugs can be utilized at the appropriate time, and that regular evaluations will be carried out. As symptoms become annoying or restrict activities, drug therapy becomes necessary. Levodopa combined with a peripheral dopa decarboxylase inhibitor (carbidopa, benserazide) is the most potent agent available. However, in many patients the best response to levodopa occurs in the first two to three years of use; furthermore, clinical fluctuations ("on-off" and "wearing-off" phenomena) occur in many patients with chronic administration. Therefore, it is reasonable to initiate drug therapy with less potent antiparkinson agents (anticholinergics and amantadine) and to reserve levodopa for annoying or disabling symptoms that are no longer suppressed by these agents.

The antiviral agent amantadine HCl (Symmetrel) has an antiparkinsonian effect in approximately two thirds of patients. The usual dosage is 100 mg twice a day, and any benefit becomes evident within two to three days. If the disease is mild, effectiveness may persist, but in more advanced stages it decreases unless levodopa has been given concomitantly. Amantadine is believed to act by enhancing the release of dopamine stored in presynaptic terminals. As the storage supply is depleted, amantadine loses it effect. If the stores are replaced by administered levodopa, the effect can be prolonged. The most common adverse effect is livedo reticularis, a medically unimportant reddish mottling of the skin present around the knees. If pronounced erythematous edema of the ankles occurs, amantadine should be discontinued. Amantadine also can cause nonfrightening visual hallucinations, usually of people and animals. Lowering the dosage usually provides relief. If amantadine is not effective within three days, it should be discontinued.

Anticholinergics are particularly useful as adjuncts to levodopa, especially to suppress tremor. They can also be used in the mild stages of parkinsonism before levodopa is administered, and are the agents of choice in drug-induced parkinsonism. Commonly employed anticholinergics are trihexyphenidyl (Artane), available in 2- and 5-mg tablets; benztropine mesylate (Cogentin), as 1- and 2-mg tablets; ethopropazine (Parsidol), as 50- and 100-mg tablets; cycrimine (Pagitane), as 1.25- and 2.5-mg tablets; procyclidine (Kemadrin), as 2- and 5-mg tablets; and biperiden (Akineton), as 2-mg tablets. Treatment should be initiated with small doses (e.g., trihexyphenidyl, 2 mg three times daily), and gradually increased until further increases yield no additional benefit or side effects occur. Peripheral anticholinergic adverse effects include blurred vision, dry mouth, anhidrosis, hyperthermia, constipation, and urinary urgency or sometimes retention. The major symptoms of central anticholinergic effects are mental disturbances, including forgetfulness, confusion, delusions, hallucinations, somnolence, and rarely coma. The last of these can be treated with physostigmine, 0.5 to 2 mg intramuscularly. Anticholinergics tend to produce mental disturbances in the elderly and can be bypassed and levodopa used instead in older patients.

When parkinsonian symptoms cannot be adequately suppressed by amantadine or anticholinergics (alone or in combination), levodopa is employed. Peripheral adverse effects (anorexia, nausea, vomiting) can be largely avoided if levodopa is taken concomitantly with a peripheral dopa decarboxylase inhibitor. In the United States this combination is marketed as Sinemet, which contains carbidopa and levodopa. The combinations available are 10/100-mg, 25/100-mg, and 25/250-mg (carbidopa/levodopa) tablets. In other countries, both carbidopa/levodopa and benserazide/levodopa combinations are available, the latter being marketed as Madopar in 20/100-mg and 50/200-mg tablets. The more decarboxylase inhibitor used, the less likely are peripheral adverse effects. However, the potency of levodopa is enhanced, increasing the possibility of central adverse effects such as abnormal involuntary movements (chorea and dystonia), confusion, hallucinations, delusions, somnolence, and postural hypotension. One method is to begin treatment with carbidopa/levodopa, 10/100 mg three times daily. If peripheral adverse reactions appear, change to 25/100-mg tablets. There is usually a latency period before maximal benefit at a given dose is encountered. The dosage can be increased gradually, utilizing half-tablets in the incremental build-up of doses, in order to "fine tune" the patient's response. A general concept is that low dosage may prevent complications seen with chronic use, including clinical fluctuations and loss of efficacy. Therefore, the patient who is retired from his occupation can be brought to a level approximately 80 to 85 per cent free of symptoms, rather than totally free, which may require higher dosages. Still-employed persons may need higher dosages to stay at work. Concomitant administration of amantadine and anticholinergics may allow for smaller doses of levodopa, and may be especially valuable to control certain symptoms, such as tremor. Levodopa can control tremor, but is especially effective in eliminating rigidity and reducing bradykinesia. Loss of postural reflexes may be ameliorated in the early but not advanced stages of the disease. With long-term treatment central adverse effects are usually more troublesome than peripheral ones. In such situations, it may be necessary to change from carbidopa/levodopa to levodopa alone. Levodopa is available in capsules and scored tablets in strengths of 100, 250, and 500 mg. Since the potency of levodopa is increased about four-fold if given as carbidopa/levodopa, levodopa alone allows for finer adjustments of the central effects of the drug.

Levodopa is contraindicated in patients with a history of malignant melanoma and in those with psychosis or profound dementia. In the presence of cardiac arrhythmias, as much as 200 mg per day of carbidopa (available as Lodosyn from Merck, Sharp and Dohme) should be given to block peripheral formation of dopamine; in addition, antiarrhythmic agents or digoxin should be used as indicated. Levodopa can be administered safely in hepatic, renal, and hematopoietic disorders. With a history of peptic ulcer, carbidopa/levodopa is preferred over levodopa alone.

In more advanced stages of parkinsonism or with chronic administration of levodopa, central adverse effects may appear with doses that are insufficient to control the symptoms of the disease. Since levodopa dosage must be reduced in this situation, adjunctive medications may be useful. In addition to amantadine and the anticholinergics mentioned above, drugs with mild anticholinergic properties can be employed. These include diphenhydramine (Benadryl), orphenadrine (Disipal), and chlorphenoxamine (Phenoxene). They are available in 50-mg strength, and a dosage of 50 mg three times daily may prove helpful. In contrast to the more powerful anticholinergic agents, these three drugs tend to be free of producing mental disturbances.

Tricyclic antidepressants are commonly employed to relieve the depressive symptoms that often accompany parkinsonism. Amitriptyline, 50 to 75 mg at bedtime, and imipramine, 25 mg three times daily, are commonly used. For tremor incompletely relieved by antiparkinson drugs and aggravated by stress or anxiety, anxiolytic agents such as diazepam provide some relief.

Direct-acting dopamine receptor agonists have less antiparkinsonian effect than Sinemet but more than amantadine and anticholinergics. Bromocriptine (Parlodel) is commercially available; other agonists (pergolide, lisuride, mesulergine) are limited currently to investigational studies. Bromocriptine is used as an adjunct to levodopa, preferably in low dosages (up to 40 mg per day), since higher dosages are frequently accompanied by adverse reactions. The most serious toxic effects are hallucinations, delusions, and confusion, and these tend to be more severe and longer lasting than those induced by levodopa. Other adverse effects seen with levodopa also occur with bromocriptine, including anorexia, nausea, vomiting, postural hypotension, and abnormal involuntary movements. In addition, erythromelalgia (St. Anthony's fire) can occur in the extremities, probably related to an ergot effect of bromocriptine, which is an ergot derivative. Erythromelalgia disappears when the drug is discontinued. Bromocriptine unfortunately tends to lose its effect with long-term use. It is probably best employed when the patient has clinical fluctuations from levodopa or when adequate dosages of levodopa are not possible.

Clinical fluctuations from levodopa therapy usually begin to occur after the drug has been administered for two years or longer and appear in at least 40 per cent of patients on long-term therapy. These troublesome fluctuations may prevent patients from working and are resistant to control. There are two predominant forms: the "on-off" phenomenon and the "wearing-off" or "end-of-dose" effect. The on-off phenomenon consists of sudden loss of the antiparkinson effect of levodopa. Symptoms of severe parkinsonism may produce immobility from severe bradykinesia and rigidity. The "off" states appear irregularly and may last up to several hours. They may occur several times daily and disappear ("on" effect) as suddenly as they occur, even without another dose of levodopa. Higher dosages of levodopa or bromocriptine can prevent these on-off episodes, but usually induce continuous and distressing dyskinesias.

The wearing-off phenomenon comes on gradually, as plasma levels of levodopa fall to low levels. The phenomenon is a pharmacokinetic effect due to reduced bioavailability of levodopa as a result of its short half-life in plasma (30 to 45 minutes). Spacing the doses more closely is a partial remedy, and some patients take levodopa every three hours, every two hours, or even more frequently to prevent the "off" periods. Unfortunately, the price is to cause a state of continual dyskinesia. Perhaps longer-acting dopamine agonists will solve this problem. Some patients with severe wearing-off phenomena are unable to miss a single dose of levodopa without being in an "off" state, and if awakened in the middle of the night are immobile. These "dopa addicts" require levodopa before retiring for the night and perhaps during the night. Patients who are free of clinical fluctuations do not usually require bedtime medication and can be maintained on three doses a day.

Drug holidays from levodopa can temporarily reverse clinical fluctuations and loss of drug efficacy. The concept is that the abstinence restores sensitivity of dopamine receptors, making them once again respond to the drug. The risks and discomfort are serious. Because of immobility and the possibility of aspiration, such levodopa withdrawal must be done in a hospital. Usually a patient is too uncomfortable to be off levodopa for longer than a few days, although ten days is the goal. Swallowing difficulty should terminate this withdrawal period in order to avoid aspiration. It is not certain that the long-term benefit from a drug holiday is sufficient to justify the risks involved.

Treatment of postencephalitic parkinsonism usually requires smaller dosages of levodopa than does idiopathic parkinsonism. Drug-induced parkinsonism responds well to anticholinergics. Striatonigral degeneration may respond to levodopa in the early stages of the disease, but then becomes resistant to therapy, as does progressive supranuclear palsy. In such diseases, in which striatal dopamine receptors are not responsive to levodopa or dopamine agonists, anticholinergics are the drugs of choice. Unfortunately, these agents offer only modest relief of symptoms compared to the usually dramatic relief of idiopathic parkinsonism by levodopa.

SURGICAL MEASURES. Stereotactic lesions of the ventrolateral thalamus can alleviate tremor and rigidity of the contralateral limbs. This approach is not useful for bradykinesia and loss of postural reflexes, which are the predominant causes of disability, nor does it halt progression of the disease. Moreover, bilateral surgery to relieve tremor on both sides usually results in impaired speech. With the introduction of levodopa therapy, surgical therapy has almost entirely been discontinued.

COURSE OF THE PARKINSONIAN SYNDROME. Although levodopa and other drugs do not alter the progression of the disease, they do increase survival time because of improved functional capacity. The mortality rate, which was three times that of the normal population, has been reduced by half since the introduction of levodopa. The symptom that becomes least responsive is loss of postural reflexes, and falling with resultant hip fracture is a potential consequence. Although chronic levodopa therapy may bring troublesome adverse effects of clinical fluctuations, dyskinesias, mental disturbances, and loss of efficacy, many patients continue to have a substantial response to the drug for a decade or more.

Earnest MP, Fahn S, Karp JH, Rowland LP: Normal pressure hydrocephalus and hypertensive cerebrovascular disease. Arch Neurol 31:262, 1974. *Discusses concept of arteriosclerotic (vascular) parkinsonism and its possible mechanism via normal pressure hydrocephalus.*

Fahn S: Secondary parkinsonism. *In* Goldensohn ES, Appel SH (eds.): Scientific Approaches to Clinical Neurology. Philadelphia, Lea & Febiger, 1977, pp 1159–1189. *A classification and review of causes of parkinsonism other than Parkinson's disease.*

Fahn S, Duffy P: Parkinson's disease. *In* Goldensohn ES, Appel SH (eds.): Scientific Approaches to Clinical Neurology. Philadelphia, Lea & Febiger, 1977, pp 1119–1158. *Thorough review of this illness.*

Hoehn MM, Yahr MD: Parkinsonism: Onset, progression and mortality. Neurology 17:427, 1967. *Provides the best data on the progression of parkinsonism prior to the introduction of levodopa therapy.*

Langston JW, Ballard P, Tetrud JW, Irwin I: Chronic parkinsonism in humans due to a product of meperidine-analog synthesis. Science 219:979, 1983. *A report describing young adults who developed acute parkinsonism after self-injection of a toxic substance known as MPTP.*

Marsden CD, Parkes JD, Quinn N: Fluctuations of disability in Parkinson's disease—clinical aspects. *In* Marsden CD, Fahn S (eds.): Movement Disorders. London, Butterworth Scientific, 1982, pp 96–122. *A detailed account of the varieties of clinical fluctuations seen in patients with parkinsonism due to the disease and due to levodopa therapy.*

Mayeux R: Depression and dementia in Parkinson's disease. *In* Marsden CD, Fahn S (eds.): Movement Disorders. London, Butterworth Scientific, 1982, pp 75–95. *A review of the literature documenting the prevalence of symptoms of depression and dementia in patients with Parkinson's disease.*

484. ESSENTIAL TREMOR
(Familial or Senile Tremor)

Essential tremor is a monosymptomatic disorder, expressed as tremor of the hands, head, and, least frequently, voice. The tremor in the hands is usually more rapid than that encountered in parkinsonism and occurs with volitional movement instead of at rest. It is aggravated by handwriting and suppressed by the use of alcohol. The age of onset is variable, typically beginning at least mildly before the age of 25 and persisting throughout life with some increase in intensity and spread to other body parts. Physical and social disability may result. There is a strong familial incidence distributed as an autosomal dominant trait. With late-life onset, the tremor is commonly called *senile tremor*. No specific pathologic lesion has been reported in the nervous system in this condition. An occasional patient may develop Parkinson's disease on top of a longstanding history of essential tremor. Beta-adrenergic blocking agents are useful in some patients, but dramatic relief of tremor is not achieved with these drugs. Propranolol* in a dosage of 120 to 240 mg per day in three or four divided doses has been most commonly used. The selective beta-1 adrenergic blocker metoprolol seems to be equally effective in doses of 50 mg three times daily. This drug has the advantage that it can be used in patients with bronchospasm or asthma. Beta-adrenergic blockers should be avoided in patients with congestive heart failure or heart block. It is probably safer to avoid the use of drugs in the elderly population. Some wine with meals offers sufficient relief while the hands are engaged in feeding. The major differential diagnosis is parkinsonism, but the lack of bradykinesia, rigidity, and postural abnormalities, as well as the presence of tremor with action instead of at rest, rules out that disorder.

Fahn S: Differential diagnosis of tremors. Med Clin North Am 56:1363, 1972. *Describes the clinical approach in diagnosing tremors and presents a useful classification.*

Newman RP, Jacobs L: Metoprolol in essential tremor. Arch Neurol 37:596, 1980. *Reports the successful use of metoprolol to control tremor in the presence of asthma.*

Young RR, Shahani BT: Pharmacology of tremor. Clin Neuropharmacol 4:139, 1979. *Reviews pharmacologic evaluations of tremor.*

485. THE CHOREAS

A large number of disorders may present with choreic movements (Table 485–1), having in common brief, involuntary contractions. It is important to determine whether the movements are fluid-like (flowing from one location to another), as in classic choreic disorders, or whether they are rhythmically repetitive in the same site (stereotypy), as in tardive dyskinesia. The presence of other neurologic deficits (gait disturbance, dementia) can assist in the diagnosis of Huntington's disease, and a detailed family history and drug history are essential for reliable diagnosis. A difficult diagnostic problem is encountered in the patient with Huntington's disease who has been treated with antipsychotic drugs. Such patients can present with a mixed picture of tardive dyskinesia and Huntington's disease.

*This use is not listed in the manufacturer's directive.

TABLE 485–1. A CLASSIFICATION OF COMMON CAUSES OF CHOREA

- I. Hereditary
  - A. Huntington's disease
  - B. Wilson's disease
  - C. Ataxia-telangiectasia
  - D. Lesch-Nyhan syndrome
  - E. Chorea-acanthocytosis
- II. Secondary
  - A. Infections
    1. Sydenham's chorea
    2. Encephalitis
  - B. Drugs
    1. Levodopa
    2. Estrogen (oral contraceptives)
    3. Phenytoin
    4. Antipsychotic drugs
  - C. Metabolic and endocrine
    1. Chorea gravidarum
    2. Thyrotoxicosis
  - D. Vascular
    1. Lupus erythematosus
    2. Polycythemia vera
    3. Hemichorea-hemiballism
- III. Unknown
  - A. Senile chorea

HEREDITARY CHOREA (Chronic Progressive Chorea, Huntington's Disease)

Huntington's disease is the most common of the hereditary choreas. It is a progressive degenerative disorder predominantly affecting the basal ganglia and the cerebral cortex. Clinically, it is manifested by a triad consisting of choreic movements, intellectual decline leading to dementia, and emotional disturbances. The disease is transmitted as an autosomal dominant trait with complete penetrance. Both sexes are equally affected, and each offspring has a 50 per cent chance of becoming affected. In the United States the prevalence ranges from 4 to 8 per 100,000 population. The disease usually begins in adulthood after childbearing, with a peak age at onset of 40 years; it can begin at any age, however, and in approximately 10 per cent onset occurs before the age of 20 (juvenile Huntington's disease). As a general rule, juvenile cases exhibit bradykinesia and rigidity, rather than chorea and hypotonia. The presence of a movement disorder is essential to the disease; emotional disturbances and cognitive disorders are common problems in the general population and hence are not sufficient by themselves for the diagnosis. Motor symptoms begin with clumsiness and the dropping of objects. The choreic movements then become apparent, typically consisting first of brief, low amplitude movements of the fingers, but spreading to involve all parts of the body (arms, legs, trunk, neck, and face). The movements can be proximal as well as distal in the limbs, and flow from one site to another. In the face they are more common in the forehead than around the mouth (the latter being more common in tardive dyskinesia). It is difficult for the patient to keep the tongue protruded for 20 seconds and to maintain a steady tight grip (causing a milkmaid grip). The chorea is more pronounced on standing and walking, and abnormal gait is characterized by hesitation and stuttering steps. Postural instability develops, often with subsequent falls. Choking is a common and sometimes fatal symptom.

Emotional disorders are common in Huntington's disease and may precede choreic movements. Personality changes, mania, hallucinations, delusions, paranoia, schizophrenia, impulsiveness, hostility, and agitation can develop, sometimes as the first sign of involvement. Most common are apathy and withdrawn behavior with a decrease in conversation and inattention to personal hygiene. Depression is frequent and leads to an increased incidence of suicide. These personality disturbances are especially troublesome for the family of the affected person. Cognitive changes tend to appear later. There is impairment of recent memory and judgment, loss of capacity to plan and organize, and intellectual decline. Dementia leads to urinary and fecal incontinence and an inability to handle activities of daily living (see also Ch. 479).

Pathologically, there is loss of neurons with reactive gliosis in many regions of the brain, particularly in the striatum and cerebral cortex. Cell loss is accompanied by depletion of neurotransmitters, the most consistent effect being a marked reduction of GABA and its synthesizing enzyme, glutamic acid decarboxylase, in the basal ganglia. There is also a loss of acetylcholine neurons and of dopamine, acetylcholine, and serotonin receptors. Treatment with GABA agonists or cholinergic agonists has not led to clinical improvement.

The differential diagnosis of chorea is long (Table 485–1), but the triad of chorea, progressive dementia, and emotional disturbances strongly suggests Huntington's disease. The diagnosis is readily apparent if a positive family history is obtained, but such a history may be lacking because a parent is unavailable, has disappeared, or has died before symptoms appeared. The lack of a positive family history in the presence of longevity and good health of the parents raises questions of paternity, spontaneous mutation, or incorrect diagnosis. Computed tomography of the head eventually will reveal atrophy of the caudate nuclei; this may assist in the diagnosis. Accurate diagnosis of affected persons and carriers is now possible by identifying a genetic marker linked to the Huntington gene.

The technique has great promise for both diagnosis and prevention by confident genetic counseling.

Treatment of Huntington's disease should extend to the family as well as the patient, since this is a hereditary disorder with potential involvement of offspring and since the mental symptoms create enormous family stress. Explaining the disease and offering nondirective genetic discussion of the inheritance pattern are important and will enable family members who are at risk for the disease or are known carriers to reach a decision about having children. Therapy is available for many of the symptoms. Presynaptic dopamine-depleting agents (reserpine and tetrabenazine) and postsynaptic dopamine antagonists (antipsychotic agents) can reduce chorea, although the latter drugs are less effective than the former and may cause tardive dyskinesia. Reserpine therapy should begin with a small dose (0.25 mg per day); the daily dosage is then increased weekly by 0.25 mg until chorea declines. As much as 8 to 10 mg per day may be required. A slow buildup in dosage will usually avoid nasal stuffiness and depression. Postural hypotension and increased apathy can occur and necessitate a reduction in dosage. Dementia is not treatable, but emotional disturbances can be ameliorated. Tricyclic antidepressants are useful for depression, and antipsychotic agents can treat psychosis.

Chorea-acanthocytosis is much less common in the United States than is Huntington's disease but is more common in Japan. It is manifested by mild chorea and tics, self-mutilation (usually of lips and tongue), loss of tendon reflexes, elevated serum creatine phosphokinase, presence of acanthocytes in the blood, and atrophy of the caudate nuclei. Other hereditary disorders that can manifest chorea are covered elsewhere: Wilson's disease in Ch. 205, ataxia telangiectasia in Ch. 492, and Lesch-Nyhan syndrome in Ch. 196.

Barbeau A, Chase TN, Paulson GW (eds.): Huntington's chorea, 1872–1972. Adv Neurol, Vol 1, 1973. *The first monograph summarizing previous studies and presenting new data, including the observation of reduced GABA levels.*

Chase TN, Wexler NS, Barbeau A (eds.): Huntington's disease. Adv Neurol, Vol 23, 1979. *Provides an update of the voluminous research that has been conducted on Huntington's disease since 1972.*

Gusella JF, Wexler NS, Conneally PM, et al.: A polymorphic DNA marker genetically linked to Huntington's disease. Nature 306:234, 1983. *Reports the localization of the gene for Huntington's disease to chromosome 4.*

Kuhl DE, Phelps ME, Markham CH, Metter EJ, Riege WH, Winter J: Cerebral metabolism and atrophy in Huntington's disease determined by 18-FDG and computed tomographic scan. Ann Neurol 12:425, 1982. *Positron emission tomography reveals hypometabolism of striatum in patients with Huntington's disease and in some at-risk individuals.*

Sakai T, Mawatari S, Iwashita H, Goto I, Kuroiwa Y: Chorea-acanthocytosis: Clues to clinical diagnosis. Arch Neurol 38:335, 1981. *Descriptions of the clinical features of chorea-acanthocytosis, which is more common in Japan than in the United States.*

Shoulson I: Care of patients and families with Huntington's disease. *In* Marsden CD, Fahn S (eds.): Movement Disorders. London, Butterworth Scientific, 1982, pp 277–290. *Describes a practical approach to the diagnosis, genetic counseling, and management of families with Huntington's disease.*

SECONDARY CHOREA

Acquired chorea has many causes (Table 485–1), which the history, examination, and laboratory studies can usually distinguish. Clinically, the choreic movements are similar in the different disorders except for tardive dyskinesia.

SYDENHAM'S CHOREA (St. Vitus' Dance). This is an acute chorea encountered primarily during childhood, with the greatest incidence between the ages of five and fifteen. Later occurrence is uncommon, but it can be associated with pregnancy (chorea gravidarum). There is a female preponderance after the age of ten. A close relationship exists with rheumatic fever, and the condition has declined substantially in recent years.

The choreic movements in this disorder are usually generalized, and only 20 per cent of patients have hemichorea. The brief, involuntary movements flow from site to site, and the patient has difficulty sitting quietly. Fidgety behavior, clumsiness, dropping of objects, dysarthria, and an awkward gait are common. Other neurologic symptoms are infrequent.

Sydenham's chorea is not fatal, and recovery occurs in two to six months. Pathologic studies have been few and have disclosed scattered lesions of vasculitis in the cortex, basal ganglia, cerebellum, and brainstem. There are no specific laboratory abnormalities. The differential diagnosis depends on eliminating other causes of chorea by appropriate history and laboratory studies.

Recurrence, with as many as two or three attacks over a period of years, occurs in almost one third of the patients. Since the disease is self-limited, specific drugs may not be necessary. If the chorea is disabling and interferes with school work, antichoreic drugs are used. Short-term treatment with perphenazine (12 to 16 mg per day in divided doses) or haloperidol (3 to 6 mg per day in divided doses) can be effective. Some patients with Sydenham's chorea may have residual deficits of valvular heart disease, behavioral problems, mild motor abnormalities, and a poor performance in psychometric testing.

HEMIBALLISM. Hemiballism is a forceful, violent form of hemichorea manifested by flinging movements of the limbs on one side of the body. The most common cause is a vascular lesion, either a hemorrhage or an infarct involving the opposite subthalamic nucleus. Tumors rarely are involved. Most often hemiballism or hemichorea develops on recovery from a hemiparesis and hemisensory deficit secondary to stroke. Occasionally the sensorimotor deficits are minor, and ballism occurs as the initial event. Like other abnormal involuntary movements, hemiballism disappears during sleep. In most instances, the intensity of hemiballism decreases gradually to hemichorea and then fades away after several weeks, but in some patients the movements persist. Severe movements can be exhausting but can be controlled with drugs such as reserpine or antipsychotic agents. Because of the self-limiting nature of hemiballism, it is reasonable to use antipsychotics for their rapid onset of action and then slowly withdraw the drug to avoid producing tardive dyskinesia.

SENILE CHOREA. Occasional patients, usually older than 60 years, present with generalized chorea resembling Huntington's disease, but with no associated dementia, emotional disturbance, positive family history, or evidence of other etiologies. Postmortem studies reveal striatal pathology identical to that of Huntington's disease. It has been speculated that such so-called senile chorea is a late-onset form of Huntington's disease in which cognitive symptoms have not developed because of the advanced age of onset. No definitive genetic studies are available.

Aron A, Freeman J, Carter S: The natural history of Sydenham's chorea. Am J Med 38:83, 1965. *One third of patients evaluated an average of 29 years after the initial episode of chorea were found to have valvular heart disease.*

Bird MT, Palkes H, Prensky AL: A follow-up study of Sydenham's chorea. Neurology 26:601, 1976. *An average of an eight-year follow-up evaluation revealed that some individuals have behavioral disorders, abnormal electroencephalograms, and poorer performance on psychometric testing.*

Johnson WG, Fahn S: Treatment of vascular hemiballism and hemichorea. Neurology 27:634, 1977. *Reports on the effectiveness of the antipsychotic drug perphenazine in eight cases of hemiballism.*

Klawans HI, Moses H, Nausieda PA, Bergen D, Weiner WJ: Treatment and prognosis of hemiballism. N Engl J Med 295:1348, 1976. *Report on the effectiveness of haloperidol and chlorpromazine in 11 cases.*

Nausieda PA, Grossman BJ, Koller WC, Weiner WJ, Klawans HL: Syndenham's chorea: An update. Neurology 30:331, 1980. *This survey points out the marked decrease in the incidence of the disorder in recent years.*

TARDIVE DYSKINESIA

This most feared complication of antipsychotic drug therapy can persist indefinitely. The disorder is associated with chronic administration of these drugs (hence the name "tardive"), but there are reports of its occurring after exposure of only several weeks. Tardive dyskinesia is more common in women and the elderly, and is more likely to occur with exposure to high dosages and longer duration of treatment. The drugs themselves mask the symptoms so that onset is not clearly recognized. Withdrawal of the drug exposes the dyskinesia, which consists of rhythmically repetitive, rapid movements that can occur in most parts of the body. The lower part of the face is involved most often; this oral-lingual-buccal dyskinesia resembles continual chewing movements, with the tongue intermittently darting out of the mouth ("fly-catcher" tongue). In the trunk the movements usually assume a repetitive flexion and extension pattern ("body-rocking"). The distal parts of the limbs may show incessant flexion-extension movements ("piano-playing" fingers and toes), whereas the proximal muscles are usually spared. On standing the patient may have repetitive movements of the legs ("marching in place"). Superficially, the gait may appear unaffected, but the arms tend to swing to a larger degree than normal and the stride may elongate. The patient may be unaware of the movements unless there is an associated akathisia (a subjective feeling of restlessness), characterized by the need to move about and walk back and forth. Sometimes patients describe feeling as if they were going to jump out of their skin. This is the most distressing symptom in the tardive dyskinesia syndrome, and resembles the acute akathisia that sometimes accompanies an initial administration of antipsychotic drugs, but disappears when the drug is withdrawn. In contrast, akathisia as it occurs in tardive dyskinesia is a chronic form that is made more severe by drug withdrawal; hence it is analogous to the dyskinesia. Both tardive akathisia and tardive dyskinesia can be suppressed by antidopaminergic drugs.

The major differential diagnoses are Huntington's disease and a focal form of facial and mandibular dystonia referred to as Meige's syndrome. Huntington's disease is particularly difficult to differentiate from tardive dyskinesia because choreic movements and emotional disturbances occur in both disorders. However, several helpful signs serve to distinguish between these two conditions (Table 485–2). Patients with known Huntington's disease also may develop tardive dyskinesia if antipsychotic drugs are used in its treatment. Meige's syndrome causes long-lasting facial movements (sustained dystonic movements), compared to the rapid, brief, and repetitive movements in tardive dyskinesia. A drug-free history eliminates tardive dyskinesia by definition.

In addition to the classic form of tardive dyskinesia described above, there are two clinical variations. One is the self-limiting "withdrawal emergent" syndrome, in which choreic movements resembling those seen in Sydenham's chorea or Huntington's disease appear when the antipsychotic drug is suddenly discontinued. There are flowing, rather than repetitive, choreic movements. The withdrawal emergent syndrome is most common in children. Reintroducing the antipsychotic drug and tapering it slowly may eliminate the symptoms. The other variant is the presence of sustained dystonic movements rather than choreic movements. This variant (tardive dystonia) is more common in young adults than in the elderly population.

TABLE 485–2. DIFFERENTIAL DIAGNOSIS OF TARDIVE DYSKINESIA AND HUNTINGTON'S DISEASE*

Clinical Features	Tardive Dyskinesia	Huntington's Disease
Akathisia	Present	Absent
Body-rocking	Present	Absent
Marching-in-place	Present	Absent
Oral-lingual-buccal dyskinesia	Present	Sometimes present
Darting tongue	Present	Rarely present
Repetitive movements	Present	Absent
Flowing movements	Absent	Present
Forehead chorea	Absent	Present
Saccadic eye movements	Normal	Abnormal
Protrusion of tongue	Maintained (normal)	Not maintained
Milkmaid grip	Absent	Present
Postural stability	Normal	Impaired
Walking	Reduces chorea	Increases chorea
Gait	Normal	Stuttering, ataxic

*Although the tabulated clinical features may be found in any individual patient, they are not always present in every patient.

Tardive dyskinesia is believed to be caused by the development of supersensitive dopamine receptors as a result of chronic blockade by antipsychotic drugs. There is no satisfactory explanation of why the disorder is often permanent. Some patients who remain drug free for several months to years have a resolution of the syndrome, and withdrawal of the offending agents is the treatment of choice. But many patients, particularly those with psychosis or severe tardive akathisia, must continue to take antidopaminergic drugs to suppress these disabling symptoms. Antipsychotic drug therapy may be required to treat psychosis. If the patient does not have psychosis, then dopamine-depleting drugs (reserpine and alpha-methylparatyrosine) that act presynaptically are the preferred agents and can relieve both the dyskinesia and akathisia. The dosages are increased slowly, as in the treatment of Huntington's chorea. The approach to treatment is diagrammed below.

Presence of Tardive Dyskinesia (TD)

- Psychosis returns → Resume antipsychotic
- No psychosis; pronounced TD or akathisia → Add reserpine
- No psychosis; no akathisia; mild TD → No medication

Levodopa administration for a few months to desensitize the dopamine receptors, followed by its withdrawal, is being evaluated as a therapeutic agent.

The incidence of tardive dyskinesia appears to be increasing owing to widespread administration of antipsychotic drugs. It is important to consider this complication before prescribing these agents. Such drugs should be used only in clinical situations in which no satisfactory alternatives exist.

Alpert M, Friedhoff AJ, Diamond F: Use of dopamine receptor agonists to reduce dopamine receptor number as treatment for tardive dyskinesia. Adv Neurol 37:253, 1983. *Report of partial success in treating tardive dyskinesia with levodopa, followed by its withdrawal after eight weeks.*

Baldessarini RJ, Tarsy D: Tardive dyskinesia. *In* Lipton J, DiMascio A, Killam KF (eds.): Psychopharmacology. A Generation of Progress. New York, Raven Press, 1978, pp 993–1004. *A concise review of the clinical features and the pharmacology of tardive dyskinesia.*

Fahn S: Treatment of tardive dyskinesia: Use of dopamine-depleting agents. Clin Neuropharmacol 6:151, 1983. *Report of control of tardive dyskinesia and tardive akathisia with the use of reserpine and alpha-methylparatyrosine.*

486. OTHER EXTRAPYRAMIDAL DISORDERS

MYOCLONUS

Myoclonic jerks are sudden, shock-like muscular contractions or inhibitions (the latter are called negative myoclonus). They can be singular or repetitive, rhythmic or arrhythmic, symmetrical or asymmetrical, synchronous or asynchronous, and generalized, segmental, or focal. Typically, myoclonic jerks occur unpredictably and irregularly. However, a form of regular and rhythmic myoclonus exists, *palatal myoclonus*, which results from infarction or degeneration involving some of the anatomic triangle that links the dentate nucleus, red nucleus, and inferior olivary nucleus. This form is categorized as myoclonus (rather than tremor) because of its synchronous (instead of alternating) contractions. Lesions in many parts of the nervous system, including spinal cord, brainstem, cerebellum, and cerebral cortex, can give rise to myoclonus. Myoclonus is most often a symptom of an irritable nervous system. It is present in many diseases (Table 486–1) but can also occur as an isolated phenomenon (essential myoclonus). When associated with objective neurologic findings, it is usually progressive. In contrast, essential myoclonus (familial or sporadic) tends to be stable and nonprogressive. Nocturnal myoclonus, now called "peri-

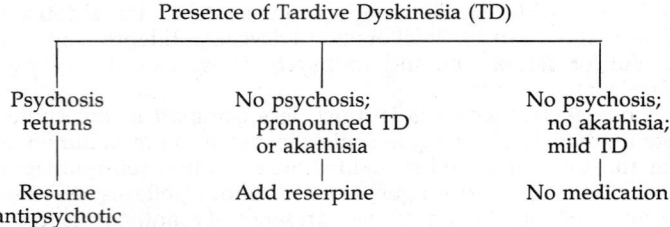

TABLE 486–1. A CLASSIFICATION OF COMMON FORMS OF MYOCLONUS

I. Benign myoclonic jerks
  A. Physiologic: sleep jerks, anxiety
  B. Essential myoclonus: familial or sporadic
  C. Periodic movements of sleep
  D. Associated with petit mal or grand mal seizures
II. Symptomatic myoclonus
  A. Myoclonus epilepsy
  B. Dementias: Creutzfeldt-Jakob, Alzheimer's
  C. Infectious: subacute sclerosing panencephalitis
  D. Lipidoses
  E. Cerebellar degenerations
  F. Hypoxia
  G. Toxins: methyl bromide, strychnine
  H. Drugs: levodopa, tricyclics
  I. Systemic illnesses: uremia, hepatic, dialysis encephalopathy
III. Rhythmic myoclonus
  A. Palatal myoclonus
  B. Ocular myoclonus

odic movements of sleep" because of its regularity, may awaken patients from sleep; it is often associated with "restless legs syndrome," dysesthesias, and mild dyskinesias while awake.

To treat myoclonic syndromes, especially posthypoxic action myoclonus, clonazepam is the drug of first choice. Because drowsiness and ataxia are common adverse effects, the dosage of clonazepam should be increased gradually until improvement or adverse effects are encountered. A dosage as high as 8 mg per day (in four divided doses) may be necessary. Valproate is another useful drug; the dosage should be increased gradually until it is effective or toxic. As much as 3000 mg per day may be necessary. The combination of clonazepam and valproate can be particularly effective. Other useful drugs include carbamazepine (up to 1000 mg per day), diazepam (up to 40 mg per day), and the serotonin precursor 5-hydroxytryptophan. The last-named drug is not available commercially in the United States.

Marsden CD, Hallett M, Fahn S: The nosology and pathophysiology of myoclonus. *In* Marsden CD, Fahn S (eds.): Movement Disorders. London, Butterworth Scientific, 1982, pp 196–248. *Most recent review of myoclonus. It presents a classification scheme based on etiology.*

TICS (Habit Spasms, Gilles de la Tourette's Syndrome)

A tic is a sudden rapid series of involuntary movements that are usually complex and coordinated. For example, an irregular sequence of movements can contain such diverse movements as eye blinking, head shaking, shoulder shrugging, and limb and facial gestures. In some instances patients describe a compelling need to make these movements. Tics can be voluntarily controlled for brief intervals, but such conscious efforts are usually followed by more intense and frequent contractions. Stress and anxiety aggravate tics, and psychotherapeutic management may diminish them.

In some individuals tics reflect recurrent nervous mannerisms appropriately called habit spasms. Other tics are caused by neurologic disorders. They may be present in the acute phase of encephalitis or as a sequela of encephalitis. Most tics are of unknown etiology and are sometimes familial. Tics can be considered in a spectrum, from transient tics of childhood, through persistent tics, to the most severe type in which vocal tics are also present. This last form is known as Gilles de la Tourette's syndrome. Vocalizations occur as various involuntary and compulsive sounds (barking, sniffing, throat clearing, yelping noises) and words or fragments of words, often obscene (coprolalia). Motor tics in Tourette's syndrome may also include obscene gestures (copropraxia). The age of onset is usually between two and fifteen years. As a general rule, there are periods of remissions and exacerbations, and the tics move from one part of the body to another. Many patients show a tendency for the tics to become less severe and more controllable with age. The presence of vocal tics, especially coprolalia, adds a new dimension to the patient's problem of adjusting in society. Patients are hesitant to be seen in public, and avoid areas where silence is required (cinema, theater, library). They are frequently misunderstood, teased, or insulted by schoolmates, teachers, and strangers. No anatomic abnormalities have been observed in the brain, but the consistency of the clinical syndrome gives every evidence that Tourette's syndrome is an organic disorder.

Haloperidol appears to be the most effective drug for treating tics and is given in divided doses up to 20 mg or more a day. Treatment is begun with a small dosage and increased slowly until control is achieved or adverse affects are obtained. Unfortunately, haloperidol affects personality ("zombie" effect) and school performance. Furthermore, there is a danger of inducing tardive dyskinesia or its variants. Other drugs should be tried initially, such as clonazepam (3 to 6 mg a day) and clonidine (up to 0.6 mg daily) in divided doses.

Friedhoff AJ, Chase TN (eds.): Gilles de la Tourette syndrome. Adv Neurol, Vol 36, 1982. *The proceedings of the first international symposium on this subject. It provides reports of many studies on tic disorders.*

Golden GS: Tics and Tourette's: A continuum of symptoms? Ann Neurol 4:145, 1978. *Describes families in which some individuals have only motor tics and others have both motor and vocal tics (Tourette's syndrome) and suggests a continuum of tic syndromes.*

Shapiro AK, Shapiro ES, Bruun RD, Sweet RD: Gilles de la Tourette Syndrome. New York, Raven Press, 1978. *Thorough review of the literature and an analysis of the large number of cases personally observed by the authors.*

ATHETOSIS (Mobile Spasms)

Clinically, athetosis falls between the rapid movements of chorea and the sustained movements of dystonia. The term is applied to constant writhing and twisting movements without fixed postures. Yet as the spectrum of torsion dystonia becomes better appreciated, athetosis increasingly seems to be part of the dystonic syndromes; athetotic dystonia may therefore be a more appropriate name. Athetosis is most frequently encountered in patients who suffered perinatal brain injury, usually from hypoxic damage (athetotic cerebral palsy). Athetosis has also been reported in kernicterus, in rare childhood degenerative diseases of the basal ganglia, in glutaric aciduria, and after hemiplegia secondary to strokes in childhood. Athetosis thus appears to be the expression of torsion dystonia caused by basal ganglia damage at an early, still developing age. In athetotic cerebral palsy pathologic studies reveal either status marmoratus of the striatum or status dysmyelinatus of the globus pallidus.

Athetosis involves the limbs (distal and proximal), trunk, neck, face, and tongue. The movements are enhanced when the patient attemps to speak ("overflow"). Speech is impaired with poor articulation, in part becuse of continual tongue movements and facial movements. Stress and attempted voluntary movements also bring out an overflow of writhing movements throughout the body. This increase of athetotic movements makes it difficult for the patient to handle daily tasks. There is no satisfactory treatment. Diazepam or anticholinergic agents may provide a little amelioration.

Dooling EC, Adams RD: The pathological anatomy of posthemiplegic athetosis. Brain 98:29, 1975. *Describes pathologically documented cases of unilateral athetosis following childhood hemiplegia.*

Leibel RL, Shih VE, Goodman SI, Bauman ML, McCabe ERB, Zwerdling RG, Bergman I, Costello C: Glutaric acidemia: A metabolic disorder causing progressive choreoathetosis. Neurology 30:1163, 1980. *A newly described metabolic error and a cause of infantile athetotic dystonia.*

Spiegel EA, Baird HW: Athetotic syndromes. *In* Vinken PJ, Bruyn GW (eds.): Handbook of Clinical Neurology, Vol 6. Amsterdam, North-Holland, 1968, pp 440–475. *The best and most thorough clinical review of athetosis in a relatively sparse literature on this subject.*

487. THE DYSTONIAS

TORSION DYSTONIA (Dystonia Musculorum Deformans, Torsion Spasms)

The torsion dystonias comprise a group of disorders in which twisting movements (torsion spasms) are characteristic. Slow torsion spasms are called athetotic dystonia or athetosis, but more often torsion spasms are rapid and are mistakenly called chorea. One characteristic feature of torsion spasms is their propensity to be maintained at the end of the movement for a second or so (dystonic movements) and even for minutes to hours (dystonic postures). Ultimately contractures can occur, leading to permanent deformity, especially in the still-growing child. Both agonist and antagonist muscles contract simultaneously in dystonia. Dystonia can be present when the patient is at rest or in the process of a volitional movement (action dystonia). In carrying out a voluntary movement, inappropriate muscles contract when they should be quiescent. Dystonic movements are sometimes broken up into a tremor pattern (dystonic tremor), which may be due to the patient's attempt to resist the abnormal pulling and maintain a more normal posture. Dystonia varies with change of posture, worsens with stress, decreases with relaxation or hypnosis, disappears with sleep, and is modified by tactile or proprioceptive input.

The torsion dystonias can be etiologically divided into primary and secondary types (Table 487–1). The first is more common and includes hereditary forms (both autosomal recessive and autosomal dominant) and those that are sporadic or idiopathic. The autosomal recessive form is found most often in Ashkenazic Jews and commonly begins between the ages of five and fifteen. The legs are typically affected first, starting with action dystonia. At rest the patient may seem normal, but when he stands or walks, one or both feet assume an equinovarus posture and the leg executes a bizarre stepping twisting movement. As the disease progresses, the other leg and other parts of the body become involved. Lordosis, scoliosis, tortipelvis, and torticollis can appear. Because of modification by proprioceptive input, walking backward may be less abnormal than walking forward. Action dystonia of the arms interferes with handwriting and other manipulations. Dystonic movements appear when the patient is at rest, and eventually dystonic postures may develop. When dystonic movements are absent, muscle tone is normal or hypotonic; hypertonia accompanies dystonic movements. Mentation, sensation, strength, and tendon reflexes remain normal. Not all patients show progression. Many tend to plateau after a period of progression.

Autosomal dominant and sporadic dystonia each follow the same pattern as the recessive form, except that the age of onset tends to be somewhat older and the disease is usually less progressive. Penetrance is usually incomplete, and there are many formes frustes in other members of the family: club foot, scoliosis, torticollis, writer's cramp, and essential tremor.

As a general rule, the younger the age of onset of dystonia, the more likely the disease is to begin in the feet and legs and to become progressive and generalized: juvenile onset tends to begin in the hands and arms and plateaus after involving several segments; adult onset tends to remain focal, the neck being the most common site (spasmodic torticollis). Other common varieties of focal dystonia are blepharospasm, facial and mandibular dystonia (Meige's syndrome), spastic dysphonia, and writer's cramp. Primary dystonia with childhood onset is also referred to as dystonia musculorum deformans.

No clear-cut pathologic lesions have been discerned in the brain in primary torsion dystonia. It is assumed that the lesion is of a chemical and physiologic nature, affecting the basal ganglia, especially the striatum, since this is the area of pathology in secondary or acquired forms of dystonia. Moreover, drugs that affect the basal ganglia (i.e., levodopa, antipsychotic agents) can induce dystonic movements and postures.

A variety of drugs have been proposed to treat torsion dystonia, but none has been consistently effective. High dosage anticholinergics are often effective and are well tolerated in children if the daily dose is increased gradually. A recommended schedule is to begin with trihexyphenidyl (Artane), 2.5 mg twice daily, and increase the daily dosage at a rate of 2.5 mg weekly. The dosage should be increased until there is satisfactory improvement or intolerable adverse effects. As much as 50 mg per day in four divided doses may be necessary. Unfortunately, most adults cannot tolerate high dosages of anticholinergics. Common adverse effects are dry mouth, blurred vision, forgetfulness, and confusion. Other compounds that may provide some benefit are carbamazepine (Tegretol, 400 to 800 mg per day), diazepam (Valium, 30 to 60 mg per day), and, rarely, levodopa (500 to 1500 mg per day). Dorsal column stimulation may help some patients. Stereotactic thalamotomies can be effective for limb dystonia, but several repeat procedures may be necessary, and bilateral surgery entails a high risk of producing a major speech deficit. Patients should not undergo such surgery unless they are well aware of the risks, have had an adequate trial of pharmacologic agents, and have intractable, disabling symptoms.

TABLE 487–1. A CLASSIFICATION OF COMMON DYSTONIC STATES

- I. Primary
  - A. Hereditary
    1. Autosomal dominant trait
    2. Autosomal recessive trait
  - B. Idiopathic
- II. Secondary
  - A. Associated with other neurologic syndromes
    1. Wilson's disease
    2. Huntington's disease
    3. Hallervorden-Spatz disease
  - B. Environmental causes
    1. Perinatal cerebral injury
    2. Encephalitis
    3. Head trauma
    4. Focal cerebrovascular injury
    5. Toxins: manganese, carbon monoxide
    6. Drugs: phenothiazines, levodopa

SPASMODIC TORTICOLLIS

Spasmodic torticollis is the most common of the various forms of focal torsion dystonia. It usually begins in adulthood and remains limited to this region of the body. Occasionally there is spread to involve the vocal cords (spastic dysphonia) and one or both arms (segmental dystonia). The patient notices a pulling sensation in the neck musculature turning the chin toward one shoulder. Usually that shoulder is elevated as well. When the symptom is mild, the patient can easily straighten the neck; when severe, the head may be held in prolonged twisted postures. In some patients the head may be flexed (antecollis), extended (retrocollis), tilted, or shifted instead of rotated or twisted. These are all examples of the same disorder and carry the name of spasmodic torticollis. A concomitant head tremor is frequent. In many patients the tremor is most pronounced when the patient attempts to keep the head straight (i.e., a dystonic tremor); in others tremor persists irrespective of the position of the head, and therefore represents essential tremor that may also be present in the hands. Placing a hand on the jaw tends to provide some relief of the torticollis.

In spasmodic torticollis, multiple and bilateral neck muscles, including the sternocleidomastoids, trapezius, and scalenus muscle, are involved in the involuntary contractions. In most patients, spasmodic torticollis persists and can be painful. In addition to pharmacologic therapy (discussed above under Torsion Dystonia) sensory biofeedback therapy has had some success in patients with spasmodic torticollis. Dorsal column stimulation is sometimes helpful. Surgical section of the spinal accessory nerve produces inconsistent relief. Initial therapy should utilize anticholinergics along with other drugs, if necessary, such as diazepam and carbamazepine. Most patients improve only mildly with drug therapy.

CRANIAL DYSTONIA

Cranial dystonia (blepharospasm, Meige syndrome) is the second most common form of adult-onset focal dystonia. It usually begins with increased blinking and then worsens, and forced contractions of the orbicularis oculi eventually develop. Frequently, other muscles innervated by the facial nerve are also involved, including those around the lips. The contractions sometimes spread to involve mandibular muscles and even the tongue and neck. When the dystonia spreads to involve the jaw muscles, the "blepharospasm-plus" has been called Meige syndrome. Bright light usually aggravates the blepharospasm, and many patients wear dark glasses, even indoors. When severe, blepharospasm can result in functional blindness, preventing many activities, such as reading, driving, watching movies, and shopping. Pharmacotherapy is frequently unsuccessful. Some patients will improve with baclofen, anticholinergics, clonazepam, or antipsychotic agents. Surgical therapy, such as sectioning or making radiofrequency lesions of the branches of the facial nerve, can be helpful; regrowth of the nerve branches frequently leads to eventual return of symptoms.

Couch JR: Dystonia and tremor in spasmodic torticollis. Adv Neurol 14:245, 1976. *Report of an analysis that indicates spasmodic torticollis to be a feature of torsion dystonia and that tremor is a forme fruste of the disease in family members.*

Eldridge R, Fahn S (eds.): Dystonia. Adv Neurol Vol 14, 1976. *Summarizes the state of the art up to the date of publication.*

Fahn S: High dosage anticholinergic therapy in dystonia. Neurology 33:1255, 1983. *Reports the successful use of very high dosage of anticholinergic agents in children with dystonia.*

Jankovic J, Ford J: Blepharospasm and orofacial-cervical dystonia: Clinical and pharmacological findings in 100 patients. Ann Neurol 13:402, 1983. *A thorough review of the clinical features of blepharospasm and associated dystonic movements.*

Lal S, Hoyte K, Kiely ME, Sourkes TL, Baxter DW, Missala K, Andermann F: Neuropharmacologic investigation and treatment of spasmodic torticollis. Adv Neurol 24:335, 1979. *Study revealed that anticholinergic drugs can be effective in reducing torticollis.*

Marsden CD: Dystonia: The spectrum of the disease. *In* Yahr MD (ed.): The Basal Ganglia. New York, Raven Press, 1976, pp 351–367. *Discusses the different forms of dystonia.*

Section Six INHERITED, CONGENITAL, AND IDIOPATHIC DEGENERATIVE DISEASES OF THE NERVOUS SYSTEM

Roger N. Rosenberg

The classic eponymic neurologic diseases discussed in this section produce characteristic pathologic changes in specific nuclei and fiber tracts in brain, spinal cord, and peripheral nerve. The disorders are usually progressive and symmetrical in their pathologic and clinical expression, and many have a clear genetic basis of inheritance or suggestion of familial involvement. The disorders involve specific regions or systems of the nervous system such as cerebellar nuclei and fiber tracts or the corticospinal or extrapyramidal motor system, resulting in specific neurologic symptoms and signs referred to as system degenerations. In most of the inherited degenerative disorders to be discussed the primary impact of disease involves the neuron, changes produced in astrocytes and oligodendrocytes being presumably of a reactive and secondary nature.

488. STRIATONIGRAL DEGENERATION

Striatonigal degeneration (Joseph's disease) is a rare disease of the nervous system inherited as an autosomal dominant disorder in persons of Portuguese or Azorean ancestry. A nongenetic form of striatonigral degeneration that resembles parkinsonism also has been described.

PATHOLOGY. The major pathologic findings are a loss of neurons and glial replacement in the corpus striatum and the zona compacta portion of the substantia nigra. The thoracic spinal cord shows degeneration of the posterior and lateral fiber tracts. There is also a moderate loss of neurons in the dentate nucleus of the cerebellum and in the nucleus ruber of the midbrain.

CLINICAL MANIFESTATIONS. The disease affects adults over 25 years old. The main neurologic findings in type I disease include extremity weakness and spasticity of all extremities, especially the legs, often with associated dystonia of the face, neck, trunk, and extremities. Patellar and ankle clonus are common, as are extensor plantar responses. The gait is slow and stiff, with a slight increase in base and lurching from side to side caused by spasticity. Affected persons have no truncal titubation. Pharyngeal weakness and spasticity cause difficulty with speech and swallowing. Of note are prominent horizontal and vertical nystagmus, the loss of the fast saccadic eye movements, hypermetric and hypometric saccades, and impairment of vertical gaze. Facial fasciculations, facial myokymia, and lingual fasciculations without atrophy are common and early manifestations. Signs of cerebellar dysfunction are prominent in cases with a late-life onset.

DIAGNOSIS. Autosomal dominant striatonigral degeneration should be considered in persons with an appropriate family history developing progressive dystonia, rigidity and spasticity of pharynx, trunk, and extremities, and associated hyperreflexia, clonus, and extensor plantar responses. The entity is distinguished from Huntington's disease by the preservation of intellect.

489. MOTOR NEURON DISEASES

The term motor neuron disease refers to a group of chronic neurologic disorders that selectively affect with varying combination and rapidity the anterior horn cells of the spinal cord and lower brainstem, plus, in some cases, those large motor neurons of the cerebral cortex that give rise to the corticospinal tract. Clinically significant sensory change or cerebellar dysfunction is absent in all instances. Cases in which upper motor neuron changes are prominent in addition to muscle fasciculation, atrophy, and weakness are called *amyotrophic lateral sclerosis* (ALS). *Progressive bulbar palsy* is a variant of ALS that produces relatively rapidly advancing upper and lower motor neuron involvement of the muscles of the jaw, pharynx, and tongue. Cases lacking signs of upper motor neuron disease and producing only a slow, progressive muscle wasting and weakness often are termed *progressive muscular atrophy* (PMA). A variety of clinical subtypes of PMA occur, some of which can produce restricted motor involvement that progresses extremely slowly over a period of many years. *Werdnig-Hoffmann disease* of infancy and young children and the *Wohlfart-Kugelberg-Welander disease* of older children and adolescents represent other variants of motor neuron disease. *Primary lateral sclerosis* is a very rare condition in which the corticospinal tracts degenerate in association with some loss of cortical neurons but no impairment of anterior horn cells. The disorder produces progressive spasticity of the extremities and bulbar muscles, unaccompanied by other neurologic abnormalities. Most autopsy studies of primary lateral sclerosis have shown disseminated sclerosis, spinal cord compression, other degenerative disorders, or high spinal neoplasms, but a few examples of the true condition do exist.

AMYOTROPHIC LATERAL SCLEROSIS

Amyotrophic lateral sclerosis (ALS) can first affect bulbar muscles, a single limb, the extremities on one side of the body, the lower or upper extremities symmetrically, or all four limbs simultaneously, depending upon the individual case. The disorder occurs mainly in the fifth, sixth, and seventh decades of life and runs a progressive course lasting from two to seven years. The bulbar form runs a more malignant course. ALS usually occurs sporadically, but familial groupings have occurred, indicating either a genetic predisposition for disease or common exposure to an unknown causative agent. Familial cases tend to come on younger and progress more rapidly than do sporadic ones. Despite extensive searches to establish ALS as an autoimmune or slow virus disease, no firm leads exist, and the cause of the motor neuron diseases remains unknown.

PATHOLOGY. The neuropathologic findings in ALS consist of degenerative changes and loss of the Betz cells in layers 3 and 5 of the precentral cerebral cortex, Brodmann's areas 4 and 6. These are absent in the more benign cases of progressive muscular atrophy. Neuronal loss also occurs in the motor cranial nuclei and the motor neurons in the anterior horns of the spinal cord. There are no characteristic features associated with the neuronal loss, and the musculature innervated by the affected motor cranial nuclei and anterior horn cells undergoes neurogenic atrophy as a result of denervation.

CLINICAL MANIFESTATIONS. ALS produces a variety of clinical patterns, all of which show muscle weakness and wasting but which vary in their rate of progression, the distribution of the major weakness, and the rapidity with which signs of upper motor neuron dysfunction occur. Patients develop a slowly progressive impairment of motor function affecting distal more than proximal structures, as evidenced by muscle atrophy involving the intrinsic muscles of the hand. Over a period of six months to a year, the process results in symmetrical muscle atrophy involving the hands, forearms, and shoulder girdle muscles. The disease may develop quite asymmetrically in some patients. Prominent and early in most patients is the occurrence of fasciculations resulting from acute and widespread denervation of entire motor units. The patient may have muscle cramps, but rarely any sensory symptoms. The deep tendon reflexes are usually preserved in the upper extremities in the early phase of disease. Signs of upper motor neuron involvement may develop at any time but almost always by the time muscle involvement has lasted as long as a year. These include spasticity, particularly in the lower extremities with associated hyperreflexia, clonus, and extensor plantar responses on one or both sides. Characteristically, the superficial abdominal reflexes and the cremasteric reflexes as well as the bladder and anal sphincters remain normal. Generalized fasciculations and muscle atrophy in most instances involve the lower extremities later than the upper. These combinations of upper and lower motor neuron deficits are characteristic of ALS. Occasionally, spasticity predominantly involves the pharynx, larynx, and extremities, and signs of muscular atrophy and fasciculations are hard to detect. In such instances, EMG testing may give the answer. The loss of the gag reflex, pharyngeal paralysis, lingual atrophy and fasciculations, and diffuse extremity atrophy and fasciculations with reduced myotatic reflexes indicate a severe bulbospinal variant of ALS (progressive muscular atrophy almost always spares the cranial nerves). ALS spares the extraocular muscles. Patients may show signs of emotional lability. Intellectual functions deteriorate in approximately 5 per cent of patients. The cerebrospinal fluid is normal. Changes of muscle denervation can be confirmed by electromyography (EMG). The motor nerve conduction velocities remain normal, however, even in the presence of severe atrophy, a finding that separates this disorder from the peripheral motor neuropathies, in which conduction velocities are reduced.

DIFFERENTIAL DIAGNOSIS. Conditions to be differentiated are primary muscle disease, peripheral nerve disorders, spinal cord compression, or tumors and conditions damaging the corticospinal tracts. None of these conditions, however, fully imitates the characteristic combination of painless, diffuse neurogenic muscle impairment plus spasticity and absent sensory change that marks severe motor neuron disease. Muscle disease can be separated by changes in serum enzymes, EMG, and biopsy. Most peripheral nerve disorders produce sensory impairment. They do not cause fasciculation, and they do cause slowing of nerve electrical conduction velocity. Cervical spinal cord or ventral spinal root compression from spondylosis or tumor often causes pain, and usually produces a combination of weakness and atrophy restricted to the arms, plus spasticity and sensory changes in the legs.

Multiple sclerosis can result in spasticity, but not muscular atrophy or fasciculation, and sensory changes are usual. Intracranial disorders can produce bilateral spasticity, but other signs of brain involvement easily distinguish the condition.

TREATMENT. This must be symptomatic and supportive, as there is no specific therapy.

WERDNIG-HOFFMANN DISEASE

Werdnig-Hoffmann disease is a progressive impairment of the motor system occurring in infancy and early childhood. The lower motor neuron is exclusively involved, paralyzing musculature innervated by motor cranial nuclei and anterior horn cells of the spinal cord. Infants and young children may present with this syndrome at birth or in the first few months of life with diffuse flaccidity, muscular atrophy, muscle fasciculations, and reduced to absent myotatic reflexes with associated respiratory and swallowing difficulties. There may be prominent lingual fasciculations and atrophy in the first few months of life. A muscle biopsy indicates neurogenic atrophy, and the cerebrospinal fluid is normal. Electromyography shows acute denervation with normal peripheral nerve conduction velocities. The disorder is inherited as an autosomal recessive trait. The cause is not known.

WOHLFART-KUGELBERG-WELANDER DISEASE

Wohlfart-Kugelberg-Welander disease is an autosomal recessive disorder in which symptoms begin during late childhood, adolescence, or early adulthood and include progressive proximal muscle atrophy, weakness, and fasciculations. It is very slowly progressive and is usually compatible with a life span into the third or fourth decade. Typical examples have been described in families in which other children have Werdnig-Hoffmann disease. Thus varying penetrance of a single gene mutation inherited in an autosomal recessive manner may produce either an aggressive form of motor neuron disease in childhood (Werdnig-Hoffmann disease) or a more benign form of motor neuron disease in later childhood and early adulthood (Wohlfart-Kugelberg-Welander disease). The onset in the first and second decades of life of proximal weakness and atrophy with fasciculations but a very slow progression without evidence of upper motor neuron involvement separates this disorder from amyotrophic lateral sclerosis. The presence of denervation without the insertional irritability characteristic of polymyositis can be determined by electromyography. Both Wohlfart-Kugelberg-Welander disease and polymyositis may present with progressive proximal weakness and atrophy; if fasciculations are not prominent, electromyography and muscle biopsy are of important differentiating value. Neurogenic denervation can be identified in biopsied muscle, thus separating it from the acquired or inherited myopathies. The cause of the disorder is unknown, and specific therapy is not available.

490. SPINOCEREBELLAR DEGENERATIONS

This term applies to a group of progressive degenerative disorders in which ataxia and dysmetria resulting from predominant involvement of the cerebellum and its pathways are combined to greater or lesser degrees, with impairment of other sensory and motor systems. All represent system degenerations, and many of the specific entities have a well established genetic basis. Although clinical signs of cerebellar involvement predominate, the extension of the disorders to involve other regions of the nervous system can produce more complex neurologic symptoms. The important and common inherited spinocerebellar degenerations include (1) Friedreich's ataxia; (2) olivopontocerebellar degeneration; (3) Roussy-Lévy syndrome; (4) Bassen-Kornzweig syndrome; (5) Refsum's syndrome; (6) Marie's ataxia; and (7) dyssynergia cerebellaris myoclonica (Table 490–1).

As classified by Greenfield, the spinocerebellar degenerations can be grouped into predominant spinal forms, spinocerebellar forms, and cerebellar forms. Further subclassification exists in the olivopontocerebellar degenerations, with at least five subtypes identified by Konigsmark and Weiner with both autosomal dominant and autosomal recessive forms of inheritance. The spinocerebellar degenerations have common neuropathologic features from the peripheral nerve through the spinal

TABLE 490–1. THE COMMON INHERITED AND ACQUIRED SPINOCEREBELLAR DEGENERATIONS

Syndrome	Age of Onset	Rate of Progression	Reflexes	Sensory Change	Cerebellar Deficit	Other Important Clinical Features
			Spinal Syndromes			
Friedreich's syndrome	First decade	Slowly progressive	Absent myotatic DTRs, extensor plantar response	Moderate loss	Severe	Dysarthria, nystagmus, moderate mental retardation; arched feet; scoliosis; cardiomegaly with fibrosis; autosomal dominant or recessive or sporadic
Hereditary spastic paraplegia	First or second decade	Slowly progressive	Hyperreflexia, clonus, extensor plantar response	Minimal loss	None	Paraplegia; impaired bowel and bladder function; may occur in families with typical Friedreich's syndrome or olivopontocerebellar degeneration; autosomal dominant or recessive or sporadic
Roussy-Lévy syndrome	First or second decade	Slowly progressive	Absent myotatic DTRs, extensor plantar response	Moderate loss	Moderate	Absence of dysarthria, peroneal muscular atrophy; intermediate between Friedreich's and Charcot-Marie-Tooth diseases; autosomal dominant or recessive
			Polyneuropathy			
Charcot-Marie-Tooth disease	First or second decade	Slowly progressive	Absent	Moderate loss	None	Predominant peroneal muscle atrophy; nerves may be hypertrophic; optic-acoustic nerve involvement occurs; usually autosomal dominant
Dejerine-Sottas disease	First or second decade	Slowly progressive	Absent	Moderate loss	None	Dysarthria, nystagmus, tremor; hypertrophic nerves; scoliosis; elevated CSF protein; usually sporadic or autosomal recessive
Ataxia telangiectasia	First decade	Slowly progressive	Reduced	Minimal loss	Severe	Telangiectatic lesions involving sclerae, face, pinna, and neck; pulmonary infections; increased incidence of lymphoma; hypogamma-IgA; autosomal recessive
Bassen-Kornzweig syndrome	First decade	Slowly progressive	Absent	Moderate loss	Severe	May have mental retardation; acanthocytosis; steatorrhea; pigmentary retinal degeneration; abetalipoproteinemia; autosomal recessive
Tangier disease	First decade	Slowly progressive	Reduced	Moderate loss	None	Enlarged, yellowish-appearing tonsils; defect in high density lipoproteins; autosomal recessive
Refsum's disease	First decade	Slowly progressive	Absent	Severe loss	Severe	Nyctalopia; pigmentary retinal degeneration; ichthyosis; cardiac conduction defects; deafness, elevated serum phytanate; defect in lipid alpha oxidase activity; autosomal recessive
			Cerebellar Syndromes			
Olivopontocerebellar degeneration	Third to fifth decade	Slowly progressive	Hyperreflexia, clonus, extensor plantar response	Moderate loss	Severe	Late development of optic atrophy and muscle atrophy; may develop a moderate dementia; CT scans show pontine and cerebellar atrophy; may be autosomal dominant or recessive
Carcinomatous cerebellar degeneration	Adult	Less than 10 years	Reduced	Moderate loss	Truncal	Truncal greater than extremity ataxia; dysarthria and nystagmus minimal; lung carcinoma most common association
Alcoholic cerebellar degeneration	Adult	Slowly progressive	Reduced	Moderate	Lower extremities and trunk	Lower extremities affected more than upper; dysarthria and nystagmus minimal; peripheral neuropathy present
Dyssynergia cerebellaris of Ramsay Hunt	Adult	Slowly progressive	Reduced	Normal	Moderate	Induced myoclonic jerks with intention; generalized seizures; sporadic

TABLE 490–2. BIOCHEMICAL DEFECTS IN THE INHERITED ATAXIAS

Associated Biochemical Defect	Clinical Type	Age of Onset	Clinical Features
		Lipid Disorders	
Autosomal recessive			
1. Storage of phytanate due to defect in alpha oxidase	Refsum's disease	20–30 years	Ataxia; retinitis pigmentosa; deafness; ichthyosis; cardiac arrhythmia; polyneuropathy
2. Abetalipoproteinemia	Bassen-Kornzweig syndrome	5–10 years	Ataxia; acanthocytosis; retinitis pigmentosa; polyneuropathy; malabsorption of fat
3. Arylsulfatase A deficiency	Juvenile onset metachromatic leukodystrophy	5–20 years	Ataxia; mild mental retardation; polyneuropathy
4. Storage of G-M2 ganglioside due to hexosaminidase A deficiency, alpha locus type	Juvenile onset atypical spinocerebellar ataxia	3 years	Progressive ataxia, spasticity, dysarthria; muscle atrophy; pes cavus; dystonic features; normal intelligence
5. Storage of G-M2 ganglioside due to hexosaminidase A deficiency, beta locus type	Juvenile onset atypical ataxia with cherry-red spots	2 years	Progressive ataxia and intention tremor; macular cherry-red spots
6. Partial deficiency of hexosaminidase A and B	Adult onset spinocerebellar degeneration	20 years	Gait and limb ataxia; head titubation; dysarthria; tremor; grimacing; chorea
X-linked recessive			
1. Storage of long chain (C24-30) fatty acids	Adrenoleukomyelo-neuropathy (Nixon-Blaw disease)	5–20 years	Cortical blindness and spasticity; skin pigmentation; childhood onset of adrenal cortical insufficiency; adult onset with ataxia and polyneuropathy
		Carbohydrate Disorders	
Autosomal recessive			
1. Pyruvate carboxylase or pyruvate dehydrogenase deficiencies or inhibitor of thiamin triphosphate formation in brain (inhibitor of thiamin pyrophosphate–ATP phosphotransferase)	Leigh's disease (subacute necrotizing encephalopathy)	Birth–5 years; rare adult form	Acute episodic extraocular muscle palsies; optic atrophy; hypotonia; ataxia; mental retardation; somnolence; hyperreflexia; extensor plantar responses; elevated serum pyruvate and lactate
2. Mitochondrial malic enzyme	Friedreich's ataxia	5–15 years	Progressive gait and limb ataxia; dysarthria; nystagmus; areflexia; extensor plantar reflex; distal sensory loss
3. Oxidative metabolism with elevated serum lactate and pyruvate	Adult onset neuromyopathy with ataxia—Kearns-Sayre syndrome	20–50 years	Retinitis pigmentosa; neuromyopathy; ophthalmoplegia; ataxia; cardiac arrhythmias; muscle biopsy shows ragged red fibers
		Disorders of Amino Acid Metabolism	
Autosomal recessive			
1. Deficiency in branched chain keto acid decarboxylase	Maple syrup urine disease and variants	Birth–5 years	Mental retardation; seizures; failure to thrive; irritability; anorexia; ataxia; maple syrup odor to urine; excretion of branched chain amino acids and keto acids
2. Hyperglycinemia	Spastic paraparesis with muscular atrophy and arm dysmetria	2–10 years	Spastic paraparesis; peroneal muscle atrophy; distal sensory loss; pes cavus; optic atrophy; arm dysmetria
3. 5-Oxoprolinuria due to deficiency of glutathione synthetase	Ataxia and defect in gammaglutamyl cycle (I) (reduced glutathione synthesis)	10 years	Progressive mental retardation; spasticity; limb and gait ataxia; tremor; hemolytic anemia with intermittent jaundice
4. Generalized aminoaciduria due to deficiency of gamma-glutamylcysteine synthetase	Ataxia and defect in gamma-glutamyl cycle (II) (reduced glutathione synthesis)	20 years	Hemolytic anemia; areflexia; gait and limb ataxia; distal sensory loss; staccato speech; acute psychosis
5. Defect in tryptophan absorption from gut; aminoaciduria	Hartnup disease	5–25 years	Intermittent ataxia; episodic, pellagra-like skin rash; progressive mental retardation; spasticity; choreoathetosis
6. Deficiency in glutamate dehydrogenase	Olivopontocerebellar degeneration	20–40 years	Progressive gait and limb ataxia; spasticity; mild extrapyramidal features; late distal amyotrophy and sensory loss; rare mental changes
		Disorder of Urea Cycle Metabolism	
Autosomal recessive			
1. Argininosuccinate synthetase deficiency	Citrullinemia, subacute type	Infancy	Vomiting; somnolence; tremor; ataxia; seizures; delay in mental and physical development; hyperammonemia
		Disorder of Immunologic Function	
Autosomal recessive			
1. Reduced serum immunoglobulins (IgA, IgG, and IgM); lymphopenia	Ataxia telangiectasia (Louis-Barr syndrome)	5–12 years	Telangiectasia of face and sclerae; Friedreich's phenotype with ataxia; dysarthria; areflexia; extensor plantar responses; oculomotor apraxia
		Disorder of Protein Metabolism (Increased Amounts of Glial Proteins)	
Autosomal dominant			
1. Increased glial acidic filamentous protein and a complex of 40,000 mw proteins in cerebellum and basal ganglia seen on 2-D gels	Joseph's disease	20–65 years	Gait ataxia often with either corticospinal and extrapyramidal findings or late onset polyneuropathy

cord and up to the cerebellum with its attendant connections. Although these disorders are well described both clinically and pathologically, only in Friedreich's syndrome, Refsum's disease, and the Bassen-Kornzweig syndrome do molecular insights exist into the cause. The similarity of neuropathologic findings in the Bassen-Kornzweig syndrome and Friedreich's syndrome despite very different molecular defects indicates the vulnerability of the spinocerebellar system to different chemical abnormalities as well as its limited neuropathologic response. A survey of biochemical defects in the inherited ataxias is presented in Table 490–2.

FRIEDREICH'S ATAXIA

This commonest form of spinocerebellar degeneration begins in childhood and is inherited mainly as an autosomal recessive or dominant disorder. Sporadic cases presumably represent "spontaneous" examples of the recessive trait. Friedreich's ataxia comprises a syndrome including several subtypes with common clinical features and pathologic changes. Established or possible causes (Table 490–2) include several inborn errors of metabolism, including disorders of lipids, diseases of oxidative metabolism, aminoacidurias, and the partial deficiency of serum immunoglobulin levels.

Blass et al. have described children in whom pyruvate oxidation was low in muscles from 4 of 7 patients with Friedreich's syndrome, in 4 of 12 patients with other ataxias, and in 8 of 19 patients with familial or idiopathic neuropathies. In those studies the degree of pyruvate dehydrogenase complex activity correlated with the severity and rapidity of the spinocerebellar disease process. For example, patients with less than 15 per cent of normal pyruvate dehydrogenase activity but with normal oxoglutarate dehydrogenase generally had severe neurologic disease and lactic acidosis beginning in infancy. Severe deficiencies of both complexes have been described in one infant with severe disease. Several patients with 20 to 30 per cent of normal pyruvate dehydrogenase activity had a milder illness in which ataxia was the most prominent sign. The patients with Friedreich's syndrome had the mildest defect, with 40 to 50 per cent of normal pyruvate dehydrogenase activity together with 50 per cent of normal oxoglutarate dehydrogenase activity. Most recently, Stumpf et al. have reported a marked reduction in activity in fibroblast cultures of the mitochondrial malic enzyme. Despite these biochemical abnormalities in some patients, in the vast majority of typical Friedreich's ataxia patients no biochemical abnormality is found.

PATHOLOGY. Demyelination with secondary gliosis affects the spinocerebellar tracts, the lateral corticospinal tracts, the posterior columns, and the peripheral nerves. Neuronal loss involves the primary sensory neurons in dorsal root ganglia as well as the cells of Clarke's column which give rise to the spinocerebellar tracts. Less often, neuronal loss affects the anterior horns of the spinal cord and cell layers in the cerebellar cortex and deep cerebellar nuclei. A diffuse and major loss of myocardial fibers with subsequent replacement by fibrosis may occur in some patients.

CLINICAL MANIFESTATIONS. Midline ataxia appears first with impairment of gait, poor coordination, and frequent falling. Gait problems may be the only sign of disease for many years, but eventually dysarthria and ataxia of arm and hand emerge. By the midpart to end of the second decade of life most patients require assistance in walking. Nystagmus is an early and prominent feature, as is the loss of fast saccadic eye movements. A few patients develop optic atrophy during the later stages of the disease. Progressive skeletal deformities include kyphoscoliosis, pes cavus, and, less consistently, a deformed and high arched palate. Distal sensory deficits, especially in the legs, develop after several years and include impairment in position sense and vibratory sensation as well as, less prominently, a reduction in pain and temperature perceptions. Additional expressions of motor dysfunction include extensor plantar responses with normal or reduced tone in trunk and extremities and absent deep tendon reflexes. Moderate weakness and the occurrence of atrophy of the extremities and occasional fasciculations are late developments. About half the patients develop cardiomegaly, murmurs, bundle branch block, T wave inversions, and complete heart block on electrocardiograms. Cardiopulmonary arrest and congestive heart failure may occur. A small percentage of patients are mentally retarded and few reach high intelligence.

DIAGNOSIS. The presence in childhood or young adolescence of insidiously beginning and slowly progressing truncal and extremity ataxia, with dysarthria and subsequent nystagmus, extensor plantar responses, and areflexia, is typical. When one adds the findings of scoliosis, pes cavus, and proprioceptive and vibratory loss in the lower extremities, hardly any other diagnosis is possible. Motor nerve conduction velocities are normal in the common neurogenic form of the disorder, but electromyography may detect denervation potentials, especially in the legs. In the hypertrophic neuropathic form of ataxia, the motor nerve conduction velocities are slowed and the peripheral nerves may be palpably enlarged with demyelination noted in peripheral nerve biopsies. The cerebrospinal fluid protein is normal. Muscle biopsies often show neurogenic atrophy but are unnecessary for diagnosis. The electrocardiogram may contain abnormalities as recorded above and the chest roentgenogram may show cardiomegaly.

DIFFERENTIAL DIAGNOSIS. Diagnosis of Friedreich's syndrome is not difficult if the case meets the aforementioned criteria. Multiple sclerosis and subacute combined degeneration of the spinal cord caused by vitamin B_{12} deficiency differ in both age of onset and clinical characteristics. Cerebellar or spinal tumors produce a more rapid course and, usually, pain. The *Roussy-Lévy syndrome,* which may not be a distinct disorder, is recognized by most authorities as having an autosomal dominant pattern. The onset occurs in childhood with ataxia, areflexia, pes cavus–clubfoot deformity, and kyphoscoliosis. It differs from Friedreich's ataxia in sparing position and vibratory sensation and by the absence of extensor plantar responses as well as of nystagmus and dysarthria. Patients with *Refsum's disease* caused by elevated serum phytanate as a result of a defect in lipid alpha-oxidase suffer the additional defects of optic atrophy, pigmentary retinal degeneration, ichthyosis, and deafness. Patients with the *Bassen-Kornzweig syndrome* have spinocerebellar signs but also prominent steatorrhea, abetalipoproteinemia, and acanthocytosis of the red blood cells.

Hereditary spastic paraplegia expresses an autosomal dominant, recessive, or sex-linked recessive trait by the occurrence of peroneal muscular atrophy, skeletal deformities, nystagmus, and prominent spastic paraplegia. The syndrome overlaps with other forms of spinocerebellar degeneration in some families.

OLIVOPONTOCEREBELLAR DEGENERATIONS

The olivopontocerebellar atrophies represent a group of adult-onset disorders manifested clinically by progressive involvement of cerebellar functions and pathologically by a reduction in neurons in the inferior olivary nuclei of the medulla, the basis pontis, the cerebellar cortex, and the deep cerebellar nuclei. Closely related are at least some examples of autonomic insufficiency of the Shy-Drager type (Ch. 478).

PATHOLOGY. Grossly, atrophy involves the cerebellum, cerebellar peduncles, and basis pontis. Microscopically, Purkinje cells, granule cells of the cerebellar cortex, and neurons from the dentate nucleus and other deep cerebellar nuclei all are severely reduced.

CLINICAL MANIFESTATIONS. Olivopontocerebellar atrophy has several variants whose principal clinical manifestations vary with the phenotype. Sporadically arising cases outnumber those with abnormal familial histories, but the pathologic changes are similar. Essential features include the development in mid-adult life of progressive ataxia, dysarthria, dysmetria, dysdiadochokinesia, nystagmus, and loss of fast saccadic eye movements. Subsequently, patients develop spasticity, optic nerve atrophy, distal sensory involvement, and late intellectual dysfunction.

In general, truncal ataxia develops initially in the second or third decades of life, and extremity ataxia and dysmetria and prominent dysarthria follow within a decade. After several years, perhaps a third of affected patients show spasticity with associated hyperreflexia, clonus, and extensor plantar responses. Nystagmus, optic nerve atrophy, and loss of fast saccadic eye movements occur frequently. A small fraction of patients display the late occurrence of muscle atrophy with fasciculations, including the facial muscles, muscles of mastication, and lingual musculature. Palatal myoclonus is an uncommon but almost pathognomonic accompaniment when it occurs. Variations in the illness include sensory deficits in a distal distribution, intellectual deterioration, signs of extrapyramidal dysfunction, external ophthalmoplegia, and early visual loss.

The olivopontocerebellar degenerations described by Holmes, Sanger-Brown, and Marie represent phenotypic variants of this general class of disease. The syndrome of *Ramsay Hunt's* dyssynergia cerebellaris myoclonica is perhaps a rare variant beginning in childhood and includes prominent, progressive ataxia and myoclonic seizures inherited as an autosomal dominant trait.

DIAGNOSIS. The olivopontocerebellar atrophies are characterized by the development early in adult life of progressive symmetrical involvement of cerebellar functions, followed in many instances by progressive and symmetrical development of spasticity in the legs. Abnormalities of eye movement, intellectual impairment, and muscle atrophy with distal sensory loss complete the clinical picture, sometimes with the addition of palatal myoclonus. Computed tomography demonstrates cerebellar atrophy, pontine atrophy, and, late in the disease, cerebral atrophy and large lateral ventricles. Motor nerve conduction velocities may be slow, and muscle denervation may be detected by electromyography. The cerebrospinal fluid is normal. Neither specific diagnostic laboratory tests nor specific treatments exist for most patients. A few patients with recessively inherited disease have had a moderate reduction in leukocyte glutamate dehydrogenase activity, as reported by Plaitakis et al. Progressive cerebellar deficits, which include truncal ataxia, nystagmus, and dysarthria, are also produced as a result of chronic malnutrition and as a remote effect of cancer, and these possibilities must be considered when a family history of cerebellar disease is lacking.

491. SYRINGOMYELIA

Syringomyelia is derived from the Greek word syrinx, which means tube, and refers to the occurrence of a cavity within the spinal cord. Such cavities usually are located in the central region at the cervical level; they often extend into the medulla (syringobulbia) and may extend inferiorly into the thoracic and lumbosacral regions of the cord. Most instances of syringomyelia occur in association with acquired spinal congenital malformations or with spinal intramedullary neoplasms, of which perhaps 25 per cent produce an associated syrinx.

PATHOLOGY. The syringomyelic cavity is usually associated with the central canal of the spinal cord but may be independent of it as well. The cavity may extend over many segments of the cervical cord and may be in direct anatomic communication with the fourth ventricle. The term hydromyelia is often used to describe those cavitary lesions of the spinal cord which do communicate with the fourth ventricle. The syringomyelic cavity dissects into and progressively replaces the gray matter of the posterior and anterior horns of the spinal cord, as well as disturbing the decussating spinothalamic pain-carrying fibers in the anterior commissure. The cavity wall is maintained by astrocytic glial and fibroblastic membranes and blood vessels. Most often, syringomyelia is associated with other congenital malformations at the cranial cervical junction, including the Arnold-Chiari malformation with herniation of the cerebellar tonsils, fusion of the cervical vertebrae (Klippel-Feil syndrome), or malformations at the lumbosacral region, including spina bifida and associated meningomyelocele. Hydrocephalus resulting from cranial cervical malformations or stenosis of the aqueduct of Sylvius occurs in some patients.

CLINICAL MANIFESTATIONS. Symptoms of syringomyelia most often begin in the second or third decade with a typically "dissociated," selective impairment in pain and temperature sensation with the preservation of the sense of touch. Earliest detected sensory changes are usually in the hands, but examination commonly discloses a similar loss in the neck, shoulders, upper chest, and back. Sensory loss is accompanied by progressive atrophy of the musculature in the upper extremities with skeletal malformations, principally kyphoscoliosis. Progressive analgesia results in severe painless ulcers, burns, and Charcot joints. Atrophy of arm, forearm, and intrinsic hand musculature, fasciculations, and areflexia develop progressively. Later upper motor neuron signs arise in the legs owing to encroachment of the syringomyelic cavity into the lateral columns of the cord. Late involvement of vibratory and position sensations in the lower extremities and an associated Romberg sign indicate that the syrinx is extending into the posterior columns of the spinal cord. A preganglionic Horner syndrome may develop owing to dissection of the syrinx into the intermediolateral cell column of the lower cervical and first thoracic segment of the spinal cord containing sympathetic neurons. The kyphoscoliosis that sometimes heralds the disease results from the asymmetrical denervation and atrophy of paravertebral muscles. The disease process is progressive, usually symmetrical, and clearly evident in adult life.

Syringobulbia refers to the development of the syringomyelic cavity into the medulla with resultant destruction of the medullary structures in the lateral tegmentum. Dissociated impairment of pain and temperature over the face, nystagmus, pharyngeal and vocal cord paralysis, and lingual atrophy are most typical. Syringobulbia is always associated with syringomyelia and is not a separate process.

DIAGNOSIS. Lepromatous neuropathy, certain rare congenital and acquired peripheral neuropathies, and intramedullary destructive lesions of the spinal cord and brainstem are the only conditions causing insidiously developing and progressive, widespread, dissociated loss of pain and temperature sensation. Leprosy can be considered if the subject has grown up in an endemic area, but neither it nor other peripheral neuropathies produce signs of spinal cord involvement. When the dissociated sensory loss is coupled with signs of long tract disease in the lower extremities or is decidedly asymmetrical in distribution and dermatomal in pattern, the differential consideration lies between congenital syrinx and intramedullary neoplasm. Pain is more frequent with tumors. Myelography, CT, or NMR imaging usually can make the distinction.

TREATMENT. Treatment generally is unsatisfactory. Surgical decompression of the distended syrinx by a laminectomy and drainage of the cavity has been claimed to slow the disease progression. Some surgeons state that the placement of muscle tissue at the junction of the fourth ventricle and the upper cervical canal with or without a ventriculocardiac shunt has stabilized the neurologic status of patients. Syrinx associated with spinal tumor is treated by treating the tumor appropriately.

492. THE PHAKOMATOSES OR NEUROCUTANEOUS SYNDROMES

NEUROFIBROMATOSIS (Von Recklinghausen's Disease)

Von Recklinghausen's disease or neurofibromatosis is a genetic disorder inherited as an autosomal dominant trait and characterized by the occurrence of pigmented skin lesions, multiple tumors of spinal or cranial nerves, tumors of the skin, and the associated occurrence of gliomas and intracranial meningiomas. There is an increased association with pheochromocytomas, cystic lung disease, renal vascular lesions causing hypertension, fibrous dysplasia of bone, gastrointestinal neurofibromas with chronic blood loss, and medullary thyroid carcinoma and other tumors of endocrine glands.

PATHOLOGY. The characteristic feature of the disease is the occurrence of multiple "neurofibromas" associated with nerves in their peripheral, intraspinal, or intracranial segments. Electron microscopic studies indicate that these tumors represent proliferation of fibroblasts or neurilemmal sheath cells (Schwann cells) in peripheral nerve. The tumors may become confluent in the region of the brachial or sacral plexus and produce large plexiform neuromas which can evolve into malignant sarcomas. Intracranial astrocytomas, ependymomas, glioblastomas, and meningiomas are also encountered with increased frequency, as are optic nerve gliomas in childhood. Stenosis of the aqueduct of Sylvius with noncommunicating hydrocephalus is also observed in this disease. The skin manifestations include pedunculated polyps, lightly colored pigmented lesions with sharp edges (referred to as café au lait spots), and depigmented lesions. Neoplasms of endocrine organs, including medullary thyroid carcinomas and pheochromocytoma with associated hypertension, have been reported in a number of patients.

Replacement of normal bone with fibroblasts and fibrocytes in a pattern similar to that of fibrous dysplasia in some patients results in overgrowth of bone with the occluding of cranial foramina and rarefaction and cyst formation. The congenital absence of a portion of the sphenoid bone resulting in pulsating exophthalmos, congenital vertebral anomalies, bone cysts, pseudoarthrosis of the tibia, local gigantism of an extremity, and scoliosis all can be encountered. Histologic abnormalities of the cerebral cortex, ectopic islands of gray matter, and focal gliosis are described and may be the basis for the increased incidence of mental retardation.

Zelkowitz et al. reported on what may be the primary basis for loss of cell contact inhibition and thus benign tumor formation. In careful studies reduced epidermal growth factor binding sites on the surface of neurofibromatosis fibroblasts were documented and may be a useful assay for genetic counseling purposes.

CLINICAL MANIFESTATIONS. Neurofibromatosis can present in a variety of ways, but the presence of multiple cutaneous neurofibromas and café au lait pigmented skin lesions represents the hallmarks.The pigmented skin lesions occur most commonly over the trunk and in the axilla. If greater than 1.5 cm in diameter and more than six in number they indicate neurofibromatosis. Nerve involvement can be solitary, involving individual nerves of the extremities, or multiple and diffuse. Multiple cranial nerves are affected as well, resulting in facial weakness, facial numbness, deafness, and visual loss with optic nerve atrophy. Multiple confluent tumors and fibrosis of the affected parts result in elephantiasis neuromatosa. A marked increase in the proliferation and overgrowth of skin and subcutaneous tissues of the skull, neck, and trunk can result in gross asymmetrical hypertrophy. Neurofibromas associated with the nerve root can invade the intervertebral foramen and result in compression of spinal cord or brainstem. Large neurofibromas of a cranial nerve can produce increased intracranial pressure resulting from hydrocephalus. Some such lesions present as a cerebellopontine angle mass lesion with ipsilateral cerebellar signs. The fifth, seventh, eighth, and tenth cranial nerves are commonly involved with neurofibromas, producing facial muscle weakness, facial numbness, weakness and atrophy of the muscles of mastication, deafness, and vertigo. Rarely, spontaneous fractures of vertebrae or long bones result because of fibrodysplasia or cystic bone formation.

The cerebrospinal fluid protein is elevated in patients having large tumors that result in cord compression. Roentgenograms of the skull and internal auditory meatus show erosion caused by adjacent tumors.

DIAGNOSIS. Neurofibromatosis is diagnosed readily by the occurrence of the characteristic neurofibromas and skin pigmented lesions. The tumors are often multiple and vary considerably in size. Most tumors are smooth, soft, and multilobulated, and can be palpated along the course of a peripheral nerve. Hypertensive patients must be evaluated for the possibility of renal artery stenosis as well as for pheochromocytoma with urinary determinations of catecholamines. Cranial nerve palsies and hydrocephalus signal the presence of an intracranial neoplasm and the need for CT brain scans or angiography for precise definition. Cerebellopontine angle meningiomas and cranial nerve or spinal nerve tumors are usually resectable and must be considered in patients manifesting progressive brainstem or spinal cord deficits. There is no treatment for neurofibromatosis other than resection of symptomatic tumors and decompression of hydrocephalus.

TUBEROUS SCLEROSIS (Bourneville's Disease)

Tuberous sclerosis (Bourneville's disease or epiloia) is a neurocutaneous disorder inherited as an autosomal dominant trait. Its triad of findings includes facial nevi (adenoma sebaceum), epilepsy, and mental retardation.

PATHOLOGY. The gross brain has many firm nodules on the surface and in the deep layers of the cortex, the underlying white matter, the basal ganglia, spinal cord, brainstem, and cerebellum. They line the lateral ventricles as projections referred to as "candle gutterings." The histologic appearance of the nodules shows a proliferation of primitive glia with multinucleated giant cells. Vascular malformations, meningiomas, gliomas, and hamartomas of the brain also occur.

The cutaneous lesions include characteristic facial "nevi" that take their origin from terminal nerves in the subcutaneous region of the skin and include a hyperplasia of connective tissue and blood vessels. Funduscopic examination can disclose similar nodules or phakomas consisting of glial elements, fibroblasts, and ganglion cells arising from the retina. Rarely an optic nerve glioma develops. Rhabdomyomas of the heart can occur, as can renal tumors and neoplasms of endocrine organs, including testis, pancreas, ovary, and thyroid.

CLINICAL MANIFESTATIONS. The clinical appearance is characteristic. Patients develop mental retardation and epilepsy during the first decade of life. The occurrence of mental retardation is evident by six years of age. Several years after the development of seizures the characteristic cutaneous facial lesions first develop in a symmetrical distribution on the malar and nasal regions and appear to be yellow or orange-red, varying in size from several millimeters to 1 cm. The occurrence of areas of roughening of the skin (shagreen patches) in the shape of small spheres caused by fibrous hyperplasia, café au lait spots, areas of depigmented nevi, and, rarely, subungual neurofibromas are characteristic of tuberous sclerosis and link it genetically to von Recklinghausen's neurofibromatosis. The concurrent neoplasms in other organs rarely cause clinical complications. Papilledema and other focal neurologic deficits signal the occurrence of a large intracranial tumor.

STURGE-WEBER DISEASE

Sturge-Weber disease produces a port wine–colored capillary hemangioma on the face, accompanied by a similar vascular malformation of the underlying meninges and cerebral cortex. The cause is unknown. No clear evidence of a hereditary cause has been established.

PATHOLOGY. The cutaneous hemangioma follows the distribution of one or more divisions of the trigeminal nerve. The underlying meninges contain a similar vascular lesion, and the capillaries of the cortex may show thickening and calcification, especially in the second and third cortical layers. The cerebral cortex may undergo atrophy with loss of nerve cells and a proliferation of glia. Cerebral calcification clearly outlines the cortical mantle in an undulating manner.

CLINICAL MANIFESTATIONS. The presence of a port wine facial nevus following the sensory dermatomal distribution of the first, second, or third portions of the trigeminal nerve is diagnostic. Generalized or focal motor seizures may occur with or without associated mental retardation. Affected patients can develop hemiplegic atrophy with shortening of the extremities contralateral to the calcified atrophic hemisphere. Exophthalmos, glaucoma, buphthalmos, optic atrophy, and other cutaneous port wine nevi and retinal angiomas can be present. There is no specific treatment; seizures are managed with anticonvulsant drugs. The stain deserves cosmetic repair, if possible.

HIPPEL-LINDAU DISEASE

Hippel-Lindau disease is a familial disorder inherited in a simple autosomal pattern producing hemangioblastomas of the cerebellar hemispheres with associated angiomas of the retina and cystic change in the kidney and pancreas. It presents in the fourth to sixth decades of life, usually not associated with cutaneous vascular lesions. The disorder can present with signs of cerebellar mass lesion, cerebellar hemorrhage, brainstem vascular malformations, or hemangioma of the retina. A clinical association with pheochromocytomas and polycythemia has been noted, especially in the patients with cerebellar hemangioblastomas. The diagnosis should be suspected in any patient with cerebellar brain tumor or cerebellar hemorrhage, especially in association with an elevated hematocrit. Diagnosis and treatment are as for other such mass lesions.

ATAXIA TELANGIECTASIA

Ataxia telangiectasia is a neurocutaneous disorder that begins in the first decade of life with prominent telangiectatic lesions involving the bulbar conjunctivae, malar eminences, ear lobes, and occasionally upper neck regions, associated with cerebellar ataxia and nystagmus. The condition is an autosomal recessive disorder. A chromosome translocation involving chromosome 14, increased chromosome breakage, and reduced lymphocyte response to phytohemagglutinin have been described and represent the only molecular clues to the pathogenesis.

PATHOLOGY. Neuropathologic changes include loss of Purkinje, granule, and basket cells in the cerebellar cortex as well as of neurons in the deep nuclei of the cerebellum. Neuronal loss is also present in the inferior olives of the medulla. The posterior columns of the spinal cord undergo demyelination, and there is a loss of anterior horn cells in the spinal cord and ganglion cells of the spinal ganglia. The most consistent defect of the lymphoid system is a poorly developed or absent thymus.

CLINICAL MANIFESTATIONS. The onset of the telangiectatic lesions occurs in the first decade of life and is associated with progressive deficits in cerebellar functions with early onset nystagmus. Truncal ataxia, extremity ataxia, dysarthria, extensor plantar responses, myoclonic jerks, areflexia, and distal sensory deficits occur in a pattern somewhat resembling that of Friedreich's syndrome. The patients have a high incidence of recurrent pulmonary infections and neoplasms of the lymphoreticuloendothelial system.

DIAGNOSIS. Ataxia telangiectasia is diagnosed by the characteristic telangiectatic lesions in association with a truncal ataxia, other cerebellar deficits, and abnormal eye movements. Serum protein electrophoresis documents a deficiency of gamma globulins, especially IgA and IgE. Cellular immune abnormalities include lymphocytopenia, a reduced response to skin test antigens, and lack of sensitization to dinitrochlorobenzene (DNCB).

Barnett HJM, Foster JB, Hudgson P: Syringomyelia. London, W. B. Saunders Company, 1974. *Comprehensive review of clinical manifestations, neuropathology, and treatment. A classic book.*

Blass JP, Kark RAP, Menon NK: Low activities of the pyruvate and oxoglutarate dehydrogenase complexes in five patients with Friedreich's ataxia. N Engl J Med 295:62, 1976. *Description of a new biochemical defect in patients with Friedreich's ataxia. First clear correlation between clinical syndrome and a defined enzyme defect.*

Brady RO: Inherited metabolic diseases of the nervous system. Science 193:733, 1976. *Excellent, comprehensive metabolic and biochemical review of genetic diseases of the nervous system.*

Crowe FW, Schull WJ, Neel JV: A Clinical Pathological and Genetic Study of Multiple Neurofibromatosis. Springfield, Ill., Charles C Thomas, 1956. *Classic clinical and neuropathologic study of the variations encountered in dominantly inherited neurofibromatosis.*

Gilman S, Bloedel J, Lechtenberg R: Disorders of the Cerebellum. Philadelphia, F. A. Davis Company, 1981. *Comprehensive book describing physiology and clinical syndromes of the cerebellum.*

Greenfield JG: The Spinocerebellar Degenerations. Springfield, Ill., Charles C Thomas, 1954. *Definitive review of the inherited and noninherited syndromes producing degeneration of the cerebellum and its pathways.*

Horton WA, Eldridge R, Brody J: Familial motor neuron disease. Neurology 26:460, 1976. *Description of genetic patterns in motor neuron disease.*

Konigsmark BW, Weiner LP: The olivopontocerebellar atrophies. Medicine 49:227, 1970. *Classic paper classifying and describing dominantly and recessively inherited degeneration of the cerebellum and its pathways.*

McFarlin PE, Strober W, Waldmann TA: Ataxia telangiectasia. Medicine 51:281, 1972. *Detailed comprehensive review of ataxia telangiectasia.Clinical and neuropathologic features are emphasized. A good background in clinical immunology is required.*

Plaitakis A, Berl S, Yahr M: Neurological disorders associated with deficiency of glutamate dehydrogenase. Ann Neurol 15:144, 1984. *Twelve of 88 tested patients with degenerative diseases producing basal ganglia or cerebellar abnormalities had 48 per cent reduction of GDH when compared with controls.*

Refsum S: Heredopathia atactica polyneuritiformis: Phytanic acid storage disease (Refsum's disease). *In* Vinken PJ, Bruyn GW (eds.): Handbook of Clinical Neurology, Chap 10, Vol 21, Part I. Amsterdam, North Holland Publishing Company, 1975, pp 181, 229. *Authoritative description of patients with Refsum's disease, including clinical, neuropathologic, and biochemical data.*

Rosenberg RN: Biochemical genetics of neurologic disease. N Engl J Med 305:1181, 1981. *Review of specific biochemical or molecular defects in inherited neurologic diseases.*

Rosenberg RN: Dominant ataxias. *In* Kety S, Rowland L, Sidman R, Matthysse S (eds.): Genetics of Neurological and Psychiatric Disorders. New York, Raven Press, 1983. *Review of clinical and basic science mechanisms in the dominant ataxias.*

Rowland LP (ed.): Human Motor Neuron Diseases. New York, Raven Press, 1982. *A good multiauthored review of the topic.*

Schwartz JF, Rowland LP, Eder H, Marks PA, Osserman EF, Hirschberg E, Anderson H: Bassen-Kornzweig syndrome. Deficiency of serum beta-lipoprotein. Arch Neurol 8:438, 1963. *Classic description of the clinical, neuropathologic, and biochemical abnormalities in Bassen-Kornzweig syndrome.*

Stumpf D, Parks J, Eguren L, Haas R: Friedreich ataxia: III. Mitochondrial malic enzyme deficiency. Neurology 32:221, 1982. *A new biochemical finding in the Friedreich syndrome.*

Zelkowitz M, Edmiston K, Stambouly J: Reduced epidermal growth factor binding sites in neurofibromatosis fibroblasts. Neurology 30:374, 1980. *New finding of epidermal growth factor binding sites as an explanation for altered tissue growth in neurofibromatosis.*

Section Seven CEREBROVASCULAR DISEASES

H. J. M. Barnett

493. INTRODUCTION

Vascular stroke represents the most common devastating disease affecting the central nervous system. In developed countries it is the third leading cause of death, ranking behind heart disease and cancer. Among white populations in the U.S. and Canada the annual incidence rate is between 1 and 2 per 1000, the death rate is between 0.5 and 1 per 1000, and the prevalence is between 4 and 6 per 1000. Blacks have an increased incidence. Encouragingly, in both North America and Western Europe the incidence of stroke is declining at a rate approaching 5 per cent per year, a change attributed to the improved control of hypertension and rheumatic fever.

Vascular stroke occurs as a result of two major causes: *ischemia* and *hemorrhage*.

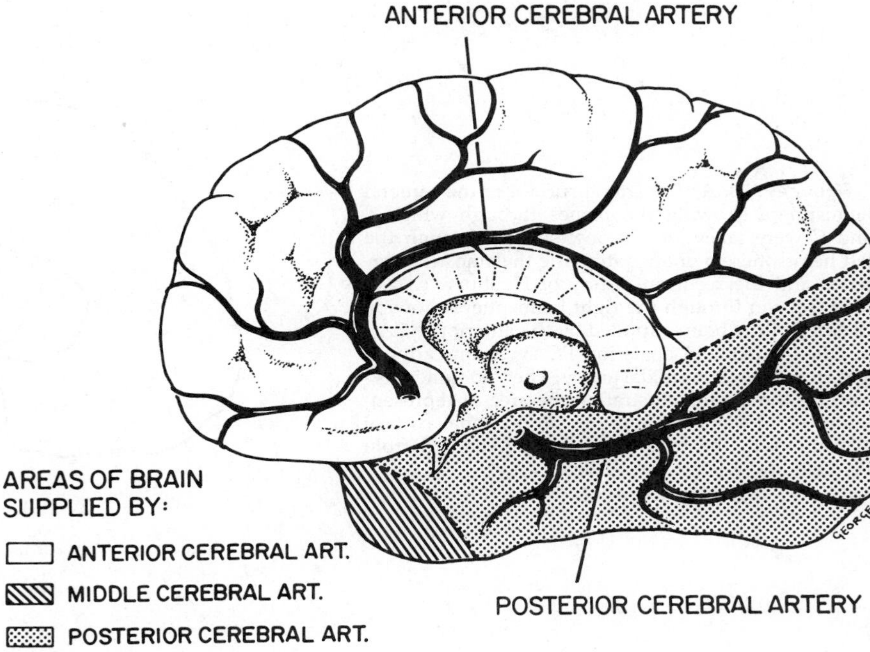

Figure 493–1. The medial surface of the cerebral hemisphere, showing the course of the anterior and posterior cerebral arteries and the medial area of brain supplied by them and the small area of medial supply of the middle cerebral artery.

ANATOMY AND SUPPLY OF THE MAJOR CEREBRAL ARTERIES

Interference with the blood supply to the brain by occlusion and stenosis, and to some degree as a consequence of arterial rupture, produces neurologic syndromes related to arterial territories rather than to specific neuroanatomic and physiologic systems. The interpretation of vascular syndromes is based on a working knowledge of these arterial territories.

Four large arteries supply the brain, the two common carotid and the two vertebral arteries. The left common carotid artery arises from the aortic arch and the right from the innominate artery in the upper thorax. The two vertebral arteries originate from the right and left subclavian arteries respectively. Each common carotid artery bifurcates in the neck at the level of the upper border of the thyroid cartilage forming the internal and external carotid arteries. No branches arise in the extracranial course of the internal carotid artery. Each internal carotid artery enters the skull through the ipsilateral foramen lacerum, passes through the cavernous sinus, and gives off the ophthalmic, anterior choroidal, and posterior communicating arteries and terminally bifurcates into the anterior and middle cerebral arteries.

ANTERIOR CEREBRAL ARTERY. As Figures 493–1 and 493–2 show, the anterior cerebral artery supplies the medial and superior surfaces of the cerebral hemisphere and the whole of the most anterior portion of the frontal lobes. This area contains the motor and sensory cortex for the foot and leg and the supplementary motor cortex. The anterior cerebral artery, through medial lenticulostriate and Heubner's arteries, also supplies several deep structures of importance, including the anterior nucleus of the thalamus with contributions to the corona radiata, the anterior limb of the internal capsule, the head of the caudate nucleus, and the putamen. The first part of either of the paired anterior cerebral arteries is vestigial or absent in 3 to 4 per cent of normal individuals, its cortical portion being supplied from the opposite normal side by the anterior communicating artery.

MIDDLE CEREBRAL ARTERY. The middle cerebral artery (Figs. 493–2 and 493–3) irrigates most of the lateral surface of the

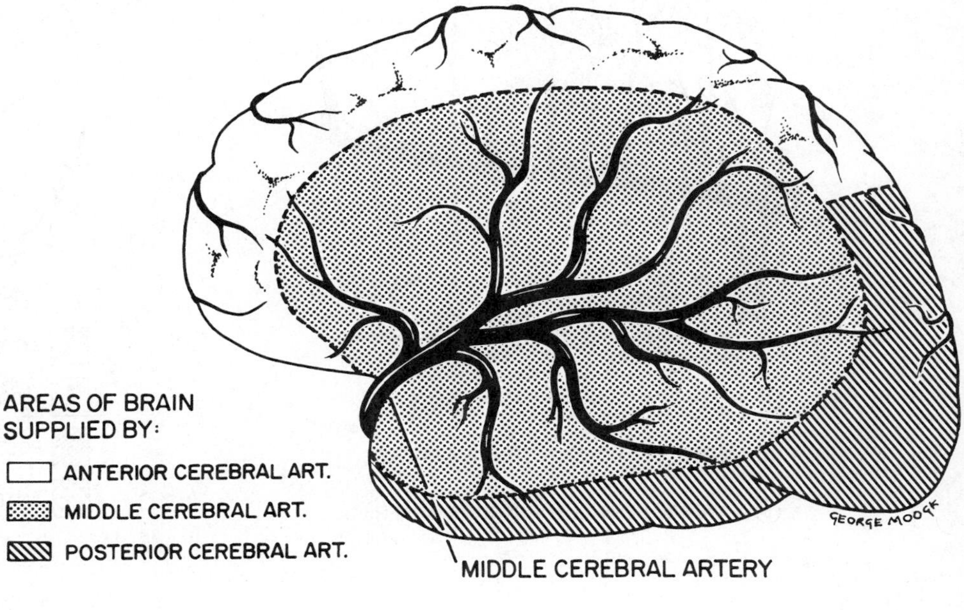

Figure 493–2. The lateral surface of the cerebral hemisphere and the course of the middle cerebral artery. The middle cerebral artery has been elevated from the Sylvian fissure to better illustrate its course. (For clarity the shadings differ from those in Figure 493–1.)

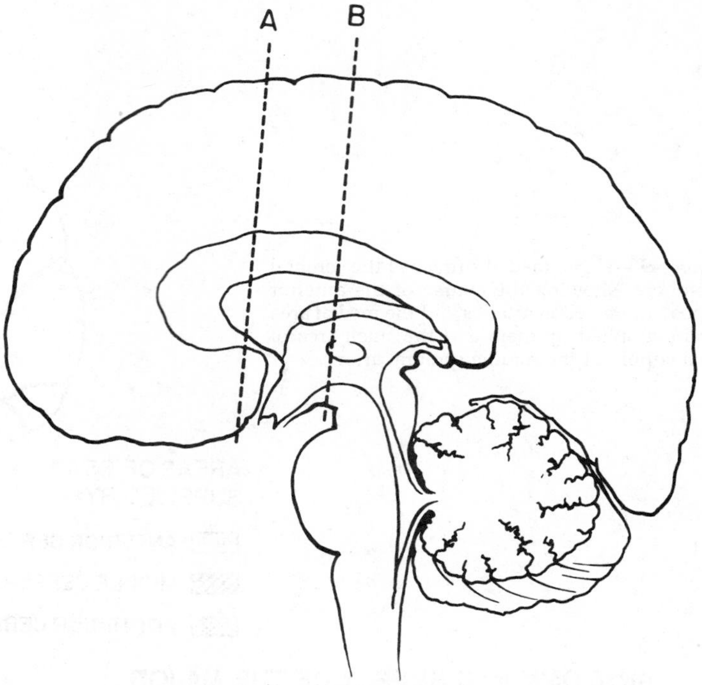

A

Figure 493–3. *A,* The lateral surface of the cerebral hemisphere showing the planes through which *B* and *C* were taken. *B,* Coronal section through the left hemisphere demonstrating the thalamostriate arteries and the recurrent artery of Heubner. *C,* Coronal section through the right hemisphere showing the area of the brain supplied by the anterior (ACA), middle (MCA), and posterior (PCA) cerebral arteries and the anterior choroidal artery. The "homunculus" overlies the cortex, illustrating the area of representation of movements and the proportional cortical allocations to the motor functions. (Adapted from Penfield and Rasmussen, 1950.)

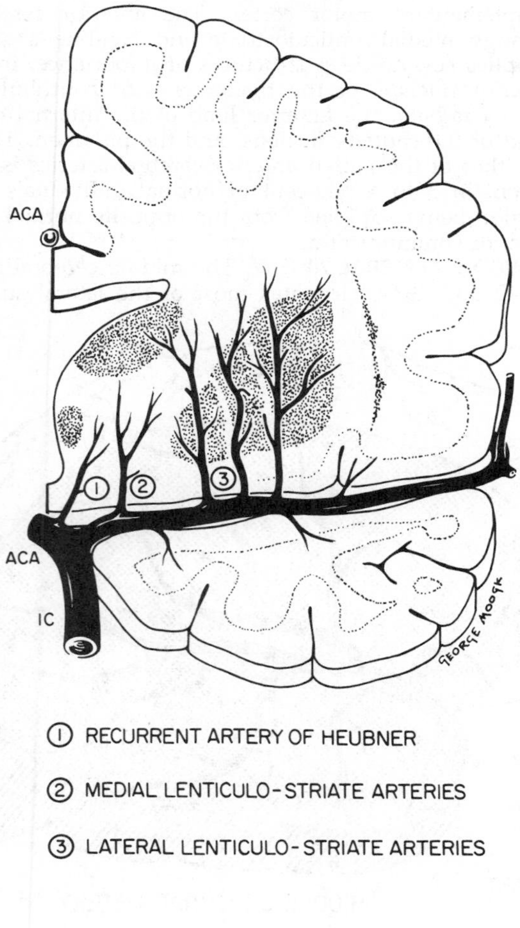

B

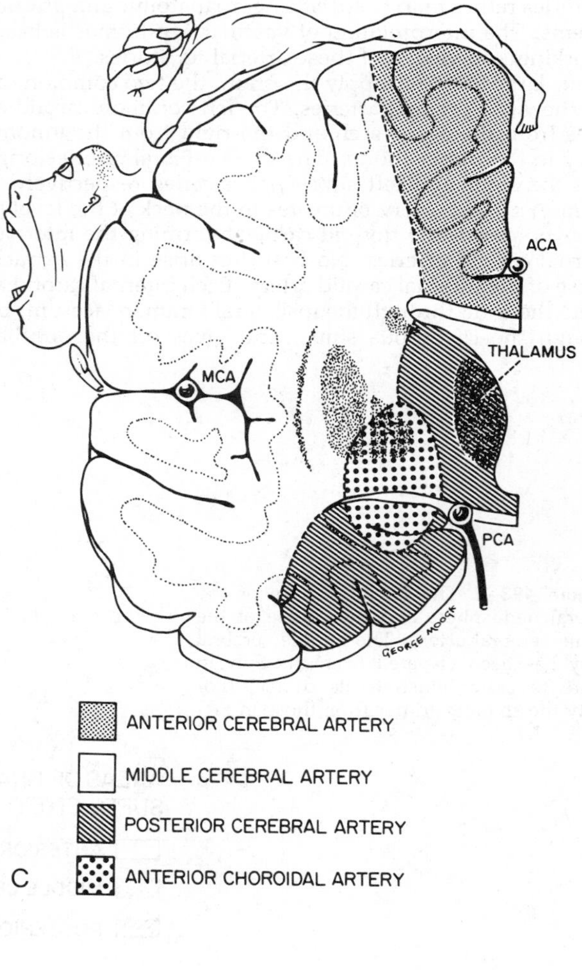

C

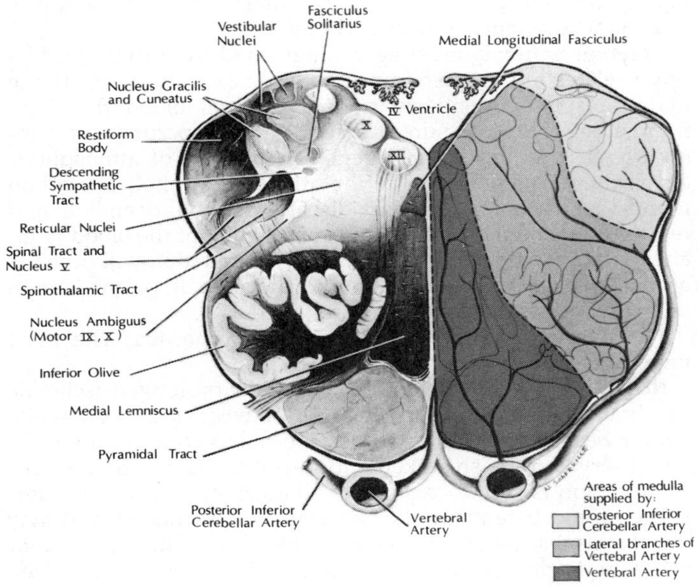

Figure 493–4. Cross-section of the medulla oblongata at the level of the hypoglossal nuclei. Short branches of the vertebral and anterior spinal arteries supply the medial medulla. Longer circumferential branches, including the posterior inferior cerebellar artery, supply the lateral portions of the medulla.

cerebral hemisphere with the exception of the occipital and frontal poles. The cortex supplied includes the primary motor and sensory areas for the face, throat, hand, and arm; the optic radiations; and, in the dominant hemisphere, the cortical areas for speech. The perforating (lenticulostriate) branches of the middle cerebral artery reach the depths of the cerebral hemisphere and contribute to the supply of the posterior limb of the internal capsule, basal ganglia, and corona radiata.

VERTEBRAL AND BASILAR ARTERIES. The vertebral arteries arise from the subclavian arteries and after a short, free course traverse the bony canals in the transverse processes from the sixth to the second cervical vertebrae and then enter the skull through the foramen magnum. The vertebral arteries have numerous branches in the neck, which anastomose with branches of the occipital artery and with the ascending and deep cervical arteries from the costocervical and thyrocervical arteries. Individual variations are common, and in approximately 10 per cent of cases one of the vertebral arteries is vestigial with the result that a single vertebral artery provides the main source of blood for the basilar artery. Immediately after entering the skull, each vertebral artery gives off a medial branch, which unites with its opposite to form the anterior spinal artery. Rostral to this point, the posterior inferior cerebellar arteries arise.

At all levels of the brainstem the ventral medial portion is supplied by short paramedian vessels. The ventrolateral portion is supplied by short circumferential branches from the vertebral or basilar arteries. The dorsal-lateral portion and the cerebellum are supplied by long circumferential branches: the posterior inferior, the anterior inferior, and the superior cerebellar arteries.

The vertebral artery lies on the lateral surface of the medulla oblongata ventrally, and from it and the anterior spinal artery short paramedian branches supply the pyramids, the inferior olives and medial lemnisci, the medial longitudinal fasciculi, and the emerging fibers of the hypoglossal nerve, as shown in Figure 493–4.

The more dorsal and lateral portion of the medulla includes the spinothalamic tract, the vestibular nuclei, the sensory nucleus of the fifth cranial nerve, descending fibers of the sympathetic nervous system, the restiform body, and the emerging fibers of the vagus and glossopharyngeal nerves; these structures are supplied by longer branches from the vertebral artery and the branches from the posterior inferior cerebellar artery. The most cephalad and dorsal segment of the medulla includes the vestibular and cochlear nuclei, which, along with the posterior portion of the cerebellum, are supplied by the posterior inferior cerebellar artery.

At the lower borders of the pons, the two vertebral arteries unite in the ventral midline to form the basilar artery. The basilar artery extends along the ventral aspect of the pons and the midbrain in the midline. From this artery short perpendicular branches enter the pons to supply paramedian structures, including the corticospinal tracts, the pontine nuclei, the medial lemnisci, the medial longitudinal fasciculi, and the pontine reticular nuclei (Fig. 493–5). The anterior inferior cerebellar artery, the long circumferential branch at this level, supplies the lateral portion of the pons, which includes the emerging seventh and eighth cranial nerves, the trigeminal nerve root, the vestibular and cochlear nuclei, and the spinothalamic tracts. It also gives branches to the most dorsal and lateral of these structures as it runs dorsally to irrigate the cerebellum.

At the midbrain level the basilar artery lies in the midline in the peduncular fossa (Fig. 493–6). Short branches pass laterally and dorsally to both sides to supply the cerebral peduncles, the emerging fibers of the third nerve, medial portions of the red nuclei, the medial longitudinal fasciculus, the oculomotor nuclei, and the midbrain reticulum. Branches of the posterior cerebral artery supply the lateral portions of the peduncles, the

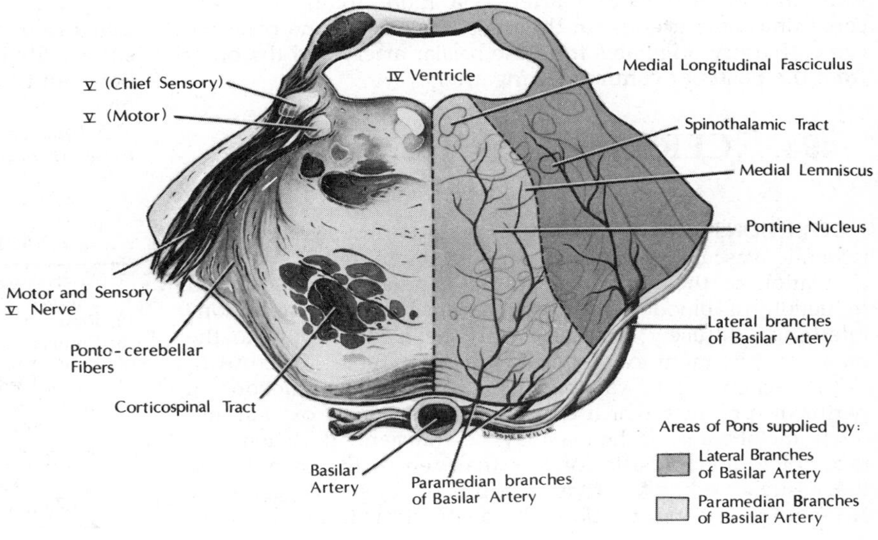

Figure 493–5. Cross-section of mid-pons. The medial portion receives blood supply from short perforating basilar artery branches. More laterally, the blood supply comes from lateral basilar artery branches.

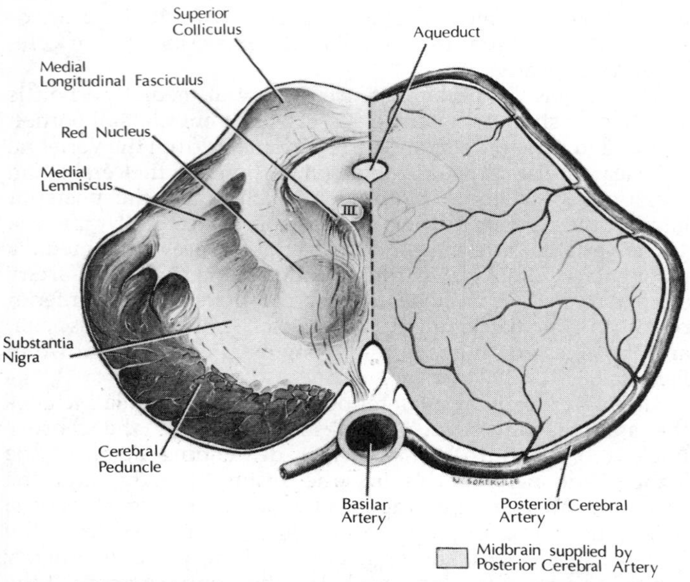

Figure 493–6. Cross-section of the midbrain. The posterior cerebra artery passes around the midbrain and gives off short branches supplying the medial, lateral, and dorsal regions.

red nuclei, and the medial lemnisci. The superior cerebellar arteries contribute to the supply of the dorsal portions of the midbrain, including the colliculi and the superior portion of the cerebellum on each side.

POSTERIOR CEREBRAL ARTERY. As shown in Figures 493–1 and 493–2, the cortical branches of the posterior cerebral artery supply the posterior pole of the lateral surface of the cerebral hemisphere and the posterior portion of the medial and inferior surfaces of the hemispheres. The cortical supply includes the calcarine cortex (the primary visual receptive area) and the hippocampus. Short perforating branches of the posterior cerebral artery supply the midbrain, including the cerebral peduncle and red nucleus, as well as the subthalamic area, the thalamus, and the posterior portion of the internal capsule, and contribute to the optic pathways and part of the hypothalamus.

Anatomic variation is common in the origin of the posterior cerebral artery. In approximately 70 per cent of cases, the origins of both posterior cerebral arteries arise from the apex of the basilar artery and small posterior communicating arteries connect to the carotid arteries. In 5 to 10 per cent of cases, the major supply of blood to the posterior cerebral arteries derives from the internal carotid artery via more robust posterior communicating arteries. In the remaining cases, one posterior cerebral artery originates from the basilar artery and the other from the posterior communicating artery.

494. CEREBRAL ISCHEMIA AND INFARCTION

DEFINITIONS AND ETIOLOGY. The signs and symptoms of ischemic vascular stroke result from interference with the circulation to the brain owing to a generalized or localized reduction of blood flow. Ischemia results from conditions interfering diffusely or locally with the blood supply to the brain, and its many causes are outlined in Table 472–2 of Ch. 472.1. Ischemia follows upon general or local reductions in perfusion pressure which deprive brain tissue of oxygen and other metabolites. Ischemia may be transient; if ischemia is incomplete and persists for less than ten to fifteen minutes, the tissue commonly survives. More prolonged or complete ischemia results in infarction, i.e., death of the tissue. Depending on the site and extent of the infarction, mild to severe neurologic disability or death will follow.

Cerebral ischemia must be distinguished from hypoxia. Hypoxia relates to the interference with the oxygen supply to the brain, despite a relatively normal cerebral blood flow and normal perfusion pressure. Cerebral hypoxia occurs for a variety of reasons, including a general reduction of atmospheric oxygen tension, pollution of the atmosphere (e.g., by carbon monoxide), chronic pulmonary disease, pulmonary emboli, and reduced or altered oxygen-carrying capability of the blood (e.g., anemia, methemoglobinemia). Ischemic infarction will occur as a consequence of severe hypoxia, although it is uncommon and relative ischemia usually is required.

The causes of cerebral ischemia are numerous. The most important are shown in Table 494–1.

NEUROPATHOLOGY OF ISCHEMIA. With prolonged ischemia the brain softens and the margins between gray and white matter become indistinct. Under the microscope the neurons are observed to be shrunken and necrotic. Frequently the area of infarction is pale, occasionally hemorrhagic. A hemorrhagic infarct is most frequent after an embolic obstruction, but may develop as a sequel to the interruption of circulation in a major artery and appears in the watershed or border zone between branches of the artery supplying the cortex or the deeper structures. An example would be the watershed infarct at the margins of the anterior and middle cerebral artery supply which may follow occlusion of the internal carotid artery. As infarcts age, the necrotic central core breaks down and is removed by phagocytic action. The area of previous necrosis (or hemorrhage) may be represented by a cavity filled with yellow fluid and a lining of glia and fibrovascular tissue, sometimes stained with hemosiderin. Areas of infarction are not unusual in postmortem examinations performed on older patients who have died of other causes. They may be numerous and exist in the absence of previous clinical symptoms.

Cerebral edema, variable in amount and dependent on the extent of the infarction, accompanies cerebral infarction. If edema is extensive, it produces distortion of the hemisphere or cerebellum with a shift medially beneath the falx, downward or upward through the tentorium cerebelli, or downward through the foramen magnum. The effects of such compression shifts are visible on CT scanning and are discussed in Ch. 472.1.

Edema and swelling resulting from infarction in the cerebellum can impede the circulation of cerebrospinal fluid and at times leads to obstructive hydrocephalus.

DEGREES OF ISCHEMIA. Partial interference with the cerebral circulation produces neither tissue ischemia nor abnormal symptoms and signs if compensatory mechanisms operate efficiently. With altered systemic blood pressure, even to hypotensive levels, autoregulation by the cerebral arteriolar bed usually is sufficient to adjust the circulation quickly and preserve the vitality and function of brain tissue. Alternatively, ischemia may be sufficiently prolonged and collateral circulation sufficiently inadequate that a major catastrophic stroke results. Between these extremes, gradations of severity may be identified:

A transient ischemic attack (TIA) is defined as a loss of neurologic function caused by ischemia, abrupt in onset, persisting

TABLE 494–1. CAUSES OF CEREBRAL ISCHEMIA

1. Arterial disease: (a) Atherothrombosis in the intra- and extracranial arteries; (b) emboli from the extracranial and larger intracranial arteries
2. Emboli of cardiac origin
3. Cardiac disease causing reduced cerebral blood flow
4. Lacunar infarction
5. Generalized cerebral hypoxia
6. Cerebral artery thrombosis due to nonarteriosclerotic vasculopathies
7. Cerebral artery thrombosis due to coagulation abnormalities (polycythemia, thrombocytosis)
8. Cerebral arterial spasm following subarachnoid hemorrhage
9. Cerebral arterial vasoconstriction associated with migraine
10. Cerebral vein and sinus thrombosis

for less than 24 hours, and clearing without residual signs. Most such TIAs last only a few minutes. If disability persists for more than 24 hours but is attended ultimately by no persisting symptoms or signs, it is conventionally called a *reversible ischemic neurologic disability* (RIND). The study of patients who have experienced TIA or RIND indicates that in approximately 15 per cent of them CT scans will detect a persistent lesion in the appropriate arterial supply. The pathogenic process by which TIA or RIND occurs is the same as that which produces clinical signs of persistent stroke, only the size of the lesion making the difference.

An ischemic event that is sufficiently severe and in an appropriate location to leave persistent disability but is short of a calamitous stroke, is defined as a *partial nonprogressing stroke* (PNS). The ultimate in severity of ischemia produces a more major degree of permanent neurologic disability, *a completed stroke.*

The disability from an ischemic event most often reaches its maximum in a few minutes. Not infrequently, however, the disability will worsen gradually or stepwise over a matter of hours to as much as a week or more: a *progressing stroke* or a *stroke-in-evolution.* When progress ceases and the clinical condition stabilizes, a PNS or a completed stroke will persist.

ATHEROTHROMBOTIC STROKE. ***Sites of Occlusion.*** Arteriosclerosis of the major extracranial arteries to the brain accounts for most strokes. The most common site for obstructive disease of the carotid artery is the region of the carotid sinus, followed by the portion within the cavernous sinus. In Caucasians, the carotid artery is responsible for atherothrombotic stroke six to seven times more frequently than is the main trunk of the middle cerebral artery. In those of Oriental race, the ratio of carotid to middle cerebral disease is reversed.

The extracranial course of the vertebral artery commonly evidences disease at its origin and at the C1–C2 level just prior to entry into the cranium. Intracranially, the most common site for vertebral artery disease and occlusion is within 1 to 2 cm of the termination of the artery, most commonly just beyond the origin of the posterior inferior cerebellar artery. Disease in the basilar artery has a predilection to involve its mid-portion (Fig. 494–1).

Anastomotic Circulation. The manifestations of stroke commonly are described in terms of the arterial territories supplied by branches of the internal carotid and vertebral-basilar arteries, i.e., as syndromes of the anterior, middle, and posterior cerebral artery, as well as of the vertebro-basilar tributaries. It is now recognized that obstruction in the more proximal, commonly the extracranial, part of the arterial supply to the brain often presents a picture indistinguishable from that of more distal obstructions. Internal carotid artery occlusion, for example, can produce no symptoms if intracranial anastomoses compensate for the obstruction. Without such protection, carotid occlusion commonly results in ischemia distributed in some part of the middle cerebral artery territory.

Collateral supply for the internal carotid artery has several potential sources: the ipsilateral basilar circulation via the posterior communicating artery; ipsilateral leptomeningeal communications between the cortical branches of the posterior cerebral artery and those of the middle and anterior cerebral arteries; the ipsilateral external carotid artery by retrograde flow through the ophthalmic artery and, of less importance, through the middle meningeal and ascending pharyngeal arteries; and, contralaterally, through the anterior communicating artery.

The vertebral artery forms anastomoses with branches of the occipital artery and branches of the ascending and deep cervical arteries arising from the thyrocervical and costocervical arteries. Vertebral artery occlusion near its origin commonly results in no symptoms because of the development of an extensive cervical anastomotic network. More serious effects are expected when the vertebral artery is occluded more distally. At any level, obstruction to one or even both vertebral arteries may be asymptomatic. Commonly a modified ischemic syndrome emerges because of the protective effect exerted by the collateral circulation.

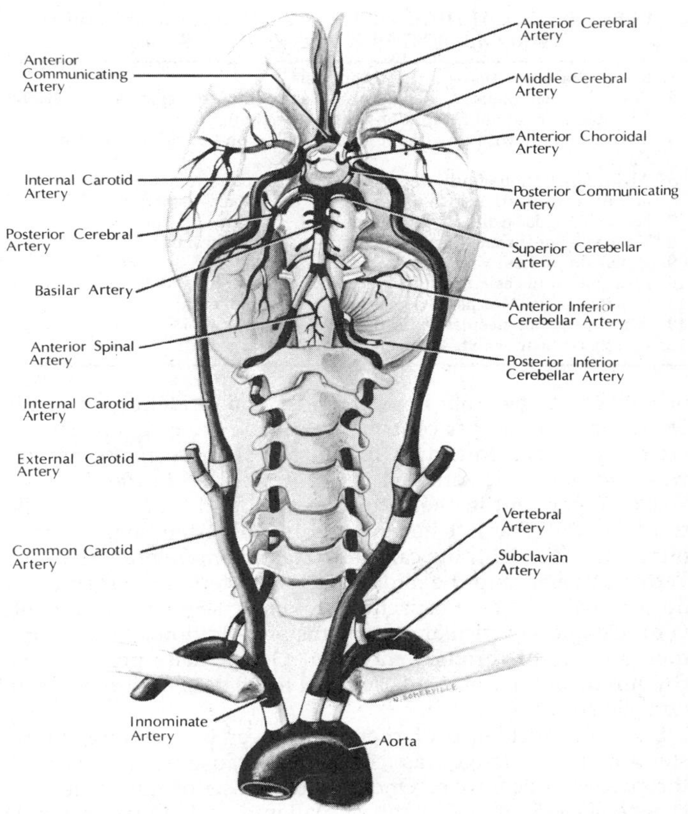

Figure 494–1. The light bands around the arteries indicate the sites of predilection for atheroma. The two most common sites to cause symptoms are the region of the carotid sinus and the intracranial portion of the carotid artery.

Basilar artery occlusion usually produces serious consequences, but the extent of the ischemia can be modified by collateral supply. In rare instances this will be sufficient to allow asymptomatic basilar artery occlusion. Mid-basilar artery occlusion or serious stenosis results in a reduction of pressure in the artery such that there is a reversal of flow with blood coming from the anterior circulation via the posterior communicating artery. The potential exists for collateral communication between the large branches of the vertebral and basilar arteries, particularly the superior, anterior inferior, and posterior inferior cerebellar arteries.

"Watershed" Infarction. Infarcts often occur in the territory where the cortical arteries overlap. The anterior and middle cerebral arteries are the major terminal branches of the internal carotid artery, and circulation may be least effective in the "marginal" or "boundary" zone or "watershed" between these branches following an occlusion of the internal carotid artery. Severe impairment of cerebral perfusion, such as occurs with cardiac arrest, tamponade, and exsanguination, especially results in infarction in these border zones. As the circulation becomes restored, blood passes into the surrounding tissues through capillaries damaged by hypoxia. Watershed infarcts tend, therefore, to be hemorrhagic.

STROKE DUE TO EMBOLI OF CARDIAC ORIGIN. Technologic advances in the past decade permit more accurate identification of cardiac sources for emboli (Table 494–2). Instead of the estimated 3 to 5 per cent of 20 years ago, the estimated incidence of stroke caused by thromboembolism originating from the heart has risen to 20 per cent. The mural thrombus forming on the endocardium in conjunction with myocardial infarction is an important source and accounts for 8 to 10 per cent of strokes. At least 5 per cent of patients with a myocardial infarction have clinical evidence of cerebral embolization. Postmortem studies

TABLE 494–2. CARDIAC LESIONS PRODUCING CEREBRAL THROMBOEMBOLIC ISCHEMIC EVENTS

1. Myocardial infarction—mural thrombosis
2. Postinfarction aneurysms and akinetic segments—stasis thrombi
3. Postinfarction atrial fibrillation—atrial thrombi
4. Mitral stenosis with or without atrial fibrillation—atrial and auricular thrombi
5. Atrial fibrillation of any cause—persistent or paroxysmal thrombi
6. Mitral regurgitation with atrial mural "jet lesions"—small mural thrombi
7. Bacterial endocarditis—valvular mycotic thrombi
8. Nonbacterial thrombotic endocarditis—valvular thrombi
9. Prolapsing mitral valve—valvular thrombi
10. Mitral annulus calcification—? degenerate valve fragments
11. Calcific aortic stenosis—? degenerate valve fragments
12. Atrial myxoma–neoplastic tissue—? attached thrombi
13. Prosthetic heart valve—attached thrombi

of patients dying from myocardial infarction identify systemic emboli in 45 to 60 per cent, half of which are cerebral. Emboli after myocardial infarction are most common in the second week. In one large series 84 per cent occurred in the first four weeks; 6 per cent in the second month, and 8 per cent in the third month. The left hemisphere is embolized slightly more often than the right, the carotid circulation more often than the vertebrobasilar, and the middle cerebral artery more than other intracranial arteries. Postischemic akinetic segments of the left ventricle and ventricular aneurysms are additional but uncommon sources of thromboembolism. Occasionally postischemic rhythm disorders, particularly atrial fibrillation, will precipitate embolic strokes.

Since the incidence of rheumatic fever is declining, mitral stenosis is no longer as common a cause as formerly of thromboembolic stroke. Once the diagnosis of mitral stenosis is established, 20 per cent of patients will suffer systemic embolism within five years, approximately half of which will involve the brain. Of those with such emboli, half will have recurrent emboli, most commonly within the first year after the initial event. The association of atrial fibrillation increases the risk of stroke. The Framingham Study disclosed that atrial fibrillation with rheumatic heart disease results in a 17-fold increase in stroke risk. Atrial fibrillation alone, without rheumatic heart disease, produces a six-fold increase in risk of stroke.

Careful cardiac history and physical examination, supplemented when indicated by ECG monitoring, two-dimensional echocardiography, wall-motion studies, and, in certain selected cases, ventricular angiocardiography, identify the less common cardiac conditions associated with cerebral thromboembolism listed in Table 494–2.

Certain valvular and mural lesions cannot be identified with certainty by physical examination, ECG, and routine radiography. These include atrial myxoma, mitral annulus calcification (a degenerative process in older subjects), and the myxomatous degeneration of the mitral valve which is the most common cause of the "ballooning" or *"prolapse"* of the *mitral valve* (PMV). Such lesions are identified by echocardiography and are being recognized increasingly as causes of ischemic events, in younger patients in the case of PMV, and in older subjects with mitral annulus calcification. The principal clinical challenge is to know when a condition like PMV, which occurs asymptomatically in 6 to 8 per cent of normal persons, is a cause of serious but common symptoms. An epidemiologic study indicated that in patients under the age of 45 who are afflicted with cerebral or retinal ischemic events, 30 per cent had no other recognizable causal factor than PMV, whereas controls matched for age and sex and without cardiac or cerebral symptoms had only a 6 to 8 per cent incidence of PMV. Familial PMV is well known, and several families are on record with strokes in younger members. Marfan's syndrome is accompanied by an increased incidence of PMV, and juveniles with this disorder have been observed with stroke when PMV was the only recognizable causative factor.

CARDIAC DISEASE CAUSING REDUCED CEREBRAL BLOOD FLOW. Disorders of cardiac output and serious hypotension result in diffuse disturbances of brain function. The most common manifestation is the syncopal Stokes-Adams attack caused by heart block, but similar clinical pictures can accompany sinoatrial node disorders, intermittent ventricular arrhythmias, or a variety of conditions producing severe orthostatic hypotension. Failing circulation produces clinical signs reflecting a diffuse reduction of cerebral perfusion, characterized by syncope, convulsions, visual blurring, nonspecific dizziness, and occasionally vertigo. Discrete focal hemispheric events, characteristic of thromboembolic ischemia, are uncommon with these hemodynamic occurrences.

LACUNAR INFARCTION. Lacunar infarction is a condition most commonly associated with longstanding hypertension in which multiple small infarcts occur in the region of the corona radiata, internal capsule, striatum, thalamus, basis pontis, and cerebellum. The distribution of the infarcts favors the territory of the penetrating branches of the middle and posterior cerebral arteries and the median branches of the basilar artery. The infarcts soften, are absorbed by phagocytosis, and leave small (1 to 3 mm diameter) residual cavities (lacunes). Similar lesions occasionally result from emboli passing distally from atheromatous lesions in the large arteries, but in most instances the pathologic cause is fibrosing hyaline degeneration ("lipohyalinosis"), followed by thrombotic occlusion in distal arteries 50 to 150 μm in diameter. The lesions are in the same small arteries which rupture in primary spontaneous intracerebral hemorrhage. It is not known why these vessels develop thrombosis in some hypertensive individuals while they become necrotic and rupture in others.

The incidence of lacunar infarction is uncertain. The Harvard Stroke Registry, a prospective study of stroke in the Boston region, estimated that 19 per cent of strokes were of lacunar origin. A decline of such cases is now evident as part of the reduction in deaths resulting from hypertension.

NONARTERIOSCLEROTIC VASCULOPATHIES. *Fibromuscular hyperplasia* is the most common nonarteriosclerotic disorder affecting the large arteries, predominantly in their extracranial course. It is of unknown etiology, first described in the renal arteries with a predilection to affect females of middle age. Although it is most commonly asymptomatic, minor or major thromboembolic events occur; the long-term prognosis is good and late recurrence of ischemic events is uncommon. An increased incidence of berry aneurysm is reported with the condition.

Dissecting aortic aneurysm consequent upon the medial necrosis related to hypertension and occurring in middle life rarely may cause obstruction to the innominate, common carotid, and subclavian arteries. Stroke developing in association with crushing pain in the chest radiating to the back and possibly into the abdomen, with obliteration of some upper or lower limb pulses, suggests this diagnosis. Affected patients who are normotensive and under middle age should be examined for features of Marfan's syndrome.

Traumatic and spontaneous dissection of carotid and vertebral-basilar arteries is a disorder distinct from aortic dissection. Dissections have been described as a sequel to trauma, including direct blows to the neck, fracture dislocations that injure the vertebral artery in its bony canal, and indirect damage such as follows neck manipulations or other violent twisting or severe cervical hyperextension movements. Most dissections develop spontaneously without recognizable disease in the arterial wall. In a minority there is detectable medial degeneration, fibromuscular dysplasia, or advanced atheroma. The condition occurs in both sexes from childhood to middle life. Internal carotid artery dissection is most common and is characterized by neck, ear, face, or head pain. A bruit is frequently audible, sometimes noted by the patient. Horner's syndrome occurs. Minor intermittent hemispheric TIAs or major strokes develop. The dissection may be bilateral, and at times is accompanied by a similar condition in the vertebral artery. Angiography reveals a long, remarkably narrowed segment of the upper cervical portion of the artery. This stenosis may persist or be combined with segmental fusiform dilatation of part of the diseased artery. In some patients, a return to near-normal or normal appearances has been noted in repeat arteriograms. A similar condition of even rarer occurrence involves the basilar artery and presents with evidence of basilar artery ischemia with or without evidence of subarachnoid hemorrhage.

Pulseless disease or *Takayasu's arteritis* is a granulomatous angiitis, involving fibrous proliferation, mononuclear infiltration, and occasional giant cells. There is a predilection for the condition to involve the media and adventitia of the arch of the aorta in young Japanese females. Occlusion or severe narrowing develops in the cranial as well as the subclavian arteries; branches of the abdominal aorta may be involved. Another inflammatory arteriopathy, particularly common in Japan, *moyamoya,* results in a progressive obliteration of the intracranial carotid arteries. In affected subjects, an extensive vascular network develops with dilatation of many small branches beyond the stenoses, and abundant small collaterals develop from the ascending pharyngeal and meningeal branches of the external carotid artery. The angiographic appearance resembles a "puff of smoke" (moyamoya). Progressive and stepwise neurologic disability is the rule, and many patients suffer abrupt worsening or death from rupture of one of the many anastomotic arteries.

A variety of uncommon pathologic processes can involve the smaller intracranial arteries and arterioles (Table 494–3).

CEREBRAL ARTERY THROMBOSIS DUE TO COAGULATION ABNORMALITIES, POLYCYTHEMIA, OR THROMBOCYTOSIS. *Coagulation abnormalities* are implicated in a variety of conditions which produce cerebral hemorrhage; they are less often associated with thrombotic events in the cerebral circulation. Some of these, such as consumption coagulopathies and thrombotic thrombocytopenic purpura (TTP), can produce combinations of hemorrhage and thrombosis in the same individual. The phenomena are confined to patients with serious systemic illness.

There are a variety of less devastating clinical states in which abnormalities of the coagulation process may be accompanied by cerebral ischemic events and stroke. Table 494–4 lists the more common conditions, none of which have been correlated with specific coagulation abnormalities. Venous thrombosis is more common in some of these conditions than is arterial occlusion. Nevertheless the gamut of ischemic phenomena, varying from TIA to devastating stroke with massive infarction, may complicate any of these conditions.

The angiographic study of patients with these conditions tends to indicate branch arterial occlusions rather than large extracranial artery lesions. However, the initiating thrombus that eventually produces the thromboembolic intracranial occlusion may begin in the large aortic branches or in the pulmonary veins and pass cephalad from these sites.

Thrombocytosis, whether alone or with other features of polycythemia, is a rare but recognized platelet abnormality sometimes accompanied by transient and major persistent cerebral and retinal ischemia.

TABLE 494–3. NONARTERIOSCLEROTIC ANGIOPATHIES CAPABLE OF CAUSING TIA AND STROKE

Large Arteries
1. Fibromuscular hyperplasia
2. Dissecting aortic aneurysm
3. Traumatic and spontaneous carotid and vertebral-basilar artery dissection
4. Takayasu's arteritis (pulseless disease)
5. Moyamoya

Smaller Arteries and Arterioles

6. Collagen vascular disease
7. Giant cell ("temporal") arteritis
8. Meningovascular syphilis
9. Allergic vasculitis
10. Congophilic angiopathy
11. Vasculitis with homocystinuria
12. Vasculopathy resulting from drug abuse
13. Vasculitis with Behçet's disease
14. Granulomatous angiitis

TABLE 494–4. CONDITIONS WITH POTENTIAL FOR ALTERED BLOOD COAGULATION PRODUCTIVE OF CEREBRAL ISCHEMIA

- The postpartum period
- Pregnancy
- Ingestion of oral contraceptives
- Manifest and occult cancer
- Postoperative and post-traumatic states
- Paroxysmal nocturnal hemoglobinuria
- Hyperviscosity syndromes
- Polycythemia rubra vera
- Sickle cell disease
- Macroglobulinemia

INTRACRANIAL VENOUS AND SINUS THROMBOSIS. In the era prior to antibiotic therapy, retrograde extension of septic thrombosis from the face to the cavernous sinus and from the mastoid and middle ear to the lateral sinus occurred relatively frequently. The results were devastating and the outcome generally fatal.

Septic venous and sinus thrombosis complicates infections of the middle ear, sinuses, and face. Lateral sinus thrombosis presents with headache and tenderness localized to the mastoid area. Extension of the inflammatory process to the jugular foramen results in dysfunction of cranial nerves IX, X, and XI. Extension toward the tip of the petrous bone results in diplopia from sixth cranial nerve involvement and in facial numbness from trigeminal nerve involvement. Thrombi from the jugular vein may produce fatal pulmonary emboli. Extension occurs into the sagittal sinus and, if sufficiently extensive, impairs venous drainage as well as absorption of cerebrospinal fluid and can result in increased intracranial pressure, papilledema, vomiting, and impaired consciousness. Persistent functional failure of the arachnoid granulations within the longitudinal sinus may be complicated by ventricular dilatation, a conditon called "otitic hydrocephalus."

Septic thrombophlebitis may spread from the nasal sinuses or infections of the face and involve the cavernous sinus. The condition is rare nowadays. The clinical features of cavernous sinus thrombosis include painful proptosis, at times bilateral, with progressive ophthalmoplegia and involvement of the first sensory division of the trigeminal nerve. Meningitis commonly occurs with coma and death in cases that are severe or far advanced prior to therapeutic intervention.

Aseptic thromboses of cerebral veins and sinuses have become more common than the septic variety since the introduction of antibiotics. Even so, the condition is uncommon but may occur spontaneously or with any of the conditions listed in Table 494–4.

Premonitory headaches and transient ischemic events herald more florid signs and symptoms in intracranial venous thromboses. Focal or generalized seizures occur in half of the cases. Major focal neurologic deficits develop and in some instances are bilateral. Mild and occasionally marked evidence of subarachnoid hemorrhage is present, and the cerebrospinal fluid may be sufficiently bloody to suggest the possibility of the rupture of an intracranial aneurysm. This subarachnoid blood comes from hemorrhagic infarction, characteristic of venous thrombosis in the brain just as it is in the retina. Diagnosis can be confirmed from the venous phase of cerebral arteriography with a failure to fill all or part of a major sinus, particularly the sagittal or the lateral sinus. The finding on head CT scan of the "delta sign," a visualization of a dark opacity in the contrast-enhanced posterior portion of the sagittal sinus at the torcula, is diagnostic. This appearance results from the stationary blood (thrombus) within the sinus.

The prognosis for aseptic cerebral phlebothrombosis is usually favorable. Even major neurologic deficits usually resolve completely, although some patients develop future epilepsy and a few develop major permanent disability or death.

SYNDROMES AND SYMPTOMS OF CEREBRAL ARTERIAL ATHEROTHROMBOSIS AND THROMBOEMBOLISM. The clinical features of ischemic infarction from intrinsic arterial disease and from embolic arterial obstruction are similar. The variability of collateral circulation makes it difficult, in the presence of a partial stroke, to state from history and physical examination alone that a main artery is occluded as opposed to one of its branches. Characteristic features of each vascular territory will be given separate consideration.

Internal Carotid Artery. The most common site for atheroma leading to stroke or threatening stroke is the carotid sinus where the common carotid artery bifurcates. Minor lesions, smooth or ulcerative stenosis, and sometimes complete occlusions can be present without any symptoms.

Internal carotid artery stenosis is frequently accompanied by transient events (TIA or RIND). The most characteristic symptom is ipsilateral monocular visual loss. Common symptoms are episodic weakness and/or sensory disturbance of the contralateral arm, leg, or face, at times causing a transient hemiplegia and hemisensory defect that returns to normal within minutes, hours, or days. The speech may be slurred, or, if the dominant hemisphere is involved, dysphasia may be present. Since an embolus may be carried from a stenosis in the proximal internal carotid artery to obstruct an important retinal or cerebral artery branch, persistent and severe signs and symptoms may occur. Consciousness is preserved during an ischemic event in carotid territory unless the ischemia initiates an uncommon convulsive episode. Vertigo, diplopia, and simultaneous bilateral visual loss are not symptoms of carotid artery disease.

Carotid artery occlusion may occur with no symptoms or signs or with no more than a single transient event, or it may be ushered in by a series of transient or minor persisting events followed by a major hemisphere stroke. Fifty per cent of cases of major strokes from carotid artery occlusion occur with no warning episodes. The motor and sensory cortex may be involved with impaired motor and sensory function of the face, arm, and leg. Speech will be lost if the dominant hemisphere is implicated. Large infarcts can cause severe brain edema with serious secondary consequences.

Approximately one third of patients with an internal carotid occlusion complain of mild to severe ipsilateral or, occasionally, contralateral frontal and orbital pain coincident with the onset. The cause is probably a consequence of distention of collateral arterial channels. Approximately 15 per cent of patients with internal carotid artery occlusion develop an ipsilateral Horner's syndrome. Some of these occur without significant evidence of cerebral ischemia, and may reflect an involvement of the vasa nervorum to the periarterial sympathetic fibers. An alternative explanation in some cases is ischemia of the cells of origin of the sympathetic pathway in the hypothalamus.

Palpation of the internal carotid artery is diagnostically inconclusive and potentially misleading. Below the upper border of the thyroid cartilage the palpable pulse is that of the common carotid artery; above this level the superficial pulsation is that of the external carotid artery. Even in the presence of a known complete occlusion of the internal carotid artery, it is often difficult to judge pulse differences. The external carotid pulse may be more apparent than usual as a result of compensatory anastomotic flow to the intracranial portion of the internal carotid artery. Total absence of the carotid pulse indicates an occlusion of the common carotid artery. This may be confirmed by noting the absence of facial and superficial temporal artery pulsations.

Bruits are common over an internal carotid stenosis and are heard loudest at the bifurcation, i.e., at the level of the upper border of the thyroid cartilage. *To identify a bruit as being of carotid origin, one must trace its disappearance down the artery, thereby separating it from transmitted heart sounds.* Carotid bruits, once identified, can subsequently disappear, reflecting a normalization of previously high blood pressure or the occlusion of a stenotic lesion. Harsh bruits usually reflect severely stenotic arteries and may be accompanied by localized palpable thrills. External carotid artery stenosis can produce a local bruit despite internal carotid occlusion. Severe intracavernous carotid stenosis may result in an orbital bruit; such bruits can also accompany severe stenosis or occlusion of the ipsilateral or contralateral internal carotid arteries, possibly from dilatation of anastomotic arteries. The absence of a bruit is not helpful as a negative finding: substantial stenosis and ulcerative disease as well as complete occlusion may be present without audible bruit.

Stenosis of an internal carotid artery is more likely to be associated with recurrent ischemic events than is an occluded artery. Nevertheless, with occlusion, recurrent ischemic events may continue from thromboembolism from the distal soft "tail" of the thrombus in the cavernous sinus portion of the carotid artery; from ulcerative atheroma in the ipsilateral, common, or external carotid arteries; or from a residual "stump" of the occluded internal carotid artery. If such a "stump" remains open, it provides a site for turbulent flow, predisposing to the accumulation of platelet-fibrin thrombus material. From these neck sources the intracranial circulation is embolized through retrograde flow in the ophthalmic artery or through meningeal and ascending pharyngeal anastomoses.

Middle Cerebral Artery. The middle cerebral territory is the most common site for cerebral infarction. The main trunk of the middle cerebral artery is occasionally the site of severe atheroma out of proportion to the other intracranial or extracranial arteries, at times in excess of that affecting the internal carotid artery. Perhaps most often, however, occlusion of the main stem of the middle cerebral artery and of its major branches reflects embolic disease. Experimental emboli placed in the carotid artery or the aorta have a predilection to lodge in the middle cerebral as opposed to other intracranial arteries. In a young person with a middle cerebral artery occlusion or occlusion of one or more of its branches, a cardiac source should be sought. In older patients, either a cardiac or an internal carotid source for thromboembolism is more probable than intrinsic disease of the middle cerebral artery. Recurrent ischemia, persistent or transient, may involve the middle cerebral artery distribution in both hemispheres or in one hemisphere and the posterior circulation, within a reasonably short period of time. Such symptoms may reflect atherothrombotic disease of two arterial systems or alert the examiner to the possibility of emboli from the heart.

The cortical distribution of the middle cerebral artery supplies the areas representing movements and higher sensory functions for the upper limb and face, sparing the leg. Dominant hemisphere involvement produces aphasia. Posterior parietal lesions may result in a lower quadrantanopia. The capsular and ganglionic branches, including particularly the lenticulostriate branches, supply a major amount of the posterior limb of the internal capsule, and infarcts in this territory produce hemiplegia with variable sensory components and with the possibility of an accompanying homonymous hemianopia—all contralateral to the lesion.

Anterior Cerebral Artery. The clinical presentation of occlusion of the anterior cerebral artery depends on the involved segment of the artery and on the availability of collateral circulation. Proximal occlusions may produce no symptoms because of adequate flow through the anterior communicating artery. At the opposite extreme, occlusion of an artery responsible for the complete supply to both anterior cerebral arteries because of a vestigial proximal portion of the opposite anterior cerebral artery results in the rare syndrome of bilateral leg paralysis, urinary incontinence, and serious personality change. Intermediate between these extremes is the usual picture of an occlusion producing partial contralateral leg weakness and sensory loss, minimal arm involvement, and a sparing of face and speech function. Voluntary control of urination is commonly disturbed; mental confusion and behavioral disorders may be encountered. Since the ganglionic branches contribute to the supply of the subcortical white matter beneath the motor speech area, dysphasic symptoms may result from occlusion of the proximal part of the anterior cerebral artery.

Vertebral-Basilar (Posterior) Circulatory System. Occlusion of one vertebral artery and even of both arteries near their origin may sometimes be accompanied by no tissue damage or symptoms because of good collateral circulation. More often, the clinical picture from unilateral vertebral artery occlusion is the lateral medullary syndrome (Wallenberg's syndrome), caused by ischemia in the supply of the posterior inferior cerebellar artery. The ipsilateral findings include limb ataxia; Horner's syndrome; loss of appreciation of facial pain and temperature (trigeminal nerve); paralysis of larynx, pharynx, and palate (tenth nerve); and nystagmus. Intense vertigo and vomiting are common at the outset. Contralateral findings consist of impaired pain and temperature sensations, sparing only the face (see Fig. 493–4).

If one vertebral artery is vestigial, the remaining one becomes the main supply of the medulla. Depending on the condition of the posterior communicating artery, it may be the origin of much of the basilar artery flow. Under these anatomic circumstances, more serious brainstem infarction can result from a single vertebral artery occlusion.

The subclavian artery is most commonly occluded proximal to the origin of the vertebral artery. When an arteriogram is done in this condition, and the opposite vertebral artery is injected with contrast, the flow in the vertebral artery in the side of the subclavian occlusion will be reversed. Contrast material flows down the vertebral artery and into the subclavian artery. Most patients tolerate this diversion without symptoms, but in occasional patients the diversion may produce symptoms of brainstem ischemia aggravated by arm exercise, a phenomenon called the "subclavian steal." It is rare and almost always associated with evidence of extensive occlusive and stenotic arterial disease in the other arteries to the brain.

Basilar Artery. Occlusion of the basilar artery results in variable amounts of infarction of pons, midbrain, cerebellum, and occipital and medial temporal lobes. Asymptomatic basilar occlusion is rare. Most such occlusions, whether thrombotic or embolic, result in patchy infarction of the anatomic structures within the artery's territory of supply. As elsewhere in the brain, the availability and adequacy of collateral circulation determine the degree and extent of infarction. The usual and frequently fatal presentation of basilar artery occlusion includes the sudden development of sustained coma from ischemia of the midbrain reticular activating system, accompanied by bilateral third nerve palsies proceeding to fixed and dilated pupils and paralysis of the face, bulbar muscles, tongue, and all extremities. Incomplete clinical pictures include combinations of bilateral corticospinal tract involvement to any or all four limbs, usually more on one side than another; ataxia in the limbs; variable sensory loss; and a variety of cranial nerve lesions which frequently are on the side opposite the major weakness ("crossed" syndromes). Horner's syndrome may be seen.

On occasion, the basilar collateral circulation is sufficient that infarction will be confined to the ventral structures on one side with a hemiparesis difficult or impossible to distinguish from a more rostral capsular or cortical lesion. Such partial brainstem lesions may result from total occlusion of the main trunk of the basilar artery but more often are the consequence of occlusion of the median and short circumferential branches of the basilar artery by atherothrombotic, lacunar, or embolic obstructions.

Posterior Cerebral Artery. The site of occlusion, anatomic variations, and the availability or lack of collateral supply determine the clinical syndromes arising from posterior cerebral artery atherothrombosis or embolism. Infarctions from proximal branch obstruction include the "thalamic syndrome" and complex midbrain syndromes, including several of the eponymic "crossed syndromes." Hemiballismus or hemichoreoathetosis, intention tremor, and ataxia may be encountered. Conjugate gaze palsies may be added to the third nerve abnormalities and may include upward gaze paresis, skew deviation, and retraction nystagmus.

Cortical branch arterial lesions result most often in homonymous hemianopia, but an upper quadrantanopia may result from interference with the lower fibers of the optic radiation in the temporal lobe. Dyslexia and a variety of visual hallucinations and distortions follow ischemia of visual association cortex.

Bilateral cortical lesions produce cortical blindness and in confused subjects are commonly accompanied by denials that the blindness exists. Sometimes central vision is preserved if the macula is represented in the posterior part of the calcarine cortex and receives leptomeningeal collateral supply from the anterior and middle cerebral cortical arteries.

Amnestic strokes result from bilateral interruptions of the posterior cerebral arteries, producing ischemia in the hippocampal formations of the temporal lobes.

Lacunar Strokes. Several acute stroke syndromes have been delineated that are associated with small vessel disease producing areas of infarction and subsequent cavitation ("lacunes"). The lacunar lesions are less than 3 mm in diameter but may be multiple and occasionally coalesce to form larger areas visible by CT scanning. The most important of the clinical syndromes related to these lacunar infarcts are "pure motor hemiplegia"; "pure sensory stroke" involving face, arm, and leg; and an "ataxic hemiparesis syndrome." Motor hemiplegia results from small discrete infarcts in the internal capsule or the basis pontis. Pure sensory stroke indicates lacunar infarction of the thalamus. Ataxic stroke indicates thrombotic obstruction of the small penetrating basilar artery branches supplying the basis pontis involving the cerebellar peduncle, as well as the corticospinal tracts in this portion of the pons. At times a distinction cannot be made between a primary motor hemiplegia from a capsular lesion and a similar picture produced by a discrete lesion in the basis pontis producing no more damage than to the corticospinal tract.

PATHOGENESIS OF THREATENED STROKE. Stroke prevention has become a realistic goal; thus it is very important to have an appreciation of the way in which stroke presents. A "threatened stroke" may be regarded as any ischemic cerebral or retinal event that causes a TIA, RIND, PNS, or progressing stroke (see previous discussions), each being conditions that can proceed to a devastating stroke. Since it is common for patients with early TIA to go on to develop RIND or PNS prior to a complete stroke, we will discuss together the pathogenesis of all the earlier warning conditions. Such warning ischemic events result from a variety of conditions, which are listed in Table 494–5.

The relative importance of these conditions in producing focal and/or generalized cerebral ischemia remains under active investigation. At the moment the order in which they are listed in Table 494–5 appears to be close to an accurate ranking of their importance.

Artery-to-Artery Emboli. The retina, in which the arterioles are visible at the bedside, provides a microcosm reflecting the circulatory dynamics and pathology of the cerebral arterioles and arteries. Patients under study for recurrent unilateral visual

TABLE 494–5. PATHOGENETIC MECHANISMS OF THREATENED STROKE

Artery-to-artery emboli
Cardiac emboli
Lacunar infarction
Hemodynamic factors
Nonarteriosclerotic vasculopathies
Mechanical interference with arteries
Coagulation abnormalities
Thrombocytosis
Cerebral venous and sinus thrombosis

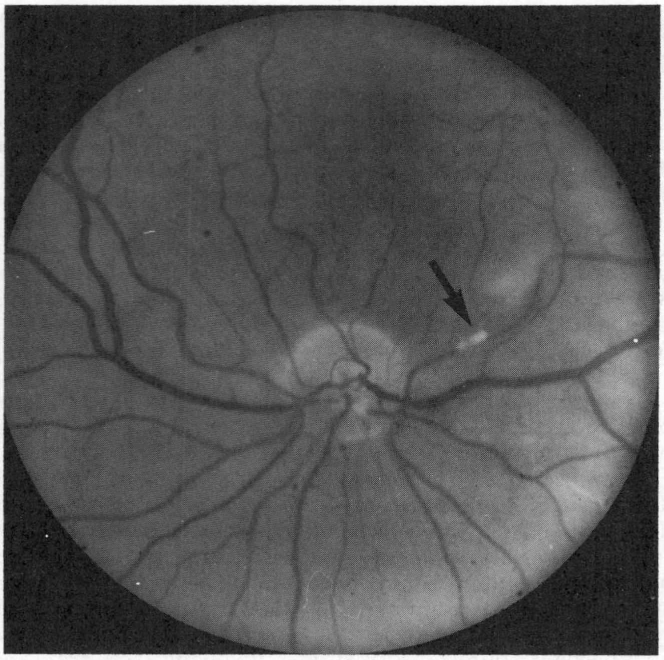

Figure 494–2. Atheromatous debris ("bright plaque") lodged in retinal arteriole in patient with history of attacks of amaurosis fugax. (From Barnett HJM: Med Clin North Am *63*:649, 1979.)

loss *(amaurosis fugax)*, a particular variety of TIA, have been observed with three kinds of material located in the retinal arterioles coincident with the development of this symptom. First, grayish-white material composed of platelets and fibrin has been noted passing in the arterioles from the central disc region out to the periphery over a 5- to 45-minute period. Second, fragments of atheromatous debris in the form of bright yellowish amorphous material have been noted. These "bright plaques" may pass through reasonably quickly or lodge and be visible for days or weeks before disappearing (Fig. 494–2). They may persist and become surrounded by white fibrous scar. Finally, pure crystals of cholesterol may be visualized, caught at the bifurcation of a retinal arteriole.

The source of platelet-fibrin emboli is to be sought in the heart valves and chambers or attached to its walls, or in the arteries which lead from it to the brain and retina. Emboli of atheromatous debris and pure cholesterol crystals come from the arteries but not from the heart. Surgeons at operation have observed both types of emboli lodging in the operative field of the exposed cortex in patients known to have irregular and ulcerative atheroma of the internal carotid or middle cerebral arteries. At postmortem examination, pathologists have identified atheromatous debris lodged within thrombi obstructing cortical and deep arteries and arterioles.

The onset of symptoms from major arterial disease may reflect the fact that the narrowing has become great enough to lead to platelet deposition in the area of turbulence beyond the stenosis. An alternative triggering mechanism is the occurrence of hemorrhage into an atheromatous plaque with a rupture into the lumen triggering off thrombosis and embolism or resulting in the formation of a roughened surface upon which platelets and fibrin are deposited. Close scrutiny of patients affected with symptoms of threatened stroke reveals that many have atheromatous lesions in the arteries leading to the territory of the threatening symptoms. Whether the significance of such emboli to TIA in the carotid artery is greater than in the vertebral-basilar territory remains an open question. One of the difficulties in proposing a difference in pathogenesis in the two major arterial systems lies in the fact that vertebral-basilar symptoms are sometimes initiated by cardiac and other systemic circulatory phenomena, and by a number of nonvascular conditions. Despite these limitations, in one study 78 per cent of cases with threatening stroke in the carotid artery territory and 82 per cent of vertebral-basilar cases had arteriographically detectable lesions appropriate to the symptoms.

Emboli of Cardiac Origin. In all age groups one must consider the heart as a source for symptoms and signs of threatening stroke. The common heart lesions resulting in major strokes also can produce minor ischemic events. Most common are mural thrombi from myocardial and endocardial infarction, mitral stenosis with and without atrial fibrillation, and atrial fibrillation from any cause. Any of these can be the ultimate cause of cerebral ischemic symptoms. More attention to the heart and improved capability of examining it adds to the number of conditions recognized to produce cerebral thromboembolism (see Table 494–2).

Lacunar Infarction. Lacunar infarcts (lacunes) are preceded by transitory symptoms in about one quarter of the cases. It is not easy to distinguish such transient events from the more usual artery-to-artery emboli, since many hypertensive individuals develop atheroma in the major arteries.

Hemodynamic Factors. Transient hemodynamic events such as cardiac arrhythmias tend to produce diffuse cerebral ischemic symptoms rather than focal ones. The evidence to support this statement comes from a variety of sources. In one study a series of 37 patients who had experienced focal TIA were exposed to a drop in blood pressure by pharmacologic and postural changes sufficient to induce syncope. Only one patient experienced focal symptoms. In a series of patients dying several days following global ischemia caused by cardiac arrest, the associated areas of cerebral infarction did not correspond to the sites of major atheromatous lesions. By contrast, old infarcts from previous cerebral events corresponded to arteriosclerosis in the appropriate arteries. A study of 290 patients who required a pacemaker because of heart block indicated that although 231 patients had suffered neurologic symptoms, only two had experienced focal ischemic events. Despite this, one sometimes encounters patients in whom a sudden impairment of cardiac output or an episode of severe hypotension (idiopathic cases, autonomic system dysfunction and disease, iatrogenic orthostatic hypotension, pulmonary emboli, carotid sinus hypersensitivity) has been accompanied by a focal ischemic event or a major stroke. Occasionally in the presence of a previously occluded major artery (internal carotid or basilar), a postural drop in blood pressure will result in symptoms that revert to normal when the patient reclines. When this happens, one usually finds that other major arteries are severely stenosed or occluded as well.

Nonarteriosclerotic Vasculopathies. Nonarteriosclerotic vasculopathies are so diverse as to make a generic description of little value. None are common, but collectively they must be recalled, especially when threatened or developed stroke takes an unusual pattern. Table 494–3 lists the conditions. Minor events in all of these disorders may precede major hemisphere or brainstem ischemic infarction. Repetitive and multiple events involving more than one hemisphere should always draw attention to the possibility of a widespread vasculopathy or to a cardiac source.

Mechanical Interference with the Course of the Cerebral Arteries. The location of the common and internal carotid arteries renders them liable to direct trauma with rupture and hemorrhage and even more to injury and subsequent thrombosis. Occasionally violent hyperextension neck injuries can stretch the carotid arteries abruptly in their extracranial course, producing intimal damage, medial dissection, and thrombosis. Similar injury can damage the vertebral artery before its entry at the C6 level into its protective bony canal in the transverse processes of the cervical vertebral bodies. At the C1-2 level, the artery is more mobile and may be levered into a hyperextended and rotated position by athletic injury, motor vehicle accident, or violent chiropractic manipulations. The trauma can lead to early thrombotic occlusion and the clinical picture of a vertebral artery ischemia, or may be followed by recurrent transient ischemic events reflecting a damaged endothelium with an irregular surface attracting thrombi and subsequent thromboembolic events.

Within the canal of the vertebral artery, there may be encroachment on the lumen of the vessel by osteophytes forming at the uncovertebral fissures, or "neurocentral joints" of the spine developing because of cervical spondylosis. Such conditions rarely cause symptoms, even when the artery must deviate around a large osteophyte. There is little movement at this site, and what there is requires lateral flexion to produce further narrowing of the affected artery. The popular concept of cervical spondylosis being a common cause of symptoms such as dizziness and vertigo is erroneous. At most this is a rare cause of ischemic events, and as a rule it occurs only after a severe neck injury.

The internal carotid artery below and adjacent to the cavernous sinus rarely may be distorted and encroached upon by tumors such as "en plaque" meningioma or extensions of nasopharyngeal cancer. Occasionally an odontoid dislocation, of traumatic origin or secondary to rheumatoid disease, will produce brainstem ischemic symptoms related to neck movement by compressing the lumen of the vertebral artery. Similarly, on very rare occasions benign tumors extending into the foramen magnum produce intermittent symptoms of vertebral artery insufficiency.

With routine activities involving neck hyperextension, elderly subjects may complain of episodes of blurred or lost vision, syncope, vertigo, or ataxia. Some of these effects may reflect vertebral artery compromise, but the mechanism is not clear.

TRANSIENT CAROTID AND VERTEBRAL-BASILAR ISCHEMIA. ***Symptoms and Signs.*** TIA, RIND, and PNS forewarn the possibility of a more significant stroke. There are some differences between the management of carotid compared with vertebral-basilar disease, and both may mimic other nonvascular conditions. Thus it is essential for the physician to be aware of the various expressions of TIA symptomatology. It must be recognized that at times a distinction cannot be made between symptoms arising from insufficiency of the internal carotid versus the vertebral-basilar arteries. Since cardiac emboli can produce similar symptoms, the occurrence of transient symptoms must not be construed as final evidence of an arterial abnormality in the carotid or the vertebral-basilar territory. The initial symptoms experienced by 311 patients with associated internal carotid disease are given in Table 494–6.

Amaurosis fugax is highly suggestive of carotid disease. The patient must be observant enough to ensure that a hemianopic disturbance is not mistaken for a monocular visual loss. The patient should be asked to cover one and then the other eye during subsequent attacks to make this distinction. Frequently the description is of a window blind coming down over the vision, obliterating the sight. Flashing or shimmering sensations only seldom emanate from retinal ischemia.

When a patient describes ipsilateral visual loss and on other occasions experiences transient loss of feeling or strength in the opposite limbs or face, there is little doubt about the carotid artery origin of the symptoms. It is rare for ocular and limb symptoms to occur simultaneously.

TABLE 494–6. SYMPTOMS OF CAROTID ARTERY DISEASE*

Symptoms	TIA AND RIND (208 Cases) (%)	PNS (103 Cases) (%)
Monocular visual	34	21
Paresis (mono-, hemi-)	59	88
Paresthesia (mono-, hemi-)	57	62
Facial paresis	22	43
Facial paresthesia	30	26
Dysphasia	21	30
Dysarthria	14	18
Headache	11	11
Binocular visual (hemianopsia)	7	10
"Dizziness"—nonspecific	6	2
Mental change	1	—
Convulsions		
Focal	—	—
Grand mal	1.5	2
Loss of consciousness	—	1
Visual hallucination	1	—

*From Barnett HJM: Clin Neurosurg 23:543, 1976.

TABLE 494–7. SYMPTOMS OF VERTEBRAL-BASILAR ARTERY DISEASE*

Symptoms	TIA or RIND (78 cases) (%)	PNS (46 Cases) (%)
Binocular visual	50	30
Vertigo	51	35
Diplopia	44	48
"Dizzy"	22	13
Ataxia	41	46
Paresthesia	44	54
Paresis	33	59
Dysarthria	21	37
Headache	18	33
Nausea and vomiting	14	17
Hearing loss	3	7
Mental change	8	8
Dysphagia	4	4
Dysphasia	3	4
Visual hallucinations	5	2
"Drop attacks"	4	4
Convulsions	—	2
Drowsiness	1	2

*From Barnett HJM: Clin Neurosurg 23:543, 1976.

Vertebral-basilar symptoms are more varied. Binocular visual loss is exceeded as a symptom only by vertigo and diplopia. The symptoms described in a series of 124 vertebral-basilar cases are outlined in Table 494–7.

The binocular visual symptoms frequently involve the entire vision, and descriptions vary from a complete blackness to a haziness of vision. At times a description is obtained of a veil over the vision with a random preservation of normal islands. Flashing and shimmering may occur as in migrainous aura. Loss of consciousness is uncommon and did not appear in our patients. Syncope, however, is a common expression of cardiac arrhythmia producing diffuse reduction in cerebral perfusion.

Motor or sensory symptoms simultaneously involving both sides of the body are highly suggestive of vertebral-basilar ischemia; so, also, is unilateral weakness or sensory loss along with evidence of cranial nerve symptomatology, especially vertigo or oculomotor dysfunction producing diplopia. The variety of symptoms experienced by patients with vertebral-basilar disease reflects the anatomic substrate subserved by the vertebral and basilar arteries and their branches. A guide to the origin of common and uncommon symptoms is given in Table 494–8.

Certain symptoms cannot be accurately localized if they occur in isolation. For example, a transient monoplegia or even a hemiplegia may arise from dysfunction of the hemisphere, either cortical or capsular, but might originate from the corticospinal tract in the ventral brainstem. Corresponding sensory phenomena may be equally difficult to localize. The occurrence or recurrence of dysarthria may be from the involvement of corticobulbar fibers coming from the nondominant hemisphere and proceeding from this area of carotid supply down to their location in the brainstem with its vertebral-basilar supply. In general, such isolated dysarthria is more likely to result from carotid than vertebral-basilar insufficiency.

Five to 10 per cent of patients with TIA experience symptoms that reflect abnormalities in both the carotid and vertebral-basilar arterial territories. Careful analysis of characteristic carotid symptoms such as amaurosis fugax or dysphasia, or of vertebral-basilar symptoms such as simultaneous bilateral long tract involvement and dysfunction of cranial nerve nuclei, helps clarify the coincidence of anterior and posterior symptomatology.

Drop attacks, in which a fully conscious older person loses the ability to remain standing, have been attributed at times to vertebral-basilar ischemia. If they are within the framework of

TABLE 494–8. CORRELATION OF VERTEBRAL-BASILAR ISCHEMIC SYMPTOMS WITH ANATOMIC STRUCTURES

Symptom	Anatomic Structure
Common symptoms:	
Bilateral visual blurring	Visual cortex—occipital lobe
Diplopia	Oculomotor nuclei—midbrain and pons
Vertigo	Vestibular nuclei—medulla and pons
Bilateral, alternating, or "crossed" motor and sensory symptoms	Long motor and sensory tracts, cranial nerve nuclei
Ataxia	Cerebellum or cerebellar connections
Less common symptoms:	
Episodic unconsciousness, drowsy state	Reticular activating structures of midbrain and rostral connections
Tinnitus and deafness	Cochlear nuclei
Dysphagia	Tenth nerve nuclei
Nausea and vomiting	Vagus nerve area
Confused episodes	Bilateral temporal lobe, upper brainstem
Amnestic episodes, transient global amnesia	Bilateral temporal lobe
Visual hallucinations	Parietal-occipital region
Symptoms less readily localized:	
Isolated monoplegia or hemiplegia and similar sensory phenomena	? Possibly carotid ? Possibly vertebral-basilar
Dysarthria	? Possibly in brainstem ? Possibly nondominant hemisphere
Drop attacks	? Pontine reticular structures ? Ventral corticospinal tract

an otherwise typical constellation of vertebral-basilar symptoms, this is an acceptable explanation for the phenomenon. It is not certain whether the symptom reflects ventral brainstem ischemia or an ischemia of the pontine portion of the reticular activating structures responsible for the regulation of postural tone. Drop attacks that recur in isolation from other symptoms cannot be ascribed to arterial disease and they provide a diagnostic enigma. Akinetic seizures and cardiac arrhythmic events enter into the differential diagnosis.

Transient global amnesia (see Ch. 478) occurs fairly frequently in older persons. When the episodes occur in conjunction with typical vertebral-basilar ischemic phenomena, their cause may be assigned properly to an ischemic origin. When impaired circulation accounts for these occurrences, it is probable that the ischemia affects bilaterally the medial temporal lobes. Less global or "transient partial amnesia" sometimes occurs and appears to be an incomplete manifestation of a similar disturbance.

Headache is common in cerebrovascular disease. It may accompany TIA and also stroke. It is most common on the side of the ischemia, frontotemporally, but may lie on the opposite side or in the occiput. As a rule such headaches are mild and nonthrobbing, lasting from a few minutes to a few hours. Thomas Willis in 1664 described a violent headache in association with an asymptomatic occlusion of the carotid artery. The designation of "Willis' headache" for the pain associated with cerebral ischemia is appropriate and, as he suggested, may be due to dilatation of anastomotic arteries.

A number of symptoms in combination with others which are appropriately attributed to carotid and vertebral-basilar disease cannot be so designated if they occur or recur in isolation. They may reflect the earliest evidence of ischemia; but if they are not accompanied by other symptoms, their exact origin must remain in doubt. More common and prosaic conditions may be the cause. The list of such indeterminate isolated symptoms includes headache, episodic loss of consciousness, amnestic episodes, drop attacks, attacks of vertigo, deafness, diplopia, and dysarthria. Even in patients with known arterial disease, with neck and orbital bruits, such isolated symptoms cannot be assigned confidently to ischemia. Frequent but stereotyped recurrence of a single symptom speaks against ischemia and requires a search for alternative mechanisms.

DIFFERENTIAL DIAGNOSIS OF TIA. Transient episodes of hemispheric, brainstem, or retinal dysfunction cannot be equated automatically with ischemia. Other conditions may mimic circulatory disturbances by exhibiting recurrent symptoms of equally abrupt onset.

Every patient presenting with the symptom of amaurosis fugax requires close scrutiny for an alternative cause other than thromboembolism. Primary ocular conditions such as muscae volitantes ("floaters"), vitreous hemorrhage, glaucoma, and retinal detachment may be mistaken. Papilledema may be associated with transient visual obscurations, as may the early phases of the ischemic optic neuropathy secondary to giant-cell ("temporal") arteritis. Migrainous auras tend to be scintillating and hemianopic, but patients often mistakenly assume they are of monocular origin. Only occasionally does migraine produce truly monocular visual symptoms.

Localized sensory ischemic events may be difficult to distinguish from focal sensory seizures. Both may occur in the same subject, since a local area of ischemia may become an epileptogenic focus. The lack of a "march" in the ischemic episode is helpful in distinguishing it from sensory epilepsy.

Benign and malignant as well as primary and metastatic brain tumors, arteriovenous malformations, subdural hematomas, and on rare occasions multiple sclerosis may produce short-lived symptoms, coming and going and mimicking ischemia. A postictal paralysis (Todd's paralysis) must not be mistaken for a transient paresis of ischemic origin. Thrombi can develop in aneurysms, and some embolize to the territory of the involved artery with carotid or vertebral-basilar symptoms indistinguishable from those resulting from arteriosclerotic lesions.

Benign positional vertigo, Menière's disease, and other peripheral vestibular causes of vertigo can be mistaken for hindbrain ischemia, since there may be accompanying ataxia. Such patients often describe visual blurring in association with severe vertigo, and they may be syncopal, increasing the resemblance of their symptoms to those of a central lesion. The occurrence and aggravation of tinnitus and deafness with vertigo are useful in alerting the physician to a peripheral vestibular origin.

Vertigo, diplopia, slurred speech, and loss of consciousness may be manifestations of "basilar artery migraine." In such patients, motor and sensory phenomena may be marked because of hemisphere involvement—"hemiplegic migraine." The diagnosis of these uncommon varieties of florid migraine must be made cautiously and seldom in the absence of an accompanying family history. The other family members must manifest an equally striking aura, with accompanying hemicrania, usually developing in late adolescence and early adult life. An important distinction is that migraine of this dramatic type rarely has its onset during the late adult years. Structural lesions are to be suspected and "hemiplegic migraine" becomes a diagnosis by exclusion in middle-aged or older subjects.

Of special importance in the differential diagnosis of vertebral basilar insufficiency are cardiac and circulatory hemodynamic crises producing diffuse disturbances of cerebral perfusion. Most patients who develop complete heart block, as well as some afflicted with a sick sinus syndrome and a variety of tachyrhythmias, experience neurologic symptoms. Sudden loss of consciousness, convulsions, vertigo, and nonspecific dizziness are the common events. Confusion, amnesia, and diplopia may be described. Focal events mimicking TIA are uncommon.

COURSE AND PROGNOSIS. ***The Prognosis of Threatened Stroke.*** Prognosis for threatened stroke patients depends on a number of factors, especially on the particular pathogenesis of the threatening symptoms. Available data are drawn largely from the group of TIA patients and indicate that after the first warning symptoms there is a 5 to 6 per cent chance per year thereafter of stroke recurring and an equal possibility of death, more often from myocardial infarction than from stroke or nonvascular causes. Some evidence indicates that the first three months after the onset of TIA carries a slightly higher risk than subsequent time periods. The prognosis for patients with TIA, RIND, and minor stroke (PNS) is nearly identical. Figures are available from the Canadian Cooperative Study with respect to the specific variety of threatening stroke caused by atherothrombosis with artery-to-artery emboli. Among the 289 patients not given effective treatment, the probability of stroke and death in the first year after diagnosis was 13 per cent, by the end of the second and third years the cumulative stroke and death figures were 22 and 30 per cent, respectively. The outlook for untreated males was worse than for untreated females.

The Prognosis of Completed Stroke. About one fourth to one fifth of patients with either thrombotic or embolic cerebral infarction die with their first attack. This figure varies somewhat with the cause of the infarction and especially with other factors such as age, cardiac status, and the degree of neurologic disability. The mortality rises sharply with increasing age: for patients over the age of 70 and those with marked neurologic defects, coma, or extensive systemic vascular disease, the initial mortality approaches 50 per cent. Infarction of the ventral portions of the brainstem after basilar artery occlusion, especially with quadriplegia, carries a poor outlook, although good medical and nursing care may preserve a vegetative or severely disabled existence for long periods.

The prognosis for cerebral infarction is better in younger patients; in those with the least evidence of vascular disease at other sites, especially cardiovascular disease; and in those who do not have hypertension, diabetes, or severe neurologic defects.

About one fifth of patients who survive a cerebral infarction from atherosclerotic vascular disease suffer another stroke within the next 12 to 24 months. However, the most significant limiting factor on survival is not recurrent stroke but cardiovascular disease. Thus in the Cornell-Bellevue stroke series, fully half of the patients who survived the initial cerebral infarction died at a later date from myocardial infarction or cardiac failure.

Recurrence of cerebral infarction is common with cerebral emboli of any cause. Estimates made over varying time periods indicate the rate of recurrent strokes caused by cerebral emboli from rheumatic heart disease to be between 30 and 70 per cent. Including extracerebral sites, nearly all patients have more than one embolus. In rheumatic heart disease, 40 per cent of the recurrences take place within the first month of the original episode and 50 to 60 per cent within the first year. Each cerebral recurrence carries a strong chance of causing death or further neurologic disability.

Course of Completed Stroke. During the first 72 hours gradual worsening of neurologic deficits and incipient or increasing impairment of consciousness are frequent. The worsening is sometimes due to extension of the cerebral infarction because of progressive and extending thrombosis or because of further emboli breaking off from a proximal arterial or cardiac source. In many instances, however, worsening is caused by the spread of edema around the necrotic area. Nowadays edema can be visualized readily by the CT scan. Other causes of lethargy and stupor in patients with cerebral infarction are the presence of fever; the injudicious use of sedatives, tranquilizers, or narcotics; circulatory failure; respiratory embarrassment; electrolyte imbalance; or combinations of these.

Patients whose course is not complicated by severe cerebral edema usually show an early improvement in neurologic function. If some voluntary movement is preserved, a good chance exists for return of more. When function improves rapidly after the onset, the outlook for a good recovery is excellent. A slow return of function over weeks or months is associated with a less complete recovery. If flaccid paralysis persists from the onset with no return of voluntary movement after 30 to 60 days, the outlook for useful recovery is poor. Substantial sensory loss impairs the chances of recovery of motor function and interferes with the process of rehabilitation. With brainstem infarction, the course is usually one of gradual improvement if the infarct is localized in the lateral medullary area. Symptoms of nausea, vertigo, diplopia, difficulty in swallowing, hoarseness of voice, and ataxia lessen and many times disappear.

Recovery from cerebral infarction and return of limb function and speech may continue slowly for as long as one to two years, but most of the improvement takes place within the first two to three months.

MANAGEMENT OF CEREBRAL ISCHEMIA. ***Investigation of Stroke, PNS, RIND, and TIA.*** The investigation as well as the treatment program is influenced by a number of factors. Patients with complete and major strokes need not be submitted to the rigorous investigation required in patients with TIA, RIND, or PNS in whom worsening can still occur. The particular variety of ischemic stroke (atherothrombotic, cardiac emboli, lacunar infarction, hemodynamic, venous infarction) influences decisions regarding treatment, as does the location in carotid as opposed to vertebral-basilar arteries. Age, the condition of the other arteries in the body, the presence of other morbid conditions, and the presence or absence of any major organ failure affect the vigor with which the physician pursues investigation and treatment.

The general examination must evaluate the condition of the systemic arteries, especially those to the lower extremities, by palpation and auscultation of the femoral pulses, evaluation of pedal pulses, and the condition of the integumentary structures of the feet. The comparability of upper limb pulses and bilateral blood pressure readings is essential, since differences may betray serious subclavian disease compromising the origins of the vertebral arteries. Bruits located over the clavicular region and the course of the carotid arteries in the neck, the mastoid area, or the orbits suggest the presence of widespread arterial disease. One must carefully evaluate the heart, including its rhythm and ECG analysis, in order to exclude a recent myocardial infarction, mitral or aortic valve disease, and atrial fibrillation.

Evidence for heart disease should be pursued extensively if there is no overt evidence of vascular disease and particularly in younger normotensive individuals with cerebral ischemia. Twenty-four-hour cardiac ECG monitoring, echocardiography, and wall-motion studies using gated acquisition techniques can be valuable. These studies carry the greatest yield in patients with a history or physical signs suggestive of heart disease. In patients lacking symptoms or signs of heart disease these studies are useful most often in patients under the age of 45 years.

Lumbar puncture is required in a few cases of stroke or TIA, particularly if meningovascular syphilis is a serious consideration. It is not a part of a routine workup in most cases of cerebral ischemia. Electroencephalography (EEG) will be useful only if seizures occur at the onset or during the subsequent course of what appears to be cerebral ischemia. In TIA the EEG is of little practical value, and with a devastating stroke the procedure contributes little to the evaluation of the patient. Doppler sonography of the carotid arteries is a noninvasive technique to detect obstructive or seriously stenotic disease. The method is prone to error. The information it imparts rarely influences the immediate management of an acute stroke but is useful as a preliminary screening test in patients with TIA, RIND, and PNS. Its use in asymptomatic disease is discussed later in this chapter. The development of computer analysis of venous-bolus angiography, a safer method of visualizing the arteries than is routine arteriography, will replace many noninvasive studies, particularly when this new technology is improved to the point of yielding better resolution.

Risk factors should be evaluated in victims of stroke, especially in those with TIA, RIND, and PNS. The presence of hypertension, fasting cholesterol and triglyceride levels, hematocrit, and cigarette smoking habits should be ascertained. Diabetes is important, and recent evidence suggests that hyperglycemic patients suffer larger and more serious cerebral infarctions than do normoglycemic patients.

Cerebral angiography should be carried out if there is diagnostic doubt and the illness cannot be differentiated from an arteriovenous malformation or a giant aneurysm by clinical criteria. Usually, however, the CT scan is more valuable in diagnosing neoplasms. Carotid angiography is indicated to search for surgically treatable lesions if the clinical picture suggests disease in the territory of the carotid artery and the general condition of the patient or the severity of the stroke does not preclude consideration of endarterectomy. Angiography is not indicated in the evaluation of most patients with stroke arising in the vertebral-basilar territory.

All cases with stroke and threatened stroke ideally should receive a CT scan. The technique distinguishes among small unsuspected hemorrhages, old and recent infarctions, and hemorrhagic infarctions and excludes unsuspected space-occupying lesions whose symptoms may imitate vascular ischemia. A negative CT scan obtained several days after the onset of persisting signs of ischemia suggests a location in the brainstem or a lacunar infarction, especially in the hypertensive patient. CT scanning has made isotope brain scanning obsolete in the study of stroke and threatened stroke.

Treatment of Threatened Stroke (TIA, RIND, PNS). Once an accurate individualized decision regarding the pathogenesis of the ischemia has been made, the possibilities for preventive treatment include risk factor management, antispasmodic drugs, antithrombotic drugs, and surgical therapy.

Risk factors are not always amenable to successful manipulation. Heredity cannot be altered. It is not certain that the reduction of high blood lipids alters the outlook once symptoms have been experienced. No data indicate that the elimination of hyperglycemia by rigid diabetic regulation reduces stroke in patients with TIA, RIND, or PNS. Control of both hyperlipidemia and diabetes mellitus is indicated, however, despite the lack of satisfactory supportive data. Cigarette smoking should be eliminated. Hypertension demands therapy, and in all age groups and both sexes the systolic and diastolic pressures must be kept at or below 160 and 90 mm Hg. An increase in hematocrit with an accompanying increase in blood viscosity has been identified as an added risk factor if above 50 and probably should be controlled with the judicious use of phlebotomy. Cardiac abnormalities, whenever amenable to therapy, require careful attention. Carotid bruits are a recognized risk factor for stroke, but evidence to date fails to prove that their investigation and surgical treatment are justified.

Antispasmodics, vasodilators, and "vasoactive" drugs have been widely used and extensively promoted, but no evidence indicates that these preparations have any value in treatment.

Antithrombotic drugs, first introduced as heparin and Coumadin derivatives, remain controversial in stroke prevention. In cases of threatened stroke from emboli arising in mural thrombi following myocardial infarction, and in mitral stenosis with and without atrial fibrillation, their use has received fairly wide acceptance. In the former instance they need not be utilized after eight weeks. In the latter condition prolonged use is customary, since most cases of rheumatic heart disease with emboli have a high incidence of recurrent events over a long period of time, particularly within the year after the initial embolus.

Many authorities advise the use of anticoagulants for recently developed TIAs in carotid and vertebral-basilar territory, recommending them for two to three months or longer if a flurry of TIAs recur and are not relieved by platelet antiaggregant therapy. The data upon which this treatment is based are equivocal and the therapy is empirical. In progressing stroke, many workers advise the use of heparin followed by a few weeks of Coumadin treatment. Controlled studies with convincing data are lacking to establish this as a scientifically proven approach, and its use remains empirical. Anticoagulants alone or combined with platelet antiaggregant agents are usually recommended in the prevention of embolization following the insertion of a prosthetic heart valve. Anticoagulants are not of value in patients with a completed stroke. The administration of anticoagulants carries a risk of fatal intracerebral or other hemorrhage, and their administration always must be rigidly controlled.

Two large and several smaller clinical trials have evaluated platelet antiaggregants in TIA, RIND, and PNS. The weight of evidence indicates that aspirin is effective in preventing stroke and death in a significant number of patients threatened with atherothrombotic stroke. The benefit to females is uncertain: one of the large trials detected a male benefit only, while the other large trial appeared to indicate no particular difference in responsiveness by gender. No benefit has yet been demonstrated for the other known platelet antiaggregants, sulfinpyrazone and dipyridamole. Theoretical evidence, however, supports the hypothesis that the combination of aspirin with dipyridamole may be superior to either drug alone. Trials are underway to establish or disprove this possibility. The optimal dosage of aspirin is unsettled. Clinical studies in stroke prevention have employed 1 to 1.5 grams daily. The balance between the dose of aspirin that suppresses the production of the aggregating thromboxane A_2 from platelets, through cyclooxygenase inhibition, and the dose that suppresses the production of antiaggregating prostacyclin by the vascular endothelial cells, through similar cyclooxygenase inhibition, is under active study. Theoretical evidence indicates that lower doses of aspirin may affect the platelet and spare the inhibition of the more beneficial prostacyclin production. In time the problem of optimal dosage will be settled by clinical trial. For the moment, the best that can be stated is that present evidence from clinical trials favors the use of 1300 mg of aspirin daily. Little information exists on the use of platelet antiaggregants in patients threatened with stroke from cardiac emboli. Some preliminary data from patients with rheumatic heart disease encourage further study.

Special consideration for anticoagulant therapy is required for cerebral vein and sinus thrombosis. Because it is an example of thrombus formation in a slow-flowing venous system, the coagulation cascade is particularly operative. In addition there is a good possibility of accompanying crural thrombosis, and a hazard exists for spread of thrombus to other veins and sinuses and for extension down the jugular vein to produce fatal pulmonary embolism. The therapeutic dilemma is that cerebral venous infarction, as in the retina, is hemorrhagic. When the diagnosis is established by a combination of clinical evidence and whatever supporting radiologic information is available, a CT scan should be employed to exclude a gross amount of blood in the subarachnoid space or in the infarcted area. If CT scanning is not available, a brisk subarachnoid hemorrhage should be excluded by a lumbar puncture. If blood is not present, heparin therapy followed by Coumadin therapy is recommended for 8 to 12 weeks. If blood is found by either technique, anticoagulation should be withheld for 72 hours. These recommendations must be accepted as empirical because no better evidence is available.

Role of Surgery in Cerebral Atherothrombotic Disease. The realization that many patients with cerebral ischemia are afflicted with disease of the extracranial arteries, combined with the development of acceptably safe cerebral angiographic procedures and the development of surgical capability to operate on arterial lesions, culminated in the first carotid endarterectomy being carried out in 1952. The role of surgery in the management of lesions of the cerebral arteries continues to be under active study. The answers are not easily obtained, and it is well to weigh the decision carefully in all cases with the following guidelines:

1. Carotid endarterectomy has become common practice for patients with specific neurologic symptoms appropriate to a stenosed and/or ulcerated atheromatous lesion in the lower cervical portion of the internal carotid artery.

2. A single major randomized study was carried out to determine the benefit of carotid endarterectomy and found no advantage for surgery. However, the study was completed

before the improved skills in angiography and surgery of the past decade were available. The results of such a study might be improved if the controlled trial were repeated.

3. Cerebral angiography and carotid endarterectomy carry a small but definite risk even in the most expert hands. If the combination of morbidity and mortality from these two procedures in a given institution exceeds 3 per cent, it is likely that the patient will fare as well by medical management alone. The risk-benefit ratio is too low to place either of these procedures in inexperienced hands.

4. A carotid endarterectomy at the usual level of the carotid sinus will be a dubious advantage if there is evidence of a stenotic or ulcerated lesion intracranially that equals or exceeds in size that in the neck area.

5. Patients with vertebral artery symptoms are not considered candidates for surgery at present. Proximal lesions in the vertebral artery may be accessible, but there is little evidence that such patients benefit by endarterectomy. Patients with vertebral-basilar symptoms do not benefit from surgery on simultaneously stenosed but asymptomatic carotid lesions.

6. Whether or not surgery is performed in suitable candidates, risk factor management and the utilization of appropriate antithrombotic treatment must not be overlooked. No controlled study to determine the benefit of endarterectomy has been pursued since the benefits of risk factor management and antihypertensive treatment have been established.

7. Carotid endarterectomy in the presence of a completed stroke or in the presence of a complete arterial occlusion appropriate to the symptoms has no demonstrated value.

Final conclusions about the role of carotid endarterectomy in extracranial symptomatic vascular disease await careful future observations. In the interim patients should be subjected to this procedure only after careful analysis of the appropriateness and significance of the symptoms and a full awareness of the angiographic and surgical risks in the particular institution concerned.

Operations purporting to revascularize the brain have been perfected technically and are being applied in a preliminary way in stroke prevention. Some enthusiasts are utilizing the procedures in the treatment of developed stroke. The operation of superficial temporal to middle cerebral artery anastomosis is innovative, but its physiologic or clinical benefits are unproven. A multicenter collaborative trial is attempting to evaluate the benefit of such anastomoses in preventing stroke in susceptible patients. No major trial is being conducted to evaluate the procedure as a means of improving the neurologic condition of the patient with a developed infarction. This is of dubious potential benefit.

The Asymptomatic Carotid Lesion. A bruit detected on routine physical examination, or stenosis revealed by carotid angiography in an artery from which no symptoms have arisen, presents unresolved management questions that are the subject of strong difference of opinion. Long-term surveillance of several large series of patients with neck bruits has determined that a bruit frequently is an index of widespread arterial disease and that such bruits are associated with an increased risk of stroke. However, the resultant stroke often develops in arteries other than the one in which the bruit exists. Bruits are more common in females than in males, but the risk for stroke in males with bruits is greater than that in females. The incidence of bruits increases with age and with the existence of hypertension. Prophylactic endarterectomy has been practiced by some surgeons as a prelude to open heart and aortic surgery if asymptomatic carotid disease is detected in the preliminary arteriograms. The weight of present evidence argues against this practice. Cerebral ischemic events after these major procedures are most often due to emboli initiated by the cardiopulmonary bypass procedure rather than to hypotension and hemodynamic focal ischemia. Until carefully conducted studies reveal convincing evidence to the contrary, we recommend not operating on asymptomatic carotid lesions and bruits.

Treatment of Completed Stroke. Treatment of cerebral infarction is designed to preserve life, limit the extent of the infarction, reduce disability, and prevent recurrences.

Stroke victims present with the same life-threatening circumstances as do patients with other serious neurologic illness. The principles of therapy are the same: the maintenance of a proper airway; adequate fluid, electrolyte, and caloric intake; and adequate urinary output. Constant vigilance is required to prevent aspiration pneumonitis and avoid necrotic skin lesions at pressure points.

The development of cerebral edema threatens to extend the brain damage. Many programs have been recommended to control its development and spread in the ischemic brain but with little success. The results of treatment with osmolar agents are disappointing, unpredictable, and short lived. Nevertheless if patients with large hemispheric infarcts deteriorate, especially if they develop reduced brainstem function, hypertonic mannitol is administered quite often despite the lack of evidence for convincing benefit. The use of corticosteroids either alone or with mannitol has been largely discredited.

Experimental evidence in animals has suggested that deep barbiturate coma given immediately after stroke onset may reduce the ultimate neuronal damage from cerebral infarction. Clinical results have not shown any advantage for the procedure, and this drastic form of treatment cannot be recommended.

Efforts to increase cerebral blood flow to limit the amount of ischemic infarction have been attempted. Vasopressor as well as vasodilator regimens have been attempted by hyperoxygenation or by producing hypercarbia, neither with evidence of benefit.

Treatment in the later and convalescent stages of stroke should be directed toward lessening the deformity and disability and requires daily passive exercise of paretic limbs, and early ambulation with appropriate assistance.

Rehabilitation. Recovery from stroke depends mainly on spontaneous neurologic recovery. It may be assisted by learning to improve function and utilize alternatives, and this requires an active rehabilitation program. Programs of retraining should begin as soon as there is no longer evidence of increasing infarction. Stabilization of the neurologic findings for 12 to 24 hours is usually sufficient evidence to permit the start of rehabilitation. All programs have as their goal the retraining of the remaining functions for maximal effectiveness. Although a few patients require and benefit from special hospital facilities for rehabilitation, most such programs can be carried out on medical services without the aid of extensive equipment. An internist or general physician who is interested in rehabilitation can direct programs of activity and exercise, and can achieve results in rehabilitating hemiplegic patients which are about as effective as those of specialized centers.

The first requirement is to increase the patient's tolerance to sitting and standing, both of which are impaired by weakness and by changes in the sense of balance. Patients are allowed to sit up and then stand for increasingly long periods, beginning with five to ten minutes several times a day. During this period daily active and passive exercises of the weakened extremities are carried out. When patients begin to stand they need firm support and often splinting or bracing of the knee on the weakened side; marked quadriceps weakness may occasionally demand a long leg brace. Ambulation is one of the main goals of rehabilitation. Gait training should begin as soon as the patient can comfortably stand for 15 to 20 minutes without fatigue. The support of parallel bars or a walker should be depended upon at first. After ambulation begins, it may be necessary to brace the foot to avoid the foot drop and inversion that commonly occur after hemiplegia. At the same time that the patient is relearning to walk, he should be trained to develop new skills with his unaffected arm and to improve the strength and function in the paretic arm. This is done by an active program of exercise and by retraining the patient in the activities of daily living such as eating, dressing and undressing, and personal hygiene. Usually the maximal effect of rehabilitation and recovery is gained in three to four months, but some patients continue to show improvement over periods lasting as long as two years. Passive exercise must be continued indefinitely for severely paralyzed patients if contractures are to be avoided.

A painful shoulder resulting from periarthritic changes is common after hemiplegia and may develop despite early passive motion of the member. Continued passive movements combined with heat and, if persistent, with subacromial steroid injection or a short course of systemic steroids will avoid additional pain and permanent fixation of the shoulder adduction movements.

For patients with cerebral infarction who have mild to moderate dysphasia, speech therapy may be helpful. It encourages patients and their families to be aggressive about the need to practice talking and gives considerable encouragement. Speech therapy does not help severe dysphasia.

HYPERTENSIVE ENCEPHALOPATHY. Hypertensive encephalopathy is an uncommon acute neurologic disorder characterized by attacks of headache, nausea, vomiting, visual impairment, focal or generalized seizures, and drowsiness, which may proceed to stupor and coma. Transient focal deficits, including hemiparesis, dysphasia, and hemianopia, may occur. The blurred vision reflects cortical or local retinal ischemic changes, but it is not necessarily associated with retinal hemorrhage or papilledema. Although the latter retinal findings are present in many of the patients, in others the only abnormality is that of narrowing, often segmental, of the arterioles. The blood pressure as a rule is severely elevated. Some patients have had longstanding raised blood pressure with recent further elevation, whereas in others a markedly elevated pressure is a new development.

Hypertensive encephalopathy can complicate acute nephritis, chronic renal disease, eclampsia, and pheochromocytoma. Hypertensive crises and encephalopathy can follow the ingestion of a combination of monamine oxidase inhibiting drugs with food high in tyramine content. The crises can result from the abrupt withdrawal of antihypertensive therapy, particularly clonidine. Excessive autonomic stimulation by bladder or gastrointestinal distention can precipitate hypertensive encephalopathy in patients with acute and chronic spinal cord injuries that can be fatal if not promptly treated.

The brain at postmortem examination in hypertensive encephalopathy sometimes appears grossly normal. In others, the organ is swollen, with evidence of tentorial and cerebellar pressure cones. The average weight of the brain may not be above normal, and edema is not a universal finding even with a history of increased intracranial pressure and papilledema. Cut section reveals small petechial hemorrhages and sometimes larger hypertensive hemorrhages. Microscopically, one finds scattered small areas of infarction accompanied, in patients with longstanding hypertension, by hyaline necrosis of the arteriolar walls.

The pathogenesis of hypertensive encephalopathy is thought to be due to a breakdown in the normal process of cerebral autoregulation, the process whereby cerebral blood flow is maintained at relatively stable levels by arteriolar changes, despite fluctuations in the mean systemic arterial pressure. The intensity and speed of elevation of blood pressure in this condition exceeds the tolerance of the regulatory mechanisms, and a combination of segmentally narrowed and segmentally dilated arterioles results. It appears that the blood-brain barrier is disturbed and that through the segmentally dilated portions of the arterioles brain edema develops. Necrotic arterioles may lead to the creation of petechial and larger hemorrhages.

Uremia closely resembles hypertensive encephalopathy in its symptoms. Once that condition is ruled out by determining that the BUN is below 100 mg per deciliter, the differential diagnosis includes the more usual complications of severe hypertension, including isolated intracerebral hemorrhage, ischemic infarction related to atherothrombosis in large arteries, and lacunar infarction. These conditions are more likely to exhibit focal clinical signs which are florid and persistent. By contrast, the focal neurologic deficits in hypertensive encephalopathy tend to be transient, mild, and multifocal. Sudden increases in intracranial pressure from obstructive hydrocephalus, brain tumor, and subdural hematoma may precipitate severe hypertension, as may acute lead encephalopathy in children. All these conditions also cause papilledema and convulsions. A careful history and attention to the condition of the retinal arterioles, heart size, and the associated conditions in which hypertensive encephalopathy develops will be valuable in differential diagnosis.

Hypertensive encephalopathy is a medical emergency. Its treatment consists of the prompt lowering of the blood pressure, taking great care to avoid dropping it to hypotensive levels. The drug of choice is sodium nitroprusside administered parenterally. The goal of the treatment is to reduce the blood pressure to acceptable levels within 30 to 60 minutes by careful titration of the parenteral drug. Although the intracranial pressure is commonly raised, it will respond to lowering of the systemic pressure and separate therapeutic measures are not required. Hypercapnia can aggravate or precipitate hypertensive encephalopathy and is to be avoided. Convulsions should be treated with intravenous diazepam, 10 to 20 mg, repeated every 30 minutes if need be until the seizures stop, taking care not to suppress respirations. The maximal dosage should be kept between 100 and 150 mg in 24 hours. An alternative is to give phenytoin (Dilantin) through a duodenal tube or intravenously in a dose of 0.5 to 1 gram per day, although that drug is less useful for immediately terminating seizures. Oral phenytoin, 300 mg daily, can be given prophylactically for a few weeks after the acute stage has passed.

Provided that the blood pressure is manageable, that other organs are not in end-stage failure, and that the cause of the hypertension is remediable, the long-term prognosis for the patient promptly recognized and treated for hypertensive encephalopathy is good. Strict, continuing supervision and regulation of the blood pressure are mandatory. Hydrochlorothiazide, beta-blockers, and alpha-methyldopa, alone or in combination, are usually the most effective drugs.

Barnett HJM: Pathogenesis of transient ischemic attacks. *In* Scheinberg P (ed.): Cerebrovascular Diseases. New York, Raven Press, 1976, pp 1-21. *The varieties of this clinical phenomenon are delineated.*

Barnett HJM: Heart in ischemic stroke—a changing emphasis. Neurol Clin 1:291, 1983. *A description of the traditional and the more recently recognized cardiac sources for cerebral ischemia.*

Bousser MG, Eschwege E, Haguenau M, Lefaucconnier JM, Thibult N, Touboul D, Touboul PJ: "AICLA" controlled trial of aspirin and dipyridamole in the secondary prevention of athero-thrombotic cerebral ischemia. Stroke 14:5, 1983. *The second large controlled trial of aspirin in stroke prevention, demonstrating a 50 per cent risk-reduction in stroke for both sexes.*

Brice JG, Dowsett DJ, Lowe RD: Haemodynamic effects of carotid artery stenosis. Br Med J 2:1363, 1964. *A landmark study which indicates that a residual lumen of the carotid artery above 2 mm does not compromise blood flow or produce a pressure gradient.*

Canadian Cooperative Study Group: A randomized trial of aspirin and sulfinpyrazone in threatened stroke. N Engl J Med 299:35, 1978. *The controlled trial which indicated the efficacy of aspirin in stroke prevention in males.*

Chester EM, Dimitris P, Agamanolis DP, Banker BQ, Victor M: Hypertensive encephalopathy: A clinicopathologic study of 20 cases. Neurology 28:928, 1978. *A detailed study of the cerebral and systemic vascular changes found in patients dying with longstanding hypertension culminating in renal failure.*

Corrin LS, Sandok BA, Houser OW: Cerebral ischemic events in patients with carotid artery fibromuscular dysplasia. Arch Neurol 38:616, 1981. *A natural history study of patients with fibromuscular dysplasia indicative of a reasonably benign prognosis.*

Easton JD, Sherman DG: Progress in cerebrovascular disease. Management of cerebral embolism of cardiac origin. Stroke 11:433, 1980. *An excellent review of the risk of stroke from cardiac lesions with a discussion of therapeutic strategies for management.*

Fisher CM: Lacunes: Small, deep cerebral infarcts. Neurology 15:774, 1965. *A paper which led to the recent revival of interest in this important complication of hypertension.*

Genton E, Barnett HJM, Fields WS, Gent M, Hoak JC: Cerebral ischemia: The role of thrombosis and antithrombotic therapy. Stroke 8:150, 1977. *A review article on antithrombotic therapy of threatened stroke.*

Heyman A, Wilkinson W, Heyden S, Helms MJ, Bartel AG, Karp HR, Tyroler HA, Hames CG: Risk of stroke in asymptomatic persons with cervical arterial bruits. A population study in Evans Country, Georgia. N Engl J Med 302:838, 1980. *A long-term surveillance study of asymptomatic carotid bruits indicates that they predict an increased risk of stroke.*

Hypertension Detection and Follow-Up Program Cooperative Group: Five-year findings of the hypertension detection and follow-up program. 1. Reduction in mortality of persons with high blood pressure including mild hypertension. JAMA 242:2562, 1979. *The importance of mild to severe untreated hypertension carefully assessed in the best study to date.*

Mohr JP, Caplan LR, Melski JW, Goldstein RJ, Duncan GW, Kistler JP, Pessin MS, Bleich HL: The Harvard cooperative stroke registry: A prospective registry. Neurology 28:754, 1978. *The report of a prospective registry to determine the incidence of the varieties of stroke in the Boston Hospitals.*

Ross Russell RW: How does blood pressure cause stroke? Lancet 2:1283, 1975. *A thoughtful commentary on the modern concepts of the pathogenesis of the arteriolar reaction in the cerebral complications of hypertension.*

Sherman DG, Hart RG, Easton JD: Abrupt change in head positon and cerebral infarction. Stroke 12:2, 1981. *An updated report on the risk of vertebral artery lesions producing stroke from neck manipulation.*

Skinhoj E, Strandgaard S: Pathogenesis of hypertensive encephalopathy. Lancet 1:461, 1973. *A good introduction to modern concepts about the pathophysiology leading to the clinical picture of hypertensive encephalopathy.*

Soltero I, Liu K, Cooper R, Stamler J, Garside D: Trends in mortality from cerebrovascular diseases in the United States, 1960 to 1975. Stroke 9:549, 1978. *A discussion of the declining incidence of stroke and the probable factors responsible for the phenomenon.*

Wiebers DO, Whisnant JP, O'Fallon WM: Reversible ischemic neurologic deficit (RIND) in a community: Rochester, Minnesota, 1955–1974. Neurology 32:459, 1982. *Describes the incidence, prevalence, and prognosis of reversible ischemic neurologic deficit (RIND) and notes the lack of substantial difference from TIA.*

Wolf PA, Kannel WB, Gordon T, McNamara PM, Dawber TR: Asymptomatic carotid bruit and risk of stroke: The Framingham Study (abstract). Stroke 10:96, 1979. *An important reference for decision-making in regard to asymptomatic carotid bruit management.*

495. INTRACRANIAL HEMORRHAGE

Intracranial hemorrhage constitutes approximately 15 per cent of acute cerebrovascular disorders, usually with drastic consequences, since it results in an abrupt increase in the intracranial contents. Perhaps a majority of patients lose consciousness at least briefly, and many die without recovering awareness. Although there are many causes of intracranial hemorrhage, the anatomic locations of the bleeding importantly influence the clinical picture, and these fall into the following general categories: (1) *Subarachnoid hemorrhage* for the most part results from bleeding from arteries on the surface of the brain, and is limited to the space between the pial and the arachnoid membranes which contains the cerebrospinal fluid. (2) *Intracerebral hemorrhage* results from rupture of vessels within the substance of the brain. (3) Surface bleeding may extend into the brain, producing a combination of *subarachnoid hemorrhage and intracerebral hemorrhage*. (4) *Intraventricular hemorrhage* results from the extension of intracerebral hemorrhage or subarachnoid blood into the ventricles.

ETIOLOGY. Bleeding from aneurysms of arteries composing the circle of Willis and bleeding from arterioles damaged by hypertension or arteriosclerosis are the two most common causes of intracranial hemorrhage. Traumatic intracranial hemorrhage, which is also common, is discussed in Ch. 516. Table 495–1 lists the usual causes of spontaneous intracranial hemorrhage.

Arterial Aneurysms. "BERRY" ANEURYSMS. These are round or saccular dilatations characteristically found at arterial bifurcations on the circle of Willis and its major branches or connections. The cause of berry aneurysms is unsettled. Muscle and elastic tissue defects in the media, possibly of congenital origin, are subjected to the physical effects of pulsatile arterial pressure aggravated by turbulence in the circulation through the aneurysm. The result is a gradual distention and thinning of the weakened segment until the wall is no longer able to contain the blood under arterial pressure. Aneurysms under 4 to 5 mm in diameter rarely rupture, whereas most aneurysms that reach 5 to 7 mm are likely to bleed, usually from the dome. Some reach a size of 2 to 3 cm or more ("giant aneurysm") before rupturing, or never rupture at all and act as a mass lesion compressing adjacent structures. Atheromatous plaques form in some aneurysms and may contribute to weakening of the wall. Larger aneurysms develop thrombi which may calcify. This process thickens the wall and may account for the growth of some to giant size without rupture.

TABLE 495–1. CAUSES OF SPONTANEOUS INTRACRANIAL HEMORRHAGE

1. Arterial aneurysms
   a. "Berry" aneurysm
   b. Fusiform aneurysm
   c. Mycotic aneurysm
   d. Aneurysm with vasculitis
2. Cerebrovascular malformations
3. Hypertensive-atherosclerotic hemorrhage
4. Hemorrhage into brain tumor
5. Systemic bleeding diatheses
6. Hemorrhage with vasculopathies
7. Hemorrhage with intracranial venous infarction

Aneurysms and subarachnoid hemorrhage are more common in association with hypertension whether idiopathic or associated with coarctation of the aorta and polycystic renal disease. Aneurysms are known to rupture under conditions associated with sudden rise in blood pressure, including severe emotional excitement, violent argument, and physical exertion (e.g., athletic competition or coitus).

Intracranial aneurysms occur in all age groups but most commonly rupture in the fifth, sixth, and seventh decades. They are slightly more common in women than in men (3:2). Approximately 85 per cent of congenital berry aneurysms develop in the anterior part of the circle of Willis derived from the internal carotid artery and its major branches (Fig. 495–1). The most common site is at the origin of the posterior communicating artery from the internal carotid artery, followed in frequency by the middle cerebral and the anterior communicating arteries. Fifteen per cent of aneurysms arise from the vertebral or basilar arteries and their branches. Aneurysms are multiple in 15 to 20 per cent of patients and are associated with arteriovenous malformation (AVM) in a small number. In subjects examined in the Cooperative Aneurysm Study, 8 per cent of the AVMs were associated with single or multiple aneurysms.

FUSIFORM ANEURYSMS. These are spindle-shaped dilatations of arteriosclerotic origin arising along the course of the large arteries. They occur most commonly on the basilar artery and less frequently on the carotid artery. When small, fusiform aneurysms are asymptomatic, but they can enlarge sufficiently to interfere with the function of surrounding structures, including the cranial nerves at the base of the brain; some compress the brainstem, others mimic cerebellopontine angle tumors, and still others simulate pituitary and suprasellar neoplasms. The underlying arteriosclerotic disease may be associated with ischemic attacks or infarction in the territory supplied by the artery and its branches. Occasionally embolism may result from thrombi forming within a large fusiform aneurysm. Fusiform aneurysms are less frequently a site of hemorrhage than are berry aneurysms; when rupture occurs, it is more often fatal since it is not amenable to direct surgical management. Extreme arteriosclerotic elongation (ectasia) of the basilar artery may be the precursor to a fusiform aneurysm. Rarely, ectasia or fusiform basilar aneurysm has been described in association with communicating hydrocephalus in which the dilated tip of the elongated basilar artery interferes with the normal cerebrospinal fluid outflow from the third ventricle and along the subarachnoid space.

MYCOTIC ANEURYSMS. Septic emboli from acute and subacute bacterial endocarditis result in arterial necrosis, which may lead to thrombosis or aneurysm formation at the site of lodgment. Such aneurysms tend to arise in a diagnostically characteristic location along the distal branches of the middle and anterior cerebral arteries rather than at the base. Frequently they are multiple.

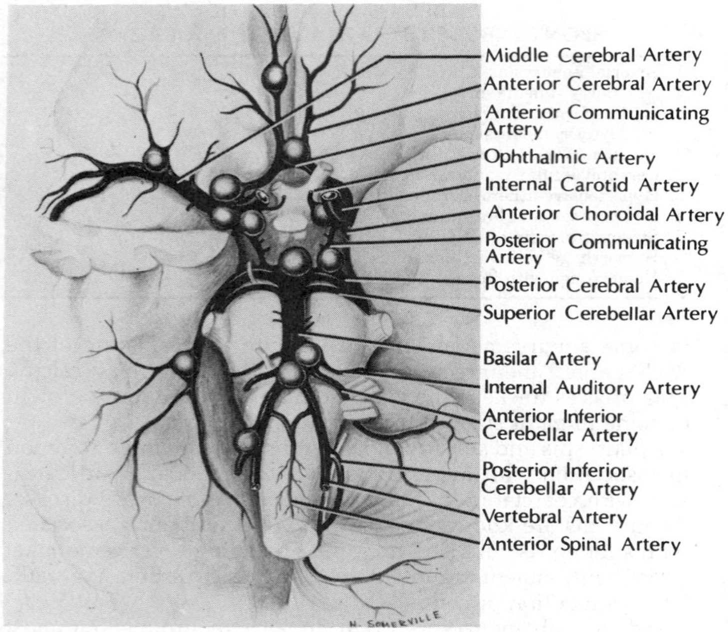

Figure 495–1. The common sites for berry aneurysms to develop at the bifurcation of arteries on the undersurface of the brain.

ANEURYSMS WITH VASCULITIS. A rare form of aneurysm is associated with collagen vascular disease, usually polyarteritis nodosa. Recently a vasculitis has been described in individuals practicing drug abuse, particularly the abuse of amphetamines. The resultant arteriopathy produces irregularly dilated segments, one of which may rupture to produce subarachnoid and intracerebral hemorrhage.

Cerebrovascular Malformations. Vascular malformations within and on the surface of the brain parenchyma constitute about 7 per cent of cases with subarachnoid hemorrhage. Four varieties are recognized: capillary telangiectasia, cavernous angioma, venous angioma, and arteriovenous malformation (AVM). Capillary telangiectasias are found most commonly as incidental postmortem findings in the brainstem; occasionally they cause bleeding into the brainstem. Venous angiomas often are the cerebrovascular abnormality associated with the Sturge-Weber syndrome. Most commonly they present with seizures; less often, with hemorrhage. Cavernous angiomas are the cause of many examples of cryptic intracerebral hemorrhage—"cryptic" since the vessels are not outlined by angiography. These lesions may be discovered at postmortem examination or during the excision of a hematoma. Their usual location is in the subcortical white matter. For unknown reasons cavernous angiomas occur twice as commonly in females as in males.

AVMs produce symptoms more commonly than the other types of cerebral vascular malformations. The malformations consist of tangled, interconnected networks of vessels in which arterial blood passes directly to the draining veins without intervening capillaries. They range in size from barely detectable lesions up to huge networks large enough to occupy an entire lobe of the brain, or to cover most of one cerebral hemisphere. They occasionally involve the cerebellum and brainstem. AVMs tend to be supplied by more than one parent artery, and the draining veins may be as large as 1 cm in diameter. It is uncertain how often AVMs rupture, but at least small bleedings appear to occur in more than 50 per cent of cases. Others declare themselves with recurrent unilateral headache of migraine type (an unusual cause for migraine, however), with epileptic seizures, or by producing a slowly increasing neurologic defect. Most AVMs do not increase much in size once they have been detected. When enlargement occurs, it is in association with small hemorrhage or with thrombosis of draining veins. Progressive neurologic disability may occur because of pressure of the abnormal arteries upon the underlying brain or possibly from shunting of blood into the malformation rather than to the underlying brain (an "intracranial steal").

Hypertensive-Arteriosclerotic Hemorrhage. At least two thirds of parenchymatous cerebral hemorrhages in adults are accompanied by clinical or pathologic evidence of systemic hypertensive vascular disease. Most of the remainder occur in subjects showing atherosclerotic vascular changes. With the increase in availability of CT scanning, small intracerebral hemorrhages in all lobes have been identified more often than were previously suspected. Most such lobar hemorrhages present as minor strokes in hypertensive or elderly patients and are initially misdiagnosed as ischemic lesions.

Hemorrhage into Brain Tumor. Primary and metastatic tumors of the brain may be the site of hemorrhage. Apoplectic onset is encountered with tumors that are benign or malignant, primary or metastatic. Hemorrhage is most common in rapidly growing malignant gliomas and very vascular secondary tumors (e.g., melanotic carcinoma; renal, thyroid, chorionic, and bronchogenic carcinoma). Bleeding complicates the clinical course in some benign brain tumors, including meningioma and pituitary adenoma, and in some slowly growing gliomas, including oligodendroglioma.

Systemic Bleeding Diatheses. Intracerebral hemorrhage complicates leukemia, aplastic anemia, thrombocytopenic purpura, hemophilia, and a variety of less common bleeding diseases. Usually there is evidence of bleeding elsewhere. The hemorrhage in the brain involves more locations than is usual in hypertensive hemorrhage, including superficial cortical areas. Multiple hemorrhages may occur, particularly in thrombotic thrombocytopenic purpura and with the consumption coagulopathies. Thrombotic infarction may accompany the hemorrhagic tendency in some instances. The primary process may lie in the vessel wall rather than in the circulating blood.

Anticoagulant therapy can be complicated by intracerebral as well as extradural, subdural, and subarachnoid hemorrhage. In the case of the intracranial surface clots, trauma is a major precipitant, but in many instances no history of injury can be obtained. When the intracerebral hematomas are in the usual locations for hypertensive hemorrhages, the relation to the anticoagulation will be uncertain and possibly incidental. By contrast a subcortical location of a hematoma is uncommon in spontaneous hypertensive hemorrhage. Extension through the pia into the subarachnoid space is common in hematoma complicating anticoagulation therapy and uncommon in spontaneous hypertension cases.

Hemorrhage with Vasculopathies. Polyarteritis nodosa is the most significant nonarteriosclerotic degenerative disease of arteries producing intracerebral hemorrhage. It may do so by causing an aneurysmal dilatation or by producing necrotic disruption of the artery. Cerebral hemorrhage with systemic lupus erythematosus is usually secondary to accompanying hypertension. Congophilic (amyloid) angiopathy is associated with intracerebral hemorrhage and occurs in older nonhypertensive patients. The usual presentation is by a sudden apoplexy with signs of cerebral hemorrhage in a patient with a recent history of progressing dementia. Such hemorrhages are often multiple and affect sites not common in hypertensive intracerebral hemorrhage. "Lobar" (white matter) hematomas in older patients are more often associated with this vascular lesion than with any other pathologic entity. When, in patients over 60 years of age, more than one lobar hematoma develops within a few days or weeks of the initial hemorrhage, the diagnosis of hemorrhage from congophilic angiopathy is reasonably certain. This amyloid degeneration of the cerebral arterioles is six times more common in women than in men and is not associated with systemic amyloidosis. Drug abuse, particularly the use of amphetamines, is associated with intracerebral hemorrhage. These hemorrhages are frontal, are occasionally ganglionic, may extend into the subarachnoid space or the ventricles, and are the accompaniment of a vasculitis in most of the cases that have been examined in detail.

Hemorrhage with Intracranial Venous Infarction. This presents most commonly in association with the complex findings described for septic or nonseptic lateral, sagittal, and cavernous sinus thrombosis (see Ch. 494). The finding of blood in cerebrospinal fluid coupled with seizures at the onset sometimes makes it difficult to distinguish between this condition and an aneurysmal rupture on clinical examination alone.

PATHOLOGIC CONSEQUENCES OF ANEURYSM RUPTURE. Aneurysms lie within the subarachnoid space, and their rupture introduces blood into this space under arterial pressure. The bleeding may be minimal and emerge through a very small tear in the sac. At the other extreme there may be sufficient bleeding to fill the basal cisterns, or to produce a hematoma locally distorting the subarachnoid space and the overlying brain. Such hemorrhages can be under sufficient pressure to cause reflux into the fourth ventricle through the foramina of Magendie and Luschka and to fill and distend the ventricles with blood. Also, aneurysms in any of the usual locations commonly send their jet of blood directly into the parenchyma of the brain. Anterior communicating artery aneurysms lying adjacent to the medial surface of the frontal lobes, and middle cerebral artery aneurysms lying within the sylvian fissure adjacent to the frontal and temporal lobes, are particularly prone to rupture into the brain. Anterior communicating aneurysms may rupture into both frontal lobes. Basilar artery aneurysms may rupture into the diencephalon or midbrain. Such intracerebral hemorrhages commonly extend through the brain substance and rupture secondarily into the ventricles.

Aneurysm rupture may include hemorrhage into the adjacent cranial nerves. The most common cranial nerve to be implicated is the third nerve, owing to rupture of an aneurysm at the point of origin of the posterior communicating artery from the internal carotid artery. Much less commonly, third nerve palsy is due to a basilar artery aneurysm. The optic nerve commonly is involved with ophthalmic artery aneurysms, and carotid aneurysms in the cavernous sinus involve the three cranial nerves acting on the muscles of the eye (III, IV, VI) and the first division of the trigeminal nerve. The distortions resulting from increased intracranial pressure commonly result in unilateral or bilateral sixth nerve palsies. Most cranial nerve palsies developing in patients with aneurysm result from bleeding in the nerve and not from compression of the nerve by the aneurysm. Large aneurysms, acting as space-occupying lesions, may damage cranial nerves progressively by compression.

Adherence of the dome of the aneurysm to the arachnoid may result in rupture into the subdural space, and a substantial quantity of subdural blood is present at postmortem examination in approximately 10 per cent of patients who die of ruptured aneurysm. Rarely, such a subdural hematoma occurs with little or no subarachnoid bleeding.

Rupture of an aneurysm produces a sudden increase in the intracranial pressure. Several mechanisms are involved. In the first place, an expanding hematoma, whether intracerebral, intraventricular, subdural, or subarachnoid, represents an abruptly enlarging space-occupying lesion. Also, blood in the basal cistern interrupts the natural flow of cerebrospinal fluid. Finally, if the pacchionian granulations become distended with blood, the reabsorption of the spinal fluid is impeded. Papilledema and subhyaloid hemorrhage in the retina follow, with coma and deterioration of brainstem function, and secondary hemorrhages develop within the midbrain.

As a late sequel to subarachnoid hemorrhage, hydrocephalus may develop or persist. The cerebrospinal fluid pressure measurements, although moderately elevated, tend to approach normal—an example of so-called "normal-pressure" hydrocephalus. Some examples of this complication are known to be sequelae to a fibrosing reaction in the basal cisterns, in particular the cisterna ambiens, producing, in effect, an extraventricular obstructive phenomenon. Others may be associated with ventricular ependymal damage and a change in the hydrodynamics of cerebrospinal fluid circulation, with accumulation of interstitial fluid in the subependymal tissue. Both causes create a form of communicating hydrocephalus.

Ischemic infarction of the brain is common in patients with subarachnoid hemorrhage. This is rarely due to arterial or venous thrombosis but is associated with segmental and at times extensive reactive narrowing of the intracranial arteries, termed vasospasm. As observed in arteriograms, cerebral vasospasm usually appears four to ten days after subarachnoid hemorrhage and develops in more than one third of patients suffering a ruptured aneurysm. In the absence of a further hemorrhage, vasospasm causes focal neurologic deterioration of 20 per cent of individuals following subarachnoid hemorrhage. Vasospasm is most marked in the territory of arteries adjacent to the bleeding point and tends to be less when the bleeding is slight. Vasoactive substances, including prostaglandins, serotonin, catecholamines, and methemoglobin, are released by the blood in the subarachnoid space and are believed to precipitate this vasospastic response. Desquamation of the endothelial cells, followed by platelet-fibrin thrombogenesis in the affected arteries, has been described. Edema, necrosis of the media, and intimal proliferation have been described as sequelae to the initial chemically induced vasospasm.

CLINICAL FEATURES OF SUBARACHNOID HEMORRHAGE. The location of the bleeding is the main determinant in the clinical presentation: aneurysms that rupture entirely into the subarachnoid space present with features of meningeal irritation or transiently increased intracranial pressure; with the formation of an intracerebral hematoma or when the blood ruptures into the ventricles, more devastating signs develop. Direct involvement of adjacent cranial nerves produces specific focal features (e.g., a third nerve palsy with posterior communicating and basilar aneurysms). Vasospasm and obstruction of the cerebrospinal fluid pathways impose new clinical signs. The most common symptom of subarachnoid hemorrhage is the sudden development of a violent headache. At the onset many patients localize the headache frontally or temporally. Soon it becomes occipital, spreads to involve the entire head and neck, and at times radiates down the spine and the backs of the legs. Arterial distortion and injury produce the first head pain, and the spreading discomfort is due to increased intracranial pressure and meningeal irritation.

The initial hemorrhage may be minor, a "warning leak" characterized by the sudden development of a headache usually severe but sometimes only moderately intense, with or without associated neck stiffness. This type of headache in an adult not prone to headache may disappear in two to three days, but demands that subarachnoid hemorrhage be considered. If hemorrhage is suspected, a diagnostic lumbar puncture must be done, since subsequent rupture is often more devastating, and in many instances fatal. The initial hemorrhage often is preceded by no other warning symptoms, but some patients complain of minor neurologic symptoms in the days or weeks prior to the major event. Although emotional excitement and physical exertion are known to precipitate the hemorrhage in some patients, they occur as well during sleep. Possibly this is because surges of increased blood pressure occur during the REM phases of sleep.

Brief loss of consciousness or seizures are common at the onset, preceded by an awareness of dizziness or vertigo and by vomiting. Persistent coma usually means massive intracerebral or intraventricular bleeding. Recovery of consciousness in a few minutes is the rule if the bleeding is confined to the subarachnoid space or is localized as a small intracerebral hematoma. The development of brainstem signs commonly indicates transtentorial compression, but occasionally indicates a posterior fossa aneurysm with rupture into the brainstem.

Neck rigidity is the most common physical sign; if severe bleeding has occurred, it produces retraction of the neck into hyperextension. Small, round hemorrhages observable by funduscopic examination over or near the optic nerve head have a "subhyaloid" or preretinal location and may be associated with the early development of papilledema. These changes reflect the fact that the optic nerve sheath is surrounded by an extension of the subarachnoid space, and an abrupt rise in the cerebrospinal fluid pressure interferes with venous return from the retina.

Cranial nerve palsies are usually the result of direct hemorrhage into the particular nerves. Secondary distortions from the mass effect of a hematoma can impair the function of cranial nerves emerging from the brainstem. Hemorrhages occurring within the brainstem account for some cranial nerve palsies.

When lateralizing signs, including hemiplegia, develop at the beginning or within a few hours, an intracerebral hematoma, a large subdural hematoma, or occasionally a subarachnoid hematoma is the usual cause. If such signs develop after several days without a fresh and violent headache, one suspects the presence of vasospasm producing ischemia and infarction. Delirium is a common and nonspecific symptom with subarachnoid hemorrhage; gradual deterioration of consciousness, after three or four days with or without an accompanying worsening of pre-existing neurologic deficits, suggests the development of hydrocephalus with increasing intracranial pressure.

Systemic signs include low-grade fever, glycosuria, albuminuria, and a peripheral white blood cell count up to 15,000. A massive outpouring of systemic catecholamines may cause multifocal micronecrosis of the myocardium, which can produce ECG abnormalities that simulate the changes of myocardial infarction. An occasional patient with subarachnoid hemorrhage develops acute pulmonary edema. Others develop the syndrome of inappropriate antidiuretic hormone secretion (SIADH).

Little other than the past history clinically distinguishes the symptoms of subarachnoid hemorrhage resulting from the rupture of an AVM from those that emanate from a ruptured aneurysm. Intracerebral bleeding is more common with AVMs since most of them lie within the brain. Accordingly, focal neurologic signs and evidence of the sudden development of a mass lesion are frequent accompaniments of a rupture. The presence of an AVM as the cause of subarachnoid hemorrhage is suggested by a history of previous focal seizures, by indolently or slowly stepwise progressing focal neurologic signs, and occasionally by recurrent unilateral throbbing headache suggesting migraine. In addition to meningeal irritation and focal neurologic signs reflecting bleeding, one finds a bruit over the orbit or skull in approximately 40 per cent of patients. Apart from occasional giant aneurysms, bruits are not audible with berry aneurysms.

LABORATORY INVESTIGATION OF SUBARACHNOID HEMORRHAGE. Cerebrospinal fluid examination by lumbar puncture is indicated in all patients with suspected subarachnoid hemorrhage unless computed tomography (CT) has been carried out and identifies blood in the subarachnoid space and/or brain and ventricles. With blood identified by CT scan little is gained by cerebrospinal fluid examination, and angiography becomes the next step in diagnosis. Furthermore, in the presence of an intracerebral hematoma lumbar puncture adds an unnecessary risk of inducing pressure coning. Small subarachnoid hemorrhages often fail to cast their shadow on the CT scan. Accordingly, in spite of a negative CT examination, if the history or signs suggest subarachnoid bleeding, a lumbar puncture is obligatory. If a CT scan is not available, lumbar puncture should be done whenever there is reasonable cause to suspect subarachnoid hemorrhage and provided that there are no signs of a mass lesion. The CT scan evidence of bleeding diminishes rapidly after the first week and should be supplemented with a lumbar puncture seeking discolored fluid, increased cells, or protein.

Confusion may result when bloody cerebrospinal fluid is encountered after a "traumatic" lumbar puncture. Even the most careful insertion of a lumbar puncture needle sometimes causes local bleeding. Usually when this occurs, the fluid dripping from the needle hub is streaked with blood and, as the fluid is collected, the amount of blood decreases in each successive tube. It is imperative, whenever cerebrospinal fluid is obtained, to compare it to water in an identical tube. Normal cerebrospinal fluid is as crystal clear and colorless as tap water. If the fluid is pink or bloody, it should be immediately centrifuged for five minutes and the supernatant visually recompared with water. Pink or yellow discoloration (xanthochromia) of the supernatant, caused by blood or the degradation of hemoglobin in the hypotonic cerebrospinal fluid, is a certain sign of subarachnoid hemorrhage. The supernatant of a freshly spun tube of blood from a traumatic tap will be clear and colorless. A repeat lumbar puncture several hours after a traumatic tap may exhibit xanthochromia. Since fresh blood left standing in cerebrospinal fluid on the way to a hospital laboratory will undergo lysis and discolor the supernatant, one should centrifuge the obtained specimen immediately.

Immediately after a subarachnoid hemorrhage, the proportion of white to red blood cells in the cerebrospinal fluid is the same as in the peripheral blood. After the lapse of 12 hours or more, the white blood count rises from the meningeal irritation; in a few days, when the red cells have become crenated, there may be as many as 500 polymorphs and lymphocytes, followed a few days later by lymphocytes alone. The protein content slowly increases to as high as 80 to 100 mg; the glucose content declines slightly at most. During the first two weeks or so, the cerebrospinal fluid pressure commonly rises to levels of 200 to 300 mm, and at times readings as high as 500 mm will be recorded owing to an associated communicating hydrocephalus.

COMPUTED TOMOGRAPHY. Immediate CT examination demonstrates blood in the subarachnoid space in about 95 per cent of cases of ruptured aneurysm or AVM. The technique will not demonstrate the high density of blood in cases in which the CT scan is delayed. Less than 30 per cent of cases of ruptured aneurysms show blood in the subarachnoid space four days after the hemorrhage. The CT scan is invaluable in the detection of intracerebral, intraventricular, subdural, and occasional subarachnoid hematomas, and has become an essential part of the optimal study of patients with subarachnoid hemorrhage. The finding of a subarachnoid clot in the CT scan in the first 24 hours following a subarachnoid hemorrhage greatly increases the likelihood that vasospasm will complicate the patient's course. Aneurysms larger than 5 mm in diameter often are directly visualized by this technique, particularly after contrast enhancement. Serial CT studies help determine whether new symptoms are related to rebleeding, ischemia secondary to vasospasm, the development of edema surrounding previous intracerebral bleeding, or hydrocephalus.

ARTERIOGRAPHY. The cerebral angiogram remains the definitive procedure to identify aneurysms and AVMs. The procedure is performed in all cases of subarachnoid hemorrhage that are considered reasonable operative risks or when diagnostic doubt exists. Four-vessel angiography is mandatory because 15 per cent of aneurysms occur in the posterior circulation, because multiple aneurysms occur in another 15 per cent of patients, and because of the association of aneurysm with AVM in a small but important number of patients. When aneurysms are multiple, the largest and most irregular is usually the source of the hemorrhage. Angiography is essential to identify areas of local or general vasospasm and occasionally may have to be repeated pre- and postoperatively when new signs develop requiring the physician to differentiate between fresh bleeding and the development of vasospasm. The CT scan complements this investigation in determining whether most of the blood is subarachnoid, intracerebral, or subdural in location.

PROGNOSIS IN SUBARACHNOID HEMORRHAGE. Subarachnoid hemorrhage from ruptured aneurysm carries a grave prognosis. It has been estimated that 28,000 individuals per year in the United States experience a subarachnoid hemorrhage caused by a ruptured aneurysm and that 10,000 die or are disabled from the initial event without referral for treatment, 9,000 die or are disabled despite treatment, and 9,000 survive without major disability. In a 30-year survey of morbidity from Rochester, Minnesota, extending from 1945 to 1975, the probability of survival for 30 days from the onset of the first subarachnoid hemorrhage was only 42 per cent. Only 39 per cent of patients survived for six months, and of these 25 per cent were disabled. The first two weeks after the initial bleeding are the most hazardous for recurrence. Very late recurrences have been described as long as 20 years after the initial bleeding. Long-term studies of prognosis, involving at least a ten-year follow-up period, indicate that if patients survive six months from subarachnoid hemorrhage, rebleeding occurs at a rate of 3.5 to 4 per cent per year and the mortality from such rebleeding is about 65 per cent.

The prognosis for bleeding from AVMs is better than that for aneurysm. Initial mortality is 10 per cent, and subsequent rebleeding occurs in approximately 20 per cent at a rate for fatal recurrence of 1 per cent per year in one major series followed for 35 years. There is a slight increase in mortality for recurrent compared with initial bleeding. Neurologic disability in the patients who have bled is higher than in surviving aneurysm patients because of the usual intracerebral location of the malformations.

TREATMENT OF BERRY ANEURYSM. The goal of aneurysm treatment is to prevent further rupture of the aneurysm while maintaining normal cerebral perfusion. The logical approach to the management of a patient with a ruptured aneurysm is to exclude the thin-walled sac from the pressure of the arterial blood while concurrently maintaining the normal patency of the parent and adjacent branch vessels. This is best accomplished by surgically placing a small metal clip or ligature across the neck of the sac. Unfortunately, it has proved to be hazardous to submit a patient to immediate or emergency surgery following subarachnoid hemorrhage. At this point in time the brain is bruised and swollen, the normal arterial autoregulation is impaired, and surgical manipulation may hasten and aggravate the evolution of vasospasm. Accordingly, many surgeons delay eight to ten days before performing craniotomy, meanwhile reducing the patient's risk of rebleeding by the judicious control of blood pressure and the giving of antifibrinolytic agents. Collaborative investigation is under way in an effort to identify patients for whom early operation appears to be the correct approach. If the aneurysm cannot be directly obliterated, surgical ligation of a proximal vessel may be effective in reducing the risk of recurrent hemorrhage by reducing the pressure and turbulence within the sac. In the anterior circulation aneurysm, where the common or the internal carotid artery or one of the major intracranial branches must be ligated, some surgeons employ a preliminary superficial temporal to middle cerebral artery anastomosis to protect against the ischemic infarction that might otherwise be expected to develop.

Recent advances in technique, including the development of the operating microscope, improved angiography, the CT scan, improved anesthesia, controlled hypotension, and the modern management of vasospasm, have reduced the morbidity and mortality of patients considered appropriate for surgery. Nevertheless, many patients die first or never become suitable candidates for surgery so that subarachnoid hemorrhage from ruptured aneurysm retains a distressingly high morbidity and mortality. The risk of dying in the first eight weeks after rupture remains at 40 per cent. The following points are important in deciding on the management of these patients:

1. The best results from direct clipping of the neck of an aneurysm are obtained in patients who have no focal neurologic signs, have had no evidence of focal bleeding for seven to ten days, and have no evidence of vasospasm in an arteriogram performed immediately prior to surgery. Unfortunately by this time about 20 per cent of hospitalized patients have died or become disabled by rebleeding, infarction, or other complications.

2. A patient deteriorating from a hematoma or hydrocephalus may require urgent surgery to remove the mass and reduce the raised intracranial pressure. Usually the aneurysm will be dealt with at the same time. Patients already in stupor or coma, however, rarely do well with surgical treatment.

3. The presence of vasospasm requires delay of surgery until the spasm disappears or it is apparent that it is causing no further neurologic worsening. Blood volume expanders such as albumin or dextran with crystalloid are recommended to treat patients with evidence of spasm so as to improve intracranial blood flow.

4. During the period of delay prior to surgery careful pharmacologic control of the blood pressure and complete rest in a quiet environment must be sought. Epsilon-aminocaproic acid,* an inhibitor of fibrinolysis, administered in a dosage of 30 to 40 grams per day intravenously is believed by many to reduce the chance of rebleeding.

5. Occasional patients develop SIADH. Fluid and electrolyte intake should be monitored appropriately. The commonest electrolyte imbalance is the result not of excess antidiuretic hormone output but of excessive administration of 5 per cent dextrose solutions, causing iatrogenic hyponatremia.

6. Patients with subarachnoid hemorrhage are best treated in centers possessing experienced teams of neurologists, neurosurgeons, and radiologists rather than by inexperienced and occasional operators. In the hands of skilled surgeons most aneurysms can be dealt with successfully, provided that the complications of vasospasm, intracerebral hemorrhage, hydrocephalus, or continuing comatose states can be prevented.

7. Giant aneurysms rebleed in 30 per cent of cases. Removal is more hazardous than with berry aneurysms even in the hands of skilled and experienced surgeons. However, no other treatment can assuredly prevent progressive and disabling neurologic signs or fatal hemorrhage.

TREATMENT OF ARTERIOVENOUS MALFORMATION. Large AVMs should not be removed if they have not bled, especially if they are in an area of the brain where a surgical approach might damage vital neurologic function. Some malformations can be dissected out and removed. Those located in the frontal or occipital poles can sometimes be safely excised by lobectomy. Ligation of the feeding vessels coupled with balloon catheter embolization and the injection of plastic polymers into the vessels of the anomaly is being carried out in a few centers. Serious complications can occur, and its indications are regarded as uncertain and its value as unproved.

*This use is not listed in the manufacturer's directive.

PATHOLOGY OF SPONTANEOUS HYPERTENSIVE-ARTERIOSCLEROTIC INTRACEREBRAL HEMORRHAGE. Intracerebral hemorrhage as a consequence of arteriolar hypertensive disease tends to occur in five locations. The first two are the most common: external capsular–putaminal hemorrhage and internal capsular–thalamic hemorrhage. Central pontine hemorrhages and cerebellar hemorrhages are less common. Least common are hemorrhages in the subcortical white matter and centrum ovale, remote from the vital structures involved with the more usual varieties.

Hypertension hastens the progress of arteriosclerosis in the larger arteries, but in many patients it produces its most devastating effects on the arterioles. The arterioles of the capsular and ganglionic (lenticulostriate) branches of the middle and posterior cerebral arteries, those supplying the central pontine structures (penetrating branches of the basilar artery), and those lying in the central cerebellum are the sites of predilection for the characteristic arteriolar changes. These distinct changes affect the small intracerebral arteries 50 to 150 μm in diameter. Microaneurysms (Charcot-Bouchard aneurysms) form with loss of lining endothelium, media, and elastic tissue, and all are replaced by fibrous tissue. Fibrin and fat constitute the hyaline tissue within the walls, and the process is described by various names, including fibrinoid necrosis and lipohyalinosis. The penetrating arteries subject to these changes are peculiar in that they do not divide into smaller branches, and the suggestion has been made that they are more vulnerable to the direct transmission of marked fluctuations of blood pressure. These same penetrating small arteries develop necrotic degeneration leading to rupturing in some hypertensive patients, whereas in others a less necrotic process leads to lipohyalinosis with thrombi and lacunes.

Hypertensive-arteriosclerotic intracerebral hemorrhages tend to be catastrophic despite their origin from an arteriole of small size. It is postulated that one arteriole ruptures, producing a small hemorrhage, and that this in turn compresses surrounding tissues. Ischemia from this compression is thought to speed the process of necrotic degeneration of adjacent arterioles, producing a "cascade" effect and an expanding area of hemorrhage. Hemorrhages in the cerebral hemisphere tend to dissect along fiber pathways and rupture into the ventricles. Relatively few extend directly into the subarachnoid space, although secondary drainage into the subarachnoid space from the ventricles is common. Pontine and cerebellar hemorrhages extend into the subarachnoid space either by direct extension or indirectly through the fourth ventricle. Massive intracerebral hemorrhage often shifts the brain tissue under the falx or downward through the tentorium, leading to secondary brainstem hemorrhage, attributed to a combination of venous obstruction and arterial ischemia. Many smaller hemorrhages remain circumscribed but may be associated with extending edema of the surrounding brain.

CLINICAL MANIFESTATIONS OF SPONTANEOUS INTRACEREBRAL HEMORRHAGE (Fig. 495–2). Intracranial bleeding develops abruptly and evolves over a period of minutes to hours. The ictus usually occurs while the patient is awake and active as compared to thrombotic obstructions, which more commonly occur during sleep. With a typical onset the patient cries out with the intensity of head pain or complains of distressing dizziness. Frequently there is a history of hypertension, and with the onset of bleeding the blood pressure can rise to excessively high levels. Cardiomegaly is common, and retinal arteriolar changes, although not always impressive, are observed within minutes to hours; 75 per cent of patients with a large hemorrhage (greater than 2 to 3 cm diameter by CT scan) will lose consciousness (Fig. 495–3). The associated physical findings depend on the size and site of the bleeding.

External Capsular–Putaminal Hemorrhage. Affected patients are likely to lose consciousness within minutes to hours and quickly develop evidence of hemiplegia. With smaller lesions there may be drowsiness without loss of awareness and the rapid evolution of a hemiplegic stroke. Conjugate deviation of the eyes to the side opposite the paretic limbs is common, but deviation toward the paralysis can occasionally reflect the irritative effects of the blood. Larger lesions compress the upper brainstem so that coma deepens, with dilated and fixed pupils, bilateral motor hypertonus, Babinski signs, and intermittent or irregular respirations.

Internal Capsular–Thalamic Hemorrhage. The onset is often not distinguishable from the more laterally located hemorrhage described above. In some instances there will be an awareness of sensory disturbances. If the patient is examined while still alert, a homonymous hemianopia may be detected because of the involvement of the optic radiation in the posterior limb of the internal capsule. The medial location of this hemorrhage and its compression of the tectal-midbrain area produce a variety of conjugate gaze palsies, including defective vertical and lateral gaze, fixed downward deviation of the eyes, unequal pupils briefly nonreactive to light, skew deviation, and retraction nystagmus.

Pontine Hemorrhage (Fig. 495–4A). Coma, accompanied by quadriplegia, decerebrate rigidity, and breathing irregularities, occurs early. The usual oculomotor sign is the finding of tiny pupils that are reactive to light; oculovestibular responses rapidly disappear. The majority of patients die after a few hours or days, but with the advent of CT scanning a larger number of nonfatal lesions are being diagnosed than were previously recognized. Most who survive are quadriparetic and severely disabled.

Cerebellar Hemorrhage (Fig. 495–4B). The clinical picture is ushered in with sudden occipital headache, diplopia, and incoordination. Early difficulty is experienced with stance and gait without prominent lateralizing ataxic signs. Vertigo is uncommon. The development is not as rapid as in pontine hemorrhage and usually evolves over several hours. Sixth nerve or conjugate lateral gaze palsies are common eye signs, but ocular bobbing and skew deviation can ensue, as can facial weakness, dysarthria, and dysphagia.

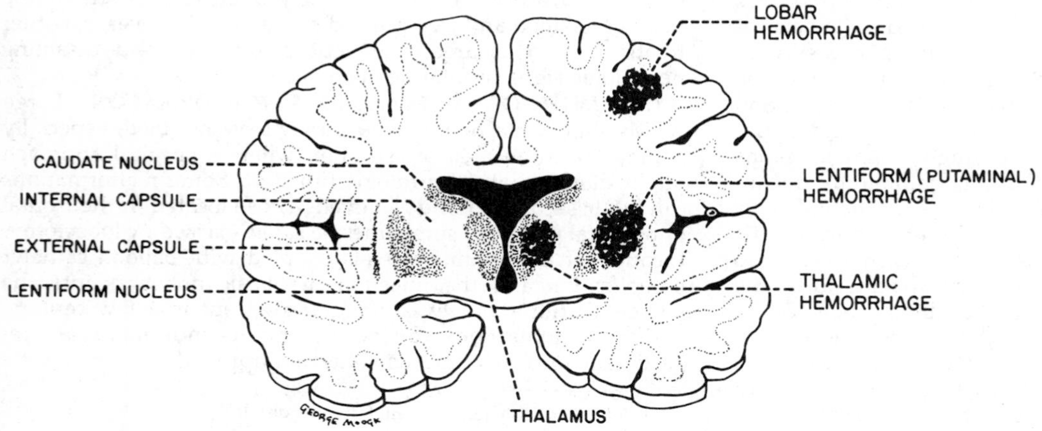

Figure 495–2. A coronal section through the cerebral hemispheres illustrating thalamic, putaminal, and lobar subcortical hemorrhages.

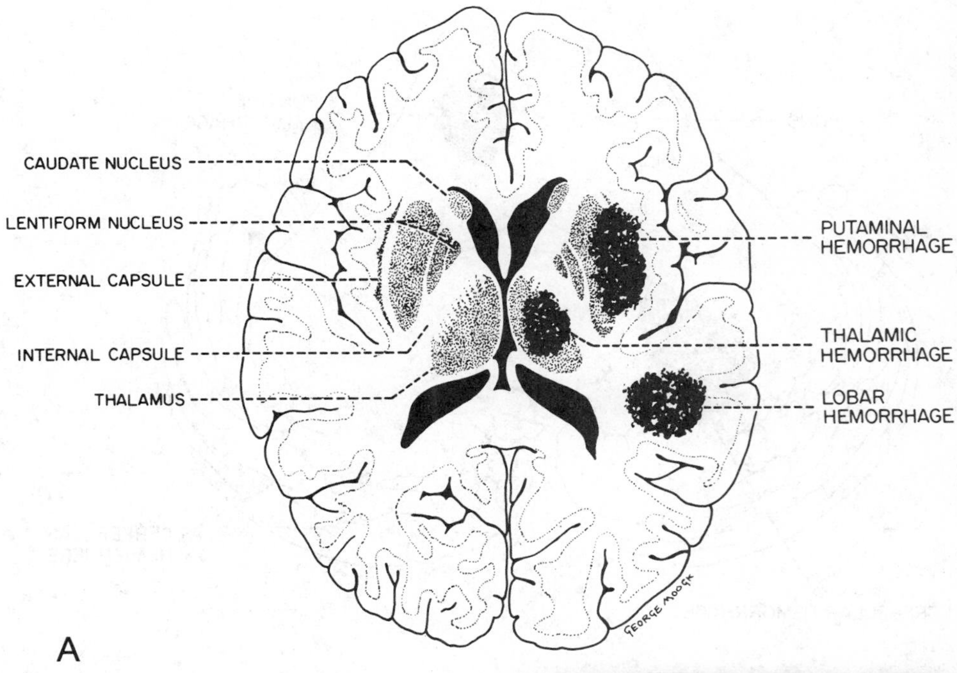

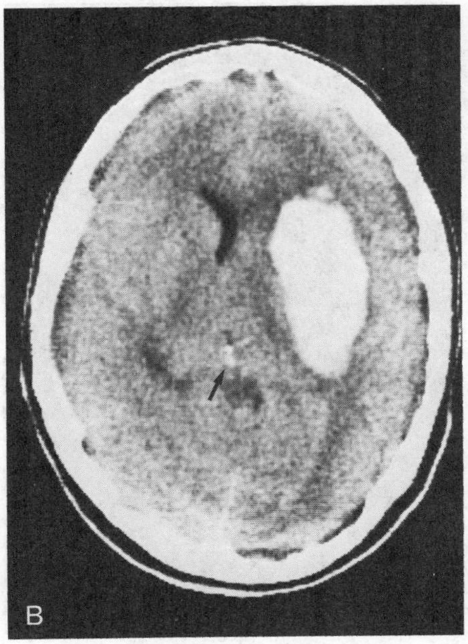

Figure 495–3. *A,* A horizontal section through the cerebral hemispheres illustrating thalamic, putaminal, and lobar hemorrhages. *B,* CT scan showing a putaminal hemorrhage. The ipsilateral lateral ventricle is obliterated by the mass effect and some blood is visible in the third ventricle (arrow).

Progressive worsening in these patients can occur either from enlargement of the hematoma and edema in surrounding tissue, producing pressure on the brainstem, or from obstruction by the mass of the fourth ventricle, leading to a subacute hydrocephalus with equally serious implications. Recognition of the condition is crucial, since surgical treatment can be lifesaving, as noted later in this chapter.

Hemorrhage in Subcortical White Matter. A small number of intracerebral hemorrhages in hypertensive individuals occur in less vital areas of the brain, generally in the centrum ovale. Such small white matter hemorrhages can produce the picture of progressing stroke. Spread of surrounding edema or further bleeding leads to clinical signs, including the development of drowsiness. However, many patients remain alert and do not develop evidence of subarachnoid bleeding. Spontaneous recovery with little or no disability is common. CT scans establish the diagnosis.

DIFFERENTIAL DIAGNOSIS OF HYPERTENSIVE HEMORRHAGE. In establishing a diagnosis of hypertensive intracerebral hemorrhage, the sudden onset and the evolution over a few minutes to hours are important. Such abrupt onsets also occur, however, with thrombosis and embolism. Headache is the predominant feature at the onset in at least one half of hemorrhages and in less than one fourth of cases of thromboembolism. Vomiting is prominent as an early symptom. Funduscopic examination will indicate extremely reduced arteriolar caliber and probably periarteriolar hemorrhages. Nuchal rigidity is common with primary intracerebral as well as subarachnoid hemorrhage. It disappears as the depth of coma increases. Restlessness and vomiting are more common with hemorrhage than with infarction. Convulsions are common with intracerebral hemorrhage, are less frequent with subarachnoid hemorrhage, and are uncommon (<10 per cent) with cerebral infarction. The most important clues to the diagnosis of hypertensive hemorrhage are the explosive onset, the history of high blood pressure, an early decline of the level of consciousness, and the detection

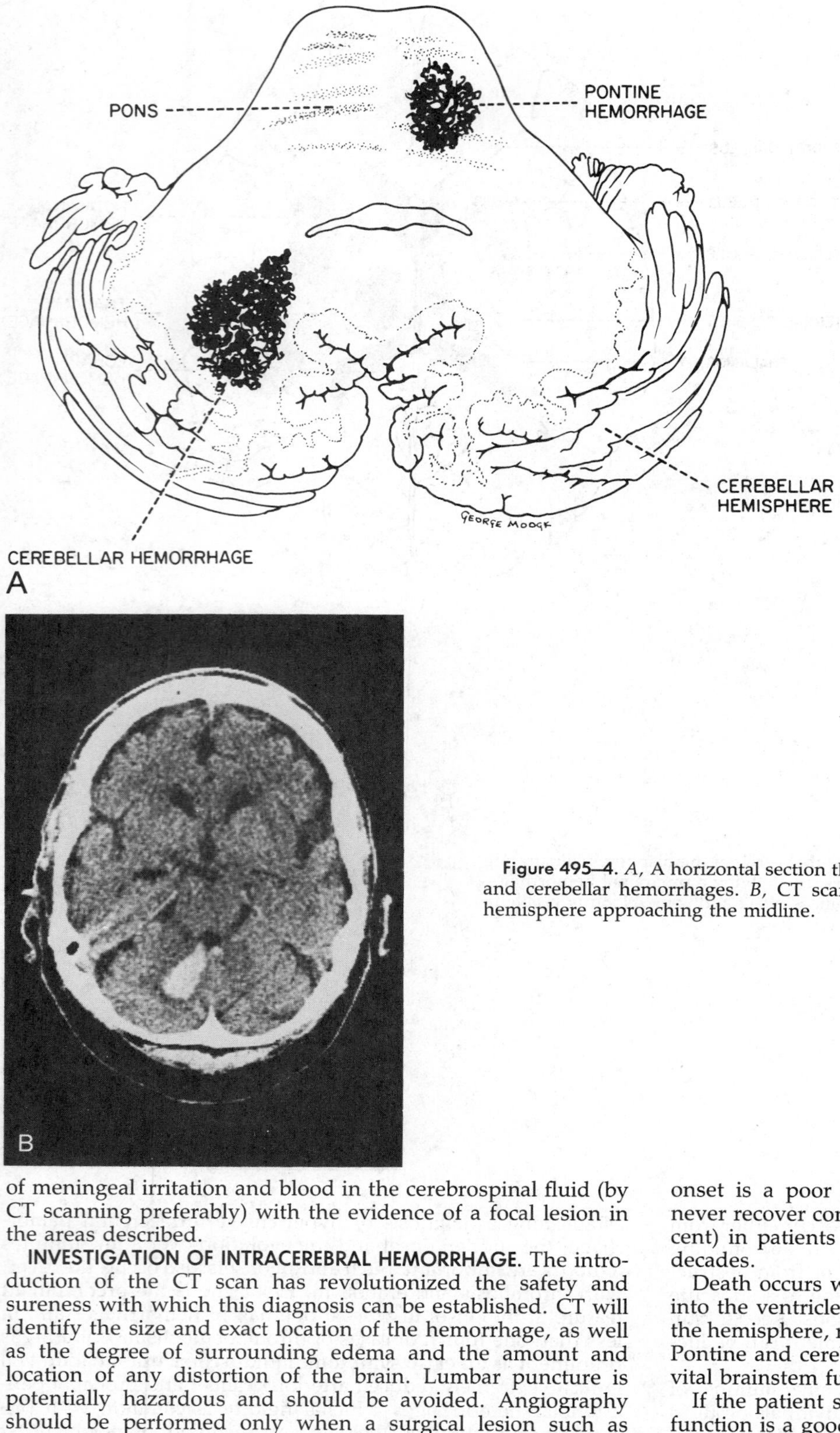

Figure 495–4. *A*, A horizontal section through the pons and cerebellum illustrating pontine and cerebellar hemorrhages. *B*, CT scan illustrating a hemorrhage in the right cerebellar hemisphere approaching the midline.

of meningeal irritation and blood in the cerebrospinal fluid (by CT scanning preferably) with the evidence of a focal lesion in the areas described.

INVESTIGATION OF INTRACEREBRAL HEMORRHAGE. The introduction of the CT scan has revolutionized the safety and sureness with which this diagnosis can be established. CT will identify the size and exact location of the hemorrhage, as well as the degree of surrounding edema and the amount and location of any distortion of the brain. Lumbar puncture is potentially hazardous and should be avoided. Angiography should be performed only when a surgical lesion such as aneurysm, AVM, or a brain tumor might exist, and in certain carefully selected cases in which surgical drainage might be considered. The possibility of a bleeding disorder requires that routine blood counts and platelet counts be performed and bleeding and prothrombin times obtained.

COURSE AND PROGNOSIS OF HYPERTENSIVE HEMORRHAGE. Hypertensive intracerebral hemorrhage carries a grave immediate prognosis. Some patients die on the day of the ictus, and 50 to 75 per cent succumb within one month. Coma at the onset is a poor prognostic sign, and most affected patients never recover consciousness. Mortality is slightly lower (40 per cent) in patients up to the fifth decade and increases in later decades.

Death occurs when a hemorrhage of sufficient size ruptures into the ventricles, causing them to become distended, or into the hemisphere, resulting in compromise of brainstem function. Pontine and cerebellar hematomas interfere most quickly with vital brainstem functions.

If the patient survives, subsequent recovery of considerable function is a good possibility. The hemorrhage resorbs slowly, and the compressed neural tissue commensurately regains much of its previous functional activity. With larger hemorrhages in which the brainstem is secondarily disrupted, functional restoration is not expected and will be accompanied by permanent sequelae. Subsequent bleeding is rare with appropriate blood pressure control.

TREATMENT OF INTRACEREBRAL HEMORRHAGE. The treatment of intracerebral hemorrhage is mostly unsatisfactory. The principles involved in the care of seriously disabled, stuporous, or comatose patients apply, with attention to the airway, fluids, and electrolytes.

Localization of the clot by history, physical signs, and, if available, CT scanning will determine the need to consider some cases for a surgical evacuation. Evacuation can benefit the small number of cases with *cerebellar hematoma* recognized before the onset of coma. If CT is available, such patients should have daily or more frequent CT scans. If signs of clinical worsening progress after admission, prompt ventricular shunting or direct removal of the clot is indicated. Signs of bilateral corticospinal tract dysfunction or reduction in level of consciousness imply that severe brainstem dysfunction has already occurred and that action has been delayed too long. Smaller intracerebellar hematomas less than 3 cm in diameter usually resolve without surgical evacuation.

Evacuation of the occasional supratentorial hematoma is considered when the lesion is larger than usual and is in the subcortical white matter, and the patient is not afflicted with calamitous hemiplegia and aphasia but is showing signs of progression with evidence of incipient deterioration of the level of consciousness. However, evacuation of most examples of hypertensive intracerebral hematoma is a futile pursuit. The most satisfactory recoveries occur in patients who have not been submitted to operation.

Too rapid lowering of the level of blood pressure while attempting to reduce the amount of bleeding may be dangerous. In the hypertensive patient the uninvolved brain requires a higher than normal perfusion pressure because of the intraluminal resistance of the widespread arteriolar disease. A dramatic reduction of blood pressure puts the patient at risk to the development of additional neurologic disability from ischemia. If the patient survives the ictus, gradual restoration of normal blood pressure and its maintenance at normal levels are mandatory.

Cole FM, Yates P: Intracerebral microaneurysms and small cerebrovascular lesions. Brain 90:759, 1967. *A study of the arteriolar changes found in hypertensive and elderly persons.*

Drake CG: Giant intracranial aneurysms: Experience with surgical treatment in 174 patients. Clin Neurosurg 26:12, 1979. *Combined with the paper by Sundt and Piepgras, a comprehensive statement is provided on the surgical approach to an uncommon but distressing clinical condition.*

Drake CG: The treatment of aneurysms of the posterior circulation. Clin Neurosurg 26:96, 1979. *A review of a very large experience in this area.*

Drake CG: Cerebral arteriovenous malformations: Considerations for and experience with surgical treatment in 166 cases. Clin Neurosurg 26:145, 1979. *A comprehensive review of the clinical features and treatment possibilities.*

Fields WS, Maslenikov V, Meyer JS, et al.: Joint study of extracranial arterial occlusion. JAMA 211:1993, 1970. *The survival data from the only major randomized trial to evaluate carotid endarterectomy in stroke prevention. Should be read with Kurtzke's critique.*

Gilbert JJ, Vinters HV: Cerebral amyloid angiopathy: Incidence and complications in the aging brain. I. Cerebral Hemorrhage. Stroke 14:915, 1983. *An update on these subcortical hemorrhages that occur in the aging brain*

Heyman A, Wilkinson W, Heyden S, Helms MJ, Bartel AG, Karp HR, Tyroler HA, Hames CG: Risk of stroke in asymptomatic persons with cervical arterial bruits. A population study in Evans County, Georgia. N Engl J Med 302:838, 1980. *A long-term surveillance study of asymptomatic carotid bruits indicates that they predict an increased risk of stroke.*

Kassell NF, Drake CG: Review of the management of saccular aneurysms. Neurol. Clin. 1:73, 1983. *A contemporary discussion on the diagnosis of saccular aneurysm, the prevention of rebleeding, the problem of vasospasm, and early versus later surgical intervention.*

Kurtzke J: Formal discussion. *In* Whisnant JP, Sandok BA (eds.): Cerebral Vascular Diseases. New York, Grune & Stratton, 1974, pp 190–193. *A succinct and impressive critique of the joint study of extracranial carotid surgery.*

Ojemann RG, Heros RC: Spontaneous brain hemorrhage. Stroke 14:468, 1983. *A recent article on spontaneous brain hemorrhage and its management.*

Ott KH, Kase CS, Ojemann RG, Mohr JP: Cerebellar hemorrhage: Diagnosis and treatment. A review of 56 cases. Arch Neurol 31:160, 1974. *A comprehensive review of a condition which must be recognized early for optimal management.*

Ropper AH, Davis KR: Lobar cerebral hemorrhages: Acute clinical syndromes in 26 cases. Ann Neurol 8:141, 1980. *A description of a series of patients with intracerebral hemorrhage located outside the usual locations common to the hypertensive patient. This paper reflects part of the new understanding of brain hemorrhage in normotensive and hypertensive patients diagnosed by CT scanning.*

Sahs AL, Perrett GE, Locksley HB, Nishioka H (eds.): Intracranial Aneurysms and Subarachnoid Hemorrhage. A Cooperative Study. Philadelphia, J. B. Lippincott Company, 1969. *The report of a cooperative study with valuable data respecting the problems of subarachnoid hemorrhage. As the preface indicates, not designed as a recipe-book for definitive therapy.*

Shenkin HA, Zavala M: Cerebellar strokes: Mortality, surgical indication and result of ventricular damage. Lancet 2:429, 1982. *A recent summary of the condition.*

Sundt TM Jr, Piepgras DG: Surgical approach to giant intracranial aneurysms. Operative experience with 80 cases. J Neurosurg 51:731, 1979.

Sundt TM Jr, Whisnant JP: Subarachnoid hemorrhage from intracranial aneurysms. Surgical management and natural history of disease. N Engl J Med 299:116, 1978. *A report of the progress being made to improve by surgery on the natural history of subarachnoid hemorrhage. The disease remains serious.*

Wolf PA, Kannel WB, Gordon T, McNamara PM, Dawber TR: Asymptomatic carotid bruit and risk of stroke: The Framingham Study (abstract). Stroke 10:96, 1979. *An important reference in decision-making respecting asymptomatic carotid bruit management.*

Section Eight INFECTIOUS AND INFLAMMATORY DISORDERS OF THE NERVOUS SYSTEM

Bacterial Diseases

496. PARAMENINGEAL INFECTIONS

Donald H. Harter

Central nervous system infections caused by pyogenic bacteria other than acute meningitis include brain abscess, collections of pus enclosed within membranes covering the brain and spinal cord (subdural empyema, cerebral epidural abscess, spinal epidural abscess, spinal subdural empyema), and dural sinus infection and thrombosis. Most of these paracranial diseases are secondary to adjacent infections of the ear, sinuses, or bones of the skull or migrate from an infection elsewhere in the body.

Availability of newer techniques, such as CT and radionuclide scans, has greatly improved the early diagnosis and, therefore, treatment of localized central nervous system infections. The new imaging techniques also permit monitoring the progress of the infection during treatment. Correct use of these methods should further reduce the mortality and morbidity from these infections in years ahead.

BRAIN ABSCESS

DEFINITION. Brain abscess describes encapsulated or free pus in the substance of the brain. Abscesses may vary in size from a microscopic focus of inflammatory cells to a major encapsulated area of necrosis occupying a major part of a cerebral hemisphere. They may be single or multiple and caused by local extension or hematogenous spread.

INCIDENCE. Brain abscess is about one sixth as frequent as bacterial meningitis and constitutes approximately 0.7 per cent of all neurosurgical operations. The condition occurs two to three times more frequently in males than in females.

PREDISPOSING FACTORS. The causes of brain abscess can be classified into those in which a primary focus of infection can be identified and those in which no extracranial focus can be found. In the majority of cases a primary focus can be found at the time of initial presentation or at necropsy. Brain abscess can arise by extension from infections within the cranium, by introduction of bacteria at the time of head trauma, or as a metastatic infection from other parts of the body. The site of primary infection can be classified into otolaryngologic causes (middle ear disease and sinus infections), metastatic infections (sepsis, pulmonary disease, and cardiac disease), or trauma.

Otogenic Abscess. About 0.5 per cent of patients with acute otitis media and 0.3 per cent of patients with chronic otitis media will develop brain abscess. Middle ear infection, even in the antibiotic era, remains the most common single causative disease. Otogenic brain abscesses are usually located in the temporal lobe or cerebellum.

Infection spreads along the path of bony erosion; final intracranial spread is precipitated by an acute exacerbation of a chronic process. Spread to the posterior fossa may be through the lateral sinus or through the internal ear with erosion of the bony labyrinth and necrosis of the horizontal semicircular canal, oval window, or promontory. Involvement of the posterior fossa occurs quickly once labyrinthine fluid is infected. Alternatively, a cholesteatoma in the mastoid antrum and attic erodes through the antral roof, leading to infection. In cerebellar abscess there is often evidence of retrograde thrombosis from the lateral, petrosal, or superior petrosal venous sinuses, but the importance of such retrograde thrombosis in the origin of otogenic abscess is uncertain. The duration of otorrhea preceding brain abscess caused by middle ear disease may vary from one month to as long as 20 years.

Infection of Paranasal Sinuses. Paranasal sinus infection accounts for about 5 to 10 per cent of all brain abscesses, usually extending directly from the frontal sinus into the anterior part of the frontal lobe. Rarely, infection of the ethmoid sinus can cause a deep temporal lobe abscess in the region of the uncus. Infection may erode the sinus wall and invade the brain directly or may spread by veins communicating with the cavernous sinus or brain.

Trauma to the Face and Skull. Brain abscess secondary to trauma is usually due to an unrepaired dural laceration in association with a compound depressed skull fracture. The abscess is always directly related to the site of injury. Penetrating gunshot wounds are often responsible for brain abscesses. In post-traumatic brain abscess a bone fragment or other foreign body may be found in the devitalized tissue. Sometimes the injury may be seemingly trivial and unsuspected. For example, penetration of the orbital roof and temporal bone by pencil tips has given rise to brain abscess. Brain abscess may also follow otolaryngologic or neurosurgical operations.

Metastatic Brain Abscess and Hematogenous Spread. Hematogenous brain abscesses usually originate from the heart, lungs, or pleura. Less frequently, septic foci in the skin, teeth, abdomen, or surgical wounds may be the origin. The incidence of metastatic abscess is always less than that of otogenic or rhinogenic abscess.

The single most important cause of metastatic brain abscess is chronic infection of the pleura or lungs, including bronchiectasis, empyema, and lung abscess. Brain abscesses metastatic from the lung often lie in frontal, parietal, or deep cortical regions but are seldom in the cerebellum. They follow a more chronic course than abscesses of cardiac origin. Metastatic abscess is believed to originate from a transient bacteremia with release of infected material into the pulmonary venous and systemic circulations. A number of these patients have had thoracic surgery.

About 10 per cent of brain abscesses are associated with congenital heart disease. Affected patients often present with the sudden onset of a focal neurologic deficit in a stroke-like manner. Paradoxical infected embolism, bacterial endocarditis, and primary thrombosis with secondary bacteremic infection have all been held responsible for the development of brain abscess. The mortality of brain abscess in association with pulmonary or cardiac disease is higher than that from abscesses of other causes.

Metastatic brain abscess of pure dental origin is rare. There is often intervening cellulitis, sinusitis, and osteomyelitis of the mandible and base of the skull, permitting direct rather than hematogenous spread. Intrauterine contraceptive devices have been incriminated as an occasional source of metastatic brain abscess.

ETIOLOGY. Comprehensive statements about the bacteriology of brain abscesses are difficult to make because of diversity in the isolation methods used. Many bacteria, notably anaerobic species, have peculiar or particular growth requirements, making them difficult to cultivate. A lack of attention to detail can lead to a failure to isolate the responsible bacteria or microorganisms in as high as 60 per cent of cases. In many instances more than a single bacterial species is isolated from a brain abscess.

For best results a gram-stained smear should be studied at the time of surgery. Aerobic and anaerobic bacterial and fungal cultures should be planted. Ideally, the bacteriologist should be on hand when the abscess is tapped in the operating room. If this is not possible, the neurosurgical team should know precisely how to inoculate suitable media as soon as the aspirate is available. Aspirated purulent material should be rapidly transported to the bacteriologic laboratory. Blood cultures should also be taken at the time of operation. Samples should be collected into a liquid anaerobic culture medium containing antibiotic inactivators.

The most common microorganisms isolated from brain abscesses are aerobic or anaerobic streptococci. Nontraumatic brain abscess has become largely a disease of streptococci, more particularly of anaerobic or microaerophilic strains. *Bacteroides* and enteric bacteria are still recovered in a number of cases. *S. pneumoniae* is now a rare cause unless the abscess is the sequel to occult cerebrospinal fluid rhinorrhea or occurs in an elderly person in association with pneumococcal pneumonia. Staphylococcal abscesses are usually due to penetrating head trauma or bacteremia. Clostridial infections are post-traumatic. Gram-negative bacilli very rarely occur alone.

Rarely *Actinomyces* and *Nocardia* species may be recovered from an abscess cavity. Actinomycotic brain abscess may be secondary to infection elsewhere, particularly the chest and oropharynx. *Nocardia asteroides* is a rare cause of cerebral abscesses which are often multiple, multilocular, and thick walled. They almost invariably are associated with pulmonary infection. Cerebral infection with *Candida albicans* can also lead to abscess formation.

PATHOLOGY. The factors leading to the development of intracerebral abscess with encapsulation in some cases and not in others are poorly understood. Localized inflammatory changes with necrosis and edema, thromboses of vessels, and collections of degenerating leukocytes represent the early response to bacterial invasion. The histologic appearance of brain abscess includes an inner layer of pus surrounding a zone of inflammatory granulation tissue, which varies in thickness. In the early acute stage, granulation tissue may be absent and the limits of the abscess defined by a zone of infiltration by polymorphonuclear leukocytes and plasma cells. Foci of perivascular cuffing are present. There is often surrounding edema of the white matter.

The acute area of local suppuration is followed in several weeks by encapsulation of the liquefied brain and accumulated pus. There is still no satisfactory explanation for the variation and progression of encapsulation from patient to patient. Virulence of the organism and ability to make granulation tissue may be involved, but what controls these factors is unknown. As encapsulation proceeds, a layer of granulation tissue merges with surrounding collagenous tissue in which there is evidence of continuing fibroblastic activity and reticulin fibers. Active fibroblasts appear to infiltrate the surrounding brain, and a zone of avascular necrosis forms. The macroscopic appearance of a dormant smooth capsule at the time of excision is not confirmed histologically, because there is active vascular hyperplasia and perivascular cuffing about the capsule. Meninges adjacent to the abscess are often infiltrated by inflammatory cells.

Multiple satellite abscesses may develop and communicate with the principal cavity. Because abscess cavities may spread through the central white matter, they often extend through the ventricular wall, producing meningitis, and may rupture into the cerebral ventricles.

CLINICAL MANIFESTATIONS. Brain abscess may happen at any time of life, but the highest incidence of the disease occurs between the second and fifth decades.

General Features. The symptoms of brain abscess are generally those of a space-occupying intracranial lesion. The illness may be acute with fever, headache, nausea or vomiting, increasing obtundation, seizures, and localizing neurologic findings. As noted, occasional cases produce a stroke-like onset. One should suspect brain abscess in the presence of chronic middle ear disease, congenital heart disease, sinusitis, or bronchiectasis. The diagnosis should also be considered in the presence of other forms of sepsis such as osteomyelitis, surgical wound infections, dental and periodontal disease, and pneumonia. Absence of a focus of infection, however, never excludes the possibility of brain abscess.

Symptoms of acute infection are often lacking unless the focus giving rise to the abscess is still active. Chills and fever at the onset of nervous system invasion may accompany an embolic lesion in the brain secondary to acute endocarditis. The body temperature may be elevated, normal, or subnormal. Approximately one third of patients lack a history of fever and remain afebrile during their illness. Most do not have fever when admitted to hospital.

Increased intracranial pressure usually develops rapidly. Headache, nausea, and vomiting are common early symptoms. Seizures, more often generalized than focal, are present in one quarter to one third of patients. The diagnosis of brain abscess can often be inferred because of past or present evidence of otitis media or sinusitis. Unexplained headache in a child with cyanotic congenital heart disease should be regarded as being due to brain abscess until proved otherwise. Headache may be localized to the side of the abscess, but it is often generalized and increases in severity as the abscess expands. Signs attributable to meningeal irritation may be present.

Increased intracranial pressure may lead to bradycardia, confusion, drowsiness, and stupor. Papilledema may be a relatively late event, but develops eventually in about half of cases. Signs of damage to the third or sixth cranial nerves may reflect an increased intracranial pressure and may not have localizing value. The course of untreated brain abscess is usually fulminating, ending fatally in five to fifteen days. In certain patients, however, the course may be prolonged and misdiagnosed as a brain tumor. Although the use of CT scanning has made localization on clinical grounds less important in many parts of the world, several distinct presentations can be recognized.

Temporal lobe abscesses tend to cause language difficulties, visual field abnormalities, or signs of uncal herniation, while *frontal lobe abscesses* are more prone to produce behavioral abnormalities or focal seizures. Both frontal and parietal lobe abscesses tend to cause contralateral motor or sensory dysfunction. Deep-lying hemispheric abscesses may be difficult to differentiate, without biopsy, from malignant brain tumors. *Cerebellar abscesses,* almost all of which extend from middle ear infections, produce ipsilateral cerebellar dysfunction, stiff neck, and, often, signs of increased intracranial pressure. Brain stem abscesses are rare and cause signs consistent with their anatomic location.

LABORATORY DIAGNOSIS. Elevation of the white blood cell count is of limited value, being above 20,000 per cubic millimeter in about 10 per cent of brain abscess patients. Lumbar puncture is unjustified when brain abscess is suspected, especially if CT scanning is available. If a lumbar puncture is inadvertently performed, cerebrospinal fluid pleocytosis greater than 5 cells per cubic millimeter is found in about two thirds of patients, a protein content greater than 100 mg per deciliter in two fifths, and a cerebrospinal fluid glucose level less than 40 mg per deciliter in about one fifth. Pressure usually is moderately elevated, and the fluid usually is sterile.

X-ray studies of the skull, including mastoids and sinuses, may disclose evidence of otitic or paranasal sepsis.

The CT scan is the most valuable test for diagnosis, and its application has had a remarkable effect in reducing the mortality of brain abscess. The most frequently observed CT appearance is a lucent area surrounded by a faint dense rim with a second lucent zone outside the rim. After intravenous administration of contrast material; dense ring enhancement is seen around an area of low attenuation with a lucent area of edema peripheral to the enhanced ring. Varying degrees of compression or shift of the ventricular system indicate mass effect (Fig. 496–1). The CT scan of patients with suspected brain abscess should be performed with and without contrast enhancement. Occasionally, one observes a patchy, nonuniform enhancement pattern consistent with preliquefactive inflammation, "cerebritis." The differential diagnosis includes septic infarcts, tumors with cyst formation, or metastatic tumors.

Ring formation represents an area of hypercellularity and hypervascularity with varying amounts of fibrous tissue. Ring enhancement is neither synonymous with a well-formed capsule nor relates to the patient's clinical condition. Ring formation may be seen in the stage prior to capsule formation and may persist after complete surgical excision and in clinically stable patients.

Arteriography adds little to the CT diagnosis of brain abscess.

In the absence of a CT scan, radionuclide brain scanning is the most reliable method of detecting supratentorial brain abscess. The scan may become positive in the early stages of focal cerebritis before true abscess or pus formation. Cerebral abscess has also been identified by radionuclide scanning after the injection of the patient's leukocytes labeled with indium-111. The EEG in brain abscess is almost always abnormal, usually indicating only the presence of a space-occupying lesion.

TREATMENT. Early diagnosis and prompt initiation of antimicrobial therapy are crucial. Once antimicrobial agents are started, parenteral corticosteroids may be used to reduce brain edema, although in any but late cases their benefit is problematic. During the stage of acute focal suppuration or cerebritis, surgical intervention is not indicated.

Recent evidence indicates that many brain abscesses can be treated by nonsurgical means if carefully monitored by CT scans. Treatment with antibiotics and other medical supportive measures alone is indicated before capsule formation has occurred or when a capsulated abscess is small and produces no shift or compression of intracranial structures. Patients who improve on medical treatment alone all show a decrease in enhancement of ring formation on CT scan and, gradually, a shrinking and disappearance of the lesion.

In all likelihood an increasing number of brain abscess patients will be nonsurgically managed in years to come. Because penicillin-susceptible organisms predominate in brain abscesses, the optimal antimicrobial regimen consists of giving 10 to 20 million units of penicillin intravenously daily in divided doses. If there is reason to suspect the presence of another organism not susceptible to penicillin, chloramphenicol or another drug can be given concurrently. If there is evidence for staphylococcal infection, adequate amounts of a penicillinase-resistant penicillin or a cephalosporin drug should be given. Antimicrobial drug therapy can be modified after the antibiotic sensitivity of the microorganism identified in abscess pus has been determined. Treatment should be continued for six weeks.

If, despite medical treatment, the patient's clinical status changes for the worse and/or the CT scan shows an increase in the size of the abscess and an increase in the intensity of ring enhancement, surgical treatment is mandatory. However, heightened ring enhancement may occur after steroids have been discontinued; if the patient shows continued clinical improvement on antibiotic therapy, close, nonsurgical observation can continue.

Possible operations include initial aspiration of the abscess cavity, followed in some cases by excision at a second operation, or primary total excision of the abscess. If the abscess is superficial and encapsulated, primary excision is the operation of choice. Persistence of a ring sign on CT scan after primary abscess excision does not imply that a residual abscess has formed. If the abscess is deep or affects a neurologically critical area, aspiration and injection of antimicrobial agents is the only operative possibility.

PROGNOSIS AND OUTCOME. Mortality from all brain abscesses remained at 30 to 40 per cent after the use of antibiotics had become common practice. The use of the CT scan to assist in diagnosis and to monitor treatment appears to have reduced this rate. Although results are still incomplete, some place current mortality as low as 5 per cent. Mortality is greatest in patients with reduced consciousness at the time of admission.

Residual neurologic damage is frequent in survivors of brain abscess. Convulsive seizures are frequent and require continuous anticonvulsant medication (see Ch. 510).

SUBDURAL EMPYEMA

DEFINITION AND CAUSE. Subdural empyema refers to an intracranial collection of pus located between the inner surface of the dura and the outer surface of the arachnoid. The most common causes are infections of the paranasal sinuses or middle ear. Other causes include rupture of an intracerebral abscess, cranial osteomyelitis, infection of a subdural hematoma, penetrating wounds of the skull, leptomeningitis, and septicemia. An acute exacerbation of sinusitis just prior to the development of subdural empyema is common.

PATHOLOGY. Infection may enter the subdural space by direct extension following erosion of osteitic areas or by indirect extension through progressive thrombophlebitis of mucosal veins and subsequent spread to dural veins, venous sinuses, and cerebral veins. The first route is more common in otitic infections, the second in paranasal infections. When the infection enters the subdural space, it elicits a prompt inflammatory response with rapid pus formation. Extension of pus depends on the primary site of infection. Dorsolateral and interhemispheric collections are common; those beneath the cerebral hemispheres are uncommon. After paranasal infection, subdural pus usually forms at the frontal poles and extends posteriorly over the convexity of the frontal lobe. It may reach into the parietal and occipital areas and along the falx and sylvian fissure. When a subdural collection occurs after ear infection, it passes posteriorly and medially over the falx to the tentorium. Pus climbs above the tentorium and extends over the occipital poles.

Thrombosis or thrombophlebitis of superficial cortical veins is a common complication, and produces hemorrhagic infarction of the area drained by the diseased vessels. The cerebral hemisphere under the pus collection is depressed and indented. Superficial layers of the cerebral cortex undergo ischemic necrosis. Microscopic studies disclose various degrees of organi-

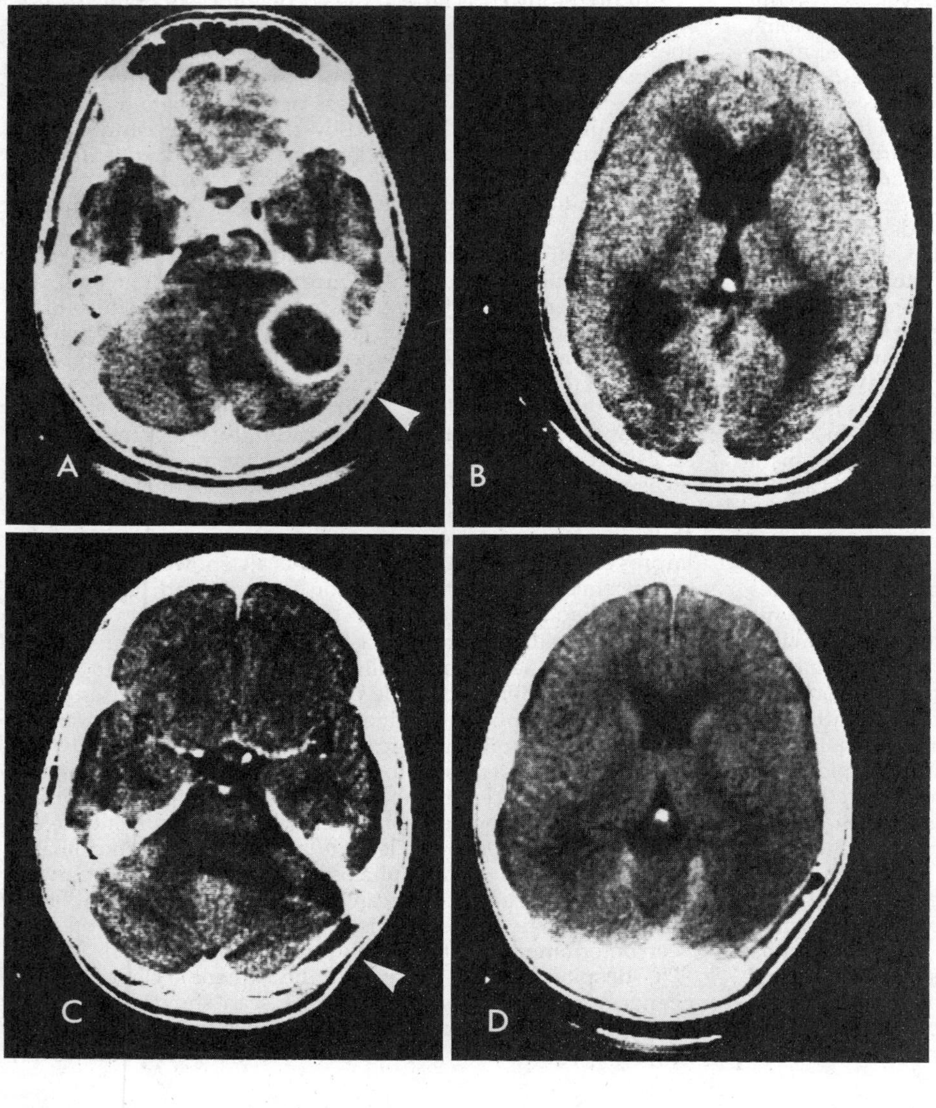

Figure 496–1. CT scan of cerebellar brain abscess in a 16-year old boy with chronic otitis media.

Initial findings: *A*, Characteristic ring appearance of the acute, untreated abscess after intravenous contrast injection. *B*, Moderate associated dilation of the lateral ventricles (hydrocephalus) due to partial obstruction of the aqueduct and fourth ventricle.

Re-examination twelve days later (after twelve days of antimicrobial therapy and ten days after removal of the well-encapsulated 3.5 cm diameter abscess): *C*, Area of abscess removal. *D*, Normal-sized lateral ventricles. The boy subsequently recovered completely.

zation of the exudate on the inner surface of the dura and infiltration of the underlying pia with inflammatory cells.

ETIOLOGY. The most common organism isolated from subdural pus is the streptococcus, often an anaerobe. Other frequent pathogens include staphylococci and gram-negative enteric organisms.

CLINICAL MANIFESTATIONS. Symptoms and signs of antecedent sinusitis, otitis, or osteomyelitis often blend into those of subdural empyema. The usual clinical onset is with high fever, headache, and vomiting, followed by impaired consciousness and signs of meningeal irritation. The patient gradually or rapidly becomes irritable and drowsy. Stiff neck and Kernig's sign are present, and the area of the abscess is characteristically tender to percussion. Progression of the infection leads to confusion, stupor, or coma. Focal neurologic signs appear, including convulsions, hemiparesis, and aphasia, and may be the result of compression of the cerebral cortex underneath the pus collection or cortical thrombophlebitis and cerebral infarction. In the later stages, the intracranial pressure may rise. The entire clinical picture may evolve in as little as a few hours or as long as ten days or more. Without treatment, death usually occurs within a few days after the onset of focal neurologic findings.

LABORATORY DIAGNOSIS. A marked peripheral leukocytosis is usually present. X-rays of the skull may show infection of the mastoid or nasal sinuses or osteomyelitis of the skull. The cerebrospinal fluid is under increased pressure and usually contains a few hundred to 1000 or more cells, an increased protein content, and a normal or near normal glucose level.

Spinal fluid is typically free of bacteria. There is potential danger in the performance of a lumbar puncture in patients with subdural empyema who have evidence of increased intracranial pressure, and the procedure should be avoided if the diagnosis can be reached or is strongly suggested by other procedures.

CT scan of the head characteristically depicts a crescent-shaped area of increased density at the periphery of the brain and mass displacement of the cerebral ventricles and midline structures. Contrast enhancement demonstrates a rim-like crescent adjacent to the cortex or a collection of pus near the falx. CT scan may be of greater reliability in showing the subdural empyema which develops in patients after drainage of a chronic subdural hematoma than in subdural empyema of other causes.

In the absence of a CT scan, cerebral arteriography is the most reliable method for detecting a subdural mass lesion. The combination of CT scanning and cerebral angiography is the current procedure of choice for demonstration of subdural empyema.

Radionuclide scan in subdural empyema is rarely sensitive enough to visualize small bilateral or parafalcial collections. It can be of help, however, in diagnosing an associated brain abscess.

TREATMENT. Subdural empyema requires prompt surgical drainage of pus by burr holes or craniotomy. Vigorous systemic therapy with penicillin (10 to 20 million units daily) and other antimicrobials as indicated is begun before surgery and continued until the infection is brought under control. Antibiotics are commonly instilled into the subdural space at the time of operation. Surgical treatment of the accompanying sinusitis, frontal osteomyelitis, or mastoiditis is usually postponed until the intracranial infection has subsided.

OUTCOME. Mortality from subdural empyema remains at between 25 and 40 per cent, usually because of delayed diagnosis. The main causes of death are thrombophlebitis associated with dural venous sinus thrombosis and massive cerebral infarction, fulminant meningitis, and multiple intracerebral abscesses. Progressive and uncontrollable cerebral edema contributes to a lethal outcome.

CEREBRAL EPIDURAL ABSCESS

Cerebral epidural (or extradural) abscess is a collection of purulent material localized to the outer layer of the dura. It occurs in relationship to adjacent osteomyelitis, mastoiditis, or paranasal sinusitis. Epidural abscess may lead to sinus thrombophlebitis, subdural empyema, leptomeningitis, or brain abscess.

Signs and symptoms are nondistinctive and apt to be masked by primary disease of the ear, nasal sinuses, or skull, or by secondary complications. There may be ipsilateral headache, fever, localized pain, tenderness on local percussion, and swelling with pitting edema. Evidence of increased intracranial pressure is rarely present. Focal neurologic signs are uncommon. In most cases the cerebrospinal fluid is sterile, contains a few lymphocytic cells, and has a mild elevation of protein content. Many cerebral epidural abscesses are diagnosed at the time of operation for a subdural empyema or a brain abscess. Treatment is with surgical drainage plus appropriate systemic antibiotic therapy.

MAJOR DURAL SINUS THROMBOSIS

The large dural sinuses may become thrombosed spontaneously, when they are infected, or when there is infection in the adjacent epidural or subdural spaces. Although any dural sinus may be involved in intracranial infection, the paired sinuses (lateral, cavernous, and petrosal) are affected most often. Spontaneous or primary sinus thrombosis tends to favor unpaired sinuses. Venous sinuses may become infected by contiguous spread from otorhinogenic foci of infection, by periphlebitis leading to the direct spread of infection through the sinus wall, by an infected draining vein, or by septic venous embolization. Inflammation may also spread from infected dural sinuses to the extradural and subdural spaces by direct extension or venous radicles, to the leptomeninges and adjacent brain, to the bloodstream, and to distant sites by embolism.

Thrombosis of major dural sinuses may result in increased intracranial pressure, multifocal regions of brain ischemia, or cerebral infarction, all because of obstruction to venous drainage from the brain.

LATERAL SINUS THROMBOSIS. Lateral sinus thrombosis is almost always a complication of acute or chronic otitis media, mastoiditis, or cholesteatoma formation. Infants and children are most commonly affected. The thrombosis may coincide with the acute attack of middle ear disease or may be delayed until the chronic stage of ear infection.

The classic symptoms of lateral sinus thrombosis are fever, headache, nausea, and vomiting. An increase of pain in the ear or cessation of aural discharge may point to sinus thrombophlebitis. Local venous distention and swelling, pain, redness, and tenderness indicate involvement of the mastoid emissary vein and may extend into the neck over the jugular vein. Pain in the neck with restriction of movement accompanies jugular vein involvement.

The intracranial pressure is typically increased and more apt to be high when the right lateral sinus is occluded, since it normally is the larger of the two. Papilledema is usually bilateral, but may be unilateral because of extension of the process to the ipsilateral cavernous sinus. Drowsiness and coma are common. Convulsive seizures occur, but focal neurologic findings are unusual.

Spread to the inferior petrosal sinus may lead to abducens nerve paralysis and trigeminal nerve involvement (Gradenigo's syndrome). Involvement of the ninth, tenth, and eleventh nerves may occur because of damage to the jugular bulb and related structures. The symptoms produced include pain on swallowing, dysphagia, dysarthria, hoarseness, weakness or spasms of the sternocleidomastoid and trapezius muscles, and changes in pulse and respiration. The incidence and mortality of lateral sinus thrombosis have been greatly reduced since the introduction and use of antibiotics for middle ear and mastoid infections. The differential diagnosis of lateral sinus thrombosis includes a flare-up of mastoiditis; a perisinus, subdural, or brain abscess; and leptomeningitis.

CAVERNOUS SINUS THROMBOSIS. Cavernous sinus thrombosis is usually due to a suppurative process in the orbit, nasal sinuses, or upper half of the face. Infection may reach the cavernous sinus by the anterior route (ophthalmic veins from orbit, frontal sinus, nasal cavity, and upper face), by the middle route (sphenoid sinus by direct spread or the pharyngeal and pterygoid plexuses from pharynx, upper jaw, and teeth), and by the posterior route (petrosal sinuses and occasionally ear and lateral sinuses). Spread by the anterior route follows the most acute course, and that by the posterior route the most protracted course. The initial infection is usually a furuncle, acute sinusitis, or ear infection. Most infections are due to *Staphylococcus aureus*.

Cavernous sinus thrombosis usually produces an illness of desperate severity with high fever, headaches, malaise, prostration, nausea, vomiting, convulsions, tachycardia, and leukocytosis. Characteristically, the sensorium remains clear until late in the infection. Local changes include chemosis, edema, and cyanosis of the upper face, particularly of the eyelids and base of the nose. These are due to obstruction of the ophthalmic vein as it enters the cavernous sinus. Superficial veins over the forehead may be distended. Swelling of the lids, haziness of the cornea, local pain, and photophobia may make examination of the eyes difficult. Ophthalmoplegia, often first affecting the sixth nerve, is common. The pupil may be dilated from parasympathetic paralysis or small and immobile if both parasympathetic and sympathetic fibers are involved. Involvement of the first division of the trigeminal nerve may lead to eye pain and hyperesthesia of the forehead. Retinal hemorrhages and papilledema are late events. Visual acuity may be normal or moderately impaired. When the infection originates in the throat, sphenoids, or ear, the evolution of the disease is less acute, and the orbit becomes less engorged.

The differential diagnosis of cavernous sinus thrombosis includes orbital tumors, meningiomas and other tumors in the region of the sphenoid, trichinosis, malignant exophthalmos, and arteriovenous aneurysms.

SUPERIOR SAGITTAL SINUS THROMBOSIS. The superior sagittal sinus is less commonly involved in septic thrombosis than the lateral or cavernous sinuses. Infections may reach the superior sagittal sinus by extension from the nasal cavities, by secondary spread from the lateral or cavernous sinuses, or by extension from osteomyelitis or an epidural or subdural infection. The site of initial thrombosis depends on the source and route of infection.

General signs of superior sagittal sinus thrombosis are prostration, fever, headache, and papilledema. Local signs include edema of the forehead and anterior part of the scalp. At times, there is engorgement of the scalp veins. The neurologic symptoms include convulsive seizures and motor paralysis. Focal seizures which alternatively involve one and then the other side of the body are characteristic. One or both legs may be weak or paralyzed, but the motor loss may be hemiplegic in distribution with the leg and proximal arm involved. Some patients develop homonymous hemianopsia or quadrantanopsia, paralysis of conjugate ocular movements, visual disorientation, alexia, apraxia, or aphasia.

DIAGNOSTIC TESTS. X-rays of the skull may provide evidence of middle ear disease, sinusitis, osteomyelitis, fracture, or other conditions associated with dural sinus thrombosis. Radionuclide dynamic and static scans sometimes show termination of radionuclide activity in the mid-portion of the sinus. CT brain scan most frequently discloses a high-density lesion (static blood) in the involved sinus on the pre-contrast scan and a filling defect in the sinus after contrast enhancement.

Cerebral angiography is the most specific diagnostic test for the demonstration of venous sinus thrombosis. Particular attention must be paid to the late filling of the venous sinuses and veins. Sagittal sinus thrombosis has been demonstrated by digital subtraction angiography.

TREATMENT. Appropriate antimicrobial drugs in high dosage and surgical drainage with the removal of infected bone and extradural or intrasinus abscess constitute the proper treatment of major sinus thrombosis secondary to infection. Ligation of the jugular vein in lateral sinus thrombosis to prevent the spread of septic emboli is usually unnecessary. Because of the frequent isolation of penicillinase-producing staphylococci, semisynthetic penicillins should be used until culture results are reported. Anticoagulants should not be used because venous thromboses tend to produce hemorrhagic brain tissue. Prognosis for recovery is fairly good when optimal treatment is given expeditiously, but residual neurologic deficits are frequent.

MALIGNANT EXTERNAL OTITIS

Malignant external otitis begins as an infection of the external auditory canal due to *Pseudomonas aeruginosa*. It affects mainly elderly patients with diabetes mellitus. The infection spreads from the outer ear to the soft tissues below the temporal bone and invades the parotid gland, temporomandibular joint, masseter muscle, and temporal bone. Necrotizing osteitis of the temporal bone develops. The high mortality rate originally reported for the condition (about 40 per cent) led to the use of the adjective "malignant" for this form of temporal bone infection.

The symptoms and signs include rapidly evolving pain in the ear, with or without purulent discharge, swelling of the parotid gland, trismus, and paralysis of the sixth to twelfth nerves. Death is usually caused by the development of meningitis.

Patients with malignant external otitis should be treated with intravenous carbenicillin and gentamicin. Minor surgical debridement is helpful. Antimicrobial treatment should be continued for about a week after apparent cure in order to avoid recurrent disease.

CEREBRAL MANIFESTATIONS OF BACTERIAL ENDOCARDITIS

Neurologic symptoms and signs occur in 25 to 30 per cent of patients with subacute bacterial endocarditis. The most common neurologic manifestation is cerebrovascular disease, which occurs in about half of the patients. Cerebral infarction, hemorrhage, or transient focal ischemic attacks are all seen and behave like similar lesions from other kinds of emboli. Another presentation consists of a subacute toxic encephalopathy, producing confusion, delirium, hallucinations, confabulation, disorientation, paranoid ideation, and other mental disturbances. Milder manifestations include drowsiness, insomnia, apathy, irritability, and personality changes. Autopsy studies suggest that these mental changes reflect the effects of multiple thromboemboli.

Mycotic aneurysms represent about 5 per cent of the neurologic manifestations. These aneurysms usually arise in the distal portion of the middle cerebral artery. They typically present with subarachnoid or intracerebral hemorrhage. Occasional mycotic aneurysms have been observed to disappear after antimicrobial therapy, but late rupture of a mycotic aneurysm after bacteriologic cure may occur. Infected embolic material carried to the nervous system may erode blood vessel walls and cause brain abscess or meningitis. There is a higher incidence of meningitis in acute bacterial endocarditis than in the subacute form. Brain abscess and embolic infarction of cerebral tissue may also complicate acute bacterial endocarditis.

SPINAL EPIDURAL ABSCESS

DEFINITION. Spinal epidural abscess describes a collection of purulent material located outside the dura mater within the spinal canal.

INCIDENCE. Epidural abscesses account for approximately one of every 20,000 admissions to United States hospitals. They make up two thirds of surgically treatable infections of the spinal cord and canal. Epidural abscesses occur at all ages, most affecting adults between 20 and 50 years of age.

PREDISPOSING FACTORS. Infections may reach the spinal epidural space by direct extension from an inflammatory process in adjacent tissues, by metastasis through the bloodstream from infections elsewhere in the body, or by perforating wounds. Bacteremia and resultant hematogenous dissemination appear to account for about one third of acute cases. Furuncles, urinary tract infections, dental infections, chronic pulmonary disease, and decubitus ulcers all have been implicated. Contamination of the epidural space by direct spread accounts for another third of acute cases and approximately one half of chronic cases in adults. The usual focus is an adjacent vertebral osteomyelitis with direct extension into the anterior epidural space. Surgical wounds, retroperitoneal abscesses, and lumbar punctures represent other potential causes. In children the usual sources of bacteremia are perineal skin infections, urinary tract infections, pharyngitis, and endocarditis.

Chronic debilitating diseases, diabetes mellitus, immunosuppressive therapy, and heroin abuse are common contributing factors. About one quarter of patients give a history of recent back trauma.

ETIOLOGY. *Staphylococcus aureus* is the most common cause and accounts for 50 to 60 per cent of epidural abscesses. Other bacteria responsible for the infection include *E. coli* and other gram-negative organisms. Hemolytic and anaerobic streptococci have also been recovered.

PATHOLOGY. Infection in the epidural space may be acute or chronic. In acute cases, there is a purulent necrosis of the epidural fat extending over several segments, or the entire length of the cord. The pus is almost always posterior to the spinal cord, but may extend to the anterior surface as well. The epidural fat is hyperemic and infiltrated with numerous polymorphonuclear leukocytes. If the infection is of low virulence, the abscess may be circumscribed and have a granulomatous appearance. Necrosis in the periphery of the cord may result from pressure of the abscess; myelomalacia of one or several cord segments may occur when spinal veins or arteries are thrombosed. Ascending and descending degeneration of the spinal cord can extend above and below the level of the necrotic lesion. In chronic infections, the dura is thickened and gray. The epidural fat is missing and replaced by granulation tissue. In the absence of pus, the granulation tissue may be mistakenly identified as a neoplasm.

CLINICAL MANIFESTATIONS. The clinical course of spinal epidural abscess proceeds in four phases: back pain, radicular pain, muscular weakness, and paralysis. Back pain is characteristically present at the level of the major pathologic process. It is usually severe and localized to a small region of the spine. Movement of the spine in the anteroposterior direction is limited, and the spinous projections overlying the disease process are tender to percussion. Fever and malaise are usually present.

Two to four days later, irritation of nerve roots leads to radicular pains in the trunk or extremities. An erroneous diagnosis of neuritis may be made at this time. Meningeal signs evolve, and headache becomes a common symptom.

The illness then progresses to cause neurologic impairment at and below the level of the lesion. If the abscess compromises the spinal cord, paraparesis and sensory loss occur, accompanied by urinary and fecal incontinence. Abscesses in the lumbosacral spine compress the cauda equina and produce painful sensations in nerve root distribution, eventually resulting in weakness, depressed stretch reflexes, and sensory impairments. There is often erythema and swelling in the area of back pain and tenderness. If appropriate treatment is not initiated, paralysis occurs within hours or at most a few days. Immediate surgery is indicated when any degree of weakness is detected, since most patients who become completely paralyzed will remain so permanently.

Evolution of a chronic epidural abscess is much slower. Fever and malaise are unusual. Weakness and paralysis may not develop for weeks or months.

LABORATORY DIAGNOSIS. The white blood cell count and erythrocyte sedimentation rate characteristically are elevated. X-rays of the spinal column may show osteomyelitis or a contiguous abscess, but are usually normal.

If spinal cord or cauda equina compression is suspected, it is wise to proceed directly with myelography. Lumbar puncture should be performed with caution when acute epidural abscess is suspected. The needle should be introduced slowly and suction applied with a syringe as the epidural space is approached. If the infection has extended to the level of the puncture, pus may be encountered; the needle should be withdrawn immediately at that point without entering and possibly infecting the subarachnoid space. Spinal fluid obtained from below the level of the abscess is xanthochromic or cloudy in appearance, with a cell count varying from a few to several hundred cells per cubic millimeter. The protein content is often between 100 and 1500 mg per deciliter. The spinal fluid sugar content is normal, and cultures of the fluid are usually sterile unless meningitis has developed. Chronic epidural abscess usually produces a complete or almost complete spinal block with an inconstant pleocytosis and an elevation of the protein content.

Myelography is abnormal in all cases. Complete extradural block is found in 80 per cent and the remainder have a partial block. Myelography should be performed by cervical subarachnoid puncture in patients in whom complete block or a lumbar abscess is suspected. Every effort should be made to define the entire extent of the abscess. Spine CT scans may someday be useful in the diagnosis of spinal epidural abscess but presently are less useful than myelography.

Acute spinal epidural abscess must be differentiated from acute or subacute meningitis, acute poliomyelitis, acute transverse myelitis or multiple sclerosis. The clinical and spinal fluid findings usually permit differentiation of these conditions. Chronic adhesive arachnoiditis and tumors within the epidural space may be confused with chronic epidural abscess; the myelogram should clarify the diagnosis.

TREATMENT. The treatment of spinal epidural abscess is immediate surgical decompression preceded and followed by appropriate antibiotic therapy. Aerobic and anaerobic cultures should be obtained at operation. The area of acute suppuration should be irrigated with an antibiotic solution. Large doses of penicillin are begun prior to surgery and continued postoperatively unless bacterial cultures and sensitivities indicate otherwise.

PROGNOSIS AND OUTCOME. Mortality from epidural abscess is near 30 per cent. The most important determinant for recovery is the patient's neurologic status at the time of operation. Total recovery occurs in patients who have no total paralysis or whose weakness has lasted less than 36 hours. One half of patients paralyzed for 48 hours or more progress to permanent paralysis or death.

SPINAL SUBDURAL EMPYEMA

Infection beneath the dura, but outside the spinal cord, is called spinal subdural empyema. The condition is very rare and has a predilection for the cervical and thoracic spinal cord. The symptoms and signs are indistinguishable from spinal epidural abscess. Coexisting meningitis is common. There is often a greater degree of spinal tenderness than in spinal epidural abscess. Sudden transverse myelitis occurs, attributable to spinal cord infarction from vascular compromise caused by the pus collection. The lesion is best demonstrated by myelography. *Staphylococcus aureus* is the most commonly isolated microorganism. Prompt antimicrobial and surgical treatment is mandatory.

Brain Abscess

Brewer ND, MacCarty CS, Wellman WE: Brain abscess: A review of recent experience. Ann Intern Med 82:571, 1975. *Describes diagnosis, microbiology, and treatment in 60 patients.*

deLouvois J: Bacteriological examination of pus from abscesses of the central nervous system. J Clin Pathol 33:66, 1980. *Discussion of the often elusive bacteriology of these conditions.*

Gruszkiewicz J, Doron Y, Peyser E, Borovich B, Schachter J, Front D: Brain abscess and its surgical management. Surg Neurol 18:7, 1982.

Nielsen H, Gyldensted C, Harmsen A: Cerebral abscess: Aetiology, and pathogenesis, symptoms, diagnosis and treatment: A review of 200 cases from 1935–1976. Acta Neurol Scand 65:609, 1982. *This and the above article emphasize the sharp reduction in mortality since CT scanning has allowed better diagnosis and monitoring.*

Rosenblum ML, Hoff JT, Norman D, Edwards MS, Berg BO: Nonoperative treatment of brain abscesses in selected high-risk patients. J Neurosurg 52:217, 1980. *Reports successful treatment by antimicrobial agents alone in eight high-risk patients followed closely by serial CT scans.*

Shaw MDM, Russell JA: Cerebellar abscess: A review of 47 cases. J Neurol Neurosurg Psychiatry 38:429, 1975. *A review of one of the largest available series, 90 per cent secondary to otogenic disease. Effective treatment required adequate radical mastoidectomy plus appropriate treatment of the abscess itself.*

Subdural Empyema

Kaufman DM, Miller MH, Steigbigel NH: Subdural empyema: Analysis of 17 recent cases and review of the literature. Medicine 54:485, 1975. *A thorough consideration of the subject.*

Kaufman DM, Litman N, Miller MH: Sinusitis: Induced subdural empyema. Neurology (New York) 33:123, 1983. *Reviews experience in 17 patients, only 5 of which had a history of sinusitis. CT exams missed the abscess in 2 of 7 patients.*

Luken MG III, Whelan MA: Recent diagnostic experience with subdural empyema. J Neurosurg 52:764, 1980. *Reviews radiographic and therapeutic aspects of primary and secondary subdural empyemas.*

Cerebral Epidural Abscess

Morello A, Hoen TI: Chronic epidural abscess and condensing osteomyelitis of the skull. Neurology 4:633, 1954. *Describes well mechanisms and pathogenesis of the condition.*

Sharif HS, Ibrahim A: Intracranial epidural abscess. Br J Radiol 55:81, 1982. *Points up potential value of CT imaging in detecting this uncommon disorder before serious neurologic damage occurs.*

Major Dural Sinus Thrombosis

Brown P: Septic cavernous sinus thrombosis. Bull Johns Hopkins Hosp. 109:68, 1961. *One of the few papers dealing directly with infected thromboses.*

Kalbag RM, Woolf AL: Cerebral Venous Thrombosis. London, Oxford University Press, 1967. *The classic monograph on the subject.*

Rao KCVG, Knipp HC, Wagner EJ: Computed tomographic findings in cerebral sinus and venous thrombosis. Radiology 140:391, 1981. *In all patients, CT revealed unusual or small ventricular hemorrhages, low density areas, and increased density of dural sinuses and tentorium.*

Malignant External Otitis

Damiani JM, Damiani KK, Kinney SE: Malignant external otitis with multiple cranial nerve involvement. Am J Otolaryngol 1:115, 1979. *A good discussion of the subject.*

Strauss M, Aber RC, Conner GH, Baum S: Malignant external otitis: Long-term (months) antimicrobial therapy. Laryngoscope 92:397, 1982. *Six patients with this often fatal syndrome were treated successfully with long-term antimicrobials plus (in two) extensive surgical debridement.*

Cerebral Manifestations of Bacterial Endocarditis

Churchill MA Jr, Geraci JE, Hunder GG: Musculoskeletal manifestations of bacterial endocarditis. Ann Intern Med 87:754, 1977. *Outlines the muscular, arthritic, and myalgic manifestations of the disorder. In 27 per cent of patients, musculoskeletal complaints were among the first symptoms.*

Pruitt AA, Rubin RH, Karchmer AW, Duncan GW: Neurologic complications of bacterial endocarditis. Medicine 57:329, 1978. *The most recent comprehensive review on the subject.*

Spinal Epidural Abscess

Altrocchi PH: Acute spinal epidural abscess vs. acute transverse myelitis. Arch Neurol 9:17, 1963. *A classic paper emphasizing the differential diagnosis of these disorders.*

Baker AS, Ojemann RG, Swartz MN, Richardson EP Jr: Spinal epidural abscess. N Engl J Med 293:463, 1975. *Reviews course and treatment of 39 patients treated in the antimicrobial era.*

Kaufman DM, Kaplan JG, Litman N: Infectious agents in spinal epidural abscesses. Neurology (New York) 30:844, 1980.

Spinal Subdural Empyema

Fraser RAR, Ratzan K, Wolpert SM, Weinstein L: Spinal subdural empyema. Arch Neurol 28:235, 1973. *A case report and review of ten examples from the literature of this uncommon disorder that can be cured only if recognized and treated early.*

497. SYPHILITIC INFECTIONS OF THE CENTRAL NERVOUS SYSTEM

Kenneth P. Johnson

A general exposition of *T. pallidum* infection is presented in Ch. 306. The following presentation is restricted to a discussion of neurosyphilis.

Neurosyphilis is the invasion and persistent infection of the leptomeninges and, in some cases, brain parenchyma with the spirochete *Treponema pallidum*. Such persistent infection may be asymptomatic or may cause a wide spectrum of neurologic abnormalities.

PATHOLOGY. A meningitis of varying severity and extent is present in every case of active neurosyphilis regardless of the neurologic syndrome. The cerebrospinal fluid (CSF) reflects this involvement even in cases of asymptomatic neurosyphilis.

Study of a few cases of *acute syphilitic meningitis* has shown a meningeal inflammatory reaction in which lymphocytes and plasma cells predominate primarily about blood vessels, often with evidence of early arteritis, although cerebrovascular accidents are rare in this stage of the disease. Reactive arachnoiditis, especially about the base of the brain, is also seen. This accounts for the cranial nerve palsies and for an impairment of CSF circulation that can sometimes result in increased intracranial pressure. A granular ependymitis is commonly present which rarely may obstruct CSF flow through the aqueduct.

In *meningovascular syphilis*, typically a more chronic disorder occurring months or a few years after the primary lesion, the inflammatory response is usually prominent. An associated arteritis (usually small vessels) predisposes to arterial occlusion and consequent infarction of neural tissue. When larger arteries become occluded, infarction of brain or spinal cord may be extensive.

In *general paresis* there is direct invasion of neural tissue by the spirochete, in addition to the meningitis. The cortical architecture is often markedly disordered. One finds meningeal thickening, atrophy of cerebral tissue (especially of frontal and temporal lobes), enlargement of ventricles, and a granularity of the ependymal surface. Microscopically, diffuse destruction and loss of neurons, especially in the cortex, are found. Special stains may demonstrate the presence of *Treponema pallidum*. Reactive gliosis with pleomorphic microglia is characteristic. Inflammation of the meninges is prominent with varying degrees of arteritis.

In *tabes dorsalis* and primary optic atrophy, the pathogenesis of the neurologic lesion is unclear. Direct invasion by the spirochete and an immunologic reaction affecting the meninges may both occur. Grossly the dorsal roots and the dorsal aspect of the spinal cord appear wasted. Secondary demyelination of dorsal columns is readily demonstrated. Involvement of anterior roots with resultant amyotrophy occurs rarely. Why the syphilitic process shows a predilection for dorsal roots is unknown.

Focal granulomatous accumulations *(gummas)* are rare; they may reach the size of clinical brain tumors and extend into the brain parenchyma from a meningeal origin. More diffuse granulomas of the dura (hypertrophic pachymeningitis) sometimes compress neural structures, especially the spinal cord.

CLINICAL SYNDROMES IN NEUROSYPHILIS. ***Asymptomatic Neurosyphilis.*** This is the most common form of neurosyphilis; it generally follows the acute infection within one to three years. As the term suggests, affected patients lack symptoms or signs of neurologic disease. The diagnosis rests on the finding in the CSF of a low-grade meningitis plus the immunologic abnormalities of syphilis. Adequate treatment prevents the development of neurologic symptoms.

Atypical Neurosyphilis. As of 1980, primary syphilis occurs in 70,000 or more persons per year in the United States and secondary syphilis in perhaps 13,000. The spirochete is known to invade the central nervous system (CNS) frequently during these early phases of infection, even though detectable neurosyphilis is rare. Probably the organism is cleared by normal host defenses. Large numbers of persons frequently receive antibiotics to which *T. pallidum* is sensitive for other conditions, but in doses inadequate to cure neurosyphilis. Therefore, many investigators fear that atypical forms of neurosyphilis may be developing following partial antibiotic therapy. Such partial treatment may also modify CSF and serologic reactivity, impairing diagnostic efficiency. Therefore, unusual or bizarre neurologic syndromes accompanied by some CSF abnormalities should at least raise the possibility of neurosyphilis. This is especially important in high risk groups such as homosexual males, in whom syphilis appears with increased frequency.

Symptomatic Neurosyphilis. MENINGITIS. An acute meningitis develops only rarely, although it seems likely that some patients with mild or even moderate symptoms go unnoticed. Symptomatic syphilitic meningitis usually occurs during the early weeks or months after infection, often during the period of the secondary rash or concurrently with a mucocutaneous relapse in a patient previously but inadequately treated. The full-blown illness usually lasts less than one month, but symptoms may persist for longer periods. Headache, vomiting, malaise, and irritability are prominent. Kernig's and Brudzinski's signs develop. Occasionally, confusion, delirium, seizures, and cranial nerve palsies (seventh and eighth nerves most common) occur. Argyll Robertson pupils do not occur in acute syphilitic meningitis. Acute syphilitic hydrocephalus with increased intracranial pressure, including papilledema, may lead to confusion with other inflammatory and neoplastic conditions. The CSF always contains an increased number of white blood cells (average about 500 per cubic millimeter—usually mononuclear, rarely polymorphonuclear), an elevated total protein (average, about 100 mg per deciliter), and normal sugar concentrations (reduced rarely). An elevated gamma globulin concentration develops in 70 per cent of cases. The serum serologic tests for syphilis (VDRL and FTS-ABS) are usually but not always positive.

The response to therapy is generally prompt, although an occasional patient will subsequently develop some other form of neurosyphilis.

MENINGOVASCULAR SYPHILIS. The incidence of this form of neurosyphilis is low, a figure of 3 per cent of syphilitic patients being recorded. Men are affected more often than women (3:1). Meningovascular syphilis occurs most commonly from two to ten years after the primary lesion. Symptoms and signs of meningitis are lacking, although headache is a frequent complaint. The neurologic deficits may develop slowly, or abruptly upon occlusion of a major vessel. Depending upon the distribution of infarction, the patient may develop hemiplegia, hemisensory defect, dysphasia, or homonymous hemianopia. Focal cerebral seizures develop occasionally. A transverse myelopathy may produce varying degrees of paraparesis, sensory loss, and impaired function of bladder and bowel. Infarction of the anterior two thirds of the cord, with resultant paraplegia and loss of pain sensation below the lesion, can follow occlusion of the anterior spinal artery. Sensory functions subserved by the posterior columns are usually preserved. Hydrocephalus and various cranial nerve palsies have been described.

A CSF lymphocytic pleocytosis (up to 100 cells per cubic millimeter) and an elevated protein concentration are characteristic. The CSF gamma globulin content is often elevated. Syphilitic reagins (VDRL) are nearly always present in the CSF as well as in the blood.

The progress of meningovascular syphilis can usually be halted by specific antibiotic treatment, but the degree of functional recovery depends upon the extent and location of the infarcts.

GENERAL PARESIS (DEMENTIA PARALYTICA, GENERAL PARALYSIS OF THE INSANE). General paresis can develop at any time from 2 to 30 (usually 10 to 25) years after the primary lesion. It appears more often in men than in women (3:1). About 60 per cent of paretics present with a progressive simple dementia; less than 20 per cent display manic symptoms and megalomania. Often faulty judgment, impaired memory (recent memory affected first), disturbed affect (depression or euphoria), or paranoia develops and progresses. The patient may complain of "nervousness," but characteristically lacks insight into the nature of his difficulty. Fine or coarse tremors, often affecting facial muscles and tongue, are present in about two thirds of the patients with fully developed general paresis. Abnormal pupillary responses, including Argyll Robertson pupil (see Tabes Dorsalis, below), impassive facies, slurred or dysarthric speech, exaggerated stretch reflexes, and extensor plantar responses are additional abnormal neurologic signs. Convulsions occur in 10 per cent of patients, and strokes may develop secondary to vasculitis.

The CSF is always abnormal, containing a modest (15 to 100) increase in mononuclear cells and an elevated total protein concentration (greater than 50 mg per deciliter in 75 per cent, and 100 mg per deciliter or higher in about 20 per cent of cases). An elevated CSF gamma globulin level is routinely found in general paresis as well as the presence of oligoclonal IgG bands. Nearly every patient has a positive VDRL and RPR (see below) test for syphilis in the CSF, and more than 90 per cent of patients have a positive blood serologic test. Incomplete, prior treatment may modify the CSF abnormalities.

General paresis, once established, evolves rapidly. If untreated, the disease is universally fatal, usually within three years. If paresis is recognized early and treated vigorously, about 80 per cent of patients will improve, but only about one half completely recover neurologic function.

TABES DORSALIS (LOCOMOTOR ATAXIA). Tabes dorsalis develops in less than 5 per cent of patients with untreated syphilis, and symptoms usually appear 10 to 20 years after the primary infection. Men are more often affected.

Dysfunction of affected posterior roots develops insidiously, usually first in the lower limbs. Impaired joint position sense results in stumbling and progressive sensory ataxia, especially in the dark when visual compensation is imperfect. Hypotonia, secondary to a lack of modulation of muscle tension by afferent fibers, accentuates the slapping gait. Paresthesias usually appear early in the disease.

Lightning pains are characteristic of tabes dorsalis but are nonspecific, occurring also in other diseases affecting dorsal roots, e.g., diabetic neuropathy. Lightning pains develop in at least 75 per cent of patients and migrate from one area of the body to another, although they are most common in the lower extremities. They are brief, sharp, burning, or aching jabs, sometimes flitting from one body region to another without predictable pattern. Involvement of thoracoabdominal nerve roots gives rise to visceral pains (gastric or visceral crises), which may simulate intrinsic visceral disease and can lead to misdiagnosis of abdominal surgical disease; in one series an estimated 25 per cent of tabetic patients had undergone inappropriate operations for tabetic pain. However, one must occasionally be wary, for the impairment of pain sensation in tabetics or the too quick assignment of lightning pain can induce disregard for true surgical emergencies.

As tabes advances, pain sensation is progressively lost and recurrent peripheral trauma goes unnoticed. Indolent ulcers of the skin develop; the toes and balls of the feet are especially vulnerable. Weight-bearing joints and adjacent bone, deprived of pain sensation, are destroyed by the constant trauma of use in 5 to 10 per cent of tabetic patients (Charcot joints).

Unless general paresis coexists, as it does in a small percentage of cases (taboparesis), tabetic patients are mentally normal. Optic atrophy complicates tabes dorsalis in about 10 per cent of cases or occurs as an isolated disorder. Argyll Robertson pupils that are small, irregular, and unequal, and respond poorly to light but constrict with accommodation, are present in most cases. Occasionally, other oculomotor functions are involved as well. Hypotonia, ataxia, and a slapping broad-based gait are common. Affection of the sensory arc accounts for the greatly diminished or absent stretch reflexes, especially the Achilles reflex. The plantar responses are normal in most cases. Loss or diminution of position and vibratory sensation is found in every case. Increased swaying when the eyes are closed and the patient is standing with feet together (Romberg's sign) results from the impaired position sense. Variable degrees of hypoesthesia and hypalgesia occur in nerve root distribution. Isolated areas of hypalgesia (Hitzig zones) sometimes affect the trunk or shoulders. Delayed perception (from one to several seconds) of pain stimuli delivered to a distal extremity provides a classic sign. Urinary bladder and bowel impairment produces incontinence and constipation in up to one third of cases. Male impotence and orthostatic hypotension are major complaints. Cystitis, hydronephrosis, and pyelonephritis are common complications of a hypotonic bladder.

The course of tabes dorsalis is unpredictable, and the response to antisyphilitic therapy varies. Patients who have had symptoms for a few months or at the most a few years, with prominent CSF abnormalities and no prior therapy, often improve with treatment. Patients with severe degeneration of dorsal roots and who suffer from painful complications usually retain many of their troubles but progress relatively little after antisyphilitic therapy ("burned out" tabes). Partial relief of pain may be achieved by analgesics, but narcotics carry a high risk of producing addiction. Benefit has been reported with anticonvulsant doses of phenytoin or carbamazepine. Urologic assistance may be required to deal effectively with uropathy. Penetrating skin ulcers and Charcot joints may similarly require surgical treatment.

Optic Atrophy. Visual impairment in syphilis may result from iritis, choreoretinitis, increased intracranial pressure, or primary optic atrophy. Optic atrophy occurs in 1 per cent of patients with untreated syphilis and is five times more common in males than in females.

Because the outer portions of the optic nerve are first affected, the initial visual impairment tends to be peripheral. Ultimately, however, the papillomacular bundle becomes involved, and impaired visual acuity with central and paracentral scotomas develops. It has been estimated that, without treatment, 50 per cent of patients go blind in two years and 90 per cent in ten years. One eye is typically affected before the other. Optic pallor is usually present by the time symptoms appear, but in the early stages it is recognizable only by the reduced vascularity. The optic atrophy of syphilis is indistinguishable from that caused by other diseases. The CSF is abnormal in most patients with active disease of the optic nerve. Intensive antisyphilitic therapy may arrest the disease process and preserve what vision remains, but return of vision cannot be anticipated.

Gumma. This rare complication of syphilis usually presents as an intracranial or intraspinal mass lesion and behaves as a slowly growing neoplasm. The correct diagnosis may be suspected from a positive serum serologic test for syphilis or from CSF abnormalities. Removal of the tumor mass, supplemented by antimicrobial therapy, alleviates symptoms and prevents spread of the disease.

Congenital Neurosyphilis. Syphilis acquired in utero after the first trimester of pregnancy tends to be a fulminant disease. Miscarriages and stillbirths are common, and a wide spectrum of clinical manifestations may be recognized in the infant or child who survives. *Neurosyphilis* develops in an estimated 10 to 20 per cent of infants and children with congenital syphilis. *Asymptomatic neurosyphilis* may be diagnosed in the early months or years of life by routine CSF examinations on children of syphilitic mothers. But, as with the acquired disease, symptoms and signs of active neurosyphilis develop only after a latent period, which in the case of *juvenile paresis* may be as long as 20 years. More often, symptoms first appear late in the first decade or during adolescence. Clinical syndromes and CSF findings mirror those found with the acquired disease, except that *tabes dorsalis* is exceedingly rare and *chorioretinitis* more common. Hydrocephalus, cranial nerve palsies (eighth cranial nerve especially), and seizures may complicate congenital syphilitic meningitis. Syphilis should be considered as a potential cause of cerebrovascular accidents in children. More than a third of all children with juvenile paresis have been retarded mentally from early life.

Non-neurologic stigmata of congenital syphilis include dental deformities (Hutchinson's teeth), saddle nose, frontal bossing of the skull, saber shins, and interstitial keratitis (usually developing during the second decade). These signs are not seen in acquired syphilis. Fortunately, the current practice of obtaining routine serologic tests on all pregnant women and on infants of syphilitic mothers has almost eliminated congenital neurosyphilis in many areas of the world. It should be remembered that the mother can acquire syphilis at any time during pregnancy and that negative serologic studies obtained early do not exclude the possibility of active syphilis later in pregnancy. Some institutions routinely test blood from the umbilical cord for the reagin of syphilis.

Early and intensive treatment of infants with congenital syphilis materially reduces the morbidity (see Treatment) from neurologic complications. Results from even optimal treatment of patients with juvenile paresis remain poor.

LABORATORY DIAGNOSIS OF NEUROSYPHILIS. Laboratory studies can be of considerable aid in the diagnosis of neurosyphilis and in the evaluation of therapy. Nevertheless, both false-positive and false-negative results may occur with all assays currently available, so that the final diagnosis requires a consideration of clinical as well as laboratory data.

Cerebrospinal Fluid Changes. Neurosyphilis always includes meningeal inflammation and its accompanying abnormalities in the CSF. Because of the chronic nature of the meningitis, the CSF changes are usually mild. A modest increase in cells, predominantly lymphocytes, numbering from 6 to 100 per cubic millimeter, is noted. The cytologic identification of plasma cells may be useful. The total CSF protein is usually elevated moderately to between 40 and 100 mg per deciliter. The CSF glucose is almost always normal.

The presence of treponemes within the CNS stimulates a local immunologic response, including the production of immunoglobulins which leak into the CSF. This is expressed as an increase in the CSF immunoglobulin G (IgG) level, which can be measured either as the IgG percentage of total protein (usually above 12 per cent) or, more specifically, by an IgG index. The index formula

$$\frac{\text{CSF IgG}}{\text{Serum IgG}} : \frac{\text{CSF albumin}}{\text{Serum albumin}},$$

which requires assessment of albumin and IgG in both serum and CSF, can be used to determine a specific increase in CSF IgG, considered by most workers to be a measure of IgG synthesis within the CNS compartment. In most laboratories an IgG index above 0.7 is considered abnormal. Specific elevation of CSF IgG is almost always noted in neurosyphilis.

In addition to quantitative IgG abnormalities, a qualitative CSF change is generally noted in neurosyphilis when concentrated CSF is assayed by agarose electrophoresis. This method demonstrates the presence of oligoclonal IgG bands which appear in perhaps 70 per cent of cases of confirmed neurosyphilis. Spirochetes have been demonstrated directly in CSF of patients with secondary syphilis by immunofluorescent methods.

Serologic Tests. The serologic tests for syphilis can be divided into two groups: those which are nontreponemal, and those which measure specific serologic reactivity to treponemal antigens. The nontreponemal tests use purified cardiolipin, which reacts with an antibody (formerly called reagin) in the serum or CSF to produce a serologic reaction. Presently, two flocculation tests, the Venereal Disease Research Laboratory (VDRL) and the rapid plasma reagin (RPR) tests, are routinely available and both can be accurately quantitated. Both are inexpensive and readily adapted to screening large numbers of specimens. Neither of these tests is as sensitive as the specific treponemal tests, and both may react in several nonsyphilitic disease states, especially the autoimmune disorders such as systemic lupus erythematosus. The specific treponemal serologic tests include the treponemal immobilization test (TPI), which is expensive, difficult to assay, and not routinely available, and the readily available indirect immunofluorescence assay, the fluorescent treponemal antibody–absorbed (FTA-ABS) test. The FTA-ABS test uses inactivated treponemes reacted with the patient's serum, which has been previously absorbed with an extract of nonpathogenic Reiter treponemes to remove nonspecific reactants. The other increasingly useful specific test is the treponemal hemagglutination test, which employs sheep or turkey erythrocytes coated with antigens of *T. pallidum*.

In practice, the nontreponemal tests are used for screening purposes and the specific treponemal tests for confirmation of diagnosis. It should be noted that the nontreponemal assays may be incorrectly reported in 5 to as many as 25 per cent of cases; therefore, if a negative result is obtained in a suspected case of neurosyphilis or a positive result is unexpectedly found, the test should first be repeated. Following confirmation of the nontreponemal assays, a specific treponemal test can be used to confirm the diagnosis.

Both the nonspecific and the specific treponemal antibody assays are positive in serum by the secondary stage of syphilis when acute meningitis and meningovascular syphilis appear. In the majority of late asymptomatic cases as well as in tabes dorsalis and general paresis, the tests are also often positive, although late CNS involvement sometimes has been reported with negative serology. The serum FTA-ABS is usually reactive even if the VDRL is negative in these late cases.

The serologic assay of CSF in neurosyphilis is still controversial. Most authorities advocate the use of the CSF VDRL test, both as an aid in the diagnosis of neurosyphilis and as a rough evaluation of therapy. The CSF VDRL is rarely falsely positive during nonsyphilitic disease states. If the test is positive, it is assumed that the patient does have invasion of the CNS by *T. pallidum*, especially if there is confirmatory clinical or CSF evidence of neurosyphilis. Usually the CSF VDRL titer falls with adequate treatment, although it may remain positive for prolonged periods. Accordingly, therapy must also be monitored by the clinical response and by a decrease in the number of CSF cells, total protein, or IgG level. The specific serologic tests often remain reactive for long periods after an apparent cure.

The specific treponemal tests, especially the CSF FTA, have yielded conflicting results in the diagnosis of neurosyphilis. Contamination of CSF with a minute amount of blood has been shown to convert a negative CSF sample to a positive one, so that CSF containing any red blood cells cannot be reliably used in a CSF FTA test. Some investigators believe that because of the extreme sensitivity of the test, even moderate amounts of antibody in the serum may cross to the CSF in the absence of true neurosyphilis. In the absence of elevated cells, protein, or IgG, no diagnostic conclusion can be made from finding a positive CSF FTA assay.

The need for evaluation of CSF during late (over one year after contact) asymptomatic syphilis remains unclear. Most authorities advocate CSF examination in all cases of a positive serum FTA-ABS test with an unclear treatment history. One recent study showed a very small yield of positive CSF findings in such patients. Nevertheless, in view of the differing treatment recommendations for late asymptomatic versus neurosyphilis patients, a CSF examination prior to therapy should probably be performed. Of course, evaluation of any patient with a positive serum FTA-ABS and any neurologic abnormality, even if not typical of the classic neurosyphilis syndromes, requires CSF assay to rule out atypical neurosyphilis.

TREATMENT OF NEUROSYPHILIS. Penicillin is the antibiotic of choice for all forms of syphilis, and no resistant strains of *T. pallidum* are known. Because the organism divides slowly and penicillin is effective during the dividing stage, prolonged therapeutic blood and CSF levels are necessary to accomplish a cure. Aqueous procaine penicillin G, 9 million units total given intramuscularly in 15 daily 600,000-unit doses, or benzathine penicillin G, given intramuscularly in three 2.4 million–unit doses at weekly intervals, has been advocated. However, some cases of neurosyphilis have progressed after such therapy, and other studies have failed to detect penicillin in CSF, especially after recommended weekly benzathine penicillin. Therefore, several authorities advocate hospitalization of all patients with neurosyphilis and treatment with 2 to 4 million units of aqueous crystalline penicillin G intravenously every four hours (12 to 24 million units per day) for ten days. As mentioned above, therapy is monitored clinically and when repeating the CSF evaluation two to six months later. CSF leukocytes should decline, as should total protein and IgG levels and, usually, the CSF VDRL titer. If CSF cell, protein, or IgG abnormalities persist unchanged, retreatment should be considered.

In cases of penicillin allergy, tetracycline HCl or erythromycin, 500 mg four times a day orally for 30 days, is usually curative.

Felman YM, Nikitas JA: Syphilis serology today. Arch Dermatol 116:84, 1980. *A detailed, comprehensive review of currently used serologic tests to detect infection with* T. pallidum *during each phase of disease.*

Holmes MD, Brant-Zawadzki MM, Simon RP: Clinical features of meningovascular syphilis. Neurology 34:553, 1984. *A short review of an acute form of neurosyphilis.*

Jaffe HW, Kabins SA: Examination of cerebrospinal fluid in patients with syphilis. Rev Infect Dis 4(Suppl.): 5842, 1982. *Current review of the assays available to analyze cerebrospinal fluid for evidence of neurosyphilis.*

Jones JE Jr, Harris RE: Diagnostic evaluation of syphilis during pregnancy. Obstet Gynecol 54:611, 1979. *Diagnosis and treatment of syphilis are necessary to prevent late maternal complications as well as congenital syphilis. A rational diagnostic approach is advocated.*

Merritt HH, Adams RD, Solomon H: Neurosyphilis. New York, Oxford University Press, 1946. *A classic lucid text on neurosyphilis, written when the various syndromes were still common and readily observable.*

Traviesa DC, Prystowsky SD, Nelson BJ, Johnson KP: Cerebrospinal fluid findings in asymptomatic patients with reactive serum fluorescent treponemal antibody absorption tests. Ann Neurol 4:524, 1978. *A study of the variations in the laboratory diagnosis of syphilis between different laboratories testing the same specimen. Text includes a helpful discussion of the use of lumbar puncture to detect neurosyphilis in asymptomatic patients.*

Venereal Disease Control Advisory Committee, Center for Disease Control, Atlanta, Georgia: Syphilis: recommended treatment schedules, 1976. Ann Intern Med 85:94, 1976. *Current official recommendations for treatment of all forms of syphilis.*

Wiggelinkhuizen J, Mason R: Congenital neurosyphilis and juvenile paresis. A forgotten entity? Clin Pediat 19:142, 1980. *A useful discussion of congenital and juvenile neurosyphilis, a disease fortunately rare but unfortunately underdiagnosed.*

Viral Infections of the Nervous System

498. INTRODUCTION

Richard T. Johnson

Most viral infections of the nervous system represent uncommon but important complications of systemic infections. With a few exceptions such as rabies or B virus *(herpes simiae)*, nervous system infections are caused by agents that often infect humans. Some of these viruses, such as polioviruses and arthropod-borne encephalitis viruses, cause clinically significant disease only on the rare occasion when the nervous system is involved. Others, such as herpes simplex and mumps virus, are frequent causes of mild disease that assumes a more serious form when the central nervous system is infected.

Experimentally, viruses have been shown to invade the nervous system by centripetal movement in peripheral nerves, by penetration across the olfactory mucosa, or by a viremia. In man most viruses that infect the nervous system spread to the brain and meninges from blood, although neural spread appears to be important in rabies, B, herpes simplex, and varicella-zoster virus infections. The infrequency of nervous system involvement can be attributed to a variety of host defense mechanisms, including cellular and humoral responses, interferon production, anatomic barriers of nonsusceptible cells, and the activity of the reticuloendothelial system, which clears viruses from the blood. Youth, severe nutritional deficiency, and defects of cellular immunity have been shown to increase the risk of nervous system infection with some viruses, but in most patients the factors that have permitted central nervous system invasion are not evident.

Viral infections of the nervous system can lead to diverse clinical signs and symptoms, varied clinical courses, and protean pathologic changes. This diversity can be explained by the following two principles: (1) the varied cell populations of the nervous system have different susceptibilities to different viruses; and (2) viral infections can have varied effects on susceptible cells. If infection is limited to the meninges covering the nervous system, signs of viral meningitis may be the only clinical manifestations. If the infection spreads to the parenchymal cells of the brain, in addition to signs of meningeal irritation, signs of encephalitis develop. Some viruses cause even more selective involvement of specific cell populations in the brain and spinal cord and thus evoke characteristic clinical symptoms and signs. For example, in poliovirus infections the selective vulnerability of anterior horn cells leads to a characteristic clinical finding of acute meningitis with lower motor neuron paralysis. On the other hand, rabies virus infections in animals tend to spare the cortical neurons involved in most types of encephalitis and infect neurons of the limbic system. Therefore, instead of obtundation, seizures, and motor or sensory deficits, the infected animal shows alertness, loss of timidity, aberrant sexual behavior, and aggressive activity. This selective infection of cells of the limbic system appears to be a diabolic adaptation of the rabies virus to specific cell populations, so that the clinical disease in animals can drive the host to transmit the virus to another host by biting. Glial cell populations may also be selectively involved, such as in progressive multifocal leukoencephalopathy in which virus infection and cell lysis appear limited to the oligodendrocytes, causing a slowly progressive demyelinating disease.

The virus-cell interaction may be quite varied. There may be *acute lysis* of the infected cell, transformation of the cell with production of neoplasm, or *chronic infection* causing cellular dysfunction, cellular degeneration, or no abnormality. In acute viral infections the clinical and pathologic abnormalities may result either from an acute viral destruction of cells, as in acute viral meningitis or encephalitis, or from the host's immunologic response to the infection, as has been postulated in postinfectious encephalomyelitis. A *latent infection* is a virus-host relationship in which the virus remains present in some form in the host without giving rise to any signs of infection, but which can, when some trigger mechanism comes into play, emerge as an acute infectious process. This appears to occur in herpes zoster and in the majority of cases of herpes simplex encephalitis. *Chronic viral infections* are those in which there is an ongoing active infection, which may give rise to a somewhat irregular or unpredictable course extending over many months or years. Chronic inflammatory disease of the central nervous system is seen with fetal infections by rubella and cytomegaloviruses. In these indolent infections virus can be recovered for long periods of time postnatally and may or may not cause continuing or evolving clinical signs of disease. *Slow infections* have a more predictable course than chronic infections. They are defined as infections with an incubation period lasting for months to years, followed by a protracted but predictable clinical course ending in death. Slow viral infections of the nervous system in man include kuru, Creutzfeldt-Jakob disease, subacute sclerosing panencephalitis, progressive rubella panencephalitis, and progressive multifocal leukoencephalopathy (see Ch. 504).

499. VIRAL MENINGITIS AND ENCEPHALITIS

Richard T. Johnson

DEFINITIONS. *Viral meningitis* is a benign, self-limited illness with clinical signs of headache, fever, and meningeal inflammation. *Viral encephalitis* is a more severe illness in which fever, headache, and meningeal inflammation are complicated by depression of the state of consciousness, seizures, and/or focal neurologic deficits suggesting inflammation within the parenchyma of the brain.

The clinical syndrome of viral meningitis is also called *aseptic meningitis* or *serous meningitis,* since some bacterial infections and chemical irritants can cause identical clinical symptoms and cerebrospinal fluid changes. Encephalitis is also called *meningoencephalitis* or *encephalomyelitis,* the latter indicating concurrent signs of spinal cord involvement.

ETIOLOGY. A variety of viruses have been associated with meningitis and encephalitis (Table 499–1). The two syndromes represent a clinical continuum and are caused by the same spectrum of viral agents. However, some viruses tend to cause predominantly benign disease such as the coxsackie- and echoviruses, which cause about half of all cases of viral meningitis but are only rarely associated with encephalitis. Other viruses tend to cause more severe disease such as arthropod-borne viruses (arboviruses) and herpes simplex virus, which are the major causes of fatal encephalitis (Table 499–2).

Enteroviruses are small, nonenveloped RNA viruses of the picornavirus family, and include polioviruses, group A and B coxsackieviruses, and echoviruses. Over 50 serotypes have been associated with meningitis and encephalitis; the serotypes most frequently recovered from patients with viral meningitis are echoviruses 3, 4, 6, 9, 11, 18, and 30, coxsackievirus A9, and coxsackieviruses B1 through 5. Echovirus 9 has been associated with the largest epidemics.

Mumps virus is a large, enveloped RNA virus of the paramyxovirus family. Mumps is the single most common cause of

TABLE 499–1. VIRUSES ASSOCIATED WITH ACUTE CENTRAL NERVOUS SYSTEM INFECTIONS IN THE UNITED STATES

RNA Viruses
- Enteroviruses
  - Polioviruses
  - Coxsackieviruses, groups A and B
  - Echoviruses
- Togaviruses
  - Eastern encephalitis*
  - Western encephalitis*
  - Venezuelan equine encephalitis*
  - St. Louis*
  - Powassan*
  - Rubella
- Reovirus
  - Colorado tick fever*
- Bunyavirus
  - California encephalitis*
- Arenavirus
  - Lymphocytic choriomeningitis
- Rhabdovirus
  - Rabies
- Myxoviruses and paramyxoviruses
  - Influenza
  - Parainfluenza
  - Mumps
  - Measles

DNA Viruses
- Herpesviruses
  - Herpes simplex, types 1 and 2
  - Varicella-zoster
  - Epstein-Barr
  - Cytomegalovirus
- Adenoviruses

*Arthropod-borne viruses (arboviruses).

TABLE 499–2. FREQUENCY OF ASSOCIATION OF AGENTS WITH ASEPTIC MENINGITIS AND ENCEPHALITIS*

Etiologic Agent	Percentage of Cases	
	Aseptic Meningitis	*Encephalitis*
Enteroviruses	40	10
Mumps	12	14
Lymphocytic choriomeningitis	6	9
Leptospira	3	2
Herpes simplex	1	10
Arboviruses	1	11
Other†	2	4

*Data from Johnson, 1982.
†Includes Epstein-Barr virus, measles, influenza, *Mycoplasma pneumoniea*, Rocky Mountain spotted fever, and fungal infections.

viral meningitis and mild encephalitis. Lymphocytic choriomeningitis virus is a small, enveloped RNA virus of the arenavirus group, which also causes both meningitis and mild encephalitis.

Herpesviruses are large, structurally complex, enveloped DNA viruses that cause a variety of neurologic diseases. Type 1 herpes simplex virus is associated with severe encephalitis in adults and represents the most common cause of endemic fatal encephalitis. Type 2 herpes simplex virus, a major cause of fatal neonatal encephalitis, seldom causes severe encephalitis in adults but has been associated with cases of meningitis. Headache and pleocytosis often accompany herpes zoster infections, but it is not known whether meningitis without radicular pain or cutaneous eruptions can be a manifestation of recrudescences of latent varicella-zoster virus infections (see Ch. 501). The Epstein-Barr virus has been related to meningitis and encephalitis, complicating approximately 1 per cent of cases of infectious mononucleosis. Cytomegalovirus, like rubella virus, is associated primarily with chronic congenital infections. However, cytomegalovirus causes encephalitis in immunocompromised patients and rarely in immunocompetent adults.

The acute neurologic disease associated with measles, vaccinia, rubella, and primary varicella (chickenpox) infections in most cases represents postinfectious encephalomyelitis. This may also be true of the encephalitis that has occasionally been reported with influenza and parainfluenza virus infections.

The arboviruses include viruses of several families (togavirus, bunyavirus, and reovirus) that are transmitted by mosquitos or ticks. More than 15 different arboviruses have been associated with encephalitis in varied geographic areas of the world; seven cause meningitis or encephalitis in the United States (Table 499–1). Over 100 cases of California virus encephalitis are reported annually over a wide geographic area. Eastern, western, St. Louis, and Venezuelan equine encephalitis viruses cause localized epidemics; St. Louis virus is the predominant cause of major epidemics.

Adenoviruses are respiratory viruses that only rarely cause meningitis or severe childhood encephalitis. Nonviral agents that cause clinical syndromes indistinguishable from viral meningitis or mild encephalitis include *Leptospira, Treponema pallidum*, the *Treponema* of Lyme disease, *Mycoplasma pneumoniae*, and *Rickettsia*.

EPIDEMIOLOGY. Over 5000 cases of aseptic meningitis and over 2000 cases of encephalitis are reported to the Centers for Disease Control annually, but this represents only a small fraction of the total number of cases per year in the United States. Both viral meningitis and encephalitis are reported with greater frequency during the later summer and early fall, and this increase results, in large part, from the seasonal dissemination of enteroviruses and arboviruses.

Epidemiologically the viruses causing meningitis and encephalitis in man fall into three categories: (1) Viruses that spread from man to man; these agents generally cause disease during a particular season of the year and often in epidemics. (2) Viruses acquired from infected animals (zoonoses); these agents may have distinct geographic distributions, and a history of animal contact in patients is often obtained. (3) Viruses spread by hematophagous arthropods and necessitating a cycle in the arthropod host; these viruses have very specific seasonal and geographic limitations.

The enteroviruses are spread by hand-to-mouth contact and to a lesser extent by respiratory spread or by fecal contamination of fomites or vectors. Virus growth is primarily in the intestinal tract. Although enteroviral infections occur throughout the year, the incidence of these infections increases dramatically in summer and early fall, often reaching epidemic proportions. Because of the mode of spread, family outbreaks are common, and the spread of virus is facilitated in families or communities with preschool children.

Mumps virus is spread by the respiratory route. Mumps occurs throughout the year, but there is a marked increase in incidence during the spring. Although the incidence of infection with mumps virus is equal between the sexes, males develop meningitis three times more frequently than females.

Lymphocytic choriomeningitis virus is the major zoonotic virus causing meningitis and encephalitis. The natural host of this virus is *Mus musculus*, the common house mouse, and the virus is present in its excreta. Man acquires the infection by contact with contaminated dust or food. Human disease is more common in winter, when the natural host tends to move indoors, increasing human exposure. Recently, lymphocytic choriomeningitis virus has also been found in hamsters, and human infections have been traced to laboratory and pet hamsters. Leptospiral infections are also acquired from both domestic and wild animals. These spirochetes are excreted in urine and contracted by man through contact with animal tissue, contaminated soil, or water polluted by animal urine.

Each of the arboviruses has a different epidemiologic cycle (see Ch. 356). In the United States, eastern, western, St. Louis, California, and Venezuelan equine encephalitis viruses are transmitted by mosquitos. Powassan virus and Colorado tick fever virus are transmitted by ticks. The seasonal occurrence of these infections is limited to seasons when the vectors are feeding. Eastern encephalitis virus is limited largely to the Atlantic and Gulf coasts and normally circulates between birds and salt marsh mosquitos, which do not bite humans. When ecologic changes alter the bird-mosquito balance, the virus can overflow into other mosquitos that feed on mammals. Regional deaths of horses or pheasants usually herald the rare human outbreaks. Western encephalitis virus is limited to the western two thirds of the country and normally circulates between mosquitos and birds; horses and humans become inadvertent hosts when bitten by infected mosquitos. This virus causes many more human infections than does eastern encephalitis virus, but only 1 in 100 of those infected develop encephalitis. St. Louis encephalitis virus causes both rural and urban disease over a large area of the United States. In the rural areas the virus has the same pattern as western encephalitis virus, but in urban areas more explosive outbreaks can occur when the virus is introduced into urban breeding mosquitos and urban birds become the intermediate hosts. California virus has a different cycle involving woodland mosquitos and small animals; birds are not involved. In recent years the virus has been related to encephalitis every year over a wide geographic area of the eastern half of the United States. Disease is confined almost entirely to children. Venezuelan encephalitis is transmitted from mosquitos to animals, and the virus has recently spread into Florida and the southwestern states. Most people infected with the virus have an influenza-like illness, but about 3 per cent develop acute meningitis or encephalitis. Powassan virus has been found in ticks in Canada and along the northern border of the United States; it is a rare cause of encephalitis in man. Colorado tick fever is found in ticks in the Rocky Mountain area; about 18 per cent of infected patients develop meningitis; encephalitis is rare.

PATHOGENESIS AND PATHOLOGY. Viruses usually replicate in cells at the site of entry. For example, after oral ingestion enteroviruses grow in the gastrointestinal tract; after respiratory spread viruses grow in the respiratory tract; or after subcutaneous or intravenous inoculation arboviruses grow in local subcutaneous, vascular endothelial, or muscle cells. Following local replication, dissemination of virus usually occurs via the blood. Despite the longstanding belief that the blood-brain barrier was impervious to viruses, it is now evident that the majority of viruses invade the central nervous system from the blood. The cerebral capillary endothelium is nonfenestrated, has tight junctions, and is surrounded by a dense basement membrane with astrocytic processes apposed to the outer surface. These structures do constitute a relative barrier to virus invasion, but experimentally viruses are found to invade the nervous system both by infection of the vascular endothelial cells with subsequent infection of surrounding glia and neurons and by passage of virus through endothelial cells. Experimentally viruses have also been found to grow in the choroid plexus and to seed virus into the cerebrospinal fluid.

Since viral meningitis by definition is a benign disease, its histopathologic correlates are unknown. In fatal encephalitis an inflammatory reaction is usually prominent in the meninges and in a perivascular distribution within the brain. Although the perivascular inflammatory reaction is composed predominantly of mononuclear cells, polymorphonuclear cells may be evident. Neural cells may show degenerative changes, and apparent phagocytosis of neurons by macrophages or microglial cells (neuronophagia) is often found.

Pathologic changes in encephalitis cannot unequivocally distinguish the agent involved. Topographic localization of lesions is of little value except in distinguishing poliomyelitis, rabies, and herpes simplex virus infections. Intranuclear inclusions are seen in herpesvirus infections and in measles virus infections, and in the latter cytoplasmic inclusions may also be found. Cytomegalovirus infections produce a characteristic pathology with the induction of cytomegalic cells containing inclusion bodies. Although fatal cases of mumps virus encephalitis are rare, pathologic studies have shown both the acute inflammatory lesions usually seen in virus encephalitis and perivenular demyelination characteristic of postinfectious encephalomyelitis.

CLINICAL MANIFESTATIONS. *Viral Meningitis.* The major clinical manifestations of viral meningitis are headache, fever, and nuchal rigidity. Signs and symptoms are often abrupt in onset and may persist from three days to two weeks. Other symptoms may include general malaise, sore throat, nausea and vomiting, drowsiness, abdominal pain, and chills and fever. The headache is often frontal or retro-orbital and associated with photophobia. Fever is seldom elevated above 40° C. Nuchal rigidity may not be as severe as that seen in bacterial meningitis and may be detectable only with extreme flexion.

Viral meningitis caused by several of the enteroviruses is often associated with rashes. The eruption usually appears at the same time as the fever and persists for four to ten days. In coxsackievirus A5, 9, and 16 and echovirus 4, 6, 9, 16, and 30 infections the rash is typically maculopapular and nonpruritic, and may be confined to the face and trunk or may involve extremities, including the palms and soles. In echovirus 9 infections the rash may be petechial, causing confusion with meningococcal infections. In group A coxsackievirus infections herpangina may develop, characterized by grayish vesicular lesions on the tonsillar fossae, soft palate, and uvula. In coxsackievirus A16 and rarely other group A serotype infections a vesicular rash may involve hands, feet, and oropharynx (hand-foot-and-mouth disease; see Ch. 345).

Mumps virus meningitis and encephalitis are associated with parotitis in approximately half the cases. However, the parotitis may precede or follow the meningitis by as much as a week. Evidence of parotitis associated with meningitis is not diagnostic of mumps virus infection, because parotitis has also been reported with group B coxsackievirus and lymphocytic choriomeningitis virus infections. Orchitis is seen in one third of postpubertal males, and tenderness of mammary tissue can be found in one third of postpubertal females with mumps virus infections. Oophoritis, pancreatitis, and thyroiditis may also be seen.

Aseptic meningitis caused by the type 2 herpes simplex virus may coincide with the eruption of genital lesions. In some cases this meningitis has been associated with radicular pain simulating lumbar or sacral root compression.

Viral Encephalitis. In addition to headache, fever, and nuchal rigidity, alterations of consciousness characterize encephalitis; mild lethargy may progress to confusion, stupor, and coma. Focal neurologic signs usually develop, and seizures are common. Motor weakness, accentuated deep tendon reflexes, and extensor plantar responses may be observed. Abnormal movements are seen in some cases of encephalitis, and rarely a tremor characteristic of Parkinson's disease may develop. The hypothalamic-pituitary area may be involved, causing severe hyperthermia or poikilothermia, diabetes insipidus, and inappropriate antidiuretic hormone secretion. Involvement of the spinal cord can lead to flaccid paralysis, depression of tendon reflexes, and paralysis of bowel and bladder. Increased intracranial pressure can cause third and sixth cranial nerve palsies.

In herpes simplex virus encephalitis, signs often include bizarre behavior, hallucinations, and aphasia, suggesting the temporal lobe localization typical of that infection (see Ch. 500).

LABORATORY FINDINGS. Blood count may be normal, show moderate leukopenia, or show a moderate leukocytosis. Epstein-Barr virus infections are suggested by large numbers of atypical mononuclear cells, as well as by positive heterophil reactions. Serum amylase may be elevated with mumps virus infections. Lymphocyte choriomeningitis virus infections are frequently associated with pulmonary infiltrates.

Cerebrospinal fluid examination is essential to establish the diagnosis of aseptic meningitis and encephalitis, but it is of little help in determining the specific virus involved. The cerebrospinal fluid may be under normal or moderately elevated pressure. The fluid is usually clear but may show xanthochromia if the protein content is over 100 mg per deciliter. Cell counts are variable, but 10 to 1000 cells are usual with a predominance of mononuclear cells. If the fluid is examined early in the course of disease, there may be no cells or a preponderance of polymorphonuclear cells. Repeat examination in 24 hours will usually show the characteristic presence of mononuclear cells. The protein content is usually elevated, and percentage of IgG may be high, suggesting intrathecal antibody synthesis. Gel immunoelectrophoresis may show oligoclonal bands of IgG, indicating the limited heterogeneity of antibody, and these bands may persist for six months or more after recovery. The glucose content in the cerebrospinal fluid is generally normal, although mild depressions are seen, particularly with mumps and lymphocytic choriomeningitis virus infections.

The electroencephalogram usually shows diffuse slowing, but shifting foci, marked asymmetry, and seizure activity may be evident in encephalitis. Diffuse slowing is not a grave sign in viral meningitis, because this abnormality can persist briefly even after the patient is asymptomatic.

Cerebral angiography, radioisotopic scans, and computed tomography of the brain may show localization of lesions of the temporal lobes in herpes simplex virus encephalitis, but these studies are of no value in differentiating other forms of encephalitis.

DIAGNOSIS AND DIFFERENTIAL DIAGNOSIS. The most important aspect of differential diagnosis is to exclude those treatable diseases which may masquerade as viral infections. These include tuberculous and fungal meningitis, parameningeal infections, brain abscess, partially treated bacterial meningitis, subacute bacterial endocarditis, amebic encephalitis, and other illnesses that may present headache, fever, and nuchal rigidity. The differential diagnosis of encephalitis is important, as specific therapy is now recommended for herpes simplex virus encephalitis (see Ch. 500).

A definitive etiologic diagnosis can be determined only by appropriate virologic laboratory studies. However, an educated clinical guess regarding the cause can be based on public health information concerning agents currently being disseminated in the area; on knowledge of the agents endemic to the area and the season of the year; and on the patient's history, including past immunizations and illnesses, possible insect bites, place of residence, travel in areas where particular infections are prevalent, health of the family, and type of dwelling place.

The coxsackievirus and echovirus infections occur sporadically throughout the year but reach epidemic proportions in the late summer and fall. Furthermore, they cause family outbreaks and protean manifestations. Thus the patient with aseptic meningitis occurring in late summer or fall who gives a history of other family members with nonspecific illness, rash, pleurodynia, or other enterovirus-associated disease probably has meningitis caused by a coxsackie- or echovirus. Transient lower motor paralysis reminiscent of poliomyelitis is also occasionally seen with these infections.

Mumps virus infections tend to occur in the spring, and a history of exposure is commonly obtained. Since there is no evidence that reinfection with mumps virus can occur, a clear-cut past history of parotitis during a mumps virus epidemic is good evidence against the patient's having mumps meningitis.

Patients with lymphocytic choriomeningitis virus infections often provide a history of living in mouse-infested houses or working in barns or other places frequented by mice. Alternatively, a history of exposure to or recent acquisition of a pet hamster should be sought. Lymphocytic choriomeningitis virus often causes a biphasic illness, with rather severe respiratory symptoms or pneumonitis preceding the abrupt onset of meningitis or encephalitis.

The mosquito-borne virus infections characteristically occur only in late summer and early fall before the frost. They vary in prevalence from year to year, depending on rainfall or other factors influencing mosquito, bird, and wildlife populations. Public health data regarding the dissemination of eastern, western, and St. Louis viruses in the population may be helpful in suggesting the diagnosis. California encephalitis virus shows little variation in frequency from year to year. Since this infection is usually acquired by children after exposure to woodland mosquitos, a history of preceding recreational woodland exposure may be obtained.

Herpesvirus infections show no seasonal distribution. In type 1 herpes simplex virus infection, a past history of cold sores, exposure to herpes labialis, or presence of labial lesions at the time of encephalitis is of no help in ruling out or suggesting the diagnosis. The diagnosis is suggested by the severity of the encephalitis and signs of localization to the temporal lobes. In contrast, onset of type 2 herpes simplex virus meningitis may coincide with the appearance of genital lesions.

Reaching a specific etiologic diagnosis in the laboratory necessitates obtaining acute and convalescent phase serum specimens. It is also useful to obtain specimens for isolation of virus (cerebrospinal fluid, stool, blood, and throat washings). Convalescent serum alone is of little value, as antibodies to most of the agents causing meningitis or encephalitis are widespread. Disease can be associated with a specific agent serologically only if a four-fold or greater increase in antibody is demonstrated between the early phase of disease and convalescence. Therefore blood should be drawn in the first few days of disease, and a subsequent serum specimen should be obtained two to six weeks later. The optimal specimens for viral isolation are dependent on the virus being sought. Arboviruses and enteroviruses can be isolated from the blood but are seldom recoverable at the time of clinical meningitis or encephalitis. During the acute disease coxsackie- and echoviruses are most readily isolated from stool or cerebrospinal fluid and, in some cases, throat washings. Lymphocytic choriomeningitis virus is most readily isolated from blood or cerebrospinal fluid. Mumps virus may be isolated from saliva, throat washings, or cerebrospinal fluid. Type 2 herpes simplex virus may also be isolated from the cerebrospinal fluid or blood. Unfortunately, type 1 herpes simplex virus can seldom be isolated from blood or cerebrospinal fluid, and definitive serologic studies require antibody determinations on spinal fluid. An early diagnosis of type 1 herpes simplex virus encephalitis still requires a brain biopsy.

TREATMENT. With the exception of vidarabine, now recommended in treatment of herpes simplex virus encephalitis, specific antiviral therapy is not available for viral meningitis or other forms of encephalitis. Treatment consists of supportive therapy and the management of the complications of encephalitis, including coma, seizures, and increased intracranial pressure.

In both viral meningitis and encephalitis bed rest is indicated. Strict isolation procedures are not essential, as most of the viruses causing meningitis and encephalitis are common in our environment. If an enteroviral infection is suspected, precautions in handling of stools and handwashing should be instituted. If measles, chickenpox, rubella, or mumps virus infections are evident, the usual isolation from susceptibles is recommended.

The headache and fever of meningitis can usually be managed with judicious doses of aspirin. Severe hyperthermia may develop in encephalitis, necessitating the use of more vigorous therapy, but it should be remembered that viruses are thermolabile. Therefore modest temperature elevations may serve as a natural defense mechanism, and attempts to reduce mild temperature elevations to normal or subnormal levels may be ill advised.

Patients with severe encephalitis are often in coma. Since these patients may make remarkable recoveries even after prolonged periods of coma, vigorous supportive therapy and avoidance of complications are essential. The airway must often be maintained by intubation or tracheostomy, and mechanical respiration may be necessary. Although intravenous fluids may suffice for brief periods, prolonged coma necessitates feeding with a nasogastric tube. Blood glucose and electrolytes should be checked frequently, because water, glucose, and salt control are frequently compromised during encephalitis. The respiratory tract, urinary tract, intravenous site, and skin are common sites of infection in comatose patients, and infections should be sought assiduously, treated vigorously, and avoided by skillful nursing, maintenance of bronchial drainage, frequent turning to avoid decubitus ulcers, and meticulous catheter care.

Although seizures frequently complicate encephalitis, prophylactic anticonvulsants are not usually recommended. If seizures develop, they can usually be managed with phenytoin and phenobarbital. If status epilepticus develops, more vigorous therapy should be instituted, remembering to treat the hypoxia and hyperthermia that complicate and aggravate status epilepticus.

Modest increases in intracranial pressure can be treated with glycerol given orally or by rectal tube. This osmotic agent is probably preferable to urea or mannitol, because it can be given over a longer period of time. Steroids should be avoided in the routine treatment of encephalitis because of their inhibitory effects on host-immune responses. However, when increased intracranial pressure is severe, the use of dexamethasone is indicated.

PROGNOSIS. Viral meningitis is a benign disease, and full recovery usually occurs within 5 to 14 days of onset, although some patients describe persistent fatigue, lightheadedness, and general asthenia that may persist for months.

The prognosis of encephalitis is dependent on the etiologic agent. The mortality rate of untreated herpes simplex virus encephalitis is approximately 70 per cent, with a high rate of sequelae in survivors. Arbovirus encephalitides have variable mortality rates; the mortality rate with eastern encephalitis is approximately 50 per cent; with St. Louis, 10 per cent; with western, 10 per cent; with Venezuelan equine, 1 per cent; and with California, less than 0.5 per cent. The mortality rates for western encephalitis are greater in children under one year of age, and for St. Louis encephalitis they are greater in the elderly. Nonfatal encephalitis caused by eastern, western, and St. Louis viruses leaves a relatively high rate of neurologic sequelae.

Encephalitis associated with mumps or lymphocytic choriomeningitis viruses is very rarely associated with death, and sequelae are infrequent. However, hydrocephalus has been reported as a late sequela of mumps meningitis and encephalitis in children.

Evans AS: Viral Infections of Humans. Epidemiology and Control. 2nd ed. New York, Plenum Medical Book Company, 1982. *A well-organized and up-to-date text with good chapters covering the epidemiology of enteroviruses, mumps, herpesviruses, arenaviruses, and arboviruses.*

Grist NR, Bell EJ, Assaad F: Enteroviruses in human disease. Prog Med Virol 24:114, 1978. *A comprehensive and well-referenced review of enteroviral diseases.*

Johnson RT: Viral Infections of the Nervous System. New York, Raven Press, 1982. *A current monograph that covers pathogenesis, epidemiology, and clinical features of acute central nervous system infections.*

Johnstone JA, Ross CAC, Dunn M: Meningitis and encephalitis associated with mumps infection. A 10 year survey. Arch Dis Child 47:647, 1972. *A concise report of clinical and laboratory data on 137 patients with mumps meningitis and encephalitis.*

500. HERPES SIMPLEX ENCEPHALITIS

Richard T. Johnson

DEFINITION. Herpes simplex encephalitis is the commonest nonepidemic fatal encephalitis. Unlike other viral encephalitides, herpes simplex encephalitis in children and adults shows unusual clinical and pathologic features of temporal and frontal lobe localization, epidemiologic and serologic evidence that most episodes represent reinfection or activation of latent infection, and unique problems of laboratory diagnosis. Early diagnosis is critical, since this is the one form of encephalitis for which effective antiviral drugs are now available. Herpes simplex encephalitis was formerly called *acute necrotizing encephalitis* or *acute inclusion-body encephalitis.*

ETIOLOGY. Encephalitis can be caused by either of the two distinct serotypes of herpes simplex virus: type 1, oral herpes; or type 2, genital herpes. Most cases of localized encephalitis are caused by type 1, with only a few caused by type 2 virus. In contrast, the diffuse, nonlocalized acute encephalitis of newborns is usually caused by a genital strain acquired during passage through the birth canal, but occasionally may be caused by type 1 virus. Aseptic meningitis and radiculitis caused by type 2 virus in adults are described in Ch. 499.

Herpes simplex viruses are large complex viruses containing double-stranded DNA coiled around core proteins. This mass is surrounded by a capsid 100 nm long, a tegument composed of fibrillar material, and finally an envelope derived from host cell nuclear membrane containing viral glycoproteins. The virion diameter is 180 nm. Since types 1 and 2 have approximately 50 per cent nucleic acid sequence homology, they share a number of common antigenic sites and biologic properties but can be differentiated by their monospecific antibodies. Herpes simplex viruses are naturally infectious only in man, but in the laboratory they have a wide host range in animals, embryonated eggs, and a variety of primate and nonprimate cell cultures.

INCIDENCE AND PREVALENCE. One thousand to two thousand cases of herpes simplex encephalitis are estimated to occur each year in the United States. The disease is seen worldwide. There is no seasonal distribution, and no sex-related preference. The disease develops at all ages, but a diphasic age distribution is evident, with persons under 20 and over 40 affected more frequently than those in the third and fourth decades of life. Predisposing factors are unknown. Most patients are otherwise in good health, although the disease can occur in immunocompromised patients.

EPIDEMIOLOGY, PATHOGENESIS, AND PATHOLOGY. Type 1 herpes simplex virus is a ubiquitous agent. Antibody develops in half the human population by age 15 and in 90 per cent by adulthood. Primary infection usually occurs during childhood by salivary or respiratory contact. This primary infection may be asymptomatic or cause gingivostomatitis, pharyngitis, or respiratory disease. During the primary infection, the virus is thought to be transported along the local sensory nerves and to establish latency in the corresponding sensory ganglia. In the case of type 1 herpes simplex virus, this is usually the trigeminal ganglia or in some persons the upper cervical or vagus ganglia. Type 2 herpes is usually acquired by venereal contact, and latency has been documented in the sacral ganglia. This latency appears to persist for life. Free infectious virus cannot be recovered from latently infected ganglia of humans or experimental animals, but virus is activated in cultures of the ganglion cells. Virus is probably sequestered as viral nucleic acid.

Activation occurs frequently. About 25 per cent of the population have activation of trigeminal ganglia infections manifested by herpes labialis or cold sores. In other asymptomatic individuals, virus can be intermittently recovered from the nasopharynx. Patients who develop encephalitis have a similar frequency of antecedent herpes labialis. This fact and serologic evidence of past infection in acute-phase sera indicate that most cases of encephalitis do not represent primary infections but are either reinfections or activations of the latent infection, with involvement of the brain.

The pathology of herpes simplex encephalitis shows a remarkable localization. The orbital surface of the frontal lobe, temporal lobe structures, and insular cortex develop hemorrhagic necrosis with inflammation and inclusion bodies. The involvement can be strikingly asymmetric. Selective vulnerability of a specific subgroup of cells fails to explain the localization, since both types 1 and 2 herpes cause diffuse encephalitis in neonates and the cells involved in localized encephalitis include both neurons and glia over a contiguous area. The findings suggest that the virus spreads from cell to cell along the base of the brain within the middle and anterior fossae.

The unique localization might be explained by the route of virus entry into the central nervous system with subsequent limitation of spread by antibody. Two such routes have been suggested. One is that primary infection or reinfection might occur across the olfactory bulbs with infection of the orbital-frontal lobes and subsequent spread to the temporal area. Alternatively, encephalitis might result from activation in the trigeminal ganglia, with spread along fibers from the ganglia that innervate pial and dural vessels.

CLINICAL MANIFESTATIONS. Herpes encephalitis can have an insidious or a fulminant course. Fever is almost invariably present, and headache is a prominent early symptom. Characteristically, 90 per cent of patients develop symptoms or findings that suggest a local lesion in one or both temporal lobes. Personality changes, hallucinations, or bizarre behavior may be evident for several days or even a week before other signs evolve, and in some cases this has led to initial hospital admission for psychiatric services. Memory may be impaired out of proportion to other cognitive functions, reflecting bilateral involvement of hippocampal systems. Generalized or focal seizures ensue in 40 per cent of patients. Hemiparesis develops in one third, frequently with a greater involvement of face and arm corresponding to the inferior frontal localization. Aphasia, superior quadrantal visual field defects, and paresthesias reflect the temporal lobe localization. In some patients there is rapid deterioration from stupor to coma without localizing signs.

DIAGNOSIS. Cerebrospinal fluid often shows increased pressure. Mononuclear cell pleocytosis usually ranges from 10 to 500 cells per milliliter, but occasionally there are either no cells or a high number of neutrophils. Red blood cells are frequent, but their presence does not indicate the diagnosis of herpetic encephalitis, nor does their absence exclude it. Protein content is usually elevated, and sugar content is usually normal or is only mildly decreased. The virus can rarely, if ever, be recovered from spinal fluid. Thus the spinal fluid examination suggests a viral encephalitis but does not differentiate a herpetic cause.

The most sensitive early test to suggest herpes encephalitis is the electroencephalogram (EEG). Unilateral or bilateral periodic discharges from the temporal leads occur in many patients, and slow wave complexes at regular two to three per second intervals are highly suggestive of the disease. Radionuclide scans may show uptake in one or both temporal lobes. Cerebral angiography usually demonstrates temporal swelling, prolonged arterial filling, and localized hypervascularity in one or both temporal lobes. Computed tomography (CT) frequently shows low-density temporal lobe lesions that may be accompanied by uptake of contrast material in the Rolandic fissure and opercular areas as well as the temporal lobe. However, the CT changes may develop later than those in the EEG or radionuclide scans.

Early definitive diagnosis of herpes simplex encephalitis depends on cerebral biopsy. To be useful in management, the biopsy should be taken as soon as clinical findings or laboratory tests indicate a viral encephalitis with frontal-temporal localization. The biopsy should be taken from an abnormal area. One cause of false negative results has been the sampling of frontal lobes or of the nondominant temporal lobe when clinical signs indicate disease in the dominant temporal lobe. Virus may be recovered from one area when it is not recoverable from others. Needle biopsy through a burr hole is probably more hazardous than craniotomy and open biopsy. In view of the frequent increase in intracranial pressure, craniotomy with decompression of the affected temporal lobe may have a therapeutic effect. This procedure also allows direct visualization of the affected area and selection of an optimal biopsy specimen. Tissue should be fixed for routine histology, frozen for immunocytochemical staining, inoculated into cell cultures for virus isolation, and possibly prepared for electron microscopy. Routine histologic studies can confirm the diagnosis of inflammatory encephalitis and rule out many other diseases, but characteristic inclusion bodies are recognized in only about one half of the biopsy virus-positive specimens. Immunocytochemical staining and electron microscopy can be done rapidly and usefully by experienced microscopists. However, both procedures are limited by a high yield of false negative results (30 per cent and 55 per cent, respectively) and a small number of false positive results because of nonspecific staining or inability to distinguish particles of Epstein-Barr virus. Virus isolation studies seldom yield false negative results but never false positive results.

A serologic diagnosis of herpes simplex encephalitis can be made with cerebrospinal fluid studies, but this cannot be sufficiently timely to guide effective antiviral therapy. Patients with herpes simplex encephalitis usually but not always develop a four-fold or greater increase in antibody to virus between acute and convalescent phase sera, but similar increases may result from nonspecific activation of virus associated with other infections. Increases in antibody in cerebrospinal fluid and elevated IgG and oligoclonal bands develop late in disease. A distorted ratio of antibody in spinal fluid and serum indicates intrathecal synthesis of virus-specific antibody. This is helpful in establishing a retrospective diagnosis of herpes simplex encephalitis and in detecting false negative biopsy results.

When herpes simplex encephalitis is suspected because of clinical findings or laboratory studies, biopsies show that only one third to one half of patients have the disease. A variety of other viruses have also been found sporadically to cause a similar localization. In 20 per cent of cases in which biopsies are done, other diseases have been found for which other treatments are indicated, including arteriovenous malformations, abscess, fungal and tuberculous infections with focal inflammation, and tumor. The cerebral biopsy is necessary to establish early diagnosis and for optimal patient management. No noninvasive diagnostic study has yet proved effective.

TREATMENT. Vidarabine is the approved drug for treatment of biopsy-proven cases of herpes simplex encephalitis. Its efficacy was originally established in a small placebo-controlled study that showed a reduction of mortality from 70 to 28 per cent. Subsequent open studies of large numbers of patients continue to show mortality of approximately 30 per cent, in contrast to mortality of 70 to 80 per cent in untreated patients or patients treated with cytosine arabinoside, an ineffective drug. When the diagnosis of herpes simplex encephalitis is suspected, biopsy should be performed and intravenous vidarabine administration started at a dose of 15 mg per kilogram daily for ten days. If there is surgical delay, the drug can be started within 24 hours prior to biopsy.

Vidarabine is a relatively nontoxic drug, but it does produce immunosuppression, is relatively insoluble, requires a fluid load, and has some degree of neurotoxicity. For these reasons the drug is contraindicated in patients with other encephalitides, and the morbidity and mortality of encephalitis patients without proven herpes infections appear to be increased if vidarabine is given indiscriminately. If the biopsy shows that the patient does not have encephalitis, vidarabine administration can be discontinued immediately. If encephalitis is found but immunocytochemical, immunocytologic, or isolation methods prove negative after five days, vidarabine should probably be discontinued. In addition to vidarabine, the other supportive treatment for acute viral encephalitis must be instituted (see Ch. 499).

Despite the efficacy of vidarabine, morbidity and mortality remain high, and the drug has undesirable side effects. Other drugs are currently being tested. Studies of vidarabine monophosphate, a more soluble derivative of the parent compound, have been halted because of unexplained greater mortality. Acyclovir is an acyclic nucleoside that has unique features for an antiviral agent because it is a selective substrate for herpes virus thymidine kinase. The drug is phosphorylated to the active compound largely in infected cells and is retained there. Once activated, the drug selectively inhibits the virus-specific DNA polymerase 10 to 20 times more than it inhibits cellular DNA polymerases. In theory, acyclovir appears superior and less toxic. Whether it is as effective as or more effective than vidarabine in treatment is being determined in controlled studies.

PROGNOSIS. For patients treated with vidarabine, the outcome depends on age and level of consciousness when therapy is begun. Ninety per cent of patients survive who are under age 30 years and only lethargic when treated, while among patients who are in coma when therapy starts mortality approaches 60 per cent, regardless of age.

Approximately half of patients who survive herpes simplex encephalitis retain debilitating sequelae, including motor and sensory deficits, aphasia, or Korsakoff's psychosis. Age and level of consciousness at the time of initiation of therapy are the major determinants. Fifty-eight per cent of patients under 30 years of age and 32 per cent of those over age 30 recover fully if treatment is initiated when they are only lethargic. In contrast, only 8 per cent survive without sequelae if therapy is delayed until after the onset of coma.

Adams H, Miller D: Herpes simplex encephalitis: A clinical and pathological analysis of twenty-two cases. Postgrad Med J 49:393, 1973. *A detailed study of a large series of patients with a careful correlation between postmortem findings and the clinical course and laboratory abnormalities.*

Baringer JR: Herpes simplex virus infection of nervous tissue in animals and man. Prog Med Virol 20:1, 1975. *A detailed review of the biology of these infections, describing their behavior in nervous tissue, their latency, and their relation to acute illness.*

Davis LE, Johnson RT: An explanation for the localization of herpes simplex encephalitis? Ann Neurol 5:2, 1979. *Speculation on the pathogenesis of the localized disease.*

Nahmias AJ, Whitley RJ, Visintine AN, Takei Y, Alford CA, the NIAID Collaborative Antiviral Study Group: Herpes simplex virus encephalitis: Laboratory evaluations and their diagnostic significance. J Infect Dis 145:829, 1982. *A current evaluation of virus identification methods and serologic tests.*

Whitley RJ, Soong SJ, Dolin R, Galasso GJ, Ch'ien LT, Alford CA, the NIAID Collaborative Antiviral Study Group: Adenine arabinoside therapy of biopsy-proven herpes simplex encephalitis. N Engl J Med 297:289, 1977. *A model placebo-controlled study showing a reduction of mortality from 70 to 28 per cent with no or only moderately debilitating neurologic sequelae in more than 50 per cent of survivors.*

Whitley RJ, Soong SJ, Hirsch MS, Karchmer AW, Dolin R, Galasso G, Dunnick JK, Alford CA, the NIAID Collaborative Antiviral Study Group: Herpes simplex encephalitis: Vidarabine therapy and diagnostic problems. N Engl J Med 304:313, 1981. *The data suggest that young patients who are only lethargic when therapy is begun have the best prognosis and that brain biopsy is rarely associated with serious complications.*

Whitley RJ, Soong SJ, Linneman C, Liu C, Pazin G, Alford CA, the NIAID Collaborative Antiviral Study Group: Herpes simplex encephalitis: Clinical assessment. JAMA 247:317, 1982. *The necessity of brain biopsy for early diagnosis is documented.*

501. HERPES ZOSTER

Richard T. Johnson

Herpes zoster is an acute viral infection of sensory ganglia and the corresponding cutaneous areas of innervation. The disease is characterized by localized pain along the distribution of the nerve and a vesicular skin eruption over a single or adjacent dermatomes. The disease is due to the same virus that causes chickenpox (varicella) (Ch. 339) and is thought to represent an acute localized recrudescent infection by the varicella virus that has remained latent in the sensory ganglia since the primary attack of chickenpox. Herpes zoster is also called shingles or zona.

ETIOLOGY. The varicella-zoster virus is a herpesvirus. The virus core measures 45 to 50 mμ and contains deoxyribonucleic acid. This is surrounded by a capsid with a diameter of 50 to 100 mμ and an outer envelope, giving a total diameter of the virion of 150 to 250 mμ. Morphologically, varicella virus resembles herpes simplex virus, with which it shares some common antigens, but it is markedly different from herpes simplex virus in its limited host range and in its loss of infectivity in most cell-free preparations. The virus is naturally pathogenic only for man, although chickenpox has been seen in anthropoid apes in zoos. There is some evidence of experimental transmission of the virus to several species of monkeys. The virus can be grown in a variety of cell cultures of human and primate origin but not in nonprimate cells. The virus is avidly cell-associated and can usually be transmitted in the laboratory only by the inoculation of infected cells, although the virus is stable in a cell-free form in the vesicular fluid.

INCIDENCE. Herpes zoster occurs at a rate of three to five cases per thousand persons per year. The disease is rare in childhood and is most frequently seen in persons over the age of 50 years. It is estimated that half the people reaching 85 years of age have suffered from at least one attack of herpes zoster. Both initial attacks and recurrences are more frequent in persons with malignancies or diabetes mellitus and in patients receiving immunosuppressant drugs or radiation therapy.

EPIDEMIOLOGY, PATHOGENESIS, AND PATHOLOGY. Chickenpox may develop after exposure to a patient with zoster, although this is less likely than development of chickenpox after exposure to chickenpox. In contrast, zoster rarely develops after exposure to chickenpox or other cases of zoster. Furthermore, chickenpox is a seasonal disease occurring mainly in the winter and spring and in epidemic proportions every two to four years. In contrast, zoster is neither seasonal nor epidemic in incidence.

The precise pathogenesis of herpes zoster is unknown, but the following hypothesis is widely accepted. Chickenpox is transmitted from man to man by respiratory spread, and in the susceptible person the virus probably disseminates throughout the body by viremia. Infection of the skin occurs through the blood, and vesicles develop most prominently over the face and trunk. It is postulated that virus then spreads centripetally via sensory nerve fibers to reside dormantly in the sensory ganglia. Virus replication is later activated. In some cases activation is associated with the development of malignancy, local x-irradiation, immunosuppressive therapy, trauma, treatment with arsenicals, neurosyphilis, or tumor entrapment of the dorsal root ganglia or nerve root. Nevertheless, in most patients there is no obvious exciting cause, and it is thought that the decline of immunity with age may promote reactivation. When virus multiplies in the ganglia, an active ganglionitis develops, causing pain along its sensory distribution. Virus then passes down the nerve and multiplies again in the skin, causing characteristic clusters of vesicles. The localized zoster lesions are most common over trigeminal or thoracic dermatomes corresponding to the areas of major eruption during the primary chickenpox infection. The more rapid secondary immune response may prevent hematogenous dissemination. Resolution and limitation of the rash of herpes zoster do not correlate well, however, with the development of antibody but appear to correlate with the collection of inflammatory cells and the presence of interferon in the vesicular fluid.

Pathologic studies of herpes zoster show an acute ganglionitis with an intense inflammatory response, cell necrosis, and occasionally hemorrhages within the ganglia. In addition, there is predominantly unilateral inflammation in the adjacent segments of the cord or brainstem, involving the posterior more than the anterior horns. Oligodendrocyte infection with focal demyelination has been described. A mild leptomeningitis is generally found that is most intense over the segments of involvement. Inflammation in the roots distal to the ganglia is also present, representing a true peripheral mononeuritis.

The skin innervated by the nerve shows degeneration of the basal and deep prickle cell layers of the epidermis. Ballooning degeneration of these cells causes the formation of the intradermal vesicles. Giant cells and eosinophilic intranuclear inclusions are found in the base of the vesicles.

CLINICAL MANIFESTATIONS. The eruption of herpes zoster is often preceded by malaise and fever for two to four days. Pain or dysesthesia along the segmental dermatome also precedes the rash by four to five days. The pain often has a superficial tingling or burning quality, but may vary from severe deep pain, suggesting appendicitis, cholecystitis, or pleurisy, to very mild itching. The pain may be intermittent or constant. Tenderness or hypesthesia may be detected along the dermatome during this pre-eruptive stage. The cutaneous lesions arise first as small, red macules, which rapidly vesiculate, becoming tense, clear vesicles on an erythematous base. On about the third day, the vesicular fluid becomes turbid as inflammatory cells collect within. Within five to ten days, the vesicles dry and crusts develop. However, in severe cases the vesicles may become confluent with a gangrenous appearance, and healing may be delayed for many weeks. During the course of the rash, the regional lymph nodes usually enlarge, and a few vesicles spread to adjacent dermatomes but seldom to the other side of the body. Pain or dysesthesia usually persists for one to four weeks; approximately 30 per cent of patients over age 40 have pain that persists for months to years. This postherpetic neuralgia is more common in the elderly when there has been a prolonged period of pain prior to cutaneous eruption and a more severe rash.

The distribution of lesions of herpes zoster corresponds to the areas of most intense rash of varicella. Although any sensory nerve distribution can be affected, two thirds of all lesions occur along thoracic dermatomes, and most of the remaining one third affect sensory branches of cranial nerves. Cranial nerve involvement tends to be more severe with greater pain, more meningeal irritation, and more serious neurologic complications. The ophthalmic division of the trigeminal nerve is the most common site of cranial involvement, accounting for 10 to 15 per cent of all cases. Usually the rash spares the eye, but occasionally keratoconjunctivitis develops. The maxillary and mandibular branches may be involved, with painful lesions involving the gums and oral epithelium. During varicella, vesicles are frequent on the buccal mucosa, which can lead to ascending infection of the petrosal as well as trigeminal ganglia. With later activation, glossopharyngeal zoster may develop with posterior pharyngeal pain and lesions in the tonsil, posterior tongue, and posterior pharyngeal wall. Similarly, the sensory fibers of the facial nerve near the external auditory meatus may carry virus to the geniculate ganglia. With activation, pain and vesicles develop in the external auditory meatus, with loss of taste in the anterior two thirds of the tongue and an ipsilateral facial palsy (Ramsay Hunt syndrome). The facial palsy is presumably due to inflammation or compression of the motor fibers of the facial nerve as they pass through the ganglion. However, with cranial zoster signs often implicate multiple cranial nerves or ganglia and suggest localized involvement of the brainstem. Ophthalmic zoster is frequently associated with abnormalities of oculomotor function, ptosis, or paralytic mydriasis and otitic zoster with severe vertigo and hearing loss.

Motor function may also be affected with herpes zoster in cervical, thoracic, and lumbar segments. The motor paralysis usually occurs within the dermatome involved by the rash, but occasionally is dissociated. Diaphragmatic paralysis with cervical zoster is usually unilateral. Asymptomatic paralysis of intercostal muscles may be found if sought. Thoracic lesions occasionally are accompanied by constipation, hypomotility, and even paralytic ileus. Urinary retention or urinary and fecal incontinence has been described with herpes zoster of sacral dermatomes. Signs of severe diffuse encephalitis, acute transverse myelitis, cerebellar ataxia, or ascending myelitis are rare and occur primarily in patients who have been receiving immunosuppressive therapy. Fatalities are infrequent.

An unusual complication of herpes ophthalmicus has recently been recognized. Days to months after the onset of vesicular lesions a sudden contralateral hemiplegia develops. Angiography may demonstrate a segmental narrowing of the carotid or cerebral arteries, scans show multifocal infarctions, occasionally bilateral angiitis develops, and in fatal cases a granulomatous arteritis with giant cells is found. The vasculitis appears to develop near the ganglia and spread distally. Whether direct viral infection or an allergic reaction causes the angiitis during convalescence from zoster is unknown.

Since the primary lesion even in uncomplicated herpes zoster is in the nervous system, cerebrospinal fluid commonly shows a pleocytosis and elevation of protein even in the absence of signs of meningeal irritation. These findings per se in the spinal fluid should not be a matter of concern.

Zoster sine herpete is typical pain in an appropriate sensory area that is not followed by the development of the characteristic vesicles. How often common transient intercostal or cranial pains represent activation of varicella virus in ganglia without spread to the skin is uncertain. An antibody response to varicella virus has been demonstrated in the absence of a rash in patients with transient intercostal pain or facial pain resembling trigeminal neuralgia and in patients with facial palsy (Bell's palsy). However, the vast majority of cases of trigeminal neuralgia and Bell's palsy are associated neither with serologic evidence of activation of the varicella nor with any other known viral infection.

Cutaneous dissemination is rare, occurring in less than 2 per cent of the cases. Dissemination is more common in patients with underlying malignancies, and about one quarter of the patients with Hodgkin's disease show a progressive spread of vesicles beyond the original one or two dermatomes of involvement. Such cutaneous dissemination, however, generally does not progress for more than six days, and spontaneous recovery occurs in most patients.

DIAGNOSIS. Characteristic development of pain and vesicular eruptions over single or adjacent dermatomes served by a segmental or cranial nerve branch usually presents no problem in differential diagnosis. However, similar zosteriform lesions can be caused by herpes simplex virus in infants.

Multinucleated giant epithelial cells with intranuclear inclusions can be found in Giemsa-stained scrapings from the base of an early vesicle, and virions can readily be found in vesicular fluid by electron microscopic examination. Neither of these tests, however, differentiates zoster from herpes simplex virus infections, although they can differentiate zoster or chickenpox from smallpox infections. Varicella and herpes simplex virus infections can be differentiated by fluorescent antibody staining of cells in scrapings from vesicles.

Virus can be isolated from vesicular fluid and, in some cases, from cerebrospinal fluid by inoculation of fluid onto cultures of human or primate cells. Serologic diagnosis can also be made, but in human sera some cross-reactions are found with herpes simplex virus, so that simultaneous serologic tests should be carried out against both viruses.

TREATMENT. Optimal treatment of acute eruption of herpes zoster is still unclear. Previously advocated treatments such as administration of protamine, vitamins, x-irradiation, vasodilators, antimicrobials, and gamma globulin are useless. In a controlled study corticosteroids decreased the incidence of postherpetic neuralgia, although they failed to alter the rate of healing or shorten the period of acute pain. However, this benefit must be weighed against the potential hazard of corticosteroids enhancing dissemination. Conversely, in controlled studies vidarabine and acyclovir have been shown to shorten the duration of acute pain and speed the healing of vesicles but not to decrease the incidence of postherpetic neuralgia.

In the young immunocompetent patient, little should be done to treat the acute eruption other than symptomatic application of powder or calamine lotion to the rash and use of analgesics for pain. In the immunocompromised patient, vidarabine or acyclovir should be given intravenously for at least five days to decrease the threat of cutaneous or visceral dissemination. In nonimmunocompromised elderly patients the risk-benefit ratio of corticosteroids is undefined, and antiviral drugs are of limited usefulness because of the need for intravenous treatment and the failure to decrease postherpetic neuralgia, the most dreaded complication in the elderly. Studies of the efficacy of oral administration of acyclovir and a re-evaluation of corticosteroids are currently in progress; these may clarify the indications for these drugs for the elderly immunocompetent patient.

There are no data to indicate the efficacy of vidarabine or acyclovir in zoster encephalomyelitis or granulomatous angiitis. Their use is rational with these potentially fatal complications, but since both conditions develop late in disease, antiviral drugs may not be effective. Because granulomatous arteritis may represent an allergic response, corticosteroids have been used in some cases but without clear-cut results.

Postherpetic Neuralgia. The development of prolonged postherpetic neuralgia after recovery from herpes zoster presents a difficult problem in management. Although the pain usually abates over a period of months to years, it is refractory to the usual analgesics. Application of cold to the area by use of an ethyl chloride spray may give transient relief. Tranquilizers or sedatives can sometimes be of help. Carbamazepine, an analgesic and anticonvulsant chemically related to the tricyclic antidepressants, is the drug of choice for postherpetic neuralgia but may be more effective when combined with other tricyclic compounds, such as amitriptyline, which more specifically block serotonin reuptake. A recent study of carbamazepine in conjunction with a similar drug, clomipramine, showed more effective pain relief than did transcutaneous nerve stimulation. Local injection of nerve root or nerve section should be avoided, since the origin of the neuralgia is in the ganglia. Surgical intervention, therefore, requires proximal nerve section or cordotomy, and results are often disappointing. In general, the patient is better served by protection from addiction or destructive surgery, treatment with analgesics and tricyclic antidepressants, and reassurance that pain usually abates with time.

PROGNOSIS. There is a popular misconception that herpes zoster does not recur. However, zoster does not give immunity to further attacks, and the likelihood of a second attack is about the same as, if not slightly greater than, that of having suffered the first. Most patients recover uneventfully, although severe vesiculation may lead to permanent scarring. Scarring of the cornea after ophthalmic involvement may result in permanent visual impairment. Motor paralysis of the local nerves recovers to adequate function levels in over 75 per cent of cases. Even in patients with encephalomyelitis, the mortality rate appears to be less than 10 per cent, and permanent sequelae are rare. The prognosis, however, must be more guarded in patients who have underlying neoplastic disease, in whom both the disease and the chemotherapeutic agents used in the treatment may increase the possibility of cutaneous and visceral dissemination.

PREVENTION. A vaccine to prevent primary chickenpox is being evaluated, but no method is known to clear latent virus from ganglia. Sera obtained from patients recuperating from herpes zoster can prevent chickenpox in children if given within 72 hours of the time of exposure. This zoster immune globulin is recommended for children on immunosuppressive therapy or with leukemia who have been exposed to chickenpox or herpes zoster. Similar measures are not recommended for disabled adults exposed to chickenpox or to zoster, although contact should be avoided in immunocompromised adults because it is in this group that occasional cases of zoster have been thought to be related to exposure to chickenpox or zoster.

Bean B, Braun C, Balfour HH: Acyclovir therapy for acute herpes zoster. Lancet 2:118, 1982. *A double-blind study of the efficacy of intravenous acyclovir therapy for zoster in otherwise healthy adults. Acyclovir did not appear to affect postherpetic neuralgia.*

Eaglstein WH, Katz R, Brown JA: The effects of early corticosteroid therapy on the skin eruption and pain of herpes zoster. JAMA 211:1681, 1970. *A double-blind study showing decrease in incidence of postherpetic neuralgia when herpes zoster in patients over age 60 is treated with corticosteroids.*

Gerson GR, Jones RB, Luscombe DK: Studies of the concomitant use of carbamazepine and clomipramine for relief of post-herpetic neuralgia. Postgrad Med J 53:104, 1977. *A controlled study showing greater efficacy of tricyclic compounds over transcutaneous stimulation in relief of pain in postherpetic neuralgia.*

Hilt DC, Buchholz D, Krumholz A, Weiss H, Wolinsky JS: Herpes zoster ophthalmicus and delayed contralateral hemiparesis due to cerebral angiitis: Diagnosis and management approaches. Ann Neurol 14:543, 1983. *A recent report of four cases with review of the English literature and thoughtful consideration of pathogenesis and therapy.*

Hope-Simpson RE: The nature of herpes zoster: A long-term study and a new hypothesis. Proc Roy Soc Med 58:9, 1965. *A classic. Simple observational data collected over 16 years from a general practice is beautifully presented to formulate the hypothesis of sensory ganglion latency and to speculate on man's evolving interrelationships with viruses.*

Jamsek J, Greenberg SB, Taber L, Harvey D, Gershon A, Couch RB: Herpes zoster-associated encephalitis: Clinicopathologic report of 12 cases and review of the literature. Medicine 62:81, 1983. *A recent article providing references on unusual neurologic complications.*

Juel-Jensen BE, MacCallum FO: Herpes Simplex, Varicella, and Zoster. Philadelphia, J. B. Lippincott Company, 1972. *This book contains a wealth of clinical data on herpes zoster, some of which has not been published elsewhere.*

McCormick WF, Rodnitzky RL, Schochet SS Jr, McKee AP: Varicella-zoster encephalomyelitis. Arch Neurol 21:559, 1969. *The best description of the neuropathology of fatal herpes zoster infections.*

502. ACUTE ANTERIOR POLIOMYELITIS

Richard T. Johnson

DEFINITION. Paralytic poliomyelitis is an acute febrile illness producing signs of meningeal irritation and flaccid motor paralysis. The term poliomyelitis means inflammation of the gray matter of the spinal cord. The disorder is characteristic of central nervous system infections with polioviruses. Mild forms of the syndrome are now often recognized with other enterovirus infections. Paralytic poliomyelitis is also called *infantile paralysis* or *acute anterior poliomyelitis.*

ETIOLOGY. Polioviruses are small, 28-nm-diameter, nonenveloped ribonucleic acid viruses that are members of the enterovirus group of the picornavirus family. There are three distinct serotypes, but they cross-react serologically, particularly types 1 and 2. Polioviruses have a restricted host range; most strains can be transmitted experimentally only to primates and cell cultures of primate origin. The host range of the polioviruses appears to be related primarily to specific cellular receptor sites for the virus; in human cells the coding for the receptor has been localized to chromosome 19. The coxsackieviruses, groups A and B, echoviruses, and related enteroviruses also can cause paralytic poliomyelitis, but unlike the polioviruses, other enteroviruses are also associated with a variety of clinical symptoms (see Ch. 341 to 347), and the resultant paralysis tends to be mild and transitory.

EPIDEMIOLOGY. Polioviruses have three distinct epidemiologic patterns. The first is endemic poliomyelitis, which occurred throughout the world until the end of the nineteenth century and is similar to the endemic disease still seen in tropical areas and developing countries. The second is the epidemic polio seen in economically advantaged countries during the first half of the twentieth century. The third is the pattern of sporadic cases seen in these countries since widespread immunization.

Descriptions of sporadic cases in children appeared in the eighteenth and early nineteenth centuries. Epidemic disease was first seen among small children in Scandinavia in the late nineteenth century and in North America and the remainder of Northern Europe in the early twentieth century. The age of patients developing paralytic poliomyelitis increased from epidemic year to epidemic year. In the great epidemic of 1916 in New York City, 9000 cases of paralysis were reported, and 80 per cent involved children under five years of age. During the epidemics of the 1950s, the peak incidence of paralysis was in children from five to nine years of age, and one third of the cases and two thirds of the deaths occurred in persons over age 15. These temperate-zone epidemics were seasonal, usually occurring in late summer and early fall. Even during epidemics when more virulent strains were circulating, the ratio of inapparent infection to disease ranged from 50:1 to 500:1.

Serologic surveys show that all three polioviruses have a worldwide distribution, and children even in population isolates have evidence of past infection with all virus types. Paralysis is age-dependent and is more frequent with advancing age. In virgin population epidemics, adults and adolescents with primary infections are ten times more likely to develop paralysis. In such epidemics almost all deaths are of patients over 20 years of age. Thus, prior to immunization programs, essentially all individuals experienced infections with all three types of virus. It is assumed that as sanitation improved virus dissemination among the very young declined, exposing a more susceptible population of older children and adults to primary infection. Quite possibly, during the time preceding epidemics of poliomyelitis children were infected with all three strains of virus at a period of infancy when they still had passive maternal antibody protection. Changes in living patterns and sanitation delayed acquisition of infection and led to an increase in the number of nonimmune persons and the appearance of the epidemic paralytic disease. As sanitation continues to improve in the developing world, more cases of paralytic poliomyelitis are seen. These cases, as expected, primarily occur in infants under three years of age. In developing tropical and semitropical countries, infections occur throughout the year, and outbreaks of disease are infrequent. Facilitation of spread in high humidity and the prevalence of other enterovirus infections that may cause interference may inhibit epidemics in these areas.

With widespread introduction of poliovirus vaccines in temperate-zone countries, the epidemic chain has been broken. In the past ten years, only 5 to 32 cases of paralytic poliomyelitis have been reported each year in the United States. Small outbreaks have occurred with the introduction of virus along the Mexican border and among religious groups where immunization is not practiced. Of the 208 cases of paralytic poliomyelitis reported between 1969 and 1982, 91 were related to vaccine viruses. Such cases occur primarily in adults in contact with children excreting vaccine virus or in children with hypogammaglobulinemia.

PATHOGENESIS AND PATHOLOGY. Humans are the only

known natural hosts of polioviruses. Virus is spread from person to person by hand-to-mouth contamination, although respiratory spread or passive transmission by insects or fomites may have a minor role. Virus is introduced orally, and initial replication occurs in lymphoid cells of the pharynx and gut. Virus can be found in the throat for several days and is excreted in feces for several weeks. After its initial replication, a viremia develops, with probable invasion of the central nervous system from the blood. There also may be neural spread from gut to spinal cord. Within the central nervous system there is selective vulnerability of motor neurons. Virus may spread from neuron to neuron by axonal transport. A possible explanation for the greater susceptibility of adults to severe paralytic and bulbar poliomyelitis is the more rapid axonal transport with maturation. Other host factors influencing paralysis include (1) excessive physical activity during the period of asymptomatic infection, which appears to favor paralysis of the exercised limbs; (2) pregnancy, which increases the risk of paralytic paralysis; (3) local injections during preceding weeks, which increase the risk of paralysis in the injected extremity; and (4) tonsillectomy, which heightens the risk of bulbar paralysis.

In fatal cases of acute poliomyelitis, inflammatory lesions are found primarily in the spinal cord when perivascular cuffing and diffuse infiltrates of mononuclear cells are present. The anterior horn cells of the spinal cord and the motor nuclei of the lower brain show the most marked abnormalities, with chromatolysis of motor neurons. Inflammatory reaction often spreads to the intermediate and posterior columns. Lesions are also found in the hypothalamus, thalamus, and brainstem, particularly in the vestibular nuclei, the deep nuclei of the cerebellum, and the reticular formation that regulates autonomic, respiratory, and circulatory functions. Lesions of the cerebral cortex are usually confined to the motor area.

CLINICAL MANIFESTATIONS. Replication of polioviruses in the intestinal tract often is not associated with any clinical signs but may cause the so-called *minor illness,* with fever, malaise, headache, and mild gastrointestinal symptoms of anorexia, nausea, vomiting, or diarrhea. This minor illness may or may not be evident three to ten days prior to obvious central nervous system involvement. Central nervous system involvement may be associated with asymptomatic meningitis, referred to as *nonparalytic poliomyelitis,* or with paralytic disease. Preceding the paralysis there are usually stiff neck, intense muscle aches, and headache with fever ranging from 38.5 to 40° C. Muscle pain and cramps may be accompanied by diffuse transient fasciculations. Paralysis may develop with great rapidity, proceeding from barely evident weakness to tetraplegia in only a few hours, or it may have a more indolent course, with additional weakness appearing over a four- to five-day period. The spread shows no consistent pattern, but paralysis is nearly always asymmetrical and at times widely scattered in its distribution. Lower extremities and lower trunk are involved most frequently. In the initial phases there may be hyperreflexia, but this is followed by flaccid paralysis with reduced or absent deep tendon reflexes. Although dysesthesias are frequent, sensory loss is rare. More than 50 per cent of adults have at least transient urinary retention.

Involvement of the brainstem is an ominous sign. This may be heralded by agitation, fear, or delirium. The ocular motor nerves are usually spared, but nystagmus with peripheral vision frequently occurs on extremes of gaze. Facial paralysis is usually restricted to one or more muscles and rarely is manifested as total facial paresis. Paralysis of swallowing is the most frequent abnormality of cranial nerve function but is usually transient. Muscle paralysis of the larynx may cause respiratory obstruction, but the greater dangers are autonomic abnormalities usually seen in adults with involvement of the reticular formation. Fulminating elevations of blood pressure, tachycardia, acute pulmonary edema, and cardiac arrhythmias are frequent with bulbar paralysis. Respiration may be ataxic, and potentially fatal sleep apnea may occur.

DIAGNOSIS AND DIFFERENTIAL DIAGNOSIS. Diagnosis in paralytic poliomyelitis is dependent on the typical clinical presentation and cerebrospinal fluid findings that document inflammation. The spinal fluid usually has a modest pleocytosis of 10 to 1000 mononuclear cells per milliliter, although early in the course of the disease there may be fewer than 10 cells or a preponderance of polymorphonuclears. Protein concentration is usually modestly elevated, and sugar content remains normal. These findings are important in the differentiation from *acute polyneuritis (Guillain-Barré syndrome).* In Guillain-Barré syndrome pleocytosis is absent or mild, and protein concentration often rises over 100 mg per deciliter, an unusual finding in poliomyelitis. More importantly, patients with polyneuritis are seldom systemically ill or febrile, and the paralysis tends to be symmetrical, in contrast to the patchy paralysis in poliomyelitis.

Paralytic poliomyelitis caused by most coxsackieviruses and echoviruses tends to have a more benign course with less serious and more transient paralysis. However, in countries with successful vaccine programs these other enteroviruses are the commonest cause of the paralytic poliomyelitis syndrome. Spinal fluid changes are similar, and definitive differentiation can only be made by isolation of virus or demonstration of antibody increases between sera from acute and convalescent phases. Furthermore, paralysis caused by nonpolio enteroviruses seldom occurs in epidemic outbreaks, with the exception of coxsackievirus A7 and two recently isolated enteroviruses.

Coxsackievirus A7 was related to several local outbreaks of paralytic disease in the Soviet Union in the 1950s and in the United Kingdom and France in the 1960s. Enterovirus 70 is the major cause of acute hemorrhagic conjunctivitis, a disease first observed in Africa in 1969. Subsequent epidemics in both Africa and Asia have probably affected more than 80 million people. Smaller outbreaks have also been reported in South and North America. Unlike other enteroviruses, this agent appears to be spread from eye to eye, and after an incubation period of only one to two days causes a febrile illness characterized by severe conjunctivitis with hemorrhage. In a small percentage of the cases a lower motor neuron paralysis resembling poliovirus infections has occurred, but curiously this paralysis usually develops several weeks after the acute illness and is often heralded by severe radicular pains. Paralysis is more common in adult males. The virus has shown a neural virulence in monkeys similar to that observed with polioviruses. Enterovirus 71 was first associated with aseptic meningitis but has shown different manifestations in different epidemics. A strain of this virus has been implicated in several outbreaks with paralytic poliomyelitis in Eastern Europe, primarily affecting young children. Fatal cases of bulbar paralysis were seen.

Epidemic neuromyasthenia (benign myalgic encephalomyelitis, Iceland disease, Royal Free disease) has some clinical similarities to poliomyelitis. Over the past 40 years, approximately 20 outbreaks have been observed of this curious disorder. Most outbreaks have involved residential communities, half of them affecting hospital staffs. The majority of cases occur in persons in the third decade of life, with women outnumbering men, although the sex ratio has been variable between outbreaks. Most outbreaks have occurred during the summer months with rapid spread, suggesting an epidemiology similar to that of poliomyelitis. However, attack rates have been higher than those seen in epidemics of paralytic poliomyelitis; for example, nearly 200 were affected at Los Angeles County Hospital in 1934 and over 300 at the Royal Free Hospital in London in 1955.

The disease begins abruptly with headache and severe muscle pains; posterior cervical lymphadenopathy and fever are variable findings. Muscle paralysis is seen in 10 to 80 per cent of patients, depending on the outbreak, but this paralysis differs from poliomyelitis since atrophy does not develop and hyperreflexia rather than hyporeflexia is found. Sensory symptoms are common, but objective sensory loss is rare. Occasionally painful muscle spasms, myoclonus, and other involuntary movements are seen, and objective signs of focal brainstem disease may be present, such as diplopia, facial paralysis, acute vertigo with nystagmus, deafness, and palatal paresis. Acute urinary retention has been described. Laboratory findings are remarkably normal. In some cases abnormal lymphocytes or an increased excretion of creatinine has been reported. The cerebrospinal fluid is usually entirely normal; 95 per cent of the cases show no pleocytosis. Variable nonspecific abnormalities have been reported on the electromyogram. The disease tends to have a protracted course. Although most patients show complete recovery within three months, relapses of weakness and myalgias are frequent, and emotional disturbances—particularly complaints of memory loss, depression, and emotional lability—may be prolonged.

Several of the early outbreaks of epidemic neuromyasthenia occurred during epidemics of paralytic poliomyelitis. An emotional etiology has been suggested by this correspondence, the high rates among young women, and the paucity of objective clinical or laboratory findings. However, something more than mass hysteria appears to be involved; the outbreaks, although widely distributed over time and place, have been remarkably stereotyped, and objective findings have been present in a significant percentage of the patients. The broad spectrum of symptoms and variable findings would make sporadic cases very difficult to diagnose, whereas in closed communities where epidemic spread of the infectious agent is facilitated, the disease would be more readily recognized. Certainly, the failure to find a pleocytosis in the spinal fluid, the inconsistency of fever, and the uniformly negative virologic studies are not conclusive evidence against a possible viral etiology.

TREATMENT. There is no specific treatment for paralytic poliomyelitis. Symptomatically, patients are treated with bed rest, aspirin, and other nonnarcotic analgesics for fever and pain and with hot packs for muscle spasm. The complications of bulbar poliomyelitis, including swallowing paralysis, respiratory failure, and cardiac abnormalities, are managed for the most part as they are in other diseases.

PROGNOSIS. During the acute illness it is impossible to predict the precise outcome. Fewer than 5 per cent of patients with paralytic poliomyelitis die with acute disease. Those over age 40 and those with bulbar involvement are at greatest risk. Muscle groups that maintain partial function at the end of the acute illness usually show good recovery. Recovery in areas of total paralysis is less certain.

Many years after paralytic poliomyelitis, a few patients, usually in their fifth or sixth decades, notice increasing weakness that is sometimes associated with muscle loss and fasciculations. The weakness is often in the area of the original paralysis. The more benign course and lack of upper motor neuron signs differentiate this late *postpoliomyelitis motor neuron disease* from *primary motor neuron disease.* It has been postulated that postpoliomyelitis disease may result from the persistence of polioviruses, but it more likely represents an aging process superimposed on a depleted anterior horn cell neuron population that may have been overloaded by the sprouting and reinnervation of larger motor units during recovery from the paralysis years before.

PREVENTION. Both live and killed poliovirus vaccines have proved successful for almost 30 years. Inactivated poliovirus vaccine used in the United States from 1955 to 1961 was effective in controlling epidemic polio, and its use has been continued with good disease control in several Northern European countries. The attenuated live oral poliovirus vaccines have been used in most of the world since 1961. Currently in the United States a trivalent oral polio vaccine (TOPV) is given in early childhood. The TOPV confers humoral and intestinal immunity similar to that of the natural infection, can be administered without trained personnel, and is inexpensive and easy to prepare. The vaccine virus is excreted in stools, and therefore inadvertent immunization is provided to many who fail to receive the vaccine. The disadvantage of TOPV is that a large percentage of paralytic poliomyelitis cases now seen in the United States are vaccine-related, either in hypogammaglobulinemic children or in adults who have been in contact with vaccine recipients. This risk has led to cogent arguments for return to use of the killed vaccine, but poor compliance and a dwindling supply of monkeys for tissue cultures and safety testing make this change impractical.

The advantages of the killed vaccine are that new preparations now produce very good and sustained immune responses and that it poses no danger of paralytic accidents. In developing countries where endemic poliomyelitis remains a problem, both vaccines have unique drawbacks. The TOPV often fails to confer immunity in tropical countries, presumably because of interference by other enteroviruses in the gut, but the killed polio vaccines pose problems in cost of production and delivery.

If an adult is traveling in areas of high endemicity or has special occupational risks and has not acquired past immunity, the killed polio vaccine is preferable. It is also indicated for immunodeficient children and their siblings.

Lyle WH, Chamberlain RN (eds.): Epidemic neuromyasthenia 1934–1977. Current approaches. Postgrad Med J 54:705, 1978. *Proceedings of a comprehensive symposium held at the Royal College of Medicine.*

Mulder DW, Rosenbaum RA, Layton DP: Late progression of poliomyelitis or forme fruste amyotrophic lateral sclerosis? Mayo Clin Proc 47:756, 1972. *A description of the problem based on the findings in 34 patients.*

Nathanson N, Martin JR: The epidemiology of poliomyelitis: Enigmas surrounding its appearance, pathogenicity, and disappearance. Am J Epidemiol 110:672, 1979. *A thoughtful essay, analyzing why poliomyelitis appeared and then disappeared as an epidemic disease in the United States during this century. The authors conclude that any change in present United States immunization practices carries considerable risk of reappearance of the disease.*

Paul JR: A History of Poliomyelitis. New Haven, Yale University Press, 1971. *A vividly told story of the social and scientific effects of one of the major "diseases of civilization."*

Robbins RC, Fox JP, Hopps HE, Horstmann DM, Quinn TC: International symposium on poliomyelitis control. Rev Infect Dis 6(Suppl 2):S301, 1984. *Proceedings of a recent conference posing the question of whether poliomyelitis can be eradicated worldwide. The disease in developing countries, current use and merits of live and killed vaccines, and the potential for better vaccines are discussed.*

Wadia NH, Katrak SM, Misra VP, Wadia PN, Miyamura K, Hashimoto K, Ogino T, Hikiji T, Kono R: Polio-like motor paralysis associated with acute hemorrhagic conjunctivitis in an outbreak in 1981 in Bombay, India: Clinical and serologic studies. J Infect Dis 147:660, 1983. *Also discusses novel modes of enterovirus transmission, problems in virus isolation, and neurovirulence in monkeys.*

503. RABIES

Michael A. W. Hattwick

DEFINITION. Rabies is an acute viral disease of warm-blooded animals, which may incidentally affect man, almost always as the result of a rabid animal bite. Human rabies is characterized by a variable incubation period, an acute neurologic illness leading rapidly to coma, and complications involving neurologic, pulmonary, and cardiovascular systems.

ETIOLOGY AND PATHOGENESIS. The rabies virus is a member of the rhabdovirus group, which includes more than 70 viruses, only three of which are reported to affect man: rabies, Duvenhage, and mokola virus. The virions are approximately 75 × 180 to 200 nm in length, contain single-stranded RNA, and are cylindrical with one conical and one flat end, giving rise to the characteristic bullet shape. Rabies virus is inactivated by drying, heating to 56° C for one hour, sunlight, ultraviolet light, and many chemical agents, including formalin, 50 to 70 per cent ethanol, strong acids, 0.1 to 1 per cent quaternary ammonium compounds, and 20 per cent soap. The virus is composed of four proteins: a glycoprotein, which is responsible for the induction of neutralizing antibodies, and is concentrated in spikes attached to the nucleocapsid core; a nucleocapsid protein, which produces complement-fixing but not neutralizing antibodies; and two membrane proteins, which are closely associated with the nucleocapsid.

Rabies virus obtained from the nervous tissue of animals which have developed the disease under natural conditions is referred to as "street virus" and is characterized by relatively long incubation periods after intracerebral inoculation (15 to 30 days or more), high infectivity after peripheral inoculation, and production of either "furious," or "dumb" (paralytic) rabies. Virus after serial passage in the brains of laboratory animals is referred to as "fixed" rabies virus and is characterized by a short incubation period after intracerebral inoculation (six to eight days), and production of paralytic rabies. Antigenic variations exist between strains of rabies virus and between rabies virus and serologically related rhabdoviruses.

After introduction by inoculation or animal bites, the virus remains near the site of inoculation for a variable time, during which replication in muscle cells may occur. Unless inactivated by natural or induced defense mechanisms, the virus subsequently enters the axoplasm of peripheral nerves, from where it travels to spinal ganglia and brain. The rabies virus spreads centrifugally soon after it reaches the central nervous system, is present in neurons throughout the body, and may be demonstrated by fluorescent antibody staining of corneal cells or skin biopsies. The virus is present in saliva in many but not all cases, and has also been identified in urine and cerebrospinal fluid. Concentrations in the brain are highest in the brainstem, basal ganglion, hippocampus, and cerebellum. Histologic examination shows perivascular lymphocytic infiltration, edema, vascular congestion, and relatively intact nerve cells. Characteristic oval cytoplasmic Negri bodies containing nucleocapsids are found in ganglia and in pyramidal cells, particularly of Ammon's horn or the cerebellum, but may be absent in 20 per cent or more of both human and animal cases.

EPIDEMIOLOGY. Rabies normally persists as an enzootic disease in warm-blooded animal species, in which it is maintained by bite transmission and possibly by transmission from mother to offspring. In areas where domestic animal rabies has been inadequately controlled, dog and cat rabies accounts for more than 90 per cent of reported cases. In other regions the majority of animal rabies cases are in wild animals. The virus is known to be maintained as an enzootic in only a few wild animal species, including, in the United States, skunks, foxes, bats, raccoons, and, elsewhere in the world, mongooses, wolves, and vampire bats. Epizootics of rabies in wild animals appear at intervals, most recently in raccoons in southeastern United States. In the United States during the 1950's, intensive dog and cat rabies control programs, including vaccination and stray animal elimination, reduced the number of annually proved rabid dogs from more than 7000 to less than 700. About 30 countries are classified as rabies free, largely because of geographical isolation and strict animal control and importation programs.

The epidemiology of human rabies closely parallels that of animal rabies; where dog rabies is inadequately controlled, most human cases result from rabid dog bites. In the United States from 1970 to 1984 27 human cases have occurred associated with a wide variety of exposures: dogs (2), a cat (1), skunks (2), bats (5), laboratories working with rabies (2), corneal transplant (1), and rabid animals in other countries (8). Six had no known exposure.

CLINICAL RABIES IN ANIMALS. Rabies virus may be present in the saliva of presymptomatic rabid animals for periods that vary with the animal species and with the rabies virus strain endemic in the area. The periods may last up to seven days for American dogs, one day for cats, four days for skunks, ten days for insectivorous bats, and possibly longer for vampire bats. Whenever a presymptomatic secretor of rabies virus has been killed and adequately examined, the brain has also contained rabies virus. Clinical rabies in animals may present either as hyperactivity (furious rabies) or as paralysis (paralytic rabies). Most animals die relatively rapidly after the onset of symptoms, although nonfatal rabies occurs.

CLINICAL RABIES IN MAN. Clinical rabies may be divided into five phases: incubation period, prodrome, acute neurologic phase, coma, and recovery.

Incubation Period. The incubation period normally ranges from 20 to 60 days, but periods as short as 10 days and as long as 19 years have been reported. Cases of rabies without any known exposure also occur. Incubation periods tend to be shorter in children than in adults, when the site of the bite is on the head rather than on the extremities, and in persons who have received postexposure treatment, possibly because of the elimination of long incubation rabies in the latter series. During the incubation period the person is asymptomatic except for symptoms related to local wound healing or postexposure treatment. Steroids have been reported to increase rabies mortality in mice and to decrease the immune response to rabies vaccine and should not be used in treating persons exposed to rabies.

Prodrome. The initial symptoms consist of malaise, anorexia, fatigue, headache, and fever. About half the patients have pain or paresthesias at the site of exposure. Apprehension, anxiety, agitation, irritability, nervousness, insomnia, and depression may be prominent; less commonly, cough, chills, sore throat, abdominal pain, nausea, vomiting, diarrhea, dysuria, pyuria, and priapism have been reported.

Acute Neurologic Phase. Two to ten days following the first symptoms, signs of nervous system involvement develop, including hyperactivity, hallucinations, disorientation, bizarre behavior, seizures, nuchal stiffness, or paralysis. Most patients develop hyperactivity, consisting of intermittent agitation, thrashing, biting, or other bizarre behavior, lasting up to five minutes. The episodes may occur spontaneously or may be precipitated by tactile, auditory, visual, or olfactory stimuli. Between episodes the patient is usually relatively lucid and cooperative, although often anxious. In half or more cases attempts to drink are followed by severe pain from spasms of the pharynx or larynx, inducing choking, gagging, and fear (hydrophobia). Hyperventilation and cardiac arrhythmias may be prominent.

Unless the patient dies abruptly, paralysis ensues and heralds impending coma. In about 20 per cent of cases paralytic symptoms dominate the clinical course (dumb rabies). Paralysis may be diffuse and symmetrical; may be maximal in the bitten extremity; or may ascend. Paralytic rabies appears to be particularly frequent after exposure to rabid bats or in persons who have received postexposure vaccination. During this period the mental status fluctuates, with increasing periods of confusion, disorientation, stupor, and finally coma. Nuchal rigidity may be present, but lumbar puncture reveals an increased number of cells in only about 50 per cent of cases. The acute neurologic phase lasts two to ten days with a longer duration in the paralytic forms and ends either with an abrupt death or with the onset of coma.

Coma Phase. In untreated cases the patient typically develops respiratory arrest shortly after the onset of coma and expires.

Recovery Phase. Intensive medical management can avert many of the complications in clinical rabies, and three cases of recovery have now been reported. In each the person had received either pre- or postexposure prophylaxis before the onset of clinical illness. In two of the three patients, a six-year-old boy and a 45-year-old woman, recovery was reported to be complete. The third case developed in a laboratory worker and the patient recovered with residual neurologic defects of speech and motor function.

COMPLICATIONS. A variety of complications have been reported, including increased intracranial pressure, cerebral edema, inappropriate secretion of ADH, diabetes insipidus, hypertension, hypotension, cardiac arrhythmias, and hypothermia. Seizures may be generalized or focal and are often accompanied by cardiac arrhythmias, cardiac arrest, or respiratory dysfunction. Hyperventilation and respiratory alkalosis are characteristic of the prodrome and early neurologic phase, whereas progressive hypoxia, hypoventilation, irregular respirations, respiratory arrest, and decreased pulmonary compliance develop later. Pneumonia, cardiovascular complications, vascular thromboses, gastrointestinal bleeding, and urinary tract infections are common late complications.

DIFFERENTIAL DIAGNOSIS. The diagnosis of clinical rabies is not difficult given a history of exposure and characteristic symptoms. If a history of exposure is not obtained, the differential diagnosis includes all forms of encephalitis. In recent years rabies has occurred after corneal transplants, and in six individuals without known history of exposure to possibly rabid animals other than hunting or working in wooded areas.

The diagnosis of rabies can be confirmed by isolation of virus from human saliva, human brain tissues, human cerebrospinal fluid, and/or urine. Attempts to isolate the virus late in the clinical course may be unsuccessful due to the development of neutralizing antibodies. Diagnosis of rabies during life occasionally can be made by utilizing fluorescent antibodies to stain rabies-infected cells obtained from corneal smears or skin biopsy specimens, although both false-positive and false-negative results occur. Diagnosis during life may also be made by measuring serum and cerebrospinal fluid antibody titers, a characteristic response occurring during the second and third weeks of illness. In unvaccinated patients neutralizing antibodies are absent until 6 to 12 days after onset and then rise rapidly to very high titers. In vaccinated patients a similar sharp rise occurs 6 to 12 days after clinical onset. Cerebrospinal fluid antibody levels rise later than do serum antibodies and are present in titers much higher than would be expected by passive transfer from the serum.

TREATMENT. Treatment of human clinical rabies consists of meticulously applied medical intensive care. Reports of human-to-human spread of rabies are rare except in the instance of corneal graft transmission. Nevertheless, rabies may be present in human saliva, cerebrospinal fluid, and urine, and treatment of persons possibly exposed to rabid patients should follow the same guidelines given for exposure to any rabid animal, as indicated below. Therapy of clinical rabies using rabies immune globulin, rabies vaccine, and human interferon has been tried, with no evidence of benefit.

PREVENTION. The most important aspect of rabies prevention is control of rabies in domestic animals. When it is not possible to prevent exposure of individuals to rabid animals or to environments containing rabies virus, prevention relies on local wound care and immunoprophylaxis. Two forms of immunoprophylaxis exist, pre- and postexposure. Both trace back to Pasteur, who showed that vaccination with inactivated rabies virus would protect against subsequent challenge with virulent rabies virus. Modern vaccines are based on growth of the virus in tissue culture, avian embryos, or suckling mice and harvested with methods that eliminate the presence of myelin components that are believed to be responsible for neurologic reactions. In the United States the only vaccines presently available are prepared on human diploid cells (HDCV), but vaccines prepared from infected mature nervous tissue (NTV) are still used in some countries.

The effectiveness of pre-exposure prophylaxis has been well established. Available studies generally indicate that individuals who have responded to pre-exposure prophylaxis with an adequate antibody response are protected against subsequent challenge by peripheral inoculation. A recent case of nonfatal rabies in an immunized laboratory worker exposed by an aerosol suggests that this protection may not extend to nonbite exposures. Protection against rabies following exposure requires both early and long-lasting immunity. The early immunity can be produced by passive antibodies or by induction of interferon. The lasting immunity must be produced by a potent vaccine. A number of studies have demonstrated that the combination of passive antibodies and active immunization with rabies vaccine is effective. In the absence of postexposure prophylaxis, the risk of human rabies following a bite on the arm or hand has been estimated as about 15 per cent for rabid dog bites and 40 per cent for rabid wolf bites. The combination of serum and vaccine prophylaxis reduces this incidence to less than 1 per cent. Both serum and vaccine are now recommended for all confirmed rabies exposures.

Pre-exposure Prophylaxis. Human diploid cell vaccine is sufficiently safe to justify immunization of individuals at high risk, such as veterinarians, animal handlers, some laboratory workers, and persons who vocationally or avocationally are likely to come in contact with rabid animals. Pre-exposure prophylaxis with HDCV consists of three 1-ml injections given intramuscularly on days 0, 7, and 21 or 28. Adequate antibody responses to this regimen have been demonstrated in all vaccinees studied. HDCV can also be given intradermally in a dose of 0.1 ml on days 0, 7, and 28. Individuals receiving intradermal pre-exposure prophylaxis should have serum tested for rabies antibodies two to three weeks following the last dose in the series. When antibody response is inadequate, an additional booster dose should be given and antibodies rechecked. Serologic testing is not required following a three-dose regimen by the intramuscular route. A person with continuing risk of inapparent or unavoidable exposure and no history of hypersensitivity reactions should have booster doses at two-year intervals. Type III hypersensitivity reactions may occur frequently after HDCV boosters, and booster doses should be given only when clearly indicated.

Postexposure Prophylaxis. Prevention of rabies in exposed individuals who have not received or responded to pre-exposure prophylaxis requires local wound therapy, passive immunization with hyperimmune rabies globulin, and rabies vaccination. The decision to initiate postexposure prophylaxis is based on the type of exposure (bite or nonbite), the animal species involved, and the condition of the animal at the time of exposure. Treatment is recommended for any bite by a known or suspected rabid dog, cat, skunk, bat, fox, coyote, raccoon, bobcat, or other carnivore unless the animal is proved nonrabid by laboratory tests. A healthy dog or cat which is available for observation should be confined for ten days, and rabies treatment given only if the animal develops rabies during the holding period. Treatment recommendations for persons exposed to a dog or cat that has escaped depend on information regarding the epizootiology of rabies in the area, which is available from local public health officials. Bites by rodents, rabbits, and hares almost never require postexposure prophylaxis. Recommendations regarding other exposures such as to livestock, laboratory specimens, or aerosol should be individually evaluated, and consultation with public health officials may be needed.

An important part of postexposure prophylaxis is local wound treatment. Rabies virus can be inactivated by soap, quarternary ammonium compounds, alcohol, and other viricidal chemicals. Local wound cleansing alone can markedly reduce the incidence of rabies in laboratory animals. Tetanus prophylaxis and appropriate antibiotic treatment for infected local wounds should be given as indicated.

Rabies immune globulin (RIG) should be administered once as soon after the exposure as possible. Up to one half of the dose of RIG should be infiltrated into the area around the wound and the rest administered intramuscularly. Human rabies immune globulin is available in 2- and 10-ml ampules containing 150 IU per milliliter and is given in a dose of 20 IU per kilogram.

Human diploid cell rabies vaccine (HDCV) is more potent than previous vaccines and is given as five 1-ml doses, 1 ml each day on days 0, 3, 7, 14, and 28. For a person who has received adequate pre-exposure prophylaxis with HDCV or has a documented adequate antibody response to another rabies vaccine, postexposure vaccination with two 1-ml doses of HDCV intramuscularly on days 0 and 3 is recommended. Serum antibody titers should be determined at the time of the last dose in persons who may be immunosuppressed due to a disease process or steroid use, who have received rabies prophylaxis with vaccines other than HDCV, or who have not had one of the above recommended regimens. If a titer of greater than 0.5 IU per milliliter of serum is not found, additional doses of vaccine should be given and the titer rechecked.

Minor complications are commonly associated with HDCV. Local pain, swelling, erythema, or induration occur in 50 per cent of vaccines. Systemic reactions including headache, malaise, fever, lymphadenopathy, nausea, or abdominal pain have been reported in 20 per cent. More serious complications with HDCV appear uncommon. Between 1974 and 1984, when nearly 2 million doses of HDCV were distributed worldwide, only two cases of associated neurologic reactions were reported. Both were Guillain-Barré–like illnesses, and the patients recovered fully. Anaphylaxis, urticaria and other allergic reactions have also occurred, but no fatal complications have been reported. Neurologic complications following vaccination with nervous tissue vaccines occur with an estimated incidence of 1 per 1630 vaccinees, and have a 15 per cent mortality rate. In most areas these complication rates are higher than the risk of rabies, and have led to the discontinuation of NTV use. Steroids should not be used to treat adverse reactions to rabies vaccine unless the reaction is life threatening, or the risk of rabies has been ruled out.

CONTROL MEASURES. The most important aspect of control is the prevention of spread between domestic animals by a combination of active vaccination and elimination of stray animals. Both killed virus and modified live rabies vaccines are available for animal use, and rabies programs can be highly effective in reducing both dog rabies and the number of associated human cases. Control of rabies in wild animals has not yet proved practical. In the absence of wild animal reservoirs and with favorable geographic conditions, rabies control programs can eradicate rabies, as has occurred in England and Japan. In such rabies-free areas preventing reintroduction of rabies requires strict importation control, including a six-month quarantine of animals with vaccination at the time of entry.

Anderson LJ, Nicholson KG, Tauxe RV, Winkler WG: Human rabies in the United States 1960–1979. Epidemiology, diagnosis, and prevention. Ann Intern Med 100:728, 1984.

Baer GM (ed.): The Natural History of Rabies, Vols I and II. New York, Academic Press, 1973. *Most comprehensive general review.*

Bernard KW, Hattwick MAW: Rabies virus. *In* Mandell GC, Douglas RC, Bennett JE (eds.): Principles and Practice of Infectious Disease. 2nd ed. New York, John Wiley & Sons, 1984. *Most current review.*

Centers for Disease Control: Rabies prevention: Recommendations of the Immunization Practices Advisory Committee. Morbid Mortal Wkly Rep 29:265, 282, 1980; updated recommendations: Morbid Mortal Wkly Rep 31:279, 1982; 32:601, 1983. Supplementary statement on pre-exposure prophylaxis by the intradermal route, 33:185, 1984. *Systemic allergic reactions following immunization with human diploid cell rabies vaccination.*

Hattwick MAW: Human Rabies. Public Health Rev 3:229, 1974. *Detailed review of human rabies.*

Hattwick MAW, Weiss TT, Stechshulte CJ, Baer GM, Gregg MB: Recovery from rabies: A case report. Ann Intern Med 76:931, 1972. *First documented nonfatal human case.*

504. SLOW VIRAL INFECTIONS OF THE NERVOUS SYSTEM

Richard T. Johnson

Slow viral infections have been related to several chronic and subacute neurologic diseases in which clinical signs of infection are lacking and in which the pathologic changes are those of degenerative or demyelinative processes. The term slow infection was originally coined in the veterinary literature to describe several transmissible diseases of sheep. Two of these sheep diseases, *scrapie* and *visna,* are the prototypes of slow infections of the nervous system. Both are transmissible. After inoculation of sheep with tissue from an affected sheep, a latent period of one to four years ensues during which the sheep appear well. This is followed by the insidious onset of neurologic signs that progress without fever for one to six months and lead inevitably to death. Scrapie is clinically characterized primarily by ataxia and visna by progressive paralysis. Pathologically the diseases are very different. The lesions of scrapie are confined to the nervous system, where there is marked proliferation of astrocytes and degeneration of neurons with vacuolization of their cytoplasms. By contrast, central nervous system lesions of visna are characterized by marked inflammation and demyelination. The agents responsible for these two slow infections of sheep are also very different. The scrapie agent has been transmitted to a variety of other animals, but the agent does not cause cytopathic changes in cell culture, and no virus-like particles have been found in infectious tissue by electron microscopy. The infectivity of this tissue remains remarkably stable on exposure to physicochemical treatments that inactivate classic viruses. Furthermore, animals naturally or experimentally infected with scrapie fail to develop any evidence of an immune response against the agent. In contrast, the visna virus is an enveloped RNA retrovirus. Although transmissible from sheep to sheep, it has not been transmitted to other animals but can be grown in a variety of tissue cultures. Of the five slow infections of the human central nervous system described below, kuru and Creutzfeldt-Jakob disease resemble scrapie pathologically, and the agents responsible for these diseases have properties similar to those described for the scrapie agent. Therefore scrapie, kuru, and Creutzfeldt-Jakob disease have been classified together as the subacute spongiform encephalopathies. Subacute sclerosing panencephalitis, progressive rubella panencephalitis, and progressive multifocal leukoencephalopathy, like visna, are due to classic viruses. These viruses have been visualized by electron microscopy, are antigenic in natural and experimental hosts, and can produce rapid cytolytic infection in some cell cultures even though they are capable of causing slow infections in man.

KURU

Kuru is an endemic disease of Melanesian tribal people inhabiting a remote area of the Eastern Highlands of central New Guinea. The disease has been seen only among the Fore linguistic group and neighboring groups with whom they have intermarried. Within this limited area, kuru, until recently, was the most common cause of death. The disease predominantly affected adult women and children over age five. Adult males were least involved. The disease begins insidiously with unsteadiness of stance and gait. A progressive symmetrical cerebellar ataxia develops over a period of months and follows a relentless, afebrile course until the patient is unable to make the slightest movement without violent ataxic tremors. Late in the course of the disease, abnormalities of extraocular movement and mental changes develop. The disease invariably leads to death in 3 to 20 months. Extensive laboratory examinations have failed to show systemic abnormalities, and the cerebrospinal fluid remains normal. Pathologic changes are confined to the brain where a marked diffuse noninflammatory increase of astrocytes and degeneration of neurons with cytoplasmic vacuolization are found. The findings are most prominent in the cerebellum and pons and, to a lesser degree, in the hypothalamus and basal ganglia.

When brain tissue from patients dying of kuru was inoculated into chimpanzees for long-term observations, a similar disease developed after incubation periods of 18 months to four years. This disease has subsequently been transmitted from chimpanzee to chimpanzee and to several other species. The agent can be transmitted with serial dilutions, proving that it replicates within the primate host. However, like scrapie, the agent of kuru has not been seen by electron microscopy, does not induce cytopathic changes in cell culture, is resistant to physical and chemical treatments that usually inactivate viruses, and fails to evoke a demonstrable immune response in humans or experimentally infected primates.

In recent years there has been a striking decline in the incidence of kuru, and the disease has disappeared among children. This decreasing incidence has coincided with the suppression of cannibalism in this primitive culture, providing circumstantial evidence that kuru was transmitted during the practice of ritual cannibalism.

CREUTZFELDT-JAKOB DISEASE

Creutzfeldt-Jakob disease is an uncommon form of rapidly progressive dementia accompanied by myoclonus, upper motor neuron paralysis, and other neurologic signs. The disease usually develops between ages 40 and 65, is worldwide in distribution, and usually occurs sporadically. However, a familial history is obtained in 10 to 15 per cent of patients, with a pattern of autosomal dominant inheritance. The dementia develops rapidly, so that deterioration from day to day or week to week is evident. Myoclonic jerks usually develop early in the disease, and often massive symmetrical myoclonic jerks of the limbs occur when the patient is startled by unexpected light or sound. Pyramidal tract signs, cerebellar ataxia, visual disturbances, and muscle wasting with fasciculations are common but inconstant features. The disease is inexorably progressive, usually reducing the patient from good health to helplessness or death in less than a year. The cerebrospinal fluid shows no abnormality, but the electroencephalogram becomes abnormal early in the disease, showing diffuse slowing with superimposed bursts of sharp waves.

Neuropathologic findings include diffuse noninflammatory loss of cortical neurons with a remarkable increase in fibrous astrocytes. Vacuoles are present in neurons and astrocytes, and this may give a spongiform appearance to the cerebral cortex. Inclusion bodies are absent. The pathologic findings are very similar to those of kuru and scrapie.

A similar disease develops in chimpanzees inoculated with brain tissue of most patients with Creutzfeldt-Jakob disease after an incubation period of 11 to 71 months. The pathologic changes in the brain resemble those of Creutzfeldt-Jakob disease. The disease has also been transmitted from chimpanzee to chimpanzee, to Old and New World monkeys, to domestic cats, to guinea pigs, and to mice. Little information is available on the agent of Creutzfeldt-Jakob disease, but the absence of virus-like particles on electron microscopic examination of infectious tissues, the failure to demonstrate cytopathic changes in cell cultures, and the absence of a demonstrable immune response suggest that the agent is similar to those causing kuru and scrapie.

The mode of spread is unknown, but the ability to transmit disease with tissues from familial cases suggests the importance of genetic factors or the possible vertical transmission of the agent. The failure to find increased incidences in medical personnel, laboratory investigators, or spouses of patients suggests a lack of significant communicability by respiratory, enteric, or sexual contact. Furthermore, the agent has not been detected in blood, sputum, or urine of patients, although it is present in extraneural tissue. On the other hand, apparent person-to-person transmission has been documented with the development of Creutzfeldt-Jakob disease in a patient 18 months after receiving a corneal transplant from another patient who proved to have the disease; by the occurrence of the disease in two young patients less than two years after cerebral corticography using the same implanted electrodes previously used in a patient with Creutzfeldt-Jakob disease; and by the occurrence of the disease in a number of patients within two years after undergoing intracranial surgery. In view of these observations, isolation of patients with Creutzfeldt-Jakob disease does not appear indicated, but careful disposal of needles and special sterilization of surgical instruments used on these patients appear mandatory. Medical personnel should avoid contamination of open sores or the conjunctiva with tissue, and no organs or corneas from patients with ill-defined neurologic diseases should be used for transplantation purposes.

No known treatment alters the relentless course of Creutzfeldt-Jakob disease.

SUBACUTE SCLEROSING PANENCEPHALITIS
(Dawson's Encephalitis, Subacute Inclusion Body Encephalitis)

This is an uncommon, subacute encephalitis that affects children or young adults between the ages of 4 and 20 years. The onset is usually insidious and is characterized by deterioration in schoolwork and behavioral disorders. This is followed in weeks or months by mental deterioration and neurologic signs, the most characteristic of which is myoclonus. The disease usually terminates after a third stage of stupor, blindness, dementia, and decorticate rigidity, which may last months to years. The cerebrospinal fluid is under normal pressure and shows no pleocytosis but an increased concentration of gamma globulin, corresponding in large part to antibodies against measles virus. During the stage of active myoclonus, the electroencephalogram usually shows a typical pattern of general suppression of activity, with periodic (8 to 15 seconds) synchronous bursts of high-voltage slow and sharp waves. Occasionally an apparent arrest of the disease process or even transient clinical improvement is seen.

In the brain perivascular infiltrates of mononuclear cells are characteristic, and eosinophilic intranuclear inclusion bodies are found in neurons and glial cells. Electron microscope studies of cerebral biopsies show virus-like particles resembling the nucleocapsids of paramyxoviruses. Astonishingly high levels of antibodies against measles virus can be demonstrated in the serums of most patients, and measles virus antigen is present in the brain. The measles virus associated with the disease is apparently defective.

The pathogenesis of subacute sclerosing panencephalitis is obscure. This disease bears little resemblance clinically or pathologically to the fulminating forms of measles virus infections, in which virus dissemination may lead to giant-cell pneumonia. Furthermore, it is distinct from parainfectious encephalomyelitis that occasionally complicates measles virus infections, in which acute neurologic disease occurs and perivascular demyelination is found in the brain and spinal cord. Epidemiologic studies have shown that subacute sclerosing panencephalitis is more common in males than females, in children of rural than of urban origin, and in patients with a history of measles during the first two years of life. These findings suggest that environmental factors and presence of residual transplacental passive immunity may play roles in inducing defective infection or precipitating disease.

Empirical treatments of patients with antiviral agents, interferon inducers, and immunosuppression and immunoenhancement therapies have provided no convincing evidence of beneficial effects. The sharp decline in cases five to seven years after the widespread use of measles vaccine attests to its preventive effect.

Rubella virus on rare occasions produces a similar chronic encephalitis called progressive rubella panencephalitis. The majority of patients bear stigmata of congenital rubella virus infections. However, after normal development or development within the limitations of the static congenital abnormalities, a chronic neurologic disease develops at 8 to 19 years of age. As in subacute sclerosing panencephalitis, the disease begins with the insidious deterioration of intellectual function, but myoclonus is variably present and cerebellar ataxia is a more prominent early finding. The disease follows an afebrile course over a period of years. Cerebrospinal fluid usually shows a mononuclear cell pleocytosis and mild protein increase with elevated gamma globulin. Antibodies to rubella virus are greatly increased in serum and cerebrospinal fluid. Neuropathologic findings include meningeal and perivascular inflammation, demyelination and gliosis in white matter, and mineralization around vessels similar to the mineralization seen in congenital rubella encephalitis. Rubella virus has been recovered from brain.

PROGRESSIVE MULTIFOCAL LEUKOENCEPHALOPATHY

This is a rare demyelinating disease of the central nervous system. It usually develops in patients having pre-existing disorders of the reticuloendothelial system such as leukemia, lymphoma, or sarcoidosis, or in those who have an acquired immune deficiency syndrome or who are immunosuppressed therapeutically or after organ transplantation. The neurologic abnormalities develop rather suddenly and follow a subacute progressive course until death. The findings usually suggest multifocal disease. Abnormalities of motor function, sensation, vision, or speech are common, and dementia frequently develops. The cerebrospinal fluid shows little if any abnormality, and the electroencephalogram shows only nonspecific slowing. Computed tomography may show multiple lucencies in the subcortical white matter. Pathologic lesions in the brain consist of multiple foci of demyelination in various stages of evolution. Oligodendrocytes are depleted within the foci, but surrounding the foci they are enlarged and contain eosinophilic intranuclear inclusions. The astrocytes within the demyelinated areas are often bizarre and contain mitotic figures. Inflammatory cells are usually not prominent.

Electron microscopic examination in almost all cases of progressive multifocal leukoencephalopathy has shown particles in the oligodendrocyte inclusions resembling small papovaviruses. Two small deoxyribonucleic acid viruses related to simian-virus 40 have been isolated from brain tissue of patients dying from progressive multifocal leukoencephalopathy. The JC virus, a new human papovavirus to which most persons have antibody since childhood, appears to be the causative agent in most cases. Viruses antigenically indistinguishable from simian-virus 40 have been related to a small number of cases. Neither of these viruses has been associated with any disease in man except progressive multifocal leukoencephalopathy. The disease apparently results from opportunistic infection of the brain by normally nonpathogenic agents. The viruses appear selectively to infect and lyse oligodendrocytes, the glial cells that maintain the myelin sheaths, and cause demyelination. The disease occurs in patients with impaired cellular immune responses, but it is not known whether it represents a primary infection of an immunologically incompetent patient or a reactivation of a latent or persistent papovavirus infection.

Evaluation of possible therapeutic agents has not been possible because of the rarity of cases and the infrequency of diagnosis during life.

OTHER NEUROLOGIC DISEASES

Since viruses can cause disease after a long incubation period, can produce disease with a subacute or relapsing course, and can give rise to noninflammatory pathologic changes, the possible role of slow or latent virus infection in a variety of neurologic diseases has been entertained.

In several chronic or relapsing inflammatory diseases of the nervous system, a viral cause has been suspected. *Chronic focal epilepsy* (epilepsia partialis continua, Kozhevnikov's epilepsy) is, in some cases, associated with a chronic focal inflammatory process in the brain. In several Soviet laboratories, tick-borne encephalitis virus has been isolated from surgically removed cerebral epileptogenic foci years after the acute encephalitis. No viruses have been isolated from similar cases in other countries. Chronic focal epilepsy can be a manifestation of focal disease processes such as neoplastic, vascular, or traumatic lesions, but chronic infection may play a role in some cases.

Recurrent acute meningitis or encephalitis occurs in three clinical syndromes of unknown cause in which latent viral infection has been suspected. *Mollaret's meningitis* is a rare, recurrent meningitis characterized by repeated attacks of headache, fever, and nuchal rigidity. Each attack is abrupt in onset and lasts for two to three days; the patient is entirely well between episodes. During attacks, the cerebrospinal fluid may contain large numbers of both polymorphonuclear and mononuclear cells and also large, poorly staining "epithelial cells," characteristic but not pathognomonic of this disease. More severe recurrent neurologic involvement can occur in *Behçet's syndrome* and in the *Vogt-Koyanagi-Harada syndrome*. Behçet's syndrome is a chronic disease characterized by recurrent oral and genital ulcers and inflammatory ocular lesions, usually taking the form of acute recurrent iritis. In about one quarter of the patients neurologic signs develop, consisting either of cranial nerve palsies, focal seizures, hemiparesis, or other focal signs or of severe depression of consciousness, coma, or meningeal signs, suggesting more diffuse neurologic involvement. Neurologic deficits usually remit and relapse but may be progressive. Neuropathologic findings include meningeal inflammatory reactions, perivascular inflammation, and focal areas of necrosis. The Vogt-Koyanagi-Harada or uveoencephalitic syndrome is characterized by depigmentation of skin and hair, inflammatory ocular lesions (usually consisting of iridocyclitis or exudative retinal detachment), and meningitis. Unlike Behçet's syndrome, neurologic involvement occurs in all cases, often precedes the ocular inflammation, and usually consists only of headache, nuchal rigidity, and a mononuclear cell pleocytosis. However, transient decrease in hearing and tinnitus may accompany the meningitis, or a severe encephalitis may develop, leaving permanent neurologic deficits. Neuropathologic findings have consisted only of a chronic arachnoiditis. Reports have been made of isolations of unidentified viruses from patients with Mollaret's, Behçet's, and Vogt-Koyanagi-Harada syndrome, but none of these claims has been entirely convincing. An allergic cause has also been postulated in each of these disorders, and consequently treatment with corticosteroids has been advocated.

Considerable interest in a possible viral cause of *multiple sclerosis* has been stimulated by epidemiologic data that indicate the role of a common exposure factor, serologic studies showing higher antibody levels against measles virus in patients with multiple sclerosis, observation of viral-like particles in brains, and unconfirmed claims of virus isolations. These data are still inconclusive. A notion that Parkinson's disease might have a viral cause has been entertained ever since the observation was made that a form of parkinsonism was a frequent sequela of encephalitis lethargica (von Economo's disease). Similarly, the possible role of a slow infection in amyotrophic lateral sclerosis and in a variety of other demyelinating and degenerative diseases has also been postulated. Although the spectrum of neurologic disease that can be potentially attributed to slow, latent, or chronic viral infections has greatly broadened in recent years, evidence is still scant for incriminating a transmissible agent in these chronic neurologic diseases.

Gajdusek DC: Unconventional viruses and the origin and disappearance of kuru. Science 197:943, 1977. *This Nobel Prize lecture recounts the story of kuru and discusses the interrelationships of the spongiform encephalopathy agents.*

Johnson RT: Selective vulnerability of neural cells to viral infections. Brain 103:447, 1980. *A review of the varied mechanisms by which viruses can cause chronic degenerative and demyelinative diseases as well as malformations and tumors of the brain. The major emphasis is on experimental diseases in animals, but chronic human diseases are covered.*

Johnson RT: Viral Infections of the Nervous System. New York, Raven Press, 1982. *This monograph summarizes known slow infections as well as the possible role of viruses in multiple sclerosis, amyotrophic lateral sclerosis, Parkinson's disease, and recurrent meningitis and encephalitis.*

Masters C, Harris JO, Gajdusek C, Gibbs CJ Jr, Bernoulli C, Asher DM: Creutzfeldt-Jakob disease: Patterns of worldwide occurrence and the significance of familial and sporadic clustering. Ann Neurol 5:177, 1978. *Recent collection of epidemiologic data on 1435 patients with Creutzfeldt-Jakob disease.*

Narayan O, Penney JB Jr, Johnson RT, Herndon RM, Weiner LP: Etiology of progressive multifocal leukoencephalopathy. Identification of papovavirus. N Engl J Med 289:1278, 1973. *This paper reports identification of papovaviruses in brains of 13 patients with progressive multifocal leukoencephalopathy. Rapid diag-*

nostic methods using fluorescent antibody staining and electron microscopic agglutination techniques are employed.

Padgett BL, Walker DL: New human papovaviruses. Prog Med Virol 22:1, 1976. *Virologic studies of JC and BK viruses are comprehensively reviewed, including discussion of the role of JC virus in progressive multifocal leukoencephalopathy.*

Roos R, Gajdusek DC, Gibbs CJ Jr: The clinical characteristics of transmissible Creutzfeldt-Jakob disease. Brain 96:1, 1973. *A summary of the clinical signs and symptoms of patients with Creutzfeldt-Jakob disease. The studies focus on transmissible cases and define the syndrome on this basis.*

Wolinsky JS: Progressive rubella panencephalitis. *In* Vinken PJ, Bruyn GW (eds.): Handbook of Clinical Neurology. Amsterdam, North-Holland Publishing Company, 1978, pp 331-341. *This chapter consolidates the limited data on the cases of progressive rubella panencephalitis. The clinical and pathologic data are particularly well covered.*

Section Nine NEUROLOGIC DISORDERS ASSOCIATED WITH ALTERED IMMUNITY OR UNEXPLAINED HOST-PARASITE ALTERATIONS

505. ACUTE TRANSVERSE MYELITIS

H. Richard Tyler

CLINICAL SYNDROME. "Transverse myelitis" refers to a clinical syndrome most often affecting the mid to upper thoracic level of the cord. There is a relatively rapid onset of severe paraparesis or paraplegia usually affecting all motor and sensory pathways distal to the lesion. It has a sharp segmental distribution, with the "clinical" lesion extending over one to three spinal segments. It occurs as a sporadic illness at any age without any seasonal incidence. About half of the patients give a history of a preceding infection or mild trauma. About one third run a low grade fever. Rarely "warning" phenomena consisting of transient paresthesias in the lower extremities precede the major syndrome by one to four weeks.

The most common presentation is initiated by radicular or localized back pain, usually affecting the thoracic region. Pain is quickly followed by bilateral paresthesia of the feet and toes and a rapidly rising sensory loss and weakness until a total paraplegia develops. Urinary and fecal incontinence and retention are prominent. Less commonly, progressive weakness of the lower extremities or retention of urine may precede other symptoms. The syndrome usually takes hours to a few days to develop. Some progression may continue in episodic or stepwise fashion for up to two weeks.

Rarely an acute spinal lesion can develop apoplectically, producing an initial flaccid state (spinal shock), which slowly evolves into a spastic paraplegia. Some patients will remain flaccid, suggesting that funicular necrosis has affected the spinal cord, not only involving the segmental level but producing descending damage in the gray matter, especially of the anterior horns.

Following this acute or subacute onset most patients enter a stable phase with no change taking place for a number of days to a few weeks. About half of the patients then undergo partial improvement, although at least some residuum, usually spastic paraparesis, is found in most. Occasionally a residual partial Brown-Séquard–like lesion with crossed sensory loss and ipsilateral motor weakness and spasticity is seen. About 50 per cent of the patients do not recover and are left with a severe spastic paraplegia. Those who recover usually have done so by three months.

"Partial" syndromes occur. One important group has an abrupt onset of symptoms and signs related to the anterior portion of the cord in the distribution of the anterior spinal artery, suggesting a vascular mechanism. In this group there can be relative preservation of the posterior column function.

In general, patients who have a rapid progression to a total paralysis and develop flaccidity below the level of the lesion have a more ominous prognosis than those who develop their syndrome subacutely over 5 to 12 days.

DIAGNOSIS. There may be enough swelling of the spinal cord in severe lesions to produce a spinal subarachnoid block acutely. Myelographically this appears as intramedullary swelling and can be difficult to distinguish from intramedullary tumor or hemorrhage. This development usually disappears in three to four weeks, but may be associated with a very high protein content and xanthochromia. The spinal fluid usually is acellular, but some cases contain up to 200 cells, usually lymphocytes. Rarely when necrosis affects the cord, a polymorphonuclear excess can be seen. Less commonly the destruction is so severe that it elicits an associated meningeal inflammation with secondary fibrosis and obliteration of the subarachnoid space. This can cause the appearance of a block by myelogram and abnormal spinal fluid and dynamics two to three months after the acute lesion. Patients who develop either an acute or delayed block may require surgical exploration to guarantee that no treatable situation is present.

PATHOLOGY. There is a destruction of all tissues of the spinal cord at the level involved. There is subsequent liquefaction of the tissue, invasion with macrophages, and scarring of the meninges to the residual tissue. Inflammatory cells, including polymorphonuclear leukocytes, and plasma cells can be seen in some of the more acute cases.

ETIOLOGY. Because of the "acute" nature of the syndrome, the suggestions as to its nature have included vascular, demyelinating, and infectious causes. In individual cases each has something to suggest its role. In most instances no cause is found and the disorder must be regarded as a "syndrome" (rather than a "disease") and capable of being produced by multiple causes. Why the thoracic cord is so selectively susceptible is unknown, but the vascular supply to the cord is probably most vulnerable in this area.

Some patients develop an acute transverse myelitis in association with segmental viral infections such as herpes zoster. With such infections the spinal cord shows a massive infiltration of inflammatory and plasma cells and an arteritis showing active inflammatory changes. Extensive tissue destruction produces a poor prognosis. In milder forms of the illness, inflammatory changes without arterial damage affect the tissue, and prognosis is better.

Because spinal cord lesions are common in multiple sclerosis, some authorities suggest that acute transverse myelitis may often represent the initial attack or a severe attack of demyelinating disease. Although the disorder is sometimes recurrent, less than 10 per cent of patients with transverse myelitis later develop signs of disseminated demyelinating disease. It should be noted that spinal lesions of multiple sclerosis rarely cause severe destructive lesions of both gray and white matter and can usually be suspected by their more gradual onset, asymmetry, and partial nature.

A vascular cause has been suggested largely because damage to a critical blood vessel supplying the spinal cord can result in the segmental destruction of the cord. In the lower thoracic area there is usually one larger radicular artery (artery of Adamkiewicz), surgical damage to which in renal, aortic, or thoracic operations can result in a syndrome of "transverse myelitis." There is an appreciable incidence of transverse myelitis in patients with systemic lupus erythematosus, which is ascribed to infarctions secondary to vascular compromise. However, in most autopsied cases of transverse myelitis, no vascular lesion has been demonstrated. Sometimes this may be a result of the failure to dissect the blood supply from its origin at the aorta to the spinal cord. Nevertheless the spinal lesion is consistent with infarction and liquefaction necrosis.

DIFFERENTIAL DIAGNOSIS. The differential diagnosis of spinal disorders that can mimic acute transverse myelitis is based on features of the illness which indicate the location, mode of progression, completeness of the transverse lesion, its symmetry or lack thereof, and any evidence of disseminated or associated lesions. Laboratory tests on spinal fluid and radiologic studies are crucial.

The most important diagnosis to consider with rapid progression of spinal symptoms is an epidural space infection of the spinal cord (acute epidural abscess) (see Ch. 496). This condition produces a surgical emergency that, if not appropriately treated, can lead to irreversible damage. Characteristically, epidural abscess occurs in a febrile patient with a warning of severe local back or radicular pain. An obvious source of infection exists in perhaps 50 per cent of cases. The onset is followed rapidly by symptoms of spinal cord dysfunction, including bladder incontinence and paraparesis. X-rays may show bone changes of osteomyelitis in as many as 20 per cent. The peripheral white count is usually elevated with a shift to the left. The sedimentation rate is almost always elevated. Spinal fluid examination usually shows an increased number of polymorphonuclear cells and a complete block. Since many of these features accompany "transverse myelitis," often myelograms and occasionally exploratory surgery must be carried out to arrive at proper diagnosis.

Spinal cord compression from other causes such as metastatic or primary tumor usually develops at a pace slower than transverse myelitis, with symptoms present over a longer period of time. Such compressions are more likely to present with asymmetrical findings and a partial Brown-Séquard syndrome. Occasionally, tumors may compress the cord rapidly over a period of hours, making differential diagnosis more difficult. However, the presence of known tumor, radiographic vertebral lesions, and findings by myelography usually resolve the problem.

Demyelinating disease, i.e., multiple sclerosis and its variants, frequently produces myelopathic findings. When these develop, they usually are painless, generally spare sensory pathways, tend to come on over two to six days rather than over hours, and rarely completely affect the cord. A rare form of demyelinating disease called Devic's disease combines severe spinal lesions with severe optic nerve lesions. This particular combination of findings has an ominous prognosis and frequently causes permanent cord dysfunction.

A partial, predominantly motor spastic paraparesis sometimes follows a known viral infection, especially measles (rubeola) or chickenpox (varicella), less often rubella and variola. The spinal signs are usually part of a more widespread perivenous demyelinating reaction.

In large poliomyelitis epidemics occasional patients present with signs of transverse myelitis accompanying other evidence of active polio infection. These patients are often left with the same severe spinal lesions, including sensory loss, that one sees with transverse myelitis. Transverse myelitis must be differentiated from the myelopathy caused by granulomatous infectious processes such as tuberculosis, coccidioidomycosis, and nocardiosis. Intramedullary abscess with actinomycosis, nocardiosis, aspergillosis, and cryptococcosis can damage the cord and produce myelitic phenomena.

Vascular diseases such as syphilis and dissecting aneurysm of the aorta have also been associated with acute spinal cord damage by affecting segmental arteries going to the spinal cord.

In patients with cancer and chronic infections such as tuberculosis, focal damage to the cord, especially in its dorsal aspect, has been described as causing myelopathy.

Subacute necrotic myelopathy of Foix and Alajouanine is characterized by a month-long progressive stepwise course. It is caused by successive infarctions associated with spinal arteriovenous malformations.

A rapidly progressing myelopathy over hours in a previously healthy person should always raise the question of spontaneous epidural or subdural bleeding. This usually occurs without known cause. In a patient taking coumarin anticoagulants or with a blood dyscrasia, one is necessarily more aware of this potential complication. The diagnosis may be made by computed tomographic body scan, which can demonstrate the mass of blood, or by exploration. Decompression of the cord is usually indicated.

Radiation myelopathy is discussed in Ch. 562.

TREATMENT. Treatment of acute transverse myelitis is supportive. The initial concern is to rule out treatable disease. Once this is done, the major concern is to prevent complications. Steroids are contraindicated because they have no beneficial effect and increase complications.

To prevent skin breakdown patients should be turned frequently, and every effort made to protect pressure points. Mattresses that distribute pressure over wide areas are preferable.

Most patients have urinary retention. A regular program of intermittent catheterizations by experienced personnel is preferable to an indwelling catheter. Fluid intake should be kept high and urinary infections treated promptly. There may be an ileus acutely. Prevention of fecal impaction is desirable. Patients with lesions that ascend into the cervical area may require mechanical ventilation.

Bed rest provides no advantages, and patients should be mobilized after the first few days if possible. Complicating venous thrombosis of the legs is common and best avoided by mobilization and passive movement.

Although some physicians give ACTH or steroids, no satisfactory evidence supports their routine use.

Berman M, Feldman S, Alter M, Zilbar N, Kehang E: Acute transverse myelitis: Incidence and etiological considerations. Neurology 31:966, 1981. *A retrospective review of the syndrome in a well controlled population with probably the best statistics available.*

Plum F, Olson ME: Myelitis and myelopathy. *In* Baker AB, Baker CH (eds.): Clinical Neurology, Vol 3. Hagerstown, Md., Harper & Row, 1978. *A complete review of the entities that can cause spinal cord damage, e.g., infection, toxins, radiation, as well as idiopathic disorders. Very complete reference list.*

Ropper AH, Poskanzer DC: The prognosis of acute and subacute transverse myelopathy based on early signs and symptoms. Ann Neurol 4:51, 1978. *An excellent review of the experience of a large general hospital with a good description of the clinical findings and follow-up of patients.*

506. CENTRAL NERVOUS SYSTEM COMPLICATIONS OF VIRAL INFECTIONS AND VACCINES

Jerry S. Wolinsky

Central nervous system (CNS) symptoms and signs arising in the course of systemic infections usually reflect direct CNS invasion by the inciting organism. Less frequently, systemic infections, especially viral infections, or the administration of certain vaccines give rise to CNS abnormalities that do not appear to depend on direct invasion of the brain but rather to reflect dysfunction as the result of presumed autoimmune or toxic mechanisms selectively. Several reasonably distinct patterns of involvement have been delineated. Two of these, *acute disseminated encephalomyelitis* and *acute hemorrhagic encephalomyelitis,* appear to be mediated by immune mechanisms and have a peripheral nervous system counterpart, *acute inflammatory polyneuropathy* or the *Guillain-Barré syndrome* (see Ch. 526). The remainder, *Reye's syndrome, acute toxic encephalopathy,* and *acute cerebellar ataxia of childhood,* are likely to be toxic in origin.

ACUTE DISSEMINATED ENCEPHALOMYELITIS (ADE)

DEFINITION. Acute disseminated encephalomyelitis (*parainfectious* or *postinfectious encephalomyelitis, acute demyelinating encephalitis, immune-mediated encephalomyelitis*) is an acute disease of the CNS that most commonly occurs in association with viral infections or as a complication of vaccination. Involvement of brain and spinal cord is usually widespread but may be limited to discrete areas such as the optic nerves, as in optic neuritis or papillitis, or to a single spinal cord level, as in acute transverse myelitis (see Ch. 506).

ETIOLOGY AND PATHOGENESIS. Predisposing factors to ADE include infection by such common agents as measles virus, herpes varicella-zoster virus, influenza virus, rubella virus, mumps virus, nonspecific upper respiratory infections, mycoplasmal pneumonia, and possibly Epstein-Barr virus. ADE also has been well documented to follow immunization for smallpox (classic *postvaccinal encephalomyelitis*), measles, and formerly rabies. Other vaccines are less well implicated in the genesis of ADE.

The neurologic complications usually occur six to ten days after the appearance of the exanthem or onset of other specific symptoms. However, ADE can occur prior to or concomitantly with systemic symptoms of infection. Characteristically, ADE begins ten days to three weeks after initiation of the vaccination regimen. Perhaps the most easily understood form of ADE is that which at one time followed vaccination against rabies with inactivated inoculum of fixed rabies virus propagated in animal brain. These early vaccines were undoubtedly contaminated with CNS proteins, including the antigens associated with myelin. Both complement-fixing antibody and specific lymphocyte blast transformation responses to crude and purified CNS antigens have been measured in blood of rabies vaccinees, and these responses were highest in those whose course of vaccination was complicated by ADE. The incidence of neuroparalytic accidents has been reported to be as high as 1:600 to 1:6000 persons vaccinated with such vaccines. Current rabies vaccines derived from virus grown in human diploid cells appear to be essentially free of neural complications (Ch. 503).

The analogy between ADE related to rabies vaccination and the animal model CNS autoimmune disease, *experimental allergic encephalomyelitis (EAE)*, is compelling. In EAE, crude brain homogenates, selected highly purified myelin components, or peptides containing the encephalogenic sequences of myelin basic protein (MBP) can, under proper conditions, induce an acute CNS perivascular inflammatory and demyelinative reaction that is histologically identical to ADE. In affected animals, clinical disease begins 10 to 14 days after sensitization and is associated with both humoral and cellular immune reponses directed against the inciting CNS antigen(s). Furthermore, EAE can be adoptively transferred to naive animals by T lymphocytes. This fact suggests that this cell type is of primary importance in the pathogenesis of the immune-mediated disorder.

The occurrence of ADE following viral infections is more difficult to understand. Encephalitis is relatively frequent following measles (1:1000 cases), but there is little evidence to implicate invasion of the CNS by measles virus as an obligate prerequisite and no compelling data available to support cross-reactivity between the antigens of measles virus and CNS proteins such as MBP. Nonetheless, very early in the course of measles ADE, specific blast transformation responses to MBP are apparent in children when the peripheral blood lymphocytes are tested in vitro and, as would be expected with any type of acute CNS demyelination, measurable quantities of MBP are released into the cerebrospinal fluid (CSF). These findings support the hypothesis that acute measles transiently alters the immune system, which in some persons results in a breakdown of tolerance to CNS antigens. This process appears to occur frequently, as reflected by a high incidence of abnormal appearing electroencephalograms (EEGs). Only occasionally is the process expressed symptomatically. Both EEG abnormalities and clinical ADE can occur after vaccination with live attenuated measles virus but at a markedly lower frequency, with ADE arising in about 1:1,000,000 persons vaccinated for measles.

INCIDENCE. Valid incidence figures for ADE are difficult to derive because clinical diagnosis is often uncertain and pathologic diagnosis the exception. Encephalitis complicates about 1:1000 cases of measles. ADE following induced vaccinia (vaccination for smallpox) is only of historical interest but occurred in the United States with a reported incidence of 2.9 per million primary vaccinations. Higher frequencies of occurrence have been reported in other countries. ADE following other childhood viral illnesses or vaccinations is distinctly uncommon. In adult cases, most examples of ADE have no identifiable antecedents.

PATHOLOGY. Neuropathologic changes consist of perivenular infiltration by lymphocytic and mononuclear cells and variable amounts of primary demyelination extending in centripetal manner from involved vessels of the white matter. The axons are relatively spared. This primary lesion can occur throughout the neuraxis but tends to be most prominent in the centrum semiovale of the cerebrum and in the pontine white matter. Attendant edema may impart a swollen appearance, but otherwise the brain appears grossly normal. The primary perivascular demyelination appears to be a potentially reversible lesion. Repair occurs through remyelination. In certain cases, large confluent lesions take on a superficial resemblance to the plaques of multiple sclerosis, differing primarily in that all lesions reflect a similar age of onset.

CLINICAL MANIFESTATIONS. The clinical disorder can resemble almost any of the acute encephalitides. In adults neurologic symptoms often first suggest the illness. With the childhood exanthemata, CNS symptoms usually begin about five days after the onset of the rash (range 0 to 24 days, with rare examples of ADE preceding the rash). The course of the preceding illness is in no way typical for patients who subsequently develop ADE. Fever or recrudescence of fever is nearly universal. Headache, with or without meningismus, and lethargy occur in from 20 to 80 per cent of cases. In about half of the cases there is one or more generalized seizure. Usually the onset of altered consciousness is abrupt, occurring within a few hours, but CNS symptoms sometimes evolve over several days. Stupor, delirium, or coma develops in severe cases. Multifocal motor and sensory deficits of varied severity are common and often asymmetrical.

The EEG is abnormal in appearance, with widespread slowing of background rhythms. The CSF in children almost invariably shows a modest mononuclear pleocytosis of 20 to 200 cells per cubic millimeter and occasionally higher. Adult CSF is sometimes acellular. The fluid contains a slight elevation of protein content, a normal glucose level, and a raised myelin basic protein level. After several days, computed tomographic scans may show scattered low density lesions in white matter, at least some of which enhance with contrast during the acute phases of the disease.

The duration of active CNS disease varies from days to weeks. The overall mortality is about 20 per cent. About 90 per cent of survivors recover completely or nearly completely, although severe residual deficits can occur. Even among the patients who recover, convalescence can be protracted for many months.

DIAGNOSIS. Diagnosis in ADE is by exclusion. First encephalitis, meningitis, or meningoencephalitis must be excluded as a direct effect of a virus or other infectious agent. In the setting of a recent exanthematous illness or vaccination, ADE is more readily implied. However, in pathologic series of clinically diagnosed ADE occurring in the course of mass vaccination programs, postmortem examination proved the majority of patients to have had other illnesses, including potentially treatable CNS infections. Differentiation of an initial severe episode of multiple sclerosis can be challenging, but subsequent recurrences eventually make the proper diagnosis clear.

TREATMENT. Treatment consists of supportive care, including the use of anticonvulsants and, when necessary, intensive care monitoring. Neither corticosteroids nor other immunosuppressive drugs have any proved benefit.

ACUTE HEMORRHAGIC LEUKOENCEPHALITIS

Acute hemorrhagic leukoencephalitis is a fulminant and fatal syndrome believed to have an immunopathogenesis similar to that of ADE. Typically, the illness arises either spontaneously or following an uneventful upper respiratory illness. Sudden headache precedes the neurologic symptoms, which include seizures and rapid progression from lethargy to coma in a matter of a few hours to several days. Major focal neurologic abnormalities are common and may suggest lateralized cerebral involvement. Systemic signs and symptoms include fever and marked peripheral leukocytosis. The accompanying CSF pleocytosis usually shows a preponderance of polymorphonuclear cells and sometimes evidence of minor degrees of hemorrhage into the subarachnoid space. More than 80 per cent of all recognized cases of acute hemorrhagic leukoencephalitis are fatal, although these findings may be biased by selective reports of postmortem studies. The brain is usually swollen, and examination shows bilateral but asymmetric abnormalities with petechial hemorrhages scattered throughout the white matter. Microscopic lesions consist of small ball and ball-ring hemorrhages with perivascular polymorphonuclear cell infiltrates and fibrin deposition in and about involved vessels, features reminiscent of hyperimmune forms of EAE. The clinical differential diagnosis includes ADE and acute viral encephalitis, especially herpes simplex encephalitis (see Ch. 500). Computed tomography may be diagnostically helpful in selected cases. Therapy is supportive, and although corticosteroids are often used they have no proved benefit.

Fenichel GM: Neurological complications of immunization. Ann Neurol 12:119, 1982. *A critical review of neurologic complications of vaccination including those reported to follow pertussis vaccines.*

Johnson RT, Griffin DE, Hirsch RL, Wolinsky JS, Roedenbeck S, de Soriano IL, Vaisberg A: Measles encephalomyelitis—Clinical and immunological studies. N Engl J Med 310:137, 1984. *A multifaceted study of ADE complicating natural measles which emphasizes possible mechanisms of disease pathogenesis.*

507. REYE'S SYNDROME

Jerry S. Wolinsky

DEFINITION. Reye's syndrome is a well delineated biphasic disease in which one of several common viral illnesses is followed by an acute and sometimes fatal encephalopathy associated with fatty infiltration and dysfunction of the liver.

ETIOLOGY AND PATHOGENESIS. Reye's syndrome most commonly occurs following influenza A, influenza B, and herpes varicella-zoster virus infections. Many other common viral illnesses have been implicated, each at a much lower frequency. Little evidence links the precipitating viral infection directly to either the central nervous system or hepatic involvement. A toxic origin is proposed for both types of involvement. The hepatic dysfunction appears to be the primary error and the direct result of a mitochondrial disturbance that causes secondary metabolic derangements including hyperammonemia, lactic acidemia, and elevated levels of serum-free fatty acids. The latter derangements have been implicated in the pathogenesis of the brain swelling and increased intracranial pressure that dominate the clinical course of severe cases. What causes the mitochondrial impairment and whether aspirin plays a potentiating role in inducing the syndrome remain to be clarified.

INCIDENCE. Reye's syndrome occurs most commonly among suburban white children between 1 and 15 years of age but has been reported in adolescents and rarely in adults. However, inner-city black infants may be especially at risk for the disease. Prospectively derived incidence figures for susceptible age groups are as high as 6.2 per 100,000 children when the syndrome is defined rigorously by highly predictive criteria.

PATHOLOGY. The liver shows a noninflammatory, panlobular, hepatocellular accumulation of lipid droplets and both histochemical and ultrastructural evidence of inflammation. At postmortem examination, swelling of astrocytic foot processes and ultrastructural changes in mitochondria similar to those seen in hepatic mitochondria may be found in the greatly swollen brain.

CLINICAL MANIFESTATIONS AND COURSE. Reye's syndrome is a biphasic disorder. As symptoms of the initial viral illness begin to wane or clear, the dramatic features of Reye's syndrome begin, usually with intractable vomiting associated with lethargy or delirium. Early diagnosis is confirmed by the findings of nonicteric hepatic dysfunction, an elevated arterial

blood ammonia level, and serum transaminase levels that exceed three times normal levels. Hepatic enlargement is present in about one half of the cases. Children under one year of age often show hypoglycemia. Signs of central nervous system deterioration include the development of generalized seizures, deepening obtundation, and the emergence of signs of central herniation (see Ch. 472). The cerebrospinal fluid is under increased pressure but is acellular, with otherwise normal constituents.

DIAGNOSIS. Diagnosis rests on the clinical findings and appropriate biochemical abnormalities. Liver biopsy may be useful in atypical cases but usually is not necessary. Central nervous system infection or the presence of known toxins, particularly salicylate, must be actively excluded.

TREATMENT. Falling mortality rates in Reye's syndrome (now approximately 10 per cent) probably reflect both better recognition and reporting of the disease and improved early supportive treatment. Affected patients require intensive care monitoring until the course of the disease is well established. Hypoglycemia and electrolyte abnormalities must be corrected. Many authorities suggest hydration with solutions of high glucose content. Conservative measures to control hyperammonemia appear warranted.

ACUTE TOXIC ENCEPHALOPATHY OF CHILDREN

A syndrome distinguishable from Reye's syndrome only by the absence of hepatic involvement and a high incidence of acute convulsions can follow both banal viral infections and vaccination. A noninflammatory brain swelling accounts for the cerebral symptoms. The findings of cerebrospinal fluid examination are normal except for increased intracranial pressure. This syndrome sometimes arises de novo and sometimes is associated with common respiratory infections. It is the most common of the central nervous system complications of rubella and occurs in about 1:6000 cases. The pathogenesis is unknown. There is no evidence to directly implicate an abnormality of cellular immune mechanisms.

Lichtenstein PK, Heubi JE, Daugherty CC, Farrell MK, Sokol RJ, Rothbaum RJ, Suchy FJ, Balistreri WF: Grade I Reye's syndrome: A frequent cause of vomiting and liver dysfunction after varicella and upper-respiratory-tract infections. N Engl J Med 309:133, 1983. *A prospective study of the incidence and course of Reye's syndrome.*

508. NEUROLOGIC COMPLICATIONS IN THE IMMUNOLOGICALLY COMPROMISED HOST

Jerry S. Wolinsky

Modern treatment of several previously fatal conditions in many instances leads to an immunocompromised state that is associated with opportunistic infections of the central nervous system (CNS). Such treatments include organ transplantation for renal, bone marrow, and cardiac failure; chemotherapy and radiotherapy of carcinoma, leukemia, and lymphomas; and immunosuppressive treatment of autoimmune diseases. The epidemic emergence of the acquired immune deficiency syndrome (AIDS) also has been associated with a marked increase in the number of unusual CNS infections likely to be encountered in routine practice.

CENTRAL NERVOUS SYSTEM INFECTIONS IN TRANSPLANT RECIPIENTS. Renal transplantation is now commonplace, and bone marrow and cardiac transplantations are performed with increasing effectiveness. Hospital-acquired bacterial species predominate in early infections in transplant recipients. Immunosuppression, especially lethal irradiation used in preparation for marrow transplantation from nonidentical donors, almost predictably gives rise to reactivation of herpes viruses: first herpes simplex viruses types 1 and 2 (HSV), then herpes varicella-zoster virus (HVZ), and finally cytomegalovirus (CMV). The systemic manifestations of each can be overwhelming, but symptomatic CNS dissemination has so far been remarkably infrequent. However, encephalitis or meningitis can complicate either HSV or HVZ infections. Also, while electroencephalographic, computed tomographic, and brain scan findings evolve as anticipated in the intact host, the characteristic cerebrospinal fluid (CSF) pleocytosis is often absent, especially in patients with severe leukopenia. CNS involvement by CMV has been pathologically documented in transplant patients but has not been associated with a recognizable clinical syndrome. At present such involvement often appears to be asymptomatic. The availability of effective antiviral chemotherapy now makes it imperative to attempt early diagnosis in cases of suspected HSV or HVZ meningoencephalitis (see Ch. 500 and 501).

Transplant patients are at greatest risk of infection by opportunistic agents after the second month of the transplant. They remain at risk while they are on most immunosuppressive regimens, if they are azotemic, and when there are ongoing graft versus host or chronic rejection reactions. *Listeria monocytogenes, Cryptococcus neoformans,* and *Aspergillus fumigatus* account for the overwhelming majority of infections. *Toxoplasma gondii, Candida* species, *Nocardia asteroides,* the rhinocerebral phycomycoses, and *Coccidioides immitis* are less frequently encountered.

The acute or subacute development of fever in the transplant patient should suggest *Listeria* meningitis even in the absence of meningeal signs. The CSF has the characteristics of a purulent meningitis, although occasionally patients with *Listeria* infection have misleading mononuclear pleocytosis (see Ch. 271). Otherwise unexplained headache of acute to chronic duration, even in the absence of a febrile response or confusion, should suggest the possibility of cryptococcal meningitis. A mononuclear pleocytosis with or without a low glucose content are the characteristic CSF findings (see Ch. 370). India ink preparations can provide immediate confirmation of diagnosis and tests for cryptococcus antigen can be more helpful than direct culture of the organism from the CSF. Since both listerial and cryptococcal meningitis represent some of the most frequently encountered and more manageable infections that affect the immunocompromised host, careful attention must be given to symptoms that suggest infection of the CNS.

Aspergillis fumigatus infections of the CNS usually are manifested as acute fulminant disease with seizures, obtundation, and frequently apoplectic onset of focal neurologic deficits. The propensity of *Aspergillis* to invade and destroy blood vessels underlies the frequent stroke-like appearance of infected patients. Low density lesions with ill-defined, poorly contrast-enhancing borders may be seen on computed tomography, but diagnosis depends on brain biopsy in the absence of systemic disease. Current diagnostic and therapeutic approaches to this CNS infection are inadequate (see Ch. 373).

CENTRAL NERVOUS SYSTEM INFECTION IN PATIENTS WITH LYMPHOMA, LEUKEMIA, OR CHRONIC IMMUNOSUPPRESSIVE THERAPY. Splenectomy, often used in the staging of Hodgkin's disease, places patients at increased risk for conventional bacterial infections that may be complicated by meningitis. In community-acquired infections, *Hemophilus influenzae* and *Streptococcus pneumoniae* species predominate. Metastatic spread from various systemic sites by a wide spectrum of bacterial organisms is a continual threat for all immunosuppressed patients. The usual signs and symptoms of CNS infection can be obscured by the anti-inflammatory effect of therapy. The use of chronic immunosuppressive therapy for leukemia, lymphoma, or presumed autoimmune disorders can be complicated by *Listeria monocytogenesis* in a manner similar to that described for transplant patients. The emergence of listerial meningitis often follows an increase in the intensity of the immunosuppressive regimen.

Cryptococcal meningitis and *Aspergillus* meningoencephalitis are significant sources of morbidity for this group of patients. Their clinical appearances parallel those seen in organ-transplant patients. Segmental zoster, occasionally with dissemination, is a well recognized problem among these patients, and CNS toxoplasmosis is occasionally encountered. Of special interest is *progressive multifocal leukoencephalopthy (PML),* which may account for up to 10 per cent of all CNS infections in this patient group. Progressive deterioration in mental status and the evolution of focal neurologic deficits in the absence of meningismus or CSF abnormalities characterize the clinical symptomatology of PML. Serial computed tomographic scans are usually diagnostic, but the recent observation that some patients with CNS infections by HVZ can have a clinical course similar to that of PML must be considered because HVZ is potentially responsive to antiviral chemotherapy.

ACQUIRED IMMUNE DEFICIENCY SYNDROME (AIDS). Recently, a new syndrome has been described characterized by the presence of severe acquired cell-mediated immune deficiency, opportunistic infections, and in some cases the development of Kaposi's sarcoma or lymphoma in selected, otherwise healthy population groups. Neurologic symptoms occur in about 30 per cent of cases, and an opportunistic CNS infection may be the mode of initial presentation for 10 per cent of all AIDS patients.

CNS toxoplasmosis is particularly prominent, accounting for about one third of all CNS infections in AIDS patients. Single or multiple toxoplasma abscesses give rise to a clinical picture that usually consists of progressive focal deficits associated with abscess location. Less frequently, confusion and lethargy with or without seizures suggest more global CNS dysfunction. Computed tomography usually shows a typical abscess pattern of a low density lesion surrounded by a well defined capsule. The appearance of the capsule usually is enhanced by contrast administration. CSF findings are variable and often normal. Serologic evidence of toxoplasmosis is often present, but specific antibody and antibody isotype titer levels frequently fail to confirm active disease. Brain biopsy, directed by CT localization, is often indicated. The presence of an abscess in an AIDS patient by itself, however, may be an adequate basis for beginning extended therapy with sulfadiazine and pyrimethamine.

A slowly progressive global deterioration of cognitive function is probably the commonest neurologic complication of AIDS. This process sometimes culminates in marked dementia with urinary incontinence in the absence of significant motor signs. The severe form may affect 10 per cent of AIDS patients. Milder degrees of deterioration are even more common. Serial CT scans often disclose increasing cerebral atrophy, and most patients show CSF pleocytosis. Postmortem findings in 50 per cent of patients are consistent with viral infection. Inclusion cells typical of CMV can be identified in some instances, but a definitive cause has not been established.

Pulmonary and systemic infections with *Mycobacterium avium-intracellulare* are frequent among AIDS patients. Instances of CNS meningoencephalitis caused by this agent should be anticipated, but so far cases have been reported infrequently. Otherwise typical PML complicates the course of about 2 per cent of AIDS patients. Cryptococcal meningitis, *Candida albicans* abscesses, coccidioidomycosis meningoencephalitis, and other infections by opportunistic agents that can invade the CNS occur at low frequencies.

As with renal transplant recipients, AIDS patients develop primary CNS lymphomas at rates far exceeding those of the normal population. These usually are immunoblastic lymphomas with variable clinical manifestations. Serial computed tomographic scans may be necessary to define abnormalities related to these diffusely infiltrating tumors. Despite the associated severe cell-mediated immune deficiency, a Guillain-Barré–like syndrome also has been recognized to complicate the courses of several AIDS patients.

Hooper DS, Pruitt AA, Rubin RH: Central nervous system infection in the chronically immunosuppressed. Medicine 61:166, 1982. *Analysis of ten years' experience with opportunistic CNS infections at a major hospital and comprehensive literature review.*

Snider WD, Simpson DM, Nielsen S, Gold JWM, Metroka CE, Posner JB: Neurological complications of acquired immune deficiency syndrome: Analysis of fifty patients. Ann Neurol 14:403, 1983. *Analysis of the experience with neural complications of AIDS at a major referral center.*

Section Ten THE DEMYELINATING DISEASES

509. THE DEMYELINATING DISEASES

Donald H. Silberberg

The demyelinating diseases are disorders that affect myelin to a greater extent than other nervous system components. In this section disorders that primarily affect central nervous system (CNS) myelin are discussed; analogous diseases of the peripheral nervous system, the demyelinating peripheral neuropathies, are discussed in Ch. 524 through 536. A few disorders, such as the neurologic complications of vitamin B_{12} deficiency and some of the leukodystrophies, affect both central and peripheral myelin.

Since central myelin is an extension of the oligodendrocyte, which manufactures the myelin sheath, most demyelinating diseases include alterations in or disappearance of this glial cell. An oligodendrocyte process wraps around a segment of an axon in a concentric fashion to form myelin. One oligodendrocyte sends processes to segments of from several to 20 or 30 axons within an area of several millimeters surrounding the oligodendrocyte. Each segment of axon myelinated by one oligodendrocyte process is 1 mm or less in length. The most active synthesis of myelin starts in utero and continues for the first two years of life; however, synthesis continues as part of brain and spinal cord growth until the adult CNS weight is achieved.

Each tightly compacted layer of mature myelin is a bimolecular lipid leaflet between parallel layers of hydrated protein, which is in close apposition to the polar groups of the lipid molecules. The lipids, which constitute about 75 per cent of the dry weight of myelin, include cerebroside, phospholipids, and cholesterol. Proteins include the distinctive molecule, myelin basic protein (the antigen capable of eliciting experimental allergic encephalomyelitis in experimental animals), proteolipid proteins, and many others detectable by electrophoretic separation but not yet well characterized. Turnover of the components of mature myelin continues at a slower rate than the rate of exchange which characterizes myelin during development. The relative contribution of the oligodendrocyte, the axon, or perhaps even nearby astrocytes to the maintenance of mature myelin is not known. What is clear is that both developing and mature myelin are readily susceptible to injury by many disease mechanisms. Myelin is commonly injured as part of many disease processes which ultimately damage neurons and other cells; the focus of this section is on those disorders which primarily damage or result in the failure of the normal development of myelin.

CLASSIFICATION. Definitive classification awaits an understanding of the causes of these disorders. Failing that, a mixed temporal-etiologic-descriptive classification must serve as the scaffold. A useful distinction is to separate what seem to be acquired disorders from those which are errors in development (Table 509–1). Multiple sclerosis will be discussed first, since it is by far the most common of these problems.

TABLE 509–1. DISORDERS SELECTIVELY AFFECTING MYELIN

I. Demyelinating diseases (acquired destruction of preformed myelin)
- A. Multiple sclerosis
  - 1. Uniphasic events presumably related to multiple sclerosis
    - a. Optic neuritis
    - b. Acute transverse myelopathy
- B. Parainfectious disorders
  - 1. Acute disseminated encephalomyelitis
  - 2. Acute hemorrhagic leukoencephalopathy
- C. Viral infections
  - 1. Progressive multifocal leukoencephalopathy
  - 2. Subacute sclerosing panencephalitis
- D. Nutritional disorders
  - 1. Combined systems disease (B_{12} deficiency)
  - 2. Demyelination of the corpus callosum (Marchiafava-Bignami)
  - 3. Central pontine myelinolysis
- E. Anoxic-ischemic sequelae
  - 1. Delayed postanoxic cerebral demyelination
  - 2. Progressive subcortical ischemic encephalopathy

II. Dysmyelinating diseases (developmental failure to form or maintain myelin)
- A. The leukodystrophies
  - 1. Metachromatic leukodystrophy
  - 2. Sudanophilic (Pelizaeus-Merzbacher disease)
  - 3. Globoid cell (Krabbe's disease)
  - 4. Adrenoleukodystrophy (Schilder's disease)
  - 5. Others (e.g., Alexander's, Canavan's, Seitelberger's disease)
- B. Aminoacidurias (e.g., phenylketonuria)
- C. Neonatal hypothyroidism

MULTIPLE SCLEROSIS

DEFINITION. Multiple sclerosis (MS) is a disorder of unknown etiology which is defined both by its clinical characteristics and by the typical scattered areas of brain, optic nerve, and spinal cord demyelination which the disease produces. Clinical diagnosis requires evidence on neurologic examination of two or more CNS white matter lesions, preferably with at least a month's interval between symptoms, in a patient of the appropriate age, in whom evidence is lacking of any other explanation for the signs and symptoms. MS usually produces its first clinical symptoms between ages 15 and 50 years. Occasional cases occur beyond these extremes, but the average age of onset is 33. Most patients recover clinically to some extent from individual bouts of demyelination, producing the classic remitting and exacerbating course, particularly early in the disease. Except for autopsy findings, presently available laboratory data may support the clinical diagnosis but cannot be used to define MS.

ETIOLOGY. Despite recognition and description of MS for over 150 years, its cause remains unknown. The tissue response has features of an immunopathologic process, with perivenular mononuclear cell infiltration and absence of any overt histopathologic evidence of an infection. Two other lines of evidence point to either an immunologic cause or immunologic participation in the MS process: (1) the frequent elevation of cerebrospinal fluid (CSF) gamma globulin, apparently synthesized by the plasma cells in areas of demyelination, and (2) changes in the proportion of lymphocyte subclasses and reactivity in the peripheral blood and CSF. These changes are, however, nonspecific and may be the consequence of demyelination induced by some other disease mechanism, rather than the cause of the demyelination.

Epidemiologic studies suggest an infectious etiology. Perhaps the best evidence for this is the outbreak of MS which occurred in the Faroe Islands during the 20 years following the start of World War II. The Faroes were occupied by British troops during the war. No cases of MS had occurred prior to the occupation. The sudden appearance of MS starting several years after the arrival of the troops strongly suggests the presence of an infectious agent. In those geographic areas where MS is prevalent, it is more common farther from the equator, which suggests the presence of an environmental factor, presumably an infectious agent. Efforts continue to recover a virus from MS tissues: to date, no reported isolation has been duplicated by others. MS is among the diseases with a strong linkage to certain HLA haplotypes. The particular haplotype varies from one population group to another. In North America, haplotype DW-2, a D locus marker, is found in about 65 per cent of MS patients, as compared with 15 per cent of control subjects. Additional evidence for an immunogenetic component in the etiology of MS is the increase in frequency of MS among close relatives of patients with MS and the fact that MS is rare among Orientals, even after emigration to the United States. A possible synthesis is that MS is an unusual consequence of infection by a common virus, or any of several viruses, with subsequent immunologic alterations in genetically susceptible individuals.

INCIDENCE AND PREVALENCE. The prevalence of MS in the northern United States and Canada and in northern Europe is about 60 per 100,000 population (Table 509–2). In Denmark the chance of an individual developing MS in a lifetime is 1 in 500. The risk is somewhat higher for women. MS is almost unknown among Orientals and among African blacks. There is no evidence for changing incidence or prevalence, except where population patterns are undergoing changes as the result of immigration.

EPIDEMIOLOGY. The epidemiology of MS has fascinated observers since the 1930's, when neurologists in northern Europe reported to their Mediterranean colleagues that MS was more common in northern cities (Table 509–2). This gradient by latitude has also been shown in the United States. In Australia and New Zealand MS is more common in the southern latitudes. Migration from high incidence areas, such as England and northern Europe, to low incidence areas, such as South Africa or Israel, permitted the observation that the immigrant who moves during childhood acquires the lower incidence of the new country. For those moving after puberty, the chance of developing MS remains what it would have been in the country of origin and follows presumptive exposure to an environmental agent by about 15 years.

The regional population figures are punctuated by many reports of clusters of an unusual number of cases in a small area, such as particular cantons in Switzerland. Many of the population studies were done before the availability of HLA typings, so that some of the observed regional differences may prove to have a genetic basis. Multiple sclerosis occurs in both members of about 50 per cent of monozygous twin pairs when the disease has been identified in one. This supports the concept that genetic susceptibility may increase the chances of developing MS, but is not sufficient to cause it and may not be required for its development.

TABLE 509–2. THE PREVALENCE OF MULTIPLE SCLEROSIS*

Area	Latitude	Prevalence per 100,000
Iceland	65° N	72
Shetland Islands	61° N	129
Oslo, Norway	60° N	80
Göteborg, Sweden	58° N	120
Carlisle, England	55° N	82
Hamburg, Germany	54° N	73
Winnipeg, Manitoba	50° N	40
Bas-Rhin, France	49° N	41
Rochester, Minnesota	44° N	64
Marseilles, France	49° N	21
Sappuro, Japan	43° N	2
Boston, Massachusetts	42° N	41
Denver, Colorado	40° N	38
San Francisco, California	38° N	30
Seoul, Korea	38° N	2
Israel	31° N	15
New Orleans, Louisiana	30° N	6
Bombay, India	18° N	2
Cairns, Australia	17° S	7
South Australia	30° S	38

*Modified from Alter M, Loewenson R, Harshe M: J Chron Dis 26:755, 1973.

PATHOLOGY. The lesions of MS consist of scattered areas of dissolution of CNS myelin, within which the axons remain intact. The border between histologically normal myelin and myelin dissolution is often sharp, or may shade from normal to thinning of myelin before bare axons occur. Some areas may show only partial myelin destruction. Lesions range in size from 1 mm to several centimeters in diameter, and occur throughout the brain, optic nerves (which are central tracts of white matter), and spinal cord. Although plaques may occur anywhere within CNS myelin, there are predilections for involvement of the optic nerves, periventricular regions within the cerebrum, and cervical spinal cord. Most if not all plaques occur near blood vessels.

Oligodendrocytes disappear from within plaques. Astrocytes proliferate and fill much of the volume vacated by myelin and oligodendroglia, forming the scar that lent the term "sclerosis" to multiple sclerosis. This produces an area that is firm to palpation on cut sections, and plaques can be seen as grayish depressed areas in fresh autopsy sections. One always finds many more plaques at autopsy than could have been suspected on the basis of the clinical history and examination. Similarly, the sensitivity and resolution provided by nuclear magnetic resonance (NMR) imaging often reveal clinically unsuspected plaques. Occasionally, typical plaques of MS are found in individuals who gave no history of neurologic abnormalities (benign MS). The acute lesion of MS may produce considerable edema, visible as cord swelling on myelography or optic nerve enlargement on computed tomography (CT scan). Electron microscope examination of plaques shows evidence of attempts at remyelination. However, this is not nearly so complete as to explain the remissions of neurologic dysfunction that characterize MS and remain unexplained.

Perivascular and mononuclear cells collect within and around plaques. Macrophages which engulf myelin breakdown products are present. Plasma cells appear to synthesize much of the excess of gamma globulin which is found in and around plaques and in CSF. Plasma cells occur throughout affected tissue, and persist in large numbers throughout a patient's lifetime, correlating with the observation that once CSF gamma globulin elevation appears, it persists. It is not known whether plasma cells and other mononuclear cells precede, accompany, or follow myelin and oligodendrocyte destruction.

LABORATORY ABNORMALITIES. *Cerebrospinal Fluid.* CSF gamma globulin elevation occurs in about 75 per cent of MS patients, more commonly after the first year following the appearance of symptoms. Normal CSF gamma globulin is less than 13 per cent of total CSF protein by most testing methods. The gamma globulin is mostly IgG, but often contains IgA and IgM as well. Separate discrete "oligoclonal" bands are seen in the gamma region on agarose or polyacrylamide gel electrophoresis in about 90 per cent of patients, including some with normal total IgG levels. These abnormalities are helpful when other causes of the phenomenon are excluded; these include CNS syphilis, subacute sclerosing panencephalitis, chronic meningitis, and any disease associated with a peripheral blood paraproteinemia. Other CSF abnormalities in MS can include elevation in total protein, usually to no more than 100 mg per deciliter, and an increase in the number of mononuclear white cells, usually to 5 to 15 per cubic millimeter, rarely to more than 50 per cubic millimeter. Myelin destruction releases myelin basic protein (MBP) into the CSF, which can be detected by radioimmunoassay. The amount present correlates with disease activity and lesion size and location; none is detectable normally, or during quiescent periods in MS patients. MBP levels rise in association with acute attacks or rapid progression. This serves as a valuable index of disease activity, but is not specific to MS. Myelin destruction from any other cause, such as acute infarction, causes a similar elevation of MBP.

Alterations in the ratio of subclasses of peripheral blood and of CSF lymphocytes occur at the time of acute exacerbations. These changes, which may indicate abnormalities of immunoregulation, are of interest to those investigating the pathogenesis of MS; at present they do not contribute to differential diagnosis.

Neurophysiologic Function Studies. The presence of myelin enhances the propagation of the nerve impulse along the axon. Loss of myelin, from any cause, slows conduction velocity. This alteration in conduction velocity can be measured by timing the appearance of an evoked potential (visual, auditory, or somatosensory) after an appropriate stimulus. Measurement of the latency of the visual evoked response (VER) is used most widely. The patient's visual system is stimulated by viewing a changing checkerboard pattern or flash stimulus with one eye at a time, and the evoked response is recorded with electroencephalogram scalp leads over the occipital cortex. The normal latency from stimulus to evoked response in most laboratories is less than 102 to 105 milliseconds. A prolonged latency indicates an abnormality in the visual system, most commonly within the optic nerve in patients with MS. An abnormality of the visual, auditory, or somatosensory evoked response is used to detect dysfunction (prolonged conduction velocity) either as an objective measurement of what has already been detected clinically or for detection of a presumed subclinical abnormality. The abnormalities detected are not specific for MS (see Role of Laboratory Aids, below).

CT and NMR Scans. Hypodense areas seen with the CT scan reflect the presence of lesion in various stages, ranging from inflammation with edema to various degrees of demyelination. Edema, which may resemble a mass lesion, often occurs acutely. During this stage, leakage of intravenously injected contrast material into the lesion area reflects abnormal leakage of the blood-brain barrier. Atrophy is seen in those instances of severe demyelination.

NMR imaging provides an even more sensitive method for detecting hypodense areas of demyelination and is becoming an important supportive aid in diagnosis.

CLINICAL MANIFESTATIONS. *Onset.* The random distribution of MS lesions leads to a great variety of initial symptoms and signs, alone or in combination. Further, it must be kept in mind that lesions occur in clinically silent areas of CNS white matter so that the first lesion that announces itself clinically may not be the first that has occurred in an individual. Common initial problems include weakness of one or more extremities, unilateral visual loss (optic neuritis), incoordination, and paresthesias (Table 509–3). Urinary frequency, incontinence, hesitancy, or retention; vertigo; hearing loss; facial, extremity, or truncal pain; dysarthria; and changes in intellectual function occur less commonly. Weakness most often affects the lower extremities and may produce a range of dysfunction from slight fatigability to paraparesis. The arm and hand may be involved alone or with the legs. Patients who develop paraparesis often develop urinary urgency and constipation. Incoordination as the result of cerebellar lesions, or loss of position sense, may occur independently of weakness and often leads to gait impairment or to tremor-like, clumsy movements of the arms and hands. Paresthesias range from the spontaneous perception of vague pins-and-needles discomfort, or girdle-like pressures, to the pain of classic trigeminal neuralgia. Loss of perception of vibration and position at the ankle and toes is common; loss of pain and touch perception is less frequent. Impairment of two-point discrimination over the palmar surface of the fingertips often accompanies cervical cord lesions.

TABLE 509–3. FIRST SYMPTOMS OF MULTIPLE SCLEROSIS IN 937 PATIENTS*

Symptom	Per Cent†
Weakness	48
Paresthesias	31
Visual loss	25
Incoordination	15
Vertigo	6
Sphincter impairment	6

*Combined series of Carter et al., 1950; Poser, 1972; and McAlpine et al., 1972.
†Many patients experience more than one symptom at onset.

Visual loss varies in degree from slight blurring with a small central scotoma, slight decrease in acuity, and a slight impairment of color perception, to no light perception. The patient often reports pain on eye movement acutely. Other visual symptoms include blurring secondary to nystagmus on primary gaze with continuing movement of the visual axis, or explicit perception of nystagmus as spontaneous movement of objects (oscillopsia). Diplopia often occurs as the result of involvement of the pontine white matter. Horizontal nystagmus of the abducting eye on lateral gaze with paresis of the adducting eye, termed *internuclear ophthalmoplegia,* is common. It is often unilateral at first, and is due to lesions involving the median longitudinal fasciculus in the pons. In rare instances, extensive midline lesions lead to alterations of consciousness.

The speed of onset of symptoms varies from minutes to days, and in patients with a chronic progressive course symptoms may appear to increase gradually over many months. The rate of recovery (remission) varies enormously, but usually occurs over the course of two to eight weeks following an acute bout.

Clinical Course. At least 70 per cent of patients experience some improvement in the days to months following their initial bout. Such recovery ranges from slight to virtual disappearance of the dysfunction which heralded the existence of a problem. Whether or not a particular patient will improve, and to what extent, is as unpredictable as whether or not more lesions will occur and when. Overall, 70 per cent or more will report typical exacerbations and remissions early in their course. However, in many patients as time goes by, the recovery from individual bouts decreases, disability results from accumulated failures to improve, and the course becomes chronically progressive.

About 30 per cent of patients develop successive disabilities without remission, often with long periods of clinical stability between periods of deterioration. This course occurs more commonly in patients experiencing their first neurologic manifestations after age 45. As a result, older onset patients seem to compress the course of events, and often develop the same degree of dysfunction within a few years that takes decades to occur in a younger onset patient.

Most patients experience additional difficulties at some time after their initial symptoms; subsequent acute bouts or chronic progression may produce signs and symptoms in any combination. Several generalizations are of interest, but help little when counseling the individual patient. Ten years after onset about 50 per cent of patients are still able to carry out their household and/or employment responsibilities. Twenty years after onset about 25 per cent have these capacities. However, a fortunate few patients never develop significant disabilities, whereas others are bedridden within months after onset. One of the major psychologic burdens which patients with MS must bear is the total uncertainty about their future, and most neurologists find it useful to emphasize the hopeful possibilities, allowing the patient's course to reveal its own manner of progression.

The average interval from clinical onset to death is 35 years. If premature death occurs, it is usually due to bacterial infection resulting from urinary retention, decubiti, or inability to handle pulmonary secretions. More rarely, primary respiratory failure from lower medullary lesions spells the terminal event.

FACTORS POSSIBLY AFFECTING THE CLINICAL COURSE. Elevation of body temperature by as little as 0.5° C will noticeably reduce neurologic function in some patients, particularly if the patient has experienced recent disease activity. Reduction in visual acuity, incoordination or weakness, and sensory or bladder dysfunction can be affected. This is the result of slowed axonal conduction induced by heating, and the alterations disappear within hours of regaining normal body temperature. For this reason, many patients' conditions worsen with the fevers of an intercurrent illness (a pseudobout). In addition, some patients seem to experience true exacerbations concomitantly with an intercurrent infection. Patients should be instructed to rest and respond to respiratory infections with more care than they might otherwise and to use aspirin to reduce fever.

There is no evidence that pregnancy makes exacerbations or progression of MS more likely. Decisions regarding childbearing should be made on the basis of the patient's overall situation, rather than on the basis of this concern alone.

DIAGNOSIS. Multiple sclerosis remains as a clinical challenge; despite the availability of increasingly complex laboratory aids, the diagnosis of clinically definite MS rests on evidence garnered from the history and physical examination alone. Physical signs on examination providing solid evidence for two or more lesions of central white matter occurring at least a month apart in a patient between age 10 and the early 50's, in the absence of any other possible etiology, are required. If the evidence for a second lesion is history alone, the diagnosis should be considered possible or probable, rather than clinically definite MS. The differential diagnosis includes cervical cord compression resulting from tumor or cervical spondylosis; cerebral, cerebellar, brainstem, and pituitary tumors; familial spinocerebellar degenerations; acute systemic lupus erythematosus (SLE); sarcoidosis; brainstem atherosclerotic cerebrovascular disease; vitamin B_{12} deficiency; chronic barbiturate or other intoxications; and psychogenic disturbances.

If all of the patient's signs can be attributed to a lesion in a single area of the nervous system, the working assumption must be that one is not dealing with MS. In patients with a persistent headache, seizures, persistent and progressive unifocal signs, or papilledema (without a central scotoma), the CT brain scan is the most sensitive screening procedure. In addition, the CT or NMR scan may show hypodense areas or mild generalized atrophy, consistent with MS. High resolution CT scan examination of the spinal canal may obviate the need for myelography to exclude cervical mass lesions.

Spinocerebellar degenerative diseases differ from MS by having associated abnormalities (such as the areflexia commonly seen with Friedreich's ataxia), by progressing slowly within a given neuroanatomic system, such as the cerebellum and its connections, and by having an abnormal family history. However, MS occurs more commonly in first degree relatives of patients with MS, so that family history alone is not sufficient to make the distinction. Neurologic presentation of SLE in young women can be distinguished by appropriate immunologic testing. The neurologic manifestations of B_{12} deficiency may precede the peripheral red blood cell abnormalities by several years; the deficiency is detected by the serum B_{12} level or Schilling test. The correct diagnosis of brainstem arterial disease in patients in their 50's can sometimes be difficult; absence of the CSF abnormalities associated with MS helps, as does the fact that all the abnormalities can be localized to a small anatomic area. The clinician's suspicion of chronic drug intoxication, often accompanied by nystagmus and ataxia, may be substantiated by appropriate blood levels, or other evidence of disturbed behavior.

The total absence of objective neurologic signs at any time, together with symptom patterns or apparent weakness or sensory loss that does not conform to known neuroanatomic systems, raises the suspicion of psychogenic illness. However, one must be wary, for many patients with urinary retention, urgency, or incontinence; ataxia; or vague sensory symptoms occurring in the early stages of MS have been misdiagnosed as psychoneurotic. Evoked response or CSF abnormalities will help exclude purely psychogenic disturbances, but must not be overinterpreted.

Role of Laboratory Aids. The rational use of laboratory abnormalities requires an awareness of their limitations. Elevation of the total CSF gamma globulin, or the appearance of an oligoclonal pattern within the gamma region on electrophoresis, is not specific for MS, although the non-MS causes can usually be readily excluded. However, these abnormalities fail to appear in 10 to 20 per cent of patients with clinically definite multiple sclerosis. Further, many patients who experience a single episode of neurologic abnormality, such as optic neuritis or transverse myelopathy, may exhibit CSF gamma globulin abnormalities, but do not develop a second clinically visible lesion after long follow-up. Thus it is not appropriate to make the diagnosis of MS with a first neurologic attack, even when one encounters CSF gamma globulin abnormalities.

Similarly, although evoked potential abnormalities serve to suggest the possibility of a lesion in that part of the CNS tested, the nonspecific nature of the electrophysiologic alterations makes it unwise to base a diagnosis on such data. A patient with paraparesis and prolonged latency of the VER may have MS, but could possibly have two tumors, pernicious anemia, systemic vasculitis, or a spinal cord tumor plus an uncorrected refractive error. Also, multiple lesions detected on CT or NMR scan may reflect another disease process. Despite these cautions, the discovery of CSF abnormalities commonly associated with MS, evoked potential evidence of a second lesion, or multiple lesions on CT or NMR scan helps greatly to focus on MS as a possible or probable diagnosis.

TREATMENT. Management of the patient with MS requires a combination of an understanding of the personal problems posed by an unpredictable disorder of unknown etiology, an awareness of the measures available to alleviate spasticity, urinary incontinence, and other dysfunctions, and a skeptical approach to "definitive" treatments which are proposed to alter the course of the illness. The fact that over 70 per cent of patients experience spontaneous improvement following an acute bout makes evaluation of proposed treatment difficult, time consuming, and expensive. Nevertheless, carefully conducted controlled trials are the only means for deciding whether or not an agent helps patients with MS. Testimonial-style reports should not be accepted as evidence until a controlled study has confirmed the findings. At present, no method for prevention of MS is known.

Dealing with patients affected by a chronic, sometimes disabling disease for which there is no specific treatment is frustrating to many physicians. Patients with MS often report that they must help alleviate their physician's depression by denying problems. Most patients respond well to an explanation of the disease, a discussion of those things which can be done, and assurance that vigorous research is underway to develop better treatment.

Acute bouts of neurologic dysfunction may be treated with short-term administration of corticosteroids. There is evidence that administration of ACTH for 10 to 14 days somewhat shortens exacerbation, although the ACTH (or other corticosteroid) does not alter the long-term course of MS. From 40 to 80 units of ACTH per day may be used; prednisone, 40 to 60 mg per day, or equivalent doses of other oral corticosteroids are often employed as alternatives. The period of treatment should not exceed three or four weeks, with appropriate precautions to avoid steroid complications. It must be emphasized that there is no evidence that corticosteroids (or any other agent) modify the MS pathogenic process. Beneficial effects are most probably due to antiedema and anti-inflammatory effects. Many responsible clinicians choose not to treat patients in this manner, believing that minimal evidence favors steroid use.

Therapeutic trials to evaluate various immunosuppressants, immunoenhancing agents, plasmapheresis, and other treatments are underway; none can be recommended at present.

Physical therapy plays an important role in several aspects of patient management, including developing alternative muscle strengths, preventing contractures, improving daily living, and providing supportive psychotherapy. A cool bath or swimming pool improves neurologic function transiently by lowering body temperature and improving axonal conduction. Occupational therapy is often a key to the patient's adjustment to MS.

Spasticity and flexor spasms can be alleviated with baclofen, or with diazepam, which inhibits central synaptic transmission. Individual responses vary sufficiently that one must start with very low doses and increase slowly if needed. Many patients depend on spasticity for support while walking, so that removal of this aid or induction of weakness or drowsiness as temporary side effects limits treatment. Occasionally, leg contractures occur despite physical therapy, and require orthopedic surgical relief for ease of handling the patient.

Bladder dysfunction is usually the result of incomplete emptying, accumulation of residual urine, and overflow frequency or incontinence and infection. Rational treatment requires careful urologic evaluation, often including urodynamic studies, in order to plan appropriate pharmacologic therapy. Uninhibited bladder contraction leading to urinary frequency or incontinence may be alleviated by controlling infection and restricting fluid intake prior to trips or several hours before sleep. Imipramine, oxybutynin chloride, or propantheline may help patients who cannot initiate urination, or cannot fully empty their bladder. Attempts to void at fixed intervals and the Credé maneuver often help. If catheterization becomes necessary, many women can learn self-catheterization in order to avoid the complications of an indwelling catheter. Long-term urinary bacterial suppressant therapy is helpful in minimizing infection in patients carrying residual urine. The possibility of an ascending urinary tract infection must be sought and treated appropriately in any patient with recurrent cystitis.

Constipation usually responds to stool softeners and laxatives. Many patients must be reassured that no harm arises from the lack of a daily bowel movement.

Painful paresthesias and dysesthesias may occur, and fortunately are usually transient. Carbamazepine, diazepam, or phenytoin will usually provide relief. Prevention of decubiti in the paraplegic or desensitized patient requires constant vigilance.

Specific psychiatric support is often needed to aid patients and their families. The incidence of marital breakup, changes in roles within the family, and financial problems is exceeded only by the frequency of frustration over the unpredictability of MS. The physician often must call on a range of associates, including social workers, community agency workers, and psychiatrists, in order to help these patients cope.

Brown FR, Beebe GW, Kurtzke JF, Loewenson RB, Silberberg DH, Tourtellotte WW: The design of clinical studies to assess therapeutic efficacy in multiple sclerosis. Neurology 29:1, 1979. *A thorough review of the many factors which must be taken into consideration in designing a study to determine whether or not a proposed treatment benefits patients with multiple sclerosis.*

Carter S, Sciarra D, Merritt HH: The course of multiple sclerosis as determined by autopsy proven cases. Res Publ Assoc Nerv Ment Dis 28:471, 1950. *A description of the clinical features of a well-characterized group of patients who came to autopsy.*

Cohen SR, Herndon RM, McKhann GM: Radioimmunoassay of myelin basic protein in spinal fluid: An index of active demyelination. N Engl J Med 295:1455, 1976. *This paper presents the first large series of patients in whom measurement of myelin basic protein in CSF was correlated with disease activity.*

Compston DA, Batchelor JR, Earl CJ, McDonald WI: Factors influencing the risk of multiple sclerosis developing in patients with optic neuritis. Brain 101:495, 1978. *An excellent study of the correlation between HLA type in patients with optic neuritis and subsequent development of multiple sclerosis.*

Hallpike JF, Adams CWM, Tourtellotte WW (eds.): Multiple Sclerosis. Pathology, Diagnosis, and Management. Baltimore, Williams & Wilkins, 1983. *A good compilation of current information and concepts.*

Kurtzke JF, Hyllested K: Multiple sclerosis in the Faroe Islands: 1. Clinical and epidemiological features. Ann Neurol 5:6, 1979. *A lucid description of the remarkable, seemingly limited epidemic of multiple sclerosis in the Faroe Islands.*

McAlpine D, Lumsden CE, Acheson ED: Multiple Sclerosis. A Reappraisal. 2nd ed. Edinburgh, Churchill Livingstone, 1972. *The major currently available monograph on multiple sclerosis. Excellent clinical and epidemiologic descriptions.*

McDonald WI, Halliday AM: Diagnosis and classification of multiple sclerosis. Br Med Bull 33:4, 1977. *An up-to-date discussion of the problems of correct diagnosis and classification of multiple sclerosis.*

Poser C, Presthus J, Horstal O: Clinical characteristics of autopsy-proved multiple sclerosis. Neurology 16:791, 1966. *A valuable analysis of the presentation and signs and symptoms which developed among a large series of patients in whom MS was proved by autopsy.*

Poser S, Raun E, Wikstrom J, Poser W: Pregnancy, oral contraceptives, and multiple sclerosis. Acta Neurol Scand 59:108, 1979. *The largest study of the possible effect of pregnancy or oral contraceptives on the course of MS; this study shows no relationship.*

Reinherz EL, Weiner HL, Hauser SL, Cohen JA, Distaso JA, Schlossman SF: Loss of suppressor T cells in active multiple sclerosis. N Engl J Med 303:125, 1980. *The first report of the use of monoclonal antibody typing of human lymphocytes in multiple sclerosis. The references include previous analyses of lymphocyte abnormalities in MS.*

Williams A, Eldridge R, McFarland H, Houff S, Krebs H, McFarlin D: Multiple sclerosis in twins. Neurology 30:1139, 1980.

MULTIPLE SCLEROSIS VARIANTS

Neuromyelitis Optica (Devic's Disease)

Neuromyelitis optica describes a syndrome characterized by the occurrence of partial or complete transverse myelopathy and optic neuritis. Loss of vision and paraplegia may occur in either disorder, and days or weeks may elapse between the onsets of the two symptom complexes. It is best considered a syndrome, in that it may occur as the result of multiple sclerosis, acute disseminated encephalomyelitis, systemic lupus erythematosus, or sarcoidosis. When this symptom complex occurs in the course of multiple sclerosis, its clinical and pathologic features are indistinguishable from those of MS.

Diffuse Sclerosis, Transitional Sclerosis

These terms describe a group of progressive neurologic disorders occurring primarily in young patients who manifest severe neurologic deficits of various types with progressive visual and mental deterioration. These are pathologists' terms, which were first used in the late nineteenth century. Schilder described three cases of what came to be known as Schilder's cerebral sclerosis, or Schilder's disease. It is likely that three separate conditions have been included as Schilder's disease, and that this eponymic designation should be discarded. Some cases represent the result of severe confluent extensions of large lesions of multiple sclerosis. Some represent white matter disease of known viral origin, such as subacute sclerosing panencephalitis and progressive multifocal leukoencephalitis (see Ch. 504). A third group includes the leukodystrophies (see later discussion). It is probable that adrenoleukodystrophy was the disorder identified by Schilder in one of his early cases.

Possibly Related Monophasic Disorders

ACUTE DISSEMINATED ENCEPHALOMYELITIS. This disorder is characterized by varying degrees of perivenous mononuclear cellular infiltration and demyelination. It appears most commonly after viral infections that do not normally affect the nervous system, or as a complication of immunization. Since an episode of acute disseminated encephalomyelitis (ADEM) closely resembles an acute attack of multiple sclerosis, it may be impossible to make the distinction until sufficient time has elapsed to determine whether or not a second bout occurs. By definition, ADEM describes those patients in whom further attacks do not occur. The distinction between ADEM and MS is blurred by the not infrequent occurrence of typical exacerbations in the course of MS, concomitant with intercurrent viral infection.

OPTIC NEURITIS. Optic neuritis denotes partial or complete loss of vision in one or both eyes, attributable to one or more optic nerve lesions of unknown etiology. If a cause is known, it is more precise to describe, for example, syphilitic optic neuropathy, or optic neuritis or neuropathy secondary to multiple sclerosis. Retrobulbar neuritis describes a lesion in the posterior two thirds of the optic nerve. The term "papillitis" indicates a lesion in the anterior portion of the optic nerve, leading to an ophthalmoscopic appearance indistinguishable from that of acute papilledema, but differing from the papilledema of increased intracranial pressure by being associated with reduction of visual acuity early in its course. The visual loss usually, but not always, includes macular vision with appearance of a central scotoma and a reduction in color perception. Pain on eye movement is frequent during the first few days of the event. Unless the patient has papillitis, ophthalmoscopic examination is normal for the first two to three weeks, after which disc pallor with loss of small vessels on the disc or more severe atrophy may develop.

Visual loss occurs over the course of hours to several days, and almost always recovers to some degree within several weeks. Blindness as the result of the optic nerve demyelination of MS rarely occurs. Optic neuritis can occur as the presenting sign of MS (see Table 509–3) or at any time during the course of the disease. Practically all MS patients exhibit optic nerve demyelination at autopsy, which underlies the usefulness of the visual evoked response. Approximately one third of patients who develop idiopathic optic neuritis will go on to develop the clinical manifestations of MS. The presence of the CSF abnormalities associated with MS makes this course somewhat more likely, but does not have firm predictive value; certainly MS may develop in the absence of CSF gamma globulin abnormalities.

The illnesses which can mimic idiopathic optic neuritis include optic nerve compression on any basis, neurosyphilis, ischemic optic neuropathy (in older patients), pernicious anemia, Leber's optic atrophy (which is hereditary), tobacco-alcohol amblyopia, and chronic papilledema with optic atrophy and visual loss, associated with prolonged increased intracranial pressure.

ACUTE TRANSVERSE MYELOPATHY. Like optic neuritis, acute transverse myelopathy may occur in isolation, or as the first sign of MS, or at any time in the course of MS. It describes partial to complete paralysis of the legs or of all four extremities, usually accompanied by sensory loss and bowel and bladder dysfunction. As described in Ch. 505, acute transverse myelopathy may be the result of any of a number of disease processes. The same cautions regarding the use of laboratory aids in attempting to predict the later development of MS apply to acute transverse myelopathy as to optic neuritis.

LEUKODYSTROPHIES

These disorders are diseases of dysmyelination, rather than demyelination, in that the normal formation of myelin is interfered with by a genetically determined biochemical defect. The classification of leukodystrophies is based on their histopathology. A biochemical defect is known for several of these disorders, but they all remain relatively rare, incurable disorders, affecting individuals from the first months of life to the 20's.

Metachromatic Leukodystrophy

This, the most common of the leukodystrophies, describes diffuse dysmyelination, usually starting in the first ten years of life. It produces personality changes leading to dementia, convulsions, cranial nerve abnormalities, and finally severe spasticity or rigidity. Death usually occurs in from two to four years, although longer survival is reported. Juvenile and adult onset cases have been reported.

The appearance of metachromatic material (staining red with toluidine blue) in the urinary sediment and in peripheral nerves usually allows diagnosis during life. The metachromatic material also collects in the liver, gallbladder, kidneys, and spleen. The CSF protein is usually elevated above 100 mg per deciliter.

Metachromatic leukodystrophy is usually inherited as an autosomal recessive trait. The pathogenesis of the widespread loss of normal myelin is accumulation of sulfatides in glial cells, in Schwann cells, within myelin lamellae, and in the cytoplasm of some nerve cells. The underlying biochemical defect is abnormally low activity of arylsulfatase A, an enzyme in the system which normally reduces the concentration of cerebroside sulfate.

Sudanophilic Leukodystrophy

This subset includes a heterogeneous group of diseases which have in common only the fact that extensive CSF myelin destruction occurs, associated with products of myelin breakdown, cholesterol esters which stain bright red with the usual fat stains. This staining quality distinguishes these diseases from the metachromatic leukodystrophies and led to the term "sudanophilic." These pathologic characteristics are found in aminoacidurias, adrenoleukodystrophy, and Pelizaeus-Merzbacher disease.

ADRENOLEUKODYSTROPHY. This disorder describes the combination of diffuse dysmyelination and myelin breakdown associated with idiopathic adrenocortical insufficiency. It occurs exclusively in males, inherited as a sex-linked recessive trait. The onset of the disorder occurs most often in childhood, but has been reported in adults, and it produces a similar progression of symptoms as described for metachromatic leukodystrophy. One of the original patients described by Schilder most probably had adrenoleukodystrophy. CSF protein is elevated in most patients. Endocrine testing reveals primary adrenal failure. Instances of adrenal failure alone have been reported in relatives of patients with adrenoleukodystrophy.

Pathologic examination reveals widespread changes in CNS myelin, and also peripheral nerve demyelination, with numerous lipid lamellar inclusions throughout the tissue. The underlying biochemical defect is not known.

PELIZAEUS-MERZBACHER DISEASE. This rare leukodystrophy affects males primarily, is inherited as a sex-linked recessive trait, and starts in early infancy. It progresses slowly, producing extensive, diffuse, symmetrical disturbances of myelin staining associated with gliosis within the cerebrum and cerebellum. The peripheral nervous system is not affected. The underlying biochemical defect is unknown. No treatment is available.

Globoid Cell Leukodystrophy (Krabbe's Disease)

This affects infants in the first two to three months of life, initially producing irritability and unexplained episodes of crying, sensitivity to light and noise, and failure to achieve developmental milestones. During the second year these children become opisthotonic, developing myoclonic jerks and atypical seizures, and optic atrophy begins. Rarer instances occur in late infancy, between two and six years of age, or in adulthood.

Neuropathologic examination reveals marked loss of myelin throughout the brain with the presence of globoid cells. These occur either as round or oval mononuclear cells the size of large glia or as larger irregular multinucleated cells. Their cytoplasm stains positively with PAS. These globoid cells contain the material which accumulates in abnormal quantities, galactocerebroside (galactosyl ceramide). The major enzymatic defect is deficiency of galactocerebroside-galactosidase. It is believed to be transmitted as an autosomal recessive trait. No treatment is known.

Spongy Degeneration of White Matter

Many disorders can produce the pathologic changes leading to this label, including aminoacidurias and other metabolic disturbances. Those instances in which no underlying metabolic defect is apparent are often called Canavan's disease. It produces the onset of weakness in early infancy, leading to spastic paraplegia, severe mental retardation, optic atrophy, and enlargement of the head. Death usually occurs by 18 months. The brain is usually larger than expected for that age. Central nervous system myelin does not stain, and there is a honeycomb-like appearance (status spongiosus) of the deeper layers of the cerebral cortex and white matter near the cortex. The majority of infantile cases occur among those descending from eastern European Jewish families. It is inherited as an autosomal recessive trait. Rarer juvenile cases are more likely to be sporadic and less likely to be from Jewish families. Spongiform degeneration is also produced by exposure to large amounts of hexachlorophine in infancy and by Creutzfeldt-Jakob disease (see Ch. 504), and can be produced experimentally in animals by intracerebral injection of ouabain, a selective blocker of ATPase.

Austin J: Metachromatic form of diffuse cerebral sclerosis: II. Diagnosis during life by isolation of metachromatic lipids from urine. Neurology 7:716, 1957. *Description, clearly written, of methods for identifying metachromatic urinary sediment in children with this disorder.*

Schaumberg H, Powers J, Raine C, Suzuki K, Richardson E: Adrenoleukodystrophy. Arch Neurol 2:577, 1975. *A thorough review of the clinical and neuropathologic features which characterize this entity, including a discussion of its relationship to "Schilder's disease."*

Seitelberger F: Pelizaeus-Merzbacher's disease. *In* Vinken P, Bruyn G (eds.): Handbook of Clinical Neurology, Vol 10. Amsterdam, North-Holland, 1970, p 150. *An excellent review of this and related degenerative diseases of myelin.*

Suzuki K, Suzuki Y: Globoid cell leukodystrophy: Deficiency of galactocerebroside-galactosidase. Proc Natl Acad Sci USA 66:302, 1970. *This report describes the detection of the enzyme deficiency underlying this rare form of leukodystrophy.*

Section Eleven THE EPILEPSIES

510. THE EPILEPSIES

Jerome Engel, Jr.

DEFINITION AND PREVALENCE. Epilepsy is the term applied to a group of disorders, perhaps better called the epilepsies, that are characterized by recurrent, spontaneous, transient paroxysms of hyperactive brain function resulting in epileptic seizures. The epileptic attack or seizure, the common denominator of all of these conditions, may appear as impaired consciousness, involuntary movement, autonomic disturbance, or psychic or sensory experiences. Epileptic disorders can be considered either primary, conditions of intrinsic nonprogressive presumably hereditary cerebral hyperexcitability, with seizures as the only manifestation of disordered brain function, or secondary, wherein the epileptic attacks are symptoms of some known pathologic process affecting the brain.

Epileptic disorders most commonly begin in early childhood but can appear at any time. Epidemiologic surveys indicate that 0.5 per cent of the United States population have active seizures, 3 per cent have had a recurrent seizure disorder at some time in their life, and 9 per cent have experienced at least one epileptic seizure. These figures may represent an underestimation since the stigma attached to epilepsy causes many individuals to deny or hide their disorder. Prevalence is greater in areas of the world where there are high rates of infection, poor perinatal care, frequent head trauma, and other opportunities for increased brain injury.

PATHOGENESIS. Most investigators now believe that the fundamental abnormality in all epileptic conditions can be traced to the cerebral cortex, including the limbic cortex (hippocampus). In chronic epilepsy, the recurrent neuronal paroxysms that underlie ictal (seizure) events are transient expressions of a more permanently physiologically disordered cortex. Even though epileptic seizures are intermittent, the epileptogenic cortical abnormality persists throughout the interictal (between seizures) period.

Epileptogenic cortex in the interictal state is characterized by the appearance of brief high-amplitude electrical discharges that usually can be recorded from the scalp by *electroencephalography (EEG).* The typical interictal EEG discharge consists of a sharp negative transient wave followed by a slower wave, referred to as a *spike-and-wave complex.* Studies of well localized cortical epileptogenic lesions (epileptic foci) in animals indicate that the EEG spike-and-wave complex reflects the summation of highly synchronized abnormal alterations in neuronal membrane potentials. These abnormal membrane events consist of large paroxysmal depolarization shifts followed by prolonged after-hyperpolarizations. The depolarization shift results in enhanced neuronal excitation, while the after-hyperpolarization represents inhibition that may prevent ictal development. Neurons in cortical areas adjacent to the epileptic focus may demonstrate paroxysmal hyperpolarization only, forming an inhibitory surround that appears to prevent epileptic spread during the interictal state. It is unclear to what degree these abnormal membrane events recorded from epileptic foci reflect inherent pathologic properties of individual epileptic neurons as opposed to disturbances in interconnections of groups of neurons.

When seizures begin in an epileptic focus, the interictal EEG spike-and-wave complex is replaced by ictal low voltage, fast, rhythmic electrical discharges. At the cellular level this change represents a breakdown of the inhibitory after-hyperpolarization and the onset of a more continuous hyperexcitable depolarized state. If the inhibitory surround is also overcome, adjacent more normal cortical areas are recruited into the ictal process by nonsynaptic means. This *ephaptic spread* can proceed in a slow and orderly fashion across the cortex to produce a gradual progression of ictal symptoms that reflect functions of the involved cortical structures. Consciousness is preserved when ictal discharges are confined to a relatively discrete area of cortex in one hemisphere.

Ictal propagation to distant brain areas can occur via long fiber tracts, leading to the development of additional symptoms. Propagation to the contralateral hemisphere, particularly to limbic structures such as the hippocampus, the amygdala, and their projections, leads to impaired consciousness. Propagation to frontal lobes and subcortical motor systems can result in progression to a tonic-clonic convulsion.

Partial seizures begin with symptoms that reflect ictal discharges in an epileptic focus involving a part of the cerebral cortex and adjacent subcortex. *Generalized seizures* begin bilaterally from the start and are caused by widespread or multiple cortical epileptogenic foci or diffusely epileptogenic cortex related to primary hereditary, toxic, or metabolic disturbances. Some seizures may be precipitated by normal synchronizing afferent influences from subcortical centers. This may be the predominant mechanism of seizure initiation in the hereditary primary generalized seizure disorders, but it appears to be the cortex and not the deeper nuclei that is primarily abnormal. For this reason, the term *corticoreticular* has replaced centrencephalic or subcortical epilepsy for these conditions.

The fundamental neuronal defects that account for epileptogenesis appear to vary from one condition to another. Common causes of acute experimental partial and generalized convulsive seizures in animals include toxic and metabolic alterations that produce membrane instability; drugs that block the action of inhibitory transmitters; and electric currents that create polarizing fields. Although these findings may explain why epileptic seizures occur in association with certain clinical conditions, they are probably not relevant to mechanisms that spontaneously generate recurrent seizures in chronic epileptic disorders. Studies of chronic epileptic foci from animals and patients and investigations of naturally occurring primary generalized epileptic disorders in animals have revealed inconsistent biochemical and anatomic disturbances at the cellular level but no definitive explanations for the ultimate epileptogenic properties.

Mechanisms responsible for the termination of epileptic seizures are even less well understood than those that start them in the first place. Seizures do not stop merely as a result of neuronal exhaustion but rather appear to self-activate inhibitory mechanisms. Neuronal function is depressed after a seizure, and there may be prominent postictal symptoms. Tonic-clonic convulsions and partial seizures with impaired consciousness are followed by diffuse EEG suppression and periods of confusion and fatigue lasting minutes to hours. Other partial seizures may be followed by transient localized EEG suppression and focal neurologic deficits, known as *Todd's paralysis,* caused by postictal dysfunction of cortical structures involved in the ictal event.

It is likely that the pathophysiologic processes discussed apply to both partial seizures and generalized tonic-clonic convulsions. The different ictal manifestations of these conditions may merely reflect the localization and extent of the cortical disturbances. However, this does not appear to be the case for all epileptic conditions. For instance, in some nonconvulsive generalized seizures (absences) ictal and interictal EEG spike-and-wave discharges are indistinguishable and respond to drugs that are different from those used to treat partial and convulsive seizures. Certain myoclonic jerks, infantile spasms, neonatal seizures, and forms of partial continuous epilepsy are unassociated with specific ictal EEG patterns and demonstrate still another spectrum of drug responsivity. Some of these latter disorders may reflect subcortical disinhibition with pathophysiologic mechanisms more similar to extrapyramidal movement disorders than to epilepsy.

ETIOLOGY. The causes of epilepsy are many, and several factors may coexist in the same patient. Commonly, it is the combination of a cerebral lesion and a genetic predisposition that determines the appearance of epileptic seizures. Systemic illness or trauma may uncover a latent epileptic condition.

Genetic factors may contribute to the development of epilepsy in three ways: (1) an individual may inherit a low threshold for seizures; (2) genetic traits underlie certain specific primary epileptic conditions; and (3) many inherited diseases of the brain are associated with structural disturbances that produce seizures.

A number of poorly understood genetic factors determine the susceptibility of individual brains to develop generalized convulsions in response to nonspecific stresses such as sleep deprivation, fever, and alcohol withdrawal. Persons who experience such convulsions do not have epilepsy as such, but they do have lowered convulsive thresholds that make them more likely to develop chronic recurrent seizures of all types if brain injury occurs for other reasons. Consequently, patients with seizures caused by pathologic processes that are clearly not familial may have family histories of epilepsy or isolated seizures.

Benign inherited primary epileptic disturbances, presumably as a result of biochemical defects and unassociated with other neurologic dysfunctions, account for 30 per cent of chronic epileptic disorders. Specific autosomal dominant genetic traits have been identified as responsible for the characteristic EEG patterns of three-per-second spike-and-wave complexes seen in the generalized disorder *(petit mal epilepsy)* and for the centrotemporal spikes seen in the partial disorders *(sylvian* or *rolandic epilepsy)*, but not all individuals with these traits have seizures. Other benign familial primary generalized epilepsies have been described with faster spike-and-wave EEG discharges and bilaterally synchronous myoclonic jerks.

Inherited neurologic diseases also can produce chronic recurrent epileptic seizures that are secondary to specific pathologic processes within the brain. These include inborn errors of metabolism such as phenylketonuria and the lipoidoses; other degenerative diseases, not only those that affect gray matter, such as the progressive myoclonus epilepsies, but also the leukodystrophies; and syndromes such as tuberous sclerosis and neurofibromatosis that are associated with the development of cerebral ectopic or alien tissue.

Congenital lesions due to pre- and perinatal injuries are commonly encountered in epileptic patients. Minor focal lesions that can give rise to partial seizures include microgyria, porencephalic cysts, areas of calcification, and atrophy. More severe trauma, anoxia, and infections such as toxoplasmosis, cytomegalic inclusion disease, rubella, herpes, and syphilis also can produce diffuse neocortical and hippocampal damage and secondary generalized seizure disorders.

Head trauma with cicatrix formation is an important cause of epileptic seizures. Chronic recurrent seizures occur in 30 per cent of patients with acute hematomas, 15 per cent of those with depressed skull fractures, and 5 per cent of those hospitalized for severe closed head trauma. Epilepsy is rare, however, after head trauma without loss of consciousness. Seizures occurring at the time of injury (contact seizures) or within the first week thereafter do not necessarily herald development of a recurrent epileptic disorder. Chronic posttraumatic seizures usually have a delayed onset, most often beginning 6 to 12 months following injury and occasionally starting even many years later.

Infectious processes involving the brain and its coverings can produce acute and chronic seizures. As with trauma, generalized seizures that occur during active meningitis and encephalitis may not indicate a recurrent epileptic condition. Acute and chronic recurrent generalized and partial seizures are seen with slow virus infections and are common late sequelae when adhesions or scars result from purulent meningitis, fungal infections, or destructive viral processes such as herpes simplex encephalitis. Partial seizures may be the first sign of focal bacterial encephalitis or abscess formation, lesions especially likely to produce chronic epilepsy. Other focal inflammatory processes such as tuberculomas and parasitic infestations, particularly cysticercosis and schistosomiasis, are common causes of partial seizures in many countries and because of increased international travel are sometimes found outside their endemic areas.

About half of all *brain tumors* located in the anterior and middle cranial fossae produce epileptic symptoms. Gliomas are most often implicated, but any neoplasm that impinges on the cortex can produce seizures. Partial seizures are common with *Sturge-Weber syndrome* and often result from small cryptogenic hamartomas, ectopias, and angiomas.

Cerebral vascular diseases produce seizures in many ways. Partial seizures are rare during acute strokes and usually reflect embolic events with bleeding into the cortex rather than thrombosis. Completed strokes, however, often produce scar tissue that can become epileptogenic months or years later. Such a process is presumed to be the most common cause of unexplained recurrent partial seizures in the elderly. Partial and generalized seizures are early symptoms of cerebral venous thrombosis, cerebral arteritis, and hypertensive encephalopathy (now rare). Partial seizures often occur with arteriovenous malformations (AVMs), and small cortical hemorrhages of any cause can produce refractory partial seizures or focal myoclonic jerks.

Systemic toxic and metabolic disturbances caused by exogenous and endogenous substances that lower seizure thresholds or produce neuronal membrane instability as well as ionic imbalance, such as hyponatremia, can give rise to generalized convulsions, but these are not considered epileptic conditions. Nevertheless, such metabolic causes occasionally can lead to status epilepticus with subsequent brain damage or death. It is important to recognize the rare reversible metabolic causes of seizures in infancy, such as hypocalcemia and pyridoxine deficiency, that can be treated easily by replacement therapy. Toxic or metabolic disturbances may occasionally cause partial seizures because of associated unsuspected focal cerebral lesions from old head injuries. These occur most commonly in alcohol and drug abusers who are undergoing withdrawal. Hyperosmolar conditions such as nonketotic hyperglycemia and uremia may also give rise to partial seizures, presumably because of brain shrinkage that tears bridging vessels and produces small areas of hemorrhage into the cortex.

Miscellaneous disorders that can cause seizures include gray matter degenerative diseases such as allergic encephalopathies and very rarely the presenile and senile dementias. Demyelinating diseases occasionally produce lesions adjacent to cortex that cause epileptic attacks: seizures occur in 3 per cent of patients with multiple sclerosis.

Mesial temporal sclerosis, consisting of largely unilateral neuronal loss often accompanied by astrocytic proliferation in the hippocampus and adjacent limbic structures, is found in over half the patients who have undergone temporal lobe resection for complex partial seizures. This may be the most common pathologic finding in epilepsy, but it remains uncertain whether the lesion is the cause or the result of seizures. Prolonged convulsive seizures are known to produce cell loss in the hippocampus, the neocortex, and the cerebellum. Some authorities believe that prolonged convulsions (lasting more than 30 minutes), such as those that occasionally accompany fever in infancy or childhood exanthems, can produce mesial temporal sclerosis and that this lesion becomes epileptogenic later in life. In any event, this form of epileptic brain damage suggests that in some situations epilepsy itself becomes a cause of progressive symptoms. Even if mesial temporal sclerosis does not actually cause seizures, it may alter their manifestations and account for some interictal behavioral disturbances. For this reason convulsive seizures should be controlled as promptly as possible.

CLINICAL MANIFESTATIONS AND CLASSIFICATION. At present epileptic seizures are classified by their clinical manifestations (Table 510–1), since precise anatomic and pathophysiologic correlates of specific ictal behaviors are still largely unknown. The classification plays an essential role in the diagnosis and management of epileptic disorders for four major reasons:

1. The diagnosis of epilepsy is often difficult because of the similarity between certain epileptic attacks and intermittent symptoms of nonepileptic disorders. Recognition that a patient's complaints are consistent with a known epileptic seizure pattern determines whether the true nature of the condition has been identified or even suspected. The classification of epileptic seizures by specific symptoms is particularly useful for this purpose.

2. Differentiation between partial and generalized seizures is of great clinical value. Partial seizures indicate the presence of a focal brain disturbance that may be a curable cause of epilepsy, such as a surgically resectable scar, or a focal progressive process that requires specific attention, such as an infection or neoplasm. Because the exact expression of a partial seizure is determined by the site of ictal onset and spread and not by the causative agent, additional clinical information is necessary to identify the nature of the underlying lesion.

3. The choice of antiepileptic drugs is determined by the seizure type rather than by the specific cause or anatomic substrate. Certain generalized seizures in particular are effectively treated by classes of pharmacologic agents that are different from those used to treat partial or generalized convulsive seizures. Consequently, the differential diagnosis between absence attacks and complex partial seizures and between myoclonus and convulsions is essential for determining appropriate drug therapy.

4. A number of epileptic syndromes have been defined on the basis of seizure manifestations and other clinical features. Although pathophysiologic mechanisms or underlying disease processes have yet to be identified for most, diagnosis of a specific syndrome usually has important therapeutic and prognostic implications. In particular, recognition of the benign inherited primary epileptic conditions such as true petit mal, juvenile epileptic myoclonus, and sylvian epilepsy may facilitate prompt control with the proper medication, spare the patient unnecessary tests, and relieve anxiety by assurance of an excellent outcome. A diagnosis of temporal lobe epilepsy in a medically intractable patient suggests that complete cure may be possible by surgical resection.

TABLE 510–1. CLASSIFICATION OF EPILEPTIC SEIZURES*

Partial seizures (focal, local)
Simple partial seizures
With motor signs
With somatosensory or special sensory symptoms
With autonomic symptoms or signs
With psychic symptoms
Complex partial seizures
Simple partial onset followed by impairment of consciousness
With impairment of consciousness at onset
Partial seizures evolving to generalized tonic-clonic convulsions (secondarily generalized)
Generalized seizures (convulsive or nonconvulsive)
Nonconvulsive seizures
Absence seizures
Atypical absence seizures
Myoclonic seizures
Atonic seizures
Convulsive seizures
Tonic-clonic seizures
Tonic seizures
Clonic seizures
Unclassified epileptic seizures

*Modified from Commission on Classification and Terminology of the International League Against Epilepsy: Epilepsia 22:489, 1981.

Partial Seizures. Although the expression of partial seizures depends on the areas of cerebral cortex that are involved, the precise anatomic origin of specific seizures cannot always be accurately inferred from ictal symptoms, since functional localization within the brain remains inexact. Moreover, epileptic manifestations may reflect dysfunction produced by propagation away from the primary lesion as much or more than from the area where the focus lies.

Partial seizures are classified as simple when consciousness is preserved. *Simple partial seizures* reflect an ictal discharge that is localized within one hemisphere. The ictal symptoms can take many forms.

Motor symptoms begin with clonic or tonic movements of a discrete body part. Areas of the body with large representation in the motor cortex, such as the face and hand, are involved most frequently. When spread occurs in an orderly fashion along the precentral gyrus, there is a progression of clonic motor symptoms from thumb or face, for example, referred to as a *Jacksonian March.* More commonly, however, ictal discharges in frontal cortex activate multiple muscle groups to produce complex versive movements such as turning of the head, eyes, or body to one side and posturing with one or more extremities. Involvement of the supplementary motor cortex classically results in adversive seizures with turning of the head and eyes away from the epileptic focus and elevation of the contralateral arm. The arm position can vary, however, and the direction in which the head turns is not a good localizing or lateralizing sign. Other simple motor manifestations include speech arrest or vocalizations when language areas are involved; eye or lid twitching, which is most often initiated from frontal or occipital foci; and inappropriate laughter unassociated with humor *(gelastic epilepsy).* Simple partial clonic or tonic motor seizures can be followed by a transient *Todd's paralysis* of involved muscles, but suspicion of an underlying progressive lesion is justified when postictal focal deficits persist after 48 hours.

Sensory symptoms occur with lesions in or connected to primary sensory cortex. Thus, localized paresthesias or numbness arise with seizures emanating from the parietal lobe, unformed luminous visions occur with lesions of the occipital lobe, and unpleasant olfactory and gustatory sensations, vertigo, and sounds result from lesions of appropriate areas of the temporal cortex. Postictal Todd's phenomena such as blindness, deafness, and anesthesia may occasionally follow simple partial seizures with sensory symptoms.

Autonomic symptoms often are due to ictal involvement of limbic structures in the mesial temporal and frontal lobes that project to the hypothalamus and brainstem and include feelings of epigastric rising or distress, nausea, or vague lightheadedness. Brief paroxysmal epigastric symptoms, including vomiting, can be the sole manifestation of an epileptic disorder *(abdominal epilepsy).* This condition has most often been identified in children, but it is rare and probably greatly overdiagnosed. In other autonomic seizures ictal signs and symptoms such as pallor, flushing, sweating, piloerection, pupillary dilatation, cardiac arrhythmia, and incontinence may be apparent.

Psychic symptoms can occur with ictal discharges in limbic and association cortex and mimic features of psychiatric disorders. These include dysmnesic symptoms such as feelings of familiarity (deja vu) and unfamiliarity (jamais vu) and forced thinking; cognitive disturbances such as dreamy states, depersonalization, and time distortion; affective symptoms such as fear and rage, which often are associated with appropriate autonomic changes, depression, and on rare occasion elation; illusions such as multiple images (polyopsia) or distortions of size (micropsia and macropsia); and hallucinations consisting of stereotyped mixed sensory experiences such as visions of well-formed recognizable faces or specific scenes accompanied by voices that can be understood, familiar smells, and emotional responses. Persistent psychic symptoms in epileptic patients may also be postictal.

Simple partial seizures are usually brief and do not interfere with daily living unless they occur frequently or evolve into other types of attacks. Simple partial seizures that consist only of experiential phenomena may be referred to as *auras* when the patient perceives them as a warning of impending more noticeable epileptic symptoms. Patients who complain only of simple partial seizures may report having many seizures a week or many a day, with each lasting a few seconds.

Partial seizures are classified as complex when they impair consciousness. Approximately 40 per cent of patients with epilepsy experience *complex partial seizures* with impaired consciousness ranging from a complete loss with unresponsiveness to mere amnesia for the ictal event. Complex partial seizures are presumed to reflect bilateral ictal involvement of limbic structures, particularly the hippocampus, amygdala, and their connections. The seizure may begin with impaired consciousness from the start, or spread of ictal discharge may result in evolution from a simple into a complex partial event. This evolution occurs most often when the simple partial seizure is caused by a lesion involving the mesial temporal lobe or a region of cerebral cortex directly connected to mesial temporal limbic areas. Autonomic auras most commonly precede complex partial seizures and include epigastric rising or distress and psychic experiences. Complex partial seizures that are preceded by olfactory auras are called *uncinate fits*. These fits may be more consistently associated with brain tumors than are other types of seizures.

The term complex partial seizure is not synonymous with *temporal lobe, psychomotor*, and *limbic seizures*. These designations have more specific anatomic implications and may involve ictal symptoms resulting from unilateral activation of mesial temporal limbic structures without impaired consciousness. Some complex partial seizures that manifest themselves solely as brief lapses in consciousness or that are associated with atypical behavior may not reflect primary activation of the limbic system. The complex partial seizure that typifies the temporal lobe or psychomotor attack begins with a motionless stare at the time consciousness is impaired, followed by purposeless movements called *automatisms*. Alimentary automatisms, such as chewing, swallowing, sucking, and lip smacking, are most common and presumably reflect amygdala involvement. Other examples of automatisms include verbal utterances of sounds or words; gestural movements such as fumbling, posturing, and picking at clothing; expressions of emotion; and ambulation. Ongoing activities such as washing dishes or even driving a car may continue automatically. Patients may undress, run, respond to commands, and demonstrate a variety of complicated automatisms that indicate a residual ability to relate to the environment despite the ictal state. In complex partial seizures that emanate from structures outside the temporal lobe, patients can display irregular thrashing movements of the extremities, scream, fall, or exhibit bizarre behavior that can be difficult to differentiate from hysteria.

Complex partial seizures usually last from a few seconds to a few minutes and are followed by confusion and amnesia for the ictal event, although most patients remember an aura. Postictal anterograde amnesia and automatisms are common, and aphasia often occurs when seizures begin in the dominant hemisphere. Other cognitive deficits and headache may be present during the postictal period. In cases of unusually prolonged or recurrent complex partial seizures, postictal anterograde memory disturbance may persist for hours or days.

Complex partial seizures and postictal symptoms can severely disrupt daily life. While it is not uncommon for patients to have many complex partial seizures a week and several auras a day, even one or two seizures a year may prevent them from driving a car or destroy a chosen career.

Both simple and complex partial seizures can evolve into *secondarily generalized tonic-clonic convulsions*. Most patients with partial seizures experience at least some secondarily generalized seizures, but generalization usually occurs infrequently and is more easily controlled by drugs than are partial ictal symptoms. Some patients, particularly those with lesions in the frontal lobes, have partial seizures that always secondarily generalize. When such secondarily generalized partial seizures begin in a silent area of the brain, initial focal symptoms may be overlooked by both the patient and observers. When neither ictal symptoms nor signs provide a clue that a seizure is secondarily generalized, postictal focal or lateralizing signs and symptoms such as reflex asymmetry, focal weakness, or aphasia may indicate a partial seizure disorder. Differentiation from true generalized convulsions in these cases is important to identify potentially progressive or treatable focal lesions.

Generalized Seizures. *Absences* are brief losses of consciousness that can be of two types. Both begin almost exclusively in childhood and take the form of a blank stare, which can also be associated with mild clonic movements of eyelids and face, more generalized jerks, alterations in motor tone, and simple automatisms. *Petit mal absences* affect about 10 per cent of epileptic children, last less than ten seconds, demonstrate a typical EEG pattern consisting of symmetrical, synchronous, and regular three-per-second (or slightly faster) spike-and-wave discharges, and begin and end abruptly without pre- or postictal EEG or clinical disturbances. These seizures are characteristic of benign genetic epileptic disorders of the primary generalized type. *Atypical absences* also occur in about 10 per cent of epileptic children, can last longer than ten seconds, demonstrate asymmetrical, asynchronous, and irregular three-per-second (or slower) spike-and-wave discharges on the EEG, and produce some degree of postictal confusion and EEG disturbance. Atypical absences often occur in patients who have other types of generalized seizures, as well as neurologic deficits, mental retardation, and a characteristic slow spike-and-wave (less than 2.5 per second) EEG pattern. This symptom complex is called the *Lennox-Gastaut syndrome* and results from multiple or diffuse brain lesions. True petit mal and atypical absences must not be confused with each other or with complex partial seizures consisting only of brief lapses of consciousness, since cause, prognosis, and treatment differ for the three seizure types.

Absences can occur spontaneously hundreds of times a day. Petit mal absences respond well to appropriate medications, tend to disappear during adolescence, and are rarely disabling. Atypical absences may be refractory to therapy and can disrupt normal function. Children with atypical absences, however, are usually hampered more by other seizures and by neurologic and mental deficits.

Myoclonic seizures are single, rapidly recurrent, bilaterally synchronous shock-like jerks of the face, trunk, and extremities that are not associated with loss of consciousness. A single myoclonic jerk that occurs while a person is falling asleep is a normal physiologic event. More frequent myoclonus implies a more serious problem. In most patients with myoclonic seizures, these events cluster shortly after waking or when falling asleep. A prolonged attack can terminate in a generalized tonic-clonic convulsion. Myoclonic seizures occur in certain rare benign genetic epileptic disorders of the primary generalized type such as *juvenile epileptic myoclonus (impulsive petit mal)* and respond well to drug therapy.

In contrast to myoclonic seizures, there are many other types of myoclonic jerks that are not generalized and should not be considered epileptic. These include (1) the asymmetrical or sporadic (involving first one area of the body and then another) jerks that are spontaneous or induced by movement or sensory stimulation and that result from anoxic, toxic, and metabolic disturbances and (2) the *progressive myoclonus epilepsies* that are associated with lesions of the diencephalon, brainstem, and cerebellar nuclei. Other myoclonic phenomena that are not epileptic seizures include regular rhythmic *palatal myoclonus* and *segmental myoclonus* that are caused, respectively, by medullary and spinal cord lesions and *benign familial (essential) myoclonus* of unknown origin.

Tonic-clonic (grand mal) convulsions occur at least once in 80 per cent of epileptic patients. Occasionally, such seizures can be epileptic responses of a normal brain to nonspecific physiologic stress or systemic disturbances. More often they represent the final form taken by partial seizures that secondarily generalize or are a manifestation of a generalized epileptic disorder. Convulsions that are not secondarily generalized from partial seizures never have auras, although patients may occasionally recognize nonspecific affective changes or experience a flurry of bilaterally synchronous myoclonic jerks some hours before a seizure occurs. The typical generalized convulsion begins with a sudden cry accompanied by loss of consciousness, falling, and bilateral tonic extensor rigidity of the trunk and extremities. After several seconds of rigidity, recurrent clonic muscular contractions are produced for one or two minutes, until the seizure ends, leaving the patient flaccid and unconscious. Cyanosis results from breath-holding during the tonic phase, and autonomic hyperactivity is prominent. The blood pressure increases abruptly, the body temperature rises, and the patient salivates and may have urinary and fecal incontinence. The tongue and the inside of the mouth often are bitten. Occasionally generalized convulsive attacks consist of either tonic or clonic activity alone.

Postictal depression can last many minutes, occasionally hours, and rarely a day or more. During this period patients gradually regain consciousness but feel exhausted, frequently complain of headache, and wish to sleep. A few remain partially confused. Focal or lateralized postictal symptoms do not occur following true generalized tonic-clonic convulsions.

Grand mal convulsions rarely occur more than a few times a year in primary generalized epileptic disorders but can occur daily in severe secondary generalized disorders. In both situations, however, the generalized seizures tend to respond well to antiepileptic drugs.

Atonic seizures (drop attacks), considered to be minor motor epileptic events, begin almost exclusively in childhood and are usually associated with diffuse lesions of the brain. The ictal episode consists of a sudden loss of tone that is too brief to determine whether alteration of consciousness has occurred. In its simplest form, the child's head drops for a second or less. In more severe forms, the patient loses tone in the entire body, collapses to the floor, and often incurs serious injuries such as concussion, broken bones, and lost teeth. This characteristic drop should be distinguished from the more gradual slump that can accompany partial seizures, the more rigid loss of balance that occurs during tonic or tonic-clonic convulsions, and the sudden impulsive falls that result from myoclonic jerks. Atonic seizures occur many times a day, are refractory to therapy, and can be the most debilitating ictal manifestation of the Lennox-Gastaut syndrome. Brief *tonic seizures* also occur as minor motor symptoms of secondary generalized epileptic disorders.

Unclassified Seizures. *Infantile spasms* begin in the first year of life as brief intermittent ictal events that take a variety of forms, ranging from subtle twitches of the mouth or nose to violent jackknife or salaam movements. They result from severe diffuse disturbances of brain function from a variety of causes, are often associated with a severely abnormal interictal EEG pattern called *hypsarrhythmia,* and have a poor prognosis. Because infantile spasms may reflect subcortical disturbances similar to myoclonus or movement disorders, they have been removed from the current classification of epileptic seizures. However, children with this EEG and clinical symptom complex *(West's syndrome)* usually develop recurrent epileptic seizures as they get older, and their illness often evolves into the Lennox-Gastaut syndrome.

Because of an immature brain, *neonatal seizures* almost never generalize. Rather, they manifest themselves subtly as jitteriness, focal or multifocal twitches, clonic movements, and posturing. The cerebral cortex in the neonatal period may not be sufficiently well developed to sustain epileptic activity, and often no correlation exists between electrographic abnormalities and behavioral seizure activity. Consequently, many of these events could also reflect disturbances that are primarily subcortical and not epileptic. Benign as well as severely disabling forms of neonatal seizures occur.

Patterns of Seizure Occurrence. Appreciation for precipitating factors and temporal patterns of certain epileptic seizures can influence approaches to management. In some of the primary generalized epileptic disorders, seizures may be induced by specific sensory stimuli, most commonly flashing light *(photosensitive epilepsy).* Reading, video games, music, and other specific complex stimuli may activate seizures in patients with rarer forms of *reflex epilepsy.* The seizures themselves range from brief absences through synchronous myoclonic jerking to occasional generalized convulsions. It is unusual for partial seizures to be induced by specific sensory stimuli, although they can be provoked by emotional stress and drowsiness. *Hyperventilation* is a potent activator of petit mal and atypical absence seizures and sometimes will precipitate other types of ictal events as well. Possibly the associated respiratory alkalosis may explain why some patients report an increased incidence of seizures during exercise. Sleep deprivation and withdrawal from alcohol and sedative drugs are well established precipitants of partial and generalized convulsive seizures in patients with chronic epilepsy. Some patients have seizures that occur only at night or only during the day. Others exhibit regular cycles of seizures over days or months or patterns of seizure clusters followed by prolonged seizure-free periods. The term *catamenial epilepsy* is used when seizures regularly recur in women around the menstrual period. Women with all forms of epileptic disorders commonly experience more frequent seizures at this time of the month, and seizures may worsen or disappear during pregnancy.

Status Epilepticus. Rapidly recurring or continuous ictal events are referred to as status epilepticus. *Epilepsia partialis continua* is a state of simple partial seizures that can last hours, days, or weeks. The focal clonic motor form resembles myoclonic jerks, while the rarer sensory and psychic forms may be difficult to differentiate from psychiatric disorders. Ictal EEG changes may be difficult to identify.

Complex partial status epilepticus is a rare condition of rapidly recurring seizures characterized by a fluctuating level of consciousness, automatic behavior, and ictal EEG discharges recorded over the temporal lobe. The condition may be confused clinically with a psychosis or metabolic disturbance and must be included in the differential diagnosis of altered states of consciousness; failure to treat it promptly can be followed by prolonged memory deficits.

Absence status or *spike wave stupor* consists of a continuous state of dulled mentation, which often has a subtle appearance. Eye blinking and other associated movements can occur, and there is a characteristic EEG pattern of diffuse spike-and-wave discharges. The condition occurs fairly often in patients with atypical absences and is also seen with a juvenile form of primary generalized petit mal epilepsy. A rare type of absence status of unknown cause also affects older adults with no previous history of epilepsy. Absence status is not a medical emergency, since no secondary brain damage occurs. The benign and adult forms respond well to antiepileptic drugs, but atypical absence status associated with diffuse lesions of the brain may be extremely difficult to control.

Major motor status epilepticus exists when generalized tonic-clonic convulsions recur so frequently that consciousness is not regained between them. This can occur with the generalized disorders but is more commonly a result of partial seizures that secondarily generalize. In the latter instance, the partial onset often is not recognized because of the severity of the attacks. Toxic and metabolic disturbances, including drug and alcohol withdrawal, can precipitate major motor status epilepticus in epileptic patients as well as in nonepileptic individuals with genetically low seizure thresholds. Major motor status epilepticus can also be a presenting symptom of acute intracranial hemorrhage and infections, as well as brain tumors and other focal processes, especially in the frontal lobes. Major motor status epilepticus is a life-threatening situation demanding immediate treatment.

Epileptic Syndromes. A number of epileptic syndromes have already been mentioned, and some of the more clinically distinctive ones are listed in Table 510–2. It is particularly valuable to recognize those syndromes that respond well to specific treatment and that are associated with a good prognosis. In this group should be included several familial conditions and temporal lobe epilepsy.

Sylvian or *rolandic epilepsy* (benign partial epilepsy of childhood with centrotemporal spikes) is a familial disorder that may be the cause of as many as 20 per cent of childhood seizures. It is characterized by nocturnal generalized convulsions and simple partial seizures that occur during the day. Typically, the partial seizures begin with perioral or lingual paresthesias, although other sensory or motor symptoms may occur, especially involving the face. The EEG demonstrates centrotemporal interictal spikes that may be unilateral or bilaterally independent. Associated neurologic deficits are lacking, and the seizures respond well to medication. The disorder almost always disappears during adolescence.

A rare benign partial epilepsy of childhood with occipital spike-and-wave discharges is characterized by seizures with visual symptoms followed by headache. This disorder may be a form of migraine.

One or more *febrile convulsions* occur in 3 to 4 per cent of otherwise healthy children between the ages of six months and five years and consist of brief tonic-clonic generalized seizures. Although febrile convulsions can be recurrent, the syndrome is so benign that it is usually not considered an epileptic disorder, and treatment is usually not necessary. A genetic basis is certain but poorly defined. Affected children outgrow their vulnerability between three and five years of age, although 5 per cent develop seizures without fever later. Against the diagnosis of benign febrile convulsions are the following: seizures lasting longer than ten minutes, focal abnormalities during or after the seizure, or an abnormal neurologic or mental status examination result. In such instances an underlying neurologic disorder is likely and treatment is required.

The primary generalized epileptic conditions of the petit mal type, mentioned earlier, account for 10 per cent of childhood epilepsies. Several varieties are recognized depending on the age of onset, frequency of EEG spike-and-wave discharges, and occurrence of myoclonic seizures. Infrequent grand mal seizures can occur in all forms, or they may occur alone. Response to appropriate medication is usually excellent, especially when onset is in early childhood. These disorders often remit in adolescence; a juvenile onset or myoclonic seizures tend to worsen the prognosis.

TABLE 510–2. CLINICALLY DISTINCTIVE EPILEPTIC SYNDROMES

	Partial Epilepsies	Generalized Epilepsies
Primary (without structural lesions; benign, genetic)	Benign partial epilepsy of childhood with centrotemporal spikes (sylvian, rolandic) Benign partial epilepsy of childhood with occipital spike waves (may be migraine)	Benign febrile convulsions (should not be considered a chronic epileptic disorder) Petit mal epilepsies; many forms, including: true petit mal, juvenile forms Juvenile epileptic myoclonus Reflex epilepsies
Secondary (with structural lesions and associated neurologic disturbances)	Temporal lobe epilepsy Epilepsia partialis continua Epileptic acquired aphasia	Lennox-Gastaut syndrome Infantile spasms Progressive myoclonus epilepsies (many forms)

True petit mal absences and grand mal seizures should not be confused with similar ictal events that occur in children with the Lennox-Gastaut syndrome as the result of diffuse or multiple lesions of the brain. Patients with primary generalized epilepsy are otherwise neurologically normal, with brief absences accompanied by regular synchronous EEG spike-and-wave discharges. Although patients with the Lennox-Gastaut syndrome can have absences identical to the primary generalized type, usually they also have or develop additional neurologic impairment, mental subnormality, multiple seizure types including drop attacks, irregular asymmetrical paroxysmal EEG discharges, and abnormal baseline EEG rhythms. In contrast to the excellent prognosis for the primary generalized epilepsies, seizures associated with the Lennox-Gastaut syndrome and other secondary generalized epileptic disorders are difficult to control. The patients often become severely handicapped by the frequent attacks as well as other static or progressive interictal neurologic deficits.

Juvenile epileptic myoclonus is a primary generalized epileptic disorder that begins in mid to late childhood with bilaterally synchronous myoclonic seizures. The paroxysms can be completely controlled with appropriate medication, and there are no other associated disturbances. The condition should not be confused with the myoclonic disorders characterized by sporadic, often stimulus-sensitive, myoclonic jerks, such as postanoxic myoclonus and the progressive myoclonus epilepsies. These last-mentioned sporadic myoclonic events are not epileptic, are extremely difficult to treat, and are usually associated with other evidence of diffuse cerebral injury.

The *progressive myoclonus epilepsies* comprise a group of familial cerebral degenerative disorders that affect both cortical and subcortical gray matter, leading to progressive neurologic deficits, dementia, sporadic multifocal myoclonic jerks, occasional epileptic myoclonus, and tonic-clonic convulsions. Whereas the epileptic myoclonus and convulsions respond well to medication, patients are severely disabled by the nonepileptic sporadic myoclonus and other handicaps. The course may be rapid with severe neurologic and mental impairment *(Lafora type)*, intermediate *(Unverricht-Lundborg type)*, or relatively slow with little mental impairment or EEG disturbance *(Ramsay-Hunt syndrome*, which is associated with cerebellar disturbances and may be considered a separate entity). A benign familial myoclonic syndrome *(essential myoclonus)* also exists.

Temporal lobe (psychomotor, limbic) epilepsy is the most common chronic epileptic syndrome and may account for 40 per cent of adult epilepsies. It is characterized by auras and complex partial seizures involving temporal lobe limbic structures either initially or occasionally by spread from other areas. Typically there are unilateral or bilateral independent anterior temporal EEG spikes. Patients may also have memory deficits and psychiatric symptomatology. Complex partial seizures, as described earlier, are often difficult to control medically but can be abolished by surgical resection. Patients with complex partial seizures that do not respond to appropriate medical therapy should be referred to a surgical facility for evaluation.

Epilepsia partialis continua also often is unresponsive to medication. This disorder occurs in adults after severe cerebral injury, such as anoxia or stroke—occasionally with brain tumors. It also can be seen in young children, particularly those with a rare unilateral chronic cerebral inflammatory disorder of unknown cause. The continuous focal motor seizures reflect widespread or multiple rather than single lesions that usually are not amenable to localized surgical resection. Seizures can be abolished by large resections such as in hemispherectomy, and this may be indicated in some children who already have hemiatrophy and hemiparesis.

Epileptic acquired aphasia syndrome is a rare partial seizure disorder of unknown cause that appears as language deterioration in young children and is associated with bilateral temporal epileptiform EEG spikes. The disorder resolves spontaneously.

DIAGNOSIS. Diagnosis in epilepsy involves searching for treatable causes when possible and recognizing epileptic conditions that indicate a specific prognosis and therapy. When a treatable cause of epilepsy is not revealed, management of the seizures is determined by correct diagnosis of the type of epileptic disorder.

History. The history is usually the most important part of the diagnostic evaluation. In order to obtain an accurate description of the typical ictal events, it is essential that someone who has witnessed the seizures accompany the patient to the interview.

The patient's own description of any auras should be recorded as well as the ictal behavioral changes observed by others. The occurrence of an aura or other focal symptoms at onset, during progression, or in the postictal period indicates a partial rather than a generalized seizure disorder. If more than one type of seizure occurs, each should be described separately. Often patients will report several seizure types, which after careful questioning are revealed to be variations of the same ictal phenomenon and not evidence for multiple lesions. For instance, when auras are not followed by further symptoms they may be recognized as one event, while the same aura that spreads to become a complex partial seizure may be reported as another phenomenon. If on occasion there is evolution to a secondarily generalized seizure without postictal recall of the aura, a careful description of the initial ictal events by an observer often will verify that the generalized convulsion is a manifestation of the same epileptogenic lesion. When patients report only seizures that are generalized from the start, an attempt should be made to determine whether convulsive and nonconvulsive ictal manifestations resemble those of benign genetic disorders, generalized disorders caused by diffuse or multiple brain lesions, or secondarily generalized partial seizures caused by a focal lesion. Clues to the differential diagnosis derive from the circumstances and age at onset of seizures and how they may have changed with time or treatment.

Drug regimens and other treatment plans can be influenced by knowledge of how often seizures occur, whether they are more common at certain times of the day or month, or whether they are related to certain precipitating factors. If the patient has been treated previously, it is important to know what drugs have been used and the specifics of their therapeutic and toxic effects.

The history can provide crucial etiologic information. In children, patterns of early development may delineate the difference between a progressive degenerative disorder and a static lesion. There may be evidence of specific predisposing factors such as perinatal injury, intracranial infections, or reactions to immunizations. A history of a prolonged childhood convulsion preceding the onset of complex partial seizures raises the possibility of mesial temporal sclerosis causing the subsequent chronic epileptic disorder. In older patients there may be hints of cerebral vascular disease or systemic cancer. A history of head trauma at any age can be relevant but must be evaluated carefully because parents and patients often recall trivial injuries of no importance occurring days or weeks prior to the first seizure. In addition, a specific injurious event such as a fall may be mistakenly interpreted as having generated traumatic epilepsy when it actually represented the first seizure.

The family history can reveal important genetic factors. The existence of relatives with similar seizures or other neurologic symptoms suggests a specific primary epileptic disorder. A family history of individuals with isolated seizures or varied epileptic conditions may indicate the inheritance of a lowered threshold for seizures. Absence of left-handedness in the family of a left-handed patient may hint at early injury of the left cerebral hemisphere.

The psychosocial history both gives important clues to diagnosis and indicates needs for more specific evaluations. Patients with benign inherited epileptic disorders should have normal school and work histories and no evidence of mental disturbance. A history of specific cognitive deficits suggests a focal lesion, while more generalized mental impairment suggests a diffuse abnormality. When the latter is progressive, more detailed laboratory, EEG, and psychometric examinations can determine whether the patient has an underlying degenerative disease, increasing dysfunction because of recurrent seizures, or toxic symptoms of overmedication.

Physical Examination. The general medical examination can uncover systemic diseases responsible for seizures. In addition to searching for toxic, metabolic, infectious, neoplastic, and cardiovascular diseases, stigmata of tuberous sclerosis, neurofibromatosis, hemangiomas, and other predisposing congenital disorders should be sought. Asymmetry (hemiatrophy) in the size of hands, feet, and face may indicate a long-standing lesion in the contralateral hemisphere.

The neurologic examination can provide evidence for a specific diagnosis or reveal focal disturbances that differentiate between partial and generalized seizure disorders. In the absence of focal features, findings of minimal brain dysfunction, such as clumsiness, posturing, and hyperreflexia, or more marked diffuse impairment indicate a secondary rather than a primary generalized seizure disorder.

The mental status examination can distinguish specific cognitive deficits caused by focal lesions from more general mental retardation or dementia. Poor attention span in patients on drug therapy may indicate medication side effects rather than structural lesions. Increasing degrees of fixed neurologic and mental impairment confer a poor prognosis for both seizure control and psychosocial adaptation.

If possible, patients should be observed during a seizure. Status epilepticus usually lasts until hospitalization, absences can be provoked by hyperventilation, reflex seizures are easily induced (it is unwise to attempt to induce tonic-clonic convulsions), and spontaneous seizures may occur in the examining room. The initial manifestations and early development should be noted. Consciousness should be assessed by repeating a phrase to determine whether the patient can recall it after the seizure is over. Even if the seizure appears to be generalized at the start, postictal examination of neurologic and mental status may reveal focal deficits that indicate a partial seizure disorder. When circumstances make direct examination impossible, try to find a reliable witness who can describe the attack.

Laboratory Studies. Epilepsy provides no diagnostic hematologic or chemical laboratory tracers, but such tests can help to diagnose underlying disease processes that give rise to seizures. One or more generalized epileptic attacks can mildly increase protein content and white cell count in the cerebrospinal fluid for 24 to 48 hours. Although up to 100 white cells per cubic millimeter have been reported after major motor status epilepticus, a lumbar puncture revealing more than 10 white cells per cubic millimeter should initiate a search for an intracranial inflammatory process. In infants and young children with seizures, it is wise to test blood and urine for metabolic disorders. In older patients with refractory focal motor seizures, hyperosmolar syndromes such as hyperglycemia and uremia should be considered. Complete blood count, liver function tests, blood urea nitrogen, and urinalysis are necessary in all patients about to begin antiepileptic drug therapy to establish a baseline for evaluating possible subsequent toxic side effects.

Radiologic Studies. A computed tomographic (CT) scan is necessary for adolescents and adults with the recent onset of seizures but may be avoided in younger children when history and other examinations indicate a primary generalized disorder or a nonprogressive lesion. Cerebral angiography should be confined to cases in which surgery is considered or a primary vascular disorder is suspected.

Psychometric Studies. Psychometric testing, including standard tests of attention, performance and verbal IQ, memory, language, and personality can help verify the existence of a focal or diffuse brain disturbance. When there is evidence that mental function is deteriorating, serial testing can quantify the change and evaluate subsequent trends of disease or therapy. An astute psychometrician should also be able to offer advice for improving psychosocial adaptation.

Electroencephalography. The EEG is the single most useful diagnostic laboratory test for epilepsy. However, overinterpretation of the EEG often generates an unwarranted diagnosis of epilepsy. A number of spike-like EEG events can be normal, and 2 per cent of the nonepileptic population may have true epileptiform spike-and-wave complexes on their EEGs but never develop seizures. Conversely, 20 per cent of patients with epilepsy do not demonstrate epileptic abnormalities on a routine interictal EEG. Whereas an EEG can help verify a clinical diagnosis of epilepsy, interictal epileptiform EEG abnormalities alone should be considered neither necessary nor sufficient information for arriving at this diagnosis. However, if a seizure occurs in the EEG laboratory, the association of an ictal EEG pattern with observed ictal clinical behavior makes possible a definitive diagnosis.

The pattern of interictal EEG abnormalities may help determine the type of epileptic disorder. Focal spike-and-wave discharges or slow waves indicate a partial epileptic disorder. A diagnosis of benign Sylvian epilepsy may be confirmed by characteristic centrotemporal spikes that are easily differentiated from the anterior temporal EEG transients of temporal lobe epilepsy. While bilaterally synchronous EEG discharges may also reflect a focal lesion (secondary bilateral synchrony), especially in the frontal lobes, such activity more often indicates a generalized epileptic disorder. Focal or diffuse slowing of baseline EEG rhythms and irregular or asymmetrical spike-and-wave complexes at a frequency of 2.5 per second or less indicate that the generalized epileptic disorder is secondary rather than primary.

Activation procedures used in the EEG laboratory include hyperventilation for absences, photic stimulation for photosensitive epilepsy, and sleep. But there are major pitfalls: hyperventilation in children and some normal adults can induce high amplitude slowing resembling spike-and-wave discharges; photomyogenic responses of facial muscles to photic stimulation can occur in normal individuals and during drug and alcohol withdrawal and should not be considered evidence of epilepsy; a number of normal sharp transients that occur during sleep and on arousal often are misinterpreted as epileptic spikes.

Nonstandard techniques, available in some laboratories, may offer additional diagnostic advantages. Nasopharyngeal and sphenoidal electrodes can clarify interictal EEG spike patterns originating in mesial temporal structures, but the same information usually can be obtained more easily from ear lobe electrodes. Special epilepsy centers exist throughout the country that offer prolonged EEG telemetry and television monitoring to provide a more precise description of specific ictal events when diagnosis is in doubt. Ambulatory EEG monitoring is being developed for outpatient evaluations.

A repeat EEG may be indicated to determine whether behavioral deterioration is due to an increase in subclinical seizure activity, an increase in drug side effects, or a progressive underlying lesion. If necessary, EEG telemetry combined with frequent antiepileptic drug level determinations or ambulatory monitoring can improve medical management by allowing dose schedules to be tailored to individual patients' needs.

The EEG is also essential for monitoring the progress of therapy for status epilepticus when clinical behavior is not a reliable guide. This is often true in stupor related to spike-and-wave discharge patterns and in complex partial status epilepticus and is always the case when anesthesia or paralysis is used to control major motor status epilepticus.

DIFFERENTIAL DIAGNOSIS. The diagnosis of epilepsy should be made only on firm clinical evidence. Such a diagnosis can have irreversible psychosocial effects resulting in the loss of a driver's license, a job, independence, and self-esteem. Consequently, a physician often does more harm by making an unjustified diagnosis than by reserving judgment until the nature of the disorder has declared itself adequately. When doubt exists injury can be minimized by warning the patient to avoid the conditions that might have precipitated the event and to be aware of potentially dangerous situations should another event occur.

Systemic Disturbances. *Syncope* is the most common systemic disturbance confused with epilepsy. Syncope can be associated with motor twitches and in rare instances may produce a tonic-clonic convulsion in susceptible individuals. This condition must be treated as syncope, not as epilepsy. Because cardiogenic syncope can cause a convulsion while seizures may be associated with cardiac arrhythmias, diagnostic monitoring of blackout spells should ideally include both ECG and EEG recordings. Other intermittent systemic disorders that can be mistaken for epilepsy include breath-holding spells in early childhood, hyperventilation syndrome, alcoholic blackouts, intermittent porphyria, hypoglycemia, pheochromocytoma, tetanus, and toxic-metabolic abnormalities.

Neurologic Disturbances. Nonepileptic episodic neurologic disturbances are most often of vascular origin. Transient ischemic attacks must be considered when intermittent neurologic symptoms occur in older patients. Drop attacks beginning in adulthood usually are caused by posterior fossa vascular disturbances or cataplexy and are almost never epileptic. Transient global amnesia also is more likely to have a vascular rather than an epileptic cause. Prodromal migraine symptoms can resemble epileptic seizures, and the subsequent headache can be mistaken for a postictal headache. The distinction between migraine and epilepsy is not always completely clear.

Sleep disorders are also commonly mistaken for epilepsy. Narcolepsy is easily diagnosed when all four of the classic symptoms are present; however, if sleep attacks, cataplexy, sleep paralysis, or hypnogogic hallucinations occur alone, they can be confused with epileptic seizures. Careful questioning usually will elicit evidence for some of the other symptoms as well. Hypersomnia, as seen in Klein-Levin and sleep-apnea syndromes, as well as dyssomnias such as somnambulism, night terrors, and enuresis must be differentiated. On rare occasions epileptic seizures can be manifested as nocturnal ambulation, fear, and urinary incontinence; all-night sleep EEG recordings may be necessary to make the correct diagnosis in such instances.

Other neurologic symptoms that can masquerade as epilepsy include intermittent vertigo from a variety of causes and the episodic uncontrolled movements that occur with *Gilles de la Tourette's syndrome,* hemiballismus, chorea, athetosis, and other extrapyramidal disorders. Although the involuntary movements of paroxysmal choreoathetosis are not epileptic, they can often be successfully treated with antiepileptic medication. The myoclonic disorders discussed earlier also should not be confused with epilepsy.

Behavioral Disturbances. It is extremely important to differentiate between true epileptic seizures and conversion reactions. Hysterical seizures (*pseudo seizures*) may be manifested in ways that have psychologic significance such as with pelvic thrusting, may involve motor symptoms that do not fit with known anatomic spread patterns, and only rarely result in injury to the patient despite risk. Nevertheless, it is impossible to make this diagnosis definitively from a description or even from observation of a seizure. Virtually any paroxysmal behavior, no matter how bizarre, could be a true epileptic seizure. The diagnosis of hysterical seizures may be made with some confidence, however, when ictal events are suggestive for the reasons just stated, EEG recordings are normal, antiepileptic medication is ineffective, and evidence of secondary gain is obtained during psychiatric interview. EEG telemetry and television monitoring of ictal events may help to substantiate the diagnosis.

There are several considerations, however, which limit conclusions drawn from telemetry. Simple partial ictal events may have no EEG correlates that can be recorded from the scalp, EEG changes that accompany motor seizures may be obscured by muscle artifact (but postictal EEG suppression is evidence that a true epileptic seizure has occurred), and repeated bilaterally synchronous myoclonic jerks unassociated with loss of consciousness may be mistaken for psychogenic events. Even if a definite diagnosis of hysterical seizure disorder can be made, many such patients have epileptic seizures as well. When hysterical seizures and real seizures coexist, EEG and television monitoring may help to differentiate the two types and provide a basis for independently assessing the results of psychiatric and medical treatment.

Some true epileptic symptoms can be confused with behavioral disturbances. Frequently occurring absences in children can be mistaken for attentional deficits, learning disabilities, and disciplinary problems, but the EEG should provide the correct diagnosis. Certain simple partial seizures with sensory or psychic symptoms may be interpreted as psychotic hallucinations. Although these epileptic experiences can have an emotional content, they usually are more stereotyped and more likely to have visual components than are psychotic hallucinations. Rarely, *fugue states* may represent continuous epileptic seizures *(poriomania)* or prolonged periods of postical confusion.

Episodic dyscontrol is a poorly defined entity consisting of intermittent periods of inappropriately violent, occasionally destructive behavior. Confusion with epilepsy is compounded by the fact that some patients with this syndrome have epileptic seizures as well. If the episodic behavior lasts only several minutes, is uncharacteristic of the patient's interictal personality, and there is amnesia for the event with appropriate remorse afterward, this may possibly reflect an epileptic disturbance. Although ictal EEG recordings have not supported this contention, an occasional patient with episodic dyscontrol may be helped by antiepileptic medication. Organized and directed violence is not seen during the epileptic seizures described earlier, and epilepsy is never the cause of premeditated criminal acts.

Epileptic Seizures That Are Not Epilepsy. Under certain circumstances generalized tonic-clonic convulsions can occur entirely as a natural reaction to physiologic stress or transient systemic injury and should not be considered evidence of an epileptic illness. These include single isolated convulsions resulting from documented precipitating events such as sleep deprivation, alcohol or sedative drug withdrawal, use of convulsant drugs, fever, and acute head trauma and recurrent convulsions induced by reversible infectious, toxic, or metabolic processes and limited to the period of systemic illness. However, a chronic epileptic condition probably exists if there is an indication of focal ictal or postictal features; if there is evidence of an intracerebral lesion; or if seizures recur in the absence of the presumed cause.

TREATMENT. Treatable causes of epileptic seizures include intracerebral mass lesions that can be surgically removed and toxic, metabolic, infectious, and vascular diseases that require medical management. A treatable cause cannot be found in most patients with chronic recurrent seizures, however, and the objective of therapy is then to maximize useful function, ideally by complete eradication of seizures without introduction of additional unwanted side effects. Adequate control is usually possible with appropriate pharmacologic, surgical, and psychosocial management. Only about half of patients treated for chronic epilepsy can expect to become seizure free indefinitely.

Pharmacologic Therapy. Although many antiepileptic drugs are available, it is prudent to become familiar with and use the few that are most effective for each of the various seizure types (Table 510–3). Pharmacologic therapy is based on obtaining an accurate diagnosis of seizure type or epileptic syndrome, selecting the single most appropriate drug for that diagnosis (monotherapy), and correlating measurements of drug levels in the serum with patient reports in order to adjust dosages and dose schedules for the best control and fewest side effects. The best control does not necessarily mean the greatest reduction in seizure frequency. In certain patients, the disability caused by some continued seizures may be less than limitations induced by therapy. For example, a few absences a day for a child is preferable to an alternative of no seizures on a dose of antiepileptic medication that produces continuous sedation and impairs school performance. Similarly, aggressive therapy is not justified for a patient with refractory epilepsy when high drug levels exacerbate existing physical and mental handicaps without producing a worthwhile improvement in the seizure pattern.

Pharmacokinetic Principles. Dose planning for individual antiepileptic drugs depends on the pharmacokinetic factors that determine the amount of available drug in the blood. The therapeutic ranges for individual antiepileptic drugs refer to the ranges of steady state levels of each drug that are effective in controlling seizures. Average or approximate pharmacokinetic variables for the commonly used antiepileptic drugs appear in Table 510–4.

The proper dose schedule for a newly introduced drug depends on balancing the need for rapid control of seizures against the avoidance of side effects. If a patient has been warned about the possible occurrence of another seizure and takes appropriate precautions, it usually is not necessary to build a drug level rapidly at the risk of producing severe side effects. It is more important that the patient accept the drug of first choice. Patients can be encouraged to remain on medication by beginning a drug regimen slowly, taking the medication with meals when nausea is anticipated, using higher doses at bedtime when sedation is anticipated, and reducing doses transiently when untoward side effects occur. Most unpleasant dose-related side effects are temporary, and an appropriate regimen eventually can be instituted. A loading dose can be given practically for some drugs (phenytoin and phenobarbital) when the risk of repeated seizures requires therapeutic levels to be rapidly achieved despite side effects. A loading dose of 1.5 (rather than 2) times the calculated total daily dose may be an adequate compromise between obtaining rapid seizure control and producing minimal side effects if the planned maintenance schedule is begun less than one half-life after the loading dose.

Although a maintenance steady-state level of a drug can be achieved with an interdose interval of approximately one half-life time, in this situation drug levels will fall below the protective range if a single dose is missed. However, a dose schedule that requires a drug to be taken too frequently may be inconvenient and reduce compliance. An interdose interval of 0.5 half-lives, which amounts to one to four times a day for the commonly used medications, is usually recommended. Therapeutic failure using recommended dose schedules may result from aberrant absorption and metabolism in some pa-

TABLE 510–3. THERAPEUTIC CLASSIFICATION OF EPILEPTIC SEIZURES

Seizure Type	Preferred Drugs
Partial seizures and generalized convulsions	Carbamazepine Phenytoin Phenobarbital Primidone Valproic acid
Absences	Ethosuximide Valproic acid Clonazepam
Myoclonus	Clonazepam Valproic acid

tients, and dose schedules must then be determined individually from measurements of serum drug levels.

The recommended therapeutic range for a given drug is based on average measures. One should use these values as a guide rather than a goal; therapeutic drug levels in individual patients may be well above or well below the average. Once an effective maintenance schedule has been achieved, determinations of trough serum drug levels, drawn just before the morning dose, provide a reliable record of long term alterations in steady state conditions. Such measurements are useful when recurrence of seizures or side effects result from decreases or increases in available drug.

ENZYME INDUCTION AND INHIBITION. The most common reasons that subtherapeutic antiepileptic drug serum levels occur after an effective maintenance schedule has been achieved are failure of patients to comply with the dose and enzyme induction. Enzyme induction refers to the increased metabolism of a drug by the liver as a result of chronic administration of that drug or addition of another drug. Because of enzyme induction, the steady state serum levels of a drug may gradually decline with time on the same dose schedule. If seizures recur and serum drug determinations reveal lower steady state levels, the amount of drug given should be increased. A common error at this point is to add a second drug that produces further enzyme induction and leads to subtherapeutic levels of both drugs. Because the antiepileptic effects usually are not cumulative but the toxic side effects are, there is an increase in both seizures and toxic symptoms.

Enzyme inhibition can also occur with addition of a new drug. Consequent reduction in metabolism causes an increase in the serum level of the first drug. In this situation, side effects that may be ascribed to the newly added second drug are actually related to toxic levels of the first. When a patient must use more than one drug, measurements of serum drug levels are essential to determine how these drugs are interacting and which may be responsible for altering seizure frequency or increasing side effects.

The best strategy for pharmacologic management is to choose the single best drug for the condition and gradually to increase the dosage over weeks or months until seizure control or intolerable side effects occur. The end point of this process must be determined clinically for each patient. If a drug is ineffective, it should be replaced with another by gradually reducing the first drug while increasing the second. An exacerbation of seizure frequency may be a transient response to withdrawal of the first drug and does not indicate that the second is ineffective. To obtain optimal control when multiple seizure types are present, the use of two drugs may be unavoidable.

Selection of Antiepileptic Drugs. PREFERRED AGENTS. While specific types of seizures respond to specific drugs (Table 510–3), many factors determine the choice of the best single drug for an individual patient. The trend today is to treat generalized convulsive and partial seizures first with either carbamazepine or the hydantoin phenytoin. The idiosyncratic hematologic side effects of carbamazepine, which were generally feared when this drug was initially introduced, have proved to be rare, and carbamazepine often is preferred over phenytoin by epileptologists. While both drugs offer the same protection, phenytoin use is associated with a high incidence of disturbing cosmetic side effects.

The barbiturates primidone and phenobarbital are also used for convulsive and partial seizures. They are less effective than carbamazepine and phenytoin, but some authorities prefer to begin with phenobarbital because it is the least expensive of the available antiepileptic drugs and has the fewest dangerous side effects. Sedation is common but may not be a problem at lower doses and may subside over time even at higher doses. Furthermore, both carbamazepine and phenytoin can dull mentation at high doses. Barbiturates are a problem in children, since these drugs commonly engender hyperkinetic activity and other undesirable behavioral disturbances. Most epileptologists now generally prefer carbamazepine for this age group because it does not seriously alter behavior. Phenobarbital should not be given to patients with depressive tendencies. It can exacerbate psychologic depression and is the most common mechanism of suicide in the epileptic population.

The drug of choice for absence seizures remains ethosuximide, since it is safer than valproic acid. Valproic acid can produce serious idiosyncratic hepatic side effects that laboratory tests may not predict. Fortunately, mortality from this complication is rare (1 per 35,000), and valproic acid is effective against a variety of seizure types. Valproic acid is the drug of choice for mixed seizure disorders because of its broad spectrum of action and for juvenile epileptic myoclonus. Valproic acid may be more effective than ethosuximide for atypical absences and also is used widely as a second choice drug for other types of seizures. Enzyme inhibition occurs with valproic acid, which greatly increases serum levels of other antiepileptic drugs. This is a particular problem with the barbiturates and sometimes results in inadvertent sedation or even coma.

The drug of choice for nonepileptic forms of myoclonus is the benzodiazepine clonazepam, although valproic acid is also effective against most myoclonic phenomena. In progressive myoclonus epilepsy, where myoclonic jerks and seizures are both present, valproic acid may be the best hope for control with monotherapy. If this is unsuccessful, clonazepam plus carbamazepine or phenytoin may be required. Clonazepam and valproic acid given together may interact to make seizures worse and produce unpleasant side effects.

SECOND LINE ANTIEPILEPTIC DRUGS. Clonazepam is a benzodiazepine currently used as an adjunctive medication for convulsive and partial seizures, although it may also be an effective

TABLE 510–4. COMMONLY USED ANTIEPILEPTIC DRUGS

Drug	Seizure Type	Adult Dose (mg/kg)	Therapeutic Range (μg/ml)	Half-life (hours)	Peak Time (hours)	Daily Doses
Carbamazepine (Tegretol)	P, GC	15–25	8–12	12	2–6	4
Phenytoin (Dilantin)	P, GC	3–8	10–30	24	4–8	2
Primidone (Mysoline)†	P, GC	10–20	5–15	12	2–4	4
Phenobarbital	P, GC	2–4	15–40	96	6–18	1
Chlorazepate (Tranxene)	P, GC	0.7–1.0	1–2*	30*	1*	2
Mephobarbital (Mebaral)	P, GC	4–10	10–30*	96*	6–18*	1
Mephenytoin (Mesantoin)	P, GC	2–10	10–40	100*	27*	1
Ethosuximide (Zarontin)	A	10–30	40–100	30‡	2–3	2
Trimethadione (Tridione)	A	20–40	500–1200*	240*	120–240*	1
Clonazepam (Clonopin)	A, M	0.03–0.3	0.01–0.05	30	1–2	2
Methsuximide (Celontin)	P, A	10–25	20–40*	40*	<3	2
Valproic acid (Depakene)	All	15–60	50–100	8	1–4	4

Modified in part from Leal KW, Troupin AS: Clin Chem 23, 1964, 1977.
*For derived metabolite.
†Substantial antiepileptic effect is obtained from derived phenobarbital.
‡For children (60 hours for adults).
Key: P = partial; GC = generalized convulsive; A = absence; M = myoclonus.

primary antiepileptic. Other drugs that may be of value if first line drugs fail include the hydantoin mephenytoin and the barbiturate mephobarbital for convulsive and partial seizures and clonazepam and trimethadione for absences. Methsuximide is effective against absence and atonic and partial seizures and can be used alone or as an adjunctive medication. Acetazolamide may be a useful adjunctive medication, particularly for ten days premenstrually through the end of menses for women with catamenial accentuation of epilepsy. Adrenocorticotropic hormone (ACTH) and adrenocorticosteroids have been found useful in the treatment of infantile spasms but not in other epileptic conditions.

Side Effects. Almost all antiepileptic drugs potentially produce undesirable side effects, and physicians should consult the *Physicians' Desk Reference* or a current textbook before first use. Common dose-related side effects of carbamazepine and the hydantoins include nausea, dizziness, diplopia, and ataxia. Sedation, impaired mentation, and hyperactivity occur most often with the barbiturates and benzodiazepines. These symptoms may abate with time. Drug-induced folic acid deficiencies may reach symptomatic levels in some patients and require vitamin supplements. Idiosyncratic side effects that usually affect skin, blood, liver, and kidneys are potentially more serious. When a new drug is introduced, complete blood counts and appropriate blood chemistry analyses should be obtained every four weeks for several months, and then monitored every 3 to 12 months as long as therapy continues. Leukopenia as low as 3000 commonly occurs with carbamazepine and does not necessarily indicate impending agranulocytosis. Moreover, an elevated serum alkaline phosphatase level alone does not indicate a hepatotoxic reaction. Mild pruritus may be treated medically. Evidence of blood dyscrasias, liver or kidney damage, or more serious skin rash requires prompt discontinuation of medication and referral to the proper specialist. Cosmetic side effects commonly associated with phenytoin include hirsutism, gingival hyperplasia, and coarsening of features; weight gain and alopecia are occasionally seen with valproic acid therapy. Carbamazepine can cause water retention and is not used for patients with congestive heart failure. A paradoxic increase in seizure frequency may result from elevated drug levels, particularly with phenytoin, and can cause seizures to recur after a period of control.

Pregnancy presents certain problems for women with epilepsy. Seizures may become more frequent, and antiepileptic drug clearance may increase, requiring higher doses of medication. Hemorrhagic disease of the newborn occurs with phenobarbital and phenytoin and can be treated with vitamin K. A two- to three-fold drug-related increase in the incidence of birth defects has been documented for phenytoin, but the nature of all antiepileptic drugs is such that they may have teratogenic effects. Phenytoin is not recommended for women of childbearing age; however, there is little to be gained from discontinuing effective medication once pregnancy has been determined, especially after the first trimester has been completed. The risk to mother and fetus from seizures may be greater than the risk of teratogenicity. Maternal drug levels can cause sedation and withdrawal in newborns but do not present a problem for breast-fed infants.

Surgical Therapy. Resective surgery has proved safe and beneficial and can cure a chronic epileptic condition when all else fails. Most surgical facilities will consider epileptic patients potential candidates for resective surgical therapy if (1) a partial seizure disorder has been documented, (2) seizures continue at a frequency that seriously interferes with daily living despite adequate levels of appropriate antiepileptic medication, and (3) there is not substantial interictal mental retardation or psychosis. Patients with complex partial seizures of temporal lobe origin are ideal candidates for surgery. Worthwhile improvement occurs in 85 per cent of such patients, and as many as two thirds may become seizure free after anterior temporal lobectomy. Common postoperative deficits include a visual superior quadrantanopsia and minor memory disturbances, the latter being more noticeable with resection in the dominant hemisphere. Local resection of an extratemporal focal epileptogenic lesion is also possible if the area of cortex can be identified precisely and removed safely. A history of generalized convulsions, a focus in the dominant hemisphere, or the presence of bilateral independent temporal spike foci on EEG do not contraindicate surgery.

Presurgical evaluation varies from center to center but generally involves localization of an epileptogenic lesion responsible for all or most of the patient's habitual seizures and determination that the abnormality can be removed without producing unacceptable neurologic deficits. Localization by surface EEG alone is possible if confirmed by independent tests of focal dysfunction such as neuropsychologic evaluations, analysis of baseline and barbiturate-induced EEG rhythms and more recently positron emission tomography. Stereotaxic depth electrode recordings can identify resectable epileptogenic lesions in some patients with complicated presentations who would not otherwise be considered surgical candidates. When necessary, the extent of the cortical excision is determined by intraoperative electrocorticography.

Section of the corpus callosum has been particularly effective in controlling drop attacks, and patients with other secondary generalized and partial seizure patterns have experienced improvement from this operation. While *hemispherectomy* is the most effective surgical procedure for epilepsy, it is only justified for children who have severely incapacitating unilateral seizures and hemiparesis. Destructive lesions and cerebellar stimulation are no longer routinely recommended.

Other Therapeutic Considerations. Patients with some types of seizures may benefit from special management. Reflex seizures induced by specific stimuli can be treated by avoiding the stimuli. For example, epileptic photosensitivity can be abolished by patching one eye or wearing colored glasses, and desensitization is possible for many forms of reflex seizures. Spread of some simple partial seizures may be aborted by strong or painful sensory stimulation administered at onset. Operant conditioning (biofeedback) sometimes can reduce seizures in some patients, but the approach is generally impractical. When seizures occur only at specific times of the day, medications can be adjusted to insure maximum levels at those times, and daily schedules can be altered so that the patient is home or in a safe environment when at risk.

Patients with all types of seizures should remain active and maintain daily habits that insure regular meals, adequate sleep, and a reduction in unnecessary stress. Alcohol or sedative drugs can be taken sparingly, but excessive use can provoke seizures during withdrawal. Patients who have seizures associated with an alteration in consciousness, particularly those that occur without warning, should be counseled to avoid hazardous situations: they should not swim alone, should shower rather than bathe, should not climb to unprotected heights, and should not operate potentially dangerous power-driven machines, including automobiles.

A *ketogenic diet* has been used as a last resort to treat children with medically intractable generalized seizures, but this does not replace antiepileptic drugs and usually has minimal or no effect on seizure frequency and severity.

Emergency Treatment. First aid for a generalized tonic-clonic convulsion consists of protecting the patient from self-injury. Clothing should be loosened, sharp objects removed from the area, and the patient's head cushioned from impact. Hard objects or fingers must not be inserted into the patient's mouth: patients do not choke on their own tongues. When the seizure is over, turn the patient's head to drain oral secretions. Have someone stay with the patient during the postictal period until full consciousness has returned. It is not necessary to call an ambulance unless the patient has never had a seizure before, the seizure lasts longer than ten minutes, another attack occurs before consciousness is regained, or there is evidence of injury, respiratory distress, or pregnancy. Patients should not be forcibly restrained during complex partial seizures but protected from surrounding hazards until ictal and postictal symptoms cease and they can care for themselves.

Major motor status epilepticus is a medical emergency requiring immediate intervention to prevent permanent brain damage or death. A recommended approach appears in Table 510–5. As soon as the airway is secured, a quick neurologic examination should be performed to appraise critical forebrain and brainstem functions. There may be evidence of an acute intracerebral lesion with herniation or other life-threatening conditions. Because the effects of diazepam are short-lived, it should be administered simultaneously with a longer-acting antiepileptic drug. Phenytoin usually is preferred, since it produces no sedative effects. This allows the patient to regain consciousness when seizures are terminated and facilitates neurologic evaluation. If seizures have not stopped 60 minutes after the institution of therapy, high intravenous doses of phenobarbital or general anesthesia are recommended; some physicians prefer to use a 4 per cent intravenous solution of paraldehyde in normal saline solution, which can be titrated to maintain the desired therapeutic effect. If these latter approaches are necessary, intubation and ventilation should be used and the progress of treatment followed with EEG recordings.

Once status has been controlled, maintenance drug therapy is instituted. The most common cause of major motor status epilepticus is a sudden reduction or discontinuation of antiepileptic drugs in patients with known seizure disorders.

Psychosocial Considerations. To some extent, psychosocial disturbances among epileptics are situational. Because most seizures occur spontaneously and unpredictably, many patients spend their lives anticipating inappropriate behavior, embarrassment, or serious injury. When patients have a sufficient warning, they may be able to remove themselves from public view or from potentially dangerous situations. In many cases, however, the fear of seizures may cause conscious or unconscious major restructuring of life patterns, with some patients almost becoming reclusive. Epileptics are frequently unable to find work if they admit to a seizure disorder, so that their opportunities for rewarding social relationships are reduced and a sense of worthlessness ensues. In most states, patients with seizures that impair consciousness are not allowed to drive. They are advised to undertake activities that could result in serious injury with caution and never alone, so that their self-confidence is further damaged. Depression and suicide are more common among epileptics than in the general population.

Although the evidence is controversial, a high incidence of aberrant personality traits, affective disorders, and psychoses are suggested among patients with epilepsy, particularly those with complex partial seizures of limbic origin. The literature variably describes *"the epileptic personality"* with words such as aggressive, emotional, overinclusive, sober, hypermoral, and hyposexual. However, the findings are by no means consistent. Even if such traits can be attributed to certain epileptic patients, it is unclear how much of this behavior results from functional disturbances caused by the underlying pathologic lesions or specific seizure activity, how much can be attributed to the effect of long-term antiepileptic drug therapy, and how much relates to the patient's long overprotection and the stigmata of being epileptic. Several authors have reported a paranoid schizophreniform psychosis in patients who have had epilepsy for many years, but the specificity of this syndrome is also debatable.

Only about one in four patients with uncontrolled epilepsy is handicapped by seizures alone. The others have physical, intellectual, and/or psychiatric disabilities that disrupt their daily lives. Epileptic seizures, perhaps more than any other neurologic symptom, are modified by internal and external influences that are under the control of the patient and other persons. For these reasons, treatment of the epileptic patient requires more than manipulation of anticonvulsant drugs, and outcome depends upon more than just seizure control. The physician must come to know the patient and the patient's family, their psychologic interactions, and their social situation. Furthermore, improving psychosocial adaptation itself often leads to a reduction in seizure frequency. To provide the comprehensive care required by patients with seizure disorders, the physican must attend to the patient as well as to his neurological disorder. The doctor must be friend as well as therapist.

TABLE 510–5. MANAGEMENT OF CONVULSIVE STATUS EPILEPTICUS

Treatment Goal	Cumulative Time Since Arrival in Emergency Room (Minutes)
Restore homeostasis	
Check for airway obstruction; check blood pressure, nasal O_2; intubate as needed	0–15
Draw blood sample for glucose, blood urea nitrogen, electrolytes, complete blood count, drug level determination	0–15
Start administering isotonic saline solution, 1000 ml, IV	
Administer glucose 50%, 50 ml, IV; thiamine, 100 mg, IM	0–15
Stop convulsive seizures	
Give diazepam, 10 mg. IV; repeat administration of 10 mg with every seizure, up to 50 mg*	15–60
Give phenytoin, 20 mg/kg, IV (< 50 mg/minute)	15–60
If seizures do not stop by 1 hour, give high doses of phenobarbital IV or general anesthesia	60–120

Modified from Wasterlain CG. *In* Engel J Jr, et al.: Ann Intern Med 97:584, 1982.

*Exceeds manufacturer's recommended dosage.

Commission on Classification and Terminology of the International League Against Epilepsy: Clinical and electroencephalographic classification of epileptic seizures. Epilepsia 22:489, 1981. *The currently accepted classification of epileptic seizures and definition of relevant terms.*

Dreifus FE, Lee SI: Epilepsy Case Studies. Garden City, Medical Examination Publishing Company, 1981. *A brief introduction to the clinical approach to epilepsy, followed by a large number of case histories illustrating specific points with questions, answers, discussions, and appropriate references.*

Engel J Jr, Crandall PH, Rausch R: The Partial Epilepsies. *In* Rosenberg RN, et al. (eds.): The Clinical Neurosciences. New York, Churchill Livingstone, 1983. *A discussion of surgical therapy for epilepsy, including presurgical evaluation and operative techniques.*

Engel J Jr, Troupin AS, Crandall PH, Sterman MB, Wasterlain CG: Recent developments in the diagnosis and therapy of epilepsy. Ann Intern Med 97:584, 1982. *A concise review of modern approaches to the management of epileptic patients. Includes recent references.*

Epilepsy Abstracts 1947–present. *Published first by* Excerpta Medica, *this monthly journal contains abstracts of all epilepsy-related papers and is an easy entrance into the literature on any subject.*

Gastaut H, Broughton R: Epileptic Seizures. Springfield, Charles C Thomas, 1972. *Complete descriptions of almost all epileptic phenomena.*

Gumnit RJ: The Epilepsy Handbook, The Practical Management of Seizures. New York, Raven Press, 1983. *An excellent practical guide for the diagnosis and treatment of patients with epilepsy. Does not include references.*

Penfield W, Jasper H: Epilepsy and the Functional Anatomy of the Brain. Boston, Little Brown, 1954. *A classic by pioneers of modern epileptology; describes epileptic phenomena and applications of clinical data to the understanding of normal brain functions.*

Schwartzkroin PA, Wyler AR: Mechanisms underlying epileptiform burst discharges. Ann Neurol 7:95, 1980. *A Review of basic research on epileptic mechanisms and an attempt to synthesize conflicting data from various experimental models.*

Solomon GE, Kutt H, Plum F: Clinical Management of Seizures. Philadelphia, W. B. Saunders Company, 1983. *This small handbook is packed with information for the practicing physician, including many illustrations, tables, and references.*

Spehlmann R: EEG Primer. Amsterdam, Elsevier/North Holland, 1981. *A simple straightforward introduction to clinical EEG.*

Temkin O: The Falling Sickness: A History of Epilepsy from the Greeks to the Beginnings of Modern Neurology. Baltimore, Johns Hopkins University Press, 1945. *A detailed account of epilepsy facts and fiction throughout history.*

Woodbury DM, Penry JK, Pippenger CE (eds.): Antiepileptic Drugs. New York, Raven Press, 1982. *A multiauthored compendium of recent concepts of pharmacologic therapy of epilepsy.*

Section Twelve INTRACRANIAL TUMORS AND STATES OF ALTERED INTRACRANIAL PRESSURE

511. INTRACRANIAL TUMORS

William R. Shapiro

Intracranial tumors include neoplasms, both benign and malignant, and space-taking lesions of chronic inflammatory origin (granulomas) that develop in brain, meninges, or skull. The present chapter concerns neoplasms; granulomas are covered elsewhere. Neoplastic tumors frequently affect the nervous system. Primary tumors of the central nervous system are the second most common cancer in children, and in adults are more common than systemic Hodgkin's disease. In 1983 in the United States there were approximately 12,000 new cases of primary central nervous system cancer. About 15 per cent of deaths from systemic cancer are directly associated with metastases of the nervous system, mostly from primaries in lung or breast, malignant melanoma, lymphomas, and leukemias.

PATHOGENESIS. ***Intracranial Neoplasms as a Form of Cancer.*** The cause of brain tumors is unknown, although genetic factors appear to be important in tumors such as hemangioblastoma, neurofibroma, and some gliomas. When a patient develops systemic cancer, his body must deal with a "cancer burden" consisting of a population of neoplastic cells in the blood or bone marrow (leukemia) or in a solid, single mass or in multiple metastatic masses (carcinoma or sarcoma). For the average adult, it is thought that a 1-kg burden of systemic tumor is lethal. In contrast, a brain tumor shares its space in the skull with the brain, which already occupies 1200 cc, and in this confined space 100 grams of tumor is almost always lethal. By the time a patient develops neurologic symptoms, the tumor is usually 30 to 60 grams in size. Benign intracranial tumors are slow growing, with few mitoses, no necrosis, and no vascular proliferation. They may arise in the meninges or as neuroectodermal tumors. Malignant tumors are characterized by more rapid growth, invasiveness, frequent mitotic figures, necrosis, vascular proliferation, and endothelial hyperplasia. However, "benign" brain tumors that cannot be entirely excised will be lethal, and "malignant" brain tumors rarely metastasize out of the central nervous system. Thus, the distinction between benign and malignant is less important for intracranial tumors than for systemic cancer.

Intracranial tumors differ from systemic cancers in several other ways. Primary neuroectodermal tumors tend to infiltrate the brain, whereas secondary metastatic brain tumors are partly encapsulated. The microenvironment of tumors in the brain—the blood-brain barrier—influences both diagnosis and therapy. The blood-brain barrier in normal brain retards entry of many compounds, including radiologic contrast agents and chemotherapeutic drugs. The blood-brain barrier appears to be intact in most benign neuroectodermal tumors, but it becomes progressively disrupted in malignant brain tumors. The breakdown of the barrier allows the entry of contrast agents and radioisotopes that permit the tumor to be perceived separately from the brain in scanning techniques. Both experimental and clinical studies suggest that the disruption of the barrier in malignant tumors also permits the entry of chemotherapeutic agents. It is not yet clear to what degree the blood-brain barrier breaks down at the growing edge of an infiltrative malignant brain tumor or within very small brain tumors; in both circumstances, the barrier may be only minimally disrupted. A second factor that distinguishes brain tumors from systemic cancer is the absence of a lymphatic system in the brain. Fluid that accumulates from leaking capillaries within the brain tumor cannot be removed except via slow diffusion toward the cerebrospinal fluid (CSF) pathways. This fluid, or "cerebral edema," itself produces symptoms by adding to the mass effect of tumors. Central nervous system tumors are also distinguished from systemic cancer by the rarity with which they metastasize to the rest of the body. Instead, they tend to infiltrate within the brain, and some have a predilection to spread along CSF pathways, producing obstruction and hydrocephalus. Perhaps the most important difference between central nervous system neoplasms and systemic cancer is that "cancer operations" are not possible in the brain. Removing generous margins of normal tissue along with such visceral tumors as lung or colonic cancer interferes with normal function to only a moderate degree. On the other hand, attempting to remove normal tissue margins in brain tumor can produce irreparable neurologic dysfunction. The surgeon removing visceral cancer operates in the surrounding normal tissue. The neurosurgeon attempting to remove a primary neuroectodermal tumor must stay within the confines of the tumor if he is to spare brain tissue. Often, he must leave tumor-infiltrated brain tissue because its removal would produce unacceptable neurologic dysfunction. Such considerations weigh heavily in the management of patients with intracranial neoplasms.

CLASSIFICATION AND PATHOLOGY. Tumors of the nervous system may be classified by pathology and by location. Table 511–1 depicts a classification of intracranial tumors by both pathology and location. Pathologically tumors are defined in terms of their tissues of origin. Neuroectodermal tumors are the most common primary parenchymal tumors of the central nervous system and occur at any age. About half are relatively benign, infiltrating astrocytomas, but they may be cystic. Neuroectodermal tumors can arise in the cerebrum in the form of astrocytomas, oligodendrogliomas, and the more malignant glioblastoma multiforme. Childhood astrocytomas tend to lie in the cerebellum and are frequently cured by surgical extirpation. Juvenile astrocytomas occur around the third ventricle, and most brainstem gliomas are infiltrating astrocytomas. Adult astrocytomas may be calcified, and some undergo malignant degeneration. The oligodendroglioma is often calcified but only rarely becomes malignant. The classic malignant parenchymal brain tumor is the glioblastoma multiforme. This tumor may arise de novo or by progressive malignant degeneration of an astrocytoma. About half of all intracranial gliomas are glioblastomas; 20 per cent are astrocytomas. In children, astrocytomas represent half of the cerebellar tumors, medulloblastomas and ependymomas making up the rest of the intracranial tumors.

Older classifications defined astrocytomas in four grades from the histologically most benign (grade I) to the most malignant (grade IV). However, a simpler classification has been shown in trials of brain tumor therapy to correlate more predictably with prognosis. *Astrocytomas* are characterized histologically by increased numbers of uniform cells resembling fibrillary gemistocytic or, less commonly, protoplasmic astrocytes; mitoses are absent. Patients harboring this tumor commonly survive four to seven years or longer. *Anaplastic astrocytomas* contain astrocytic elements with considerable nuclear pleomorphism, markedly increased cellular density, increased mitotic figures, endothelial hyperplasia, but no necrosis. These tumors are associated with survival of 1.5 to 2.5 years. *Glioblastoma multiforme* is characterized by heterogeneous cell populations with bizarre pleomorphic nuclei that make it difficult to identify their astrocytic origin. There is prominent endothelial hyperplasia and areas of focal necrosis that often resemble palisades. Survival with this tumor exceeds a year in only a minority of patients.

Intracranial ependymomas occur primarily in children as fourth ventricle masses that obstruct the CSF pathways. Medulloblastomas arise from a primitive neuroectodermal cell, usually in the cerebellum, and may seed throughout the CSF. They are highly malignant, although sensitive to radiation therapy and chemotherapy.

Mesodermal tumors are represented most commonly by the benign meningioma. Meningiomas arise in certain favored sites: along the dorsal surface of the brain, the base of the skull, the

TABLE 511–1. CLASSIFICATION OF INTRACRANIAL TUMORS

	Location and Macroscopic Characteristics	Microscopic Characteristics
Neuroectodermal		
Astrocytoma	Diffuse infiltration, especially cerebrum and brainstem; microcystic or macrocystic, especially in cerebellum; occasionally calcifies	Astrocytic proliferation and infiltration; may convert to glioblastoma multiforme
Oligodendroglioma	Circumscribed, globular mass, often cystic and often calcifies	Diffuse, cellular, wide perinuclear halos; rarely becomes malignant
Glioblastoma multiforme (malignant astrocytoma)	Variegated, infiltrative; occasionally cystic, necrotic, or hemorrhagic	Cellular pleomorphism, necrosis, palisading; endothelial hyperplasia, mitoses present
Ependymoma	Most often fourth ventricle, demarcated	Regular, polygonal cells that form rosettes; rarely malignant
Medulloblastoma	Most commonly arises in vermis of cerebellum in children	Highly cellular, hyperchromatic nuclei; seeds the meninges via CSF
Mesodermal meningioma	Arises from dura on dorsal surface, along base of brain, from falx, sphenoid ridge	Benign, variable pattern; rarely converts to malignant tumor
Cranial nerves		
Acoustic schwannoma (acoustic neurilemoma), trigeminal neurilemoma	Nodular mass on cranial nerve	Benign, Schwann cell proliferation
Neurofibroma	Nodular mass on cranial nerve	Schwann cell and fibroblast proliferation
Pituitary tumors		
Adenomas	Sellar and suprasellar masses of various sizes	Chromophobic, acidophilic, and basophilic; all may be secretory or nonsecretory
Craniopharyngioma	Sellar or suprasellar, often calcified and cystic	Derived from Rathke's pouch
Pineal tumors	Germinomas, may produce endocrinopathy	May seed via CSF
Metastatic tumors	Parenchymal, skull, meningeal	Depends on nature of primary tumor
Vascular tumors	Arteriovenous malformation	Non-neoplastic
	Hemangioblastoma (von Hippel-Lindau syndrome)	Neoplastic
Congenital tumors	Craniopharyngioma, chordoma, dermoid, teratoma	
Granuloma and parasitic cysts	Tuberculoma, toruloma (cryptococcosis), sarcoidosis, cysticercosis	

falx cerebri, the sphenoid ridge, or within the lateral ventricles. Although these tumors are benign, they often reach large size before they are discovered and may be difficult to remove. The most common cranial nerve tumor is the acoustic schwannoma (neurilemoma, neuroma). Such tumors have been discovered earlier in recent years through the advent of refined auditory tests and computed tomographic (CT) scans and are frequently removable via a translabyrinthine approach. The pituitary tumors include the adenomas and the craniopharyngiomas. Pituitary adenomas may appear as intrasellar masses extending into an extrasellar location. The advent of advanced radiologic techniques has made it easier to diagnose microadenomas of the pituitary. Craniopharyngiomas are developmental tumors derived from Rathke's pouch and may be intrasellar or suprasellar in location; they are frequently calcified and often cystic. Pineal tumors occur primarily in children and rarely truly originate from the pineal gland; most commonly they are germinomas and may produce endocrinopathies. Metastatic tumors may invade the brain parenchyma, the skull, or the meninges; their pathology depends on the primary tumor. The benign colloid cyst usually grows in the anterior third ventricle. Vascular tumors include arteriovenous malformations, which are not truly neoplastic, and the hemangioblastomas, which are. The latter tumors, when located in the brainstem or cerebellum, may be part of the von Hippel–Lindau syndrome that includes hemangioblastomas elsewhere in the body. Congenital tumors include the craniopharyngiomas, chordomas (that arise from the primitive notochord), dermoids, and teratomas. Granulomas and parasitic cysts come from tuberculomas, cryptococcosis (toruloma), sarcoidosis, and cysticercosis.

PATHOPHYSIOLOGY. Brain tumors produce *generalized symptoms* because of their expanding size and *focal symptoms* by direct compression on or infiltration into specific areas of the brain. As tumors grow, they raise the intracranial pressure because the volume of the intracranial cavity is fixed. The total mass effect is a sum of both the tumor size and the cerebral edema the tumor produces. Large tumor masses obstruct the CSF pathways, producing enlargement of the upstream ventricular system. As the primary or secondary mass produced by the tumor enlarges, brain tissue may be displaced through the fixed intracranial openings, producing various herniation syndromes as discussed in Ch. 472.

Focally, the mass of the tumor compresses and infiltrates the surrounding brain tissue. Edema, produced within a parenchymal brain tumor, increases the total size of the mass. Cerebral edema may also be produced by compression by an extra-axial tumor, in which case the edema comes from the brain itself. Focal symptoms occur as the tumor compresses surrounding brain, producing distortion and ischemia; such symptoms may be reversible if the pressure is relieved before tissue necrosis occurs. In addition, tumor tissue may infiltrate along nerve fiber tracts, interfering with neurologic function. Cyst formation within tumors provides another mechanism that compresses adjacent normal brain.

CLINICAL MANIFESTATIONS. The symptoms and signs of intracranial tumor depend on the size of the tumor and on its rate of growth. The characteristic clinical feature of intracranial neoplasms is that they produce progressive symptoms. The rate of progression ranges from an acute apoplectic onset such as follows hemorrhage into an intracranial neoplasm, or a seizure disorder associated with cortical stimulation to a slowly progressive mental deterioration associated with slower growing neoplasms.

Headache occurs frequently as a general manifestation of an intracranial neoplasm and most commonly accompanies rapidly growing tumors. Of special importance are headaches that have recently begun or changed in character, are worse in the morning or awaken the patient at night, or are of a recurrent nature. The occurrence of a headache in a patient not otherwise prone to headaches or a recent change in headache pattern in patients known to have headaches should alert the physician to a possible intracranial expanding lesion.

Papilledema occurs in only about one fourth of patients with intracranial neoplasms, and its absence does not exclude such pathology. It is more likely to accompany tumors that obstruct CSF flow and may be accompanied by visual phenomena, especially acute visual obscurations and "graying out." Papilledema is part of the "pseudotumor cerebri" syndrome described below.

Generalized convulsions, along with focal seizures (see below), occur in 35 per cent of patients with cerebral tumors. They are more likely to accompany slower-growing tumors than the more rapid malignant neoplasms. They are more likely to occur following alcohol use or withdrawal of barbiturates or other sedative drugs. The onset of generalized convulsions in the adult or focal seizures at any age should alert the physician to the possibility of a structural lesion. Intracranial tumors produce generalized major motor seizures and various forms of focal seizures. Minor temporal lobe seizures that occasionally resemble petit mal attacks may accompany temporal lobe tumors. Other lesions of the temporal lobe may give rise to psychomotor seizures that may be associated with olfactory hallucinations (uncinate fits), disorders of visual or auditory perception, or episodes of "déjà vu" phenomena or of automatic behavior. Jacksonian seizures usually imply a lesion of the motor or sensory cortex.

Mental changes are frequent manifestations of intracranial tumor. They are often subtle in quality and gradual in onset and may not attract the attention of coworkers or family members until the patient's behavior changes substantially. Mental changes may include impersistence in routine tasks, increased irritability, emotional lability, inertia, faulty insight and forgetfulness, reduction in the range of mental activity, indifference to social practices, reduced initiative and spontaneity, and blunted affect. The patient may complain of fatigue, tiredness, dizziness, and lethargy. If the tumor continues to grow, such symptoms progress to confusion, dementia, and eventually stupor. Changes in personality may be described in psychologic terms but should be recognized as symptoms of structural brain disease rather than functional anxiety or depression.

Nausea and vomiting may occur as a result of direct or reflex stimulation of the emetic center of the medulla. This most often accompanies increased intracranial pressure, particularly with brainstem displacement secondary to herniation or bleeding into the CSF. Vomiting that occurs without preceding nausea may be projectile.

Vasomotor and autonomic changes that accompany expanding intracranial tumors include bradycardia and hypertension, as well as respiratory abnormalities associated with brainstem compression. Rarely, patients with brain tumor may have gastric ulceration (Cushing's ulcer) that may produce hemorrhage. Fortunately, however, the adrenal corticosteroids used for treating the edema of brain tumors rarely contribute to such hemorrhages. Other autonomic changes associated with hypothalamic compression include fever, hypothermia, hyperthermia, disturbances in eating and drinking, and occasionally more specific abnormalities such as diabetes insipidus, inappropriate antidiuretic hormone secretion, hypopituitarism, and precocious puberty.

False localizing signs may accompany prolonged elevation of intracranial pressure. They include unilateral or bilateral lateral rectus palsy from sixth nerve traction and compression, hemiplegia ipsilateral to a cerebral tumor from compression of the opposite cerebral peduncle against the tentorium, and visual field defects ipsilateral to the tumor from compression of the opposite posterior cerebral artery.

Focal clinical manifestations of intracranial tumors depend on localized impairment of nervous tissue function, and therefore vary with the location of the process. Of specific interest are focal seizures which sometimes accompany cerebral tumors. They imply specific cortical irritation from either a benign or a malignant condition. Visual loss—reduced visual acuity, field defects, or diplopia—implies involvement of the visual apparatus from a local eye problem to the occipital cortex or to the oculomotor nerves. Hearing impairment may mean reduced auditory acuity or the occurrence of tinnitus, and may be associated with vertigo. Speech disturbances may be transient or progressive and include dysphasia and dysarthria. Motor signs include postural disturbances, incoordination, weakness, and tremor. Sensory disturbances include unusual pains, paresthesias, or numbness. Ataxia may accompany local tumors in the posterior fossa or occasionally in the frontal lobes. Anosmia may be associated with infrafrontal meningiomas. Neuroendocrine disturbances may accompany pituitary and pineal tumors. Cerebral hemorrhage into a tumor, usually choriocarcinoma, testicular tumors, melanomas, glioblastomas, and, more rarely, other primary tumors, may produce an associated subarachnoid hemorrhage.

TUMOR SYNDROMES. Tumors of the cerebral hemispheres are characterized by progressive, focal neurologic deficits and commonly by generalized or focal convulsive seizures. Tumors of the *frontal lobe*, being in a "silent area," often first cause impairment of judgment and of intellectual function. Tumors involving the motor pathways produce contralateral hemiplegia. A tumor of the medial surface of the frontal lobe may cause urinary urgency or, occasionally, precipitate incontinence. Mental changes and ataxic gait are common when the tumor spreads across the corpus callosum to both frontal lobes. Tumors of the dominant hemisphere are frequently associated with disturbances in language.

Parietal lobe tumors may produce either generalized convulsions or sensory focal seizures. Cutaneous tactile, pain, and temperature senses are usually spared, but stereognosis and the cortical sensory modalities (position sense, two-point discrimination) are impaired contralaterally. Contralateral homonymous hemianopia, apraxia, and anosognosia (nonrecognition of bodily defects) may also be present with tumors in the nondominant hemisphere. Denial of illness is characteristic, especially if obtundation is present. Speech disturbances, agraphia, and finger agnosia may occur when the tumor involves the dominant hemisphere. Thalamic invasion produces contralateral cutaneous sensory impairment.

Temporal lobe tumors, particularly in the nondominant hemisphere, are often relatively "silent" except when they cause convulsive seizures. A tumor deep in the temporal lobe may cause contralateral hemianopia, psychomotor seizures, or convulsive seizures, preceded by an olfactory aura or visual hallucinations of complex formed images. Tumors involving the surface of the dominant temporal lobe produce mixed expressive and receptive aphasia or dysphasia, chiefly anomia.

Occipital lobe tumors usually cause contralateral quadrantic defects in the visual field or a hemianopia with sparing of central vision. Associated seizures may be preceded by an aura of flashing lights, but not formed images.

Cranial, extradural, or subdural metastatic tumors, by compression or invasion of the underlying brain tissue, produce the same localizing signs as those caused by primary tumors.

Tumors of the *pituitary* and suprasellar region produce neurologic and endocrinologic abnormalities. Pituitary adenomas may present as intrasellar secretory or nonsecretory masses, or masses with extrasellar extension. Secretory adenomas produce hormones that cause specific endocrinopathies. For example, adenomas that overproduce growth hormone lead to gigantism prior to puberty and acromegaly after puberty. Basophilic adenoma produces ACTH, leading to Cushing's syndrome. Chromophobe adenomas once were believed not to secrete hormones, but now are known to be responsible for most of the endocrinopathies caused by pituitary tumors. The most common endocrine hypersecretion is prolactin, producing amenorrhea and galactorrhea in women and, less frequently, impotence and gynecomastia in men. Many secretory tumors are microadenomas found only after an endocrine abnormality is discovered.

Enlarging pituitary adenomas cause headache; as the tumor grows out of the sella, it compresses the optic chiasm, nerve, or tracts and the hypothalamus. The most common visual field defect is bitemporal hemianopia, but unilateral optic atrophy, contralateral hemianopia, or any combination of the three may occur. Hypothalamic compression usually causes diabetes insipidus from injury to the supraoptic-pituitary tract. The tumor may destroy functioning glandular tissue and cause pituitary deficiency. Skull x-rays show a characteristic balloon-shaped appearance of the sella, but microadenomas may produce no more than laterally placed focal bulging of the sellar floor, visible only on x-ray tomograms.

Other tumors in the region of the sella turcica (e.g., meningiomas, craniopharyngiomas, metastases, dermoid cysts) or aneurysms may compress the optic chiasm, invade the sella, and produce symptoms similar to those of chromophobe adenoma.

Pineal tumors (usually germinomas) occur at any age but are most common in childhood. Precocious puberty may result, especially in boys. The tumor compresses the aqueduct of Sylvius, causing hydrocephalus, papilledema, and other signs of increased intracranial pressure. The pretectum rostral to the superior colliculi is also compressed, resulting in paralysis of upward gaze, ptosis, and loss of pupillary light and accommodation reflexes.

Gliomas of the brainstem are usually astrocytomas, of which about one half eventually become anaplastic. Symptoms result from destruction of nuclear masses or unilateral or bilateral paralysis of the fifth, sixth, seventh, and tenth cranial nerves and paralysis of lateral gaze. Damage to the motor or sensory pathways causes hemiplegia, hemianesthesia, or cerebellar disturbance (ataxia, nystagmus, intention tremor). Increased intracranial pressure appears late in brainstem tumors.

Posterior fossa tumors: Tumors of the fourth ventricle and cerebellum (usually medulloblastomas, ependymomas, or occasionally a metastasis) interfere with CSF circulation, and symptoms of increased pressure appear early. Ataxic gait, intention tremor, and other signs of cerebellar dysfunction follow.

Cerebellopontine angle tumors, particularly acoustic schwannomas, are characterized by tinnitus, unilateral hearing impairment, and sometimes vertigo. Pressure on the adjacent cranial nerves, brainstem, and cerebellum produces loss of corneal reflex, facial palsy and anesthesia, palatal weakness, signs of cerebellar dysfunction, and, rarely, contralateral hemiplegia or anesthesia. Loss of vestibular response to caloric stimulation, enlargement of the porus acusticus as shown by skull x-ray, and a high CSF protein content suggest an acoustic schwannoma.

Diffuse meningeal neoplasm (meningeal carcinomatosis): Carcinomas, gliomas, sarcomas, melanomas, and lymphomas may diffusely infiltrate the leptomeninges and subarachnoid space to produce a syndrome of chronic meningitis, which may simulate chronic meningitis caused by fungi, tuberculosis, sarcoidosis, and meningovascular syphilis. Characteristically, there is involvement of more than one central nervous system region, i.e., brain, cranial nerves, spinal cord and nerves. Common manifestations include headache, mental changes, cranial nerve palsies, weakness and areflexia, and minimal or no signs of meningeal irritation. The CSF findings generally establish the diagnosis. The pressure may be normal or elevated, sugar content is often below 45 mg per deciliter, protein content is usually elevated, and cell counts may reveal an increased number of mononuclear cells or cytologic evidence of malignant cells. Cultures are negative. Biochemical tumor markers (β-glucuronidase) are frequently present.

Optic nerve gliomas may develop in the intraorbital, retroorbital, or chiasmatic region of the optic nerve, the first being most common. These tumors usually occur in early childhood, with uniocular loss of vision as the most common presenting symptom. Proptosis is seen in about a third of the cases. Uniocular optic atrophy or papilledema may be noted. X-ray evidence of enlargement of the optic foramen is common. The tumor is most often a slowly growing astrocytoma, may be associated with neurofibromatosis, and will occasionally invade the hypothalamus.

Tumors of the skull: Benign osteomas rarely reach a size sufficient to compress underlying brain. Malignant tumors arising in the paranasal sinuses or nasopharynx directly invade the base of the skull and cause chronic facial pain and multiple cranial nerve involvement. Tumors of the glomus jugulare (nonchromaffin paraganglioma) arise near the jugular bulb and often lead to progressive deafness and a bloody discharge in the external auditory canal. Other lesions that give x-ray evidence of bone destruction and that must be differentiated include Paget's disease, Hand-Schüller-Christian disease, eosinophilic granuloma, and cholesteatoma (epidermoids). As noted, metastases are common to the skull and will occasionally invade through the dura to produce subdural effusions indistinguishable in their manifestations from subdural hematoma.

DIAGNOSIS. Computed tomography and now nuclear magnetic resonance (NMR) scanning permit the diagnosis of most intracranial tumors at a level of safety not achievable by invasive techniques. Such tumors produce abnormalities in the normal structures and may be visualized directly or after the intravenous infusion of iodide-containing contrast material (see Fig. 511–1). Skull tumors are seen as eroded regions of bone. Parenchymal lesions may distort the normal ventricular structures and produce cerebral edema visible as low density regions in the brain's parenchyma. After intravenous contrast enhancement, the tumor may be visualized as a hyperdense region, frequently ring-like, around a central radiolucent area. The more malignant the tumor, the more densely enhanced will it appear. The degree of enhancement is a function of the breakdown of the blood-brain barrier rather than of the presence of tumor cells themselves, and therefore is much more likely to occur with more malignant tumors. Low density lesions may imply cysts, necrotic tumor, or cerebral edema. Ventricular enlargement occurs secondary to obstruction of CSF pathways. CT has almost eliminated the need for pneumoencephalography in the diagnosis of brain tumor, although contrast-enhanced arteriography may be necessary as an aid to guiding surgical treatment. In the latter technique, the tumors are visualized as displacing normal blood vessels and often demonstrate abnormal vasculature within the tumor itself.

Routine skull x-rays are usually not needed when high-quality CT scanning is available. Similarly, electroencephalography and isotope encephalography have been largely replaced by CT scanning as a screening test for brain tumor.

Lumbar puncture and examination of CSF rarely contribute to the diagnosis of intracranial neoplasm except for diffuse meningeal carcinomatosis. Lumbar puncture is contraindicated in the presence of raised intracranial pressure associated with a mass lesion producing incipient herniation. A CSF examination for meningeal carcinomatosis should be deferred until after CT is used to search for solid intracranial neoplasms.

DIFFERENTIAL DIAGNOSIS. The characteristic clinical feature of intracranial neoplasm is progressive neurologic dysfunction traceable to a focal neurologic origin. The onset may be abrupt, as when a hemorrhage or seizure occurs, or may be insidious as the brain tumor grows. Any neurologic disease producing similar symptoms can be confused with intracranial neoplasm; a neoplasm should be ruled out while considering other diagnoses. Computed tomography is the procedure of choice. The importance of considering other neurologic syndromes in differential diagnosis lies in emphasizing the clinical differences that should lead the physician to search for intracranial neoplasm.

Benign intracranial hypertension is described in detail elsewhere (Ch. 513). Patients develop headache and papilledema but usually have no focal signs, and CT demonstrates no mass lesions. Patients with stroke characteristically present with acute onset of neurologic dysfunction, although occasionally a "stuttering" onset may be confused with the insidious history of tumor. Patients with subdural hematoma may have headache, drowsiness, papilledema, and hemiparesis; the diagnosis can be suspected on clinical grounds but requires CT or arteriography for certainty. Patients with dementia from Alzheimer's disease usually have minimal motor abnormalities. The problem of differentiating tumor from granuloma or abscess is more difficult. Cysticercosis is suggested by exposure to an endemic area and by the presence of eosinophilic pleo-

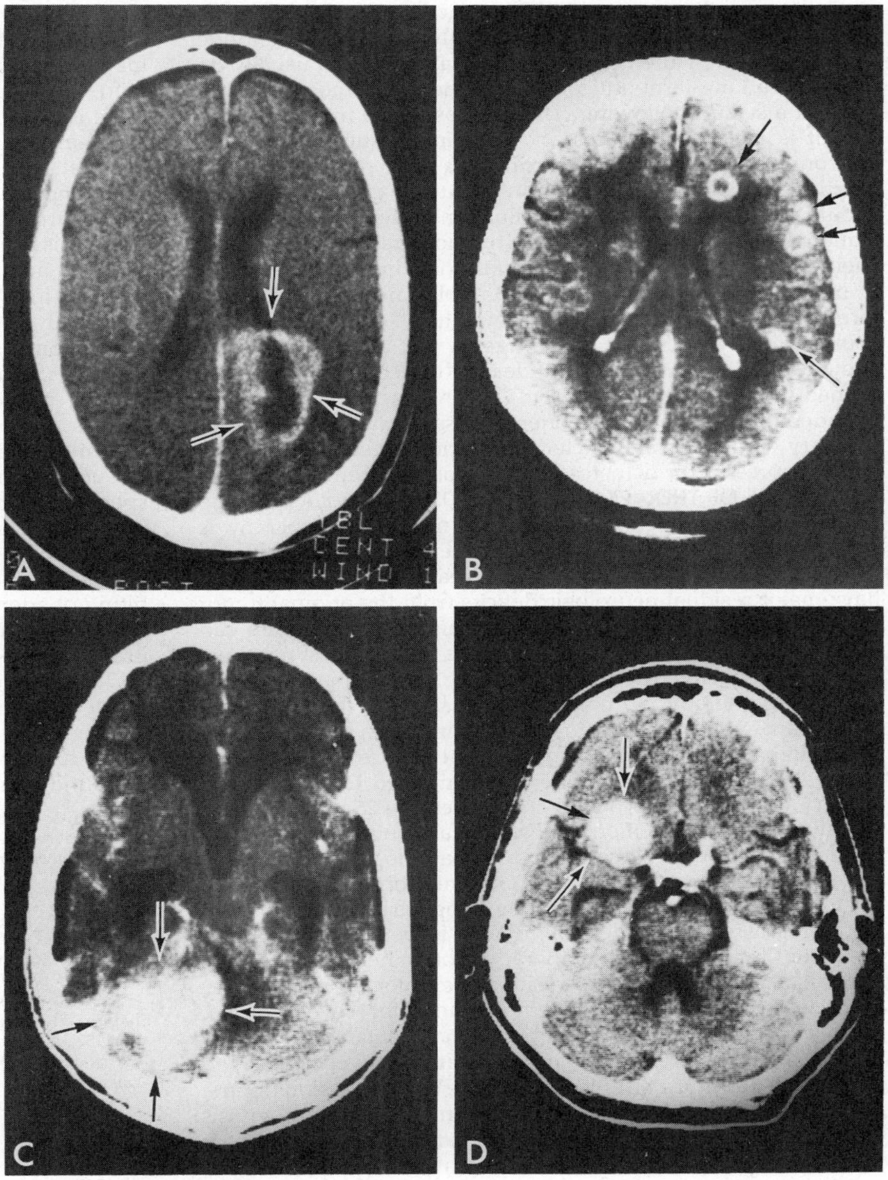

Figure 511–1. Computed tomographic scans of patients with intracranial tumors. *(A)* Glioblastoma multiforme of the medial parieto-occipital lobes. Note the ring enhancement with central region of hypodensity (arrows). *(B)* Multiple metastatic brain tumors from carcinoma of the lung. Each enhanced mass represents a brain tumor (arrows). *(C)* Medulloblastoma of the right and mid-cerebellum. Note the displacement and encroachment of the fourth ventricle and hydrocephalus (arrows). *(D)* Sphenoid wing meningioma. The lesion is diffusely contrast enhanced (arrows).

cytosis in the CSF. Although CT scans are usually characteristic, a differential diagnosis between tumor and brain abscess can sometimes be difficult and may require biopsy.

TREATMENT. ***Surgery.*** The principles of treating intracranial neoplasm include its removal if possible, its palliation if unresectable. Surgery for intracerebral tumors has several goals: (1) diagnosis, which can be established in life only by surgical tissue removal; (2) treatment of symptoms, especially those arising from increased intracranial pressure; (3) debulking of tumor as a form of anticancer therapy; and (4) permitting time for radiation and early chemotherapy. Surgery for meningiomas should be aimed at total removal and cure if possible, and subtotal removal to relieve symptoms if total removal is not possible. For infratentorial parenchymal tumors, surgery is necessary for diagnosis and to open CSF pathways. Surgery for benign cerebellar or acoustic schwannomas is potentially curative. For acoustic schwannoma, surgery may be accomplished by a translabyrinthine approach if the tumors are small, or by suboccipital craniectomy if the tumors are larger. Surgery for metastatic brain tumors should be considered in selective circumstances if the metastatic tumor is single or if systemic disease is minimal or well controlled. Pituitary tumors are usually removed by transsphenoidal resection, although, if they are large, a transfrontal craniotomy may be necessary.

Radiation Therapy. Radiation is utilized primarily for malignant tumors. The radiation therapy is delivered through whole-head or large-field ports for a total dose of up to 6000 rads in six to seven weeks. Radiation therapy has been recommended as a form of treatment in low grade astrocytomas and oligodendrogliomas, although the efficacy of such therapy has not been demonstrated by prospective trials. For such tumors, the radiation is usually limited to the region of the tumor at total doses of 5000 to 5500 rads. Radiation therapy is the therapy of choice for most metastatic brain tumors. Radiation therapy is frequently recommended for large pituitary tumors after surgery.

Medical Therapy. Corticosteroid hormone therapy usually will relieve cerebral edema if present. Steroids almost always improve general clinical manifestations, but are less effective against specific clinical manifestations. Dexamethasone in doses of 16 to 32 mg per day is recommended, although attempts should be made to reduce the doses slowly to a level of relatively stable symptoms. Anticonvulsants are given to patients who have seizures, and any patient who develops generalized or focal seizures should be placed on anticonvulsants for three to five years or permanently, if attacks continue postoperatively. Patients who do not have seizures usually do not require long-term anticonvulsant therapy. Since the likelihood of a seizure following clean neurosurgical intervention is low, it is usually not necessary to maintain such patients on anticonvulsants. Seizures occurring late after primary therapy for intracranial neoplasms imply recurrence of tumor and should immediately lead to re-evaluation of the patient's status. National cooperative trials have demonstrated that several chemotherapeutic agents are useful in the adjunctive treatment of malignant astrocytomas. Two examples are bis-chloroethyl-nitrosourea (BCNU) and methyl-cyclohexyl-chloroethyl-nitrosourea (methyl-CCNU). These agents are highly toxic and should only be administered under the direction of physicians trained in their use.

Endocrine replacement is often necessary after treatment of pituitary adenomas and includes anterior pituitary hormones and vasopressin for diabetes insipidus as required.

OUTCOME OF THERAPY AND PROGNOSIS. For *malignant neuroectodermal tumors,* e.g., glioblastoma multiforme, therapy is palliative, almost never curative. Patients are often able to return to gainful employment for a year or two, unless they have major residual neurologic deficits from the original tumor or from the surgery. Late radiation damage to the brain can occur and may be responsible for the return of symptoms, although tumor recurrence accounts for most patient worsening. Chemotherapy is immunosuppressive and bone marrow depressant, and may lead to systemic infection and bleeding. For malignant astrocytomas, most recent studies give a median survival time of 52 weeks following combined treatment with surgery, radiation, and BCNU chemotherapy; 25 to 30 per cent of patients survive 18 months. Factors favoring longer survival include age younger than 50, histopathology of anaplastic astrocytoma rather than glioblastoma multiforme, and minimal postoperative neurologic deficit. The prognosis for more benign intracerebral neuroectodermal tumors is better than for the malignant tumors. Radiation therapy is often helpful. Although patients may have minimal residual neurologic deficits, they frequently return to gainful employment for several years. Seizures are likely, but control is usually obtained. Patients may survive for three to seven years with relatively preserved neurologic deficit until tumor recurrence or progression occurs. Childhood medulloblastoma carries a much better prognosis with the advent of whole neuraxis radiation therapy; five-year survival rates of 50 to 60 per cent are now being reported.

Following therapy of *metastatic brain tumors,* short-term results are often good. With a combination of steroids and either radiation therapy alone or a combination of surgery and radiation therapy, two thirds to three fourths of patients show substantive amelioration of presenting symptoms. Many patients are able to return to work for short periods of time. The median survival of such patients is approximately six months, with survival at a year limited to 10 to 15 per cent of the patients. Most patients do not die of their metastatic nervous system disease but rather of their primary or systemic cancer. There are occasional long-term survivors of more than two years. *Meningeal carcinomatosis* treated with combination radiation therapy and intrathecal chemotherapy often responds when the primary tumor is lymphoma or carcinoma of the breast. Both neurologic deficits and the CSF may improve for periods of up to a year or more. Affected patients usually die of their systemic disease.

Meningiomas are often curable. There may be residual neurologic deficits, including seizures, but overall the prognosis for survival is excellent, and that for neurologic recovery is good to very good. After surgery for meningiomas, most patients return to full-time employment. Meningiomas rarely recur and rarely become malignant, and most patients can be expected to survive a normal lifespan. The prognosis of patients with *acoustic schwannomas* depends on the size of the tumor. For small acoustic schwannomas and especially those removed by translabyrinthine approach, the results are excellent, with a low mortality and a high percentage of cures. Eighth nerve deficits, including hearing loss and some vestibular difficulty, may hinder overall functional capacity. Facial paresis is common, and occasionally functionally disturbing. In contrast, there is a 10 to 20 per cent mortality with surgical resection for large tumors and considerable morbidity. Many patients have residual neurologic deficits, including hearing loss, facial paresis, and hydrocephalus.

Pituitary tumors and *craniopharyngiomas* carry a fairly good prognosis. Fifty to 60 per cent of macroscopically obvious pituitary adenomas come to attention because of visual failure, whereas in 20 per cent headaches are the initial symptom. Less commonly, an endocrine abnormality is noted, although microadenomas, occurring primarily in women, are usually diagnosed because of infertility, galactorrhea, or amenorrhea. Rarely, pituitary apoplexy can occur. Adult craniopharyngiomas similarly have a good prognosis, although recurrence is somewhat more common than in children following therapy of such tumors. Pituitary tumors may be removed by transsphenoidal microsurgery or craniotomy. They may also be treated by irradiation alone or irradiation after surgery. Surgery is indicated if vision is threatened, but the method of treatment of microadenomas is controversial. Hyperprolactinemia from pituitary adenomas may be effectively treated with bromocriptine, but resection or irradiation is necessary to treat the tumor itself.

Other intracranial tumors generally have a good prognosis, depending on their location. *Cholesteatomas* and *colloid cysts* are usually easily removed with little neurologic deficit, although some tumors may not be resectable because of danger to surrounding normal brain.

Bloom HJG: Medulloblastoma in children: Increasing survival rates and further prospects. Int J Radiat Oncol Biol Phys 8:2023, 1982. *A concise review of the problem of therapy in this disease by a recognized authority. Well referenced.*

Cairncross JG, Kim J-H, Posner JB: Radiation therapy for brain metastases. Ann Neurol 7:529, 1980. *One of the largest series of such cases yet reported.*

Fishman RA: Brain edema. N Engl J Med 293:706, 1975. *An excellent review of the mechanisms of cerebral edema.*

Russell DS, Rubinstein LJ: Pathology of Tumours of the Nervous System. 4th ed. Baltimore, Williams & Wilkins Company, 1977. *An excellent, well illustrated textbook of tumors of the nervous system.*

Shapiro WR: Treatment of neuroectodermal brain tumors. Ann Neurol 12:231, 1982. *A review of the treatment of adult primary brain tumors; includes results of national cooperative trials of surgery, radiation therapy, and chemotherapy.*

Walker MD: Brain and peripheral nervous system tumors. In Holland JF, Frei E (eds.): Cancer Medicine. 2nd ed. Philadelphia, Lea & Febiger, 1982, p 1603. *A good review of the clinical presentation of central nervous system tumors.*

Wasserstrom WR, Glass JP, Posner JB: Diagnosis and treatment of leptomeningeal metastases from solid tumors: Experience with 90 patients. Cancer 49:759, 1982. *A definitive review of wide-ranging experience with this disease, including its diagnosis and treatment.*

512. INTRACRANIAL HYPOTENSION

David A. Rottenberg

Cerebrospinal fluid (CSF) pressure measured at lumbar puncture in the lateral decubitus position normally ranges from 70 to 200 mm CSF (5 to 15 mm Hg). Low (or zero) lumbar CSF pressure may be recorded in patients with chronic subdural hematoma or spinal subarachnoid block. Such low pressure recordings may be associated with normal or raised intracranial pressure in the absence of free communication between the ventriculocisternal and lumbar CSF compartments. Intracranial hypotension with low lumbar CSF pressure is usually a consequence of prior lumbar puncture, craniospinal CSF fistula, or profound dehydration. The term *aliquorrhea*—spontaneous or "primary" intracranial hypotension—has been used to describe those rare cases in which, in the absence of known or discernible CNS injury or disease, self-limited symptoms and signs of low spinal fluid pressure develop.

The clinical syndrome of low spinal fluid pressure is characterized by severe throbbing frontal and occipital headache, which appears within 30 seconds after the patient assumes an erect posture and which subsides completely when he lies down. Associated complaints may include dizziness, nausea, stiff neck, and photophobia. The disorder often arises 3 to 21 days after lumbar puncture, and the symptoms described are uncommonly followed by diplopia and a rapidly evolving (unilateral or bilateral) abducens palsy. In most instances, the palsy resolves completely within six weeks to six months. Rarely, auditory symptoms such as buzzing, popping, humming, roaring or frank hearing loss may supervene.

Symptoms and signs of intracranial hypotension probably result from CSF leakage, loss of the normal CSF "cushion," and caudal displacement of the brain within the cranial vault. Traction on pain-sensitive intracranial structures, including cerebral veins and venous sinuses dilated in a compensatory manner, and stretching of the abducens nerve over the apex of the petrous temporal bone probably account for the observed headache and diplopia. Auditory symptoms and signs may reflect a functionally important fall in intralabyrinthine pressure. Treatment is largely symptomatic, since the manifestations of the low spinal fluid pressure syndrome are almost always transient. When symptoms are persistent, disabling, or both, an *epidural "blood patch"* may be indicated. This procedure involves the injection of 10 ml of the patient's own blood into the epidural space to seal a presumed dural leak. Rarely, in very long-lasting cases surgical exploration has exposed the dural leak and closed it. As regards symptomatic intracranial hypotension following lumbar puncture, the use of a small (22-gauge) needle diminishes the risk of headache and abducens paralysis. Contrary to popular belief, bed rest has no effect on the incidence or duration of post-lumbar-puncture headache.

MacRobert RG: The cause of lumbar puncture headache. JAMA 70:1350, 1918. *A classic description of lumbar puncture headache. No better illustrations of the causative mechanism have ever been published.*

Vandam LD, Dripps RD: Long-term follow-up of patients who received 10,098 spinal anesthetics. JAMA 161:586, 1956. *This prospective study of over 10,000 spinal anesthetizations documents the incidence of headache associated with lumbar puncture and describes the syndrome of decreased intracranial pressure.*

513. INTRACRANIAL HYPERTENSION

David A. Rottenberg

Cerebrospinal fluid (CSF) pressure in excess of 250 mm CSF is usually a manifestation of serious underlying neurologic disease. Although intracranial hypertension is most often observed in the setting of a rapidly expanding intracranial mass lesion, CSF outflow obstruction or cerebral venous congestion as well as a variety of systemic and central nervous system disorders may be pathophysiologically associated with increased intracranial pressure (ICP) (Table 513–1). It should be emphasized that lumbar CSF pressure may not accurately reflect ICP. In patients with intracranial mass lesions and brain hernias, lumbar CSF pressure may be normal or low despite grossly elevated supratentorial CSF pressure. Kinking of the aqueduct of Sylvius or impaction of the temporal lobes into the tentorial incisura or of the cerebellar tonsils into the foramen magnum can prevent the transmission of ICP into the lumbar subarachnoid space.

There are no pathognomonic symptoms or signs of intracranial hypertension. Nevertheless, the observation of frequently associated symptoms and signs such as headache, papilledema, unilateral pupillary dilatation, oculomotor or abducens paresis, irregular respirations, and so forth should indicate possible raised intracranial pressure. Most of the signs and symptoms traditionally associated with intracranial hypertension are related to traction on cerebral blood vessels, distortion of pain-sensitive dura mater, impending herniation with intermittent vascular compression, midline shifts, or axial distortion of the brainstem and are not caused by increased ICP per se. Papilledema, when present, is the most reliable sign of intracranial hypertension; however, many patients with raised ICP fail to develop papilledema, and in some patients with pseudotumor cerebri (see later discussion), papilledema develops and then subsides spontaneously although CSF pressure remains elevated. Moreover, papilledema is not synonymous with raised ICP. Ocular hypotony, bilateral optic neuritis, orbital venous stasis, retrobulbar tumors, and granulomatous inflammation or cystic lesions of the optic nerve sheath may produce papilledema in the absence of intracranial hypertension. Retinal venous pulsations, when present, imply that CSF pressure is normal or not significantly elevated, but the absence of spontaneous venous pulsations is not helpful diagnostically. A variety of nonepileptic paroxysmal phenomena (crescendo headache, visual obscurations, photopsia, chalastic-hypertonic fits, impairment of consciousness, sensory hallucinations) have been described in relation to spontaneous elevations of ICP, often referred to as *plateau waves*. The occurrence of plateau waves during sleep may explain why nighttime deterioration and early morning headache are frequently reported by patients with raised ICP.

The initial treatment of any patient with increased ICP whose neurologic status is deteriorating is aimed at reducing the volume of the intracranial contents in an attempt to prevent irreversible brain damage (Table 513–2). Once the patient's condition has stabilized, additional treatment modalities are employed in an effort to consolidate the gains of emergency therapy and to allow the physician ample opportunity to deal with the underlying pathologic process. Almost always, ICP is not the actual cause of the patient's distress but a reflection of a pre-existing pathologic process; the definitive treatment of intracranial hypertension is ultimately determined by the nature of the underlying pathologic process.

TABLE 513–1. PATHOGENESIS OF INCREASED INTRACRANIAL PRESSURE

Perturbation	Proximate Cause	Clinical Example
Increased dural sinus venous pressure	Sinus compression or occlusion	Sagittal sinus thrombosis Otitic hydrocephalus Brain tumors
	Increased sinus blood flow	CO_2 retention Arteriovenous malformation
	Increased peripheral venous pressure	Internal jugular vein occlusion Superior vena cava syndrome Congestive heart failure
Increased CSF outflow resistance	Ventricular outflow obstruction	Brain tumors Aqueductal stenosis
	Obliteration of the cisternal and/or convexity subarachnoid space	Meningitis Extra- or subdural masses Cerebral masses or edema
	Plugging of the arachnoid villi	Subarachnoid hemorrhage Infectious polyneuritis Spinal cord tumors
Increased rate of CSF formation	Increased choroidal CSF formation	Choroid plexus papilloma
	Increased extrachoroidal CSF formation	Hypo-osmolality Cerebral edema

TABLE 513–2. EMERGENCY TREATMENT OF IMPENDING HERNIATION IN ACUTELY DECOMPENSATING PATIENTS

Therapy	Dosage or Procedure
Osmotherapy	Mannitol, 0.5 to 2.0 grams per kilogram intravenously over 15 minutes followed by 25 grams as needed
Corticosteroids	Dexamethasone, 100-mg intravenous push followed by 100 mg daily in divided doses
Hyperventilation	Lower P_{CO_2} to 25 to 30 mm Hg

Ethelberg S, Jensen VA: Obscurations and further time-related paroxysmal disorders in intracranial tumors; syndrome of initial herniation of parts of the brain through the tentorial incisure. Arch Neurol Psychiatr 68:130, 1952. *A fascinating account of pseudoparoxysmal phenomena in patients with intracranial tumors.*

Lundberg N: Continuous recording and control of ventricular fluid pressure in neurosurgical practice. Acta Psychiatr Neurol Scand (Suppl) 149:1, 1960. *An encyclopedic account of ventricular CSF pressure measurement and monitoring. The clinical significance of plateau waves is nowhere better discussed.*

Rottenberg DA, Posner JB: Intracranial pressure control. *In* Cottrell JE, Turndorf H (eds.): Anesthesia and Neurosurgery. St. Louis, C. V. Mosby Company, 1980, pp 89–118. *This well-referenced chapter provides a quantitative description of the CSF system. Some familiarity with the subject is helpful.*

514. PSEUDOTUMOR CEREBRI

David A. Rottenberg

DEFINITION. Pseudotumor cerebri is a syndrome of increased intracranial pressure in the absence of localizing neurologic signs, intracranial mass lesion, or cerebrospinal fluid (CSF) outflow obstruction in an alert, otherwise healthy appearing patient. Pseudotumor (also called *benign intracranial hypertension, serous meningitis,* or *otitic hydrocephalus*) can be associated with a variety of systemic and iatrogenic disorders. The illness is usually brief and benign, lasting weeks to several months. However, recurrent and chronic cases have been reported, and permanent visual loss rarely may occur in spite of vigorous medical or surgical treatment. Chronically increased intracranial pressure may give rise to the "primary empty sella syndrome," which refers to a globular enlargement of the sella turcica caused by an incompetent diaphragma sellae.

CLINICAL MANIFESTATIONS. Pseudotumor cerebri may be manifested as asymptomatic papilledema. More common early symptoms include headache, nausea and vomiting, visual disturbances (blurring, obscurations of vision, scotomata), retro-ocular pain, diplopia, tinnitus, and vertigo. Bilateral papilledema, the cardinal feature, is almost invariably present and may be associated with peripapillary retinal hemorrhages, exudates, or both. Visual loss, the only serious complication of pseudotumor, may occur either early or late in the course of the disease. Hypertension may be a risk factor for visual loss, but obscurations of vision do not predict subsequent visual failure. Characteristically, visual field testing reveals enlarged blind spots. Generalized constriction of the peripheral isopters and inferior nasal quadrantopsia are less frequently observed, as are central and paracentral scotomata. Diplopia, caused by unilateral or bilateral abducens palsy, may develop as a false localizing sign. The remainder of the neurologic examination results are normal. As regards the diagnosis of papilledema, it is important to distinguish *pseudopapilledema*—defined as an anomalous elevation of the optic disc—from true papilledema, which is prima facie evidence of increased intracranial pressure. Anomalous elevation of the optic papilla, which may be associated with identifiable hyaline bodies *(drusen),* should suggest the diagnosis of *retinitis pigmentosa.* In patients with ophthalmologically visible hyaline bodies, static perimetry frequently reveals a range of visual field abnormalities, including enlargement of the blind spot, nerve fiber bundle defects (particularly in the inferior nasal field), and general constriction.

PATHOPHYSIOLOGY. Pseudotumor cerebri is generally believed to be a self-limited disease in which CSF pressure returns to normal as clinical symptoms remit. However, clinical improvement is not always accompanied by a reduction in CSF pressure, and there is a subgroup of pseudotumor patients whose pressure remains persistently elevated after neurologic signs and symptoms have resolved. The course of such cases implies that clinical symptoms may be independent of the absolute magnitude of CSF pressure and that chronically raised intracranial pressure may be totally asymptomatic. Also, despite persistently elevated CSF pressure, most patients with chronic pseudotumor do not become hydrocephalic. This observation suggests that whatever mechanism "resets" CSF pressure above normal does not necessarily predispose to the development of communicating hydrocephalus. Although pseudotumor cerebri may occur without obvious precipitants in the setting of general good health, its occasional relationship to drug administration and steroid withdrawal and its reported association with a variety of endocrine disorders suggest the existence of a final common mechanism rather than a multitude of distinct pathogenetic mechanisms.

Chronically increased intracranial pressure necessarily implies an increase in dural sinus venous pressure, an increase in CSF outflow resistance, an increase in the rate of CSF formation, or some combination of these factors. One or more of these mechanisms must elevate CSF pressure in pseudotumor patients. Pathogenetic hypotheses that postulate an increase in brain bulk consequent to an increase in cerebral blood volume or in brain water content (interstitial brain edema) do not provide an adequate explanation for the intracranial hypertension of pseudotumor.

ASSOCIATED DISORDERS. The typical patient with pseudotumor is 20 to 40 years old, female, and obese. The frequency of menstrual irregularities in obese female pseudotumor patients may simply reflect the increased incidence of menstrual irregularities in obese females of child-bearing age. The association of pseudotumor with head trauma, middle ear disease, internal jugular vein ligation, oral contraceptive use, pregnancy, and polycythemia vera can be explained on the basis of cerebral venous sinus thrombosis and/or increased sagittal sinus venous pressure. Corticosteroid therapy, steroid withdrawal, hypoparathyroidism, hypervitaminosis and hypovitaminosis A, and a variety of commonly prescribed drugs (nalidixic acid, nitrofurantoin, tetracycline, and sulfonamides) have been considered as precipitating causes. In some cases an effect on the arachnoid villi and CSF outflow resistance has been postulated.

DIAGNOSIS. The diagnosis of idiopathic pseudotumor cerebri in a patient with papilledema but without localizing neurologic signs is one of exclusion. Intracranial masses (tumors, hematomata, infections) and CSF outflow obstruction must be ruled out by appropriate neuroradiologic studies, including transmission computed tomography (CT) or nuclear magnetic resonance scanning (NMR), or both. Cerebral angiography is occasionally necessary in order to rule out dural venous sinus or cortical venous thrombosis. Skull films, electroencephalography and/or pneumoencephalography are seldom indicated. Lumbar puncture, which is usually deferred until CT or NMR scanning has revealed a normal or small ventricular system, is required in order to confirm the diagnosis of increased intracranial pressure. Lumbar spinal fluid pressure is elevated, frequently above 300 mm CSF, but the composition of the fluid is normal; the protein content is usually in the low normal range, below 20 mg per dl. Laboratory evidence of hypothalamic-hypophyseal insufficiency may be present, but the diagnostic significance of subclinical endocrinopathy in obese patients with increased intracranial pressure remains to be established. Pseudopapilledema can be distinguished from true disc edema by means of stereoscopic color fundus photography and fluorescein angiography.

TREATMENT. Whereas papilledema may persist for many years without visual impairment, visual failure may occur without warning, often early in the course of the disease. Thus, if the aim of treatment is to prevent visual loss, all pseudotumor patients ideally should be treated from the time of diagnosis. Unfortunately, there is no convincing evidence that any of the frequently recommended treatment modalities are efficacious, and the high rate of spontaneous remission complicates the evaluation of various therapies. At present, four general approaches to symptomatic treatment are used: (1) repeated lumbar puncture, (2) ventriculosystemic shunting, (3) medical treatment (with corticosteroids, glycerol, diuretics, acetazolamide), and (4) incision of the optic nerve sheath.

Although repeated (weekly) lumbar puncture may provide transient relief of symptoms and document the occurrence of remission, there is no convincing evidence that this therapeutic approach is beneficial. Subtemporal decompression, once the mainstay of neurosurgical treatment, has been abandoned because of significant morbidity and mortality in the absence of established benefit. This procedure has been replaced by ventriculosystemic or lumboperitoneal shunting, the efficacy of which has not been determined. The use of glycerol, chlorthalidone, and acetazolamide has been advocated by various authors. Corticosteroids (especially prednisone) have been the mainstay of medical treatment in many clinics, although there is evidence to suggest that systemic corticosteroid administration, by raising intraocular pressure, may increase the risk of visual loss. Incision of the optic nerve sheath for the relief of papilledema is of unproved value and is performed infrequently because of the risk of postoperative blindness.

In conclusion, repeated lumbar puncture and the administration of diuretics (such as furosemide) are relatively safe and may provide temporary symptomatic relief. The use of corticosteroids, which can provoke pseudotumor cerebri in susceptible individuals and may raise intraocular pressure, seems to be contraindicated. The normal or small ventricles of patients with pseudotumor provide difficult targets for shunt catheters; thus, lumboperitoneal shunting is preferable to ventriculosystemic shunting and should be considered the treatment of last resort in patients with disabling symptoms or failing vision, or both.

Ahlskog JE, O'Neill BP: Pseudotumor cerebri. Ann Intern Med 97:249, 1982. *A critical review of the clinical syndrome of pseudotumor cerebri. The section on patient management is particularly noteworthy.*

Bulens C, De Vries WAEJ, Van Crevel H: Benign intracranial hypertension. J Neurol Sci 40:147, 1979. *A careful clinical evaluation of 36 pseudotumor patients with long-term follow-up.*

Corbett JJ, Savino PJ, Thompson HS, Kansu T, Schatz NJ, Orr LS, Hopson D: Visual loss in pseudotumor cerebri. Arch Neurol 39:461, 1982. *This paper provides a detailed and definitive discussion of the only serious complication of pseudotumor cerebri, visual loss.*

515. HYDROCEPHALUS

David A. Rottenberg

Hydrocephalus refers to the net accumulation of cerebrospinal fluid (CSF) within the cerebral ventricles and the consequent enlargement of the ventricles. Although acute obstructive hydrocephalus usually produces a sudden increase in intraventricular pressure, CSF pressure is frequently normal (or low) in patients with chronic hydrocephalus. It is useful to distinguish between "noncommunicating" and "communicating" hydrocephalus; the former is produced by lesions that obstruct the CSF circulation at or proximal to the foramina of Luschka and Magendie, the latter by obstruction of the basal cisterns or convexity subarachnoid space such that the ventricular system communicates with the spinal subarachnoid space. It is also useful to distinguish hydrocephalus associated with cerebral atrophy ("hydrocephalus ex vacuo") from congenital or acquired disorders of the cerebrospinal fluid system

DIAGNOSIS. Ventriculomegaly is readily diagnosed by means of computed tomographic (CT) or nuclear magnetic resonance (NMR) scanning. The diagnosis of hydrocephalus, however, must take into account the increase in ventricular volume that accompanies normal aging and the presence or absence of cerebral atrophy. Enlargement of the temporal horns and an inability to visualize the sylvian and interhemispheric fissures or cerebral sulci, plus the presence of periventricular lucencies, favor the diagnosis of hydrocephalus. A normal or small fourth ventricle in the presence of enlarged lateral and third ventricles suggests aqueductal stenosis.

ACUTE HYDROCEPHALUS. Sudden complete ventricular outflow obstruction leads to acute hydrocephalus, coma, and death. Partial obstruction is more common and only moderately less dangerous. Acute obstructive hydrocephalus may arise as a complication of head injury, spontaneous subarachnoid hemorrhage, cerebellar hemorrhage or infarction, acute exudative meningitis, viral encephalitis, colloid cyst of the third ventricle, and decompensation of large intracranial tumors or hematomas. Chronic hydrocephalus in the adult is most frequently caused by aqueductal stenosis or the complications of subarachnoid hemorrhage; other reported causes and associations include hindbrain (Chiari) malformations, spinal cord tumors, ectasia and elongation of the basilar artery, granulomatous meningitis, and meningeal carcinomatosis. In many instances, the cause of chronic symptomatic hydrocephalus ("normal-pressure hydrocephalus") cannot be determined. It should be noted that unequivocally asymptomatic hydrocephalus may be found in approximately 4 per cent of patients over the age of 60 who consult a neurologist for assorted neurologic complaints and undergo CT scanning.

CLINICAL MANIFESTATIONS. The patient with acute hydrocephalus has severe headache, lethargy, signs of increased intracranial pressure (papilledema and/or abducens palsy), and signs of the causative lesion. Hyperactive reflexes and bilateral extensor plantar responses are almost invariably present. Ventricular CSF pressure is markedly increased, but this increase may not be transmitted to the lumbar subarachnoid space. Patients with chronic communicating hydrocephalus, including normal-pressure hydrocephalus, have a progressive dementia, characterized by forgetfulness and psychomotor retardation, an unsteady gait, and urinary incontinence. Apathy, hypophonia, and bilateral pyramidal and extrapyramidal signs may be present. The lumbar CSF pressure is usually normal or near normal in range.

TREATMENT. Acute hydrocephalus responds dramatically to ventricular drainage and CSF diversion. Treatment of the primary lesion is the treatment of choice. Temporary ventricular decompression or ventriculosystemic shunt may be necessary in some cases. Medical treatment (with acetazolamide) for long-term symptomatic hydrocephalus is not efficacious. Ventricular shunting also has been employed for patients with chronic communicating hydrocephalus. Unfortunately not all respond, and there are no reliable clinical or neuroradiologic predictors of shunt response. Absence of cerebral atrophy and temporary psychomotor improvement after lumbar puncture seem to correlate with, but do not guarantee, benefit from a shunt operation.

Adams, RD, Fisher CM, Hakim S, Ojemann RTG, Sweet WH: Symptomatic occult hydrocephalus with "normal" cerebrospinal-fluid pressure. N Engl J Med 273:117, 1965. *This classic account of normal pressure hydrocephalus is still worth reading.*

Milhorat TH: Acute hydrocephalus. N Engl J Med 283:857, 1970. *A concise account of an uncommon but serious and eminently treatable illness.*

Vassilouthis J, Richardson AE: Ventricular dilatation and communicating hydrocephalus following spontaneous subarachnoid hemorrhage. J Neurosurg 51:341, 1979. *A retrospective study of 210 patients in whom subarachnoid hemorrhage was confirmed by lumbar puncture. The authors distinguish between early and delayed ventricular enlargement and discuss the clinical consequences of both syndromes.*

Section Thirteen INJURY TO THE HEAD AND SPINE

Donald P. Becker

516. HEAD INJURIES

GENERAL CONSIDERATIONS

Head injuries in Western nations are a major contributing factor in half of the deaths that result from physical trauma. Trauma is the leading cause of death in Western nations in persons of ages 1 to 44 years, and head injury clearly is a major medical problem. While 50,000 Americans die each year as a direct consequence of traumatic brain injury, another 50,000 to 60,000 survive severe head injury with varying degrees of disability. Each year about a million Americans seek medical care for a head injury that involves the brain.

The brain injury represents the most serious sequel to head trauma. Brain injuries from head trauma range from mild, in which a person is momentarily stunned and sees "stars," to severe, in which extensive brainstem damage rapidly leads to death. Brain injuries produce various degrees of pathologic damage, ranging from cellular and subcellular reversible injury to shearing and tearing of brain cells and even disruption of brain tissue by contusion, brain hemorrhage, or laceration. The lesions vary in location and degree from patient to patient. Following the initial brain damage, the brain may be further damaged by secondary hypoxemia from respiratory embarrassment, cerebral ischemia from elevated intracranial pressure, or brain shift caused by accumulation of an intracranial hematoma or brain swelling. The physician must seek to define, in each patient, the locations, extent, and nature of the brain damage and plan management accordingly.

MECHANISMS OF BRAIN INJURY AND TRAUMATIC UNCONSCIOUSNESS

DIFFUSE BRAIN MOVEMENT INJURY. The most common mechanism is brain movement and deformation within the skull—the "acceleration-deceleration" injury. In deceleration injury, the rapidly moving head is suddenly stopped, as in an auto-tree collision. The skull movement is immediately arrested but the gelatinous and viscoelastic brain continues to move during a 20-millisecond time period. The brain may also rotate in the skull around the axis of the brainstem. Different loci of the brain substance are deformed to different degrees, and internal shearing and stress forces can traumatize and disrupt cells and their processes in depths of the brain. If blood vessels are not disrupted, there may be no intracerebral hemorrhage, even with severe injury leading to early death. The immediate loss of consciousness results from the deformation affecting the brainstem and its reticular activating system.

In acceleration injury, the head is suddenly accelerated, as occurs, for example, during the boxer's upper cut when the head jolts back and inertial forces strike the still unmoving brain against the accelerating skull. If the brainstem cells have been severely traumatized, he may remain unconscious for days or longer. If the brainstem trauma was mild, he may be unconscious for just a few seconds or less than a minute. In this case most of the traumatized brain cells are presumed to recover.

CONCUSSION. This term describes head trauma associated with brief unconsciousness but no physical signs in sensorimotor systems or by radiographic test to indicate residual structural brain damage. Brief vegetative paralysis may occur at the moment of impact, as noted in the later discussion. The physiologic basis for the loss of consciousness and rapid recovery is not well understood, but sudden diffuse neurotransmitter release has been postulated.

DIRECT BRAIN INJURY. The other major mechanism of brain damage is direct tissue injury under the site of impact. Extensive local brain injury can occur even among patients who remain alert. For example, a crushing injury to the fixed head can drive a large plate of skull inward, destroying the right posterior parietal and occipital lobes, yet the patient need not lose consciousness despite a left homonymous hemianopsia and neurologic signs of injury to the right sensory associative cortex. With the head fixed, only the directly traumatized cerebrum is damaged; the brainstem is not deformed, and there is no loss of consciousness.

Gunshot wounds cause brain damage along the tract of the missile and extending radially outward from the path in proportion to the size and velocity of the missile. The shock wave will cause loss of consciousness if it reaches the brainstem with sufficient force.

CLINICAL APPEARANCE OF THE PATIENT

MILD BRAIN INJURY. Most are caused by acceleration or deceleration brain movement. The mildest form is represented by visual disturbance ("seeing stars") and a sensation of being dazed or stunned that lasts seconds to several minutes. The next degree is immediate unconsciousness. Boxers present a classic example. With a clean knockout blow there is prompt flaccidity, accompanied by apnea and bradycardia, with widely dilated pupils that are unresponsive to light. Rarely, a generalized seizure follows the blow. Oculovestibular reflexes may be lost transiently. In experimental animals given this "mild" injury, there are simultaneous transient arterial hypertension and slowing of the electroencephalogram. The signs and symptoms usually resolve over 30 to 60 seconds, and the individual progressively becomes oriented.

The duration of postconcussion signs and symptoms is variable and related to the intensity of the blow and degree of brain deformity. Recovery from mild injury takes place in 3 to 5 minutes. With stronger blows the physiologic response can be prolonged, and apneic periods lasting 8 to 12 minutes following the blow have been recorded in humans, with subsequent excellent recovery. Nevertheless, a major cause of death from acute head injury is prolonged apnea leading successively to hypoxemia, arterial hypertension, hypotension, and cardiac arrest. Early artificial respiration by a well-trained rescue worker undoubtedly saves some lives.

Most persons who lose consciousness probably suffer at least some irreversible injury to brain cells. Although most of the traumatized cells rapidly regain normal function, some recover only over a protracted period of time and others never. The "punchdrunk" boxer shows evidence of the cumulative effect of recurrent brain damage, part of which is a progressive communicating hydrocephalus. Affected persons are dysarthric, absent-minded, and argumentative. They have difficulty concentrating and a poor memory for recent events and walk on a wide base, with a stiff, spastic gait.

Within minutes after the injury, patients with mild brain trauma are characteristically alert and oriented. They can usually describe what they were doing up to the moments before the injury and have little or no retrograde amnesia. They rarely remember the blow itself and often cannot remember events that occurred for up to ten minutes after the accident. This period of memory loss following the injury is called the time of *antegrade amnesia* or *post-traumatic amnesia*.

MODERATE BRAIN INJURY. Patients with moderate brain injury characteristically remain lethargic or stuporous after emerging from periods of unconsciousness lasting five to ten minutes or more. They are often intermittently restless and sometimes combative but return to sleep if undisturbed. They may speak in short sentences or phrases or repeatedly say the same word. Most are sufficiently in contact to follow at least a simple single-stage command. Some have symptoms of a mild to moderate delirious reaction. Although a mild focal neurologic deficit such as a hemiparesis or visual field defect may exist, these patients do *not* show signs of motor posturing such as decorticate or decerebrate positioning of the limbs spontaneously or in response to noxious stimuli.

Patients with moderate brain injury usually make a reasonably satisfactory recovery, even when they have suffered subarachnoid hemorrhage, cerebral contusions, or a small intracerebral hematoma. A few have reduced mental performance, reflecting the presence of permanent brain damage.

Over a period of several days to one to two weeks, such patients gradually recover orientation and alertness. Mild focal neurologic deficits usually disappear. However, during the acute stages these patients are potentially vulnerable to secondary brain insults from respiratory insufficiency and hypoxemia, the growth of an intracranial blood clot, or development of brain edema, and they require close observation and carefully applied medical care.

SEVERE BRAIN INJURY. Such patients do not regain consciousness for at least 20 minutes and often much longer after injury. When seen at hospital, they do not speak understandable words or follow simple commands. This state remains after cardiopulmonary resuscitation. Other serious neurologic signs are common, and prognosis is related largely to evidence of brainstem injury. Motor posturing (decorticate and decerebrate responses) indicating extensive deep cerebral injury occurs in 30 per cent. Decerebrate (extensor) posturing carries a poorer prognosis than decorticate posturing. Impaired eye movements to the doll's head maneuver (oculocephalic test) or ice water irrigation of the ear canal (oculovestibular test) are seen in 40 per cent of patients in this group and represents brainstem damage or, less often, inner ear or cranial nerve III, IV, VI, or VIII injury. Bilateral pupillary unresponsiveness to light also signifies brainstem damage. Bilateral decerebrate (extensor) posturing with impaired or absent oculocephalic responses implies a very extensive brain injury involving both the hemispheres and brainstem. Most such patients (80 per cent) die, and the survivors can be expected to remain severely disabled or vegetative, even in the absence of an intracranial hematoma or elevated intracranial pressure.

Patients with decerebrate motor posturing but *normal* eye movements have a less extensive brain injury and sometimes make a good recovery. Likewise, patients with normal motor responses to noxious stimuli, but who have impaired eye movements or fixed pupils, occasionally make a good recovery because of the more limited extent of the brain damage. Patients with severe head injury who have normal withdrawal or normal flexor response of their limbs to noxious stimuli can be expected to make a good recovery *unless* they harbor an intracranial mass lesion that causes a major brain shift or elevates intracranial pressure to levels over 40 mm Hg for a prolonged period or unless they develop systemic complications such as septic shock or pulmonary edema.

The presence of flaccidity or paralysis of all four limbs to noxious stimuli may be caused by a concomitant spinal cord injury, but even if related to the brain injury, flaccidity is an ominous sign.

About 40 per cent of patients with severe brain injury harbor an intracranial hematoma causing brain compression and displacement as well as a high intracranial pressure. Such patients almost always require prompt surgery to evacuate the mass lesion. If the physician waits for signs of neurologic deterioration, further permanent brain damage will usually occur. Patients who show with bilateral decerebrate posturing, impaired eye movements, and pupils fixed to light can, on rare occasions, recover if they are harboring a subdural or epidural hematoma and the clot is quickly evacuated.

PATIENTS SHOWING PROGRESSIVE NEUROLOGIC DETERIORATION. The conditions of patients with mild, moderate, or severe brain injury may progressively worsen. If the vital signs and blood oxygen levels are satisfactory, such early deterioration usually comes from an expanding intracranial hematoma, usually in the subdural or epidural space, but sometimes from an intracerebral hematoma. A less frequent cause is progressive brain swelling. Unless checked by prompt treatment, such expanding masses threaten to produce potentially fatal uncal or central transtentorial herniation with signs and symptoms as outlined in Ch. 472. It is imperative that the signs of impending transtentorial herniation be recognized because rapid appropriate treatment with osmotic diuretics and surgical evacuation of a mass can save life and, perhaps more important, brain function.

SKULL FRACTURES

Fractures of the calvarium may indicate the general site and severity of the blow, but their occurrence often bears little relationship to the severity of the underlying brain injury. Autopsy demonstrates an intact skull in 30 per cent of patients who die from severe head injury. Patients with no fracture may have extensive brain injury. Linear, nondisplaced skull fractures may gain clinical importance if the crack extends across the groove of the middle meningeal artery in the temporal bone. Bleeding from this artery is a common cause of an *extradural hematoma*. This clot commonly causes brain compression within a few hours of injury. However, most patients with a linear fracture of the temporal bone do not develop an epidural hematoma, and some patients who accumulate epidural blood clots do *not* have radiographically visible fractures of the temporal bone. Thus knowledge of the presence or absence of a linear fracture is of limited help in directing the care of the individual patient. Modern diagnostic facilities with computed tomographic (CT) scanning have largely replaced plain skull x-rays in the evaluation of head injuries.

Fractures across the base of the skull produce a potential for complications. The dura over the base of the skull is thin and firmly adherent to the bone and can be easily lacerated. If the fracture traverses an air sinus or the middle or external ear canal, external communication risks producing intracranial infection, particularly meningitis. Clinical signs of communication include cerebrospinal fluid (CSF) rhinorrhea or otorrhea or the presence of intracranial air visible on radiography. When a fracture occurs on the floor of the anterior fossa, blood usually seeps into the loose periorbital tissue, producing the appearance of "raccoon eyes." With fractures of the floor of the middle fossa, subcutaneous blood may accumulate over the mastoid bone just behind the ear (*Battle's sign*). Although opinions differ, the evidence indicates that antibiotics used prophylactically do not reduce the incidence of meningitis. Traumatic CSF rhinorrhea or otorrhea usually stops spontaneously or after treatment with repeated lumbar punctures. CSF leaks that persist for longer than seven to nine days should be surgically repaired.

The cranial nerves exit via the skull base and any may be traumatized by a basal skull fracture. Post-traumatic cranial nerve palsies involving II, III, IV, VII, and VIII almost invariably reflect the presence of a fracture. A fracture may damage the olfactory and abducens nerves, but these cranial nerves have a long intracranial course and also can be traumatized by brain movement and deformation.

In *depressed skull fracture* the outer table of one or more of the segments is displaced below the level of the inner table of the surrounding intact skull. The bone position on x-ray represents the end point; the fragments usually have penetrated more deeply at the moment of impact and then "bounced" back. Open depressed fractures require cleansing and debridement of the wound to prevent infection. Post-traumatic epilepsy can be a problem. When such fractures are complicated by a lacerated dura mater, a seizure in the first week after injury, or a period of post-traumatic antegrade amnesia for over 24 hours, the incidence of chronic epilepsy reaches 60 per cent. Patients who have a dural laceration but a short period of post-traumatic amnesia and no early seizures have a 15 per cent chance of developing post-traumatic epilepsy.

CLINICAL PATHOLOGY, INTRACRANIAL PRESSURE (ICP), AND CEREBRAL BLOOD FLOW

With severe brain injury rotational brain movement is so great that grossly visible intracerebral hemorrhagic lesions can be created at the moment of trauma. Contusions and lacerations occur for the most part on the anterior and inferior surfaces of the frontal lobes and in the anterior and middle portions of the temporal lobes. Memory deficits resulting from temporal lobe injury, emotional deficits from the frontal lesions, and intellectual and behavioral impairment from both are common residual abnormalities. Focal motor, cortical sensory, or visual defects are less common. Intracerebral hematomas in the depths of the brain can develop from vascular disruption. Large hematomas in the brainstem are usually fatal.

Following brain trauma, further damage can occur because of a growing blood clot or brain swelling. The brain almost always swells around a contusion and in some cases diffusely in both hemispheres, a process thought to be caused by impairment of normal cerebrovascular autoregulation. When vascular autoregulation is impaired, the cerebral vessels lose their normal resistance tone and dilate in response to the head of arterial blood pressure, which passes downstream toward the capillary bed. In the face of normal or elevated arterial blood pressure, the brain becomes full and engorged with blood, much like an erectile organ.

Cerebrovascular engorgement, brain edema, or a growing blood clot or contusion can, alone or in combination, raise ICP well above the normal level of up to 10 mm Hg, and the pressure can eventually reach levels that impair blood flow. If cerebrovascular autoregulation is preserved, ICP must reach levels of 60 mm Hg or more before blood flow is reduced to levels that hamper tissue nutrition. In patients with severe head injury, autoregulation is usually impaired to at least some degree. In this situation, brain tissue flow may fall to critical levels when the ICP reaches only 20 to 30 mm Hg. If cerebral blood flow declines below 20 ml per 100 grams per minute, neurologic worsening follows, producing gradual or abrupt deterioration of neurologic signs. Such deterioration can occur with ICP values as low as 25 or 30 mm Hg. Although opinions differ, many neurosurgeons believe that brain ischemia stemming from elevated ICP is an important problem in severe head injury. Most patients who have a large intracranial mass have elevated ICP during their postoperative course.

Expanding intracranial hematomas can cause neurologic deterioration, because they elevate ICP, cause diffuse reduction in brain blood flow, and cause shifts, distortion, and local compression of brain tissue. Other delayed brain insults result from systemic complications, including hypoxemia from pulmonary or upper respiratory airway insufficiency, arterial hypotension from septic shock or sudden gastrointestinal hemorrhage, severe hyponatremia, and myocardial infarction. Most comatose patients who die after arriving at hospital do so because of severe elevation of ICP or as an immediate result of one of the systemic insults.

MANAGEMENT

Patients with mild to moderately severe head injuries require close monitoring to prevent medical complications and to guard against the potential delayed effects of intracranial hemorrhage or cerebral edema. With severe mechanical brain injury, carefully planned treatment in experienced hands appears to reduce mortality by 20 per cent and to improve recovery. The rapid transfer of the patient from the accident scene to an appropriately equipped hospital is equally important. Delays in transport or at a receiving hospital can be devastating. Patients with subdural hematoma who arrive at their final hospital in less than two hours fare twice as well as those who are admitted five or more hours after the accident.

IMMEDIATE MANAGEMENT. On arrival in the emergency room, approximately 35 per cent of comatose patients with severe head injury are hypoxemic (Pa_{O_2} <60 mm Hg), 15 per cent are hypotensive (systolic pressure <95 mm Hg), and 10 per cent are anemic (hematocrit <30 per cent). These abnormalities can worsen the already damaged brain and should be corrected during emergency care.

At the Scene of the Accident. Care must be taken to avoid flexing the patient's spine while moving the patient. The patient should be placed promptly in the supine, horizontal, neutral position. The three-quarter prone position should *not* be used. In the supine position, the patient can be examined and the airway dealt with directly. The mouth should be cleared.

If the patient is apneic or hypoventilating, assisted ventilation is indicated, using mouth-to-mouth assistance or positive pressure ventilation with an oral airway and Ambu bag. When the rescue team arrives, face mask positive pressure, an esophageal occlusive airway, or endotracheal intubation can be applied, depending on local expertise. One hundred per cent oxygen should be administered and continued during transportation to the hospital. Serious scalp bleeding can usually be controlled with firm pressure against the bone. Rescue workers can be taught to use the *Glasgow Coma Scale (GCS)* to assess the level of brain function (Table 516–1). Painful stimulus is administered by firmly pressing one of the victim's fingernails at the base. The GCS assessment plus examination of pupil size and reactivity to light provides an adequate emergency measure of brain function.

Transport. Provided that one has a skilled emergency crew, the patient should be transferred without delay to an optimal care hospital where CT scanning and neurosurgical care are available. Distance traveled is not the primary consideration. The only indication for transport to a local receiving hospital is profound shock (blood pressure <60 to 70 mm Hg).

For ideal care during transport of comatose patients, the following steps should be followed: insert an intravenous catheter, 16-gauge, for the possible administration of agents to maintain circulation. Initially, use a saline solution, Ringer's lactated solution, 100 ml per hour. Administer nasal oxygen at 3 to 5 liters per minute. If the patient is intubated, deliver oxygen at 100 per cent concentration. Place a nasogastric tube and empty the stomach by suction. Place a cervical collar or sandbags to protect the neck. Many recommend administration of a single intravenous dose of steroids equivalent to 50 mg of dexamethasone or 250 mg of methylprednisolone, but there is little evidence that this has a beneficial effect. Make repeated assessment of pupils, eye opening, and motor and verbal response during transport. Repeatedly check the pulse, blood pressure, and breathing. Osmotic agents such as mannitol should be given when there is progressive neurologic deterioration consistent with a growing mass and tentorial herniation.

Emergency Room Care. VENTILATION. Patients not talking and not following commands should be intubated. Respiratory insufficiency in the comatose patient can occur suddenly and unexpectedly from upper airway obstruction, generalized sei-

TABLE 516–1. GLASGOW COMA SCALE

Eye opening	
Spontaneous	4
To sound	3
To pain	2
None	1
Motor response	
Obeys commands	6
Localizes pain	5
Normal flexion (withdrawal)	4
Abnormal flexion (decortication)	3
Extension (decerebration)	2
None	1
Verbal response	
Oriented	5
Confused conversation	4
Inappropriate words	3
Incomprehensive sounds	2
None	1

zures, or soft tissue swelling in the neck. When positive pressure ventilation is initiated early, progressive respiratory failure only rarely occurs, although ventilation often must be maintained for several days. Also, CT scanning and other diagnostic procedures are improved with patient immobility; an intubated, ventilated patient can be temporarily paralyzed with pancuronium bromide.

CIRCULATION. If the patient is hypotensive, the arterial blood pressure should be brought into the normal range (mean pressure, 80 to 100 mm Hg).

Acute hypotension may result from the primary brain insult, but this should be transient or should promptly reverse with administration of intravenous fluids. Most often, hypotension reflects blood loss, and the blood volume must be rapidly expanded with appropriate agents.

A central venous pressure line should be inserted and blood drawn for a coagulation screen, blood count, and availability for typing and cross-matching, determination of electrolyte levels, SMA 12, blood alcohol, and arterial Po_2, Pco_2, and pH. A serum and urine toxicology screen is done if drug overdose or abuse is suspected.

If the circulation is satisfactory, administration of intravenous fluids is begun at 125 ml per hour of 5 per cent dextrose in 0.45 per cent saline solution. The patient should be kept well hydrated and not hemoconcentrated. As long as the serum sodium level does not fall, normal or even excessive hydration will not cause brain edema. Hyponatremia, however, can accentuate brain edema and intracranial hypertension.

EXAMINATION. The emergency room examination should include visual observation of the entire body, the extremities for possible fractures, and the pelvis for stability, as well as an evaluation of the abdomen, chest, and cardiovascular system.

Neurologic examination includes the GCS, plus appropriate evaluation of brainstem function. The pupils are evaluated for size, reactivity, shape, and position. If the cervical spine is in proper alignment, the oculocephalic reflexes are tested; otherwise, oculovestibular reflexes (cold calorics) are obtained. The motor system is evaluated for weakness and muscle tone, reflexes are tested for symmetry and response, a sensory examination is attempted, and the superficial reflexes are tested. (See Ch. 472 for evaluation of the comatose patient.)

TRIAGE ACCORDING TO SEVERITY OF INJURY. For purposes of defining initial management, patients can be grouped as having mild, moderate, or severe injury, as described earlier.

Mild Injury (Grade I). The concern is that Grade I patients may develop delayed damage from extradural or subdural hematoma. Most such patients can be observed at home if results of their initial examination are normal, with warnings to the family to awaken the patient during the first night to check responsiveness. If there is severe headache, vomiting, or lethargy, a 24-hour period of hospital observation is advisable. CT scan rather than skull films is the procedure of choice.

Moderate and Severe Injury (Grades II and III). Standard radiographs are obtained in the emergency room and include skull: anteroposterior and lateral (cross table); cervical spine: lateral (cross table); and chest: anteroposterior (semi-upright if possible). Other x-rays are taken as indicated by the physical examination. A diagnostic peritoneal lavage to detect cryptic abdominal hemorrhage is recommended if the patient has been hypotensive, hemoglobin level is below 10 grams per deciliter, or the patient has had violent body trauma.

A CT head scan is recommended in all Grade II and III patients, promptly in those with Grade III status. Assignment to the operating room or intensive care unit can then be made on the basis of the findings.

Because up to 40 per cent of comatose patients with severe brain injury show a major intracranial mass, the radiographic indications for surgical evacuation are important. If there is a clearly identifiable extra-axial lesion of increased (or decreased) density and the midline can be seen to be shifted on the CT scan, by 5 mm or more, many neurosurgeons believe that surgery is indicated. Intra-axial hematomas producing comparable shifts also are considered surgical problems. Small intra- or extra-axial lesions without midline shift and no contralateral balancing lesion can be managed without surgery. However, frequent neurologic examinations are recommended in order to guide therapy and determine if evacuation of a mass is ultimately required. Some surgeons believe that all such patients deserve ICP monitoring.

If immediate access to CT is not available, Grade III patients should have an angiogram or a ventriculogram. A ventriculogram provides rapid information about the position of the midline and the ICP level. Midline shifts of 5 mm or more are an indication for craniotomy.

INTENSIVE CARE AND MEDICAL MANAGEMENT. ***Neurologic Monitoring and General Graphic Display.*** A 24-hour clinical chart describing the neuro-ophthalmologic findings and the status of motor responses and voluntary motor strength provides an excellent graphic description of the brain-injured patient's course. The same side of the graphic neurologic examination sheet can contain graphs or spaces for recording hourly pulse rate, arterial blood pressure, ICP (when appropriate), body temperature, respiratory state and rate, and central venous pressure. Indications and techniques for intracranial pressure recording are discussed in the references.

Other important variables include hemoglobin and hematocrit levels, white blood counts, arterial blood gases, serum electrolytes, and other pertinent metabolic measurements. A radial arterial indwelling catheter can be used to monitor arterial blood pressure and to obtain blood samples. A transducer will keep the system patent, and this method can usually be used for three to five days. Urine specimens, CSF specimens (when available), and tracheal aspirate should be sent for bacterial culture at regular intervals.

Fluid and Electrolyte Management. Central venous pressure should be maintained at 8 to 12 cm H_2O or pulmonary wedge pressure at 5 to 10 cm H_2O. Urinary output measured via an indwelling bladder catheter should be about 30 ml per hour. Higher or lower outputs imply either improper fluid administration or some other specific medical abnormality. Fluid therapy usually recommended is dextrose, 5 per cent in 0.45 per cent saline solution, plus 20 mEq of KCl per 1000 ml. About 3000 ml per day is usually given to adults, but gastric, third space, and diarrheal losses must be replaced. Serum and urine electrolyte levels should be checked daily.

Many patients with head injuries transiently develop hyponatremia caused by inappropriate secretion of antidiuretic hormone (ADH). This may occur as early as the second day after injury. The treatment is fluid restriction and slow administration of 5 per cent dextrose and isotonic saline solution. Severe hyponatremia may require hypertonic intravenous saline solution; sometimes steroid hormones that cause sodium retention are used. If the central venous pressure is low and the patient is volume depleted, then the hyponatremia may be caused by inappropriate antidiuretic hormone release. Treatment consists of giving hypertonic saline solution and *no* fluid restriction.

If the patient cannot eat after five days, feeding via nasogastric tube can usually begin. Earlier efforts risk producing aspiration or vomiting. Total parenteral nutrition (TPN) can be started the day following injury. There is preliminary evidence that TPN, given to match metabolic needs, can reduce nitrogen loss and muscle wasting, can stimulate recovery of the immune system, and may reduce mortality. Since hyperglycemia may predispose to a potentially harmful cerebral lactic acidosis, blood sugar concentration should be maintained below 180 milligram per cent.

Ventilation. Most authorities recommend using controlled ventilation for all comatose head injury patients, employing a volume respirator initially set in adults at a rate of 12 per minute with a tidal volume varying between 750 and 900 ml (13 ml per kilogram of body weight). The slow rate permits adequate venous blood return to the heart, and the large volume helps re-expand collapsed alveoli. Minute volume is adjusted to bring the $Pa{CO_2}$ in a range of 25 to 30 mm Hg and oxygen flow to maintain a $Pa{O_2}$ above 70 mm Hg. To "phase" the patient onto the ventilator and avoid respiratory distress, intramuscular chlorpromazine, intravenous morphine, or pancuronium bromide (Pavulon), 2 to 4 mg intravenously, can be used as needed. Ventilator control is continued until the patient begins to follow commands or becomes neurologically stable. Most patients are maintained on this regimen for three to four days, but it can be used successfully for as long as two to three weeks.

Medications and General Care. Although seizures are infrequent following closed head injury, convulsions can precipitate a second brain insult by increasing ICP, causing respiratory distress, or increasing cerebral metabolism. To reduce this risk, phenytoin sodium and phenobarbital are usually begun on admission. Despite the lack of evidence that steroids are beneficial, they are often given to severely head-injured patients as dexamethasone or methylprednisolone every six hours. Cimetidine, 300 mg every six hours to inhibit gastric acid secretion, and antacids can reduce the likelihood of serious gastric bleeding.

Elevation of the head 10 to 20 degrees, turning and changing position every hour, frequent pulmonary toilet, pulmonary physical therapy, long-leg antiembolic stockings, standard catheter care, connecting a nasogastric tube to suction, instilling artificial tears every four hours, oral hygiene, and range of motion exercises of all extremities are all standard.

The role of ICP management and the controversial question of using barbiturate anesthesia in management are discussed in the appropriate references.

RECOVERY FROM HEAD INJURY

Most recovery from traumatic brain injury occurs in the first six months, but some neurologic improvement can continue for 12 to 18 months. Improvement thereafter is usually due to retraining or learning of special skills. Few patients with severe brain injury fully recover their neurologic and psychologic faculties. Even patients with mild brain injury frequently have annoying subjective symptoms that last up to one to two years or longer.

The location and extent of the initial and secondary brain injuries determine the quality of the ultimate outcome. Focal residual neurologic deficits such as hemiparesis or hemianopsia are relatively uncommon. Unfortunately, deficits and alterations in intellectual function, memory, and behavior are frequent and reflect injury to the frontal and temporal lobes and limbic structures. Most patients who survive severe brain injury recover independence; 80 per cent are able to function without assistance in daily living. Of the remainder, 15 per cent end up severely disabled, and a further 5 per cent are severely demented or vegetative.

Rehabilitation after head injury should include neuropsychologic testing and therapy tailored to specific handicaps in the motor, emotional, behavioral, and mental spheres. Endogenous depression is common and may be related to a reduced level of brain biogenic amines. Drug treatment with antidepressants is often effective. Family counseling is critical.

POSTCONCUSSIVE SYNDROME. Many patients who suffer brain injury experience annoying symptoms that may last for months and, rarely, years. Those who had a mild or moderate injury and are thus expecting an early complete recovery complain the most. Often, there are no obvious abnormal neurologic signs, and the physician is at a loss to explain the complaints. The symptoms usually include headache, irritability, and a feeling of lightheadedness or dizziness but not true vertigo. Other complaints include difficulty with concentration, worry and apprehension, a preoccupation with self, a lack of interest in others' affairs, mild difficulty with memory, intolerance to loud noises and alcohol, insomnia, and loss of sexual interest. Quick movements or turning the head up or sideways may bring on lightheadedness or a dazed, weak feeling. Perhaps as many as half of these patients show mild, subtle neurologic signs such as abnormal electronystagmography.

The anatomic basis for the postconcussive syndrome is not known. Presumably, many patients have had an injury to the vestibular apparatus. Associated neck injuries (whiplash) are often a part of the complex. Neural connections between damaged neck muscles and the brainstem may be a contributing cause. Minimal brainstem injury could conceivably be responsible for some of the symptoms. The syndrome is so frequent and the complaints so consistent that it must have a consistent biologic substrate, but whether this is structural, neuropharmacologic, or psychologic remains a mystery. The symptoms are not merely a reflection of compensation claims or pending litigation, although such concerns undoubtedly influence the length and degree of the complaints. The most important aspect of treatment is firm and immediate reassurance that the symptoms are not unusual, have no serious implications, and will eventually disappear. The patient who is told there is no reason for his complaints becomes even more preoccupied with his symptoms. Diazepam, 5 mg three or four times a day, helps some patients. Recovery is the rule but may take as long as several years in some cases.

CHRONIC SUBDURAL HEMATOMA

Chronic subdural hematoma presents a problem apart from acute traumatic brain injury. The clinical syndrome develops remotely in time from the original trauma. The effects of the lesion on the brain relate primarily to brain shift, although focal cortical compression, elevated ICP, and cerebral vascular insufficiency with brain ischemia occasionally contribute to the pathogenesis of the symptoms. Subdural hematoma is a disorder that follows mild more often than severe head injury and occurs more frequently among the alcoholic, the elderly, and those receiving anticoagulants. The minor head injury may not be remembered by the patient or his family. Headache is common and may be present almost from the time of injury. After two or three weeks subtle mental changes may occur and the patient may become somewhat lethargic with a loss of initiative. Following this stage, at about six weeks after injury, the patient may develop waxing and waning of the level of consciousness. A slight paresis with a Babinski sign may be seen. If untreated, patients may then progressively develop signs and symptoms of tentorial herniation (see Ch. 472). Obtundation, somnolence, confusion, and memory loss are the most frequent early signs. The clinical diagnosis can be difficult. Before the days of widely available radiographic contrast studies, many patients thought to be psychotic and confined to mental institutions were found at autopsy to have chronic subdural hematomas. Seizures are uncommon and are associated with a poor outcome.

The clinician must consider chronic subdural hematoma in the differential diagnosis of any new mental disturbance or focal neurologic deficit in the patient who is 40 years or older and in all patients with chronic alcoholism. CT scanning will clarify the diagnosis in nearly all instances. The hematoma will appear less dense than brain in most cases. However, early in development some chronic subdural hematomas may be isodense with brain on CT, and all that may be seen is a shift of the ventricular system. Smaller hematomas may resolve spontaneously, but for larger lesions surgical drainage by twist drill or burr holes is the treatment of choice.

Becker DP, Miller JD, Young HF: Diagnosis and treatment of head injury in adults. *In* Youmans JR (ed.): Neurological Surgery. 2nd ed. Philadelphia, W. B. Saunders Company, 1982. *This chapter presents a comprehensive, detailed, and practical description of head injury management.*

Bricolo A, Turazzi S, Feinotto G: Prolonged post-traumatic unconsciousness: Therapeutic assets and liabilities. J Neurosurg 52:625, 1980. *Coma and emergence from unconsciousness is a complex phenomenon. This article is the most well documented modern view on unconsciousness after head injury. The references are well selected.*

Gadisseux P, Ward JD, Young HF, Becker DP: Nutrition and the neurosurgical patient. J Neurosurg 60:219, 1984. *Fulfilling nutritional requirements in comatose traumatized patients can make a difference in outcome. Contains an excellent bibliography.*

Jennett B, Teasdale GM: The Management of Head Injuries. Philadelphia, F. A. Davis Company, 1981. *A comprehensive manuscript giving detailed statistics on the relation of outcome to early signs and to varied treatments.*

Russell RR: The Traumatic Amnesias. London, Oxford University Press, 1971. *A short, lucid, and delightfully written treatise covering brain injury mechanisms and memory loss in head injury.*

Rutherford WH, Merrett JD, McDonald JR: Sequelae of concussion caused by minor head injuries. Lancet 1:1, 1977. *This brief paper places the postconcussive syndrome into perspective. The authors discuss the interplay between symptoms from organic brain damage and post-traumatic neurosis.*

517. INJURIES TO THE SPINE

GENERAL CONSIDERATIONS

The spinal column surrounds and encases the spinal cord, nerve roots, and cauda equina. This part of the anatomy, made up of the vertebral bodies, intervertebral discs, ligaments, and vertebral joints, provides the major support for the body as well as flexibility for the neck and back. Injury to the spine can cause severe pain, impair spinal support and flexibility, and create deformity. It is, however, potential or actual injury to the nervous system so intimately enclosed by the spinal column that presents the greatest hazard.

Spinal cord injury has a low incidence but a high residual morbidity. Each year in the United States, approximately 8000 new cases are admitted to hospital. There are about 200,000 individuals who have survived traumatic spinal cord injury living in America today, half quadriplegic and half paraplegic. Slightly more are rendered quadriplegic at the time of injury, but a higher, early death rate renders the ratio equal. Half of the initially quadriplegic and 60 per cent of the paraplegic patients remain completely paralyzed below the level of their spinal lesions. Only 17 per cent recover enough function to walk. Eighty per cent are under age 40, and half of the injuries occur in the 15- to 25-year age group.

MECHANISMS OF INJURY TO SPINE AND SPINAL CORD

Physical forces generally deform the spinal column in one of four ways: flexion injuries can fracture the vertebral body and cause acute disc rupture; extension deformation often fractures posterior bony elements (laminae and spinous processes) and disrupts the strong and stabilizing longitudinal ligaments that run along the anterior and posterior surfaces of the vertebral bodies; compression injuries cause explosion fractures of the vertebral body and tear surrounding ligaments; and rotational injuries can disrupt the entire ligamentous structures. Flexion or extension injuries usually have a major rotational element which combines to produce extensive ligamentous and bony injury.

If there is deformation and dislocation of the spinal column at the time of injury, the spinal cord can be injured at that moment. If the spinal column remains dislocated, an additional insult of continuing pressure on the spinal cord and nerve roots may compound the problem. The maximal vertebral displacement that actually occurs at the moment of impact is greater than that seen on the initial x-ray, since the bone rebounds back toward normal position.

The cervical spine is the least protected and most flexible portion of the vertebral column. It is relatively fixed to the thoracic spine below and its top end supports the head. This makes it vulnerable, and only moderate trauma can cause a fracture or fracture dislocation. The cervical spinal canal normally is at least 30 per cent larger in diameter than the spinal cord. Individuals who have normal or large canals can often tolerate a considerable vertebral dislocation and show no spinal cord deficit. In contrast, patients with narrow canals or older individuals with osteoarthritic ridging causing a narrow canal can develop major spinal cord deficits from flexion or extension injury with minimal or no spinal column malalignment. Relatively low energy forces can displace the cervical spinal column. The result is that a relatively larger number of partial or reversible cord injuries occur in the cervical region. In contrast, the vast majority of thoracic cord injuries are complete and irreversible. The thoracic spine has additional fixation from the ribs and is the least flexible area of the spine. Tremendous force is required to malalign the thoracic spine; if dislocation occurs, the spinal cord is subjected to a major impact. Additionally, the thoracic canal is normally small in relation to the spinal cord diameter, and malalignment that does not relocate is likely to cause continued compression of the cord.

The lumbar column is heavily constructed and gains additional support from the bulky paraspinal muscles. Here, also, massive energy forces are required to dislocate the spine. The lumbar canal widens relative to the neural structures it contains. The spinal cord usually ends opposite the top of the L2 vertebra. Below this level are the cauda equina, which can tolerate much higher levels of trauma and compression than the spinal cord. So, although incomplete neural lesions of the thoracic cord are a rarity, incomplete neural lesions at the thoracolumbar junction and lumbar and cervical region are fairly common.

COMPLETE AND INCOMPLETE SPINAL CORD INJURY

Whether the neurologic deficit came on *immediately* and whether it is *complete* below the level of injury are the most notable factors in spinal cord injury. Patients with complete functional transection rarely recover, especially if they remain transected upon arrival at the hospital and stay so after realignment of the spinal canal. A patient may be rendered immediately "transected" from a cervical injury and then begin to recover function within minutes of the injury. This is considered to be a *concussive,* reversible membrane injury to the cervical cord. Such patients invariably show recovering neurologic function by the time they reach the hospital. An even rarer patient may be completely functionless on admission with a malaligned cervical spinal fracture dislocation and may begin to recover almost immediately after early spinal realignment. In such a case the cord injury was mild and the compressive forces were at the threshold of irreversible injury.

An *incomplete* spinal cord injury is one in which the patient shows *any voluntary* movement or preserved sensation below the level of the lesion. This may include no more than touch or pin sensation in the perianal region (termed sacral sparing; the sacral sensory fibers run in the most peripheral aspect of the spinal cord at the cord equator). The distinction is important because some patients with incomplete lesions eventually show remarkable functional improvement in motor and sensory function. All the compact bundles of ascending and descending long fiber tracts in the white matter of the spinal cord tend to be damaged to the same degree. If one bundle or part of a fiber tract retains function across the injury site, there is a good chance that the remaining tracts have only been severely concussed and not disrupted or contused. Reports in the literature and elsewhere of spectacular recoveries following "complete" lesions with no distal normal neurologic function even after 6 to 24 hours probably represent failure of the examiners to test sensory function sufficiently, especially perianal function. Retained distal reflex function does *not* define an incomplete lesion. Bulbocavernous reflex, full penile erection in males, anal wink, cremasteric reflex, reflex leg withdrawal, or downgoing toe movement to noxious stimuli can all represent reflex activity in an isolated cord. Spinal shock, defined as loss of all reflex activity below the lesion, is usually present for three to six weeks after complete lesions, but in civilian spinal cord trauma, it may not develop at all. This is especially true with cervical cord damage.

The center gray matter is the most sensitive and vulnerable to physical blows to the spinal cord. As the force of the blow increases, increasing damage extends radially outward into the more lateral ascending and descending long white matter fiber tracts that carry information from brain to body and vice versa.

SPINAL CORD INJURY NEUROLOGIC SYNDROMES

The *central cord syndrome* represents the clinical correlate of the cord damage from injury force just above the concussive blow. With increasing trauma, the lesion extends from central gray matter into the medial portion of the cord white matter. This medial location is where voluntary myelinated motor fibers to the arms are located (motor fibers to the legs are more peripheral). The characteristic clinical syndrome is identified by lower motor neuron changes in the arms combined with spasticity in the legs, with the arms being weaker than the legs. Sensory modalities are variably involved, depending upon extent of injury into the posterior columns and anterolateral columns, but pain and temperature sensation is characteristically reduced in the hands. Urinary retention incontinence is often present (voluntary urinary bladder function is also transmitted in medially placed myelinated fibers). Striking neurologic recovery may be seen over time, although some permanent handicap in arm and hand function often remains.

In the *anterior cord syndrome,* voluntary motor function and pain and temperature sensation are absent, but distal position sense, light touch, and vibratory sensation remain. The anterior and lateral columns of the cord are dysfunctional, but the posterior columns are intact. Anterior cord compression or a lesion involving the anterior spinal artery may be the culprit. Prognosis for good recovery in these cases is less common than that in the *posterior cord syndrome,* in which the opposite clinical picture is present.

Recovery with *Brown-Séquard's syndrome* lies between the aforementioned extremes. Affected patients have dysfunction of half of the cord (the meridian defined in the sagittal plane), with distal motor weakness ipsilateral to the lesion and distal pain and temperature loss contralateral to the lesion. They may also have ipsilateral loss of position and vibratory sense if the injury represents a true "hemisection" of the cord. Improvement is the rule, but some permanent deficit almost always remains.

All the syndromes seen with incomplete spinal cord lesions may be associated with continuing compression of the cord from bony spicules, herniated discs, or displaced vertebrae that remain dislocated after the initial blow.

Most patients with incomplete lesions show progressive improvement, but on occasion neurologic worsening develops. Early after injury progressive loss of function is almost always due to continued or increased compression of the spinal cord by a protruded disc, bone spicules, or distortion of the spinal canal.

The level of the injury is critical. Complete lesions involving the cervical spine cause quadriplegia. If the lesion is above the C4 cord level, the mortality rate is high because diaphragmatic breathing control (via C3–5 cervical roots to the phrenic nerve) is impaired. Patients with complete lesions in the C6 cord region may retain some biceps function but can lack important arm extension, wrist extension, and finger flexion. If the injury is at C7–T1 spine level (C8 cord level), hand intrinsic function is impaired, but since the patient usually retains wrist extension, linkage splints applied to the wrist and fingers will give finger pincer function. Spinal cord injuries that are complete after 24 hours do not show distal motor or sensory functional improvement, but neurologic function related to the level of injury may improve. Thus, a patient with a complete injury at C7 cord level might initially lack wrist extension and finger movement and have weak triceps functions, yet over time may regain improved triceps function and recovery of wrist extension.

PATIENT MANAGEMENT

EMERGENCY AND EARLY MANAGEMENT. Careful placement of the patient in a neutral supine position at the accident site and maintenance of that position during transport are now being employed by most rescue teams. During transport, the head should be kept in alignment with the spine and the spine not flexed during any movement. Nasal oxygen should be administered and artificial ventilation and cardiovascular support provided as needed.

In the emergency room cardiorespiratory resuscitation is often required. Tracheostomy should be avoided; if intubation is necessary, nasotracheal or endotracheal intubation should be performed. Following a major cervical or upper thoracic cord injury, signs of peripheral sympathetic nervous system denervation are common. Characteristically, patients have bradycardia, hypotension, and perhaps hypothermia. Immediately following the impact, there occurs a brief and temporary three- to four-minute episode of marked arterial hypertension secondary to cord sympathetic massive discharge. The hypotension that then follows the initial hypertensive phase can be reversed with alpha-adrenergic agonists such as metaraminol, and also responds to intravenous fluid administration. Hypoxemia is common after cervical and upper thoracic cord trauma. The thoracic intercostal muscles are paralyzed, and diaphragmatic breathing initially may be inadequate to support adequate ventilation. Associated lung, chest, and abdominal injuries are frequent. After resuscitation a baseline neurologic examination can be completed and appropriate spine x-rays obtained. The goals of treatment are to realign the spinal column, restore spinal canal diameter, stabilize the spine, and prevent a secondary or delayed cord injury.

Cervical Spine Injuries. Fracture-dislocations should be promptly reduced. These injuries often are unstable and threaten to produce worse cord damage. Skull tongs that can be placed without the necessity of a scalp incision or skull drill holes are now available. These metal tongs (prototype, Gardner-Wells) with sharp points are placed just above the pinna, and fix firmly to the skull. Initially, weights are applied at 5 pounds per interspace (a C3–4 dislocation would have 15 to 20 pounds). Weights are increased progressively under x-ray control (a radiograph and neurologic examination are checked after each 5- to 10-pound addition of weight). With careful and judicious use of diazepam (Valium) or, in unusual cases when ventilation is controlled, neuromuscular junction blockade, most dislocations can be reduced with less than 60 pounds. Following reduction, further management concerning the need for restoration of canal diameter is controversial. Patients whose neurologic deficits remain complete do not ordinarily improve with surgical decompression of the spinal cord, and those whose are incomplete generally improve. All agree that the patient who demonstrates neurologic worsening should have the canal diameter defined and restored. The modern view that many specialists espouse is that the canal diameter should be defined radiologically in *all* cases and any pressure on the cord removed surgically so as to give the spinal cord maximal chance for recovery. Clinical evidence to support this aggressive approach is not available.

Myelography with or without CT will define diameter and cord position. If extrinsic cord compression is present and surgery is to be performed, the operation must be tailored to the location of the intraspinal pressure and the type of ligamentous rupture. Anterior compression is best removed via an anterior approach to the spine.

Thoracolumbar Injuries. An open operation is almost always required to reduce thoracic and lumbar fracture dislocations. This should usually be preceded by myelography and possibly CT. Surgical reduction and stabilization can often be accomplished with intraoperative traction on the laminae, using Harrington metal rods. Permanent fusion is accomplished with intraoperative bone grafting at the injury site in operated cases.

MEDICAL CARE. Over 40 per cent of patients with spinal cord injury have serious medical complications. Cardiovascular-pulmonary complications are the most lethal, urinary complications the most common, and skin breakdown from pressure the most intractable to treatment. Prompt diagnosis and treatment of complications are the predominant factors in early management. Medical care during the acute phase should follow the principles defined in Ch. 516.

Cardiorespiratory. Because the intercostal muscles are paralyzed with higher lesions, vital capacity is impaired, and breathing is diaphragmatic-abdominal. Pressure on the abdomen must be avoided when the patient is prone. Patients often hyperventilate and reduce their Pa_{CO_2}. Ventilatory reserve is reduced, and a small pulmonary insult can cause hypoxemia.

The cardiovascular system may be very unstable. Arterial tone is diminished because of the traumatic sympathectomy, and venous tone decreased because of muscle paralysis. Peripheral pooling in the vascular compartment is profound. Severe bradycardia can be life threatening. Anticholinergics such as atropine will help reverse this, but occasionally a cardiac pacemaker is temporarily needed. Although the hypotension will temporarily respond to alpha agonists such as norepinephrine, volume expansion with colloids and saline is imperative. Monitoring of the central venous pressure or wedge pressure and heart rate helps one gauge requirements. Venous stasis is responsible for a high incidence of venous thrombosis and pulmonary embolism. Antiembolic stockings, continuous passive leg movement, and subclinical heparinization may reduce this complication.

Gastrointestinal. Paralytic ileus is common, and nasogastric suction is advisable for a minimum of 48 hours. Hyponatremia is common secondary to high sodium loss via nasogastric suction, diarrhea and urinary loss, or loss into the gut in association with the adynamic ileus. Total parenteral nutrition, begun early, may minimize the complications of inanition. With extensive paralysis, metabolic and caloric requirements may be reduced below normal. Once eating begins, daily stool softeners and laxative suppositories given every other day will help the patient develop spontaneous reflex defecation.

Skin. After two hours of pressure, anesthetic skin begins to develop ischemic changes that can lead to ulcer formation. Skin over the sacrum, ischial tuberosities, trochanters, and heels is prone to pressure sores. A program designed to prevent skin pressure should begin as soon as possible after admission.

Spinal Cord Injury Beds. Rotating bed frames that incorporate traction devices are commonly used to change patient position. Recently, a bed that moves continuously and essentially places the patient in perpetual motion has been introduced. It is expensive and has not yet been widely applied, but the reported reduction of pulmonary complications, decubitus ulcers, and venous thromboembolism is impressive and attests to the need for frequent turning, pulmonary toilet, range of motion passive exercises to extremities, and early mobilization. Halo traction for external cervical spine stabilization has permitted earlier mobilization for many patients.

Genitourinary Tract. A Foley catheter should remain in the urinary bladder for ten days, during which time chemoprophylaxis is recommended. After the tenth day, it is a good policy to discontinue straight drainage and begin an every-four-hour intermittent catheterization program, preferably done by the patient. Reflex spontaneous voiding may sometimes be achieved, but one must monitor the patient for possible ureteral reflux, which can lead to hydroureter, hydronephrosis, and renal damage. In the male, reflex penile erections are not uncommon, and can often be brought on by tactile stimulation. Ejaculation can also be induced in some patients. Both males and females can often participate in satisfying sexual activity and, on occasion, become parents.

Pain, Spasticity, and Reflex Dysautonomia. Severe pain and spasticity with flexor spasms may affect the lower extremities. Baclofen, a gamma-aminobutyric acid analogue, dantrolene, and diazepam alone or in combination often control these symptoms. Surgical procedures such as rhizotomy, myelotomy, and neurectomy are seldom required. Reflex dysautonomia characterized by acute onset of sweating above the injury level, hypertension, headache, and leg spasms may occur spontaneously, but more often reflect an overdistended urinary bladder, gastric dilatation, sexual activity, or an infected hypertrophic spastic bladder.

REHABILITATION. Direct and straightforward discussions with patient and family should begin immediately regarding the diagnosis and prognosis. Early, honest communication usually creates an optimal attitude for expeditious institution of a rehabilitative program. The common psychologic response to spinal cord injury is initial denial, followed by anger and then depression. The patient must be encouraged to cope and move quickly to retraining. Physical therapy, occupational therapy, and respiratory therapy should begin early. Physical restoration is not the only goal of a rehabilitative program. The total process includes psychologic, social, sexual, and vocational rehabilitation. Most patients can be brought back into competitive society. Life expectancy following spinal cord transection for those who survive the initial hospitalization period is just 10 per cent less than for the population at large, but lifelong follow-up care is a necessary part of the medical program. The major impediments to success are renal failure, decubitus ulcers, and psychosocial problems.

Cooper PR, Maravilla KR, Sklar FH, et al.: Halo immobilization of cervical spine fractures. Indications and results. J Neurosurg 50:603, 1979. *Halo immobilization is now in common use. Indications, complications, and contraindications are clearly outlined.*

Guttmann L: Spinal Cord Injuries, Comprehensive Management and Research. 2nd ed. Oxford, Blackwell Scientific Publications, 1976. *This is the most comprehensive publication on spinal cord injury. Sir Ludwig pioneered the development of spinal cord injury centers, which deal with care from injury through rehabilitation. The clinical descriptions of medical syndromes and ultimate results are superb.*

Maynard FM, Reynolds GG, Fountain S, et al.: Neurological prognosis after traumatic quadriplegia. J Neurosurg 50:611, 1979. *A careful assessment of how patients recover with modern care. The neurologic findings and recovery in patients are well documented.*

Yashon D: Spinal Injury. New York, Appleton-Century-Crofts, 1978. *Modern diagnosis and management as practiced in the United States are clearly outlined in a practical manner. Common complications are discussed lucidly, and each chapter is well referenced.*

Young HF, Becker DP: Complications of spine surgery and trauma. *In* Greenfield LJ (ed.): Complications in Surgery and Trauma. Philadelphia, J.B. Lippincott Company, 1984. *Complications of spinal trauma and their management are covered in a comprehensive yet concise fashion.*

Section Fourteen MECHANICAL LESIONS OF NERVE ROOTS AND SPINAL CORD

Jerome B. Posner

Several lesions of the vertebral column, its contents, or its surroundings cause symptoms by distorting or compressing the spinal cord or its exiting nerve roots. With the exception of herniated intervertebral discs, these mechanical lesions of nerve roots or spine are not common, but their most frequent symptom, neck or back pain, is very common indeed, and the physician must consider these lesions in the differential diagnosis of many patients. Furthermore, if untreated, many of these disorders lead to more serious symptoms of sensory loss, paralysis, and incontinence—abnormalities that can often be reversed by early diagnosis and appropriate treatment. A general approach to the patient suffering from neck or back pain is considered in Ch. 481. This section begins with a discussion of the differential diagnosis of muscle, nerve root, and spinal disorders and proceeds to consideration of mechanical lesions of spine and nerve roots. Individual disorders of the peripheral nerves are considered in Section Fifteen and those of the muscle and neuromuscular junction in Section Sixteen.

518. DIFFERENTIAL DIAGNOSIS OF MUSCLE, NERVE ROOT, AND SPINAL DISORDERS

INTRODUCTION. In order for an organism to move, perceive its environment, and maintain homeostasis in a changing environment, signals from peripheral receptors must reach the brain, and signals originating in brain effectors must reach appropriate end-organs. Three different *peripheral common pathways* subserve the functions of motion, sensation, and homeostasis. Some knowledge of the anatomy and physiology of these three common pathways (motor, sensory, and autonomic) is required for the physician to make an intelligent differentiation among lesions of the individual elements of these pathways.

ANATOMY AND PHYSIOLOGY. The *lower motoneuron* is anatomically and physiologically the most well defined of the peripheral common pathways. It consists of the cell body of an anterior horn cell of the spinal cord and its axon that travels through a nerve root, a nerve plexus, and a peripheral nerve to end at the myoneural junction and innervate a number of voluntary muscle fibers. The anterior horn cells consist of large alpha motoneurons destined to innervate extrafusal skeletal muscle fibers that control motion and small gamma motoneurons that innervate intrafusal muscle fibers that control tone. The anterior horn cells of a spinal segment and their emerging axons form a nerve root arranged so that each segment innervates a specific group of muscles called a myotome. In the thoracic and abdominal area, the nerve roots continue as peripheral nerves to innervate intercostal and abdominal muscles in the myotomal pattern. Elsewhere, however, as the nerve roots leave the spinal canal, they intermix and rearrange themselves to form nerve plexuses and later peripheral nerves, both of which innervate muscles in a pattern different from that of a single nerve root (see accompanying table). Branches to specific muscles leave the nerve trunk at specific points along its course, allowing one to determine the site of a nerve lesion by the pattern of muscles paralyzed or spared. For example, damage to the radial nerve in the humeral groove (a common site of compression) paralyzes the brachioradial muscle and the wrist and finger extensors but spares the triceps muscle. A lesion of the radial nerve in the axilla involves the triceps muscle as well. When a motor nerve reaches the muscle that it will innervate, each large heavily myelinated alpha motoneuron fiber (12 to 20 μ in diameter) breaks up into several small, nonmyelinated twigs, each twig reaching an individual extrafusal muscle fiber. Each nerve fiber innervates between 10 (in the ocular muscles) and 1000 (in proximal limb muscles) muscle fibers. The muscle fibers innervated by an individual nerve fiber are scattered throughout the muscle bundle, but become grouped because of reinnervation if there is longstanding disease of the lower motoneuron (see Ch. 471 and 489).

The peripheral common pathway for sensation, the *lower sensory neuron*, is less well defined. It begins with either specialized or nonspecialized receptors that supply a small area of tissue (pacinian corpuscles that measure mechanical deformation are an example of a specialized receptor, and free nerve endings in the skin are examples of unspecialized ones). The receptors transduce mechanical, chemical, and other forms of energy into a depolarization of the sensory nerve ending, which generates an action potential in the peripheral sensory axon. The pattern of the peripheral sensory axon recapitulates that of the motor axon in that it travels first in a peripheral nerve, rearranges itself into nerve plexuses (except in the abdomen and thorax), and then enters the spinal canal as a sensory root. The area of skin supplied by each sensory root is called a dermatome (see Table 518–1). The cell body of the peripheral sensory neuron, unlike the lower motoneuron, is not in the spinal cord but in the dorsal root ganglion, usually lying within the intervertebral foramen. Sensory neurons range in size from the large, heavily myelinated I-A fibers (12 to 22 μ), afferent from muscle spindles; through type II fibers (5 to 12 μ) that subserve light touch and proprioception, and the small, myelinated type III fibers (2 to 5 μ) that subserve temperature and sharp, pricking pain; to the small unmyelinated C-fibers (0.1 to 1.3 μ) that subserve poorly localized noxious, burning pain (see Ch. 481). Each dorsal root ganglion cell possesses a branched axon, the first branch reaching the periphery and the second branch extending from the dorsal root ganglion to enter the dorsolateral portion of the spinal cord. Many large myelinated axons ascend in the dorsal columns without synapsing to reach the cuneate and gracile nuclei of the lower brainstem. These long ascending axons often send branches to synapse at segmental levels as well. Other large, myelinated axons synapse in the posterior gray matter of the spinal cord and then ascend in the spinocerebellar tracts to bring sensory information to the cerebellum. Small, unmyelinated axons synapse in the posterior horn of the spinal cord and then cross in the anterior commissure to ascend in the spinothalamic tract.

Lower autonomic neurons are of two types, sympathetic and parasympathetic. (Strictly speaking, lower autonomic neurons as defined here are not the same as lower motor and sensory neurons, since the sympathetic and parasympathetic fibers which leave the spinal cord synapse once in the periphery before reaching their end-organ. However, the analogy is useful in determining differential diagnoses in patients with disease of the autonomic nervous system.) *Lower sympathetic neurons* begin in the interomediolateral cell column of the spinal cord from T1 through L3. They exit the spinal cord in the ventral root but leave the spinal nerve in the paravertebral region to enter the paravertebral chain of ganglia that extend from the base of the skull to the coccyx. Sympathetic fibers may either synapse in a paravertebral ganglion or travel farther from the spinal cord to synapse in a prevertebral ganglion (e.g., the celiac or superior mesenteric). The synaptic mediator is acetylcholine. From both the paravertebral and prevertebral ganglia, long postganglionic axons travel along either spinal nerves or blood vessels to reach and synapse on the effector organ. The synapse may be on smooth muscle (e.g., pupillary fibers, blood vessels, respiratory tree, gut, and urinary bladder) or on glandular structures such as lacrimal, salivary, and adrenal glands. The synaptic mediator in most postganglionic sympathetic fibers is norepinephrine, but in some, such as sweat glands, the mediator is acetylcholine. Other mediators have been postulated.

Parasympathetic neurons arise either in the special visceral nuclei of the brainstem (including the oculomotor complex, the superior and inferior salivary nuclei, and the vagus nuclei) or in the lateral horns of the second, third, and fourth sacral spinal segments. They exit the central nervous system with cranial nerves (the oculomotor, facial, glossopharyngeal, and vagus) or sacral roots 2, 3, and 4. The preganglionic parasympathetic fibers travel with cranial or spinal nerves until they synapse in a ganglion near the organ they will innervate (e.g., the ciliary ganglion of the eye). Postganglionic fibers then synapse on smooth muscle or glandular structures of the organ destined for innervation. Both the preganglionic and the postganglionic parasympathetic fibers are cholinergic.

GENERAL CHARACTERISTICS OF PERIPHERAL COMMON PATHWAY LESIONS. Lesions of the peripheral common motor, sensory, and autonomic pathways have characteristics that distinguish them from lesions of their respective supranuclear pathways of the brain and spinal cord. Lesions of individual portions of each pathway (particularly with respect to the motor system) also have characteristics that distinguish them from lesions elsewhere in the same pathway. The former characteristics are considered first and the latter in succeeding paragraphs. As a general rule in neurology, when the nervous system is involved at several levels, only the most distal level can be discerned reliably by clinical examination. For example, in the presence of severe muscle disease, one usually cannot determine if the motor nerves supplying these muscles are normal, and in the presence of motor nerve disease one often cannot determine if the corticospinal tracts or motor areas of the brain are intact.

The general characteristics of primary muscle and lower motoneuron dysfunction include weakness, atrophy (rarely pseudohypertrophy [see Ch. 524 and 537]), diminished muscle tone (myotonia is an exception), hypo- or areflexia, and relatively preserved dexterity. The last is particularly important in distinguishing upper from lower motoneuron lesions; with lower motoneuron lesions, skilled movements are preserved until the patient becomes profoundly weak. With upper motoneuron lesions, skilled movements are invariably involved to a greater extent than is gross strength. Patients with lower motoneuron lesions are fully cognizant of the fact that they are weak. Patients with upper motoneuron lesions, particularly when proprioceptive functions are also impaired, may be unaware of their deficit.

The general characteristics of involvement of the lower sensory neuron include loss of one or more primary modalities of sensation (touch, pain, temperature, proprioception), with relative preservation of the integrative sensory modalities, i.e., stereognosis, graphesthesia. In lower sensory motoneuron disorders, stereognosis and graphesthesia may be impaired, but only in proportion to the loss of primary modalities. The opposite is sometimes true with upper sensory neuron lesions. In lower sensory neuron lesions caused by local mechanical disease of a root, plexus, or nerve, all primary sensory modalities are usually lost to a similar degree. (There are exceptions: during the development of compressive nerve lesions, the largest fibers suffer disproportionately, leading to early light touch and proprioceptive loss with *relative* preservation of pain; local anesthetic injection into a nerve affects small pain fibers first.) In some metabolic or inflammatory lesions of the lower sensory neuron (e.g., nutritional neuropathy, Guillain-Barré polyneuropathy), individual fiber types may be selectively involved, leading to the loss of one modality of primary sensation and preservation of the others, but in these instances the pattern of sensory change is almost always bilateral, symmetrical, and of a distal stocking-glove or dermatomal distribution. Sensory loss involving one half of the body if organic in origin always implies an upper sensory neuron lesion.

Only a few features distinguish lower autonomic neuron lesions from upper autonomic neuron lesions. The outstanding one is *denervation hypersensitivity,* the response of a denervated target organ to concentrations of transmitter or transmitter-like substances lower than necessary to stimulate an innervated organ. For example, a parasympathetically denervated pupil constricts when exposed to 0.125 per cent pilocarpine, a parasympathetic agent; a normal pupil will usually not respond. Denervation hypersensitivity is most marked when the lesion involves postganglionic fibers; it is less when preganglionic, lower autonomic neuron fibers are impaired; the response is virtually nonexistent when upper autonomic neuron fibers are damaged.

A second feature of postganglionic lower autonomic neuron lesions is failure of the end-organ to respond to a chemical substance which promotes release of transmitter from nerve terminals. For example, in sympathetically denervated pupils, if the lesion is in the postganglionic fibers, hydroxyamphetamine hydrobromide 1 per cent, which acts at the presynaptic nerve terminal to stimulate release of norepinephrine, will fail to dilate the pupil; a normal pupil will dilate when exposed to this drug.

CHARACTERISTICS OF MUSCLE LESIONS. These diseases are discussed in Ch. 537 to 539. Like lower motoneuron lesions, disease of muscle is characterized by weakness, atrophy, and diminished tendon reflexes. In general, diseases of muscle affect proximal muscles more profoundly than distal ones, and deep tendon reflexes are preserved until the patients become quite weak. Muscle disease, particularly if it is acute and inflammatory, can be accompanied by pain and tenderness in the muscles, but other sensory symptoms or signs are absent. The electromyogram of muscle disease is characteristic in that the potentials are of small amplitude and short duration, with a normal number of motor units recruited on attempted volitional movement (complete interference pattern). Fibrillation potentials, which are characteristic of nerve disorders, may occasionally be seen in muscle disease, particularly polymyositis (see Ch. 451). The intracellular muscle enzyme creatine phosphokinase may be elevated in the serum. Muscle biopsy is also characteristic, demonstrating random loss of muscle fibers with central migration of nuclei. Sometimes specific histochemical changes characterize a particular muscle disorder.

DISEASES OF THE MYONEURAL JUNCTION. These diseases are discussed in Ch. 537 to 539. In general, myoneural junction diseases are characterized by intermittent and fluctuating weakness (particularly in myasthenia gravis, but also in the myasthenic syndrome), by fatigability, and by a characteristic muscle distribution (bulbar and respiratory muscles are predominantly affected by myasthenia gravis and botulism, proximal extremity muscles by the myasthenic syndrome). Responses to cholinergic test substances or electrical studies of neuromuscular transmission are necessary to establish the diagnosis. There are no sensory changes, although some patients with the myasthenic syndrome complain of paresthesias.

DISEASES OF THE PERIPHERAL NERVES. These diseases are discussed in Ch. 524 to 536. Lesions of peripheral nerves are characterized by the distribution of sensory loss, motor weakness, and autonomic dysfunction, as well as by the early loss of deep tendon reflexes. Because most peripheral nerves are mixed sensory and motor, patients with lesions of peripheral nerves usually suffer both sensory loss and motor dysfunction. Some exceptions occur if the nerve or the portion of the nerve involved is exclusively or almost exclusively sensory or motor. (For example, radial nerve palsies may produce weakness alone when the autonomous area of sensory distribution is so small that the overlap from other nerves allows normal sensation; carpal tunnel syndromes may produce solely sensory changes in the median nerve distribution because the motor twig is not compressed.) If autonomic fibers travel with the nerve, autonomic changes may also develop in the same distribution. These can consist of signs of autonomic hyperactivity (e.g., hyperhidrosis, decreased temperature) or reduced activity (e.g. hypohidrosis, warmth, swelling, discoloration, shiny skin, and failure of wrinkling on immersion in water). Involvement of peripheral nerves can be of several types, each of which has characteristic pathologic and electrographic changes (see Ch. 471). In general, when peripheral nerves or more proximal portions of the lower motoneuron are involved, the electromyogram is characterized by long duration, high amplitude action potentials with a reduced number of motor units recruited on volitional movement, and by spontaneous activity in the muscle, consisting of fibrillations and fasciculations. Muscle biopsy in peripheral nerve involvement reveals grouped atrophy, but several months are usually required for these changes to become evident.

PLEXUS AND ROOT INVOLVEMENT. Involvement of nerve plexuses and roots is distinguished from dysfunction of muscle by the same characteristics that distinguish peripheral nerve from muscle lesions. Plexus and root lesions differ from peripheral nerve lesions by the distribution of sensory and autonomic changes. Knowledge of the differences among root, plexus, and peripheral nerve innervation of various structures is required to make this distinction (see Table 518–1).

SPINAL CORD LESIONS. Spinal cord lesions can be distin-

TABLE 518–1. DIFFERENTIAL DIAGNOSIS OF LESIONS OF NERVE ROOTS AND PERIPHERAL NERVES*

						Nerve
	C2–3	*C5*	*C6*	*C7*	*C8*	*T1*
Pain	Back of head, lateral face, behind ear	Lateral border of arm and medial scapula	Lateral forearm, thumb, and index finger	Posterior arm, lateral hand, mid-forearm, and medial scapula	Medial forearm and hand	Deep aching in shoulder and axilla to olecranon
Sensory loss	Posterior scalp, pinna, lateral face	Lateral border of upper arm	Lateral forearm, including thumb	Mid-forearm and middle finger	Medial forearm and little finger	Axilla down to olecranon
Reflex loss	None	Biceps	Supinator	Triceps	Finger stretch	None
Motor deficit	Usually none	Deltoid, supraspinatus, infraspinatus, rhomboids	Biceps, brachioradialis, brachialis (pronators and supinators of forearm)	Latissimus dorsi, pectoralis major, triceps, wrist extensors, wrist flexors	Finger flexors, finger extensors, flexor carpi ulnaris (thenar muscles in some patients)	*All* small hand muscles (in some thenar muscles via C8)
Some causative lesions	Tumor, injury	Brachial neuritis, cervical disc or spondylosis, upper plexus injury	Cervical disc or spondylosis	Cervical disc or spondylosis	Pancoast tumor, rare in disc lesions or spondylosis, metastatic tumor, thoracic outlet syndrome	Pancoast tumor, cervical rib, outlet syndromes, metastatic carcinoma in deep cervical nodes
Autonomic changes	Gustatory sweating					Horner's syndrome

				Peripheral
	Axillary	*Musculocutaneous*	*Radial*	*Median*
Pain	Across shoulder tip	Lateral forearm	Dorsum of thumb and index finger	Thumb, index and middle finger, often spreads up forearm
Sensory loss	Small area over deltoid	Lateral forearm	Dorsum of thumb and index finger (if any)	Lateral palm and lateral fingers
Reflex loss	Nil	Biceps jerk	Triceps jerks and supinator jerk	Finger jerks (flexor digitorum sublimis)
Motor deficit	Deltoid (teres minor cannot be evaluated)	Biceps, brachialis (coracobrachialis weakness not detectable)	Triceps, wrist extensors, finger extensors, brachioradialis, supinator of forearm	Wrist flexors, long finger flexors (thumb, index and middle fingers), pronators of forearm, abductor pollicis brevis
Some causative lesions	Fractured neck of humerus, dislocated shoulder, deep intramuscular injections	Very rarely damaged	Crutch palsy, Saturday night palsy, fractured humerus in supinator muscle	Carpal tunnel syndrome, direct trauma to wrist

*Modified from Patten JT: Neurological Differential Diagnosis. New York, Springer-Verlag, 1977.

TABLE 518–1. DIFFERENTIAL DIAGNOSIS OF LESIONS OF NERVE ROOTS AND PERIPHERAL NERVES (*Continued*)

Roots

T4	*T10*	*L2*	*L3*	*L4*	*L5*	*S1*	*S2–4*
Anterior chest and/or upper back	Midback and/or anterior abdomen	Across thigh	Across thigh	Down to medial malleolus	Back of thigh, lateral calf, dorsum of foot	Back of thigh, back of calf, lateral foot	Buttocks, genitalia, back of thigh
Usually none (upper back and chest at nipple level)	Usually none (midback and abdomen at umbilicus level)	Often none	Often none	Medial leg	Dorsum of foot	Behind lateral malleolus	Buttocks, genitalia
None	Decreased abdominal reflex	None	Adductor reflex	Knee jerk	None	Ankle jerk	Bulbocavernosus
Not discernible	None	Hip flexion, adduction of thigh	Knee extension, adduction of thigh	Inversion of foot	Dorsiflexion of toes and foot (latter L4 also)	Plantar flexion and eversion of foot	Bladder and bowel
Intravertebral or paravertebral tumor, herpes zoster	Intravertebral and paravertebral tumor, herpes zoster	Neurofibroma, meningioma, neoplastic disease; disc lesions very rare (except L4 < 5 per cent *all*)			Disc lesions, metastatic malignancy, neurofibromas, meningioma		Tumor, midline disc
Chest wall, piloerection, hyperhidrosis, unilateral gynecomastia, galactorrhea	Chest wall, piloerection, hyperhidrosis, retrograde ejaculation	Alterations in temperature and color of all or parts of the leg or thigh					Incontinence, impotence, urinary retention

Nerves

Ulnar	*Obturator*	*Femoral*	*Sciatic, Peroneal Division*	*Sciatic, Tibial Division*
Ulnar supplied fingers and palm distal to wrist, pain occasionally along course of nerve	Medial thigh	Anterior thigh and medial leg	Often painless	Often painless
Medial palm and fifth and medial half of ring finger, but often none at all	Often none		Often just dorsum of foot	Sole of foot
Nil	Adductor reflex	Knee jerk	None	Ankle jerk
All small hand muscles excluding abductor pollicis brevis, flexor carpi ulnaris, long flexors of ring and little fingers	Adduction of thigh	Extension of knee	Dorsiflexion, inversion and eversion of the foot (plus lateral hamstrings)	Plantar flexion and inversion of foot (plus medial hamstrings)
Elbow: trauma, bedrest, fractured olecranon; wrist: local trauma, ganglion of wrist joint	Pelvic neoplasm, pregnancy	Diabetes, femoral hernia, femoral artery aneurysm, posterior abdominal neoplasm, psoas abscess	Pressure palsy at fibula neck, hip fracture or dislocation, penetrating trauma to buttock, misplaced injection	Very rarely injured, even in buttock; peroneal division more sensitive to damage

guished from lesions of the rest of the final common pathway in part because spinal lesions are usually accompanied by signs of upper motoneuron disease as well as lower motoneuron disease and in part because of the relatively unique signs of lower motoneuron disease of the spinal cord. In the motor system, involvement of the anterior horn cells produces not only weakness, atrophy, and reflex diminution but also fasciculations (i.e., spontaneous firing of individual bundles of muscle that can be observed through the overlying skin). Fascicular twitchings occur with other lesions of the lower motoneuron as well, but less commonly than in anterior horn cell disease. In addition, in most spinal cord disease, the corticospinal tracts are involved, leading to spasticity, hyperactive reflexes, and extensor plantar responses. Extensor plantar responses may be present even when other signs of corticospinal tract disease are masked by the concomitant lower motoneuron disease.

In the sensory system, because the spinothalamic tract subserves pain and temperature sensation on the contralateral side of the body and the dorsal columns subserve proprioception on the ipsilateral side, dissociation between pin and temperature sensation on the one hand and proprioception and vibration on the other suggests spinal cord disease. When the spinocerebellar pathways are involved selectively, ataxia is the prominent complaint. If other pathways are spared, deep tendon reflexes may be normal or even hyperactive. The crossing of several pathways in the spinal cord gives additional clues that localize disease processes to the spinal cord. Lower and upper motoneuron disease confined to one side of the body, whether or not accompanied by vibratory and position sense loss, with absence of pain and temperature sensation on the contralateral part of the body (so-called *Brown-Séquard's syndrome*) suggests disease of one half of the spinal cord. Bilateral lower and upper motoneuron disease dysfunction, with bilateral loss of pain and temperature but sparing of light touch and position sense, suggests involvement of the anterior two thirds of the spinal cord, probably by occlusion of the anterior spinal artery or one of its branches. Profound absence of position sense, more marked in the upper than the lower extremities, with relative preservation of vibration sense suggests a posteriorly placed lesion of the upper cervical cord compressing the posterior columns. Anterior compressive lesions of the cord such as occur with herniated discs often produce bilateral and symmetrical upper motoneuron corticospinal tract dysfunction accompanied by profound loss of vibratory sense, relative sparing of position sense, and almost total sparing of pain, temperature, and touch sensation. The explanation for these findings is not certain. Some have suggested that the effect is due to mechanical deformation of the heavily myelinated fibers of the posterior columns and corticospinal tracts when the spinal cord is pushed but still tethered by the denticulate ligaments.

PAIN. Pain is a common but not an invariable accompaniment of lesions of peripheral common pathways. Pain and tenderness in muscles may appear with polymyositis and other inflammatory diseases of the muscle. They are generally absent from most myopathies and the dystrophies. Peripheral nerves that are compressed or entrapped often cause pain both locally and in the distribution of that nerve. Pain may also precede other symptoms of sensory change in nutritional neuropathy. Pain is a prominent finding in mechanical compressive lesions of nerve plexuses and roots, and may be present long before clinical sensory or motor findings indicate dysfunction of the neural structure. Such pain is commonly constant and relatively severe, but frequently can be relieved by postural maneuvers which serve to decompress the neural structure. Thus, patients with lumbar discs may be free of pain when they are lying down or standing and bending forward, because both positions make the intervertebral foramen larger. The same patient may be uncomfortable when sitting or standing in a hyperlordotic position, because both of these positions increase the pressure in the disc and make the intervertebral foramen smaller.

MANAGEMENT OF PERIPHERAL COMMON PATHWAY LESIONS. In patients presenting with symptoms of peripheral common pathway dysfunction, particularly weakness, atrophy, loss of tendon reflexes, and signs of lower sensory and autonomic neuron dysfunction, appropriate management depends on diagnosis. The physician should first endeavor by history and physical examination to localize the lesion to one of the structures of the peripheral common pathway. Such a localization is usually made clinically, on the basis of the history and neurologic findings, but may require the support of laboratory tests. The most important tests for diagnosing abnormalities of peripheral structures are electrodiagnostic studies and muscle and nerve biopsy; the most important tests for examining central structures are CT scan and myelography. Once the lesion is localized, the physician should consider in a systematic fashion the lesions that may involve that structure. These are detailed in later chapters. Each disease of each of the structures of the final common pathway produces characteristic signs, symptoms, and pathologic changes.

When a definite diagnosis has been made, appropriate treatment can be instituted if the disorder diagnosed has an appropriate treatment, e.g., thymectomy, steroids, possibly plasmapheresis, and anticholinesterase agents for myasthenia gravis. In the absence of an appropriate treatment, the physician must attempt to keep the patient as functional as possible given the degree of disability. This includes the use of analgesic drugs to relieve pain if present, the use of assistive devices such as short leg braces in patients with foot drop, a wheelchair for patients who cannot walk, scrupulous attention to skin and joint care in patients with sensory loss in areas subject to trauma, and a fairly active program by skilled physical therapists who can train the patient not only to strengthen the muscles that remain but to learn to substitute one muscle for another. With appropriate training, many otherwise bedridden patients can lead a full life in a wheelchair, using other assistive devices. Since many of the diseases of the lower motoneuron are progressive, frequent monitoring of the patient's neurologic status, with special attention to respiratory function, may help in planning activities that he is capable of carrying out. These disorders are usually disabling but do not affect cognitive functions, and patients frequently become desperate, demanding the latest "cure" that has appeared in the newspapers or that is being tried in some distant clinic around the world. The physician has an important role to play in helping the patient evaluate the likelihood that the new therapy will be effective and in continuing to give supportive therapy so that the patient does not feel abandoned. Paradoxically, it might seem, this approach is much easier for patients with terminal cancer than those with neuromuscular disease. In cancer, a variety of new and experimental drugs are available that even to the scientist appear to have a rational basis. In many of the neuromuscular diseases, the nature of the illness is so obscure that one has no rational basis for choosing even an experimental drug. It is in this setting that unlikely remedies (such as snake venom) appear and the physician's emotional support can be particularly helpful.

Aids to the Investigation of Peripheral Nerve Injuries. London, Her Majesty's Royal Stationery Office, 1953. *A paperback pictorial essay that should be carried in every physician's bag. Photographs demonstrate how to test muscles, and drawings illustrate the sensory and motor distribution of nerve roots and nerves.*

Patten J: Neurological Differential Diagnosis. New York, Springer-Verlag, 1977. *A monograph describing with schematic drawings the localization and differential diagnosis of common neurologic lesions.*

519. INTERVERTEBRAL DISC DISEASE

HERNIATED DISC. Herniated intervertebral discs are the most common identifiable cause of neck or low back pain (see Ch. 481). Between each two vertebral bodies is a fibrocartilaginous intervertebral disc. The disc consists of a soft inner nucleus pulposus (a remnant of the notochord) surrounded by thicker fibrous tissue (the anulus fibrosus). The nucleus pulposus is gelatinous in structure and acts as a shock absorber between adjacent vertebral bodies. With advancing age, the nucleus pulposus loses fluid, volume, and resiliency, and the entire disc structure becomes more susceptible to trauma and compression. Tears develop in the anulus fibrosus as a result of repeated minor trauma, and eventually, if the tears become large enough, a portion of the soft nucleus pulposus herniates through the anulus. Asymptomatic herniation may occur into the center of the vertebral bodies bordering the disc (Schmorl's nodules). However, if the disc material herniates into the vertebral canal, it compresses nerve endings and nerve roots, causing pain and other symptoms. Generally, the disc herniates lateral to the posterior longitudinal ligament, thus compressing spinal roots as they enter the intervertebral foramen. Occasionally the disc herniates more centrally, compressing either the spinal cord in the cervical or thoracic area or the cauda equina in the lumbar area. Some authors use the term herniated disc to mean that the disc maintains continuity with the nucleus pulposus, and extruded disc to mean that the disc fragment within the spinal canal has lost continuity with the disc itself. The signs and symptoms of herniated discs are caused by compression of the disc on either nerve roots or the spinal cord. The specific signs and symptoms depend in part on whether the predominant compression is spinal cord or nerve root, and in part on the level at which the neural structures are compressed. The most common sites of disc herniation are in the lumbar area, between L4 and L5 and between L5 and S1. The L5 and S1 roots are those commonly compressed by lumbar disc herniation. (Because of the anatomy of the exiting roots, a laterally herniated disc between L4 and L5 compresses the L5 root, and a disc between L5 and S1, the S1 root.) L3–L4 herniations are less common. In the cervical area, the common herniations occur between C5 and C6 (C6 root) and C6 and C7 (C7 root). Less commonly, herniations appear between C3 and C4, C4 and C5, and C7 and T1. The C7 root is the one most commonly compressed by cervical disc herniation. Thoracic discs are rare, but when they occur they usually compress the spinal cord as well as the emerging root because most of the thoracic vertebral canal is occupied by spinal cord. Although clinical localization in diagnosis of disc disease is usually quite accurate, at times an extruded disc fragment may be large enough to affect several roots, or may migrate from the disc space in which it herniated, causing signs at a distance from the original herniation.

The most common symptom of a herniated disc is pain. The pain from disc disease is of two types: local and radicular. Local pain is felt as a dull aching in the neck or back, with an associated stiffness of those structures, frequently occurring episodically in response to minor trauma (or no discernible trauma at all) months or years prior to the development of radicular pain. The exact pathogenesis of the local pain in disc disease is not known, but some believe that it results from compression of the sinu-vertebral nerve, a recurrent branch of the nerve root that supplies the dura mater. Radicular pain may occasionally be the first sign of disc disease, but is far more likely to follow repetitive bouts of local pain. Radicular pain is generally sudden in onset, often following minor trauma such as a twist, turn, or unusual bend. Radicular pain is perceived as sharp and well localized, and may radiate from the back along the entire distribution of the involved root or affect only a portion of the root. Both local and radicular pain have the characteristics of being exacerbated by activity and relieved by rest.

With cervical disc herniation, most patients hold their necks stiffly and resist passive movement. Lateral bending either to or away from the side of the herniated disc frequently exacerbates both the local and radicular pain. The patient may be more comfortable with his neck slightly flexed but is usually comfortable only in the recumbent position. Patients with lumbar disc disease are most comfortable lying, most uncomfortable sitting, and a little less uncomfortable standing. The back is held stiffly, so that the normal lumbar lordotic curve is no longer apparent, and pain is usually exacerbated by extension of the back. Slow forward bending sometimes relieves the pain. Muscle spasm is prominent with both cervical and lumbar disc disease. Raising the intraspinal pressure, as by coughing, sneezing, or straining, increases the pain sharply. Stretching the compressed root also aggravates the pain. In the upper extremities, extending the arm and laterally flexing the neck away from the extended arm often reproduces radicular pain. In the lower extremities, raising the extended leg with the patient in the recumbent position frequently reproduces the pain of an L5 or S1 radiculopathy and, if the pain is felt on the opposite side as well (crossed straight leg raising), the sign is very suggestive of herniated disc disease. Symptoms of L4 radiculopathy can often be reproduced by extending the hip (stretching the femoral nerve) when the patient is lying in the prone position. Often tenderness is present along the entire distribution of the nerve(s) supplied by the compressed root as well as in muscles supplied by the root. In patients with cervical disc disease, palpation or light percussion of the brachial plexus and the supraclavicular fossa or axilla often causes pain. In patients with lumbar disc disease, palpation over the femoral nerve (L4) in the groin or over the sciatic nerve (L5–S1) in the calf, thigh, or buttocks often causes severe pain. Occasionally tenderness in the calf (the posterior tibial nerve) is so striking as to suggest that the patient is suffering from thrombophlebitis rather than disc herniation. Other neurologic signs that commonly accompany disc disease include paresthesias and sensory loss in the distribution of the involved root and motor weakness in the myotome supplied by that root. The most important single sign is a diminished or absent reflex, giving objectively verifiable evidence of neurologic disease.

If an intervertebral disc herniates medially rather than laterally, it may spare the root and involve the spinal cord directly. When this occurs, there may be little or no pain or pain in a bilateral radicular distribution. Sometimes the pain is felt at a site far distant from the disc herniation as a result of compression of long sensory tracts in the spinal cord. The signs and symptoms of cord involvement are the same as those of compression of the spinal cord by other mass lesions. The corticospinal tracts are involved early, leading to spastic weakness and hyperreflexia below the site of the compression. Large myelinated dorsal column fibers are more sensitive than spinothalamic fibers, leading to an early loss of position and particularly vibration sense, with relative sparing of pin and temperature sensation. In contradistinction to diseases that arise within the spinal cord themselves, compressive lesions tend to spare bladder and bowel function until late. (The exception is when the compression occurs either at the conus medullaris or in the cauda equina.)

The diagnosis of herniated disc is deduced from the characteristic clinical symptoms and findings. In many patients with radiculopathy, findings are minimal and it is the history that must establish the diagnosis. The differential diagnosis of herniated disc disease when there are signs of spinal cord or root dysfunction includes the several mass lesions that can compress roots or spinal cord; these are described in Ch. 518. When the patient complains of back pain, with or without a radicular component, but has no motor, sensory, or reflex changes to suggest the site of a radiculopathy, the differential diagnosis includes pain arising from pain-sensitive nerve endings in the muscles, ligaments, and joints of the vertebral bodies and the paravertebral structures. These structures must be examined carefully to determine which of them is responsible. A high-resolution computed tomographic (CT) scan often establishes the diagnosis.

There is controversy about the management of herniated discs. Most physicians believe that the first step is bedrest. Some investigators have reported that adrenocorticosteroids, either taken orally or injected into the epidural space, may hasten resolution of pain and other symptoms. A short course of oral steroids is safe, but there is no unequivocal evidence that it is efficacious. Steroids injected into the epidural or subarachnoid space, particularly those in depot form, may produce severe inflammatory reactions and are inadvisable. Surgery is indicated when (1) bedrest fails, and the patient is incapacitated by severe, intractable pain; (2) a centrally placed lumbar disc compresses the cauda equina, producing urinary dysfunction; (3) motor weakness, e.g., foot drop, is severe and progresses on bedrest; or (4) acute cervical or thoracic discs cause substantial myelopathy. Myelography may be performed before surgical extirpation to localize the site of disc herniation and to determine whether other disc lesions or tumors are present as well, but in many cases the CT scan alone suffices. The best operation removes the involved disc, leaving as much bone as possible intact. Fusion of the lumbar spine is rarely necessary. Lumbar disc operations are done posteriorly via a laminotomy. Cervical disc operations may be done either posteriorly to decompress the cord or anteriorly to remove the disc without disturbing posterior bony elements. The surgical approach for myelopathy should probably be anterior if the disc is in the cervical area and lateral if the disc is in the thoracic area.

A relatively new technique of disc dissolution by the injection of the enzyme chymopapain directly into a lumbar disc space has received enthusiastic support from some centers. The technique is still being subjected to clinical trials, and what role it will play in the therapeutic armamentarium remains uncertain.

SPONDYLOSIS. Spondylosis is a term applied to chronic degenerative disease of intervertebral discs associated with reactive changes in the adjacent vertebral bodies. Spondylotic changes in the neck and low back increase with increasing age and are almost invariably present in the elderly. Spondylosis is usually asymptomatic except when the reactive tissue compresses a nerve root or the spinal cord. When this occurs, the signs and symptoms are similar to those of herniated disc disease, but the onset is less abrupt and the treatment often more difficult. In both the cervical and lumbar areas, spondylosis is more likely to produce spinal cord or cauda equina symptoms if the sagittal diameter of the spinal canal is congenitally narrow. The symptoms are much more likely to develop in middle life if a marginally adequate canal is further impinged upon by osteophytes. The signs and symptoms of *cervical spondylosis* result from compression either of the spinal cord or its emerging roots and are thus similar to those of herniated discs. Most patients suffer either radiculopathy or myelopathy, but not both. Pain is common in patients with spondylotic radiculopathy but usually less acute and severe than that with herniated discs. Because the onset is more insidious, pain may not be a prominent feature, and muscle spasm may be absent. However, the vertebral degenerative changes in the neck lead to limitation of movement in all directions. The classic picture of cervical spondylotic myelopathy is one of little or no pain but slowly developing weakness, atrophy, and fasciculations in the upper extremities, particularly the small muscles of the hand, and spastic paraparesis with decreased proprioception in the legs. At first the findings may suggest a diagnosis of amyotrophic lateral sclerosis. However, in cervical spondylosis there are sensory changes, particularly vibration loss in the lower extremities, and in amyotrophic lateral sclerosis there are fasciculations in areas different from the anterior horn cells compressed at the cervical level (e.g., the tongue). The differential diagnosis also includes other compressive lesions of root and spinal cord.

Plain x-rays of the cervical spine confirm the presence of cervical spondylosis, but many patients without symptoms have similar x-ray findings. Evidence that spondylosis is symptomatic is found by measuring the sagittal diameter of the cervical canal. When the diameter is less than 10 mm, cord compression is almost a certainty. If the diameter is over 13 mm, it is unlikely that cord compression is occurring, but a soft disc or tumor not seen on the x-ray may be impinging on the cord. The CT scan sometimes helps to delineate accurately the size of the cervical canal, and myelography determines the site of the lesion and the degree of obstruction.

The natural history of cervical myelopathy and radiculopathy is not well established. It is known that many patients experience long periods of pain relief and remission or stabilization of neurologic symptoms. Such spontaneous improvement often makes it difficult to evaluate the effect of a particular treatment. Many physicians prefer, once having established the diagnosis, to begin conservative treatment with a period of bedrest accompanied by cervical traction and stabilization of the neck with a soft collar. If these approaches are successful, they should be continued. However, if the patient develops progressive neurologic signs in the face of conservative treatment, surgical therapy is indicated. Most neurosurgeons believe that if the spinal cord compression occurs at one or two segments, anterior removal of the disc material with spinal fusion is the preferred course. If more than a few segments are involved, laminectomy with foraminotomy is preferred.

In some patients with cervical spondylosis (or with congenital narrowing of the cervical spinal canal, or both), neurologic symptoms are exacerbated by exercise, with pain, numbness, and weakness appearing when a particular extremity is exercised. The pathogenesis is thought to be compression of the spinal cord so severe that the blood supply to the area cannot increase during its activity, leading to ischemia of cord and root structures (pseudoclaudication).

The considerations described above under cervical spondylosis also apply to *lumbar spondylosis*. The symptoms of lumbar spondylosis are similar to those of herniated disc, often occurring at multiple levels. One outstanding difference is the frequent presence of pseudoclaudication from cauda equina compression in patients with spinal stenosis from either spondylosis or congenital narrowing. Typically, symptoms and signs are evoked or accentuated by walking, and include pain, paresthesias, and weakness in the lower extremities. All of the symptoms may disappear when the patient ceases walking, even though he remains in the standing position. At times, however, the symptoms may be exacerbated by prolonged standing and relieved only by sitting or lying down. Pseudoclaudication of the cauda equina may be distinguished from intermittent vascular claudication in several ways. In vascular disease, the pulses in the lower extremities are usually absent or become absent as the patient begins exercise. With vascular disease, the symptoms are usually reproducible and stereotypic, i.e., the patient can predict the exact distance he can walk at a given speed before symptoms develop. Symptoms of cauda equina pseudoclaudication are less stereotypic, so that on some days patients can walk much longer distances than others. The reason for this variability is not known. In patients with pseudoclaudication the neurologic examination may be normal when the patient is at rest, but neurologic signs, particularly reflex absence, may appear as the patient exercises. In patients with pseudoclaudication the lumbar canal is narrowed on either lateral x-ray or CT scan, and there is a substantial block to the passage of myelographic dye. With severe lumbar stenosis, conservative treatment usually fails and decompressive laminectomy is the treatment of choice.

520. NEOPLASMS OF THE SPINAL CANAL

Neoplastic growths that cause nerve root or spinal cord compression can be paravertebral, extradural, intradural, or intramedullary. The majority of neoplasms that cause spinal cord compression are extradural and metastatic. Most extradural neoplasms originate in the vertebral body surrounding the spinal cord and compress spinal roots or cord without invading them. Most intradural neoplasms also cause symptoms by compressing spinal roots or cord without invading, but unlike extradural neoplasms the majority are benign and slow growing. Intramedullary neoplasms cause symptoms by both invading and compressing spinal structures; the tumors may be either benign or malignant.

PARAVERTEBRAL TUMORS. Neoplastic lesions that begin in or metastasize to the paravertebral space often cause serious and perplexing neurologic problems. The tumor may extend longitudinally within the paravertebral space, progressively compressing nerve roots as it grows. At times, the tumor may grow through an intervertebral foramen and compress not only the nerve root but also the spinal cord. Rarely, spinal cord symptoms may be caused by paravertebral tumors compromising radicular arteries that supply the spinal cord. If the tumor is more lateral than the immediate paravertebral space, the brachial, lumbar, or sacral plexus may be compressed, causing symptoms similar to root compression but with a different pattern of sensory and motor loss. The symptoms of extravertebral tumor begin insidiously with severe, unremitting pain, often with a burning quality and usually localized just lateral to the spine, radiating in a band-like pattern in the distribution of the involved dermatome(s). If the lesion involves abdominal or thoracic roots, motor and sensory changes are usually not appreciated by either the patient or the examiner. Autonomic changes may be a prominent or the only neurologic sign. Hyperhidrosis occurring in a band coinciding with the site of the pain strongly suggests the diagnosis. When the tumor involves cervical or lumbar roots, the pain may be soon followed by numbness in fingertips or toes, with accompanying weakness and reflex diminution, depending on the roots involved. Autonomic changes, including anhidrosis or hyperhidrosis, may affect the arm or leg. Horner's syndrome and/or diaphragmatic paralysis often accompany cervical or upper thoracic paravertebral tumors. The diagnosis is best established by computed tomographic (CT) scan at the level suggested by the clinical findings. The CT scan can also determine whether the lesion has grown through the intervertebral foramen or has eroded vertebral bodies. Myelography should also be performed to assess the extent of intravertebral tumor.

The differential diagnosis of paravertebral tumor includes a variety of other disorders that cause paravertebral pain with or without compression of nerve roots. *Psychophysiologic muscle tension syndromes* often cause low back or neck paravertebral pain. In some instances, there may be radiation of the pain, usually in a nondermatomal distribution. On examination there is often marked tenderness of muscles, and sometimes one can find trigger points identified by either their hardness to palpation or their ability to reproduce patients' symptoms when they are compressed. Relief of pain in these instances can be produced by injecting the trigger point with saline solution or a local anesthetic. Temporary relief of pain after such injection does not imply that structural disease is absent; the trigger points may be a reaction to spinal or nerve root disease. In muscle tension syndrome, autonomic, sensory, or motor changes are never present. Disease of kidneys and other viscera lying in the retroperitoneal space may cause pain similar to that of paravertebral tumors, but the pain usually does not radiate and is not associated with autonomic, motor, or sensory changes. Percussion of the involved viscera reproduces the pain that is described as a dull ache rather than a neurogenic burning pain. Spontaneous or induced *entrapment neuropathies* not caused by tumor occasionally mimic the symptoms of paravertebral tumor. Chronic pain after a thoracotomy *(postthoracotomy pain)* probably results from entrapment of nerve roots at the time of surgery, perhaps with neuroma formation. The pain characteristically appears shortly after surgery and may be unremitting for many years. Motor, sensory, or autonomic changes are rare. The pain can sometimes be relieved by paravertebral anesthetic blocks.

The management of paravertebral masses depends on the diagnosis. In patients known to have cancer, particularly lymphomas or carcinomas of the breast or lung, the tumor can be assumed to be metastatic and should be treated with radiation therapy and, if available, chemotherapy. If the patient has no history of cancer, a biopsy is required and, depending on the site of the lesion, resection may be attempted both to establish a diagnosis and to decompress the nerve roots. Once the diagnosis is established by biopsy, further therapy such as radiation or chemotherapy may be indicated.

EXTRADURAL TUMORS. Extradural neoplasms compress spinal roots and cord in one of three ways. Either they arise in vertebrae surrounding the spinal cord and grow into the epidural space or they arise in the paravertebral space and grow through the intervertebral foramen to compress the cord laterally. Rarely, tumors may arise in the epidural space itself, without involving either vertebral or paravertebral structures. Most extradural neoplasms are metastatic from carcinomas of the breast, lung, prostate, or kidney or from malignant melanoma. Some extradural neoplasms arise de novo in the vertebral bodies (e.g., chordoma, osteogenic sarcoma, myeloma, chondrosarcoma). A minority of extradural neoplasms are benign (e.g., chordoma, osteoma, osteoid osteoma, angioma). Because extradural neoplasms usually arise in and destroy bone before producing spinal cord compression, local pain is the first symptom and may precede the development of either radicular pain or other symptoms of spinal cord compression by weeks or months, depending on the rate of growth of the tumor. Rarely, extradural neoplasms may be painless and the first symptoms may be those of spinal cord dysfunction. The first spinal cord symptoms other than pain are usually those of corticospinal tract disease with weakness, spasticity, and hyperreflexia, followed by paresthesias and loss of vibration and position sense. Unless the lesion compresses the conus medullaris or the cauda equina, bladder and bowel dysfunctions are late signs. As with other causes of spinal cord compression, extradural neoplasms cause symptoms first distally and later proximally. Thus, even thoracic and cervical neoplasms generally cause weakness and numbness in the legs before trunk and upper extremity muscles are involved. The diagnosis of extradural spinal cord compression must be suspected by the history of pain followed by signs and symptoms of spinal cord dysfunction and confirmed by radiographic study. In about 85 per cent of patients suffering from extradural spinal cord compression, there are bone lesions at the site of compression on plain radiographs. In the few patients with negative plain radiographs, x-ray tomography, radionuclide bone scan, or CT scan may demonstrate a bone lesion. The diagnosis of extradural spinal cord compression and its localization require myelography. A myelogram not only establishes the site of cord compression but also determines that the compression is extradural rather than intradural or intramedullary. The differential diagnosis of extradural neoplasms includes inflammatory disease of bone and epidural abscess (e.g., vertebral tuberculosis, bacterial osteomyelitis), acute or subacute epidural hematomas (see Ch. 505), herniated intervertebral discs, spondylosis, and, very rarely, extramedullary hematopoiesis (in patients with severe and chronic anemias) or epidural lipomatosis (in patients on chronic steroid therapy). Often a definitive diagnosis can be made only by biopsy of the lesion either during the course of a decompressive laminectomy or by percutaneous needle biopsy of the involved vertebral body.

The treatment of extradural neoplasms depends on the cause. Most neoplasms that cause extradural spinal cord compression are malignant and progress rapidly. Once spinal cord symptoms begin, paraplegia may develop in a matter of hours to days. Complete paraplegia is irreversible, whereas patients with mild to moderate spinal cord signs often can maintain or regain spinal cord function. Thus, the early diagnosis and vigorous emergency treatment of extradural spinal cord compression is mandatory. The diagnosis and localization are established by myelography. The treatment of patients known to be suffering from cancer who develop typical signs and symptoms of spinal cord compression from extradural metastases is radiation therapy. Therapy should begin with corticosteroids (dexamethasone, 16 to 100 mg daily) to decrease spinal cord edema, and radiation therapy should begin immediately upon establishing the diagnosis. If chemotherapeutic agents are available, they should be used in conjunction with steroids and radiation therapy for the treatment of metastatic or primary malignant tumors of the extradural space. In patients not known to be suffering from a primary cancer, metastatic disease is the most common cause of extradural spinal cord compression, but in these instances a definitive diagnosis must be made by biopsy. Such patients should begin corticosteroid therapy followed by surgery with removal of as much tumor as possible for both diagnostic and therapeutic purposes. If a malignant neoplasm is encountered at operation, radiation therapy should be begun as soon after the surgery as is practical. In a few patients in whom radiation therapy and chemotherapy are ineffective, resection of the vertebral body involved by tumor may delay the development of paraplegia. In some patients with extradural tumors and destruction of the vertebral body, subluxation may compress the cord and may be relieved by surgery. Benign extradural tumors require surgery.

INTRADURAL EXTRAMEDULLARY TUMORS. Most intradural tumors are benign. Meningiomas and neurofibromas are the two most common types. Teratomas, arachnoid cysts, and lipomas are less common causes. *Meningiomas* occur in middle-aged and elderly women, predominantly in the thoracic region of the spinal cord. Another common site of meningiomas is at the foramen magnum. Meningiomas are benign, slow growing, and usually located on the posterior aspect of the spinal cord. Pain is the first symptom in the majority of patients, but in about 25 per cent the meningioma is painless, the first symptom being gradually developing signs of spinal cord compression. Because they are often located on the posterior aspect of the cord, paresthesias and sensory changes beginning distally in the lower extremities are a frequent early symptom and are often mistaken for peripheral neuropathy. As the disease progresses, however, corticospinal tract signs indicate the spinal origin of the symptoms. Even when spinal cord signs and symptoms are obvious, the lack of pain may lead one to suspect a degenerative or demyelinating disease such as multiple sclerosis rather than a neoplasm. In patients with meningiomas, the lumbar puncture reveals an elevated spinal fluid protein content higher than that in degenerative or demyelinating diseases. Myelography usually establishes the diagnosis of a tumor. When the tumors are located posteriorly, if small or near the foramen magnum, they may be difficult to identify on the usual prone myelogram. If a meningioma is suspected and routine myelography is negative, the spinal needle should be removed and the patient fluoroscoped in the supine position in order to visualize adequately the posterior aspect of the subarachnoid space. The treatment of spinal cord compression from meningiomas is surgical removal. Because the tumor grows so slowly and the cord has an opportunity to adapt to compression, even patients with severe neurologic disability often make a full recovery after the lesion is removed.

The second common cause of intradural spinal cord compression is *neurofibroma*. Because these tumors usually arise from the dorsal root, radicular pain is often the first symptom preceding signs of spinal cord compression by months or years. When spinal cord compression develops, it progresses slowly. Some patients with spinal neurofibromas suffer from neurofibromatosis. That diagnosis may be suspected either by a positive family history or by the cutaneous stigmata of the disease. A neurofibroma may extend on either side of the intervertebral foramen, involving the root both in the paravertebral space and within the spinal canal. As neurofibromas grow through the intervertebral foramen, they enlarge it, a finding appreciated by an appropriately positioned radiograph. The cerebrospinal fluid protein is almost always elevated. The diagnosis is established by myelography, and surgical extirpation of the lesion usually leads to complete recovery.

Occasionally *metastatic tumors* involving the leptomeninges present with intradural extramedullary mass lesions. Pain is almost always a prominent early symptom, and spinal cord compression develops more rapidly than it does with the more benign intradural tumors. In addition, malignant cells are frequently encountered in the spinal fluid. Spinal fluid glucose may be low in addition to the protein being elevated. The treatment of intradural malignant neoplasms is radiation therapy and chemotherapy, since complete surgical extirpation is almost always impossible. Because the tumor has almost always seeded the entire subarachnoid space, radiation therapy, if it is to have more than temporary effect, must be supplemented by chemotherapy or be delivered to the entire neuraxis.

INTRAMEDULLARY TUMORS. The most common intramedullary spinal tumors are astrocytomas (usually benign) and ependymomas. Other tumors which occasionally cause intramedullary spinal lesions are hemangioblastomas, lipomas, and hematogenous metastases. Pain is an early symptom of most intramedullary tumors, and signs of spinal cord dysfunction progress rapidly or slowly, depending on the growth characteristics of the tumor. Intramedullary tumors are often associated with syringomyelia, the syrinx sometimes being at a distance from the primary tumor and producing its own symptoms of spinal dysfunction. The so-called characteristic signs of intramedullary spinal cord lesions (dissociated sensory loss, sacral sparing, and early onset of bladder and bowel dysfunction) are not reliable enough clinically to distinguish intramedullary from extramedullary lesions; that diagnosis must be established by myelography and in the future probably by nuclear magnetic resonance scan. In some patients with long-standing benign intramedullary lesions, plain radiographs of the spine may show widening of the spinal canal and erosion of the pedicles. Myelography reveals an enlarged spinal cord, sometimes with complete block to the passage of myelographic contrast material. If a syrinx is suspected, a CT scan performed six hours after myelography with water-soluble contrast material usually reveals contrast material in the syrinx. The differential diagnosis of intramedullary tumors includes intramedullary abscesses and syringomyelia without tumor. A definitive diagnosis is established by biopsy. Successful surgical removal of intramedullary tumors is possible, particularly with ependymomas and hemangioblastomas but sometimes with gliomas as well. Highly skilled and experienced surgeons are necessary for tumors to be removed without increasing neurologic symptoms. If the tumor cannot be totally excised, postoperative radiation therapy often delays recurrence.

Ependymomas have a predilection to involve the lower end of the spinal cord and the filum terminale. An unusual symptom sometimes produced by such tumors is hydrocephalus. The patient may present with headache, papilledema, and enlarged cerebral ventricles without cauda equina signs or with only minor signs such as mild sacral sensory loss or an absent ankle jerk. The pathogenesis of the hydrocephalus is believed to be the plugging of pacchionian granulations by protein exuded from the tumor into the spinal fluid. The diagnosis is suspected in a patient with papilledema and hydrocephalus because the spinal fluid protein is very high; myelography establishes the diagnosis.

521. INFLAMMATORY DISEASES OF THE SPINAL CANAL

Inflammatory diseases that compress nerve roots and spinal cord can arise in extradural, intradural, or intramedullary areas. Extradural inflammatory lesions include tuberculosis or other bacterial osteomyelitis with extradural extension and primary extradural bacterial abscesses. These entities are discussed in Ch. 496. Intradural but extramedullary inflammatory diseases include bacterial, fungal, and parasitic meningitis; inflammatory disease of the leptomeninges of unknown cause such as sarcoidosis or Behçet's syndrome; and reactions to foreign substances such as myelographic contrast material, spinal anesthetics, or steroids. Occasionally, leptomeningeal infiltration with tumor or subarachnoid hemorrhage causes an inflammatory response of the leptomeninges that mimics subacute or chronic infection. All of these inflammatory intradural lesions can lead to spinal arachnoiditis. *Spinal arachnoiditis* is characterized by neck and back pain and by radicular pain in the distribution of the roots involved in the inflammatory process. Dysfunction of multiple roots, particularly in the lumbosacral area, is common; occasional patients go on to develop signs of spinal cord dysfunction, which may progress to paraplegia. The diagnosis of spinal arachnoiditis is established by myelography. A myelogram reveals spotty and irregular collections of contrast material with impairment of the flow through the subarachnoid space. Sometimes there is a complete block to the passage of the myelographic contrast material. The spinal fluid may contain an increased cellular response and a decreased glucose concentration. The protein concentration is usually elevated. Sometimes a specific infectious organism can be identified either by microscopic examination or by culture. There is no treatment for spinal arachnoiditis unless a specific infective agent is identified that can be treated with appropriate chemotherapy.

Intramedullary infectious processes include bacterial and parasitic abscesses and acute transverse myelitis. These entities are discussed under the appropriate chapter headings.

522. VASCULAR DISORDERS OF THE SPINAL CANAL

Extradural, intradural, and intramedullary vascular disorders all can cause spinal cord compression. The most common and most serious extradural vascular disease is *spinal epidural hematoma.* Hemorrhage into the spinal epidural space may occur spontaneously or be associated with trauma, a bleeding diathesis, or a vascular malformation. It is particularly common in patients being treated with anticoagulants. It may occasionally follow lumbar puncture, particularly in patients with bleeding abnormalities. Hemorrhage usually arises from the epidural venous plexus and tends to collect over the dorsum of the spinal cord covering several segments. The clinical picture is characterized by the sudden onset of severe localized back pain and the rapid development of spinal cord dysfunction, often leading to complete paraplegia in several hours. If the patient has a known bleeding disorder, the clinical diagnosis is easily established. In patients without known bleeding or clotting disorders the differential diagnosis includes acute epidural abscess and acute transverse myelopathy. Although occasional patients recover from paraparesis related to epidural spinal cord compression spontaneously, the majority require emergency surgical evacuation if the spinal cord function is to be saved. The more rapidly the paralysis develops and the longer the delay in decompression, the less likely is the patient to recover.

Intradural but extramedullary vascular lesions are usually caused by hemorrhage from *vascular malformations* on the surface of the spinal cord. Spinal subarachnoid hemorrhage is characterized by the sudden onset of back pain, often with a radicular component with or without the development of signs of spinal cord compression. A lumbar puncture reveals evidence of subarachnoid hemorrhage with red cells, xanthochromic spinal fluid, and usually an elevated protein concentration. In the absence of spinal cord signs, the differential diagnosis includes spontaneous intracerebral subarachnoid hemorrhage. The diagnosis of spinal subarachnoid hemorrhage is usually suspected clinically because symptoms begin with back pain in spinal subarachnoid hemorrhage and headache in intracerebral hemorrhage. Arteriovenous anomalies of the subarachnoid space and spinal cord can often be identified on myelography by the characteristic worm-like appearance of the surface of the spinal cord. Supine myelography may be necessary. More direct identification of the vascular anomaly requires selective spinal angiography. Because spinal angiography can

be risky, it should be considered only if surgery is contemplated. Some subarachnoid vascular malformations can be successfully removed after their feeding vessels are identified by angiography.

Vascular malformations may be present within the substance of the spinal cord as well as on its surface. They may thus give rise to intramedullary hemorrhage (hematomyelia) as well as subarachnoid hemorrhage. The sudden development of partial or complete transverse myelopathy is the most common onset. If there is bleeding into the subarachnoid space, pain in the neck and back and other signs of meningeal irritation occur.

Arteriovenous malformations may also compress the spinal cord or give rise to hemodynamic changes that result in spinal ischemia. In such cases, distortion and compression of the cord by enlarged, abnormal vessels occur only gradually, and patients present with slowly progressive symptoms of spinal cord dysfunction. Transient exacerbation of symptoms may occur in association with menstrual periods or pregnancy.

Complete or partial recovery of function can follow episodes of spinal cord ischemia or even small hemorrhages. The unchanging localization of the attacks and the prominence of pain help differentiate those symptoms caused by arteriovenous malformations from other recurrent neurologic disorders such as multiple sclerosis. In some patients a spinal bruit may be heard by auscultation over the site of the malformation. Angiography with regional catheterization of radicular vessels is necessary to establish the diagnosis and as a preliminary step to surgical treatment. Advances in microsurgery have increased considerably the chances for satisfactory removal of spinal vascular malformations. Embolization of the malformation or ligation of feeding arteries has been performed when the lesion cannot be removed surgically.

523. CONGENITAL ANOMALIES OF THE CRANIOVERTEBRAL JUNCTION, SPINE, AND SPINAL CORD

Congenital anomalies of the spine are common and are often encountered on radiographs of patients suffering from neck or low back pain. Some congenital anomalies such as *spina bifida occulta* are so common as to be considered variants of normal and are probably never responsible in and of themselves for low back pain. Other congenital anomalies such as the *Klippel-Feil syndrome* (congenital fusion of two or more cervical vertebrae) are not responsible for neck pain or other neurologic symptoms except when associated with coexisting congenital anomalies of the central nervous system. Congenital abnormalities of the spine that are common and usually asymptomatic but that must be considered potential causes of neck or back pain include *facet tropism* (misalignment of the facets on the two sides of the corresponding vertebral body; several authorities believe that this increases rotational stress on the facet joints and may cause back pain); *transitional vertebrae,* such as in sacralization of a lumbar vertebra or lumbarization of a sacral vertebra, altering spinal mechanics and resulting in instability and stress and sometimes producing back pain; and *spondylolisthesis* (forward slipping of one vertebral body onto another, caused by a defect between the articular facets). A third group of congenital anomalies of the spine consists of those that are likely to cause not only neck or back pain but also neurologic disability. These include *basilar impression,* which is often associated with *Arnold-Chiari malformation* (see later discussion). Severe spinal *scoliosis* or *kyphosis,* congenital *stenosis* of the lumbar or cervical spinal canal, anterior and lateral spinal *meningoceles,* and *diastematomyelia* are other causes of back pain and neurologic disability. Diastematomyelia is a bony abnormality that divides the spinal canal, leading to duplication of the spinal cord. It is usually associated with evidence of spina bifida on plain x-rays, and sometimes the bony septum can be identified as well. Patients who become symptomatic in adulthood almost always have some cutaneous abnormality, especially hypertrichosis over the sacral area. The disorder may be associated with other congenital abnormalities of the central nervous system as well.

ARNOLD-CHIARI MALFORMATION

INFANTILE FORM. The Arnold-Chiari malformation is characterized by downward displacement of the cerebellum through the foramen magnum of the skull and by similar caudal elongation of the medulla. The infantile form is commonly associated with other midline defects such as spina bifida and meningocele, hydrocephalus caused by aqueductal or fourth ventricular obstruction, and other congenital malformations of the brain and cord. The infantile form of the Arnold-Chiari malformation usually occurs because of hydrocephalus in the early months of life, with evidence of spina bifida or frank paraparesis resulting from meningomyelocele. Therapy is directed toward surgical relief of the hydrocephalus with a ventricular shunting procedure and repair of the meningomyelocele. Prognosis is poor for patients with extensive defects.

ADULT FORM. The malformation may be asymptomatic until adult life, when the patient gradually develops symptoms and signs of dysfunction of the cerebellum, lower cranial nerves, pyramidal tracts, and posterior columns. Downbeat nystagmus is a characteristic sign. At times the initial signs may be those of hydrocephalus secondary to obstruction of the cerebrospinal fluid pathways or to coexisting syringomyelia of the cervical spinal cord and medulla (see Ch. 491 and 513). Commonly, there is x-ray evidence of fusion of the cervical vertebrae, platybasia, or basilar impression, but computed tomographic or nuclear magnetic resonance scans can establish the diagnosis even when there are no coexisting bony abnormalities. The Arnold-Chiari malformation in adults may simulate syndromes produced by tumors near the foramen magnum and by multiple sclerosis. Surgical enlargement of the foramen magnum and decompression of the cervicomedullary junction are beneficial in selected cases.

BASILAR IMPRESSION AND PLATYBASIA

Basilar impression refers to abnormal invagination of the cervical spine into the base of the posterior fossa of the skull. The diagnosis is made from lateral roentgenograms of the skull when there is excessive protrusion of the tip of the odontoid process of the axis above Chamberlain's line, that is, a line drawn from the back of the hard palate to the posterior margin of the foramen magnum. Other radiologic criteria are also useful. *Platybasia* refers to flattening of the base of the skull, wherein lateral roentgenograms of the skull reveal flattening of the angle between the orbital plates of the anterior fossa and the clivus, the sloping anterior floor of the posterior fossa. The angle is normally 135 degrees and becomes 145 degrees or more in platybasia. Platybasia alone is asymptomatic.

These malformations, which commonly coexist or may exist alone, are usually developmental in origin, and there may be hereditary transmission. Occasionally, these deformations of the base of the skull may result from metabolic bone diseases such as rickets, osteitis deformans, osteomalacia, or osteogenesis imperfecta. The congenital form may be associated with the Klippel-Feil syndrome, Arnold-Chiari malformation, and other congenital malformations of the altas and axis, such as fusion of the atlas to the base of the skull, malpositioning of the odontoid process, or atlantoaxial subluxation. Minor degrees of deformity of the base of the skull give rise to no symptoms. The neck appears shortened, and its movements may be limited. With more severe invagination, there may be signs of impaired function of the cerebellum, lower cranial nerves, pyramidal tracts, and posterior columns. Syringomyelia and syringobulbia may also be present. Increased intracranial pressure may develop owing to obstruction of the foramina of the fourth ventricle and the basal cisterns. The clinical manifestations must be differentiated from those caused by neoplasms in the region of the foramen magnum and multiple sclerosis. When neurologic signs are progressive, surgical decompression of the posterior fossa and upper cervical cord may be indicated.

Aminoff MJ: Spinal Angiomas. Oxford, Blackwell Scientific Publications, 1976. *A comprehensive text on spinal vascular anomalies.*

Austin GM (ed.): The Spinal Cord. 3rd ed. New York, Igaku-Shoin, 1983. *The third edition of a comprehensive, multi-authored monograph describing the clinical findings and management of many disorders of the spinal cord, including lumbar and cervical disc disease.*

Vinken PJ, Bruyn GW: Tumours of the spine and spinal cord, I & II. Handbook of Clinical Neurology, Vol. 19, 20. New York, American Elsevier Publishing Company, 1975, 1976. *Comprehensive descriptions of benign and malignant tumors and herniated discs.*

Vinken PJ, Bruyn GW: Congenital malformations of the spine and spinal cord. Handbook of Clinical Neurology, Vol 32. New York, American Elsevier Publishing Company, 1978. *Comprehensive essays on congenital anomalies of the spine and spinal cord, including chapters on stenosis of the lumbar and cervical spinal canal and spondylodysplasia.*

Section Fifteen DISEASES OF THE PERIPHERAL NERVOUS SYSTEM

524. INTRODUCTION AND BASIC TERMINOLOGY

Herbert H. Schaumburg

The structure and function of the peripheral nervous system (PNS) appear deceptively simple when compared with the central nervous system (CNS). Actually, however, PNS diseases represent a confusing jumble of conditions whose only common thread appears to be PNS dysfunction. Thus, while the anatomic diagnosis of peripheral neuropathy is readily established in nearly 100 per cent of cases by symptoms and signs, the correct cause is determined in less than one half of cases except in a few special centers. Recent clinical and experimental studies suggest a simple, anatomic classification of most PNS disorders (see Ch. 525) insuring that a working knowledge of the common peripheral neuropathies can be easily mastered. However, since common diseases (diabetes or malignancy) produce more than one type of anatomic reaction in the PNS and most physicians are "etiology oriented," this chapter is organized according to individual diseases, stressing their common anatomic and pathophysiologic features whenever possible.

Certain terms associated with peripheral nerve disease have, by common usage, acquired set connotations. These include:

Neuropathy (peripheral neuropathy). This is the usual term for any disorder of peripheral nerves and replaces the term *peripheral neuritis.*

Polyneuropathy (symmetrical polyneuropathy). This designates a generalized process resulting in widespread and symmetrical effects on the peripheral nervous system.

Focal or multifocal neuropathy (mononeuropathy, mononeuropathy multiplex). These terms indicate local involvement of one or more individual peripheral nerves.

Dysesthesia. This term, like paresthesia, is poorly defined; it is commonly used to describe an unpleasant sensation produced by an ordinarily painless stimulus.

Paresthesia. This term indicates a spontaneous aberrant sensation such as pins and needles or tingling.

Hypoesthesia. This term refers to diminished sensation.

Hyperesthesia. This condition is an excessive response to sensory stimulus, even when the sensory threshold is elevated.

525. ANATOMIC CLASSIFICATION OF NEUROPATHY

Herbert H. Schaumburg

SYMMETRICAL GENERALIZED NEUROPATHY (POLYNEUROPATHY)

DISTAL AXONOPATHY (dying-back neuropathy). This is the most common morphologic reaction of the peripheral nervous system (PNS) to toxins and probably underlies many metabolic and hereditary neuropathies.

The pathologic features include initial degeneration of the distal ends of large and long axons; the myelin sheath breaks down concomitantly with axonal disintegration. Axonal degeneration appears to advance slowly proximally toward the nerve cell body. Schwann cells and their connective tissue tubes remain in distal nerves, facilitating appropriate peripheral regeneration (Fig. 525–1).

Many prominent clinical phenomena closely correlate with the morphologic profile. Gradual onset reflects chronic metabolic disease or prolonged intoxication, stocking-glove sensorimotor loss reflects distal axonal degeneration in long nerves (sciatic, ulnar), normal cerebrospinal fluid protein reflects the sparing of proximal sited nerve roots, and slow recovery corresponds to the indolent rate of axonal repair.

MYELINOPATHY. The term myelinopathy, when applied to the PNS, refers to conditions in which the lesion primarily affects myelin or the myelinating (Schwann) cell. The Guillain-Barré syndrome is the only frequently encountered disease that primarily affects PNS myelin. It is likely that the demyelination of spinal roots and nerves in this disorder results from an immune-system–mediated attack on PNS myelin.

The cardinal pathologic features, depicted in Figure 525–2, include primary destruction of the myelin sheath with the axon usually left intact. Demyelination initially affects multiple sites in nerves. The Schwann cell subsequently divides and rapidly remyelinates the axon to restore function.

Many prominent clinical findings correlate closely with the morphologic profile. Onset and recovery are rapid, reflecting the speed of demyelination and remyelination. Initial changes may be distal or proximal or may affect cranial nerves. Generalized weakness and reflex loss are dominant features, reflecting the vulnerability of long myelinated fibers, and the cerebrospinal fluid protein is usually elevated because inflammation in spinal roots results in leakage of protein into the surrounding subarachnoid space.

NEURONOPATHY. This term describes conditions in which the initial morphologic or biochemical changes occur in the neuron cell body. If the changes are intense, the affected neuron dies and there is permanent total motor or sensory dysfunction in the affected segment. The neuronopathies are a heterogeneous, poorly understood group of conditions and, in the broadest sense, include many disorders of motor, sensory, and autonomic neurons. Infectious neuronopathies include familiar conditions such as poliomyelitis (motor neuronopathy) and herpes

TABLE 525–1. CLASSIFICATION OF PERIPHERAL NEUROPATHY

A. Symmetrical generalized polyneuropathy
   - Distal axonopathy (associated with drugs, industrial chemicals, metabolic diseases, deficiency syndromes)
   - Myelinopathy (associated with diphtheria, Guillain-Barré syndrome, genetic leukodystrophies)
   - Neuropathy (associated with motor neuron diseases, herpes zoster neuronitis, carcinomatous sensory neuronopathy)

B. Focal and multifocal neuropathies (mononeuropathy)
   - Ischemia
   - Trauma
   - Infiltration (granulomatous, malignancy)

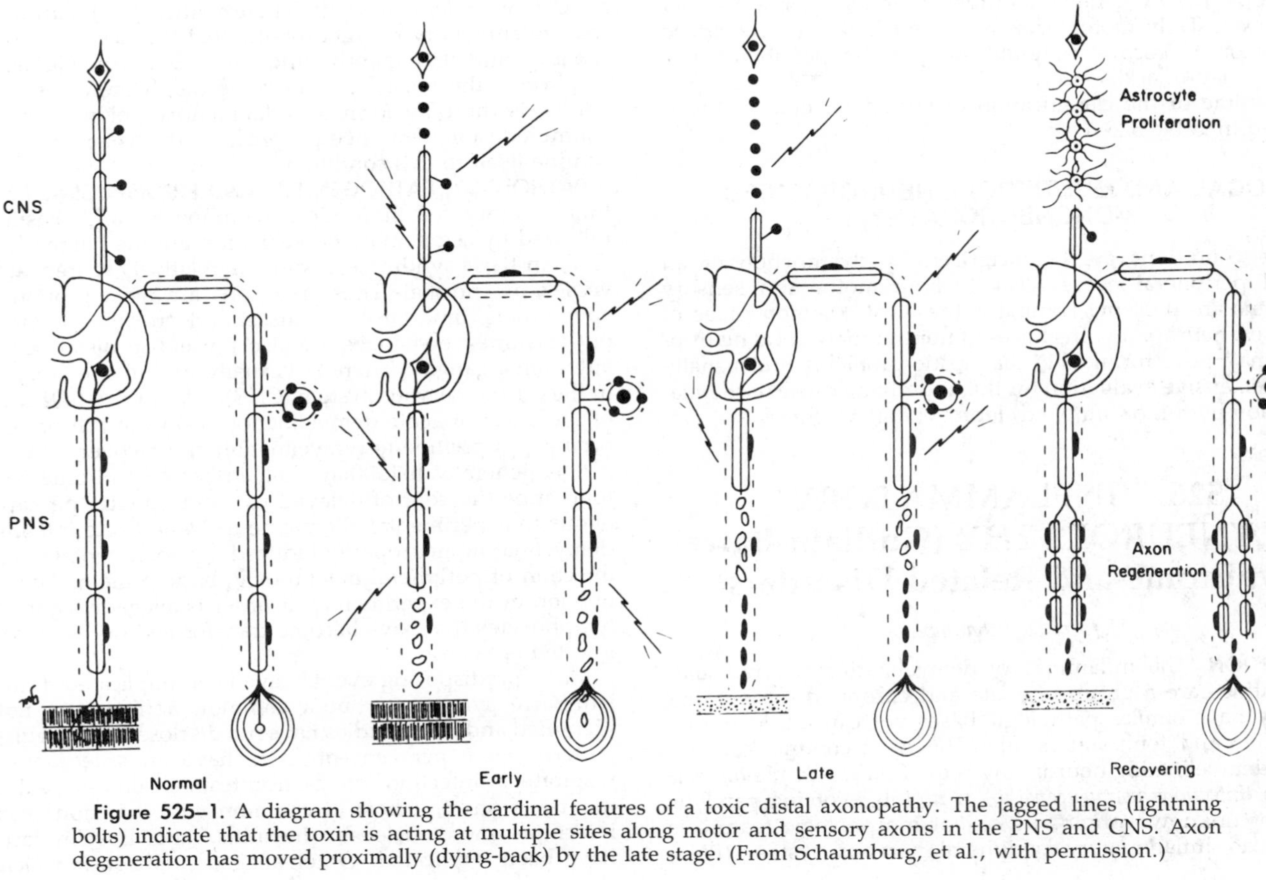

Figure 525–1. A diagram showing the cardinal features of a toxic distal axonopathy. The jagged lines (lightning bolts) indicate that the toxin is acting at multiple sites along motor and sensory axons in the PNS and CNS. Axon degeneration has moved proximally (dying-back) by the late stage. (From Schaumburg, et al., with permission.)

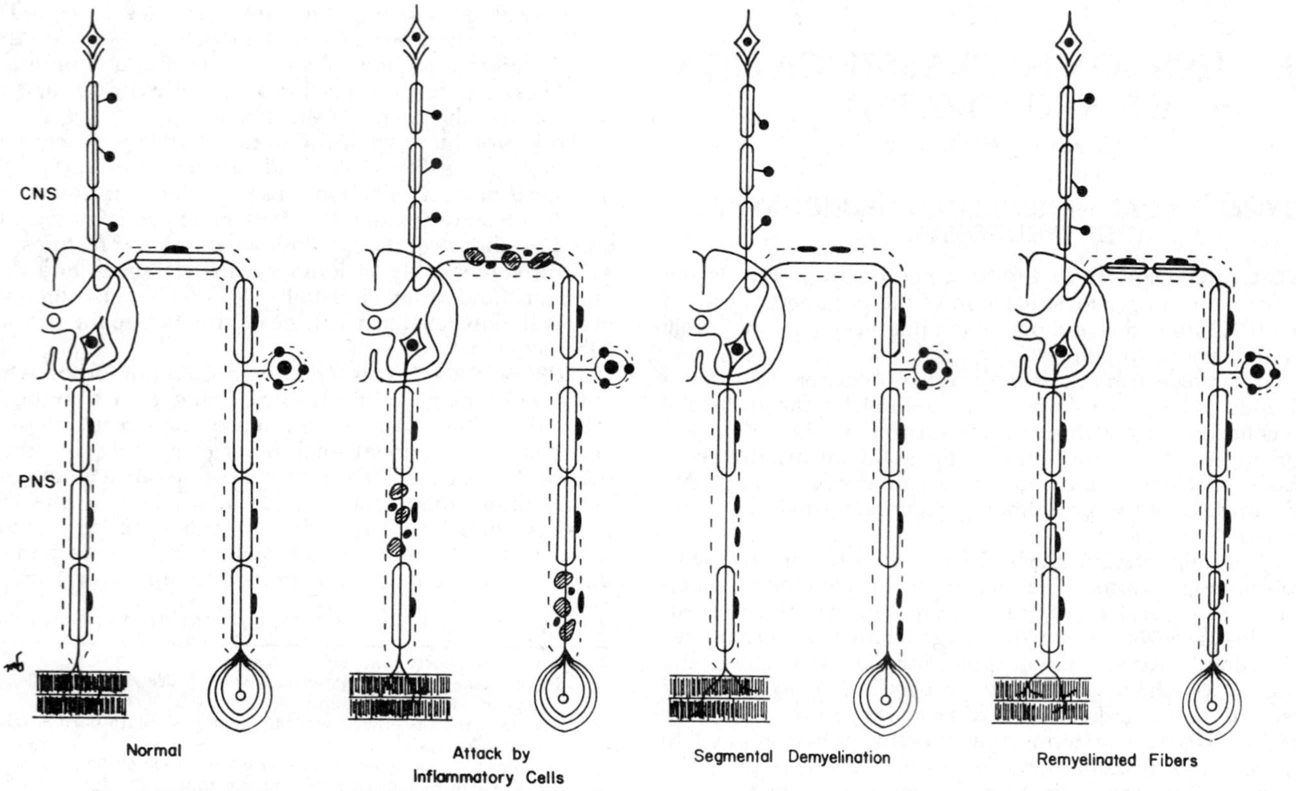

Figure 525–2. A diagram of the cardinal pathologic features of an inflammatory myelinopathy. Axons are spared as is CNS myelin. After the attack, the remaining Schwann cells divide and remyelinate the denuded segments of axons. (From Schaumburg, et al., with permission.)

zoster ganglionitis (sensory neuronopathy). Some hereditary and toxic neuropathies probably are best conceptualized as neuronopathies. In general, a diffuse peripheral nerve disorder that is exclusively motor or sensory and that is characterized by little or no recovery should suggest the possibility of a primarily neuronal disorder.

An outline of the classification of peripheral neuropathy is provided in Table 525–1.

FOCAL AND MULTIFOCAL NEUROPATHIES (MONONEUROPATHY)

These conditions are characterized by dysfunction of an isolated peripheral nerve. Usually both motor and sensory symptoms are present. Trauma is the most common cause of monofocal neuropathy. Instances of nontraumatic focal neuropathies may pose formidable diagnostic problems and usually require extensive evaluation for the underlying cause (ischemia, infiltration by tumor, amyloid, leprosy, among others).

526. INFLAMMATORY POLYNEUROPATHY (Guillain-Barré Syndrome and Related Disorders)

Herbert H. Schaumburg

DEFINITION. The inflammatory demyelinating polyradiculoneuropathies are a group of acute and chronic disorders that probably have similar pathologic bases but can differ in anatomic sites and temporal profile. The most common inflammatory demyelinating neuropathy is the *Guillain-Barré syndrome (acute postinfectious polyneuropathy)*, a rapidly evolving paralytic illness of unknown origin. Its salient morphologic feature is widespread inflammatory peripheral nervous system (PNS) demyelination, presumably secondary to a hypersensitivity reaction. Other less common forms of inflammatory neuropathy are chronic inflammatory polyneuropathy (CIP), chronic recurrent inflammatory polyneuropathy (CRIP), acute sensory neuropathy, and acute pandysautonomia. Since the Guillain-Barré syndrome, the most frequent acute paralytic illness in young adults, is the only form of inflammatory polyneuropathy encountered in general medical practice, this chapter will largely confine itself to this condition.

PATHOLOGY, PATHOGENESIS, AND PREDISPOSING FACTORS. Inflammatory cell infiltration (lymphocytes and plasma cells) followed by segmental demyelination are the hallmarks of the Guillain-Barré syndrome. Axons are relatively spared and blood vessels are normal. These reactions are most pronounced in spinal roots, limb girdle plexuses, and proximal nerve trunks, but less intense changes are also present in distal nerves and autonomic ganglia. There is virtually no inflammatory change in the central nervous system (CNS). Within two to three weeks of the onset of acute demyelination Schwann cell proliferation occurs as a prelude to remyelination and recovery.

It is generally held that Guillain-Barré syndrome is an autoimmune disorder of delayed hypersensitivity, perhaps analogous to experimental allergic neuritis, an acute inflammatory demyelinating neuropathy induced in experimental animals by injection of peripheral myelin or P_2 basic protein. The demyelination in the experimental disorder is allegedly controlled by lymphocytes that have become transformed in response to the injected antigen.

Many predisposing events have been implicated in the Guillain-Barré syndrome, but a common antigen has not been identified and HLA studies have not disclosed any predisposing pattern. Sixty per cent of cases have an antecedent upper respiratory infection or gastrointestinal illness within one month of onset; a host of common viral infections including infectious mononucleosis, hepatitis, and Epstein-Barr virus have been implicated. Other alleged predisposing factors include vaccination against rabies and swine flu, surgery, pregnancy, and malignancy (especially lymphoma).

CLINICAL FEATURES. This is a worldwide illness and occurs throughout the year. It has a bimodal age distribution, with the majority of cases in young adults and a second lesser peak in incidence in the 45 to 64 age group.

The Guillain-Barré syndrome is a rapidly progressive, largely reversible, predominantly motor neuropathy. The cardinal clinical features are progressive and usually symmetrical weakness, combined with hyporeflexia. Weakness usually begins in the distal lower limbs and spreads upward (ascending paralysis); however, this pattern is not inevitable and patients may have weakness of the proximal upper limbs or face. Most weakened individuals do not appear systemically ill, and constitutional signs such as fever, chills, and weight loss are unusual.

The eventual degree of paralysis varies, encompassing a broad spectrum that includes the occasional individual who never progresses beyond a mild footdrop to others with extreme weakness of all extremities and of the face. Severe involvement may lead to flaccid quadriplegia with inability to breathe, swallow, speak, or move the eyes. Limb weakness is generally symmetrical and early muscle atrophy uncommon. Tendon reflexes are usually absent.

The presence of facial weakness helps to distinguish the Guillain-Barré syndrome from most other neuropathies, apart from those related to sarcoidosis. Rarely, limb ataxia, paralysis of eye movements, and diffuse hyporeflexia may be the sole manifestations (*Miller Fisher syndrome*). Central nervous system involvement is not part of this illness. Increased intracranial pressure and papilledema may rarely occur late.

Sensory symptoms, usually distal paresthesias, are present in most cases, rarely persist or progress (in contrast to the weakness), and generally are not accompanied by signs of a profound loss of sensation. Mild impairment of distal position and vibration sensation and slight loss of pinprick sensation over the toes are common.

Autonomic dysfunction accompanies many cases and probably reflects involvement of the myelinated preganglionic fibers and the ganglia. Orthostatic hypotension and hypertension are frequent, may result from denervation supersensitivity, are difficult to treat, and can complicate the management of patients with respiratory compromise. Individuals who appear otherwise clinically stable can die suddenly following unexplained fluctuation in blood pressure or cardiac dysrhythmias.

Cerebrospinal fluid (CSF) and electrodiagnostic studies are helpful. The CSF protein concentration is usually normal during the first three days of illness; it then steadily rises and may reach levels in excess of 500 mg per deciliter. The CSF protein level may remain elevated for several months, even after recovery is underway. Mononuclear cells, usually less than 10 per millimeter, are present in up to one half of the cases.

Early in the illness, distal motor nerve conduction may be normal. Presumably, in such cases the disease process is confined to spinal roots and proximal nerves. If the demyelination affects distal nerves as well, more profound slowing of motor conduction, characteristic of segmental demyelination, occurs. Analysis of the F response, a measurement of proximal motor conduction, may be of value in patients suspected to have Guillain-Barré syndrome who display normal distal motor conduction.

Differential diagnosis is not difficult, especially since the decline of poliomyelitis and diphtheria in North America. Hypokalemia, tick paralysis, botulism, acute myelitis, and cervical spine fracture should be ruled out rapidly.

COURSE AND PROGNOSIS. Rapid progression of weakness is characteristic of the Guillain-Barré syndrome. Paralysis is maximal by one week in more than half, by three weeks in 80 per cent, and by one month in 90 per cent. In the remaining 10 per cent of cases, weakness may progress for variable intervals up to eight weeks.

Recovery usually begins with two to four weeks after progression ceases. The pattern is variable, normally proceeding at a steady pace. Within six months 85 per cent of patients are ambulatory. Occasionally individuals experience more rapid recovery and are able to return to work within two months following quadriparesis. Rare cases show little or no improvement.

Although in time most patients recover almost complete function, the illness is not benign. The overall mortality is 5 per cent, and more than 50 per cent of all patients retain evidence of damage to the peripheral nervous system. Sixteen per cent remain significantly handicapped by weakness. Few features of the initial clinical illness are of help in predicting the eventual outcome. In general, individuals who experience only mild distal extremity weakness and subsequently improve within weeks of the first signs do best.

TREATMENT. Patients suspected of having the Guillain-Barré syndrome must be admitted to the hospital even if the involvement is minimal, since the neuropathy may evolve rapidly and unpredictably. In general, such patients should be admitted to a unit where respiratory care is available, to remain until their condition stabilizes or improves. The tidal volume, oxygen saturation, vital capacity, blood pressure, and ability to cough and swallow should be closely monitored, since they can change without warning.

If a need for mechanical ventilation is anticipated (as determined by the degree of respiratory effort, the vital capacity, and the blood gases), it should be instituted early without waiting for decompensation.

Autonomic dysfunction may produce pupillary disturbances, neuroendocrine disturbance, peripheral pooling of blood, poor venous return, cardiac arrhythmias, and low cardiac output. Beat to beat (R-R) variation of the heart rate during normal and deep breathing is a reliable index. Pharmacologic manipulation of blood pressure in Guillain-Barré syndrome patients is perilous and should be avoided unless absolutely necessary.

Some patients will be unable to swallow or to gag. Feeding should be done through a small nasogastric tube. The patient should be sitting when food is given and for 30 to 60 minutes thereafter to minimize the risk of aspiration.

If patients with the Guillain-Barré syndrome can be carried through the acute stage of progressive paralysis (usually two to three weeks), strength will gradually return. Since most patients achieve good recovery after months of weakness, the importance of extremely fastidious supportive care in the acute stage cannot be overstressed. Glucocorticoids and plasmapheresis are not indicated.

ACUTE INFLAMMATORY SENSORY POLYNEUROPATHY (Postinfectious Sensory Neuropathy or Neuronopathy)

This disorder is presumed to represent a sensory polyradiculopathy and is probably the counterpart of the motor polyradiculoneuropathy of Guillain-Barré. There are no histopathologic studies; it is suggested that inflammatory demyelination of the dorsal roots has also involved adjacent dorsal root ganglion cells. Thus this disease may be conceptualized as a combined myelinopathy-neuronopathy disorder to explain the rapid onset and poor recovery of many cases.

As in the motor variety of the disease, a preceding infection may antedate the neurologic syndrome by several weeks. Typically the onset is acute or subacute and marked by combinations of sensory dysfunction and pain. The sensory dysfunction is most commonly described as unsteadiness in gait or clumsiness in the use of the hands. Even more incapacitating are painful dysesthesias that develop in some patients. Varying combinations of lancinating pain, prickling hyperesthesia, constricting bandlike sensations, and burning or coldness of skin may be described. Any region of the body may be affected, and the disorder involves proximal as well as distal dermatomes. Lower limbs tend to be affected more than upper, and the various modalities of sensation may be affected to different degrees. Patients often exhibit sensory ataxia, and because of the severe impairment of joint position the limbs may be held in distorted positions. Tendon reflexes are often diminished or absent.

Concurrent minor involvement of motor and autonomic function may occur. Cerebrospinal fluid changes are similar to those in the motor variety of the illness. Motor nerve conduction velocity may be within normal limits; by contrast, nerve action potentials cannot be elicited from stimulation of sensory nerve fibers, either because the afferent fibers have degenerated or because the action potential is so dispersed.

Prognosis for recovery in sensory polyneuropathy is poor. Symptoms of cutaneous hyperpathia often persist or recur for many years. Sensory ataxia usually improves but may not recover completely. This persistence of the neurologic deficit probably reflects irreversible damage of spinal ganglion neurons.

ACUTE INFLAMMATORY AUTONOMIC NEUROPATHY (Postinfectious Pandysautonomia)

Acute inflammatory autonomic neuropathy is a poorly understood, rare condition that may be the autonomic counterpart of the motor and sensory varieties already described. Pathologic studies are unavailable. The onset and time course are similar to those in the motor and sensory neuropathies. Principal symptoms include postural hypotension, cramping abdominal pain, and varying amounts of diarrhea and constipation. Hypotension may be so severe that the patient cannot sit up without losing consciousness. Affected subjects reportedly improve with time, but few long-term follow-up studies are available.

CHRONIC RELAPSING INFLAMMATORY NEUROPATHY (CRIP) AND CHRONIC INFLAMMATORY POLYNEUROPATHY (CIP)

DEFINITION, PATHOLOGY, AND PATHOGENESIS. Affected individuals initially have an illness similar to the Guillain-Barré syndrome, although usually with a more gradual onset, but subsequently undergo either a chronic relapsing (CRIP) or a chronic progressive course (CIP). The salient histologic features of both chronic forms are remarkably similar to those of the Guillain-Barré syndrome. It is claimed that onion-bulb formation (concentric rings of Schwann cell processes around a demyelinated axon) is a prominent feature of CRIP and that lymphocytic infiltration is more common in CIP. It is generally considered that CRIP and CIP represent clinical variants of the same condition and may have a pathogenetic mechanism in common with the Guillain-Barré syndrome.

CLINICAL FEATURES. Both conditions are rare. The temporal relationship to antecedent infections is much less frequent than for the Guillain-Barré syndrome.

The cardinal symptoms and signs reflect predominant motor involvement. Weakness of the extremities, intercostal muscles, and lower cranial nerves all occur in CIP and CRIP.

Sensory complaints are almost as common as weakness, and objective signs of sensory loss are more frequent in the chronic disorders than in the Guillain-Barré syndrome. Hyporeflexia or areflexia have been observed in almost all patients.

The development and course of illness are considered the salient features that distinguish between CRIP and CIP. CRIP and CIP generally each have a protracted onset and an indolent progression. The occurrence of subsequent relapsing episodes suggests CRIP, while steady progression suggests CIP. In many instances these guidelines become blurred. For example, it may be impossible to distinguish between a fluctuation in the course of progressing CIP and a relapse in the course of CRIP. This factor, in concert with the histopathologic similarities, suggests that CIP and CRIP are variants of the same condition.

The course of CRIP may vary considerably in the interval between relapses, the severity of episodes, and the rate and degree of recovery. Subsequent attacks usually resemble the initial one, and disability varies considerably. With treatment, improvement is generally good between episodes. Life-threatening episodes with respiratory insufficiency are more common early in the illness. The degree of disability following repeated attacks is variable, and the attacks often cease after a few years.

The course of CIP is usually stepwise but may be gradual. If untreated, this condition may become disabling or fatal; the prognosis is uncertain.

The CSF protein level is elevated at some stage of the illness in almost every case of CIP or CRIP but may fluctuate to normal levels in either condition. Slowed nerve conduction, sometimes profound, in both motor and sensory nerves is characteristic of CIP and CRIP, although this is not always present. Nerve biopsy may be extremely helpful in diagnosis if a diseased area can be located. The histologic picture is characteristic for these disorders. The differential diagnosis of CRIP is seldom a problem after several episodes have occurred. The differential diagnosis of CIP is sometimes extremely difficult. Unless a nerve biopsy displays characteristic changes, CIP may be indistinguishable from some hereditary disorders (see Ch. 530).

TREATMENT. Glucocorticoids are often efficacious in both disorders. Plasma exchange may produce marked improvement in CRIP but does not appear effective in CIP. This technique offers a useful alternative for individuals who cannot tolerate long-term corticosteroids or other immunosuppressive therapy.

527. THE DIABETIC NEUROPATHIES

Herbert H. Schaumburg

A variety of peripheral nerve disorders may occur in diabetes mellitus, reflecting the multiple causes of nerve degeneration in this disorder. Diabetic neuropathies may be classified as either mononeuropathies or symmetrical polyneuropathies, but neuropathy is frequent in diabetes and mixed syndromes often occur. For instance, an individual with symmetrical sensory polyneuropathy may develop acute third nerve palsy (a mononeuropathy). See Table 527–1.

SYMMETRICAL POLYNEUROPATHY

PATHOLOGY AND PATHOGENESIS. Pathologic studies in individuals with advanced distal sensory neuropathy show nonspecific changes that include mixtures of axonal loss and segmental demyelination. The pathogenesis of the symmetrical polyneuropathies and the clinical features, which often selectively involve particular fiber types, favor a metabolic basis, but the inconsistent relationship of severity of neuropathy to control of blood glucose does not support this hypothesis. Other biochemical mechanisms currently suggested endorse either accumulation of nerve sorbitol or depletion of nerve myoinositol.

CLINICAL FEATURES AND TREATMENT. ***Distal Primary Sensory Neuropathy.*** This is the commonest type of diabetic peripheral nerve disorder, estimated to be present in about 40 per cent of individuals with diabetes of 25 years' duration. It is present in less than 10 per cent of patients at the time of diagnosis (which it may antedate) and is uncommon in children.

It may be asymptomatic, with abnormal signs first detectable

TABLE 527–1. CLASSIFICATION OF DIABETIC NEUROPATHIES

Symmetrical polyneuropathies
Distal primary sensory neuropathy
Autonomic neuropathy
Rapidly reversible neuropathy
Mononeuropathy and multiple mononeuropathies
Cranial neuropathies
Focal nerve lesions (other than cranial)
Proximal painful lower limb neuropathy (diabetic amyotrophy)

on routine examination, or there may be a variety of symptoms. There appear to be three consistent patterns:

1. A "large-fiber" pattern with paresthesias in legs, absent ankle jerks, and impaired senses of light touch, vibration, and position in the lower limbs. Slight distal weakness is common and the hands may become involved.

2. A "small-fiber" pattern with dull aching pain and impaired senses of cutaneous pain, touch, and temperature sensation. Position and vibration sense, deep tendon reflexes, and strength are usually spared. Autonomic nervous system dysfunction may accompany this variant.

3. A rare "pseudotabetic" pattern associated with long-term diabetes. Severe impairment of cutaneous and deep senses permits ulceration of the feet and distal joint deformity. Romberg's sign is present, tendon reflexes are absent in the legs, and hypotension and Argyll Robertson pupils may be observed.

The course is variable in sensory neuropathy. Most often it fluctuates and then plateaus at a steady level. The pseudotabetic variety of the illness has an especially bad prognosis. Electrodiagnostic tests usually reveal changes in sensory conduction and variable alteration in motor conduction. The cerebrospinal fluid protein level is usually elevated, sometimes to a very high level.

There is no specific treatment. Diabetic neuropathies of all types are more likely to develop and patients recover less well if the metabolic state is poorly supervised. Simple analgesics rarely help the severe pain that accompanies sensory neuropathy. Trial treatment with phenytoin, carbamazepine, phenothiazine, and tricyclic antidepressants is advocated. Persons with pain and temperature insensitivity of hands and feet are vulnerable to many injuries that potentially can cascade into ulceration, cellulitis, lymphangitis, osteomyelitis, and osteolysis. Similar abnormalities are seen in syphilitic tabes, leprosy, inherited amyloidosis, and other inherited and acquired neuropathies, with the aforementioned sensory loss. The goal in treatment is to prevent the onset of tissue damage or, when it has occurred, to promote healing and prevent further damage. Persons with loss of pain and temperature sensation should not engage in most forms of manual labor or perform potentially bruising tasks with the hands and feet. Repeated inspection of hands and feet is necessary. If any bruise or ulcer appears, weight bearing or rough use should be stopped until healing occurs. Shoes should be wide and well constructed. The insides of the shoes must be inspected to remove retained objects or nails. Such patients should soak the feet in lukewarm water for 15 minutes twice daily and cover them lightly with petrolatum lotion to retain moisture in the softened skin.

Autonomic Neuropathy. Diabetic autonomic neuropathy generally is associated with symmetrical sensory neuropathy and occasionally predominates. Autonomic involvement may be asymptomatic or can cause incapacitating disability. Three types of dysfunction are prominent: gastrointestinal, cardiovascular, and genitourinary. The common gastrointestinal disturbances are gastroparesis, episodic nocturnal diarrhea, and colonic dilatation. Cardiovascular manifestations include impaired vasomotor reflexes (postural hypotension), elevated heart rate, and loss of respiratory sinus arrhythmia. Genitourinary disturbances are especially distressing and include disordered micturition with large residual volume, retrograde ejaculation, and impotence. Impotence is sometimes the initial manifestation of autonomic neuropathy. It usually steadily worsens and rarely, if ever, is improved by control of hyperglycemia, the use of testosterone, or penile implants.

Treatment of autonomic disturbances is difficult. Diabetic diarrhea may be helped by codeine phosphate or diphenoxylate, but not all cases respond favorably. A single 250-mg dose of tetracycline, if given at the outset, sometimes aborts the attack. Simple cases of postural hypotension may be helped by support stockings. More severe cases may require supplemental sodium in the diet plus sodium-retaining steroids.

Rapidly Reversible Neuropathy. Newly diagnosed untreated diabetics may display asymptomatic slowing of nerve conduction velocity. This slowing is rapidly reversed by lowering blood sugar concentration to normal levels. It seems unlikely that this phenomenon is associated with structural breakdown in peripheral nerve fibers, and it is not known whether such individuals are at greater risk of developing persistent symptomatic neuropathy.

MONONEUROPATHY AND MULTIPLE MONONEUROPATHY

PATHOLOGY AND PATHOGENESIS. It is widely held that isolated peripheral nerve lesions in diabetics have a vascular basis. Several clinical facts support this notion: they have an abrupt onset, often recover spontaneously, and are most common in the elderly. Three autopsy studies, two of oculomotor palsy and one of femoral neuropathy, have demonstrated focal vascular lesions within the area of nerve damage.

CLINICAL FEATURES AND TREATMENT. *Cranial Nerve Lesions.* Isolated or multiple palsies of extraocular muscle nerves or lower cranial nerves may be the first indication of diabetes in asymptomatic older adults. The third nerve is most frequently affected. Onset is usually abrupt and is associated with an intense, retro-orbital aching sensation. Sparing of the pupillomotor fibers in diabetic third-nerve palsy helps distinguish this condition from lesions that compress the nerve, such as aneurysm. Satisfactory recovery of nerve function usually occurs within several weeks.

Isolated Peripheral Nerve Lesions (Other Than Cranial). Almost every isolated peripheral nerve can be affected by diabetic mononeuropathy. Lesions of the ulnar, radial, sciatic, peroneal, tibial, and lateral cutaneous nerves of the thigh are especially common. Diabetic nerves are especially vulnerable to compression, and lesions frequently appear at such sites. Onset is abrupt and usually painful. Recovery is usually good in distally sited lesions and less satisfactory if the lesions are proximal. Treatment includes physical therapy and use of appropriate orthotic devices.

Proximal Lower Extremity Motor Neuropathy (Diabetic Amyotrophy). This syndrome usually appears after middle age. Cardinal findings include progressive, painful, asymmetrical weakness of thigh muscles, loss of knee jerks, and a few sensory abnormalities. The spinal fluid protein level is usually elevated, and the motor changes are usually bilateral, differentiating the condition from acute nerve root disease. Recovery is gradual. There is considerable variation in all of the clinical features, and many patients display distal weakness as well. As a result, the term diabetic amyotrophy has come to encompass a spectrum of illnesses that range from ischemic femoral or lumbar plexus neuropathy to symmetrical proximal metabolic neuropathy. Treatment includes major analgesics for relief of the severe self-limited pain and physical therapy directed at the thigh and hip flexor muscles.

528. NEUROPATHY ASSOCIATED WITH UREMIA

Herbert H. Schaumburg

DEFINITION AND ETIOLOGY. Uremic polyneuropathy can be associated with chronic renal insufficiency of any cause. The cause is unknown. It is widely held that uremic neuropathy is related to dialyzable toxins or metabolites normally excreted by the kidneys. The responsible agent has a molecular weight exceeding that of urea or creatinine.

PATHOLOGY. Axonal degeneration is characteristic of this disorder, and the distribution suggests that it is a distal axonopathy. The nature of the axonal change is nonspecific.

CLINICAL FEATURES. Initially, sensory symptoms predominate, with especially frequent tingling paresthesias of the leg. Occasionally a "burning foot" or "restless leg" syndrome accompanies uremic polyneuropathy. Muscle cramps in the distal extremities are common. Diminished sensation in distal limbs is the most consistent feature, usually in combination with hyporeflexia and moderate weakness.

Uremic neuropathy has an insidious onset, and subclinical cases are common. Most cases progress over several months to reach a plateau despite worsening of the renal state. The prognosis of untreated uremic neuropathy is poor.

TREATMENT. Successful renal transplantation both prevents and reverses uremic polyneuropathy. Patients with mild cases display prompt relief of paresthesias and a steady return of strength. Recovery is more prolonged in advanced cases and is not always complete. Chronic hemodialysis is less helpful and often ineffective in reversing the neuropathy.

529. NEUROPATHY ASSOCIATED WITH ENDOCRINE DISEASES (OTHER THAN DIABETES)

Herbert H. Schaumburg

Hypothyroidism is associated with both mononeuropathy and symmetrical polyneuropathy. Clumsiness and limb ataxia of uncertain origin are common and usually are attributed to cerebellar disease. Thyroid replacement therapy ameliorates the carpal or tarsal tunnel syndrome and the diffuse symmetrical neuropathy.

Acromegaly produces entrapment neuropathies at wrist and elbow and a distal symmetrical polyneuropathy. Proximal muscle weakness occurs independently of the peripheral neuropathies and may make the clinical profile confusing. The carpal tunnel syndrome presumably results from compression by acral soft-tissue hyperplasia and osteoarthritis. Improvement follows removal of the pituitary tumor, and surgery of the carpal ligament is seldom necessary. Symmetrical polyneuropathy usually occurs late in the illness and bears no relationship to plasma levels of growth hormone. No studies have been made of the effect of removal of the pituitary adenoma on neuropathy.

530. HEREDITARY NEUROPATHIES

Herbert H. Schaumburg

GENERAL. These represent a group of slowly progressive disorders probably caused by inborn errors of metabolism. They are characterized by the type of inheritance, by their natural history, and by which population of neurons is involved. Predominant involvement of lower motor neurons (progressive muscular atrophy) is called *inherited motor neuropathy;* involvement of sensory neurons is *hereditary sensory neuropathy (HSN);* involvement of both motor and sensory neurons is *hereditary motor and sensory neuropathy (HMSN);* and involvement of autonomic neurons is *dysautonomia.*

Expression of clinical symptoms in inherited neuronal disorders varies widely from patient to patient. Functional disability is frequently less than might be expected from the neurologic signs. Certain of these disorders (HMSN Type I, HMSN Type II) are common and probably account for many cases of cryptogenic neuropathy. The number of correct diagnoses increases considerably when the patient's asymptomatic relatives are examined clinically and by nerve conduction studies.

HEREDITARY MOTOR AND SENSORY NEUROPATHY

These disorders, previously described by various eponyms (Charcot-Marie-Tooth disease, Roussy-Lévy syndrome, Dejerine-Sottas disease) are now numerically subdivided into Types I, II, and III. Table 530–1 outlines the salient features of these conditions.

TABLE 530–1. THE HEREDITARY MOTOR AND SENSORY NEUROPATHIES (HMSN)

Nomenclature	Heredity	Clinical Features	Pathology and Pathogenesis
HMSN Type I (peroneal muscle atrophy) (hypertrophic form of Charcot-Marie-Tooth disease)	Autosomal dominant	Common; many mild cases; childhood onset; slow progression; predominantly motor; deformed feet (pes cavus); extreme distal lower limb atrophy; very slow motor nerve conduction	Possibly a distal axonopathy but much segmental demyelination and remyelination ("onion bulbs"); nerves may be enlarged
HMSN Type II (neuronal form of Charcot-Marie-Tooth disease or peroneal muscle atrophy)	Autosomal dominant	Less common than Type I; onset in second decade; nerve conduction almost normal; otherwise, identical to Type I	Possibly a motor and sensory neuronopathy syndrome; loss of fibers; little remyelination (no "onion bulbs")
HMSN Type III (Dejerine-Sottas disease)	Autosomal recessive	Rare; infantile onset; short stature, scoliosis, pes cavus; steady progression to severe disability; very slow nerve conduction	Few studies; enlarged nerves; many "onion bulbs"; pathogenesis unclear

DISORDERS OF PERIPHERAL SENSORY NEURONS

Patients with disorders of peripheral sensory neurons characteristically suffer from pain, cutaneous injury from lack of sensation, unsteady movement from kinesthetic sensory loss, or combinations of these conditions. Frequently they also have autonomic dysfunction. The nature of these symptoms and the associated sensory loss correspond reasonably well with the populations of fibers affected. Thus patients with loss of pain and temperature sensation and with autonomic impairment have degeneration mostly of unmyelinated and small myelinated fibers, whereas patients with loss of touch-pressure sensation have degeneration of large myelinated fibers of cutaneous nerves. In advanced disease this selectivity of involvement by fiber size tends to be lost.

HEREDITARY SENSORY NEUROPATHY, TYPE I. Hereditary sensory neuropathy, Type I, is a dominantly inherited sensory radicular neuropathy. It has been variously termed as perforating ulcers of the feet, mutilating acropathy, acrodystrophic neuropathy, and hereditary sensory radicular neuropathy. The severity varies widely. Sensory loss is usually more severe over the feet and legs than in the hands and forearms, and some patients have lancinating pains. Pain and temperature sensation are affected more than touch-pressure sensation. Nerve conduction of motor fibers is usually normal, as is life expectancy in most cases. Late in the disorder, perforating ulcers of the foot may develop, especially in patients with poor foot care.

HEREDITARY SENSORY NEUROPATHY, TYPE II. This is a recessively inherited disorder, also called congenital sensory neuropathy, that usually manifests itself in infancy or childhood with a mutilating acropathy characterized by paronychia, whitlows, ulcers of the fingers and plantar surfaces of the feet, and, frequently, unrecognized fractures of the extremities. Sensory loss affects all types of cutaneous and sometimes kinesthetic sensation and is most marked distally in all four limbs. Tendon reflexes are usually absent.

HEREDITARY SENSORY NEUROPATHY, TYPE III (DYSAUTONOMIA OF RILEY-DAY). Familial dysautonomia is a recessively inherited disorder of Jewish infants and children. It affects peripheral autonomic neurons, peripheral sensory neurons, peripheral motor neurons, and probably other central nervous system neurons. Characteristics are onset in infancy, poor feeding, repeated episodes of vomiting and pulmonary infections, autonomic disturbances, and premature death. Autonomic abnormalities include defective lacrimation, defective temperature control, skin blotching, excessive perspiration, hypertension, and postural hypotension. There is also insensitivity to pain, areflexia, corneal insensitivity, and absence of the fungiform papillae of the tongue. A congenital abnormality of nerve growth factor is postulated.

531. TOXIC NEUROPATHY Pharmaceutical Agents

Herbert H. Schaumburg

GENERAL. New pharmaceutical agents are constantly being implicated as causes of peripheral neuropathy. Except for isoniazid, pyridoxine, and vincristine, few careful experimental studies of these substances have been conducted. Clinical reports are the sole basis for many of the alleged drug-induced neuropathies. Since following prolonged use most agents appear to produce an insidious-onset distal axonopathy, there is frequently little in the clinical diagnostic profile that helps to identify the offending agent. The most important diagnostic factor in these disorders is a meticulous history of drug use. Table 531–1 lists pharmaceutical agents that are associated with generalized neuropathy. Treatment consists of withdrawing the drug if symptoms are prominent or progressive.

TABLE 531–1. PHARMACEUTICAL AGENTS ASSOCIATED WITH GENERALIZED NEUROPATHY

Chloramphenicol
Dapsone*
Disulfiram
Dichloracetate
Ethionamide
Gold
Gluthethimide
Hydralazine
Isoniazid†
Lithium
Metronidazole-misonidazole
Nitrofurantoin*
Nitrous oxide
Platinum (cis-platinum)†
Pyridoxine†
Sodium cyanate
Thalidomide†
Vincristine

*Predominantly motor.
†Predominantly sensory.

532. TOXIC NEUROPATHY Occupational, Biological, and Environmental Agents

Herbert H. Schaumburg

GENERAL. Many potential toxic chemicals are deployed in the work place and general environment, and several have been implicated as causes of peripheral neuropathy, usually of the distal axonopathic type. Since the various agents result in similar clinical syndromes, a careful occupational and environmental history is often the most important clue for diagnosis. The various agents are listed in Table 532–1, with prominent clinical features included in parentheses. *Buckthorn* and *diphtheritic neuropathies,* which are demyelinating conditions, are listed as the sole examples of diseases in which biologic toxins are consistently associated with neuropathy. Diphtheria is further discussed in Ch. 276.

TABLE 532–1. AGENTS CAUSING SYMPTOMS ASSOCIATED WITH TOXIC NEUROPATHY

Acrylamide (truncal ataxia)
Arsenic (sensory, brown skin, Mees' lines)
Buckthorn toxin
Carbon disulfide
Cyanide
Dimethylaminopropionitrile (urinary complaints)
Dichlorophenoxyacetic acid
Biologic toxin in diphtheritic neuropathy (pharyngeal neuropathy)
Ethylene oxide
n-Hexane
Lead (wrist drop, abdominal colic)
Lucel-7 (cataracts)
Methyl bromide
Organophosphates (cholinergic symptoms, delayed onset of neuropathy)
Thallium (pain, alopecia, Mees' lines)
Trichlorethylene (facial numbness)

533. MISCELLANEOUS DISEASE-SPECIFIC NEUROPATHIES

Herbert H. Schaumburg

NEUROPATHY ASSOCIATED WITH MALIGNANCY AND DYSPROTEINEMIA

Direct compression of nerves by metastic tumors occurs within the spinal canal or invertebral foramina and behind tight fascial sheaths. Bronchogenic, renal, prostatic, and breast carcinomas are especially prone to such metastases. The direct and nonmetastatic neurologic effects of cancer are described in Ch. 174.

Polyneuropathy is more common in multiple myeloma than in most other malignancies; furthermore, subclinical neuropathy appears to be frequent. Recent evidence has made it increasingly apparent that the benign gammopathies are also associated with polyneuropathy. Accordingly, the gradual development of a painful sensorimotor or sensory neuropathy in a male in middle age or later should lead to the suspicion of dysproteinemia or myeloma. These conditions are described in Chapter 174.

AMYLOID NEUROPATHY

Extracellular deposition of the fibrous protein amyloid is associated with peripheral neuropathy in both hereditary (non-immunoglobulin-derived) amyloidosis and nonhereditary (immunoglobulin-derived) amyloidosis.

Hereditary amyloidosis is frequent only in endemic regions such as Portugal and Japan. Rare variants have also been described in Iowa and Indiana. In the Portuguese variety, which is inherited as an autosomal dominant trait, the disorder usually begins in the third, fourth, and fifth decades and affects predominantly small sensory and autonomic fibers. Lumbosacral dermatomes show a syringomyelia-like loss of pain and thermal discrimination with preservation of touch-pressure sensation. Loss of potency in the male, postural hypotension, and bladder and bowel incontinence are common in advanced stages. The disorder tends to progress over a decade or so. Biopsied sural nerves show an endoneurial reduction in unmyelinated and small myelinated fibers with nodular deposits of amyloid among the nerve trunks.

Nonhereditary amyloidosis may be divided into primary and secondary varieties. The peripheral neuropathy of primary amyloidosis also affects the distal aspects of the lower extremities more than the upper and includes small fibers as much as or more than larger ones. When typical symptoms of neuropathy are associated with enlargement of the heart, nephropathy, and enlargement of the tongue, the diagnosis of primary amyloidosis should be strongly suspected and can be confirmed by histologic examination of rectal mucosa, kidney, carpal ligament, muscle, gingivae, nerve, or bone marrow. No effective treatment for the neuropathy is available.

Patients with multiple myeloma who develop a symmetrical carpal tunnel syndrome should be investigated for systemic amyloidosis.

NEUROPATHY ASSOCIATED WITH NECROTIZING ANGIITIS AND RHEUMATOID ARTHRITIS

No fewer than nine disorders are associated with vasculitis and ischemic neuropathy. These include: polyarteritis nodosa, rheumatoid arthritis, systemic lupus erythematosus (SLE), hypersensitivity angiitis, allergic granulomatosis (Churg-Strauss syndrome), Sjögren's syndrome, Wegener's granulomatosis, and cranial arteritis (temporal arteritis).

Only polyarteritis nodosa, rheumatoid arthritis, and lupus erythematosis are encountered with any frequency in clinical practice. Although the fundamental expression of these conditions varies considerably, they all produce similar clinical and pathologic syndromes of ischemic mononeuritis multiplex. The pathogenesis of nerve fiber destruction in each condition presumably relates to focal ischemia from arteriolar occlusion. The clinical features are similar to those depicted for the mononeuropathies associated with diabetes (Ch. 527).

Rheumatoid arthritis, in addition to producing a vascular mononeuropathy, may also cause entrapment neuropathy (reflecting prolonged immobilized postures and nerve compression by articular deformity) and a chronic symmetrical sensory neuropathy. This latter disorder develops with long-term rheumatoid arthritis and is characterized by mild, distal, symmetrical sensory loss. Although frequently painful, the condition is generally benign and improves spontaneously. Corticosteroid treatment is not indicated.

INFECTIOUS AND GRANULOMATOUS NEUROPATHY (HERPES ZOSTER, LEPROSY, AND SARCOIDOSIS)

HERPES ZOSTER. This viral disorder affects sensory ganglia of cranial or spinal nerves to produce characteristic disorders, which are discussed in Ch. 501.

LEPROSY. This remains one of the most common neuropathies on a worldwide scale. It is discussed in Ch. 300.

SARCOIDOSIS. Peripheral neuropathy of uncertain pathogenesis develops in 5 per cent of cases. Both multiple mononeuropathy and symmetrical polyneuropathy occur. A mixture of localized granulomatous infiltration and vascular compromise is probably the cause.

Mononeuropathy can affect either the spinal or the cranial nerves. Most cranial neuropathy with sarcoid involvement occurs as an acute facial (Bell's) palsy that is indistinguishable from the idiopathic variety unless it causes an isolated bilateral facial paralysis that is almost pathognomonic. Simultaneous bilateral involvement is rare. Lower cranial nerves are less commonly involved. Severe paralysis is common and incomplete recovery the rule, even with corticosteroid therapy.

Distal symmetric polyneuropathy is a rare complication of sarcoidosis. Little is known about the specific cause, prognosis, or natural history of this neuropathy. Paradoxically, this form of neuropathy is usually not accompanied by prominent evidence of systemic disease.

ACUTE PHYSICAL INJURY. The results of recent experimental studies suggest a simple classification for acute nerve injury in which the clinical features, including prognosis, closely approximate the nature of the acute injury. Basically there are three different types (classes 1 through 3). In mild injury (class 1) axonal integrity is maintained but myelin may be damaged. In more severe injury (class 2) axonal continuity is lost but the connective tissue framework of the nerve is maintained. In the most severe injuries (class 3), nerve fibers and connective tissue are damaged to varying degrees. Table 533–1 depicts the types of nerve injury and their corresponding anatomic and clinical features.

NEUROPATHY ASSOCIATED WITH ALCOHOLISM, NUTRITIONAL DEFICIENCY, AND MALABSORPTION

See Ch. 482.

TABLE 533–1. TYPES OF NERVE INJURY

Type	Anatomic Lesion	Clinical Features	Course and Prognosis
Class 1	Either (A) transient conduction block due to ischemia or (B) demyelination	(A) Mild sensory loss and weakness (ischemic type) from transient abnormal posture (legs crossed) (B) Prolonged compression (Saturday night palsy) with paralysis and moderate sensory loss below site of lesion	(A) Rapid complete recovery (B) Gradual (lasting weeks) complete recovery
Class 2	Axonal interruption; connective tissue intact	Closed crush and percussion injury; loss of motor, sensory, and autonomic function below site of lesion; surgical exploration not indicated	Very slow recovery; prognosis best with distal lesions
Class 3	Transection of axons and connective tissue sheaths	Severe stretch injuries (heavy blows, motorcycle accidents) or penetrating wounds; total loss of all motor, sensory, and autonomic function; surgical intervention indicated for penetrating wounds	Little recovery even with surgical repair; poor prognosis

534. ACUTE PHYSICAL INJURY AND CHRONIC COMPRESSION-ENTRAPMENT NEUROPATHIES

Herbert H. Schaumburg

The pathophysiologic features of chronic compressions and entrapment are still debated. It is widely held that demyelination initially occurs and, if the condition persists, axonal destruction may follow. Several clinical forms are common, including carpal tunnel syndrome, ulnar palsy, meralgia paresthetica, and cervical rib form.

CARPAL TUNNEL SYNDROME. The median nerve becomes compressed at the wrist as it passes deep within the tissue to the flexor retinaculum. The usual symptoms include numbness, tingling, and burning sensations in the hand and fingers. The pain sometimes radiates up the forearm as far as the elbow or even as high as the shoulder or root of the neck. These sensations are occasionally restricted to the radial fingers but may affect all the digits. Pain and paresthesias are most prominent at night and often wake the patient from sleep. They may be relieved by shaking the hand. The hand tends to feel numb and useless on waking in the morning, but these sensations subside after brief use. The symptoms may recur following use or when the patient is sitting with the hands immobile. Such symptoms may persist for many years without objective signs of median nerve damage. In other patients, weakness of the thumb muscles develops in association with atrophy of the lateral aspect of the thenar eminence. Sensory loss may appear over the tips of the fingers. Occasionally, patients have motor symptoms of median nerve deficit in the hand without paresthesias, or motor and sensory signs may be discovered incidentally in the absence of symptoms, particularly in older individuals.

Most cases of carpal tunnel compression occur in middle-aged and often obese females. In younger women it is commonly associated with excessive use of the hands, and it may develop in males after unaccustomed use of the hands, such as in house-painting. The disorder may be caused by tenosynovitis at the wrist, by involvement of the wrist joint in rheumatoid arthritis, or as a consequence of osteoarthritis of the carpus, perhaps in relation to an old fracture. Other predisposing causes are pregnancy, myxedema, acromegaly, infiltration of the transverse carpal ligament in primary amyloidosis, and chronic hemodialysis treatments. Diagnosis is based on clinical symptoms, the finding of Tinel's sign over the median nerve in the tunnel, and demonstration of conduction block at the wrist by motor nerve velocity studies. Individuals with muscle weakness and wasting or prominent sensory loss should undergo decompression of the nerve by section of the transverse carpal ligament. In patients with paresthesias alone or when the cause is probably tenosynovitis at the wrist, a reduction in hand activity may be sufficient to allow the symptoms to subside. Injection into the carpal tunnel of a long-acting corticosteroid preparation sometimes gives temporary relief, as does splinting of the wrist to reduce movement. When troublesome symptoms persist, decompression is advisable.

For most patients with paresthesias, symptoms are relieved by decompression. Sensory impairment and cutaneous hyperesthesia, however, may persist postoperatively, and there may not be recovery after prolonged denervation of the thenar muscles.

ULNAR PALSY. The ulnar nerve may be injured at the elbow, especially in persons with a shallow ulnar groove, those who rest their weight on their elbows excessively, and those who are cachectic and lie in bed. Injury may occur years following a previously malunited supracondylar fracture of the humerus with bony overgrowth *(tardive ulnar palsy)*. Contrary to the findings in the carpal tunnel syndrome, muscle weakness and atrophy characteristically predominate over sensory symptoms and signs. Patients notice atrophy of the first dorsal interosseous muscle or difficulty in performing fine manipulation. There may be numbness of the small finger, the contiguous half of the proximal and middle phalanges of the ring finger, and the ulnar border of the hand. Treatment in mild cases consists of prevention of further injury. A doughnut cushion for the elbow may be helpful. Mobilizing and transplanting the nerve to a position in front of the medial epicondyle sometimes prevents further progression.

LATERAL CUTANEOUS NERVE OF THE THIGH. *Meralgia paresthetica* is an entrapment neuropathy resulting from compression of this nerve as it passes under the inguinal ligament. Although the cause often remains unexplained, obese persons wearing tight girdles, individuals with gun belts, and those with pendulous abdomens are especially prone to develop numbness or burning sensations over the lateral thigh. Sometimes prolonged standing or walking provokes the symptoms. Weight reduction may help, and in many cases the condition subsides spontaneously. Surgical decompression is rarely necessary.

CERVICAL RIB AND THORACIC OUTLET SYNDROME. Angulation of the brachial plexus over an abnormal rib or fibrous band can damage its lower fibers and lead to weakness and wasting of the small hand muscles. Numbness and pain may occur along the inner border of the forearm and hand. Surgical removal of the rib or fibrous band sometimes abolishes the pain and paresthesias, but the small muscles of the hand often fail to recover strength. Cervical rib compression is uncommon, and most patients with paresthesias of the fingers prove to have either root compression from a cervical disc or a carpal tunnel syndrome.

535. BELL'S PALSY, BRACHIAL NEURITIS, AND TRIGEMINAL NEUROPATHY

Herbert H. Schaumburg

BELL'S PALSY (Idiopathic Facial Paralysis)

PATHOLOGY AND PATHOGENESIS. Neither the pathology nor the pathogenesis of this common illness are known. It is likely that mild cases with rapid recovery represent segmental demyelination and that axonal degeneration occurs in instances with prolonged dysfunction.

CLINICAL FEATURES. Idiopathic unilateral facial paralysis may develop rapidly within a few hours or evolve over one or two days and is often accompanied by pain behind the ipsilateral ear and excess tearing. Numbness of the face is a common complaint but inevitably refers to a proprioceptive sensation that accompanies weakness. Global facial muscle weakness is the hallmark of this condition. Hyperacusis, diminished lacrimation, and abnormal taste sensation are present to variable degrees. Untreated, 80 to 85 per cent of all patients with Bell's palsy recover completely or almost so. In a smaller number, persistent facial weakness ensues. Rarely, motor recovery fails completely. Aberrant regeneration is frequent. There may be embarrassing synkinetic movements (chewing producing eye winking) or excessive lacrimation.

Patients who are going to recover completely usually begin to show improvement during the first two weeks, while those destined to have permanent residual disability show no changes in status for three or more months. Except when paralysis is incomplete, there is little in the acute clinical profile to indicate prognosis. In patients who have complete paralysis from the onset, reliance must be placed on careful observation and electrodiagnostic tests of nerve excitability (performed at about one week after the onset).

Most authorities recommend treatment with prednisone, 1 mg per kilogram daily in two divided doses for four days, with dosage tapered to a total of 5 mg per day within ten days. It is claimed that prednisone therapy should be instituted as soon as possible if it is to have an effect in decreasing residual paralysis and synkinetic movements. In any event, pain usually subsides promptly. The unusual residual of a severe facial paralysis has a distressing cosmetic effect. Hypoglossal-facial nerve anastomosis will restore facial tone and is the operation of choice.

ACUTE BRACHIAL NEURITIS (Idiopathic Brachial Plexus Neuropathy)

PATHOLOGY AND PATHOGENESIS. There have been no thorough pathologic examinations of this condition, and the pathogenesis is unknown. Biopsy of cutaneous nerves has revealed nonspecific axonal degeneration. In most cases there is no common antecedent illness, immunization, or toxic exposure; some cases follow surgical procedures. The clinical profile is identical to that in certain serum vaccine paralyses, and a common immunologic basis has been suggested.

CLINICAL FEATURES. The condition arises as an acute, painful, and usually monophasic illness characterized by brachial plexus dysfunction. It is especially common in males aged 18 to 40. A cardinal feature is sudden severe shoulder girdle-scapular pain, occasionally extending into the arm or hand. The pain persists for a few days to a week and then subsides concomitantly with or shortly after the appearance of weakness, although it sometimes persists for several weeks. The serratus anterior is the single most commonly affected muscle. Distal weakness occurs less frequently. Rarely, the entire arm and ipsilateral diaphragm are affected. Uncommonly, weakness may appear in the other arm. Tendon reflexes are diminished in the involved extremity, but sensory loss is slight or negligible, being most commonly found at the apex of the shoulder. Involvement is usually restricted to muscles innervated by the brachial plexus. Weakness and atrophy of involved muscles lasts for months in many cases, but total recovery occurs in 90 per cent within two or three years. Treatment consists of physical therapy and orthotic devices to prevent joint damage. Corticosteroid therapy has no demonstrated value. There are occasional recurrences.

TRIGEMINAL NEUROPATHY

Rare cases are encountered of a slowly progressive bilateral sensory loss confined to the territory of the trigeminal nerve. This may lead to tissue destruction, particularly around the nostrils, as a result of repeated picking and scratching. Drug toxicity with trichloroethylene or stilbamidine may cause this syndrome. Sjögren's syndrome, systemic sclerosis, and trigeminal neurilemomas should be excluded. Some cases have been found at autopsy to have infiltration of the trigeminal ganglion with amyloid. The explanation for other cases is obscure.

536. NERVE BIOPSY IN PERIPHERAL NERVE DISEASE

Jerry G. Kaplan

Nerve biopsy is most useful in identifying the cause of multiple mononeuropathy syndromes (amyloidosis, sarcoidosis, leprosy, and vasculitis) and demyelinating neuropathies. Conditions readily diagnosed on clinical grounds, such as diabetic neuropathy and Guillain-Barré syndrome, do not require biopsy. Biopsy is seldom helpful in distal axonopathies, since most display similar nonspecific findings.

Either the sural nerve at the ankle or the radial nerve at the wrist may be sampled under local anesthesia. Tissue should be processed for routine histopathologic study, electron microscopy, and nerve fiber teasing. The latter technique is especially useful because it allows the rapid examination of long segments of individual fibers. Ideally, nerve biopsy should be performed only in institutions with considerable experience in using these techniques by a surgeon accustomed to handling such tissues.

Chapter 471 gives a description of diagnostic electrical studies in nerve or muscle disease.

Asbury AK, Arnason BG, Adams RD: The inflammatory lesion in idiopathic polyneuritis: Its role in pathogenesis. Medicine 48:173, 1969. *The classic comprehensive description of the role of the inflammatory cell in Guillain-Barré syndrome.*

Asbury AK, Johnson PC: Pathology of Peripheral Nerves. Philadelphia, W. B. Saunders Co., 1970. *A concise, clearly written book covering the salient aspects of peripheral neuropathy.*

Dyck PJ, Oviatt KF, Lambert EH: Intensive evaluation of unclassified neuropathies yields improved diagnosis. Ann Neurol 10:222, 1981. *A description of the increased diagnostic yield when a patient with neuropathy is studied in a special center.*

Dyck PJ, Thomas PK, Lambert EH: Peripheral Neuropathy. Philadelphia, W. B. Saunders Company, 1984. *A multiauthored and authoritative reference for peripheral nerve disease.*

Moore PM, Cupps T: Neurological complications of vasculitis. Ann Neurol 14:155, 1983. *A comprehensive review of the protean neurologic complications of these disorders, especially the neuropathies.*

Raff MC, Asbury AK: Ischemic mononeuropathy and mononeuropathy multiplex in diabetes mellitus. N Engl J Med 279:17, 1968. *A paper that clearly demarcated the role of small-vessel disease in diabetic mononeuropathy.*

Schaumburg HH, Spencer PS, Thomas PK: Disorders of Peripheral Nerves. Philadelphia, F. A. Davis Company, 1983. *A short lucidly written monograph providing a good introduction to this complex subject.*

Spencer PS, Schaumburg HH: Experimental and Clinical Neurotoxicology. Baltimore, Williams & Wilkins, 1980. *A multiauthored comprehensive text with special emphasis on the peripheral nervous system.*

Sunderland S: Nerves and Nerve Injuries. New York, Churchill Livingstone, Inc., 1978. *A monumental monograph on nerve injury; the standard reference.*

Section Sixteen DISEASES OF MUSCLE AND NEUROMUSCULAR JUNCTION

Lewis P. Rowland

537. INTRODUCTION

DEFINITIONS. The *motor unit* comprises four elements: the motor neuron, its peripheral axon, the terminal branches and corresponding neuromuscular junctions, and the many muscle fibers innervated by the particular nerve cell. The major symptom of most diseases of the motor unit is *weakness*.

The word *atrophy* means, literally, "lack of nourishment." It has come to mean wasting of muscle, or loss of muscle bulk from any cause, and it is also used to denote single muscle fibers that are smaller than normal when viewed microscopically. When used in the name of a disease, atrophy always implies that the muscle wasting is secondary to a neural disorder, e.g., infantile spinal muscular atrophy, progressive spinal muscular atrophy, or peroneal muscular atrophy. To avoid ambiguity, it is therefore appropriate in examining patients to use "wasting" rather than "atrophy" to describe diminution in muscle bulk unless the cause is known to be neurogenic. *Myopathies* include disorders characterized by weakness or some other symptom of muscle dysfunction that is not due to emotional or neurogenic cause. Some authors speak of "primary" or "secondary" myopathies, but there is little evidence that any muscle disease is really "primary," in the sense that there is an abnormality in muscle and nowhere else. In some myopathies, as in thyrotoxic myopathy, the fundamental disorder is elsewhere, and this could be true even in genetically determined diseases. The *dystrophies* are a subgroup of myopathy with three special characteristics: heritable transmission, progressive weakness, and histologic evidence of degeneration of muscle with no evidence of abnormally stored material or structural abnormality of the fibers.

DIFFERENTIAL DIAGNOSIS OF MUSCLE DISEASE

The differential diagnosis of muscle disease can be broken down into several considerations: (1) the nature of the symptoms, (2) combinations of muscles affected, (3) age of the patient, (4) findings on examination, (5) tempo of disease, (6) genetics, and (7) results of laboratory studies.

SYMPTOMS. *Weakness* implies lack of normal strength or power. However, patients with pathologically weak muscles usually complain of the consequences of weakness, not weakness itself. That is, they have difficulty walking or rising from low seats if leg muscles are affected. They may lose manual dexterity for buttoning clothes or writing, or have difficulty lifting or raising the arms. Or, if cranial muscles are affected, there may be *dysarthria* (slurred speech), *dysphagia* (difficulty swallowing), *diplopia* (double vision), or *ptosis* (a droopy eyelid). In contrast, explicit complaint of loss of strength is less likely to be a manifestation of disease; a fading athlete may be growing older, losing prowess, but he or she is not sick. Complaints of fatigue, constant tiredness, and an urge to rest are likely to be manifestations of emotional depression but not muscle disease.

In muscle diseases, it has also been traditional to explain the weakness in solely morphologic terms; many muscle fibers show evidence of degeneration and are ultimately replaced by fat and connective tissue. However, clinical weakness often seems disproportionately more severe than the histologic evidence indicates. Conversely, many fibers may be morphologically abnormal (for instance, muscle fibers may be severely distorted by stored glycogen in McArdle's disease), but the patient may not be weak at all. Therefore, we presume that functional alterations of muscle, as well as the morphologic changes, also contribute to the weakness of muscle disease.

Other symptoms of muscle disease are less common than weakness. Aching muscles *(myalgia)* may result from vigorous exercise of specific muscles that are "untrained" or "out of condition," or may occur more diffusely in patients with polymyositis or dermatomyositis, or during attacks of myoglobinuria. Myalgia is attributed to stimulation of pain-sensitive nerves within muscle by edema or toxic metabolites but has not been formally studied. In *myoglobinuria,* the red muscle pigment is released from muscle into blood serum in amounts sufficient to darken the urine overtly. Oxidized myoglobin appears rust-colored or brown, rather than red. Limb weakness, myalgia, and malaise often accompany attacks of frank myoglobinuria, the causes of which will be discussed later. *Myotonia* refers to a painless condition of impaired relaxation of muscle after a forceful contraction; for instance, patients may have difficulty letting go after trying to unscrew a bottle cap or turn a recalcitrant doorknob. Myotonia occurs in several different diseases, but the common physiologic abnormality seems to be repetitive depolarization of muscle fibers. It is most common in specific genetic disorders but may affect otherwise normal individuals who are taking diazacholesterol or other drugs that affect the lipid composition of muscle cell membranes.

Muscle cramps are another kind of involuntary and sustained muscle spasm, but differ from myotonia in that sustained voluntary effort is not a precipitating factor and because the sudden forceful shortening of a cramp is painful.

When any one of these symptoms (other than weakness) is prominent, the differential diagnosis is narrowed to a relatively few conditions. The differential diagnosis of weakness, however, involves much of clinical neurology. We are not here concerned with cerebral causes of weakness (likely to be expressed by hemiparesis) or other upper motor neuron disorders (which may cause weakness or incoordination of all four limbs) because they are immediately separated from diseases of the lower motor neuron or motor unit by the characteristic exaggeration of tendon reflexes, clonus, and Hoffmann and Babinski signs. Neurogenic and myopathic diseases of the motor unit, however, must be distinguished from each other, and the distinction is not always easy. The following criteria help.

CHARACTERISTIC COMBINATIONS OF MUSCLES AFFECTED IN DIFFERENT SYNDROMES. A few conditions can be recognized at a glance because of the characteristic appearance of the patient, imparted to some extent by the particular set of muscles affected. Perhaps the most specific is the long, lean face of myotonic dystrophy—long and lean because the temporalis and masseter muscles are small; the appearance is made even more characteristic because there may be ptosis of the eyelids (caused by weakness of the levators) and eversion of the lips (caused by weakness of facial muscles). Dysarthria (resulting from weakness of oropharyngeal muscles) and thin neck (resulting from smallness of sternomastoid muscles) contribute to the appearance.

In myasthenia gravis, many of the same muscles are affected. Ptosis of the eyelids, facial weakness, dysarthria, and dysphagia are common but the appearance differs. In contrast to those with myotonic dystrophy, patients with myasthenia are more likely to have diplopia and ophthalmoparesis, asymmetric ptosis (often unilateral), and do not have the long, lean face or thin neck. The only other myopathic conditions likely to be confused with these disorders of cranial muscles are the *ocular myopathies,* described later. Among neurogenic diseases, only motor neuron disease causes diffuse and symmetrical weakness of cranial muscles, but the eyelids and ocular movements are spared, and only oropharyngeal muscles are affected prominently.

When limb muscles are affected predominantly, there are few characteristic combinations that distinguish neurogenic from myopathic disease, a distinction that often must be made by laboratory tests. Even when specific combinations are engrafted in the names of conditions (such as "facioscapulohumeral muscular dystrophy" or "scapuloperoneal syndromes"), the cause may be either neurogenic or myopathic. In both of these sets of disorders, *"winging of the scapula"* (visible protrusion of the scapula away from the chest wall) is prominent.

In general, two rules apply: (1) Distal limb weakness is more likely to be due to neurogenic disorder, but some cases are myopathic. (2) Proximal limb weakness is more likely to be myopathic, but this is an even less reliable criterion because there are so many exceptions. Probably the only syndromes of proximal limb weakness that are evident on inspection are facioscapulohumeral muscular dystrophy and Duchenne dystrophy. In the latter, however, it is not just the distribution of weakness that identifies the disorder, for the patient is always a young boy and the severity of weakness is appropriate to his age; by about age 12 he will not be able to walk. Before he stops walking, his calves are likely to appear disproportionately large *("pseudohypertrophy").*

AGE AT ONSET OF WEAKNESS. Duchenne dystrophy is not the only diagnosis that depends on age. In the neonatal period, at least three neuromuscular disorders may appear: neonatal myasthenia gravis (in children of myasthenic mothers), myotonic muscular dystrophy, and botulism. "Congenital myasthenia gravis" and "congenital myopathies," despite the names, usually become evident later in the first year or two of life. In the first year of life, almost all cases of limb weakness of neuromuscular origin (not cerebral) are due to infantile spinal muscular atrophy (Werdnig-Hoffmann disease); peripheral neuropathy and early-onset myopathies are only rarely expressed before age two years.

After infancy, children and adults experience the gamut of neuromuscular diseases, involving areas from the motor neuron through the peripheral nerve and neuromuscular junction to muscle, although the names and tempo may differ at different ages. Among the diagnostic clues that depend upon age are the following: (1) Among the muscular dystrophies, the Duchenne form is one of early childhood, almost always evident before age three years. Facioscapulohumeral and limb-girdle forms usually begin in adolescence. The only muscular dystrophies that begin after age 35 are some cases of the autosomal dominant forms (myotonic muscular dystrophy, facioscapulohumeral dystrophy, and ocular myopathies). (2) Dermatomyositis occurs in children (and with roughly equal frequency in all decades of life into old age). Polymyositis, in contrast, rarely occurs before adolescence. (3) Charcot-Marie-Tooth disease and other hereditary neuropathies begin in childhood or adolescence, rarely later.

SIGNS ON EXAMINATION. When there is solely proximal limb weakness, both neurogenic and myopathic disorders can cause the same triad of manifestations: weakness, wasting, and loss of reflexes. Some signs are indicative of neurogenic disease: (1) *Fasciculation,* visible twitching of portions of a muscle, occurs in chronic motor neuron diseases, rarely in peripheral neuropathy, and probably never in myopathy (with the possible exception of a severe form of thyrotoxic myopathy that is no longer seen in these days of prompt diagnosis of hyperthyroidism). (2) *Glove-stocking patterns of cutaneous sensory loss* imply peripheral neuropathy. (3) *Combinations of upper and lower motor neuron signs* in the same limbs are virtually pathognomonic of amyotrophic lateral sclerosis. Similarly, the combination of distal limb weakness, fasciculation, and other lower motor neuron signs in the arms or cranial muscles with upper motor neuron signs in the legs bespeaks amyotrophic lateral sclerosis.

When, as is too often the case, there are no clear signs of neurogenic disease and there is only chronic proximal limb weakness, the differential diagnosis depends upon laboratory tests, as described below.

Few signs can be regarded as pathognomonic of myopathy. *"Pseudohypertrophy"* of the calves, or disproportionate enlargement of these or other muscles, is characteristic of Duchenne dystrophy but occurs occasionally in other myopathies and also in some cases of neurogenic disease. Myotonia is characteristically myopathic, but other disorders (that are different electromyographically) may be similar clinically. The combination of myotonia and muscular enlargement is restricted to myotonia congenita. Only the concomitant appearance of myoglobinuria and weakness or the entire constellation of signs that indicate myotonic muscular dystrophy can be regarded as definitely myopathic.

TEMPO OF DISEASE. Recognition and definition of neurogenic and myopathic diseases are often based upon tempo. For instance, periodic paralysis is just that—attacks of weakness that come on in moments or hours and last for hours or days. Between attacks, the patient may be normal or there may be chronic weakness that is less severe than in the periodic attacks.

The periodic pattern differs from the fluctuations seen in myasthenia gravis, which may be of three kinds: (1) There may be minute-to-minute variation, especially for ptosis of the eyelids. (2) There may be variations during the course of a single day, or from day to day. (3) There may be longer and more dramatic fluctuations in severity, exacerbations or periods of improvement. The extremes are represented by "myasthenic crisis," which is defined by the need for respiratory assistance, or "remissions," in which symptoms disappear for weeks, months, or years, only to return again. No other neuromuscular disease fluctuates the way myasthenia gravis does.

Both myasthenia and periodic paralysis, when first starting, may appear to be acute illnesses, but there are not many other acute neuromuscular disorders. Among the myopathies, polymyositis may become severe in a few days or weeks, and attacks of myoglobinuria may be accompanied by severe weakness in a day or two. But most myopathies are chronic. Among neurogenic diseases, the Guillain-Barré syndrome usually reaches peak severity in a few days or within two weeks. A similar pattern is followed by brachial plexus neuropathies, toxic neuropathies, and botulism, but most acquired neuropathies are slower in evolution, taking months to reach maximal severity, and most genetic neuropathies progress for years.

GENETICS. Genetic patterns influence diagnosis in two ways. First, a family history of affected relatives may alert the clinician (or the patient) to a known diagnosis, or the pattern of inheritance may suggest the diagnosis. Second, when a diagnosis of genetic disorder is made, other members of the family may then be identified as carriers of recessive genes (by biochemical markers) or as affected by a dominant disorder (by clinical examination). In the near future, it is expected that the application of recombinant DNA techniques will aid in the identification of specific heritable diseases in individual patients and their relatives.

LABORATORY TESTS. Many diseases can be identified without recourse to any laboratory test. Other conditions may also be diagnosed clinically, but laboratory tests are used to confirm the diagnosis, to be certain that some other condition is not masquerading. That is why muscle biopsy and EMG are done in myotonic disorders or Duchenne dystrophy, for example, although these procedures are essentially superfluous for diagnosis if the serum creatine kinase (CK) concentration is very high.

Some conditions are virtually defined by laboratory tests. For instance, changes in muscle biopsy define the "structurally specific" congenital myopathies (such as central core disease or nemaline disease), mitochondrial myopathies, and lipid-storage myopathies, all of which are named after the specific abnormal structure. Changes in muscle biopsy may also aid in the diagnosis of sarcoid, amyloidosis, toxoplasmosis, trichinosis, or periarteritis nodosa. But all of these are rare, and the most common use of both muscle biopsy and EMG is to determine whether or not weak muscle is denervated.

In general both EMG and biopsy give concordant results. Discordant or contradictory results occur in 5 to 10 per cent of cases and are of two types: (1) If the EMG is consistent with denervation but the biopsy shows "myopathic" changes, most centers would give primacy to the EMG because the muscle biopsy may show myopathic changes in unequivocally denervating disorders, as in survivors of paralytic poliomyelitis. (2) If the reverse is found—"myopathic EMG" and denervating changes in the biopsy—no diagnosis is possible, a conflict only rarely experienced.

Several pairs of diseases are defined by EMG and muscle biopsy. In each of these pairs the clinical syndromes are similar, and, unless there is overt fasciculation, the clinician cannot distinguish the neurogenic and myopathic forms. In assigning a diagnosis to any of these pairs, EMG signs of denervation make one diagnosis, and either lack of these neurogenic signs or a "myopathic" EMG pattern makes the other diagnosis (Table 537–1).

Diagnostic Use of Muscle Biopsy. SIGNS OF DENERVATION. Normally, histochemical stains show two major types of muscle fibers. One type stains strongly for glycolytic enzymes, the other for oxidative enzymes. In some muscles there is only one fiber type, but in most human muscles both types are represented in a "checkerboard" pattern. This biochemical differentiation parallels physiologic differences of fast- and slow-twitch fibers. Furthermore, all of the muscle fibers innervated by the same neuron are of the same fiber type. Studies have shown that the muscle fibers of a normal single motor unit are not usually grouped together but the fibers of several units are intermingled.

The diagnostic signs of denervation in human biopsies are based upon these principles and concepts of "collateral sprouting" in reinnervation. In partially denervated muscle, surviving terminal axons send branches to adjacent muscle fibers which have lost the original innervation. By this process, the size of functioning units is larger than normal, and contiguous muscle fibers are of the same histochemical type (fiber-type grouping) instead of the normal checkerboard appearance. Atrophic fibers may also appear in groups (group atrophy), and this may be a consequence of later denervation of an augmented motor unit. Another histochemical sign of denervation, defined by its appearance, is the "target fiber," which is found only in neurogenic disorders but is not understood. All of these histologic signs tend to affect muscle focally so that lack of morphologic change in a small sample does not exclude a neurogenic disorder.

SIGNS OF MYOPATHY. In contrast to the group lesions of denervation, myopathic changes often occur randomly. More specifically "myopathic" changes include evidence of degeneration and regeneration of muscle fibers. Degenerating fibers lose their normal striations and become fragmented and subject to invasion by macrophages. Early in the process, there is disproportionate variation of fiber size. The smaller fibers are thought to be recently regenerated or to result from fiber-splitting. The large fibers are larger than usual, occur more often in chronic disorders, and may be due to compensatory

TABLE 537–1. PAIRS OF DISEASES THAT ARE DISTINGUISHED BY EMG AND MUSCLE BIOPSY

Age	Neurogenic	Myopathic
Infancy	Infantile spinal muscular atrophy	Severe congenital myopathy
Childhood and adolescence	Juvenile spinal muscular atrophy	Limb-girdle muscular dystrophy Facioscapulohumeral muscular dystrophy Quadriceps myopathy
Adults	Motor neuron disease	Distal myopathy

work hypertrophy of surviving fibers when diseased fibers cannot participate in the work of the muscle. In muscular dystrophies, macrophages are few, except in scattered fibers, and there is little perivascular monocytic response, but these signs of "inflammation" may be prominent in polymyositis. In both the dystrophies and polymyositis, regeneration is heralded by a basophilic appearance in sections stained with hematoxylin and eosin, presumably because of increased content of RNA in newly formed fibers that are actively making new proteins. In advanced myopathy, muscle fibers are replaced by fat and connective tissue; this may be evident earlier in some dystrophies, but the end-stage is similar in either neurogenic or myopathic disease.

OTHER HISTOCHEMICAL ALTERATIONS. The "congenital myopathies" are identified by, and defined by, physical structures such as nemaline rods, fingerprint structures, and central cores. These structures are "specific" only in appearance, since little is known about the pathogenesis of any of them. Histochemical methods also allow the identification of accumulations of glycogen or lipid, observations that may lead to specific biochemical diagnosis by appropriate biochemical tests on muscle homogenates.

SPECIFIC DIAGNOSIS BY MUSCLE BIOPSY. None of the preceding uses of muscle biopsy is definitive; even accumulations of glycogen or lipid require further biochemical analysis. The only truly specific diagnoses that can be made from a biopsy are sarcoid, periarteritis nodosa, amyloidosis, and parasitic infestation (trichinosis, cysticercosis, toxoplasmosis). By using special histochemical stains, it is possible to identify conditions caused by genetic lack of phosphorylase or phosphofructokinase, but these and other specific enzyme disorders should be verified by enzyme assay of homogenates. Special studies may aid in the diagnosis of Lafora's disease and neuronal ceroid lipofuscinosis.

ROLE OF ELECTRON MICROSCOPY. Ultrastructural study of muscle has engaged a major research effort, but the electron microscope has no role in routine diagnosis.

RESEARCH APPLICATIONS OF MUSCLE BIOPSY. Research laboratories throughout the world are using biopsied muscle specimens for biochemical analysis, physiologic study, or muscle culture. Muscle diseases are almost all resistant to specific therapy and hope for ultimate treatment lies in this kind of research. Because of this, because diagnostic biopsy provides only limited information that is not likely to affect therapy, and because it is difficult to justify more than one standard biopsy, it seems reasonable to make a plea for regional muscle biopsy centers. At present, biopsies are done in most community hospitals, and by the time the patient reaches a research center it is difficult to suggest a second biopsy for purely research purposes.

Electromyography. The distinction between neurogenic and myopathic disease depends upon the electrical activity of a muscle at rest and during weak contractions. Attention is paid to the frequency, amplitude, and duration of motor unit potentials. Details of the electromyogram and its diagnostic usefulness in muscle disorders are given in Ch. 471.

Biochemical Studies. The most common biochemical test used in the diagnosis of muscle disease is the measurement of serum activity of sarcoplasmic enzymes, especially CK, but also other enzymes. In myopathic diseases, these enzyme activities are characteristically high; the enzyme proteins in serum are thought to enter blood from necrotic muscle or because of altered permeability of muscle surface membranes. CK determination is often regarded as the most sensitive, and it may be—in the sense that CK is often abnormal when other enzymes are normal. However, the increased sensitivity in detecting myopathies comes at a price, because CK is also often abnormal in chronic motor neuron diseases, thus losing the ability to discriminate myopathic and neurogenic diseases. In most hospitals, routine blood chemistry determinations are now automated and include other enzyme activities such as GOT, GTP, and LDH. The concentrations of these serum enzymes also rise in patients with muscle disease and only rarely in neurogenic disease. When there is no obvious heart or liver disease, therefore, these other enzymes may be useful in neuromuscular diagnosis. Still other enzyme assays (such as aldolase or pyruvate kinase) or radioimmunoassay for myoglobin are favored in some institutions but have no special advantage in the diagnosis of muscle disease. Similarly, isoenzyme analysis has no particular advantage; even the MB or "cardiac" isoenzyme of CK may appear in the serum in Duchenne dystrophy or polymyositis, not because the heart is involved but presumably because this isoenzyme dominates in immature muscle skeletal muscle fibers, and regenerating fibers are plentiful in these diseases.

Specific biochemical diagnosis is restricted to the glycogen and lipid storage diseases and the analysis of myoglobinuria, as discussed later. These biochemical studies are indicated when histochemical stains show accumulation of fat or glycogen in syndromes of limb weakness, and in all cases of nontraumatic myoglobinuria.

Brooke MH: A Clinician's View of Neuromuscular Diseases. Baltimore, Williams & Wilkins Company, 1977. *A favorite of students because of the lively and accurate descriptions of clinical syndromes.*

Buchthal F, Schmallbruch H: Motor unit of mammalian muscle. Physiol Rev 60:90, 1980. *A modern statement of the organization of the motor unit, with attention to physiology and morphology.*

Dubowitz V: Muscle Disorders in Childhood. Philadelphia, W. B. Saunders Company, 1978. *A comprehensive review of common and rare syndromes by a single author who is an experienced clinician. The many excellent illustrations include instructive photographs of patients and muscle biopsies.*

Goodgold J, Eberstein A: Electrodiagnosis of Neuromuscular Diseases. 3rd ed. Baltimore, Williams & Wilkins Company, 1983. *A popular, well-illustrated, and clear introduction to the theory and practice of electromyography and nerve conduction studies.*

Mastaglia FL, Walton JN: Skeletal Muscle Pathology. Edinburgh, Churchill-Livingstone, 1982. *Lucid descriptions and beautiful illustrations cover the common and the exotic conditions.*

Vinken PJ, Bruyn GW, Ringel SP (eds.): Diseases of Muscle. Handbook of Clinical Neurology. Vols. 40, 41. Amsterdam, North-Holland Publishing Company, 1979. *Individual chapters by different authors cover every conceivable disorder in great detail.*

Walton JN (ed.): Diseases of Voluntary Muscle. 4th ed. Edinburgh, Churchill-Livingston, 1981. *A multiauthored and authoritative book, with attention to basic science as well as clinical aspects. The four editions attest to the book's status as the standard reference.*

538. INHERITED DISEASES

MUSCULAR DYSTROPHIES

DEFINITION. Muscular dystrophies are inherited myopathies, characterized primarily by progressively severe weakness. In the absence of known biochemical abnormality, they are distinguished from similar diseases by lack of histologic evidence of any metabolic storage material, or by changes other than those of degeneration and regeneration of muscle or tissue reactions to these processes.

ETIOLOGY. Although it is generally believed that inherited diseases must be due to a missing or structurally abnormal protein (either an enzyme or a structural protein), this abnormality has not been identified in any form of dystrophy. Increasing biochemical and ultrastructural evidence implicates the muscle surface membrane as the site of fundamental disorder. There is evidence of dysfunction of enzymes that are an integral part of the membrane, and there are gaps in the plasma membrane that permit the entry of large molecules such as horseradish peroxidase, a protein, or procion yellow, a dye. Biochemical study of isolated membranes has been limited, however, because only small amounts of tissue are available in a biopsy and the membrane preparations include fat and connective tissue. In red blood cell membranes and cultured fibroblasts no consistent abnormality has been discovered.

Pathologic and biochemical abnormalities can be detected in muscle, and there is no clear evidence of neural abnormality in traditional terms. There is still debate about the possible role of altered motor neurons, and some writers postulate a debatable vascular cause, functional ischemia of muscle.

CLASSIFICATION. No classification of the muscular dystrophies is entirely satisfactory, but clinical and genetic analysis provides the best approach at present. The classification in Table 538–1 is based upon the clearly identifiable features of Duchenne dystrophy, facioscapulohumeral dystrophy, and myotonic muscular dystrophy. Limb-girdle dystrophy is probably not a single disease but encompasses cases that do not fall into the other categories. The techniques of molecular genetics should give more precise classifications.

INCIDENCE. None of the muscular dystrophies is common. Incidence rates vary from 5 per million births for facioscapulohumeral dystrophy to about 250 per million for Duchenne dystrophy. The mutation rate of Duchenne dystrophy is high, 7×10^{-5}, and about two thirds of the cases appear sporadically, with no other affected individual in the family.

PATHOLOGY. Pathologic abnormalities are restricted to skeletal muscle, sometimes involving cardiac muscle. The brain, spinal cord, and peripheral nerves are devoid of histologic change, although some authors have implicated the brain because of a seemingly high incidence of mental retardation in children with Duchenne dystrophy. Terminal pneumonia may cause changes in the lungs, and there may be a variety of associated diseases not directly linked to the dystrophy. In myotonic muscular dystrophy, baldness and testicular atrophy are integral parts of the disease in men, and corneal opacities affect both sexes.

The abnormalities in muscle seem to involve all fibers in random fashion. Early, there is scattered evidence of necrosis and regeneration, with prominent variation in fiber size, including many fibers much larger than normal and many fibers that appear hyalinized. Later, fibers disappear, to be replaced by fibrous connective tissue and fat. "Pseudohypertrophy" is probably due to both "true" hypertrophy (large fibers) and increased accumulation of fat and connective tissue. In myotonic dystrophy, unusual figures form "ring fibers" (with one fiber running at right angles, encircling the other fibers in the same bundle) and "sarcoplasmic masses," or accumulations of sarcoplasm that are free of myofilaments. However, these abnormalities occur occasionally in other diseases and are not pathognomonic of myotonic dystrophy. In Duchenne dystrophy, the myocardium may be affected by similar changes, but cardiac symptoms are rarely evident in life, a discrepancy that has been attributed to the sedentary life imposed upon the patients by advanced muscular weakness. Myopathic changes in the heart are common in myotonic dystrophy. There is no good evidence that smooth muscle is regularly affected in any form of dystrophy.

Ultrastructural investigations suggest an early, and perhaps primary, abnormality of the muscle surface membrane, but it is not clear how this might be related to the progressive degeneration of muscle. The postulated abnormality of the surface membranes may allow an inappropriate influx of calcium, and this could have several deleterious effects, including local hypercontraction of myofilaments near the sites of calcium entry (overstretching and disrupting myofilaments in adjacent sarcomeres), stealing of intracellular ATP (because mitochondrial calcium uptake is an energy-dependent process), or activating of intracellular proteases. The initiating event in the degenerative process is not known; disruption of myofibrillar structure, alterations of mitochondria, and degeneration of tubules and sarcoplasmic reticulum all seem to proceed together.

CLINICAL MANIFESTATIONS. The symptoms and signs of all forms of the muscular dystrophies are related to weakness alone, except that additional systems are involved in myotonic dystrophy. In other forms, the symptoms depend upon the distribution of weakness and the age at onset. In *Duchenne dystrophy* weakness is primarily proximal at onset, and symptoms begin early. By definition, girls are not affected. (However, girls with chromosomal abnormalities may have the disorder; study of these unusual cases identified the location of the Duchenne gene as Xp21.) There are no symptoms in the first year of life, but walking may be somewhat delayed beyond 18 months. Once the child walks, some abnormality is usually evident to an experienced observer (either a parent with a previously affected child or a skilled physician). The boys tend to waddle or walk on their toes, or fall frequently and have difficulty rising. They are probably never able to run, because they have difficulty raising their knees. These symptoms become more evident as the children grow older, and even the most unsuspecting parent becomes aware of some abnormality by age five. Teachers sometimes may detect the difficulty when the child starts school. Some cases are averred to start between ages five and ten, but these must be exceptional. It is difficult to examine individual muscles of a young child, but the waddling gait, the typical method of rising from the ground by "climbing up" himself (*Gowers' sign*), enlargement of calf or other muscles, and inability to run are characteristic. Myotatic reflexes may be normal at first, but by three years the knee jerks are usually lost, and later the ankle jerks disappear. As the child grows, increased growth and coordination may com-

TABLE 538–1. CLASSIFICATION OF HUMAN MUSCULAR DYSTROPHIES

	Duchenne Dystrophy	Facioscapulohumeral Dystrophy	Limb-Girdle Dystrophy	Myotonic Dystrophy
Genetic pattern	X-linked, recessive	Autosomal, dominant	Autosomal, recessive	Autosomal, dominant
Age at onset	Before age 5	Adolescence	Adolescence	Early or late
First symptoms	Pelvic	Shoulders	Pelvic	Distal; hands or feet
Pseudohypertrophy	+	0	0	0
Predominant weakness, early	Proximal	Proximal	Proximal	Distal
Progression	Relatively rapid; incapacitated in adolescence	Slow	Variable	Slow
Facial weakness	0	+	0	Occasional
Ocular, oropharyngeal weakness	0	0	0	Occasional
Myotonia	0	0	0	+
Cardiomyopathy	0 or late	0	0	Arrhythmia, conduction block
Associated disorders	None (?mental retardation)	None	None	Cataracts; testicular atrophy and baldness in men
Serum enzymes	Very high	Slight or no increase	Slight or no increase	Slight or no increase
Prevalence (per million population)	38	5	20	25
Incidence (per million births)	251	5	47	–
Mutation rate	9×10^{-5}	5×10^{-7}	3×10^{-5}	10×10^{-6}

pensate temporarily for the concurrent progressive weakness and wasting, but the disease always prevails. There is increased difficulty walking. Going up grades or stairs first requires aid, then becomes impossible. Weakness of the trunk muscles leads to increased lordosis and a protuberant abdomen. Then the arms become weak. Finally, in early adolescence, the child becomes unable to walk. This may be accelerated by a period of inactivity after an injury or an orthopedic operation. Contractures appear, at first in the feet, as the gastrocnemius muscles tighten. When the child stops walking, flexion contractures limit motion of the knees, and scoliosis becomes more a problem with prolonged sitting. Ultimately respiration becomes shallow and the child is increasingly subject to pulmonary infection. Sooner or later, one of these infections is fatal, usually in the third decade. Although muscles are ravaged from the neck down, the cranial muscles are entirely spared. Congestive heart failure and abnormalities of cardiac rhythm are rare.

Becker dystrophy has manifestations similar to those of Duchenne dystrophy, including X-linked inheritance, but the onset is later in childhood or in adolescence, and the tempo is slower and more variable. This form may also be devastating, but some patients are able to function, albeit with limitations, well into adult life. The clinical similarities include pseudohypertrophy of calf muscles and increased serum content of creatine kinase (CK) and other sarcoplasmic enzymes. However, although the two forms are similar, they are genetically separate; there are no mildly affected individuals in typical Duchenne families, nor are young children affected severely in Becker families. In some sporadic cases and in some families it is difficult to decide whether the disorder is Duchenne dystrophy of relatively late appearance or Becker dystrophy of relatively early appearance. The distinction awaits recognition of the specific genes or specific biochemical abnormalities in the two or more forms.

Still a third X-linked recessive form is called *Emery-Dreifuss muscular dystrophy*. It differs from the Duchenne type in later age at onset and benign course and from both Duchenne and Becker types because pseudohypertrophy is not found and serum enzymes are normal or only minimally increased. Additionally, the Emery-Dreifuss form has two characteristics that are not found in either of the other X-linked dystrophies: cardiac arterial standstill and contractures at knees, elbows, and neck. The cardiac disorder poses a threat of sudden death and requires treatment by pacemaker.

The manifestations of *limb-girdle dystrophy* are also similar because weakness of muscles of the pelvic girdle usually initiates the syndrome, but symptoms start in late childhood or adolescence. Girls are affected as often as boys, and pseudohypertrophy is rare. Waddling gait, difficulty in walking and climbing, and frequent falls are common. Occasionally, symptoms begin in the shoulder girdle. In either case, there is usually weakness in all four limbs by the time the patient seeks medical attention. Severity, age at onset, and rate of progression vary considerably, suggesting that this category contains more than one disease.

Facioscapulohumeral dystrophy is distinct. Symptoms vary in severity so that some affected individuals never have any disability (but can be recognized by the signs), whereas others become incapacitated early; there are all grades in between. The first symptoms are apt to be related to difficulty in raising the arms or to prominence of the scapulae. Weakness of the legs may affect pelvic girdle muscles, or equally prominent weakness of the anterior tibial muscles may lead to a steppage gait. Weakness of trunk muscles may lead to prominent scoliosis. The face is always involved on examination; the perioral muscles may be more affected than those of the upper face, but ultimately patients have difficulty in closing the eyes. The sternal head of the pectoral muscle is affected earlier than the clavicular head, a selectivity that can be detected on testing the individual muscles, and leads to a peculiar appearance of the axillary folds when the arms are dependent, because the anterior axillary fold of normal people is formed by the sternal portion of the pectoral muscle. As a result, the anterior axillary fold normally extends upward and outward from the chest to the head of the humerus, but in patients with this form of muscular dystrophy the anterior fold may seem to rise straight up or even reverse, rising medially toward the clavicle. Winging of the scapulae can be seen when the patient leans against a wall with the arms extended, and the weakness of shoulder girdle muscles leads to an unusual appearance because, viewed from the front, the superior margin of the scapula is higher than the clavicle.

Myotonic muscular dystrophy diverges from the preceding types in several respects. (1) The distribution of weakness differs in that cranial muscles are often affected and limb weakness is initially more marked in distal muscles. Thus weakness of the hands precedes shoulder weakness, and footdrop or steppage gait precedes symptoms of pelvic muscle weakness. *Ptosis, facial weakness,* and *dysarthria* are signs not seen in the other forms of dystrophy. Moreover, there is almost always selective weakness and smallness of the sternomastoids. The masticatory muscles either are poorly developed or waste early (even when not symptomatically weak), causing a characteristic long, lean facial appearance. (2) Myotonia, or difficulty in relaxation, may be symptomatic, and after a firm grip the patient may have difficulty letting go. Myotonia may cause other symptoms in patients with myotonia congenita (see below), but in the dystrophy only the hands are affected by this kind of stiffness. Myotonia of grip may be evident on examination, and can also be elicited by percussing the thenar eminence. In normal persons this evokes a rapid twitch, whereas in patients with myotonia, a sustained contraction of the adductor pollicis muscle persists for several seconds, only gradually relaxing. Similar responses to percussion may be elicited in the finger extensors or tongue but the response is difficult to demonstrate in other muscles. Although myotonia is a dramatic sign and a symptom that can be relieved by drugs, it is not the symptom that causes the major disability in myotonic dystrophy; weakness is the problem. (3) Other systems are involved in this pleomorphic disorder; cataracts appear sooner or later in all patients, and are sometimes the only sign of the disease; most of the men (but not the women) have frontal baldness; testicular atrophy affects most of the men, but often after they have already sired children to perpetuate the disease (there is no definite evidence of gonadal insufficiency in affected women); the basal metabolic rate is often low, but other tests of thyroid function are normal (extrathyroidal hypometabolism). The incidence of diabetes mellitus may be increased. Glucose metabolism is often abnormal but analysis has been difficult and controversial; insulin resistance may be due to decreased affinity of insulin receptors. (4) Conduction defects are common in the electrocardiogram and may lead to clinically significant arrhythmia or congestive heart failure.

Certain rare forms of muscular dystrophy are named after the prominent manifestations. *Ocular muscular dystrophy* is a slowly progressive disorder in which ptosis of the eyelids and progressive immobility of the eyes are the cardinal features. The pupils are spared, and both eyes are usually affected symmetrically so that diplopia is uncommon. Other muscles of the head, neck, and limbs may also be affected, varying from family to family. This syndrome raises problems of definition; some cases probably are myopathic in origin, but this kind of ophthalmoplegia is often associated with other manifestations that are clearly neurogenic (such as spinocerebellar degeneration or peripheral neuropathy). The final distinction is often difficult or impossible to make because, in ocular muscles, the conventional electromyographic and biopsy criteria of myopathy are not valid. In some patients with myopathic ophthalmoplegia, structural and biochemical abnormalities may be found in limb muscles. Abnormally large mitochondria are present in increased numbers; this can be seen dramatically in electron microscopy, and the numbers are sufficient to stain fibers red in the trichrome stain for light microscopy, leading to the appellation "ragged red fibers." In these cases there is apt to be an accumulation of glycogen, but the biochemical cause of this has not been ascertained.

Distal myopathy, as the name implies, affects distal leg and hand muscles first. It is probably the rarest form of dystrophy, and can be identified only by characteristic signs of myopathy in electromyography and muscle biopsy.

In the *scapuloperoneal syndrome* distal weakness in the legs resembles that of neurogenic peroneal muscular atrophy, but sensory loss is lacking, and there is proximal weakness in the shoulder girdle similar to that of facioscapulohumeral dystrophy. Some of these cases are myopathic and some neurogenic as distinguished by electromyography, muscle biopsy, and serum enzymes. In either case, autosomal dominant inheritance and a relatively slow progression seem characteristic.

DIAGNOSIS. The clinical picture of Duchenne dystrophy entails little diagnostic confusion. In its first stages, some children are merely regarded as clumsy, and some receive orthopedic care because of toe-walking; otherwise the diagnosis becomes obvious. As noted, the trait is transmitted as a sex-linked recessive, and once a case is recognized, members of the family rapidly detect the signs in subsequently affected youngsters. Once a family is known, affected individuals can be identified in the neonatal period because the serum enzymes are already markedly abnormal. Limb-girdle and facioscapulohumeral dystrophy must be differentiated from neurogenic diseases, from congenital myopathies, and from polymyositis, as will be discussed below. Myotonic dystrophy may be confused with endocrine disorders or, because of the distal weakness, with neuropathy or amyotrophy, or with hypothyroidism or gonadal disorders. Ocular myopathy must be differentiated from myasthenia gravis; there is no fluctuation of symptoms in the myopathy, and the weakness does not respond to cholinergic drugs.

The familial cases of progressive ophthalmoplegia (ocular muscular dystrophy) also have to be distinguished from an unusual syndrome that seems to be sporadic and has only once been reported to affect siblings. This form, *the Kearns-Sayre syndrome,* is identified by the triad of progressive ophthalmoplegia, pigmentary degeneration of the retina, and onset before age 15. Almost all patients with these three features will be found to have evidence of heart block on the electrocardiogram and cerebrospinal protein content of more than 100 mg per deciliter. More than half of these patients also have short stature, hearing loss, and evidence of corticospinal tract or cerebellar disease.

The differential diagnosis of the myopathies also depends upon the age of the patient. In childhood and adolescence, the major problems involve peroneal muscular atrophy (Charcot-Marie-Tooth) and "muscular atrophy simulating muscular dystrophy" (Wohlfart-Kugelberg-Welander). In adults, amyo trophic lateral sclerosis is the major problem. At all ages, polyneuritis must be considered.

MOLECULAR GENETICS. The chromosomal site of the gene for Duchenne dystrophy is known to be on the short arm of the X chromosome, and flanking probes are already available. It is anticipated that even closer probes will be available in 1985. The method then could be used for prenatal diagnosis and for precise identification of carriers.

The gene for Becker dystrophy was long thought to be on the long arm of the X chromosome because it seemed to be linked to the gene for colorblindness. However, molecular probes suggest that the Becker gene is allelic to the Duchenne gene; this would account for the similarity of these diseases. With better probes, it should be possible to identify young boys while they are still walking, and this would give more accurate prognosis.

The gene for myotonic muscular dystrophy is on chromosome 19, as determined by linkage studies and molecular probes. If better probes can be found, it would be possible to identify which at-risk members of the family will have the disease and which will be spared. It will also be possible to determine whether the syndrome is heterogeneous and comprises more than one form.

TREATMENT. There is no specific treatment for any form of dystrophy. Physical therapy, exercises, splints, braces, and corrective orthopedic surgery are applied in different centers with varying degrees of enthusiasm. Some claim that walking can be prolonged into late adolescence in Duchenne dystrophy. The most poignant decisions concern the use of antimicrobial drugs or supported respiration for young men paralyzed from the neck down and with no hope of ultimate recovery. The myotonia of myotonic dystrophy can be relieved by phenytoin (0.3 to 0.6 gram daily) or by quinine (0.3 to 1.5 grams daily), but this is rarely the problem, and nothing can be done for the weakness. Cataracts are treated surgically upon appropriate indication, and cardiac arrhythmias and congestive heart failure are managed accordingly.

PROPHYLAXIS. Genetic counseling offers the only possibility to control muscular dystrophy at present. Carriers of Duchenne dystrophy may often but not always be identified by abnormally increased serum enzyme activity (higher than normal, but not as high as in affected boys). In some centers, antenatal detection of sex allows selective prophylactic abortion. There is presently no way to determine whether a male fetus is affected, however. The development of methods to measure CK in fetal blood unfortunately did not predict reliably whether the fetus was affected. Fetal blood sampling may ultimately provide the way to identify the true biochemical abnormality in the fetus, assuming that it will be the same in both muscle and erythrocytes, an assumption that is not proved. Birth control ought to be effective in dominantly inherited diseases such as facioscapulohumeral and myotonic dystrophy, but many cases are relatively mild and the risk is acceptable to some families. The high rates of mutation do not encourage optimism that genetic restriction can be the ultimate goal.

Bradley WG: The limb-girdle syndromes. Handb Clin Neurol 40:433, 1979. *A thoughtful review of a common syndrome that illustrates the difficulty of separating myopathies from neurogenic disorders.*

Harper PS: Myotonic Dystrophy. Philadelphia, W. B. Saunders Company, 1979. *A modern classic; thorough in coverage, thoughtful in analysis, and written in a lively style.*

Munsat TL: The classification of human myopathies. Handb Clin Neurol 40:275, 1979. *Overview of the problem of identifying different muscle diseases, introducing a multiauthored summary of all of the dystrophies.*

Roses AD, Pericak-Vance MA, Yamaoka LH, Stubblefield E, Stajich J, Vance JM, Roses MJ, Carter DB: Recombinant DNA strategies in genetic neurological diseases. Muscle Nerve 6:339, 1983. *A primer of modern genetic approaches to muscular dystrophies and other diseases in which the gene product is not known.*

Rowland LP: Biochemistry of muscle membranes in Duchenne muscular dystrophy. Muscle Nerve 3:3, 1980. *A detailed review of the evidence for and against the theory that the genetic lesion in this disease affects muscle surface membranes.*

Rowland LP, Layzer RB: X-linked muscular dystrophies. Handb Clin Neurol 40:349, 1979. *A review of the four different forms of X-linked muscular dystrophy.*

Stuart CA, Armstrong RM, Provow SA, Plishker GA: Insulin resistance in myotonic dystrophy. Neurology 33:679, 1983. *A review and study of an unresolved endocrine problem in myotonic muscular dystrophy.*

OTHER INHERITED BIOCHEMICAL DISORDERS: METABOLIC MYOPATHIES, MITOCHONDRIAL MYOPATHIES, AND FAMILIAL MYOGLOBINURIA

DEFINITION. The muscular dystrophies may ultimately prove to be disorders of metabolism, but that is speculative and the term "metabolic myopathy" is now used only for diseases in which there are more or less clearly defined abnormalities of glycogen, lipid, or energy metabolism. Although some of these conditions are described in greater detail in other chapters, it is necessary to mention them here because they enter into the differential diagnosis of syndromes of proximal limb weakness or myoglobinuria.

GLYCOGEN STORAGE MYOPATHIES

These diseases, described in detail in Ch. 179, were the first heritable diseases of muscle in which the biochemical defect was discerned. Of the several forms, the only ones that do not affect muscle are type 1 (lack of glucose-6-phosphate dehydrogenase) and type 6 (lack of liver phosphorylase).

Pompe's disease, the infantile form of glycogen storage disease type 2, is associated with *lack of acid maltase.* It affects both motor neurons and muscle, causing a clinical disorder that resembles Werdnig-Hoffmann disease, from which it is distinguished by glossomegaly and cardiomegaly with congestive heart failure. It is uniformly fatal by one year of age. In another group of acid maltase deficiencies the disease starts later in childhood or even in adult years. The syndrome is one of proximal limb and diaphragm weakness that resembles either limb-girdle dystrophy or polymyositis. The only clinical clues to the nature of the disease are the prominence of respiratory failure and the presence of myotonic discharges in the electromyogram (although there is no clinical myotonia). Histologically, there is a vacuolar myopathy, which can be shown to be due to deposition of glycogen in skeletal muscle. In the infantile form, but not in late-onset forms, cardiac muscle is affected and motor neurons in the brain and spinal cord are also swollen and distorted by abnormal accumulation of glycogen. Lack of acid maltase is demonstrated by biochemical assay of muscle homogenates or in the urine.

Type 3 glycogen storage disease, caused by *lack of the debrancher enzyme system,* is usually manifest by hepatomegaly and hypoglycemia, but skeletal muscle may be involved with the liver, or even alone. This disorder may also resemble limb-girdle dystrophy or polymyositis. Diagnosis is suspected on the basis of histochemical study of muscle and proved by biochemical analysis. Types 5 and 7, resulting from *lack of phosphorylase (McArdle's disease)* or *phosphofructokinase (Tarui's disease)* are causes of recurrent myoglobinuria, as described earlier and in Ch. 179.

LIPID STORAGE AND MITOCHONDRIAL MYOPATHIES

There is no adequate classification of mitochondrial myopathies because the specific biochemical abnormalities are unknown. For the same reason it is not known how many of these disorders are inherited and how many are acquired. For convenience, they may be separated into four categories: (1) a group identified only by morphologic abnormality, (2) abnormalities of muscle lipid metabolism, (3) abnormalities of pyruvate oxidation or electron transport, and (4) myoglobinuria. See Table 538–2.

MORPHOLOGICALLY ABNORMAL MITOCHONDRIA. In these conditions the mitochondria are too numerous, too large, or contain abnormal crystalline inclusions. Histochemical examination with the light microscope reveals a colorful pattern in muscle fibers as a result of accumulations of large mitochondria. In trichrome stain, the muscle fibers are blue and the mitochondria at the periphery are a striking red, giving rise to the popular term *"ragged red fibers."* The histologic abnormality is associated with a diversity of clinical syndromes, and there is no apparent relationship between the mitochondrial abnormality and the symptoms. For instance, the histologic changes are seen in both congenital and later-life syndromes of proximal limb weakness. The same changes are almost always present in patients with two very different kinds of ocular myopathy, including those with the specific constellation of manifestations that characterize the Kearns-Sayre syndrome (described earlier) and those with nothing more than restricted external ophthalmoplegia. Even vague fatigue states or cramps may be associated with abnormal mitochondria. In some of these nonspecific syndromes, there may be a persistent but slight increase in venous blood lactate content, not enough to cause acidosis. In others, there is profound lactic acidosis, as described below in disorders of pyruvate metabolism. Results of biochemical studies of mitochondria are either normal or show minor and nonspecific deviations from controls. There is no effective therapy.

LIPID STORAGE MYOPATHIES. In some syndromes of proximal limb weakness, there is gross accumulation of lipid *within* muscle fibers (in contrast to the fat that is deposited *between* fibers in Duchenne dystrophy), which can be identified by simple histochemical stains. Usually there are mitochondrial abnormalities as well. The accumulation of lipid in some cases can be attributed to very low levels of muscle carnitine, a compound necessary for the esterification and transport of long-chain fatty acids into mitochondria. Fatty acid oxidation

TABLE 538–2. MITOCHONDRIAL MYOPATHIES

Common Name	Clinical Manifestations	Morphologic	Biochemical Abnormality
Morphologic abnormality			
Nonspecific mitochondrial myopathy	Proximal limb weakness (early or late), cramps, fatigue syndrome	Ragged red fibers, giant mitochondria, increased number of mitochondria, crystalline conclusions	Slight or no increase in venous lactate
Ocular myopathy	Progressive ophthalmoplegia with or without limb weakness	Same	Same
Kearns-Sayre syndrome	Ophthalmoplegia, pigmentary degeneration of retina, heart block, high CSF protein, neural disorders	Same	Same
Lipid storage myopathy			
Muscle carnitine deficiency	Limb weakness	As above, plus lipid storage	Carnitine low in muscle, normal in serum
Systemic carnitine deficiency	Limb weakness plus hepatic encephalopathy	Same, plus lipid storage	Carnitine low in muscle, serum, and liver
Triglyceride storage disease	Ichthyosis, steatorrhea, limb weakness	Lipid storage in muscle, white blood cells	No specific abnormality
Disordered energy metabolism			
Pyruvate dehydrogenase deficiency Cytochrome deficiencies	Limb weakness plus encephalopathy in infants	Lipid storage, ragged red fibers	Lactic acidemia; lack of one of three components of PDH or cytochrome
Luft's disease	Euthyroid hypermetabolism	Same	Partial uncoupling of mitochondrial respiration and phosphorylation
MELAS*	Myopathy, encephalopathy, strokes in childhood	Same	Lactic acidosis, biochemical disorder not known
Fukuhara syndrome	Ataxia, myoclonus, seizures	Same	Lactic acidosis, biochemical disorder not known
Myoglobinuria			
DiMauro's disease	Recurrent myoglobinuria	Usually normal	Lack of carnitine palmityl transferase
Malignant hyperthermia	Fever, muscle stiffness, lactic acidosis, myoglobinuria, cardiac arrhythmia	Normal	Abnormal muscle response to caffeine; increased muscle adenyl cyclase

*MELAS = mitochondrial encephalomyopathy, lactic acidosis, and stroke.

is impaired and triglycerides accumulate. There is no predictable clinical pattern except that progression may be slightly more rapid than in most muscular dystrophies or there may be periods of improvement or worsening, or respiratory muscles may be affected—all characteristics that might lead to suspicion of polymyositis rather than muscular dystrophy. There are at least two types of carnitine deficiency. In one *(muscle carnitine deficiency)*, the content of carnitine in muscle is about 10 per cent of normal, but the serum content of carnitine is normal and symptoms are confined to limb weakness. In the second type *(systemic carnitine deficiency)*, serum and liver carnitine contents are reduced in addition to muscle, and symptoms include attacks of hepatic encephalopathy that may be fatal. Oral carnitine therapy has helped some patients, and, for unknown reasons, prednisone may help. Some cases are familial in a pattern that suggests an autosomal recessive trait; the sporadic cases could also be inherited, but some may be acquired. In the third syndrome of proximal limb weakness and lipid storage in muscle, carnitine determinations are normal and the cause of lipid accumulation is not known.

One other lipid storage myopathy can be recognized by four characteristics that seem to go together: congenital ichthyosis, lifelong steatorrhea, lipid storage myopathy, and accumulation of triglycerides in white blood cells and cultured fibroblasts or cultured muscle. The cause is not known.

DISORDERS OF PYRUVATE METABOLISM OR ELECTRON TRANSPORT. A block in the oxidation of pyruvate would affect such a fundamental metabolic process that it ought to be incompatible with life. In fact, genetic lesions affecting each of the three component enzymes of the pyruvate dehydrogenase complex have been identified. These syndromes usually appear in the newborn period and affect brain as well as muscle; the resulting encephalopathy and severe lactic acidosis are rapidly fatal. Less severe but similar syndromes affect older children with encephalopathy, proximal limb weakness, lactic acidemia, and lipid storage myopathy. Although a disorder of mitochondrial oxidation of pyruvate is suspected, the nature of the disorder is not clear because the pyruvate dehydrogenase enzymes are normal.

There are also infantile syndromes of severe myopathy that seem to be due to inherited abnormalities of the cytochromes.

A most dramatic mitochondrial disorder is *Luft's disease*, described in only two unrelated adults with euthyroid hypermetabolism. Heat intolerance was manifest by constant sweating and fever that resulted from uncoupling of mitochondrial respiration and phosphorylation of unknown cause, with no satisfactory treatment.

FAMILIAL MYOGLOBINURIA. Sporadic myoglobinuria is described in Ch. 539. In some persons, however, repeated attacks from childhood suggest a genetic disorder, and sometimes more than one individual in a family is affected. Some of these familial cases are due to lack of muscle phosphorylase or phosphofructokinase. The patterns of myoglobinuria are similar in both disorders, but phosphofructokinase deficiency is accompanied by hemolytic anemia as well as the myopathy. These disorders can be recognized by the ischemic work test in which contracture is induced and venous lactate fails to rise, by histochemical evidence of glycogen accumulation in muscle, and finally by biochemical assays for the appropriate enzymes (see Ch. 179).

In three recognized disorders of glycolysis, there is no storage of glycogen, but recurrent myoglobinuria is seen. The affected enzymes are phosphoglycerate kinase (DiMauro), phosphoglycerate mutase (DiMauro), and lactate dehydrogenase (Kanno). They are distinguished from other forms of recurrent myoglobinuria only by biochemical analysis.

In the most common form of inherited myoglobinuria (*DiMauro's disease*), the missing enzyme is carnitine palmityl transferase, which plays a vital role in the oxidation of long-chain fatty acids. It might be expected that lack of this enzyme would result in the same syndrome that accompanies carnitine deficiency. However, in DiMauro's disease, there is neither persistent limb weakness nor consistent lipid storage; the only symptoms are recurrent attacks of myoglobinuria. In still other cases of familial recurrent myoglobinuria, no abnormality has been found in either lipid or glycogen metabolism.

In all of these familial syndromes, episodic myoglobinuria is the main and usually the only manifestation. Permanent proximal limb weakness is rare. Renal failure, however, may complicate an attack of myoglobinuria of any cause. The only way to prevent attacks is to limit physical activity, avoiding prolonged or unusually vigorous exercise. The limits are soon learned by affected individuals.

MALIGNANT HYPERTHERMIA. Malignant hyperthermia is a rare problem defined by a catastrophic reaction to general anesthesia. In the course of preparing for surgery, the patient receives a muscle relaxant (usually succinylcholine) and a general anesthetic (usually halothane). Soon the muscles become very stiff and body temperature begins to rise rapidly. Severe metabolic acidosis caused by lactic acidemia follows, and there may be myoglobinuria. Cardiac arrhythmias and renal failure may ensue. When the syndrome was first recognized, the incidence was said to be about 1 in every 50,000 general anesthesias, and the mortality rate was about 75 per cent. Now, however, anesthesiologists are alert to the possibility. By stopping the operation, ending anesthesia, cooling rapidly, neutralizing the acidosis, and, perhaps, giving dantrolene, the malignant element can be removed. Similar syndromes are seen in patients who take psychoactive drugs (*malignant neuroleptic syndrome*) and in heat stroke, but these syndromes are not seen in families with malignant hyperthermia.

In some families, the condition seems to be inherited as an autosomal dominant trait, but in most cases the event is sporadic and there is likely to be more than one kind of susceptibility. Patients with central core disease and Duchenne muscular dystrophy may be at special risk. It is suspected that patients inherit an abnormal susceptibility to either succinylcholine or halothane (or other agents), to which they react by excessive and prolonged release of calcium in muscle and that this is followed by the other manifestations.

Treatment of the acute attack requires prompt intervention to institute symptomatic measures. Prevention is difficult because it is so hard to identify those at risk. Some patients who have actually had attacks have congenital structural abnormalities (such as cryptorchidism or pedal abnormalities), or they may have high serum creatine kinase activity between attacks, or there may be minor abnormalities of nonspecific nature in muscle biopsy. Several patients have had histologic evidence of central core disease. However, none of these characteristics has proved a reliable guide, and immediate relatives of patients should have physiologic tests of excised muscle with caffeine or biochemical studies of adenylate cyclase or phosphorylase activity. If either physiologic or biochemical test results are abnormal, a warning bracelet should be worn by the individual. Even if these tests give normal results, all immediate relatives of patients who have had attacks should be identified to anesthesiologists before elective surgery. Patients with central core disease or Duchenne dystrophy also require caution for elective surgical procedures, especially in early childhood.

Prophylaxis may be possible. If there is sufficient evidence of risk, the individual may be given dantrolene by mouth for 24 hours before elective surgery. In a multicenter study, the mean dose was 2.5 mg per kilogram of body weight, but this does not guarantee protection.

DiMauro S: Metabolic myopathies. Handb Clin Neurol 41:175, 1979. *Clearly written review of myopathies resulting from disorders of glycogen or lipid metabolism and mitochondrial abnormalities.*

DiMauro S, Trevisan C, Hays A: Disorders of lipid metabolism in muscle. Muscle Nerve 3:369, 1980. *Review of a rapidly evolving field.*

Gronert GA: Malignant hyperthermia. Anesthesiology 53:395, 1980. *Comprehensive review of a clinical problem of growing importance.*

Penn AS: Myoglobin and myoglobinuria. Handb Clin Neurol 41:259, 1979. *A thorough review of the many causes of myoglobinuria.*

Rowland LP, DiMauro S: Glycogen storage diseases of muscle: Genetic problems. Res Proc Assoc Nerv Ment Dis 60:239, 1983. *A review of the heterogeneity of these syndromes.*

Scarlato G, Cerri C (eds.): Mitochondrial Pathology in Muscle Diseases. Padua, Piccin Medical Books, 1983. *Chapters cover this evolving field, including infantile disorders of pyruvate metabolism, other identified biochemical abnormalities of mitochondrial function, and clinically identified disorders such as the Kearns-Sayre and Fukuhara Syndromes.*

Willner JH, Nakagawa M: Controversies in malignant hyperthermia. Semin Neurol 3:275, 1983. *A critical review of the methods used to detect susceptibility to this baffling syndrome.*

CONGENITAL MYOPATHIES

DEFINITION. These are rare diseases characterized by weakness that is usually mild but persists throughout life, usually remaining stationary or progressing imperceptibly.

ETIOLOGY. The cause is not known. A few of these disorders are familial and suspected of having a genetic basis, but so many cases are sporadic that other causes are not excluded, and there are no clear clues.

PATHOLOGY. These diseases are defined in terms of pathology, and most of them have been delineated within the past 20 years since the introduction of histochemical techniques to study muscle biopsy. The names of the diseases reflect the predominant anatomic disorder.

In *central core disease,* the central portion of the muscle fiber appears rather amorphous, in contrast to the fibrillar appearance of the surrounding normal portion. In cross-section, the central portion appears blue when stained with Gomori's trichrome, in striking contrast to the red periphery. The central areas lack all oxidative enzyme activity, and there are no mitochondria in this region. In *nemaline myopathy* or *rod myopathy,* small threadlike or rod bodies are scattered throughout the fiber. The rods are barely visible in conventional hematoxylin and eosin stains, but can be seen readily in phase contrast or with the trichrome stain. In electron microscopy the structures seem to originate in the Z-band, and circumstantial evidence suggests that they are composed of tropomyosin. *Myotubular myopathy* designates the appearance of myofibers that resemble a stage in the early development of fetal muscle, with nuclei located centrally rather than at the periphery and surrounded by a halo of apparently empty space. Because the pathogenesis of this appearance is uncertain, some investigators prefer the name *centronuclear myopathy.* As indicated above, some *mitochondrial myopathies* are associated with only morphologic abnormalities of these organelles (with no recognizable functional abnormality) in a syndrome of congenital and static limb weakness.

CLINICAL MANIFESTATIONS. Some congenital myopathies lack specific morphologic signs; such disorders have been called *severe nonspecific congenital myopathy* or, if associated with severe mental retardation, *congenital muscular dystrophy of Fukuyama.* (Because the syndrome is not progressive, "myopathy" may be the preferable word.) Nonspecific myopathic changes are also seen in patients with multiple congenital abnormalities of joints, *arthrogryposis multiplex congenita.* Some cases of arthrogryposis show histologic changes that imply a neurogenic cause.

These disorders are only exceptionally symptomatic in the first year of life, except that the onset of walking may be delayed. Later, symptoms of proximal limb weakness become evident: waddling gait, difficulty in climbing stairs, frequent falls, scoliosis, and weakness of the arms. Sometimes, onset of the syndrome in adults makes it unlikely that the morphologic changes were congenital, and some acquired but unknown cause is suspected. In none of the structurally defined congenital myopathies is it possible to link the morphologic abnormality to a biochemical or physiologic cause of the weakness.

The hallmark of arthrogryposis is congenital fixation of joints, often with other skeletal abnormalities. The disorders may be mild or severe but are always static.

GENETICS. Most cases of congenital myopathy are sporadic, but some patterns of inheritance suggest autosomal dominant or autosomal recessive transmission. Arthrogryposis syndromes are likely to be autosomal dominant if there is more than one case in a family, but most are sporadic.

DIAGNOSIS AND TREATMENT. Proximal limb weakness in a young child is usually myopathic in origin, but must be distinguished from the neurogenic Wohlfart-Kugelberg-Welander syndrome and from polyneuritis. Myopathic abnormalities in the electromyogram, an abnormal family history, an incidence in girls, and especially the histologic abnormalities define the individual entities. The serum enzymes may be normal or slightly increased. In some clinics most cases of apparently congenital myopathy fail to meet the specific histologic criteria, showing only nonspecific myopathic changes in biopsy. There is no better designation for these cases than "congenital myopathy," but it is likely that there is more than one cause.

In infancy, the major cause of weakness is a form of motor neuron disease (*Werdnig-Hoffmann disease*). Among infants with multiple congenitally fixed joints (arthrogryposis multiplex), some prove to have myopathic disease as defined by muscle biopsy and electromyography. In some cases, neonatal difficulty in swallowing is followed by delayed onset of walking, possibly persistent weakness, obesity, childhood diabetes, mental retardation, and a characteristic facial appearance (*Prader-Willi syndrome*), but there is no abnormality on muscle biopsy or electromyogram.

Bender, AN: Congenital myopathies. Handb Clin Neurol 41:1, 1979. *A thorough review of the congenital myopathies that are identified by morphologic abnormality.*

Brooke MH, Carroll JE, Ringel SP: Congenital hypotonia revisited. Muscle Nerve 2:84, 1979. *A skeptical view of the practice of "defining" disease solely on the basis of morphologic change.*

Brown LM, Robson MJ, Sharrard WJW: The pathophysiology of arthrogryposis multiplex congenita neurologica. J Bone Joint Surg 62-B:291, 1980. *A clinical analysis, with discussion of orthopedic treatment.*

Dubowitz V: Muscle Disorders in Childhood. Philadelphia, W. B. Saunders Company, 1978. *Congenital myopathies are placed in the perspective of other neuromuscular diseases of childhood by an experienced clinician and investigator.*

Edstrom L, Wroblewski R, Mair WGP: Genuine myotubular myopathy. Muscle Nerve 5:604, 1982. *Detailed analysis of one dramatic form of congenital myopathy.*

Hall JG, Reed SD, Greene G: The distal arthrogryposes: Delineation of new entities—review and nosologic discussion. Am J Hum Genet 11:185, 1982. *An interesting attempt to classify hereditary arthrogryposis syndromes according to association with other congenital malformations.*

Mastaglia FL, Walton JN: Skeletal Muscle Pathology. Edinburgh, Churchill-Livingstone, 1982. *Illustrations and discussion of the congenital disorders are provided in this excellent text.*

MYOTONIA CONGENITA
(Thomsen's Disease)

DEFINITION. Myotonia congenita is a rare disorder characterized by difficulty in relaxation of skeletal muscle after forceful contraction, present from early childhood.

There are occasional sporadic cases, but most are inherited in a pattern corresponding to an autosomal dominant trait. In a few families, the disease seems to be autosomal recessive. The abnormality must be inherent within the muscle, because myotonic phenomena may be elicited after all neural influences are abolished by spinal anesthesia, block of motor nerves by local anesthesia, or blockade of the neuromuscular junction by intra-arterial injection of d-tubocurarine. Myotonia is abolished by the intramuscular administration of procaine. In human myotonia congenita, as in a genetic myotonia of goats, there seems to be an abnormality of chloride conductance in muscle, and this could account for the tendency to discharge repetitively. The disorder in myotonic muscular dystrophy seems to differ, and it is possible that the biochemical abnormality is different in each of the several forms of inherited human myotonia.

CLINICAL MANIFESTATIONS. The difficulty in relaxation is widespread. Difficulty in relaxing the grip may lead to prominent and sometimes embarrassing symptoms. Ocular muscles may be affected, so that the eyes seem momentarily "stuck" in one position, or the eyelids may remain closed after forceful closure. Sometimes oropharyngeal muscles are affected, with difficulty in speaking or swallowing. Startle reactions may induce stiffness of the legs, thwarting sudden attempts to catch a bus or run from home plate. There is no weakness, and one characteristic is the unusual muscular development of many patients, causing a Herculean appearance. The myotonia can be elicited by tapping any muscle in severely affected cases. Reflexes are unaltered.

DIAGNOSIS. The major problem is in distinguishing the disorder from myotonic muscular dystrophy. Here the only symptoms and signs are related to myotonia. There is no weakness, cataract, baldness, or gonadal atrophy. So-called "transitional cases" are probably patients in families with myotonic muscular dystrophy who are only mildly affected and show only myotonia before the other manifestations.

TREATMENT. For many years, quinine was the staple treatment in doses of 0.3 to 1.5 grams daily. Recently, phenytoin has proved equally effective and less apt to cause disagreeable side effects in therapeutic doses of 0.3 to 0.6 gram daily. Procainamide has also been used, in doses of 4 to 6 grams daily, but this drug is prone to induce lupus erythematosus and is therefore avoided.

Harper PS: Myotonic Dystrophy. Philadelphia, W. B. Saunders Company, 1979. *The standard reference for this multisystem disorder and related conditions.*

Howeler CJ, Busch HFM, Bernini LF, Van Loghem E, Khan PM, Nijienhuis LE: Dystrophia myotonica and myotonia congenita concurring in one family. Brain 103:497, 1980. *These two disorders are ordinarily distinct and only rarely occur in the same family—a paradox awaiting the techniques of molecular genetics for solution.*

Lipicky RJ: Myotonic syndromes other than myotonic muscular dystrophy. Handb Clin Neurol 40:533, 1979. *Analysis of myotonic syndromes by a leading physiologist who has been investigating the basic mechanisms.*

Roses AD, Harper PS, Bossen EH: Myotonic muscular dystrophy. Handb Clin Neurol 40:485, 1979. *Comprehensive review of clinical and biochemical aspects.*

FAMILIAL PERIODIC PARALYSIS

DEFINITION. Periodic paralysis is characterized by recurrent attacks of flaccid weakness usually associated with abnormally high or low serum potassium concentrations. Many cases are familial. In sporadic cases the abnormality may be due to aberrations of potassium metabolism.

ETIOLOGY AND PATHOGENESIS. Familial cases are distributed in a pattern consistent with autosomal dominant inheritance. Hypokalemia during attacks was the first metabolic abnormality to be recognized, with no loss of potassium in urine. It was presumed that potassium shifted from extracellular to intracellular compartments, especially muscle. This has been difficult to prove, and the anticipated hyperpolarization of the muscle membrane potential has not been substantiated by direct measurement with intracellular electrodes. Abnormalities of glucose metabolism have been suspected, because attacks can be precipitated by infusions of glucose and insulin, by eating a large meal, or by administration of epinephrine. However, biochemical studies have failed to pinpoint the abnormality.

In other families, the serum potassium rises during attacks, which can be induced by ingestion of potassium. This variety is therefore called *hyperkalemic periodic paralysis* and is generally considered to be the mirror image of the hypokalemic type, with potassium presumably shifting out of muscle and into blood during attacks. There are clinical differences between the two forms of periodic paralysis, but there are so many areas of overlap and so many common features that it is difficult to decide just how many genetically distinct forms there really are.

PATHOLOGY. In both forms of periodic paralysis there may be vacuoles within muscle fibers. These may be numerous or scanty, and it is not clear whether they are more frequent in paralyzed muscle. Most electron microscopists believe that the vacuoles are derived from the sarcoplasmic reticulum, but others think they originate in the T-system in areas of necrotic muscle. Glycogen seems to be increased in amount in ultrastructural studies, but the results of biochemical analysis have been inconsistent. There is no evidence that other organs are affected in either form of the disease. The heart is usually spared pathologically.

CLINICAL MANIFESTATIONS. In the hypokalemic variety, attacks tend to start in late childhood or adolescence, frequently occur at night, are apt to be severe, and last for a day or more. In the hyperkalemic variety, attacks start at an early age, occur much more frequently, tend to be milder, and may last minutes or hours. Moreover, patients with hyperkalemic periodic paralysis usually have some evidence of myotonia, often limited to percussion myotonia of the tongue. Lid-lag and Chvostek's sign are identified with the hyperkalemic type. These clinical distinctions may break down in application to individual cases and are only crude guides. Moreover, many features are common to both types: dominant pattern of inheritance, susceptibility to attacks during periods of rest after vigorous exercise, ability to ward off attacks by mild exercise after a mild attack has begun, persistent weakness between attacks, vacuoles in muscle, lack of clear relation between serum potassium concentration and severity of paresis, induction of local weakness by cooling, and protection against attacks by acetazolamide. Some patients are affected by attacks in which the serum potassium may be either high or low.

Typical attacks start with weakness of the legs, followed by weakness of the arms. Cranial muscles are affected in severe attacks only, and respiratory insufficiency is exceptional. The attacks may be mild and brief, or severe and prolonged, with all gradations in between. During severe attacks, the myotatic reflexes are lost, and the muscles are electrically inexcitable. Attacks are rarely apoplectic in onset and usually take an hour or more to develop, except that attacks beginning in sleep may be fully developed when the patient awakes. Paresthesias and myalgia may be prominent at the onset, or may be completely lacking. Some patients are aware of oliguria during the attack and diuresis afterward.

The serum potassium is in the range of 2.5 to 3.5 mEq per liter in hypokalemic attacks, and 5.0 to 7.0 mEq per liter in the hyperkalemic type. Between attacks serum potassium values may be normal. The electrocardiogram is altered as would be predicted from the serum values, with low T waves in hypokalemia and peaked T waves in hyperkalemia.

In the hyperkalemic form, some members of the family may be found to have myotonia without any history of periodic paralysis.

In both types of the disease, there may be persistent weakness between attacks, most often proximal, sometimes distal. Experience with acetazolamide therapy indicates that even long-lasting weakness may be reversible, regardless of pathologic changes in muscle. A few patients with intermittent normokalemic or hyperkalemic paralysis have had persistent cardiac arrhythmia, especially bigeminy, and bouts of ventricular tachycardia. The cardiac disorder is neither temporally related to attacks of limb weakness nor related to serum potassium content.

DIAGNOSIS. Periodic paralysis can be recognized by the history of typical attacks; no other disease causes this pattern of recurrent weakness. In myasthenia gravis, weakness may come and go, but less abruptly and with a duration of weeks rather than hours or days; remissions are less frequent so that it is less "periodic." Polymyositis may be transient, but episodes are rarely shorter than several weeks or months. Attacks of myoglobinuric weakness could conceivably be confusing if the pigmenturia were not recognized, but myalgia and malaise are so prominent that it is rarely mistaken for periodic paralysis. Hysterical attacks might be confusing.

If the patient is seen during the attack and the serum potassium level is abnormal, other causes of hypo- or hyperkalemia must be considered. Low serum potassium concentrations with paralysis are also encountered in hyperaldosteronism; potassium-losing nephritis; potassium depletion caused by laxative abuse, diuretics, or diarrhea; and thyrotoxicosis. *Thiazide* and *thalidone diuretics* are likely to be an increasingly frequent cause of hypokalemic weakness; in one series, about 25 per cent of randomly chosen patients receiving these drugs had serum potassium content below normal. Hyperkalemia is most often due to renal insufficiency, but may also occur in adrenal insufficiency, after administration of spironolactone, or as a manifestation of aldosterone deficiency.

Thyrotoxicosis can cause a variant of periodic hypokalemic paralysis closely resembling the familial variety. The condition especially occurs in young Chinese and Japanese men in their third or fourth decade, but other Asians and women have occasionally been affected. The clinical manifestations of hyperthyroidism are usually not prominent, although tachycardia and even cardiac arrhythmias are frequent. Attacks are commonly precipitated by exercises or heavy carbohydrate meals. Serum potassium is low. Effective treatment of the thyrotoxicosis abolishes this form of periodic paralysis.

A family history of periodic paralysis is useful in diagnosis, but sporadic cases may be indistinguishable from the familial disorder. If the patient is not having a spontaneous attack when studied, the only way to distinguish the two forms is to provoke an attack. The techniques to be described have been used in numerous centers with many patients, without serious complications. But induced attacks may be frightening to patient and physician, and should be left to experienced investigators. Facilities for supported respiration should be immediately available. Appropriately informed consent is mandatory. Because of the uncertainty of clinical distinction, it is advisable to start with glucose (100 grams) given intravenously in one hour with 20 units of regular insulin either in the infusion or given subcutaneously. Hypoglycemic symptoms should be anticipated, and the electrocardiogram should be monitored. Hypokalemia is induced as the blood sugar falls, usually within one hour after the infusion is completed. If an attack is induced, it can be terminated with administration of 7 to 10 grams of potassium chloride (KCl) or about 90 to 130 mEq of mixed potassium salts by mouth. Whether or not an attack is induced by glucose and insulin, but especially if it is not, the patient should then be challenged with potassium. This poses problems because it is not clear how much potassium constitutes an adequate challenge. The author starts with 3 grams of KCl by mouth (or 40 mEq of mixed potassium salts). If this fails, the dose is gradually increased on successive days to a maximum of 8 or 10 grams of KCl (about 100 or 125 mEq of potassium salts). Patients with hyperkalemic paralysis have attacks with serum potassium levels between 5 and 8 mEq per liter.

Other members of the family should be investigated clinically and electromyographically for evidence of myotonia.

TREATMENT. Acute attacks of hypokalemic paralysis are best treated with oral KCl, 5 to 10 grams (65 to 130 mEq of potassium). Relief of weakness usually commences within 30 minutes but may take several hours, and some attacks are peculiarly refractory.

Hyperkalemia may be relieved by infusions of glucose and insulin. Chlorothiazide and calcium gluconate have also been reported to be effective. In severe attacks, weakness may persist even after the serum potassium has returned to normal concentrations.

The traditional method used to protect patients against hypokalemic paralysis was, until recently, a low-sodium diet supplemented by oral KCl, or perhaps by spironolactone or dexamethasone. Then, acetazolamide in small doses, sometimes only 250 per mg daily, sometimes more, was found to be effective prophylaxis in the hyperkalemic type. Subsequently, it was found that similar doses of acetazolamide were equally effective in the hypokalemic variety, so a single drug is beneficial in both forms. How it exerts this effect is not known. The best-known effects of this compound relate to its ability to inhibit carbonic anhydrase, but muscle lacks this enzyme, and no definite systemic effects of the drug have been recognized in the doses used, but respiratory acidosis may be responsible.

Engel AG: Hypokalemic and hyperkalemic periodic paralysis. *In* Goldensohn ES, Appel SH (eds.): Scientific Approaches to Clinical Neurology. Philadelphia, Lea & Febiger, 1977, pp 1742–1761. *Research on this interesting problem has not progressed rapidly. This is still a valid statement of what is known about the disordered physiology, with a comprehensive review of clinical aspects.*

Griggs RC, Resnick J, Engel WK: Intravenous treatment of hypokalemic periodic paralysis. Arch Neurol 90:539, 1983. *Intravenous therapy is rarely necessary; when it is, mannitol solutions are preferred instead of glucose for administered potassium.*

Riggs JE, Griggs RC: Diagnosis and treatment of the periodic paralysis. *In* Klawans H (ed.): Clinical Neuropharmacology, Vol 4. New York, Raven Press, 1979, pp 123–138. *Practical guidelines for diagnosis and treatment.*

MYOSITIS OSSIFICANS

This rare disorder is most dramatic in its consequences, producing the "stone man" of circus sideshows. Symptoms usually begin in early childhood, with transient and localized swellings of the neck and back. Ultimately there is progressive rigidity of the neck, trunk, and limbs. Palpable plates are discernible beneath the rigid parts. Severely affected patients may be able to stand and walk, and yet unable to bend so that they must be raised from bed with assistance. The bars beneath the skin are visible roentgenographically. Microscopically, muscle is replaced by bone and connective tissue. Whether the primary disorder is in the fibroblasts (leading to abnormal ossification) or in the muscle itself is not resolved. Muscle biopsy early in the disease may show widespread necrosis and inflammation, but serum enzymes are not always elevated, nor is the electromyogram always myopathic. Few cases are familial, but the disorder is believed to be inherited because digital abnormalities are almost always present in both the patients and other members of the family in a pattern suggesting an autosomal dominant inheritance. Microdactyly commonly affects the great toe, and clinodactyly (curved digits) may affect the hands. There is no detectable systemic abnormality of calcium and phosphate metabolism, and there has been no effective therapy.

Bassett CAL, Donath A, Macagno F, Preisig R, Fleisch H, Francis MD: Diphosphonates in the treatment of myositis ossificans. Lancet 2:845, 1969. *Evaluation of this treatment still fails to prove its worth.*

Connor JM, Smith R: The cervical spine in fibrodysplasia ossificans progressiva. Br J Radiol 55:492, 1982. *Fusion of cervical vertebrae, a congenital anomaly, may be a universal finding in these patients, even when there is no ossification of adjacent muscle.*

Smith R: Myositis ossificans progressiva. A review of current problems. Semin Arthritis Rheum 4:369, 1975. *The most modern and detailed review of this condition.*

539. SPORADIC DISORDERS

ACQUIRED MYOPATHIES

Several acquired myopathies, particularly when they present with little or no systemic symptoms or evidence of inflammation, enter the differential diagnosis of the muscular dystrophies. Most common are dermatomyositis and polymyositis, but the other disorders listed in the following paragraphs require consideration as well.

DERMATOMYOSITIS-POLYMYOSITIS. Polymyositis without cutaneous lesions is the commonest syndrome likely to be confused with muscular dystrophy. The syndrome probably has several causes and is discussed in Ch. 454. In the absence of a telltale rash, the criteria listed in Table 539–1 help to differentiate the disorder from the primary myopathies. The following paragraphs describe several additional acquired myopathies that must be distinguished from polymyositis.

TABLE 539–1. FEATURES SUGGESTING POLYMYOSITIS RATHER THAN DYSTROPHY

No family history of similar disease
Rapid onset, with weeks or months to maximum disability
Any spontaneous unequivocal improvement
Dysphagia and neck weakness common
Arthralgia or Raynaud's symptoms common
Inflammatory reaction in muscle biopsy
Signs of irritability (spontaneous activity) in the EMG
Age over 35 at onset

CARCINOMATOUS MYOPATHY. Muscle weakness without rash may occur in patients with carcinoma of the lung or of any other primary site. Myeloma, macroglobulinemia, and other gammopathies may also be associated with myopathy. The tumor itself may or may not be symptomatic, and treatment of the tumor may or may not affect the muscular symptoms.

COLLAGEN DISEASES. Proximal limb weakness may occur in the course of systemic lupus erythematosus, progressive systemic sclerosis, rheumatoid arthritis, Sjögren's syndrome, or rarely, periarteritis nodosa or giant cell arteritis. In these circumstances, the myopathy is treated as part of the general disorder.

ENDOCRINE DISEASE. *Thyrotoxic myopathy* is a well-recognized but now rare syndrome. Usually there is clinical evidence of hyperthyroidism, but not always ("apathetic hyperthyroidism"). Signs of hypermetabolism are especially apt to be lacking in elderly patients. The myopathy disappears when the patient is rendered euthyroid by treatment. Similarly, weakness may complicate *hypothyroidism,* and sarcoplasmic enzyme levels in serum may rise so much that polymyositis is suspected. Another muscle syndrome of hypothyroidism is *Hoffmann's syndrome,* a peculiar difficulty in relaxing muscles that lack the characteristic electromyographic abnormalities of myotonia, that is therefore called "*pseudomyotonia.*" This, too, disappears with appropriate replacement therapy.

Hyperparathyroidism and hyperadrenocorticism may also be responsible for weakness that looks like any other proximal myopathy. Weakness may be part of hyperpituitarism, but acromegalic features always overshadow the myopathy. Myalgia, with or without weakness, may be a prominent symptom in patients with osteomalacia, and the muscular disorder may respond dramatically to administration of vitamin D. If the endocrine disorder is not clinically overt and the myopathy is pronounced, the condition may simulate polymyositis. However, serum enzyme levels are not usually increased.

INFECTIONS. Structures resembling viral particles have been seen with the electron microscope in cases of polymyositis, and sometimes there are acute myopathic disorders in individuals with serologically proved influenza or other viral infections, or with encephalomyelitis assumed to be viral in origin. In one special form, children with congenital agammaglobulinemia develop dermatomyositis, and echovirus can be isolated from cerebrospinal fluid. Other infections or infestations that can be associated with clinical polymyositis are trichinosis, toxoplasmosis, cysticercosis, schistosomiasis, and trypanosomiasis.

SARCOIDOSIS. Sarcoidosis is a significant cause of polymyositis. Usually there is other evidence of the disease, but sometimes the first symptoms are due to weakness, and in a few cases only muscle seems to be involved. Myalgia may be severe in these patients.

DRUGS. A variety of drugs used to treat more common disorders may themselves cause muscular weakness, especially triamcinolone and other fluorinated adrenal steroids (but probably all steroids), vincristine, chloroquine, bretylium, emetine, ipecac, carbenoxolone, guanethidine, thiazide diuretics and other kaluretics, epsilon-aminocaproic acid, penicillamine, and clofibrate. Repeated injections of narcotics and other drugs may lead to fibrosis of muscle that simulates a diffuse myopathy.

ALCOHOLIC MYOPATHY. The clearest myopathic disorder in alcoholic persons is acute myoglobinuria. Some of these individuals, and some who never have an attack of pigmenturia, also suffer from proximal limb weakness, especially affecting the legs. The serum creatine kinase is often elevated. The problem in some of these patients, however, is that they also suffer from the typical polyneuritis of alcoholism, and it then becomes difficult to prove that the muscular weakness is not also secondary to a neurogenic disorder. Too few patients have been evaluated to know whether abstinence and a good diet will reverse the persistent weakness.

CHRONIC HYPOKALEMIA. Chronic hypokalemia from any cause may be associated with the syndrome of polymyositis: weakness of relatively abrupt onset, muscle necrosis in biopsy, and high serum enzymes. This is most commonly seen in patients taking thiazide diuretics, but may also occur in hypokalemic states caused by chronic diarrhea. Hypokalemia may also contribute to some cases of alcoholic myopathy.

Alpert JN, Groff AE, Bastian FO, Blum MA: Acute polymyositis caused by sarcoidosis: Report of a case and review of the literature. Mt Sinai J Med 46:486, 1979. *Description of one cause of polymyositis.*

Askari A, Vignos PJ Jr, Moskowitz RW: Steroid myopathy in connective tissue disease. Am J Med 61:485, 1976. *Paradoxically, steroid therapy of muscle disease may also cause weakness. This paper reviews the problem but may underestimate the difficulty of resolving it.*

Bohan A, Peter JB, Bowman RL, Pearson CM: A computer-assisted analysis of 153 patients with polymyositis and dermatomyositis. Medicine 56:255, 1977. *A standard reference for questions about the controversial classification of these diseases.*

Callen JP: The value of malignancy evaluation in patients with dermatomyositis. J Am Acad Dermatol 6:253, 1982. *There appears to be little value if there is no evidence of malignancy on physical examination or from blood counts, chest films, and stool guaiac tests.*

Floyd M, Ayar DR, Barwick DD, Hudgson P, Weightman D: Myopathy in chronic renal failure. Q J Med 43:509, 1974. *The standard discussion of the problem.*

Gamboa ET, Eastwood AB, Hays AP, Maxwell J, Penn AS: Isolation of influenza virus from muscle in myoglobinuric polymyositis. Neurology 29:1323, 1979. *First description of viral isolation in polymyositis.*

Lane RJM, Mastaglia FL: Drug-induced myopathies in man. Lancet 2:562, 1978. *Comprehensive listing of iatrogenic causes of muscle disease.*

Magid SK, Kagen LJ: Serologic evidence for acute toxoplasmosis in polymyositis-dermatomyositis. Am J Med 75:313, 1983. *Toxoplasmosis is a documented cause of acute polymyositis. Whether it is a common cause of chronic syndromes, as suggested by serologic data, is uncertain.*

Perkoff GT: Alcoholic myopathy. Ann Rev Med 22:125, 1971. *The best review of the subject.*

Rowland LP, Clark C, Olarte M: Therapy for dermatomyositis and polymyositis. Adv Neurol 17:63, 1977. *A critical review of reported therapies.*

Schott GD, Wills MR: Muscle weakness in osteomalacia. Lancet 1:626, 1976. *A clear description of an often unrecognized problem.*

Stern LA, Fagan JM: The endocrine myopathies. Handb Clin Neurol 40:235, 1979. *Thorough review of myopathies associated with endocrine disorders.*

Whitaker JN: Inflammatory myopathy: A review of etiologic and pathogenetic factors. Muscle Nerve 5:573, 1982. *A thorough review of reported cellular and humoral abnormalities in these syndromes, emphasizing the paucity of definitive evidence.*

SPORADIC MYOGLOBINURIA

DEFINITION. Sporadic myoglobinuria comprises a group of disorders characterized by injury of muscle and excretion of myoglobin in the urine in amounts sufficient to discolor the urine. *Rhabdomyolysis* has been proposed as a more precise term, but it is never used except when there is gross myoglobinuria and is therefore of dubious value.

PATHOGENESIS. Sensitive radioimmunoassays for myoglobin show small amounts of myoglobin in normal serum. Like serum enzymes, the serum content of myoglobin may increase in myopathies or after myocardial infarction, and under these circumstances myoglobin may pass into the urine, although not in amounts sufficient to darken. (Oxidized myoglobin in the urine is more likely to appear brown than red.) The clinical syndrome of "myoglobinuria" refers to gross pigmenturia and implies more acute and more massive destruction of muscle.

Sometimes the cause of overt myoglobinuria is evident, as in *crush injuries.* Similar pressure injuries may occur in comatose persons who lie on one side without moving for prolonged periods. This kind of injury is perhaps more apt to occur when there are other causes of *metabolic depression;* for instance, in coma after suicidal ingestion of barbiturates or carbon monoxide intoxication, or prolonged unconsciousness in the snow. A similar effect may be induced by *arterial occlusion* by tourniquet or embolism, or even by prolonged knee-chest posture under anesthesia.

In other patients, the cause is less discernible. In every series of patients with myoglobinuria, a disproportionate number are *alcoholics,* but why this should occur is not known. Sometimes there has been exposure to a known *membrane toxin,* such as the bite of the Malayan sea snake. In some addicts, heroin (or an adulterant) seems to cause myoglobinuria. Or there may be *metabolic alterations* that do not ordinarily cause this kind of trouble, such as diarrhea with hypokalemia; potassium depletion caused by diuretics, amphotericin, or licorice; diabetic acidosis; or systemic infection with fever. In many attacks, however, not even these clues prevail.

The most common cause of myoglobinuria is probably unusually *vigorous exercise* by an otherwise normal person. Most cases have been reported by military physicians, and designations include such titles as the "squat-jump syndrome" or "march hemoglobinuria." When large numbers of recruits endure these tortures, a certain number will have attacks of myalgia followed by pigmenturia. Why these individuals have attacks and others are spared is not clear, but this seems to be a "normal" variation. In civilians, cases have been caused by the excess muscular activity of an initiation rite into a club or fraternity, and isolated attacks have occurred after the vigorous muscular activity induced by succinylcholine before it achieves relaxation. With the spread of running for fun and health, cases of myoglobinuria have been reported in joggers and marathon athletes.

In *malignant hyperthermia*, there is a rapid rise in temperature, widespread muscular rigidity, hyperkalemia, and metabolic acidosis, with a fatal outcome in about 75 per cent. The offending agents are usually halothane and succinylcholine. Increased serum activities of sarcoplasmic enzymes are the rule, and often there is myoglobinuria. The intense muscular contraction may be the proximate cause of myoglobinuria in this syndrome, but the widespread metabolic disorder probably contributes. Spontaneous convulsions and electroconvulsive therapy have also been followed by myoglobinuria. The only genetic causes presently recognized are deficiencies of phosphorylase, phosphofructokinase, carnitine palmityl transferase, phosphoglycerate kinase, phosphoglycerate mutase, or lactate dehydrogenase.

CLINICAL MANIFESTATIONS. In attacks other than those caused by local crushing or arterial occlusion, the clinical picture is similar. Affected muscles are apt to be the ones subject to greatest physical strain (the legs in squat-thrusts, the arms after chinning or push-ups, the arms and legs after wrestling matches). The muscles ache, may be swollen, and are weak. Sometimes there is so much edema that local vascular abnormalities are suspected. There may be fever and considerable malaise. Symptoms persist for several days even though pigmenturia rarely lasts more than 48 hours. Recovery may be gradual. Cranial muscles are rarely involved, and although respiratory failure is uncommon it is a hazard. The most important threat to life is renal injury due to excretion of heme. There may be red cells or myoglobin in the urine as well as casts. Oliguria is followed by azotemia and hyperkalemia.

DIAGNOSIS. The diagnosis of myoglobinuria can be made on clinical grounds and with relatively simple tests, but precise identification of the pigment depends upon either absorption spectrophotometry and electrophoresis on starch gel, acrylamide, or cellulose acetate, or more recently, immunochemical methods. The urine may appear red-brown because of hemoglobin, myoglobin, or porphyrins. The latter would not give a positive test result with benzidine (or other heme-reacting reagents), and would give a positive Watson-Schwartz test result for porphobilinogen. Besides, the neurologic disorder of porphyria is neuropathy, not an acute myopathy. If the urine gives a positive test for heme and contains no or few erythrocytes, the pigment is either myoglobin or hemoglobin. If it is hemoglobin, the serum would be pink (after a hemolytic reaction), whereas the color of the serum in myoglobinuria is normal. (This distinction depends upon the affinity of serum haptoglobin for hemoglobin and not for myoglobin. Hemoglobin is not excreted until haptoglobin is saturated by visible amounts of the pigment, whereas myoglobin is excreted at much lower concentrations.) Furthermore, in attacks of myoglobinuria, the muscular weakness and myalgia are distinctive, and serum enzymes are greatly increased, whereas they are not in hemolysis.

Myoglobinuria should be considered a possible cause in all cases of acute renal failure of uncertain etiology. If the serum content of sarcoplasmic enzymes is very high (e.g., creatine kinase values to 10,000 to 50,000 units, with a method giving normal maximal values of 50 units), myoglobinuria must be the cause.

TREATMENT. If there is no renal injury, myoglobinuria is not threatening. The hazards of renal injury are not directly correlated to the amount of pigment excreted, and other factors are probably involved. Once an attack starts, it is useful to encourage excretion of dilute urine by administration of mannitol or other osmotic diuretics; some authorities favor alkalinizing agents, although it has not been clearly demonstrated that these treatments protect the kidneys. Few patients are left with residual weakness, but in some the syndrome is characterized by prolonged weakness punctuated by attacks of myoglobinuria.

Gabow PA, Kaehny WD, Kelleher SP: The spectrum of rhabdomyolysis. Medicine 61:141, 1982. *A thorough review of myoglobinuria from the view of the nephrologist.*

Gamboa ET, Eastwood AB, Hays AP, Maxwell J, Penn AS: Isolation of influenza virus from muscle in myoglobinuric polymyositis. Neurology 29:1323, 1979. *Viral infections may cause myoglobinuria.*

Knochel JP, Barcenas C, Cotton JR, Fuller TJ, Haller R, Carter NW: Hypophosphatemia and rhabdomyolysis. J Clin Invest 62:1240, 1978. *Detailed analysis of metabolic abnormalities that may cause myoglobinuria in alcoholics.*

Rowland LP: Myoglobinuria. Can J Neurol Sci (in press), 1984. *A review of contemporary problems from the view of a neurologist focusing on muscle rather than on the kidney.*

MYASTHENIA GRAVIS

DEFINITION. Myasthenia gravis is a disease of unknown cause, due to circulating antibodies to acetylcholine receptors, and manifested by weakness that has special characteristics: predilection for ocular and other cranial muscles, tendency to fluctuate in severity, no signs of neural lesion, and amelioration of weakness by cholinergic drugs.

ETIOLOGY. Although the initiating event is not known, it seems clear that myasthenic weakness results from the presence of circulating antibodies to acetylcholine receptor (AChR). Rabbits and other species can be immunized with purified AChR. When antibodies appear in the blood, weakness results, which has all the essential properties found in the human disease. Also, as in human myasthenia, there are morphologic changes at the neuromuscular junction, especially simplification of the postjunctional folds, with loss of functional AChR sites, and antibody can be demonstrated on the postjunctional membrane by immunocytochemical methods. As a result, the postjunctional membrane becomes less sensitive to the application of acetylcholine or other agonists.

Soon after experimental autoimmune myasthenia gravis was discovered, similar antibodies to AChR were found demonstrated in the blood of patients with myasthenia gravis. In a transient syndrome of infants born to myasthenic mothers, the symptoms disappeared when the antibodies disappeared. When purified IgG from patients was injected into mice, characteristics of myasthenia were induced in the animals, and if the plasma (but not lymphocytes) of patients was removed by plasmapheresis or thoracic duct drainage, the symptoms were ameliorated. For all these reasons, the antibodies seem to be responsible for the symptoms of the disease.

Some questions remain. Foremost is the nature of the events that initiate the formation of the antibodies. Also, it is not clear what role sensitized lymphocytes play, for there is evidence of altered cellular immunity, too. There are questions about the antibodies themselves, for they seem to be directed to antigenic sites on the AChR other than the combining site for acetylcholine. Simple blockade of AChR by steric hindrance is one possible mechanism, but the antibodies also seem to accelerate the loss of AChR, and other mechanisms of interference are possible. In intercostal muscle from patients with the disease, miniature end-plate potentials are reduced in amplitude and there is decreased sensitivity to cholinergic agonists.

Other evidence of an autoimmune disorder includes the following: abnormalities of the thymus gland in most patients, either germinal centers or thymoma; accumulation of lymphocytes in muscle and other organs; increased coincidence with other autoimmune diseases; and increased frequency of nonspecific autoantibodies against nuclear antigens (ANA), striation-binding muscle antigens, and thyroid antigens.

NEUROMUSCULAR DISORDER. The symptoms of myasthenia gravis resemble those of curare intoxication. This observation led to the use of curare antagonists in treatment, and several drugs currently in use are inhibitors of the enzyme cholinesterase. These drugs also partially repair a physiologic defect that can be detected in patients by relatively simple techniques. When the ulnar nerve of normal individuals is stimulated at rates of 20 per second or less, the action potential of the hypothenar muscles is sustained at a constant amplitude. In patients with myasthenia, however, there is a rapid decline in the height of the evoked potentials. If the patient is then given neostigmine, the amplitude of the evoked potentials is restored to normal. This abnormality has been regarded as characteristic and is consistent with the reduced amplitude of miniature end-plate potentials found in intercostal muscle. Microelectrode studies of excised intercostal muscle have also demonstrated reduced sensitivity of the end-plates to cholinergic agonists.

The use of repetitive stimulation for diagnostic purposes has disadvantages because it causes some discomfort to the patient and because decrementing responses can be encountered in diseases other than myasthenia gravis. Attention has therefore been given to single-fiber electromyography (SFEMG), but this technique may be neither more convenient for the examiner nor more comfortable for the patient. In SFEMG, the intervals are measured between discharges of different fibers within the same motor unit. These intervals vary normally, a variation called "jitter," and the temporal limits have been defined. In myasthenia, jitter increases; when the intervals are very long, expected potentials do not appear, a phenomenon called "blocking," and the number of blockings increases in myasthenia. These abnormalities are attributed to slowing of and uncertainty of neuromuscular transmission.

INCIDENCE AND PREVALENCE. The prevalence of myasthenia gravis is about 33 per million population and the annual incidence of new cases is about 2 to 5 per million. Cases occur in all decades of life, most frequently at about age 40. Among young adults, the disease affects women about three times more frequently than men. Among children and older persons, however, men and women are affected equally. There are a few familial cases, perhaps somewhat more than by chance, and there may be increased incidence of thyroid or other autoimmune disease in relatives of patients with myasthenia. Some genetic predisposition is suggested by a disproportionate frequency of particular transplantation antigen haplotypes in affected individuals, and these may differ in those with thymoma and in younger patients with no tumor.

PATHOLOGY. Pathologic changes in myasthenia gravis are limited to muscle and thymus. Skeletal muscles may appear normal but often contain collections of lymphocytes around blood vessels. Some cases show degeneration of muscle fibers, and the inflammatory cellular response may be extensive. Rarely, similar lesions are encountered in the myocardium. With the electron microscope, there is simplification of the postjunctional folds and widening of the synaptic cleft. Using labelled α-bungarotoxin, loss of AChR sites can be demonstrated and, with immunocytochemical methods, IgG and complement are seen on postsynaptal membranes.

The thymus gland is often abnormal. Encapsulated tumors (thymoma) occur in about 15 per cent of cases, almost all after age 30. About 25 per cent of these tumors invade locally, but distant metastases are virtually unknown and local invasiveness is rarely a cause of symptoms. Lymphocytic proliferation, in the form of germinal centers, is seen in thymus glands of almost all other patients, but sometimes the gland appears normal, and in some older individuals the gland is so involuted that it cannot be found. Patients dying of this disease usually have some pulmonary disorder (edema, atelectasis, infection) resulting from the terminal events. It has not been shown that myasthenia occurs more frequently in patients with cancer than might be expected on the basis of chance.

CLINICAL MANIFESTATIONS. The most common presenting symptoms relate to weakness of eye muscles, causing ptosis or diplopia. At the onset these symptoms may last only a few days, then disappear, only to return weeks or months later. Ptosis frequently varies even in the course of a single day. Diplopia may be noted in particular directions of gaze. Difficulty in chewing, dysarthria, and dysphagia are common. Limb weakness is often proximal, so that patients have difficulty climbing stairs, rising from chairs, or lifting heavy objects or raising the arms overhead. However, distal weakness is not uncommon, and the initial symptoms may be related to the strength of the hands or fingers. Selective respiratory weakness is unusual. There is no alteration of consciousness, no pain, and, in untreated patients, no cramps or muscular twitching. Difficulty in chewing and swallowing may lead to loss of weight, but specific wasting of muscle occurs only in patients with severe chronic weakness.

On examination there is evidence of weakness of the appropriate muscle groups. If any sensory abnormality is found, there must be some other disorder, alone or in combination with myasthenia. Similarly, hyperactive reflexes and Babinski signs imply some other disorder, as does complete loss of reflexes. Weakness is responsible for all the signs of myasthenia. Ptosis may be unilateral or bilateral. Most often, there is asymmetrical weakness of several ocular muscles in a pattern that cannot be explained by disorder of a particular ocular motor nerve. In addition, there is frequently weakness of eye closure because of paresis of the orbicularis oculi. Muscles of the lower face are involved later. Lingual and palatal weakness is evident in patients with dysarthria, causing a nasal twang and indistinct speech. In advanced cases, patients support the chin with one hand to help them talk, a maneuver almost pathognomonic of myasthenia. Neck weakness may be mild or severe enough to cause difficulty in holding the head erect. Limb weakness may be mild or so severe that the patient cannot walk or even turn in bed. Ventilatory insufficiency occurs only in severely affected patients and usually in generalized disease, but some patients with oropharyngeal weakness may be unable to breathe unassisted even though limb muscles are strong. A normal neurologic examination is inconsistent with the diagnosis of myasthenia gravis if the patient is symptomatic at the time and is not taking anticholinesterase drugs.

COURSE. The nature of the disease in a given patient is established within weeks or months of onset, with fluctuations afterward. If after one year, or certainly after two years, myasthenia is still restricted to ocular muscles, it is unlikely to become generalized; purely ocular myasthenia may account for 20 per cent of all cases.

SPECIAL FORMS OF MYASTHENIA. ***Neonatal Myasthenia.*** Infants born to myasthenic women may have a transient syndrome of weakness. The most prominent symptom is difficulty in sucking and swallowing. This may be the sole manifestation, or there may also be noticeable reduction in spontaneous movement and in the vigor of the baby's cry. Only rarely is there respiratory difficulty, but unrecognized neonatal myasthenia has been fatal in exceptional cases. The condition can be identified by the intramuscular injection of neostigmine (0.1 to 0.25 mg), followed by improved sucking, a louder cry, better response to the Moro reflex, and stronger spontaneous movements. Small doses of cholinergic drugs may be administered therapeutically, but more often all that is needed is a nasogastric tube to ensure adequate nutrition. Symptoms subside within a week or, at most, a month.

Congenital Myasthenia. Myasthenia gravis may commence at any age. But a few children seem to have had ophthalmoplegia from birth, with or without other signs of myasthenia. The mothers do not have symptoms of myasthenia (in contrast to mothers of children with neonatal myasthenia). Although presumably congenital, this disorder rarely causes concern until after the first year of life, when the ophthalmoplegia is recognized as having always been present. Many children with congenital myasthenia have no demonstrable antibodies to AChR. Some investigators therefore believe this is a distinct syndrome of "hereditary myasthenia," which they distinguish from the more common "acquired autoimmune" form. Whether this is a reliable distinction is not certain. With standard tests, congenital myasthenia behaves physiologically and pharmacologically like forms of later onset, and it fluctuates in typical fashion. Moreover, antibodies are not found in all cases of later onset, and some familial cases are not congenital, beginning in adolescence or later.

Thyrotoxicosis. About 5 per cent of patients with myasthenia have thyrotoxicosis at some time. Usually the two disorders occur simultaneously, but sometimes hyperthyroidism is evident for weeks or months before there are myasthenic symptoms. Only rarely does myasthenia come long before the thyrotoxicosis, and patients who appear euthyroid do not ordinarily have laboratory evidence of thyroid overactivity. Treatment of the two disorders is directed according to the usual indications for each.

DIAGNOSIS. The diagnosis of myasthenia usually is obvious by history and examination and is immediately confirmed by the response to cholinergic drugs. For adults, 10 mg of edrophonium is given by vein, 2 to 3 mg at a time. If there is no increase in muscle strength within 30 seconds, a second dose of 3.0 mg is given and the patient's condition re-evaluated. If there is still no response, the remainder of the dose is given. This drug is preferred when cranial muscles are being tested because the response is prompt and dramatic. Cranial weakness cannot be simulated voluntarily, and placebo injections are unnecessary.

If it is desired to evaluate limb strength, the injection of neostigmine has advantages because the effect lasts longer, permitting more leisurely testing. The adult dose is 1.5 mg intramuscularly, and it is usually combined with atropine, 0.5 mg, to avoid the muscarinic symptoms of abdominal cramps and sweating. When limb strength is evaluated, it is sometimes advisable to evaluate placebo responses by giving the atropine 30 minutes before the neostigmine. In all cases of myasthenia gravis there is some response to these drugs, but the response is sometimes slight, and the test may have to be repeated on several occasions to provide convincing evidence.

To provide confirmatory evidence, the electromyographic response to nerve stimulation may be studied. The characteristic decline in amplitude of the evoked potential may be normal when the disease is restricted to the eyes. As noted above, SFEMG is finding increasing use in diagnosis. Rarely, it is desirable to administer d-tubocurarine, but this involves hazards and should probably be left to research centers; d-tubocurarine should never be given without appropriate precautions to support respiration.

Detection of antibodies to AChR has become an important diagnostic criterion, but also has limitations. With the most sensitive assay (using human antigen), about 85 per cent of patients are "positive" and there are virtually no false positives. With other commonly used antigens (such as denervated rat muscle), even more test results are negative in patients with unequivocal myasthenia. There are no special characteristics of the patients with negative antibody test results, except perhaps that patients with ocular and congenital forms are more likely to lack antibodies. A negative test result does not exclude the diagnosis.

In evaluating patients with known or suspected myasthenia, it is useful to perform a standard series of laboratory studies. In addition to repetitive nerve stimulation and tests for AChR antibodies, the possible presence of thymoma is assessed. These tumors are almost always evident in standard radiograms of the chest supplemented by oblique views. Lateral laminagrams are even more revealing, but still not quite 100 per cent accurate. Computed tomography (CT) invariably shows the tumor, but it is also prone to false-positive interpretations of soft tissue images that are not thymomas. Invasive studies such as thymic venography, mediastinal pneumography, or isotope scans have no additional value. Thyroid function should be tested, and it is useful to evaluate immunologic disorders by serum protein electrophoresis, LE cell preparation, latex fixation test for rheumatoid factor, and antinuclear antibodies. Tests for muscle antibodies or lymphocyte sensitivity are performed in special centers.

The differential diagnosis requires special consideration. Probably the most frequent error in diagnosis concerns patients with emotional fatigue states and hysterical weakness. There are no cranial muscle symptoms in these patients (except globus hystericus), whereas cranial muscles are involved in virtually all myasthenics. Their symptoms are not those of weakness but of exhaustion, and in tests of strength against resistance there is apt to be marked variation in effort, or dramatic giving way.

Acute oculomotor paralysis occurs in four diseases: myasthenia gravis, botulism, acute cranial polyneuropathy, and acute Wernicke's encephalopathy. Each has its special hazards and treatments and deserves thoughtful consideration in such cases. Amyotrophic lateral sclerosis and peripheral neuropathy may be confused with myasthenia when these disorders affect cranial muscles, but signs indicative of a neurogenic disorder distinguish them from myasthenia. Polymyositis may be confusing, but ocular muscle paresis is not found. There is some debate about the specificity of the therapeutic effect of cholinergic drugs, but for practical purposes it may be taken that an authentic (not placebo), convincing (not equivocal), and reproducible (not seen by one examiner only) effect is found only in myasthenia gravis.

TREATMENT. Therapeutic efforts fall into two categories: those which affect symptoms without influencing the course of the disease (cholinergic drugs), and those designed to induce remission of the disease itself (thymectomy, steroids, immunosuppressive drugs). Plasmapheresis can be considered an intermediate form of therapy, with effects lasting longer than those of cholinergic drugs but not as prolonged as, for instance, the optimal effect of thymectomy. Management starts as soon as the diagnosis is made, using cholinergic drugs. Then decisions are made regarding other forms of treatment.

In treating myasthenia, the clinician is faced with a variety of choices that include anticholinesterase drugs, corticosteroids, immunosuppressive drugs, thymectomy, and plasma exchange. Authorities disagree about the preferred sequence of choices, but the following guidelines may be useful:

1. Treatment should start with anticholinesterase therapy because improvement is prompt and use of these drugs entails little risk. However, cholinergic drugs alone rarely restore normal function, and, except in very mild cases or those restricted to ocular muscles, some other form of therapy is also indicated.

2. For all patients, the severity of symptoms and risks of therapy must be weighed in considering thymectomy or the use of steroids or immunosuppressive drugs. For this reason, thymectomy is rarely performed in patients with solely ocular myasthenia. For the same reason, some authorities hesitate to use steroids or immunosuppressive drugs in ocular myasthenia, in which risks might outweigh advantages. However, for some individuals (police officers, actors, or those who work on roofs or other heights), the disabling effects of ocular myasthenia might warrant the risks of steroid therapy.

3. Because of the advances in surgical technique, anesthesia, and respiratory support, the risks of thymectomy in major centers have been reduced to almost nil. Additionally, complete remission or significant improvement is seen in about 85 per cent of patients after thymectomy. Therefore, the operation is done increasingly for all patients with generalized myasthenia.

It seems logical to refer these patients to centers where sufficient numbers are seen to deal with specific questions of myasthenic management.

4. Although some investigators have recommended treatment with steroids before thymectomy (so that the resulting improvement would make postoperative care easier), this policy has been contested and may be supplanted by use of plasma exchange to prepare patients for thymectomy.

5. If these guidelines prove to be appropriate, steroid therapy would be reserved for patients with severe disability after thymectomy, or who are otherwise not candidates for thymectomy. Although it has not been demonstrated that the risks of immunosuppressive drugs (azathioprine, cyclophosphamide) are actually greater than the risks of steroids, most authorities in this country reserve these drugs for patients who fail to improve after both thymectomy and steroid therapy.

Cholinergic Drug Therapy. The major drugs used to treat myasthenia gravis are inhibitors of cholinesterase, neostigmine and pyridostigmine. It is best to use only one drug; there is no benefit from combinations of two or more. Neostigmine is provided in 15 mg tablets, and pyridostigmine in 60 mg tablets; these are essentially interchangeable. The choice is arbitrary because there is no evidence that the maximal benefit achieved by one is more than that of the other. Most patients prefer pyridostigmine because it is less apt to cause abdominal cramps and diarrhea or noticeable peaks and valleys of strength. Pyridostigmine is also provided in a slow-release capsule (Timespan) of 180 mg, said to provide 60 mg immediately and the remainder in 8 to 12 hours. Some clinicians use the prolonged-action preparation throughout the day, but because of uncertainties of release, it seems advisable to use this only at bedtime for patients who would otherwise have to awaken at night or who are very weak on waking in the morning. (For patients who cannot swallow pills, both drugs may be administered parenterally, and pyridostigmine may be given as a syrup. The intramuscular dose is about one tenth of the oral dose, and the intravenous dose is one thirtieth of the oral dose.) Decisions about optimal dosage are sometimes difficult. Some authorities advocate the use of edrophonium to evaluate oral drug therapy; a test dose of 2 mg is given intravenously. If the patient's condition improves, oral therapy has been too little. If there is aggravation of weakness, oral therapy has been too much. Other authorities find this an unreliable guide, and we do not use this technique. If edrophonium is not used, there is nothing but clinical observation to guide the therapist. For mild cases, two tablets of either neostigmine or pyridostigmine three times daily, with meals, is useful. If there is inadequate response, the dose may be increased, first by shortening the interval between doses, then by increasing the quantity of drug with each dose. Problems arise because these drugs never completely reverse symptoms. Therefore the dose should be increased only so long as there is clear-cut response, and it should not be increased beyond the amount giving some perceptible benefit. Doses exceeding 120 mg every two hours are almost never necessary.

Overtreatment itself can cause weakness; cholinesterase inhibitors may cause a depolarizing block at the neuromuscular junction. This probably does not occur with oral treatment in the amounts recommended.

Drugs advocated as "adjuvants" include potassium chloride, ephedrine, and guanidine, but their true value is unproved and guanidine may cause aplastic anemia.

Steroids and Immunosuppressive Drugs. Prednisone now enjoys widespread popularity in the treatment of myasthenia, but it has never been put to an adequately controlled prospective therapeutic trial. Some investigators report improvement in as many as 80 per cent of patients treated, with virtually no side effects. Others are less enthusiastic about beneficial effects and are more concerned about deleterious effects. Some treat virtually all patients; others restrict therapy to those with incapacitating disease. It is agreed that the minimal early dose should be about 50 mg daily for an adult, often given as 100 mg on alternate days. For patients who are seriously ill, larger doses may be used. Initiation of steroid therapy may cause an exacerbation of myasthenia. Therefore, in less emergent situations, it seems advisable to start with a prednisone dosage of 25 mg on alternate days and gradually increase to the full dose in a week or two. Some use prednisone preparation for thymectomy; others reserve steroids until some interval after thymectomy. If there is no beneficial response, it is not clear how long prednisone should be continued before deeming the trial a failure; a minimum of three months at full dosage seems reasonable. No matter how used, steroid drugs should be initiated with close supervision and probably in hospital because of the danger of temporarily increasing the weakness.

The mechanism of action of steroids in myasthenia is not known, but current theories favor an immunosuppressive role. More specific immunosuppressive drugs such as azathioprine, methotrexate, or cyclophosphamide have also been used. There is no indication that these drugs are any better than prednisone, and evaluation of them is probably best performed in research centers.

Surgical Treatment. Thymectomy is followed by significant improvement in about 85 per cent of patients with myasthenia and no tumor. Patients with thymoma fare worse whether the tumor is excised or not.

All patients with generalized myasthenia may be considered for thymectomy, but most clinicians are reluctant to recommend the operation for patients with solely ocular symptoms, for preadolescent children, or for the elderly. However, in each of these categories individual circumstances might warrant thymectomy. Because the effects of thymectomy are not seen for months or years, it should not be regarded as an emergency procedure.

In preparing patients for operation, the usual oral dosage cholinergic medication is maintained until the day of surgery, and then stopped abruptly. Endotracheal intubation is used throughout the thymectomy and maintained for assisted respiration in the immediate postoperative period. Induction of anesthesia requires no special precautions, but many anesthesiologists prefer to dispense with muscle relaxants. Parenteral steroids in appropriate dosage should be given to patients who have been taking prednisone in the preoperative period.

After the operation, depending upon circumstances, the endotracheal tube may be removed in a few hours or the next day. If there are any complications and the endotracheal tube must remain in place, it ultimately becomes necessary to consider tracheostomy, but this is necessary in few cases. Specific cholinergic drug therapy is withheld if there is postoperative fever or any other obvious complication; when these complications have been controlled, pyridostigmine therapy may be restarted at a level of one half the preoperative dose.

Plasmapheresis. Plasmapheresis is safe, and beneficial effects are seen in almost all patients. However, plasma exchange is expensive because of the instruments, supplies, and personnel involved. It requires several hours and a trip to the hospital. The benefits may be slight or great and may last days or months without relation to antibody titer. It is not clear that concomitant use of prednisone or azathioprine enhances or prolongs improvement. Conversely, it has not been shown that the long-range effects of steroids or immunosuppressive therapy are enhanced or accelerated by plasma exchange. To determine whether plasma exchange can shorten the duration of myasthenic crisis or neonatal myasthenia would require a controlled clinical trial. For all of these reasons, the ultimate role of plasma exchange in treating myasthenia remains to be clarified; it is being evaluated in many centers, and guidelines may soon be forthcoming. In the meantime it is being used only for patients with severe symptoms that have resisted other therapeutic approaches or in preparation for thymectomy.

Crisis. Patients with myasthenia gravis may suddenly develop difficulty breathing that is severe enough to require artificial ventilation. This may be induced by systemic infection or major surgical procedures, but often there is no apparent cause. Patients with oropharyngeal weakness are especially liable to this threat, perhaps because of aspiration. Whenever there is doubt about the adequacy of ventilation or the state of the airway, endotracheal intubation should be used for short periods of respiratory support. The insertion of a cuffed tube makes intermittent positive pressure breathing feasible and also reduces the hazard of aspiration. Patients are best transferred to a respiratory intensive care unit. Cholinergic drugs are stopped. After several days, usually after fever (a common concomitant of crisis) has started to subside, drugs may be started once again, at half the precrisis dosage. The cause of crisis is not clear, but it is usually transient and will subside if the patient can be kept alive. The mortality rate of crisis was formerly about 50 per cent, but since the advent of intensive care units, few patients die, and these are mostly elderly persons with complicating cardiac and renal disease.

A few patients require assisted ventilation for prolonged periods. For these patients, a trial of either plasmapheresis or steroid therapy seems warranted.

PROGNOSIS. The course of myasthenia is variable. The disease may be restricted to ocular muscles for many years, with no threat to life. Other patients are disabled to a variable degree by oropharyngeal or limb weakness, and a few are crippled. Crisis occurs in about 10 per cent of the cases. The overall mortality from myasthenia itself is probably less than 5 per cent, and although myasthenia was formerly the main hazard, intercurrent and unrelated disease is now more often the cause of death.

Drachman DB: The biology of myasthenia gravis. Ann Rev Neurosci 4:195, 1981. *Thoughtful review of the pathogenesis of myasthenic manifestations.*

Engel AG: Myasthenia gravis. Handb Clin Neurol 41:95, 1979. *Comprehensive discussion of clinical aspects and pathophysiology of myasthenia.*

Grob D (ed.): Myasthenia gravis. Pathophysiology and management. Ann NY Acad Sci 277:1, 1981. *Covers every conceivable aspect of the pathogenesis and treatment of myasthenia.*

Keesey J, Bein M, Mink J, Sample F, Sarti D, Mulder D, Herrmann C Jr, Peter JB: Detection of thymoma in myasthenia gravis. Neurology 30:233, 1980. *Discussion of the value and limitation of computed tomography in detecting thymoma.*

Lindstrom J, Dau P: Biology of myasthenia gravis. Ann Rev Pharmacol Toxicol 20:337, 1980. *Detailed review of the immunology of myasthenia.*

Lindstrom JM, Lambert EH: Content of acetylcholine receptor and antibodies bound to receptor in myasthenia gravis, experimental autoimmune myasthenia gravis and Eaton-Lambert syndrome. Neurology 26:130, 1978. *A detailed review of the pathophysiology of these disorders.*

Lisak RP, Barchi RL: Myasthenia Gravis. Philadelphia, W. B. Saunders, 1982. *An immunologist and a neuroscientist combine efforts to give a lucid and comprehensive review of theory and practice.*

Pascuzzi RM, Coslett HB, Johns TR: Long-term corticosteroid treatment of myasthenia gravis: Report of 116 patients. Ann Neurol 15:291, 1984. *A review of extensive clinical experience.*

Rodriguez M, Gomez MR, Howard FM, Taylor WF: Myasthenia gravis in children: Long-term follow-up. Ann Neurol 13:504, 1983. *Therapeutic decisions may be especially difficult in children with myasthenia; guidelines are presented in this analysis.*

Rowland LP: Controversies about the treatment of myasthenia gravis. J Neurol Neurosurg Psychiat 43:644, 1980. *Intended to be an impartial but critical review of the controversies that influence clinicians in the choice of therapy.*

EATON-LAMBERT SYNDROME (Myasthenic Syndrome)

DEFINITION. The Eaton-Lambert syndrome is a "facilitating" disorder of neuromuscular transmission in which the amplitude of the first muscle action potential evoked by stimulation of the nerve is reduced, and with repetitive stimulation the amplitude of the action potential increases to more than three times the original height.

PATHOGENESIS. The first cases were associated with oat-cell carcinoma of the lung, but cases have been found with other tumors, with other diseases, and sometimes with no complicating disorder. Microelectrode studies indicate that the defect is due to impaired release of acetylcholine at the nerve terminals. Antibodies to components of nerve terminals may be responsible.

CLINICAL MANIFESTATIONS. The first evidence may be prolonged apnea after curarization for surgery. Formal testing with d-tubocurarine also indicates that patients are unduly sensitive. Other patients may have symptoms of limb weakness, but cranial muscle weakness is never prominent. The response to cholinergic drugs is usually equivocal at best. Pain in the limbs and dry mouth may be prominent. Movements may be peculiarly slow, and tendon reflexes may be lost. In tests of strength the patient may seem to get stronger with continued effort. Myotatic reflexes are frequently depressed.

DIAGNOSIS. The signs listed above diverge sufficiently from myasthenia to avoid confusion; only limb weakness and curare sensitivity are similar. The remainder of the syndrome resembles polymyositis, and polyneuritis would also have to be considered. The diagnosis is made by the response to repetitive stimulation. Antibodies to AChR have not been found in typical cases. When the diagnosis of Eaton-Lambert syndrome has been established, special efforts should be made to find the underlying tumor.

TREATMENT. Guanidine promotes the release of acetylcholine, and the drug is effective in daily doses of 35 mg per kilogram of body weight, given orally. This drug may suppress bone marrow, however, and great caution must be taken so that guanidine should probably not be used unless the neuromuscular disorder is disabling. 4-Aminopyridine is also effective in promoting release of acetylcholine, but it is also hazardous and may cause seizures. Steroid therapy may be beneficial. Plasmapheresis may be beneficial. Any tumor should be treated appropriately.

Eaton LM, Lambert EH: Electromyography and electric stimulation of nerves in diseases of motor unit: Observations in myasthenic syndrome associated with malignant tumors. JAMA 163:1117, 1957. *The classic description of the Eaton-Lambert syndrome.*

Elmqvist D, Lambert EH: Detailed analysis of neuromuscular transmission in a patient with myasthenic syndrome sometimes associated with bronchogenic carcinoma. Mayo Clin Proc 43:689, 1968. *The original electrophysiologic analysis of the Eaton-Lambert syndrome.*

Lange DJ: The Eaton-Lambert syndrome: Current concepts of pathogenesis and treatment. Neurol Neurosurg Update 4:1, 1983. *A comprehensive review of pathogenesis, diagnosis, and treatment.*

Newsom-Davis JN, Murray NMF: Plasma exchange and immunosuppressive drug treatment in the Lambert-Eaton myasthenic syndrome. Neurology 34:480, 1984. *Treatments based on the theory that the syndrome is caused by autoantibodies.*

UNUSUAL CAUSES OF NEUROMUSCULAR BLOCK

Botulism and *tick paralysis* are described in Ch. 279 and 424. Both cause a syndrome of flaccid quadriplegia with paresis of cranial muscles and must be differentiated from polyneuritis, myasthenia gravis, and periodic paralysis. In neither is there a sensory disorder, but autonomic fibers may be affected in botulism, especially pupilloconstrictor fibers (resulting in a dilated, fixed pupil). The electromyogram in botulism may resemble that in the Eaton-Lambert syndrome, an observation that may be diagnostically important.

Several *aminoglycoside antimicrobial drugs* interfere with the release of acetylcholine, and may cause clinical syndromes. The offending drugs include neomycin, streptomycin, colistin, polymyxin, and kanamycin. The most common manifestation is postoperative apnea without other evidence of paralysis. This is most apt to occur in patients with renal failure, presumably with unusually high blood levels of the antimicrobial drug. In occasional cases, however, there may be flaccid quadriplegia. Administration of calcium and guanidine may be helpful, but the essence of management is supportive treatment and use of a safer antimicrobial.

Cornblath DR, Sladky JT, Sumner AJ: Clinical electrophysiology of infantile botulism. Muscle Nerve 6:448, 1983. *Analysis of 25 cases in one hospital.*

Swift TR: Disorders of neuromuscular transmission other than myasthenia gravis. Muscle Nerve 4:334, 1981. *A comprehensive review of theoretical and practical aspects of these syndromes.*

SYNDROMES OF MUSCULAR OVERACTIVITY: CRAMPS AND RELATED DISORDERS

Cramps, caused by painful, abrupt shortening of muscle, affect almost everyone at some time or other. Electromyographic investigation indicates that motor units fire at a rate of about 300 per second, much higher than the most vigorous voluntary contraction. It is presumably the high rate of discharge that causes the palpable muscle tautness and the pain. The pain can be relieved by stretching the affected muscle, or by massage. The stimulus responsible for cramps is not known; relief by stretching suggests that some central mechanism is involved, since this is the stimulus for receptors in muscle that inhibit discharge of the motor neuron to the same muscle. Certain conditions are associated with a propensity to cramps: denervation (especially amyotrophic lateral sclerosis), pregnancy, and electrolyte disorders (especially water intoxication and hyponatremia). Cramps attributed to hypo-osmolarity are seen in some patients treated with maintenance hemodialysis and respond to treatment with hypertonic solutions of glucose or sodium.

Cramps occur most commonly in otherwise normal individuals, and some people are more susceptible than others for unknown reasons, with or without a family history of cramps. Others occur only at night, and can be prevented by quinine sulfate, 0.3 gram orally at bedtime. Others occur frequently during the day, occasionally so often that the individual is effectively crippled. Phenytoin, 0.3 to 0.6 gram daily, may be helpful to these patients, but some are resistant to this and to other drugs that may be tried, including diazepam and diphenhydramine. Patients with *"benign fasciculation"* (lacking weakness, wasting, or other signs of motor neuron disease) seem especially prone to have frequent cramps.

Tetany is a special form of cramp, identified by its predilection for flexor muscles of the hand and fingers, its association with laryngospasm, and its relationship to hypocalcemia. Tetany can be painful. It differs from other cramps electromyographically because of the characteristic rhythmic grouping of discharging potentials. Hyperventilation tetany is likely to be overlooked as a cause of cramps or laryngospasm.

Contracture is the term reserved for the painful shortening of muscles in glycogen storage diseases, in which the muscles are electrically silent although maximally shortened.

Myokymia has been used to describe a variety of apparently different disorders characterized by cramps in association with spontaneous twitching of muscle. In some cases there are prolonged trains of spontaneous potentials, whereas in others there is grouping of potentials. Some of these patients have difficulty in relaxing grip, but, unlike myotonia, the muscular activity is abolished by neuromuscular blocking agents, indicating a neural rather than a muscular origin. Hyperhidrosis is prominent in some patients and is secondary to the increased muscular activity.

Continuous shortening of the muscle would lead to abnormal postures and abnormally increased resistance to passive movement. These abnormalities, of course, are often due to central neurologic disorders. In recent years, however, an increasing number of patients have been described because of fluctuating rigidity of axial and limb muscles. For want of a better name, and lacking understanding of the pathogenesis, this has been called the *stiff man syndrome.* The diagnosis requires that there be no signs of cerebral or spinal cord disease, and there must be continuous electromyographic activity despite authentic attempts to relax. Ordinary cramps may be superimposed upon the persistent stiffness. Diazepam, 30 to 60 mg daily, may bring dramatic relief.

A variety of other names have been applied to these syndromes, including *Isaac's syndrome, quantal squander, armadillo disease, neuromyotonia,* and *continuous muscle fiber activity.* Some cases of brief duration may be related to mild cases of tetanus. It will take some time to sort out the variety of causes. If these unusual forms can be analyzed, we may yet understand why an otherwise normal individual occasionally has a cramp.

Auger RG, Daube JR, Gomez MR, Lambert EH: Hereditary form of sustained muscle activity of peripheral nerve origin causing generalized myokymia and muscle stiffness. Ann Neurol 15:13, 1984. *A description of an unusual form of the syndrome with an excellent discussion of differential diagnosis.*

Gordon EE, Januszko DM, Kaufman L: A critical survey of stiff man syndrome. Am J Med 42:582, 1967. *Whatever this disease is, this paper describes it.*

Hudson AJ, Brown WF, Gilbert JJ: The muscular pain–fasciculation syndrome. Neurology 28:1105, 1978. *Review of an old problem; also called "benign fasciculation."*

Layzer RB: Motor unit hyperactivity states. Handb Clin Neurol 40:259, 1979. *Comprehensive and lucid description of cramps and related disorders.*

Milutinovich J, Graefe V, Follette WC, Scribner BH: Effect of hypertonic glucose on the muscular cramps of hemodialysis. Ann Intern Med 90:926, 1979. *Cramps are common in patients treated with hemodialysis; this describes one approach to management.*

Sheehy MP, Marsden CD: Writers cramp—a focal dystonia. Brain 105:461, 1982. *A comprehensive discussion and description of the problem.*

Van den Bergh P, Bulcke JA, Dom R: Familial muscle cramps with autosomal dominant transmission. Eur Neurol 19:207, 1980. *Familial susceptibility to cramps is being recognized more frequently.*

Part XXIV
EYE DISEASES

John W. Gittinger, Jr.

540. INTRODUCTION

Because many systemic diseases manifest in the eyes, ophthalmoscopy is a necessary skill for the physician. The pupil of the eye is a window opening onto the arterioles and venules of the retina, the optic disc, and the pigmented tissues of the fundus. In addition, the pupil, innervated by both sympathetic and parasympathetic nerves, provides an index of autonomic function.

The second, third, fourth, fifth, sixth, and seventh cranial nerves subserve vision. Ocular motility is the most precisely documented of complex motor acts. Similarly, the intracranial visual pathways—optic nerve, chiasm, and tract, geniculate body, superior colliculus, optic radiations, striate cortex, and visual association areas—are the paradigm of sensory processing in the nervous system.

The discussion that follows highlights the interrelationship between ocular and systemic disease, beginning with a brief review of the two common ophthalmic disorders—cataract and glaucoma—and then turning to ocular entities and ocular manifestations of medical disorders likely to present to nonophthalmic physicians.

Leigh RJ, Zee DS: The Neurology of Eye Movements. Philadelphia, F. A. Davis Company, 1983. *The current understanding of neural control of eye movements.*

Moses RA: Adler's Physiology of the Eye; Clinical application. 7th ed. St. Louis, C. V. Mosby Company, 1981. *A clinically oriented review of basic physiologic mechanisms.*

541. CATARACT

A cataract is an opacity of the lens that manifests as painless, gradual loss of vision. Cataracts are described according to their location—nuclear (deep in the lens), cortical (more superficial), and subcapsular (immediately beneath the capsule). Cataracts are classified as immature, mature, or hypermature. An immature cataract has some clear cortex; a mature cataract is totally opaque: the pupil appears white—leukocoria. A hypermature cataract has liquefied cortex that leaks through the capsule and may excite destructive inflammation. Immature cataracts are usually removed for visual reasons. A mature or hypermature cataract in an eye with potential for useful vision should be removed to prevent irreversible damage.

Etiology

Congenital cataracts are a feature of rubella embryopathy and often are associated with other congenital malformations. Acquired cataracts may result from trauma, radiation, or metabolic disorder. In some cases of Wilson's disease, orange copper deposits appear on the anterior capsule—the sunflower cataract. Chlorpromazine administration may result in a brown or white dusting on the anterior lens surface. Red, green, and blue opacities in the lenticular cortex characterize myotonic dystrophy but are occasionally encountered in its absence. All of these colorful cataracts have diagnostic, but little visual, significance.

Hypocalcemia may be cataractogenic. Cataracts occur in disorders of carbohydrate metabolism: hypoglycemia, galactosemia, and diabetes mellitus. Diabetics do not necessarily have an increased incidence of cataracts, but theirs progress rapidly, perhaps because of variations in lens hydration as the result of changing sugar concentrations in the aqueous humor.

Systemic corticosteroids promote formation of posterior subcapsular cataracts. Because of the path light takes through the lens, posterior subcapsular cataracts reduce vision more than similar, eccentric opacities. Central posterior opacities get in the way of light most often when the pupil is small, as in bright light or with near work. Difficulties with driving and reading are the first complaints of patients with posterior subcapsular cataracts.

Most cataracts have no known etiology. The common nuclear sclerotic cataract, or senile cataract, is often familial, but no specific factors have been proven to accelerate or retard its development.

Treatment

The treatment for cataract is surgical removal. With the exception of mature and hypermature cataracts and of immature cataracts that have swollen sufficiently to threaten to precipitate angle-closure glaucoma (see below), most cataracts are removed for visual reasons. Considerations in planning cataract extraction are the patient's visual needs, the potential for visual improvement, and the risks of surgery. A person who drives will require surgery when the better eye is worse than 20/40, the legal minimum for a driver's license in most states. By contrast, an elderly patient with 20/200 vision and limited visual needs may be perfectly happy without intervention. Care must be taken to identify intercurrent ocular disease; removal of the lens of an eye with advanced glaucoma or macular degeneration does not necessarily improve vision.

The risk of cataract surgery itself is relatively small. Despite the possibility of intraocular hemorrhage, postoperative infection, corneal decompensation, or problems with wound healing, the chances for a good visual outcome are excellent. Even successful cataract surgery increases the likelihood of subsequent retinal detachment, and a small percentage of eyes develop prolonged cystoid macular edema with reduced acuity.

General anesthesia constitutes a major portion of the risk when it is used. Cataract surgery can usually be performed under local anesthesia, and this should be considered the method of choice in medically fragile patients.

Spaeth GL: Ophthalmic Surgery; Principles and Practice. Philadelphia, W. B. Saunders Company, 1982. *A clear and concise presentation of the current state of ophthalmic surgery. Indications, techniques, and complications are discussed.*

542. GLAUCOMA

Glaucoma is a group of disorders in which elevated intraocular pressure damages the optic nerve. The major types of glaucoma are open-angle, angle-closure, congenital, and secondary.

The dynamics of aqueous humor control intraocular pressure. The aqueous humor is derived from blood by a process of secretion and ultrafiltration in the ciliary body. Aqueous humor then passes from the posterior chamber through the pupil to fill the anterior chamber, the space between the back of the cornea and the plane of the iris and pupil. The aqueous humor is reabsorbed through the trabecular meshwork, located in the angle between the cornea and the iris, to enter Schlemm's canal, which connects with the venous system.

Open-angle Glaucoma

In chronic open-angle glaucoma, the most common glaucoma, a block in aqueous humor reabsorption exists at the level of the trabecular meshwork. Intraocular pressure rises above its normal maximum of 21 mm Hg and gradually destroys axons and supporting tissue on the optic disc.

The prevalence of open-angle glaucoma varies with the population studied and the diagnostic criteria employed. A conservative estimate of unequivocal glaucoma in American and European adults is 0.5 per cent. A much larger percentage of these adults sustains increased intraocular pressure without signs of optic nerve damage—*ocular hypertension.* The patient with ocular hypertension is considered a glaucoma suspect.

Open-angle glaucoma is ordinarily asymptomatic until well advanced. Only rarely does the elevated intraocular pressure cause corneal edema, with the attendant perception of halos around lights. Pain is not characteristic of open-angle glaucoma. Initial visual loss in chronic open-angle glaucoma is confined to the peripheral field, especially in the nasal area and the area surrounding fixation. Visual acuity remains normal until late in the course of the disease.

Diagnosis is made by measurement of intraocular pressure, examination of the optic disc, and testing of the visual fields. Gonioscopy, the visualization of the angle structures under high magnifications with special contact lenses, allows distinction of an angle-closure from an open-angle mechanism.

The treatment of open-angle glaucoma is primarily medical. Topical administration of parasympathomimetics (pilocarpine and carbachol), beta-adrenergic blockers (timolol), and sympathomimetics (epinephrine) decreases intraocular pressure. When these medications—individually and in combination—are ineffective in arresting progressive disc damage and visual field loss, indirect parasympathomimetics (echothiophate) and carbonic anhydrase inhibitors (acetazolamide and methazolamide) are prescribed.

If maximum tolerated medical therapy fails to halt progression, surgery is indicated. *Laser trabeculoplasty* opens aqueous outflow channels by burning the surface of the trabecular meshwork. If all else fails, a surgical fistula can be created between the anterior chamber and the subconjunctival space, allowing direct absorption of aqueous humor by subconjunctival and episcleral vessels. This operation is called a filtering procedure.

The management of open-angle glaucoma and that of systemic hypertension have many similarities. In both, the prevention of complications depends upon early recognition, careful follow up, and patient compliance with therapeutic regimens. Routine measurement of intraocular pressures (*tonometry*) at general physical examinations is often advocated, but careful ophthalmoscopy with referral of patients whose central excavation ("cup") exceeds one-third of the disc's area may be an equally effective screen.

Angle-closure Glaucoma

When aqueous outflow is mechanically impeded owing to a shallow anterior chamber, the resulting increase in intraocular pressure is angle-closure glaucoma. Intraocular pressure is normal until resistance to aqueous flow through the pupil—pupillary block—bows the iris forward to obstruct the resorptive surfaces in the angle. The pressure then rises precipitously, often to above 50 mm Hg.

Acute angle-closure glaucoma is generally monocular. The eye is red and painful, and the pupil about 6 mm and fixed. Vision is decreased. The patient is diaphoretic and nauseated and often vomits.

Typical angle-closure glaucoma is easy to recognize. Occasionally, chronic or subacute angle-closure mimics open-angle glaucoma. Gonioscopy is then necessary to distinguish between the two mechanisms. The elderly often do not develop the full set of clinical signs and symptoms. One should always consider angle-closure glaucoma when the patient presents with a fixed, mid-dilated pupil and decreased vision.

Angle-closure can be precipitated in predisposed eyes by dilating the pupils. The risk of pharmacologic dilation is assessed by noting the depth of the anterior chamber. Eyes with shallow anterior chambers are at risk for angle-closure. This distinction is not always easy to observe, and in some cases an experienced ophthalmologist may not be able to determine whether an angle will close with dilation. The risk of dilation increases with age, and everyone over the age of 50 whose anterior chamber is less than full depth should be considered to have the potential for angle-closure. This does not mean, however, that most patients should not be dilated, but rather that dilation should be performed with a relatively short-acting mydriatic agent such as tropicamide or hydroxyamphetamine. The patient should then be observed until the effects of the mydriatic are known.

A nonophthalmologist should probably not routinely dilate adult outpatients. Children and inpatients should be dilated if there is no other contraindication such as recent head trauma, an iris-fixated intraocular lens, or impending general anesthesia. With these exceptions, the diagnostic benefits of dilation outweigh the risk of precipitating angle-closure. Should angle-closure glaucoma develop, it can be recognized and promptly treated.

An acute angle-closure attack is a medical emergency. Initial management consists of administration of parenteral acetazolamide, oral glycerol or intravenous mannitol, and topical pilocarpine, and perhaps timolol. Once the attack has been broken, the anatomic predisposition can be effectively eliminated by creating a communication between the posterior and anterior chamber through the peripheral iris, either with a laser—*laser iridotomy*—or with surgical iridectomy. The anterior segment abnormality that underlies angle-closure glaucoma is bilateral, and prophylactic surgery on the other eye is usually indicated.

Congenital Glaucoma

Congenital glaucoma is an open-angle glaucoma that is the result of dysgenesis of the angle structures. Increased intraocular pressure enlarges the immature eye (*buphthalmos*), and a corneal diameter greater than 12 mm suggests congenital glaucoma. Progressive corneal enlargement ruptures the deeper layers of the cornea, with resulting corneal edema and loss of transparency. The cornea of a child with advanced congenital glaucoma is enlarged, with a ground-glass translucency.

Treatment of congenital glaucoma is both surgical and medical. Congenital glaucoma is fortunately rare; the prognosis for preservation of vision is only fair.

Secondary Glaucoma

Secondary glaucoma develops as the consequence of another ocular disease. Examples of secondary glaucomas are angle-closure glaucoma precipitated by intumescence of the lens, glaucoma developing as a result of formation of new vessels in the angle, and glaucoma in a chronically inflamed eye. Severe blunt trauma to the eye damages angle structures, predisposing to the subsequent development of open-angle glaucoma.

The treatment of secondary, lens-induced angle-closure glaucoma is surgical removal of the lens. Most other secondary glaucomas are managed in much the same way as primary open-angle glaucoma. Neovascular glaucoma is difficult to treat, and most eyes ultimately lose all useful vision. If the stimulus to neovascularization is ischemia, ablation of ischemic tissues by photocoagulation may halt progression. If neovascularization continues, medical control will become ineffective. Filtering procedures generally fail because exuberant tissue growth closes the surgical fistula, a problem that may be circumvented by the implantation of a plastic valve connecting the anterior chamber and the subconjunctival space. Destruction of the ciliary body by an externally applied liquid nitrogen probe—*cyclocryotherapy*—controls intraocular pressure, but seldom preserves useful vision.

Any glaucoma where all light perception has been lost is called *absolute glaucoma.* Enucleation is the definitive treatment for a blind, painful eye.

Chandler PA, Grant WM: Glaucoma. Philadelphia, Lea & Febiger, 1979. *A well-written exposition of one approach to glaucoma. Glaucoma syndromes are especially well covered.*

Kolker AE, Hetherington J Jr: Becker-Shaffer's Diagnosis and Therapy of the Glaucomas. St. Louis, The C. V. Mosby Company, 1983. *The best one-volume compendium on this subject. The illustrations are numerous and clear.*

543. DISC SWELLING AND OPTIC ATROPHY

The optic disc marks the transition from retina to optic nerve. The central retinal artery and vein pass through the disc and bifurcate on its surface. There is considerable variation in the disc's ophthalmoscopic appearance. Vessels enter the interior of the eye through the nasal half of the disc. A central excavation or cup occupies a variable portion of its substance; vessels are often seen curving over the edge of this cup.

Over one million axons originate in the ganglion cells of the retina and pass through each optic disc. Although these axons are nearly transparent, in the light of a bright ophthalmoscope they form fine reflective striations on the disc's surface and the immediately surrounding retina. Disc swelling is a consequence of ischemia, infarction, infiltration, or local changes in tissue pressures.

Papilledema

Disc swelling from increased intracranial pressure is termed papilledema; nevertheless, it does not represent purely extracellular edema. Instead, the increased intracranial pressure results in an accumulation of axoplasm, the cytoplasm of the axons, in and around the disc. Normally the axoplasm circulates along the axon—axoplasmic flow. Increased intracranial pressure causes axoplasmic stasis at the level of the lamina cribosa, the perforated plate of sclera through which the axons leave the eye. This stasis appears ophthalmoscopically as a protrusion of the disc, with swelling most obvious just adjacent to the disc's normal borders. When the increase in intracranial pressure is rapid, the veins are engorged, and hemorrhages appear on the disc or adjacent retina.

Papilledema is usually bilateral, but may be asymmetrical. Visual acuity remains normal in acute papilledema. Only in long-standing papilledema does secondary optic atrophy, with decreased vision, ensue (see below).

Pseudopapilledema

Because the common causes of papilledema include intracranial tumor and hemorrhage, its recognition and differential diagnosis are important. Various other disc appearances may be confused with papilledema. Hyperopic (farsighted) eyes are small, with axonal crowding at the disc. Drusen of the optic nerve, which are depositions of hyaline material in the prelaminar optic nerve, appear as swollen discs in young persons. Such anomalous discs are often discovered incidentally. One clue to their nature is the frequent absence of the physiologic cup, for in true papilledema the cup is preserved until the disc swelling is far advanced.

Papillitis

Papillitis is an anterior form of optic neuritis. In the majority of acute optic neuritides the disc appears normal—*retrobulbar optic neuritis*. In papillitis, the disc is swollen and may be hemorrhagic, an appearance ophthalmoscopically indistinguishable from papilledema. Unlike papilledema, however, acuity is characteristically reduced, and papillitis is often truly unilateral.

Ischemic Optic Neuropathy

Papillitis is largely a disease of the young. In older persons, disc swelling and loss of vision suggest infarction—ischemic optic neuropathy. Often only the superior or inferior half of the disc is involved, with consequent loss of function in the inferior or superior visual field. Most instances of ischemic optic neuropathy are idiopathic, but the disorder may be the initial manifestation of giant cell or temporal arteritis, a disease of the elderly. In such cases the erythrocyte sedimentation rate is usually elevated; symptoms of this generalized arteritis include malaise, fever, headache, scalp tenderness, and painful chewing.

Other Causes of Disc Swelling

Another cause of disc swelling is severe hypertension. The relative roles of local vascular changes and of increased intracranial pressure in the pathogenesis of the disc swelling that defines malignant hypertension are uncertain. Decreased intraocular pressure, encountered after ocular surgery or injury, also produces disc swelling. The disc is rarely swollen during an attack of angle-closure glaucoma, because the sudden increase in intraocular pressure allegedly obstructs axoplasmic flow.

Infiltration of the optic nerve heads is encountered in leukemia, metastatic carcinoma, and sarcoid. Cryptococcal invasion of the optic nerve is associated with disc swelling in some cases of cryptococcal meningitis.

Optic Atrophy

Optic atrophy results from death of the axons in the retina and optic nerve. Disc pallor and optic atrophy are not synonymous; some pallor is a feature of normal discs. The optic nerve's axons originate in the ganglion cell layer of the retina, pass through the optic disc, nerve, chiasm, and tract, and terminate in the lateral geniculate body and brain stem. A large majority of these axons synapse in the lateral geniculate body of the thalamus; axons subserving the pupillary light reflex leave the optic tract to synapse in upper brain stem centers. A lesion anywhere from the retina through the optic tract will cause optic atrophy. Lesions behind the lateral geniculate in early life may cause trans-synaptic degeneration and optic atrophy.

Optic atrophy may be classified as primary, secondary, and glaucomatous. *Primary optic atrophy* refers to progressive pallor without loss of disc substance, a sign of wallerian degeneration as the result of compression, vascular injury, or axonal death from toxic or metabolic disturbances. *Secondary optic atrophy* develops after disc swelling, as in chronic papilledema. Vascular and glial changes may give the disc an irregular, milky gray appearance with ill-defined borders. The distinction is not absolute; some cases in which the process is clearly "secondary" have a crisp, white disc. *Glaucomatous optic atrophy* denotes loss of disc substance, already referred to as increased cupping. Again, nature rejects arbitrary classifications, and enlarged cups are occasionally observed with compressive optic neuropathy.

Optic atrophy is difficult to recognize in children, in whom the discs may have a pale appearance normally. In adults with nuclear sclerotic cataracts, the pallor is masked by the lens acting as a yellow filter. The diagnosis of optic atrophy should not be made unless there is evidence of alteration in visual function: decreased acuity or field—or, in infants, nystagmus.

In the final analysis, optic atrophy is not a clinical finding but a pathologic entity. In retinitis pigmentosa there is a primary dystrophy of the rods and cones. The ganglion cells remain intact, but there are secondary vascular and gliotic changes with a waxy pallor of the disc, but not a true optic atrophy. Disc pallor is a finding to be evaluated in the context of the entire ophthalmologic and neurologic examination.

Miller NR: Walsh and Hoyt's Clinical Neuro-Ophthalmology. 4th ed. Baltimore, Williams & Wilkins Company, 1982, Vol 1, pp 175–271, 329–342. *The most recent revision of a classic monograph. The pages cited contain a comprehensive review of the entities discussed briefly here.*

544. OCULAR INFLAMMATION

Uveitis

Uveitis is any inflammation of the uveal tract—the iris, ciliary body, and choroid. There are two major clinical types of uveitis: anterior and posterior. Anterior uveitis, also known as *iritis* or *iridocyclitis*, has as its hallmark cells in the anterior chamber. Curiously, it is the rare case of iritis that displays any recognizable iris abnormality. Posterior uveitis may take the form of *chorioretinitis.* The choroid and retina are so intimately connected that it is difficult to have inflammation of one without the other.

Acute anterior uveitis presents with congestion of the eye, often in a perilimbal distribution described as ciliary flush. Frequently, the eye is painful, vision reduced, and the pupil small and poorly reactive. The diagnosis is confirmed on slit lamp examination by the presence of free cells in the aqueous humor, visible as bright points as the slit beam passes through the anterior chamber. In more severe inflammation, *keratitic precipitates,* cellular aggregates on the back of the cornea, appear. The slit beam itself is seen passing through the normally optically empty anterior chamber, its light dispersed by the protein and other solutes leaking into the aqueous from inflamed vessels, a phenomenon called *flare.*

Most cases of anterior uveitis are idiopathic. Rarely, anterior uveitis can be a manifestation of a systemic inflammatory disease such as sarcoid, or an infection such as syphilis or tuberculosis. In such cases the inflammation may be marked, with large, oily keratitic precipitates classically described as resembling mutton fat. This variant of anterior uveitis is *granulomatous iritis.*

Uveitis and Arthritis

Juvenile rheumatoid arthritis and ankylosing spondylitis are especially apt to be associated with uveitis. The uveitis of ankylosing spondylitis is an acute, usually self-limited, anterior uveitis. Young men with this disorder may have recurrent episodes that respond to standard treatments (see below). A great majority are HLA-B27 positive. By contrast, the uveitis accompanying juvenile rheumatoid arthritis is chronic and may initially be subclinical. The young women with the pauciarticular form of juvenile rheumatoid arthritis who develop uveitis often have white and quiet eyes. With time, however, adhesions, called posterior synechiae, form between the iris and lens, leading to a potential secondary pupillary block glaucoma or occlusion of the pupil. The inflammation may cause cataract formation and ectopic calcification in the corneal epithelium—band keratopathy. Physicians treating seronegative pauciarticular arthritis should schedule slit lamp and dilation examinations several times a year. Posterior synechiae are visible with a hand light after instillation of mydriatics as the pupil does not fully dilate and has an irregular, scalloped border.

Reiter's Disease

The triad of arthritis, urethritis, and conjunctivitis suggests Reiter's disease. This develops most often in men between the ages of 20 and 40 as a nonbacterial urethritis followed by polyarthritis and ocular inflammation. The initial ocular manifestation is usually a mucopurulent conjunctivitis, followed in many cases by an anterior uveitis. Keratitis and episcleritis also occur. As in ankylosing spondylitis, with which it shares similarities, HLA-B27 is often positive. Reiter's disease is usually self-limited.

Behçet's Syndrome

Uveitis (or retinitis) is also a cardinal feature of Behçet's syndrome. Behçet's original description of oral and genital ulceration combined with ocular inflammation has been expanded to include many other manifestations of Behçet's syndrome. In some cases a layer of white cells forms in the lower portion of the anterior chamber (*hypopyon*). Hypopyon iritis is characteristic of Behçet's syndrome. In other patients the primary manifestation may be a retinal vasculitis and vitritis. Rarer neuro-ophthalmic manifestations such as cranial nerve palsies or homonymous hemianopias are part of a wider central nervous system involvement.

Uveomeningitis—The Vogt-Koyanagi-Harada Syndrome

Another systemic disease with characteristic ocular inflammation is uveomeningitis (the Vogt-Koyanagi-Harada syndrome). This disease affects the uvea, retina, meninges, and skin and is especially common in Orientals. Manifestations include meningeal signs, alopecia, poliosis, vitiligo, tinnitus, and dysacousis. There may be an anterior or a posterior uveitis with exudative retinal detachment.

Reticulum Cell Sarcoma

A steroid-responsive exudative process simulating uveitis occurs in adults over the age of 40 and represents a lymphoreticular neoplasia (variously called reticulum cell sarcoma, histiocytic sarcoma, or—when the brain is involved—microglioma). Diagnosis may be made from the cytology of a vitreous aspirate, and treatment with radiation has palliative value.

Leukemia

An apparent iritis developing during a course of treatment for leukemia may represent infiltration of the anterior segment. Diagnosis and therapy are similar to reticulum cell sarcoma.

Treatment

The treatment of uveitis consists largely of topical or, when the inflammation is prolonged or severe, systemic immunosuppression. Prednisolone or dexamethasone topically, or prednisone orally, is the preferred drug. Cytotoxic immunosuppressive agents are sometimes used in chronic, intractable uveitis. Mydriatic-cycloplegics in anterior uveitis reduce discomfort and retard posterior synechiae formation.

James DG, Spiteri MA: Behçet's disease. Ophthalmology 89:1279, 1982. *A review of Behçet's disease's multiple manifestations with excellent color illustrations.*

Kanski JJ: Anterior uveitis in juvenile rheumatoid arthritis. Arch Ophthalmol 95:1794, 1977. *A description of the ocular findings in 160 children with seronegative rheumatoid arthritis and uveitis evaluated in a rheumatology unit.*

Ohno S, Char DH, Kimura SJ, O'Connor GR: Vogt-Koyanagi-Harada syndrome. Am J Ophthalmol 83:735, 1977. *An analysis of 51 patients with uveomeningitis.*

Rosenthal AR: Ocular manifestations of leukemia: A review. Ophthalmology 90:899, 1983. *This paper covers the retinal, orbital, optic nerve, and uveal manifestations of leukemia.*

Sloas HA, Starling J, Harper DG, Cupples HP: Update of ocular reticulum cell sarcoma. Arch Ophthalmol 99:1048, 1981. *A case report occasioning a thorough review.*

Smith RE, Nozik RM: Uveitis: A Clinical Approach to Diagnosis and Management. Baltimore, Williams & Wilkins Company, 1983. *The most current of the monographs on uveitis. Many entities are briefly discussed.*

545. OCULAR INFECTIONS

Ocular infections (or inflammations) are most sensibly grouped according to their locations. The most common and most superficial infection is a *blepharoconjunctivitis.* Infection of the lacrimal gland is a *dacryoadenitis;* infection of the lacrimal drainage system, a *dacryocystitis.* When the cornea is involved, the infection is called *keratitis. Uveitis, scleritis,* and *episcleritis,* which are seldom infectious, are discussed elsewhere. Infection or inflammation inside the eye is an *endophthalmitis.* An infectious *vitritis* is usually called an endophthalmitis, e.g., *Candida* endophthalmitis. Some *chorioretinitis* is infectious.

Conjunctivitis

Inflammation of the mucous membranes of the eye is conjunctivitis. Isolated lid involvement is blepharitis. Most often these contiguous structures are both inflamed—blepharoconjunctivitis—but the term conjunctivitis is conventionally applied (just as iritis is for iridocyclitis). The etiologies for the conjunctivitides include allergic, viral, bacterial, chlamydial, and chemical. Mild acute viral conjunctivitis, with a watery discharge and lids that are sealed closed upon awakening, usually requires only symptomatic treatment—warm or cool compresses and a topical vasoconstrictor to whiten the eye. Antibiotics have no clear efficacy. Any severe or chronic conjunctivitis should be managed by an ophthalmologist.

Gonococcal Conjunctivitis

Purulent conjunctivitis is usually bacterial and amenable to antibiotics. An important variety is gonococcal conjunctivitis, a disease of the newborn (*gonococcal ophthalmia neonatorum*) and of sexually active adults. The eye is markedly inflamed with a copious discharge and swollen lids, a picture described as hyperpurulent conjunctivitis.

The discharge should be Gram stained and cultured on Thayer-Martin medium. Treatment consists of parenteral penicillin, or an equivalent antibiotic, and saline lavage of ocular secretions. There is debate as to the necessity and efficacy of topical antibiotics. Untreated gonococcal infection can penetrate the intact eye and destroy it; treatment should be immediately initiated if there is a reasonable suspicion of the diagnosis.

Chlamydial Conjunctivitis

In some parts of the world, chronic chlamydial conjunctivitis leads to conjunctival scarring and corneal vascularization, a disease known as *trachoma*. The resulting corneal blindness is an important international public health problem. In developed countries, chlamydial infection manifests as a subacute conjunctivitis, frequently with associated urethritis. Although a keratitis may be present, severe corneal damage does not ensue. Chlamydial conjunctivitis, also called *inclusion blennorrhea* because of the cytoplasmic inclusions found in Giemsa-stained conjunctival scrapings, is difficult to eradicate in adults unless treated with systemic tetracycline or erythromycin.

Herpesvirus hominis Keratitis

Viral keratitis is a common and potentially serious consequence of infection with *Herpesvirus hominis*. The corneal involvement may be recognized by the characteristic *dendrite*, a branching epithelial ulcer. Topical antivirals promote healing, but recurrence is frequent, with increasing risk of corneal stromal involvement and scarring. Topical steroids activate epithelial herpes infections and should not be used without ophthalmological consultation.

Corneal Ulcers

Bacterial and fungal infections of the cornea are a serious threat to vision. Corneal ulcers tend to develop in the context of ocular trauma or contact lens wear, after surgery, or with pre-existing corneal disease. Corneal ulceration appears as an area of white, gray, or yellow infiltrate that stains with fluorescein. Such patients should be referred promptly to an ophthalmologist for further evaluation and treatment.

Endophthalmitis

Infection inside the eye is seen most often following accidental or surgical perforation of the eye. Epidemics have been reported following use of contaminated solutions in intraocular surgery. Only rarely do infections elsewhere metastasize to the eye.

Bacterial endophthalmitis must be treated very aggressively if there is to be any chance of preserving vision. When the infection is recognized, cultures and smears are taken from the anterior chamber and vitreous cavity by aspiration, and a course of systemic, topical, and periocular antibiotics is begun. The choice of antibiotics depends upon what organisms, if any, are found on the Gram stain.

Candida Endophthalmitis

Candida albicans is the most prevalent organism causing metastatic (endogenous) endophthalmitis. Fungemia after prolonged use of intravenous catheters or parenteral drug abuse results in colonization of the eye, with multiple white, fluffy chorioretinal infiltrates. These often involve the macula, reducing central vision. Careful direct ophthalmoscopy through a dilated pupil is indicated in patients at risk. Most *Candida* endophthalmitis requires systemic administration of antifungal agents, although spontaneous resolution has been observed.

Infectious Chorioretinitis

CONGENITAL TOXOPLASMOSIS. A common type of infectious chorioretinitis is *toxoplasmosis*, acquired in utero. This protozoan parasite can remain dormant in large, pigmented chorioretinal scars for many years and then become active, with white infiltration at the border of the scar and an overlying vitritis. If a previously uninvolved macula is threatened, treatment with pyrimethamine and sulfa or with clindamycin may be indicated.

CYTOMEGALOVIRUS CHORIORETINITIS. Cytomegalovirus chorioretinitis appears in immunosuppressed hosts as a discrete area of white or yellow retinal opacification with associated hemorrhage or vascular sheathing. The ophthalmoscopic picture may resemble that of a branch retinal vein occlusion (see below), but in this instance, one eye often has multiple foci and there is a tendency for bilaterality.

Diagnosis can be made clinically and by culture of throat and urine. Dosages of immunosuppressive drugs should be reduced, if possible. The efficacy of treatment with the antiviral agent adeninine arabinoside is uncertain.

OTHER INFECTIOUS CHORIORETINITIDES. Syphilis and tuberculosis are now rarely encountered as chorioretinitis. *Herpesvirus* retinitis resembles that of cytomegalovirus. Cryptococcal meningitis may have an associated chorioretinitis.

Parke DW II, Jones DB, Gentry LO: Endogenous endophthalmitis among patients with candidemia. Ophthalmology 89:789, 1982. *A prospective study of 38 patients with fungemia. Over one third of patients with* Candida *had ocular lesions.*

Pollard RB, Egbert PG, Gallaher JG, Merigan TC: Cytomegalovirus retinitis in immunosuppressed hosts. I. Natural history and effects of treatment with adenine arabinoside. II. Ocular manifestations. Ann Intern Med 93:655, 1980. *Reports of a large case series. The possible role of adenine arabinoside in treatment is discussed.*

Vastine D: Infections of the ocular adnexa and cornea. *In* Peyman GA, Sanders DR, Goldberg MF (eds.): Principles and Practice of Ophthalmology. Philadelphia, W. B. Saunders Company, 1980, pp 281–355. *This well-referenced and comprehensive review appears in one of the recently published major textbooks of ophthalmology.*

546. ORBITAL DISEASE AND TUMORS

Graves' Orbitopathy

The orbitopathy of Graves' disease consists of inflammation and infiltration of orbital tissues, with characteristic enlargement and scarring of the extraocular muscles. The varied clinical manifestations include lid retraction, exophthalmos, and limitation of eye movement.

Graves' orbitopathy frequently develops in persons previously treated for hyperthyroidism. When the orbitopathy first appears, the patient may be hyperthyroid, euthyroid, or hypothyroid. A classic Graves' orbitopathy in the absence of a demonstrable thyroid abnormality, even to sophisticated testing, is referred to as *ophthalmic Graves' disease.* Computed tomography demonstrating enlarged ocular muscles is probably the most sensitive diagnostic maneuver.

Graves' orbitopathy is the most frequent cause of both unilateral and bilateral exophthalmos. Retraction of the upper lid to expose sclera above the cornea exaggerates the appearance of exophthalmos and predisposes to a major complication, corneal exposure. Tethering of the eye by fibrotic muscles produces a mechanical ophthalmoplegia. Movement up and out is often restricted; pure loss of abduction mimicking sixth nerve palsy occurs. Ophthalmoplegia is not necessarily accompanied by obvious exophthalmos.

Enlargement of the ocular muscles at the apex of the orbit may lead to another major complication of Graves' orbitopathy—compressive optic neuropathy. Severe exposure or major visual loss from compressive optic neuropathy is an indication for treatment. Systemic steroids will reduce exophthalmos and relieve optic nerve compression temporarily. Surgical decompression of the orbit by one of several routes is one definitive therapy; orbital irradiation is also used. Direct surgery on the ocular muscles relieves diplopia and permanent lid retraction.

Pseudotumor of the Orbit

Orbital pseudotumor is an idiopathic inflammation that falls within the spectrum of lymphoproliferative disorders. Its clinical manifestations are pain, exophthalmos, and limitation of eye movement. There may also be erythema and swelling of the lids. Orbital pseudotumors thus mimic orbital infection, true tumors, and the orbitopathy of Graves' disease. The major site of inflammation is muscle (myositis), nerve (perineuritis), sclera (scleritis), or lacrimal gland (dacryoadenitis).

If the inflammation is posterior to the orbital apex in the walls of the cavernous sinus, the painful ophthalmoplegia that results is called the *Tolosa-Hunt syndrome*. Orbital pseudotumor merges pathologically and clinically with orbital lymphoma, which in turn merges with systemic lymphoma.

Initial evaluation of a patient with clinical signs and symptoms of orbital pseudotumor should include orbital ultrasonography and computed tomography. A trial of high dose systemic corticosteroids is usually indicated prior to biopsy. Orbital biopsy is not a trivial undertaking and should be reserved for steroid-unresponsive or recurrent processes. Some histologically benign infiltrations do not respond to corticosteroids. Biopsy in such cases reveals fibrous tissue—*sclerosing pseudotumor*. Occasionally, a patient with a histologically benign pseudotumor subsequently develops a systemic lymphoma.

A necrotizing vasculitis, Wegener's granulomatosis, must also be included in the differential diagnosis of orbital pseudotumor, especially when the inflammation is bilateral. Most cases of Wegener's granulomatosis involve contiguous sinus structures, but local ocular forms of the disease have been reported. The combination of progressive proptosis and sinus disease also suggests orbital aspergillosis, especially in residents of warmer climates.

Rhabdomyosarcoma

Rhabdomyosarcoma is the commonest malignant tumor of the orbit during the first decade of life and occurs during the second and third decades. The initial presentation is usually ptosis with lid infiltration and proptosis. Progression may be extremely rapid, the clinical picture mimicking trauma or cellulitis. Biopsy and prompt treatment with irradiation and chemotherapy results in a high percentage of survival, although vision in the eye on the side of the tumor is seldom preserved.

Other Orbital Tumors

The variety of primary, secondary, and metastatic tumors in the orbit is large. Most present with exophthalmos, visual loss, and limitation of eye movement. High degrees of malignancy are rare with meningiomas, gliomas, hemangiomas/lymphangiomas, and dermoids. Carcinomas of the lacrimal or meibomian glands represent a serious threat to life, and some cases require the most terrible of all ophthalmologic surgery—*exenteration*, removal of the orbital contents. Carcinoma from contiguous sinuses invades the orbit, and breast carcinoma is especially likely to metastasize to the orbit.

Rootman J, Nugent R: The classification and management of acute orbital pseudotumors. Ophthalmology 89:1040, 1982. *A personal series detailing the presentation and management of 17 cases of acute pseudotumor. The value of computed tomography and the effectiveness of steroids are emphasized.*

Sergott RC, Glaser JS: Graves' ophthalmopathy. A clinical and immunologic review. Surv Ophthalmol 26:1, 1981. *A comprehensive review of the subject.*

547. INTRAOCULAR TUMORS

Retinoblastoma

Retinoblastoma, a malignancy of the retina, is the most common intraocular tumor of childhood (and one of the more common tumors at any site). One third are bilateral. About 6 per cent of retinoblastomas are inherited as an autosomal dominant disease; half of these are bilateral. Ninety per cent of retinoblastomas are discovered before the child is three.

Retinoblastomas present in several ways. Perhaps the most important is as childhood strabismus, a condition ordinarily considered benign. Any child with strabismus should have a fundus examination to rule out retinoblastoma. The most common presentation is *leukocoria*, a white pupillary reflex. This manifestation is shared with mature cataract, retinopathy of prematurity, toxoplasmosis, *Toxocara* endophthalmitis, and other anomalies and disorders of the interior of the eye. Retinoblastoma should also be considered in a child with a detached retina and glaucoma, or with neovascularization of the anterior segment (suggested by spontaneous hyphema). Retinoblastomas tend to calcify, and CT and ultrasound scans help in making the differential diagnosis.

Early treatment improves survival and approaches 100 per cent if the tumor is small and unilateral. Enucleation (removal of the eye and attached optic nerve) and radiation are the primary therapeutic modalities. Children with a history of retinoblastoma have an increased incidence of osteosarcomas and other tumors, which are not necessarily found in the fields of previous radiotherapy.

Malignant Melanoma

Primary melanomas develop in the conjunctiva or choroid, and skin melanomas have a predilection for metastasis to the eye and orbit. Malignant melanomas of the choroid are the most common primary intraocular tumor of adulthood. Most occur in middle-aged Caucasians.

The prognosis of malignant melanoma of the choroid depends upon size, cytology, and the presence or absence of extrascleral extension. Choroidal malignant melanomas often metastasize to the liver.

The differential diagnosis of a pigmented intraocular mass includes benign choroidal nevus, senile disciform macular degeneration (also known as central exudative hemorrhagic retinopathy), peripheral exudative hemorrhagic chorioretinopathy, choroidal hemangioma, and hypertrophy or hyperplasia of the retinal pigment epithelium. Many eyes have been removed because of the suspicion of malignant melanoma when the pathology revealed a benign condition.

Enucleation is the traditional treatment for malignant melanoma of the choroid. Many pigmented choroidal tumors are now followed without intervention, especially when they are found incidentally in the seeing eyes of elderly patients. The effect of enucleation on life expectancy is currently being debated.

Metastatic Carcinoma to the Eye

Once considered rare, metastatic cancer is now the most common ocular malignancy of adulthood, with an incidence exceeding that of choroidal melanoma. Most are carcinomas invading the choroid, the commonest being carcinoma of the breast. Although ocular metastases appear late in the course of breast carcinoma, they may be the first sign of disseminated disease. Next in frequency are carcinomas of the lung, followed by kidney, gastrointestinal tract, testis, and prostate. With lung or renal carcinoma, the primary site may be inapparent at the time the metastasis is detected.

If tumor is identified elsewhere, removal of the eye is seldom indicated. Enucleation should be performed only if the eye is completely blind and painful, as palliative radiotherapy often preserves vision.

Abramson DH, Notterman RB, Ellsworth RM, Kitchin FD: Retinoblastoma treated in infants in the first six months of life. Arch Ophthalmol 101:1362, 1983.

Lennox EL, Draper GJ, Sanders BM: Retinoblastoma: A study of natural history and prognosis of 268 cases. Br Med J 3:731, 1975. *Two reviews of large series treated in Great Britain and the United States.*

Mewis L, Young SE: Breast carcinoma metastatic to the choroid. Ophthalmology 89:147, 1982. *The current status of detection and treatment.*

Yanoff M, Fine BS: Ocular Pathology; A Text and Atlas. 2nd ed. Philadelphia, Harper Medical, 1982. *A comprehensive textbook with many clinicopathologic correlations.*

548. RHEUMATOID AND CONNECTIVE TISSUE DISEASES

To a neurologist, the eye is an anterior extension of the brain; to a rheumatologist, the eye is a joint. Medicine and ophthalmology come together in the diagnosis and management of rheumatoid and connective tissue disorders. Uveal manifestations are discussed in conjunction with uveitis; the toxicity of drugs used in treatment, in a chapter on drug side effects; and the retinal changes, under ocular vascular disease. This chapter will deal with scleritis and episcleritis and keratoconjunctivitis sicca.

Episcleritis and Scleritis

Inflammation of the collagenous shell of the eye is divided into superficial (*episcleritis*) and deep (*scleritis*). The transparent, avascular cornea is continuous with the opaque, vascular sclera and may be secondarily involved.

Episcleritis resembles a localized conjunctivitis. The inflammation is deeper, however, and the dilated vessels do not blanch with topically applied phenylephrine 2.5 per cent, as in a pure conjunctivitis. Episcleritis usually is self-limited (although it may be recurrent) and does not permanently damage the eye. Most episcleritis is idiopathic, but it may be encountered in rheumatoid arthritis, polyarteritis nodosa, Wegener's granulomatosis, systemic lupus erythematosus, dermatomyositis, progressive systemic sclerosis, and relapsing polychondritis.

Scleritis is more likely than episcleritis to accompany a systemic disease, although the list of associations is about the same for the two disorders. Any portion of the sclera may be affected. The differential is especially difficult with posterior scleritis, which may present as ocular pain or as an exudative retinal detachment. Anterior scleritis is often a prolonged, indolent inflammation with eventual permanent structural alteration of tissues. Pain, which may be severe, is often a prominent feature.

In the initial phase the inflammation is localized and may be nodular or diffuse. With prolonged inflammation, scleral thinning results in a localized bluish discoloration as the underlying choroid becomes visible. Scleral necrosis with perforation is possible; this is especially frequent in rheumatoid arthritis. The adjacent cornea may melt away.

Management of scleritis is difficult. Local steroid injections may predispose to perforation. Systemic corticosteroids and other antirheumatic drugs are useful in some patients. The ocular process often closely parallels the activity of the underlying disease, and the best approach to the patient is a systemic one.

Keratoconjunctivitis Sicca

Corneal inflammation as the result of drying is referred to as *keratoconjunctivitis sicca*. Keratoconjunctivitis sicca, a dry mouth (xerostomia), and a connective tissue disorder constitute *Sjögren's syndrome*. The underlying pathophysiology appears to be an autoimmune reaction in the lacrimal and salivary glands. Sjögren's syndrome is common in patients, especially middle-aged women, with rheumatoid arthritis. The possibility of a dry eye should be considered with complaints of burning, irritation, or excessive secretions. Unfortunately, these symptoms are notoriously nonspecific.

Diagnosis depends upon demonstration of tear hyposecretion (usually by decreased wetting of a strip of litmus or filter paper placed between the lower lid and the eye in the inferior cul-de-sac) and corneal and conjunctival epithelial damage. Once epithelial cells start to slough, the corneal surface will take up the vital dye fluorescein instilled into the conjunctival sac. Devitalized cells that have not yet been sloughed stain with rose bengal, making this dye even more sensitive than fluorescein as a test for keratitis sicca.

Treatment consists of tear replacement and reduction of tear turnover. Various preparations of artificial tears are available. All share the disadvantage that they must be instilled very frequently to be effective. Longer lasting ointments blur vision. Other therapeutic maneuvers include occlusion of the lacrimal puncta to reduce tear outflow and placement of contact lenses, moisture chambers, or goggles over the eyes to decrease evaporation. Such measures are reserved for severe keratitis.

Watson PG, Hazleman BC: The Sclera and Systemic Disorders. London, W. B. Saunders Company Ltd., 1976. *A monograph on the subject.*

549. OCULAR VASCULAR DISEASE

Systemic Hypertension and Arteriosclerosis

Despite widely held notions to the contrary, the retinal vascular abnormalities in hypertension are nonspecific and variable. They can, nonetheless, be important both diagnostically and therapeutically. The effects of blood pressure on the retinal vessels depend upon both its absolute level and its duration. Although essential hypertension is a disease of arterioles, the retinal vascular bed lacks sympathetic innervation, and the fundus changes must be considered secondary.

Arteriolar narrowing is both the commonest and the most difficult hypertensive change to differentiate as abnormal. The normal ratio of the diameters of the arteriolar and venous blood columns is 2:3 or 3:4. A decrease in this ratio can best be appreciated in the smaller branches away from the disc.

Other findings include microaneurysms, hemorrhages, lipid deposits, and edema. Retinal and disc edema usually follows a rapid increase in systemic blood pressure. Disc edema defines the entity *malignant hypertension*. By contrast, opacification (or sclerosis) of the vessel walls—described ophthalmoscopically as copper or silver wiring—occurs with longstanding hypertension.

Thickening of the arteriolar wall explains arteriovenous crossing changes—AV nicking and venous dilation distal to the crossing. Cotton-wool spots are signs of local ischemia; hemorrhages and hard exudates are signs of vascular leakage. Microaneurysms indicate irreversible structural alterations in the capillary beds. Vascular occlusions (see below) and ischemic optic neuropathy are potential consequences of hypertensive vascular changes.

Some classifications distinguish arteriosclerotic from hypertensive changes, but this division is difficult to justify clinically or pathophysiologically. The only pure arteriosclerotic change is atheroma of the retinal arterioles. This is seen as a yellow-white plaque in the central retinal artery or its first branches, where the arteries still have an internal elastic lamina. These plaques must be differentiated from calcific or lipid emboli, which are usually smaller or more peripheral. Hypertension accelerates atherosclerosis, but atherosclerosis does not require hypertension.

Diabetic Retinopathy

The retinal vessels react in a limited number of ways. Diabetic retinopathy shares many features with hypertensive retinopathy. Diabetes is simply the most common of the vascular retinopathies.

The pathophysiologic defect in diabetic retinopathy appears to be at the level of the retinal capillaries. Progressive degeneration of the cells of the capillary walls results in leakage, diffuse and focal expansion (microaneurysms), and closure of these small vessels. The ischemic retina in the focal areas of nonperfusion probably elaborates factors stimulating new vessel and fibrous ingrowth. (A retinopathy similar to that of diabetes is produced by radiation, usually radiotherapy given as part of the treatment for head and neck cancers. The radiation damages capillary cells.)

Diabetic retinopathy is classified as *background* or *proliferative*. Background retinopathy is further subdivided into *simple* background—with microaneurysms, dot/blot hemorrhages, and hard exudates—and a *preproliferative* form. In preproliferative background retinopathy there is beading of veins, cotton-wool spots, and many hemorrhages. Also characteristic is intraretinal new vessel pathology, so-called *intraretinal microvascular anomalies* (IRMA).

In proliferative retinopathy, neovascularization appears on the disc and elsewhere, especially along the major vascular arcades. There may be fibrovascular proliferation and vitreous hemorrhages. Proliferative diabetic retinopathy confers a poor visual prognosis.

Background retinopathy alone reduces visual acuity when there is edema or exudation in the macula. There are more new cases of blindness from background retinopathy with macular edema than from proliferative retinopathy, because backround retinopathy is so much more prevalent. The incidence of diabetic retinopathy increases with the duration of the disease. Background retinopathy with macular edema is common in adult-physiology diabetics over age 50.

Treatment

Good control appears to retard the progression of diabetic retinopathy. There is now proof that ablation of ischemic retina by panretinal photocoagulation helps preserve central vision in patients with early proliferative retinopathy, making this the current treatment of choice. Advanced proliferative retinopathy may require major intraocular surgery—*pars plana vitrectomy.* In such cases the visual prognosis is guarded even with intervention, but an estimated 50 to 75 per cent of operated patients experience some visual improvement.

Other Vascular Retinopathies

RETINOPATHY OF COLLAGEN VASCULAR DISEASE. Retinopathy in systemic lupus erythematosus is common but nonspecific. The most frequent findings are retinal hemorrhages and cotton-wool spots. Cotton-wool spots are localized areas of axoplasmic stasis caused by ischemia, which may indicate active vasculitis. Although occasionally referred to as "soft exudates," cotton-wool spots are not exudations. Patients with lupus often have hypertensive retinopathy (see above).

Central nervous system involvement in lupus may be associated with optic and chiasmal neuropathy, papilledema, ocular motor cranial nerve palsies, and hemianopias. A migraine-like syndrome is also a feature of CNS lupus.

RETINOPATHY OF HEMATOLOGIC DISEASE. Anemia and thrombocytopenia predispose to retinal and subconjunctival hemorrhages. When these are the result of leukemia, the hemorrhages often have a white center—the classic *Roth spot.* Roth spots are encountered in a number of situations, including septic embolism from subacute bacterial endocarditis, and are therefore nonspecific.

Leukemia is one cause of hyperviscosity retinopathy, characterized by venous tortuosity and dilation, retinal hemorrhages, and vascular occlusions. A chronically elevated leukocyte count also predisposes to capillary drop out and microaneurysm formation, but proliferative retinopathy is rare. Other causes of hyperviscosity retinopathy are Waldenström's macroglobulinemia, multiple myeloma, polycythemia, and sickle cell anemia. In extreme cases sludging of blood in the veins is visible ophthalmoscopically.

PERIPHERAL RETINAL NEOVASCULARIZATION. Diabetic retinopathy affects largely the posterior pole of the eye. The retinopathy of prematurity (retrolental fibroplasia) and sickle cell disease have their major impact on the peripheral retina. The etiology of the retinopathy of sickle cell disease is multiple occlusions of capillaries by abnormal blood constituents. In the retinopathy of prematurity, high levels of oxygen prevent the normal growth of vessels into the retinal periphery of the developing eye, resulting in an ischemic stimulus when ambient oxygen levels return to normal. High levels of oxygen are also directly toxic to vessels.

The ocular and systemic manifestations of sickling hemoglobinopathies correlate poorly. In patients with sickle cell anemia, proliferative retinopathy is rare. Peripheral neovascularization is more common in sickle cell hemoglobin C disease (SC) and sickle cell thalassemia (S-thal). Patients with sickle cell trait usually have no ocular symptoms, although hypoxia encountered at high altitudes may precipitate hemorrhages and vascular occlusions.

The ocular findings in sickle hemoglobinopathies include small, dark red, comma-shaped conjunctival vascular segments, best seen on the inferior bulbar conjunctiva after instillation of a topical vasoconstrictor. Ischemic infarction of iris segments is also observed. In addition to the "sea fan" peripheral neovascularization, other characteristic retinal findings include hemorrhages that have a salmon pink coloration from hemoglobin breakdown products—salmon patch hemorrhages—and black chorioretinal scars with irregular borders in the equatorial periphery—the black sunburst sign.

Treatment of Peripheral Neovascularization

About one fifth of proliferative sickle retinopathy regresses spontaneously. The rest, if untreated, will progress to retinal detachment and vitreous hemorrhage. Treatment consists of photocoagulation or transscleral cryotherapy or diathermy.

Retinal Vascular Occlusions

CENTRAL RETINAL ARTERY OCCLUSION (CRAO). The central retinal artery is a branch of the ophthalmic artery, in turn a branch of the internal carotid artery. Occlusion of the central retinal artery causes sudden, usually nearly complete, visual loss in one eye. Ophthalmoscopy reveals arteriolar narrowing and venous stasis (most obvious as segmentation of the venous blood column—"boxcar" pattern).

Within hours the fundus picture changes as the infarcted superficial layers of the retina lose their normal transparency to assume a milky-white translucency. Because the thin retina over the fovea receives its oxygen from the underlying choroid, this region retains its normal reddish-pink color. This contrasts with surrounding tissue, producing an appearance described as a cherry red macula. (A similar appearance is encountered in certain lipid storage diseases, where abnormal metabolic products partially opacify the ganglion cell layer.)

Eventually arterial flow is restored, the edema resolves, and the fundus appearance returns to near normal. The disc, which is initially normal because it derives its blood supply from the surrounding choroid, gradually becomes pale and atrophic. After several weeks it is difficult to distinguish a central retinal artery occlusion from other causes of optic atrophy.

Acute central retinal artery occlusion is an emergency. Prompt action may dislodge an embolus and restore circulation in time to prevent retinal death and to preserve vision. For a nonophthalmologist this action consists of firm, intermittent pressure on the globe. This ballotment alternately raises and lowers intraocular pressure. Ophthalmologists use other measures: retrobulbar injection of anesthetic and anterior chamber paracentesis to lower the pressure in the ocular vascular bed. Inhalation of a mixture of 95 per cent oxygen and 5 per cent carbon dioxide is recommended by some. Rarely does any treatment save vision.

In a number of eyes, portions of the retina are supplied by vessels arising from the choroidal circulation. Retina supplied by such cilioretinal arteries will be spared if the central retinal artery alone is occluded. In a few eyes, the island of spared retina encompasses the disc, macula, and intervening retina; visual acuity remains normal even in the presence of a CRAO. Most eyes with CRAO are deprived of useful vision.

CRAO's are the result of emboli (atheromatous, myxomatous, and material from diseased or artificial heart valves), of local small vessel disease, or of carotid occlusion. A CRAO is sometimes the initial sign of giant cell arteritis or polyarteritis nodosa. CRAO has been reported in patients with sickle cell trait after trauma or other stress.

BRANCH RETINAL ARTERY OCCLUSION (BRAO). Branch arterial occlusions present as sudden visual loss that leaves only a portion of the field affected. Ophthalmoscopically there is a wedge-shaped area of infarcted retina spreading outward from an arteriolar bifurcation.

In contrast to central retinal artery occlusions, branch retinal artery occlusions are almost always embolic in origin. By far the commonest source of emboli in older adults is the ipsilateral carotid artery. In children and young adults, migraine, coagulation abnormalities, increased intraocular pressure, and oral contraceptives may predispose to vascular occlusions.

CENTRAL RETINAL VEIN OCCLUSION (CRVO). The dramatic ophthalmoscopic findings of dilated, tortuous veins, extensive retinal hemorrhages, and disc swelling in one eye have classically been called a central retinal vein occlusion. Actually there is evidence that such *hemorrhagic retinopathy* is the consequence of both arterial ischemia and venous disease.

A CRVO presents as sudden unilateral visual loss in older adults, but unlike a CRAO, a CRVO is not an emergency, as there is no accepted immediate therapy. There are also no specific accompanying diseases, although hypertension and diabetes are loosely associated, and hypercoagulable states must be considered.

Visual prognosis varies. In the fully developed form usually encountered in older persons, vision is poor and generally remains so. Panretinal photocoagulation appears to decrease the risk of subsequent neovascular glaucoma. A less severe ophthalmoscopic picture is encountered in younger patients. Acuity in such *partial central retinal vein occlusion* or *venous stasis retinopathy* is only slightly reduced, and the visual prognosis is good. Ischemic oculopathy after carotid occlusion produces a similar retinopathy; retinal arterial pressures measured by ophthalmodynamometry or ocluopneumoplethysmography will be low in such cases.

BRANCH RETINAL VEIN OCCLUSIONS. Patients with branch vein occlusions complain of blurred vision. In the fundus, hemorrhages and cotton-wool spots spread out in a wedge from an arteriovenous crossing. As in CRVO, there are few specific systemic associations. Neovascular glaucoma is rare, but vision may be persistently reduced by macular edema. Branch retinal vein occlusion must be distinguished from viral retinitis.

Asdourian GK: Peripheral retinal neovascularization—differential diagnosis. *In* Peyman GA, Sanders DR, Goldberg MF (eds.): Principles and Practice of Ophthalmology. Philadelphia, W. B. Saunders Company, 1980, pp 1277–1298. *A clear review of clinical manifestations and pathogenesis.*

Brown GC, Magorgal LE, Shields JA, et al.: Retinal arterial obstruction in children and young adults. Ophthalmology 88:18, 1981. *A report of 27 cases of BRAO or CRAO in patients under 30 years of age.*

Gold D, Feiner L, Henkind P: Retinal arterial occlusive disease in systemic lupus erythematosus. Arch Ophthalmol 95:1580, 1977. *A discussion of the retinal findings.*

Kearns TP: Differential diagnosis of central retinal vein obstruction. Ophthalmology 90:475, 1983. *This paper is one of four in the same issue that describes the work-up, differential, and management of CRVO.*

Lessell S: The neuro-ophthalmology of systemic lupus erythematosus. Docum Ophthalmol 47:13, 1979. *This paper is hard to find but well worth the effort. The most complete review of the ocular manifestations other than retinopathy.*

Little HL, Jack RL, Patz A, Forsham PH: Diabetic Retinopathy. New York, Thieme-Stratton Inc., 1983. *A collection of 31 position papers on various aspects of diabetic retinopathy.*

550. THE EYE AND MEDICATIONS

Drugs with Ocular Side Effects

ANTICHOLINERGICS. A variety of systemic drugs have ocular side effects. Any medication with anticholinergic properties can dilate the pupil and diminish accommodation (the ability to focus at close range). The possibility of angle-closure is the basis for the caution that such medications are contraindicated in glaucoma. Patients on therapy for open-angle glaucoma are at little risk, as mydriasis will not usually affect intraocular pressure. If the patient has known angle-closure, previous iris surgery all but eliminates the danger of dilation. Only when there is a potential for angle-closure are such drugs contraindicated, and this is usually unrecognized. Of the systemic anticholergic drugs, transdermal scopolamine alone can dilate and fix pupils and paralyze accommodation even in young persons.

CORTICOSTEROIDS. Systemically administered corticosteroids are cataractogenic. Prolonged administration of high dosages of corticosteroids often leads to the formation of posterior subcapsular cataracts. Topical corticosteroids increase intraocular pressure in genetically predisposed persons. Topical steroids also activate *Herpesvirus* keratitis and should be administered only under the supervision of an ophthalmologist.

QUININE AND CHLOROQUINE. Quinine—used for malaria and muscle cramps, as an abortifactant, and to dilute street heroin—may cause acute blindness, with narrowing of the retinal arterioles. An overdose increases the probability of toxic effects, but rare persons are sensitive even to therapeutic doses. The symptoms of quinine toxicity include dizziness, tinnitus, and hearing loss. Central vision may improve, with persistent constriction of peripheral field and evolution of optic atrophy.

The synthetic antimalarials chloroquine and hydroxychloroquine, used for the treatment of systemic lupus erythematosus and rheumatoid arthritis, have a specific retinal toxicity. This usually appears only after prolonged administration of the drugs in doses exceeding 250 mg per day for chloroquine and 400 mg per day for hydroxychloroquine. Reduced visual acuity is the usual initial symptom, but the parafoveal retina is most affected. The chloroquine binds to pigmented tissues, exerting a toxic effect on the retinal pigment epithelium with loss of pigmentation in a target-like or bull's eye pattern around the fovea. Discontinuation of the drug may result in improvement, but if the process is moderately advanced, visual loss may be progressive.

Chloroquine and hydroxychloroquine also cause whorl-like corneal epithelial deposits, which reduce acuity and produce halos around lights. Such deposits bear no direct relationship to the retinal toxicity and disappear after discontinuation of the drug.

THIORIDAZINE. Phenothiazines are potentially toxic to retina and retinal pigment epithelium, producing a coarse pigmentary degeneration. Of those now in common use, only thioridazine has clinically significant toxicity, and then only with dosages exceeding 1 gram per day for prolonged periods.

ETHAMBUTOL. Various drugs have been implicated in optic neuropathies. Only with ethambutol is the incidence of such side effects high enough that monitoring is considered mandatory. The physician administering ethambutol should perform monthly checks of acuity and color vision, especially when dosages exceed 15 mg per kilogram.

Oculocutaneous Disorders

A variety of related disorders (including erythema multiforme, Stevens-Johnson syndrome, and toxic epidermal necrolysis, or Lyell's syndrome) arise as idiosyncratic responses to drugs or infections. Their ocular manifestations are a bullous conjunctival eruption followed by a cicatricial conjunctivitis. Adhesions, called symblepharons, may obliterate the conjunctival sacs. The alterations in conjunctival architecture prevent the normal production and distribution of tears. A severe dry eye may be the most disabling sequela of these disorders.

Early treatment with topical steroids (and perhaps antibiotics to prevent secondary infection) is sometimes effective in limiting damage. Sweeping the conjunctival fornices several times a day with a sterile glass rod inhibits symblepharon formation.

Systemic Side Effects of Topical Ocular Medications

Medications in solution are easily absorbed from the nasal mucosa, and systemic side effects are more likely with drops than ointments. Dilation of the pupil with 10 per cent phenylephrine solution has been known to precipitate severe hypertension, especially in infants and the elderly. Topical epinephrine increases ventricular extrasystoles in some patients. Timolol maleate causes bronchospasm in asthmatics.

Topical anticholinergics such as atropine, scopolamine, and cyclopentolate may contribute to confusional states in the elderly. Cyclopentolate is occasionally a cause of acute hallucinations and even psychosis in the young. Pilocarpine, used in large doses in the treatment of acute angle-closure glaucoma, has resulted in cholinergic overdose—nausea, vomiting, salivation, and gastrointestinal cramps. As these are also symptoms of the angle-closure attack itself, such toxicity may not be immediately recognized, leading to continued administration and cardiovascular collapse.

Echothiophate iodide, an organophosphate used in the treatment of some forms of childhood strabismus and of open-angle glaucoma, predisposes to cholinergic crisis, mimicking an acute surgical abdomen. Also, patients receiving echothiophate have impaired metabolism of succinylcholine. Use of succinylcholine during the induction of general anesthesia in a patient receiving echothiophate has caused death.

Carbonic Anhydrase Inhibitors

Acetazolamide and methazolamide inhibit aqueous production and are used systemically to reduce intraocular pressure when topical medications are inadequate. Most patients experience paresthesias; their absence is thought by some to indicate noncompliance. Carbonic anhydrase inhibitors also induce a systemic acidosis, with a syndrome of malaise and anorexia, depression, and weight loss that responds to concurrent administration of sodium bicarbonate. Acetazolamide increases the incidence of urolithiasis. The combination of a carbonic anhydrase inhibitor and a thiazide diuretic depletes body potassium. Carbonic anhydrase inhibitors should not be given to people with known allergy to sulfonamides.

Adler AG, McElwain GE, Merli GJ, Martin JH: Systemic effects of eye drops. Arch Intern Med 142:2293, 1982. *A brief review that serves as a cautionary tale.*

Fraunfelder FT, Meyer SM: Drug-Induced Side Effects and Drug Interactions. 2nd ed. Philadelphia, Lea & Febiger, 1982. *A compendium based on a collection of reports of side effects.*

Grant WM: Toxicology of the Eye. 2nd ed. Springfield, Charles C Thomas, 1974. *An enormous review with component parts that are still coherent and readable.*

Part XXV
SKIN DISEASES

Marie-Louise Johnson

551. INTRODUCTION

The skin is our interface with the world, and more. It is the glassine bag through which physiologic and chemical changes are perceived; the self-substance that is invaded and traumatized from within and without; an organ that responds and repairs, that shares the burdens of growing up and growing old, of environmental insults, and of systemic disease.

As an organ system it is unique. It stretches before the examiner patently obvious with significant data waiting to be read. The student attuned to palpating and auscultating forgets to look. He misses basic physiologic facts about his patient, perhaps significant signals of serious disease. Further, when the patient draws attention to a skin change, the student is uncertain as to what it may be or its importance. If the patient is sufficiently persistent, or the examiner sufficiently compulsive, a consultation can be obtained, usually with dispatch during medical school and house staff training. But later, when the examiner is removed from the medical center and the logistics and economics of the consultation must be reckoned, decisions are made on shaky foundations. The risk of ignoring the mortal and promoting morbidity is increased as much as is the cost of care through unnecessary referral. Such decisions are not infrequent; some 30 per cent of Americans have a dermatologic problem that should be seen by a physician; further, 52 per cent of all problems related to the skin present to internists, pediatricians, and generalists.

This is not to say that every practicing physician needs to be a dermatologist. It does suggest that every doctor involved in patient care should be comfortable recognizing and treating *common* skin problems, ten of which constitute 76 per cent of the burden of skin disease as established by population survey (Table 551–1).

Part XXV reviews pathophysiologic mechanisms that will prepare the observer for an informed assessment of the skin. Once there is confidence in identifying the morbid processes observed, the facts can be interpreted and the diagnosis elaborated. Without awaiting a confirmed impression, however, the patient can be made more comfortable; thus Ch. 554 will emphasize principles of therapy as well as precautions and proscriptions. Finally, the more common dermatologic conditions will be reviewed, as well as those that have implications for systemic illness, and those which in their management utilize medications and modalities of therapy uncommon to other disciplines. Our aim is to ensure an ease of recognition and management for the common dermatoses; to provide a useful guide to the identification and assessment of cutaneous signs of systemic disease; and, finally, to sharpen suspicion and enhance understanding of the risk and challenge of the more significant dermatologic diagnoses as judged by morbidity and mortality. In no way are the following chapters an attempt to substitute for a text in dermatology; hence frequent reference will be made to the literature, especially to selected texts and review articles, where the reader can further his knowledge.

TABLE 551–1. PREVALENCE OF COMMON DERMATOLOGIC DISEASE IN THE UNITED STATES*

	Rate per 1000	Numbers (in 1000's)
Fungus infections	81.1	15,733
Tinea pedis	38.7	7509
Tinea unguium	21.8	4232
Tinea versicolor	8.4	1623
Tinea cruris	6.7	1301
Acne vulgaris	68.1	13,217
Cystic acne	1.9	375
Acne scars	1.7	321
Seborrheic dermatitis	28.2	5476
Verruca vulgaris	8.5	1684
Folliculitis	8.0	1553
Atopic dermatitis	6.9	1332
Lichen simplex chronicus	4.5	882
Hand eczema	1.6	311
Dyshidrotic eczema	2.1	405
Psoriasis	5.5	1070
Vitiligo	4.9	957
Herpes simplex	4.2	824

*Persons 1 to 74 years of age—noninstitutionalized.

Johnson ML, Roberts J: Skin conditions and related need for medical care among persons 1–74 years, United States 1971–1974. Vital and Health Statistics Series II, No 212 (1979). *Because this study had by direct examination gathered data on a large and representative sampling of the noninstitutionalized American population, it provides the most extensive and reliable source for information about the prevalence and morbidity of dermatologic problems.*

Stern RS, Johnson ML, DeLozier J: Utilization of physician services for dermatologic complaints. Arch Dermatol 113:1062, 1977. *A good look at who goes where for dermatologic services based on national survey data.*

General Dermatology Reference Texts

Braverman IM: Skin Signs of Systemic Disease. 2nd ed. Philadelphia, W. B. Saunders Company, 1981. *An excellent review of cutaneous signs that should evoke from the internist or generalist concern of systemic disease.*

Fitzpatrick TB, Eisen AZ, Wolff K, Freedberg IM, Austen KF (eds.): Dermatology in General Medicine. 2nd ed. New York, McGraw-Hill Book Company, 1979. *A solid, readable, complete text with great strength in pigmentation.*

Fitzpatrick TB, Eisen AZ, Wolff K, Freedberg IM, Austen KF (eds.): Dermatology in general medicine. Update. New York, McGraw-Hill Book Company, 1983. *An expansion and "tidying up" of the text of the same title.*

Moschella SL, Pillsbury DM, Hurley HJ Jr: Dermatology, 2 vols. Philadelphia, W. B. Saunders Company, 1975. *A detailed text with historical insights and helpful treatment advice.*

Rook A, Wilkinson DS, Ebling FG: Textbook of Dermatology, 2 vols. 3rd ed. Oxford, Blackwell Scientific Publications, 1979. *With the greatest detail and finest prose, the Rook book is quite "compleat."*

552. PATHOPHYSIOLOGY

The skin is an essential organ. Deprived of significant amounts, as by burn and trauma, we cannot survive. Excessive losses of fluid and electrolytes are difficult to replace, and without the natural barrier to organisms infection is hard to contain.

But the disruptions of the integument are not always so gross. To understand challenges that have targeted effects, to interpret disease processes that show characteristic anatomic change or deposits of immune proteins at selected sites, some detailed information about the structure and function of the skin is required.

ANATOMIC CONSIDERATIONS

The living envelope which enfolds us contributes 16 per cent or so to the body weight of the average adult. It is composed of two mutually dependent layers of distinct developmental origin: the outer *epidermis* from the ectoderm and the inner *dermis* from the mesoderm, both cushioned on the fat-containing subcutaneous tissue, the *panniculus adiposus* (Fig. 522–1). Mesenchymal structures such as collagen, blood vessels, and fat originate from the mesoderm.

The stratified cellular epidermis is derived by a division of a basal layer of cells which forms successive sheets moving outward as keratinocytes synthesizing the insoluble protein keratin. From the *stratum germinativum* the columnar basal cell resting on a basement membrane generates, by mitosis, daughter cells, one or both of which progress to the surface, becoming more polyhedral as they go; still nucleate, they are bound at the tufts called desmosomes, to which are fixed cytoplasmic filaments constituting by their quill-like appearance the *stratum spinosum* (Fig. 552–2). In the course of 14 days the matured daughter cell will have flattened from a polyhedral form to a pancake, acquiring keratohyaline granules that in the aggregate

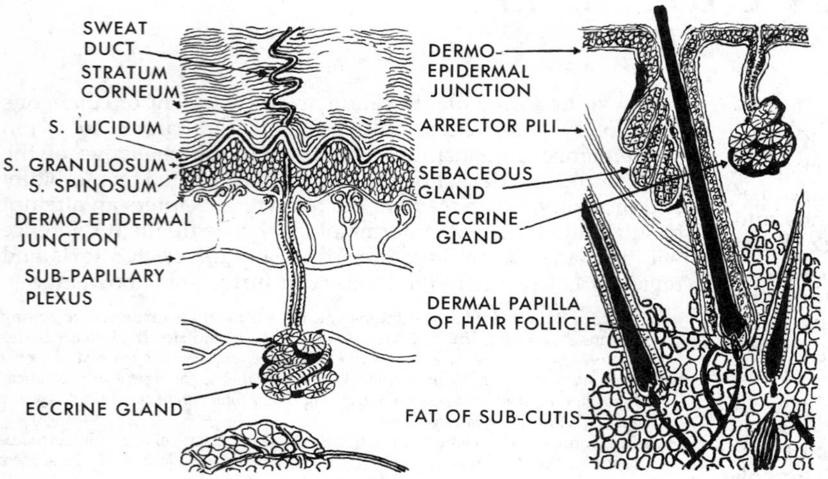

Figure 552–1. Structure of the skin.

suggest the label *stratum granulosum*. Eventually it will lose its nucleus to become part of the *stratum corneum*. In another 14 days, by wear and programmed replacement from beneath, it will be shed completely; this slough of skin is continuous and imperceptible in the normal individual, with a turnover time of four weeks from basal cell to extinction. Anatomically there is some variation. The stratum corneum has its greatest thickness on the palms and soles, for example, and in these areas epidermal turnover is prolonged.

The differentiation of the migratory epidermal cells involves the formation of one or more fibrous proteins known collectively as keratin. The process, complete in the stratum corneum, yields mature keratin, a system of filaments embedded in a continuous matrix within a thickened cell membrane. As the stratum corneum, keratin serves as a rate-limiting membrane affecting the passage of ions and molecules. It is the protective layer against harmful chemicals; it also admits selected substances, including topical allergens as well as topical therapy. It freely admits water, up to four times its weight, and it freely yields water to the environment as insensible perspiration. Transport across the membrane is enhanced by increased temperature, by the lipid solubility of the solute, and by increased hydration of the stratum corneum itself.

Pathologic processes that disorder the differentiation of epidermal cells toward keratin may manifest themselves as blocking the transport of insensible water, the admission of topical therapy, or even the clinical appearance of casings or scale, be it retained or overproduced keratin. Further, in the loss of the

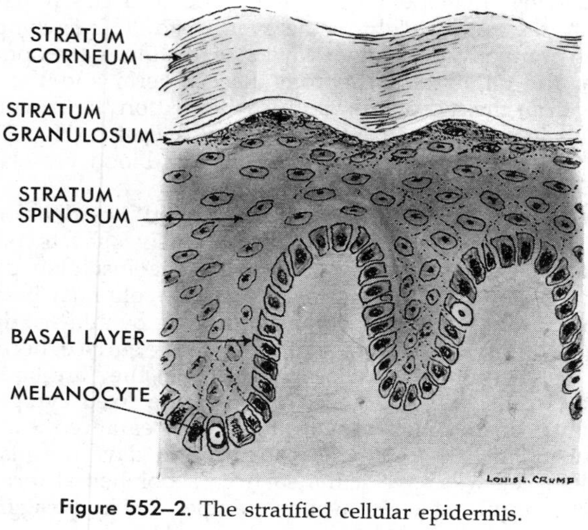

Figure 552–2. The stratified cellular epidermis.

spinous adherence of cells at desmosomes, the intercellular spaces trap fluid to the consequent development of blisters.

Although the pathogenesis may vary, the disrupted cell is the keratinocyte—that general name for the epidermal cell derived from the basal layer. In the epidermis, however, there are also *melanocytes* which originate in the neural crest of the embryo and retain migratory capabilities in the adult. They transfer pigment to the epidermal cells through their dendritic processes. Malfunction can mean absence of pigment or pigment production to the extreme, both potential cosmetic disasters. Also present in the epidermis are Langerhans' cells, of long recognition, of debated origin and function, and of recent focus for their suspected role in contact dermatitis and delayed hypersensitivity. As dendritic nonkeratinocytes, probably originating from the mesenchyme, Langerhans' cells are found in the basal and suprabasal layers of the epidermis, and at times in the dermis. They can also be seen in stratified squamous epithelia as of the buccal and vaginal mucosa, and rather ubiquitously in lymph nodes, thymus, spleen, and other organs. Immunocompetent cells involved in the uptake and processing of antigenic material, they are the receptors for the initial cutaneous response to external antigens.

Beneath the epidermis is the principal mass of skin, the dermis, a mixture of fibrous protein and collagen embedded in mucopolysaccharide along with water, elastic fibers, nerves, blood vessels, lymph channels, glands, appendages, and a few cells, largely fibroblasts, mast cells, and histiocytes. Actually eccrine sweat glands and the pilosebaceous apparatus, although dermal in location, are of ectodermal origin and formed from embryonic invaginations into the mesoderm. Because the stratum corneum covers only the most superficial part, transport through these structures is more rapid. Undoubtedly the pilosebaceous and sweat glands contribute heavily to the transport of molecular substances through the skin.

MECHANICAL CONSIDERATIONS

The mechanical properties of skin are important from the standpoint of toughness and resistance to forces of disruption, to shearing, but also as they relate to wound healing, to the aging process, or to inherited disorders in which structural elements are defective. Strength and flexibility are significant attributes, and the extracellular components of the dermis are important contributors. *Collagen* fibers, for example, give high tensile strength, and their loose mesh permits the mobility of joints. The return of collagen to the unstressed state depends on the elastic restoring forces of *elastin*. In old age the degradation of the elastic fiber network leaves the collagen mesh without the support to restore fully its original configuration, and wrinkled skin is the surface evidence. The ground substance, which is less well understood, through its viscous and elastic properties, resists compression and accepts molding, thus serving to reduce point pressure on more sensitive skin structures.

PHYSIOLOGIC CONSIDERATIONS

The skin cannot survive without oxygen and nutrients. Although the prime provider role of blood vessels is dramatically underscored in its disruption, as with gangrenous toes and stubborn leg ulcers, the skin compared to other organs is low in metabolic requirements. Like the kidney, its blood flow is far in excess of nutritional need, and its vascular system is adapted to mechanisms that meet other demands such as the regulation of body heat. In normal and warm environments blood flow is greater in the digits and other acral skin areas, achieved in part through the arteriovenous shunt of the glomus body, a dermal vessel peculiar to the acral areas. At normal environmental temperatures and low work levels, dermal blood flow is the only thermoregulatory mechanism required to maintain a constant body temperature. Increase in the metabolic rate of the body will increase skin blood flow. Posterior hypothalamic centers in the brain control dermal blood flow through deep vasoconstrictor mechanisms of the sympathetic nervous system.

Apart from nutrition and thermal regulation, dermal blood vessels participate in the inflammatory response and demonstrate recognizable pathologic changes in specific diseases. Reacting to a noxious stimulus, transient vasoconstriction will be followed by dilatation with a ten-fold increase in blood flow, an increase in vessel permeability, and a consequent escape of fluid into the interstitial space. There is a relaxing of precapillary sphincters which become refractory to vasoconstrictor stimuli, and finally, initiation of the cellular response. With certain traumatic stimuli to normal skin in disease states, the dermal response may be a vascular proliferation or constriction, or even development of the complete lesion of the disease, the isomorphic response as seen in collagen diseases, psoriasis, and lichen planus.

SWEAT GLANDS

Eccrine

The thermoregulatory mechanism depends significantly on the eccrine sweat gland, which produces and transports to the skin surface a hypotonic solution for evaporation and cooling. Given sufficient thermal stimulation, an individual through his 2 to 3 million sweat glands can produce 2 to 3 liters of sweat per hour for a short interval. Each gland is a simple tubule with a coiled secretory segment deep in the dermis and a straight duct extending up to become spiraled terminally before it pierces the stratum corneum. It is well supplied with blood vessels, and, in its secretory part, with unmyelinated nerve endings, anatomically sympathetic but functionally parasympathetic.

Lesions develop with anatomic blockage of the sweat duct. A rupture in the mid-dermis nearer the secretory part stimulates little dermal response, although the trapped sweat may be visible in the skin. Like a deep millet seed, it is called descriptively *miliaria profunda.* Rupture more distally near the papillary plexus ensures proximity to blood vessels and nerve endings, which provokes redness and itching because of reactive dilatation of the capillaries and stimulation of the *c* fibers of the nerves. Clinically it is known as *miliaria rubra* or, more commonly, *prickly heat.* Inability of sweat to escape at the surface leaves a superficial drop of sweat with few symptoms, scattered dew drops in transparent casings; it is important only to be recognized for what it is—*miliaria crystallina.* In all physiologic entrapments of sweat the therapy is to reduce the activity of the gland, remove blockage at the duct orifice, and counteract the local irritant effects of escaped intradermal sweat. Cooling will reduce the need to sweat; mild keratolytics such as 1 per cent salicylic acid in alcohol will free the eccrine sweat pores of retained keratin and lipid, and anti-inflammatory agents such as topical steroids will reduce erythema and pruritus.

Sweat is formed not by passive filtration but by active metabolic processes, with lactate produced in the secretory segment and sodium resorbed in the ductal segment. Sweat appearing on the skin is usually lower in sodium and chloride and higher in lactate than interstitial fluid from which it is derived. The maximal capacity to resorb sodium is only one quarter the capacity to secrete. Hence at times of profuse sweating, significant amounts of sodium can be lost. True adaptation can be seen with repeated intense thermal stress, leading to a conservation of sodium through a mechanism that may involve increased adrenal aldosterone secretion and enhanced reabsorption in the ductal segment.

An increase in body heat arouses temperature-sensitive centers in the hypothalamus and serves as a potent stimulus for generalized sweating. Pyrogens raise the hypothalamic temperature threshold for inducing sweating, and fever is the consequence, the heat produced through shivering if the ambient temperature is low. When the receptor function returns to normal levels and body temperature is then perceived as too high, profuse sweating ensues.

The palms and soles have large eccrine sweat gland populations. Although they respond poorly to thermal stimulation, they do respond immediately and profusely to psychogenic stimuli. Palmar sweat as an index of emotional stress is used in the polygraph or lie-detector test.

The physical aspects of heat loss and retention have their obvious dramatic roles in the desert and polar regions, but they also have an important and certainly more extensive role in prophylactic skin care and management of dermal pathology. Heat may be lost or gained relative to environmental temperature by radiation, conduction, or convection. Ordinary metabolic heat from organs and muscle is transported by the blood to the skin, where it is lost through radiation and convection by adjustments in cutaneous circulation effecting perhaps small changes in skin surface temperature. The balance is maintained readily and without sweat. With excessive metabolic heat the regulated blood flow through skin is accelerated; the increased vascular surface area permits heat to be lost to the lower ambient temperature of the air, to colder solid or liquid surfaces as to rocks or lake water, and through the evaporation of water or sweat from the skin.

At rest in a 35° C, windy dry environment, an elevated body temperature will lose heat not by radiation or convection but through evaporation calculated as 150 grams of sweat per hour to remain stable. With exercise and consequent increase in metabolic heat, and with an extreme environmental temperature to 46° C, 830 grams of sweat per hour would be needed for stabilization. In a hot humid environment with evaporation restricted, profuse sweat drips rather than evaporating and the heat load is difficult to dissipate, with risk of severe hyperthermia, dehydration, and sodium depletion, which may be followed by collapse, failure of the eccrine apparatus, and fatal heat stroke; the victim's skin is flushed, warm, and dry. In hot environments it is vital to replace salt and water losses continuously and to promote cooling by evaporation with air currents, nonrestrictive clothing, and cool water immersion.

The conservation of body heat, less dramatic physiologically, is a more common phenomenon, since there is greater risk to life from unexpected or prolonged exposure to cold. Survival in water of 0° C unprotected is no more than 30 minutes. Actually one primary physiologic defense to cold, to shut down the cutaneous circulation, thus increasing the distance heat must be conducted to be lost at the surface, is inadequate for most environmental cold. We rely heavily on shelter and clothing. In pathologic conditions with inflammation, body heat loss can be impressive even with common protection at average temperatures, and the comfort of patients is compromised by their constant sense of chill. It is recognizing heat loss as it manifests the pathologic process and modifies the therapeutic management that is most important for our consideration in dermatology.

The Pilosebaceous-Apocrine Apparatus

The hair unit, including sebaceous and apocrine glands, develops in utero over the entire skin surface except the palms and soles. One would never see a furuncle, for example, an abscess of a hair follicle, on the palm, sole, or glans penis, unless the patient had had a skin graft from a hairy site. Before birth the apocrine portion of the hair-gland apparatus atrophies in most complexes, but persists as a full pilosebaceous-apocrine apparatus in the axillae and genital area, occasionally at the areolae of the breast, and about the umbilicus. The breast is actually a modified apocrine gland, as are the ceruminous glands of the ear and Moll's glands of the eyelid. At puberty apocrine glands enlarge to produce an oily, colorless substance, which remains odorless until bacterial decomposition results in a characteristic body odor. Individuals vary in the intensity of odor related to apocrine gland size and personal hygiene. Short chain fatty acids and ammonia are the major odorogenic products of bacterial degradation, but other unidentified substances in the sweat or on the skin could contribute to individual variations in the malodorous emanations.

A rare individual may have colored apocrine sweat, apocrine chromhidrosis, which can be axillary or exceptionally facial or, even more rarely, of the scalp, according to where vestigial apocrine glands are functional. Apart from concern and the need for reassurance, the nuisance of stained underclothing is a common complaint in those with axillary chromhidrosis. Most frequently yellow, the pigment can be green, blue, or blue-black and is attributed to one or more lipofuscins produced, for reasons unknown, within the apocrine gland. The staining must be distinguished from that resulting from surface pigments of corynebacteria or piedra, which thrive in the axilla and lend their pigment to colorless sweat after it leaves the sweat duct. The latter staining can be controlled with shaving and topical antimicrobial agents; true chromhidrosis cannot. Patients with ochronosis may stain axillary secretions or skin brown but have homogentisic acid in the urine.

As with eccrine sweat, apocrine secretions can be plugged, disrupting the duct, breaking into the dermis, and triggering intense pruritus with erythema. The problem, often provoked by emotional stimuli to apocrine excretion through adrenergic sympathetic discharge, is really an apocrine miliaria and is known as *Fox-Fordyce disease.* Usually involving the axillae, often the genital area, and occasionally the periareolar glands, the trapped apocrine sweat raises small discrete rounded lesions with a consequent relative apocrine anhidrosis. Therapy of variable success is aimed at reducing stimuli to apocrine sweating, limiting maceration from eccrine sweat, and counteracting the inflammatory response with topical and injectable steroids.

As distressing and persistent as apocrine miliaria may be, the severe disease of apocrine glands is the chronic, suppurative, and cicatricial problem known as *hidradenitis suppurativa.* It may involve the axillae exclusively, as it often does in women, or the anogenital area, or both; in some affected individuals it is associated with severe scarring acne, occasionally with cicatrizing perifolliculitis of the scalp, or a pilonidal cyst. Although an isolated axillary or inguinal lesion might be mistaken for an abscess, multiple lesions or recurrences, especially an associated acne or scalp problem, should suggest the diagnosis. Once made, vigorous antimicrobial therapy with topical preparations and systemic antibiotics is indicated to reduce smoldering infection and minimize sinus tract formation. Early surgery may reduce the number of glands at risk and abort a potentially devastating disease (Fig. 552–3).

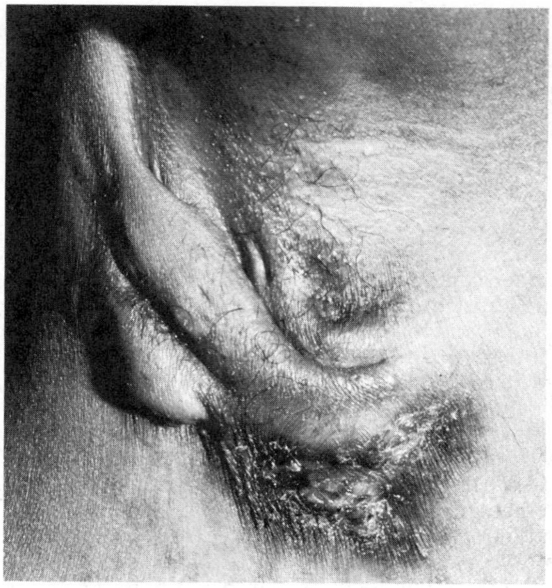

Figure 552–3. Hidradenitis suppurativa, axilla.

The *sebaceous gland* specialized for lipid synthesis is widely distributed over the body but concentrated in the scalp, face, upper back, and chest. Each hair follicle is associated with sebaceous glands, but the converse is not true. Some sebaceous glands without associated hairs open directly onto the surface and are known as sebaceous follicles; others, by reason of anatomic localization and modification, are singled out for special identification. In the buccal mucosa and at the vermilion border of the lip, for example, they are known as Fordyce's spots; around the female areola, as Montgomery's tubercles; at the prepuce, as Tyson's glands; and on the eyelids, as meibomian glands. As sebaceous glands they share in the pathophysiologic mechanisms to be considered; as normal anatomic structures they should not be confused with skin pathology.

The sebaceous gland depends upon and is extremely receptive to androgenic hormones. Maternal androgens ensure full development and function at birth. The vernix caseosa covering the neonate is mostly sebum. Normally the gland then atrophies until the child's pubertal hormones stimulate it once more. Sebaceous gland activity in children can result from congenital adrenal hyperplasia or anabolic hormone therapy as given in aplastic anemia. Disorders of androgen excess in adult women are associated with increased sebaceous gland activity. Androgen insufficiency in either sex such as hypogonadism or adrenal insufficiency is associated with decreased activity. Androgens increase the sebaceous gland size, increase the secretion of sebum, and increase sebaceous gland mitotic rate. Estrogens decrease gland size and secretion but do not decrease the mitotic rate. Their effect may be from the suppression of androgens primarily at sites of androgen synthesis rather than at the glandular level. In women, adrenal androgens in addition to gonadal androgens are a source of sebaceous stimulation. Progesterone in physiologic amounts has no effect, and the role of the pituitary is most likely indirect through tropic hormones. With severe caloric deprivation sebum secretion levels decrease.

The function of sebaceous gland lipid is in question. Although variously touted as a barrier to microbes or other hostile environment, as a regulator of percutaneous absorption, and as a vitamin D precursor, all these roles have been challenged. Further, skin conditions characterized by dry skin, such as ichthyosis or asteatosis, are allegedly associated with decreased sebum production, but without supporting data.

What is known is that sebaceous gland maturation, which begins at age eight to ten and continues through adolescence, remains fairly unchanged through adult life until it decreases some time past the fifth decade in women and the seventh decade in men. Patients with Parkinson's disease and postmenopausal women with breast cancer have statistically higher rates of sebum secretion than the average. Because the distribution of sebum levels overlaps with normal values, an individual reading has limited diagnostic importance.

The final portion of the pilosebaceous apparatus to be considered is the hair, and any understanding of hair implies some knowledge of its *growth cycle* and *pattern*. *Hair growth* can be reckoned in three phases: *telogen* when it is resting in its cornified sac, *anagen* when it is actively growing, and *catagen* when it is involuting. Throughout telogen, the resting hair is high in the follicle at the level of the arrector pili muscle, a stubby hair bulb resembling a club, and is inactive mitotically. When anagen begins, there is a burst of mitosis and downward growth. The newly formed hair shaft dislodges the old resting hair bulb, the club hair. With a hand lens a fallen or plucked hair can be determined from root inspection as having been resting or actively growing. Catagen is the brief respite when mitosis ceases and the hair pulls upward in the dermis and hair shaft to become a club hair. In the adult most hairs, 85 per cent, are in anagen at any given time, 14 per cent in telogen, and 1 per cent in catagen.

Hair growth cycles vary with *hair type*, of which there are several in humans. Vellus hair is fine, soft, short, nonpigmented, and common to "nonhairy" areas of the body. Its anagen phase is short and telogen long. A terminal hair is coarse, long, pigmented, and located in "hairy" areas—scalp, beard, eyebrow, eyelash, axilla, and pubes. The ratio of the duration of anagen to telogen in terminal hairs varies. It is short and equal for eyebrows, but for scalp hair anagen is long, two to six years, and telogen short, about three months. Hair length depends upon duration of active growth compared to that of resting.

Acute disease, high fever, and gross metabolic illness can all markedly affect the hair cycle. Classic postfebrile hair loss tends to be diffuse, with the loss first noted two to three months after the fever. The suggested mechanism is that the altered physiologic state stuns the actively growing follicles into a resting state. Following the ordinary physiologic pattern, the hair rests for three months, then is shed at the time new growth begins, a phenomenon called *telogen effluvium*. Excessive hair fall may continue over a month or more. Stress as from anesthesia, normal delivery, or psychic shock may do the same. Malabsorption or the serious malnutrition of kwashiorkor often has an associated severe hair loss. Debilitated chronically ill patients may lose hair, too, but more often they merely note change in texture. Depletion of dietary protein, anemia, and iron deficiency can be correlated with damaged hair shafts, suggesting insults insufficient to trigger the resting phase but enough to deform the hair. Complete disruption can follow more severe deprivation.

Interference with essential amino acid incorporation, as suggested for the effect of thallium ingestion, leads to a fracture of the hair shaft within the follicle. Once used for depilation in the therapy of scalp fungus, hair shedding occurs about one week after treatment. In an unsuspected (or intended) ingestion of rat poison containing thallium, hair loss should be anticipated, a so-called *anagen effluvium*, since the fall occurs during the active phase of the follicle cycle. Similar alopecias are seen with the antimitotic agents used in chemotherapy. Hair fall following exposure to X-irradiation occurs at a dose of no more than 300 R because of the exquisite sensitivity of the germinal layers of the hair follicle. Only growing hairs are affected; hence scalp and beard where most hairs are in anagen show the greatest fall, which occurs spontaneously in two weeks and regrows in two to three months. Permanent epilation depends on dose; 1200 R or so is usually required for permanent destruction of the hair follicles of the scalp. The damage can be dose related, for if mitosis is merely impaired, not halted, the hair shaft may not be disrupted but merely narrowed, as with methotrexate therapy for psoriasis or colchicine for gout. Heparin and coumarin, although they, too, show some mitotic inhibition, have their full effect through shunting anagen follicles into telogen until occasionally as many as half the follicles are at rest. At two to three months after the initiation of anticoagulant therapy, hair will fall; the cosmetic significance of the alopecia will depend upon the original density of hair growth and the percentage of follicles in telogen.

In many instances hair loss may be anticipated or its cause immediately identified. Even with the sparse or absent scalp hair of congenital ectodermal defects, the diagnosis is apparent from the history, perhaps reinforced by pedigree, and the physician feels no compulsion to justify the defect. With alopecia areata, however, there is a difference. Of obscure etiology, it is a problem of increased incidence in patients with autoimmune disease, Addison's disease, diabetes mellitus, or vitiligo. It commonly presents as one or two small circumscribed bald areas, usually of the scalp, which may not progress but in some few patients will increase in size, coalesce, and extend until all scalp hair is lost (alopecia totalis) or all body hair (alopecia universalis). Exclamation point hairs, 3 mm or so in length and tapered toward the skin surface, are diagnostic if present. As hair regrows it may, at first, be devoid of pigment; even the alopecic skin itself may share in the pigment loss. Most patients with alopecia areata will do well; four out of five will get full regrowth of hair. Initially the course is unpredictable but deserves guarded optimism. However, when the alopecia is extensive, recurs, is associated with nail dystrophy, or lasts more than a year, the prognosis for recovery is not good.

In the instances of hair loss cited thus far, the scalp, on inspection, appears as normal skin devoid of some or all hair. There is no scarring. When inflammatory and infiltrative diseases affect the scalp so as to produce hair loss, the basic lesion is grossly evident. The hair is lost because of the pathologic process disrupting and perhaps destroying the hair follicle. This is true even with traction alopecia when the pull of hair styles or the self-plucking of hairs, consciously or unconsciously as in trichotillomania, leads to the permanent damage of the hair follicles and occasionally their destruction.

As to *growth pattern*, the hair follicles common to both sexes that produce the same type of hair in pre- and postpubertal individuals are not hormone dependent. Others, common to both sexes, are androgen dependent, such as the conversion of vellus to terminal hair in the axillae, the lower pubic triangle, and the temporal area of the scalp. In males responding to higher concentration of androgens there is a conversion from vellus to terminal hair in the follicles of the beard, ears, nasal tip, sternum, and upper pubic triangle. At the same time on a genetic basis some terminal hair may change to vellus in the vertex and frontal regions of the scalp, with slow recession of the anterior hair line to produce male pattern baldness. Similar pattern loss occurs in women but rarely progresses to the total bare crown seen in men. In both, hereditary factors influence the time of onset, pattern, and severity, with androgen playing an undisputed role. Castration interrupts pattern baldness in males, and masculinizing diseases of women produce baldness subject to genetic predisposition.

Hypertrichosis and Hirsutism

Excessive hair growth may be genetically determined, as in a nevus, or from repeated local trauma, as with weights carried on the shoulders. It may be generalized and appear after encephalitis or with the onset of multiple sclerosis. It is seen in dermatomyositis and is induced by drugs such as phenytoin. Although the reason for the increased hair may be obscure, an association can be made with a genetic determinant or recognized problem.

Hirsutism, however, a term used mainly for the excessive growth of coarse terminal hair occurring in women in the adult male distribution, is more of a diagnostic challenge. In most, the hair growth is idiopathic without underlying pathology. Genetic and racial differences are considerable, and their recognition may help differentiate a familial problem from an underlying masculinizing process. If there is no menstrual abnormality, no male pattern balding, no increase in muscle mass or deepening of the voice, and a normal pelvic examination, the problem should probably not be pursued further. On the other hand, diffuse vellus hairs occurring suddenly over the face of women past 40 should arouse suspicion of underlying malignancy.

Aging and Actinic Damage

With age, the epidermis thins and the skin appendages atrophy. Hair becomes sparse and sebaceous secretions decrease, with consequent susceptibility to dryness, chapping, and fissuring. The dermis diminishes with loss of elastic and collagen fibers—hence loss of elasticity and support for dermal vessels easily visualized and readily ruptured (senile purpura).

Sunlight exposure wreaks far greater destruction on the skin than time itself, however, as the contrast between covered and exposed skin clearly shows, even in the skin of the elderly. It intensifies and augments the aging process. Sun-damaged skin is thin, wrinkled, and variably hyperpigmented with fine thread-like telangiectatic vessels and small erythematous scaling patches of actinic keratoses. Yellow papules in a reticulated pattern may occur on the nose and forehead. Comedones and follicular cysts appear in the periorbital region. The back of the neck becomes thickened. Histologically collagen is replaced by amorphous or granular material of slightly basophilic stain on hematoxylin and eosin preparation. Called elastotic, it gives its name to the clinical observation of thinning and sagging, senile elastosis.

553. THE EXAMINATION OF THE SKIN

The traditional approach to the medical patient is to elicit the chief complaint and elaborate the history before seeking supportive clinical findings. The dermatologist on the contrary looks first, with an eye trained to see and recognize, his hand lens being more important than his stethoscope. He has the advantages of concurrent review—the history of the present illness often being written for him in the skin—markers of genetic predisposition, and even something of the patient's physiologic age and exposure to the elements and to actinic radiation. It is all there: the ectoderm and the mesoderm; the blood vessels and the nerves; the collagen, the elastin, the ground substance. It is there and sharing, perhaps, in an inflammatory, metabolic, or even neoplastic change that is widespread in the body but comes to focus first in the skin. Dermatology is a visual specialty, and its excitement derives from the direct and patent entry into general medicine that the skin provides, and from the clarity with which pathologic processes can be assessed and followed. It is a showcase for reaction patterns and for responses to therapy.

For the examination of the skin, to see *what* is there and *all* that is there is the only cardinal rule. Good lighting is essential. Nonglaring north light is best for both lesion configuration and true color, but a mix of fluorescent bulbs to simulate daylight is acceptable. It can never be too bright, but the capability of side lighting in a darkened room is also useful for detecting minimally raised and depressed lesions.

The skin should be observed from head to toe in a routine repetitive way so that no orifice or appendage is overlooked. For the writer, the horizontal patient completely disrobed and covered with a sheet is easiest to examine in a systematic way. In the *supine* position the frontal scalp is examined first, then the face, with special attention to the eyes (conjunctiva, iris and pupil, eyelids), followed by the ears, nose, lips, mouth (observing mucosa and dentition), pharynx, neck, thorax, abdomen, genital area, anterior legs, and then the fingernails, forearms, and arms, anterior and posterior. With the patient changed to the *prone* position and the knees flexed, the feet, toenails, and webs can be examined easily, next the posterior aspect of the legs, the perianal and sacral area, the back, lower and upper, nuchal area, and then the full scalp to complete the round. By uncovering only limited areas of the body at a time the patient is mostly covered and comfortable throughout the examination. If the presenting complaint has been only a finger wart, the surprised patient is usually reassured that his integument has been assessed for present or potential pathology and good preventive medicine has been practiced.

After having surveyed the entire skin surface, *generalized observation* warrants first notation. A blue man with argyria, the result of silver deposits in sweat glands and elastic fibers, may present with a fungus infection. Although the pigmentation may be untreatable and permanent, it nonetheless is an important part of his dermatologic assessment. So, too, is the *pattern of a problem.* Skin change following a dermatome distribution is significant. At a distance a segmental color change over the thorax might suggest a diagnostic differential between herpes zoster and nevus, but on close inspection viral vesicles would resolve the diagnosis. The limitation of the specific viral lesions to a dermatome makes the presumptive diagnosis. It underscores the importance of the pattern of appearance—important for description and the diagnostic process, as well as for the record for others to interpret.

The examiner, then, must be aware of the whole skin and the pattern of the problem before focusing on specific lesions. He will have noted signs of aging, trauma, pigment response, general turgor, nutrition, and hygiene. He will attempt to assess the pathology he notes with reference to configuration and anatomic location. Distribution may follow innervation, as in the dermatome, or vascular patterns, as in the reticulated changes in mottled skin of chilled swimmers, cutis marmorata. The pathology may be localized or generalized, perhaps universal, involving the entire integument, including hair and nails. Most important, the examiner will try to assess what physical change has occurred in the skin. Is it flushed or blanched? If red, is it the hot bright red of infection or the cool blue red of a connective tissue disorder? He will attempt to make a microscopic judgment and decide whether the skin surface is normal or thickened, raised or flat, infiltrated with cells and at what level, filled with fluid, filled with pus, freely movable, bound down, atrophic, excoriated, or ulcerated.

Often the consultation request proffers dermatologic terms that bear no relation to the lesion described. It is far better to call an urticarial lesion a hive, or a lesion resembling a mosquito bite, than to define it as an erythematous papule, which is interpreted differently by the indoctrinated. Terms are useful in descriptive interchange, but if they defeat the honest analysis of the pathophysiologic process, their value is lost.

Despite this conviction, it is necessary to provide some guide to the description of pathologic changes in skin (Fig. 553–1). A defined lesion that leaves the epidermis and dermis unchanged except in color is a *macule.* Stroking the lesion and adjacent normal skin with eyes closed resolves any doubt; the macule cannot be distinguished. If the surface is raised in a circumscribed way by an infiltrate of cells or change in anatomic thickness, the lesion is a *papule* and should be further described as rounded or flat-topped, perhaps as angular, smooth, or verrucuous (the roughness of a wart), and by color. If penetration of the process into the dermis gives greater substance and depth, the lesion is *nodular* rather than papular. Either may be a sac for entrapped cellular debris and secretions, a *cyst,* suspected by the palpation of a soft center.

For wheals or hives, edema in the upper dermis produces raised rounded or plateau-like evanescent lesions known as *urticaria,* which, according to size, may be ordinary or giant. Trapped fluid in the skin produces a *vesicle* if the blister is less than 0.5 cm, a *bulla* if larger. The anatomic level of the fluid and its cellular content will affect translucency and stability. Significant vesicles may be so numerous as to become confluent and indistinguishable as vesicles, presenting instead as a weeping denuded area. Superficial bullae also rupture easily and in the mouth are rarely seen intact. Ones that occur more deeply, such as friction blisters, can persist, and some may be so overlayered with skin that it is difficult to distinguish them from a papule. When the fluid-filled sac contains abundant neutrophils, with or without bacteria, it is considered a *pustule.* If it occurs anatomically related to a pilosebaceous apparatus, it is a follicular pustule, usually conical, and with a protruding hair.

When skin is abnormal and raised over a relatively large but circumscribed area, the term *plaque* is used. If the skin surface is denuded, it may just be a superficial *erosion;* if the defect penetrates into the dermis, it is an *ulcer.* Coagulated blood elements can provide a *crust* for such lesions. When the deeper ones heal, there will be scar, pink and vascularized at first, then *atrophic,* i.e., white and avascular. Healing could occur with an exuberant pink raised hypertrophic scar that subsequently flattens or perhaps persists as a fibrous, rubbery cicatrix, a *keloid.* Even without recognized injury the skin may become depressed, with the normal skin markings and appendages diminished or effaced. Such *atrophy* can be part of a pathologic process or may result from such topical therapy as steroids.

In contrast to atrophic change, the skin in certain conditions may be thickened with accentuation of the normal epidermal pattern, as is caused by rubbing, *lichenification;* or the thickness may be from *scale,* flaking keratin, that may be loose or adherent, thick as an oyster shell (ostraceous), or fine as cigarette paper; scale may be dry or greasy and slough in a localized desquamation or generalized exfoliation.

Finally, the descriptive process will reflect pigment, its presence or absence, and the vascular changes that affect skin color,

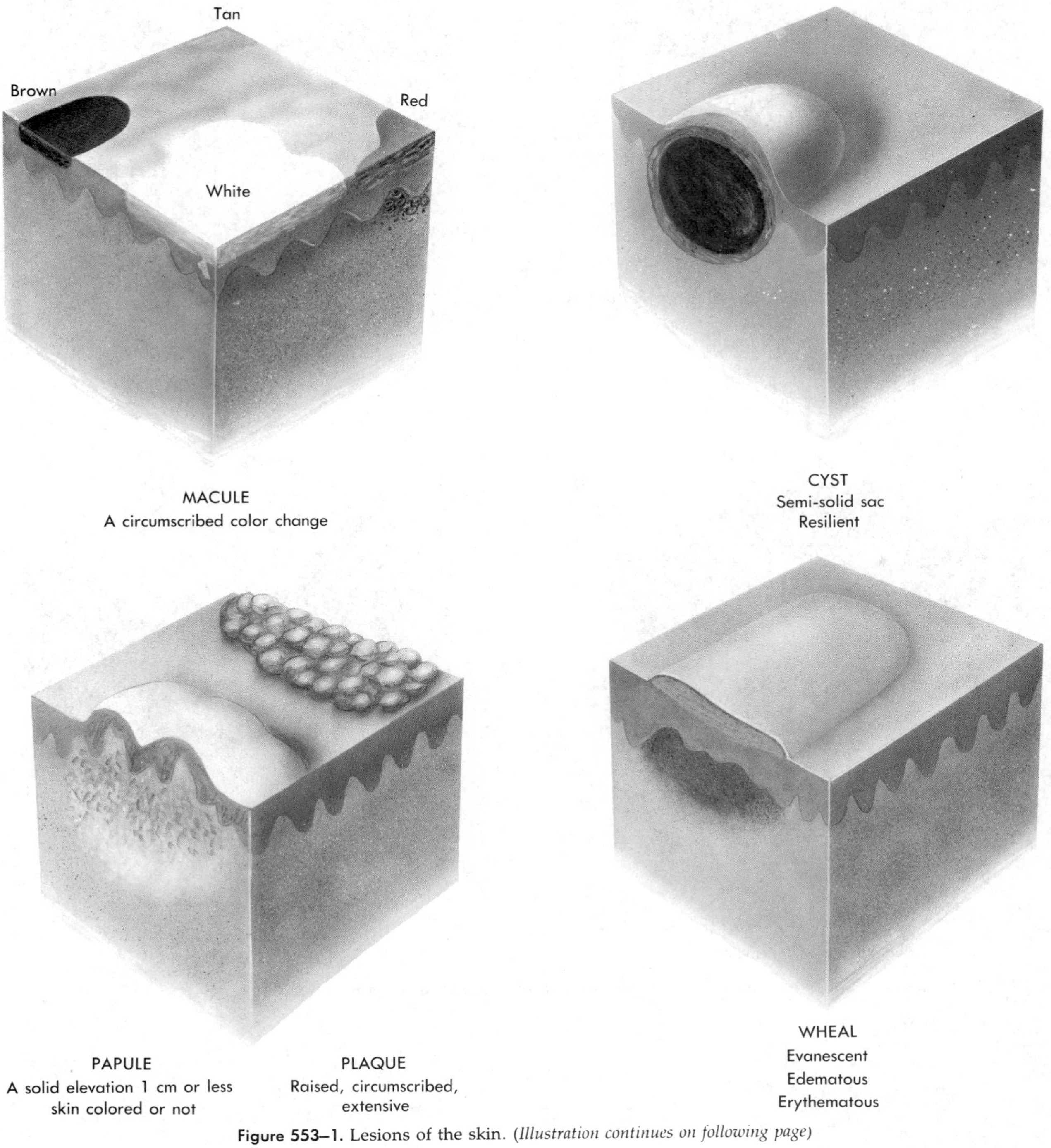

Figure 553–1. Lesions of the skin. *(Illustration continues on following page)*

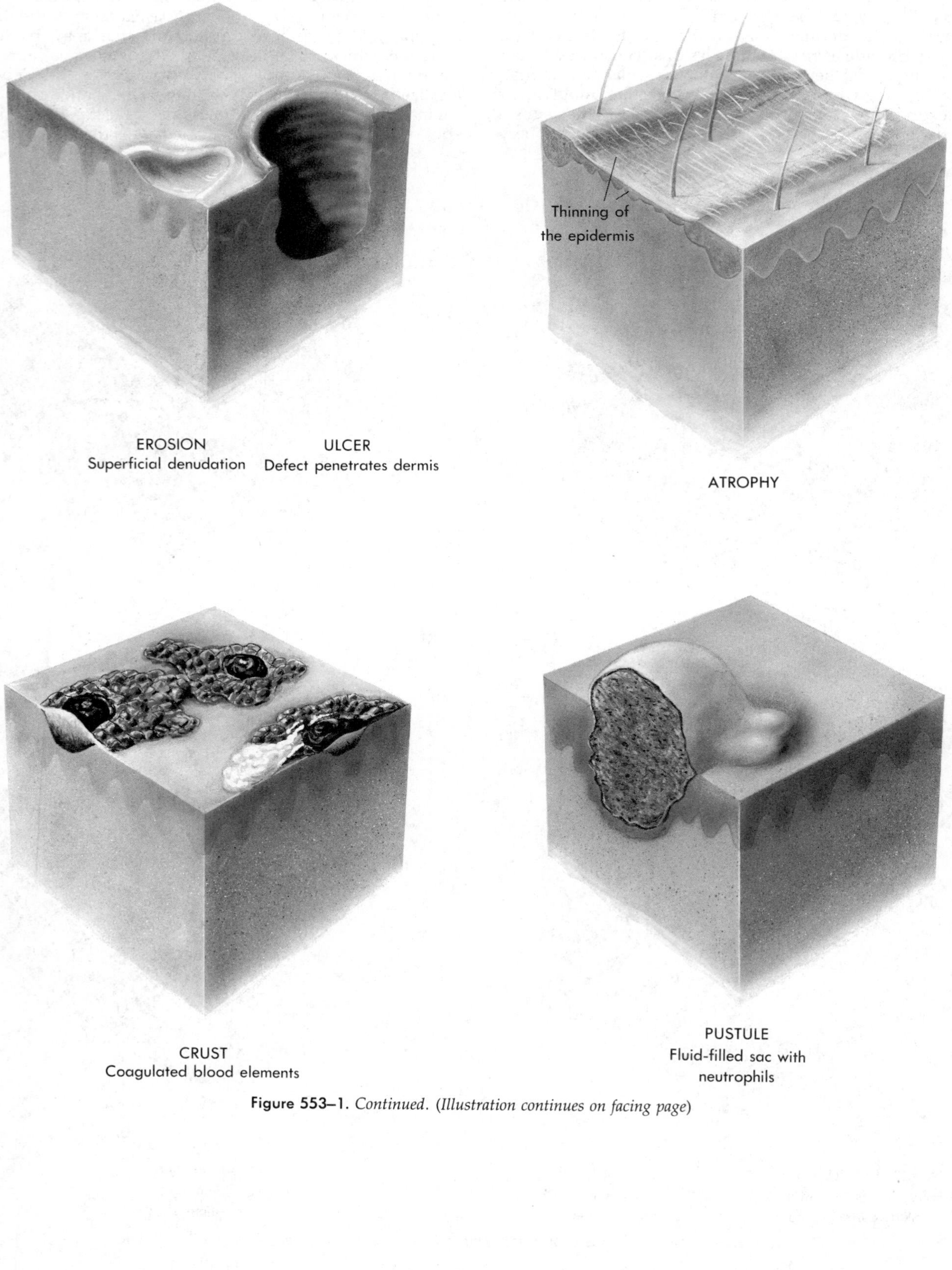

Figure 553–1. *Continued. (Illustration continues on facing page)*

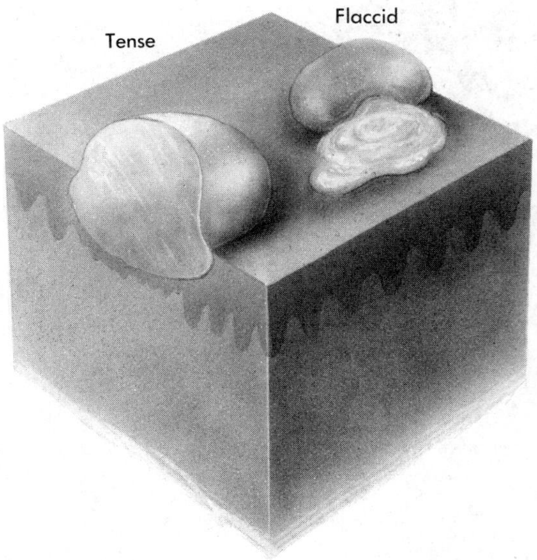

BULLAE
Fluid-filled
0.5 cm or larger

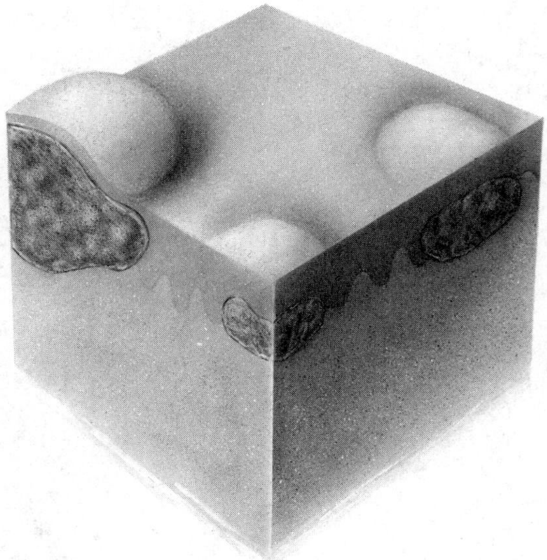

NODULE
Solid deeper lesion

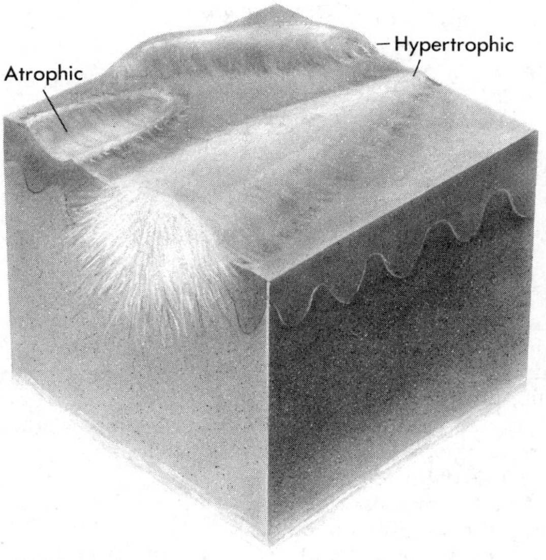

SCAR

Figure 553–1. *Continued. (Illustration continues on following page)*

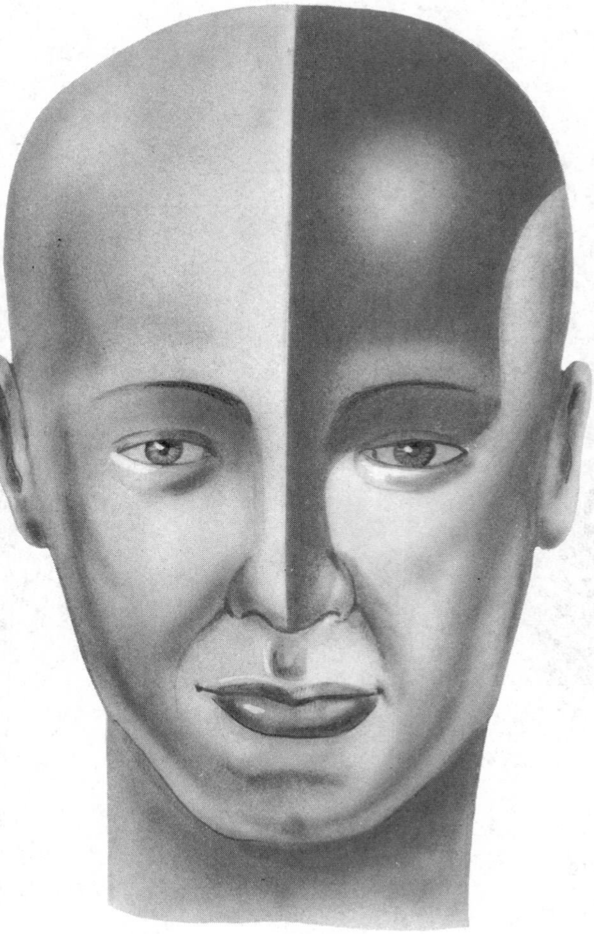
ZOSTERIFORM

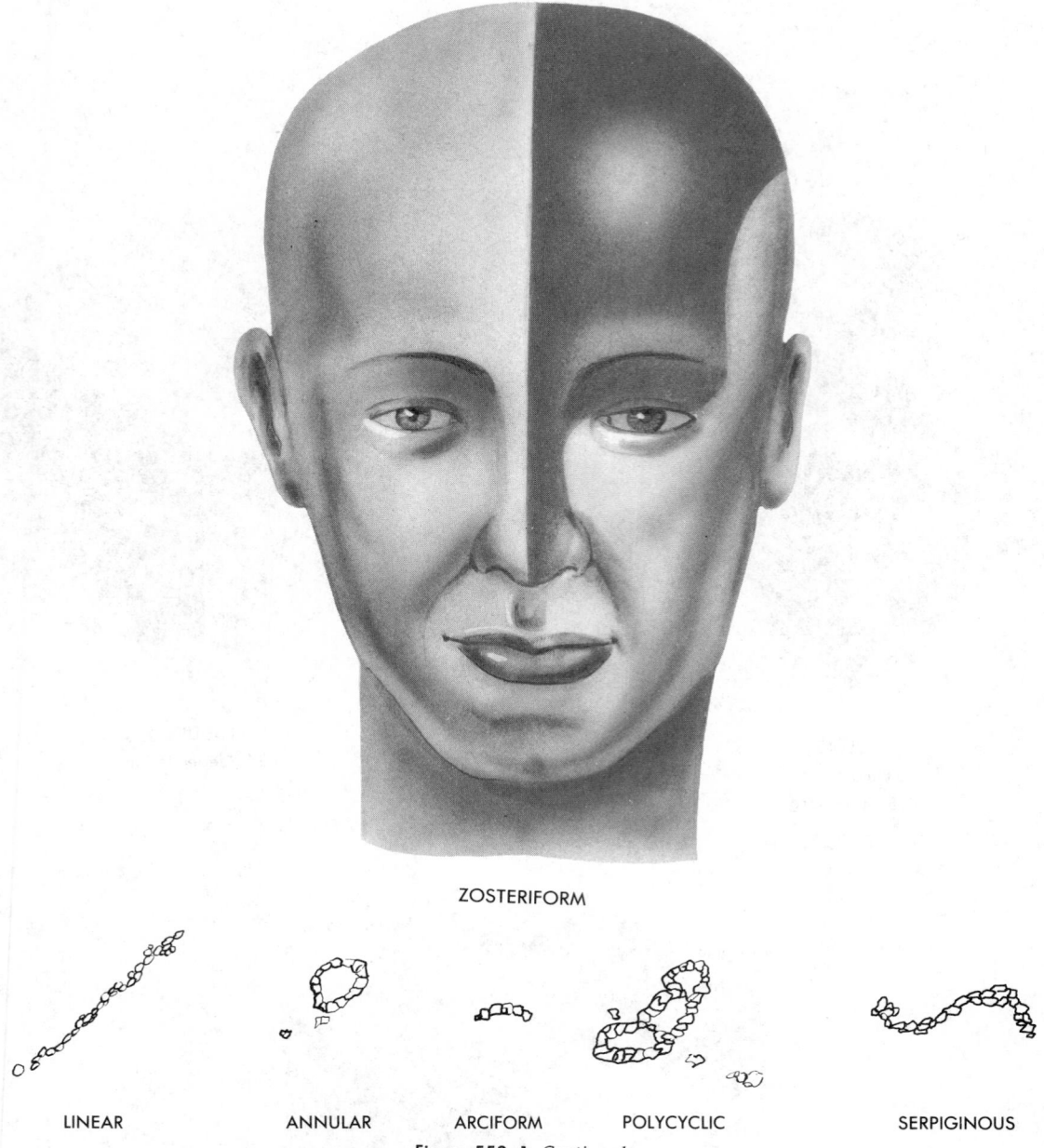

LINEAR
ANNULAR
ARCIFORM
POLYCYCLIC
SERPIGINOUS

Figure 553–1. *Continued.*

not only physiologically because of blood flow, but because of anatomic considerations. Lips, red or blue, are transparent to blood color because of a thin to absent stratum corneum. New vessel growth or suffusion can produce hemangiomas. Superficial wispy dilated vessels, *fine telangiectasia,* one of the stigmata of solar damage, may, without the hand lens, be mistaken for erythema; coarse telangiectasia would not, but should be identified for its association with acrosclerosis, for example, and roentgen damage where it is found with atrophy and pigmentary change. The trick is to see what is present in the skin without prejudice and to tabulate the data without premature interpretation.

With the distribution of lesions noted and their pattern of arrangement determined, whether in a dermatome (zosteriform) or linear (/), annular (○), arciform (∩), polycyclic (∞), or serpiginous (~), the individual lesion can be assessed according to the broad description given. The eye may detect different kinds of lesions which in fact may be the same at different stages of development, or a primary lesion that has been subjected to the trauma of scratching or secondary infection or perhaps to an adverse reaction to therapy. The search for the representative lesion should yield the most typical and the most recent.

SUPPORTING TESTS

TZANCK SMEAR (Fig. 553–2). If the primary lesion is a vesicle or bulla, a rapid cytologic examination known as the Tzanck test can be helpful. The vesicle or bulla is unroofed with a sterile scissors and the base curetted lightly with the blunt side of a scalpel. A smear is made and stained with Wright's or Giemsa's stain to reveal the multinucleated epidermal giant cells of a viral infection or the rounded acantholytic cells devoid of their intercellular bridges, a phenomenon present in certain blistering diseases and in viral vesicles as well, but not in friction blisters or burns or in the vesicles of contact dermatitis.

THE KOH TEST AND CULTURE. Should the primary problem be a circumscribed scaling dermatitis of the sort that suggests a

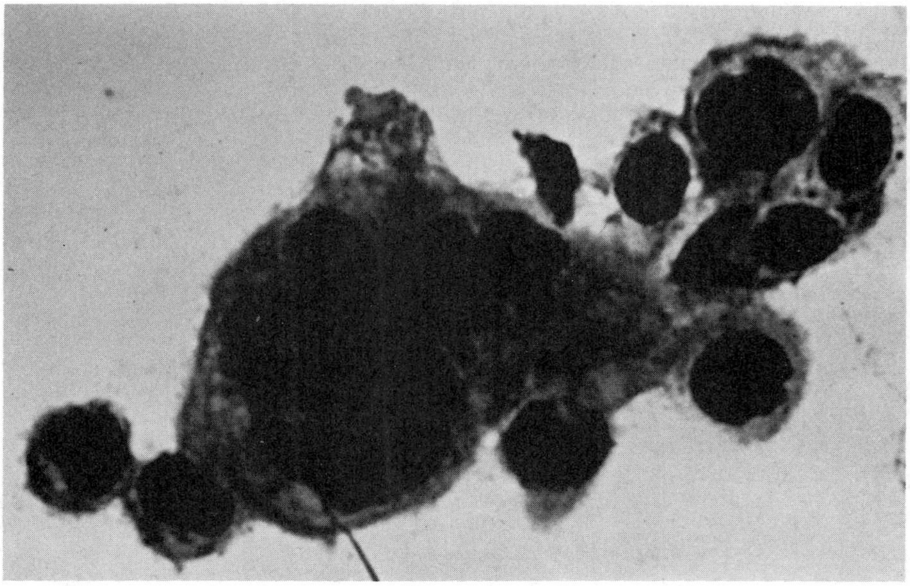

Figure 553–2. Positive Tzanck smear, herpes simplex.

diagnosis of fungus, a very simple examination for the presence of mycelia should be done. After heating a sample of scale with 10 per cent potassium hydroxide to dissolve the keratin (and a drop of methylene blue to improve visualization), fungal elements, if present, can be observed by direct microscopic examination (Fig. 553–3). The scale should be cultured in Sabouraud's medium to establish the identity of the fungus involved. If repeated attempts to visualize hyphae and grow fungus are negative, the diagnosis of mycotic infection is certainly in question.

WOOD'S LIGHT. Examination under long wave ultraviolet light will be helpful in detecting hair and skin infected with fungi that fluoresce at 360 nm; it is important for diagnosis and for plucking infected hairs for culture.

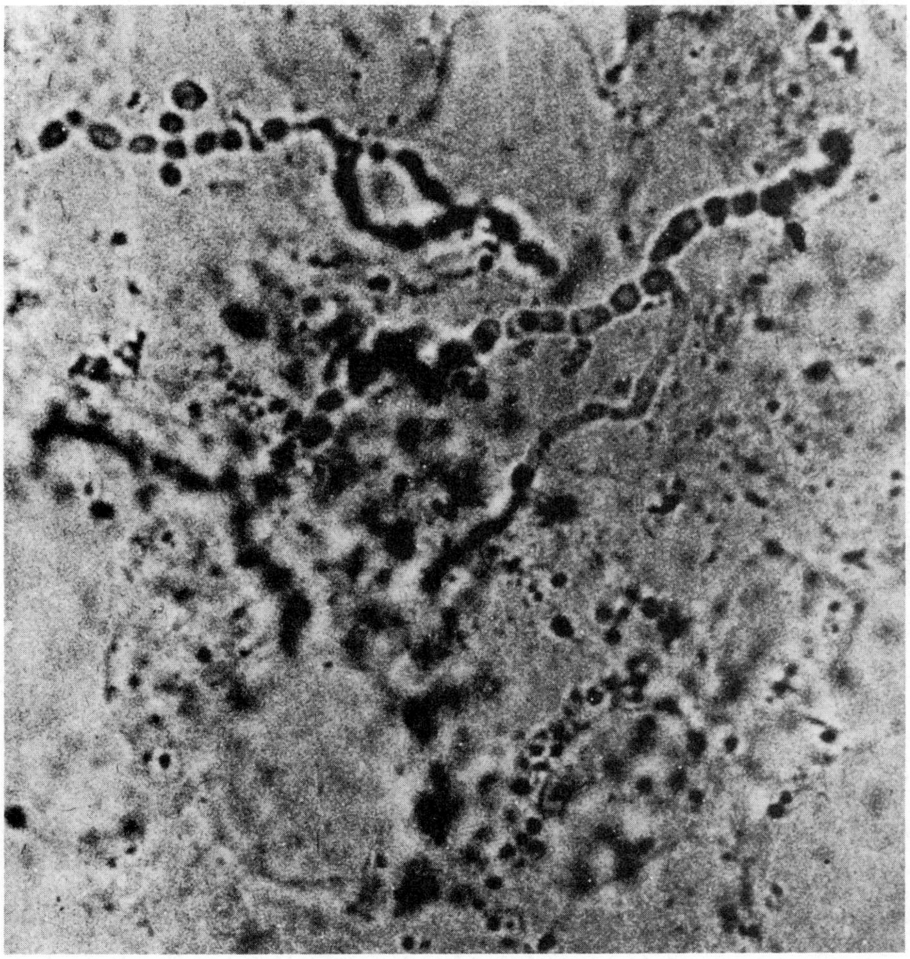

Figure 553–3. KOH preparation, high power.

Wood's filter, made of nickel oxide and silica fitted to a high pressure mercury lamp, is opaque to all light under 320 nm and above 400 nm. Inspection under Wood's light is also useful in differentiating between hypo- and depigmented areas of skin, an important diagnostic clue, and in detecting porphyrins in the urine of patients suspected of having porphyria.

BACTERIOLOGIC CULTURES. When the primary lesion is a pustule, bacteriologic cultures should be taken, especially if it is suspected that a micrococcus may be the etiologic agent. The nephritogenic strains of the *Streptococcus* are associated with glomerulonephritis, and certain strains of *Staphylococcus pyogenes* as well as the *Streptococcus* can produce a severe infection with bright erythema and extensive desquamation.

DIASCOPY. If it is unclear whether the redness of a macule is erythema from dilated capillaries or the purpura of extravasated blood, observation under firm pressure through clear glass or plastic will reveal the difference. The purpura is not compressible to pallor. Pressure with a glass slide is also useful in detecting the "apple jelly" glassy fawn-colored papules of granulomatous disease such as occur in the mycobacterial infections of lupus vulgaris and swimming pool granuloma, or even in sarcoidosis and lymphoma.

BIOPSY. Of all that may be done to aid the assessment of the primary lesion, the very best is to re-examine it with the clinical eye, using magnification greater than the hand lens, and to see

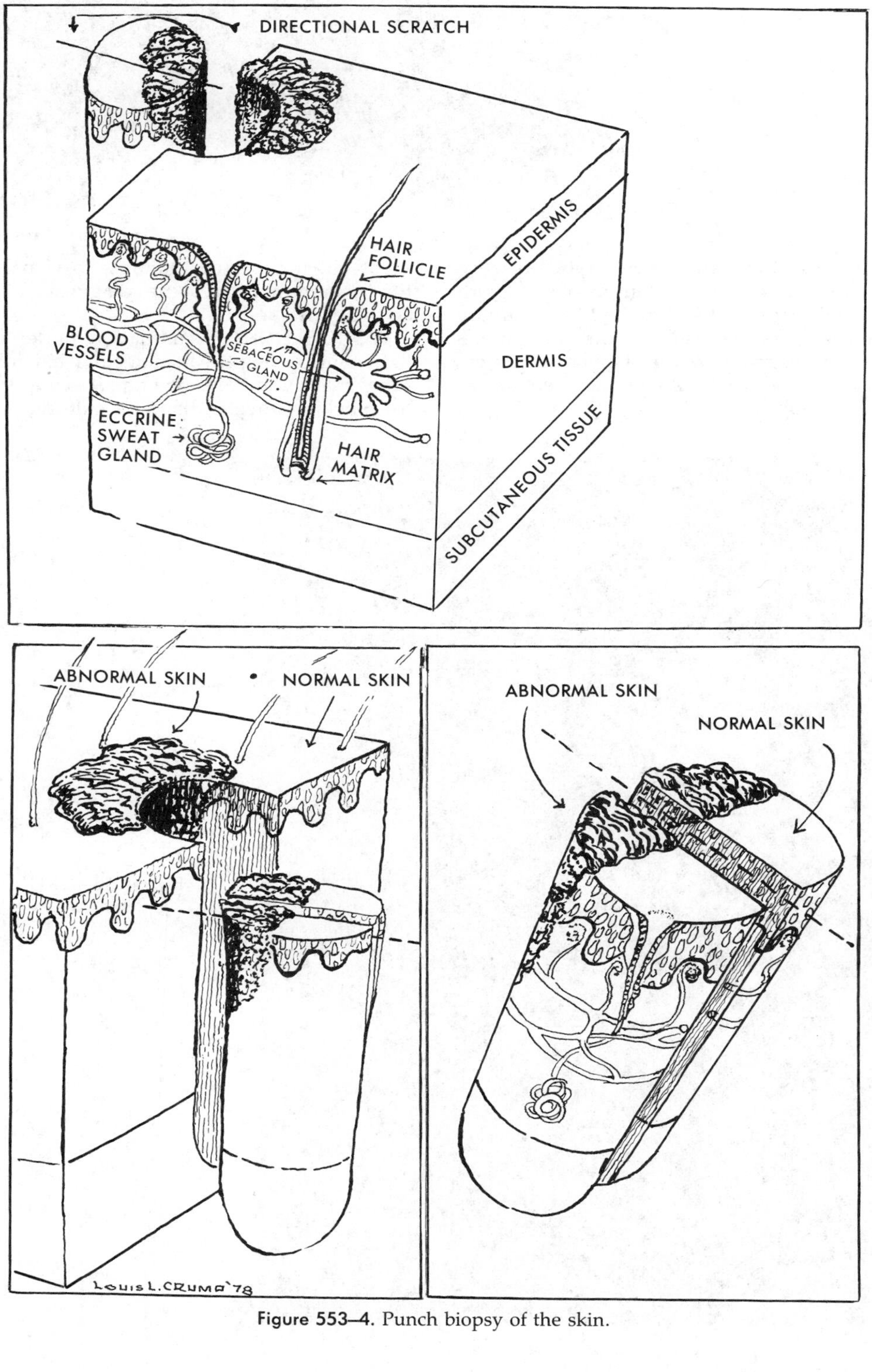

Figure 553–4. Punch biopsy of the skin.

it in cross-section. The biopsy has no magic other than the wonderment of seeing precisely what is going on at every level of the skin. For this to be pertinent, we must be looking at a representative lesion, and for best comparisons we should see it against the patient's normal skin for that area.

For the most complete histopathologic assessment, especially if for reasons of concern or cosmetics the lesion is to be removed, an elliptical excision is best. One procedure removes the lesion, secures tissue for diagnosis, and leaves a defect easily sutured. Of greater speed and ease is the punch biopsy, which at 2 mm is hardly more than a venipuncture but permits adequate tissue to be removed and examined. After anesthetizing the site with deep rather than superficial infiltration to avoid histologic distortion, a tubular blade bears through the skin by slight rotary motion, clockwise and back, to the depth of the subcutis. By light external pressure with a curved iris scissors astride the plug, the specimen lifts without the distorting pressure of forceps and can be easily clipped at its base through the loose subcutaneous tissue. The plug gently lifted to absorbent paper attaches upright, the fat adherent to the paper, the epidermis on top. Such orientation and some detailed instruction for fixing and sectioning is needed by even the most experienced technician who is unaccustomed to handling small specimens.

To enhance the value of the biopsy by contrast with normal tissue, the excision should, if possible, cut through normal and abnormal tissue, but here the laboratory will need a diagram (Fig. 553–4), and in addition a prebiopsy directional scratch on the skin sample made with a scalpel to establish the direction for histopathologic sectioning. Rotating the sections 90 degrees could provide all lesion or, most distressing, all normal skin.

For the punch biopsy suturing is not necessary for hemostasis; a Gelfoam plug to fill the defect or Monsel's solution (ferric subsulfate solution) on an applicator stick will suffice, but the cosmetic result will not be as fine as with a suture. Anatomic location and convenience of suture removal will influence the choice.

554. PRINCIPLES OF THERAPY

Before considering more detailed diagnostic formulations, it is possible to look at therapy as it seeks to correct the pathologic situation observed. Specific metabolic changes and cell infiltrates, as with lymphomas, will require a particular treatment regimen for management, but, apart from these, there is a broad group of pathologic changes that can be reversed and symptoms alleviated by therapeutic maneuvers directed toward restoration to the normal state.

The skin that is undergoing an *inflammatory* response with coalescent allergic or viral vesicles, so that it quite figuratively "weeps," requires a reduction of heat and a drying of the serous ooze through evaporation and coagulation of serum proteins. Superimposed infection will require antimicrobial therapy; debridement may be indicated. All of this can be accomplished with the wet dressing.

WET DRESSINGS

OPEN WET DRESSINGS. The prototype is a piece of undyed finely woven cloth, cotton or linen, thoroughly wet with clear water, wrung out so as not to drip, and then applied to the skin. Considered solely for its physical effects, the water evaporates, cooling and drying the underlying skin. As the cloth dries and is removed to be reimmersed, it cleanses. To get maximal benefit from evaporation, the dressing should not be more than a layer or two thick and should be changed every 15 to 30 minutes, depending on the ambient temperature and humidity. If permitted to dry completely and become adherent, the debriding effect will be greater, perhaps damaging. Remoistening the dressing in place may be needed to facilitate removal.

The wet dressing described can be initiated anywhere, even on a camping trip. In ordinary practice, however, the effectiveness of the wet dressing can be enhanced by medications added to the water. A mild protein precipitant, aluminum acetate, serves to coagulate bacterial and serum protein. As a 5 per cent preparation it is known as Burow's solution, and it must be further diluted for use. Appropriate concentrations, indications, and modes of prescribing various medications are shown for convenience in Table 554–1. If infection is a complication, potassium permanganate or silver nitrate should be in the wet dressing, but with precautions; potassium permanganate is a poison and must be kept from children's reach. Both preparations stain the skin and everything else they touch. Patient compliance will be improved by forewarnings. To use rubber gloves to protect nails from becoming brown, for example, and to use disposable containers for mixing solutions and plastic liners for sinks and tubs if porcelain is old or porous will reduce the burden of therapy. One further caution concerns the maneuver of removing the wet dressing to reimmerse the cloth rather than basting on new solution. Although important to enhance the cleansing effect, it is absolutely essential with potassium permanganate and silver nitrate, in which evaporation can permit the solute to increase in the dressing to concentrations sufficient to cause irritation or chemical burn.

The question is often raised about the use of antimicrobial agents in wet dressings. Apart from the risk of sensitization which limits the topical use of penicillin and neomycin, the quantities needed for adequate concentration in the dressing would make their use exceedingly inefficient and wasteful. The same might be said for enzymic preparations for debridement. Although the physical effects of the wet dressing would be helpful to reduce erythema and free tissue, the manipulations of the wet dressings would deactivate the enzymes prematurely. When required, they are best used separately as creams or gels.

Wet dressings, if needed at all, are needed three to four hours a day divided according to the patient's schedule. Although best split into four to five treatments of equal duration, two or three ten-minute dressings with the balance in the evening or whenever the patient is free are preferable to one solid four-hour block in the evening. Use of long narrow wrappers the length of a forearm or whole leg, just wide enough to circumvent it once, pinned top, bottom, and in between, obviates winding as with an Ace bandage, and hence is fast. Knowing that the dressing can be secured and ordinary work continued gives the patient a sense of release from an imprisoning routine. Dermatologic treatments can be time consuming and a nuisance; patients would much rather swallow a pill. The physician's attention to convenience and realistic scheduling may mean the difference between treatment and no treatment.

TABLE 554–1. USE OF WET DRESSINGS

Condition	Ingredient	Effect	Prescribed	Prepared Preparation H_2O	Approximate Final Concentration
Eczematous	AlAc (Burow's solution)	Protein coagulation	Tablets or powder packets	1 tab/packet 500 ml 1 tab/packet 1000 ml	1:20 1:40
Mild infection	$AgNO_3$	Antimicrobial (especially gram-negative)	10% stock solution 25% stock solution	10 ml 1000 ml 5 ml 1000 ml	1:1000 1:800
Infection	$KMnO_4$	Antimicrobial	Tab 300 mg	1 tab 1500 ml 1 tab 3000 ml	1:5000 1:10,000

BATHS AND SOAKS. Should the need for wet dressings be extensive—head to toe or even half that—it requires little imagination to sense the chilling experience of lying naked under a wet sheet. It matters little that the initial temperature of the wet dressing was warm. Actually the solution need be of no set temperature. It should neither chill nor scald and is best at a temperature that the patient finds comfortable. However, evaporation from a wet dressing over an extensive surface of inflamed skin will soon cause chill. The useful alternative is to immerse the total body in water of selected temperature which permits regulated cooling; if starch powders are added to the bath, there will be an after-film and a drying effect. With infections potassium permanganate can be added to the tub. To protect against undissolved crystals burning the skin, tablets crushed with a hammer in fibrous paper should be dissolved in a small container and the solution decanted into the bath. When infection or necrotic debris is a problem in a limited area, such as the draining sinus tracts of a diabetic toe, foot immersion in appropriate medication serves as a limited therapeutic bath. Because there is the mechanical need to force the solution to the depths of the tract, such irrigation is difficult to achieve except with immersion. The same can be said for the treatment of pilonidal cysts and for many anogenital problems.

CLOSED WET DRESSINGS. The need for the open wet dressing or immersion soak will diminish as inflammation subsides, lesions dry, and draining infection is controlled. Further, not all lesions are benefited by cooling and drying. A patient with much retained keratin of the palms or soles or even generalized scaling may need maceration rather than drying. Another with an early abscess may need heat to focalize the infection. For these problems the *open* wet dressing can be covered with an impervious material to induce maceration and heat retention and to enhance penetration of a specific medication; it thereby becomes known as a *closed* wet dressing, prescribed because of need for its physical effects. Compared to the open dressing, its use is infrequent. However, it can be inadvertently created when a fastidious nurse or patient covers the open wet dressing with plastic to protect the bedclothing or furniture. The routine instructions for open wet dressings should include a warning about covering with plastic. Although it is unlikely that any significant harm has come from the extended or untimely use of open wet dressings, the inadvertent or injudicious use of occlusion can lead to a phenomenon in which a pruritic papular eruption occurs at the site of active dermatitis and then distally in body folds, and may even progress to become generalized. Unfortunately termed "autosensitization," the phenomenon is nonetheless very real.

TOPICAL THERAPY

In the general approach to therapy, wet dressings are but the beginning. Topical medications are the mainstay. Their array can be bewildering if some basic principles of selection are overlooked. They must be sorted out by active ingredients, but equal importance must be given to the vehicle that contains the active preparation.

BASES. Topicals vary in their base from lotions, through creams, to ointments. Beginning at one side of the spectrum with the simplest shake lotion, talc in water, there is a progression of relative concentrations of oil and water bases in the first of which water is the continuous phase with dispersed oil droplets. These are the water-washable bases, easy to apply and easy to wash away. They are nongreasy and vanish into the skin. As the oil-water ratio reverses and oil becomes the continuous phase with water dispersed, the preparation is more lubricating, leaves a film on the skin, and is cosmetically less elegant. At the far end of this spectrum is 100 per cent inert oil such as mineral oil or petrolatum.

Confusion about bases derives from mislabeling as lotions preparations that are other than powder and water, and from forgetting that the fluid state has little to do with the composition of the base. Water in oil and oil in water bases may pour or not. The same is true with inert oil. Mineral oil pours; petrolatum does not. A cream may be either an oil in water (water-washable) or water in oil; an ointment may be water in oil or inert oil. Both cream and ointment must be further defined if a prescription is to be compounded. Writing for the right medication in an unspecified inert oil base may result in having a preparation in mineral oil streaming down the patient's face.

BASE SELECTION. The selection of the base depends on the need for its physical properties. A powder in water such as the classic calamine lotion permits evaporation and cooling with some drying from the powder, suggestive surely of an open wet dressing. Petrolatum by contrast conserves heat, promotes maceration, and recalls completely the closed wet dressing. The inert oil has one additional role that may be overlooked, that of protection. One would not swim the English Channel without a covering of grease.

In between these two extremes there is a spectrum of possibilities permitting some cooling but adding lubrication. Choice will weigh need and cosmetic acceptance. When a medication is to be applied to the face or scalp, a greasy base would be unsightly and underutilized. If it is an antimicrobial, for example, known to penetrate better in an ointment base, the physician will nonetheless opt for a vanishing cream, recognizing the value of compliance and preferring therapy with less penetration over no therapy at all.

Having made a judgment about the base required, a separate selection is made for the active ingredients. Some compromises may be required. Steroids, for example, may be needed and a lotion base indicated, but because lotions are easily spilled and too lavishly applied, the same steroid in a nonpouring water-washable base may prove as effective and more economical. Similarly, when lubrication is needed, the ointment base of a steroid may serve just as well without the steroid and at a fraction of the cost. In such a situation a steroid cream used sparingly and rubbed well into the skin can be overlayered with a lubricating ointment for better utilization of both.

TOPICAL STEROIDS. Although specific medications will be included under consideration of the specific diseases, some of broad use are more conveniently considered together—for example, the steroids. It is difficult to imagine dermatology without them. As topical therapy their local anti-inflammatory action is a major stroke toward restoration of the skin to normal. By vasoconstriction they halt the edema and cellular infiltrates that contribute to pruritus and local discomfort. By breaking the itch-scratch cycle with its consequent tissue damage, they permit healing. By modifying the full effect of the antigen-antibody complexes in delayed hypersensitivity reactions, they abort the intensity of the inflammatory response and permit the situation to defuse over time with the erosion of the antigen. Here, they are curative in the sense that they erase the effects of the reaction until the reaction no longer occurs. When steroids alleviate the symptoms of a specific infection, as with some yeasts and fungi, they are not curative and infection will persist unless overcome by the host's defenses. The same is true with certain opportunistic organisms that overtake an area of active dermatitis. The response of the dermatitis to steroids with consequent restoration of the skin may discourage the invader. With more aggressive organisms and in the immunocompromised patient eradication will depend on specific antimicrobial therapy.

Hydrocortisone is the "Model A" of topical steroids. In a 1 per cent concentration it is still a useful preparation and continues to serve as a norm for comparing potency of the subsequently synthesized fluorinated corticosteroids, powerful anti-inflammatory agents at concentrations as low as 0.01 per cent. Less potent than the fluorinated steroids, prednisolone and methylprednisone are also less frequently used; concentration for concentration, they are more effective than hydrocortisone.

The adverse effects reported with steroids relate almost

exclusively to the fluorinated compounds, no doubt because of their high potency and because of their frequent use under occlusion (an impervious dressing analogous to the closed wet dressing which enhances absorption). Epidermal and dermal atrophy can be a pronounced adverse effect; decreased collagen synthesis and reduced stromal support for blood vessels lead to telangiectasia, purpura, and striae. A perioral dermatitis has also been reported with the fluorinated steroids, as well as aggravation of facial erythema, restricting absolutely the extended use of these compounds for the face. Further, the provoking of elevated intraocular pressure warrants a strong proscription against the prolonged application of any topical steroids near the eyes.

The reality of systemic absorption of topical steroids presents an additional hazard. Lowering of the plasma cortisol level is seen with as little as 20 per cent of the body under occlusion. The risk of rebound after discontinuing steroids in those skin diseases characterized by the phenomenon cannot be overlooked. Despite all side effects, steroids, systemically and topically, are supremely useful therapy, saving life and the quality of life.

Systemic steroids are used for three major groups of dermatologic patients. First are the severely ill with a life-threatening disease known to be responsive to corticosteroids. Initial doses will be high, 80 to 100 mg of daily prednisone or equivalent; if response is poor, the dose may be doubled. In the second group are those with an acute but severe self-limiting problem which the steroids will control or suppress during a predicted activity. Intermediate doses of 40 to 60 mg of prednisone will be initiated, and a planned but *supervised* taper would be extended over one to two weeks. Last are the patients with chronic problems who because of exacerbation or other stresses need a respite. For them the doses will be low, no more than 15 to 20 mg of prednisone, with a concurrent focus on increased supportive topical therapy so that the systemic treatment can be phased out.

SUNSCREENS. Although topical protection from ultraviolet light might be considered under photosensitivity, the carcinogenic and aging effects of actinic radiation for all skin, but especially for skin with little or no protective melanin, warrant placement here to emphasize a general usefulness as good preventive medicine. Its recommendation should be adjunctive to sun avoidance. Selecting activities, clothing, and times of the day to reduce the opportunity and intensity of ultraviolet light exposure is the best protection. Precautions are equally important on cloudy days.

The action of topical photoprotectives is to reduce penetration of photoactive nonionizing radiation to the viable epidermal cells beneath the keratin. Such protection can be achieved by absorbing or reflecting the radiation potentially damaging to normal, light-complexioned skin or abnormal skin peculiarly sensitive to light. No sunscreen enhances tanning. Rather, if an incomplete block, it permits melanin production relative to the radiation transmitted and the inherent capacity of the partially protected skin to respond.

Most sunscreens are designed to protect against the shorter burning rays of ultraviolet light in the wavelength range of 290 to 320 nm, UVB. Most effective for this is p-aminobenzoic acid used as a 5 per cent concentration in 50 to 70 per cent ethyl alcohol. Other non-PABA chemical sunscreens such as the benzophenones and cinnamates are also useful, although the protection factor may not be as high. If protection is required against the longer wavelengths of UVA, 320 to 400 nm, or visible light, 400 to 760 nm, then physical sunscreens are needed such as titanium dioxide, zinc oxide, kaolin, or iron oxide—all available as heavy creams or pastes. Unfortunately, such opaque protectors are not nearly so acceptable as the clear and milky lotions that protect against UVB. Because certain photodermatoses are evoked by UVA, even visible light, and because UVA may also contribute to skin aging and carcinogenesis, the physical sunscreens have a significant role for selected patients.

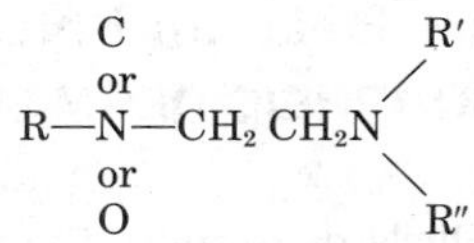

Figure 554–1. The three antihistamine linkages.

ANTIHISTAMINES. Before leaving the general considerations of dermatologic therapy, antihistamines deserve mention. Used often for their soporific and tranquilizing effect, they are still helpful in blocking one or more of the effects of histamine. No one antihistamine blocks all the effects. Those antagonists for the histamine H_2-receptor can be arranged biochemically in three major groups according to the linkage of their side arm through a C or N or O (Fig. 554–1). The selection of an effective agent for a given patient may be from any one group (Table 554–2) or from a combination of groups, but is unlikely to be enhanced by combining antihistamines within the group. If response to one antihistamine is minimal or poor, another from another group should be added or substituted. Evidence that blood vessels of human skin have H_2 as well as H_1-receptors has led to the evaluation of an H_2-receptor antagonist such as cimetidine in combination with an H_1-antagonist, and the combination has proved effective in the treatment of some cases of chronic urticaria unresponsive to standard antihistamines.

555. THE DIFFERENTIAL DIAGNOSIS

With the primary lesion assessed, a representative site biopsied, and perhaps general therapy initiated to reduce discomfort, the dermatologic diagnosis, if not immediately obvious, can be elaborated. There are broad classifications and wide-ranging considerations which help frame a diagnostic grid so that a reasonable differential can be narrowed. The skin has only a finite number of ways to respond, and many diagnoses have predilections for selected anatomic areas, suggesting their identity by their location. Further, the bulk of dermatologic problems is distributed among no more than a dozen diagnoses, so the framework need not be too cumbersome.

In the examination of the skin, noting the pattern of lesions has been stressed, but the value of the pattern has not been exploited. With a look to commonly encountered problems by anatomic region it is possible to check the supporting evidence that might be expected in a given diagnosis.

TABLE 554–2. SELECTED ANTIHISTAMINES GROUPED BY MOLECULAR LINKAGE

Carbon	Nitrogen	Oxygen
Alkylamines	**Ethylenediamines**	**Ethanolamines**
Chlorpheniramine (DL mixture) (Chlor-Trimeton)	Tripelennamine (Pyribenzamine)	Diphenhydramine (Benadryl)
Chlorpheniramine (D form) (Polaramine)	Pyrilamine (Neo-Antergan)	Bromodiphenhydramine (Ambodryl)
Parabromdylamine (Dimetane)		Dimenhydrinate (Dramamine)
		Carbinoxamine Maleate (Clistin)
Piperazines	**Phenothiazines**	
Meclizine (Bonamine)	Promethazine (Phenergan)	
Hydroxyzine (Atarax)		

The Head and Neck

SEBORRHEIC DERMATITIS

In the scalp, if there is scale and erythema but no evidence of atrophy or hair follicle disruption, the most likely diagnosis is that of seborrheic dermatitis. There may be pattern baldness and the complaint of hair thinning, but the observed pathology is a greasy scale, covering a yellow-red marginated base. The problem is common; it is shared by 12 million Americans, of whom 5.5 million have it severely enough to warrant medical consultation. Although usually a problem limited to the scalp or perhaps by extension to the retroauricular fold, it can involve the eyebrows and skin between, the eyelids in blepharitis, or the pinna in otitis externa, as well as the alae nasi, axillae, anterior thorax, periumbilical area, and genital area with focus in the crural and intergluteal folds. Obese patients with a predisposition to seborrheic dermatitis can have severe erythema and maceration in all intertriginous areas. An occasional individual can progress to a generalized exfoliative dermatitis.

The differential diagnosis in the adult is fairly limited. If scalp scaling is severe, laminated, and adherent, psoriasis must be considered. In fact, seborrheic dermatitis of such severity may be a forme fruste of psoriasis. Axillary and genital erythema raise the question of infection of the body folds with *Candida albicans* or *Corynebacterium*, but the presence of scalp lesions and the inability to demonstrate causative organisms support the diagnosis of seborrheic dermatitis. Even with positive routine cultures as for *Candida*, characteristic scalp lesions and other stigmata of seborrheic dermatitis (periumbilical erythema and scale) may suggest the diagnosis. Unresponsiveness to antiseborrheic therapy and discreteness of lesions would suggest the possibility of histiocytosis. In fact, the high prevalence of seborrheic diathesis may extend features of seborrheic dermatitis to an associated eruption. Lupus erythematosus has been observed in a seborrheic distribution with a greasiness to the lupus scale. Present, too, however, were atrophy, telangiectasia, and follicular plugging, classic for lupus erythematosus but not part of seborrheic dermatitis. In Parkinson's disease in which sebaceous glands are enlarged and sebum production is increased, seborrheic dermatitis is frequently a problem. Although treatment with L-dopa lowers sebum production, there is not always correlation of the degree of sebum suppression and neurologic improvement. Seborrheic dermatitis has been noted unilaterally in association with neurologic lesions, and with sympathetic nerve regeneration it has disappeared.

The tendency to develop seborrheic dermatitis in those genetically predisposed cannot be altered, but its manifestations can be suppressed, often by a simple acceptable routine. To reduce risk of progression and to delay hair fall, active treatment ought to be encouraged. Therapy should control inflammation and scaling, thereby reducing pruritus and oiliness. Medicated shampoos containing antimicrobial agents and salicylic acid may be all that is needed. Frequent shampooing is important, daily at first, although it need not always be with the medicated preparation. Topical steroid in lotion bases applied to the scalp two or three times daily will reduce erythema. If scale is marked, however, no medication will penetrate; warm oil soaks under plastic occlusion with or without salicylic acid will loosen the scale.

Once control has been achieved and the scalp appears normal, therapy may be reduced gradually until a minimal maintenance is determined: topical steroids every other day or less often; medicated shampoos alternating with regular shampoos in a determined repetitive pattern. As a rule, maintenance requirements will increase in winter.

For seborrheic dermatitis of areas other than the scalp, a similar routine is effective. The maceration of scale in body folds obviates the need for oil occlusion. In fact, warmth and erythema may suggest wet dressings as an initial therapy. These, combined with topical steroid, will usually control the problem, but ultraviolet light, cautiously administered, often hastens resolution.

It is also important to recognize conditions associated with seborrheic dermatitis. Severe *acne vulgaris*, for example, is always associated with some seborrheic dermatitis and so is *acne rosacea*.

ACNE

Diagnostically, acne will not be a problem. Its stigmata have become a hallmark of adolescence, and the advertising media have brought into sharp focus the characteristic erythematous papules and pustules of the pilosebaceous apparatus, the comedones open and closed (blackheads and whiteheads). When acne appears suddenly and for the first time in the 30-year-old or menopausal woman, everyone is surprised, the diagnosis is doubted, and there is uneasiness about underlying pathology. Newer investigative techniques that permit assessment of blood levels of free testosterone and dehydroepiandrosterone sulfate indicate that these may be elevated in such patients. At the present time, however, unless there are other clinical indications of virilization or endocrine dysfunction, the diagnosis of acne should merely be a challenge to active and adequate therapy, not to hormonal evaluation.

This is not to take acne lightly as a diagnosis. So prevalent in the second decade as to be considered almost a normal physiologic phenomenon, acne vulgaris defaces youth at a most vulnerable and insecure time. Further, it can persist throughout life and be severe and disfiguring, as in the conglobate form, causing marked morbidity and debility. Even severe cases that resolve can leave such destructive scarring that the psychologic burden never lifts.

There is other acne that is aggravated or perhaps frankly caused by oil, such as mechanics experience in their work, and by medications such as halogens and systemic steroids. Industrial exposure to the chlorinated hydrocarbons will almost invariably produce acne in exposed workers (chloracne). For these, improving the environment, removing the oil, discontinuing the bromides or iodides, or reducing the steroid dosage will be therapeutically advantageous. However, in most instances treating acne successfully relies on patient compliance derived mostly from an understanding of the pathophysiologic process. The patient should know that the aim of therapy is to foster the free drainage of the pilosebaceous unit, to avoid rupture, and to limit bacterial growth. The hydrolysis of the triglycerides of sebum by cutaneous bacteria yields fatty acids which have an inflammatory effect on the follicle, and which then, with its disruption, pass into the surrounding tissue as a primary irritant. The abnormality in acne is at the follicular dyskeratosis that plugs the duct. Comedones, open and closed, must be dislodged, and surface bacteria, especially *Corynebacterium acnes*, suppressed.

The patient should be instructed in the need for simple cleansing every four to six hours to stun bacteria and discourage their logarithmic growth. Washing with soap will do, or a mild alcohol preparation carried or kept in a locker may be used. A topical antimicrobial preparation should be applied twice daily, benzoyl peroxide 5 or 10 per cent, for example, or the antimicrobial clindamycin, tetracycline, or erythromycin 1 or 2 per cent in an alcohol base. Plugged follicles will respond to topical retinoic acid, presumably through the labilization of lysosomes in the keratinizing cells of the follicles. A brisk erythematous response is often induced that may necessitate a reduction in the concentration or frequency of application of the vitamin A acid. Further, the concern for enhanced damage from solar radiation, or the possibility of a co-carcinogenic effect as suggested by experiments in hairless albino mice, contraindicates its use in summer or in light-complexioned individuals. For these as for all patients with acne, the mechanical removal of comedones and the incision and drainage of pustules and cysts foster resolution.

Systemic broad-spectrum antimicrobials in low to moderate

doses given over long periods have proved a useful management for more severe acne, and, contrary to the expectations of some, have not been complicated by microbial resistance or superinfections. The tetracyclines, although commonly used, carry risk of dental discoloration, photosensitivity, and even pregnancy through drug interaction with oral contraceptives. Because they are incorporated into growing bones and teeth, they should not be prescribed from the fourth fetal month through age 12. There is also the possibility of subsequent mobilization from bone under stress, as in pregnancy, with consequent risk of maternal hepatitis or fetal absorption. All patients of the childbearing age should be cautioned if prolonged therapy is anticipated. Photosensitivity, impossible to predict, must be considered in the event of untoward reaction. Erythromycin is a useful alternative; compared to tetracycline, gastrointestinal distress may be more prevalent with erythromycin, but ingestion with meals and consumption of supplemental *Lactobacillus* as from yogurt reduce such symptoms. More severe acne may require more extensive surgical procedures, higher doses of antimicrobials, intralesional steroid, or even systemic steroid. Estrogens have been used in selected women with stubborn severe acne with good results, but used as cyclic estrogen progestin therapy they have all the attendant risk of anovulatory preparations given for contraception. X-ray has no part in the management of acne. The question of diet is invariably raised, but there is no evidence to support a role for diet as either cause or aggravation. Of proven value in cystic acne but with risk not fully assessed, oral isotretinoin (13-*cis*-retinoic acid and a probable metabolite of vitamin A) alters sebaceous gland differentiation, reducing sebum production in ways not clear but not as an antiandrogen. Within four weeks after treatment is begun, erythema and pustules are reduced. When treatment is stopped, usually after four months, sebum production returns toward pretreatment levels, yet the cystic acne continues in remission or even improves. The clinical toxic effects are similar to those of vitamin A, are dose dependent in incidence and severity, and are reversible when therapy is stopped. This includes pseudotumor cerebri or benign intracranial hypertension manifest by papilledema, headache, nausea, vomiting, and visual disturbances, which warrant an immediate stop to therapy and a neurologic assessment. Laboratory abnormalities seem limited to occasional elevations of liver function test results that return to pretreatment levels even as therapy is continued, and to elevations in blood lipids, especially triglycerides, that return to pretreatment levels after therapy. Current studies of treatment of dyskeratoses indicate the possibility of greater hepatic dysfunction with the prolonged use of isotretinoin over a period of years. Of primary importance is the fact that isotretinoin is teratogenic. Patients must not conceive while on therapy or for a month or more thereafter. Nor are blood banks to accept blood for transfusion from patients on isotretinoin therapy lest a recipient be or become pregnant. Clearly a useful adjunct for the treatment of recalcitrant persistent cystic acne, isotretinoin should not be prescribed without thoughtful review, detailed explanation, strict contraception, and close clinical and laboratory monitoring.

ACNE ROSACEA

Characteristically appearing in the central one third of the face, acne rosacea occurs more commonly in women of 30 to 50 years, but more severely in men; it can be seen in both sexes at any age. Comedones are lacking, and the acne pustules are associated with telangiectasia and persistent flush; spices, alcohol, hot drinks, and temperature extremes that foster flushing aggravate the condition. Rhinophyma (Fig. 555–1) is associated with longstanding rosacea, but ocular involvement (blepharitis, conjunctivitis, episcleritis, and keratitis) can be far more serious. Therapy as outlined for acne vulgaris can be helpful for the pustular component of rosacea, but the flush and telangiectasia remain. Foods and situations that provoke flushing should be avoided. For both acne vulgaris and acne rosacea, control of the seborrheic dermatitis is important for management.

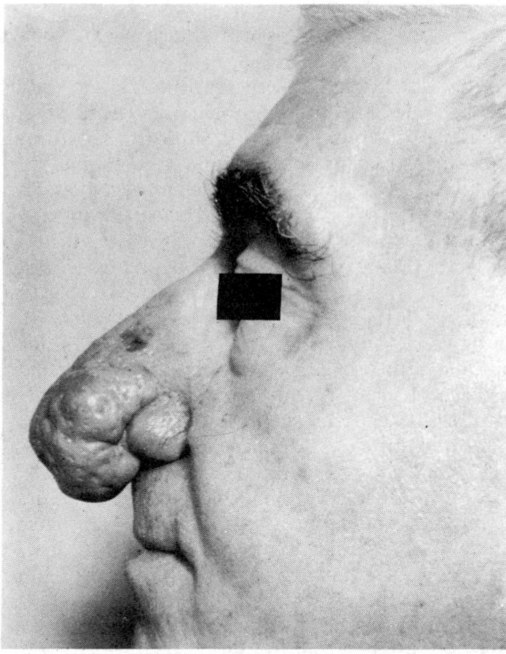

Figure 555–1. Rhinophyma.

LESIONS OF THE MOUTH

Pathology of the buccal mucosa and lips is often overlooked unless the patient offers a specific complaint or corroborative evidence is sought for a suspected diagnosis based on a distant lesion. When oral inspection is routine and the mucosa under dentures never excluded, a wide range of normal and pathologic change will be recognized.

Pigmentation, for example, most marked on the gingiva, buccal mucosa, hard palate, tongue, and soft palate, has an intensity commensurate with that of the skin and increases from childhood to adult life. Racial variation is considerable. Melanocytic nevi, usually compound, and less common in the mouth than on the skin, can be seen in all races, but most often in blacks. Exogenous pigment can be deposited from the silver amalgam of dental fillings through an accidental tattoo or by diffusion. A dark blue-black lesion of the lip, which might be deeply placed pigment but blanches on diascopy, is a benign phlebectasia. Relatively common past middle life, phlebectasia of the oral mucosa, tongue, and scrotum can be associated with similar lesions of the jejunum and may be a cause of gastrointestinal bleeding.

Vascular nevi of the lips and buccal mucosa are recognized from infancy or childhood. They can cause obstructive problems as well as bleeding because of friability. The less obvious punctate telangiectasia of Osler-Rendu-Weber disease is not often seen before puberty, but almost always involves the mucous membranes occurring in the mouth, nasal septum, nasopharynx, and throughout the gastrointestinal tract. The lesions of the tongue are diagnostic, for within the fungiform papillae is a single, dilated vessel that may lead to an expanded papilla.

The most common problems of the mouth, however, derive from infection and trauma. Periodontal and periapical disease are associated not only with bacteremia but also with local erosions and, in the most severe form, with acute necrotizing ulcerative gingivitis. Attention to oral hygiene, the removal of bacterial plaque, and the massaging of gingivae will restore tissue turgor and resistance to infection. Even the gum hypertrophy associated with phenytoin therapy can be controlled with scrupulous cleansing.

The diagnostic challenge of erosions of the mouth must include in the differential diagnosis the primary chancre of syphilis, herpes simplex infection, aphthous stomatitis, the blistering diseases such as pemphigus, and mechanical trauma as from ill-fitting prostheses. *Extragenital chancres* are not uncommon, and the lips and adjacent buccal cavity are the most common places to find them. Because of the numerous nonsyphilitic treponemas of the mouth, a positive dark field examination is not definitive of infection with *T. pallidum* and serologic confirmation is required.

Lesions of *herpes simplex, Herpesvirus hominis,* subtype 1 primarily, but also subtype 2 especially if a primary infection, may have extensive buccal erosions with gingivostomatitis and systemic symptoms. Recurrent lesions, which can be intraoral but are much more common on the lips, usually present as grouped vesicles of 1 to 3 mm; a positive Tzanck smear will show the multinucleated giant cells. Some 85 per cent of patients report prodromal symptoms of burning, tingling, or pruritus a few hours before the vesicular eruption. With such lead time, an attack may be aborted using topical steroid or 5-iodo-2-deoxyuridine applied frequently, every hour or two. Once the vesicles have erupted, the clinical infection, although short-lived, runs its course. Drying agents and antimicrobial preparations to thwart secondary bacterial infection should limit the problem to five to seven days. Acyclovir, which inhibits the multiplication of herpes simplex virus types 1 and 2, reduces morbidity in primary infections and viral shedding but not morbidity in recurrences. Because of the emergence of resistant virus, the use of acyclovir should be reserved for life-threatening herpetic infections, primary or secondary, which occur in the immunocompromised host.

Aphthous stomatitis or canker sores are recurrent, painful ulcerations of the oral mucosa. Although aphthae can be the first clinical manifestation of pernicious anemia and perhaps of folic acid or iron deficiency, most recurrent aphthae are of unknown cause. They are more common in women, and familial occurrence of a severe variety has been reported. An association between jejunal mucosal abnormalities and aphthae is suggested. Immunoglobulins, i.e., IgE-bearing lymphocytes, are reportedly increased.

No specific treatment is available for aphthae, but topical anesthetics such as viscous lidocaine or the antihistamine diphenhydramine held in the mouth just before mealtime, numb the pain and ease alimentation. Suspensions of antibiotic such as tetracycline, 250 mg per 5 ml held against the sores for two minutes before swallowing four or five times per day, promote healing. The antibiotic can be combined with the diphenhydramine. Steroids in the dental preparation Orabase are difficult to keep in place. To concentrate steroid locally, a cortisone tablet, 5 mg whole or halved, can dissolve in the ulcer; intralesional steroid can be injected. Such therapy can be used for all painful erosions of the mouth when anesthesia, infection control, and reduction of the inflammatory response will promote healing. It will be of benefit for oral erosions of the blistering diseases while the diagnosis is being elaborated, and will ease the discomfort of mechanical erosions from dentures and bridges while the cause is being corrected.

Friable white tissue, with or without erosion but along the bite line, suggests a chewing of the cheek and consequent damage to the mucosa. Lacy infiltrates or friable mucosa away from the bite line may suggest lichen planus, lupus erythematosus, or perhaps a white sponge nevus; the distinction from leukoplakia is difficult but important, and the lesion needs assessment. Stigmata of disease elsewhere are helpful; a biopsy is in order, but may not be definitive. The microscopic study, however, can rule out epithelial dysplasia. Requiring equally close surveillance and perhaps biopsy is smoker's palate, a papular, gray-white, palatal mucosa, the result of inflamed, plugged salivary glands, each papule bearing the red dot of a ductal orifice. The process seen in habitual pipe smokers is precancerous, but may show regression if smoking is stopped.

Any lesion of the buccal mucosa or lips that is not identified, especially one that is enlarging or eroded, should be biopsied. Actinic damage involves the lips, the lower more than the upper, with characteristic atrophy and fine scale and occasionally induration. Malignant change must always be suspect. Angular stomatitis, fissuring at the labial commissures, may be associated with *Candida albicans* infection, but most often is the result of chronic irritation with bacterial and yeast infection, opportunistic and secondary. The redundancy of tissue with aging but more with the gum and bone resorption of the edentulous, aggravated perhaps by ill-fitting prostheses, leads to chronic ulceration. When sleeping, such patients frequently salivate to macerate further one commissure or both.

Intensive topical therapy should reduce secondary infection with appropriate antimicrobial agents, the inflammation with steroid, and the risk of continuing irritation by sealing with a protective film such as zinc oxide paste, at least at night. If the defect is slow to respond, a biopsy should be taken; chronic ulcerations predispose to malignant change. If the physical fact of redundancy precludes healing, surgical revision is indicated.

The Thorax

In the course of the regional examination, note is constantly made of the isolated pigmentary lesions (see Ch. 556) and the stigmata of aging and actinic exposure (see Ch. 552). The present larger focus is the pattern of appearance of eruptions.

DRUG ERUPTION

Symmetrical, scaling, erythematous macules or papules on the thorax, if of sudden onset, would suggest a drug eruption (Fig. 555–2). Itching need not be present but would support the impression.

PITYRIASIS ROSEA

Should the lesions be oval with a collarette of fine scale and follow skin cleavage lines (Fig. 555–3), the diagnosis of pityriasis rosea is likely. In this self-limited eruption, which is not uncommon and is often seen in young adults, there is occasionally recognition of a larger antecedent lesion, the herald patch. Usually on the trunk it can be several centimeters in size, erythematous, and scaling. It is often mistaken for fungus; the negative KOH test result would correct that error. When the generalized eruption appears, the immediate reflex of the knowing examiner is to look again at the pharynx and palms lest luetic lesions be overlooked. Secondary syphilis is always in the differential diagnosis, and a serologic test should be obtained; but without systemic symptoms, coryza, or palmar and plantar lesions, syphilis is an unlikely cause of the eruption. Pityriasis rosea lasts six to eight weeks; although most patients are asymptomatic, one in five will complain of pruritus.

LICHEN PLANUS

Lichen planus, of characteristic color but sparse scale must, nevertheless, be included in the differential diagnosis of scattered scaling lesions of the thorax, especially if there are lesions on the flexor aspect of the wrists, lower legs, or genitalia. Most often the typical polygonal flat-topped papule with a lilac hue and, on close inspection, the delicate whitish lines of Wickham's striae can be found. The classic lesion is diagnostic, and the histology supports the diagnosis. Mouth lesions are seen in half the patients, a lacy white network involving the buccal mucosa and lips. Ulcerative, erosive, hypertrophic, and atrophic variants have been described, and lichen planus–like eruptions have been induced by certain drugs, heavy metals,

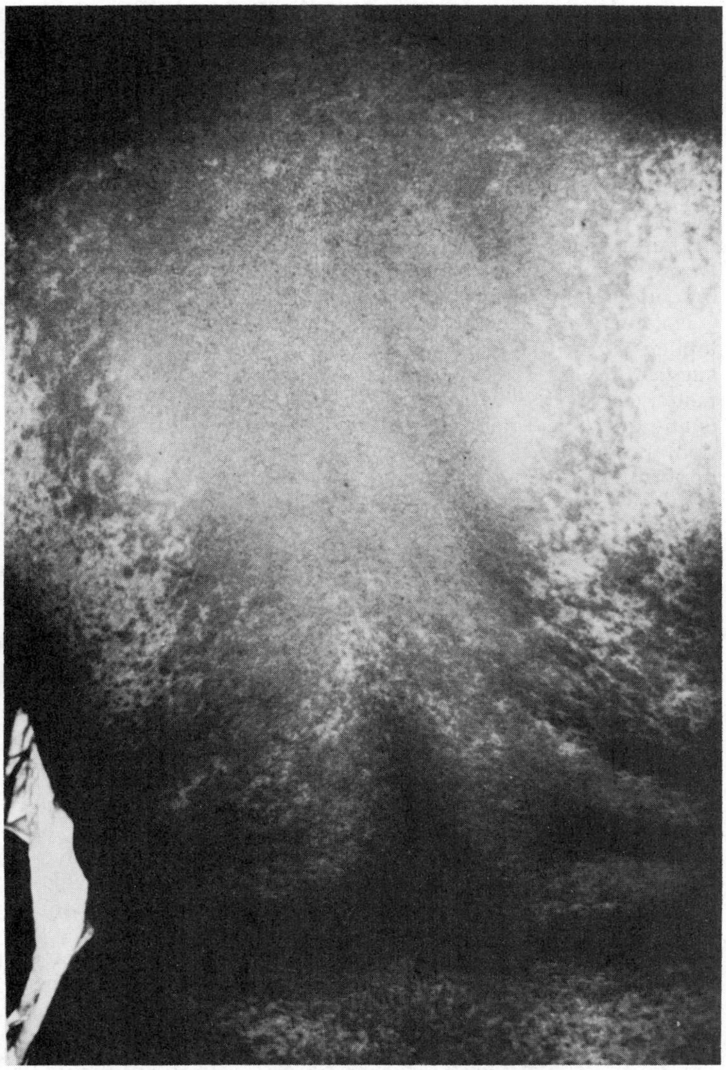

Figure 555–2. Drug eruption.

and color photo developers. The drugs include streptomycin, methyldopa, gold, phenothiazine, and the antimalarials chloroquine and quinacrine.

The etiology remains obscure, but the known association with drugs and chemicals and the observation of deficiency of glucose-6-phosphate dehydrogenase in lichen planus skin support a hypothesis that certain susceptible enzyme-deficient individuals respond to various chemicals and other environmental factors with lichen planus–like lesions. Eruptions resembling lichen planus have also been observed with polymyositis and lymphoma.

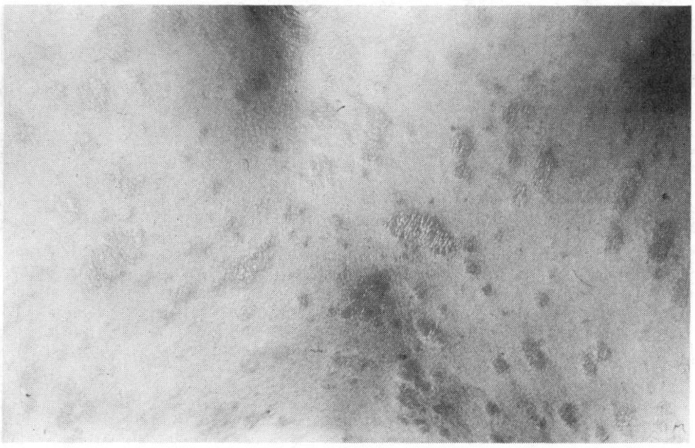

Figure 555–3. Pityriasis rosea.

PSORIASIS

Psoriasis, although classically presenting with plaques over the elbows and knees, can appear suddenly over the thorax as small, scattered papulosquamous lesions described as guttate. If these are the first manifestations of the disease, the finding of supporting stigmata may be essential. Characteristic silvery micaceous scale would be a helpful clue, and so, too, would be severe scaling of the scalp. Pitting of the fingernails with lifting and flaring is supportive, and a change suggestive of an oil droplet underneath the nail is pathognomonic. Nails can be greatly thickened. Historical or current evidence of scaling plaques of the elbows or knees, erythema or fissuring of the intergluteal fold, and associated arthritis of the distal interphalangeal joints all leave the diagnosis hard to challenge. In severe cases much of the skin may be involved (Fig. 555–4). In some there can be erosive, inflammatory joint disease, usually polyarticular and occasionally severe, even mutilating. Appearing in 4.5 per cent of psoriatic patients with no serologic evidence of lupus erythematosus or rheumatic factors, it is recognized as psoriatic arthritis.

In the United States more than one million people have psoriasis, and of these more than 11 per cent have experienced disability of such severity as to compromise employment and effectiveness. The disease can begin at any age and has its peak appearance in the third decade. Its severity, course, and remissions are unpredictable. It is inherited in a pattern still unclear. There are studies relating two HLA antigens and psoriasis. One, Bw17, is a useful genetic marker for that group of psoriatic patients with a high rate of affected relatives and a mean age of onset under 20 years (18.2 years). Those with HLA-B13 have little heritable tendency and milder disease.

Patients whose psoriasis requires therapy, or patients who demand it, are usually referred to a dermatologist, for, in general, physicians do not appreciate the discomfort and dis-

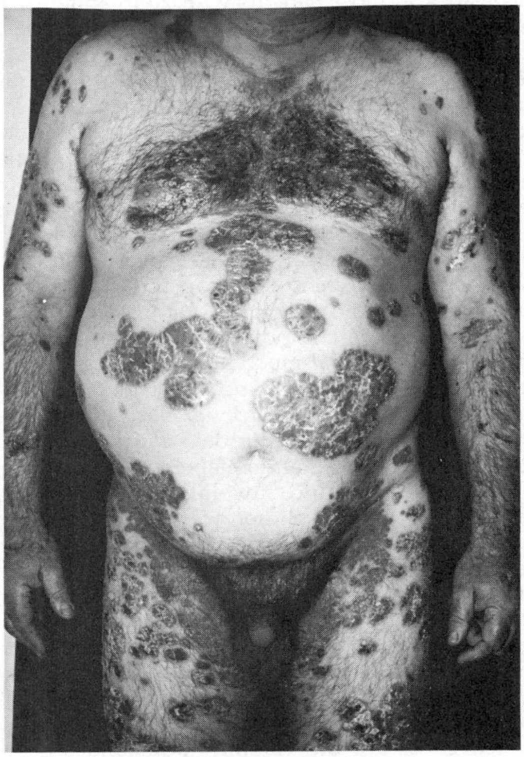

Figure 555–4. Psoriasis.

figurement of the disease and the potential for severity, arthritis, generalized exfoliation, or even death. Lesions are often dismissed as untreatable, or sometimes are subjected to an overkill with systemic therapy and attendant significant side effects. Systemic corticosteroids, for example, can induce prompt resolution of psoriatic lesions, but suppression requires ever-increasing doses. When therapy is tapered, there is a rebound phenomenon, with extension of lesions possibly to exfoliation. If systemic steroids are used for other valid reasons in patients with psoriasis, the risk of aggravated psoriasis should be recognized and weighed in the decision for initiating therapy.

Psoriasis is without cure but is responsive to treatments which can induce remission of many months to years and maintenance therapy that can help sustain the remission. Corticosteroids applied topically under occlusion or given intralesionally promote blanching and flattening of lesions. If the impetus to remit is enhanced by the use of tar and ultraviolet light through the Goeckerman regimen, the chance of steroid rebound will lessen and a true remission may be realized. Black coal tars are applied directly to the skin in sufficient amounts to penetrate, and then are wiped clean so as not to filter out the long range ultraviolet light, which evokes a phototoxic reaction. Increasing exposures to ultraviolet light are given on a set schedule—as often as twice daily for inpatients, perhaps once or twice weekly for outpatients. The duration of exposure is pushed to tolerance of erythema but not burn, lest the Koebner phenomenon, the isomorphic response by which tissue injury induces new lesions, activate a psoriatic flare. Within three to four weeks the most extensive psoriasis is usually resolved. Continuing use of light and tar, alone or together if possible, at reduced intervals helps preserve the favorable response. Variations of the Goeckerman method have included the use of anthralin paste with dressings after the baths and light.

Long wave ultraviolet light (UVA) has also been used from a high intensity source through photosensitization with oral psoralens which potentiate the effect of light. Experience with PUVA (psoralens plus UVA) suggests good resolution of the psoriatic lesions in most patients with 20 treatments, but with a need for maintenance therapy in a significant percentage. Treatment requires traveling to a center and risk of burn or eye damage from normal sunlight before and after therapy until the psoralen is metabolized. The importance of long-term assessment is recognized because of the laboratory inducement of skin malignancies and cataracts in albino mice on high dose psoralens and intense exposure to UVA. In fact, from the multicenter study where PUVA has been on protocol, there are data to show an increased prevalence of cutaneous malignancy, with more squamous cell carcinoma relative to basal cell carcinoma. Whether such tumor will follow the more benign course of actinically induced malignancy rather than the biologic aggressiveness of radiation-induced tumor remains to be seen.

The effect of the topical modalities utilizing ultraviolet light is believed to be through mitotic arrest and the consequent return toward normal of the psoriatic cell turnover time, which is at an accelerated three to four days rather than the normal 27 to 28 days. Surely the antimetabolites have this effect on mitosis and thereby induce involution of psoriatic lesions. Arsenic used as Fowler's solution was an early cellular poison for psoriasis, and its previous use in a given patient is an important historical fact to alert the examiner to search for sequelae of arsenic ingestion. Aminopterin, amethopterin or methotrexate, and azaribine have also been used for therapy, methotrexate being the most widely used and the only one still accepted. Its prescription in psoriasis is limited to grave situations and to rigid guidelines set by the Psoriasis Task Force, National Program for Dermatology. Of less risk and of promising effectiveness are the vitamin A analogues. A new oral aromatic retinoid etretinate on protocol in the United States and available in Germany causes psoriatic lesions to enlarge and disappear. Clinical toxic effects are similar to those of vitamin A and laboratory abnormalities similar to those experienced with isotretinoin.

Because patient care is so often fragmented among specialists and because not all patients appreciate the gravity of therapy, it is important for any physician to inquire about every treatment regimen prescribed for his patient. The psoriasis in a patient with clear skin on methotrexate may escape detection. In the same way the dermatologist should know if the patient whose skin cancer he is about to curette and electrodesiccate is on anticoagulation and has a pacemaker.

Isolated psoriatic lesions, especially if circinate, and psoriasis limited to the seborrheic areas such as axillae or groin may suggest the differential diagnosis of fungus infection. For that matter, so would the "herald patch" of pityriasis rosea. If there is any question, scrapings should be taken for KOH examination and culture. Not uncommonly, ubiquitous organisms are opportunistic. Patients *can* have two diagnoses, but the KOH test result and cultures sooner or later must support the clinical impression of fungus.

FUNGUS INFECTIONS

Scaling lesions of the thorax, with macular patches of all sizes and shapes, varying in color from white to tan to brown, represent *tinea versicolor* (Fig. 555–5). Extending sometimes to the neck, face, and arms, it is asymptomatic and is usually just a cosmetic bother. Wood's light examination aids visualization because of skin pigment change and because of the brick-red fluorescence of the causative organism, *Malassezia furfur (Pityrosporon orbiculare)*, which is not readily cultured. Scraping of the lesion removes scale and leaves normal skin beneath. Direct microscopic examination of the scale shows short hyphal filaments and grape-like clusters of budding forms (Fig. 555–6). The therapy prescribed is usually the common fungicides. Any preparation with sodium thiosulfate, haloprogin, or tolnaftate, for example, is useful, as is clotrimazole or miconazole. The

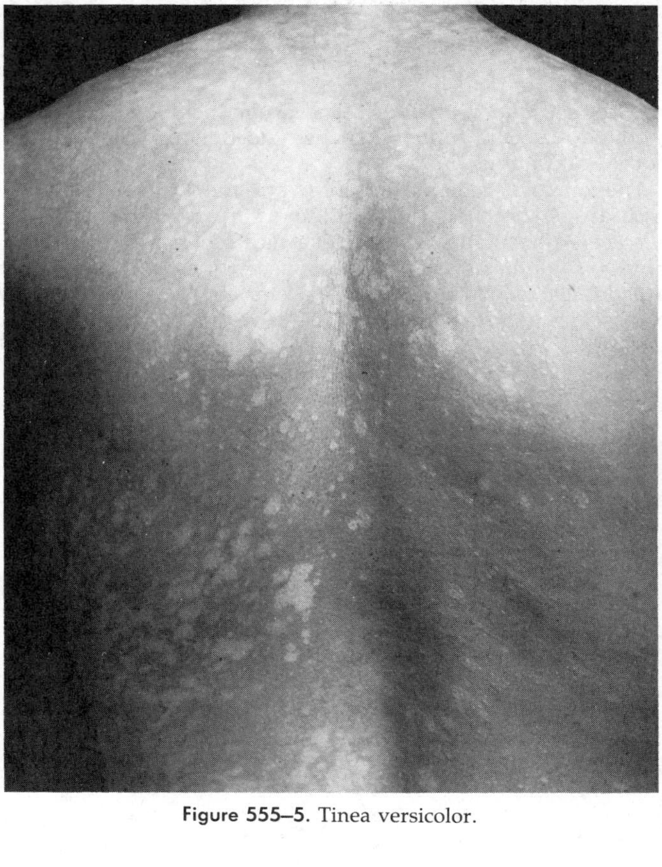

Figure 555–5. Tinea versicolor.

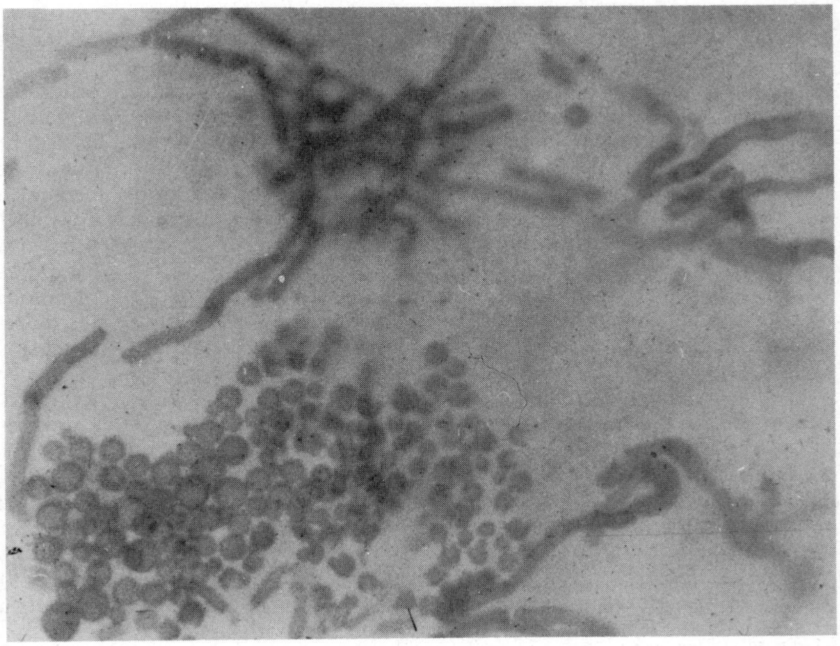

Figure 555–6. *Malassezia furfur.*

problem tends to recur, but can be prevented by daily scrubs with a keratolytic antimicrobial soap. No systemic therapy is indicated.

In general, if scaling lesions show hyphal elements and the appropriate cultures are positive but if another diagnosis is still suspected, the basic problem may not be fungus. A course of antifungal therapy should resolve the question; if it is a secondary invader, it will disappear, leaving the underlying pathology.

Traditionally, fungus is considered anatomically, from head to foot. Tinea capitis, so common to children, is hardly ever seen in adults except for a rare *Trichophyton tonsurans* infection. Occasionally parents of children with infected scalps can have glabrous or smooth, nonhairy skin involvement, having come in contact with the child's infection, but such anthropophilic fungi provoke little in tissue reaction. Animal fungi by contrast can stimulate a brisk reaction. From the broken hair "black dot" infection of *T. tonsurans* the spectrum extends through the red scaling dermatophytosis of groin and foot characteristic of *Trichophyton* and *Epidermophyton* infections to the boggy, bumpy tumefaction, raised, red, and tender, of a *Microsporum* infection such as *M. gypseum, M. canis,* or even *M. audouini.* These kerions resemble bacterial abscesses and initially can be misdiagnosed and mistreated. The importance of the direct and immediate examination for fungus by the KOH preparation cannot be overemphasized.

Scaling lesions of the trunk or body folds, if KOH-positive for hyphal elements, are tinea until proved otherwise. In areas where fungus has been associated with the continued maceration of wet clothing, as from occupation or wet swim trunks, plaques and nodules may develop; the history of maceration is important. Therapy which can be specific topically and systemically is less effective when good local care is neglected. Tub baths for adequate cleansing, removal of wet garments promptly, and use of drying powders can all be helpful.

Scaling lesions of the hands and feet offer a wider differential, since contact and chronic irritant dermatitis are so common. The differential diagnosis will be considered below. Persistent inflammation of nail beds and the presence of psoriatic lesions in the nail plate can deform nails without fungal infection. However, the opportunities for fungi to infect macerated keratin further the confusion. Scrapings for fungal study should be taken from glabrous skin and nails as well as finger and toe webs. Too often oral griseofulvin is prescribed for scaling lesions without benefit of confirmatory KOH examination and culture. Rarely it may be considered for a therapeutic trial despite negative test results but never without them. It is useful against most dermatophytes but inactive against deep fungi and *Candida* species. It works best for fungal infection of the scalp, trunk, or groin.

When griseofulvin is given as 1 gram per day after a fatty meal to enhance absorption, pruritus, if a symptom, should disappear in 24 to 48 hours. Glabrous skin involvement should clear in seven to fourteen days. Dystrophic, infected nails, however, will require continuing therapy for as long as the pregriseofulvin keratin is retained, i.e., as long as it takes for replacement—three to four months for fingernails, six months or longer for toenails. Interrupting therapy will permit reinfection from retained infected keratin. Even throughout constant therapy and thereafter, a topical antifungal agent should be used.

The lengthy duration of required treatment should give the physician pause about committing a patient to a half year or more of a medication that can have unpleasant neurologic, hematologic, and gastrointestinal side effects. Further, once cleared, the chance of reinfection is considerable because of the ubiquitous organisms and the selected inability of some individuals to resist such infections.

A useful alternative to prolonged treatment is to clear glabrous skin with a short oral course of griseofulvin while instituting a vigorous topical program that ideally will contain the infection in the nails and keep the skin free of disease. Should there be a relapse at a future date, the oral course can be repeated. Most mild to moderate tinea infections require only topical medication such as tolnaftate, haloprogin, miconazole, or clotrimazole.

YEAST INFECTIONS

Yeast infections of the skin mimic fungal infections as in the groin, but most often the erythema is a bit brighter, the scale is more macerated, and there will be telltale satellite lesions at the periphery of the patch. When *Candida* infects webs or paronychia—a common hazard of the prolonged water immersion experienced by bartenders and janitors—or when it involves the mouth or vagina as a sequela of systemic antimicrobial therapy, perhaps a signal of diabetes—the lesions are more characteristic. The erythematous base is often raw with a cheesy exudate, and there may be pruritus, but more often tenderness and pain occur.

Therapy to reduce erythema and itching is helpful in initiating symptomatic relief, and eradication of the underlying predisposing factors is mandatory, but specific topical anticandidal medications, such as nystatin, amphotericin, or the broader-spectrum clotrimazole, are also indicated and would be prescribed, as might be expected, in a water-washable or lotion base, never occlusive. The sexual partner of a patient with balanitis or vulvovaginitis should be alerted to the possibility of infection and treated if the patient's problem is slow to clear or recurrent. Vaginal suppositories of nystatin are available, as well as oral suspension for direct application to mouth lesions.

Candida albicans is usually the infecting species, but several others of the same genus, *Candida tropicalis,* for example, may be the agent under predisposing conditions, especially with paronychial infections. Since they are common organisms of the gastrointestinal tract, the chance for reinfection with *Candida* organisms is ever present. Precautions should include adequate cleansing and drying of the body folds routinely but especially after defecation, and the adding of an anticandidal preparation to any topical antibacterial medication that is to be used in the anogenital area. Neither nystatin nor amphotericin B is sufficiently absorbed from the gastrointestinal tract to be of value as systemic therapy; but taken orally, either agent will reduce the *Candida* population of the intestine. This may be indicated if topical control fails in the vulvovaginitis of *Candida*-induced pruritus among those on contraceptives or long-term antimicrobial therapy. Stubborn *Candida* infections respond well to the new oral antimicrobial agent ketoconazole, but risk of hepatotoxicity should limit its use to recalcitrant problems.

Despite the tendency to chronicity and recurrence, and despite the acute discomfort of the active infection, most candidiasis is responsive to therapy. Occasionally severe infection can have quite generalized erythematous crusting and be associated with horny excrescences on granulomatous bases. Labeled chronic mucocutaneous candidiasis, this intractable infection may appear at birth or early childhood and may be associated with endocrinopathy such as hypoparathyroidism, hypoadrenalism, and diabetes, or with congenital thymic disorders affecting lymphocyte function and cell-mediated immunity. There are data to suggest that chronic mucocutaneous candidiasis results from a deficiency of migration inhibitory factor or from the presence of an inhibitor to this factor or other mediator of delayed hypersensitivity. Despite endocrinopathy and the compromised immune status in the presence of severe extensive mucocutaneous infection, systemic candidiasis develops rarely—all the more surprising because in general medicine systemic manifestations of *Candida* infection are not that unusual.

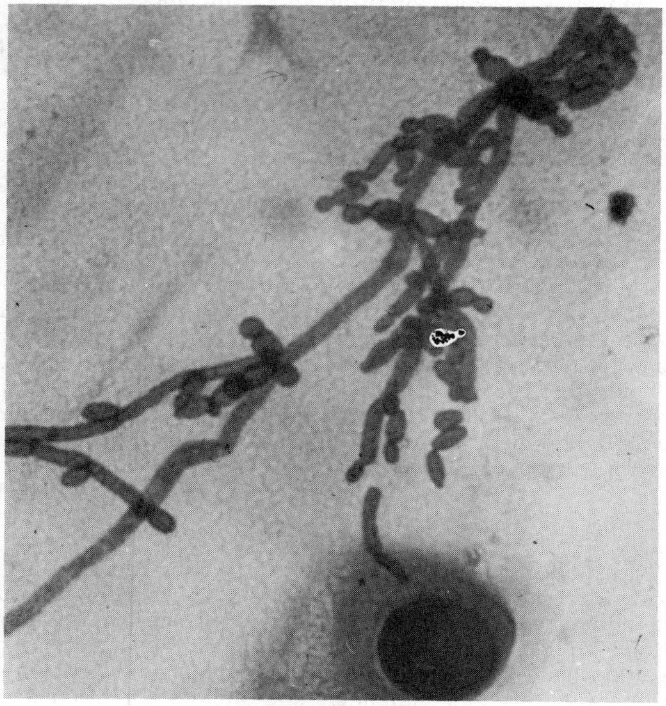

Figure 555–7. *Candida albicans.*

In systemic infection, bronchopulmonary and pulmonary candidiasis are the most common manifestations seen as complications of chronic primary pulmonary disease, especially in the diabetic or those on systemic corticosteroids or antimicrobial agents. Candidemia, with or without seeding, is a complication of surgery associated with prolonged use of indwelling catheters, and of those conditions requiring long-term therapy with immunosuppressive agents and antimetabolites.

Because of the frequent finding of *Candida* in and on the body, establishing *Candida* as a cause of a particular problem requires the demonstration of budding yeasts and filaments in the scraping or biopsy from the lesion in question (Fig. 555–7), a generous and repeated growth of the organism or culture, and a fit of the lesions to what might be anticipated for a *Candida* infection.

Dermatitis of the Hands and Feet

The problem of redness and scaling of the hands and feet can be exasperating to clinician and patient alike. Hands and feet have similar and sympathetic reaction patterns. A dermatitis on one may produce an "id" on the other. Both are subjected to trauma and both are exposed to abundant contactants, greater in variety on the hands perhaps, but greater in intensity on the feet in their enclosed pressure casings.

Thus far, a consideration of psoriasis and of fungus has included hands and feet, but the differential has not been extended for those from whom no fungus could be isolated and no stigmata of psoriasis identified. Erythema and scale of long standing, a chronic dermatitis, might mean a continuing contact dermatitis or the late manifestations of atopic dermatitis, or perhaps might be part of an ill-defined group of reaction patterns that are quite characteristic in their manifestations but of obscure etiology.

CONTACT DERMATITIS

Of all the dermatitides of the hands and feet, contact dermatitis is perhaps the most important. Irritants and allergic sensitizers commonly involve hands and feet. If the offending substance can be identified, avoidance or protection can restore a patient to normal. If the problem is ignored or the offender escapes detection and the dermatitis smolders, a chronicity is established that may totally disable the patient.

Any dermatitis that presents acutely with erythema and vesicles warrants intense restorative therapy and an undaunted search for the cause. Plants and airborne contactants can leave their linear vesicles or exposure pattern as a clue; the distribution in a hand or foot problem may not be that revealing. Nonetheless, history taking and patch testing may narrow the field. Screening trays are available to test to common allergens, to medications, to the components of shoes, and to cosmetics, and for every patient it is possible to test with the part of his own environment that is suspect, a part of the lining of a shoe, as an example. For hands rather than feet, photosensitivity may be checked to establish if the minimal erythema dose for the individual is lowered or if a photo-contact reaction can be demonstrated in association with medications or soaps.

If the offending irritant or allergen is identified, the source of the patient's exposure and other occult and unsuspected sources can be established to ensure protection. Fisher's text is the definitive reference for elaborating a suspected contact dermatitis and then sorting out the cross-reactions and tabulating where the allergen is to be found. Contact dermatitis placed first in prevalence among 75,000 consecutive visits to the Skin and Cancer Clinic of New York University. There were 11,100 visits for contact and an additional 4600 for chronic dermatitis of obscure etiology. The importance of recognition and identification cannot be overstated.

ATOPIC DERMATITIS

In that same pool of diagnoses atopic dermatitis placed seventh, a disease determined by heredity and characterized by a lower threshold to pruritus. With scratching, the skin becomes spongiotic and weeps, the eczematous form seen more often in the young. At any age rubbing can produce lichenification with accentuation of skin markings. Across the United States, 0.7 per cent of the population has this inherited diathesis of sufficient severity that a physician's consultation is warranted. Most cases contributing to the burden of the problem occur in infancy or childhood. After a period of quiescence from age two or three, it can recur in late childhood, in adolescence, or in early adult life, tending to localize in flexural areas of the neck, antecubital and popliteal folds, often about the eyelids, behind the ears, and at the wrists. Of those who are afflicted in adulthood, occasionally to the fifth decade, chronic hand and foot eczema is a common expression of the problem. At any age, a pruritic dermatitis in the "atopic distribution" should raise the possibility of the diagnosis. Such patients will have a personal history of atopic dermatitis and a personal or family history of atopy, asthma, hay fever, or perhaps urticaria, which is part of the complex but of more obscure relationship.

The atopic diathesis is manifest in the skin by a blanching response to injections of acetylcholine or methacholine, in contrast to normal skin in which vasodilatation results in erythema. The skin of the atopic has been shown to contain up to 60 times the concentration of acetylcholine of skin in nonatopic rashes, as well as an excess of cholinesterase. Sweat glands in the atopic have an increased sensitivity to acetylcholine rather like that produced by a partial beta receptor blockade. Atopic skin also differs from normal in its exquisite sensitivity to epinephrine and norepinephrine. In fact the "grainy" skin of patients with atopic dermatitis has been ascribed to a permanent state of piloerection mediated by norepinephrine.

The role of allergy in atopic dermatitis is not completely elaborated. Immediate urticarial reactions to skin tests with common antigens are frequently observed. The skin-sensitizing antibody can be transferred by serum to another subject and has been identified as a distinct immunoglobulin, IgE. Some patients with atopic dermatitis will have excessive serum levels of IgE but with little correlation between the serum level and the severity of the dermatitis. Further, high levels of IgE have been reported in nonatopic conditions. T-cell function is said to be deficient in atopic dermatitis, whether depressed by elevated IgE levels or de novo with the IgE rise in response to reacting B cells.

The major implications of these documented facts are that atopic skin responds to slight trauma with vasoconstriction and pruritus, leading to a weeping vesicular dermatitis acutely, and then more chronically to dry lichenified skin. Wet dressings, if indicated, will physically reduce erythema and weeping, and topical steroids and systemic antihistamines will alter the pruritus and inflammatory response. Dry or lichenified skin may suggest lubrication, but the inability to sweat may be aggravated by occlusive lubricants which, with retained heat, may increase pruritus. Should secondary pyogenic or fungal infection be present, specific therapy may be needed to control it. Restoring the integrity of the skin will thwart opportunistic organisms.

One major risk of atopic dermatitis derives from the depression of T-cell function which makes the patient more susceptible to widespread viral infection with vaccinia, herpes simplex, and, of less concern, molluscum contagiosum and verruca vulgaris. Even without active dermatitis, infection with herpes simplex can lead to a generalized vesicular eruption with high fever and significant mortality. With the control of variola, there is no longer a public health requirement for vaccination, which is absolutely contraindicated in the atopic patient and all close contacts. Protection from latent herpes simplex virus is not so easy to achieve.

Any acute flare in the dermatitis of an atopic should be inspected closely for vesicles. If they are present, to differentiate viral vesicles from the eczematous process of atopy, a Tzanck smear should be done in search of multinucleated giant cells indicative of viral infection. If such cells are found, the patient warrants close assessment and continued expectant observation. Widespread infection can occur; its severity will dictate therapy. Corticosteroids, topically and systemically, would be contraindicated because of the risk of viral dissemination, but all other topical therapy to promote resolution of the atopic dermatitis should be undertaken. Specific therapy with idoxuridine has not proved to be of much help with cutaneous infection. Acyclovir intravenously is effective and safe for the patient but should be used only if the severity of the problem warrants the risk of evoking resistant strains of herpes simplex virus, which are occurring with ever increasing frequency. Because contained viral infections can also occur in the atopic, all that may be needed is good supportive care.

Infection with the virus of verruca vulgaris or with molluscum contagiosum, even though generalized, merely requires a good topical regimen. Although some physicians would anesthetize and curette all lesions from the start, a trial of salicylic acid in flexible collodion or plaster, with self-peeling or paring by the patient, is less traumatic with less risk of scar. Destroying the epidermal cells in which the virus lives is all that is needed, but repetition and persistence are required to ensure extinction. The diagnosis of both these viral problems is usually obvious once one has seen a common verruca or an umbilicated shiny flesh-colored papule from which a core can be easily shelled. Both verruca vulgaris and molluscum contagiosum are seen most commonly in children, and both can be seen as venereal problems in young adults, but they are of greatest challenge and concern when widespread in the immunosuppressed patient or the atopic individual.

One further risk borne by the severe atopic is that of developing cataracts, which may be minimal or blinding. Occurring most frequently in the second and third decades, they are a serious complication of the atopic diathesis and may be further aggravated by corticosteroid therapy.

Canales L, Middlemas RO III, Louro JM, South MA: Immunological observations in chronic mucocutaneous candidiasis. Lancet 2:567, 1969. *Of interest for pedigree and for the focused study of an immune deficiency disease through the detailed assessment of one patient.*

Chilgren RA, Quie PG, Meuwissen HJ, Hong R: Chronic mucocutaneous candidiasis: Deficiency of delayed hypersensitivity, and selective local antibody defect. Lancet 2:688, 1977. *An update and further focus on delayed hypersensitivity.*

Farber EM, Cox AJ (eds.): Psoriasis: Proceedings of the Second International Symposium. New York, Yorke Medical Books, 1977. *The latest research and ruminations on psoriasis are published after each International Symposium.*

Fisher A: Contact Dermatitis. 2nd ed. Philadelphia, Lea & Febiger, 1973. *The cookbook for detecting the offending allergen in contact dermatitis.*

Fredriksson T, Petersson U: Severe psoriasis: Oral therapy with new retinoid. Dermatologica 157:238, 1978. *The dawn of a new era in the treatment of psoriasis.*

Montes LF, Pittman CS, Moore WJ, Taylor CG, Cooper MD: Chronic mucocutaneous candidiasis. JAMA 221:156, 1972. *The spontaneous clearing of resistant mucocutaneous candidiasis present from infancy after the detection and treatment of hypothyroidism at age seven is of interest for the implications for delayed hypersensitivity and anergy.*

556. SIGNIFICANT DERMATOLOGIC SIGNS OF DISEASE

In assessing the skin for pathology the diagnostic range extends to systemic implications of cutaneous signs. The integument nourished by blood with a markedly elevated bilirubin is a dramatic indicator of pathology. Because serologic tests can detect preclinical icterus, the clinical fact of jaundice loses its edge. However, there is an array of metabolic substances, abnormal or in excess of normal, that settle in the skin and await recognition. Lipids and amyloid are good examples. Pathologic processes such as vasculitis can affect both viscera and skin, and malignancy can extend or metastasize to both. There are also physiologic symptoms of pruritus or weakness and skin changes of ichthyosis or weeping dermatitis that relate to occult malignancy and respond to therapy directed at the malignancy. But most curious of all are the congenital aberrations and pigmentary hallmarks associated with specific systemic disease in an established but obscure relationship.

The purpose of the present chapter is to review these various skin stigmata so that they may be identified by the examiner, providing him with some broad indications of the kinds of problems with which they may be associated. Then, grouped with a special organ system as the key, selected skin signs are tabulated and ranked for potential value in suspecting or establishing a diagnosis (see Tables 556–4 to 556–7).

Acanthosis Nigricans

A brown-black velvety skin change, verrucous and creased, and localized in the axillae, nuchal folds, or groin is readily recognized as acanthosis nigricans (Fig. 556–1). Blending into normal adjacent skin, it is characteristically bilateral and symmetrical. Affecting any body fold and favoring flexural surfaces, it may rarely be generalized. Histologically there is epidermal thickening and folding over a hypertrophic papillary layer. Because acanthosis nigricans can occur with malignancy, with hormonal dysfunction, or as an inherited disorder, it is a clinical sign of note; yet neither the clinical nor the histologic appearance helps in the differential diagnosis of associated pathology.

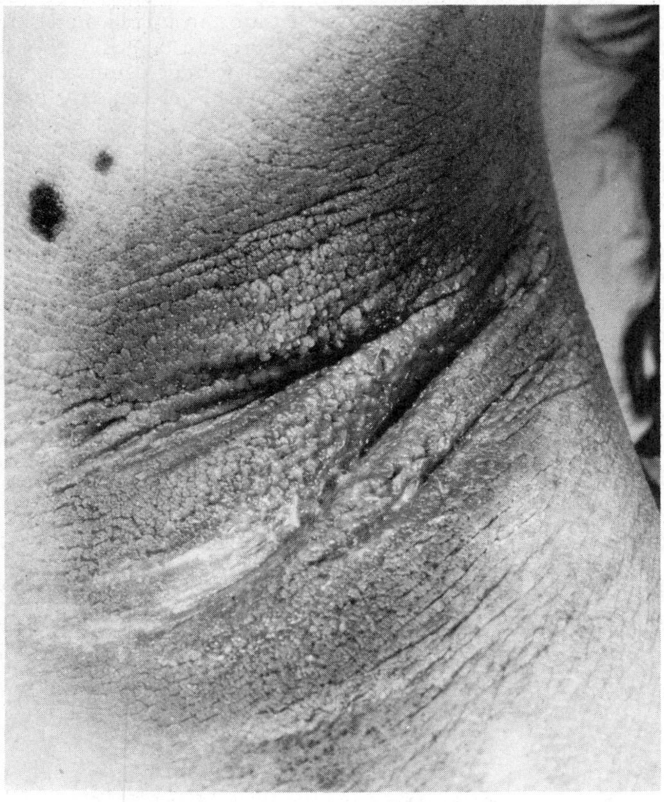

Figure 556–1. Acanthosis nigricans.

When found with visceral malignancy, usually an adenocarcinoma, the acanthosis nigricans has been labeled "malignant," a poor choice of terminology, for the skin change is in no way malignant.

Unassociated with malignancy, acanthosis nigricans is found with developmental, hormonal, and metabolic pathology, and after the administration of certain drugs and hormonal agents. In the inherited form benign cutaneous changes are considered nevoid genodermatoses present from birth or childhood with the possibility of spread or intensification at puberty. In the juvenile idiopathic type with cushingoid obesity, the onset is frequently at puberty. Acanthosis nigricans is found with adrenal insufficiency, Cushing's syndrome, acromegaly, Stein-Leventhal syndrome, and various pituitary and hypothalamic tumors or other lesions involving the base of the brain. It has been postulated that a pituitary peptide hormone secreted under hypothalamic control may stimulate papillary dermal hypertrophy. Crude preparations of MSH have been shown to induce acanthosis nigricans in a patient with melanoma, with MSH-like peptides the most likely agent. Diethylstilbestrol, corticosteroids, and nicotinic acid have also been implicated in the cutaneous phenomenon, and there are reports of appearance and disappearance correlated with the use of oral contraceptives. In insulin-resistant diabetes associated acanthosis nigricans tends to remit as the glucose intolerance lessens. Correlation is made with the antibody titer to insulin receptors.

Although there is no local therapy for acanthosis nigricans, the early recognition of the cutaneous sign, especially in the adult, warrants an immediate and thorough search for underlying pathology, especially tumor. The associated malignancies tend to be aggressive and rapidly fatal. Extension of the acanthosis nigricans is an ominous sign.

Banuchi SR, Cohen L, Lorinca AL, Morgan J: Acanthosis nigricans following diethylstilbestrol therapy: Occurrence in patients with childhood muscular dystrophy. Arch Dermatol 109:545, 1974. *Development of acanthosis nigricans in two of six children receiving diethylstilbestrol for childhood muscular dystrophy brings into question the role of estrogens in this uncommon disorder.*

Givens JR, Kerber IJ, Wiser WL, Andersen RN, Coleman SA, Fish SA: Remission of acanthosis nigricans associated with polycystic ovarian disease and a stromal luteoma. J Clin Endocrinol Metab 38:347, 1974. *The study of a case in which the suppression of luteinizing hormone and the hyperandrogenism associated with improvement of the acanthosis nigricans is important in light of the above.*

Kahn CR, Flier JS, Bar RS, Archer JA, Gorden P, Martin MM, Roth J: Syndromes of insulin resistance and acanthosis nigricans: Insulin receptor disorders in man. N Engl J Med 294:739, 1976. *Another link of hormonal abnormalities and circulating antibodies to acanthosis nigricans.*

Lerner AB: On the cause of acanthosis nigricans. N Engl J Med 281:706, 1969. *Hypothesizes that acanthosis nigricans is caused by the release of a peptide from either the pituitary gland or a nonpituitary neoplasm.*

Nordlund JJ, Lerner AB: Cause of acanthosis nigricans (letter). N Engl J Med 293:200, 1975. *Proof of the hypothesis cited above was demonstrated in a patient with melanoma.*

Ichthyosis

An integument that is rough and dry with retained scale but free of erythema suggests a "fish skin" designation (Fig. 556–2). On close inspection there may be fine scale with keratin-plugged follicles, or large polyhedral scales loosely adherent. The palms and soles may be normal, or may be thickened with accentuation of normal creases.

INHERITED. If the condition has been present from birth or childhood, perhaps only clinically apparent in dry winter months, the diagnosis is likely to be one of the *ichthyosiform dermatoses*, an inherited disorder in which excessive amounts of keratin are retained at the skin surface. Through an analysis of clinical and anatomic findings as well as a consideration of the cellular kinetics and genetic aspects, distinctions are made among the four more common types, of which ichthyosis vulgaris is the most common (Table 556–1). These ichthyoses

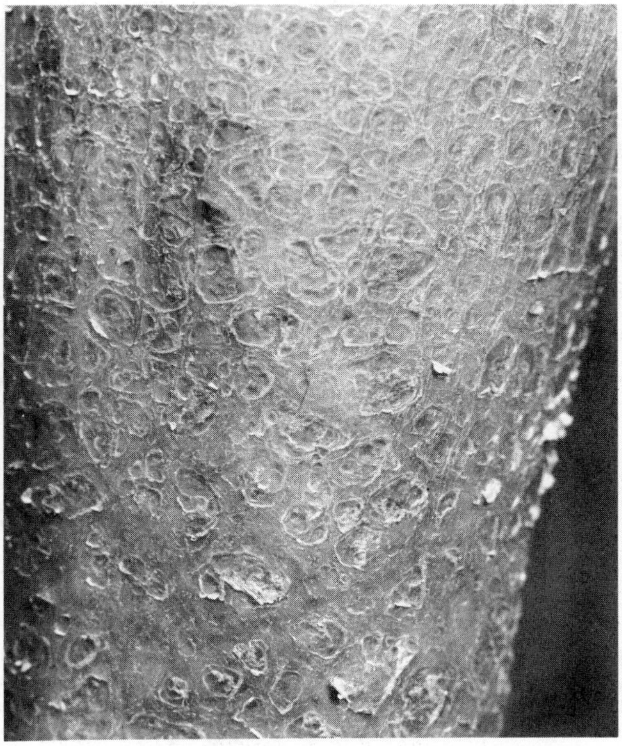

Figure 556–2. Ichthyosis.

are important to be recognized for what they are and to be differentiated from the ichthyosis-like dermatoses of abnormal lipid metabolism and the acquired ichthyosis of malignancy. Recently a biochemical deficiency of steroid sulfatase and aryl sulfatase C has been found underlying X-linked ichthyosis.

METABOLIC. Except for an inherited metabolic disorder as in Refsum's disease, the ichthyosis of abnormal lipid metabolism will appear later in life and be associated temporally with a drug that inhibits lipid synthesis, such as the butyrophenones or triparanol. So too, the dryness and scale of hypothyroidism, which may have a yellow cast because of carotenemia; it will appear with the disease and be supported by laboratory evidence of decreased thyroid function.

MALIGNANCY. The onset of ichthyosis in an adult without drug inducement or metabolic disorder is of grave significance, suggesting an underlying malignant process. Hodgkin's disease is found most frequently, but also other lymphomas, multiple myeloma, and carcinoma of the breast. As with *acanthosis nigricans,* the regression and recurrence of the tumor may be reflected in the activity of the dermatosis.

For those attuned to this significant cutaneous sign, the question of possible malignancy is often raised when the observation is of minimal dryness and polyhedral scale over the legs, arms, or abdomen of the older patient. Winter dryness at any age, but especially in the lipid-deprived skin of the elderly, is prone to pruritus and ichthyosiform change. If the problem is mild, limited, and historically of long standing or winter occurrence, the dermatosis observed is probably not a sign of tumor and should respond to simple lubrication. More intensive therapy would be to increase environmental moisture and free retained keratin with special lubricants, especially those containing urea, 15 to 30 per cent.

Frost P, Van Scott EJ: The ichthyosiform dermatoses. Classification based on anatomical and cellular kinetic observations. Arch Dermatol 94:113, 1966. *A classic sorting among recognized dermatological entities to separate and group by clinical and histologic data as well as cellular kinetics.*

Steinberg D, Vroom FQ, Engel WK, Cammermeyer J, Mize CE, Avigan J: Refsum's disease—a recently characterized lipoidosis involving the nervous system. Combined Clinical Staff Conference at the NIH. Ann Intern Med 66:365, 1967. *Although Refsum's disease is a rare inherited syndrome, it underscores the association of ichthyosis with multiple congenital ectodermal defects and a disturbance of lipid metabolism.*

Acquired Erythrodermas

ICHTHYOSIFORM

Generalized dryness and scaling with erythema in a universal distribution may be total body psoriasis. The plaque-like quality of the lesions is no longer discerned, but nail stigmata and severe scalp involvement, as well as an antecedent diagnosis of psoriasis, may aid the differential. An explosive ichthyosiform erythroderma may be a manifestation of mycosis fungoides (see Ch. 557.5).

Localized ichthyosiform or psoriasiform erythroderma may be of equal significance. *Bowen's disease,* a sharply demarcated red-brown plaque moderately thickened with scale, loose or adherent, is sometimes misdiagnosed as psoriasis. It commonly occurs on covered areas of the body, and since it can be a sequela of arsenic ingestion, patients treated in the past with Fowler's solution for psoriasis may have both psoriasis and Bowen's disease. They may also have the stigmata of arseniasis: arsenical keratoses, discrete hyperkeratotic papules of the palms and soles, plus the raindrop hyperpigmentation over the thorax. Bowen's disease is a cutaneous premalignancy, and the diagnosis can be established by biopsy. Although most Bowen's disease remains as intraepidermal carcinoma in situ for many years, it may transform into invasive squamous cell carcinoma. Any unremitting erythematous scaling lesion of long duration, especially if slowly enlarging, should be regarded with suspicion.

PAGET'S DISEASE

Paget's disease is another example. A sharply defined plaque of erythema, often eczematous with crusting or even erosion, it can be psoriasiform. Classically of the breast, it involves the nipple and areola unilaterally, perhaps only a portion, and is associated with underlying malignancy, most often a ductal adenocarcinoma. It appears usually, but not exclusively, in women; the mean age is 55 years. Extramammary Paget's disease, frequently of the anogenital area, occurs in both sexes at about the same age, but more often in women. It is without the invariable association of malignancy, which is found in less than half the patients. The malignancies that do occur derive most often from cutaneous apocrine structures.

Histologically Paget cells lie within the epidermis. Large round cells with large nuclei and abundant cytoplasm, they can be confused with nevus cells and those of Bowen's disease, although mucin stains are helpful in the differential. The histopathology is definitive and underscores the importance of biopsy for any persistent psoriasiform or eczematous lesion anywhere, but especially of the breast. In the patient with skin that is otherwise normal, the lesion of Paget's disease is obvious

TABLE 556–1. COMMON ICHTHYOSIFORM DERMATOSES

	Inheritance	Onset	Distribution	Clinical Associations	Kinetics
Lamellar ichthyosis	Autosomal recessive	Birth	Body, palms, soles	Ectropion	Increased
Epidermolytic hyperkeratosis	Autosomal dominant	Birth	Predominant flexural involvement	Blisters	Increased
X-linked ichthyosis (steroid sulfatase deficiency)	X-linked	Birth	Trunk	Corneal opacities	Normal
Ichthyosis vulgaris	Autosomal dominant	Childhood	Spares flexural areas	Atopy	Normal

and the course clear. It is the patient with other psoriasiform and eczematous dermatitis who is at risk of having Paget's disease overlooked. Any suspicious lesion of the areola should be treated intensively for a week or two with high potency steroid; if the skin does not return to normal, the lesion should be biopsied.

ACRODERMATITIS ENTEROPATHICA

This condition is occasionally misdiagnosed as psoriasis, and more often as candidiasis because of periorificial dermatitis, but it can present with reddened ichthyosiform plaques. It is a persistent dermatitis about the mouth, with acral involvement that begins as vesicles but is soon crusted, thickened, and perhaps superinfected with bacteria or *Candida,* and may be associated with diarrhea. The symptoms are due to zinc deficiency and are seen when there is hyperalimentation without attention to trace metal supplements in the course of malabsorptive disorders, but the disorder is of greater interest as an inherited defect. With its onset in childhood and poor prognosis without therapy, the adult form of acrodermatitis enteropathica, even if not controlled, will have been identified. Two thirds of patients have a family history of the disease, and an autosomal recessive inheritance is suggested. The affected children tend to be slow in growth and development, and to have a deficiency in cell-mediated immunity. They are reported to have increased IgA and deficient or "absent" thymus, and to lack germinal centers and plasmacytosis of lymph nodes and spleen. In the bowel, in the fasting state, jejunal cytoplasmic inclusions are found by electron microscopy. Plasma zinc levels are low, but also decreased are serum lipids and arachidonic acid. Prostaglandin synthesis is defective. Zinc supplements will dramatically reverse all clinical manifestations of the disease within a few days, even in adult patients plagued with the disease from childhood. Abnormalities of the intestinal mucosa were noted to revert to normal on oral zinc therapy.

Although it is not clear that the defect in zinc uptake is the primary lesion, prostaglandin "zinc-binding ligand" is necessary for zinc absorption. Aspirin, which inhibits prostaglandin synthesis, impairs zinc absorption in rats. Arachidonic acid, decreased in acrodermatitis enteropathica, is known to be a prostaglandin precursor. There is the further evidence of clinical benefit from a dietary supplement of zinc or prostaglandin. Curiously, human milk has PGE_2 as a zinc ligand; cow's milk has none, fitting the frequently observed onset of the disease at weaning. Because calcium ingestion can impede zinc absorption in the gastrointestinal tract, as can soy milk protein, the prescribing of zinc supplements should include precautions about calcium, soy proteins, and aspirin.

Evans GW, Johnson PE: Defective prostaglandin synthesis in acrodermatitis enteropathica (letter). Lancet 1:52, 1977. *A succinct assessment of the recognized role of zinc and prostaglandin in acrodermatitis enteropathica, the report of the isolation of a low-molecular weight zinc binding ligand from human milk, and the neat conclusion that the zinc-prostaglandin complex in human milk explains the observed clinical efficacy of human breast milk in the treatment of acrodermatitis enteropathica.*

Hirsch FS, Michel B, Strain WH: Gluconate zinc in acrodermatitis enteropathica. Arch Dermatol 112:475, 1976. *From clinical observations of two patients much is deduced about the effectiveness and best use of gluconate zinc.*

Kelly R, Davidson GP, Townley RRW, Campbell PE: Reversible intestinal mucosal abnormality in acrodermatitis enteropathica. Arch Dis Child 51:219, 1976. *The reassurance of the documented reversibility of the pathology of the intestinal mucosa was an important impetus to further the search for more effective therapy.*

Michaelson G: Zinc therapy in acrodermatitis enteropathica. Acta Derm Venereol 54:377, 1974. *The search is always for the cause, but without finding it the course may be altered. After 18 years of difficult and discouraging management of acrodermatitis enteropathica, an observed low serum zinc value suggested treatment with zinc sulfate with prompt and impressive good results.*

EXFOLIATIVE ERYTHRODERMA

When the skin is normal rather than thickened but generally red with fine scale, the term exfoliative erythroderma (Fig. 556–3) is used. It can be the eventuality of any extensive eruption; when seen, of itself, it gives few clues to the etiology. Drug allergy, contact dermatitis, an eczematous process, seborrheic dermatitis or psoriasis, the lymphomas and leukemias, or any extensive inflammatory insult to the skin may be the cause. Older patients are more predisposed to the phenomenon, and it is most difficult to clear in them; it may smolder for months or years.

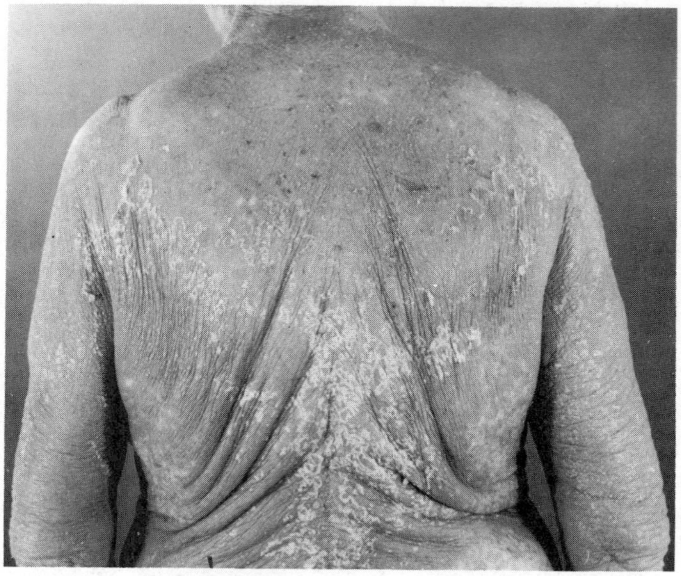

Figure 556–3. Exfoliative erythroderma.

The best treatment is prevention. Any acute dermatitis of whatever etiology should be quieted with wet dressings and topical steroids, with antihistamines or other sedation, and with rest. The specific cause should be sought, although it may remain obscure. If the eruption continues to progress, systemic steroids or immune suppression should be considered. If generalized exfoliation has occurred, initial efforts should be conservative and supportive, but systemic therapy will probably be needed.

PHOTOSENSITIVITY

The skin of the normal individual will react to sunlight in a range of responses that are modified by pigmentary protection, geographic location, solar and solstice time, and duration of exposure. The data derived would be a base line of normal and predictable responses, however varied or unpleasant, from no reaction through erythema to blistering; cumulatively one could anticipate actinic damage (see Ch. 552) and malignancy (see Ch. 557). Here, however, consideration is given only to responses that deviate from the normal as modified by genetic, chemical, allergic, or nutritional factors.

The patient with an abnormal light reaction could present with an exaggerated sunburn in a patterned exposure with the outline of protective clothing, but more often there is merely the subtle sparing of the submental area of the chin or the eyelids, perhaps with accentuation at the "V" of the neck. Frequently the lesions are not as diffuse as a burn but are characterized by papules or urticaria, or even an eczematous response.

To sort out the etiology, light must be suspected from historical or physical evidence and from any recognized predisposition to sun sensitivity. Seasonal recurrences, especially in the spring or early summer, would arouse suspicion. The evoked reaction may be to light alone, to light in association with abnormal metabolites as in the porphyrias, or to light plus chemicals and medications applied to the skin or ingested.

Light Alone

Adverse reactions to light alone are rare and may all have a genetic predisposition. *Xeroderma pigmentosum,* for example, inherited as an autosomal recessive problem, has a defect in DNA repair or replication. The light-exposed skin undergoes severe early solar damage with erythema, spotty pigmentation, atrophy, and neoplasm. From infancy there is photophobia and a prolonged erythematous response to sun. In albinism, too, there is photophobia and increased sun sensitivity, but the skin, except for lacking the protective shield of pigment, is normal. Repair is normal. The defect in the tyrosinase function of the melanocyte leaves the albino with a sunburn susceptibility comparable to that of the lightest-complexioned Celt.

But more than an exaggerated response to sun damage, light alone can evoke a polymorphous light eruption. Common among certain North American Indians, and reported in families and identical twins, it is without indication of genetic factors in most patients. As the name polymorphous photodermatitis implies, the eruption is a mixture of papules and vesicles which may become confluent. It occurs at any age but usually has its onset in young adulthood with no evidence of sex predisposition or protection from melanin; it is seen in a range of patients of all races from the lightly to the heavily pigmented. Pursuing a chronic course, it flares each spring until some sun tolerance develops in summer. Selected sun protection and topical steroids are the mainstay of therapy.

Light Plus

METABOLITES. With the porphyrias, of which there are at least seven types, light reacts with circulating porphyrins present in the cutaneous tissue to produce both acute and chronic change. The onset of photosensitivity in childhood and the associated severe scarring, hair loss, and discolored teeth readily suggest the diagnosis of congenital erythropoietic porphyria. Even the milder symptoms of burning, edema, and waxy scars of congenital erythropoietic protoporphyria will suggest light as a damaging factor. The manifestations of photosensitivity in the adult onset porphyrias are more subtle, however. The appearance of skin fragility with bullae and erosions localized to the dorsa of the hands, possibly involving the forehead or scalp of the balding older patient, is frequently missed as a sign of porphyria cutanea tarda (Fig. 556–4). Such patients excrete urinary uroporphyrins and some coproporphyrins and can be shown to be photosensitive to those wavelengths of light which the porphyrin molecule absorbs best: 400 to 410 nm in the blue-violet region, and 500 to 600 nm in the orange. Their sun-exposed skin becomes prematurely aged, with associated hypertrichosis characteristically found at the outer canthus of the eyes. Therapy by phlebotomy to reduce hepatic iron stores and porphyrin production, and the use of sun screens to filter out the damaging light rays give most patients with acquired porphyria sustained remissions from the dermatologic manifestations of the disease.

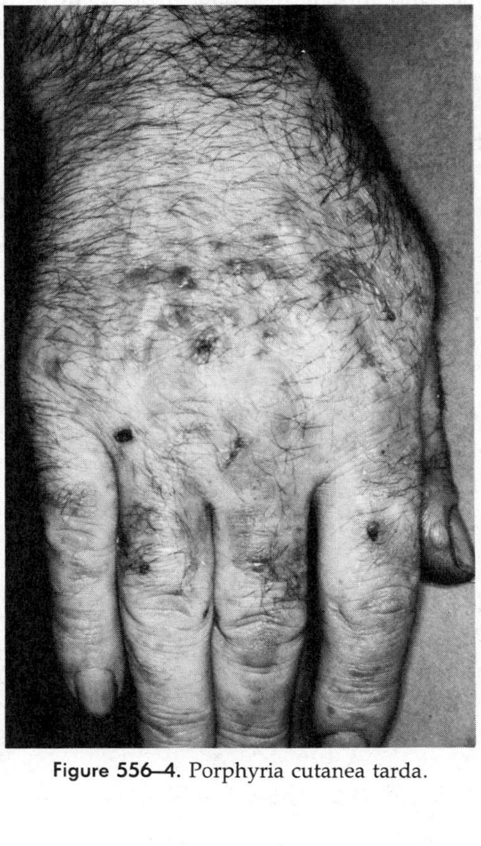

Figure 556–4. Porphyria cutanea tarda.

Photosensitivity is also observed with the aminoacidurias. In Hartnup disease, for example, in which there is a transport defect of tryptophan, with hydroxykynureninuria and tryptophanuria, minimal exposure to sun can lead to erythema, edema, and even vesiculation. At least for Hartnup disease, the eruption is associated with a cellular deficiency of nicotinamide. As in nutritional pellagra, high doses of nicotinamide improve the dermatitis. The observation that patients deficient in nicotinamide excrete increased amounts of certain porphyrins and indican has led to the suggestion for all these photosensitivity responses that sunlight induces photochemical reactions in the skin that lead to tissue destruction and antigen formation.

EXOGENOUS AGENTS. Of even greater diagnostic challenge are the many phototoxic and photoallergic reactions encountered. *Phototoxicity* occurs without recognized immune mechanisms. It is the kind of reaction seen in patients receiving systemic antimicrobial therapy such as Declomycin or sulfonamides; dyes such as acridine, methyl violet, or eosin; psychotherapeutic drugs such as phenothiazine; the sulfonylurea hypoglycemic agents; the thiazide diuretics; and the antifungal agent griseofulvin. Upon exposure to light there is burning, followed by prompt erythema and edema reaching a maximum intensity in 12 to 24 hours, and then by desquamation and hyperpigmentation. The initial reaction is common to a large number of people upon first exposure. The sensitivity will not persist, and future exposure to ultraviolet light will be normal.

Photoallergy differs in that reactions, although occasionally prompt and urticarial, can appear after 24 hours or more. They occur in only a small number of exposed individuals, are often persistent, and show cross-photosensitization; with photo patch testing there may be flares at previous reaction sites. Few oral ingestants contribute to the phenomenon, although sulfanilamide, sulfadiazine, and sulfisoxazole have been implicated as being both phototoxic and photoallergic. The bulk of photoallergy is through topical exposure, whether airborne or applied, and such reactions should be known as *photoallergic contact dermatitis.* It is postulated that light acts upon the offending chemical to form a haptene that binds protein, accounting for persistence and recurrence.

Therapy for all photodermatitis is the treatment for burn and contact dermatitis. With phototoxicity, if there is merely marked erythema, or if the reaction is noted early, topical steroids with occlusion will encourage vasoconstriction and reduce the overall intensity of the reaction. With photoallergy antihistamine may be helpful. Whether phototoxic or photoallergic, the offending agent must be sought to be identified and avoided, along with its cross-reactants.

Brodthager H: Polymorphous light eruption. *In* Urbach F (ed.): The Biologic Effects of Ultraviolet Radiation. Oxford, Pergamon Press, 1969. *A review of the physical effects of ultraviolet light.*

Cleaver JE: Defective repair replication of DNA in xeroderma pigmentosum. Nature 218:652, 1968. *The problem of radiation-induced malignancy came into sharper focus with the demonstration of a defect in DNA repair replication by fibroblasts from patients with xeroderma pigmentosum.*

Cleaver JE: Xeroderma pigmentosum: Variants with normal DNA repair and normal sensitivity to ultraviolet light. J Invest Dermatol 58:124, 1972. *Following the above, however, the reporting of variants of xeroderma pigmentosum, with the classic predisposition to cutaneous malignancy but with fibroblasts indistinguishable from normal cells in repair replication, would caution against inferences about DNA repair and carcinogenesis.*

Urbach F, Davies RE, Forbes PD: Ultraviolet radiation and skin cancer in man. *In* Montagna W (ed.): Advances in Biology of Skin Carcinogenesis. Oxford, Pergamon Press, 1966. *The basics for ultraviolet radiation and cutaneous malignancy in man.*

Light-Sensitive Diseases

Lupus erythematosus, known for its photosensitivity, is characterized by the isomorphic response whereby exposure to sunlight will evoke lesions of lupus erythematosus in the skin. In the patient with recognized disease the untoward response will be accepted and skin lesions, however mildly erythematous or urticarial, will be clinically identified as the disease. In a patient without antecedent diagnosis, however, an urticarial response to sunlight may be overlooked as a first manifestation of a collagen disease. Persistence of the hive, bluing of the erythema, development of scale, and follicular plugging should suggest the diagnosis, and histopathologic evidence should support it.

Pigmentary Disturbances

Color changes in the skin and mucous membrane are common and occasionally important. The wide range of normal hues and markings that racial diversity confers makes it necessary to review continuously the full array of normal possibilities through attention to the multiple banal lesions in every patient examined.

Melanin contributes significantly to the color of eyes, hair, and skin. It is most conspicuous in its heavy concentration or total absence. Brown to black eumelanin is a high molecular weight, relatively insoluble polymer, a polyquinone. In man it is derived from the phenolic precursors tyrosine and 3,4-dihydroxyphenylalanine (dopa). Tyrosinase, a copper-containing enzyme, catalyzes the oxidation of tyrosine in the cytoplasm of the melanocyte. Formed melanin is then transferred to keratinocytes; thus skin color derives from pigment in the epidermal cells as well as the melanocytes. When deep in the skin, melanin can appear blue or slate colored because of light scatter of the Tyndall effect.

Although melanocyte distribution is varied throughout the body, with twice higher concentrations in the skin of the head and forearms than in the rest of the skin (excepting the scrotum and foreskin), there are no differences in distribution or total numbers among races. Genotypic variations that underlie racial differences are within the ultrastructure of the melanocyte relating to the production and distribution of melanosomes following ultraviolet light irradiation or other stimulation. In situations in which generalized pigmentation is induced, the pigment pattern will reflect the melanocyte concentration.

HYPERPIGMENTATION

Ephelides

Increased concentrations of melanin may be localized or diffuse. The circumscribed melanoses commonly observed include *ephelides* or freckles, the small flat macules of less than 0.5 cm that first appear on sun-exposed areas at about age four and tend to fade in later life. Long wave ultraviolet light, 300 to 400 nm, will darken them. The melanocytes of ephelides are not increased in number but are more arborized and more active in melanin production.

Lentigines

These small flat macular lesions resemble ephelides clinically but are histologically distinct because of increased numbers of normal-appearing melanocytes. Evoked by aging and solar damage, they come in later life—so-called "liver spots," the *senile lentigo*.

A separate group unrelated to light, in fact occasionally involving mucous membranes, appearing at any age and genetically determined, is the *nevoid lentigines*. Associated with inherited syndromes such as the "leopard" syndrome and Moynihan's syndrome, they are present from birth and are found with a wide range of defects and mental retardation. In Peutz-Jeghers syndrome, the perioral mucous membrane and digital lentigines are associated with small bowel polyps, especially of the jejunum. These histologically distinct hamartomas arising from the muscularis mucosae have little malignant propensity in the small bowel, but when also present in the colon the risk of malignancy is increased.

Freckles of the axillae, especially when seen with irregular hyperpigmented mottling of the skin elsewhere, are known as Crowe's sign of neurofibromatosis. The pigment changes are believed to be a variant of café-au-lait spots, the large tan uniformly pigmented macules that may be present at birth anywhere on the skin or may appear later. Café-au-lait spots larger than 1.5 cm and more numerous than six are suggested as presumptive evidence of neurofibromatosis. They are also seen in other neurocutaneous syndromes such as tuberous sclerosis. In Albright's syndrome the circumscribed hypermelanotic macules may appear in a linear, rarely segmental pattern on one side or the other without crossing the midline. They occur on the forehead, nuchal and sacral areas, and buttocks. Their distribution rather than their clinical appearance or histology distinguishes them from the café-au-lait lesions of neurofibromatosis.

Pigmented Nevi

Pigmented nevi, often called moles, are formed of clusters of melanocytes and are rarely present from birth. They are divided clinically and histologically into four groups: the nevus spilus, and junctional, compound, and dermal nevi or moles. The nevus spilus (Fig. 556–5) is a small oval macule from tan to dark brown or black, usually of uniform color. Hyperpigmentation of the keratinocyte is intense, and there may be elongation of the rete ridges. The melanocytes are normal, not nested. Histologic differentiation is also used for the further classification of the moles or nevi, often called nevus cell nevi to distinguish them from the epidermal and connective tissue nevi. Junctional nevi have nevus cell nests above the basement membrane, compound nevi have them in both the epidermis and dermis, and intradermal nevi have them in the dermis

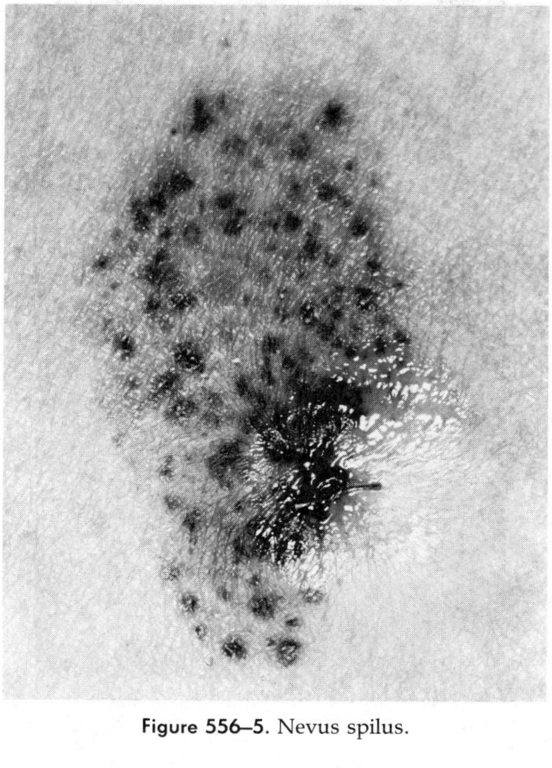

Figure 556–5. Nevus spilus.

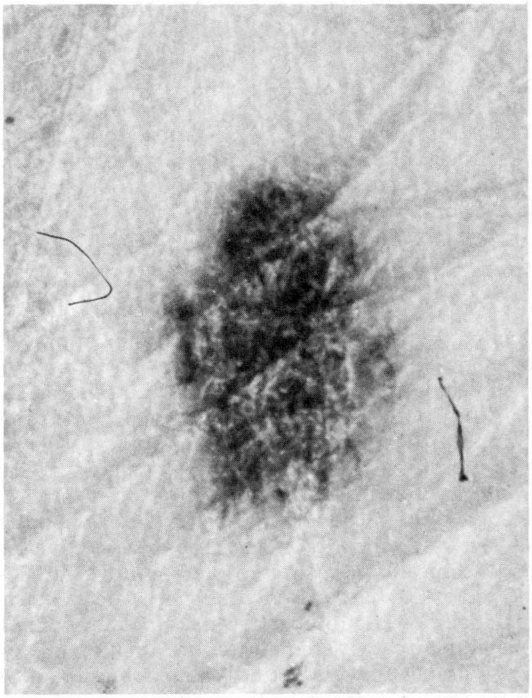

Figure 556–6. Junctional nevus.

alone. Junctional nevi tend to be flat and pigmented, dark brown to black, with the pigment orderly and the skin markings preserved (Fig. 556–6). Compound and intradermal nevi (Fig. 556–7) may be dome shaped, polypoid, or even verrucoid. They may be deeply pigmented but mostly are light or even skin colored.

Occasionally a depigmented area may develop around a nevus cell nevus, sometimes with eventual obliteration of the nevus. Occurring primarily in children and young adults, the *"halo nevus"* has been associated with vitiligo and noted in melanoma.

Not nevi but sometimes confused with them are *seborrheic keratoses*, the benign keratotic tumor of aging. Their distribution, growth, and depth of pigment are sunlight related, and their numbers can be legion. Beginning as yellow to light brown flat lesions with a verrucous or velvety surface, they can develop from less than 1 cm to several centimeters, become dark brown with a greasy keratotic scale, and assume a "tacked on" appearance.

Their importance is in differentiating them from nevi or not overlooking a changing nevus among them; also, they have been reported in their explosive appearance or sudden enlargement to be associated with underlying malignancy (the sign of Leser-Trélat).

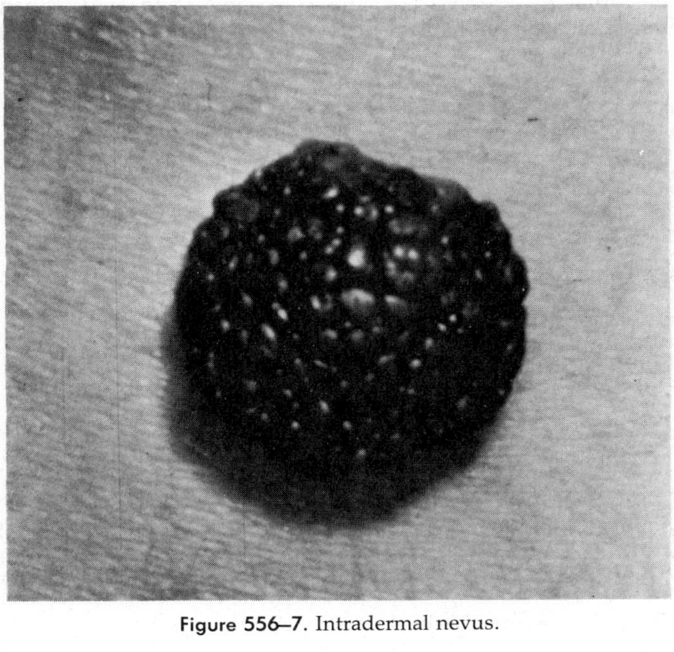

Figure 556–7. Intradermal nevus.

Pigment in Patterns

Whorls of pigmentation, zebra stripes, and angular flecks and sprays, occurring in no known neural or anatomic configuration and crossing the midline, should suggest *incontinentia pigmenti* (Fig. 556–8). The macules are dark brown or slate colored and intensely pigmented in childhood. With gradual fading they leave few dermatologic residua in later adult life. However, the patterned pigmentation should warn the examiner of the possibility of ectodermal defects and the need for genetic counseling. Although incontinentia pigmenti is of unknown etiology, the evidence suggests genetic transmission of the disease as an autosomal dominant with expression mainly in females or as an X-linked trait lethal for males. It presents with an inflammatory vesicobullous phase with little or no pigment change, and evolves either through a verrucous papillomatous phase or directly to the distinctive pigmentation. One or more of the stages may be present at birth or may begin in the first weeks of life. Despite the extent of the inflammatory lesion, the patient is afebrile. There may be pronounced eosinophilia of the blood and vesicle fluid.

The importance of recognizing the pigmentary stigma is the identification of a significant genodermatosis and the association of the diagnosis with other ectodermal abnormalities in 60 per cent of patients. Eyes, teeth, central nervous system, and cutaneous appendages are affected. Eye problems include strabismus, nystagmus, blue sclerae, optic atrophy, exudative chorioretinitis, papillitis, congenital retinal folds, and retrobulbar glioma. With the dental abnormalities, permanent dentition is compromised. There are impacted and missing teeth, pegged

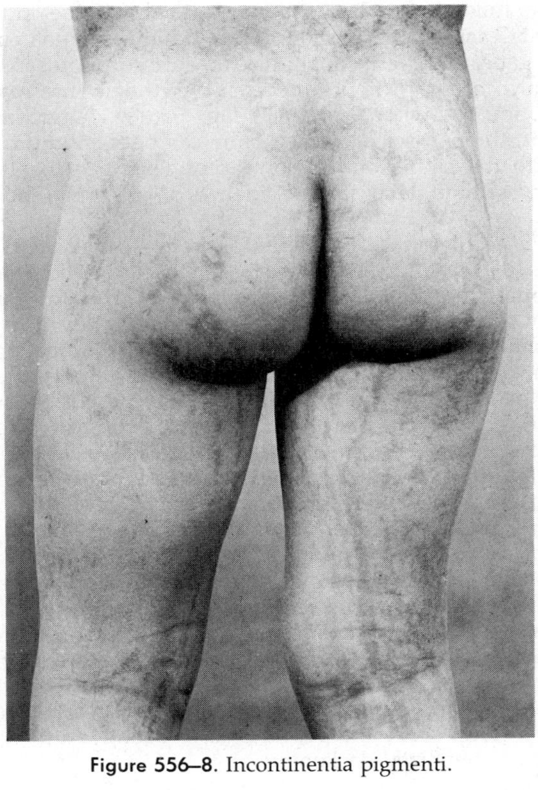

Figure 556–8. Incontinentia pigmenti.

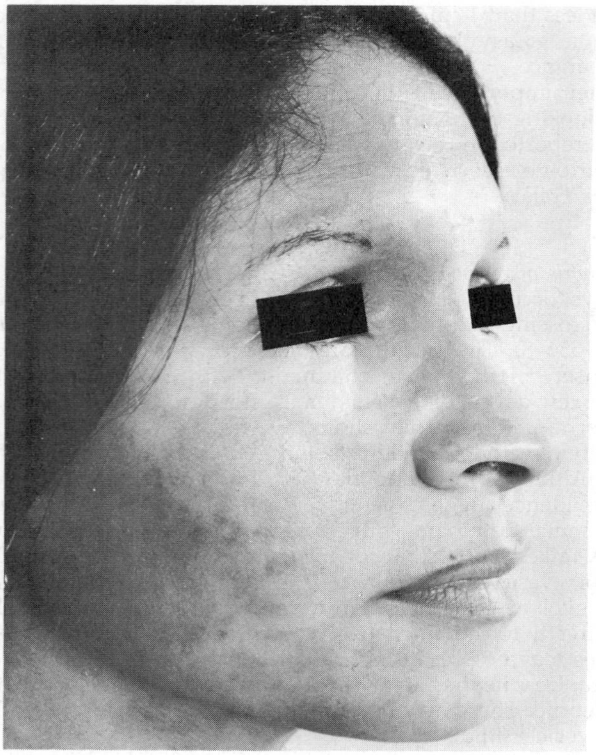

Figure 556–9. Melasma.

teeth, and malformed crowns. Neurologically, seizures and spastic paralysis are seen, and there may be mental retardation, deafness, and homonymous hemianopsia. Occasionally there are cardiac abnormalities and skeletal deformities, including syndactyly and shortened extremities.

Other Hyperpigmentations

Blotchy pigmentation of the skin without discrete lesions may be seen following inflammation, especially if the individual pigments easily. Thus it may follow trauma such as cuts and burns, generalized eruptions, or exposure to photosensitizers. It can also occur without antecedent erythema in a mask-like distribution known as *melasma* (Fig. 556–9). Aggravated by sunlight, the patterned pigmentation can be seen in pregnancy and with the taking of oral contraceptives, but it is also seen in men without laboratory evidence of abnormal hormonal levels.

Generalized hyperpigmentation is often associated with abnormalities of the endocrine system but can also be related to nutritional, metabolic, or chemical factors and to drugs. In primary adrenocortical insufficiency the pituitary activity increases in response to the decreased cortisol. With melanocyte-stimulating hormone (MSH) elaborated in excess by the pituitary along with the corticotropin (ACTH), there is consequent darkening of the skin. An MSH-producing tumor of the pituitary would have the same effect. If increased ACTH were also produced, the stimulation of the adrenal might make the initial clinical impression that of Cushing's syndrome. Without appreciation for the central lesions the adrenals might be removed.

Diffuse melanosis is seen in the cachectic and with metabolic problems such as hemochromatosis and biliary cirrhosis. It has been noted with inorganic arsenical poisoning and with a number of drugs, including busulfan and long-term high dose chlorpromazine. In malignancies such as melanoma, melanin may be deposited directly in the dermis. With certain tumors, as of the lung, MSH-like peptides have been identified which stimulate generalized darkening.

HYPOPIGMENTATION

Localized

In assessing a circumscribed area of leukoderma, the distinction between hypomelanosis and amelanosis is crucial and should be confirmed by Wood's light examination, which shows the amelanotic lesion as ivory white. If by historical data it can be determined that normal amounts of pigment were never present in the lesion, a developmentally determined nevoid lesion is suggested as distinct from the progressive pigmentary losses of varying cause.

Tuberous Sclerosis

A polygonal hypomelanosis, an ovoid lesion rounded at one end and tapered at the other like the leaf of a mountain ash, is seen from birth in 85 per cent of patients with tuberous sclerosis (Fig. 556–10). Found in the skin over trunk and limbs, the lesions range in size from a few millimeters to several centimeters. They appear before the other skin signs and can be of signal value in the differential diagnosis of seizures. By age four, 90 per cent of patients will have developed *adenoma sebaceum*—actually angiofibromas without sebaceous gland involvement. Clinically these are red-pink nodules with a smooth surface found at the nasolabial folds, over the cheeks and chin, and occasionally on the forehead and scalp. In the lumbosacral area the shagreen patch, a circumscribed area of subepidermal fibrosis, is almost always found. Skin-colored and slightly raised, it resembles studded leather. The ungual fibromas, soft pink papules growing out from the nail bed, are the fourth skin sign of tuberous sclerosis and appear first at puberty. Intraoral fibromas are also seen, and there can be increased pigmentation as manifested in bronzing of the skin and café-au-lait macules.

Because the classic triad of tuberous sclerosis, the seizures, mental retardation, and adenoma sebaceum, is so emphasized, the importance of subtle signs pathognomonic of the diagnosis is sometimes ignored.

DEPIGMENTATION

Partial Albinism

Areas of amelanosis in otherwise normal skin have a limited differential diagnosis. In partial albinism or piebaldism, the lack of pigment is unchanged from birth with melanocytes absent in the white areas. It is inherited as a simple autosomal dominant; there is frequently an associated white forelock. In contrast with vitiligo, there are often normally pigmented macules in hypomelanotic areas. Piebaldism associated with perceptual deafness is considered Woolf's syndrome. When there is also lateral displacement of inner canthi and of lacrimal

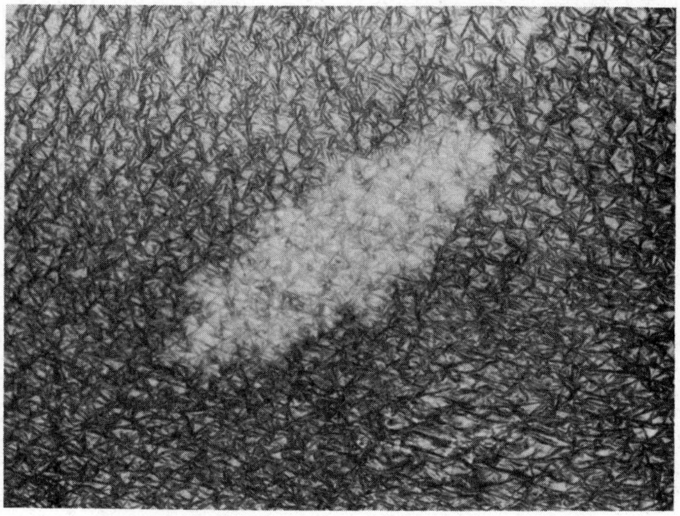

Figure 556–10. Tuberous sclerosis ash leaf.

puncta, prominence of the nasal root and the medial eyebrows, and heterochromic irides, it is considered Waardenburg's syndrome with a neural crest abnormality proposed as the cause.

Vitiligo

Vitiligo can be present from infancy but usually is not. Half the patients note the onset before the third decade. Pigment is lost in exposed areas, about body orifices, over pressure points, and from the axillae, genitalia, hair, and nevi (halo nevus). Occurring in 0.5 per cent of the population of the United States, vitiligo is inherited as an autosomal dominant trait with variable expression. Familial early graying is frequently found. Melanocytes, present from birth, persist in the vitiliginous areas for a time but eventually disappear. Autoimmune mechanisms have been suggested for the melanocyte destruction, and also the failure to protect against toxic intermediates generated during melanogenesis.

Individuals with vitiligo are usually healthy, but the prevalence of vitiligo is higher than expected among patients with diseases suspected of autoimmune pathogenesis: pernicious anemia, thyroid dysfunction, Addison's disease, and alopecia areata. Circulating antibody for gastric parietal cell antigens, thyroglobulin, and adrenal antigens has been demonstrated in patients with vitiligo, with and without endocrine pathology or pernicious anemia. In adult onset diabetes, vitiligo is encountered five times more frequently than in controls. Further, a number of ocular syndromes with uveitis, as well as gastritis, gastric cancer, IgA deficiency, and melanoma, are reported with vitiligo.

When vitiligo is *universal* and includes the hair, eye color remains. Even without a history of pigment loss, such a totally depigmented patient is readily distinguished from the albino. There is no photophobia. Biopsy would also differentiate between the two, for melanocytes are present in normal numbers in the albino; the pathology is in the enzyme tyrosinase which is defective or absent.

Albinism

Albinism, an inherited defect in melanin synthesis, affects skin, hair, and eyes to varying degrees according to the completeness of the defect, permitting classification of at least six types of oculocutaneous albinism and three of ocular albinism (Table 556–2). Skin and eye color may be diluted over a considerable range, with some individuals having yellow or yellow-brown hair with pigmented irides and some tanning on sun exposure. Eye symptoms may be minimal. Related to the severity of the defect and to the intensity and frequency of actinic exposure, the cumulative dosage of radiation will produce cutaneous malignancy. In a Nigerian study, no albino over the age of 20 was without such change.

Neurofibromas

Clinical neurofibromatosis of the skin (Fig. 556–11) is no diagnostic challenge. With its multiple skin-colored pedunculated tumors and subcutaneous nodules along nerve sheaths, the cosmetic disfigurement is vivid and remembered. If the disease is early, or not fully expressed, or even without the disease at all, an individual may have a solitary neurofibroma, an organoid overgrowth of Schwann cells and endoneurium that presents clinically as a smooth, flesh-colored, dome-shaped papule, soft to firm, looking rather like an intradermal nevus. A doughy feel and the ability to invaginate the lesion could aid the differential diagnosis. When seen in association with the café-au-lait spots (Fig. 556–12) and axillary freckles as described above, the diagnosis should be made.

Neurofibromatosis of von Recklinghausen is a dominantly inherited disorder with systemic manifestations in the nervous system, bone, and soft tissues as well as skin. Half the cases are sporadic, presumably representing new mutations, but once expressed they will transmit the disease as a mendelian dominant. It occurs in one of 3000 births and has a prevalence of 0.04 per cent.

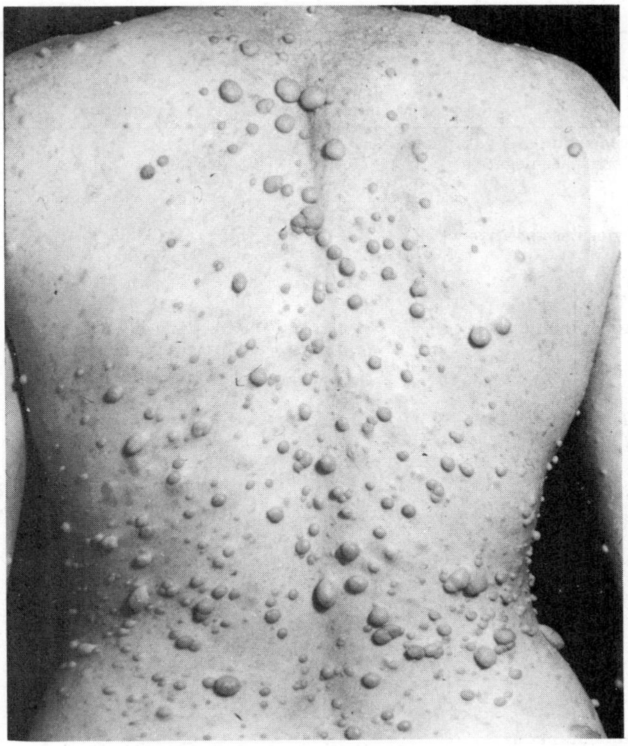

Figure 556–11. Neurofibromatosis—von Recklinghausen's disease.

The pigmentary stigmata of neurofibromatosis can be present at birth, and 90 per cent of patients with the disease will have them. The tumors, with rare exceptions, begin to develop after birth but before puberty, becoming more numerous throughout life. They may arise in all tissues, including bone and lung, in which they cause cystic lesions. Bone lesions, occurring in half the patients, are quite variable, and may represent growth

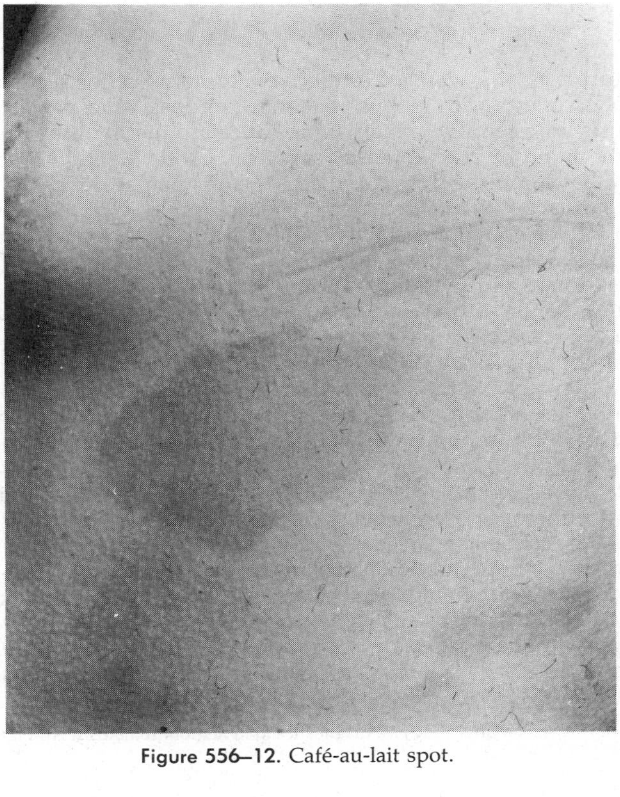

Figure 556–12. Café-au-lait spot.

TABLE 556–2. ALBINISM

			Skin		Hair		
	Inheritance	Frequency	Color	Pigmented Nevi Freckles		Color	Red Reflex
Oculocutaneous Albinism							
Tyrosinase-negative	AR*	1 in 34,000	pink/wte	none	white	gray-blue	present
Tyrosinase-positive	AR	blk: 1 in 15,000 wte: 1 in 40,000	wte-cream	present	wte-yellow red-darkens	blue-yellow brown	present but may be absent in dark races
Yellow-mutant	AR	rare—Amish, Polish, German-American; Blacks (American, Ceylonese, African)	wte at birth, slgt tan pos	present	wte-birth red/yellow 6 mos	blue at birth; darkens	present
Hermansky-Pudlak syndrome	AR	rare—cases from Puerto Rico; Southern Holland; Madras	cream-lgt normal	present	wte-red dk brown	blue-gray to brown	wte—present blk—absent
Cross-McKusick-Breen syndrome (oculocerebral hypopigmentation syndrome)	AR	extremely rare—3 in Amish family	pink/wte	present	wte-lt yel	gray-blue	?, cataracts
Chédiak-Higashi syndrome	AR	rare in most countries; none in blacks	pink/wte	present	blond-dk brown-steel gray	blue to brown	present but diminishes with time
Oculocutaneous Albinoidism	AD†		pink/wte	?	wte blond	blue	present
Ocular Albinism							
Vogt	X-linked	uncommon	normal	present	normal	blue	
Forsius-Eriksson	X-linked	less common	normal	present	normal	blue	
Autosomal recessive	AR	10 families	normal	present	normal	blue	present

*AR = Autosomal recessive.
†AD = Autosomal dominant.

disturbances as well as erosion by tumor. Scoliosis, severe kyphoscoliosis with gibbus formation, lordosis, and pseudoarthrosis are seen. Of greater significance are the neurofibromas in the brain or cranial nerves, eye, or bowel. Mental capacity may be diminished by the disease, and mental deficiency is not unusual. Bilateral acoustic neuromas lead to deafness; gliomas of the optic nerve present with exophthalmia and decreased visual acuity. There may be nodules of the iris and hamartomas of the retina.

In patients with pheochromocytoma, 5 to 10 per cent have neurofibromatosis.

Although the quality of life is severely compromised in von Recklinghausen's disease, the prognosis for survival is fairly good. Mesenteric and colonic neurofibroma may cause obstruction or result in bleeding. There is risk of malignancy—5 to 16 per cent in various series. The malignant tumors may be neurofibrosarcomas, histologically malignant nonmetastasizing brain tumors, liposarcomas, rhabdomyosarcomas, or undifferentiated sarcomas. The dangers for patients with neurofibromatosis are hypertension and sudden enlargement of a tumor. Blood pressure should be checked regularly and tumors with growth spurts biopsied. In younger patients, or those with limited numbers of lesions, continuing excisions of neurofibromas of the head and arms may contain the cosmetic disfigurement.

Crowe FW: Axillary freckling as a diagnostic aid in neurofibromatosis. Ann Intern Med 61:1142, 1964. *A subtle cutaneous sign of note.*

Fienman NL, Yakovac WC: Neurofibromatosis in childhood. J Pediat 76:339, 1970. *Underscoring the possibility and importance of early detection for counseling and because of the risk of malignancy.*

Person JR, Perry HO: Recent advances in phakomatoses. Int J Dermatol 17:1, 1978. *An excellent review.*

Schenkein I, Beuker ED, Helson L, Axelrod F, Dancis J: Increased nerve-growth-stimulating activity in disseminated neurofibromatosis. N Engl J Med 290:613, 1974. *This brief report is important for its observations and for provoking the challenging editorial that appeared in the same issue, cited below.*

Snyder SH: Nerve growth in neurofibromatosis (editorial). N Engl J Med 290:626, 1974.

Pseudoxanthoma Elasticum

A change in the skin of the neck and axilla that is reticular and sometimes telangiectatic, with small 1- to 3-mm tan-yellow papules resembling chicken skin, should bring pseudoxanthoma elasticum to mind. The problem is an inherited disorder of elastic tissue, occurring in both autosomal recessive and autosomal dominant forms that involve the skin, vascular system, and eyes. The earliest histologic change is the deposits of calcium on elastic fibers that seem otherwise normal. Fragmentation of these fibers in the skin, blood vessels, and Bruch's membrane produces the characteristic clinical features. Prevalence rates are estimated at 0.001 to 0.006 per thousand, and females are affected more frequently than males.

The skin lesions develop in the second decade or later and are progressive. Characteristically seen at the sides of the neck, in axilla, and in groin, they may be found in the flexural areas

TABLE 556–2. ALBINISM (*Continued*)

Eyes								
Nystagmus	*Photophobia*	*Visual Acuity*	*Pigment in Fundus*	*Other*	Hair Bulb Incubation (Tyrosine)	Defect	Melanosome Maturation by Stage	Complications or Associated Problems
Oculocutaneous Albinism								
marked	severe	legally blind	none	—	negative	no tyrosinase	I–unmelanized II	skin malignancy basal cell ca squamous cell ca
present but less	present but variable	severe defect in children; may improve with age	none; some with age	pigment cartwheel pupil, limbus	positive	no access of enzyme to tyrosine	I, II, some III, rare IV	skin malignancy basal cell ca squamous cell ca
present but variable	present but variable	marked defect; may improve with age	none; some with age	pigment cartwheel effect	neg to pos ?	unknown ? pheomelanogenesis	I, II, III	unknown
present but variable	present, may be severe	normal or slight decrease	none; some with age	may have pigment cartwheel	positive	pleiotropic effect—single gene mutation	I, II, III	storage-pool defect platelets; ceroid-like material in RE system, oral mucosa, urine
marked	—	blind	?, cataracts	?, cataracts	weakly positive	decreased melanocytes	I, II, III, IV	oligophrenia, athetosis, severe mental retardation
absent or slight	absent or slight	normal or slight decrease	some; increase with age	normal or cartwheel effect	positive	giant melanosomes, lethal defect in leukocytes	I, II, III, IV	infections; hematologic and neurologic abnormalities; lymphoreticular malignancy
no	no	normal or slight decrease	punctate		positive	unknown	unknown	none
present	severe	marked decrease	reduced		positive			
latent	absent or slight	color blind			positive			
present	severe	marked decrease			positive			

of arms and legs or about the umbilicus, and may involve the breast and penis or even the mucosal surfaces of the mouth, vagina, rectum, and stomach. Initially, and in mild cases, the small papules are best seen in stretched skin. In some, the lesions may have a serpiginous distribution with points of perforation. Eventually, there will be thickening of the skin and redundancy with exaggerated folds.

The combination of skin and eye changes is found most often (60 per cent); eye changes only are found in 30 per cent; skin changes only are found least frequently (10 per cent). Nearly all patients (80 per cent) have some vascular abnormality. This condition is presented in detail in Ch. 202.

Altman LK, Fialkow PJ, Parker F, Sagebiel RW: Pseudoxanthoma elasticum, an underdiagnosed genetically heterogenous disorder with protean manifestations. Arch Intern Med 134:1048, 1974. *A fine summary review with a clinical and histologic study of nine probands and the detection of seven previously unrecognized cases, underscoring the subtle and unsuspected presence of this disorder.*

McKee PH, Cameron CHS, Archer DB, Logan WC: A study of four cases of pseudoxanthoma elasticum. J Cut Pathol 4:146, 1977. *A light and electron microscopic focus on the histologic changes of pseudoxanthoma elasticum in an effort to elucidate its pathogenesis. Data support the theory that the basic lesion lies within the elastic fiber.*

Pope FM: Historical evidence for the genetic heterogeneity of pseudoxanthoma elasticum. Br J Dermatol 92:493, 1975.

Nodose Lesions of the Leg

The differential diagnosis of tender erythematous nodules of the lower legs is not so much of the lesion itself, which is a reaction pattern, but of the number of significant diagnoses that are characterized by such lesions. The cutaneous nodules vary in size, number, and location, appear suddenly or gradually, and disappear over weeks or months with or without scar or ulceration. They are sorted out according to their onset, course, distribution, and associations.

ERYTHEMA NODOSUM

Appearing acutely is the classic erythema nodosum, recognized as a clinical entity since 1798 and associated with a variety of infections and drug reactions. It is considered a hypersensitivity vasculitis; the ordinary presentation is of bilateral pretibial red nodules, occasionally with lesions of the extensor aspect of the arms. Rare in children and the elderly, it is most common between 15 and 23 years and is found in females three times more often than in males. According to the country and prevailing infections, it will be reported with tuberculosis, leprosy, sarcoid, streptococcal pharyngitis, pertussis, measles, primary atypical pneumonia, lymphogranuloma venereum, gonorrhea, syphilis, and also the superficial and deep fungus infections. It is seen in chronic ulcerative colitis and, less frequently, in regional enteritis or as a reaction to drugs such as iodides, bromides, sulfonamides, arsphenamine, contraceptives, and others.

The onset is often associated with fever and arthralgia, and occasionally with gastrointestinal upsets. It is a self-limited disease with a three- to five-week course and resolution without scarring. Recurrences and relapses occur in fewer than 10 per cent of patients. Any hematologic or roentgenographic abnormalities observed would be those of the underlying disease, to

Text continues on page 2266.

TABLE 556–3. CUTANEOUS LESIONS IN INFECTIOUS DISEASE

	Cutaneous Lesion	Systemic Component	Agents
Viral Diseases			
Rubella	Faint flush in 25%; centripetal spread of small, irregular pink macules and papules; petechiae on soft palate	Fever, malaise, headache, sore throat, adenopathy, mild respiratory infection, arthritis in adult women	Myxovirus
Varicella	Centrifugal spread of maculopapular lesions which vesiculate; may have mucosal lesions	Fever, malaise, pruritus	Herpesvirus
Variola	Erythematous macular eruption becomes vesicular with umbilication; most prominent in bathing trunk area; rash may be petechial	Fever, headache, vomiting	Poxvirus variolae
Hand, foot, and mouth disease	Vesicular eruption on margins of palms, soles, dorsa of hands, feet, lips, and buccal mucosa	Fever, malaise, abdominal pain	Coxsackievirus A5, A16, A10
Rubeola	Erythematous maculopapules; spreads from head to trunk to limbs; Koplik spots, blue-gray to white areas on tonsils may be seen	Fever, malaise, coryza, conjunctivitis, photophobia, adenopathy, encephalitis	Myxovirus
Bacterial Diseases			
Rheumatic fever	Subcutaneous nodules over bony prominences; erythema marginatum on trunk and limbs; erythema papillatum on flexor surfaces	Fever, carditis, chorea, arthritis	Group A hemolytic *Streptococcus*
Scarlet fever	Red pharynx with large tonsils, white exudate; 1 to 2 mm papules spread from neck to feet; rash most prominent in body folds	Fever, sore throat, lymphadenopathy, hematuria	Group A beta-hemolytic *Streptococcus*
Gonococcemia	Vesiculopustular lesions on extremities; may be purpuric	Fever, migratory arthritis, tenosynovitis, bacteremia (endocarditis)	*Neisseria gonorrhoeae*
Meningococcemia	Vesiculopustular lesion, which may be petechial on extremities or trunk, purpura fulminans	Myalgia, fever, encephalitis, hypotension, vomiting, septic arthritis, pericarditis, endocarditis, pneumonia, bacteremia	*Neisseria meningitidis*
Bacterial Diseases (*Continued*)			
Bacterial endocarditis	Petechiae, subungual splinter hemorrhages, Osler's nodes on fingers, hands, toes; Janeway lesions (palms and soles)	Fever, murmur, splenomegaly, bacteremia	Several, including viridans streptococci, *Staphylococcus*
Typhoid fever	1 to 3 mm slightly raised pink papules in groups of 10 to 20 lesions on upper part of abdomen and lower part of chest or midback (rose spots)	Headache, fever, aching, constipation	*Salmonella typhi*
Bartonellosis	Soft, round, hemangiomatous nodules and papules on neck, hands, and extensor surfaces	Fever, myalgias, malaise, headache, gastrointestinal irritability, anemia	*Bartonella bacilliformis*
Tularemia	Red, tender papule develops into vesiculopustule and then necrotic ulcer—usually on hand; some have maculopapular or petechial exanthem	Headache, malaise, myalgias, fever, adenopathy (regional)	*Francisella tularensis*
Diphtheria	Primary: cutaneous—tender pustular lesion to ulcer with gray membrane; does not extend below fascia, bluish rolled margins on lower extremities; secondary: infection of wound—purulent exudate or superinfection of eczematized skin; pharynx gray-white, pseudomembrane on tonsils	Fever, myocarditis, polyneuritis, croup, malaise, sore throat, dyspnea	*Corynebacterium diphtheriae*
Anthrax	95% have papule to vesicle with brawny gelatinous nonpitting edema surrounding the area (usually exposed surface)	Fever, malaise, pulmonary symptoms	*Bacillus anthracis*
Ritter's disease (SSSS)	Intense erythema of face and body, profuse desquamation, leaving raw, red, moist surface; bullae may be present	Refusal of feeding, vomiting, diarrhea, hypotension	Staphylococci phage type 71

Table continues on facing page.

TABLE 556–3. CUTANEOUS LESIONS IN INFECTIOUS DISEASE (*Continued*)

	Cutaneous Lesion	Systemic Component	Agents
Rickettsial Diseases			
Rocky Mountain spotted fever	Centripetal spread of maculopapular eruption; may become purpuric (initially on palms and soles)	Fever, chills, headache, myalgia, arthralgia, splenomegaly, hypotension, myocarditis	*Rickettsia rickettsii*
Boutonneuse fever	Tache noir—site of tick bite, small ulcer with black center and red halo; generalized red, maculopapular eruption; involves palms and soles	Fever, headache, regional lymphadenopathy	*R. conorii*
Epidemic typhus	Pink macules initially in axilla, to trunk, to extremities; may become petechial	Fever, chills, headache, malaise, weakness	*R. prowazekii*
Endemic typhus	Maculopapular eruption, primarily on trunk; does not become purpuric	Fever, chills, headache, malaise, nausea and vomiting	*R. mooseri*
Fungal Diseases			
Blastomycosis	Verrucous lesion with central healing and a serpiginous border on one side on exposed surfaces; small ulcers; 25% mucous (oral or nasal) lesions—only one half of these from a contiguous skin lesion	Fever, anorexia; bone, pulmonary, cerebral, liver, spleen, adrenal, and gastrointestinal tract may be involved	*Blastomyces dermatitidis*
Cryptococcosis	10–15% have cutaneous lesions; papules or nodules with surrounding erythema, also ulcers, pustules, and purple plaques	Pulmonary, one third renal involvement; 80% meningitis	*Cryptococcus neoformans*
Mucormycosis	Orbital, nasal sinus, or oropharyngeal form; red to gangrenous skin or mucosal changes with purulent drainage and swelling	Local pain, proptosis, CNS involvement	Phycomycetes
Fungal Diseases (*Continued*)			
Actinomycosis	25% cervicofacial; swelling over lower face or neck with indurated draining lesion; 15% thoracocutaneous lesion or subcutaneous abscess; 60% abdominal sinus or abscess	Osteomyelitis	*Actinomyces israelii*
Disseminated coccidioidomycosis	Subcutaneous cellulitis, abscesses, draining sinus tracts	Fever, malaise, chest pain, cough, anorexia, pulmonary fibrosis	*Coccidioides immitis*
Paracoccidioidomycosis	Painful ulcerative lesions—usually on face; abscesses with sinus tract	Cough, chest pain; bone, adrenal, CNS, and spleen involved	*Paracoccidioides brasiliensis*
Mycobacterial Diseases			
Tuberculosis	Lupus vulgaris (90% on head and neck), scrofuloderma—usually in cervical area; tuberculosis verrucosa cutis	Pulmonary, bone, and more widespread	*Mycobacterium tuberculosis*
Leprosy	Hypopigmented, slightly erythematous macules; nodules mainly on face; loss of eyebrows and lashes; raised hypopigmented plaques	Thickened peripheral nerves; sensory abnormalities	*Mycobacterium leprae*
Treponemal Disease			
Syphilis	Primary: chancre, eroded papule—usually on genitalia; secondary: erythematous macules and papules diffuse and on palms and soles, alopecia, condylomata lata; tertiary: locally destructive, partial spontaneous healing	Primary: adenopathy; secondary: malaise, fever, headache, adenopathy; tertiary: cardiac, neurologic involvement	*Treponema pallidum*

TABLE 556–4. CUTANEOUS LESIONS ASSOCIATED WITH GASTROINTESTINAL DISEASE

Diseases	Lesion and Description	Gastrointestinal Disorders and Symptoms	Other
Disorders Associated with Gastrointestinal Bleeding			
Degos' disease	Pink papules → small white scar with peripheral telangiectasias; spares palms, soles, and face	Cramps, vomiting, enteritis, bowel perforation, hemorrhage	CNS involvement
Osler-Weber-Rendu syndrome	Telangiectasias (multiple), especially upper half of body	Hemorrhage, hepatic arteriovenous anastomoses, hepatomegaly, cirrhosis	Epistaxis
Syndrome of phlebectasia of jejunum, oral cavity, and scrotum	Fordyce lesions (scrotum), caviar spots (tongue), phlebectasia (buccal mucosa and lips)	Hemorrhage and ulcer symptoms	
Blue rubber bleb disease	Cutaneous hemangiomas (predominantly on trunk and arms)	Hemorrhage; lesions involve liver and spleen	Lesions in CNS, lung, kidney, adrenal
Ehlers-Danlos syndrome	Easy bruising, fragile skin, pseudotumors at pressure points, stretchability of skin	Hiatal hernia, diverticula, rupture of bowel, hemorrhage	Pneumothorax, CNS bleeding, hyperextensible joints
Pseudoxanthoma elasticum	1- to 3-mm yellowish papules in plaques associated with telangiectasia, especially on neck and flexures; soft lax skin in folds at neck, axilla, umbilicus, face, antecubital fossa, groin	Hemorrhages	Angioid streaks of retina; vascular abnormalities, hypertension
Kaposi's sarcoma	Dark blue–purple macules → nodules initially on extremities; also hands, ears, nose	10% visceral involvement, hemorrhage, perforation, intestinal obstruction	Epidemic variety associated with AIDS
Henoch-Schönlein purpura	Erythematous macules which become papules, urticarial, purpuric, or necrotic (external aspects of limbs, buttocks, and occasionally face)	75% of patients > 2 years old have abdominal complaints: colic, vomiting, diarrhea, melena, hematemesis	Arthritis; renal involvement; fever
Polyarteritis nodosa	Tender nodules in groups along superficial arteries—may be cutaneous or subcutaneous; purpuric plaques, gangrene, Osler's nodes, and splinter hemorrhages have been noted	Pain, peritonitis; infarcts in bowel, liver, spleen; hemorrhage, pancreatitis, steatorrhea, gangrene of bowel	Multisystem: hypertension, myocardial infarction, renal thrombosis; neurologic—encephalopathy, convulsions, neuritis; arthralgia; myopathy
Disorders Associated with Gastrointestinal Polyposis			
Gardner's syndrome	Epidermal and sebaceous cysts, inclusion cysts; primarily on face and scalp	45% incidence of malignancy of colonic polyps	Osteomas, desmoid tumors
Peutz-Jeghers-Touraine syndrome	2- to 5-mm brown-black macules on lips, face, buccal mucosa, hands	Polyps with predilection for jejunum and ileum (malignancy proximal to ligament of Treitz)	
Cronkhite-Canada syndrome	Diffuse hyperpigmentation affecting palms, volar surface of fingers, face, and neck; alopecia (patchy → complete); dystrophic nails	Diarrhea, acquired polyps of gastrointestinal tract	
Disorders Associated with Dysphagia			
Scleroderma	Raynaud's, tense, smooth, hardened, and bound-down skin, starting with hands → upper extremities, face, trunk; cutaneous calcification; resorption of terminal phalanges; matlike telangiectasias	Dysphagia, malabsorption	Pulmonary fibrosis, arthritis
Plummer-Vinson syndrome	Angular stomatitis, brittle nails, koilonychia, atrophic tongue	Dysphagia due to strictures in esophagus	Anemia, iron deficiency
Epidermolysis bullosa	Trauma results in blisters which heal with scarring	Dysphagia due to strictures in esophagus	
Behçet's disease	Recurrent oral and genital ulcerations; pyoderma of groin and genitalia; sterile pustules at puncture sites	Dysphagia	Photophobia, uveitis, CNS abnormality

Table continues on facing page.

TABLE 556–4. CUTANEOUS LESIONS ASSOCIATED WITH GASTROINTESTINAL DISEASE (*Continued*)

Diseases	Lesion and Description	Gastrointestinal Disorders and Symptoms	Other
Disorders Associated with Diarrhea or Malabsorption			
Carcinoid	Flushing and patchy cyanosis and telangiectasia on face and upper trunk; hyperpigmented, hyperkeratotic lesions on legs, trunk, forearms, without hyperkeratosis on forehead, back, wrists, thighs	Diarrhea, metastatic lesions of carcinoid	Asthma, valvular heart disease, arthritis
Ulcerative colitis	3 to 34% have skin lesions; pyoderma gangrenosum (1 to 10%), purpura, aphthae, erythema nodosum, erythema multiforme, perianal fistula, and abscess (10 to 20%), pyostomatitis vegetans	Diarrhea, hemorrhage	Arthritis
Systemic mastocytosis	Flushing (secondary histamine release); generalized multiple reddish-brown or yellow macules, papules or nodules, or erythroderma	Symptoms in 23%—abdominal pain, cramps, diarrhea	(Mast cell leukemia is a possible complication)
Hartnup disease	Dry, scaly, well-marginated, affecting light-exposed area; stomatitis and glossitis	Diarrhea	Cerebral ataxia; renal aminoaciduria
Acrodermatitis enteropathica	Alopecia, pustular eruption around orifices and bullous or verrucous on extremities	Diarrhea	Zinc deficiency
Dermatitis herpetiformis	Papular and vesicular lesions with severe pruritus over extensor surfaces; symmetrical, chronic with recurrences; mucous membranes clear	Gluten enteropathy	
Reiter's syndrome	Mucocutaneous lesions, 80% keratosis blennorrhagica of palms and soles; hyperkeratosis of scalp; onycholysis, shedding and dystrophies of nails; scrotal and penile erosions; balanitis circinata sicca	Dysentery may precede other symptoms	Nonspecific urethritis, conjunctivitis, asymmetric arthritis
Crohn's disease	20% (15 to 50%) perineal ulceration with fistula formation; occasional pyoderma gangrenosum; 20% abdominal wall sinuses	Diarrhea, obstruction, perforation	Arthritis, iritis
Dermatogenic enteropathy	Erythroderma due to psoriasis, eczema or other etiology	Steatorrhea (malabsorption)	
Malabsorption syndrome	90% stomatitis; 50% angular stomatitis, purpura, petechiae; 10 to 20% have dermatitis, either erythematous or scaling like seborrheic dermatitis or psoriasis; in others, eczema, ichthyosis, asteatosis; alopecia, Beau's lines in nails, koilonychia; hyperpigmentation: melasmic, addisonian, or pellagroid	Diarrhea	
Pellagra	Hard, rough, cracked blackish and brittle epidermis of fingers, face, neck (Casal's necklace), dorsa of hands, arms, feet; fissures on palms and soles; earlier, may have blisters	Diarrhea; 50% achlorhydria	Dementia
Disorders Associated with Liver Disease			
Laennec's cirrhosis	Spider angiomas in 75%; palmar erythema; men—sparse axillary, pubic, and pectoral hair; Dupuytren's contracture; purpura; opaque white nails in 25%	Cirrhosis, hemorrhage from esophageal varices	Ascites, varices, testicular atrophy, gynecomastia
Biliary cirrhosis	Jaundice, melanotic hyperpigmentation generalized but more prominent on exposed areas; xanthelasma; tuberous xanthomas over extensor and pressure areas; flat xanthomas in palmar creases and scars	Biliary cirrhosis	Pruritus
Total lipoatrophy	Loss of subcutaneous fat; hypertrichosis, xanthomas, axillary and inguinal folds, associated with hyperpigmentation and linear epidermal thickenings (in congenital form)	Hepatic failure hematemesis, hepatomegaly	↑ Bone growth; diabetes; hyperlipemia; enlarged genitalia; renal, neurologic, and cardiac disorders
Hemochromatosis	15 to 20% gingival, palatal, buccal, and conjunctival hyperpigmentation—pigment most noticeable on flexures; loss of pubic and axillary hair	Cirrhosis	Diabetes, hypogonadism
Symptomatic porphyria	Bullous lesions on exposed parts of body; milia; hypertrichosis; onycholysis; conjunctival injection	Chronic liver dysfunction	
Disorders Associated with Pancreatic Disease			
Necrolytic migratory erythema	Symmetrical dermatitis initially eczematous over perineum, buttocks, and extremities → central blister with crusting, followed by hyperpigmentation, stomatitis	Glucagon-secreting tumor of pancreas	Weight loss, depression, anemia
Weber-Christian disease	Tender subcutaneous nodules on upper thighs and buttocks which resolve with depressed atrophic areas	Ileus, perforation	Fever, malaise
Nodular fat necrosis	Recurrent crops of red, painful, inflammatory subcutaneous nodules 0.5 to 5 cm initially on legs, especially lower; in 2 to 3% of patients with pancreatic disease, heal without atrophy	Pancreatitis or pancreatic neoplasm	Fever, eosinophilia, synovitis
Grey Turner's sign	Bruise-like discoloration of skin of left flank	Pancreatitis or other abdominal hemorrhage	
Cullen's sign	Bruise around umbilicus	Acute pancreatitis or ruptured common bile duct or perforated duodenal ulcer	
Miscellaneous Disorders			
Familial angioedema	Recurrent swelling of skin and mucous membranes	Nausea, vomiting, colic	Urinary symptoms, deficient in C1 esterase inhibitor
Familial Mediterranean fever	40% (8 to 45%) have erysipelas-like erythema on feet or lower legs	95 to 98% have abdominal pain	Fever, chest pain, arthralgia, renal amyloidosis
Acanthosis nigricans	Gray-brown to black pigmentation with thickened skin covered by small papillomas over axilla, sides of neck, groin, anogenital region; thickened palms; nails may be brittle or ridged	Gastric adenocarcinoma	Endocrinopathy Insulin resistance

TABLE 556–5. DISEASES WITH RENAL AND CUTANEOUS MANIFESTATIONS

Diseases	Cutaneous Manifestations	Renal Manifestations	Other
Tumors			
Hypernephroma	Solitary vascular lesions—tend to be pedunculated	Hypernephroma	
Tuberous sclerosis	60 to 70% skin lesions; adenoma sebaceum; periungual fibroma, shagreen patch, ash leaf spots, poliosis	Benign renal hamartomas, hematuria	Mental retardation (60–70%), epilepsy (70%), eye lesions (8 to 40%), rhabdomyoma
Anomalies of Development			
Oral-facial-digital syndrome	Short upper lip; hypertrophied frenula of lips and tongue; multilobed tongue; clefts of hard and soft palate; sparse hair; numerous milia	Polycystic kidneys	Polycystic liver; 50% mentally retarded; dental caries; brachydactyly and syndactyly
Neurofibromatosis	Neurofibromas, nodules in relation to peripheral nerves; 5 to 15% sarcomatous change in neurofibroma; café-au-lait spots; axillary freckles; oral tumors	60% oligophrenia; defect of renal tubules; osteomalacia; renal artery stenosis	Spinal deformities, endocrine and neurologic abnormalities, hypertension
Metabolic Disorders			
Sarcoidosis	Lupus pernio, plaques, maculopapular eruptions, erythema nodosum	25% hypercalciuria; nephrocalcinosis; polyuria, nocturnal polydipsia; 1 to 3% renal failure	Anemia, joint pain, adenopathy, CNS involvement, pulmonary fibrosis
Metastatic calcinosis	Nodules or plaques from 0.5 to 5 cm symmetrically on extremities and trunk—discharge of chalk-like material from lesions	Deposits in kidney of Ca^{++}	Blood vessels of muscles, stomach, lungs, and large blood vessels have deposits of Ca^{++}
Systemic amyloidosis, urticaria, and deafness syndrome	Urticaria	Nephropathy secondary to amyloid	Chills, malaise, deafness
Gout	Subcutaneous nodules, pink and most common on helix of ear, bursae of elbow, digits of hands and feet; chalky drainage	Renal calculi	
Cold agglutinins	Acrocyanosis	Hematuria	Anemia; may be associated with *Mycoplasma* pneumonia, reticulosarcoma, or lymphoma
Multiple myeloma	Plasmacytoma, petechial bleeding at perianal and periocular sites	Proteinuria, nephrolithiasis	Anemia; 10 to 20% amyloid; bone destruction; frequent infection; neuropathy
Diabetes mellitus	Necrobiosis lipoidica diabeticorum, granuloma annulare, carotenemia, lipodystrophy, frequent cutaneous infections	Kimmelstiel-Wilson disease; papillary necrosis	Heart, vascular, neurologic disease
Fabry's disease	Dry skin, dark red or black macule or papule in groups, especially on thighs, scrotum, and periumbilical	Hypertension, albuminuria, hematuria, uremia	Coronary artery disease, cerebrovascular attacks, eye lesions
Alcaptonuria	Skin discoloration (bluish-black) of nose tip, ear, extensor tendons, and costochondral junctions	Renal disease accelerates other abnormal findings; homogentisic acid in urine	Arthropathy
Hartnup disease	Stomatitis, glossitis; dry scaly eruption in light-exposed areas	Aminoaciduria	Diarrhea, cerebellar ataxia, psychiatric problems
Familial Mediterranean fever	40% erysipelas-like erythema	Death from renal amyloidosis	Fever, abdominal and chest pain, arthralgia, synovitis
Glomerulitis			
Hypersensitivity angiitis	Palpable purpura, urticaria, necrotic ulcerations	Necrotizing glomerular nephritis	Cardiac, neurologic, pulmonary, and joint involvement
Henoch-Schönlein purpura	See Table 556–4	40% microscopic hematuria (worse in adults)	Edema of feet and hands; polyarthritis; abdominal pain; fever, headache, anorexia
Scleroderma	See Table 556–4	Hypertension; 60% have abnormal BUN and creatinine	Arthritis, edema of hands; dysphagia; pulmonary fibrosis; malabsorption
Systemic lupus erythematosus	70 to 85% cutaneous lesions—butterfly erythema; maculopapular rash primarily above waist; chronic discoid lesions; alopecia; mucosal ulcers; periungual erythema; bullae; ecchymoses	50% renal disease (proteinuria-hematuria); 10% have nephrotic syndrome	Fever, fatigue, arthritis, pericarditis, neurologic involvement, pleural involvement
Polyarteritis nodosa	See Table 556–4	Cortical infarction, glomerulosclerosis, thrombosis	Malaise, fever, weight loss, abdominal pain, neurologic and cardiac involvement, arthralgia, myopathy
Nail-patella syndrome	Nails absent or hypotrophic	Chronic glomerulonephritis, renal dysplasia	Skeletal abnormalities; decrease in size or absence of patella
Wegener's granulomatosis	Early—papulonecrotic or vesicular lesions, symmetrically distributed over elbows, knees, buttocks; Later—erythematous, purpuric or vesicular lesions become generalized and oral ulcerations appear	Focal necrotizing glomerulitis, renal failure	CNS involvement; destruction of paranasal sinus, nasopharynx, and lung
Miscellaneous Disorders			
Osler-Weber-Rendu syndrome	Telangiectasias on upper half of body	Hematuria	Hemorrhages, epistaxis; cirrhosis of liver, arteriovenous anastomoses
Pseudoxanthoma elasticum	Yellow papules 1 to 3 mm in confluent plaques on neck and flexures; skin soft and lax	Hypertension from involvement of renal arteries	Gastrointestinal hemorrhage, circulatory abnormalities, arterial degeneration
Partial lipodystrophy	Loss of subcutaneous fat from face spreading downward	Nonspecific renal abnormalities; increased incidence	
Erythema multiforme	Erythematous macules, bullae, and target lesions symmetrical on distal extremities	Transient albuminuria	Infections or allergies possibly related
Sickle cell disease	Leg ulcers at early age; increased pigment in lower leg	Acute pyelonephritis, hematuria	Fever, abdominal pain, osteomyelitis, bone pain
Congenital ichthyosis, mental retardation, dwarfism, and renal impairment	Nonbullous congenital ichthyosiform erythroderma, most marked on back and extensor surfaces	Elevated BUN and creatinine, 50% of glomerular filtration rate	Mental retardation, dwarfism

TABLE 556–6. CUTANEOUS LESIONS IN DISORDERS WITH A HEMATOLOGIC COMPONENT

Diseases	Cutaneous Lesions	Hematologic Component	Other
Fanconi's syndrome	85% generalized olive-brown pigmentation most prominent on lower trunk, in flexures, and on neck with macules of hyper- and hypopigmentation	Hypoplastic anemia, neutropenia, thrombocytopenia, increased incidence of leukemia	Short broad hands, microcephaly, mental retardation, hypogonadism, aplasia of radii
Dyskeratosis congenita	Nail dystrophy; reticulate gray-brown pigmentation of neck, thighs, trunk; face and hands, atrophic skin; bullae on hands and feet secondary to trauma; leukoplakia on mucous membranes	Myeloid aplasia, refractory anemia, pancytopenia, blood dyscrasias, possible Fanconi's anemia	Dental abnormalities; mental and physical growth retarded
Sickle cell anemia	Leg ulcers at early age; increased pigment of lower leg	Anemia with typical red cells	Fever, abdominal pain, bone osteomyelitis
Cold agglutinin syndrome	Acrocyanosis, ulceration, gangrene	Anemia (hemolytic)	Hematuria, may be associated with *Mycoplasma* pneumonia, lymphoma, or reticulosarcoma
Gardner-Diamond syndrome	Recurrent painful erythematous and purpuric lesions	Autoerythrocyte sensitization	Psychiatric disturbances may be present
Chédiak-Higashi syndrome	Light color hair, skin, retinas, and translucent irides	Lethal defect in leukocytes	Frequent infections
Job's syndrome	Red, scaly, crusted lesions over scalp, ears, periorbital, skin, groin; cold staphylococcal abscesses	Defect in polymorphonuclear neutrophil function	Recurrent pneumonia; liver, spleen, and lymph nodes enlarged
Leukemia cutis	Erythroderma, papules, nodules, nonspecific infection, purpura, urticaria	Chronic lymphocytic leukemia most common type to develop lesions (11% of patients with acute myeloblastic or monocytic leukemia, as compared to 1.3% of acute lymphoblastic leukemia, developed leukemia cutis)	
Sézary's syndrome	Pruritus and generalized erythroderma, dystrophic nails, alopecia; thickening and convolution of skin, especially on face	Variant of mycosis fungoides or leukemia form of it	Adenopathy
Systemic mastocytosis	See Table 556–4	Mast cell leukemia	23% flushing, diarrhea, abdominal pain
Pernicious anemia	Glossitis, vitiligo, cheilitis (pallor, hyperpigmentation, jaundice)	Anemia, B_{12} deficiency	
Plummer-Vinson syndrome	Koilonychia, glossitis, cheilitis	Microcytic hypochromic anemia	Dysphagia, cancer of upper gastrointestinal tract
Methemoglobinemia	Violet or brownish skin color	Intrinsic defect in red cell enzyme of altered structure of hemoglobin	Inherited, acquired from medications (dapsone)
von Willebrand's disease	Albinism; ecchymoses or hematomas	Deficiency of factor VIII (long bleeding time)	
Polycythemia	Ruddy cyanosis; erythromelalgia; gangrene	May be primary or secondary; primary associated with elevated red blood cells, white blood cells, platelets; secondary with elevated red blood cells	Splenomegaly in primary form
Congenital erythropoietic porphyria	Photosensitivity and vesiculobullous eruption in light-exposed areas; hypertrichosis, alopecia; scarring marked	Hemolytic anemia; fluorescence of red blood cells	Splenomegaly; erythrodontia; nausea and vomiting on exposure to sunlight
Erythropoietic protoporphyria	Photosensitivity resulting in swelling and erythema and burning sensation; may have vesicular eruption in center of face with small scars; skin over knuckles thickened	High concentration of protoporphyrin in red blood cells—may have fluorescence of red blood cells	Cholecystitis, cholelithiasis
Paroxysmal cold hemoglobinuria	Pain and acrocyanosis; urticaria	Hemolysis on warming	Seen in syphilis, viral infections; chills, fever, aching, asthma
Multiple myeloma	Plasmacytoma; petechial bleeding at perianal, periocular areas	Plasma cell leukemia (eventual anemia, thrombocytopenia)	Proteinuria, nephrolithiasis, amyloidosis, bone destruction, neuropathies, frequent infections
Strawberry hemangioma (multiple)	Most common on head; superficial lesions red; deeper components dark blue or purple; grow rapidly after birth; ulceration and spontaneous involution.	May have thrombocytopenia	Cardiac hypertrophy due to high output; neurologic manifestations of lesions in CNS
Systemic lupus erythematosus	See Table 556–5	Anemia, thrombocytopenia	Fever, fatigue, arthritis, renal disease; serositis, neurologic disease

TABLE 556–7. DISEASES WITH BOTH CUTANEOUS AND RHEUMATIC COMPONENTS

Diseases	Cutaneous Lesions	Rheumatic Component	Other
Stevens-Johnson syndrome	Vesiculobullous and urticarial lesions; target lesions on mucous membranes and distal extremities	Arthralgias	Fever, malaise, nausea, vomiting, myalgias, chest pain, sore throat, eye involvement
Reiter's syndrome	See Table 556–4	Asymmetric arthritis of weight-bearing joints; tendinitis, fasciitis, ankylosing spondylitis	Urethritis, conjunctivitis (dysentery)
Behçet's disease	See Table 556–4	Arthralgia, noninflammatory joint effusions	Iritis or uveitis, fever, malaise, phlebitis, gastrointestinal ulcers, pericarditis, neurologic involvement
Rocky Mountain spotted fever	See Table 556–3	Arthralgia	Fever, chills, myalgia, headache
Gonococcemia	See Table 556–3	Migratory arthritis, tenosynovitis, septic arthritis	Fever, pharyngitis, urethritis
Rubella	See Table 556–3	Arthritis noted in adult women—elbows, knees, phalangeal joints, wrists	Fever, malaise, headache, sore throat, adenopathy
Meningococcemia	See Table 556–3	Septic arthritis	Myalgia, fever, hypotension, pneumonia, pericarditis, endocarditis
Diseases Associated with Hypersensitivity States			
Henoch-Schönlein purpura	See Table 556–4	Polyarthritis—knees, elbows, ankles, hands	Fever, anorexia, headache, abdominal pain; edema of hands and feet in children; 40% microscopic hematuria
Serum sickness	90% of skin lesions in this syndrome are urticarial; morbilliform and scarlatiniform eruptions are less common; rarely erythema multiforme, erythema nodosum	Arthralgias and arthritis; migratory distal large joints	Fever, lymphadenopathy
Hypersensitivity angiitis	See Table 556–5	May be associated with rheumatoid arthritis	Kidneys, lungs, gastrointestinal tract, heart, peripheral nerves; also affected by angiitis
Polyarteritis nodosa	See Table 556–4	Arthralgia	50% fever, malaise, weight loss, abdominal pain, hemiplegia, polyneuritis, renal, cardiac, gastrointestinal involvement
Erythema nodosum	Tender erythematous nodules on lower legs	Arthralgia	Fever, chills, malaise
Miscellaneous			
Psoriasis	Silvery scales on erythematous plaques; most common on scalp, knees, elbows	1–32% have arthritis, erosive polyarticular joint disease	
Reticulohistiocytoma	Small, firm, pink moderately pruritic papules or nodules on hands, face, scalp, ears, lips, trunk	Destructive polyarthritis with shortening of fingers	May involve lymph nodes, marrow, and endocardium
Sarcoidosis	See Table 556–5	50% polyarthralgia	70% of those with skin lesions have intrathoracic involvement
Systemic lupus erythematosus	See Table 556–5	Migratory arthritis (small joints of hands, wrists, elbows, shoulders, knees, and ankles)	Renal, cardiac, neurologic complications
Erythema elevatum diutinum	Multiple nodules and plaques on extensor surfaces of extremities; may resemble xanthomas but most are purple-red	Associated polyarthritis	
Scleroderma	See Table 556–4	Resorption of bone, dissociation of terminal phalanges	Pulmonary fibrosis, malabsorption, dysphagia
Ehlers-Danlos syndrome	See Table 556–4	Hyperextensibility of joints	Gastrointestinal bleeding, rupture of bowel

which the therapy should be directed. In more than a quarter of the cases, however, no etiology can be determined.

The histopathologic changes in the skin are nonspecific and are completely reversible. The venous walls can be edematous and the fat lobules show disintegration, but there is no leukocytoclastic or lymphocytic angiitis.

ACUTE FEBRILE NEUTROPHILIC DERMATOSIS

The same is true of the rare, self-limiting acute febrile neutrophilic dermatosis of Sweet. Characterized by high persistent fever with painful nodules and plaques occurring asymmetrically over the extremities, face, and neck, it is often noted to follow an upper respiratory infection and is considered a probable hypersensitivity reaction. However, it has also been observed with unsuspected malignancy, especially acute myelogenous leukemia, and as such may be considered a cutaneous marker of malignant change or immunologic dysfunction. The disease is reported most in middle-aged women, in whom it is associated with leukocytosis and an elevated sedimentation rate. Histopathologic examination of the skin lesions shows vasodilatation and endothelial swelling, with infiltration of polymorphonuclear leukocytes in the upper and mid-dermis. There is no suppuration and no scarring.

NODULAR LIQUEFYING PANNICULITIS

In this condition, by contrast, there are foci of fat necrosis with preservation of cell membranes but with basophilic granular changes of the cytoplasm, as well as loss of nuclear staining in the fat septum to produce characteristic ghost-like cells. The recurrent crops of red painful nodules 0.5 to 5 cm, which appear on the legs but occasionally elsewhere, can be noted to soften and drain a viscous aseptic material as evidence of fat liquefaction. Associated with pancreatitis or occasionally with acinous adenocarcinoma of the pancreas, the fat necrosis has been attributed to the action of the pancreatic enzyme lipase on the subcutaneous fat. Occurrences may be associated with episodes of abdominal pain, polyarthritis, and fever. The problem is rare. The differential diagnosis is that of other nodular lesions of the leg rather than Weber-Christian disease, a nonsuppurative panniculitis in which the nodular lesions are primarily on the trunk and thighs, and are associated with fever and recurrence.

ERYTHEMA INDURATUM

This chronic recurring nodular vasculitis of the lower legs is not rare, at least in Europe or Japan. It is found predominantly in women from the teens to old age; there are peak appearances in adolescence and at the menopause. Histologically panniculitis and vasculitis are seen, along with a granulomatous reaction that may be nonspecific or tuberculoid.

The lesions occur mostly on the posterior rather than anterior aspect of the lower legs and, rarely, on the thighs. The nodules, painful to pressure, may ulcerate with subsequent scarring, or resorb, leaving an atrophic depressed surface. Traditionally associated with tuberculosis, active disease is hardly ever found. Most observers now designate a group of nodose lesions as nodular vasculitis and distinguish between those associated with tuberculous infection (erythema induratum of Bazin) and those not.

The usual course of the problem is protracted and subject to remission and exacerbations. If there is antecedent or current evidence of tuberculosis infection, antituberculous therapy may be beneficial.

Cutaneous Correlations with Specific Organ Systems

Throughout Ch. 556, the focus has been on the lesion observed to identify and differentiate it from similar clinical presentations. Since multiple etiologies can generate the same lesion, a further focus is directed to the manifestations of internal malignancy in Ch. 557. Here, we will redistribute the dermatologic manifestations according to infection and disorders of specific systems. Infectious disease produces a variety of cutaneous responses, some primary, many secondary. They are grouped in Table 556–3* according to the etiologic agent, whether viral, bacterial, rickettsial, or fungal. The progression of lesions is indicated where applicable. In Table 556–4* are the gastrointestinal problems associated with dermatologic diagnoses and lesions that may have as a complication gastrointestinal bleeding or polyposis, or that may be associated with dysphagia or diarrhea, or with hepatic or pancreatic disease. In the same way renal, hematologic, and rheumatic disorders are presented, with a synopsis of the skin pathology, in Tables 556–5 to 556–7*, respectively. The data given are not all discussed in the text, but the standard general dermatologic references cited in Ch. 551 will provide depth of detail.

*Tables 556–3 to 556–7 were compiled with Dr. Virginia Fallon-Pellicci.

557. SELECTED SIGNIFICANT DERMATOLOGIC DIAGNOSES

The Blistering Diseases

The concentrated accumulation of fluid in the skin sufficient to replace the pre-existent tissue structure and produce a visible vesicle or bulla can be the result of forces as divergent as friction and infection, or may be from causes completely obscure. For blisters of unknown etiology categorization yields to microscopic morphologic grouping and to further sorting according to the clinical expression of disease. It is among these, the blisters known to be other than infectious, chemical, or traumatic, that the searchlight of immunofluorescence has been disclosing immune complexes to correlate with clinical disease and its course. Antibodies, circulating and tissue-fixed, whether cause or effect of the observed pathology, are important indicators that must be fully assessed.

In this chapter we shall assume that historical information and close observation will have enabled the examiner to identify blisters associated with solar and thermal burn, with infections such as herpes simplex, or with vesicants such as cantharidin used in the treatment of warts but found in certain stinging insects and flies. It is the differential diagnosis of the one or several blisters on a fairly normal base that is to be considered. In the physical examination, the distribution of the lesions and any extension to mucous membranes or eyes would have been noted. The tenseness of the bulla would have been assessed to estimate the morphologic depth of cleavage and whether this split is easily revealed or extended by light pressure or rubbing as one would skin a ripe peach (Nikolsky's sign).

Bullae that are flaccid on normal-appearing skin which is easily denuded, favoring a truncal location with associated mouth erosions, should suggest pemphigus. If the bullae are few and unroofed so that only superficial erosions are observed, there will still be a history of blisters. The presence of an erythematous base or of other nonbullous papular to urticarial lesions might mean erythema multiforme. Taut preserved bullae are found in pemphigoid and dermatitis herpetiformis, although in the latter the more common presentation is vesicular with marked pruritus and a characteristic distribution over the extensor aspect of the limbs, the shoulders, and the buttocks. The further diagnostic assessment and the support from biopsy and immunofluorescence studies are shown in Table 557–1, which is best perused after a review of the specific diseases.

PEMPHIGUS

Pemphigus is a cluster of blistering entities characterized histologically by acantholysis (see Ch. 553) with resultant fluid accumulation within bullae, and immunologically by the unexplained presence of circulating autoantibodies to an intercellular epidermal antigen. Of unknown etiology, it is found throughout the world, in both sexes, and in all races, with a reported higher incidence in Jews. The onset commonly occurs between 40 and 60 years. It has been seen in children and in families as fogo selvagem, or Brazilian wildfire, and in patients undergoing penicillamine therapy for rheumatoid arthritis. Such penicillamine-induced pemphigus, temporally related to treatment, is indistinguishable from spontaneous pemphigus clinically, histopathologically, or by immunofluorescence. Broadly, and according to the intraepidermal level of the acantholytic blister, pemphigus is divided into suprabasilar pemphigus vulgaris and, if more superficial and just under the corneum, subcorneal pemphigus foliaceus.

Pemphigus vulgaris, which had a 95 per cent mortality before the advent of steroids, can still present acutely and run a swiftly fatal course despite therapy. More often it is a controlled but chronic problem of varying severity. Occasionally it remains localized for months with lesions of the mouth or scalp, perhaps axilla or groin; within a year or so it can be predicted to become generalized. Those presenting with mouth lesions tend to have a poorer prognosis, and some 30 to 40 per cent of all those diagnosed will succumb to the disease or side effects of therapy. The Nikolsky sign is present in uninvolved as well as involved skin, and areas readily traumatized become sloughed. When this extends to the pharynx and larynx, hoarseness is a clinical sign. In general, lesions tend to favor the seborrheic areas—the scalp; the periocular, paranasal, and perioral areas; the presternum; the mid-back; the area around the umbilicus; and the groin. Denuded intertriginous lesions may tend to become vegetative through heaped peripheral collarettes of epidermis and crust, lending a descriptive name to the clinical subdivision of *pemphigus vegetans.* It is further classified into Neumann and Hallopeau types; the former affects younger patients, and the latter tends to follow a more benign course. Noted for pustules extending peripherally, both these pemphigus variants are characterized by vegetative lesions containing eosinophilic abscesses. Both variants can be fatal.

Pemphigus foliaceus is a milder disease, with finer, smaller lesions and more crust and scale; it almost always spares the mouth. It affects mainly the older patient, occasionally children, and is believed to occur in a localized variant as pemphigus

TABLE 557–1. THE BLISTERING DISEASES: CORRELATIONS WITH HISTOLOGY AND IMMUNOFLUORESCENCE

	Pemphigus	Pemphigoid	Erythema Multiforme	Dermatitis Herpetiformis
Histology				
Blister	Intraepidermal	Subepidermal	At basal layer	Subepidermal
Special	Acantholysis	Eosinophils predominate in papillary dermis	Vacuolar alteration at basal layer, necrotic keratinocytes	Neutrophils at tips of dermal papillae
Tzanck test	Acantholytic cells	Negative	Negative	Negative
Immunofluorescence				
Indirect	Positive—intercellular*	Positive—basement membrane	Negative	Negative
Direct	Positive—intercellular	Positive—basement membrane	Negative	Positive—granular deposits in papillary dermis, less often along basement membrane
Treatment	Corticosteroids Immunosuppressives Cyclophosphamide Azathioprine Gold	Corticosteroids ?Immunosuppressives	Supportive ?Corticosteroids	Sulfones Gluten-free diet

*Antibody levels correlate with disease activity.

erythematosus and as an endemic problem in Brazil, where it affects immigrants as well as Brazilians. In the era before steroids some 40 per cent succumbed.

Therapy for pemphigus includes corticosteroids, immunosuppressives, and gold in combinations which will vary according to the form and severity of the disease and the current persuasion of the practitioner. For active widespread disease, most will treat initially with high dose steroids (100 to 150 mg of prednisone or equivalent) to suppress the disease; if there is failure to respond, the dosage will be increased, perhaps doubled. When no new bullae form for several days, a slow taper is begun by first gradually reducing to zero the dosage for alternate days. If it is clear that prolonged or high dose corticosteroid therapy will be required, many elect to begin immunosuppressive therapy from the start: methotrexate, azathioprine,* or cyclophosphamide.* Gold therapy,* too, is being used with new interest, and in some patients is reported to be effective even without initial corticosteroid control. Of note is the unexplained but beneficial effect of ACTH infusion on those whose disease is uncontrolled by more than 200 mg of prednisone or equivalent. The management of pemphigus also includes therapeutic baths, protective ointments and powders, and intralesional injection of corticosteroids when bullae are few. Disease activity can be correlated with the titer of indirect immunofluorescent intercellular antibody.

A benign suprabasilar acantholytic disease is Hailey-Hailey disease, an incompletely penetrant autosomal dominant genodermatosis also known as *benign familial chronic pemphigus*. Small flaccid vesicles are noted about the neck and in body folds where they are aggravated by heat and humidity. The disease is rarely widespread and rarely involves the mouth. Two of three patients will have a family history of the problem. All can expect prolonged spontaneous remission.

PEMPHIGOID

Pemphigoid is a chronic and comparatively benign blistering disease in which subepidermal bullae *without* acantholysis present clinically as large, tense, irregular blisters frequently on an erythematous base. It is often associated with or preceded by pruritus and an urticarial, perhaps eczematous eruption. Serum IgG antibody to basement membrane of skin, capable of fixing complement, occurs at the site of pathologic change and suggests an autoimmune pathogenesis. However, the disease cannot be transferred passively and, unlike pemphigus vulgaris, antibody levels do not correlate with disease activity.

Pemphigoid is a problem of the elderly; it is chronic and subject to exacerbations and remissions. Lesions, which may occur anywhere, favor the abdomen, groin, inner aspect of the thighs, and flexor aspect of the forearms. Mucosal lesions occur but are small; they heal readily with minor discomfort and, unlike pemphigus vulgaris, are no threat to nutrition.

In *benign mucosal pemphigoid* subepidermal bullae without acantholysis form on the mucous membranes, less often the skin, with the possibility of severe residual scarring. Women are afflicted twice as often as men, but both may have involvement of the conjunctivae as well as the oral cavity, pharynx, larynx, esophagus, genitalia, and anus. Secondary fibrous bands may lead to dysphagia, hoarseness, blindness, and stenotic anogenital orifices. Response to steroid therapy—topical, intralesional, and systemic—is poor.

Lever WF, Schaumburg-Lever G: Immunosuppressants and prednisone in pemphigus vulgaris. Therapeutic results obtained in 63 patients between 1961 and 1975. Arch Dermatol 113:1236, 1977. *A review of treatment results of a series of 63 patients over a decade and a half. Important to know for the assessment of therapy and outcome.*

Penneys NS, Eaglstein WH, Frost P: Management of pemphigus with gold compounds. A long-term follow-up report. Arch Dermatol 112:185, 1976. *The place of gold in the management of pemphigus is still debated, but a review of long-term follow-up is important.*

Rosenberg FR, Sanders S, Nelson CT: Pemphigus: A 20-year review of 107 patients treated with corticosteroids. Arch Dermatol 112:962, 1976. *Again in the consideration of long-term management for a chronic problem, experience with a therapeutic modality over years is helpful.*

DERMATITIS HERPETIFORMIS

Dermatitis herpetiformis is grouped with the blistering diseases. It can occasionally have bullae, but presents most often with intense pruritus and with excoriated papules or grouped vesicles in classic distribution over buttocks, shoulders, elbows and knees, and sometimes scalp, face, and ears. Histologically papillary microabscesses occur with aggregates of neutrophils leading to dermoepidermal separation and widespread destruction of the basement membrane. Direct immunofluorescent staining of uninvolved paralesional skin is positive at the dermoepidermal junction. Although IgG and IgM may be identified, as well as complement at the tips of the dermal papillae, IgA is the immunoglobulin most predominant; in fact, without it the diagnosis of dermatitis herpetiformis is in question. Since IgA does not fix complement by the direct pathway beginning with C1q, some other mechanism is necessary to implicate IgA. There is rather convincing evidence to suggest activation of the alternative pathway of complement through IgA aggregates, not unlike that which is known to occur in myeloma. Conventional complexes have been demonstrated, but circulating immunoglobulin and significant serum complement levels have not been detected.

*Investigational drugs for this purpose.

Dermatitis herpetiformis appears between the second and fifth decades. It occurs in men twice as often as women. Of special interest, however, is its association with malabsorptive enteropathy. As in celiac disease, disaccharidase and dipeptidase activities are decreased, and there is villous atrophy of the small intestine most apparent in the proximal jejunum. In patients diagnosed as having dermatitis herpetiformis with IgA deposits at the dermoepidermal junction of the skin, 19 of 23 had total or partial villous atrophy. As in the celiac syndrome they had autoantibodies to thyroid, reticulin, and parietal cells, as well as atrophic gastritis and overt pernicious anemia. Comparisons of histocompatibility indicate that HLA antigens A1 and B8 have a high frequency in dermatitis herpetiformis when contrasted to normals, and even higher in adult celiac disease. No correlation can presently be made with HLA type and the presence or absence of intestinal involvement from the data at hand, but to identify villous atrophy may take more than one biopsy.

Whether dermatitis herpetiformis is a reaction pattern and whether the activity and extent of skin lesions can be correlated with observed enteropathy are not yet known. Three reports in as many years which document jejunal lymphoma complicating a clinical dermatitis herpetiformis, characterized by IgA skin deposits and intestinal villous atrophy, warrant careful consideration. Further, the riddle of antireticulin antibody titers and the degree of villous atrophy must be solved. There is a cross-reactivity reported between fraction III of gluten and reticulin. However, the anticipated favorable response to the gluten-free diet, important in the management of celiac disease, has not been noted consistently in dermatitis herpetiformis and is challenged. In a match of diet, HLA type, and mucosal abnormality in a series of 44 patients, 22 with celiac disease and 22 with dermatitis herpetiformis, milk antibody titer was used as an index of mucosal abnormality. It was similar in both groups, but antigluten antibody was consistently higher in celiac disease, suggesting that the antigluten response may not be part of the enteropathy of dermatitis herpetiformis. One patient with both diseases finds that her dermatitis herpetiformis is not benefited by the gluten-free diet that controls her celiac disease.

The classic case of dermatitis herpetiformis is not difficult to diagnose, and at its onset the severe pruritus and paucity of lesions might be confused only with scabies, which the telltale burrow and mite would differentiate. Halogens have been known to aggravate the disease or even to provoke it, and thus may provide a clue. A skin patch test with 20 per cent KI is frequently positive and has been known to induce characteristic lesions with IgA deposition. One last and perhaps definitive test is the therapeutic response to sulfapyridine or diaminodiphenylsulfone, each of which has a dramatic beneficial effect that suppresses pruritus and lesions in 12 to 24 hours. The individual dose required to maintain the patient must be titrated. The end-point is surprisingly sharp. Because the medications must be continued for long periods, there is considerable risk of hematologic or perhaps carcinogenic effects (sulfone), or hepatic and renal side effects (sulfa); hence treatment must be monitored closely.

Baker PG, Palmer RK: Autoantibodies in patients with coeliac disease and dermatitis herpetiformis. Lancet 1:750, 1976. *The study of the immune response in patients with celiac disease and dermatitis herpetiformis provides another means of differentiating between the two and another step toward elaborating the pathogenesis of both.*

Charlesworth EN, Backe JT, Garcia RL: Iodide-induced immunofluorescence in dermatitis herpetiformis. Arch Dermatol 112:555, 1976. *The observed provocation of immunofluorescent histologic findings under an epidermal patch test of potassium iodide gives a further piece of the puzzle in this disease related to celiac disease and gluten sensitivity but by contrast aggravated by iodides.*

Fausa O, Larsen TE, Husby G, Thune P: Gastro-intestinal investigations in dermatitis herpetiformis. Acta Derm Venereol 55:203, 1975. *A further effort to distinguish between dermatitis herpetiformis and celiac disease on the basis of gastrointestinal studies.*

O'Donoghue DP, Lancaster-Smith M, Johnson GD, Kumar PJ: Gastric lesion in dermatitis herpetiformis. Gut 17:185, 1976. *A closer focus at the gastric pathology and the presence of parietal cell antibody in the sera.*

Scott BB, Losowsky MD: Gluten antibodies in coeliac disease and dermatitis herpetiformis. Gut 17:398, 1976. *Gluten antibody levels, being higher in coeliac disease than in dermatitis herpetiformis, suggested a fundamental difference in the immunologic abnormality.*

Silk DBA, Mowat NAC, Riddell RH, Kirby JD: Intestinal lymphoma complicating dermatitis herpetiformis. Br J Dermatol 96:555, 1977. *Perhaps more than chance.*

HERPES GESTATIONIS

Should an extremely pruritic vesiculobullous disease occur in pregnancy, the most likely diagnosis is *herpes gestationis.* If the pregnancy is early and unsuspected, the grouped vesicles and intense pruritus might suggest dermatitis herpetiformis, but the lesions lack symmetry and pigmentation, are frequently bullous and occasionally urticarial, and resemble erythema multiforme more than any other diagnosis. Histopathologically they are subepidermal bullae with abundant eosinophils indistinguishable from those of bullous pemphigoid. The possibility of a toxic or allergic reaction to fetal or placental protein or their metabolites, or to hormones, has been considered but remains unproved. With exacerbations and remission the disease is likely to persist throughout the pregnancy and perhaps into the puerperium, especially if the onset is just ante partum. It can recur with the menses for a year or more after delivery and is likely to recur with subsequent pregnancies.

The problem for the mother is only one of discomfort, but for the fetus it is significant, with threat of abnormalities or death. Recent experience with successful outcome using systemic steroids would give a more optimistic, although guarded, prognosis.

Pruritus in pregnancy with erythematous papules in the absence of blisters may represent the rare papular dermatitis of Spangler that is generalized, intensely pruritic, difficult to control, and also associated with fetal risk. In the more benign prurigo gestationis of Besnier, without threat to the fetus, the pruritic papules occur mostly over the extremities in the last trimester and are usually amenable to topical therapy. In the differential diagnosis both conditions suggest drug eruptions and excoriations from other causes of pruritus, rather than any of the blistering diseases. Perhaps the most common pruritic disease of pregnancy, often misdiagnosed as a drug eruption or even erythema multiforme, is the *pruritic urticarial papules and plaques of pregnancy* (PUPPP), an intensely pruritic eruption characterized by erythematous urticarial plaques and papules that present on the abdomen and extend to the thighs, buttocks, and occasionally the arms, beginning in the third trimester. The histology is that of a superficial, occasionally mid-dermal perivascular and lymphocytic infiltrate with some edema of the papillary dermis. The response of symptoms to topical steroids is usually quite adequate and the eruption disappears at delivery, although it may recur. There is no risk to the infant.

ERYTHEMA MULTIFORME

Erythema multiforme is a reaction pattern in the skin and mucous membranes, an angiitis which in the upper corium leads to symptomless erythematous lesions, perhaps edematous or bullous, that darken with age, leaving the concentric rings of an "iris" or "target" lesion. Acute appearances and recurrences have been associated with recognized infections such as herpes simplex and, more recently, *Mycoplasma pneumoniae,* as well as with vaccinations, drugs, malignancy, deep x-ray therapy, and even infectious mononucleosis, but a third of the cases defy explanation. The expression of erythema multiforme may range from minor disease with a few scattered lesions to major illness with extensive bullous erosions, life-threatening fever, and prostration. The syndrome described and named erythema exudativum multiforme by Hebra in 1866 was not familiar to Stevens and Johnson, who reported "a new eruptive fever with stomatitis and ophthalmia" in 1922, giving their names to the extreme expression of the disease.

In the severe form, erythema multiforme can be associated with mild prodromal symptoms suggestive of an upper respiratory infection that would be unremarkable except for the very sudden and dramatic eruption that ensues. The eyes are involved almost as often as the mouth and vagina. Endoscopy reveals erosions of the esophagus and colon, leading to gastrointestinal symptoms. Nephritis and uremia may be a further complication. Its course lasts two to four weeks or longer, and is prone to recur. Although systemic steroids are usually used in severe cases, the improvement is not as prompt as expected in steroid-responsive blistering diseases and can be questioned. An underlying cause of erythema multiforme must always be sought, particularly with recurrent disease. Although most patients are between 10 and 30, in those over 50 years old a search for malignancy is warranted.

TOXIC EPIDERMAL NECROLYSIS

This eruption resembles scalded skin and may not be in the clinical differential of classic erythema multiforme, but the reaction pattern is analogous. Both diseases probably represent part of a continuous disease spectrum. Toxic epidermal necrolysis has a prodrome followed by the appearance of erythema and the loss of skin in sheets, with a threat of death and liability of recurrence. Two forms are recognized: one occurring mainly in young children with associated staphylococcal infections of phage Type 71, and the other affecting adults or older children and associated with drugs or other infections and conditions. When toxic epidermal necrolysis is induced by staphylococcal toxins, the epidermal cleavage is in the malpighian or granular layer, in contrast to the subepidermal split of toxic epidermal necrolysis from other causes. The prognosis is good. It is now separately labeled the staphylococcal scalded skin syndrome (SSSS), the histology reflecting the effect of toxin on the intercellular region of the lower granular layer without significant cytotoxic change in adjacent cells. The usefulness of corticosteroids and antimicrobial agents in the course of the epidermal change has not been demonstrated; but with the delay in developing a humoral response to staphylococcal toxin, and risk of contagion, specific prompt antimicrobial therapy is indicated. In toxic epidermal necrolysis of other causes, the epidermal cleavage occurs just above or at the basal layer as a result of basal cell disintegration. Although nonstaphylococcal infections, immunizations, and vaccinations have been implicated, the reaction is more often precipitated by drugs such as the sulfonamides, phenylbutazone, penicillin, hexametaphosphate, tetracycline, mithramycin, barbiturates, aspirin, amidopyrine, procaine, phenolphthalein, allopurinol, dapsone, gold salts, and hydantoin. Even a gin and tonic has caused toxic epidermal necrolysis, presumably from the quinine, and it has been reported following inhalation of acrylonitrile, a pesticide. Since the full thickness of the epidermis is separated in toxic epidermal necrolysis, the serum loss is greater and the prognosis is more guarded. Unlike staphylococcal scalded skin syndrome the mucous membranes are often involved, and associated membranoproliferative glomerulonephritis has been noted.

The clear histologic distinction between staphylococcal scalded skin syndrome and toxic epidermal necrolysis of other causes makes the biopsy an important diagnostic tool for differentiation and prognosis. By using the Nikolsky sign to advantage, skin peeled from a fresh wound of staphylococcal scalded skin syndrome shows, on frozen section, the stratum corneum with focally adherent granular cells. The Tzanck smear from the denuded base has broad cells with a low nucleus-to-cytoplasm ratio. In toxic epidermal necrolysis the full thickness of the epithelium is found on the frozen peeled specimen and the Tzanck preparation shows inflammatory cells, basal cells, and a high nucleus-to-cytoplasm ratio. Further, direct immunofluorescent staining in toxic epidermal necrolysis has shown intercellular fixation of immunoglobulins and complement at the basal cell layer, suggesting that drugs bind to intercellular epidermal protein and that the basal cells are the site of damage. Therapy is supportive with close attention to fluid balance, but corticosteroids or even renal dialysis may be required.

Mucocutaneous Lymph Node Syndrome (Kawasaki's Disease)

A recently recognized entity, first reported in 1967 in children, but now documented in adults, the mucocutaneous lymph node syndrome is included here because of the ocular and conjunctival involvement, the mucous membrane erythema and erosions, and the severe prostration with fever, rash, and lymphadenopathy. Of obscure etiology and unresponsive to recognized therapy, it can be associated with myocardial involvement and death from coronary artery occlusion.

Of epidemic prevalence in Japan, where more than 10,000 cases have been recorded, the diagnostic criteria of the syndrome have been met by children the world over—Hawaii, North America, England, Greece, Korea—and now by adults. Of the 633 American cases reported to the Center for Disease Control by 1981, the mean age was 4.2 years, ranging from 7 months to 27 years. Those affected present with ulcerative gingivitis, rhinitis, and fever which can last one to two weeks. There is acute nonsuppurative enlargement of cervical lymph nodes. On the third day or so of illness, a generalized macular eruption appears with intense bright erythema and edema of the palms and soles, followed by desquamation of the skin of fingers and toes. Proteinuria, pyuria, diarrhea, aseptic meningitis, and mild icterus may be observed, with leukocytosis and a shift to the left, slight anemia, and perhaps an elevated transaminase. Thrombocytosis even to 1 million platelets is seen. There are complaints of photophobia and arthralgia. The diagnosis is made only when a patient has five of the following six criteria: fever for more than five days, conjunctival injection, mouth lesions, desquamation of the peripheral extremities, erythematous rash, and lymph node enlargement. Diligent search for causative microorganisms and detailed study of paired serologic specimens have been unrewarding.

Although the course is usually benign and self-limited, sudden death has been reported in 1 to 2 per cent of patients; electrocardiograms have suggested myocarditis or pericarditis in 70 per cent of cases. Further, abnormal coronary angiograms were noted in more than half of 20 patients studied three weeks to four years after their illness. With a view of preventing coronary aneurysm, several treatment schedules were assessed, including steroids alone, with anticoagulants, with aspirin, and then aspirin and antibiotics alone. The steroid-treated group fared significantly less well and, from these data, steroids are contraindicated.

Darby CP, Kyong CU: Mucocutaneous lymph node syndrome. JAMA 236:2295, 1976. *Alerting the United States to clinical "findings" observed and reported primarily but not exclusively in Japan.*

Kato H, Koike S, Yokoyama T: Kawasaki disease: Effect of treatment on coronary artery involvement. Pediatrics 63:175, 1979. *A further review with additional cases.*

Kawasaki T, Kosaki F, Okawa S, Shigematusu I, Yanagawa HL: A new infantile acute febrile mucocutaneous lymph node syndrome (MLNS) prevailing in Japan. Pediatrics 54:271, 1974. *The initial report in the American literature.*

Melish ME, Hicks RV, Reddy V: Kawasaki syndrome: Update. Hosp Prac 17:99, 1982. *Kawasaki's disease may be more prevalent than first supposed.*

Behçet's Disease

So often considered in the differential diagnosis of erythema multiforme because of oral and genital erosions with inflammatory ocular disease, Behçet's disease should be mentioned here although it is reviewed in depth in Ch. 464. A chronic and frequently multisystem disease, it is characterized by the triad cited and often by joint and bowel disease, with vasculitis important to the pathogenesis. Of uncommon occurrence despite alleged under-reporting, it appears regularly in the differential diagnosis of aphthae, recurrent severe herpes simplex, and Reiter's syndrome. The variability in expression of the entity, however, and the lack of minimal criteria or specific diagnostic tests for irrefutable identification leave clinical considerations unconfirmed.

Oral and genital ulcerations are usually the first symptoms, followed within days, months, or years by the uveitis and other clinical signs that may express an associated thrombophlebitis or vasculitis. Fever, malaise, and arthralgia are usually present during periods of active disease. The ocular pathology produces the most disability.

The mucosal lesions may be superficial erosions or deep punched-out ulcers, with necrosis leading to pain, with dysphagia and fetor if of the mouth, and to perforation of the labia minora in the genital area. If the colon is involved, discrete mucosal ulcers can be observed with intervening normal bowel; thus it is differentiated from the continuous inflammatory change of ulcerative colitis.

Cutaneous lesions occur in some 80 per cent of cases: follicular pustules, furuncles, inflammatory dermal nodules, acneiform lesions, cellulitis, and other forms of pyoderma. Of interest, and perhaps of diagnostic significance, sterile pustules occur after intradermal injection of normal saline or even a needle prick. The histology of induced sterile pustules shows mild to intense perivascular round cell infiltrates at 24 hours, with an occasional cluster of polymorphonuclear leukocytes. On immunofluorescent study, no deposits of immunoglobulins, complement, fibrinogen, or albumin are noted, although circulating alpha$_2$ globulin, gamma globulin, IgA, IgG, and IgM have been elevated.

Therapy for the basic disease process is probably not helpful. Corticosteroids systemically and topically may reverse some of the inflammatory processes, but the condition is known for its natural clinical fluctuations. Immunosuppressive therapy, azathioprine and cyclophosphamide, is used to reduce the need of corticosteroids.

Mast Cell Disease

Mast cell disease is a group of entities of which the common denominator is the spindle-shaped, dendritic connective tissue mast cell which aggregates in excessive numbers in the skin and occasionally in other organs. Symptoms relate to the pharmacologic effect of the histamine released by the degranulated mast cell and to the disruption of the organ structure and strength, as in bones, by mast cell infiltrates.

Several schemata distinguish among the clinical manifestations of mastocytosis. The cells may appear in the skin alone, or with systemic involvement, rarely as systemic infiltrates without skin lesions. The classic mast cell infiltrate appears as a small, discrete, reddish brown pigmented macule that becomes hive-like when stroked (Darier's sign), the released histamine having provoked a wheal. Such *urticaria pigmentosa* is the most common form of mastocytosis, occurring primarily in children, with half the patients clearing and almost all improving before adult life. Occasionally in infants there may be a single nodular lesion, a larger aggregate of cells known as a *mastocytoma.* Stroking for urtication can induce systemic effects of flushing and colic, with sufficient local edema to produce vesicles and bullae. Rarely is there *diffuse mastocytosis* with the skin so widely infiltrated as to become thickened, doughy, and lichenified. When the diffuse form is seen in children or when the urticaria pigmentosa has its onset in adulthood, noncutaneous organ involvement must be suspected. Any tissue where the mast cell is found can be affected. The central nervous system is thus excluded, leaving bone, liver, spleen, and gastrointestinal tract as sites of predilection in *systemic mastocytosis* (see Ch. 438). Here the associated macular lesions of the skin may acquire persistent telangiectasia, or may become more papular, suggestive of leukemia cutis. A small percentage of patients with systemic mastocytosis actually develop leukemia, which can be mast cell leukemia but is usually not.

Urticaria pigmentosa without systemic involvement accounts for 90 per cent of persons affected with mast cell disease. These and the balance of patients with systemic mastocytosis dem-

onstrating cutaneous involvement all have skin lesions readily recognized by the trained eye and provable by biopsy. The nests of mast cells are diagnostic. When selecting a lesion for histology, however, care must be taken lest the granules be discharged and thus rendered invisible by stroking or other manipulation prior to biopsy. Brisk skin cleansing must be avoided, and anesthesia should be injected at a distance and deeply. After fixation in 10 per cent formalin or absolute alcohol and staining with Giemsa, toluidine blue, or methylene blue, the characteristic basophilic metachromatic granules will be seen in the cytoplasm of the mast cell.

The symptomatology of mast cell disease varies with the site and extent of organ involvement. If it is confined to the skin, more than half the patients are asymptomatic. A third or so complain of pruritus, flushing, and headache often induced by the mechanical degranulation of the mast cell, as with hot baths and exercise, or by the pharmacologic degranulation, as with codeine and aspirin. In more extensive involvement patients may experience diarrhea and peptic ulcer, usually without acid hypersecretion.

Those mast cell lesions present at birth or appearing in childhood and limited to the skin have an excellent prognosis. In fact mast cell disease confined to skin and bone is compatible with life and minimal morbidity. Solitary lesions can be excised. Therapy otherwise relates to symptomatology, the avoidance of maneuvers and situations that lead to mast cell degranulation, or the selection of time for such discharge when it interferes least with the patient's life style and can be anticipated with antihistamine coverage.

Malignancy

Skin can undergo malignant change, and it can support the metastatic malignant growth of other organs. Even more, it can respond to the systemic presence of malignancy in ways that challenge the implication of the malignant cell and process. Considered here are the common *cutaneous malignancies,* often radiation induced; then *mycosis fungoides,* an uncommon neoplastic disease but a distinct histopathologic and clinical entity first manifested in the skin; Kaposi's sarcoma because of its recent epidemic presentation with the acquired immune deficiency syndrome; and finally *melanoma.*

THE COMMON CUTANEOUS MALIGNANCIES

The individual at highest risk for developing skin cancer is the light-complexioned, blue-eyed freckler who has had considerable ultraviolet light exposure, whether geographically determined or influenced by occupation and avocation. The effect of such natural radiation will be augmented by any x-irradiation ever received, or by any exposure to carcinogens such as the oral inorganic arsenicals or to chronic cutaneous infection, ulceration, or burn.

Basal Cell Epithelioma

The most common cancer of the skin by far is the basal cell epithelioma, which affects the white population but rarely blacks or Orientals. The prevalence in the United States is 3.9 per 1000, or 757,000 cases. The average patient is over 40 years of age, but basal cell epithelioma can be seen in young adults or even children. Men are more often affected than women (2.2:1.7). The clinical lesion is a raised nodule with a pearly translucent border showing telangiectatic vessels (Fig. 557–1). It may be ulcerated and, more rarely, pigmented. Some lesions remain unchanged for years; others can be ulcerated and invasive from the first clinical observation. When removed completely by any destructive measure—excision, desiccation and curettage, even x-ray—the subsequent morbidity of the enlarging eroding lesion is thwarted. Proximity to sensitive structures and the capacity to burrow compel early recognition.

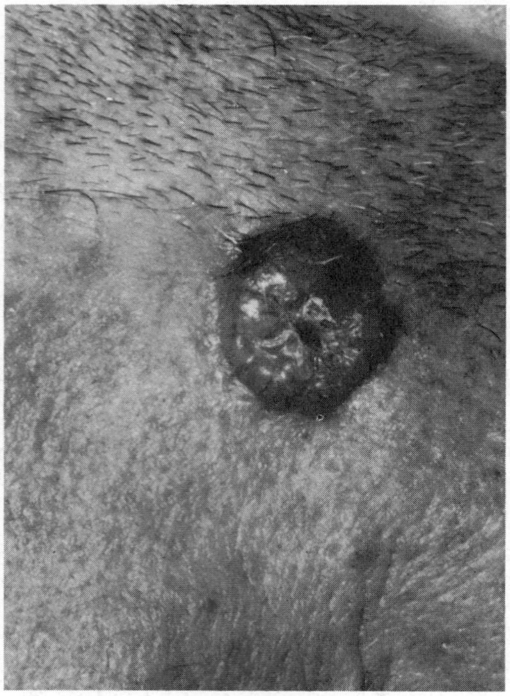

Figure 557–1. Basal cell epithelioma.

The clinical diagnosis is readily confirmed by biopsy. Therapy should be selected to ensure removal with minimal cosmetic compromise and without increasing risk through long-term radiation effects. X-ray therapy, for example, which induces cutaneous malignancy in 15 to 20 years and augments all other radiation effects, should be reserved for the feeble and elderly. Recurrent lesions, or those proximal to the eye, at the inner canthus, for example, where neither should normal tissue be sacrificed nor risk of recurrence permitted, are best treated by the microscopically monitored removal of the last malignant cell through the tedious staging of Mohs' chemosurgery; fixed or frozen tissue is charted, and each shaved specimen is checked for the persistence of the readily recognized basophilic cell.

Basal cell epitheliomas usually appear singly, but may not, and the individual who has developed one is prone to develop others. The areas most struck by sunlight in the erect individual are the surfaces prone to actinic damage and consequent cutaneous malignancy: cheeks, forehead, and nasolabial fold. Certain basal cell lesions, such as the sclerosing waxy morphea type occurring on the head and neck or the superficial spreading type seen on the trunk, may confound the inexperienced, but biopsy will usually be definitive. Nevoid tumors such as trichoepithelioma can occasionally be confused with keratotic basal cell epithelioma, especially if solitary. Multiple basal cell tumors appearing in childhood should alert the observer to the basal cell nevus syndrome and its associated abnormalities of skin, bone, central nervous system, eye, and gonads.

Squamous Cell Carcinoma

Induced by the same factors as basal cell epithelioma but with a fraction of the prevalence, squamous cell carcinoma arises in the light-exposed areas from keratinizing epidermal cells. The typical patient is more than 60 years old and male with a history of considerable sun exposure (Fig. 557–2). The tumors arising on sun damaged skin are, when compared to other squamous cell carcinoma, less aggressive, and less likely to metastasize, except perhaps for those of the ear and lip which, even when small, can metastasize to local lymph nodes. Squamous cell tumors induced by x-ray or arsenicals, or arising in burn scars, or in chronic granulomas such as lupus vulgaris, are of greater concern and have a poorer prognosis. Commencing in chronic ectodermal change as they do, they may go unnoticed or unappreciated until extensive and metastatic. Ordinarily squamous cell carcinoma appears as a slowly enlarging nodule with an inflamed, indurated base growing more rapidly than a basal cell tumor. Therapy is urgent complete removal. The prognosis is guarded for lesions of the lip, especially of the vermilion border, and for all lesions with metastases. Patients treated for cutaneous malignancy must be assessed periodically for recurrence and for new tumor. Those who have had one skin cancer are at risk of developing others even when the initiating factors are not apparent. They should be cautioned about this and about the need for surveillance, as well as the harmful effects of continued sun exposure.

MYCOSIS FUNGOIDES
(Cutaneous T-Cell Lymphoma)

Mycosis fungoides is a chronic fatal disease of the reticuloendothelial system, a T-cell lymphoma which initially and primarily involves skin but can involve lymph nodes and viscera. It is distinguishable from Hodgkin's disease and other malignant lymphomas. Clinically there is an erythematous pretumor stage which progresses to thickened, indurated, plaque-like lesions, and ultimately tumor. The early premycotic stage may last from months to years, with scaling and erythema persisting to the end; uncommonly, the presenting complaint can be a tumefaction. The disease is not rare, accounting for perhaps 1 per cent of deaths from lymphoma; it occurs in all races, usually in those from 40 to 60 years, but has been seen in teenagers.

A psoriasiform or eczematous dermatitis, chronic, persistent, and pruritic, that is not caused by drug or contactant should bring mycosis fungoides into the differential diagnosis. Fixed giant hive-like lesions or plaques are further clinical indicators, as is lymphadenopathy. Often, histopathologic confirmation of the diagnosis is delayed for years past the clinical impression of mycosis fungoides. Biopsies from plaques or tumors, however, provide the histologic features that establish the diagnosis: Pautrier's microabscesses, atypical cells nested within the epidermis; an infiltrate of atypical mononuclear cells; and hyperchromatic larger cells with irregular nuclei, the "mycosis cells." After the appearance of tumor, lymphadenopathy, or ulceration, the median survival is less than two to five years; with the appearance of all three, the median survival is less than one year.

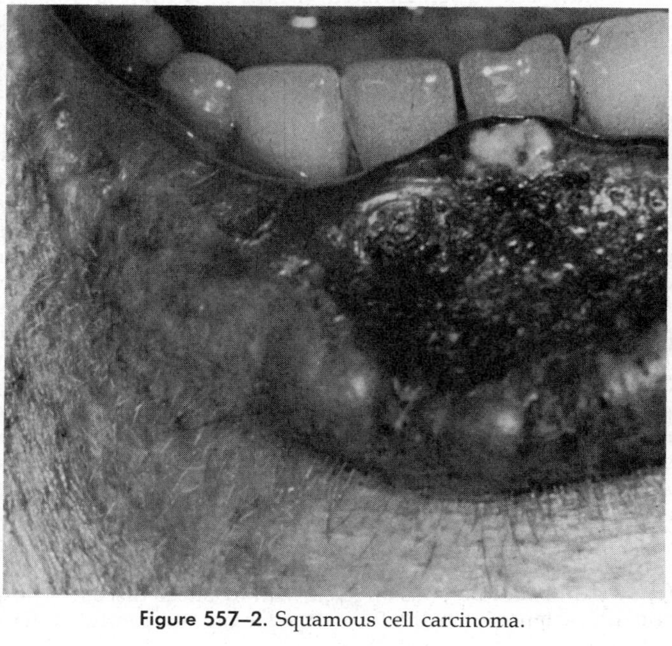

Figure 557–2. Squamous cell carcinoma.

Extracutaneous dissemination of mycosis fungoides, once thought rare, is no longer considered uncommon; visceral involvement is noted in two thirds of patients (61 to 82 per cent) at autopsy. Lung, liver, and spleen are the more common sites, but nearly every organ or tissue may be involved with atypical cells. Any lymph node involvement indicates the likelihood of spread to other extracutaneous sites. Staging for prognosis will have impetus as treatment protocols are developed. However, one third of patients who succumb to mycosis fungoides have disease limited to the skin.

Therapy for this uniformly fatal disease has been palliative. Pruritus, dermatitis, and tumor are treated at each stage as they appear. Corticosteroids have been used, as well as chemotherapeutic agents such as cyclophosphamide and chlorambucil, and also the antimetabolites azaribine and methotrexate. Bleomycin is a promising cytotoxic antibiotic because of its concentration in the skin (and lung). Electron beam therapy is of advantage for the remission of lesions if not the disease, as is conventional x-ray and, more recently, a simultaneous combined treatment with x-irradiation plus chemotherapy. Skin painting with nitrogen mustard or by intralesional injection has given favorable results, as have psoralens with high intensity ultraviolet light. To date, however, no protocol or series has been adequate to provide the definitive data for the proper treatment of this devastating disease.

No consideration of mycosis fungoides is complete without mention of Sézary's syndrome. Probably a variant of mycosis fungoides, it is characterized by an extensive exfoliative erythroderma with intense pruritus, lymphadenopathy, and large mononuclear cells in the skin and blood. Elevated leukocyte counts are found in most patients; all have a lymphocytosis, with atypical cells varying in size from 10 to 20 μ recognized as Sézary cells by their folded, lobulated nucleus and rim of PAS-positive, diastase-resistant cytoplasm. A "small cell" variant has been described. Studies of the ultrastructure of these abnormal lymphocytes have identified them in cutaneous infiltrates of mycosis fungoides. In Sézary's syndrome these abnormal thymus-derived cells constitute more than 40 per cent of purified lymphocyte fractions from the peripheral blood. In patients affected, immune mechanisms are generally not impaired.

Although Sézary's syndrome might be looked upon as the erythrodermatous phase of mycosis fungoides, it does not respond well to palliative therapy, even electron beam irradiation. Reduction of the intravascular neoplastic T-cells by leukapheresis to effect a mobilization and reduction of tissue infiltrates gives a new and innovative but not yet fully assessed approach to the management.

Edelson RL (ed.): Cutaneous T-cell lymphoma (special issue). J Dermatol Surg Oncol 6:357, 1980. *An excellent review.*

Epstein EH, Levin DL, Croft JD, Lutzner MA: Mycosis fungoides. Survival, prognostic features, response to therapy and autopsy findings. Medicine 51:61, 1972. *An important reference point for weighing the value and morbidity of therapy.*

Thomas LE, Rappaport H: Mycosis fungoides and its relationship to other malignant lymphomas. *In* Rebuck JW, et al. (eds.): The Reticuloendothelial System. Baltimore, Williams & Wilkins Company, 1975.

Van Scott EJ, Haynes HA: Cutaneous lymphoma. *In* Fitzpatrick TB (ed.): Dermatology in General Medicine. New York, McGraw-Hill Book Company, 1971, pp 556–573.

KAPOSI'S SARCOMA

Into the same limelight of uncommon but lethal cutaneous tumor has moved Kaposi's sarcoma, with new and fascinating connections to second primary malignancies and opportunistic infections that implicate reduced immune competence and the possible role of infectious agents and environmental factors. A rare neoplasm of multifocal origin, Kaposi's sarcoma presents as red-purple to blue-brown macules, plaques, and nodules of the skin and other organs. The cutaneous lesions may be firm or compressible, solitary or numerous, and may even appear initially as a dusky stain, especially about the toes.

Reporting an "idiopathic multiple pigmented sarcoma" of the skin, Moritz Kaposi in 1872 recognized that these round-

cell and spindle-cell sarcomas were also to be found in viscera and seemed to occur predominantly in older men, leading to their demise. In Europe and North America, where it is more frequently seen among Jews and those of Mediterranean descent, the lesions commonly affect the lower extremities, are indolent, and often are associated with chronic lymphedema, indicating tumor infiltration of the lymphatics. Men are affected 10 to 15 times more often than women, are usually in their seventh decade, and have an average survival time of approximately 10 years, although some live much longer. The incidence of such Kaposi's sarcoma variously reported for the United States is less than 0.1 per 100,000 population and fewer than 0.02 per cent of all malignancies.

In tropical Africa, however, there is an endemic belt at an altitude of 1200 to 1500 meters where the disease accounts for 3 to 9 per cent of all malignancies, afflicting the black population while sparing white people and Indians. It is found among the young with a peak incidence in the first decade, with most patients less than 20 years of age, and with survival of less than three years. Visceral rather than cutaneous involvement and marked lymphadenopathy are the predominant clinical signs in these African children, who exhibit a unique form of Kaposi's sarcoma found in no other population.

The selective geographic distribution of the lymphadenopathic type of Kaposi's sarcoma is remarkably similar to that of Burkitt's lymphoma. With the electron microscopic studies that affirm an association between cytomegalovirus and Kaposi's sarcoma, another parallel is made with Burkitt's lymphoma, the malignancy so closely linked to the Epstein-Barr virus. In the acquiring of Kaposi's sarcoma, therefore, it would seem that infectious agents and immune status are of significance, as well as genetic and environmental factors. Kaposi's sarcoma has been observed to complicate systemic lupus erythematosus being treated with immunosuppression and to appear along with tumors of lymphoreticular origin in the immunosuppressed recipients of renal transplants. It is known to coexist with other primary malignancies. However, its appearance as an aggressive lethal tumor in the young male homosexual without underlying disease is the stunning observation of grave concern. Those affected have a mean age in the fourth decade. Their skin lesions are generalized in distribution and are smaller, softer, and lighter in color than the classic firm, indurated lesions of the legs. Mucous membrane tumors or symptomatic visceral or lung lesions may appear before the hemorrhagic sarcomas of the skin. Average survival time from onset of the disease is less than two years.

Such fulminant Kaposi's sarcoma is appearing alone or with *Pneumocystis carinii* pneumonia and other opportunistic infections in increasing numbers in a population comprising male homosexuals and drug abusers with geographic clustering in New York and California, a population that has experienced a variety of sexually transmitted diseases and demonstrates the presence of antibodies to cytomegalovirus implicated as a causal agent in the induction of the immunosuppressed state (see Ch. 430). The documented infectivity of contaminated blood products and seminal fluid has extended the risk to transfusion recipients and the heterosexual partners of bisexual individuals. Among those cases reported to the CDC since June, 1981, Kaposi's sarcoma was the presenting disease in almost half. A small painless red nodule of the skin, easily overlooked, can signal a profoundly compromised immune state and grave prognosis. There is no adequate therapy.

Friedman-Kien A, Laubenstein L, Rubenstein P, Buimovici-Klein E, Marmor M, Stahl R, Springland I, Soo Kim K, Zollar-Pazner S: Disseminated Kaposi's sarcoma in homosexual men. Ann Intern Med 96:693, 1982.

Hardwood A, Osoba D, Hofstader S, Goldstein M, Cardella C, Holecek M, Kunynetz R, Giammarco R: Kaposi's sarcoma in recipients of renal transplants. Am J Med 67:759, 1979.

Hardy M, Goldfarb P, Levine S, Dattner A, Muggia F, Levitt S, Weinstein E: De novo Kaposi's sarcoma in renal transplantation. CA 38:144, 1976.

Haverkos HW, Curran JW: The current outbreak of Kaposi's sarcoma and opportunistic infections. CA 32:330, 1982. *Impressive data and review of the challenge of why these diseases are occurring now and in the population afflicted.*

Hymes K, Cheung T, Greene J, Prose N, Marcus A, Ballard H, William D, Laubenstein L: Kaposi's sarcoma in homosexual men—a report of eight cases. Lancet 2:98, 1981.

Klein M, Pereira F, Kantor I: Kaposi sarcoma complicating systemic lupus erythematosus treated with immunosuppression. Arch Dermatol 110:602, 1974.

Myers B, Kessler E, Levi J, Pick A, Rosenfeld J, Israel P: Kaposi sarcoma in kidney transplant recipients. Arch Intern Med 133:307, 1974.

Safai B, Good RA: Kaposi's sarcoma: A review and recent developments. CA 31:2, 1981. *An excellent review of the facets that suggest Kaposi's sarcoma as a potential model for a virus-associated human cancer.*

Safai B, Mike V, Giraldo G, Beth E, Good R: Association of Kaposi's sarcoma with second primary malignancies. CA 45:1472, 1980.

MELANOMA

Melanoma is a neoplasm of melanocytes that has the potential for invasion and metastasis. It contributes little to the burden of cutaneous malignancy by case load (fewer than 3 percent of new skin cancers), but by mortality it accounts for two thirds of the deaths from skin cancer, and at an appreciably young age. In fact, those who develop any malignancy between ages 35 and 40 are at greater risk only for cancer of the lung, breast, or cervix.

Along with other skin cancer, melanoma shows a currently increasing incidence, highest in Caucasians, and influenced adversely by ultraviolet light exposure as judged by the anatomic distribution of lesions and by occupational and geographical factors. As with other skin cancers, patients who develop melanoma are apt to have a light complexion and light-colored eyes, and to sunburn readily. They may have a family predisposition to the development of melanoma, or they may have had one primary melanoma which places them at greater risk of having a second primary.

Three out of four melanomas that develop in the skin undergo progressive change over an extended period from not less than six months to many years, thereby providing the informed examiner with a prolonged opportunity to recognize and remove surgically the potentially lethal lesion for probable cure. Change in texture, color, or size of a pre-existing nevus arouses suspicion of melanoma, but even without such signs there are clinical characteristics that make a pigmented lesion suspect. Any brown-black spot with areas of red or red-purple, plus white, whether gray-white or pink-white, and blue, should be examined histopathologically. There is further suspicion of melanoma if the borders of the lesion are irregular, appear notched or smudged, and have pigment streaming from the pigmented edge. Of grave concern is the lesion with a surface that is elevated or ulcerated and devoid of skin markings.

Regarding all melanotic lesions with red, white, and blue as possible melanoma and hence in need of definitive histopathologic diagnosis, one may gather a few vascular lesions and a rare pigmented basal cell epithelioma, but would also net a significant number of early melanomas when most are at a curative stage. This underscores the importance of examining the entire integument carefully, in good light, and with hand lens magnification, for all suspicious pigmented lesions. It presumes confidence in recognizing the common benign pigmented lesions of the skin reviewed in Ch. 556.

Primary cutaneous melanoma can be classified according to clinicohistologic type, the level of invasion, the thickness of the lesion, and the density of the inflammatory response. With the establishment of criteria for sorting among the various clinical presentations, realistic comparisons can be made, prognoses given, and the value of therapeutic measures assessed. Clinically, several types are recognized and the histology correlated.

Lentigo maligna (Fig. 557–3) begins as a small tan macular lesion, a circumscribed precancerous melanosis, the melanotic freckle of Hutchinson. Usually a lesion of the elderly, it can occur in the 20's. Over years, or even decades, it may enlarge by lateral growth, with the margins becoming irregular and the color modified to brown-black and pink-white. Eventually there will be dermal invasion, the vertical growth phase, associated with a papular or nodular surface. Melanotic freckles are mostly seen on the face but may occur anywhere on the skin where there has been significant sunlight exposure. The radial growth phase of 5 to 7 cm and measured in years provides the long lead time for therapy before active malignant invasion. Unfortunately, the benignity of appearance and the confusion of the smaller early lesion with a solar lentigo often delay definitive treatment until size alone precludes simple excision.

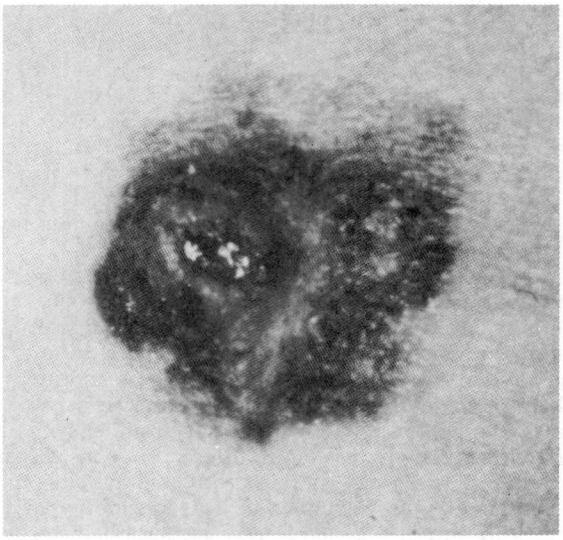

Figure 557–3. Lentigo maligna.

Superficial spreading melanoma occurs in younger individuals; it may appear anywhere in the body, characteristically on the upper back in both sexes and on the legs of women (Fig. 557–4). Fairly regular in outline, sometimes notched, lesions range in color from tan to black, often with the telltale mix of red, white, and blue. Initially barely palpable, these, too, become papular or nodular with the vertical growth phase.

Nodular melanoma, as might be suspected from the terminology, does not have a discernible radial growth phase but, from the first, is observed as a nodule or plaque, dark brown or black, with a gray or blue cast (Fig. 557–5). It is invasive from the start, and the prognosis is never as good as with other melanomas. Further, the nodular variety can occasionally be amelanotic and extremely difficult to diagnose clinically.

The clinicohistologic grouping recognizes an *acral lentiginous melanoma* of the palms, soles, and terminal phalanges, which is similar in its benign clinical appearance to *lentigo maligna melanoma,* but which, like it and like *superficial spreading melanoma,* can develop a vertical growth phase. It also distinguishes nodular melanoma of the mucous membranes, occurring more frequently in blacks and Orientals, and a miscellaneous group of melanomas that arise in various nevi, the central nervous system, and the viscera.

In all melanomas there is correlation between the depth of the histologic invasion and the prognosis. Clark and his coworkers have designated intraepidermal malignancy as Level I, invasion of the papillary dermis as Level II, filling the papillary dermis and impinging upon but not invading the reticular dermis as Level III, reaching into the reticular dermis as Level IV, and reaching into the subcutaneous tissue as Level V. Correlated with these levels is an increasing mortality: 8.3 per cent for Level II; 35.2 per cent for Level III: 46.1 per cent for Level IV; and 52 per cent for Level V. Breslow measures depth of tumor invasion with an ocular micrometer and finds 100 per cent five-year survival in those with a melanoma depth less than 0.75 mm; 74 per cent with a depth of 0.76 to 1.50 mm; 79 per cent at 1.51 to 2.25 mm; 44 per cent at 2.26 to 3.0

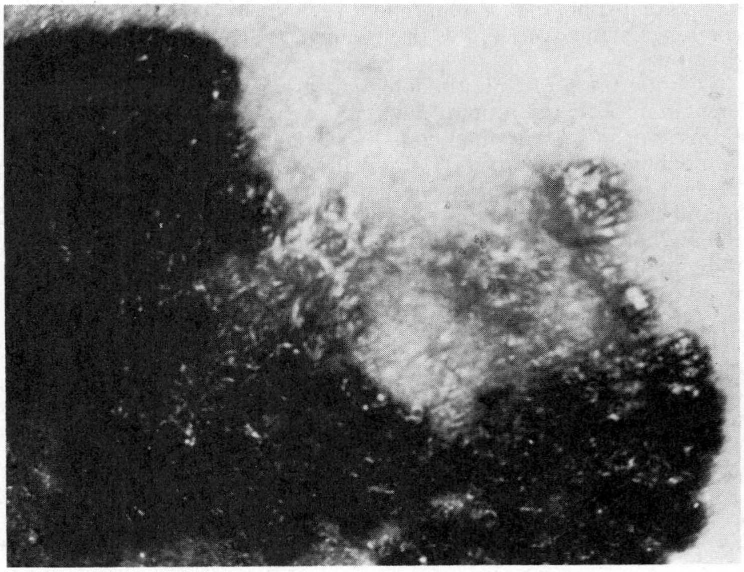

Figure 557–4. Superficial spreading melanoma.

mm; and 22 per cent at depths over 3 mm. Current histopathologic reporting gives both Clark levels and Breslow measurements, useful for clinical correlations, cooperative studies, and predictive value. There is also a difference in survival according to the clinical type of melanoma, with lentigo maligna melanoma having the longest survival, followed by superficial spreading melanoma, and, poorest, nodular melanoma.

Prognosis, in addition to a consideration of the type of melanoma, its size, and depth of invasion, is also dependent on the age and sex of the patient, the anatomic location of the tumor, and the presence or absence of metastases and of pigment. With similar lesions women fare better than men, and lesions of the leg or of the head or neck permit longer survival than those of the trunk. Absence of pigment portends a poor prognosis. So may pregnancy, although this is not certain for a given patient. In a study of women with melanoma there was no indication of benefit to the melanoma patient from termination of the pregnancy, oophorectomy, adrenalectomy, or hypophysectomy. Survival of those with localized disease was unchanged when compared to nonpregnant melanoma patients at the same stage. Those with nodal disease and pregnant did less well. They and those whose lesions had been activated during gestation should be cautioned against subsequent pregnancies.

The question of melanoma arising in pre-existing nevi is always posed. Congenital nevi account for fewer than 0.1 per cent of the nevi of the average young adult, but they are usually larger than acquired nevi and, since present from birth, are likely to be identified by the patient or his family. The risk of malignant change in such nevi is probably proportional to the numbers of aggregated melanocytes—hence the size of the lesion. Giant pigmented congenital nevi (the giant hairy or bathing trunk nevi) have an incidence of malignant change variously reported from 15 to 42 percent. Although melanoma is rare before puberty, almost half of those occurring in childhood arise in such giant congenital nevi. However, of all patients who develop melanoma, only one in four will recall a pre-existing pigmented lesion present from childhood, a figure supported by the 20 per cent of melanoma lesions that have histologic evidence of associated nevus.

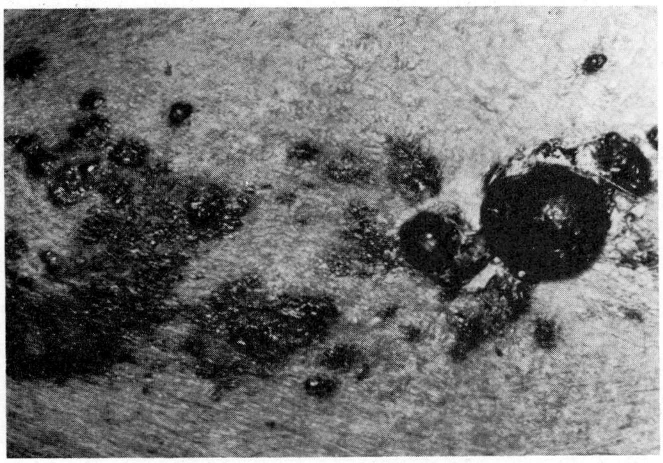

Figure 557–5. Nodular melanoma.

The removal of giant congenital nevi is indicated for malignant risk as well as cosmetic disfigurement, but often it is not surgically feasible. For small congenital nevi there are no data to support significant risk. If one accepts the relationship of size to risk, such aggregates of melanocytes must pose greater risk per unit area than normal skin. There is probably value in considering the removal of all congenital nevi larger than 1 cm after weighing the possibility of cosmetic disfigurement and such factors as complexion, eye color, and anatomic location.

When the sheer number of observed nevi preclude prophylactic excision and there is great variability among the nevi, the patient may well have the "B-K mole syndrome," characterized by myriad heritable melanocytic nevi and grave risk of multiple primary melanomas. One patient had six. In 25 individuals with one or more primary cutaneous melanoma, all from six families, 17 were examined and 15 had the syndrome. The prototypic "mole" is 1 cm in diameter, irregular in outline, and haphazardly colored tan, brown, black, and pink. Although appearing flat, it has a small palpable dermal component. These dysplastic nevi may be as few as 10 or more than 100, concentrating in a horsecollar distribution but found on the extremities as well. Unlike the ordinary noncongenital nevus, they appear later in childhood and after age 35. When observed in a group of four or five there is a striking difference among them, but it is by their histology with their atypical melanocytes that they can be identified. The melanomas that arise are biologically aggressive.

Melanoma, capable of persisting for years before active metastatic spread, can signal its presence by metastases with the primary lesion undiscoverable. In such cases (15 per cent in two large series) the occult primary melanoma may have undergone spontaneous regression, since melanoma, even visceral metastatic disease, has been known to disappear without therapy.

Perhaps parts of this phenomenon are the areas of depigmentation observed around nevi, and occasionally around the primary or metastatic cutaneous lesions of patients with melanoma. Such leukoderma is clinically indistinguishable from that present in halo nevi of the individual *without* melanoma, in whom the depigmentation can progress to the obliteration of the pigmented nevus clinically and histopathologically. In such individuals, free of malignancy, circulating anti-melanoma antibodies have been reported.

With suspected melanoma, an unequivocal diagnosis is mandatory. Clinical diagnoses can be quite wrong, and histopathologically certain pigmented lesions such as the Spitz nevus (benign juvenile melanoma) can be misread or confused with melanoma. A biopsy must be done and the histology reviewed.

The suspected lesion should be excised with a 5- to 10-mm border and penetration to the subcutaneous fat. If the size of the lesion precludes simple excision, an incisional biopsy is justified without concern over dissemination of tumor.

With confident histologic confirmation, a wide surgical excision is indicated. With a lesion less than 1 mm in depth, a 1-cm margin around the lesion is adequate. Depending upon the type and level of penetration of the tumor, further surgery or therapy may be suggested. Systemic and regional chemotherapy have been used and, more recently, immunotherapy with vaccinia and BCG.

Clark WH Jr, Reimer RR, Greene M, Ainsworth AM, Mastrangelo MJ: Origin of familial malignant melanomas from heritable melanocytic lesions: "B-K mole syndrome." Arch Dermatol 114:732, 1978. *The dysplastic nevus is another signal in our early warning system for melanoma.*

Day CL Jr, Mihm MC Jr, Sober AJ, Fitzpatrick TB, Malt RA: Narrower margins for clinical stage I malignant melanoma. N Engl J Med 306:479, 1982.

Kopf AW, Bart RS, Rodriguez-Sains, BA: Malignant melanoma: A review. J Dermatol Surg Oncol 3:41, 1977. *A thorough review.*

Mihm MC Jr, Fitzpatrick TB, Brown MML, Raker JW, Malt RA, Kaiser JS: Early detection of primary cutaneous malignant melanoma. A color atlas. N Engl J Med 289:989, 1973. *The ABC's of early detection.*

Part XXVI
OCCUPATIONAL AND ENVIRONMENTAL MEDICINE

558. PRINCIPLES OF OCCUPATIONAL MEDICINE

Charles E. Becker

Occupational medicine is concerned with the physical and emotional safety and health of workers. It encompasses issues of public concern, particularly the quality of air and water, the degree of environmental pollution, and the complex mosaic of legal, economic, social, and ethical questions that are raised whenever human action produces human disorders.

Among the 100 million workers in the United States today, approximately 100,000 deaths per year are attributed to the workplace. Yet there are only 8000 physicians whose self-determined primary specialty is occupational medicine, and only 800 of these have subspecialty board certification. Primary-care internists, family physicians, and emergency physicians constitute the "front line" for identification of work-related disorders, therefore, and must learn to target the medical history and to recognize classic signs and symptoms of occupational and environmental disorders.

Occupational medicine deals almost exclusively with diagnosis and prevention, not treatment. The diagnosis of an occupational disease may be difficult, since occupational diseases (1) may simulate many other disorders, (2) often lack unique pathology, and (3) may be marked by a long latency period between exposure and the manifestation of the disease.

Problems from chemical contamination do not always remain exclusively in the workplace; they may extend into the community: polychlorinated biphenyls (PCBs) in Japan; dioxin in Seveso, Italy; radiation exposure at Three Mile Island; mercury contamination in Minamata Bay; lead pollution in cities and around smelting plants; and nervous system, liver, and reproductive toxicity from chlordecone (Kepone) in Virginia. These events give rise to important political, social, and economic considerations that emphasize the need for specialized training in occupational medicine.

Competency in occupational medicine is best acquired from a base of general training in internal medicine, with extended knowledge and experience in epidemiology, industrial hygiene, and toxicology. The relationship between workplace-environmental exposures and disease centers on four basic concepts: recognition, prevention, exacerbation, latent manifestation. Workplace-associated diseases are presumed to be preventable when recognized and fully understood. Since the signs and symptoms of occupational diseases may be identical to those of many other diseases, a high level of suspicion is required for the recognition that allows prevention. Rather than causing an illness, occupational environmental conditions may, in fact, exacerbate or compound a pre-existing condition. For example, a patient with toxicity from aminoglycoside antibiotics may have additional otologic injury from loud noises occurring at work. Although some environmental and occupational diseases become manifest acutely, many have a long latency period and may extend from the workplace into the family or society and thus pose important considerations in diagnostic and preventive strategies.

In occupational medicine there are four basic categories of hazard: physical, biologic, psychologic, and chemical. Physical hazards may include vibration, heat, noise, radiation, and trauma. Occupational injuries account for approximately 14,000 deaths, 245 million lost work days, and $25 billion in direct and indirect costs annually in the United States. Biologic hazards include the well-known occupational risks of hepatitis or tuberculosis, for example. Psychologic hazards of stress and work-shift changes are complex and will be discussed subsequently. Chemical hazards involve exposure to solvents, dusts, vapors, and gases. It is important here to distinguish between toxicity and hazard. *Toxicity* is the inherent capability of a material to cause injury to a living cell. *Hazard* is the chance of a resultant injury from use of such a material in a given setting. Asbestos, for example, is a useful fire retardant construction material with known basic toxicity that may become hazardous during repair or demolition work or fire, which may cause its release into the air.

In occupational medicine one is also concerned with the difference between exposure and dose. Exposure is determined by surveillance of the environment with the knowledge that a toxic agent(s) has had the potential of being delivered into the body. For example, environmental measurements of lead can provide an index of exposure. Dose, however, can be assessed only by biologic monitoring of blood, urine, and hair, and indices of enzyme systems that may be affected. In the case of lead, the total dose delivered is dependent on the amount that is respirable and the amount absorbed from the gastrointestinal tract.

This chapter outlines some of the basic concepts and a few selected disorders encompassed in occupational medicine. Other chapters in this section describe at length occupational diseases of the lung (Ch. 559) and of the skin (Ch. 561) and a variety of chemical and physical sources of injury. Some chapters in other parts of the book contain useful information related to the discipline: toxic nephropathies (Ch. 81.3), epidemiology of cancer (Ch. 170), painful back and painful shoulders (Ch. 458 and 459), and neuropathies associated with the workplace (Ch. 565).

THE OCCUPATIONAL-ENVIRONMENTAL HISTORY

"When you come to a patient's house, you should ask him what sort of pains he has, what caused them, how many days he has been ill, whether the bowels are working and what sort of food he eats." So said Hippocrates in his work, *Affections*. I may venture to add one more question: "What occupation does he follow?" (*Diseases of Workers*, Preface, Bernardino Romazzini [1633–1714]).

Table 558–1 lists key elements of an occupational and environmental history that may be added to the data base collected on all patients. In every problem-oriented assessment of a current illness, individual problem lists should include such questions concerning the occupational health history as, Are symptoms associated with work, or do they improve during vacations and weekends? Are other workers similarly affected? Is there or has there been direct exposure to dust, fumes, and chemicals? Have there been work-related injuries? Is periodic testing and medical surveillance or routine industrial hygiene sampling of the workplace performed? A careful work history should include a chronologic list of all previous jobs with a reasonably detailed description of the work site, the scope of a typical work day, and such pertinent factors as protective equipment, ventilation, and pre-employment examinations.

A specific listing of the total number of days missed on each job and the reasons for the absences may be useful. Has a worker compensation claim been filed in the past? Does the worker perform additional jobs, i.e., is he or she moonlighting? A patient may not relate work to health, and so the physician should obtain initially, on each examination, specific answers to common occupational problems, for example, Have you ever been exposed to loud noises, excessive vibration, or heat? Do you work with asbestos? Have you been exposed to radioactive chemicals? Have you had previous chemical exposure? During the military, what were your duties?

TABLE 558–1. KEY ELEMENTS OF AN OCCUPATIONAL AND ENVIRONMENTAL HISTORY

Present illness (for each element of problem list)
Symptoms related to work
Other employees similarly affected
Current exposure to dusts, fumes, chemicals, biologic hazards
Prior first report of work injury
Work history
Description of all prior jobs; typical work day; change in work process
Work site
Ventilation; medical and industrial hygiene surveillance; employment examinations; protective measures
Union health and safety; moonlighting; days missed work last year, why; prior worker compensation claims
Past history
Exposure to noise, vibration, radiation, chemicals, asbestos
Environmental history
Present and prior home and work locations
Jobs of "significant others"
Hazardous wastes/spills exposure
Air pollution
Hobbies: painting, sculpture, welding, woodworking
Home insulation-heating
Home and work cleaning agents
Pesticide exposure
Do you wear seat belts?
Do you have firearms at home or work?
Review of systems
Specific emphasis
Shift changes; boredom; reproductive history

The environmental health history should include information about industries located in the neighborhood, exposure to hazardous waste or toxic spills, jobs of the spouse, degree of air pollution, and types of hobbies and recreational activities that also may contribute to health-related problems, such as painting, sculpturing, welding, or woodworking.

In addition, it may be important to elicit a description of home insulation or heating as well as exposure to cleaning agents and insecticides. Special questions should be directed toward unique workplace problems such as working hours and job schedule (Do these affect your sleep pattern? Are you bored on the job?). The reproductive history is essential: the number of miscarriages, children, stillbirths, previous pregnancies; difficulty in conceiving; and changes in libido and menses.

Signs and Symptoms of Occupational and Environmental Disorders

Because occupational and environmental diseases have a long latency and may be synergistic with other causes for disease, the clinician should always consider that the signs and symptoms may be caused by occupational or environmental conditions. Sometimes it may be useful to identify all the signs and symptoms that could be associated with disease of the environment or the workplace. A useful handbook by Daugaard provides such a guide to signs and symptoms of both acute and chronic occupational diseases compiled from standard works on toxicology and occupational medicine. For instance, knowledge of exposure to certain substances may implicate or suggest the cause: chlorinated hydrocarbons and acne, arsenic and thallium and alopecia; solvent exposure and anosmia; chlorinated hydrocarbons and arrhythmias; and aniline dyes and bladder or other cancers.

Reproductive hazards, noise–induced hearing abnormalities, and work-shift changes will be discussed as important occupational entities not covered specifically by other chapters in this section.

REPRODUCTIVE HAZARDS

Seven per cent of all newborns in the United States have birth defects, approximately 70 per cent of which are of unknown cause. The relationship between exposure to environmental and occupational agents and consequent development of male and female reproductive abnormalities is an area of intense study and interest. Animal studies have demonstrated the transmission to subsequent generations of chemically induced abnormalities of sperm and at a rate determined by mendelian principles. These observations have sparked interest in predicting and thereby preventing reproductive hazards from environmental agents. Short-term bioassays for mutagenesis, such as the Ames test, have been used to screen for teratogenic agents to predict reproductive outcome. These relatively inexpensive and rapid initial screening tests of chemicals can be performed in animals or bacteria. Agents encountered in the environment or the workplace can clearly cause reproductive hazards, i.e., testicular toxicity of dibromochloropropane (DBCP) recognized in California chemical workers in 1977. Male workers with sterility suffered no systemic illness and were working in an environment that was alleged to be safe. Previous laboratory tests in animals had suggested reproductive hazards from this chemical. The controversy surrounding this event sparked great interest in this subject. To date, the following environmental and occupational agents have been shown to cause adverse reproductive effects in men: anesthetic gases, carbon disulfide, diethylstilbestrol, toluene diamine, ethylene dibromide, chlordecone, and ionizing radiation. A much stronger data base is required to assess environmental effects on pregnancy outcome, spontaneous abortion, and stillbirth.

NOISE-INDUCED HEARING LOSS

More than five million people in the United States have noise-induced hearing loss. This most common form of hearing loss is associated with damage to, and loss of, hair cells in the organ of Corti. Early or moderately advanced, noise-induced hearing loss is associated with normal hearing in the low frequencies but gradually increasing loss of hearing at higher frequencies (with a maximum of 3,4, or 6 kHz). There may be some return toward normal function at 8 kHz. The audiometric shape of this curve is not pathognomonic because other otologic disorders, e.g., that caused by aminoglycoside antibiotic therapy, can result in an identical audiogram. Some of the hearing loss attributed to aging (presbycusis) may be due to the nearly ubiquitous noise pollution in modern society. Epidemiologic studies suggest that aging individuals in a nonindustrialized society have much better hearing preservation than older Americans. Major individual differences in susceptibility to noise-induced hearing loss occur. Men are much more susceptible to noise-induced hearing loss than women. Smoking and lack of skin pigmentation may also be risk factors for noise-induced hearing loss. Hearing impairment from occupational and environmental factors is a major and entirely preventable public health problem.

WORK SHIFT CHANGES

Twenty per cent of American workers work evenings or nights. In some industries, such as automobile production, petrol chemicals, and textile manufacturing, shift workers number nearly 50 per cent. There is growing evidence to suggest clinically significant health effects from shift work. Twenty per cent of workers are unable to tolerate shift work, tolerance for which also diminishes with increasing age. Daily physiologic variations known as circadian rhythms are distorted by shift work, which in turn alters the quality of sleep and causes important disturbances of the gastrointestinal tract and other organs. Diabetes mellitus and epilepsy may be aggravated by shift work, and the risk of accidents may be increased. Shift workers tend to have an increased number of subjective health complaints in general and may have enhanced risk factors complicating management of other medical disorders.

CONCLUSIONS

Strictly speaking, all diseases that are not genetic in origin are "environmental." Even genetic disorders are not totally endogenous, since they most frequently alter the ability of the host to accommodate to the environment. Broadly conceived, even the infectious diseases and nutritional disorders are environmental in origin. In practice, however, the term *environmental medicine* is used in a much more restrictive sense to reflect the chemical and physical hazards to which an individual is exposed and the injuries that may result from that exposure. Occupational medicine is that subset of environmental medicine directly concerned with the hazards of the workplace. The following chapters will describe in greater detail some of the specific hazards and injuries incident to modern occupations. The topics selected cannot be inclusive, since the boundaries of occupational and environmental medicine are indistinct, merging into the traditional domains of internal medicine, epidemiology, toxicology, surgery, orthopaedics, and many other clinical and basic science disciplines.

Daugaard J: Symptoms and Signs in Occupational Disease: A Practical Guide. Copenhagen, Munksgaard, 1978. *A thorough catalog of symptoms and signs of occupationally related conditions.*

Lauwerys RR: Industrial chemical exposure: Guidelines for biological monitoring. Davis, Calif., Biomedical Publications. *A paperback book with a practical guide to methods of assessment of exposure to toxic chemicals.*

Levy BS, Wegman TH: Occupational Health: Recognizing and Preventing Work-Related Disease. Boston, Little, Brown and Company, 1983. *A useful and easy-to-read paperback text by multiple authors encompassing a broad curriculum of occupational medicine; limited bibliography.*

Rom WN: Environmental and Occupational Medicine. Boston, Little Brown and Company, 1983. *A hard-bound, detailed text, well referenced, with strong emphasis on occupational lung disorders.*

559. OCCUPATIONAL LUNG DISEASE

Robert J. Mason

The air we exhale is cleaner than the air we inhale. The 15,000 liters of air we inhale per day to meet our metabolic needs contains a heterogeneous aerosol of dusts, vapors, and microorganisms. The net result is that people living in an urban environment inhale about 2 mg of dust each day. Of course, cigarette smokers and people who work in certain dusty environments inhale more. Elaborate protective mechanisms for filtering air and clearing deposited particles have evolved to protect the delicate alveolar-capillary membrane; in certain occupational settings, however, the defenses are inadequate and occupational pulmonary disease develops. The major factors that determine if disease will occur are the biologic properties of the inhaled material, the dose of the inhaled material (concentration and duration of exposure), and the defenses of the individual (genetic, physical, immunologic, concurrent illness).

Because of the diversity of industrial dusts and vapors, there can be a variety of clinical presentation for occupational pulmonary diseases (Table 559–1). The clinical presentation of almost all nonoccupational pulmonary diseases can be mimicked by an occupational disease. The key to diagnosis of occupational pulmonary disease is suspicion by the examining physician and an appropriate occupational history. The major problem is that the relation of the occupation to the illness may not be obvious: (1) There may be a long delay between initial exposure and impairment of pulmonary function or development of a carcinoma. (2) Symptoms may not occur at work. In some forms of occupational asthma, for example, the main symptoms occur after work, especially at night. (3) Exposure alone does not itself necessarily prove the etiology of the disease. Workers who have been exposed to an occupational hazard may have a nonoccupationally related disease.

TABLE 559–1. DIVERSITY OF OCCUPATIONAL PULMONARY DISEASES

Interstitial parenchymal disease
Asbestosis, coal workers' pneumoconiosis, silicosis, berylliosis, hypersensitivity pneumonitis
Pulmonary edema
Smoke inhalation, acute toxic fumes (NO_2, chlorine)
Pleural disease
Asbestos-related plaques and effusions, mesothelioma
Bronchitis
Grain dust, heavy dust exposures (coal workers)
Asthma
Toluene diisocyanate, platinum salts, formalin, flour, cotton dust, western red cedar
Bronchogenic carcinoma
Uranium, asbestos, chromates, nickel, chloromethyl ether
Infectious disease
Anthrax (wood sorters, imported hides)
Coccidioidomycosis (construction workers, archeologists)
Mycobacterial disease (silicosis)
Psittacosis (pet shop owners, taxidermists)
Echinococcus (sheep and dog handlers)
Q fever (tanners and sheep handlers)

It is important to differentiate occupational pulmonary diseases from other pulmonary diseases in order to provide specific treatment and to assist in obtaining financial compensation for the patient when warranted. Removal of the patient from the hazardous environment may be the only treatment that reduces symptoms or prevents deterioration. When an occupational pulmonary disease is diagnosed, fellow workers need to be notified and their status evaluated, and preventive measures need to be applied as appropriate. An index case of an occupationally related disease should be thought of conceptually as a case of tuberculosis so that appropriate public health measures are instituted and the conditions of the patient's working colleagues are evaluated.

Our major efforts should be directed toward preventing occupational diseases, but the means of prevention and the establishment of safe levels of exposure are difficult and complex. This is because individuals vary in their susceptibility to adverse effects, because it may take many years to assess the effect of a given exposure, and because establishment of levels of exposure has major economic consequences. Epidemiologic surveys can provide data for establishing exposure levels that should pose minimal risk for the general population. It is, however, the sensitive individual who is most adversely affected. How can these sensitive individuals be identified, how should they be advised, and should the standards be set low enough to avoid any risk even to sensitive individuals? Only a few traits of sensitive individuals are known, for example, bronchial hyper-reactivity for some types of occupational asthma, and cigarette smoking for most forms of occupationally related bronchogenic cancer. Ways of identifying sensitive individuals for different occupational hazards are needed so that the relative risks are known, the patients advised, and appropriate standards set.

Dosman JA, Cotton DJ: Occupational Pulmonary Disease; Focus on Grain Dust and Health. New York, Academic Press, 1980. *The proceedings of an international symposium on grain dust and health. Excellent introductory chapters on general occupational pulmonary disease by the leaders in this field. The discussion of grainhandlers' respiratory diseases forms the bulk of the text, but the problems are pertinent to all other forms of occupational pulmonary disease.*

Hunter D: The Diseases of Occupations. London, Hodder and Stroughton, 1978. *A wonderful historic perspective and a wealth of clinical information presented in a delightful style.*

Parkes WR: Occupational Lung Disorders. London, Butterworths, 1982. *An excellent, comprehensive, well-referenced text.*

Weil H, Ziskind MM: Occupational pulmonary diseases. *In* Fishman AP (ed.): Pulmonary Diseases and Disorders. New York, McGraw-Hill Book Company, 1980, pp 754–792. *Well written and well referenced, the next stop for additional reading on almost any aspect of occupational pulmonary disease.*

DEPOSITION AND CLEARANCE OF INHALED MATERIALS

DEPOSITION. The site of deposition is the most likely area for initial injury and production of symptoms. In general, this depends upon the aerodynamic size of the inhaled particles, the anatomy of the respiratory system, and the breathing pattern of the individual.

The first barrier for inhaled materials during quiet breathing is the nose, which removes essentially all particles larger than 10 μ. However, during exercise, because of the increased volume of ventilation and mouth breathing, up to 20 per cent of particles 10 to 20 μ in diameter pass the nose, mouth, and pharynx and are deposited in the large airways. This is an important consideration for workers in strenuous occupations in dusty environments or for exercising atopic children during pollen season. The second site of deposition is the ciliated epithelium of large and small airways. The number of particles deposited increases at high flow rates, during rapid shallow breathing, or in areas of disease, e.g., bronchiectasis. As the inhaled air passes into smaller and smaller bronchioles the rate of flow decreases and particles sediment. The third site of deposition is the alveolar surface, where deposition is by diffusion, aided by the relatively long residence time of the suspended particles and short distance to the alveolar wall. Slow, deep breathing favors alveolar deposition. The *respirable fraction* consists of particles (from 0.5 to 5 μ) that are most likely to be deposited in alveoli or very small airways and produce parenchymal lung disease. Particles larger than 10 μ are usually removed by the upper airway, and therefore they are considered more innocuous and less pathogenic. How then do asbestos fibers, which may be 25 μ long, penetrate so deeply into the lung? The explanation is that their site of deposition is based on aerodynamic diameter and not length.

CLEARANCE. Pulmonary clearance can be divided into three phases, depending on where the particles are deposited. (1) Particles that lie on the mucous blanket over the ciliary epithelium are normally cleared rapidly, within an hour. The cilia propel the mucus toward the pharynx, and the particles are swallowed or expectorated. This process could be severely impaired by viral infections that damage ciliated cells, extensive squamous metaplasia, genetic defects in ciliary function (ciliary dyskinesis syndromes), or alterations in the physical properties of mucus. (2) Particles deposited in the alveolar region distal to the ciliated airways are ingested by macrophages and then over a period of hours to days the particle-laden macrophages move to the small airways and are transported up the ciliary escalator. (3) Free particles that traverse the respiratory epithelium are ingested by interstitial macrophages and cleared by unknown pathways over months to years. Some ingested particles stay in the interstitium in the lung parenchyma, some are transported to regional lymph nodes, and others eventually make their way back to the airways and are cleared by the ciliated epithelium. The rate of clearance from the interstitium is thought to be dependent on the solubility of the ingested material. The rate of clearance is much slower in smokers than in nonsmokers. The ultimate fate of and tissue reaction to different dusts are determined mainly by the interaction of the dusts and the macrophages, but the precise cellular mechanisms and host factors that facilitate clearance or stimulate fibrosis are unknown.

Brain JD, Valberg PA: Deposition of aerosol in the respiratory tract. Am Rev Respir Dis 120:1325, 1979.

DIAGNOSIS AND ASSESSMENT OF HAZARDS

HISTORY. A detailed occupational history is the key to the diagnosis of an occupationally related illness (Table 558–1). People change jobs frequently. Furthermore, there may be a long interval between exposure and disease, especially for development of lung cancer. Therefore, all part-time and full-time jobs and hobbies must be recorded, preferably by recording the first job and then listing all subsequent jobs chronologically. Attention must be given to precisely what kind of job the worker did, which hazardous agents were present, whether they were in high or low concentration, whether or not protective clothing or masks were used, whether the workplace was monitored for exposure levels, and whether or not other workers developed similar illnesses. A useful clue for occupational asthma or bronchitis is the abatement of symptoms during vacations away from the job. Some work-related diseases may not be obvious. A nine-month exposure to asbestos in a shipyard during World War II may account for the mesothelioma or bronchogenic carcinoma arising 30 years later. Hobbies can also be important, e.g, pigeon breeding can lead to hypersensitivity pneumonitis, archeology to coccidioidomycosis, furniture and bathtub refinishing to occupational asthma. Exposure may also be indirect. Asbestos-related illness has been reported in family members exposed to work clothes of an asbestos worker and in households near asbestos-manufacturing plants. Similarly, sensitive individuals may be affected by very low concentrations of toluene diisocyanate originating from a neighborhood plant.

ROENTGENOGRAPHIC TECHNIQUES. Chest roentgenographs are especially useful for evaluating parenchymal and pleural disease. The standard description of abnormalities is based on the ILO U/C classification. Its purpose is to convey assessment of roentgenographs in a standard way for epidemiologic studies and not to make an etiologic assessment in terms of type of dust, fibrosis, or infection. Parenchymal opacities are assessed for size, shape, profusion, and extent. Newer radiographic techniques such as computed axial tomography are useful in individual cases for defining specific abnormalities such as pleural disease after asbestos exposure.

PULMONARY FUNCTION TESTING. Pulmonary function tests are useful for detailed assessment of an individual patient and for epidemiologic investigations of population groups. The detailed pulmonary function studies of an individual patient are, in general, the same for occupational or nonoccupational disease. The only major exception is for patients with suspected occupational asthma. In this case, specific bronchial provocation tests can be done under careful supervision in a defined laboratory environment to evaluate sensitivity to particular substances (see below). Individual patients can also be assessed for bronchoconstriction before, during, and after work. This type of testing has been useful for evaluating byssinosis. Because symptoms may occur only at work during strenuous exertion, evaluation should be carried out not only when the patient is at rest but also during exercise.

Simple measurement of FEV (forced expiratory volume in one second) has proven to be reproducible, sufficiently sensitive to detect clinical disease, and predictive for identifying patients who are likely to get progressive disease. Tests of small airways disease and maldistribution, i.e., flow at low lung volumes, comparison of flow volume curves during exhalation of helium-oxygen mixtures and air, and the single-breath nitrogen test, are more sensitive, but additional studies will be required to document their utility. Pre-employment and serial pulmonary function studies will help identify workers with pre-existing disease and those who develop abnormalities that antedate symptoms. In general, individuals who show evidence of disease the earliest are the ones likely to develop progressive disease and should be advised about their disease and alternative employment.

PATHOLOGY. Most occupational diseases can be diagnosed without biopsy. If biopsy is necessary, an open lung biopsy is preferred so that the types of dust retained in the lung can be identified by chemical analysis or by newer techniques of energy-dispersive x-ray analysis and x-ray diffraction.

ASSESSMENT OF HAZARDS. The description of the job usually identifies the offending substance, but direct measurements of the air the worker breathes will help quantitate the hazard and ensure that control measures are effective. Particulates are usually collected by filtration and weighed; vapors can be measured continuously. Federal and private organizations have established threshold limit values for different substances based on a time-weighted average concentration for an 8-hour working day, 40-hour working week, and a 40-year working span. Threshold limit values do not address the problems of high peak levels of short duration or the sensitive individual.

DISEASES PRODUCED BY INORGANIC MATERIALS

Coal Worker's Pneumoconiosis

DEFINITION. Coal worker's pneumoconiosis (CWP) is the parenchymal lung disease produced by the deposition of coal dust and the host response to the retained dust. Classification is based on roentgenographic appearance. Simple CWP is based on the profusion of small, round opacities up to 1 cm in diameter; complicated CWP is defined by the presence of one or more opacities greater than 1 cm in diameter. In addition to parenchymal disease, inhalation of coal dust also causes industrial bronchitis (see below).

OCCUPATIONAL EXPOSURE. Although first reported in the nineteenth century, lung disease associated with coal mining did not become a major occupational pulmonary disease until the 1930's, when machinery for underground mining was developed. The development of simple CWP is related to the dust exposure and the amount of coal dust retained in the lungs. The highest dust concentrations occur at the coal face, where the coal is cut and detached, and dust levels fall progressively as the coal is transported to the surface. Workers who cut into rock strata or work on the shuttle car system, which uses sand on the rails to improve traction, are exposed to silica as well as coal dust. The current dust standard is 2 mg per cubic meter. A recent study of United States miners reported a prevalence of 10 per cent simple CWP and 0.4 per cent complicated CWP. These studies are difficult to interpret because some of the severely affected miners have left the trade and because the prevalence data relate to exposure levels 20 to 30 years ago, which were much higher than the current standard. The economics of energy production and the large supply of unmined coal ensure that CWP will remain a clinical problem for many years.

In the 1977 Black Lung Benefits Reform Act, total disability is defined as inability to do regular work in or around the mine or coal preparation facility due to breathing impairment caused by pneumoconiosis. Total disability may be determined on the basis of roentgenographic evidence, pulmonary function impairment, or both. As a result, coal workers may be compensated for chronic airway obstruction due to cigarette smoking at a much higher rate than are workers in other industries with chronic airway obstruction.

PATHOLOGY AND PATHOGENESIS. ***Simple Coal Worker's Pneumoconiosis.*** The distinctive lesion of simple coal worker's pneumoconiosis is the *coal macule*, discrete, small, black nodules that are typically more profuse in the upper lobes. These lesions consist of dust-laden macrophages, fibroblasts, extracellular dust, and cell debris and a loose collection of reticulin fibers. These macules are sometimes associated with focal centrilobular emphysema (localized dilatation of the respiratory bronchioles) but are not thought to produce clinically significant respiratory impairment.

Complicated Coal Worker's Pneumoconiosis. Rarely the macules enlarge and coalesce to produce large, rubbery aggregates of black tissue greater than 1 cm in diameter, typically in a posterior segment of an upper lobe or the superior segment of a lower lobe. Progressive massive fibrosis, arbitrarily defined as a lesion with a diameter exceeding 3 cm, may result from one or more of four factors: (1) the presence of silica in addition to the coal dust, (2) a very high concentration of coal dust, (3) typical or atypical mycobacterial infections, and (4) poorly defined immunologic host factors. Some patients have antinuclear antibodies, high levels of rheumatoid factor, and antibodies to lung connective tissue components.

CLINICAL MANIFESTATIONS. *Simple CWP* produces no signs or symptoms. Diagnosis is made roentgenographically. Lesions progress very slowly; side-by-side comparisons are usually useful only if the chest films were obtained at least five years apart. Pulmonary function abnormalities are minimal. It takes about 30 years of underground mining to produce even a small decrease in FEV_1. The single-breath diffusing capacity is normal. The major determinant for pulmonary function abnormalities in coal miners is the presence or absence of cigarette smoking.

Complicated CWP may produce dyspnea on exertion and may progress to severe respiratory insufficiency due to obstructive and restrictive lung disease, cor pulmonale, pulmonary hypertension, and right ventricular failure. Rare patients have melanoptysis, which is the sudden coughing up of a small amount of jet black fluid. *Caplan's syndrome* is the association of large, peripheral, round lung opacities in coal miners with rheumatoid arthritis. The nodules may increase in size rapidly, e.g., within a few weeks, may cavitate, and are usually associated with active joint disease, high titers of rheumatoid factor, and the presence of subcutaneous nodules. However, the pulmonary nodules may appear before the clinical manifestation of rheumatoid arthritis. The nodules, which may appear up to ten years before joint disease, resemble nodules of rheumatoid lung disease; both have a center of necrotic tissue and a surrounding cellular zone of epithelial cells, lymphocytes, plasma cells, and other inflammatory cells. Vasculitis is commonly associated. Compared to progressive massive fibrosis, the nodules contain relatively little dust. Syndromes similar to that described by Caplan for coal workers have been described in patients with silicosis and asbestosis. The pathogenesis of Caplan's syndrome is thought to be an interaction, as yet undefined, of rheumatoid lung disease with the inhaled dust and its cellular response.

Coal dust can also produce chronic bronchitis that is manifested by cough and sputum production but minimal changes in pulmonary function. The bronchitic symptoms vary directly in relation to dust exposure, but there is poor correlation to radiographic category of parenchymal lung disease (CWP). The bronchitis ceases after the worker leaves the dusty environment. Cigarette smoking is thought to be at least five times more important than coal dust in producing airway obstruction.

DIAGNOSIS AND DIFFERENTIAL DIAGNOSIS. The diagnosis of CWP is based on the history of exposure and radiographic abnormalities. Simple CWP does not produce breathlessness, and, therefore, symptomatic patients with simple CWP should be studied for nonoccupational pulmonary disease. Patients with progressive massive fibrosis and associated mycobacterial infection may have minimal fever, weight loss, or other constitutional symptoms. Diagnosis of mycobacterial infection is made by sputum examination, culture, and occasionally biopsy. Patients respond to standard treatment regimens. The incidence of lung cancer is not increased in patients with simple or complicated CWP. Progressive massive fibrosis may be difficult to distinguish from bronchogenic carcinoma, especially if serial chest films are not available. Features that favor progressive massive fibrosis are the variable radiodensity of the lesion, irregular opacities at the periphery, calcification within the lesion, and a recent history of expectoration of jet black fluid if cavitation is present.

TREATMENT, PROGNOSIS, AND PREVENTION. The presence of simple CWP is not a sufficient reason for someone who has worked in the mines for many years to discontinue mining. However, a documented increase in the size of the opacities or presence of complicated CWP should exclude the worker from all dusty trades. When the exposure ceases, simple CWP will remain stable or decrease, but complicated CWP may progress. Prevention of CWP can be achieved only by dust control.

Morgan WKC, Lapp NL: Respiratory disease in coal miners. Am Rev Respir Dis 113:531, 1976. *A detailed, comprehensive review.*

Morgan WKC, Lapp NL, Seaton D: Respiratory disability in coal miners. JAMA 243:2401, 1980. *Pulmonary impairment and black lung legislation.*

Silicosis

DEFINITION. Silicosis is the parenchymal lung disease produced by inhalation of respirable particles of crystalline silica, SiO_2, and the tissue reaction to the retained dust. Quartz is the most common form of crystalline silica in nature; cristobalite and tridymite are other forms of crystalline silica, which occur rarely in nature but are produced by heating quartz in smelting and steel making or by heating diatomite, an amorphous form of silica. Silicates such as asbestos, kaolin, and talc are less fibrogenic and produce different pneumoconioses.

OCCUPATIONAL EXPOSURE. Silicosis occurs in workers in numerous occupations, including mining, quarrying, tunneling, stone cutting, sandblasting, and foundry work. The most tragic exposure in the United States was during the excavation of a tunnel at Gauley Bridge, West Virginia, in the 1930's, when 476 workers died of silicosis, and another 1500 contracted the disease. Since that time dust control and substitution of other abrasives for sand have decreased the incidence of fulminant disease.

PATHOLOGY AND PATHOGENESIS. The rate of development of clinical disease is dependent on the amount of inhaled silica. Three forms of silicosis can be distinguished: (1) chronic silicosis, in which exposure extends for more than 15 years before symptoms and radiographic changes occur; (2) accelerated silicosis, in which changes occur in 5 to 15 years; and (3) acute silicosis, in which changes occur within 5 years.

Chronic silicosis is characterized by small, silica-containing, upper lobe nodules composed of concentric swirls of hyalinized collagen, which is surrounded by a cellular capsule composed of macrophages, plasma cells, and fibroblasts. Hilar lymph nodes may contain similar nodules. Massive conglomerate lesions form by coalescence of the smaller nodules and may obliterate or distort some of the conducting airways and vasculature. The lesions seldom cavitate in the absence of tuberculosis.

Accelerated silicosis, which is seen in sandblasters, is similar to chronic silicosis but progresses more rapidly, commonly to massive fibrosis. Typical and atypical mycobacterial infections are frequent. In *acute silicosis*, which is rare, there is an eosinophilic coagulum in the alveolar spaces that stains with the periodic acid–Schiff stain and appears similar to alveolar proteinosis.

The good correlation between the fibrogenic potential of different types of silica in vivo and the cytotoxic effects of these dusts on macrophages in vitro suggests the following mechanism. Free silica is ingested by the macrophage but tends to disrupt its phagolysosome and is released extracellularly. More macrophages are recruited to the area of inflammation, and the cycle is slowly repeated. Collagen is formed and then becomes hyalinized. Macrophages produce factors that stimulate fibroblast proliferation and collagen formation. The precise role of these macrophage factors in the pathogenesis of silicosis is still unknown.

CLINICAL MANIFESTATIONS. Simple and complicated silicosis are defined radiographically as described for coal worker's pneumoconiosis. Simple silicosis generally produces no signs or symptoms; when people with simple silicosis cough and produce sputum, these symptoms can usually be attributed to cigarette smoking or inhalation of other dust. In complicated silicosis, dyspnea on exertion, recurrent infections, weight loss, and general weakness are frequent. The physical findings correlate with the severity of the complicated silicosis.

Radiographic studies in simple silicosis show nodules predominantly in the upper lung fields, which may become calcified. In complicated silicosis, large masses develop that may appear as an "angel's wing" pattern. As the fibrosis proceeds and lesions contract, adjacent areas of lung become overexpanded and appear radiolucent. Pleural reactions over the dense conglomerate lesions are frequent. The hilar lymph nodes are commonly enlarged and may develop the typical egg shell calcification of silicosis (Fig. 559–1).

Pulmonary function is normal in simple silicosis. As the disease progresses, restrictive, obstructive, and mixed types of abnormalities occur. The vital capacity, single-breath diffusion capacity, and compliance are reduced. Hypoxia occurs initially during exercise and later at rest. Because of the wide spectrum of clinical and radiographic disease, there is also a wide spectrum of pulmonary function abnormalities.

DIAGNOSIS AND DIFFERENTIAL DIAGNOSIS. The diagnosis of silicosis is based on a history of inhalation of respirable free silica and radiographic abnormalities. The major clinical problems are infectious complications and the possibility of concurrent collagen vascular disease. There is no increase in cancer of the lung. Historically the most important infectious complication was tuberculosis. Recently half of the mycobacterial infections have been reported to be caused by atypical organisms, either *Mycobacterium kansasii* or *M. avium intracellulare*, depending on the geographic area. Fungal, nocardial, and pyogenic bacterial infections also occur frequently. In the accelerated silicosis of sandblasters, more than 40 per cent of the individuals have antinuclear antibodies, and about 10 per cent have clinical manifestations of collagen vascular diseases such as rheumatoid arthritis, scleroderma, and systemic lupus erythematosus. It is uncertain if patients with accelerated disease should be treated with anti-inflammatory or immunosuppressive drugs with the hope of preventing progression of their lung disease. The link between the inflammatory and heightened immune response and subsequent fibrosis is unknown, but is potentially a site for treatment.

Coalescence of nodules and enlarging opacities may indicate spontaneous progression of silicosis, a complicating infectious process, or coexisting carcinoma. Because of expanding lesions, a history of mixed dust exposure, or the suspicion of infectious disease, carcinoma, or sarcoidosis, an open lung biopsy may be required. Silica can be seen as doubly refractile particles with polarized light. In mixed dust exposure, energy dispersive x-ray analysis can identify silicon and elements associated with silicates (calcium, magnesium, and iron).

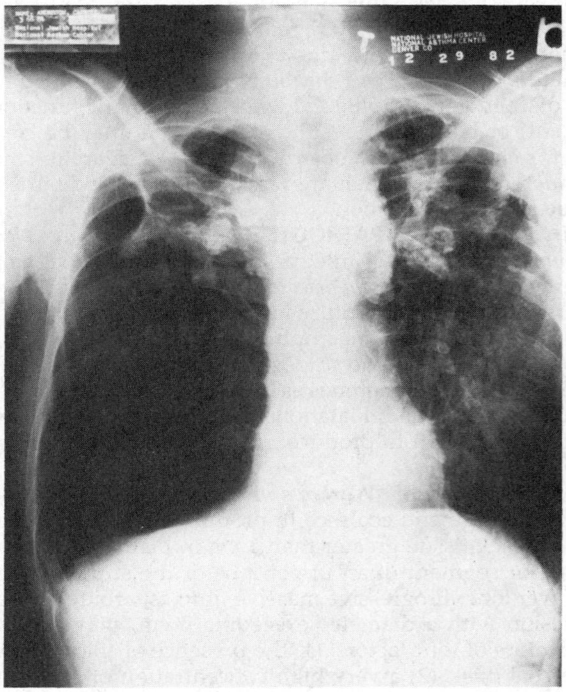

Figure 559–1. Patient with silicosis, classic egg shell lymph node calcification, and multiple cavities in the right upper lobe due to *Mycobacterium avium intracellulare* infection. Note the upper lung zone fibrosis, retraction, and secondary overdistention of the lower lobes.

Treatment, Prognosis, and Prevention. There is no proven treatment for silicosis. As in other forms of pneumoconiosis, the earlier the symptoms or radiographic abnormalities appear, the worse the prognosis. If symptoms occur within ten years of exposure, progression is likely, and the prognosis is grim. Pre-employment examination should include a tuberculin skin test and chest film. Patients with silicosis and a positive tuberculin reaction should be treated for at least a year with isoniazid. Patients with active tuberculosis should be treated with standard drugs. In areas where *M. kansasii* is common the initial regimen should include three drugs (Ch. 298). Short-course therapy should be avoided, and treatment regimens should be longer than those for patients without silicosis. Prevention of silicosis is by avoiding dust exposure and by substitution when possible. For example, "sandblasting" is now commonly performed with metal grit and coal ash instead of sand.

Dauber JH: Silicosis. *In* Fishman AP (ed.): Update: Pulmonary Diseases and Disorders. New York, McGraw-Hill Book Company, 1982, pp. 149–166. *Excellent summary of pathogenesis.*
Ziskind M, Jones RN, Weill H: Silicosis. Am Rev Respir Dis 113:643, 1976.

Asbestos-Related Diseases

DEFINITIONS. Inhalation of asbestos fibers can produce fibrosis and tumors. The most common disease is interstitial pulmonary fibrosis, which is termed asbestosis. Asbestos fibers may also produce benign pleural effusions and fibrosis, pleural plaques, mesotheliomas of pleura and peritoneum, lung cancer, and cancers of the gastrointestinal tract. The types of disease, especially pleural disease, depend on the type of fiber. Asbestos fibers, a group of naturally occurring fibrous silicates of different chemical composition, are classified as serpentine (chrysotile) or amphibole (crocidolite, amosite, and anthophyllite). Chrysotile is a magnesium silicate, forms soft, flexible, curly fibers, accounts for over 90 per cent of the world's asbestos production, and rarely produces mesotheliomas. The amphiboles form straight, brittle fibers, have a greater potential for penetrating deep into the lung, and are more likely to produce pleural disease. Some amphiboles (e.g., crocidolite) are strongly implicated in the induction of mesotheliomas; others (e.g., anthophyllite) are associated with a high frequency of pleural plaques but not mesotheliomas. In general, increased fiber length (over 10 μ) is associated with increased fibrogenicity and oncogenicity. Since different types of asbestos tend to produce different asbestos-related diseases, the exposure to different types of fibers should be defined and recorded as completely as possible.

OCCUPATIONAL EXPOSURE. The major occupational exposures to asbestos occur in mining, milling, work in shipyards, insulation work, demolition of old buildings, construction, and production of asbestos cement. Two worker groups that have had high exposure to respirable asbestos and a high prevalence of disease are insulation and shipyard workers. During World War II, more than two million people were employed in U.S. shipyards, and, because of the long interval (20 to 40 years) between exposure and the development of disease, many of these individuals have only recently come to medical attention. Not only is there a long latent period, but the exposure may be brief or indirect. Workers exposed to amosite for only 6 to 12 months have an increased incidence of lung cancer. People who live near manufacturing plants or who handled clothing of asbestos workers have been reported to get asbestosis and mesotheliomas.

The incidence of asbestos-related diseases should decrease as dust control measures and work practices improve. The current threshold limit value is 2 fibers per cubic centimeter as a time-weighted average for eight hours. Much of our data on the incidence of disease are from insulation and shipyard workers who were employed from 1930 to 1950 when it is estimated that the level of exposure may have been as high as 50 to 500 fibers per cubic centimeter. It is difficult, therefore, to predict exactly how much the current standards will reduce the incidence of disease. In the past when exposure levels were high, the dose was the major determinant in production of disease. With the low current levels of exposure, host factors may become more important than the actual dose in predicting who will develop disease.

PATHOLOGY AND PATHOGENESIS. Asbestos produces interstitial fibrosis and pneumonitis, predominantly in the lower lobes. Because of the large individual variation in response among workers, host factors for amplifying or suppressing the fibrotic response are likely to be very important. Similarly, host factors may regulate movement of fibers within the lung parenchyma and the rate of dissolution of inhaled fiber, which may be important in the pathogenesis of parenchymal and pleural disease.

Ferruginous bodies are the pathologic hallmark of asbestos exposure. These bodies, which are 2 to 5 μ wide and 20 to 150 μ long, usually contain an amphibole fiber as a core, surrounded by an exterior composed of protein and iron pigments. The core can also be a different silicate or even a vegetable fiber. The presence of ferruginous bodies indicates past exposure to asbestos, but it does not establish the etiology of disease. Up to 50 per cent of urban dwellers have ferruginous bodies in their lungs at autopsy. However, the number of fibers found correlates with the intensity of the past exposure and therefore the presence of disease. Fibers can be collected by bronchoalveolar lavage.

Pleural reactions occur in two independent types: (1) a diffuse exudative reaction that involves both pleural surfaces and may eventually obliterate the pleural space and (2) discrete pleural plaques on the parietal pleura. Benign pleural effusions are commonly the first manifestation of asbestos-related pulmonary disease and occur within ten years of initial exposure. The pathology of the exudative lesion is not distinctive and accounts for some "idiopathic" pleural effusions. The pleural plaques are discrete, raised white lesions that occur over the lower ribs and diaphragm and are not associated with pleural adhesions. These plaques are composed of relatively acellular collagenous connective tissue, which contains uncoated asbestos fibers, mostly amphiboles, and may calcify.

Malignant mesotheliomas of the pleura are bulky, slow-growing tumors that spread by local extension and enclose the lung and mediastinum and present clinically with the symptoms of chest wall pain and weight loss (see Ch. 68). They vary histologically and can be difficult to diagnose even with an open pleural biopsy, because some of these tumors appear like metastatic adenocarcinomas. There is a high incidence in insulation workers and a low incidence in Canadian miners of chrysotile asbestos. Miners of a thinner type of crocidolite in Northwest Cape, South Africa, have a higher incidence of mesothelioma than miners of a thicker type of crocidolite in the Transvaal. These epidemiologic features imply that thin, straight fibers with a small aerodynamic diameter are most likely to penetrate deep into the lung and produce mesotheliomas. Mesotheliomas are not associated with cigarette smoking.

CLINICAL MANIFESTATIONS. Asbestosis presents like other forms of pulmonary fibrosis. The first symptoms are dyspnea on exertion and a nonproductive cough. Symptoms usually develop several years after radiographic changes appear. On physical examination, patients have end-inspiratory, crisp crackles that are heard best over the lower lobes. In advanced disease, clubbing of the fingers may be present.

Radiologic studies in asbestosis reveal small linear opacities in the lower lung fields as the initial abnormalities. These may extend to the pleura and resemble Kerley B lines. As the disease progresses the lung volumes decrease, and there is distortion of the pulmonary architecture. Pleural plaques, fibrosis, or effusions may also be present. Pleural plaques can be best seen on oblique views, but care must be used to differentiate true plaques from companion shadows that are produced by muscle attachments in normal individuals. The extent of the pleural disease is best detemined with computed tomography (Fig. 559–2).

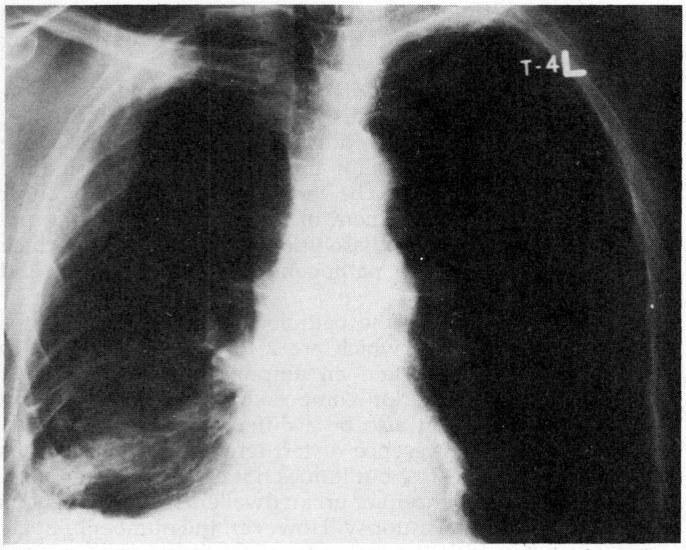

Figure 559–2. Patient with asbestosis and linear parenchymal marking, pleural calcifications, and an extensive right pleural reaction. There is also some pericardial calcification.

Pulmonary function tests classically show restrictive patterns typical of pulmonary fibrosis. The lung volumes, compliance, and single-breath diffusing capacity are all reduced. Because of the high prevalence of cigarette smoking in asbestos workers and the distortion of the airways in advanced disease, airway obstruction may also be present. Although asbestos can produce peribronchial inflammation and fibrosis, asbestos is not thought to produce clinically significant obstructive lung disease in the absence of obvious restriction and distortion of lung architecture.

DIAGNOSIS. The diagnosis of asbestosis requires a history of exposure and radiographic evidence of parenchymal lung disease, especially linear opacities in the lower lung fields. Patients usually also have dyspnea on exertion, end-inspiratory rales over the lower lobes, radiographic evidence of pleural disease, and pulmonary function impairment. If a biopsy is necessary to exclude other interstitial lung diseases or for other medical reasons, it should be an open lung biopsy, and the tissue should be examined for coated and uncoated fibers. Fibers can also be recovered and quantitated in bronchoalveolar lavage fluid.

Patients with asbestos exposure have an increased incidence of lung, laryngeal, and gastrointestinal cancer. Cigarette smoking together with asbestos exposure increases the risk of developing lung cancer about 60-fold over nonexposed, nonsmoking controls. In individuals not exposed to asbestos, smoking alone increases the risk about tenfold. The risk of lung cancer in nonsmoking asbestos workers is much smaller than in smokers, but it is greater than the risk in nonsmoking, nonexposed controls. The diagnosis of lung cancer is made by standard cytologic procedures and biopsy. The cell types of bronchogenic cancer due to asbestosis and cigarette smoking are not different from the cell types of other types of lung cancer. It remains to be shown how effective analysis of prospective serial roentgenograms and sputum cytology will be for detection and management of lung cancer in patients with asbestosis or a history of heavy exposure to asbestos.

TREATMENT, PROGNOSIS, AND PREVENTION. Asbestosis and its related diseases are for the most part not treatable. Most effort has to be made to prevent the diseases by reducing exposure and by encouraging workers to refrain from cigarette smoking. Those who work with asbestos should give up smoking; those who are young and cannot stop smoking should avoid trades that entail exposure to asbestos. It would be helpful to be able to identify those individuals who are likely to develop pulmonary fibrosis. Unfortunately the only available clue to those who will develop clinical asbestosis is the appearance of radiographic abnormalities during their working life. Workers who have an abnormal chest film when they leave their trade are the ones who are most likely to develop severe asbestosis.

Aisner J, Wiernik P (eds.): Asbestos related neoplasms. Semin Oncol 8:241, 1981. *Thorough discussion of pathogenesis, pathology, natural history, and options for therapy and palliation.*

Becklake M: Asbestos-related fibrosis of the lungs (asbestosis) and pleura. *In* Fishman AP (ed.): Update: Pulmonary Diseases and Disorders. New York, McGraw-Hill Book Company, 1982, pp 167–192. *A complete current review.*

Craighead JE, Mossman BT: The pathogenesis of asbestos associated diseases. N Engl J Med 306:1446, 1982.

Selikoff IJ, Hammond EC (eds.): Health hazards of asbestos exposure. Ann NY Acad Sci Vol. 330, 1979. *A wealth of information. The article by Hammond et al. on asbestos exposure, cigarette smoking, and death rates provides first data on possible carcinogenic effect of asbestos in nonsmokers (four cases).*

Disease Caused by Other Silicates

Nonasbestos silicates may also produce pneumoconioses. Talc, a hydrous magnesium silicate, may produce pulmonary fibrosis and pleural plaques. The pulmonary lesions tend to be more nodular than those seen in asbestosis. Talc is commonly extracted from rock that also contains silica and asbestos. Therefore, miners usually have exposure to mixed dusts. The particle size of talc used for cosmetics is large, 10 to 40 μ, and therefore personal use is unlikely to produce pneumoconiosis. Talc is found in pulmonary granulomas in intravenous drug abusers. Other silicates, i.e., kaolin, slate, and portland cement, rarely produce lung disease in the absence of free silica.

Disease Caused by Hard Metals and Other Inorganic Dusts

Dusts containing elements with high atomic numbers absorb roentgen rays and produce dramatic radiographic abnormalities. Most of these dusts are considered nonfibrogenic and produce minimal symptoms or pulmonary function abnormalities. Progressive disease strongly suggests mixed dust exposure that includes silica. The classic examples are *stannosis* (from tin oxide) and *baritosis* (from barium sulfate). Iron oxides accumulate in lungs of arc welders and hematite miners and, in the absence of inhalation of quartz or asbestos, produce abnormal chest films but minimal fibrosis or functional impairment.

Beryllium Disease

Beryllium disease differs from other occupational pulmonary diseases in that beryllium and its compounds become distributed throughout the body and produce a systemic illness. The acute fulminant form, caused by brief intense exposure, is characterized by bronchiolitis, pneumonia, and pulmonary edema. The mortality is as high as 10 per cent. The chronic form, which begins 5 to 15 years after exposure, presents as diffuse granulomatous pneumonitis, which progresses to pulmonary fibrosis and respiratory insufficiency. The hilar nodes may calcify.

Beryllium disease was initially associated with the manufacture of fluorescent lights, but this form of exposure ceased after beryllium was removed from fluorescent lights in 1949. Currently, exposures occur in the milling of beryllium metal alloys, which are used in the aerospace industry, in the manufacture of x-ray tubes, and in nuclear physics. Beryllium is quite toxic at even low concentration, and disease has been reported in people who handled clothes of exposed workers.

The diagnosis is made by the history of exposure and by demonstration of a granulomatous tissue reaction. Noncaseating granulomas may be found in skin, liver, spleen, and lymph nodes as well as in the lungs. Tissue and urine can be analyzed for beryllium content, though the concentration of beryllium in the urine indicates exposure only and does not correlate well with disease activity. Lymphocyte transformation in vitro by beryllium salts has been reported to differentiate beryllium disease from simple exposure and from other granulomatus diseases. However, beryllium disease remains difficult to differentiate from sarcoidosis (Ch. 67). Involvement of the uvea, salivary glands, or central nervous system strongly favors the diagnosis of sarcoidosis. Prolonged treatment with glucocorticoids is useful in suppressing beryllium disease in many patients.

Metal Fume Fever

Metal fume fever is a benign, self-limited, acute illness produced by inhalation of fumes of the metals zinc, copper, and magnesium. The syndrome occurs in people who weld galvanized metals in an enclosed, poorly ventilated space. Several hours after exposure, workers experience cough, dry throat, and tightness in the chest. These symptoms are followed by fever, chills, myalgias, and leukocytosis. The illness lasts only one day. Tolerance develops, and the worker may return to the same job without recurrence. However, the syndrome may recur after exposure following a layoff.

DISEASES PRODUCED BY ORGANIC MATERIALS

Hypersensitivity Pneumonitis

Inhalation of organic dusts produces inflammation in the lung parenchyma (hypersensitivity pneumonitis) or obstructive disease of the conducting airways (occupational asthma and bronchitis). Hypersensitivity pneumonitis, also termed extrinsic allergic alveolitis, will be discussed only briefly in this section because it is discussed in detail in Ch. 62. The classic example of hypersensitivity pneumonitis is *farmer's lung disease,* which is produced by inhalation of *Micropolyspora faeni* or *Thermoactinomyces vulgaris* in dust from moldy hay. Symptoms of chill, nonproductive cough, dyspnea, and malaise occur four to eight hours after exposure. Physical findings include fever, tachypnea, tachycardia, and rales. Evidence of obstructive airway disease such as wheezing or prolonged expiration is typically absent. The chest roentgenogram reveals bilateral, irregular parenchymal infiltrates. Patients with a chronic form of hypersensitivity pneumonitis may have pulmonary fibrosis and respiratory failure without a clear history of episodic disease. Other examples of hypersensitivity pneumonitis include *bagassosis* (from dried sugar cane), *suberosis* (from cork dust), *sequoiosis* (from redwood saw dust), *cheese washer's lung* (from moldy cheese), and *pigeon breeder's lung* (from bird droppings). The pathogenesis involves both humoral and cell-mediated immunity (type III and IV immunologic reactions). Patients have precipitating IgG against the pertinent fungal or avian antigens. Diagnosis is made by history, serum precipitins, Arthus skin reaction, in vitro lymphocyte transformation and lymphokine production, and occasionally by bronchial provocation tests or open lung biopsy. Treatment is by avoidance of the antigen when possible and with glucocorticoids when necessary.

Syndromes related to air treatment systems are common and have been lumped under the term *humidifier fever.* In some instances the clinical presentation is a classic hypersensitivity pneumonitis with fever, infiltrates, and identification of a source of aerosolization of *Micropolyspora faeni* or thermophilic actinomyces. However, in other cases the presentation is more like occupational asthma with cough, wheeze, chest tightness, and fever, but no pulmonary infiltrate. In these latter cases the causative agents include ameba, protozoa, fungi, and bacteria that have contaminated water for aerosolization. The successful treatment usually requires thorough cleaning of the air conditioning system and ducts.

Diseases produced by inhalation of toxic gas (e.g., chloride, sulfur dioxide, ammonia) are discussed in Ch. 560.

Occupational Asthma

DEFINITION. Asthma is broadly defined as a disease characterized by increased responsiveness of the airways to various stimuli and manifested by slowing of forced expiration that changes in severity either spontaneously or as a result of therapy (see Ch. 59). This definition allows for numerous syndromes that all result in bronchoconstriction but that may be produced by a variety of factors mediated through different mechanisms. In Table 559–2 there is a list of a few of the different forms of occupational asthma; a more complete list and description of the individual types of occupational asthma can be found in the references. Occupational asthma occurs in two different population groups. One group has pre-existing asthma that is exacerbated by an occupational dust or fume, and the other group has no previous history of asthma and first develops symptoms after the occupational exposure. Patients with known asthma tend to leave the industry if they become severely symptomatic. If their symptoms are mild they remain in the work force and may account for some of the heterogeneity in clinical studies. Individuals with pre-existing asthma are likely to be more sensitive, may have different clinical manifestations, and may react differently to components in the occupational fumes or dusts than individuals without pre-existing asthma.

TABLE 559–2. TYPES OF OCCUPATIONAL ASTHMA*

Material	Industry	Etiology *IgE*	Etiology *Other*	Onset of Typical Reaction
Animal dander	Veterinarians Laboratory workers	+	0	Immediate only
Green coffee bean	Food industry	+	0	Immediate only
Enzymes from *Bacillus subtilis*	Detergent industry	+	?	Immediate and late
Complex salts of platinum	Metal refining	+	?	Immediate and late
Flour, grain	Bakers, grain handlers	+	?	Immediate and late
Toluene diisocyanate (TDI)	Polyurethane industry	?	+	Dual and late
Western red cedar	Saw mills	?	+	Dual and late
Resin core solder	Electronics industry	0	+	Dual and late
Formalin	Medical	0	+	Immediate and late
Cotton dust	Cotton mills (byssinosis)	0	+	Late

*The cause and mechanisms of different types of occupational asthma are still being investigated and remain speculative.

The time of onset of reactions varies for different workers in a given industry, and it is likely that the precise combination of mechanisms that cause the airway obstruction will also vary for individual workers within a given industry.

The onset of reaction is immediate if it occurs within 30 minutes and late if it occurs after 30 minutes, usually 2 to 6 hours after exposure. Dual reactions include both immediate and late components. The type of reactions of patients with asthma due to western red cedar, toluene diisocyanate, and liquid core solder fluxes is similar in that about half have late reactions, half dual reactions, and less than 10 per cent immediate reactions only.

+ = probable; ? = possible; 0 = unlikely.

OCCUPATIONAL EXPOSURE. Patients with immediate reactions can usually identify the offending agents, which may include both particulate dusts and gaseous fumes. For those with delayed reactions, identification of the offending material may be much more difficult. The sensitization and cause of the respiratory disease may not originate in the actual workplace of the patient. There have been reports of toluene diisocyanate produced in one factory affecting sensitive individuals in a neighboring workplace.

PATHOGENESIS. The pathogenesis of most cases of occupational asthma, especially the kinds with delayed symptoms, is not known. At least four different mechanisms for producing occupational asthma have been suggested:

1. *Production of specific IgE (or perhaps a sensitizing IgG) against an inhaled antigen.* The sensitization will usually occur within

one year of exposure; the affected individual is likely to be atopic; and exposure to the antigen evokes immediate symptoms, which are produced by a type I immunologic reaction, and in some individuals, a late reaction as well. Prick skin tests and the radioallergosorbent tests are almost always positive. Examples of asthma produced by this mechanism include baker's asthma and reactions to animal dander, green coffee beans, and castor beans.

2. *Direct damage to the airway epithelium and stimulation of irritant receptors that produce bronchospasm through parasympathetic reflexes.* Damage to the airway epithelium might allow penetration of inhaled materials into the submucosa, which would enhance their immunologic and inflammatory effects, and induction of nonspecific bronchial hyper-reactivity to other inhaled dusts and fumes. Viral infections and ozone have been shown to produce transient bronchial hyper-reactivity to histamine in normal subjects. Bronchial hyper-reactivity is considered to explain in part how acute episodic asthma can develop into a more persistent, chronic form that produces symptoms even in the absence of the sensitizing agent. Examples of reactions that could be caused by epithelial damage and inflammation include those due to toluene diisocyanate, platinum salts, western red cedar, formalin, resin core soldering flux, and aminoethyl ethanolamine.

3. *Production of substances that are generated slowly or are slow to react,* i.e., production of leukotrienes, platelet-activating factor (PAF), C5a and C3a for immune complex reactions and complement activation, and other chemotactic factors for polymorphonuclear leukocytes.

4. *The pharmacologic properties of the inhaled material,* i.e., release of mediators from mast cells (cotton dust), complement activation (western red cedar), or increased parasympathetic tone by inhibition of acetylcholinesterase (organic phosphate insecticides).

A great deal more investigation is necessary to define the precise mechanisms in different forms of occupational asthma.

CLINICAL MANIFESTATIONS. In general, the symptoms of cough, sputum production, and chest tightness are more common than wheezing. Cough is a symptom of airway irritation or obstruction, and patients with persistent cough, especially one that decreases when the worker has been away from work for three or four days, should be examined for the possibility of occupational asthma. In recording the history, it is important to identify all symptoms, and for each symptom to determine at what time of day, during what type of work, and where in the workplace the symptom occurs. Patients with immediate reactions can usually identify the eliciting substance. The symptoms occur at work and increase during the working day. Patients with late reactions may have symptoms that occur only after work, especially at night. Sometimes the only clue that these late symptoms are work related is that they decrease after the person is away from the workplace for several weeks.

Physical examination away from work may be normal. It is important to examine the patient at work or while symptoms are present for signs of airway obstruction. Some agents produce dermatitis, e.g., platinum salts and formalin. Chest roentgenograms are normal except for diseases that can progress to chronic obstructive lung disease, e.g., byssinosis.

DIAGNOSIS AND DIFFERENTIAL DIAGNOSIS. The diagnosis is made by history, pulmonary function tests, and immunologic tests. It is important to establish if the symptoms are only work related, because, if they are, the diagnosis is established, and the possibility of prevention by changing jobs can be strongly considered.

Pulmonary function studies are extremely useful for establishing the diagnosis. Routine spirograms obtained away from work may be normal. However, evaluations before, during, and after work may be diagnostic. The most important diagnostic tools are a peak flowmeter and a symptom diary. In general, measurements that allegedly determine the extent of small airway function and distribution of inspired air (frequency dependence of dynamic lung compliance, single-breath nitrogen test with determination of the alveolar plateau and closing volume, and comparison of maximal expiratory flow curves during exhalation of helium and air) show abnormalities before the FEV_1 is abnormal. However, the clinical importance and predictive value of these tests will have to await additional studies in patients with occupational asthma. Most patients with occupational asthma show bronchial hyper-reactivity to histamine or methylcholine, but it is not known if the hyper-reactivity is a cause or a result of the occupational disorder. Results of this test may be positive in an individual whose baseline studies are normal. However, byssinosis and toluene diisocyanate asthma have been reported not to show bronchial hyper-reactivity to histamine.

A specific bronchial provocation test is the single most diagnostic test. For this test the patient performs his exact work with actual industrial materials under careful supervision in a controlled laboratory setting, and measurements of pulmonary function are serially recorded. Inhalation challenges can also be performed with aerosolized material or in an environmental chamber. Bronchial provocation tests with inert substances (lactose) and with different types of dusts found in the work environment can help identify the inciting factor and exclude nonspecific bronchial hyper-reactivity. Extreme care must be used in selecting the doses of inhaled materials, and observation of the patient should be extended to cover late reactions. In patients with late or complex reactions and for substances for which there is no satisfactory skin test or antigen for the radioallergosorbent assay, bronchial provocation may be the only means of making the diagnosis with certainty, e.g., toluene diisocyanate.

Prick skin tests are useful for evaluating immediate hypersensitivity, but there are many false positive findings and perhaps some false negative ones.

TREATMENT, PROGNOSIS, AND PREVENTION. As in other forms of occupational disease, prevention has priority over treatment. Sometimes symptoms disappear if the worker moves to another area of the workplace and does different work. If this is not satisfactory, the worker may have to change jobs. Symptoms can be relieved by treating the airway obstruction with beta adrenergic agonists, theophylline, or cromolyn, but the disease will likely persist. It is not known if the long-term prognosis of those whose symptoms are controlled medically and who remain exposed to the sensitizing material is different from those who move to a new environment. In a few patients, such as those with baker's asthma, the symptoms disappear with time, perhaps because a blocking antibody (IgG) is produced. In some occupations, prevention can be achieved by changing the process or eliminating the antigen (detergents that contain proteases from *Bacillus subtilis*).

Bernstein IL: Occupational asthma. Clin Chest Med 2:255, 1981. *Review of clinical types, diagnosis, and therapy.*

Boushey HA, Holtzman MJ, Sheller JR, Nadel JA: Bronchial hyperreactivity. Am Rev Respir Dis 121:389, 1980. *A detailed state-of-the-art review of an important mechanism in occupational asthma.*

INDUSTRIAL BRONCHITIS

Although most bronchitis is still attributable to cigarette smoking, prolonged exposure to high levels of dust can produce industrial bronchitis. Two population groups that are clinically affected are coal workers and grain handlers. In coal workers, large particles (5 to 10 μ) are thought to be deposited on the epithelium of the proximal airways and to produce clinical bronchitis that only slightly decreases the FEV_1, does not produce emphysema, has no effect on life expectancy, and remits after the dust exposure is gone. In grain handlers, the cause and long-term effect of the clinical bronchitis is not as well characterized because the disease is more complex. A variety of components of grain dust (grain antigens, fungal antigens, grain weevils, mites, animal antigens, and bacterial endotoxins as well as inert dust) have been implicated in the production of symptoms, and these components probably elicit more of an inflammatory and immunologic reaction in the chronic bronchitis of grain handlers that the reaction produced by coal dust.

Morgan WKC: Industrial bronchitis. Br J Indust Med 35:285, 1978. *Detailed discussion of a complex issue.*

OCCUPATIONALLY RELATED LUNG CANCER

Certain minerals and chemicals are associated with a high incidence of lung cancer. There is a long delay (15 to 25 years) between exposure and the development of clinical cancer. But it is not known how to identify those individuals who are most likely to develop lung cancer or how clinically useful serial chest films and sputum cytology are in the detection and subsequent course of lung cancer. Materials that are thought to be responsible for the development of lung cancer include arsenic, asbestos (lung cancer and mesothelioma), carbonyl nickel (squamous cell carcinoma), chloromethyl ethers (oat cell carcinoma), chromates, coal tars, emissions from coke ovens, mustard gas, uranium, and other sources of radiation (oat cell carcinoma). The concept that specific occupational exposures are associated with specific cell types of lung cancer is controversial. The assessment of causality for lung cancer in patients who smoke cigarettes and have an occupational exposure is one of the most vexing problems for compensation.

Frank AL: Occupational Lung Cancer. *In* Harris CC (ed.): Pathogenesis and Therapy of lung cancer. New York, Marcel Dekker, Inc., 1978, pp 25–51.

560. PHYSICAL, CHEMICAL, AND ASPIRATION INJURIES OF THE LUNG

James D. Crapo

The lung has an extremely large and delicate surface exposed to the environment. Extensive defense mechanisms exist to protect the lung from inhaled pathogens and toxic substances. Under normal conditions, air is fully humidified and warmed to body temperature and all large particulate substances are cleared by the upper airways. These defenses are not adequate to handle many physical and chemical substances that cause lung injury. This chapter deals with a variety of lung injuries that are initiated by external factors rather than being due to an intrinsic defect or failure of the respiratory system and its defenses.

PHYSICAL DISORDERS

Thermal Injuries

About 25 per cent of patients with major burns have pulmonary complications, and these complications now account for the majority of burn-related deaths. Thermal injury to the lung is associated with three groups of complications: (1) *Immediate reaction*—direct thermal injury to upper airways, leading to upper airway obstruction, carbon monoxide poisoning, and smoke inhalation (potent bronchoconstrictors and edemagenic substances). (2) *Adult respiratory distress syndrome* (ARDS) developing 24 to 48 hours after the thermal injury. (3) *Late onset pulmonary complications,* which include pneumonia, atelectasis, thromboembolism, and chest-wall restriction caused by circumferential thoracic burns.

Few burns actually cause thermal injury to the lung parenchyma; the large capacity of the upper airways to humidify and modify the temperatures of inhaled air protects the alveolar tissue. Exceptions are steam burns and explosions in an enclosed space.

The initial symptoms are tachypnea, cough, dyspnea, wheezing, cyanosis, hoarseness, and stridor (an ominous sign). During the next 12 to 48 hours the patient may become increasingly hypoxic; lung compliance may decrease, and pulmonary edema may develop in the presence of normal pulmonary capillary wedge pressure. Roentgenograms of the chest may show no significant changes or a pattern of diffuse, patchy infiltrates. The major complication is infection, usually caused by *Pseudomonas aeruginosa* or *Staphylococcus aureus.* The lung defenses against infection are compromised by thermal injury to the airway epithelium and often by an endotracheal or tracheostomy tube. The pathway of infection may be either by inhalation of airborne organisms or by hematogenous spread from the burn.

The constituents of smoke are potent mucosal irritants and bronchoconstrictors and contribute to the upper and lower lung lesions. Typical constitutents of smoke include oxides of nitrogen, sulfur and lead, ammonia, hydrochlorides, chlorine, and aldehydes. Acrolein, found in wood smoke, is a potent mucosal irritant which contributes to upper airway obstruction and to pulmonary edema. Carbon monoxide poisoning from inhaled smoke is discussed in Chemical Injury to the Lung.

The adult respiratory distress syndrome commonly develops 24 to 48 hours after the initial symptoms subside. The causes of adult respiratory distress syndrome in the burn patient are controversial, but possibilities include a chemical pneumonitis caused by constituents in smoke, a circulating burn toxin, disseminated intravascular coagulation, microembolism, or central neurogenic pulmonary edema. The extent of surface thermal injury does not correlate with the degree of respiratory distress that subsequently develops.

Late onset pulmonary burn complications—atelectasis, thromboembolism, and pneumonia—are discussed in Ch. 61, 65, and 260 to 266, respectively.

THERAPY. Carbon monoxide poisoning and upper airway obstruction are the most immediate life-threatening complications in the patient presenting with major burns or with the history of smoke or steam inhalation. The patient should be closely observed for evidence of these complications and given high levels of inspired oxygen. Fiberoptic bronchoscopy may help detect laryngeal and tracheobronchial inflammation and evidence of smoke contamination in the lower airways. Arterial blood gases should be monitored and prompt intubation or tracheostomy performed if evidence of significant airway obstruction develops. Corticosteroids may be helpful to treat edema of the upper airways, but must be used with caution since one of the major complications of both skin and lung thermal injury is infection. Prophylactic antibiotics are of no value in preventing pneumonia and may predispose to infection with resistant organisms. Careful pulmonary toilet, humidification, and sterile suctioning should be used to reduce the risk of pneumonia. Repeated bronchoscopy is often necessary to remove mucous plugs and thereby prevent segmental atelectasis and infection.

Crapo RO: Smoke-inhalation injuries. JAMA 246:1694, 1981. *A review of the clinical presentation and treatment of smoke inhalation injuries.*
Pruitt BA, Goodwin CW: Current treatment of the extensively burned patient. Surg Annu 15:331, 1983. *A general review of the approach to the burned patient; 97 references.*
Trunkey DD: Inhalation injury. Surg Clin North Am 58:1133, 1978. *A detailed review of pulmonary damage caused by smoke inhalation; 16 references.*

Radiation Injury (See also Ch. 562)

The predominant factors determining the incidence of radiation pneumonitis are the total radiation dose, the number of fractions, and the duration of time over which the total dose is given. Some chemotherapeutic drugs may potentiate damage from radiation. A total lung dose of less than 2000 rads generally is not associated with severe radiation pneumonitis, whereas a total dose in excess of 4000 rads, even if distributed over as many as 30 fractions, has virtually a 100 per cent risk of radiation pneumonitis.

HISTOPATHOLOGIC CHANGES. The reaction of the lung to radiation injury can be divided into three phases: (1) The acute phase, occurring one to two months after radiation, is characterized by vascular damage, congestion, edema, and mononuclear cell infiltration. Alveolar Type II cells and alveolar macrophages are increased in number. (2) The subacute phase occurs two to nine months later. The alveolar walls become infiltrated with mononuclear inflammatory cells and fibroblasts. (3) The chronic or fibrotic phase generally occurs more than nine months after irradiation. Capillary sclerosis and alveolar fibrosis are its predominant histologic features.

CLINICAL PRESENTATION. Signs of bronchial irritation may appear immediately after radiation therapy and/or evidence of esophagitis shortly thereafter, but patients may have no symptoms for 6 to 12 weeks, at which time mild cough appears. If large volumes of lung have been irradiated, or if high radiation doses over short periods have been given, dyspnea, tachypnea, and fever, sometimes high and spiking, can develop. These symptoms can be extremely severe, and will either progress to severe dyspnea and death or gradually subside, leaving varying degrees of respiratory impairment resulting from chronic lung fibrosis. The permanent changes of fibrosis take 6 to 24 months to evolve, and then usually remain stable after two years if no further exposure occurs. Auscultation of the chest is usually normal, although rales, signs of consolidation, and rubs may be found. Clubbing does not develop after radiation injury. Laboratory findings include a mild leukocytosis and an increased erythrocyte sedimentation rate. If the irradiated area is extensive, arterial hypoxemia may be found. Radiographic changes generally appear one to three months following treatment. After therapeutic thoracic irradiation the affected areas are generally demarcated by a sharp edge limited to the margins of the portal of irradiation and have a "ground glass appearance"—a hazy increase in density with indistinct pulmonary markings. In the later phases of the radiation injury, fibrosis and contraction of the irradiated region are the predominant radiographic findings.

Pulmonary function testing shows no change until clinical symptoms appear, at which time a restrictive ventilatory defect is present. Capillary sclerosis is associated with a decrease in blood flow to the affected region and a decrease in carbon monoxide transfer capacity. Severe radiation injury is associated with a decrease in lung compliance and hypoxemia.

Complications of radiation pneumonitis include small pleural effusions and occasionally spontaneous pneumothorax. The cough may be severe enough to cause rib fractures.

The differential diagnosis of acute radiation pneumonitis is usually complicated by the immunocompromised state of many of the patients, by the presence of bacterial, fungal, and protozoan pneumonias, particularly *Pneumocystis carinii*, or by the signs and symptoms of the neoplasm being treated. Radiation pneumonitis has not been documented in parts of the lung outside the radiation portal.

TREATMENT. The best management of radiation pneumonitis is to avoid it when possible. The patient who develops radiation pneumonitis requires supportive care, including medication for cough suppression and often oxygen delivered by nasal catheter or mask for hypoxemia. Corticosteroids (prednisone, 1 mg per kilogram of body weight) are effective at the start of pneumonitis. On occasion the response may be dramatic, with complete resolution of symptoms within 24 hours. Corticosteroids should be tapered as rapidly as possible. There is no evidence that corticosteroids given at the time of irradiation have any protective effect. They are also ineffective in the late fibrotic phases of the disease.

Antibiotics have been tried both prophylactically and when pneumonitis develops. There is no evidence that this treatment modifies the clinical course; therefore antibiotic therapy should be reserved for patients in whom the findings suggest significant infection to be present. Since the lesion involves occlusion and thrombosis of many small blood vessels, anticoagulation has been suggested but without experimental evidence of its effectiveness.

Catane R, Schwade JG, Turris AT, Webber BL, Muggia FM: Pulmonary toxicity after radiation and bleomycin: A review. Radiat Oncol Biol Phys 5:1513, 1979. *The synergistic effects of these two agents are reviewed; 32 references.*

Gross NJ: Pulmonary effects of radiation therapy. Ann Intern Med 86:81, 1977. *An excellent and thorough review with 112 references.*

Disorders of the Lung Caused by Barometric Pressure

Altitude

The major physiologic effects of reduced atmospheric pressure are due to the resulting low partial pressure of oxygen. At 10,000 feet (3048 meters) the alveolar P_{O_2} is approximately 60 mm Hg, and some individuals will manifest impairment of recent memory, judgment, and the ability to perform complex calculations, and demonstrate an increased heart rate and increased pulmonary ventilation. The time required for these symptoms to begin is partially related to age, physical fitness, and acclimatization. At 12,000 feet (3658 meters) the alveolar P_{O_2} is 52, and dyspnea, headache, nausea, and decreased visual acuity may occur. At 18,000 feet (5486 meters) the alveolar P_{O_2} is 40, and unacclimatized individuals will lose consciousness after several hours of exposure. At 22,000 feet (6706 meters) the alveolar P_{O_2} is 30, and almost all acutely exposed individuals become unconscious after sufficient time. The rapid change in physiologic functions that begins to occur at about 10,000 feet is due to the shape of the oxygen-hemoglobin dissociation curve, which has a steep downslope below a P_{O_2} of approximately 60 mm Hg. A small drop in P_{O_2} below this level results in a relatively large decrease in arterial saturation.

In general, commercial aircraft cabins are maintained at a pressure greater than or equal to that encountered at 8000 feet so that no supplemental oxygen is required. Some patients with reduced cardiac reserve or with chronic obstructive lung disease may have difficulty tolerating even a small drop in arterial oxygen saturation and may require supplemental oxygen during flights. Aircraft regulations require that the flight crew receive supplemental oxygen when the cabin pressure drops below that at 10,000 feet, and that passengers receive supplemental oxygen should the cabin pressure drop below that at 15,000 feet.

ACUTE MOUNTAIN SICKNESS. This syndrome occurs in unacclimated persons who rapidly ascend to a high altitude. Symptoms can occur at altitudes as low as 7000 to 8000 feet in particularly susceptible individuals, usually those in poor physical condition, and during a rapid ascent requiring significant physical exertion. The symptoms are headache, exertional dyspnea, malaise, anorexia, nausea, vomiting, diarrhea, and abdominal pain. Judgment may be impaired. Inability to sleep is a common problem. Cyanosis, Cheyne-Stokes breathing, and tachycardia are commonly present. In untreated individuals, these signs and symptoms subside gradually over a period of several days. The treatment is oxygen therapy or descent to a lower altitude. The disorder is thought to be related to an increase in ventilation stimulated by hypoxia and resulting in hypocapnia and respiratory alkalosis. Acetazolamide, 250 mg every eight hours prior to and during the ascent to altitude, can prevent symptoms, presumably by increasing renal excretion of bicarbonate and reducing the extent of the respiratory alkalosis. Furosemide, 80 mg every 12 hours, has also produced relief of symptoms.

CHRONIC MOUNTAIN SICKNESS (MONGE'S DISEASE). Chronic mountain sickness occurs in people living at high altitudes, usually at over 14,000 feet, for many years. These "highlanders" have a blunted respiratory drive in response to hypoxia and have a lower minute ventilation at high altitudes than do those who normally reside at lower altitudes. Chronic mountain sickness is characterized by what appears to be an exaggerated adaptive response to altitude. This includes erythrocytosis with hemoglobin levels as high as 25 grams per deciliter, a decreased minute ventilation with an elevated P_{CO_2}, low arterial oxygen saturation, and an impaired sensitivity of the respiratory center to hypoxia. Clinical manifestations are similar to those of polycythemia rubra vera and include cyanosis, dyspnea, cough, palpitations, headache, giddiness, muscular weakness, pain in the extremities, sensory and motor changes, and episodic stupor. The only therapy is to move the patient to a lower altitude. Subacute forms of this illness also occur in which the marked cyanosis and alveolar hypoventilation are absent. A similar syndrome, brisket disease, has been described in cattle.

HIGH ALTITUDE PULMONARY EDEMA. Acute pulmonary edema is a potentially fatal complication of rapid ascent to altitudes of greater than 9000 feet. The mechanism is unknown, but clearly hypoxia is the provoking cause. Symptoms begin after 6 to 36 hours at high altitude and may follow an episode of acute mountain sickness. Rales, cyanosis, orthopnea, and hemoptysis commonly develop unless oxygen is administered or the patient is rapidly moved to a lower altitude.

At autopsy the lungs are typically heavy, congested, and edematous and have hyaline membranes in the small airways and alveoli. The cause of hyaline membrane formation is not known; this is not a characteristic finding in death caused by other forms of hypoxia. During a large military airlift in India, approximately 6 of each 1000 persons flown to an altitude of 11,500 feet developed this syndrome.

Hemodynamic studies have shown elevations of the pulmonary artery pressure with a normal pulmonary venous pressure. The pulmonary edema may be due to an increase in pulmonary capillary pressure in small regions of the pulmonary capillary bed, or to increased permeability in lung capillaries.

Increased Barometric Pressure

Pressure increases approximately 1 atmosphere for each 33 feet of descent in water. Direct body contact with increased barometric pressure under water is most commonly encountered during breathhold diving, when continuous consumption of oxygen and production of CO_2 lead to hypoxia and hypercapnia. The increasing serum carbon dioxide concentration causes an almost irresistible drive to breathe. Since hypoxia is a mild stimulation for ventilation, it is relatively easy to continue holding one's breath in the presence of profound hypoxia. A common hazardous error made by swimmers is to hyperventilate prior to a dive in an effort to increase the time of breath holding. This depletes the body of carbon dioxide stores, but does not significantly increase oxygen stores. In these circumstances hypoxia can cause unconsciousness before accumulation of carbon dioxide forces the termination of the dive. This is thought to account for many deaths in swimming pools. Decompression during ascent from a breathhold dive can cause a marked fall in alveolar Po_2, leading to the diver's losing consciousness just as the surface is reached.

DECOMPRESSION SICKNESS. Decompression sickness was first described in the last century in caisson workers in tunnel construction, where compressed air was used to exclude water and mud. The increase in military, commercial, and sport diving has made decompression sickness a relatively common clinical problem. When ordinary air is breathed under increased ambient pressure, inert gas, commonly nitrogen, dissolves in tissue and blood, reaching saturation equilibrium at the greater partial pressures. Upon rapid decompression to sea level, the inert gas may come out of solution to form intravascular bubbles. The onset of symptoms tends to be gradual, beginning minutes to hours after the termination of a dive. Manifestations include "bends" (deep pain in joints, aggravated by exercise), pruritus, cyanosis, substernal chest pain, dyspnea, nonproductive cough, evidence of spinal cord injury, confusion, blurred vision, visual field defects, paralysis, dysphasia, headache, vertigo, and seizures. In severe cases the symptoms may rapidly progress to shock and death. Symptoms of mild or early decompression sickness resemble and are often confused with acute alcohol intoxication.

The treatment of decompression sickness is recompression with a gradual return to sea level pressures over a period of days to weeks. Recompression decreases bubble size and permits their gradual resorption during the "ascent" to surface pressures.

Air embolism can occur in scuba divers who ascend without exhaling. Intrapulmonary gas expands and the high pressure may rupture a portion of the lung and introduce gas into the systemic circulation, mediastinum, pleura, or subcutaneous tissues. Gas bubbles may form arterial emboli to the brain and result in sudden unconsciousness, focal or generalized seizures, visual field loss or blindness, weakness, paralysis, hypoesthesia, or confusion. The therapy is rapid recompression similar to that employed to treat decompression sickness. Gas embolism has been reported during ascents of as little as 2.2 meters and is thought to be one of the most common causes of accidental death in divers.

THERAPEUTIC HYPERBARIC OXYGEN. Hyperbaric oxygen has been clearly proven to be beneficial in treating only a limited number of illnesses: acute carbon monoxide poisoning, acute cyanide poisoning, clostridial myonecrosis, decompression sickness, air embolism, and osteoradionecrosis. The hazards of oxygen toxicity limit the dose of oxygen that can be delivered by hyperbaric techniques. Central nervous system toxicity, usually in the form of convulsions, occurs at oxygen pressures greater than 2.5 atmospheres if the exposure is maintained for a sufficient length of time. Thus, hyperbaric oxygen therapy is limited to a maximum of two to three atmospheres of oxygen and durations of no more than one to three hours.

Kidd DJ, Elliott DH: Decompression disorders in divers. *In* Bennett PB, Elliott DH (eds.): The Physiology and Medicine of Diving and Compressed Air Work. Baltimore, Williams & Wilkins Company, 1975, pp 471–495. *A good text and a good chapter on the problems encountered in decompression.*

Singh I, Khanna PK, Srivastava MC, Lal M, Roy SB, Subramanyam CSV: Acute mountain sickness. N Engl J Med 280:175, 1969. *A good review.*

Strauss RH: Diving medicine. Am Rev Respir Dis 119:1001, 1979. *A comprehensive state-of-the-art review on all aspects of diving medicine.*

CHEMICAL INJURY TO THE LUNG

Toxic Inhaled Gases

A large number of gases and chemicals, to which exposures most frequently occur in an industrial setting, can cause both an acute and sometimes a chronic injury to the respiratory system.

A few agents cause an *"asthma-like" reaction* with cough, chest pain, and wheezing. Toluene di-isocyanate and other isocyanates (liberated as gas during the reaction of isocyanates with polyol in the manufacture of polyurethane foams), aluminum soldering flux, and platinum salts are typical examples. Reaginic and precipitating antibodies against platinum salts and soldering flux have been found in symptomatic individuals, suggesting an immunologic basis for the reaction. An allergic basis for the reaction to toluene di-isocyanate has not been demonstrated. The symptoms usually subside after removal from exposure; however, chronic lung injury may occur if the exposure is prolonged.

A number of highly irritating gases cause an *acute chemical pneumonitis.* Such gases include chlorine (used in the chemical and plastic industries and to disinfect water), ammonia (used in refrigeration), sulfur dioxide (used in paper manufacture and smelting of sulfide containing ores), ozone (generated in welding and in photochemical smog), nitrogen dioxide (released from decomposed corn silage), and phosgene (used in production of aniline dyes).

The prototype for injury of this type is *silo-filler's disease* (nitrogen dioxide). During the initial exposure there may be no symptoms, there may be tracheobronchitis with cough and shortness of breath, or there may be the immediate onset of acute pulmonary edema. Signs of ocular and oropharyngeal mucous membrane irritation may be present. The symptoms may rapidly progress, but commonly the initial symptoms resolve and are followed by a period of minimal symptoms (cough) lasting up to 48 hours. Fever, myalgias, dyspnea, and progressive hypoxemia then occur and the radiographic picture is that of pulmonary edema. These severe symptoms may resolve only to recur two to five weeks later and may lead to progressive pulmonary insufficiency with a picture of bronchiolitis obliterans. Treatment with corticosteroids (prednisone, 1 mg per kilogram per day) may dramatically improve the acute illness. Bronchodilators, mechanical ventilation, and supplemental oxygen may be necessary. Since there may be a period of temporary improvement following the initial exposure, observation for a period of 48 hours is advisable.

The clinical response caused by each irritant gas varies, but appears to be closely related to the degree of acute irritation it causes and to its water solubility. The less irritating gases, such as ozone and the oxides of nitrogen, phosgene, mercury, and nickel carbonyl, can be inhaled for prolonged periods of time and thereby cause injury throughout the respiratory system. Highly irritating and soluble gases, such as ammonia and hydrochloric acid, are less likely to be inhaled deeply and tend to result in immediate injury to the upper airways and have potential for obstruction secondary to mucosal edema. Less soluble gases, such as chlorine, cadmium, zinc chloride, osmium tetroxide, and vanadium, can cause injury to the entire tracheobronchial tree and do not commonly present with upper airway obstruction. Bronchiolitis and pulmonary edema are common, ultimately leading to bronchiolitis obliterans. The long-term consequences vary with the gas. Cadmium, for example, can cause diffuse emphysema and severe airway obstruction but only minimal fibrosis.

Different mechanisms are involved in the injury caused by these gases. Most of them cause injury by acting as a strong acid, a strong base, or an oxidant. Gases of chemicals that are strong acids or bases in water solution, such as hydrogen chloride, sulfuric acid, sulfur dioxide, and ammonia, tend to react more in the upper airways where they change tissue pH and thereby cause cell damage.

Chester EH, Kaimal PJ, Payne CB, Kohn PM: Pulmonary injury following exposure to chlorine gas. Chest 72:247, 1977. *Discussion of the response of two patients and a review of literature suggest that corticosteroid therapy may be beneficial.*
Horvath EP, doPico GA, Barbee RA, Dickie HA: Nitrogen dioxide-induced pulmonary disease. J Occup Med 20:103, 1978. *A well-written report of five cases and a review of the literature.*
Summer W, Haponik E: Inhalation of irritant gases. Clin Chest Med 2:273, 1981. *A comprehensive review of gases that are toxic to the lung; 74 references.*

Pulmonary Oxygen Toxicity

Oxygen is used in extremely high concentrations in large numbers of patients in intensive care units, often with endotracheal intubation and mechanical ventilation. The toxic effects of hyperoxic atmospheres may not infrequently outweigh the potential therapeutic benefits. Superoxide, an unstable free radical produced by the single electron reduction of oxygen, is produced as a normal byproduct of oxidative metabolism in almost every plant and animal tissue that uses oxygen as an electron sink. Superoxide dismutase is a protective enzyme that catalyzes the dismutation and therefore the detoxification of the superoxide free radical. If not scavenged by superoxide dismutase, this free radical can react with hydrogen peroxide to form the hydroxyl free radical (OH•) and free radical chain reactions can be initiated, resulting in the destruction of cell lipids and proteins. This "free radical injury" is the presumed chemical basis for oxygen toxicity (Fig. 560–1).

In the adult the major target tissue of oxygen injury is the pulmonary capillary endothelium. Other body organs are protected by the consumption of oxygen and the characteristics of the binding of oxygen to hemoglobin. The mixed venous Po_2 is maintained at about 40 to 50 torr even when the patient is breathing 100 per cent oxygen.

At autopsy the lungs are atelectatic, congested, and edematous and have hyaline membranes. The most serious injury appears to be destruction of the capillary bed with resultant interstitial and alveolar edema, hypoxemia, and sometimes death. Alveolar epithelium is also injured, causing hyperplasia of Type II cells. An acute tracheobronchitis also occurs, and histologic changes have been found in the ciliated epithelium and Clara cells in the small airways.

The typical presentation in the adult is that of an acutely ill patient who is receiving oxygen in high concentrations and mechanical ventilation for a lung injury that makes the onset of pulmonary oxygen toxicity difficult to detect. Lung compliance progressively falls; the patient develops tachypnea, substernal pain, and increased cough. The alveolar-arterial oxygen gradient gradually widens with progressive hypoxemia. Increasing concentrations of oxygen are needed to maintain adequate oxygenation of arterial blood, and the cycle progresses to pulmonary edema, respiratory failure, and death.

The earliest symptoms of oxygen toxicity are due to acute tracheobronchitis. A dry, hacking cough and substernal pain may occur within six to twelve hours while breathing pure oxygen. Nausea, vomiting, and paresthesias follow. Vital capacity decreases, and there is an increase in the respiratory rate.

The flow of tracheal mucus decreases after short exposures

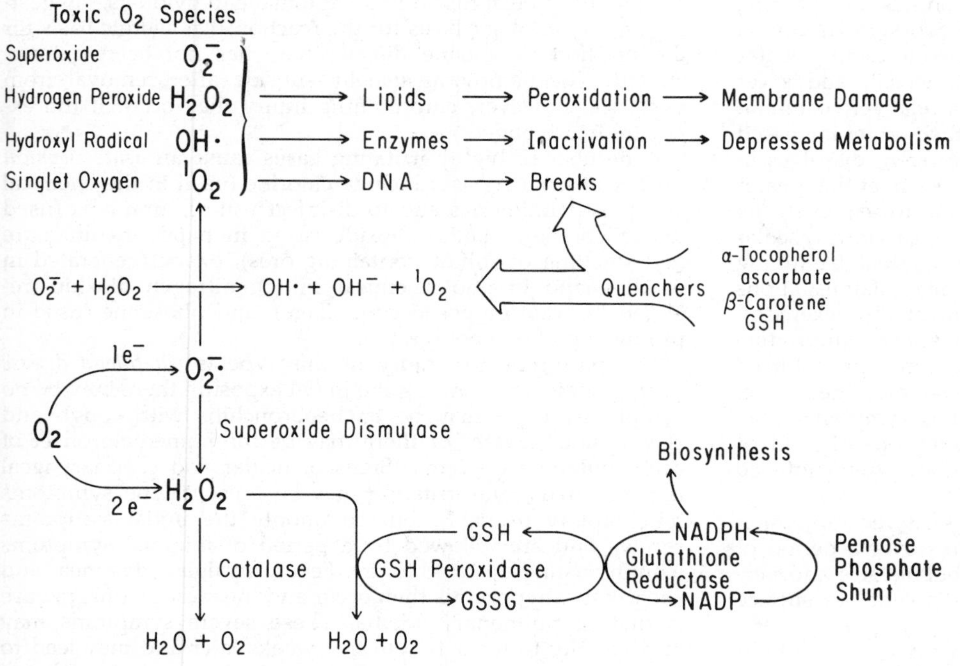

Figure 560–1. Toxic oxygen species and antioxidant defense systems. The incomplete reduction of oxygen produces superoxide and/or hydrogen peroxide. These species can react together in the presence of metal salts to form the hydroxyl radical and singlet oxygen. Free radical chain reactions can be initiated in lipid membranes, with enzymes and DNA also attacked by these reactive O_2 species. Quenchers interact with the oxygen species or with oxidized tissue components to block further tissue oxidation and to terminate free radical chain reactions. The antioxidant defense systems, superoxide dismutase, catalase, and glutathione peroxidase, function to detoxify superoxide and hydrogen peroxide, thus preventing the formation of other toxic O_2 species and the subsequent reactions with tissue. Glucose-6-phosphate dehydrogenase is the rate limiting enzyme in the pentose phosphate shunt and thereby controls the availability of NADPH. This cofactor is essential both for the reduction of glutathione and for the biosynthetic pathways critical for repair processes. Net tissue injury represents the balance between the rate of production of partially reduced oxygen species, the rate at which these species are scavenged, and the rate of repair of any injury that occurs.

to excess oxygen, probably reflecting functional injury of airway epithelium. These patients are therefore more susceptible to mucus impaction and to infection caused by failure to clear inhaled pathogens adequately.

The only proven therapy is prevention of the insult by using high oxygen concentrations judiciously. Corticosteroids have no proven benefit and may actually enhance the lung injury caused by hyperoxia. It is usually impossible clinically to distinguish early oxygen toxicity because of the severity of the original lung insult. The physician often faces a dilemma in which increasing concentrations of oxygen are essential for immediate survival but its administration contributes to deterioration of the patient a short time later. Alternative methods to improve tissue oxygen delivery without using high inspired partial pressures of oxygen should be used whenever possible. These include transfusion of packed red cells to raise the serum hemotocrit to even supranormal levels, measures to improve cardiac output, and measures to decrease the tissue oxygen demand by reducing fever or intense agitation.

The safe maximal concentration of oxygen is not known. Many recommend the range of 40 to 50 per cent oxygen as safe because little injury has been demonstrated in normal animals or human volunteers breathing 40 to 50 per cent oxygen for prolonged periods. The diseased lung may be more susceptible to oxygen injury, however. Rather than identify an arbitrary oxygen concentration that should not be exceeded, rational therapy is to use only enough oxygen to provide adequate arterial blood saturation—an arterial P_{O_2} of 60 torr. Patients should not continuously be given 40 to 50 per cent oxygen under the assumption that this concentration is harmless. If the patient survives oxygen toxicity, some residual damage to the lung parenchyma may remain, with septal fibrosis replacing areas where the pulmonary capillary bed was destroyed by the hyperoxia.

Crapo JD, Barry BE, Foscue HA, Shelburne J: Structural and biochemical changes in rat lungs occurring during exposures to lethal and adaptive doses of oxygen. Am Rev Respir Dis 122:123, 1980. *A detailed description of oxygen-induced injury in experimental animals.*

Deneke SM, Fanburg BL: Normobaric oxygen toxicity of the lung. N Engl J Med 303:76, 1980. *A comprehensive and well-written review.*

Frank L, Massaro D: Oxygen toxicity. Am J Med 69:117, 1980. *A current review with an excellent discussion of current and future studies aimed at modifying oxygen injury.*

Freeman BA, Crapo JD: Free radicals and tissue injury. Lab Invest 47:412, 1982. *A review of the mechanisms of production of free radicals and their role in tissue injury; 173 references.*

Carbon Monoxide Poisoning

Carbon monoxide is commonly produced by internal combustion engines, by poorly vented heating devices, and by gas refrigerators. Lower levels can exist in automobile repair shops, in areas in high automobile traffic density, and in arc welding. Natural gas is free of carbon monoxide, but its incomplete combustion by a faulty heating apparatus can produce carbon monoxide. The most common source of human exposure to carbon monoxide is smoking; cigarette smokers commonly have carboxyhemoglobin concentrations of 3 to 8 per cent. Endogenous carbon monoxide is normally produced from cleavage of the α-methylene bridge in the catabolism of heme, which results in a normal blood carboxyhemoglobin concentration of 0.5 to 0.8 per cent.

Carbon monoxide injures by causing tissue hypoxia. Carbon monoxide has an affinity for hemoglobin which is 218 times greater than that of oxygen. Thus, even small amounts of inspired carbon monoxide will have profound effects on the oxygen-carrying capacity of blood. An alveolar carbon monoxide tension of 0.5 torr and an arterial oxygen tension of 100 torr will produce blood concentrations of 50 per cent carboxyhemoglobin and 50 per cent oxyhemoglobin. In addition, carbon monoxide shifts the oxyhemoglobin saturation curve to the left and changes its shape, resulting in a further decrease in oxygen unloading in tissues.

The clinical picture of carbon monoxide poisoning is dependent upon the blood concentration of carboxyhemoglobin. Levels of less than 10 per cent carboxyhemoglobin produce few clinical

symptoms. At 10 to 30 per cent carboxyhemoglobin, headaches and nausea occur and there may be mild dysfunction of the central nervous system with decreased visual acuity and impaired cognitive functions. Thirty to 40 per cent carboxyhemoglobin is associated with severe headaches, dyspnea on exertion, dizziness, nausea, vomiting, dimness of vision, ataxia, and possible collapse. Levels greater than 50 per cent carboxyhemoglobin cause tachypnea, convulsions, coma, and death from profound shock and respiratory and cardiovascular failure.

The diagnosis is confirmed by the determination of blood carboxyhemoglobin concentration. Carboxyhemoglobin has a characteristic cherry red color which can produce the classic bright red skin color in patients poisoned by carbon monoxide. This is in fact rare during life and is seen most often after death.

TREATMENT. The patient must be immediately removed from the contaminated environment. The specific therapy is administration of oxygen. Breathing normal air will result in a 50 per cent clearance of blood carbon monoxide in approximately five hours. Administration of 100 per cent oxygen at sea level will achieve a 50 per cent reduction of carboxyhemoglobin in 80 minutes, whereas oxygen at 3 atmospheres of pressure will achieve the same clearance in approximately 25 minutes. The use of 95 per cent oxygen–5 per cent carbon dioxide will hasten oxygenation, largely by lowering the pH (Bohr effect). In the acutely ill patient the presence of metabolic acidosis is a contraindication to further reductions in pH by administration of carbon dioxide. The level of carboxyhemoglobin is not the sole determinant of the need for therapy. Patients with neurologic abnormalities should be considered for treatment with hyperbaric oxygen even if carboxyhemoglobin levels are low.

Patients who do not become comatose usually recover without permanent sequelae. Among those who survive more severe intoxication, some have residual neurologic symptoms such as seizures, dysphasia, parkinsonism, or mental impairment. Some resolution of neurologic symptoms will occur over a period of weeks, and maximal recovery should be expected within two years of the acute episode.

Dinman BD: The management of acute carbon monoxide intoxication. J Occup Med 16:662, 1974. *A good clinical review.*

Jackson DL: Accidental carbon monoxide poisoning. JAMA 243:772, 1980. *A brief review of the effects and treatment of carbon monoxide poisoning.*

Unsworth IP: Acute carbon monoxide poisoning. Anaesth Intens Care 2:329, 1974. *A good discussion of the management of patients with carbon monoxide toxicity.*

ASPIRATION-RELATED INJURIES

Injury to the respiratory system by aspiration can be categorized by the nature of the aspirate: (1) *Infectious material.* Contamination of the lungs by aspiration of oropharyngeal bacterial flora is discussed in Ch. 63. (2) *Toxic or inflammatory substances.* Aspiration of gastric acid is the most commonly occurring example in an adult population; hydrocarbon aspiration occurs predominantly in children but is encountered in adults. Both these injuries can cause fulminant illness. By contrast, lipids (mineral oil, vegetable and animal fats) most often provoke a chronic inflammatory reaction. (3) *Inert matter.* The injury of drowning is predominantly secondary to asphyxia. Food particles can cause a fibrotic, granulomatous lesion or, if large enough to occlude the larynx or trachea, sudden death by asphyxiation ("café coronary").

Aspiration Pneumonitis

Aspiration pneumonitis refers to the caustic injury to the respiratory system caused by gastric acid. This is in contrast to "aspiration pneumonia," an infectious process caused by the contamination of the tracheobronchial tree by oropharyngeal flora. Aspiration of gastric acid can occur during vomiting or during regurgitation, and in the latter instance the event may go unnoted—i.e., "silent aspiration." The normal protective mechanisms of the upper airway include epiglottic closure during deglutition, glottic closure on contact with solids or fluids, the cough reflex, and the esophageal sphincters. Altered states of consciousness, anesthesia and surgery, neuromuscular disease, gastrointestinal disease, and medical devices (nasogastric tubes or uncuffed tracheostomy tubes) impair these defenses. The use of low pressure, high volume cuffs on endotracheal tubes serves to reduce the high incidence of aspiration of gastric contents in patients with predisposing disorders.

The main factors determining the extent of illness caused by gastric acid aspiration are as follows: (1) *pH of the aspirate.* The acidity of the material is the most important cause of lung injury, with a critical pH ≤ 2.5 inducing severe pneumonitis from acid aspiration. (2) *The presence of food particles.* Aspiration of gastric foodstuff has been shown to cause a severe pneumonitis and peribronchial inflammatory reaction in the absence of a low pH. (3) *Volume of the aspirate.* Aspiration of more than 0.4 ml per kilogram of body weight of gastric acid is sufficient to cause pneumonitis. (4) *Distribution of the aspirate.* Many patients who aspirate immediately begin to cough, which may expel the aspirate and thereby partially protect the lung from injury or may enhance dispersion of the acid over a greater area and turn a potentially localized lesion into a diffuse one. (5) *Contamination of the gastric contents with fecal matter,* as in intestinal obstruction. Such a soiling of the tracheobronchial tree is associated with a marked increase in mortality, but death presumably ensues from infection, not from acid injury.

PATHOPHYSIOLOGY. After intratracheal instillation, acid is rapidly distributed in the lungs, and can reach the pleura in 12 to 18 seconds. It is rapidly neutralized by bronchial secretions; in less than 30 minutes the pH at the bronchial surface will have returned to normal. The acid causes a chemical burn of the bronchi, bronchioles, and alveolar walls, with subsequent exudation of fluid into the lungs. Plasma volume may decrease by as much as 35 per cent in severe injury without fluid replacement, and cardiac output and systemic arterial blood pressure may fall. Pulmonary capillary wedge pressure is normal or low, indicating a nonhydrostatic cause of the pulmonary edema. The characteristics of phospholipids in the alveolar surface lining layer (surfactant) are altered, causing increased surface forces, and promoting early airway and alveolar closure. Lung compliance decreases secondary to the increase in interstitial fluids and the alteration of surface forces. These disturbances of airways, alveoli, and vascular elements cause profound imbalance of the normal ventilation-perfusion relationships. Hypoxemia is invariably present and usually severe. Increased right-to-left shunting is commonly present.

CLINICAL MANIFESTATIONS. Some patients aspirate a large volume of gastric acid and almost immediately become apneic and hypotensive and die. More commonly a patient aspirates stomach contents and, with various amounts of coughing, survives the initial crisis, but later develops a fulminant illness marked by dyspnea, cough, and pink, frothy sputum. Alternatively aspiration may be secondary to regurgitation and not accompanied by immediate coughing and agitation. With this so-called silent aspiration the patient presents with acute respiratory failure but with no obvious reason for the precipitous deterioration in function. Within two to five hours after aspiration of gastric acid, tachypnea, rales, and rhonchi occur, and wheezing, cyanosis, and hypotension may be present. Fever of 38 to 39° C in the first 36 hours occurs in about 50 per cent of patients.

Laboratory tests are nonspecific. A moderate leukocytosis with left shift develops early. Arterial blood gases, the best variable to follow, show hypoxemia, and the arterial oxygen tension does not reach predicted levels after the patient has been breathing 100 per cent oxygen for several minutes, indicating increased right-to-left shunting of blood. The arterial P_{CO_2} may be slightly elevated, normal, or mildly reduced, and pH will vary reciprocally. Abnormalities on chest roentgenograms are extremely variable, and there is no characteristic pattern. Extent of radiographic abnormalities does not correlate with clinical outcome. Although the distribution of the acid in some cases is preferentially to areas dependent at the time of aspiration, frequently the abnormalities are diffuse, presumably from enhanced dispersion of the acid during coughing. On radiographs taken early in the course, the majority of patients have perihilar or basilar infiltrates, usually bilateral or multicentric, with bilaterally symmetrical infiltrates in only about 40 per cent of cases. Pleural effusions and cavitation of infiltrates are not seen in uncomplicated cases. Bronchoscopic findings are diagnostic if food particles or gastric debris is seen in the trachea or bronchi. Subsegmental mucosal erythema in a suspected case is a supportive but not diagnostic finding.

The key to the accurate diagnosis of aspiration pneumonitis is a high index of suspicion for this entity in any patient with an abrupt respiratory deterioration, especially a patient with a condition that places him at increased risk of gastric acid aspiration. The differential diagnosis includes cardiogenic pulmonary edema, pulmonary embolus, bacterial pneumonia, and many of the causes of the adult respiratory distress syndrome such as sepsis, hypotension, amniotic fluid embolism, and increased intracranial pressure.

TREATMENT. Treatment of the individual whose aspiration was witnessed begins with the prompt establishment of an adequate airway. The airway should be suctioned to remove any particulate matter. A single lavage of 10 ml of saline may be used; larger volumes have been shown to increase the extent of injury in rabbits. Intratracheal instillation of sodium bicarbonate or of steroids is of no value.

General supportive measures include fluid replacement with crystalloid or colloid solution. Supplemental oxygen is given to maintain $Pa_{O_2} > 60$ torr. Bronchodilators (intravenous aminophylline) may help. Associated pulmonary edema is not cardiogenic in origin and is usually associated with intravascular volume depletion. Therefore, there is no place for the routine use of digitalis or diuretics.

Antibiotics should not be used prophylactically for acid aspiration since they do not reduce morbidity or mortality and they increase the risk of subsequent infection with a resistant organism. The acid-damaged respiratory tract has an increased susceptibility to bacterial infection. In a patient who has been improving after aspiration, new deterioration, especially after the first three days, with increasing fever, leukocytosis, worsening hypoxemia, new infiltrates on chest x-ray, and the production of purulent sputum is suggestive of a secondary bacterial pneumonia. Management of the patient who has aspirated gastric contents that had been contaminated with fecal matter would include the early use of antibiotics providing activity against anaerobes and gram-negative organisms.

The role of systemic corticosteroids in aspiration pneumonitis is controversial. There have been no controlled human trials. Early anecdotal reports supported their use, but more recent retrospective and prospective but uncontrolled series totaling approximately 250 patients have failed to show any improvement in morbidity or mortality.

Positive-pressure ventilation is helpful, particularly when it is initiated early after the aspiration. Arterial oxygen tensions improve and mortality rates decrease with its use. Positive end-expiratory pressure (PEEP) to improve oxygenation has been beneficial in other forms of adult respiratory distress syndrome and is commonly used in the management of gastric acid aspiration. Caution should be used in applying PEEP, since in the acid-injured lung a marked increase in lung extravascular water content can occur, especially if PEEP >15 cm water is applied.

Aspiration pneumonitis carries a high mortality rate despite treatment, and because it largely occurs in a defined population at increased risk, efforts should be made at prevention. Elevation of the head of the bed will retard regurgitation. In intubated patients placement of a nasogastric tube to keep the stomach decompressed should be considered. Aspiration may occur even in the presence of a cuffed endotracheal tube. Elective general anesthesia should be given with the stomach empty, after at least a 12-hour fast. If anesthesia must be undertaken with a full stomach, consideration should be given to rapid induction and intubation while employing cricoid pressure. In recognition of the critical role of the degree of acidity of the aspirate, the pH of gastric contents can be raised by a single dose of cimetidine (300 to 400 mg orally two to four hours before surgery, given with minimal water) or by a single 10 ml dose orally of antacid, best given after premedication.

OUTCOME. Mortality from aspiration pneumonitis is high, reaching 28 to 62 per cent of cases. Factors associated with highest risk of death are age greater than 50 years, the early development of shock or apnea, severe and prolonged hypoxemia, pH of gastric contents $\leq$ 1.75 at the time of aspiration, and the development of secondary bacterial pneumonia. Most but not all survive the early moments. After the initial deterioration (24 to 36 hours), some then show steady improvement, with radiographic resolution within a week. Some have a second episode of deterioration, an event which should suggest a new problem such as bacterial infection, pulmonary embolism, heart failure, or another aspiration. Still others pursue a relentlessly worsening course to death. Few data exist regarding long-term clinical follow-up, but it is thought that pulmonary fibrosis of varying degrees ensues in some of these patients.

Newman GE, Effman EL, Putman CE: Pulmonary aspiration complexes in adults. Curr Prob Diagn Radiol 11(4):1–47, 1982. *A thorough review of the mechanisms, diagnosis, and treatment of aspiration; 65 references.*

Schwartz, DJ, Wynne JW, Gibbs CP, Hood CI, Kuck EJ: The pulmonary consequences of aspiration of gastric contents at pH values greater than 2.5. Am Rev Respir Dis 121:119, 1980. *Aspiration of gastric food particles will cause a severe pneumonitis in dogs even when the pH is 5.9.*

Drowning

Drowning accounts for about 7000 deaths annually in the United States, mostly in children and young adults. It is one of the three leading causes of accidental death. Pathophysiologically, drowning can be of four types: (1) *"Wet" drowning*—initial laryngospasm but early relaxation and subsequent aspiration of copious amounts of fluid. The majority of drownings are of this sort. (2) *"Secondary" drowning*—death occurs 15 minutes to 72 hours after extraction from the water, and is due to a form of adult respiratory distress syndrome. (3) *"Dry" drowning*—asphyxiation secondary to intense glottic spasm which persists beyond the point of apnea, so that when the muscles relax, no water is aspirated. This accounts for 10 to 20 per cent of drownings. (4) *Immersion syndrome*—cardiac arrest secondary to the intense parasympathetic discharge of the diving reflex.

The most important consequences of near-drowning are severe hypoxemia and metabolic acidosis. The difference between fresh water and salt water near-drowning appears to be of little significance. Life-threatening electrolyte disturbances caused by water aspiration in humans are rare, and the salt content of the aspirate is relatively unimportant. Hypoxemia is caused by occlusion of airways with fluid and particulate debris in the water, by changes in surfactant activity, by direct injury to the alveolar septa, and by bronchospasm. There is a marked increase in right-to-left shunting and an increase in physiologic dead space. Severe metabolic acidosis develops in most cases, presumably secondary to anaerobic metabolism in the asphyxiating victim, especially with the violent struggling that normally occurs. Cardiac arrhythmias, conduction disturbances, and central nervous system injury can occur in this setting. Cerebral edema is far more common than actual brain infarction.

Autopsies of drowned persons demonstrate wet, heavy lungs with varying amounts of hemorrhage and edema and some disruption of alveolar walls. In about 70 per cent, vomitus, sand, mud, and aquatic vegetation have been aspirated. Specimens from victims dying from "secondary drowning" show desquamation of alveolar epithelial cells, hemorrhage, hyaline membrane formation, acute inflammatory infiltrates, and foreign body reactions to particulate matter. Cerebral necrosis and edema are seen; changes of acute tubular necrosis are found sometimes in the kidneys.

CLINICAL MANIFESTATIONS, TREATMENT, AND OUTCOME OF NEAR-DROWNING. The initial appearance of the patient can vary widely, from coma to agitated alertness. Cyanosis, coughing, and the production of frothy pink sputum are common. Tachypnea, tachycardia, and a low grade fever in the first few hours are seen if the patient did not become hypothermic during submersion. Rales, rhonchi, and, less often, wheezes are heard. Neurologic signs vary between patients and can fluctuate in any given patient but usually derive from bihemispheric cerebral dysfunction. Signs of associated trauma should be sought.

Laboratory studies reveal mild hypokalemia, hypernatremia, and hyperchloremia, none of life-threatening magnitude. There may be a moderate leukocytosis. Hematocrit (Hct) and hemoglobin usually are normal on first measurement; in fresh water aspiration the Hct sometimes falls slightly in the first 24 hours. An increase in serum free hemoglobin is seen more often, without significant changes in Hct. Rarely the picture of disseminated intravascular coagulation has been reported in near-drowning. Arterial blood gases, usually obtained after preliminary resuscitation, show severe hypoxemia and metabolic acidosis. The most common electrocardiographic changes are sinus tachycardia and nonspecific S-T segment and T wave changes, which revert to normal within hours; however, other, more ominous abnormalities may occur—ventricular arrhythmias, complete heart block, or myocardial infarction. The chest x-ray may be normal initially in spite of severe respiratory disturbances. It often shows patchy infiltrates, and sometimes a classic pulmonary edema pattern is seen.

Treatment of the near-drowning victim begins with the establishment of an adequate airway and, if necessary, emergency cardiopulmonary resuscitation. Oxygen in high concentrations is necessary, since hypoxemia is present in essentially all victims. Even the patient who quickly becomes apparently normal should be hospitalized for 24 hours to watch for a subsequent picture of adult respiratory distress syndrome. During transportation to a hospital, supplemental oxygen should be continued, and precautions taken for potential cervical spine injury and other critical trauma.

In the hospital, subsequent therapy is dictated largely by the arterial blood gases and the degree of respiratory failure. Continuous positive airway pressure or PEEP is particularly helpful. Prophylactic antibiotics have not been shown to be beneficial. The use of corticosteroids for the pulmonary lesions of near-drowning remains controversial, and there have been no controlled prospective human studies of that therapy; animal models and retrospective studies in man have failed to demonstrate any benefit.

If there is evidence of cerebral edema, intracranial pressure (ICP) monitoring can be used to guide therapy. In the event of increased ICP, PEEP should be minimized, since it increases ICP. Hyperventilation to maintain a Pa_{CO_2} of 25 to 30 torr will decrease cerebral blood flow and ICP. Mannitol or glycerol should be used. Corticosteroids (e.g., dexamethasone, 16 mg intravenously initially, then 4 mg intravenously every four hours) are beneficial for the central nervous system injury. Seizures, shivering, or random nonpurposeful movements can increase ICP and should be aborted with pancuronium bromide. If these maneuvers fail to lower ICP, then barbiturates (e.g., pentobarbital, 3 mg per kilogram) every hour intravenously to obtain a serum level of 2.5 to 4 mg per deciliter can be tried.

Outcome in near-drowning is best judged by the neurologic status. The shorter the interval between extraction from the water to first spontaneous gasp, the better the prognosis for recovery without chronic neurologic sequelae, which include mental subnormality, minimal brain dysfunction, spastic quadriplegia, extrapyramidal syndromes, optic and cerebral atrophy, and peripheral neuromuscular damage. Between 5 and 20 per cent of children who survive near-drowning have such residual deficits. Survival without neurologic damage is better in children who are hypothermic when recovered, and occurs even after 40 minutes of submersion. Similar information regarding adults is lacking.

Conn AW, Edmonds JF, Barber GA: Near-drowning in cold fresh water: Current treatment regimen. Can Anaesth Soc J 25:259, 1978. *This paper describes a treatment protocol designed to minimize brain edema, including deliberate hypothermia, hyperventilation, muscle paralysis, barbiturates, and corticosteroids.*

Hoff BH: Multisystem failure: A review with special reference to drowning. Crit Care Med 7:310, 1979. *An excellent, thoroughly complete review of the evaluation and care of the nearly drowned patient with attention to all critical organ systems.*

Modell JH, Graves SA, Ketover A: Clinical course of 91 consecutive near-drowning victims. Chest 70:231, 1976. *Clinical details from this study refute the importance of a distinction between fresh vs. salt water immersion and provide guidelines for assessment.*

Redding JS: Drowning and near drowning. Can the victim be saved? Postgrad Med 74:85, 1983. *A review of current therapy.*

Hydrocarbon Pneumonitis

Hydrocarbon pneumonitis results from the direct toxic effects of volatile hydrocarbons on the respiratory epithelium and vasculature. It occurs in individuals who have ingested the hydrocarbons, but results almost exclusively from aspiration into the respiratory tract rather than from absorption from the gastrointestinal tract and systemic distribution. It does not occur from "sniffing" the compounds. The problem occurs most often in children, particularly below the age of five years, in whom it is usually accidental. It is an uncommon problem in adults, occurring most often in industrial accidents, in patients attempting suicide, in siphoning of gasoline, and in uninformed alcoholics seeking an ethanol substitute.

Different hydrocarbons cause respiratory injury of varying extent, the critical parameters being the viscosity and volume of the aspirate. The lower the viscosity or the larger the volume, the worse the lesion. Being lipid solvents, all these compounds are directly toxic to respiratory tissues. The lungs of children dying from hydrocarbon pneumonitis demonstrate hemorrhage, pulmonary edema, atelectasis, hyaline membrane formation, and necrosis of airway epithelium and alveolar septa. In animal models the acute inflammation begins to resolve by the third day, and is followed by a proliferative response of alveolar lining cells, an increase in intra-alveolar macrophages, and a mononuclear cell infiltration in perivascular and peribronchiolar tissues. By six weeks there is partial clearing of these changes, although the alveolar walls remain thickened. These compounds have systemic toxicity, and in fatal cases degenerative changes in the liver and kidneys have been seen.

CLINICAL MANIFESTATIONS. Aspiration usually occurs at the time of hydrocarbon ingestion. There may be choking and coughing, with a burning sensation in the mouth and throat. A history of vomiting after hydrocarbon ingestion is obtained in less than half the patients. Dyspnea, tachypnea, tachycardia, and high fever quickly ensue. Sputum may be bloody. Lethargy is common, but more severe disturbances of consciousness such as confusion, coma, and seizures also occur. Auscultation is frequently normal, but rales and rhonchi may be present.

The chest radiograph is particularly helpful, since even before auscultation becomes abnormal, infiltrates frequently occur, developing as quickly as 20 to 30 minutes after aspiration of some types of hydrocarbons but later in others. The distribution of the multiple, fluffy, ill-defined infiltrates is preferentially in the dependent areas of the lungs, predominantly on the right side, but occurs bilaterally in about one fourth of cases. Some patients present a picture of bilateral perihilar infiltrates, a "pulmonary edema" pattern. Pleural effusions, pneumothorax, and pneumomediastinum occur but are uncommon. Pneumatoceles can form later, especially in children.

Laboratory tests give nonspecific results. A moderate leukocytosis with left shift is common. Arterial hypoxemia of various degrees develops owing to shunting and to ventilation-perfusion mismatching.

The differential diagnosis is that of respiratory distress of abrupt onset, frequently in a patient with an impaired sensorium at the time of presentation. In the adult this is often an alcoholic. Gastric acid aspiration, an intracranial catastrophe, cardiogenic pulmonary edema, pulmonary embolism, and acute bacterial pneumonia can all present similarly. The correct diagnosis requires the history of hydrocarbon ingestion or aspiration. The diagnosis is also suggested by the odor of the patient's breath and by extensive radiographic abnormalities in a patient with a clear chest by auscultation.

TREATMENT. Emesis to remove residual hydrocarbons is contraindicated. Gastric lavage by nasogastric tube may induce vomiting and should be performed only in the patient who has ingested a large volume of hydrocarbons and then only after placement of a cuffed endotracheal tube. Supplemental oxygen should be given to maintain Pa_{O_2} >60 torr. Mechanical ventilation and PEEP may be necessary. There are no data to show that the routine use of antibiotics modifies the course. The use of systemic corticosteroids is supported by anecdotal reports of improvement after their use in children and adults. Prednisone, 1 mg per kilogram per day, or its equivalent should be used during the acute illness, with termination as the patient improves.

OUTCOME. Hydrocarbon pneumonitis in adults is rare, so that morbidity and mortality estimates are not available. In children death occurs in as many as 10 per cent of cases, but most children have a prompt clinical recovery. Bronchiectasis, recurrent bronchitis, and/or pulmonary fibrosis ensue in an unknown portion of cases. After recovery from the initial illness, children frequently are asymptomatic and have normal chest examinations and radiographs. However, pulmonary function abnormalities suggestive of small airway (<2 mm diameter) disease have been found in asymptomatic patients as late as 8 to 14 years after the hydrocarbon pneumonitis.

Gurwitz D, Kattan M, Levison H, Culham JAG: Pulmonary function abnormalities in asymptomatic children after hydrocarbon pneumonitis. Pediatrics 62:789, 1978. *This study of 17 children several years after hydrocarbon pneumonitis demonstrated obstructive changes in small airways that may predispose to later clinically important respiratory diseases.*

Lipoid Pneumonia

Lipoid pneumonia is a chronic inflammatory reaction of the lungs that results from the aspiration of vegetable, animal, or most commonly mineral oils. This material differs greatly from the excessive accumulation of endogenous lipids in the lungs occurring in fat embolism, cholesterol pneumonitis, pulmonary alveolar proteinosis, and the lipid storage diseases.

The most frequently implicated agent is a mineral oil, which is used as a laxative and to reduce dysphagia, either in clear liquid form or as petroleum jelly. Mineral oil is bland and when introduced into the pharynx can enter the bronchial tree without eliciting the cough reflex. It also mechanically impedes the ciliary action of the airway epithelium. Risk of mineral oil aspiration is increased in the debilitated or senile patient, in those having neurologic disease that interferes with deglutition, and in patients with esophageal disease. Mineral oil taken as nose drops to relieve nasal dryness has caused lipoid pneumonia, and in earlier years was a frequent cause of the illness. Smoking blackfat tobacco, a Kentucky tobacco to which mineral oils are added for flavoring and as humectants, has caused lipoid pneumonia. Inhalation of mineral oil mists by airplane and automobile mechanics has been implicated as a cause of the problem. Aspiration of vegetable (e.g., castor, olive) or animal (e.g., cod liver oil, milk, butter, egg yolk) fats has been an infrequent cause.

Mineral oils, which are relatively inert, cannot be hydrolyzed in the body and provoke a chronic inflammatory reaction which may not become clinically overt until years later. The fat is emulsified in the alveolar spaces, where macrophages accumulate and phagocytize it. Some macrophages disintegrate, releasing their lysosomal enzymes and fat. The alveolar septa become thickened and edematous, containing lymphocytes and lipid-laden macrophages. Oil droplets are seen in the pulmonary lymphatics and hilar nodes. Later, fibrosis develops and the normal lung architecture is effaced. It is usual in a single specimen to find both the early inflammatory and the later fibrotic picture, in keeping with repetitive aspirations over many months or years. If nodular, the lesion may grossly resemble tumor and is called a paraffinoma.

CLINICAL MANIFESTATIONS, DIAGNOSIS, AND TREATMENT. Most patients are asymptomatic, coming to a physician's attention because of an abnormal chest radiograph, or the lesion is found unexpectedly at autopsy. When patients are symptomatic, the complaints are nonspecific, with cough and exertional dyspnea being the most frequent. Chest pain (sometimes pleuritic), hemoptysis, fever (usually low grade), chills, night sweats, and weight loss may occur. The physical examination may be completely normal, or fever, tachypnea, dullness on percussion of the chest, bronchial or bronchovesicular breath sounds, rales, and rhonchi may be found. Clubbing is rare. Cor pulmonale uncommonly develops.

The erythrocyte sedimentation rate may be prolonged. In mild lipoid pneumonia arterial blood gases may be normal at rest but show hypoxemia after exercise. In more severe disease, resting hypoxemia, hypocapnia, and mild respiratory alkalosis develop. Pulmonary function testing reveals a restrictive ventilatory defect; static compliance of the lungs is decreased. The only specific laboratory finding is the presence in sputum of macrophages with clusters of vacuoles 5 to 50 μ in diameter that stain deep orange with Sudan IV, and extracellular droplets that similarly stain.

Radiographically, the earliest abnormalities are air space infiltrates, unilateral or bilateral, localized or diffuse, but most often in the dependent portions of the right lung. Air bronchograms may be seen. Hilar adenopathy and pleural reaction are rare. As fibrosis develops, there is volume loss and the appearance of linear and nodular infiltrates. A solid lesion may develop which closely resembles bronchogenic carcinoma.

The differential diagnosis is extensive, particularly in the late phase when multiple other causes of pulmonary fibrosis must be considered. Sarcoidosis, mycobacterial and fungal infection, chronic hypersensitivity pneumonitis, primary lung carcinoma, bronchiectasis, pneumoconiosis, pulmonary alveolar proteinosis, and pulmonary hemosiderosis are some of the major diseases that are a part of the differential diagnosis. The key to the correct diagnosis before biopsy is the history of chronic use of an oil or a lipid-based product, orally or intranasally, or an occupational exposure to oil mists. The presence of lipid-laden macrophages in the sputum confirms the diagnostic impression.

Once the diagnosis has been made and the aspiration stopped, the subsequent course is variable. Some patients will have no change in symptoms. Others will have improvement in some or all parameters, whereas a few patients continue to deteriorate with worsening pulmonary function and cor pulmonale.

Discontinuation of the use of the offending lipid is essential. Since the only way the body can dispose of mineral oil is by expectoration, the patient should be instructed in coughing exercises to be performed many times each day for months. Expectorants have not been shown to help. Systemic corticosteroids are recommended by some: prednisone, 40 mg orally each day at the beginning and then decreased to 10 mg daily until stabilization of clinical and radiographic signs (which might involve months of therapy). The use of steroids has been based on improvements seen in a very few patients in uncontrolled, anecdotal trials. The rationale has been that the cellular reaction, rather than the oil itself, is the destructive factor. Because of the well-recognized side effects from prolonged use of systemic corticosteroids, their use for lipoid pneumonia should be limited to those patients who have significant symptoms, and then for as brief a period as possible, to "buy time" while decreasing the lipid burden by expectoration.

Blöndal T, Hartvig P, Bengtsson A, Wilander E: An unnecessary case of paraffin oil pneumonia. Acta Med Scand 213:227, 1983. *The problems in diagnosis of mineral oil pneumonia are illustrated in a current case report.*

Heckers H, Melchar FW, Dittmar K, Knorpp K, Nekarda K: Long-term course of mineral oil pneumonia. Lung 155:101, 1978. *This case report documents persistence of oil in expectorated sputum for months after stopping the oil use and the sequential improvement in physiologic parameters.*

561. OCCUPATIONAL DISEASES OF THE SKIN

Edward A. Emmett

Occupational skin diseases are a group of heterogeneous conditions that share a common occupational etiology. They account for about one half of reported occupational disease in the United States. Occupational contact dermatitis, the prototypical disorder, makes up about 95 per cent of all occupational skin disease; infections, about 2.5 per cent; and a large number of different, infrequent diseases, the remainder. The relative frequency of each of these diseases in any location depends largely on the pattern of industrialization.

Almost all occupational skin disease is due to external contact with chemical, physical, and biologic agents. The cause is often multifactorial. In relatively few instances are systemically (rather than locally) absorbed agents responsible.

OCCUPATIONAL CONTACT DERMATITIS

DEFINITION. Occupational contact dermatitis is an erythematous or eczematous response of the skin as a result of local contact with one or more irritating, allergenic, or photosensitizing chemical agents.

ETIOLOGY. Many chemicals from a wide variety of classes—alkalies, acids, volatile organic solvents, metallic salts, organic prepolymers, and many others—are capable of inducing contact dermatitis. The cause is often multifactorial; in addition to one or more chemicals, friction, abrasion, changes in temperature and humidity, and ultraviolet radiation may play a role. Superinfection may occur. Severe and persistent occupational contact dermatitis is more frequent in those with an atopic diathesis.

INCIDENCE AND PREVALENCE. Workers' compensation reports put the incidence in the United States at about 1.4 per 1000 full-time workers per year, although, because of substantial under-reporting, the true incidence is estimated to be from 10 to 50 times higher.

EPIDEMIOLOGY. The incidence of occupational contact dermatitis is generally highest in the agricultural and manufacturing industries. The highest risks occur in poultry dressing plants, meat packing plants, fabrication of rubber products, leather tanning and finishing, manufacture of ophthalmic goods, plating and polishing, production of frozen fruits and vegetables, internal combustion engine manufacture, machining operations, and in canning and curing of seafoods, but virtually no industry is immune.

PATHOGENESIS. Contact dermatitis may result from direct local irritation, cell-mediated immune reactions, or photosensitivity.

Direct local irritation may be immediate, as in irritation from strong acids or alkalies, or may be delayed and occur only after repeated or prolonged local application as cumulative insult dermatitis. The latter can occur from one or more relatively mildly irritating substances that are termed marginal irritants.

Allergic contact dermatitis occurs as a result of sensitization to specific haptens through a process of cell-mediated immunity. The hapten combines with protein in the skin to form a complete antigen that is processed and presented to T lymphocytes by epidermal Langerhans cells, specialized macrophages that form an intraepidermal network. Among the most frequent allergens are poison ivy/oak; rubber additives, particularly accelerators and antioxidants; monomers of plastics and resins, such as epoxies, acrylates, and diisocyanates; nickel, chromium salts; paraphenylenediamine and derivatives; and formaldehyde. There are many more possible allergens; the number of substances reported to cause allergic contact dermatitis is very large.

Chemical photosensitivity results from the photochemical excitation of an ultraviolet (UV)-absorbing molecule with resultant tissue damage. In a photoirritant reaction there is direct damage to cellular components, for example, when psoralens in the presence of long UV bind covalently to DNA. Coal tar pitch, certain aromatic dyes, and UV absorbers used in printing processes also cause photoirritation. In the rarer photoallergic reaction, photochemical alteration of the inciting chemical forms an allergen in the skin, leading to a cell-mediated immune reaction.

A major part of the resistance to environmental chemicals is provided by the epidermal barrier in the stratum corneum. Damage to this barrier by trauma, inflammation, or skin disease or by altering barrier conditions, for example by occlusion, seems to play an important role in the development of contact dermatitis.

CLINICAL MANIFESTATIONS. The clinical presentation is dominated by dermatitis that is confined, at least initially, to the region of contact. The morphology varies according to the concentration and duration of the exposure, the pathogenesis, and individual constitutional differences, although there is much overlap. Acute irritant dermatitis is characterized by erythema (perhaps by edema), papules and vesicles, or in the more extreme instance by one or more large bullae filled with purulent fluid. Postinflammation hyperpigmentation and hypopigmentation may occur; necrosis may leave scars. The cause of acute irritant dermatitis is usually obvious because of the rapidity with which the reaction develops.

Cumulative insult dermatitis may develop only after a long period of contact. On the hands it tends to start under rings or watchbands and to be somewhat patchy in distribution. Individual susceptibility is probably important. Initially, drying and fissuring may be seen with subsequent development of an eczematous response with papules and vesicles. Excoriations and lichenification are frequent if the process persists. Relapse may occur on relatively brief exposure to mild irritants, even when the dermatitis is clinically healed, especially if the epidermal barrier has not yet been reestablished.

Allergic contact dermatitis most often presents as an acute or chronic eczematous reaction with erythema, papules and vesicles, scaling, and pruritus. Characteristically there is a latent period of at least seven to ten days before the development of dermatitis following first exposure to the allergen. Recurrence usually occurs 24 to 72 hours after an eliciting exposure. Certain allergens, for example, epoxy resin monomers, have a tendency to produce severe acute reactions with significant edema.

Localization is important for diagnosis. Over 90 per cent of occupational contact dermatitis involves the hands, sometimes in conjunction with other sites. Where the eruption is due to contact with objects or contaminated surfaces, the pattern of contact will determine localization. Reaction to immersion of the hands in liquids generally involves the dorsum of the hands and palmar aspects of the wrists. Photosensitivity reaction on exposed sites may be distinguished from airborne contact dermatitis by the relative sparing of shaded areas such as the eyelids or behind the ears.

DIAGNOSIS. A good occupational history is the cornerstone of diagnosis. It is most useful to get a description of the worker's daily activities, including nonoccupational activities, with particular attention to contact of the skin with chemicals. The localization of the eruption at its onset, initial appearance of lesions, nature of progression, and circumstances of remissions and recurrences are important to the determination of occupational etiology. A personal or family history or both will confirm the presence of atopy, in which there is increased susceptibility to irritants, changes in heat and humidity, and other factors. A complete examination of the skin will help rule out dermatoses other than contact dermatitis, including id reactions of the hands secondary to dermatophytosis of the feet. Allergic contact dermatitis is confirmed by diagnostic patch testing; photoallergy, by photopatch testing. Patch testing is relatively easy to perform, but the interpretation requires skill. There is no clinically useful confirmatory test for irritant contact dermatitis.

Other information may be necessary to make a precise diagnosis and formulate appropriate management. Toxicity information on industrial compounds can be obtained from Material Safety Data Sheets, which reveal the composition and properties of industrial materials. Recent regulations in the United States make these available to most employees and their physicians. A visit by the physician to the workplace allows the physician to view the work firsthand. If such a visit is made, opportunity for skin contact with hazardous agents should be explored as well as the use of protective measures.

Epidemologic surveys to establish the prevalence of dermatitis in workers at similar jobs and industrial hygiene surveys to characterize the nature and amount of chemical exposure may occasionally be helpful. Public health authorities, university centers for occupational and environmental health, and sometimes concerned employers may be able to assist in such investigations.

TREATMENT. Symptomatic treatment is similar to that for dermatitis of other types. Acute contact dermatitis is treated with cold wet dressings of Burow's solution. Systemic steroids in rapidly tapering doses are indicated in severe acute widespread disabling eruptions; topical steroids and emollients, for dry and chronic eczema. Superinfection requires appropriate systemic antibiotics. Antihistamines may be given for sedation and are mildly antipruritic. The patient should be given careful instruction to avoid casual exposures, and should be alerted to the fact that even when the skin has apparently healed the barrier may not have returned to normal. A temporary or permanent change of job tasks may be necessary. If a permanent job change is necessary, vocational rehabilitation should be considered. Some states require reporting of occupational diseases.

PROGNOSIS. The prognosis of occupational contact dermatitis is surprisingly poor, especially if effective treatment is not given early and if the dermatitis is prolonged. The reasons for this are not entirely clear; however, surveys have shown that a high percentage of individuals still have dermatitis several years later, in many cases despite a change of employment. Those with atopy appear to have the worst prognosis. In allergic contact dermatitis the prognosis is dependent on the ease with which the allergen can be avoided.

PREVENTION. Preventive measures serve both to prevent recurrences and to halt the development of novel disease. These include elimination or substitution for strong irritants and sensitizers; education of workers as to skin care; avoidance of overly harsh skin cleansers; prompt reporting and treatment of dermatitis; engineering controls to minimize skin contact with potential hazards; appropriate impervious protective clothing; good personal hygiene with rapid effective removal of contaminants; and counseling of individuals with predisposing conditions, such as atopy, regarding career selection.

OTHER OCCUPATIONAL DERMATOSES

A relatively large number of other dermatoses can result from occupational exposure. In large part, management is dependent upon diagnostic recognition and on discontinuing further exposures, using measures outlined above.

Chemical burns result from corrosive agents that produce necrosis, ulceration, and subsequent scarring. Prompt removal of these agents (such as strong acids, alkalies, phenol, alkyl metal compounds, and metal chlorides) from skin, eyes, and mucous membranes is essential. Water is generally best for removal; quicklime, tin tetrachloride, and titanium tetrachloride should be removed with mineral oil. Specific antidotes are few; these include topical or injected calcium gluconate for hydrofluoric acid burns.

Urticaria may occur from local contact or systemic absorption with agents that elicit an immediate hypersensitivity reaction or directly release histamine and other vasoactive substances.

Fiberglass dermatitis causes intense pruritus; there may be no visible changes or it may be accompanied by excoriations, pinpoint petechial papules, or both. Microscopy of a cellophane tape stripped from the skin, which had been treated with 10 per cent potassium hydroxide, reveals the fibers.

Relatively deep indolent *ulcers* of skin and mucous membranes result from contact with arsenic, chromates, and lime.

Chemical acne and folliculitis may result from contact with greases and oils, coal tar pitch, creosote, and a number of cosmetics (acne cosmetic) and from ingestion of bromides, iodides, and isoniazid. These forms of acne typically commence with comedones or inflammatory papules.

Chloracne is due to halogenated aromatic compounds with specific molecular shape, including dioxin and related chlorinated aromatic hydrocarbons. The illness is characterized by small straw-colored cysts and comedones that first involve the malar crescent and behind the ear and may not spread beyond these areas. Inflammatory pustules, abscesses, and large cysts may be seen in severe cases. Chloracne is the first and most constant finding in chronic dioxin poisoning. More variable findings may include porphyrinuria, hyperpigmentation, hypertrichosis, central and peripheral nervous system effects, alteration of lipid metabolism, and mild hepatotoxicity. Experimentally observed effects include teratogenicity, immunosuppression, and tumor induction.

Cutaneous granulomas occur as slightly erythematous grouped flesh-colored papules, with or without inflammatory changes, from foreign body reactions at the site of contact with talc and silica or as an immunologic response to beryllium and zirconium.

Chemical leukoderma, which may mimic vitiligo but which is confined to the areas of skin contact, may result from a number of phenols and catechols, including hydroquinone, monobenzyl, and monomethyl ethers of hydroquinone (used as rubber additives) and *p*-tertiary butyl and amyl phenols (in disinfectants).

Basal and squamous cell carcinomas and keratoacanthomas result from prolonged exposures to ultraviolet radiation, ionizing radiation, polycyclic aromatic hydrocarbons (including coal tar pitches and related products), and arsenic. Exposures to arsenic may be associated with various internal malignant neoplasms.

INFECTIONS AND INFESTATIONS

The development of infections and infestations frequently depends on occupational factors, individual susceptibility, and the geographic distribution of the causal organism. Occupational associations include the following:

Viral. Herpes simplex (dentists, medical personnel), milkers' nodules and papular stomatitis (veterinarians, milk handlers), orf (farmers, shepherds, abattoir workers), viral warts (butchers), Rift Valley fever (shepherds).

Bacterial. Staphylococcal infections of hands (abattoir workers and butchers), erysipeloid (fish, fowl, rabbit, and pig handlers), anthrax (wool, hair, and hide handlers), tularemia (farmers), nontuberculous mycobacterial infections (aquarium workers and pet shop attendants). Bacterial and yeast infections and tinea versicolor are prominent with heat, humidity, occlusion, and lack of hygiene.

Fungal. Dermatophyte infections are more frequent in farm workers, surveyors, zoo attendants, animal care technicians, and certain others. Particular examples include tinea verrucosum (farmers); infection due to *Trichophyton rubrum* (miners), *Microsporum canis* (pet shop workers), *Trichophyton violaceum* (wrestlers), and *Candida albicans* (those in wet work, particularly

those in contact with sugar and fruit); sporotrichosis (mine workers); chromomycosis (agricultural workers); and actinomycosis (agricultural workers).

Protozoal. South American leishmaniasis (foresters).

Helminths. Creeping eruption (plumbers, gardeners, farm workers in the tropics), ankylostomiasis (miners), schistosomiasis and cercarial dermatitis (rice planters and canal workers).

In addition, bites and stings of arthropods and other creatures are common in those who work out of doors and in certain other occupations.

Emmett EA: Occupational skin disease. J Allergy Clin Immunol 72:649, 1983. *A brief review of important occupational dermatoses with current references and emphasis on the approach to a patient with suspected occupational skin disease.*

Maibach HI, Gellin GA: Occupational and Industrial Dermatology. Chicago, Yearbook Medical Publishers, 1982. *A multiauthor text that broadly covers occupational dermatoses and dermatotoxicology and describes the skin diseases of a number of specific occupations.*

562. RADIATION INJURY

Theodore L. Phillips

DEFINITIONS

Radiation injury may be defined as any somatic or genetic disruption of function or form caused by electromagnetic waves or accelerated particles. Common sources of such injury include ultraviolet radiation from the sun and man-made sources, microwave radiations from radar and ovens and other appliances, high-intensity ultrasound and ionizing radiations from natural and man-made sources.

Ultraviolet radiation, produced by the sun, is largely absorbed by the atmosphere of the earth. It has very short penetration in tissue and is thus of concern only for exposed body surfaces. It causes injury through direct chemical effects in molecules with high absorbance for the given wavelength. Ultrasound and microwave radiations exert their effects through the generation of heat during absorption.

Radiations with wavelengths shorter than light have an additional property, the ability to displace electrons from their normal orbits with production of charged particles. As these particles traverse tissue, they form ions and free radicals that then react with biologically important molecules, leading to cell injury and death. The ability of the high-energy ray to penetrate and cause large amounts of biologic damage after deposition of small amounts of energy makes it of concern to the physician.

Ionizing radiations, both natural and man made, are of two types: (1) photons or waves and (2) accelerated particles. The *photons* do not cause direct injury but cause damage through the interactions that occur with orbital electrons that become charged particles in tissue. Ionizing photons, called gamma rays, are given off by many types of nuclear decay. Man-made ionizing rays, called x-rays, occur when an accelerated electron is stopped rapidly in a dense material.

Accelerated particles include protons from solar radiation, heavy nuclei in cosmic rays, and beta and alpha particles given up in nuclear decay. These particles are charged and cause direct ionization. Neutrons are also given off in nuclear decay and are found in cosmic radiation. They cause damage through secondary reactions in tissue in which protons are produced, which then cause ionization.

Radiation dose is defined in terms of energy deposition. Previously the unit was the rad, 100 ergs per gram, but it is now the *gray* (abbreviated *Gy*), defined as equal to 100 rads or 1 joule per kilogram. Radioactivity is defined in terms of the rate of decay or disintegration. The *curie,* a unit based on the radioactivity of a gram of radium, is still used, but in the new SI unit system the unit is the *bequerel*. Because radiations differ in the density of the ionization they cause, the biologic effects vary. Densely ionizing radiations, such as heavy particles and neutrons, will have greater biologic effects. Thus the *rem* is a unit used for safety considerations in which a "quality factor" is applied to a quantity similar to a centigray (one hundredth of a gray).

Absorption of charged particles and their range in tissue are determined by their charge and mass. Particles with high charge and mass give up their energy rapidly and penetrate only short distances, unless they are of extremely high energy. Photons are absorbed exponentially by electron or nuclear interactions, and thus some radiation can penetrate long distances. Because photons diverge as they leave the source, the dose will decrease as the square of the distance from the source, as it does for light.

Injury from radiation may be either thermal (dealt with elsewhere in this book) or ionizing. Ionizing radiation injury expressed within a few hours or days is termed acute.

Low radiation doses that do not produce acute or delayed organ dysfunction are termed low level. Such small doses (1 gray or less) can produce genetic and carcinogenic effects in the population and are also of great concern.

ETIOLOGY

BIOLOGY OF ULTRAVIOLET RADIATION. Very short wave light photons are capable of generating chemical changes in DNA and other molecules, the most important of which is the production of pyrimidine dimers. Although they may be excised and repaired, if unrepaired these lesions lead to reproductive cell death and desquamation after skin irradiation. Ultraviolet exposure also causes immediate effects such as vasodilatation and erythema. The short penetration and the absorption by melanin limit human injury to the superficial layers of the skin.

CELLULAR BIOLOGY OF IONIZING RADIATIONS. When the electrons generated by photons or charged particles traverse a cell they cause the formation of ion pairs in both cell water and the DNA. During such events, radicals are formed with unpaired outer electrons. These radicals react with DNA or occur in the DNA itself. A radical may be repaired by reduction with SH groups or fixed by oxidation or electron transfer. If a free radical persists, it leads to a break in the DNA molecule. Single-strand breaks are generally repaired, but if two occur side by side a double-strand break occurs. Unrepaired double-strand breaks lead to chromosome aberrations that can be lethal to the cell or cause mutations and carcinogenesis.

Chromosome injury is expressed at the time of cell division. Most mammalian cells die of mitotic death. Deletions and dicentric chromosomes lead to loss of genetic information at each cell division. Some cells survive a few divisions but will be incapable of sustained reproduction. Intermitotic death occurs in some lymphocytes and gonadal cells, even after low radiation doses, but most cells will survive 10 to 30 Gy with no obvious damage until mitosis occurs. Intermitotic death is poorly understood but may be related to interference with RNA synthesis in cells with scant cytoplasmic organelles.

DOSE-RESPONSE RELATIONSHIPS. The percentage of cells that will survive after exposure to ionizing radiation decreases logarithmically with dose. There are two components to the injury, reparable and irreparable. Low-level effects are generally less than one would expect based on observations at high doses. Cells can repair radiation damage very effectively. Repair is primarily of single- and double-strand DNA breaks and requires only a few hours to complete.

The radiation dose required to reduce survival to 10 per cent is quite uniform in mammalian cells. The most sensitive cells require 1 Gy (100 rads) to reduce survival to 10 per cent and the most resistant about 3 Gy. Changes in sensitivity by a factor of 3 occur under hypoxia and as cells traverse the mitotic cycle.

INCIDENCE AND PREVALENCE

BACKGROUND RADIATION. Both ionizing and ultraviolet radiations are ubiquitous in the universe because of the fusion processes in stars. Gamma rays, x-rays, and highly energetic particles are emitted by stars and by nuclear decay of isotopes produced by stellar processes. On the earth, radiation comes from isotopes in the ground and construction materials and from the sun and other sources in space. The dose of radiation that one receives from this natural radiation depends on the altitude and the geologic nature of the region. Most people receive annually between 40 and 90 units known as millirems, which are one hundred thousandth of a Gy. Frequent flights at high altitude can cause a large increase in this dose. Such exposures do not cause clinically detectable syndromes, but may add to the incidence of genetic diseases and cancer.

MEDICAL EXPOSURE. Shortly after the discovery of x-rays by Röntgen in 1895 and the subsequent discovery of radioactivity, the first medical injuries occurred. The early workers were unaware of the cell-killing properties of the rays until damage to hands, eyes, and bone marrow was evident. After World War II the full hazards of radiation exposure were recognized, and exposures were strictly limited. Currently injury of the acute and chronic types is rare after medical exposure of personnel, but is of course a major side effect of radiation therapy.

Radiation is used in the treatment of 50 to 60 per cent of patients with malignant disease, and thus 300,000 to 400,000 patients are exposed and will be seen annually by general physicians as well as radiation oncologists. Although every precaution is taken to avoid clinically important late or delayed effects, acute reactions to radiation therapy are common. Since most tumors require doses for cure close to organ tolerance, the risk of injury is always present.

Injury due to inadvertent or accidental exposure of medical radiation workers is uncommon, but occasional cases will be seen either to the whole body or to hands or face during equipment repair or operational accidents. Workers and patients, as well as the general public, are also exposed to low-level radiation either while obtaining diagnostic studies or working in medical radiation environments. Permissible exposures have been reduced to 5 rem for workers and 500 millirem annually for the public, with half that exposure highly recommended. These rules keep medical exposure to the population as a whole to less than half the background level.

INDUSTRIAL AND MILITARY EXPOSURE. High-level radiation to the largest populations occurred at the Hiroshima and Nagasaki fission weapon explosions in World War II. Although most casualties were due to blast and burns, 40 to 50 per cent of the survivors had radiation injury. Frequent medical evaluations of this population have identified late effects, including several hundred cases of leukemia and other malignant diseases. Atomic weapons testing has led to inadvertent exposure of 300 or more persons, with about 25 per cent showing clinically detectable effects. The fallout from nuclear tests has also added a few millirem to the universal annual background radiation exposure.

Ingestion or inhalation of long-lived isotopes is also potentially injurious. About 5000 persons have been exposed to radium ingestion, and at least 400 malignant tumors have occurred, with increased incidence in the sinuses and in bone. Inhalation of plutonium and other alpha emitters is also a potential problem in the nuclear industry.

EPIDEMIOLOGY

Radiation injury is not caused by a vector, and the source and nature of the exposure should be obvious. It is not always so, however, and epidemiologic techniques are required. Persons may be exposed at work or in the environment without awareness, and clinical symptoms must be identified for an exposure to be suspected. In other cases psychologically deranged persons may have access to radioactive materials and ingest them or expose themselves but deny the exposure.

It is extremely important to determine the nature of the exposure and reconstruct the dose distribution to predict the level of the injury and the required treatment. In addition, the relationship between low-level exposures and subsequent genetic and carcinogenic effects can be learned only by careful dosimetry and long-term clinical follow-up.

PATHOGENESIS

CELL KINETICS AND RADIATION EFFECTS. A few cell types express injury and cell death that will be observed within a few hours after exposure because of intermitotic death. Most cells will live until one or more mitoses have passed. Most cells do not die in mitosis, although failure of cell separation due to dicentric chromosomes can be lethal. They will live out their normal life span, and their injury will become apparent only when depopulation occurs, since the dying cells cannot be replaced because of mitotic death.

Some cells, such as mature muscle cells and neurons, do not normally divide and will persist for many years after radiation exposure. Other cells, such as the functional stromal cells in the renal tubules and the liver, are replaced slowly, and eventually depopulation will occur. The capillary system exhibits slow replacement of the endothelial cells. The number of patent capillaries is slowly reduced after radiation doses of 5 Gy or more, which leads to secondary depletion of the nondividing cells such as neurons.

SPECIFIC TISSUE RADIOBIOLOGY. The tissues of the body can be divided into those critical to life and those whose injury by radiation may cause morbidity but is not fatal. The critical tissues for survival are discussed below. The doses quoted are for single exposure to high-energy photons. Because of sublethal damage repair, doses two to four times higher are required for the same effect after fractionated exposures.

Bone Marrow. Because of the short life span and rapid renewal of most peripheral blood and marrow cells, this organ shows the most evident and acute clinical syndrome. Small lymphocytes die an intermitotic death with depletion in a few hours. Depletion of platelets and granulocytes is maximal at three weeks. The normal survival of red blood cells is about 100 days so depletion is late. There is a dynamic balance among the declining numbers of mature cells living out their lives, delay in replacement because of a reduced stem cell pool and regeneration.

The marrow will regenerate after a single exposure up to 6 Gy and can be repopulated by transplantation after doses up to 10 Gy. Above that dose, damage to the vascular supply prevents regeneration.

Intestine. The mature surface and villus cells of the intestinal mucosa are replaced by the division of cells in the crypts that migrate up the villus. In contrast to this rapid renewal system, the muscular wall contains a slowly renewing capillary network. Doses as low as 1 Gy can reduce crypt cell survival to 50 per cent but histopathologically detectable injury requires 10 Gy or more. After 15 Gy the cell kill in the crypt is sufficient to cause complete loss of the villus and in some cases denudation. At this dose, depopulation peaks in four to eight days; regeneration by the surviving crypt cells is complete two weeks after exposure. Higher local doses will cause these acute changes, but will also lead to late injury in the muscular layer and serosa due to capillary injury; this late injury results in fibrotic responses and obstruction.

Central Nervous System. There are no rapid renewal systems in the CNS, but the glial cells and the endothelial cells cycle slowly and can show injury. The neurons are not injured except secondarily or by doses of 50 Gy or more. Very large exposures of 15 to 50 Gy can produce acute functional changes and, at the highest doses, immediate death. After 15 Gy, changes begin in four to five months and develop further over one to two years. There is focal necrosis and calcification, demyelinization, and gliosis, especially in the white matter.

Skin. After exposure to 3 to 9 Gy the skin may show transient vasodilatation, cessation of mitosis in the basal layer, and thinning of the prickle cell layer. At doses above 20 Gy, denudation and ulceration occur before repopulation begins from either surviving basal cells or cells at the periphery of the exposed area. Although there is usually healing to a normal-appearing epidermis, the cells of the hair follicles and sweat glands are often completely destroyed and will not regenerate if the dose was more than 10 to 15 Gy. Late vascular damage expression can cause a second wave of ulceration as well as telangiectasis.

Lung. In the lung, both the type II pneumocytes and the capillary cells as well as the mucosal cells of the bronchial tree are slowly regenerating. About 90 days after a dose of 10 Gy, acute pneumonitis will occur with capillary occlusion and endothelial cell loss. It is preceded by depletion of surfactant and type II cells. Secondary influx of alveolar macrophages is seen. This acute phase is followed over the ensuing nine months by replacement of the vessels and alveoli by collagen. Acute pneumonitis is reversible only at the lowest dose, 8 to 11 Gy in a single exposure.

Heart. The cardiac muscle cells do not proliferate; therefore, almost all radiation changes occur primarily in the endothelium of the capillaries. Four to six months after exposure to 15 Gy or more the capillaries become occluded, with dose-related reduction in their number. This can lead to loss of the muscle cell as well if all four or even three of the capillaries that surround each muscle cell are lost. At similar doses there is also injury to the pericardium with effusion and fibrotic thickening of the wall.

Liver. The hepatocytes are normally replaced very slowly, but injury to the liver can induce a wave of cell division. There is also continuous replacement of the sinusoidal endothelium in the lobules. Six weeks after 10 Gy, central lobular occlusion occurs with secondary hepatocyte loss and portal hypertension.

Kidney. After 10 Gy there is a reduction in the number of tubule cells and a flattening in the tubule lining. Whole nephrons are lost over a period of 4 to 18 months after exposure. At the same time the endothelium is lost, and many capillaries are occluded. At one year and beyond, damage in the glomerulus, with loss of foot processes and thickening of the basement membrane, can be seen. All of these processes may progress over as long as ten years. Secondary hypertension is common.

Gonads. In contrast to most other tissues there is little sparing of gonadal injury during fractionated exposure, making the gonads quite sensitive to complete depopulation of the reproductive cells. Sterilization can occur after as little as 5 to 10 Gy, and prolonged hypospermia after a few Gy. The hormone-secreting cells of the gonads are much more resistant, but, of course, ovarian hormone secretion is dependent on ovulation and is obliterated by sterilization.

CARCINOGENESIS AND MUTAGENESIS. Much smaller doses than those discussed above will cause changes in some of the chromosomes in all exposed tissues. At a dose of 1 Gy, half of the cells may contain at least one abnormal chromosome. Most of the injuries are deletions or will be expressed at mitosis as dicentrics or rings. Many, but not all, of these will result in reproductive cell death. Although radiation does not cause extensive sister chromatid exchanges, it does cause point mutations as well as deletions and rearrangements, all of which can be mutagenic and in some cases carcinogenic. Thus even one hundredth of a Gy can cause a small number of mutations that will lead to expression as malignant disease or abnormal offspring if a large enough population is observed.

CLINICAL MANIFESTATIONS

ACUTE WHOLE-BODY EXPOSURES. The classic acute whole-body radiation syndrome is usually seen after reactor accidents, malfunction of large treatment or research accelerators or industrial irradiation facilities, and after nuclear explosions. It is also seen after total-body irradiation for bone marrow transplantation and treatment of cancer.

The initial symptoms relate directly to the radiation dose. After 2 Gy of high-energy photons, about half of the patients will exhibit nausea and vomiting two to six hours after exposure, and after 3 Gy the incidence is 100 per cent. With doses above 3 Gy the syndrome may be divided into three types:

1. The *hematologic syndrome* occurs in patients receiving up to 10 or 12 Gy. At these doses, although the small intestine is affected, there is usually little or no diarrhea and the bowel is not denuded. The chief effects are in the bone marrow, although patients surviving the acute phase can develop lung or renal injury months to years later. In the hematologic syndrome the patient will experience the prodromal symptoms of nausea and vomiting in most serious cases, often associated with malaise and weakness. These symptoms subside over the first 24 hours and may be followed by salivary gland swelling. If the dose has been less than 5 Gy there will then be a quiescent period of two to three weeks. At that point, depopulation of the marrow and the resultant granulocyte and platelet suppression will lead to infection and hemorrhage. Purpura, petechiae, and fevers are common. Skin erythema and desquamation can occur, particularly if local areas of higher dose exist. Epilation occurs if the patient survives, but is temporary. If the dose is 3 Gy or below, recovery is usual and can occur at doses up to 5 or 6 Gy with medical support.

2. The *gastrointestinal syndrome* occurs at doses of 13 to 30 Gy. When the dose exceeds that needed to denude the small bowel, the gastrointestinal syndrome will occur before the hematologic syndrome, and since it is usually fatal, will be dominant. After initial symptoms similar to the hematologic syndrome, a brief asymptomatic period will ensue, although malaise and diarrhea may be persistent. Five to seven days after exposure, severe diarrhea and fluid loss occur, followed by infection with enteric bacteria. It is not possible to survive this syndrome, even with modern bone marrow transplantation techniques.

3. The *cardiovascular–central nervous system syndrome* occurs at doses greater than 20 to 30 Gy and is uniformly fatal. After 20 to 50 Gy the patient will experience immediate nausea, vomiting, and diarrhea. This is followed rapidly by ataxia, sweating, prostration, and shock. Huge doses, such as 30 to 500 Gy, can cause immediate death, which is due to generalized CNS dysfunction.

LOCAL OR REGIONAL RADIATION INJURY. The clinical syndromes following whole-body irradiation are all associated with acute effects that subside within two months of exposure. Local or regional exposures to very high doses can occur without immediate death, however, and thus late effects can be seen. The signs and symptoms to be expected after local or regional radiation exposure can be deduced from the pathogenesis section and will be summarized here.

Local irradiation of the bone marrow usually leads to no detectable clinical syndrome. The peripheral white and red cell counts will be depressed, but more than half the marrow must be exposed to doses greater than 4 Gy before any clinical symptoms similar to the acute whole body syndrome will occur. With doses over 10 Gy in a single exposure or 25 Gy fractionated exposure there will be prolonged aplasia of the marrow in the irradiated area. This will lead to clinical symptoms of marrow aplasia if additional radiation exposure, infection, or cytotoxic chemotherapy takes place.

Abdominal irradiation can lead to signs and symptoms from the liver, kidney, and small bowel. The stomach and colon can be injured by doses over 50 Gy of fractionated radiotherapy. Radiation hepatopathy results in ascites six to eight weeks after the exposure with other signs of portal hypertension. Renal injury leads to edema and proteinuria six to eight months later. Hypertension, occasionally severe, can be seen one to ten years after exposure, as can the symptoms of renal failure. The acute small-bowel or gastrointestinal syndrome can occur after abdominal exposure, but it is usually not fatal after local exposures. Delayed injury to the small bowel results in signs of intestinal obstruction or occasional malabsorption or diarrhea. Gastric irradiation produces signs of hypochlorhydria, and at 15 Gy can lead to large ulcers of the greater curvature.

Local radiation of the CNS predominantly produces late signs. Whole-brain irradiation with 10 Gy in a single exposure causes edema with transient nausea and vomiting. Doses of 15 Gy to 20 Gy can be fatal in 6 to 18 months with generalized dementia. More focal irradiation can produce a mass lesion with focal signs, headache, and vomiting.

Injury to the skin results from almost all local or regional exposures. This leads to transient erythema the first day. After three weeks, erythema, dry desquamation, or moist desquamation can occur. Epidermolysis and chronic ulceration occur early after a single exposure of over 25 Gy and with more delayed onset after 18 Gy. The subcutaneous tissues are also damaged. The skin may be ulcerated and heal at first, but reulcerate 2 to 20 years later because of progressive fibrosis and vascular damage in the subcutaneous tissue.

Thoracic irradiation can lead to symptoms due to either cardiac or pulmonary damage. Pulmonary damage is first seen three to four months after a single exposure or six weeks to two months after fractionated exposure. The patient experiences fever, dyspnea, and cyanosis. If the acute phase is survived, there will be chronic signs of pulmonary constriction and fibrosis. Somewhat higher doses cause acute pericarditis with symptoms similar to viral pericarditis with fever, malaise, and some dyspnea about 7 to 24 months after irradiation. Paradoxical pulse and cardiac tamponade with large effusions can be seen. Myocardial infarcts and chronic myocarditis are sometimes seen.

Gonadal irradiation in the male rarely leads to symptoms. Oligospermia will occur after low doses and aspermia after higher doses about six weeks after exposure. The duration will depend on the dose, but can be as long as two years. Ovarian effects usually occur by the next cycle and result in amenorrhea, which is rarely reversible, after doses of 5 Gy in a single exposure or 20 Gy in fractionated exposures.

SYSTEMIC EXPOSURE TO RADIONUCLIDES. Systemic radioisotopes cause symptoms and signs similar to external exposure, if one takes into account the distribution of the isotope and the dose to each organ. In each case there is whole-body exposure and specific-organ exposure that depends on concentration of the isotope in the organ and the nature and energy of the radioactivity. Ingestion of ^{131}I, for example, leads to whole-body exposure and high doses in normal thyroid. There can be symptoms of nausea and vomiting and the hematologic syndrome, followed by hypothyroidism and pharyngitis. Plutonium, usualy present in the air, concentrates in the pulmonary macrophages, causing local fibrosis and malignant disease. For each isotope, it is necessary to know the distribution to predict the symptoms.

DELAYED EFFECTS OF LOW-LEVEL EXPOSURE. These effects are purely genetic and carcinogenic. If an exposure does not lead to sterilization, genetic damage can persist in the sperm or egg. Experiments have shown point mutations in mice, but they have been difficult to prove in humans because of the background of about 10 per cent spontaneous abortions. Carcinogenesis occurs, and the symptoms will be related to the organ in which the tumor develops.

DIAGNOSIS

General Principles

It is essential that any facility likely to deal with radiation injuries have a trained team on call. The physician should obtain a clear history of the exposure, including the nature of the radiation, the distance from the source, and any documentation such as monitors or badges and witnesses. A preliminary

TABLE 562–1. SYMPTOMS, THERAPY AND PROGNOSIS AFTER RADIATION INJURY IN MAN

Dose range	0–1 Gy	1–2 Gy	2–6 Gy	6–10 Gy	10–20 Gy
Therapeutic needs	None	Observation	Specific treatment	Possible treatment	Palliative
Vomiting	None	5–50%	3 Gy = 100%	100%	100%
Time delay, nausea, and vomiting	—	3 hr	2 hr	1 hr	30 min
Main organ damaged	None	Lymphocytes	Bone marrow	Bone marrow	Small bowel
Symptoms and signs	—	Mod. leukopenia	Leukopenia, purpura, hemorrhage, epilation	Leukopenia, purpura, hemorrhage, epilation	Diarrhea, fever, electrolyte imbalance
Critical period	—	—	4–6 wk	4–6 wk	5–14 days
Therapy	Psychotherapy	Observation	Transfusion granulocytes, platelets; antibiotics	Transfusion; antibiotics; bone marrow transplant	Fluids and salts; possible marrow transplant
Prognosis	Excellent	Excellent	Guarded	Guarded	Poor
Lethality	None	None	0–80%	80–100%	100%
Time of death	—	—	2 months	1–2 months	2 wk
Cause of death	—	—	Infection, hemorrhage	Hemorrhage, infection	Enteritis, infection

estimate of the dose should be made from the history as well as the symptoms. Symptoms of malaise, nausea, and vomiting indicate an exposure over 1 Gy, and occur in all patients who have been exposed to 3 Gy or more (Table 562–1).

The physical examination should pay particular attention to the skin, conjunctiva, mucous membranes, and salivary glands. After high local doses there may be acute erythema. A patient who comes in two to three weeks after exposure may show signs of infection or hemorrhage.

Laboratory tests include an immediate complete blood count with differential count. The total lymphocyte count directly reflects the dose received in whole-body exposures within 24 hours. Elevation of the granulocyte count can occur transiently at 24 to 48 hours. If possible, a lymphocyte culture should be done by a cytogeneticist to determine the number of chromosome aberrations, which allows calculation of the dose received. Pulmonary function tests are useful after thoracic irradiation, as are lung scans and chest roentgenograms. Hematologic counts are essential one to three weeks after exposure to follow the pancytopenia and to direct therapy. In the gastrointestinal syndrome there may be findings of dehydration and electrolyte imbalances.

Specific Findings

WHOLE-BODY EXPOSURE. The granulocyte count may rise transiently to 10,000 or more 24 to 48 hours after exposure, while the lymphocyte count falls close to zero with doses of 3 Gy or more. The granulocyte count hits a nadir at four weeks and then returns toward normal at eight weeks. The lymphocyte count may remain low for many years.

LOCAL OR REGIONAL EXPOSURE. Clinical findings after such exposure vary widely and reflect the injury to the specific organ involved. CNS damage will be reflected in an abnormal neurologic examination, signs of edema, and enhancing areas on the CT scan months to years after irradiation. The cerebrospinal fluid is generally normal.

Radiation injury to the thorax is usually detected on the chest roentgenogram. Initially there are areas of patchy or confluent pneumonitis that conform to the shape of the exposed area. This progresses to stranded fibrosis and retraction toward the apex, hilum, or mediastinum. Cardiac injury may lead to transient ECG abnormalities, pericarditis with effusion detectable on ultrasound scans, and signs of myocardial ischemia.

Abdominal exposure leads to changes detectable in function tests for kidney and liver. High doses to the pancreas can lead to diabetes and a decrease in pancreatic enzymes. Chronic diarrhea can occur; it is due to malabsorption and bile salt irritation.

SYSTEMIC EXPOSURE TO RADIOISOTOPES. Large doses of gamma ray–emitting isotopes can cause symptoms and signs similar to those seen in the acute whole-body syndrome or local skin or mucosal injury. The most important diagnostic tests that must be obtained are radioactivity counts and spectroscopy to establish the nature of the isotope(s) and the predicted dose and its localization. Urine and blood samples and, if possible, a whole-body count in a suitable counter should be obtained.

GENETIC OR MUTAGENIC EFFECTS. The low doses usually associated with these effects do not cause changes in standard laboratory tests. Lymphocyte cultures are very sensitive and can predict the size of the exposure and the risk. Sperm counts will reflect the dose to the testis but not the genetic damage.

TREATMENT

ACUTE WHOLE-BODY EXPOSURE. The initial symptoms of whole-body exposure can be treated with antiemetics, and the profound weakness seen at doses above 3 Gy can be reduced by a short course of intravenous corticosteroids. Further therapy is not needed for patients who have received 2 Gy or less. Above that and up to 10 Gy, survival is possible with active medical management. Support similar to that used for the pancytopenic leukemia patient is needed at the higher doses. This includes reverse isolation or life-island type of support. Antibiotics should be used if the granulocyte count is below 1000 per microliter or if there is infection, in which case granulocyte transfusions should be used as well. Platelet transfusions should be given if the platelet count is below 10,000 per microliter. The diarrhea seen at lower doses is usually mild but may require intravenous fluid and electrolyte replacement.

Bone marrow transplantation can be a useful adjunct at doses of 5 Gy or more. Bone marrow samples and peripheral blood for tissue typing should be obtained early, before depletion occurs. Techniques similar to those used for leukemia should be employed (Ch. 156).

Exposures above 10 Gy, which will lead to the gastrointestinal or CNS syndromes, are uniformly fatal. Palliative support is indicated with fluids and the treatment of infection or hemorrhage.

LOCAL OR REGIONAL EXPOSURE. The most common injury requiring treatment will be in the skin. Dry or moist desquamation occurs and can be ameliorated by cleansing with an antibacterial soap. Crusts should be soaked off and the open areas dressed with petroleum jelly or bacitracin ointment. Large areas can benefit from temporary use of lanolin closed dressings, which should be changed daily; the area should be washed before each redressing (Table 562–2).

Most other local injuries cannot be treated specifically. The electrolyte imbalances seen with nausea and vomiting must be corrected. Severe hypokalemia can occur. Radiation pneumonitis can be reversed at borderline doses with prednisone 60 mg per day tapered over the ensuing month. The acute symptoms of pericarditis can be relieved by aspirin or other anti-inflammatory agents. Delayed effects of doses of 20 Gy or more may require skin grafts, resection of necrotic bone, and other surgical procedures, including resection of necrotic brain tissue.

SYSTEMIC EXPOSURE TO RADIONUCLIDES. After the victim has been given urgent first aid and decontaminated if there is

TABLE 562–2. ORGAN DAMAGE, DYSFUNCTION, TREATMENT AND PROGNOSIS AFTER LOCAL IRRADIATION

Organ	Acute Lesion	Delayed Lesion	Clinical Signs	Treatment	Prognosis
Bone marrow	Pancytopenia	Vascular occlusion Myelofibrosis	Infection Hemorrhage	Antibiotics Transfusion	Good if % of total marrow irradiation small
Intestine	Flattened villi	Fibrosis, obstruction	Diarrhea	Fluid, electrolyte acute Resection for obstruction	Good for acute Obstruction can be fatal
CNS	Edema	Necrosis	Headache Focal neurologic	 Resection	Poor Fair
Skin	Desquamation	Ulcer, necrosis	Pain, oozing	Cleansing, ointments, graft	Good
Lung	Pneumonitis	Fibrosis	Cough, fever, cyanosis Dyspnea	Corticosteroids	Good at low dose Good if small volume
Heart	Pericarditis	Carditis	Fever, dyspnea	Anti-inflammatory, pericardiocentesis	Fair
Liver	Central venous thrombosis	Fibrosis	Ascites	Diuretics	Fair
Kidney	Tubular degeneration	Fibrosis	Proteinuria Hypertension, renal failure	Dialysis Transplant	Fair

surface contamination, the dose and nature of the exposure should be determined, making use of a whole-body counter if possible. Large body burdens should be treated by specific methods designed to remove the isotope or block uptake. After iodine exposure, stable iodine should be given as 5 drops of potassium iodide. One gram of soluble phosphate should be given to patients ingesting ^{32}P. Radium ingestion can be treated with magnesium sulfate or epsom salts, 10 grams in 100 ml of water. Strontium exposure is treated with 100 ml of aluminum phosphate gel.

Pulmonary exposures can be treated by bronchial lavage, expectorants, and DTPA (diethylenetriaminepentaacetic acid) aerosol mist. DTPA products are available from the United States Department of Energy for experimetal use and cause chelation of heavy metals.

Gastrointestinal absorption can be reduced with use of mild laxatives. Sodium alginate and aluminum hydroxide gel may reduce strontium uptake.

Certain heavier isotopes, including plutonium, americium, yttrium, lanthanum, cerium, scandium, zinc, and other fission products can be partially removed from the body by DTPA (0.5 to 1 gram given intravenously as soon as possible after exposure and repeated once in 250 ml of normal saline).

PROGNOSIS

ACUTE RADIATION SYNDROMES. Survival with little or no treatment outside good hygiene and treatment of infections can be expected after exposures to 3 Gy or less. Between 3 and 6 Gy, effective therapy with antibiotics, platelets, and granulocytes allows a high survival rate. Leukemic patients show 80 per cent survival after 10 Gy whole-body exposure at a dose rate of 4 Gy per hour when bone marrow transplantation is used. The use of all available methods will allow a high rate of survival after 5 Gy and some survival after acute exposures to 10 Gy. Survival has not been achieved in those patients exhibiting the gastrointestinal or CNS syndromes, probably because irreversible lung, kidney, and marrow damage have occurred.

LOCAL RADIATION EFFECTS. Acute skin reactions usually heal completely. If the exposure has been over 20 Gy, late ulceration can be expected. Most delayed radiation injury is irreversible and slowly progressive as depopulation of stromal and capillary cells occurs.

SYSTEMIC EXPOSURE. The prognosis will depend on the whole-body dose and the nature of the isotope. Large whole-body doses will result in a prognosis similar to that for whole-body external exposure. Thyroid ablation will occur after 50 to 100 millicuries of ^{125}I, and bone marrow ablation after smaller doses of ^{32}P.

GENETIC AND MUTAGENIC EFFECTS. Estimates of the risk of genetic and mutagenic effects are based on extrapolations from higher doses, generally 1 Gy or more, and are thus subject to the dose-response model used. Current best estimates place the additional risk of death from cancer at 77 to 226 per million persons per cumulative centigray of exposure. The risks are higher in the pediatric population and are much higher in the fetus and embryo, particularly in the first trimester.

PREVENTION

Because radiation injury always has an irreversible component, prevention is essential. The largest population exposure is from natural background and can be limited only by moving to a location with low background at low altitude.

The largest controllable additional exposure is medical. This can be limited by careful selection of diagnostic tests. Optimum techniques, collimation, and shielding of the gonads must be employed. The design of facilities must limit the exposure to public and monitored personnel to less than recommended levels. Proper training of workers using radiation is essential. Radiation treatment must be carried out by highly skilled specialists who limit the dose to tumor areas as much as possible.

Hall EJ: Radiation and Life. Elmsford NY, Pergamon Press, 1976. *An introductory overview of radiation in the environment for the student and lay person.*

Hall EJ: Radiobiology for the Radiologist. 2nd ed. Hagerstown, MD, Harper & Row, 1978. *The best introductory text on the biologic effects of radiation for the medical worker.*

Johns HE, Cunningham JR: The Physics of Radiology. 4th ed. Springfield, IL, Charles C Thomas, 1983. *The most comprehensive text in the field of medical radiation physics.*

Principles and General Procedures for Handling Emergency and Accidental Exposures of Workers. ICRP publication 28, Annals of the ICRP 2:1, 1978. *Detailed instructions and useful references for physicians who may be required to deal with victims of accidental exposure.*

Protection Against Ionizing Radiation from External Sources Used in Medicine. ICRP Publication 33, Annals of the ICRP 9:1, 1982. *The basic international manual that sets dose limits, protection standards, and monitoring standards. Essential for anyone employing radiation equipment.*

Shapiro J: Radiation Protection—A Guide for Scientists and Physicians. 2nd ed. Cambridge, Mass., Harvard University Press, 1981. *The standard text for those using ionizing radiations in medicine, with particular emphasis on radionuclides. Covers biology, physics, and protection aspects.*

Thames HD, Withers HR, Peters LJ, et al.: Changes in early and late radiation responses with altered dose fractionation: Implications for dose-survival relationships. Int J Radiation Oncol Biol Phys 8:219, 1982. *A detailed review of the factors influencing acute and late radiation injury. Some background in radiobiology needed.*

The Effects on Populations of Exposures to Low levels of Ionizing Radiations. Washington, National Academy of Sciences—National Research Council, 1980. *A detailed presentation and analysis of radiation exposure information and the incidence of malignancy induction with projections for large populations.*

563. ELECTRIC INJURY

Basil A. Pruitt, Jr.

INCIDENCE AND PREVALENCE. Electricity produces a spectrum of injury ranging from sudden death caused by cardiopulmonary arrest to immediate tissue injury and necrosis caused by transformation of electric energy into heat. Delayed organ damage may also occur; its pathogenesis is incompletely defined. The number of electric injuries occurring annually in the United States and other industrialized countries has paralleled the use of electricity. It is estimated that in the United States more than 1100 deaths occur from high voltage electricity and up to 300 from lightning injury each year. The incidence of electric injury is unknown, but the percentage of patients with high voltage electric injury admitted to burn centers in this country ranges from 0.04 to 6.7 per cent.

PATHOGENESIS. The effects of electricity on tissue depend upon current, voltage, type of current, i.e., direct or alternating and the frequency of the latter, pathway of the current, duration of contact, and environmental conditions. High-tension is arbitrarily defined as voltage above 1000, apparently because the likelihood of sudden death and remote tissue injury is much less with lower voltage. However, any voltage above 40 should be considered potentially dangerous. In general, alternating current is considered more dangerous than direct current, in part because of the tetanic effect of the former, which may "lock" the patient to the source of electricity, and its likelihood of producing cardiac and/or pulmonary arrest. Injurious tissue effects decrease as the frequency of alternating current increases above 60 cycles per second, which is extremely dangerous to the heart and respiratory center. The points of contact and the current pathway through the body are important in determining tissue damage; passage of current through the heart or respiratory center is particularly dangerous. Current flow from a hand to the feet of only 100 ma is capable of producing ventricular fibrillation. The longer the duration of passage of the electric current, the greater will be the tissue damage, emphasizing the need for rapid separation of the victim from the source of electricity. Environmental conditions influence the resistance at the point of contact; dry thickened palmar skin is more resistant to the passage of current than is similar thickness skin when moistened by perspiration or other liquid.

In high voltage electric injury, heat is the principal mediator of tissue damage, and such damage is related to both voltage and duration of application. Because all body tissues and fluids are conductive, the body should be considered as a volume conductor. Heat is produced in this conductor as a function of voltage drop and current flow per unit cross-sectional area, i.e., current density. This characteristic accounts for the rarity of major injury to the trunk and the frequency of severe injury to the digits and extremities in high-tension electric injury. The skin is severely injured and chars at the points of contact, where current density is highest. Charring of the skin may also occur from arcing across flexor surfaces of joints, and arcing can also ignite the patient's clothing and thereby produce associated flame burns. Below 1000 volts, when arcing and contact point charring occur, resistance rises rapidly and limits subsequent current passage and tissue heating; in this sense, such electric injury is self-limiting. Above 1000 volts, arcing is intense, and relatively constant levels of current are maintained with an associated marked increase in tissue destruction. The heated tissue cools unevenly, the superficial portions cooling more rapidly than the deeper portions. Since tissue injury caused by thermal energy depends upon both temperature and duration of exposure, the deeper tissues are more liable to severe injury. These characteristics of tissue as a volume conductor and a volume radiator influence surgical treatment in patients with high voltage electric injury.

Low voltage direct current may also produce tissue damage, and focal injury has occurred at the contact sites of ground plates used with electrosurgical devices. Prolonged application of direct current of as little as 3 volts to such grounding plates can cause tissue injury either directly or as a result of electrolysis of the conductive materials used to ensure contact of the grounding plates and the skin surface.

CLINICAL MANIFESTATIONS. Cardiopulmonary arrest is relatively common in patients who have sustained high voltage electric injuries. Cardiac arrhythmias may occur after resuscitation and persist for a variable period thereafter or develop as late as 24 to 48 hours post-injury. The risk of renal failure is also great in patients with electric injury for two reasons. First, the extent of deep tissue injury may not be appreciated, which leads to underestimation of fluid needs, inadequate resuscitation, and oliguria. Second, the deep tissue injury may liberate myoglobin, which may precipitate in the renal tubules unless a brisk urinary output is maintained. Hyperkalemia may also occur as a result of extensive tissue destruction and reach sufficient levels to interfere with cardiac function.

The effects of electric injury on the deep tissues of a limb may produce sufficient edema beneath the investing fascia of an involved muscle compartment to impair nutrient blood flow and to reduce flow to distal unburned tissue, requiring fasciotomy to relieve pressure and restore circulation.

BURNS OF THE ORAL COMMISSURE IN CHILDREN. Burns of the oral commissure are frequently sustained by children, usually less than three years of age, as a consequence of sucking on the end of a live extension cord or biting the cord of a light or small appliance. Although these burns often have the pearly white appearance of an avascular full thickness burn and initially appear to be significantly deforming, most heal with minimal cosmetic defects when treated conservatively with periodic debridement of only nonviable tissue. Following spontaneous healing, residual functional or cosmetic defects can be repaired electively.

REMOTE ORGAN INJURY. Instances of intestinal perforation, focal pancreatic necrosis, focal gallbladder necrosis, and direct liver injury have been reported, but are uncommon.

Deficits of cerebral, cerebellar, spinal cord, and peripheral nerve function may be evident immediately following electric injury or may be delayed in onset. In all patients with high voltage electric injury, a thorough neurologic examination must be performed on admission and at scheduled intervals thereafter, and any nerve deficits must be fully documented. Return of function following direct nerve damage is uncommon. In general, immediate and early deficits involving nerves not directly injured (motor nerves appear to be more sensitive to current injury than sensory nerves) show spontaneous resolution. Late appearing peripheral nerve deficits may be part of a polyneuritic syndrome involving nerves far removed from the points of electric contact. The immediate symptoms of spinal cord injury are considered to result from direct neuronal insult and are more often transient than are those of later onset, which are more apt to be permanent. Spinal cord deficits of delayed onset may take the form of quadriplegia, hemiplegia, or localized nerve deficits with signs of ascending paralysis, transverse myelitis, or an amyotrophic-lateral-sclerosis-like syndrome.

Delayed hemorrhage from moderate to large-sized blood vessels has occurred in many patients with high voltage electric injury and is ascribed by some to "arteritis" caused by electric injury per se. It has been our experience that such hemorrhage has occurred only when debridement has been inadequate or when the vessel wall underwent desiccation and necrosis secondary to exposure following debridement.

Fractures of long bones may result from falls following the electric shock, and compression fractures of vertebral bodies may result from tetanic contractions of the paraspinous muscles. Both types of fractures should be ruled out by indicated roentgenograms.

The opinions or assertions contained herein are the private views of the author and are not to be construed as official or as reflecting the views of the Department of the Army or the Department of Defense.

DELAYED ORGAN DAMAGE. Recurrent gastrointestinal dysfunction has been reported within 12 to 18 months following high voltage electric injury in up to three fourths of such patients. Cataracts are common sequelae of high voltage electric injury and are most frequent in patients in whom the contact point has been on the head or neck. The formation of such cataracts may be quite rapid or may occur three or more years following high voltage electric injury.

TREATMENT. Cardiopulmonary resuscitation must be begun immediately in any patient with cardiopulmonary arrest following electric injury. All patients who have sustained high voltage electric injury should undergo continuous electrocardiographic (ECG) monitoring for at least 48 hours beyond the last ECG evidence of dysrhythmia, if such occurs. In those patients with high urinary hemochromogen concentrations, an hourly urinary output of 75 to 100 ml should be maintained. If the patient remains oliguric despite the administration of more than the estimated fluid resuscitation needs or the hemochromogens do not clear promptly, 12.5 grams of mannitol should be added to each liter of intravenous fluid given until the pigment has cleared from the urine. Hyperkalemia should be treated by administration of hypertonic glucose, insulin, calcium salts, ion exchange resins, or hemodialysis, depending upon its severity (Ch. 76).

The clinical indications for fasciotomy and surgical exploration of a limb include stony hardness of a muscle compartment to palpation, cyanosis of distal unburned skin, impaired capillary refilling of distal unburned skin or nails, and absent or diminished pulsatile flow in distal arteries on ultrasonic flowmeter examination. If large vessel pulses are intact but significant deep tissue injury is otherwise indicated by clinical signs, arteriography is helpful in determining the need for operation. Arteriographic evidence of large vessel thrombosis merely confirms clinical findings, but luminal irregularity, "beading," or narrowing may be identified in severely injured vessels that will subsequently be occluded by thrombosis, when the arteriogram is performed early following injury. Moreover, "pruning" (a decrease in the density of muscular nutrient arteries in a limb) helps define the level of amputation needed to remove muscle that has sustained inapparent but irreversible damage. ^{133}Xenon wash-out studies have also been used to assess the need for amputation. Muscle flow of less than 1 ml per minute per 100 grams of tissue has been proposed as the level below which amputation is required. An intramuscular compartment pressure of greater than 30 mm Hg, as measured by a wick-type catheter, has also been used as an indication for the need of immediate post-injury wound decompression. Technetium-99m pyrophosphate scintigraphy performed within 24 hours following injury has been suggested as a means to determine the extent of muscle damage, i.e., frankly necrotic tissue showed no perfusion and uninjured tissue showed normal perfusion, while areas of increased uptake of the radioactive material showed variable degrees of partial necrosis requiring operative exposure and debridement of a variable amount of tissue. Since repeated debridement was often required in patients in whom the scintigraphic findings of partial necrosis were present, the clinical reliability, accuracy, and usefulness of that diagnostic method remain uncertain.

Tissue damaged by high voltage electric injury should be explored as soon as the patient is hemodynamically stable. The viability of vital structures and deep muscle is assessed, with necrotic tissue debrided to reduce the risk of infection and eliminate a source of hyperkalemia. Extensive muscle necrosis and destruction of vital structures, such as nerves, tendons, and vessels, speak for amputation at a level proximal to the area of tissue death. Operative wounds following debridement or amputation are left open, and the patient is rescheduled for exploration of the wounds 24 to 72 hours later, at which time further debridement of any residual necrotic tissue is carried out. If no, or only minimal, debridement is required, the amputation wound can be closed by a sausage type of delayed primary closure.

Vascularized free muscle flaps may be used for immediate coverage of deep electric injuries in which the tissues exposed following debridement, e.g., bone or tendon, do not have sufficient blood supply to support a skin graft.

In those patients in whom electric injury is confined to the skin and subcutaneous tissue, bacterial control is best achieved by the use of Sulfamylon burn cream, the active ingredient of which (mafenide acetate) can diffuse into the nonviable tissue to exert its antimicrobial action.

LIGHTNING INJURY. A lightning bolt may have a voltage in the neighborhood of 1 billion volts and induce currents ranging from 12,000 to 200,000 amperes. Its duration is characteristically brief, ranging from one hundredth to one thousandth of a second. The temperature in a lightning bolt may be as high as 30,000° K, but dissipates in a few microseconds. Cardiopulmonary arrest is common in patients struck by lightning and may be secondary to either asystole or fibrillation. Immediate cardiopulmonary resuscitation is life-saving in such patients, and persistent or recurrent ECG abnormalities are rare, although later signs of acute myocardial damage have been reported. Recovery of lightning-struck patients who have apparently been without signs of life for 15 or more minutes speaks for the immediate institution of cardiopulmonary resuscitation. Coma and neurologic deficits are common immediately after injury, but may resolve in a matter of hours. Myoglobinuria, although infrequent, is treated as described previously. The cutaneous burns are characteristically superficial and present a "splashed-on" appearance of arborescent and spidery character. Signs of vasoconstriction and mottling of the skin, previously considered characteristic of lightning injury, typically relent with adequate resuscitation. Prompt treatment of the sequelae of lightning injury, including immediate cardiopulmonary resuscitation, has significantly decreased the mortality associated with this injury, and two thirds of lightning-injured patients now survive.

Apfelberg DB, Masters FW, Robinson DW: Pathophysiology and treatment of lightning injuries. J Trauma 14:453, 1974. *Four cases of lightning injury are discussed with the clinical manifestations of this injury related to the pathophysiologic changes caused by lightning.*

Holliman CJ, Saffle JR, Kravits M, Warden GD: Early surgical decompression in the management of electrical injuries. Am J Surg 144:733, 1982. *The management of electric burns of the extremities is detailed, and the use of radionuclide scanning in assessing extent of muscle injury is described.*

Hunt JL, Mason AD Jr, Masterson TS, Pruitt BA Jr: The pathophysiology of acute electric injuries. J Trauma 16:335, 1976. *The experimental studies reported confirm that an electric injury is simply a thermal burn. The fact that tissue acts as a volume conductor is identified, as is the self-limiting nature of electric injury.*

Levine NS, Atkins A, McKell DW Jr, Peck SD, Pruitt BA Jr: Spinal cord injury following electric accidents; case reports. J Trauma 15:459, 1975. *Report of two patients with spinal cord injury following electric injury with a review of the spectrum and natural history of the neurologic sequelae of high voltage injury.*

Pruitt BA Jr: The burn patient: I. Initial care. *In* Ravitch MM (ed.): Current Problems in Surgery. Chicago, Year Book Medical Publishers, 1979, pp 43–52. *A thorough description of techniques of diagnosis and treatment of high voltage electric injury.*

Sances A Jr, Myklebust JB, Larson SJ, Darin JC, Swiontek T, Prieto T, Chilbert M, Cusick JF: Experimental electrical injury studies. J Trauma 21:589, 1981. *Experimental studies of electric injury relate tissue damage to voltage, current flow, and tissue characteristics, including cross-sectional area.*

564. DISORDERS DUE TO HEAT AND COLD

James P. Knochel

To maintain a normal body temperature requires that heat gain equal heat loss. Heat is produced by metabolism or gained from the environment. Thermoregulation is heavily dependent upon blood flow to cutaneous vessels. Cutaneous flow is regulated by hypothalamic centers. Vasoconstriction reduces and vasodilatation increases delivery of heated blood to the skin. Heat is exchanged between the skin and the environment by radiation, conduction, or convection. If heat loss is inadequate by these means, active sweating begins, and cooling occurs by vaporization of sweat. If heat gain is necessary, metabolic heat production rises by a voluntary increase of physical activity or involuntarily by shivering. Body heat thus produced is retained by cutaneous vasoconstriction. *Acclimatization*, a term defining critical cardiovascular, endocrine, exocrine, and other physiologic adaptations to heat stress, requires one to two weeks to develop. Such adaptations permit one to work comfortably and safely under conditions of heat stress that were previously intolerable.

DISORDERS DUE TO HEAT

HEAT CRAMPS. Workers who sweat profusely and replace sweat losses with water but inadequate salt may experience excruciating muscle cramps. They are more common in acclimatized and physically fit men whose bodies are able to produce voluminous quantities of sweat. The cramps tend to occur in muscles used while working and often do not appear until the person relaxes after work. Cooling the muscles during a cold shower is likely to bring on an attack. Cramps in the abdominal wall may suggest a perforated viscus. Mild hyponatremia is a consistent finding. Severe cramps may cause rhabdomyolysis and modest serum elevations of muscle enzymes (creatine phosphokinase). Salted liquids taken orally or saline given intravenously leads to rapid improvement. Heat cramps are preventable by replacement of sweat with a solution containing about 2.5 grams (one-half teaspoon) NaCl per liter of water, or merely by increasing dietary salt intake.

HEAT EXHAUSTION. Heat exhaustion is a common disorder that occurs after sustained heat stress of three or more days. Its cause is water or salt depletion or both.

Primary water loss heat exhaustion is particularly dangerous since it increases the risk of heat stroke. This form is seen most often in the elderly, infirm, obtunded, or very young who are unable to communicate their thirst. It is also seen in active persons who take salt supplements without adequate water. Deliberate efforts should be made to ensure water intake by patients in nursing homes where summertime room temperatures are often too high to prevent progressive, subtle dehydration. Symptoms of heat exhaustion resulting from predominant water loss include intense thirst, fatigue, weakness, anxiety, and impaired judgment. Signs may include dehydration, hyperventilation, paresthesias, tetany, agitation, hysteria, muscular incoordination, and psychotic behavior. Body temperature may rise to 38.9°C. Delirium, rising temperature, coma, and frank heatstroke may occur in advanced cases. Laboratory findings include hemoconcentration, hypernatremia, and oliguria.

Salt depletion heat exhaustion occurs mainly in unacclimatized persons in whom losses of thermal sweat are replaced with water but not adequate salt. Dehydration, weight loss, and thirst are absent in the pure form. Sweating and urinary output remain normal. Prominent symptoms include profound weakness, fatigue, severe headache, giddiness, and muscle cramps. In some patients, anorexia, myalgia, nausea, vomiting, and diarrhea may masquerade as a viral illness. Such patients appear haggard, with pale, clammy skin. Hypotension and tachycardia are common. Fever is notably absent.

Treatment of heat exhaustion should be individualized, depending upon symptoms and findings. Since kidney function is usually normal, most patients can be treated with lightly salted fluids, rest, and elimination of heat stress. Hypernatremic dehydration should be treated with isotonic dextrose at a rate sufficient to reduce serum sodium about 2 mEq per liter per hour. It is seldom necessary to administer hypertonic salt solutions to patients with hyponatremic heat exhaustion.

HEATSTROKE. Heatstroke is a catastrophic illness requiring immediate treatment for survival. It is convenient to subclassify heatstroke into two forms, classic and exertional.

Classic heatstroke occurs especially in the poor, the elderly, the chronically ill, alcoholics, patients with advanced heart disease, and the obese. Hot, humid weather of three or more days' duration usually precedes epidemics of this disorder. Deaths due to myocardial infarction and congestive heart failure in patients with cardiovascular disease increase sharply during heat waves because of increased demands placed upon the heart by heat stress. Certain medications also increase the propensity to develop heatstroke. These include drugs that depress sweating (anticholinergics, beta blockers, antihistamines), diuretics, and drugs that may increase heat production (amphetamines, neuroleptics). Rarely, patients with classic heatstroke may recall a prodrome resembling heat exhaustion or cessation of sweating. Once sweating stops, body temperature mounts and collapse soon follows. Typical findings include profound central nervous system dysfunction, especially coma or bizarre behavior; hot, dry, flushed skin; and hyperpyrexia. Rectal temperature exceeds 40.6°C and may reach 44°C or more. Hypotension is common. It is probably due to redistribution of blood from the central to the peripheral circulation since it often responds to cooling alone. Convulsive seizures, fasciculations, and muscle rigidity are absent until active cooling is under way.

Exertional heatstroke is more likely to develop in laborers, farmers, military recruits, football players, long distance runners, and those who work in boiler rooms or foundries. They display physical findings in the acute phase similar to those of patients with classic heatstroke, with one common exception: About half of these patients continue to sweat. If this occurs, the skin may be deceptively cool despite a high core temperature.

Other major differences between classic and exertional heatstroke become apparent from laboratory measurements. In the classic form, respiratory alkalosis is usual, and circulatory collapse may cause modest increases of lactate, a particularly ominous sign. In contrast, *lactic acidosis* is the rule in exertional heatstroke, may exceed 20 mmol per liter, and is not a foreboding finding in this condition. Although serum creatine phosphokinase activities may be slightly increased in classic heatstroke (usually not greater than 1000 to 2000 IU per liter), clinically important rhabdomyolysis is exceptionally rare unless heatstroke occurs in an individual who has a pre-existing myopathy, such as a chronic alcoholic. Major *rhabdomyolysis* and its associated complications such as hyperkalemia, hyperphosphatemia, hypocalcemia out of proportion to hypoalbuminemia, hyperuricemia, and myoglobinuria are almost invariable findings in exertional heatstroke. Both forms of heatstroke may be complicated by *hemorrhage* (resulting from *disseminated intravascular coagulation*, fibrinolysis, clotting factor deficiency due to hepatic injury, or *thrombocytopenia* due to bone marrow injury); *jaundice; acute renal failure; pancreatitis; brain damage; peripheral neuropathy; myocardial necrosis and arrhythmias;* and pulmonary capillary damage with *adult respiratory distress syndrome.* Hypokalemia in heatstroke usually results from respiratory alkalosis, but it may represent potassium deficiency in those who have performed hard work in the heat for one or two weeks. Hypoglycemia may also occur.

Treatment of heatstroke depends upon anticipation, prompt recognition, and rapid cooling. The importance of educating paramedical personnel, nurses, athletes, coaches, and trainers to prevent, accurately recognize, and initiate immediate cooling cannot be overestimated. Common mistakes include administration of fluids to comatose patients or delay of cooling.

Proper emergency management includes removal from direct sunlight, removal of clothing, wetting the body surface, and fanning to move air and thereby promote vaporization. When such simple measures are undertaken on the spot, some victims awaken. Most require aggressive cooling in the hospital. A thermistor probe temperature device should be inserted high in the rectum to ensure recording of core temperature.

Conventional cooling techniques include immersion in ice water while the skin is rubbed briskly or placing the patient on a stretcher, rubbing the skin with ice bags while keeping the skin wet, and moving air over the skin to promote vaporization of the water. Rapid cooling by ice water immersion may cause cutaneous vasoconstriction, shivering, and convulsions. Current experimental studies suggest that immersion in cool water (11°C) may facilitate cooling with equal speed by avoiding cutaneous vasoconstriction.

Hypotension often responds to cooling alone, but if it persists, 0.5 liter of normal saline should be infused. If additional quantities are necessary, one must guard against circulatory congestion. Hypotension not responding to such quantities of saline suggests myocardial injury or serious rhabdomyolysis, and vasopressor support may be necessary. The stomach should be emptied, since vomiting and aspiration often occur during cooling. Cooling should be stopped when core temperature reaches 39°C to avoid progressive hypothermia.

Steroids are unnecessary. Hypokalemia and hypophosphatemia are very common in the acute phase but usually resolve quickly without treatment. Glucose may be necessary for hypoglycemia. Although lactic acidosis usually responds to volume expansion, if it persists in the absence of hypotension, 44 to 88 mEq of $NaHCO_3$ may be helpful. Other complications described earlier should be anticipated, and appropriate measures taken as necessary.

MALIGNANT HYPERTHERMIA. This rare but serious disorder, representing an idiosyncratic reaction to general anesthesia, is discussed in Ch. 538.

MINOR DISORDERS RELATED TO HEAT STRESS. *Heat edema* is a transient, benign disorder that occurs during initial exposure to hot weather. It appears to result from aldosterone-mediated salt and water retention (a physiologic adaptation) and usually disappears spontaneously with continued heat exposure. It seldom, if ever, requires treatment. Diuretics should not be administered. *Miliaria* (heat rash) is caused by sweat gland occlusion. Its medical importance is enhanced, since it may impair sweat formation and evaporative heat loss.

Heat syncope occurs when a healthy person squats for a minute and then suddenly stands, upon which a sensation of transient dizziness or visual blurring may occur. Such symptoms are exaggerated by salt and water losses induced by sweating and by heat-induced vasodilatation of the superficial blood vessels and may cause syncope in an individual unacclimatized to heat. When acclimatization occurs, the associated retention of salt and water corrects the problem. Besides syncope, findings usually include slight tachycardia and moist skin. Fever is absent. Recovery occurs rapidly if the patient is allowed to remain supine. Removal from the heat and administration of lightly salted liquids are helpful.

Hart GR, Anderson RJ, Crumpler CP, Shlkin A, Reed G, Knochel JP: Epidemic classical heat stroke: Clinical characteristics and course of 28 patients. Medicine 61:189–197, 1982. *A detailed presentation of classic heatstroke, emphasizing the important roles of medications that impair heat loss and pre-existent disease in its pathogenesis. It also presents a detailed analysis of laboratory abnormalities commonly observed in this illness.*

Jones TS, Liang AP, Kilbourne EM, et al.: Morbidity and mortality associated with the July 1980 heat wave in St. Louis and Kansas City, Mo. JAMA 247:3327–3331, 1982. *A report illustrating increased death rates during heat waves.*

Knochel JP: Environmental heat illness. Arch Intern Med 133:841–864, 1974. *A general review of heat stress injuries and description of exertional heatstroke.*

Knochel JP, Reed G: Disorders of heat regulation. *In* Maxwell MH, Kleeman CR, Narins RG (eds.): Clinical Disorders of Fluid and Electrolyte Metabolism. 4th ed. New York. McGraw-Hill Book Company. In press. *A review of environmental heat illness, pharmacologic and endocrine hyperthermia, malignant hyperthermia, and hypothermic disorders.*

HYPOTHERMIA

Hypothermia, defined as a core temperature of less than 35°C, is a medical emergency that occurs in both temperate and cold environments. Its prompt recognition is critical to avoid serious morbidity or death. When body temperature declines, heat production increases by shivering, and heat loss is reduced by decreasing cutaneous blood flow. Reduction of core temperature decreases the rate of chemical reactions so that cooling proceeds until a new equilibrium is established between the body and its environment.

TABLE 564–1. CAUSES OF HYPOTHERMIA

Exposure plus:
- I. Central nervous system disease
  - Brain tumor, injury, seizure
  - Cord transection
  - Hypoglycemia
  - Thiamin deficiency
  - Uremia
  - Hepatic failure
- II. Interference with vasoconstriction
  - Drugs
    - Alcohol
    - Phenothiazines
  - Sepsis
  - Erythroderma
- III. Interference with muscle movement
  - Paralysis, paresis
  - Extremes of age
  - Drugs
    - Alcohol
    - Phenothiazines
  - Hypothyroidism
- IV. Mixed causes
  - Starvation
  - Adrenal insufficiency
  - Hypothyroidism
  - Hypopituitarism

From Fitzgerald FT, Jessop C: Accidental hypothermia: A report of 22 cases and review of the literature. Adv Intern Med 27:127, 1982. Reprinted with permission.

As hypothermia develops, cerebral blood flow declines. The resulting fall in nutrient availability is offset by a reduction in brain metabolism. This fall in metabolic demand permits successful cerebral resuscitation of hypothermic patients even after prolonged periods of anoxia and circulatory arrest.

PATHOGENESIS. The causes of hypothermia seen in clinical practice are summarized in Table 564–1. Advanced age, disorders causing hypometabolism, central nervous system disease, malnutrition, a variety of drugs, and exposure commonly cause hypothermia. In elderly persons, hypothermia, hyperventilation, hypotension, and thrombocytopenia are common signs of bacteremia and sepsis.

CLINICAL MANIFESTATIONS. A decline in mental status, ataxia, tremulous speech, and hyperreflexia appear as temperature falls to about 32°C. At lower temperatures, hyporeflexia, stupor, dysarthria, and sluggish pupillary responses appear. Shivering usually stops below 32°C. Muscle rigidity becomes prominent. Established hypothermia reduces heart rate, blood pressure, peripheral vascular resistance, cardiac output, and central venous presure. Creatine phosphokinase (MB isoenzyme) may increase with severe hypothermia without evidence of myocardial infarction, suggesting myocardial cellular damage. Cardiac arrhythmias are very common. Atrial arrhythmias are usually benign. Ventricular ectopic beats may herald ventricular fibrillation, an imminent danger if core temperature becomes less than 28°C. Stimulation, such as urethral catheterization, movement, endotracheal intubation, and vascular catheterization, also predisposes to the development of this arrhythmia. Osborn waves, characterized by a widening of the base of the QRS complex and J point deflection, are the most characteristic ECG findings. They can be seen with hypothermia from any cause and do not herald the onset of ventricular fibrillation. Early tachypnea and respiratory alkalosis are replaced by progressive hypoventilation. Advancing hypothermia leads to carbon dioxide retention and respiratory acidosis. Shivering increases lactic acid production and hypoxia in muscles and may cause severe lactic acidosis.

In early hypothermia, hypokalemia may be caused by respiratory alkalosis. Additional cooling corrects hypokalemia by reducing sodium-potassium transport. During therapeutic rewarming, sodium-potassium exchange accelerates, such that hypokalemia may become important and contribute to arrhythmias. Hypophosphatemia may also occur during the recovery phase of hypothermia.

TREATMENT. Significant hypothermia is a medical emergency. When it is suspected, an estimate of core temperature should be obtained, by inserting a thermistor probe high into the rectum. Esophageal temperature probes are difficult to place properly and may precipitate ventricular arrhythmias or fibrillation.

Airway patency must be insured in comatose patients and steps taken to prevent aspiration of gastric contents. A large intravenous catheter should be inserted, and thiamin and glucose given immediately in appropriate situations. Stimulation of the patient should be minimized to avoid precipitating ventricular fibrillation. Blood pressure, pulse, temperature, electrocardiogram, neurologic status, and urine output should be monitored frequently during rewarming.

A warming rate of about 0.5°C per hour is generally accepted as optimal. Most shivering patients will spontaneously rewarm at a rate equal to or greater than this. *Passive* rewarming and blankets for hemodynamically stable, moderately hypothermic patients is ideal. This method will allow a rise of 0.5 to 1°C per hour if the initial core temperature is greater than about 27°C. It is especially effective in patients with acute hypothermia without underlying disease. *Active* rewarming becomes necessary in patients with severe hypothermia or cardiopulmonary arrest or both. This is especially important in patients with ventricular fibrillation or asystole because the hypothermic myocardium is resistant to mechanical or pharmacologic intervention until temperatures are above 28°C to 30°C.

"Rewarming shock" and accentuated lactic acidosis have been most commonly encountered with active external rewarming techniques, i.e., heat applied to the surface of the body with hot water bottles or immersion in warm water. To avoid these problems, rapid rewarming of core blood has been attempted by several means in patients with severe hypothermia or cardiac arrest. Most patients with hypothermia will tolerate warm intravenous fluids and heated oxygen. If rapid rewarming is required, peritoneal lavage with solutions warmed to about 40°C is effective.

Supportive measures may be very important. Because of the wide diversity of electrolyte derangements in hypothermic patients, no general recommendations can be made regarding fluid management other than warming the fluid to 37 to 40°C before administration. Plasma volume expanders may be given if the central venous pressure is low. Oxygen and bicarbonate should be given if serious metabolic acidosis exists. Subsequent metabolic alkalosis and its adverse effects on oxyhemoglobin dissociation, calcium, and ventricular irritability must be avoided. As patients are rewarmed, metabolic acidosis may worsen as lactate is washed out of previously hypoxic tissues. Recognition and treatment of this phenomenon are important to reduce the risk of ventricular fibrillation and cardiovascular collapse. Severe respiratory impairment with significant carbon dioxide retention should be treated with assisted ventilation. Ventilatory adjustments should be made with respect to reduced carbon dioxide production. Hypoglycemia should be suspected in any patient with hypothermia. Hyperglycemia should be treated only if severe and potentially life threatening. Vasopressors should be avoided if possible because of their ability to induce ventricular arrhythmias. Drugs with significant myocardial depressing effects such as quinidine and propranolol should be avoided. Thyroxine should be given only if significant hypothyroidism is suspected.

Fitzgerald FR, Jessop C: Accidental hypothermia: A report of 22 cases and review of the literature. Adv Intern Med 27:127, 1982. Reuler JB: Hypothermia: Pathophysiology, clinical settings, and management. Ann Intern Med 89:519, 1978. *These two articles are excellent clinical reviews of hypothermia as seen in medical practice, with discussions of differential diagnosis, clinical manifestations, and treatment.*

Wong KC: Physiology and pharmacology of hypothermia. West J Med 138:227, 1983. *This is a recent general overview of the physiologic consequences of hypothermia, with 74 references.*

565. TRACE METAL POISONING

Donald B. Louria

Many trace elements, both metals and nonmetals, are capable of causing human disease. In some cases poisoning is a consequence of workplace exposure. In others the disease results from use of prescription or nonprescription medicines or as an adverse effect of medical procedures such as hemodialysis or insertion of prosthetic devices. Occasionally trace element poisoning results from attempts at suicide or homicide. Increasingly the source of poisoning is the food we eat, the liquids we drink, or the air we breathe; some soil or water has naturally high concentrations of potential toxins such as arsenic, but more often the environmental contamination is man made.

Over the past few decades, increased awareness of the health consequences of industrial substances, more stringent federal and state regulations, and fear of lawsuits have resulted in a healthier workplace. On the other hand, technologic advances have increased the use of trace elements, often with inadequate safety precautions until adverse effects are recognized. Furthermore, the majority of the potentially exposed work force is employed by small industries that may not have plant physicians or insist on proper worker protection.

We know a great deal about overwhelming exposure that results in acute illness, but our knowledge of the subtle consequences of chronic, low level trace element exposure is still grossly inadequate. This is well illustrated by lead exposure. Acute lead poisoning in children or adults is readily diagnosed, but we are only beginning to understand the consequences of increased body lead burdens in the absence of the anemia, colic, or clinically apparent encephalopathy.

The interrelationships between and among trace elements are also poorly understood. For example, copper smelter workers are exposed not only to copper but also to lead, zinc, arsenic, gold, silver, cadmium, and mercury; in these workers pneumonitis or other acute illnesses may result from two or more metals acting in concert. In other instances excesses or deficits of a trace element may act indirectly by inducing deficiency or toxicity of another trace element.

LEAD

ETIOLOGY. In the past lead poisoning was ascribed to pica (abnormal ingestion) among children living in dilapidated houses with peeling layers of lead-based paints. In the last two decades lead intoxication has occurred with increasing frequency in less socioeconomically deprived areas of the cities, as well as in more affluent suburbs. This may in part be related to environmental contamination from leaded gasoline; several studies relate environmental lead contamination to traffic density patterns. Contaminated soil is also a well-described source of lead.

In the United States, hundreds of occupations entail potentially significant exposure. Lead and other metal smelter workers or miners, welders, storage battery workers, and pottery makers are particularly heavily exposed. Workers in auto manufacturing, ship building, paint manufacture, and printing industries are also at substantial risk.

Lead-soldered kettles and cans and lead-glazed pottery can release lead when acidic fluids are stored or cooked in them. Demolition workers and those employed in firing ranges have become poisoned from intensive aerosol exposure. The concentration of lead in printing inks is significant; poisoning even occurred after repeated burning of newspapers and magazines in a fireplace. In the southern United States, moonshine whiskey is an important cause of poisoning. The stills are connected with lead solder, and old lead-containing radiators are used as condensers; 20 to 90 per cent of moonshine samples contain lead in the potentially toxic range.

In past centuries lead was added to wine to sweeten it, a deception that was eventually made punishable by death; recently, addition of lead to aphrodisiacs and various herbal and folk medicines has resulted in poisoning. Retained bullets can result in lead poisoning, especially if host metabolic changes favor lead mobilization or if a joint is involved, since synovial fluid appears to be a good solvent for lead.

Gasoline sniffing for hedonistic purposes can produce lead poisoning; the organic tetraethyl lead appears to have a proclivity for the nervous system.

In a sense we are all lead poisoned; prior to the industrial revolution the total body burden of lead was about 2 mg, whereas currently in industrialized societies the whole body content is about 200 mg. One hundred and fifty to 250 μg per day is ingested, 5 to 10 per cent of which is absorbed; in children the percentage is higher and absorption is facilitated by iron, calcium, magnesium, and perhaps zinc deficiency. Aerosol exposure is especially likely to result in poisoning, since approximately 40 per cent of inhaled lead is absorbed.

CLINICAL MANIFESTATIONS. The major toxic effects of lead are referable to the abdomen, the blood, and the nervous system.

Gastrointestinal Tract. The exact pathogenesis of lead colic remains uncertain; in part it appears to be due to a direct effect of lead on smooth muscle. The crampy, diffuse, often intractable abdominal pain may be accompanied by nausea, vomiting, anorexia, constipation, or occasionally diarrhea. The pain may be confined to the epigastric, periumbilical, or other areas of the abdomen and may simulate a variety of surgical and nonsurgical diseases. Lead-induced megacolon has been reported.

Blood. Lead interferes with a variety of red cell enzyme systems, including delta-aminolevulinic acid dehydratase and ferrochelatase. The former is needed for the conjugation of levulinic acid to form porphobilinogen; the latter facilitates the incorporation of iron into protoporphyrin IX (see Fig. 134–3). The red cell abnormalities include punctate basophilic stippling and clover leaf morphology. Anemia is frequent and may be normocytic normochromic, owing to decreased red cell life span, or microcytic hypochromic.

Nervous System. Either the brain or peripheral nerves may be involved. The CNS symptoms at first are vague and are often mistakenly disregarded; these manifestations include irritability, incoordination, memory lapses, labile affect, sleep disturbances, restlessness, listlessness, paranoia, headache, lethargy, and dizziness. In more serious cases manifestations include syncopal-like attacks, disorientation, flaccidity, more intense headache, severe mental impairment, ataxia, vomiting, cranial nerve palsies, localized neurologic signs, psychosis, somnolence, seizures, blindness, and coma. Severe lead encephalopathy is not restricted to children. Occasionally the brain manifestations mimic a space-occupying lesion. The cerebrospinal fluid may show an increased protein content, a modest pleocytosis (predominantly lymphocytic), and rarely diminished glucose levels. Papilledema has been reported, as have grayish deposits surrounding the optic disc and optic atrophy. Frank encephalopathy is an ominous prognostic sign in regard to both mortality and persistent brain damage. Most children who experience two or more bouts of clinically evident encephalopathy have neurologic residua.

The peripheral nerve involvement, seen more often in adults than in children, is almost always exclusively motor and involves muscle groups used extensively. Wrist drop and foot drop are seen most often; the former, depending on type of occupation, may be asymmetrical and there may be paresthesias.

The spinal cord may also be involved, manifestations having some similarity to those of amyotrophic lateral sclerosis.

Tetraethyl lead poisoning causes euphoria, nervousness, insomnia, hallucinations, convulsions, and sometimes frank psychosis.

The question of subtle brain damage in the absence of clinical evidence of encephalopathy remains controversial. Some studies suggest that inordinate body burdens of lead may result in mentation difficulties, emotional lability, intelligence and memory deficits, impaired psychomotor function, and behavioral aberrations in both children and adults, even in the absence of overt evidence of poisoning.

Other Clinical Manifestations. In adults the kidneys are often involved (see Ch. 81.3), the characteristic lesion being interstitial nephritis; as the disease progresses, glomerular filtration rate falls. In children, Fanconi's syndrome, characterized by glycosuria, aminoaciduria, and phosphaturia, may occur transiently; and occasionally, asymptomatic renal failure supervenes. Lead poisoning appears to be responsible for some cases of renal failure associated with either gout or hypertension.

Occasionally arrhythmias and cardiomegaly have been reported as have abnormalities of liver function. A gingival blue, blue-black, or gray line is found in up to 20 per cent of adult patients but is infrequent in children.

Lead readily crosses the placenta and is thought to be responsible for an increased incidence of spontaneous abortion and miscarriage. Some studies suggest lead poisoning may result in hypospermia and other sperm abnormalities. Teratogenic effects occur in lead-treated animals, but congenital abnormalities have not been convincingly documented in man. Lead exposure may also result in transient chromosomal breakage.

DIAGNOSIS. The interference with delta-aminolevulinic acid dehydratase results in marked increase in delta-aminolevulinic acid in the urine. Urinary coproporphyrin levels are also increased. Lead interferes with incorporation of iron into heme and zinc then replaces the iron to form zinc protoporphyrin (ZPP). The latter or its hydrolysis product erythrocyte protoporphyrin (EP) can be measured rapidly fluorometrically; both EP and ZPP are reliable indicators of lead poisoning. False-positive EP and ZPP elevations occur in patients suffering from iron deficiency anemia or erythropoietic protoporphyria. Table 565–1 lists some indications of undue lead absorption.

Blood aminolevulinic acid dehydratase activity can also be measured directly. Blood lead levels are readily determined by atomic absorption spectrophotometry or anodic stripping voltometry; specimens can be obtained by either venipuncture or finger stick; the latter technique suffers from low specificity because of skin contamination. Urine lead concentrations can also be measured; if concentrations are normal, increased body burdens can still be detected by measuring urinary lead excretion after administration of calcium disodium edetate (Table 565–2). In children a blood level of 60 μg per deciliter or greater is considered evidence of definite lead poisoning; and concentrations of 30 μg per deciliter or greater, evidence of excessive absorption. For adults, who show less enzyme inhibition at a given blood lead concentration, the permissible industrial concentration is currently up to 50 μg per deciliter.

Additional industrial exposure should probably not be permitted if blood levels exceed 50 μg per deciliter or if there is any increase in EP or ZPP.

TREATMENT. Three agents are used that form tight complexes with lead and thus promote its elimination from tissues (Table

TABLE 565–1. POSITIVE SCREENING TESTS INDICATING UNDUE LEAD ABSORPTION

Whole blood lead	Children	> 30 μg/dl
	Adults	> 40 μg/dl
Whole blood erythrocyte protoporphyrin or zinc protoporphyrin	Children	> 50 μg/dl
	Adults	> 70 μg/dl
Urine delta-aminolevulinic acid		> 3 mg/m²/24 hours
Reduction in erythrocyte delta-aminolevulinic acid dehydratase activity		< 15–20% of normal activity

TABLE 565–2. $CaNa_2$ EDTA LEAD MOBILIZATION TEST

	Children	Adults
Normal premobilization test	< 100 µg/day	< 150 µg/day
	Normal	
Post-$CaNa_2$ EDTA 50 mg/kg IM or IV or 500–1000 mg/m^2 (children); or 1 gm IM* × 2, 12 hours apart (adults)	< 1 µg Pb/mg $CaNa_2$ EDTA† administered over 24-hour collection period	< 650 µg/day
	Increased Body Burden	
	> 1 µg Pb/mg $CaNa_2$ EDTA administered	> 1000 µg/day

*Procaine must be used with intramuscular injections.
†EDTA = edetate.

565–3). Dimercaprol (British anti-lewisite, BAL) is given in oil intramuscularly; calcium disodium edetate (calcium versenate) can be given either intramuscularly or intravenously; and D-penicillamine is administered by mouth. Chelation should be undertaken only after careful consideration in those with milder evidences of poisoning, because each of the agents is associated with potentially severe adverse effects. Occasionally chelation may be complicated by acute renal failure. Because most of the body lead is stored in the bones, clinical improvement and reduction in blood lead levels (or reduction in EP or ZPP) may be followed by increases in blood lead concentrations and clinical evidence of repoisoning owing to mobilization of lead from bone. In such cases chelating agents should again be administered.

Treatment is ordinarily successful in extra-CNS disease, but is not predictably effective in patients with encephalopathy. Various degrees of mentation deficits may remain in both children and adults. Among adults the frequency of residual brain deficits is not clearly established.

Batuman V, Landy E, Maesaka JK, Wideen RP: Contribution of lead to hypertension with renal impairment. N Engl J Med 309:17, 1983.
Batuman V, Maesaka JK, Haddad B, et al: The role of lead in gout nephropathy. N Engl J Med 304:520, 1981. *These two articles present reasonably compelling evidence that renal dysfunction associated with either hypertension or gout may be related to lead intoxication in a small but important percentage of such cases.*
Browder AA, Joselow MM, Louria DB: The problem of lead poisoning. Medicine 52:121, 1973. *A thorough review with 150 references.*
Chisholm JJ Jr, Barltrop D: Recognition and management of children with increased lead absorption. Arch Dis Child 54:249, 1979. *An updated summary of environmental aspects, pathogenesis, and treatment of lead poisoning.*
Needleman HL, Gunnoc C, Leviton A, et al.: Deficits in psychologic and classroom performance of children with elevated dentine lead levels. N Engl J Med 300:689, 1979. *This important, although controversial, article gives substantial support for the notion that subtle lead poisoning can result in significant psychosocial defects. Based on comparison of 58 children with high dentine levels and 100 with low levels.*
Wedeen RP, Maesaka JK, Weiner B, et al.: Occupational lead nephropathy. Am J Med 59:630, 1975. *This meticulous assessment of glomerular and tubular function in six asymptomatic and two symptomatic adults strongly suggests that lead-induced nephropathy in occupationally exposed adults occurs far more frequently than previously recognized.*
Whitfield CL, Ch'ien LT, Whitehead JD: Lead encephalopathy in adults. Am J Med 52:289, 1972. *Twenty-three adults exposed to moonshine developed encephalopathy, manifestations ranging from confusion to coma, seizures, and death. This article emphasizes that encephalopathy can be a major problem in adults. Chelation therapy appeared to be effective.*

TABLE 565–3. CHELATION REGIMENS

	Children*	Adults*	Duration
$CaNa_2$ EDTA	50 mg/kg/day IM† or IV, or 1500 mg/m^2/24 hours (severe disease); 500–1000 mg/m^2/day (mild-moderate intoxication)	1.0 gram IV in 5% dextrose twice daily, or 2.0 grams/day IM in divided doses; longer-term, 1 gram IM 3 × per week† until lead burden reduced to satisfactory levels	Three to five days
BAL	3 mg/kg/dose IM, or 500–1000 mg/m^2/24 hours IM	2.5 mg/kg/dose IM	Two days if with $CaNa_2$ EDTA; three days if used alone
	(Given in divided doses every four hours first day, every six hours thereafter)		
Penicillamine	30 mg/kg/day PO	1.0–1.5 grams/day PO	Until blood lead and FEP‡ levels approach normal

*$CaNa_2$ EDTA and BAL are used together for severe illness.
†Procaine must be used for IM injections of $CaNa_2$ EDTA.
‡FEP, free erythrocyte protoporphyrin.

MERCURY

ETIOLOGY. Mercury has been used for at least 2000 years. At present more than 60 occupations involve mercury exposure. These include chloralkali work; manufacture of pesticides, insecticides, and fungicides; manufacture of mercury-containing instruments, lamps, neon lights, batteries, paper, paint, dye, electrical equipment, and jewelry; and dentistry.

In addition to occupational or industrial exposure, poisoning has resulted from inadvertent contamination of grains by mercury-containing pesticides; and accidental or intentional ingestion or injection of elemental mercury or mercury-containing compounds. In the past mercury was administered medicinally as a component of cathartics, teething powders, and anthelmintics. Mercury compounds are now rarely used as diuretics.

CLINICAL MANIFESTATIONS AND TREATMENT. The biologic effects, tissue distribution, and toxicity of mercury depend on the form in which it is introduced into the body. Mercury possesses a strong affinity for sulfhydryl, amine, phosphoryl, and carboxyl groups and inactivates a wide variety of enzymes. Mercury poisoning can be conveniently divided into four categories.

Metallic Mercury. Elemental mercury is a liquid at environmental temperatures but vaporizes with agitation as well as gentle heating. Bulk mercury is used in dental amalgams; up to 10 per cent of dental offices have been found to have excessive mercury vapor levels; and accidental spillage has occurred occasionally in homes or offices. The greatest exposure to metallic mercury is in industry. Heavy aerosol exposure to mercury produces chills, fever, cough, chest pain, and hemoptysis; roentgenograms show diffuse pulmonary infiltrates. Inhaled elemental mercury is readily absorbed from the alveoli; thereafter the target tissue is the brain. With mild exposure the manifestations are likely to be subtle and diagnosis difficult. Insomnia, nervousness, impaired judgment, memory deficits, emotional lability, headache, fatigue, loss of sexual drive, and depression are early manifestations and are often mistakenly ascribed to psychogenic causes. These symptoms have been referred to as micromercurialism. Abdominal cramps, dermatitis, and diarrhea may also occur, and the victim may complain of a metallic taste. As the poisoning becomes more severe, persistent involuntary tremors of the extremities are noted. Thereafter other signs of mercury poisoning may appear, including amblyopia, polyneuropathy, erythroderma, acrodynia, swollen gums with a blue line around the teeth, sialorrhea, and paresthesias. The major manifestation of mercury vapor exposure may be renal damage, including the nephrotic syndrome. A clinical picture simulating the mucocutaneous lymph node syndrome (Kawasaki's) has also been described.

Blood and urine levels may be unreliable, and clear evidence of poisoning may be documented only after administration of drugs that augment mercury excretion in the urine.

In most cases improvement occurs after removal from exposure or treatment with either dimercaprol (BAL) or N-acetyl penicillamine.

The effects of ingestion of even large amounts of metallic mercury range from no clinical disturbance to local gastrointestinal irritation to central nervous system damage. Aspiration of liquid mercury is also usually benign, although roentgenologic visualization of mercury globules may be evident for many years. After intravenous injection of mercury there may be no abnormalities other than roentgenologic densities or an illness ranging from mild to lethal with hepatic, renal, lung, and central nervous system dysfunction.

The wide range of clinical findings after elemental mercury exposure appears to relate in part to the rate of oxidation to mercuric salts and the rapidity of their subsequent excretion through the kidneys, saliva, and urine.

Inorganic Mercury. Exposure to $HgCl_2$ and Hg_2Cl_2 occurs primarily in industry and results from ingestion. $HgCl_2$ is far more toxic than Hg_2Cl_2. The major manifestations are renal and include proteinuria, granular casts in the urinary sediment, and pyuria from tubular damage. In some cases severe oliguria, and even anuria, may occur. Additionally, diarrhea, abdominal pain, hepatic dysfunction, and lesser evidences of central nervous system disease may be found (micromercurialism). Rhabdomyolysis with striking muscle enzyme elevation and acrodynia have also been reported. In this type of mercury poisoning BAL or penicillamine is usually effective.

Organomercurials with Rapid Metabolism to Inorganic Mercury. Included are phenyl and methoxyethyl mercury salts found in diuretics and fungicides. Toxicity is limited and usually renal.

Short Chain Alkyl Mercury Compounds. Methyl mercury is far more toxic than ethyl or diethyl mercury; the latter produces primarily renal abnormalities.

Methyl mercury is well absorbed from the intestinal tract, is widely distributed in the body, readily passes through the placenta into the fetus and also into breast milk. About 10 per cent localizes in the brain, and the ensuing damage is largely irreversible. Major epidemics have resulted from industrial contamination of water with subsequent biotransformation of elemental and inorganic mercury into methyl mercury, followed by ingestion by fish and then by man. Other epidemics have resulted from use of grains contaminated by organic mercurial pesticides or animal ingestion of seeds treated with mercury. The epidemics in the Minamata and Niigata regions of Japan, Iraq, Guatemala, Pakistan, and the United States have resulted in a high death rate and an appalling residue of permanent brain damage. In addition to the milder symptoms listed under elemental mercury poisoning, central nervous system manifestations include severe paresthesias, dysarthria, ataxia, visual field constriction, hearing loss, blindness, microcephaly, spasticity, paralysis, and coma. Some of the children of methyl mercury–poisoned mothers show various degrees of cerebral palsy–like abnormalities and mental retardation, and some die.

Chang LW: Neurotoxic effects of mercury—a review. Environ Res 14:329, 1977. *A very useful review with good clinical-pathologic correlations.*

Elhassani SB: The many faces of methylmercury poisoning. J Toxicol Clin Toxicol 19:875, 1982–1983. *A very nice, thorough review with 133 references.*

Joselow MM, Louria DB, Browder AA: Mercurialism: Environmental and occupational aspects. Ann Intern Med 76:119, 1972. *A useful summary with 149 references.*

Magos L: Mercury and mercurials. Br Med Bull 31:241, 1975. *A concise, valuable summary of the clinical manifestations and tissue localization after exposure to different chemical forms of mercury.*

ARSENIC

ETIOLOGY. Arsenic is ubiquitous in nature; it is present in the earth's crust in concentrations of 2 to 5 parts per billion. It is found in inordinately high concentrations in some well waters, particularly in Taiwan. It is used in the glass, pigment, and bronze-plating industries; in wood preservation; in a variety of metal alloys; in veterinary medicines; in some herbicides, insecticides, and rodenticides; in fire salts to produce multicolored flames; and by farmers and vintners. American industry uses about one half of the world's production of arsenic trioxide. Arsenic poisoning has also resulted from using certain herbal preparations and from the ingestion of illegal (moonshine) whiskey.

Elemental arsenic is not toxic even if ingested in substantial dosage. There are three toxic forms of arsenic: pentavalent salts, trivalent salts, and arsine gas. The arsenic in the earth's crust and in most foods is in the pentavalent form. Trivalent arsenic, which is far more toxic, accumulates in the body more readily than the pentavalent form. Arsenic gas (arsine) is extraordinarily toxic; it is formed by the hydrolysis of metallic arsenide or by the action of acids or nascent hydrogen on arsenical compounds, especially in the refining of certain metals. Arsine can be liberated in sewage plants, and in one small cluster of cases eight children were poisoned while cleaning out a cattle dip in Australia.

CLINICAL MANIFESTATIONS. The toxic potential of arsenicals relates to their ability to combine with sulfhydryl groups and thereby interfere with multiple enzyme systems. The evidences of *acute toxicity* are generally similar in those poisoned by either the respiratory or the gastrointestinal route, but the onset of clinical illness is much more rapid after arsine gas exposure, usually appearing within one to twelve hours. The initial manifestations usually include nausea, vomiting, weakness, colicky abdominal pain, and profuse diarrhea. The patient may complain of a metallic taste and there may be a garlic odor to the breath, but the latter is not pathognomonic of arsenic poisoning, occurring also in selenium, tellurium, and phosphorus poisonings. In arsine poisoning there may be a temperature elevation of up to 39° C.

Because arsenic preferentially binds to red blood cells, hemolytic anemia and hemoglobinuria occur early and red cell ghosts may be seen in the peripheral blood. Leukopenia occurs frequently, but in some cases moderate leukocytosis is found and both monocytosis and eosinophilia have been described.

Shortly after the initial red cell binding, arsenic can be found in liver, spleen, heart, kidneys, brain, and intestinal tract. Skin, nails, and hair do not contain arsenic until two to four weeks after exposure.

Other manifestations that may occur in the first week include jaundice, hematuria, hepatomegaly with hepatic enzyme abnormalities; electrocardiographic abnormalities; a cardiomyopathy that can be lethal; evidence of encephalopathy, including headache, irritability, delusions, and hallucinations; and respiratory muscle paralysis. Renal failure may occur consequent to the hemoglobinuria or as a result of cortical necrosis. Megaloblastic changes may be seen in the bone marrow. Optic neuritis with visual field constriction has been reported after pentavalent arsenic exposure.

The most prominent manifestation after the first week of illness is symmetrical polyneuropathy. At first sensory manifestations predominate, the patient complaining of a burning sensation in a stocking-glove distribution. Motor involvement follows almost immediately with diminished or absent reflexes and severe weakness. Prolonged encephalopathy and/or psychosis have been reported in a few instances.

In cases of subacute poisoning, Aldrich-Mees lines (transverse white bands) may be seen in the nails; like the garlic odor, these may be seen in other trace element intoxications. Erythroderma and exfoliative dermatitis may also supervene.

Chronic exposure is associated with several abnormalities. The most characteristic of these are the cutaneous lesions, particularly hyperpigmentation (arsenic melanosis) and hyperkeratoses located primarily on the palms and soles. Alopecia and so called raindrop depigmentation may also occur. In about 5 to 10 per cent of those chronically exposed, skin cancers appear after latent periods of 5 to more than 25 years; these tend to be multiple, are situated mainly on the trunk and upper extremities, and show either intraepithelial squamous cell (Bowen's disease) or basal cell morphology on histologic examination. In the United States the most frequent cause of such skin lesions in past years was the medicinal use of Fowler's solution, an inorganic trivalent arsenical. Currently most cases arise after occupational exposure, but a small number have been ascribed to chronic exposure to well water with high arsenic content.

Epidemiologic studies on gold ore miners, vineyard workers, laborers in sheep dip factories, and smelter workers show a clear increase in the incidence of squamous cell carcinoma of the lung, the risk of bronchogenic cancer correlating with the intensity and duration of arsenic trioxide exposure.

Several types of liver disease may occur; these include postnecrotic cirrhosis, hepatocellular carcinoma, and hemangioendothelioma. Additionally, portal fibrosis and/or sinusoidal collagenosis may be found, and this can lead to a form of noncirrhotic portal hypertension with splenomegaly and esophageal varices but normal hepatic artery wedge pressure. Like the skin cancers, the liver abnormalities may occur many years after exposure to arsenic has been discontinued, and the exposure period can have been relatively brief.

A severe form of peripheral arteriosclerosis in Taiwan called blackfoot disease has been attributed to chronic arsenic exposure, but the data are currently inconclusive. Arsenic exposure is also thought to induce chromosomal aberrations, but the significance of these abnormalities is not clear.

DIAGNOSIS. If the diagnosis is suspected, there is a qualitative urine test (Gutzeit test) employing sulfuric acid, zinc, and silver nitrate. Arsenic concentrations can be measured in blood, urine, hair, or nails by atomic absorption spectrophotometry or neutron activation techniques.

TREATMENT. The treatment of choice is dimercaprol (BAL), but it should be given within the first 24 hours after exposure. If the BAL is given later, it is less likely that improvement will be observed, and in most cases the peripheral neuropathy is refractory to treatment. Exchange transfusion shortly after the onset of acute illness has also been reported to be beneficial.

The neuropathy and renal failure may slowly resolve completely, or there may be residual abnormalities that range from mild to severe.

Gerhardt RE, Crecelius EA, Hudson JB: Moonshine-related arsenic poisoning. Arch Intern Med 140:211, 1980. *Twelve cases of arsenic poisoning are reviewed; in one half, illicit whiskey appeared to be the source.*

Schoolmeester WL, White DR: Arsenic poisoning. South Med J 73:198, 1980. *A fine comprehensive review with 102 references. Includes ten illustrative case reports.*

TRACE ELEMENTS WHOSE TOXICITY IS IN LARGE PART ASSOCIATED WITH HEMODIALYSIS

ZINC. The normal adult body zinc content is 1.5 to 3.0 grams. Daily intake ranges from 5 to 35 mg. Zinc is bound to metallothioneins synthesized in the liver and is excreted by both the urine and the gastrointestinal tract. Particularly high concentrations are found in the uveal tract, choroid plexus, and prostate; substantial amounts are also found in bone, brain, skeletal muscles, and other tissues of the eye.

Zinc has a strong affinity for red cells and plasma proteins. Consequently there is no loss across dialysis membranes; instead, blood zinc concentrations may increase markedly during hemodialysis. There appear to be two well-documented zinc sources: adhesive plaster (containing zinc oxide) used to prevent dialysis coils from unwinding, and the water of the dialysis fluid. Even if water has an initially low zinc content, galvanized iron pipes or tanks may release substantial amounts. This can be prevented by using deionized water or by reverse osmosis. Zinc may also be taken by mouth for a variety of reasons or may be administered intravenously.

The manifestations of zinc toxicity do not necessarily correlate well with plasma or whole blood zinc levels. Nausea, vomiting, anorexia, lethargy, irritability, abdominal pain, and anemia are the most frequent manifestations. The mechanisms responsible for the anemia are not well understood, but in many cases the anemia may be microcytic and associated with evidence of copper deficiency. Zinc can decrease copper absorption in the gut and also promote urinary copper excretion. Fever may accompany zinc toxicity. Other manifestations may include diarrhea, muscle pain, hyperamylasemia with or without pancreatitis, intestinal bleeding, thrombocytopenia, oliguria, hypotension, and renal failure with tubular necrosis. Injection of large amounts of zinc has resulted in death. Intestinal manifestations may supervene after either orally or parenterally induced zinc intoxication.

Welders, smelter workers, and solderers are exposed to aerosolized zinc and may experience zinc fume fever, characterized by chills, fever, myalgias, a metallic taste, cough, nausea, lethargy, and occasionally hemoptysis. There may be diffuse roentgenologic infiltrates and pulmonary dysfunction. Ordinarily all manifestations disappear rapidly after cessation of exposure. If more prolonged pulmonary dysfunction occurs, it is thought to result from the effects of other metals to which the workers are simultaneously exposed.

ALUMINUM. First described in 1972, aluminum-induced dialysis dementia is an often fatal disease. The tap water is usually to blame. Some waters naturally contain high concentrations of aluminum. In other cases aluminum sulfate had been added to the community water supply to remove organic materials. In still other cases the dialysis fluid appeared to be less responsible than aluminum-containing gels administered by mouth to reduce phosphate levels. However, if oral aluminum hydroxide is administered to nondialyzed patients suffering from renal failure, the encephalopathy syndrome occurs very rarely. Dialysis encephalopathy occurs only after repeated dialyses, usually spanning at least several months. Use of parenteral nutrition solutions containing aluminum can also be followed by aluminum poisoning.

Early manifestations include malaise, memory loss, and a characteristic speech disturbance. As the disease progresses, dysarthria, asterixis, myoclonic twitches, dementia, somnolence, and seizures occur. The electroencephalogram shows slowing, together with bursts of delta activity and high voltage, symmetric spikes. Among those who die, aluminum levels are markedly increased in the gray matter.

Other manifestations include anemia, myalgias, proximal myopathy, and severe skeletal pain caused by profound osteodystrophy that is unresponsive to vitamin D and is followed by fractures. Aluminum is deposited at the calcified bone-osteoid junction and bone formation is impaired.

Although frequently lethal, in some cases the encephalopathy has regressed after intake of oral aluminum is stopped or the aluminum content of the dialysis water is reduced or following renal transplantation. Treatment with deferoxamine, which complexes with aluminum, may be beneficial.

It has been suggested that Alzheimer's disease and other types of senile dementia may be related to brain aluminum deposition, but available data are unconvincing.

Those involved in aluminum processing or manufacturing, pottery or explosive making, or welding may be exposed to aluminum aerosols. Pulmonary granulomas, fibrosis, and in some cases postfibrosis emphysema may supervene. In bauxite smelters this is known as Shaver's disease.

COPPER. Since the late 1960's, copper tubing in dialysis equipment has been known to release copper when exposed to acid water. Copper levels may also be inordinately high in the dialysis water if the water is supplied through copper plumbing. Copper is a potent red cell poison, damaging cell membranes and inhibiting a variety of red cell enzymes. Major manifestations of toxicity include hemolysis and gastrointestinal disturbances. Nausea, vomiting, diarrhea, abdominal pain, fever, chills, hemolytic anemia, jaundice, hemoglobinuria, and severe myalgias all occur frequently. Myoglobinemia, necrotizing pancreatitis, and hepatic necrosis may also occur. There may be profound leukocytosis.

Copper poisoning during dialysis is fortunately readily avoidable, since copper is no longer a component of the tubing.

Copper poisoning may also occur after intentional or accidental ingestion. There may be a metallic taste, vomiting, and abdominal pain. In more severe cases hematemesis, melena, hepatic necrosis, and shock supervene.

In Wilson's disease rapid increases in circulating copper concentrations may be followed by acute hemolytic anemia.

These exposed to metallic copper industrially may develop transient pulmonary manifestations (metal fume fever). These disappear rapidly when exposure is stopped.

COBALT. Patients with renal failure may have elevated tissue cobalt levels. In a small number of cases, cardiomegaly and myocardial dysfunction have been attributed to the myocardial cobalt content. In some cases cobaltous chloride has been given by mouth to patients on maintenance hemodialysis to combat anemia. This has been associated with increased blood and myocardial cobalt levels and suggestive evidence of cardiomyopathy.

In the past cobalt had been used to increase red cell production. Toxicity included nausea, vomiting, anorexia, tinnitus, peripheral neuropathy, goiter resulting from blockage of iodine uptake, neurogenic deafness, hyperlipidemia, optic atrophy, and renal tubular damage.

Cobalt was added to beer in the 1960's as a foam stabilizer. This resulted in extraordinary cardiomyopathy, often accompanied by pericardial effusion. Mortality from heart failure or arrhythmias ranged from 5 to 47 per cent (see Ch. 51).

Persons exposed to cobalt industrially may occasionally develop cardiomyopathy. Workers exposed to finely powdered cobalt may also develop pulmonary interstitial fibrosis and cor pulmonale. Cobalt is often a component of alloys that are used in joint prostheses. Cases have been reported of joint pains, spontaneous dislocation of the prosthesis, and bone necrosis starting nine months to four years postoperatively, apparently caused by a reaction to the cobalt in the alloy.

OTHER METALS. In one group of dialysis patients *nickel* toxicity occurred when nickel leached from a stainless steel water heater tank into the dialysis fluid. Manifestations included nausea, vomiting, weakness, and headache. Symptoms developed within a few hours after dialysis and disappeared within 48 hours.

Tissue *tin* concentrations, especially in the liver, are increased in patients undergoing hemodialysis. However, tin levels are even higher in uremic patients who have not been dialyzed. No definite clinical disease has been associated with these increased body tin burdens.

Patients undergoing maintenance hemodialysis are often treated with *iron* for anemia. In such patients parenteral and occasionally oral iron administration may be followed by hemosiderosis and occasionally hemochromatosis. Serum ferritin concentrations exceed 500 ng per milliliter. A proximal myopathy has been described. The severity of the tissue iron overload and the likelihood of hemochromatosis may be related to the histocompatibility antigens A-3, B-7, and B-14. Iron overload has been complicated by porphyria cutanea tarda and by a variety of infections, including those due to species of *Yersinia* and *Vibrio* and to the yeast *Trichosporon cutaneum.* Treatment with deferoxamine may reduce the body iron burden.

Aggett PJ, Harrison JT: Current status of zinc in health and disease states. Arch Dis Child 54:909, 1979. *This is a superb review with 110 references. Only a small section is devoted to toxicity.*

Bogden JD, Oleske JM, Weiner B, et al.: Elevated plasma zinc concentrations in renal dialysis patients. Am J Clin Nutr 33:1088, 1980. *A careful study of two dialysis units that demonstrates clearly significant leakage of zinc from some coils.*

Manifold IH, Platts MM, Kennedy A: Cobalt cardiomyopathy in a patient on maintenance haemodialysis. Br Med J 2:1609, 1978. *A 17-year-old woman given oral cobalt for anemia.*

O'Hare JA, Callaghan NM, Murnaghan DJ: Dialysis encephalopathy. Clinical, electroencephalographic and interventional aspects. Medicine 62:129, 1983. *A marvelous summary article and a careful analysis of 14 patients who developed encephalopathy 16 to 92 months after starting dialysis.*

Ott SM, Maloney NA, Klein GL, et al: Aluminum is associated with low bone formation in patients receiving chronic parenteral nutrition. Ann Intern Med 98:910, 1983. *The toxicity of aluminum to bone is clearly shown in 14 patients receiving casein hydrolysate.*

Petrie JJB, Row PG: Dialysis anaemia caused by subacute zinc toxicity. Lancet 1:1178, 1977. *Ten patients on home dialysis were studied; nine developed anemia from zinc released from galvanized iron piping.*

Sandstead HH: Trace elements in uremia and hemodialysis. Am J Clin Nutr 33:1501, 1980. *A very good review article in which the author urges caution in ascribing the dialysis encephalopathy syndrome solely to aluminum.*

Taylor A, Marks V: Cobalt: A review. J Hum Nutr 32:165, 1978. *A nice review with 73 references.*

Webster JD, Parker TF, Alfrey A, et al.: Acute nickel intoxication by dialysis. Ann Intern Med 92:631, 1980. *Nausea, vomiting, weakness, and headache were the predominant manifestations among 37 patients. Symptoms remitted three to thirteen hours after dialysis was concluded.*

CADMIUM

ETIOLOGY. Over 10 million pounds of cadmium are used industrially every year in the United States. The metal is a component of alloys; it is used in the manufacture of electrical conductors and in electroplating; and it is present in ceramics, pigments, dental prosthetics, plastic stabilizers, and storage batteries. It is also a byproduct of zinc smelting and is used in the photographic, rubber, motor, and aircraft industries. Smelters, metal processing furnaces, and the burning of coal and oil are responsible for much of the cadmium in air.

CLINICAL MANIFESTATIONS. *Acute intoxication* from cadmium fumes produces a characteristic clinical picture. Four to ten hours after exposure dyspnea, cough, and substernal discomfort supervene, often accompanied by prominent myalgias and fatigue. In more severe cases wheezing, hemoptysis, and progressive dyspnea caused by pulmonary edema may occur.

In most cases, the pulmonary manifestations resolve rapidly but pulmonary function abnormalities may not disappear for months; in these cases vital capacity is reduced and there is a restrictive defect. Occasionally pulmonary edema is lethal. Autopsy and experimental studies show alveolar cell metaplasia and proliferation of Type II pulmonary cells.

Ingestion of large amounts of cadmium results in nausea, vomiting, and abdominal pain, often accompanied by weakness, prostration, and myalgias. The onset of the gastroenteritis occurs one half to five hours after ingestion and lasts for less than 24 hours.

Chronic cadmium exposure by aerosol for at least ten years has resulted in emphysema in a small number of cases. The emphysema is not accompanied by bronchitis and may appear many years after industrial exposure has stopped. Workers exposed for at least ten years also may suffer olfactory nerve damage; in some cases this progresses to total anosmia. The most frequent long-term consequence of aerosol or oral exposure is proteinuria. After prolonged and heavy contact, cadmium urinary excretion continues for years and is associated with damage to the proximal tubule. The major urinary protein is a low molecular weight β_2 microglobulin.

On occasion the proteinuria may be accompanied by glycosuria and aminoaciduria. Only infrequently is the proteinuria and tubular damage followed by progressive renal failure. An exception to the relatively benign course of the renal damage is the disease in Japan known as itai-itai (ouch-ouch), which affected almost exclusively multiparous women of ages 40 to 70 who lived in an area contaminated by industrial cadmium waste. Manifestations included striking back and joint pains, a waddly gait, osteomalacia, bone deformities, and fractures, all presumably secondary to cadmium-induced renal tubular damage. The occurrence of the disease primarily in middle-aged multiparous women remains unexplained; presumably concomitant nutritional deficiencies played an important role. In other areas of Japan greater cadmium intake produced no such manifestations.

Animal studies have suggested that cadmium administration can produce hypertension; there is no satisfactory evidence documenting an association of cadmium with hypertension in man. Some studies on workers exposed to cadmium have suggested an increased risk of lung or prostatic carcinoma, but the data are not convincing.

One of the most intriguing aspects of cadmium distribution in the body is its relation to metallothioneins, low molecular weight metal binding proteins with high cysteine content. The cadmium appears to induce production of the proteins in the liver and kidneys and probably in the intestines. The thioneins may act to prevent absorption of ingested cadmium and may play a role in storage and detoxification of cadmium in the liver and kidneys, the two tissues of maximal cadmium concentrations.

Brenner I: Cadmium toxicity. World Rev Nutr Diet 32:165, 1978. *Interactions with calcium, zinc, copper, and selenium are emphasized. Additionally there is a detailed analysis of the role of metallothioneins. Contains 183 references.*
Lauwery RR, Roels AA, Buchet JP, Bernard A, Stanescu D: Investigations on the lung and kidney function of workers exposed to cadmium. Environ Health Persp 28:137, 1979. *Three epidemiologic studies were conducted on more than 200 workers. The kidney was affected to a much greater extent than the lungs. Both tubular and glomerular aberrations were found, mainly in persons with substantially increased blood and urine cadmium concentrations.*

NICKEL

ETIOLOGY. Nickel is used widely industrially in various alloys, iron shell castings, ball bearings, and heart and joint prostheses. It is also used in nickel plating; as a catalyst; in magnetic tapes, dyes, and paints; and in acrylic plastics. It is found in petroleum and coal, in diesel fuels, and in soil and air. Municipal incinerators may contribute to the ambient air nickel concentrations.

Nickel is a potent contact allergen; the most frequent adverse effect for man is nickel dermatitis, which may be both persistent and severe. Serious systemic reactions have occurred in allergic persons given fluids intravenously through a nickel-containing needle. Prosthetic heart and joint valves have failed because of a reaction to the nickel in the prosthesis. In cases of recalcitrant nickel dermatitis, restriction in dietary nickel may be helpful.

CLINICAL MANIFESTATIONS AND TREATMENT. By far the most toxic of the nickel compounds is nickel carbonyl, created by a reaction between nickel and carbon monoxide. Industrial aerosol exposure is followed immediately by headache, drowsiness, substernal pain, nausea, and vomiting. This is followed by a latent period of one to five days, after which the victim experiences fever, chills, dyspnea, a feeling of chest tightness, cough that is sometimes productive of blood-tinged sputum, muscle pains, weakness, and fatigue. Hepatic enzyme concentrations may be considerably elevated. In severe cases cyanosis, progressive respiratory difficulties, and convulsions ensue, and death may follow in 4 to 23 days. At autopsy the lungs show hemorrhage, atelectasis, fibroblastic proliferation, and hyaline membrane formation. The treatment of choice is diethyl dithiocarbamate (Dithiocarb); dimercaprol (BAL) is an alternative but less effective therapeutic agent. Although overwhelming pneumonitis caused by nickel carbonyl is now rare, milder pulmonary toxicity in occupations such as welding probably occurs quite commonly and goes unrecognized under the general rubric of metal fume fever. Nickel exposure may also be followed by Löffler's syndrome.

CARCINOGENESIS. Nickel is considered a potent respiratory tract carcinogen. Studies of nickel refinery workers in the 1950's showed a fivefold increase in risk of lung cancer and a 150-fold increase in the risk of nasal cancer. Recent studies also indicate a substantially increased risk of larynx cancer. Among one group of Norwegian nickel workers, one third of all cancers involved the lungs and an additional 10 per cent involved the sinuses. Those occupations most at risk among nickel workers are roasting, smelting, and electrolysis. Workers developing lung, laryngeal, and nasal cancers have usually been exposed for at least ten years. Biopsies of nasal mucosa show potentially precancerous epithelial dysplasia in a substantial percentage of nickel workers. The cancer risk is so great that workers heavily exposed for over ten years should probably have annual nasal mucosa biopsies as well as sputum cytologic studies and roentgenologic examinations every four to six months in an attempt at secondary prevention. The incidence of respiratory tract cancer in nickel workers is dependent on both the extent of nickel exposure and the effects of cocarcinogens, in particular cigarette tobacco. Some data suggest that nickel in tobacco may play a role in cigarette-induced lung cancer and that nickel compounds attached to asbestos fibers may contribute to the neoplastic potential of asbestos; conversely, asbestos contamination of nickel may augment nickel carcinogenicity.

Sunderman FW Jr: A review of the metabolism and toxicity of nickel. Ann Clin Lab Sci 7:377, 1977. *An excellent review by one of the world's leading authorities (with 177 references).*

Sunderman FW Sr: Efficacy of sodium diethyldithiocarbamate (Dithiocarb) in acute nickel carbonyl poisoning. Ann Clin Lab Sci 9:1, 1979. *The data presented strongly suggest that this is currently the agent of choice.*

OTHER TOXIC METALS

Thallium

ETIOLOGY AND PATHOGENESIS. Thallium is used in optical lenses, jewelry, low temperature thermometers, semiconductors, luminescent tubes, dyes and pigments, scintillation counters, and fireworks. It forms a stainless alloy with silver, a corrosion-resistant alloy with lead, and may be a byproduct of lead and zinc production. In some areas it is still a component of rodenticides, pesticides, and insecticides. Thallium can enter the body through the respiratory tract, gastrointestinal tract, or skin. Like many other trace metals thallium has a strong affinity for sulfhydryl groups and thus interferes with many enzyme systems. Additionally, it enters the cell, exchanging for intracellular potassium.

CLINICAL MANIFESTATIONS. Poisoning can be acute and overwhelming after suicidal ingestion or it can be chronic and subtle. In acute poisoning manifestations include nausea, vomiting, abdominal pain, diarrhea that may be bloody, insomnia, myalgias, fever, hyperhidrosis, excessive thirst, delirium, seizures, coma, and respiratory failure. At least 10 per cent of acutely poisoned persons die.

Among those who survive at least a week or in those exposed to smaller amounts of thallium, the most predictable manifestations are a combined sensory and motor, often painful, peripheral neuropathy and alopecia. Although the head alopecia is total, the facial, axillary, and pubic hair are spared as is the inner one third of the eyebrows. Motor manifestations may predominate, and the ascending, predominantly motor paralysis may mimic Guillain-Barré syndrome. Abdominal colic, nausea, and vomiting occur frequently in both the acute and subacute forms of thallium toxicity and may so dominate the clinical picture that a diagnosis of acute appendicitis is made. Other manifestations of subacute intoxication include dementia, headache, fatigue, sleep disorders, intractable thirst, hallucinations, blindness caused by optic neuritis, impotence, amenorrhea, a blue discoloration of the gingivae, centrilobular hepatic necrosis, renal tubular necrosis, orthostatic hypotension, and myoclonic twitches. Multiple cranial nerves may be involved, but the eighth nerve is almost always spared. The electrocardiogram may show arrhythmias and changes similar to those associated with hypokalemia.

DIAGNOSIS. Thallium can be measured in blood and urine, but blood levels are often deceptively low even during clinically apparent poisoning. Since thallium is excreted in the urine, thallium determinations on 24-hour specimens are more reliable. A qualitative urine test is available. Urine is mixed with 0.4 per cent sodium bismuth in 20 per cent nitric acid and 10 per cent sodium iodide; if thallium is present, a red precipitate forms.

In some cases there is no history of occupational, environmental, or intentional exposure. Unexplained abdominal pain, neurologic abnormalities, and alopecia suggest the diagnosis.

TREATMENT. Treatment consists of hemodialysis, which can remove up to half the thallium body burden, potassium, forced diuresis, and administration of Prussian blue. Prussian blue, given by mouth, absorbs thallium so that fecal thallium concentrations increase. The half-life of thallium in the body is about one month, and repeated dialyses are usually needed. Hemoperfusion may also help. During potassium administration thallium is displaced from its intracellular site, and this may cause transient exacerbations of clinical manifestations. Barbiturates may increase the severity of the disease, and their use should be avoided.

PROGNOSIS. As many as 30 per cent of those poisoned suffer some residual effects. The neuropathy may persist for many months before resolving, and some are left with variable amounts of dementia, neuropathy, ataxia, visual impairment, and myoclonus.

Selenium

ETIOLOGY. Selenium is well absorbed from both the gastrointestinal tract and the lungs. The amount normally ingested varies markedly, depending on the local soil selenium content and on the geographic provenance of foods consumed. Grains, pork, kidney, seafoods, garlic, mushrooms, radishes, beef, egg yolk, and chicken frequently contain substantial amounts of selenium. The element is widely used in pigment, glass, electronics, ceramics, and steel industries.

CLINICAL MANIFESTATIONS. Both deficiency and toxicity syndromes are well described in animals. Deficiency, resulting from foraging on grains grown in soil deficient of selenium, produces white muscle disease, a diffuse, often severe myopathy. Excess caused by chronic ingestion of grains containing more than 10 parts per million of selenium results in two syndromes, alkali disease and the staggers. The former is milder and is characterized by anemia, emaciation, alopecia, and hoof deformity. The staggers is manifested by visual difficulties, anemia, liver cell degeneration, paralysis, and respiratory failure. In sheep, excessive selenium intake can produce severe cardiomyopathy.

In man a *selenium deficiency syndrome* has not been clearly defined. However, in the Republic of China diffuse cardiomyopathy has been associated with low soil and blood selenium levels, and the incidence of the disease allegedly has been strikingly reduced by selenium supplementation.

Selenium toxicity syndromes in man can be divided into acute and chronic poisoning. Subjects with inordinate exposure to selenium fumes experience one or more of the following abnormalities: intestinal disturbances, giddiness, apathy, lassitude, pallor, nervousness, depression, hair and nail loss, a garlic odor to the breath, and a metallic taste. Sore throat, dyspnea, and cough may also be noted. Symptoms usually disappear after removal from the occupational exposure. Among those ingesting excessive selenium the following symptoms and signs have been reported: nausea, vomiting, anorexia, fatigue, sore throat, emotional lability, a metallic taste, a garlic odor to the breath, a bronze color to the skin, hepatic dysfunction, and diffuse dermatitis. Increased selenium burdens may be associated with an increased prevalence of dental caries.

EPIDEMIOLOGY. Subacute and chronic selenium toxicity will likely be seen with an increasing frequency because selenium is being promoted as a nonprescription supplement. Epidemiologic data suggest an inverse relationship between selenium blood levels and the incidence of certain cancers, particularly of the intestinal tract. In experimental studies oral selenium in dosage of 0.1 to 2.0 parts per million diminishes the frequency of or delays the appearance of a variety of spontaneous or induced tumors.

In experimental animals selenium potentiates the immune response. Additionally, it is being used without adequate documentation in patients with cystic fibrosis on the assumption that the disease is related in part to selenium deficiency. There are as yet no convincing data to recommend that selenium supplements be taken by ostensibly healthy adults as a cancer preventive or as an immunopotentiator.

Manganese

Manganese toxicity occurs primarily in miners who have been exposed to manganese dioxide aerosols for prolonged periods. The manifestations, known as manganic madness, are limited to the central nervous system. The manganese is concentrated primarily in the basal ganglia and cerebellum accounting for the extrapyramidal Parkinson-like facies, the rigidity, and the difficulty in walking. Other manifestations include compulsive behavior (including singing, dancing, fighting, and running), explosive and involuntary laughter, headache, muscular weakness, tremors, dystonia, hypotonia, retropulsion and propulsion, dementia, speech disturbances, irritability, hypersomnia, and memory defects. In some cases psychosis may be the dominant feature. There is no effective therapy. After removal from manganese exposure or following attempts to reduce the body manganese load by treatment with calcium versenate or L-dopa, the mental aberrations usually improve but the neurologic abnormalities persist. Manganese contamination of dialysates or ingestion has been associated with abdominal pain, liver dysfunction, and evidence of pancreatitis.

Barium

Barium compounds are used in printing; in the production of paints, glass, paper, leather, soap, and rubber; in ceramics, plastic, steel, oil, textile, and dye industries; as fuel additives; and in insecticides, rodenticides, and depilatories. There are two major adverse effects. After accidental or intentional ingestion of large amounts, abdominal pain, vomiting, and increased peristalsis occur. If enough is absorbed, potassium is displaced intracellularly resulting in profound hypokalemia, which in turn may produce flaccid paralysis, potentially dangerous cardiac arrhythmias, renal failure, and respiratory paralysis. Treatment consists of administration of potassium and forced diuresis to promote barium excretion.

The other adverse effect from contact with barium is a benign pneumoconiosis that may supervene after one or more years of aerosol exposure. Chest roentgenograms show extensive, very dense, bilateral nodules up to 4 to 5 mm in diameter. There is no prominent fibrosis and no clinically significant disease; the nodules often regress after occupational exposure is stopped.

Boron

There are few reports of boron toxicity. Ingestion of boric acid can result in nausea, vomiting, diarrhea, anemia, seizures, a variety of skin eruptions characterized by intense erythema, desquamation, and exfoliation, and striking alopecia. Additionally, occupational aerosol exposure to diborane (B_2H_6) in high energy fuels can produce acute pulmonary edema that resolves after the exposure is discontinued.

Antimony

Industrial antimony toxicity is very rare, as are intentional ingestion or inadvertent poisoning from release of antimony from inexpensive enamelware. Manifestations of acute poisoning include nausea, abdominal pain, weakness, headache, vomiting, diarrhea, myalgias, and circulatory collapse. Gaseous SbH_3 (stibine) is as toxic as arsine, producing CNS toxicity and hemolysis. After antimonial injection for medicinal purposes, adverse effects include nausea, vomiting, cough, and muscle and joint pain. Hepatic dysfunction can occur, as can cardiac arrhythmias, including Adams-Stokes syndrome. Antimony is also considered one of the metals capable of causing metal fume fever.

Chromium

Chromium is used extensively in metal and galvanizing industries and in the manufacture of dyes, enamel, and paints. There is substantial epidemiologic evidence that chromate exposure is associated with an increased incidence of lung cancer. Additionally, chromium-exposed workers may show evidence of proximal renal tubule dysfunction and may suffer nasal septum perforations.

Molybdenum

In animals molybdenum produces diarrhea, anemia, alopecia, diminished growth, and bone and joint abnormalities. No clearly defined molybdenum toxicity syndrome has been reported in man.

Platinum

The major adverse effects observed in platinum workers are allergic pulmonary reactions, including bronchial asthma.

Plutonium

In experimental models, plutonium, because of its radioactivity, is a potent carcinogen. Workers have been generally well protected, and it seems unlikely that occupational exposure will be found to be a major problem. Some still controversial epidemiologic studies have suggested that accidental community exposure has resulted in an increase in frequency of certain cancers and fetal malformations.

Tellurium

Used particularly in rubber, metallurgic, and electronics industries, tellurium can cause giddiness, headache, nausea, a metallic taste, and a garlic smell to the breath. In animals tellurium causes neuropathy, but this has not been convincingly demonstrated in man.

Tin

Tin can be released into beverages or foods from tin cans; ingestion can produce nausea, vomiting, abdominal pain, and diarrhea. Such toxicity occurs infrequently. Additionally, there have been occasional reports of encephalopathy following industrial exposure to organic tin compounds; this was characterized by headache, vomiting, visual defects, and paresis. Aerosol exposure to tin may result in stannosis, a mild pneumoconiosis in which there may be dense bilateral infiltrates but usually no pulmonary dysfunction.

Vanadium

Vanadium is used in alloys and in the steel and chemical industries. Its inhalation can result in neurasthenia, anorexia, vertigo, throat pain, nasal irritation (even nasal hemorrhage), and acute bronchitis characterized by a cough that is sometimes accompanied by a whoop. The nasal mucosa of vanadium-exposed workers shows vascular hyperemia and round cell infiltration.

Doig AT: Baritosis: A benign pneumoconiosis. Thorax 31:30, 1976. *Nine cases are described. Despite dense infiltrates, no significant clinical disease or physiologic abnormalities occurred.*

Ghezzi R, Bozza Marrubini M: Prussian blue in the treatment of thallium intoxication. Vet Human Toxicol 21 (Suppl):64, 1979. *Five cases of rodenticide poisoning are reported. Clinical manifestations are summarized. Prussian blue increased fecal thallium and effected clinical improvement.*

Gordon AS, Prichard JS, Freedman MH: Seizure disorders and anemia associated with chronic borax intoxication. Can Med Assoc J 108:719, 1973. *Two infants poisoned by use of pacifiers dipped in borax.*

Louria DB, Joselow MM, Browder AA: The human toxicity of certain trace elements. Ann Intern Med 76:307, 1972. *A review of 12 metals with 154 references.*

Nordberg GF: Factors influencing metabolism and toxicity of metals: A consensus report. Environ Health Persp 25:3, 1978. *This marvelous analysis covers the toxicity and interactions with other metals of arsenic, cadmium, lead, and mercury. Highly recommended. Contains 312 references.*

Saddique A, Peterson CD: Thallium poisoning: A review. Vet Hum Toxicol 25:16, 1983. *A very good review indeed, with 48 references.*

Thallium poisoning. Clinical Conferences of the Johns Hopkins Hospital. Johns Hopkins Med J 142:27, 1978. *A single case accompanied by an excellent discussion of clinical manifestations and treatment.*

Yang G, Wang S, Zhou R, et al: Endemic selenium intoxication of humans in China. Am J Clin Nutr 37:872, 1983. *An extraordinary disease characterized by nail and hair loss and probably by skin and nervous system abnormalities was first described in Hubei Province of China. Stony coal with very high selenium content was the source, the incidence of the disease reaching almost 50 per cent in heavily affected villages.*

Part XXVII
LABORATORY REFERENCE RANGE VALUES OF CLINICAL IMPORTANCE

566. REFERENCE RANGES AND LABORATORY VALUES OF CLINICAL IMPORTANCE*

Norbert W. Tietz

Reference ranges are valuable guidelines for the clinician, but they should not be regarded as absolute indicators of health and disease. There are several reasons for using reference ranges with caution, some of which are listed in Ch. 20. Most importantly, values for "healthy" individuals often overlap significantly with values for persons afflicted with disease. In addition, laboratory values may vary significantly because of methodological differences and mode of standardization. This is especially true for immunological tests, which utilize antibodies that may have different characteristics. As a result, laboratory values in individual institutions may differ from those listed in this chapter.

The values in this chapter are primarily for adults in the fasting state. Values for other age groups, when included, are clearly identified.

All laboratory values are given in conventional and international units. In general, the international units given conform to the SI system (Système International d'Unités). However, in some cases the recommendations of the International Union of Pure and Applied Chemistry (IUPAC) and the Commission on World Standards of the World Association of Societies of Pathology (COWS of WASP) are used, since it is felt that these have found wider acceptance in clinical laboratories and offer advantages over the units recommended in the SI system.

Throughout this chapter we have used the prefixes for units as approved by the CGPM (Conférence Générale des Poids et Mésures), 1964, and the International Congress of Clinical Chemistry, 1966. The pertinent prefixes denoting the decimal factors are listed below.

PREFIXES DENOTING DECIMAL FACTORS

Prefix	*Symbol*	*Factor*
mega	M	10^6
kilo	k	10^3
hecto	h	10^2
deka	da	10^1
deci	d	10^{-1}
centi	c	10^{-2}
milli	m	10^{-3}
micro	μ	10^{-6}
nano	n	10^{-9}
pico	p	10^{-12}
femto	f	10^{-15}

*The material in this chapter was partially extracted from: *Clinical Guide to Laboratory Tests*, NW Tietz, ed.: Philadelphia, W. B. Saunders Company, 1983. The main contributors are RV Blanke and RA Blouin: Drugs and Toxicology; C Hougie: Coagulation; HP Lehmann: International Units; J Leonard: Endocrinology; W Mertz and RV Blanke: Trace Metals; DA Nelson: Hematologhy; SE Ritzmann: Proteins; and HE Sauberlich: Vitamins. A portion of the values was generated in the clinical laboratories of the University of Kentucky Medical Center. Other sources are listed under references for this chapter.

ABBREVIATIONS

For convenience and to preserve space we have used standard abbreviations commonly used in laboratory medicine. Less common abbreviations and some nonstandard abbreviations are given below.

AU	Arbitrary Units
BMD	Boehringer Mannheim Diagnostics, Inc.
EU	Ehrlich Unit
G-D	General Diagnostics
GPIMH	Guinea Pig Intestinal Mucosal Homogenate
ICSH	International Committee for Standardization in Hematology
IFA	Immunofluorescent Assay
IRP-2-hMG	2nd International Reference Preparation of Human Menopausal Gonadotropin
IU	International Unit (of hormone activity)
NEFA	Nonesterified Fatty Acids (Free Fatty Acids)
Occup.	Occupational
P-5'-P	Pyridoxal-5'-Phosphate
RIA	Radioimmunoassay
RID	Radialimmunodiffusion
RT	Room Temperature
U	International Unit (of enzyme activity)
WHO	World Health Organization

ACKNOWLEDGMENT. We thankfully acknowledge the assistance of Nancy M. Logan, B.A., and Susan C. Blandford in the preparation of this material.

Beutler E: Hemolytic Anemia in Disorders of Red Cell Metabolism. New York, Plenum Publishing Company, 1978.

Brown SS, Mitchell FL, Young DS (eds.): Chemical Diagnosis of Disease. Amsterdam, Elsevier/North-Holland Biomedical Press, 1979.

Conn HF, Conn RB (eds.): Current Diagnosis. 6th ed. Philadelphia, W. B. Saunders Company, 1980.

Gilman AG, Goodman L, Gilman A (eds.): The Pharmacological Basis of Therapeutics. 6th ed. New York, The Macmillan Company, 1980.

Henry JB (ed.): Todd-Sanford-Davidsohn Clinical Diagnosis and Management by Laboratory Methods. 16th ed. Philadelphia, W. B. Saunders Company, 1979.

Mabry C, Tietz NW: Tables of normal laboratory values. *In* Nelson WE, Vaughan VC, McKay RJ, Behrman RE (eds.): Nelson Textbook of Pediatrics. 12th ed. Philadelphia, W. B. Saunders Company, 1983.

Miale JB: Laboratory Medicine: Hematology. 5th ed. St. Louis, C. V. Mosby Company, 1977.

Tietz NW (ed.): Fundamentals of Clinical Chemistry. 2nd ed. Philadelphia, W. B. Saunders Company, 1976.

Tietz NW, Blackburn RH (eds.): Reference Ranges and General Information. Clinical Laboratories, A. B. Chandler Medical Center, University of Kentucky, Lexington, Kentucky, 1984.

Tietz NW (ed.): Clinical Guide to Laboratory Tests. Philadelphia, W. B. Saunders Company, 1983.

Williams WJ, Beutler E, Erslev AJ, Rundles RW: Hematology. 2nd ed. New York, McGraw-Hill Book Company, 1977.

CLINICAL CHEMISTRY, TOXICOLOGY, SEROLOGY

Test	Specimen	Reference Range	Reference Range (International Units)
Acetoacetate			
Semiquantitative	Serum or plasma (fluoride/oxalate)	Negative (< 3 mg/dL)	Negative (< 0.3 mmol/L)
	Urine	Negative	Negative
Acetone			
Semiquantitative	Serum or plasma (fluoride or oxalate)	Negative (< 3 mg/dL)	Negative (< 0.5 mmol/L)
Quantitative		0.3–2.0 mg/dL	0.05–0.34 mmol/L
Semiquantitative	Urine	Negative	Negative
Adrenocorticotropic hormone (ACTH)	Plasma (EDTA)	Adult 0800 h: 25–100 pg/mL 1800 h: < 50 pg/mL	 25–100 ng/L < 50 ng/L
Adrenocorticotropic Hormone Stimulation Test (Prolonged Infusion) *Dose: 500 μg Cortrosyn/d × 3*	Urine, 24 h	17–KGS: 2- to 4-fold rise 17–KS: 2-fold rise 17–OHCS: 2- to 5-fold rise Cortisol: 25–50 μg/dL	17–KGS: 2- to 4-fold rise 17–KS: 2-fold rise 17–OHCS: 2- to 5-fold rise Cortisol: 0.7–1.4 μmol/L
Adrenocorticotropic Hormone Stimulation Test (Rapid Test) *Dose: 250 μg Cortrosyn IM*	Serum; fasting, 30 and 60 min after stimulation	Cortisol Baseline: > 5.0 μg/dL After Cortrosyn: 2× baseline	 Baseline: < 0.14 μmol/L After Cortrosyn: 2× baseline
Alanine Aminotransferase (ALT, GPT)	Serum	*U/L* Newborn/Infant: 5–28 Adult: 8–20 > 60 y, M: 7–24 F: 7–16	*U/L* 5–28 8–20 7–24 7–16
Albumin *Nephelometric, colorimetric*	Serum	Adult: 3.5–5.0 g/dL > 60 y: 3.4–4.8 g/dL Avg. ~ 0.3 g/dL higher in ambulatory individuals	35–50 g/L 34–48 g/L Avg. ~ 3 g/L higher in ambulatory individuals
Nephelometric, rate	CSF	10–30 mg/dL	100–300 mg/L
	Urine	< 80 mg/d at rest < 150 mg/d ambulatory	< 80 mg/d < 150 mg/d
Aldolase	Serum	*U/L* 1.0–7.5 (30°C) 0.3–3.0 (at bed rest) 1.5–12.0 (37°C)	*U/L* 1.0–7.5 (30°C) 0.3–3.0 (at bed rest) 1.5–12.0 (37°C)
Aldosterone	Plasma (heparin, EDTA) or serum	*ng/dL* 3–11 y: 5–70 11–15 y: < 5–50 Adult, *average sodium diet* supine: 3–10 upright, F: 5–30 M: 6–22	*nmol/L* 0.14–1.9 < 0.14–1.4 0.08–0.3 0.14–0.8 0.17–0.61
		2–3× higher during pregnancy; adrenal vein: 200–800	 5.5–22
		Low sodium diet: value increases 2– to 5– fold; Florinef suppression: < 4 ng/dL ACTH or angiotensin stimulation, 1 h: 2– to 5–fold increase	 < 0.1 nmol/L

CLINICAL CHEMISTRY, TOXICOLOGY, SEROLOGY (*Continued*)

Test	Specimen	Reference Range	Reference Range (International Units)
	Urine, 24 h	*Total Urinary Na nmol/d* / *Plasma Renin activity ng AI/mL/h* / *Urinary aldosterone μg/d* < 20 / 5–24 / > 35–80 50 / 2–7 / 13–33 100 / 1–5 / 5–24 150 / 0.5–4 / 3–19 200 / / 1–16 250 / / 1–13 (assuming normal serum Na, K, and extracellular vol)	*Urinary aldosterone nmol/d* > 97–220 36–91 14–66 8–53 3–44 3–36
δ-Aminolevulinic Acid (δ-ALA)	Serum	15–23 μg/dL; lower in children	1.1–1.8 μmol/L
	Urine	1.3–7.0 mg/d	9.9–53.4 μmol/d
Ammonia Nitrogen *Resin or enzymatic*	Serum or plasma (Na-heparin)	*μg N/dL* Newborn: 90–150 < 1 mo: 29–70 Adult: 15–45	*μmol N/L* 64–107 21–50 11–32
	Urine, 24 h	140–1500 mg/d	10–107 mmol/d
Amobarbital	Serum	Therap. conc.: 1–5 μg/mL Toxic conc.: > 10 μg/mL	4–22 μmol/L > 44 μmol/L
Amylase *(Beckman; BMD)*	Serum	Adult: 25–125 U/L > 70 y: 20–160 U/L	25–125 U/L 20–160 U/L
	Urine, timed specimen	1–17 U/h	1–17 U/h
Androstenedione	Serum	*ng/dL(mean ± 1SE)* *M* / *F* Cord: 85 ± 27 / 93 ± 28 1–3 mo: 34 ± 11 / 19 ± 4 Adult: 107 ± 25 / 151 ± 38	*nmol/L (mean ± 1 SE)* *M* / *F* 2.9 ± 0.94 / 3.2 ± 1.0 1.2 ± 0.4 / 0.66 ± 0.14 3.74 ± 0.87 / 5.27 ± 1.33
Angiotensin I	Peripheral venous plasma (KEDTA)	11–88 pg/mL	11–88 ng/L
Angiotensin II	Plasma (KEDTA)	Arterial blood: 2.4 ± 1.2 ng/dL Venous blood: 50–75% of arterial blood concentration	24 ± 12 ng/L Fraction of arterial blood conc.: 0.50–0.75
Anion Gap **[Na − (Cl^- + HCO_3^-)]**	Plasma (heparin)	7–14 mmol/L	7–14 mmol/L
Antidiuretic Hormone–Water Deprivation Stimulation Test (Miller Test)	Serum (0600 h) and hourly urine for osmolality; when urine osmolality plateaus after fluid restriction, measure serum osmolality and ADH	Max. urine osmolality before vasopressin admin. more than serum osmolality; at end of test, serum osmolality: < 300 mOsmol/kg; urine osmolality: > 500 mOsmol/kg; ADH levels: see table under hADH; 1 h after vasopressin admin. < 5% increase in urine osmolality over previous specimen	
Antihyaluronidase Titer (AH Titer)	Serum	≤ 128 units/mL	≤ 128 units/mL
Antistreptolysin-O Titer (ASO Titer)	Serum	≤ 166 Todd Units; 170–330 Todd Units in school-aged children	
α_1-Antitrypsin	Serum	Newborn: 145–270 mg/dL Adult: 78–200 mg/dL	1.45–2.70 g/L 0.78–2.00 g/L
Arsenic	Whole blood (heparin)	*μg/dL* 0.2– 6.2 Chronic poisoning: 10–50 Acute poisoning: 60–93	*μmol/L* 0.03–0.82 1.33–6.65 7.98–12.37
	Urine, 24 h	5–50 μg/d	0.067–0.665 μmol/d
Ascorbic Acid, see *Vitamin C*			
Aspartate Aminotransferase (AST, SGOT, 30°C)	Serum	*U/L* Infant: 15–60 Adult: 8–20 < 60 y, M: 11–26 F: 10–20 With P-5′-P: 12–29	*U/L* 15–60 8–20 11–26 10–20 12–29

CLINICAL CHEMISTRY, TOXICOLOGY, SEROLOGY (*Continued*)

Test	Specimen	Reference Range	Reference Range (International Units)
Base Excess	Whole blood (heparin)	*mmol/L* Newborn: (−10)–(−2) Infant: (−7)–(−1) Child: (−4)–(+2) Adult: (−2)–(+3)	*mmol/L* (−10)–(−2) (−7)–(−1) (−4)–(+2) (−2)–(+3)
Bicarbonate	Serum	Art.: 21–28 mmol/L Ven.: 22–29 mmol/L	Art.: 21–28 mmol/L Ven.: 22–29 mmol/L
Bile Acids, Total	Serum, fasting Serum, 2 h postprandial	0.3–2.3 μg/mL 1.8–3.2 μg/mL	0.74–5.64 μmol/L (conv. factor 4.41–7.84 μmol/L based on cholic acid, M.W. 408.6)
	Feces	120–225 mg/d	294–551 μmol/d
Bilirubin			
Total	Serum	*Premature mg/dL* / *Full Term mg/dL* Cord: < 2.0 / < 2.0 0–1 d: < 8.0 / < 6.0 3–5 d: < 16.0 / < 12.0 Thereafter: < 2.0 / 0.2–1.0	*Premature* / *Full Term* *μmol/L* < 34 / < 34 < 137 / < 103 < 274 / < 205 < 34 / 3.4–17.1
	Urine	Negative	Negative
Conjugated (direct)	Serum	0–0.2 mg/dL	0–3.4 μmol/L
C-Peptide	Serum	*ng/mL* Adult: ≤ 4.0 > 60y, M: 1.5–5.0 F; 1.4–5.5	*μg/L* ≤ 4.0 1.5–5.0 1.4–5.5
C-Reactive Protein	Serum	Cord blood: 10–350 ng/mL Adult: 68–8200 ng/mL	10–350 μg/L 68–8200 μg/L
Calcium, Ionized (iCa)	Serum, plasma or whole blood (heparin)	*mg/dL* Cord 5.5 ± 0.3 Newborn, 3–24 h: 4.3–5.1 24–48 h: 4.0–4.7 Adult: 4.48–4.92 or 2.24–2.46 mEq/L 2.25–2.60 mEq/L >60 y:	*mmol/L* 1.37 ± 0.07 1.07–1.27 1.00–1.17 1.12–1.23 1.13–1.30
Calcium, Total	Serum	*mg/dL* Child: 8.8–10.8 Adult: 8.4–10.2 M, > 60 y: 8.4–10.0	*mmol/L* 2.2–2.70 2.1–2.55 2.1–2.50
	Urine, 24 h	*Ca in Diet* *mg/d* Free Ca: 5–40 Low to average: 50–150 Average (20 mmol/d): 100–300	*mmol/d* 0.13–1.0 1.25–3.8 2.5–7.5
	CSF	2.1–2.7 mEq/L or 4.2–5.4 mg/dL	1.05–1.35 mmol/L 1.05–1.35 mmol/L
	Feces	Avg.: 0.64 g/d	16 mmol/d
Carbon Dioxide, Partial Pressure (Pco_2), at sea level	Whole blood (heparin)	*mm Hg* Newborn: 27–40 Infant: 27–41 Adult, M: 35–48 F: 32–45	*kPa* 3.6–5.3 3.6–5.5 4.7–6.4 4.3–6.0
Carbon Dioxide, Total (Tco_2)	Serum, plasma (heparin)	*mmol/L* Cord: 14–22 Newborn: 13–22 Infant: 20–28 Child: 20–28 Adult: 22–28 > 60 y: 23–31	*mmol/L* 14–22 13–22 20–28 20–28 22–28 23–31
Carbon Monoxide	Whole blood (EDTA)	Nonsmokers: < 2% HbCO Smokers: < 10% HbCO Toxic: > 20% HbCO Lethal: > 50% HbCO	*HbCO Fraction:* < 0.02 < 0.10 >0.20 > 0.5

CLINICAL CHEMISTRY, TOXICOLOGY, SEROLOGY (*Continued*)

Test	Specimen	Reference Range	Reference Range (International Units)
Carboxyhemoglobin, see *Carbon Monoxide*			
Carcinoembryonic Antigen (CEA)	Serum	Nonsmokers: 0–3.0 ng/mL	0–0.3 μg/L
		Smokers: 0–5.0 ng/mL	0–5.0 μg/L
β-Carotene	Serum	*μ/dL*	*μmol/L*
		Infant: 20–70	0.37–1.30
		Child: 40–130	0.74–2.42
		Adult: 60–200	1.12–3.72
Carotene Absorption Test	Serum	Increase by ≥ 35 μg/dL	Increase by ≥ 0.65 μmol/L
Catecholamines,	Urine, 24 h		
HPLC		< 110 μg/d	< 650 nmol/d (conv. factor based on norepinephrine, M.W. 169.18)
Fluorometric		< 280 μg/d	< 1655 nmol/d
Catecholamines, Fractionated	Urine, 24 h		
		Norepinephrine *μg/d*	*nmol/d*
		1–4 y: 0–29	0–170
		4–10 y: 8–65	47–380
		10–15 y: 15–80	89–470
		Adult: 0–100	0–590
		Epinephrine *μg/d*	*nmol/d*
		1–4 y: 0–6.0	0–33
		4–10 y: 0–10.0	0–55
		10–15 y: 0.5–20	2.7–110
		Adult: 0–15	0–82
		Dopamine *μg/d*	*nmol/d*
		1–4 y: 40–260	260–1700
		> 4 y: 65–400	425–2610
Catecholamines, Free	Plasma (EDTA and sodium metabisulfite)	*pg/ml*	*pmol/L*
		Epinephrine, random: < 88	< 480
		Norepinephrine, random: 104–548	615–3240
		Dopamine, random: < 136	< 888
Cerebrospinal Fluid Pressure	CSF	50–180 mm water	50–180 mm water
Cerebrospinal Fluid Volume	CSF	Child: 60–100 mL	0.06–0.10 L
		Adult: 100–160 mL	0.1–0.16 L
Ceruloplasmin	Serum	*mg/dL*	*mg/L*
RID		Newborn: 1–30	10–300
		6 mo–1 y: 15–50	150–500
		1–12 y: 30–65	300–650
		Thereafter: 15–60	150–600
Chloride	Serum or plasma (heparin)	98–106 mmol/d	98–106 mmol/d
	CSF	118–132 mmol/L	118–132 mmol/L
	Urine, 24 h	*mmol/d*	*mmol/d*
		Infant: 2–10	2–10
		Child: 15–40	15–40
		Thereafter: 110–250 (vary greatly with Cl intake)	110–250
	Sweat	*mmol/L*	*mmol/L*
		Normal (homozygote): 3–35	0–35
		Marginal: 30–60	30–60
		Cystic fibrosis: 60–200	60–200
Cholesterol, Total	Serum or plasma (EDTA)	*mg/dL*	*mmol/L*
		Cord: 45–100	1.17–2.59
		Newborn: 53–135	1.37–3.50
		Infant: 70–175	1.81–4.53
		Child: 120–200	3.11–5.18
		Adolescent: 120–210	3.11–5.44
		Adult: 140–310	3.63–8.03
		Recommended (desirable) range for adults: 140–220	3.63–5.70

CLINICAL CHEMISTRY, TOXICOLOGY, SEROLOGY (*Continued*)

Test	Specimen	Reference Range	Reference Range (International Units)
Chorionic Gonadotropin, β-Subunit (β-HCG)	Serum or plasma (EDTA)	*mIU/mL*	*mIU/mL*
		M, and nonpregnant female: <3.0	< 3.0
		F, postconception,	
		7–10 d: > 3.0	> 3.0
		30 d: 100–5000	100–5000
		40 d: > 2000	> 2000
		10 wks: 50,000–140,000	50,000–140,000
		> 16 wks: 10,000–50,000	10,000–50,000
		Trophoblastic disease: $> 100,000$	$> 100,000$
Complement			
Total hemolytic complement activity	Plasma (EDTA)	75–160 U/mL or $> 33\%$ of plasma CH_{50}	75–160 kU/L or fraction of plasma CH_{50}: > 0.33
Total complement decay rate (functional)	Plasma (EDTA)	~ 10–20%	*Fraction decay rate* ~ 0.10–0.20
		Deficiency: $> 50\%$	> 0.50
Classic pathway components:		*mg/dL*	*mg/L*
C1q	Serum	6.5 ± 0.7	65 ± 7
C1r	Serum	2.5–3.8	25–38
C1s (C1 esterase)	Serum	2.5–3.8	25–38
C2	Serum	2.8 ± 0.6	28 ± 6
C3 (β₁ C-globulin)	Serum	80–155	800–1550
C4 (β₁ E-globulin)	Serum	13–37	130–370
C5 (β₁ F-globulin)	Serum	6.4 ± 1.3	64 ± 13
C6	Serum	5.6 ± 0.8	56 ± 8
C7	Serum	4.9–7.0	49–70
C8	Serum	4.3–6.3	43–63
C9	Serum	4.7–6.9	47–69
Alternative pathway components:			
C4 binding protein	Serum	18–32	180–320
Factor B (C3 proactivator)	Serum	20–45	200–450
Properdin	Serum	2.8 ± 0.4	28 ± 4
Regulatory proteins			
β_1H-globulin (C3b inactivator accelerator)	Serum	56.1 ± 7.8	561 ± 78
C1 inhibitor (esterase inhibitor)	Plasma (EDTA)	17.4–24.0	174–240
C1 inhibitor by complement decay rate (functional)	Plasma (EDTA)	~ 10–20%	*Fraction decay rate* ~ 0.10–0.20
		Deficiency: $>50\%$	> 0.50
C3b inactivator (KAF)	Serum	4.0 ± 0.7 mg/dL	40 ± 7 mg/L
S protein	Serum	41.8–60.0 mg/dL	418–600 mg/L
Copper	Serum	*μg/dL*	*μmol/L*
		Birth-6 mo: 20–70	3.14–10.99
		6 y: 90–190	14.13–29.83
		Adult, M: 70–140	10.99–21.98
		F: 80–155	12.56–24.34
		Pregnancy at term: 118–302	18.53–47.41
	Erythrocytes (heparin)	90–150 μg/dL	14.13–23.55 μmol/L
	Urine, 24 h	15–30 μg/d	0.24–0.47 μmol/d
Coproporphyrin	Urine, 24 h	34–234 μg/d	51–351 nmol/d
	Feces, 24 h	< 30 μg/g dry wt	< 45 nmol/g dry wt
		400–1200 μg/d	600–1800 nmol/d
Corticobinding Globulin (CBG), see *Transcortin*			
Corticosterone	Serum or plasma (heparin, EDTA, or oxalate)	0.13–2.3 μg/dL	3.75–66 nmol/L
Cortisol	Serum or plasma (heparin)	0800 h: 5–23 μg/dL	138–635 nmol/L
		1600 h: 3–15 μg/dL	82–413 nmol/L
		2000 h: $\leq 50\%$ of 0800 h	Fraction of 0800h: ≤ 0.50
Cortisol, Free	Urine, 24 h	*μg/d*	*nmol/d*
		Child: 2–27	5.5–74
		Adolescent: 5–55	14–152
		Adult: 10–100	27–276

CLINICAL CHEMISTRY, TOXICOLOGY, SEROLOGY (*Continued*)

Test	Specimen	Reference Range	Reference Range (International Units)
Creatine Kinase (CK)			
Total, 30°C	Serum	*U/L* Newborn: 10–200 Adult, M: 12–80 F: 10–55 > 60 y, M: 20–110 F: 16–80 > 70 y, M: 22–90 F: 16–80 Ambulatory, M: 25–90 F: 10–70 Higher after exercise	*U/L* 10–200 12–80 10–55 20–110 16–80 22–90 16–80 25–90 10–70
Isoenzymes	Serum	Fraction 2 (MB) < 4–6% of total (method dependent)	Fraction of total: < 0.04–0.06
Creatinine *Jaffe, kinetic or enzymatic*	Serum or plasma	*mg/dL* Cord: 0.6–1.2 Child: 0.3–0.7 Adult, M: 0.6–1.2 F: 0.5–1.1	*μmol/L* 53–106 27–62 53–106 44–97
Jaffe, manual	Serum or plasma	0.8–1.5 mg/dL	70–133 μmol/L
	Urine, 24 h	*mg/d/kg* Child; 8–22 Adult, M: 14–26 F: 11–20 Declines with age to 10 mg/kg/d at age 90	*μmol/d/kg* 71–195 124–230 97–177
		or: *mg/d* M: 800–1800 F: 600–1600	*mmol/d* 7–16 5.3–14.0
Creatinine Clearance (Endogenous)	Serum or plasma, and urine	< 40 y, M: 97–137 mL/min/1.73m^2 F: 88–128 mL/min/1.73m^2 Decreases ~ 6.5 mL/min/1.73 m^2 per decade	0.93–1.32 mL/s/m^2 0.85–1.23 mL/s/m^2
Dehydroepiandrosterone Sulfate (DHEA-SO_4)	Serum or plasma (heparin or EDTA)	*μg/mL* Newborn: <300 1–4 d: <20 Child: 0.60–2.54 Adult, M: 1.99–3.34 F, Premeno-pausal: 0.82–3.38 Postmeno-pausal: 0.11–0.61 Pregnancy, Term: 0.23–1.17	*μmol/L* <780 <52 1.6–6.6 5.2–8.7 2.1–8.8 0.3–1.6 0.6–3.0
11-Deoxycortisol (Compound S)	Plasma (heparin, EDTA or oxalate)	*μg/dL* < 1 without metyrapone > 7 after metyrapone	*nmol/L* *< 30* *> 200*
Dexamethasone Suppression Test (Standard)			
Low dose, adult: 0.5 mg q 6 h × 8	Serum, 0800 h Control, day 2, day 3	Cortisol: suppression on day 3 to < 50% of baseline or to < 5 μg/dL	Cortisol: suppression on day 3, fraction of baseline: < 0.50 or < 138 nmol/L
	Urine, 24 h Day 1, 2, and 3	17-KGS: suppression on day 2 to < 7.5 mg/d	17-KGS: suppression on day 2 to < 26 μmol/d
		17-OHCS: suppression on day 2 to < 4.5 mg/d	17-OHCS: suppression on day 2 to < 12.4 μmol/d
		Free cortisol: < 50% of baseline	Free cortisol: fraction of baseline, < 0.50
High dose, adult: 2.0 mg q 6 h × 8		Cortisol, 17-KGS, 17-OHCS: suppression on day 3 to < 50% of baseline	Cortisol, 17-KGS, 17-OHCS: suppression on day 3, fraction of baseline: < 0.50

CLINICAL CHEMISTRY, TOXICOLOGY, SEROLOGY (*Continued*)

Test	Specimen	Reference Range		Reference Range (International Units)
Dexamethasone Single Dose Overnight Suppression Test				
Dose: 1 mg orally at 2300 h or 2400 h	Serum for cortisol, 0800 h following morning	Suppression to 5–10 μg/dL or to < 50% of baseline		Suppression to 138–276 nmol/L or fraction of baseline: < 0.50
			ng/mL	*nmol/L*
Digoxin	Serum, plasma (heparin, EDTA); collect at least 12 h after dose	Therap. conc.,		
		CHF:	0.8–1.5	1.0–1.9
		Arrhythmias:	1.5–2.0	1.9–2.6
		Toxic conc.,		
		Adult:	> 2.5	> 3.2
		Child:	> 3.0	> 3.8
Estradiol	Serum or plasm (heparin *or EDTA*)		*pg/mL*	*pmol/L*
		Adult, M:	8–36	29–132
		F,		
		Follicular:	10–90	37–330
		Midcycle:	100–500	370–1835
		Luteal:	50–240	184–880
		Postmenopausal:	10–30	37–110
	Urine, 24 h		*μg/d*	*nmol/d*
		Adult, M:	0–6	0–22
		F,		
		Follicular:	0–3	0–11
		Ovulatory peak:	4–14	15–51
		Luteal:	4–10	15–37
		Postmenopausal:	0–4	0–15
Estriol (E_3), Free	Serum	*Weeks of gestation*	*μg/L*	*nmol/L*
		25–28:	3.5–12.5	12–43.3
		30–32:	4.5–16.0	16–55.5
		34:	5.5–18.5	19–64.2
		36:	7.0–25.0	24–86.8
		37:	8.0–28.0	28–97.2
		38:	9.0–32.0	31–111
		39:	10.0–34.0	35–118
		40–41:	10.5–25.0	36–86.7
Estriol (E_3), Total	Serum		*ng/mL*	*nmol/L*
		Pregnancy (wks),		
		24–28:	30–170	104–590
		28–32:	40–220	140–760
		32–36:	60–280	208–970
		36–40:	80–350	280–1210
		Adult, M and non-pregnant F:	<2	<7
	Urine, 24 h		*mg/d*	*μmol/d*
		Pregnancy (wks),		
		30:	6–18	21–62
		35:	9–28	31–97
		40:	13–42	45–146
		Decrease of > 40% of previous value suggests fetus at risk		Fraction of previous value of < 0.60 suggests fetus at risk
Estrogens, Total	Serum		*pg/mL*	*ng/L*
		M:	40–115	40–115
		F, cycle-days,		
		1–10:	61–394	61–394
		11–20:	122–437	122–437
		21–30:	156–350	156–350
		Prepubertal and postmenopausal:	≤40	≤40
			μg/d	*μg/d*
	Urine, 24 h	M:	5–25	5–25
		F,		
		Preovulation:	4–25	4–25
		Ovulation:	28–100	28–100
		Luteal peak:	22–80	22–80
		Pregnancy, term:	< 45,000	< 45,000
		Postmenopausal:	< 10	< 10
Estrogen Receptor Assay (ERA)	0.5–1 g tissue		*fmol/mg protein*	*nmol/kg protein*
		Negative:	< 3.0	< 3.0
		Borderline positive:	3–10	3–10
		Positive:	> 10.0	> 10.0

CLINICAL CHEMISTRY, TOXICOLOGY, SEROLOGY *(Continued)*

Test	Specimen	Reference Range		Reference Range (International Units)	
Estrone (E_1)	Serum		*pg/mL*	*pmol/L*	
		M, Pubertal stage,			
		I:	11	41	
		II:	16	59	
		III:	21	78	
		Adult:	30–170	111–630	
		F, Pubertal stage,			
		I:	0–29	0–107	
		II:	10–35	37–130	
		III:	15–45	55–166	
		IV:	20–80	74–296	
		Follicular:	20–150	74–555	
	Urine, 24 h		*μg/d*	*nmol/d*	
		Adult, M:	3–8	11–30	
		F,			
		Ovulatory peak:	11–31	41–115	
		Luteal:	10–23	37–85	
		Postmenopausal:	1–7	3.7–26.0	
			mg/dL	*mmol/L*	
Ethanol	Serum, whole blood (oxalate)	Toxic:	50–100	10.9–21.7	
		Depression of CNS:	> 100	> 21.7	
		Fatalities reported:	> 400	> 86.8	
Fat, Fecal	Feces, 72 h		*g/d*	*g/d*	
		Infant, breast-fed:	< 1	< 1	
		0–6 y:	< 2	< 2	
		Adult:	< 7	< 7	
		Adult (fat-free diet):	< 4	< 4	
Fatty Acids, Nonesterified (Free)	Serum or plasma (heparin)		*mg/dL*	*mmol/L*	
		Adult:	8–25	0.30–0.90	(conv. factor based on oleic acid, M.W. 282.47)
		Child and obese adult:	< 31	< 1.10	
Fatty Acids, Total	Serum	190–420 mg/dL		7–15 mmol/L	
Ferritin	Serum		*ng/mL*	*μg/L*	
		Newborn:	25–200	25–200	
		1 mo:	200–600	200–600	
		2–5 mo:	50–200	50–200	
		6 mo–15 y:	7–140	7–140	
		Adult, M:	15–200	15–200	
		F:	12–150	12–150	
α_1-Fetoprotein	Serum	Adult: < 30 ng/mL		< 30 μg/L	
		Mean: 2.6 ± 1.6 (1 SD) ng/mL		2.6 ± 1.6 (1 SD) μg/L	
		Fetal: peak of 200–400 mg/dL in first trimester		Peak of 2–4 g/L in first trimester	
		1 y: < 30 ng/mL		< 30 μg/L	
	Amniotic fluid	(see below)			

Weeks	*mg/dL* median	*mg/dL* ± 2 log SD	*mg/L* median	*mg/L* ± 2 log SD
11–12	2.4	1.0–5.0	24	10–50
13–14	2.3	1.3–4.1	23	13–41
15–16	1.8	0.9–3.5	18	9–35
17–18	1.5	0.6–3.3	15	6–33
19–20	1.0	0.5–2.5	10	5–25
21–25	0.7	0.4–1.4	7	4–14
26–30	0.6	0.3–1.0	6	3–10
31–35	0.2	0.05–0.7	2	0.5–7.0
36–40	0.1	0.02–0.3	1	0.2–3.0

Test	Specimen	Reference Range	Reference Range (International Units)
Fibrinogen, see *Hematology section*			
FIGLU *Dose: 5 g histidine q 4 h × 3*	Urine, 24 h, after initial dose of histidine	< 35 mg/d	< 200 μmol/d
Folate	Serum	1.8–9 ng/mL	4.1–20.4 nmol/L
		> 60 y: 1.8–12 ng/mL	4.1–27.2 nmol/L
	Erythrocytes (EDTA)	150–450 ng/mL packed cells	340–1020 nmol/L packed cells
		< 60 y: 95–500 ng/mL packed cells	215–1132 nmol/L packed cells
Folate Absorption Test	Urine, 24 h	45 ± 7% of dose	Fraction of dose: 0.45 ± 0.07

CLINICAL CHEMISTRY, TOXICOLOGY, SEROLOGY (*Continued*)

Test	Specimen	Reference Range	Reference Range (International Units)
Follicle-Stimulating Hormone (FSH)	Serum or plasma (heparin)	*mIU/mL*	*IU/L*
		Adult, M: 4–25	4–25
		F,	
		Premenopausal: 4–30	4–30
		Midcycle peak: 10–90	10–90
		Pregnancy: low to undetectable	low to undetectable
		Postmenopausal: 40–250	40–250
	Urine, 24 h	*IU/d (IRP-2-hMG)*	*IU/d (IRP-2-hMG)*
		Birth-1 y, F: < 0.5–1.4	< 0.5–1.4
		1–8 y, M: < 0.5–4.5	< 0.5–4.5
		F: < 0.5–4.0	< 0.5–4.0
		9–10 y, M: 1–5	1–5
		F: 1–4	1–4
		11–12 y, M: 1.5–5	1.5–5
		F: 1–8	1–8
		13–14 y, M: 2–12	2–12
		F: 1–10	1–10
		Adult, M: 4–18	4–18
		F: 3–12	3–12
		Higher in males > 60 y	Higher in males > 60 y
Free Thyroxine Index (FT_4I)	Serum	*FT_4 Index* 1.2–5.0	
with normalized T_3RU		1–3 d: 9.3–26.6	
		1–4 wk: 7.6–20.8	
		1–4 mo: 7.4–17.9	
		4–12 mo: 6.1–14.5	
		1–6 y: 5.7–13.3	
		6–10 y: 5.5–10.0	
		> 10 y: 5.5–10.0	
		Borderline low: 4.8	
		Borderline high: 14.0	
Free Triiodothyronine, see *Triiodothyronine, Free*			
Fructose	Serum	1–6 mg/dL	55.5–333.0 μmol/L
	Urine	< 60 mg/d	< 333 μmol/d
Gastric Secretion Rate	Total gastric contents, six 15 min spec.	BAO: 0–5 mmol/h	0–5 mmol/h
		PAO: 5–20 mmol/h (post pentagastrin)	5–20 mmol/h (post pentagastrin)
		BAO/PAO: 0.20	0.20
Gastrin	Serum	< 60 y: < 100 pg/mL	< 100 ng/L
		> 60 y: upper 15% of population: 100–800 pg/mL	upper 15% of population: 100–800 ng/L
Gastrin-Calcium Infusion Stimulation Test	Serum	Gastrin: Slight or no increase Z.E. syndrome: > 450 pg/mL	Gastrin: Slight or no increase Z.E. syndrome: > 450 ng/L
Gastrin-Secretin Stimulation Test	Serum, fasting, at 15 min intervals for 1 h	No response or slight suppression	No response or slight suppression
IV dose: 5 U secretin/kg		Z.E. syndrome: Increase > 110 pg/mL if base level 80–500 pg/mL; increase > 1400 pg/mL if basal level is high	Z.E. syndrome: Increase > 110 ng/L if base level 80–500 ng/L; increase > 1400 ng/mL if basal level is high
Glucose	Serum	*mg/dL*	*mmol/L*
		Cord: 45–96	2.5–5.3
		Premature: 20–60	1.1–3.3
		Neonate: 30–60	1.7–3.3
		Newborn,	
		1 d: 40–60	2.2–3.3
		> 1 d: 50–80	2.8–4.4
		Child: 60–100	3.3–5.5
		Adult: 70–105	3.9–5.8
		> 60 y: 80–115	4.4–6.4
	Whole blood (heparin)	Adult: 65–95	3.6–5.3
	CSF	Adult: 40–70	2.2–3.9
Quantitative, enzymatic	Urine	< 0.5 g/d	< 2.8 mmol/d
Qualitative	Urine	Negative	Negative

CLINICAL CHEMISTRY, TOXICOLOGY, SEROLOGY (Continued)

Test	Specimen	Reference Range	Reference Range (International Units)
Glucose, 2 h Postprandial	Serum	< 120 mg/dL Diabetes: see *Glucose Tolerance Test, Oral*	<6.7 mmol/L
Glucose Tolerance Test (GTT) with Cortisone *Dose: 50 mg, 8.5 and 2 h before test*	Plasma (fluoride oxalate); fasting, 1, 1½, 2 h after glucose ingestion	*Glucose* *mg/dL* Fasting: 70–105 1 h: < 200 1½ h: < 200 2 h: < 140	*mmol/L* 3.9–5.8 < 11 < 11 < 7.8

Glucose Tolerance Test (GTT), Oral — Serum

		mg/dL		*mmol/L*	
Adult,		*Normal*	*Diabetic*	*Normal*	*Diabetic*
Fasting:		70–105	> 140	3.9–5.8	> 7.8
60 min:		120–170	≥ 200	6.7–9.4	≥ 11
90 min:		100–140	≥ 200	5.6–7.8	≥ 11
120 min:		70–120	≥ 140	3.9–6.7	≥ 7.8

Test	Specimen	Reference Range	Reference Range (International Units)
IV	Serum	5 min: ~ 250 mg/dL 90 min: at or below fasting concentration or K = > 1.5%	5 min: ~13.9 mmol/L
γ-Glutamyltransferase (GGT), 37°C, aca	Serum	M: 9–50 U/L F: 8–40 U/L	M: 9–50 U/L F: 8–40 U/L
Glycerol, Free	Plasma	3–10 y: 0.56–2.14 mg/dL 11–80 y: 0.29–1.72 mg/dL	0.061–0.232 mmol/L 0.032–0.187 mmol/L
Gold	Serum	< 10 μg/dL Therap. range: 38–500 μg/dL	< 0.51 μmol/L Therap. range: 1.93–25.40 μmol/L
	Urine, 24 h	< 1 μg/d	< 5 nmol/d
Gonadotropins, see *Pregnancy Tests* and *Chorionic Gonadotropin, β-subunit*			

Growth Hormone (HGH, Somatotropin) — Serum or plasma (EDTA, heparin)

	ng/mL	*μg/L*
Cord:	10–50	10–50
Newborn:	10–40	10–40
Child:	< 1–10	< 1–10
	(occasional values up to 20)	
Adult, M:	< 2	< 2
F:	< 10	< 10
> 60 y, M:	0.4–10	0.4–10
F:	1–14	1–14

Test	Specimen	Reference Range	Reference Range (International Units)
Growth Hormone–Arginine Stimulation Test *Dose, adult: 30 g arginine HCl IV within 30 min; child: 0.5 g/kg*	Serum, fasting, 30 min intervals for 2 h	Fasting: < 5 ng/mL; rise to > 7 ng/mL during test (peak range 8–35 ng/mL) at 30–60 min	Fasting: < 5 μg/L; rise to > 7 μg/L during test (peak range 8–35 μg/L) at 30–60 min
Growth Hormone–Glucagon Stimulation Test *Dose: 1 mg glucagon IM or SC*	Serum, fasting, then hourly for 3–4 h	> 7 ng/mL after stimulation or > 5 ng/mL rise above baseline	> 7 μg/L after stimulation or > 5 μg/L rise above baseline
Growth Hormone–L-Dopa Stimulation Test *Dose, adult: 500 mg L-dopa, orally; child: 10 mg/kg*	Serum, fasting, 30, 60, 90, 120, and 180 min after L-dopa	Peak: > 7 ng/mL or > 5 ng/mL rise above baseline	> 7 μg/L or > 5 μg/L rise above baseline
Haptoglobin, see *Hematology section*			

HDL-Cholesterol (HDLC) — Serum or plasma (EDTA)

	mg/dL		*nmol/L*	
	M	F	M	F
Mean, adult:	45	55	1.17	1.42
Cord:	5–50	5–50	0.13–1.30	0.13–1.30
< 19 y:	30–65	30–70	0.78–1.68	0.78–1.81
20–29 y:	30–70	30–75	0.78–1.81	0.78–1.94
40 + y:	30–70	30–85	0.78–1.81	0.78–2.20
Values for blacks, ~ 10 mg/dL higher				

	HDLC, % of total cholesterol:		*Fraction HDLC of total cholesterol*	
CHD Risk	M	F	M	F
Dangerous:	< 7	< 12	< 0.07	< 0.12
High:	7–15	12–18	0.07–0.15	0.12–0.18
Average:	15–25	18–27	0.15–0.25	0.18–0.27
Below average:	25–37	27–40	0.25–0.37	0.27–0.40
Protection probable:	> 37	> 40	> 0.37	> 0.40

CLINICAL CHEMISTRY, TOXICOLOGY, SEROLOGY (*Continued*)

Test	Specimen	Reference Range	Reference Range (International Units)
Hemoglobin A_{1c}	Whole blood (heparin, EDTA or oxalate)		
Electrophoresis		5.6–7.5% of total Hb	Fraction of Hb: 0.056–0.075
Column		6–9% of total Hb	Fraction of Hb: 0.06–0.09
Homovanillic Acid (HVA)	Urine, 24 h	Child: 3–16 µg/mg creatinine Adult: < 15 mg/d	1.9–10 mmol/mol creatinine < 82 µmol/d
17-Hydroxycorticosteroids (17-OHCS)	Urine, 24 h	*mg/d* 0–1 y: 0.5–1.0 Child: 1.0–5.6 Adult, M: 3.0–10.0 F: 2.0–8.0 or: 3–7 mg/g creatinine	*µmol/d* 1.4–2.8 2.8–15.5 8.2–27.6 5.5–22 or: 0.9–2.5 mmol/mol creatinine (conv. factor based on hydrocortisone, M.W. 362)
5-Hydroxyindole Acetic Acid (5-HIAA)			
Qualitative	Fresh random urine	Negative	Negative
Quantitative	Urine, 24 h	2–8 mg/d	10.5–42 µmol/d
17-Hydroxyprogesterone (17-OHP)	Serum	*ng/mL* M, Pub. stage I: 0.1–0.3 Adult: 0.2–1.8 F, Pub. stage I: 0.2–0.5 Follicular: 0.2–0.8 Luteal: 0.8–3.0 Postmenopausal: 0.04–0.5	*nmol/L* 0.3–0.9 0.6–5.4 0.6–1.5 0.6–2.4 2.4–9.0 0.12–1.5
Immunoglobulin A (IgA)	Serum	*mg/dL* Cord: 0–5 Newborn: 0–2.2 4–6 mo: 3–82 6 mo–2 y: 14–108 2–6 y: 23–190 6–12 y: 29–270 12–16 y: 81–232 Adult: 76–390	*mg/L* 0–50 0–22 30–820 140–1080 230–1900 290–2700 810–2320 760–3900
Immunoglobulin D (IgD)			
RID	Serum	Newborn: None detected Adult: 0–8 mg/dL	None detected 0–0.44 µmol/L
Immunoglobulin E (IgE)			
RID	Serum	*IU/mL* Adult: 0–380 < 60 y, M: 0–250 F: 0–175	*kIU/mL* 0–380 0–250 0–175
Immunoglobulin G (IgG)			
Nephelometric	Serum	*mg/dL* Cord: 760–1700 Newborn: 700–1480 ½–6 mo: 300–1000 6 mo–2 y: 500–1200 2–6 y: 500–1300 6–12 y: 700–1650 12–16 y: 700–1550 Adult: 600–1600 (higher in blacks)	*g/L* 7.6–17 7–14.8 3–10 5–12 5–13 7–16.5 7–15.5 6–16
	CSF	0.5–5 mg/dL	5–50 mg/L
Immunoglobulin G/Albumin Ratio	CSF and serum	0.3–0.6	0.3–0.6
Immunoglobulin G Synthesis Rate	CSF and serum	(−9.9) to (+3.3) mg/d	(−9.9) to (+3.3) mg/d

CLINICAL CHEMISTRY, TOXICOLOGY, SEROLOGY *(Continued)*

Test	Specimen	Reference Range	Reference Range (International Units)
Immunoglobulin M (IgM)	Serum	*mg/dL*	*mg/L*
		Cord: 4–24	40–240
		Newborn: 5–30	50–300
		½–6 mo: 15–109	150–1090
		6 mo–2 y: 43–239	430–2390
		2–6 y: 50–199	500–1990
		6–12 y: 50–260	500–2600
		12–16 y: 45–240	450–2400
		Adult: 40–345	400–3450
		Results vary with std. preparation	
	CSF	0–1.3 mg/dL	0–13 mg/L
		μIU/mL	*mIU/L*
Insulin (12 h Fasting)	Serum	Newborn: 3–20	3–20
		Adult: 6–24	6–24
		< 60 y: 6–35	6–35
Insulin with Oral Glucose Tolerance Test	Serum	*Min* *Insulin, μIU/mL*	*mIU/L*
		0: 6–24	6–24
		30: 25–231	25–231
		60: 18–276	18–276
		120: 16–166	16–166
		180: 4–38	4–38
Insulin Tolerance Test			
Dose: 0.1–0.15 U/kg IV	Serum	*Glucose:* Decrease ~50% of the fasting level by 30 min and return to normal fasting limits by 90–120 min	Fractional decrease in glucose ~0.50 of the fasting level by 30 min and return to normal fasting limits by 90–120 min
		HGH: Increase of > 5 ng/mL within 60 min of hypoglycemia or > 20 ng/mL	*HGH:* Increase of > 5 μg/L within 60 min of hypoglycemia or > 20 μg/mL
		Cortisol: Increase of > 6 μg/dL with peak of > 20 μg/dL	Cortisol: Increase of > 165 nmol/L with peak of > 552 nmol/L
Intrinsic Factor, see *Vitamin B_{12} Intrinsic Factor*			
Inulin Clearance Test	Serum and urine	*Mean (±2 SD) mL/min* *M* / *F*	
		20–29 y: 132 (90–174) 119 (84–156)	
		30–39 y: 128 (88–168) 116 (82–150)	
		40–49 y: 120 (78–162) 114 (82–146)	
		50–59 y: 110 (68–152) 104 (66–142)	
		60–69 y: 97 (57–137) 94 (58–130)	
		70–79 y: 82 (42–122) 83 (45–121)	
		80–89 y: 67 (39–105) 67 (39–105)	
Iron	Serum	*μg/dL*	*μmol/L*
		Newborn: 100–250	17.90–44.75
		Infant: 40–100	7.16–17.90
		Child: 50–120	8.95–21.48
		Adult, M: 50–160	8.95–28.64
		F: 40–150	7.16–26.85
Iron-Binding Capacity, Total (TIBC)	Serum	*μg/dL*	*μmol/L*
		Infant: 100–400	17.90–71.60
		Thereafter: 250–400	44.75–71.60
Iron Saturation	Serum	20–55%	Fraction of iron saturation 0.20–0.55
17-Ketogenic Steroids (17-KGS)	Urine, 24 h	*mg/d*	*μmol/d* (conv. factor based on DHEA, M.W. 288)
		0–1 y: < 1.0	< 3.5
		1–10 y: < 5	< 17
		11–14 y: < 12	< 42
		Adult, M: 5–23	17–80
		F: 3–15	10–52
		> 70 y, M: 3–15	10–52
		F: 3–13	10–45
Ketone bodies			
Qualitative	Serum	Negative (0.5–3.0 mg/dL)	Negative (5–30 mg/L)
	Urine, random	Negative	Negative

CLINICAL CHEMISTRY, TOXICOLOGY, SEROLOGY (*Continued*)

Test	Specimen	Reference Range	Reference Range (International Units)
17-Ketosteroids (17-KS), Total			
		mg/d	*μmol/d*
Zimmerman reaction	Urine, 24 h	14 d–2 y: < 1	< 3.5 (conv. factor based on DHEA, M.W. 288)
		2–6 y: < 2	< 7
		6–10 y: 1–4	3.5–14
		10–12 y: 1–6	3.5–21
		12–14 y: 3–10	10–35
		14–16 y: 5–12	17–42
		Adult,	
		M, 18–30: 9–22	31–76
		M, > 30: 8–20	28–70
		F: 6–15	21–52
		Decreases with age	Decreases with age
Chromatography	Urine, 24 h	Adult, M: 5.0–12.0	Adult, M: 17–42
		F: 3.0–10.0	F: 10–35
LDL-Cholesterol (LDLC)	Serum or plasma (EDTA)	*mg/dL* *M* *F*	*mmol/L* *M* *F*
		Cord blood: 10–50 10–50	0.26–1.30 0.26–1.30
		0–19 y: 60–140 60–150	1.55–3.63 1.55–3.89
		20–29 y: 60–175 60–160	1.55–4.53 1.55–4.14
		30–39 y: 80–190 70–170	2.07–4.92 1.81–4.40
		40–49 y: 90–205 80–190	2.33–5.31 2.07–4.92
		50–59 y: 90–205 90–220	2.33–5.31 2.33–5.70
		60–69 y: 90–215 100–235	2.33–5.57 2.59–6.09
		≥ 70 y: 90–190 95–215	2.33–4.92 2.46–5.57
		Recommended (desirable) range for adults: 65–175 mg/dL	1.68–4.53
L-Lactate	Whole blood (heparin)	*mg/dL*	*mmol/L*
		Venous: 4.5–19.8	0.5–2.2
		Arterial: 4.5–14.4	0.5–1.6
		Inpatients,	
		Venous: 8.1–15.3	0.9–1.7
		Arterial: < 11.3	< 1.25
Lactate Dehydrogenase (LDH), 30°C			
		U/L	*U/L*
Total (L → P)	Serum	Newborn: 160–450	160–450
		Neonate: 300–1500	300–1500
		Infant: 100–250	100–250
		Child: 60–170	60–170
		Adult: 45–90	45–90
		> 60 y: 55–100	55–100
		150–320	150–320
Total (P → L)	CSF	~ 10% of serum value	~ 0.10 fraction of serum value
Isoenzymes Electrophoresis (Agarose)	Serum	%	*Fraction of total:*
		Fraction 1: 14–26	0.14–0.26
		Fraction 2: 29–39	0.29–0.39
		Fraction 3: 20–26	0.20–0.26
		Fraction 4: 8–16	0.08–0.16
		Fraction 5: 6–16	0.06–0.16
Lactate/Pyruvate Ratio	Whole blood (heparin)	10/1	10/1
Lead	Whole blood (heparin)	*μg/dL*	*μmol/L*
		Child: < 30	< 1.45
		Adult: < 40	< 1.93
		Toxic: ≥ 100	≥ 4.83
	Urine, 24 h	< 80 μg/L	< 0.39 μmol/L
Lipase	Serum		
Tietz method		< 1.0 unit/mL	< 278 U/L
BMD turbidimetric		Adult: 10–150 U/L	10–150 U/L
		> 60 y: 18–180 U/L	18–180 U/L
Lithium	Serum, plasma, whole blood (heparin, EDTA)	Therap. conc.: 0.6–1.2 mEq/L	0.6–1.2 mmol/L
		Toxic conc.: > 2 mEq/L	> 2 mmol/L

CLINICAL CHEMISTRY, TOXICOLOGY, SEROLOGY (*Continued*)

Test	Specimen	Reference Range	Reference Range (International Units)
Luteinizing Hormone (LH)	Serum or plasma (heparin)	*mIU/mL* M, 10–13 y: 4–12 12–17 y: 6–16 15–18 y: 7–19 Adult: 6–23 F, 9–14 y: 2.0–14.0 12–18 y: 3.0–29.0 F, Follicular phase: 5–30 Midcycle: 75–150 Luteal: 3–30 Postmenopausal: 30–130	*IU/L* 4–12 6–16 7–19 6–23 2.0–14.0 3.0–29.0 5–30 75–150 3–30 30–130
	Urine	*IU/d* 11–13 y: 0.48–11.28 13–15 y: 2.6–27.6 15–17 y: 4.6–24.0 Adult, M: 13–60 F, Follicular phase: 7.2–23.5	*IU/d* 0.48–11.28 2.6–27.6 4.6–24.0 13–60 7.2–23.5
Lysozyme	Serum, plasma (EDTA)	5–15 μg/mL	5–15 mg/L
Magnesium	Serum	1.3–2.1 mEq/L higher in females during menses	0.65–1.05 mmol/L
	Urine, 24 h	6.0–10.0 mEq/d	3.00–5.00 mmol/d
Mercury	Whole blood (EDTA)	< 5.0 μg/dL	< 0.25 μmol/L
	Urine, 24 h	< 20 μg/L Toxic: > 150 μg/L	< 0.1 μmol/L > 0.75 μmol/L
Metanephrine, Total	Urine, 24 h	*μg/mg creatinine* < 1 y: 0.001–4.60 1–2 y: 0.27–5.38 2–5 y: 0.35–2.99 5–10 y: 0.43–2.70 10–15 y: 0.001–1.87 15–18 y: 0.001–0.67 Adult: 0.05–1.20	*mmol/mol creatinine* 0.0006–2.64 0.15–3.09 0.20–1.72 0.25–1.55 0.0006–1.07 0.0006–0.38 0.03–0.69
Methanol	Whole blood (fluoride/oxalate)	< 0.15 mg/dL Toxic: > 20 mg/dL	< 0.05 mmol/L > 6.24 mmol/L
	Urine	Occup. exposure: < 5.0 mg/dL	< 1.6 mmol/L
	Breath	< 0.8 ppm Occup. exposure: > 2.5 ppm	< 0.02 mmol/L > 0.08 mmol/L
Metyrapone (Metopyrone) Stimulation Test	Serum	11-Deoxycortisol: > 7.0 μg/dL Cortisol: < 8 μg/dL	11-Deoxycortisol: > 200 nmol/L Cortisol: < 220 nmol/L
Dose, adult: 750 mg q 4 h × 6; child: 300 mg/m²	Urine, 24 h	17-KGS: 2.5- to 3-fold rise, but at least 10 mg/d 17-KS: > 2× base level 17-OHCS: 3–5× base level	17-KGS: 2.5- to 3-fold rise but at least 35 μmol/d* 17-KS: > 2× base level 17-OHCS: 3–5× base level *(conv. factor based on DHEA, M.W. 288)
Single-Dose Metyrapone Test *Dose: 30 mg/kg orally with milk or snack at midnight*	Serum for 11-deoxycortisol determination at 0800 h following morning	> 7 μg/dL	> 200 nmol/L
Microsomal Antibodies, Thyroid, see *Thyroid Microsomal Antibodies*			
Myelin Basic Protein	CSF	< 4 ng/mL	< 4 μg/L
Myoglobin	Serum	*μg/mL ± 1 SD* M: 49 ± 17 F: 35 ± 14 Increases slightly with age	*μg/mL* 49 ± 17 35 ± 14
	Urine, random	Negative	Negative
Nitrogen, Total	Feces	Infant: 0.11–0.52 g N/d Adult: < 2 g N/d	7.9–37 mmol N/d < 143 mmol N/d

CLINICAL CHEMISTRY, TOXICOLOGY, SEROLOGY (*Continued*)

Test	Specimen	Reference Range	Reference Range (International Units)
Normetanephrine, Total	Plasma (EDTA and sodium metabisulfite)	Normotensive: 1.2 ng/mL ± 0.1 (SEM)	6.5 nmol/L ± 0.55
Osmolality	Serum	Child, adult: 275–295 mOsmol/kg	
	Urine, random	50–1400 mOsmol/kg, depending on fluid intake After 12 h fluid restriction: > 850 mOsmol/kg	
	Urine, 24 h	~ 300–900 mOsmol/kg	
Oxalate	Serum	1–2.4 μg/mL Ethylene glycol poisoning: > 20 μg/mL	11–27 μmol/L Ethylene glycol poisoning: > 228 μmol/L
	Urine, 24 h	8–40 μg/d Ethylene glycol poisoning: > 150 μg/d	90–456 μmol/L Ethylene glycol poisoning: > 1710 μmol/d
Oxygen, Partial Pressure (Po_2)	Whole blood (heparin), arterial	83–100 mm Hg (decreases with age and high altitude)	11–14.4 kPa
Oxygen Saturation	Whole blood (heparin), arterial	95–99%	Fraction saturated: 0.95–0.99
Po_2, see *Oxygen, Partial Pressure*			
Pentobarbital	Serum, plasma (heparin, EDTA); collect at trough conc.	*μg/mL* Therap. conc., hypnotic: 1–5 Therap. coma: 20–50 Toxic conc.: > 10	*μmol/L* 4–22 88–221 > 44
pH	Whole blood (heparin), arterial	7.35–7.45 Must be corrected for body temperature	H^+ concentration: 36–44 nmol/L
	Urine, random	Newborn/neonate: 5–7 Thereafter: 4.5–8 (average ~ 6)	0.1–10 μmol/L 0.01–32 μmol/L (average ~ 1.0 μmol/L)
Phenobarbital	Serum, plasma (heparin, EDTA); collect at trough conc.	μg/mL Therap. conc.: 15–40 Toxic conc., slowness, ataxia, nystagmus: 35–80 Coma with reflexes: 65–117 Coma without reflexes: > 100	*μmol/L* 65–172 151–345 280–504 > 430
Phenytoin (Dilantin)	Serum, plasma (heparin, EDTA); collect at steady-state trough conc.	Therap. conc.: 10–20 μg/mL Toxic conc.: > 20 μg/mL	40–79 μmol/L > 79 μmol/L
Phosphatase, Acid			
Prostatic (RIA)	Serum	< 3.0 ng/mL	< 3.0 μg/L
Roy, Brower, and Hayden, 37°C		0.11–0.60 U/L	0.11–0.60 U/L
Phosphatase, Alkaline *(p-nitrophenyl phosphate, carbonate buffer, 30°C)*	Serum	*U/L* Infant: 50–165 Child: 20–150 Adult: 20–70 > 60 yr: 30–75	*U/L* 50–165 20–150 20–70 30–75
Bowers and McComb, 30°C		25–90 U/L	25–90 U/L
IFCC, 30°C		M: 30–90 U/L F: 20–80 U/L	30–90 U/L 20–80 U/L
Phosphorus, Inorganic	Serum	*mg/dL* Cord: 3.7–8.1 Child: 4.5–5.5 Thereafter: 2.7–4.5 > 60 y, M: 2.3–3.7 F: 2.8–4.1	*nmol/L* 1.2–2.6 1.45–1.78 0.87–1.45 0.74–1.2 0.90–1.3
	Urine, 24 h	Adult, On diet containing 0.9–1.5 g P and 10 mg Ca/kg: < 1.0 g/d On nonrestricted diet: 0.4–1.3 g/d	Adult, On diet containing 29–48 mmol P and 0.25 mmol Ca/kg: < 32 mmol/d On nonrestricted diet: 13–42 mmol/d

CLINICAL CHEMISTRY, TOXICOLOGY, SEROLOGY *(Continued)*

Test	Specimen	Reference Range	Reference Range (International Units)
Porphobilinogen (PBG)			
Quantitative	Urine, 24 h	0–2.0 mg/d	0–8.8 μmol/d
Qualitative	Urine, fresh random	Negative	Negative
Potassium	Serum	*mEq/L*	*mmol/L*
		Newborn: 3.7–5.9	3.7–5.9
		Infant: 4.1–5.3	4.1–5.3
		Child: 3.4–4.7	3.4–4.7
		Thereafter: 3.5–5.1	3.5–5.1
	Plasma (heparin)	3.5–4.5 mmol/L	3.5–4.5 mmol/L
	Urine, 24 h	25–125 mEq/d; varies with diet	25–125 mmol/d; varies with diet
Pregnancy Tests			
Chorionic Gonadotropin (HCG) Tube Test			
Qualitative	Serum or urine	Negative Positive by 4th–8th d after expected menstrual period	Negative Positive by 4th–8th d after expected menstrual period
Semi-quantitative		Peak values up to 120,000 mIU/mL	Peak values up to 120,000 IU/L
Chorionic Gonadotropin, (β-HCG), see *Chorionic Gonadotropin, β-Subunit*			
Radio Receptor Assay (RRA); Qualitative	Serum	Negative; pregnancy can be detected 10 d after conception	Negative; pregnancy can be detected 10 d after conception
Pregnanediol	Urine, 24 h	*mg/d*	*μmol/d*
		< 2 y: < 0.1	< 0.3
		6–9 y: < 0.5	< 1.6
		M, 10–15 y: 0.1–0.7	0.3–2.2
		Adult: 0.6–1.5	1.9–4.7
		F, 10–15 y: 0.1–1.2	0.3–3.7
		Adult,	
		Follicular: < 1.0	<3.1
		Luteal: 2–7	6.2–22
		Postmenopausal: 0.2–1.0	0.6–3.1
		Week of pregnancy:	
		16: 5–21	16–65
		20: 6–26	19–81
		24: 12–32	37–100
		28: 19–51	59–160
		32: 22–66	69–206
		36: 13–77	41–240
		40: 23–63	72–197
Pregnanetriol	Urine, 24 h	*mg/d*	*μmol/d*
		2 wk–2 y: 0.02–0.2	0.06–0.6
		2–5 y: < 0.5	< 1.5
		5–15 y: < 1.5	< 4.5
		> 15 y: < 2.0	< 5.9
Pregnenolone	Serum	Adult: 0.3–2 ng/ml	0.9–6.3 nmol/L
Progesterone	Serum	*ng/mL*	*nmol/L*
		M, Pubertal stage I: 0.11–0.26	0.35–0.83
		Adult: 0.12–0.3	0.38–1
		F, Pubertal stage I: 0–0.3	0–1
		II: 0–0.46	0–1.5
		III: 0–0.6	0–2
		IV: 0.05–13.0	0.16–41
		Follicular; 0.02–0.9	0.06–2.9
		Luteal: 6.0–30.0	19–95
Progesterone Receptor Assay (PRA)	Tumor tissue	*fmol/mg protein*	*nmol/kg protein*
		Normal, or benign and non-responsive tumor: ≤ 5	≤ 5
		Positive: > 10	> 10
Prolactin (hPRL)	Serum	*ng/mL*	*μg/L*
		Adult, M: < 20	< 20
		F,	
		Follicular phase: <23	< 23
		Luteal phase: 5–40	5–40
		Pregnancy,	
		1st trimester: < 80	<80
		2nd trimester: < 160	<160
		3rd trimester: < 400	< 400
		Newborn: > 10-fold adult levels	

CLINICAL CHEMISTRY, TOXICOLOGY, SEROLOGY *(Continued)*

Test	Specimen	Reference Range	Reference Range (International Units)
Protein			
Total	Serum	*g/dL*	*g/L*
		Premature: 3.6–6.0	36.0–60.0
		Newborn: 4.6–7.0	46.0–70.0
		≥ 3 y: 6.0–8.0	60.0–80.0
		Ambulatory: 6.4–8.3	64.0–83.0
		Recumbent: 6.0–7.8	60.0–78.0
		> 60 y: slight lower (~0.2)	~ 2
		~ 0.5 g higher in ambulatory patients	~ 5 g higher in ambulatory patients
Electrophoresis		*g/dL*	*g/L*
		Albumin,	
		Adult: 3.5–5.0	35–50
		> 60 y: 3.7–4.7	37–47
		α_1-Globulin,	
		Adult: 0.1–0.3	1–3
		> 60 y: 0.2–0.5	2–5
		α_2-Globulin,	
		Adult: 0.6–1.0	6–10
		> 60 y: 0.5–1.1	5–11
		β-Globulin,	
		Adult: 0.7–1.1	7–11
		> 60 y: 0.5–1.2	5–12
		γ-Globulin,	
		Adult: 0.8–1.6	8–16
		> 60 y: 0.6–1.6	6–16
Total	Urine, 24 h	1–14 mg/dL	10–140 mg/L
		50–80 mg/d at rest	50–80 mg/d at rest
		< 250 mg/d after intense exercise	< 250 mg/d after intense exercise
Electrophoresis		*Average % of Total Protein*	*Fraction of Total*
		Alb. 37.9	0.379
		α_1 27.3	0.273
		α_2 19.5	0.195
		β 8.8	0.088
		γ 3.3	0.033
Total	CSF		
Column		Lumbar: 8–32 mg/dL	80–320 mg/L
Turbidimetry		Lumbar,	
		Adult: 15–45 mg/dL	150–450 mg/L
		Newborn: 40–120 mg/dL	400–1200 mg/L
Electrophoresis		*% of Total*	*Fraction of Total*
		Prealbumin: 2–7	0.02–0.07
		Albumin: 56–76	0.56–0.76
		α_1-Globulin: 2–7	0.02–0.07
		α_2-Globulin: 4–12	0.04–0.12
		β-Globulin: 8–18	0.08–0.18
		γ-Globulin: 3–12	0.03–0.12
Electrophoresis	Synovial fluid	Albumin: 63	0.63
		α_1-Globulin: 7	0.07
		α_2-Globulin: 7	0.07
		β-Globulin: 9	0.09
		γ-Globulin: 14	0.14
		Fibrinogen: 0	0
Protoporphyrin	Whole blood (heparin or EDTA)	< 50 μg/dL RBC	< 0.89 μmol/L RBC
	Feces, 24 h	≤ 60 μg/g dry wt or < 1500 μg/d	≤ 0.11 mmol/kg dry wt or < 2.67 μmol/d
Pyruvic Acid	Whole blood (heparin)	0.3–0.9 mg/dL	0.03–0.10 mmol/L
Renal Plasma Flow (RPF)	Plasma and urine	M: 560–830 mL/min	
		F: 490–700 mL/min	
		or: 390 mL/min/m² body surface	
		> 40 y: decreases ~ 75 mL/decade	
Renin	Plasma (EDTA)	*Normal sodium diet:*	
		ng/h/mL ± 1 SE	*μg/h/L ± 1 SE*
		Supine: 1.6 ± 1.5	1.6 ± 1.5
		Standing (4 h): 4.5 ± 2.9	4.5 ± 2.9
		Low sodium:	
		Supine: 3.2 ± 1.1	3.2 ± 1.1
		Standing (4 h): 9.9 ± 4.3	9.9 ± 4.3

CLINICAL CHEMISTRY, TOXICOLOGY, SEROLOGY (*Continued*)

Test	Specimen	Reference Range	Reference Range (International Units)
Riboflavin (Vitamin B_2)	Urine, random, fasting	*μg/g creatinine* Adult: 80–269 Pregnancy: 90–120	*μmol/mol creatinine* 24–81 27–36
Salicylates	Serum, plasma (heparin, EDTA); collect at trough conc.	Therap. conc.: 150–300 μg/mL Toxic conc.: > 300 μg/mL	1086–2172 μmol/L > 2172 μmol/L
Schilling Test (Intrinsic Factor Test) *Dose: 0.5– 1.0 μCi ^{58}Co-Vitamin B_{12}*	Urine, 24 h	> 7.5% of dose	Fraction of dose: 0.075
Secobarbital	Serum	Therap. conc.: 1–2 μg/mL Toxic conc.: > 5 μg/mL	4.2–8.4 μmol/L > 21.0 μmol/L
Sediment	Urine, fresh random		
Casts		Hyaline: occasional (0–1) casts/hpf RBC: not seen WBC: not seen Tubular epithelial: not seen Transitional and squamous epithelial: not seen	Hyaline: occasional (0–1) casts/hpf RBC: not seen WBC: not seen Tubular epithelial: not seen Transitional and squamous epithelial: not seen
Cells		RBC: 0–2/hpf WBC, Adult, M: 0–3/hpf F and child: 0–5/hpf Epithelial: few; more frequent in newborn Bacteria, Unspun: no organisms/oil immersion field Spun: < 20 organisms/hpf	RBC: 0–2/hpf WBC, M: 0–3/hpf F and child: 0–5/hpf Epithelial: few; more frequent in newborn Bacteria, Unspun: no organisms/oil immersion field Spun: < 20 organisms/hpf
Semen Analysis (Sperm Count)	Ejaculate	Volume: 2–6 mL Sperm count: > 20 million/mL Motility: > 50% Morphology: ≥ 60% normal forms	Volume: 0.002–0.006 L Sperm count: > 20 × 10^9/L Motility: Fraction of total: > 0.50 Morphology: Fraction of total: ≥ 0.60 normal forms
Sodium	Serum or plasma (heparin)	*mEq/L* Newborn: 134–146 Infant: 139–146 Child: 138–145 Thereafter: 136–146	*mmol/L* 134–146 139–146 138–145 136–146
	Urine, 24 h	40–220 mEq/d (diet dependent)	40–220 mmol/d
	Sweat	10–40 mEq/L	10–40 mmol/L
Specific Gravity	Urine, random	Adult: 1.002–1.030 After 12 h fluid restriction: > 1.025	Adult: 1.002–1.030 After 12 h fluid restriction: > 1.025
	Urine, 24 h	1.015–1.025	
Testosterone, Free	Serum		

Testosterone, Free (Serum)	ng/dL (mean ± 1 SE)	% of total (mean ± 1 SE)	pmol/L (mean ± 1 SE)	% of total (mean ± 1 SE)
Cord, M:	1.0 ± 0.4	2.9 ± 0.6	34.7 ± 14	0.029 ± 0.006
Cord, F:	0.89 ± 0.29	3.0 ± 0.5	31 ± 10	0.03 ± 0.005
1–15 d, M:	0.8 ± 0.8	1.3 ± 0.2	27.8 ± 27.8	0.013 ± 0.002
1–15 d, F:	0.14 ± 0.06	1.2 ± 0.2	4.9 ± 2	0.012 ± 0.002
Prepubertal, M:	0.04 ± 0.01	0.7 ± 0.2	1.4 ± 0.3	0.007 ± 0.002
Prepubertal, F:	0.04 ± 0.01	0.7 ± 0.1	1.4 ± 0.3	0.007 ± 0.001
Adult, M:	7.9 ± 2.3	1.4 ± 0.3	274 ± 80	0.014 ± 0.003
Adult, F:	0.31 ± 0.07	0.9 ± 0.2	10.8 ± 2.4	0.009 ± 0.002

Test	Specimen	Reference Range	Reference Range (International Units)
Testosterone, Total	Serum	*ng/dL*	*nmol/L*
		Prepubertal,	
		M: 6.6 ± 2.5	0.23 ± 0.09
		F: 6.6 ± 2.5	0.23 ± 0.09
		Adult, M: 572 ± 135	19.8 ± 4.7
		F: 35 ± 10	1.3 ± 0.3
	Urine	*Pubertal stage* — *μg/kg body weight*	*nmol/kg body weight*
		I, M: 0.25	0.87
		F: 0.16	0.55
		II, M: 0.34	1.18
		F: 0.16	0.55
		III, M: 0.37	1.28
		F: 0.16	0.55
		μg/d	*nmol/d*
		20–50 y,	
		M: 50–135	173–470
		F: 2–12	7–42
		< 50 y,	
		M: 40–60	139–210
		F: 2–8	7–28
Thiopental	Serum, plasma (heparin, EDTA); collect at trough conc.	*μg/mL*	*μmol/L*
		Therap. conc.,	
		Hypnotic: 1.0–5.0	4.1–20.7
		Therap. coma: 30–100	123.9–413
		Anesthesia: 7–130	29–537
		Toxic conc.: > 10	> 41
Thyroglobulin (Tg)	Serum	< 50 ng/mL	< 50 μg/L
Thyroid Antibodies	Serum	Adult: ≤ 1:10 dilution	Adult: ≤ 1:10 dilution
		Child: ≤ 1:4	Child: ≤ 1:4
Thyroid Microsomal Antibodies	Serum	Nondetectable (hemagglutination) or < 1:10 (IFA)	Nondetectable (hemagglutination) or < 1:10 (IFA)
Thyroid-Stimulating Hormone (hTSH)	Serum or plasma	*μIU/mL*	*mIU/L*
		Cord: 3–12	3–12
		Child: 4.5 ± 3.6	4.5 ± 3.6
		Adult: 2–10	2–10
		> 60 y, M: 2–7.3	2–7.3
		F: 2–16.8	2–16.8
Thyroid-Stimulating Hormone—Response to TRH	Serum	30 min after stimulation: *μU/mL*	30 min after stimulation: *mIU/L*
		Child: 11–35	Child: 11–35
		Adult, M: 15–30	Adult, M: 15–30
		F: 20–40	F: 20–40
Thyroid Uptake of Radioactive Iodine	Activity over thyroid gland		Fractional uptake:
		2 h: < 6%	2 h: < 0.06
		6 h: 3–20%	6 h: 0.03–0.20
		24 h: 8–30%	24 h: 0.08–0.30
Thyroid Uptake of $^{99m}TcO_4^-$	Activity over thyroid gland	Uptake ratio: < 1.15 in euthyroid	< 1.15
Thyrotropin-Releasing Hormone	Plasma	5–60 pg/mL	50–60 ng/L
Thyrotropin-Releasing Hormone Stimulation Test *Dose, adult: 500 μg TRH IV*	Serum	TSH within 30 min, < 40y: > 6 μIU/mL rise; > 40 y, M: > 2 μIU/mL rise; hPRL: 3- to 5-fold rise above baseline (diminishes with age)	TSH within 30 min, < 40 y: > 6 μIU/mL rise; > 40 y, M: > 2 μIU/mL rise; hPRL: 3- to 5-fold rise above baseline (diminishes with age)
Thyroxine (T_4), Total	Serum	*μg/dL*	*nmol/L*
		Cord: 8–13	103–167
		Newborn: 11.5–24	148–310
		Neonate: 9–18	116–232
		Infant: 7–15	90–194
		1–5 y: 7.3–15	94–194
		5–10 y: 6.4–13.3	83–172
		Thereafter: 5–12	65–155
		> 60 y, M: 5.0–10.0	65–129
		F: 5.5–10.5	71–135
		Pregnancy, last 5 mo: 6.1–17.6	79–227
Thyroxine-Binding Globulin (TBG)	Serum	15.0–34.0 μg/mL	15.0–34.0 mg/L
Thyroxine Ratio, Effective (ETR)		0.86–1.13	0.86–1.13
Thyroxine, Free (FT_4)	Serum	0.8–2.4 ng/dL	10–31 pmol/L

CLINICAL CHEMISTRY, TOXICOLOGY, SEROLOGY (Continued)

Test	Specimen	Reference Range	Reference Range (International Units)
Thyroxine Index, Free, see *Free Thyroxine Index*			
Thyroxine/TBG Ratio	Serum	0.2–0.5 T_4 (μg/dL)/TBG (μg/mL)	2.7–6.4 T_4 (nmol/L)/TBG (mg/L)
Transferrin	Serum	Adult: 220–400 mg/dL > 60 y: 180–380 mg/dL	2.20–4.0 g/L 1.80–3.80 g/L
Transketolase			
Ribose/sedoheptulose, 37°C	Whole blood (heparin)	9–12 μmol/h/mL whole blood 2.1–2.4 μmol/h/10^9 red cells	150–200 U/L whole blood 0.035–0.040 nU/red cell

Trigylcerides (TG)
Serum, after ≥ 12 h fast

	mg/dL M	mg/dL F	mmol/L M	mmol/L F	
Cord blood:	10–98	10–98	0.11–1.11	0.11–1.11	(conv. factor
0–5 y:	30–86	32–99	0.34–0.97	0.36–1.12	based on
6–11 y:	31–108	35–114	0.35–1.22	0.40–1.29	triolein,
12–15 y:	36–138	41–138	0.41–1.56	0.46–1.56	M.W. 885)
16–19 y:	40–163	40–128	0.45–1.84	0.45–1.45	
20–29 y:	44–185	40–128	0.50–2.09	0.45–1.45	
30–39 y:	49–284	38–160	0.55–3.21	0.43–1.81	
40–49 y:	56–298	44–186	0.63–3.37	0.50–2.10	
50–59 y:	62–288	55–247	0.70–3.25	0.62–2.79	

Values decrease slightly above age 60

Levels for blacks: 10–20 mg/dL lower

Recommended (desirable) levels for adults:
M: 40–160 mg/dL
F: 35–135 mg/dL

Values decrease slightly above age 60

Levels for blacks: 0.11–0.23 mmol/L lower

Recommended (desirable) levels for adults:
M: 0.45–1.81 mmol/L
F: 0.40–1.53 mmol/L

Triiodothyronine (T_3-RIA)
Serum

	ng/dL	nmol/L
Cord:	30–70	0.46–1.08
Newborn:	75–260	1.16–4.00
1–5 y:	100–260	1.54–4.00
5–10 y:	90–240	1.39–3.70
10–15 y:	80–210	1.23–3.23
Thereafter:	115–190	1.77–2.93
> 60 y, M:	105–175	1.62–2.69
F:	108–205	1.66–3.16

Triiodothyronine, Free
Serum

	mean pg/dL	mean pmol/L
Cord:	130 ± 10 (SE)	2.00 ± 0.15 (SE)
1–3 d:	410 ± 20	6.31 ± 0.31
6 wk:	400 ± 20	6.16 ± 0.31
Adult (20–50 y):	230–660	3.54–10.10

Triiodothyronine Index, Free
Serum

1–5 y:	165
5–10 y:	150
10–15 y:	130

Triiodothyronine Resin Uptake Test (T_3RU)
Serum

		Fractional uptake:	
Newborn:	25–37%	Newborn:	0.25–0.37
Adult:	24–34%	Adult:	0.24–0.34
> 60 y:	23–32%	> 60 y:	0.23–0.32

Triolein-^{131}I Absorption Test
Plasma — > 1.7% of administered dose/L after 4–6 h — Fraction of administered dose: > 0.017/L

Dose: 50 μCi in milk — Feces, 72 h — < 5% of administered dose in 72 h specimen — Fraction of administered dose: < 0.05/72 h

Tubular Reabsorption of Phosphate (TRP)
Urine, 4 h (0800–1200 h) and serum — 82–95% — Fraction reabsorbed: 0.82–0.95

Urea Nitrogen
Serum or plasma

	mg/dL	mmol urea/L
Cord:	21–40	3.5–6.6
Premature (1 wk):	3–25	0.5–4.2
Newborn:	4–12	0.7–2.0
Infant/child:	5–18	0.8–3.0
Adult:	7–18	1.2–3.0
> 60 y:	8–21	1.3–3.5

Higher after high protein intake

Urine — 12–20 g/d — 200–333 mmol urea/d

Urea Nitrogen/Creatinine Ratio
Serum — 12/1 to 20/1
Varies with diet and methods used — 12/1 to 20/1

Test	Specimen	Reference Range	Reference Range (International Units)
Uric Acid			
Phosphotungstate	Serum	*mg/dL* Adult, M: 4.5–8.2 F: 3.0–6.5 > 60 y, M: 4.2–8.0 F: 3.2–7.3	*μmol/L* 268–488 178–387 250–476 190–434
Uricase		Child: 2.0–5.5 Adult, M: 3.5–7.2 F: 2.6–6.0	119–327 208–428 155–357
	Urine, 24 h	*mg/d* Free purine diet M: < 420 F: slightly lower Low purine diet, M: < 480 F: < 400 High purine diet: < 1000 Average diet: 250–750	*mmol/d* < 2.48 < 2.83 < 2.36 < 5.90 1.48–4.43
Urinary Sediment, see *Sediment*			
Urobilinogen	Urine, 2 h Urine, 24 h	0.1–0.8 EU/2 h 0.5–4.0 EU/d	0.1–0.8 EU/2 h 0.5–4.0 EU/d
	Feces	75–275 EU/100 g 74–400 EU/d 40–280 mg/d	770–2750 EU/kg 75–400 EU/d 67–473 μmol/d
Uroporphyrin	Urine, 24 h	< 50 μg/d	< 60 nmol/d
	Feces, 24 h specimen	10–40 μg/d	12–48 nmol/d
	Erythrocytes (heparin or EDTA)	Negative	Negative
Vanillylmandelic Acid (Vanilmandelic Acid)	Urine, 24 h	*mg/d* Newborn: < 1.0 Infant: < 2.0 Child: 1–5 Adolescent: 1–5 Thereafter: 2–7 or 1.5–7 μg/mg creatinine	*μmol/d* < 5.1 < 10.1 5.1–25.3 5.1–25.3 10.1–35.4 or 0.86–4 mmol/mol creatinine
Viscosity	Serum	1.10–1.22 Centipoise	1.10–1.22 Centipoise
Vitamin A	Serum	30–65 μg/dL	1.05–2.27 μmol/L
Vitamin A Tolerance Test	Serum	3 and/or 6 h: 200–600 μg vit. A/dL	7–21 μmol/L
Dose: 5000 U vit. A in oil/kg orally			
Vitamin B_2, see *Riboflavin*			
Vitamin B_6	Plasma (EDTA)	3.6–18 ng/mL	14.6–72.8 nmol/L
Vitamin B_{12}	Serum	100–700 pg/mL > 60 y: 110–800 pg/mL	74–516 pmol/L 81–590 pmol/L
Vitamin B_{12} Intrinsic Factor	Gastric juice	50–400% enhancement of ^{57}Co-B_{12} uptake by GPIMH	Fractional increase in ^{57}Co-B_{12} uptake by GPIMH: 0.50–4.00
Vitamin C	Plasma (oxalate, heparin, or EDTA)	0.6–2.0 mg/dL	34–114 μmol/L
	Buffy coat (heparin)	20–53 μg/10^8 WBC	11.4–30.1 amol/cell
Vitamin C Saturation Test	Urine, 24 h	60–80% of test dose excreted	Fraction test dose excreted: 0.60–0.80
Vitamin D_3, 25-hydroxy	Plasma (heparin)	Summer: 15–80 ng/mL Winter: 14–42 ng/mL	37.4–200 nmol/L 34.9–105 nmol/L
Vitamin D_3, 1.25–dihydroxy	Serum	25–45 pg/mL	60–108 pmol/L
Vitamin E	Serum	5.0–20 μg/mL	11.6–46.4 μmol/L
Xylose Absorption Test	Whole blood (Na-fluoride)	*mg/dL* Child, 1 h (5 g dose): > 20 Adult, 2 h (25 g dose): > 25	*mmol/L* > 1.33 > 1.67
	Urine, 5h	Child: 16–33% of ingested dose	Fraction ingested dose: 0.16–0.33
		Adult, *g/5 h* 5 g dose: > 1.2 25 g dose: > 4.0 > 65 y: > 3.5	*mmol/5 h* > 8.00 > 26.64 > 23.31

HEMATOLOGY AND COAGULATION

Test	Specimen	Reference Drugs	Reference Range (International Units)
Activated Partial Thromboplastin Time (APTT)	Whole blood (Na citrate); remove plasma immediately	25–35 s (differs with method)	25–35 s
Microtechnique (Miale)	Capillary blood (siliconized micropipets; Na citrate)	Infant: < 90 s Reaches adult levels by 2–6 mo	< 90 s
Bleeding Time (BT)			
Ivy	Blood from skin pucture	Normal: 2–7 min Borderline: 7–11 min	2–7 min 7–11 min
Simplate (G-D)		2.75–8 min	2.75–8 min
Blood Volume	Whole blood (heparin)	M: 52–83 mL/kg F: 50–75 mL/kg	M: 0.052–0.083 L/kg F: 0.050–0.075 L/kg
Bone Marrow, Differential Count	Bone marrow aspirate	*% (mean)*	*Number fraction (mean)*
Myeloblasts		0.3–5.0 (2.0)	0.003–0.05 (0.02)
Promyelocytes		1.0–8.0 (5.0)	0.01–0.08 (0.05)
Myelocytes: Neutrophilic		5.0–19.0 (12.0)	0.05–0.19 (0.12)
Eosinophilic		0.5–3.0 (1.5)	0.005–0.03 (0.015)
Basophilic		0.0–0.5 (0.3)	0.00–0.005 (0.003)
Metamyelocytes		13.0–32.0 (22.0)	0.13–0.32 (0.22)
Polymorphonuclear neutrophils		7.0–30.0 (20.0)	0.07–0.30 (0.20)
Polymorphonuclear eosinophils		0.5–4.0 (2.0)	0.005–0.04 (0.02)
Polymorphonuclear basophils		0.0–0.7 (0.2)	0.00–0.007 (0.002)
Lymphocytes		3.0–17.0 (10.0)	0.03–0.17 (0.10)
Plasma cells		0.0–2.0 (0.4)	0.00–0.02 (0.004)
Monocytes		0.5–5.0 (2.0)	0.005–0.05 (0.02)
Reticulum cells		0.1–2.0 (0.2)	0.001–0.02 (0.002)
Megakaryocytes		0.03–3.0 (0.1)	0.0003–0.03 (0.001)
Pronormoblasts		1.0–8.0 (4.0)	0.01–0.08 (0.04)
Normoblasts		7.0–32.0 (18.0)	0.07–0.32 (0.18)
Clot Lysis, 37°C	Whole clotted blood	48–72 h	48–72 h
Clot Retraction			
Screen	Whole blood (no anticoagulant)	Retraction begins at 1 h, maximum at 24 h	Retraction begins at 1 h, maximum at 24 h
Clotting Time			
Lee-White, 37°C	Whole blood (no anticoagulant)	5–8 min	5–8 min
Clotting Time, Plasma	Plasma (citrate)	Platelet-rich plasma: 100–150 s	Platelet-rich plasma: 100–150 s
Differential Count, see *Bone Marrow Differential Count; Leukocyte Differential Count;* and *Synovial Fluid Differential Count*			
Eosinophil Count	Whole blood (EDTA); capillary blood	50–350 cells/μL (mm³)	50–350 × 10⁶ cells/L
Erythrocyte Count (RBC Count)	Whole blood (EDTA)	*millions of cells/μL (mm³)* 2–14 y: 3.7–5.2 Adult M: 4.3–5.9 F: 4.0–5.2	*× 10¹² cells/L* 3.7–5.2 4.3–5.9 4.0–5.2
Erythrocyte Sedimentation Rate (ESR)			
Westergren, modified	Whole blood (EDTA)	*mm/h* Child: 0–10 Adult: M, < 50 y: 0–15 > 50 y: 0–20 F, < 50 y: 0–20 > 50 y: 0–30	*mm/h* 0–10 0–15 0–20 0–20 0–30
Wintrobe		Child: 0–13 Adult: M, 0–9 F, 0–20	0–13 0–9 0–20
Zeta (ZSR)		41–54%	41–54 AU

HEMATOLOGY AND COAGULATION (*Continued*)

Test	Specimen	Reference Drugs	Reference Range (International Units)
Ferritin, see *Chemistry section*			
Fibrin Degradation Products			
Agglutination (Thrombo-Wellco test)	Whole blood; special tube containing thrombin and proteolytic inhibitor	< 10 μg/mL	< 10 mg/L
	Urine: 2 mL in special tube (see above)	< 0.25 μg/mL	< 0.25 mg/L
Staphylococcal clumping	Whole blood, collected with thrombin and ε-aminocaproic acid	< 10 μg/mL	< 10 mg/L
Fibrin Lysis Time	Plasma	> 60 min	> 60 min
Fibrinogen	Plasma (Na citrate)	200–400 mg/dL	2.00–4.00 g/L
Glucose-6-phosphate Dehydrogenase (G-6-PD) in Erythrocytes	Whole blood (ACD, EDTA, or heparin)	12.1 ± 2.09 U/g Hb (1 SD)	0.78 ± 0.13 MU/mol Hb (1 SD)
WHO and ICSH methods			
Haptoglobin (Hp)	Serum; avoid hemolysis		
RID		83–267 mg/dL	830–2670 mg/L
Hemoglobin-binding capacity		40–180 mg Hb/dL	6.20–27.90 μmol Hb/L
Nephelometry		26–185 mg/dL	260–1850 mg/L
Hematocrit (HCT, Hct) *Calculated from MCV and RBC (electronic displacement or laser)*	Whole blood (EDTA)	*% of packed red cells (V red cells/V whole blood × 100)* 1–3 d (cap): 45–67 2 mo: 28–42 6–12 y: 35–45 12–18 y, M; 37–49 F: 36–46 18–49 y, M: 41–53 F: 36–46	*Volume fraction (V red cells/V whole blood)* 0.45–0.67 0.28–0.42 0.35–0.45 0.37–0.49 0.36–0.46 0.41–0.53 0.36–0.46
Hemoglobin (Hb)	Whole blood (EDTA)	*g/dL* 1–3 d (cap): 14.5–22.5 2 mo: 9.0–14.0 6–12 y: 11.5–15.5 12–18 y, M: 13.0–16.0 F: 12.0–16.0 18–49 y, M: 13.5–17.5 F: 12.0–16.0	*mmol/L* 2.25–3.49 (conv. factor based on hemoglobin, M.W. 64,000) 1.40–2.17 1.78–2.40 2.02–2.48 1.86–2.48 2.09–2.71 1.86–2.48
	Plasma (heparin, ACD, or EDTA)	1–4 mg/dL	0.16–0.62 μmol/L
	Serum	< 3 mg/dL with butterfly setup and 18 g needle	< 0.47 μmol/L with butterfly setup and 18 g needle
	Urine, fresh, random	Negative	Negative
Hemoglobin Electrophoresis	Whole blood (EDTA, citrate or heparin)	HbA > 95% HbA_2 1.5–3.5% Lower in infants < 1 y HbF < 2%	*Mass fraction* HbA > 0.95 HbA_2 0.015–0.035 HbF < 0.02
Hemoglobin F *Alkali denaturation (White)*	Whole blood (EDTA)	*% HbF* 1 day: 77.0 ± 7.3 6 mo: 4.7 ± 2.2 Adult: < 2.0	*Mass fraction HbF* 0.77 ± 0.073 0.047 ± 0.022 < 0.020
Hemoglobin H (HbH)	Whole blood (ACD, EDTA, or heparin)	No precipitation at 40 min	No precipitation at 40 min
Isopropanol precipitation			
Leukocyte Count (WBC Count)	Whole blood (EDTA)	*× 1000 cells/μL (mm³)* Birth: 9.0–30.0 24 h: 9.4–34.0 1 mo: 5.0–19.5 1–3 y: 6.0–17.5 4–7 y: 5.5–15.5 8–13 y: 4.5–13.5 Adult: 4.5–11.0	*Cells × 10⁹/L* 9.0–30.0 9.4–34.0 5.0–19.5 6.0–17.5 5.5–15.5 4.5–13.5 4.5–11.0
	CSF	0–5 mononuclear cells/μL	0–5 × 10^6 cells/L

HEMATOLOGY AND COAGULATION (*Continued*)

Test	Specimen	Reference Drugs	Reference Range (International Units)
Leukocyte Differential Count	Whole blood (EDTA)	% — *Cells/µL (mm³)*	*Number fraction* — *Cells × 10⁶/L*
Myelocytes		0 — 0	0 — 0
Neutrophils-'bands'		3–5 — 150–400	0.03–0.05 — 150–400
Neutrophils-'segs'		54–62 — 3000–5800	0.54–0.62 — 3000–5800
Lymphocytes		25–33 — 1500–3000	0.25–0.33 — 1500–3000
Monocytes		3–7 — 285–500	0.03–0.07 — 285–500
Eosinophils		1–3 — 50–250	0.01–0.03 — 50–250
Basophils		0–0.75 — 15–50	0–0.0075 — 15–20
Leukocyte Differential Count	CSF	%	*Number fraction*
Lymphocytes		62 ± 34	0.62 ± 0.34
*Monocytes**		36 ± 20	0.36 ± 0.20
Neutrophils		2 ± 5	0.02 ± 0.05
Histocytes		Rare	Rare
Ependymal cells		Rare	Rare
Eosinophils		Rare	Rare
*Includes pia-arachnoid mesothelial cells			
Mean Corpuscular Hemoglobin (MCH)	Whole blood (EDTA)	*pg/cell*	*fmol/cell*
		0.5–6 y: 23–30	0.36–0.46
		6–18 y: 25–35	0.39–0.54
		Adults 26–34	0.40–0.53
Mean Corpuscular Hemoglobin Concentration (MCHC)	Whole blood (EDTA)	*% Hb/cell or gHb/dL RBC* Adult and child: 31–36	*mmol Hb/L RBC* 4.81–5.58
Mean Corpuscular Volume (MCV)	Whole blood (EDTA)	*fL (µm³)*	*fL*
		1–3 d (cap): 95–121	95–121
		0.5–2 y: 70–86	70–86
		6–12 y: 77–95	77–95
		12–18 y, M: 78–98	78–98
		F: 78–102	78–102
		18–49 y, M: 80–100	80–100
		F: 80–100	80–100
Methemoglobin (MetHb)	Whole blood (EDTA, heparin, or ACD)	0.06–0.24 g/dL or 0.78 ± 0.37% of total Hb	9.3–37.2 µmol/L 0.008 ± 0.0037 (mass fraction)
Partial Thromboplastin Time (PTT)	Whole blood (Na citrate)		
Nonactivated		60–85 s (Platelin)	60–85 s
Activated		25–35 s (differs with method)	25–35 s
Plasma Volume	Plasma (heparin)	M: 25–43 mL/kg F: 28–45 mL/kg	M: 0.025–0.043 L/kg F: 0.028–0.045 L/kg
Platelet Count (Thrombocyte Count)	Whole blood (EDTA)	*× 10³/µL (mm³)*	*× 10⁹/L*
		Newborn: 84–478	84–478
		(After 1 wk, same as adult)	
		Adult: 150–400	150–400
Prothrombin Consumption (PCT, Serum Prothrombin Time)	Whole blood (no anticoagulant)	>30 s or >80% consumed in 1 h	>30 s >0.80 (fraction consumed)
Prothrombin Time	Whole blood (Na citrate)		
One-stage (Quick)		In general: 11–15 s (varies with type of thromboplastin)	11–15 s
		Newborn: prolonged by 2–3 s	prolonged by 2–3 s
Two-stage modified (Ware and Seegers)		18–22 s	18–22 s
RBC Count, see *Erythrocyte Count*			
Red Cell Volume	Whole blood (heparin)	M: 20–36 mL/kg F: 19–31 mL/kg	M: 0.020–0.36 L/kg F: 0.019–0.031 L/kg
Reticulocyte Count	Whole blood (EDTA, heparin, or oxalate)	Adult: 0.5–1.5% of erythrocytes or 25,000–85,000 cells/uL (mm³)	0.005–0.015 (number fraction) 25,000–85,000 × 10⁶ cells/L
Sulfhemoglobin	Whole blood (EDTA, heparin, or ACD)	≤ 1.0% of total Hb	< 0.010 of total Hb (mass fraction)

HEMATOLOGY AND COAGULATION (*Continued*)

Test	Specimen	Reference Drugs	Reference Range (International Units)
Synovial Fluid Differential Count	Synovial fluid		
		%	*Number fraction*
Polymorphonuclear cells		0–25	0–0.25
Monocytes		0–71	0–0.71
Lymphocytes		0–78	0–0.78
Clasmatocytes		0–26	0–0.26
Unclassified		0–21	0–0.21
Synovial cells		0–12	0–0.12
Thrombin Time	Whole blood (Na citrate)	Control time ± 2 s when control is 9–13 s	Control time ± 2 s when control is 9–13 s
Thromboplastin Time, activated, see *Activated Partial Thromboplastin Time (APTT)*			

Index

Note: In this index, the expression "vs." has been used to denote "differential diagnosis." Italics indicate illustration and t indicates tables.